The 5-Minute Clinical Consult Standard 2016

24th EDITION

The 5-Minute Clinical Consult Standard 2016

24th EDITION

Print + 10-Day Web Trial Access

Editor-in-Chief

Frank J. Domino, MD
Professor and Director of Predoctoral Education
Department of Family Medicine and Community Health
University of Massachusetts Medical School
Worcester, Massachusetts

Associate Editors

Robert A. Baldor, MD, FAAFP
Professor and Vice-Chairman, Educational Affairs
Department of Family Medicine and Community Health
University of Massachusetts Medical School
Worcester, Massachusetts

Jeremy Golding, MD, FAAFP
Professor of Family Medicine and Obstetrics & Gynecology
University of Massachusetts Medical School
Quality Officer
Department of Family Medicine and Community Health
University of Massachusetts Memorial Health Care
Hahnemann Family Health Center
Worcester, Massachusetts

Mark B. Stephens, MD, MS, FAAFP, CAPT, MC, USN
Professor and Chair
Department of Family Medicine
Uniformed Services University
Bethesda, Maryland

Consulting Dermatology Editor

Mary Maloney, MD
Professor of Medicine and Director of Dermatologic Surgery
University of Massachusetts Medical School
Worcester, Massachusetts

Assistant Consulting Dermatology Editor

Lorena Ceci, MSIV
University of Massachusetts Medical School
Worcester, Massachusetts

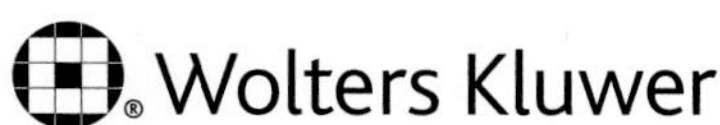

Philadelphia • Baltimore • New York • London
Buenos Aires • Hong Kong • Sydney • Tokyo

5MinuteConsult

Acquisitions Editor: Rebecca Gaertner
Product Development Editor: Leanne Vandetty
Production Project Manager: Priscilla Crater
Senior Manufacturing Coordinator: Beth Welsh
Strategic Marketing Manager: Stephanie Kindlick
Design Coordinator: Teresa Mallon
Production Service: Absolute Service, Inc.

Two Commerce Square
2001 Market Street
Philadelphia, PA 19103 USA
LWW.com

Printed in China

Library of Congress Cataloging-in-Publication Data available from the Publisher upon request.

ISBN-13: 978-1-4963-0863-4
ISBN-10: 1-4963-0863-8

To purchase additional copies of this book, call our customer service department at (800) 638-3030 or fax orders to (301) 223-2320. International customers should call (301) 223-2300.

10 9 8 7 6 5 4 3 2 1

CCS0415

This edition of *The 5-Minute Clinical Consult* is dedicated to the men and women of the United States Armed Forces (their families and those who care for them). Their bravery, professionalism, and tireless devotion to duty allow us all to comfortably rest under the warm blanket of freedom each and every night.

Patty, Trevor, and Abby–I love you.

MARK STEPHENS, MD

PREFACE

If your actions inspire others to dream more, learn more, do more and become more, you are a leader.

–John Quincy Adams

This is a book of diseases, diagnostic methods, and treatment recommendations. Much of the work provided by primary care providers is focused on helping the patient help themselves to be healthier. Diet, exercise, safety, and prevention are the interventions that provide the greatest number of people with the greatest return on longevity and its enjoyment.

In our role, we do more than diagnose and treat disease. Yet, when you listen to a patient's story, or touch them, their burden is in some way lifted. We are a place for patients to turn when they are in need, sometimes when they have no place else to turn.

Our role is more than preventing and treating illness. We are leaders. Asking a recently widowed person how they will get through tomorrow is more than a condolence, it is a therapeutic intervention. Prompting an "at-risk" teen to use contraception, avoid drugs, or consider higher education, are all therapeutic interventions. Dropping an email to your state legislator about a pressing issue affecting your patient population, or stating publically your opinion about important community issues are all components of your position and role, and more valued than you probably imagine.

This year's *5-Minute Clinical Consult* is here to assist in fulfilling our role as a healthcare provider. In each patient interaction, in addition to bringing your clinical expertise, remember how others view you, as a leader, and the power of your words and actions. Encourage them to dream more, learn more, do more, and to be more.

Welcome to *The 5-Minute Clinical Consult 2016*. Our editorial team has collaborated with hundreds of authors so that you may deliver your patients the best care. Each topic provides you with quick answers you can trust, where and when you need them most, either in print or online at www.5MinuteConsult.com.

This highly organized content provides you with:

- Differential diagnosis support from our expanded collection of algorithms
- Current evidence-based designations highlighted in each topic
- 600+ commonly encountered diseases in print, with an additional 1,400 online topics, including content from *The 5-Minute Pediatric Consult* and *Rosen & Barkin's 5-Minute Emergency Medicine Consult*
- FREE point-of-care CME and CE: 1/2 hour credit for every digital search
- Thousands of images to help support visual diagnosis of all conditions
- Video library of procedures, treatment, and physical therapy
- A to Z Drug Database from Facts & Comparisons®
- Laboratory test interpretation from *Wallach's Interpretation of Diagnostic Tests*
- More than 3,000 patient handouts in English and Spanish
- ICD-9 and ICD-10 codes and *DSM-5* criteria; additionally, SNOMED codes are available online.

Our website, www.5MinuteConsult.com delivers quick answers to your questions. It is an ideal resource for patient care. Integrating *5-Minute* content into your workflow is easy and fast. And, our patient education handouts can assist in helping you meet Meaningful Use compliance.

If you purchased the Premium Edition your access includes 1 year FREE; the Standard Edition includes a free 10-day trial! The site promises an easy-to-use interface, allowing smooth maneuverability between topics, algorithms, images, videos, and patient education materials, as well as more than 1,400 online-only topics.

Evidence-based health care is the integration of the best medical information *with* the values of the patient and your skill as a clinician. We have updated our EBM content and its visibility, so you can focus on how to best apply it in your practice.

We have solved the health maintenance challenge by including the link to the U.S. Preventive Services Task Force calculator. Enter a patient's gender and age, and you are presented with the best recommendations to keep that specific patient healthy.

The algorithm section includes both diagnostic and treatment algorithms. This easy-to-use graphic method helps you evaluate an abnormal finding and prioritize treatment. They are also excellent *teaching tools*, so share them with the learners in your office.

In our role as clinicians, caring for those who are ill or helping to prevent illness, we use tests and prescribe treatments, hoping they improve outcomes. As importantly, our words and actions, even a shared smile, can make a huge difference. Thank you for being a leader in your practice and community.

The 5-Minute Clinical Consult editorial team values your observations, so please share your thoughts, suggestions, and constructive criticism through our website, www.5MintueConsult.com.

Frank J. Domino, MD
January 1, 2015

EVIDENCE-BASED MEDICINE

WHAT IS EVIDENCE-BASED MEDICINE?

Remember when we used to treat every otitis media with antibiotics? These recommendations came about because we applied logical reasoning to observational studies. If bacteria cause an acute otitis media, then antibiotics should help it resolve sooner, with less morbidity. Yet, when rigorously studied (via a systematic review), we found little benefit to this intervention.

The underlying premise of evidence-based medicine (EBM) is the evaluation of medical interventions, and the literature that supports those interventions, in a systematic fashion. EBM hopes to encourage treatments proven to be effective and safe. And when insufficient data exists, it hopes to inform you on how to safely proceed.

EBM uses as end points of real patient outcomes; morbidity, mortality and risk. It focuses less on intermediate outcomes (bone density) and more on patient conditions (hip fractures).

Implementing EBM *requires* 3 components: the best medical evidence, the skill and experience of the provider, and the values of the patients. Should this patient be screened for prostate cancer? It depends on what is known about the test, on what you know of its benefits and harms, your ability to communicate that information, and that patient's informed choice.

This book hopes to address the first EBM component, providing you access to the best information in a quick format. Although not every test or treatment has this level of detail, many of the included interventions here use systematic review literature support.

The language of medical statistics is useful in interpreting the concepts of EBM. Below is a list of these terms, with examples to help take the confusion and mystery out of their use.

Prevalence: *proportion of people* in a population who have a disease (in the United States, 0.3% [3 in 1,000] people older than the age of 50 years have colon cancer)

Incidence: How many *new cases of a disease* occur in a population during an interval of time; for example, "the estimated incidence of colon cancer in the United States is 104,000 in 2005."

Sensitivity: percentage of people with disease who test positive; for mammography, the sensitivity is 71–96%.

Specificity: percentage of people without disease who test negative; for mammography, the specificity is 94–97%.

Suppose you saw ML, a 53-year-old woman, for a health maintenance visit, ordered a *screening* mammogram, and the report demonstrates an irregular area of microcalcifications. She is waiting in your office to receive her test results; what can you tell her?

Sensitivity and specificity refer to characteristics of people who are *known to have disease* (sensitivity) or those that are *known not to have disease* (specificity). But, what you have is an abnormal test result. To better explain this result to ML, you need the positive predictive value.

Positive predictive value (PPV): percentage of *positive* test results that are truly positive; the PPV for a woman aged 50–59 years is approximately 22%. That is to say that only 22% of abnormal screening mammograms in this group truly identified cancer. The other 78% are false positives.

You can tell ML only 1 out of 5 abnormal mammograms correctly identify cancer; the 4 are false positives, but the only way to know which mammogram is correct is to do further testing.

The corollary of the PPV is the negative predictive value (NPV), which is the percentage of negative test results that are truly negative.

The PPV and NPV tests are population-dependent, whereas the sensitivity and specificity are characteristics of the test, and have little to do with the patient in front of you. So when you receive an abnormal lab result, especially a screening test such as mammography, understand their limits based on their PPV and NPV.

Treatment information is a little different. In discerning the statistics of randomized, controlled trials of interventions, first consider an example. The Scandinavian Simvastatin Survival Study (4S) (*Lancet.* 1994;344[8934]:1383–1389) found using simvastatin in patients at high risk for heart disease for 5 years resulted in death for 8% of simvastatin patients versus 12% of those on placebo; this results in a relative risk of 0.70, a relative risk reduction of 33%, and a number needed to treat of 25.

There are two ways of considering the benefits of an intervention with respect to a given outcome. The absolute risk reduction is the difference in the percentage of people with the condition before and after the intervention. Thus, if the incidence of MI was 12% for the placebo group and 8% for the simvastatin group, the absolute risk reduction is 4% (12% − 8% = 4%).

The relative risk reduction reflects the improvement in the outcome as a percentage of the original rate and is commonly used to exaggerate the benefit of an intervention. Thus, if the risk of MI were reduced by simvastatin from 12 to 8%, then the relative risk reduction would be 33% (4%/12% = 33%); 33% sounds better than 4%, but the 4% is the absolute risk reduction and reflects the true outcome.

Absolute risk reduction is usually a better measure of *clinical* significance of an intervention. For instance, in one study, the treatment of mild hypertension was been shown to have relative risk reduction of 40% over 5 years (40% fewer strokes in the treated group). However, the absolute risk reduction was only 1.3%. Because mild hypertension is not strongly associated with strokes, aggressive treatment of mild hypertension yields only a small clinical benefit. Don't confuse relative risk reduction with relative risk.

Absolute (or attributable) risk (AR): the percentage of people in the placebo or intervention group who reach an end point; in the simvastatin study, the absolute risk of death was 8%.

Relative risk (RR): the risk of disease of those treated or exposed to some intervention (i.e., simvastatin) divided by those in the placebo group or who were untreated

–If RR <1.0, it reduces risk–the smaller the number, the greater the risk reduction.

–If RR >1.0, it increases the risk–the greater the number, the greater the risk increase.

Relative risk reduction (RRR): the relative decrease in risk of an end point compared to the percent of that end point in the placebo group

If you are still confused, just remember the RRR is an overestimation of the actual effect.

Number needed to treat (NNT): This is the number of people who need to be treated by an intervention to prevent one adverse outcome. A "good" NNT can be a large number (>100) if risk of serious outcome is great. If the risk of an outcome is not that dangerous, then lower (<25) NNTs are preferred.

The NNT should be compared to a similar statistic, the number needed to harm (NNH). This is the number of people who have to be given treatment before one excess side effect or harm occurs. When the NNT is compared to the NNH, you and the patient can judge whether the benefit of the intervention is great enough to outweigh the risk of harm.

EVIDENCED-BASED GRADING:

To help you interpret diagnostic and treatment recommendations within *The 5-Minute Clinical Consult*, we have graded the best information within the text, and highlighted this content.

An "A" grade means the reference is from the highest quality resource, such as a systematic review. A *systematic review* is a summary of the medical literature on a given topic that uses strict, explicit methods to perform a thorough search of the literature and then provides a critical appraisal of individual studies, concluding in a recommendation. The most prestigious collection of systematic reviews is from the Cochrane Collaboration (www.cochrane.org).

A "B" grade means the data referenced comes from high-quality randomized controlled trials performed to minimize bias in their outcome. Bias is anything that interferes with the truth; in the medical literature, it is often unintentional, but it is much more common than we appreciate. In short, always assume some degree of bias exists in any research endeavor.

A "C" grade implies the reference used does not meet the A or B requirements; they are often treatments recommended by consensus groups (such as the American Cancer Society). In some cases, they may be the standards of care. But implicit in a group's recommendation is the bias of the author or the group that supports the reference. For example, the American Urological Society's recommendation around screening for prostate cancer may be motivated by their narrow scope and financial benefit. Compare this to the recommendations of the U.S. Preventive Services Task Force (www.ahrq.gov), which recommends against screening for prostate cancer.

BIAS:

Bias is anything that interferes with the truth. There are many types of bias that should be considered by the publishers of medical information. Below describes a number of bias types that often affect our care without us knowing it is present:

Publication bias occurs when research is not published; this is often when a study finds data that does *not* support an intervention. The motivation to publish information that "didn't work" is low. It is estimated that up to 40% of all medical research never gets published. When you read of an effective intervention," wonder if other studies did not show benefit and went unpublished.

Comparator bias occurs when research compares an intervention to placebo, when placebo is not the standard of care. Knowing a new antibiotic is more effective than placebo for treating a condition is not helpful if you typically use a drug or procedure. Why not release research comparing the new drug to the standard of care? Sometimes the new treatment is no better than the current standard. And if a study was done to see if the new is better than the old, and not published, you have an example of publication bias.

Selection bias involves choosing study populations that might be different than the average patient or just reporting a just subset of study participants from a study. Either will result in the data being skewed because it can only be applied to small subset of people.

Attrition bias and the concept of intention to treat. Attrition bias is when researchers do not fully acknowledge and address how a study deals with participants who do not adhere to the research protocol or drop out completely. Intention to treat analysis hopes to diminish attrition bias by statistically considering the nonadhering or dropped out patients as unsuccessfully benefiting from the intervention.

Commercial (funder) bias involves who paid for the research being done, and do they have a vested interest in the outcome. If the developer of a new drug does a large study, or a researcher has a personal financial interest in seeing a study succeed, they may consciously or unconsciously alter what is reported in a study. The data may be accurate, but until this is studied by less vested interests, some feel its outcome cannot be clinically applied.

Have you been annoyed how one week you learn of a randomized controlled trial that supports a treatment, to be followed the next week with a contradictory article? Statisticians have figured out how to resolve this using something called a systematic review.

A Systematic Review gathers all the literature on a topic, say using antibiotics to treat otitis media, and combines the data to determine if the sum of all the trials tells a different story than any single trial. The large number of participants in this type of research results in a much more statistically (and clinically) significant conclusion than any single paper. Want more? Check this out: http://musculoskeletal.cochrane.org/what-systematic-review.

A **Meta-Analysis** is a quantitative systematic review and demonstrates its outcomes in the form of a forest plot. The bottom line with interpretation of a forest plot is to look for the diamond on the bottom. If it is to LEFT of the vertical line, it means risk of an outcome was reduced by the intervention. If it is fully to the RIGHT, then risk of that outcome was increased. And if the diamond touches the vertical line, it means there was no statistical influence of the intervention on the outcome.

I hope this brief introduction to EBM has been informative, clear, and helpful. If any of the information above seems unclear, or if you have a question, please contact us via www.5MinuteConsult.com.

ACKNOWLEDGMENTS

This is the 24th edition of *The 5-Minute Clinical Consult*, a comprehensive point-of-care tool to assist in the care of patients. From beginning to end, one cannot find a more current and easy-to-use collection of clinically useful content.

Developing and maintaining a book and website of this magnitude requires an equally broad effort from its supporting team. I wish to thank the dedication and tireless efforts of many: executive editor, Rebecca Gaertner; product development editors, Leanne Vandetty and Kristina Oberle; marketing manager, Stephanie Kindlick; and publisher, Lisa McAllister. And, the editorial team would like to welcome Morrison and Vera!

This 2016 edition is the direct result of the dedication and insights of our associate editors. I wish to thank Drs. Robert Baldor, Jeremy Golding, and Mark Stephens for their hard work, and overwhelming commitment to *The 5-Minute Clinical Consult*. And to Dr. Jill Grimes for her continued support while away.

I wish to especially thank my wife, Sylvia, and my daughter, Molly, who have given greatly for this book.

The challenge of completing a book covering this broad a spectrum of medicine requires insights and skills far beyond my own. Many thanks to my mentors Bob Baldor and Mark Quirk who have been an enormous support—always there to encourage, reassure, and impart wisdom.

Many in the academic and health care worlds are due thanks for support, insight, and friendship: Daniel Lasser, Alan Chuman, Michele Pugnaire, Karen Rayla, Phil Fournier, Erik Garcia, Jeff Stovall, Jim Comes, Len Levin, Judy Norberg, J. Herb Stevenson, Robert Jenal, Michael Kidd, Zainab Nawab, Sanjiv and Amita Chopra, Vasilios (Bill) Chrisostomidis, James (Jay) Broadhurst, Danuta Antkowiak, Atreyi Chakrabarti, Kerry Morse, Kate Peasha, Amanda Deary-Reardon, the staff of Shrewsbury Family Medicine, Mark Powicki, Steve Messineo, and the faculty and students of the University of Massachusetts Medical School.

Medicine is a challenge I have fortunately not had to meet alone. Thanks to my parents, Frank and Angela (Jean); my brother John and his family, Marylou, Cate, and Jane; Frank, Mary Anne, Diane, and David Christian; the Diana and Hymie Lipschitz family; and the Bob and Ruth Pabreza family; they are responsible for who I am and my success in life.

I am blessed with the best of friends; without them, I would not be a physician. Thanks to Bob Bacic, Ron Jautz, Richard Onorato, John Horcher, Auguste Turnier, Bob Smith, Paul Saivetz, Bob and Nancy Gallinaro, Drew and Jill Grimes, Louay Toma, Laurie, Alan, Daniel, Jenny and Matt Bugos, Alan Ehrlich, Andy Jennings, Bill Demianiuk, Mark Steenbergen, John and Kathleen Polanowicz, Phil and Carol Pettine, Mark Shelton, Steve Bennett, Vicki Triolo, and Michael Bernatchez.

–Frank J. Domino, MD

CONTRIBUTING AUTHORS

Basmah Abdalla, MD
Nephrology Fellow
University of Massachusetts
Worcester, Massachusetts

Thomas L. Abell, MD

Arthur M. Schoen, MD
Chair in Gastroenterology
University of Louisville
Louisville, Kentucky

George M. Abraham, MD, MPH
Associate Chief of Medicine
Saint Vincent Hospital
Professor of Medicine
University of Massachusetts Medical School
Worcester, Massachusetts

Sherly Abraham, MD, FAAFP
Residency Program Director
Family Medicine Department
The Brooklyn Hospital Center
Brooklyn, New York

Reem Abu-Sbaih, DO
Assistant Professor
Department of Osteopathic Manipulative Medicine
New York College of Osteopathic Medicine
Old Westbury, New York

Ghazwan Acash, MD, FCCP
Assisstant Professor of Medicine
Tufts Medical School
Department of Pulmonary and Critical Care
Lahey Clinic
Burlington, Massachusetts

Yadira E. Acevedo, MD
Director of Medical Education
Faculty, Family Medicine Residency Program
Middlesex Hospital
Middletown, Connecticut

Joseph R. Adams, DO†
Department of Family Medicine
Martin Army Community Hospital
Fort Benning, Georgia

Lanier H. Adams, DO†
Department of Family Medicine
Eisenhower Army Medical Center
Fort Gordon, Georgia

Rae Adams, MD
Associate Professor of Family and Community Medicine
Texas A&M Health Science Center College of Medicine
Bryan, Texas

Ehiozogie Adu
Brooklyn, New York

Sumera R. Ahmad, MD
Department of Pulmonary and Critical Care
UMass Memorial Medical Center
Worcester, Massachusetts

Yasir Ahmed, MD
Penn State Hershey Eye Center
Penn State College of Medicine
Hershey, Pennsylvania

Mariam Akhtar, MD
Georgia Regents University
Augusta, Georgia

Jowhara Al-Qahtani, MD
General Surgery Resident
Maimonides Medical Center
Brooklyn, New York

Abdullah A. Al-Shahrani, MBBS
Medical Research Fellow
Division of Gastroenterology and Liver Diseases
The George Washington University
Washington, DC

Ben P. Alencherry, MD
Division of Gastroenterology and Liver Diseases
The George Washington University
Washington, DC

Andrew G. Alexander, MD
Assistant Clinical Professor of Family Medicine
University of California Riverside School of Medicine
Riverside, California

Mohammed Algodi, MD
Clinical Study Supervisor
Cardiology
Montefiore Medical Center
Bronx, New York

Fozia Akhtar Ali, MD
Family & Community Medicine
The University of Texas Health Science Center at San Antonio
San Antonio, Texas

Jason B. Alisangco, DO, FAAFP†
Family Medicine Department
Fort Belvoir Community Hospital
Fort Belvoir, Virginia

Aliyi Aliyi, MD
Resident
Georgia Regents University
Augusta, Georgia

Andrew Allegretti, MD
Clinical Fellow in Medicine
Division of Nephrology
Massachusetts General Hospital
Harvard Medical School
Boston, Massachusetts

Richard W. Allinson, MD
Associate Professor
Department of Surgery
The Texas A&M University System Health Sciences Center
Senior Staff Physician
Baylor Scott & White Clinic
Waco, Texas

Ziad Alnabki, MD
University of Louisville
Louisville, Kentucky

Melanie Dawn Altizer, MD
Assistant Professor
Deptartment of Obstetrics and Gynecology
Carilion Clinic
Roanoke, Virginia

Bree Alyeska, MD
Resident
Department of Emergency Medicine
University of Massachusetts Medical Center
Worcester, Massachusetts

Roger Allan Anderson, MD†
Staff Ophthalmologist
Department of Ophthalmology
Madigan Army Medical Center
Tacoma, Washington

Tanya E. Anim, MD
Fellow in Women's Health with Obstetrics Focus
Florida Hospital Family Medicine Residency Program
Winter Park, Florida

Arvind R. Ankireddypalli, MD
Attending Physician
Department of Family Medicine
The Brooklyn Hospital Center
Brooklyn, New York

David Anthony, MD, MSc
Assistant Professor of Family Medicine
The Warren Alpert Medical School of Brown University
Providence, Rhode Island

Kashif S. Anwar, MD
Department of Family Medicine
Robinson Memorial Hospital
Kent, Ohio

Paul M. Arguin, MD
Chief, Domestic Malaria Unit
Centers for Disease Control and Prevention
Atlanta, Georgia

Michael Arnold, MD, CDR, MC†
United States Naval Hospital
United States Navy
Naples, Italy

Armand Asarian, MD

Aneel A. Ashrani, MD, MS
Assistant Professor
Division of Hematology
Department of Internal Medicine
Mayo Clinic
Rochester, Minnesota

Shumaila Athar, MD
Department of Family Medicine
The University of Texas Southwestern Medical Center
Dallas, Texas

Carlos Atore, MD
Family Medicine Resident
The University of Texas Southwestern Austin
Austin, Texas

Stephen E. Auciello, MD
Resident Physician
Family Medicine Residency Program
OhioHealth Riverside Methodist Hospital
Columbus, Ohio

Gerard P. Aurigemma, MD
Professor of Medicine and Radiology
University of Massachusetts Medical School
Director, Noninvasive Cardiology
University of Massachusetts Memorial Medical Center
Worcester, Massachusetts

Philip Aurigemma, MD
Department of Orthopedics
University of Massachusetts Medical School
Worcester, Massachusetts

Swati B. Avashia, MD, FAAP
Assistant Professor, Internal Medicine, Pediatrics, Holistic Medicine
Family Medicine Residency Program
The University of Texas Southwestern Austin
Austin, Texas

Thomas R. Avonda, MD
Assistant Professor
Department of Family Medicine
East Tennessee State University
Johnson City, Tennessee

Nida S. Awadallah, MD
Assistant Clinical Professor
Department of Family Medicine
Rose Family Medicine Residency
University of Colorado
Denver, Colorado

Jennifer L. Ayres, PhD
Director of Behavioral Health Services
Family Medicine Residency Program
The University of Texas Southwestern Medical Center Austin
Austin, Texas

Holly L. Baab, MD
Assistant Director
Bayfront Family Medicine Residency
St. Petersburg, Florida

Sultan M. Babar, MD
Department of Family Medicine
Brody School of Medicine
East Carolina University
Greenville, North Carolina

Franklyn C. Babb, MD, FAAFP
Assistant Professor, Family Medicine
Clerkship Director
Department of Family and Community Medicine
Texas Tech University Health Sciences Center
Lubbock, Texas

Megan Babb, DO
Resident
Mercy Family Health Center
Sacramento, California

Kavita Babu, MD
Associate Professor
Department of Emergency Medicine
Division of Medical Toxicology
University of Massachusetts Memorial Medical Center
Worcester, Massachusetts

Elisabeth L. Backer, MD
Clinical Associate Professor
Department of Family Medicine
University of Nebraska Medical Center
Omaha, Nebraska

Melissa Badowski, PharmD
Clinical Assistant Professor
Section of Infectious Diseases
Department of Pharmacy Practice and Science
University of Illinois at Chicago, College of Pharmacy
Chicago, Illinois

Mirza Z. Baig, MD

Jennifer Bailey, DO, FAAP
Assistant Professor
Clinical Sciences
West Virginia School of Osteopathic Medicine
Lewisburg, West Virginia

Robert A. Baldor, MD, FAAFP
Professor and Vice-Chairman, Educational Affairs
Department of Family Medicine and Community Health
University of Massachusetts Medical School
Worcester, Massachusetts

Katherine L. Ball, MD
Department of Family Medicine
University of Washington
Seattle, Washington

Laura S. Ball, DO†
General Medical Officer
Family Medicine
Martin Army Community Hospital
Fort Benning, Georgia

Jonathan R. Ballard, MD, MPH, MPhil
Assistant Professor
Department of Family and Community Medicine
University of Kentucky College of Medicine
Lexington, Kentucky

Rahul Banerjee, MD
Internal Medicine Residency
Perelman School of Medicine
University of Pennsylvania
Philadelphia, Pennsylvania

Brent J. Barber, MD
Associate Professor, Pediatric Cardiology
University of Arizona College of Medicine
Tucson, Arizona

Wendy Brooks Barr, MD, MPH, MSCE
Associate Residency Director
Lawrence Family Medicine Residency
Assistant Professor of Family Medicine
Tufts University School of Medicine
Lawrence, Massachusetts

John P. Barrett, MD, MPH, MS, COL, USA†
Department of Family Medicine
Madigan Army Medical Center
Tacoma, Washington

Michael C. Barros, PharmD, BCPS, BCACP
Clinical Assistant Professor of Pharmacy Practice
Temple University School of Pharmacy
Philadelphia, Pennsylvania

Erin Bassett-Novoa, MD

Kay A. Bauman, MD, MPH
Medical Director
New Mexico Department of Corrections
Professor
Department of Family and Community Medicine
University of New Mexico School of Medicine
Albuquerque, New Mexico

Dennis J. Baumgardner, MD
Department of Family Medicine
Aurora University of Wisconsin Medical Group
University of Wisconsin School of Medicine and Public Health
Center for Urban Population Health
Milwaukee, Wisconsin

Hillery Bavani, DO, CPT, USA†
Family Medicine Resident
Martin Army Community Hospital
Fort Benning, Georgia

Jeffrey Baxter, MD
Assistant Professor
Department of Family Medicine and Community Health
University of Massachusetts Medical School
Worcester, Massachusetts

Cheryl Bayart, MD, MPH
PGY3
Department of Dermatology
Cleveland Clinic Foundation
Cleveland, Ohio

Sheryl Beard, MD
Senior Associate Program Director
Via Christi Family Medicine Residency Program
Clinical Assistant Professor
University of Kansas School of Medicine–Wichita
Wichita, Kansas

Kelly H. Beers, DO
New York Institute of Technology College of Osteopathic Medicine
Old Westbury, New York

Adriane E. Bell, MD†
Faculty
Family Medicine Residency Program
Tripler Army Medical Center
Honolulu, Hawaii

Hershey S. Bell, MD, MS, FAAFP
Vice President of Academic Affairs and Dean
Lake Erie College of Osteopathic Medicine School of Pharmacy
Erie, Pennsylvania and Bradenton, Florida

Paul P. Belliveau, PharmD, RPh
Professor of Pharmacy Practice
Department of Pharmacy Practice
Massachusetts College of Pharmacy and Health Sciences University
Worcester, Massachusetts

Ileana Bembenek, MD
Family Medicine Residency of Southwest Washington
Vancouver, Washington

Paul Beninger, MD, MBA

Crystal Benjamin, MD, MPH
Resident Physician, Family Medicine
University of Massachusetts Medical School
Fitchburg, Massachusetts

Sheldon Benjamin, MD
Professor of Psychiatry and Neurology
Department of Psychiatry
University of Massachusetts Medical School
Worcester, Massachusetts

Terrell Benold, MD
Clinical Assistant Professor
Department of Family Medicine
Dell Medical School, The University of Texas
Austin, Texas

Lionel Bercovitch, MD
Director of Pediatric Dermatology
Hasbro Children's Hospital
Professor of Dermatology
The Warren Alpert Medical School of Brown University
Providence, Rhode Island

Jasmine S. Beria, DO, MPH
Department of Medicine
Mount Sinai St. Luke's and Roosevelt Hospitals
New York, New York

Louis J. Berk, MD
Assistant Clinical Instructor
Department of Family Medicine
State University of New York-Downstate Medical Center
Brooklyn, New York

Jamie L. Berkes, MD
Assistant Professor of Medicine
Medical Director of Liver Transplant
Loyola University
Maywood, Illinois

Bettina Bernstein, DO
Clinical Assistant Professor
Department of Psychiatry
Philadelphia College of Osteopathic Medicine, Philadelphia Campus
Clinical Affiliate
Department of Child and Adolescent Psychiatry
Children's Hospital of Philadelphia
Philadelphia, Pennsylvania

John F. Bertagnolli, Jr., DO
Associate Professor of Family Medicine
Rowan University School of Osteopathic Medicine
Stratford, New Jersey

Neela Bhajandas, PharmD
Clinical Assistant Professor of Pharmacy
Temple University School of Pharmacy
Philadelphia, Pennsylvania

Varun Kumar Bhalla, MD
Pediatric Surgical Critical Care Fellow
Children's National Health System
Washington, DC

Nirmanmoh Bhatia, MD
Department of Medicine
University of Louisville
Louisville, Kentucky

Amit Bhojwani, DO
Otolaryngology/FPS Resident
Rowan University School of University
Stratford, New Jersey

Kenneth M. Bielak, MD, FACSM, FAAFP, CAQ-SM
Professor
Director of Primary Care Sports Medicine
Department of Family Medicine
Graduate School of Medicine
University of Tennessee Health Science Center
Knoxville, Tennessee

Ghazaleh Bigdeli, MD, FCCP
Pulmonary Rehab Associates
Youngstown, Ohio

Barton L. Blackorby, MD†
Resident Ophthalmologist
Department of Ophthalmology
Madigan Army Medical Center
Tacoma, Washington

Joceyln F. Blackwell, MD, MAJ, MC†
Carl R. Darnall Army Medical Center
Fort Hood, Texas

James D. Blake, MD

Lewis S. Blevins, Jr., MD
Professor of Neurological Surgery and Medicine
Director
California Center for Pituitary Disorders at University of California San Francisco
San Francisco, California

Elise Bognanno, MD

Aaron R. Bolduc, MD
Surgery Department
Georgia Regents University
Augusta, Georgia

Kimberly Bombaci, MD

Nancy A. Bono, DO, FACOFP
Associate Professor/Chair of Family Medicine
New York Institute of Technology College of Osteopathic Medicine
Old Westbury, New York

Katrina A. Booth, MD
Assistant Professor
Division of Gerontology, Geriatrics, and Palliative Care
The University of Alabama at Birmingham
Birmingham, Alabama

Bryan C. Bordeaux, DO, MPH
Clinical Instructor
Department of Population Medicine
Harvard Medical School
Boston, Massachusetts

Marie L. Borum, MD, EdD, MPH
Professor of Medicine
Director
Division of Gastroenterology and Liver Diseases
The George Washington University
Washington, DC

Douglas J. Bosin, DO
Traditional Intern
Allegiance Health
Jackson, Michigan

Emily Bouley, MD
University of Massachusetts Medical School
Worcester, Massachusetts

Crystal C. Bowe, MD, MPH
Family Medicine Physician
Caromont Medical Group
Gastonia, North Carolina

Andrew Boylan, MD

Rachel Bramson, MD
Associate Professor
Department of Community and Family Medicine
College of Medicine
Texas A&M Health Science Center
Bryan, Texas

Doreen B. Brettler, MD
Director, New England Hemophilia Center
Professor of Medicine
Department of Medicine
University of Massachusetts Medical Center
Worcester, Massachusetts

Ekaterina Brodski-Quigley, MD, EdM

Emma Brooks, MD
Assistant Professor
Department of Family Medicine
Oregon Health Sciences University
Portland, Oregon

Christine M. Broszko, MD

Benjamin P. Brown, MD
Resident
Department of Obstetrics and Gynecology
University of Chicago Medical Center
Chicago, Illinois

Jimmy J. Brown, DDS, MD, FACS
Chief, Head and Neck Surgery
Georgia Regents University
Augusta, Georgia

Michael L. Brown, MD
Division of Psychiatry and Psychology
Baylor Scott & White Healthcare College Station
Assistant Professor
Department of Psychiatry and Behavioral Sciences
Texas A&M University Health Science Center College of Medicine
College Station, Texas

Samuel Luke Brown, DO
Emergency Medicine Resident
Dartmouth-Hitchcock Medical Center
Lebanon, New Hampshire

Theodore R. Brown, DO, MPH, FAAFP†
Command Surgeon
National Defense University Health and Fitness Directorate
Fort Lesley J. McNair
Washington, DC

Karen Browning, MD
Obstetrics and Gynecology Resident
Women & Infants Hospital
Brown University
Providence, Rhode Island

Matthew E. Bryant, MD†

Shima Syed, MD
Department of Family Medicine
Dwight D. Eisenhower Army Medical Center
Fort Gordon, Georgia

Carl Bryce, MD†
Family Medicine Resident
Nellis Air Force Base
Las Vegas, Nevada

Nitin Budhwar, MD
Associate Professor
Department of Family and Community Medicine
The University of Texas Southwestern Medical Center
Dallas, Texas

Han Q. Bui, MD, MPH†
Naval Medical Clinic Quantico
Quantico, Virginia

Christopher W. Bunt, MD, FAAFP†
Assistant Professor
Department of Family Medicine
Uniformed Services University
Bethesda, Maryland

Tiffany Burca, DO
Family Medicine Residency
University of Nebraska Medical Center
Omaha, Nebraska

Kristina G. Burgers, MD†
Faculty Family Physician
Department of Family Medicine
Madigan Army Medical Center
Tacoma, Washington

John R. Burk, MD
Texas Pulmonary and Critical Care Consultants, PA
Fort Worth, Texas

Harold J. Bursztajn, MD
Associate Clinical Professor of Psychiatry
Cofounder, Program in Psychiatry and the Law
Beth Israel Deaconess Medical Center
Psychiatry of Harvard Medical School
President of the American Unit of the UNESCO Bioethics Chair
Boston, Massachusetts

Blake R. Busey, DO†
Family Medicine Physician
Department of Family Medicine
Womack Army Medical Center
Fort Bragg, North Carolina

Jason N. Butler, DO, MS†
Resident
Womack Family Medicine Residency
Womack Army Medical Center
Fort Bragg, North Carolina

Nancy Byatt, DO, MBA, FAPM
Assistant Professor of Psychiatry and Obstetrics & Gynecology
UMass Memorial Medical Center/UMass Medical School
Worcester, Massachusetts

Stephen D. Cagle, Jr., MD, Capt, USAF, MC†
Nellis Air Force Base
Las Vegas, Nevada

Mitchell A. Cahan, MD, MBA, FACS
Associate Professor of Surgery
University of Massachusetts Medical School
Worcester, Massachusetts

Elizabeth M. Cain, MD, FAAFP
Assistant Professor of Family Medicine
Assistant Program Director
Louisiana State University Rural Family Medicine Residency Program
Bogalusa, Louisiana

Katherine M. Callaghan, MD
Assistant Professor of Obstetrics and Gynecology
UMass Memorial Medical Center
Worcester, Massachusetts

Ryan J. Callery, MD
Assistant Professor of Obstetrics and Gynecology
UMass Memorial Medical Center
Worcester, Massachusetts

Maya Campara, PharmD, BCPS
Clinical Assistant Professor
Clinical Pharmacist
Transplant Department of Pharmacy Practice
University of Illinois at Chicago
Chicago, Illinois

Nathan Cardoos, MD
Primary Care Sports Medicine
Department of Family Medicine
University of Massachusetts
Worcester, Massachusetts

Jennifer L. Carey, MD
Assistant Professor
Department of Emergency Medicine
University of Massachusetts Medical School
Worcester, Massachusetts

Patrick M. Carey, DO, MAJ, USA†
Family Medicine Department
Fort Belvoir Community Hospital
Fort Belvoir, Virginia

Samuel B. Carli, MD
Portland, Oregon

Amanda M. Carnes, MD†
Department of Family Medicine
Womack Army Medical Center
Fort Bragg, North Carolina

Matthew C. Carpenter, MD
Family Physician
Rose Family Medicine
University of Colorado
Denver, Colorado

Noel J.M. Carrasco, MD, FAAP
Professor
A.T. Still University School of Osteopathic Medicine in Arizona
Mesa, Arizona

Laurie A. Carrier, MD
Director of Behavioral Health and Integrated Care
Heartland Health Centers
Northwestern University
Department of Family and Community Medicine
Feinberg School of Medicine
Chicago, Illinois

Ana I. Casanegra, MD, RPVI, FSVM
Assistant Professor, Department of Medicine
Cardiovascular Section
University of Oklahoma Health Sciences Center
Oklahoma City, Oklahoma

Casandra Cashman, MD
Assistant Director
Community Health Network
Family Medicine Residency
Indianapolis, Indiana

Mary Cataletto, MD, FAAP, FCCP
Winthrop University Hospital
Mineola, New York

Rodrigo Cavallazi, MD

Jeanne Cawse-Lucas, MD
Assistant Professor of Family Medicine
University of Washington School of Medicine
Seattle, Washington

Lorena Ceci, MSIV
University of Massachusetts Medical School
Worcester, Massachusetts

Jan Cerny, MD, PhD, FACP
Assistant Professor of Medicine
Division of Hematology/Oncology
Department of Medicine
Director, Leukemia Program
University of Massachusetts Medical School
Associate Director
Cancer Research Office
UMass Memorial Cancer Center
Worcester, Massachusetts

Olga M. Ceron, MD
Assistant Professor
Department of Ophthalmology
University of Massachusetts Medical School
Worcester, Massachusetts

Cindy J. Chambers, MD, MAS, MPH
Department of Dermatology
UC Davis Health System
Sacramento, California

Jacquelyn Chambers, MD

Ronald G. Chambers, Jr., MD, FAAFP
Program Director
Methodist Family Medicine Residency
Sacramento, California

Aditya Chandrasekhar, MD, MPH
Instructor, Harvard Medical School
Fenway Health/Beth Israel Deaconess Medical Center
Boston, Massachusetts

Felix B. Chang, MD, DABMA, ABIHM
Clinical Associate Professor
Department of Family Medicine
University of Massachusetts School of Medicine
Hospital Medicine
Director, Inpatient Service
UMass Fitchburg Family Medicine Residency Program
Hospitalist
UMass Memorial Medical Group
Leominster, Massachusetts

Jennifer G. Chang, MD, Maj, USAF, MC†
Family Medicine Faculty Physician
Family Medicine Residency Clinic
Offutt Air Force Base, Nebraska

Joann Y. Chang, MD
Resident Physician
Long Beach Memorial Family Medicine
Long Beach, California

Millicent King Channell, DO, MA, FAAO
Associate Professor
Departments of Family Medicine and Osteopathic Manipulative Medicine
Rowan University
Stratford, New Jersey

Jason Chao, MD, MS
Professor
Department of Family Medicine and Community Health
Case Western Reserve University
University Hospitals Case Medical Center
Cleveland, Ohio

Arka Chatterjee, MD
Chief Fellow
Division of Cardiovascular Disease
University of Alabama at Birmingham
Birmingham, Alabama

Bimal P. Chaudhari, MD, MPH
Medical Genetics Resident
Center for Medical Genetics
Magee-Womens Hospital of UPMC
Division of Medical Genetics
Department of Pediatrics
Children's Hospital of Pittsburgh
Pittsburgh, Pennsylvania

Sarah H. Cheeseman, MD
Division of Infectious Diseases and Immunology
UMass Memorial Health Care
Clinical Professor of Medicine, Pediatrics, Microbiology, and Applied Physiologic Systems
University of Massachusetts Medical School
Worcester, Massachusetts

Amy Chen, MD, PhD
Assistant Professor
Department of Neurology
University of Rochester
Rochester, New York

Moses H. Cheng, MAJ, MC, USA†
Department of Family Medicine
Naval Hospital Camp Pendleton
Camp Pendleton, California

Suma Chennubhotla, MD
Department of Internal Medicine
University of Louisville
Louisville, Kentucky

Rebecca M. Cherner, DO
Associate Professor, Family Medicine
Nova Southeastern University College of Osteopathic Medicine
Davie, Florida

Sonia Nagy Chimienti, MD
Clinical Associate Professor of Medicine
Medical Director
Solid Organ Transplantation and Transplant Infectious Diseases
UMass Memorial Medical Center
University of Massachusetts Medical School
Worcester, Massachusetts

Manasi Chitre, MD

Zoya Chittireddy, MD
Internal Medicine
North Shore-LIJ
Forest Hills, New York

Binny Chokshi, MD
Pediatric Chief Resident
Children's National Health System
Washington, DC

Tayseer Husain Chowdhry, MD, MA
Department of Surgery
Georgia Regents University
Augusta, Georgia

Vasilios Chrisostomidis, DO
Assistant Professor
Department of Family Medicine and Community Health
University of Massachusetts Medical School
Worcester, Massachusetts

Ashley K. Christiani, MD
Associate Program Director
Kaiser Permanente Napa-Solano Family Medicine Residency Program
Vallejo, California

Alia Christy, MD, MS
Assistant Professor, Medicine
Temple University School of Medicine
Philadelphia, Pennsylvania

Felicia Chu, MD
Assistant Professor
Department of Neurology
University of Massachusetts Medical School
Worcester, Massachusetts

Tara Chute, MD
Resident Physician
Department of Obstetrics and Gynecology
University of Massachusetts Memorial Campus
Worcester, Massachusetts

Brian Ciampa, MD
Gastroenterology Fellow
Department of Gastroenterology
The George Washington University Hospital
Washington, DC

Amanda Vick Clark, MD
Resident
University of Alabama at Birmingham
Birmingham, Alabama

S. Lindsey Clarke, MD, FAAFP
Professor (Greenwood/Family Medicine)
Medical University of South Carolina Area Health Education Consortium
Self Regional Healthcare Family Medicine Residency Program
Greenwood, South Carolina

David M. Clive, MD
Professor of Medicine
Department of Medicine
University of Massachusetts Medical School
Worcester, Massachusetts

Kara M. Coassolo, MD
Maternal Fetal Medicine
Lehigh Valley Health Network
Allentown, Pennsylvania

Jason Cohn, DO, MS
Academic Medicine Scholar
New York Institute of Technology College of Osteopathic Medicine
Old Westbury, New York

Timothy J. Coker, MD†
Assistant Program Director
Ehrling Bergquist Family Medicine Residency
Offutt Air Force Base, Nebraska

Brian R. Coleman, MD
Associate Professor
University of Oklahoma
Department of Family Medicine
Oklahoma City, Oklahoma

Sarah Coles, MD
Clinical Educator
Family Medicine
Banner Good Samaritan Family Medicine Residency
Phoenix, Arizona

Irene C. Coletsos, MD
Associate Professor of Psychiatry
University of Massachusetts Medical School
Worcester, Massachusetts

Jeffrey W. Collins, DO
Good Samaritan Regional Medical Center
Corvallis, Oregon

Rebecca Collins, DO, MPH, FAAFP
Medical Director
NYMC Phelps Family Medicine Residency Program
Open Door Family Medical Centers, Inc.
Ossining, New York

Jamie N. Colombo, DO
Pediatric Resident
Department of Pediatrics
University of Arizona
Tucson, Arizona

Stephen J. Conner, MD†

Stephanie L. Conway, PharmD, RPh
Assistant Professor of Pharmacy Practice
Massachusetts College of Pharmacy and Health Sciences University
Worcester, Massachusetts

Jiadi Cook, MD
Geriatric Fellow
Thomas Jefferson University Hospital
Philadelphia, Pennsylvania

Maryann R. Cooper, PharmD, BCOP
Assistant Professor of Pharmacy Practice
Massachusetts College of Pharmacy and Health Sciences
University School of Pharmacy-Worcester/Manchester
Manchester, New Hampshire

Macario C. Corpuz, MD, MBA, FAAFP
Medical Staff
St. Vincent Medical Group
Worcester, Massachusetts

Danton Spohr Correa, MD, PhD
Attending Surgeon, Department of Surgery
Federal University of Santa Catarina Medical School
Florianopolis, Santa Catarina, Brazil

Paul Crawford, MD†
Program Director
Nellis Family Medicine Residency
Las Vegas, Nevada
Associate Professor
Department of Family Medicine
Uniformed Services University
Bethesda, Maryland

Alan Cropp, MD, FCCP
Department of Pulmonary Medicine
St. Elizabeth Hospital Health Center
Youngstown, Ohio

Steven J. Crosby, MA, RPh, FASCP
Assistant Professor of Pharmacy Practice
Department of Pharmacy Practice
Massachusetts College of Pharmacy and Health Sciences University
Boston, Massachusetts

Katie M. Crowder, Maj, USAF, MC†
Family Physician
Medical Director
Family Health Clinic
Hickam Air Force Base, Hawaii

Mary Anne de la Cruz Estacio, DO
Family Medicine Resident
The University of Texas Health Science Center at San Antonio
San Antonio, Texas

Sandra Cuellar, PharmD, BCOP
University of Illinois Hospital & Health Sciences System
Department of Pharmacy
Chicago, Illinois

Hongyi Cui, MD, PhD, FACS, FICS
Assistant Professor of Surgery
Department of General and Laparoscopic Surgery
University of Massachusetts Medical School
Associate Director, Acute Care Surgery
University of Massachusetts Memorial Medical Center
Worcester, Massachusetts

William Dabbs, MD
Clinical Educator
Family Medicine
Banner Good Samaritan Family Medicine Residency
Phoenix, Arizona

Julie Dahl-Smith, DO, FAAFP, DABMA
Associate Professor
Associate Director
Residential Educational Program
Osteopathic Program Director
Department of Family Medicine
Medical College of Georgia
Georgia Regents University
Augusta, Georgia

Anthony Dambro, MD†
Camp Lejeune Family Medicine Residency
Camp Lejeune, North Carolina

Daniela Darrah, MD

Akhil Das, MD, FACS
Assistant Professor
Department of Urology
Thomas Jefferson University
Philadelphia, Pennsylvania

Jessica Davis, MD
Department of Internal Medicine
The George Washington University
Washington, DC

Robert C. Day, MD
PGY1
Obstetrics and Gynecology
Kaiser Permanente
Santa Clara, California

Sondra M. De Antonio, MD
Adjunct Assistant Professor
Neurology
Internal Medicine Department
Rowan University School of Osteopathic Medicine
Stratford, New Jersey

Garreth C. Debiegun, MD, FACEP
Department of Emergency Medicine
Maine Medical Center
Portland, Maine
Assistant Professor
Tufts University School of Medicine
Boston, Massachusetts

Alexei DeCastro, MD
Assistant Professor
CAQ Sports Medicine Director
MUSC/Trident Family Medicine Residency
Department of Family Medicine
Medical University of South Carolina
Charleston, South Carolina

Jeremy D. DeFoe, DO†
Resident
Department of Family Medicine
Dwight D. Eisenhower Army Medical Center
Fort Gordon, Georgia

Konstantinos E. Deligiannidis, MD, MPH
Assistant Professor of Family Medicine and Community Health
University of Massachusetts Medical School
Worcester, Massachusetts

John Delzell, Jr., MD, MSPH
Herbert Wertheim College of Medicine
Florida International University
Miami, Florida

Deborah M. DeMarco, MD
Senior Associate Dean for Clinical Affairs
Professor of Medicine
Division of Rheumatology
University of Massachusetts Medical School
Worcester, Massachusetts

LeeAnne Denny, MD
Clinical Educator
Banner Good Samaritan Hospital
Phoenix, Arizona

David DeNofrio, MD
Medical Director
Advanced Heart Failure Program
Cardiology Division
Tufts Medical Center
Boston, Massachusetts

Gautam J. Desai, DO, FACOFP, CPI
Professor, Department of Family and Community Medicine
Kansas City University of Medicine and Biosciences
Kansas City, Missouri

Tarina Desai, MD
Family Medicine
The University of Texas Health Science Center at San Antonio
San Antonio, Texas

Richard F. DeSouza, MD
Clinical Instructor of Medicine
Yale School of Medicine
Attending Physician/Hospitalist
Yale New-Haven Hospital
New Haven, Connecticut

Richard D. Detheridge, MD[†]
Resident
Department of Family and Community Medicine
Dwight D. Eisenhower Army Medical Center
Fort Gordon, Georgia

Mathew J. Devine, DO
Associate Medical Director
Highland Family Medicine
Family Medicine Department
University of Rochester
Rochester, New York

William W. Dexter, MD, FACSM
Sports Medicine Program
Maine Medical Center
Portland, Maine

Lisa M. Diaz, DO

Howard Dickey-White, MD, FACEP
Chief Medical Officer
4M Medical Management
Akron, Ohio

Mary DiGiulio, DO[†]
Fort Gordon, Georgia

Robert J. Dimeff, MD
Professor
Orthopedics Surgery, Pediatrics, and Family & Community Medicine
The University of Texas Southwestern Medical Center
Dallas, Texas

Michael K. Ditkoff, MD, FACS
Department of Otolaryngology–Head & Neck Surgery
North Shore University Hospital
Manhasset, New York

Jason E. Domagalski, MD, FAAFP
Associate Program Director
Family Medicine Residency
University of California
Riverside Health Clinic
Palm Springs, California

Frank J. Domino, MD
Professor and Director of Predoctoral Education
Department of Family Medicine and Community Health
University of Massachusetts Medical School
Worcester, Massachusetts

Grace Donohue, MD
Family Practice Resident, PGY3
Bayfront Health St. Petersburg
St. Petersburg, Florida

Tammy Donoway, DO, FAAFP[†]
Assistant Residency Program Director
Department of Family Medicine
Womack Army Medical Center
Fort Bragg, North Carolina

John N. Dorsch, MD
Associate Professor
Department of Family and Community Medicine
University of Kansas School of Medicine–Wichita
Wichita, Kansas

Kristin D'Orsi, DO
Resident
Department of Obstetrics and Gynecology
University of Massachusetts Medical School
Worcester, Massachusetts

Hobie Dotson, PsyD
Licensed Clinical Psychologist
Assistant Professor
University of Kentucky
Hazard, Kentucky

Elizabeth Dougherty, MD
Internal Medicine/Pediatrics Resident
Maine Medical Center
Portland, Maine

Kathleen Downey, MD
Associate Clinical Professor
Family and Community Medicine
UC Primary Care–Wyoming
Cincinnati, Ohio

Karen Draper, MD

Anahita Dua, MD

Jacqueline Dubose, MD

Maurice Duggins, MD
Clinical Associate Professor
Department of Family and Community Medicine
Kansas University School of Medicine–Wichita
Associate Director, Via Christi Family Medicine Residency Program
Wichita, Kansas

Kaelen C. Dunican, PharmD
Associate Professor
Department of Pharmacy Practice
Massachusetts College of Pharmacy and Health Sciences University
Worcester, Massachusetts

Maegen Dupper, MD

Nedim Durakovic, MD
Resident Physician
Department of Otolaryngology
Washington University School of Medicine
St. Louis, Missouri

Cheryl Durand, PharmD
Assistant Professor of Pharmacy Practice
Massachusetts College of Pharmacy and Health Sciences University
Manchester, New Hampshire

Omar Durani, MD
Family and Community Medicine
The University of Texas Southwestern
Dallas, Texas

William Jerry Durbin, MD
Professor of Pediatrics and Internal Medicine
University of Massachusetts Medical School
Worcester, Massachusetts

Nathalie Duroseau
New York Institute of Technology College of Osteopathic Medicine
Old Westbury, New York

Phillip Marks Ecker, MD
Dermatologist
Minnesota Dermatology, PA
Plymouth, Minnesota

Samuel Ecker, DO
Dermatology Resident
Larkin Community Hospital
Miami, Florida

Alan M. Ehrlich, MD
Assistant Professor of Family Medicine
University of Massachusetts Medical School
Worcester, Massachusetts

Jordan Eisenstock, MD
Departments of Neurology and Psychiatry
University of Massachusetts Memorial Healthcare
Assistant Professor
University of Massachusetts Medical School
Director of Neurorehabilitation
Fairlawn Rehabilitation Hospital
Worcester, Massachusetts

William G. Elder, PhD
Professor
Family and Community Medicine
University of Kentucky
Lexington, Kentucky

Nancy Elliott, MD, FACS
Montclair Breast Center
Montclair, New Jersey

Taiwona Elliot, DO

Carrie Lynn Ellis, DVM, MS
Associate Veterinarian
Animal Hospital on Mt. Lookout Square
Cincinnati, Ohio

Robert Ellis, MD
Associate Professor
Department of Family and Community Medicine
University of Cincinnati
Cincinnati, Ohio

Pamela Ellsworth, MD
Professor of Urology
Vice Chair
Department of Urology
Chief
Division of Pediatric Urology
UMass Memorial Medical Center
University of Massachusetts Medical School
Worcester, Massachusetts

Fallon Enfinger, PharmD, CDE
Assistant Professor of Pharmacy Practice
Lake Erie College of Osteopathic Medicine School of Pharmacy
Bradenton, Florida

Katelin Engerer, MD
Dartmouth-Hitchcock Medical Center
Lebanon, New Hampshire

Petagaye English, DO, MS
Family Medicine Resident, PGY2
University Hospitals Richmond Medical Center
Cleveland, Ohio

Justin Thomas Ertle, BS, MD
PGY1
Internal Medicine
The George Washington University
Washington, DC

Jorge Luis Escobar Valle, MD
Internal Medicine Resident
University of Massachusetts
Worcester, Massachusetts

William A. Fabricius, MD
Hematology-Oncology Division
Department of Medicine
University of Massachusetts Medical School
Worcester, Massachusetts

Kristyn T. Fagerberg, MD
Private Practice
West Hills Family Health Center
Austin, Texas

Margaret Fairhurst, DO
Internal Medicine Resident
University Hospitals Regional Medical Center
Richmond Heights, Ohio

Nathan Falk, MD
Director, Primary Care Sports Medicine
University of Nebraska Medical Center
Omaha, Nebraska

Pang-Yen Fan, MD
Professor of Medicine
University of Massachusetts Medical School
Worcester, Massachusetts

Farimah Farahani, DO
Obstetrics and Gynecology Department
Virginia Tech Carilion School of Medicine
Roanoke, Virginia

Matthew V. Fargo, MD, MPH†
Family Medicine Program Director
Dwight D. Eisenhower Army Medical Center
Fort Gordon, Georgia

Rami Farhat, DO
Graduate Medical Education
Meadowlands Hospital Medical Center
Secaucus, New Jersey

Edwin A. Farnell, IV, MD†
Associate Program Director
Family Medicine Residency
Dwight D. Eisenhower Army Medical Center
Fort Gordon, Georgia

Umer Farooq, MD, MBBS
Staff Addiction Psychiatrist
Pine Rest Christian Mental Health Services
Grand Rapids, Michigan

Olusola Fasusi, MD

John W. Faught, MD
Program Director
Family Medicine Residency Program
Martin Army Community Hospital
Fort Benning, Georgia

Rhonda A. Faulkner, PhD
Director of Behavioral Medicine
Department of Family Medicine
Saint Joseph Hospital-UIC Master Affiliate
Chicago, Illinois

Kinder Fayssoux, MD
Eisenhower Medical Center
La Quinta, California

Jeffery P. Feden, MD, FACEP
Assistant Professor
Department of Emergency Medicine
The Warren Alpert Medical School of Brown University
Providence, Rhode Island

Ryan B. Feeney, PharmD
Community Staff Pharmacist
Philadelphia, Pennsylvania

Patricia Feito, MD
Family Medicine
Bayfront Health St. Petersburg
St. Petersburg, Florida

Neil J. Feldman, DPM, FACFAS
Owner
Central Massachusetts Podiatry, PC
Worcester, Massachusetts

Edward Feller, MD, FACP, FACG
Clinical Professor of Medicine
Adjunct Professor of Health Services, Policy and Practice
The Warren Alpert Medical School of Brown University
Providence, Rhode Island

Jennifer Fernandez, MD
Associate Program Director
Family Medicine Residency Program
Carolinas Health Care System-Union
Monroe, North Carolina

Kathleen Ferrer, MD, FAAP, AAHIVS
Children's National Medical Center
Department of Pediatrics
The George Washington University School of Medicine
Washington, DC

Scott A. Fields, MD, MHA
Professor and Vice Chair
Department of Family Medicine
Oregon Health and Science University
Portland, Oregon

Sara J. Fine, MD
University of Massachusetts Medical School
Worcester, Massachusetts

Stanley Fineman, MD
Adjunct Associate Professor
Department of Pediatrics
Emory University School of Medicine
Atlanta, Georgia

Jonathon M. Firnhaber, MD
Assistant Professor
Department of Family Medicine
East Carolina University
Greenville, North Carolina

Julietta Fiscella, MD, CPE, FCAP
Director of Pathology and Laboratory Medicine
University of Rochester Medicine/ Highland Hospital
Chair of Quality and Compliance
University of Rochester Medical Center Labs
Rochester, New York

Joshua Fischer, MD, PHD

Marc Fisher, MD
Department of Neurology
University of Massachusetts Medical School
Worcester, Massachusetts

Timothy P. Fitzgibbons, MD, PhD
Assistant Professor of Medicine
Cardiovascular Division
University of Massachusetts Medical School
Worcester, Massachusetts

Jonathan M. Flacker, MD, AGSF
Chief, Section of Geriatrics and Gerontology
Emory University School of Medicine
Atlanta, Georgia

Theodore B. Flaum, DO, FACOFP
Assistant Professor
Department of Osteopathic Manipulative Medicine
New York Institute of Technology College of Osteopathic Medicine
Old Westbury, New York

Joseph A. Florence, MD
Director of Rural Programs
Department of Family Medicine
James H. Quillen College of Medicine
East Tennessee State University
Johnson City, Tennessee

Emily K. Flores, PharmD, BCPS
Associate Professor of Pharmacy Practice
Bill Gatton College of Pharmacy
Adjunct Faculty
Department of Family Medicine
James Quillen College of Medicine
East Tennessee State University
Johnson City, Tennessee

Mary K. Flynn, MD
Assistant Professor
Department of Family Medicine and Community Health
University of Massachusetts Medical School
Worcester, Massachusetts

Harry W. Flynn, Jr., MD
Bascom Palmer Eye Institute
Miami, Florida

Jay Fong, MD
Assistant Professor
Department of Pediatrics
University of Massachusetts Medical Center
Worcester, Massachusetts

Joao C.S. Fontoura, Jr., MD
Department of Medicine and Pediatrics
University of South Florida
Tampa, Florida

Emily Forbes, DO
New York Institute of Technology College of Osteopathic Medicine
Old Westbury, New York

Brian Ford, MD[†]
Resident
Family Medicine
Naval Hospital Camp Pendleton
Camp Pendleton, California

William Fosmire, MD
Clinical Instructor
Saint Joseph Family Medicine Residency
Denver, Colorado

Lorna Fountain, MD
Associate Director
Family Medicine Residency
Bayfront Health
St. Petersburg, Florida

Phillip Fournier, MD
Associate Professor of Family Medicine and Community Medicine
University of Massachusetts Medical School
UMass Memorial Health Care
Worcester, Massachusetts

Robert L. Frachtman, MD, FACG
Austin Gastroenterology, PA
Austin, Texas

Mony Fraer, MD, FACP, FASN
Assistant Professor
Internal Medicine and Nephrology
University of Iowa Hospital and Clinics
Iowa City, Iowa

Brian Frank, MD
Assistant Professor
Family Medicine
Oregon Health and Science University
Portland, Oregon

Minjin Fromm, MD
Assistant Professor
Department of Orthopedics and Physical Rehabilitation
University of Massachusetts Medical School
Worcester, Massachusetts

Tara Futrell, MD
Sports Medicine
University of Massachusetts Medical School
Worcester, Massachusetts

Noah D. Futterman, DO
Emergency Medicine Resident
Robert Wood Johnson University Hospital
New Brunswick, New Jersey

Heidi L. Gaddey, MD[†]
Program Director
Family Medicine Residency
Ehrling Bergquist Clinic
Offutt Air Force Base, Nebraska

Steven W. Gale, MD[†]
Family Medicine Resident
Offutt Air Force Base
University of Nebraska Medical Center
Omaha, Nebraska

Curtis L. Galke, DO, FAAFP
Assistant Professor
Family and Community Medicine
The University of Texas Health Science Center at San Antonio
Associate Program Director, Family Medicine Residency
UTHSCSA-RGV-DHR
Edinburg, Texas

Sumanth Gandra, MD, MPH
Fellow
Center for Disease Dynamics, Economics & Policy
Washington, DC

Jennifer J. Gao, MD
Hematology and Oncology Fellow
National Cancer Institute
National Institutes of Health
Bethesda, Maryland

Andrew Gara, MD
University of Massachusetts Medical School
Worcester, Massachusetts

William T. Garrison, PhD
Professor of Pediatrics
University of Massachusetts Medical School
Worcester, Massachusetts

Brian Garrity, DO

Jewell V. Gaulding, MD
Resident, Internal Medicine
The Christ Hospital
Cincinnati, Ohio

Gerald Gehr, MD
Assistant Professor of Medicine
Dartmouth Medical School
Hanover, New Hampshire

Felix Geissler MD, PhD
Global Medical Affairs
Sanofi Oncology
Cambridge, Massachusetts

Bethany Gentilesco, MD

Paul George, MD, MHPE
Assistant Professor of Family Medicine
The Warren Alpert Medical School of Brown University
Providence, Rhode Island

Travis C. Geraci, MD
Resident
Department of Surgery
Brown University/Lifespan
Providence, Rhode Island

Fereshteh Gerayli, MD, FAAFP
Professor, Family Medicine
Johnson City Family Medicine Residency Program
East Tennessee State University
Quillen College of Medicine
Johnson City, Tennessee

Tiana M. Germann, MD
Family Medicine Resident
SUNY Stony Brook
Stony Brook, New York

Mahmoud Ghaderi, DO

Amaninderapal S. Ghotra, MD
Department of Internal Medicine
Division of General Internal Medicine
Palliative Medicine and Medical Education
University of Louisville
Louisville, Kentucky

Lawrence M. Gibbs, MD†
Assistant Clinical Professor
St. Louis University
Belleville Family Medicine Residency
Belleville, Illinois

Kory L. Gill, DO, FAAFP
Program Director
Department of Family and Community Medicine
Family Medicine Residency
Texas A&M Health Science Center College of Medicine
Bryan/College Station, Texas

Nora Gimpel, MD
Associate Professor
The University of Texas Southwestern Medical Center at Dallas
Dallas, Texas

Chad Van Ginkel, MD, MPH
Resident Physician
Department of Emergency Medicine
The Warren Alpert Medical School of Brown University
Providence, Rhode Island

Jonathan Giordano, DO, MSc
Department of Emergency Medicine
Maimonides Medical Center
Brooklyn, New York

Jason P. Glass, MD
Division of Gastroenterology and Liver Diseases
The George Washington University
Washington, DC

Gerald Gleich, MD

Ankur Goel, MD
Department of General Surgery
Georgia Regents University
Augusta, Georgia

Dori Goldberg, MD
Assistant Professor of Medicine
Division of Dermatology
University of Massachusetts Medical School
Worcester, Massachusetts

Jeremy Golding, MD, FAAFP
Professor of Family Medicine and Obstetrics & Gynecology
University of Massachusetts Medical School
Quality Officer
Department of Family Medicine and Community Health
University of Massachusetts Memorial Health Care
Hahnemann Family Health Center
Worcester, Massachusetts

Michael Golding, MD
Headquarters Senior Psychiatrist
California Department of Corrections
Elk Grove, California

Matthew J. Goldman, MD
Department of Family Medicine
University Hospitals Case Medical Center
Cleveland, Ohio

Rayna Goldstein, MD
Mount Sinai Hospital
New York, New York

Walter K. Goljan, MD
Webster Square Medical Center
Worcester, Massachusetts

Mercedes E. Gonzalez, MD, FAAD
Pediatric Dermatology of Miami
Miami, Florida

Herbert P. Goodheart, MD
Associate Clinical Professor
Department of Dermatology
Mount Sinai College of Medicine
New York, New York

Bharat Gopal, MD, MPH
Coordinator of Research
Carle Family Medicine Residency
Urbana, Illinois

Geetha Gopalakrishnan, MD
Associate Professor of Medicine
The Warren Alpert Medical School of Brown University
Providence, Rhode Island

Dónal Kevin Gordon, MD
Residency Program Director
Cedar Rapids Family Medicine Residency
Cedar Rapids, Iowa

Edward A. Gotfried, DO, FACOS
Assistant Professor
Department of Osteopathic Medicine
New York Institute of Technology College of Osteopathic Medicine
Old Westbury, New York

Parag Goyal, MD
Division of Cardiology
Department of Medicine
Weill Cornell Medical Center
New York-Presbyterian Hospital
New York, New York

Shami Goyal, MD
University of Pittsburgh Physicians
Department of Family Medicine
UPMC Matilda Theiss Health Center
Pittsburgh, Pennsylvania

Geoffrey M. Graeber, MD

Scott F. Graham, MD
Assistant Director
Bayfront Family Medicine Residency
St. Petersburg, Florida

Jane M. Grant-Kels, MD
Professor of Dermatology, Pathology, and Pediatrics
Chair, Department of Dermatology
Director of Dermatopathology
Director of the Cutaneous Oncology Program and Melanoma Center
Dermatology Residency Director
Assistant Dean of Clinical Affairs
University of Connecticut Health Center
Farmington, Connecticut

Meredith Gray, MD
Resident
Virginia Tech Carilion Department of Obstetrics and Gynecology
Roanoke, Virginia

Michael J. Gray, MD, MA, MS, ATC
Attending Physician
Emergency Care Center
Harrington Hospital
Southbridge, Massachusetts

Jonathan Green, MD
General Surgery Resident
Department of General Surgery
University of Massachusetts Medical School
Worcester, Massachusetts

Ronya L. Green, MD, MPH
Faculty Physician
Methodist Charlton Family Medicine Residency Program
Dallas, Texas

Ellen M. Greenblatt, BSc, MDCM
Medical Director
Centre for Fertility and Reproductive Health
Mount Sinai Hospital
Associate Professor
University of Toronto
Toronto, Ontario, Canada

David A. Greenwald, MD
Associate Division Director
Division of Gastroenterology
Montefiore Medical Center
Professor of Clinical Medicine
Albert Einstein College of Medicine
Bronx, New York

Charles K. Grigsby, MD
Resident, Surgery
Georgia Regents University
Augusta, Georgia

Pamela L. Grimaldi, DO, FAAFP
Medical Staff, Family Medicine
Saint Vincent Hospital
Worcester, Massachusetts

Andrew Grimes, MD
Medical Director
Capitol Anesthesiology Association
Austin, Texas

Jill A. Grimes, MD, FAAFP
Clinical Instructor
Department of Family Medicine
University of Massachusetts Medical School
Worcester, Massachusetts
Attending Physician
The University of Texas Health Services
Austin, Texas

Kristin Grindstaff, DO
Community Health Network
Family Medicine Residency
Indianapolis, Indiana

Matthew K. Griswold, MD
Resident, Emergency Medicine
University of Massachusetts
Worcester, Massachusetts

Scott P. Grogan, DO, MBA, FAAFP[†]
Department of Family and Community Medicine
Dwight D. Eisenhower Army Medical Center
Fort Gordon, Georgia

Michael W. Groves, MD, FACS
Assistant Professor
Department of Otolaryngology–Head and Neck Surgery
Medical College of Georgia
Georgia Regents University
Augusta, Georgia

Adarsh K. Gupta, DO, MS, FACOFP
Associate Professor
Department of Family Medicine
Stratford, New Jersey

Neena R. Gupta, MD
Assistant Professor of Pediatrics
Medical Director, Pediatric Kidney Transplant Program
Division of Pediatric Nephrology
University of Massachusetts Memorial Children's Medical Center
Worcester, Massachusetts

Sergey G. Gurevich, MD
Department of Medicine
New York-Presbyterian Hospital
New York, New York

Reem Hadi, MD
Family Medicine
The University of Texas Health Science Center at San Antonio
San Antonio, Texas

Laura Hagopian, MD, FAWM
Resident Physician
Department of Emergency Medicine
Boston Medical Center
Boston, Massachusetts

Ildiko Halasz, MD
VA Boston Healthcare System
Primary Care Clinic
West Roxbury, Maryland

Steven J. Halm, DO, FAAP, FACP
Associate Professor
Clinical Sciences
Medical Director of the Clinical Evaluation Center
West Virginia School of Osteopathic Medicine
Lewisburg, West Virginia

Phillip Benson Ham, III, MD, MS
General Surgery Resident
Department of General Surgery
Medical College of Georgia
Georgia Regents University
Augusta, Georgia

Jennifer L. Hamilton, MD, PhD, FAAFP
Assistant Professor
Department of Family, Community, and Preventive Medicine
Drexel University College of Medicine
Philadelphia, Pennsylvania

Ihab Hamzeh, MD, FACC
Division of Cardiology
Department of Medicine
Baylor College of Medicine
Houston, Texas

Edward Han, PharmD
Adjunct Assistant Professor
Department of Pharmacy Practice
Massachusetts College of Pharmacy and Health Sciences University
Worcester, Massachusetts

Jessica Handel, DO
Associate Program Director
St. Elizabeth Family Medicine Residency
St. Elizabeth Health Center
Youngstown, Ohio

Komal Hanif, MD
PGY1
Family Medicine
St. Louis University
Belleville, Illinois

Thomas J. Hansen, MD
Chief Academic Officer
Advocate Health Care
Downers Grove, Illinois

David M. Hardy, MD
Vascular Surgery Fellow
Department of Vascular Surgery
Cleveland Clinic
Cleveland, Ohio

Allison Hargreaves, MD

Dausen J. Harker, MD

Lisa M. Harris, DO, MAJ, MC, FS†
Family Medicine Faculty Physician
Womack Army Medical Center
Fort Bragg, North Carolina

Amena Hashmi, DO
Family Physician
Plano, Texas

Robyn M. Hatley, MD
Professor of Surgery and Pediatrics
Department of Surgery
Children's Hospital of Georgia
Georgia Regents Health System
Augusta, Georgia

Fern R. Hauck, MD, MS

Spencer P. Bass, MD
Twenty-First Century Professor of Family Medicine
Professor of Public Health Sciences
Department of Family Medicine
University of Virginia
Charlottesville, Virginia

Aaron Hauptman, MD
Resident
The University of Texas Southwestern Austin
Austin, Texas

Matthew Kendall Hawks, MD†
Resident Physician
Family Medicine
Nellis Air Force Base
Las Vegas, Nevada

James W. Haynes, MD
Associate Professor
Program Director
Department of Family Medicine
University of Tennessee College of Medicine
Chattanooga, Tennessee

Kevin Heaton, DO, CAQSM
Primary Care Sports Medicine
Access Sports Medicine and Orthopaedics
Exeter, New Hampshire

Brandon David Hecht, DO†
Family Medicine Resident
Dwight D. Eisenhower Army Medical Center
Augusta, Georgia

Robyn Heidenreich, MD
Family Medicine Resident, PGY2
Loma Linda University
Loma Linda, California

Janet O. Helminski, PT, PhD
Professor
College of Health Sciences
Midwestern University
Downers Grove, Illinois

Scott T. Henderson, MD
Director, Medical Services
Student Health Center
University of Missouri
Columbia, Missouri

Jaroslaw T. Hepel, MD
Assistant Professor
Department of Radiation Oncology
Rhode Island Hospital
Brown University
Providence, Rhode Island
Department of Radiation Oncology
Tufts Medical Center, Tufts University
Boston, Massachusetts

Nicolas Hernandez, MD
Family Medicine Senior Resident Physician
UMass Family Residency Program
Fitchburg, Massachusetts

Pablo I. Hernandez Itriago, MD, MS, FAAFP
Assistant Clinical Professor
Department Family Medicine
Boston University
Boston, Massachusetts

David N. Herrmann, MBBCh
Professor of Neurology and Pathology
University of Rochester
Rochester, New York

Brian Hertz, MD
Kaiser Permanente
San Rafael, California

Jessica Heselschwerdt, MD
Family Medicine Resident Physician
Department of Family Medicine
The University of Texas Southwestern Austin
Austin, Texas

Mary Annette Hess, PhD, FNP-BC, CNS
Assistant Professor
School of Nursing
University of Alabama at Birmingham
Birmingham, Alabama

David G. Hicks, MD
Professor
Department of Pathology and Laboratory Medicine
Director
Surgical Pathology Unit
University of Rochester Medical Center
Rochester, New York

Michael P. Hirsh, MD
Department of Surgery
University of Massachusetts Medical School
Worcester, Massachusetts

Crystal L. Hnatko, DO†
Family and Sports Medicine
Kaiser Permanente
Vacaville, California
Family Medicine Residency Faculty Physician
U.S. Air Force Reserves
David Grant Medical Center
Travis Air Force Base, California

Brian Ho, MD

Brandi Hoag, DO
Director
St. Vincent Ambulatory Care Center
Worcester, Massachusetts

Abigail Weil Hoffman, MD
General Surgery Resident
Georgia Regents University
Augusta, Georgia

Holly Milne Hofkamp, MD
Assistant Professor
Department of Family Medicine
Oregon Health & Science University
Portland, Oregon

Christopher Hogan, MD
Director of Trauma and Acute Care Surgery
Doctors Hospital
Augusta, Georgia

Thomas S. Hoke, MD
Primary Care
Sports Medicine Fellow
Maine Medical Center
Portland, Maine

Roger P. Holland, MD, PhD†
Department of Family and Community Medicine
Dwight D. Eisenhower Army Medical Center
Fort Gordon, Georgia

N. Wilson Holland MD, FACP, AGSF†
Associate Professor of Medicine
General Medicine and Geriatrics
Emory University School of Medicine
Staff Physician, Geriatric Clinics
Acting Designated Education Officer (DEO)
Atlanta Veterans Affairs Medical Center
Decatur, Georgia

Steven B. Holsten, Jr., MD, FACS
Associate Professor of Surgery
Georgia Regents University
Augusta, Georgia

Laurie Hommema, MD
Program Director
Riverside Family Medicine
Riverside Methodist Hospital
Columbus, Ohio

Amer Homsi, MD
General Surgery Resident
Department of Surgery
The Brooklyn Hospital Center
Brooklyn, New York

J. David Honeycutt, MD†
Nellis Air Force Base Family Medicine Residency
Nellis Air Force Base, Nevada

Vincent F. Honrubia, MD, FACS
South Texas Sinus Institute
Doctor's Hospital at Renaissance
Edinburgh, Texas

Michael P. Hopkins, MD, MEd
Chairman and Professor
Department of Obstetrics and Gynecology
Northeast Ohio Medical University
Rootstown, Ohio
Program Director
Department of Obstetrics and Gynecology
Aultman Hospital
Canton, Ohio

James M. Horowitz, MD, FACC
Assistant Professor of Medicine
Associate Director, Cardiac Care Unit
Division of Cardiology
New York Presbyterian Hospital–Weill Cornell Medical Center
New York, New York

Evan R. Horton, PharmD
Assistant Professor
Department of Pharmacy Practice
School of Pharmacy
Massachusetts College of Pharmacy and Health Sciences University
Worcester, Massachusetts

Robert W. Hostoffer, DO, FACOP, FACOI, FAAP, FCCP
Associate Professor of Pediatrics
Case Western Reserve University
Cleveland, Ohio

James E. Hougas, III, MD

Steven A. House, MD, FAAFP
Associate Professor
University of Louisville
Department of Family and Geriatric Medicine
Program Director University of Louisville/ Glasgow Family Medicine Residency Program
Glasgow, Kentucky

Laura Howe, MD
Department of Internal Medicine
University of Arizona
Tucson, Arizona

Kattie Hoy, MD†
Family Medicine Faculty Physician
Family Medicine Residency Clinic
Eglin Hospital
Eglin Air Force Base, Florida

Garrett W. Huck, MD, Capt, USAF†
Nellis Air Force Base Family Medicine Residency
Nellis Air Force Base, Nevada

Heather J. Hue, MD, MPH
Hematology & Medical Oncology
Lone Tree, Colorado

Dennis E. Hughes, DO, FAAFP, FACEP
Emergency Department
Cox Health
Branson, Missouri

Karen A. Hughes, MD, FAAFP
Family Medicine Residency Program
North Mississippi Medical Center
Tupelo, Mississippi

Michael D. Hughes, MD
Assistant Clinical Professor
Family Medicine
UC Riverside School of Medicine/UC Riverside Health
Palm Springs, California

Karen Hulbert, MD
Associate Professor
Department of Family and Community Medicine
The Medical College of Wisconsin
Milwaukee, Wisconsin

Jennifer L. Hunt, MD
Ridgecrest, California

James Hurlburt, DO
Family Medicine Resident
Texas A&M Family Medicine Residency
Bryan, Texas

John C. Huscher, MD
Associate Program Director
Family Medicine
Norfolk Rural Training Track
University of Nebraska Medical Center
Norfolk, Nebraska

Zeeshan Hussain, MD
Resident
Internal Medicine
University of Louisville
Louisville, Kentucky

Eric F. Hussar, MD
Family Physician
Susquehanna Family Medicine
Medical Director
Hope Within Community Health Center
Lancaster County, Pennsylvania

Carol Hustedde, PhD
Assistant Professor
Department of Family and Community Medicine
University of Kentucky
Lexington, Kentucky

Benjamin Hyatt, MD
Assistant Professor of Medicine
Division of Gastroenterology
University of Massachusetts Medical School
UMass Memorial Medical Center
Worcester, Massachusetts

Sara Hyatt, DO
New York Institute of Technology College of Osteopathic Medicine
Old Westbury, New York

Robert J. Hyde, MD, MA
Assistant Professor of Medicine
Section of Emergency Medicine
Geisel School of Medicine
Dartmouth-Hitchcock Medical Center
Lebanon, New Hampshire

Brenda W. Iddins, DNP, FNP-BC
University of Alabama at Birmingham
Birmingham, Alabama

P. Charles Inboriboon, MD, MPH FACEP
Assistant Professor of Emergency Medicine
University of Missouri Kansas City
Truman Medical Center
Kansas City, Missouri

Christine K. Jacobs, MD, FAAFP
Associate Professor
Saint Louis University School of Medicine
St. Louis, Missouri

Neha Jakhete, MD
Department of Medicine
Johns Hopkins Hospital
Baltimore, Maryland

Catherine A. James, MD
Assistant Professor
Department of Pediatrics
University of Massachusetts Medical School
Attending Physician in Pediatric Emergency Medicine
UMass Memorial Medical Center
Worcester, Massachusetts

Daniel S. Jamorabo, MD
University of Massachusetts Memorial Medical Center
Worcester, Massachusetts

Kyu K. Jana, MD
Assistant Professor
The University of Texas Medical Branch
Galveston, Texas

Maissaa Janbain, MD
Tulane School of Medicine
New Orleans, Louisiana

Adam Janicki, MD
Department of Emergency Medicine
The Warren Alpert Medical School of Brown University
Rhode Island Hospital
Providence, Rhode Island

Carrie Janiski, DO, MS, ATC
Resident Physician
Osteopathic Manipulative Medicine
University of New England College of Osteopathic Medicine
Biddeford, Maine

Elizabeth Janopaul-Naylor, MD
Resident
Cambridge Health Alliance
Psychiatry Residency of Harvard University
Cambridge, Massachusetts

Courtney I. Jarvis, PharmD
Associate Professor
Department of Pharmacy Practice
Massachusetts College of Pharmacy and Health Sciences University Worcester/Manchester
Worcester, Massachusetts

Salmaan Jawaid, MD
Pediatric Resident
Department of Internal Medicine
University of Massachusetts Medical Center
Worcester, Massachusetts

Razia Jayman-Aristide, MD
Associate Program Director
Internal Medicine
Forest Hills Hospital—Northshore-LIJ
Forest Hills, New York

Melissa S. Jefferis, MD, FAAFP
Riverside Family Medicine Residency
Columbus, Ohio

Cynthia Jeremiah, MD
Assistant Professor
Department of Family Medicine
UMass Memorial Medical Center
Worcester, Massachusetts

Pim Jetanalin, MD
Assistant Professor
Department of Rheumatology/Internal Medicine
University of Missouri–Kansas City
Kansas City, Missouri

Zaiba Jetpuri, DO, MBA
Assistant Professor
Family Medicine Department
The University of Texas Southwestern Medical Center
Dallas, Texas

Anub G. John, MD
Resident
Internal Medicine
University of Louisville
Louisville, Kentucky

Isaiah Johnson, MD

Julia V. Johnson, MD
Professor and Chair
Department of Obstetrics and Gynecology
University of Massachusetts Medical School
Worcester, Massachusetts

Julie Ann Johnston, MD
Faculty
Lawrence Family Medicine Residency
Lawrence, Massachusetts
Clinical Instructor
Department of Family Medicine
Tufts University School of Medicine
Boston, Massachusetts

Koryn Johnston, DO

Brandon Q. Jones, MD†
Family Medicine Physician
Nellis Family Medicine Residency
Nellis Air Force Base, Nevada

Marci D. Jones, MD
Associate Professor
Department of Orthopedic Surgery
University of Massachusetts
Worcester, Massachusetts

Stacy Jones, MD
Capitol Anesthesiology Association
Austin, Texas

Melody A. Jordahl-Iafrato, MD
Assistant Professor
Department of Family and Community Medicine
University of Arizona College of Medicine
Tucson, Arizona

Maurice F. Joyce, MD, EdM
Resident, Department of Anesthesiology
Tufts Medical Center
Boston, Massachusetts

Patrick Wakefield Joyner, MD, MS, LCDR†
Bone & Joint/Sports Medicine Institute
Naval Medical Center Portsmouth
Portsmouth, Virginia

Tya-Mae Y. Julien, MD
Gastroenterology and Hepatology
Baylor Regional Medical Center Plano
Plano, Texas

Manjula Julka, MD, FAAFP
Associate Professor and Medical Director
Dr. John L. and Louise Roan Professorship in Family Medicine
Family Medicine-Primary Care
The University of Texas Southwestern Medical Center
Dallas, Texas

Tipsuda Junsanto-Bahri, MD
Chair
Basic Biomedical Sciences
Assistant Professor
Pathology
Touro College of Osteopathic Medicine
New York, New York

Jenna Kahn, MD
Transitional Year Intern
Newton Wellesley Hospital
Newton, Massachusetts

Achyut B. Kamat, MD, FACEP
Clinical Associate Professor
Department of Emergency Medicine
The Warren Alpert School of Medicine of Brown University
Providence, Rhode Island

Amar Kapur, DO, CPT, MC, USA[†]
Medical Director
JBER—Soldier Centered Medical Home
Fort Richardson, Alaska

Rahul Kapur, MD, CAQSM
Associate Professor
Family Medicine and Sports Medicine
University of Pennsylvania
Department of Family Medicine and Community Health
Penn Sports Medicine Center
Philadelphia, Pennsylvania

Atil Y. Kargi, MD
Program Director
J. Maxwell McKenzie Fellowship Program
Assistant Professor of Medicine
Division of Endocrinology, Diabetes, and Metabolism
Department of Medicine
Miller School of Medicine
University of Miami
Miami, Florida

Deirdre L. Kathman, DO
Fellow
Division of Pulmonary, Allergy, and Critical Care Medicine
University of Massachusetts Medical School
Worcester, Massachusetts

Anubhav Kaul, MD
Associate Professor, Family Medicine
Loma Linda University
Loma Linda, California

Neha Kaushik, MD
Resident Physician
Department of Family and Community Medicine
Penn State Milton S. Hershey Medical Center
Hershey, Pennsylvania

Clara M. Keegan, MD, FAAFP
Clinical Assistant Professor
Department of Family Medicine
University of Vermont Medical Center
Burlington, Vermont

Jennifer Tickal Keehbauch, MD
Associate Professor, Family Medicine
Loma Linda University
Loma Linda, California

Brendan P. Kelly, MD
Baystate Children's Hospital
Assistant Professor of Pediatrics and Medicine
Tufts University School of Medicine
Springfield, Massachusetts

Christina Kelly, MD, FAAFP

Glenn Kershaw, MD
Professor of Clinical Medicine
University of Massachusetts Medical School
Attending Nephrologist
Renal Medicine
UMass Memorial Medical Center
Worcester, Massachusetts

Robert M. Kershner, MD, MS, FACS
Eye Physician and Surgeon
Professor and Chairman
Department of Ophthalmic Medical Technology
Medical Director
Associate in Science OMT Program
Palm Beach State College
Bioscience Technology Complex
Palm Beach Gardens, Florida

Sujin Key, PharmD
Postdoctoral Fellow
Department of Pharmacy Practice
Massachusetts College of Pharmacy and Health Sciences University
Boston, Massachusetts

Anila Khaliq, MD
Faculty
Family Medicine Residency Program
St. Elizabeth Medical Center
Utica, New York

Komel Khaliq, MBBS

Mahpara Khaliq, MD
Department of Internal Medicine and Pediatrics
Stony Brook University Medical Center
Stony Brook, New York

Muhammad Imran Khan, MD
Karachi, Pakistan

Omar Khan, MD, MHS, FAAFP
Associate Vice-Chair
Department of Family & Community Medicine
Medical Director
Community Health and Eugene du Pont Preventive Medicine & Rehabilitation Institute
Institute Director
Global Health Residency Track
Christiana Care Health System
Wilmington, Delaware

Rabeea Khan, MD
Department of Ophthalmology
Kresge Eye Institute
Detroit, Michigan

Sana Khan, DO
Resident Physician
Family Medicine
Houston Methodist Hospital
Houston, Texas

Vikesh Khanijow, MD
Fellow
Gastroenterology
The George Washington University Hospital
Washington, DC

Cameron M. Kielhorn, DO

Andrew Kim, MD
Dermatology Resident
Department of Dermatology
UConn Health
Farmington, Connecticut

Daniel Y. Kim, MD, FACS
Chairman, Department of Otolaryngology–Head & Neck Surgery
University of Massachusetts
Worcester, Massachusetts

Gemma Kim, MD
Assistant Professor
Family Medicine
UC Riverside School of Medicine
Riverside, California

Tae Kim, MD
Assistant Professor
Family Medicine
UC Riverside School of Medicine
Riverside, California

Walter M. Kim, MD, PhD
Research/Clinical Fellow
Division of Gastroenterology
Brigham and Women's Hospital
Boston, Massachusetts

Brian James Kimbrell, MD, FACS
Trauma Medical Director/Surgical Critical Care Director
Blake Medical Center
Bradenton, Florida
Assistant Clinical Professor
University of South Florida
Tampa, Florida

Jaime Kimmel, PharmD
Oncology Pharmacy Resident, PGY2
University of Illinois
Chicago, Illinois

Franklin King, MD

Stella O. King, MD, MHA
Clinical Assistant Professor
Department of Family Medicine
University at Buffalo
Buffalo, New York

Ray S. King, MD, PhD
Department of Surgery
Medical College of Georgia
Georgia Regents University
Augusta, Georgia

Rebecca G. Kinney, MD
University of Washington
Missoula, Montana

Cecilia M. Kipnis, MD[†]
Family Medicine–Obstetrics
Naval Hospital Jacksonville
Jacksonville, Florida

Jeffrey T. Kirchner, DO, FAAFP, AAHIVS
Clinical Associate Professor
Temple University School of Medicine
Philadelphia, Pennsylvania

Brandon Kirsch, MD
Department of Dermatology
Mayo Clinic
Jacksonville, Florida

Gloria J. Klapstein, PhD
Associate Professor
Department of Basic Sciences
College of Osteopathic Medicine
Touro University California
Vallejo, California

J. Michael Klatte, MD
Assistant Professor of Pediatrics
Department of Pediatrics
Division of Pediatric Infectious Diseases
Tufts University School of Medicine
Baystate Medical Center
Springfield, Massachusetts

Jacob W. Kleinman, MD
Resident Physician
Department of Emergency Medicine
University of Pittsburgh Medical Center
Pittsburgh, Pennsylvania

Anton Klochkov, DO
Traditional Rotating Intern
Coney Island Hospital
Brooklyn, New York

Laura K. Klug, PharmD
Assistant Professor of Pharmacy Practice and Family Medicine
Department of Pharmacy Practice
Creighton University
Omaha, Nebraska

Ryan R. Knapp, MD, MS
Lebanon, New Hampshire

Sandra L. Knaur, APRN, BC
Texas Pulmonary and Critical Care Consultants of Texas, PA
Fort Worth, Texas

Sharon L. Koehler, DO, FACS
Assistant Professor
Department of Medicine
Division of Surgery
New York Institute of Technology College of Osteopathic Medicine
Old Westbury, New York

Aaron Kofman, MD
The Warren Alpert Medical School of Brown University
Providence, Rhode Island

Nathalee Kong, MD
Department of Medicine
Massachusetts General Hospital
Boston, Massachusetts

Scott E. Kopec, MD
Associate Professor of Medicine
Division of Pulmonary, Allergy, and Critical Care
University of Massachusetts Medical School
Worcester, Massachusetts

Kelly G. Koren, MD[†]
Staff Physician
Department of Family Medicine
Fort Belvoir Community Hospital
Fort Belvoir, Virginia

Adam W. Kowalski, MD

Rudolph M. Krafft, MD, FAAFP
Director
Family Medicine Residency
St. Elizabeth Health Center
Youngstown, Ohio

Sathya S. Krishnasamy, MD
Associate Professor of Medicine
Division of Endocrinology, Metabolism and Diabetes
University of Louisville
Louisville, Kentucky

Merrill Krolick, DO, FACC, FACP, FSCAI
Interventional Cardiology
The Heart Institute at Largo
Largo Medical Center
Largo, Florida

David C. Krulak, MD, MPH, MBA, FAAFP
Pensacola, Florida

Edward James Kruse, DO
Associate Professor of Surgery
Department of Surgery
Surgical Oncology Section
Georgia Regents University
Augusta, Georgia

David W. Kruse, MD
CAQ Primary Care Sports Medicine
Orthopaedic Specialty Institute
Orange, California

Rebecca Kruse-Jarres, MD, MPH
Associate Professor of Medicine
Section of Hematology/Oncology
Tulane University
New Orleans, Louisiana

Archana Kudrimoti, MBBS, (MD), MPH
Assistant Professor
Department of Family and Community Medicine
University of Kentucky
Lexington, Kentucky

Ajoy Kumar, MD, FAAFP
Chair
Department of Family Medicine
Bayfront Health
Assistant Director
Bayfront Family Medicine Residency
St. Petersburg, Florida

Barrett J. Kumar, DO, MSBA
Department of Internal Medicine
University Hospitals - Regional Hospitals
Cleveland, Ohio

Jason Kurland, MD
Assistant Professor of Medicine
UMass Memorial Medical Group
Division of Renal Medicine
University of Massachusetts Medical School
Worcester, Massachusetts

Daniel B. Kurtz, PhD
Associate Professor of Biology
Utica College
Utica, New York

SreyRam Kuy, MD, MHS
Department of Surgery
Louisiana State University Health Sciences Center at Shreveport
Shreveport, Louisiana
Overton Brooks Veterans Affairs Medical Center
Washington, DC

Melinda Y. Kwan, DO, MPH
Urgent Care Physician
Urgent Care Department
Southwest Medical Associates
Las Vegas, Nevada

LaShell LaBounty, DO
Family Medicine Resident
Saint Louis University Family Medicine Residency
Belleville, Illinois

Patricia May Lacsina, MD
Department of Family and Community Medicine
The University of Texas Health Science Center at San Antonio
San Antonio, Texas

Nanette Lacuesta, MS, MD
Assistant Program Director
Riverside Methodist Hospital Family Medicine Residency Program
OhioHealth
Columbus, Ohio

Youmna Lahoud, MD
Rheumatology Department
University of Massachusetts
Worcester, Massachusetts

Aaron Lambert, MD
Assistant Clinical Professor
Department of Family Medicine
East Carolina University
Greenville, North Carolina

Rahele Lameh, MD
Community Faculty
Family Medicine Department
The University of Texas Southwestern Dallas
Dallas, Texas

Stephen K. Lane, MD, FAAFP
Scituate, Massachusetts

Jeffrey B. Lanier, MD, FAAFP[†]
Martin Army Community Hospital
Family Medicine Residency Program
Fort Benning, Georgia

Eduardo Lara-Torre, MD
Vice-Chair for Academic Affairs
Residency Program Director
Carilion Clinic
Associate Professor
Departments of Obstetrics and Gynecology and Pediatrics
Virginia Tech Carilion School of Medicine
Roanoke, Virginia

Deborah A. Lardner, DO, DTM&H
Assistant Professor
Department of Family Medicine
College of Osteopathic Medicine
New York Institute of Technology
Old Westbury, New York

Richard A. Larson, MD
Professor of Medicine
Section of Hematology/Oncology
University of Chicago
Chicago, Illinois

Shane L. Larson, MD[†]
Staff Family Physician and Flight Surgeon
Department of Primary Care
Fort Carson, Colorado

Lakshmi Devi Nelson Lattimer, MD
Gastroenterology
The George Washington University
Washington, DC

Emily S. Lau, MD
Internal Medicine Resident
Department of Medicine
Brigham and Women's Hospital
Boston, Massachusetts

Justin P. Lavin, Jr., MD, FACOG
Chairman
Department of Obstetrics and Gynecology
Akron General Medical Center
Professor Emeritus of Obstetrics and Gynecology
Northeastern Ohio Medical University
Akron, Ohio

Ashik Lawrence, MD

Naomi Lawrence-Reid, MD
Children's Hospital at Montefiore
Bronx, New York

Miles C. Layton, DO, MAJ, MC, USA[†]
Martin Army Community Hospitals
Fort Benning, Georgia

Mary Le, MD

James J. Ledwith, Jr., MD, FAAFP
Residency Director
University of Massachusetts Fitchburg Family Medicine Residency Program
University of Massachusetts Medical School
Fitchburg, Massachusetts

Alison Lee, MD
Resident
Maine Medical Center
Portland, Maine

Amy L. Lee, MD
Assistant Professor
Department of Family Medicine
Tufts University School of Medicine
Boston, Massachusetts

Andrew G. Lee, MD
Professor of Ophthalmology, Neurology, and Neurosurgery
Weill Cornell Medical College
Chair of Ophthalmology
Houston Methodist Hospital
Adjunct Professor of Ophthalmology
Baylor College of Medicine
Clinical Professor of Ophthalmology
The University of Texas Medical Branch (UTMB) Galveston
The University of Texas MD Anderson Cancer Center
Adjunct Professor of Ophthalmology
University of Iowa Hospitals and Clinics
Houston, Texas

Bianca Lee
College of Osteopathic Medicine
New York Institute of Technology
Old Westbury, New York

Damon F. Lee, MD
Assistant Director, Office of Student Affairs
Assistant Clinical Professor
Department of Family Medicine and Community Health
John A. Burns School of Medicine
University of Hawaii
Honolulu, Hawaii

Daniel T. Lee, MD, MA
Clinical Professor of Family Medicine
David Geffen School of Medicine
University of California Los Angeles
Santa Monica, California

Ernestine M. Lee, MD, MPH
Assistant Director
Allopathic Family Residency
Florida Hospital
Family Medicine Program
Assistant Professor
University of Central Florida College of Medicine
Clinical Assistant Professor
Florida State University College of Medicine
Winter Park, Florida

Ginny H. Lee, MD
Department of Emergency Medicine
Summa Health System
Akron, Ohio

Hobart Lee, MD
Assistant Professor
Department of Family Medicine
Loma Linda University
Loma Linda, California

Jennifer Lee, DO
Family Medicine Resident
Greenbrier Valley Medical Center
Lewisburg, West Virginia

Justin Lee, MD
Clinical Assistant Professor
Family and Sports Medicine
Brody School of Medicine
East Carolina University
Greenville, North Carolina

Woo Jung Lee, MD, MS
Clinical Gastroenterology University of Connecticut School of Medicine Fellow
Department of Medicine
Division of Gastroenterology
The George Washington University
Washington, DC

F. Stuart Leeds, MS, MD
Assistant Professor
Department of Family Medicine
Boonshoft School of Medicine
Wright State University
Dayton, Ohio

Jaclyn E. A. Legg, DO, MA
Psychiatry Resident
University of Kansas Medical Center
Kansas City, Kansas

Leslie Lemanek, MD†
Dwight D. Eisenhower Army Medical Center
Augusta, Georgia

Carrie G. Lenneman, MD, MSCI
Assistant Professor
Cardiovascular Medicine
University of Louisville
Louisville, Kentucky

Maya Leventer-Roberts, MD, MPH
Pediatric Environmental Health Fellow
Department of Preventive Medicine
Icahn School of Medicine at Mount Sinai
New York, New York

Jay H. Levin, MD
Department of Neurology
Rhode Island Hospital
The Warren Alpert Medical School of Brown University
Providence, Rhode Island

Nikki A. Levin, MD, PhD
Associate Professor of Medicine
Division of Dermatology
UMass Memorial Health Care
University of Massachusetts Medical School
Worcester, Massachusetts

David C. Levine, MD, FACS
Assistant Dean
Clinical Education
Assistant Professor of Surgery
College of Osteopathic Medicine
New York Institute of Technology
Old Westbury, New York

Gary I. Levine, MD
Associate Professor
Department of Family Medicine
The Brody School of Medicine
East Carolina University
Greenville, North Carolina

Brent J. Levy, MD
Chief Resident
Emergency Medicine
Dartmouth-Hitchcock Medical Center
Lebanon, New Hampshire

Douglas P. Lewis, MD
Associate Director
Via Christi Family Medicine Residency
Associate Director
Via Christi Adult Cystic Fibrosis Specialty Clinic
Assistant Clinical Professor
University of Kansas School of Medicine–Wichita
Wichita, Kansas

James H. Lewis, MD, FACP, FACG, AGAF
Professor of Medicine
Division of Gastroenterology
Georgetown University Hospital
Washington, DC

Anjie Li, MD
Department of Obstetrics and Gynecology
University of Massachusetts
Worcester, Massachusetts

Rung-chi Li, DO, PhD
Internal Medicine
The Christ Hospital
Cincinnati, Ohio

Charmiane Lieu, MD
Resident Physician, PGY4
Department of Emergency Medicine
The Warren Alpert Medical School of Brown University
Providence, Rhode Island

Jennifer Lin, DO
Family Medicine Resident
University of Massachusetts
Fitchburg, Massachusetts

Jonathan T. Lin, MD
Resident
Department of Medicine
Mount Sinai Hospital
New York, New York

Xueting Lin, PharmD, RPh
Postdoctoral Fellow
Regulatory Affairs
Massachusetts College of Pharmacy and Health Sciences University
Boston, Massachusetts

Adriana C. Linares, MD, MPH, DrPH
Clinician/Teacher
Family Medicine
Peacehealth Southwest Medical Center
Vancouver, Washington

Mary Segraves Lindholm, MD
Clinical Associate Professor
Department of Family Medicine and Community Health
University of Massachusetts Medical School
Worcester, Massachusetts

Janelle M. Lindow, DO†
Transitional Year Resident
Dwight D. Eisenhower Army Medical Center
Fort Gordon, Georgia

Melanie J. Lippmann, MD
Assistant Professor
Emergency Medicine
The Warren Alpert Medical School of Brown University
Rhode Island Hospital
The Miriam Hospital
Providence, Rhode Island

Kenneth Liu, PharmD
Postdoctoral
U.S. Medical Affairs at Genzyme, a Sanofi Company Adjunct Faculty
Massachusetts College of Pharmacy and Health Sciences University
Cambridge, Massachusetts

Kimberly E. Liu, MD, MSL
Assistant Professor
University of Toronto
Toronto, Ontario, Canada

Jenifer R. Lloyd, DO
Program Director
Dermatology Residency
Department of Dermatology
University Hospitals - Regional Hospitals Richmond Campus
Richmond Heights, Ohio

Paul Locus, MD
Faculty
Memorial Hermann Family
Medicine Residency Program
Clinical Assistant Professor
Department of Family and Community Medicine
Texas A&M Health Science Center College of Medicine
Sugar Land, Texas

David E. Longstroth, MD
Inpatient Hospitalist
Registrar
Family Medicine and Surgery Departments
Contra Costa Regional Medical Center
Martinez, California

Gisela M. Lopez Payares, MD
Department of Family and Community Medicine
The University of Texas Health Science Center at San Antonio
San Antonio, Texas

Mary L. Lopresti, DO
University of Massachusetts
Worcester, Massachusetts

Bency K. Louidor-Paulynice, MD
Family Medicine
University of Massachusetts Medical School
Worcester, Massachusetts

Zhen Lu, MD
Chief Medical Director
Pacific Urgent Care & Family Medicine
Orange, California

John R. Luksch, DO
Chief Resident, PGY3
Department of Family Medicine
Rowan University School of Osteopathic Medicine
Stratford, New Jersey

Marie Luksch, DO
Resident
Department of Family Medicine
Rowan University School of Osteopathic Medicine
Straford, New Jersey

Alicia Lydecker, MD
Department of Emergency Medicine
University of Massachusetts
Worcester, Massachusetts

Angela Lye, PharmD
Postdoctoral Fellow
Clinical Documentation
Massachusetts College of Pharmacy and Health Sciences University
Cambridge, Massachusetts

Ann M. Lynch, PharmD, RPh, AE-C
Associate Professor
Pharmacy Practice
Massachusetts College of Pharmacy and Health Sciences University
Worcester, Massachusetts

Jonathan MacClements, MD, FAAFP
Professor
Assistant Dean
Graduate Medical Education
Dell Medical School
The University of Texas at Austin
Austin, Texas

Marina MacNamara, MD, MPH
Resident Physician
Family Medicine Residency Program
Mountain Area Health Education Center
Asheville, North Carolina

Douglas W. MacPherson, MD, MSc(CTM), FRCPC
Department of Pathology and Molecular Medicine
McMaster University
Hamilton, Ontario, Canada
Migration Health Consultants, Inc.
Qualicum Beach, British Columbia, Canada

Michelle Magid, MD
Clinical Associate Professor
Department of Psychiatry
The University of Texas Southwestern Austin
Clinical Assistant Professor
The University of Texas Medical Branch
Clinical Assistant Professor
Texas A&M Health Science Center
Austin, Texas

Jeffrey D. Mailhot, MD
Assistant Professor of Medicine
Division of Dermatology
University of Massachusetts Medical School
Worcester, Massachusetts

Suzana K. Everett Makowski, MD, MMM, FACP, FAAHPM
Assistant Professor
Medicine
Co-Chief
Palliative Care
Department of Medicine
University of Massachusetts Medical School
Worcester, Massachusetts

Maricarmen Malagon-Rogers, MD
Associate Professor
Family Medicine
Pediatric Nephrology
University of Tennessee Graduate School of Medicine
Knoxville, Tennessee

Melanie J.S. Malec, MD
Physician
Department of Family Medicine
Lake Health Hospital System
Chardon, Ohio

Uzma Malik, MD
Glen Cove, New York

Samir Malkani, MD, MRCP (UK)
Associate Clinical Professor
Medicine
University of Massachusetts Medical School
Worcester, Massachusetts

Michael A. Malone, MD
Assistant Professor
Department of Family and Community Medicine
Penn State College of Medicine
Hershey, Pennsylvania

Mary Maloney, MD
Professor of Medicine and Director of Dermatologic Surgery
University of Massachusetts Medical School
Worcester, Massachusetts

Lee A. Mancini, MD, CSCS*D, CSN

Alison Mancuso, DO
Assistant Professor
Department of Family Medicine
Rowan University School of Osteopathic Medicine
Stratford, New Jersey

Krishna Manda, MD, MRCP
Renal Medicine
University of Massachusetts Memorial Health Care
Worcester, Massachusetts

Mark J. Manning DO, MsMEL
Chief
General Obstetrics and Gynecology
Assistant Professor
Department of Obstetrics and Gynecology
University of Massachusettes Medical School
Worcester, Massachusetts

Kenia Mansilla-Rivera, MD
Director
Medical Student Education
Assistant Professor
Department of Family Medicine
University of Connecticut School of Medicine
Farmington, Connecticut

Eric Ji-Yuan Mao, MD
Gastroenterology Fellow
The Warren Alpert Medical School of Brown University
Providence, Rhode Island

Rachel Marinch, MD
Resident Physician, PGY2
Department of Family Medicine
Exempla Saint Joseph Hospital
Denver, Colorado

Robert A. Marlow, MD, MA
Professor of Clinical Family Medicine
Department of Family, Community and Preventive Medicine
University of Arizona College of Medicine—Phoenix
Phoenix, Arizona
Associate Director/Director of Research
Family Medicine Residency Program
Scottsdale Healthcare
Scottsdale, Arizona

Wendy K. Marsh, MD, MSc
Associate Professor
Department of Psychiatry
University of Massachusetts
Worcester, Massachusetts

Cara Marshall, MD
Faculty
Lawrence Family Medicine Residency
Lawrence, Massachusetts

Kathleen J. Martin, MD, FAAP
Chair
Pediatrics
Department of Clinical Sciences
West Virginia School of Osteopathic Medicine
Lewisburg, West Virginia

Michelle T. Martin, PharmD, BCPS, BCACP
Clinical Pharmacist
University of Illinois Hospital and Health Sciences System
Clinical Assistant Professor
Department of Pharmacy Practice
College of Pharmacy
University of Illinois at Chicago
Chicago, Illinois

Stephen A. Martin, MD, EdM
Assistant Professor
Department of Family Medicine and Community Health
University of Massachusetts Medical School
Worcester, Massachusetts

Marni Martinez, APRN

Carlos Martínez-Balzano, MD
Division of Lung, Allergy and Critical Care Medicine
University of Massachusetts Medical School
Worcester, Massachusetts

Mohamad Masoumy, MD, MS
Chief General Surgery Resident
Department of Surgery
Medical College of Georgia
Georgia Regents University
Augusta, Georgia

Jerin Mathew, MD

Donnah Mathews, MD, FACP
Attending Physician
Department of Medicine
Rhode Island Hospital
Assistant Professor, Clinician Educator
The Warren Alpert School of Medicine of Brown University
Providence, Rhode Island

Daniel R. Matta, MD
Second-Year Resident
Bayfront Health Family Medicine Residency
St. Petersburg, Florida

George H. Maxted, MD
Associate Program Director
Tufts University Family Medicine Residency
Cambridge Health Alliance
Malden, Massachusetts

Beth Mazyck, MD
Associate Clinical Professor
Family Medicine
University of Massachusetts Medical School
Fitchburg, Massachusetts

Casey McCann, MD

Kelly McCants, MD

Margaret J. McCormick MS, RN
Clinical Associate Professor
Nursing
Towson University
Towson, Maryland

Michelle McCreary, MD

Kristina McGraw, DO
Assistant Professor
Family Medicine
West Virginia School of Osteopathic Medicine
Lewisburg, West Virginia

Tamara McGregor, MD
Associate Professor
University of Texas Southwestern Medical Center
Department of Family and Community Medicine
Department of Internal Medicine, Palliative Care
Dallas, Texas

Christopher S. McGuire, MD, MPH†
Resident
Family Medicine
Martin Army Community Hospital
Fort Benning, Georgia

Bridget E. McIlwee, DO
PGY2
Department of Dermatology
Texas College of Osteopathic Medicine
University of North Texas
Fort Worth, Texas

Elizabeth C. McKeen, MD
Clinical Instructor in Pediatrics
Harvard Medical School
Boston, Massachusetts

Marc W. McKenna, MD
Clinical Associate Professor of Family and Community Medicine Program Director
Department of Family Medicine
Chestnut Hill Hospital
Philadelphia, Pennsylvania

Donna-Marie McMahon, DO, FAAP
Assistant Professor
Medicine
Division of Pediatrics
College of Osteopathic Medicine
New York Institute of Technology
Old Westbury, New York

Roger L. McRoberts, III, MD
Assistant Professor
Psychiatry
The University of Texas Southwestern Austin
Austin, Texas

Melissa Meghpara, OMS IV, BA
College of Osteopathic Medicine
New York Institute of Technology
Old Westbury, New York

Michelle L. Mellion, MD
Assistant Professor
Department of Neurology
The Warren Alpert Medical School of Brown University
Rhode Island Hospital
Providence, Rhode Island

Daniel E. Melville, MD
Destination Health™
Southlake, Texas

Donna I. Meltzer, MD
Department of Family Medicine
SUNY Stony Brook
Stony Brook, New York

Julissa Mendoza, MD†
Resident Physician
Department of Family Medicine
Dwight D. Eisenhower Army Medical Center
Fort Gordon, Georgia

Caleb J. Mentzer, DO
Resident
Department of General Surgery
Medical College of Georgia
Georgia Regents University
Augusta, Georgia

Miesha Merati, DO
Dermatology Fellow
Skin and Cancer Associates
Plantation, Florida

Michael G. Mercado, MD, FAAFP†
Naval Hospital Camp Pendleton
Camp Pendleton, California

Brendan Merchant, MD
Cardiology Fellow
University of Massachusetts
Worcester, Massachusetts

Nessa S. Meshkaty, MD
Infectious Disease Department
Baystate Medical Center
Springfield, Massachusetts

Theo E. Meyer, MD, DPhil
Professor
Department of Cardiovascular Medicine
University of Massachusetts Medical School
Director, Cardiac Cath Lab
Department of Cardiology
UMass Memorial Medical Center
Worcester, Massachusetts

Christina Mezzone, DO, MS
College of Osteopathic Medicine
New York Institute of Technology
Old Westbury, New York

Alyssa Miceli, DO
College of Osteopathic Medicine
New York Institute of Technology
Old Westbury, New York

Tracy O. Middleton, DO
Clinical Professor and Chair
Department of Family Medicine
Midwestern University
Arizona College of Osteopathic Medicine
Glendale, Arizona

Elise Mikaloff, DO, CPT, MC†
Womack Family Medicine Residency
Fort Bragg, North Carolina

Mariya Milko, DO
Internal Medicine Resident, PGY1
Department of Internal Medicine
Largo Medical Center
Largo, Florida

Heidi S. Millard, MD
Assistant Clinical Faculty
University of California Riverside School of Medicine
Riverside, California

James P. Miller, MD
Medical Director
Pediatric Surgery
Cook Children's Medical Center
Fort Worth, Texas

John Michael Miller, II, MD
House Officer
Department of Family Medicine
University of Mississippi Medical Center
Jackson, Mississippi

Suzanne Minor, MD, FAAFP
Clerkship Director
Family Medicine
Assistant Professor
Division of Family Medicine
Department of Humanities, Health, and Society
Herbert Wertheim College of Medicine
Florida International University
Miami, Florida

Mark Minot, MD

Jeffrey F. Minteer, MD
Program Director
Washington Health System Family Medicine Residency
Washington, Pennsylvania

Saadia Mohsin, MD
Resident Physician
Family Medicine
Summa Barberton Hospital
Barberton, Ohio

Maria Montanez, MD

Justin B. Moore, MD, FACP
Division of Endocrinology
Department of Internal Medicine
University of Kansas School of Medicine–Wichita
Wichita, Kansas

Wynne S. Morgan, MD
Child Psychiatry Fellow
Department of Psychiatry
University of Massachusetts Medical School
Worcester, Massachusetts

Kelvin A. Moses, MD, PhD
Assistant Professor
Department of Urologic Surgery
Vanderbilt University
Nashville, Tennessee

Timothy F. Mott, MD†
Assistant Professor
Family Medicine
Uniformed Services University of Health Sciences
Bethesda, Maryland

Wael S. Mourad, MD
Assistant Professor
Department of Community and Family Medicine
University of Missouri–Kansas City School of Medicine
Truman Medical Center Lakewood
Kansas City, Missouri

Sarah E. Mowry, MD
Assistant Professor
Department of Otolaryngology
Georgia Regents University
Augusta, Georgia

Mohammad Ansar Mughal, MD
Assistant Professor
University Health System
San Antonio, Texas

Shani Muhammad, MD
Family Medicine Physician
Fresno, California

Joshua Mularella, DO
Assistant Professor
Department of Emergency Medicine
Upstate Medical University
Syracuse, New York

Herbert L. Muncie, Jr., MD
Professor
Family Medicine
Department of Family Medicine
Louisiana State University Health Sciences Center
New Orleans, Louisiana

Amanda B. Murchison, MD
Assistant Professor
Department of Obstetrics and Gynecology
Virginia Tech Carilion School of Medicine
Roanoke, Virginia

Gregory Murphy, MD
University of Connecticut
Farmington, Connecticut

Rachel Myers, MD
Family Medicine
The University of Texas Health Science Center at San Antonio
San Antonio, Texas

Catherine Mygatt, MD
Chief Resident
Lawrence Family Medicine Residency
Lawrence, Massachusetts

Aung Myint, DO
PGY2
Internal Medicine
Department of Medicine
The George Washington University Hospital
Washington, DC

Jennifer Mytar, DO
PGY1
Internal Medicine
The Christ Hospital
Cincinnati, Ohio

Urooj Najm, MBBS

Anne Nash, MD

Papia Nasiri, MD
Second-Year Resident Physician
Department of Family and Community Medicine
Penn State Milton S. Hershey Medical Center
Hershey, Pennsylvania

Eddie Needham, MD, FAAFP
Program Director
Florida Hospital Family Medicine Residency Program
Clinical Associate and Professor
Florida State University College of Medicine
Associate Professor
University of Central Florida College of Medicine
Winter Park, Florida

Michael O. Needham, MD, CPT, MC, USA†
Family Medicine Residency Program
Dwight D. Eisenhower Army Medical Center
Fort Gordon, Georgia

Jordan W. Neighbors, DO
Department of Surgery
Maricopa Medical Center
Phoenix, Arizona

Tara J. Neil, MD
Associate Director
Via Christi Family Medicine Residency Program
Clinical Assistant Professor
Department of Family and Community Medicine
University of Kansas School of Medicine–Wichita
Wichita, Kansas

Holli K. Neiman-Hart, MD, FAAFP
Family Medicine Residency
West Virginia University
Morgantown, West Virginia

Eric D. Nelson, MD
Pediatric Urologist
Assistant Professor of Urology
Connecticut Children's Medical Center
Hartford, Connecticut
University of Connecticut School of Medicine
Farmington, Connecticut

Sandra N. New, DrNP

Anne Newbold, DO
Department of Emergency Medicine
Midwestern University
Swedish Covenant Hospital
Chicago, Illinois

Jelaun K. Newsome, DO†
Family Medicine
Womack Army Medical Center
Fort Bragg, North Carolina

Dana Nguyen, MD, FAAFP†
Assistant Professor
Department of Family Medicine
Uniformed Services University
Bethesda, Maryland

Tam Nguyen, MD, FAAFP
Program Director
Family Medicine Residency Program
San Joaquin General Hospital
French Camp, California

Yummy Nguyen, MD

Stacey Nickoloff, DO
Program Director
Family Medicine Residency Program
Presence Resurrection Medical Center
Chicago, Illinois

Maria De La Luz Nieto, MD
Clinical Fellow and Instructor
Division of Urogynecology and Reconstructive Pelvic Surgery
University of North Carolina at Chapel Hill
Chapel Hill, North Carolina

Elise Taylor Nissen, MD
Family Medicine Resident, PGY1
Kaiser Napa-Solano
Vallejo, California

Thomas Noh, MD
Department of Neurological Surgery
Henry Ford Hospital
Detroit, Michigan

Rocio Nordfeldt, MD
Assistant Professor
Family Medicine Department
University of Massachusetts Medical School
Leominster, Massachusetts

David R. Norris, MD
Assistant Professor
Department of Family Medicine
University of Mississippi Medical Center
Jackson, Mississippi

Bakr Nour, MD, PhD, FACS
Professor and Vice-Chair
Department of General Surgery
Weill Cornell Medical College in New York City
Associate Dean
Clinical Affairs
Weill Cornell Medical College in Qatar
Al Rayyan, Qatar

Laura Novak, MD
Hospital Residency Program
Summa Barberton
Barberton, Ohio

Rathna Nuti, MD
Resident
The University of Texas Southwestern Dallas
Dallas, Texas

Theodore X. O'Connell, MD
Program Director
Family Medicine Residency Program
Kaiser Permanente Napa-Solano
Assistant Clinical Professor
Department of Family and Community Medicine
University of California San Francisco School of Medicine
Assistant Clinical Professor
Department of Family Medicine
David Geffen School of Medicine at UCLA
Los Angeles, California

John B. O'Donnell, MD, MS
Director
Preclinical Curriculum
College of Human Medicine
Michigan State University
Grand Rapids, Michigan

David T. O'Gurek, MD
Assistant Professor
Department of Family and Community Medicine
Temple University School of Medicine
Philadelphia, Pennsylvania

Heather O'Mara, DO[†]
Staff
Family Medicine Residency Clinic
Womack Army Medical Center
Fort Bragg, North Carolina

M. Allison Ogden, MD
Associate Professor
Department of Otolaryngology
Washington University School of Medicine in St. Louis
St. Louis, Missouri

Annie Oh, MD
Assistant Professor
Hospital and Health Sciences Systems
University of Illinois
Chicago, Illinois

Jin Sol Oh, MD
General Surgery Resident
Department of Surgery
Georgia Regents University
Augusta, Georgia

Arthur Ohannessian, MD
Assistant Clinical Professor
Department of Family Medicine
David Geffen School of Medicine at UCLA
Los Angeles, California

Smriti Ohri, MD
Assistant Professor
Family Medicine
Oregon Health and Science University
Portland, Oregon

Amy Okpaku, DO
Assistant Professor
Family & Community Medicine
The University of Texas Southwestern Austin
Austin, Texas

Jacqueline L. Olin, MS, PharmD, BCPS, CPP, CDE, FASHP
Associate Professor of Pharmacy
Wingate University School of Pharmacy
Wingate, North Carolina

Folashade Omole, MD, FAAFP
Professor and Vice-Chair
Academic Affairs
Director
Residency Program
Department of Family Medicine
Morehouse School of Medicine
East Point, Georgia

Jill SM Omori, MD
Associate Professor
Department of Family Medicine and Community Health
Office of Medical Education
John A. Burn School of Medicine
University of Hawaii
Honolulu, Hawaii

Imola K. Osapay, MD

Sean M. Oser, MD, MPH
Assistant Professor of Family and Community Medicine
Department of Family and Community Medicine
Pennsylvania State University College of Medicine
Hershey, Pennsylvania

Tamara K. Oser, MD
Assistant Professor of Family and Community Medicine
Department of Family and Community Medicine
Pennsylvania State University College of Medicine
Hershey, Pennsylvania

Chidinma Osineme, MD
Faculty, Physician
Family Medicine and Obstetrics
Virginia Tech Carilion Family Medicine Residency Program
Assistant Professor
Virginia Tech Carilion School of Medicine
Vice-Section Chief
Department of Family Medicine
Carilion Clinic, Roanoke Memorial Hospital
Roanoke, Virginia

Aimee Ostick, MD
Residency Faculty
Family Medicine
Kaiser Permanente
Woodland Hills, California

Brian Ostick, MD, FACEP
Director
Valley Presbyterian Emergency Department
Valley Presbyterian Hospital
Van Nuys, California

Cindy England Owen, MD
Assistant Professor and Associate Program Director
Division of Dermatology
University of Louisville
Louisville, Kentucky

Linda Paniagua, MD
Emergency Department
The University of Texas Health Science Center at Houston
Houston, Texas

Kelly Pagidas, MD
Women and Infants Hospital
Providence, Rhode Island

Kate R. Parese, PharmD, RPh
Postdoctoral Fellow
Global Pharmacovigilance and Epidemiology
Genzyme, a Sanofi Company
Cambridge, Massachusetts

Jon S. Parham, DO, MPH
Associate Professor
Department of Family Medicine
Graduate School of Medicine
University of Tennessee
Knoxville, Tennessee

Douglas S. Parks, MD
Associate Professor of Family Medicine
University of Wyoming Family Medicine Residency
Cheyenne, Wyoming

Michael Passafaro, DO, DTM&H, FACEP, FACOEP
Assistant Professor
Division of Emergency Medicine
Center for Global Health
College of Osteopathic Medicine
New York Institute of Technology
Old Westbury, New York

Monica Passi, MD
The George Washington University Hospital
Washington, DC

Birju B. Patel, MD, FACP, AGSF
VISN 7 Co-Consultant for Outpatient Geriatrics
Director
Geriatric Primary Care Clinic
Director
Mild Cognitive Impairment Clinic, Atlanta Veterans Affairs Medical Center
Assistant Professor of Medicine
Division of General Medicine and Geriatrics
Department of Medicine
Emory University School of Medicine
Atlanta, Georgia

Krunal Patel, MD
Resident, Internal Medicine
University of Massachusetts Medical School
Worcester, Massachusetts

Lena A.N. Patel, MD
Medical Resident
Family Medicine
Bayfront Family Medicine Residency
St. Petersburg, Florida

Mahesh C. Patel, MD
Assistant Professor
Division of Infectious Diseases, Immunology, and International Medicine
Department of Internal Medicine
University of Illinois at Chicago
Attending Physician
The University of Illinois Hospital & Health Sciences System
Chicago, Illinois

Mohita Patel, MD
University of Texas Southwestern Clinical Center
Dallas, Texas

Nihal Patel, MD
Hepatology Fellow
Division of Gastroenterology and Hepatology
Department of Medicine
Montefiore Medical Center
Bronx, New York

Nupam A. Patel, MD

Rishin Patel, MD
Chief Resident
Family Practice
Barberton Citizens Hospital
Barberton, Ohio

Vaishali M. Patel, MD

Abhijeet Patil, MD, MS
Assistant Professor
Department of Family Medicine and Geriatric Medicine
UMass Memorial and Fitchburg Family Medicine Residency Program
Fitchburg, Massachusetts

Joseph E. Patruno, MD
Lehigh Valley Health Network
University of South Florida School of Medicine
Allentown, Pennsylvania

Candace Y. Pau, MD
Department of Family Medicine
Kaiser Permanente Napa-Solano
Vallejo, California

Charles Pavia, PhD
Associate Professor of Microbiology
Departments of Medical Education and Biomedical Sciences
College of Osteopathic Medicine
New York Institute of Technology
Old Westbury, New York

Erica Pearce, PharmD, BCPS, BCACP
Assistant Professor of Pharmacy Practice
Division of Ambulatory Care
Department of Pharmacy Practice
St. Louis College of Pharmacy
St. Louis, Missouri

Maryse A. Pedoussaut, MD
Assistant Professor
Division of Medicine and Society
Department of Humanities, Health, and Society
Herbert Wertheim College of Medicine
Florida International University
Miami, Florida

Helio Pedro, MD
Section Chief, Genetics
Hackensack University Medical Center
Hackensack, New Jersey

Rebecca L. Peebles, DO

Rade N. Pejic, MD, MMM
Assistant Professor of Family Medicine
Tulane University School of Medicine
New Orleans, Louisiana

Rod Pellenberg, MD

Randall Pellish, MD
Assistant Professor of Medicine
Program Director
Gastroenterology Fellowship
Department of Medicine
University of Massachusetts Medical School
Worcester, Massachusetts

Ellen E. Anderson Penno, MD, MS, FRCSC, Diplomate ABO
Western Laser Eye Associates
Calgary, Alberta, Canada

Brian P. Peppers, DO, PhD
Pediatrics
University Hospitals - Regional Hospitals
Richmond Heights, Ohio

Ruben Peralta, MD, FACS
Director of Trauma and Critical Care Fellowship Program
Senior Consultant in Surgery, Emergency, Trauma and Critical Care Medicine
Vice-Chair QPS Program
Department of Surgery
Associate Director of Trauma ICU
Department of Surgery
Hamad General Hospital
Department of Medical Education
Hamad Medical Corporation
Doha, Qatar

T. Ray Perrine, MS, MD, FAAFP
Faculty
Family Medicine Residency Center
North Mississippi Medical Center
Tupelo, Mississippi

Christine S. Persaud, MD
Assistant Professor
Department of Orthopaedic Surgery and Rehabilitation Medicine
Medical Director
Division of Sports Medicine
SUNY Downstate Medical Center
Brooklyn, New York

Bobby Peters, MD, FAAEM
Clinical Assistant Professor
Emergency Department
University of Iowa Hospitals and Clinics
Iowa City, Iowa

Hugh Peterson, MD, FACP
Associate Professor
Department of Medicine
School of Medicine
University of Louisville
Louisville, Kentucky

Tatiana Petrikova, BS, MD
Family Medicine
Summa Barberton Hospital
Barberton, Ohio

Christopher Khanh Thien Pham, DO[†]
Martin Army Community Hospital
Family Medicine Residency Program
Fort Benning, Georgia

Ho Phong Pham, MD

Phung Dinh Phan, DO, CPT, USA[†]
Doctor of Osteopathy
Resident Physician
Womack Family Medicine Residency
Fort Bragg, North Carolina

Karen Sue Phelps, MD[†]
Family Medicine Residency
Dwight D. Eisenhower Army Medical Center
Fort Gordon, Georgia

Teny Anna Philip, MD
Department of Community and Family Medicine
The University of Texas Health Science Center at San Antonio
San Antonio, Texas

Jeffrey Phillips, MD
Family Doctors, LLC
Swampscott, Massachusetts

Kantima Phisitkul, MD
Clinical Assistant Professor
Division of Nephrology
Department of Internal Medicine
University of Iowa Hospital and Clinics
Iowa City, Iowa

Jonathan Piercy, MD
Assistant Professor of Family and Community Medicine
East Kentucky Family Medicine Residency Program
University of Kentucky
Hazard, Kentucky

Warren W. Piette, MD
Chair
Division of Dermatology
John H. Stroger, Jr. Hospital of Cook County
Professor
Department of Dermatology
Rush Medical School
Chicago, Illinois

Tanika M. Pinn, MD
Family and Sports Medicine
Assistant Professor
Department of Family and Community Medicine
Meharry Medical College
Nashville, Tennessee

Maria A. Pino, PhD, MS, RpH
Assistant Professor of Pharmacology
Department of Basic Biomedical Science
Touro College of Osteopathic Medicine
New York, New York

Walter L. Pipkin, MD
Associate Professor of Surgery and Pediatrics
Children's Hospital of Georgia
Georgia Regent's University
Augusta, Georgia

Jennifer Pisani, PharmD

Maria M. Plummer, MD
Assistant Professor
Department of Medical Education
College of Osteopathic Medicine
New York Institute of Technology
Old Westbury, New York

Phyllis Pollack, MD
Associate Clinical Professor of Pediatrics
University of Massachusetts Medical School
Worcester, Massachusetts

Anna C. Porter, MD
Assistant Professor of Medicine
Section of Nephrology
Department of Medicine
University of Illinois at Chicago
Chicago, Illinois

Stacy Potts, MD, MEd
Associate Professor
Department of Family Medicine and Community Health
University of Massachusetts
Worcester, Massachusetts

Anne Powell, MD

Jennifer Luo Powell, DO
Resident Physician
Department of Family Medicine
University of Massachusetts
Worcester, Massachusetts

Robert Powell, DO, MS

James E. Powers, DO, FACEP
Associate Dean for Clinical Affairs
Associate Professor of Emergency Medicine
Edward Via College of Osteopathic Medicine, Virginia Campus
Blacksburg, Virginia

Pia Prakash, MD
Department of Gastroenterology and Liver Diseases
The George Washington University
Washington, DC

Tharani Vadivelu Prasad, MD
Resident
Department of Family and Community Medicine
The University of Texas Health Science Center at San Antonio
San Antonio, Texas

Jane C. Preotle, MD
Assistant Professor of Emergency Medicine
The Warren Alpert Medical School of Brown University
Rhode Island Hospital and The Miriam Hospital
Providence, Rhode Island

Colleen M. Prinzivalli, PharmD, BCPS, CGP
Director of Clinical Pharmacy Services
Dovetail Health
Needham, Massachusetts

Barbara J. Provo, MSN, FNP-BC, CWON
Nurse Practitioner
Vascular Surgery
Froedtert Hospital & Medical College of Wisconsin
Milwaukee, Wisconsin

George G.A. Pujalte, MD, FACSM
Sports Medicine
Departments of Family Medicine, and Orthopedics
Mayo Clinic Health System
Waycross, Georgia

Samantha L. Pyle, MD, MAJ, MC[†]
Family Medicine Residency Staff
Martin Army Community Hospital
Fort Benning, Georgia

Sascha Qian, MD
Resident Physician
Department of Anesthesiology
New York-Presbyterian Hospital–Columbia
New York City, New York

Juan Qiu, MD, PhD
Associate Professor
Department of Family and Community Medicine
Pennsylvania State University College of Medicine
Penn State Hershey Medical Group Colonnade and Endoscopy Center
State College, Pennsylvania

Kelli Quercetti, DO

Diane M. Radford, MD, FACS, FRCSEd
Breast Surgical Oncologist
Mercy Clinic
St. Louis, Missouri

Megan Radmer, DO
Resident Physician
Broward Health Medical Center
Fort Lauderdale, Florida

Naureen Bashir Rafiq, MBBS, MD
Creighton University Medical Center
Bellevue, Nebraska

Alysha M. Rahman, MD
Family Medicine
Summa Barberton Hospital
Barberton, Ohio

Kyle Rahrig, DO
Family Medicine Resident
Family Practice
Resurrection Medical Center
Chicago, Illinois

Jyoti Ramakrishna, MD
Chief
Pediatric Gastroenterology and Nutrition
Floating Hospital for Children
Tufts Medical Center
Boston, Massachusetts

Kalyanakrishnan Ramakrishnan, MD
Department of Family and Preventive Medicine
University of Oklahoma Health Sciences Center
Oklahoma City, Oklahoma

Muthalagu Ramanathan, MD
Department of Hematology/Oncology
UMass Memorial Medical Center
Worcester, Massachusetts.

Alexis Ramirez, MD
University of Massachusetts Medical School
Worcester, Massachusetts

Laura K. Randolph, DO, MS
Chief Resident
Aultman Hospital
Clinical Instructor
Obstetrics and Gynecology Department
Northeast Ohio Medical University
Canton, Ohio

Swathi A.N. Rao, MD
Endocrinology Fellow
University Hospitals Case Medical Center
Cleveland, Ohio

Wasiq Faraz Rawasia, MD
Cardiovascular Medicine Fellow
University of Louisville
Louisville, Kentucky

Nischal Raya, MD

Tyler R. Reese, MD†
Family Medicine Residency Program
Tripler Army Medical Center
Honolulu, Hawaii

Jennifer Reidy, MD, MS, FAAHPM
Co-Chief
Division of Palliative Care
University of Massachusetts Memorial Medical Center
Assistant Professor
University of Massachusetts Medical School
Worcester, Massachusetts

Kathryn Reilly, MD
University of Oklahoma Health Sciences Center
Oklahoma City, Oklahoma

Emmanuel Reyes-Ramos, MD
The George Washington University
Washington, DC

Alliam Regan, MD
Internal Medicine Resident
Clinical Associate
Tufts University School of Medicine
Baystate Medical Center
Springfield, Massachusetts

Kristen A. Reineke-Piper, MD†
Faculty Physician
Scott Air Force Base
St. Louis University Family Medicine Residency
Belleville, Illinois

Lisa Requena, DO, MPH
Chief Resident
Department of Family Medicine
Broward Health Medical Center
Fort Lauderdale, Florida

Emily Reus, MD
Resident
UMass Memorial Medical Cente
Worcester, Massachusetts

Harlan G. Rich, MD, FACP, AGAF
Associate Professor of Medicine
The Warren Alpert Medical School of Brown University
University Medicine Foundation, Inc.
Director of Endoscopy
Rhode Island Hospital
Providence, Rhode Island

Andrew Richardson, MD
Family Medicine Resident
Texas A&M Family Medicine Residency Program
Bryan, Texas

Angela M. Riegel, DO†
Family Medicine Faculty
Offutt Air Force Family Medicine Residency
Offutt Air Force Base, Nebraska

Sonia Rivera-Martinez, DO, FACOFP
Assistant Professor
Department of Family Medicine
College of Osteopathic Medicine
New York Institute of Technology
Old Westbury, New York

Anthony F. Rizzo, DO
Family Medicine Resident
Presence Resurrection Medical Center
Chicago, Illinois

Ramona Roach-Davis, DNP, FNP-BC

Farhana Rob, DO
Family Medicine Resident
Memorial Family Medicine Residency Program
Sugar Land, Texas

Michele Roberts, MD, PhD
Clinical Genetics
Anatomic and Clinical Pathology
Paxton, Massachusetts

Scott W. Rodi, MD, MPH, FACEP
Chief and Medical Director
Section of Emergency Medicine
Associate Professor of Medicine
Geisel School of Medicine at Dartmouth
Clinical Director
Center for Rural Emergency Services and Trauma
Dartmouth-Hitchcock Medical Center
Lebanon, New Hampshire

Theodore Rogers, DO†
Family Medicine Resident
Naval Hospital Camp LeJeune
Jacksonville, North Carolina

Ashley Alexandra Roselle, DO, CPT†
Family Medicine Department
Womack Army Medical Center
Fort Bragg, North Carolina

Noah K. Rosenberg, MD
The Warren Alpert Medical School of Brown University
Department of Emergency Medicine
Providence, Rhode Island

Noah M. Rosenberg, MD
Chief Resident
Department of Family Medicine and Community Health
University of Massachusetts Memorial Medical Center
Worcester, Massachusetts

Montiel Teresa Rosenthal, MD
Associate Clinical Professor and Director of Maternity Services
Department of Family and Community Medicine
The Christ Hospital
University of Cincinnati Family Medicine Residency Program
University of Cincinnati College of Medicine
Cincinnati, Ohio

Steven E. Roskos, MD
Associate Professor
Department of Family Medicine
College of Human Medicine
Michigan State University
East Lansing, Michigan

David A. Ross, MD
Resident Physician
Department of Family Medicine and Community Health
University of Pennsylvania
Philadelphia, Pennsylvania

Michael J. Ross, MD
Associate Professor of Medicine
Division of Nephrology
Icahn School of Medicine at Mount Sinai
New York, New York

Steven Rougas, MD, MS, MEd
Assistant Professor of Emergency Medicine
The Warren Alpert Medical School of Brown University
Providence, Rhode Island

Michael P. Rowane, DO, MS, FAAFP, FAAO
Associate Clinical Professor of Family Medicine and Psychiatry
Director of Medical Education
Case Western Reserve University
University Hospitals Regional Hospitals
University Hospitals Case Medical Center
Richmond Heights, Ohio

Mark R. Rowe, DO†
Resident
Family Medicine Residency Program
Mike O'Callaghan Federal Medical Center
Nellis Air Force Base, Nevada

Sani Mathew Roy, MD
Pediatric Endocrinology Fellow
Division of Endocrinology and Diabetes
The Children's Hospital of Philadelphia
Philadelphia, Pennsylvania

Vibin Roy, MD
Instructor
Family and Community Medicine
Jefferson Medical College
Philadelphia, Pennsylvania

Anna Rudnicki, MD
Assistant Professor of Medicine
Division of Pulmonary, Allergy, and Critical Care
Department of Medicine
University of Massachusetts Medical School
Worcester, Massachusetts

Stephanie M. Ruest, MD
Pediatric Resident
Boston, Massachusetts

Lloyd A. Runser, MD, MPH, FAAFP†
Faculty
Womack Family Medicine Residency
Womack Army Medical Center
Fort Bragg, North Carolina

Travis C. Russell, MD, FAWM†
Core Faculty
Nellis Family Medicine
Nellis Air Force Base, Nevada

Emilio A. Russo, MD
Assistant Professor
Department of Family Medicine
Louisiana State University
Bogalusa, Louisiana

Veronica J. Ruston, DO†
Family Medicine Resident
Ehrling-Bergquist Clinic
Offutt Air Force Base, Nebraska

Anup K. Sabharwal, MD, MBA, FACE, CCD
Division of Endocrinology, Diabetes, and Metabolism
Herbert Wertheim College of Medicine
Florida International University
Miami, Florida

Daniel W. Saltzman, DO
Resident
Department of Emergency Medicine
Rutgers-Robert Wood Johnson Medical School
New Brunswick, New Jersey

Afshin Sam, MD
Department of Medicine
University of Arizona
Tucson, Arizona

Kathryn Samai, PharmD, BCPS
Assistant Professor
School of Pharmacy
Lake Erie College of Osteopathic Medicine
Bradenton, Florida

Adam K. Saperstein, MD, FAAFP†
Assistant Professor
Department of Family Medicine
Uniformed Services University of the Health Sciences
Bethesda, Maryland

Paul Savel, MD†
Faculty
Womack Family Medicine Residency
Womack Army Medical Center
Fort Bragg, North Carolina

Shailendra K. Saxena, MD, PhD
Assistant Professor
Department of Family Medicine
Creighton University School of Medicine
Omaha, Nebraska

Durr-e-Shahwaar Sayed, DO
Faculty Physician
Inspira Health Network
Glassboro, New Jersey

Payam Sazegar, MD
Assistant Clinical Professor
Department of Family and Community Medicine
University of California San Francisco
San Francisco, California

Matthew J. Schear, DO, MS
Department of Osteopathic Manipulative Medicine
College of Osteopathic Medicine
New York Institute of Technology
Old Westbury, New York

Edward Scheiner, DO

Fred J. Schiffman, MD
Sigal Family Professor of Humanistic Medicine
The Warren Alpert Medical School of Brown University
Providence, Rhode Island

Jonathan Schimmel, MD
Brown University
Rhode Island Hospital
Providence, Rhode Island

Benjamin N. Schneider, MD
Assistant Professor
Department of Family Medicine
Oregon Health & Science University
Portland, Oregon

Brian Joseph Schneider, MD
PGY3
Division of Medicine, Pediatrics
University of Massachusetts Medical School
Worcester, Massachusetts

Lisa M. Schroeder, MD
Assistant Director
Summa Barberton Family Practice Residency Program
Barberton, Ohio

Jennifer Schwartz, MD
Steward Medical Group
Boston, Massachusetts

Christopher J. Scola, MD
Assistant Clinical Professor of Medicine
University of Connecticut School of Medicine
Chief, Rheumatology Division
Hartford Hospital
Hartford, Connecticut

Ingrid U. Scott, MD, MPH
Professor of Ophthalmology and Public Health Sciences
Penn State Hershey Eye Center
Penn State College of Medicine
Hershey, Pennsylvania

Stephen Scott, MD, MPH
Associate Dean for Student Affairs
Weill Cornell Medical College in Qatar
Doha, Qatar

Gail Scully, MD, MPH
University of Massachusetts Memorial Medical Center
University of Massachusetts Medical School
Worcester, Massachusetts

David Sealy, MD
Professor
Medical University of South Carolina
Director, Greenwood Area Health Education Center
Primary Care Sports Medicine Fellowship
Self Regional Healthcare Family Medicine Residency
Greenwood, South Carolina

Margaret Seaver, MD, MPH
Palliative Medicine Service
Lahey Hospital and Medical Center
Burlington, Masschusetts

L. Michelle W. Seawright, DO†
Naval Hospital Camp Lejeune
Camp Lejeune, North Carolina

Sheila M. Seed, PharmD, MPH, RPh
Associate Professor
Department of Pharmacy Practice
Massachusetts College of Pharmacy and Health Sciences University
Worcester, Massachusetts

Amy Seery, MD
Assistant Professor
Department of Family and Community Medicine
University of Kansas School of Medicine–Wichita
Wichita, Kansas

Jamie A. Seidl, DO†
Family Medicine Resident
Dwight D. Eisenhower Army Medical Center
Fort Gordon, Georgia

Anna Serur, MD, FACS, FASCRS
Chief
Colon and Rectal Surgery
Maimonides Medical Center
Brooklyn, New York

Jessica T. Servey, MD, Col, USAF, MC†
Assistant Dean for Faculty Development
Associate Professor of Family Medicine
Uniformed Services University of the Health Sciences
Bethesda, Maryland

Chirag N. Shah, MD, FACEP
Assistant Professor
Department of Emergency Medicine
Rutgers Robert Wood Johnson Medical School
New Brunswick, New Jersey

Samir A. Shah, MD, FACG, FASGE, AGAF
Clinical Professor of Medicine
The Warren Alpert Medical School of Brown University
Chief of Gastroenterology
Department of Medicine
The Miriam Hospital
Providence, Rhode Island

Kevin C. Shannon, MD, MPH, FAAFP
Associate Professor
Department of Family Medicine
Loma Linda University School of Medicine
Loma Linda, California

Musa A. Sharkawi, MB, BCh, BAO
Resident Physician
Department of Internal Medicine
Lahey Hospital and Medical Center
Burlington, Massachusetts

Radhika Sharma, MD
Physician
Obstetrics and Gynecology Resident
Aultman Hospital/NEOMED
Canton, Ohio

Sanjeev Sharma, MD
Associate Professor
Creighton University School of Medicine
Omaha, Nebraska

Victoria R. Sharon, MD, DTMH
Assistant Professor of Dermatology and Dermatologic Surgery
Department of Dermatology
University of California Davis
Sacramento, California

Cameron M. Shawver, DO†
Nellis Air Force Base Family Medicine Residency
Mike O'Callaghan Federal Medical Center
Las Vegas, Nevada

Karen Sheflin, DO
Assistant Professor
Department of Family Medicine
College of Osteopathic Medicine
New York Institute of Technology
Old Westbury, New York

Paula A. Shelton, MD
Family Medicine
The University of Texas Health Science Center at San Antonio
San Antonio, Texas

Tisamarie B. Sherry, MD, PhD
Internal Medicine Resident
Department of Medicine
Brigham and Women's Hospital
Boston, Massachusetts

Nicole Shields, MD
Assistant Professor of Family Medicine
DeBusk College of Osteopathic Medicine
Lincoln Memorial University
Harrogate, Tennessee

Jeffrey Shih, MD
Assistant Professor of Medicine
Advanced Heart Failure and Transplantation
Cardiovascular Medicine
University of Massachusetts
Tufts Medical Center
Worcester, Massachusetts

Sonya Shipley, MD
Assistant Professor of Family Medicine
University of Mississippi Medical Center
Jackson, Mississippi

Justin R. Shirley MD, CPT†
Family Medicine
Womack Army Medical Center
Fort Bragg, North Carolina

Matthew W. Short, MD†
Associate Director, Medical Education
Graduate Medical Education
Madigan Army Medical Center
Tacoma, Washington

Suzanne Shurtz, MLIS, AHIP
Associate Professor
Medical Sciences Library
Texas A&M University
College Station, Texas

Natalie S. Shwaish, MD
Resident Physician
Department of Pediatrics
University of Arizona
Tucson, Arizona

Aamir Siddiqi, MD
Director of Clinical Services
Norris Health Center
University of Wisconsin—Milwaukee
Milwaukee, Wisconsin

Najm Hasan Siddiqui, MD
Hospitalist Physician
Parkview Medical Center
Pueblo, Colorado

Julia Siegel, BA
MD Candidate
University of Massachusetts Medical School
Worcester, Massachusetts

Samuel N. Sigoloff, DO, CPT, MC, USA†
Martin Army Community Hospital
Fort Benning, Georgia

Kimberly Sikule, MD
Family Medicine Residency
University of Massachusetts Worcester
Worcester, Massachusetts

Hugh J. Silk, MD, MPH
Clinical Associate Professor
Department of Family Medicine and Community Health
University of Massachusetts Medical School
Worcester, Massachusetts

Matthew A. Silva, PharmD, RPh, BCPS
Professor of Pharmacy Practice
Massachusetts College of Pharmacy and Health Sciences University
Worcester, Massachusetts

Tiffany A. Moore Simas, MD, MPH, MEd
Associate Professor of Obstetrics & Gynecology and Pediatrics
Department of Obstetrics & Gynecology
University of Massachusetts Medical School
University of Massachusetts Memorial Health Care
Worcester, Massachusetts

Ashley Simela, DO
Orthopedic Spine Surgeon
Cedars Sinai Medical Center
West Hollywood, California

Lauren M. Simon, MD, MPH, FAAFP, FACSM
Associate Professor of Family Medicine
Director
Primary Care Sports Medicine
Loma Linda University
Loma Linda, California

Marvin H. Sineath, Jr., MD, CAQSM†
Family Medicine Residency
Sports Medicine Director
Nellis Air Force Base, Nevada

Nick Singh, MD

Avani Sinha, MD
The Warren Alpert Medical School of Brown University
Providence, Rhode Island

Nga Yan Siu, DO, MS
College of Osteopathic Medicine
New York Institute of Technology
Old Westbury, New York

Maja Skikic, MD
Resident in Psychiatry
Department of Psychiatry
Vanderbilt University Medical Center
Nashville, Tennessee

Brian G. Skotko, MD, MPP
Co-Director
Down Syndrome Program
Division of Medical Genetics
Massachusetts General Hospital
Boston, Massachusetts

Glenn Skow, MD, MPH
Chief Medical Officer
Fayette County Hospital
Vandalia, Illinois

Jason C. Sluzevich, MD
Assistant Professor of Dermatology
Mayo Clinic
Jacksonville, Florida

Adam J.T. Smith, MD, PhD
Resident Physician
Department of Radiation Medicine
University of Kentucky
Lexington, Kentucky

Andrew Smith, MD

Dennis Smith, DO
Program Director
North Mississippi Medical Center
Family Medicine Residency Program
Tupelo, Mississippi

Kayla J. Smith, MD
Georgia Regents University
Augusta, Georgia

Lee P. Smith, MD
Chief
Division of Pediatric Otolaryngology
Cohen Children's Medical Center
Assistant Professor of Otolaryngology
Hofstra North Shore-LIJ School of Medicine
Forest Hills, New York

Miriam A. Smith, MD, MBA

John C. Smulian, MD, MPH
Division of Maternal Fetal Medicine
Department of Obstetrics and Gynecology
Lehigh Valley Health Network
Allentown, Pennsylvania
University of South Florida-Morsani College of Medicine
Tampa, Florida

Matthew Snyder, DO†
Military Program Director
St. Louis University Family Medicine Residency
Belleville, Illinois

L. Michael Snyder, MD
Professor
Department of Medicine and Pathology
University of Massachusetts Medical School
UMass Memorial Medical Center
Chief Medical Officer
Quest Diagnostics MA, LLC
Worcester, Massachusetts

Leah Soley, MD

D'Ann Somerall, DNP, MAEd, FNP-BC
Assistant Professor
Family Caregiving and Systems
University of Alabama at Birmingham School of Nursing
Birmingham, Alabama

William E. Somerall, Jr., MD, MEd
Visiting Associate Professor School of Nursing
University of Alabama at Birmingham
Birmingham, Alabama

David B. Sommer, MD, MPH

Alexandra Sophocles, MD
University of Massachusetts Medical Center
Worcester, Massachusetts

Adam J. Sorscher, MD
Assistant Professor
Department of Community and Family Medicine
Geisel Medical School at Dartmouth
Lebanon, New Hampshire

Andres F. Sosa, MD
Assistant Professor of Medicine
Interventional Pulmonary
Division of Lung, Allergy and Critical Care Medicine
UMass Memorial Medical Center
Worcester, Massachusetts

Marie Anne Sosa, MD
Assistant Professor of Medicine
Division of General Medicine
Division of Nephrology
University of Massachusetts School of Medicine
Worcester, Massachusetts

Sara Soshnick, DO, MS
College of Medicine
New York Institute of Technology
Old Westbury, New York

Alison Southern, MD, MS, FACEP
Associate Program Director
Department of Emergency Medicine
Summa Akron City Hospital
Akron, Ohio

Charles Sow, MD, MSCR

Mikayla Spangler, PharmD, BCPS
Assistant Professor
Department of Family Medicine
Department of Pharmacy Practice and School of Medicine
School of Pharmacy and Health Professions
Creighton University
Omaha, Nebraska

Craig Spergel, DO
Internal Medicine Resident, PGY2
Department of Internal Medicine
Largo Medical Center
Largo, Florida

Jacoby D. Spittler, DO
Department of Obsetrics and Gynecology
Akron General Medical Center
Akron, Ohio

Kellie A. Sprague, MD
Assistant Professor of Medicine
Tufts Medical Center/Tufts University School of Medicine
Boston, Massachusetts

Dana Sprute, MD, MPH, FAAFP
Associate Professor of Family & Community Medicine
Family Medicine Residency Program
The University of Texas Southwestern Austin
Austin, Texas

Rama Challapalli Sri, MD
Nephrology Fellow, PGY5
University of Massachusetts Medical School
Worcester, Massachusetts

Aaron K. Starbuck, MD, ABFM†
Teaching Faculty
Department of Family Medicine
Martin Army Community Hospital
Fort Benning, Georgia

Stephen Staub, MD†
Family Physician
Naval Hospital Camp LeJeune
Jacksonville, North Carolina

Laura Steadman, EdD, CRNP, MSN, RN
Assistant Professor
School of Nursing
Adult/Acute Health
Chronic Care and Foundations
University of Alabama at Birmingham
Birmingham, Alabama

Daniel J. Stein, MD, MPH
Resident Physician
Department of Internal Medicine
University of Virginia Health System
Charlottesville, Virginia

Kim Michal Stein, MD
Resident Physician
University of Virginia Health System
Charlottesville, Virginia

Noah A. Steinberg, PA-C†
United States Army
Bagram, Afghanistan

Mark B. Stephens, MD, MS, FAAFP, CAPT, MC, USN†
Professor and Chair
Department of Family Medicine
Uniformed Services University
Bethesda, Maryland

Nathaniel Stepp, DO, LCDR, USN†
Family Medicine Physician
Family Medicine Residency Staff
Naval Hospital Camp Lejeune
Camp Lejeune, North Carolina

J. Herbert Stevenson, MD
Director of Sports Medicine
Director of the Sports Medicine Fellowship Program
Associate Professor
Department of Family Health
Joint Appointment Department of Orthopedics
University of Massachusetts
Worcester, Massachusetts

Sheila O. Stille, DMD
Associate Professor
Department of Surgical Dentistry
Assistant Director General Practice Residency
University of Colorado School of Dental Medicine
Aurora, Colorado

Marcus F. Stoddard, MD
Professor of Medicine
Director
Non-invasive Cardiology Division
Cardiovascular Medicine
University of Louisville
Louisville, Kentucky

Jeffrey G. Stovall, MD
Associate Professor
Department of Psychiatry
Vanderbilt University School of Medicine
Nashville, Tennessee

Celeste Straight, MD
Resident Physician
Department of Obstetrics and Gynecology
University of Massachusetts Medical School
Worcester, Massachusetts

Rishi Esvy Subbarayan, MD
Vascular Surgery Fellow
Department of Vascular Surgery
Medical College of Wisconsin
Milwaukee, Wisconsin

Karyn M. Sullivan, PharmD, MPH
Associate Professor of Pharmacy Practice
Massachusetts College of Pharmacy and Health Sciences University
Worcester, Massachusetts

Heather Summe, MD
Division of Dermatology
University of Massachusetts Memorial Health Center
Worcester, Massachusetts

Shima Syed, MD†
Staff Physician
Department of Family and Community Medicine
Dwight D. Eisenhower Army Medical Center
Fort Gordon, Georgia

Alfonso Tafur, MD, MS, RPVI
Assistant Professor of Medicine
Department of Medicine—Cardiovascular
Oklahoma University Health Sciences Center
Oklahoma City, Oklahoma

Denisse V. Tafur, MD
Guayaquil, Ecuador

Komal Talati, MD
Radiology Resident
Department Radiology
Beth Israel Deaconess Medical Center
Boston, Massachusetts

Irene J. Tan, MD, FACR
Associate Professor of Clinical Medicine
Department of Medicine, Section of Rheumatology
Temple University School of Medicine
Philadelphia, Pennsylvania

Weizhen Tan, MD
Clinical Fellow in Nephrology
Boston Children's Hospital
Boston, Massachusetts

Michael Tarpey, MD

Paul A. Tate, Jr., MD†
Womack Army Medical Center
Family Medicine Residency
Fort Bragg, North Carolina

Eugene M. Tay, MD, MS
Clinical Assistant Professor
Department of Family Medicine
College of Human Medicine
Michigan State University
Grand Rapids, Michigan

Danielle Taylor, DO, MS
Obstetrics and Gynecology Resident, PGY3
Akron General Medical Center
Akron, Ohio

James L. Taylor, PharmD
Ambulatory Clinical Pharmacist
Family Medicine Residency Program
North Mississippi Medical Center
Tupelo, Mississippi

David Tegay, DO, FACMG, FACOI
Associate Professor and Chair
Department of Medicine
College of Osteopathic Medicine
New York Institute of Technology
Old Westbury, New York

Meaghan Tenney, MD
Assistant Professor
Section of Gynecologic Oncology
Department of Obstetrics and Gynecology
University of Chicago Medicine
Chicago, Illinois

Jose-Luis Terrazas, MD
Administrative Chief Resident—Department of Obstetrics and Gynecology
University of South Florida School of Medicine
Tampa, Florida
Lehigh Valley Health Network
Allentown, Pennsylvania

Michael J. Terzella, DO
Assistant Professor
Department of Osteopathic Manipulative Medicine
College of Osteopathic Medicine
New York Institute of Technology
Old Westbury, New York

Nimmy Thakolkaran, MD
Resident
Department of Family Medicine
Mount Sinai Hospital
Chicago, Illinois

Pardeep Thandi, MD
Emergency Medicine
The Brooklyn Hospital Center
Brooklyn, New York

Margaret E. Thompson, MD
Associate Professor
Family Medicine
College of Human Medicine
Michigan State University
Grand Rapids, Michigan

Richard C. Tibbetts, MD
Intern, Internal Medicine
University of Massachusetts Medical School
Worcester, Massachusetts

Bryan Tischenkel, MD
PGY2 in Anesthesiology
Columbia University
New York-Presbyterian Hospital
New York, New York

Adam Z. Tobias, MD, MPH, FACEP
Assistant Professor of Emergency Medicine
University of Pittsburgh School of Medicine
Pittsburgh, Pennslyvania

Elizabeth M. Tocci
University of Massachusetts Medical School
Worcester, Massachusetts

Rachelle E. Toman, MD, PhD
Medical Director and Associate Program Director
Georgetown University-Providence Hospital
Family Medicine Residency
Washington, DC

Sebastian T. C. Tong, MD, MPH
Family Medicine Resident
Greater Lawrence Family Health Center
Lawrence, Massachusetts

Moshe S. Torem, MD
Professor of Psychiatry
Northeast Ohio Medical University
Rootstown, Ohio

John R. Torro, MD
Faculty Development Fellow
Lawrence Family Medicine Residency
Lawrence, Massachusetts

Carmen Tran, MD
Resident, Internal Medicine
The University of Texas at Tyler
Good Shepherd Medical
Longview, Texas

Hayden Tran, DO, MS
Physician
Hospital Medicine
Marietta Memorial Hospital
Marietta, Ohio

Huy Tan Tran, MD, LCDR, MC, USN†
Family Medicine Resident
Naval Hospital Camp Pendleton
Camp Pendleton, California

Kashyap Trivedi, MD
Hertz and Associates in Gastroenterology
Los Alamitos, California

Rupal Trivedi, MD
Assistant Professor
Family & Community Medicine
St. Louis University
St. Louis, Missouri

Zoltan Trizna, MD, PhD
Austin, Texas

Katherine M. Tromp, PharmD
Assistant Professor
Lake Erie College of Osteopathic Medicine School of Pharmacy
Bradenton, Florida

Artsiom Tsyrkunou, MD, MPH
Hillcrest Family Practice
Berkshire Medical Center
Pittsfield, Massachusetts

Annie Marian Tubman, MD
Family Medicine Resident
Family Medicine of Southwest
Vancouver, Washington

Deepali Nivas Tukaye, MD, PhD
Fellow, Cardiovascular Medicine
Department of Medicine/Division of Cardiology
The Ohio State University—Wexner Medical Center
Columbus, Ohio

Bradley M. Turner, MD, MPH, MHA
Assistant Professor
University of Rochester
Rochester, New York

Auguste Turnier, MD
Internist/Gastroenterologist, Private Practice
Haddonfield, New Jersey

John K. Uffman, MD, MPH
Pediatric Surgery
Cook Children's Medical Center
Fort Worth, Texas

Katherine S. Upchurch, MD
Clinical Professor of Medicine
University of Massachusetts Medical Group
Clinical Chief
Divison of Rheumatology
University of Massachusetts Memorial Medical Group
Worcester, Massachusetts

Onameyore Utuama, MD, MPH
Morehouse School of Medicine Family Medicine Residency
Atlanta, Georgia

Diana P. Vaca, MD
Newark, New Jersey

Santiago O. Valdes, MD, FAAP
Pediatric Cardiology
Baylor College of Medicine
Texas Children's Hospital
Houston, Texas

Anthony Valdini, MD, MS, FACP, FAAFP
Clinical Professor of Family Medicine and Community Health
University of Massachusetts School of Medicine
Lawrence, Massachusetts

Olga Valdman, MD
Assistant Professor
Department of Family Medicine
University of Massachusetts Medical School
Worcester, Massachusetts

Virginia Van Duyne, MD
Assistant Professor
Associate Residency Director of Women's Health Education
Department of Family Medicine and Community Health
University of Massachusetts Worcester Family Medicine Residency Program
Family Health Center of Worcester
Worcester, Massachusetts

Tricia Elaine VanWagner, MD[†]
Department Head, Sports Medicine
Associate Sports Medicine Fellowship Director
Naval Hospital Camp Pendleton
Camp Pendleton, California

Sharlin Varghese, MD
Assistant Professor
Department of Pathology and Laboratory Medicine
University of Rochester Medical Center
Rochester, New York

Kathleen M. Vazzana, DO
Academic Medicine Scholar
College of Osteopathic Medicine
New York Institute of Technology
Old Westbury, New York

Nandhini Veeraraghavan, MD
Faculty
Family Medicine Residency
Sacred Heart Hospital
Allentown, Pennsylvania

Suman Vellanki, MD
Family Medicine Resident
Summa Barberton Hospital
Barberton, Ohio

Bryon Veynovich, DO

Alicia Huff Vinyard, DO
General Surgery Resident Physician
Georgia Regents University
Augusta, Georgia

Siva Vithananthan, MD, FACS
Associate Professor of Surgery (Clinical)
The Warren Alpert Medical School of Brown University
Providence, Rhode Island

Stacey Vitiello, MD
Breast Imaging Specialist
Montclair Breast Center
Montclair, New Jersey

Kirsten Vitrikas, MD, FAAFP[†]
Program Director
David Grant Medical Center
Family Medicine Residency
Travis Air Force Base, California

Katherine Vlasica, DO
Attending Physician
Emergency Medicine
Saint Joseph's Regional Medical Center
Paterson, New Jersey

John T. Vogel, DO, CPT, USAF[†]
Family Medicine Residency Clinic
David Grant Medical Center
Travis Air Force Base, California

Kenton I. Voorhees, MD
Vice Chair for Education
Professor of Clinical Practice
Department of Family Medicine
University of Colorado School of Medicine
Aurora, Colorado

Puja Vora, MD

Yongkasem Vorasettakarnkij, MD, MSc
Clinical Instructor and Consultant
Department of Medicine
Faculty of Medicine
Chulalongkorn University
Cardiovascular Magnetic Resonance Imaging Cardiac Center
King Chulalongkorn Memorial Hospital
Thai Red Cross Society
Bangkok, Thailand

Kamal C. Wagle, MD, MPH
Assistant Professor
Family & Community Medicine
Baylor College of Medicine
Houston, Texas

Joseph R. Wagner, MD
Director of Robotic Surgery
Department of Urology
Hartford Healthcare
Hartford, Connecticut

Cynthia M. Waickus, MD, PhD
Associate Professor
Department of Family Medicine
Rush Medical College
Chicago, Illinois

Anne Walsh, MMSc, PA-C, DFAAPA
Instructor of Clinical Family Medicine
Department of Family Medicine
Keck School of Medicine
University of Southern California
Los Angeles, California

Nathaniel J. Walsh, MD
Georgia Regents University
Department of Surgery
Augusta, Georgia

Katrina E. Walters, MD, FAAFP, FM†
Director
Obstetrics Fellowship Program
Department of Family and Community Medicine
Carl R. Darnall Army Medical Center
Fort Hood, Texas

Annie R. Wang, MD
Department of Dermatology
The Warren Alpert Medical School of Brown University
Providence, Rhode Island

Hsin-Yi Janey Wang, MD
Family Medicine
The University of Texas Health Science Center at San Antonio
San Antonio, Texas

Jeff Wang, MD, MPH
UMass/Fitchburg Family Medicine Residency
University of Massachusetts Medical School
UMass Memorial Health Care
Worcester, Massachusetts

Ryan Wargo, PharmD, BCACP
Assistant Professor of Pharmacy Practice
Lake Erie College of Osteopathic Medicine School of Pharmacy
Bradenton, Florida

Donald E. Watenpaugh, PhD
Adjunct Professor
Department of Integrative Physiology
University of North Texas Health Science Center
Fort Worth, Texas

Andrea N. Watson, DO, MS
Assistant Professor
Department of Family Medicine
College of Osteopathic Medicine
New York Institute of Technology
Old Westbury, New York

Jill T. Wei, MD
Department of Family Medicine
David Geffen School of Medicine at UCLA
Santa Monica, California

Eilene Weibley, MD
Bayfront Family Medicine Residency
St. Petersburg, Florida

Patrice M. Weiss, MD, FACOG
Chair and Professor
Carilion Clinic/Virginia Tech Carilion School of Medicine
Roanoke, Virginia

Frederick C. Weitendorf, RPH, RN
ICCU Clinical Pharmacist
Department of Pharmacy
Robley Rex VA Medical Center
Louisville, Kentucky

Mark Weitzel, DO
Otolaryngology Department
Philadelphia College of Osteopathic Medicine
Philadelphia, Pennsylvania

Jennifer Greene Welch, MD
Assistant Professor of Pediatrics
The Warren Alpert Medical School of Brown University
Providence, Rhode Island

Jeremy Blake Wells, MD
Chief Resident
Department of Family Medicine
University of Mississippi Medical Center
Jackson, Mississippi

Katie L. Westerfield, DO†
Faculty, Family Medicine Residency
Martin Army Community Hospital
Fort Benning, Georgia

Tyler Wheeler, MD
Family Practice Center, PC
Atlanta, Georgia

Vernon Wheeler, MD, FAAFP

Chris Wheelock, MD
PeaceHealth Southwest Washington Clinical Assistant Professor
Family Medicine
University of Washington
Vancouver, Washington

Ebony Whisenant, MD
Florida International University
Miami, Florida

Kimara Whisenant, MD
Bako Pathology
Atlanta, Georgia

Brett White, MD
Newport Family Medicine
Newport Beach, California

Christopher White, MD, JD
Assistant Professor of Psychiatry & Family Medicine
University of Cincinnati College of Medicine
Cincinnati, Ohio

Margaret Whitney, MD

Rebecca M. Wight, MD
Department of Surgery
University of Massachusetts Medical School
Worcester, Massachusetts

Susanne Wild, MD
Clinician Educator
Banner Good Samaritan Family Medicine Center
Clinical Assistant Professor
Department of Family and Community Medicine
University of Arizona College of Medicine
Phoenix, Arizona

Joshua Scott Will, DO†
Chief, Department of Women's Health and Newborn Care
Martin Army Community Hospital
Fort Benning, Georgia

Midhuna William, MD
PGY2
Family Medicine
Carilion Clinic/Virginia Tech School of Medicine
Roanoke, Virginia

Faren H. Williams, MD, MS
Chief, Physical Medicine & Rehabilitation
Clinical Professor
Department of Orthopedics and Physical Rehabilitation
University of Massachusetts Medical School
Worcester, Massachusetts

Michelle Williams, MD
Bayfront Health Family Medicine Residency
St. Petersburg, Florida

Paul N. Williams, MD
Assistant Professor of Clinical Medicine
Section of General Internal Medicine
Temple University Hospital
Philadelphia, Pennsylvania

Alan J. Williamson, MD†
Medical Director
Family Health Clinic
Ehrling Bergquist Clinic
Offutt Air Force Base, Nebraska

Shenelle Wilson, MD
Section of Urology
Department of Surgery
Georgia Regents University
Augusta, Georgia

Amy B. Wilson-LaMothe, PharmD, BCPS
Assistant Professor of Pharmacy Practice
Massachusetts College of Pharmacy and Health Sciences University
Worcester, Massachusetts

Norton Winer, MD
Assistant Clinical
Professor of Neurology
Case Western Reserve University School of Medicine
Cleveland, Ohio

Robyn D. Wing, MD
Pediatric Emergency Medicine Fellow
Department of Emergency Medicine
The Warren Alpert Medical School of Brown University/Hasbro Children's Hospital
Providence, Rhode Island

James Winger, MD
Associate Professor of Family Medicine
CAQ, Primary Care Sports Medicine
Loyola Stritch School of Medicine
Maywood, Illinois

Fawn Winkelman, DO
Board-Certified in Osteopathic Family Medicine
Fort Lauderdale, Florida

Aaron M. Winnick, MD, FACS
Department of Surgery
Maimonides Medical Center
Brooklyn, New York

Christopher M. Wise, MD
W. Robert Irby Professor of Medicine
Division of Rheumatology, Allergy, and Immunology
Department of Medicine
Virginia Commonwealth University Health System
Richmond, Virginia

Amy L. Wiser, MD
Assistant Professor
Department of Family Medicine
Oregon Health & Science University School of Medicine
Portland, Oregon

Jeffrey D. Wolfrey, MD
Chair, Department of Family Medicine
Banner Good Samaritan Medical Center
Clinical Professor
Department of Family and Community Medicine
University of Arizona College of Medicine
Phoenix, Arizona

Kimberly Wollett, MD
Family Medicine Resident, PGY3
Bayfront Health St. Petersburg
St. Petersburg, Florida

Wendy Hin-Wing Wong, MD, MPH
Department of Emergency Medicine
The Warren Alpert Medical School of Brown University
Providence, Rhode Island

J. Andrew Woods, PharmD, BCPS
Assistant Professor of Pharmacy
Wingate University School of Pharmacy
Internal Medicine Clinical Pharmacy Specialist
Carolinas Medical Center—Main
Charlotte, North Carolina

Dawna H. Woodyear, MD
Assistant Professor
University of Pittsburgh School of Medicine
Department of Family and Community Medicine
Medical Director
University of Pittsburgh Medical Center Matilda Theiss Health Center
Pittsburgh, Pennsylvania

Bart D. Worthington, DO, MS†
Family Medicine Resident
St. Louis University Family Medicine Residency—Belleville
Belleville, Illinois

Frances Y. Wu, MD
Assistant Director
Somerset Family Medicine Residency Program
Robert Wood Johnson Medical Center at Somerset
Somerville, New Jersey

Roger Y. Wu, MD, MBA
Resident Physician
Department of Emergency Medicine
The Warren Alpert Medical School of Brown University
Rhode Island Hospital
Providence, Rhode Island

Kristen M. Wyrick, MD†
Assistant Professor of Family Medicine
Department of Family Medicine
Uniformed Services University
Bethesda, Maryland

Ewa M. Wysokinska, MD
Willmar Cancer Center
Willmar, Minnesota

Michael Y. Yang, MD
Resident
Department of Family Medicine
Chestnut Hill Hospital
Philadelphia, Pennsylvania

Tianjiang Ye, MD
Resident
Department of Emergency Medicine
The Warren Alpert Medical School of Brown University
Providence, Rhode Island

James R. Yon, MD
General Surgery Resident
Department of General Surgery
Georgia Regents University
Augusta, Georgia

Robert A. Yood, MD
Chief of Rheumatology
Reliant Medical Group
Clinical Professor of Medicine
University of Massachusetts Medical School
Worcester, Massachusetts

Edward L. Yourtee, MD, FACP
Chief Medical Officer
Parkland Medical Center
Derry, New Hampshire

David H. Yun, MD

Edlira Yzeiraj, DO, MS
Internal Medicine
Cleveland Clinic
Cleveland, Ohio

Christine Clarice Zacharia, MD, MS
Endocrinology Fellow
Department of Endocrinology
The Warren Alpert Medical School of Brown University
Providence, Rhode Island

Isabel Zacharias, MD
Staff Physician
Department of Gastroenterology
UMass Memorial Medical Center
Worcester, Massachusetts

Amy M. Zack, MD, FAAFP
Family Medicine Physician
Associate Program Director, Family Medicine
Department of Family Medicine
MetroHealth Medical Center/Case Western Reserve University
Cleveland, Ohio

Isheeta Zalpuri, MD
Psychiatry Resident
University of Massachusetts
Worcester, Massachusetts

Matthew Zanghi, MD

Katrina Darlene Zedan, MSPAS, PA-C
South Texas Sinus Institute
San Antonio, Texas

Steven M. Zeddun, MD
Assistant Professor of Medicine
Division of Gastroenterology and Liver Diseases
The George Washington University
Washington, DC

Youhua Zhang, MD, PhD
Assistant Professor
Department of Biomedical Sciences
College of Osteopathic Medicine
New York Institute of Technology
Old Westbury, New York

Ruslan Zhuravsky, DO
PGY4
Otolaryngology and Facial Plastic Surgery
Rowan School of Osteopathic Medicine
Stratford, New Jersey

Derek G. Zickgraf, DO[†]
Family Physician and Brigade Surgeon
8th Military Police Brigade
Schofield Barracks, Hawaii

Russell S. Zide, MD, FSVM
Departments of General Internal Medicine and Cardiovascular Medicine
Lahey Hospital and Medical Center
Burlington, Massachusetts

Peter J. Ziemkowski, MD
Associate Dean for Student Affairs
Associate Professor
Department of Family and Community Medicine
Western Michigan University School of Medicine
Kalamazoo, Michigan

Gennine M. Zinner, RNCS, ANP
Nurse Practitioner
Boston Health Care for the Homeless Program
Massachusetts General Hospital Institute of Health Professions
Boston, Massachusetts

Kimberly Zoberi, MD
Department of Family Medicine
St. Louis University School of Medicine
St. Louis, Missouri

Susan Zweizig, MD
Director
Division of Gynecologic Oncology
Department of Obstetrics and Gynecology
University of Massachusetts
Worcester, Massachusetts

[†]The views expressed are those of the authors and do not reflect the official policy of the Department of the Army, Department of the Navy, the Department of Defense, or the United States Government.

CONTENTS

Topics

Diagnosis and Treatment: An Algorithmic Approach

This section contains flowcharts (or algorithms) to help the reader in the diagnosis of clinical signs and symptoms and treatment of a variety of clinical problems. They are organized by the presenting sign, symptom, or diagnosis.

These algorithms were designed to be used as a quick reference and adjunct to the reader's clinical knowledge and impression. They are not an exhaustive review of the management of a problem, nor are they meant to be a complete list of diseases.

ABDOMINAL PAIN, CHRONIC

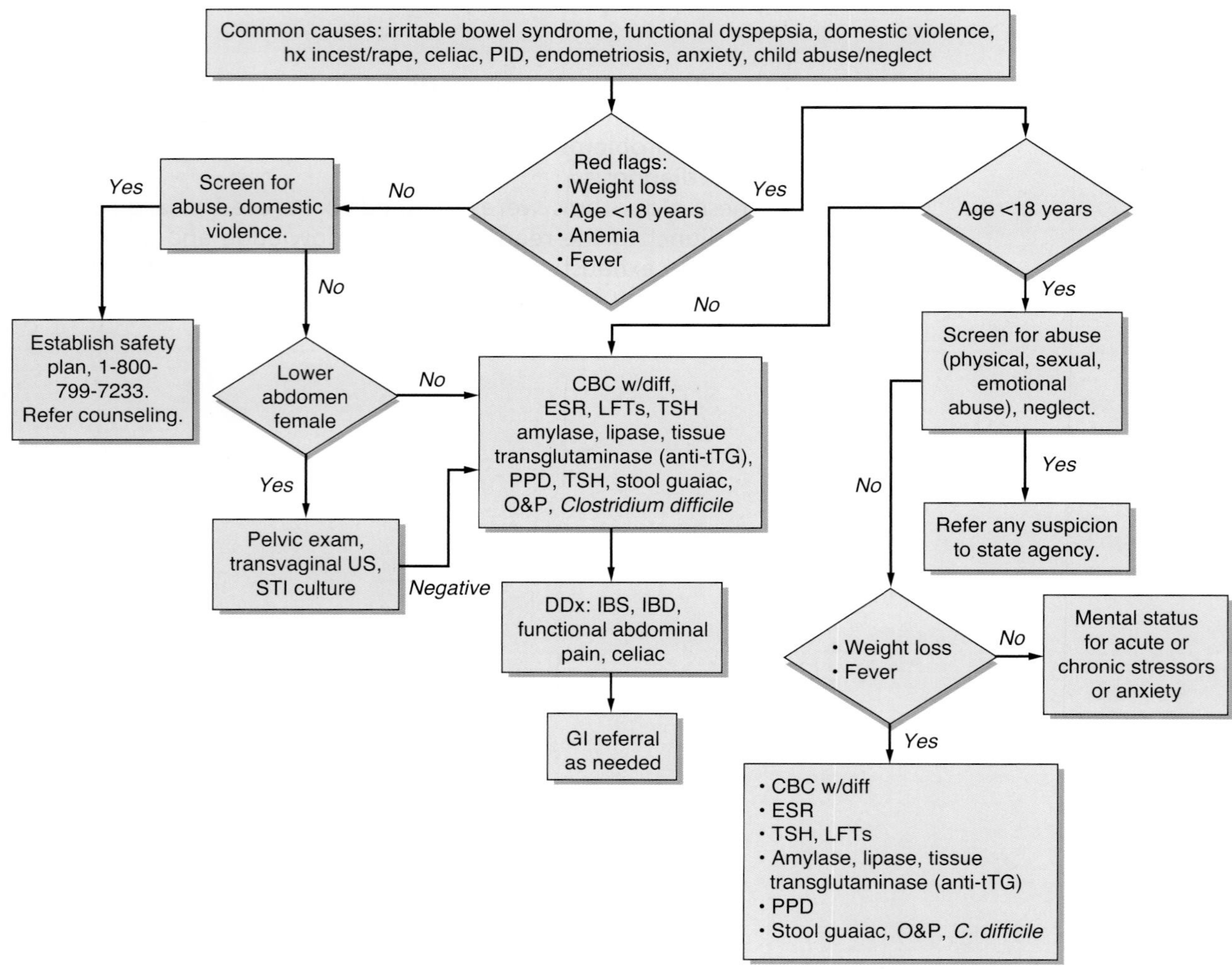

Frank J. Domino, MD and Bree Alyeska, MD

Camilleri M. Management of patients with chronic abdominal pain in clinical practice. *Neurogastroenterol Motil.* 2006;18(7):499–506.

ABDOMINAL PAIN, LOWER

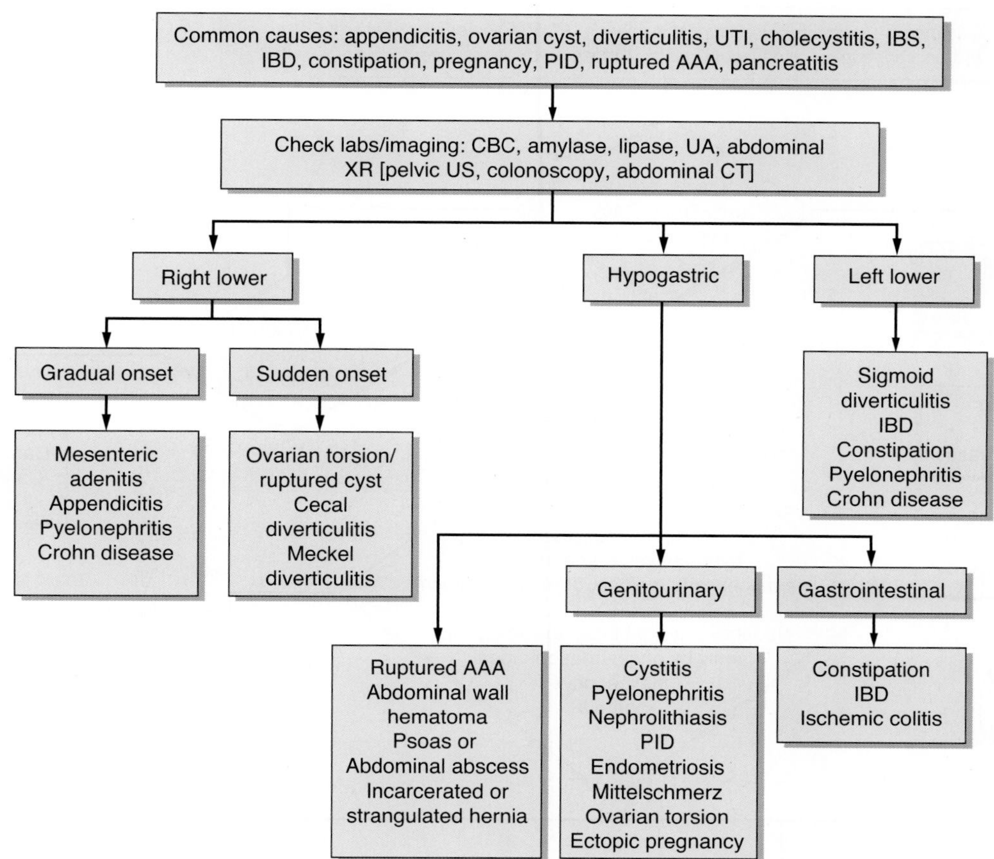

Nihal Patel, MD and Siva Vithananthan, MD, FACS

Heading RC. Prevalence of upper gastrointestinal symptoms in the general population: a systematic review. *Scand J Gastroenterol Suppl.* 1999;231:3–8.

ABDOMINAL PAIN, UPPER

Common Causes: GERD, functional dyspepsia, PUD, Pancreatitis, biliary dysfunction, angina, esophageal/gastric cancer, medications, pneumonia

Acute severe pain radiating to back, hypotension?

- *Yes* → Stabilize patient, Ultrasound, CT chest/abd → Aortic dissection, AAA, severe acute pancreatitis
- *No* → Suspicion of cardiac disease?
  - *Yes* → Cardiac Evaluation Cardiac Enzymes EKG → Angina, MI, pericarditis
  - *No* → GI Alarm Symptoms?

    Bleeding: tachycardia, hypotension, hematemesis, Hematochezia, melena, drop in hematocrit

    Neoplasia: weight loss, age >50 years family hx of gastroesophageal malignancy, anemia
    - *Yes* → Endoscopy → PUD, esophageal/gastric carcinoma
    - No alarm symptoms
      - LUQ pain → Fever, tenderness → Splenic abscess, splenic infarct
      - RUQ pain → CMP, LFTs, GGT, RUQ ultrasound
        - Elevated bilirubin, elevated alk phos, fever, jaundice → Cholangitis
        - Elevated AST/ALT elevated bilirubin, hepatomegaly on ultrasound → Acute Hepatitis, Budd-Chiari syndrome
        - Associated with meals, +/– Elevated WBC/fever, + Murphy Sign → Cholecystitis, biliary colic
      - Epigastric pain
        - Indigestion, bloating → PUD, gastroparesis, gastritis, GERD, IBS
        - Pain radiates to back, severe for hours, hx of alcohol abuse, gallstones → Elevated amylase & lypase → Pancreatitis
        - Heartburn, acid taste in mouth, worse at night → GERD
      - Poorly localizable
        - Symptoms that do not resolve with PPI → Functional dyspepsia, IBS
        - Pulmonary sym Cough, Fever Chest X-ray → Pneumonia

Nischal Raya, Brian Ciampa, MD, and Marie L. Borum, MD, EdD, MPH

Yamamoto W, Kono H, Maekawa M, Fukui T. The relationship between abdominal [pain regions and specific diseases: an epidemiologic approach to clinical practice. *J Epidemiol.* 1997;7:27.

ACETAMINOPHEN POISONING, TREATMENT

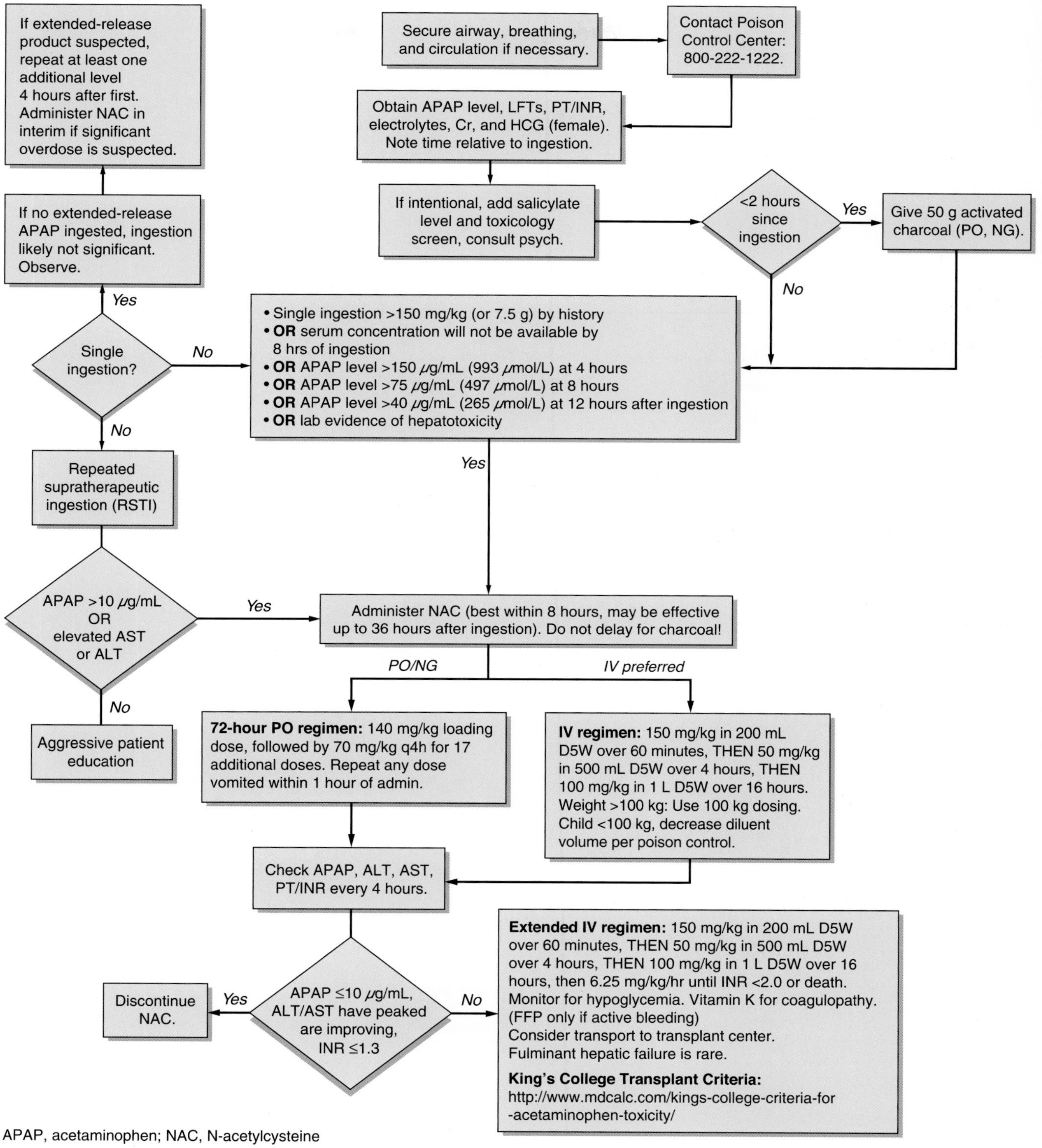

Secure airway, breathing, and circulation if necessary.

Contact Poison Control Center: 800-222-1222.

Obtain APAP level, LFTs, PT/INR, electrolytes, Cr, and HCG (female). Note time relative to ingestion.

If intentional, add salicylate level and toxicology screen, consult psych.

<2 hours since ingestion — *Yes*: Give 50 g activated charcoal (PO, NG). *No*: proceed to criteria below.

Single ingestion? — *Yes*: If no extended-release APAP ingested, ingestion likely not significant. Observe. → If extended-release product suspected, repeat at least one additional level 4 hours after first. Administer NAC in interim if significant overdose is suspected.

No (to the right):

- Single ingestion >150 mg/kg (or 7.5 g) by history
- **OR** serum concentration will not be available by 8 hrs of ingestion
- **OR** APAP level >150 μg/mL (993 μmol/L) at 4 hours
- **OR** APAP level >75 μg/mL (497 μmol/L) at 8 hours
- **OR** APAP level >40 μg/mL (265 μmol/L) at 12 hours after ingestion
- **OR** lab evidence of hepatotoxicity

No (below): Repeated supratherapeutic ingestion (RSTI) → APAP >10 μg/mL OR elevated AST or ALT — *No*: Aggressive patient education. *Yes*: Administer NAC.

Yes: Administer NAC (best within 8 hours, may be effective up to 36 hours after ingestion). Do not delay for charcoal!

PO/NG: **72-hour PO regimen:** 140 mg/kg loading dose, followed by 70 mg/kg q4h for 17 additional doses. Repeat any dose vomited within 1 hour of admin.

IV preferred: **IV regimen:** 150 mg/kg in 200 mL D5W over 60 minutes, THEN 50 mg/kg in 500 mL D5W over 4 hours, THEN 100 mg/kg in 1 L D5W over 16 hours. Weight >100 kg: Use 100 kg dosing. Child <100 kg, decrease diluent volume per poison control.

Check APAP, ALT, AST, PT/INR every 4 hours.

APAP ≤10 μg/mL, ALT/AST have peaked are improving, INR ≤1.3 — *Yes*: Discontinue NAC. *No*:

Extended IV regimen: 150 mg/kg in 200 mL D5W over 60 minutes, THEN 50 mg/kg in 500 mL D5W over 4 hours, THEN 100 mg/kg in 1 L D5W over 16 hours, then 6.25 mg/kg/hr until INR <2.0 or death. Monitor for hypoglycemia. Vitamin K for coagulopathy. (FFP only if active bleeding)
Consider transport to transplant center.
Fulminant hepatic failure is rare.

King's College Transplant Criteria:
http://www.mdcalc.com/kings-college-criteria-for-acetaminophen-toxicity/

APAP, acetaminophen; NAC, N-acetylcysteine

Christine K. Jacobs, MD, FAAFP

Hodgman MJ, Garrard AR. A review of acetaminophen poisoning. *Crit Care Clin.* 2012;28(4):499–516.

ACID PHOSPHATASE ELEVATION

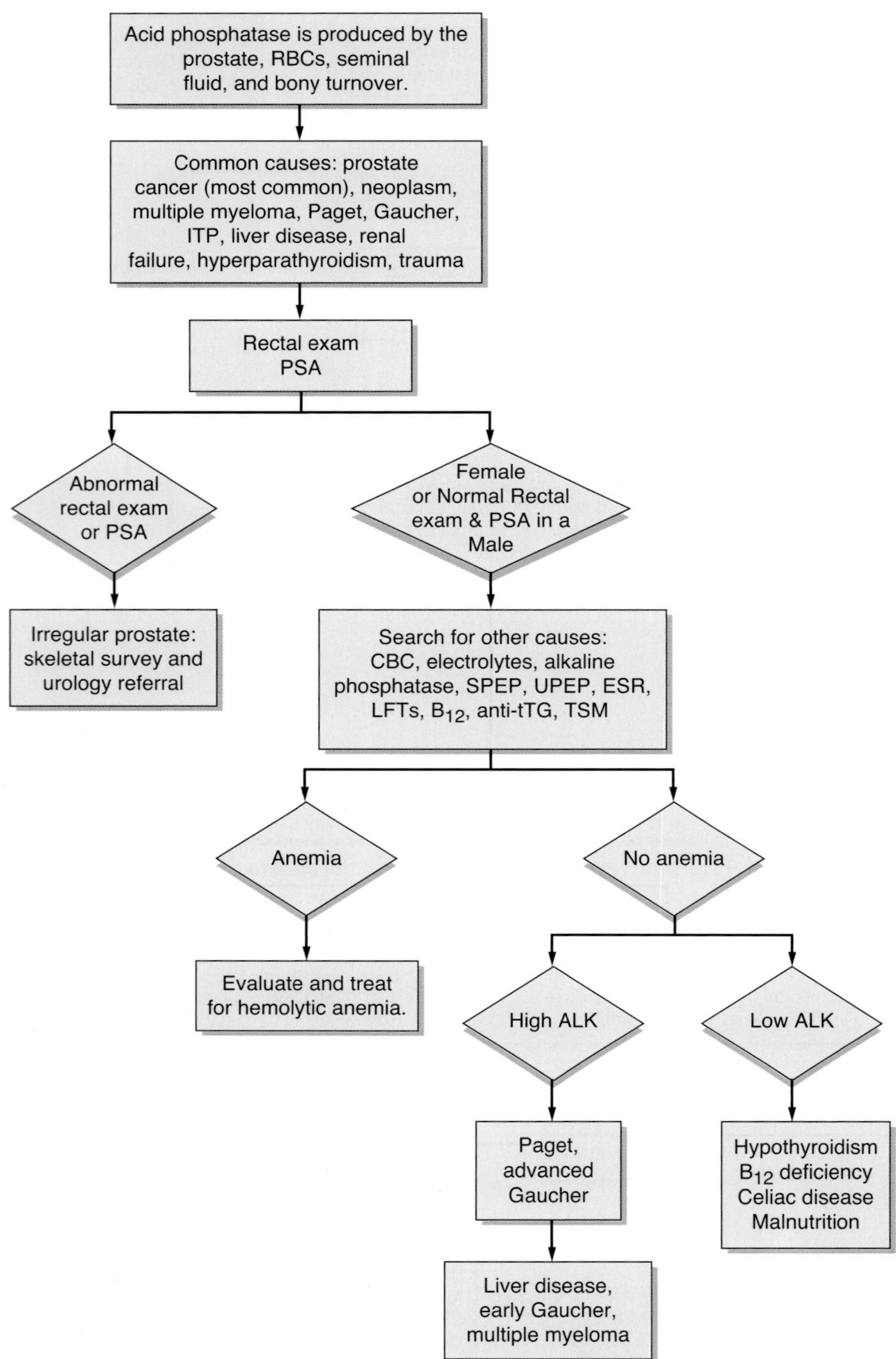

Laura Hagopian, MD, FAWM and L. Michael Snyder, MD

Scarnecchia L, Minisola S, Pacitti MT, et al. Clinical usefulness of serum tartrate-resistant acid phosphatase activity determination to evaluate bone turnover. *Scand J Clin Lab Invest.* 1991;51(6):517–524.

ACIDOSIS

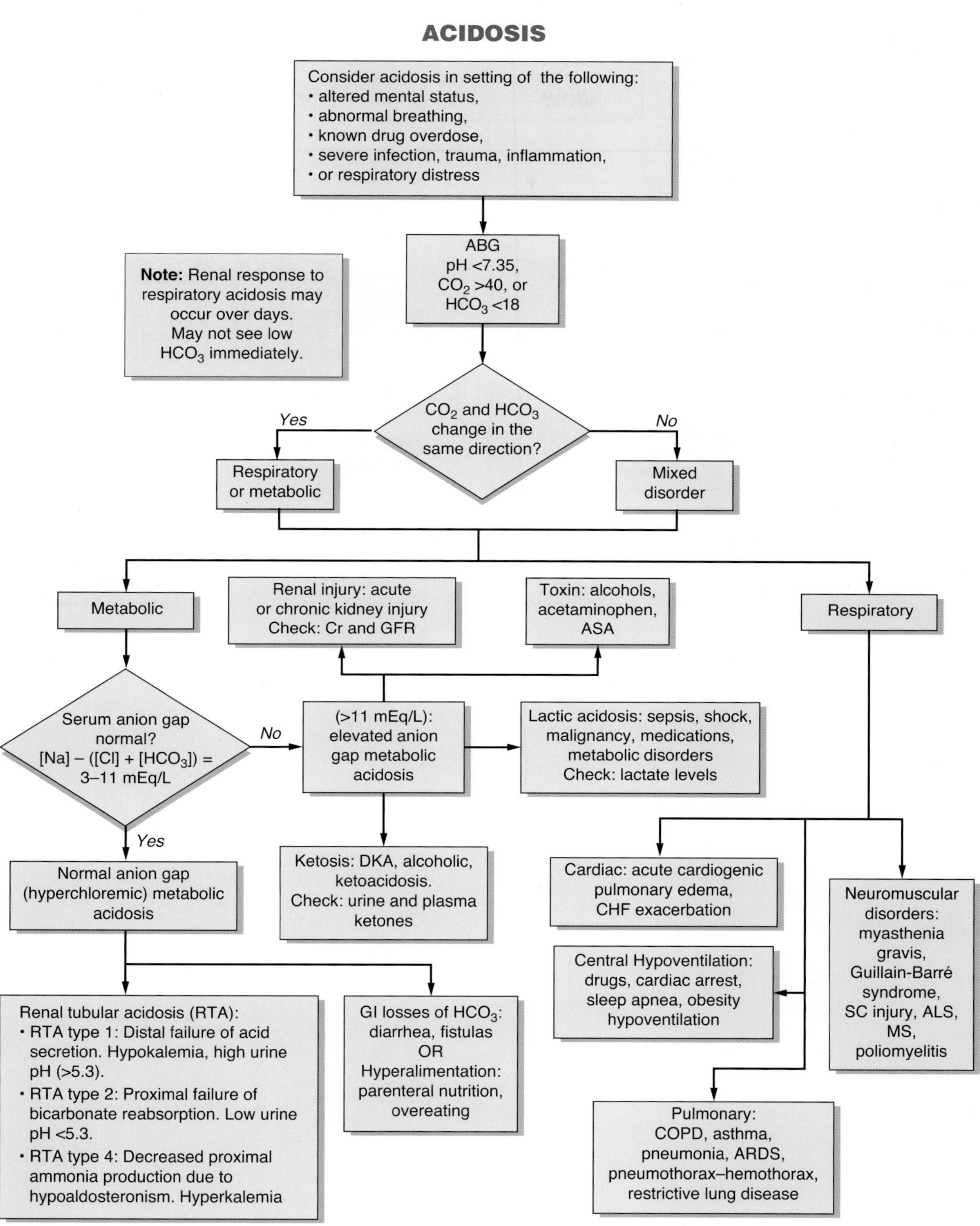
Consider acidosis in setting of the following:
• altered mental status,
• abnormal breathing,
• known drug overdose,
• severe infection, trauma, inflammation,
• or respiratory distress
ABG
pH <7.35,
CO_2 >40, or
HCO_3 <18
Note: Renal response to respiratory acidosis may occur over days. May not see low HCO_3 immediately.
CO_2 and HCO_3 change in the same direction?
Yes
No
Respiratory or metabolic
Mixed disorder
Metabolic
Renal injury: acute or chronic kidney injury Check: Cr and GFR
Toxin: alcohols, acetaminophen, ASA
Respiratory
Serum anion gap normal? [Na] – ([Cl] + [HCO_3]) = 3–11 mEq/L
No
(>11 mEq/L): elevated anion gap metabolic acidosis
Lactic acidosis: sepsis, shock, malignancy, medications, metabolic disorders Check: lactate levels
Yes
Normal anion gap (hyperchloremic) metabolic acidosis
Ketosis: DKA, alcoholic, ketoacidosis. Check: urine and plasma ketones
Cardiac: acute cardiogenic pulmonary edema, CHF exacerbation
Neuromuscular disorders: myasthenia gravis, Guillain-Barré syndrome, SC injury, ALS, MS, poliomyelitis
Central Hypoventilation: drugs, cardiac arrest, sleep apnea, obesity hypoventilation
Renal tubular acidosis (RTA):
• RTA type 1: Distal failure of acid secretion. Hypokalemia, high urine pH (>5.3).
• RTA type 2: Proximal failure of bicarbonate reabsorption. Low urine pH <5.3.
• RTA type 4: Decreased proximal ammonia production due to hypoaldosteronism. Hyperkalemia
GI losses of HCO_3: diarrhea, fistulas OR Hyperalimentation: parenteral nutrition, overeating
Pulmonary: COPD, asthma, pneumonia, ARDS, pneumothorax–hemothorax, restrictive lung disease

Katelin Engerer, MD and Robert J. Hyde, MD, MA

Kaplan LJ, Frangos S. Clinical review: acid-base abnormalities in the intensive care unit—part II. *Crit Care*. 2005;9:198–203.

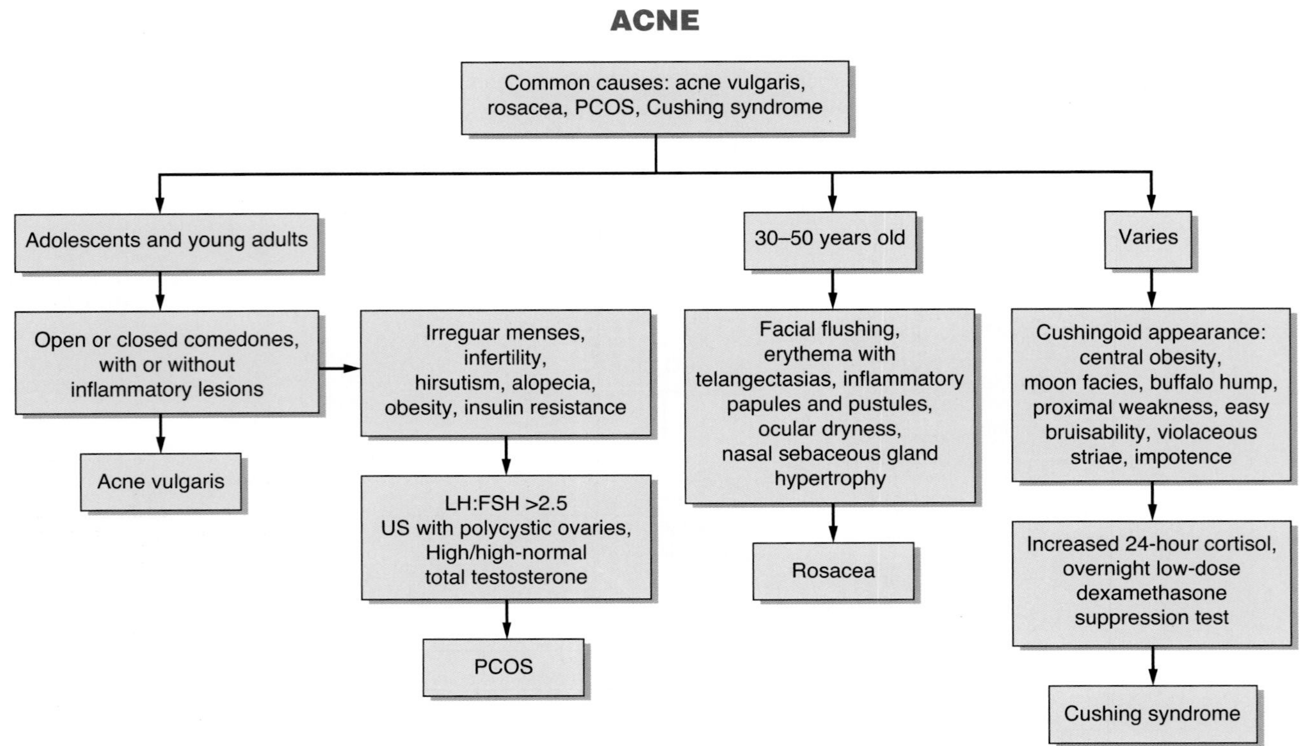

Elise Bognanno, MD and Frank J. Domino, MD

Titus S, Hodge J. Diagnosis and treatment of acne. *Am Fam Physician.* 2012;86(8):734–740.

ALCOHOL WITHDRAWAL, TREATMENT

History: Duration and quantity of alcohol intake, time since last drink, previous episodes of alcohol withdrawal, concurrent substance use, preexisting medical and psychiatric conditions, prior detoxification admissions, prior seizure activity, living situation, social supports, stressors, triggers, etc

Physical: VS (fever, tachycardia, tachypnea, hypertension). **CIWA** (see below), MSE, (arousal, orientation, hallucinations), HEENT (diaphoresis, scleral icterus), CV (arrhythmias, M/R/G), eval s/sx liver failure (asciles, varices, caput medusae, asterixis, palmar erythema), neuro (nystagmus, tremor, seizure activity).

Include assessment of conditions likely to *complicate, exacerbate,* or *precipitate* alcohol withdrawal: arrhythmias, CHF, CAD, dehydration, GI bleeding, infections, liver disease, pancreatitis, neurologic deficits.

Clinical Institute Withdrawal Assessment of Alcohol Scale (CIWA)
- Nausea and vomiting 0–7; (7-constant nausea, frequent dry heaves/vomiting)
- Tremor 0–7; (7-severe, even with arms not extended)
- Paroxysmal sweats 0–7; (7-drenching sweats)
- Anxiety 0–7; (7-acute panic state)
- Agitation 0–7; (7-constantly thrashing about or pacing)
- Tactile disturbances 0–7; (4–7 for hallucinations, 1–3 for pruritus or paresthesias)
- Auditory disturbances 0–7; (4–7 for hallucinations, 1–3 for increased sensitivity)
- Visual disturbances 0–7; (4–7 for hallucinations, 1–3 for increased sensitivity)
- Headache, fullness in head 0–7
- Orientation and clouding of sensorium 0–4:
  Cannot do serial additions or is uncertain about date
  Disoriented to date but within 2 calendar days
  Disoriented to date by >2 days
  Disoriented to place or person

Mild withdrawal; CIWA 0–7 (onset 5–8 hr after cessation or significant decrease in consumption): anxiety, restlessness, agitation, mild nausea, decreased appetite, sleep disturbance, facial sweating, mild tremulousness, fluctuating tachycardia and hypertension, possible mild cognitive impairment

Good candidate for outpatient therapy:
- Not pregnant
- No comorbid illnesses requiring hospitalization
- No history of seizures
- Not a suicide risk
- Low risk of delirium tremens
- No history of unsuccessful outpatient detoxification
- Good access to follow-up
- Tolerating oral medication

Treat as outpatient
- 100 mg thiamine PO daily, 1 g folic acid PO daily for 5 days
- Evaluate daily until symptoms decrease
- Assess BP, heart rate, and CIWA-Ar score at each follow-up visit
- Perform alcohol breath analysis randomly
- Facilitate entry into a long-term outpatient therapy program (e.g., Alcoholics Anonymous)
- Do not give Rx for benzodiazepine
- **If patient misses an appointment or resumes drinking, refer to addiction specialist or inpatient treatment facility.**

Outpatient therapy contraindicated: pregnant, history of seizures, or withdrawal seizures, chronic or acute comorbid illness requiring inpatient observation, lack of ability to follow-up
High risk of delirium tremens:
- Age >30 years
- Heavy drinking >8 years
- Drinking >100 g ethanol daily
- Random BAC >200 mg/dL
- Elevated MCV
- Cirrhosis

Moderate withdrawal; CIWA 8–14 (onset 24–72 hr after cessation): marked restlessness and agitation, moderate tremulousness with constant eye movement, diaphoresis, nausea, vomiting anorexia, diarrhea

- Admit to inpatient detoxification program
- Private room if possible
- Vital signs q4h
- CIWA q1-3h
- Institute seizure precautions
- IV fluids

Diazepam 20 mg PO q1–2h until CIWA<8, **OR** Diazepam 2–5 mg IV/min-maximum 10–20 mg q1h
If severe liver disease, severe asthma or respiratory failure, elderly, debilitated, or low serum albumin:
Lorazepam SL, Po 1–2 mg q2–4h PRN
Long-acting benzodiazepines (diazepam) have rapid onset of action and provide smooth treatment course with fewer breakthrough symptoms.
Short-acting (lorazepam) may have lower risk when there is concern about prolonged sedation, e.g., elderly patients or those with severe hepatic insufficiency

Severe withdrawal/delirium tremens; CIWA >15 (onset 72-96 hr after alcohol cessation): marked tremulousness, fever, drenching sweats, severe hypertension and tachycardia, delirium

- Admit to ICU for inpatient detoxification
- Vital signs q30 min
- CIWA q1h
- NPO, IV fluids
- Lateral decubitus position, restrain if necessary
- Glucose, Na, K, PO4, Mg replacement as needed

Diazepam 5–20 mg IV q10 min until calm, then q1h to maintain light somnolence for duration of delirium
If severe liver disease, severe asthma or respiratory failure, elderly, debilitated, or low serum albumin:
Lorazepam 1–4 mg q10 min until calm, then q1h to maintain light somnolence for duration of delirium

Labs: Tox screen/BAL to assess need for and timing of withdrawal regimen; electrolytes, phos, Mg with severe withdrawal [B and folate repleted regardless of levels], amylase/lipase if sx pancreatitis, PT, PTT if suspect liver failure; CBC if suspect infection
Imaging: Head CT if history of trauma or mental status changes out of range expected for degree of withdrawal. Seizure workup if no history of withdrawal seizures. Head CT and EEG if local neurologic signs or prolonged postictal state

Thiamine 100 mg IM/IV/PO q24h • 5 days; up to 1,000 mg/d if oculogyric crisis
- Sympatholytic adjunctive therapy: Atenolol 50–100 mg q24

Beta blockers and clonidine maybe used only in conjunction with benzodiazepines because they *may mask symptoms of alcohol withdrawal and artificially lower CIWA score* and reduce peripheral signs and symptoms of alcohol withdrawal but have not been shown to prevent or treat delirium or seizures.
- Phenothiazines for hallucinosis: Haloperidol 2–5 mg IM/PO q1–4h max 5 mg/d used only in conjunction with benzodiazepines. May lower seizure threshold; use with extreme caution.

Discharge planning
- CIWA scores <8–10 for 24 hr
- Begin 1:1 or group therapy
- Discharge to treatment center, day program, home
- Facilitate entry into Alcoholics Anonymous
- Do not discharge with benzodiazepine prescription
- Nutrition/social work consult

Paul A. Tate, Jr., MD and Paul Savel, MD

Muncie HL, Yasinian Y, Oge L. Outpatient management of alcohol withdrawal syndrome. *Am Fam Physician*. 2013;88(9):589–595.

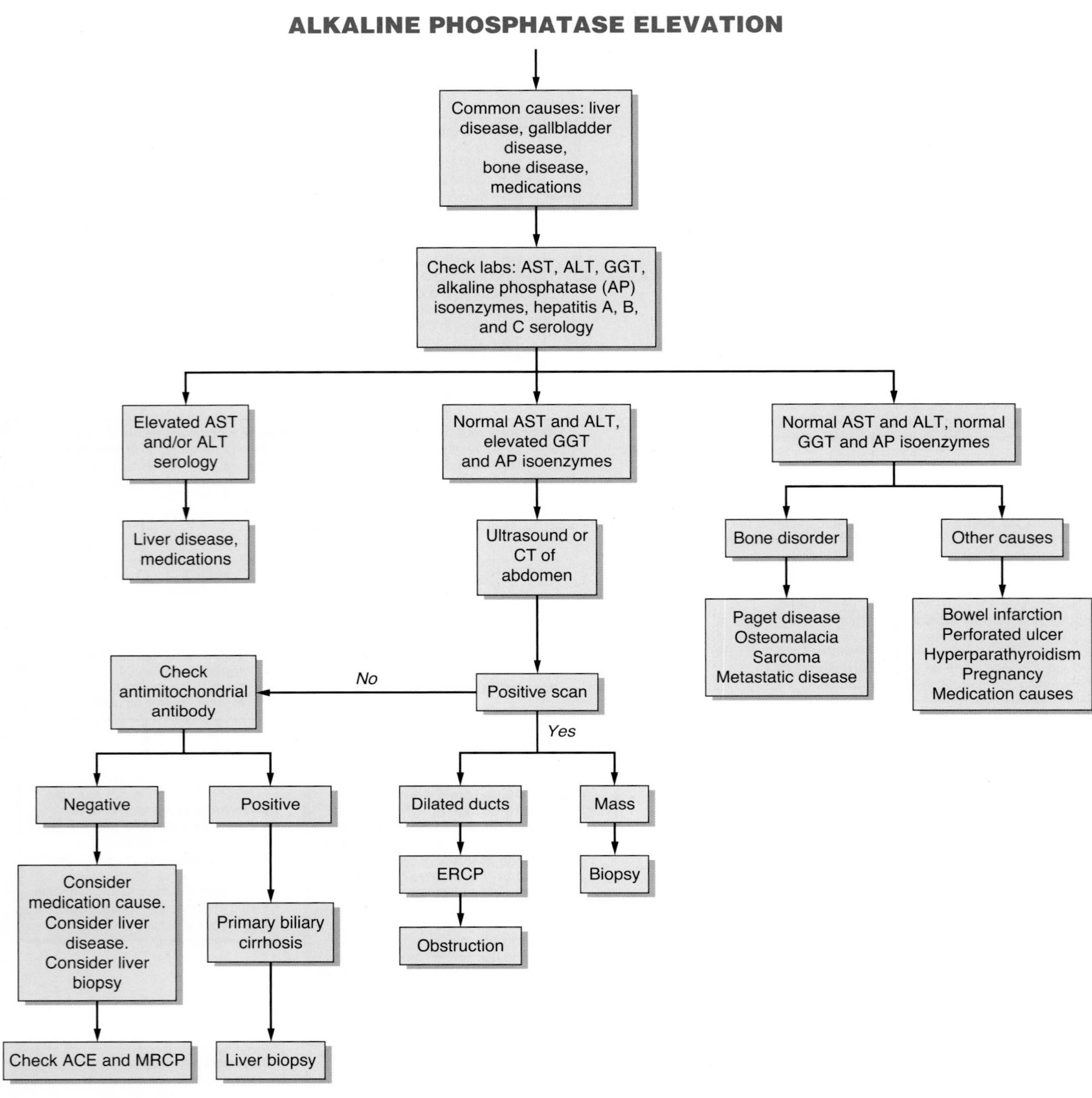

Reem Hadi, MD and Fozia Akhtar Ali, MD

Siddique A, Kowdley KV. Approach to a patient with elevated serum alkaline phosphatase. *Clin Liver Dis*. 2012;16(2):199–229.

AMENORRHEA, SECONDARY

Absence of menses >3 months in woman with regular periods
OR
Absence of menses >6 months in a woman with irregular periods

→ Common causes: pregnancy, ectopic pregnancy, anorexia/starvation, infection, PCOS, ovarian failure (menopause), pituitary adenoma, hypothyroidism

→ Urine hCG

- (+) → Intrauterine pregnancy, ectopic pregnancy
- (−) → Vaginal/bimanual exam; FSH, LH, TSH, prolactin, BMP
  - Stress; Weight loss; Extreme exercise → Eating disorders
  - Acne, hirsutism, BMI >30, deepening of voice, LH/FSH ratio >2 → Check labs: DHEA-S, testosterone (increased) → PCOS
  - ↑ FSH; ↑ LH → Hot flashes; Sleep difficulty; Decreased libido → Menopause
  - Medications: Oral contraceptives; Metoclopramide; Antipsychotics
  - Galactorrhea → Increased serum prolactin → Pituitary MRI → Pituitary adenoma
  - Elevated TSH → Hypothyroidism
  - ↑ Creatinine → Renal disease
  - Normal labs → GYN exam, transvaginal US
    - (−) → Obtain the following: cortisol, serum testosterone → Cushing disease; Androgen tumor
    - (+) → Asherman syndrome; Cervical stenosis

Maria Montanez, MD and Fozia Akhtar Ali, MD

Master-Hunter T, Heiman DL. Amenorrhea: evaluation and treatment. *Am Fam Physician*. 2006;73(8):1374–1382.

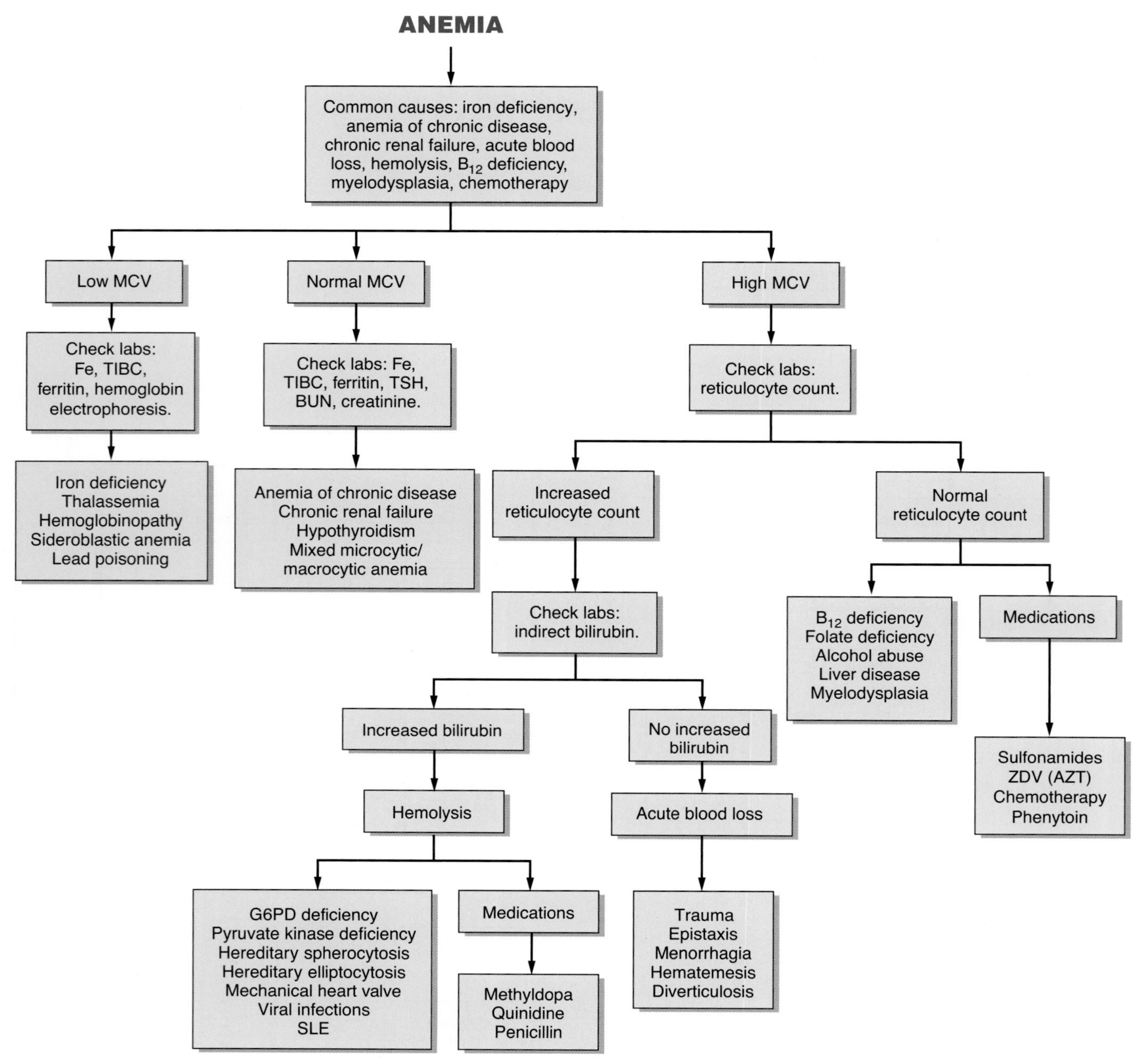
ANEMIA
Common causes: iron deficiency, anemia of chronic disease, chronic renal failure, acute blood loss, hemolysis, B12 deficiency, myelodysplasia, chemotherapy
Low MCV
Normal MCV
High MCV
Check labs: Fe, TIBC, ferritin, hemoglobin electrophoresis.
Check labs: Fe, TIBC, ferritin, TSH, BUN, creatinine.
Check labs: reticulocyte count.
Iron deficiency
Thalassemia
Hemoglobinopathy
Sideroblastic anemia
Lead poisoning
Anemia of chronic disease
Chronic renal failure
Hypothyroidism
Mixed microcytic/ macrocytic anemia
Increased reticulocyte count
Normal reticulocyte count
Check labs: indirect bilirubin.
B12 deficiency
Folate deficiency
Alcohol abuse
Liver disease
Myelodysplasia
Medications
Increased bilirubin
No increased bilirubin
Sulfonamides
ZDV (AZT)
Chemotherapy
Phenytoin
Hemolysis
Acute blood loss
G6PD deficiency
Pyruvate kinase deficiency
Hereditary spherocytosis
Hereditary elliptocytosis
Mechanical heart valve
Viral infections
SLE
Medications
Methyldopa
Quinidine
Penicillin
Trauma
Epistaxis
Menorrhagia
Hematemesis
Diverticulosis

Robert A. Baldor, MD, FAAFP and Alan M. Ehrlich, MD

Smith DL. Anemia in the elderly. *Am Fam Physician*. 2000;62(7):1565–1572.

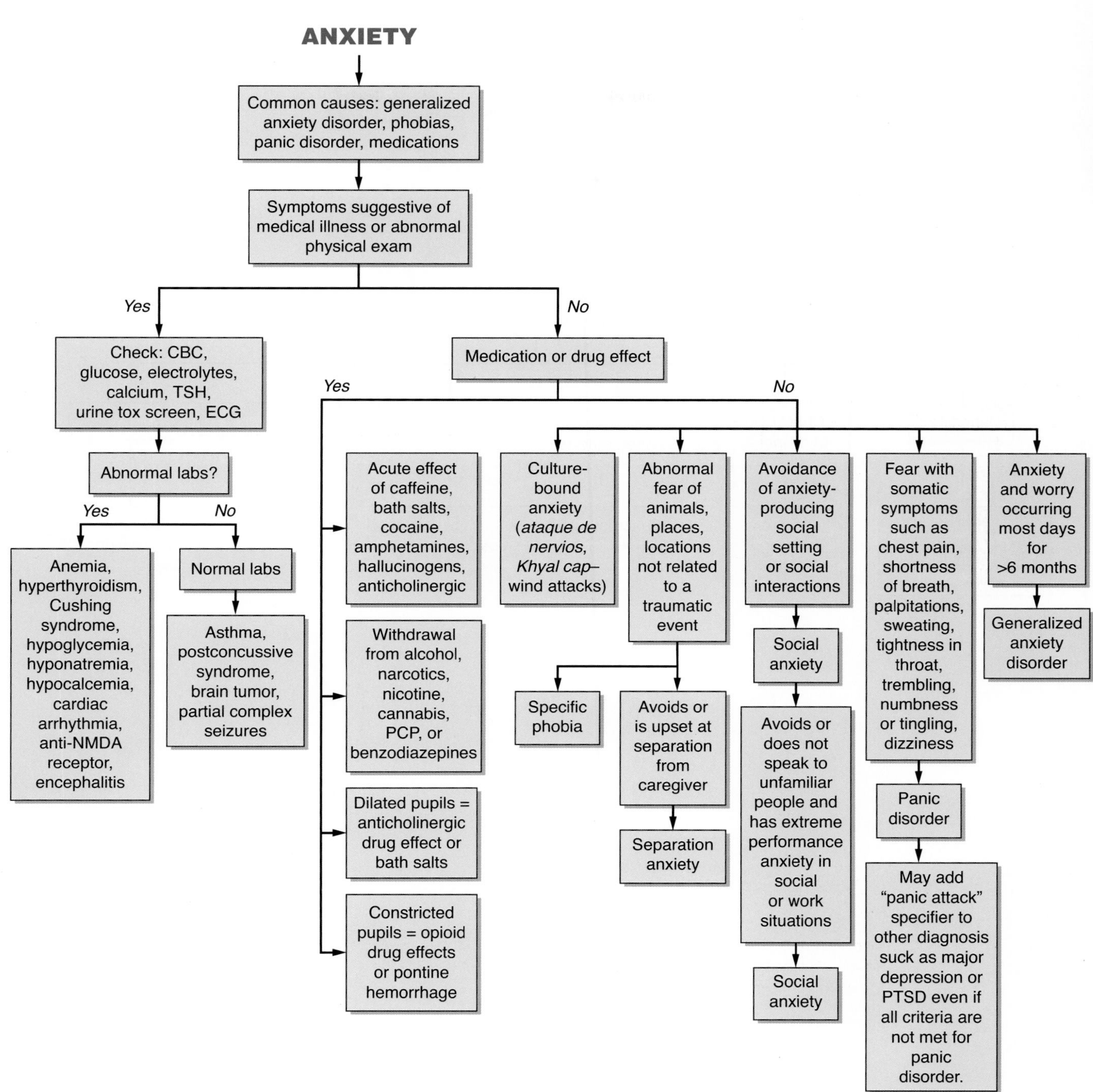

Bettina Bernstein, DO

Bienvenu OJ, Wuyek LA, Stein MB. Anxiety disorders diagnosis: some history and controversies. *Curr Top Behav Neurosci.* 2010;2:3–19.

AST ELEVATION

Common causes: hemolysis, liver disease, myocardial infarction, CHF, acute renal failure, biliary obstruction, pancreatitis, muscle disorders, medications

↓

Check: LFTs, consider CBC, BUN, creatinine, hepatitis serologies, CPK, amylase, CXR, ultrasound/CT of abdomen.

↓

- Jaundice → Liver disease, Biliary obstruction, Hemolysis, Viral hepatitis
- Chest pain or dyspnea → Myocardial infarction, CHF
- Abdominal pain, Elevated amylase → Pancreatitis
- Edema → CHF, Acute renal failure
- Muscle disorder or injury
- Liver toxicity → Alcohol, Medications

Robert A. Baldor, MD, FAAFP and Alan M. Ehrlich, MD

Giboney PT. Mildly elevated liver transaminase levels in the asymptomatic patient. *Am Fam Physician.* 2005;71(6):1105–1110.

ASTHMA EXACERBATION, PEDIATRIC ACUTE

Initial evaluation: brief history of present illness, physical exam
Asthma history: emergency department visits, hospital and ICU admissions, home medications, frequency of oral steroid use, history of intubation, rapidly progressive episodes, food allergy
Physical exam: auscultation, use of accessory muscles, ability to speak, heart rate, oxygen saturation

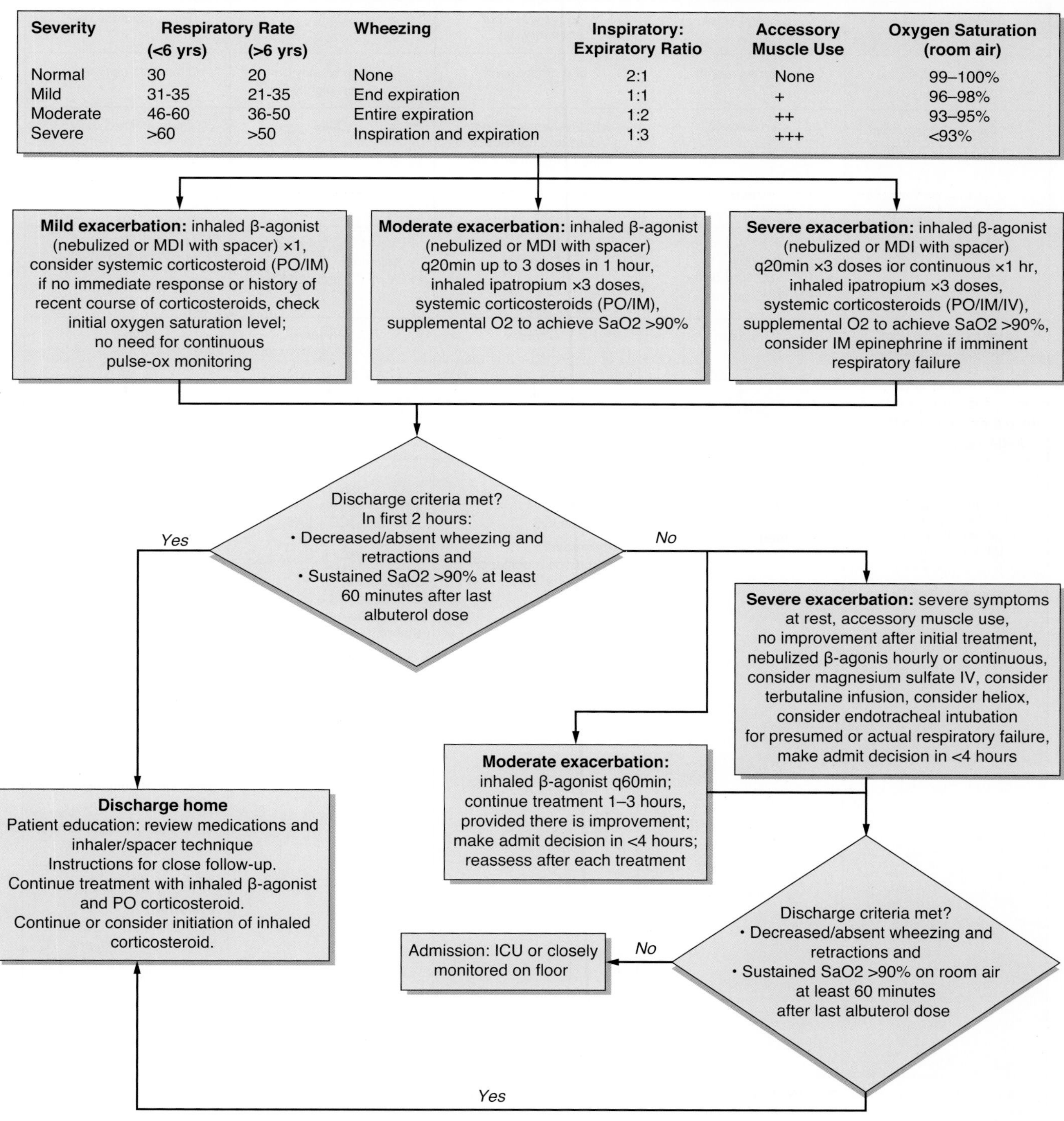

Severity	Respiratory Rate (<6 yrs)	Respiratory Rate (>6 yrs)	Wheezing	Inspiratory: Expiratory Ratio	Accessory Muscle Use	Oxygen Saturation (room air)
Normal	30	20	None	2:1	None	99–100%
Mild	31-35	21-35	End expiration	1:1	+	96–98%
Moderate	46-60	36-50	Entire expiration	1:2	++	93–95%
Severe	>60	>50	Inspiration and expiration	1:3	+++	<93%

Mild exacerbation: inhaled β-agonist (nebulized or MDI with spacer) ×1, consider systemic corticosteroid (PO/IM) if no immediate response or history of recent course of corticosteroids, check initial oxygen saturation level; no need for continuous pulse-ox monitoring
Moderate exacerbation: inhaled β-agonist (nebulized or MDI with spacer) q20min up to 3 doses in 1 hour, inhaled ipatropium ×3 doses, systemic corticosteroids (PO/IM), supplemental O2 to achieve SaO2 >90%
Severe exacerbation: inhaled β-agonist (nebulized or MDI with spacer) q20min ×3 doses ior continuous ×1 hr, inhaled ipatropium ×3 doses, systemic corticosteroids (PO/IM/IV), supplemental O2 to achieve SaO2 >90%, consider IM epinephrine if imminent respiratory failure
Discharge criteria met? In first 2 hours: • Decreased/absent wheezing and retractions and • Sustained SaO2 >90% at least 60 minutes after last albuterol dose
Yes
No
Severe exacerbation: severe symptoms at rest, accessory muscle use, no improvement after initial treatment, nebulized β-agonis hourly or continuous, consider magnesium sulfate IV, consider terbutaline infusion, consider heliox, consider endotracheal intubation for presumed or actual respiratory failure, make admit decision in <4 hours
Moderate exacerbation: inhaled β-agonist q60min; continue treatment 1–3 hours, provided there is improvement; make admit decision in <4 hours; reassess after each treatment
Discharge home Patient education: review medications and inhaler/spacer technique Instructions for close follow-up. Continue treatment with inhaled β-agonist and PO corticosteroid. Continue or consider initiation of inhaled corticosteroid.
Discharge criteria met? • Decreased/absent wheezing and retractions and • Sustained SaO2 >90% on room air at least 60 minutes after last albuterol dose
No
Admission: ICU or closely monitored on floor
Yes

Catherine A. James, MD

National Asthma Education and Prevention Program. Expert panel report 3 (EPR-3): guidelines for the diagnosis and management of asthma-summary report 2007. *J Allergy Clin Immunol.* 2007;120(5)(Suppl):S94–S138.

ASTHMA, INITIAL TREATMENT

Management of chronic asthma
Classification of asthma severity in youth ≥12 years of age and adults

Components of severety	Intermittent	Mild persistent	Moderate persistent	Severe persistent
Daytime symptoms	≤2 days/week	>2 days/week but not every day	Daily	Throughout the day
Nighttime awakenings	≤2 times/month	3 or 4 times/month	>1 time weekly but not nightly	Often 7 times weekly
Short-acting β_2-agonist use for symptom control	≤2 days/week	>2 days/week but not daily and not more than 1 time on any day	Daily	Several times daily
Interference with normal activity	None	Minor limitation	Some limitation	Extremely limited
Lung function	• Normal FEV_1 between exacerbations • FEV_1 >80% predicted • FEV_1/FVC normal	• FEV_1 >80% predicted • FEV_1/FVC normal	• FEV_1 >60%, but <80% predicted • FEV_1/FVC reduced 5%	FEV_1 <60% Predicted; FEV_1/FVC reduced >5%
Astma exacerbations requiring oral steroids	0–1 year	≥2/year	≥2/year	≥2/year

Recommended step for initiating treatment	Step 1	Step 2	Step 3	Step 4, 5, or 6
Preferred and alternative pharmacotherapy based on step	***Preferred:*** Short-acting β_2-agonist as needed	***Preferred:*** Low-dose ICS ***Alternative:*** Leukotriene modifier or theophylline	***Preferred:*** Low-dose ICS + LABA or medium-dose ICS ***Alternative:*** Low-dose ICS + leukotriene modifier, theophylline or zileuton	**Step 4** ***Preferred:*** Medium-dose ICS + LABA ***Alternative:*** Medium-dose ICS + leukotriene modifier, theophylline or zileuton Identify triggers (cold air, dust, allergic exposures/pets), and control exposures. **Step 5** ***Preferred:*** High-dose ICS + LABA, and consider omalizumab for patients with allergies Identify triggers, and control exposures. **Step 6** ***Preferred:*** High-dose ICS + LABA + oral corticosteroid, and consider omalizumab for patients with allergies Identify patients at risk for reactions to aspirin and NSAIDs, and avoid exposure.
At each step discuss patient education, environmental control, and management of comorbidities.				

Michael C. Barros, PharmD, BCPS, BCACP, Colleen M. Prinzivalli, PharmD, BCPS, CGP, and Alia Christy, MD, MS

Elward KS, Pollart SM. Medical therapy for asthma: updates from the NAEP Pguidelines. *Am Fam Physician.* 2010;82(10):1242–1251.

ASTHMA, MAINTENANCE

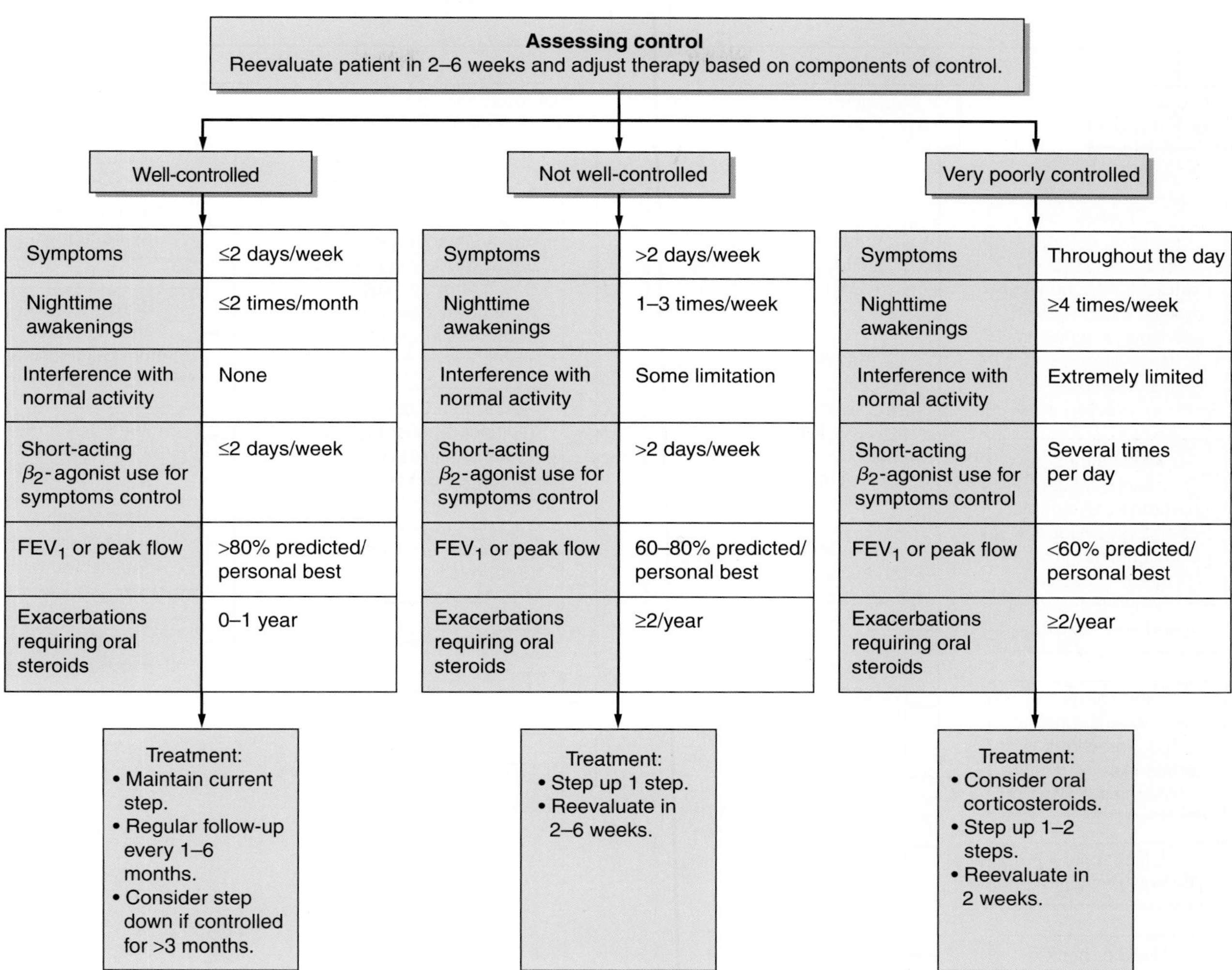

FEV_1, forced expiratory volume in 1 second

Michael C. Barros, PharmD, BCPS, BCACP, Colleen M. Prinzivalli, PharmD, BCPS, CGP, and Alia Christy, MD, MS

Elward KS, Pollart SM. Medical therapy for asthma: updates from the NAEPP guidelines. *Am Fam Physician.* 2010;82:1242–1251.

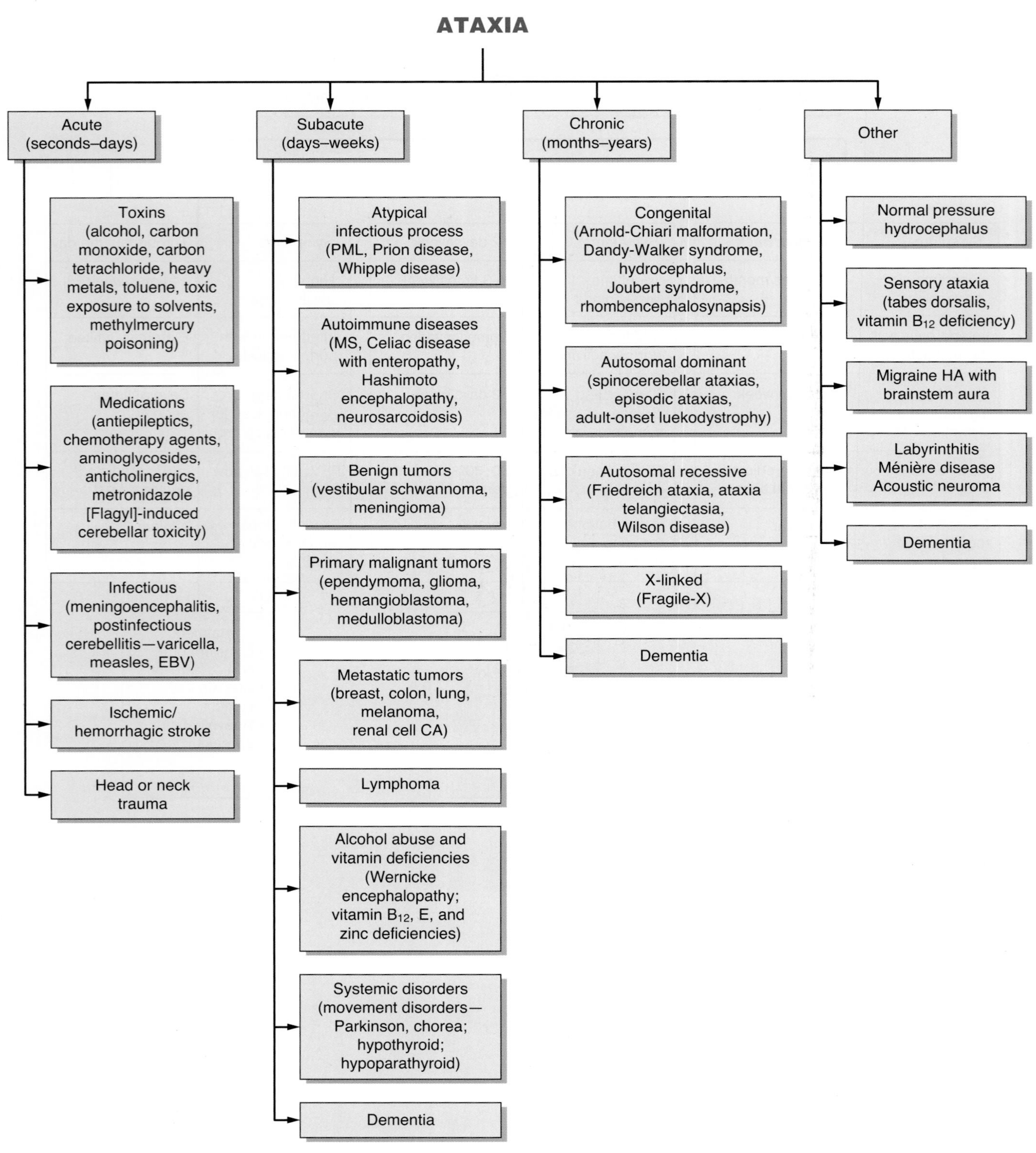

Fozia Akhtar Ali, MD and Teny Anna Philip, MD

Brunberg JA; Expert Panel on Neurologic Imaging. Ataxia. *AJNR Am J Neuroradiol.* 2008;29(7):1420–1422.

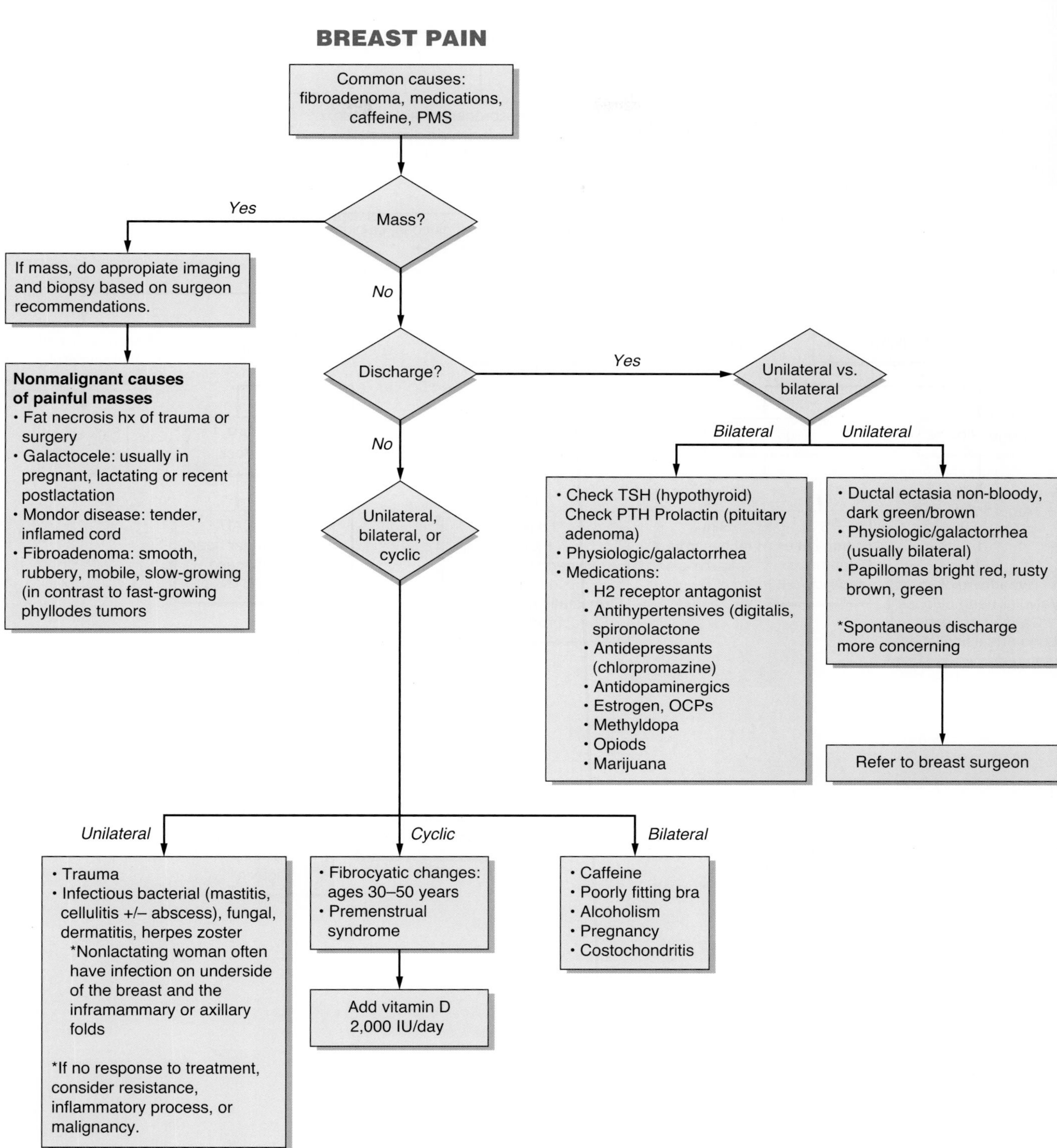
BREAST PAIN
Common causes: fibroadenoma, medications, caffeine, PMS
Mass?
Yes
If mass, do appropiate imaging and biopsy based on surgeon recommendations.
Nonmalignant causes of painful masses
• Fat necrosis hx of trauma or surgery
• Galactocele: usually in pregnant, lactating or recent postlactation
• Mondor disease: tender, inflamed cord
• Fibroadenoma: smooth, rubbery, mobile, slow-growing (in contrast to fast-growing phyllodes tumors
No
Discharge?
Yes
Unilateral vs. bilateral
Bilateral
Unilateral
• Check TSH (hypothyroid) Check PTH Prolactin (pituitary adenoma)
• Physiologic/galactorrhea
• Medications:
• H2 receptor antagonist
• Antihypertensives (digitalis, spironolactone
• Antidepressants (chlorpromazine)
• Antidopaminergics
• Estrogen, OCPs
• Methyldopa
• Opiods
• Marijuana
• Ductal ectasia non-bloody, dark green/brown
• Physiologic/galactorrhea (usually bilateral)
• Papillomas bright red, rusty brown, green
*Spontaneous discharge more concerning
Refer to breast surgeon
No
Unilateral, bilateral, or cyclic
Unilateral
Cyclic
Bilateral
• Trauma
• Infectious bacterial (mastitis, cellulitis +/– abscess), fungal, dermatitis, herpes zoster
*Nonlactating woman often have infection on underside of the breast and the inframammary or axillary folds
*If no response to treatment, consider resistance, inflammatory process, or malignancy.
• Fibrocyatic changes: ages 30–50 years
• Premenstrual syndrome
Add vitamin D 2,000 IU/day
• Caffeine
• Poorly fitting bra
• Alcoholism
• Pregnancy
• Costochondritis

Mohamad Masoumy, MD, MS, Varun Kumar Bhalla, MD, and Edward James Kruse, DO

Salzman B, Fleegle S, Tully AS. Common breast problems. *Am Fam Physician.* 2012;86(4):343–349.

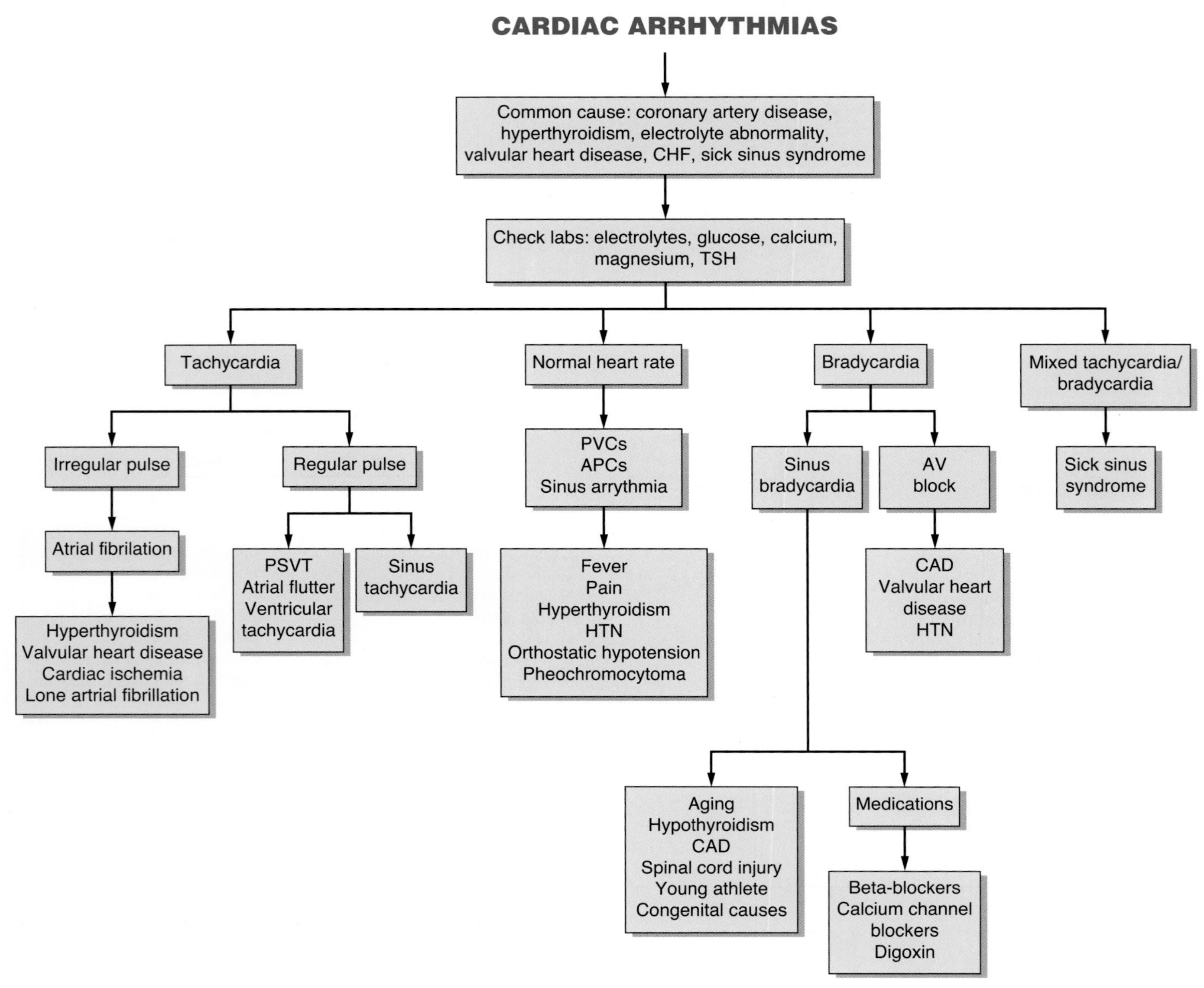

Amaninderapal S. Ghotra, MD, Suma Chennubhotla, MD, and Kelly McCants, MD

Link MS. Clinical practice. Evaluation and initial treatment of supraventricular tachycardia. *N Engl J Med.* 2012;367:1438–1448.

CERVICAL HYPEREXTENSION INJURY

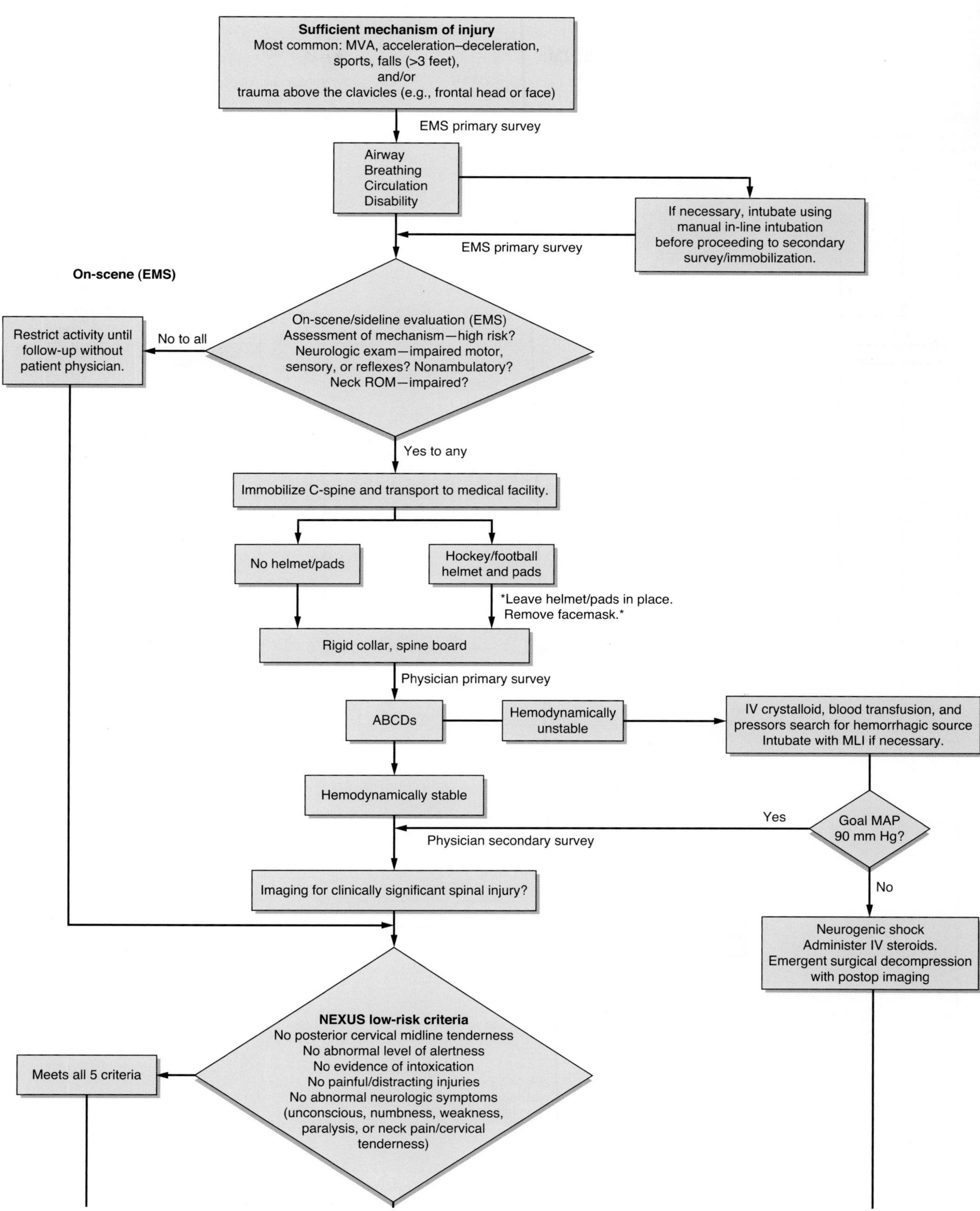

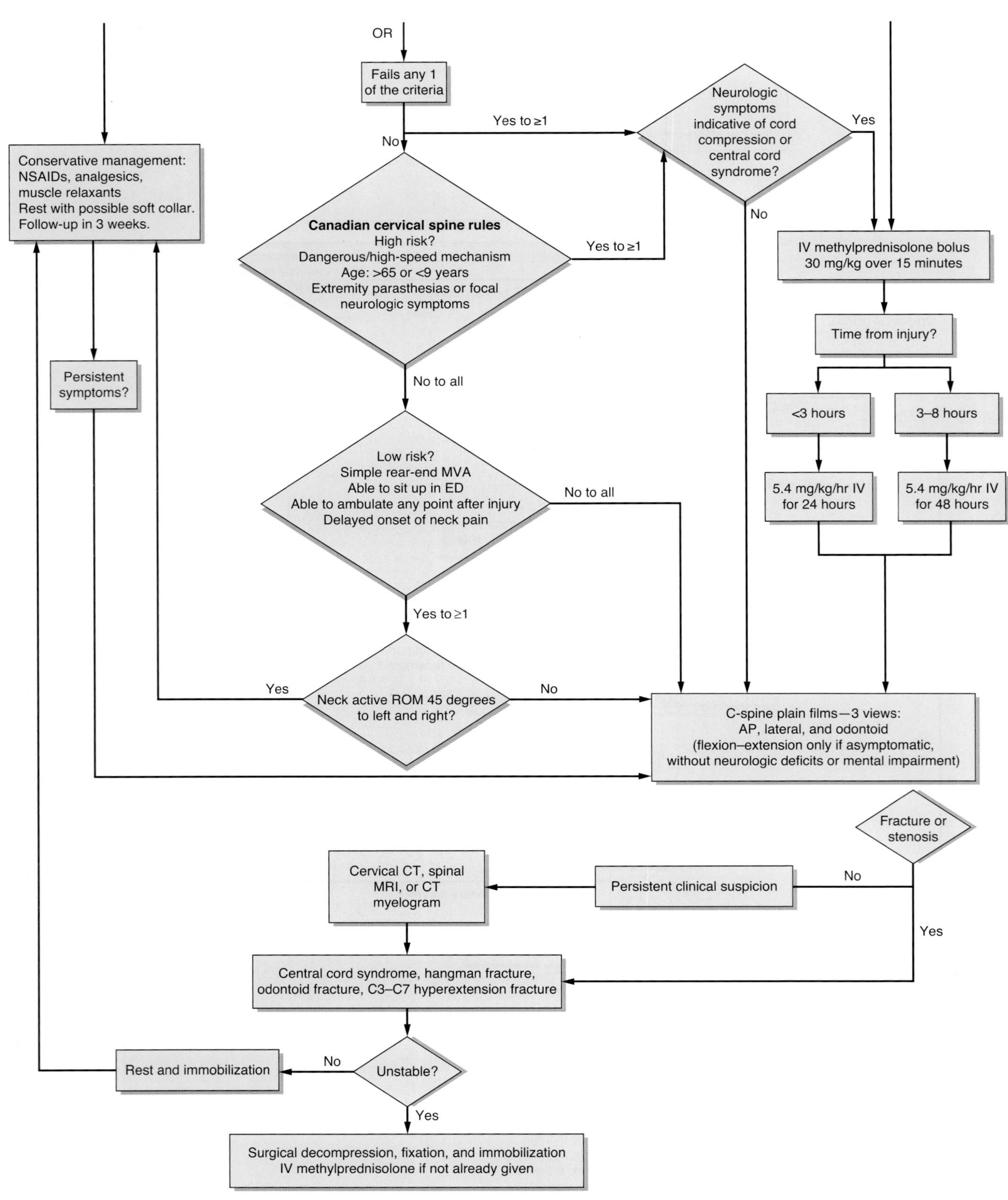

Bobby Peters, MD, FAAEM

Pimentel L, Diegelmann L. Evaluation and management of acute cervical spine trauma. *Emerg Med Clin North Am*. 2010;28(4):719–738.

CHEST PAIN/ACUTE CORONARY SYNDROME

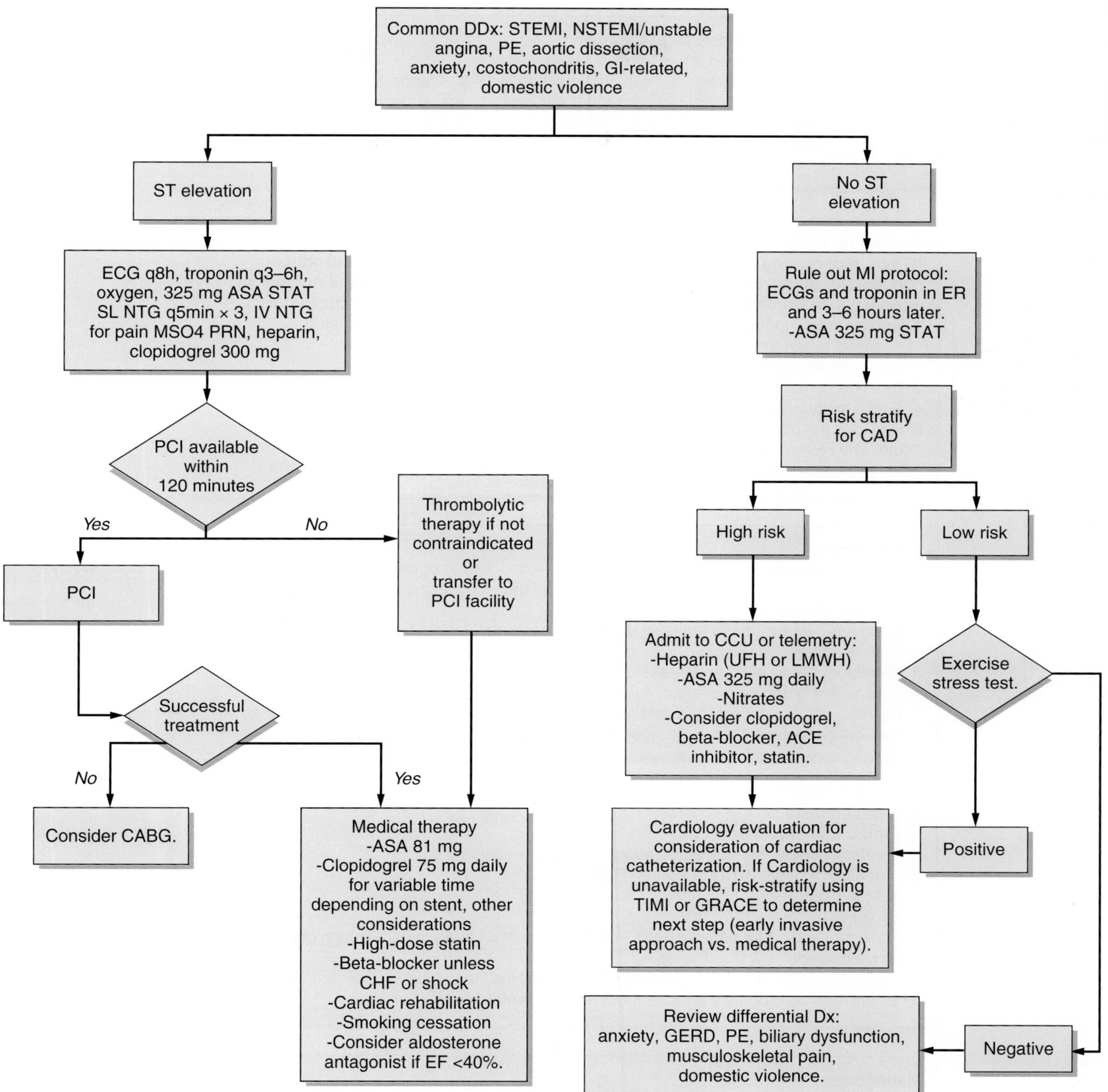

Jeremy Golding, MD, FAAFP

Amsterdam EA, Wenger NK, Brindis RG, et al. 2014 AHA/ACC guideline for the management of patients with non–ST-elevation acute coronary syndromes: executive summary: a report of the American College of Cardiology/American Heart Association Task Force on Practice Guidelines. *Circulation*. 2014;130:2354–2394.

CHILD ABUSE

Be suspicious for nonaccidental trauma if
- A vague or no explanation for an injury
- An important detail of caregiver's explanation changes significantly.
- Caregiver's or patient's story is inconsistent with pattern, age, or severity of injury.
- Different witnesses provide different explanations for the injury.
- Explanation is inconsistent with child's physical and/or developmental capabilities.
- Caregiver(s) refuse to permit child to be interviewed alone.

↓

Medical history
(When interviewing children, ask open-ended questions that do not introduce concepts of abusive acts/abuser. Avoid leading questions and limit the number of interviews. Document direct quotes of child and caretaker as part of the history.)
1. Routine past medical history (trauma, congenital/chronic illnesses, prematurity, neonatal abstinence syndrome, developmental delay)
2. Family history (bleeding, bone, metabolic, genetic)
3. Developmental history
4. Social history (substance abuse, job loss, new partner, other stressors)
5. Previous hospitalizations/ED visits for injury

*Note: The history taking is the most important part of the child abuse exam—documenting who, what, when, where, and how the stories differ between caregivers and patient.

↓

Physical exam
1. General assessment—child's alertness, demeanor, degree of pain, growth chart parameters, evidence of neglect (severe dental caries, diaper dermatitis, neglected wound care, cachexia)
2. Complete head-to-toe exam (skin: bruises, lacerations, burns, bites) noting patterned injuries, shape, and depth.
3. Consider photographs and/or sketches of physical signs.
4. Complete a neurologic exam.
5. If sexual abuse suspected, a detailed genital exam should be performed by a trained medical professional within 72 hours of suspected incident.

↓

Diagnostic tests
(As indicated based on exam)
1. "Skeletal survey" for suspected abuse in children <2 years old
2. Hematologic tests (CBC, platelets, PT/PTT/INR)
3. Retinal exam
4. CT (head)
5. Additional testing for osteogenesis imperfecta or other bone mineralization disorders as suspected

*Note: Obtain neuroimaging in children if nonaccidental head injury suspected, and consider in all children <6 months with suspected nonaccidental trauma.

↓

Management
1. Referral to investigative agencies/child-protection agencies according to state-specific mandated reporting laws (800-442-4453). Health care providers are mandated to report all suspected abuse/neglect. State reporting statutes and other resources are available from the Child Welfare Information Gateway (www.childwelfare.gov).
2. Referral to appropriate medical providers (such as pediatric trauma center)
3. Medicolegal documentation
4. Safety plan in place before discharge and appropriate follow-up plan

Jennifer Bailey, DO, FAAP and Kathleen J. Martin, MD FAAP

Kellogg N. Evaluation of suspected child physical abuse. *Pediatrics.* 2007;119(6):1232–1241. doi:10.1542/peds.2007-0883

CHRONIC JOINT PAIN AND STIFFNESS

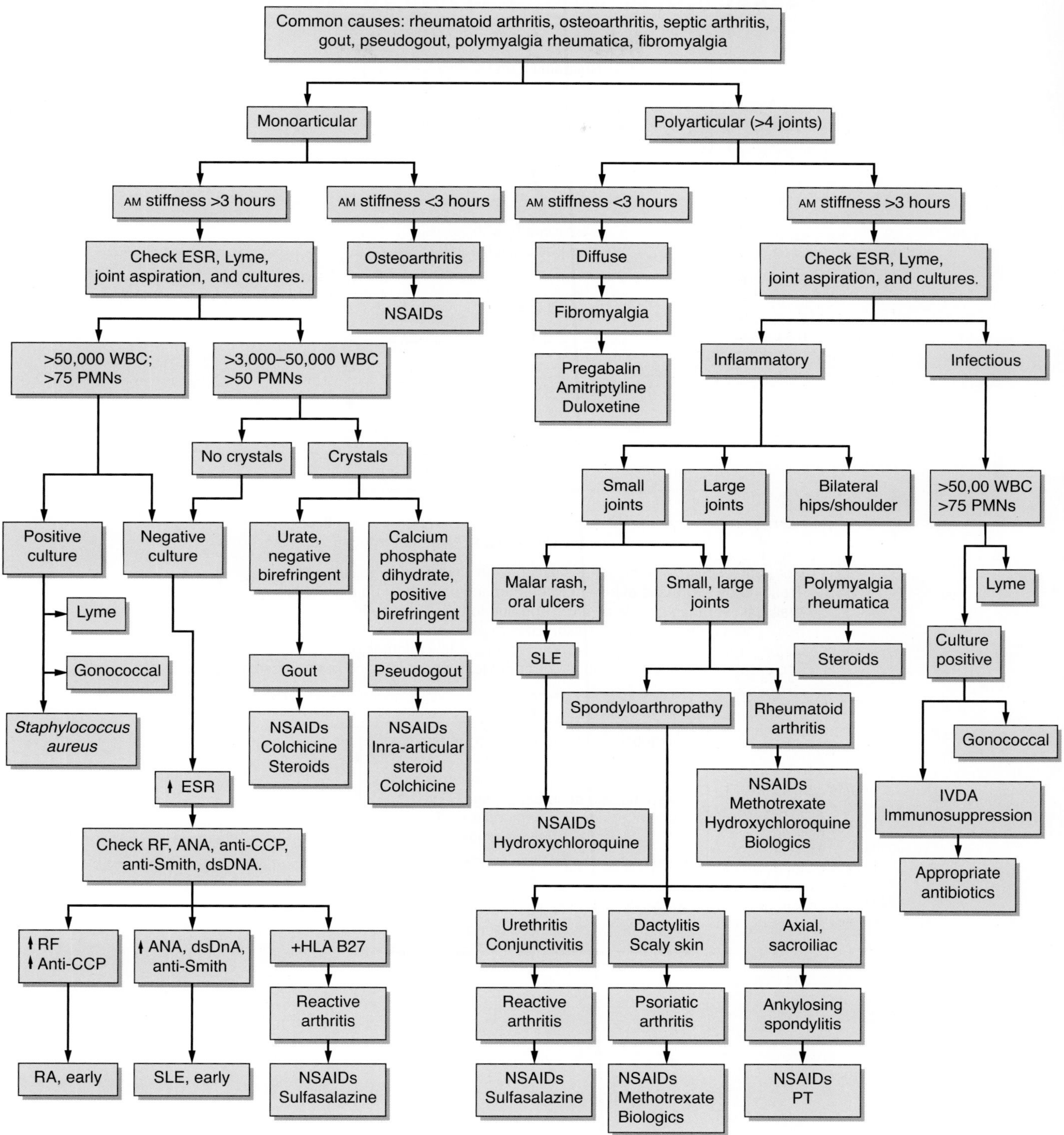

Kimberly Sikule, MD and J. Herbert Stevenson, MD

Mies Richie A, Francis ML. Diagnostic approach to polyarticular joint pain. *Am Fam Physician*. 2003;68(6):1151–1160.

CHRONIC OBSTRUCTIVE PULMONARY DISEASE (COPD), DIAGNOSIS AND TREATMENT

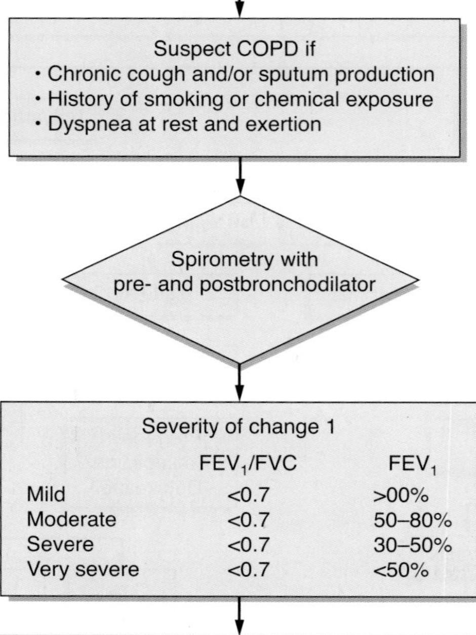

	FEV_1/FVC	FEV_1
Mild	<0.7	>00%
Moderate	<0.7	50–80%
Severe	<0.7	30–50%
Very severe	<0.7	<50%

Functional Dyspnea Scale

0	Not troubled with breathlessness except with strenuous exercise
1	Troubled by shortness of breath when hurrying or walking up a slight hill
2	Walks slower than people of same age due to breathlessness or has to stop for breath when walking at own pace on the level
3	Stops for breath after walking ~100 m or after a few minutes on the level
4	Too breathless to leave the house or breathless when dressing or undressing

Diagnosis confirmed, initiate preventative measures:
Influenza vaccine (yearly), pneumococcal vaccine one dose before age 65 years, one after age 65 years, at least 5 years after previous dose

Aggressive smoking cessation counseling if actively smoking

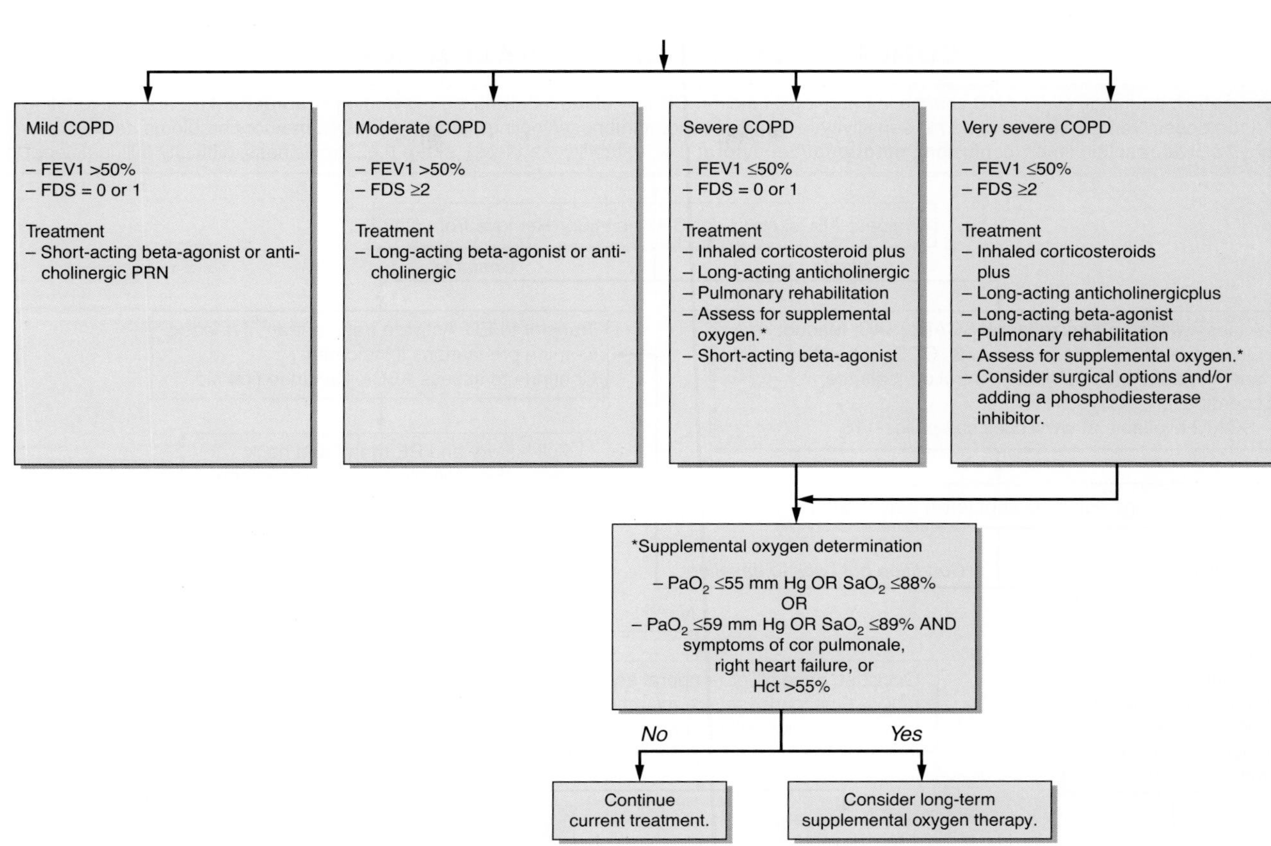
Mild COPD
– FEV1 >50%
– FDS = 0 or 1
Treatment
– Short-acting beta-agonist or anticholinergic PRN
Moderate COPD
– FEV1 >50%
– FDS ≥2
Treatment
– Long-acting beta-agonist or anticholinergic
Severe COPD
– FEV1 ≤50%
– FDS = 0 or 1
Treatment
– Inhaled corticosteroid plus
– Long-acting anticholinergic
– Pulmonary rehabilitation
– Assess for supplemental oxygen.*
– Short-acting beta-agonist
Very severe COPD
– FEV1 ≤50%
– FDS ≥2
Treatment
– Inhaled corticosteroids plus
– Long-acting anticholinergicplus
– Long-acting beta-agonist
– Pulmonary rehabilitation
– Assess for supplemental oxygen.*
– Consider surgical options and/or adding a phosphodiesterase inhibitor.
*Supplemental oxygen determination
– PaO_2 ≤55 mm Hg OR SaO_2 ≤88%
OR
– PaO_2 ≤59 mm Hg OR SaO_2 ≤89% AND symptoms of cor pulmonale, right heart failure, or Hct >55%
No
Yes
Continue current treatment.
Consider long-term supplemental oxygen therapy.

Scott E. Kopec, MD

Global Initiative for Chronic Obstructive Lung Disease. Global strategy for the diagnosis, management and prevention of chronic obstructive pulmonary disease. http://www.goldcopd.org/

CONCUSSION, SIDELINE EVALUATION

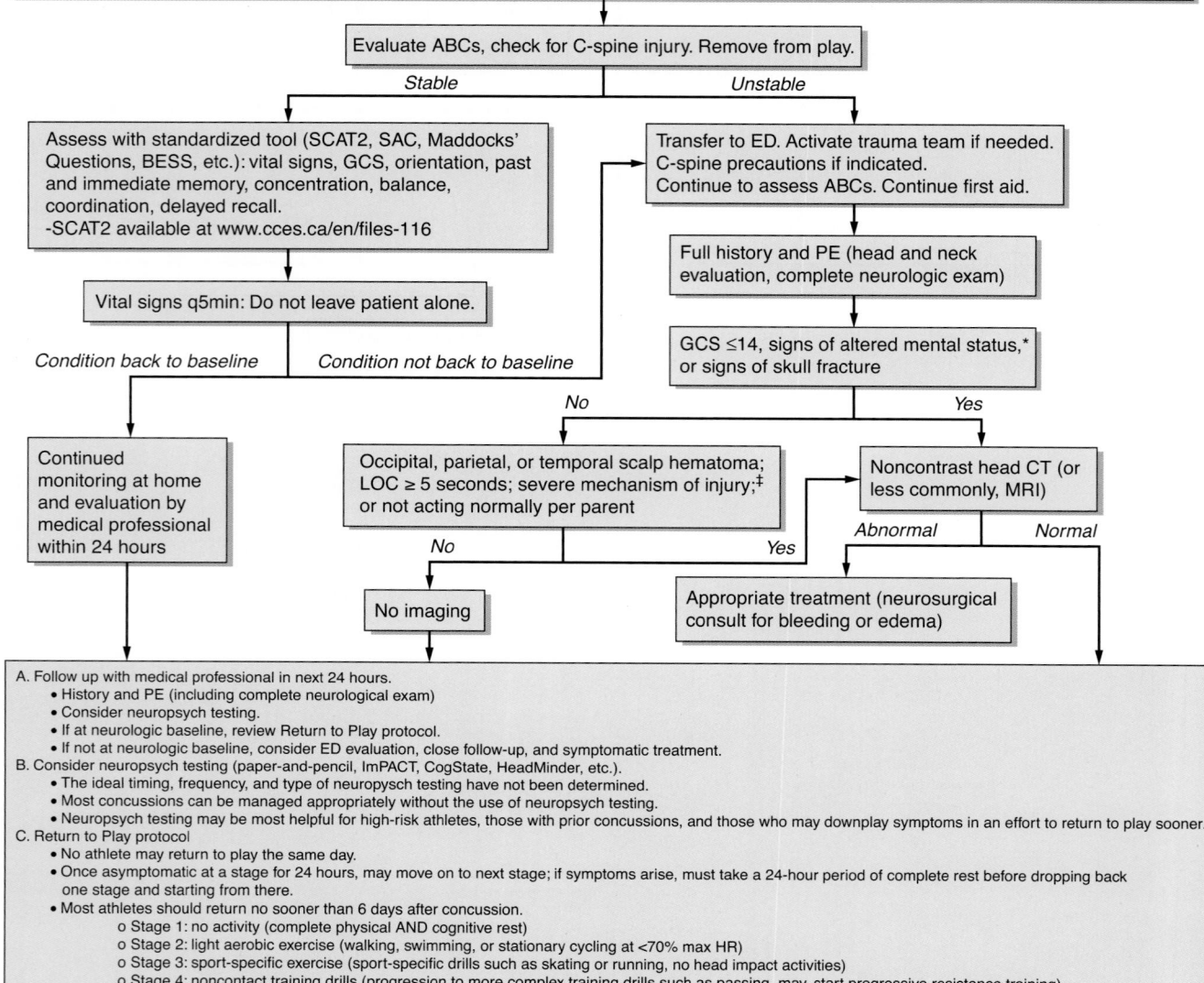

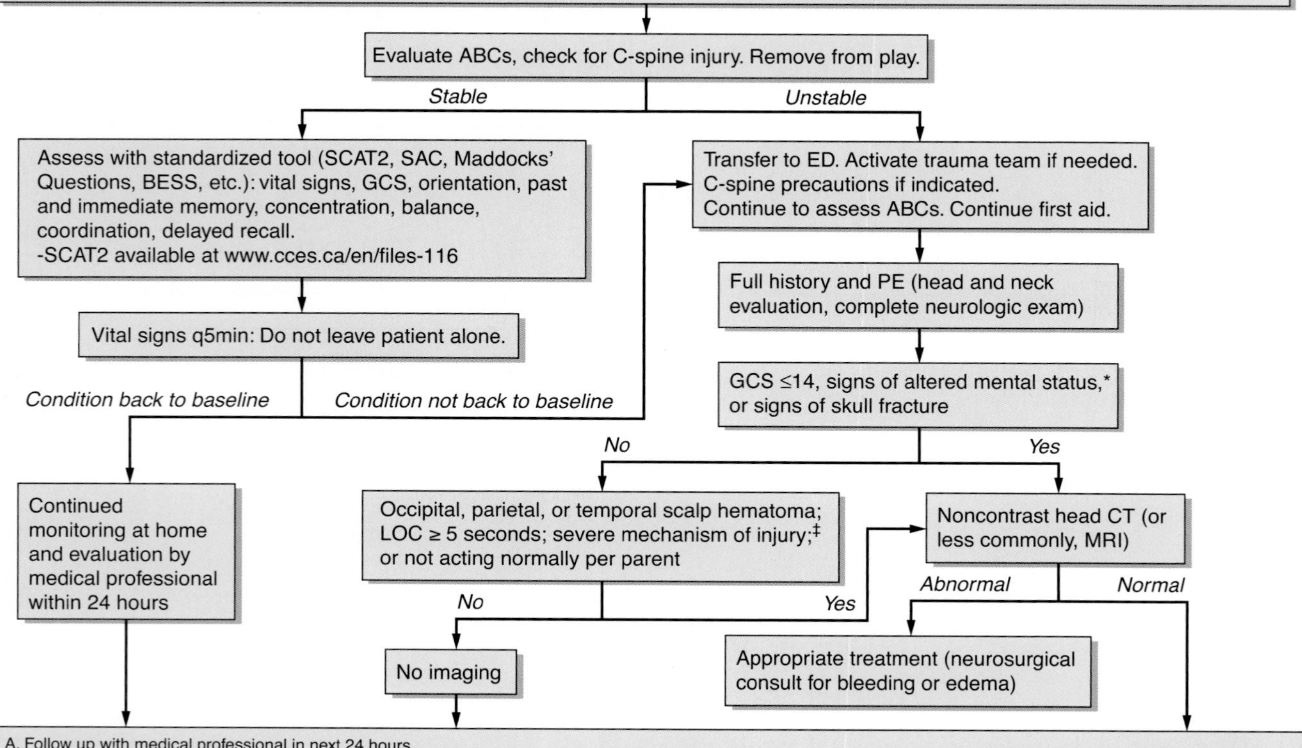
Concussion: traumatic event AND change in neurologic function OR one of the following signs/symptoms: **somatic** (HA, nausea/vomiting [N/V], dizziness, vertigo, visual problems, sensitivity to light or sound, numbness/tingling), **cognitive** (LOC, memory problems, feeling “foggy,” slower reaction times, confusion), **emotional/behavioral** (i.e., irritability, sadness), **sleep** (i.e., drowsiness, difficulty falling asleep)
Evaluate ABCs, check for C-spine injury. Remove from play.
Stable
Unstable
Assess with standardized tool (SCAT2, SAC, Maddocks' Questions, BESS, etc.): vital signs, GCS, orientation, past and immediate memory, concentration, balance, coordination, delayed recall.
-SCAT2 available at www.cces.ca/en/files-116
Transfer to ED. Activate trauma team if needed. C-spine precautions if indicated. Continue to assess ABCs. Continue first aid.
Full history and PE (head and neck evaluation, complete neurologic exam)
Vital signs q5min: Do not leave patient alone.
Condition back to baseline
Condition not back to baseline
GCS ≤14, signs of altered mental status,* or signs of skull fracture
No
Yes
Continued monitoring at home and evaluation by medical professional within 24 hours
Occipital, parietal, or temporal scalp hematoma; LOC ≥ 5 seconds; severe mechanism of injury;‡ or not acting normally per parent
Noncontrast head CT (or less commonly, MRI)
Abnormal
Normal
No
Yes
No imaging
Appropriate treatment (neurosurgical consult for bleeding or edema)

A. Follow up with medical professional in next 24 hours.
- History and PE (including complete neurological exam)
- Consider neuropsych testing.
- If at neurologic baseline, review Return to Play protocol.
- If not at neurologic baseline, consider ED evaluation, close follow-up, and symptomatic treatment.

B. Consider neuropsych testing (paper-and-pencil, ImPACT, CogState, HeadMinder, etc.).
- The ideal timing, frequency, and type of neuropysch testing have not been determined.
- Most concussions can be managed appropriately without the use of neuropsych testing.
- Neuropsych testing may be most helpful for high-risk athletes, those with prior concussions, and those who may downplay symptoms in an effort to return to play sooner.

C. Return to Play protocol
- No athlete may return to play the same day.
- Once asymptomatic at a stage for 24 hours, may move on to next stage; if symptoms arise, must take a 24-hour period of complete rest before dropping back one stage and starting from there.
- Most athletes should return no sooner than 6 days after concussion.
    - o Stage 1: no activity (complete physical AND cognitive rest)
    - o Stage 2: light aerobic exercise (walking, swimming, or stationary cycling at <70% max HR)
    - o Stage 3: sport-specific exercise (sport-specific drills such as skating or running, no head impact activities)
    - o Stage 4: noncontact training drills (progression to more complex training drills such as passing, may start progressive resistance training)
    - o Stage 5: full contact practice
    - o Stage 6: return to game play (should also be free of any medicines that could mask symptoms of concussion)
- Please note initial cognitive rest and a graded resumption of typical cognitive activity is also important. Patients may require accommodations such as a shortened school day, reduced academic workload, extended time for tests, and so on, when recovering from a concussion.

D. Symptom management: If concussive symptoms (typically HA, sleep, cognitive, and mood disturbances) are persistent and interfering with function, consider symptomatic treatment.
- In the acute setting, ASA and NSAIDs should be used with caution due to increased risk of intracranial bleeding. Acetaminophen and physical modalities are OK.
- If HA persists for a few days, consider typical abortive treatment. There is no established role for pharmacotherapy in the acute treatment of concussion-induced sleep, cognitive, or mood disturbances.
- If symptoms persist beyond a few weeks, consider referral to specialist (neurology, sports medicine, etc.). Multidisciplinary approach is often needed.
- If symptoms do not resolve despite appropriate evaluation and treatment, consider terminating athletic season or athletic career (no clear guidelines have been established; this decision should be made on a case-by-case basis).

**Signs of altered mental status: agitation, somnolence, repetitive questioning, or slow response to verbal communication.*
‡Severe mechanism of injury: motor vehicle crash with patient ejection, death of another passenger, or rollover; pedestrian or bicyclist without helmet struck by motorized vehicle; falls of >3 ft for patients <2 years old or >5 ft for patients ≥2 years old; or head struck by high-impact object.

Michelle McCreary, MD and Frank J. Domino, MD

Kuppermann N, Holmes JF, Dayan PS, et al. Identification of children at very low risk of clinically-important brain injuries after head trauma: a prospective cohort study. *Lancet.* 2009;374:1160–1170.

CONGESTIVE HEART FAILURE: DIFFERENTIAL DIAGNOSIS

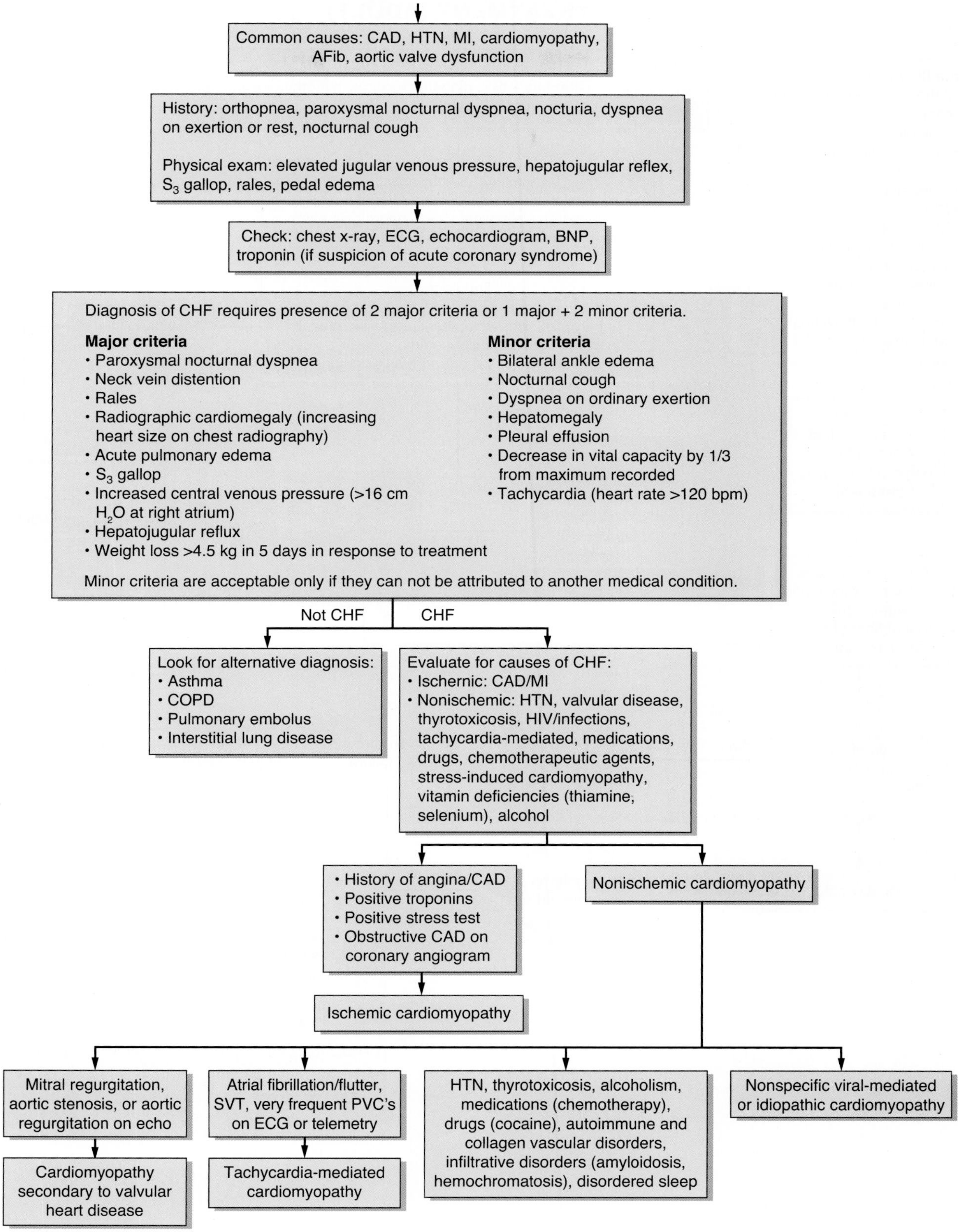

Common causes: CAD, HTN, MI, cardiomyopathy, AFib, aortic valve dysfunction

↓

History: orthopnea, paroxysmal nocturnal dyspnea, nocturia, dyspnea on exertion or rest, nocturnal cough

Physical exam: elevated jugular venous pressure, hepatojugular reflex, S_3 gallop, rales, pedal edema

↓

Check: chest x-ray, ECG, echocardiogram, BNP, troponin (if suspicion of acute coronary syndrome)

↓

Diagnosis of CHF requires presence of 2 major criteria or 1 major + 2 minor criteria.

Major criteria
- Paroxysmal nocturnal dyspnea
- Neck vein distention
- Rales
- Radiographic cardiomegaly (increasing heart size on chest radiography)
- Acute pulmonary edema
- S_3 gallop
- Increased central venous pressure (>16 cm H_2O at right atrium)
- Hepatojugular reflux
- Weight loss >4.5 kg in 5 days in response to treatment

Minor criteria
- Bilateral ankle edema
- Nocturnal cough
- Dyspnea on ordinary exertion
- Hepatomegaly
- Pleural effusion
- Decrease in vital capacity by 1/3 from maximum recorded
- Tachycardia (heart rate >120 bpm)

Minor criteria are acceptable only if they can not be attributed to another medical condition.

Not CHF →

Look for alternative diagnosis:
- Asthma
- COPD
- Pulmonary embolus
- Interstitial lung disease

CHF →

Evaluate for causes of CHF:
- Ischernic: CAD/MI
- Nonischemic: HTN, valvular disease, thyrotoxicosis, HIV/infections, tachycardia-mediated, medications, drugs, chemotherapeutic agents, stress-induced cardiomyopathy, vitamin deficiencies (thiamine, selenium), alcohol

↓

- History of angina/CAD
- Positive troponins
- Positive stress test
- Obstructive CAD on coronary angiogram

↓

Ischemic cardiomyopathy

Nonischemic cardiomyopathy

↓

Mitral regurgitation, aortic stenosis, or aortic regurgitation on echo → Cardiomyopathy secondary to valvular heart disease

Atrial fibrillation/flutter, SVT, very frequent PVC's on ECG or telemetry → Tachycardia-mediated cardiomyopathy

HTN, thyrotoxicosis, alcoholism, medications (chemotherapy), drugs (cocaine), autoimmune and collagen vascular disorders, infiltrative disorders (amyloidosis, hemochromatosis), disordered sleep

Nonspecific viral-mediated or idiopathic cardiomyopathy

Nirmanmoh Bhatia, MD and Carrie G. Lenneman, MD, MSCI

King M, Kingery J, Casey B. Diagnosis and evaluation of heart failure. *Am Fam Physician.* 2012;85(12):1161–1168.

CONSTIPATION, DIAGNOSIS AND TREATMENT (ADULT)

Rome III criteria
- 2 of the following for 12 weeks in past 6 months:
  - <3 stools/week
  - For 25% of time, any of the following:
    - Hard stools
    - Straining
    - Manual assist
    - Sense of incomplete evacuation
    - Sense of anorectal blockade
- Rare loose stools without laxative use

Common causes: primary—functional, slow transit, pelvic floor dysfunction; secondary—IBS, diabetes mellitus, hypothyroidism, hypercalcemia, pregnancy, obstruction, medication side effect

History and physical: diet, fluid intake, exercise, Rome III criteria, digital rectal exam, abdominal exam, neurologic exam

Red flags: unintentional weight loss, hematochezia, family Hx IBD or colon cancer, positive fecal occult, anemia, new onset in age >50 years, change in stool size, neurologic findings

Yes → Colonoscopy

No → Medication Hx: anticholinergics, opiates, calcium channel blockers, antidepressants, antacids

Yes → Consider medication effect: Adjust and/or begin with empiric treatment.

No → Diagnostic testing: CBC, glucose, creatinine, calcium, TSH

Positive → Anemia (→ Colonoscopy); Hypothyroidism; Hypercalcemia; Diabetes mellitus

Negative → Empiric treatment: Increase exercise and water intake; trial of fiber of bulk-forming laxatives

Symptoms improved?
- *Yes* → Functional constipation
- *No* → Add polyethylene glycol and/or stimulant laxative.

Symptoms improved?
- *Yes* → Functional constipation
- *No* → Treatment failure → Diagnostic testing: colonic transit time study (CTT), balloon expulsion test (BET), anorectal manometry (AM)

Abnormal CTT → Slow transit constipation → Treatments earlier, enemas, biofeedback

Normal CTT, abnormal BET, abnormal AM → Pelvic floor dysfunction → Treatments earlier, biofeedbacks, also Botox, surgery

Jacquelyn Chambers, MD and Robert A. Baldor, MD, FAAFP

Longstreth GF, Thompson WG, Chey WD, et al. Functional bowel disorders. *Gastroenterology.* 2006;130(5):1480–1491.

CONSTIPATION, TREATMENT (PEDIATRIC)

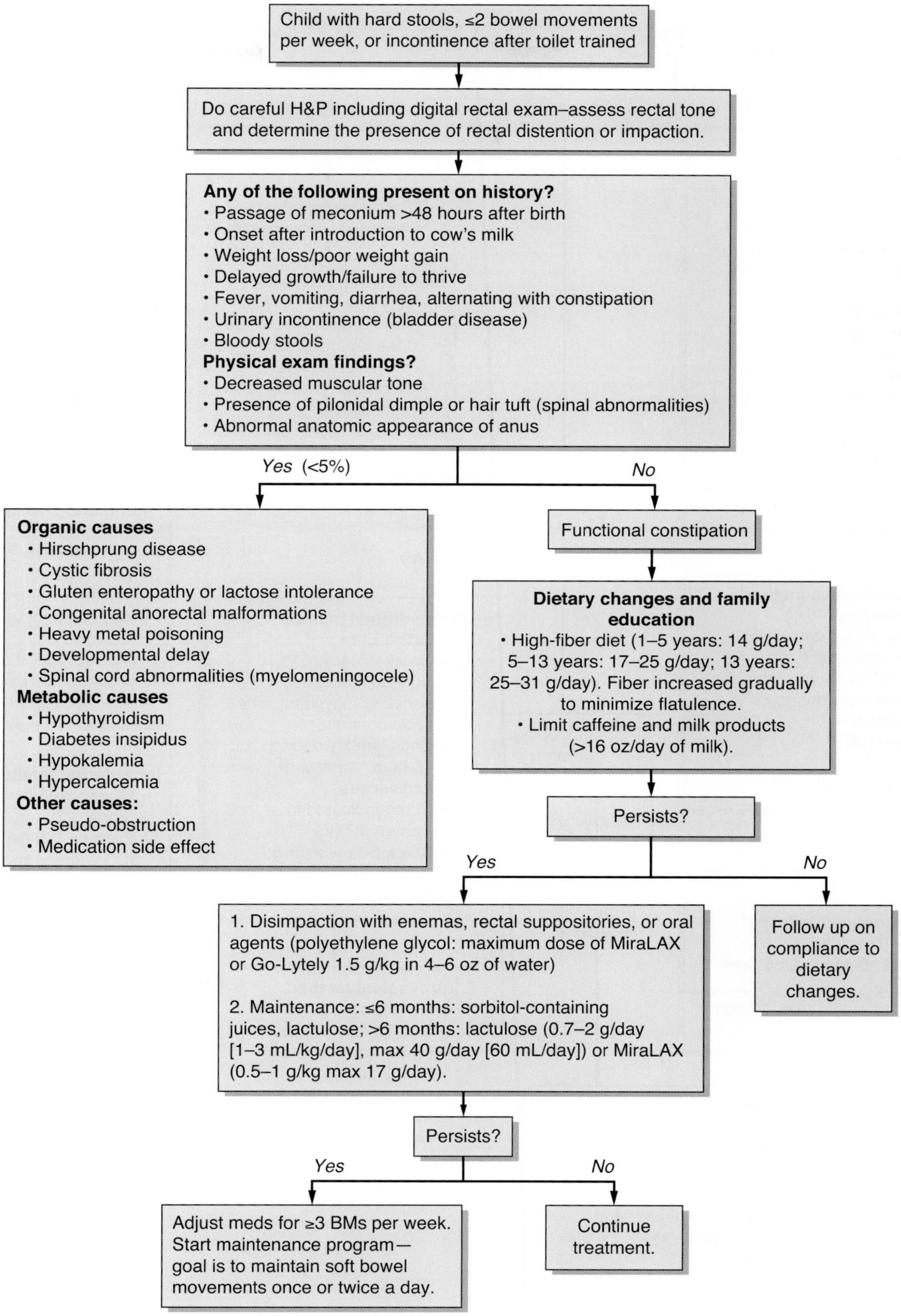

Child with hard stools, ≤2 bowel movements per week, or incontinence after toilet trained

↓

Do careful H&P including digital rectal exam–assess rectal tone and determine the presence of rectal distention or impaction.

↓

Any of the following present on history?
- Passage of meconium >48 hours after birth
- Onset after introduction to cow's milk
- Weight loss/poor weight gain
- Delayed growth/failure to thrive
- Fever, vomiting, diarrhea, alternating with constipation
- Urinary incontinence (bladder disease)
- Bloody stools

Physical exam findings?
- Decreased muscular tone
- Presence of pilonidal dimple or hair tuft (spinal abnormalities)
- Abnormal anatomic appearance of anus

Yes (<5%) →

Organic causes
- Hirschprung disease
- Cystic fibrosis
- Gluten enteropathy or lactose intolerance
- Congenital anorectal malformations
- Heavy metal poisoning
- Developmental delay
- Spinal cord abnormalities (myelomeningocele)

Metabolic causes
- Hypothyroidism
- Diabetes insipidus
- Hypokalemia
- Hypercalcemia

Other causes:
- Pseudo-obstruction
- Medication side effect

No →

Functional constipation

↓

Dietary changes and family education
- High-fiber diet (1–5 years: 14 g/day; 5–13 years: 17–25 g/day; 13 years: 25–31 g/day). Fiber increased gradually to minimize flatulence.
- Limit caffeine and milk products (>16 oz/day of milk).

↓

Persists?

Yes →

1. Disimpaction with enemas, rectal suppositories, or oral agents (polyethylene glycol: maximum dose of MiraLAX or Go-Lytely 1.5 g/kg in 4–6 oz of water)

2. Maintenance: ≤6 months: sorbitol-containing juices, lactulose; >6 months: lactulose (0.7–2 g/day [1–3 mL/kg/day], max 40 g/day [60 mL/day]) or MiraLAX (0.5–1 g/kg max 17 g/day).

↓

Persists?

Yes → Adjust meds for ≥3 BMs per week. Start maintenance program—goal is to maintain soft bowel movements once or twice a day.

No → Continue treatment.

No →

Follow up on compliance to dietary changes.

Tarina Desai, MD and Fozia Akhtar Ali, MD

Constipation Guideline Committee of the North American Society for Pediatric Gastroenterology, Hepatology and Nutrition. Evaluation and treatment of constipation in infants and children: recommendations of the North American Society for Pediatric Gastroenterology, Hepatology and Nutrition. *J Pediatr Gastroenterol Nutr.* 2006;43(3):e1–e13.

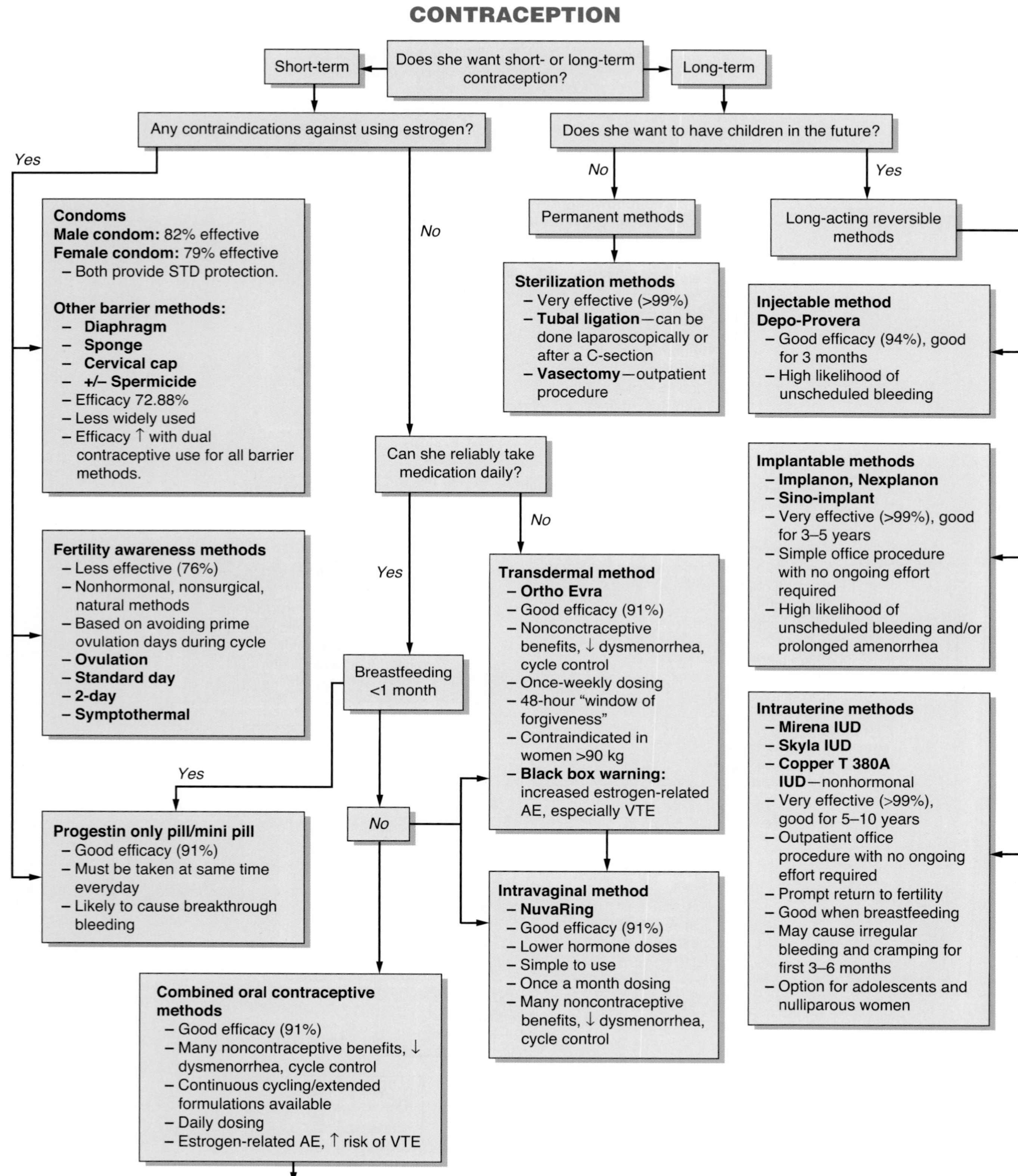
CONTRACEPTION
Short-term
Does she want short- or long-term contraception?
Long-term
Any contraindications against using estrogen?
Does she want to have children in the future?
Yes
No
No
Yes
Permanent methods
Long-acting reversible methods
Condoms
Male condom: 82% effective
Female condom: 79% effective
– Both provide STD protection.
Other barrier methods:
– Diaphragm
– Sponge
– Cervical cap
– +/– Spermicide
– Efficacy 72.88%
– Less widely used
– Efficacy ↑ with dual contraceptive use for all barrier methods.
Sterilization methods
– Very effective (>99%)
– Tubal ligation—can be done laparoscopically or after a C-section
– Vasectomy—outpatient procedure
Injectable method
Depo-Provera
– Good efficacy (94%), good for 3 months
– High likelihood of unscheduled bleeding
Can she reliably take medication daily?
No
Yes
Implantable methods
– Implanon, Nexplanon
– Sino-implant
– Very effective (>99%), good for 3–5 years
– Simple office procedure with no ongoing effort required
– High likelihood of unscheduled bleeding and/or prolonged amenorrhea
Fertility awareness methods
– Less effective (76%)
– Nonhormonal, nonsurgical, natural methods
– Based on avoiding prime ovulation days during cycle
– Ovulation
– Standard day
– 2-day
– Symptothermal
Transdermal method
– Ortho Evra
– Good efficacy (91%)
– Nonconctraceptive benefits, ↓ dysmenorrhea, cycle control
– Once-weekly dosing
– 48-hour "window of forgiveness"
– Contraindicated in women >90 kg
– Black box warning: increased estrogen-related AE, especially VTE
Breastfeeding <1 month
Yes
No
Intrauterine methods
– Mirena IUD
– Skyla IUD
– Copper T 380A IUD—nonhormonal
– Very effective (>99%), good for 5–10 years
– Outpatient office procedure with no ongoing effort required
– Prompt return to fertility
– Good when breastfeeding
– May cause irregular bleeding and cramping for first 3–6 months
– Option for adolescents and nulliparous women
Progestin only pill/mini pill
– Good efficacy (91%)
– Must be taken at same time everyday
– Likely to cause breakthrough bleeding
Intravaginal method
– NuvaRing
– Good efficacy (91%)
– Lower hormone doses
– Simple to use
– Once a month dosing
– Many noncontraceptive benefits, ↓ dysmenorrhea, cycle control
Combined oral contraceptive methods
– Good efficacy (91%)
– Many noncontraceptive benefits, ↓ dysmenorrhea, cycle control
– Continuous cycling/extended formulations available
– Daily dosing
– Estrogen-related AE, ↑ risk of VTE

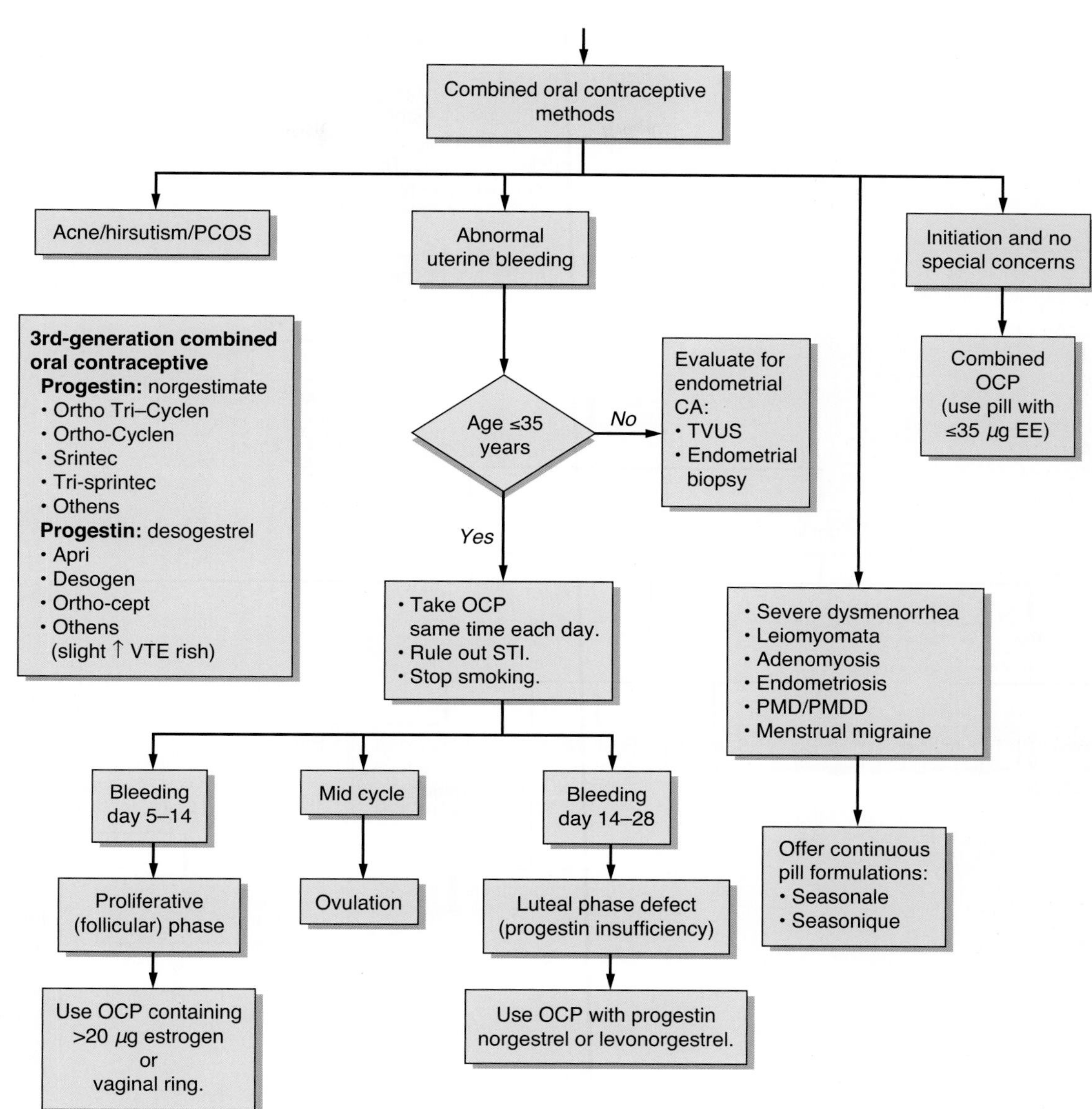

Mary Le, MD and Anne Powell, MD

Blenning CE, Paladine H. An approach to the postpartum office visit. *Am Fam Physician*. 2005;72(12):2491–2496.

COUGH, CHRONIC

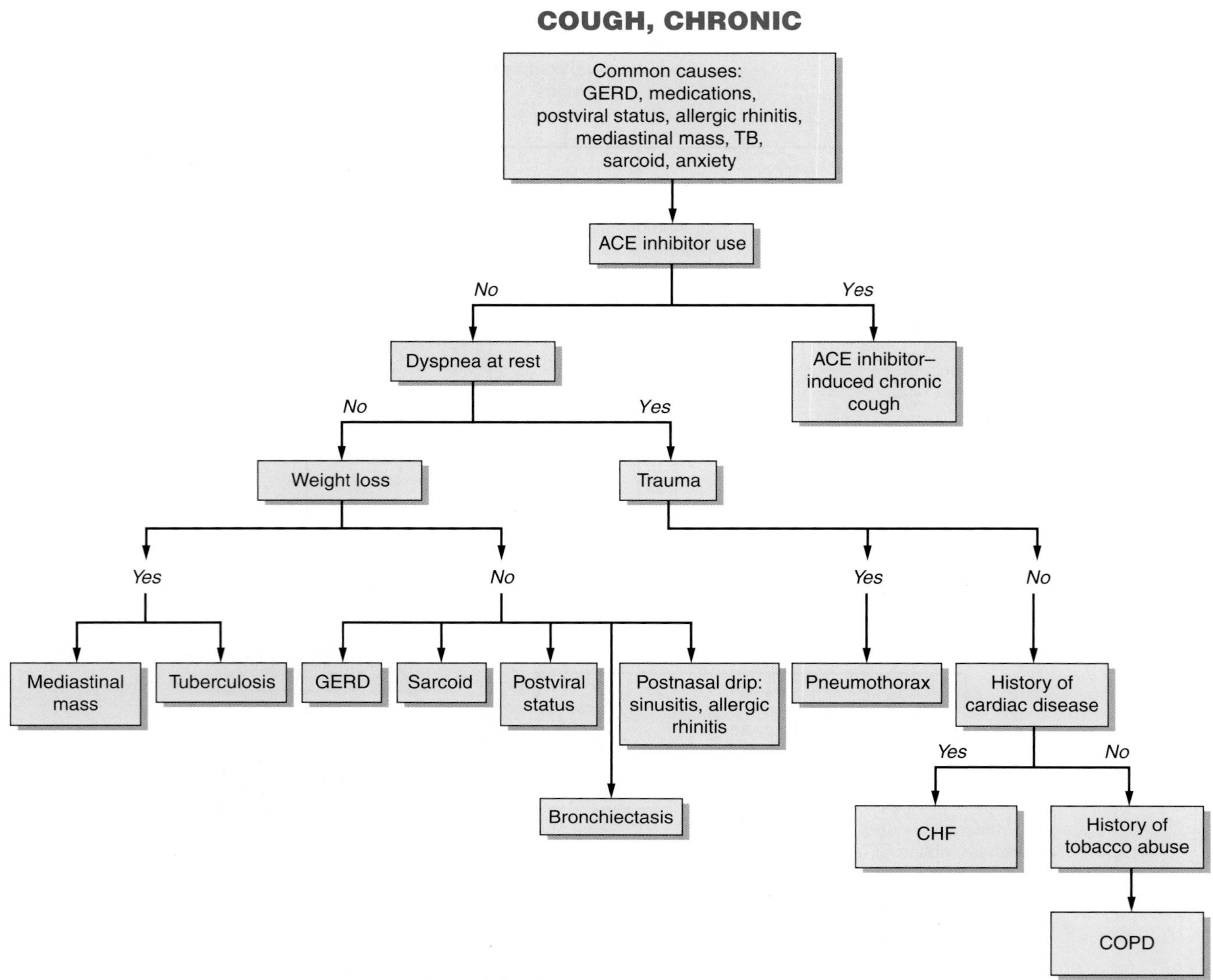

Robert A. Baldor, MD, FAAFP and Alan M. Ehrlich, MD

Pratter MR. Unexplained (idiopathic) cough: ACCP evidence-based clinical practice guidelines. *Chest.* 2006;129(1)(Suppl):220S–221S.

DEEP VENOUS THROMBOSIS, DIAGNOSIS, AND TREATMENT

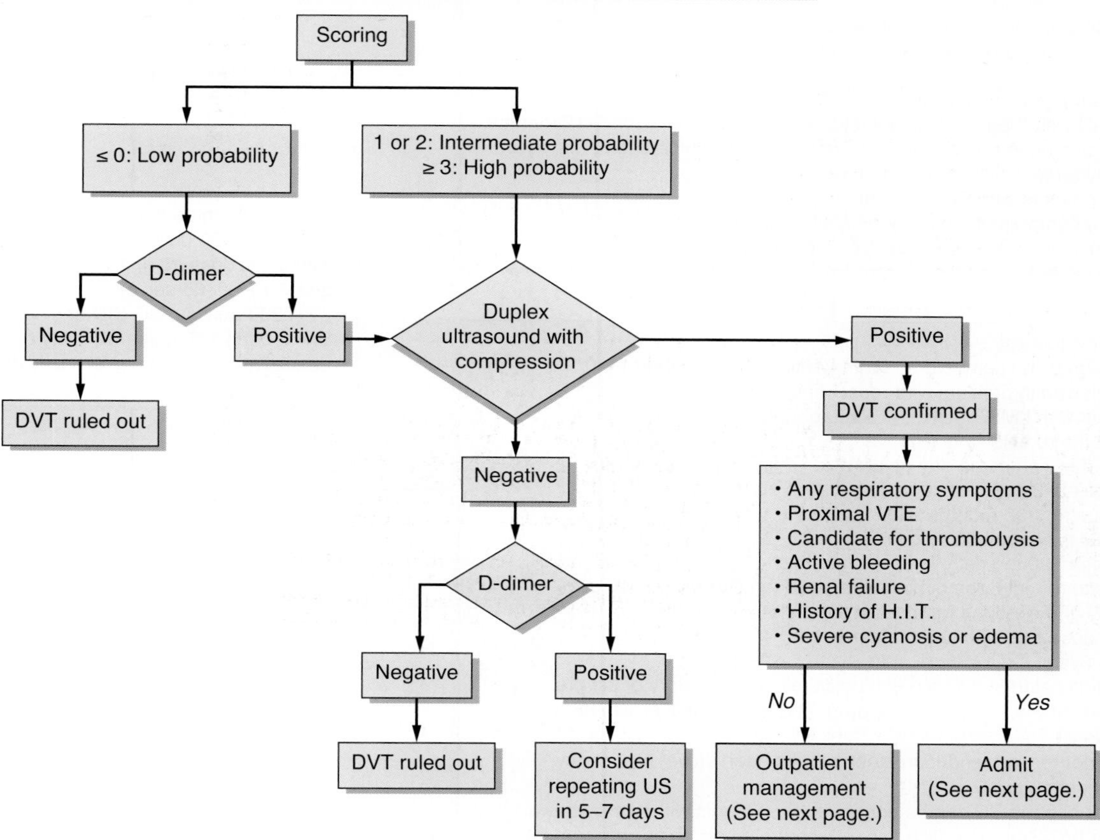
Determine Wells score
• Active cancer +1
• Calf swelling >3 cm +1
• Collateral superficial veins +1
• Pitting edema +1
• Previous DVT +1
• Pain along venous system +1
• Paralysis or recent immobilization (cast) +1
• Recently bedridden for >3 days or general anesthesia +1
Scoring
≤ 0: Low probability
1 or 2: Intermediate probability
≥ 3: High probability
D-dimer
Negative
Positive
DVT ruled out
Duplex ultrasound with compression
Positive
DVT confirmed
Negative
D-dimer
Negative
Positive
DVT ruled out
Consider repeating US in 5–7 days
• Any respiratory symptoms
• Proximal VTE
• Candidate for thrombolysis
• Active bleeding
• Renal failure
• History of H.I.T.
• Severe cyanosis or edema
No
Yes
Outpatient management (See next page.)
Admit (See next page.)

Deep Vein Thrombosis, Treatment

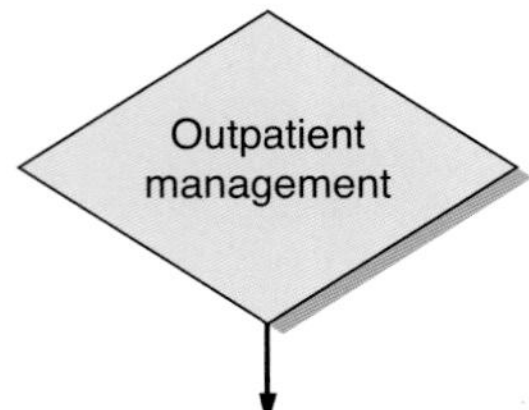

Inpatient management indications

Low-molecular weight heparin (LMWH):
- Enoxaparin 1 mg/kg SC BID or
- Dalteparin 200 international units/kg SC daily for patients with cancer
- LMWH is the preferred treatment in pregnancy

Rivaroxaban (factor Xa inhibitor):
- 15 mg BID with food for 3 weeks followed by 20 mg daily for 6–12 months
- Contraindicated in patients with active pathological bleeding or history of severe hypersensitivity reaction to the drug
- Avoid in patients with CrCl <30 mL/min
- Use not recommended in pregnancy or breastfeeding
- Current use is limited due to cost and lack of reversal agent

Inpatient management indications:
- Massive DVT
- Symptomatic PE
- High risk bleeding with anticoagulation therapy
- Comorbid conditions

- IV unfractionated heparin (UFH): 80 units/kg bolus or 5,000 units → continuous infusion with initial dose 18 units/kg/hour → Titrate to goal PTT 60–85 sec or
- UFH 250 units/kg SC BID or
- Enoxaparin 1.5 mg/kg SC daily or
- Fondaparinux 5–10 mg SC daily depending on weight

Maintenance therapy
- Hypercoagulation test before starting anticoagulation therapy
- UFH preferred in patients with renal impairment
- Treatment with LMWH, UFH, or fondaparinux is recommended for at least 5 days **AND** until INR ≥ 2 for 2 consecutive days
- Start Warfarin on same day as LMWH, UFH, and fondaparinux
  - Goal INR 2–3
  - Continue for 3–6 months after 1st DVT
  - Warfarin is contraindicated in pregnancy
- Rivaroxaban 20 mg daily for 6–12 months
- Dabigatran (direct thrombin inhibitor): 150 mg BID after 7–10 days of LMWH and continue for at least 6 months
  - Adjust dose for CrCl <50 mL/min
  - Do not use in CrCl <15 mL/min
  - Contraindicated in active pathological bleeding, history of severe hypersensitivity reaction to the drug, and mechanical prosthetic heart valve.
  - Use is not recommended in bioprosthetic heart valve, pregnancy, and breastfeeding.
- LMWH or heparin SC can be continued for patients with allergy to warfarin.
- Consider IVC filter for individuals with contraindication to anticoagulation.

Bency K. Louidor-Paulynice, MD and Kimberly Bombaci, MD

Wells P, Forgie M, Rodger M. Treatment of venous thromboembolism. *JAMA*. 2014;311:717–728.

DEHYDRATION, PEDIATRIC

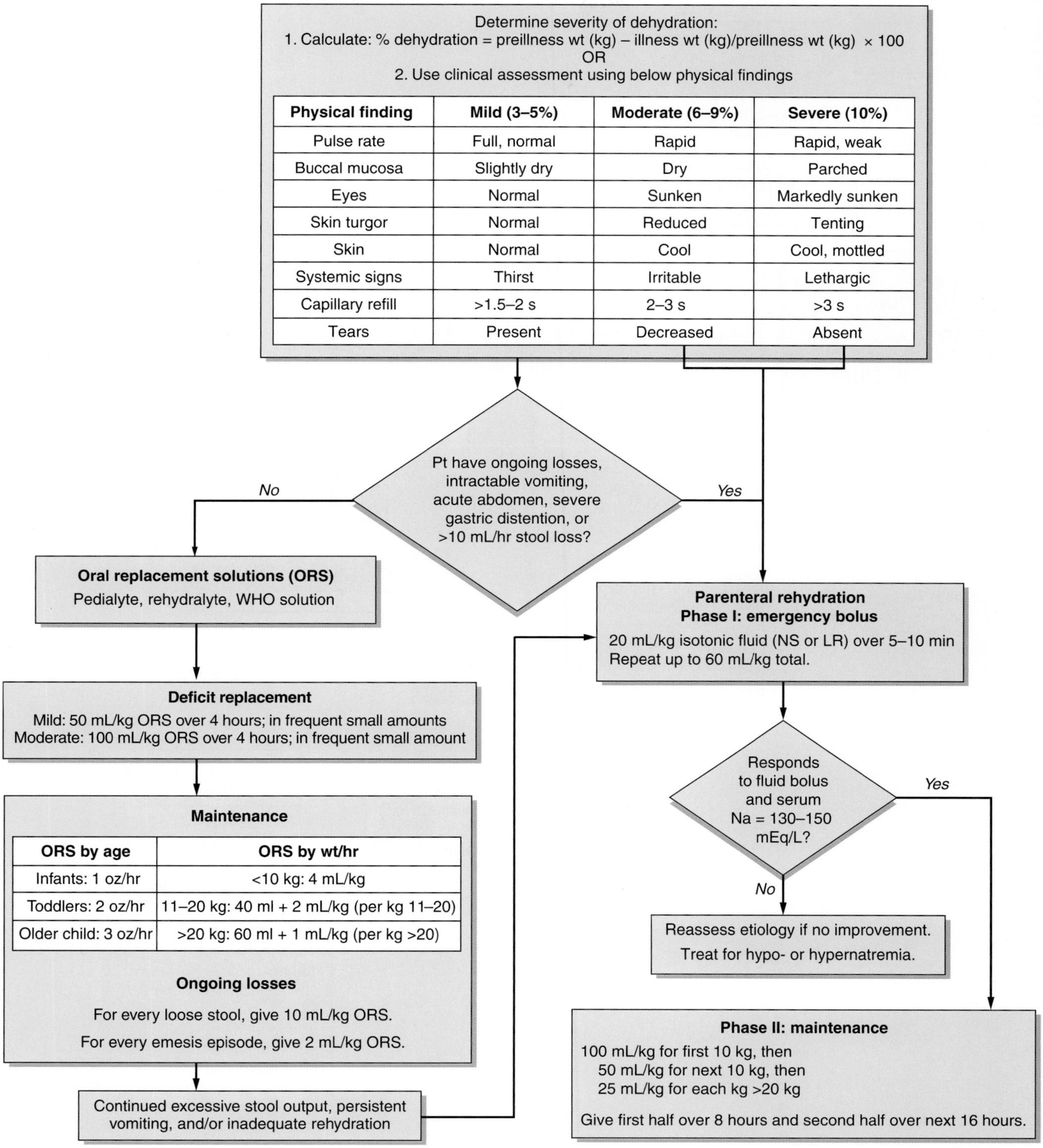

Determine severity of dehydration:
1. Calculate: % dehydration = preillness wt (kg) – illness wt (kg)/preillness wt (kg) × 100
OR
2. Use clinical assessment using below physical findings

Physical finding	Mild (3–5%)	Moderate (6–9%)	Severe (10%)
Pulse rate	Full, normal	Rapid	Rapid, weak
Buccal mucosa	Slightly dry	Dry	Parched
Eyes	Normal	Sunken	Markedly sunken
Skin turgor	Normal	Reduced	Tenting
Skin	Normal	Cool	Cool, mottled
Systemic signs	Thirst	Irritable	Lethargic
Capillary refill	>1.5–2 s	2–3 s	>3 s
Tears	Present	Decreased	Absent

Pt have ongoing losses, intractable vomiting, acute abdomen, severe gastric distention, or >10 mL/hr stool loss?

No

Oral replacement solutions (ORS)
Pedialyte, rehydralyte, WHO solution

Deficit replacement
Mild: 50 mL/kg ORS over 4 hours; in frequent small amounts
Moderate: 100 mL/kg ORS over 4 hours; in frequent small amount

Maintenance

ORS by age	ORS by wt/hr
Infants: 1 oz/hr	<10 kg: 4 mL/kg
Toddlers: 2 oz/hr	11–20 kg: 40 ml + 2 mL/kg (per kg 11–20)
Older child: 3 oz/hr	>20 kg: 60 ml + 1 mL/kg (per kg >20)

Ongoing losses

For every loose stool, give 10 mL/kg ORS.

For every emesis episode, give 2 mL/kg ORS.

Continued excessive stool output, persistent vomiting, and/or inadequate rehydration

Yes

Parenteral rehydration
Phase I: emergency bolus
20 mL/kg isotonic fluid (NS or LR) over 5–10 min
Repeat up to 60 mL/kg total.

Responds to fluid bolus and serum Na = 130–150 mEq/L?

No

Reassess etiology if no improvement.
Treat for hypo- or hypernatremia.

Yes

Phase II: maintenance
100 mL/kg for first 10 kg, then
50 mL/kg for next 10 kg, then
25 mL/kg for each kg >20 kg

Give first half over 8 hours and second half over next 16 hours.

L. Michelle W. Seawright, DO and Nathaniel Stepp, DO, LCDR, USN

Tschudt M, Arcara K. *Harriet Lane Handbook*. 19th ed. Philadelphia: Elsevier; 2012:271–291.

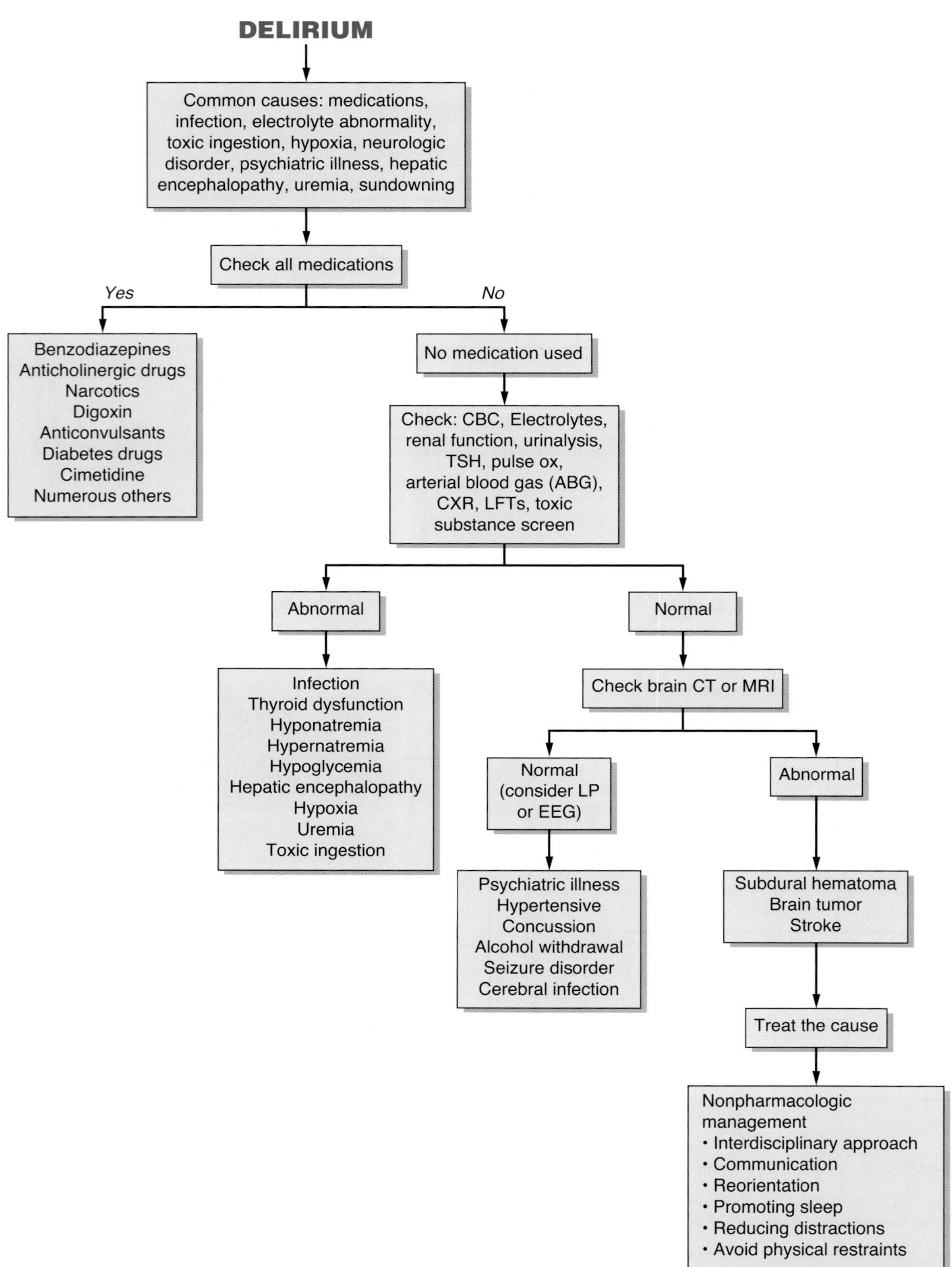
DELIRIUM
Common causes: medications, infection, electrolyte abnormality, toxic ingestion, hypoxia, neurologic disorder, psychiatric illness, hepatic encephalopathy, uremia, sundowning
Check all medications
Yes
No
Benzodiazepines
Anticholinergic drugs
Narcotics
Digoxin
Anticonvulsants
Diabetes drugs
Cimetidine
Numerous others
No medication used
Check: CBC, Electrolytes, renal function, urinalysis, TSH, pulse ox, arterial blood gas (ABG), CXR, LFTs, toxic substance screen
Abnormal
Normal
Infection
Thyroid dysfunction
Hyponatremia
Hypernatremia
Hypoglycemia
Hepatic encephalopathy
Hypoxia
Uremia
Toxic ingestion
Check brain CT or MRI
Normal (consider LP or EEG)
Abnormal
Psychiatric illness
Hypertensive
Concussion
Alcohol withdrawal
Seizure disorder
Cerebral infection
Subdural hematoma
Brain tumor
Stroke
Treat the cause
Nonpharmacologic management
• Interdisciplinary approach
• Communication
• Reorientation
• Promoting sleep
• Reducing distractions
• Avoid physical restraints

Kamal C. Wagle, MD, MPH

Inouye SK, Westendorp RG, Saczynski JS. Delirium in elderly people. *Lancet*. 2014;383(9920):911–922.

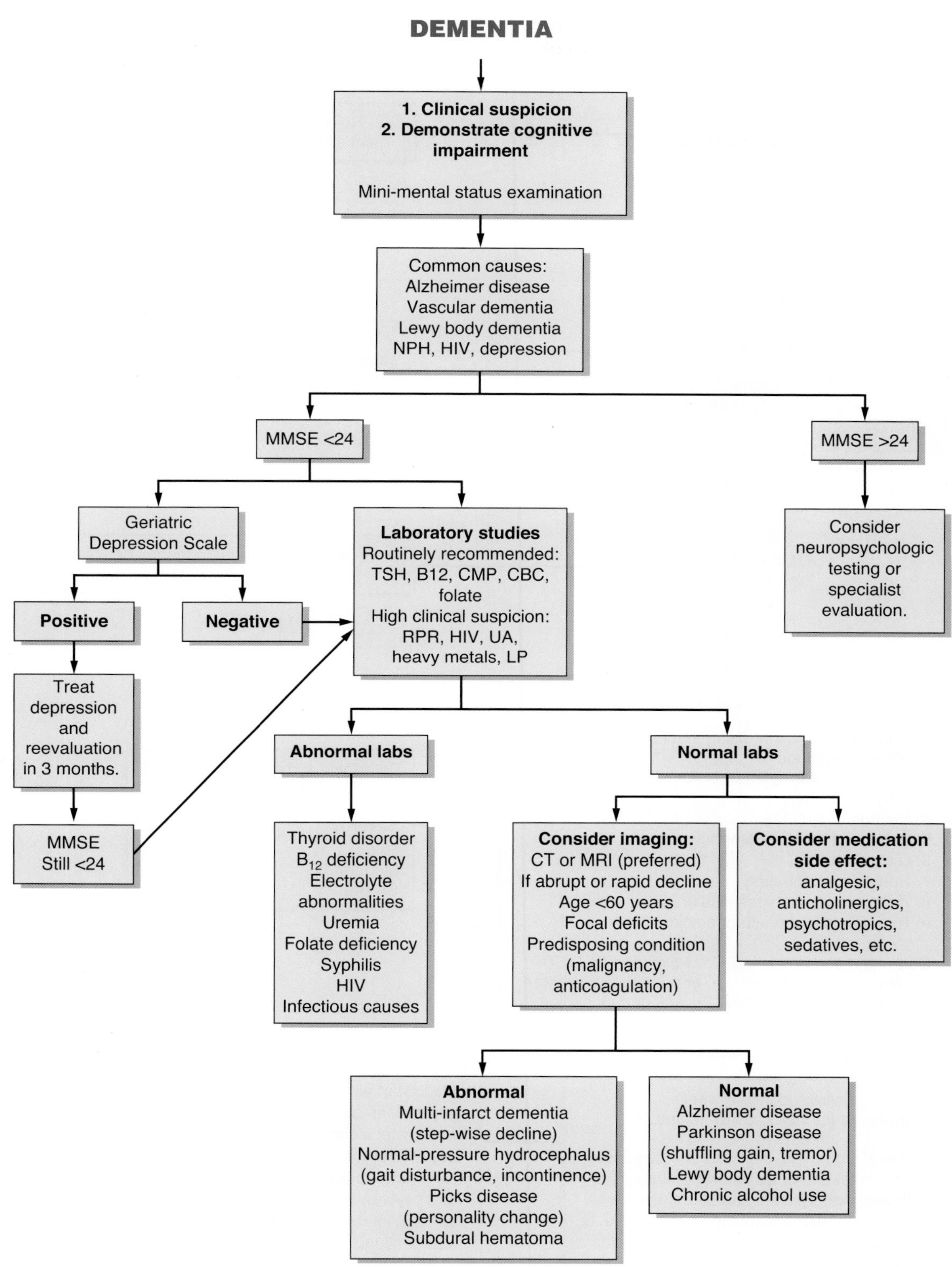

Kristin Grindstaff, DO and Casandra Cashman, MD

Adelman AM, Daly MP. Initial evaluation of the patient with suspected dementia. *Am Fam Physician.* 2005;71(9):1745–1750.

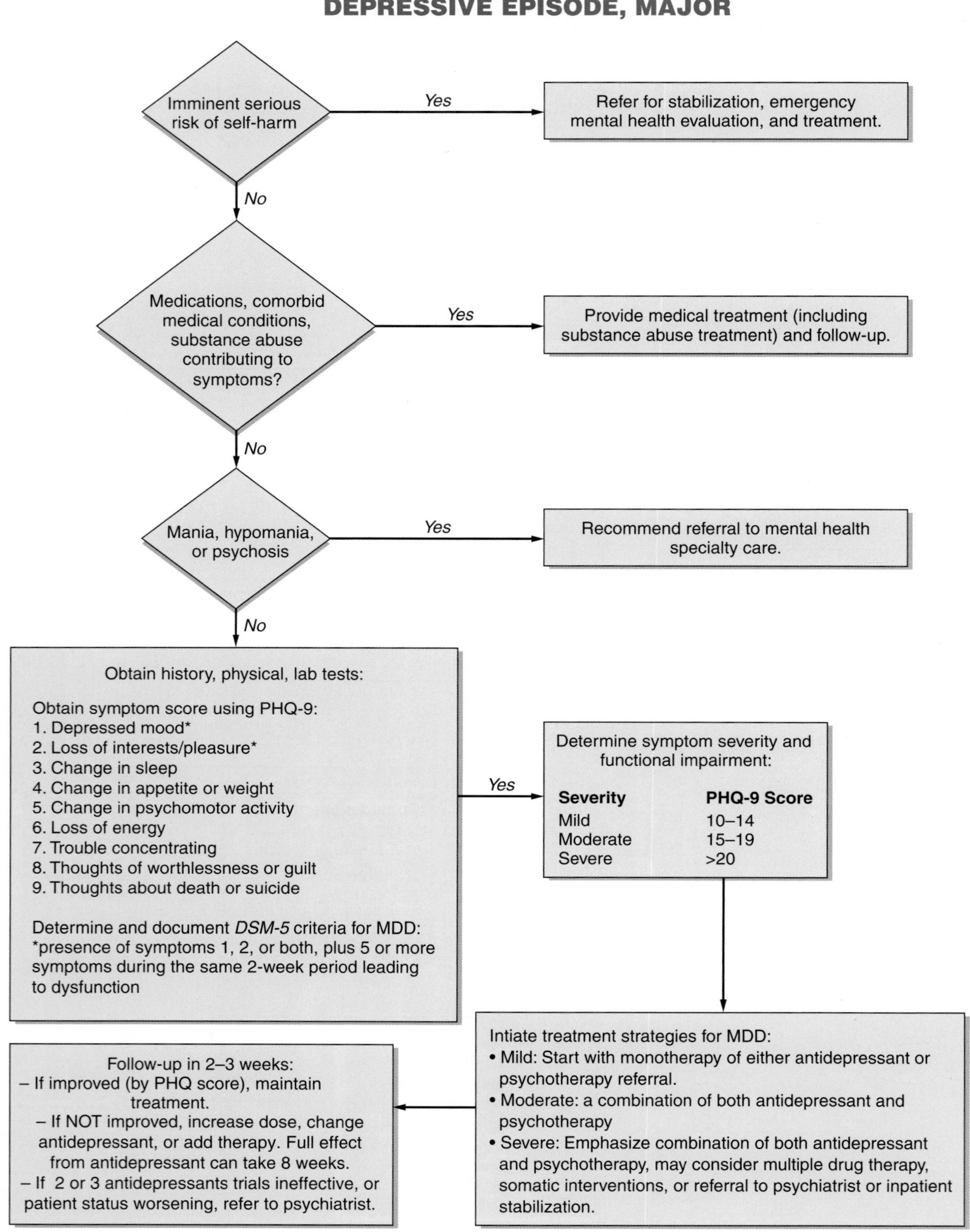

DEPRESSIVE EPISODE, MAJOR
Imminent serious risk of self-harm
Yes
Refer for stabilization, emergency mental health evaluation, and treatment.
No
Medications, comorbid medical conditions, substance abuse contributing to symptoms?
Yes
Provide medical treatment (including substance abuse treatment) and follow-up.
No
Mania, hypomania, or psychosis
Yes
Recommend referral to mental health specialty care.
No
Obtain history, physical, lab tests:
Obtain symptom score using PHQ-9:
1. Depressed mood*
2. Loss of interests/pleasure*
3. Change in sleep
4. Change in appetite or weight
5. Change in psychomotor activity
6. Loss of energy
7. Trouble concentrating
8. Thoughts of worthlessness or guilt
9. Thoughts about death or suicide
Determine and document DSM-5 criteria for MDD: *presence of symptoms 1, 2, or both, plus 5 or more symptoms during the same 2-week period leading to dysfunction
Yes
Determine symptom severity and functional impairment:
Severity PHQ-9 Score
Mild 10–14
Moderate 15–19
Severe >20
Intiate treatment strategies for MDD:
• Mild: Start with monotherapy of either antidepressant or psychotherapy referral.
• Moderate: a combination of both antidepressant and psychotherapy
• Severe: Emphasize combination of both antidepressant and psychotherapy, may consider multiple drug therapy, somatic interventions, or referral to psychiatrist or inpatient stabilization.
Follow-up in 2–3 weeks:
– If improved (by PHQ score), maintain treatment.
– If NOT improved, increase dose, change antidepressant, or add therapy. Full effect from antidepressant can take 8 weeks.
– If 2 or 3 antidepressants trials ineffective, or patient status worsening, refer to psychiatrist.

Wendy K. Marsh, MD, MSc

US Department of Veterans Affairs. *VA/DoD Clinical Practice Guideline for Management of Major Depressive Disorder.* Washington, DC: Department of Veteran Affairs; 2010.

DIABETIC KETOACIDOSIS (DKA), TREATMENT

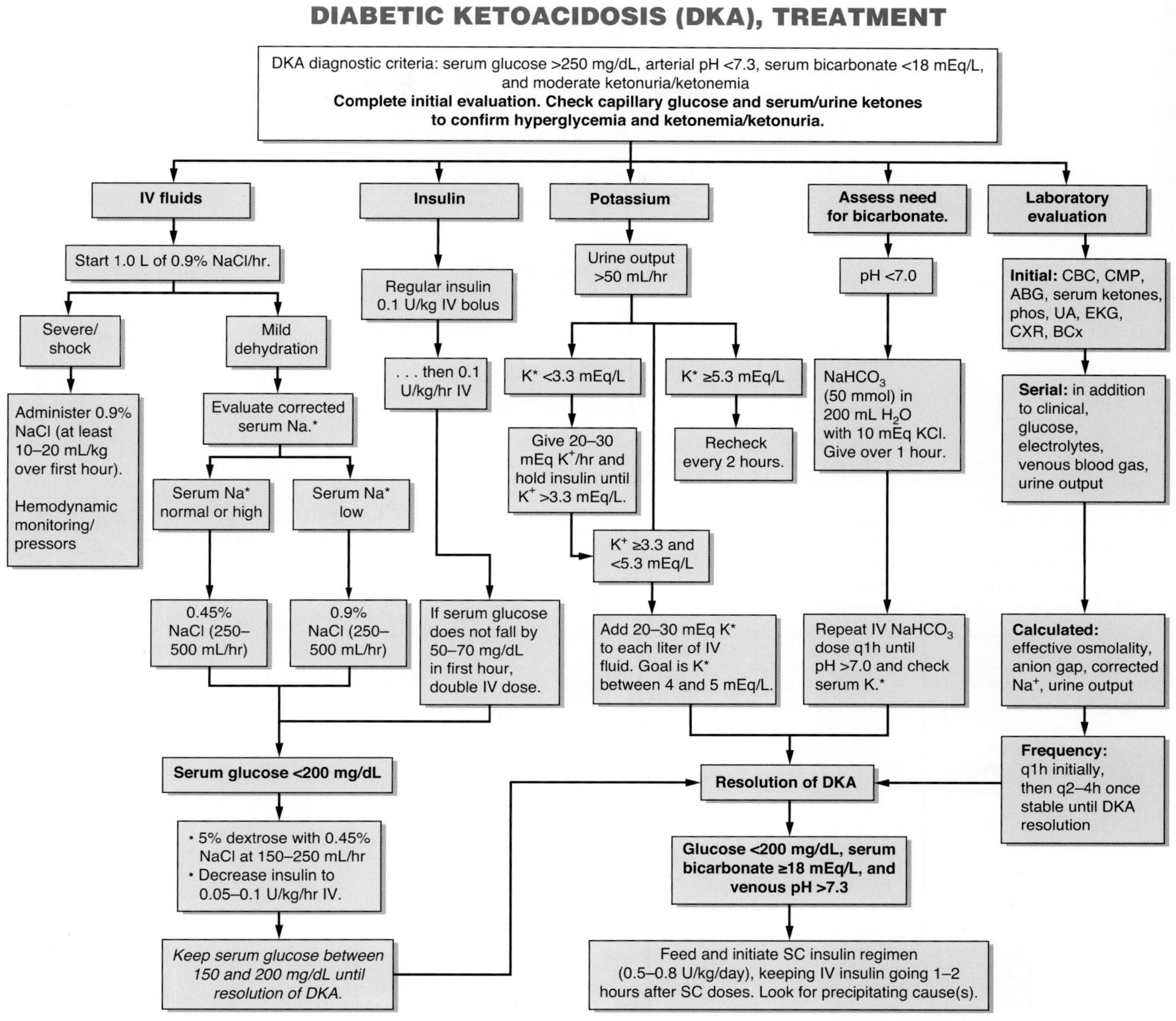
DKA diagnostic criteria: serum glucose >250 mg/dL, arterial pH <7.3, serum bicarbonate <18 mEq/L, and moderate ketonuria/ketonemia
Complete initial evaluation. Check capillary glucose and serum/urine ketones to confirm hyperglycemia and ketonemia/ketonuria.
IV fluids
Start 1.0 L of 0.9% NaCl/hr.
Severe/ shock
Administer 0.9% NaCl (at least 10–20 mL/kg over first hour).
Hemodynamic monitoring/ pressors
Mild dehydration
Evaluate corrected serum Na.*
Serum Na* normal or high
0.45% NaCl (250–500 mL/hr)
Serum Na* low
0.9% NaCl (250–500 mL/hr)
Insulin
Regular insulin 0.1 U/kg IV bolus
. . . then 0.1 U/kg/hr IV
If serum glucose does not fall by 50–70 mg/dL in first hour, double IV dose.
Serum glucose <200 mg/dL
• 5% dextrose with 0.45% NaCl at 150–250 mL/hr
• Decrease insulin to 0.05–0.1 U/kg/hr IV.
Keep serum glucose between 150 and 200 mg/dL until resolution of DKA.
Potassium
Urine output >50 mL/hr
K* <3.3 mEq/L
Give 20–30 mEq K+/hr and hold insulin until K+ >3.3 mEq/L.
K* ≥5.3 mEq/L
Recheck every 2 hours.
K+ ≥3.3 and <5.3 mEq/L
Add 20–30 mEq K* to each liter of IV fluid. Goal is K* between 4 and 5 mEq/L.
Assess need for bicarbonate.
pH <7.0
NaHCO3 (50 mmol) in 200 mL H2O with 10 mEq KCl. Give over 1 hour.
Repeat IV NaHCO3 dose q1h until pH >7.0 and check serum K.*
Laboratory evaluation
Initial: CBC, CMP, ABG, serum ketones, phos, UA, EKG, CXR, BCx
Serial: in addition to clinical, glucose, electrolytes, venous blood gas, urine output
Calculated: effective osmolality, anion gap, corrected Na+, urine output
Frequency: q1h initially, then q2–4h once stable until DKA resolution
Resolution of DKA
Glucose <200 mg/dL, serum bicarbonate ≥18 mEq/L, and venous pH >7.3
Feed and initiate SC insulin regimen (0.5–0.8 U/kg/day), keeping IV insulin going 1–2 hours after SC doses. Look for precipitating cause(s).

Frank J. Domino, MD and Emily Bouley, MD

Trachtenbarg DE. Diabetic ketoacidosis. *Am Fam Physician.* 2005;71(9):1705–1714.

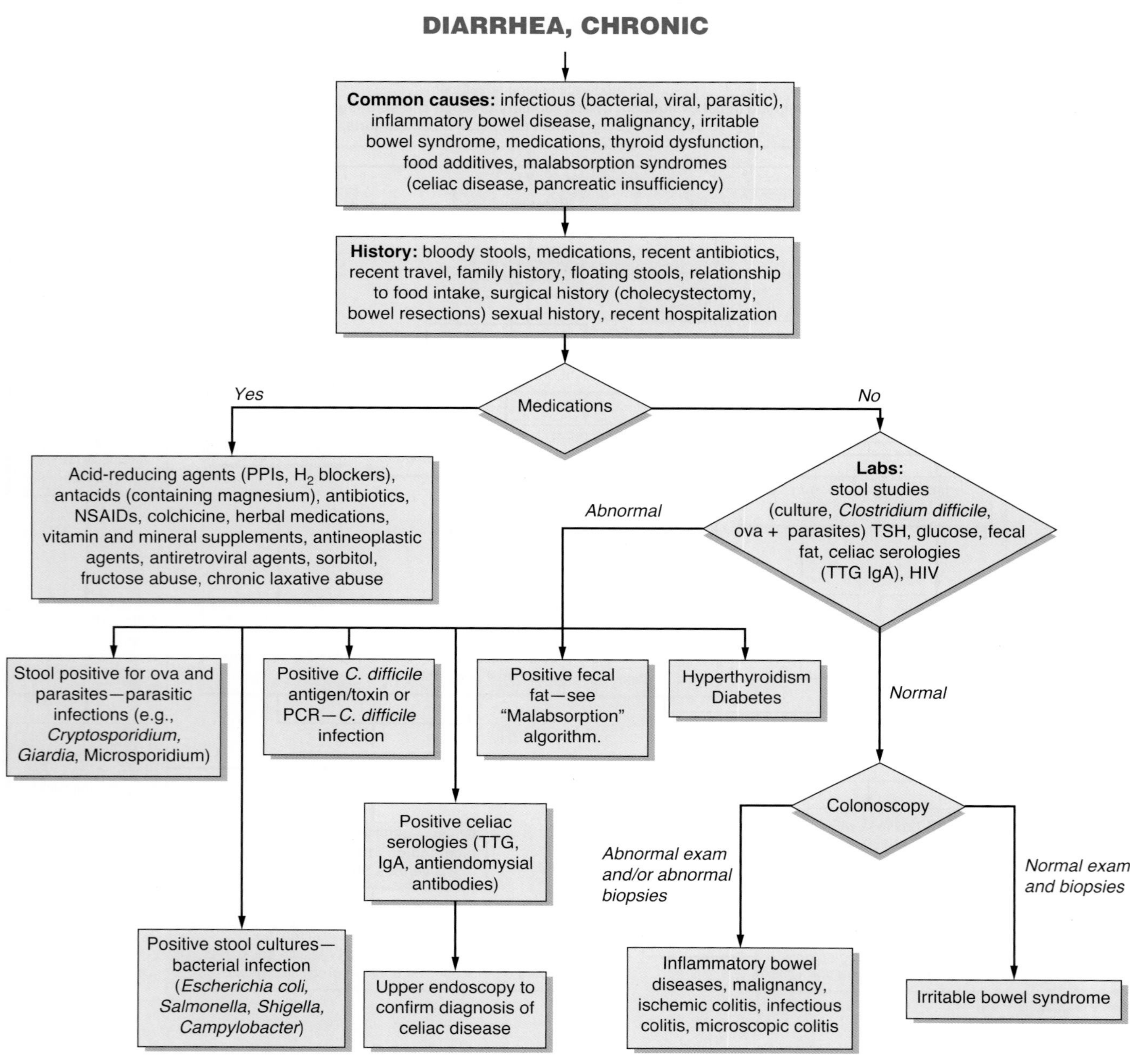
DIARRHEA, CHRONIC
Common causes: infectious (bacterial, viral, parasitic), inflammatory bowel disease, malignancy, irritable bowel syndrome, medications, thyroid dysfunction, food additives, malabsorption syndromes (celiac disease, pancreatic insufficiency)
History: bloody stools, medications, recent antibiotics, recent travel, family history, floating stools, relationship to food intake, surgical history (cholecystectomy, bowel resections) sexual history, recent hospitalization
Medications
Yes
No
Acid-reducing agents (PPIs, H2 blockers), antacids (containing magnesium), antibiotics, NSAIDs, colchicine, herbal medications, vitamin and mineral supplements, antineoplastic agents, antiretroviral agents, sorbitol, fructose abuse, chronic laxative abuse
Labs: stool studies (culture, Clostridium difficile, ova + parasites) TSH, glucose, fecal fat, celiac serologies (TTG IgA), HIV
Abnormal
Normal
Stool positive for ova and parasites—parasitic infections (e.g., Cryptosporidium, Giardia, Microsporidium)
Positive C. difficile antigen/toxin or PCR—C. difficile infection
Positive fecal fat—see "Malabsorption" algorithm.
Hyperthyroidism
Diabetes
Positive celiac serologies (TTG, IgA, antiendomysial antibodies)
Positive stool cultures—bacterial infection (Escherichia coli, Salmonella, Shigella, Campylobacter)
Upper endoscopy to confirm diagnosis of celiac disease
Colonoscopy
Abnormal exam and/or abnormal biopsies
Normal exam and biopsies
Inflammatory bowel diseases, malignancy, ischemic colitis, infectious colitis, microscopic colitis
Irritable bowel syndrome

Lakshmi Devi Nelson Lattimer, MD, and Marie L. Borum, MD, EdD, MPH

Fine KD, Schiller LR. AGA technical review on the evaluation and management of chronic diarrhea. *Gastroenterology.* 1999;(6):1464–1486.

DISCHARGE, VAGINAL

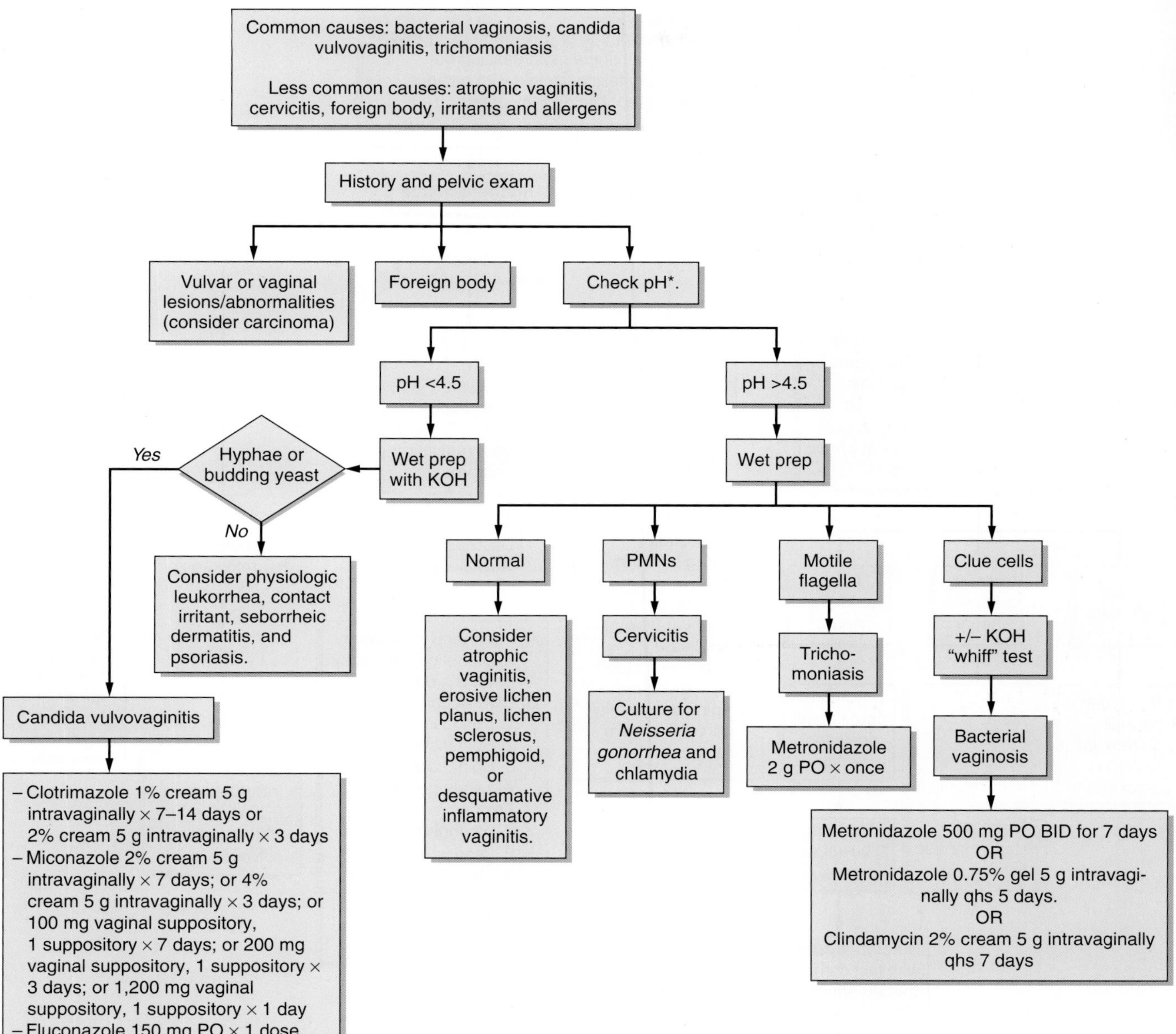

*pH is inaccurate if any blood is present and is less accurate at the extreme of ages.

Nicole Shields, MD

Hainer BL, Gibson MV. Vaginitis. *Am Fam Physician*. 2011;83(7):807–815.

DIZZINESS

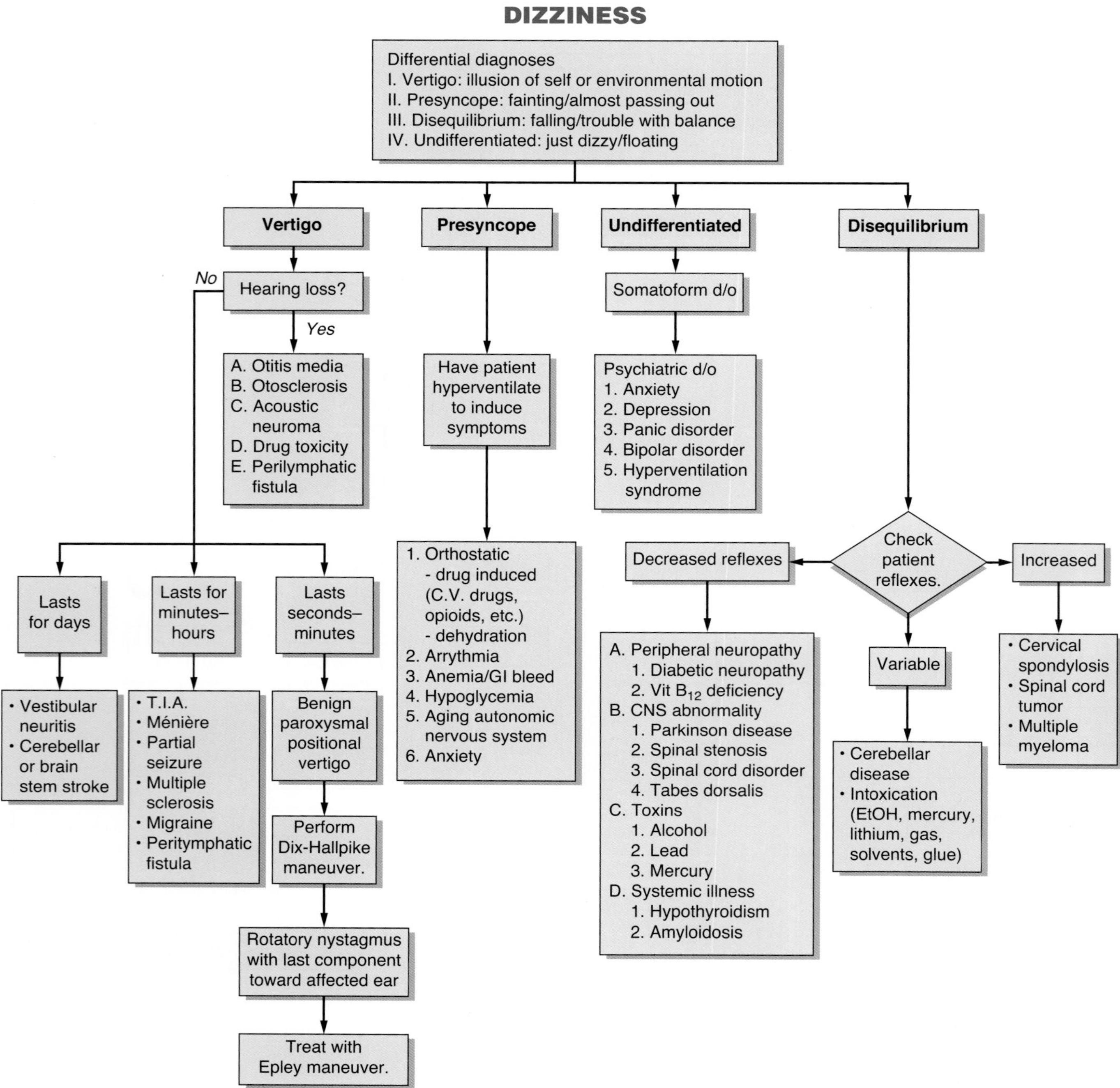

Julie Dahl-Smith, DO, FAAFP, DABMA, Aliyi Aliyi, MD, and Jacqueline Dubose, MD

Post RE, Dickerson LM. Dizziness: a diagnostic approach. *Am Fam Physician*. 2010;82(4):361–368.

DYSPEPSIA

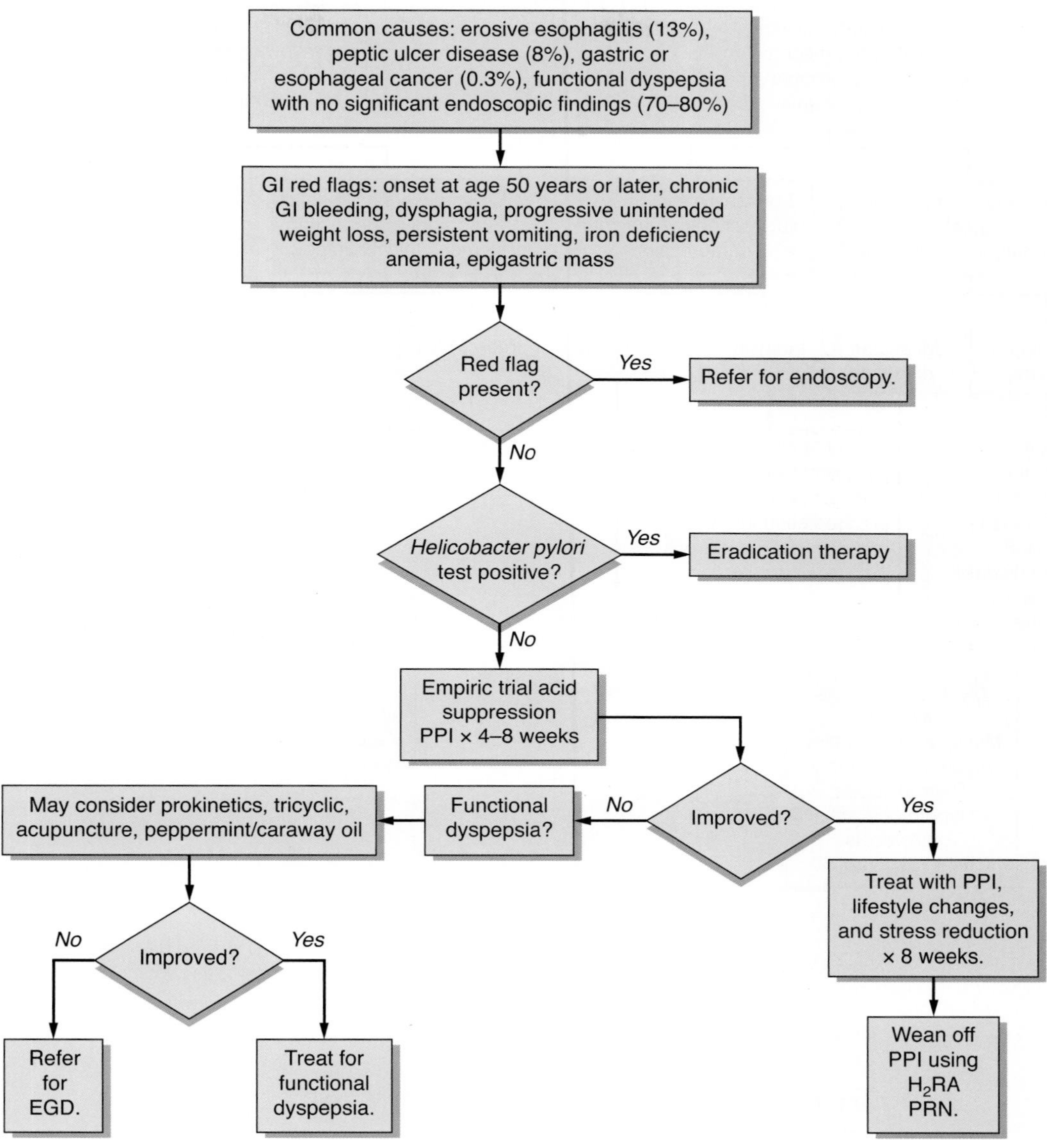

Jennifer L. Hamilton, MD, PhD, FAAFP

Ford AC, Moayyedi P. Dyspepsia. *BMJ*. 2013;347:f5059.

DYSPHAGIA

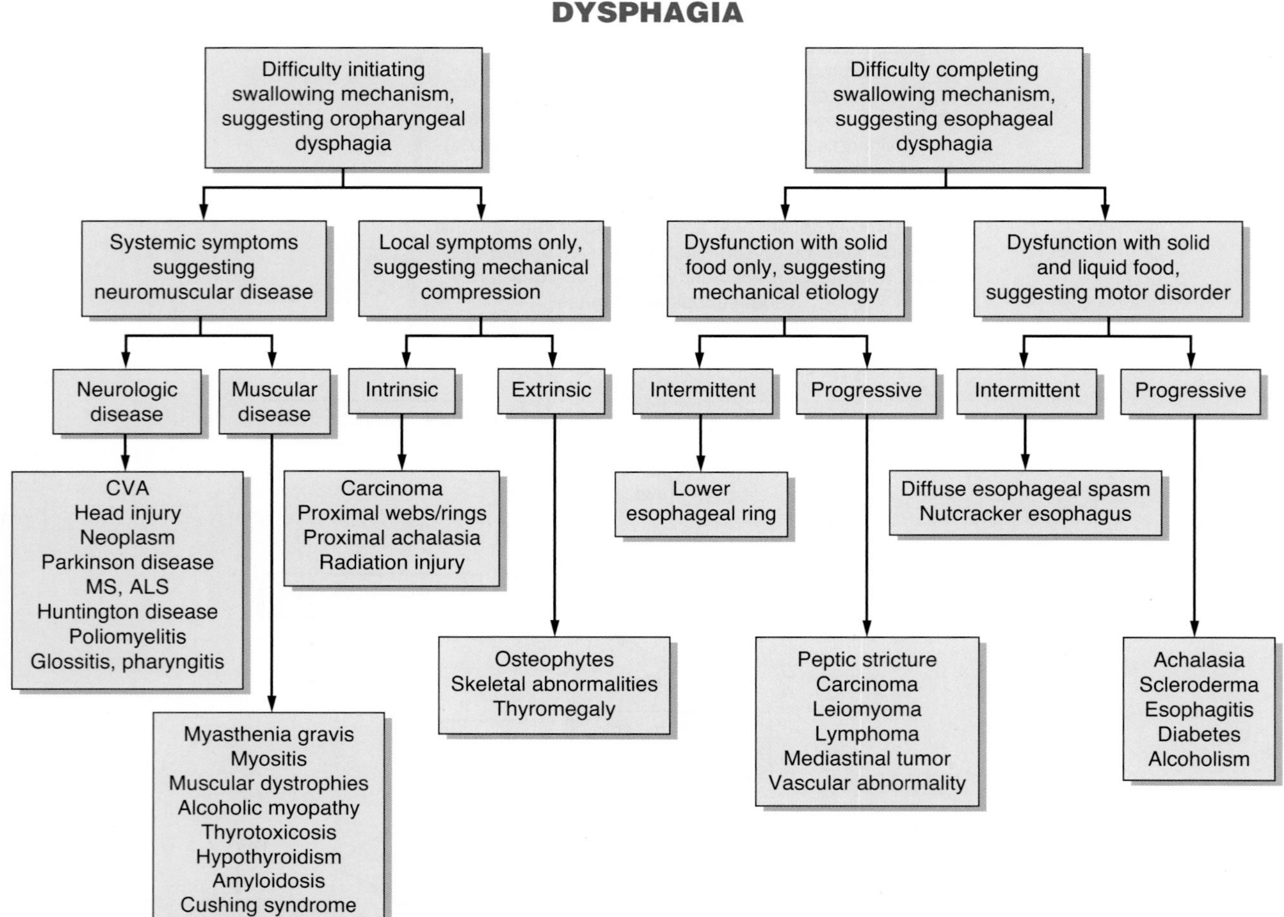

Parag Goyal, MD

Lind CD. Dysphagia: evaluation and treatment. *Gastroenterol Clin North Am*. 2003;32(2):553–575.

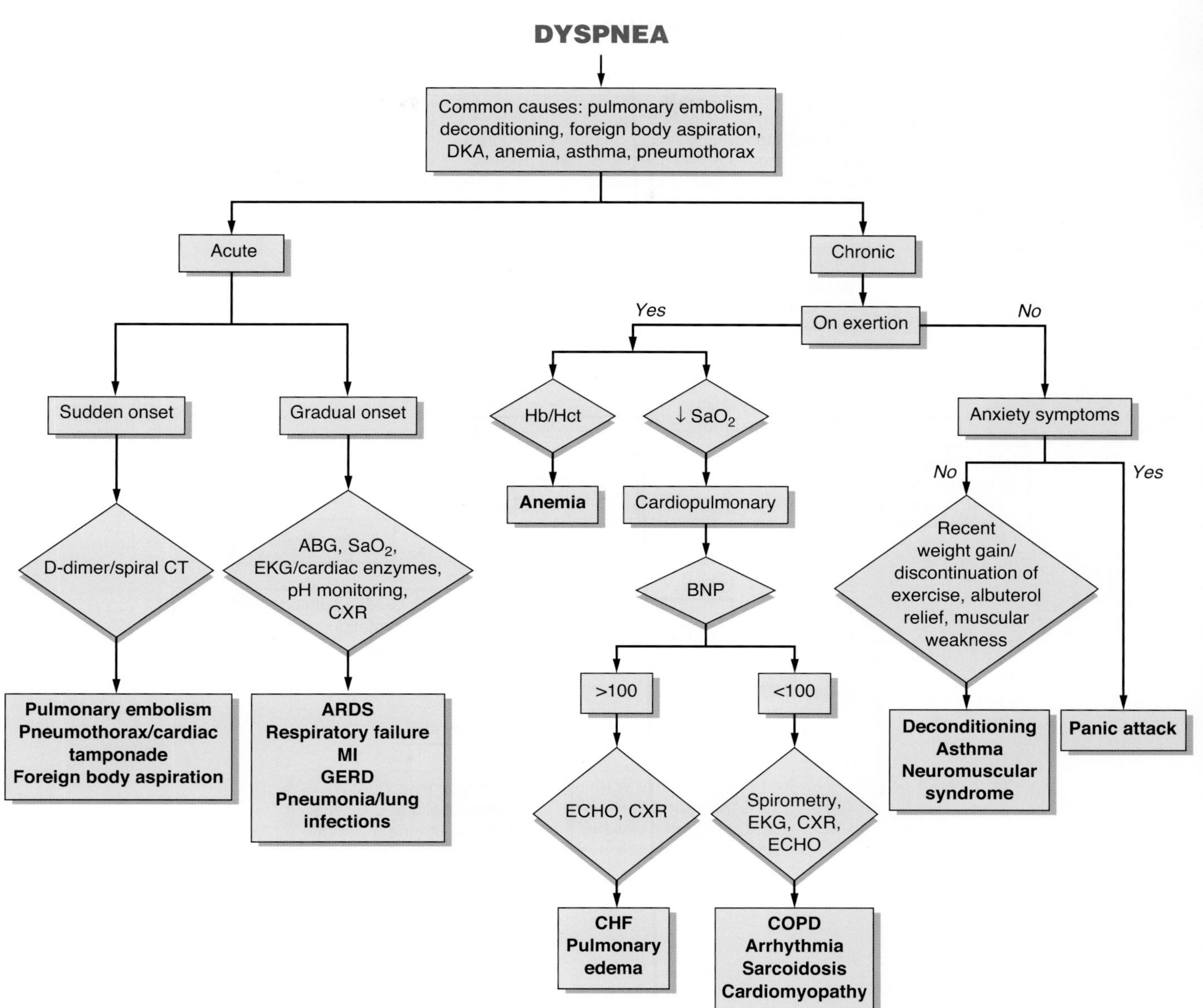

Onameyore Utuama, MD, MPH, Folashade Omole, MD, FAAFP, and Charles Sow, MD, MSCR

Parshall MB, Schwartzstein RM, Adams L, et al. American Thoracic Society Committee on Dyspnea. An official American Thoracic Society statement: update on the mechanisms, assessment, and management of dyspnea. *Am J Respir Crit Care Med.* 2012;185(4):435–452.

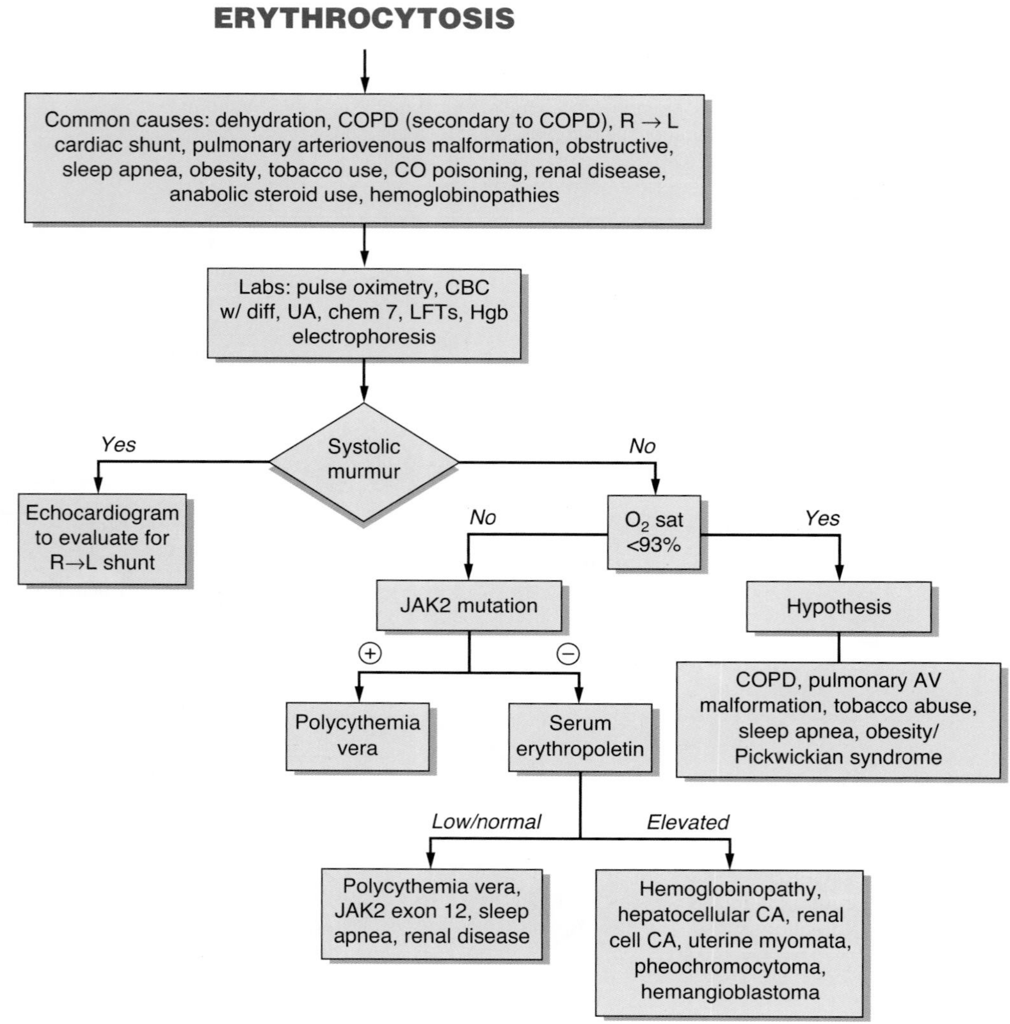

Alexis Ramirez, MD and L. Michael Snyder, MD

Tefferi A. JAK2 mutations in polycythemia vera–molecular mechanisms and clinical applications. *N Engl J Med.* 2007;356(5):444–445.

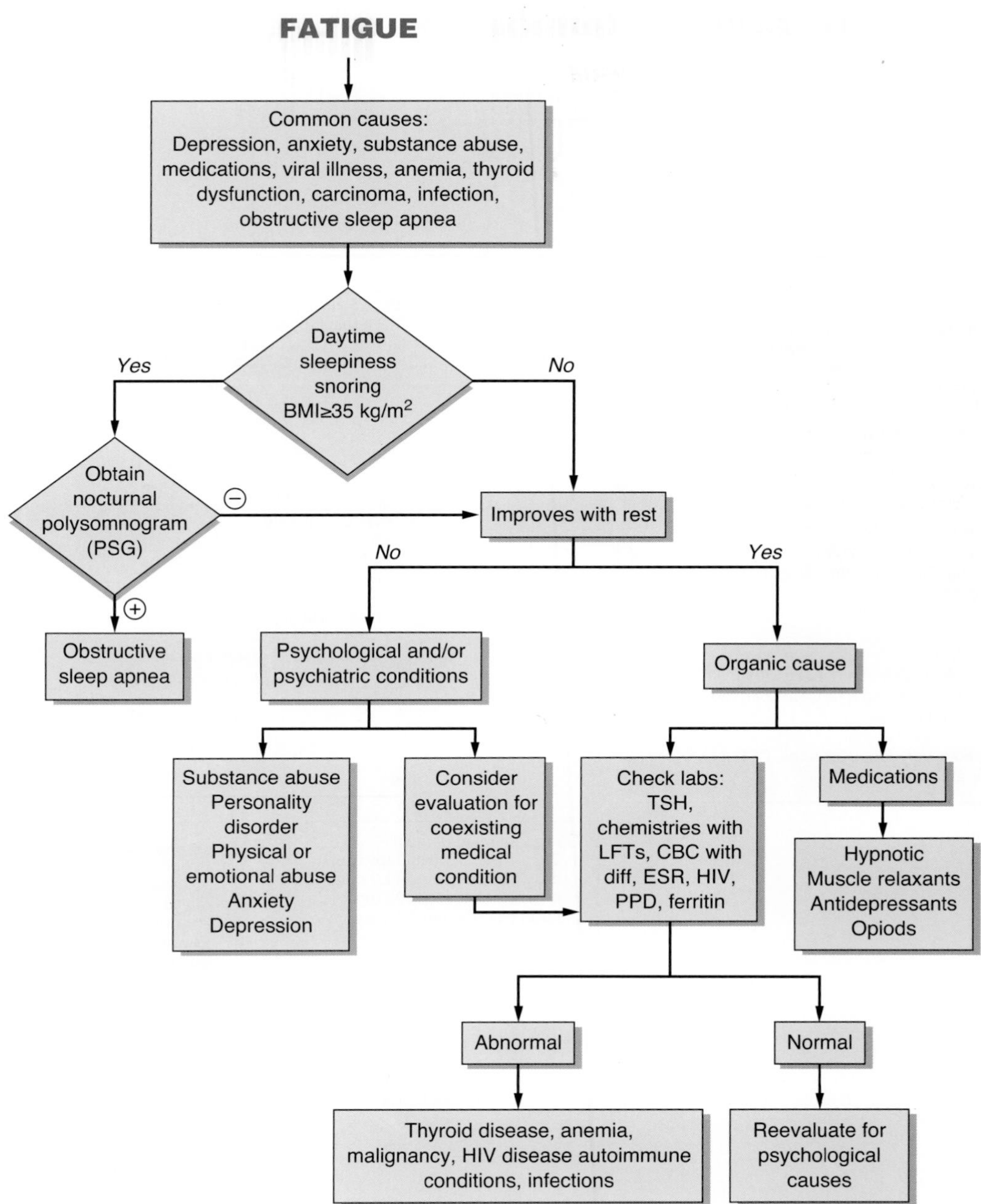

Bharat Gopal, MD, MPH

Rosenthal, TC, Majeroni BA, Pretorius R, et al. Fatigue: An overview. *Am Fam Physician.* 2008:78(10). 1173–1179.

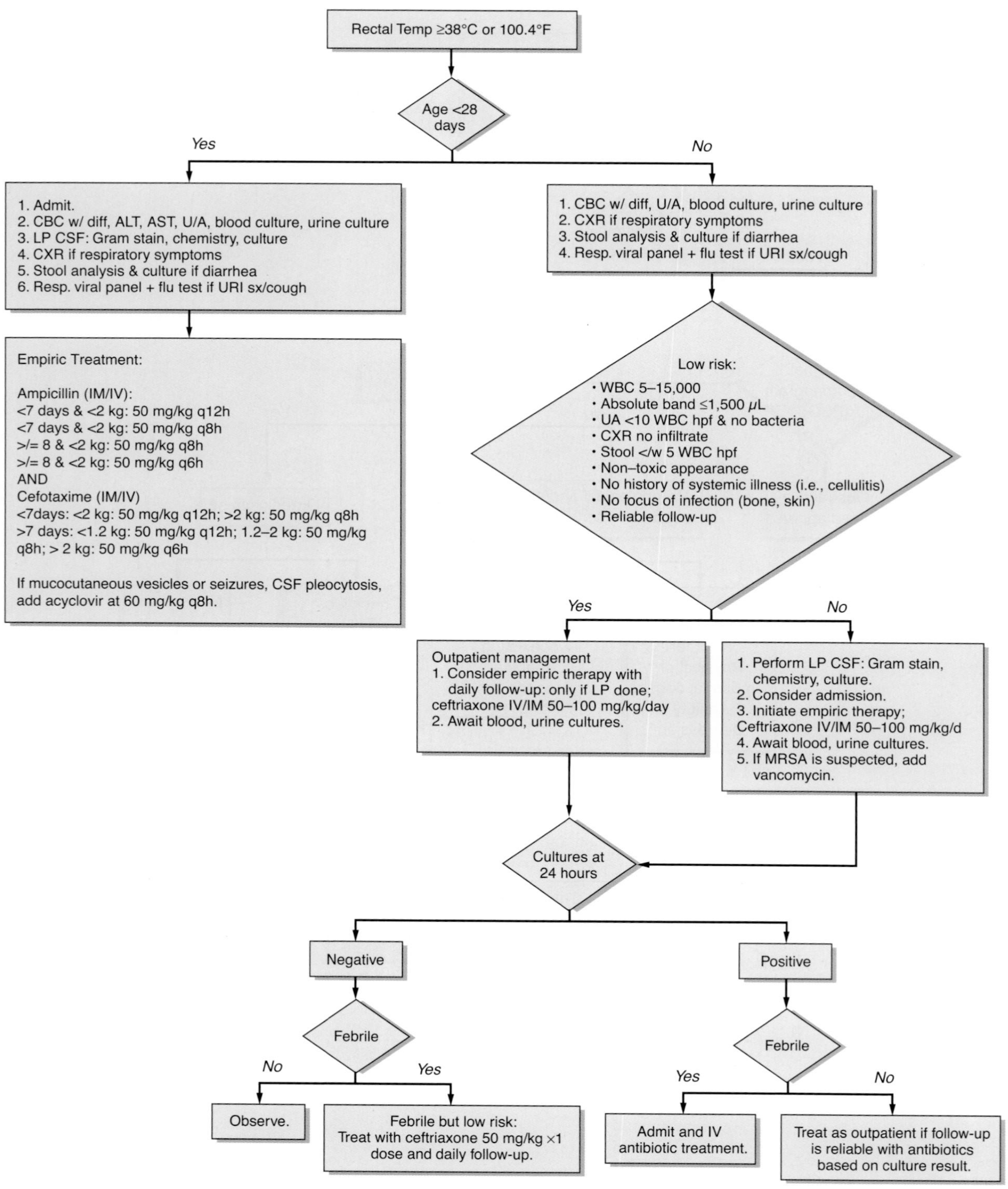
FEVER IN THE FIRST 3 MONTHS OF LIFE
Rectal Temp ≥38°C or 100.4°F
Age <28 days
Yes
No
1. Admit.
2. CBC w/ diff, ALT, AST, U/A, blood culture, urine culture
3. LP CSF: Gram stain, chemistry, culture
4. CXR if respiratory symptoms
5. Stool analysis & culture if diarrhea
6. Resp. viral panel + flu test if URI sx/cough
Empiric Treatment:
Ampicillin (IM/IV):
<7 days & <2 kg: 50 mg/kg q12h
<7 days & <2 kg: 50 mg/kg q8h
>/= 8 & <2 kg: 50 mg/kg q8h
>/= 8 & <2 kg: 50 mg/kg q6h
AND
Cefotaxime (IM/IV)
<7days: <2 kg: 50 mg/kg q12h; >2 kg: 50 mg/kg q8h
>7 days: <1.2 kg: 50 mg/kg q12h; 1.2–2 kg: 50 mg/kg q8h; > 2 kg: 50 mg/kg q6h
If mucocutaneous vesicles or seizures, CSF pleocytosis, add acyclovir at 60 mg/kg q8h.
1. CBC w/ diff, U/A, blood culture, urine culture
2. CXR if respiratory symptoms
3. Stool analysis & culture if diarrhea
4. Resp. viral panel + flu test if URI sx/cough
Low risk:
• WBC 5–15,000
• Absolute band ≤1,500 μL
• UA <10 WBC hpf & no bacteria
• CXR no infiltrate
• Stool </w 5 WBC hpf
• Non–toxic appearance
• No history of systemic illness (i.e., cellulitis)
• No focus of infection (bone, skin)
• Reliable follow-up
Yes
No
Outpatient management
1. Consider empiric therapy with daily follow-up: only if LP done; ceftriaxone IV/IM 50–100 mg/kg/day
2. Await blood, urine cultures.
1. Perform LP CSF: Gram stain, chemistry, culture.
2. Consider admission.
3. Initiate empiric therapy; Ceftriaxone IV/IM 50–100 mg/kg/d
4. Await blood, urine cultures.
5. If MRSA is suspected, add vancomycin.
Cultures at 24 hours
Negative
Positive
Febrile
No
Yes
Observe.
Febrile but low risk: Treat with ceftriaxone 50 mg/kg ×1 dose and daily follow-up.
Febrile
Yes
No
Admit and IV antibiotic treatment.
Treat as outpatient if follow-up is reliable with antibiotics based on culture result.

Robyn D. Wing, MD and William Jerry Durbin, MD

American College of Emergency Physicians Clinical Policies Committee, American College of Emergency Physicians Clinical Policies Subcommittee on Pediatric Fever. Clinical policy for children younger than three years presenting to the emergency department with fever. *Ann Emerg Med.* 2003;42(4):530–545.

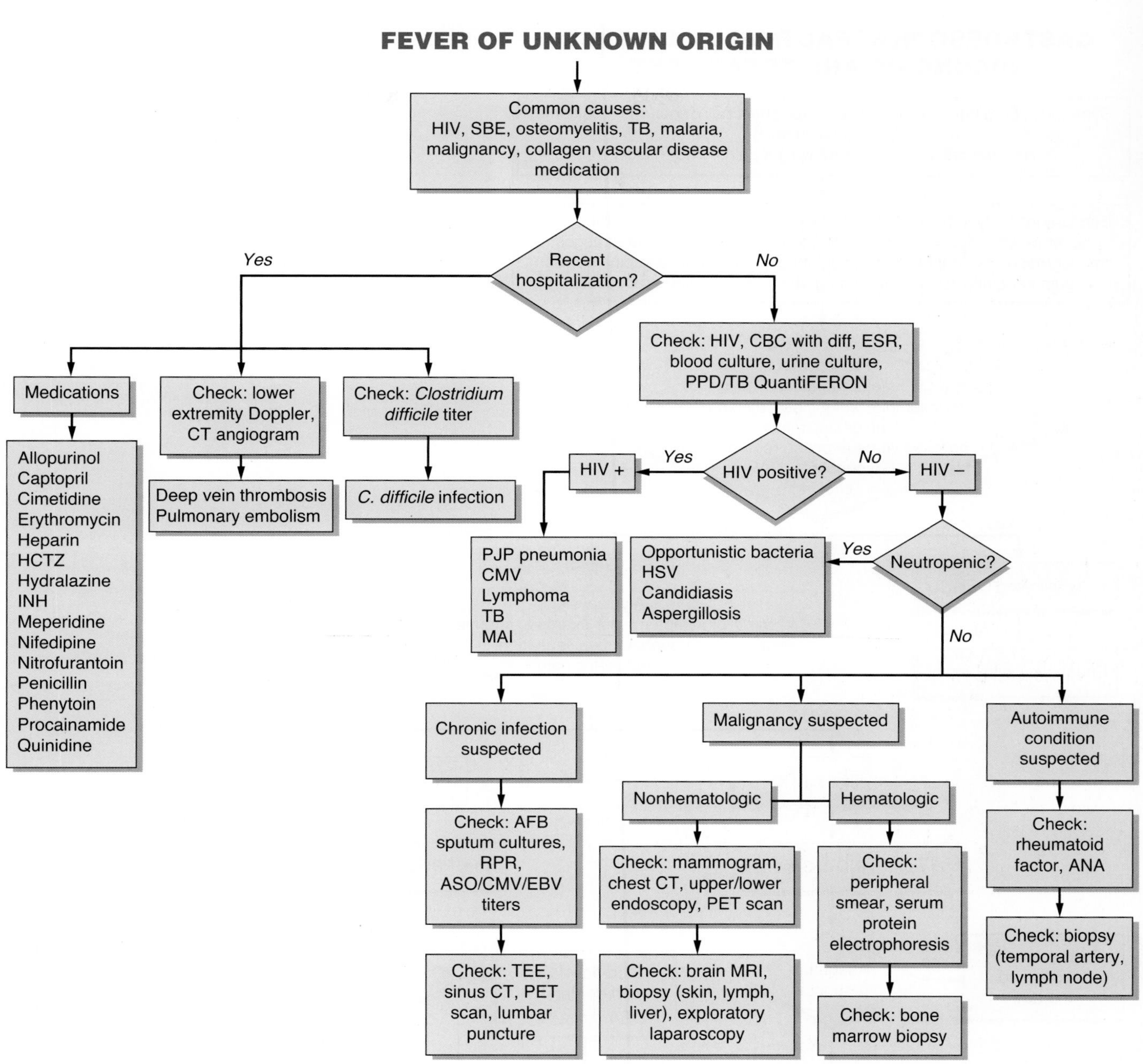

Rachelle E. Toman, MD, PhD, Joshua Fischer, MD, PhD, and Koryn Johnston, DO

Roth AR, Basello GM. Approach to the adult patient with fever of unknown origin. *Am Fam Physician.* 2003;68(11):2223–2228.

GASTROESOPHAGEAL REFLUX DISEASE, DIAGNOSIS AND TREATMENT

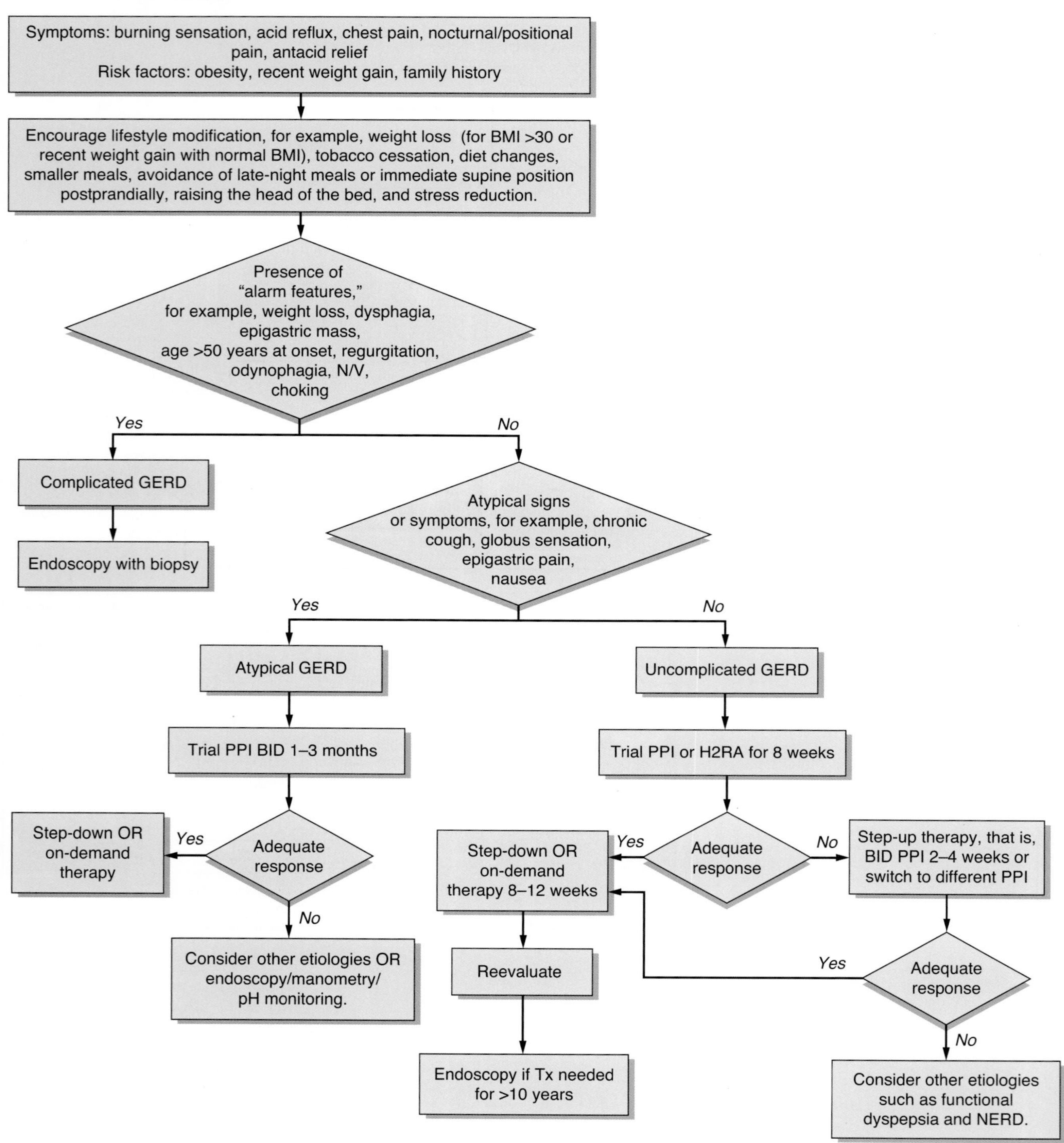

Suma Chennubhotla, MD, Amaninderapal S. Ghotra, MD, and Thomas L. Abell, MD

Katz PO, Gerson LB, Vela MF. Guidelines for the diagnosis and management of gastroesophageal reflux disease. *Am J Gastroenterol.* 2013;108(3):308–328.

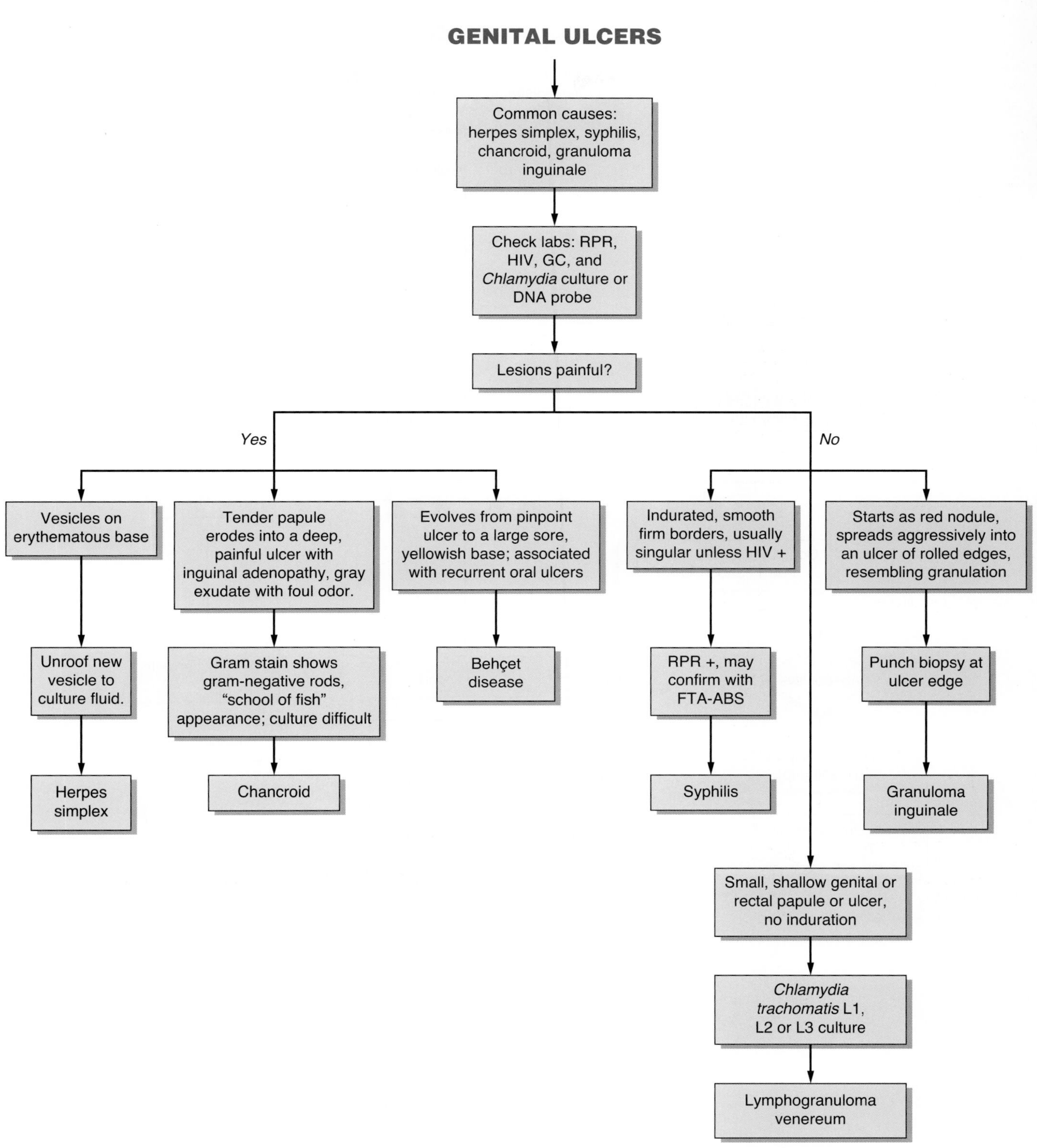

Chidinma Osineme, MD and Midhuna William, MD

Roett M, Mayor M, Uduhiri K. Diagnosis and management of genital ulcers. *Am Fam Physician.* 2012:85(3):254–262.

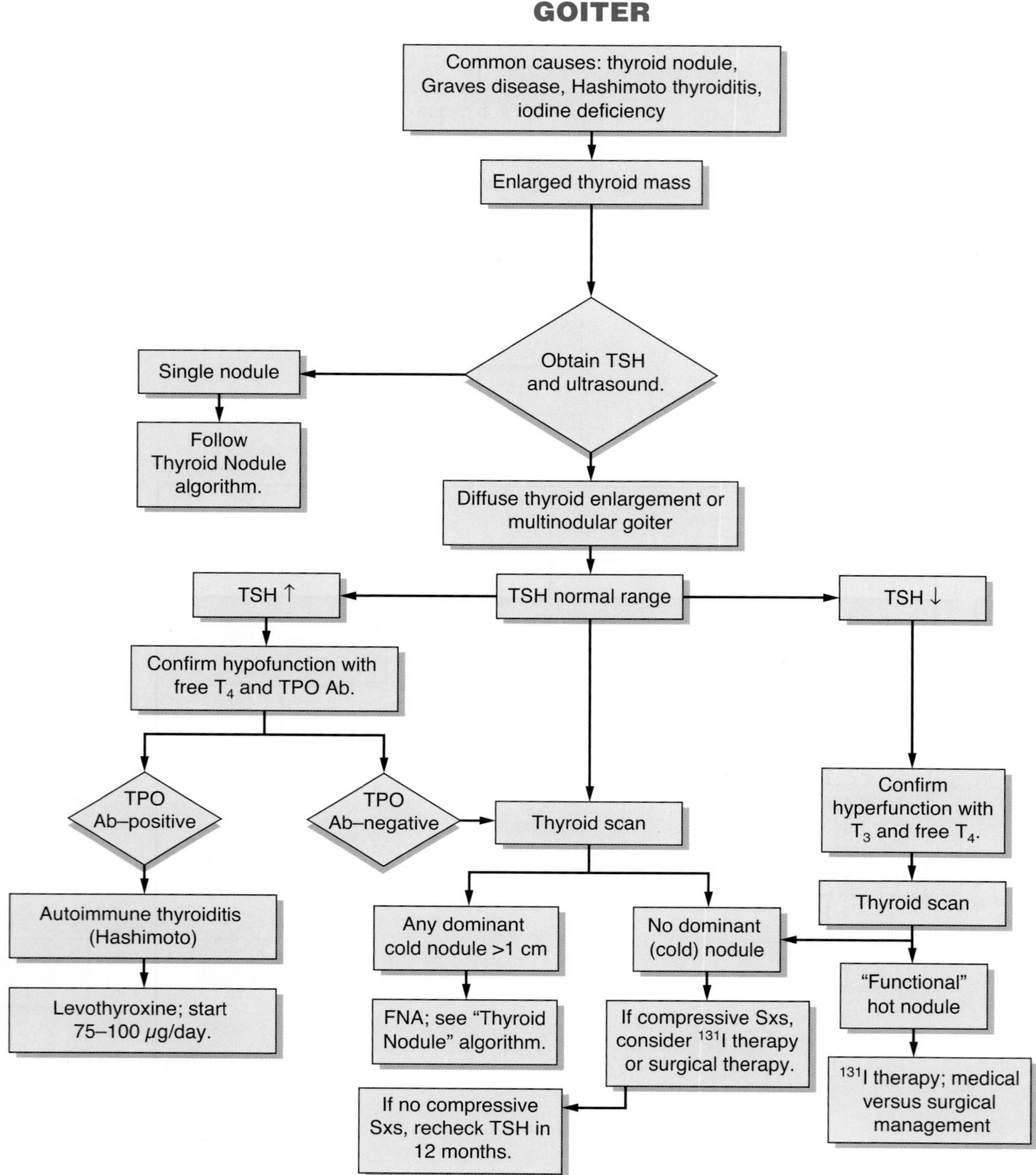

Noah A. Steinberg, PA-C and Scott P. Grogan, DO, MBA, FAAFP

Gharib H, Papini E, Paschke R, et al. American Association of Clinical Endocrinologists, Associazione Medici Endocrinologi, and European Thyroid Association medical guidelines for clinical practice for the diagnosis and management of thyroid nodules. *Endocr Pract.* 2010;16(Suppl 1):1–43.

HEAD INJURY, DIAGNOSIS AND MANAGEMENT

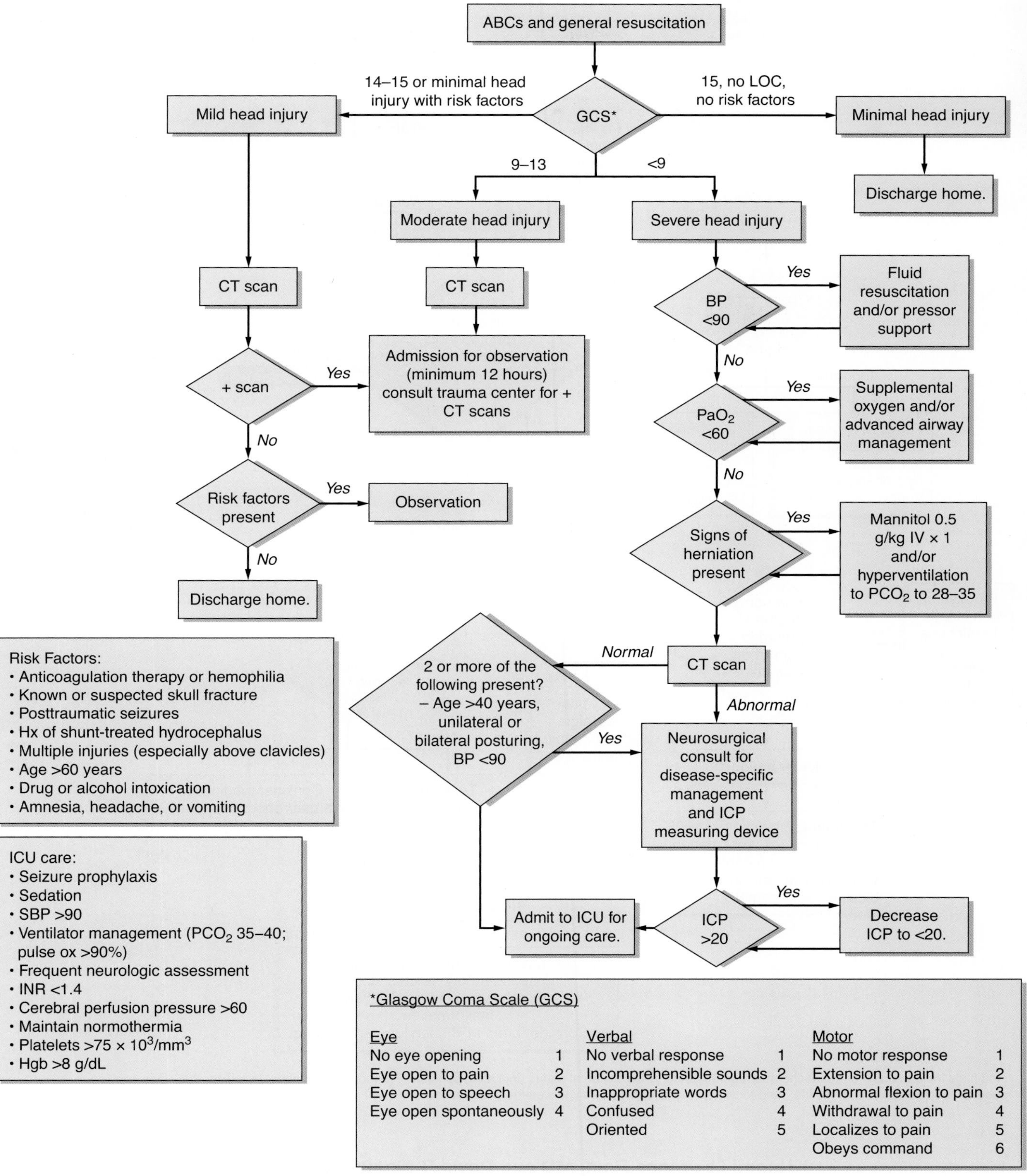

Eye		Verbal		Motor	
No eye opening	1	No verbal response	1	No motor response	1
Eye open to pain	2	Incomprehensible sounds	2	Extension to pain	2
Eye open to speech	3	Inappropriate words	3	Abnormal flexion to pain	3
Eye open spontaneously	4	Confused	4	Withdrawal to pain	4
		Oriented	5	Localizes to pain	5
				Obeys command	6

Michael J. Gray, MD, MA, MS, ATC

Swadron SP, LeRoux P, Smith WS, et al. Emergency neurological life support: traumatic brain injury. *Neurocit Care*. 2012;17:S112–S121.

HEADACHE, CHRONIC

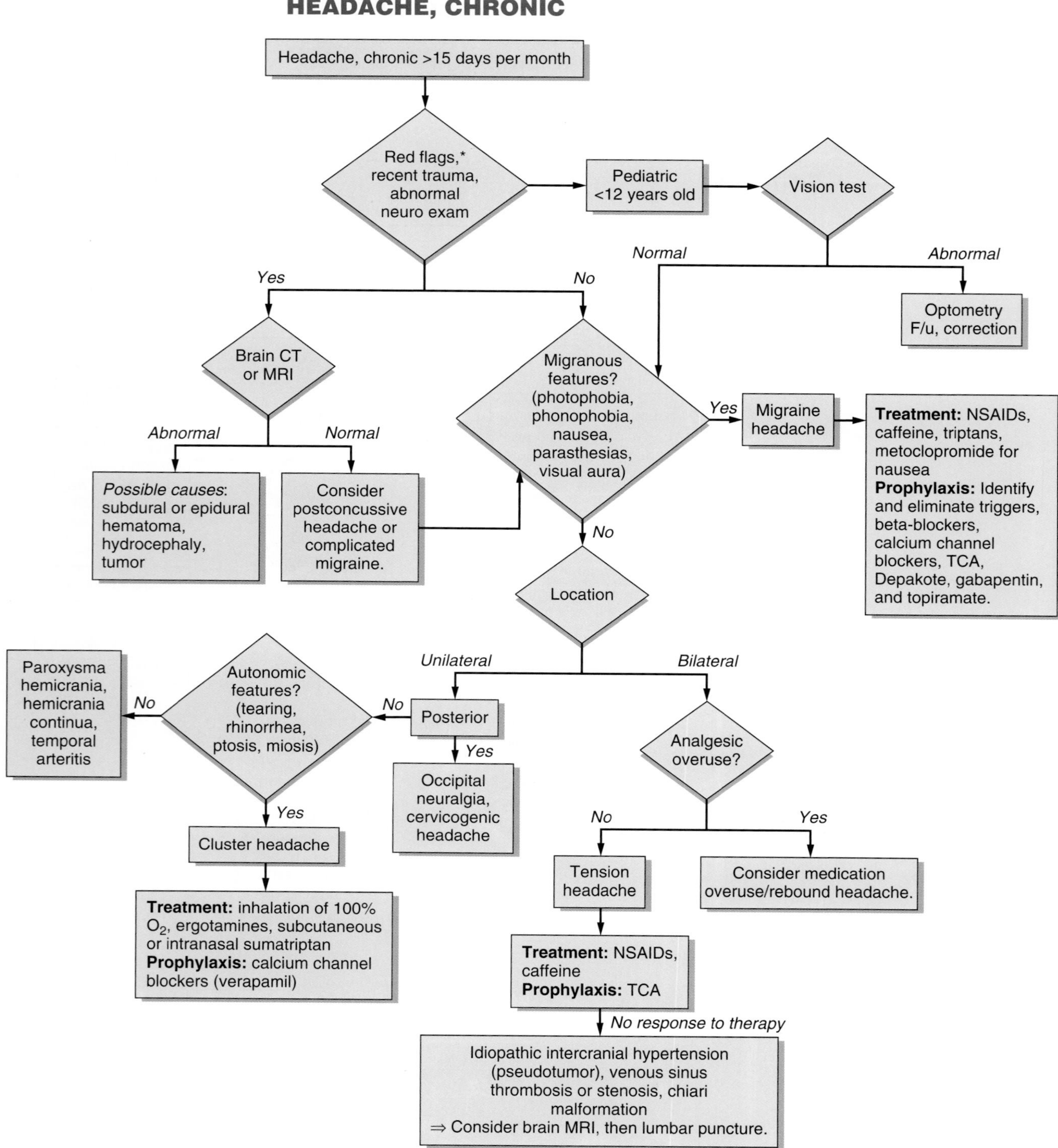

*Red flags include onset of headache after age 50 years, altered mental status (including confusion, personality changes), papilledema, report of "worst headache of my life," and focal neurologic deficits such as weakness or ataxia.

Naomi Lawrence-Reid, MD and David B. Sommer, MD, MPH

National Guidelines Clearinghouse. *Diagnosis and Treatment of Headache*. http://www.guideline.gov/content.aspx?id=14440&search=chronic+headache. Accessed 2014; Sobri M, Lamont AC, Alias NA, et al. Red flags in patients presenting with headache: clinical indications for neuroimaging. *Br J Radiol*. 2003;76(908):532–535.

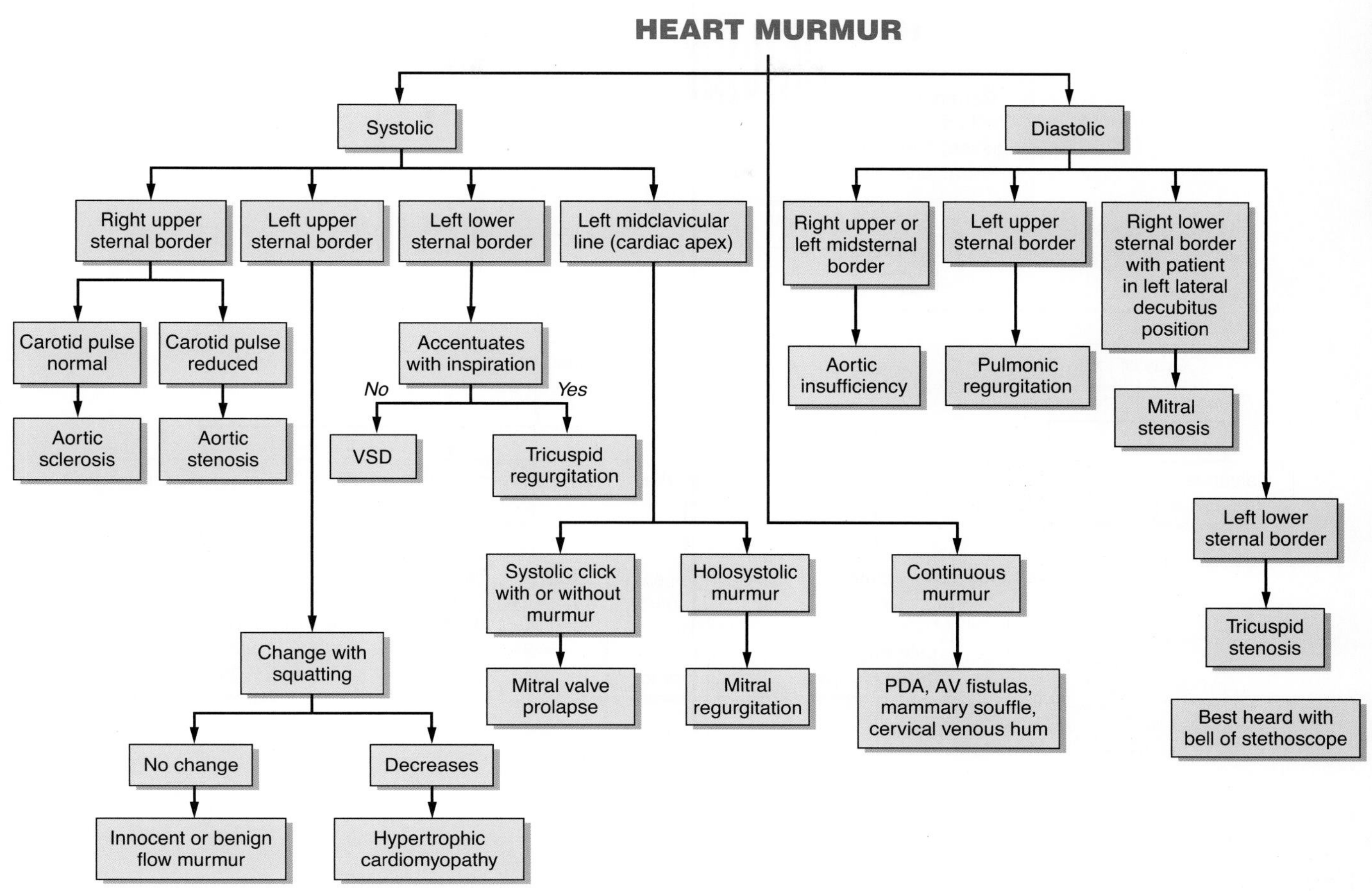

Nirmanmoh Bhatia, MD, Amaninderapal S. Ghotra, MD, and Marcus F. Stoddard, MD

Bonow RO, Carabello BA, Chatterjee K, et al. 2008 Focused update incorporated into the ACC/AHA 2006 guidelines for the management of patients with valvular heart disease: a report of the American College of Cardiology/American Heart Association Task Force on Practice Guidelines (Writing Committee to Revise the 1998 Guidelines for the Management of Patients With Valvular Heart Disease): endorsed by the Society of Cardiovascular Anesthesiologists, Society for Cardiovascular Angiography and Interventions, and Society of Thoracic Surgeons. *Circulation* 2008;118(15):e523–e661.

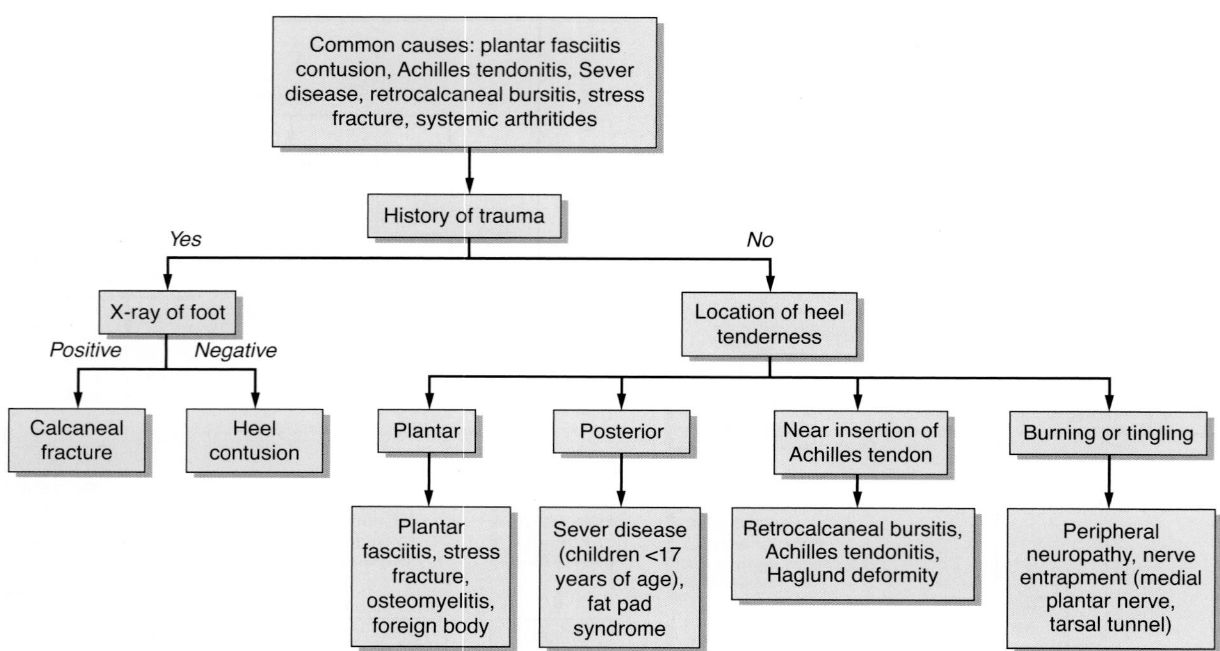

Alexei DeCastro, MD

Tu P, Bytomski J. Diagnosis of heel pain. *Am Fam Physician.* 2011;84(8):909–916.

HEMATEMESIS (BLEEDING, UPPER GASTROINTESTINAL)

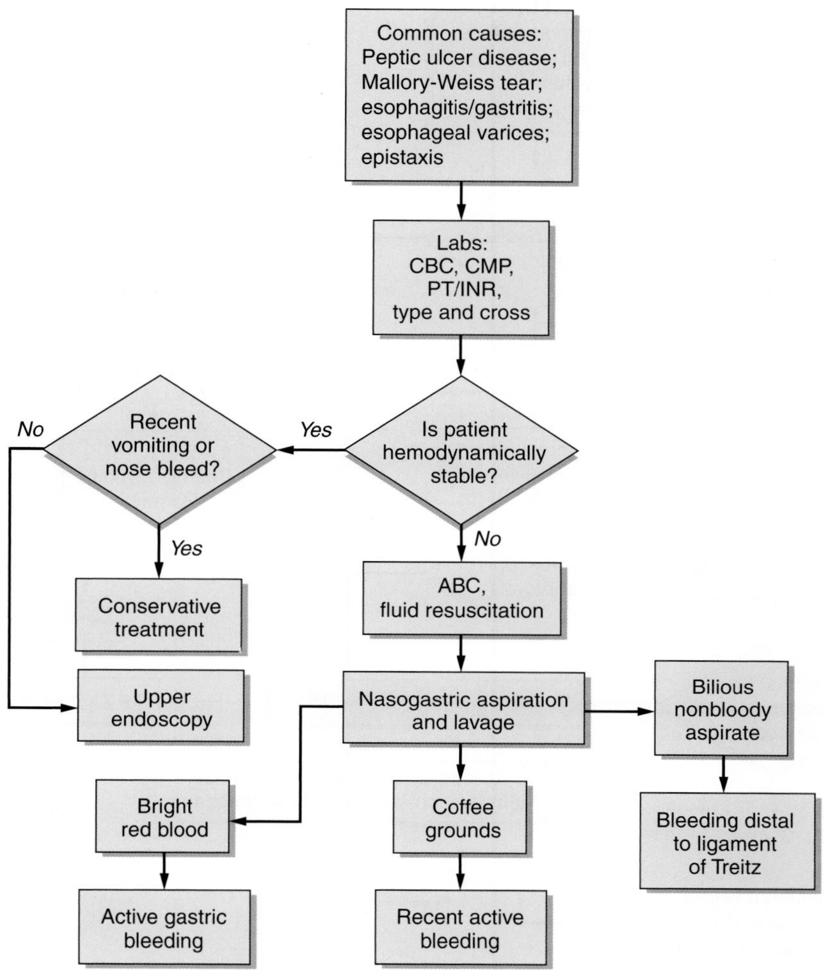

Sanjeev Sharma, MD

Barkun A, Fallone CA, Chiba N, et al. A Canadian clinical practice algorithm for the management of patients with nonvariceal upper gastrointestinal bleeding. *Can J Gastroenterol.* 2004;18(10):605–609.

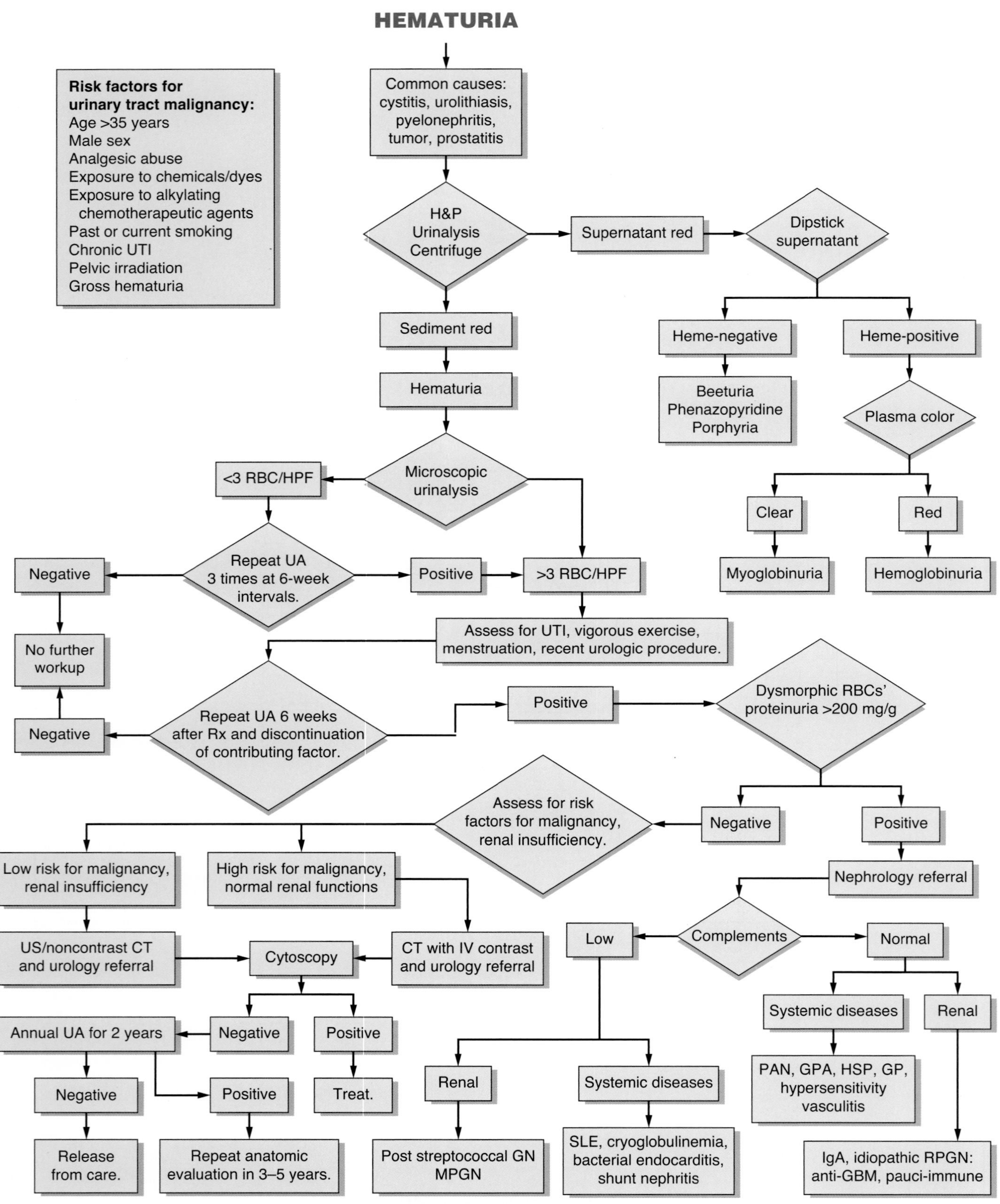

Krishna Manda, MD, MRCP, Nathalee Kong, MD, and Marie Anne Sosa, MD

Sharp VJ, Barnes KT, Erickson BA. Assessment of asymptomatic microscopic hematuria in adults. *Am Fam Physician.* 2013;88(11):747–754.

HEPATOMEGALY

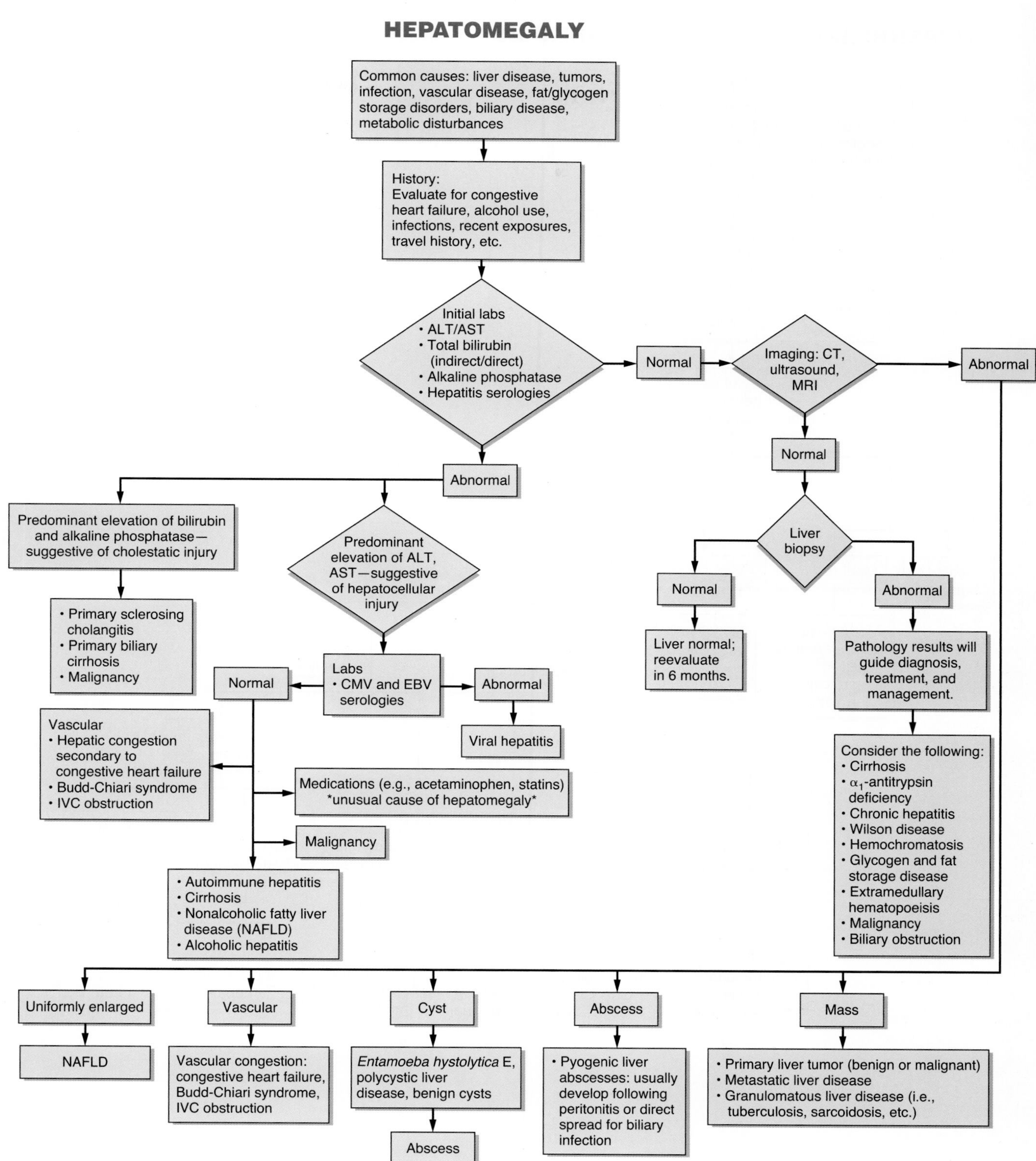

Neha Jakhete, MD and Marie L. Borum, MD, EdD, MPH

Starr SP, Raines D. Cirrhosis: diagnosis, management, and prevention. *Am Fam Physician.* 2011;84(12):1353–1359.

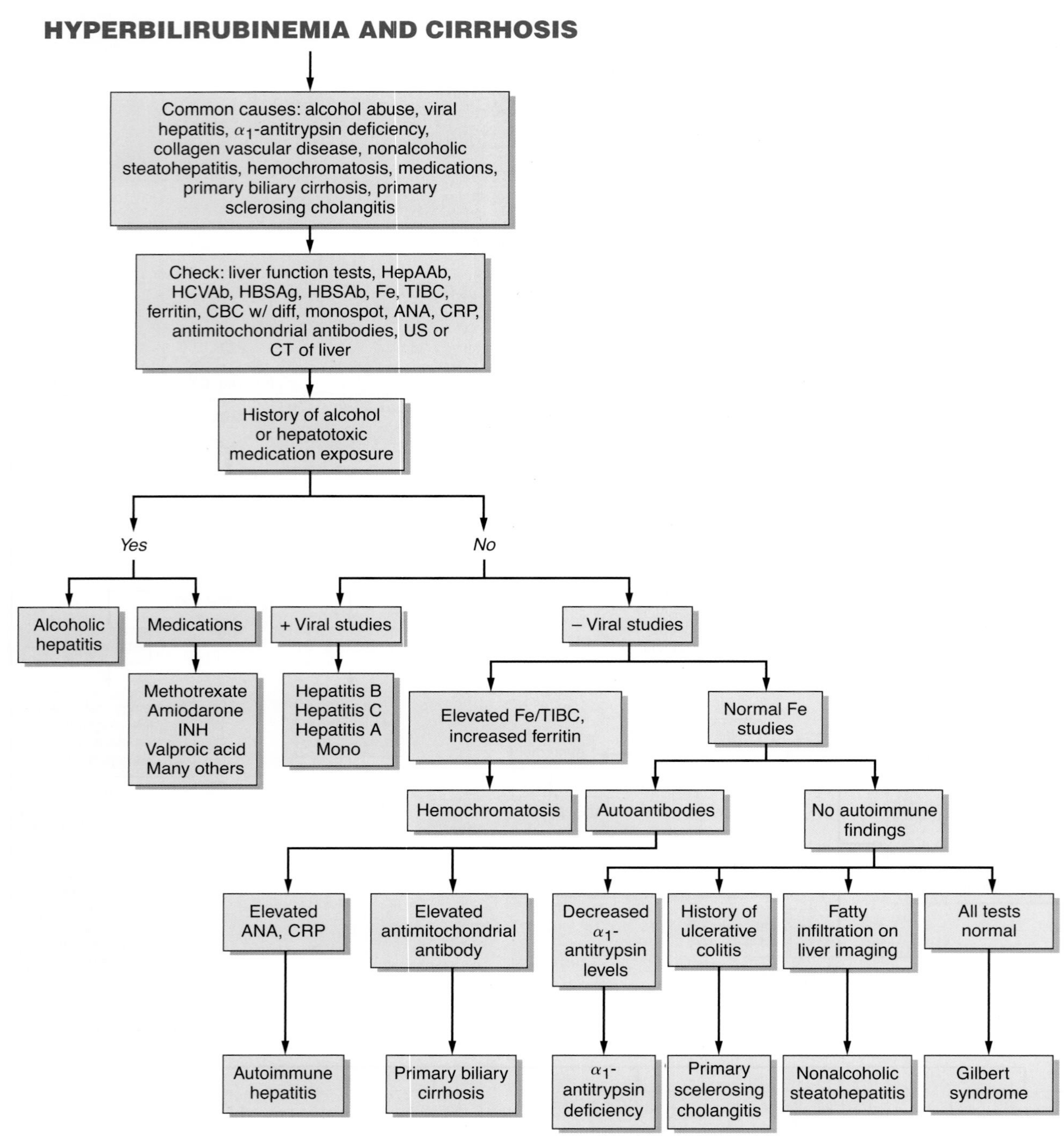

Robert A. Baldor, MD, FAAFP and Alan M. Ehrlich, MD

Porter ML, Dennis BL. Hyperbilirubinemia in the term newborn. *Am Fam Physician*. 2002;65(4):599–606.

HYPERCALCEMIA

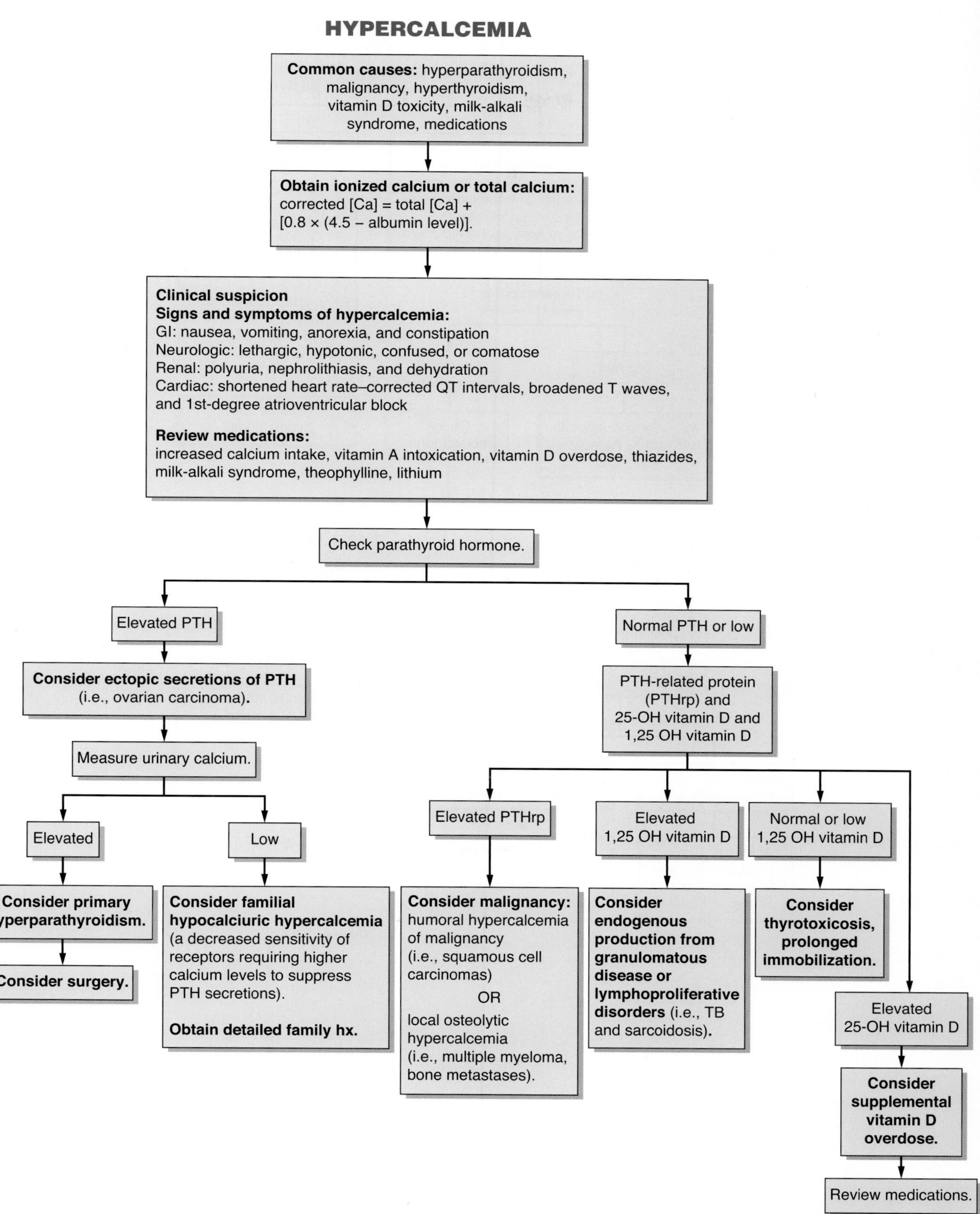
Common causes: hyperparathyroidism, malignancy, hyperthyroidism, vitamin D toxicity, milk-alkali syndrome, medications
Obtain ionized calcium or total calcium: corrected [Ca] = total [Ca] + [0.8 × (4.5 – albumin level)].
Clinical suspicion
Signs and symptoms of hypercalcemia:
GI: nausea, vomiting, anorexia, and constipation
Neurologic: lethargic, hypotonic, confused, or comatose
Renal: polyuria, nephrolithiasis, and dehydration
Cardiac: shortened heart rate–corrected QT intervals, broadened T waves, and 1st-degree atrioventricular block
Review medications:
increased calcium intake, vitamin A intoxication, vitamin D overdose, thiazides, milk-alkali syndrome, theophylline, lithium
Check parathyroid hormone.
Elevated PTH
Consider ectopic secretions of PTH (i.e., ovarian carcinoma).
Measure urinary calcium.
Elevated
Consider primary hyperparathyroidism.
Consider surgery.
Low
Consider familial hypocalciuric hypercalcemia (a decreased sensitivity of receptors requiring higher calcium levels to suppress PTH secretions).
Obtain detailed family hx.
Normal PTH or low
PTH-related protein (PTHrp) and 25-OH vitamin D and 1,25 OH vitamin D
Elevated PTHrp
Consider malignancy: humoral hypercalcemia of malignancy (i.e., squamous cell carcinomas)
OR
local osteolytic hypercalcemia (i.e., multiple myeloma, bone metastases).
Elevated 1,25 OH vitamin D
Consider endogenous production from granulomatous disease or lymphoproliferative disorders (i.e., TB and sarcoidosis).
Normal or low 1,25 OH vitamin D
Consider thyrotoxicosis, prolonged immobilization.
Elevated 25-OH vitamin D
Consider supplemental vitamin D overdose.
Review medications.

Deborah A. Lardner, DO, DTM&H and Michael Passafaro, DO, DTM&H, FACEP, FACOEP

Kacprowicz RF, Lloyd JD. Electrolyte complications of malignancy. *Emerg Med Clin North Am.* 2009;27(2):257–269.

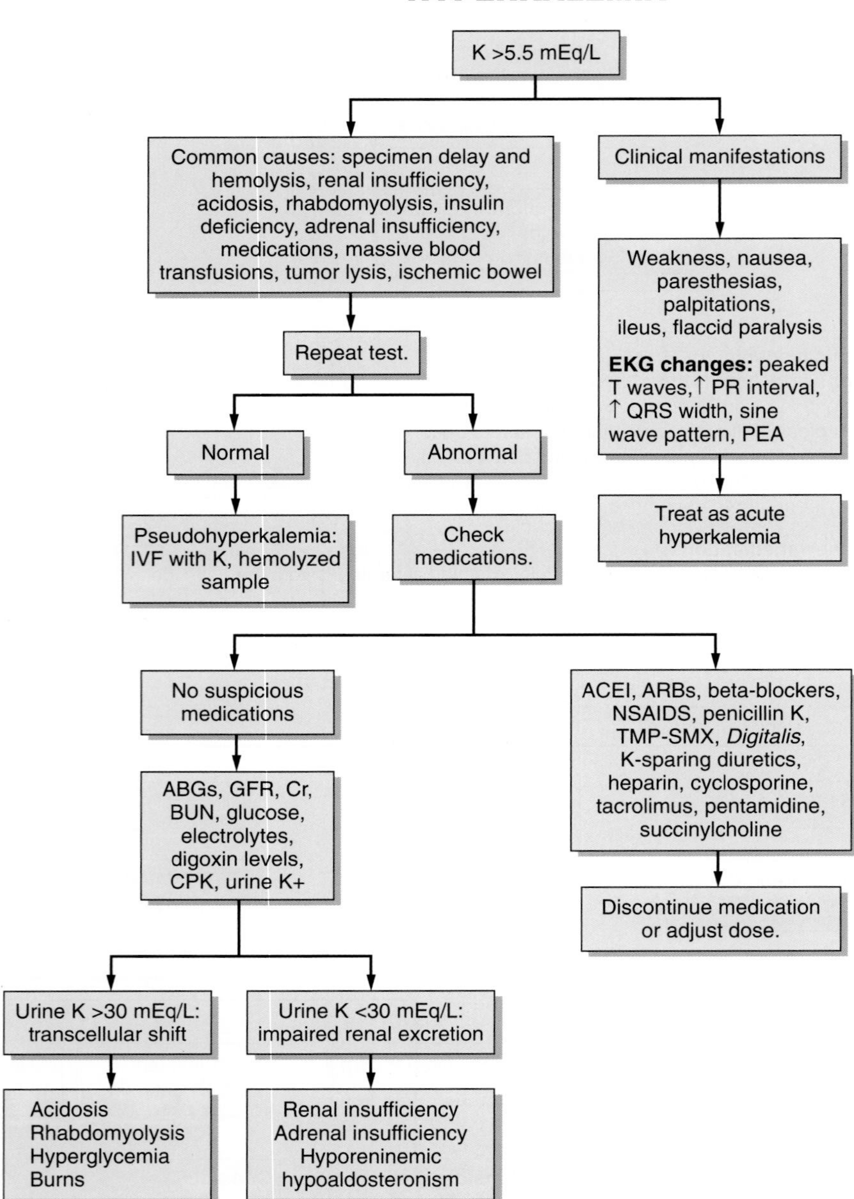
HYPERKALEMIA
K >5.5 mEq/L
Common causes: specimen delay and hemolysis, renal insufficiency, acidosis, rhabdomyolysis, insulin deficiency, adrenal insufficiency, medications, massive blood transfusions, tumor lysis, ischemic bowel
Clinical manifestations
Weakness, nausea, paresthesias, palpitations, ileus, flaccid paralysis
EKG changes: peaked T waves, ↑ PR interval, ↑ QRS width, sine wave pattern, PEA
Treat as acute hyperkalemia
Repeat test.
Normal
Abnormal
Pseudohyperkalemia: IVF with K, hemolyzed sample
Check medications.
No suspicious medications
ACEI, ARBs, beta-blockers, NSAIDS, penicillin K, TMP-SMX, Digitalis, K-sparing diuretics, heparin, cyclosporine, tacrolimus, pentamidine, succinylcholine
Discontinue medication or adjust dose.
ABGs, GFR, Cr, BUN, glucose, electrolytes, digoxin levels, CPK, urine K+
Urine K >30 mEq/L: transcellular shift
Urine K <30 mEq/L: impaired renal excretion
Acidosis
Rhabdomyolysis
Hyperglycemia
Burns
Renal insufficiency
Adrenal insufficiency
Hyporeninemic hypoaldosteronism

Rocio Nordfeldt, MD and Felix B. Chang, MD, DABMA, ABIHM

Palmer BF. A physiologic-based approach to the evaluation of a patient with hyperkalemia. *Am J Kidney Dis.* 2010;56(2):387–393.

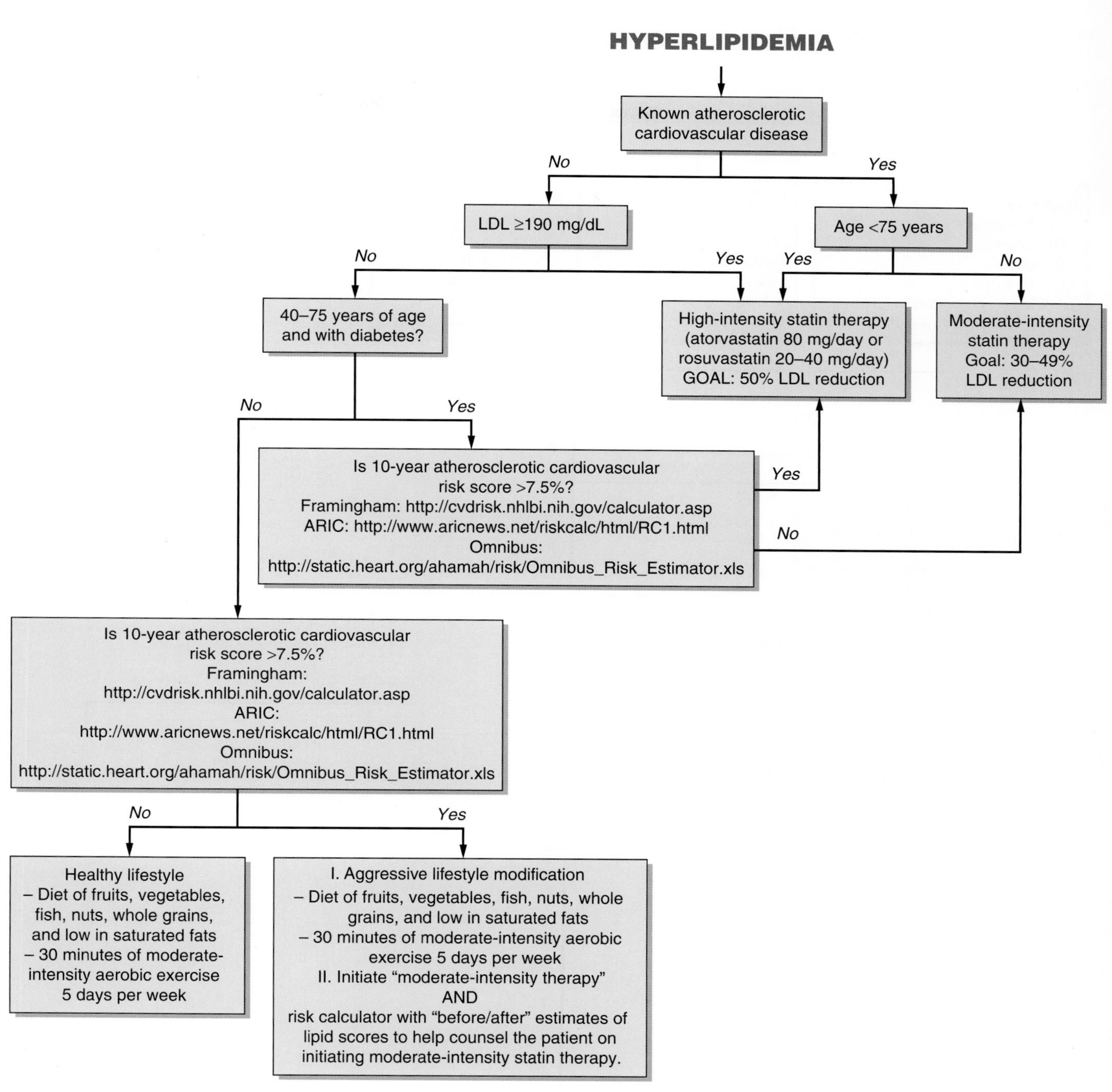

Rade N. Pejic, MD, MMM and Frank J. Domino, MD

Stone NJ, Robinson J, Lichtenstein C, et al. 2013 ACC/AHA guideline on the treatment of blood cholesterol to reduce atherosclerotic cardiovascular risk in adults: a report of the American College of Cardiology/American Heart Association Task Force on Practice Guidelines. *Circulation.* 2014;129(25)(Suppl 2):S1–S45.

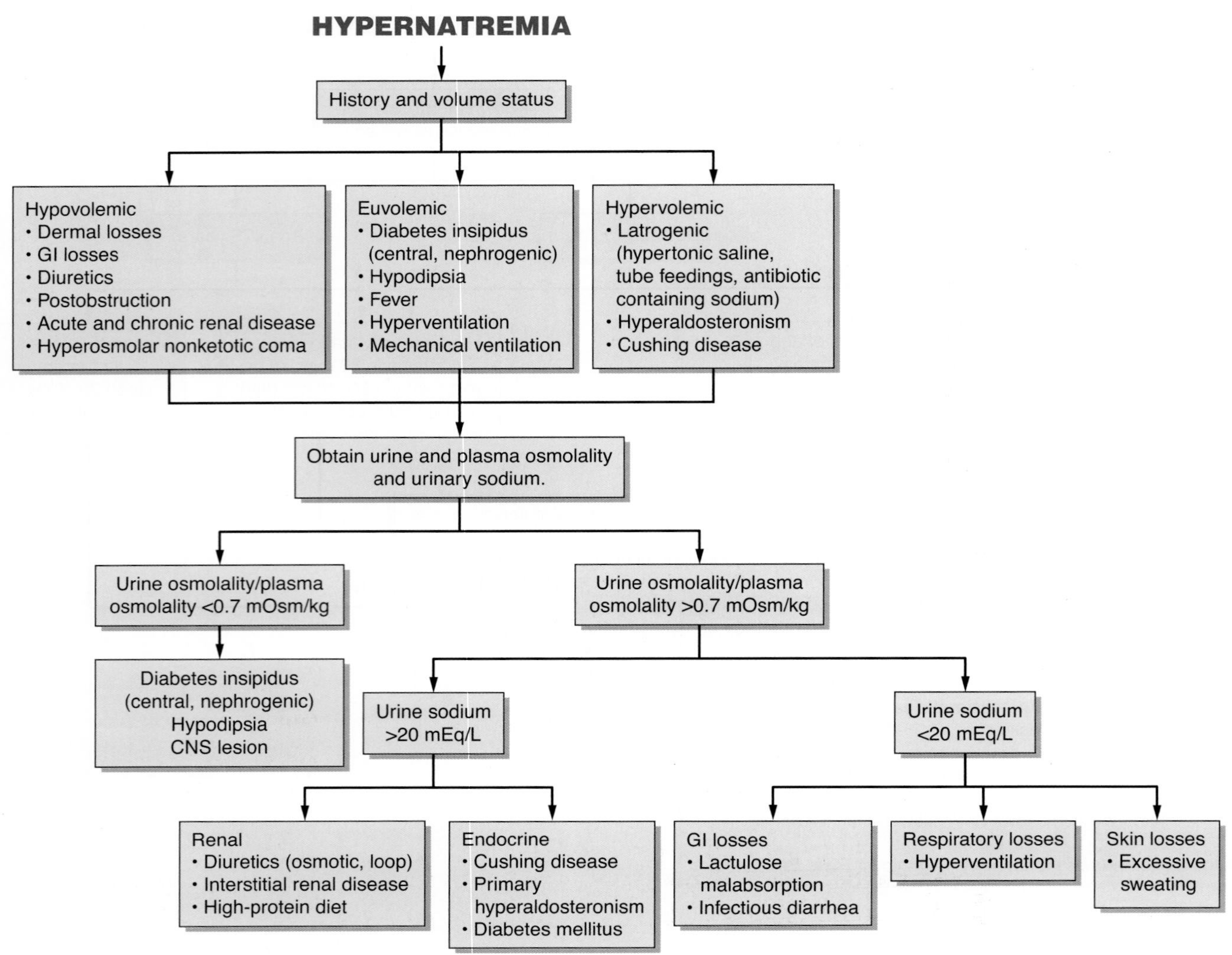
HYPERNATREMIA
History and volume status
Hypovolemic
• Dermal losses
• GI losses
• Diuretics
• Postobstruction
• Acute and chronic renal disease
• Hyperosmolar nonketotic coma
Euvolemic
• Diabetes insipidus (central, nephrogenic)
• Hypodipsia
• Fever
• Hyperventilation
• Mechanical ventilation
Hypervolemic
• Latrogenic (hypertonic saline, tube feedings, antibiotic containing sodium)
• Hyperaldosteronism
• Cushing disease
Obtain urine and plasma osmolality and urinary sodium.
Urine osmolality/plasma osmolality <0.7 mOsm/kg
Urine osmolality/plasma osmolality >0.7 mOsm/kg
Diabetes insipidus (central, nephrogenic) Hypodipsia CNS lesion
Urine sodium >20 mEq/L
Urine sodium <20 mEq/L
Renal
• Diuretics (osmotic, loop)
• Interstitial renal disease
• High-protein diet
Endocrine
• Cushing disease
• Primary hyperaldosteronism
• Diabetes mellitus
GI losses
• Lactulose malabsorption
• Infectious diarrhea
Respiratory losses
• Hyperventilation
Skin losses
• Excessive sweating

Timothy J. Coker, MD

Reynolds RM, Padfield PL, Seckl JR. Disorders of sodium balance. *BMJ.* 2006;332(7543):702–705.

HYPOALBUMINEMIA

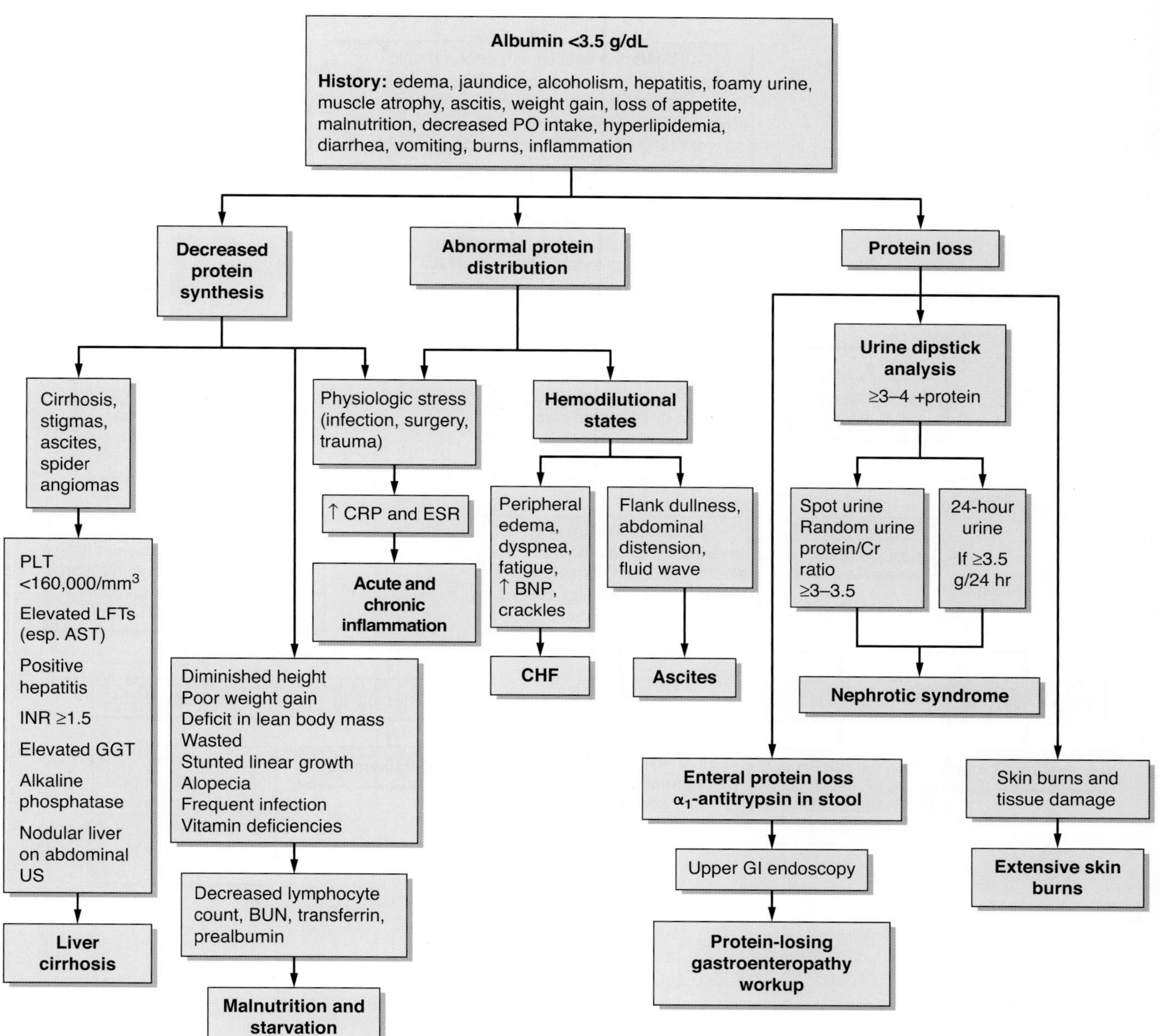

Crystal Benjamin, MD, MPH and Felix B. Chang, MD, DABMA, ABIHM

Kodner C. Nephrotic syndrome in adults: diagnosis and management. *Am Fam Physician*. 2009;80(10):1129–1134.

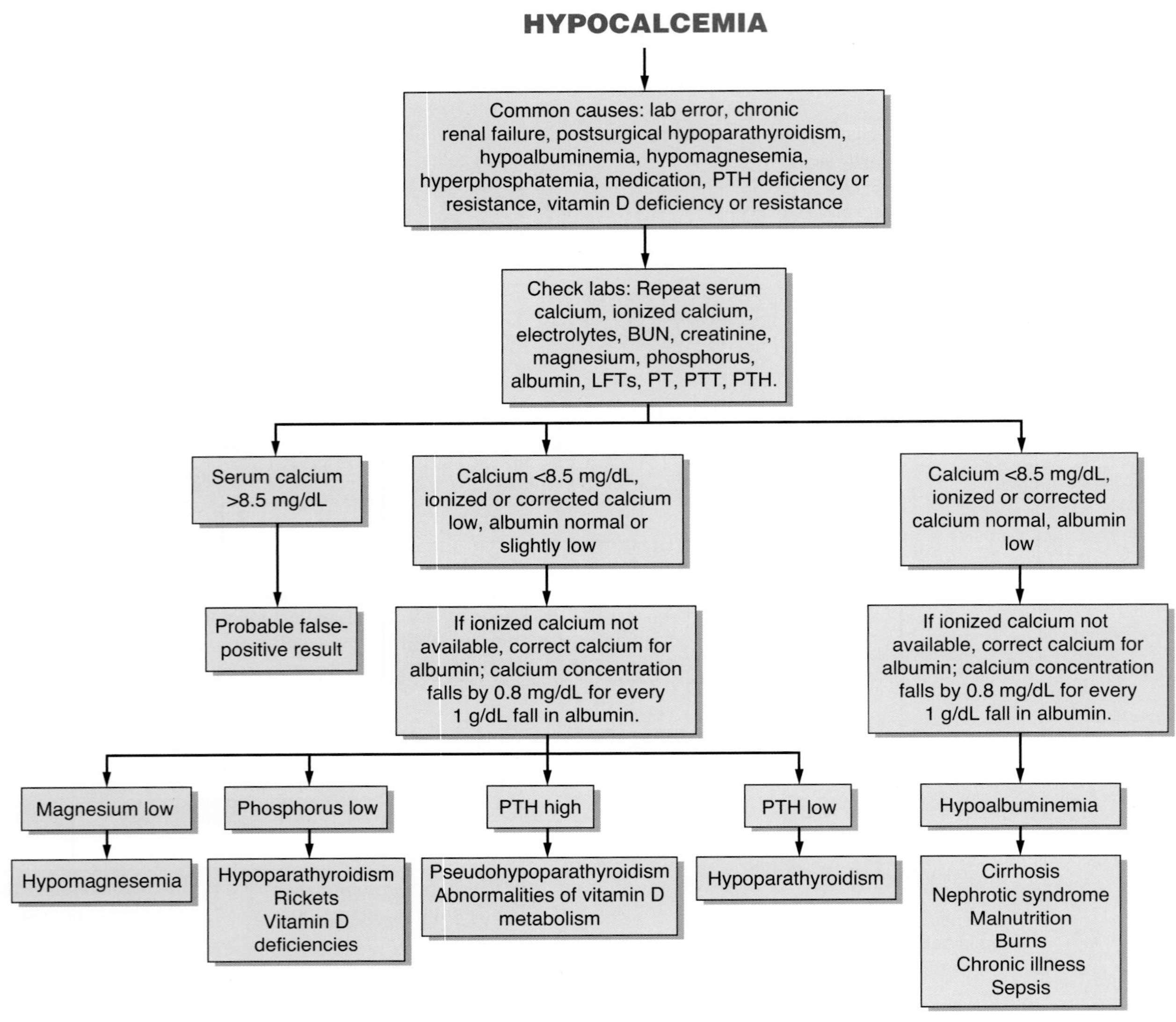
HYPOCALCEMIA
Common causes: lab error, chronic renal failure, postsurgical hypoparathyroidism, hypoalbuminemia, hypomagnesemia, hyperphosphatemia, medication, PTH deficiency or resistance, vitamin D deficiency or resistance
Check labs: Repeat serum calcium, ionized calcium, electrolytes, BUN, creatinine, magnesium, phosphorus, albumin, LFTs, PT, PTT, PTH.
Serum calcium >8.5 mg/dL
Probable false-positive result
Calcium <8.5 mg/dL, ionized or corrected calcium low, albumin normal or slightly low
If ionized calcium not available, correct calcium for albumin; calcium concentration falls by 0.8 mg/dL for every 1 g/dL fall in albumin.
Calcium <8.5 mg/dL, ionized or corrected calcium normal, albumin low
If ionized calcium not available, correct calcium for albumin; calcium concentration falls by 0.8 mg/dL for every 1 g/dL fall in albumin.
Magnesium low
Hypomagnesemia
Phosphorus low
Hypoparathyroidism
Rickets
Vitamin D deficiencies
PTH high
Pseudohypoparathyroidism
Abnormalities of vitamin D metabolism
PTH low
Hypoparathyroidism
Hypoalbuminemia
Cirrhosis
Nephrotic syndrome
Malnutrition
Burns
Chronic illness
Sepsis

Tiffany Burca, DO and Timothy J. Coker, MD

Michels TC, Kelly KM. Parathyroid disorders. *Am Fam Physician.* 2013;88(4):249–257.

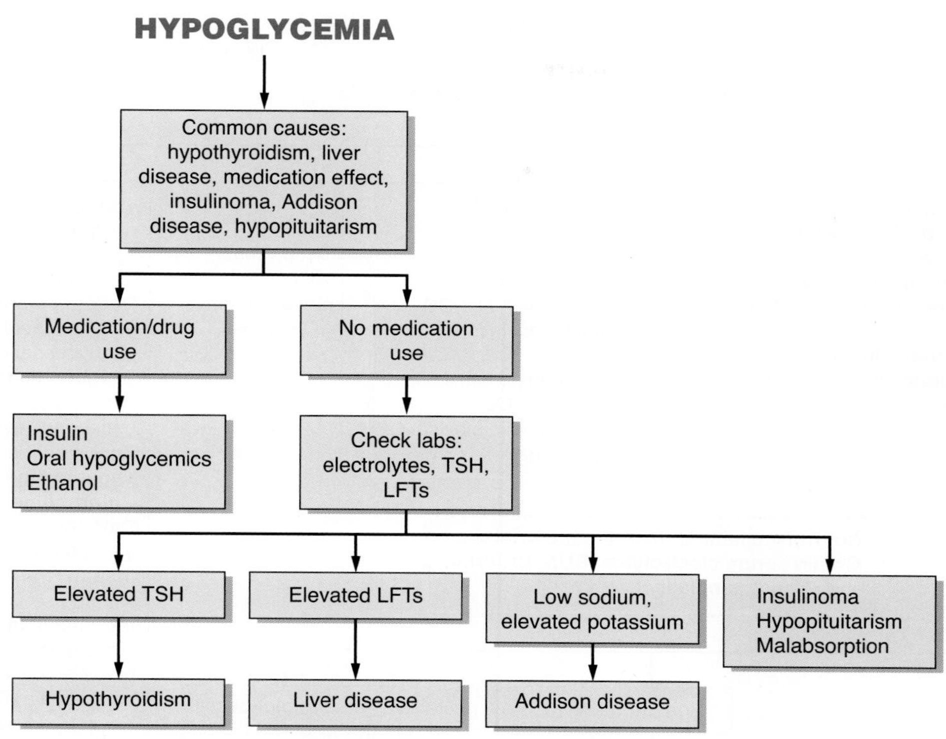

Robert A. Baldor, MD, FAAFP and Alan M. Ehrlich, MD

Murad MH, Coto-Yglesias F, Wang AT, et al. Clinical review: drug-induced hypoglycemia: a systematic review. *J Clin Endocrinol Metab.* 2009;94(3):741–745.

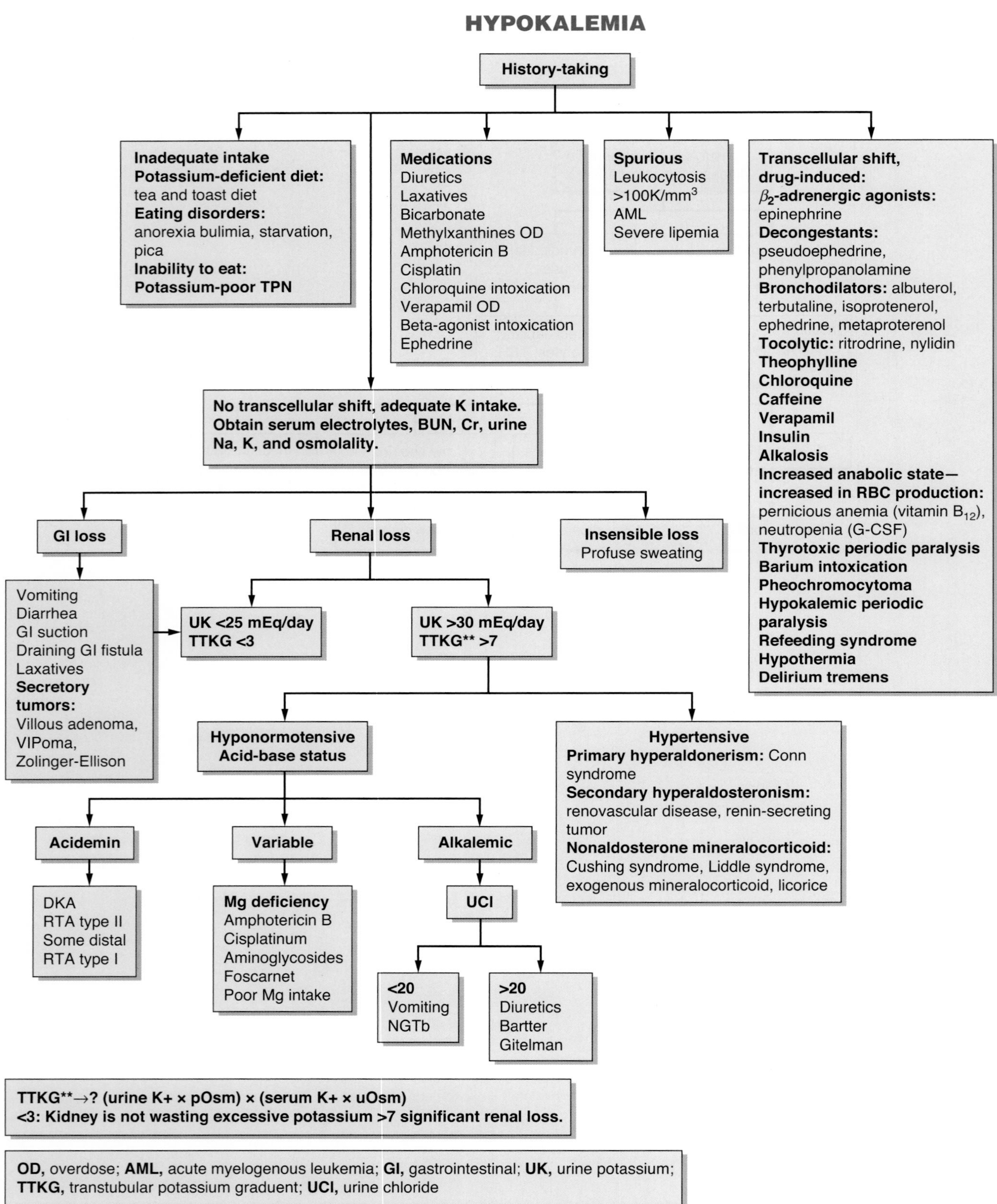

Nicolas Hernandez, MD and Felix B. Chang, MD, DABMA, ABIHM

Unwin RJ, Luft FC, Shirley DG. Pathophysiology and management of hypokalemia: a clinical perspective. *Nat Rev Nephrol.* 2011;7(2):75–84.

HYPONATREMIA

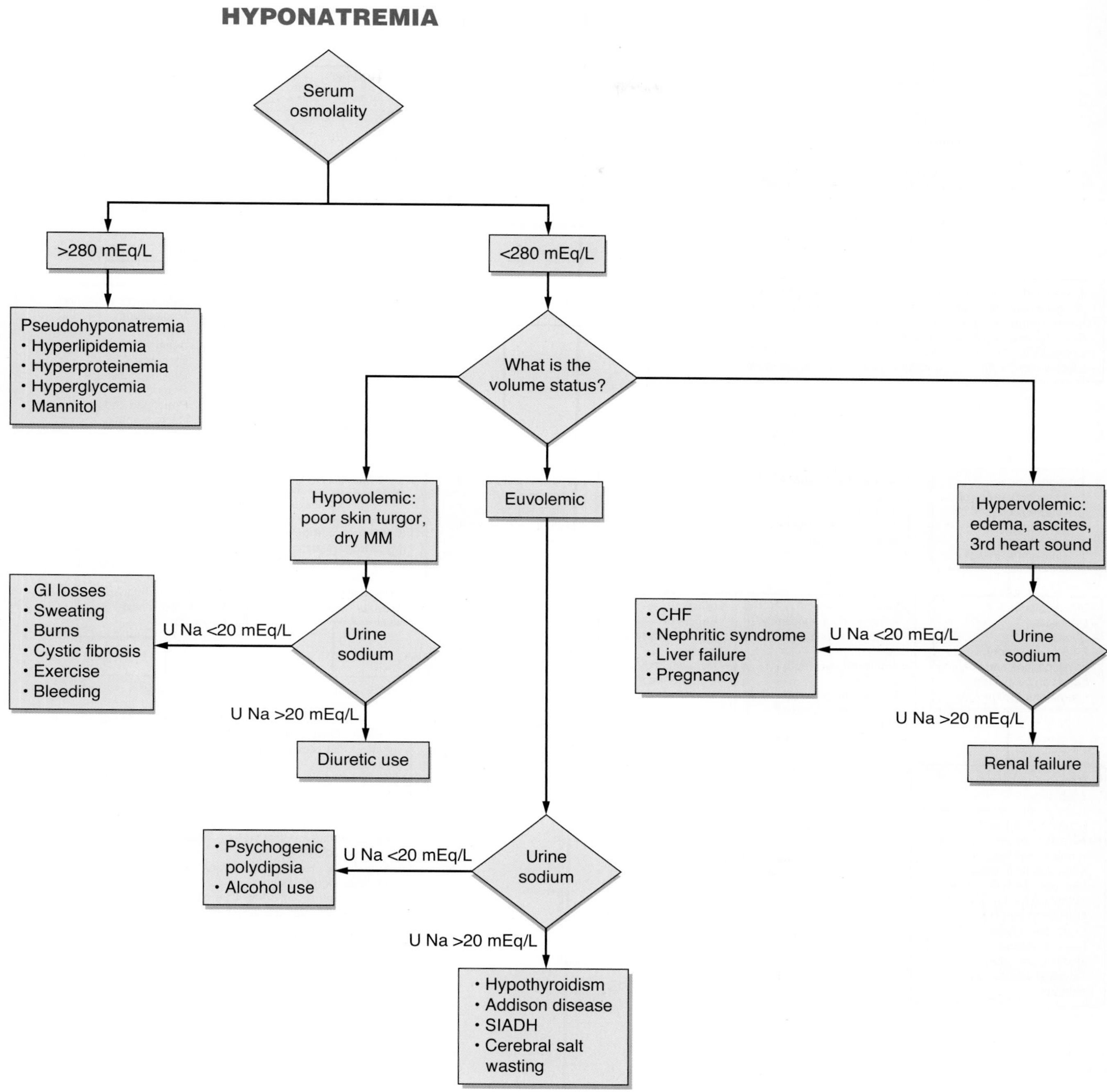

Sultan M. Babar, MD and Aaron Lambert, MD

Lien YH, Shapiro JI. Hyponatremia: clinical diagnosis and management. *Am J Med.* 2007;120(8):653–658.

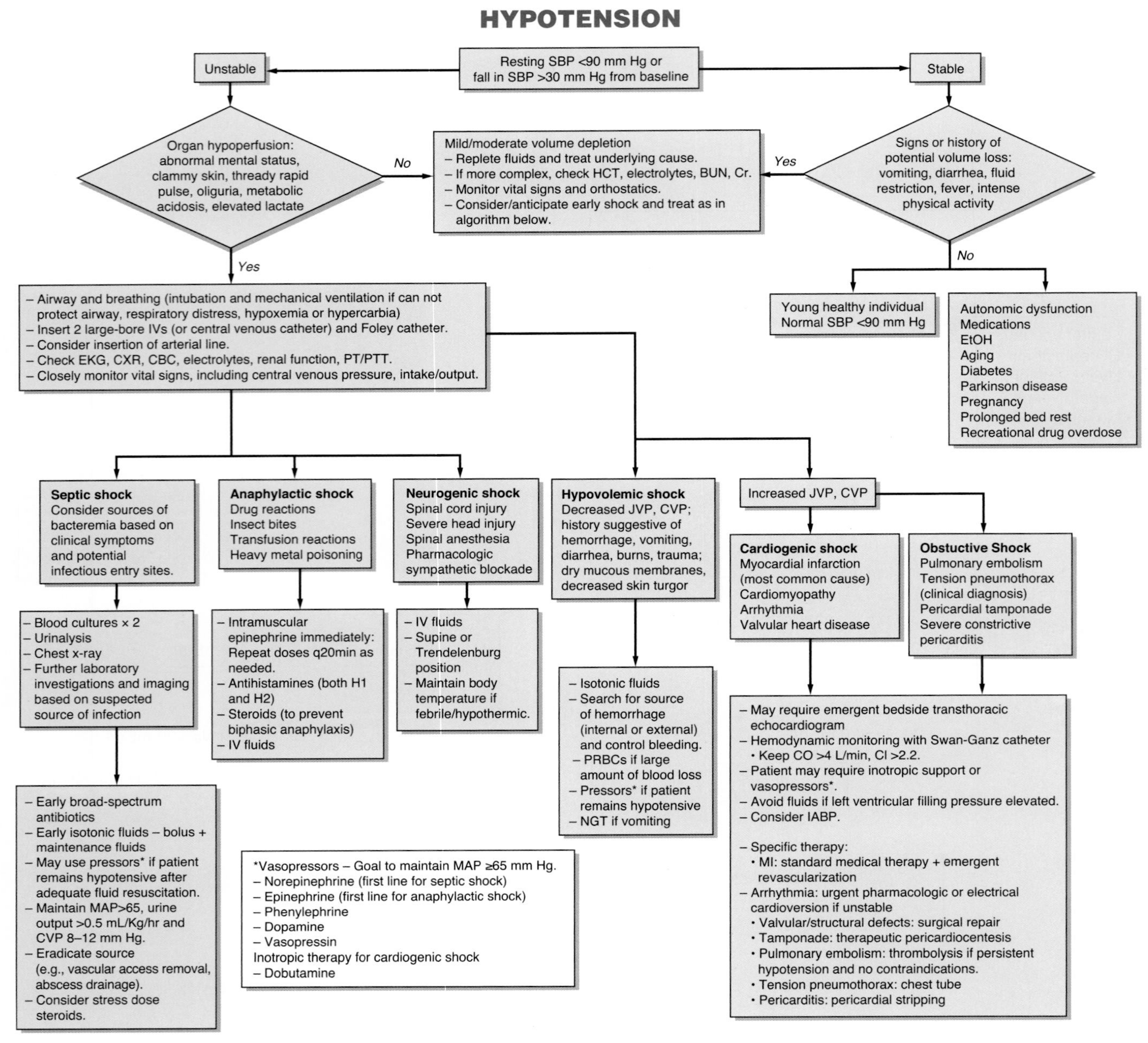

Musa A. Sharkawi, MB, BCh, BAO and Ghazwan Acash, MD, FCCP

Rivers E, Nguyen B, Havstad S, et al. Early goal-directed therapy in the treatment of severe sepsis and septic shock. *N Engl J Med.* 2001;345:1368–1377

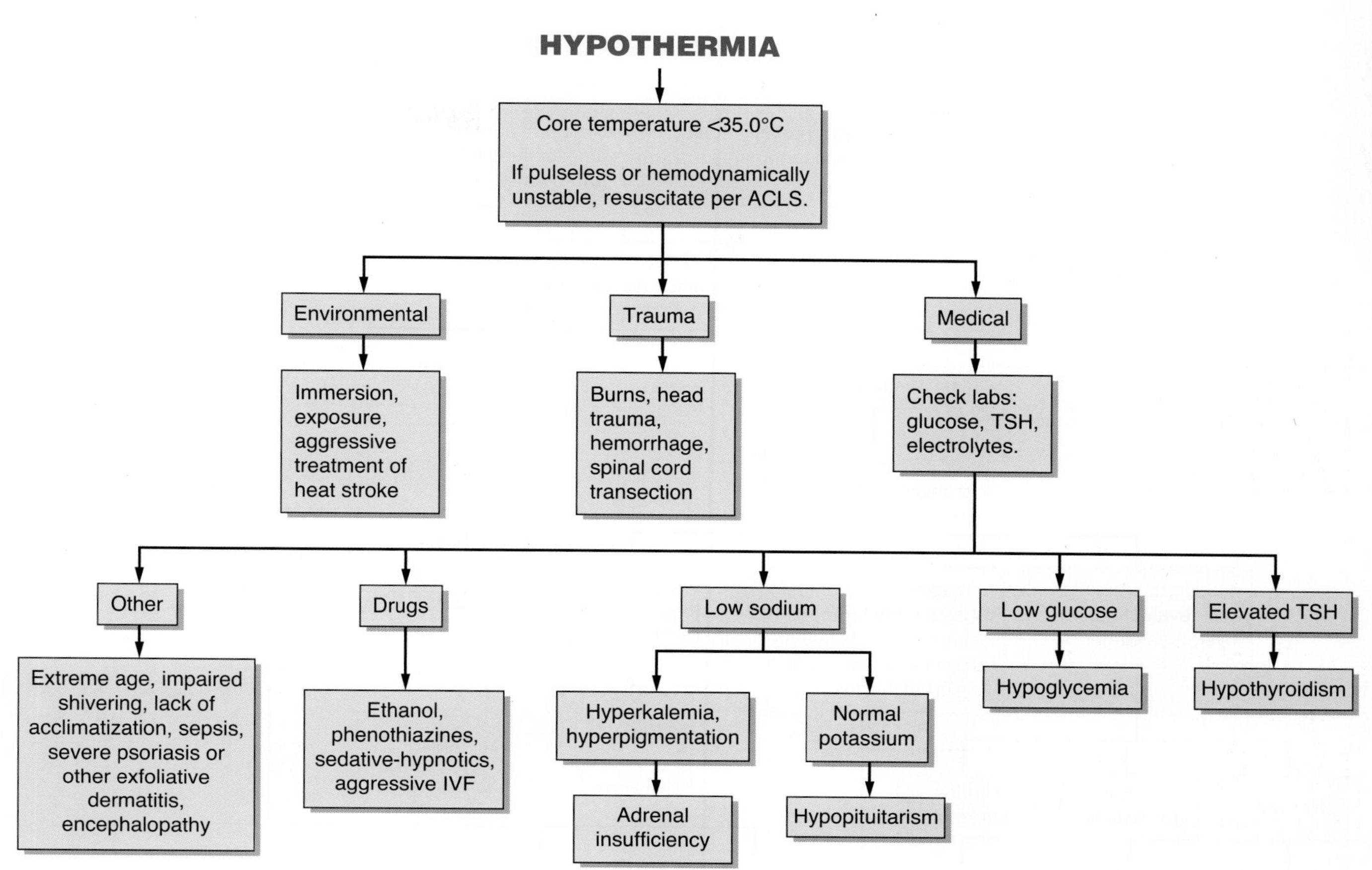

Joshua Mularella, DO

Smith DL. Anemia in the elderly. *Am Fam Physician*. 2000;62(7):1565–1572.

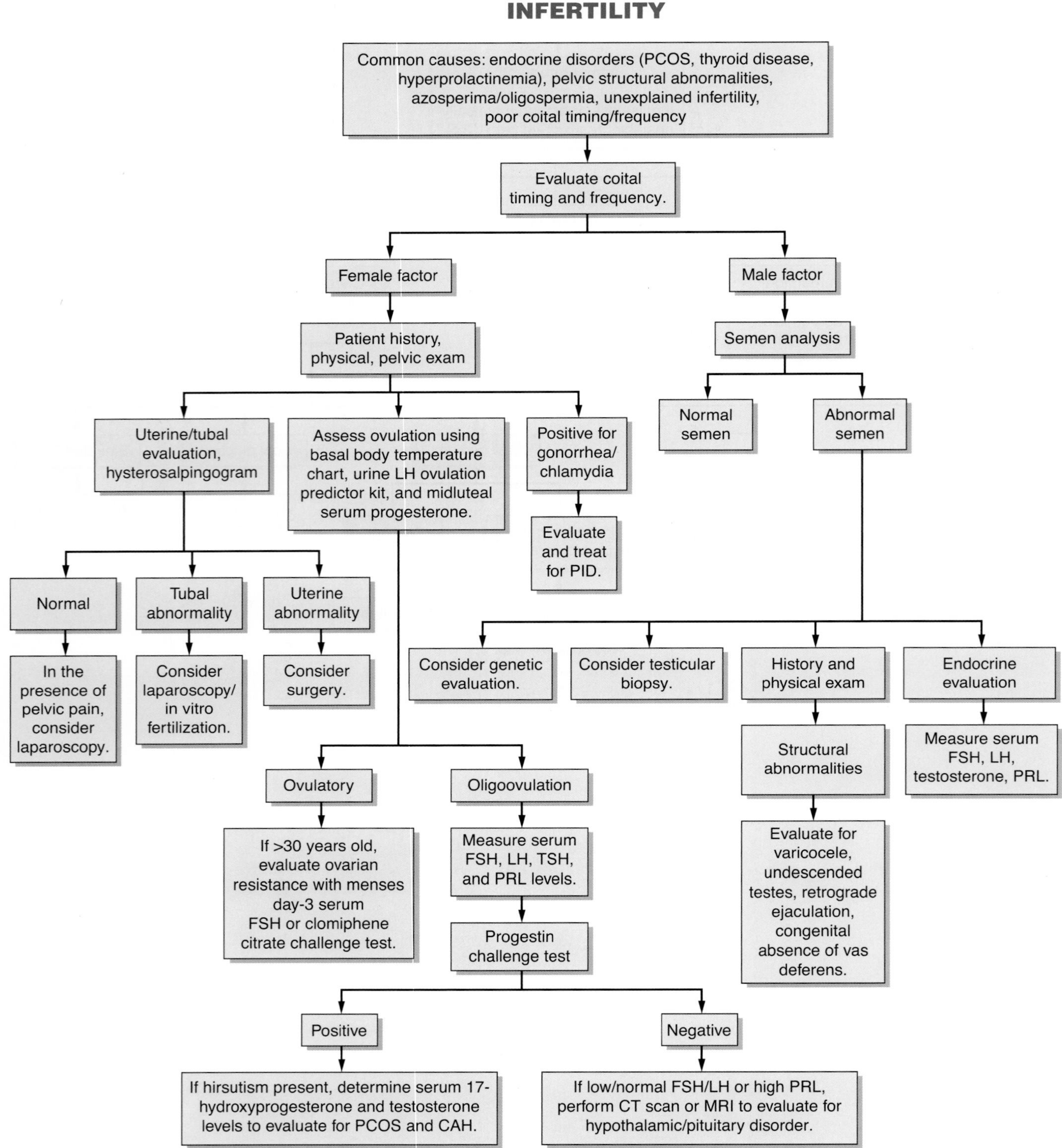
INFERTILITY
Common causes: endocrine disorders (PCOS, thyroid disease, hyperprolactinemia), pelvic structural abnormalities, azosperima/oligospermia, unexplained infertility, poor coital timing/frequency
Evaluate coital timing and frequency.
Female factor
Male factor
Patient history, physical, pelvic exam
Semen analysis
Uterine/tubal evaluation, hysterosalpingogram
Assess ovulation using basal body temperature chart, urine LH ovulation predictor kit, and midluteal serum progesterone.
Positive for gonorrhea/ chlamydia
Normal semen
Abnormal semen
Evaluate and treat for PID.
Normal
Tubal abnormality
Uterine abnormality
In the presence of pelvic pain, consider laparoscopy.
Consider laparoscopy/ in vitro fertilization.
Consider surgery.
Consider genetic evaluation.
Consider testicular biopsy.
History and physical exam
Endocrine evaluation
Structural abnormalities
Measure serum FSH, LH, testosterone, PRL.
Ovulatory
Oligoovulation
If >30 years old, evaluate ovarian resistance with menses day-3 serum FSH or clomiphene citrate challenge test.
Measure serum FSH, LH, TSH, and PRL levels.
Progestin challenge test
Evaluate for varicocele, undescended testes, retrograde ejaculation, congenital absence of vas deferens.
Positive
Negative
If hirsutism present, determine serum 17-hydroxyprogesterone and testosterone levels to evaluate for PCOS and CAH.
If low/normal FSH/LH or high PRL, perform CT scan or MRI to evaluate for hypothalamic/pituitary disorder.

Sara J. Fine, MD and Julia V. Johnson, MD

Jose-Miller AB, Boyden JW, Frey KA. Infertility. *Am Fam Physician*. 2007;75(6):849–856.

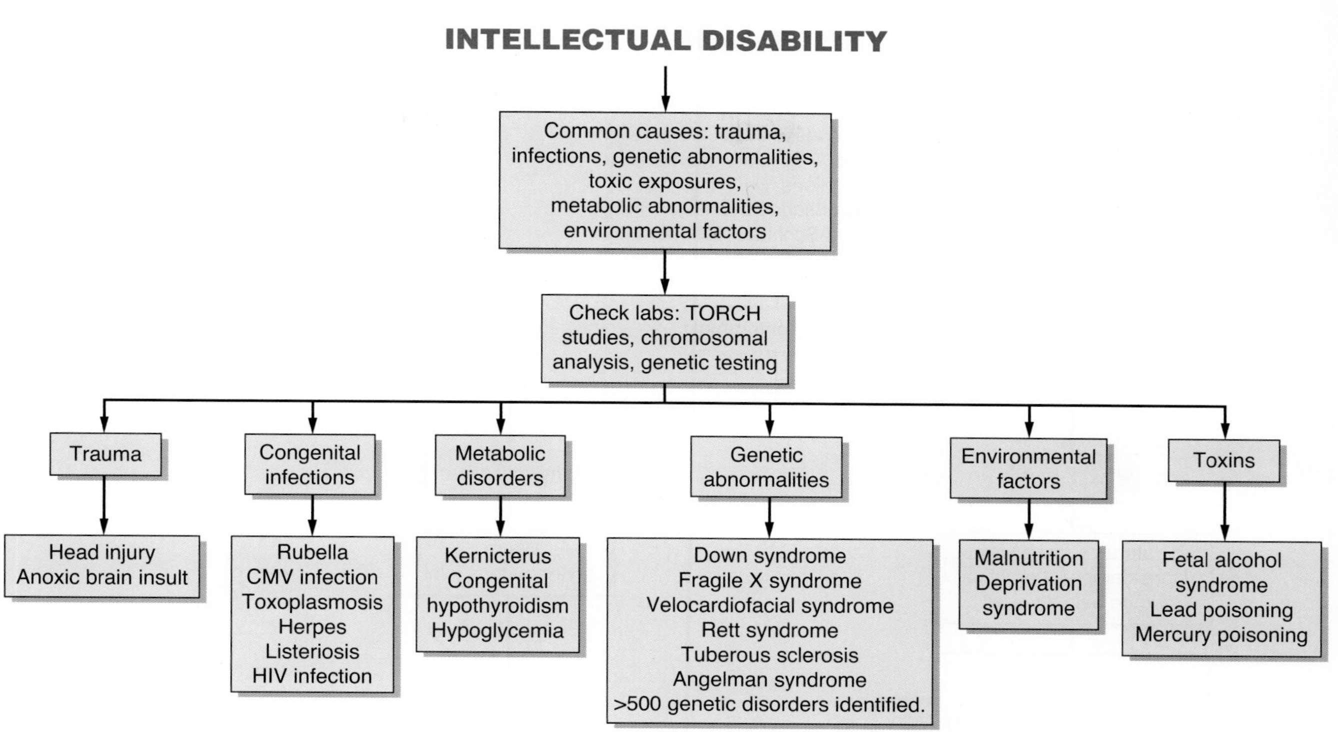

Crystal C. Bowe, MD, MPH

Carbone PS, Farley M, Davis T. Primary care for children with autism. *Am Fam Physician.* 2010;81(4):453–460.

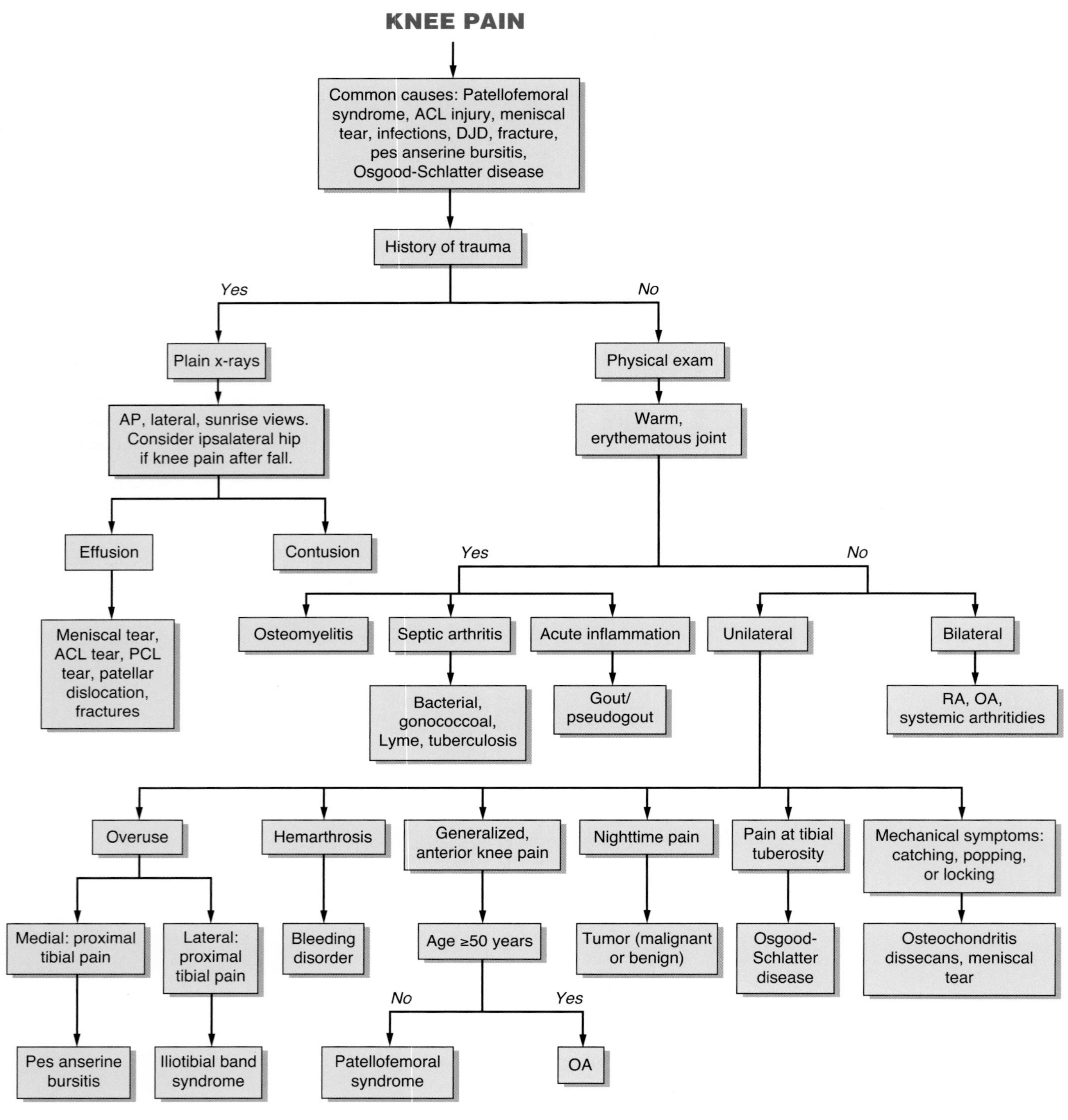

Alexei DeCastro, MD

Calmbach WL, Hutchens M. Evaluation of patients presenting with knee pain: part I. History, physical examination, radiographs, and laboratory tests. *Am Fam Physician*. 2003;68(5):907–912.

LACTATE DEHYDROGENASE ELEVATION

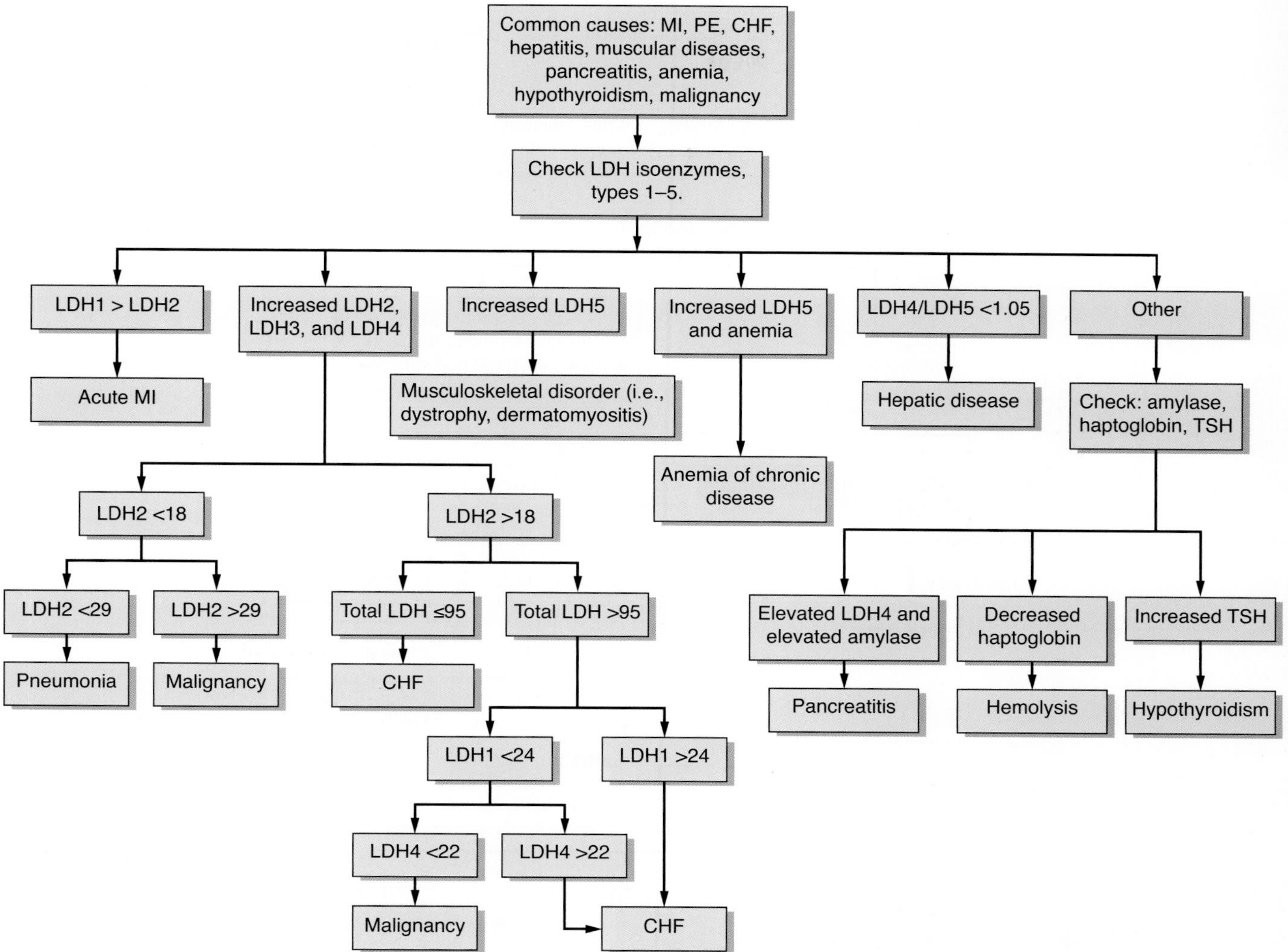

Curtis L. Galke, DO, FAAFP

Lossos IS, Breuer R, Intrator O, et al. Differential diagnosis of pleural effusion by lactate dehydrogenase isoenzyme analysis. *Chest.* 1997;111(3):648–651.

LEAD TOXICITY, DIAGNOSIS AND TREATMENT (ADULT)

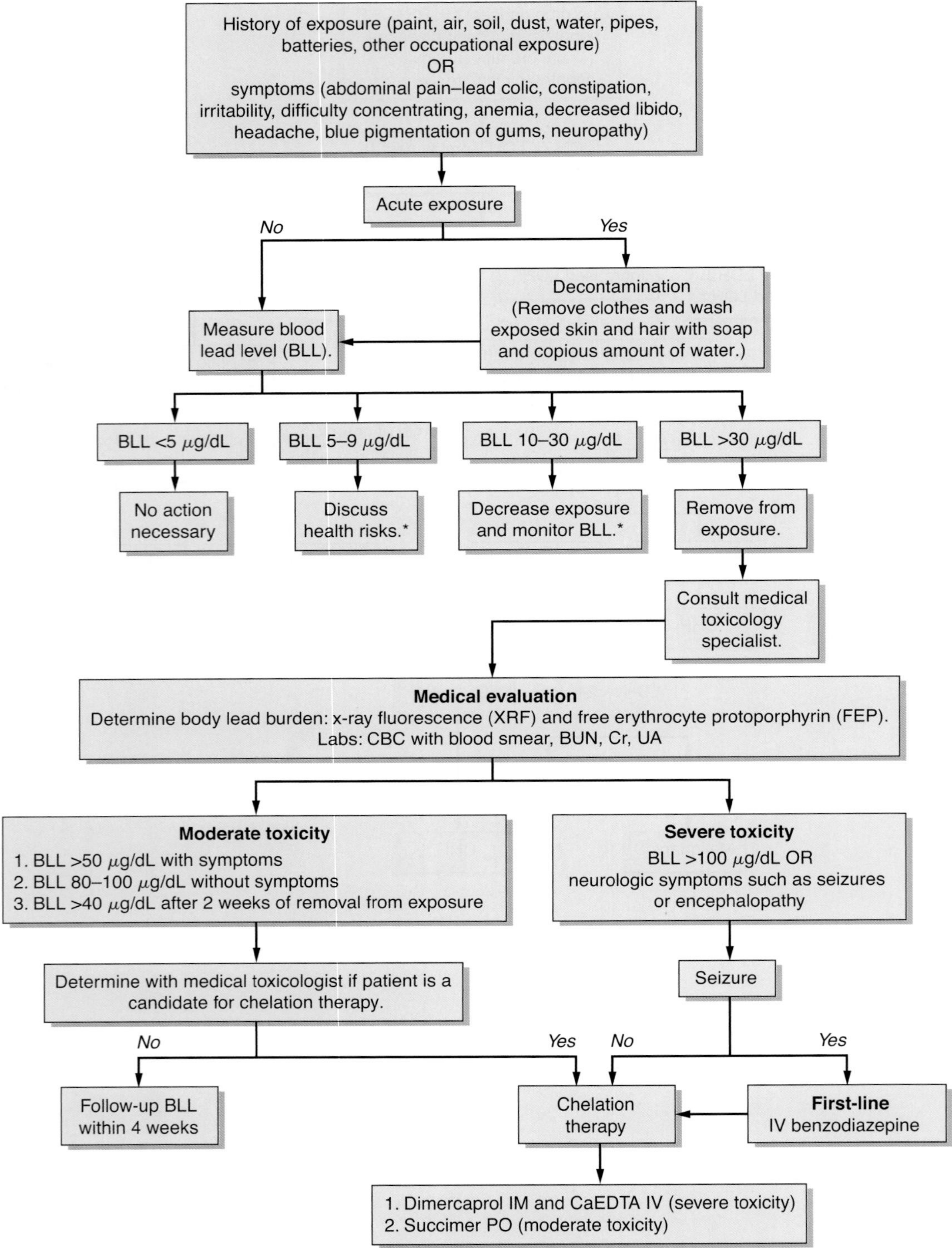

* If pregnant, reduce lead exposure for BLL 5–9 μg/dL and remove lead exposure for BLL >10 μg/dL.

Han Q. Bui, MD, MPH

Kosnett MJ, Wedeen RP, Rothenberg SJ, et al. Recommendations for medical management of adult lead exposure. *Environ Health Perspect.* 2007;115(3):463–471.

LOW BACK PAIN, CHRONIC

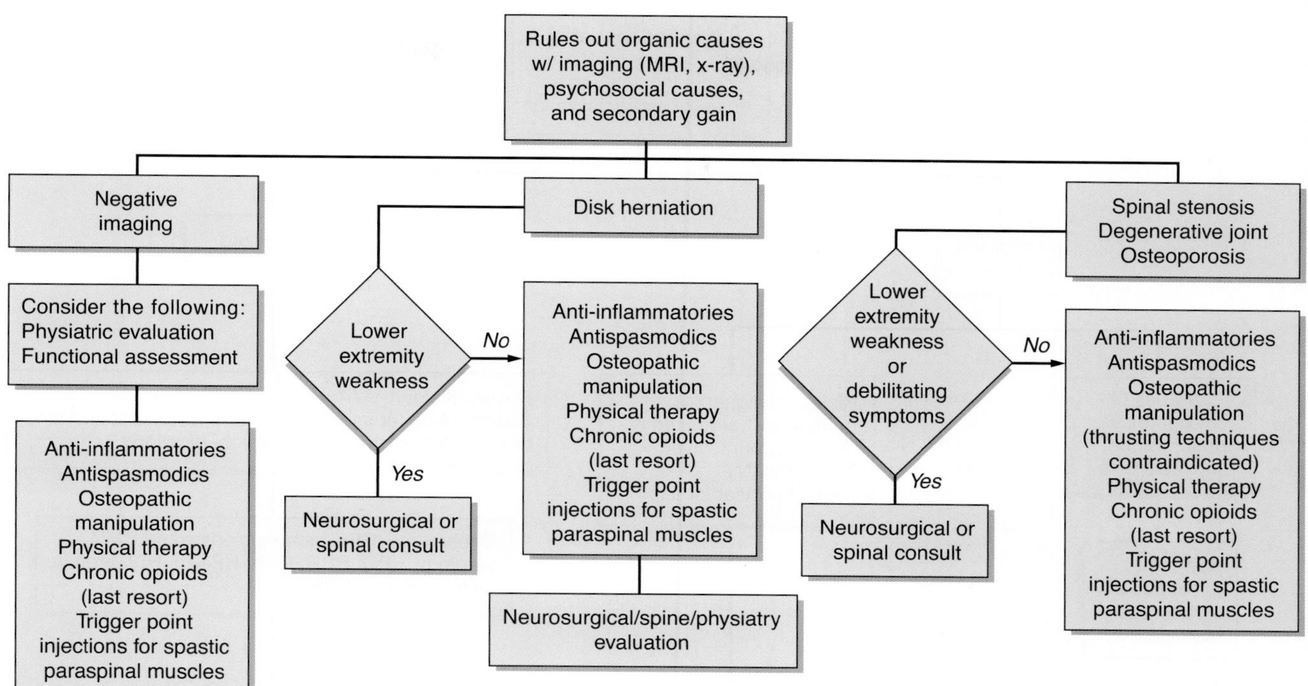

Ashley Simela, DO

Carey TS, Freburger JK, Holmes GM, et al. A long way to go: practice patterns and evidence in chronic low back pain care. *Spine*. 2009;34(7):718–724.

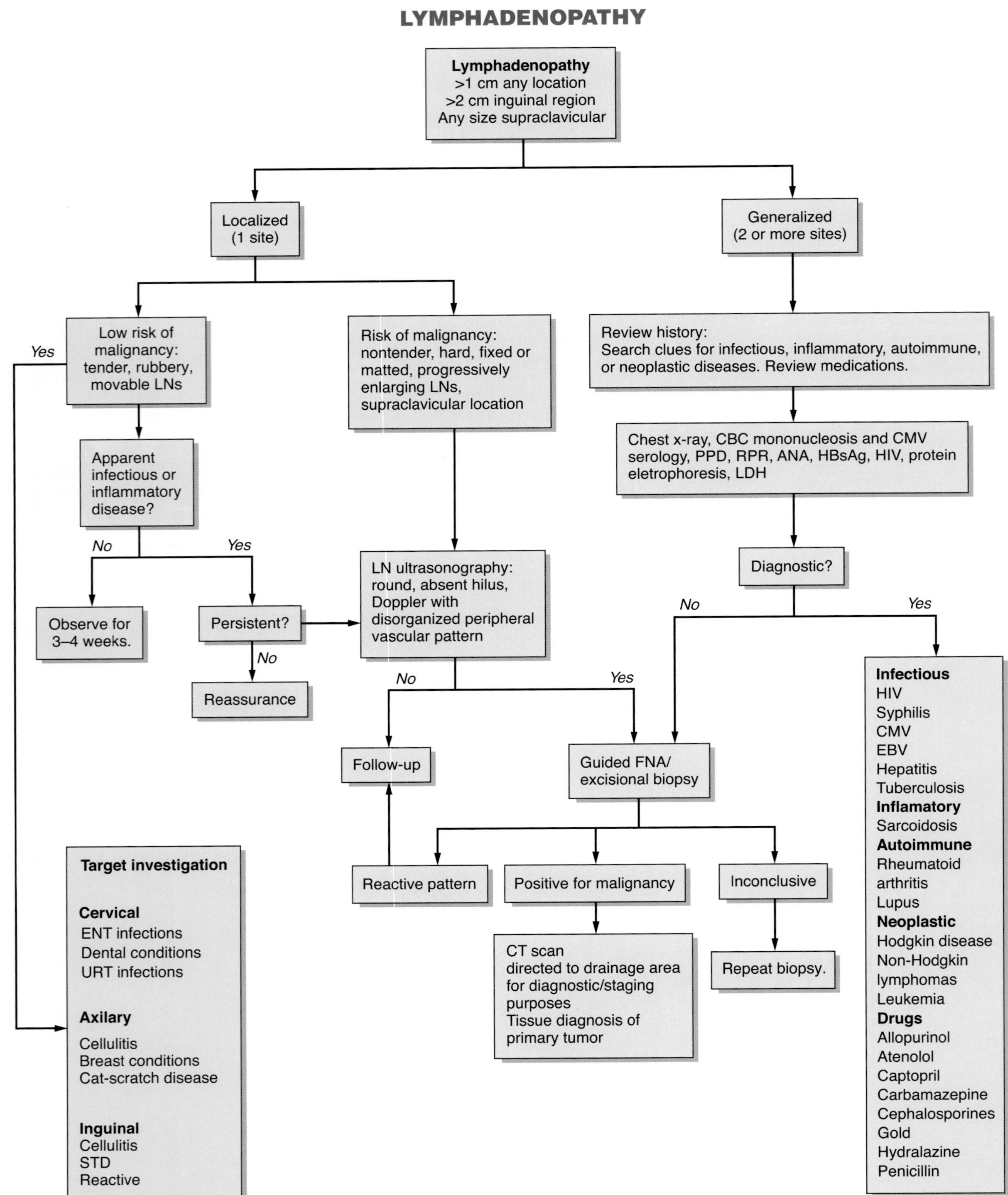

Danton Spohr Correa, MD, PhD and Felix B. Chang, MD, DABMA, ABIHM

Motyckova G, Steensma DP. Why does my patient have lymphadenopathy or splenomegaly? *Hematol Oncol Clin North Am.* 2012;26(2):395–408.

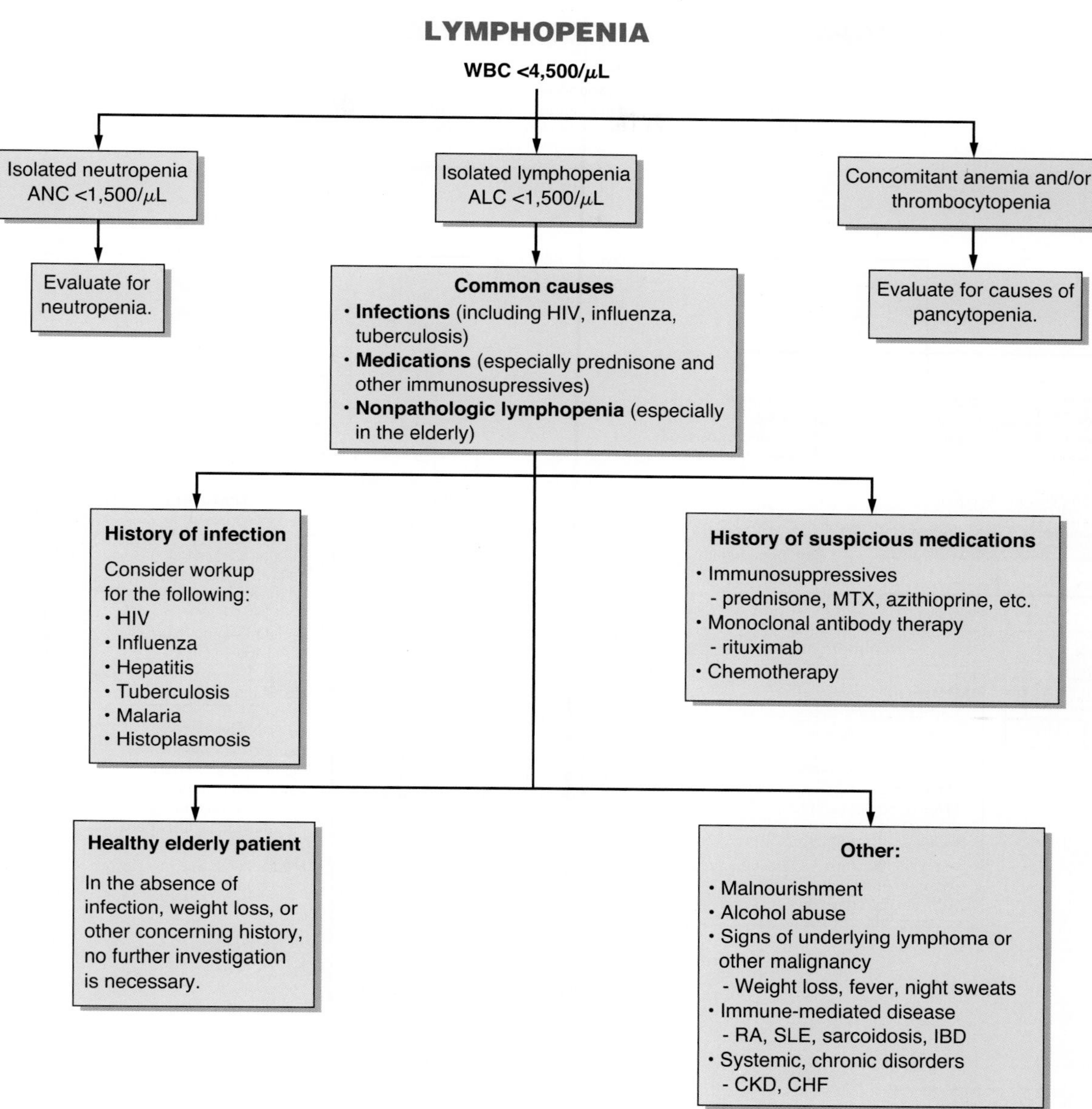

Andrew Smith, MD and Erin Bassett-Novoa, MD

Brass D, Mckay P, Scott F. Investigating an incidental finding of lymphopenia. *BMJ.* 2014;348:g1721.

MENOPAUSE, EVALUATION AND MANAGEMENT

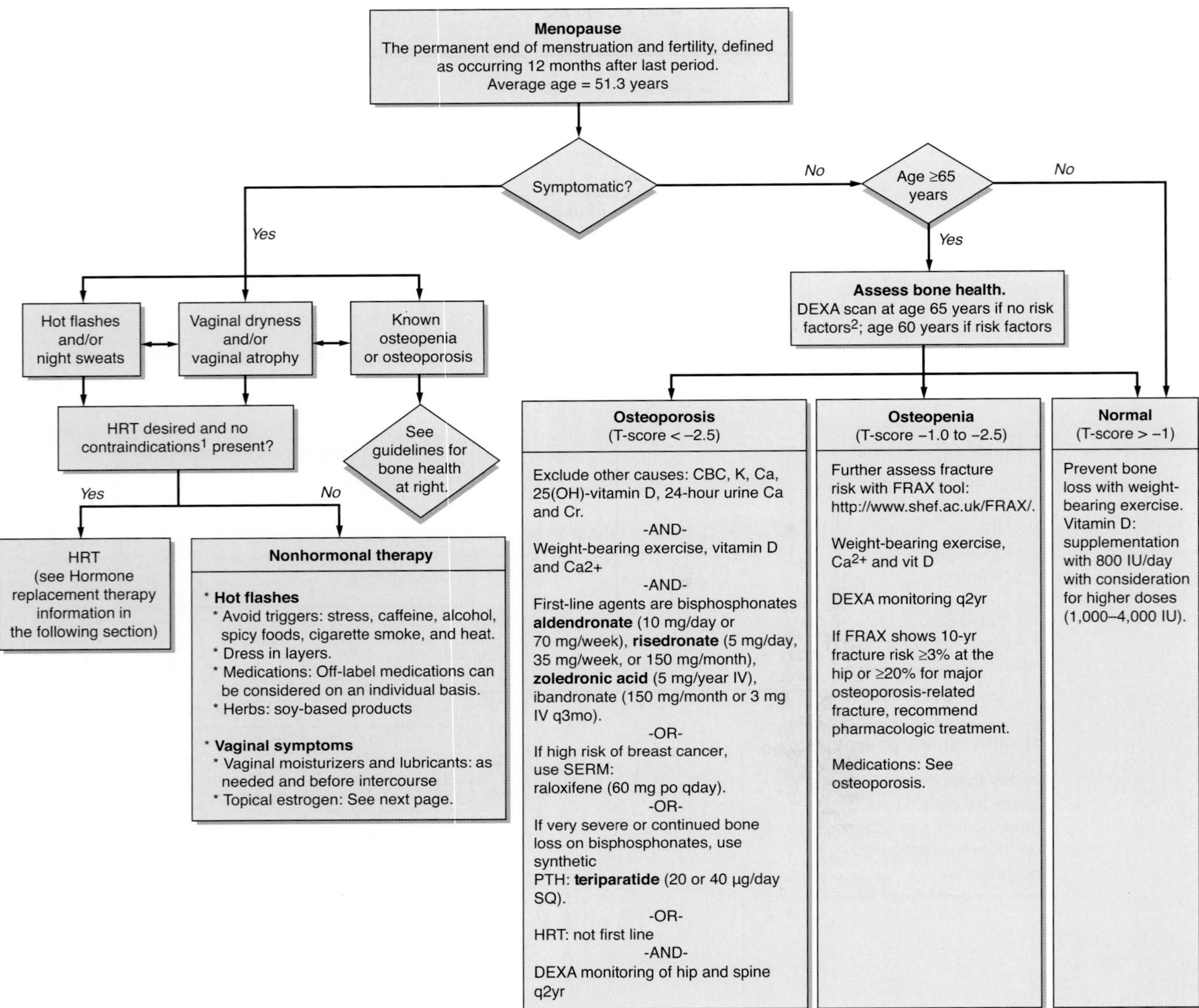

Menopause
The permanent end of menstruation and fertility, defined as occurring 12 months after last period.
Average age = 51.3 years
Symptomatic?
Yes
No
Age ≥65 years
No
Yes
Assess bone health.
DEXA scan at age 65 years if no risk factors2; age 60 years if risk factors
Hot flashes and/or night sweats
Vaginal dryness and/or vaginal atrophy
Known osteopenia or osteoporosis
HRT desired and no contraindications1 present?
See guidelines for bone health at right.
Yes
No
HRT (see Hormone replacement therapy information in the following section)
Nonhormonal therapy
* Hot flashes
* Avoid triggers: stress, caffeine, alcohol, spicy foods, cigarette smoke, and heat.
* Dress in layers.
* Medications: Off-label medications can be considered on an individual basis.
* Herbs: soy-based products
* Vaginal symptoms
* Vaginal moisturizers and lubricants: as needed and before intercourse
* Topical estrogen: See next page.
Osteoporosis
(T-score < −2.5)
Exclude other causes: CBC, K, Ca, 25(OH)-vitamin D, 24-hour urine Ca and Cr.
-AND-
Weight-bearing exercise, vitamin D and Ca2+
-AND-
First-line agents are bisphosphonates aldendronate (10 mg/day or 70 mg/week), risedronate (5 mg/day, 35 mg/week, or 150 mg/month), zoledronic acid (5 mg/year IV), ibandronate (150 mg/month or 3 mg IV q3mo).
-OR-
If high risk of breast cancer, use SERM: raloxifene (60 mg po qday).
-OR-
If very severe or continued bone loss on bisphosphonates, use synthetic PTH: teriparatide (20 or 40 μg/day SQ).
-OR-
HRT: not first line
-AND-
DEXA monitoring of hip and spine q2yr
Osteopenia
(T-score −1.0 to −2.5)
Further assess fracture risk with FRAX tool: http://www.shef.ac.uk/FRAX/.
Weight-bearing exercise, Ca2+ and vit D
DEXA monitoring q2yr
If FRAX shows 10-yr fracture risk ≥3% at the hip or ≥20% for major osteoporosis-related fracture, recommend pharmacologic treatment.
Medications: See osteoporosis.
Normal
(T-score > −1)
Prevent bone loss with weight-bearing exercise.
Vitamin D: supplementation with 800 IU/day with consideration for higher doses (1,000–4,000 IU).

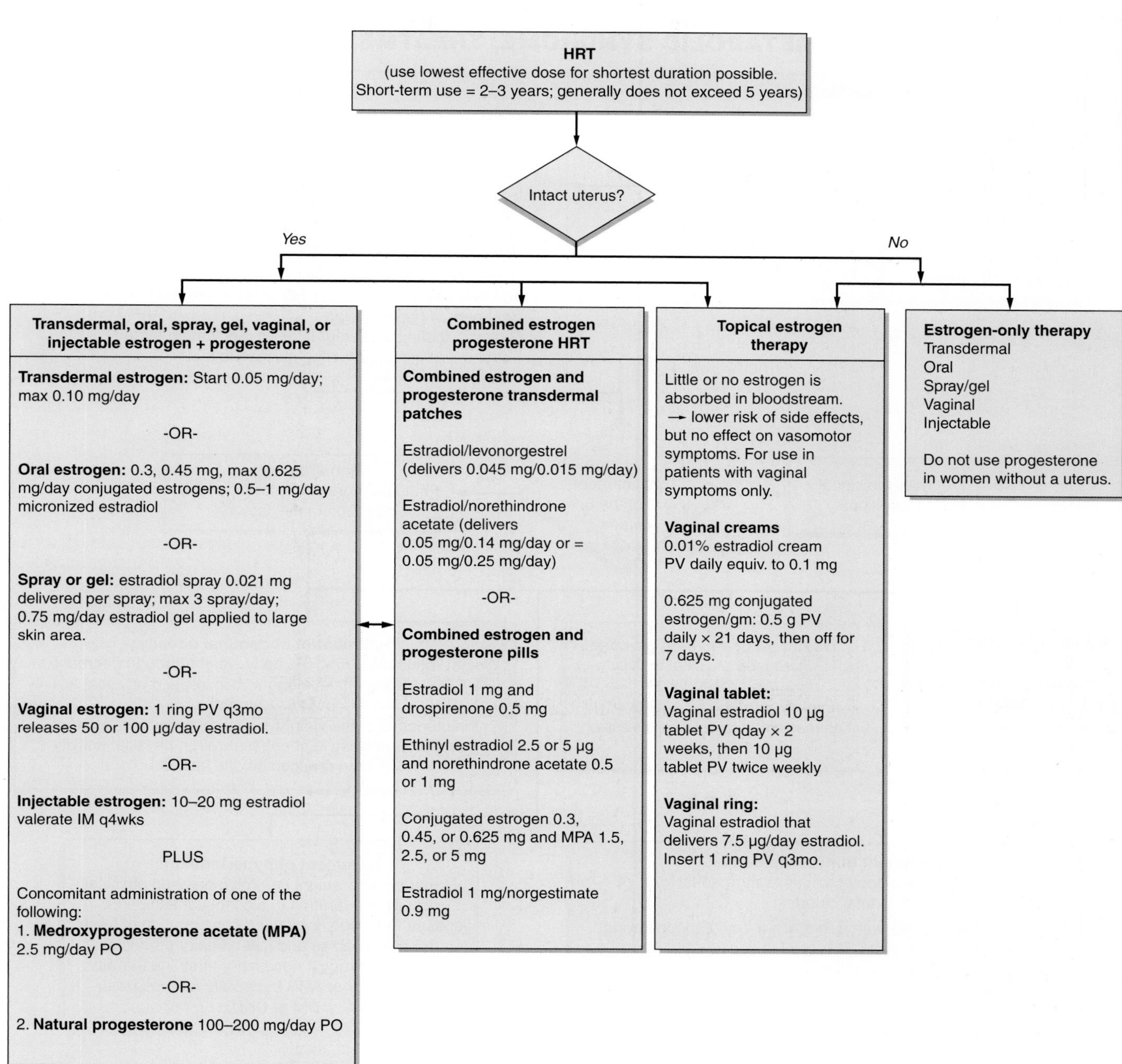

HRT
(use lowest effective dose for shortest duration possible.
Short-term use = 2–3 years; generally does not exceed 5 years)
Intact uterus?
Yes
No
Transdermal, oral, spray, gel, vaginal, or injectable estrogen + progesterone
Transdermal estrogen: Start 0.05 mg/day; max 0.10 mg/day
-OR-
Oral estrogen: 0.3, 0.45 mg, max 0.625 mg/day conjugated estrogens; 0.5–1 mg/day micronized estradiol
-OR-
Spray or gel: estradiol spray 0.021 mg delivered per spray; max 3 spray/day; 0.75 mg/day estradiol gel applied to large skin area.
-OR-
Vaginal estrogen: 1 ring PV q3mo releases 50 or 100 µg/day estradiol.
-OR-
Injectable estrogen: 10–20 mg estradiol valerate IM q4wks
PLUS
Concomitant administration of one of the following:
1. Medroxyprogesterone acetate (MPA) 2.5 mg/day PO
-OR-
2. Natural progesterone 100–200 mg/day PO
Combined estrogen progesterone HRT
Combined estrogen and progesterone transdermal patches
Estradiol/levonorgestrel (delivers 0.045 mg/0.015 mg/day)
Estradiol/norethindrone acetate (delivers 0.05 mg/0.14 mg/day or = 0.05 mg/0.25 mg/day)
-OR-
Combined estrogen and progesterone pills
Estradiol 1 mg and drospirenone 0.5 mg
Ethinyl estradiol 2.5 or 5 µg and norethindrone acetate 0.5 or 1 mg
Conjugated estrogen 0.3, 0.45, or 0.625 mg and MPA 1.5, 2.5, or 5 mg
Estradiol 1 mg/norgestimate 0.9 mg
Topical estrogen therapy
Little or no estrogen is absorbed in bloodstream. → lower risk of side effects, but no effect on vasomotor symptoms. For use in patients with vaginal symptoms only.
Vaginal creams
0.01% estradiol cream PV daily equiv. to 0.1 mg
0.625 mg conjugated estrogen/gm: 0.5 g PV daily × 21 days, then off for 7 days.
Vaginal tablet:
Vaginal estradiol 10 µg tablet PV qday × 2 weeks, then 10 µg tablet PV twice weekly
Vaginal ring:
Vaginal estradiol that delivers 7.5 µg/day estradiol. Insert 1 ring PV q3mo.
Estrogen-only therapy
Transdermal
Oral
Spray/gel
Vaginal
Injectable
Do not use progesterone in women without a uterus.

Karen Browning, MD and Kelly Pagidas, MD

Hutzinger A. Practice Guidelines. AHRQ releases evidence report on managing menopause-related symptoms. *Am Fam Physician.* 2005;72(4):709–710.

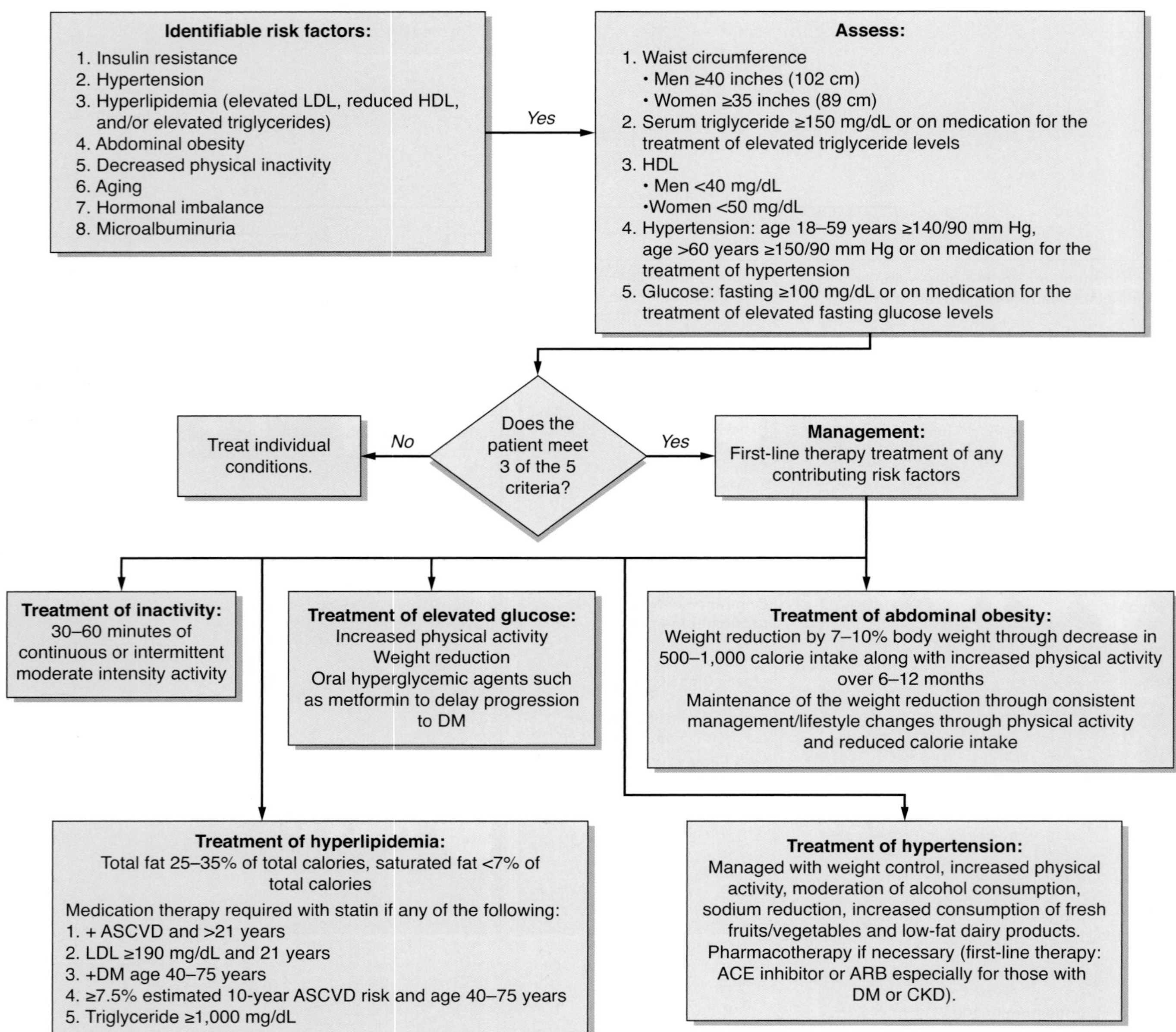

METABOLIC SYNDROME, TREATMENT
Identifiable risk factors:
1. Insulin resistance
2. Hypertension
3. Hyperlipidemia (elevated LDL, reduced HDL, and/or elevated triglycerides)
4. Abdominal obesity
5. Decreased physical inactivity
6. Aging
7. Hormonal imbalance
8. Microalbuminuria
Yes
Assess:
1. Waist circumference
• Men ≥40 inches (102 cm)
• Women ≥35 inches (89 cm)
2. Serum triglyceride ≥150 mg/dL or on medication for the treatment of elevated triglyceride levels
3. HDL
• Men <40 mg/dL
•Women <50 mg/dL
4. Hypertension: age 18–59 years ≥140/90 mm Hg, age >60 years ≥150/90 mm Hg or on medication for the treatment of hypertension
5. Glucose: fasting ≥100 mg/dL or on medication for the treatment of elevated fasting glucose levels
Does the patient meet 3 of the 5 criteria?
No
Treat individual conditions.
Yes
Management:
First-line therapy treatment of any contributing risk factors
Treatment of inactivity:
30–60 minutes of continuous or intermittent moderate intensity activity
Treatment of elevated glucose:
Increased physical activity
Weight reduction
Oral hyperglycemic agents such as metformin to delay progression to DM
Treatment of abdominal obesity:
Weight reduction by 7–10% body weight through decrease in 500–1,000 calorie intake along with increased physical activity over 6–12 months
Maintenance of the weight reduction through consistent management/lifestyle changes through physical activity and reduced calorie intake
Treatment of hyperlipidemia:
Total fat 25–35% of total calories, saturated fat <7% of total calories
Medication therapy required with statin if any of the following:
1. + ASCVD and >21 years
2. LDL ≥190 mg/dL and 21 years
3. +DM age 40–75 years
4. ≥7.5% estimated 10-year ASCVD risk and age 40–75 years
5. Triglyceride ≥1,000 mg/dL
Treatment of hypertension:
Managed with weight control, increased physical activity, moderation of alcohol consumption, sodium reduction, increased consumption of fresh fruits/vegetables and low-fat dairy products.
Pharmacotherapy if necessary (first-line therapy: ACE inhibitor or ARB especially for those with DM or CKD).

Julie Dahl-Smith, DO, FAAFP, DABMA and Mariam Akhtar, MD

Armstrong C. AHA and NHLBI review diagnosis and management of the metabolic syndrome. *Am Fam Physician.* 2006;74(6):1039–1047.

MIGRAINE, TREATMENT

Suspected migraine headache

POUND:
Pulsatile quality
One-day duration (4–72 hours)
Unilateral location
Nausea or vomiting
Disabling intensity

With or without photophobia or phonophobia

↓

Possible secondary headache?

↓

Sudden onset	Age >55 years
Worst headache ever	Seizures
Increasing frequency	Fever, scalp tender
Worsening intensity	Systemic disease
Awakens from sleep	History trauma
Focal neurologic signs	Weight loss
Altered mental status	Myalgia
Precipitated by valsalva	Exertion, bending

Yes → Consider alternate diagnosis and workup as directed by history and physical.

No → Meets criteria for migraine?

- No → Consider other headache syndrome.
- Yes → Move to quiet, dark room. IV rehydration Antiemetics PRN
  - Hydroxyzine
  - Metoclopramide
  - Prochlorperazine
  - Caffeine

→ Classify severity as mild, moderate, severe, or status *(drugs can be used singularly or in compatible combinations).*

Mild
- Acetaminophen/ASA/caffeine
- Lidocaine nasal
- Midrin
- NSAIDs
- **5-HT agonist (triptans): almotriptan, eletriptan, sumatriptan, zolmitriptan, nazatriptan, rizatriptan, frovatriptan

→ Success? Yes → Headache resolved. No → Moderate

Moderate
- Mild treatments
- *DHE
- Ergotamine tartrate

→ Success? Yes → Headache resolved. No → Severe

Severe
- Mild and moderate treatments
- Chlorpromazine
- Depacon
- Ketorolac IM
- Magnesium sulfate IV

→ Success? Yes → Headache resolved. No → Consider consultation with headache specialist.

↓

Status: >72 hours duration
- *DHE or chlorpromazine, valproate sodium IV or magnesium sulfate IV or prochloperazine

→ Success? Yes → Headache resolved. No → Ketorolac or opiates

→ Success? Yes → Headache resolved. No → Dexamethasone

→ Success? Yes → Headache resolved. No → Consult headache specialist.

Headache resolved. →
- Assess for hormone-related migraine.
- Consider prophylactic treatments as appropriate.

***Dihydroergotamine mesylate**
DHE must NOT be given to
- Pregnant or breastfeeding
- History of ischemic heart disease
- History of Prinzmetal angina
- Severe peripheral vascular disease
- Onset of chest pain after test dose
- Elevated blood pressure
- Within 24 hours of pain or ergot derivatives
- Basilar migraine headache patients (any 3: diplopia, dysarthria, tinnitus, vertigo, temporary hearing loss, mental confusion)
- Cerebrovascular disease

****5-HT (triptans)**
- Avoid in patients with vascular disease, uncontrolled hypertension, and hemiplegic migraine.

Ellen E. Anderson Penno, MD, MS, FRCSC, Diplomate ABO

Gilmore B. Michael M. Treatment of acute migraine headache. *Am Fam Physician.* 2011;83(3):271–280.

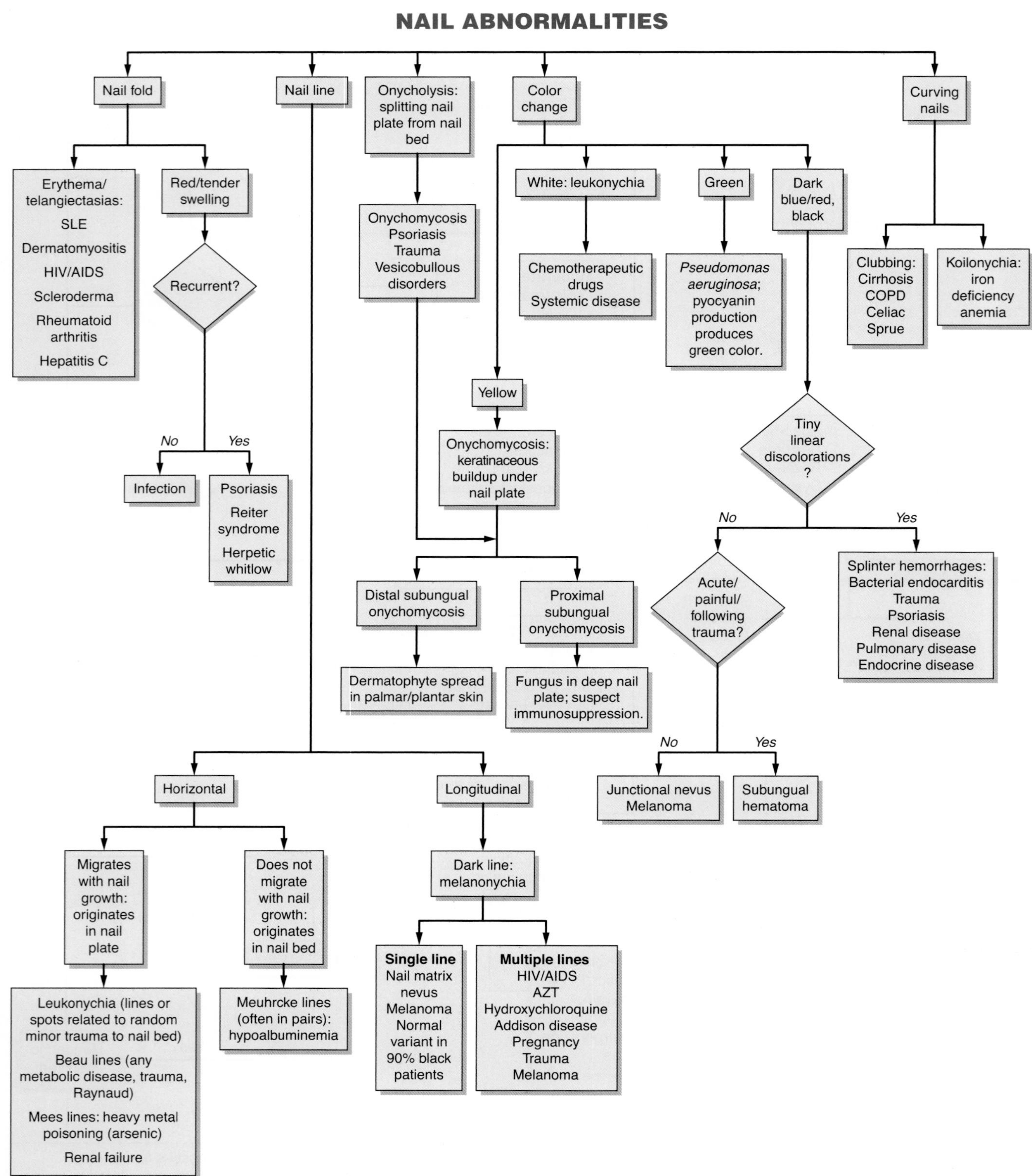

Miesha Merati, DO and Jenifer R. Lloyd, DO

Tully AS, Trayes KP, Studdiford JS. Evaluation of nail abnormalities. *Am Fam Physician*. 2012;85(8):779–787.

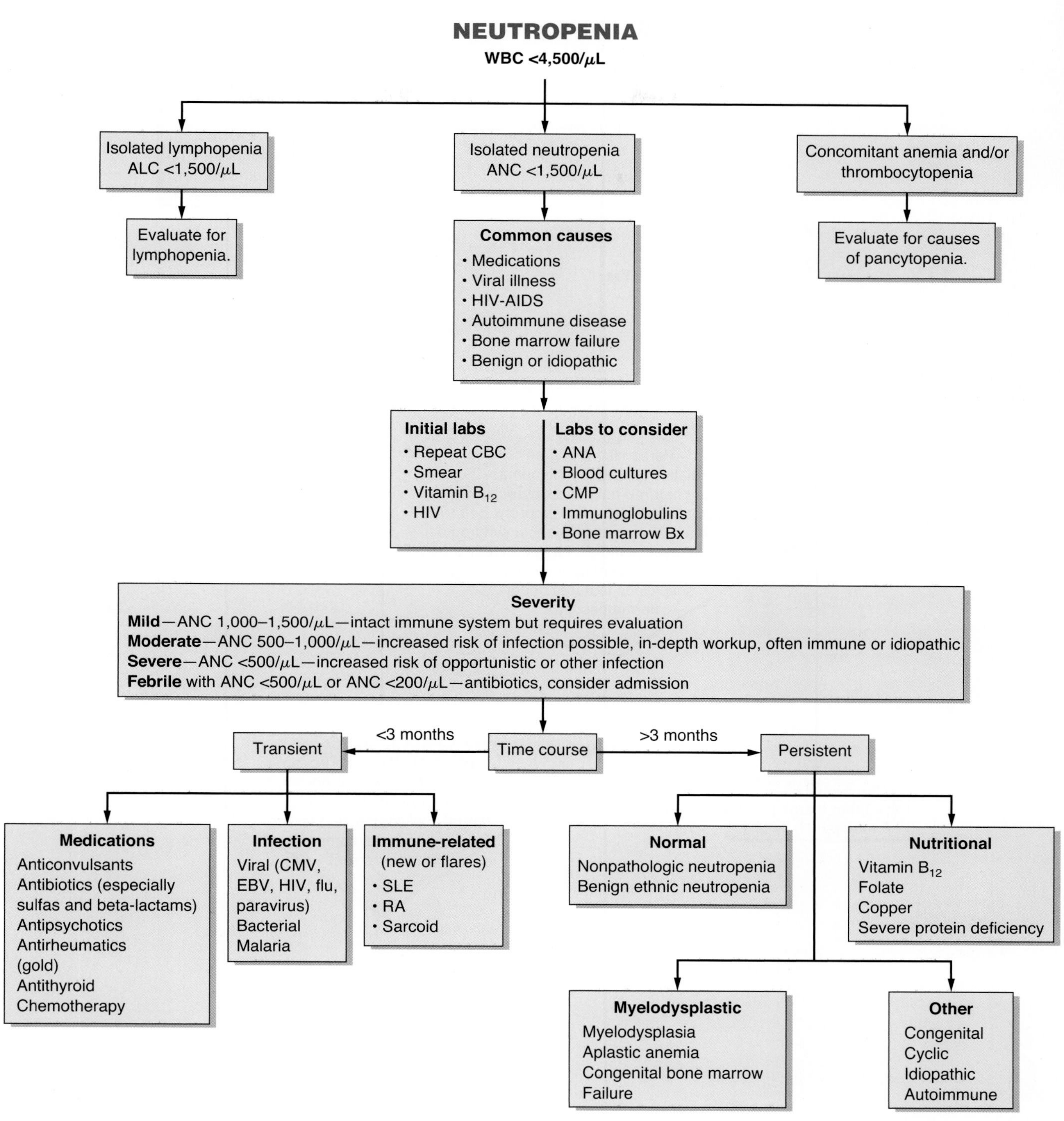

Andrew Smith, MD and Erin Bassett-Novoa, MD

Newburger PE, Dale DC. Evaluation and management of patients with isolated neutropenia. *Semin Hematol.* 2013;50(3):198–206.

NEVUS, ABNORMAL

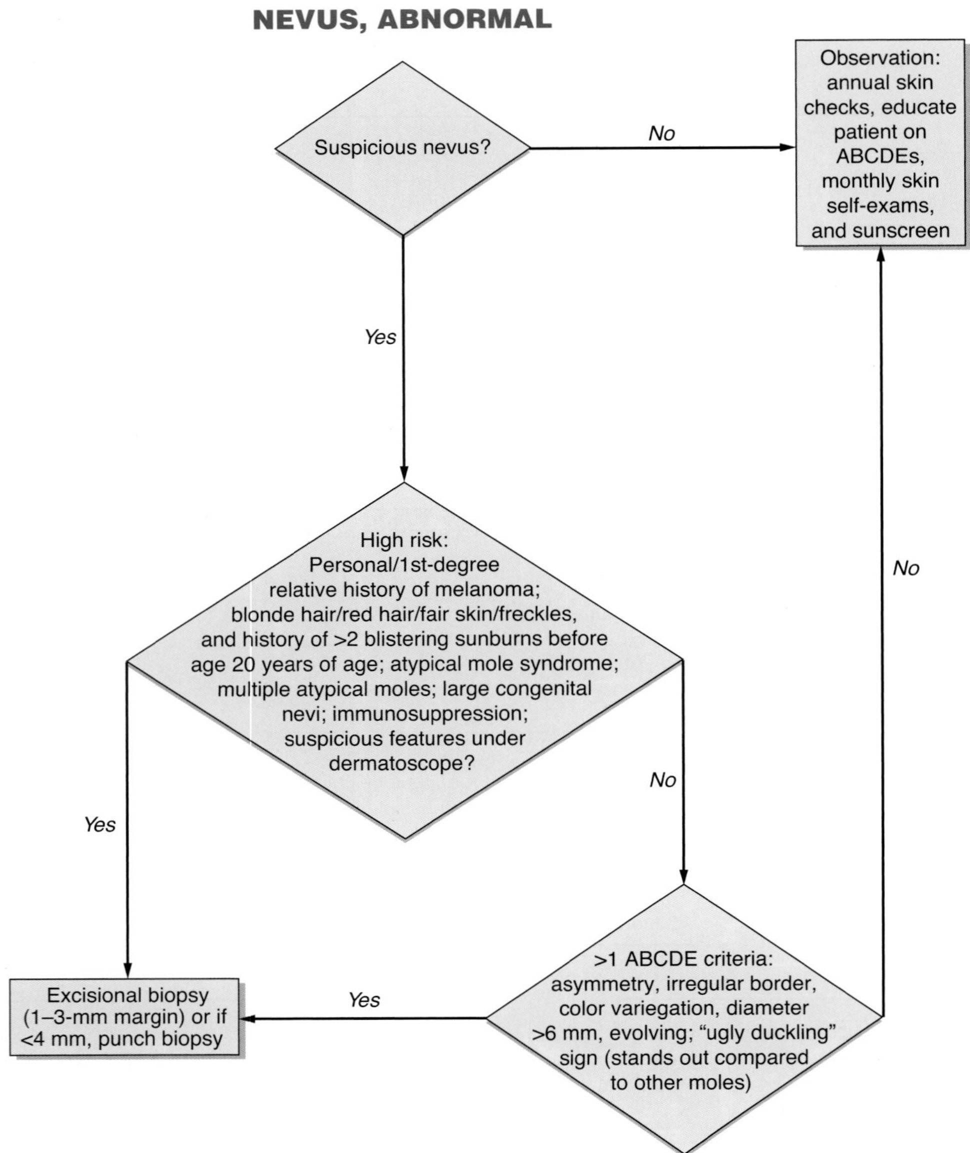

Miesha Merati, DO and Jenifer R. Lloyd, DO

Shenenberger DW. Cutaneous malignant melanoma: a primary care perspective. *Am Fam Physician.* 2012;85(2):161–168.

OPIOID DEPENDENCE

Screen all patients for opioid abuse/dependence every 12 months. Tools: CAGE AID

(Cut down drug use, annoyed by criticism of drug use, guilty about drug, used drug in morning to steady nerves, or get rid of hangover?)

↓

Meet *DSM-5* criteria for substance abuse?

1. Substance use leading to impairment or distress, at least 2 of the following, within a 12-month period:
    1. Failure to fulfill major role obligations at work, school, or home
    2. Recurrent substance use in physically hazardous situations
    3. Recurrent substance-related legal problems
    4. Continued substance use despite having recurrent social or interpersonal problems
2. The symptoms have never met the criteria for substance dependence for this class of substance.

- *No* → Counseling
- *Yes* → Urine drug screen, pregnancy test, LFTs, HBV, HCV, HIV testing. Any psychosocial and medical comorbidities?
    - *Yes* → Treat any preexisting medical conditions.
    - *No* → Risk of withdrawal? (http://www.naabt.org/documents/cows induction flow sheet.pdf); if >12 years of age, consider admission. If ≤12 years of age, is patient ready to change?
        - *No* → Provide support, refer to treatment program, offer no enabling prescriptions.
        - *Yes* → Type of treatment indicated: Is the patient: dependent only on oral opioids, has history of dependence (<1 year), has no major psychiatric comorbidity, and is socially stable with a supportive network? → If pregnant, use methadone.
            - *Yes* →
                - Office-based
                    1. Buprenorphine/naloxone
                    2. Rapid naloxone with clonidine and/ or buprenorphine/naloxone
                    3. Clonldine
                    - Failure? → Opioid treatment program
                - Hospital-based
                    1. Methadone
                    2. Buprenorphine/naloxone
                    3. Rapid naloxone with clonidine and/ or buprenorphine
            - *No* → Consider maintence therapy in patients with long history of abuse or repeated failed attempts.
                - Opioid treatment program:
                    1. Methadone
                    2. Naltrexone
                    3. Buprenorphine/naloxone
                - Office-based Buprenorphine/naloxone
                    - Failure? → Opioid treatment program

Andrea N. Watson, DO, MS and Nathalie Duroseau

Krantz MJ, Mehler PS. Treating opioid dependence. Growing implications for primary care. *Arch Intern Med.* 2004;164(3):277–288.

PAIN, CHRONIC

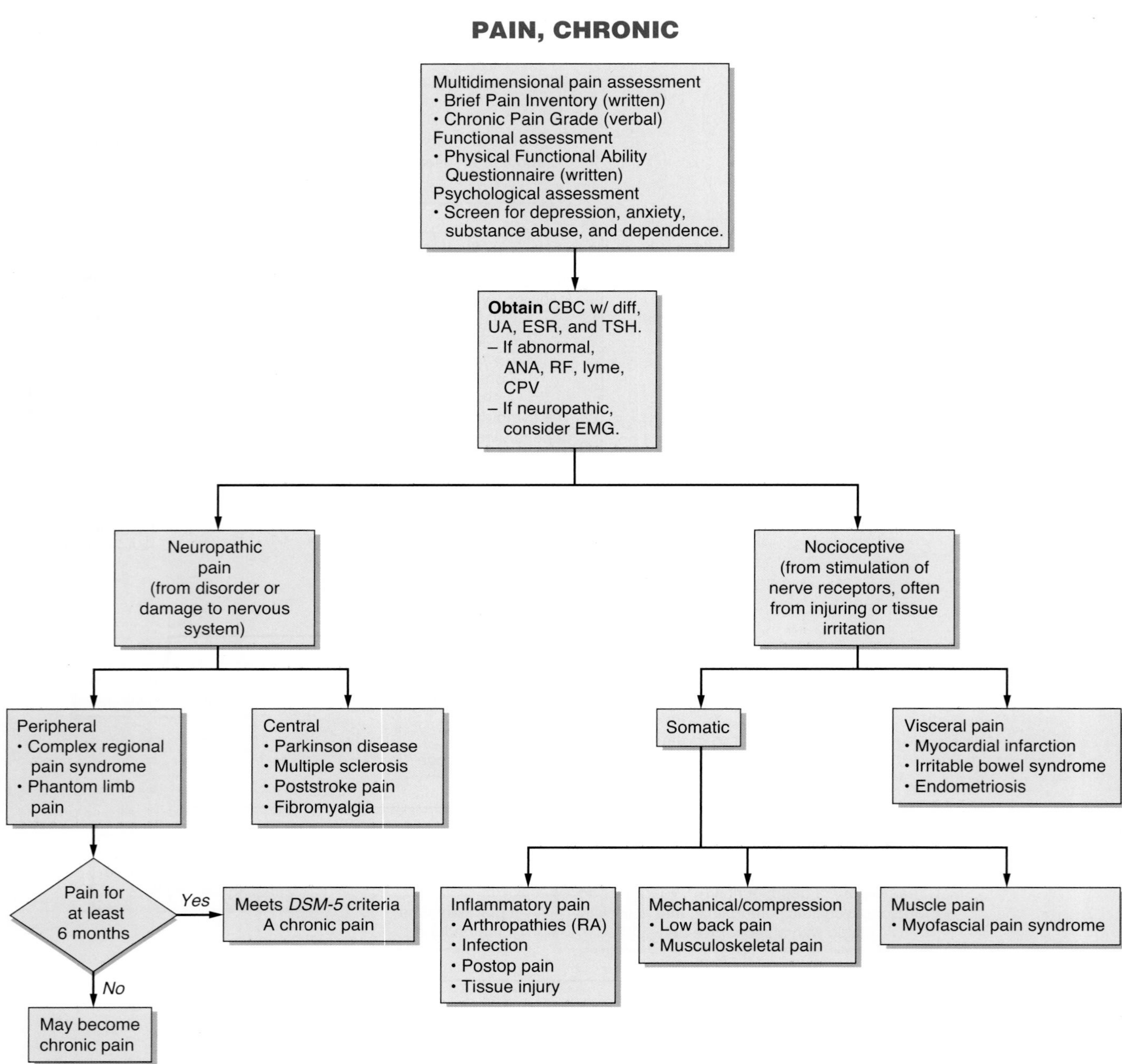

Ashik Lawrence, MD, Anubhav Kaul, MD, and Margaret Seaver, MD, MPH

Institute for Clinical Systems Improvement. *Health Care Guideline: Assessment and Management of Chronic Pain.* 5th ed. Bloomington, MN: Institute of Clinical System Improvement; 2011.

PAIN, CHRONIC, TREATMENT

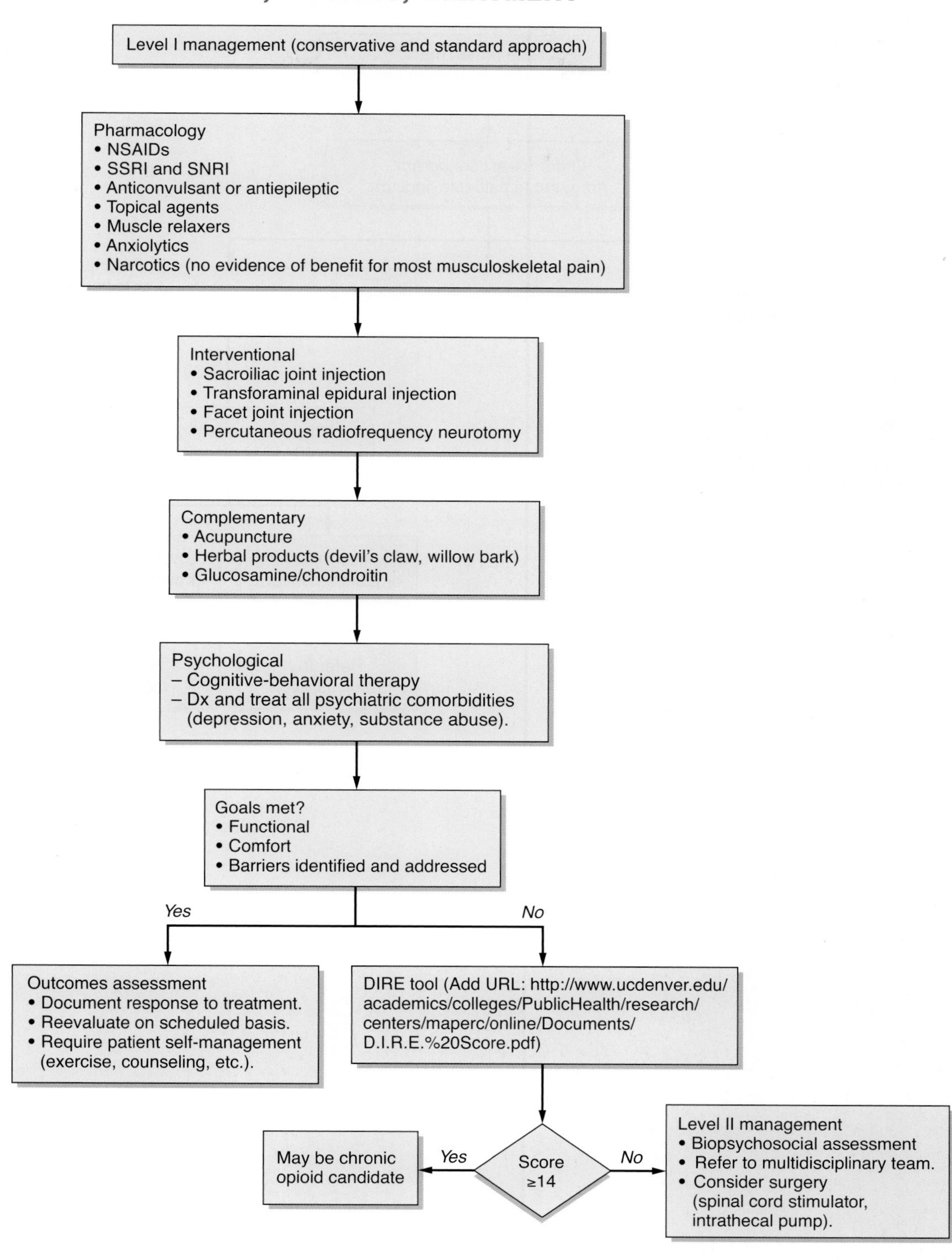

Ashik Lawrence, MD, Anubhav Kaul, MD, and Margaret Seaver, MD, MPH

Institute for Clinical Systems Improvement. *Health Care Guideline: Assessment and Management of Chronic Pain.* 5th ed. Bloomington, MN: Institute of Clinical System Improvement; 2011.

PALPABLE BREAST MASS (AGE <30 YEARS OR PREGNANT OR LACTATING)

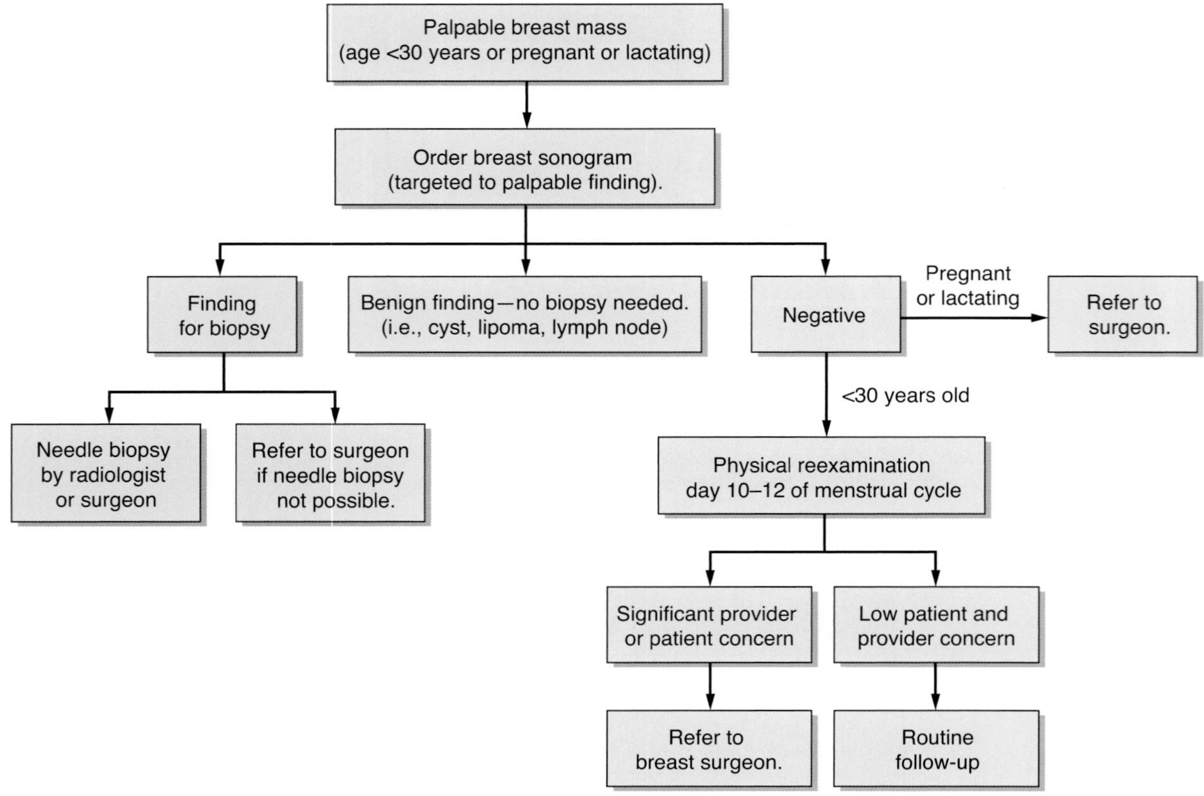

Stacey Vitiello, MD and Nancy Elliott, MD, FACS

Salzman B, Fleegle S, Tully AS. Common breast problems. *Am Fam Physician.* 2012;8(4):343–349.

PALPABLE BREAST MASS (AGE ≥30 YEARS)

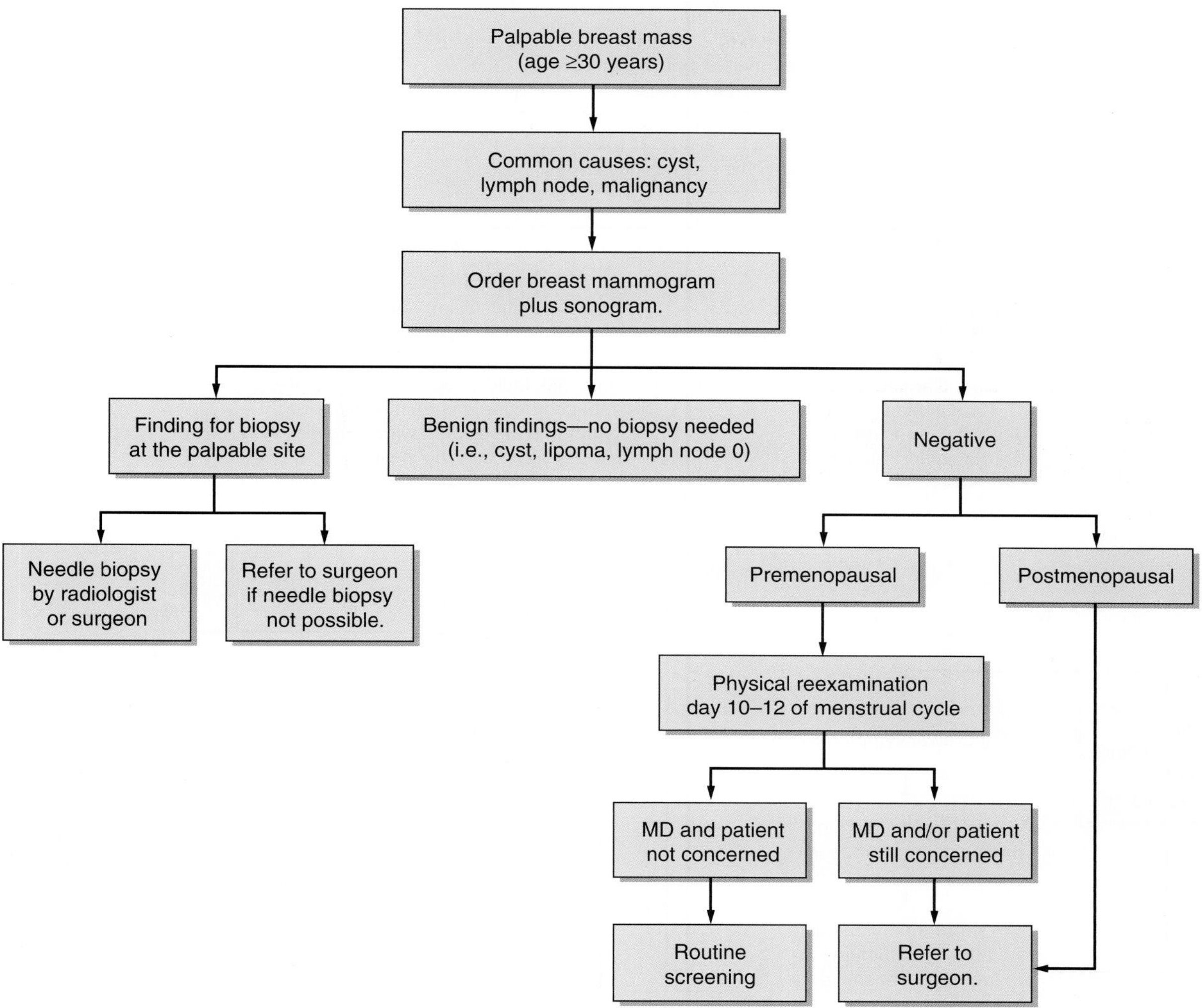

Stacey Vitiello, MD and Nancy Elliott, MD, FACS

Salzman B, Fleegle S, Tully AS. Common breast problems. *Am Fam Physician*. 2012;86(4):343–349.

PALPITATIONS

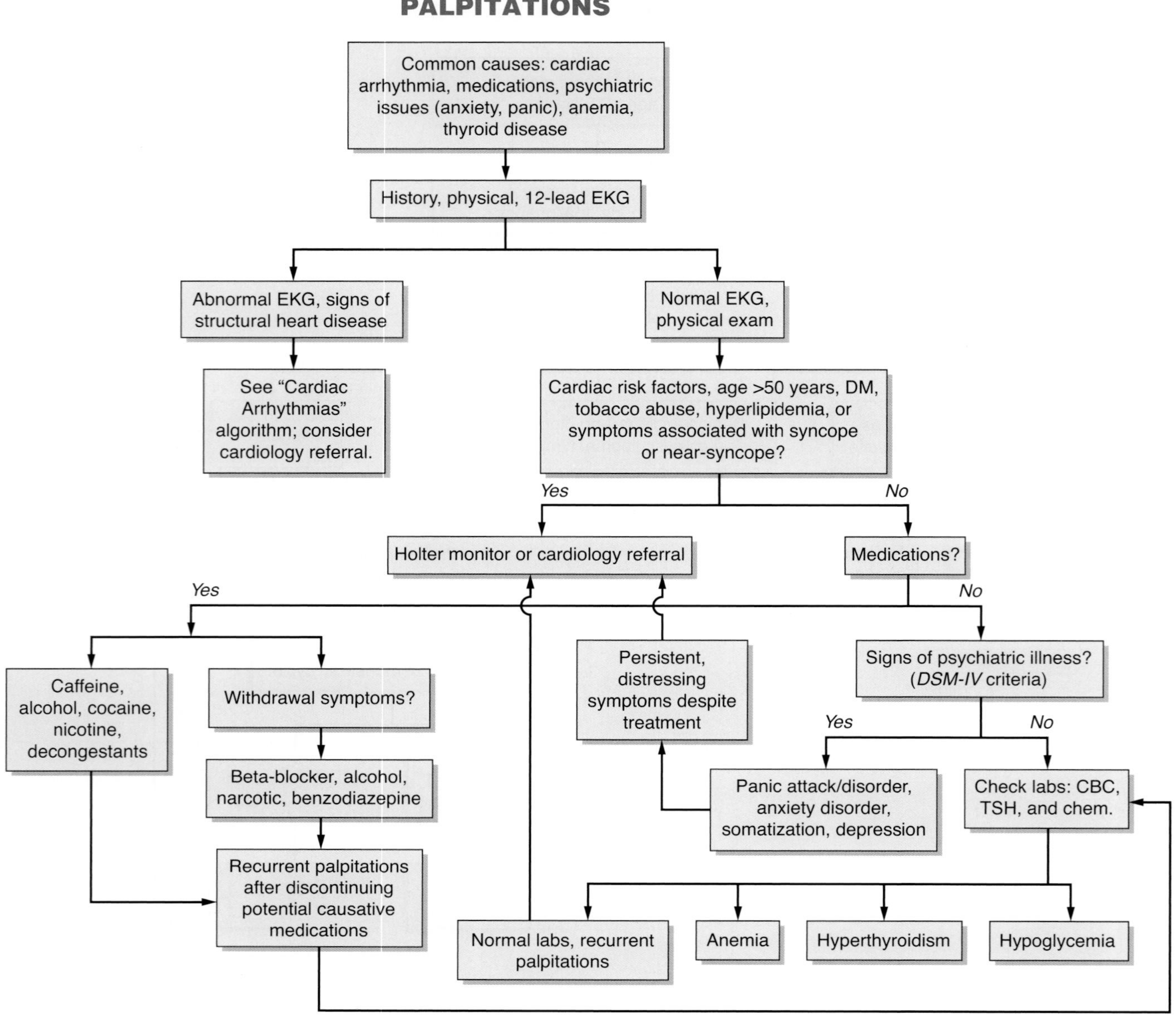

Elizabeth Dougherty, MD and Frank J. Domino, MD

Wexler RK, Pleister A, Raman, S. Outpatient approach to palpitations. *Am Fam Physician*. 2011;84(1):63–69.

PAP, NORMAL AND ABNORMAL IN NONPREGNANT WOMEN AGES 25 YEARS AND OLDER

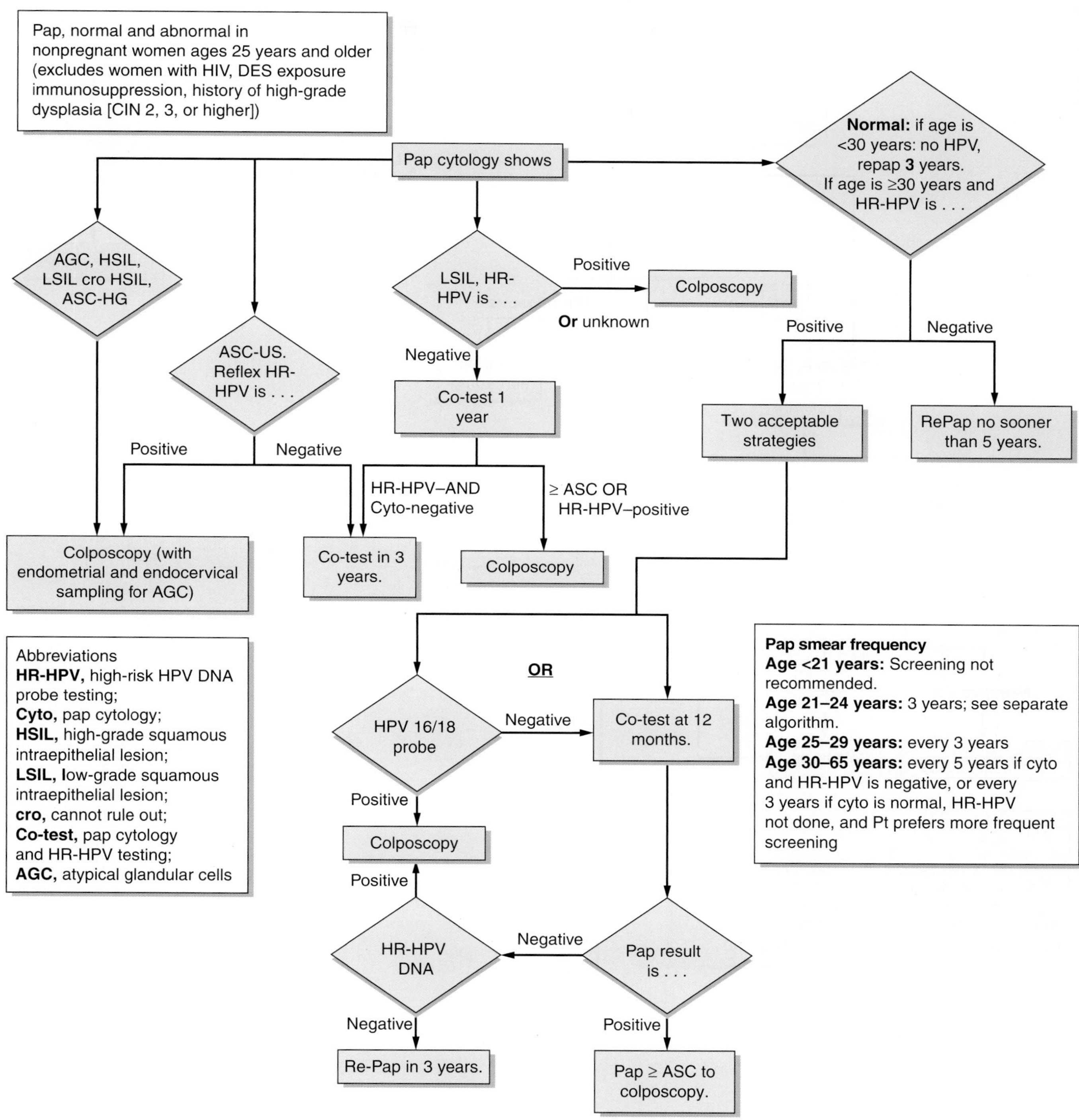

Abbreviations
HR-HPV, high-risk HPV DNA probe testing;
Cyto, pap cytology;
HSIL, high-grade squamous intraepithelial lesion;
LSIL, low-grade squamous intraepithelial lesion;
cro, cannot rule out;
Co-test, pap cytology and HR-HPV testing;
AGC, atypical glandular cells

Pap smear frequency
Age <21 years: Screening not recommended.
Age 21–24 years: 3 years; see separate algorithm.
Age 25–29 years: every 3 years
Age 30–65 years: every 5 years if cyto and HR-HPV is negative, or every 3 years if cyto is normal, HR-HPV not done, and Pt prefers more frequent screening

Jeremy Golding, MD, FAAFP

Adapted from American Society for Colposcopy and Cervical Pathology. Algorithms: updated consensus guidelines for managing abnormal cervical cancer screening tests and cancer precursors. http://www.asccp.org/portals/9/docs/algorithms%207.30.13.pdf. Accessed 2014.

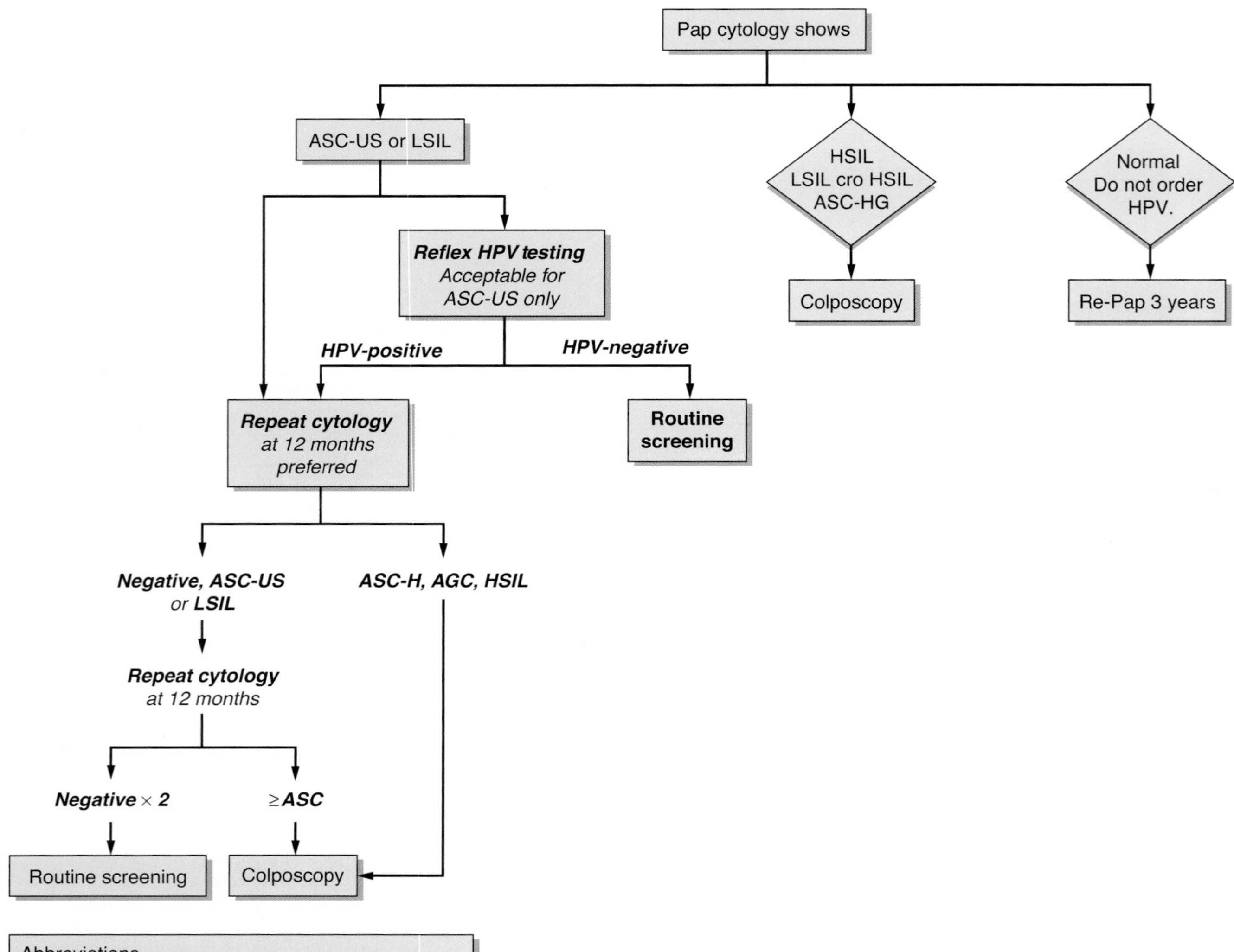

Jeremy Golding, MD, FAAFP

Adapted from American Society for Colposcopy and Cervical Pathology. Algorithms: updated consensus guidelines for managing abnormal cervical cancer screening tests and cancer precursors. http://www.asccp.org/portals/9/docs/algorithms%207.30.13.pdf. Accessed 2014.

PARKINSON DISEASE, TREATMENT

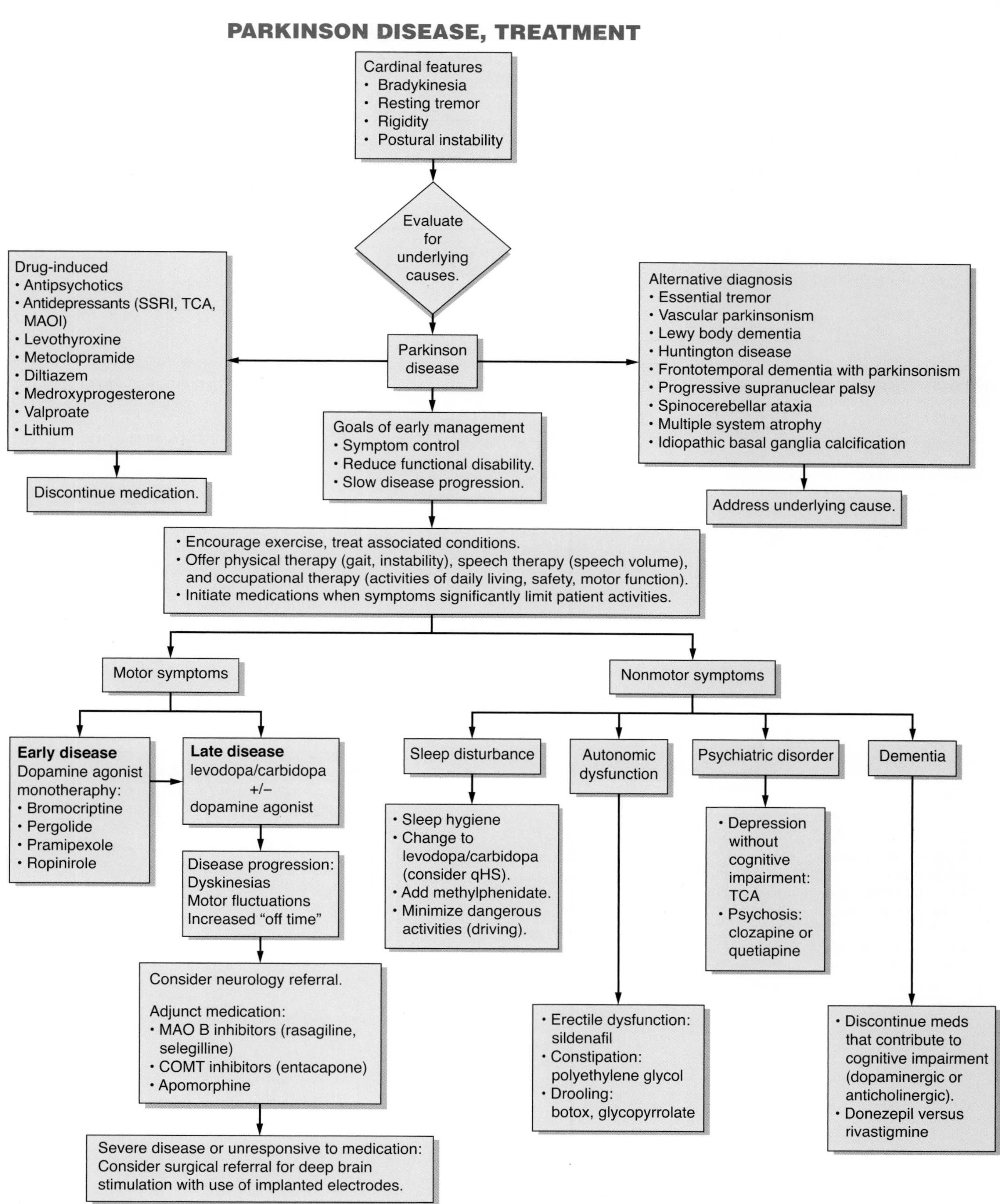

Sarah Coles, MD and William Dabbs, MD

Gazewood JD, Richards DR, Clebak K. Parkinson disease: an update. *Am Fam Physician.* 2013;87(4):267–273.

PEDIATRIC EXANTHEMS, DIAGNOSTIC

URI symptoms present?

- *No* → **Roseola (sixth disease, exanthem subitum)**
  - Rash: Erythematous maculopapular rash develops as fever resolves; starts on trunk and progresses to neck, extremities, (rarely) face
  - Prodrome: fever
  - Enanthem: erythematous macules on soft palate
  - Peak prevalence: 7–13 months
- *Yes* → Enanthem (involvement of mucous membranes)?
  - *No* → Vesicular?
    - *No* → **Erythema infectiosum (fifth disease)**
      - Rash: intensely red malar rash followed in 1–2 days by reticular erythematous maculopapular rash on trunk, extremities, and buttocks; recrudescence can last up to months.
      - Prodrome: generally mild, may have 1–4 days of headache, chills, URI symptoms
      - Enanthem: none
    - *Yes* → **Varicella (chickenpox)**
      - Rash: Macules form on trunk and spread to face and extremities; progress quickly in clusters to papules then tear-dropped shaped vesicles ("dew drops on a rose petal") that crust over or umbilicate
      - Prodrome: 1–2 days of fever, malaise, anorexia
      - Enanthem: Rarely, vesicles can lead to erosions of hard palate.
  - *Yes* → Vesicular?
    - *Yes* → **Coxsackie (hand-foot-mouth disease)**
      - Rash: Erythematous macules and papules ~2–3 mm found on palmar surface of hand, plantar surface of feet, and oral mucosa; progresses quickly through vesicular phase to form central gray ulcer
      - Prodrome: 12–36 hours of cough, fever, malaise, anorexia, abdominal pain
      - Enanthem: occurs with exanthem as painful ulcerative lesions commonly found on tongue, hard palate, and buccal mucosa
    - *No* → Koplik spots (white papules on buccal muscos)?
      - *No* → Fast-spreading rash?
        - *No* → **Rubella (third disease, German measles)**
          - Rash: erythematous maculopapular rash with downward progression from face
          - Prodrome: 1–7 days of malaise, painful lymphadenopathy
          - Enanthem: Forchheimer spots
        - *Yes* → **Scarlet fever (second disease)**
          - Rash: rapidly progressing erythematous macules and pinpoint, blanchable papules ("goose pimples") with sandpaper texture, greatest intensity at skin folds
          - Prodrome: 1–2 days of fever, sore throat, vomiting, abdominal pain
          - Enanthem: progression from white to red strawberry tongue
          - Perform rapid strep testing, a throat culture, and initiate treatment.
      - *Yes* → **Measles (first disease, rubeola)**
        - Rash: erythematous maculopapular rash with downward progression from face and brownish hue during resolution
        - Prodrome: 3–4 days of conjunctivitis, coryza, fever, cough
        - Enanthem: Koplik spots

Phillip Fournier, MD

Dyer JA. Childhood viral exanthems. *Pediatr Ann.* 2007;36(1):21–29.

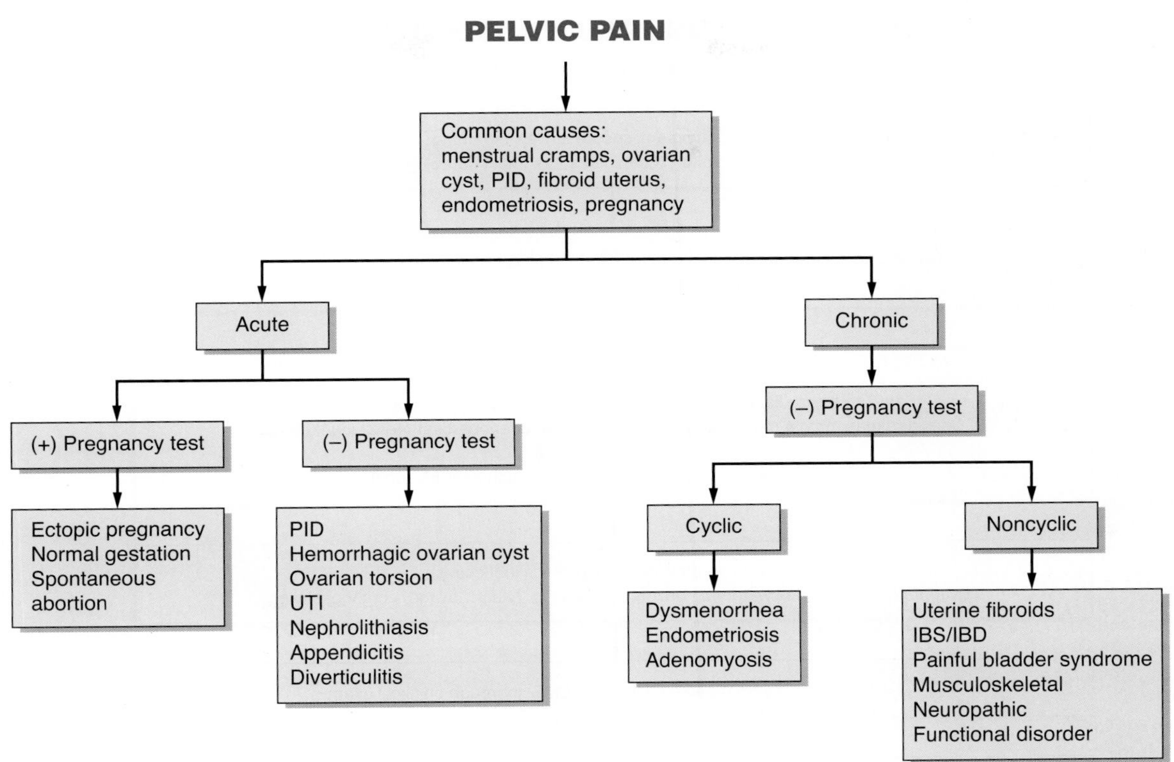

Meredith Gray, MD and Isaiah Johnson, MD

Howard FM. Chronic pelvic pain. *Obstet Gynecol.* 2003;101(3):594–611.

POISON EXPOSURE AND TREATMENT

POISON EXPOSURE

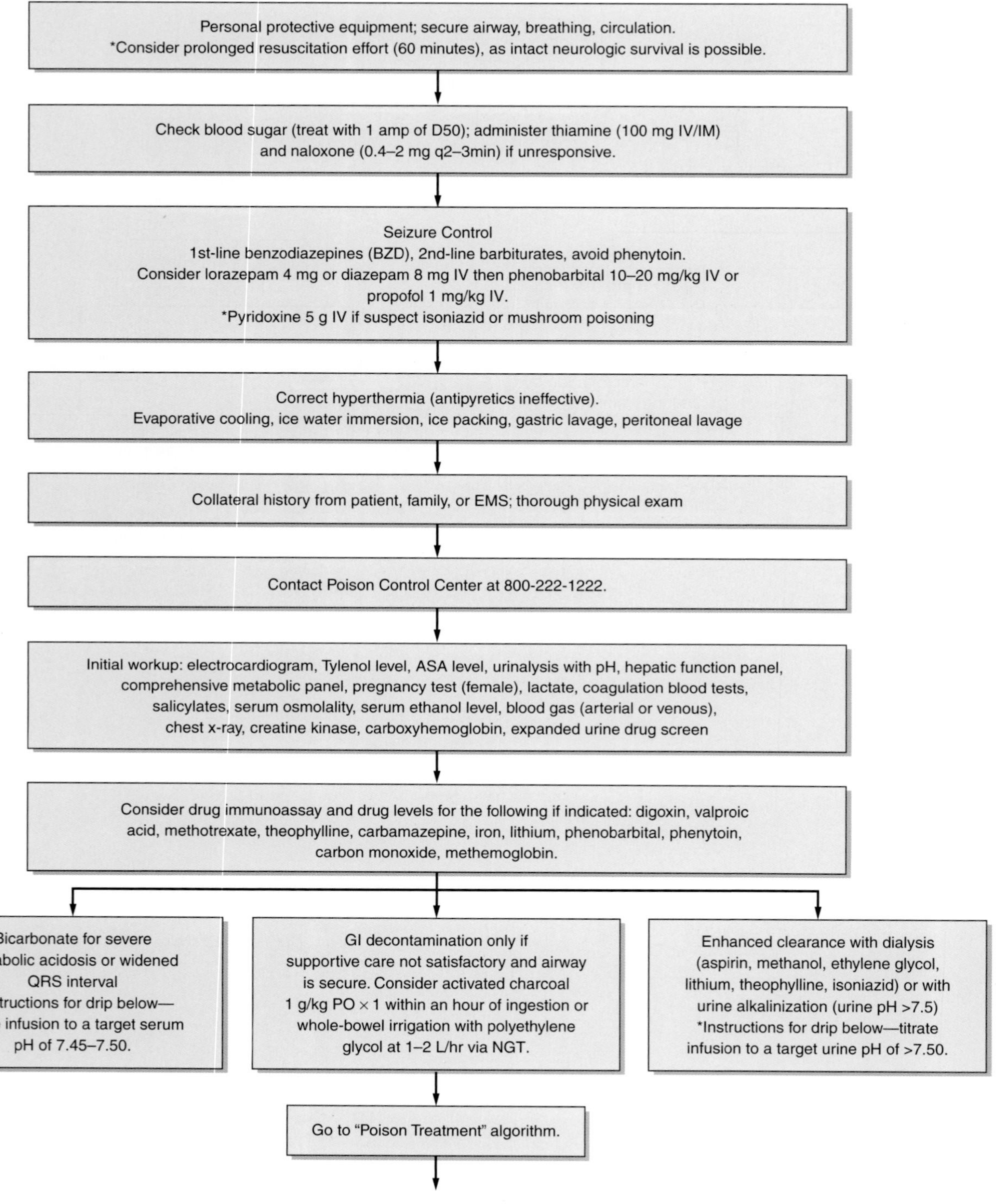

Personal protective equipment; secure airway, breathing, circulation.
*Consider prolonged resuscitation effort (60 minutes), as intact neurologic survival is possible.
Check blood sugar (treat with 1 amp of D50); administer thiamine (100 mg IV/IM) and naloxone (0.4–2 mg q2–3min) if unresponsive.
Seizure Control
1st-line benzodiazepines (BZD), 2nd-line barbiturates, avoid phenytoin.
Consider lorazepam 4 mg or diazepam 8 mg IV then phenobarbital 10–20 mg/kg IV or propofol 1 mg/kg IV.
*Pyridoxine 5 g IV if suspect isoniazid or mushroom poisoning
Correct hyperthermia (antipyretics ineffective).
Evaporative cooling, ice water immersion, ice packing, gastric lavage, peritoneal lavage
Collateral history from patient, family, or EMS; thorough physical exam
Contact Poison Control Center at 800-222-1222.
Initial workup: electrocardiogram, Tylenol level, ASA level, urinalysis with pH, hepatic function panel, comprehensive metabolic panel, pregnancy test (female), lactate, coagulation blood tests, salicylates, serum osmolality, serum ethanol level, blood gas (arterial or venous), chest x-ray, creatine kinase, carboxyhemoglobin, expanded urine drug screen
Consider drug immunoassay and drug levels for the following if indicated: digoxin, valproic acid, methotrexate, theophylline, carbamazepine, iron, lithium, phenobarbital, phenytoin, carbon monoxide, methemoglobin.
Bicarbonate for severe metabolic acidosis or widened QRS interval
*Instructions for drip below—titrate infusion to a target serum pH of 7.45–7.50.
GI decontamination only if supportive care not satisfactory and airway is secure. Consider activated charcoal 1 g/kg PO × 1 within an hour of ingestion or whole-bowel irrigation with polyethylene glycol at 1–2 L/hr via NGT.
Enhanced clearance with dialysis (aspirin, methanol, ethylene glycol, lithium, theophylline, isoniazid) or with urine alkalinization (urine pH >7.5)
*Instructions for drip below—titrate infusion to a target urine pH of >7.50.
Go to "Poison Treatment" algorithm.

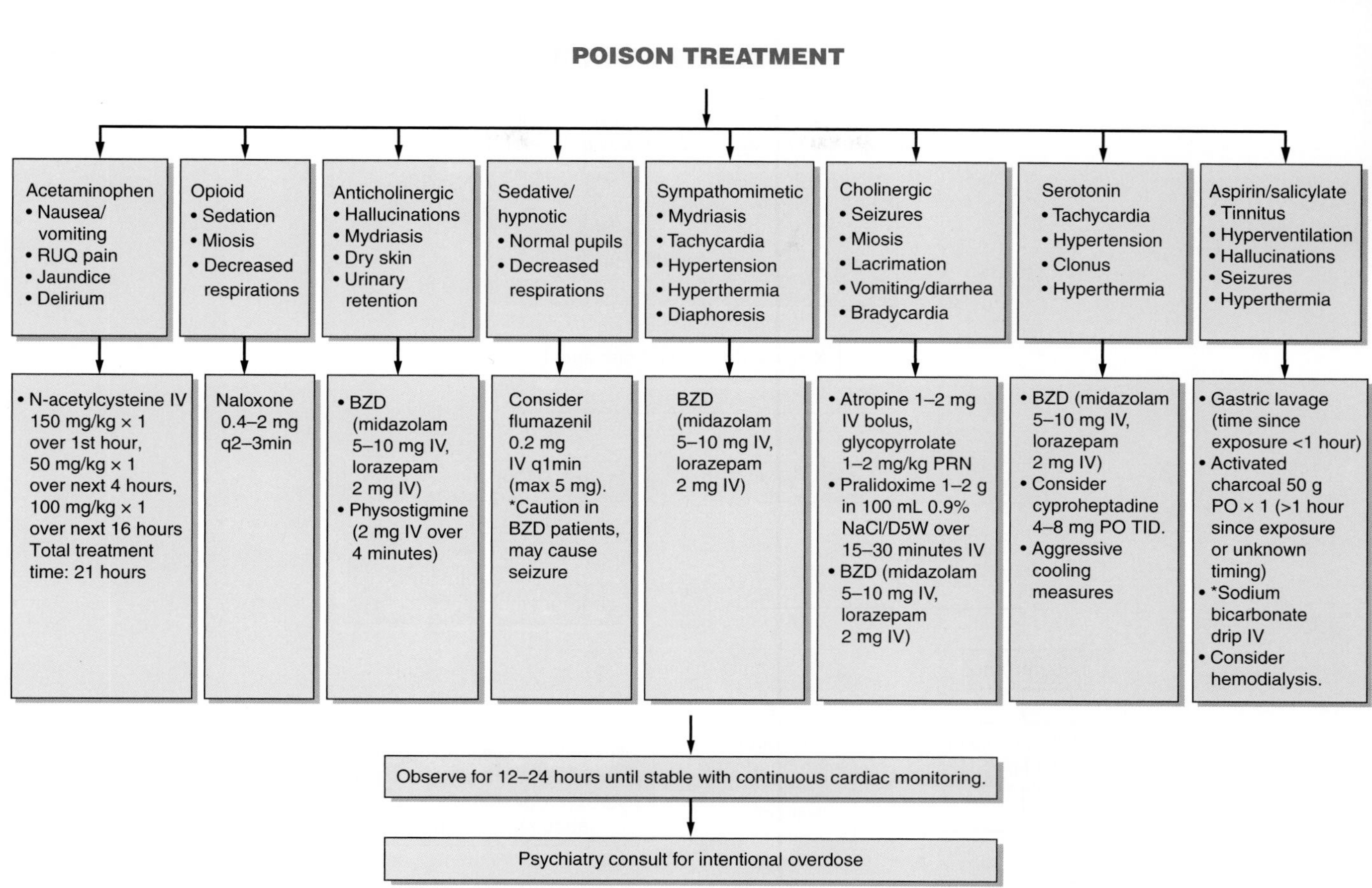

*To mix a bicarbonate drip: 150 mEq (3 amps) $NaHCO_3$ in 1 L of D5W, then start at a rate of 150–200 mL/hr.

Pediatric dosing (adult doses in algorithm)

- Activated charcoal (0.5–1 g/kg PO)
- Atropine (0.02 mg/kg IV)
- Bicarbonate (1–2 mEq/kg IV*)
- Chlorpromazine (not recommended)
- Cyproheptadine (0.25 mg/kg/day divided BID or TID)
- Dextrose (2.5 mL/kg of 10% or 1 mL/kg of 25% IV)
- Flumazenil (5 μg/kg IV)
- Glycopyrrolate (0.025 mg/kg IV)
- Lorazepam (0.05–0.1 mg/kg IV)
- Midazolam (0.1 mg/kg IV)
- Phenobarbital (10–20 mg/kg IV)
- Physostigmine (10–30 μg/kg IV)
- Polyethylene glycol (250–500 mL/hr PO/NG)
- Pralidoxime (20–40 mg/kg IV)
- Pyridoxine (same as adults)
- Naloxone (0.1 mg/kg IV q2–3min)
- Thiamine (not routinely given)

Michelle Williams, MD and Scott F. Graham, MD

Chun LJ, Tong MJ, Busuttil RW, et al. Acetaminophen hepatotoxicity and acute liver failure. *J Clin Gastroenterol.* 2009;43(4):342–349. http://www.ncbi.nlm.nih.gov/entrez/query.fcgi?db=pubmed&cmd=Retrieve&dopt=Abstract&list%5Fuids=19169150&. Accessed 2014; Dargan PI, Wallace CI, Jones AL. An evidence based flowchart to guide the management of acute salicylate (aspirin) overdose. *Emerg Med J.* 2002;19(3):206–209. http://www.ncbi.nlm.nih.gov/pubmed/11971828?dopt=Abstract. Accessed 2014.

PRECOCIOUS PUBERTY

Signs of secondary sexual development in boys >9 years and girls >8 years

→ Common causes: medication, pituitary tumor, congenital, adrenal hyperplasia, adrenal tumor, ovarian tumor, pseudoprecocious puberty

→ X-ray to determine bone age

- Bone age > chronologic age
  - → Basal LH levels
    - <5 mIU/mL → GnRH stimulation test, LH, FSH
      - LH, FSH increased. → Gonadotropin-dependent (central) precocious puberty → Estradiol, testosterone, TSH, MRI of brain
        - CNS lesion
        - Abnormal TSH → Chronic primary hypothyroidism
        - Negative → Idiopathic precocious puberty
      - Absent LH response → Gonadotropin-independent (peripheral) precocious puberty
    - >5 mIU/mL → Gonadotropin-independent (peripheral) precocious puberty → Testosterone, estradiol, LH, FSH, cortisol, DHEA, DHEA-S, 17-hydroxyprogesterone, hCG (males), abdominal and pelvic US
      - → In ♀, US + for ovarian cyst(s) or tumor
      - Elevated hCG in ♂ → Germ cell tumor
      - Very high levels of testosterone in ♂ → Leydig cell tumor
      - Elevated17-hydroxyprogesterone → Congenital adrenal hyperplasia
      - Pubertal values of testosterone in ♂ and estradiol in ♀, with bone and skin findings → McCune Albright syndrome
      - Elevated DHEA, DHEA-S, findings on imaging → Adrenal tumor or cancer
      - Elevated testosterone in ♂ and estradiol in ♀ → Exogenous sex steroids
- Bone age = chronologic age
  - → Incomplete precocious puberty (premature adrenarche or thelarche)

Nicole Shields, MD

Berberoğlu M. Precocious puberty and normal variant puberty: definition, etiology, diagnosis and current management. *J Clin Res Pediatr Endocrinol.* 2009;1(4):164–174.

PREOPERATIVE EVALUATION OF NONCARDIAC SURGICAL PATIENT

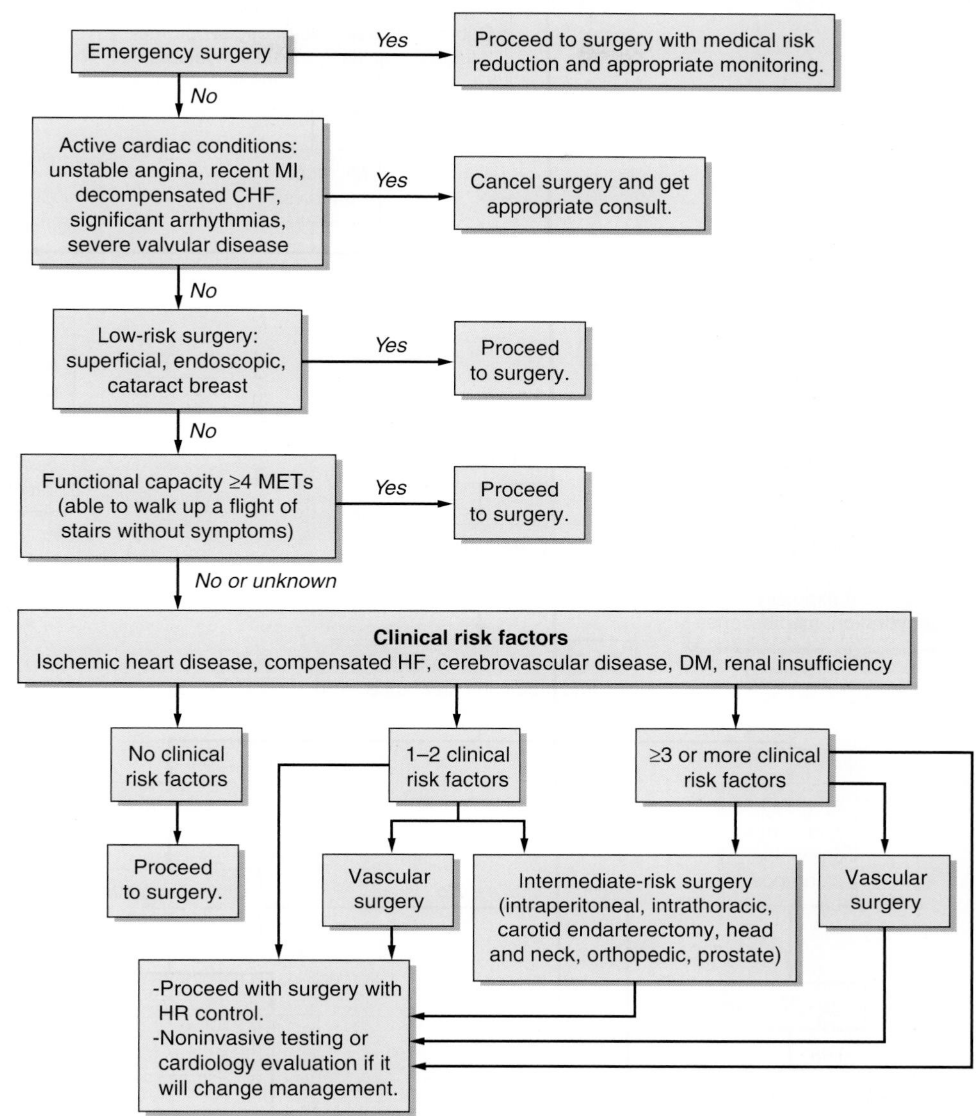

Andrew Grimes, MD and Stacy Jones, MD

Fleisher LA, Beckman JA, Brown KA, et al. ACC/AHA 2007 guidelines on perioperative cardiovascular evaluation and care for noncardiac surgery: a report of the American College of Cardiology/American Heart Association Task Force on Practice Guidelines (Writing Committee to revise the 2002 Guidelines on Perioperative Cardiovascular Evaluation for Noncardiac Surgery): developed in collaboration with the American Society of Echocardiography, American Society of Nuclear Cardiology, Heart Rhythm Society, Society of Cardiovascular Anesthesiologists, Society for Cardiovascular Angiography and Interventions, Society for Vascular Medicine and Biology, and Society for Vascular Surgery. *Circulation*. 2007;116(17):e418–e499.

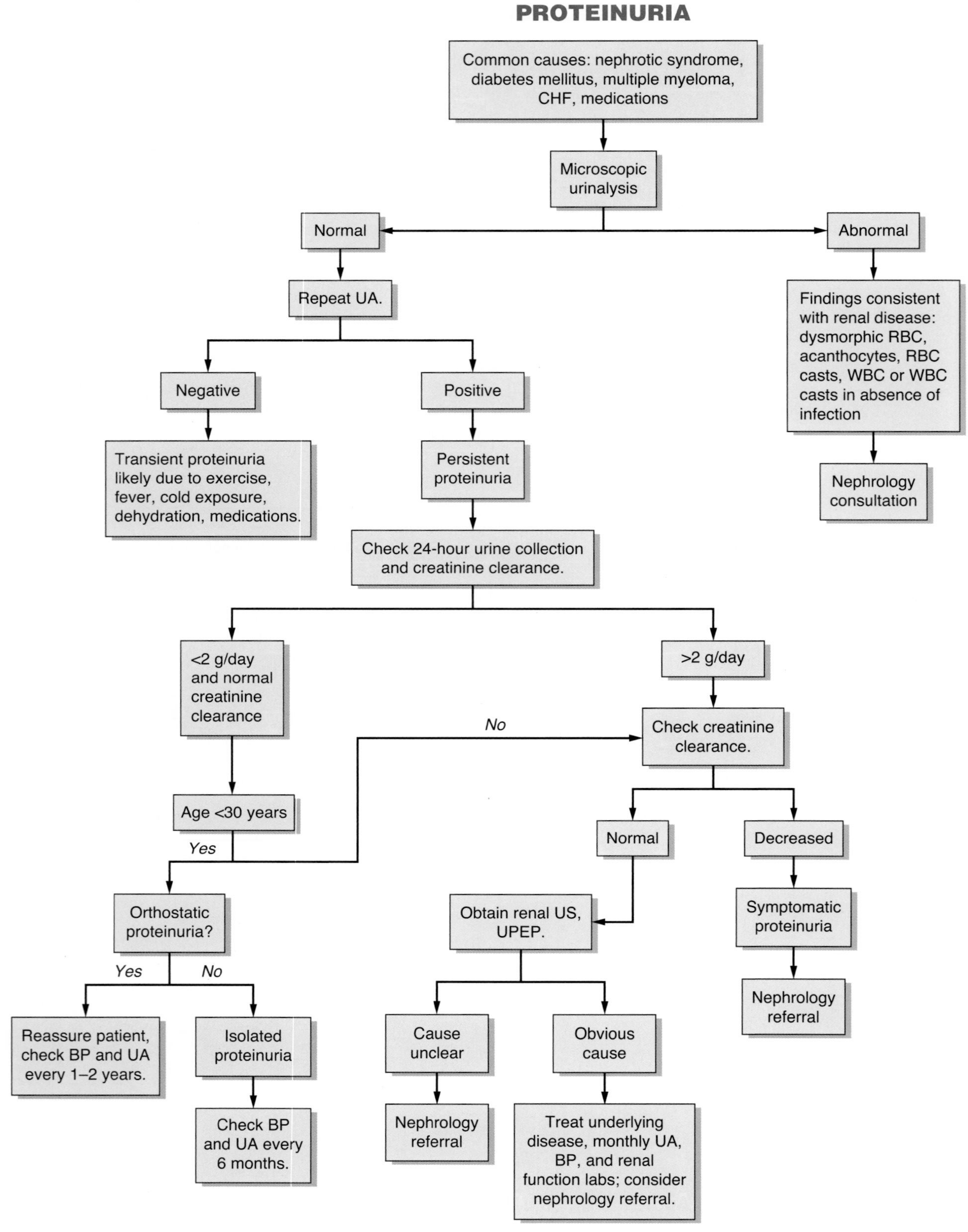

Jennifer Fernandez, MD

Simerville JA, Maxted WC, Pahira JJ. Urinalysis: a comprehensive review. *Am Fam Physician.* 2005;71(6):1153–1162.

PULMONARY EMBOLISM, DIAGNOSIS

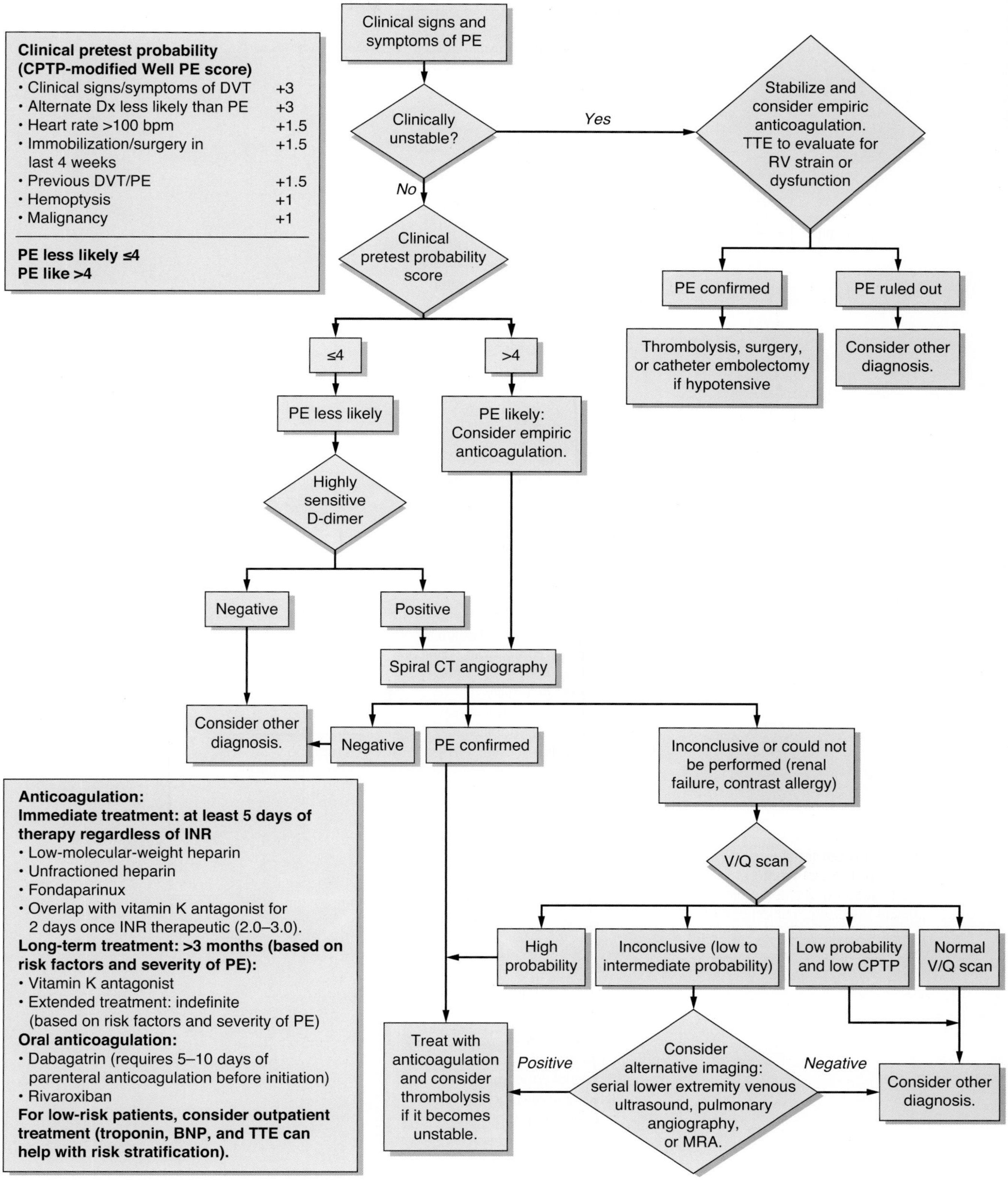

Clinical pretest probability (CPTP-modified Well PE score)

• Clinical signs/symptoms of DVT	+3
• Alternate Dx less likely than PE	+3
• Heart rate >100 bpm	+1.5
• Immobilization/surgery in last 4 weeks	+1.5
• Previous DVT/PE	+1.5
• Hemoptysis	+1
• Malignancy	+1

PE less likely ≤4
PE like >4

Clinical signs and symptoms of PE

Clinically unstable?

Yes → Stabilize and consider empiric anticoagulation. TTE to evaluate for RV strain or dysfunction
- PE confirmed → Thrombolysis, surgery, or catheter embolectomy if hypotensive
- PE ruled out → Consider other diagnosis.

No → Clinical pretest probability score
- ≤4 → PE less likely → Highly sensitive D-dimer
  - Negative → Consider other diagnosis.
  - Positive → Spiral CT angiography
- >4 → PE likely: Consider empiric anticoagulation. → Spiral CT angiography

Spiral CT angiography
- Negative → Consider other diagnosis.
- PE confirmed → Treat with anticoagulation and consider thrombolysis if it becomes unstable.
- Inconclusive or could not be performed (renal failure, contrast allergy) → V/Q scan
  - High probability → Treat with anticoagulation and consider thrombolysis if it becomes unstable.
  - Inconclusive (low to intermediate probability) → Consider alternative imaging: serial lower extremity venous ultrasound, pulmonary angiography, or MRA.
    - *Positive* → Treat with anticoagulation and consider thrombolysis if it becomes unstable.
    - *Negative* → Consider other diagnosis.
  - Low probability and low CPTP → Consider other diagnosis.
  - Normal V/Q scan → Consider other diagnosis.

Anticoagulation:
Immediate treatment: at least 5 days of therapy regardless of INR
- Low-molecular-weight heparin
- Unfractioned heparin
- Fondaparinux
- Overlap with vitamin K antagonist for 2 days once INR therapeutic (2.0–3.0).

Long-term treatment: >3 months (based on risk factors and severity of PE):
- Vitamin K antagonist
- Extended treatment: indefinite (based on risk factors and severity of PE)

Oral anticoagulation:
- Dabagatrin (requires 5–10 days of parenteral anticoagulation before initiation)
- Rivaroxiban

For low-risk patients, consider outpatient treatment (troponin, BNP, and TTE can help with risk stratification).

Musa A. Sharkawi, MB, BCh, BAO and Russell S. Zide, MD, FSVM

Kearon C, Kahn SR, Agnelli G, et al. Antithrombotic therapy for venous thromboembolic disease: American College of Chest Physicians Evidence-Based Clinical Practice Guidelines (9th edition). *Chest.* 2012;141(2)(Suppl):419S–494S.

PULMONARY EMBOLISM, TREATMENT

Probability of pulmonary embolism above treatment threshold

Coagulation contraindicated:
- Prior intracranial bleed
- Ischemic stroke <3 months
- Suspected aortic dissection
- Active bleeding diathesis
- Recent brain or spinal surgery
- Closed head or facial trauma

Yes → IVC filter

No → Massive pulmonary embolism? (SBP <90 mm Hg for >15 minutes)

Yes → Thrombolysis contraindicated?

Yes → Embolectomy, per local expertise

No → Thrombolysis → Clinical improvement?

No → Embolectomy, per local expertise

Yes → History of heparin-induced thrombocytopenia?

Massive pulmonary embolism? *No* → Benefits of thrombolysis outweigh risks based on evidence of following clinical factors:
1. Hemodynamic instability,
2. Worse respiratory insufficiency,
3. Severe RV strain, and/or
4. Major myocardial necrosis?

Yes → Thrombolysis contraindicated?

No → History of heparin-induced thrombocytopenia?

Yes → Consider fondaparinox, lepirudin, or argatroban. (Caution use of lepirudin in liver disease; caution use of argatroban in kidney disease.)

No → Administer parenteral heparin-based product + vitamin K antagonist, with at least 5 days of concomitant therapy and INR >2 × 24 hours prior to discontinuing heparin product.

Parag Goyal, MD

Jaff MR, McMurtry MS, Archer SL, et al. Management of massive and submassive pulmonary embolism, iliofemoral deep vein thrombosis, and chronic thromboembolic pulmonary hypertension: a scientific statement from the American Heart Association. *Circulation.* 2011;123(16):1788–1830.

RASH, FOCAL

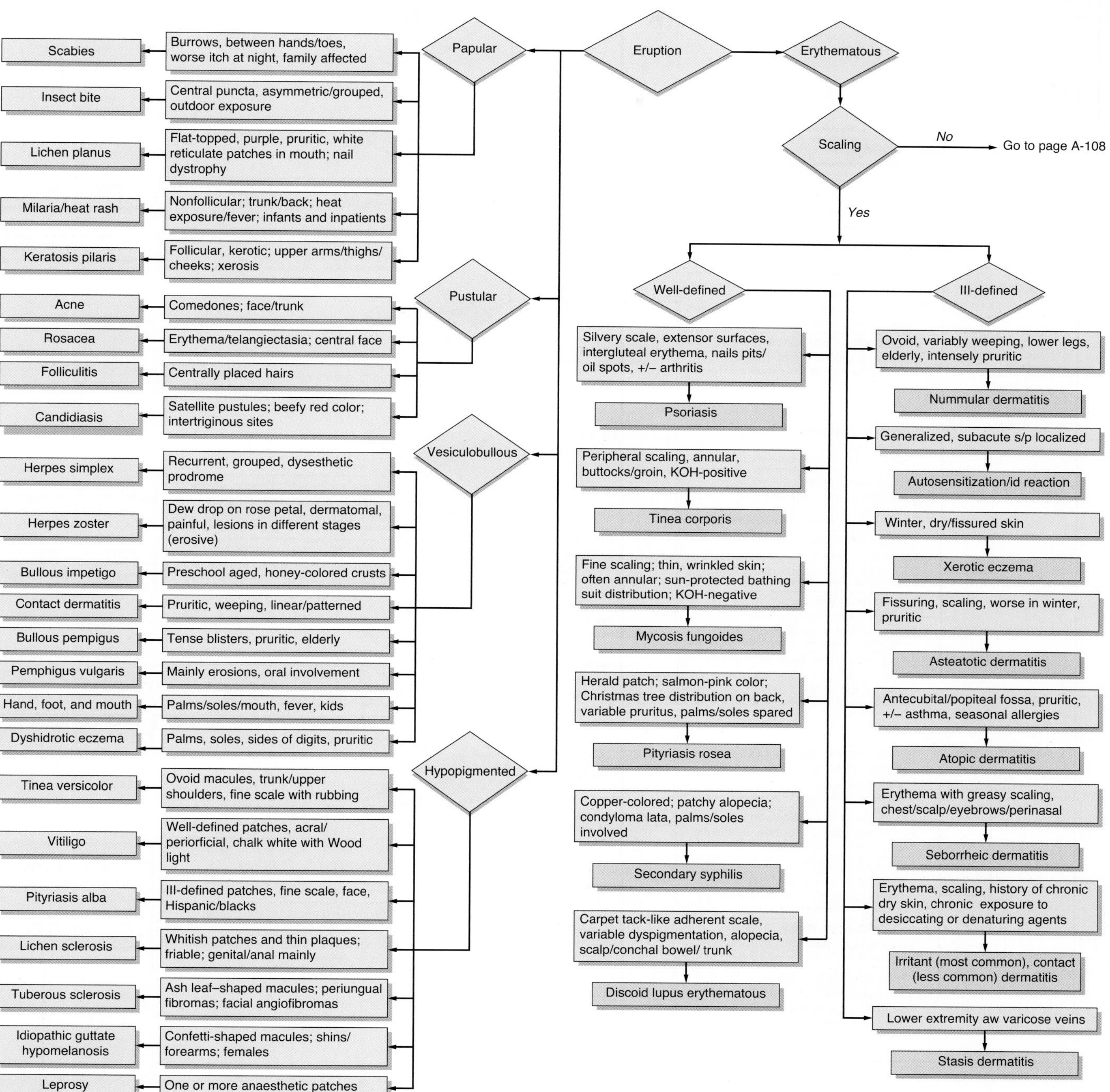

7 classes of topical steroids based on ability to constrict capillaries. Class 1, strongest; Class 7, weakest

Class 1	Class 2	Class 3	Class 4	Class 5	Class 6	Class 7
Clobetasol propionate 0.05% (Dermovate)	Flucinonide 0.05% (Lidex)	Triamcinolone acetonide 0.5% (Kenalog)	Hydrocortisone valerate 0.2% (Westcort)	Fluticasone propionate 0.05% (Cutivate)	Alclometasone dipropionate 0.05% (Aclovate)	Hydrocortisone 2.5% (Hytone)
Betamethasone dipropionate 0.25% (Diprolene)	Halcinonide 0.05% (Cyclocort)	Mometasone furoate 0.1% (Elocon)	Triamcinolone acetonide 0.1% (Kenalog)	Desonide 0.05% (Tridesilon)	Fluocinolone acetonide 0.01% (Dermasmooth)	Hydrocortisone 1%
Halobetasol proprionate 0.5% (Ultravate, Halox)	Desoximetasone 0.25% (Topicort)	Fluticasone propionate 0.005% (Cutivate)	Hydrocortisone butyrate 0.1% (Locoid)	Fluocinolone acetonide 0.025% (Synalar)	Triamcinolone acetonide 0.025% (Kenalog)	

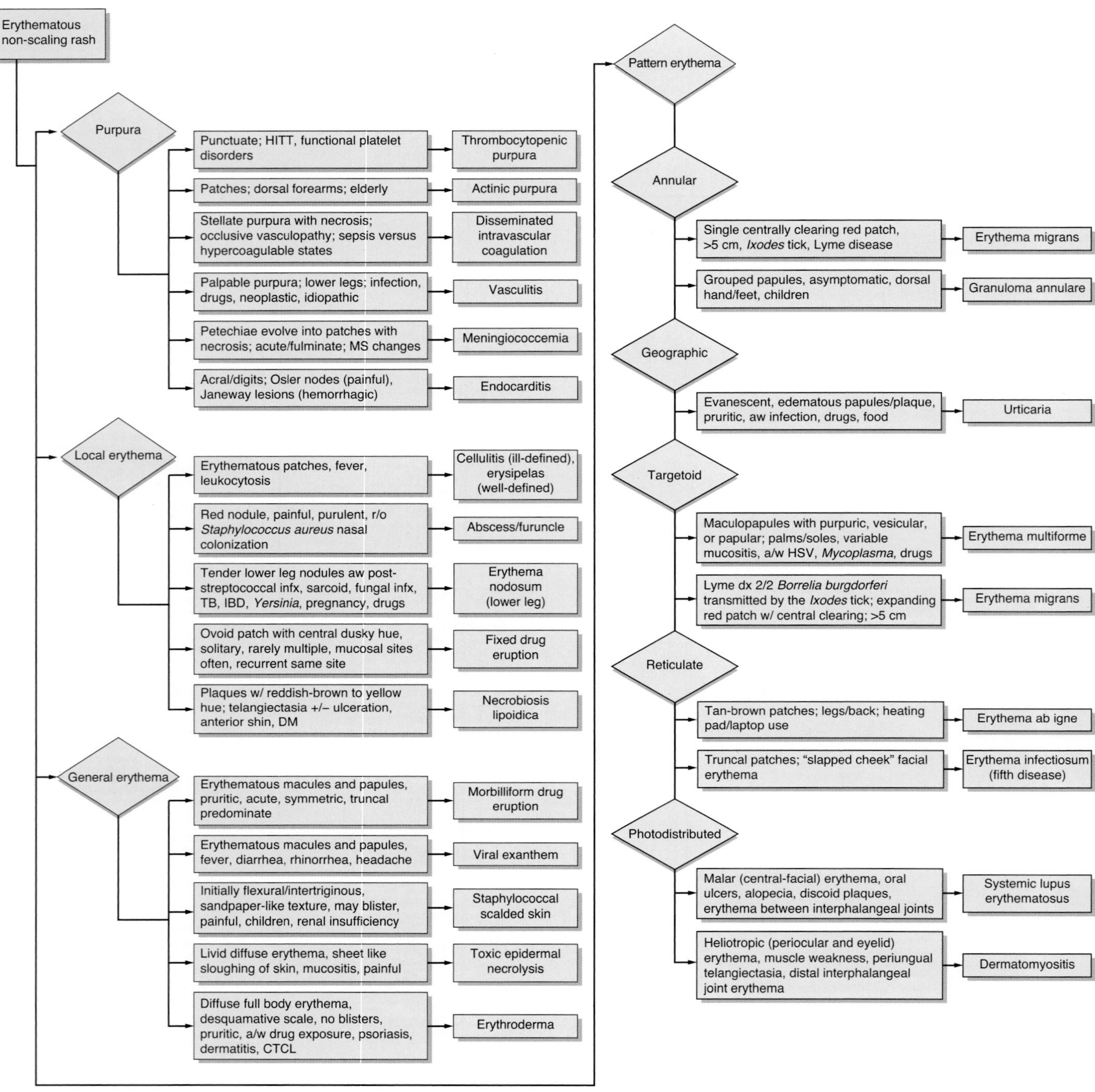

7 classes of topical steroids based on ability to constrict capillaries. Class 1, strongest; Class 7, weakest						
Class 1	**Class 2**	**Class 3**	**Class 4**	**Class 5**	**Class 6**	**Class 7**
Clobetasol propionate 0.05% (Dermovate)	Flucinonide 0.05% (Lidex)	Triamcinolone acetonide 0.5% (Kenalog)	Hydrocortisone valerate 0.2% (Westcort)	Fluticasone propionate 0.05% (Cutivate)	Alclometasone dipropionate 0.05% (Aclovate)	Hydrocortisone 2.5% (Hytone)
Betamethasone dipropionate 0.25% (Diprolene)	Halcinonide 0.05% (Cyclocort)	Mometasone furoate 0.1% (Elocon)	Triamcinolone acetonide 0.1% (Kenalog)	Desonide 0.05% (Tridesilon)	Fluocinolone acetonide 0.01% (Dermasmooth)	Hydrocortisone 1%
Halobetasol proprionate 0.5% (Ultravate, Halox)	Desoximetasone 0.25% (Topicort)	Fluticasone propionate 0.005% (Cutivate)	Hydrocortisone butyrate 0.1% (Locoid)	Fluocinolone acetonide 0.025% (Synalar)	Triamcinolone acetonide 0.025% (Kenalog)	

Brandon Kirsch, MD and Jason C. Sluzevich, MD

Ely W, Seabury Stone M. The generalized rash: part I. Differential diagnosis; The generalized rash: part II. Diagnostic approach. *Am Fam Physican*. 2010;81(6):726–739.

RECTAL BLEEDING AND HEMATOCHEZIA

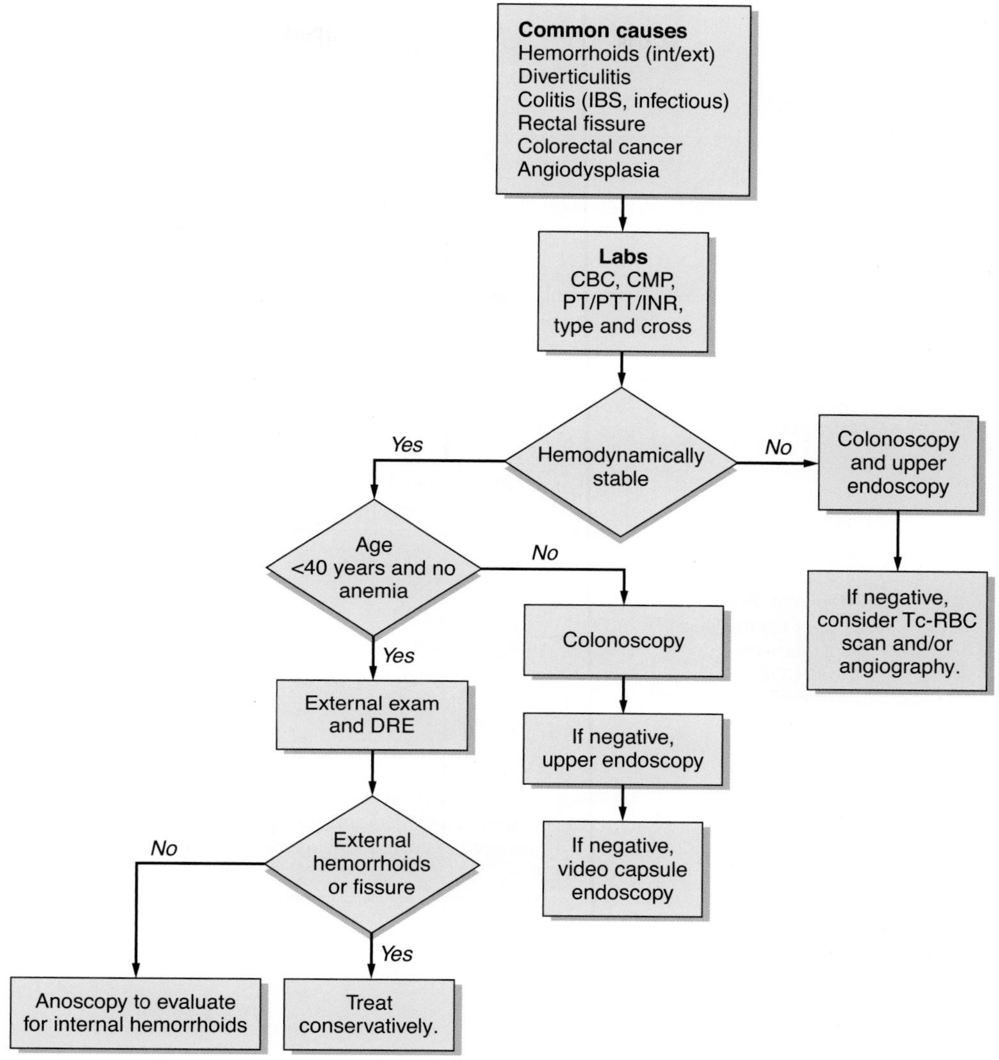

Mohammad Ansar Mughal, MD

Hoedema RE, Luchtefeld MA. The management of lower gastrointestinal hemorrhage. *Dis Colon Rectum*. 2005;48(11):2010–2024.

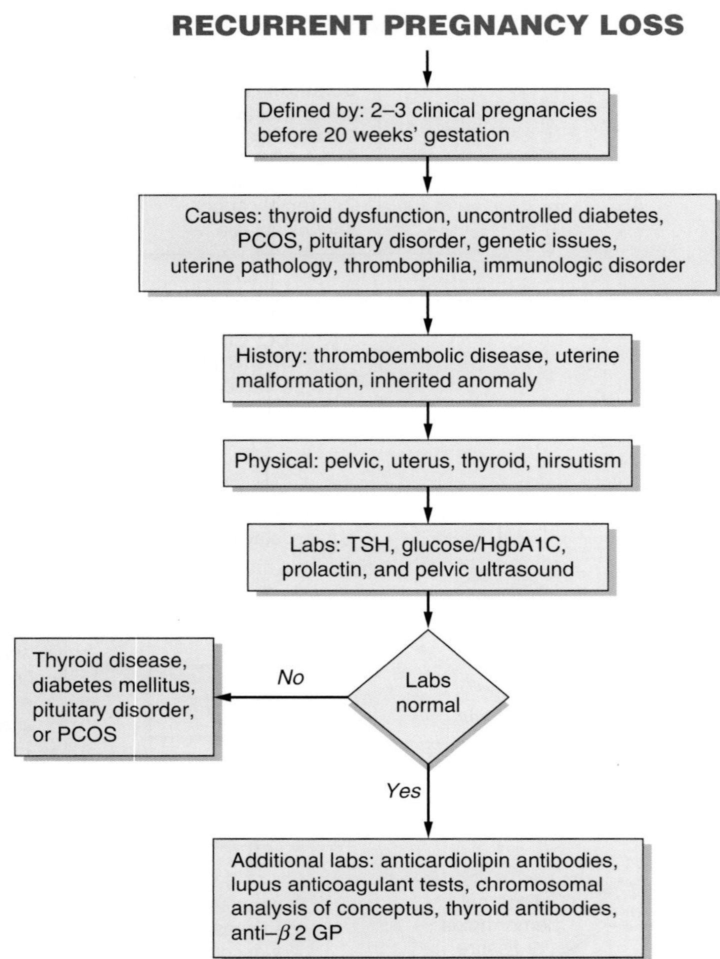

Aaron K. Starbuck, MD, ABFM

Alijotas-Reig J, Garrido-Gimenez C. Current concepts and new trends in the diagnosis and management of recurrent miscarriage. *Obstet Gynecol Surv.* 2013;68(6):445–466.

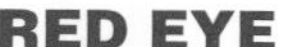

Common causes: conjunctivitis, episcleritis, scleritis, subconjunctival hemorrhage, uveitis, acute angle-closure glaucoma

- Pain?
  - *Yes* → Hyperemia?
    - *Focal* → Scleritis*
      Accompanied by photophobia
    - *Diffuse* → Discharge?
      - *No/minimal* → Uveitis**
        Constricted, sluggish pupil with blurred vision
      - *Yes, tearing* → Acute angle-closure glaucoma
        Sudden onset, pupil mid-dilated and nonreactive
  - *No* → Foreign body sensation?
    - *Yes* → Discharge?
      - *Watery* → Itching?
        - *Intense* → Allergic conjunctivitis
        - *Mild* → Viral conjunctivitis
      - *Prolific, mucoid* → Bacterial conjunctivitis
    - *No* → Discharge?
      - *Yes, watery* → Episcleritis
        Rapid, focal hyperemia, no photophobia
      - *No* → Subconjunctival hemorrhage
        Asymptomatic

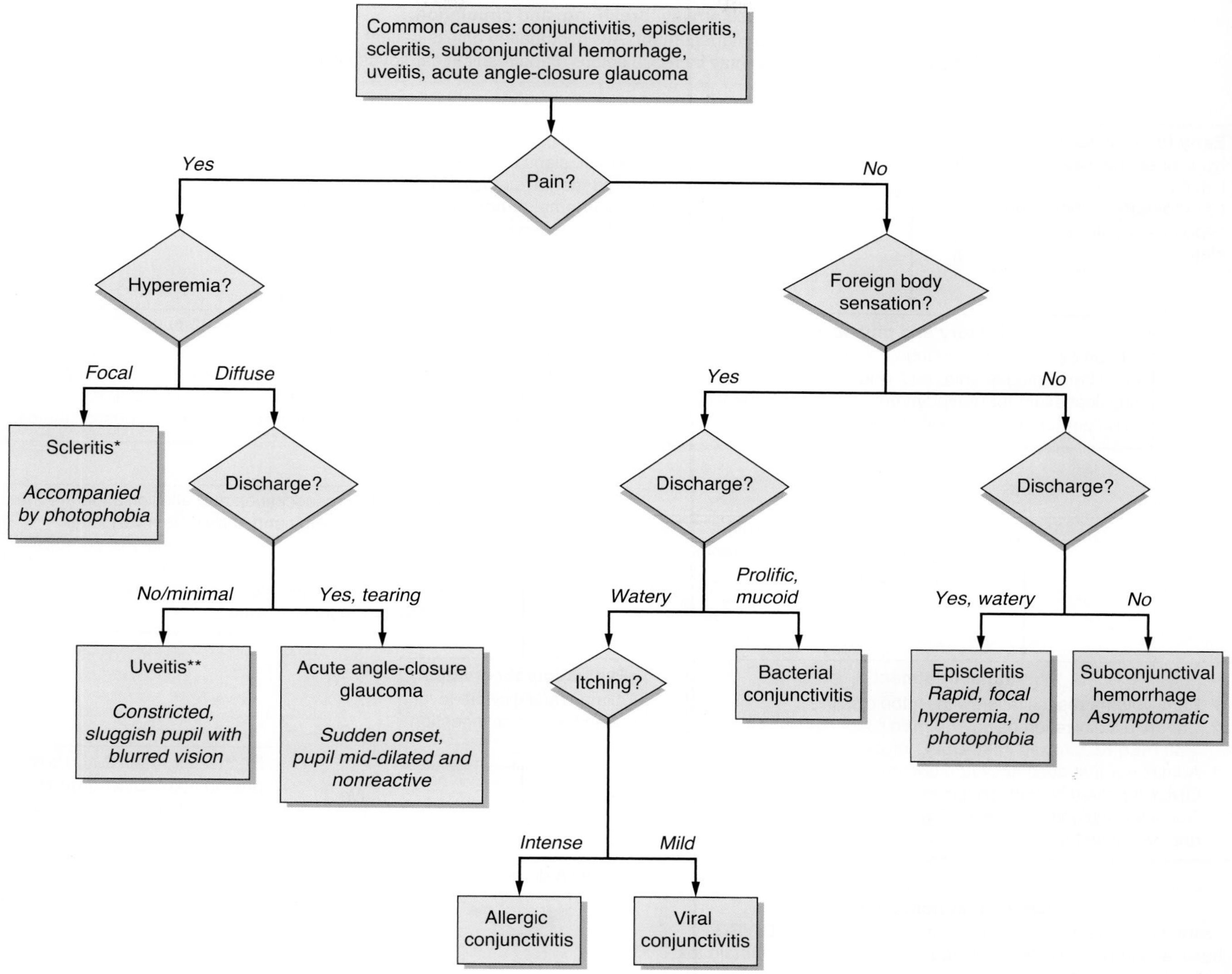

*Urgent ophthalmologic consultation
**Ophthalmologic consultation within 24 hours

Kelly G. Koren, MD

Mahmood AR, Narang AT. Diagnosis and management of the acute red eye. *Emerg Med Clin N Am.* 2008;26(1):35–55.

SALICYLATE POISONING, ACUTE, TREATMENT

Assess airway, breathing, and circulation.
Provide appropriate ABC management. Avoid intubation unless patient is unable to protect airway. Intubation may increase acidosis and result in cardiovascular collapse.

Early toxicity: tachypnea, hyperpnea, nausea, vomiting, tinnitus, vertigo
Late toxicity: hyperthermia, hypotension, altered mental status

Does the patient exhibit signs of severe toxicity (altered mental status/coma, seizure, pulmonary edema, or need for endotracheal intubation and mechanical ventilation)?

Yes →

Initiate emergent hemodialysis
Begin volume resuscitation and alkalinization using 150 mEq (3 amps) NaHCO3 + 40 mEq KCL in 1L D5W unless prohibited by cerebral/pulmonary edema. Administer 25g (1 amp) D50 for altered mental status. Do not delay treatment for diagnostic studies.

No →

History and physical
Obtain careful history of ingestion (time, reported ingestion, coingestants, etc.) and perform thorough physical exam for hemodynamic instability, alterations in respiratory pattern, and changes in mental status.

Is the patient asymptomatic, stable, and known to have ingested <150 mg/kg?

Yes →

Evaluation/observation
Obtain first salicylate level, noting time since ingestion occurred.

ASA detectable?

No → Recheck if within 2 hours of presentation. Discharge after 6 hours observation if patient remains asymptomatic, and levels are nondetectable.

Yes → Recheck levels q2h until persistently within therapeutic range, trending down, or nondetectable. Routinely reassess for changes in clinical status, and initiate treatment if indicated.

Note: Volume resuscitation and alkalinization are the mainstays of therapy and should be given to all symptomatic patients unless pulmonary or cerebral edema is present. Respiratory alkalosis (pH >7.5) is NOT a contraindication to therapy. Do not delay for charcoal or diagnostic studies.

No →

Initial treatment
1. Early volume resuscitation with isotonic saline
2. Urinary alkalinization using 150 mEq (3 amps) NaHCO3 + 40 mEq KCL mixed in 1L D5W, infused at 2–3 mL/kg/hr.
3. Administer first dose activated charcoal at 1g/kg (max 50g) ONLY if patient is alert, cooperative, and can tolerate. Consider additional doses of 25g q3h if patient can tolerate and has bowel sounds on exam.

Obtain diagnostic studies
Labs: salicylate level (note time since ingestion), ABG/VBG, basic electrolytes, BUN Creatinine, LFTs, coags, UA. Obtain tox screen if polysubstance overdose suspected.
Imaging: chest radiograph (to evaluate for pulmonary edema). Consider head CT for altered mental status to evaluate for cerebral edema or alternative causes of mental status changes.

Presence of salicylate level >100 mg/dL, arterial pH <7.3, pulmonary or cerebral edema, renal failure, or has patient deteriorated?

Yes → Initiate hemodialysis.

No →

Maintenance therapy and evaluation
1. Continue bicarbonate infusion to maintain urine output of 1–2 mL/kg/hr.
2. Measure urine pH hourly and titrate infusion to goal pH of 7.5–8.
3. Measure serum K hourly and replete if <4.5 mEq/L.
4. Measure ABG or VBG hourly and decrease rate of bicarbonate drip if serum pH exceeds 7.6.
5. Measure serum salicylate level q2h until salicylate level begins to decline and acid-base status is normal.

Disposition
Treatment should be continued with frequent clinical assessment for improvement. Treatment and testing may be stopped ONLY when patient is asymptomatic, acid-base status is stable, AND salicylate level has fallen into therapeutic range (10–30 mg/dL).

Alicia Lydecker, MD, Matthew K. Griswold, MD, and Kavita Babu, MD

Chyka PA, Erdman AR, Christianson G. Salicylate poisoning: an evidence-based consensus guideline for out-of-hospital management. *Clin Toxicol (Phila).* 2007;45(2):95–131.

SEIZURE, NEW ONSET

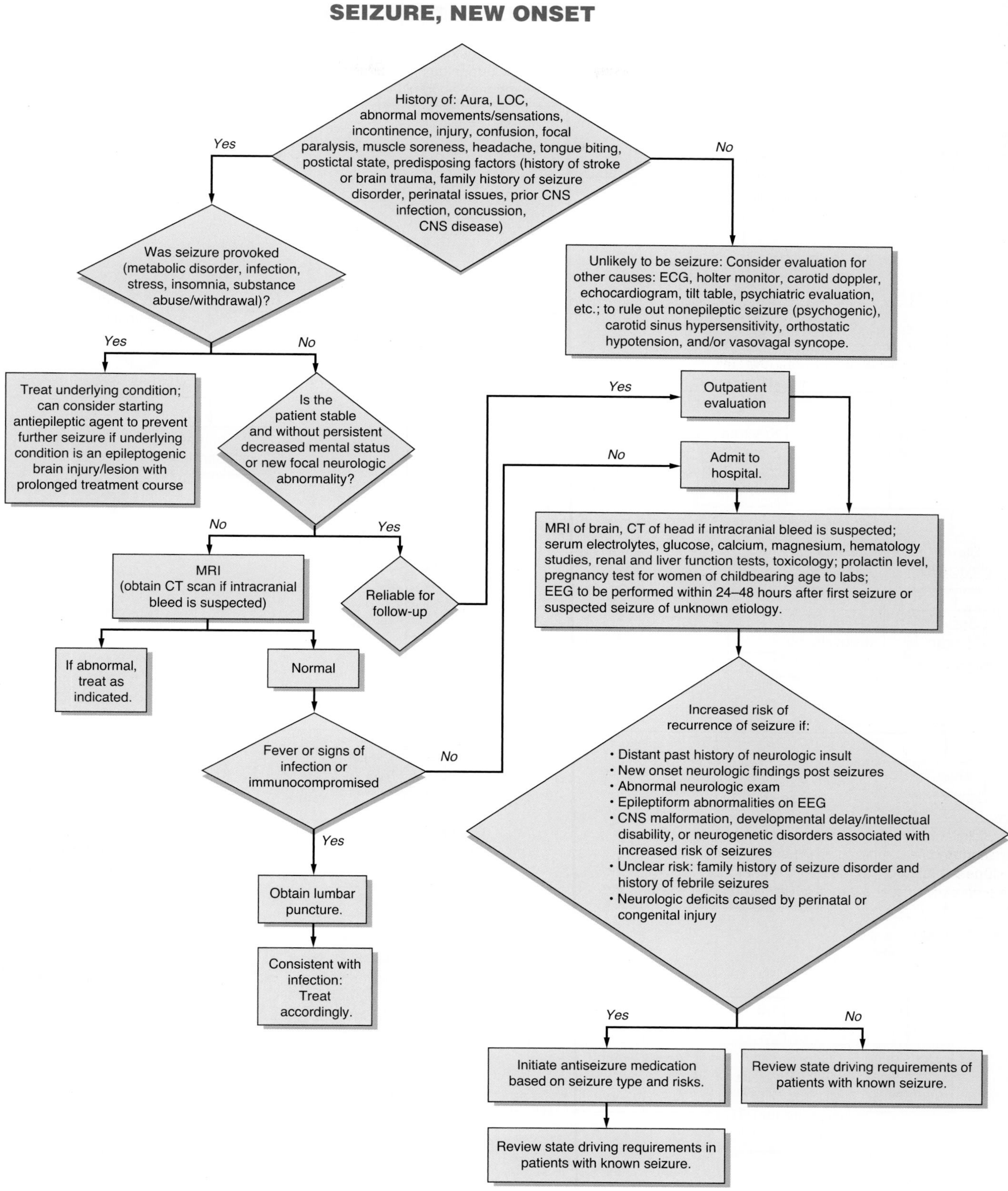
History of: Aura, LOC, abnormal movements/sensations, incontinence, injury, confusion, focal paralysis, muscle soreness, headache, tongue biting, postictal state, predisposing factors (history of stroke or brain trauma, family history of seizure disorder, perinatal issues, prior CNS infection, concussion, CNS disease)
Yes
No
Was seizure provoked (metabolic disorder, infection, stress, insomnia, substance abuse/withdrawal)?
Unlikely to be seizure: Consider evaluation for other causes: ECG, holter monitor, carotid doppler, echocardiogram, tilt table, psychiatric evaluation, etc.; to rule out nonepileptic seizure (psychogenic), carotid sinus hypersensitivity, orthostatic hypotension, and/or vasovagal syncope.
Yes
No
Treat underlying condition; can consider starting antiepileptic agent to prevent further seizure if underlying condition is an epileptogenic brain injury/lesion with prolonged treatment course
Is the patient stable and without persistent decreased mental status or new focal neurologic abnormality?
Yes
Outpatient evaluation
No
Admit to hospital.
No
Yes
MRI (obtain CT scan if intracranial bleed is suspected)
Reliable for follow-up
MRI of brain, CT of head if intracranial bleed is suspected; serum electrolytes, glucose, calcium, magnesium, hematology studies, renal and liver function tests, toxicology; prolactin level, pregnancy test for women of childbearing age to labs; EEG to be performed within 24–48 hours after first seizure or suspected seizure of unknown etiology.
If abnormal, treat as indicated.
Normal
Fever or signs of infection or immunocompromised
No
Yes
Obtain lumbar puncture.
Consistent with infection: Treat accordingly.
Increased risk of recurrence of seizure if:
• Distant past history of neurologic insult
• New onset neurologic findings post seizures
• Abnormal neurologic exam
• Epileptiform abnormalities on EEG
• CNS malformation, developmental delay/intellectual disability, or neurogenetic disorders associated with increased risk of seizures
• Unclear risk: family history of seizure disorder and history of febrile seizures
• Neurologic deficits caused by perinatal or congenital injury
Yes
No
Initiate antiseizure medication based on seizure type and risks.
Review state driving requirements of patients with known seizure.
Review state driving requirements in patients with known seizure.

Daniel R. Matta, MD and Scott F. Graham, MD

Wilden JA, Cohen-Gadol AA. Evaluation of first nonfebrile seizures. *Am Fam Physician*. 2012;86(4):334–340.

SHOULDER PAIN, DIAGNOSIS

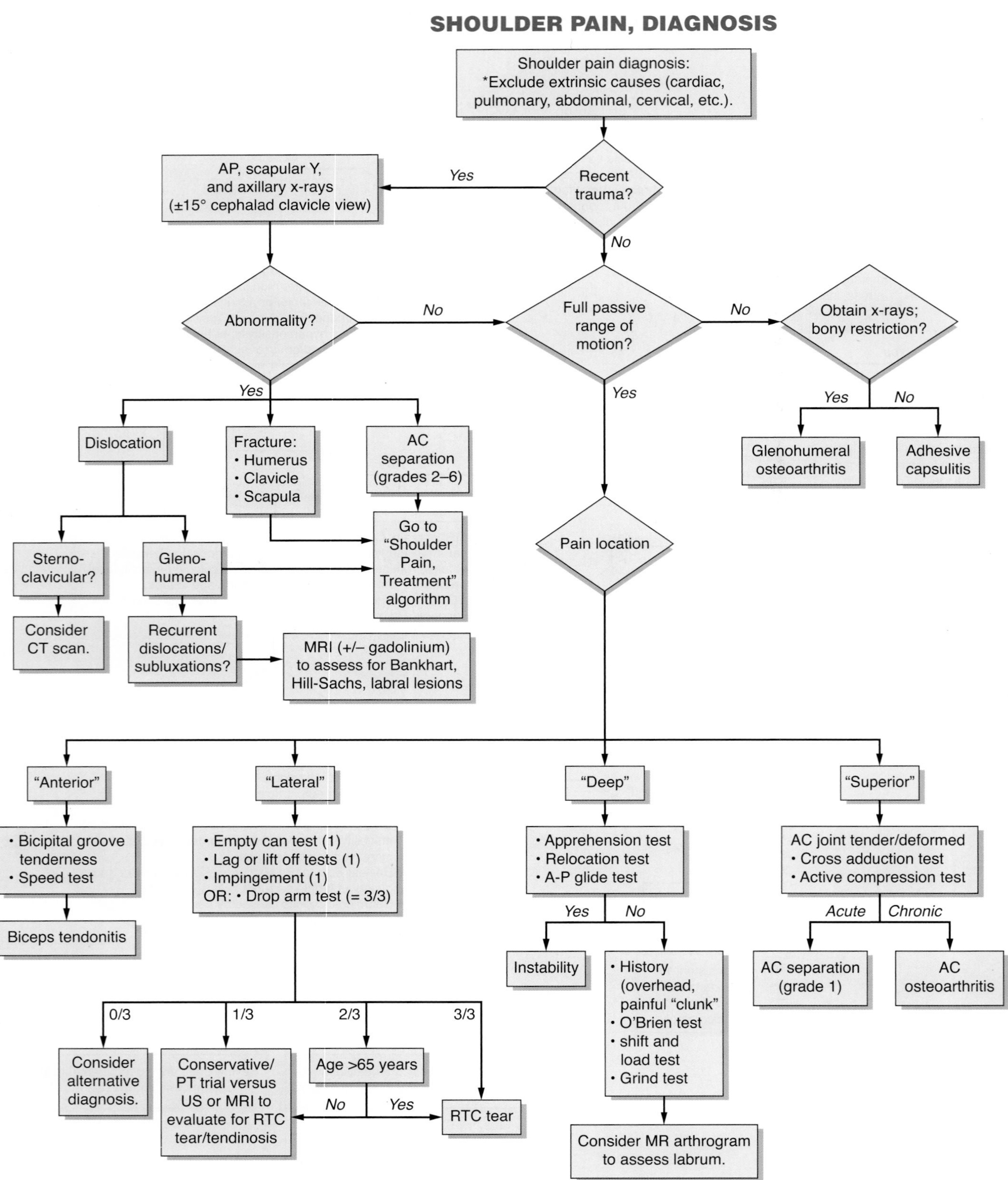

Thomas S. Hoke, MD, and William W. Dexter, MD, FACSM

Hegedus EJ, Goode AP, Cook CE, et al. Which physical examination tests provide clinicians with the most value when examining the shoulder? Update of a systemic review with meta-analysis of individual tests. *Br J Sports Med.* 2012;46(14):964–978.

SHOULDER PAIN, TREATMENT

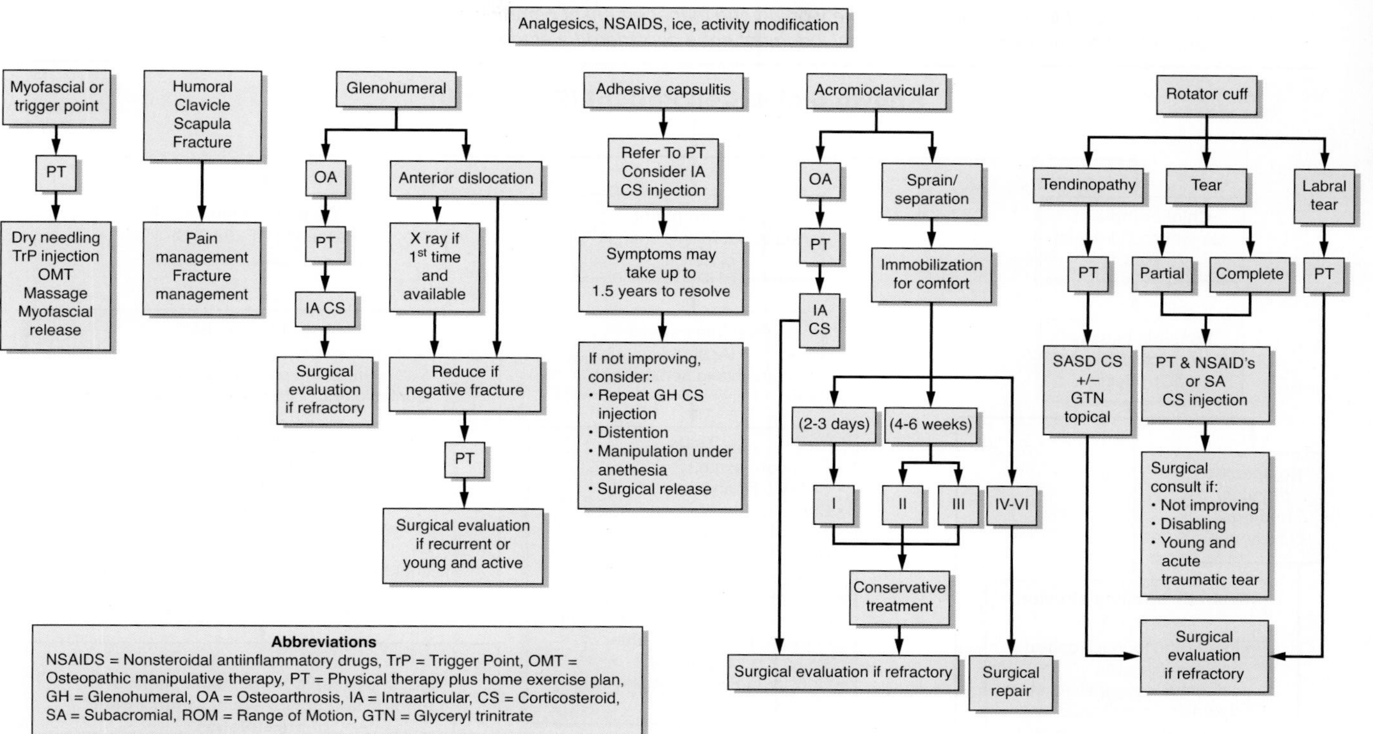

Alison Lee, MD and William W. Dexter, MD, FACSM

Song A, Higgins LD, Newman J, et al. Glenohumeral Corticosteroid Injections in Adhesive Capsulitis: A Systematic Search and Review. PM R. 2014 Jul 1. pii: S1934–1482(14)00306–2.

SICKLE CELL ANEMIA, ACUTE, EVALUATION AND MANAGEMENT

This algorithm is meant to assist clinicians in the workup and management of common complications of sickle cell disease. It should not replace a physician's clinical judgment or be considered a standardized protocol for all patients.

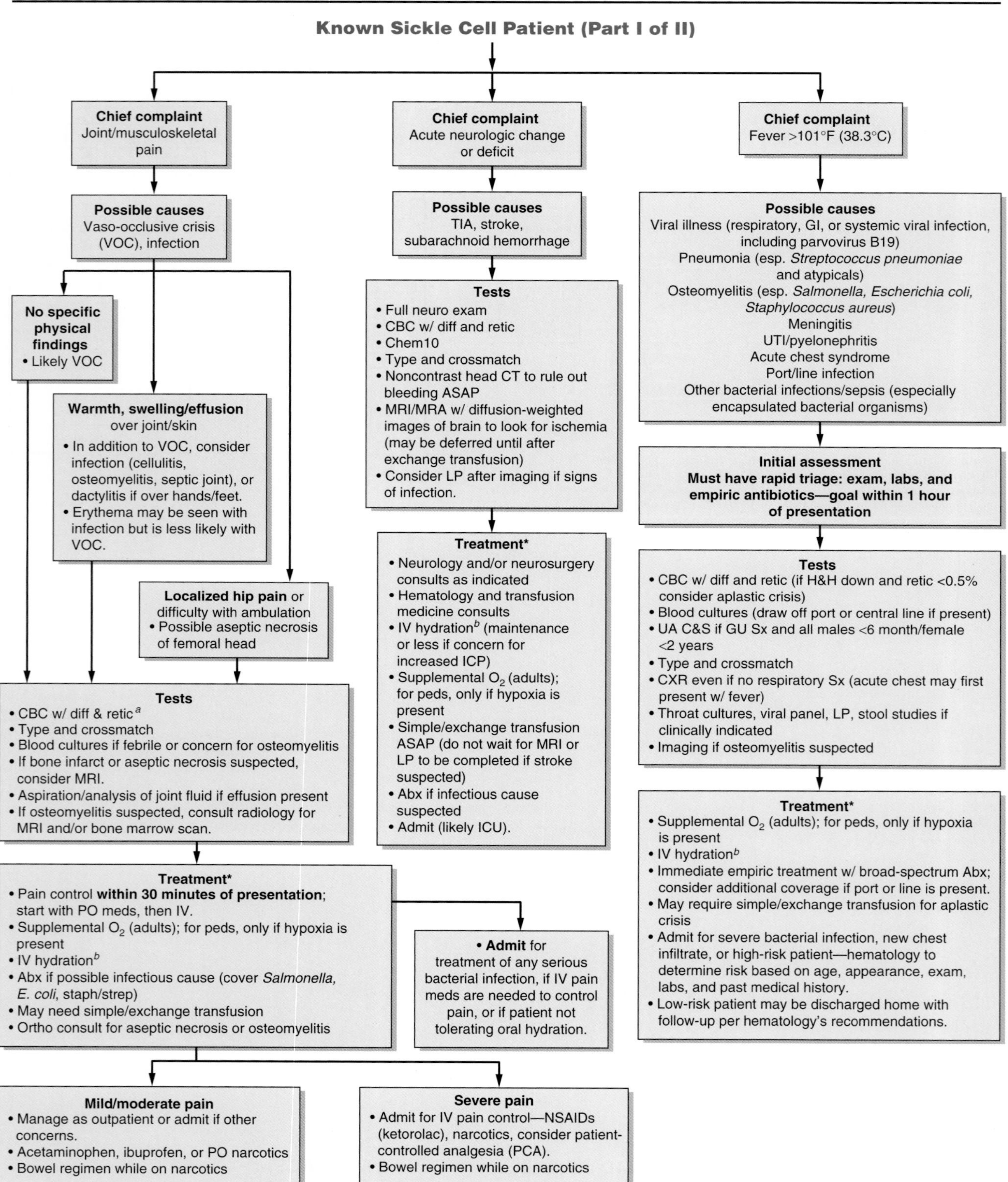

Known Sickle Cell Patient (Part I of II)
Chief complaint Joint/musculoskeletal pain
Possible causes Vaso-occlusive crisis (VOC), infection
No specific physical findings • Likely VOC
Warmth, swelling/effusion over joint/skin • In addition to VOC, consider infection (cellulitis, osteomyelitis, septic joint), or dactylitis if over hands/feet. • Erythema may be seen with infection but is less likely with VOC.
Localized hip pain or difficulty with ambulation • Possible aseptic necrosis of femoral head
Tests • CBC w/ diff & retic [a] • Type and crossmatch • Blood cultures if febrile or concern for osteomyelitis • If bone infarct or aseptic necrosis suspected, consider MRI. • Aspiration/analysis of joint fluid if effusion present • If osteomyelitis suspected, consult radiology for MRI and/or bone marrow scan.
Treatment* • Pain control within 30 minutes of presentation; start with PO meds, then IV. • Supplemental O_2 (adults); for peds, only if hypoxia is present • IV hydration[b] • Abx if possible infectious cause (cover Salmonella, E. coli, staph/strep) • May need simple/exchange transfusion • Ortho consult for aseptic necrosis or osteomyelitis
• Admit for treatment of any serious bacterial infection, if IV pain meds are needed to control pain, or if patient not tolerating oral hydration.
Mild/moderate pain • Manage as outpatient or admit if other concerns. • Acetaminophen, ibuprofen, or PO narcotics • Bowel regimen while on narcotics
Severe pain • Admit for IV pain control—NSAIDs (ketorolac), narcotics, consider patient-controlled analgesia (PCA). • Bowel regimen while on narcotics
Chief complaint Acute neurologic change or deficit
Possible causes TIA, stroke, subarachnoid hemorrhage
Tests • Full neuro exam • CBC w/ diff and retic • Chem10 • Type and crossmatch • Noncontrast head CT to rule out bleeding ASAP • MRI/MRA w/ diffusion-weighted images of brain to look for ischemia (may be deferred until after exchange transfusion) • Consider LP after imaging if signs of infection.
Treatment* • Neurology and/or neurosurgery consults as indicated • Hematology and transfusion medicine consults • IV hydration[b] (maintenance or less if concern for increased ICP) • Supplemental O_2 (adults); for peds, only if hypoxia is present • Simple/exchange transfusion ASAP (do not wait for MRI or LP to be completed if stroke suspected) • Abx if infectious cause suspected • Admit (likely ICU).
Chief complaint Fever >101°F (38.3°C)
Possible causes Viral illness (respiratory, GI, or systemic viral infection, including parvovirus B19) Pneumonia (esp. Streptococcus pneumoniae and atypicals) Osteomyelitis (esp. Salmonella, Escherichia coli, Staphylococcus aureus) Meningitis UTI/pyelonephritis Acute chest syndrome Port/line infection Other bacterial infections/sepsis (especially encapsulated bacterial organisms)
Initial assessment Must have rapid triage: exam, labs, and empiric antibiotics—goal within 1 hour of presentation
Tests • CBC w/ diff and retic (if H&H down and retic <0.5% consider aplastic crisis) • Blood cultures (draw off port or central line if present) • UA C&S if GU Sx and all males <6 month/female <2 years • Type and crossmatch • CXR even if no respiratory Sx (acute chest may first present w/ fever) • Throat cultures, viral panel, LP, stool studies if clinically indicated • Imaging if osteomyelitis suspected
Treatment* • Supplemental O_2 (adults); for peds, only if hypoxia is present • IV hydration[b] • Immediate empiric treatment w/ broad-spectrum Abx; consider additional coverage if port or line is present. • May require simple/exchange transfusion for aplastic crisis • Admit for severe bacterial infection, new chest infiltrate, or high-risk patient—hematology to determine risk based on age, appearance, exam, labs, and past medical history. • Low-risk patient may be discharged home with follow-up per hematology's recommendations.

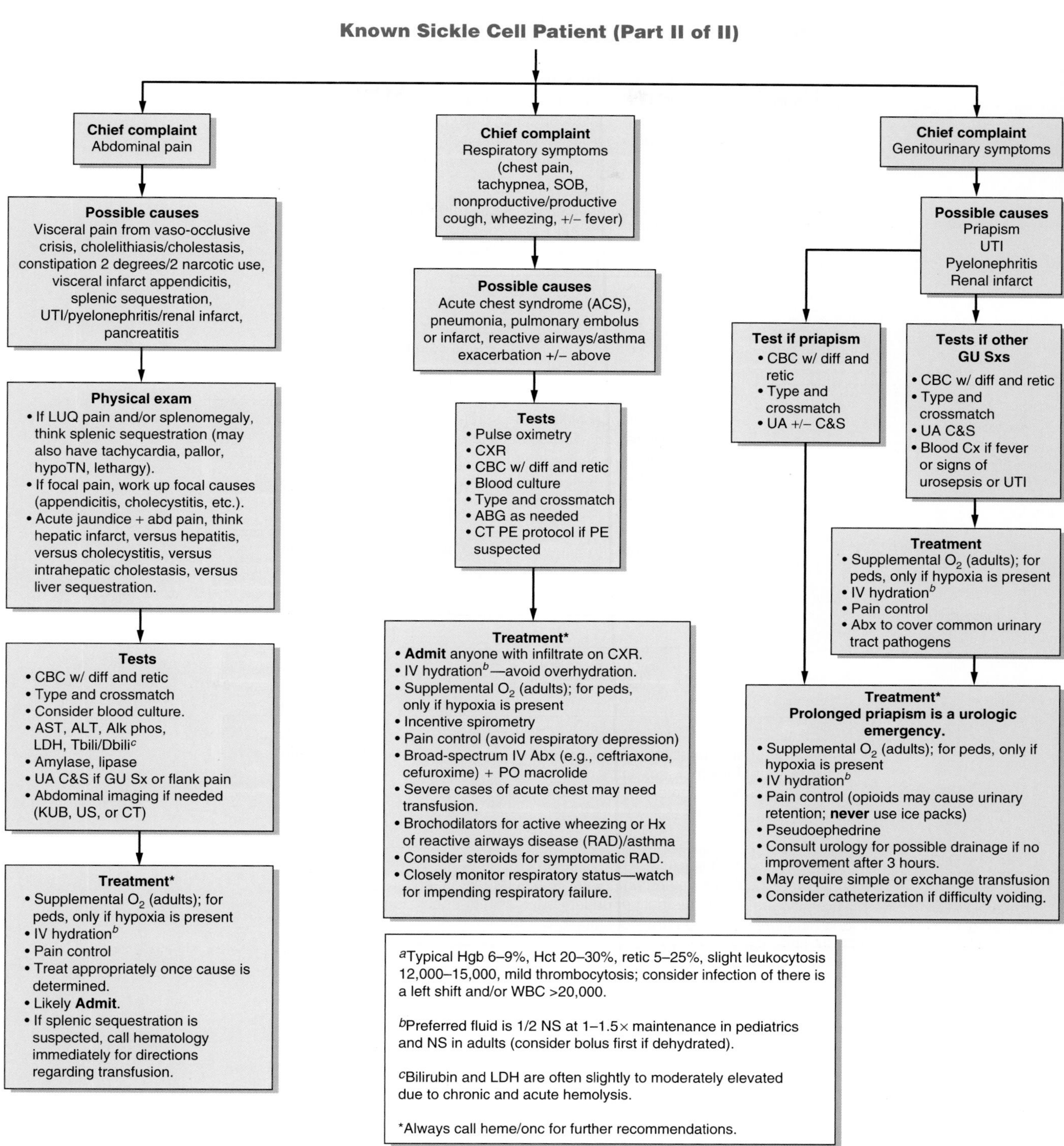

Known Sickle Cell Patient (Part II of II)
Chief complaint
Abdominal pain
Possible causes
Visceral pain from vaso-occlusive crisis, cholelithiasis/cholestasis, constipation 2 degrees/2 narcotic use, visceral infarct appendicitis, splenic sequestration, UTI/pyelonephritis/renal infarct, pancreatitis
Physical exam
• If LUQ pain and/or splenomegaly, think splenic sequestration (may also have tachycardia, pallor, hypoTN, lethargy).
• If focal pain, work up focal causes (appendicitis, cholecystitis, etc.).
• Acute jaundice + abd pain, think hepatic infarct, versus hepatitis, versus cholecystitis, versus intrahepatic cholestasis, versus liver sequestration.
Tests
• CBC w/ diff and retic
• Type and crossmatch
• Consider blood culture.
• AST, ALT, Alk phos, LDH, Tbili/Dbili[c]
• Amylase, lipase
• UA C&S if GU Sx or flank pain
• Abdominal imaging if needed (KUB, US, or CT)
Treatment*
• Supplemental O_2 (adults); for peds, only if hypoxia is present
• IV hydration[b]
• Pain control
• Treat appropriately once cause is determined.
• Likely Admit.
• If splenic sequestration is suspected, call hematology immediately for directions regarding transfusion.
Chief complaint
Respiratory symptoms (chest pain, tachypnea, SOB, nonproductive/productive cough, wheezing, +/– fever)
Possible causes
Acute chest syndrome (ACS), pneumonia, pulmonary embolus or infarct, reactive airways/asthma exacerbation +/– above
Tests
• Pulse oximetry
• CXR
• CBC w/ diff and retic
• Blood culture
• Type and crossmatch
• ABG as needed
• CT PE protocol if PE suspected
Treatment*
• Admit anyone with infiltrate on CXR.
• IV hydration[b]—avoid overhydration.
• Supplemental O_2 (adults); for peds, only if hypoxia is present
• Incentive spirometry
• Pain control (avoid respiratory depression)
• Broad-spectrum IV Abx (e.g., ceftriaxone, cefuroxime) + PO macrolide
• Severe cases of acute chest may need transfusion.
• Brochodilators for active wheezing or Hx of reactive airways disease (RAD)/asthma
• Consider steroids for symptomatic RAD.
• Closely monitor respiratory status—watch for impending respiratory failure.
Chief complaint
Genitourinary symptoms
Possible causes
Priapism
UTI
Pyelonephritis
Renal infarct
Test if priapism
• CBC w/ diff and retic
• Type and crossmatch
• UA +/– C&S
Tests if other GU Sxs
• CBC w/ diff and retic
• Type and crossmatch
• UA C&S
• Blood Cx if fever or signs of urosepsis or UTI
Treatment
• Supplemental O_2 (adults); for peds, only if hypoxia is present
• IV hydration[b]
• Pain control
• Abx to cover common urinary tract pathogens
Treatment*
Prolonged priapism is a urologic emergency.
• Supplemental O_2 (adults); for peds, only if hypoxia is present
• IV hydration[b]
• Pain control (opioids may cause urinary retention; never use ice packs)
• Pseudoephedrine
• Consult urology for possible drainage if no improvement after 3 hours.
• May require simple or exchange transfusion
• Consider catheterization if difficulty voiding.
[a]Typical Hgb 6–9%, Hct 20–30%, retic 5–25%, slight leukocytosis 12,000–15,000, mild thrombocytosis; consider infection of there is a left shift and/or WBC >20,000.
[b]Preferred fluid is 1/2 NS at 1–1.5× maintenance in pediatrics and NS in adults (consider bolus first if dehydrated).
[c]Bilirubin and LDH are often slightly to moderately elevated due to chronic and acute hemolysis.
*Always call heme/onc for further recommendations.

Stephanie M. Ruest, MD and Doreen B. Brettler, MD

New England Pediatric Sickle Cell Consortium. Practice guidelines. http://www.nepscc.org/nepscc.html. Accessed 2014.

SUICIDE, EVALUATING RISK FOR

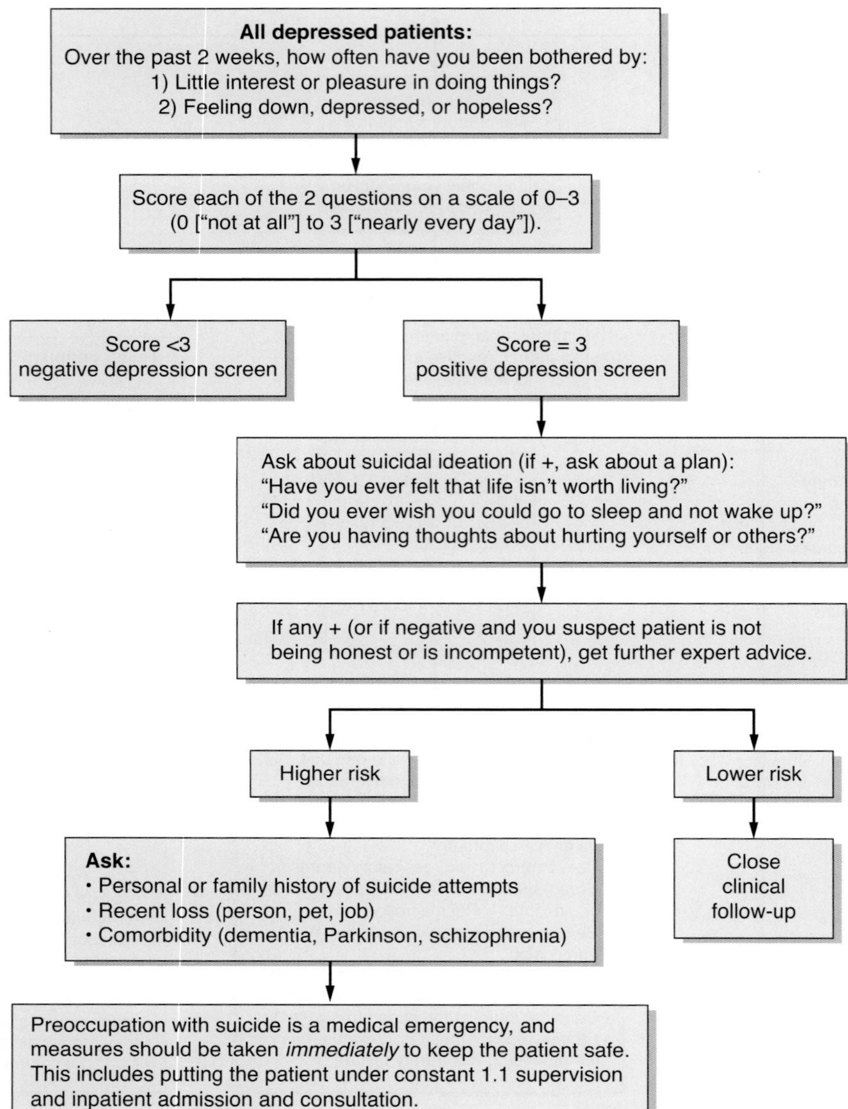

All depressed patients:
Over the past 2 weeks, how often have you been bothered by:
1) Little interest or pleasure in doing things?
2) Feeling down, depressed, or hopeless?
Score each of the 2 questions on a scale of 0–3
(0 ["not at all"] to 3 ["nearly every day"]).
Score <3
negative depression screen
Score = 3
positive depression screen
Ask about suicidal ideation (if +, ask about a plan):
"Have you ever felt that life isn't worth living?"
"Did you ever wish you could go to sleep and not wake up?"
"Are you having thoughts about hurting yourself or others?"
If any + (or if negative and you suspect patient is not
being honest or is incompetent), get further expert advice.
Higher risk
Lower risk
Ask:
• Personal or family history of suicide attempts
• Recent loss (person, pet, job)
• Comorbidity (dementia, Parkinson, schizophrenia)
Close
clinical
follow-up
Preoccupation with suicide is a medical emergency, and
measures should be taken *immediately* to keep the patient safe.
This includes putting the patient under constant 1.1 supervision
and inpatient admission and consultation.

Irene C. Coletsos, MD, and Harold J. Bursztajn, MD

Posner K, Oquendo MA, Gould M, et al. Columbia Classification Algorithm of Suicide Assessment (C-CASA): classification of suicidal events in the FDA's pediatric suicidal risk analysis of antidepressants. *Am J Psychiatry.* 2007;164(7):1035–1043.

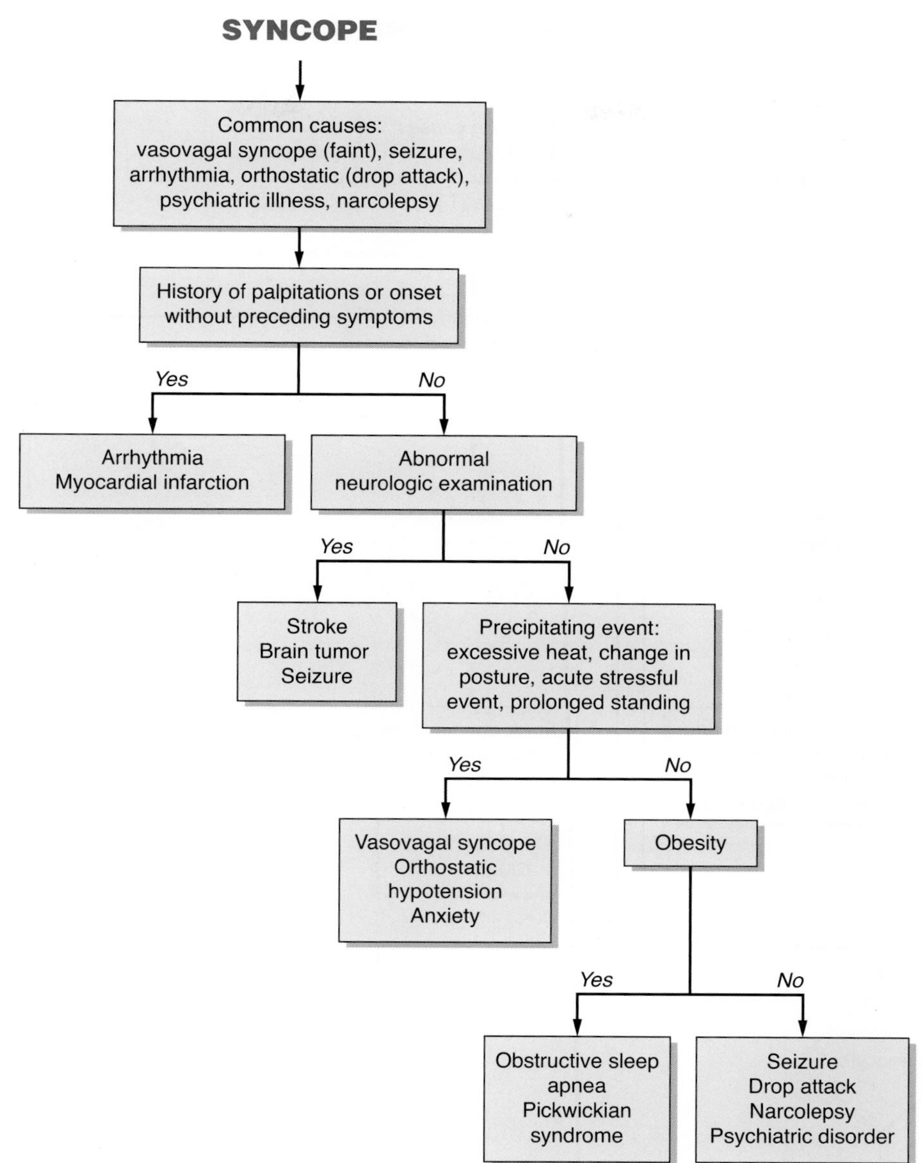

Amaninderapal S. Ghotra, MD, Nirmanmoh Bhatia, MD, and Kelly McCants, MD

Task Force for the Diagnosis and Management of Syncope, European Society of Cardiology (ESC), European Heart Rhythm Association (EHRA), et al. Guidelines for the diagnosis and management of syncope (version 2009). *Eur Heart J.* 2009;30:2631–2671.

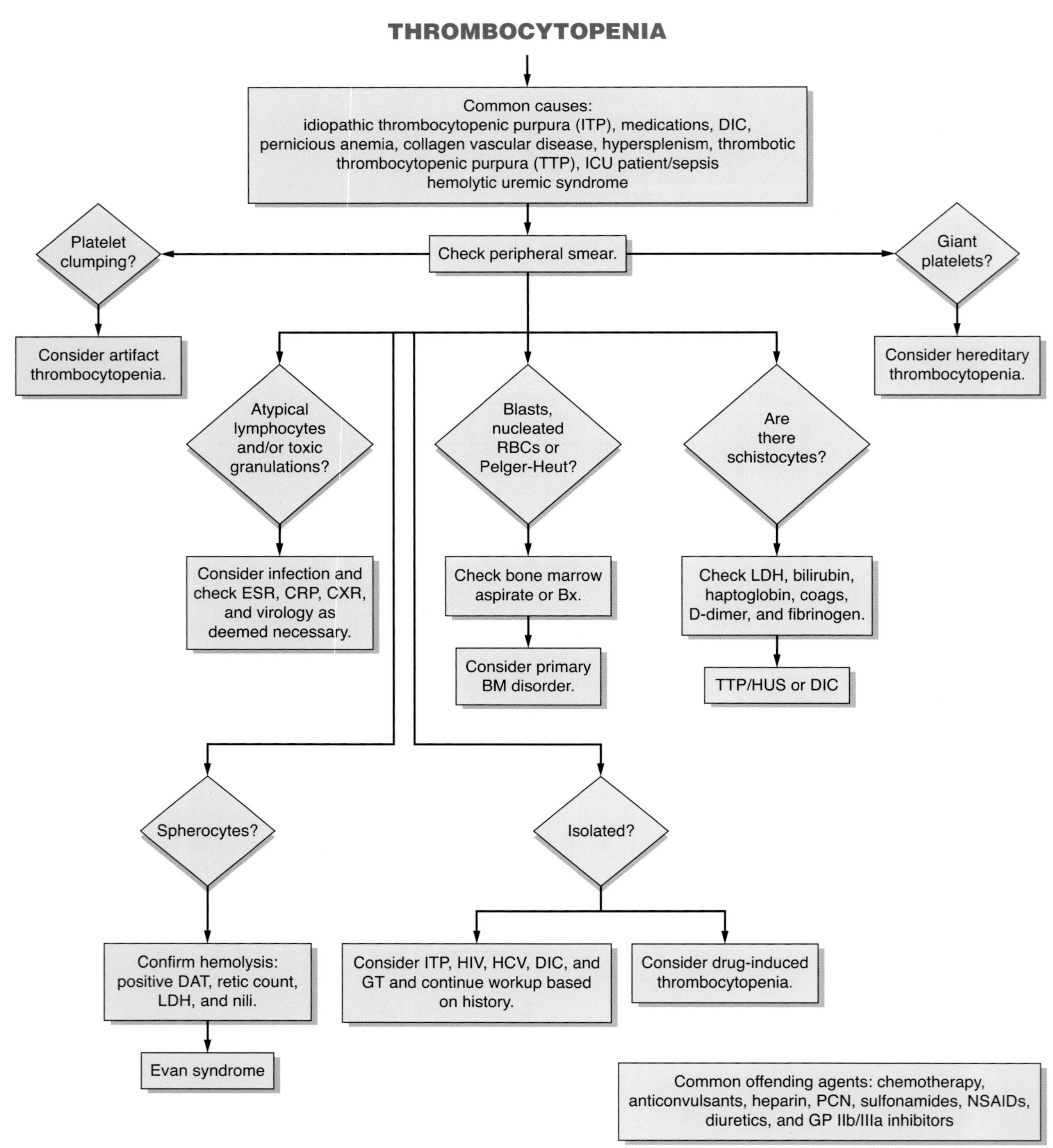

Nupam A. Patel, MD and Samuel B. Carli, MD

Reese JA, Li X, Hauben M, et al. Identifying drugs that cause acute thrombocytopenia: an analysis using 3 distinct methods. *Blood.* 2010;116:2127–2133.

THYROID NODULE

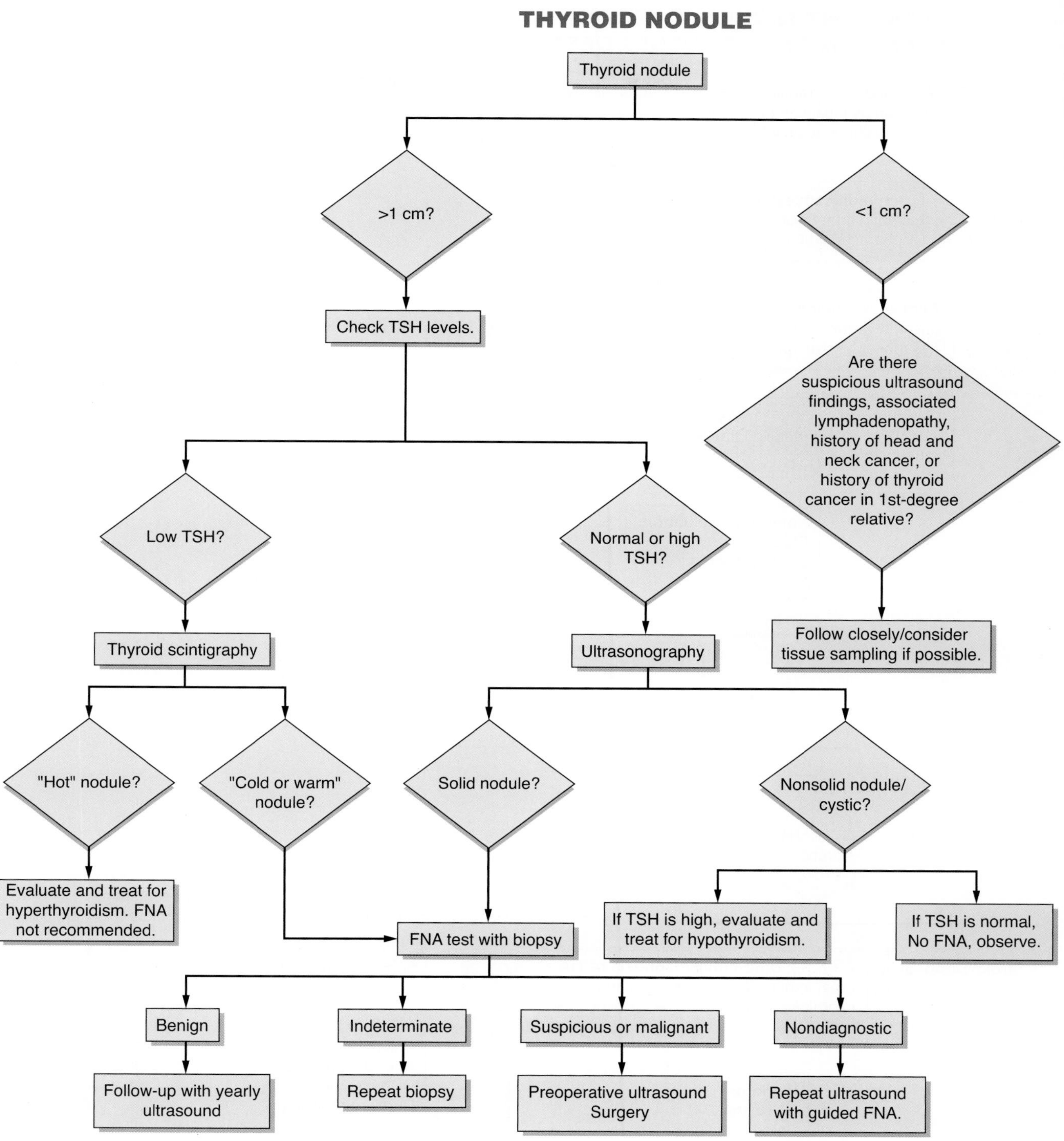

Maria M. Plummer, MD and Ehiozogie Adu

American Thyroid Association Guidelines Taskforce on Thyroid Nodules and Differentiated Thyroid Cancer, Cooper DS, Doherty GM, et al. Revised American Thyroid Association management guidelines for patients with thyroid nodules and differentiated thyroid cancer. *Thyroid.* 2009;19(11):1167–1214.

TRANSIENT ISCHEMIC ATTACK AND TRANSIENT NEUROLOGIC DEFECTS

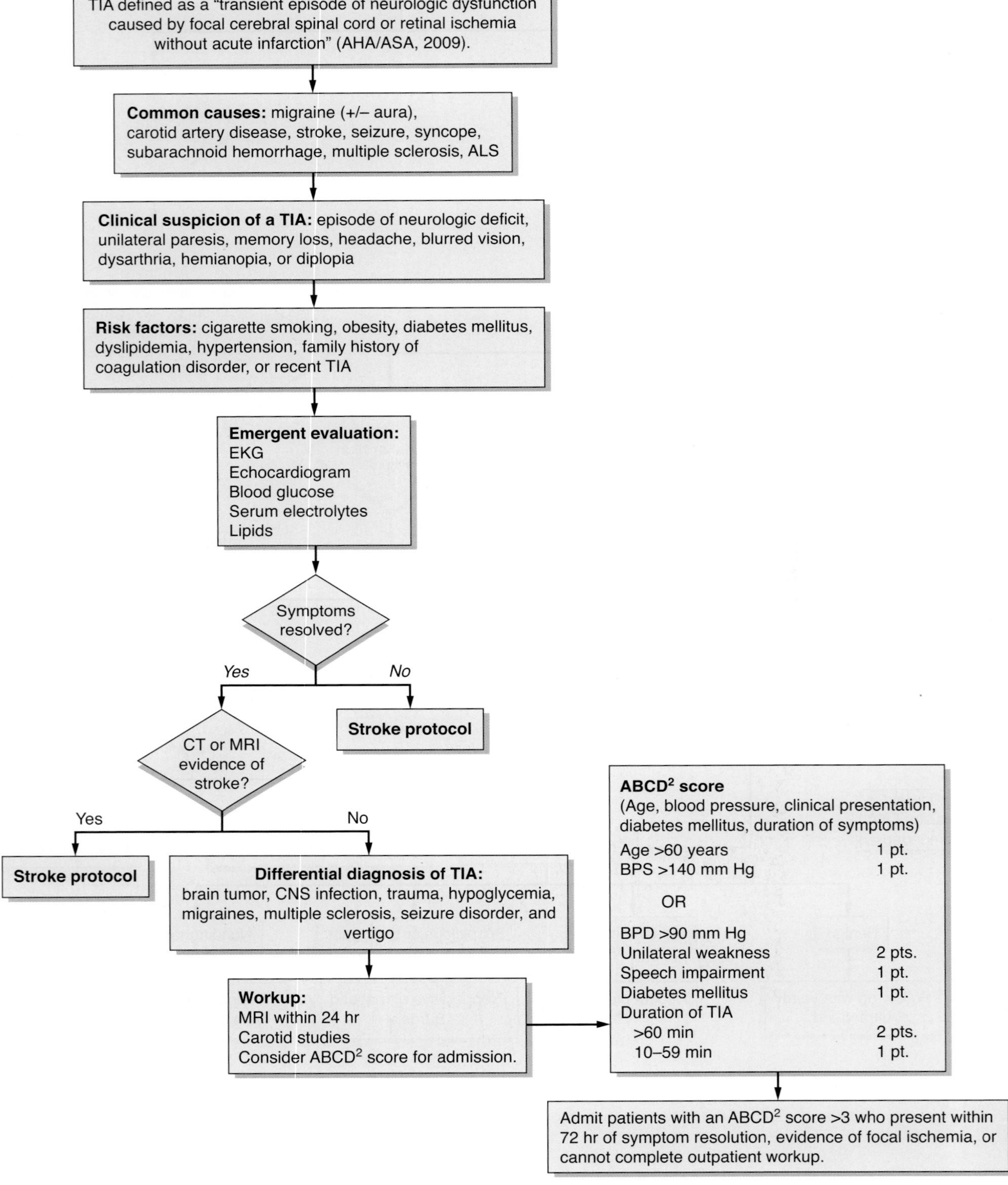

TIA defined as a "transient episode of neurologic dysfunction caused by focal cerebral spinal cord or retinal ischemia without acute infarction" (AHA/ASA, 2009).
Common causes: migraine (+/– aura), carotid artery disease, stroke, seizure, syncope, subarachnoid hemorrhage, multiple sclerosis, ALS
Clinical suspicion of a TIA: episode of neurologic deficit, unilateral paresis, memory loss, headache, blurred vision, dysarthria, hemianopia, or diplopia
Risk factors: cigarette smoking, obesity, diabetes mellitus, dyslipidemia, hypertension, family history of coagulation disorder, or recent TIA
Emergent evaluation: EKG Echocardiogram Blood glucose Serum electrolytes Lipids
Symptoms resolved?
Yes
No
Stroke protocol
CT or MRI evidence of stroke?
Yes
No
Stroke protocol
Differential diagnosis of TIA: brain tumor, CNS infection, trauma, hypoglycemia, migraines, multiple sclerosis, seizure disorder, and vertigo
Workup: MRI within 24 hr Carotid studies Consider ABCD² score for admission.
ABCD² score
(Age, blood pressure, clinical presentation, diabetes mellitus, duration of symptoms)
Age >60 years 1 pt.
BPS >140 mm Hg 1 pt.
OR
BPD >90 mm Hg
Unilateral weakness 2 pts.
Speech impairment 1 pt.
Diabetes mellitus 1 pt.
Duration of TIA
>60 min 2 pts.
10–59 min 1 pt.
Admit patients with an ABCD² score >3 who present within 72 hr of symptom resolution, evidence of focal ischemia, or cannot complete outpatient workup.

Deborah A. Lardner, DO, DTM&H and Michael Passafaro, DO, DTM&H, FACEP, FACOEP

Simmons BB, Cirignano B, Gadegbeku AB. Transient ischemic attack: part I. Diagnosis and evaluation. *Am Fam Physician.* 2012;86(6):521–526.

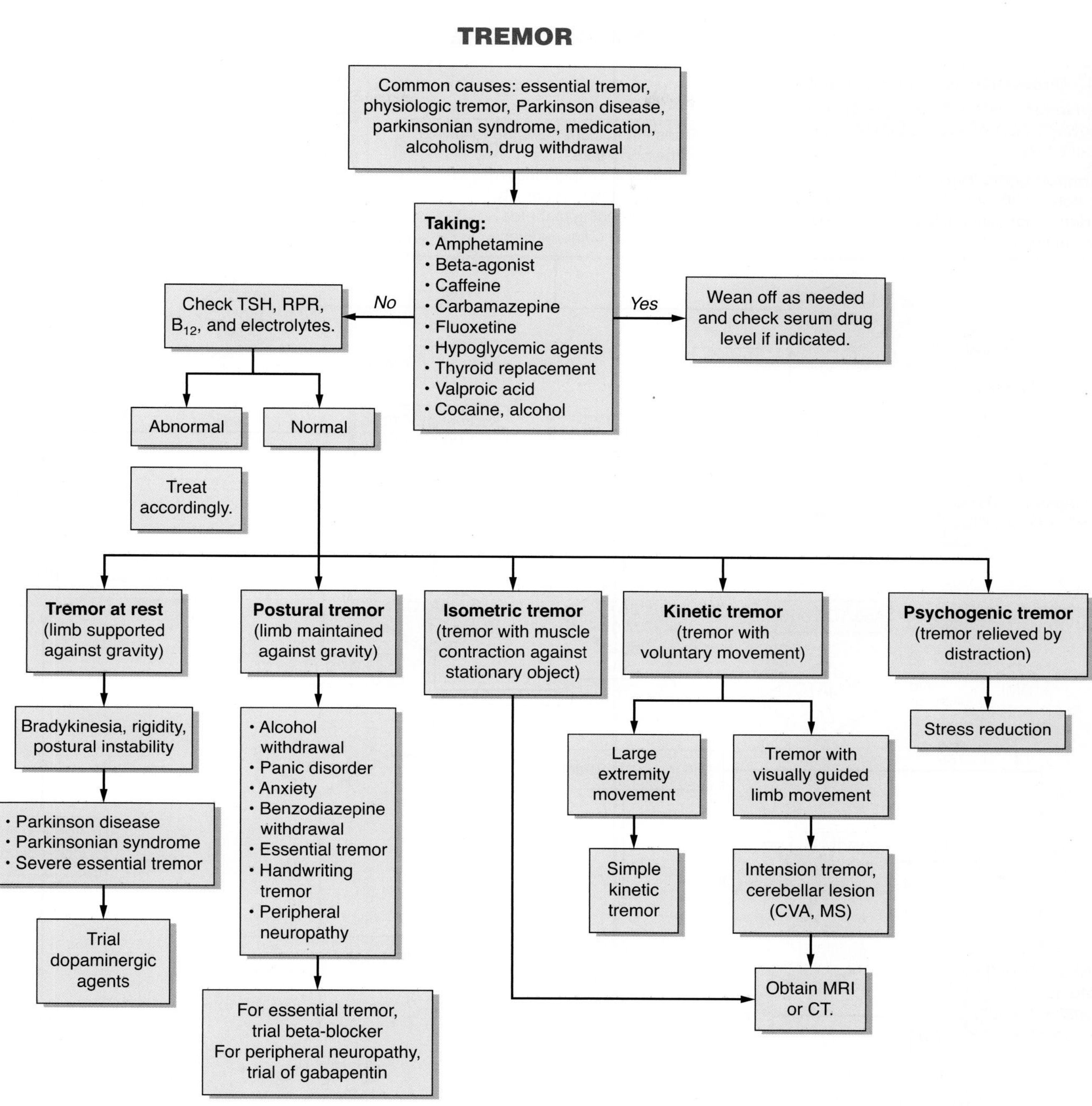

Kenneth Liu, PharmD, Steven J. Crosby, MA, RPh, FASCP, and Ildiko Halasz, MD

Crawford P, Zimmerman EE. Differentiation and diagnosis of tremor. *Am Fam Physician*. 2011;83(6):697–702.

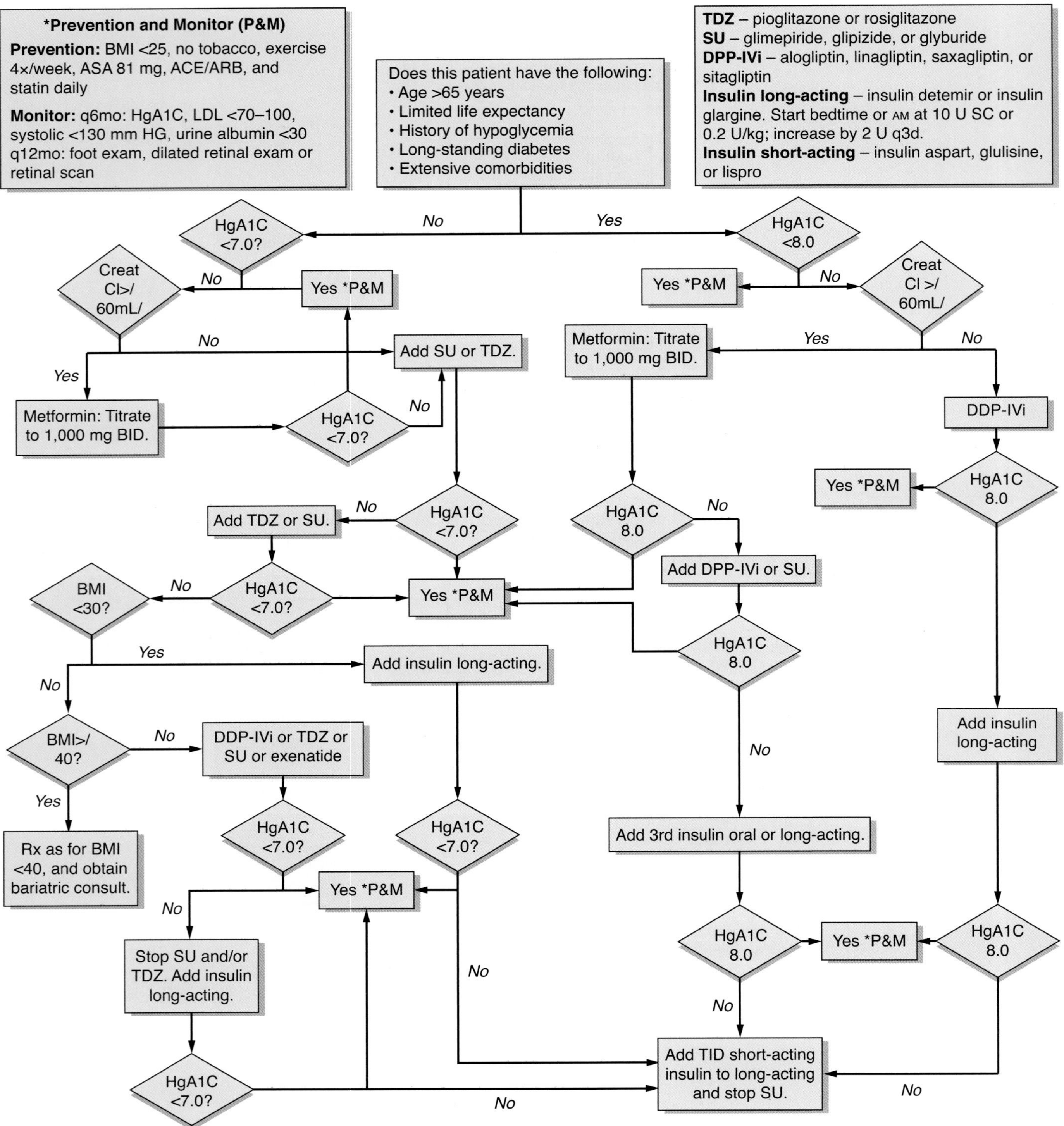

Andrew G. Alexander, MD

American Diabetes Association. Standards of medical care in diabetes—2015. *Diabetes Care*. 2015;38(1):S1–S94.

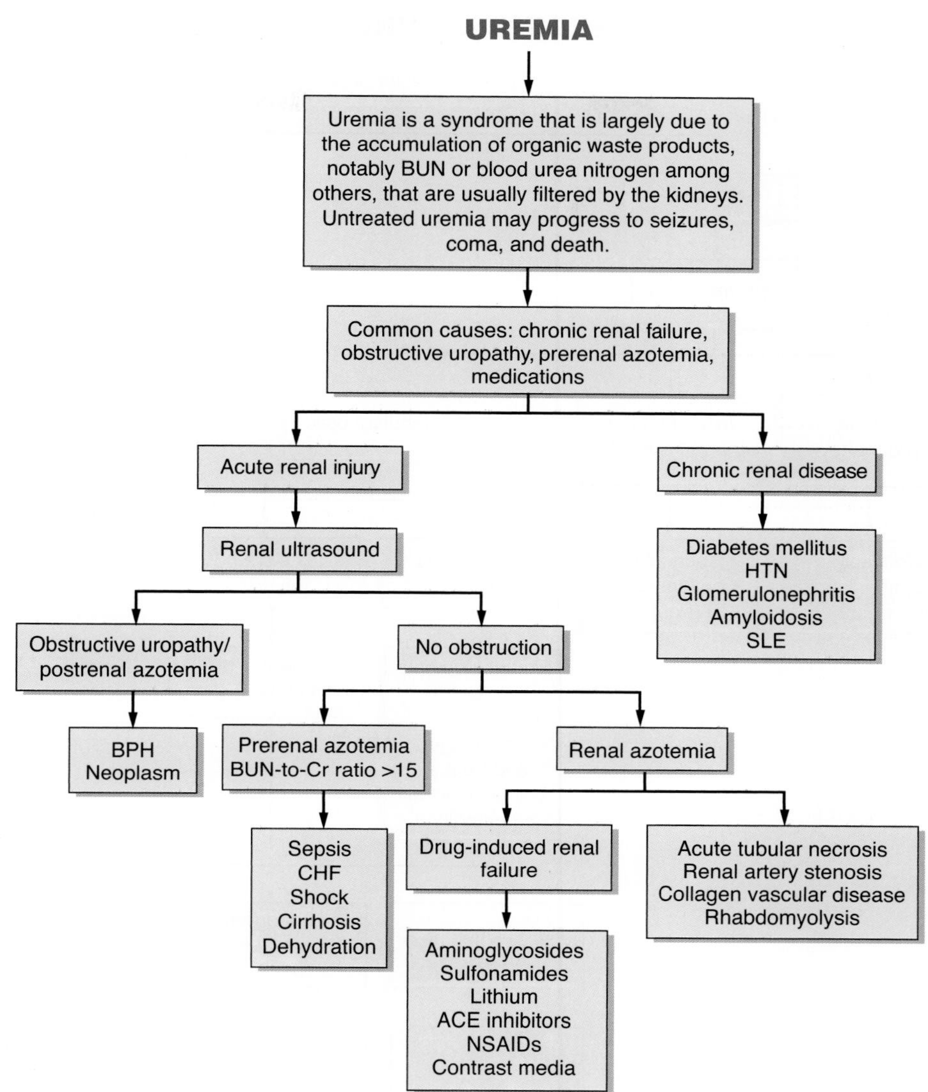

Steven A. House, MD, FAAFP

Rahman M, Shad F, Smith MC. Acute kidney injury: a guide to diagnosis and management. *Am Fam Physician.* 2012;86(7):631–639.

VAGINAL BLEEDING DURING PREGNANCY

- 1st trimester of pregnancy
  - Stable
    - Perform TVUS.
      - Viable intrauterine pregnancy (threatened abortion)
        - Establish prenatal care.
      - Ectopic pregnancy
        - Counsel on options and treat.
      - Incomplete or missed abortion
        - Counsel on options and treat.
      - Nondiagnostic
        - hCG >1,500 mIU/mL
          - Treat as ectopic or perform curettage and treat as ectopic if no villi on pathology.
        - hCG <1,500 mIU/mL
          - Repeat hCG in 48 hours.
            - Normal increase (double)
              - Perform TVUS when hCG >1,500 mIU/mL; manage as above once TVUS diagnostic.
            - Abnormal decrease or decline
              - Treat as ectopic or perform curettage and treat as ectopic if no villi on pathology.
            - Normal decrease
              - No treatment
  - Unstable
    - Resuscitate and proceed to OR.
      - Heavy vaginal bleeding
        - Suction D&C for likely SAB versus incomplete AB
      - Acute abdomen
        - Laparoscopy versus ex-lap for likely ectopic

- 2nd or 3rd trimester of pregnancy
  - Perform US.
    - Placenta previa
      - If delivery indicated proceed with C-section.
    - Placental abruption
      - Consider delivery based on maternal-fetal status.
    - Normal US and NST-reactive
      - Continue with routine prenatal care.

Emily Reus, MD and Mark J. Manning, DO, MsMEL

Garcia CR, Barnhart KT. Diagnosing ectopic pregnancy: decision analysis comparing six strategies. *Obstet Gynecol.* 2001;97(3):464–470.

VAGINAL BLEEDING, ABNORMAL

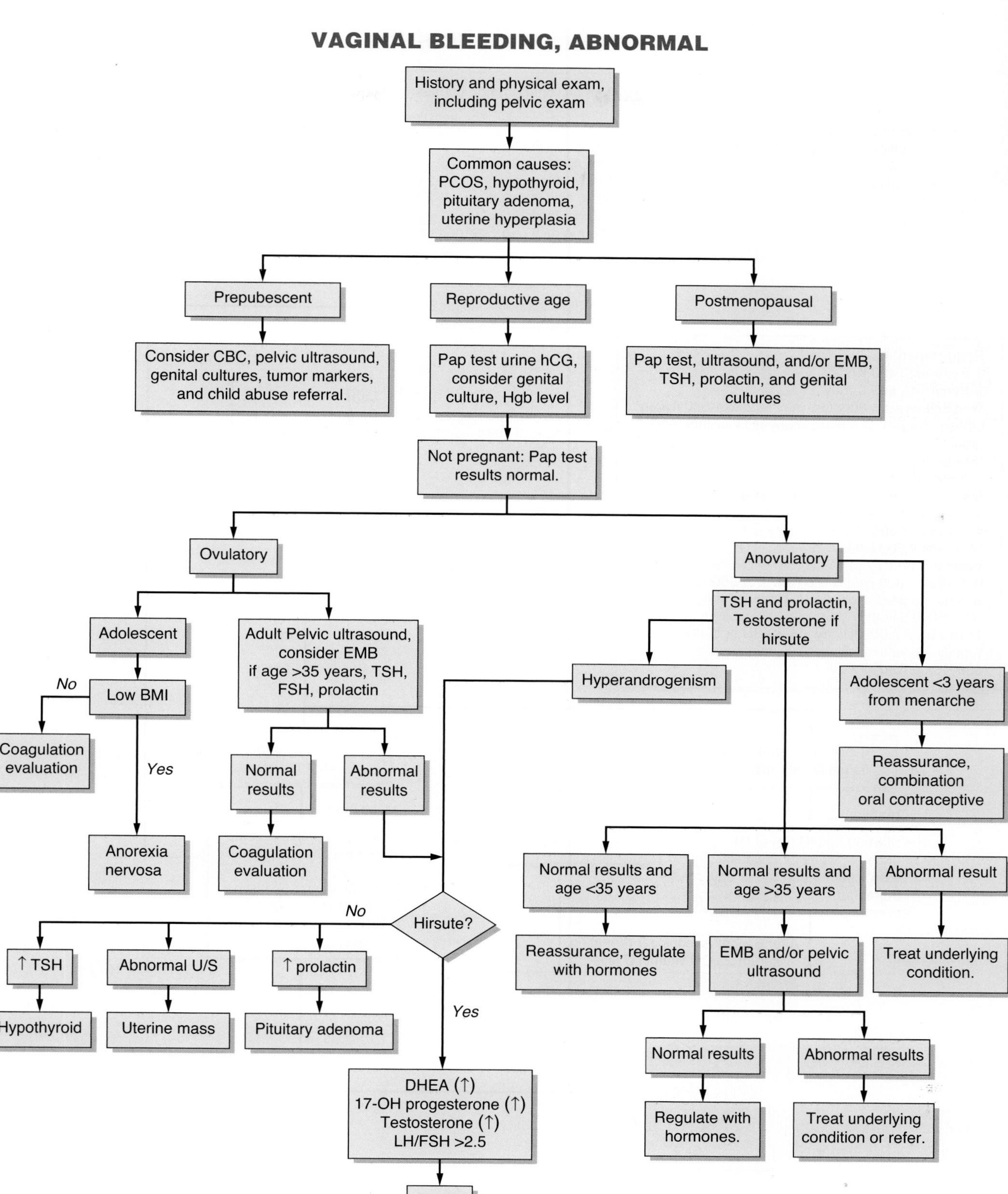

EMB—endometrial biopsy

Tanya E. Anim, MD and Jennifer Tickal Keehbauch, MD

Sweet MG, Schmidt-Dalton TA, Weiss PM, et al. Evaluation and management of abnormal uterine bleeding in premenopausal women. *Am Fam Physician.* 2012;85(1):35–43.

VITAMIN D DEFICIENCY

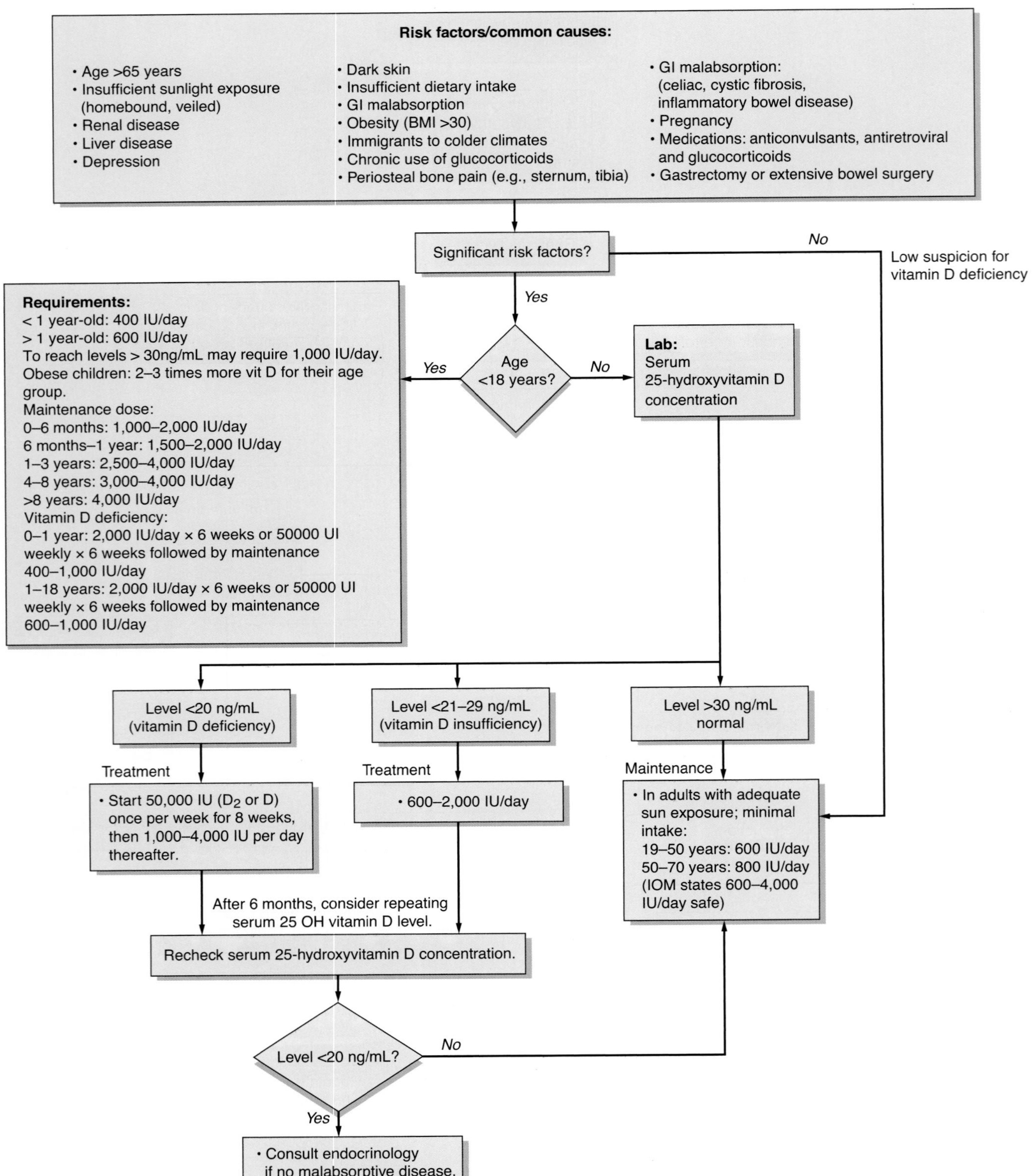

Gisela M. Lopez Payares, MD and Fozia Akhtar Ali, MD

Holick MF, Binkley NC, Bischoff-Ferrari HA, et al. Evaluation, treatment and prevention of vitamin D deficiency: an Endocrine Society clinical practice guideline. *J Clin Endocrinol Metab*. 2011;96(7):1911–1930.

WEIGHT LOSS, UNINTENTIONAL

Weight loss, unintentional >5% last 6 months.

→ Adequate food intake? 25–30 kcal/kg/day

- *Yes*
  - Increased expenditure
    → Fever, Sweats, Tachycardia, Tremors
    → TSH, glucose, PPD, HIV
    → **Endocrine** Hyperthyroidism, Diabetes; **Infectious** HIV, Tuberculosis; **Chronic disease** Cardiac, Pulmonary, Renal; **Increased activity level**
  - Increased loss
    → Chronic diarrhea/ loose stools
    → Malabsorption?
    → • Antitransglutaminase • Antiendomysium • Fecal fat study • Stool O&P • Upper GI endoscopy • Colonoscopy; If all negative, check the following: • Upper GI/barium follow-through • Endoscopic capsule
    → Celiac disease, Pancreatic insufficiency, *Giardia*, Inflamatory bowel disease, Whipple disease, GI resections or bypasses
- *No*
  → Food available?
  - *Yes*
    - Difficulty ingesting food?
      - Oral? → Poorly fitting dentures, Poor dentition, Periodontal disease, Xerostomia
      - GI? → Disphagia, Odynophagia, Vomiting, Abd pain, Distension, Constipation
        → Upper GI endoscopy, Esophageal manometry, Upper GI series, Occult fecal blood, Barium enema, Colonoscopy
        → Cancer, Peptic stricture, Caustic stricture, Esophageal diverticula, Extrinsic compression, Gastric volvulus, Inflammatory bowel disease
      - Neuro? → Memory loss, Cognitive impairment, Sensory/motor deficit
        → CNS imaging
        → Dementia, Alzheimer, Parkinson, Stroke
    - Loss of appetite?
      - Psych? → Mood instability, Distorted body image
        → Depression, Anxiety, Bulimia, Anorexia
      - Drugs? → Polypharmacy, Fluoxetine, Alcohol, Amphetamines, Cocaine, Opiates, Topirimate
  - *No*
    → Social evaluation
    → Financial issues, Inability to obtain preferred foods

Danton Spohr Correa, MD, PhD and Felix B. Chang, MD, DABMA, ABIHM

Bouras EP, Lange SM, Scolapio JS. Rational approach to patients with unintentional weight loss. *Mayo Clin Proc.* 2001;76(9):923–929.

ABNORMAL (DYSFUNCTIONAL) UTERINE BLEEDING

Stephen D. Cagle, Jr., MD, Capt, USAF, MC • Matthew Snyder, DO

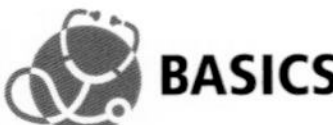

BASICS

DESCRIPTION

- Abnormal uterine bleeding (AUB) is irregular menstrual bleeding (usually heavy, prolonged, or frequent); it is a diagnosis of exclusion after establishment of normal anatomy and the absence of other medical illnesses.
- The International Federation of Gynecology and Obstetrics (FIGO) revised the terminology system and now uses AUB rather than dysfunctional uterine bleeding (DUB).
- Commonly associated with anovulation

EPIDEMIOLOGY

Adolescent and perimenopausal women are affected most often.

Incidence

5% of reproductive age women will see a doctor in any given year for DUB.

Prevalence

10–30% of reproductive age women have DUB.

ETIOLOGY AND PATHOPHYSIOLOGY

- Anovulation accounts for 90% of AUB.
  - Loss of cyclic endometrial stimulation
  - Elevated estrogen levels stimulate endometrial growth.
  - No organized progesterone withdrawal bleed
  - Endometrium eventually outgrows blood supply, breaks down, and sloughs from uterus.
  - 6–10% will have PCOS.
- Adolescent AUB is usually due to an immature hypothalamic-pituitary-ovarian (HPO) axis that leads to anovulatory cycles.
- AUB can be broadly divided into anovulatory bleeding (usually irregular and unpredictable menses) or ovulatory bleeding (usually heavy regular menses) after pathologic causes of abnormal bleeding have been ruled out.
  - Pregnancy: ectopic pregnancy, threatened or incomplete abortion, or hydatidiform mole
  - Reproductive pathology and structural disorders
    - Uterus: leiomyomas, endometritis, hyperplasia, polyps, trauma
    - Adnexa: salpingitis, functional ovarian cysts
    - Cervix: cervicitis, polyps, STIs, trauma
    - Vagina: trauma, foreign body
    - Vulva: lichen sclerosus, STIs
- Malignancy of the vagina, cervix, uterus, and ovaries
- Systemic diseases
  - Inflammatory bowel disease
  - Hematologic disorders (e.g., von Willebrand disease, thrombocytopenia)
  - Advanced or fulminant liver disease
  - Chronic renal disease
- Diseases causing anovulation
  - Hyperthyroidism/hypothyroidism
  - Adrenal disorders
  - Pituitary disease (prolactinoma)
  - Polycystic ovarian syndrome (PCOS)
  - Eating disorders
- Medications (iatrogenic causes)
  - Anticoagulants
  - Steroids
  - Tamoxifen
  - Hormonal medications: intrauterine devices
  - Selective serotonin reuptake inhibitors (SSRIs)
  - Antipsychotic medications
- Other causes of AUB
  - Excessive weight gain
  - Increased exercise
  - Stress

Genetics

Unclear but can include inherited disorders of hemostasis

RISK FACTORS

Risk factors for endometrial cancer (which can cause AUB)

- Age >40 years
- Obesity
- PCOS
- Diabetes mellitus
- Nulliparity
- Early menarche or late menopause (>55 years of age)
- Hypertension
- Chronic anovulation or infertility
- Unopposed estrogen therapy
- History of breast cancer or endometrial hyperplasia
- Tamoxifen use
- Family history: gynecologic, breast, or colon cancer

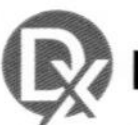

DIAGNOSIS

HISTORY

- Menstrual history
  - Onset, severity (quantified by pad/tampon use, presence and size of clots), timing of bleeding (unpredictable or episodic)
  - Menorrhagia with onset of menarche is suggestive of a coagulation disorder.
  - Menopausal status
  - Association with other factors (e.g., coitus, contraception, weight loss/gain)
- Gynecologic history: gravidity and parity, STI history, previous pap smear results
- Review of systems (exclude symptoms of pregnancy and of bleeding disorders, bleeding from other orifices, stress, exercise, recent weight change, visual changes, headaches, galactorrhea)
- Medication history: Evaluate for use of aspirin, anticoagulants, hormones, and herbal supplements (1,2).

ALERT

Postmenopausal bleeding is any bleeding that occurs >1 year after the last menstrual period; cancer must always be ruled out (2)[C].

PHYSICAL EXAM

Discover anatomic or organic causes of DUB

- Evaluate for
  - Body mass index (obesity)
  - Pallor, vital signs (anemia)
  - Visual field defects (pituitary lesion)
  - Hirsutism or acne (hyperandrogenism)
  - Goiter (thyroid dysfunction)
  - Galactorrhea (hyperprolactinemia)
  - Purpura, ecchymosis (bleeding disorders)
- Pelvic exam
  - Evaluate for uterine irregularities and Tanner stage.
  - Check for foreign bodies.
  - Rule out rectal or urinary tract bleeding.
  - Include Pap smear and tests for STIs (2)[C]

Pediatric Considerations

Premenarchal children with vaginal bleeding should be evaluated for foreign bodies, physical/sexual abuse, possible infections, and signs of precocious puberty.

DIFFERENTIAL DIAGNOSIS

See "Etiology."

DIAGNOSTIC TESTS & INTERPRETATION

Initial Tests (lab, imaging)

- Everyone: urine human chorionic gonadotropin (hCG; rule out pregnancy and/or hydatiform mole) and complete blood count (CBC) (1)
- If anovulation suspected: thyroid stimulating hormone (TSH) level, prolactin level (1)
- Consider other tests based on differential diagnosis.
  - Follicle-stimulating hormone (FSH) level to evaluate for hypo- or hypergonadotropism
  - Coagulation studies and factors if coagulopathy is suspected (1)
  - 17-hydroxyprogestrone if congenital adrenal hyperplasia suspected
  - Testosterone and/or DHEA-S if PCOS
  - Screening for STI
- Endometrial biopsy (EMB) should be performed as part of the initial evaluation for postmenopausal uterine bleeding and in premenopausal women with risk factors for endometrial carcinoma (1)[A].
- TVUS, sonohysterography, and hysteroscopy may be similarly effective in detection of intrauterine pathology in premenopausal women with AUB (1)[A],(2)[C].
- If normal findings following imaging in patients without known risk factors for endometrial carcinoma, a biopsy should be performed if not done so previously (2)[C].

Diagnostic Procedures/Other

- Pap smear to screen for cervical cancer if age >21 years (2)[C]
- EMB should be performed in
  - Women age >35 years with AUB to rule out cancer or premalignancy
  - Postmenopausal women with endometrial thickness >5 mm
  - Women aged 18–35 years with AUB and risk factors for endometrial cancer (see "Risk Factors")
  - Perform on or after day 18 of cycle, if known; secretory endometrium confirms ovulation occurred.
- Dilation and curettage (D&C)
  - Perform if bleeding is heavy, uncontrolled, or if emergent medical management has failed.
  - Perform if unable to perform EMB in office (2)[C].
- Hysteroscopy if another intrauterine lesion is suspected.

Test Interpretation

Pap smear could reveal carcinoma or inflammation indicative of cervicitis. Most EMBs show proliferative or dyssynchronous endometrium (suggesting anovulation) but can show simple or complex hyperplasia without atypia, hyperplasia with atypia, or endometrial adenocarcinoma.

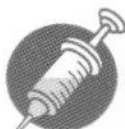

TREATMENT

Attempt to rule out other causes of bleeding prior to instituting therapy.

GENERAL MEASURES

NSAIDs (naproxen sodium 500 mg BID, mefenamic acid 500 mg TID, ibuprofen 600–1,200 mg/day) (1)[B]

- Decreases amount of blood loss compared with placebo, with no one clearly superior NSAID
- Diminishes pain

MEDICATION

First Line

- Acute, emergent, nonovulatory bleeding
  - Conjugated equine estrogen (Premarin): 25 mg IV q4h (max 6 doses) or 2.5 mg PO q6h should control bleeding in 12–24 hours (3)[A]
  - D&C if no response after 2–4 doses of Premarin or sooner if bleeding >1 pad/hour (2)[C]
  - Then change to oral contraceptive pill (OCP) or progestin for cycle regulation, that is, IUD (4)[A]
- Acute, nonemergent, nonovulatory bleeding
  - Combination OCP with ≥30 μg estrogen given as a taper. An example of a tapered dose: 4 pills/day for 4 days; 3 pills/day for 3 days; 2 pills/day for 2 days, daily for 3 weeks then 1 week off, then cycle on OCP for at least 3 months.
- Nonacute, nonovulatory bleeding (ranked in order based on decision analysis as best option based on efficacy, cost, side effects, and consumer acceptability Svs.Med) (4)[A]
  - Levonorgestrel intrauterine device (Mirena) is most effective form of progesterone delivery and is not inferior to surgical management.
  - Progestins: medroxyprogesterone acetate (Provera) 10 mg/day for 5–10 days each month. Daily progesterone for 21 days per cycle results in significantly less blood loss.
  - OCPs: 20–35 μg estrogen plus progesterone
- Do not use estrogen if contraindications, such as suspicion for endometrial hyperplasia or carcinoma, history of deep vein thrombosis (DVT), or the presence of smoking in women >35 years of age (relative contraindication), are present.
- Precautions
  - Failed medical treatment requires further workup.
  - Consider DVT prophylaxis when treating with high-dose estrogens (2)[C].

Second Line

- Leuprolide (varying doses and duration of action); gonadotropin-releasing hormone (GnRH) agonist
- Danazol (200–400 mg/day for a maximum of 9 months) is more effective than NSAIDs but is limited by androgenic side effects and cost. It has been essentially replaced by GnRH agonists.
- Antifibrinolytics such as tranexamic acid (Lysteda) 650 mg, 2 tablets TID (max 5 days during menstruation) (1)[A]
- Metformin or Clomid alone or in combination in women with PCOS who desire ovulation and pregnancy (5)[A]

ISSUES FOR REFERRAL

- If an obvious cause for vaginal bleeding is not found in a pediatric patient, refer to a pediatric endocrinologist or gynecologist (6).
- Patients with persistent bleeding despite medical treatment require reevaluation and referral to a gynecologist (6).

ADDITIONAL THERAPIES

- Antiemetics if treating with high-dose estrogen or progesterone (2)[C]
- Iron supplementation if anemia (usually iron deficiency) is identified

SURGERY/OTHER PROCEDURES

- Hysterectomy in cases of endometrial cancer if medical therapy fails or if uterine pathology found
- Endometrial ablation is less expensive than hysterectomy and is associated with high patient satisfaction; failure of primary medical treatment is not necessary (1,4)[A].
  - This is a permanent procedure and should be avoided in patients who desire continued fertility.

INPATIENT CONSIDERATIONS

Admission Criteria/Initial Stabilization

Significant hemorrhage causing acute anemia with signs of hemodynamic instability; with acute bleeding, replace volume with crystalloid and blood, as necessary (1)[A].

Nursing

Pad counts and clot size can be helpful to determine and monitor amount of bleeding.

Discharge Criteria

- Hemodynamic stability
- Control of vaginal bleeding (2)[C]

ONGOING CARE

FOLLOW-UP RECOMMENDATIONS

- Once stable from acute management recommend follow-up evaluation in 4–6 months for further evaluation (4)
- Routine follow-up with a primary care or OB/GYN provider

Patient Monitoring

Women treated with estrogen or OCPs should keep a menstrual diary to document bleeding patterns and their relation to therapy.

DIET

No restrictions, although a 5% reduction in weight can induce ovulation in anovulation caused by PCOS (7)[C].

PATIENT EDUCATION

- Explain possible/likely etiologies.
- Answer all questions, especially those related to cancer and fertility.
- http://www.acog.org/For_Patients

PROGNOSIS

- Varies with pathophysiologic process
- Most anovulatory cycles can be treated with medical therapy and do not require surgical intervention.

COMPLICATIONS

- Iron deficiency anemia
- Uterine cancer in cases of prolonged unopposed estrogen stimulation

REFERENCES

1. Sweet MG, Schmidt-Dalton TA, Weiss PM, et al. Evaluation and management of abnormal uterine bleeding in premenopausal women. *Am Fam Physician*. 2012;85(1):35–43.
2. Committee on Practice Bulletins—Gynecology. Practice bulletin no. 128: diagnosis of abnormal uterine bleeding in reproductive-aged woman. *Obstet Gynecol*. 2012;120(1):197–206.
3. DeVore GR, Owens O, Kase N. Use of intravenous Premarin in the treatment of dysfunctional uterine bleeding—a double-blind randomized control study. *Obstet Gynecol*. 1982;59(3):285–291.
4. Marjoribanks J, Lethaby A, Farquhar C. Surgery versus medical therapy for heavy menstrual bleeding. *Cochrane Database Syst Rev*. 2006;(2):CD003855.
5. Radosh L. Drug treatments for polycystic ovary syndrome. *Am Fam Physician*. 2009;79(8):671–676.
6. Ely JW, Kennedy CM, Clark EC, et al. Abnormal uterine bleeding: a management algorithm. *J Am Board Fam Med*. 2006;19(6):590–602.
7. Schroeder BM. ACOG releases guidelines on diagnosis and management of polycystic ovary syndrome. *Am Fam Physician*. 2003;67(7):1619–1622.

ADDITIONAL READING

- Farquhar C, Ekeroma A, Furness S, et al. A systematic review of transvaginal ultrasonography, sonohysterography and hysteroscopy for the investigation of abnormal uterine bleeding in premenopausal women. *Acta Obstet Gynecol Scand*. 2003;82(6):493–504.
- Kouides PA, Conard J, Peyvandi F, et al. Hemostasis and menstruation: appropriate investigation for underlying disorders of hemostasis in women with excessive menstrual bleeding. *Fertil Steril*. 2005;84(5):1345–1351.
- Lethaby A, Irvine G, Cameron I. Cyclical progestogens for heavy menstrual bleeding. *Cochrane Database Syst Rev*. 2008;(1):CD001016.
- Lethaby AE, Cooke I, Rees M. Progesterone or progestogen-releasing intrauterine systems for heavy menstrual bleeding. *Cochrane Database Syst Rev*. 2005;(4):CD002126.
- Lethaby A, Farquhar C, Cooke I. Antifibrinolytics for heavy menstrual bleeding. *Cochrane Database Syst Rev*. 2000;(4):CD000249.
- Lethaby A, Shepperd S, Cooke I, et al. Endometrial resection and ablation versus hysterectomy for heavy menstrual bleeding. *Cochrane Database Syst Rev*. 2000;(2):CD000329.

SEE ALSO

- Dysmenorrhea; Menorrhagia
- Algorithm: Menorrhagia

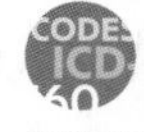

CODES

ICD10

- N93.9 Abnormal uterine and vaginal bleeding, unspecified
- N93.8 Other specified abnormal uterine and vaginal bleeding
- N91.2 Amenorrhea, unspecified

CLINICAL PEARLS

- AUB is irregular bleeding that occurs in the absence of pathology, making it a diagnosis of exclusion.
- Anovulation accounts for 90% of AUB.
- An EMB should be performed in all women >35 years of age with AUB to rule out cancer or premalignancy, and it should be considered in women aged 18–35 years with AUB and risk factors for endometrial cancer.

ABNORMAL PAP AND CERVICAL DYSPLASIA

Fozia Akhtar Ali, MD • Tharani Vadivelu Prasad, MD

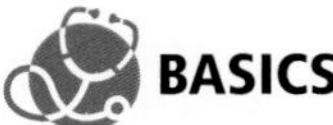

BASICS

DESCRIPTION

- Cervical dysplasia: Premalignant cervical disease that is also called cervical intraepithelial neoplasia (CIN). Precancerous epithelial changes in the transformation zone of the uterine cervix almost always associated with human papillomavirus (HPV) infections.
- Cervical intraepithelial neoplasia (CIN) encompasses a range of histologic diagnoses:
  - CIN I: Mild dysplasia. Low-grade lesion. Cellular changes are limited to the lower 1/3 of the squamous epithelium.
  - CIN II: Moderate dysplasia. High-grade lesion. Cellular changes are limited to the lower 2/3 of the squamous epithelium.
  - CIN III or carcinoma in situ: Severe dysplasia. High-grade lesion. Cellular changes involve the full thickness of the squamous epithelium.
- System(s) affected: reproductive

ALERT

Incidence of cervical cancer has decreased by >50% in the last 30 years due to cervical cytology screening.

Pediatric Considerations

Cervical cancer is very rare before age 21 years. Screening women younger than age 21 years (regardless of sexual history) does not reduce cervical cancer incidence and mortality compared with beginning screening at age 21 years. Screenings of adolescents lead to unnecessary evaluation and overtreatment of cervical lesions, which are highly likely to spontaneously regress (1)[A].

Geriatric Considerations

- Women age >65 years who have had adequate prior screening and no history of CIN 2+ in the last 20 years should not be screened for cervical cancer. Adequate prior screening is defined as 3 consecutive negative cytology results or 2 consecutive negative HPV results within 10 years before cessation of screening (with the most recent test within the last 5 years).
- Routine screening should continue for at least 20 years after spontaneous regression or appropriate management of a high-grade precancerous lesion, even if this extends screening past age 65 years.

Pregnancy Considerations

- Squamous intraepithelial lesions can progress during pregnancy but often regress postpartum.
- Colposcopy only to exclude the presence of invasive cancer in high-risk women.
- Endocervical curettage is contraindicated during pregnancy (2).
- Unless cancer is identified or suspected, treatment of cervical intraepithelial neoplasia is contraindicated during pregnancy.

EPIDEMIOLOGY

- Cervical cancer is the 3rd most common cancer among women worldwide and ranks 14th for cancer deaths in women (3).
- Predominant age: Can occur at any age, but incidence of CIN III peaks between ages 25 and 29; invasive disease peaks 15 years later. Cervical cancer most commonly occurs in women aged 35–55 years.

Incidence

The American Cancer Society estimates that, in 2014, 12,360 women will be diagnosed with invasive cervical cancer and 4,020 women will die from cervical cancer (4). Large declines in incidence rates over the past decades have begun to taper off. From 2006 to 2010, cervical cancer incidence rates have been stable in women younger than 50 years and decreasing by 3.1% per year in women 50 years and older.

Prevalence

- ~80% of sexually active women will have acquired a genital HPV infection by 50 years of age.
- Overall, 26.8% of women are HPV positive. Point prevalence of HPV positivity is highest in those 18–22 years of age (as high as 70%), falling off rapidly as women enter their 30s.

PATHOPHYSIOLOGY

HPV DNA is found in virtually all cervical carcinomas and precursor lesions worldwide.

- High-risk HPV types: 16, 18, 31, 33, 35, 45, 52, and 58 are common oncogenic virus types for cervical cancer.
- HPV16 is the most carcinogenic HPV genotype and accounts for 55–60% of all cervical cancers.
- HPV18 is the next most carcinogenic HPV genotype. HPV18 causes a greater proportion of glandular cancers, adenocarcinoma and adenosquamous carcinoma, than squamous cell carcinoma.
- Most HPV infections are transient, becoming undetectable within 1–2 years. Persistent infections are what place women at significant risk for developing precancerous lesions.
- Low-risk types: HPV viral types 6, 11, 42, 43, and 44 are considered common low-risk types and may cause genital warts. HPV6 and 11 (cause 90% of benign anogenital warts) can lead to low-grade squamous intraepithelial lesion (LSIL) and CIN 1.

RISK FACTORS

- Previous or current HPV infection
- HIV infection and other immunosuppressive conditions
- In utero exposure to diethylstilbestrol
- Previous treatment of a high-grade precancerous lesion or cervical cancer
- Cigarette smoking
- Early age at first coitus (<20 years) and multiple sexual partners
- Some correlation with low socioeconomic status, high parity, oral contraceptive use, and poor nutrition

GENERAL PREVENTION

- Immunization: Immunization decreases high-risk HPV infections and cervical pathology for at least 5–7 years but has not yet been shown to decrease cervical cancer.
  - Ideally, HPV immunization of girls, boys, and women should be initiated prior to first intercourse
    - Gardasil (quadrivalent: HPV4)
      - Reduces dysplasia due to HPV types 16 and 18 (70% of cervical cancer) and types 6 and 11 (anogenital warts)
      - 3 doses at 0, 2, and 6 months, approved for use in females ages 9–26 years. Only the quadrivalent vaccine is approved for males (ages 9–26 years) for prevention of anogenital warts.
    - Cervarix (bivalent: HPV2): Reduces dysplasia due to HPV 16 and 18 infection and CIN. 3 doses at 0, 1, and 6 months, approved for use in females ages 10–25 years.
- Safe sex practices: condom use
- Screening
  - Pap smear is the main screening test for cervical cellular pathology.
  - Screening recommendations by age and source (see algorithm "Pap, Normal and Abnormal in Nonpregnant Women [Ages 25 and Older]" and separate algorithm [Ages 21—24])
    - <21 years: so not screen (5) (USPSTF/ASCCP/ACS/ASCP/ACOG)
  - Frequency of screening recommendation: USPSTF/ASCCP/ACS/ASCP generally agree by age and screen
    - 21–29 years: Screen with cytology (Pap smear) every 3 years (5)[A]. Do not screen with HPV testing alone or combined with cytology (5).
    - 30–65 years: Screen with cytology every 3 years (acceptable) or co-testing (cytology/HPV testing) every 5 years (preferred).
    - >65 years (who have had adequate prior screening and are not high risk): Do not screen (5).
- Special circumstances: Women after hysterectomy with removal of the cervix and with no history of CIN 2+: do not screen (6)[A].

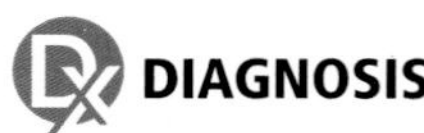

DIAGNOSIS

HISTORY

Usually asymptomatic until there is invasive disease. Patients may present with vaginal discharge, abnormal vaginal bleeding, postcoital bleeding, pelvic pain, cervical mass, or bladder obstruction.

PHYSICAL EXAM

Pelvic exam occasionally reveals external HPV lesions. Examine for exophytic or ulcerative cervical lesions, with or without bleeding.

DIFFERENTIAL DIAGNOSIS

Acute or chronic cervicitis; cervical glandular hyperplasia; cervical polyp; cervical fibroid; HPV infection; invasive cervical malignancy; uterine malignancy

DIAGNOSTIC TESTS & INTERPRETATION

- Current evidence indicates no clinically important differences between conventional cytology and liquid-based cytology in detecting cervical cancer precursors (6)[A]. Conventional Pap smear involves a cervical sample plated on a microscope slide with fixative. Thin prep is a liquid-based collection and thin-layer preparation.
- Sensitivity of a single Pap smear for HSIL ~60–70%; specificity of ~90%. Pap smears done routinely at recommended intervals increases the sensitivity further.
- HPV viral typing: High-risk HPV subtype testing is more sensitive but less specific for identifying women with prevalent CIN 3+.
- Co-testing: HPV typing in combination with Pap smear for women ≥30
- Cytology report component: specimen type (conventional Pap smear or liquid based), adequacy (presence of endocervical cells), and categorization (negative for intraepithelial lesion or malignancy or epithelial cell abnormality; i.e., squamous/glandular)

- Bethesda system (cytologic grading) epithelial cell abnormalities
  - Squamous cell
    - ASC (atypical squamous cells) (ASC-US [of undetermined significance], ASC-H [cannot exclude high-grade squamous intraepithelial lesion])
    - HPV, mild dysplasia, CIN1
    - Moderate/severe dysplasia CIS, CIN II, and CIN III
  - Glandular cell
    - AGC (**a**typical **g**landular **c**ells)
      - AGCs: not otherwise specified
      - AGCs: favor neoplasia
    - AIS (adenocarcinoma in situ)
    - Adenocarcinoma

Diagnostic Procedures

Algorithms differ for women age 21–24 years; see "ASCCP Guideline" (2) and algorithm "Pap, Normal and Abnormal in Nonpregnant Women Ages 21–24." Below recommendations for ages as noted.

- HPV positive, cytology negative (30 years of age and older)
  - Option 1: HPV DNA typing: if HPV 16 or 18 +, proceed to colposcopy; if negative, repeat co-testing at 1 year (6)[B]
  - Option 2: Repeat co-testing at 1 year: if ASC or HPV positive, proceed to colposcopy; if negative, repeat co-testing at 3 years
- ASC-US: (>24 years of age)
  - Option 1: HPV testing (preferred)
    - if HPV +, proceed to colposcopy (2)[B]
    - if HPV negative, repeat co-testing at 3 years (2)[B]
  - Option 2: Repeat cytology at 1 year (acceptable) (2)
    - if repeat cytology ASC or greater, proceed to colposcopy
    - if repeat cytology is negative, proceed to routine screening in 3 years
- ASC-H: colposcopy required
- LSIL: (>24 years of age)
  - LSIL with negative HPV test: repeat co-testing at 1 year (preferred)
    - If repeat co-testing is negative, repeat co-testing in 3 years.
    - If co-testing is positive, proceed to colposcopy
  - LSIL with no HPV test or positive HPV test: Proceed to colposcopy (2).
- HSIL: LEEP or colposcopy (2)[B]
- Atypical glandular cells: colposcopy with endocervical sampling and endometrial sampling (if 35 years or older or at risk for endometrial neoplasia) (2)[A]
- Atypical endometrial cells: Endometrial and endocervical sampling
  - If negative, perform colposcopy
- Women with no lesion on colposcopy or CIN I (preceded by "lesser abnormalities" such as ASC-US, LSIL, HPV 16+, 18+, and persistent HPV)
  - Follow-up without treatment: co-testing at 12 months
  - If both HPV and cytology are negative, age appropriate retesting 3 years later
  - If either positive, proceed to colposcopy. If persistent CIN I for at least 2 years, proceed to treatment with ablative or excisional methods.
- Ages 21–24: Management is slightly different than above, see "ASCCP Guidelines" (2), or algorithm "Pap, Normal and Abnormal in Nonpregnant Women Ages 21–24."

Test Interpretation

Atypical squamous or columnar cells; coarse nuclear material; increased nuclear diameter; koilocytosis (HPV hallmark)

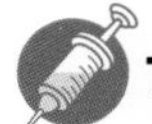

TREATMENT

ASCCP guidelines: Evidence-based management algorithms guide Pap smear and postcolposcopic diagnostics and therapeutics and are available online at http://www.asccp.org/Guidelines (2).

GENERAL MEASURES

Office evaluation and observation; promote smoking cessation; promote protected intercourse; promote immunization

MEDICATION

- Infective/reactive Pap smear: Treat trichomoniasis, symptomatic candida or shift in flora suggestive of bacterial vaginosis found on Pap smear results.
- Condyloma acuminatum: may be treated with cryotherapy or podophyllin topically q1–2wk or podofilox 0.5% applied BID × 3 days then off 4 days, repeated for 1–4 weeks OR trichloroacetic acid, applied topically by a physician and covered for 5–6 days OR imiquimod cream 3×/wk at bedtime up to 16 weeks

SURGERY/OTHER PROCEDURES

- Persistent CIN 1, CIN 2, or 3: Ablative or excisional methods. If inadequate colposcopy for CIN 2 or 3 or recurrent CIN 2 or 3, diagnostic excisional procedure is done. For adenocarcinoma in situ, hysterectomy is preferred.
- Cryotherapy, laser ablation, LEEP/large loop excision of transition zone, or cold-knife conization all effective but require different training and with different side effects for patient. If cervical malignancy, see "Cervical Malignancy."

ONGOING CARE

FOLLOW-UP RECOMMENDATIONS

After treatment (excision or ablation) of CIN 2 or 3, women may reenter routine screening only after negative co-testing at 12 and 24 months. Screening should be continued for 20 years (6)[B].

DIET

Promote increased intake of antioxidant-rich foods.

PATIENT EDUCATION

HPV vaccination, smoking cessation, protected intercourse, regular screening with pap smear per guidelines

PROGNOSIS

- Progression of CIN to invasive cervical cancer is slow, and the likelihood of regression is high: up to 43% of CIN2 and 32% of CIN3 lesions may regress. CIN3 has a 30% probability of becoming invasive cancer over a 30-year period, although only about 1% if treated.
- CIN3 becomes invasive (7). Lesions discovered early are amenable to treatment with excellent results and few recurrences.
- One- and 5-year relative survival rates for cervical cancer patients are 87% and 68%, respectively. The 5-year survival rate for patients diagnosed with localized disease is 91% (4).

COMPLICATIONS

Aggressive cervical surgery may be associated with cervical stenosis, cervical incompetence, and scarring affecting cervical dilatation in labor.

REFERENCES

1. Yang KY. Abnormal pap smear and cervical cancer in pregnancy. *Clin Obstet Gynecol*. 2012;55(3): 838–848.
2. Massad S, Eienstein MH, Warner KH. 2012 updated consensus guidelines for the management of abnormal cervical cancer screening tests and cancer precursors. *J Low Genit Tract Dis*. 2013;17(5): S1–S27.
3. American Cancer Society. Cancer facts and figures 2013. American Cancer Society Web site. http://www.cancer.org/acs/groups/content/@epidemiologysurveilance/documents/document/acspc-036845.pdf. Accessed May 21, 2013.
4. American Cancer Society. Cancer facts and figures 2014. American Cancer Society Web site. http://www.cancer.org/acs/groups/content/@research/documents/webcontent/acspc-042151.pdf. Accessed July 21, 2014.
5. U.S. Preventive Services Task Force. Cervical cancer: screening. U.S. Preventive Services Task Force Web site. http://www.uspreventiveservicestaskforce.org/uspstf11/cervcancer/cervcancerrs.pdf. Accessed July 23, 2014.
6. American College of Obstetricians and Gynecologists. *ACOG Practice Bulletin No. 131: Screening for Cervical Cancer*. Washington, DC: American College of Obstetricians and Gynecologists; 2012.
7. McCredie MR, Sharples KJ, Paul C, et al. Natural history of cervical neoplasia and risk of invasive cancer in women with cervical intraepithelial neoplasia 3: a retrospective cohort study. *Lancet Oncol*. 2008;9(5):425–434.

SEE ALSO

- Cervical Malignancy; Condyloma Acuminata; Trichomoniasis; Vulvovaginitis, Prepubescent
- Algorithm: Pap (Abnormal), >21 Years of Age; Pap (Abnormal), Pap, Use of HPV DNA Co-Testing in Women Over 30

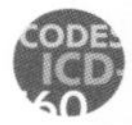

CODES

ICD 10

- R87.619 Unspecified abnormal cytological findings in specimens from cervix uteri
- N87.9 Dysplasia of cervix uteri, unspecified
- N87.1 Moderate cervical dysplasia

CLINICAL PEARLS

- HPV is present in virtually all cervical cancers (99.7%), but most HPV infections are transient.
- Vaccine should be offered prior to onset of any sexual activity for maximum effectiveness.
- Know and adhere to recognized screening guidelines to avoid the harms of overscreening.

ABORTION, SPONTANEOUS (MISCARRIAGE)

Clara M. Keegan, MD

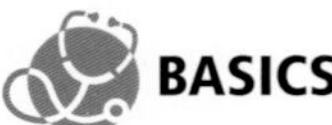

BASICS

DESCRIPTION

- Spontaneous abortion (SAb) (miscarriage) is the failure or loss of a pregnancy before 14 weeks' gestational age (WGA).
- Related terms
  - Anembryonic gestation: gestational sac on ultrasound (US) without visible embryo after 6 WGA
  - Complete abortion: entire contents of uterus expelled
  - Ectopic pregnancy: pregnancy outside the uterus
  - Embryonic or fetal demise: Cervix closed, embryo or fetus present in the uterus without cardiac activity.
  - Incomplete abortion: abortion with retained products of conception, generally placental tissue
  - Induced or therapeutic abortion: evacuation of uterine contents or products of conception medically or surgically
  - Inevitable abortion: cervical dilatation or rupture of membranes in the presence of vaginal bleeding
  - Recurrent abortion: ≥3 consecutive pregnancy losses at <15 WGA
  - Threatened abortion: vaginal bleeding in the 1st trimester of pregnancy
  - Septic abortion: a spontaneous or therapeutic abortion complicated by pelvic infection; common complication of illegally performed induced abortions
- Synonym(s): miscarriage; early pregnancy loss
  - Missed abortion and blighted ovum are used less frequently in favor of terms representing the sonographic diagnosis.

EPIDEMIOLOGY

Predominant age: increases with advancing age, especially >35 years; at age 40 years, the loss rate is twice that of age 20 years.

Incidence

- Threatened abortion (1st-trimester bleeding) occurs in 20–25% of clinical pregnancies.
- Between 10 and 15% of all clinically recognized pregnancies end in SAb, with 80% of these occurring within 12 weeks after last menstrual period (LMP) (1).
- When both clinical and biochemical (β-hCG detected) pregnancies are considered, about 30% of pregnancies end in SAb.
- One in four women will have a SAb during her lifetime (1).

ETIOLOGY AND PATHOPHYSIOLOGY

- Chromosomal anomalies (50–65% of cases)
- Congenital anomalies
- Trauma
- Maternal factors: uterine abnormalities, infection (toxoplasma, other viruses, rubella, cytomegalovirus, herpesvirus), maternal endocrine disorders, hypercoagulable state

Genetics

~50–65% of 1st-trimester SAbs have significant chromosomal anomalies, with 50% of these being autosomal trisomies and the remainder being triploidy, tetraploidy, or 45X monosomies.

RISK FACTORS

Most cases of SAb occur in patients without identifiable risk factors; however, risk factors include the following:

- Chromosomal abnormalities
- Advancing maternal age
- Uterine abnormalities
- Maternal chronic disease (antiphospholipid antibodies, uncontrolled diabetes mellitus, polycystic ovarian syndrome, obesity, hypertension, thyroid disease, renal disease)
- Other possible contributing factors include smoking, alcohol, cocaine use, infection, and luteal phase defect.

GENERAL PREVENTION

- Insufficient evidence supports the use of aspirin and/or other anticoagulants, bed rest, hCG, immunotherapy, progestogens, uterine muscle relaxants, or vitamins for general prevention of SAb, before or after threatened abortion is diagnosed.
- By the time hemorrhage begins, 1/2 of pregnancies complicated by threatened abortion already have no fetal cardiac activity.
- Recurrent abortion: Women with a history of ≥3 prior SAbs may benefit from progestogens (OR 0.39, 95% CI 0.21–0.72) (2)[A].
- Antiphospholipid syndrome: The combination of unfractionated heparin and aspirin reduces risk of SAb in women with antiphospholipid antibodies and a history of recurrent abortion (RR 46%, 95% CI 0.29–0.71) (3)[A].

DIAGNOSIS

HISTORY

- The possibility of pregnancy should be considered in a reproductive-age woman who presents with nonmenstrual vaginal bleeding.
- Vaginal bleeding
  - Characteristics (amount, color, consistency, associated symptoms), onset (abrupt or gradual), duration, intensity/quantity, and exacerbating/precipitating factors
  - Document LMP if known: allows calculation of estimated gestational age
- Abdominal pain/uterine cramping, as well as associated nausea/vomiting/syncope
- Rupture of membranes
- Passage of products of conception
- Prenatal course: toxic or infectious exposures, family or personal history of genetic abnormalities, past history of ectopic pregnancy or SAb, endocrine disease, autoimmune disorder, bleeding/clotting disorder

PHYSICAL EXAM

- Orthostatic vital signs to estimate hemodynamic stability
- Abdominal exam for tenderness, guarding, rebound, bowel sounds (peritoneal signs more likely with ectopic pregnancy)
- Speculum exam for visual assessment of cervical dilation, blood, and products of conception (confirms diagnosis of SAb)
- Bimanual exam to assess for uterine size–dates discrepancy and adnexal tenderness or mass

DIFFERENTIAL DIAGNOSIS

- Ectopic pregnancy: potentially life-threatening; must be considered in any woman of childbearing age with abdominal pain and vaginal bleeding
- Physiologic bleeding in normal pregnancy (implantation bleeding)
- Subchorionic bleeding
- Cervical polyps, neoplasia, and/or inflammatory conditions
- Hydatidiform mole pregnancy
- hCG-secreting ovarian tumor

DIAGNOSTIC TESTS & INTERPRETATION

Initial Tests (lab, imaging)

- Quantitative hCG
  - Particularly useful if intrauterine pregnancy (IUP) has not been documented by US
  - Serial quantitative serum hCG measurements can assess viability of the pregnancy. Serum hCG should rise at least 53% every 48 hours through 7 weeks after LMP. An inappropriate rise, plateau, or decrease of hCG suggests abnormal IUP or possible ectopic pregnancy.
- CBC with differential
- Rh type
- Cultures: gonorrhea/chlamydia
- US exam to evaluate fetal viability and to rule out ectopic pregnancy (4)[A]
  - hCG >2,000 mIU/mL necessary to detect IUP via transvaginal US (TVUS), >5,500 mIU/mL for abdominal US
  - TVUS criteria for nonviable intrauterine gestation: 7-mm fetal pole without cardiac activity or 25-mm gestational sac without a fetal pole, IUP with no growth over 1 week, or previously seen IUP no longer visible
  - Structures and timing: with TVUS, gestational sac of 2–3 mm generally seen around 5 WGA; yolk sac by 5.5 WGA; fetal pole with cardiac activity by 6 WGA

Follow-Up Tests & Special Considerations

- In the case of vaginal bleeding with no documented IUP and hCG <2,000 mIU/mL, follow serum hCG levels weekly to zero.
- If levels plateau, consider ectopic pregnancy or retained products of conception. If levels are very high, consider gestational trophoblastic disease.
- If initial hCG level does not permit documentation of IUP by TVUS, follow serum hCG in 48 hours to document appropriate rise.
- Repeat US once hCG is at a level commensurate with visualization on US (see above).
- Provide patient with ectopic precautions in interim: worsening abdominal pain, dizziness/syncope, nausea/vomiting.
- In a pregnancy of unknown location with hCG rise <53% in 48 hours, offer methotrexate for treatment of presumed ectopic pregnancy.

Diagnostic Procedures/Other

- Fetal heart tones can be auscultated with Doppler starting between 10 and 12 WGA in a viable pregnancy.
- In threatened abortion, fetal cardiac activity at 7–11 WGA is 90–96% predictive of continued pregnancy.

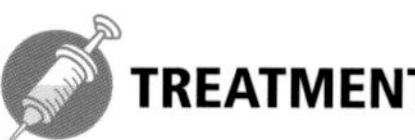

TREATMENT

GENERAL MEASURES

- Discuss contraception plan at the time of diagnosis of SAb, as ovulation can occur prior to resumption of normal menses.
- "Watchful waiting" is 90% effective for incomplete abortion, although it may take several weeks for the process to be complete (1)[A].

MEDICATION

- Long-term conception rate and pregnancy outcomes are similar for women who undergo expectant management, medical treatment, or surgical evacuation.
- Postinfection rates are lower with medical versus surgical management.

First Line

- Misoprostol: most common agent for inducing passage of tissue in missed or incomplete abortion
  - Off-label use; has not been submitted to the FDA for consideration for use in treatment of early pregnancy failure. Recognized by the World Health Organization as a life-saving medication for this indication
  - Efficacy: complete expulsion of products of conception in 71% by day 3, 84% by day 8
  - Efficacy depends on route of administration, gestational age of pregnancy, and dose.
  - Recommended dose is 800 μg vaginally; alternate regimens include the World Health Organization (WHO) regimen of 600 μg sublingually q3h for up to 3 doses; multidose regimens and oral dosing (including buccal and sublingual) may result in increased side effects.
- Common adverse effects include abdominal pain/cramping, nausea, and diarrhea. Pain increases at higher doses but is manageable with oral analgesia. There is no increase in nausea/diarrhea with a higher dose.
- Recommended for stable patients who decline surgery but do not want to wait for spontaneous passage of products of conception

Second Line

- Rh-negative patients should be given Rh immunoglobulin (RhoGAM) 50 μg IM following a SAb.
- Women with evidence of anemia should receive iron supplementation.

ISSUES FOR REFERRAL

Patients should be monitored for up to 1 year for the development of pathologic grief. There is insufficient evidence to support counseling to prevent development of anxiety or depression related to grief following SAb.

SURGERY/OTHER PROCEDURES

- Uterine aspiration (suction dilation and curettage [D&C] or manual vacuum aspiration [MVA]) is the conventional treatment.
- Indications: septic abortion, heavy bleeding, hypotension, patient choice
- Risks (all rare): anesthesia (usually local), uterine perforation, intrauterine adhesions, cervical trauma, infection that may lead to infertility or increased risk of ectopic pregnancy
- When compared with expectant management, surgical intervention leads to fewer days of vaginal bleeding, with a lower risk of incomplete abortion and heavy bleeding but a higher risk of infection (5)[A].
- Vacuum aspiration (manual or electric) is considered preferable to sharp curettage, as aspiration is less painful, takes less time, involves less blood loss, and does not require general anesthesia. The WHO supports use of suction curettage over rigid metal curettage.
- Although data from induced abortions suggest that antibiotic prophylaxis with doxycycline 100 mg BID reduces the already rare risk of postprocedure infection, data are insufficient to support use of antibiotics after aspiration for SAb (6)[A].

COMPLEMENTARY & ALTERNATIVE MEDICINE

A systematic review of Chinese herbal medicine alone and in conjunction with Western medicine showed benefit over Western medicine alone in achieving continued viability at 28 weeks (number needed to treat [NNT] = 4.8 pregnancies with combined therapy). However, the available studies did not meet international standards for reporting quality (7)[C].

INPATIENT CONSIDERATIONS

Admission Criteria/Initial Stabilization

If the patient has orthostatic vital signs, initiate resuscitation with IV fluids and/or blood products, if needed.

IV Fluids

Hemodynamically unstable patients may require IV fluids and/or blood products to maintain BP.

ONGOING CARE

FOLLOW-UP RECOMMENDATIONS

All patients should be offered follow-up in 2–6 weeks to monitor for resolution of bleeding, return of menses, and symptoms related to grief, as well as to review the contraception plan.

Patient Monitoring

- If SAb occurs in setting of previously documented IUP and abortion is completed with resumption of normal menses, it is not necessary to check or follow serum hCG to 0.
- If pregnancy is not immediately desired, offer effective contraception. Immediate insertion of an intrauterine device is both acceptable and safe.
- If pregnancy is desired, provide preconception counseling. There is no evidence that it is necessary to wait a certain number of cycles before attempting conception again.

DIET

NPO if patient is to undergo D&C under general anesthesia

PATIENT EDUCATION

- Pelvic rest for 1 week after D&C or MVA
- Advise patients to call with excessive bleeding (soaking two pads per hour for 2 hours), fever, pelvic pain, or malaise, which could indicate retained products of conception or endometritis.
- A patient fact sheet on miscarriage is available through the American Academy of Family Physicians at http://www.aafp.org/afp/2011/0701/p85.html.

PROGNOSIS

- Prognosis is excellent once bleeding is controlled.
- Recurrent abortion: Prognosis depends on etiology. Up to 70% rate of success with subsequent pregnancy

COMPLICATIONS

- D&C or MVA: uterine perforation, bleeding, adhesions, cervical trauma, and infection that may lead to infertility or increased risk of ectopic pregnancy. Bleeding and adhesions more common with D&C than with MVA; all complications rare.
- Retained products of conception

REFERENCES

1. Prine LW, MacNaughton H. Office management of early pregnancy loss. *Am Fam Physician*. 2011;84(1):75–82.
2. Haas DM, Ramsey PS. Progestogen for preventing miscarriage. *Cochrane Database Syst Rev*. 2013;10:CD003511.
3. Empson M, Lassere M, Craig J, et al. Prevention of recurrent miscarriage for women with antiphospholipid antibody or lupus anticoagulant. *Cochrane Database Syst Rev*. 2005;(2):CD002859.
4. Doubilet PM, Benson CB, Bourne T, et al. Diagnostic criteria for nonviable pregnancy early in the first trimester. *N Engl J Med*. 2013;369(15):1443–1451.
5. Nanda K, Lopez LM, Grimes DA, et al. Expectant care versus surgical treatment for miscarriage. *Cochrane Database Syst Rev*. 2012;3:CD003518.
6. May W, Gülmezoglu AM, Ba-Thike K. Antibiotics for incomplete abortion. *Cochrane Database Syst Rev*. 2007;(4):CD001779.
7. Li L, Dou L, Leung PC, et al. Chinese herbal medicines for threatened miscarriage. *Cochrane Database Syst Rev*. 2012;5:CD008510.

ADDITIONAL READING

- Murphy FA, Lipp A, Powles DL. Follow-up for improving psychological well being for women after a miscarriage. *Cochrane Database Syst Rev*. 2012;3:CD008679.
- Neilson JP, Gyte GM, Hickey M, et al. Medical treatments for incomplete miscarriage. *Cochrane Database Syst Rev*. 2013;3:CD007223.
- Okusanya BO, Oduwole O, Effa EE. Immediate post-abortal insertion of intrauterine devices. *Cochrane Database Syst Rev*. 2014;7:CD001777.
- Tunçalp O, Gülmezoglu AM, Souza JP. Surgical procedures for evacuating incomplete miscarriage. *Cochrane Database Syst Rev*. 2010;(9):CD001993.

SEE ALSO

- Ectopic Pregnancy
- Algorithm: Abortion, Recurrent

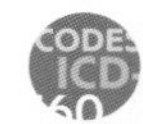

CODES

ICD10

- O03.9 Complete or unspecified spontaneous abortion without complication
- O03.4 Incomplete spontaneous abortion without complication
- O02.1 Missed abortion

CLINICAL PEARLS

- Any pregnant woman with abdominal pain and/or vaginal bleeding must be evaluated to rule out ectopic pregnancy, which is potentially life threatening.
- As all options have similar long-term outcomes, patient preference should determine whether management is expectant, medical, or surgical.

ACL INJURY

Tara Futrell, MD • J. Herbert Stevenson, MD

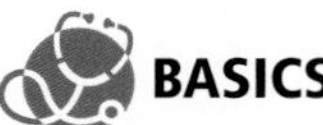

BASICS

DESCRIPTION

- The anterior cruciate ligament (ACL) is a major stabilizer of the knee that prevents excessive anterior translation and internal rotation of the tibia in relation to the femur.
  – During dynamic movement, the ACL and posterior cruciate ligament (PCL) work together to stabilize the knee.
- ACL injuries are common and can occur through multiple mechanisms. >70% of ACL injuries are caused by noncontact forces.
- Although partial tears occur, complete ACL tears are more common.
- Due to differences in pelvic architecture and lower extremity alignment, female athletes are at 2–5 times higher at risk of ACL tear.
- ACL injury is associated with early onset of knee osteoarthritis.

EPIDEMIOLOGY

Incidence

- 250,000 ACL injuries annually in the United States
- Female incidence 2–5-fold > male (1)
- Greater incidence of noncontact ACL injuries in sports requiring cutting, pivoting, and rapid deceleration, such as basketball and soccer (1)

Prevalence

- Young athletes (15–25 years) sustain >50% of all ACL injuries (1)[B].
- >2/3 of patients with complete ACL tear have associated meniscal and/or articular cartilage injury.

Pediatric Considerations

- Rule out physeal injuries in the skeletally immature patients.
- The incidence of ACL tears in patients with open physes has increased in recent years.
- ACL injury rates increase for both boys and girls after age 11 years.

ETIOLOGY AND PATHOPHYSIOLOGY

- Noncontact mechanisms: torsional or hyperextension forces creates anterior translation of the tibia relative to the femur that creates excessive stress across the ACL with resultant rupture.
- Direct trauma: most often a valgus blow to the knee with resultant trauma to ACL, medial collateral ligament, and lateral meniscus ("unhappy triad")

Genetics

A genetic predisposition has been identified.

RISK FACTORS

- Female athletes have increased risk likely due to multiple variables.
  – Hormonal influence
    ○ Alterations in hormonal balance hypothesized to increase risk, but no conclusive evidence linking menstrual phase to ACL injury risk.
  – Anatomic gender differences
    ○ Increased Q angle, increased genu valgum, narrower femoral notch size, smaller ACL
    ○ Neuromuscular imbalances (increased quadriceps activation, decreased hamstring activity during landings)
  – Movement patterns (sudden deceleration, change-of-direction cutting movements, landing from a jump in hyperextension)

GENERAL PREVENTION

- Neuromuscular training with proprioceptive, plyometric, and strength exercises may reduce noncontact ACL injuries by 72% in female athletes if performed more than once per week for >6 weeks (2)[C].
- Prophylactic knee bracing not shown to prevent ACL injury.

COMMONLY ASSOCIATED CONDITIONS

- Meniscal tear
- Collateral ligament tear
- PCL tear
- Tibia or femur fractures
- Osteochondral injury
- Early-onset degenerative joint disease

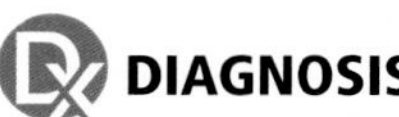

DIAGNOSIS

HISTORY

May recall mechanism

- Noncontact
  – Sudden deceleration
  – Cutting, sudden change in direction
  – Landing from a jump in extension
- Contact with player, object
- May recall sudden pop or snap
- Sudden pain and giving way
- Marked effusion/hemarthrosis within 4–12 hours
- "Pop" with deceleration or twisting movement associated with early effusion and inability to continue with participation are highly suggestive of ACL tear.

PHYSICAL EXAM

- Inspect for malalignment (fracture, dislocation).
- Palpate for effusion.
- Decreased range of motion (ROM)
  – Deficits may be secondary to pain, effusion, mechanical blocks (meniscal tear, loose body, torn ACL stump).
- Joint instability
- Difficulty bearing weight
- Evaluate extensor mechanism integrity
- Special maneuvers (Lachman; anterior drawer; pivot shift)
- Lachman test: most sensitive and highly specific diagnostic test for ACL injury, especially in acute setting (3)[B]
  – Knee placed in 20–30 degrees of flexion. Tibia is translated anteriorly, whereas the femur is stabilized with the opposite hand. Increased anterior translation compared with uninjured knee indicates injury. Lack of a solid endpoint indicates rupture.
- Pivot shift test: less sensitive, but more than Lachman test: specific for ACL tear (3)[B]
  – Knee placed in extension. Knee is flexed while valgus and internal rotation stress is applied. A positive test is anterior subluxation at 20–40 degrees of flexion.
- Anterior drawer test (3)[B]
  – Low sensitivity for ACL integrity, especially in acute setting
- Posterior drawer test assesses PCL integrity.
- McMurray test assesses for meniscal tears.
- Valgus/varus stress test for medial collateral ligament/lateral collateral (MCL/LCL) integrity

DIFFERENTIAL DIAGNOSIS

- Fracture
- Meniscal injury
- Patellar dislocation/subluxation
- Tendon disruption
- PCL injury
- Collateral ligament injury

DIAGNOSTIC TESTS & INTERPRETATION

Initial Tests (lab, imaging)

- Radiographs to rule out associated bony injury
- Anterior-posterior (AP), lateral, and tunnel views
  – Segond fracture: avulsion fracture of the lateral capsular margin of the tibia
  – Tibial eminence avulsion fracture
  – Fracture of proximal tibia or distal femur
  – Osteochondral injuries

Follow-Up Tests & Special Considerations

- MRI is the gold standard for imaging ligamentous and intra-articular structures. The sensitivity of MRI is 87–94%, specificity 88–93% (4).
- Secondary signs of ACL injury on MRI include bone contusion of the anterior femoral condyle and/or posterior tibial plateau, anterior translation of the tibia, an uncovered or displaced posterior horn of the lateral meniscus, PCL buckling, or a Segond fracture (an avulsion fracture of the lateral tibial condyle).

Diagnostic Procedures/Other

Surgical management should be considered in the active population, young or old.

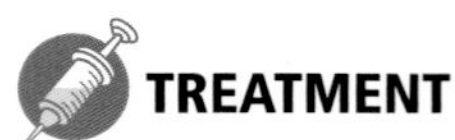

TREATMENT

GENERAL MEASURES

- Acute injury: protection, relative rest, ice, compression, elevation, medications, modalities (PRICEMM) therapy
- Crutches may be useful until patient is able to ambulate without pain.
- Locked knee brace may be used initially for comfort. Use with caution and transition to a hinged knee brace as soon as possible to avoid quadriceps atrophy and stiffness.
- Aspiration of large effusion may alleviate pain and increase ROM.

MEDICATION

First Line

- Nonsteroidal anti-inflammatory drugs (NSAIDs)
  – Acute ligament sprains
    ○ Ibuprofen: 200–800 mg TID
    ○ Naproxen: 250–500 mg BID
- Acetaminophen: 3 g/day divided TID
- Opioids for severe pain (e.g., acetaminophen-hydrocodone)

ISSUES FOR REFERRAL

The decision to manage ACL tears surgically or nonsurgically ("conservatively") can be difficult.Surgical management should be considered in the active population or if the injury interferes with activities of daily living.

- Physical therapy is essential whether an athlete chooses nonsurgical or surgical treatment. Proper rehabilitation is time-consuming (6–12 months) and hard work. Physical therapy focuses on restoring ROM, strength, and proprioception.
- Preoperative phase
  - Increase ROM and quadriceps strength, minimize inflammation
- Early postoperative phase: weeks 2–4
  - ROM: Full extension is the most important goal. Rehabilitation begins immediately.
  - Progress to full-weight bearing
- Intermediate postoperative phase: weeks 4–12
  - ROM: full flexion, hyperextension
  - Quadriceps and hamstring strengthening proprioceptive training, normalize gait
- Late postop phase: >3 months postop
  - Straight-line running
  - Increase speed, duration over 6–8 weeks
  - Progress to cutting and sport-specific drills
  - Strength and proprioceptive training

Geriatric Considerations

Management is based on anticipated activity level, associated injuries, coexisting medical conditions, and acute versus long-standing ACL deficiency.

SURGERY/OTHER PROCEDURES

- Surgical versus conservative management depends on patient's activity level, age, associated injuries, and presence of osteoarthritis.
- There is insufficient evidence to recommend surgery versus conservative management in skeletally immature patients.
- No significant difference in patient-reported knee function or muscle strength between surgical and nonsurgical patients (5)[B].
- In young, active adults with acute ACL tears, rehabilitation plus early ACL repair was not superior to a strategy of initial rehabilitation with delayed repair if rehabilitation alone failed. Rehabilitation alone results in an overall reduction of ACL reconstructions (5)[B].
- Reconstruction techniques
  - Bone-patella tendon-bone autograft
  - Hamstring autograft
  - Allograft tendon (from cadaver)
- No consistent significant differences in outcome between patellar tendon and hamstring tendon autografts
- Concomitant meniscal tears are repaired at the time of ACL reconstruction.

INPATIENT CONSIDERATIONS

Admission Criteria/Initial Stabilization

Outpatient

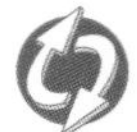

ONGOING CARE

FOLLOW-UP RECOMMENDATIONS

- ROM exercises to regain full flexion and extension
- Advance activity as tolerated

Patient Monitoring

Assess functional status, rehabilitative exercise compliance, and pain control at follow-up visit.

PROGNOSIS

- Athletes typically are out of competitive play for 6–9 months after injury to undergo ACL reconstructive surgery and rehabilitation.
- High prevalence of OA, even in those with early ACL reconstruction
- Delaying surgical repair of torn ACL increases risk of secondary meniscal injury.

COMPLICATIONS

- Instability
- Secondary meniscal and articular cartilage injury
- Early-onset degenerative arthritis
- Surgical risks
  - Infection, pulmonary embolism (PE), subsequent ACL graft rupture, laxity due to failure of graft remodeling

REFERENCES

1. Beynnon B. Vacekp P, Newell MK, et al. The effects of level of competition, sport and sex on the incidence of first time noncontact anterior cruciate ligament injury. *Am J Sports Med*. 2014;42(8):1806–1812.
2. Acevedo RJ, Rivera-Vega A, Miranda, G, et al. Anterior cruciate ligament injury: identification of risk factors and prevention strategies. *Curr Sports Med Rep*. 2014:13(3):186–191.
3. Jain DK, Amaravati R, Sharma G. Evaluation of the clinical signs of anterior cruciate ligament and meniscal injuries. *Indian J Orthop*. 2009;43(4): 375–378.
4. Vincken PW, ter Braak BP, van Erkell AR, et al. Effectiveness of MR imaging in selection of patients for arthroscopy of the knee. *Radiology*. 2002;223(3):739–746.
5. Grindem H, Eitzer I, Engbretsen L. et al. Nonsurgical or surgical treatment of ACL injuries: knee function, sports participation, and knee reinjury: the Delaware-Oslo ACL cohort study. *J Bone and Joint Surg*. 2014;96(15):1233–1241.

ADDITIONAL READING

- Cascio BM, Culp L, Cosgarea AJ. Return to play after anterior cruciate ligament reconstruction. *Clin Sports Med*. 2004;23(3):395–408, ix.
- Christiansen BA, Anderson MJ, Lee CA, et al. Musculoskeletal changes following non-invasive knee injury using a novel mouse model of post-traumatic osteoarthritis. *Osteoarthr Cartil*. 2012;20(7):773–782.
- Frobell RB, Roos EM, Roos HP, et al. A randomized trial of treatment for acute anterior cruciate ligament tears. *N Engl J Med*. 2010;363(4):331–342.
- Hewett TE, Di Stasi SL, Myer GD. Current concepts for injury prevention in athletes after anterior cruciate ligament reconstruction. *Am J Sports Med*. 2013;41(1):216–224.
- Hewett TE, Ford KR, Myer GD. Anterior cruciate ligament injuries in female athletes: part 2, a meta-analysis of neuromuscular interventions aimed at injury prevention. *Am J Sports Med*. 2006;34(3):490–498.
- Linko E, Harilainen A, Malmivaara A, et al. Surgical versus conservative interventions for anterior cruciate ligament ruptures in adults. *Cochrane Database Syst Rev*. 2005;(2):CD001356.
- Mohtadi NG, Chan DS, Dainty KN, et al. Patellar tendon versus hamstring tendon autograft for anterior cruciate ligament ruptures in adults. *Cochrane Database Syst Rev*. 2011;(9):CD005960.
- Silvers HJ, Mandelbaum BR. Prevention of anterior cruciate ligament injury in the female athlete. *Br J Sports Med*. 2007;41(Suppl 1):i52–i59.
- Spindler KP, Kuhn JE, Freedman KB, et al. Anterior cruciate ligament reconstruction autograft choice: bone-tendon-bone versus hamstring: does it really matter? A systematic review. *Am J Sports Med*. 2004;32(8):1986–1995.
- White K, Di Stasi SL, Smith AH, et al. Anterior cruciate ligament- specialized post-operative return-to-sports (ACL-SPORTS) training: a randomized control trial. *BMC Musculoskelet Disord*. 2013;14:108.

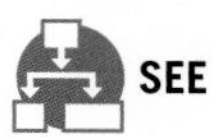

SEE ALSO

Algorithm: Knee pain

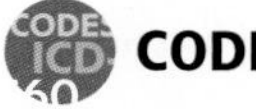

CODES

ICD10

- S83.519A Sprain of anterior cruciate ligament of unsp knee, init
- M23.619 Oth spon disrupt of anterior cruciate ligament of unsp knee
- S83.511A Sprain of anterior cruciate ligament of right knee, init

CLINICAL PEARLS

- Lachman test is the most sensitive and specific test for diagnosing acute ACL injury.
- Bone contusion of the anterior femoral condyle and/or posterior tibial plateau on MRI is highly suggestive of ACL tear even if it appears intact on imaging.
- 2/3 of complete ACL tears have associated meniscal or articular injuries.
- The decision for surgical ACL repair (vs. conservative treatment) should be based on patient age, activity level, and associated symptoms.

ACNE ROSACEA

Adarsh K. Gupta, DO, MS, FACOFP

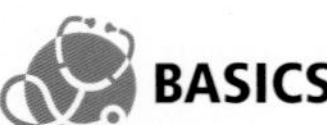

BASICS

DESCRIPTION

- Rosacea is a chronic condition characterized by recurrent episodes of facial flushing, erythema (due to dilatation of small blood vessels in the face), papules, pustules, and telangiectasia (due to increased reactivity of capillaries) in a symmetric, facial distribution. Sometimes associated with ocular symptoms (ocular rosacea).
- System(s) affected: skin/exocrine
- Synonym(s): rosacea

Geriatric Considerations

- Uncommon >60 years of age
- Effects of aging might increase the side effects associated with oral isotretinoin used for treatment (at present, data are insufficient due to lack of clinical studies in elderly patients ≥65 years).

EPIDEMIOLOGY

Prevalence

- Predominant age: 30–50 years
- Predominant sex: female > male. However, males are at greater risk for progression to later stages.

ETIOLOGY AND PATHOPHYSIOLOGY

- No proven cause
- Possibilities include the following:
  - Thyroid and sex hormone disturbance
  - Alcohol, coffee, tea, spiced food overindulgence (unproven)
  - Demodex follicular parasite (suspected)
  - Exposure to cold, heat, hot drinks
  - Emotional stress
  - Dysfunction of the GI tract

Genetics

People of Northern European and Celtic background commonly afflicted

RISK FACTORS

- Exposure to cold, heat, hot drinks
- Environmental trigger factors: sun, wind, cold

GENERAL PREVENTION

No preventive measures known

COMMONLY ASSOCIATED CONDITIONS

- Seborrheic dermatitis of scalp and eyelids
- Keratitis with photophobia, lacrimation, visual disturbance
- Corneal lesions
- Blepharitis
- Uveitis

DIAGNOSIS

HISTORY

- Usually have a history of episodic flushing with increases in skin temperature in response to heat stimulus in mouth (hot liquids), spicy foods, alcohol, sun (solar elastosis)
- Acne may have preceded onset of rosacea by years; nevertheless, rosacea usually arises de novo without preceding history of acne or seborrhea.
- Excessive facial warmth and redness are the predominant presenting complaints. Itching is generally absent.

PHYSICAL EXAM

- Rosacea has typical stages of evolution:
  - The rosacea diathesis: episodic erythema, "flushing and blushing"
  - Stage I: persistent erythema with telangiectases
  - Stage II: persistent erythema, telangiectases, papules, tiny pustules
  - Stage III: persistent deep erythema, dense telangiectases, papules, pustules, nodules; rarely persistent "solid" edema of the central part of the face (phymatous)
- Facial erythema, particularly on cheeks, nose, and chin. At times, entire face may be involved.
- Inflammatory papules are prominent; pustules and telangiectasia may be present.
- Comedones are absent (unlike acne).
- Women usually have lesions on the chin and cheeks, whereas nose is commonly involved in men.
- Ocular findings (mild dryness and irritation with blepharitis, conjunctival injection, burning, stinging, tearing, eyelid inflammation, swelling, and redness) are present in 50% of patients.

DIFFERENTIAL DIAGNOSIS

- Drug eruptions (iodides and bromides)
- Granulomas of the skin
- Cutaneous lupus erythematosus
- Carcinoid syndrome
- Deep fungal infection
- Acne vulgaris
- Seborrheic dermatitis
- Steroid rosacea (abuse)
- Systemic lupus erythematosus

DIAGNOSTIC TESTS & INTERPRETATION

Diagnosis is based on physical exam findings.

Test Interpretation

- Inflammation around hypertrophied sebaceous glands, producing papules, pustules, and cysts
- Absence of comedones and blocked ducts
- Vascular dilatation and dermal lymphocytic infiltrate

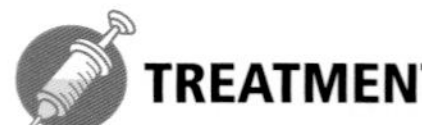

TREATMENT

GENERAL MEASURES

- Proper skin care and photoprotection are important components of management plan (1)[B]. Use of mild, nondrying soap is recommended; local skin irritants should be avoided.
- Reassurance that rosacea is completely unrelated to poor hygiene
- Treat psychological stress if present.
- Avoid oil-based cosmetics:
  - Others are acceptable and may help women tolerate symptoms.
- Electrodesiccation or chemical sclerosis of permanently dilated blood vessels
- Cyclosporine 0.05% ophthalmic emulsion may be more effective than artificial tears for rosacea of the eyes.
- Possible evolving laser therapy
- Support physical fitness.

MEDICATION

First Line

- Topical metronidazole preparations once (1% formulation) or twice (0.75% formulations) daily for 7–12 weeks was significantly more effective than placebo in patients with moderate to severe rosacea. A rosacea treatment system (cleanser, metronidazole 0.75% gel, hydrating complexion corrector, and sunscreen SPF30) may offer superior efficacy and tolerability to metronidazole (2)[A].
- Azelaic acid (Finacea) is very effective as initial therapy; azelaic acid topical alone is effective for maintenance (3)[A].
- Doxycycline 40-mg dose is at least as effective as 100-mg dose and has a correspondingly lower risk of adverse effects but is much more expensive (4)[A].
- Precautions: Tetracyclines may cause photosensitivity; sunscreen is recommended.
- Significant possible interactions:
  - Tetracyclines: Avoid concurrent administration with antacids, dairy products, or iron.
  - Broad-spectrum antibiotics: may reduce the effectiveness of oral contraceptives; barrier method is recommended.

Second Line

- Topical erythromycin
- Topical clindamycin (lotion preferred)
- Possible use of calcineurin inhibitors (tacrolimus 0.1%; pimecrolimus 1%). Pimecrolimus 1% is effective to treat mild to moderate inflammatory rosacea (5)[A].
- Permethrin 5% cream; similar efficacy compared to metronidazole (6)[B]
- Topical steroids should not be used, as they may aggravate rosacea.
- For severe cases, isotretinoin PO for 4 months

Pediatric Considerations

Tetracyclines: not for use in children <8 years

Pregnancy Considerations

- Tetracyclines: not for use during pregnancy
- Isotretinoin: teratogenic; not for use during pregnancy or in women of reproductive age who are not using reliable contraception; requires registration with iPLEDGE program

ADDITIONAL THERAPIES

Surgery/Other Procedures

Laser treatment is an option for progressive telangiectasias or rhinophyma.

ONGOING CARE

FOLLOW-UP RECOMMENDATIONS

Outpatient treatment

Patient Monitoring

- Occasional and as needed
- Close follow-up for women using isotretinoin

DIET

Avoid alcohol, excessive sun exposure, and hot drinks of any type.

PROGNOSIS

- Slowly progressive
- Subsides spontaneously (sometimes)

COMPLICATIONS

- Rhinophyma (dilated follicles and thickened bulbous skin on nose), especially in men
- Conjunctivitis
- Blepharitis
- Keratitis
- Visual deterioration

REFERENCES

1. Del Rosso JQ, Thiboutot D, Gallo R, et al. Consensus recommendations from the American Acne & Rosacea Society on the management of rosacea, part 3: a status report on systemic therapies. *Cutis*. 2014;93(1):18–28.
2. Van Zuuren EJ, Kramer SF, Carter BR, et al. Effective and evidence-based management strategies for rosacea: summary of a Cochrane systematic review. *Br J Dermatol*. 2011;165(4):760–781. doi:10.1111/j.1365-2133.2011.10473.x.
3. Thiboutot DM, Fleischer AB, Del Rosso JQ, et al. A multicenter study of topical azelaic acid 15% gel in combination with oral doxycycline as initial therapy and azelaic acid 15% gel as maintenance monotherapy. *J Drugs Dermatol*. 2009;8(7):639–648.
4. Del Rosso JQ, Webster GF, Jackson M, et al. Two randomized phase III clinical trials evaluating anti-inflammatory dose doxycycline (40-mg doxycycline, USP capsules) administered once daily for treatment of rosacea. *J Am Acad Dermatol*. 2007;56(5):791–802. doi:10.1016/j.jaad.2006.11.021.
5. Kim MB, Kim GW, Park HJ, et al. Pimecrolimus 1% cream for the treatment of rosacea. *J Dermatol*. 2011;38(12):1135–1139. doi:10.1111/j.1346-8138.2011.01223.x.
6. Koçak M, Yağli S, Vahapoğlu G, et al. Permethrin 5% cream versus metronidazole 0.75% gel for the treatment of papulopustular rosacea. A randomized double-blind placebo-controlled study. *Dermatology*. 2002;205(3):265–270.

ADDITIONAL READING

- Leyden JJ. Efficacy of a novel rosacea treatment system: an investigator-blind, randomized, parallel-group study. *J Drugs Dermatol*. 2011;10(10):1179–1185.
- Liu RH, Smith MK, Basta SA, et al. Azelaic acid in the treatment of papulopustular rosacea: a systematic review of randomized controlled trials. *Arch Dermatol*. 2006;142(8):1047–1052.

SEE ALSO

- Acne Vulgaris; Blepharitis; Dermatitis, Seborrheic; Lupus Erythematosus, Discoid; Uveitis
- Algorithm: Acne

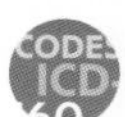

CODES

ICD10

- L71.9 Rosacea, unspecified
- L71.8 Other rosacea

CLINICAL PEARLS

- Rosacea usually arises de novo without any preceding history of acne or seborrhea.
- Rosacea may cause chronic eye symptoms, including blepharitis.
- Avoid alcohol, sun exposure, and hot drinks.
- Medication treatment resembles that of acne vulgaris, with oral and topical antibiotics.

ACNE VULGARIS

Gary I. Levine, MD

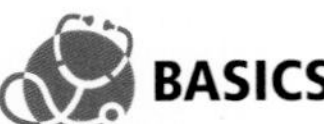

BASICS

DESCRIPTION

- Acne vulgaris is a disorder of the pilosebaceous units. It is a chronic inflammatory dermatosis notable for open/closed comedones, papules, pustules, or nodules.
- Systems affected: skin/exocrine

Geriatric Considerations

Favre-Racouchot syndrome: comedones on face and head due to sun exposure

Pregnancy Considerations

- May result in a flare or remission of acne
- Erythromycin can be used in pregnancy; use topical agents when possible.
- Isotretinoin is teratogenic; pregnancy Category X
- Avoid topical tretinoin as it may cause retinoid embryopathy; class C (1).
- Contraindicated: isotretinoin, tazarotene, tetracycline, doxycycline, minocycline

Pediatric Considerations

- Neonatal acne (neonatal cephalic pustulosis) (2)
  - Newborn to 8 weeks, lesions limited to face, responds to topical ketoconazole 2% cream (3)
- Infantile acne
  - Newborn to 1 year, lesions on face, neck, back, and chest, no Rx required (3)
- Early–mid childhood acne
  - 1–7 years; rare, consider hyperandrogenism (3)
- Preadolescent acne
  - 7–11 years; common, 47% of children, usually due to adrenal awakening
- Do not use tetracycline in those <8 years of age (2,3).

EPIDEMIOLOGY

- Predominant age: early to late puberty, may persist into 4th decade
- Predominant sex
  - Male > female (adolescence)
  - Female > male (adult)

Prevalence

- 80–95% of adolescents affected. A smaller percentage will seek medical advice.
- 8% of adults aged 25–34 years; 3% at 35–44 years

ETIOLOGY AND PATHOPHYSIOLOGY

- Androgens (testosterone and dehydroepiandrosterone sulfate [DHEA-S]) stimulate sebum production and proliferation of keratinocytes in hair follicles (4).
- Keratin plug obstructs follicle os, causing sebum accumulation and follicular distention.
- *Propionibacterium acnes*, an anaerobe, colonizes and proliferates in the plugged follicle.
- *P. acnes* promote chemotactic factors and proinflammatory mediators, causing inflammation of follicle and dermis.

Genetics

- Familial association in 50%
- If a family history exists, the acne may be more severe and occur earlier.

RISK FACTORS

- Increased endogenous androgenic effect
- Oily cosmetics
- Rubbing or occluding skin surface (e.g., sports equipment such as helmets and shoulder pads), telephone, or hands against the skin
- Polyvinyl chloride, chlorinated hydrocarbons, cutting oil, tars
- Numerous drugs, including androgenic steroids (e.g., steroid abuse, some birth control pills)
- Endocrine disorders: polycystic ovarian syndrome, Cushing syndrome, congenital adrenal hyperplasia, androgen-secreting tumors, acromegaly
- Stress
- High glycemic load and possibly high-dairy diets may exacerbate acne (4,5)[B].
- Severe acne may worsen with smoking.

COMMONLY ASSOCIATED CONDITIONS

- Acne fulminans, pyoderma faciale
- Acne conglobata, hidradenitis suppurativa
- Pomade acne
- SAPHO syndrome (synovitis, acne, pustulosis, hyperostosis, and osteitis)
- Acne
- Behçet syndrome, Apert syndrome
- Dark-skinned patients: 50% keloidal scarring and 50% acne hyperpigmented macules

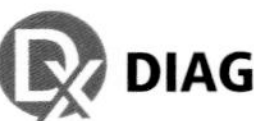

DIAGNOSIS

HISTORY

- Ask about duration, medications, cleansing products, stress, smoking, exposures, diet, and family history.
- Females may worsen 1 week prior to menses.

PHYSICAL EXAM

- Closed comedones (whiteheads)
- Open comedones (blackheads)
- Nodules or papules
- Pustules ("cysts")
- Scars: ice pick, rolling, boxcar, atrophic macules, hypertrophic, depressed, sinus tracts
- Grading system (American Academy of Dermatology, 1990) (4)
  - Mild: few papules/pustules; no nodules
  - Moderate: some papules/pustules; few nodules
  - Severe: numerous papules/pustules; many nodules
  - Very severe: acne conglobata, acne fulminans, acne inversa.
- Most common areas affected are face, chest, back, and upper arms (areas of greatest concentration of sebaceous glands) (4).

DIFFERENTIAL DIAGNOSIS

- Folliculitis: gram negative and gram positive
- Acne (rosacea, cosmetica, steroid-induced)
- Perioral dermatitis
- Chloracne
- Pseudofolliculitis barbae
- Drug eruption
- Verruca vulgaris and plana
- Keratosis pilaris
- Molluscum contagiosum
- Sarcoidosis
- Seborrheic dermatitis
- Miliaria

DIAGNOSTIC TESTS & INTERPRETATION

Initial Tests (lab, imaging)

Only indicated if additional signs of androgen excess; if so: free testosterone, DHEA-S, LH, and FSH (6)

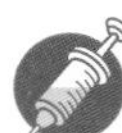

TREATMENT

- Comedonal (grade 1): keratinolytic agent (7)[A] (see as follows for specific agents)
- Mild inflammatory acne (grade 2): benzoyl peroxide ± topical antibiotic + keratinolytic agent
- Moderate inflammatory acne (grade 3): add systemic antibiotic to grade 2 regimen
- Severe inflammatory acne (grade 4): as in grade 3, or isotretinoin (7)[A]
- Topical retinoid plus a topical antimicrobial agent is 1st-line treatment for more than mild disease (8).
- Topical retinoid + antibiotic (topical or PO) is better than either alone for mild/moderate acne (7)[A].
- Topical retinoids are 1st-line agents for maintenance. Avoid long-term antibiotics for maintenance.
- Avoid topical antibiotics as monotherapy.
- Recommended vehicle type
  - Dry or sensitive skin: cream or ointment
  - Oily skin, humid weather: gel, solution, pledget, or wash
  - Hair-bearing areas: lotion, hydrogel, or foam
- Apply topical agents to entire affected area, not just visible lesions.
- Mild soap daily to control oiliness; avoid abrasives
- Avoid drying agents with keratinolytic agents.
- Gentle cleanser and noncomedogenic moisturizer help decrease irritation.
- Oil-free, noncomedogenic sunscreens
- Stress management if acne flares with stress

MEDICATION

ALERT

Most prescription topical medications are expensive. Review cost

- Keratinolytic agents (alpha-hydroxy acids, salicylic acid, azelaic acid) (side effects include dryness, erythema, and scaling; start with lower strength; increase as tolerated) (6,7)[A].
- Tretinoin (Retin-A, Retin A Micro, Avita), varying strengths and formulations: apply at bedtime; wash skin and let skin dry 30 minutes before topical application
  - Retin-A Micro and Avita are less irritating; produce less phototoxicity
  - May cause an initial flare of lesions; may be eased by 14-day course of oral antibiotics
  - Avoid in pregnant and lactating women.
- Adapalene (Differin): 0.1%, apply topically at night
  - Effective; less irritation than tretinoin or tazarotene (7)[A]
  - May be combined with benzoyl peroxide
- Tazarotene (Tazorac): apply at bedtime
  - Most effective and most irritating; teratogenic
- Azelaic acid (Azelex, Finevin): 20% topically, BID
  - Keratinolytic, antibacterial, anti-inflammatory
  - Reduces postinflammatory hyperpigmentation in dark-skinned individuals
  - Side effects: erythema, dryness, scaling, hypopigmentation
  - Less effective in clinical use than in studies
- Salicylic acid: 2%, less effective and less irritating than tretinoin
- Alpha-hydroxy acids: available over-the-counter

- Topical antibiotics and anti-inflammatories
  - Topical benzoyl peroxide (6,7)[A]
    - 2.5% as effective as stronger preparations
    - Gel penetrates better into follicles.
    - When used with tretinoin, apply benzoyl peroxide in morning and tretinoin at night.
    - Side effects: irritation; may bleach clothes; photosensitivity
- Topical antibiotics (6,7)[A]
  - Erythromycin 2%
  - Clindamycin 1%
  - Metronidazole gel or cream: apply once daily
  - Azelaic acid (Azelex, Finevin): 20% cream: enhanced effect and decreased risk of resistance when used with zinc and benzoyl peroxide
  - Benzoyl peroxide-erythromycin (Benzamycin): especially effective with azelaic acid
  - Benzoyl peroxide-clindamycin (BenzaClin, DUAC, Clindoxyl)
  - Benzoyl peroxide-salicylic acid (Cleanse & Treat, Inova): similar in effectiveness to benzoyl peroxide-clindamycin
  - Sodium sulfacetamide (Sulfacet-R, Novacet, Klaron): useful in acne with seborrheic dermatitis or rosacea
  - Dapsone (Aczone) 5% gel: may cause yellow/orange skin discoloration when mixed with benzoyl peroxide
- Oral antibiotics: use for at least 6–8 weeks after initiation, discontinue after 12–18 weeks' duration; indicated when acne is more severe, trunk involvement, unresponsive to topical agents, or at greater risk for scarring (6,7,9)[A]
  - Tetracycline: 500–1,000 mg/day divided BID; high dose initially, taper in 6 months. Side effects: photosensitivity, esophagitis
  - Minocycline: 100–200 mg/day, divided daily–BID; side effects include photosensitivity, urticaria, gray-blue skin, vertigo, hepatitis
  - Doxycycline: 50–200 mg/day, divided daily—BID; side effects include photosensitivity
  - Erythromycin: 500–1,000 mg/day; divided BID–QID; decreasing effectiveness as a result of increasing *P. acnes* resistance
  - Trimethoprim-sulfamethoxazole (Bactrim DS, Septra DS): 1 daily or BID
  - Azithromycin (Zithromax): 500 mg 3 days/week × 1 month, then 250 mg every other day × 2 months
- Oral retinoids
  - Isotretinoin: 0.5–1 mg/kg/day divided BID to maximum 2 mg/kg/day divided BID for very severe disease; 60–90% cure rate; usually given for 12–20 weeks; maximum cumulative dose = 120–150 mg/kg; 20% of patients relapse and require retreatment (4,6,7)[A]
    - Side effects: teratogenic, pancreatitis, excessive drying of skin, hypertriglyceridemia, hepatitis, blood dyscrasias, hyperostosis, premature epiphyseal closure, night blindness, erythema multiforme, Stevens-Johnson syndrome, suicidal ideation, psychosis
    - Avoid tetracyclines or vitamin A preparations during isotretinoin therapy.
    - Monitor for pregnancy, psychiatric/mood changes, CBC, lipids, glucose, and liver function tests at baseline and every month.
    - Must be registered and adhere to manufacturer's iPLEDGE program (www.ipledgeprogram.com)
- Medications for women only
  - Oral contraceptives (4,6,7)[A],(10)
    - Norgestimate/ethinyl estradiol (OrthoTricyclen), norethindrone acetate/ethinyl estradiol (Estrostep), drospirenone/ethinyl estradiol (Yaz, Yasmin) are approved by USFDA for this indication.
    - Levonorgestrel/ethinyl estradiol (Alesse) and most combined contraceptives effective.
- Spironolactone (Aldactone); 25–200 mg/day; antiandrogen; reduces sebum production

ISSUES FOR REFERRAL

Consider referral/consultation to dermatologist:

- Refractory lesions despite appropriate therapy
- Consideration of isotretinoin therapy
- Management of acne scars

ADDITIONAL THERAPIES

- Acne hyperpigmented macules (11)
  - Topical hydroquinones (1.5–10%)
  - Azelaic acid (20%) topically
  - Topical retinoids
  - Corticosteroids: low dose, suppresses adrenal androgens (6)[B]
  - Dapsone 5% gel (Aczone): topical, anti-inflammatory use in patients older than 12 years of age
- Light-based treatments
  - Ultraviolet A/ultraviolet B (UVA/UVB), blue or blue/red light, pulse dye laser, KTP laser, infrared laser
  - Photodynamic therapy for 30–60 minutes with 5-aminolevulinic acid × 3 sessions is effective for inflammatory lesions.
    - Greatest use when used as adjunct to medications or if can't tolerate medications

SURGERY/OTHER PROCEDURES

- Comedo extraction after incising the layer of epithelium over closed comedo (6)[C]
- Inject large cystic lesions with 0.05–0.3 mL triamcinolone (Kenalog 2–5 mg/mL); use 30-gauge needle to inject and slightly distend cyst (6)[C].
- Acne scar treatment: retinoids, steroid injections, cryosurgery, electrodessication, micro/dermabrasion, chemical peels, laser resurfacing

COMPLEMENTARY & ALTERNATIVE MEDICINE

- Topical tea tree oil is effective but slow onset (6)[B].
- Nicotinamide 4% gel (Nicam): as effective as clindamycin in moderate inflammatory acne

ONGOING CARE

FOLLOW-UP RECOMMENDATIONS

Use oral or topical antibiotics for 3 months; taper as inflammatory lesions resolve. Do not use topical and oral antibiotic together.

Patient Monitoring

- Pretreatment and monthly lipids, psychiatric/mood changes, glucose, liver function tests, and pregnancy tests when on isotretinoin
- Consider antibiotic resistance (60% overall) or gram-negative folliculitis if treatment fails.

DIET

Special diets do not diminish acne (5,6)[B].

PATIENT EDUCATION

- There may be a worsening of acne during first 2 weeks of treatment.
- Results are typically seen after a minimum of 4 weeks of treatment

PROGNOSIS

Gradual improvement over time (usually within 8–12 weeks after beginning therapy)

COMPLICATIONS

- Acne conglobata: severe confluent inflammatory acne with systemic symptoms
- Facial scarring and psychological distress, including anxiety and depression (4)

REFERENCES

1. Pugashetti R, Shinkai K. Treatment of acne vulgaris in pregnant patients. *Dermatol Ther*. 2013;26(4):302–311.
2. Friedlander SF, Baldwin HE, Mancini AJ, et al. The acne continuum: an age-based approach to therapy. *Semin Cutan Med Surg*. 2011;30(3)(Suppl):S6–S11.
3. Admani S, Barrio V. Evaluation and treatment of acne from infancy to preadolescence. *Dermatol Ther*. 2013;26(6):462–466.
4. Dawson AL, Dellavalle RP. Acne vulgaris. *BMJ*. 2013;346:f2634.
5. Burris J, Rietkerk W, Woolf K. Acne: the role of medical nutrition therapy. *J Acad Nutr Diet*. 2013;113(3):416–430.
6. Strauss JS, Krowchuk DP, Leyden JJ, et al. Guidelines of care for acne vulgaris management. *J Am Acad Dermatol*. 2007;56(4):651–663.
7. Feldman S, Careccia RE, Barham KL, et al. Diagnosis and treatment of acne. *Am Fam Physician*. 2004;69(9):2123–2130.
8. Thiboutot D, Gollnick H, Bettoli V, et al. New insights into the management of acne: an update from the global alliance to improve outcomes in acne group. *J Am Acad Dermatol*. 2009;60(5)(Suppl):S1–S50.
9. Del Rosso JQ, Kim G. Optimizing use of oral antibiotics in acne vulgaris. *Dermatol Clin*. 2009;27(1):33–42.
10. Heymann WR. Oral contraceptives for the treatment of acne vulgaris. *J Am Acad Dermatol*. 2007;56(6):1056–1057.
11. Woolery-Lloyd HC, Keri J, Doig S. Retinoids and azelaic acid to treat acne and hyperpigmentation in skin of color. *J Drugs Dermatol*. 2013;12(4):434–437.

ADDITIONAL READING

- Bhate K, Williams HC. Epidemiology of acne vulgaris. *Br J Dermatol*. 2012;168(3):474–485.
- Titus S, Hodge J. Diagnosis and treatment of acne. *Am Fam Physician*. 2012;86(8):734–740.
- Williams HC, Dellavalle RP, Garner S. Acne vulgaris. *Lancet*. 2012;379(9813):361–372.

SEE ALSO

- Acne Rosacea
- Algorithm: Acne

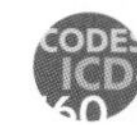

CODES

ICD10

- L70.0 Acne vulgaris
- L70.4 Infantile acne
- L70.1 Acne conglobata

CLINICAL PEARLS

- Expect worsening for the first 2 weeks of treatment. Full results for changes in therapy take 8–12 weeks.
- Decrease topical frequency from BID to every day or to every other day for irritation.

ACOUSTIC NEUROMA

Jason Cohn, DO, MS • Kelli Quercetti, DO • Mahmoud Ghaderi, DO

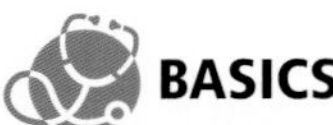

BASICS

DESCRIPTION
- Acoustic neuromas (vestibular schwannomas) are slow-growing, benign intracranial, extra-axial tumors originating from the vestibulocochlear nerve:
  - Originate from Schwann cells of the nerve sheath
  - Usually arise in the internal auditory canal near the cerebellopontine angle
  - Most are unilateral; bilateral seen in neurofibromatosis type 2.
- Patients commonly present with hearing loss, tinnitus, and disequilibrium. Rarely associated facial paralysis, brain stem compression, and even death

EPIDEMIOLOGY
- 6–10% of all intracranial tumors
- 80–90% of cerebellopontine angle tumors
- 95% of cases are unilateral.
- Present most commonly in the 5th–6th decades
- Female predominance
- 5% of acoustic neuromas are a result of neurofibromatosis 2.
- Bilateral acoustic neuroma occurring in neurofibromatosis 2 present before age 30 years.

Incidence
- 1/100,000 per year
- Asymptomatic lesions may be more common.

Prevalence
3,000 diagnosed annually in the United States

ETIOLOGY AND PATHOPHYSIOLOGY
- Compression of acoustic and facial nerve when located within internal acoustic canal
- Compression of brain stem, 4th ventricle, and trigeminal nerve when tumor is at the cerebellopontine angle
- Vestibular schwannomas are related to the NF2 gene and its product merlin. Merlin acts as a tumor suppressor and as a mediator of contact inhibition. Thus, deficiencies in both NF2 genes lead to vestibular schwannoma development.

Genetics
- Unknown for unilateral acoustic neuroma
- Neurofibromatosis type 2: bilateral acoustic neuromas
  - Autosomal dominant
  - Gene located on chromosome 22q1.

RISK FACTORS
- High-dose ionizing radiation
- Pregnancy and epilepsy may increase risk.
- 1 study demonstrated that smoking cigarettes may decrease the risk. However, this reduced risk was not observed in a subsequent study involving subjects receiving nicotine only in the form of snuff. Therefore, this protective mechanism may be due to tobacco or other ingredients found in cigarettes rather than nicotine.
- No proven increase in risk of acoustic neuroma with regular use of a mobile phone.

COMMONLY ASSOCIATED CONDITIONS
- Neurofibromatosis type 2
- Pregnancy may accelerate the growth of the tumor.

DIAGNOSIS

HISTORY
- Common
  - Sensorineural hearing loss (unilateral), often progressive
  - Loss of speech discrimination
  - Tinnitus
  - Disequilibrium is common, but vertigo is less common.
- Less common
  - Weakness/loss of facial muscle functions
  - Headache with hydrocephalus and increased intracranial pressure
  - Trigeminal nerve dysfunction when tumor is large and compressing on cranial nerve 5 (CN V)
  - Ataxia due to cerebellar or brain stem compression from large tumor

PHYSICAL EXAM
- Exclude other causes of hearing loss (e.g., middle-ear effusion, infection, cerumen (wax), cholesteatoma, or tympanic membrane perforation) with otoscopic exam.
- Neurologic exam of cranial nerves
- Weber and Rinne tests to screen for sensorineural hearing loss versus conductive hearing loss
- Contralateral ear exam in patients <30 years; suspect neurofibromatosis type 2 (at risk for bilateral hearing loss).

DIFFERENTIAL DIAGNOSIS
- Cerebellopontine lesions
  - Meningioma
  - Glioma
  - Facial nerve schwannoma
  - Epidermoid cyst
  - Hemangioma
  - Arachnoid cyst
- Sensorineural hearing loss
  - Presbycusis (age-related)
  - Ménière disease
  - Ototoxicity (medications or excessive noise exposure)
  - Viral illness (i.e., labyrinthitis)
  - Autoimmune disease
  - Congenital
  - Cerebellar pathology

DIAGNOSTIC TESTS & INTERPRETATION

Initial Tests (lab, imaging)
- MRI with gadolinium (gold standard)
  - 100% specificity. Detects tumors starting at 2 mm
- Noncontrast T2 weighted fast spin-echo MRI
  - 98% specificity. Less expensive than MRI with gadolinium
  - CT scan detects tumors as small as 1 cm. Up to 37% false-negative findings. Provides good information about surrounding bony structures of the tumor

Diagnostic Procedures/Other
- Pure tone and speech audiometry (asymmetric, high-frequency sensorineural hearing loss)
- Speech discrimination
- Stacked auditory brain stem response (ABR): 95% sensitivity and 88% specificity. Can detect tumors <1 cm
- Standard ABR: can only detect tumors >1 cm
- Distortion-product otoacoustic emission tests can differentiate cochlear schwannomas from vestibular schwannomas. Retrocochlear hearing loss correlates more with cochlear schwannomas (1)[C].

Test Interpretation
- Well-demarcated and encapsulated mass attached to neural structures without direct invasion
- The mass may be dense or cystic.
- Diagnostic microscopy: densely packed spindle cells (Schwann cells) mixed in with myxoid and collagenous matrix
  - Zones of alternatively dense and sparse areas of Antoni type A and B patterns of tissue
  - Palisading nuclei (Verocay bodies)
  - S-100 antibody immunoreactivity

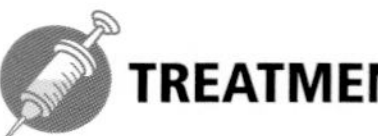

TREATMENT

GENERAL MEASURES
- Treatment options include observation, stereotactic radiosurgery, fractionated radiotherapy, and microsurgery.
- Without intervention, 16–26% of patients require additional treatment, with 54–63% preserving functional hearing.
- With radiosurgery, only 2–4% of patients require additional treatment and hearing preservation is accomplished in 44–66%.
- With fractionated radiotherapy, 3–7% of patients will require additional treatment; hearing preservation is reported at 59–94% of patients, although long-term outcomes are not known.
- Up to 57% of acoustic neuromas may not grow or shrink without treatment.
- Up to 70% of extracanalicular tumors may never have a growth rate exceeding 2 mm per year.

Pediatric Consideration
Acoustic neuromas in children typically grow at slower rates compared to adults; this affects treatment outcomes. For example, gamma knife surgery had a 35.3% tumor control rate at 3 years. In addition, useful hearing preservation was 67% and 53% at 1 and 5 years after gamma knife surgery, respectively (2)[B].

MEDICATION
A greater understanding of molecular tumorigenesis has yielded novel therapies. Reduced morbidity and mortality by decreasing tumor burden, tumor volume, hearing loss, and cranial nerve deficits. Suggested therapies
- Bevacizumab induces regression of progressive schwannomas by >40% and improves hearing.
- An inhibitor of VEGF synthesis, PTC299, is currently in phase II trials as a potential agent to treat vestibular schwannoma.
- In vitro studies have shown that trastuzumab (an ErbB2 inhibitor) reduces vestibular schwannoma cell proliferation.

ISSUES FOR REFERRAL

If an asymptomatic tumor becomes symptomatic, intervention is indicated.

ADDITIONAL THERAPIES

Geriatric Considerations

Conservative management is suitable for elderly patients with contraindications to surgery and radiotherapy:

- Conservative therapy is more likely to preserve hearing than radiotherapy or surgery.
- Of patients, 69% with 100% speech discrimination at diagnosis have maintained good hearing, even after 10 years of observation.
- Stereotactic radiosurgery
  - Gamma knife single-dose stereotactic radiosurgery
    - Performed on an outpatient basis
    - Alternative for those with smaller tumor (<3 cm) or contraindications to microsurgery
    - Shown to have better tumor control rates than conservative management
    - Lower dose radiation has fewer complications but unclear whether this is as effective as high-dose radiation in tumor control.
    - Higher dose radiation significantly influences hearing preservation rates.
    - Complications (radiation damage): trigeminal, and/or facial nerve neuropathy, hydrocephalus
  - Fractionated stereotactic radiosurgery
    - Conformal radiation delivers a higher dose of radiation within the tumor and less damage to surrounding healthy tissue.
    - Required multiple treatments and total radiation dose is higher than single-dose radiation.
    - Suitable for all sizes of tumor

SURGERY/OTHER PROCEDURES

- Surgery is recommended definitive treatment.
- Lowest rate of recurrence, with up to 97.5% complete tumor removal
- 3 standard operating microscope approaches
  - Retromastoid/retrosigmoid: can be used for all acoustic tumors, especially tumors located mostly outside the internal auditory canal and adjacent to the brain stem. May require retraction of cerebellum
  - Middle cranial fossa: for small tumors with aim of preserving hearing. Involves retraction of temporal lobe and has higher risk of facial nerve injury
  - Translabyrinthine: for larger tumors. Hearing not preserved. Completely exposes the distal internal auditory canal and has more favorable facial nerve results. A fat graft must be used, with chance of complications, such as infections and bleeding.
  - Transpetrous approaches are safe for acoustic neuroma removal, and the postoperative complication rate is low.
  - The retrolabyrinthine approach seems to be a good hearing preservative approach, regardless of tumor volume.

- In 1 study, 79.1% of surgeries involved a translabyrinthine approach, with the remainder being combined retrosigmoid and transtemporal (10.4%), middle fossa (6.0%) and stereotactic radiosurgery (4.5%). The highest complication rate was seen in the combined retrosigmoid and transtemporal approach cohort (3)[B].

ONGOING CARE

FOLLOW-UP RECOMMENDATIONS

- Yearly MRI follow-up for slow-growing tumors is advised.
- MRI and audiometric follow-up for those treated by surgical excision, radiotherapy, and conservative management.

- In 1 study, composite quality of life (cQOL) score 0–5 years out of surgery was significantly highest among patients receiving stereotactic radiosurgery compared to those either having microsurgery or those being observed over time. However, after 5 years these differences were not seen (4)[B].

Patient Monitoring

- Preoperative practice of physical activity promotes the neuroplasticity of neural networks involved in motor learning, which allows benefit of physical therapy more rapidly and efficiently.
- Physical activity allows the implementation of new sensorimotor and behavioral strategies leading to an improvement of balance control.

COMPLICATIONS

- Mass effects: cranial nerve compression, hydrocephalus, brain stem compression, cerebellar tonsil herniation
- Surgical complications: hearing loss, CSF leakage, facial nerve injury, headaches, meningitis

- In 1 study, 22.4% of patients experienced postoperative complications; most commonly facial weakness (13.4%), CSF leak (6.0%), and infection (3.0%) (3)[B].
- In a larger study, 28.2% of patients experienced complications; most commonly nervous system complications not elsewhere specified (15.2%) and facial paralysis (8.7%). Other complications included hydrocephalus, CSF leak, dysphagia, among others (5)[A].

REFERENCES

1. Kagoya R, Shinogami M, Kohno M, et al. Distortion-product otoacoustic emission tests evaluate cochlear function and differentiate cochlear and vestibular schwannoma. *Otolaryngol Head Neck Surg*. 2013;148(2):267–271.
2. Choi JW, Lee JY, Phi JH, et al. Clinical course of vestibular schwannoma in pediatric neurofibromatosis Type 2. *J Neurosurg Pediatr*. 2014;13(6):650–657.
3. Olshan M, Srinivasan VM, Landrum T, et al. Acoustic neuroma: an investigation of associations between tumor size and diagnostic delays, facial weakness, and surgical complications. *Ear Nose Throat J*. 2014;93(8):304–316.
4. Robinett ZN, Walz PC, Miles-Markley B, et al. Comparison of long-term quality-of-life outcomes in vestibular schwannoma patients. *Otolaryngol Head Neck Surg*. 2014;150(6):1024–1032.
5. Mahboubi H, Ahmed OH, Yau AY, et al. Complications of surgery for sporadic vestibular schwannoma. *Otolaryngol Head Neck Surg*. 2014;150(2):275–281.

ADDITIONAL READING

- Arthurs BJ, Fairbanks RK, Demakas JJ, et al. A review of treatment modalities for vestibular schwannoma. *Neurosurg Rev*. 2011;34(3):265–277; discussion 277–279.
- Combs SE, Welzel T, Schulz-Ertner D, et al. Differences in clinical results after LINAC-based single-dose radiosurgery versus fractionated stereotactic radiotherapy for patients with vestibular schwannomas. *Int J Radiat Oncol Biol Phys*. 2010;76(1):193–200.
- Fong B, Barkhoudarian G, Pezeshkian P, et al. The molecular biology and novel treatments of vestibular schwannomas. *J Neurosurg*. 2011;115(5):906–914.
- Gauchard GC, Parietti-Winkler C, Lion A, et al. Impact of pre-operative regular physical activity on balance control compensation after vestibular schwannoma surgery. *Gait Posture*. 2013;37(1):82–87.
- INTERPHONE Study Group. Acoustic neuroma risk in relation to mobile telephone use: results of the INTERPHONE international case-control study. *Cancer Epidemiol*. 2011;35(5):453–464.
- Maniakas A, Saliba I. Conservative management versus stereotactic radiation for vestibular schwannomas: a meta-analysis of patients with more than 5 years' follow-up. *Otol Neurotol*. 2012;33(2):230–238.
- Palmisano S, Schwartzbaum J, Prochazka M, et al. Role of tobacco use in the etiology of acoustic neuroma. *Am J Epidemiol*. 2012;175(12):1243–1251.
- Repacholi MH, Lerchl A, Röösli M, et al. Systematic review of wireless phone use and brain cancer and other head tumors. *Bioelectromagnetics*. 2012;33(3):187–206.
- Smouha EE, Yoo M, Mohr K, et al. Conservative management of acoustic neuroma: a meta-analysis and proposed treatment algorithm. *Laryngoscope*. 2005;115(3):450–454.
- Stangerup SE, Caye-Thomasen P, Tos M, et al. The natural history of vestibular schwannoma. *Otol Neurotol*. 2006;27(4):547–552.
- Stangerup SE, Thomsen J, Tos M, et al. Long-term hearing preservation in vestibular schwannoma. *Otol Neurotol*. 2010;31(2):271–275.

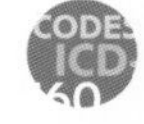

CODES

ICD10

D33.3 Benign neoplasm of cranial nerves

CLINICAL PEARLS

- The most common presenting signs and symptoms are unilateral sensorineural hearing loss, poor speech discrimination, and tinnitus.
- MRI with gadolinium is the diagnostic gold standard.
- Neurofibromatosis type 2 should ruled out in patients presenting with bilateral acoustic neuromas.
- The commonly used treatment options include observation, stereotactic radiosurgery, fractionated radiotherapy, and microsurgery.

ACUTE CORONARY SYNDROMES: STEMI

Tarina Desai, MD • Fozia Akhtar Ali, MD

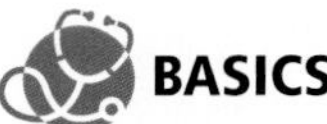

BASICS

DESCRIPTION

Acute myocardial infarction (AMI) is the rapid development of myocardial necrosis resulting from a sustained and complete absence of blood flow to a portion of the myocardium. ST-segment elevation myocardial infarction (STEMI) occurs when coronary blood flow ceases following thrombotic occlusion of a large coronary artery (usually) affected by atherosclerosis, causing transmural ischemia. This is accompanied by release of serum cardiac biomarkers and ST elevation (and likely a Q wave when infarction occurs) on an ECG.

EPIDEMIOLOGY

Incidence

In the United States, estimated annual incidence of MI is 600,000 new and 320,000 recurrent attacks. In 2009, ~683,000 patients were discharged from U.S. hospitals diagnosed with acute coronary syndromes (ACS).

Prevalence

- Leading cause of morbidity and mortality in the United States
- ~7.5 million people in the United States are affected by MI.
- Prevalence increases with age and is higher in men (5.5%) than in women (2.9%).

ETIOLOGY AND PATHOPHYSIOLOGY

- Atherosclerotic coronary artery disease (CAD)
- Nonatherosclerotic
  - Emboli: for example, thrombi from left ventricle or atrium
  - Mechanical obstruction: chest trauma, dissection of aorta or coronary arteries
  - Increased vasomotor tone, variant angina
  - Arteritis, others: hematologic (disseminated intravascular coagulation [DIC]), aortic stenosis, cocaine, IV drug use, severe burns, prolonged hypotension
- Atherosclerotic lesions may be smooth and concentric or rough, eccentric, and fissured. Plaques that are rough and eccentric are more unstable, thrombogenic, and prone to rupture.

RISK FACTORS

Advancing age, hypertension, tobacco use, diabetes mellitus, dyslipidemia, family history of premature onset of CAD, sedentary lifestyle

GENERAL PREVENTION

Smoking cessation, healthy diet, weight control, regular physical activity, maintain goal BP

COMMONLY ASSOCIATED CONDITIONS

Abdominal aortic aneurysm, extracranial cerebrovascular disease, atherosclerotic peripheral vascular disease

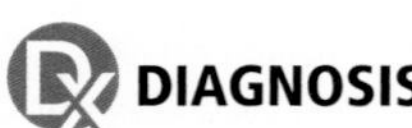

DIAGNOSIS

HISTORY

- Classically, sudden-onset of chest heaviness/tightness, with or without exertion, lasting at least minutes
- Pain/discomfort radiating to neck, jaw, interscapular area, upper extremities, and epigastrium
- Previous history of myocardial ischemia (stable or unstable angina, MI, coronary bypass surgery, or percutaneous coronary intervention [PCI])
- Assess risk factors for CAD, history of bleeding, noncardiac surgery, family history of premature CAD.
- Medications: Ask if recent use of phosphodiesterase-5 inhibitors (If recent use, avoid concomitant nitrates.)
- Alcohol and drug abuse (especially cocaine)

PHYSICAL EXAM

- General: restless, agitated, hypothermia, fever
- Neurologic: dizziness, syncope, fatigue, asthenia, disorientation (especially in the elderly)
- Cerebrovascular (CV): dysrhythmia, hypotension, widened pulse pressure, S_3 and S_4, jugular venous distention (JVD)
- Respiratory: dyspnea, tachypnea, crackles
- GI: abdominal pain, nausea, vomiting
- Musculoskeletal: pain in neck, back, shoulder, or upper limbs
- Skin: cool skin, pallor, diaphoresis

Geriatric Considerations

Elderly patients may have an atypical presentation, including silent or unrecognized MI, often with complaints of syncope, weakness, shortness of breath, unexplained nausea, epigastric pain, altered mental status, delirium. Patients with diabetes mellitus may have fewer and less dramatic chest symptoms.

DIFFERENTIAL DIAGNOSIS

Unstable angina, aortic dissection, pulmonary embolism (PE), perforating ulcer, pericarditis, dysrhythmias, gastroesophageal reflux disease (GERD) and spasm, biliary/pancreatic pain, hyperventilation syndrome

DIAGNOSTIC TESTS & INTERPRETATION

ALERT

The third universal definition for MI issued in 2012 by the American College of Cardiology, American Heart Association, European Society of Cardiology, and World Heart Federation revises older definitions of MI. It establishes the level of troponin necessary to diagnose MI in various clinical situations (e.g., after cardiac and noncardiac procedures). According to the definition, an MI diagnosis requires a cardiac troponin (I or T) level above the 99th percentile of a normal reference population, plus one or more of the following:

- Symptoms of ischemia
- New significant ST-/T-wave changes or left bundle branch block
- Pathologic Q waves on ECG
- New loss of viable myocardium or regional wall motion abnormality, as observed on imaging
- Intracoronary thrombus diagnosed by angiography or autopsy

Initial Tests (lab, imaging)

- Coronary angiography
- 12-lead ECG: ST-segment elevation in a regional pattern ≥1 mm ST elevation, ± abnormal Q waves. ST depression ± tall R wave in V_1/V_2 may be STEMI of posterior wall. Absence of Q waves represents partial or transient occlusion or early infarction. New ST- or T-wave changes indicative of myocardial ischemia or injury. Consider right-sided and posterior chest leads if inferior MI pattern (examine V_3R, V_4R, V_7–V_9).
- ECG with continuous monitoring
  - 2D and M-mode echocardiography is useful in evaluating regional wall motion in MI and left ventricular function.
  - Portable echo can clarify diagnosis of STEMI if concomitant left bundle branch block (LBBB).
  - Useful in assessing mechanical complications and mural thrombus

Follow-Up Tests & Special Considerations

- Serum biomarkers:
  - Troponin I and T (cTnI, cTnT) rise 3–6 hours after onset of ischemic symptoms.
  - Elevations in cTnI persist for 7–10 days, whereas those in cTnT persist for 10–14 days after MI.
  - Myoglobin fraction of creatine kinase (CK-MB): rises 3–4 hours after onset of myocardial injury; peaks at 12–24 hours and remains elevated for 2–3 days; CK-MB adds little diagnostic value in assessment of possible ACS to troponin testing.
  - Myoglobin: early marker for myocardial necrosis; rises 2 hours after onset of myocardial necrosis, reaches peak at 1–4 hours, and remains elevated for 24 hours; myoglobin adds little diagnostic value in assessment of possible ACS to troponin testing.
- Fasting lipid profile, CBC with platelets, electrolytes, magnesium, BUN, serum creatinine, and glucose; international normalized ratio (INR) if anticoagulation contemplated; brain natriuretic peptide (BNP) is elevated in acute MI; may or may not indicate heart failure

Pregnancy Considerations

Findings mimicking acute MI in pregnancy: ST-segment depression after anesthesia, increase in CK-MB after delivery, and mild increase in troponin I levels in preeclampsia and gestational hypertension

Diagnostic Procedures/Other

High-quality portable chest x-ray; transthoracic and/or transesophageal echocardiography, contrast chest CT scan or MRI may occasionally be of value acutely. Coronary angiography is definitive test.

ALERT

Isosmolar contrast medium or low-molecular-weight contrast medium other than ioxaglate or iohexol is indicated in patients with chronic kidney disease undergoing angiography who are not having chronic dialysis.

Test Interpretation

Myocardial necrosis and atherosclerosis, if etiologic

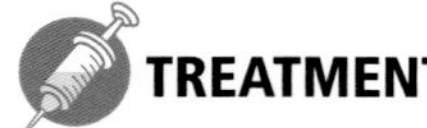

TREATMENT

GENERAL MEASURES

- Admit to telemetry/coronary care unit (CCU) with continuous ECG monitoring and bed rest. anxiolytics, if needed; stool softeners
- Antiarrhythmics, as needed, for unstable dysrhythmia; deep vein thrombosis (DVT) prophylaxis
- Continuation of aspirin and clopidogrel or prasugrel or ticagrelor, BB, ACE inhibitors (or ARB if ACE-intolerant), lipid-lowering therapy, tight BP control, progressively increased physical activity, smoking cessation, annual influenza vaccine
- Elicit symptoms or signs of depression, and treat with an SSRI or psychotherapy if present.

MEDICATION

Medication recommendations based on 2009 ACC/AHA (1) focused guideline updates [A] and [B] level recommendations and 2012 ESC STEMI guidelines (2)[A,B]

First Line

- Supplemental oxygen 2–4 L/min for patients with arterial oxygen saturation <90% or respiratory distress
- Nitroglycerin (NTG) sublingual 0.4 mg q5min for total of 3 doses, followed by nitroglycerin IV if ongoing pain and/or hypertension and/or management of pulmonary congestion if no contraindications exist (systolic <90 mm Hg or 30 mm Hg below baseline, right ventricle (RV) infarct, use of sildenafil within 24 hours or within 48 hours of tadalafil)
- Morphine sulfate 2–4 mg IV with increments of 2–8 mg IV repeated at 5–15-minute intervals to relieve pain or pulmonary congestion
- Antiplatelet agents:
  - Aspirin (ASA), non–enteric-coated, initial dose 162–325 mg chewed (1)[A]
  - A loading dose of a thienopyridine is recommended for patients with STEMI for whom PCI is planned.
    - 600 mg of clopidogrel should be given as early as possible before or at the time of primary or nonprimary PCI.
    - Prasugrel 60 mg should be given as soon as possible for primary PCI. Do not use in patients likely to undergo coronary artery bypass graft (CABG) or with active bleeding, history of transient ischemic attack (TIA) or stroke, or additional risk factors for bleeding (body weight <60 kg or concomitant use of medications that increase risk of bleeding). (Generally, not recommended for patients age ≥75 years.)
    - Ticagrelor 180 mg loading dose
    - Duration of therapy with a thienopyridine varies. At least 12 months for patients receiving drug-eluting stent (DES) during PCI for ACS and up to 12 months for patients receiving bare-metal stent (BMS). Consider earlier discontinuation if risk of morbidity due to bleeding outweighs the benefits of therapy. May continue clopidogrel or prasugrel or ticagrelor for longer than 15 months in patients undergoing DES placement. Discontinue clopidogrel for at least 5 days or prasugrel at least 7 days prior to planned CABG.
  - For patients with STEMI undergoing nonprimary PCI:
    - Continue clopidogrel in a patient who has received fibrinolytic therapy and has been given clopidogrel.
    - Administer loading dose of clopidogrel 600 mg if patient received a fibrinolytic without a thienopyridine or ticagrelor 180 mg or once the coronary anatomy is known and PCI is planned, administer a loading dose of prasugrel as soon as possible but not later than 1 hour after PCI. Administer loading dose of clopidogrel 300 mg in patients <75 years of age who received fibrinolytic therapy or who did not receive reperfusion therapy.
    - Clopidogrel 75 mg should be given with aspirin in patients with STEMI regardless of reperfusion therapy.
- β-Blocker (BB) within 24 hours, if no contraindications exist (signs of congestive heart failure [CHF], low output state)
- Glycoprotein IIb/IIIa receptor antagonists at time of primary PCI in selected patients: abciximab, eptifibatide, or tirofiban
- ACE inhibitors should be initiated orally within 24 hours of STEMI in patients with anterior infarction, HF, or ejection fraction (EF≤0.40) unless contraindicated.

PCI versus fibrinolysis: Goal is to keep total ischemic time within 120 minutes. Door to needle time should be within 30 minutes or door to balloon time within 90 minutes.

- Coronary reperfusion therapy
  - Primary PCI
    - Symptom onset of ≤12 hours
    - Symptom onset of ≤12 hours and contraindication to fibrinolytic therapy irrespective of time delay
    - Cardiogenic shock or acute severe HF irrespective of time delay from onset of MI
    - Evidence of ongoing ischemia 12–24 hours after symptom onset
    - If substantial risk for intracranial hemorrhage (ICH)
    - Age <75 years with STEMI or LBBB who develop shock within 36 hours of AMI
- Fibrinolysis
  - If EMS has fibrinolytic capability and the patient qualifies for therapy, prehospital fibrinolysis should be started within 30 minutes of EMS arrival on scene.
  - If presenting at a hospital without PCI capability and cannot be transferred to a PCI-capable facility to undergo PCI within 90 minutes of first medical contact
  - If no contraindications, administer within 12 hours, but not beyond 24 hours, of onset of symptoms to patients with STEMI in ≥2 contiguous leads and/or new or presumably new left bundle branch block (LBBB).
    - Alteplase (rt-PA): 15-mg IV bolus, followed by 0.75 mg/kg (up to 50 mg) IV over 30 minutes, then 0.5 mg/kg (up to 35 mg) over 60 minutes; maximum 100 mg over 90 minutes
    - Reteplase (r-PA): 10 units IV bolus over 2 minutes, give 2nd bolus 30 minutes later.
    - Tenecteplase (TNK-tPA): 30–50 mg (based on weight) IV bolus over 5–10 seconds
  - Combination reperfusion with abciximab and half-dose r-PA or TNK-tPA
  - Use anticoagulants (unfractionated heparin [UFH], enoxaparin, or fondaparinux) as ancillary therapy to reperfusion therapy for minimum 48 hours and duration of admission (up to 8 days). Avoid UFH if >48 hours of anticoagulant required. Recommend supportive anticoagulant regimens in patients proceeding to primary PCI who have been treated with ASA and thienopyridine. Administer additional boluses of UFH as needed to maintain therapeutic clotting time levels in patients who received prior treatment with UFH. Bivalirudin recommended as a supportive measure for primary PCI in patients with or without prior treatment with UFH.

Second Line

- Long-acting nondihydropyridine calcium channel blocker (CCB) when BB is ineffective or contraindicated if eEF is normal; use of immediate-release nifedipine is contraindicated in patients with STEMI.
- See chapter on "Heart Failure, Chronic" for additional medication management.

SURGERY/OTHER PROCEDURES

Intra-aortic balloon pump for cardiogenic shock; PCI of the left main coronary artery with stents as an alternative to CABG in patients with favorable anatomy and comorbid conditions that may increase risk of adverse surgical outcomes if CABG chosen

INPATIENT CONSIDERATIONS

Admission Criteria/Initial Stabilization

All patients with STEMI should be admitted to a CCU for evaluation and treatment. Transfer high-risk patients who receive fibrinolytic therapy as primary reperfusion therapy at a non–PCI-capable facility to a PCI-capable facility as soon as possible. Also admit suspected acute MI, ACS/positive cardiac markers or ST deviations, hemodynamic abnormalities.

IV Fluids

Right ventricular infarction may need fluid resuscitation for hypotension.

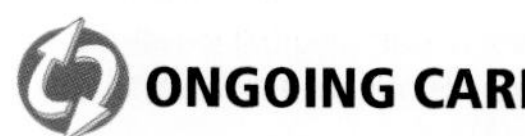

ONGOING CARE

FOLLOW-UP RECOMMENDATIONS

Follow up in 3–6 weeks of discharge. Identify high-risk patients for implantable cardioverter defibrillator (ICD) placement (especially those with EF <30%).

DIET

NPO for first 4–12 hours due to risk of emesis or aspiration; request dietary consult if lipid, weight, or glucose issues.

PATIENT EDUCATION

May resume sexual activity within 10 days, consistent with current exercise capacity. Driving can resume 1 week after discharge. Low-fat diet

COMPLICATIONS

Heart failure, myocardial rupture/left ventricular aneurysm, pericarditis, dysrhythmias, acute mitral regurgitation, severe depression (common)

REFERENCES

1. O'Gara PT. 2013 ACC/AHA guideline for the management of ST-elevation myocardial infarction and ACC/AHA/SCAI guidelines on percutaneous coronary intervention. *J Am Coll Cardiol*. 2013;127:529–555.
2. Task Force on the Management of ST-Segment Elevation Acute Myocardial Infarction of the European Society of Cardiology; Steg PG, James SK, Atar D, et al. ESC guidelines for the management of acute myocardial infarction in patients presenting with ST-segment elevation. *Eur Heart J*. 2012;33(20):2569–2619.

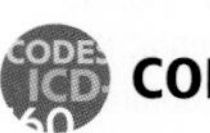

CODES

ICD10

- I24.9 Acute ischemic heart disease, unspecified
- I21.3 ST elevation (STEMI) myocardial infarction of unspecified site
- I21.09 STEMI involving oth coronary artery of anterior wall

CLINICAL PEARLS

Discontinue clopidogrel at least 5–7 days before elective CABG. Do not administer nitrates to patients who have recently used PDE-5 inhibitors.

ACUTE CORONARY SYNDROMES: UNSTABLE ANGINA AND NSTEMI

Brendan Merchant, MD • Louis J. Berk, MD

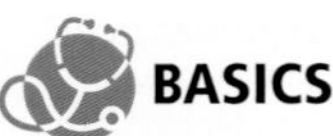

BASICS

DESCRIPTION

- Unstable angina (UA) and non–ST-segment elevation myocardial infarction (NSTEMI) are acute coronary syndromes (ACS) without ST-segment elevation.
- NSTEMI is defined by the rise and fall of cardiac biomarker values (preferably cardiac troponin) higher that the 99th percentile upper reference limit and accompanied by one of the following: symptoms of ischemia, new ST-segment T-wave changes, development of pathologic Q waves on ECG, or imaging evidence of new regional wall motion abnormality (1).
- UA, although clinically indistinguishable from NSTEMI (in an appropriate clinical setting, new-onset anginal chest pain, or change in typical anginal pattern, or development of angina at rest, or change in typical anginal equivalent), can be differentiated from NSTEMI by a lack of elevation in cardiac biomarkers based on 2 or more samples collected at least 6 hours apart. Just as with NSTEMI, nonspecific ECG changes, such as ST-segment depressions or T-wave inversions, may be present (1).

EPIDEMIOLOGY

- Incidence of UA/NSTEMI increases with age (2).
- Presentation of coronary events in women is, on average, 10 years later than in men, with comparable rates of occurrence (2)

Incidence

Age-adjusted coronary heart disease (CHD) incidence rates (per 1,000 person-years): white men, 12.5; black men, 10.6; white women, 4.0; and black women, 5.1 (2).

Prevalence

For adults ≥20 years of age: 8.3% for men and 6.1% for women (2)

ETIOLOGY AND PATHOPHYSIOLOGY

- Platelet-rich thrombus forming on a disrupted plaque
- Dynamic obstruction triggered by intense spasm of a coronary artery, for example, Prinzmetal angina or coronary spasm induced by cocaine or methamphetamine abuse
- Progressive mechanical limitation of coronary flow
- Coronary arterial inflammation
- Coronary dissection/rupture and thrombogenesis
- Myocardial oxygen demand exceeds supply
- UA/NSTEMI is usually caused by acute rupture of an atherosclerotic plaque, causing thrombosis and partial or total occlusion of a coronary artery (1).

RISK FACTORS

- Age
- Hypertension
- Tobacco use
- Diabetes mellitus
- Dyslipidemia
- Family history of early coronary artery disease (CAD)
- Sedentary lifestyle
- Overweight/obesity
- Psoriasis and other systemic inflammatory conditions

GENERAL PREVENTION

- Smoking cessation, healthy diet, weight control, physical activity
- If risk factors are present: BP control, lipid-lowering therapy, daily aspirin (in select patients)

COMMONLY ASSOCIATED CONDITIONS

- Cardiovascular disease (atherosclerotic, aneurysmal, autoimmune, peripheral)
- Other forms of heart disease (myocardial, valvular, high-output states)

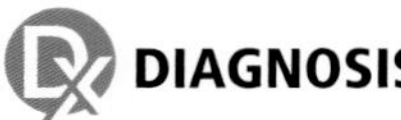

DIAGNOSIS

HISTORY

- Chest heaviness/tightness, with or without exertion, and increasing in frequency
- Pain or discomfort radiating to the neck, jaw, interscapular area, upper extremities, or epigastrium
- Associated symptoms of dyspnea, nausea, diaphoresis, light-headedness, dysphoria
- History of myocardial ischemia (stable or unstable angina, MI, coronary bypass surgery, or percutaneous coronary intervention [PCI])
- Family history of CAD or MI
- Risk factors for CAD and bleeding
- Use of phosphodiesterase-5 inhibitors (e.g., sildenafil) and concomitant nitrates
- Use of cocaine or amphetamines
- Medications and recent medication changes

PHYSICAL EXAM

- General: abnormal vital signs including tachycardia or bradycardia, hypertension or hypotension, widened pulse pressure, tachypnea, fever
- Neurologic: dizziness, syncope, fatigue, weakness, altered mental status
- Cardiovascular: dysrhythmia, jugular venous distention (JVD), new murmur, rub or gallop, diminished peripheral pulses, carotid bruits
- Respiratory: tachypnea, increased work of breathing, crackles
- Musculoskeletal: Sharp pain reproducible with movement or palpation is unlikely to be cardiac.
- Skin: cool skin, pallor, diaphoresis, signs of dyslipidemia (xanthomas, xanthelasma)

DIFFERENTIAL DIAGNOSIS

- Aortic dissection
- Pulmonary embolism
- Pleuropericarditis
- Perforating ulcer
- Gastroesophageal reflux disease (GERD) and spasm
- Esophageal perforation
- Biliary or pancreatic pain
- Dysrhythmia

Geriatric Considerations

Elderly patients, as well as women and those with diabetes, may have an atypical presentation without classic anginal symptoms.

DIAGNOSTIC TESTS & INTERPRETATION

Initial Tests (lab, imaging)

- 12-lead ECG (1)[A]: applies to both UA and NSTEMI
  - ST-segment depression and/or T-wave inversion:
    - ≥1-mm ST depression in ≥2 contiguous leads
    - T-wave inversions, other changes
    - ST depression and/or tall R wave in V_1/V_2 with upright T waves may indicate transmural STEMI of posterior wall.
    - If initial ECG is nondiagnostic but symptoms persist with suspicion for ACS, perform serial ECGs at 15–30-minute intervals.
- Serum biomarkers (negative by definition in UA)
  - NSTEMI is strictly defined as a rise and fall in serum biomarkers (usually troponin I or T, as they are more sensitive for detecting NSTEMI) exceeding the 99th percentile of a normal reference population. Troponin concentration rises 3–6 hours after onset of ischemic symptoms but can be delayed to 8–12 hours (troponin T is not specific in patients with renal dysfunction).
  - CK-MB increases 3–4 hours after onset of myocardial injury.
  - Myoglobin: early marker for myocardial necrosis; increases 2 hours after onset of myocardial necrosis
  - Patients with negative biomarkers within 6 hours of the onset of symptoms should have biomarkers remeasured 8–12 hours from onset of symptoms.
- Chest x-ray
- Consider transthoracic echocardiography if not recently performed (1)[B].

Follow-Up Tests & Special Considerations

- Patients with ischemia are recommended to undergo an assessment of left ventricle (LV) function to identify impaired function and/or need for appropriate medications such as ACE inhibitors, beta-blockers, and aldosterone antagonists.
- Fasting lipid profile
- CBC, basic metabolic panel, activated partial thromboplastin time (aPTT)
- Other laboratory tests:
  - Lactate dehydrogenase: increases within 24 hours, peaks 3–6 days, baseline 8–12 days (not routinely ordered)
  - Leukocytes: increase within several hours after MI, peak in 2–4 days
  - Brain natriuretic peptide (BNP): increases with MI, may not indicate heart failure

Pregnancy Considerations

Findings mimicking NSTEMI in pregnancy: ST depression after anesthesia, increase in CK-MB after delivery, and mild increase in troponin in preeclampsia and gestational hypertension. Spontaneous coronary dissection is a rare cause of ST elevation in pregnancy.

Diagnostic Procedures/Other

- Coronary angiography (discussed under "Treatment")
- If serial cardiac enzymes are negative and symptoms have resolved, consider stress testing, including either standard exercise treadmill test (ETT), stress echocardiography, or stress nuclear study (1)[B].
- Transesophageal echocardiography, contrast chest CT scan, or MRI generally are reserved for differentiating acute coronary syndrome and other causes of chest pain from aortic dissection.

Test Interpretation

- Subendocardial myocardial necrosis may be present.
- Atherosclerosis

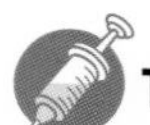

TREATMENT

GENERAL MEASURES

- Bed/chair rest with continuous ECG monitoring
- Antiarrhythmics as needed
- Anxiolytics as needed
- Deep vein thrombosis prophylaxis
- Continuation of aspirin, clopidogrel or prasugrel or ticagrelor, beta-blockers, ACE inhibitors (or ARBs if ACE intolerant), lipid-lowering therapy
- Tight BP control
- Treatment for depression PRN (common post-MI)
- Cardiac rehabilitation and increased physical activity
- Smoking cessation
- Annual influenza vaccine

MEDICATION

First Line

- Aspirin, nonenteric-coated, initial dose of 162–325 mg PO or chewed to all patients (1)[A]
  - In patients planned for PCI who are not at high risk for complex disease requiring coronary artery bypass graft (CABG) surgery, administer clopidogrel, loading dose 300–600 mg followed by 75 mg/day (1)[A]; or prasugrel, loading dose 60 mg followed by 10 mg/day (1)[B]; or ticagrelor, loading dose 180 mg followed by 90 mg BID (1)[B]. (Ticagrelor increases the risk of fatal intracranial hemorrhage [ICH] compared with clopidogrel and should be avoided in those with a prior history of ICH [1]).
  - Patients unable to take aspirin should receive a loading and maintenance dose of either clopidogrel, ticagrelor, or prasugrel.
- Nitroglycerin (NTG) sublingual 0.4 mg every 5 minutes for total of 3 doses, then assess need for IV NTG (1)[C]
- Supplemental oxygen 2–4 L/min, maintaining arterial oxygen saturation >90% (1)[B]
- Morphine sulfate 2–4 mg IV (with increments of 2–8 mg IV repeated at 5–15-minute intervals (1)[A]
- Oral beta-blocker (cardioselective agent such as metoprolol or atenolol preferred) in patients without signs of heart failure, cardiogenic shock, or other contraindications (1)[B]
- Risk stratify using the TIMI or GRACE score to select use of early invasive approach (within 12–24 hours of admission) versus medical therapy.
- Risks and benefits of the early invasive approach:
  - 33% relative risk reduction for both the end points of refractory angina and rehospitalization at 6–12 months (2)[A]
  - 27% and 22% relative risk reduction in rates of MI at 6–12 months and 3–5 years, respectively (2)[A]
  - Doubled risk of procedure-related MI and increased risk of minor periprocedural bleeding (1)[A]
- Invasive management
  - Benefits are more pronounced in higher risk patients, such as those with ECG changes or diabetes (2).
- Subsequent recommendations (1)[A]: For patients with elevated risk for clinical events or refractory angina or hemodynamic or electrical instability, initiate anticoagulant: enoxaparin or unfractionated heparin (UFH) or bivalirudin. Prior to angiography, add GP IIb/IIIa inhibitor (eptifibatide or tirofiban) or thienopyridine (clopidogrel or ticagrelor).
- Medical management
  - For low-risk or selected intermediate-risk patients; based on patient or physician preference; or in chronic renal insufficiency stage IV: Initiate anticoagulant therapy: enoxaparin or UFH or fondaparinux; enoxaparin or fondaparinux preferable. Initiate clopidogrel, prasugrel, or ticagrelor (1)[B].
- Contraindications: Prasugrel and ticagrelor are contraindicated in patients >75 years or those with history of CVA/TIA or increased bleeding risk.

Second Line

- ACE inhibitor in patients with pulmonary congestion or left ventricular ejection fraction (EF) ≤40%. Substitute ARB for ACE-intolerant patients (1)[A].
- Nondihydropyridine calcium channel blocker (CCB) (verapamil or diltiazem) to reduce myocardial oxygen demand when beta-blockers are contraindicated if normal EF (1)[B]. Use oral long-acting CCB only after beta-blockers and nitrates have been fully used (1)[C].
- Long-term nitrate therapy for recurrent angina/ischemia or heart failure (1)[C].
- Sublingual NTG at discharge (1)[C]
- Lipid-lowering therapy: high-dose statin (preferred due to nonlipid benefit on vascular function) (1)[A], niacin, or fibrate (1)[C]

ISSUES FOR REFERRAL

Cardiology consultation is appropriate for likely UA/NSTEMI, particularly regarding the complexities of anticoagulation/antiplatelet therapy.

SURGERY/OTHER PROCEDURES

- Coronary reperfusion
  - PCI with stent placement
  - CABG surgery
- Intra-aortic balloon pump for severe ischemia, hypotension, refractory pain

INPATIENT CONSIDERATIONS

Admission Criteria/Initial Stabilization

- All patients with definite or suspected acute MI, ongoing pain, positive cardiac markers, ST deviations, hemodynamic abnormalities, probable or definite ACS
- Bed rest with continuous ECG monitoring, assess for reperfusion therapy, relieve ischemic pain, treat life-threatening complications, admit to coronary care unit.

ONGOING CARE

FOLLOW-UP RECOMMENDATIONS

- Follow-up within 2–6 weeks (low risk) and 14 days (high risk).
- Refer to cardiac rehabilitation.

DIET

- Diet low in saturated fat, cholesterol, and sodium
- Request dietary consult.

PATIENT EDUCATION

- Education on new medications, diet, exercise, smoking cessation, lifestyle modification
- Resume exercise, sexual activity after outpatient reevaluation

PROGNOSIS

UA/NSTEMI patients have lower in-hospital mortality than those with STEMI but a similar or worse long-term outcome.

COMPLICATIONS

- Cardiogenic shock
- Heart failure
- Myocardial rupture
- Ventricular aneurysm
- Dysrhythmia
- Acute pulmonary embolism
- Acute thromboembolic stroke
- Pericarditis/Dressler syndrome
- Depression (increases mortality risk)
- Hyperglycemia

REFERENCES

1. Anderson JL, Adams CD, Antman EM, et al. 2012 ACCF/AHA focused update incorporated into the ACC/AHA 2007 guidelines for the management of patients with unstable angina/non-ST-elevation myocardial infarction: a report of the American College of Cardiology Foundation/American Heart Association Task Force on Practice Guidelines. *J Am Coll Cardiol*. 2013;61(23):e179–e347.
2. Roger VL, Go AS, Lloyd-Jones DM, et al. Heart disease and stroke statistics–2012 update: a report from the American Heart Association. *Circulation*. 2012;125(1):e2–e220.

ADDITIONAL READING

- Hoenig MR, Aroney CN, Scott IA. Early invasive versus conservative strategies for unstable angina and non-ST elevation myocardial infarction in the stent era. *Cochrane Database Syst Rev*. 2010;(3):CD004815.
- 2012 Writing Committee Members, Jneid H, Anderson JL, et al. 2012 ACCF/AHA focused update of the guideline for the management of patients with unstable angina/non–ST-elevation myocardial infarction (updating the 2007 guideline and replacing the 2011 focused update): a report of the American College of Cardiology Foundation/American Heart Association Task Force on practice guidelines. *Circulation*. 2012;126(7):875–910.

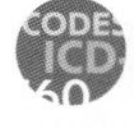

CODES

ICD10

- I24.9 Acute ischemic heart disease, unspecified
- I20.0 Unstable angina
- I21.4 Non-ST elevation (NSTEMI) myocardial infarction

CLINICAL PEARLS

- Discontinue NSAIDs, nonselective or selective cyclooxygenase (COX)-2 agents, except for ASA, due to increased risks of mortality, reinfarction, hypertension, heart failure, and myocardial rupture.
- Discontinue clopidogrel or prasugrel or ticagrelor 5–7 days before elective CABG.
- Do not use nitrate products in patients who recently used a phosphodiesterase-5 inhibitor (24 hours of sildenafil or 48 hours of tadalafil).
- Duration of antithrombotic therapy after NSTEMI depends on type of stent received and medications administered.
- Avoid beta-blockers in cocaine user.

ACUTE KIDNEY INJURY

Jason Kurland, MD

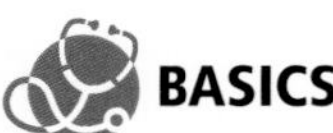

BASICS

DESCRIPTION

Abrupt loss of kidney function, defined as a rise in serum creatinine of ≥0.3 mg/dL or a 50% increase within 48 hours, resulting in retention of nitrogenous waste as well as electrolyte, acid–base, and volume homeostasis abnormalities, with or without oliguria (urine output <500 mL/day) (1)

EPIDEMIOLOGY

Incidence

5% of hospital and 30% of ICU admissions have a diagnosis of acute kidney injury (AKI). 25% of patients develop AKI while in the hospital, and 50% of those cases are iatrogenic. Development of AKI in the inpatient setting is associated with a >4-fold increased risk of death (2).

ETIOLOGY AND PATHOPHYSIOLOGY

Can be divided into 3 categories: prerenal, intrarenal, and postrenal

- Prerenal (~55%)
  - Hypotension; volume depletion (GI losses, excessive sweating, dehydration, hemorrhage); renal artery stenosis/embolism; burns; heart failure; liver failure
  - Secondary to decreased renal perfusion (often due to hypovolemia) leading to a decrease in glomerular filtration rate (GFR); reversible if factors decreasing perfusion are corrected; otherwise, it can progress to an intrarenal pathology known as *ischemic acute tubular necrosis*
- Intrarenal (~40%)
  - Acute tubular necrosis (ATN) (from prolonged prerenal state, radiographic contrast material, aminoglycosides, NSAIDs, or other nephrotoxic substances); glomerulonephritis (GN); acute interstitial nephritis (drug-induced); arteriolar insults; vasculitis; accelerated hypertension; cholesterol embolization (common after arterial procedures); intrarenal deposition/sludging (uric acid nephropathy and multiple myeloma [Bence-Jones proteins])
- Postrenal (~5%)
  - Extrinsic compression (e.g., benign prostatic hypertrophy [BPH], carcinoma, pregnancy), intrinsic obstruction (e.g., calculus, tumor, clot, stricture, sloughed papillae), decreased function (e.g., neurogenic bladder)
  - Secondary to extrinsic (e.g., BPH) or intrinsic (e.g., stones) obstruction of the urinary collection system

Genetics

No known genetic pattern

RISK FACTORS

- Chronic kidney disease (CKD)
- Comorbid conditions (e.g., diabetes, hypertension, heart failure, liver failure) (3)
- Advanced age
- Radiographic contrast material exposure
- Nephrotoxic medications (e.g., aminoglycoside antibiotics, NSAIDs, ACE inhibitors)
- Volume depletion (e.g., sepsis, hemorrhage, dehydration)
- Surgery
- Rhabdomyolysis
- Solitary kidney (risk in nephrolithiasis)
- BPH
- Malignancy (e.g., multiple myeloma)

GENERAL PREVENTION

See "Treatment; General Measures."

COMMONLY ASSOCIATED CONDITIONS

Hyperkalemia, hyperphosphatemia, hypercalcemia, hyperuricemia, hydronephrosis, BPH, nephrolithiasis, congestive heart failure (CHF), uremic pericarditis, cirrhosis, chronic renal insufficiency, malignant hypertension, vasculitis, drug reactions, sepsis, severe trauma, burns, transfusion reactions, recent chemotherapy, rhabdomyolysis, internal bleeding, dehydration

DIAGNOSIS

HISTORY

- General: PO intake, urine output, body weight, baseline creatinine (to assess magnitude of change), and medication use
- Prerenal: thirst, orthostatic dizziness
- Intrarenal: nephrotoxic medications, radiocontrast material, other toxins
  - Fever, arthralgias, and pruritic rash suggest *allergic interstitial nephritis (AIN)*, although systemic effects are not always seen in this pathology (only ~10% present with this triad).
  - Edema, hypertension, and oliguria with nephritic urine sediment (RBCs and RBC casts) point to *glomerulonephritis* or *vasculitis*
  - Livedo reticularis, SC nodules, and ischemic digits despite good pulses suggest *atheroembolization*.
  - Flank pain suggests *occlusion of the renal artery or vein*.
- Postrenal: Colicky flank pain that radiates to the groin suggests a *ureteric obstruction* such as a stone; nocturia, frequency, and hesitancy suggest *prostatic disease*; suprapubic and flank pain are usually secondary to *distension* of the bladder and collecting system; ask about anticholinergic drugs that could lead to *neurogenic bladder*.
- Uremic Sx: lethargy, nausea/vomiting, anorexia, pruritus, restless legs, sleep disturbance, hiccups

PHYSICAL EXAM

- Signs of uremia: mental status changes, seizures, asterixis, myoclonus, pericardial friction rub, peripheral neuropathies
- Prerenal signs: tachycardia, decreased jugular venous pressure (JVP), orthostatic hypotension, dry mucous membranes, decreased skin turgor; look for stigmata of associated comorbid conditions such as liver and heart failure, as well as sepsis.
- Intrinsic renal signs: pruritic rash, livedo reticularis, SC nodules, ischemic digits despite good pulses
- Postrenal signs: suprapubic distension, flank pain, enlarged prostate

DIFFERENTIAL DIAGNOSIS

See "Etiology."

DIAGNOSTIC TESTS & INTERPRETATION

Initial Tests (lab, imaging)

- Urinalysis: dipstick for blood and protein; microscopy for cells, casts, and crystals
- Casts: transparent hyaline casts—prerenal etiology; pigmented granular/muddy brown casts—ATN; WBC casts—acute interstitial nephritis; RBC casts—GN
- Urine eosinophils: ≥1% eosinophils by Hansel stain suggestive of acute interstitial nephritis (sensitivity, 67%; specificity, 83%)
- Urine electrolytes in an oliguric state
  - $FE_{Na} = [(U_{Na} \times P_{Cr})/(P_{Na} \times U_{Cr})] \times 100$, where U = urine, P = plasma, Na = sodium, Cr = creatinine; FE_{Na} <1%, likely prerenal; >2%, likely intrarenal
  - If patient is on diuretics, use FE_{urea} instead of FE_{Na}: $FE_{urea} = [(U_{urea} \times P_{Cr})/(P_{BUN} \times U_{Cr})] \times 100$; FE_{urea} <35% suggests prerenal etiology (4)[B].
- CBC, BUN, creatinine, electrolytes (including Ca/Mg/Phos), consider arterial blood gases (ABGs)
- Common lab abnormalities in AKI
  - Increased: K^+, phosphate, Mg, uric acid
  - Decreased: hematocrit (Hct), Na, Ca
- Calculate creatinine clearance (CrCl) to ensure that medications are dosed appropriately.
  - Cockcroft-Gault equation for CrCl (mL/min) = (140–age) × (weight in kilograms) × (0.85 if female)/(72 × serum creatinine)
  - Note that estimating equations of CrCl/GFR are only valid when renal function (serum Cr) is at steady-state; anuria implies CrCl of 0.
  - Renal ultrasound (US): first-line; excludes postrenal causes if negative; identifies kidney size, hydronephrosis, and nephrolithiasis
  - Doppler-flow renal US: rules out renal artery stenosis/thrombosis
  - Abdominal x-ray (kidney, ureter, bladder [KUB]): identifies calcification, renal calculi, and kidney size
- Several novel biomarkers, such as urinary IL-18, NGAL (neutrophil gelatinase associated lipocalin), KIM-1 (kidney injury molecule), and plasma cystatin C, are currently being validated for their role in the initial evaluation and management of AKI (5)[C].

Follow-Up Tests & Special Considerations

- Consider CKD (if suspect rhabdomyolysis) and immunologic testing (if suspect GN/vasculitis)
- More advanced imaging techniques should be considered if initial tests do not reveal etiology.
  - Radionucleotide renal scan: evaluates renal perfusion, function (GFR), and presence of obstructive uropathy and extravasation
  - CT scan: limited use due to need for radiographic contrast material, which can worsen AKI, although noncontrast helical scan is test of choice for suspected lithiasis
  - MRI: Acute tubulointerstitial nephritis can show an increased T2-weighted signal. Gadolinium contrast contraindicated if GFR <30 mL/min due to risk of nephrogenic systemic fibrosis.

Diagnostic Procedures/Other

Cystoscopy with retrograde pyelogram evaluates for bladder tumor, hydronephrosis, obstruction, and upper tract abnormalities and poses no threat of radiocontrast toxicity.

Test Interpretation

Kidney biopsy: last resort if patient does not respond to therapy or other tests do not reveal a diagnosis; most useful for evaluation of intrinsic AKI of unclear cause, such as AIN, GN, vasculitis, or renal transplant rejection

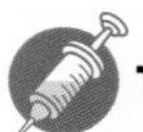

TREATMENT

GENERAL MEASURES

Identify and correct all prerenal and postrenal causes.

- Stop nephrotoxic drugs and renally dose others.
- Strictly record intake/output and daily weights.
- Optimize cardiac output to maintain renal perfusion.
- Follow nutrition suggestions and be aware of infections; treat aggressively if they occur.
- Avoid aspirin to reduce bleeding tendency.
- Indications for initiation of hemodialysis in patients with AKI: volume overload, severe or progressive hyperkalemia, or severe metabolic acidosis refractory to medical management; advanced uremic complications (pericarditis, encephalopathy, bleeding diathesis)

MEDICATION

First Line

- Focus on treating the underlying cause and associated complications.
- Monitor and adjust fluids and electrolytes to prevent fluid overload, hyperkalemia, hyperphosphatemia, and hypermagnesemia.
  - If patient is oliguric and not volume overloaded, a *fluid challenge* may be appropriate with diligent monitoring for volume overload.
- Furosemide is ineffective in preventing and treating AKI (6)[A] but can judiciously be used to manage volume overload and/or hyperkalemia.
- Dopamine, natriuretic peptides, insulin-like growth factor, and thyroxine also have no benefit in the treatment of AKI.
- Fenoldopam, a dopamine agonist, has been equivocal in decreasing risk of RRT and mortality in setting of AKI; not currently recommended for use, large RCT in progress (7)[C]
- Hyperkalemia with ECG changes: give IV calcium gluconate, isotonic sodium bicarbonate (only if acidemic, and avoid use of hypertonic "amps" of $NaHCO_3$), glucose with insulin (to drive K^+ into cells); Kayexalate and/or furosemide (to increase K^+ excretion); hemodialysis if severe/refractory
- Oliguric patients should have a fluid restriction of 400 mL + yesterday's urine output (if they are euvolemic).
- Metabolic acidosis (particularly pH <7.2): Sodium bicarbonate can be given; be aware of volume overload, hypocalcemia, hypokalemia.
- Effective strategies for AKI prevention: IV isotonic hydration, once-daily dosing of aminoglycosides (8)[A], use of lipid formulations of amphotericin B, use of iso-osmolar nonionic contrast media
- Risk of contrast-induced AKI may be reduced by avoidance of hypovolemia: isotonic saline 1 mL/kg/hour morning of procedure and continued until next morning or isotonic $NaHCO_3$ 3 mL/kg/hour × 1 hour before and 1 mL/kg/hour × 6 hours after contrast administration (9)[B]. N-acetylcysteine, although previously recommended, shown to have no benefit in recent large-scale RCT (10)[A].

Second Line

- Tamsulosin or other selective α-blockers for bladder outlet obstruction secondary to BPH
- Dihydropyridine calcium channel blockers may have a protective effect in posttransplant ATN.

ISSUES FOR REFERRAL

- Nephrology should be consulted for all cases as soon as patient is found with AKI.
- Urology consults for obstructive nephropathy

SURGERY/OTHER PROCEDURES

- Relief of obstruction with retrograde ureteral catheters/percutaneous nephrostomy
- Hemodialysis catheter placement

COMPLEMENTARY & ALTERNATIVE MEDICINE

Many supplements not approved by the FDA can be nephrotoxic.

INPATIENT CONSIDERATIONS

Admission Criteria/Initial Stabilization

Most patients with AKI will require admission; consider discharge in a stable patient with mild AKI and a clearly identified, reversible cause.

- ABCs of resuscitation
- Evaluate for and treat potentially life-threatening complications: hyperkalemia, metabolic acidosis, volume overload, advanced uremia.
- If volume depleted, give isotonic IV fluids.
- Place a Foley catheter.

IV Fluids

Isotonic fluids should be used in to treat hypovolemia.

Nursing

Place a Foley catheter; strict recording of intakes and outputs and daily weights.

Discharge Criteria

- Stabilization of renal function and a concrete plan for continued treatment, if necessary
- Some patients may require dialysis until renal recovery.

ONGOING CARE

FOLLOW-UP RECOMMENDATIONS

Patient Monitoring

As needed

DIET

- Total caloric intake should be 20–30 kcal/kg/day to avoid catabolism (7).
- Restrict Na^+ to 2 g/day (unless hypovolemic).
- Consider K^+ restriction (to 2–3 g/day) if hyperkalemic.
- If hyperphosphatemic, consider use of phosphate binders, although no evidence of benefit in AKI.
- Avoid magnesium and aluminum-containing compounds.

PATIENT EDUCATION

Keep well-hydrated. Avoid nephrotoxic drugs, such as NSAIDs and aminoglycosides.

PROGNOSIS

- Depending on the cause, comorbid conditions, and age of patient, mortality ranges from 5 to 80%.
- In cases of prerenal and postrenal failure, very good rates of recovery are positively correlated with shorter duration of AKI. Intrarenal etiologies usually take more time to recover. Overall, average recovery takes from days to months.

COMPLICATIONS

Death, sepsis, infection, seizures, paralysis, peripheral edema, CHF, arrhythmias, uremic pericarditis, bleeding, hypotension, anemia, hyperkalemia, uremia

REFERENCES

1. Lameire N. The pathophysiology of acute renal failure. *Crit Care Clin*. 2005;21(2):197–210.
2. Wang HE, Muntner P, Chertow GM, et al. Acute kidney injury and mortality in hospitalized patients. *Am J Nephrol*. 2012;35(4):349–355.
3. Hilton R. Acute renal failure. *BMJ*. 2006;333(7572):786–790.
4. Lameire N, Van Biesen W, Vanholder R. Acute renal failure. *Lancet*. 2005;365(9457):417–430.
5. McCullough PA, Kellum JA, Mehta RL, et al, eds. ADQI consensus on AKI biomarkers and cardiorenal syndromes. *Contrib Nephrol*., 2013;182:45–64.
6. Ho KM, Sheridan DJ. Meta-analysis of furosemide to prevent or treat acute renal failure. *BMJ*. 2006;333(7565):420.
7. International Society of Nephrology. Summary of recommendation statements. *Kidney Int Suppl*. 2012;2(Suppl 1):8.
8. Venkataraman R, Kellum JA. Prevention of acute renal failure. *Chest*. 2007;131(1):300–308.
9. Merten GJ, Burgess WP, Gray LV, et al. Prevention of contrast-induced nephropathy with sodium bicarbonate: a randomized controlled trial. *JAMA*. 2004;291(19):2328–2334.
10. ACT Investigators. Acetylcysteine for prevention of renal outcomes in patients undergoing coronary and peripheral vascular angiography: main results from the randomized Acetylcysteine for Contrast-induced nephropathy Trial (ACT). *Circulation*. 2011;124(11):1250–1259.

SEE ALSO

- Glomerulonephritis, Acute; Hepatorenal Syndrome; Hyperkalemia; Prostatic Hyperplasia, Benign (BPH); Renal Failure, Chronic; Reye Syndrome; Rhabdomyolysis; Sepsis
- Algorithm: Anuria or Oliguria

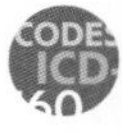

CODES

ICD10

- N17.9 Acute kidney failure, unspecified
- N17.0 Acute kidney failure with tubular necrosis
- N00.9 Acute nephritic syndrome with unsp morphologic changes

CLINICAL PEARLS

- Can be divided into 3 categories: prerenal, intrarenal, and postrenal
  - Prerenal: decreased renal perfusion (often from hypovolemia) leading to a decrease in GFR; reversible if factors decreasing perfusion are corrected
  - Intrarenal: intrinsic kidney damage; ATN is the most common cause via ischemic/nephrotoxic injury to the kidney
  - Postrenal: secondary to extrinsic/intrinsic obstruction of the urinary collection system
- Recognize the need for emergent hemodialysis: severe hyperkalemia, metabolic acidosis, or volume overload refractory to conservative therapy; uremic pericarditis, encephalopathy, or neuropathy; and alcohol and drug intoxications.

ADDISON DISEASE

Richard F. DeSouza, MD

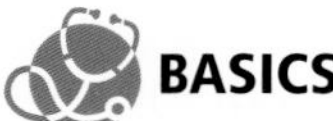

BASICS

DESCRIPTION

- Primary adrenal gland insufficiency, which results from partial or complete destruction of the adrenal cells with inadequate secretion of glucocorticoids and mineralocorticoids
- ~80% of cases are caused by an autoimmune process, followed by tuberculosis (TB), AIDS, systemic fungal infections, and adrenoleukodystrophy
- Addison disease (primary adrenocortical insufficiency) can be differentiated from secondary (pituitary failure) and tertiary (hypothalamic failure) causes because mineralocorticoid function usually remains intact in secondary and tertiary causes.
- Addisonian (adrenal) crisis: acute complication of adrenal insufficiency (circulatory collapse, dehydration, hypotension, nausea, vomiting, hypoglycemia); usually precipitated by an acute physiologic stressor(s) such as surgery, illness, exacerbation of comorbid process, and/or acute withdrawal of long-term corticosteroid therapy
- First described by Dr. Thomas Addison in 1855 (1)
- System(s) affected: endocrine/metabolic
- Synonym(s): adrenocortical insufficiency; corticoadrenal insufficiency; primary adrenocortical insufficiency

EPIDEMIOLOGY

- Predominant age: all ages; typical age of presentation is 30–50 years
- Predominant sex: females > males (slight)
- No racial predilection

Incidence

0.6:100,000

Prevalence

4–6:100,000

ETIOLOGY AND PATHOPHYSIOLOGY

- Autoimmune adrenal insufficiency (~80% of cases in the United States)
- Infectious causes: TB (most common infectious cause worldwide), HIV (most common infectious cause in the United States), Waterhouse-Fredrickson syndrome, fungal disease
- Bilateral adrenal hemorrhage and infarction (for patients on anticoagulants, 50% are in the therapeutic range)
- Antiphospholipid syndrome
- Lymphoma, Kaposi sarcoma, metastasis (lung, breast, kidney, colon, melanoma); tumor must destroy 90% of gland to produce hypofunction
- Drugs (e.g., ketoconazole, fluconazole, etomidate)
- Surgical adrenalectomy, radiation therapy
- Sarcoidosis, hemochromatosis, amyloidosis
- Congenital enzyme defects (deficiency of 21-hydroxylase enzyme is most common), neonatal adrenal hypoplasia, congenital adrenal hyperplasia, familial glucocorticoid insufficiency, autoimmune polyglandular autoimmune syndromes 1 and 2, adrenoleukodystrophy
- Idiopathic
- Destruction of the adrenal cortex resulting in deficiencies in cortisol, aldosterone, and androgens

Genetics

- Autoimmune polyglandular syndrome (APS) type 2 genetics are complex. It is associated with adrenal insufficiency, type 1 diabetes, and Hashimoto disease. It is more common than APS type 1.
- APS type 1 is caused by mutations of the autoimmune regulator gene. Nearly all have the following triad: adrenal insufficiency, hypoparathyroidism, and mucocutaneous candidiasis before adulthood.
- Adrenoleukodystrophy is an X-linked recessive disorder resulting in toxic accumulation of unoxidized long-chain fatty acids.
- Increased risk with cytotoxic T-lymphocyte antigen 4 (CTLA-4)

RISK FACTORS

- 40% of patients have a 1st- or 2nd-degree relative with associated disorders.
- Chronic steroid use, then experiencing severe infection, trauma, or surgical procedures
- Exposure to gastric infection is the most important risk factor for adrenal crisis in those with Addison disease.

GENERAL PREVENTION

- No preventive measures known for Addison disease; focus on prevention of complications
  - Anticipate adrenal crisis and treat before symptoms begin.
- Elective surgical procedures require upward adjustment in steroid dose.

COMMONLY ASSOCIATED CONDITIONS

- Diabetes mellitus
- Graves disease
- Hashimoto thyroiditis
- Hypoparathyroidism
- Hypercalcemia
- Ovarian failure
- Pernicious anemia
- Myasthenia gravis
- Vitiligo
- Chronic moniliasis
- Sarcoidosis
- Sjögren syndrome
- Chronic active hepatitis
- Schmidt syndrome

DIAGNOSIS

HISTORY

- Weakness, fatigue
- Dizziness
- Anorexia, nausea, vomiting
- Abdominal pain
- Chronic diarrhea
- Depression (60–80% of patients)
- Decreased cold tolerance
- Salt craving

PHYSICAL EXAM

- Weight loss
- Low BP, orthostatic hypotension
- Increased pigmentation (extensor surfaces, hand creases, dental-gingival margins, buccal and vaginal mucosa, lips, areola, pressure points, scars, "tanning," freckles)
- Vitiligo
- Hair loss in females

DIFFERENTIAL DIAGNOSIS

- Secondary adrenocortical insufficiency (pituitary failure)
  - Withdrawal of long-term corticosteroid use
  - Sheehan syndrome (postpartum necrosis of pituitary)
  - Empty sella syndrome
  - Radiation to pituitary
  - Pituitary adenomas, craniopharyngiomas
  - Infiltrative disorders of pituitary (sarcoidosis, hemochromatosis, amyloidosis, histiocytosis X)
- Tertiary adrenocortical insufficiency (hypothalamic failure)
  - Pituitary stalk transection
  - Trauma
  - Disruption of production of corticotropic-releasing factor
  - Hypothalamic tumors
- Other
  - Myopathies
  - Syndrome of inappropriate antidiuretic hormone
  - Heavy metal ingestion
  - Severe nutritional deficiencies
  - Sprue syndrome
  - Hyperparathyroidism
  - Neurofibromatosis
  - Peutz-Jeghers syndrome
  - Porphyria cutanea tarda
  - Salt-losing nephritis
  - Bronchogenic carcinoma
  - Anorexia nervosa

DIAGNOSTIC TESTS & INTERPRETATION

Initial Tests (lab, imaging)

- Basal plasma cortisol and adrenocorticotropic hormone (ACTH) (low cortisol and high ACTH indicative of Addison disease) (2,3)[A]
- Standard ACTH stimulation test: Cosyntropin 0.25 mg IV, measure preinjection baseline and 60-minute postinjection cortisol levels (patients with Addison disease have low to normal values that do not rise).
- Insulin-induced hypoglycemia test
- Metapyrone test
- Autoantibody tests: 21-hydroxylase (most common and specific), 17-hydroxylase, 17-alpha-hydroxylase (may not be associated), and adrenomedullin
- Circulating very-long-chain fatty acid levels if boy or young man
- Low serum sodium
- Elevated serum potassium
- Elevated BUN, creatinine, calcium, thyroid-stimulating hormone (TSH)
- Low serum aldosterone
- Hypoglycemia when fasting
- Metabolic acidosis
- Moderate neutropenia
- Eosinophilia
- Relative lymphocytosis
- Anemia, normochromic, normocytic

Follow-Up Tests & Special Considerations
- Plasma ACTH levels do not correlate with treatment and should not be used for routine monitoring of replacement therapy.
- TSH: Repeat when condition has stabilized
  - Thyroid hormone levels may normalize with the treatment of Addison disease.
- Drugs that may alter lab results: digitalis
- Disorders that may alter lab results: diabetes

Diagnostic Procedures/Other
- Abdominal CT scan: small adrenal glands in autoimmune adrenalitis; enlarged adrenal glands in infiltrative and hemorrhagic disorders
- Abdominal radiograph may show adrenal calcifications.
- Chest x-ray may show small heart size and/or calcification of cartilage.
- MRI of pituitary and hypothalamus if secondary or tertiary cause of adrenocortical insufficiency is suspected
- CT-guided fine-needle biopsy of adrenal masses may identify diagnoses.

Test Interpretation
- Atrophic adrenals in autoimmune adrenalitis
- Infiltrative and hemorrhagic disorders produce enlargement with destruction of the entire gland.

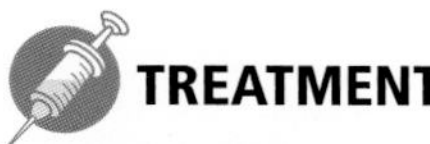

TREATMENT

GENERAL MEASURES
Consider the 5 Ss for the management of adrenal crisis:
- Salt, sugar, steroids, support, and search for a precipitating illness (usually infection, trauma, recent surgery, or not taking prescribed replacement therapy)

MEDICATION
First Line
- Chronic adrenal insufficiency
  - Glucocorticoid supplementation (4)[A]
    - Dosing: hydrocortisone 15–20 mg (or therapeutic equivalent) PO each morning upon rising and 10 mg at 4–5 PM each afternoon; dosage may vary and is usually lower in children and the elderly
    - Precautions: hepatic disease, fluid disturbances, immunosuppression, peptic ulcer disease, pregnancy, osteoporosis
    - Adverse reactions: immunosuppression, osteoporosis, gastric ulcers, depression, hyperglycemia, weight gain, glaucoma
    - Drug interactions: concomitant use of rifampin, phenytoin, or barbiturates
  - Mineralocorticoid supplementation
    - Dosing: fludrocortisone 0.05–0.2 mg/day PO
  - May require salt supplementation
- Addisonian crisis
  - Hydrocortisone 100 mg IV followed by 10 mg/hr infusion or hydrocortisone 100 mg IV bolus q6–8h
  - IV glucose, saline, and plasma expanders
  - Fludrocortisone 0.05 mg/day PO (may not be required; high-dose hydrocortisone is an effective mineralocorticoid)
- Acute illnesses (fever, stress, minor trauma)
  - Double the patient's usual steroid dose, taper the dose gradually over a week or more, and monitor vital signs and serum sodium.
- Supplementation for surgical procedures
  - Administer hydrocortisone 25–150 mg or methylprednisolone 5–30 mg IV on the day of the procedure in addition to maintenance therapy; taper gradually to the usual dose over 1–2 days.

Second Line
Addition of androgen therapy:
- Dehydroepiandrosterone (DHEA) 25–50 mg PO once daily may be considered in women to improve well-being and sexuality (5)[A].

INPATIENT CONSIDERATIONS
Admission Criteria/Initial Stabilization
- Presence of circulatory collapse, dehydration, hypotension, nausea, vomiting, hypoglycemia
- ICU admission for unstable cases

Addisonian crisis:
- Airway, breathing, and circulation management
- Establish IV access; 5% dextrose and normal saline.
- Administer hydrocortisone 100 mg IV bolus q6–8h; replacement with fludrocortisone is not necessary (high-dose hydrocortisone is an effective mineralocorticoid).
- Correct electrolyte abnormalities.
- BP support for hypotension
- Antibiotics if infection suspected

IV Fluids
IV saline containing 5% dextrose and plasma expanders

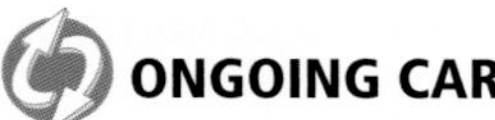

ONGOING CARE

FOLLOW-UP RECOMMENDATIONS
Patient Monitoring
- Verify adequacy of therapy: normal BP, serum electrolytes, plasma renin, and fasting blood glucose level
- Periodically assess for the development of long-term complications of corticosteroid use, including screening for osteoporosis, gastric ulcers, depression, and glaucoma.
- Lifelong medical supervision for signs of adequate therapy and avoidance of overdose

DIET
Maintain water, sodium, and potassium balance.

PATIENT EDUCATION
- National Adrenal Diseases Foundation, Great Neck, NY 11021, (516) 487-4992 (http://www.nadf.us)
- Patient should wear or carry medical identification about the disease and the need for hydrocortisone or other replacement therapy.
- Instruct patient in self-administration of parenteral hydrocortisone for emergency situations.

PROGNOSIS
Requires lifetime treatment: Life expectancy approximates normal with adequate replacement therapy; without treatment, the disease is 100% lethal.

COMPLICATIONS
- Hyperpyrexia
- Psychotic reactions
- Complications from underlying disease
- Over- or underuse of steroid treatment
- Hyperkalemic paralysis (rare)
- Addisonian crisis

REFERENCES

1. Addison T. *On the Constitutional and Local Effects of Disease of the Suprarenal Capsules*. London, United Kingdom: Highley; 1855.
2. Husebye ES, Allolio D, Arlt W, et al. Consensus statement on the diagnosis, treatment and follow-up of patients with primary adrenal insufficiency. *J Intern Med*. 2014; 274(2):104–115.
3. Michels A, Michels N. Addison disease: early detection and treatment principles. *Am Fam Physician*. 2014; 89(7):563–568.
4. Coursin DB, Wood KE. Corticosteroid supplementation for adrenal insufficiency. *JAMA*. 2002;287(2): 236–240.
5. Arlt W, Callies F, van Vlijmen JC, et al. Dehydroepiandrosterone replacement in women with adrenal insufficiency. *N Engl J Med*. 1999;341(14):1013–1020.

ADDITIONAL READING

Nieman LK, Chanco Turner ML. Addison's disease. *Clin Dermatol*. 2006;24(4):276–280.

SEE ALSO
Algorithm: Adrenocortical Insufficiency

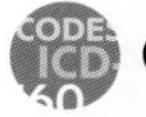

CODES

ICD10
- E27.1 Primary adrenocortical insufficiency
- A18.7 Tuberculosis of adrenal glands
- E27.2 Addisonian crisis

CLINICAL PEARLS
- 80% of cases are caused by an autoimmune process; the average age of diagnosis in adults is 40 years.
- Consider the 5 Ss for the management of Addison disease: salt, sugar, steroids, support, and search for an underlying cause.
- The goal of steroid replacement therapy should be the lowest dose that alleviates patient symptoms while preventing adverse drug events.
- Plasma ACTH levels do not correlate with treatment and should not be used for routine monitoring for efficacy of replacement therapy.
- Long-term use of steroids predisposes patients to the development of osteoporosis; screen accordingly and encourage calcium and vitamin D supplementation.

ADENOVIRUS INFECTIONS

Scott F. Graham, MD • Lena A.N. Patel, MD

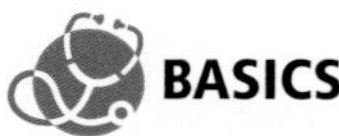

BASICS

DESCRIPTION

- Acute febrile illnesses characterized by inflammation of various mucous membranes including the conjunctivae, and the respiratory and GI tracts. Typically self-limited
- Adenovirus infections occur in epidemic and endemic situations:
  - Common types
    - Acute febrile respiratory illness, affects primarily children
    - Acute respiratory disease, affects adults
    - Viral pneumonia, affects children and adults
    - Acute pharyngoconjunctival fever, affects children, particularly after summer swimming
    - Acute follicular conjunctivitis, affects all ages
    - Epidemic keratoconjunctivitis, affects adults
    - Intestinal infections leading to enteritis, mesenteric adenitis, and intussusception
  - Conjunctivitis, sometimes called "pink eye"
- System(s) affected: cardiovascular; GI; hematologic/lymphatic/immunologic; musculoskeletal; nervous; pulmonary; renal/urologic; ophthalmologic

Geriatric Considerations

Complications more likely in elderly populations

Pediatric Considerations

Viral pneumonia in infants and neonates may be fatal.

EPIDEMIOLOGY

- Predominant age: <10 years, but epidemics in all ages
- Predominant sex: male = female
- Occurs worldwide and throughout the year but more frequently in warmer months

Incidence

- Very common infection, estimated at 2–5% of all upper respiratory infections (URIs) and >10% of URIs in children
- Most individuals show evidence of prior adenovirus infection by age 10 years.
- As many as half, the infections with adenovirus are subclinical or asymptomatic.
- 15–70% of conjunctivitis worldwide

ETIOLOGY AND PATHOPHYSIOLOGY

- Adenovirus (DNA viruses 60–90 nm in size, 6 species [A–F] with over 50 known serotypes)
- Transmission
  - Aerosol droplets, fecal–oral, contact with contaminated fomites
  - Virus can survive long periods on skin and environmental surfaces.
  - Incubation period is 5–9 days (1).
- Most common known pathogens
  - Types 1, 2, 3, 4, 5, 7, 14, and 21 cause upper respiratory illness and pneumonia.
  - Types 3, 7, and 21 cause pharyngoconjunctival fever.
  - Types 31, 40, and 41 cause gastroenteritis.
  - Types 8, 19, 37, 53, and 54 cause epidemic keratoconjunctivitis.
  - Types 5, 7, 14, and 21 cause the most severe illnesses.

RISK FACTORS

- Large number of people gathered in a confined area (e.g., military recruits, college students, daycare centers, summer camps, community swimming pools)
- Immunocompromised persons are at risk for severe disease.

GENERAL PREVENTION

- Live, enteric-coated oral type 4 and type 7 adenovirus vaccine available for military recruits (or other personnel at high risk ages 17–50 years); reduces incidence of acute respiratory disease (2)
- Frequent hand washing
- Decontamination of environmental surfaces using chlorine, bleach, formaldehyde, or heat
- Vigorous hand washing and use of gloves when examining patients with epidemic keratoconjunctivitis; add droplet precautions if suspected adenoviral respiratory infection.
- Health care providers with suspected adenoviral conjunctivitis should avoid direct patient contact for 14 days after onset (in 2nd eye).

COMMONLY ASSOCIATED CONDITIONS

- Otitis media
- Conjunctivitis
- Bronchiolitis
- Viral enteritis
- Less frequent syndromes seen primarily in immunocompromised individuals include meningoencephalitis, hepatitis, myocarditis, pancreatitis, genital infections, intussusception and mesenteric adenitis hemorrhagic cystitis, and interstitial nephritis.

DIAGNOSIS

HISTORY

Depends on type (See "Differential Diagnosis"). Common symptoms with most respiratory forms (3),(4)

- Headache
- Malaise
- Sore throat
- Cough
- Coryza
- Fever (moderate to high)
- Vomiting
- Diarrhea
- Abdominal pain
- Ear pain
- Urinary symptoms/hematuria
- Eye redness and pain
- Irritative voiding symptoms (bladder involvement)

PHYSICAL EXAM

- Fever
- Tonsillitis, usually with exudates
- Cervical lymphadenopathy
- Otitis media
- Conjunctivitis

DIFFERENTIAL DIAGNOSIS

- Depends on clinical presentation
- The following are the primary characteristics of the major adenovirus infections:
  - Acute respiratory illness
    - Mostly in children
    - Incubation period: 2–5 days
    - Malaise, fever, chills, headache, pharyngitis, hoarseness, dry cough
    - Fever lasting 2–4 days
    - Illness subsiding in 10–14 days
    - DDx: rhinovirus, influenza, parainfluenza, RSV
  - Viral pneumonia
    - Sudden onset of high fever, rapid infection of upper and lower respiratory tracts, skin rash, diarrhea
    - Occurs mostly in children aged a few days up to 3 years
    - DDx: bacterial pneumonia, RSV, influenza, parainfluenza
  - Acute pharyngoconjunctival fever
    - Spiking fever lasting several days, headache, pharyngitis, conjunctivitis, rhinitis, cervical adenitis
    - Conjunctivitis, usually unilateral
    - Subsides in 1 week
    - DDx: bacterial conjunctivitis, enterovirus, herpes simplex virus (HSV)
  - Epidemic keratoconjunctivitis
    - Usually unilateral onset of ocular redness and edema, periorbital edema, periorbital swelling, local discomfort suggestive of foreign body
    - Lasts 3–4 weeks
    - DDx: bacterial conjunctivitis, enterovirus, HSV
  - Viral enteritis
    - Nausea/vomiting, diarrhea, abdominal pain
    - DDx: bacterial enteritis, bowel obstruction

DIAGNOSTIC TESTS & INTERPRETATION

Initial Tests (lab, imaging)

- Diagnosis only needs to be confirmed in severe cases and epidemics.
- Viral cultures from respiratory, ocular, or fecal sources
  - Pharyngeal isolate suggests recent infection.
- Adenovirus-specific ELISA; rapid but less sensitive than culture (5)[A]
- Adenovirus DNA detection through polymerase chain reaction (PCR)
- Rapid pathogen screening, adeno-detector, is available for detecting adenoviral conjunctivitis (sensitivity, 89%; specificity, 94%); results in 10 minutes (6)[B]
- Antigen detection in stool for enteric serotypes
- Serologic procedures, such as complement fixation, with a 4-fold rise in serum antibody titer, identify recent adenoviral infection.
- Radiographs: bronchopneumonia in severe respiratory infections

Diagnostic Procedures/Other

Biopsy (lung or other) may be needed in severe or unusual cases; usually only in immunocompromised patients

Test Interpretation

- Varies with each virus
  - Severe pneumonia may be reflected by extensive intranuclear inclusions.
- *Bronchiolitis obliterans* may occur.

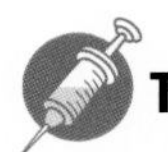

TREATMENT

GENERAL MEASURES

- Treatment is supportive and symptomatic.
- Infections are usually benign and of short duration.

MEDICATION

First Line

- Acetaminophen 10–15 mg/kg PO for analgesia (avoid aspirin)
- Antivirals and immunotherapy are reserved for immunocompromised individuals and patients with severe disease:
  - No controlled trials showing benefit of any antiviral agents against human adenovirus infection; however, cidofovir (1 mg/kg every other day) is most commonly used.
  - For adenoviral conjunctivitis, topical ganciclovir 0.15% ophthalmic gel has been suggested for "off-label" use.

COMPLEMENTARY & ALTERNATIVE MEDICINE

Echinacea has not been shown to be better than placebo for treatment of viral URIs (7)[B].

INPATIENT CONSIDERATIONS

Admission Criteria/Initial Stabilization

Severely ill infants or immunocompromised patients with severe illness

Nursing

Hospitalized patients with adenoviral infections should be placed on contact precautions; add droplet precautions for those with respiratory illness.

ONGOING CARE

FOLLOW-UP RECOMMENDATIONS

Rest during febrile phases

Patient Monitoring

For severe infantile pneumonia and conjunctivitis, daily physical exam until well

DIET

No special diet

PATIENT EDUCATION

- Avoid aspirin in children.
- Give instructions for saline nasal spray, cough preparations, frequent hand washing, and surface cleaning.

PROGNOSIS

- Self-limited, usually without sequelae
- Severe illness and death in neonates and in immunocompromised hosts can occur; severe pneumonia in children under 2 years can have a mortality rate as high as 16%.

COMPLICATIONS

Few, if any, recognizable long-term problems

REFERENCES

1. Lessler J, Reich NG, Brookmeyer R, et al. Incubation periods of acute respiratory viral infections: a systematic review. *Lancet Infect Dis*. 2009;9(5):291–300.
2. Lyons A, Longfield J, Kuschner R, et al. A double-blind, placebo-controlled study of the safety and immunogenicity of live, oral type 4 and type 7 adenovirus vaccines in adults. *Vaccine*. 2008;26(23):2890–2898.
3. Dominguez O, Rojo P, de Las Heras S, et al. Clinical presentation and characteristics of pharyngeal adenovirus infections. *Pediatr Infect Dis J*. 2005;24(8):733–734.
4. Centers for Disease Control and Prevention. Adenovirus symptoms. http://www.cdc.gov/adenovirus/about/symptoms.html. Accessed 2014.
5. Goto E. Meta-analysis of evaluating diagnostic accuracy of adenoclone (ELISA) for adenoviral infection among Japanese people. *Rinsho Byori*. 2010;58(2):148–155.
6. Kaufman HE. Adenovirus advances: new diagnostic and therapeutic options. *Curr Opin Ophthalmol*. 2011;22(4):290–293.
7. Barrett BP, Brown RL, Locken K, et al. Treatment of the common cold with unrefined echinacea. A randomized, double-blind, placebo-controlled trial. *Ann Intern Med*. 2002;137(12):939–946.

ADDITIONAL READING

- Houlihan C, Valappil M, Waugh S, et al. Severe adenovirus infection: an under-recognized disease with limited treatment options. *JICS*. 2012;13(4), October.
- Majeed A, Naeem Z, Khan DA, et al. Epidemic adenoviral conjunctivitis report of an outbreak in a military garrison and recommendations for its management and prevention. *J Pak Med Assoc*. 2005;55(7):273–275.
- Pihos AM. Epidemic keratoconjunctivitis: a review of current concepts in management. *J Optom*. 2013;06:69–74.
- Spurling GKP, Del Mar CB, Dooley L, et al. Delayed antibiotics for symptoms and complications of respiratory infections. *Cochrane Database Syst Rev*. 2004;(4):CD004417.

SEE ALSO

Conjunctivitis, Acute; Intussusception; Pneumonia, Viral

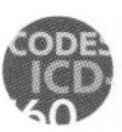

CODES

ICD10

- B34.0 Adenovirus infection, unspecified
- B30.1 Conjunctivitis due to adenovirus
- J12.0 Adenoviral pneumonia

CLINICAL PEARLS

- Can present like streptococcus pharyngitis with white exudates and cervical adenitis but negative strep test
- Most common cause of strep-negative tonsillitis in young children
- Diagnosis only needs to be confirmed in severe cases and epidemics.
- Average incubation time is 5–6 days.
- Adenovirus conjunctivitis is highly contagious; cold compresses may help relieve symptoms.

ADHESIVE CAPSULITIS (FROZEN SHOULDER)

Lanier H. Adams, DO • Brandon David Hecht, DO

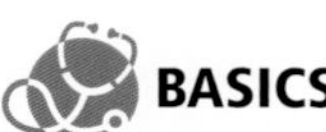

BASICS

DESCRIPTION

- A poorly understood condition marked by the painful, gradual loss of both active and passive glenohumeral (GH) motion in >1 plane due to a progressive fibrosis/contracture of the GH joint capsule
- The clinical course of adhesive capsulitis (AC) follows a predictable progression
  - Stage 1, freeze/pain: subacute onset of diffuse vague pain, lasting 2–9 months
  - Stage 2, frozen/adhesive: insidious onset of stiffness, lasting 4–12 months
  - Stage 3, thaw/recovery: gradual resolution over 5–24+ months. Resolution may be protracted (symptoms lasting >36 months) and incomplete but rarely results in a functional limitation.
- AC also categorized as primary (idiopathic) and secondary (underlying or associated condition)
- System(s) affected: musculoskeletal
- Synonym(s): pericapsulitis; scapulohumeral periarthritis

EPIDEMIOLOGY

- Predominant age: 40–60 years
- Predominant sex: female > male

Prevalence

- General population: 2–5%
- Diabetics type 1 and type 2: 10–20%

ETIOLOGY AND PATHOPHYSIOLOGY

- Synovial inflammation and capsular fibrosis resulting in contracture of the rotator interval, coracohumeral ligament, and anterior shoulder capsule restricting movement of the shoulder
- A poorly understood chronic inflammatory response with fibroblastic proliferation, possibly immunomodulated

Genetics

No known genetic predispositions

RISK FACTORS

- Sedentary vocation or lifestyle
- Age >40 years
- History of AC: 20–30% will develop the condition in contralateral shoulder.
- Minor injury: 20–30% of those with AC will report recent minor trauma to the shoulder.
- Systemic diseases: endocrinopathies, autoimmune disorders, atherosclerotic disease (see "Commonly Associated Conditions")

GENERAL PREVENTION

No current evidence regarding prevention

COMMONLY ASSOCIATED CONDITIONS

- Idiopathic AC can be associated with a history of Dupuytren contractures.
- Secondary AC is associated with diabetes types 1 and 2, thyroid disease, autoimmune diseases, rotator cuff injury or minor shoulder trauma, surgery or immobilization of shoulder, prior cerebrovascular accident, or myocardial infarction.

DIAGNOSIS

HISTORY

- Insidious onset of progressive, diffuse shoulder pain followed by the complaint of gradual onset of stiffness
- Pain predominates early in the course of the disease:
  - Night pain often interrupts sleep.
  - Debilitating pain: achy at rest and sharper with movement, poorly localized
  - Muscle spasm/pain in the neck, shoulder, acromioclavicular joint, and posterior thorax due to scapular overcompensation (can also cause shoulder impingement)
- Stiffness predominates as pain begins to wane in later stages of disease:
  - Difficulties with activities of daily living (ADLs)
    - Inability to reach overhead or into back pocket
- Weakness
- Preceding injury, illness, or immobilization (secondary AC)

PHYSICAL EXAM

- Limited active and passive shoulder range of motion (ROM) in >1 plane of motion: Document ROM for forward flexion, abduction, and external and internal rotation for all patients with shoulder complaints at each visit.
- Diffuse shoulder tenderness with deep palpation
- Loss of natural arm swing with gait
- Normal strength (weakness may be present if pain inhibits effort, but objective strength testing reveals 5/5 strength in all planes)
- Special tests (Neer, Hawkins, etc.) are not diagnostic.
- No neurovascular deficits.

DIFFERENTIAL DIAGNOSIS

- Rotator cuff strain/tear/impingement syndrome
- GH or acromioclavicular joint osteoarthritis (OA)
- Cervical strain/radiculopathy/OA
- Myofascial pain syndromes
- Calcific tendonitis
- Fracture, dislocation
- Bony neoplasm/metastases

DIAGNOSTIC TESTS & INTERPRETATION

Initial Tests (lab, imaging)

No lab is diagnostic for primary (idiopathic) AC. If suspected, labs may be indicated to rule out any underlying systemic diseases associated with secondary AC: Hbg A1C, TSH, etc.

- Plain radiograph (anteroposterior [AP], axillary, supraspinatus outlet views) to rule out OA, calcific tendinitis, avascular necrosis, osteomyelitis, fracture, dislocation, and tumor
- Radiographs typically normal but may demonstrate disuse osteopenia of the proximal humerus in late AC.
- If suspicious for secondary AC, consider MRI to evaluate for a characteristic thickening of the axillary pouch and to rule out other shoulder disorders.

Follow-Up Tests & Special Considerations

- Serial exams advised in patients who present with nonspecific shoulder pain and normal radiographs eluding a specific diagnosis. At follow-up visits, the diagnosis of AC is supported if progressive motion restriction is identified in >1 plane of motion.
- Early in stage 1, pain is the predominant feature and restriction of motion may be difficult to identify. At 8-week follow-up, the patient may not complain of stiffness, but the loss of passive ROM may be easier to identify on exam.
- Early on, AC is difficult to distinguish from subacromial bursitis. The loss of passive external rotation may be the only finding that differentiates early AC from subacromial bursitis. The only other condition that may cause insidious loss of passive external rotation is GH arthritis.

Diagnostic Procedures/Other

Diagnostic subacromial anesthetic injection can help to differentiate AC from rotator cuff pathologies:

- Resolution of pain and restoration of ROM after subacromial injection suggests rotator cuff pathology or other cause of subacromial bursitis.
- Intact muscle strength with persistent active and passive ROM deficits and a firm mechanical end point are consistent with AC.

Test Interpretation

If performed, surgical arthroscopy classically demonstrates capsular thickening and synovial inflammation with adhesions to the humerus.

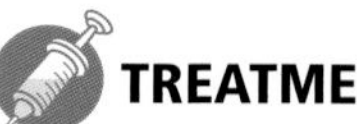

TREATMENT

- Treatment is driven by the stage of AC at presentation. Conservative therapy is recommended initially (the first 4–6 months).
- Therapy includes any combination of physical therapy, oral medications, and joint/bursal injections (1)[A].
- Structured physical therapy is superior to home exercises (2)[A].
- Patient education should include explanation of the following:
  - Expectations for a protracted recovery (months to years) characterized by resolution of pain prior to the return of function
  - Full ROM may never be recovered; however, functional limitations are uncommon.

GENERAL MEASURES

- Goal of all therapies: control pain, preserve mobility, and allow for restful sleep.
- Codman pendulum exercises: Lean forward onto table or chair with unaffected arm bending at the waist; let the affected arm dangle. Swing the affected arm slowly by moving the torso. Try smaller and then bigger circles (clockwise and counterclockwise).
- Climbing the wall: Put the hand flat on a wall in front of you; use the fingers to "climb" the wall; pause 30 seconds every few inches. Repeat the exercise after turning 90 degrees to wall (abduction).
- Heat and/or ice: may temporarily improve pain and secondary spasm
- Address underlying causes of secondary AC (see "Associated Conditions").
- Patient reassessment must be ongoing to reinforce expectations and determine patient's goals.

MEDICATION

First Line

- NSAIDs: widely used in the treatment of AC and thought to be most beneficial in stage 1 when pain is the predominant feature. If contraindicated, reasonable alternatives include acetaminophen or opioid analgesics. Concomitant use of NSAIDs with oral or injectable corticosteroids has no added benefit.
- Oral corticosteroids: rarely used in clinical practice, but evidence demonstrates short-term improvement in pain and ROM (up to 6 weeks) most likely beneficial early in the course of the disease (stage 1 and early stage 2)
  - Prednisolone: 30 mg/day for 3 weeks (alternatively 10 mg × 4 weeks, then 5 mg × 2 weeks)
- Subacromial (SA) corticosteroid injection: At any stage, SA injection in conjunction with physical therapy provides short-term (16 weeks) benefit in pain and ROM.
- Intra-articular (IA) corticosteroid injection: Like SA injections, IA injections have demonstrated short-term (16 weeks) improvement in pain and ROM if used in conjunction with physical therapy.
  - May require serial injection and requires technical expertise
  - Equal efficacy to scheduled NSAID therapy (3)[A]

Second Line

Tricyclic antidepressants (amitriptyline) have been used as neuromodulators. No evidence exists to support use in AC.

ISSUES FOR REFERRAL

- 7–12% of cases will not respond to nonoperative treatment.
- Orthopedic surgical referral should be considered if patient is considering a more invasive treatment option and the patient has not responded adequately to conservative treatment within 4–6 months.

ADDITIONAL THERAPIES

- Physical therapy: additive effect when used in conjunction with other treatments (NSAIDs, injections, manipulation under anesthesia [MUA], surgical release), but there is no evidence to support the use of physical therapy alone in the treatment of AC (1,2)[A].
- Iontophoresis (electromotive drug administration) is generally not recommended in this condition.
- Although not commonly used, supervised neglect is a plausible treatment option for some patients.
- Capsular hydrodilation (arthrography distention): IA injection of large-volume saline with steroid or hyaluronic acid has demonstrated some short-term improvements (12 weeks) in pain and function (4)[A].
- IA hyaluronic acid: A systematic review showed non-inferiority to IA corticosteroid when used in conjunction with physical therapy (5)[A].
- Suprascapular nerve block: Early evidence suggests short-term improvement in pain.
- Low-power laser therapy: superior to placebo (1)[A]
- Botox: Evidence suggests no benefit.

ALERT

Indications for more invasive options remain highly subjective and need to be individualized to each patient.

SURGERY/OTHER PROCEDURES

- Arthroscopic capsular release: most common surgical method for treating recalcitrant AC
  - Short-term benefits: improved pain and function
  - Long-term benefits: mixed findings (similar vs. superior to conservative therapy)
- MUA: Outcomes are similar to those with athroscopic capsular release. Contraindicated in post-traumatic/postsurgical AC (6)[A].
- Transcatheter arterial embolization: Early evidence suggests benefit (7)[B].

COMPLEMENTARY & ALTERNATIVE MEDICINE

- Acupuncture: Insufficient evidence exists for a definitive conclusion about the effectiveness of acupuncture for AC.
- Osteopathic manipulative technique: Evidence is lacking.

INPATIENT CONSIDERATIONS

Initial Stabilization

Outpatient care

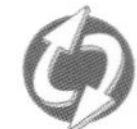

ONGOING CARE

FOLLOW-UP RECOMMENDATIONS

Reinforce the natural course of the disease and discuss the various treatment options as the patient progresses through different stages of the disease. Many patients are more likely to request invasive procedures (injections, capsular distension, MUA, surgery) when stiffness starts to affect ADLs.

Patient Monitoring

Frequent reinforcement of the natural history of AC along with patient encouragement are often needed for successful recovery. A multidisciplinary team approach to patient care helps in this regard.

DIET

No restrictions

PATIENT EDUCATION

Long-term course of treatment until resolution of symptoms; stretching and ROM exercises daily during and after improvement

PROGNOSIS

- Although AC is considered self-limiting, up to 50% of patients will have permanent restrictions of ROM (usually external rotation).
- Rare functional disability results.

COMPLICATIONS

Surgical complications and complications due to MUA can be disabling but are uncommon.

REFERENCES

1. Jain TK, Sharma NK. The effectiveness of physiotherapeutic interventions in treatment of frozen shoulder/adhesive capsulitis: a systematic review. *J Back Musculoskelet Rehabil*. 2014;27(3):247–273.
2. Russel S, Jariwala A, Conlon R, et al. A blinded, randomized, controlled trial assessing conservative management strategies for frozen shoulder. *J Shoulder Elbow Surg*. 2014;23(4):500–507.
3. Dehghan A, Pishgooei N, Salami MA, et al. Comparison between NSAID and intra-articular corticosteroid injection in frozen shoulder of diabetic patients; a randomized clinical trial. *Exp Clin Endocrinol Diabetes*. 2013;121(2):75–79.
4. Park KD, Nam HS, Lee JK, et al. Treatment effects of ultrasound-guided capsular distention with hyaluronic acid in adhesive capsulitis of the shouler. *Arch Phys Med Rehabil*. 2013;94(2):264–270.
5. Harris JD, Griesser MJ, Copelan A, et al. Treatment of adhesive capsulitis with intra-articular hyaluronate: a systematic review. *Int J Shoulder Surg*. 2011;5(2):31–37.
6. Grant JA, Schroeder N, Miller BS, et al. Comparison of manipulation and arthroscopic capsular release for adhesive capsulitis: a systematic review. *J Shoulder Elbow Surg*. 2013;22(8):1135–1145.
7. Okuno Y, Oguro S, Iwamoto W, et al. Short-term results of transcatheter arterial embolization of abnormal neovessels in patients with adhesive capsulitis: a pilot study. *J Shoulder Elbow Surg*. 2014;23(9):e199–e206. doi.org/10.1016/j.jse.2013.12.014

ADDITIONAL READING

- Ewald A. Adhesive capsulitis: a review. *Am Fam Physician*. 2011;83(4):417–422.
- Favejee MM, Huisstede BM, Koes BW. Frozen shoulder: the effectiveness of conservative and surgical interventions–systematic review. *Br J Sports Med*. 2011;45(1):49–56.
- Maund E, Craig D, Suekarran S, et al. Management of frozen shoulder: a systematic review and cost-effectiveness analysis. *Health Technol Assess*. 2012;16(11):1–264.
- Rill BK, Fleckenstein CM, Levy MS, et al. Predictors of outcome after nonoperative and operative treatment of adhesive capsulitis. *Am J Sports Med*. 2011;39(3):567–574.

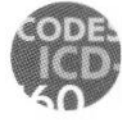

CODES

ICD10

- M75.00 Adhesive capsulitis of unspecified shoulder
- M75.02 Adhesive capsulitis of left shoulder
- M75.01 Adhesive capsulitis of right shoulder

CLINICAL PEARLS

- Early-stage AC is nearly indistinguishable from rotator cuff pathology. Restriction of external ROM suggests AC.
- Diagnostic subacromial bursa injection may help differentiate early AC from impingement syndrome. (In AC, ROM deficits persist and strength is intact after injection.)
- Normal radiographs in the setting of progressive restriction of motion in >1 plane confirms AC.
- Initial AC treatment is conservative: NSAIDs; oral, bursal, or intra-articular corticosteroids; physical therapy; and appropriate patient education.
- Depending on the patient, invasive treatment options can be considered after 4–6 months of conservative therapy (about 10% of cases). Options include capsular distention, MUA, and arthroscopy.

ADOPTION, INTERNATIONAL

Theodore R. Brown, DO, MPH, FAAFP

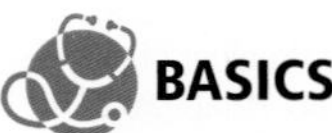

BASICS

DESCRIPTION

Although international adoptions have decreased in the past 10 years, they still represent a significant portion of the roughly 135,000 yearly U.S. adoptions. The demographics of those children and their homelands have shifted significantly during that time. The diverse birth countries, disease exposures, and unknown health histories of these children make them a population that requires special attention. And although specialty clinics are becoming more prevalent, many adoptive parents will look to their primary care provider for their adoption health care needs.

EPIDEMIOLOGY

Incidence

- 7,092 children were adopted internationally in 2013.
- Approximately 5% of all U.S. adoptions are international, decreased from 17% in 2004.
- In 2013, the most common countries of origin for internationally adopted children were the following in descending order: China, Ethiopia, Ukraine, Haiti, Democratic Republic of Congo, Uganda, Russia, Nigeria, Philippines, and Bulgaria.
- In 2013, 8% of internationally adopted children were <1 year of age, 54% were ages 1–4 years, 29% were ages 5–12 years, and 9% were ≥13 years. 55% were girls.

RISK FACTORS

- Unknown birth, medical, and vaccination histories
- Possible exposure to toxins and/or inadequate nutrition in utero
- Exposures to infectious diseases not commonly seen in the United States (1)
- Previous living conditions
  - Overcrowding
  - Institutionalization (orphanages)
  - Environmental toxins
- History of neglect, deprivation, or abuse
- For adoptive family, risks associated with required foreign travel (2)

GENERAL PREVENTION

- Required to be examined by a U.S. State Department physician in their native country before immigration to the United States. This is a limited examination targeted at identifying diseases that would exclude qualifying for a visa.
- Should be examined by a U.S. physician within 2 weeks of arrival or sooner if indicated (2)
- A follow-up visit 4–6 weeks after their postadoption appointment is recommended.
- All internationally adopted children should be screened for hearing, vision, growth, and developmental delays (3).
- Travel medicine visit for all family members traveling to adopted child's country (2)
- A preadoption visit between the adoptive family and physician can be helpful in clarifying medical diagnoses, reviewing available medical records as well as photos and/or video that can help to confirm/refute specific diagnoses (1).

COMMONLY ASSOCIATED CONDITIONS

- 60% of international adoptees have a mild to moderate medical or developmental issue (4).
  - 20% have no issue; 20% have a severe problem.
- Infectious diseases, including the following:
  - Hepatitis A/B
  - Intestinal parasites
  - Tuberculosis (TB), primarily latent
  - Syphilis, including inadequately treated
  - HIV
  - *Helicobacter pylori*
- Emotional or behavioral problems
- Developmental delay
- Fetal alcohol syndrome
- Feeding difficulties, malnutrition, rickets
- Anemia
- Congenital conditions (e.g., cleft lip/palate, orthopedic deformities)
- Prematurity or low birth weight
- Inadequate immunizations
- Lead poisoning
- Sensorineural and conductive hearing loss
- Strabismus, blindness

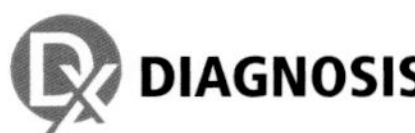

DIAGNOSIS

HISTORY

- Immunization records and titers (records that are "too perfect" should be reviewed carefully)
  - Some vaccinations (e.g., *Haemophilus influenzae* type B [Hib], pneumococcal, varicella) not routine in other countries
  - Measles vaccination may be documented as "MMR," even if not vaccinated against mumps and rubella (5)[C].
- Birth/prenatal history, including exposures
- Known family history of birth parents
- Prenatal and perinatal disease or toxin exposures
- Documented history of emotional or nutritional deprivation, or physical or sexual abuse
- Duration of time, if any, spent in orphanage
- Growth charts when available: Earliest sign of malnutrition is failure to gain weight, followed by slowed linear growth, and finally, lagging head circumference.
- Development, behavior, attachment, parent stress, and parent–child interactions should also be routinely monitored.

PHYSICAL EXAM

- Comprehensive unclothed physical exam, paced to child's comfort; particular attention to
  - Growth parameters
  - General appearance; presence of features suggestive of genetic disorder, syndromes or congenital defects
  - Skin for infection or signs of prior abuse (4)[C]
  - Genitalia for signs of abuse or ritual cutting
  - Neurologic findings
  - May be child's first comprehensive exam; remain sensitive to child's cues and consider translator for older children.
- Evaluate for signs of dental decay, and refer for prompt treatment.
- Developmental assessment, especially for those with unknown date of birth (1)[C]

DIAGNOSTIC TESTS & INTERPRETATION

- Developmental screening: validated developmental screening tools at each visit to screen for potential developmental delay and to assess improvement, decline, and need for additional services
- Age-appropriate hearing and vision screening

Initial Tests (lab, imaging)

- Obtain (1,6)[C],(2,7)[A]
  - Hepatitis A (Hep A IgM, Hep A IgG)
  - Hepatitis B (HBsAg, HBsAb, HBcAb)
  - Hepatitis C (enzyme immunoassay [EIA])
  - HIV 1,2 antibody testing/ELISA
  - Syphilis: nontreponemal (RPR, VDRL, or ART) and treponemal (MHA-TP, FTA-ABS, or TPPA)
  - Tuberculin skin test (TST) in all ages or interferon-gamma release assay ages ≥5 years
  - 3 stool specimens for ova and parasites, specific request for *Giardia intestinalis* and *Cryptosporidium* species testing of one sample
  - CBC with indices and differential
  - Blood lead concentration for ages ≤6 years
  - Thyroid-stimulating hormone (TSH)
  - Urinalysis
  - Hemoglobinopathy/blood disorder screen: sickle cell, thalassemia, glucose-6-phosphate dehydrogenase (G6PD) deficiency
- Consider based on clinical presentation:
  - Stool cultures for bacterial pathogens (for children with diarrhea) (1)[C]
  - *H. pylori* testing (for children with dyspepsia, abdominal pain, or anemia) (6)[C]
  - Ca^{++}, PO_4, alkaline phosphate, and 25 vitamin D level (if signs of rickets) (1)[C]
  - >12 months of age: for Chagas disease via *Trypanosoma cruzi*, serologic testing in adoptees from endemic countries (Mexico, Central and South America)
  - >24 months of age: for lymphatic filariasis in those with eosinophilia if from endemic countries (7)[A]

Follow-Up Tests & Special Considerations

Follow-up testing

ALERT

If initially negative, repeat of HIV, Hep B, Hep C, and TST testing are recommended at 6 months. Negative tests may represent a "window" period or be falsely negative due to malnutrition in the case of TST (6)[C].

- HIV: If antibody positive in children <18 months, confirm with DNA PCR (may represent maternal antibody) (2)[A].
- Hep C: Confirm positive tests with recombinant immunoblot assay (RIBA) and/or HCV RNA PCR. An initial positive in children <18 months may be due to maternal antibody; repeat after 18 months of age.
- Positive TST should NOT be attributed to bacille Calmette-Guérin (BCG) vaccine and must be investigated. If active disease is ruled out, treat for latent TB (6)[C].
- GI tract signs or symptoms occurring years after immigration: test for intestinal parasites.
- Eosinophilia >450 cells/mm^3 with negative stool ova and parasites: serologic testing for *Schistosoma*; add *Strongyloides* for adoptees from sub-Saharan African, Latin American, and Southeast Asian countries (1)[C].
- Developmental screening: Repeat at each visit and follow progress. 50–90% of all internationally adopted children are delayed on adoption; however, most of them have normal cognition at long-term follow-up (3)[C].
- Social history screening: Behavioral concerns may first present during adolescence, even for children adopted in infancy.
- Serial evaluations to age 12 months for children with history of treated congenital syphilis: ophthalmologic, audiologic, neurologic, and developmental (6)[C]

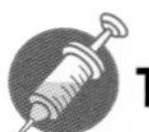

TREATMENT

GENERAL MEASURES

- Regular diet for children who arrive malnourished
- Monitor linear growth.
- If developmental delay is diagnosed, consider early services (e.g., Early Intervention) or referral to developmental specialist.
- Recommend local support groups for parents.
- Attention to parental interactions: Postadoption depression may occur.

MEDICATION

- Immunizations per CDC schedule (http://www.cdc.gov/vaccines/schedules/) with catch-up as needed
- If absent/incomplete records or immunogenicity of vaccines administered are in question, treat as unimmunized.
- Multiple approaches to children vaccinated outside the United States are acceptable (7)[A]:
  - Repeating questionable vaccinations negates the need to obtain serologic tests.
  - To minimize/avoid vaccine administration, check antibody titers (for those >12 months).
- Adoptive parents, caretakers, and household members should be up to date on Tdap, Hep A, Hep B, and measles (2)[A],(4)[C].

ISSUES FOR REFERRAL

- Referrals are often necessary for diagnostic and treatment expertise; however, they should be minimized and planned carefully to ensure adjustment to the new home (1)[C].
  - Elective surgical procedures should likewise be deferred until the child has grown accustomed to his or her new home (3)[C].
- Individual or family counseling considered for all adoptive families for adjustment support
- Internationally adopted children may exhibit self-stimulating behaviors (e.g., rocking, head banging); may be related to prior sensory deprivation. These behaviors typically decrease with time, and no treatment is necessary if otherwise developing normally. If in doubt, refer to developmental pediatrics or occupational therapy.
  - If a child continues to have disruptive behaviors, or would rather self-soothe than seek nurturing human interaction, consider a thorough developmental evaluation.
  - Persistent behavioral issues in the parent–child interactions should be evaluated by a pediatric psychologist or psychiatrist (3)[C].
- Vision (strabismus in 10–25% of previously institutionalized adoptees): Refer to pediatric ophthalmology.
- Hearing (higher rates of conductive and sensorineural hearing loss): Refer to audiology and/or ENT for concerns; questionable screening results or if slow to acquire language skills (3)[C]
- Pediatric dental evaluation by 12 months of age, sooner if signs of dental pathology (1)[C]

ONGOING CARE

FOLLOW-UP RECOMMENDATIONS

Patient Monitoring

- Regular well-child visits, particularly within first months of entry into the United States
- Close monitoring of developmental milestones, behavior, and individual attachment

DIET

- Regular diet
- Up to 68% fall >2 standard deviations below the mean for one/more growth parameters; most begin to follow a curve <2 deviations from the mean in 9–12 months (3).

PATIENT EDUCATION

- Eating: Allow access to as much healthy food as the child wants, as often as he or she wants it, so the child can learn self-regulatory behaviors of eating that may not have been learned in an institution (hunger, satiety) and can build trust with the parent(s) who feed him or her.
- Toileting: Although some children may simply not be trained yet, others who were may regress and have accidents in their new home. Time, positive reinforcement, and avoiding punishment will resolve this issue as the child becomes comfortable with his or her new surroundings.
- Sleeping: Children must learn to trust their new home and parents, and thus this is not a time for aggressive sleep rules. Parents should be present, physically and emotionally, just enough to let the child knows that he or she is safe, establishing, and then gently reinforcing a bedtime ritual on arrival.
- Language: The adoptive family should learn key phrases in the child's native language prior to adoption. A translator should be available for school-aged children for the first few weeks; avoid the perception on the child's part that a translator's presence signifies potential return to his or her country.
- Adopted children may experience grieving of lost family, relationships, and culture, which is common, expected, and healthy behavior; encourage parents to acknowledge and work through this loss with their children, and consider formal counseling, if needed (3).
- Children and families should be encouraged to learn about the culture of the birth country and the ethnic group of origin. This includes forming relationships with others of the same racial or ethnic group (4).

PROGNOSIS

- Degree of recovery of developmental delays is likely dependent on duration of time spent in an institution.
  - Likelihood of long-term developmental, behavioral, or academic problems increases with adoption age.
  - Rate of recovery appears to exceed rate of normal development over a period of years and continues indefinitely (2).
  - There is a good chance that delays can be reversed in children adopted before the age of 2 years (5).
- Some children may regress in previously acquired skills (1).
- When child reaches adolescence, he or she will commonly want to search for his or her biologic family (4).
- Adoption medicine is an evolving specialty, with an ever-increasing number of resources available, including the American Academy of Pediatrics' Council on Foster Care, Adoption, & Kinship Care (http://www2.aap.org/sections/adoption/index.html).

REFERENCES

1. Jones VF, High PC, Donoghue E, et al. Comprehensive health evaluation of the newly adopted child. *Pediatrics*. 2012;129(1):e214–e223.
2. Centers for Disease Control and Prevention. *CDC Health Information for International Travel 2014*. New York, NY: Oxford University Press; 2014.
3. Schulte EE, Springer SH. Health care in the first year after international adoption. *Pediatr Clin North Am*. 2005;52(5):1331–1349, vii.
4. Barratt MS. International adoption. *Pediatr Rev*. 2013;34(3):145–146.
5. Grogg SE, Grogg BC. Intercountry adoptions: medical aspects for the whole family. *J Am Osteopath Assoc*. 2007;107(11):481–489.
6. Miller LC. International adoption: infectious diseases issues. *Clin Infect Dis*. 2005;40(2):286–293.
7. American Academy of Pediatrics. Medical evaluation of internationally adopted children for infectious diseases. In: Pickering LK, ed. *Red Book: 2012 Report of the Committee on Infectious Diseases*. 29th ed. Elk Grove Village, IL: American Academy of Pediatrics; 2012.

ADDITIONAL READING

- Centers for Disease Control and Prevention. General recommendations on immunization: recommendations of the Advisory Committee on Immunization Practices (ACIP). *MMWR Morb Mortal Wkly Rep*. 2011;60(2):27–29.
- Hawk B, McCall RB. CBCL behavior problems of post-institutionalized international adoptees. *Clin Child Fam Psychol Rev*. 2010;13(2):199–211.
- U.S. Department of State, Bureau of Consular Affairs. The Hague Convention on Intercountry Adoption: a guide for prospective adoptive parents. http://travel.state.gov/content/dam/aa/pdfs/PAP_Guide_1.pdf. Accessed 2014.
- Weitzman C, Albers L. Long-term developmental, behavioral, and attachment outcomes after international adoption. *Pediatr Clin North Am*. 2005;52(5):1395–1419, viii.

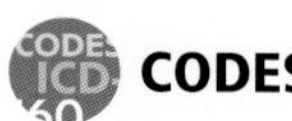

CODES

ICD10

Z02.82 Encounter for adoption services

CLINICAL PEARLS

- Initial labs: Hep B, Hep A, Hep C, HIV 1 and 2, syphilis, CBC, TSH, lead, G6PD deficiency, hemoglobin electrophoresis; TST (or IGRA ages ≥5 years), ova and parasites (3 stool specimens, including single specimen for *G. intestinalis* and *Cryptosporidium parvum* antigens), urinalysis
- If initially negative, repeat of HIV, Hep B, Hep C, and TST testing are recommended at 6 months. Negative tests may represent a "window" period or be falsely negative due to malnutrition in the case of TST.
- Immunizations per CDC schedule with catch-up (http://www.cdc.gov/vaccines/schedules/) as needed. Ensure that adoptive family, caretakers are current on Tdap, Hep A, Hep B, measles.
- Internationally adopted children may exhibit self-stimulating behaviors (e.g., rocking, head banging); may be related to prior sensory deprivation. These behaviors typically decrease with time, and no treatment is necessary if otherwise developing normally. If in doubt, refer to developmental pediatrics or occupational therapy.
- Adoption medicine is an evolving specialty, with an ever-increasing number of resources available, including the American Academy of Pediatrics' Council on Foster Care, Adoption, & Kinship Care (http://www2.aap.org/sections/adoption/index.html).

ALCOHOL ABUSE AND DEPENDENCE

Gennine M. Zinner, RNCS, ANP

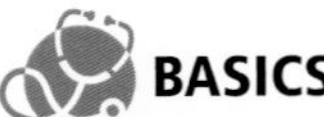

BASICS

DESCRIPTION

- Any pattern of alcohol use causing significant physical, mental, or social dysfunction; key features are tolerance, withdrawal, and persistent use despite problems.
- Alcohol abuse: maladaptive pattern of alcohol use manifested by ≥1 of the following:
  - Failure to fulfill obligations at work, school, or home
  - Recurrent use in hazardous situations
  - Recurrent alcohol-related legal problems
  - Continued use despite related social or interpersonal problems
- Alcohol dependence: maladaptive pattern of use manifested by ≥3 of the following:
  - Tolerance
  - Withdrawal
  - Using more than intended
  - Persistent desire or attempts to cut down/stop
  - Significant amount of time obtaining, using, or recovering from alcohol
  - Social, occupational, or recreational activities sacrificed for alcohol use
  - Continued use despite physical or psychological problems
- National Institute on Alcohol Abuse and Alcoholism criteria for "at-risk" drinking: men: >14 drinks a week or >4 per occasion; women: >7 drinks a week or >3 per occasion
- System(s) affected: nervous, gastrointestinal (GI)
- Synonym(s): alcoholism; alcohol abuse; alcohol dependence

Geriatric Considerations

- Common and underdiagnosed in elderly; less likely to report problem; may exacerbate normal age-related cognitive deficits and disabilities
- Multiple drug interactions
- Signs and symptoms may be different or attributed to chronic medical problem or dementia.
- Common assessment tools may be inappropriate.

Pediatric Considerations

- Children of alcoholics are at increased risk.
- In 2004, 28% of persons 12–20 years reported use in past month, 1 in 5 binge drink; binge drinkers are 7 times more likely to report illicit drug use.
- Negative effect on maturation and development
- Early drinkers are 4 times more likely to develop a problem than those who begin >21 years.
- Depression, suicidal or disorderly behavior, family disruption, violence or destruction of property, poor school or work performance, sexual promiscuity, social immaturity, lack of interests, isolation, moodiness

Pregnancy Considerations

- Alcohol is teratogenic, especially during the 1st trimester; women should abstain during conception and throughout pregnancy.
- 10–50% of children born to women who are heavy drinkers will have fetal alcohol syndrome.
- Women experience harmful effects at lower levels and are less likely to report problems.

EPIDEMIOLOGY

- Predominant age: 18–25 years, but all ages affected
- Predominant sex: male > female (3:1)

Prevalence

- Lifetime prevalence: 13.6%
- 20% in primary care setting
- 48.2% of 21-year-olds in the United States reported binge drinking in 2004.

ETIOLOGY AND PATHOPHYSIOLOGY

- Multifactorial: genetic, environment, psychosocial
- Alcohol is a CNS depressant, facilitating γ-aminobutyric acid (GABA) inhibition and blocking *N*-methyl-D-aspartate receptors.

Genetics

50–60% of risk is genetic.

RISK FACTORS

- Family history
- Depression (40% with comorbid alcohol abuse)
- Anxiety
- Other substance abuse
- Tobacco
- Male gender
- Low socioeconomic status
- Unemployment
- Peer/social approval
- Family dysfunction or childhood trauma
- Posttraumatic stress disorder
- Antisocial personality disorder
- Bipolar disorder
- Eating disorders
- Criminal involvement

GENERAL PREVENTION

Counsel with family history and risk factors

COMMONLY ASSOCIATED CONDITIONS

- Cardiomyopathy, atrial fibrillation
- Hypertension
- Peptic ulcer disease/gastritis
- Cirrhosis, fatty liver, cholelithiasis
- Hepatitis
- Diabetes mellitus
- Pancreatitis
- Malnutrition
- Upper GI malignancies
- Peripheral neuropathy, seizures
- Abuse and violence
- Trauma (falls, motor vehicle accidents [MVAs])
- Severe psychiatric disorders (depression, bipolar, schizophrenia): >50% of patients with these disorders have a comorbid substance abuse problem.

DIAGNOSIS

HISTORY

- Behavioral issues
  - Anxiety, depression, insomnia
  - Psychological and social dysfunction, marital problems
  - Social isolation/withdrawal
  - Domestic violence
  - Alcohol-related legal problems
  - Repeated attempts to stop/reduce
  - Loss of interest in nondrinking activities
  - Employment problems (tardiness, absenteeism, decreased productivity, interpersonal problems, frequent job loss)
  - Blackouts
  - Complaints about alcohol-related behavior
  - Frequent trauma, MVAs, emergency department visits
- Physical symptoms
  - Anorexia
  - Nausea, vomiting, abdominal pain
  - Palpitations
  - Headache
  - Impotence
  - Menstrual irregularities
  - Infertility

PHYSICAL EXAM

- Physical exam may be completely normal.
- General: fever, agitation, diaphoresis
- Head/eyes/ears/nose/throat: plethoric face, rhinophyma, poor oral hygiene, oropharyngeal malignancies
- Cardiovascular: hypertension, dilated cardiomyopathy, tachycardia, arrhythmias
- Respiratory: aspiration pneumonia
- GI: stigmata of chronic liver disease, peptic ulcer disease, pancreatitis, esophageal malignancies, esophageal varices
- Genitourinary: testicular atrophy
- Musculoskeletal: poorly healed fractures, myopathy, osteopenia, osteoporosis, bone marrow suppression
- Neurologic: tremors, cognitive deficits (e.g., memory impairment), peripheral neuropathy, Wernicke-Korsakoff syndrome
- Endocrine/metabolic: hyperlipidemias, cushingoid appearance, gynecomastia
- Dermatologic: burns (e.g., cigarettes), bruises, poor hygiene, palmar erythema, spider telangiectasias, caput medusae, jaundice

DIFFERENTIAL DIAGNOSIS

- Other substance use disorders
- Depression
- Dementia
- Cerebellar ataxia
- Cerebrovascular accident (CVA)
- Benign essential tremor
- Seizure disorder
- Hypoglycemia
- Diabetic ketoacidosis
- Viral hepatitis

DIAGNOSTIC TESTS & INTERPRETATION

- CAGE Questionnaire: (Cut down, Annoyed, Guilty, and Eye opener): >2 "yes" answers is 74–89% sensitive, 79–95% specific for alcohol use disorder; less sensitive for white women, college students, elderly. Not an appropriate tool for less severe forms of alcohol abuse (1)[A]
- AUDIT: Alcohol Use Disorders Identification Test: 10 items, if >4: 70–92% sensitive, better in populations with low incidence of alcoholism (2)[A]: http://www.nams.sg/addictions/Alcohol/Pages/Self-Assessment-Tool.aspx
- Single question for unhealthy use screening: "How many times in the last year have you had X or more drinks in 1 day?" (X = 5 for men, 4 for women); 81.8% sensitive, 79% specific for alcohol use disorders (3)[C]

Initial Tests (lab, imaging)

- CBC; liver function tests (LFTs); electrolytes; BUN/creatinine; lipid panel; thiamine; folate; hepatitis A, B, and C serology
- Amylase, lipase (if GI symptoms present)

- Serum levels increased in chronic abuse:
  - AST/ALT ratio >2.0
  - γ-glutamyl transferase (GGT)
  - Carbohydrate-deficient transferrin
  - Elevated mean corpuscular volume (MCV)
  - Prothrombin time
  - Uric acid
  - Triglycerides and cholesterol (total)
- Often decreased
  - Calcium, magnesium, potassium, phosphorus
  - BUN
  - Hemoglobin, hematocrit
  - Platelet count
  - Serum protein, albumin
  - Thiamine, folate
- Blood alcohol concentration
  - >100 mg/dL in outpatient setting
  - >150 mg/dL without obvious signs of intoxication
  - >300 mg/dL at any time
- CAT scan or MRI of brain: cortical atrophy, lesions in thalamic nucleus and basal forebrain
- Abdominal ultrasound (US): ascites, periportal fibrosis, fatty infiltration, inflammation

Test Interpretation

- Liver: inflammation or fatty infiltration (alcoholic hepatitis), periportal fibrosis (alcoholic cirrhosis occurs in only 10–20% of alcoholics)
- Gastric mucosa: inflammation, ulceration
- Pancreas: inflammation, liquefaction necrosis
- Heart: dilated cardiomyopathy
- Immune system: decreased granulocytes
- Endocrine organs: elevated cortisol levels, testicular atrophy, decreased female hormones
- Brain: cortical atrophy, enlarged ventricles

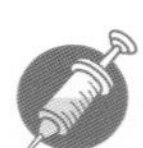

TREATMENT

- For management of acute withdrawal, please see "Alcohol Withdrawal."
- For outpatient withdrawal treatment, see "Alcohol Withdrawal, Treatment" or http://www.aafp.org/afp/2005/0201/p495.html

GENERAL MEASURES

- Brief interventions and counseling by clinicians have proven efficacy for problem drinking (4)[B].
- Treat comorbid problems (sleep, anxiety, etc.); use caution if prescribing medications with cross tolerance to alcohol (benzodiazepine).
- Group programs and/or 12-step programs may have benefit in helping patients accept treatment.
- Research shows the benefit of referring patients with alcohol dependence to an addiction specialist or treatment program (2)[A].

MEDICATION

First Line

- Adjuncts to withdrawal regimens:
  - Naltrexone: 50–100 mg/day PO or 380 mg IM once every 4 weeks; opiate antagonist reduces craving and likelihood of relapse (IM route may enhance compliance and thus efficacy) (2,5)[A].
  - Acamprosate (Campral): 666 mg PO TID beginning after completion of withdrawal; reduces relapse risk. If helpful, recommended to use for 1 year (6)[A].
  - Topiramate (Topamax): 25–300 mg/day PO or divided BID; enhances abstinence (2)[B] (not approved by FDA for use in alcohol dependence; off-label use)
- Supplements to all
  - Thiamine: 100 mg/day (1st dose IV prior to glucose to avoid Wernicke encephalopathy)
  - Folic acid: 1 mg/day
  - Multivitamin daily
- Contraindications
  - Naltrexone: pregnancy, acute hepatitis, hepatic failure
  - Monitor LFTs.
- Precautions: organic pain, organic brain syndromes
- Significant possible interactions: alcohol, sedatives, hypnotics, naltrexone, and narcotics

ALERT
Treat acute symptoms if in alcohol withdrawal; give thiamine 100 mg/day with 1st dose prior to glucose.

Second Line

- Disulfiram: 250–500 mg/day PO; unproven efficacy; may provide psychologic deterrent
- Selective serotonin reuptake inhibitors may be beneficial if comorbid depression exists.

ISSUES FOR REFERRAL

Addiction specialist, 12-step or long-term program, psychiatrist

INPATIENT CONSIDERATIONS

Assess medical and psychiatric condition (CIWA >8).

Admission Criteria/Initial Stabilization

- Correct electrolyte imbalances, acidosis, hypovolemia (treat if in alcohol withdrawal).
- Thiamine: 100 mg IM, followed by 100 mg PO; folic acid: 1 mg/day
- Benzodiazepines used to lower risk of alcohol withdrawal, seizures

ONGOING CARE

FOLLOW-UP RECOMMENDATIONS

Patient Monitoring

- Outpatient detoxification: daily visits (not recommended for heavy alcohol abuse)
- Early outpatient rehabilitation: weekly visits
- Detoxification alone is not sufficient.

PATIENT EDUCATION

- American Council on Alcoholism: (800) 527-5344 or http://www.aca-usa.com (treatment facility locator, educational information)
- National Clearinghouse for Alcohol and Drug Information: (800) 729-6686 or http://www.health.org
- Center for Substance Abuse Treatment: (800) 662-HELP or http://www.csat.samhsa.gov
- Alcoholics Anonymous: http://www.aa.org
- Rational Recovery: http://www.rational.org
- Secular Organizations for Sobriety: http://www.cfiwest.org/sos/index.htm
- http://www.alcoholanswers.org/list: an evidence-based Web site for those seeking credible information on alcohol dependence and online support forums

PROGNOSIS

- Chronic relapsing disease; mortality rate more than twice general population, death 10–15 years earlier
- Abstinence benefits survival, mental health, family, employment
- 12-step programs, cognitive behavior, and motivational therapies are often effective during 1st year following treatment.

COMPLICATIONS

- Cirrhosis (women sooner than men)
- GI malignancies
- Neuropathy, dementia, Wernicke-Korsakoff syndrome
- CVA
- Ketoacidosis
- Infection
- Adult respiratory distress syndrome
- Depression
- Suicide
- Trauma

REFERENCES

1. Dhalla S, Kopec JA. The CAGE questionnaire for alcohol misuse: a review of reliability and validity studies. *Clin Invest Med*. 2007;30(1):33–41.
2. Willenbring ML, Massey SH, Gardner MB. Helping patients who drink too much: an evidence-based guide for primary care physicians. *Am Fam Physician*. 2009;80(1):44–50.
3. Smith PC, Schmidt SM, Allensworth-Davies D, et al. Primary care validation of a single-question alcohol screening test. *J Gen Intern Med*. 2009;24(7):783–788.
4. McQueen J, Howe TE, Allan L, et al. Brief interventions for heavy alcohol users admitted to general hospital wards. *Cochrane Database Syst Rev*. 2011;(8):CD005191.
5. Pettinati HM, Gastfriend DR, Dong Q, et al. Effect of extended-release naltrexone (XR-NTX) on quality of life in alcohol-dependent patients. *Alcohol Clin Exp Res*. 2009;33(2):350–356.
6. Rösner S, Hackl-Herrwerth A, Leucht S, et al. Acamprosate for alcohol dependence. *Cochrane Database Syst Rev*. 2010;(9):CD004332.

ADDITIONAL READING

National Institute on Alcohol Abuse and Alcoholism. Helping patients who drink too much: a clinician's guide. http://www.niaaa.nih.gov/guide. Accessed 2014.

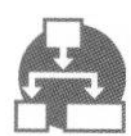

SEE ALSO

Substance Use Disorders, Alcohol Withdrawal

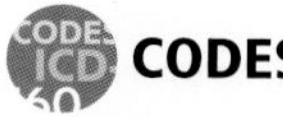

CODES

ICD10

- F10.10 Alcohol abuse, uncomplicated
- F10.20 Alcohol dependence, uncomplicated
- F10.239 Alcohol dependence with withdrawal, unspecified

CLINICAL PEARLS

- CAGE Questionnaire: >2 "yes" answers is 74–89% sensitive, 79–95% specific for alcohol use disorder; less sensitive for white women, college students, elderly. Not an appropriate tool for less severe forms of alcohol abuse
- Single question for unhealthy use screening: "How many times in the last year have you had X or more drinks in 1 day?" (X = 5 for men, 4 for women); 81.8% sensitive, 79% specific for alcohol use disorders
- National Institute on Alcohol Abuse and Alcoholism criteria for "at-risk" drinking: men >14 drinks a week or >4 per occasion; women: >7 drinks a week or >3 per occasion

ALCOHOL WITHDRAWAL

Neela Bhajandas, PharmD • Paul N. Williams, MD

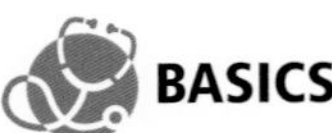

BASICS

DESCRIPTION

Alcohol withdrawal syndrome (AWS) is a spectrum of symptoms that results from abrupt cessation of alcohol in a dependent patient. Symptoms can begin within 5 hours of the last drink and persist for 5–10 days, ranging in severity.

EPIDEMIOLOGY

Each year, 8.2 million Americans meet diagnostic criteria for alcohol dependence. Data suggest that 2–9% of patients seen in a family physician's office have alcohol dependence. It is more prevalent among men, whites, Native Americans, younger and unmarried adults, and those with lower socioeconomic status; only 24% of those with dependence are ever treated. <5% of U.S. adults will experience withdrawal, but 8% of hospitalized patients exhibit signs and symptoms of withdrawal.

ETIOLOGY AND PATHOPHYSIOLOGY

- Consumption of alcohol potentiates the effect of the inhibitory neurotransmitter γ-aminobutyric acid (GABA). With chronic alcohol ingestion, this repeated stimulation downregulates the inhibitory effects of GABA.
- Concurrently, alcohol ingestion inhibits the stimulatory effect of glutamate on the CNS, with chronic alcohol use upregulating excitatory NMDA glutamate receptors.
- When alcohol is abruptly stopped, the combined effect of a downregulated inhibitory neurotransmitter system (GABA-modulated) and upregulated excitatory neurotransmitter system (glutamate-modulated) results in brain hyperexcitability when no longer suppressed by alcohol; clinically seen as AWS

Genetics

There is some evidence for a genetic basis of alcohol dependence.

RISK FACTORS

- High tolerance, prolonged use, high quantities
- Previous alcohol withdrawal episodes, detoxifications, alcohol withdrawal seizures, and delirium tremens (DTs)
- Serious medical problems
- Concomitant benzodiazepine (BZD) dependence

Geriatric Considerations

Elderly dependent on alcohol are more susceptible to withdrawal, and chronic comorbid conditions place them at higher risk of complications from withdrawal.

Pregnancy Considerations

Hospitalization or inpatient detoxification is usually required for treatment of acute alcohol withdrawal.

GENERAL PREVENTION

- Routinely screen all adults for alcohol misuse (1)[B].
- Screen with the **CAGE** or similar questionnaire:
  - Feeling the need to **C**ut down
  - **A**nnoyed by criticism about alcohol use
  - **G**uilt about drinking/behaviors while intoxicated
  - "**E**ye opener" to quell withdrawal symptoms
  - Useful to detect problematic alcohol use, positive screen is ≥2 "yes" responses.
- 10-question AUDIT screening test is also useful to identify problem drinking.
- The "5 A's" is a screening tool used in primary care settings (Assess, Advise, Agree, Assist, Arrange).

COMMONLY ASSOCIATED CONDITIONS

- General: poor nutrition, electrolyte abnormalities (hyponatremia, hypomagnesemia, hypophosphatemia), thiamine deficiency, and dehydration
- GI: hepatitis, cirrhosis, varices, GI bleed
- Heme: splenomegaly, thrombocytopenia, macrocytic anemia
- Cardiovascular: cardiomyopathy, hypertension, atrial fibrillation, other arrhythmias
- CNS: trauma, seizure disorder, generalized atrophy, Wernicke-Korsakoff syndrome
- Peripheral nervous system: neuropathy, myopathy
- Pulmonary: aspiration pneumonitis or pneumonia; increased risk of anaerobic infections
- Psychiatric: depression, posttraumatic stress disorder, bipolar disease, polysubstance abuse

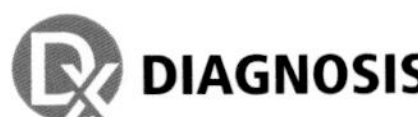

DIAGNOSIS

- *Diagnostic and Statistical Manual of Mental Disorders* AWS criteria are diagnosed when ≥2 of the following present within a few hours to several days after the cessation or reduction of heavy and prolonged alcohol ingestion 2[C]:
  - Autonomic hyperactivity (sweating, tachycardia)
  - Increased hand tremor
  - Insomnia
  - Psychomotor agitation
  - Anxiety
  - Nausea
  - Vomiting
  - Grand mal seizures
  - Transient (visual, auditory, or tactile) hallucinations or illusions
- These should cause clinically significant distress or impair functioning and not be secondary to an underlying medical condition or mental disorder.
- There are 3 stages of AWS:
  - Stage 1 (minor withdrawal; onset 5–8 hours after cessation)
    - Mild anxiety, restlessness, and agitation
    - Mild nausea/GI upset and decreased appetite
    - Sleep disturbance
    - Sweating
    - Mild tremulousness
    - Fluctuating tachycardia and hypertension
  - Stage 2 (major withdrawal; onset 24–72 hours after cessation)
    - Marked restlessness and agitation
    - Moderate tremulousness with constant eye movements
    - Diaphoresis
    - Nightmares
    - Nausea, vomiting, diarrhea, anorexia
    - Marked tachycardia and hypertension
    - Alcoholic hallucinosis (auditory, tactile, or visual) may have mild confusion but can be reoriented.
  - Stage 3 (DTs; onset 72–96 hours after cessation)
    - Fever
    - Severe hypertension, tachycardia
    - Delirium
    - Drenching sweats
    - Marked tremors
    - Persistent hallucinations
- Alcohol withdrawal–associated seizures are often brief, generalized tonic–clonic seizures, and can occur 6–48 hours after last drink.

HISTORY

Essential historical information should be as follows:

- Duration and quantity of alcohol intake, time since last drink
- Previous episodes/symptoms of alcohol withdrawal, prior detox admissions
- Concurrent substance use
- Preexisting medical and psychiatric conditions, prior seizure activity
- Social history: living situation, social support, stressors, triggers, etc.

PHYSICAL EXAM

Should include assessment of conditions likely to complicate or that are exacerbated by AWS

- Cardiovascular: arrhythmias, heart failure, coronary artery disease
- GI: GI bleed, liver disease, pancreatitis
- Neuro: oculomotor dysfunction, gait ataxia, neuropathy
- Psych: orientation, memory (may be complicated by hepatic encephalopathy)
- General: hand tremor (6–8 cycles per second), infections

DIFFERENTIAL DIAGNOSIS

- Cocaine intoxication
- Opioid, marijuana, and methamphetamine withdrawal
- Anticholinergic drug toxicity
- Neuroleptic malignant syndrome
- ICU delirium
- Liver failure
- Sepsis, CNS infection, or hemorrhage
- Mania, psychosis
- Thyroid crisis (3)[C]

DIAGNOSTIC TESTS & INTERPRETATION

Initial Tests (lab, imaging)

- Blood alcohol level, urine drug screen
- CBC; comprehensive metabolic panel
- CNS imaging if acute mental status changes

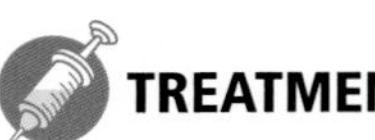

TREATMENT

- The goal is to prevent and treat withdrawal symptoms (e.g., seizures, DTs, cardiovascular events). This is done primarily with BZDs, which reduce the duration of symptoms and raise the seizure threshold:
  - Exclude other medical and psychiatric causes.
  - Provide a quiet, protective environment.
  - The Clinical Institute Withdrawal Assessment for Alcohol Scale revised (CIWA-Ar) is useful for determining medication dosing and frequency of evaluation for AWS. Severity of symptoms are rated on a scale from 0 to 7, with 0 being without symptoms and 7 being the maximum score (except orientation and clouding of sensorium, scale 0–4):
    - Nausea and vomiting
    - Tremor
    - Paroxysmal sweats
    - Anxiety
    - Agitation
    - Tactile disturbances
    - Auditory disturbances
    - Visual disturbances
    - Headache or fullness in head
    - Orientation and clouding of sensorium
- Frequent reevaluation with CIWA-Ar score is crucial.

MEDICATION

First Line

- BZD monotherapy remains the treatment of choice (4)[A]; it is associated with fewer complications compared with neuroleptics (5)[A].
- BZD should be chosen by the following considerations:
  - Agents with rapid onset control agitation more quickly (e.g., IV diazepam [Valium]).
  - Long-acting BZDs (diazepam, chlordiazepoxide [Librium]) are more effective at preventing breakthrough seizures and delirium management.
  - Short-acting BZDs (lorazepam [Ativan], oxazepam [Serax]) are preferable when prolonged sedation is a concern (e.g., elderly patients or other serious concomitant medical illness) and preferable when severe hepatic insufficiency may impair metabolism (5)[A].
- BZD dosages will vary by patients. Given as symptom-triggered or fixed-schedule regimens. Symptom-triggered regimens have been found to require less BZD amounts and reduce hospitalization time (3)[A].
- Symptom-triggered regimen: Start with chlordiazepoxide 50–100 mg PO, repeat CIWA-Ar hourly and if score is ≥8, give additional dose of chlordiazepoxide 50 mg PO. Continue to reevaluate with CIWA-Ar hourly until adequate sedation achieved (score chlordiazepoxide with respective doses of diazepam, lorazepam, or oxazepam (3)[C].

Second Line

- Thiamine: 100 mg daily IV or IM for at least 3 days (5)[C]
  - Note that IV glucose administered before treatment with thiamine may precipitate Wernicke encephalopathy and Korsakoff psychosis.
- β-Blockers (e.g., atenolol [Tenormin]) and α_2-agonists (e.g., clonidine [Catapres]) help to control hypertension and tachycardia and can be used with BZDs (3)[C]. Not used as monotherapy, due to their inability to prevent DTs and seizures. May worsen underlying delirium.
- Carbamazepine: Not recommended as 1st-line therapy; associated with reduced incidence of seizures, but more studies are needed.
- If the patient exhibits significant agitation and alcoholic hallucinosis, an antipsychotic (4,6)[C] (haloperidol [Haldol]) can be used, but this requires close observation, as it lowers the seizure threshold (3)[C].

ADDITIONAL THERAPIES

Peripheral neuropathy and cerebellar dysfunction merit physical therapy evaluation.

INPATIENT CONSIDERATIONS

Patients in withdrawal stages 1 and 2 can be treated as outpatients unless medical comorbidities require inpatient care. A reliable and supportive social environment should be in place with frequent follow-up.

Admission Criteria/Initial Stabilization

- CIWA score >15, or severe withdrawal
- Concurrent acute illness requiring in patient care
- Poor ability to follow up or no reliable social support
- Pregnancy
- Seizure disorder or history of severe alcohol-related seizures
- Suicide risk
- Concurrent BZD dependence
- Age >40 years old
- Prolonged heavy drinking >8 years
- Consumes >1 pint of alcohol or 12 beers per day
- Random blood alcohol level >200 mg/dL
- Elevated MCV, BUN
- Cirrhosis, liver failure

Discharge Criteria

CIWA scores of <10 on 3 consecutive determinations

ONGOING CARE

FOLLOW-UP RECOMMENDATIONS

- Discharge arrangements include transfer to a treatment facility (e.g., sober house or residential program), outpatient substance abuse counseling, peer support groups (Alcoholics Anonymous), and the use of adjuvant treatment such as disulfiram (Antabuse), acamprosate (Campral), or naltrexone (ReVia, Vivitrol).
- Disulfiram: Irreversibly inhibits aldehyde dehydrogenase, blocking alcohol metabolism, leading to an accumulation of acetaldehyde; therefore, it reinforces the individual's desires to stop drinking by providing a disincentive associated with increased acetaldehyde:
  - 250–500 mg/day PO × 1–2 weeks; maintenance 250 mg/day PO
  - Contraindications: Concomitant use of metronidazole and ethanol-containing products, psychosis, severe myocardial disease, and coronary occlusion
- Acamprosate (666 mg PO TID): Glutamate and GABA modulator indicated to reduce cravings:
  - Contraindications: renal impairment (CrCl <30 mL/min)
- Naltrexone (50 mg/day PO; 380 mg IM every 4 weeks): Opiate receptor antagonist, theorized to attenuate pleasurable effects of alcohol and reduce craving. Initiate therapy after patient is opioid-free for at least 7 days:
  - Contraindications: acute hepatitis/liver failure, concomitant opioid therapy

Patient Monitoring

Frequent follow-up to monitor for relapse

PATIENT EDUCATION

- Alcoholics Anonymous: www.aa.org
- SMART Recovery (Self-Management and Recovery Training): www.smartrecovery.org (not spiritually based)
- National Institute on Alcohol Abuse and Alcoholism: www.niaaa.nih.gov
- FamilyDoctor.Org: alcoholism (Spanish resources available)

PROGNOSIS

Mortality from severe withdrawal (DTs) is 1–5%.

COMPLICATIONS

Occurs more frequently in individuals who have prior episodes of withdrawal or concomitant illnesses

REFERENCES

1. U.S. Preventive Services Task Force. Screening and behavioral counseling interventions in primary care to reduce alcohol misuse: U.S. Preventive Services Task Force recommendation statement. *Ann Intern Med*. 2013;159(3):210–218.
2. American Psychiatric Association. *Diagnostic and Statistical Manual of Mental Disorders*. 5th ed. Arlington, VA: American Psychiatric Association; 2013.
3. Mayo-Smith MF. Pharmacological management of alcohol withdrawal: a meta-analysis and evidence-based practice guideline. *JAMA*. 1997;278(2):144–151.
4. Amato L, Minozzi S, Vecchi S, et al. Benzodiazepines for alcohol withdrawal. *Cochrane Database Syst Rev*. 2010;(3):CD005063.
5. Amato L, Minozzi S, Davoli M. Efficacy and safety of pharmacological interventions for the treatment of the alcohol withdrawal syndrome. *Cochrane Database Syst Rev*. 2011;(6):CD008537.
6. Minozzi S, Amato L, Vecchi S, et al. Anticonvulsants for alcohol withdrawal. *Cochrane Database Syst Rev*. 2010;(3):CD005064.

ADDITIONAL READING

Sarff M, Gold JA. Alcohol withdrawal syndromes in the intensive care unit. *Crit Care Med*. 2010;38(9)(Suppl):S494–S501.

SEE ALSO

Substance Use Disorders

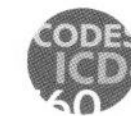

CODES

ICD10

- F10.239 Alcohol dependence with withdrawal, unspecified
- F10.230 Alcohol dependence with withdrawal, uncomplicated
- F10.231 Alcohol dependence with withdrawal delirium

CLINICAL PEARLS

- The *kindling phenomenon* has postulated that long-term exposure to alcohol affects neurons, resulting in increased alcohol craving and progressively worse withdrawal episodes (also known as *allostasis*).
- The CIWA-Ar is a useful tool for managing the symptoms and treatment of alcohol withdrawal.
- Any BZD dose should be patient-specific, sufficient to achieve and maintain a "light somnolence" (e.g., sleeping but easily arousable), and should be tapered off carefully even after AWS resolves.
- Administer thiamine before patient receives glucose, so as not to precipitate Wernicke encephalopathy.
- There should be frequent outpatient follow-up to monitor for relapse.
- Counsel patients taking disulfiram to avoid over-the-counter products that contain alcohol (i.e., mouthwashes).
- Avoid administering diazepam and lorazepam intramuscularly (i.e., IM diazepam or IM lorazepam) because of erratic absorption.

ALOPECIA

Amy M. Zack, MD, FAAFP

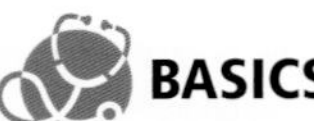

BASICS

DESCRIPTION

- Alopecia: absence of hair from areas where it normally grows
  - Anagen phase: growing hairs, 90% scalp hair follicles at any time, lasts 2–6 years
  - Catagen phase: regression of follicle, <1% follicles, lasts 3 weeks
  - Telogen phase: Resting phase lasts 2–3 months, 50–150 telogen hairs shed per day.
- Classified as scarring (cicatricial), nonscarring, or structural
- Scarring (cicatricial) alopecia
  - Inflammatory disorders leading to *permanent* hair loss and follicle destruction
  - Includes lymphocytic, neutrophilic, and mixed subtypes
- Nonscarring alopecia
  - Lack of inflammation, no destruction of follicle
  - Includes focal, patterned, and diffuse hair loss such as androgenic alopecia, alopecia areata, telogen effluvium, anagen effluvium, syphilitic hair loss
- Structural hair disorders
  - Brittle or fragile hair from abnormal hair formation or external insult

EPIDEMIOLOGY

- Androgenic alopecia: onset in males between 20 and 25 years of age. Onset in females prior to 40 years of age, affecting as many as 70% of women older than 65 years of age
- Alopecia areata: onset usually prior to 30 years of age; men and women are equally affected. Well-documented genetic predisposition

Incidence

Incidence greatest in Caucasians, followed by Asians, African Americans, and Native Americans. In females, 13% premenopausal, with as many as 70% females older than 65 years of age

Prevalence

- Androgenic alopecia: in males, 30% Caucasian by 30 years of age, 50% by 50 years of age, and 80% by 70 years of age
- Alopecia areata: 1/1000 with lifetime risk of 1–2%
- Scarring alopecia: rare, 3–7% of all hair disorder patients

ETIOLOGY AND PATHOPHYSIOLOGY

- Scarring (cicatricial) alopecia
  - Slick smooth scalp without follicles evident
  - Inflammatory disorders leading to permanent destruction of the follicle; it is not known what causes inflammation to develop.
  - Three major subtypes based on type of inflammation: lymphocytic, neutrophilic, and mixed
  - Primary scarring includes discoid lupus, lichen planopilaris, dissecting cellulitis of scalp, among others.
  - Secondary scarring from infection, neoplasm, radiation, surgery, and other physical trauma, including tinea capitis
- Nonscarring alopecia
  - Focal alopecia
  - Alopecia areata
    - Patchy hair loss, usually autoimmune in etiology, T-cell–mediated inflammation resulting in premature transition to catagen then telogen phases
    - May occur with hair loss in other areas of the body (alopecia totalis [entire scalp]), alopecia universalis (rapid loss of all body hair)
    - Nail disease frequently seen
    - High psychiatric comorbidity (1)
  - Alopecia syphilitica: "moth-eaten" appearance, secondary syphilis
  - Postoperative, pressure-induced alopecia: from long periods of pressure on one area of scalp
  - Temporal triangular alopecia: congenital patch of hair loss in temporal area, unilateral or bilateral
  - Traction alopecia: patchy, due to physical stressor of braids, ponytails, hair weaves
- Pattern hair loss
  - Androgenic alopecia: hair transitions from terminal to vellus hairs
  - Male pattern hair loss: androgen-mediated hair loss in specific distribution; bitemporal, vertex occurs where androgen sensitive hairs are located on scalp (2)
    - Increased androgen receptors, increased 5-alpha reductase leads to increased testosterone conversion in follicle to dihydrotestosterone (DHT). This leads to decreased follicle size and vellus hair (2).
    - Norwood Hamilton Classification type I–VII
    - Female pattern hair loss: thinning on frontal and vertex areas. (Ludwig Classification, grade I–III). Females with low levels of aromatase have more testosterone available for conversion to DHT (3).
    - Polycystic ovarian syndrome, adrenal hyperplasia, and pituitary hyperplasia all lead to androgen changes and can result in alopecia.
  - Drugs (testosterone, progesterone, danazol, adrenocorticosteroids, anabolic steroids)
- Trichotillomania: intentional pulling of hair from scalp. May present in variety of patterns
- Diffuse alopecia
  - Telogen effluvium: sudden shift of many follicles from anagen to telogen phase resulting in decreased hair density but not bald areas
    - May follow major stressors, including childbirth, injury, illness. Occurs 2–3 months after event
    - Can be chronic with ongoing illness, including SLE, renal failure, IBS, HIV, thyroid disease, pituitary dysfunction
    - Adding or changing medications (oral contraceptives, anticoagulants, anticonvulsants, SSRIs, retinoids, β-blockers, ACE inhibitors, colchicine, cholesterol-lowering medications, etc.)
    - Malnutrition from malabsorption, eating disorders; poor diet can contribute
  - Anagen effluvium
    - Interruption of the anagen phase without transition to telogen phase. Days to weeks after inciting event
    - Chemotherapy is most common trigger.
    - Radiation, poisoning, and medications can also trigger.
- Structural hair disorders
  - Multiple inherited hair disorders including Menkes disease, monilethrix, and so forth. These result in the formation of abnormal hairs that are weakened.
  - May also result from chemical or heat damaging from hair processing treatments

Genetics

- Family history of early patterned hair loss is common in androgenic alopecia, also in alopecia areata.
- Rare structural hair disorders may be inherited.

RISK FACTORS

- Genetic predisposition
- Chronic illness including autoimmune disease, infections, cancer
- Physiologic stress including pregnancy
- Poor nutrition
- Medication, chemotherapy, radiation
- Hair treatments, braids, weaves

GENERAL PREVENTION

Minimize risk factors where possible.

COMMONLY ASSOCIATED CONDITIONS

- See "Etiology and Pathophysiology."
- Vitiligo—4.1% patients with alopecia areata (AA), may be the result of similar autoimmune pathways (4).

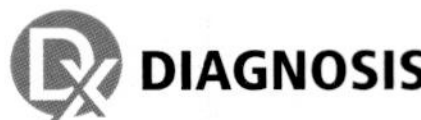

DIAGNOSIS

HISTORY

- Description of hair loss problem: rate of loss, duration, location, degree of hair loss, other symptoms including pruritus, infection, hair care, and treatments
- Medications
- Medical illness including chronic disease, recent illness, surgeries, pregnancy, thyroid disorder, iron deficiency, poisonings, exposures
- Psychological stress
- Dietary history and weight changes
- Family history of hair loss or autoimmune disorders

PHYSICAL EXAM

- Pattern of hair loss
  - Generalized, patterned, focal
  - Assess hair density, vellus versus terminal hairs, broken hair
- Scalp scaling, inflammation, papules, pustules
- Presence of follicular ostia to determine class of alopecia
- Hair pull test
  - Pinch 25–50 hairs between thumb and forefinger and exert slow, gentle traction while sliding fingers up.
    - Normal: 1–2 dislodge
    - Abnormal: ≥6 hairs dislodged
    - Broken hairs (structural disorder)
    - Broken-off hair at the borders patch that are easily removable (in alopecia areata)
- Hair loss at other sites, nail disorders, skin changes
- Clinical signs of thyroid disease, lupus, or other diseases
- Clinical signs of virilization: acne, hirsutism, acanthosis nigricans, truncal obesity

DIFFERENTIAL DIAGNOSIS

Search for type of alopecia and then for reversible causes.

DIAGNOSTIC TESTS & INTERPRETATION

Initial Tests (lab, imaging)

- No testing may be indicated depending on clinical appearance.
- Nonandrogenic alopecia
  - TSH, CBC, ferritin
  - Consider: LFT, BMP, zinc, VDRL, ANA, prolactin all depending on clinical history and exam
- Androgenic alopecia: especially in females
  - Consider free testosterone and dehydroepiandrosterone sulfate.

Diagnostic Procedures/Other

- Light hair-pull test: Pull on 25–50 hairs; ≥6 hairs dislodged is consistent with shedding (effluvium, alopecia areata).
- Direct microscopic exam of the hair shaft
  - Anagen hairs: elongated, distorted bulb with root sheath attached
  - Telogen hairs: rounded bulb, no root sheath
  - Exclamation point hairs: club-shaped root with thinner proximal shaft (alopecia areata)
  - Broken and distorted hairs may be associated with multiple hair dystrophies.
- Biopsy: most important in scarring alopecia
- Ultraviolet light fluorescence and potassium hydroxide prep (to rule out tinea capitis)

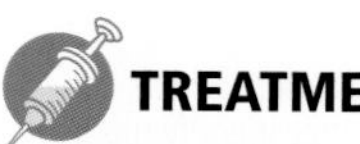

TREATMENT

GENERAL MEASURES

- Stop any possible medication causes if possible; this will often resolve telogen effluvium (5)[C].
- Treat underlying medical causes (e.g., thyroid disorder, syphilis).
- Traction alopecia: Change hair care practices; education.
- Trichotillomania: often requires psychological intervention to induce behavior change

MEDICATION

- *Nonscarring*
  - Androgenic alopecia: Treatment must be continued indefinitely. Can use in combination
  - Minoxidil (Rogaine): 2% topical solution (1 mL BID) for women, 5% topical solution (1 mL BID) or foam (daily) for men. Works in 60% of cases (2,3)[A]
    - Unclear mechanism of action; appears to prolong anagen phase (2)[A]
    - Adverse effects: skin irritation, hypertrichosis of face/hands, tachycardia. Category C in pregnancy (2,3)[A]
  - Finasteride (Propecia): 1 mg/day for men and women (off label) (6,7)[A]
    - 5-alpha reductase inhibitor, reduces DHT in system, increases total and anagen hairs, slows transition of terminal to vellus hairs
    - Works best on vertex, least in anterior, temporal areas (2)[A]
    - Adverse effects: loss of libido, gynecomastia, depression. Caution in liver disease. Absolutely no use or contact during pregnancy, category X, reliable contraception required in female use (7)[A]
  - Spironolactone (Aldactone): 100–200 mg/day (off-label) (3)[C]
    - Aldosterone antagonist, antiandrogen; blocks the effect of androgens, decreasing testosterone production
    - Adverse effects: dose-dependent, hyperkalemia, menstrual irregularity, fatigue; category D in pregnancy
  - Ketoconazole: decreases DHT levels at follicle, works best with minoxidil in female androgenic alopecia (7)[A]
  - Alopecia areata: no FDA-approved treatment; high rate of spontaneous remission in patchy AA
- Intralesional steroids
  - Triamcinolone: 2.5–5 mg/mL (3,7)[C]
    - First line if <50% scalp involved
    - Inject 0.1 mL into deep dermal layer at 0.5–1 cm intervals with ½ in 30-gauge needle, every 4–6 weeks. Maximum 20 mg/session (1)[C]
    - Adverse effects: local burning, pruritus, skin atrophy
  - Topical steroids: very limited evidence for efficacy
  - Betamethasone: 0.1% foam shows limited hair regrowth (1)[C].
    - Adverse effects: folliculitis, high relapse rate after discontinuation
  - Systemic glucocorticoids: use in extensive AA. May induce regrowth but requires long-term monthly treatment to maintain growth (1)[B]
    - Adverse effects: hyperglycemia, adrenal insufficiency, osteoporosis, cataracts, obesity
    - Psychiatric: SSRIs, psychiatric care, support groups
  - Tinea capitis: see "Tinea (Capitis, Corporis, Cruris)"

SURGERY/OTHER PROCEDURES

- Hair transplantation
- Wigs, hairpieces, extensions
- Surgical: graft transplantation, flap transplantation, or excision of the scarred area; used primarily in scarring alopecia
- Laser therapies to promote growth: lacks evidence (2)[A]

COMPLEMENTARY & ALTERNATIVE MEDICINE

- Many herbal medications are available; no clear evidence at this time.
- Volumizing shampoos can help remaining hair look fuller.

ONGOING CARE

DIET

If nutritional deficit noted, supplementation may be necessary.

PATIENT EDUCATION

National Alopecia Areata Foundation: www.naaf.org

PROGNOSIS

- *Androgenic alopecia*: Prognosis depends on response to treatment.
- *Alopecia areata*: often regrows within 1 year even without treatment. Recurrence common. 10% have severe, chronic form. Poor prognosis more likely with long duration, extensive hair loss, autoimmune disease, nail involvement, and young age.
- *Telogen effluvium*: maximum shedding 3 months after the inciting event and recovery following correction of the cause. Usually subsides in 3–6 months but takes 12–18 months for cosmetically significant regrowth. Rarely, permanent hair loss, usually with long-term illness
- *Anagen effluvium*: Shedding begins days to a few weeks after the inciting event, with recovery following correction of the cause. Rarely, permanent hair loss
- *Traction alopecia*: excellent prognosis with behavior modification
- *Cicatricial alopecia*: hair follicles permanently damaged; prognosis depends on type of alopecia and available treatments
- *Tinea capitis*: excellent prognosis with treatment

REFERENCES

1. Alkhalifah A. Alopecia areata update. *Dermatol Clin*. 2013;31(1):93–108.
2. Banka N, Bunagan MJ, Shapiro J. Pattern hair loss in men: diagnosis and medical treatment. *Dermatol Clin*. 2013;31(1):129–140.
3. Rathnayake D, Sinclair R. Innovative use of spironolactone as an antiandrogen in the treatment of female pattern hair loss. *Dermatol Clin*. 2010;28(3):611–618.
4. Kumar S, Mittal J, Mahajan B. Colocalization of vitiligo and alopecia areata: coincidence or consequence? *Int J Trichology*. 2013;5(1):50–52.
5. Harrison S, Bergfeld W. Diffuse hair loss: its triggers and management. *Cleve Clin J Med*. 2009;76(6):361–367.
6. BMJ Best Practice. http://bestpractice.bmj.com/best- practice/monograph/223/basics/epidemiology.html. Accessed May 30, 2013.
7. Atanaskova Mesinkovska N, Bergfled W. Hair: what's new in diagnosis and management? Female pattern hair loss update: diagnosis and treatment. *Dermatol Clin*. 2013;31(1):119–127.

ADDITIONAL READING

Otberg N. Primary cicatricial alopecias. *Dermatol Clin*. 2013;31(1):155–166.

SEE ALSO

- Tinea (Capitis, Corporis, Cruris); Syphilis; Systemic Lupus Erythematosus; Polycystic Ovarian Syndrome; Lichen Planus; Hyperthyroidism
- Algorithm: Alopecia

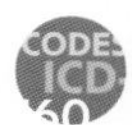

CODES

ICD10

- L65.9 Nonscarring hair loss, unspecified
- L64.9 Androgenic alopecia, unspecified
- L63.9 Alopecia areata, unspecified

CLINICAL PEARLS

- History and physical are necessary in determining type of alopecia for appropriate treatment.
- Treatment of underlying medical condition or removal of triggering medication will often resolve hair loss.
- Educating the patient about the nature of the condition and expectations is key to care.
- Alopecia can affect the psychological condition of the patient, and it may be necessary to address this in any type of hair loss.

ALZHEIMER DISEASE

Jill A. Grimes, MD, FAAFP

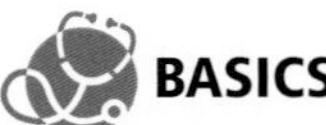

BASICS

DESCRIPTION

- Alzheimer disease (AD) is the most common cause of dementia in the elderly.
- Degenerative neurologic disease with progressive impairment in ≥2:
  - Memory, executive function, attention, language, or visuospatial skills
  - With significant interference in ability to function in work, home, or social interactions
- *New diagnostic criteria* released in 2011 emphasize full spectrum of disease (1)[A]:
  - Preclinical AD (*research purposes only*: biomarkers present; subtle decline evident to patient, but cognitive tests in "normal" range)
  - Mild cognitive impairment (MCI): Social, occupational, and functional skills are preserved despite significant decline in cognition.
  - Alzheimer dementia
- System(s) affected: nervous
- Synonym(s): presenile dementia; senile dementia of the Alzheimer type

Geriatric Considerations

Asymptomatic screening is not recommended.

EPIDEMIOLOGY

- Predominant age: >65 years
- 2/3 females, 1/3 males in United States

Incidence

1 in 8 Americans age >65 years (13%); nearly 50% once >85 years

Prevalence

>5.2 million in United States

- 200,000 younger onset (<65 years)

ETIOLOGY AND PATHOPHYSIOLOGY

- Unknown, but involves amyloid beta accumulation initially, then synaptic dysfunction, neurodegeneration, and eventual neuronal loss
- Age, genetics, systemic disease, behaviors (smoking), and other host factors may influence the response to amyloid beta and/or the pace of progression toward the clinical manifestations of AD.

Genetics

- Positive family history in 50%, but 90% of AD is sporadic:
  - APOE4 increases risk, but full role unclear
- Familial/autosomal dominant AD accounts for <5% AD:
  - Amyloid precursor protein (APP), presenilin-1 (PS-1), and presenilin-2 (PS-2)

RISK FACTORS

- Aging, family history, APOE4, Down syndrome
- Cardiovascular and carotid artery disease
- Smoking (2–4-fold increase)
- Head trauma

GENERAL PREVENTION

- NSAIDs estrogen, and vitamin E do NOT delay AD; insufficient evidence for statins (2)[A].
- Intellectual challenge (puzzles) and regular physical exercise may offer preventive benefit.
- Control vascular risk factors (e.g., hypertension); lowering cholesterol may retard pathogenesis of AD.
- Ginkgo biloba may be beneficial for cognition but not activities of daily living.
- Physical activities and omega-3 fatty acids may help to prevent or delay cognitive decline.
- Ultrasound (US) may help to identify asymptomatic patients at increased risk with chronic brain hypoperfusion secondary to cardiovascular or carotid artery pathology.

COMMONLY ASSOCIATED CONDITIONS

- Down syndrome
- Depression

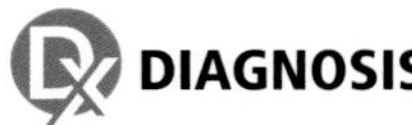

DIAGNOSIS

Degenerative neurologic disease with *progressive impairment in ≥2 areas*:

- Memory, executive function, attention, language, or visuospatial skills AND
- Significant interference in ability to function in work, home, or social interactions

HISTORY

- Include family members in interview (for accuracy and for behavioral assessment).
- Progressive and disruptive memory loss
- Depression, anhedonia, or apathy
- Intellectual decline, difficulty with calculations, multiple missed appointments
- Loss of interest, social withdrawal
- Date or time confusion
- Occupational dysfunction or personality change
- Restlessness and sleep disturbances

PHYSICAL EXAM

- Neurologic exam to rule out other causes
- Folstein Mini-Mental State Exam (MMSE): copyrighted but available (http://www.aafp.org/afp/20010215/703.html)
- Counting coins test: "If I gave you a nickel, quarter, dime, and penny, how much is that?"
- No focal neurologic signs
- Short-term memory loss
- Acalculia (e.g., cannot balance checkbook)
- Agnosia: inability to recognize objects
- Apraxia: inability to carry out movements
- Confabulation
- Delusions
- Impaired abstraction
- Decreased attention to hygiene
- Visuospatial distortion
- Late signs: psychotic features, mutism

DIFFERENTIAL DIAGNOSIS

- Depression
- Vascular dementia, multi-infarct dementia
- Lewy body disease
- Dementia associated with Parkinson disease
- Normal pressure hydrocephalus
- Creutzfeldt-Jakob disease
- End-stage multiple sclerosis
- Brain tumor: primary or metastatic
- Subdural hematoma
- Progressive multifocal leukoencephalopathy
- Metabolic dementia (hypothyroidism)
- Drug reactions, alcoholism, other addictions
- Dementia pugilistica
- Toxicity from liver and kidney failure
- Vitamin and other nutritional deficiencies
- Vasculitis
- Neurosyphilis

DIAGNOSTIC TESTS & INTERPRETATION

Neuropsychological testing: Order if clinical picture is confusing or to help determine level of independence for skills such as balancing checkbooks, driving, or managing medicines.

Initial Tests (lab, imaging)

- To help rule out other causes of dementia
  - CBC, ESR
  - Chemistry panel
  - Thyroid-stimulating hormone
  - Folate and B_{12} levels
  - Venereal disease reaction level (VDRL) or rapid plasma reagin (RPR)
  - HIV antibody (selected cases)
  - APOE4 or biomarker testing *is not routine*.
- **Imaging**: Controversy exists; may identify moderate cortical atrophy or ventricular enlargement.
  - Consider MRI or CT scan if
    - Cognitive decline is recent and rapid; age <60 years; history of stroke; gait disturbance or focal neurologic signs
    - Cancer, urinary incontinence, bleeding disorder, or current use of anticoagulants
  - Single-photon emission computed tomography (SPECT) and positron emission tomography (PET): only if diagnostic uncertainty after CT or MRI; *insufficient evidence to use alone*
  - Medicare pays for PET to distinguish AD from frontotemporal dementia under specific requirements; *this should not be routine*.

Follow-Up Tests & Special Considerations

Genetic testing for APOE4 or for familial AD types; discuss with genetic counselor

Test Interpretation

- Gross: diffuse cerebral atrophy in hippocampus, amygdala, and some subcortical nuclei
- Microscopic
  - Neuritic senile plaques
  - Neurofibrillary tangles
  - Pyramidal cell loss
  - Decreased cholinergic innervation (other neurotransmitters variably decreased)
  - Degeneration of locus ceruleus and basal forebrain nuclei of Meynert; amyloid angiopathy

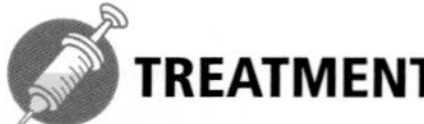

TREATMENT

GENERAL MEASURES

- Optimize treatment of associated comorbid conditions (including hearing and vision loss).
- Analyze environment for safety and security, and avoid sudden changes in environment.
- Assess spouse/caregiver burnout.
- Advance directives, living will, power of attorney

MEDICATION

First Line

2014 meta-analysis shows cholinesterase inhibitors (ChEIs) and memantine are "able to stabilize or slow decline in cognition, function, behavior, and global change" (3)[A].

- Debate continues regarding the clinical significance and cost-effectiveness of AD medication.

- ChEIs (4)[A]
  - Equally effective; all have potential for GI side effects; monitor for bradycardia/syncope; associated with abnormal dreams
  - When used for at least 6 months, provide mild benefit in cognition, daily function, and behavior. (No deterioration over 6–12 months is evidence of efficacy.)
  - Shown to reduce nursing home placement by 20% after 25 months of treatment
  - Best in mild to moderate disease (Folstein MMSE scores 10–24); drugs *may* be effective in Lewy body dementia.
  - Donepezil (Aricept): start at 5 mg/day PO; may increase to 10 mg/day after 1 month
  - Tablets or orally disintegrating tablets; generic available
  - Caution with digoxin or beta-blockers (can cause 3rd-degree heart block)
  - Aricept 23-mg tablet approved in 2010
  - Rivastigmine (Exelon): start at 1.5 mg PO BID, increase by 1.5 mg BID every 2 weeks; maintenance 6–12 mg/day total
  - Capsule, solution, or patch (patch greatly reduces side effects)
  - Indicated for both AD and Parkinson dementia
  - Galantamine (Razadyne): start at 4 mg BID for 4 weeks, then increase by 4 mg BID every month with goal of 16–24 mg/day dose
  - Tablets, solution, extended-release (ER) capsule, and transdermal formulations (ER and transdermal have daily dosing)
- *N*-methyl-D-aspartate (NMDA) receptor antagonists (for moderate to severe AD; MMSE 5–14)
  - Monotherapy or in combination with acetylcholinesterase inhibitors
  - Memantine (Namenda): start at 5 mg/day, with starter pack titrating to target dose of 10 mg BID after 4 weeks
  - Often improves behavioral issues
  - Beneficial for cognition and physician's global impression; increases risk of somnolence, weight gain, confusion, hypertension, nervous system disorders, and falling (5)[A]
- For depression (occurs in 1/3 of patients), SSRIs preferred first line.
- Insomnia
  - Trazodone 25–100 mg at bedtime, zolpidem (Ambien) 5 mg at bedtime, zaleplon (Sonata) 5–10 mg at bedtime, ramelteon (Rozerem) 8 mg at bedtime
  - Avoid diphenhydramine in elderly due to negative cognitive effects and risk of urinary retention (males).
- Moderate anxiety/restlessness: Consider low-dose, short-acting benzodiazepines, buspirone, or SSRIs (efficacy unproven).
- Severe aggressive agitation
  - Behavioral techniques and environmental modification help more than medications for wandering, restlessness, uncooperativeness, hoarding, and irritability:
    - Consider changing environment, rewards, behavioral redirection, hearing aids, and bright light therapy.
  - Memantine (Namenda): start at 5 mg/day, with starter pack titrating to target dose of 10 mg BID after 4 weeks
  - Antipsychotics (both conventional and atypical) are associated with increased mortality and acute care hospital admissions in elderly patients with dementia.
  - Antiepileptic agents (carbamazepine valproate, lamotrigine) have been used for their mood stabilizing properties.
- Precautions
  - Avoid anticholinergic drugs, such as tricyclic antidepressants and antihistamines.
  - Ginkgo biloba: Avoid anticoagulants and aspirin.
  - Benzodiazepines may produce paradoxical excitation or daytime drowsiness.
  - Triazolam (Halcion) can produce confusion, memory loss, and psychotic behavior.
  - Benzodiazepines may increase serum phenytoin concentration.
  - Cimetidine may increase benzodiazepine concentration.
  - Donepezil (Aricept): use with caution with anticholinergic medication, in sick sinus syndrome, or history of peptic ulcers
  - Paroxetine increases donepezil levels.

Second Line

Vitamin E, statins, estrogen, and NSAIDs should not be routinely recommended due to lack of evidence and safety concerns (1)[A].

ISSUES FOR REFERRAL

- Assess driving safety (vision, spatial relations, hearing, judgment):
  - http://www.nhtsa.gov/people/injury/olddrive/Driving%20Safely%20Aging%20Web/
- Support groups for patient and family: Alzheimer Association: http://www.alz.org

ADDITIONAL THERAPIES

- Exercise to reduce restlessness
- Cognitive challenge; traditional and computerized training both effective
- Occupational, music, aroma, and pet therapy

COMPLEMENTARY & ALTERNATIVE MEDICINE

- Huperzine A 400 mg (herbal ChEIs) may improve cognition with minimal side effects (6)[A].
- Ginkgo biloba extracts (120 mg/day) show conflicting efficacy in treatment of AD but may be beneficial.
- Coenzyme Q10 is not effective.

ONGOING CARE

FOLLOW-UP RECOMMENDATIONS

Patient Monitoring

- Schedule regular follow-up (3 months) to assess medical complications, provide support for family, and assess need for placement.
- Serial mental status testing is potentially helpful, but bedside tests (Folstein MMSE) offer wide variability and lack of sensitivity.

PATIENT EDUCATION

- Alzheimer Association: http://www.alz.org/
- Explain progressive nature of the disease and start advance directives planning as early as possible.

PROGNOSIS

Poor: Average survival from diagnosis is 4–8 years (diagnosis is often delayed).

COMPLICATIONS

- Behavioral: hostility, agitation, wandering, falls
- Metabolic: infection, dehydration, drug toxicity
- "Sundowning" (increase full-spectrum lights), depression (1/3 of patients), suicide

REFERENCES

1. McKhann GM, Knopman DS, Chertkow H, et al. The diagnosis of dementia due to Alzheimer's disease: recommendations from the National Institute on Aging-Alzheimer's Association workgroups on diagnostic guidelines for Alzheimer's disease. *Alzheimers Dement*. 2011;7(3):263–269.
2. McGuinness B, O'Hare J, Craig D, et al. Cochrane review on "statins for the treatment of dementia." *Int J Geriatr Psychiatry*. 2013;28(2):119–126.
3. Tan CC, Yu JT, Wang HF, et al. Efficacy and safety of donepezil, galantimine, rivastigmine, and memantine for the treatment of Alzheimer's disease: a systematic review and meta-analysis. *J Alzheimers Dis*. 2014;41(2):615–631.
4. Birks J. Cholinesterase inhibitors for Alzheimer's disease. *Cochrane Database Syst Rev*. 2006;(1):CD005593.
5. Yang Z, Zhou X, Zhang Q. Effectiveness and safety of memantine treatment for Alzheimer's disease. *J Alzheimers Dis*. 2013;36(3):445–458.
6. Xing SH, Zhu CX, Zhang R, et al. Huperzine A in the treatment of Alzheimer's disease and vascular dementia: a meta-analysis. *Evid Based Complement Alternat Med*. 2014;2014:363985.

ADDITIONAL READING

- Schindler SE, McConathy J, Ances BM, et al. Advances in diagnostic testing for Alzheimer disease. *Mo Med*. 2013;110(5):401–405.
- Wang C, Yu JT, Wang HF, et al. Meta-analysis of peripheral blood apolipoprotein E levels in Alzheimer's disease. *PLoS One*. 2014;9(2):e89041.
- Wang C, Yu JT, Wang HF, et al. Pharmacological treatment of neuropsychiatric symptoms in Alzheimer's disease: a systematic review and meta-analysis. [published online ahead of print May 29, 2014]. *J Neurol Neurosurg Psychiatry*. doi:10.1136/jnnp-2014-308112

SEE ALSO

Substance Use Disorders; Hypothyroidism, Adult; Depression

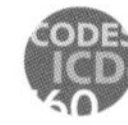

CODES

ICD10

- G30.9 Alzheimer's disease, unspecified
- G30.0 Alzheimer's disease with early onset
- G30.1 Alzheimer's disease with late onset

CLINICAL PEARLS

- Daily intellectual stimulation, such as puzzles, and moderate physical exercise may help prevent AD.
- Imaging studies have low yield in patients with a history typical of AD.
- Encourage families to join a chapter of the Alzheimer Association and to pursue advanced directive planning early in the course of the disease.
- Atypical antipsychotic medications increase mortality.

AMENORRHEA

Heidi L. Gaddey, MD

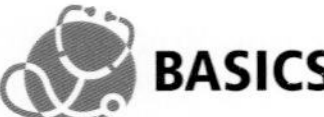

BASICS

DESCRIPTION

- Primary amenorrhea
  - No menses by age 13–14 years with absence of secondary sexual characteristics *OR*
  - No menses by age 15–16 years with normal secondary characteristics
- Secondary amenorrhea: absence of menses for 3 months in a woman with previously normal menstruation or 6 months in a woman with a history of irregular cycles
- System(s) affected: endocrine/metabolic; reproductive

Pregnancy Considerations

Pregnancy is by far the most common cause of secondary amenorrhea.

EPIDEMIOLOGY

Prevalence

- Primary amenorrhea: <1% of female population
- Secondary amenorrhea: 3–5% of female population
- No evidence for race and ethnicity affecting prevalence

ETIOLOGY AND PATHOPHYSIOLOGY

- Primary amenorrhea
  - Hypothalamic–pituitary abnormalities
    - Constitutional delay of puberty
    - Functional hypothalamic amenorrhea
    - Eating disorder
    - Stress/exercise
    - Central lesions (tumors, hypophysitis, granulomas)
    - Pituitary dysfunction (hyperprolactinemia, abnormal secretion of follicle-stimulating hormone [FSH], luteinizing hormone [LH], or GnRH)
    - Thyroid dysfunction
  - Gonadal abnormalities
    - Chromosomal abnormalities (androgen insensitivity syndrome)
    - Euchromosomal gonadal agenesis or dysgenesis (Turner syndrome, Swyer syndrome, and pure gonadal dysgenesis)
    - Polycystic ovarian syndrome (PCOS)
    - Abnormal gonadotropin function
    - Autoimmune gonadal failure
    - Idiopathic gonadal failure
  - Anatomic abnormalities
    - Imperforate hymen
    - Transverse vaginal septum
    - Congenital absence of the cervix
    - Müllerian agenesis
- Secondary amenorrhea
  - Pregnancy
  - Thyroid disease
  - Hyperprolactinemia (altered metabolism, ectopic production, breastfeeding/stimulation, hypothyroidism, medications, empty sella syndrome, pituitary adenoma)
  - If pregnancy, thyroid disease, and hyperprolactinemia are ruled out, consider the following:
    - Normogonadotropic amenorrhea: Hyperandrogenic anovulation (acromegaly, androgen-secreting tumors, Cushing disease, exogenous androgens, nonclassical congenital adrenal hyperplasia, PCOS); outflow tract obstruction (Asherman syndrome, cervical stenosis, fibroids, or polyps)
    - Hypergonadotropic hypogonadism: normal menopause; premature ovarian failure (autoimmune, chemotherapy, galactosemia, fragile X premutation and other genetic causes, 17-hydroxylase deficiency, idiopathic, mumps oophoritis, pelvic radiation)
    - Hypogonadotropic hypogonadism: eating disorders, CNS tumors, chronic illness, cranial radiation, excessive weight loss/exercise/malnutrition, hypothalamic or pituitary destruction, Sheehan syndrome
- Pathophysiology varies, depending on etiology.
- Primary amenorrhea should be evaluated in the context of presence or absence of secondary sexual characteristics.
- Can result from dysfunction in hypothalamic-pituitary-gonadal axis, anatomic abnormalities, or another endocrine gland disorder

Genetics

May occur with Turner syndrome or testicular feminization

RISK FACTORS

- Obesity
- Overtraining (prolonged, excessive exercise)
- Eating disorders
- Malnutrition
- Anovulatory disorders
- Psychosocial crisis
- Treatment with antipsychotic medications

GENERAL PREVENTION

Maintenance of proper body mass index (BMI) and healthy lifestyle with respect to food and exercise

COMMONLY ASSOCIATED CONDITIONS

- Premature ovarian failure may be associated with autoimmune abnormalities (autoimmune thyroiditis, type 1 diabetes).
- Polycystic ovarian syndrome is associated with insulin resistance and obesity.
- Decreased exposure to estrogen may increase risk for osteopenia or osteoporosis.

DIAGNOSIS

HISTORY

- Review of systems, including recent weight changes, symptoms of early pregnancy or menopause, virilizing changes, cyclic pelvic pain, galactorrhea, headaches, vision changes, fatigue, palpitations
- Growth and pubertal development history, including age of breast development, pubertal growth spurt, and adrenarche
- History of chronic illness, trauma, surgery, medications, prior chemotherapy or radiation
- Psychiatric history
- Social history, including diet and exercise history, drug abuse, and sexual history

PHYSICAL EXAM

- General appearance
- Vital signs, height, weight, growth percentile and BMI, hypotension, bradycardia, hypothermia (anorexia nervosa)
- HEENT exam: evidence of dental erosions, trauma to palate (bulimia), visual field defect, funduscopic changes, cranial nerve findings (prolactinoma), webbed neck (Turner syndrome), thyromegaly
- Skin exam: evidence of androgen excess (acne, hirsutism), acanthosis nigricans (PCOS), fine downy hair on body (anorexia nervosa)
- Breast: state of development, evidence of galactorrhea (prolactinoma)
- Pelvic exam: presence or absence of pubic hair (if sparse: androgen insensitivity or deficiency); clitoromegaly (androgen excess); distention or bulging of external vagina (imperforate hymen); thin, pale vaginal mucosa without rugae (estrogen deficiency and ovarian failure); presence of cervical mucus (evidence for estrogen production); blind vaginal pouch (müllerian agenesis, androgen insensitivity syndrome); ovarian enlargement (tumors, PCOS, autoimmune oophoritis)

DIAGNOSTIC TESTS & INTERPRETATION

Initial Tests (lab, imaging)

- Primary amenorrhea
  - Serum prolactin (PRL) and thyroid-stimulating hormone (TSH)
  - If no secondary sexual characteristics, measure serum FSH and LH.
    - FSH/LH <5 IU/L suggests primary hypothalamic or pituitary etiology.
    - FSH >20 and LH >40 IU/L suggests gonadal failure, and karyotype analysis should be performed.
  - If secondary sexual characteristics present, evaluate for anatomic abnormalities. If uterus is absent or abnormal, perform karyotype analysis, testosterone level, and dehydroepiandrosterone (DHEA-S).
- Secondary amenorrhea
  - Exclude pregnancy with HCG.
  - Serum TSH: Elevated in hypothyroidism, decreased in hyperthyroidism
  - Consider (low yield): serum chemistry, CBC, urinalysis to rule out underlying disease
  - PRL:
    - >100 ng/mL suggests empty sella syndrome or pituitary adenoma; perform MRI for evaluation.
    - <100 ng/mL: Evaluate for other etiologies, of which medications are most common.
- If PRL and TSH are normal, perform progestin challenge (see "Treatment").
  - If withdrawal bleed: normogonadotropic amenorrhea related to hyperandrogenic chronic anovulation, most commonly PCOS
  - If no withdrawal bleed: Follow-up with estradiol priming (see "Diagnostic Procedures/Other" and "Treatment") and repeat progestin challenge:
    - If no bleed: Consider outflow tract obstruction.
    - If bleed occurs: Check FSH/LH: elevated in hypergonadotropic hypogonadism, decreased in pituitary tumors or hypogonadotropic hypogonadism
- If virilizing signs and significant acne present, measure free testosterone, DHEA-S, and 17-OH progesterone levels. Initiate evaluation for androgen-secreting tumor if testosterone >200 ng/dL.
- Imaging is not generally indicated as a first-line approach.
- US may show ovarian cysts (PCOS), presence or absence of uterus, and endometrial thickness.

- An MRI of the pelvis can clarify any uterine or vaginal anomalies suggested by US or if pediatric patient is unable to tolerate transvaginal US probe.
- An MRI of the sella turcica if prolactinoma suspected (elevated PRL >100), and consider with functional hypothalamic amenorrhea (other adenomas)

Follow-Up Tests & Special Considerations

- Women <30 years with ovarian failure (see below) should have karyotype analysis and be investigated for premutations of FMR1 gene (fragile X syndrome) and for adrenal antibodies.
- If absence of uterus or foreshortened vagina, karyotype analysis should also be performed.
- Laparoscopy: diagnosis of streak ovaries (Turner syndrome) or polycystic ovaries
- Hysterosalpingogram: Rule out Asherman syndrome and other etiologies of outflow obstruction.

Diagnostic Procedures/Other

- If constitutional delay suspected, obtain bone age.
- If hypothalamic amenorrhea from functional suppression suspected, consider dual-energy x-ray absorptiometry (DEXA) scan to assess for bone loss (1).

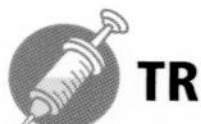

TREATMENT

GENERAL MEASURES

Treatment depends on the underlying cause.

MEDICATION

- Progesterone challenge and replacement: medroxyprogesterone (Provera): 10 mg/day for 10 days will result in withdrawal bleed if hypothalamic–pituitary–gonadal axis is intact although experts disagree (2).
- Estrogen replacement: Cycling with a combination oral contraceptive (containing 35 or 50 μg of estrogen) or conjugated estrogen (Premarin) 0.625 mg for 25 days with progesterone added as above for the last 10 days will result in a withdrawal bleed if the uterus and lower genital tract are normal.
- Use of hormonal therapies will not correct the underlying problem. Other drugs might be required to treat specific conditions (e.g., bromocriptine for hyperprolactinemia).
- Use of hormonal replacement therapy is *not* recommended for long-term management of amenorrhea in older women.
  - It may be safe for symptom management in young women.
  - Give to maintain secondary sex characteristics and to prevent osteoporosis in adolescents and young women (3)[A].
- Combination estrogen/progesterone contraceptives (oral contraceptive pills [OCPs], patch, ring) replace estrogen and prevent pregnancy.
  - Have a positive effect on bone mineral density in oligo-/amenorrheic women but not in functional hypothalamic amenorrhea (4)[A]
  - Can decrease hirsutism in PCOS
- Calcium supplementation: 1,500 mg/day if cause is hypoestrogenism
- Because PCOS is related to insulin resistance, metformin (Glucophage) has been used (start at 500 mg BID) to correct metabolic abnormalities, improve ovulation, and restore normal menstrual patterns. Of note, treatment with metformin has shown an increase in clinical pregnancy rates but not in live birth rates (5)[A].
- Functional hypothalamic amenorrhea appears to improve with administration of exogenous leptin (still under investigation) (6)[C].
- Contraindications to estrogen administration
  - Pregnancy, thromboembolic disease, previous myocardial infarct or cerebrovascular accident, estrogen-dependent malignancy, severe hepatic impairment or disease
- Precautions
  - Patients with amenorrhea who desire pregnancy should not be given hormone replacement therapy but should receive treatment for infertility based on the specific cause.

ISSUES FOR REFERRAL

Many causes of amenorrhea require referral to specialists in ob/gyn, endocrine, surgery, and/or psychiatry.

SURGERY/OTHER PROCEDURE

- Hymenectomy for primary amenorrhea if due to imperforate hymen
- Lysis of adhesions in Asherman syndrome is often effective in restoring regular menses and fertility.
- If karyotype is XY, gonads must be removed due to increased risk of tumors.
- Patients with congenital short vagina can undergo surgery to create a functioning vagina.

ONGOING CARE

FOLLOW-UP RECOMMENDATIONS

If overtraining is suspected, activity level should be reduced by 25–50%.

Patient Monitoring

- Depends on the cause and treatment chosen
- If hormonal replacement is used, discontinue after 6 months to assess spontaneous resumption of menses.

DIET

- Correct overweight or underweight by dietary management and behavior modification.
- If PCOS is the etiology, a weight-loss diet will help restore ovulation.

PATIENT EDUCATION

- Educate the patient on the circumstances and complications of her condition and its underlying etiology.
- Specific educational resources are helpful (e.g., prenatal classes and menopause support groups).
- Discuss the expected duration of amenorrhea (temporary or permanent), effect on fertility, and the long-term sequelae of untreated amenorrhea (e.g., osteoporosis, vaginal dryness).
- Appropriate contraceptive advice should be given because fertility returns before menses.
- Additional support may be needed if the amenorrhea is associated with a reduction in, or loss of, fertility.

PROGNOSIS

Reflects the underlying cause. In functional hypothalamic amenorrhea, 1 study demonstrated 83% reversal rate in presence of obvious contributing factor.

COMPLICATIONS

- Estrogen-deficiency symptoms (e.g., hot flashes, vaginal dryness) and osteoporosis in prolonged hypoestrogenic amenorrhea
- Increased risk of endometrial cancer in patients whose amenorrhea is secondary to anovulation with estrogen excess (obesity, PCOS)
- Premature ovarian failure may increase cardiovascular risk.

REFERENCES

1. Gordon CM. Clinical practice. Functional hypothalamic amenorrhea. *N Engl J Med*. 2010;363(4):365–371.
2. Klein D. Poth M. Amenorrhea: an approach to diagnosis and management. *Am Fam Physician*. 2013;87(11):781–788.
3. Marjoribanks J, Farquhar CM, Roberts H, et al. Long term hormone therapy for perimenopausal and postmenopausal women. *Cochrane Database Syst Rev*. 2012;7:CD004143.
4. Liu SL, Lebrun CM. Effect of oral contraceptives and hormone replacement therapy on bone mineral density in premenopausal and perimenopausal women: a systematic review. *Br J Sports Med*. 2006;40(1):11–24.
5. Tang T, Lord JM, Norman RJ, et al. Insulin-sensitising drugs (metformin, rosiglitazone, pioglitazone, D-chiro-inositol) for women with polycystic ovary syndrome, oligo amenorrhoea and subfertility. *Cochrane Database Syst Rev*. 2012;5:CD003053.
6. Chou SH, Chamberland JP, Liu X, et al. Leptin is an effective treatment for hypothalamic amenorrhea. *Proc Natl Acad Sci U S A*. 2011;108(16):6585–6590.

ADDITIONAL READING

- Practice Committee of American Society for Reproductive Medicine. Current evaluation of amenorrhea. *Fertil Steril*. 2008;90(Suppl 5):S219–S225.
- Santoro N. Update in hyper- and hypogonadotropic amenorrhea. *J Clin Endocrinol Metab*. 2011;96(11):3281–3288.

SEE ALSO

Algorithms: Amenorrhea, Primary; Amenorrhea, Secondary; Delayed Puberty; Thyroid Disorders; Osteoporosis

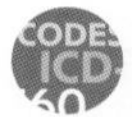

CODES

ICD10

- N91.2 Amenorrhea, unspecified
- N91.0 Primary amenorrhea
- N91.1 Secondary amenorrhea

CLINICAL PEARLS

- First evaluate whether amenorrhea is primary or secondary and exclude pregnancy. TSH and PRL are usual first blood tests.
- Progestin challenge may cause withdrawal bleeding in women with an intact hypothalamic-pituitary-gonadal axis.

AMYOTROPHIC LATERAL SCLEROSIS

Ajoy Kumar, MD, FAAFP • Ryan Wargo, PharmD, BCACP • Kimberly Wollett, MD

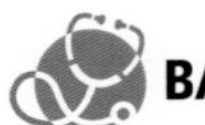

BASICS

Amyotrophic lateral sclerosis (ALS) is a progressive neurodegenerative disease of the brain and spinal cord. Characterized by loss of motor neurons, it is relentless in progression and is currently incurable.

DESCRIPTION

- Average survival ranges from 2 to 5 years from the time of diagnosis.
- 50% live >3 years, 25% live >5 years, 10% live >10 years, 5% live up to 20 years.
- Sporadic ALS form is 90–95% of all cases of the disease. It includes a number of overlapping syndromes, such as pseudobulbar palsy, progressive bulbar palsy, progressive muscular atrophy, and primary lateral sclerosis.
- Familial ALS is an autosomal dominant or autosomal recessive disease, which is clinically similar to sporadic ALS but probably represents a distinct entity pathologically and biochemically.
- Guam ALS and Parkinson-dementia complex are ALS-like syndromes often, but not always, associated with Parkinson syndrome and dementia. Guam ALS is prevalent among the Chamorro Indians of Guam and rare in the United States.
- System(s) affected: nervous
- Synonym(s): motor neuron disease (MND); Lou Gehrig disease; ALS

ALERT

- Infantile and juvenile spinal muscular atrophies are conditions distinct from ALS, both clinically and pathologically.
- Symptoms of ALS may inappropriately be attributed to age.

Pregnancy Considerations

- Uncommon among affected individuals
- If pregnancy did occur, the only foreseeable difficulties would be related to weakness.

EPIDEMIOLOGY

Incidence

- In United States, 5,600 newly diagnosed per year
- Rate = 2/100,000 per year

Prevalence

- Estimated 3,000 Americans may have the disease at any given time.
- No racial, ethnic, or socioeconomic boundaries
- Predominant age: uncommon before age 40 years
- Predominant sex: male > female in sporadic ALS:
  - After 70 years: male = female

ETIOLOGY AND PATHOPHYSIOLOGY

- Sporadic ALS: Unknown cause, but elevated levels of glutamate have been found in serum and CSF.
- Familial ALS: Neurodegenerative disease passed on directly or indirectly by skipping generation (1).
- Guam ALS and Parkinson-dementia complex: possible relationship to ingestion of the cycad nut or to some other environmental toxin
- Degeneration of the upper motor neuron (UMN) and lower motor neuron (LMN) with gliosis replacing lost neurons; leads to spinal cord atrophy, thin ventral roots, and loss of large myelinated fibers in motor nerves
- Progressive weakness of both skeletal and smooth muscles that leads to progressive loss of function related to movement, speech, swallowing, and breathing

Genetics

- Currently 18 types of genetic mutations
- Familial ALS, most common (5% of cases); can be autosomal dominant or autosomal recessive; X-linked cases have been reported.
- Gene locus has been localized to the long arm of chromosome 21 and encodes the superoxide dismutase (SOD1) enzyme in 20% of familial ALS cases.
- Mutation in the gene encoding fused in sarcoma (FUS) was identified in familial ALS type 6.
- Mutations in the angiogenin gene (ANG) have been recently discovered to be associated with sporadic ALS.
- Mutations in transcription of RNA activating protein (TARDP) region encoding TAR DNA-binding protein TDP-43 have also been identified in familial and sporadic ALS.
- *FIG4* gene accounts for 3% of familial ALS.
- C9ORF72 repeat expansions found in 2011 is a major cause of ALS.

RISK FACTORS

- Family history
- Age >40 years and <60 years
- Smoking

GENERAL PREVENTION

Genetic counseling is advised if there is a family history of ALS; however, sporatic ALS is not associated with genetic transmission.

DIAGNOSIS

- Diagnosis can be established according to Revised El Escorial World Federation of Neurology criteria.
- The presence of
  - Evidence of LMN degeneration by clinical, electrophysiologic, or neuropathologic examination
  - Evidence of UMN degeneration by clinical examination
  - Progressive spread of symptoms or signs within a region or to other regions, as determined by history or examination
- The absence of
  - Electrophysiologic and pathologic evidence of other disease processes that might explain the signs of LMN and/or UMN degeneration
  - Neuroimaging evidence of other disease processes that might explain the observed clinical and electrophysiologic sign
- The newer Awaji criteria may offer higher sensitivity and earlier diagnosis of ALS (2)[C].

HISTORY

ALS is suggested when symptoms are consistent with UMN and LMN dysfunction that worsens over time. Symptoms include the following:

- Loss of muscle strength and coordination
- Difficulty opening and closing the jaw, drooling
- Voice change, hoarseness
- Muscle cramps and stiffness, difficulty breathing, difficulty swallowing, paralysis (2)[C]

PHYSICAL EXAM

Variable combinations of

- Unexplained weight loss
- Limb weakness with variable symmetry and distribution
- Gait disorder (steppage-waddling)
- Slurring of speech
- Inability to control affect (inappropriate laughing, crying, yawning)
- Focal atrophy of muscle groups (initially in a myotomal distribution)
- Fasciculations (other than calves)
- Hyperreflexia (including jaw jerk—Hoffmann sign)
- Babinski sign, present in 50% of patients
- Spasticity
- Sialorrhea
- Spares cognitive, oculomotor, sensory, and autonomic functions

DIFFERENTIAL DIAGNOSIS

- Multifocal motor neuropathy
- Cervical radiculomyelopathy
- Cervical spondylosis
- Lead intoxication
- Spinal muscular atrophy (adult form)
- Primary lateral sclerosis
- Familial spastic paraparesis
- Benign fasciculations
- Lyme disease
- Spinal multiple sclerosis
- Tropical spastic paraparesis
- Myasthenia gravis
- Hyperthyroidism
- Paraneoplastic syndromes

DIAGNOSTIC TESTS & INTERPRETATION

Initial Tests (lab, imaging)

- No simple reliable laboratory test or imaging test is available that confirms the diagnosis. Creatinine kinase levels may be elevated.
- Rule out other conditions (i.e., check serum protein electrophoresis [SPEP]/urine protein electrophoresis [UPEP], TSH, PTH, B_{12}, 24-hour urine for heavy metals, HIV, human T-lymphotropic virus [HTLV], Lyme, syphilis, tick-borne encephalitis):
  - Elevated levels of glutamate in CSF and serum
  - Anti-monosialoganglioside autoantibodies in low titer commonly found (of unclear significance)
  - Possibly reduced levels of nerve growth factor
- MRI is used to exclude other possible diagnoses:
  - MRI is usually normal in ALS, although increased signal in the corticospinal tracts on T2-weighted and FLAIR images and hypointensity of the motor cortex on T2-weighted images have been reported.
  - Should be performed in all areas rostral to clinical findings
  - Experimental MR spectroscopy testing is underway (2)[C].

Diagnostic Procedures/Other

- Electromyography (EMG): EMG findings include evidence of ongoing denervation, fibrillation or positive sharp waves, and chronic partial reinnervation implying frequently unstable, increased duration motor unit action potentials with a reduced interference pattern.
- Nerve conduction studies: usually elicit normal values in recordings from relatively unaffected muscles. However, during disease progression, compound motor action potential (CMAP) amplitude elicited by distal stimulation may induce greater physiologic phase cancellation, such as a pathologic conduction block.
- Motor unit number estimation: attractive end point measure in clinical drug trials in ALS because it directly assesses loss of LMNs and is sensitive to disease progression

- Muscle biopsy: not a routine part of the diagnostic evaluation of ALS but may be performed if myopathy is suspected on clinical, electrodiagnostic, or serologic grounds (2)[C]
  - Muscle biopsy will show groups of shrunken angulated muscle fibers (grouped atrophy) that are darkly staining amid other groups of fibers with a uniform fiber type (fiber type grouping); however, these are nonspecific findings of chronic denervation with reinnervation.

Test Interpretation

- Loss of Betz cells in the motor cortex
- Atrophic or absent anterior horn cells of spinal cord
- Atrophic or absent neurons within the motor nuclei of the medulla and pons
- Degeneration of the lateral columns of the spinal cord
- Atrophy of the ventral roots
- Grouped atrophy of muscle (motor units)

TREATMENT

GENERAL MEASURES

- Multidisciplinary care should be available as this may extend survival, decrease medical complications, and improve quality of life (3)[C].
- Outpatient may ultimately need nursing home placement or hospice (3)[C].
- Supportive care is necessary for complicating emergencies (aspiration, respiratory failure). Use of a respirator is a major ethical dilemma (3)[C]. Consideration should be given to those with selective respiratory dysfunction.
- Discussion of advance directives, focusing on patient's specific values about which interventions are to be used, is critical to meeting the patient's needs (3)[C].
- Prosthetic devices

MEDICATION

Riluzole: 50 mg PO BID: the only FDA-approved drug for ALS. It produces a slight prolongation in life expectancy by decreasing the release of glutamate, and it slows the disease progression (4)[A].

ALERT

Riluzole withhold should be considered for patients developing fatigue. Monitor LFTs for hepatic dysfunction and CBC for neutropenia (4)[A].

ISSUES FOR REFERRAL

- Early exam by a neurologist can confirm diagnosis of ALS.
- Tracheostomy or gastrostomy tube placement may be performed by surgeon or gastroenterologist (3)[C].
- Pulmonologist and respiratory therapist for ventilator assistance and management of concurrent infections and tracheostomy
- Referral to ongoing clinical trials may be beneficial (ClinicalTrials.gov).
- Palliative care management is beneficial to both patient and patient's family at end stage (3)[C].

ADDITIONAL THERAPIES

- These drugs may be used to relieve severe spasticity:
  - Baclofen: 5 mg PO TID initially, followed by gradual increase of 5 mg/day every 4–7 days; not to exceed 80 mg/day divided QID (3)[C]
  - Tizanidine: 4–8 mg PO q8h PRN; not to exceed 36 mg/day (3)[C]
- Treatment for refractory sialorrhea:
  - Botulinum toxin B (3)[B]
  - Low-dose radiation therapy to the salivary glands (3)[C]

SURGERY/OTHER PROCEDURES

- Percutaneous endoscopic gastrostomy (PEG) tube should be considered with early signs of malnutrition to stabilize weight and prolong survival (3,5)[C]
- Noninvasive ventilation (NIV) can lengthen survival and improve quality of life (5)[C].
- Elective tracheostomy should be considered in patients with early signs of respiratory difficulty (5)[C].

COMPLEMENTARY & ALTERNATIVE MEDICINE

- Currently, insufficient evidence to recommend disease-modifying treatment other than Riluzole
- Research offering therapy with stem cells is evolving, providing a new approach in cellular replacement and support for patients (6)[C].
- Several therapy options are under current investigation, including ceftriaxone, dexpramipexole, memantine, tamoxifen, and insulin-like growth factor.
- Therapeutic trials of the efficacy of antioxidants (vitamin E and vitamin C and β-carotene), nerve growth factor, gabapentin, myotrophin, thyrotropin-releasing hormone, and creatine have been undertaken. Reports are not encouraging.

ONGOING CARE

FOLLOW-UP RECOMMENDATIONS

Patients should be involved in regular exercise and a physical therapy program (7)[C].

Patient Monitoring

- Initially every 3 months; frequency to be increased as needed for symptomatic therapy
- Patients with a presumed diagnosis of ALS should have neuroimaging and electrodiagnostic studies (7)[C].
- Screening for cognitive and behavioral impairment (3)[B]

DIET

- Evaluate swallowing to quantify any dysphagia.
- Modify the patient's diet to prevent aspiration.
- Consider a gastrostomy tube when patient cannot swallow fluids or soft foods (7)[C].

PATIENT EDUCATION

Printed material for patients (and reference lists for physicians) available from:

- The Muscular Dystrophy Association: (520) 529-2000; (800) 572-1717; http://www.mdausa.org
- The ALS Association: (800) 782-4747; http://www.alsa.org
- Families of Spinal Muscular Atrophy: http://www.fsma.org

PROGNOSIS

- Median survival of patients with ALS is 3–5 years from diagnosis.
- Patients who predominantly manifest progressive muscular atrophy have a better prognosis.
- There have been reports of spontaneous arrest of the disease.

COMPLICATIONS

- Aspiration pneumonia
- Pulmonary embolism
- Nutritional deficiency
- Complications from wheelchair-bound or bedridden states, including decubitus ulcers and skin infections

REFERENCES

1. Andersen PM, Borasio GD, Dengler R; EALSC Working Group. Good practice in the management of amyotrophic lateral sclerosis: clinical guidelines. An evidence-based review with good practice points. EALSC Working Group. *Amyotroph Lateral Scler*. 2007;8(4):195–213.
2. Andersen PM, Abrahams S, Borasio GD, et al. EFNS guidelines on the clinical management of amyotrophic lateral sclerosis (MALS)—revised report of an EFNS task force. *Eur J Neurol*. 2012;19(3):360–375.
3. Miller RG, Brooks BR, Swain-Eng RJ, et al. Quality improvement in neurology: amyotrophic lateral sclerosis quality measures. Report of the Quality Measurement and Reporting Subcommittee of the American Academy of Neurology. *Neurology*. 2013;81(24):2136–2140.
4. Bensimon G, Lacomblez L, Meininger V. A controlled trial of riluzole in amyotrophic lateral sclerosis. ALS/Riluzole Study Group. *N Engl J Med*. 1994;330(9):585–591.
5. Miller RG, Jackson CE, Kasarskis EJ, et al. Practice parameter update: the care of the patient with amyotrophic lateral sclerosis: drug, nutritional, and respiratory therapies (an evidence-based review): report of the Quality Standards Subcommittee of the American Academy of Neurology. *Neurology*. 2009;73(15):1218–1226.
6. Kim SU, de Vellis J. Stem cell-based cell therapy in neurological diseases: a review. *J Neurosci Res*. 2009;87(10):2183–2200.
7. Miller RG, Jackson CE, Kasarskis EJ, et al. Practice parameter update: the care of the patient with amyotrophic lateral sclerosis: multidisciplinary care, symptom management, and cognitive/behavioral impairment (an evidence-based review: report of the Quality Standards Subcommittee of the American Academy of Neurology. *Neurology*. 2009;73(15):1227–1233.

ADDITIONAL READING

- Inghilleri M, Iacovelli E. Clinical neurophysiology in ALS. *Arch Ital Biol*. 2011;149(1):57–63.
- Kiernan MC, Vucic S, Cheah BC, et al. Amyotrophic lateral sclerosis. *Lancet*. 2011;377(9769):942–955.
- Morren JA, Galvez-Jimenez N. Current and prospective disease-modifying therapies for amyotrophic lateral sclerosis. *Expert Opin Investig Drugs*. 2012;21(3):297–320.
- Pastula DM, Moore DH, Bedlack RS, et al. Creatine for amyotrophic lateral sclerosis/motor neuron disease. *Cochrane Database Syst Rev*. 2010;(6):CD005225.

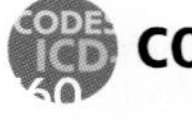

CODES

ICD10

- G12.21 Amyotrophic lateral sclerosis
- G12.22 Progressive bulbar palsy

CLINICAL PEARLS

- ALS is a progressive upper and lower motor neuron degenerative disease.
- Diagnosis is made by history, physical exam, EMG, and NCS.
- Riluzole is the only available treatment that might increase survival.

ANABOLIC STEROID ABUSE

Justin R. Shirley, MD, CPT • Tammy Donoway, DO, FAAFP

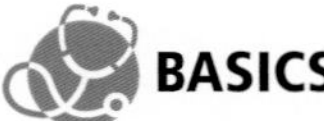

BASICS

Anabolic steroid abuse is the misuse of testosterone and closely related compounds (often in supratherapeutic dosages) to increase lean muscle mass and improve athletic performance.

DESCRIPTION

- Anabolic-androgenic steroids (AAS) are used medically to treat endocrine disorders such as primary or secondary hypogonadism. These agents increase muscle strength and lean muscle mass, which can alter physical appearance. This has led to the abuse of AAS (1). Examples of AAS include exogenous testosterone, synthetic androgens, synthetic androgen receptor modulators, androgen precursors, and other androgen stimulators.
- Multiple street names ("roids" or "juice"). AAS are administered orally, transdermally, topically, or intramuscularly (2).
- When used in supraphysiologic doses, AAS contribute to muscle building and masculinization.
- Individuals typically "stack" steroids, using a cocktail of multiple agents at high doses and then discontinuing use for a period of weeks to reduce side effects and avoid detection (2).
- Side effects of AAS use are typically dose dependent, and many will reverse after use is discontinued (3).
- AAS use is not associated immediate "high" as with other drugs of abuse. Dependence, however, has been increasingly recognized (4).
- AAS use is prohibited by the World Anti-Doping Agency (WADA) list. In 2010, AAS accounted for 60% of positive results in WADA laboratories (1). Testosterone, stanozolol, and nandrolone were the most frequent AAS identified (1).
- There is no evidence that AAS abuse or dependence develops from the therapeutic use of AAS.

EPIDEMIOLOGY

Incidence

Rates are difficult to estimate as AAS use is typically concealed (3).

Prevalence

- Epidemiologic studies suggest that the lifetime prevalence of AAS use in men is at least 3% (3).
- In power sports or weight lifting, the prevalence has been estimated at 10–50% (5).
- Past estimates suggest there are up to 3 million AAS users in the United States at any one time (3).
- Usage rates in men exceed those in women (4).

ETIOLOGY AND PATHOPHYSIOLOGY

- Natural testosterone is produced in small amounts in the adrenal gland and ovaries and in large amounts by the testes.
- AAS exert their anabolic effects through increased protein production, particularly in muscle cells.
- In addition, AAS decrease catabolism by blocking the effects of cortisol.
- Administration of exogenous testosterone suppresses the hypothalamic-pituitary-gonadal (HPG) axis, causing testicular atrophy and suppressed spermatogenesis. Users often concurrently use human chorionic gonadotropin (hCG) to mitigate this side effect (6).
- In addition, aromatase inhibitors are concurrently used to counteract gynecomastia, which occurs with exogenous AAS use due to peripheral conversion of testosterone to estradiol.
- AAS use may also lead to accelerated cartilage formation and premature closure of the epiphyses when used in adolescents (2).
- Muscle mass decreases after cessation of AAS use.

Genetics

Genetic variations in enzymatic and androgen receptor activity may impact the pharmacodynamic effects of AAS and their subsequent anabolic and toxic effects (1).

RISK FACTORS

- Male gender (5)
- Age 20–30 years old (5)
- Participation in power sports, weight lifting (5)
- Residing in a developed country (6)
- Consumption of legal performance-enhancing substances (5)
- Use of alcohol and/or illicit drugs (5)
- Lower education level (3)

GENERAL PREVENTION

- The U.S. Preventive Services Task Force states that there is insufficient evidence to recommend screening for anabolic steroid abuse (7).
- Individuals (particularly those at risk for AAS use) should be counseled about the negative side effects associated with anabolic steroid abuse (7).

COMMONLY ASSOCIATED CONDITIONS

- Major depressive disorder (8)
- Body dysmorphic disorder (8)
- Substance abuse (5)

DIAGNOSIS

- History and physical exam are central to detecting AAS abuse.
- WADA incorporates the Athlete Biological Passport (ABP) as part of a comprehensive anti-doping program. By monitoring selected biologic variables over time, this will reveal the physiologic effects of doping more specifically than detecting the individual doping substance itself (9).

HISTORY

- Review of patient risk (age, sports participation, body dysmorphism). If patients endorse use, query about the specific product used as well as the duration, dosage, frequency, and route of usage.
- Ask about side effects, including impotence, mood disturbance, and amenorrhea in females.
- Ask about use of concurrent substances, including OTC supplements, illegal drugs, alcohol, and prescription drug use (5,8)[C].
- Social situation, including stressors and current support system
- Preexisting medical and psychiatric conditions (8)[C]
- Body image: Screen for features of muscle dysmorphia and body-checking behavior (6,8)[C].
- Assess for suicidality.

PHYSICAL EXAM

- General
  - Increased muscle mass
  - Decreased body fat
  - Deepening of voice and hirsutism in women
  - Decreased height velocity change in adolescents (2)
- Cardiovascular: hypertension
- Breast: gynecomastia
- Gastrointestinal: hepatomegaly
- Integumentary: acne, male pattern baldness, evidence of injection sites over the buttocks, thighs, or deltoids
- Genitourinary: testicular atrophy, clitoromegaly
- Psychiatric: anxiety, depression, mania, psychosis

DIFFERENTIAL DIAGNOSIS

- Cushing syndrome
- Congenital adrenal hyperplasia
- Adrenal neoplasm
- Polycystic ovarian syndrome
- Precocious puberty
- Drug-induced hirsutism

DIAGNOSTIC TESTS & INTERPRETATION

Initial evaluation should focus on side effects of anabolic steroid usage and any comorbid medical conditions. Laboratory studies are not routinely performed as they are limited by the timing of consumption. Results are often affected by advanced administration techniques in sophisticated users.

Initial Tests (lab, imaging)

- Urine testosterone:epitestosterone (T:E) ratio
- T:E ratio greater than 3:1 may indicate abuse of AAS (1)[C].
- The WADA ABP tracks athletes' urine for an individuals' "steroid profile," which can be followed longitudinally (1,9)[C].
- Fasting lipid profile and liver function tests AAS abuse is associated with (2)[C]
  - LDL increase
  - HDL decrease
  - AST, ALT, and gamma-glutamyltranspeptidase elevation
- No imaging studies are required unless the patient is symptomatic or there is other evidence of liver dysfunction.
- Small studies have demonstrated a difference in echocardiogram results among AAS users compared to nonusers. Echocardiography may be considered as clinically indicated. Routine echocardiography for all AAS users is not currently recommended (2).

Diagnostic Procedures/Other

- Renal function is difficult to assess given increased muscle mass and frequent ingestion of creatine supplements (10).
- Urinalysis to screen for proteinuria (10)[C]

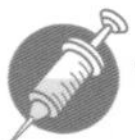

TREATMENT

- Treatment is limited by the fact that AAS abusers rarely seek assistance (6).
- AAS abuse/dependence is complicated by
  - High frequency of comorbid body image disorders including muscle dysmorphia (6,8)
  - Few patients develop marked depressive symptoms upon withdrawal of AAS (4,8).
  - Neurologic basis for dependence (possibly related to opioid receptors) needs to be overcome for sustained abstinence (4,8).

GENERAL MEASURES

Goal of therapy is to have patients acknowledge that anabolic steroid usage is detrimental to their health. The first step is cessation of AAS use in the short term followed by long-term abstinence (6).

- Minimize withdrawal side effects and treat any comorbid psychiatric or substance abuse conditions (8)[C]. The primary side effect of withdrawal is

often psychologic as patients struggle with loss of muscle mass.
- Assure adequate social support and coping mechanisms (8)[C].

MEDICATION
- Medications are limited to treating any underlying psychiatric illness and the clinical manifestations of hypogonadism (6)[C].
- Naltrexone, which blocks opioid-mediated positive reinforcement behaviors, has shown promise in animal studies (6).
- Available studies on medication usage are limited by small sample size.

First Line
Depressive symptoms and body dysmorphism can be treated pharmacologically. SSRIs are often the 1st-line agents of choice (6)[C]. Cognitive-behavioral therapy may also help patients identify and change negative thinking patterns (6)[C].

Second Line
- hCG may be used (through endocrinology consultation) to help accelerate endogenous testicular testosterone production (6)[C]. Hypogonadal treatment in young men should be tailored to maximize fertility potential (3)[C].
- Clomiphene supplementation may be used to stimulate pituitary function (3)[C].
- Less frequently, tamoxifen and phosphodiesterase inhibitors, such as sildenafil, are used to improve the symptoms of hypogonadism (3)[C].
- Severe depression that is refractory to medication and is associated with anabolic steroid discontinuation has been treated successfully with electroconvulsive therapy.

ISSUES FOR REFERRAL
- Endocrinology: prolonged hypothalamic-pituitary-gonadal-axis suppression, management of persistent symptoms of hypogonadism
- Psychiatry: psychosis, grandiosity, suicidal ideation

ADDITIONAL THERAPIES
- Cognitive-behavioral therapy
- Couples therapy
- Family therapy

INPATIENT CONSIDERATIONS
- Inpatient psychiatric hospitalization should be considered for those with significant mood alterations or those who pose an immediate threat to themselves or others.
- Inpatient treatment may be required for other complications of AAS abuse such as symptomatic cardiomyopathy or severe liver dysfunction.

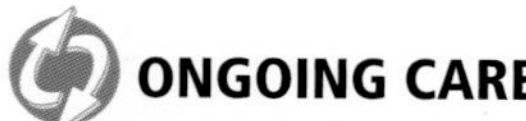

ONGOING CARE

Patients who abuse AAS should follow-up with their primary care physician and other specialists (e.g., behavioral health specialist or addiction specialist) based on the clinical picture.

FOLLOW-UP RECOMMENDATIONS
Determined by side effects and comorbid psychiatric illness

PATIENT EDUCATION
- Substance Abuse and Mental Health Services Administration: findtreatment.samhsa.gov or 1-800-662-HELP
- National Center for Drug Free Sport, Inc: www.drugfreesport.com or 816-474-8655
- World Anti-Doping Agency: www.wada-ama.org/

PROGNOSIS
Most side effects resolve when AAS are discontinued and prognosis is generally good. Long-term side effects are not completely understood. Approximately 30% of patients who abuse anabolic steroids become chronic users. AAS use is more often problematic and recalcitrant to treatment when polypharmacy is present (including concomitant use of legal dietary and sports supplements).

COMPLICATIONS
- Testicular atrophy
- Profound hypogonadism
- Decreased sperm count
- Decreased fertility index
- Impotence
- Premature epiphyseal closure in adolescents
- Hypertension
- Myocardial infarction
- Cardiomyopathy (unclear causation)
- Sudden cardiac death
- Thrombosis
- Dyslipidemia
- Depression
- Substance abuse
- Suicide
- Violent behavior
- Anxiety
- Paranoia
- Hepatotoxicity
- Cholestasis
- Hepatocarcinoma
- Tendon rupture
- Hepatitis C, HIV, blood-borne illnesses
- Local site infections

REFERENCES

1. Rane A, Ekstrom L. Androgens and doping tests: genetic variation and pit-falls. *Br J Clin Pharmacol*. 2012;74(1):3–15.
2. Kersey RD, Elliot DL, Goldberg L, et al; National Athletic Trainers' Association. National Athletic Trainers' Association position statement: anabolic-androgenic steroids. *J Athl Train*. 2012;47(5):567–588.
3. Coward R, Rajanahally S, Kovac J, et al. Anabolic steriod induced hypogonadism in young men. *J Urol*. 2013;190(6):2200–2205.
4. Kanayama G, Hudson JI, Pope HG Jr. Illicit anabolic-androgenic steroid use. *Horm Behav*. 2010;58(1):111–121.
5. Dodge T, Hoagland MF. The use of anabolic androgenic steroids and polypharmacy: a review of the literature. *Drug Alcohol Depend*. 2011;114(2–3):100–109.
6. Kanayama G, Brower KJ, Wood RI, et al. Treatment of anabolic-androgenic steroid dependence: emerging evidence and its implications. *Drug Alcohol Depend*. 2010;109(1–3):6–13.
7. Moyer V; U.S. Preventive Services Task Force. Primary care behavioral interventions to reduce illicit drug and nonmedical pharmaceutical use in children and adolescents: U.S. Preventive Task Force recommendation statement. *Ann Intern Med*. 2014;160(9):634–639.
8. Hildebrandt T, Lai J, Langenbucher JW, et al. The diagnostic dilemma of pathological appearance and performance enhancing drug use. *Drug Alcohol Depend*. 2011;114(1):1–11.
9. Mazzoni I, Barroso O, Rabin O. The list of prohibited substances and methods in sport: structure and review process by the world anti-doping agency. *J Anal Toxicol*. 2011;35(9):608–612.
10. Herlitz LC, Markowitz GS, Farris AB, et al. Development of focal segmental glomerulosclerosis after anabolic steroid abuse. *J Am Soc Nephrol*. 2010;21(1):163–172.

ADDITIONAL READING

- Angoorani H, Narenjiha H, Tayyebi B, et al. Amphetamine use and its associated factors in body builders: a study from Tehran, Iran. *Arch Med Sci*. 2012;8(2):362–367.
- Eaton DK, Kann L, Kinchen S, et al. Youth risk behavior surveillance—United States, 2009. *MMWR Surveill Summ*. 2010;59(5):1–142.
- Lundmark J, Gårevik N, Thörngren JO, et al. Nonsteroidal anti-inflammatory drugs do not influence the urinary testosterone/epitestosterone glucuronide ratio. *Front Endocrinol (Lausanne)*. 2013;4:51.

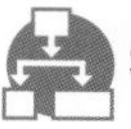

SEE ALSO

Substance Use Disorders

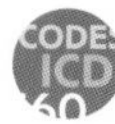

CODES

ICD10
F55.3 Abuse of steroids or hormones

CLINICAL PEARLS

- Anabolic steroid use is common and is not limited to elite athletes.
- Suspect anabolic steroid abuse in at-risk patients with suspicious clinical side effects.
- Discuss steroid use in an unbiased manner.
- Treating symptoms of withdrawal helps individuals remain abstinent.
- Psychosis, mania, violence, or severe depression are serious behavior consequences associated with AAS abuse.

ANAL FISSURE

Anne Walsh, MMSc, PA-C, DFAAPA • Kashyap Trivedi, MD

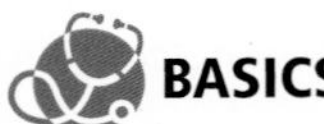

BASICS

DESCRIPTION

Anal fissure (fissure in ano): longitudinal tear in the lining of the anal canal distal to the dentate line, most commonly at the posterior midline. Characterized by a knifelike tearing sensation upon defecation, often associated with bright red blood per rectum. This very common benign anorectal condition is often confused with hemorrhoids. May be acute (<6 weeks) or chronic (>6 weeks) in duration

EPIDEMIOLOGY

- Affects all ages. Common in infants 6–24 months; not common in older children, suspect abuse or trauma. Elderly less common due to lower resting pressure in the anal canal.
- Sex: male = female; women more likely to get anterior midline tears (25% vs. 8%).

Incidence

Exact incidence is unknown. Patients often treat with home remedies and do not seek medical care.

Prevalence

- 80% of infants, usually self-limited
- 20% of adults, most of whom do not seek medical advice

ALERT

- Lateral fissure: Rule out infectious disease.
- Atypical fissure: Rule out Crohn disease.

ETIOLOGY AND PATHOPHYSIOLOGY

High resting pressure within the anal canal (usually as a result of constipation/straining) leads to ischemia of the anoderm, resulting in splitting of the anal mucosa during defecation and spasm of the exposed internal sphincter.

Genetics

None known

RISK FACTORS

- Constipation (25% of patients)
- Diarrhea (6% of patients)
- Passage of hard or large-caliber stool
- High resting tone of internal anal sphincter (prolonged sitting, obesity)
- Trauma (sexual abuse, childbirth, mountain biking)
- Inflammatory bowel disease (Crohn disease)
- Infection (chlamydia, syphilis, herpes, tuberculosis)

GENERAL PREVENTION

All measures to prevent constipation and prolonged sitting on toilet

COMMONLY ASSOCIATED CONDITIONS

Constipation, irritable bowel syndrome, Crohn disease, tuberculosis, leukemia, and HIV

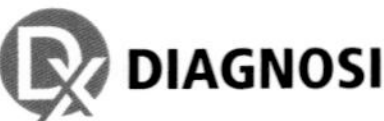

DIAGNOSIS

HISTORY

- Severe, sharp rectal pain, often with and following defecation but can be continuous; some patients will see bright red blood on the stool or when wiping
- Occasionally, anal pruritus or perianal irritation

PHYSICAL EXAM

- Gentle spreading of the buttocks with close inspection of the anal verge will reveal a smooth-edged tear in the anodermal tissue, typically posterior midline, occasionally anterior midline, rarely eccentric to midline.
- Minimal edema, erythema, or bleeding may be seen.
- Chronic fissures may demonstrate rolled edges, hypertrophic papillae at proximal end, and a sentinel pile (tag) at distal end.

DIFFERENTIAL DIAGNOSIS

- Thrombosed external hemorrhoid: swollen, painful mass at anal verge
- Perirectal abscess: tender, warm erythematous induration or fluctuance
- Perianal fistula: abnormal communication between rectum and perianal epithelium with purulent drainage
- Pruritus ani: shallow excoriations rather than true fissure

DIAGNOSTIC TESTS & INTERPRETATION

Diagnostic Procedures/Other

- Avoid anoscopy/sigmoidoscopy initially unless necessary for other diagnoses.
- Rarely, due to pain, some patients may require exam under anesthesia in order to confirm the diagnosis.

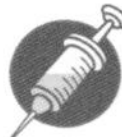

TREATMENT

The goal of treatment is to avoid repeated tearing of the anal mucosa with resultant spasm of the internal anal sphincter by decreasing the patient's high sphincter tone and addressing its underlying cause.

GENERAL MEASURES

- Wash area gently with warm water; consume high-fiber diet; avoid constipation, maintain healthy weight.
- Medical therapy for chronic fissures usually initiated in a stepwise manner: nitrates, calcium channel blockers, botulinum toxin (1)[B]

MEDICATION

First Line

Acute fissures—most heal spontaneously with supportive measures:

- Stool softeners (docusate) daily
- Osmotic laxatives if needed (polyethylene glycol)
- Fiber supplements (e.g., psyllium, methylcellulose, inulin) and increased fluid intake
- Topical analgesics (2% lidocaine gel)
- Topical lubricants/emollients (Balneol cream)
- Sitz baths (sit in hot water bath for 20 minutes 2–3 times daily)

Second Line

Chronic fissures—require medical therapy:

- Chemical sphincterotomy
  - Topical nitroglycerin ointment 2% diluted to 0.2–0.4% applied QID; nitroglycerin 0.4% ointment available commercially (Rectiv): marginally but significantly better than placebo in healing (48.6% vs. 37%); late recurrence common (50%) (1)[A]; effect is to reduce resting anal pressure through the release of nitric oxide
  - Calcium channel blockers (e.g., nifedipine, diltiazem), oral or topical: no better than nitrates but with fewer side effects; effect is to relax the internal sphincter muscle, thereby reducing the resting anal pressure (2)[A]
  - Botulinum toxin 4 mL (20 units) injected into the internal sphincter muscle: no better than topical nitrates but with fewer side effects; effect is to inhibit the release of acetylcholine from nerve endings to inhibit muscle spasm (3)[B]

ISSUES FOR REFERRAL

- Late recurrence is common (50%) particularly if the underlying issue remains untreated (constipation, irritable bowel, etc.).
- Medical therapy usually is tried for 90–120 days prior to colorectal surgery referral.

ADDITIONAL THERAPIES

Anococcygeal support (modified toilet seat) may offer some advantage in chronic fissures to avoid surgery.

SURGERY/OTHER PROCEDURES

- Reserved for failure of medical therapy; involves division of the internal sphincter muscle
- Lateral internal sphincterectomy is the surgical procedure of choice (4)[B].
- Risk for fecal incontinence: 45% short term, 6–8% long term
- Anal stretching/dilation: unlikely to benefit; has been abandoned as treatment (5)[A]

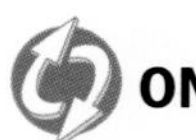

ONGOING CARE

DIET

High fiber (>25 g/day; augment with daily fiber supplements); increase fluid intake

PATIENT EDUCATION

- Avoid prolonged sitting or straining during bowel movements; drink plenty of fluids; avoid constipation; lose weight if obese.
- Avoid use of triple antibiotic ointment and long-term use of steroid creams to anal area.

PROGNOSIS

Most acute fissures heal within 6 weeks with conservative therapy. Medical therapy is less likely to be successful for chronic anal fissures; 40% failure rate (6)[A].

COMPLICATIONS

Fecal incontinence and incontinence to flatus, primarily associated with surgery (30% postop), which may become permanent (14% long term)

REFERENCES

1. Altomare DF, Binda GA, Canuti S, et al. The management of patients with primary chronic anal fissure: a position paper. *Tech Coloproctol*. 2011;15(2):135–141.
2. Samim M, Twigt B, Stoker L, et al. Topical diltiazem cream versus botulinum toxin A for the treatment of chronic anal fissure: a double-blind randomized clinical trial. *Ann Surg*. 2012;255(1):18–22.
3. Madalinski MH. Identifying the best therapy for chronic anal fissure. *World J Gastrointest Pharmacol Ther*. 2011;2(2):9–16.
4. Mousavi SR, Sharifi M, Mehdikhah Z. A comparison between the results of fissurectomy and lateral internal sphincterotomy in the surgical management of chronic anal fissure. *J Gastrointest Surg*. 2009;13(7):1279–1282.
5. Nelson RL, Chattopadhyay A, Brooks W, et al. Operative procedures for fissure in ano. *Cochrane Database Syst Rev*. 2011;(11):CD002199. doi:10.1002/14651858.
6. Shao WJ, Li GC, Zhang ZK. Systematic review and meta-analysis of randomized controlled trials comparing botulinum toxin injection with lateral internal sphincterotomy for chronic anal fissure. *Int J Colorectal Dis*. 2009;24(9):995–1000.

ADDITIONAL READING

- Gee T, Hisham RB, Jabar MF, et al. Ano-coccygeal support in the treatment of idiopathic chronic posterior anal fissure: a prospective randomized controlled pilot trial. *Tech Coloproctol*. 2013;17(2):181–186.
- Sinha R, Kaiser AM. Efficacy of management algorithm for reducing need for sphincterotomy in chronic anal fissures. *Colorectal Dis*. 2012;14(6):760–764.
- Sugerman DT. JAMA patient page. Anal fissure. *JAMA*. 2014;311(11):1171.
- Yiannakopoulou E. Botulinum toxin and anal fissure: efficacy and safety systematic review. *Int J Colorectal Dis*. 2012;27(1):1–9.

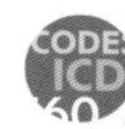

CODES

ICD10

- K60.2 Anal fissure, unspecified
- K60.0 Acute anal fissure
- K60.1 Chronic anal fissure

CLINICAL PEARLS

- Avoid anoscopy or sigmoidoscopy initially unless necessary for other diagnoses.
- Best chance to prevent recurrence is to treat the underlying cause (e.g., chronic constipation).
- No medical therapy approaches the cure rate of surgery for chronic fissure.

ANEMIA, APLASTIC

Muthalagu Ramanathan, MD • Jan Cerny, MD, PhD, FACP

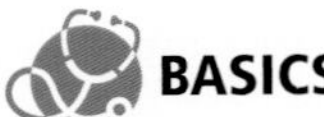

BASICS

DESCRIPTION

- Pancytopenia due to hypocellular bone marrow without infiltrates or fibrosis. Classified as acquired (much more common) and congenital.
- Acquired aplastic anemia: insidious onset; due to exogenous insult triggering an autoimmune reaction; often responsive to immunosuppression
- Congenital forms: rare, mostly presents in childhood (exception is atypical presentation of Fanconi syndrome in adults; 30s for males and 40s for females)
- The occurrence of specific mutations in genes of the telomere complex in acquired aplastic anemia has blurred the distinction between the congenital and acquired forms.
- System(s) affected: heme/lymphatic/immunologic
- Synonym(s): hypoplastic anemia; panmyelophthisis; refractory anemia; aleukia hemorrhagica; toxic paralytic anemia

ALERT

- Early intervention for aplastic anemia greatly improves the chances of treatment success.
- Hematopoietic growth factors require close monitoring in newly diagnosed patients.

Geriatric Considerations

The elderly are often exposed to large numbers of drugs and therefore may be more susceptible to acquired aplastic anemia.

Pediatric Considerations

- Congenital forms of aplastic anemia require different treatment regimens than acquired forms.
- Acquired aplastic anemia is seen in children exposed to ionizing radiation or treated with cytotoxic chemotherapeutic agents.

Pregnancy Considerations

- Pregnancy is a real but rare cause of aplastic anemia. Symptoms may resolve after delivery and with termination.
- Complications in pregnancy can occur from low platelet counts and paroxysmal nocturnal hemoglobinuria-associated aplastic anemia.

EPIDEMIOLOGY

- Predominant age: (1) biphasic 15–25 years (more common) and >60 years
- Predominant sex: male = female

Incidence

- 2–3 new cases per million per year in Europe and North America
- The incidence is 3-fold higher in Thailand and China versus the Western world.

ETIOLOGY AND PATHOPHYSIOLOGY

- Idiopathic (~70% of the cases)
- Drugs: phenylbutazone, chloramphenicol, sulfonamides, gold, cytotoxic drugs, antiepileptics (felbamate, carbamazepine, valproic acid, phenytoin)
- Viral: HIV, Epstein-Barr virus (EBV), nontypeable postinfectious hepatitis (not A, B, or C), parvovirus B19 (mostly in the immunocompromised), atypical mycobacterium
- Toxic exposure (benzene, pesticides, arsenic)
- Radiation exposure
- Immune disorders (systemic lupus erythematosus, eosinophilic fascitis, graft vs. host disease)
- Pregnancy (rare)
- Congenital (Fanconi anemia, dyskeratosis congenita, Shwachman-Diamond syndrome, amegakaryocytic thrombocytopenia)
- The immune hypothesis: Activation of T cells with associated cytokine production leading to destruction or injury of hematopoietic stem cells. This leads to a hypocellular bone marrow without marrow fibrosis (2).
- The activation of T cells likely occurs because of both genetic and environmental factors. Exposure to specific environmental precipitants, diverse host, genetic risk factors, and individual differences in characteristics of immune response likely account for variations in its clinical manifestations and patterns of responsiveness to treatment.
- Telomerase deficiency leads to short telomeres. This leads to impaired regenerative capacity and hence a reduction in marrow progenitors and qualitative deficiency in the repair capacity of hematopoietic tissue.
- Reduction of natural killer cells in the bone marrow

Genetics

- Telomerase mutations found in a small number of patients with acquired and congenital forms. These mutations render carriers more susceptible to environmental insults.
- Mutations in genes called TERC and TERT were found in pedigrees of adults with acquired aplastic anemia who lacked the physical abnormalities or a family history typical of inherited forms of bone marrow failure. These genes encode for the RNA component of telomerase.
- HLA-DR2 incidence in aplastic anemia is twice that in the normal population.

RISK FACTORS

- Treatment with high-dose radiation or chemotherapy
- Exposure to toxic chemicals
- Use of certain medications
- Certain blood diseases, autoimmune disorders, and serious infections
- Tumors of thymus (red cell aplasia)
- Pregnancy, rarely

GENERAL PREVENTION

- Avoid possible toxic industrial agents.
- Use safety measures when working with radiation.

DIAGNOSIS

HISTORY

- Solvent and radiation history, family, environmental, travel, and infectious disease history
- Patients are often asymptomatic but may have frequent infections, fatigue, shortness of breath, headache, or bleeding/bruising.

PHYSICAL EXAM

- Mucosal hemorrhage, petechiae
- Pallor
- Fever
- Hemorrhage, menorrhagia, occult stool blood, melena, epistaxis
- Dyspnea
- Palpitations
- Progressive weakness
- Retinal flame hemorrhages
- Systolic ejection murmur
- Weight loss
- Signs of congenital aplastic anemia
  - Short stature
  - Microcephaly
  - Nail dystrophy
  - Abnormal thumbs
  - Oral leukoplakia
  - Hyperpigmentation (café au lait spots) or hypopigmentation

DIFFERENTIAL DIAGNOSIS

Includes other causes of bone marrow failure and pancytopenia

- Marrow replacement
  - Acute lymphoblastic leukemia
  - Lymphoma
  - Hairy cell leukemia (increased reticulin and infiltration of hairy cells)
  - Large granular lymphocyte leukemia
  - Fibrosis
- Megaloblastic hematopoiesis
  - Folate deficiency
  - Vitamin B_{12} deficiency
- Paroxysmal nocturnal hemoglobinuria, hemolytic anemia (dark urine), pancytopenia, and venous thrombosis (classically hepatic veins)
- Systemic lupus erythematosus
- Prolonged starvation or anorexia nervosa (bone marrow is gelatinous with loss of fat cells and increased ground substance)
- Transient erythroblastopenia of childhood
- Drug-induced agranulocytosis that may be reversible on withdrawal of drug
- Overwhelming infection
  - HIV with myelodysplasia
  - Viral hemophagocytic syndrome

DIAGNOSTIC TESTS & INTERPRETATION

Screening tests to exclude other etiologies

- CBC and absolute reticulocyte count
- Blood smear exam
- Cytogenetic studies of peripheral lymphocytes if <35 years of age to exclude Fanconi anemia
- Liver function test
- Viral serology: hepatitis A, B, C; EBV; cytomegalovirus (CMV); HIV
- Vitamin B_{12} and folate levels
- Autoantibody screening antinuclear antibody (ANA) and anti-DNA
- Flow cytometry looking for glycosylphosphatidylinositol (GPI), negative neutrophils and RBCs for detecting paroxysmal nocturnal hemoglobinuria
- Fetal hemoglobin in children
- Red cell adenosine deaminase (pure red cell aplasia)
- Cytogenetic analysis of bone marrow

Initial Tests (lab, imaging)

- CBC: pancytopenia, anemia (usually normocytic), leukopenia, neutropenia, thrombocytopenia
- Decreased absolute number of reticulocytes
- Increased serum iron secondary to transfusion
- Normal total iron-binding capacity (TIBC)
- High mean corpuscular volume (MCV) >104
- CD 34+ cells decreased in blood and marrow

- Urinalysis: hematuria
- Abnormal liver function tests (hepatitis)
- Increased fetal hemoglobin (Fanconi)
- Increased chromosomal breaks under specialized conditions (Fanconi)
- Molecular determination of abnormal gene (Fanconi)
- CT of thymus region if thymoma-associated RBC aplasia suspected
- Radiographs of radius and thumbs (if congenital anemia suspected)
- Renal ultrasound (to rule out congenital anemia or malignant hematologic disorder)
- Chest x-ray to exclude infections such as mycobacterial infection

Diagnostic Procedures/Other

Bone marrow aspiration and biopsy

Test Interpretation

- Normochromic RBC
- Bone marrow
  - Decreased cellularity (<10%): no fibrosis, no malignant cells seen.
  - Decreased megakaryocytes
  - Decreased myeloid precursors
  - Decreased erythroid precursors
  - Prominent fat spaces and marrow stroma, polyclonal plasma cells

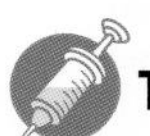

TREATMENT

Early treatment increases the chance of success. 2 major options: immunosuppressive therapy (1) and hematopoietic stem cell transplantation. Treatment decisions are based on age of the patient, severity of disease, and availability of a human leukocyte antigen (HLA)–matched sibling donor for transplantation.

GENERAL MEASURES

- Supportive measures: RBC and platelet transfusions. Use only irradiated leuko-reduced or CMV-negative blood initially if patient is a candidate for hematopoietic stem cell transplantation.
- Antibiotics, antifungals, antivirals when appropriate, especially if ANC <200 cells/μL
- Oxygen therapy for severe anemia
- Good oral hygiene
- Control menorrhagia with norethisterone or oral contraceptive pills
- Avoid/discontinue causative agents/isolation if necessary.
- HLA testing on all patients and their immediate families
- Transfusion support (judiciously prescribed RBCs for severe anemia; platelets for severe thrombocytopenia)
  - Transfuse when
    - Hb <8 g/dL or if Hb <9 g/dL and symptomatic ± CHF (congestive heart failure)
    - Platelet count is $<10 \times 10^9$ or if $<20 \times 10^9$ with fever

MEDICATION

First Line

- Corticosteroids (methylprednisolone) are often given with immunosuppressive regimens
- Immunosuppressive therapy (3)
  - A combination of antithymocyte globulin (ATG) plus cyclosporine. ATG eliminates lymphocytes, and cyclosporine blocks T-cell function.
- ATG
  - Horse serum containing polyclonal antibodies against human T cells
  - 1st choice treatment for patients >40 years of age and for younger patients without a compatible donor. Consider in patients 30–40 years of age.
  - May be used as a single agent but has better response in combination with cyclosporine
- Cyclosporine following initial ATG therapy for minimum of 6 months (4)
  - Monitor through blood levels. Normal values for assays vary.
  - Granulocyte colony-stimulating factor (G-CSF)
    - May be used in conjunction with ATG and cyclosporine
    - Shows faster neutrophil recovery but survival is not improved.
    - Treatment is costly and is disputed in 2 randomized trials.
  - Note: Relapses may occur after the initial response to the immunosuppressive therapy if cyclosporine is discontinued too early. Restarting cyclosporine can lead to a response in up to 25% of patients.
- Stem cell transplant: matched sibling allogeneic stem cell transplant for age <20 years and absolute neutrophil count (ANC) <500 or age 20–40 years and ANC <200

Second Line

- Rabbit ATG + cyclosporine
- Campath
- Androgen in a subset of patients who have anemia as a predominant feature
- Matched unrelated donor stem cell transplant
- Clinical trials: thrombopoietin (TPO) receptor agonists (5) http://patientrecruitment.nhlbi.nih.gov/AplasticAnemia.aspx

SURGERY/OTHER PROCEDURES

- First-line hematopoietic stem cell transplantation is recommended for patients with an HLA-identical donor and severe aplastic anemia when age <20 years and ANC <500 or age 20–40 years and ANC <200. Consider in patients 40–50 years of age in good general medical condition.
- Patients >40 years of age have higher rates of graft versus host disease and graft rejection.
- Unrelated donor transplants should be considered for patients age <40 years without HLA-matched sibling donor who failed first-line immunosuppressive therapy.
- Thymectomy for thymoma

INPATIENT CONSIDERATIONS

Nursing

If neutropenic, use antiseptic mouthwash such as chlorhexidine.

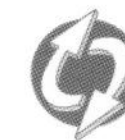

ONGOING CARE

DIET

If neutropenic, avoid foods that can expose patient to bacteria, such as uncooked foods.

PATIENT EDUCATION

- Stay away from people who are sick; avoid large crowds.
- Wash your hands often.
- Brush and floss your teeth; get regular dental care to reduce risk of infections.
- Pneumonia vaccine and annual flu shot.
- Printed patient information available from Aplastic Anemia & MDS International Foundation, Inc., 800-747-2828. Web site: www.aamds.org/aplastic

PROGNOSIS

- Hematopoietic stem cell transplantation with HLA-matched sibling
  - Age <16 years, 91% at 5 years
  - Age >16 years, 70–80% at 5 years
- Immunosuppressive therapy using ATG and cyclosporine: overall survival of 75%; 90% among responders at 5 years

COMPLICATIONS

- Infection (fungal, sepsis)
- Graft versus host disease in bone marrow transplant recipients (acute 18%; chronic 26%)
- Side effects of immunosuppressant medications
- Hemorrhage
- Transfusion hemosiderosis
- Transfusion hepatitis
- Heart failure
- Development of secondary cancer: leukemia or myelodysplasia (15–19% risk at 6–10 years)
- Refractory pancytopenia

REFERENCES

1. Bacigalupo A, Passweg J. Diagnosis and treatment of acquired aplastic anemia. *Hematol Oncol Clin North Am*. 2009;23(2):159–170.
2. Townsley DM, Desmond R, Dunbar CE, et al. Pathophysiology and management of thrombocytopenia in bone marrow failure: possible clinical applications of TPO receptor agonists in aplastic anemia and myelodysplastic syndromes. *Int J Hematol*. 2013;98(1):48–55.
3. Brodsky RA, Jones RJ. Aplastic anaemia. *Lancet*. 2005;365(9471):1647–1656.
4. Beuno C, Roldan M, Anguita E, et al. Bone marrow mesenchymal stem cells from aplastic anemia patients preserve functional and immune properties and do not contribute to the pathogenesis of the disease. *Haematologica*. 2014;99(7):1168–1175.
5. Scheinberg P, Young NS. How I treat acquired aplastic anemia. *Blood*. 2012;120(6):1185–1196.

SEE ALSO

- Myelodysplastic Syndromes; Systemic Lupus Erythematosus (SLE)
- Algorithm: Anemia

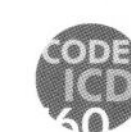

CODES

ICD10

- D61.9 Aplastic anemia, unspecified
- D61.89 Oth aplastic anemias and other bone marrow failure syndromes
- D61.01 Constitutional (pure) red blood cell aplasia

CLINICAL PEARLS

- Acquired aplastic anemia has an insidious onset and is caused by an exogenous insult triggering an autoimmune reaction. This form is usually responsive to immunosuppressive therapy.
- Immunosuppressive therapy using ATG and cyclosporine: overall survival of 75%; 90% among responders at 5 years.

ANEMIA, AUTOIMMUNE HEMOLYTIC

Heather J. Hue, MD, MPH • Rahul Banerjee, MD • Emily S. Lau, MD

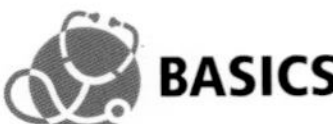

BASICS

DESCRIPTION

- Autoimmune hemolytic anemia (AIHA): premature or accelerated destruction of RBCs in the presence of anti-RBC autoantibodies (1,2)
- Classified into 3 main groups (1,2)
  - Warm AIHA (antibodies optimally bind at 37°C): mainly IgG-mediated; triggers are either idiopathic or secondary to an underlying process
  - Cold AIHA (antibodies optimally bind at 4–18°C): mainly IgM-mediated (IgG or IgA possible); includes cold agglutinin syndrome and paroxysmal cold hemoglobinuria
  - Mixed AIHA (antibodies bind from 4–37°C): primarily IgM-mediated, linked to lymphomas; has features of both warm and cold AIHA
- Drug-induced AIHA: related to drug exposure, behaves similarly to warm AIHA (mainly IgG-mediated) (1,2)

EPIDEMIOLOGY

Incidence

- Adults: 10–30 cases per million, female > male (2)
  - Warm AIHA: 70–80% cases, age of onset: 40–60 years
  - Cold AIHA: 20–30% cases, age of onset: >65 years
- Pediatric: 0.2–1 cases per million, male > female (2,3)
  - Warm AIHA: average age of onset: 4 years; 40% of cases associated with Evans syndrome
- Cold AIHA: typically after *Mycoplasma* or Epstein-Barr virus (EBV) infection (1)
- Mixed AIHA: 10% of cases, mainly in adults (1)

ETIOLOGY AND PATHOPHYSIOLOGY

- General concepts (1,2)
  - IgG, IgA, and IgM target RBC antigens, resulting in direct opsonization and/or the triggering of complement fixation.
  - Antibody-triggered complement fixation can lead to cell opsonization (via C3b) or cell lysis (via the C5–C9 membrane attack complex).
  - Result: intravascular or extravascular hemolysis
- Extravascular hemolysis: macrophage-mediated phagocytosis or lymphocyte-mediated cytotoxicity (1,2)
  - Mediator: opsonization of RBCs by autoantibody binding and/or antibody-induced complement fixation (e.g., C3b)
  - Phagocytosis: primarily within spleen (IgG-opsonized) or liver (IgM-opsonized)
- Intravascular hemolysis: direct destruction of circulating RBCs within bloodstream (1,2)
  - Mediator: Membrane attack complex insertion triggered by complement fixation (as a result of autoantibody-RBC binding).
  - Not as common as extravascular hemolysis because of protective RBC surface proteins (specifically, CD55 and CD59)
- Pathogenicity of autoantibodies depends on circulating antibody titer, antibody class, avidity for RBC antigens, and ability to fix complement.
- Clinical symptoms depend on rate of hemolysis, ability of body to process breakdown products, and bone marrow capacity to regenerate RBCs.
- Warm AIHA (extravascular hemolysis) (1,2)
  - Pathophysiology: autoantibody formation (typically IgG targeting Rh peptide or RBC band 3 on RBCs) leading to extravascular hemolysis
  - Causes
    - Idiopathic: 50% of cases
    - Acquired lymphoproliferative disorders: chronic lymphocytic leukemia (CLL), lymphomas, Castleman disease
    - Autoimmune disorders: systemic lupus erythematosus (SLE), rheumatoid arthritis (RA), ulcerative colitis (UC)
    - Infections: herpesviruses (e.g., EBV or CMV), influenza, *Brucella*
    - Organ transplantation (especially heart/lung)
  - Predisposing risk factors for anti-RBC autoantibody formation
    - Common variable immunodeficiency (CVID)
    - Allogeneic stem cell transplant
- Cold AIHA (intravascular hemolysis) (1,4,5)
  - Pathophysiology: autoantibody formation (typically IgM targeting I-i peptide on RBCs) leading primarily to intravascular hemolysis
    - IgM binds RBCs at low temperatures (e.g., acral areas) and can trigger permanent complement fixation even if IgM later detaches at warmer temperatures.
  - Intravascular hemolysis possible in states of CD55/CD59 deficiency; also common in paroxysmal cold hemoglobinuria
  - Causes
    - Idiopathic cold agglutinin syndrome
    - Infections: *Mycoplasma*, EBV (rarer: CMV, *Legionella*, *Chlamydia*)
    - Lymphoproliferative disorders and plasma cell dyscrasias
  - Paroxysmal cold hemoglobinuria (PCH) (1,2)
    - Rare type of cold AIHA historically linked to syphilis in adults; in children, linked to varicella or measles infection/vaccination
    - Mediator: Donath-Landsteiner antibodies (IgG, not IgM) against P antigen on RBCs
    - Primarily intravascular hemolysis
- Mixed AIHA (1,2)
  - Mediated by autoantibodies with wide range of binding temperatures, linked to lymphoma
- Drug-induced AIHA (extravascular hemolysis) (1,6)
  - Pathophysiology: RBC opsonization by antidrug antibodies or immune complexes; rarely, de novo anti-RBC antibody production
  - Causes
    - Antimicrobials: ribavirin, cephalosporins, penicillin, piperacillin, quinine
    - Antineoplastics: fludarabine, cladribine, oxaliplatin, alkylating agents
    - Others: methyldopa, interferon, NSAIDs, sulfa drugs, procainamide

Genetics

- No genetic component in majority of cases (1)
- Inherited: autoimmune lymphoproliferative syndrome (rare disorder of lymphocyte apoptosis involving *Fas* or *FasL* genes) (1,3)

RISK FACTORS

Malignancy, lymphoproliferative disorders, infection, autoimmune disorders, CVID, medications (1,2)

COMMONLY ASSOCIATED CONDITIONS

- Warm AIHA (1,2,3)
  - CLL, SLE, RA, UC, idiopathic thrombocytopenic purpura (ITP) (Evans syndrome)
- Cold AIHA (1,4,5)
  - *Mycoplasma* or EBV infection
  - Lymphoproliferative diseases
- Plasma cell dyscrasias (1)

DIAGNOSIS

HISTORY

- Symptoms of anemia: fatigue/weakness, palpitations, dyspnea, dizziness (1,2)[C]
- Symptoms of hemolysis: jaundice (± dark urine in intravascular hemolysis, e.g., PCH) (1,2)[C]
- Temperature-related symptoms: discoloration, rash, or pain in acral surfaces (cold AIHA) (1,2,4)[C]
- Predisposing factor assessment (1,2)[C]
  - Recent infections or medication use
  - History or risk factors for underlying causes
  - Concurrent lymphoproliferative disorder or plasma cell dyscrasia

PHYSICAL EXAM

- Signs of anemia: tachycardia, conjunctival pallor, flow murmur (1,2)[C]
- Signs of hemolysis: scleral icterus, splenomegaly, and/or hepatomegaly from extravascular hemolysis (1,2)[C]
- Temperature-related signs: blue-gray discoloration or livedo reticularis on acral surfaces (cold AIHA) (1,2,4)[C]
- Predisposing factor assessment (1,2)[C]
  - Fevers (infection, autoimmune, malignancy)
  - Lymphadenopathy, splenomegaly, or hepatomegaly (infection, malignancy)

DIFFERENTIAL DIAGNOSIS

- Allo-antibody syndromes (pregnancy, post-RBC transfusion, post–stem cell transplant) (1,2)[C]
- Microangiopathic hemolytic disorders (e.g., thrombotic thrombocytopenic purpura [TTP]) (1,2)[C]
- Other hemolytic anemias (e.g., G6PD deficiency or paroxysmal nocturnal hemoglobinuria) (1,2)[C]
- Other anemias (e.g., aplastic, megaloblastic)
- Other hemoglobin disorders (e.g., thalassemia, sickle-cell anemia) (1)[C]
- Evans Syndrome (if ITP also present) (1,3)[C]

DIAGNOSTIC TESTS & INTERPRETATION

Initial Tests (lab, imaging)

- CBC and blood smear (1,2,4)[B]
  - Anemia, ± mild leukocytosis
  - Blood smear examination: anisocytosis, polychromasia (reticulocytosis), macrocytosis
  - Warm AIHA-specific: spherocytes
  - Cold AIHA-specific: agglutinated RBCs
- Hemolytic workup (1,2,4)[B]
  - Reticulocyte count, elevated lactate dehydrogenase (LDH), decreased haptoglobin
  - Bilirubinemia: unconjugated (indirect) but can be conjugated (direct) in extravascular hemolysis
  - Hemoglobinuria in cases of intravascular hemolysis (e.g., PCH)
- Gold standard: direct antiglobulin test (DAT), also known as the Coombs reaction (1,2,4)[B]
  - Warm AIHA: DAT+ for IgG ± C3d
  - Cold AIHA: DAT+ for C3d alone, although weak IgG signal in 20% of patients
    - Confirmatory test: cold agglutinin titers (with incubation at 4°C) at least 1:64
  - Mixed AIHA: DAT+ for IgG and C3d
  - PCH: Test for Donath-Landsteiner antibody.

Follow-Up Tests & Special Considerations

Targeted workup based on clinical suspicion for underlying associated conditions (SLE, CLL, EBV, *Mycoplasma*) (1)[C]

Diagnostic Procedures/Other

Bone marrow biopsy not routinely required (1,2)[C].

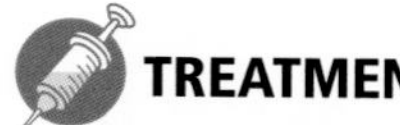

TREATMENT

GENERAL MEASURES

- Treatment of underlying condition if identified (1,2)[C]
- Avoidance or discontinuation of triggering agents (cold weather or fluids for cold AIHA, offending medication for drug-induced AIHA) (1,2)[C]
- Vitamin supplementation (folate, calcium/vitamin D if on long-term steroids) (1,2)[C]

MEDICATION

First Line

- Warm/mixed AIHA (2,7)[B]
  - Glucocorticoids
    - Effective but 3–12 months required for complete response
    - Side effects include weight gain, hyperglycemia, depression, osteoporosis.
    - Dosing: oral prednisone 1 mg/kg for 3–4 weeks, or IV methylprednisolone 250–1,000 mg/day for 1–3 days if continued hemolysis
  - Danazol
    - Most effective when given with prednisone
    - Black-box warning in pregnancy, androgenic side effects in females
    - Long-term hepatotoxicity risk
    - Dosing: 400–800 mg PO daily
- Cold AIHA (2,4,5)[B]
  - Glucocorticoids have low efficacy.
  - Rituximab
    - Partial response in 54–58% of patients
    - Side effects uncommon but include hypotension, fevers, infection.
    - Dosing: 375 mg/m^2 IV infusion repeated periodically
  - Fludarabine
    - Synergistic with rituximab but higher immunosuppression risk when used together

Second Line

- Warm/mixed AIHA (2,7)[C]
  - Rituximab
    - 25–100% response rates in both primary and secondary warm AIHA
    - Delayed efficacy, with weeks to months required before maximum response
    - Dosing: 375 mg/m^2 IV infusion weekly × 4 doses
  - Other agents in refractory illness
    - Cyclophosphamide, azathioprine, cyclosporin A, intravenous immunoglobulin (IVIG) mycophenolate, sirolimus
  - IVIG
    - Indication: glucocorticoid-refractory or transfusion-dependent patients; presplenectomy temporizing measure
    - Potentially synergistic with glucocorticoids
    - Dosing: 400–1,000 mg/kg IV daily × 5 days
- Cold AIHA (2,7,8)[C]
  - Chlorambucil or cyclophosphamide
  - No benefit from immunosuppressive drugs
  - Investigational agents
    - Darbepoetin as transfusion-sparing strategy
    - Eculizumab, C1 esterase inhibitor

SURGERY/OTHER PROCEDURES

- RBC transfusions (2,4,9)[C]
  - Supportive measure to improve oxygenation; minimize transfusion quantity when possible
  - Warm AIHA
    - Urgent setting: Transfuse with typed and crossed blood; however, 33% risk of exacerbating hemolysis due to alloantibodies to minor RBC antigens.
    - Nonurgent setting: extended RBC pretransfusion workup, including RBC phenotyping and antibody detection
    - Hemopure (nonnephrotoxic variant of bovine hemoglobin) has been used with success in patients who will not accept transfusions.
  - Cold AIHA
    - Typed and crossed blood transfusions; extended testing generally not required
    - All RBC compatibility tests should be performed at 37°C.
    - Use prewarmed blood products (or in-line blood warmer) to avoid hemolytic crises.
- Splenectomy (1,2,5)[C]
  - 38–70% success rate in warm/mixed AIHA
  - Not effective in cold AIHA
  - Pediatric considerations: splenectomy not recommended given typically self-limited course
  - Laparoscopic approach preferred due to significant difference in mortality (1.6% vs. 6%)

ALERT

Vaccinate against encapsulated bacteria (*Streptococcus pneumoniae, Neisseria meningitidis, Haemophilus influenzae*) before splenectomy (at least 2 weeks).

INPATIENT CONSIDERATIONS

Admission Criteria

- Symptomatic patients (tachycardia, dyspnea)
- Unstable patients (significant anemia or hemolysis with end-organ damage) (1,2,7)[C]
- Patients requiring surgery or patients requiring stabilization with transfusions (2,7)[C]

ALERT

Use prewarmed IV fluids in cold AIHA to avoid major hemolytic crises.

Discharge Criteria

- Cessation or reduction in hemolysis (2,7)[C]
- Uneventful posttransfusion or operative course (2,7)[C]

ONGOING CARE

FOLLOW-UP RECOMMENDATIONS

Patient Monitoring

- Serial hemoglobin measurements to evaluate degree of anemia and/or ongoing hemolysis (2,7)[C]
- Avoidance of hypothermic fluids, blood products, or surgeries for cold AIHA (2,7)[C]

PATIENT EDUCATION

Behavior modification in cold AIHA (2,4,5)[C]

PROGNOSIS

- Primary AIHA: good with appropriate lifestyle changes and pharmacologic treatment (1,2)[C]
- Secondary AIHA: dependent on prognosis of underlying disorder (1)[C]

COMPLICATIONS

- End-organ damage related to severe anemia (1,2,7)
- Hepatic or splenic dysfunction (1,2,7)
- Morbidity from underlying diseases (1,4)
- Treatment side-effects (see above) (2,7)

REFERENCES

1. Bass GF, Tuscano ET, Tuscano JM. Diagnosis and classification of autoimmune hemolytic anemia. *Autommun Rev*. 2014;13(4–5):560–564.
2. Michel M. Warm autoimmune hemolytic anemia: advances in pathophysiology and treatment. *Presse Med*. 2014;43(4, Pt 2):e97–e104.
3. Aladjidi N, Leverger G, Leblanc T, et al. New insights into childhood autoimmune hemolytic anemia: a French national observational study of 265 children. *Haemotologica*. 2011;96(5): 655–663.
4. Berensten S, Tjønnfjord GE. Diagnosis and treatment of cold agglutinin mediated autoimmune hemolytic anemia. *Blood Rev*. 2012;26(3):107–115.
5. Swiecicki PL, Hegerova LT, Gertz MA. Cold agglutinin disease. *Blood*. 2013;122(7):1114–1121.
6. Garratty G. Immune hemolytic anemia caused by drugs. *Expert Opin Drug Saf*. 2012;11(4):635–642.
7. Jaime-Perez JC, Rodriguez-Martinez M, Gomez-de-Leon A, et al. Current approaches for the treatment of autoimmune hemolytic anemia. *Arch Immunol Ther Exp (Warsz)*. 2013;61(5):385–395.
8. Wouters D, Stephan F, Strengers P, et al. C1-esterase inhibitor concentrate rescues erythrocytes from complement-mediated destruction in autoimmune hemolytic anemia. *Blood*. 2013;121(7):1242–1244.
9. Jordan SD, Alexander E. Bovine hemoglobin: a nontraditional approach to the management of acute anemia in a Jehovah's Witness patient with autoimmune hemolytic anemia. *J Pharm Pract*. 2013;26(3):257–260.

ADDITIONAL READING

- Liu B, Gu W. Immunotherapy treatments of warm autoimmune hemolytic anemia. *Clin Dev Immunol*. 2013;2013:561852.
- Michel M. Classification and therapeutic approaches in autoimmune hemolytic anemia: an update. *Exp Rev Hematol*. 2011;4(6):607–618.

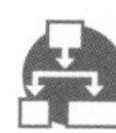

SEE ALSO

- Lymphoma, Non-Hodgkin's; Leukemia; Systemic Lupus Erythematosus (SLE)
- Algorithm: Anemia

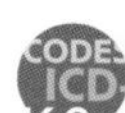

CODES

ICD10

- D59.1 Other autoimmune hemolytic anemias
- D59.0 Drug-induced autoimmune hemolytic anemia

CLINICAL PEARLS

- AIHA is a rare cause of anemia; diagnosis requires evidence of hemolytic anemia and a positive direct antiglobulin test (Coombs).
- In AIHA secondary to an underlying process (e.g., CLL, SLE, EBV, *Mycoplasma*), treatment of the underlying process determines prognosis.
- For primary warm AIHA, corticosteroids are first-line; alternatives include rituximab, IVIG, and splenectomy.
- For primary cold AIHA, avoidance of hypothermic conditions (weather, fluids, surgery) is preventative.

ANEMIA, CHRONIC DISEASE

Carmen Tran, MD • Matthew J. Goldman, MD • Hayden Tran, DO, MS

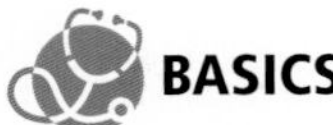

BASICS

DESCRIPTION

- Otherwise known as anemia of chronic inflammation
- During chronic systemic infection, inflammation, or malignancy, the production of proinflammatory mediators causes the inhibition of erythropoiesis as well as the imbalance in iron homeostasis (1).
- Anemia of chronic disease (ACD) is characterized as a normocytic, normochromic, hypoproliferative anemia and classically has low serum iron levels, elevated ferritin levels, and an elevated total iron-binding capacity (TIBC) (1).

EPIDEMIOLOGY

Incidence

ACD is the second most common anemia, after iron deficiency anemia (IDA), due to the high rate of infectious diseases in developing countries as well as the high rate of inflammatory and malignant disorders in developed countries (1).

Prevalence

For isolated causes of anemia, ACD was found in a large number of adults, especially those >65 years of age and with cancer (1,2)[A].

ETIOLOGY AND PATHOPHYSIOLOGY

- Production of red blood cell is decreased due to a reduction in iron use and functional iron deficiency through the following mechanism below.
- In general, the severity of the anemia will correspond with the severity of the underlying disease (1).
- Proinflammatory cytokines such as interleukins, tumor necrosis factor (TNF), and interferons create changes in iron homeostasis in several ways (1,3):
  - Dysregulating iron homeostasis
  - Diminishes proliferation as well as differentiation of red blood cell progenitor cells
  - Diminished erythropoietin response
  - Increased erythrocyte phagocytosis and apoptosis
- The production of interleukin-6 (IL-6), a proinflammatory cytokine, acts to increase the production of an iron-regulating hormone called Hepcidin from the hepatocytes (3–6).
  - Hepcidin acts to decrease both iron absorption within the gastrointestinal tract (GIT) as well as the release of iron from macrophages. Increased retention of iron within the reticuloendothelial cells also occurs (5,6).
  - Hepcidin accomplishes these by specifically negatively regulating ferroportin (5,6).
  - This downregulation results in low serum iron levels and inhibited erythropoiesis known as iron-restricted erythropoiesis.
  - As a result, iron delivery to erythroid progenitor cells within bone marrow is reduced and erythropoiesis is dimished, causing anemia.
- Erythropoietin (EPO) production and the response to EPO by erythroid bone marrow is suppressed by proinflammatory cytokines such as interleukin-1 (IL-1),TNF, and interferon gamma (IFN-γ) (1).
- Increased production of hemolysins causing increased erythrocyte apoptosis

COMMONLY ASSOCIATED CONDITIONS

- Chronic systemic diseases
  - Rheumatoid arthritis (RA), systemic lupus erythematosus (SLE), sarcoidosis, temporal arteritis, inflammatory bowel disease (IBD), systemic inflammatory response syndrome (SIRS)
- Hepatic disease or failure
- Congestive heart failure or coronary artery disease
- Chronic kidney disease (CKD)
- Acute or chronic infections
  - Viral
    - HIV
  - Bacterial
    - Abscess, subacute bacterial endocarditis, tuberculosis, osteomyelitis
  - Fungal
  - Parasitic
- Malignancies
  - Lymphomas, myelomas, carcinomas
- Cytokine dysregulation
  - Anemia of aging
- Hypometabolic states
  - Protein malnutrition, thyroid disease, panhypopituitarism, diabetes mellitus, Addison disease

DIAGNOSIS

HISTORY

- The spectrum of causes for ACD is so broad that there is no classical presentation.
- ACD symptoms resemble those of the causative infectious, inflammatory, or malignant process without any source of occult bleeding; often mild and general for anemic symptoms, such as fatigue, dizziness, and palpitations (1)
- ACD is often discovered incidentally on a routine CBC with differential.
- Those with a cardiovascular condition may experience symptoms of angina, shortness of breath, and reduced exercise capacity with a moderate hemoglobin (Hgb) level (10–11 g/dL).

PHYSICAL EXAM

Physical exam findings are associated with the causative underlying condition.

DIFFERENTIAL DIAGNOSIS

- IDA
- Anemia of CKD
- Drug-induced marrow suppression or hemolysis
- Endocrine disorders
- Thalassemia
- Sideroblastic anemia
- Dilutional anemia

DIAGNOSTIC TESTS & INTERPRETATION

Initial Tests (lab, imaging)

- Hgb (1)
  - Typically, 8.5–9.5 g/dL; may be 10–12 g/dL within 2 days of an acute bacterial infection
  - May produce a drop in Hgb levels of 2–3 g/dL within 2 days due to hemolysis
  - An Hgb of <8 g/dL typically suggest a second underlying cause for the anemia.
- Hematocrit (Hct) (1)
  - Rarely <60% of baseline (unless in the presence of kidney failure)
- Mean corpuscular volume (MCV)
  - Usually normal
  - Usually between 80 and 100 fL
  - Microcytosis (<80 fL) may occur.
- RBC morphology
  - Normocytic and normochromic
  - Increased protoporphyrin levels
- Serum ferritin levels (1)
  - Elevated
  - Typically 30–200 μg/L
  - Serum ferritin levels <30 μg /L is suggestive of coexisting iron deficiency.
- Serum iron levels
  - Low due to increased retention and decreased release from the RES
  - <50
- TIBC
  - Extremely low
  - <300
- Serum transferrin levels (1)
  - Low
- Transferrin saturation levels
  - Extremely low
  - Typically 10–20%
- Absolute reticulocyte count
  - Inappropriately low (reticulocyte index <20,000–25,000/μL) due to reduced erythropoiesis
    - Serum B_{12} and folate
      - Diminished due decreased absorption or lacking in diet

Diagnostic Procedures/Other

- Distinguishing ACD from absolute IDA (1,6)
  - Determining the type of anemia is necessary when ACD is associated with a cause of iron deficiency (e.g., hemodialysis, chronic blood loss).
    - Administration of iron will typically correct IDA but will leave ACD unresolved.
  - Bone marrow biopsy with iron stain
    - Gold standard for diagnosis; necessary to establish a diagnosis if pancytopenia is present, as serum tests do not provide a diagnosis; there is progression of the anemia; or there is no response to empirical treatment
    - Localized iron within macrophages of the bone marrow is indicative of ACD.
    - Absent iron staining is indicative of IDA.
  - Reticulocyte Hgb concentration of <28 pg (3)
  - Soluble serum transferrin (sTfR):log ferritin (1)
    - Ratio used to reflect erythropoiesis within bone marrow as well as to differentiate ACD from IDA
    - ACD without IDA, ACD with IDA, or IDA without ACD can be determined from this ratio.
  - Functional test
    - The response of Hgb to oral or parenteral iron
- Although a known cause of anemia may be present, iron, B_{12}, and folate deficiencies should still be ruled out.

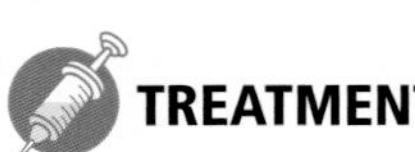

TREATMENT

GENERAL MEASURES

- Primary management should address the disorder causing the ACD (1).
  - This is the preferred treatment.
  - Treatment of the underlying disorder will generally restore basal Hgb levels as well as the normal production of erythrocytes.
- In some cases, where treatment of the underlying disease (e.g., cancer, end-stage kidney disease) is not possible, symptomatic anemia will require treatment.
  - Two dominant forms of treatment are transfusions and EPO (1).
  - Studies have shown that ACD is frequently responsive to EPO in pharmacologic doses (1).
    - Epoetin-α
    - Darbepoetin

  - Evaluation of iron status and repletion of iron must be performed for maximal effects from EPO.
  - Indication for recombinant EPO is an Hgb of <10 g/dL.
- Coexisting iron deficiency or folic acid (FA) deficiency should be considered severe cases of anemia.
  - A reduced dietary intake of iron or FA is common among patients who are chronically ill.
  - Patients who regularly undergo hemodialysis will often lose both iron and FA during treatment.

MEDICATION

- Epoietin-α (1,4,7)
  - Indications
    - EPO concentration <500 mU/mL (some recommend <100 mU/mL)
    - Hgb is < 10g/dL.
    - Fatigue or exertional intolerance
    - Anemia due to IBD, RA, hepatitis C
    - Chemotherapy in patients with a solid malignancy (palliative therapy)
    - CKD (eGFR <60 mL/min)
  - Dosing and schedule
    - Individualized in order to maintain an Hgb level between 10 and 12 g/dL; usually reached within 4–6 weeks when iron levels are adequate; ~90% of patients respond.
    - When target Hgb level is obtained, EPO dose can be decreased; if Hgb level decreases with EPO therapy, consider iron deficiency or infection.
    - Dialysis patients, CKD-associated: start 50–100 U/kg SC/IV 3×/week; use lowest dose to maintain Hgb level sufficient to reduce RBC transfusion need.
    - Nondialysis patients: start 50–100 U/kg SC/IV 3×/week for patients with Hgb <10 g/dL and when rate of decline indicates RBC transfusion need; use lowest dose to maintain Hgb level sufficient to reduce RBC transfusion need.
    - Patients with cancer who are undergoing chemotherapy: 150 U/kg SQ 3×/week or 40,000 units 1×/wk use in cancer patients restricted to certified prescribers and facilities; contact via www.esa-apprise.com or call 1-866-284-8089; due to evidence of tumor progression in patients with cancer who are undergoing chemotherapy, EPO administration must be approached with caution.
  - Adverse affects:
    - Increased risk of cardiovascular complications and mortality in CKD patients
    - Increased risk of thromboembolism
    - Rare red cell aplasia
    - Elevated risk of mortality with possible tumor progression in cancer patients
  - Specific benefits
    - Usually well tolerated; safe
- Darbepoetin-α (7,8): Limited use in humans
  - Longer-acting, molecularly modified EPO preparation with a half-life 3–4× longer than recombinant human EPO reduces the frequency of injections to weekly or biweekly.
  - Dosing and schedule
    - CKD-associated; conversion from epoetin, >1 year old; Start: see package insert based on current epoetin therapy; administer SC/IV q1–2wk; for patients with Hgb <10 g/dL; IV route preferred in hemodialysis patients; use the lowest dose to maintain Hgb level sufficient to reduce RBC transfusion need.
  - Adverse affects
    - Increased risk of thromboembolism
- Epoetin-α or darbepoetin-α dose adjustments
  - Follow FDA-approved labeling.
  - Treatment beyond 6–8 weeks without appropriate rise of Hgb (>1–2 g/dL) is not recommended.

ADDITIONAL THERAPIES

- Iron (1,2)
  - Indications
    - Coexisting iron deficiency
    - Resistance to EPO
  - Adverse affects
    - Gastrointestinal side effects (oral)
    - Systemic and/or local reactions (parenteral)
  - Benefits
    - Relatively safe
    - Inexpensive
- Transfusions (1,4)
  - Indications
    - Cardiac ischemia with an Hgb <10 g/dL
    - Chest pain, SOB, reduced exercise capacity, and/or EKG changes
    - Lack of response to medical therapy
  - Possible adverse affects
    - Infection
    - Volume overload
    - Transfusion reaction
  - Specific benefits
    - Rapid correction of anemia
  - In general, patients without serious pulmonary of cardiovascular disease may tolerate Hg levels > 8 g/dL and would only require intervention when the level falls below.
  - Transfusion is typically justifiable when the Hgb level is <7 g/dL.
  - Patients with underlying physiologic compromise such as cardiac or pulmonary disease, elderly patients, or patients who have symptoms interfering with daily functioning may require an Hgb level maintained above 10 g/dL.
  - When an infection occurs during EPO therapy, it is best to cease EPO therapy and rely on transfusion therapy instead until infection is properly treated.

ONGOING CARE

FOLLOW-UP RECOMMENDATIONS

Referral to a hematologist is not always warranted.

Patient Monitoring

- Hgb should be raised to near 12 g/dL at which dosages should be managed to maintain that level of Hgb (1).
- Baseline and periodic monitoring of iron, TIBC, transferrin saturation, and/or ferritin levels may be of value.
  - Iron repletion may be indicated for patients requiring EPO therapy (1).

PATIENT EDUCATION

- Patients receiving medical therapy should be advised about the following possible risks:
  - Mortality, cardiovascular complications, blood clots, progression of tumor
  - Patients can access more information at www.esa-apprise.com or by calling 1-866-284-8089.

PROGNOSIS

ACD does not typically progress.

COMPLICATIONS

Adverse affects of EPO (7):

- Heightened risk of mortality and/or cardiovascular complications in CKD patients
- Heightened risk of mortality and/or tumor progression in cancer patients
- Elevated risk of thromboembolism
- Arterial thrombotic episodes

REFERENCES

1. Weiss G, Goodnough LT. Anemia of chronic disease. *N Engl J Med*. 2005;352(10):1011–1023.
2. Knight K, Wade S, Balducci L. Prevalence and outcomes of anemia in cancer: a systematic review of the literature. *Am J Med*. 2004;116(Suppl 7A):11S–26S.
3. Roy CN. Anemia of inflammation. *Hematology Am Soc Hematol Educ Program*. 2010;2010:276–280.
4. Goodnough LT, Nemeth E, Ganz T. Detection, evaluation, and management of iron-restricted erythropoiesis. *Blood*. 2010;116(23):4754–4761.
5. Ganz T. Hepcidin and iron regulation, 10 years later. *Blood*. 2011;117(17):4425–4433.
6. Cheng PP, Jiao XY, Wang XH, et al. Hepcidin expression in anemia of chronic disease and concomitant iron-deficiency anemia. *Clin Exp Med*. 2011;11(1):33–42.
7. Rizzo JD, Somerfield MR, Hagerty KL, et al. Use of epoetin and darbepoetin in patients with cancer: 2007 American Society of Hematology/American Society of Clinical Oncology clinical practice guideline update. *Blood*. 2008;111(1):25–41.
8. Bloomfield M, Jaresko G, Zarek J, et al. Guidelines for using darbepoetin alfa in patients with chemotherapy-induced anemia. *Pharmacotherapy*. 2003;23(12, Pt 2):110S–118S.

SEE ALSO

- Anemia, Iron Deficiency
- Normocytic Anemia
- Microcytic Anemia
- Iron Studies

ADDITIONAL READING

Epoetin: for better or for worse? *Lancet Oncol*. 2004;5:1.

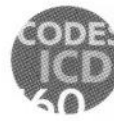

CODES

ICD10

- D63.8 Anemia in other chronic diseases classified elsewhere
- D63.0 Anemia in neoplastic disease
- D63.1 Anemia in chronic kidney disease

CLINICAL PEARLS

- ACD is one of the most common anemias clinically seen.
- One of the most common diagnostic problems, encountered within the clinical setting, is making the distinction between ACD and IDA.
  - Iron values will usually make a clear distinction.
- Iron should be given to all patients treated with EPO.

ANEMIA, IRON DEFICIENCY

Vibin Roy, MD

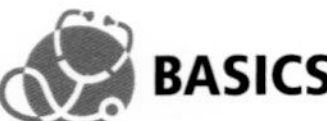

BASICS

DESCRIPTION

- Deficiency in red blood cells, hemoglobin, or blood volume due to decreased iron stores
- Onset may be acute (rapid blood loss) or chronic (nutrition derangement or slow blood loss).
- System(s) affected: heme, lymphatic, immunologic
- Synonym(s): anemia of chronic blood loss; hypochromic, microcytic anemia; chlorosis

Geriatric Considerations

60% of anemias occur in people >65 years of age.

Pediatric Considerations

Problematic in infants whose major source of nutrition is unfortified cow's milk and/or juices

Pregnancy Considerations

Iron supplements (15–30 mg/day) are recommended during pregnancy.

EPIDEMIOLOGY

- Iron deficiency anemia (IDA) is the most common cause of anemia in the world (1).
- Predominant age: all ages but especially toddlers and menstruating women
- Predominant sex: female > male
- More likely in the poor and in underimmunized children

Incidence

- Adults: men 2%, women 15–20% annually
- Infants and toddlers: 3–5% annually
- Pregnant patients: unclear; maybe as high 20% (pseudoanemia common during pregnancy as plasma volume expands faster than red cell mass) (2,3)

Prevalence

- Infants and children age <12 years: 4–7%
- Men: 2–5%
- Women: 9–16% (18–50% in menstruant blood donors) (2,3)

ETIOLOGY AND PATHOPHYSIOLOGY

Depletion of iron stores leads to decrease in both reticulocyte count and production of hemoglobin.

- Blood loss (e.g., menses, GI bleeding, trauma)
- Poor iron intake
- Poor iron absorption (e.g., atrophic gastritis, post-gastrectomy, celiac disease)
- Increased demand for iron (e.g., infancy, adolescence, pregnancy, and breastfeeding)

RISK FACTORS

- Premenopausal woman
- Frequent blood donor
- Pregnancy and breastfeeding
- Strict vegan diet
- Use of NSAIDs

GENERAL PREVENTION

- Screen asymptomatic pregnant women and children at 1 year of age (1).
- Supplementation in asymptomatic children aged 6–12 months if at risk for IDA (e.g., malnutrition, abuse, cow's milk <12 months)

COMMONLY ASSOCIATED CONDITIONS

- GI tract malignancy, peptic ulcer disease (PUD), *Helicobacter pylori* infection, irritable bowel disease
- Hookworm or other parasitic infestations
- Hypermetrorrhagia
- Pregnancy
- Obesity treated with gastric bypass surgery

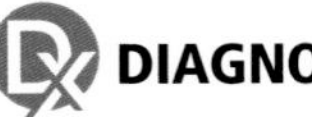

DIAGNOSIS

HISTORY

- Asymptomatic in most cases
- Weakness, fatigue, and/or malaise
- Exertional dyspnea
- Angina in patients with coronary artery disease
- Headaches or inability to concentrate
- Melena
- Pica

PHYSICAL EXAM

- Pallor
- Cheilosis
- Tachycardia
- Tachypnea
- Koilonychia (spoon-shaped, brittle nails)

DIFFERENTIAL DIAGNOSIS

- GI bleeding (e.g., gastritis, PUD, carcinoma, varices)
- Chronic intravascular hemolysis (e.g., paroxysmal nocturnal hemoglobinuria, malfunctioning prosthetic valve)
- Defective iron usage (e.g., thalassemia trait, sideroblastosis, G6PD deficiency)
- Defective iron reutilization (e.g., infection, inflammation, cancer, other chronic diseases)
- Hypoproliferation (e.g., decreased erythropoietin from hypothyroidism, renal failure)

DIAGNOSTIC TESTS & INTERPRETATION

Initial Tests (lab, imaging)

- Asymptomatic men and postmenopausal women should not be screened for IDA. Testing should be performed in patients with signs and symptoms of anemia, and a complete evaluation should be performed if iron deficiency is confirmed (1,3).
- Hemoglobin: <13 g in men and <12 g in women. Patients with higher premorbid hemoglobin (e.g., those with chronic hypoxemia, smokers, those who live at high altitudes) may be anemic at higher hemoglobin levels.
- Mean corpuscular volume (MCV): <80 fL
- Ferritin: <30 ng/mL, noninvasive test for diagnosis in adults but may miss some deficient patients because ferritin is an acute-phase reactant. Ferritin values >100 ng/mL generally exclude anemia (1).
- Total iron-binding capacity (TIBC): increased
- Transferrin saturation: <9%
- CBC with differential, peripheral smear, reticulocyte count, and index. A peripheral smear usually shows hypochromia and microcytosis, but may be normal, and reticulocyte production index is low. (2)
- Consider testing for G6PD deficiency: Assay at least 6 weeks after the last drop in hemoglobin.
- Rule out thalassemia.
  - Review prior CBCs for persisting mild anemia and marked micro-ovalocytosis, elevated hemoglobin A2 or hemoglobin F, family history, and especially high or high normal RBC count.
  - A low RBC count in patients with chronic bleeding helps to distinguish it from the thalassemia trait, where the count is high or high-normal.
  - Microcytosis with ovalocytosis and anemia unresponsive to iron suggests the thalassemia trait.
- MCV may be normal in mild anemia or hidden by the population of larger cells (e.g., reticulocytes or macrocytes). Red cell distribution width (RDW) will be increased if a mixed population of cells is present (e.g., mixed iron deficiency anemia and B_{12} deficiency).
- An empiric trial of iron at 3 mg/kg/day may be the best way to diagnose decreased iron stores in infants and children; reticulocytes become elevated in 7–10 days or hemoglobin increases >1 g/dL weekly, indicating iron deficiency.
- Drugs that may alter lab results: iron supplements or multivitamin–mineral preparations that contain iron
- Disorders that may alter lab results are the following:
  - Elevated ferritin: acute or chronic liver disease, Hodgkin disease, acute leukemia, solid tumors, fever, acute inflammation, renal dialysis
  - Elevated hemoglobin: smoking, chronic hypoxemia, long-term residency at high altitude
  - Stool guaiac; if high index of suspicion of GI bleed, perform GI endoscopy. Under appropriate circumstances, check stool for ova and parasites.
  - Rule out poor reutilization: trial of iron, bone marrow aspiration, and iron stain
  - Rule out colorectal cancer and gastric carcinoma, especially in the elderly.

Diagnostic Procedures/Other

- GI (upper and lower) endoscopy to evaluate for bleeding sites in following cases (1,4)[C]:
  - premenopausal women with negative GYN workup and/or lack of response to iron
  - men and postmenopausal women
- Bone marrow aspiration confirms diagnosis but is rarely performed.

Test Interpretation

- Absent or decreased marrow iron stores
- Marrow: hyperplastic, micronormoblastic

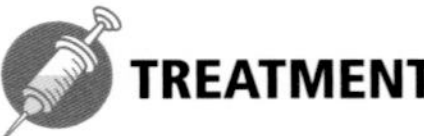

TREATMENT

GENERAL MEASURES

- Search for underlying cause and correct, if possible.
- Avoid transfusions, except in rare cases.

MEDICATION

- Ferrous sulfate 325 mg TID or ferrous gluconate 324 mg 1–2 tablets TID or ferrous fumarate 324 mg 1 tablet BID on an empty stomach 1 hour before meals (1)[C].
  - Reduce dose as needed for GI symptoms, which affect 25% of patients receiving standard iron therapy, or the dose can be taken with meals, which may reduce the delivery of iron by 50%. Constipation will occur in ~1/4 patients using various iron formulations.
  - Drugs that increase gastric pH (e.g., proton pump inhibitors, H_2 antagonists) also reduce iron absorption.
  - Special oral iron formulations (including enteric-coated iron) and compounds are expensive and reduce symptoms only to the degree that they reduce the delivery of iron.
- Liquid iron preparations are useful for children, with a recommended dose of 3 mg/kg/day; can also be used in adults when tablets are not absorbed or low tolerance requires a dose reduction.
- Foods and beverages containing ascorbic acid (vitamin C) enhance iron absorption when taken simultaneously with the iron (1,3).

- Continued bleeding and untreated hypothyroidism are causes for "failure to respond" to iron.
- Formula to determine elemental iron needed:
  - Elemental Iron in mg for adults and children over 15 kg (33 lbs):
    - Dose (mL) = 0.0442 (Desired Hb − Observed Hb) × LBW + (0.26 × LBW)
  - Desired Hb = the target Hb in g/dL
  - Observed Hb = the patient's current hemoglobin in g/dL
  - LBW = lean body weight in kg
  - For males: LBW = 50 kg + 2.3 kg for each inch of patient's height over 5 feet
  - For females: LBW = 45.5 kg + 2.3 kg for each inch of patient's height over 5 feet
  - Normal hemoglobin (males and females)
    - over 15 kg (33 lbs). . . . . 14.8 g/dL
    - 15 kg (33 lbs) or less . . . . 12.0 g/dL
- Consider parenteral iron for patients with a hemoglobin level <6 g/dL, malabsorption, chronic kidney disease, or if higher oral doses and use of vitamin C fail (1).
- Numerous parenteral iron formulations approved for use are the following:
  - Anaphylaxis to parenteral iron therapy has occurred; a test dose for iron dextran recommended prior to first dose; ferric gluconate or iron sucrose may be safer alternatives to iron dextran. Dimercaprol increases risk of nephrotoxicity.
  - Dosing is product dependent; refer to individual product for suggested dosing
- Reserve blood transfusion for severe acute blood loss or severely symptomatic patients (e.g., demand ischemia due to anemia). Hemoglobin threshold varies by risk factors and clinical scenario (1,5)[C].
- Contraindications (oral iron) (3)
  - Tetracycline concomitantly
- Significant possible interactions (oral iron)
  - Allopurinol
  - Antacids
  - Penicillamine
  - Fluoroquinolones
  - Tetracyclines
  - Vitamin E
- Precautions
  - Iron preparations may cause dark stools and constipation.
  - Iron overdose is highly toxic; patients should be instructed to keep tablets and liquids out of the reach of small children.

ISSUES FOR REFERRAL

- Adult men and postmenopausal women with IDA should be screened for possible GI malignancy.
- Pregnant women with a hemoglobin (Hgb) level <9 g/dL
- Failure to respond to a 4–6-week trial of oral iron therapy
- Nonpregnant women or other patients with an Hgb level <6 g/dL

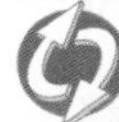

ONGOING CARE

FOLLOW-UP RECOMMENDATIONS

Patient Monitoring

- Regularly after Hgb returns to normal (to detect recurrences)
- Hgb increases 1 g/dL every 3–4 weeks.
- Iron stores may take up to 4 weeks to correct after Hgb returns to normal.

DIET

- Do not consume milk or other dairy products, antacids, fluoroquinolones, or tetracycline within 2 hours of iron supplement ingestion.
- Limit tea, coffee, and caffeinated beverages.
- Limit milk to 16 oz/day (adults).
- Emphasize protein and iron-containing foods (meat, beans, and leafy green vegetables).
- Taking iron with orange juice or ascorbic acid may increase absorption but decreases GI tolerability.
- Increase fluid and dietary fiber to decrease likelihood of constipation during iron replacement therapy.

PATIENT EDUCATION

National Heart, Lung & Blood Institute, Communications & Public Information Branch, National Institutes of Health, Building 31, Room 41–21, 9000 Rockville Pike, Bethesda, MD 20892; (301) 251–1222.

PROGNOSIS

- Can be resolved with iron therapy if the underlying cause can be discovered and appropriately treated.
- Treat subclinical hypothyroidism and IDA together when these conditions coexist. Failure to treat hypothyroidism results in poor response to iron therapy.

COMPLICATIONS

- Neglecting to identify hidden bleeding points, particularly a bleeding malignancy
- Maternal iron deficiency negatively affects mother–child interactions. Iron supplementation protects against these negative effects.

REFERENCES

1. Short MW, Domagalski JE. Iron deficiency anemia: evaluation and management. *Am Fam Physician*. 2013;87(2):98–104.
2. Killip S, Bennett JM, Chambers MD. Iron deficiency anemia. *Am Fam Physician*. 2007;75(5):671–678.
3. Johnson-Wimbley TD, Graham DY. Diagnosis and management of iron deficiency anemia in the 21st century. *Therap Adv Gastroenterol*. 2011;4(3):177–184.
4. Zhu A, Kaneshiro M, Kaunitz JD. Evaluation and treatment of iron deficiency anemia: a gastroenterological perspective. *Dig Dis Sci*. 2010;55(3):548–559.
5. Murphy MF, Wallington TB, Kelsey P, et al; British Committee for Standards in Haematology, Blood Transfusion Task Force. Guidelines for the clinical use of red cell transfusions. *Br J Haematol*. 2001;113(1):24–31.

ADDITIONAL READING

- Chertow GM, Mason PD, Vaage-Nilsen O, et al. On the relative safety of parenteral iron formulations. *Nephrol Dial Transplant*. 2004;19(6):1571–1575.
- Chertow GM, Mason PD, Vaage-Nilsen O, et al. Update on adverse drug events associated with parenteral iron. *Nephrol Dial Transplant*. 2006;21(2):378–382.
- Cinemre H, Bilir C, Gokosmanoglu F, et al. Hematologic effects of levothyroxine in iron-deficient subclinical hypothyroid patients: a randomized, double-blind, controlled study. *J Clin Endocrinol Metab*. 2009;94(1):151–156.
- de Benoist B, McLean E, Egli I, et al, eds. *Worldwide Prevalence of Anaemia 1993–2005. WHO Global Database on Anaemia*. Geneva, Switzerland: World Health Organization; 2008. http://whqlibdoc.who.int/publications/2008/9789241596657_eng.pdf. Accessed on October 19, 2011.
- Dubois RW, Goodnough LT, Ershler WB, et al. Identification, diagnosis, and management of anemia in adult ambulatory patients treated by primary care physicians: evidence-based and consensus recommendations. *Curr Med Res Opin*. 2006;22(2):385–395.
- Mabry-Hernandez IR. Screening for iron deficiency anemia–including iron supplementation for children and pregnant women. *Am Fam Physician*. 2009;79(10):897–898.
- Melamed N, Ben-Haroush A, Kaplan B, et al. Iron supplementation in pregnancy—does the preparation matter? *Arch Gynecol Obstet*. 2007;276(6):601–604.
- Murray-Kolb LE, Beard JL. Iron deficiency and child and maternal health. *Am J Clin Nutr*. 2009;89:946S–950S.
- Tefferi A, Hanson CA, Inwards DJ. How to interpret and pursue an abnormal complete blood cell count in adults. *Mayo Clin Proc*. 2005;80(7):923–936.

SEE ALSO

Algorithm: Anemia

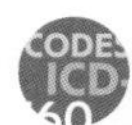

CODES

ICD10

- D50.9 Iron deficiency anemia, unspecified
- D62 Acute posthemorrhagic anemia
- D50.0 Iron deficiency anemia secondary to blood loss (chronic)

CLINICAL PEARLS

- IDA due to poor dietary intake is the most common type of anemia in in the world.
- Blood loss and reduced iron stores due to malabsorption or poor utilization are major risk factors for IDA.
- Premenopausal women and children are at the greatest risk for IDA.
- Recommend no cow's milk to any child age <12 months.
- Oral iron supplementation is the standard treatment option for patients with IDA.

ANEMIA, SICKLE CELL

Rami Farhat, DO • Tipsuda Junsanto-Bahri, MD

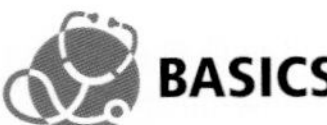

BASICS

DESCRIPTION

- Hereditary, chronic hemoglobinopathy marked by chronic hemolytic anemia, periodic acute episodes of painful "crises," and increased susceptibility to infections
- The heterozygous condition (Hb A/S), sickle cell trait, is usually asymptomatic without anemia.
- Among the compound heterozygotes, sickle-hemoglobin C disease (HbSC) and $S\beta+$ thalassemia are clinically similar to the heterozygous condition, whereas, $S\beta°$ thalassemia is clinically similar to the homozygous condition.
- Synonym(s): sickle cell disease (SCD); Hb SS disease

Pediatric Considerations

- Sequestration crises and hand–foot syndrome seen typically in infants/young children
- Adolescence/young adulthood
  - Frequency of complications and organ/tissue damage increases with age (except for strokes, which occur mostly in childhood).
  - Psychological complications: body image, interrupted schooling, restriction of activities; stigma of disease; low self-esteem

Pregnancy Considerations

- Complicated, especially 3rd trimester and delivery
  - Fetal mortality 35–40%. Fetal survival is >90% if the fetus reaches the 3rd trimester (1)[B].
  - High prevalence of small for gestational age (SGA) babies
- Increased risk of preterm delivery, pain, toxemia, infection, pulmonary infarction, phlebitis
- Partial exchange transfusion in 3rd trimester may reduce maternal morbidity and fetal mortality, but this is controversial.
- Chronic transfusions have been effective in diminishing pain episodes in pregnant women. However, this method should be used with caution due to risk of alloimmunization.

EPIDEMIOLOGY

Prevalence

- ~90,000 Americans have sickle cell anemia (SCA) and 10% of African Americans carry the trait. ~1/500 African Americans and 1/1,000 Hispanics have homozygous SCA. Each year in the United States, about 1/400 African American infants are born with SCD.
- Lesser risk: Middle East, Mediterranean area, and populations in India may be affected.

ETIOLOGY AND PATHOPHYSIOLOGY

- Substitution of valine for glutamic acid in 6th amino acid of hemoglobin β-chain. Mutation → RBCs change from biconcave to sickle shape when deoxygenated due to poor solubility of mutated hemoglobin chain.
- Sickle RBCs are inflexible, causing increased blood viscosity, stasis, obstruction of small arterioles and capillaries, and ischemia.
- Chronic anemia; crises:
  - Vaso-occlusive crisis: tissue ischemia and necrosis; progressive organ failure/tissue damage from repeated episodes
  - Hand–foot syndrome: Vessel occlusion/ischemia affects small blood vessels in hands or feet.
  - Aplastic crisis: suppression of RBC production by severe infection (e.g., parvoviral and other viral infections)
  - Suppression of RBC production
  - Hyperhemolytic crisis: accelerated hemolysis with reticulocytosis; increased RBC fragility/shortened lifespan
  - Sequestration crisis: splenic sequestration of blood (only in young children as spleen is later lost to autoinfarction)
- Susceptibility to infection: impaired/absent splenic function leading to decreased ability to clear infection; defect in alternate pathway of complement activation.
- Increased red cell destruction causes an inability to maintain adequate hemoglobin levels and results in anemia and fatigue.
- Sickle cells exhibit increased adhesion and decreased ability to maneuver through small vessels, leading to vaso-occlusion.

Genetics

Autosomal recessive. Homozygous condition, Hb SS; heterozygous condition, Hb A/S. The heterozygote condition can also be combined with other hemoglobinopathies, the most common of which are HbC and β thalassemia.

RISK FACTORS

- For vaso-occlusive crisis ("painful crisis"): hypoxia, dehydration, fever, infection, acidosis, cold, anesthesia, strenuous physical exercise, smoking
- For aplastic crisis (suppression of RBC production): severe infections, human parvovirus B19 infection, folic acid deficiency.
- Hyperhemolytic crisis (accelerated hemolysis with reticulocytosis) (existence is controversial): acute bacterial infections, exposure to oxidant drugs

GENERAL PREVENTION

- Prevention of crises:
  - Avoid hypoxia, dehydration, cold, infection, fever, acidosis, and anesthesia.
  - Prompt management of fever, infections, pain
  - Hydration
  - Avoid alcohol and smoking.
  - Avoid high-altitude areas.
- Minimizing trauma: Aseptic technique is imperative.

DIAGNOSIS

Diagnosis is often made by newborn screening programs.

HISTORY

- Often asymptomatic in early months of life due to presence of fetal hemoglobin
- In those >6 months of age, earliest symptoms are irritability and painful swelling of the hands and feet (hand–foot syndrome). May also see pneumococcal sepsis or meningitis, severe anemia and acute splenic enlargement (splenic sequestration), acute chest syndrome, pallor, jaundice, or splenomegaly.
- Major manifestations in older children include anemia, severe or recurrent musculoskeletal or abdominal pain, aplastic crisis, acute chest syndrome, splenomegaly or splenic sequestration, and cholelithiasis.
- Painful crises in bones, joints, abdomen, back, and viscera account for 90% of all hospital admissions.
- Acute chest syndrome: tachycardia, fever, bilateral infiltrates caused by pulmonary infarctions

PHYSICAL EXAM

Fever, pale skin and nail beds, mild jaundice

DIFFERENTIAL DIAGNOSIS

Anemia: other hemoglobinopathies

DIAGNOSTIC TESTS & INTERPRETATION

Initial Tests (lab, imaging)

- Screening test: Sickledex test
  - Hb electrophoresis (diagnostic test of choice); sickle cell anemia (FS pattern)
    - 80–100% Hb S, variable amounts of Hb F, and no Hb A1
    - Sickle cell trait (FS pattern): 30–45% Hb S, 50–70% Hb A1, minimal Hb F
- Hemoglobin ~5–10 g/dL; RBC indices: mean corpuscular volume (MCV) normal to increased; mean corpuscular hemoglobin concentration (MCHC) increased; HgSS, reticulocytes 3–15%
- Leukocytosis; bands in absence of infection, platelets elevated; peripheral smear: sickled RBCs, nucleated RBCs, Howell-Jolly bodies
- Serum bilirubin mildly elevated (2–4 mg/dL); ferritin very elevated in multiply transfused patients; serum lactate dehydrogenase (LDH) elevated
- Fecal/urinary urobilinogen high
- Haptoglobin absent or very low
- Urine analysis: hemoglobinuria, hematuria (sickle cell trait may have painless hematuria), increased albuminuria (monitor for progressive kidney disease)
- Need for imaging depends on clinical circumstances:
  - Bone scan to rule out osteomyelitis
  - CT/MRI to rule out CVA; high index of suspicion required for any acute neurologic symptoms other than mild headache.
  - Chest x-ray: may show enlarged heart; diffuse alveolar infiltrates in acute chest syndrome
  - Transcranial Doppler: start at age 2 years; repeat yearly. Transcranial Doppler ultrasound identifies children age 2–16 years at higher risk of stroke.
  - ECG to detect pulmonary hypertension and echocardiogram every other year from age 15 years and older.

Test Interpretation

Hyposplenism due to autosplenectomy is common; hypoxia/infarction in multiple organs

TREATMENT

GENERAL MEASURES

- Painful crises: hydration, analgesics; oxygen regardless of whether the patient is hypoxic (2)[A]
- Retinal evaluation starting at school age to detect proliferative sickle retinopathy (2)[A]
- Occupational therapy, cognitive and behavioral therapies, support groups
- All standard childhood vaccinations should be administered accordingly.
- Special immunizations
  - Influenza vaccine yearly starting at age 2 years
  - Conjugated pneumococcal vaccine (PCV13) at ages 2, 4, and 6 months; booster at 12–15 months
  - 23-valent polysaccharide vaccine (PPSV23) at 2 years; booster 3–5 years after first dose
  - Patients younger than 5 years of age with incomplete vaccination history should receive catch-up doses accordingly.
  - PPSV23 should be administered at least 8 weeks after most recent dose of PCV13.

- Meningococcal vaccine (MCV4): age 2–18 months: MCV4 at ages 2, 4, 6, and 12 months; age 19–23 months: two doses of MCV4 separated by 3 months; >2 years of age, two doses of MCV4 separated by 2 months; boosters recommended every 5 years. G-CSF use is contraindicated as it may lead to vaso-occlusive episodes and multiorgan failure.

MEDICATION

First Line

- Supplemental oxygen
- Painful crises (mild, outpatient) (3)[A]
  – Nonnopioid analgesics (ibuprofen)
- Painful crises (severe, hospitalized)
  – Parenteral opioids (e.g., morphine on fixed schedule); patient-controlled analgesia (PCA) pump may be useful.
- Hydroxyurea for prevention of painful acute chest syndrome, vaso-occlusive episodes, and very severe anemia. Start with 15 mg/kg/day single daily dose; titrate upward every 12 weeks (max dose of 30 mg/kg/day) if blood counts satisfactory (avoid severe neutropenia)
- Acute chest syndrome: may deteriorate quickly; aggressive management with oxygen, analgesics, antibiotics, simple or exchange transfusion
- Empiric antibiotics to cover *Streptococcus pneumoniae*, *Haemophilus influenzae*, *Mycoplasma pneumoniae*, and *Chlamydia pneumoniae* (cephalosporins or azithromycin) (3)[A]. If osteomyelitis, cover for *Staphylococcus aureus* and *Salmonella* (e.g., ciprofloxacin). If apparent pneumonia not promptly responding to antibiotics, consider diagnosis of acute chest syndrome and initiate simple or exchange transfusion.
- Prophylactic penicillins indicated in infants and children starting at 2 months: For children younger than 5 years of age, a dose of 125 mg BID is recommended. Unless the patient has a history of severe pneumococcal sepsis, administration may be stopped at 5 years. If a history of pneumococcal sepsis is present, a dose of 250 mg BID is suggested; if high risk remains, continue until puberty. Rising pneumococcal resistance to penicillin may change future recommendations.
- Precautions: Avoid high-dose estrogen oral contraceptives; consider Depo-Provera.

Second Line

Folic acid: 0–6 months: 0.1 mg/day; 6–12 months: 0.25 mg/day; 1–2 years: 0.5 mg/day; >2 years of age: 1 mg/day

ADDITIONAL THERAPIES

Transfusions and additional therapies (3)[A]:

- Transfusion for aplastic crises, severe complications (i.e., CVA), prophylactically before surgery, and treatment for acute chest syndrome; prophylactic transfusions for primary or secondary stroke prevention in children (3)[A]
- Preoperative transfusions have been shown to reduce the risk of perioperative complications.
- Avoid blood hyperviscosity.
- Consider chelation with deferasirox, an oral agent, if the patient is multiply transfused (after age 2 years). Red cell exchange transfusion minimizes risk of iron overload.

SURGERY/OTHER PROCEDURES

- Targeted fetal hemoglobin induction treatment (4)[A]
- Hematopoietic stem cell transplant (HSCT) (5)[A]: curative, but with significant morbidity and mortality; limited to individuals <16 years old.

INPATIENT CONSIDERATIONS

Admission Criteria/Initial Stabilization

Severe pain, suspected infection or sepsis, evidence of acute chest syndrome

IV Fluids

The preferred maintenance IV fluid is 1/2 NS, as NS may theoretically increase the risk of sickling.

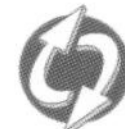

ONGOING CARE

FOLLOW-UP RECOMMENDATIONS

Patient Monitoring

- Treat infections early. Parents/patients: Any temperature of ≥101°F (38.3°C) requires immediate medical attention.
- For patients who receive chronic transfusions, monitor for hepatitis and hemosiderosis.
- Periodic eye evaluations: starting age 5 years to detect proliferative sickle retinopathy (3)[A]
- Biannual examination for hepatic, renal, and pulmonary dysfunction
- Baseline pulmonary evaluation at each visit to assess for wheezing, shortness of breath, or cough as these may be indicators of disease severity and pulmonary hypertension
- Consider venous thromboembolism (VTE) prophylaxis as there is an increased incidence of thromboembolism (6)[A].

DIET

- Folic acid supplementation; avoid alcohol (leads to dehydration); maintain hydration
- Multivitamin without iron is recommended; as there is high incidence of vitamin D deficiency and decreased bone marrow density in SCD patients.

PATIENT EDUCATION

- SickleCellKids.org—Education Web site for children with sickle cell anemia: SickleCellKids.org
- Sickle Cell Disease.org: http://www.sicklecelldisease.org
- American Sickle Cell Anemia Association: http://www.ascaa.org

PROGNOSIS

- In adulthood, fewer crises, but more complications. Median age of death is 42 years for men and 48 years for women. Causes: infections, thrombosis, pulmonary emboli, pulmonary hypertension, and renal failure
- Anemia occurs in infancy; sickle cell crises at 1–2 years of age; some children die in their 1st year.

COMPLICATIONS

- Alloimmunization, bone infarct and osteomyelitis, aseptic necrosis of femoral head
- CVA (peak age 6–7 years), impaired mental development, even without history of stroke
- Cholelithiasis/abnormal liver function
- Chronic leg ulcers, poor wound healing
- Impotence, priapism, hematuria/hyposthenuria, renal concentrating and acidifying defects
- Retinopathy, splenic infarction (by age 10 years)
- Acute chest syndrome (infection/infarction) leading to chronic pulmonary disease
- Infections (pneumonia, osteomyelitis, meningitis, pyelonephritis); sepsis (leading cause of morbidity and mortality)
- Hemosiderosis (secondary to multiple transfusions).
- Substance abuse related to chronic pain

REFERENCES

1. Costa VM, Viana MB, Aguilar RA. Pregnancy in patients with sickle cell disease: maternal and perinatal outcomes [published online ahead of print June 26, 2014]. *J Matern Fetal Neonatal Med*. doi:10.3109/14767058.2014.928855
2. Brousse V, Makani J, Rees DC. Management of sickle cell disease in the community. *BMJ*. 2014;348:g1765.
3. Chou ST. Transfusion therapy for sickle cell disease: a balancing act. *Hematol Am Soc Educ Program*. 2013;2013:439–446.
4. Manwani D, Frenette PS. Vaso-occlusion in sickle cell disease: pathophysiology and novel targeted therapies. *Blood*. 2013;122(24):3892–3898.
5. Hsieh MM, Fitzhugh CD, Weitzel RP, et al. Nonmyeloablative HLA-matched sibling allogeneic hematopoietic stem cell transplantation for severe sickle cell phenotype. *JAMA*. 2014;312(1):48–56.
6. Naik RP, Streiff MB, Lanzkron S. Sickle cell disease and venous thromboembolism: what the anticoagulation expert needs to know. *J Thromb Thrombolysis*. 2013;35(3):352–358.

ADDITIONAL READING

- Cober MP, Phelps SJ. Penicillin prophylaxis in children with sickle cell disease. *J Pediatr Pharmacol Ther*. 2010;15(3):152–159.
- Howard J, Malfroy M, Llewelyn C, et al. The transfusion alternatives preoperatively in sickle cell disease (TAPS) study: a randomised, controlled, multicentre clinical trial. *Lancet*. 2013;381(9870):930–938.
- Machado RF, Farber HW. Pulmonary hypertension associated with chronic hemolytic anemia and other blood disorders. *Clin Chest Med*. 2013:34(4): 739–752.

SEE ALSO

Algorithm: Anemia

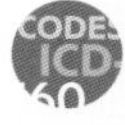

CODES

ICD10

- D57.1 Sickle-cell disease without crisis
- D57.3 Sickle-cell trait
- D57.00 Hb-SS disease with crisis, unspecified

CLINICAL PEARLS

- Almost 90,000 Americans have SCA and, ~1/500 African Americans and 1/1,000 Hispanics have SCA; 10% carry the trait
- The preferred maintenance IV fluid is 1/2 NS, as NS may theoretically increase the risk of sickling.
- Painful crises in bones, joints, abdomen, back, and viscera account for 90% of all hospital admissions.
- Acute chest syndrome: tachycardia, fever, bilateral infiltrates caused by pulmonary infarctions

ANEURYSM OF THE ABDOMINAL AORTA

Michael J. Gray, MD, MA, MS, ATC

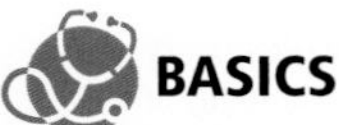

BASICS

DESCRIPTION

- An infrarenal aorta ≥3 cm in diameter is considered aneurysmal (1–5).
- Types
  - Fusiform aneurysm: involves the whole circumference or wall of the artery
  - Saccular aneurysm: does not involve the full circumference; often appears as an asymmetrical bleb or blister on side of aorta. Clinical presentation relates to aneurysm location, size, type, and comorbid factors affecting patient. The majority are asymptomatic. May present with rupture, embolism, or thrombosis. Treatment and indications for surgical repair are dictated by risk of rupture, risk of surgical repair, and estimated patient life expectancy.
- System(s) affected: cardiovascular; neurologic; heme/lymphatic/immunologic
- Synonym(s): aortic aneurysms; AAA

Geriatric Considerations

Incidence of AAA, risk of rupture, and operative morbidity and mortality all rise with age.

Pediatric Considerations

Rare in children; may be associated with umbilical artery catheters, connective tissue diseases, arteritides, or congenital abnormalities

EPIDEMIOLOGY

- Frequency increases >50 years of age.
- Predominant sex: male > female (5:1) (1)

Incidence

- >15,000 deaths per year in United States
- 10th leading cause of death in men 65–75 years
- 3.9–7.2% males older than 50 years (3)
- 1.0–1.3% females older than 50 years (3)
- Females with 2–4 times increased risk of rupture (6)

Prevalence

- Depends on risk factors associated with AAA
- Prevalence of AAAs 2.9–4.9 cm in diameter ranges from 1.3% for men aged 45–54 years to 12.5% for men 75–84 years. Data for women are 0% and 5.2%, respectively; however, when detected, women presented at an older age and were more likely to present with a ruptured AAA. Female sex is an independent risk factor for *death* from AAA (2).

ETIOLOGY AND PATHOPHYSIOLOGY

- Vascular inflammatory degenerative disease, with major role of matrix metalloproteinases and inflammatory markers that result in aortic medial degeneration (4,6)
- Gradual and/or sporadic expansion of aneurysm and accumulation of mural thrombus (4)
- Mural thrombus can contribute to an area of localized hypoxia, thus further weakening the aneurysm (4).
- Aneurysms tend to expand over time. (Laplace law: T [wall tension] = pressure × radius. Wall tension directly related to BP and radius of artery.) When wall tension exceeds wall tensile strength, rupture occurs (2,4).
- Average small AAA (<5.5 cm) grows at rate of 2.6–3.2 mm/year. Larger aneurysms grow faster rate as do aneurysms in current smokers; otherwise no identifiable risk factors to assess which small AAAs will advance to require further intervention.
- Annual growth rate of 2.2 mm/year average for small aneurysms but increased in smokers; decreased in diabetics (4)
- 60–80% of AAAs between 40 and 49 mm will enlarge and require surgery in 5 years.
- Degenerative: atherosclerotic (80%); other causes: inflammatory diseases (5%), trauma, connective tissue disorders, infection (*Brucella*, *Salmonella*, staph, tuberculosis)

Genetics

- Familial aggregations exist: Aneurysms may develop at an earlier age.
- 2× risk of AAA if 1st-degree relative with AAA (1,2,6)
- 12–19% of patients with repair had 1st-degree relative with AAA (2).
- Marfan syndrome
- Ehlers-Danlos syndrome
- Polycystic kidney disease
- Tuberous sclerosis

RISK FACTORS

Older age, male, Northern European ethnicity, family history, smoking, hypertension (HTN), hyperlipidemia, peripheral vascular disease, peripheral aneurysms, chronic obstructive peripheral disease (COPD), obesity (2,4,6)

GENERAL PREVENTION

- Address cardiovascular disease risk factors.
- Follow screening guidelines: US screening for detection of AAA in male patients, 65–75 years, who have ever smoked.

COMMONLY ASSOCIATED CONDITIONS

- HTN, myocardial infarction (MI), heart failure, carotid artery, and/or lower extremity peripheral arterial disease
- Screening for thoracic aneurysm should also be considered.

DIAGNOSIS

- Screening: recommended 1-time US for AAA in men 65–75 years who have EVER smoked (3)[B], selective offer 1-time US in men 65–75 years who have NEVER smoked (3)[C]
- U.S. Preventive Services Task Force recommends against routine screening for women who have NEVER smoked and states that there is insufficient evidence to make a recommendation for women 65–75 years old who have EVER smoked.
- Most often asymptomatic: discovered during exams for other complaints (1)
- Symptomatic: embolization, thrombosis, vague abdominal or back pain, syncope, lower extremity paralysis
- Rupture

ALERT

- The triad of shock, pulsatile mass, and abdominal pain always suggests rupture of AAA, and immediate surgical evaluation recommended (2)[B].
  - Shock may be absent if rupture is contained.
  - Palpable pulsatile mass may be absent in up to 50% of patients with rupture.
  - Pain may radiate to the back, groin, flank (mimics urolithiasis), buttocks, or legs.
- Unusual presentations:
  - Primary aortoenteric fistula: erosion/rupture of AAA into duodenum
  - Aortocaval fistula: erosion/rupture of AAA into vena cava or left renal vein: 3–6%
  - Inflammatory aneurysm: encasement by thick inflammatory rind; can cause chronic abdominal pain, weight loss, and elevated ESR. Surrounding viscera densely adherent

HISTORY

Abdominal or back pain; AAA risk factors

PHYSICAL EXAM

- Pulsatile supraumbilical mass
- Only 30–40% of AAA detected by physical exam (6)
- Physical exam will only detect 76% of aneurysms >5 cm (6).
- 14% of AAA associated with femoral or popliteal aneurysms, and 62–85% of patients with femoral or popliteal aneurysms will have a AAA (6); therefore recommended AAA evaluation for all patients with known femoral or popliteal aneurysms (2)[B]
- Vague abdominal tenderness: may radiate to the back or flank
- Encroachment by aneurysm
  - Vertebral body erosion, gastric outlet obstruction, ureteral obstruction
  - Lower extremity ischemia secondary to embolization of mural thrombus
- Rupture leads to tachycardia, hypotension, evidence of shock and anemia, possible flank contusion (Grey-Turner sign) (6).

DIAGNOSTIC TESTS & INTERPRETATION

Initial Tests (lab, imaging)

- If rupturing AAA is considered: complete blood chemistry (chemistries, coags, type and cross), ECG
- US: simplest and least expensive diagnostic procedure
- Multiple studies have demonstrated high sensitivity (94–100%) and specificity (98–100%) of US (3,6).
- Although effective in detecting AAA, US is a poor test to show leakage or rupture if bleeding is into the retroperitoneal space.
- Surveillance of asymptomatic aneurysm
  - 2.6–2.9 cm: Screen at 5-year intervals (6)[C].
  - 3.0–3.9 cm: Screen at 3-year intervals (2)[B],(6)[C].
  - 4.0–5.4 cm: Screen every 6–12 months (2)[A].
- CT scans are preferred preoperative study (caution with IV contrast in renal failure).
- MRI/MRA can visualize AAA but is often not possible in emergent situations.
- Aortography: does not define outer dimensions of aneurysm
- Abdominal x-rays can be diagnostic if calcifications exist; not a diagnostic tool of choice (1,2)
- Ongoing research is exploring alternative diagnostic measurements, including measurement of total aortic volume versus single axial diameter measurement and measurement of total thrombus burden associated with AAA because this appears to have a greater risk association (2,4).

Follow-Up Tests & Special Considerations

Evaluation for coronary artery disease is appropriate prior to elective AAA repair (i.e., cardiac clearance), including stress test, echocardiography, and ECG if appropriate (1).

Diagnostic Procedures/Other

ALERT
Use clinical judgment: Patients with known AAA having abdominal or back pain symptoms may be rupturing despite a negative CT scan.

DIFFERENTIAL DIAGNOSIS
- Other abdominal masses
- Other causes of abdominal or back pain (e.g., peptic ulcer disease, renal colic, diverticulitis, appendicitis, incarcerated hernia, bowel obstruction, GI hemorrhage, arthritis, metastatic disease, myocardial infarction)

TREATMENT

GENERAL MEASURES
- Treat atherosclerotic risk factors (2,5)[C].
- Medical optimization of cardiac, renal, and pulmonary conditions
- Smoking cessation (increased rate of expansion of 20–25% with continued smoking) and exercise (2,5)[B]
- Emergent treatment in unstable or symptomatic patients is immediate vascular surgery consultation, adequate IV access and resuscitation, type and cross for multiple units, and rapid bedside US.
- Less acute treatment of AAA/prevention of rupture is elective repair and risk factor modification.

MEDICATION
- Beta-blockers should be used perioperatively in absence of contraindications (2,6)[A]; bronchodilators should be used for 2 weeks prior to repair for patients with COPD (6)[C].
- Statin therapy may be effective in decreasing the growth rate of small AAA according to a meta-analytic study. More data and trials are still needed (6)[C].
- Aspirin may inhibit expansion by inhibiting thrombus growth.
- Doxycycline and beta-blockers may also inhibit expansion, but further studies are needed. Early animal studies indicate possible role for ACE-I/ARBs, mast cell stabilizers, prostaglandin inhibitors, and novel gene therapy (6).

SURGERY/OTHER PROCEDURES
Current recommendations
- Elective
  - 5.5-cm diameter is threshold for repair in "average" patient (2)[B].
  - Younger, low-risk patients with long life expectancy may prefer early repair.
  - Women or AAA with high risk of rupture: Consider elective repair at 4.5–5 cm.
  - Consider delayed repair in high-risk patients.
  - 5% perioperative mortality for open elective repair (2)
- High risk of rupture
  - Expansion >0.6 cm/year
  - Smoking/COPD severe/steroids
  - Family history; multiple relatives
  - Hypertension poorly controlled
  - Shape nonfusiform
- High-risk patients for elective repair
  - Risk factors for open repair include age >70 years, COPD, chronic renal insufficiency (CRI), suprarenal clamp site, with 1-year mortality if no risk factors present of 1.2% and 67% for all 4 risk factors present.
  - Other poor prognostic factors include inactive/poor stamina, congestive heart failure, significant coronary artery disease, liver disease, family history of AAA.
  - Consider coronary revascularization prior to aneurysm repair if coronary artery disease (6)[B].
  - Discontinue thienopyridine (clopidogrel and others); use 10 days prior to AAA repair, and restart immediately postoperatively (6)[C].
  - Transfusion to hematocrit >28.0 if elective open repair planned (6)[C]
- Emergent/symptomatic repair: traditionally, open repair; however, candidates with appropriate anatomy can have endovascular repair, with an estimated mortality of 32% for endovascular versus 44% open.
- Open repair versus endovascular repair (EVAR)
  - Open repair or EVAR in patients who are good or average surgical candidates (6)[B]
  - Open repair for patients who are unable to comply with the recommended periodic long-term surveillance (6)[B]
  - EVAR for patients at high surgical risk due to significant cardiac, pulmonary, or renal disease, but no significant mortality improvement compared with no therapy (6)[B]
  - EVAR tends to have improved procedural mortality (1.8% vs. 4.3%), but long-term mortality over 6 years is similar (7.5 deaths/patient-years for EVAR vs. 7.7 deaths/patient-years for open repair), and EVAR patients require lifelong follow-up for monitoring (2,3).

INPATIENT CONSIDERATIONS
Risk of abdominal compartment syndrome after repair, 4–12%; usually associated with large fluid resuscitation

ONGOING CARE

FOLLOW-UP RECOMMENDATIONS
CT or MRI evaluation of the graft for EVAR surveillance at 1 month, 6 months, then annually (2)[B]

Patient Monitoring
BP and fasting lipid values: Control as for atherosclerotic disease (6)[C].

DIET
Low-fat, low-salt, and low-caffeine diet; nutrition optimized prior to elective repair; parenteral nutrition started within 7 days postoperatively if unable to have enteral feeds

PATIENT EDUCATION
Smoking cessation, aerobic exercise

PROGNOSIS
- Annual risk of rupture: (1)
  - <4-cm diameter: ~0% 4–4.9 cm: ~0.5–5%
  - 5–5.9 cm: ~3–15% 6–6.9 cm: ~10–20%
  - 7–7.9 cm: ~20–40% >8 cm: 30–50%
- Patients with AAAs measuring ≥5.5 cm should undergo repair as should all patients with symptomatic AAA. Recommended routine surveillance at 1 year and every 5 years following repair (2)
- Only ~18% of patients with ruptured AAA survive.
- Despite a 5:1 ratio of AAA between males and females, women have higher AAA-associated mortality and morbidity, regardless of open or endovascular repair (2).
- 59–83% mortality if rupture occurs prior to hospitalization (3).

COMPLICATIONS
- Nonoperative: rupture, dissection, thromboembolization. Elective operative (conventional): death 2–8%, all cardiac 10–12% (MI 2–8%) (6)
- 5.1% of patients with EVAR repair required reintervention compared with 1.7 for open repair group.
- Pneumonia 5%, renal insufficiency 5–12%, bleeding 2–6%, DVT 5–8%, stroke 1–2%, rare <1% include graft thrombosis, graft infection, ureteral injury (6)

REFERENCES

1. Aggarwal S, Qamar A, Sharma V, et al. Abdominal aortic aneurysm: a comprehensive review. *Exp Clin Cardiol*. 2011;16(1):11–15.
2. Hirsch AT, Haskal ZJ, Hertzer NR, et al. ACC/AHA 2005 practice guidelines for the management of patients with peripheral arterial disease: a collaborative report. *Circulation*. 2006;113(1):e563–e601.
3. LeFevre ML; U.S. Preventative Services Task Force. Screening for abdominal aortic aneurysm: U.S. Preventative Services Task Force recommendation statement. *Ann Intern Med*. 2014;161(4):281–290.
4. Moxon JV, Parr A, Emeto TI, et al. Diagnosis and monitoring of abdominal aortic aneurysm: current status and future prospects. *Curr Probl Cardiol*. 2010;35(10):512–548.
5. Rooke TW, Hirsch AT, Misra S, et al. 2011 ACCF/AHA focused update of the guideline for the management of patients with peripheral artery disease (updating the 2005 guideline). *J Am Coll Cardiol*. 2011;58(19):2020–2045.
6. Chaikof EL, Brewster DC, Dalman RL, et al. The care of patients with an abdominal aortic aneurysm: the Society for Vascular Surgery practice guidelines. *J Vasc Surg*. 2009;50(4)(Suppl):S2–S49.

ADDITIONAL READING

Sweeting MJ, Thompson SG, Brown LC, et al. Meta analysis of individual patient data to examine factors affecting growth rupture of small abdominal aortic aneurysms. *Br J Surg*. 2012;99(5):655–665.

SEE ALSO

Aortic Dissection; Ehlers-Danlos; Giant Cell Arteritis; Marfan Syndrome; Polyarteritis Nodosa; Turner Syndrome

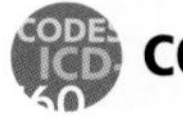

CODES

ICD10
- I71.4 Abdominal aortic aneurysm, without rupture
- I71.3 Abdominal aortic aneurysm, ruptured

CLINICAL PEARLS
- US is procedure of choice for screening for AAA in any male >65 years with any history of tobacco use.
- Suspect AAA for any elderly patient with back, abdominal, or groin pain. Triad of hypotension/shock, pulsatile abdominal mass, and abdominal/back pain always suggests rupture, which requires emergent evaluation for surgery.
- 5.5 cm is threshold diameter for elective surgical treatment (with some exceptions).

ANGIOEDEMA

Michelle T. Martin, PharmD, BCPS, BCACP • Jamie L. Berkes, MD

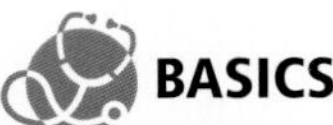

BASICS

DESCRIPTION

- Angioedema (AE) is an acute, localized swelling of skin, mucosa, and submucosa caused by extravasation of fluid into the affected tissues. It often resolves in hours to days, but it can be life-threatening if the upper airway is involved.
- Hereditary AE (HAE) and acquired angioedema (AAE) are diseases of the complement cascade that result in recurrent episodes of AE of the skin, upper airway, and GI tract.
- Synonym(s): angioneurotic edema; Quincke edema

EPIDEMIOLOGY

- Predominant age
  - Allergen, medication, or other triggers can affect all ages.
  - HAE: infancy to 2nd decade of life
  - AAE: Typically patients in 4th decade of life
- Predominant gender: male = female (except type III HAE, which affects more women than men)

Prevalence

- AE occurs in ~15% of the population over a lifetime.
- AE: 0.1–2.2% of patients receiving ACE inhibitors: African Americans have a 4–5 times greater risk of ACE inhibitor–induced AE than Caucasians.
- HAE: 1:10,000–50,000 population in the United States

ETIOLOGY AND PATHOPHYSIOLOGY

- Idiopathic
- Medication induced
  - ACE inhibitors cause 10–25% of AE cases, mostly occurring within the 1st month of use. However, onset may be delayed by years.
  - Angiotensin-receptor blockers (ARBs) also can cause AE but more rarely than ACE inhibitors.
- Allergic triggers
  - Food allergens such as shellfish, nuts, eggs, milk, wheat, soy
  - Medications such as aspirin, NSAIDs, antibiotics, narcotics, and oral contraceptives
  - Latex, venom
- Physically induced: cold, heat, pressure, vibration, trauma, emotional stress, ultraviolet light
- Hereditary or acquired C1 INH deficiency
- Thyroid autoimmune disease–associated AE
- Type I hypersensitivity reaction
- Increase in vascular permeability secondary to IgE-mediated mast cell–stimulated histamine release or from activation of the complement system and an elevation in bradykinin (HAE)
- Attacks of HAE are triggered by prolonged mechanical pressure, cold, heat, trauma, emotional stress, menses, illness, and inflammation:
  - Type I HAE, the most common form, caused by decreased production of C1 esterase inhibitor (C1 INH), has autosomal dominant inheritance.
  - Type II HAE has functionally impaired C1 INH and autosomal dominant inheritance.
  - Type III (HAE-FXII) involves mutations in coagulation factor XII gene (occurs more frequently in women, often estrogen dependent, associated with estrogen administration); also, type III HAE-unknown exists.
- AAE is a rare condition:
  - Type I is associated with lymphoproliferative diseases or paraneoplastic diseases.
  - Type II is due to autoimmune disorders (anti-C1 INH antibody).
  - Affected patients have circulating antibodies directed either against specific immunoglobulins expressed on B cells (type I) or against C1 INH (type II).
  - AAE typically presents later in life (>40 years), and patients lack family history of AE.

Genetics

- HAE types I and II are autosomal dominant, whereas type III is dominant X-linked.
- HAE occurs in 25% of patients as a result of spontaneous genetic mutations.

RISK FACTORS

- Consuming medications and foods that can cause allergic reactions
- Preexisting diagnosis of HAE or AAE

GENERAL PREVENTION

- Avoid known triggers.
- Do not use ACE inhibitors in patients with C1 INH deficiency.

COMMONLY ASSOCIATED CONDITIONS

- Quincke disease (AE of the uvula)
- Urticaria

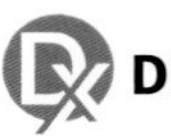

DIAGNOSIS

HISTORY

- Identify potential triggers, including medication history, recent exposure to allergens, physical elements, or trauma.
- In comparison with urticaria, AE typically is nonpruritic, but it can cause a burning sensation.
- Family history

PHYSICAL EXAM

- Acute onset of asymmetric localized swelling, usually of the face (eyelids, lips, ears, nose), tongue, larynx, and, less often, of the extremities or genitalia.
- GI tract involvement may manifest as intermittent unexplained abdominal pain.

ALERT

10–35% of patients present with severe respiratory compromise requiring endotracheal intubation.

DIFFERENTIAL DIAGNOSIS

Urticaria (with AE in 40–50% of patients); allergic contact dermatitis; connective tissue disease: lupus, dermatomyositis; anaphylaxis; cellulitis, erysipelas; lymphedema; diffuse SC infiltrative process

DIAGNOSTIC TESTS & INTERPRETATION

Initial Tests (lab, imaging)

- If AE with urticaria and/or anaphylaxis, check for allergen-specific IgE to verify suspected trigger. Serum tryptase is elevated during acute AE (1)[C].
- Without a clear etiology and recurrence in AE and urticaria, check CBC and ESR:
  - Macrocytosis implies a pernicious anemia.
  - Eosinophilia may imply atopy or, rarely, a parasitic infection.
  - Elevated ESR may imply systemic disorders (1)[C].
- In recurrent AE without a clear etiology and without urticaria, consider ordering serum C4 level:
  - Low serum C4 is a sensitive but nonspecific screening test for hereditary and acquired C1 INH deficiency.
  - If C4 is normal, determine C1 INH level and function and recheck C4 during an acute attack.
  - If C4 level and C1 INH level and function are still normal, consider other causes (i.e., medications or HAE type III) for AE (2)[C].
  - If C4 level, C1 INH level, and C1 INH function are low, this indicates HAE type I.
  - HAE type II is characterized by low C4 and low C1 INH function, but C1 INH level can be normal or elevated (2)[C].
- C1q is decreased in ~75% of AAE but is usually normal in all types of HAE (2)[C].
- Abdominal radiographs and CT scan can demonstrate GI AE or ileus.
- C1 INH deficiency may occur in association with internal malignancy, so AE rarely can be a paraneoplastic disease. Imaging (CT scan, radiography, etc.) then would be done as part of a neoplastic workup for patients with AAE.

Follow-Up Tests & Special Considerations

If C4 and C1q are low (as in AAE), neoplastic and autoimmune workup is warranted. CBC, a peripheral smear, protein electrophoresis, immunophenotyping of lymphocytes, and imaging studies are often undertaken to rule out hematologic malignancies or cancer (1)[C].

Diagnostic Procedures/Other

Skin biopsy (may be nonspecific)

Test Interpretation

- Edema of deep dermis and SC tissue
- Variable perivascular and interstitial infiltrate

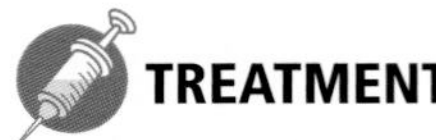

TREATMENT

GENERAL MEASURES

Intubation if airway is threatened

MEDICATION

First Line

- Acute allergic AE (with airway compromise)
  - Epinephrine 1:1,000, 0.3 mL IV or SC (1)[C]
  - Glucocorticoids (hydrocortisone 200 mg IV or Solu-Medrol 40 mg IV) (1)[C]
  - Diphenhydramine 50 mg IV
  - If medication induced, stop the causative agent.
- Idiopathic recurrent AE
  - 1st-generation antihistamines for acute AE (cause drowsiness)
  - Older children and adults: hydroxyzine (Vistaril) 5 mg/5 mL, 25-mg tablets 10–25 mg TID, or diphenhydramine (Benadryl) 25–50 mg q6h (3)[C]
  - Children <6 years of age: diphenhydramine 12.5 mg (elixir) q6–8h (5 mg/kg/day) (2)[C]
  - 2nd-generation H_1 blockers: fexofenadine (Allegra) 180 mg/day BID, cetirizine (Zyrtec) 10 mg/day, desloratadine (Clarinex) 5 mg/day (3)[C]; use with caution in pregnancy and in the elderly.

- HAE chronic prophylaxis
  - A nanofiltered plasma-derived C1 INH (pdC1 INH) concentrate (Cinryze) dosed at 1,000 units/10 mL IV, rate of 1 mL/min (for 10 min) q3–4d. Administration setting options include clinic, home health care, and after proper training, home self-administration (4,5)[B].
  - Attenuated androgens increase hepatic production of C1 INH: oral danazol 50–200 mg/day or oral stanozolol 2 mg/day; use lowest effective dose. Side effects include, but are not limited to, headache, weight gain, liver dysfunction, hirsutism, and menstrual disturbances. Monitor CBC, liver function tests, creatinine kinase, lactic dehydrogenase, fasting lipid profile, and urinalysis at baseline and q6mo. Abdominal US to be performed annually or q6mo if dose of danazol >200 mg/day. Danazol is not to be used in children, during first 2 trimesters of pregnancy, during lactation, and in patients with hepatitis or cancer (2)[C].
- HAE short-term prophylaxis
  - Minor procedures (dental work): If C1 INH is available, no prophylaxis; otherwise danazol 2.5–10 mg/kg/day (max 600 mg/day), stanozolol 4–6 mg/day, for 5 days prior to and 2–5 days after event (2)[C]
  - Major procedures (including intubation): C1 INH 1 (max 6) hour prior with additional dose on hand during procedure. If unavailable, danazol 2.5–10 mg/kg/day (max 600 mg/day) and solvent-/detergent-treated plasma (SDP). If SDP unavailable, use fresh frozen plasma (FFP) 10 mL/kg; 2–4 units (400–800 mL) for an adult 1–6 hours prior
- Acute HAE treatment
  - C1 INH concentrate IV, dosed at 1,000 units if <50 kg; 1,500 units if 50–100 kg; 2,000 units if >100 kg (2)[C]
  - Pasteurized human pdC1 INH (Berinert), dosed at 20 units/kg (available in 500 units/10 mL, max infusion rate of 4 mL/min IV via peripheral vein (4,6)[B]. DO NOT SHAKE (will denature the protein). Worsening of HAE pain was reported as the most severe adverse event.
  - Ecallantide (Kalbitor), a kallikrein inhibitor, is dosed in patients aged ≥16 years at 30 mg SC with 3 separate 10 mg/mL injections in the abdomen, thigh, or upper arm, and a 2nd 30-mg dose may be repeated within 24 hours if needed (4,7)[B]. Injection-site rotation not necessary but must be 2 inches away from attack site. A black box warning of anaphylaxis (potential adverse event) mandates administration in health care setting.
  - Icatibant (Firazyr), a bradykinin receptor-2 antagonist, is dosed at 30 mg SC over at least 30 seconds in the abdomen in patients aged ≥18 years and supplied in a prefilled 10 mg/mL (3 mL) syringe for home administration. Subsequent doses of 30 mg may be repeated in 6-hour intervals (max 90 mg/24 hours) (4,8)[B].
  - Antihistamines and glucocorticoids typically do not benefit patients with HAE. Epinephrine can offer transient stabilization/improvement in laryngeal AE but is not sufficient for full treatment and does not alter the course of attack.
- New therapies are under investigation for acute HAE treatment:
  - Other C1 INH replacement therapy: a recombinant human C1 INH isolated from the milk of transgenic rabbits (Rhucin), dosed 50 units/kg IV. Treatment is approved in Europe: Ruconest (9)[C].
  - Cinryze is awaiting FDA approval for use during acute attacks (4)[C].
- Acute AAE treatment
  - C1 INH concentrate and FFP
  - Treatment of underlying lymphoproliferative disease is often curative in AAE type I.
  - Immunosuppressive therapy to suppress antibody production
  - Clinical trials under way with recombinant human C1 INH (Rhucin) (4)[C].

Second Line

- HAE chronic prophylaxis: If pdC1 INH is unavailable and if patient cannot tolerate attenuated androgens, antifibrinolytic agents (plasmin inhibitors) such as tranexamic acid (not approved by the FDA in United States) 25–50 mg/kg/day divided BID or TID (3–6 g/day max) or ε-aminocaproic acid could be used. They are less effective than attenuated androgens and have many side effects. On rare occasions, they have been linked to (but not proven to cause) thrombophlebitis, embolism, or myositis (2)[C].
- Acute HAE: FFP if C1 INH concentrate is not available, but it can potentially worsen attack.
- Idiopathic AE: Oral doxepin (Sinequan) may be effective for AE (10–25 mg at bedtime).
- H2RA: Oral ranitidine (Zantac) 150 mg/day BID

SURGERY/OTHER PROCEDURES

Tracheostomy if progressive laryngeal edema prevents endotracheal intubation

INPATIENT CONSIDERATIONS

Admission Criteria/Initial Stabilization

Ensure patent airway. If anaphylaxis, epinephrine (1:1,000) SC 0.3–0.5 mg q10–15min

IV Fluids

Given if needed to stabilize patient

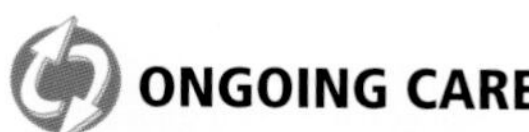

ONGOING CARE

FOLLOW-UP RECOMMENDATIONS

Patient Monitoring

- Diagnostic workup if symptoms are severe, persistent, or recurrent
- Protect airway if mouth, tongue, or throat is involved.

DIET

Avoid known dietary allergens.

PATIENT EDUCATION

Educate on avoidance of triggers (i.e., food, medication, other physical stimuli), types of treatment, when to seek emergency care, and wearing Medic Alert bracelet.

PROGNOSIS

- AE symptoms often resolve in hours to 2–4 days. If airway is compromised, AE can be life-threatening.
- Patients with HAE have an average of 20 attacks/year; each may last 3–5 days. Prophylaxis can decrease the frequency of events and number of missed days of school or work.

COMPLICATIONS

Anaphylaxis

REFERENCES

1. Temiño VM, Peebles RS. The spectrum and treatment of angioedema. *Am J Med*. 2008;121(4):282–286.
2. Zuraw BL, Bernstein JA, Lang DM, et al; American Academy of Allergy, Asthma and Immunology; American College of Allergy, Asthma and Immunology. A focused parameter update: hereditary angioedema, acquired C1 inhibitor deficiency, and angiotensin-converting enzyme inhibitor-associated angioedema. *J Allergy Clin Immunol*. 2013;131(6):1491–1493.
3. Frigas E, Park M. Idiopathic recurrent angioedema. *Immunol Allergy Clin North Am*. 2006;26(4):739–751.
4. Altman KA, Naimi DR. Hereditary angioedema: a brief review of new developments. *Curr Med Res Opin*. 2014;30(5):923–930.
5. Zuraw BL, Busse PJ, White M, et al. Nanofiltered C1 inhibitor concentrate for treatment of hereditary angioedema. *N Engl J Med*. 2010;363(6):513–522.
6. Craig TJ, Levy RJ, Wasserman RL, et al. Efficacy of human C1 esterase inhibitor concentrate compared with placebo in acute hereditary angioedema attacks. *J Allergy Clin Immunol*. 2009;124(4):801–808.
7. Cicardi M, Levy RJ, McNeil DL, et al. Ecallantide for the treatment of acute attacks in hereditary angioedema. *N Engl J Med*. 2010;363(6):523–531.
8. Lumry WR, Li HH, Levy RJ, et al. Randomized placebo-controlled trial of the bradykinin B_2 receptor antagonist icatibant for the treatment of acute attacks of hereditary angioedema: the FAST-3 trial. *Ann Allergy Asthma Immunol*. 2011;107(6):529–537.
9. Riedl MA, Bernstein JA, Li H, et al; Study 1310 Investigators. Recombinant human C1-esterase inhibitor relieves symptoms of hereditary angioedema attacks: phase 3, randomized, placebo-controlled trial. *Ann Allergy Asthma Immunol*. 2014;112(2):163–169.

SEE ALSO

Urticaria; Anaphylaxis

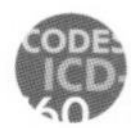

CODES

ICD10

- T78.3XXA Angioneurotic edema, initial encounter
- D84.1 Defects in the complement system

CLINICAL PEARLS

- AE is an acute, localized swelling of skin, mucosa, and submucosa caused by extravasation of fluid into the affected tissues. It often resolves in hours to days, but it can be life-threatening if the upper airway is involved.
- HAE and AAE are diseases of the complement cascade that result in recurrent episodes of AE of the skin, upper airway, and GI tract.
- Trigger identification and avoidance are key in the prevention of AE.
- Patients with a history of allergies and AE should be prescribed an epinephrine autoinjector.

ANKLE FRACTURES

Wendy Hin-Wing Wong, MD, MPH • Jeffrey P. Feden, MD, FACEP

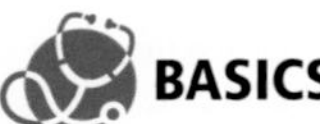

BASICS

- Bones: tibia, fibula, talus
- Mortise: tibial plafond (horizontal surface of the tibia), medial malleolus, and lateral malleolus
- Ligaments: syndesmotic, lateral collateral, and medial collateral (deltoid) ligament

DESCRIPTION

- Two common classification systems are useful for describing fractures but do not always predict instability of fracture (1)[B].
  - Danis-Weber system: based on level of the fibular fracture in relationship to the syndesmosis
    - Type A: below syndesmosis (of tibiofibular joint). Usually stable (30% of ankle fractures)
    - Type B (most common): at syndesmosis. Can be stable or unstable (63%)
    - Type C: above syndesmosis. Usually unstable (7%)
  - Lauge-Hansen (LH): based on foot position and direction of applied force relative to the tibia
    - Supination-adduction (SA)
    - Supination-external rotation (SER): most common, 40–75% of fractures
    - Pronation-abduction (PA)
    - Pronation-external rotation (PER)
- Stability-based classification (1)[B]
  - Stable
    - Isolated lateral malleolar fractures (Weber A/B) without talar shift and has negative stress test
    - Isolated nondisplaced medial malleolar fractures
  - Unstable
    - Bi- or trimalleolar fractures
    - High fibular fractures (Weber C) or lateral malleolar fracture with medial injury and positive stress test
    - Lateral malleolar fracture with talar shift/tilt (bimalleolar equivalent)
    - Displaced medial malleolus fractures
- Pilon fracture: tibial plafond fracture due to axial loading mechanism (unstable)
- Maisonneuve: fracture of proximal 1/3 of fibula associated with ankle fracture (unstable); high risk of peroneal nerve injury

Pediatric Considerations

- Ankle fractures are more common than sprains in children compared to adults because ligaments are stronger than physis.
- Talar dome: osteochondral fracture of talar dome; suspect in child with nonhealing ankle "sprain" or recurrent effusions.
- Tillaux: isolated Salter-Harris III of distal tibia with growth plate involvement
- Triplane fracture: Salter-Harris IV with fracture lines oriented in multiple planes: 2-, 3-, and 4-part variants

EPIDEMIOLOGY

- Ankle fractures = 9% of all adult and 5% of all pediatric fractures
- Predominant age: Average is 46 years.
- Predominant sex: peak incidence in women 45–64 years and men 8–15 years

Incidence

- 107–184 per 100,000 people per year
- 3-fold increase in incidence predicted from 2000 to 2030 in adults >60 years old

ETIOLOGY AND PATHOPHYSIOLOGY

- Most common: falls (38%), inversion injury (32%), sports-related (10%)
- Foot typically plantar flexed (less stable)
- Axial loading: tibial plafond or pilon fracture

RISK FACTORS

- Age, fall and fracture history, polypharmacy, or intoxication
- Obesity, sedentary lifestyle
- Sports, physical activity
- History of smoking or diabetes
- Alcohol or slippery surfaces

GENERAL PREVENTION

- Nonslip, flat, protective shoes
- Fall precautions in elderly

COMMONLY ASSOCIATED CONDITIONS

- Most ankle fractures are isolated injuries, but 5% have associated fractures, usually ipsilateral lower limb.
- Ligamentous or cartilage injury (sprains)
- Ankle or subtalar dislocation
- Other axial loading or shearing injuries (i.e., vertebral compression or contralateral pelvic fractures)

DIAGNOSIS

HISTORY

- Location of pain, timing, and mechanism of injury
- Weight-bearing status after injury
- History of ankle injury or surgery
- Tetanus status
- Assess for safety and fall risk (particularly in the elderly).

PHYSICAL EXAM

- Examine skin integrity (open vs. closed fracture).
- Assess point of maximal tenderness.
- Assess neurovascular status, pulses, motor/sensory exam, and ability to bear weight.
- Evaluate for compartment syndrome.
- Consider associated injuries (secondary survey).
- Assess ankle stability: anterior drawer test for the anterior talofibular ligament (ATFL), talar tilt test for lateral and medial ligaments, and squeeze test and external rotation stress test for the tibiofibular syndesmosis.

DIFFERENTIAL DIAGNOSIS

- Ankle sprain
- Other fractures: talus, 5th metatarsal, calcaneus

DIAGNOSTIC TESTS & INTERPRETATION

- Plain films: 1st-line for suspected fractures (2)[A]
- Ottawa Ankle Rules (OAR): Overall sensitivity of 98% in adults, increasing to 99.6% if applied within the first 48 hours after trauma (3)[A].
- OAR suggest films in patients aged 18–55 years only if
  - Tenderness at the posterior edge or tip of the medial malleolus, *OR*
  - Tenderness at the posterior edge or tip of the lateral malleolus, *OR*
  - Inability to bear weight both immediately and in the ED for four steps, *OR*
  - Tenderness at navicular or 5th metatarsal (Ottawa Foot Rules)
- If symptoms persist beyond 48–72 hours, obtain x-rays.
- In children >1 year old, OAR sensitivity is 98.5%.
- OAR not valid in intoxicated patients, patients with multiple injuries, or sensory deficits (diabetics with neuropathy)
- 3 standard views
  - Anteroposterior (AP)
  - Lateral: instability depicted by talar dome and distal tibia incongruity
  - Mortise (15–25-degree internal rotation view): Look for parallel lines between joint spaces; space between the medial malleolus and talus should not be >4 mm.
  - Additional stress view may demonstrate instability: increased medial clear space with manual external rotation (4)[A]

Pediatric Considerations

- Tenderness over distal fibula with normal films should be considered Salter-Harris I.
- Stress views unnecessary in children may cause physeal damage (5)[C].
- Salter-Harris V often missed, diagnosed when leg length discrepancy or angular deformity after Salter-Harris I; rare, 1% of fractures (5)[C]

Follow-Up Tests & Special Considerations

- CT recommended for operative planning in trimalleolar, Tillaux, triplane, pilon fractures, or fractures with intra-articular involvement (2)[A].
- MRI not routinely indicated; does not increase sensitivity of detecting complex ankle fractures (6)[C]
  - MRI useful for chronic instability, osteochondral lesions, occult fractures, unexpected stiffness in children

Diagnostic Procedures/Other

- Ultrasound for soft tissue injury associated with displaced fractures (2)[A]
- Bone scan or MRI for stress fracture (7)[A]

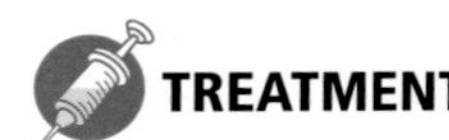

TREATMENT

GENERAL MEASURES

- Immobilize in temporary cast/splint and protect with crutches/non–weight bearing
  - 1–2 weeks to allow decreased swelling, if not open or irreducible fracture (8,9)[C]
- Ice and elevate the extremity; pain due to swelling best controlled with elevation (10)[A]
  - Compression stockings offer no benefit for swelling (11)[A].
- Closed ankle fractures: stable versus unstable
  - Stable = nonoperative (2)[A]
  - Unstable = surgery
  - Lateral shift of talus ≥2 mm or displacement of either malleolus by 2–3 mm = surgery (8)[C]
  - In adults with displaced fractures: insufficient evidence if surgery or nonoperative management produces superior long-term outcomes
- Syndesmosis injury = nonoperative
- Fracture-dislocations: Reduce quickly (12)[C].
  - Do not wait for imaging if neurovascular compromise or obvious deformity.
  - Flex hip and knee 90 degrees for easier reduction.
  - Post reduction: neurovascular exam and x-rays

MEDICATION

First Line

- NSAIDs and/or acetaminophen for pain (2)[A]
- Initial IM pain injection (i.e., ketorolac ≥50 kg adult: 60 mg single dose or 30 mg q6hr, max 120 mg daily; children 2–16 years old, <50 kg or ≥ age 65 years: 1 mg/kg or 30 mg single dose or 15 mg q6hr, max 60 mg daily)
- For suspected open fractures: tetanus booster, broad-spectrum cephalosporin and aminoglycoside within 3 hours post injury (8)[C]

Second Line

- Opioid analgesics as adjunctive therapy (2)[A]

ISSUES FOR REFERRAL

- ED consultation for neurovascular compromise, tenting of skin or open fracture, displaced or unstable fracture, compartment syndrome
- All other fractures: orthopedic follow-up within 1 week and remain non–weight-bearing

ADDITIONAL THERAPIES

- Nonoperative = cast immobilization
  - No difference in type of immobilization (air-stirrup, cast, orthosis) (11)[A]
  - Weight bearing 50% with crutches for 6 weeks, then full weight bearing (10)[A]
  - If removable cast, gentle range of motion exercises at 4 weeks (10)[A]
- Open ankle fractures (2%)
  - Remove gross debris/contamination in ED.
  - Surgical emergency, OR within 24 hours: Usually wounds heal by secondary intention, external fixation if inadequate soft tissue coverage.

SURGERY/OTHER PROCEDURES

- Surgical options
  - Open reduction internal fixation (ORIF); preferred in athletes (7)[A], more cost effective in unstable fractures (4)[A]
  - External fixation may be preferred in extreme tissue injury or comminuted fractures; may have more malunion compared to ORIF, but no difference in wound complications
- Timing of surgery
  - Immediately if neurovascular compromise, open fracture, unsuccessful reduction, tissue necrosis (8)[C]
  - Otherwise delay >5 days post injury because inflammation can affect wound healing (8)[C].
- Length of recovery: usually 6–8 weeks

Pediatric Considerations

- Salter-Harris I and II = nonoperative
  - Distal tibia: long leg cast for 4–6 weeks, then short leg cast for 2–3 weeks (6)[C]
  - Distal fibula: posterior splint or ankle brace 3–4 weeks, weight bearing. If displaced, then short leg cast 4–6 weeks, non–weight bearing (6)[C]
  - Limit reduction attempts because detrimental to growth plate (5,6)[C].
  - No reduction recommended if presenting ≥1 week post injury (6)[C].
  - Intra-articular displacement of ≥2 mm in child with >2 years growth remaining = ORIF (5)[C]
- Salter-Harris III and IV:
  - Distal tibia: if >2 mm displacement = ORIF (5)[C]
  - Distal fibula: rare, usually stable after tibial reduction (5)[C]
  - Tillaux and triplane: ORIF if displaced ≥2 mm (5,6)[C]

Geriatric Considerations

- Higher surgical risk due to age/comorbidities
- Osteoporosis increases risk of implant/fixation failure but not a risk factor for fracture.
- Risks from surgery/anesthesia: wound healing problems, pulmonary embolism, mortality, amputation, reoperation

INPATIENT CONSIDERATIONS

Admission Criteria/Initial Stabilization

Admit to the hospital if

- Emergency surgery required
- Patient nonadherence, lack of social support, inability to maintain non–weight-bearing status, significant associated injuries
- Concerning mechanism of injury (i.e., syncope, myocardial infarction, head injury)

Nursing

Non–weight bearing, maintain splint/cast, apply ice, keep leg elevated, pain control, assist in ADLs.

Discharge Criteria

- Ambulates with walker or crutches
- Medical workup (if needed) completed
- Orthopedic follow-up arranged

ONGOING CARE

FOLLOW-UP RECOMMENDATIONS

Patient Monitoring

- Orthopedic follow-up: serial x-rays
  - In children, monitor for sclerotic lines on x-ray (Parker-Harris growth arrest lines) to indicate growth disturbance (6)[C].
- Immobilization for 4–6 weeks, then progressive activity, weight bearing, with removable splint or boot (11)[A]
- Physical therapy: no difference in outcomes between stretching, manual therapy, exercise program (11)[A]

DIET

- NPO if surgery is being considered

PATIENT EDUCATION

- Ice and elevate for 2–3 weeks, use crutches/cane as instructed, prevent splint/cast from getting wet.
- Notify physician if swelling increases, paresthesias, pain, or change in color of extremity

PROGNOSIS

- Good results can be achieved without surgery if fracture is stable.
  - Most return to activity within 3–4 months.
- Most athletes return to preinjury sports activity (7)[A].
- Increasing age, *NOT* injury severity, associated with worsening mobility after fracture (13)[B]

COMPLICATIONS

- Displaced fracture or instability
- Delayed union, malunion, or nonunion (0.9–1.9%)
- Postsurgical wound problems: loss of fixation, further surgery, amputation
- Deep venous thrombosis
- Complex regional pain syndrome, extensor retinaculum syndrome in children (6)[C]
- Infection (osteomyelitis)
- Posttraumatic arthritis, degenerative joint disease, growth arrest in children

REFERENCES

1. Pakarinen HJ, Flinkkil TE, Ohtonen PP, et al. Stability criteria for nonoperative ankle fracture management. *Foot Ankle Int*. 2011;32(2):141–147.
2. Ankle and foot disorders. In: Hegmann KT, ed. *Occupational Medicine Practice Guidelines. Evaluation and Management of Common Health Problems and Functional Recovery in Workers*. 3rd ed. Elk Grove Village, IL: American College of Occupational and Environmental Medicine; 2011.1–268. http://www.guideline.gov/content.aspx?id=36625&search=%22ankle+fractures%22. Accessed June 29, 2014.
3. Polzer H, Kanz KG, Prall WC, et al. Diagnosis and treatment of acute ankle injuries: development of an evidence-based algorithm. *Orthop Rev (Pavia)*. 2012;4(1):e5.
4. Slobogean GP, Marra CA, Sadatsafavi M, et al. Is surgical fixation for stress-positive unstable ankle fractures cost effective? Results of a multicenter randomized control trial. *J Orthop Trauma*. 2012;26(11):652–658.
5. Kay RM, Matthys GA. Pediatric ankle fractures: evaluation and treatment. *J Am Acad Orthop Surg*. 2001;9(4):268–278.
6. Parrino A, Lee MC. Ankle fractures in children. *Curr Orthop Pract*. 2013;24:617–624.
7. Del Buono A, Smith R, Coco M, et al. Return to sports after ankle fractures: a systematic review. *Br Med Bull*. 2013;106:179–191.
8. Mandi DM. Ankle fractures. *Clin Podiatr Med Surg*. 2012;29(2):155–186.
9. Clare MP. A rational approach to ankle fractures. *Foot Ankle Clin*. 2008;13(4):593–610.
10. Work Loss Data Institute. *Ankle & Foot (Acute & Chronic)*. Encinitas, CA: Work Loss Data Institute; 2013. http://www.guideline.gov/content.aspx?id=47571&search=ankle+fracture. Accessed June 29, 2014.
11. Lin CW, Donker NA, Refshauge KM, et al. Rehabilitation for ankle fractures in adults. *Cochrane Database Syst Rev*. 2012;11:CD005595.
12. Mordecai S, Al-Hadithy N. Management of ankle fractures. *BMJ*. 2011;343:d5204.
13. Keene D, James G, Lamb SE, et al. Factors associated with mobility outcomes in older people post-ankle fracture: an observational cohort study focusing on peripheral vessel function. *Injury*. 2013;44(7):987–993.

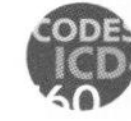

CODES

ICD10

- 82.899A Oth fracture of unsp lower leg, init for clos fx
- S82.309A Unsp fracture of lower end of unsp tibia, init for clos fx
- S82.66XA Nondisp fx of lateral malleolus of unsp fibula, init

CLINICAL PEARLS

- Ottawa Ankle Rules are nearly 100% sensitive in determining need for x-rays.
- Assess neurovascular status, pulses, motor/sensory function, ability to bear weight, associated injuries.
- Assess joint above (Maisonneuve).
- Normal x-rays with tenderness in children are considered as Salter-Harris type I fracture.

ANKYLOSING SPONDYLITIS

Damon F. Lee, MD

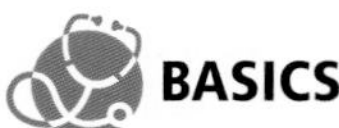

BASICS

DESCRIPTION

- Ankylosing spondylitis (AS) is the prototypical axial spondyloarthropathy (axSpA) characterized by inflammatory arthritis of the axial skeleton and radiologic evidence of sacroiliitis.
- System(s) affected: musculoskeletal; eyes; cardiac; neurologic; pulmonary
- Synonym(s): Marie-Strümpell disease; "bamboo spine"

EPIDEMIOLOGY

- Onset usually in early 20s; rarely occurs after age 40 years
- Male > female (approximately 2–3:1)

Incidence

Age- and gender-adjusted rate of 6.3–7.3/100,000 person-years

Prevalence

~0.55% for AS and ~1.4% for all axSpA in the United States (1)

ETIOLOGY AND PATHOPHYSIOLOGY

- Interaction between genetic factors triggering autoinflammation at sites of bacterial (previously hypothesized to be *Klebsiella* species) or mechanical stress (2)
- Inflammation at the insertion of tendons, ligaments, and fasciae to bone (enthesopathy), causing erosion, remodeling, and new bone formation
- Inflammation-independent pathways of bony changes have also been hypothesized (2).

Genetics

- 80–90% of patients with AS are HLA-B27–positive.
- Other genetic associations include genes for endoplasmic reticulum aminopeptidase 1 (ERAP1), interleukin 23 receptor (IL23R), and gene deserts on chromosome 2p15 and 21q22 (2).

RISK FACTORS

- HLA-B27
  - 1–8% of HLA-B27–positive adults have AS.
- Positive family history
  - HLA-B27–positive child of a parent with AS has a 10–30% risk of developing the disease.

COMMONLY ASSOCIATED CONDITIONS

- Uveitis/iritis (up to 40%)
- Enthesopathy: Achilles tendonitis, plantar fasciitis
- Dactylitis (sausage digit) from oligoarthritis
- Peripheral spondyloarthritis (SpA): psoriatic arthritis, reactive arthritis, inflammatory bowel disease (IBD)-related arthritis, juvenile idiopathic arthritis
- Aortitis and cardiac conduction defects

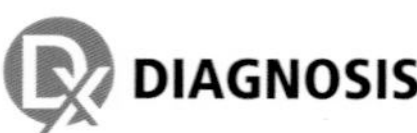

DIAGNOSIS

HISTORY

- Inflammatory back pain
  - Insidious onset
  - Duration >3 months
  - Morning stiffness in spine lasting >1 hour
  - Night time awakenings secondary to back pain
  - Increased pain and stiffness with rest, improvement with activity
- Alternating buttock/hip pain is common.
- Constitutional symptoms (fatigue, weight loss, low-grade fever)
- Chest pain with inspiration due to enthesitis at costochondral junction and diminished chest wall expansion
- Symptoms associated with or a history of enthesopathy (Achilles pain, plantar fascia pain); dactylitis (oligoarthritis); iritis (painful, red eye, photophobia, vision changes)

PHYSICAL EXAM

- Sacroiliac joint tenderness; loss of lumbar lordosis, and cervical spine rotation
- Diminished range of motion in the lumbar spine in all 3 planes of motion
- Modified Wright-Schober test for lumbar spine flexion is abnormal:
  - Mark patient's back over the L5 spinous process (or at dimples of Venus) and measure 10 cm above and 5 cm below this point. Normal is at least 5 cm of expansion between these 2 marks on maximal forward flexion.
- Thoracocervical kyphosis (rarely occurs before 10 years of symptoms)
- Occiput–wall distance increased (distance between occiput and wall when standing with back flat against a vertical surface; zero is normal).
- Measurement of respiratory excursion of chest wall
  - Normal is >5 cm of maximal respiratory excursion of chest wall measured at 4th intercostal space; <2.5 cm is consistent with AS.
- Tenderness over sites of tendon insertions (e.g., Achilles, plantar fascia)
- Peripheral oligoarthritis/dactylitis seen mostly with peripheral SpA
- Cauda equina syndrome rarely occurs in late disease.
- Extra-articular manifestations: uveitis, psoriasis, IBD
- Aortic regurgitation murmur (1%)

DIFFERENTIAL DIAGNOSIS

- Nonradiographic axial SpA (features of AS without x-ray evidence of sacroiliitis; MRI detects changes earlier than plain films)
- Other SpA
- Osteoarthritis of the axial spine
- Diffuse idiopathic skeletal hypertrophy (DISH)
- Osteitis condensans ilii: benign sclerotic changes in the iliac portion of the SI joint after pregnancy
- Infectious arthritis or discitis, especially unilateral sacroiliitis: tuberculosis, brucellosis, bacterial (particularly in IV drug users)

DIAGNOSTIC TESTS & INTERPRETATION

Initial Tests (lab, imaging)

- Up to 10% of Caucasian population and 4% of African American population are HLA-B27–positive. Therefore, gene testing is not necessary as part of initial evaluation, especially with a suspicious history and exam.
- ESR and C-reactive protein (CRP) may be mildly elevated or normal; if high, it correlates with disease activity and prognosis.
- Absence of rheumatoid factor
- Mild normochromic anemia (15%)
- Synovial fluid: mild leukocytosis
- SI joints: Oblique projection is preferred for imaging the SI joints with plain films.
  - X-ray changes may not be apparent for up to 10 years after disease onset. MRI is more sensitive; showing increased signal from the bone and bone marrow suggests osteitis and edema.
  - Sequential plain radiographic changes over time: widening, erosions, sclerosis on both sides of joint not extending >1 cm from articular surface, and (lastly) ankylosis of sacroiliac joint
- Spine
  - Early plain radiograph changes: "shiny corners" due to osteitis and sclerosis at site of annulus fibrosus attachments to the corners of vertebral bodies with "squaring" due to erosion and remodeling of vertebral body; contrast-enhanced MRI is more sensitive for detecting early changes.
  - Late changes: ossification of annulus fibrosis resulting in bony bridging between vertebral bodies (syndesmophytes) giving classic "bamboo spine" appearance; ankylosis of apophyseal joints, ossification of spinal ligaments, and/or spondylodiscitis also occurs.
- Peripheral joints
  - Asymmetric pericapsular ossification, sclerosis, loss of joint space, and erosions may occur.

Diagnostic Procedures/Other

- ECG: conduction defects; echocardiogram: aortic valvular abnormalities
- Dual energy x-ray absorptiometry scan may reveal osteopenia/osteoporosis.

Test Interpretation

- Erosive changes and new bone formation at bony attachment of the tendons and ligaments result in ossification of periarticular soft tissues.
- Synovial hypertrophy and pannus formation, mononuclear cell infiltrate into subsynovium and subchondral bone marrow inflammation in the SI joint with erosions, followed by granulation tissue formation, and finally obliteration of joint space by fusion of joint and sclerosis of para-articular bone

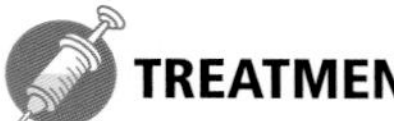

TREATMENT

GENERAL MEASURES

Aggressive physical therapy is the most important nonpharmacologic management.

- Posture training and spinal range-of-motion exercises are essential.
- Firm bed; sleep in supine position without a pillow
- Breathing exercises 2–3×/day
- Smoking cessation

MEDICATION

First Line

Nonsteroidal anti-inflammatory drugs (NSAIDs) are first line for pain and stiffness in AS (3)[C].

- NSAIDs provide rapid and dramatic symptomatic relief, which may be diagnostic. No single NSAID preferred. Higher doses tend to be more efficacious.
- Continuous NSAID therapy may slow radiographic disease progression but may not be superior to intermittent therapy in terms of symptom control (4)[A].
- Precautions
  - Consider CVD, GI and renal risks.
  - Consider GI prophylaxis (PPIs or misoprostol) while on NSAIDs in those with hx of PUD, gastritis, or age >60 years; consider using COX-2 inhibitor.
  - Use with caution in patients with a bleeding diathesis or patients receiving anticoagulants.
- Injection of intra-articular corticosteroids into SI joints and prostheses can provide transient relief, but systemic corticosteroids are usually ineffective.

Pregnancy Considerations

Infants exposed to NSAIDs in 1st trimester may have a higher incidence of cardiac malformations (5)[A].

Second Line

- Biologic agents: tumor necrosis factor (TNF)-α antagonists
  - Recommended for high disease activity or when a trial of 2 NSAIDs over 4 weeks have failed (3)[C]
  - FDA-approved agents for AS include etanercept (recombinant TNF receptor fusion protein), infliximab (chimeric monoclonal IgG1 antibody to TNF-α), adalimumab (fully humanized IgG1 monoclonal antibody to TNF-α), and golimumab (human IgG1 kappa monoclonal antibody to TNF-α).
  - All 4 approved agents have similar efficacy in managing axial signs and symptoms without a difference in adverse effects (6)[A].
  - No definitive evidence for TNF-α blockers with regards to disease remission, prevention of radiologic progression or prevention of extra-articular manifestations (7).
  - Monoclonal TNF-α blockers are preferred when IBD is involved (3)[C].
  - Further investigation as to the effectiveness of TNF blocker therapy with NSAIDs is needed (8).
- Precautions with TNF-α blockers
  - Anti-TNFs increase the risk of serious bacterial, mycobacterial, fungal, opportunistic, and viral infections.
  - Screen for and treat latent tuberculosis before initiating treatment.
  - Screen for hepatitis B.
  - Monitor for reactivation of tuberculosis and invasive fungal infections, such as histoplasmosis, in all patients, especially with travel to (or residence in) endemic areas.
  - Lymphomas, nonmelanoma skin cancers, and other malignancies have been reported in patients receiving anti-TNFs.
  - Immunizations (especially live vaccines) should be updated before initiating anti-TNFs because live vaccines are contraindicated once patients receive anti-TNFs.
- Disease-modifying antirheumatic drugs (DMARDs), such as methotrexate and sulfasalazine, are ineffective for axial disease; sulfasalazine may be effective for peripheral arthritis (3)[C].

ISSUES FOR REFERRAL

- Physical therapy can assist with treatment plan (including home regimens).
- Coordinate care with rheumatology for diagnosis, monitoring, and management (anti-TNF therapy).
- Management of aortic regurgitation, uveitis, spinal fractures, pulmonary fibrosis, hip joint involvement, renal amyloidosis, and cauda equina syndrome may require referral to appropriate specialty.

ADDITIONAL THERAPIES

- Bisphosphonate medications if osteopenia or osteoporosis is present
- Monitoring and management of CVD risk factors and comorbidities

SURGERY/OTHER PROCEDURES

- Crucial to evaluate for C-spine ankylosis/instability before intubation in patients with AS undergoing surgery.
- Total hip replacement should be considered to restore mobility and to control pain.
- Vertebral osteotomy can improve posture for patients with severe cervical or thoracolumbar flexion.

ONGOING CARE

FOLLOW-UP RECOMMENDATIONS

Patient Monitoring

- Symptom control and maintenance of spinal mobility and function are primary goals of treatment.
- Monitor posture and range of motion with 6–12 month visits; increase frequency if higher disease activity.
- Bath Ankylosing Spondylitis Disease Activity Index (BASDAI) or Ankylosing Spondylitis Disease Activity Score (ASDAS) can be used to measure disease activity and effects of inflammation.

PATIENT EDUCATION

- Maintain physical activity and posture to prevent disability.
- Swimming, tai chi, walking, and maintenance of active lifestyle are excellent activities.
- Avoid trauma/contact sports.
- Appropriate ergonomic modification at workplace
- Counsel about risk of spinal fracture.
- MedicAlert bracelet (helpful if intubation required)
- Arthritis Foundation: http://www.arthritis.org
- Spondylitis Association of America: http://www.spondylitis.org

PROGNOSIS

- Extent and rapidity of progression of ankylosis are highly variable.
- Progressive limitation of spinal mobility necessitates lifestyle modification.

COMPLICATIONS

- Spine
  - Spinal fusion causing kyphosis
  - Cervical spine fracture or subluxation carries high mortality rate; fracture can occur at any level of ankylosed spine.
  - Cauda equina syndrome (rare)
- Pulmonary: restrictive lung disease, upper lobe fibrosis (rare)
- Cardiac: conduction defects at atrioventricular (AV) node, aortic insufficiency, aortitis, pericarditis (extremely rare)
- Eye: uveitis and cataracts
- Renal: IgA nephropathy, amyloidosis (<1%)
- GI: microscopic, subclinical ileal, and colonic mucosal ulcerations in up to 50% of patients, mostly asymptomatic

REFERENCES

1. Reveille JD, Weisman MH. The epidemiology of back pain, axial spondyloarthritis and HLA-B27 in the United States. *Am J Med Sci*. 2013;345(6):431–436.
2. Dougados M, Baeten D. Spondyloarthritis. *Lancet*. 2011;377(9783):2127–2137.
3. Braun J, van den Berg R, Baraliakos X, et al. 2010 update of the ASAS/EULAR recommendations for the management of ankylosing spondylitis. *Ann Rheum Dis*. 2011;70(6):896–904.
4. Guellec D, Nocturne G, Tatar Z, et al. Should non-steroidal anti-inflammatory drugs be used continuously in ankylosing spondylitis? *Joint Bone Spine*. 2014;81(4):308–312.
5. Adams K, Bombardier C, van der Heijde DM. Safety of pain therapy during pregnancy and lactation in patients with inflammatory arthritis: a systematic literature review. *J Rheumatol Suppl*. 2012;90:59–61.
6. Machado MA, Barbosa MM, Almeida AM, et al. Treatment of ankylosing spondylitis with TNF blockers: a meta-analysis. *Rheumatol Int*. 2013;33(9):2199–2213.
7. Gensler L, Inman R, Deodhar A. The "knowns" and "unknowns" of biologic therapy in ankylosing spondylitis. 2010. *Am J Med Sci*. 2012;343(5):360–363.
8. Sieper J. Treatment challenges in axial spondyloarthritis and future directions. *Curr Rheumatol Rep*. 2013;15(9):356. doi:10.1007/s11926-013-0356-9.

ADDITIONAL READING

- Baraliakos X, van den Berg R, Braun J, et al. Update of the literature review on treatment with biologics as a basis for the first update of the ASAS/EULAR management recommendations of ankylosing spondylitis. *Rheumatology*. 2012;51(8):1378–1387.
- Sieper J. Developments in therapies for spondyloarthritis. *Nat Rev Rheumatol*. 2012;8(5):280–287.
- Sieper J, Rudwaleit M, Baraliakos X, et al. The Assessment of Spondyloarthritis International Society (ASAS) handbook: a guide to assess spondyloarthritis. *Ann Rheum Dis*. 2009;68(Suppl 2): ii1–ii44.
- van den Berg R, Baraliakos X, Braun J, et al. First update of the current evidence for the management of ankylosing spondylitis with non-pharmacological treatment and non-biologic drugs: a systematic literature review of the ASAS/EULAR management recommendations in ankylosing spondylitis. *Rheumatology*. 2012;51(8):1388–1396.

SEE ALSO

Arthritis, Psoriatic; Arthritis, Rheumatoid (RA); Crohn Disease; Reactive Arthritis (Reiter Syndrome); Ulcerative Colitis

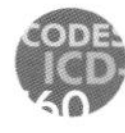

CODES

ICD10

- M45.9 Ankylosing spondylitis of unspecified sites in spine
- M08.1 Juvenile ankylosing spondylitis
- M45.8 Ankylosing spondylitis sacral and sacrococcygeal region

CLINICAL PEARLS

- Diagnosis of AS is suggested by: a history of inflammatory back pain, with evidence of limited chest wall expansion and restricted spinal movements in all planes; radiographic evidence of sacroiliitis and a good therapeutic response to NSAIDs
- HLA-B27 testing helps to support the diagnosis if clinical features are less definitive.
- Physical therapy helps to maintain posture and mobility and is an important treatment modality.
- NSAIDs and TNF-α blockers are the mainstays of pharmacologic treatment of AS.

ANORECTAL FISTULA

Nihal Patel, MD • David A. Greenwald, MD

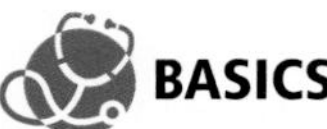

BASICS

DESCRIPTION

- An anorectal fistula is an open communication between an anal abscess and the perirectal skin.
- Most commonly, anorectal fistulas form due to drainage of an abscess of the anal crypt glands.
- The classification of fistulas grades severity and guides treatment.
- Five categories exist:
  - Submucosal or superficial: The fistula tracks beneath the submucosa and does not involve the sphincter mechanism (not classified under original Parks' classification).
  - Intersphincteric: The fistula travels along the intersphincteric plane (Parks' type 1).
  - Transsphincteric: The fistula traverse through the internal and external sphincter (type 2).
  - Suprasphincteric: The fistula originates at the dentate line and loops over the external sphincter, to the ischiorectal fossa (type 3).
  - Extrasphincteric (rare): high in the anal canal, (proximal to dentate line), does not involve sphincter complex (type 4)
- Fistulas can also be classified as low or high:
  - Low fistulas involve the distal 1/3 of the external sphincter muscle.
  - High fistulas involve more of the external sphincter muscle.
- Fistulas may be simple or complex:
  - Simple fistulas are low and include superficial, intersphincteric, or low transsphincteric fistulas. They also involve only 1 communicating tract and are not associated with inflammatory bowel disease (IBD) or other organs (bladder).
  - Complex fistulas are higher along the gastrointestinal (GI) tract, have multiple tracts, involve other organs, are recurrent, or are associated with IBD or radiation.
  - System(s) affected: GI, skin/exocrine
  - Synonym(s): fistula-in-ano; anal fistula

EPIDEMIOLOGY

- True prevalence is unknown because anorectal pain is commonly attributed to symptomatic hemorrhoids.
- Mean age of presentation for anal abscess and fistula is 40 years (range 20–60).
- Predominant sex: males twice as likely to develop an abscess and/or fistula compared with females
- Lifetime risk of developing fistula in Crohn disease patients is 20–40%.

ETIOLOGY AND PATHOPHYSIOLOGY

- Inspissated debris in an obstructed anal crypt gland results in suppuration and abscess formation along the path of least resistance in the perianal and perirectal spaces (cryptoglandular theory).
- Abscess rupture or drainage leads to an epithelialized track or fistula formation in ~1/3 of patients.
- Other causes for fistula formation include IBD such as Crohn disease.
- Radiation proctitis in patients undergoing pelvic radiation predisposes patients to fistula formation.
- Immunocompromised patients rarely develop primary perianal actinomycosis, which can cause fistula-in-ano.
- Anorectal mucosal laceration due to rectal foreign bodies or trauma can result in abscess and fistula formation.

RISK FACTORS

- Inflammatory bowel disease (Crohn disease)
- Pelvic radiation
- Perianal trauma
- Previous anorectal abscess
- Pelvic carcinoma or lymphoma
- Ruptured anal hematoma
- Abscess formation due to acute appendicitis, salpingitis, or diverticulitis
- Tuberculosis (rare)
- Syphilis
- Lymphogranuloma venereum
- Immunocompromised state (actinomycosis)

GENERAL PREVENTION

- Perianal hygiene
- Prevention or prompt treatment of anorectal abscess. Management of commonly associated conditions or risk factors.

COMMONLY ASSOCIATED CONDITIONS

- Anorectal abscess
- IBD (Crohn disease)
- Diabetes
- Chronic steroid treatment

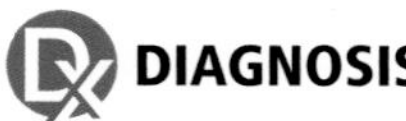

DIAGNOSIS

HISTORY

- Diagnosis based on perianal pain, purulent perianal drainage, and perirectal skin lesions
- Intermittent rectal pain worse with defecation or sitting may also be described.
- Perianal drainage may be malodorous and may be accompanied by pruritus.

PHYSICAL EXAM

- Excoriations or inflammation of perianal skin
- Perineal or perianal external exam may reveal visible orifice. Anorectal abscess may also be palpated as an indurated or fluctuant tender perianal mass or small tender palpable lesion on rectal exam at level of anal crypt.
- May also present as induration if opening is incomplete or blind
- Anoscopy may reveal an internal orifice.
- Fever most common with abscesses, generally not common with fistulas
  - Goodsall rule is commonly cited to assist in determining course of the fistula tract (more predictive with posterior external anal openings):
    - If external opening is *anterior* to an imaginary line drawn transversely through anal canal, fistula usually runs directly (radially) into anal canal.
    - If external opening is within 3 cm of anal verge and *posterior* to line, fistula leads to a curved tract, with an internal opening in posterior commissure (except for a long anterior fistula).
    - In children, tract is usually straight.

DIFFERENTIAL DIAGNOSIS

- Pilonidal sinus
- Hidradenitis suppurativa
- Hemorrhoids
- Anal fissure, ulcer, or sores
- Infected inclusion cyst
- Urethroperineal fistulas
- Ischiorectal or high muscular abscess
- Rule out: Crohn disease, carcinoma, lymphoma, tuberculosis, chronic *Chlamydia trachomatis* infection, actinomycosis in immunocompromised, acute untreated pelvic inflammatory condition

DIAGNOSTIC TESTS & INTERPRETATION

Initial Tests (lab, imaging)

- Imaging helps define perianal anatomy.
- MRI and endoscopic ultrasound are preferred imaging tests in the evaluation of perianal fistulas.
- MRI has ~80–90% overall concordance with surgical examination under anesthesia; accuracy improves with dedicated pelvic MRI to allow better resolution.
- Angulation of fistula from internal opening correlates with the type of fistula (acute angle likely high transsphincteric; obtuse angle likely lower fistula)
- Fistulography (insertion of catheter into external opening of fistula and injection of radiographic contrast material) is *not* preferred and generally not accurate when evaluating perianal disease.
- Fistulography is reserved for patients who may have a fistula between the rectum and another organ (such as bladder).
- CT is limited in evaluating perianal fistula tracts; more helpful when looking for large perianal abscesses and inflammation

Follow-Up Tests & Special Considerations

- Rule out inflammatory bowel disease (Crohn disease) if suspected.
- Consider testing for syphilis for recurrent fistulas in sexually active patients.

Diagnostic Procedures/Other

- Anoscopy or sigmoidoscopy
- Colonoscopy and esophagogastroduodenoscopy if Crohn disease suspected

- Probing into the tract may be done under anesthesia prior to surgery to determine course of fistula.
- Injection of dilute methylene blue or hydrogen peroxide intraoperatively may help identify internal opening.

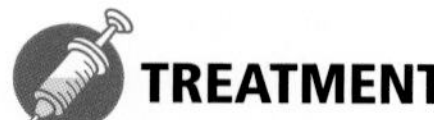

TREATMENT

GENERAL MEASURES

- Surgical treatment is definitive (1)[A].
- Optimal surgical treatment based on correct fistula classification
- Goals of treatment include resolving the inflammatory process, maintaining continence, and preventing recurrence.
- Sitz baths 3–4 times per day until definitive surgery

MEDICATION

- Medical management with antibiotics and immunosuppressive agents plays a role in the treatment of fistulas due to Crohn disease, particularly if patients are minimally symptomatic.
- Studies have shown improvement (reduced pain, discharge, and induration) and healing in up to 80% of patients with 8 weeks of treatment using oral metronidazole in patients with Crohn disease.
- Use of infliximab has also been shown to be effective in healing perianal Crohn fistulas but has been associated with a high rate of recurrence.
- Antibiotics may be indicated if patients have signs of sepsis or an active infection with a concurrent anorectal abscess.
- Surgery may be reserved for Crohn patients who fail long-term medical therapy.

SURGERY/OTHER PROCEDURES

- Choice of surgical procedure is a balance between achieving cure, avoiding recurrence, and maintaining fecal incontinence (2)[A].
- Low transsphincteric and intersphincteric simple fistulas can be treated with simple fistulotomy or fibrin sealant (fistula plug) (3)[A].
- Fistula plugs can be used as initial treatment for high transsphincteric fistulas. If the fistula recurs, then an advancement flap may be performed.
- Complex fistulas should be treated with an endorectal advancement flap, which closes the internal opening of the fistula with a mobilized flap of healthy mucosal and submucosal tissue.
- Fistulotomy opens the entire fistula tract (unroofing) (4)[B].
  - Fistula tract is cauterized or curetted and tract is marsupialized to promote healing.
  - Lower rates of recurrence compared to incision and drainage alone
  - Fistulotomy results in incontinence in about 12% of patients with simple fistulas, compared with almost 50% of patients with complex fistulas.
- Setons may be placed for complex fistulas treated with fistulotomy and, for those that involve >30% of the external sphincter, are proximal to the dentate line, or are categorized as high transsphincteric fistulas
- A seton is a reactive suture or elastic that is used for drainage (noncutting seton) or to allow scarring of the tract (cutting seton). Cutting setons are tightened at regular intervals to allow slow cutting through the tract and causing scarring.
- Postoperative: Patients discharged on day of procedure. Sitz baths several times per day (sit in warm bath 20 minutes 3–4 times per day and after bowel movements)
- Aggressive bowel regimen to prevent constipation
- Patients undergoing anal fistulotomy may benefit postoperatively from the use of topical application of sucralfate.

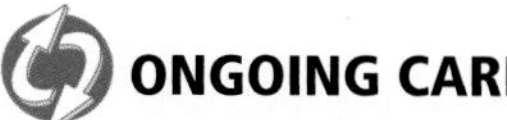

ONGOING CARE

FOLLOW-UP RECOMMENDATIONS

Resumption of activity as tolerated after surgery

Patient Monitoring

Anoscopy at 3–6 months following procedure. Frequent follow-up to ensure complete healing and assess continence.

DIET

High-fiber diet

PROGNOSIS

Postoperative healing:

- 4–5 weeks for perianal fistulas
- 12–16 weeks for deeper fistulas
- Postoperative healing may occur within 2–3 weeks in children.
- Healing may be significantly delayed in patients with Crohn disease.

COMPLICATIONS

- Fecal incontinence
- Constipation
- Rectovaginal fistula
- Delayed wound healing
- Low-grade carcinoma may develop in long-standing fistulas.
- Recurrent anorectal fistula if fistula is incompletely treated

REFERENCES

1. Whiteford MH, Kilkenny J III, Hyman N, et al. Practice parameters for the treatment of perianal abscess and fistula-in-ano (revised). *Dis Colon Rectum*. 2005;48(7):1337–1342.
2. Malik AI, Nelson RL. Surgical management of anal fistulae: a systematic review. *Colorectal Dis*. 2008;10(5):420–430.
3. Cirocchi R, Farinella E, La Mura F, et al. Fibrin glue in the treatment of anal fistula: a systematic review. *Ann Surg Innov Res*. 2009;3:12.
4. Rizzo JA, Naig LA, Johnson EK. Anorectal abscess and fistula-in-ano: evidence-based management. *Surg Clin North Am*. 2010;90(1):45–68.

ADDITIONAL READING

- A ba-bai-ke-re MM, Wen H, Huang HG, et al. Randomized controlled trial of minimally invasive surgery using acellular dermal matrix for complex anorectal fistula. *World J Gastroenterol*. 2010;16(26):3279–3286.
- Gupta PJ, Heda PS, Shrirao SA, et al. Topical sucralfate treatment of anal fistulotomy wounds: a randomized placebo-controlled trial. *Dis Colon Rectum*. 2011;54(6):699–704.
- Jacob TJ, Perakath B, Keighley MR. Surgical intervention for anorectal fistula. *Cochrane Database Syst Rev*. 2010;(5):CD006319.
- Lewis RT, Maron DJ. Anorectal Crohn's disease. *Surg Clin North Am*. 2010;90(1):83–97.
- Mishra A, Shah S, Nar AS, et al. The role of fibrin glue in the treatment of high and low fistulas in ano. *J Clin Diagn Res*. 2013;7(5):876–879.
- Niyogi A, Agarwal T, Broadhurst J, et al. Management of perianal abscess and fistula-in-ano in children. *Eur J Pediatr Surg*. 2010;20(1):35–39.

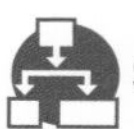

SEE ALSO

Anorectal Abscess; Crohn Disease

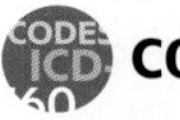

CODES

ICD10

- K60.5 Anorectal fistula
- K60.3 Anal fistula
- K60.4 Rectal fistula

CLINICAL PEARLS

- Suspect anorectal fistula when a patient complains of perianal pain, perianal purulent drainage, and perirectal skin lesions.
- Surgery is the mainstay of treatment unless patients have fistulas related to Crohn disease.
- MRI or endoscopic ultrasound are the imaging modalities of choice to define the anatomy of anorectal fistulas.

ANOREXIA NERVOSA

Umer Farooq, MD, MBBS • Najm Hasan Siddiqui, MD

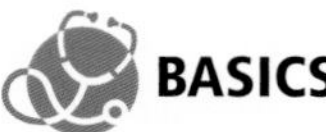

BASICS

DESCRIPTION

- Restriction of energy intake leading to significantly low in the context of age, sex, developmental trajectory, and physical health, with associated fear of weight gain and body image disturbance. Significantly low weight is defined as weight that is less than minimally normal/expected.
- *Diagnostic and Statistical Manual of Mental Disorders, V,* divides anorexia into 2 types:
  - Restricting type: not engaged in binge eating or purging behaviors for last 3 months
  - Binge eating/purging type: regularly engages in binge eating or purging behaviors (last 3 months)
- System(s) affected: cardiovascular, endocrine, metabolic, gastrointestinal, nervous, reproductive
- Severity of anorexia nervosa (AN) is based on BMI (per *DSM-5*):
  - Mild: BMI $\geq$ 17 kg/m^2
  - Moderate: BMI 16–16.99 kg/m^2
  - Severe: BMI 15–15.99 kg/m^2
  - Extreme: BMI less than 15 kg/m^2

EPIDEMIOLOGY

- Predominant age: 13–20 years
- Predominant sex: female > male (10–20 times more common in females)
- Global distribution

Incidence

8–19 women/2 men per 100,000 per year

Prevalence

- 0.9% in women
- 0.3% in men (higher in gay and bisexual men)

ETIOLOGY AND PATHOPHYSIOLOGY

- Complex relationship among genetic, biologic, environmental, psychological, and social factors that results in an unrealistic perception of fatness
- Subsequent malnutrition leads to disorder of multiple organs.
- Serotonin, norepinephrine, and dopamine neuronal systems are implicated.

Genetics

- Underlying genetic vulnerability likely but not well understood, some evidence of higher concordance rates in monozygotic twins than in dizygotic
- 1st-degree female relative with eating disorder increases risk 6–10-fold.

RISK FACTORS

- Female gender
- Adolescence
- Body dissatisfaction
- Perfectionism
- Negative self-evaluation
- Academic and other achievement pressure
- Severe life stressors
- Participation in sports or artistic activities that emphasize leanness or involve subjective scoring: ballet, running, wrestling, figure skating, gymnastics, cheerleading, weight lifting
- Type 1 diabetes mellitus
- Family history of substance abuse, affective disorders, or eating disorder

GENERAL PREVENTION

Prevention programs can reduce risk factors and future onset of eating disorders (1)[A]:

- Target adolescents and young women 15 years of age or older.
- Encourage realistic and healthy weight management strategies and attitudes.
- Decrease body dissatisfaction.
- Promote self-esteem.
- Reduce focus on thin as ideal.
- Decrease anxiety/depressive symptoms and improve stress management.

COMMONLY ASSOCIATED CONDITIONS

- Mood disorder (major depression)
- Social phobia, obsessive-compulsive disorder
- Substance abuse disorder
- High rates of cluster C personality disorders

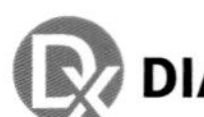

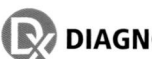

DIAGNOSIS

HISTORY

- Patient unlikely to self-identify problem (lack of insight into the illness), corroborate with family
- Fear of weight gain and/or distorted body image
- Report feeling fat even when emaciated
- Preoccupation with body size, weight control
- Onset may be insidious or stress-related.
- Elaborate food preparation and eating rituals
- Extensive exercise
- Amenorrhea (primary or secondary)
- Weakness, fatigue, cognitive impairment
- Cold intolerance
- Constipation, bloating, early satiety
- Growth arrest, delayed puberty
- History of fractures (decreased bone density)

PHYSICAL EXAM

- May be normal
- Vital signs: hypothermia, bradycardia, orthostatic hypotension, body weight <85% of expected
- Cardiac: dysrhythmias, midsystolic click of mitral valve prolapse
- Skin/extremities: dry skin; lanugo hair on extremities, face, and trunk; hair loss; edema
- Neurologic and abdominal exams: to rule out other causes of weight loss and vomiting

DIFFERENTIAL DIAGNOSIS

- Hyperthyroidism, adrenal insufficiency
- Inflammatory bowel disease, malabsorption
- Immunodeficiency, chronic infections
- Diabetes
- CNS lesion
- Bulimia, body dysmorphic disorder
- Depressive disorders with loss of appetite
- Anxiety disorder, food phobia
- Conversion disorder

DIAGNOSTIC TESTS & INTERPRETATION

- Psychological self-report screening tests may be helpful, but diagnosis is based on meeting the *DSM-5* criteria.
- Most findings are related directly to starvation and/or dehydration. All findings may be within normal limits.
- Psychological self-report screening tools:
  - Eating Attitudes Test
  - Eating Disorder Inventory
  - Eating Disorder Screen for Primary Care

Initial Tests (lab, imaging)

- CBC: anemia, leukopenia, thrombocytopenia
- Low serum luteinizing hormone, follicle-stimulating hormone; low serum testosterone in men
- Thyroid function tests: low thyroid-stimulating hormone with normal T_3/T_4
- Liver function tests: abnormal liver enzymes
- Chem 7: altered BUN, creatinine clearance; electrolyte disturbances
- Hypoglycemia, hypercholesterolemia, hypercortisolemia, hypophosphatemia
- Low sedimentation rate
- 12-lead electrocardiogram to assess for prolonged QT interval
- Dual-energy x-ray absorptiometry of bone to assess for diminished bone density, only if underweight for >6 months

Test Interpretation

- Osteoporosis/osteopenia, pathologic fractures
- Sick euthyroid syndrome
- Cardiac impairment

ALERT

AN may exist concurrently with chronic medical disorders such as diabetes and cystic fibrosis.

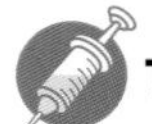

TREATMENT

GENERAL MEASURES

- Initial treatment goal geared to weight restoration; most managed as outpatients (OPs)
- OP treatment:
  - Interdisciplinary team (primary care physician, mental health provider, dietician)
  - Average weekly weight gain goal: 0.5–1.0 kg, with stepwise increase in calories
  - Cognitive-behavioral therapy, interpersonal psychotherapy, family-based therapy
  - Focus on health, not weight gain alone.
  - Build trust and a treatment alliance.
  - Involve the patient in establishing diet and exercise goals.
  - Challenge fear of uncontrolled weight gain; help the patient to recognize feelings that lead to disordered eating.
  - In chronic cases, goal may be to achieve a safe weight rather than a healthy weight.
- Inpatient treatment:
  - If possible, admit to a specialized eating disorders unit.
  - Assess risk for refeeding syndrome (weight loss >10% in 2–3 months; current weight <70% ideal body weight).
  - Monitor vital signs, electrolytes, cardiac function, edema, and weight gain.
  - Initial supervised meals may be necessary.
  - Stepwise increase in activity
  - Tube feeding or total parenteral nutrition is used only as a last resort.
  - Supportive symptomatic care as needed
- Most patients should be treated as OPs using an interdisciplinary team.
- Behavioral therapies (e.g., cognitive-behavioral, interpersonal, or family therapy) should be offered (2–4)[A].
- CBT has demonstrated effectiveness as a means of improving treatment adherence and minimizing dropout among patients with AN (5)[A].

MEDICATION

First Line

- No medications are available that effectively treat patients with AN, but pharmacotherapy may be used as an adjuvant to cognitive-behavioral therapies (4,6)[A].
- If medications are used, start with low doses due to increased risk for adverse effects.
- SSRIs may:
  - Help to prevent relapse after weight gain
  - Treat comorbid depression or obsessive-compulsive disorder
  - Use of atypical antipsychotics is being studied with mixed findings to date. Olanzapine is potentially beneficial as an adjuvant treatment of underweight individuals in the inpatient settings.
- Attend to black box warnings concerning antidepressants.

Second Line

- Management of osteopenia:
  - Primary treatment is weight gain.
  - Elemental calcium 1,200–1,500 mg/day plus vitamin D 800 IU/day
  - No indication for bisphosphonates in AN
  - Weak evidence for use of hormone-replacement therapy
- Psyllium (Metamucil) preparations to prevent constipation

ISSUES FOR REFERRAL

Patients with AN require an interdisciplinary team (primary care physician, mental health provider, nutritionist). An important step in management is to arrange OP mental health therapist.

INPATIENT CONSIDERATIONS

Admission Criteria/Initial Stabilization

- Suggested physiologic values: heart rate <40 beats/min, BP <90/60 mm Hg, symptomatic hypoglycemia, potassium <3 mmol/L, temperature <97.0°F (36.1°C), dehydration, other cardiovascular abnormalities, weight <75% of expected, rapid weight loss, lack of improvement while in OP therapy
- Suggested psychological indications: poor motivation/insight, lack of cooperation with OP treatment, inability to eat, need for nasogastric feeding, suicidal intent or plan, severe coexisting psychiatric disease, problematic family environment

Pediatric Considerations

- Children often present with nausea, abdominal pain, fullness, and inability to swallow.
- Additional indications for hospitalization: heart rate <50 beats/min, orthostatic BP, hypokalemia or hypophosphatemia, rapid weight loss even if weight not <75% below normal
- Children and adolescents should be offered family-based treatment.

Geriatric Considerations

Late-onset AN (>50 years of age) may be long-term disease or triggered by death of loved one, marital discord, or divorce.

Discharge Criteria

Discharge when medically stable. Arrange OP appointment with mental health provider and primary care provider.

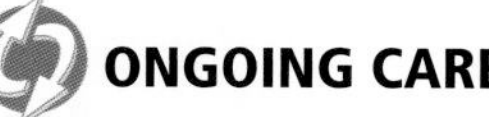

ONGOING CARE

FOLLOW-UP RECOMMENDATIONS

- Close follow-up until patient demonstrates forward progress in care plan
- Family and individual therapy extremely important for the long-term benefits/outcomes
- CBT is very helpful for the treatment of AN and may be helpful for the prevention of relapse.
- Emphasize importance of moderate activity for health, not thinness.

Patient Monitoring

- Level of exercise activity
- Weigh weekly until stable, then monthly.
- Depression, suicidal ideation

DIET

- Dietary consult while pt is inpt.
- Nutritional education programs

PATIENT EDUCATION

- Provide patients and families with information about the diagnosis and its natural history, health risks, and treatment strategies.
- The National Alliance on Mental Illness: http://www.nami.org/helpline/anorexia.htm

PROGNOSIS

- Prognosis: ~50% recover, 30% improve, 20% are chronically ill
- Outcomes in men likely better than for women
- Mortality: 3%
- Suicide is the cause of death in 1 in 5 individuals who died with AN.

COMPLICATIONS

- Refeeding syndrome
- Cardiac arrhythmia, cardiac arrest
- Cardiomyopathy, congestive heart failure
- Delayed gastric emptying, necrotizing colitis
- Seizures, Wernicke encephalopathy, peripheral neuropathy, cognitive deficits
- Osteopenia, osteoporosis

Pregnancy Considerations

- Fertility may be affected.
- Behaviors may persist, decrease, or recur during pregnancy and the postpartum interval.
- Increased risk for preterm labor, operative delivery, and infants with low birth weight; anemia, genitourinary infections, and labor induction should be managed as high risk.

REFERENCES

1. Stice E, Shaw H, Marti CN. A meta-analytic review of eating disorder prevention programs: encouraging findings. *Ann Rev Clin Psychol*. 2007;3:207–231.
2. Hay P, Bacaltchuk J, Claudino A, et al. Individual psychotherapy in the outpatient treatment of adults with anorexia. *Cochrane Database Syst Rev*. 2003;(4):CD003909.
3. Fisher CA, Hetrick SE, Rushford N. Family therapy for anorexia nervosa. *Cochrane Database Syst Rev*. 2010;(4):CD004780.
4. Bulik CM, Berkman ND, Brownley KA, et al. Anorexia nervosa treatment: a systematic review of randomized controlled trials. *Int J Eat Disord*. 2007;40(4):310–320.
5. Galsworthy-Francis L, Allan S. Cognitive behavioural therapy for anorexia nervosa: a systematic review. *Clin Psychol Rev*. 2014;34(1):54–72.
6. Claudino AM, Hay P, Lima MS, et al. Antidepressants for anorexia nervosa. *Cochrane Database Syst Rev*. 2006;(1):CD004365.

ADDITIONAL READING

- American Psychiatric Association. *Practice Guideline for the Treatment of Patients with Eating Disorders*. 3rd ed. Arlington, VA: American Psychiatric Publishing; 2006.
- Dalle Grave R. Eating disorders: progress and challenges. *Eur J Intern Med*. 2011;22(2):153–160.
- National Collaborating Centre for Mental Health. *Eating Disorders: Core Interventions in the Treatment and Management of Anorexia Nervosa, Bulimia Nervosa and Related Eating Disorders*. Leicester, United Kingdom: British Psychological Society; 2004.

SEE ALSO

- Amenorrhea; Osteoporosis; Bulimia Nervosa
- Algorithm: Weight Loss

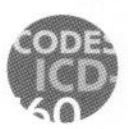

CODES

ICD10

- F50.00 Anorexia nervosa, unspecified
- F50.01 Anorexia nervosa, restricting type
- F50.02 Anorexia nervosa, binge eating/purging type

CLINICAL PEARLS

- "Are you satisfied with your eating patterns?" and/or "Do you worry that you have lost control over how you eat?" may help to screen those with an eating problem.
- Studies have shown patients with AN will not accept medications unless combined with psychotherapy.
- To care for a patient with AN, an interdisciplinary team that includes a medical provider, a dietician, and a behavioral health professional is the most accepted approach.
- Family analysis is necessary for the patients with AN to determine what kind of therapy would be most helpful.
- 3 months amenorrhea is no longer the criteria needed for the diagnosis of AN.

ANTIPHOSPHOLIPID ANTIBODY SYNDROME

Ho Phong Pham, MD • Dausen J. Harker, MD

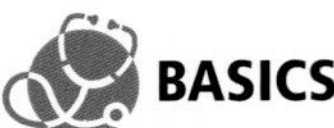

BASICS

DESCRIPTION

Antiphospholipid antibody syndrome (APS) is an autoantibody-mediated thrombophilic disorder characterized by recurrent arterial or venous thrombosis and/or recurrent fetal loss in the presence of antiphospholipid antibodies (APAs). The APAs enhance clot formation by interacting with phospholipid-binding plasma proteins. The resulting APS can cause significant morbidity and mortality in both pregnant and nonpregnant individuals:

- Types of APS (based on clinical presentation)
  - Primary: occurs without associated underlying disease
  - Secondary: associated with autoimmune diseases (systemic lupus erythematosus [SLE] is most common). Transient APAs linked to certain infections, drugs, and malignancy.
  - Catastrophic APS (CAPS) a.k.a Asherson syndrome (<1%)
    - Most severe form of disease; characterized by thrombotic microangiopathy and associated with multiorgan failure
    - High mortality if treatment is delayed
    - Severe thrombocytopenia, hemolytic anemia, and DIC are additional features.
  - Associated clinical manifestations: livedo reticularis, cardiac valvular disease, thrombocytopenia, nephropathy, hemolytic anemia, coronary artery disease, and cognitive impairment

Pregnancy Considerations

- Complications include maternal thrombosis (stroke, venous thromboembolism [VTE]), fetal death, preeclampsia and placental insufficiency, fetal growth retardation, and preterm birth.
- Low-dose aspirin and low-molecular-weight heparin (LMWH) or unfractionated heparin are the drugs of choice in pregnancy.
- Prophylactic-dose heparin is recommended in the postpartum period (unless patient is on therapeutic anticoagulation) given high risk of thrombosis during this time.With adequate treatment, >70% with APS deliver viable infant.

EPIDEMIOLOGY

- The prevalence of APAs increases with age but is not necessarily associated with a higher risk of thrombosis.
- For APS, female > male

Incidence

- In patients with positive APAs without prior risk of thrombosis, the annual incident risk of thrombosis is 0–3.8%. This risk is up to 5.3% in those with triple positivity (anticardiolipin antibodies, lupus anticoagulant, and anti–β2-glycorotein 1 (GP1) antibodies positive).
- 10–15% of recurrent abortions are attributable to APS.

Prevalence

APAs are present in 1–5% of the general population and in ~40% of those with SLE. A higher prevalence is seen in those with VTE and stroke.

ETIOLOGY AND PATHOPHYSIOLOGY

- Anti–β2 glycoprotein-1 antibodies play a central role in the pathogenesis of APS. The procoagulant effect is mediated by various possible mechanisms:
  - Endothelial effects: inhibition of prostacyclin production and loss of annexin V cellular shield
  - Platelet activation resulting in adhesion and aggregation
  - Interference of innate anticoagulant pathways (such as inhibition of protein C)
  - Complement activation
- Pregnancy-related complications are also a result of autoantibody-mediated effects:
  - Interference with expression of trophoblastic adhesion molecules resulting in abnormal placentation and placental thrombosis
- Proposed mechanisms: excess production of natural antibodies, molecular mimicry due to infections, exposure of phospholipid antigens during platelet activation, cardiolipin peroxidation, and genetic predisposition
- A "second hit" by environmental factors may be required to produce thrombosis.

Genetics

Most cases of APS are acquired. There are a few studies of familial occurrence of anticardiolipin antibodies and lupus anticoagulant (LAC). A valine 247/leucine polymorphism in β2-glycoprotein I could be a genetic risk for the presence of anti-β2GPI antibodies and APS.

RISK FACTORS

- Age >55 years in males, >65 in females
- Cardiovascular risk factors (hypertension, diabetes, obesity, smoking, combined oral contraceptive use)
- Inherited thrombophilia
- Surgery, immobilization, pregnancy

GENERAL PREVENTION

Risk factor modification: Control HTN and diabetes; smoking cessation; avoidance of oral contraceptives in high-risk patients; start thromboprophylaxis in established cases.

COMMONLY ASSOCIATED CONDITIONS

- Autoimmune diseases: SLE (most common), scleroderma, Sjögren syndrome, dermatomyositis, and rheumatoid arthritis
- Malignancy
- Infections: viral, bacterial, parasitic, and rickettsial
- Certain drugs associated with APA production without increased risk of thrombosis; phenothiazines, hydralazine, procainamide, and phenytoin
- HELLP syndrome (hemolysis, elevated liver enzymes, and low platelet count in association with pregnancy)
- Sneddon syndrome (APS variant syndrome with livedo reticularis, HTN, and stroke)

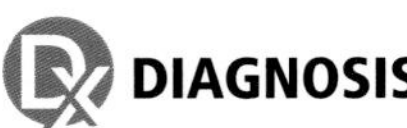

DIAGNOSIS

Sapporo criteria, revised 2006:

- At least one of the following clinical criteria:
  - Vascular thrombosis
    - ≥1 clinical episodes of arterial, venous, or small vessel thrombosis, occurring within any tissue or organ and confirmed by unequivocal imaging studies or histopathology
  - Complications of pregnancy (any one of the following):
    - ≥3 consecutive spontaneous abortions before the 10th week of pregnancy, unexplained by maternal/paternal chromosomal abnormalities or maternal anatomic/hormonal causes
    - ≥1 unexplained deaths of morphologically normal fetuses at ≥10th week of gestation
    - ≥1 premature births of morphologically normal newborn babies at ≤34th week of pregnancy due to severe preeclampsia, eclampsia, or placental insufficiency
- *AND* the presence of at least one of three laboratory findings (confirmed on ≥2 occasions at least 12 weeks apart):
  - Lupus anticoagulant (LAC) detected in blood
  - Anticardiolipin IgG and/or IgM antibodies present at moderate or high levels in the blood (>40 GPL or MPL or 99th percentile) via a standardized ELISA
  - Anti–β2-GP1 IgG and/or IgM antibodies in blood at a titer >99th percentile by standardized ELISA

HISTORY

- History of VTE or arterial thrombosis (stroke, MI)
- History of fetal loss or other obstetric complications
- Bleeding from thrombocytopenia if severe or acquired factor II deficiency
- Personal or family history of autoimmune disease

PHYSICAL EXAM

- Signs of venous thrombosis in extremities
- Skin manifestations, including a vasculitic rash in the form of palpable purpura or livedo reticularis or lower extremity ulcers
- Livedo reticularis
- Cardiac murmurs
- Focal neurologic or cognitive deficits

DIFFERENTIAL DIAGNOSIS

- Thrombophilic conditions
  - Inherited: deficiency of protein C, protein S, antithrombin III; mutation of factor V Leiden, prothrombin gene mutation
  - Acquired: neoplastic and myeloproliferative disorders, hyperviscosity syndromes, nephrotic syndrome
- Embolic disease secondary to atrial fibrillation, LV dysfunction, endocarditis, cholesterol emboli
- Heparin-induced thrombocytopenia
- Atherosclerosis
- CAPS: hemolytic-uremic syndrome, TTP, or malignant hypertension

DIAGNOSTIC TESTS & INTERPRETATION

- LAC assay, and ELISA for anticardiolipin antibodies and anti–β2-GP1 antibodies are diagnostic tests of choice.
- The LAC assay combines at least 2 out of 3 screening tests (prolongation of aPTT, dilute Russell viper venom time [dRVVT], and kaolin clotting) with 2 confirmatory tests.
- Anti–β2-GP1 antibodies are important in the pathogenesis of thrombosis. A positive LAC assay recognizes antibodies against β2-GP1 and prothrombin.
- The clinical significance of other autoantibodies (annexin V, phosphatidylserine, and phosphatidylinositol) remains unclear.

Initial Tests (lab, imaging)

- CBC, PT/INR, aPTT, LAC, anticardiolipin antibodies, anti–β2-GP1 antibodies (3)[B]
- Further testing for secondary causes such as SLE when clinically suspected
- Imaging is based on clinical picture, suspected sites of thrombosis, and organ involvement.

Follow-Up Tests & Special Considerations

- The results of LAC are difficult to interpret in patients treated with warfarin. Unfractionated heparin or LMWH and fondaparinux do not affect the LAC assay.
- Repeat testing at 12 weeks for persistence of APA.

Diagnostic Procedures/Other

Biopsy of the affected organ system may be necessary to distinguish from vasculitis.

Test Interpretation

Usual finding is thrombosis and minimal vascular or perivascular inflammation:

- Acute changes: capillary congestion and noninflammatory fibrin thrombi
- Chronic changes: ischemic hypoperfusion, atrophy, and fibrosis

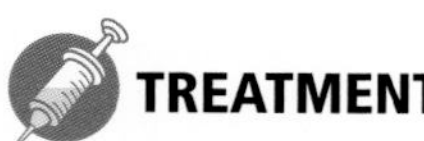

TREATMENT

MEDICATION

First Line

- Primary thromboprophylaxis: Low-dose aspirin is indicated in asymptomatic carriers of APAs with SLE and in pregnancy. It may be considered in other asymptomatic carriers. Hydroxychloroquine is recommended in all antiphospholid-positive SLE patients.
- Secondary thromboprophylaxis: All symptomatic, nonpregnant patients with APS need indefinite anticoagulation. The target INR depends on the severity and type of thrombosis:
  - Venous thrombosis (1st episode): warfarin with target INR of 2.0–3.0
  - Arterial thrombosis or recurrent venous thrombosis despite anticoagulation: warfarin with target INR 3.0–4.0
  - LMWH and fondaparinux are alternatives.
- New oral anticoagulants such as rivaroxaban, apixaban, and dabigatran; all have been approved for treatment of DVT/PE; studies in APS are lacking, a prospective randomized controlled trial of warfarin versus rivaroxaban in patients with thrombotic APS and with a target INR or 2.5 is underway.
  - Rituximab may be an option in severe cases, possibly in those with hematologic and microthrombotic/microangiopathic manifestations (1,2)[B].
- Danaparoid, fondaparinux, and argatroban can be considered in APS patients with heparin-induced thrombocytopenia.
- Newer oral anticoagulants (dabigatran, apixaban, and rivaroxaban) may be alternatives to warfarin with few drug interactions and no need for monitoring. The presence of APA interferes with hemostatic mechanisms and can interfere with anticoagulants. Ongoing phase III trials will help evaluate the role of new oral anticoagulants.
- Statins can decrease proinflammatory and prothrombotic state in APS. At this time, although they are not recommended in the absence of hyperlipidemia, APA-positive patients with recurrent thrombosis while adequately anticoagulated may benefit from statin therapy.
- B-cell inhibition may help in recalcitrant APS cases.
- Complement inhibition may be useful in cases refractory to anticoagulation, but further evaluation is needed.
- Peptide therapy may be a future treatment for APA-positive patients.
- Vitamin D deficiency/insufficiency should be corrected in all APA-positive patients but its role in APS needs further study.
- CAPS: Anticoagulants and high-dose steroids may suffice in less severe cases. Aggressive treatment with either IVIG or plasmapheresis is often required in this life-threatening condition. These measures have improved survival to 66%.
- Treatment in pregnancy as follows:
  - For women with no prior history of thrombosis and ≥2 early miscarriages, either 81 mg ASA alone or in combination with unfractionated heparin (5,000–10,000 units SC q12h) or LMWH (prophylactic dose). In those with a previous late pregnancy loss (>10 weeks' gestation) or preterm (<34 weeks) delivery due to severe preeclampsia, a combination of ASA and heparin is recommended.
  - In those with a history of thrombosis, low-dose ASA plus either therapeutic low-dose heparin (dosed every 8–12 hours to maintain mid-interval aPTT or factor Xa levels) or LMWH (therapeutic dose)
  - Refractory cases: Up to 30% of patients have recurrent pregnancy loss despite the use of ASA and heparin. There is no role for warfarin due to risk of teratogenicity (early pregnancy) and fetal bleeding (late pregnancy). Such cases are best managed in consultation with a maternal-fetal medicine specialist.

SURGERY/OTHER PROCEDURES

Patients with thrombosis may require thrombectomy or an IVC filter (depending on site) when anticoagulation is contraindicated.

ONGOING CARE

FOLLOW-UP RECOMMENDATIONS

Patient Monitoring

- Standard guidelines for monitoring to maintain INR at goal with warfarin therapy
- Close monitoring is required during pregnancy.

DIET

Heart-healthy diet. Patients on warfarin should avoid foods rich in vitamin K (kale, spinach, sprouts, greens).

PATIENT EDUCATION

- Compliance with warfarin therapy to keep INR at goal
- Awareness of drug and diet interactions with warfarin
- Avoid oral hormonal contraceptives.

PROGNOSIS

- Pulmonary HTN, neurologic involvement, myocardial ischemia, nephropathy, gangrene of extremities, and catastrophic APS are associated with a worse prognosis.
- 30% risk of recurrent thrombosis in the absence of adequate anticoagulation

COMPLICATIONS

- Pregnancy complications and pulmonary HTN are associated with higher morbidity and mortality.
- Thrombotic complications are the most common cause of death.

REFERENCES

1. Arachchillage DJ, Cohen H. Use of new oral anticoagulants in antiphospholipid syndrome. *Curr Rheumatol Rep*. 2013;15(6):331.
2. Erkan D, Aguiar CL, Andrade D, et al. 14th International Congress on Antiphospholipid Antibodies: task force report on antiphospholipid syndrome treatment trends. *Autoimmun Rev*. 2014;13(6):685–696.
3. Giannakopoulos B, Passam F, Ioannou Y, et al. How we diagnose the antiphospholipid syndrome. *Blood*. 2009;113(5):985–994.
4. Ruiz-Irastorza G, Crowther M, Branch W, et al. Antiphospholipid syndrome. *Lancet*. 2010;376(9751):1498–1509.

ADDITIONAL READING

- Baker WF Jr, Bick RL, Fareed J. Controversies and unresolved issues in antiphospholipid syndrome pathogenesis and management. *Hematol Oncol Clin North Am*. 2008;22(1):155–174, viii.
- Branch D, Holmgren C, Goldberg J. Practice bulletin no. 132: Antiphospholipid syndrome. *Obstet Gynecol* 2012;120(6):1514–1521.
- Branham K, Thomas M, Nelson-Piercy C, et al. First-trimester low-dose prednisolone in refractory antiphospholipid antibody-related pregnancy loss. *Blood*. 2011;117(25):6948–6951.
- Miyakis S, Lockshin MD, Atsumi T, et al. International consensus statement on an update of the classification criteria for definite antiphospholipid syndrome (APS). *J Thromb Haemost*. 2006;4(2):295–306.
- Ruiz-Irastorza G, Crowther M, Branch W, et al. Antiphospholipid syndrome. *Lancet*. 2010;376(9751):1498–1509.

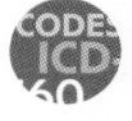

CODES

ICD10

- D68.61 Antiphospholipid syndrome
- D68.69 Other thrombophilia
- D68.62 Lupus anticoagulant syndrome

CLINICAL PEARLS

- APS can be either primary, secondary, or present as a severe microvascular disease known as CAPS.
- Both clinical and laboratory criteria are required for diagnosis. The latter must be confirmed on two separate occasions at least 12 weeks apart.
- Thrombotic manifestations of APS can be either venous or arterial. Patients require lifelong anticoagulation.

ANTITHROMBIN DEFICIENCY

Ryan Wargo, PharmD, BCACP • Patricia Feito, MD • Holly L. Baab, MD

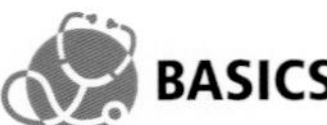

BASICS

DESCRIPTION

- Antithrombin is a glycoprotein that inhibits thrombin by forming an irreversible complex.
- There are 2 active sites: one that binds to heparin and one that binds to thrombin/target enzyme. Antithrombin can also inhibit factors Xa, IXa, and XIa. This process is catalyzed by the presence of heparin.
- Patients deficient in antithrombin have an increased incidence of venous thrombosis, including deep vein thrombosis (DVT) of the lower extremity. Arterial thrombosis is much less common in patients deficient in antithrombin.
- System(s) affected: cardiovascular, nervous, pulmonary, reproductive, hematologic, lymphatic/ immunologic hemic/lymphatic/immunologic
- Synonym(s): antithrombin III deficiency

EPIDEMIOLOGY

- Predominant age: Mean age of 1st thrombosis is in 2nd decade, usually after puberty.
- Predominant sex: male = female
- No racial or ethnic predisposition

Incidence

1/20 to 1/200 with thrombophilia (1)

Prevalence

1/2,000 to 1/20,000 of normal individuals (1)

ETIOLOGY AND PATHOPHYSIOLOGY

- Hereditary deficiency (1)
  - Type I deficiency is characterized by low levels of antigen (decreased synthesis). Plasma levels of antithrombin are often <50%.
  - Type II deficiency is found when the antithrombin molecule is dysfunctional (decreased function).
  - Type II deficiencies are due to mutations in either the active center of antithrombin that binds the target enzyme or the heparin-binding site.
  - No patients homozygous for defects in the active center have been described, suggesting that this is a lethal condition. Patients heterozygous for mutations in the heparin-binding site rarely have thrombotic episodes.
- Acquired deficiency (1)
  - Many clinical conditions are associated with antithrombin deficiency, such as those listed under special considerations, but limited evidence suggests these deficiencies contribute to increased thrombosis.

Genetics

Autosomal dominant

RISK FACTORS

- Oral contraceptives, pregnancy, and the use of hormone replacement therapy (HRT) increase the risk of venous thrombosis in patients with antithrombin deficiency.
- Patients with antithrombin deficiency and another prothrombotic state, such as factor V Leiden or the prothrombin G20210A mutation, have increased rates of thrombosis.

Pregnancy Considerations

Increases thrombotic risk in patients with antithrombin deficiency and specific complications may include preeclampsia, eclampsia, placental abruption, HELLP, premature birth, and recurrent pregnancy loss.

GENERAL PREVENTION

Patients with antithrombin deficiency without a history of thrombosis do not require prophylactic treatment.

COMMONLY ASSOCIATED CONDITIONS

Venous thromboembolism

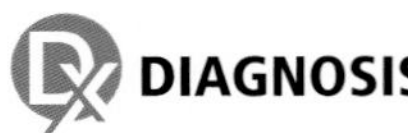

DIAGNOSIS

HISTORY

- Previous thrombosis
- Family history of thrombosis
- Family history of antithrombin deficiency

PHYSICAL EXAM

Signs consistent with a deep or superficial venous thrombosis or pulmonary embolism

DIFFERENTIAL DIAGNOSIS

- Factor V Leiden
- Protein C deficiency
- Protein S deficiency
- Dysfibrinogenemia
- Dysplasminogenemia
- Homocystinemia
- Prothrombin G20210A mutation
- Elevated factor VIII levels

DIAGNOSTIC TESTS & INTERPRETATION

Initial Tests (lab, imaging)

- For evaluation of a new clot in a patient at risk: CBC with peripheral smear, PT/INR, aPTT, thrombin time, lupus anticoagulant, antiphospholipid antibodies, factor VIII, anticardiolipin antibody, anti-B2 glycoprotein I antibody, activated protein C resistance, protein S antigen and resistance, antithrombin III assay, fibrinogen, factor V Leiden, prothrombin G20210A, homocysteine
- Testing should be done off heparin and at least 2 weeks after the 3–6 months course of oral anticoagulation.
- Another test to consider in the workup of antithrombin deficiency:
  - Antithrombin-heparin cofactor assay measures the ability of heparin to bind to antithrombin, which neutralizes the action of thrombin and factor Xa. This is an indirect measure of factor Xa and thrombin inhibition, the factor Xa inhibition activity being more specific. This assay will detect all currently recognized subtypes of hereditary antithrombin deficiency.
- Drugs that may alter lab results: Heparin (increased clearance), estrogen, and L-asparaginase (decreased synthesis) can lower antithrombin levels.

Follow-Up Tests & Special Considerations

- The role of family screening for antithrombin deficiency is unclear because most patients with this mutation do not have thrombosis. Screening may be offered to pregnant women with a family history of factor protein S deficiency considering using oral contraceptives or pregnancy.
- Antithrombin levels are low in:
  - DIC
  - Sepsis
  - Burns
  - Severe trauma
  - Acute thrombosis
  - Pregnancy or postpartum
  - Liver disease
  - Nephrotic syndrome
  - Malignancy
  - Myeloproliferative disorders
- Antithrombin levels could be elevated by oral contraceptive pills.
- US to diagnose DVT if clinically indicated
- If DVT diagnosis in question, a negative D-dimer will help to rule out DVT.
- Spiral CT or V/Q scan to diagnose pulmonary embolism (PE) if clinically indicated
- V/Q scan may be difficult to interpret in patients with other lung disease.

Test Interpretation

Venous thrombosis

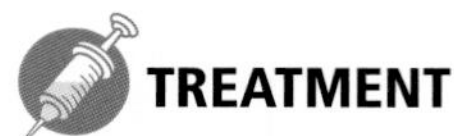

TREATMENT

GENERAL MEASURES

Routine anticoagulation for asymptomatic patients with antithrombin deficiency is not recommended (2,3,4)[C].

MEDICATION

First Line

- Patients with antithrombin deficiency and a first thrombosis should be anticoagulated initially with unfractionated heparin followed by oral anticoagulation with warfarin (5)[C].
- Heparin can be stopped after 5 total days of therapy provided the INR is 2–3 (5)[C].
- Oral anticoagulant should be started with the initial administration of heparin. Warfarin (Coumadin) 10 mg/day PO for the first 2 days, then adjusted to INR of 2–3. Patients should be maintained on warfarin for at least 6 months (5)[C].
- Recurrent thrombosis requires indefinite anticoagulation.
- Contraindications:
  - Active bleeding precludes anticoagulation; risk of bleeding is a relative contraindication to long-term anticoagulation.

- Precautions:
  - Observe patient for signs of embolization, further thrombosis, or bleeding.
  - Avoid IM injections.
  - Periodically check stool and urine for occult blood and monitor CBCs, including platelets.
  - Heparin-thrombocytopenia and/or paradoxical thrombosis with thrombocytopenia
- Significant possible interactions:
  - Agents that intensify the response to oral anticoagulants: Common anti-infective agents that potentially increase the effect of warfarin include ciprofloxacin, clarithromycin, erythromycin, metronidazole, trimethoprim-sulfamethoxazole, and azole antifungals. Additional interacting agents include alcohol, allopurinol, amiodarone, anabolic steroids, androgens, cimetidine, chloral hydrate, disulfiram, all NSAIDs, sulfinpyrazone, tamoxifen, thyroid hormone, vitamin E, ranitidine, salicylates, and acetaminophen.
  - Agents that diminish the response to oral anticoagulants: aminoglutethimide, antacids, barbiturates, carbamazepine, cholestyramine, diuretics, griseofulvin, rifampin, oral contraceptives
  - See "Diet."

Second Line

- Argatroban: 0.4–0.5 μg/kg/min. Case reports describing the use of this direct thrombin inhibitor in patients with antithrombin deficiency have been published (5)[C].
- Antithrombin III (ATnativ, Thrombate III): 50–100 IU/min IV titrated to antithrombin level desired. Precise role in therapy remains unclear (4)[C].
- Low-molecular-weight heparin (LMWH) is difficult to manage in this population but is preferred during pregnancy (5)[C].

ISSUES FOR REFERRAL

- Recurrent thrombosis on anticoagulation
- Difficulty anticoagulating
- Genetic counseling

ADDITIONAL THERAPIES

- Patients with severe antithrombin deficiency may require plasma replacement of thrombin in order for heparin to be effective.
- Compression stockings for prevention

SURGERY/OTHER PROCEDURES

Thrombectomy may be indicated in complicated cases.

INPATIENT CONSIDERATIONS

Admission Criteria/Initial Stabilization

Complicated thrombosis, such as pulmonary embolism. Heparin initial bolus of 80 U/kg followed by infusion of 18 U/kg/hr. Frequent monitoring of the partial thromboplastin time (PTT) is important, as ~50% of patients deficient in antithrombin require >40,000 U of heparin daily to adequately prolong PTT.

Discharge Criteria

Stable on anticoagulation

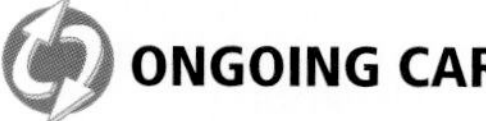

ONGOING CARE

FOLLOW-UP RECOMMENDATIONS

Patient Monitoring

Warfarin use requires periodic INR measurements (monthly after initial stabilization) with a goal of 2–3.

DIET

Foods high in vitamin K may interfere with anticoagulation on warfarin. Consider nutrition consultation.

PATIENT EDUCATION

- Patients should be educated about:
  - Use of oral anticoagulant therapy
  - Avoidance of NSAIDs while on warfarin
- The role of family screening is unclear, as most patients with this mutation do not have thrombosis. In a patient with a family history of factor V Leiden, consider screening during pregnancy or if considering oral contraceptive use.

PROGNOSIS

- The odds ratio of thrombosis in a patient with antithrombin deficiency is much higher than in patients with other thrombophilic conditions. The recurrence rate is similarly high.
- There is no difference in clinical severity between patients with type I defects and type II mutations.
- Overall, prognosis is good, if appropriately anticoagulated.

COMPLICATIONS

Recurrent thrombosis (requires indefinite anticoagulation)

REFERENCES

1. Maclean PS, Tait RC. Hereditary and acquired antithrombin deficiency: epidemiology, pathogenesis and treatment options. *Drugs*. 2007;67(10):1429–1440.
2. Dager WE, Gosselin RC, Owings JT. Argatroban therapy for antithrombin deficiency and mesenteric thrombosis: case report and review of the literature. *Pharmacotherapy*. 2004;24(5):659–663.
3. De Stefano V, Rossi E. Testing for inherited thrombophilia and consequences for antithrombotic prophylaxis in patients with venous thromboembolism and their relatives. A review of the guidelines from Scientific Societies and Working Groups. *Thromb Haemost*. 2013;110(4):697–705.
4. Rodgers GM. Role of antithrombin concentrate in treatment of hereditary antithrombin deficiency. An update. *Thromb Haemost*. 2009;101(5):806–812.
5. Guyatt GH, Akl EA, Crowther M, et al. Executive summary: Antithrombotic Therapy and Prevention of Thrombosis, 9th ed: American College of Chest Physicians Evidence-Based Clinical Practice Guidelines. *Chest*. 2012;141(2 Suppl):7S–47S.

ADDITIONAL READING

- Van Cott EM, Laposata M, Prins MH. Laboratory evaluation of hypercoagulability with venous or arterial thrombosis: venous thromboembolism, myocardial infarction, stroke, and other conditions. *Arch Pathol Lab Med*. 2001;126(11):1281–1295.
- Vinazzer H. Hereditary and acquired antithrombin deficiency. *Semin Thromb Hemost*. 1999;25(3):257–263.

SEE ALSO

Deep Vein Thrombophlebitis (DVT)

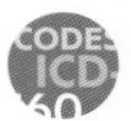

CODES

ICD10

D68.59 Other primary thrombophilia

CLINICAL PEARLS

- Antithrombin levels will be low on heparin and during acute thrombosis.
- Diagnosis can be difficult. Conditions causing low levels of antithrombin III, such as pregnancy, liver disease, sepsis, and DIC, must be ruled out.
- Testing should be done off heparin and at least 2 weeks after the 3–6 month course of oral anticoagulation.
- For pregnant women with antithrombin deficiency but no prior history of VTE, antepartum and postpartum vigilance are recommended. Postpartum prophylaxis with prophylactic or intermediate-dose LMWH or vitamin K antagonists with target INR 2–3 for 6 weeks is only recommended if there is positive family history of VTE.

ANXIETY

Mary K. Flynn, MD

BASICS

DESCRIPTION

- Persistent, excessive, and difficult-to-control worry associated with significant symptoms of motor tension, autonomic hyperactivity, and/or disturbances of sleep or concentration.
- System(s) affected: nervous (resulting in increased sympathetic tone and increased catecholamine release); may have secondary effects on other symptoms such as cardiac (tachycardia) and GI (nausea, irregular bowels)

EPIDEMIOLOGY

Prevalence

- 12-month prevalence rate: 2–3%
- Lifetime prevalence rate: 5%
- Onset can occur any time in life but is typically adulthood; median age of onset in the United States is 31 years.
- Predominant sex: female > male (2:1) (1)

ETIOLOGY AND PATHOPHYSIOLOGY

Mediated by abnormalities of neurotransmitter systems (i.e., serotonin, norepinephrine, and γ-amino butyric acid [GABA])

Genetics

- Strongly linked to depression in heritability studies
- A variant of the serotonin transporter gene (*5HT1A*) may contribute to both conditions; other genes (such as that for glutamic acid decarboxylase) also may play a role.

RISK FACTORS

- Caucasian race
- Adverse life events: stress, medical illness, disability, unemployment, and childhood physical and mental abuse
- Family history
- Lack of social support
- Depression
- Lesbian/bisexual women at increased risk (1)

GENERAL PREVENTION

Regular exercise is associated with decreased anxiety and depression.

COMMONLY ASSOCIATED CONDITIONS

- Major depressive disorder (>60%), dysthymia, bipolar disorder
- Alcohol/drug abuse
- Cigarette smoking in adolescence
- Panic disorder, agoraphobia, simple phobia, social anxiety disorder, anorexia nervosa

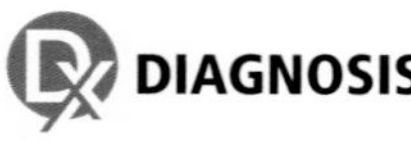

DIAGNOSIS

HISTORY

Diagnosis is primarily made through history taking. *DSM-5* criteria are as follows:

- History and evaluation should carefully identify generalized anxiety disorder (GAD) from other anxiety disorders.
- Symptoms of excessive anxiety and worry must occur more often than not for at least 6 months.
- At least 3 additional criteria are required for diagnosis of GAD in adults; only 1 is required in children.
  - Restlessness or feeling keyed up or on edge
  - Easily fatigued
  - Difficulty concentrating or mind going blank
  - Irritability
  - Muscle tension
  - Sleep disturbances (difficulty falling or staying asleep)
  - Difficulty controlling worry
- Persistent worry must cause significant distress or impairment in social, occupational, or other areas of functioning.
- Focus of anxiety and worry is not consistent with or limited to the occurrence of other types of psychiatric disorders and is not directly related to posttraumatic stress disorder (PTSD).
- All other causes of anxiety and worry have been eliminated (see "Differential Diagnosis").
- Patient may report symptoms of dyspnea, palpitations, diaphoresis, nausea, or diarrhea or may experience tremor (2).

PHYSICAL EXAM

No specific physical findings, but patient may be noted to be irritable or easily startled; observable findings of bitten nails, a tremor, or clammy hands may also be present.

DIFFERENTIAL DIAGNOSIS

- Cardiovascular: ischemic heart disease, valvular heart disease (mitral valve prolapse), cardiomyopathies, arrhythmias, congestive heart failure
- Respiratory: asthma, chronic obstructive pulmonary disease, pulmonary embolism
- CNS: stroke, seizures, dementia, migraine, vestibular dysfunction, neoplasms
- Metabolic and hormonal: hyper- or hypothyroidism, pheochromocytoma, adrenal insufficiency, Cushing syndrome, hypokalemia, hypoglycemia, hyperparathyroidism
- Nutritional: thiamine, pyridoxine, or folate deficiency; iron deficiency anemia
- Drug-induced anxiety: alcohol, sympathomimetics (cocaine, amphetamine, caffeine), corticosteroids, herbals (ginseng)
- Withdrawal: alcohol, sedative-hypnotics
- Psychiatric: other disorders (e.g., panic disorder, obsessive-compulsive disorder, PTSD, social phobia, adjustment disorder, and somatization disorder)

DIAGNOSTIC TESTS & INTERPRETATION

Initial Tests (lab, imaging)

- Laboratory tests are normal. Initial tests should include thyroid-stimulating hormone, CBC, basic metabolic panel, and ECG.
- See "Differential Diagnosis" for other conditions to consider, especially in patients with many physical symptoms.
- GAD-2: 2-question self-reporting scale (22% positive predictive value [PPV]/78% negative predictive value [NPV])

Diagnostic Procedures/Other

Psychological testing

- GAD-7: 5 additional questions; provides more detailed information for treatment (29% PPV/71% NPV); also may be indicative of panic disorder (GAD-7: 29% PPV/71% NPV).
- Hamilton Anxiety Scale (HAM-A), Anxiety Disorders Interview Schedule (ADIS-IV)
- In pediatric populations: ADIS-IV Parent and Child Version, Multidimensional Anxiety Scale for Children (MASC), Screen for Child Anxiety Related Emotional Disorders (SCARED)

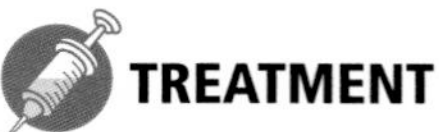

TREATMENT

GENERAL MEASURES

- Assess for suicidality given increased risk.
- Identify and treat coexisting substance abuse and other psychiatric conditions.

MEDICATION

First Line

- SSRI and SNRI antidepressants are well tolerated, do not cause abuse/dependence, and treat comorbid depression. Data to compare between agents are limited (3)[A].
  - SSRIs
  - Paroxetine (Paxil): initially 10–20 mg/day; may titrate to a maximum of 50 mg/day (no added benefit more than 20 mg/day)
  - Escitalopram (Lexapro): initially 10 mg/day; may titrate to a maximum of 20 mg/day
  - Sertraline (Zoloft): initially 25 mg/day; may titrate to a maximum of 200 mg/day
- Selective-norepinephrine reuptake inhibitors (SNRIs)
  - Duloxetine (Cymbalta): initially 30 mg/day; may titrate to a maximum of 120 mg/day
  - Venlafaxine XR (Effexor XR): initially 37.5–75 mg; may titrate up by 75 mg every 4 days to a maximum of 225 mg/day

Second Line

- Benzodiazepines (highly efficacious in the short-term, but less effective long-term) (3)[A]
  - Clonazepam (Klonopin): 0.25 mg BID; may increase to 4 mg/day divided BID
  - Diazepam (Valium): 2–5 mg BID–QID; may increase to a maximum of 40 mg/day
  - Lorazepam (Ativan): 0.5 mg BID–TID; may increase to 6 mg/day divided TID
- Hydroxyzine (Vistaril, Atarax): CNS depressant, antihistamine, anticholinergic; decreased risk of dependence compared with benzodiazepines: usual dose: 50–100 mg PO QID; limit use in the elderly
- Azapirones: buspirone (BuSpar): less risk of dependence, although may be less effective. 15 mg/day divided BID–TID initially; maximum of 60 mg/day divided BID–TID (3)[A]
- Quetiapine (Seroquel): optimal dose 150 mg/day. Second-generation antipsychotic. Efficacious but less well-tolerated than SSRIs (3,4)[A].
- Pregabalin (Lyrica): has shown promise in decreasing anxiety scores and preventing relapse at 75–300 mg BID; may cause less sexual dysfunction and sleep disruption than SSRIs (3)[A]
- Tricyclic antidepressants (TCAs): imipramine (Tofranil): initially 25–50 mg/day; maximum of 300 mg/day, 100 mg/day in the elderly

Geriatric Considerations

- Avoid TCAs and long-acting benzodiazepines; benzodiazepines may cause delirium.
- Pregabalin may cause dizziness and somnolence.

Pediatric Considerations

- Black box warning (SSRIs): Antidepressants increase the risk of suicidal thinking and behavior in children, adolescents, and young adults.
- However, studies have also shown increase in suicide attempts in adolescents after SSRI use decreased.

- Medications other than SSRIs have not been well-tested in pediatric populations.
- Anxiety often exists comorbid with ADHD.

Pregnancy Considerations

- Buspirone: Category B: secreted in breast milk; inadequate studies to assess risk
- Benzodiazepines: Category D: may cause lethargy and weight loss in nursing infants; avoid breast-feeding if the mother is taking chronically or in high doses
- SSRIs: if possible, taper and discontinue. After 20 weeks' gestation, there is increased risk of pulmonary hypertension; mild transient neonatal syndrome of CNS; and motor, respiratory, and GI signs. Studies regarding risk of autism show mixed results. Most are Category C:
  - Paroxetine: Category D: conflicting evidence regarding the risk of congenital cardiac defects and other congenital anomalies
- Hydroxyzine: Category C: Case reports of neonatal withdrawal exist.

ALERT

Precautions

- Benzodiazepines: age >65 years, hepatic insufficiency, respiratory disease/sleep apnea, renal insufficiency, suicidal tendency, contraindicated with narrow-angle glaucoma, precaution with open-angle glaucoma; sudden discontinuation, especially of alprazolam, increases seizure risk. Long-term use has potential for tolerance and dependence; use with caution in patients with history of substance abuse.
- Buspirone: hepatic and/or renal dysfunction; monoamine oxidase inhibitor (MAOI) treatment
- TCAs: advanced age, glaucoma, benign prostate hypertrophy, hyperthyroidism, cardiovascular disease, liver disease, urinary retention, MAOI treatment
- SSRIs: use caution in those with comorbid bipolar disorder; may trigger mania. Avoid with medications that may increase risk of serotonin syndrome

ISSUES FOR REFERRAL

Concomitant depression or other comorbidities may warrant a psychiatric evaluation in light of increased suicide risk.

ADDITIONAL THERAPIES

- Psychological treatments are effective in treating GAD: number needed to treat (NNT) = 2 (5)[A].
- Cognitive-behavioral therapy (CBT): Most well-studied psychological treatment may improve comorbid conditions such as depression.
- Relaxation training: historical treatment of choice
- Psychodynamic psychotherapy: Treatment is focused on patient discovering and verbalizing unconscious content of the psyche.
- Insufficient evidence to compare efficacy of the various treatment types at this time (5)[A]

COMPLEMENTARY & ALTERNATIVE MEDICINE

- Patients frequently engage in complementary and alternative medicine (CAM); providers should be familiar with common therapies.
- Probable benefit but more study needed on several complementary therapies, including acupuncture, yoga, tai chi, and aromatherapy (6)[A].
- Kava: Some evidence for benefit over placebo in mild to moderate anxiety, but concern regarding potential hepatotoxicity persists. Safety is potentially affected by many factors, including manufacturing quality, plant part used, dose, and interactions with other substances (6)[A].
- Limited evidence to support other herbal medicines and St. John's wort likely not effective (6)[A]
- Strong evidence to support regular physical activity to relieve anxiety symptoms (6)[A]

INPATIENT CONSIDERATIONS

Patients at risk of suicide should be treated as inpatients; consider as well for patients with comorbid substance use.

ONGOING CARE

FOLLOW-UP RECOMMENDATIONS

Patient Monitoring

- Follow up within 2–4 weeks from starting new medications.
- Medications should be continued past the initial period of response and probably for at least 6 months (3)[A].
- Monitor mental status on benzodiazepines and avoid drug dependence.
- Monitor BP, heart rate, and anticholinergic side effects of TCAs.
- Monitor all patients for suicidal ideation but especially those on SSRIs, SNRIs, and imipramine.

DIET

- Limit caffeine intake.
- Avoid alcohol (drug interactions, high rate of abuse, potential for increased anxiety).

PATIENT EDUCATION

- Regular exercise, especially yoga, may be beneficial for both anxiety and comorbid conditions.
- Continue with meditation, CBT, and other therapies that provide relief.
- Moderate caffeine use; avoid alcohol and nicotine if possible.

PROGNOSIS

- Probability of recovery is approximately 40–60%, but relapse is common.
- Comorbid psychiatric disorders and poor relationships with spouse or family make relapse more likely (1).

REFERENCES

1. Weisberg RB. Overview of generalized anxiety disorder: epidemiology, presentation, and course. *J Clin Psychiatry*. 2009;70(Suppl 2):4–9.
2. American Psychiatric Association. *Diagnostic and Statistical Manual of Mental Disorders*. 5th ed. Arlington, VA: American Psychiatric Association; 2013.
3. Baldwin DS, Waldman S, Allgulander C. Evidence-based pharmacological treatment of generalized anxiety disorder. *Int J Neuropsychopharmacol*. 2011;14(5):697–710.
4. Depping AM, Komossa K, Kissling W, et al. Second-generation antipsychotics for anxiety disorders. *Cochrane Database Syst Rev*. 2010;(12):CD008120.
5. Cujipers P, Sijbrandij M, Koole S, et al. Psychological treatment of generalized anxiety disorder: a meta-analysis. *Clin Psychol Rev*. 2014;34(2):130–140.
6. Sarris J, Moylan S, Camfield DA, et al. Complementary medicine, exercise, meditation, diet, and lifestyle modification for anxiety disorders: a review of current evidence. *Evid Based Complement Alternat Med*. 2012;2012:809653.

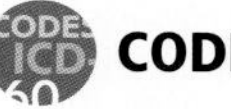

SEE ALSO

- Panic Disorder, Insomnia, Social Anxiety Disorder
- Algorithms: Depression, Adult; Anxiety

CODES

ICD10

- F41.9 Anxiety disorder, unspecified
- F41.1 Generalized anxiety disorder
- F41.8 Other specified anxiety disorders

CLINICAL PEARLS

- Psychiatric comorbidities, especially depression, are extremely common with GAD; patients are at increased risk for suicidality.
- SSRIs are the treatment of choice, although they require up to 4 weeks for full effect.
- Benzodiazepines may be used initially but should be tapered and withdrawn if possible.
- Psychological therapy should be used in conjunction with medications if patients are agreeable.
- CAM use is common, and certain therapies may be effective.

AORTIC VALVULAR STENOSIS

Nirmanmoh Bhatia, MD • Amaninderapal S. Ghotra, MD • Marcus F. Stoddard, MD

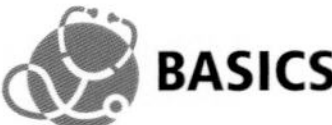

BASICS

DESCRIPTION

Aortic stenosis (AS) is a narrowing of the aortic valve area causing obstruction to left ventricular (LV) outflow. The disease has a long asymptomatic latency period, but development of severe obstruction or onset of symptoms such as syncope, angina, and congestive heart failure (CHF) are associated with a high mortality rate without surgical intervention.

EPIDEMIOLOGY

- Most common valvular disease in developed countries
- Predominant age
  - <30 years: congenital
  - 30–65 years: congenital or rheumatic fever
  - >65 years: degenerative calcification of aortic valve

Prevalence

- Affects 1.3% of population 65–74 years old, 2.4% 75–84 years old, 4% >84 years old (1)
- Bicuspid aortic valve: 1–2% of population. Bicuspid aortic valve predisposes to development of AS at an earlier age (1).

ETIOLOGY AND PATHOPHYSIOLOGY

- Progressive stiffening of aortic valve results in LV outflow obstruction. Obstruction causes increased afterload and decreased cardiac output.
- Increase in LV pressure is required to preserve cardiac output; this leads to development of concentric left ventricular hypertrophy (LVH). LVH preserves ejection fraction but adversely affects heart functioning:
  - LVH impairs coronary blood flow during diastole by compression of coronary arteries and reduced capillary ingrowth into hypertrophied muscle.
  - LVH results in diastolic dysfunction by reducing ventricular compliance.
- Diastolic dysfunction necessitates stronger left atrial (LA) contraction to augment preload and maintain stroke volume. Loss of LA contraction by atrial fibrillation can induce acute deterioration.
- Angina: Myocardial demand is elevated due to increased LV pressure. Myocardial supply is compromised due to LVH.
- Syncope (exertional): can be multifactorial from inability to augment cardiac output due to the fixed obstruction to LV outflow, ventricular arrhythmias, or, most commonly, abnormal vasodepressor reflexes
- Heart failure: Eventually, LVH cannot compensate for increasing afterload, resulting in high LV pressure and volume, which are accompanied by an increase in LA and pulmonary pressures.
- Degenerative calcific changes to aortic valve (2)
  - Mechanism involves mechanical stress to valve leaflets as well as atherosclerotic changes to the valve tissue. Bicuspid valves are at higher risk for mechanical stress.
  - Early lesions: subendothelial accumulation of oxidized LDL and macrophages and T lymphocytes (inflammatory response)
  - Disease progression: Fibroblasts undergo transformation into osteoblasts. Protein production of osteopontin, osteocalcin, and bone morphogenic protein-2 (BMP-2), which modulates calcification of leaflets
- Congenital: unicuspid valve, bicuspid valve, tricuspid valve with fusion of commissures, hypoplastic annulus
- Rheumatic fever: chronic scarring with fusion of commissures

RISK FACTORS

- Congenital unicommissural valve or bicuspid valve (1)
  - Unicommisural valve: most cases detected during childhood
  - Bicuspid valve: predisposes to development of AS earlier in adulthood (4th–5th decade) compared to tricuspid valve (6th–8th decade)
- Rheumatic fever (1)
  - Prevalence of chronic rheumatic valvular disease has declined significantly in the United States.
  - Most cases are associated with mitral valve disease.
- Degenerative calcific changes
  - Most common cause of acquired AS in the United States
  - Shares same risk factors as coronary artery disease (CAD) due to similar pathophysiology that includes the following: hypercholesterolemia, hypertension, smoking, male gender, age, and diabetes mellitus

COMMONLY ASSOCIATED CONDITIONS

- CAD (50% of patients)
- Hypertension (40% of patients): results in "double-loaded" left ventricle (dual source of obstruction from AS and hypertension)
- Aortic regurgitation (common in calcified bicuspid valves and rheumatic disease)
- Mitral valve disease: 95% of patients with AS from rheumatic fever (RF) also have mitral valve disease.
- LV dysfunction and CHF
- Acquired von Willebrand disease: Impaired platelet function and decreased vWF results in bleeding (ecchymosis and epistaxis) in 20% of AS patients. Severity of coagulopathy is directly related to severity of AS.
- Gastrointestinal arteriovenous malformations (AVMs)

DIAGNOSIS

HISTORY

- Primary symptoms: angina, syncope, and heart failure (3). Angina is most frequent symptom. Syncope is often exertional. Heart failure symptoms include fatigue, exertional dyspnea, orthopnea, paroxysmal nocturnal dyspnea, and shortness of breath.
- Palpitations
- Neurologic events (transient ischemic attack or cerebrovascular accident) secondary to embolization
- Geriatric patients may have subtle symptoms such as fatigue and exertional dyspnea.
- Note: Symptoms do not always correlate with valve area (severity of AS) but most commonly occur when aortic valve area is <1 cm^2.

PHYSICAL EXAM

- Auscultation (3)
  - Harsh, systolic crescendo–decrescendo murmur best heard at 2nd right sternal border, radiates into carotid arteries. Peak of murmur correlates with severity of stenosis: Later peaking murmur suggests greater severity.
  - High-pitched diastolic blow suggests associated aortic regurgitation.
  - Paradoxically split S_2 or absent A_2. Note: Normally split S2 reliably excludes severe AS.
  - S_4 due to stiffening of left ventricle
- Other associated signs (3) include *Pulsus parvus et tardus*: decreased and delayed carotid upstroke. LV heave. Findings of CHF: crackles at lung bases, lower extremity edema

DIFFERENTIAL DIAGNOSIS

- Mitral regurgitation: either primary (such as mitral valve prolapse or a flail mitral valve) or secondary to underlying CAD or dilated cardiomyopathy. Usually an apical, high-frequency, pansystolic murmur, often radiates to axilla.
- Hypertrophic obstructive cardiomyopathy: also systolic crescendo–decrescendo murmur but best heard at left sternal border and may radiate into axilla. Murmur intensity increases by changing from squatting to standing and/or by Valsalva maneuver.
- Discrete fixed subaortic stenosis: 50–65% has associated cardiac deformity (patent ductus arteriosus [PDA], ventricular septal defect [VSD], coarctation of aorta).
- Aortic supravalvular stenosis: Williams syndrome, homozygous familial hypercholesterolemia

DIAGNOSTIC TESTS & INTERPRETATION

Initial Tests (lab, imaging)

- Chest x-ray (CXR) (1)
  - May be normal in compensated, isolated valvular AS
  - Boot-shaped heart reflective of concentric hypertrophy
  - Poststenotic dilatation of ascending aorta and calcification of aortic valve (seen on lateral PA CXR)
- ECG: often normal ECG (ECG is nondiagnostic), or may show LVH, LA enlargement, and nonspecific ST- and T-wave abnormalities
- Echo indications
  - Initial workup
    - Doppler echocardiogram is a mainstay of diagnosis.
    - Assesses the severity of AS
    - Assesses LV wall thickness, size, function
  - In known AS and changing signs/symptoms
  - In known AS and pregnancy due to hemodynamic changes of pregnancy
- Echo findings
  - Aortic valve morphology, thickening, calcifications
  - Decreased aortic valve excursion
  - Aortic valve area
  - Transvalvular gradient across aortic valve
  - LVH and diastolic dysfunction
  - LV ejection fraction
  - Wall-motion abnormalities suggesting CAD
  - Evaluate for concomitant aortic valve insufficiency or mitral valve disease.

- AS severity based on echo values (assumes normal cardiac output)
  - Normal: area: 3–4 cm^2; mean pressure gradient: 0 mm Hg; jet vel. <2.5 m/s
  - Mild: area: 1.5–2 cm^2; mean pressure gradient: <25 mm Hg; jet vel. 2.5–2.9 m/s
  - Moderate: area: 1–1.5 cm^2; mean pressure gradient: 25–40 mm Hg; jet vel. 3–4 m/s
  - Severe: area: <1 cm^2; mean pressure gradient: >40 mm Hg; jet vel. >4 m/s
  - Extremely severe: area <0.6 cm^2; mean pressure gradient >60 mm Hg; jet vel. >5 m/s
- Patients with severe AS and low cardiac output may have a relatively low transvalvular pressure gradient (i.e., mean pressure gradient <30 mm Hg).

Diagnostic Procedures/Other

- Exercise stress testing
  - Asymptomatic patients (4)[B]: helpful to uncover subtle symptoms or changes, abnormal BP (increase <20 mm Hg), and ECG changes (ST depressions). 1/3 of patients develop symptoms with exercise testing; STOP testing at this point.
  - Symptomatic patients (4)[B]: DO NOT perform exercise stress testing, as it may induce hypotension or ventricular tachycardia.
  - CHF patients (4)[B]: Dobutamine stress echocardiography is reasonable to evaluate patients with low-flow/low-gradient AS and LV dysfunction.
- Cardiac catheterization
  - Perform prior to aortic valve replacement in patients with suspected CAD (4)[B]. Determines need for coronary artery bypass graft (CABG). If unambiguous diagnosis of AS, perform only coronary angiography.
  - Use if noninvasive testing is inconclusive or if there is discrepancy between severity of symptoms and findings on ECG
  - Measures transvalvular flow, transvalvular pressure gradient, and effective valve area
  - Hemodynamic measurements with infusion of dobutamine can be useful for evaluation of patients with low-flow/low-gradient AS and LV dysfunction.

Test Interpretation

- Aortic valve: nodular calcification on valve cusps (initially at bases), cusp rigidity, cusp thickening, and fibrosis
- LVH, myocardial interstitial fibrosis
- 50% incidence of concomitant CAD

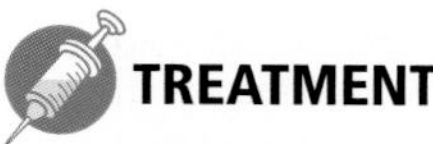

TREATMENT

MEDICATION

- NO medical therapy for severe or symptomatic AS
- Prevention: Currently no recommended medical therapy. Statins have been thought to slow progression if initiated during mild disease. However, this has not been supported by large, randomized controlled trials.
- Antibiotic prophylaxis against recurrent RF is indicated for patients with rheumatic AS (penicillin G 1,200,000 U IM q4wk, duration varies with age and history of carditis).
- Antibiotic prophylaxis is no longer indicated for prevention of infective endocarditis (4).
- Comorbidities: hypertension: angiotensin-converting enzyme (ACE) inhibitors, start with low dose and increase cautiously. Be cautious of vasodilators, which may cause hypotension.

SURGERY/OTHER PROCEDURES

- The only proven treatment for AS is valve replacement.
- Indications for aortic valve replacement (AVR) surgery
  - Symptomatic and severe AS (4)[B]
  - Asymptomatic, severe AS
    - Requires aortic root surgery or other valve surgery (4)[C]
    - Requires CABG (4)[C]
    - Ejection fraction positive stress test (4)[C]
    - Risk of rapid progression (moderate to severe calcification, age, CAD) (4)
  - In addition, it is reasonable to perform AVR in patients with moderate stenosis and undergoing CABG or other valve surgery (4)[B].
  - AVR may be considered for patient with asymptomatic, extremely severe AS (4)[C] or mild AS and CABG and high risk of rapid progression (4)[C]; however, this is controversial.

ALERT

Note: If the aortic valve area is >1.5 cm^2 and the gradient is <15 mm Hg, there is no benefit from AVR.

- Transcatheter aortic valve replacement (TAVR) may be indicated in patients with symptomatic, severe AS who are considered high surgical risk (5).
- Percutaneous balloon valvuloplasty may have role as bridge to valve replacement in hemodynamically unstable or high-risk patients (4)[C] but is not recommended as an alternative to valve replacement.
  - May be used as palliative therapy for patients who are not surgical candidates (4)[C].
  - Indicated in young adults and others without calcified valves and no AR if
    - Symptoms of angina, syncope, CHF, and peak gradients >50 mm Hg on catheterization (4)[C]
    - ST- or T-wave changes in the left precordial leads and catheter peak gradient >60 mm Hg (4)[C].
    - Patient plays competitive sports or may become pregnant and has catheter peak gradient >50 mm Hg (4)[C].

ONGOING CARE

FOLLOW-UP RECOMMENDATIONS

- Advise patients to immediately report symptoms referable to AS.
- Asymptomatic patients: yearly history and physical (4)[C]
- Serial ECHO: yearly for severe AS, every 1–2 years for moderate AS, every 3–5 years for mild AS (4)[B]

PATIENT EDUCATION

Physical activity limitations

- Asymptomatic mild AS: no restrictions
- Asymptomatic moderate to severe AS: Avoid strenuous exercise. Consider exercise stress test prior to starting exercise program.

PROGNOSIS

- 25% mortality/year in symptomatic patients who do not undergo valve replacement; average survival is 2–3 years without AVR surgery.
- Median survival in symptomatic AS (3): heart failure: 2 years; syncope: 3 years; angina: 5 years
- Perisurgical mortality: AVR surgery has 4% mortality rate; AVR + CABG has 6.8% mortality rate.
- Adverse postoperative prognostic factors: age, heart failure (HF) New York Heart Association (NYHA) class III/IV, cerebrovascular disease, renal dysfunction, CAD

REFERENCES

1. Carabello BA, Paulus WJ. Aortic stenosis. *Lancet*. 2009;373(9667):956–966.
2. Otto CM. Calcific aortic stenosis–time to look more closely at the valve. *N Engl J Med*. 2008;359(13): 1395–1398.
3. Grimard BH, Larson JM. Aortic stenosis: diagnosis and treatment. *Am Fam Physician*. 2008;78(6): 717–724.
4. Bonow RO, Carabello BA, Kanu C, et al; American College of Cardiology/American Heart Association Task Force on Practice Guidelines; Society of Cardiovascular Anesthesiologists; Society for Cardiovascular Angiography and Interventions, et al. ACC/AHA 2006 guidelines for the management of patients with valvular heart disease: a report of the American College of Cardiology/American Heart Association Task Force on Practice Guidelines. *Circulation*. 2006;114(5):e84–e231.
5. Smith CR, Leon MB, Mack MJ, et al. Transcatheter versus surgical aortic-valve replacement in high-risk patients. *N Engl J Med*. 2011;364(23):2187–2198.

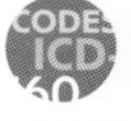

CODES

ICD10

- I35.0 Nonrheumatic aortic (valve) stenosis
- I06.0 Rheumatic aortic stenosis
- Q23.0 Congenital stenosis of aortic valve

CLINICAL PEARLS

- AS is diagnosed on physical exam by a systolic crescendo–decrescendo murmur, and delayed and diminished pulses.
- Symptomatic AS most commonly presents as angina, syncope, and heart failure.
- Symptomatic AS has a very poor prognosis, unless treated with surgical intervention.

ARTERITIS, TEMPORAL

Cynthia M. Waickus, MD, PhD

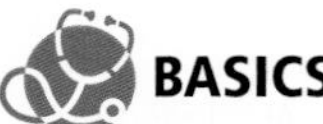

BASICS

DESCRIPTION

- Technically termed giant cell arteritis (GCA)
- A chronic, generalized, cellular and humoral immune-mediated vasculitis of large- and medium-sized vessels, predominantly affecting the cranial arteries originating from the aortic arch, although vascular involvement may be widespread. Inflammation of the aorta is observed in 50% of cases (1).
- Frequent features include fatigue, headaches, jaw claudication, loss of vision, scalp tenderness, polymyalgia rheumatica (PMR), and aortic arch syndrome (decreased or absent peripheral pulses, discrepancies of blood pressure, arterial bruits) (2).

EPIDEMIOLOGY

- The mean age of onset is approximately 70 years; rare younger than age 50 years.
- Women are affected about 3 times as often as men.
- Most common vasculitis in individuals of Northern European decent
- Rare in Asians and African Americans

Incidence

- Prevalence in individuals >50 years: 1 in 500 (1,3,4)
- Cyclic incidence: peaking every 5–7 years

ETIOLOGY AND PATHOPHYSIOLOGY

- The exact etiology of GCA remains unknown, although current theory suggests that advanced age, ethnicity, and specific genetic predisposition lead to a maladaptive response to endothelial injury, intimal hyperplasia, and ultimately vascular stenosis.
- Temporal arteritis (TA) is a chronic, systemic vasculitis primarily affecting the elastic lamina of medium- and large-sized arteries. Histopathology of affected arteries is marked by transmural inflammation of the intima, media, and adventitia, as well as patchy infiltration by lymphocytes, macrophages, and multinucleated giant cells. Mural hyperplasia can result in arterial luminal narrowing, resulting in subsequent distal ischemia (1,3,4).
- Current theory regarding the etiology of TA is that a maladaptive response to endothelial injury leads to an inappropriate activation of T cell–mediated immunity via immature antigen-presenting cells. The subsequent release of cytokines within the arterial vessel wall can attract macrophages and multinucleated giant cells, which form granulomatous infiltrates and gives diseased vessels their characteristic histology. This also leads to an oligoclonal expansion of T cells directed against antigens in or near the elastic lamina. Ultimately, this cascade results in vessel wall damage, intimal hyperplasia, and eventual stenotic occlusion (4,5).
- In recent years, GCA and polymyalgia rheumatica (PMR) have increasingly been considered to be closely related conditions (2,3).

Genetics

The gene for HLA-DRB1–04 has been identified as a risk factor for TA, and polymorphisms of ICAM-1 have also been implicated (5).

RISK FACTORS

- Increasing age >70 years is the greatest risk factor.
- Genetic predisposition
- Environmental factors influence susceptibility (5,6,7).
- Heavy smoking and atherosclerotic disease are risk factors for females but not for males.

COMMONLY ASSOCIATED CONDITIONS

Polymyalgia rheumatica (PMR) may develop either before or after the arteritis (3,6).

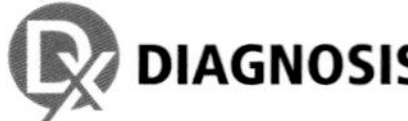

DIAGNOSIS

HISTORY

- Most common presenting symptom is headache (2/3 of patients) (1,2,6)[A].

- Scalp tenderness or sensitivity
- Jaw claudication (presence of symptom significantly increases likelihood of a positive biopsy)
- Claudication of upper extremities
- Constitutional symptoms (fever, fatigue, weight loss)
- Symptoms of polymyalgia rheumatica (shoulder and hip girdle pain and stiffness)
- Any visual disturbances (amaurosis fugax, diplopia)
- Vision loss (20% of patients)
- Distal extremity swelling/edema
- Upper respiratory symptoms

PHYSICAL EXAM

- Temporal artery abnormalities (beading, prominence, tenderness)
- Typically appear "ill"
- Decreased peripheral pulses in the presence of large vessel diseases
- Funduscopic exam shows pale and edema of the optic disk, scattered cotton wool patches, and small hemorrhages.
- Unlike other forms of vasculitis, GCA rarely involves the skin, kidneys, and lungs.

DIFFERENTIAL DIAGNOSIS

- *Classification Criteria:*
  - Age >70 years
  - New localized headache
  - Temporal artery abnormality (tenderness to palpation, decreased or absent pulses)
  - ESR >50 mm/hr
  - Abnormal temporal artery biopsy showing vasculitis with predominance of mononuclear cell infiltration or granulomatous inflammation
- Three or more of the above symptoms: 95% sensitivity/91% specificity for GCA diagnosis (The American College of Rheumatology criteria for the classification of GCA)

DIAGNOSTIC TESTS & INTERPRETATION

Initial Test (lab, imaging)

- ESR >50 mm/hr (86% sensitivity), although nonspecific (27%); infrequently, may be normal (2,6)[A]

- C-reactive protein (CRP) >2.45 mg/dL is a more sensitive marker of inflammation (97% sensitivity) and is associated with increased odds of a positive biopsy result.
- Platelet count $>400 \times 10^3$
- A normal ESR and/or CRP renders the diagnosis of GCA unlikely.
- Acute-phase reactants (fibrinogen, interleukin-6) are frequently elevated, but very nonspecific, and reserved for diagnostically difficult cases.
- Mild anemia: very nonspecific but may be associated with a lower rate of ischemic complications.
- Color Doppler US of the temporal artery may identify vascular occlusion, stenosis, or edema ("halo sign"); it is low cost and noninvasive but also very operator dependent and does not significantly improve on the clinical exam. It may aid in the diagnosis of larger vessel involvement (8).
- MRI and MRA allow for noninvasive evaluation of both the vessel lumen and the vessel wall and assess mural thickness (edema) and lumen diameter (occlusion). The information may aid in diagnosis, but results are affected by prior glucocorticoid treatment, perhaps indicating more value in assessing the disease course or relapse. Cost, logistics, and lack of validity data preclude its routine usefulness.
- Positron emission tomography (PET), like MRI/MRA and color Doppler, may be useful in diagnostically difficult cases to quantify the inflammatory burden and early in the course of disease, as the metabolic changes occur prior to structural vascular damage, but it also lacks studies to support its use (9).

Follow-Up Tests & Special Considerations

- Development of aortic aneurysms (late and potentially serious complication of GCA) can lead to aortic dissection.
- Due to the risk of irreversible vision loss, treatment with high-dose steroids should be started on strong clinical suspicion of temporal arteritis, prior to the temporal biopsy being done.

Diagnostic Procedures/Other

- Gold standard diagnostic study: histopalogic examination of the temporal artery biopsy specimen
- Overall sensitivity is 87%.
- The temporal artery is chosen because of its accessibility in the systemic disease, but any accessible cranial artery may be chosen.
- Length of biopsy specimen should be at least 2 cm to avoid false-negative results, as skip lesions may occur.
- Diagnostic yield of biopsy may be increased if procedure is coupled with imaging (high-resolution MRI or color Doppler ultrasound).
- Bilateral temporal artery biopsy should not be performed unless the initial histopathology is negative and the suspicion for GCA remains high.
- May be negative in up to 42% of patients, especially in large vessel disease
- Biopsy results are not affected by prior glucocorticoids, so treatment should not be delayed.

Test Interpretation

- Inflammation of the arterial wall, with fragmentation and disruption of the internal elastic lamina
- Multinucleated giant cells are found in <50% of cases and are not specific for the disease.
- Temporal arteritis occurs in three histologic patterns: classic, atypical, and healed.

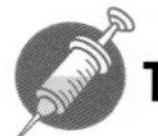

TREATMENT

MEDICATION

First Line

Glucocorticoids:

- Prolonged treatment with glucocorticoids has been the mainstay of treatment and should be initiated immediately when the diagnostic suspicion for GCA is high (2)[A],(10)[B].
- Because of the risk of irreversible vision loss, treatment with high-dose steroids should be started on strong clinical suspicion of temporal arteritis, prior to the temporal biopsy being done.
- The typical dose of prednisone is 60 mg/day (or 1 mg/kg/day). Steroids should not be in the form of alternate day therapy, as this is more likely to lead to a relapse of vasculitis.
- The initial dose of steroids is continued for 2–4 weeks and slowly tapered over 9–12 months. Tapering may require ≥2 years.
- Oral steroids are at least as effective as IV steroids, except in the treatment of acute visual loss where IV steroids appear to offer significant benefit over oral steroids.
- It has been suggested that low-dose aspirin might be effective for patients with GCA (11)[B].
- Patients on corticosteroids should be placed on therapy to minimize osteoporosis unless there are contraindications.

Second Line

- Methotrexate as an adjunct to glucocorticoid therapy may have a modest effect in decreasing the relapse rate of temporal arteritis (12)[B],(13,14)[A].
- Therapies directed at TNF and IL-6 blockade as adjunct to steroids have not shown significant benefit (14,15)[B].

ONGOING CARE

FOLLOW-UP RECOMMENDATIONS

Sun avoidance and protection of the head and the face from photodamage may eventually prove to be important preventive measures for TA.

Patient Monitoring

- TA is typically self-limited and lasts several months or years.
- Overall, TA does not seem to decrease longevity. Nevertheless, it may lead to serious complications such as visual loss, which occurs in about 15–20% of patients.
- Another complication of GCA is the development of aortic aneurysms, usually affecting the ascending aorta. Yearly chest x-rays may be useful to identify this problem.
- About 50% of the patients with GCA will eventually develop polymyalgia rheumatica (stiffness of shoulder and hip girdle).

DIET

Calcium and vitamin D supplementation

PATIENT EDUCATION

- Consequences of discontinuing steroids abruptly (adrenal insufficiency, disease relapse)
- Risks of long-term steroid use (infection, hyperglycemia, weight gain, impaired wound healing, osteoporosis, hypertension)
- Possibility of relapse and importance of reporting new headaches and vision changes to provider immediately

PROGNOSIS

- Life expectancy is not affected by the disease unless severe aortitis is present.
- Once vision loss has occurred, it is unlikely to be recovered, but treatment resolves the other symptoms and prevents future vision loss and stroke.
- In most patients, glucocorticoid therapy can eventually be discontinued without complications. In a few patients, however, the disease is chronic and prednisone must be continued for years.
- Disease relapse is a distinct possibility.

COMPLICATIONS

- Vision loss with delayed diagnosis
- Glucocorticoid-related toxicity

REFERENCES

1. Ezeonyeji AN, Borg FA, Dasgupta B. Delays in recognition and management of giant cell arteritis: results from a retrospective audit. *Clin Rheumatol*. 2011;30(2):259–262.
2. Waldman CW, Waldman SD, Waldman RA. Giant cell arteritis. *Med Clin North Am*. 2013;97(2):329–35.
3. Cantini F, Niccoli L, Storri L, et al. Are polymyalgia rheumatica and giant cell arteritis the same disease? *Semin Arthritis Rheum*. 2004;33(5):294–301.
4. Gonzalez-Gay MA, Vazquez-Rodriguez TR, Lopez-Diaz MJ, et al. Epidemiology of giant cell arteritis and polymyalgia rheumatica. *Arthritis Rheum*. 2009;61(10):1454–1461.
5. Weyand CM, Goronzy JJ. Immune mechanisms in medium and large-vessel vasculitis. *Nat Rev Rheumatol*. 2013;9(12):731–740.
6. Kermani TA, Warrington KJ. Recent advances in diagnostic strategies for giant cell arteritis. *Curr Neurol Neurosci Rep*. 2012;12(2):138–144.
7. Crowson CS, Matteson EL, Myasoedova E, et al. The lifetime risk of adult-onset rheumatoid arthritis and other inflammatory autoimmune diseases. *Arthritis Rheum*. 2011;63(3):633–639.
8. Arida A, Kyprianou M, Kanakis M, et al. The diagnostic value of ultrasonography-derived edema of the temporal artery wall in giant cell arteritis: a second meta-analysis. *BMC Musculoskelet Disord*. 2010;11:44.
9. Besson FL, Parienti JJ, Bienvenu B, et al. Diagnostic performance of ^{18}F-fluorodeoxyglucose positron emission tomography in giant cell arteritis: a systematic review and meta-analysis. *Eur J Nucl Med Mol Imaging*. 2011;38(9):1764–1772.
10. Villa-Forte A. Giant cell arteritis: suspect it, treat it promptly. *Cleve Clin J Med*. 2011;78(4):265–270.
11. Lee MS, Smith SD, Galor A, et al. Antiplatelet and anticoagulant therapy in patients with giant cell arteritis. *Arthritis Rheum*. 2006;54(10):3306–3309.
12. Mahr AD, Jover JA, Spiera RF, et al. Adjunctive methotrexate for treatment of giant cell arteritis: an individual patient data meta-analysis. *Arthritis Rheum*. 2007;56(8):2789–2797.
13. Kotter I, Henes JC, Wagner AD, et al. Does glucocorticoid-resistant large-vessel vasculitis (giant cell arteritis and Takayasu arteritis) exist and how can remission be achieved? A critical review of the literature. *Clin Exp Rheumatol*. 2012;30(1)(Suppl 70):S114–S129.
14. Borchers AT, Gershwin ME. Giant cell arteritis: a review of classification, pathophysiology, geoepidemiology and treatment. *Autoimmun Rev*. 2012;11(6–7):A544–A554.
15. Yates M, Loke YK, Watts RA, et al. Prednisolone combined with adjunctive immunosuppression is not superior to prednisolone alone in terms of efficacy and safety in giant cell arteritis: meta-analysis. *Clin Rheumatol*. 2014;33(2):227–236.

ADDITIONAL READING

Mukhtyar C, Guillevin L, Cid MC, et al. EULAR recommendations for the management of large vessel vasculitis. *Ann Rheum Dis*. 2009;68(3):318–323.

SEE ALSO

Depression; Fibromyalgia; Headache, Cluster; Headache, Tension; Polymyalgia Rheumatica; Polymyositis/Dermatomyositis

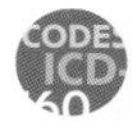

CODES

ICD10

- M31.6 Other giant cell arteritis
- M31.5 Giant cell arteritis with polymyalgia rheumatica

CLINICAL PEARLS

- Due to the risk of irreversible vision loss, treatment with high-dose steroids (prednisone 60 mg/day) should be started immediately in patients suspected of temporal arteritis.
- Temporal artery biopsy is the gold standard for diagnosis. Temporal artery biopsy is not likely to be affected by a few weeks of treatment.
- Treatment consists of a very slow steroid taper. Bone protection therapy and low-dose aspirin should be considered.
- Normal ESR level = value of age/2 for men and age + 10/2 for women

ARTHRITIS, JUVENILE IDIOPATHIC

Donna-Marie McMahon, DO, FAAP • Kathleen M. Vazzana, DO

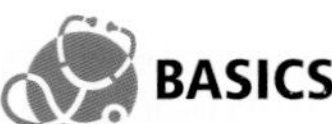

BASICS

DESCRIPTION

- Juvenile idiopathic arthritis (JIA): most common chronic pediatric rheumatologic disease
  - Causes significant short- and long-term disability
- General characteristics
  - Age of onset: <16 years
  - Signs of arthritis: joint swelling, restricted range of motion, warmth, redness, or pain
  - At least 6 weeks of symptoms
- 7 (International League of Associations for Rheumatology) subtypes, determined by clinical characteristics in the 1st 6 months of illness (1):
  - Systemic (Still disease): 10%; preceded by febrile onset of at least 2 weeks with rash, serositis, hepatosplenomegaly, or lymphadenopathy (1)
  - Polyarticular rheumatoid factor (RF) (+): 5–10%; ≥5 joints involvement 1. Large and small joints. RF positive on 2 tests at least 3 months apart (2)
  - Polyarticular RF (−): 10–30%; ≥5 (large and small) joints involved (1); RF negative (2)
  - Oligoarticular: 30–60%; involvement of 1–4 joints; risk for chronic uveitis in ANA (+) females (1) and axial skeletal involvement in older boys (2). Types: (a) monoarthritis (50%): knee, ankle, elbow; (b) extended type = >4 joints after first 6 months
  - Psoriatic arthritis: 5%; arthritis with psoriasis or arthritis with >2 of the following: dactylitis, nail changes, psoriasis in a 1st-degree relative (1)
  - Enthesitis arthritis: 1–7%; oligo- or polyarthritis in small or large joints and enthesis plus 2 of the following: sacroiliac or lumbosacral pain, Reiter syndrome family history or presence of acute anterior uveitis, HLA-B27 (+), ankylosing spondylitis, inflammatory bowel disease (1)[C]
  - Undifferentiated arthritis: Arthritis that does not fulfill above categories or in ≥2 categories (2)
- System(s) affected: musculoskeletal, hematologic, lymphatic, immunologic
- Synonyms: juvenile chronic arthritis; juvenile arthritis; juvenile rheumatoid arthritis (JRA); Still disease (2)

EPIDEMIOLOGY

- Male = female (1); onset: throughout childhood; 54% of cases occur in children 0–5 years (3).
- Polyarticular RF (+): female > male, 3:1 (2); onset: late childhood or adolescence (1)
- Polyarticular RF (−): female > male, 3:1; onset: early peak: 2–4 years, late peak: 6–12 years (2)
- Oligoarticular: female > male, 5:1; onset: 2–4 years (2)
- Psoriatic: female > male; 1:0.95 (2); onset: early peak: 2–3 years; late peak: 10–12 years (1)
- Enthesitis: female > male, 1:7; onset: early peak: 2–4 years; late peak: 6–12 years (2)
- Affected patients have an increased risk of developing cancer, although short-term risk is low (4).

Incidence

2–20/100,000 children <16 years/year in developed nations

Prevalence

16–150/100,000 children <16 years in developed nations (1)

ETIOLOGY AND PATHOPHYSIOLOGY

Multifactorial, including the following:

- Immunodysregulation
- Genetic predisposition
- Environmental triggers, possibly infectious
  - Rubella or parvovirus B19 (5)
  - Heat shock proteins (5)
- Immunoglobulin or complement deficiency

Genetics

- Human leukocyte antigen (HLA) class I and II alleles
- HLA-A2 = early onset oligoarthritis in females
- HLA-DRB1*11 increases risk of systemic and oligo-JIA.
- HLA-B27 increases risk of enthesitis-related arthritis.
- HLA-DR4 is associated with polyarthritis RF (+) (5).

RISK FACTORS

Female gender

GENERAL PREVENTION

No known preventive measures

COMMONLY ASSOCIATED CONDITIONS

Other autoimmune disorders, chronic anterior uveitis (iridocyclitis), nutritional impairment, growth issues (5)

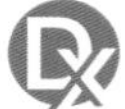

DIAGNOSIS

Clinical diagnostic criteria: age of onset <16 years and >6 weeks duration of objective arthritis (defined as swelling or restricted range of motion of a joint accompanied by heat, pain, or tenderness with no other form of childhood arthritis) in ≥1 joints

HISTORY

- Arthralgias, fever, fatigue, malaise, myalgias, weight loss, morning stiffness, rash
- Limp if lower extremity involvement
- Arthritis for ≥6 weeks

PHYSICAL EXAM

- Arthritis: swelling, effusion, limited range of motion, tenderness, pain with motion, warmth
- Rash, rheumatoid nodules, lymphadenopathy, hepato- or splenomegaly, enthesitis, dactylitis

DIFFERENTIAL DIAGNOSIS

- Musculoskeletal: Legg-Calve-Perthes, toxic synovitis, growing pains, Perthes disease
- Infectious: septic arthritis, osteomyelitis, viral infection, mycoplasmal infection, Lyme disease
- Reactive arthritis: postinfectious, rheumatic fever, Reiter syndrome
- Inflammatory bowel disease: Crohn disease or ulcerative colitis
- Hemoglobinopathies; rickets
- Malignancy: leukemia, bone tumors (osteoid osteoma), neuroblastoma
- Vasculitis, Henoch-Schönlein purpura, Kawasaki disease
- Systemic lupus erythematosus, dermatomyositis, mixed connective tissue disease, sarcoidosis, systemic sclerosis, collagen disorders
- Farber disease
- Trauma: accidental or nonaccidental; abuse

DIAGNOSTIC TESTS & INTERPRETATION

Initial Tests (lab, imaging)

- CBC: leukocyte count normal or markedly elevated (systemic), lymphopenia, reactive thrombocytosis, anemia
- Joint-fluid aspiration/analysis: exclude infection
- ESR and C-reactive protein may be elevated.
- Antinuclear antibodies (ANA) positive (>1:80): 40% (polyarticular, oligoarticular, psoriatic early onset); increased risk of uveitis
- RF (+): 2–10% (usually polyarticular); poor prognosis
- HLA-B27 positive: enthesitis-related arthritis
- Diagnostic radiography, MRI, US, and CT; no one modality has superior diagnostic value (6)[A].
- Radiograph of affected joint(s): **early** radiographic changes: soft tissue swelling, periosteal reaction, juxta-articular demineralization; **later** changes include joint space loss, articular surface erosions, subchondral cyst formation, sclerosis, joint fusion
- If orthopnea, obtain ECG to rule out pericarditis
- Radionuclide scans: for infection, malignancy
- MRI can assess synovial hypertrophy and cartilage degeneration. Also used to monitor clinical responsiveness to treatment in peripheral joints.

Follow-Up Tests & Special Considerations

- RF & ANA present in mixed connective tissue disease (7)[B].
- When interpreting results of dual energy x-ray photon absorptiometry scans, it is important to use pediatric, not adult, controls as normative data.

Diagnostic Procedures/Other

- **Synovial biopsy**: indicated if synovial fluid cannot be aspirated or if infection is suspected in spite of negative synovial fluid culture

Test Interpretation

Synovial biopsy→ synovial cells hyperplasia, hyperemia, infiltration of small lymphocytes and mononuclear cells

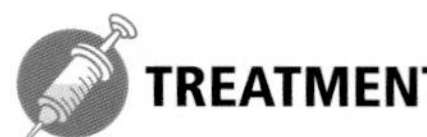

TREATMENT

GENERAL MEASURES

- Goal is to control active disease and extra-articular manifestations to achieve clinical remission.
- All patients require regular (every 3–4 months for oligo-JIA and in ANA-positive patients) ophthalmic exams to uncover asymptomatic eye disease, at least for 1st 3 years following diagnosis.
- Moist heat, sleeping bag, or electric blanket to relieve morning stiffness
- Splints for contractures
- Aerobic exercise: weight bearing or aquatic therapy to improve functional capacity (8)

MEDICATION

First Line

4 or fewer joints

- NSAIDs: adequate in ~50%, symptoms often improve within days, full efficacy 2–3 months
- Drugs for children include the following:
  - Ibuprofen (Motrin, Advil, Nuprin): 30–50 mg/kg/day, divided QID, max dose 2,400 mg/day
  - Naproxen (Naprosyn, Aleve): 10 mg/kg/day divided BID, max dose 1,250 mg/day
  - Tolmetin sodium: 20 mg/kg/day; TID or QID, max dose 30 mg/kg/day
  - Diclofenac: 2–3 mg/kg, divided TID, max dose 50 mg TID
  - Indomethacin: 1–2 mg/kg/day, divided BID to QID, max of 4 mg/kg/day
  - Contraindications to NSAIDs: known allergies
  - Precautions: may worsen bleeding diatheses; use caution with all NSAIDs in renal insufficiency and hypovolemic states; take with food.
  - Significant possible interactions: NSAIDs may lower serum levels of digitalis and anticonvulsants and blunt the effect of loop diuretics. NSAIDs may increase serum methotrexate levels.

- Intra-articular long-acting corticosteroids: immediately effective, local treatment. Improve synovitis, joint damage, and contractures and prevent leg length discrepancy (7)[B].
  - Indication: patients with oligoarthritis who have failed a 2-month NSAID trial or with poor prognosis factors (9)[C]
  - Ex: triamcinolone hexacetonide
- ≥5 Joints
  - If high disease activity or a failed 1–2 month NSAID trial→ methotrexate (9)[C]

Second Line

- 30–40% of patients require addition of disease-modifying antirheumatic drugs (DMARDs), including methotrexate, sulfasalazine, leflunomide, and tumor necrosis factor (TNF) antagonists (etanercept, infliximab, adalimumab); newer biologic therapies, including IL-1 and IL-6 receptor antagonists, currently under investigation
- Methotrexate: 10 mg/m^2/wk PO or SC (7)[B]
  - Plateau of efficacy reached with 15 mg/m^2/wk; further increase in dosage is not associated with therapeutic benefit (10)[A].
- Sulfasalazine: oligoarticular and HLA-B27 spondyloarthritis (7)[B]
- Etanercept (Enbrel): 0.8 mg/kg (max of 50 mg/dose) given SC q1wk or 0.4 mg/kg SC twice a week (max of 25 mg/dose)
- Infliximab: 5 mg/kg q6–8wk
- Adalimumab: if weight 15 kg—<30 kg, 20 mg SC q2wk; if weight ≥30 kg, 40 mg SC q2wk
- Tocilizumab: IL-6 antibody demonstrating efficacy in phase III open label trials; ongoing studies to evaluate efficacy and appropriate dosing (7)[B]
- Anakinra: IL-1 receptor antibody under investigation with phase II and III clinical trials for systemic JIA (7)[B]
- Begin treatment with TNF-α inhibitors in children with a history of arthritis in ≤4 joints and significant active arthritis despite treatment with methotrexate or arthritis in ≥5 joints and any active arthritis following an adequate trial of methotrexate (9)[C].
- Begin treatment with anakinra in children with systemic arthritis and active fever whose treatment requires a 2nd medication in addition to systemic glucocorticoids (9)[C].
- Analgesics for pain control, including narcotics

ISSUES FOR REFERRAL

- Consult pediatric rheumatologist to help manage JIA.
- Orthopedic surgeon: if needed
- Ophthalmology consult for suspected uveitis
- Physical therapy to maintain range of motion, improve muscle strength and prevent deformities
- Occupational therapy to maintain and improve appropriate age-related functional activities
- Behavioral health if difficulty coping with disease

SURGERY/OTHER PROCEDURES

- Total hip and/or knee replacement for severe disease
- Soft tissue release if splinting/traction unsuccessful
- Correct limb length or angular deformities
- Synovectomy is rarely performed.

INPATIENT CONSIDERATIONS

Admission Criteria/Initial Stabilization

- Patient loses ambulatory ability.
- Signs/symptoms of pericarditis
- Persistent fever
- Need for surgery

Discharge Criteria

Resolution of fever and swelling or serositis

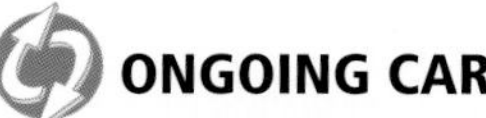

ONGOING CARE

FOLLOW-UP RECOMMENDATIONS

Patient Monitoring

Determined by medication

- NSAIDs: periodic CBC, urinalysis, liver function tests (LFTs), renal function tests
- Aspirin and/or other salicylates: transaminase and salicylate levels, weekly for 1st month, then every 3–4 months
- Methotrexate: monthly LFTs, CBC, BUN, creatinine

DIET

Regular diet with special attention to adequate calcium, iron, protein, and caloric intake

PATIENT EDUCATION

- Ongoing education of patients and families with attention to psychosocial needs; school issues, educational needs; behavioral strategies for dealing with pain and noncompliance; use of health care resources; support groups
- Printed and audiovisual information available from local arthritis foundation

PROGNOSIS

- 50–60% ultimately remit, but functional ability depends on adequacy of long-term therapy (disease control, maintaining muscle and joint function)
- Poor prognosis: active disease at 6 months, polyarticular disease, extended pauciarticular disease course, female gender, RF (+), ANA (+), persistent morning stiffness, rapid appearance of erosions, hip involvement

COMPLICATIONS

- Blindness, band keratopathy, glaucoma, short stature, micrognathia if temporomandibular joint involvement, debilitating joint disease, disseminated intravascular coagulation, hemolytic anemia
- On NSAIDs: peptic ulcer, GI hemorrhage, CNS reactions, renal disease, leukopenia
- On DMARDs: bone marrow suppression, hepatitis, renal disease, dermatitis, mouth ulcers, retinal toxicity (antimalarials, rare)
- On TNF antagonists: higher risk of infection
- Osteoporosis, avascular necrosis
- On methotrexate: folate supplementation decreases hepatic/GI symptoms, may reduce stomatitis (11)[A]
- Macrophage activation syndrome: decreased blood cell precursors secondary to histiocyte degradation of marrow

REFERENCES

1. Restrepo R, Lee EY. Epidemiology, pathogenesis, and imaging of arthritis in children. *Orthop Clin North Am*. 2012;43(2):213–225.
2. Prince FH, Otten MH, van Suijlekom-Smit LW. Diagnosis and management of juvenile idiopathic arthritis. *BMJ*. 2010;341:c6434.
3. Behrens EM, Beukelman T, Gallo L, et al. Evaulation of the presentation of systemic onset juvenile rheumatoid arthritis: data from the Pennsylvania Systemic Onset Juvenile Arthritis Registry. *J Rheumatol*. 2008;35(2):343348.
4. Beukelman T, Haynes K, Curtis JR, et al. Rates of malignancy associated with juvenile idiopathic arthritis and its treatment. *Arthritis Rheum*. 2012;64(4):1263–1271.
5. Weiss JE, Ilowite NT. Juvenile idiopathic arthritis. *Rheum Dis Clin North Am*. 2007;33(3):441–470.
6. McKay GM, Cox LA, Long BW. Imaging juvenile idiopathic arthritis: assessing the modalities. *Radiol Technol*. 2010;81(4):318–327.
7. Kahn P. Juvenile idiopathic arthritis—current and future therapies. *Bull NYU Hosp Jt Dis*. 2009;67(3):291–302.
8. Klepper S. Making the case for exercise in children with juvenile idiopathic arthritis: what we know and where we go from here. *Arthritis Rheum*. 2007;57(6):887–890.
9. Beukelman T, Patkar NM, Saag KG, et al. 2011 American College of Rheumatology recommendations for the treatment of juvenile idiopathic arthritis: initiation and safety monitoring of therapeutic agents for the treatment of arthritis and systemic features. *Arthritis Care Res*. 2011;63(4):465–482.
10. Takken T, van der Net J, Helders P. Methotrexate for treating juvenile idiopathic arthritis. *Cochrane Database Syst Rev*. 2001;(4):CD003129.
11. Shea B, Swinden MV, Tanjong Ghogomu E, et al. Folic acid and folinic acid for reducing side effects in patients receiving methotrexate for rheumatoid arthritis. *Cochrane Database Syst Rev*. 2013;(5):CD000951.
12. Kemper AR, Van Mater HA, Coeytaux RR, et al. Systematic review of disease-modifying antirheumatic drugs for juvenile idiopathic arthritis. *BMC Pediatr*. 2012;12:29.

ADDITIONAL READING

Chang HJ, Burke AE, Glass RM. JAMA patient page. Juvenile idiopathic arthritis. *JAMA*. 2010;303(13):1328.

CODES

ICD10

- M08.90 Juvenile arthritis, unspecified, unspecified site
- M08.80 Other juvenile arthritis, unspecified site
- M08.00 Unsp juvenile rheumatoid arthritis of unspecified site

CLINICAL PEARLS

- JIA is the most common form of arthritis in children.
- JIA should be included in the differential diagnosis for a limping child.
- High-titer RF correlates with disease severity; positive RF titers confer poorer prognosis.
- DMARDs improve JIA-associated symptoms (12)[A].

ARTHRITIS, PSORIATIC

Lorena Ceci, MSIV • Nikki A. Levin, MD, PhD

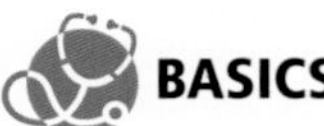

BASICS

Psoriatic arthritis (PsA) is a chronic, destructive, seronegative arthropathy seen most commonly in patients with long-standing psoriasis.

DESCRIPTION

- PsA is a seronegative spondyloarthropathy characterized by inflammatory arthritis and enthesitis.
- 5 patterns of arthritis in PsA
  - Asymmetric oligoarthritis: involves <5 small or large joints
  - Distal interphalangeal (DIP) joint predominant: osteoarthritis-like, often associated with nail changes
  - Symmetric polyarthritis: may be indistinguishable from rheumatoid arthritis (RA), is typically milder
  - Spondyloarthritis: asymmetric and discontinuous, unlike ankylosing spondylitis (AS)
  - Arthritis mutilans: destructive, resorptive arthritis; producing "opera-glass" or telescoping digit
- Psoriasis is present to varying degrees.
  - Course of arthritis and extent of psoriasis do not appear to correlate.
  - Other extra-articular features, such as iritis, are less common.
  - Damaging joint disease may occur in 40–57%.

EPIDEMIOLOGY

- Peak onset age: 30–50 years
- Predominant gender: female = male
- Polyarthritis is more common in women.
- Spondylitis in up to 25%, more common in men
- Psoriasis typically precedes arthritis by an average of 12 years. Arthritis may precede psoriasis in up to 15% (more often in children). Arthritis and psoriasis also may present simultaneously.
- Psoriasis occurs in 2–3% of the U.S. population; 6–42% of these individuals develop PsA (1).

Prevalence

Prevalence: 1–2/1,000 population (1)

ETIOLOGY AND PATHOPHYSIOLOGY

- Unknown. Probably multifactorial: immunologic, genetic, environmental factors
- CD4+/CD8+ T cells; tumor necrosis factor α (TNF-α); interleukins 1 (IL-1), 6, 8, and 10; and matrix metalloproteases present in synovial fluid (2)
- Osteoclast precursor cell upregulation

Genetics

- 30–40% concordance in identical twins
- HLA-B27 in 15–50% with PsA (spondylitis pattern) versus 90% in AS
- Other HLA associations in psoriatic arthritis: HLA-B7, HLA-B38, HLA-B39, HLA-Cw6

RISK FACTORS

- Psoriasis
- Family history of PsA

GENERAL PREVENTION

There are no known prevention strategies. It is unknown if early systemic treatment of psoriasis prevents PsA.

COMMONLY ASSOCIATED CONDITIONS

Psoriasis

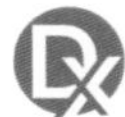

DIAGNOSIS

- A history of inflammatory arthritis, dactylitis, or enthesitis in a patient with existing psoriasis is usually adequate to establish the diagnosis. Differentiation from other inflammatory arthropathies, such as RA, can be difficult.
- The CASPAR criteria may be used to screen patients for PsA. The sensitivity and specificity of the CASPAR criteria are 91.4% and 98.7%.
- A patient must have inflammatory articular disease (joint, spine, or entheseal) with ≥ 3 points from the following 5 categories (3):
  - Evidence of current psoriasis, a personal history of psoriasis, or family history of psoriasis (2 points)
  - Typical psoriatic nail dystrophy, including onycholysis, pitting, and hyperkeratosis (1 point)
  - A negative rheumatoid factor (RF), preferentially by ELISA (1 point)
  - Current or past history of dactylitis (1 point)
  - Radiologic evidence of new bone formation (excluding osteophyte formation) on plain radiographs of the hand or foot (1 point)

HISTORY

- History of psoriasis
- Morning stiffness of hands, feet, or low back for >30 minutes
- Swelling, pain, or redness of affected joints
- Low back or buttock pain
- Ankle or heel pain
- Dactylitis or uniform swelling of an entire digit

PHYSICAL EXAM

- Affected peripheral joints may have overlying erythema, warmth, and swelling:
  - Synovitis
  - Dactylitis
  - Swelling of tendons (e.g., Achilles tendon) and tenderness at insertion sites (e.g., calcaneus)
  - Limited range of motion of axial skeleton
  - Pain with stress on the sacroiliac joint
- Well-demarcated pink-to-red erythematous plaques with a white silvery scale; common locations include scalp, ears, trunk, buttocks, elbows and forearms, knees and legs, and palms and soles.
- Nails may be dystrophic with pits, oil spots, crumbling, leukonychia, and red lunulae.

DIFFERENTIAL DIAGNOSIS

- Reactive arthritis
- Psoriasis and RA
- Psoriasis and osteoarthritis
- Psoriasis and polyarticular gout
- Psoriasis and AS

DIAGNOSTIC TESTS & INTERPRETATION

History and physical exam may adequately diagnose PsA. Plain radiographs may demonstrate characteristic changes. Imaging allows assessment of current damage, disease progression, and response to therapy.

Initial Tests (lab, imaging)

- RF and cyclic citrullinated peptide (anti-CCP) antibody are usually negative.
- HLA-B27 may be positive. HLA-B27 is noted in 50–70% with axial disease and $<15\%$ with peripheral disease.
- Antinuclear antibodies are usually negative.
- Acute-phase reactants (ESR and C-reactive protein) may be elevated.
- Juxta-articular new bone formation (periostitis) and marginal joint erosions that may progress centrally to form the "pencil-in-cup" erosions are the most characteristic plain radiographic features.
- Baseline plain radiographs of affected joints

Follow-Up Tests & Special Considerations

Follow-up radiographs; interval based on severity

Diagnostic Procedures/Other

Diagnosis is typically clinical.

Test Interpretation

Diagnosis is clinical, and biopsy of either skin or synovium is not usually required.

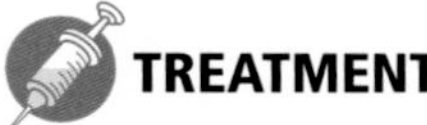

TREATMENT

GENERAL MEASURES

Physical therapy and/or occupational therapy may be beneficial in all stages of disease.

- Treatment algorithms in PsA are based on severity of joint symptoms, extent of structural damage, and extent and severity of psoriasis (4)[A].

MEDICATION

First Line

- NSAIDs may be considered for control of symptoms with mild disease. Intra-articular glucocorticoid injections may be given.
- There are no systematic trials of NSAIDs for PsA treatment. NSAIDs doses are typically directed toward suppressing mild inflammation, and selection should consider patient preference and dosing schedule. Sample doses of select NSAIDs are as follows: ibuprofen 400–800 mg PO TID–QID, naproxen 250–500 mg PO BID–QID, meloxicam 7.5–15 mg/day PO (5)[A].

Second Line

- Patients with moderate to severe arthritis should be started on disease-modifying antirheumatic drugs (DMARDs), which can reduce or prevent joint damage and preserve joint integrity and function.
- First-line DMARDs recommended for therapy are sulfasalazine, leflunomide, methotrexate, and cyclosporine. No evidence supports the use of combination DMARD therapy.

ALERT

- Anti-TNF agents should not be used in the setting of active infection, including in patients with TB and hepatitis B infection, with concurrent live vaccinations, with New York Heart Association (NYHA) class III–IV congestive heart failure, with malignancy, or with history of demyelinating disease.
- Ustekinumab should not be used in patients with active infection, mycobacterial or *Salmonella* infection, with concurrent live vaccinations including Bacillus Calmette-Guérin vaccination, or with history of malignancy.

Pregnancy Considerations

- Teratogenic medications (e.g., category X methotrexate, leflunomide).
- Adalimumab, etanercept, golimumab, infliximab, and ustekinumab are currently listed as Category B medications.

ISSUES FOR REFERRAL

- Rheumatology
- Dermatology

SURGERY/OTHER PROCEDURES

Joint fusion or replacement for advanced destruction

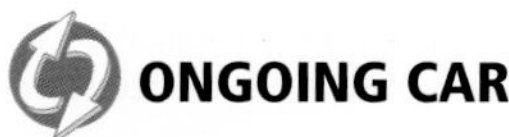

ONGOING CARE

FOLLOW-UP RECOMMENDATIONS

Epidemiologic evidence suggests a relationship between psoriasis, the metabolic syndrome, myocardial infarction, and stroke. Periodic measurement of BP, fasting lipids and glucose, cholesterol, and body mass index is recommended (6).

PATIENT EDUCATION

- Stress noncontagious nature of condition.
- For a listing of sources for patient education materials favorably reviewed on this topic, physicians may contact the following:
  - National Psoriasis Foundation, 6600 SW 92nd Ave., Suite 300, Portland, OR 97223. Also see http://www.psoriasis.org/i-have-psoriatic-arthritis.
  - Arthritis Foundation, 2970 Peachtree Road NW, Suite 200, Atlanta, GA 30305, 404-237-8771. Also see http://www.arthritis.org/conditions-treatments/disease-center/psoriatic-arthritis/.
  - American College of Rheumatology, 2200 Lake Boulevard NE, Atlanta, GA 30319, 404-633-3777. Also see http://www.rheumatology.org/practice/clinical/patients/diseases_and_conditions/psoriaticarthritis.asp.

PROGNOSIS

- Course: insidious and chronic joint disease and recurring and remitting chronic skin disease
- More favorable than for RA (except for patients who develop arthritis mutilans)

COMPLICATIONS

- Chronicity
- Disability
- Psychosocial impact of psoriasis

REFERENCES

1. American Academy of Dermatology Work Group, Menter A, Korman NJ, et al. Guidelines of care for the management of psoriasis and psoriatic arthritis: section 6. Guidelines of care for the treatment of psoriasis and psoriatic arthritis: case-based presentations and evidence-based conclusions. *J Am Acad Dermatol*. 2011;65(1):137–174.
2. Gottlieb A, Korman NJ, Gordon KB, et al. Guidelines of care for the management of psoriasis and psoriatic arthritis: section 2. Psoriatic arthritis: overview and guidelines of care for treatment with an emphasis on the biologics. *J Am Acad Dermatol*. 2008;58(5):851–864.
3. Taylor W, Gladman D, Helliwell P, et al. Classification criteria for psoriatic arthritis: development of new criteria from a large international study. *Arthritis Rheum*. 2006;54(8):2665–2673.
4. Menter A, Korman NJ, Elmets CA, et al. Guidelines of care for the management of psoriasis and psoriatic arthritis. Section 3. Guidelines of care for the management and treatment of psoriasis with topical therapies. *J Am Acad Dermatol*. 2009;60(4):643–659.
5. Ritchlin CT, Kavanaugh A, Gladman DD, et al. Treatment recommendations for psoriatic arthritis. *Ann Rheum Dis*. 2009;68(9):1387–1394.
6. Gottlieb AB, Dann F. Comorbidities in patients with psoriasis. *Am J Med*. 2009;122(12):1150.e1–e9.
7. Prey S, Paul C, Bronsard V, et al. Assessment of risk of psoriatic arthritis in patients with plaque psoria a systematic review of the literature. *J Eur Acad Dermatol Venereol*. 2010;24(suppl 2):31–35.

ADDITIONAL READING

- Donahue KE, Jonas D, Hansen RA, et al. *Drug Therapy for Psoriatic Arthritis in Adults: Update of a 2007 Report*. Rockville, MD: Agency for Healthcare Research and Quality; 2012.
- Tillett W, McHugh N. Treatment algorithms for early psoriatic arthritis: do they depend on disease phenotype? *Curr Rheumatol Rep*. 2012;14(4):334–342.
- Winchester R, Minevich G, Steshenko V, et al. HLA associations reveal genetic heterogeneity in psoriatic arthritis and in the psoriasis phenotype. *Arthritis Rheum*. 2012;64(4):1134–1144.

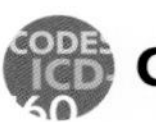

CODES

ICD10

- L40.50 Arthropathic psoriasis, unspecified
- L40.51 Distal interphalengeal psoriatic arthropathy
- L40.53 Psoriatic spondylitis

CLINICAL PEARLS

- Severity of psoriasis may correlate with the likelihood of developing arthritis; however, severity of psoriasis does not correlate with severity of arthritis; 24% of psoriasis patients develop PsA (7)[A].
- The polyarticular pattern of PsA may mimic RA; however, the presence of enthesitis and psoriasis characterize PsA.
- Axial skeleton involvement in PsA is asymmetric and discontinuous, in contrast to axial involvement in AS.

ARTHRITIS, RHEUMATOID (RA)

Blake R. Busey, DO

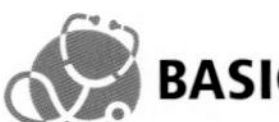

BASICS

DESCRIPTION

- Chronic systemic autoimmune inflammatory disease with symmetric polyarthritis and synovitis
- Progressive chronic inflammation leads to large and small joint destruction, deformity, decline in functional status, and premature morbidity/mortality.
- System(s) affected: musculoskeletal, skin, hematologic, lymphatic, immunologic, muscular, renal, cardiovascular, neurologic, pulmonary

Geriatric Considerations

- Increased contribution of age-related comorbidities; pericarditis, septic arthritis, Sjögren syndrome are more common
- Decreased medication tolerance; increased incidence of hydroxychloroquine-associated maculopathy, D-penicillamine rash, and sulfasalazine-induced nausea/vomiting

Pregnancy Considerations

- Use effective contraception in patients taking disease-modifying antirheumatic drugs (DMARDs).
- Modify medication regimen for pregnant or breastfeeding patients.
- 50–80% of patient improve during pregnancy because of immunologic tolerance but relapse in 6 months. First episode may occur in pregnancy or postpartum.

EPIDEMIOLOGY

Incidence

- 25–30/100,000 cases for males
- 50–60/100,000 cases for females
- Peak age is 35–50 years.

Prevalence

U.S. population: 1%

ETIOLOGY AND PATHOPHYSIOLOGY

- Pathogenesis is postulated to be triggered by an insult (e.g., infection) that precipitates an initial autoimmune reaction; systemic disorder primarily affecting synovial tissues where antibody-complement complex activation leads to synovial hypertrophy and joint inflammation. Pathogenesis is mediated by abnormal B- and T-cell interactions and overproduction of cytokines such as TNF and IL-6.
- Multifactorial disease with genetic, host (hormonal, immunologic), and environmental (socioeconomic, smoking) factors

Genetics

- RA is 50% attributable to genetic causes.
- Monozygotic twin concordance 15–20%, suggesting that nongenetic roles also contribute to development of RA
- HLA DR4 and DRB1, STAT4, and CD40+ persons have increased relative risk.

RISK FACTORS

- Family history: 1st-degree relatives have 2–3-fold increased risk.
- Smokers have a relative risk of 1.4–2.2 for developing RA.
- Pregnancy and breastfeeding for 24 months lowers risk.

COMMONLY ASSOCIATED CONDITIONS

Accelerated atherosclerosis, pericarditis, amyloidosis, Felty syndrome (RA, splenomegaly, neutropenia), interstitial lung disease, pulmonary nodules, rheumatoid nodules, vasculitis, lymphomas

DIAGNOSIS

HISTORY

- Constitutional symptoms: fatigue, malaise, weight loss, low-grade fevers (1,2)[A],(3)[C]
- Articular symptoms: tender/swollen joints, early morning stiffness (at least 60 minutes), and difficulty with activities of daily living (ADL) (1,2)[A],(3)[C].
- Extra-articular involvement: skin, pulmonary, cardiovascular, and ocular symptoms. Onset is typically insidious. Patients rarely present with abrupt onset of symptoms and extra-articular manifestations (1,2)[A], (3)[C].

PHYSICAL EXAM

- Evaluate for swollen, boggy, or tender joints:
  - Small joints: metacarpophalangeal (MCP), proximal intraphalangeal (PIP), wrist, 2nd–5th metatarsophalangeal (MTP), and thumb interphalangeal (IP) joints. Pain and decreased ROM; usually symmetric and affected first
  - Large joints: shoulders, elbows, hips, knees, and ankles
- Joint deformity, nodules, and fusion are late findings.
- Extra-articular findings associated with RA:
  - Splenomegaly, lymphadenopathy, subcutaneous nodules, peripheral neuropathy, and atlantoaxial joint instability. Axial migration of dens into foramen magnum may contribute to occipital headaches.

DIFFERENTIAL DIAGNOSIS

Sjögren syndrome, systemic lupus erythematosus (SLE), systemic sclerosis, adult Still disease, psoriatic arthritis, polymyalgia rheumatica (older), seronegative polyarthritis, erosive osteoarthritis, crystal arthropathy, septic arthritis, rheumatic fever, chronic Lyme disease, viral-induced arthritis (parvovirus B19, hepatitis C [with cryoglobulinemia]), occult malignancy, vasculitis (Behçet syndrome), inflammatory bowel disease (3)[B]

DIAGNOSTIC TESTS & INTERPRETATION

Initial Tests (lab, imaging)

- CBC: Mild anemia and thrombocytosis are common and associated with disease activity (3)[C].
- ESR and C-reactive protein (CRP) are nonspecific inflammatory markers used to assess disease activity (1)[A].
- Rheumatoid factor (RF): >1:80 in 70–80% of patients with RA (most commonly IgM Ab) (1)[A]
- Anticyclic citrullinated peptide antibodies (anti-CCP antibodies). Specificity >90% (1)[A]
- Antinuclear antibody: present in 20–30%
- Electrolytes, creatinine, liver function, and urinalysis to assess comorbid states, establish baseline, and to assist with medication management (4)[C]
- Radiographic findings help establish diagnosis and monitor treatment (2)[C].
- Plain film radiographs are preferred for RA:
  - Initial radiographs of the hands, wrists, and feet
  - Hallmark is a lack of bony remodeling and symmetric joint space narrowing.
  - Earliest pattern of erosions is loss of cortical distinctness, followed by dot-dash pattern of cortical bone loss. Marginal erosions at cortical bone within joint capsule not covered by cartilage result in "mouse-ear" erosions.

Follow-Up Tests & Special Considerations

- Who should be screened?
- The 2010 American College of Rheumatology/European League Against Rheumatism (ACR/EULAR) classification criteria
- Patients with symptoms in at least 1 joint and definite clinical synovitis which is not explained by another disease
- A score of ≥6 is needed for the classification of definite RA:
  - Joint score
    - 1 large joint: 0
    - 2–10 large joints: 1
    - 1–3 small joints (with or without large joints; distal interphalangeal [DIP], 1st MCP, and 1st MTP joints are excluded from assessment.): 2
    - 4–10 small joints (with or without large joints): 3
    - >10 joints (at least 1 small joint): 5
  - Serology score: At least 1 test is needed: negative RF (rheumatoid factor) and negative ACPA (anti-citrullinated protein antibody): 0; low positive RF or low positive ACPA: 2; high positive RF or high positive ACPA: 3
  - Acute-phase reactants score: At least 1 result is needed. Normal CRP and normal ESR: 0; abnormal CRP or ESR: 1
  - Duration of symptoms score (self-reported): <6 weeks: 0; ≥6 weeks: 1
- Patients with a score <6/10 are not classifiable as having RA, therefore reevaluation may be necessary over time (3)[C].
- Joint erosions, nodules, deformity, and fusion are late findings for RA (3)[C].

Diagnostic Procedures/Other

- Joint aspiration can be performed to exclude crystal arthropathy and septic arthritis.
- Synovial fluid
  - Gram stain, cell count, culture, crystal analysis, and overall appearance
  - Yellowish-white, turbid, poor viscosity in RA
  - WBC increased (3,500–50,000 WBC/mm^3)
  - Protein: ~4.2 g/dL (42 g/L)
  - Serum-synovial glucose difference ≥30 mg/dL (≥1.67 mmol/L)

Test Interpretation

Synovial tissue is expanded by recruitment and retention of inflammatory cells, with formation of villous projections and pannus that invade and destroy cartilage and bone.

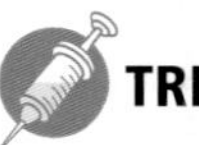

TREATMENT

Goals: control disease activity and progression, relieve pain, maintain or improve function, prevent or correct impairments, and promote self-management

GENERAL MEASURES

- Early, aggressive treatment prevents structural damage and disability (1)[A],(2–4)[C].
- Periodical evaluation of disease activity and extent of synovitis (1)[A]
- Arthritis self-management education (1)[A]

MEDICATION

- Early therapy with DMARDs is the standard of care to slow disease progression and induce remission (1)[A].
- Tuberculin testing and hepatitis B and C testing recommended prior to starting DMARDs (4)[C]
- Symptomatic therapy in addition to DMARDs
  - NSAIDs: naproxen (500 mg BID) or ibuprofen (800 mg TID) for symptomatic relief. If poor response to initial NSAID after 2 weeks, try alternative NSAID (1)[A]
  - If still poor response, can try prednisone (5–30 mg/day); should taper off NSAID or prednisone as soon as effective control of disease activity with DMARD is achieved (1)[A].
- DMARDs

History of hepatitis, malignancy, and heart failure (HF) may alter 1st-line therapy (4)[C].

- Nonbiologic DMARDs
  - DMARD should be started within 3 months of making the diagnosis of RA (1)[A].
  - Due to their greater convenience, lower toxicity profiles, and quicker onset of action, initial therapy is a nonbiologic DMARD: methotrexate, sulfasalazine, and leflunomide have comparable efficacy (1)[A].
  - Methotrexate (MTX) (Rheumatrex): 7.5–25 mg/week PO. DMARD with the most predictable benefit; many significant side effects, but the addition of folate reduces toxicity; 3–6-month trial. Monitor CBC every month × 3 months, renal and liver function every 8–12 weeks. Give with folic acid 1 mg PO daily. Contraindicated in renal and hepatic diseases, pregnancy, and breastfeeding (1)[A].
  - Sulfasalazine (SSZ): 500 mg/day, increase to 2 g/day over 1 month; max: 2–3 g/day; 6-month trial. Monotherapy for low disease activity. Monitor CBC, liver enzymes every 2 weeks × 3 months, then every month × 3 months, then every 3 months. Screen for G6PD deficiency.
  - Leflunomide (Arava): loading dose 100 mg/day × 3 days, then 10–20 mg/day. GI side effects and potentially teratogenic; contraindicated in pregnancy. Monitor CBC, LFTs, and, phosphate monthly for the first 6 months. Stop use if ALT > 3× upper limit normal.
  - Antimalarials: hydroxychloroquine (HCQ) (Plaquenil) 400 mg QHS for 2–3 months, then 200 mg at bedtime; 6-month trial is usual. Usually used to treat milder forms or in combination with other DMARDs. Ophthalmologic exam every 6–12 months due to potential maculopathy. Adjust dose in renal insufficiency.
- Biologic DMARDs
  - TNF inhibitors: IV infliximab (Remicade), SC adalimumab (Humira), and SC etanercept (Enbrel). No evidence that one is superior. The combination with MTX appears to be the most effective. Optimal dosage and duration of treatment unclear. Low toxicity; costly. Check purified protein derivative (PPD) prior to treatment and periodic CBC. Risk of lymphoma, and CHF (1)[A].
  - 2 long-acting anti-TNF agents, certolizumab pegol (Cimzia) and golimumab (Simponi), have been also approved in moderate to severe disease.
  - Abatacept (Orencia) and Anakinra (Kineret) are no longer considered cost-effective or efficacious treatment for RA (1)[A].
  - Rituximab (Rituxan) is recommended with or without MTX for active moderate to severe RA with inadequate response to other DMARDs or failed anti-TNF agent (1)[A].
- For guidelines on biologics, refer to "2012 Update of the 2008 American College of Rheumatology Recommendations for the Use of Disease-Modifying Antirheumatic Drugs and Biologic Agents in the Treatment of Rheumatoid Arthritis."
- Avoid use of Zostavax while on biologic DMARD therapy (4)[C].
- Flare-ups
  - Intra-articular steroids: if disease is well controlled after ruling out intra-articular infection (1)[A]

ADDITIONAL THERAPIES

- Capsaicin cream: apply 3–4 times per day. Best results seen after 2–4 weeks of continuous use.
- Interdisciplinary care and management including physical therapy to minimize the consequences of loss of function, joint damage, maladaptive coping, and social isolation (1,4,5)[A]
- Recommended vaccinations
  - Pneumococcal, HPV, hepatitis B, influenza, varicella zoster (4)[C]

SURGERY/OTHER PROCEDURES

Surgical treatment including synovectomy, tendon reconstruction, joint fusion, and joint replacement may be considered to prevent disability in RA unresponsive to therapy or in advanced RA (1)[A].

COMPLEMENTARY & ALTERNATIVE MEDICINE

- Omega-3 may be of small benefit (1)[A],(6)[B].
- Gamma linolenic acid and *Tripterygium wilfordii* may have potential benefits (1)[A],(3)[B].

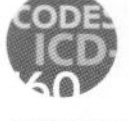

ONGOING CARE

The goals of comprehensive, interdisciplinary care are to stop the disease process, reduce pain, manage symptoms such as fatigue and stiffness, preserve joint integrity and function, and maintain social and occupational roles and quality of life.

FOLLOW-UP RECOMMENDATIONS

- Encourage full activity, avoiding heavy work or exercise during active (flare) phases. Emphasize exercise, mobility, and reduction of joint stress.
- Promote general health care and psychosocial well-being.

Patient Monitoring

Address risk factors and evaluate for cardiovascular disease and osteoporosis. Disease Activity Score 28 (DAS28) questionnaire for disease activity periodically and Health Assessment Questionnaire (HAQ) for functional status yearly.

DIET

Most beneficial diet for symptom control include gluten-free and vegetarian. Some benefits have been noted for "allergen-free," elemental, and Mediterranean diets. The Mediterranean diet is encouraged as RA patients are at increased cardiovascular disease risk.

PATIENT EDUCATION

American College of Rheumatology patient education overviews: http://www.rheumatology.org/practice/clinical/patients/diseases_and_conditions/ra.asp

PROGNOSIS

- Poor prognostic findings
  - Persistent moderate to severe disease; early or advanced age at disease onset
  - Many affected joints; swelling and pain in affected joints, positive MCP squeeze test, and PIP and MCP symmetric involvement
- 50% cannot function in their primary jobs within 10 years of onset.

REFERENCES

1. National Collaborating Centre for Chronic Conditions (UK). *Rheumatoid Arthritis: National Clinical Guideline for Management and Treatment in Adults* (NICE Clinical Guidelines, No. 79.). London, UK: Royal College of Physicians; 2009 Feb.
2. Aletaha D, Neogi T, Silman AJ, et al. 2010 rheumatoid arthritis classification criteria: an American College of Rheumatology/European League Against Rheumatism collaborative initiative. *Arthritis Rheum*. 2010;62(9):2569–2581.
3. Wasserman, A. Diagnosis and management of rheumatoid arthritis. *Am Fam Physician*. 2011;84(11):1245–1252.
4. Singh JA, Furst DE, Bharat A, et al. 2012 update of the 2008 American College of Rheumatology ecommendations for the use of disease-modifying antirheumatic drugs and biologic agents in the treatment of rheumatoid arthritis. *Arthritis Care Res (Hoboken)*. 2012;64(5):625–639.
5. Richards BL, Whittle SL, Buchbinder R. Neuromodulators for pain management in rheumatoid arthritis. *Cochrane Database Syst Rev*. 2012;1:CD008921.
6. Geusens P, Wouters C, Nijs J, et al. Long-term effect of omega-3 fatty acid supplementation in active rheumatoid arthritis. A 12-month, double-blind, controlled study. *Arthritis Rheum*. 1994;37(6):824–829.

CODES

ICD10

- M06.9 Rheumatoid arthritis, unspecified
- M05.60 Rheu arthritis of unsp site w involv of organs and systems
- M05.00 Felty's syndrome, unspecified site

CLINICAL PEARLS

- Rheumatoid arthritis occurs in 1% of the U.S. population.
- Females have more articular disease; males have more systemic presentations.
- RA is an idiopathic, chronic, systemic inflammatory disease characterized by symmetric polyarthritis and synovitis.
- >75% improve during pregnancy because of immunologic tolerance but relapse within 6 months.
- Plain films are the imaging modality of choice in RA.
- Treatment with DMARDs (MTX ideally) within 3 months of diagnosis slows disease progression and may lead to more remissions.
- Atlantoaxial joint involvement leads to instability; avoid unnecessary manipulation of the cervical spine.

ARTHRITIS, SEPTIC

Tianjiang Ye, MD • Jeffrey P. Feden, MD, FACEP

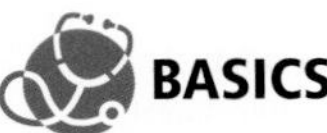

BASICS

DESCRIPTION

- Direct bacterial invasion of the joint space
- Systems affected: musculoskeletal
- Synonyms: suppurative arthritis; infectious arthritis; pyarthrosis; pyogenic arthritis; bacterial arthritis

EPIDEMIOLOGY

- Occurs at any age; higher incidence in very young and elderly
- Incidence:
  - 4–10/100,000 annual case rate (1)
- Prevalence: in patients presenting with monoarticular arthritis, 27% have nongonococcal septic arthritis (2)
- Gender differences:
  - Gonococcal: female > male
  - Nongonococcal: male > female

ETIOLOGY AND PATHOPHYSIOLOGY

- Many different pathogenic organisms
- Nongonococcal:
  - *Streptococcus aureus* (Most common organism in adults)
    - MRSA risk: elderly, intravenous drug users (IVDU), postsurgical
  - *Streptococcus* spp. (2nd most common in adults)
  - Gram-negative rods (GNR): usually in IVDU, trauma, extremes of age, immunosuppressed
- *Neisseria gonorrhea* (most common in young, sexually active adults)
- Other: lyme, fungal, Mycobacterium
- Risk by specific age (3,4):
  - <1 month: *S. aureus*, group B strep (GBS), GNR
  - 1 month–4 years: *S. aureus*, *Streptococcus pneumoniae*, *Neisseria meningitidis*
  - 16–40 years: *N. meningitidis*, *S. aureus*
  - >40 years: *S. aureus*
- Specific high-risk groups:
  - Rheumatoid arthritis: *S. aureus*
  - IVDU: *S. aureus*, GNR, opportunistic pathogens
  - Neonates: GBS
  - Immunocompromised: gram-negative bacilli, fungi
  - Trauma patients with open injuries: mixed flora
- Pathogenesis:
  - Hematogenous spread is most common.
  - Direct inoculation by microorganisms secondary to trauma or iatrogenic cause (i.e., joint surgery)
  - Adjacent spread from another infection site (i.e., osteomyelitis)
- Pathophysiology:
  - Microorganisms initially enter via synovial membrane and spread to the synovial fluid.
  - Resulting inflammatory response elicits cytokines and destructive proteases leading to joint damage.
  - Microbial surface components recognizing adhesive matrix molecules (MSCRAMMs) on bacteria may play a key role in septic arthritis (5).

RISK FACTORS

- Age >80 years
- Low socioeconomic status
- Alcoholism
- Cellulitis and skin ulcers
- Prior violation of joint capsule
  - Prior orthopedic surgery
  - Intra-articular steroid injection
  - Trauma
- History of previous joint disease
  - Inflammatory arthritis (rheumatoid arthritis [RA]: 10-fold increased risk)
  - Osteoarthritis
  - Crystal arthritides
- Systemic illness
  - Diabetes mellitus, liver disease, HIV, malignancy, end-stage renal disease/hemodialysis, immunosuppresion, sickle cell anemia
- Risks for hematogenous spread
  - IVDU, severe sepsis/systemic infection

GENERAL PREVENTION

- Prompt treatment of skin and soft tissue infections
- Control of risk factors
- Immunization

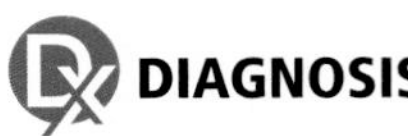

DIAGNOSIS

HISTORY

- Typically presents with combination of joint pain, swelling, warmth, and decreased range of motion
- Nongonococcal arthritis: predominantly monoarticular (80%)
  - Typically large joints (knees in 50% of cases)
  - Most patients report a history of fever.
  - IV drug users may develop infection in axial joints (e.g. sternoclavicular joint).
  - Prosthetic joints may show minimal findings and present with draining sinus over the joint.
  - Patients on chronic immunosuppressive drugs and those receiving steroid joint injections may present atypically (no fever or joint pain).
- Pediatric considerations
  - Infants may present with refusal to move limb which may be mistaken as neurologic problem.
  - Hip joint pain may refer to the knee or thigh.
- Gonococcal:
  - Bacteremic phase: migratory polyarthritis, tenosynovitis, high fever, chills, pustules (dermatitis-arthritis syndrome)
  - Localized phase: nonoarticular, low-grade fever

PHYSICAL EXAM

- Poor sensitivity and specificity in general
- Limited range of motion
- Joint effusion and tenderness
- Erythema and warmth over affected joint
- Pain with passive range of motion
- Hip and shoulder involvement may reveal severe pain on range of motion with less obvious joint swelling on exam.
- Pediatric consideration: Infants with septic hip will typically sit with hip flexed and externally rotated.

DIFFERENTIAL DIAGNOSIS

- Crystal arthritis: gout, pseudogout, calcium oxalate, cholesterol
- Infectious arthritis: fungi, spirochetes, rheumatic fever, HIV, viral
- Inflammatory arthritis: RA, spondyloarthropathy, systemic lupus erythematosus, sarcoidosis
- Osteoarthritis
- Trauma: meniscal tear, fracture, hemarthrosis
- Other: bursitis, cellulitis, tendinitis

DIAGNOSTIC TESTS & INTERPRETATION

Initial Tests (lab, imaging)

- Serum tests:
  - WBC count is neither sensitive nor specific when used alone.
  - ESR with cutoff of >15 mm/hr has sensitivity up to 94% but poor specificity (6)[B].
  - CRP >20 mg/L has sensitivity of 92% (6)[B].
  - Serum procalcitonin >0.4 ng/mL has 85% sensitivity and 87% specificity for septic arthritis but needs further study (7)[B].
  - Synovial lactate is a potential biomarker (8)[C].
  - Blood cultures are positive in 50% of cases.
- Other tests:
  - Disseminated gonococcus: culture blood, cervix, urine, urethra in addition to joint fluid
  - Suspected Lyme arthritis: send serum Lyme titers
- Synovial fluid analysis (key to diagnosis):
  - Should be obtained in suspected cases prior to antibiotic therapy (9)[A]
  - Send for gram stain, cultures, cell count/differential, and crystal analysis.
  - Use blood culture bottles to increase yield.
  - >50,000 WBCs/HPF with >90% polymorphonuclear leukocytes is suspcious; however, *synovial WBC* (sWBC) *count alone is insufficient to rule in or rule out septic arthritis* (3)[A].
  - The presence of crystals (e.g., urate or calcium pyrophosphate) *does not exclude infectious arthritis* (10)[B].
  - Joint fluid: for Gram stain (positive in 50%); culture (positive in 50–70%) should be sent with understanding of limitations.
  - Prosthetic joint: WBC count unreliable for indicating septic arthritis. A lower number of sWBCs may indicate infection.
- Pediatrics: No single lab test distinguishes septic arthritis from transient synovitis.
  - The combination of fever, non–weight bearing, and elevated ESR and CRP is suspicious, but synovial fluid should still be obtained.
- Imaging: helpful to identify effusion; not helpful in differentiating septic from other forms of arthritis
  - X-ray:
    - Nondiagnostic for septic arthritis but can screen for other pathology such as trauma, soft tissue swelling, osteoarthritis, or osteopenia
    - Nonspecific changes of inflammatory arthritis may be appreciated (i.e., erosions, joint destruction, joint space loss)
  - Ultrasound:
    - Accurately identifies joint space to help guide arthrocentesis
    - Recommended for aspiration of the hip
  - MRI:
    - Highly sensitive for effusion; increasing role to help distinguish between transient synovitis and septic arthritis in children (11)[B]
  - Other imaging techniques:
    - CT is not routinely indicated.
    - Bone scans are not performed unless there is concurrent suspicion of osteomyelitis.

Diagnostic Procedures
- Arthrocentesis in all suspected cases (prior to initiation of antibiotics whenever possible)
- Arthrocentesis should avoid contaminated tissue (e.g., overlying cellulitis).

Test Interpretation
Synovial biopsy shows polymorphonuclear leukocytes and possibly the causative organism.

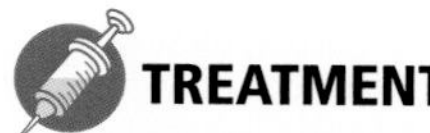

TREATMENT

GENERAL MEASURES
- All patients should be admitted for parenteral antibiotics and monitoring. Antibiotics should begin immediately after appropriate cultures sent.
- Removal of purulent material is *required*:
  - Pediatric consideration: Surgical drainage and irrigation is recommended for septic hip due to high risk of avascular necrosis (12)[B].
- If prosthetic joint is involved, antibiotics and consultation with orthopedic surgeon for replacement arthroplasty, resection arthroplasty, or débridement should be strongly considered (13)[B].
- Continue treatment for 1–2 weeks after total resolution of all signs of inflammation, for a total of 4–6 weeks for most organisms.
  - Exception: gonococcal (2–3 weeks)
- Intra-articular antibiotics not recommended (14)[B]
- IV dexamethasone in conjunction with antibiotics may reduce long-term sequelae and improve recovery time in pediatric patients (15)[A].

MEDICATION

First Line
- Initial antibiotic choice is guided by gram stain or most likely organism based on age and clinical history.
- Nongonococcal (16)[A]:
  - Gram-positive cocci:
    - Vancomycin 15 to 20 mg/kg twice to three times daily or linezolid 600 mg twice daily
  - Gram-negative bacilli:
    - Cefepime 2 g twice daily or ceftriaxone 2 g daily or ceftazidime 2 g three times daily or cefotaxime 2 g three times daily
    - For cephalosporin allergy: Consider treatment with ciprofloxacin 400 mg three times daily.
  - Negative Gram stain:
    - Vancomycin 15 to 20 mg/kg twice to three times daily plus 3rd-generation cephalosporin until cultures and susceptibilities return
  - Duration of therapy: typically 2 weeks of IV and an additional 2–3 weeks PO while monitoring therapeutic response
- Gonococcal (17)[A]:
  - Ceftriaxone 1 g IV/IM daily for 7–14 days (and at least 24–48 hours after symptoms resolve)
  - May require concurrent drainage of affected joint
  - Concomitant treatment for *Chlamydia* (doxycycline 100 mg twice daily or azithromycin 1g daily).
- Other considerations:
  - Narrow antibiotic therapy based on culture and sensitivities
  - *Salmonella* should be considered in pediatric patients with a history of sickle cell disease: Consider 3rd-generation cephalosporin.
  - If Lyme arthritis considered: doxycycline 100 mg PO twice daily or amoxicillin 500 mg PO three times daily for 28 days if no neurologic involvement, otherwise treat with ceftriaxone 2 g IV daily (18)[A]

ISSUES FOR REFERRAL
- Infectious disease and orthopedic consultations are strongly encouraged.
- Involvement of prosthetic joint mandates orthopedic consultation.
- IVDU; immunosuppression warrants infectious disease consultation to guide therapy.

SURGERY/OTHER PROCEDURES
- Drainage should be considered in all cases.
- Other treatment options include repeat needle aspiration, arthrscopy, or arthrotomy.
- Initial drainage strongly considered with shoulder, hip, and prosthetic joints

ONGOING CARE

FOLLOW-UP RECOMMENDATIONS

Patient Monitoring
- Monitor synovial fluid to verify decreasing WBC and sterile fluid after initial treatment.
- If no improvement within 24 hours, reevaluate and consider arthroscopy.
- Follow up 1 week and 1 month after stopping antibiotics to ensure no relapse.

PROGNOSIS
- Early treatment allows for better functional outcome.
- Delayed recognition/treatment leads to high morbidity and mortality.
- Elderly, concurrent rheumatoid arthritis, *S. aureus* infections, and infection of hip and shoulder increases chances of poor outcome.

COMPLICATIONS
- Mortality rate estimated at 11% (2)
- Limited joint range of motion
- Secondary osteoarthritis
- Flail or fused or dislocated joint
- Sepsis, septic necrosis
- Sinus formation
- Ankylosis
- Osteomyelitis, postinfectious synovitis
- Shortening of limb (in children)

REFERENCES

1. Geirsson AJ, Statkevicius S, Vikingsson A. Septic arthritis in Iceland 1990–2002: increasing incidence due to iatrogenic infections. *Ann Rheum Dis*. 2008;67(5):638–643.
2. Mathews CJ, Weston VC, Jones A, et al. Bacterial septic arthritis in adults. *Lancet*. 2010;375 (9717):846–855.
3. Margaretten ME, Kohlwes J, Moore D, et al. Does this adult patient have septic arthritis? *JAMA*. 2007;297(13):1478–1488.
4. Morgan DS, Fisher D, Merianos A, et al. An 18-year clinical review of septic arthritis from tropical Australia. *Epidemiol Infect*. 1996;117(3):423–428.
5. Shirtliff ME, Mader JT. Acute septic arthritis. *Clin Microbiol Rev*. 2002;15(4):527–544.
6. Hariharan P, Kabrhel C. Sensitivity of erythrocyte sedimentation rate and C-reactive protein for the exclusion of septic arthritis in emergency department patients. *J Emerg Med*. 2011;40(4):428–431.
7. Maharajan K, Patro DK, Menon J, et al. Serum procalcitonin is a sensitive and specific marker in the diagnosis of septic arthritis and acute osteomyelitis. *J Orthop Surg Res*. 2013;8:19.
8. Lenski M, Scherer MA. The significance of interleukin-6 and lactate in the synovial fluid for diagnosing native septic arthritis. *Acta Orthop Belg*. 2014;80(1):18–25.
9. Guidelines for the initial evaluation of adult patient with acute musculoskeletal symptoms. American College of Rheumatology Ad Hoc Committee on Clinical Guidelines. *Arthritis Rheum*. 1996;39(1):1–8.
10. Baer PA, Tenenbaum J, Fam AG, et al. Coexistent septic and crystal arthritis. Report of four cases and literature review. *J Rheumatol*. 1986;13(3):604–607.
11. Yang WJ, Im SA, Lim GY, et al. MR imaging of transient synovitis: differentiation from septic arthritis. *Pediatr Radiol*. 2006;36(11):1154–1158.
12. Fabry G, Meire E. Septic arthritis of the hip in children: poor results after a late and inadequate treatment. *J Pediatr Ortho*. 1983;3(4):461–466.
13. Mittal Y, Fehring TK, Hanssen A, et al. Two-stage reimplantation for periprosthetic knee infection involving resistant organisms. *J Bone Joint Surg Am*. 2007;89(6):1227–1231.
14. Goldenberg DL, Reed JI. Bacterial arthritis. *N Engl J Med*. 1985;312(12):764–771.
15. Macchiaiolo M, Buonuomo PS, Mennini M, et al. Question 2: should steroids be used in the treatment of septic arthritis? *Arch Dis Child*. 2014;99(8): 785–787. doi:10.1136/archdischild-2013-305617.
16. Liu C, Bayer A, Cosgrove SE, et al. Clinical practice guidelines by the infectious diseases society of America for the treatment of methicillin-resistant *Staphylococcus aureus* infections in adults and children. 2011;52(3):e18–e55. doi:10.1093/cid/ciq146.
17. Centers for Disease Control and Prevention, Workowski KA, Berman SM. Sexually transmitted diseases treatment guidelines, 2006. *MMWR*. 2006;55(RR-11):42–49.
18. Wormser GP, Dattwyler RJ, Shapiro ED, et al. The clinical assessment, treatment, and prevention of lyme disease, human granulocytic anaplasmosis, and babesiosis: clinical practice guidelines by the Infectious Diseases Society of America. Clin Infect Dis. 2006;43(9):1089–1134.

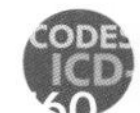

CODES

ICD10
- M00.9 Pyogenic arthritis, unspecified
- M00.869 Arthritis due to other bacteria, unspecified knee
- M00.859 Arthritis due to other bacteria, unspecified hip

CLINICAL PEARLS
- Arthrocentesis and synovial fluid analysis are mandatory in suspected cases of septic arthritis.
- Early IV antibiotics and drainage of infected joint spaces are critical to the successful management of septic arthritis.
- Crystalline disease can coexist with septic arthritis.
- Initial antibiotic therapy is guided by age, history, and Gram stain for likely organism.

ARTHROPOD BITES AND STINGS

James E. Powers, DO, FACEP

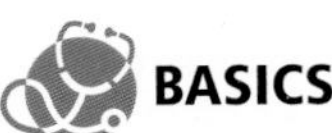

BASICS

DESCRIPTION

Arthropods make up the largest division of the animal kingdom; 2 classes, insects and arachnids, have the greatest medical impact on humans. Arthropods affect humans by inoculating poison or irritative substances through a bite or sting, by invading tissue, or by contact allergy to their skin, hairs, or secretions. The greatest medical importance is transmission of infectious microorganisms that may occur during insect feeding. Sequelae to arthropod bites, stings, or contact may include the following:

- Local redness with itch, pain, and swelling: common, usually immediate and transient
- Large local reactions increasing over 24–48 hours
- Systemic reactions with anaphylaxis, neurotoxicity, organ damage, or other systemic toxin effects
- Tissue necrosis or secondary infection
- Infectious disease transmission: presentation may be delayed weeks to years

EPIDEMIOLOGY

Incidence

- Difficult to estimate, as most encounters unreported
- ~50 deaths per year in the United States from fatal anaphylactic reaction to *Hymenoptera* stings
- Unrecognized anaphylactic reactions to *Hymenoptera* stings may be cause of 1/4 of sudden and unexpected deaths outdoors (1).

Prevalence

Widespread, with regional and seasonal variations

ETIOLOGY AND PATHOPHYSIOLOGY

- Arthropods: 4 medically important classes
  - Insects: *Hymenoptera* (bees, wasps, hornets, fire ants), mosquitoes, bed bugs, flies, lice, fleas, beetles, caterpillars, and moths
  - Arachnids: spiders, scorpions, mites, and ticks
  - Chilopods (centipedes)
  - Diplopods (millipedes)
- 4 general categories of pathophysiologic effects: toxic, allergic, infectious, and traumatic
  - Toxic effects of venom: local (tissue inflammation or destruction) versus systemic (neurotoxic or organ damage)
  - Allergic: Antigens in saliva may cause local inflammation. Exaggerated immune responses may result in anaphylaxis or serum sickness.
  - Trauma: Mechanical injury from biting or stinging causes pain, swelling, and portal of entry for bacteria and secondary infection. Retention of arthropod parts can cause a granulomatous reaction.
  - Infection: Arthropods are vectors and can transmit bacterial, viral, and protozoal diseases.

Genetics

Family history of atopy may be a factor in the development of more severe allergic reactions.

RISK FACTORS

- Previous sensitization is a key to most severe allergic reactions, but exposure history may not be recalled.
- Although most arthropod contact is inadvertent, certain activities, occupations, and travel increase risk.
- Greater risk for adverse outcome in young, elderly, immune compromised, or those with unstable cardiac or respiratory status

GENERAL PREVENTION

- Avoidance of common arthropod habitats, where possible
- Insect repellents (not effective for bees, spiders, scorpions, caterpillars, bed bugs, fleas, ants)
  - N,N-diethyl-meta-toluamide (DEET)
    - Most effective broad-spectrum repellent against biting arthropods (2)
    - Formulations with higher concentrations (20–50%) are 1st-line choice when visiting areas where arthropod-borne diseases are endemic (2).
    - Concentrations >30% give longer duration of effect
    - Safe for children >6 months of age and pregnant and lactating women (2)
  - Icaridin (formerly known as *picardin*)
    - Use of concentrations <20% may require more frequent application to maintain effectiveness.
  - P-menthane3,8-diol (PMD): component of lemon eucalyptus extract
    - Recommended alternative repellent to DEET at concentrations >20% (2)
    - May be used in children >6 months of age (2)
  - IR3535: less effective in most studies
  - Other botanical oils (citronella etc.): less effective than DEET; not for disease-endemic areas
- Barrier methods: clothing, bed nets
  - Use of light-colored pants, long-sleeved shirts, and hats may reduce arthropod impact.
  - Permethrin: Synthetic insecticide derived from chrysanthemum plant should not be applied to skin, but permethrin-impregnated clothing provides good protection against arthropods.
  - Mosquito nets: Insecticide-treated nets are advised for all travelers to disease-endemic areas at risk from biting arthropods (2).
  - WHO-recommended nets are Permanet 2.0 (Vestergaard), Olyset (Sumitomo), and Interceptor (BASF) (2).
- Desensitization 75–95% effective for *Hymenoptera*-specific venom
  - Skin tests are needed to determine sensitivity.
  - Refer to allergist/immunologist if candidate
- Fire ant control (but not elimination) possible
  - Baits; sprays, dusts, aerosols; biologic agents
- Risk of tick-borne diseases decreased by prompt removal of ticks within 24 hours of attachment.

DIAGNOSIS

HISTORY

- Sudden onset of pain or itching with visualization of arthropod
- Many cases unknown to patient or asymptomatic initially (bed bugs, lice, scabies, ticks). Consider in patients presenting with localized erythema, urticaria, wheals, papules, pruritus, or bullae.
- May identify insect by its habitat or by remnants brought by patient
- History of prior exposure useful but not always available or reliable
- Travel, occupational, social, and recreational history important

PHYSICAL EXAM

- If stinger is still present in skin, remove by flicking or scraping away from skin.
- Anaphylaxis is a clinical diagnosis. Essential to examine for signs and symptoms of anaphylaxis (3,4)
  - Erythema, urticaria, angioedema
  - Itching/edema of lips, tongue, uvula; drooling
  - Persistent vomiting
  - Respiratory distress, wheeze, repetitive cough, stridor, dysphonia
  - Hypotension, dysrhythmia, syncope, chest pain
- If anaphylaxis not present, exam focuses on the sting or bite itself. Common findings include local erythema, swelling, wheals, urticaria, papules, or bullae; excoriations from scratching.
- Thorough exam to look for arthropod infestation (lice, scabies) or attached ticks. Body lice usually found in seams of clothing. Skin scraping to identify scabies.
- Signs of secondary bacterial infection after 24–48 hours: increasing erythema, pain, fever, lymphangitis, or abscess
- Delayed manifestations of insect-borne diseases

DIFFERENTIAL DIAGNOSIS

- Urticaria and localized dermatologic manifestations:
  - Contact dermatitis, drug eruption, mastocytosis, bullous diseases, dermatitis herpetiformis, tinea, eczema, vasculitis, pityriasis, erythema multiforme, viral exanthem, cellulitis, abscess, impetigo, folliculitis, erysipelas, necrotizing fasciitis
- Anaphylactic-type reactions
  - Cardiac, hemorrhagic, or septic shock; acute respiratory failure, asthma; angioedema, urticarial vasculitis; flushing syndromes (catecholamines, vasoactive peptides); panic attacks, syncope
  - Differential diagnosis of the acute abdomen should include black widow spider bite.

DIAGNOSTIC TESTS & INTERPRETATION

Initial Tests (lab, imaging)

Seldom needed; basic lab parameters usually normal. Some findings may help confirm diagnosis of anaphylaxis:

- Plasma histamine levels elevated briefly after mast cell activation
- Serum tryptase within 15 minutes–3 hours after onset of symptoms with second sample 24 hours later (4)

Follow-Up Tests & Special Considerations

- Severe envenomations may affect organ function and require monitoring of lab values (CBC, comprehensive metabolic panel, prothrombin time/international normalized ratio)
- Labs for arthropod-borne diseases, as indicated
  - Ticks: Lyme disease, Rocky Mountain spotted fever, relapsing fever, ehrlichiosis, babesiosis, tularemia
  - Flies: tularemia, leishmaniasis, African trypanosomiasis, bartonellosis, loiasis
  - Chigger mites: scrub typhus
  - Body lice: epidemic typhus, relapsing fever
  - Kissing bugs: Chagas disease
  - Mosquitoes: malaria, yellow fever, dengue fever, West Nile virus, equine encephalitis, chikungunya
- Refer to allergist for formal testing with history of anaphylaxis, significant systemic symptoms, progressively severe reactions (3,4)

Diagnostic Procedures/Other

Various skin tests and immunologic tests available to try to predict anaphylactic risk

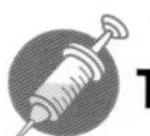

TREATMENT

ALERT
- The more rapidly anaphylaxis develops, the more likely the reaction is to be severe and potentially life-threatening. Most deaths due to anaphylaxis occur within 30–60 minutes of sting.
- Epinephrine should be given as soon as diagnosis of anaphylaxis is suspected. Delayed injection of epinephrine is associated with fatal anaphylaxis (3,4).
- Antihistamines and steroids do not replace epinephrine in anaphylaxis, and no direct outcome data regarding their effectiveness in anaphylaxis are available (3,4).
- Airway management critical if angioedema

GENERAL MEASURES
Local wound care, ice compress, elevation, analgesics

MEDICATION
First Line
- For arthropod bites/stings **with anaphylaxis**:
  - There are no randomized controlled trials on treatments, so the following recommendations are all based on expert opinion consensus (4)[C].
  - Epinephrine: **Most important:** IM injection in midanterolateral thigh (vastus lateralis muscle):
    - IM injection: epinephrine 1:1,000 (1 mg/mL): adult: 0.3–0.5 mg per dose; pediatric: give 0.01 mg/kg to a maximum dose of 0.5 mg per dose, can repeat every 5–15 minutes (4)
  - Positioning: supine with legs elevated
  - Oxygen 6–8 L/min up to 100%, as needed
  - IV fluids: Establish 1–2 large-bore IV lines. Normal saline rapid bolus 1–2 L IV; repeat as needed (pediatrics 20–30 mL/kg)
  - H_1 antihistamines: diphenhydramine 25–50 mg IV (pediatrics 1–2 mg/kg)
  - β_2 agonists: albuterol for bronchospasm nebulized 2.5–5 mg in 3 mL
  - Emergency treatment of refractory cases: consider epinephrine infusion, dopamine, glucagon, vasopressin, large-volume crystalloids (3,4)
- Arthropod bites/stings without anaphylaxis
  - Tetanus booster, as indicated
  - Oral antihistamines
    - Diphenhydramine
    - Cetirizine
    - H_2 blockers: ranitidine
  - Oral steroids: consider short course for severe pruritus; prednisone or prednisolone 1–2 mg/kg once daily
  - Topical intermediate-potency steroid cream or ointment × 3–5 days
    - Desoximetasone 0.05%
    - Triamcinolone 0.1%
    - Fluocinolone 0.025%
  - Wound care: antibiotics *only* if infection
  - Other specific therapies:
    - Scorpion stings: Treat excess catecholamine release (nitroprusside, prazosin, β-blockers). Diazepam for muscle spasms. Atropine for hypersalivation (5). Only one FDA-approved scorpion antivenom in United States and should be administered in conjunction with toxicologist. Black widow bites: Treat muscle spasms with diazepam and opioid analgesics PO or IV (5). Antivenom: Available but should be administered in conjunction with toxicologist.
    - Poison control should be consulted for questions regarding management of envenomation. 1-800-222-1222.
  - Fire ants: characteristically cause sterile pustules. Leave intact: Do not open or drain.
  - Brown recluse spider: pain control, supportive treatment; surgical consult if débridement needed
  - Ticks: early removal. Review guidelines for disease prophylaxis.
  - Pediculosis: head, pubic, and body lice
    - First line: permethrin 1% (Nix) topical lotion. Apply to affected area, wash off in 10 minutes.
    - Alternatives: pyrethrin or malathion 0.5% lotion, ivermectin (not FDA approved for pediculosis) orally
    - Repeat above treatment in 7–10 days.
    - For eyelash infestation: Apply ophthalmic-grade petroleum jelly BID for 10 days.
  - *Sarcoptes scabii* scabies
    - Permethrin 5% cream: Apply to entire body. Wash off after 8–14 hours. Repeat in 1 week.
    - Ivermectin: 200 μg/kg PO once; repeat in 2 weeks (not FDA approved for this use)
    - Crotamiton 10% cream or lotion less efficacious; apply daily for 2 days after bathing

Second Line
Second-line options for **anaphylaxis**:
- Ranitidine
- Methylprednisolone 1 mg/kg for 3–4 days or hydrocortisone 200 mg (4)

ISSUES FOR REFERRAL
Refer to allergist with history of anaphylaxis, severe systemic symptoms, or progressively severe reactions

SURGERY/OTHER PROCEDURES
Débridement and delayed skin grafting may be needed for brown recluse spider and other bites.

COMPLEMENTARY & ALTERNATIVE MEDICINE
- Some stings may be treated with a paste of 3 tsp of baking soda and 1 tsp water.
- None well tested

INPATIENT CONSIDERATIONS
Admission Criteria/Initial Stabilization
Anaphylaxis, vascular instability, neuromuscular events, pain, GI symptoms, renal damage/failure

ONGOING CARE

FOLLOW-UP RECOMMENDATIONS
- Immunotherapy as recommended by allergist/consultant for anaphylaxis or serious reactions; venom immunotherapy cornerstone of treatment for *Hymenoptera*.
- Patient-administered epinephrine must be provided to patients with anaphylaxis. Consider "med-alert" identifiers (3,4).

Patient Monitoring
- Monitor for delayed effects, including infectious diseases from arthropod vectors.
- Serum sickness reactions, vasculitis (rare)

PATIENT EDUCATION
Avoidance and prevention

PROGNOSIS
- Excellent for local reactions
- For systemic reactions, best response with early intervention to prevent cardiorespiratory collapse

COMPLICATIONS
- Scarring
- Secondary bacterial infection
- Arthropod-associated diseases as mentioned earlier
- Psychological effects, phobias

REFERENCES

1. Diaz JH. Recognition, management, and prevention of hymenopteran stings and allergic reactions in travelers. *J Travel Med*. 2009;16(5):357–364.
2. Moore, SJ, Mordue, AJ, Logan JG. Insect bite prevention. *Infect Dis Clin N Am*. 2012;26(3): 655–673.
3. Simons FE, Ardusso L, Bilo MB, et al. 2012 update: World Allergy Organization guidelines for the assessment and management of anaphylaxis. *Curr Opin Allergy Clin Immunol*. 2012;12(4):389–399.
4. De Bisschop M, Bellou A. Anaphylaxis. *Curr Opin Crit Care*. 2012;18(4):308–317.
5. Quan D. North American poisonous bites and stings. *Crit Care Clin*. 2012;28(4):633–659.

ADDITIONAL READINGS

- Centers for Disease Control and Prevention. Protection against mosquitoes, ticks, & other insects & arthropods. http://wwwnc.cdc.gov/travel/yellowbook/2014/chapter-2-the-pre-travel-consultation/protection-against-mosquitoes-ticks-and-other-insects-and-arthropods. Accessed 2014.
- Centers for Disease and Prevention. FAQ. Insect repellent use & safety. http://www.cdc.gov/westnile/faq/repellent.html. Accessed 2014.
- Sicherer SH, Leung DY. Advances in allergic skin disease, anaphylaxis, and hypersensitivity reactions to foods, drugs, and insects in 2012. *J Allergy Clin Immunol*. 2013;131(1):55–66.
- Studdiford JS, Conniff KM, Trayes KP, et al. Bedbug infestation. *Am Fam Physician*. 2012;86(7): 653–658.
- Swanson DL, Vetter RS. Bites of brown recluse spiders and suspected necrotic arachnidism. *N Engl J Med*. 2005;352(7):700–707.
- Warrell DA. Venomous bites, stings, and poisoning. *Infect Dis Clin North Am*. 2012; 26(2):207–223.

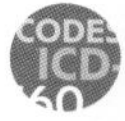

CODES

ICD10
- T63.481A Toxic effect of venom of arthropod, accidental, init
- T63.301A Toxic effect of unsp spider venom, accidental, init
- T63.484A Toxic effect of venom of oth arthropod, undetermined, init

CLINICAL PEARLS
- Urgent administration of epinephrine is a key to anaphylaxis treatment.
- Local treatment and symptom management are sufficient in most insect bites and stings.

ASCITES

Robert Powell, DO, MS • Mark B. Stephens, MD, MS, FAAFP, CAPT, MC, USN

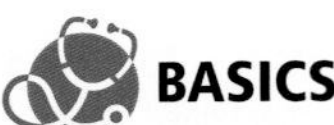

BASICS

DESCRIPTION
Accumulation of fluid in the peritoneal cavity; may occur in conditions that cause generalized edema

EPIDEMIOLOGY
- Children: nephrotic syndrome and malignancy most common
- Adults: cirrhosis, heart failure, nephrotic syndrome, peritonitis most common
- ~85% of all cases of ascites are caused by liver disease and cirrhosis.

Incidence
~50–60% of patients with cirrhosis will develop ascites within 10 years.

Prevalence
10% of patients with liver cirrhosis have ascites.

ETIOLOGY AND PATHOPHYSIOLOGY
- Acute liver failure
- Hepatitis (alcoholic, viral, autoimmune, drugs)
  - Peritoneal infection and inflammation
  - Bacterial infection (foreign body, fistula), tuberculosis, fungal disease, parasitic infection
  - Perforated viscus
  - Granulomatous peritonitis (e.g., sarcoidosis)
- Metabolic disease
  - Cirrhosis or prehepatic and posthepatic portal hypertension
  - Nephrotic syndrome
  - Myxedema
  - Protein malnutrition (hypoalbuminemia <2 g/dL)
- Cardiac congestion
  - Congestive heart failure (CHF), constrictive pericarditis
- Trauma
  - Pancreatic or biliary fistula
  - Lymphatic tear (chylous ascites), hemoperitoneum (trauma, ectopic pregnancy, tumor)
- Malignancy
  - Peritoneal seeding: ovarian, colon, pancreas, others
  - Primary peritoneal carcinoma, leukemia, or lymphoma
- Mixed (>1 of the above causes, e.g., cirrhosis and cancer)
- May develop as a consequence of sustained portal hypertension (portal pressure >12 mm Hg). Interactions of biochemical mediators (e.g., nitric oxide) lead to decreased systemic vascular resistance, splanchnic arterial vasodilation, reduced effective circulating arterial blood volume, and reduced renal perfusion.
- Renal hypoperfusion contributes to activation of systemic vasoconstrictors and antinatriuretic mechanisms, stimulating the sympathetic nervous system and renin-angiotensin-aldosterone system, ultimately culminating in sodium and water retention leading to ascites and edema.

DIAGNOSIS

HISTORY
Progressive abdominal distention which may be painless or painful; weight gain, dyspnea/orthopnea, edema, early satiety, and nausea. Those with spontaneous bacterial peritonitis may present with fever, abdominal tenderness, and altered mentation. Those with underlying malignancy may present with weight loss.

PHYSICAL EXAM
- Abdominal distention, flank dullness, shifting dullness, fluid wave
- Edema (penile/scrotal, pedal), pleural effusion, rales
- Stigmata of cirrhosis (palmar erythema, spider angiomata, abdominal wall collaterals)
- Other signs of advanced liver disease: jaundice, muscle wasting, gynecomastia, leukonychia
- Signs of underlying malignancy: cachexia, umbilical nodule

DIAGNOSTIC TESTS & INTERPRETATION

Initial Tests (lab, imaging)
- Diagnostic paracentesis for ascitic fluid analysis should be obtained in all new-onset, new-to-treatment, or hospitalized patients with ascites (1)[B] to assess for infection:
  - Paracentesis has a complication rate of 1% (despite high prevalence of abnormal coagulation parameters). Ascitic fluid analysis should include the following:
    - Cell count and differential:
      - Polymorphonuclear leukocytes: ≥250 cells/mm^3 suggests infection.
    - Albumin in both serum and ascites: serum-to-ascites albumin gradient (SAAG):
      - <1.1 g indicates exudate (i.e., inflammatory, biliary/pancreatic, carcinomatosis):
        - Neoplasm, myxedema, tuberculosis, pancreatitis, biliary pathology
      - ≥1.1 g indicates transudate/portal hypertension:
        - Etiologies include cirrhosis, CHF, constrictive pericarditis, Budd-Chiari syndrome, nephrotic syndrome, protein malnutrition/hypoalbuminemia.
    - Fluid culture, if diagnostic paracentesis (not necessary in therapeutic paracentesis) or
      - If infection suspected (*cirrhotic patients with ascites can fail to mount adequate fever or significant leukocytosis*)
      - Fluid cultures are positive in 50–90% of cases.
    - Amylase, especially if bowel perforation, choledocholithiasis, or pancreatitis suspected
    - Triglyceride if fluid appears milky
    - Lactate dehydrogenase (LDH) from fluid and serum: An ascitic fluid–to–serum LDH ratio >1.0 can indicate infection or tumor.
    - Gram stain, acid-fast stain, fungal cultures/smears, and cytology to evaluate for peritoneal infection or carcinomatosis
- Blood tests:
  - BUN/creatinine, electrolytes, and other labs as indicated by underlying condition (e.g., liver enzymes, tumor markers)
- Abdominal ultrasound: to confirm ascites; highly sensitive, cost-effective, involves no radiation, and available at bedside
- CT scan to rule out intra-abdominal pathology (e.g., portal vein thrombosis, especially in setting of markedly elevated aminotransferases)
- MRI best for evaluation of liver disease or confirmation of portal vein thrombosis

Diagnostic Procedures/Other
Laparoscopy: preferred when CT and fluid cytology are nondiagnostic
- Helps to determine cause of ascites if unrelated to portal hypertension (SAAG <1.1)
- Allows for direct visualization and biopsy of peritoneum, liver, and intra-abdominal lymph nodes
- Preferred for evaluating suspected peritoneal tuberculosis or malignancies

Test Interpretation
Cytology may reveal malignant cells: adenocarcinoma (ovary, breast, GI tract); rarely, primary peritoneal carcinoma are most commonly associated with ascites.

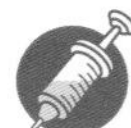

TREATMENT

For all patients:
- Daily record of weight
- Restrict dietary sodium to 2 g/day (1)[A].
- Water restriction (1–1.5 L/day) generally not helpful; only necessary if serum sodium <120–125 mEq/L (1)[C]
- Creatinine >2.0 mg/dL: decrease diuretic doses, peritoneal paracentesis.
- Abstinence from alcohol and adequate nutrition if liver disease (1)[A]
- Baclofen may be used to reduce alcohol craving/consumption (1)[C].

MEDICATION

ALERT
Carefully approach diuresis; aggressive diuresis can induce prerenal acute kidney injury, encephalopathy, and hyponatremia. Monitor creatinine and electrolytes closely. Serum creatinine >2 mg/dL or serum sodium <120 mmol/L should prompt withdrawal of diuretics.

NSAIDs may worsen or initiate oliguria or azotemia, and should be avoided.

Use of ACE inhibitors and angiotensin receptor blockers (ARBs) may be harmful in patients with cirrhosis/ascites due to an increased risk of hypotension and renal failure (1)[C]; ACE inhibitors and ARBs should be avoided in refractory ascites (1)[B].

Consider discontinuing beta-blockers in patients with refractory ascites or worsening hypotension or azotemia (1)[B].

First Line
- Sodium restriction
- Diuretics: Mainstay of treatment are sodium restriction and diuretics, to induce a negative sodium balance:
  - Spironolactone 100–400 mg daily PO; typical initial dose is 100–200 mg given in AM:
    - Diuretic of choice due to its antialdosterone effects. Can be used as single agent in minimal ascites
  - Furosemide 40–160 mg daily PO; typical initial dose is 40 mg given in AM:
    - Antinatriuretic effect helps to achieve negative sodium balance. Not a 1st-line diuretic but is an effective adjunct to potentiate maximum effects of spironolactone with better natriuresis
  - May use spironolactone and furosemide together (maintaining a 100:40 ratio) for maximum efficacy. Most patients eventually require combination therapy.
    - Doses should be sufficient to obtain net sodium loss in urine:
      - Spot urine sodium in mEq/L × estimated urine output (1 L if no information) should equal estimated dietary sodium. Increase diuretics daily until this goal is attained. Measure serum electrolytes before dose change.
      - Follow daily weight. Emphasize sodium restriction.

- Diuretic-intractable ascites (10% of patients): persistent or worsening ascites despite maximum doses of spironolactone (400 mg/day) and furosemide (160 mg/day) and sodium restriction *or* progressive rise in creatinine to 2.0
  - *Ensure compliance with dietary sodium restriction with* 24-hour urine sodium excretion: If <78 mEq/day, patient is compliant with 2-g dietary sodium restriction.
  - Therapeutic paracentesis or serial large-volume paracentesis (LVP)
    - Complications: infection, hemodynamic collapse, acute renal failure
    - Replace albumin when removing >5 L of ascites: 5.5–8 g albumin for each liter removed has been shown to decrease renal dysfunction, hyponatremia post paracentesis, and overall morbidity (2)[A], although limited studies directly compare albumin doses.
    - Continue diuretics at 1/2 previous doses.

Second Line

- Most commonly used in cases of GI intolerance or allergic reactions
- Alternatives to spironolactone: amiloride up to 40 mg/day; triamterene up to 200 mg/day in divided doses
- Alternatives to furosemide: torsemide up to 100 mg/day; ethacrynic acid 50 mg IV (may be effective when oral drugs cannot be used)
- Vaptans may have a beneficial effect on hyponatremia and ascites, but the data do not support their routine use in ascites (3)[A].

ISSUES FOR REFERRAL

Referral for liver transplant should be considered in patients with decompensated liver disease, whether or not ascites is present/controlled. Liver transplant is the definitive treatment for portal hypertension (HTN) (1)[B].

SURGERY/OTHER PROCEDURES

- Transjugular intrahepatic portosystemic shunt (TIPS)
  - Transjugular conduit from the liver to the hepatic vein for intractable ascites; placed under fluoroscopy (4)[A]
    - At time of placement, measure portal pressure; should drop ≥20 mm Hg or to <12 mm Hg, and ascites should be readily controlled with diuretics. Yearly US to confirm functional shunt.
    - 4 weeks after TIPS, urinary sodium and serum creatinine improve significantly and can normalize after 6–12 months in combination with diuretics (4). Dilation/replacement may be required after >2 years.
    - Encephalopathy is a complication. TIPS is superior to paracentesis to control ascites, but no difference in mortality (4)[A].
- Peritoneovenous shunt (LeVeen or Denver shunt): A shunt drains ascites directly into the inferior vena cava.
  - Clinical trials show poor long-term shunt patency, no survival advantage compared with medical therapy. Complications include the following:
    - Bacteremia, bowel obstruction, and variceal bleed as a result of rapid volume overload from ascitic fluid into systemic circulation
    - Usually reserved for patients with refractory ascites who are not candidates for TIPS or liver transplant, and who have numerous abdominal scars, making repeated paracentesis unsafe (1)[A]
- Percutaneous endoscopic gastrostomy should be avoided in patients with ascites due to an associated high mortality rate following this procedure (1)[B].

COMPLEMENTARY & ALTERNATIVE MEDICINE

Avoid herbs and other dietary supplements (risk drug interactions, hepatotoxicity, coagulopathy).

ONGOING CARE

PROGNOSIS

- Prognosis varies depending on underlying cause. Ascites is rarely life-threatening in itself but can be a sign of life-threatening disease (e.g., cancer, end-stage liver disease).
- Conservative therapy usually successful if cause is reversible or treatable (e.g., infection).

COMPLICATIONS

- Spontaneous bacterial peritonitis (SBP)
  - Ascitic fluid polymorphonuclear (PMN) leukocyte count ≥250 cells/mm^3, positive culture
    - Broad-spectrum antibiotics: cefotaxime 2 g q8h or similar 3rd-generation cephalosporin is treatment of choice for suspected SBP. Covers 95% of flora (including *Escherichia coli*, *Klebsiella*, pneumococci) (1)[A]
    - Lifetime antibiotic prophylaxis with norfloxacin or trimethoprim-sulfamethoxazole (TMP-SMX) is indicated in some patients who survive an episode of SBP (1)[A]. Reduced incidence of SBP, delayed development of hepatorenal syndrome, and improved survival in (5)[C]
    - Suspect primary bacterial peritonitis (PBP) due to bowel perforations when ascitic fluid >250 cells/mm^3 (often >5,000 cells/mm^3), and any 2 of the following:
      - Ascitic fluid total protein >1 g/dL (often >3 g/dL)
      - Ascitic fluid glucose <50 mg/dL (or 2.8 mmol/L)
      - Ascitic fluid LDH that is 3-fold greater than serum LDH
- Hepatorenal syndrome: diagnosed when possible causes of acute renal failure are excluded, and at least 2 days of diuretic withdrawal and maximal intravascular volume expansion with albumin
  - Urine volume <500 mL/day, rising BUN, and creatinine >1.5 mg/dL, fractional excretion of sodium <1%, and decreased urine sodium excretion (<20 mEq/L, indicates significant sodium avidity)
    - Stop diuretics and begin intravascular volume expansion, preferably with colloid (5–20 g IV albumin/day) (6)[B].
    - Consider vasoactive drugs, such as octreotide 200 μg SC TID and midodrine 12.5 mg PO TID, either alone or together, in addition to colloid volume expanders in rapidly progressive (type I) renal failure (1)[B].
    - Liver transplant is definitive treatment.
    - May need hemodialysis to control azotemia and correct electrolyte imbalance while awaiting transplant
    - Cellulitis is increasingly common in obese patients with brawny edema and should be treated with diuretics and appropriate antibiotics (1)[B].

REFERENCES

1. Runyon BA. Management of adult patients with ascites due to cirrhosis: update 2012. http://www.aasld.org/practiceguidelines/Documents/ascitesupdate2013.pdf. Accessed on November 28, 2014.
2. Bernardi M, Caraceni P, Navickis RJ, et al. Albumin infusion in patients undergoing large-volume paracentesis: a meta-analysis of randomized trials. *Hepatology*. 2012;55(4):1172–1181.
3. Watson H, Jepsen P, Wong F, et al. Satavaptan treatment for ascites in patients with cirrhosis: a meta-analysis of effect on hepatic encephalopathy development. *Metab Brain Dis*. 2013;28(2):301–305.
4. Rössle M, Gerbes AL. TIPS for the treatment of refractory ascites, hepatorenal syndrome, and hepatic hydrothorax: a critical update. *Gut*. 2010;59(7):988–1000.
5. Fernández J, Navasa M, Planas R, et al. Primary prophylaxis of spontaneous bacterial peritonitis delays hepatorenal syndrome and improves survival in cirrhosis. *Gastroenterology*. 2007;133(3):818–824.
6. Sussman AN, Boyer TD. Management of refractory ascites and hepatorenal syndrome. *Curr Gastroenterol Rep*. 2011;13(1):17–25.

ADDITIONAL READING

- Dahl E, Gluud LL, Kimer N, et al. Meta-analysis: the safety and efficacy of vaptans (tolvaptan, satavaptan, and lixivaptan) in cirrhosis with ascites or hyponatraemia. *Aliment Pharmacol Ther*. 2012;36(7):619–626.
- Perumalswami PV, Schiano TD. The management of hospitalized patients with cirrhosis: the Mount Sinai experience and a guide for hospitalists. *Dig Dis Sci*. 2011;56(5):1266–1281.

SEE ALSO

- Cirrhosis of the Liver; Congestive Heart Failure: Differential Diagnosis; Nephrotic Syndrome; Hepatorenal Syndrome
- Algorithm: Hyperbilirubinemia and Cirrhosis

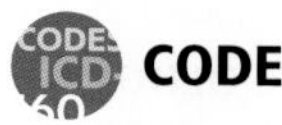

CODES

ICD10

- R18.8 Other ascites
- R18.0 Malignant ascites
- K70.31 Alcoholic cirrhosis of liver with ascites

CLINICAL PEARLS

- Most common cause of "diuretic-intractable ascites" is noncompliance with dietary sodium restriction.
- ACE inhibitors, ARBs, and beta-blockers should be avoided in patients with ascites.
- Cellulitis of the abdominal wall or lower extremity is an increasing problem in obese patients with ascites.
- Cirrhosis remains the most common cause of ascites.

ASTHMA

Urooj Najm, MBBS • Najm Hasan Siddiqui, MD

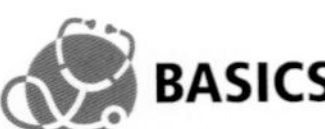

BASICS

DESCRIPTION

- Chronic, reversible inflammatory airway disease characterized by recurrent attacks of breathlessness and wheezing
- Four major classifications of asthma severity used primarily to initiate therapy (1,2):
  - Intermittent: symptoms ≤2 days/week, nighttime awakenings ≤2×/month, short-acting β-agonist use ≤2 days/week, no interference with normal activity, and normal forced expiratory volume in 1 second (FEV_1) between exacerbations with FEV_1 (predicted) >80% and FEV_1/forced vital capacity (FVC) >80%
  - Mild persistent: symptoms >2 days/week but not daily, nighttime awakenings 3–4×/month, short-acting β-agonist use >2 days/week but not daily, minor limitations in normal activity, and FEV_1 (predicted) >80% and FEV_1/FVC >80%
  - Moderate persistent: daily symptoms, nighttime awakenings ≥1×/week but not nightly, daily use of short-acting β-agonist, some limitation in normal activity, and FEV_1 (predicted) 60–80% and FEV_1/FVC 75–80%
  - Severe persistent: symptoms throughout the day, nighttime awakenings often 7×/week, short-acting β-agonist use several times a day, extremely limited normal activity, and FEV_1 (predicted) <60% and FEV_1/FVC <75%

EPIDEMIOLOGY

Prevalence

- Affects 5–10% of population
- One of the most common chronic diseases of childhood, affecting 7 million children
- In children, more common in boys than girls
- In adults, more common in women than men, African Americans than Caucasians

Pregnancy Considerations

In the United States, maternal asthma complicates approximately 4–8% of all pregnancies.

Geriatric Considerations

Prevalence of asthma in seniors (age >65 years) is 5.3%.

ETIOLOGY AND PATHOPHYSIOLOGY

- Airway inflammation begins with inflammatory cell infiltration, sub-basement fibrosis, mucus hypersecretion, epithelial injury, smooth muscle hypertrophy, angiogenesis that then leads to intermittent airflow obstruction, and bronchial hyperresponsiveness.
- Remodeling of airways may occur (1).

Genetics

- Inheritable component with complex genetics and environment interaction
- A gene-by-environment interaction occurs in which the susceptible host is exposed to environmental factors that are capable of generating immunoglobulin (Ig) E and sensitization occurs.

RISK FACTORS

- Host factors: genetic predisposition, gender, race, BMI
- Environmental: viral infections, animal and airborne allergens, tobacco smoke, and so on
- Exercise, obesity, and emotional stress
- Aspirin or NSAIDs hypersensitivity or β-blockers
- Food allergies and asthma → increased risk for fatal anaphylaxis from those foods.

GENERAL PREVENTION

- Eliminate or modify exposure to asthma triggers (e.g., allergens, smoking, aspirin, NSAIDs).
- Consider allergen immunotherapy.
- Treat comorbidities such as allergic rhinitis.
- Annual influenza vaccine (inactivated influenza vaccine) for age <6 months
- Patients at risk for anaphylaxis should carry an EpiPen.

COMMONLY ASSOCIATED CONDITIONS

- Atopy: eczema, allergic conjunctivitis, allergic rhinitis
- Obesity (associated with higher asthma rates)
- Sinusitis
- Gastroesophageal reflux disease (GERD)
- Obstructive sleep apnea (OSA)
- Allergic bronchopulmonary aspergillosis (rare)
- Stress/depression

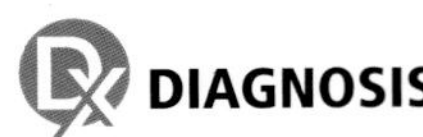

DIAGNOSIS

It is important to classify asthma severity.

HISTORY

- Question frequency of symptoms and rescue inhaler use.
- Symptoms include the following:
  - Cough (particularly if worse at night)
  - Wheeze
  - Chest tightness/difficulty breathing

PHYSICAL EXAM

- May be normal
- Focus on
  - General appearance: signs of respiratory distress such as use of accessory muscles
  - Upper respiratory tract: rhinitis, nasal polyps, swollen nasal turbinates
  - Lower respiratory tract: wheezing, prolonged expiratory phase
  - Skin: eczema

DIFFERENTIAL DIAGNOSIS

- In children
  - Upper airway diseases (allergic rhinitis or sinusitis)
  - Large airway obstruction (foreign body aspiration, vocal cord dysfunction, vascular ring or laryngeal web, laryngotracheomalacia, lymph nodes, or tumor)
  - Small airway obstruction (viral bronchiolitis, cystic fibrosis, bronchopulmonary dysplasia, heart disease)
  - Other causes (recurrent cough *not* due to asthma, aspiration/GERD)
- In adults
  - Chronic obstructive pulmonary disease, congestive heart failure, pulmonary embolism, benign or malignant tumor, pulmonary infiltration with eosinophilia, Churg-Strauss syndrome, drugs such as an ACE inhibitor, vocal cord dysfunction

DIAGNOSTIC TESTS & INTERPRETATION

Initial Tests (lab, imaging)

- Blood tests not required but may find eosinophilia or elevated serum IgE levels
- Spirometry: Normal test does not rule out asthma. It measures the FVC and the FEV_1. A reduced predicted ratio of FEV_1/FVC with reversibility (increase of 200 mL or 12% of FEV_1/FVC) after using a short-acting bronchodilator establishes the diagnosis.
- Bronchoprovocation (methacholine, histamine, cold air, or exercise) is used to simulate bronchoconstriction, which is very useful in atypical presentation/normal baseline spirometry. Abnormal test is not entirely specific for asthma, but normal test excludes asthma.
- Peak expiratory flow rates are inappropriate for diagnosis. Typically used for monitoring of symptoms in diagnosed asthma patients.
- Chest x-ray is used to exclude alternative diagnoses and to evaluate patients for complicating cardiopulmonary processes.

Follow-Up Tests & Special Considerations

Asthma action plan: Patients monitor their own symptoms and/or peak flow measurements.

Diagnostic Procedures/Other

- Allergy skin testing is not useful for diagnosis of asthma but may be considered to evaluate atopic triggers.
- Sweat testing if diagnosis of cystic fibrosis
- Arterial blood gases is indicated for patients with respiratory distress and hypoxia.

Test Interpretation

Inflammatory cell infiltration, edema, goblet cell hyperplasia, smooth muscle hyperplasia, thickened basement membrane

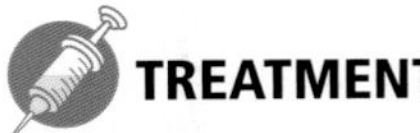

TREATMENT

GENERAL MEASURES

- Identify triggers and control exposures.
- Identify patients at risk for reactions to aspirin and NSAIDs and avoid exposure.
- All patients requiring inhaled agents should be prescribed with spacer (holding chamber) device.

MEDICATION

First Line

- Short-acting β-agonist (SABA) for quick relief of acute symptoms and to prevent exercise-induced bronchospasm (1)[A]:
  - SABA include albuterol and levalbuterol (Xopenex) (3).
- Anticholinergic agent
  - Ipratropium bromide: used in combination with SABA for acute treatment, mainly in the ED (1)[A]
- Systemic corticosteroids can be used
  - In all patients with acute asthma exacerbations (4)[A]
  - In moderate to severe asthma as adjunct
  - Prednisolone 1–2 mg/kg/day or equivalent for up to 7 days in adults and for 3 days in children with no need for tapering (4)[A]

ALERT

- HFA inhalers provide smaller particle size, better lung deposition, and less oropharyngeal deposition.
- All metered-dose inhalers (MDIs) need to be primed before use.
- Reserve nebulized delivery of medication for those unable to use spacer (e.g., infants, those intubated).
- All short-acting agents are pregnancy Category C.

Second Line

For long-term control:

- Inhaled corticosteroids (ICS)
  - Most potent and effective long-term controller therapy for children and adults with persistent asthma and persistent asthma during pregnancy (1)[A]
  - Advice patients to rinse their mouth after inhalation to reduce adverse effects (1)[B].
  - Long-acting β_2-agonists (LABA)
    - Salmeterol or formoterol
    - Should not be used as monotherapy (1)[A]; doing so leads to an increased risk of severe outcomes, including death
  - Combination products, including a LABA and ICS, are available and are indicated if ICS alone do not provide control; preferred in moderate and severe persistent disease (1,3)[A]. This is not recommended to treat acute symptoms or exacerbation (1)[A].
  - Leukotriene receptor agonists: alternative, not preferable, for mild and moderate persistent asthma (1)[A]
    - Montelukast or zafirlukast (patients ≥5 years)
  - Lipoxygenase pathway inhibitor: alternative, not preferred for adjunctive treatment in adults (1)[A]: zileuton (patients ≥12 years)
  - Theophylline: not preferred as adjunctive therapy with inhaled corticosteroids (1)[A]. Monitoring of serum theophylline level is essential.
  - Cromolyn sodium and nedocromil are also alternatives; not preferred options for mild persistent asthma (1)[A]; can also be used before exercise and exposure to allergens for prevention of asthma
  - Immunomodulators
    - Omalizumab: adjunctive; not preferred therapy for patients ≥12 years with allergies and severe persistent asthma (1)[B]

ISSUES FOR REFERRAL

Referral to an asthma specialist (either a pulmonologist or an allergist) should be considered when

- Diagnosis unclear
- Additional asthma education needed
- Comorbidities: rhinitis, GERD, sinusitis, OSA
- Specialized testing (e.g., bronchoprovocation, skin testing)
- Specialized treatments (e.g., immunotherapy, anti-IgE therapy)
- Poorly controlled, moderate to severe persistent asthma in adults
- Moderate to persistent asthma in children
- Poorly controlled asthma: multiple emergency room visits for asthma

Pregnancy Considerations

- Poorly controlled asthma results in low birth weight, increased prematurity, and perinatal mortality.
- Albuterol is the preferred SABA, and budesonide is the preferred ICS due to excellent safety profile (1).
- Other ICS agents are pregnancy Category C, but no data indicate their unsafety in pregnancy (1). Montelukast and zafirlukast are Category B but are not studied extensively in pregnancy.

ADDITIONAL THERAPIES

- Allergen immunotherapy when clear relationship between symptoms and exposure to an unavoidable allergen
- Omalizumab (Xolair): anti-IgE therapy, approved for patients >12 years with moderate to severe asthma

INPATIENT CONSIDERATIONS

Admission Criteria/Initial Stabilization

No single measure is predictive:

- Dyspnea/hypoxia
- Poor or no response to SABA
- Peak expiratory flow (PEF) or FEV_1 <40%
- Decision for admission should be based on duration and severity of symptoms, severity of airflow obstruction, response to ED treatment, course and severity of prior exacerbations, access to medical care and medication, and adequacy of home condition (1).
- Supplemental oxygen to correct hypoxemia
- Repeated doses or continuous administration of SABA (1)[A]
- Ipratropium bromide may be used in the ED but is not for inpatient treatment (1)[B].
- Systemic corticosteroids for acute exacerbations (1)[A]
- Adjunctive therapy with $MgSO_4$ or helium–oxygen mixture (heliox) may be considered in severe cases (1)[B].

IV Fluids

- Avoid aggressive hydration in older children and adults.
- Monitor electrolytes.

Nursing

- Careful respiratory monitoring, including vital signs, pulse oximetry, response and duration of response to SABA, and, when possible, an objective measure of lung function such as PEF or FEV_1
- Asthma education

Discharge Criteria

- Minimal or absent asthma symptoms
- Hypoxia has resolved.
- FEV_1 or PEF ≥70% predicted or personal best
- Bronchodilator response sustained ≥60 minutes

ONGOING CARE

FOLLOW-UP RECOMMENDATIONS

Smoking cessation counseling or elimination of secondhand smoke, if applicable

Patient Monitoring

- Quality-of-life measures: impact on activities, sleep, ED visits/hospitalizations, and so forth
- Pharmacotherapy: efficacy, compliance, side effects, technique
- Peak flow to evaluate if cough is due to exacerbation in those with known asthma

DIET

Food allergies and sulfites (in food and wine) can precipitate symptoms for some patients.

PATIENT EDUCATION

- Patients' care plan and inhaled medication technique at every visit
- American Academy of Allergy, Asthma & Immunology: 800-822-2762 or www.aaaai.org
- American Lung Association: www.lungusa.org
- Asthma and Allergy Foundation of America: 800-727-8462 or www.aafa.org
- Mattress and pillow covers DO NOT improve outcomes and should not be recommended.

PROGNOSIS

- Prognosis is good for male patients, nonsmokers, and children with mild disease.
- Asthma worsens in 1/3 of women during pregnancy and improves in another 1/3.

COMPLICATIONS

- Atelectasis
- Pneumonia
- Air leak syndromes: pneumomediastinum, pneumothorax
- Medication-specific side effects/adverse effects/interactions
- Respiratory failure
- Death: ~50% of asthma deaths occur in the elderly (age >65 years), and mortality is increasing in that population (5).

REFERENCES

1. National Heart, Lung, and Blood Institute. *National Asthma Education and Prevention Program Expert Panel Report 3: Guidelines for the Diagnosis and Management of Asthma*. Washington, DC: National Institutes of Health; 2007. NIH publication 08-5846.
2. Reddel HK, Taylor DR, Bateman ED, et al. An official American Thoracic Society/European Respiratory Society statement: asthma control and exacerbations: standardizing endpoints for clinical asthma trials and clinical practice. *Am J Respir Crit Care Med*. 2009;180(1):59–99.
3. Fanta CH. Asthma. *N Engl J Med*. 2009;360(10):1002–1014.
4. Doherty S. Prescribe systemic corticosteroids in acute asthma. *BMJ*. 2009;338:b1234.
5. Stupka E, deShazo R. Asthma in seniors: part 1. Evidence for underdiagnosis, undertreatment, and increasing morbidity and mortality. *Am J Med*. 2009;122(1):6–11.

ADDITIONAL READING

Dombrowski MP, Schatz M; ACOG Committee on Practice Bulletins-Obstetrics. ACOG practice bulletin: clinical management guidelines for obstetrician-gynecologists number 90, February 2008: asthma in pregnancy. *Obstet Gynecol*. 2008;111(2, Pt 1): 457–464.

SEE ALSO

Algorithm: Asthma Exacerbation, Pediatric Acute

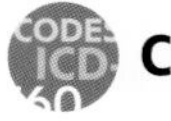

CODES

ICD10

- J45.909 Unspecified asthma, uncomplicated
- J45.901 Unspecified asthma with (acute) exacerbation
- J45.20 Mild intermittent asthma, uncomplicated

CLINICAL PEARLS

- SABA is the most effective rescue therapy for acute asthma symptoms.
- ICSs are the preferred long-term control therapy for patients of all ages.
- Peak flow is an inexpensive and easily available monitoring device once the diagnosis of asthma has been established.

ATELECTASIS

Frank J. Domino, MD

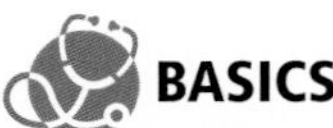

BASICS

DESCRIPTION

- Atelectasis is defined as incomplete expansion of lung tissue.
- The collapse of lung tissue and resultant loss of lung volume and function are due to various causes broadly defined in two groups:
  - Obstructive: blockage of an airway
  - Nonobstructive: loss of contact between the parietal and visceral pleurae, replacement of lung tissue by scarring or infiltrative disease, surfactant dysfunction, and parenchymal compression
- Symptoms and signs are determined by the rapidity with which the bronchial occlusion occurs, the size of the lung area affected, and the presence or absence of lung disease and comorbidities.
- Reduced respiratory gas exchange, leading to hypoxemia if severe

EPIDEMIOLOGY

- Affects all ages; mean age of presentation is 60 years.
- Male = female. No racial predilection.

Incidence

- Round atelectasis (see "Imaging") is high in asbestos workers (65–70%).
- Incidence of lobar atelectasis depends on the collateral ventilation within each individual lung lobe.

Prevalence

Postoperative atelectasis is extremely common, affecting up to 90% of patients.

ETIOLOGY AND PATHOPHYSIOLOGY

- Obstructive (resorptive) atelectasis (most common); causes intrinsic respiratory blockage
  - Due to luminal blockage (foreign body, mucus plug, asthma, cystic fibrosis, trauma, tumor) or airway wall abnormality (congenital malformation, emphysema)
  - Distal to the obstruction, air is reabsorbed from the alveoli into the deoxygenated venous system, causing complete collapse of the alveolar tissue.
- Nonobstructive atelectasis
  - Passive atelectasis: results from pleural membrane separation of the visceral and parietal layers
    - Pleural effusion, pneumothorax
  - Compression atelectasis: alveoli compression leading to diminished resting volume (functional residual capacity [FRC]):
    - Space-occupying lesions, lymphadenopathy, cardiomegaly, abscess, chest wall pressure
  - Adhesive atelectasis: surfactant dysfunction, resulting in increased surface tension and alveoli collapse
    - Respiratory distress syndrome, acute respiratory distress syndrome (ARDS), radiation exposure, smoke inhalation, uremia
  - Cicatrization: pleural or parenchymal scarring
    - Granulomatous disease, toxic inhalation, drug-induced fibrosis (e.g., amiodarone), radiation exposure
  - Replacement atelectasis: diffuse tumor manifestation resulting in complete lobar collapse
    - Bronchioalveolar cell carcinoma
- Rounded atelectasis: distinct form of atelectasis following asbestos exposure
- Other
  - Hypoxemia due to pulmonary embolus
  - Muscular weakness (anesthesia, neuromuscular disease)
- Obstructive atelectasis
  - There are 3 collateral ventilation systems in each lobe: the pores of Kohn, canals of Lambert, and fenestrations of Boren. The patency and formation of the systems depends on multiple factors including age, lung disease, and FiO_2.
  - Age: Due to the late development of collaterals in children, atelectasis is frequently diagnosed after foreign body aspiration.
  - Emphysema: The fenestra of Boren in emphysematous patients often become enlarged; this enlargement can lead to a delay in atelectasis despite an obstructing lesion or mass.
  - FiO_2: Oxygen rapidly dissociates from the alveoli to deoxygenated vessels in an obstructed airway. The 79% nitrogen in atmospheric air has a much slower rate of dissociation from the alveoli and thereby prevents collapse by maintaining a positive pressure inside the alveoli. With increased FiO_2, the concentration of nitrogen is decreased, predisposing the patient to a rapid development of atelectasis at the onset of obstruction.

RISK FACTORS

- General anesthesia
  - Positive fluid balance, ≥4 units blood transfusion, use of nasogastric tube, long-acting muscle relaxants, hypothermia, postoperative epidural anesthesia, ventilator settings with high tidal volume and plateau pressure
- Common postoperatively, particularly following thoracic or upper abdominal surgery, neurosurgery, orofacial and neck surgery, surgery >3 hours in duration, emergency surgery, and vascular surgery
- Risk factors for developing atelectasis after surgery:
  - Age >60 and <6 years, chronic obstructive pulmonary disease (COPD), obstructive sleep apnea, CHF, alcohol abuse, pulmonary hypertension, albumin <3.5 g/dL, hemoglobin <10 g/dL, BMI >27 kg/m^2, ASA class II+ functional dependence in activities of daily living (ADL), heart failure, smoking
- Intensive care and prolonged immobilization
- Brock syndrome: recurrent right middle lobe collapse secondary to airway disease, infection, or a combination thereof. The right middle lobe airway is long and thin and has the poorest drainage and clearance of all the lobes, resulting in trapped mucus.

GENERAL PREVENTION

- Encourage activity; breathing exercises, frequent changes in body position, coughing, and early mobilization. However, further large randomized controlled trials are needed before conclusions can be made regarding the effect of chest physiotherapy and incentive spirometry on postoperative pulmonary complications and mortality.
- Ventilator settings during anesthesia with high tidal volumes (Vt >10 mL/kg), high plateau pressures (>30 cm H_2O), and without positive end-expiratory pressure (PEEP) are associated with postoperative pulmonary complications such as pneumonia and respiratory failure:
  - Ventilator-induced lung injury can be minimized by using low Vt and plateau pressures at sufficient PEEP, while maintaining lower FiO_2 during anesthetic induction and intraoperatively.
- Application of continuous positive airway pressure (CPAP) during anesthesia induction and reversal of anesthesia-induced atelectasis after intubation by a recruitment maneuver may decrease postoperative pulmonary complications.

COMMONLY ASSOCIATED CONDITIONS

- COPD and asthma
- Trauma
- ARDS, neonatal respiratory distress syndrome, pulmonary edema, pulmonary embolism
- Neuromuscular disorders (muscular dystrophy, spinal muscular atrophy, spinal cord injury), cystic fibrosis
- Respiratory syncytial virus (RSV), bronchiolitis
- Bronchial stenosis, pulmonic valve disease, pulmonary hypertension
- Pneumonia, pleural effusion, pneumothorax

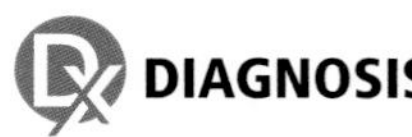

DIAGNOSIS

HISTORY

- Frequently asymptomatic
- Tachypnea and sudden-onset dyspnea
- Nonproductive cough
- Pleuritic pain on affected side
- History of smoking, radiation, asbestos, or other air pollutants

PHYSICAL EXAM

- Hypoxia, cyanosis
- Tracheal or precordial impulse displacement toward the affected side
- Bronchial breathing if airway is patent or absent breath sounds if airway is occluded
- Diminished chest expansion
- Wheezing may be heard with focal obstruction, dullness to percussion over the involved area.

DIFFERENTIAL DIAGNOSIS

The differential is found under "Etiology."

DIAGNOSTIC TESTS & INTERPRETATION

Initial Tests (lab, imaging)

- CBC and sputum culture if infection is suspected
- ABG: Despite hypoxemia, the partial pressure of carbon dioxide in $PaCO_2$ level is usually normal or low.
- Chest x-ray (CXR), posterior-anterior and lateral
  - Raised diaphragm, flattened chest wall, movement of fissures and mediastinal structures toward the atelectatic region
  - Unaffected lung may show compensatory hyperinflation.
  - Wedge-shaped densities: obstructive atelectasis
  - Small, linear bands (Fleischner lines) often at lung bases: discoid (subsegmental or plate) atelectasis
  - Lobar collapse
    - Direct signs: displacement of fissures and opacification of the collapsed lobe
  - Indirect signs: displacement of the hilum, mediastinal shift toward the side of collapse, loss of volume on ipsilateral hemithorax, elevation of ipsilateral diaphragm, crowding of the ribs, compensatory hyperlucency of the remaining lobes, and silhouetting of the diaphragm or the heart border
  - Right upper lobe collapse may display the Golden inverted S sign, suggesting neoplastic shift of the minor fissure.
  - Air bronchograms: Evidence of pleural fluid or air may indicate compressive atelectasis.
  - Adhesive atelectasis may present as a diffuse reticular granular pattern, progressing to a pulmonary edema pattern and finally to bilateral opacification in severe cases.

- Pleural-based round density on CXR: round atelectasis
- Complete atelectasis of an entire lung: opacification of the entire hemithorax and an ipsilateral shift of the mediastinum

Follow-Up Tests & Special Considerations

Albumin level: Low serum albumin level (<3.5 g/L) is a powerful marker of increased risk for postoperative pulmonary complications, including atelectasis.

- Chest CT or MRI may be indicated to visualize airway and mediastinal structures and to identify cause of atelectasis.
- Pulmonary function tests (PFTs) may detect restrictive disease, decreased respiratory muscle pressures, or airflow obstruction.

Diagnostic Procedures/Other

Bronchoscopy to assess airway patency in unexplained or refractory cases

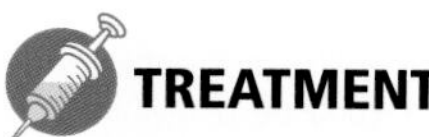

TREATMENT

GENERAL MEASURES

- If known, treat the underlying cause.
- Ensure patient is lying on the unaffected side to promote drainage:
  - Maximize patient mobility and encourage frequent coughing and deep breathing every hour.
- Incentive spirometry
  - Evidence has not shown that incentive spirometry prevents postoperative pulmonary complications in CABG (1)[A].
- Initiate intubation and mechanical ventilation with PEEP in severe respiratory distress or hypoxemia:
  - Lower tidal volume (6 mL/kg) and lower end-inspiratory values (<30 mm Hg) are associated with reduced mortality.
  - PEEP 15–20 mL may be necessary to maintain arterial O_2 saturation in surfactant-impaired states.
- Postsurgical measures include positive airway pressure, continuous or intermittent.

MEDICATION

First Line

Therapies directed at basic cause:

- Antibiotics for infection
- Chemo/radiation therapy for tumor
- Steroids for asthma
- Analgesia for pain control to permit deep inspiration and coughing

Pediatric Considerations

- RhDNase may be effective in clearing mucinous secretions in persistent atelectasis in children.
- Chest physiotherapy including percussion, drainage, deep insufflation, and saline lavage is a common treatment in the prevention and treatment of atelectasis in the hospital setting. However, caution is required when interpreting the possible positive effects of chest physiotherapy as the numbers of babies studied are small, the results are not consistent across trials, data on safety are insufficient, and applicability to current practice may be limited.
- The application of continuous distending pressure has been shown to have some benefits in the treatment of preterm infants with respiratory distress syndrome. Continuous distending pressure has the potential to reduce lung damage particularly if applied early, before atelectasis has occurred (2)[A].

Second Line

Bronchofibroscopy in aspiration of inspissated secretions in atelectasis has been efficacious in several studies. However, counterevidence continues to question its efficacy in the treatment of atelectasis.

Pediatric Considerations

In obstructive atelectasis, bronchoscopy remains controversial. In the presence of a mucus plug or cast, bronchoscopy may be beneficial.

SURGERY/OTHER PROCEDURES

Only for resectable underlying disease (e.g., tumor, severe lymphadenopathy), bronchoscopy

INPATIENT CONSIDERATIONS

Admission Criteria/Initial Stabilization

Ensure adequate oxygenation (may start with 100% FiO_2 then taper) and humidification.

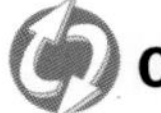

ONGOING CARE

FOLLOW-UP RECOMMENDATIONS

Patient Monitoring

- Varies with cause and patient status
- In simple atelectasis associated with asthma or infection, outpatient visits are adequate.

PATIENT EDUCATION

Maximize patient mobility and encourage frequent coughing and deep breathing every hour.

PROGNOSIS

- Spontaneous resolution usually occurs within 24 hours but can persist for days after surgery.
- The prognosis of lobar atelectasis secondary to endobronchial obstruction depends on treatment of the underlying malignancy.
- Surgical therapy is needed only for resectable causes or if chronic infection and bronchiectasis supervene.

COMPLICATIONS

- Pneumonia
- Acute atelectasis
  - Hypoxemia and respiratory failure
  - Postobstructive drowning of the lung
- Chronic atelectasis
  - Bronchiectasis
  - Pleural effusion and empyema

REFERENCES

1. Freitas ER, Soares BG, Cardoso JR, et al. Incentive spirometry for preventing pulmonary complications after coronary artery bypass graft. *Cochrane Database Syst Rev*. 2007;(3):CD004466.
2. Ho JJ, Henderson-Smart DJ, Davis PG. Early versus delayed initiation of continuous distending pressure for respiratory distress syndrome in preterm infants. *Cochrane Database Syst Rev*. 2002;(2):CD002975.

ADDITIONAL READING

- Brower RG. Consequences of bed rest. *Crit Care Med*. 2009;37(10)(Suppl):S422–S428.
- Deng J, Zheng Y, Li C, et al. Plastic bronchitis in three children associated with 2009 influenza A(H1N1) virus infection. *Chest*. 2010;138(6):1486–1488.
- Ferreyra G, Long Y, Ranieri VM, et al. Respiratory complications after major surgery. *Curr Opin Crit Care*. 2009;15(4):342–348.
- Flenady VJ, Gray PH. Chest physiotherapy for preventing morbidity in babies being extubated from mechanical ventilation. *Cochrane Database Syst Rev*. 2002;(2):CD000283.
- Guimarães MM, El Dib R, Smith AF, et al. Incentive spirometry for prevention of postoperative pulmonary complications in upper abdominal surgery. *Cochrane Database Syst Rev*. 2009;(3):CD006058.
- Hendriks T, de Hoog M, Lequin MH, et al. DNase and atelectasis in non-cystic fibrosis pediatric patients. *Crit Care*. 2005;9(4):R351–R356.
- McCunn M, Sutcliffe AJ, Mauritz W, et al. Guidelines for management of mechanical ventilation in critically injured patients. *Trauma Care*. 2004;14(4):147–151.
- Qaseem A, Snow V, Fitterman N, et al. Risk assessment for and strategies to reduce perioperative pulmonary complications for patients undergoing noncardiothoracic surgery: a guideline from the American College of Physicians. *Ann Intern Med*. 2006;144(8):575–580.
- Tusman G, Böhm SH, Warner DO, et al. Atelectasis and perioperative pulmonary complications in high-risk patients. *Curr Opin Anaesthesiol*. 2012;25(1):1–10.
- Wu KH, Lin CF, Huang CJ, et al. Rigid ventilation bronchoscopy under general anesthesia for treatment of pediatric pulmonary atelectasis caused by pneumonia: a review of 33 cases. *Int Surg*. 2006;91(5):291–294.

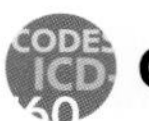

CODES

ICD10

J98.11 Atelectasis

CLINICAL PEARLS

- Bronchogenic carcinoma, which may present with atelectasis, must be excluded in all patients >35 years.
- In complete atelectasis of an entire lung, the mediastinal ipsilateral shift separates atelectasis from massive pleural effusion.
- Low serum albumin is a powerful predictor of postoperative pulmonary complications, including atelectasis.
- Anesthesia-induced atelectasis occurs in almost all anesthetized patients.

ATRIAL FIBRILLATION AND ATRIAL FLUTTER

Youhua Zhang, MD, PhD • Bianca Lee

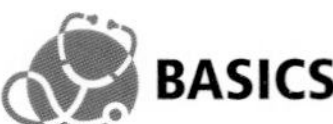

BASICS

This topic covers both atrial fibrillation (AFib) and atrial flutter (AFlut).

DESCRIPTION

- AFib: Paroxysmal or continuous supraventricular tachyarrhythmia characterized by rapid, uncoordinated atrial electrical activity and an irregularly irregular ventricular response. In most patients, the ventricular rate is rapid because the atrioventricular (AV) node is bombarded with very frequent atrial electrical impulses (400–600 bpm).
- AFlut: Paroxysmal or continuous supraventricular tachyarrhythmia with rapid but organized atrial electrical activity. The atrial rate is typically between 250 and 350 bpm and is often manifested as "saw-tooth" flutter (F) waves on the ECG, particularly in the inferior leads and V_1. AFlut commonly occurs with 2:1 or 3:1 AV block, so the ventricular response may be regular and typically at a rate of ~150 bpm.
- AFib and AFlut are related arrhythmias, sometimes seen in the same patient. Distinguishing the two is important as there may be implications for management.
- Clinical classifications:
  - Paroxysmal: self-terminating episodes, usually <7 days
  - Persistent: sustained >7 days, usually requiring pharmacologic or DC cardioversion to restore sinus rhythm
  - Permanent: Sinus rhythm cannot be restored or maintained. It is a shared decision between patient and clinician as to when to cease further attempts to restore and/or maintain sinus rhythm.
- Lone AFib occurs in patients <60 years (with possible genetic predisposition) who have no clinical or echocardiographic evidence of cardiovascular disease, including hypertension (HTN).

EPIDEMIOLOGY

- Incidence/prevalence increases significantly with age.
- Young patients with AFib, particularly lone AFib, are most commonly males.

Incidence

- AFib: from <0.1%/year <40 years to >1.5%/year >80 years
- Lifetime risk: 25% for those ≥40 years
- AFlut is less common.

Prevalence

- Estimated at 0.4–1% in general population, with 2.2 million patients in America
- Increase with age, up to 8% in those ≥80 years

ETIOLOGY AND PATHOPHYSIOLOGY

- Cardiac: HTN, ischemic heart disease, heart failure, valvular heart disease, cardiomyopathy, pericarditis, and infiltrative heart disease
- Pulmonary: pulmonary embolism (PE), chronic obstructive pulmonary disease (COPD), obstructive sleep apnea, pneumonia
- Ingestion: ethanol, caffeine
- Endocrine: hyperthyroidism, diabetes
- Obesity
- Postoperative: cardiac, pulmonary, or esophageal
- Idiopathic: lone AFib
- Patients with paroxysmal episodes are usually associated with premature atrial beats and/or bursts of tachycardia, originating in pulmonary vein ostia or other sites.
- Many patients with AFib are thought to have some degree of atrial fibrosis or scarring. This is often subclinical and usually not detectable with current cardiac imaging techniques but plays an important role in the pathogenesis of the arrhythmia.
- Autonomic (vagal and sympathetic) tone may play a role in triggering the arrhythmia.
- The presence of AFib is associated with electrical and structural remodeling processes that promote arrhythmia maintenance in the atria, termed "AFib begets AFib."

Genetics

Familial forms are rare but do exist. There are ongoing efforts to identify the genetic underpinnings of such cases.

RISK FACTORS

Age, HTN, and obesity are the most important risk factors for both AFib and AFlut.

GENERAL PREVENTION

Adequate control of HTN may prevent development of AFib due to hypertensive heart disease and is the most significant modifiable risk factor for AFib. Weight reduction may decrease the risk of AFib in obese patients. Ethanol consumption may trigger AFib in some.

COMMONLY ASSOCIATED CONDITIONS

HTN and other cardiac diseases

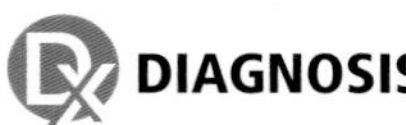

DIAGNOSIS

HISTORY

Symptoms vary from none to mild (palpitations, lightheadedness, fatigue, poor exercise capacity) to severe (angina, dyspnea, syncope).

PHYSICAL EXAM

- AFib: irregularly irregular heart rate and pulse, frequently tachycardiac
- AFlut: similar to AFib but may have regular pulse

DIFFERENTIAL DIAGNOSIS

- Multifocal atrial tachycardia
- Sinus tachycardia with frequent atrial premature beats
- Paroxysmal supraventricular tachycardia (Wolff-Parkinson-White [WPW], atrioventricular nodal reentry tachycardia [AVNRT])

DIAGNOSTIC TESTS & INTERPRETATION

- AFib: The ECG is diagnostic, with findings of low-amplitude fibrillatory waves without discrete P waves and an irregularly irregular pattern of QRS complexes. There is often tachycardia in the absence of heart rate–controlling medications (1).
- AFlut: The ECG is again diagnostic. Saw-tooth flutter waves are the classic sign, generally best seen in the inferior leads, although ventricular rate may need to be slowed to see the waves. QRS complexes may be regular or irregular; there is usually tachycardia (1).
- Ambulatory rhythm monitoring (e.g., telemetry, Holter monitoring, event recorders) is helpful in diagnosing paroxysmal AFib or AFlut and monitoring for recurrence (1)[C].

Initial Tests (lab, imaging)

TSH, electrolytes, CBC, PT/INR (if anticoagulation is contemplated); digoxin level (if appropriate)

Follow-Up Tests & Special Considerations

- Occasional Holter monitoring and/or exercise stress testing to assess for adequacy of rate and/or rhythm control
- Chest x-ray (CXR) for cardiopulmonary disease
- ECG for signs of cardiac hypertrophy, ischemia, and/or other arrhythmias
- Transesophageal echocardiogram to detect left atrial appendage thrombus if cardioversion is planned
- Sleep study may be useful if sleep apnea is suspected.

Test Interpretation

- Atrial dilatation and fibrosis
- Atrial thrombus, especially in atrial appendage
- Valvular/rheumatic disease
- Cardiomyopathy

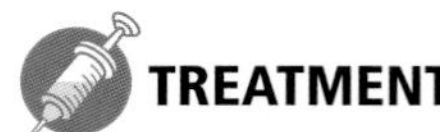

TREATMENT

MEDICATION

- 2 primary issues in the management of AFib and/or AFlut:
  - Decisions on heart rate control (control ventricular rate while allowing AFib to continue) or rhythm control (terminate AFib and restore normal sinus rhythm)
  - Anticoagulation therapy to prevent thromboembolism (primarily stroke)
- Anticoagulation guidelines (the same for AFib and AFlut) (1,2)[C]:
  - Unless contraindicated, patients with AFib or AFlut with any high-risk factors for stroke (prior transient ischemic attack [TIA]/cerebrovascular accident [CVA]/thromboembolism) should receive long-term warfarin therapy to maintain an INR of 2.0–3.0 (1,3)[A]. Patients with mechanical valves should maintain an INR >2.5 (2)[B]. For patients with AFib and mitral stenosis, a target INR range of 2.0–3.0 is recommended (2)[B].
  - Dabigatran (Pradaxa), a direct thrombin inhibitor, and apixaban (Eliquis) and rivaroxaban (Xarelto), factor Xa inhibitors, have recently been approved as alternatives to warfarin for the prevention of 1st and recurrent stroke in patients with nonvalvular AFib (1,3)[B]. The selection of an antithrombotic should be individualized; consider the risks of each agent, cost, patient preference, and tolerability. ALERT: Renal function should be evaluated prior to initiation of direct thrombin or factor Xa inhibitors (1)[B]. Dosing of such agents may in fact need individualized adjustment.
  - $CHADS_2$ scoring (**C**HF [1 point], **H**TN [1 point], **A**ge ≥75 [1 point], **D**M [1 point], prior **S**troke or TIA [2 points])
    - Patients with a score ≥2 (high risk) should receive anticoagulation unless contraindicated (2,3)[A]. In patients with a prior history of stroke or TIA who are unable to take anticoagulants, aspirin alone is recommended (3)[A].
    - Patients with a score of 1 (intermediate risk) should be treated with anticoagulation or aspirin (81–325 mg/day) (3)[A].
    - In patients with a score of 0 (low risk) (including most patients with lone AFib), aspirin (81–325 mg/day) or no treatment is recommended (3)[A].
  - Combination therapy of clopidogrel and aspirin is not recommended for patients with a hemorrhagic contraindication to warfarin (3)[B].
  - CHA_2DS_2VASc index further refines the risk calculation of $CHADS_2$ with the addition of **V**ascular disease (defined as history of MI, PAD, or complex aortic plaque), **A**ge 65–74 years (1 point; 2 points for age ≥75 years), female **S**ex **c**ategory (1 point)

(1–3). Anticoagulation generally recommended for score ≥2 (1)[B].
  - Anticoagulation recommendations are independent of AFib pattern (paroxysmal, persistent, and permanent) (1,2)[B] although ongoing efforts to better understand who may be at greater and lesser risk of thromboembolism continue.
- 4 classes of medications are available to achieve ventricular rate control: β-blockers (i.e., metoprolol), nondihydropyridine calcium channel blockers (i.e., verapamil, diltiazem), digoxin, and amiodarone. Optimal target for ventricular rate has not been firmly established, but there is evidence that aggressive control of the ventricular rate (<80 bpm) offers no benefit beyond more modest rate control (i.e., resting heart rate <110 bpm) (1,4)[B].
- Preventing rapid ventricular response (RVR) rates using AV nodal blocking medications is also often effective at controlling a patient's symptoms associated with AFib or AFlut. Patients in whom rate control cannot be achieved or who continue to have persistent symptoms despite reasonable heart rate control may require attempts at restoration of sinus rhythm.
- Of note, ventricular rate control can often be difficult to achieve in AFlut due to the more organized nature of the atrial electrical activity. For this reason, conversion to sinus rhythm is often the preferred strategy, and catheter ablation is also considered as a 1st-line treatment in recurrent AFlut (1).
- Restoration of sinus rhythm using electrical or pharmacologic cardioversion may significantly reduce the symptom burden of AFib or AFlut in many patients and may also be useful for controlling ventricular rate. Cardioversion does not impact the long-term risk/benefit ratio of anticoagulation:
  - Cardioversion is most often performed electrically, but may also be achieved using antiarrhythmic drug therapy in some instances, by experienced clinicians (1)[A].
  - If duration of AFib is >48 hours or unknown, anticoagulate for ≥3 weeks before cardioversion to reduce the risk of stroke. Alternatively, once anticoagulation is established, a transesophageal echo may be performed to exclude the presence of left atrial thrombus, allowing cardioversion to proceed. After cardioversion, anticoagulation should be continued for ≥4 weeks in all patients in whom duration of AFib/AFlut is >48 hours, as the postcardioversion period is a time of increased stroke risk (1,2)[B].
- Randomized clinical trials (AFFIRM and RACE) comparing the outcomes of rate versus rhythm control found no difference in morbidity, mortality, and stroke rates in patients assigned to one therapy or the other (1).
- Chronic PO antiarrhythmic therapy to suppress AFib recurrence is available for appropriately selected patients. Expert consultation is recommended owing to the complexities of safe antiarrhythmic drug selection.

ISSUES FOR REFERRAL

Management of AFib or AFlut refractory to standard medical therapy (i.e., unable to achieve adequate rate control with medication or development of significant bradycardia with treatment) may require the use of more aggressive treatments. These may include pacemaker implantation (to allow for more intensive pharmacologic blocking of the AV node) or an ablation procedure. AFlut in particular is often very amenable to ablation; thus, consideration should be given to early expert referral in appropriate patients. Antiarrhythmic drug therapy can often be very effective but should be prescribed by experienced practitioners.

SURGERY/OTHER PROCEDURES

- Electrophysiologic study and ablation may be considered for patients with either AFib or AFlut. In the case of AFlut, ablation is often a relatively straightforward procedure generally viewed as a 1st-line therapy due to its high rate of success in appropriate candidates. Ablation of AFib is a much more complex procedure with a more variable success rate; it continues to evolve. Thus, it is typically reserved for drug refractory patients.
- Cardiac surgery (e.g., the maze procedure, ligation of the left atrial appendage) may be considered in patients planning to undergo cardiac surgery for other reasons. Surgical therapy in isolation is rarely indicated for AFib or AFlut.

INPATIENT CONSIDERATIONS

Admission Criteria/Initial Stabilization

- Patients with significant symptoms, RVR, AFib/AFlut triggered by an acute process (e.g., MI, CHF, PE), or in whom antiarrhythmic therapy is being started likely require admission to the hospital for a period of stabilization.
- Outpatient management is reasonable for low-risk patients with controlled ventricular rates.
- Acute therapy for symptomatic or hemodynamically compromised patients with AFib or AFlut:
  - IV β- or nondihydropyridine calcium channel blockers for control of ventricular rate. Once hemodynamically stable, oral medications may be administered (1)[B].
- Commonly used therapies in the acute setting include (1,5):
  - Metoprolol: 2.5–5.0 mg IV bolus over 2 minutes; up to 3 doses
  - Diltiazem: 0.25 mg/kg IV bolus over 2 minutes, then 5–15 mg/hr
  - Some patients will be far more responsive to 1 class of agents than another. For this reason, if rate control is difficult to achieve, switching drug classes may be useful.
- Urgent cardioversion should be performed in hemodynamically unstable patients (1)[B]. It is somewhat unusual for AFib or AFlut alone to cause marked hemodynamic insult; thus, the possibility of a concurrent process should be considered in this setting.
- Consider the initiation of PO anticoagulation therapy. Inpatients may be "bridged" with IV or SC heparin or SQ low-molecular-weight heparin (LMWH) while waiting for warfarin to become effective (1)[C].

Discharge Criteria

Adequate rate or rhythm control without symptoms; long-term plan for anticoagulation established

ONGOING CARE

Many patients may benefit from elective expert consultation. In patients with no significant symptoms, if ventricular rate control or sinus rhythm is easily achieved and the choice of thromboembolic prevention is clear, management in a primary care setting may be appropriate.

FOLLOW-UP RECOMMENDATIONS

Patient Monitoring

- Adequate anticoagulation levels (if warfarin is employed) should be determined at least weekly during initiation and monthly when stable (1)[A]. Ventricular rate control should be assessed on a regular basis.

DIET

Patients on warfarin should attempt to consume a stable amount of vitamin K.

PROGNOSIS

Anticoagulation reduces the annual embolic stroke rate from ~5–6% per year to 1–2% for most patients. AFib and AFlut may increase morbidity and mortality, but the overall prognosis is a function of underlying heart disease and adherence with therapy. Reported risk of anticoagulation varies but lies between 1% and 4% per year for major hemorrhage.

COMPLICATIONS

- Embolic stroke
- Peripheral arterial embolization
- Bleeding with anticoagulation
- Tachycardia-induced cardiomyopathy with prolonged periods of inadequate rate control

REFERENCES

1. January CT, Wann LS, Alpert JS, et al. AHA/ACC/HRS 2014 guidelines for the management of patients with atrial fibrillation. *Circulation*. 2014;129:5–84.
2. You JJ, Singer DE, Howard PA, et al. Antithrombotic therapy for atrial fibrillation: antithrombotic therapy and prevention of thrombosis: American College of Chest Physicians Evidence-Based Clinical Practice Guidelines. *Chest*. 2012;141(2)(Suppl):e531S–e575S.
3. Furie KL, Goldstein LB, Albers GW, et al. Oral antithrombotic agents for the prevention of stroke in nonvalvular atrial fibrillation: a science advisory for healthcare professionals from the American Heart Association/American Stroke Association. *Stroke*. 2012;43(12):3442–3453.
4. Wann LS, Curtis AB, January CT, et al. 2011 ACCF/AHA/HRS focused update on the management of patients with atrial fibrillation (updating the 2006 guideline): a report of the American College of Cardiology Foundation/American Heart Association Task Force on Practice Guidelines. *Circulation*. 2011;123(1):104–123.
5. Neumar RW, Otto CW, Link MS, et al. Part 8: adult advanced cardiovascular life support: 2010 American Heart Association Guidelines for Cardiopulmonary Resuscitation and Emergency Cardiovascular Care. *Circulation*. 2010;122(18 Suppl 3):S729–S767.
6. Charlton B, Redberg R. The trouble with dabigatran. *BMJ*. 2014;349:g4681.

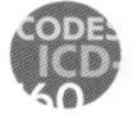

CODES

ICD10

- I48.91 Unspecified atrial fibrillation
- I48.92 Unspecified atrial flutter
- I48.0 Paroxysmal atrial fibrillation

CLINICAL PEARLS

- Primary decision in persistent AFib is whether to strive for rate control or rhythm control. Younger patients often do better with a rhythm control strategy, whereas older patients often do well with rate control. Decision is complex.
- Anticoagulate most patients with paroxysmal or persistent AFib/AFlut without contraindication

ATRIAL SEPTAL DEFECT

Daniel J. Stein, MD, MPH • Stephen K. Lane, MD, FAAFP

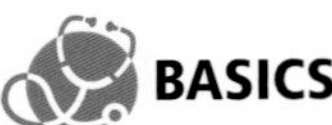

BASICS

DESCRIPTION

- Anatomy
  - Opening in the atrial septum allowing flow of blood between the two atria
  - Patent foramen ovale is similar but is not open most of the time, causes no hemodynamic disturbance, and is not considered an atrial septal defect (ASD) (no tissue defect).
- Types (by location in the interatrial septum) (1)
  - 75%: Ostium secundum defect occurs in the fossa ovalis region.
  - 15%: Ostium primum defect occurs in the inferior septum; often associated with cleft mitral valve and failure of endocardial cushion development.
  - 10%: Sinus venosus defect occurs in the superior-posterior septum near the orifice of the superior vena cava; usually associated with partial anomalous right upper pulmonary venous return.
- Hemodynamic effects
  - Left-to-right shunting in late ventricular systole and early diastole
  - Degree depends on size of the defect and relative pressures of the two ventricles.
  - Causes excessive blood flow through the right-sided circulation, ultimately leading to reactive pulmonary hypertension and heart failure
- Systems affected: cardiovascular; pulmonary

Pediatric Considerations

- Most cases of ASD are detected and corrected in the pediatric population.
- The smaller the defect and the younger the child, the greater the chance of spontaneous closure.

EPIDEMIOLOGY

Incidence

- Predominant age: present from birth, may be diagnosed at any age
- Slight female predominance (2)
- No race predilection
- 6–10/10,000 births (2)

Prevalence

Accounts for 10% of congenital heart defects and 25–30% of congenital heart defects detected in adulthood

ETIOLOGY AND PATHOPHYSIOLOGY

- Flow across ASD usually left-to-right shunt because of higher left-sided pressures:
  - Minimal right-to-left shunting in early ventricular systole, especially during inspiration
  - Increased right-sided pressure/pulmonary hypertension can cause reversal of shunt flow (Eisenmenger syndrome) with resulting cyanosis and clubbing.
- Symptoms typically occur due to right ventricular and pulmonary vascular volume overload and right-sided heart failure.

Genetics

- Most cases are spontaneous.
- 5% with chromosomal abnormalities; other rare mutations exist
- 25% prevalence in Down syndrome

RISK FACTORS

- Other congenital heart defects
- Family history (~7–10% recurrence)
- Thalidomide, alcohol exposure in utero, smoking, maternal age >35 years, and elevated blood glucose have been associated with increased risk (2).

COMMONLY ASSOCIATED CONDITIONS

- ASDs may occur as a component of other complex cardiac structural defects.
- Important to exclude anomalous pulmonary venous return
- Occasionally can indicate underlying genetic syndromes, for example: Holt-Oram (ASD present in 66%), Ellis-von-Creveld, or VACTERL Association
- Overall, ~70% isolated (1)

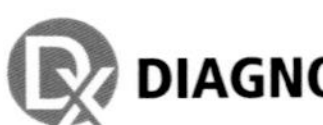

DIAGNOSIS

HISTORY

- Initially often asymptomatic
- Infants/children may be small for age, even in the absence of other symptoms. Patients will generally improve with surgical treatment.
- Most common symptoms are dyspnea on exertion, palpitations, and easy fatigability.
- Consider if history of right-sided heart failure (more advanced, only 10% at diagnosis), frequent respiratory tract infections, stroke, or unexplained end-organ infarcts due to paradoxical emboli
- Should be considered in children with other congenital heart defects, Down syndrome

PHYSICAL EXAM

- Signs vary according to extent of shunting.
- Cardiac auscultation
  - *Fixed, widely split S_2 (key physical finding)*
  - May also have
    - Systolic ejection murmur (pulmonic flow murmur)
    - Low-pitched diastolic rumble (tricuspid flow murmur)
    - Diastolic murmur (pulmonic regurgitation)
    - Systolic murmur (mitral regurgitation)
- Right ventricular heave
- Palpable pulmonary artery pulse at left upper sternal border
- If heart failure has developed, may hear a 4th heart sound (right-sided)
- Signs of Eisenmenger syndrome:
  - Cyanosis and clubbing
  - Jugular venous distention and edema

DIFFERENTIAL DIAGNOSIS

- Other congenital heart disease
- Right bundle branch block (for widely split S_2)

DIAGNOSTIC TESTS & INTERPRETATION

Initial Tests (lab, imaging)

- Echocardiography is 1st-line testing as it allows for characterization of the defect, does not involve radiation, is often diagnostic, and can be used to quantify hemodynamic significance (1)[C].
- Generally start with transthoracic Doppler imaging of the entire atrial septum (sensitivity is ~89% of secundum, ~100% of primum, and ~44% of sinus venosus ASDs), with progression to TEE if TTE is nondiagnostic
- Patients with right ventricular overload by transthoracic echocardiography (TTE) but an otherwise negative study should have further testing
- Oximetry: Cyanosis may suggest Eisenmenger syndrome (right-to-left shunting).
- ECG is not typically diagnostic, but findings include the following:
  - Right axis deviation
  - Right atrial enlargement (tall P in inferior leads)
  - Right ventricular conduction delay
  - Q wave in lead V_1
  - Right bundle branch block
  - Leftward axis, inverted P wave in lead III (sinus venosus)
  - Leftward axis (ostium primum)

Follow-Up Tests & Special Considerations

- Bubble contrast enhancement may be helpful.
- Transesophageal echocardiography (TEE) may be required to define ASD morphology and to locate the pulmonary veins; often used prior to percutaneous closure. TEE has excellent sensitivity and specificity.

Diagnostic Procedures/Other

- Cardiac catheterization (1)[C]
  - Demonstrates right ventricle enlargement, location/fraction of the shunt, size of the ASD, any valvular disease, and overall anatomy
  - Used to assess pulmonary vascular resistance if pulmonary hypertension is suspected, particularly if surgery is planned
  - Generally not used in young patients for initial diagnosis, more often reserved for use when
    - Part of a planned interventional closure
    - Evaluating other disease simultaneously (e.g., coronary artery disease)
    - Visualization by other methods insufficient
- Cardiac magnetic resonance: a noninvasive follow-up to echo that allows viewing the defect/pulmonary veins and measurement of shunt fraction and right ventricular function—particularly useful for sinus venosus defects (2)
- Exercise testing: useful to quantify symptoms not consistent with clinical findings or to document change over time (1)[C]
- Chest x-ray: may demonstrate right ventricular and pulmonary artery enlargement, increased pulmonary vascular markings
- Cardiac CT scans can also define ASDs but with significant radiation exposure.

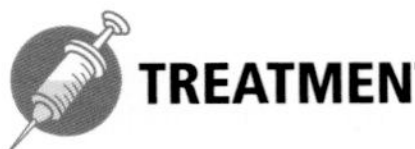

TREATMENT

GENERAL MEASURES

- 75% of small secundum ASDs (<8 mm) will close spontaneously by 18 months of age; however, close follow-up is warranted (3).
- The likelihood of spontaneous closure is mainly determined by defect diameter: >10 mm at time of diagnosis is unlikely to spontaneously close (4).
- Primum and sinus venosus defects do not generally close and generally require surgical closure (2).

MEDICATION

First Line

- Treatment of secondary atrial fibrillation/supraventricular tachycardia with anticoagulation and cardioversion, followed by anticoagulation with maintenance of sinus rhythm if possible, or rate control if this fails (1)[A]
- Respiratory tract infections should be treated promptly.
- Treatment of heart failure (diuretics, oxygen, digoxin, etc.)

Second Line

- No antibiotic prophylaxis is recommended for unrepaired ASDs.
- Antibiotic prophylaxis against infective endocarditis during dental or other oral procedures is recommended for 6 months by the American Heart Association (AHA) after a device or patch is placed (5)[B]:
  - In patients with repaired ASD who have a residual defect at or adjacent to the device, prophylaxis is recommended indefinitely.
  - If prophylaxis is indicated, for dental procedures, amoxicillin 2 g (adults) or 50 mg/kg (children). Other options include cephalosporins (e.g., ceftriaxone 1 g [adults] or 50 mg/kg [children] IM or IV) or clindamycin 600 mg PO (adults) or 20 mg/kg PO (children) or azithromycin 500 mg PO (adults) or 15 mg/kg (children) in patients who are penicillin-sensitive (6).
- To prevent thrombus formation after device deployment, aspirin 325 mg daily for 6 months and clopidogrel 75 mg for at least 1 month

ISSUES FOR REFERRAL

Appropriate health care: referral to a cardiologist and possibly cardiac surgeon for evaluation

SURGERY/OTHER PROCEDURES

- In children, many secundum defects <6 mm close by age 5 years. Closure is generally indicated in children with
  - Defect >8 mm (unlikely to close) in children older than 2 years of age (to allow time for spontaneous closure, even though uncommon)
  - Defects of any size in a child older than 5 years with related symptoms
- Closure for secundum defects is delayed until at least 2 years of age except for symptomatic defects (poor growth or exercise intolerance—rare) because of the high rate of spontaneous closure.
- Management of <8 mm asymptomatic secundum defects in children older than 5 years of age is controversial and follows adult guidelines for flow ratio (see below).
- In adults, secundum closure via percutaneous transcatheter device or surgery to reduce subsequent morbidity and mortality, if:
  - Right side heart enlargement regardless of symptoms (1)[B]
  - Pulmonary systemic flow ratio is 2:1 (or >1.5:1 and <21 years old according to the AHA)
  - Symptoms such as documented orthodeoxia/platypnea or paradoxical embolism (1)[C]
- Flow ratio can be measured with Doppler echo (lab specific) or cardiac catheterization.
- Surgical repair is standard for a sinus venosus, coronary sinus, or primum ASD (1),(2)[B]. These defects rarely close spontaneously and are not considered amenable to percutaneous closure.
- Percutaneous transcatheter device closure of secundum ASDs is standard and has largely replaced surgery except when other interventions are planned or anatomy is not favorable (7)[A].
- Secundum ASDs that are suitable for percutaneous closure should be ~35 mm in stretched balloon diameter and should have a sufficient rim of surrounding atrial tissue.
- Closure is not indicated for patients who have developed irreversible severe pulmonary hypertension without continued shunting or those who never develop symptoms and have an ASD <5 mm.
- Overall, closing small asymptomatic secundum ASDs is controversial and not often done.
- Radiofrequency ablation, either before or after closure, can be considered for patients with refractory atrial fibrillation (8).

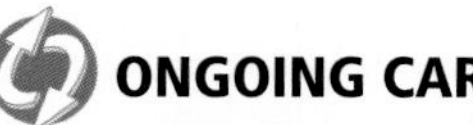

ONGOING CARE

FOLLOW-UP RECOMMENDATIONS

Echocardiography can be used to monitor both repaired and unrepaired ASDs.

Patient Monitoring

- In otherwise asymptomatic healthy children, follow until defect has closed or become negligible in size.
- Appropriate evaluation and management for atrial tachyarrhythmias in patients with long-term follow-up (1)[C]
- If ASD repaired as an adult, periodic long-term follow-up indicated (1)[C]
- ASDs repaired in childhood generally do not have late complications.
- In female patients with unrepaired ASD and Eisenmenger syndrome, pregnancy is not recommended due to increased risk of maternal and fetal mortality (1)[C].
- Pregnancy is well tolerated in patients with repaired ASD and small unrepaired ASDs.
- Scuba diving and high-altitude travel must be approached with caution in patients with unrepaired ASDs; consultation is recommended.

PATIENT EDUCATION

For patient education materials on this topic, consult the following:

- American Heart Association: http://www.heart.org
- Mayo Clinic information: http://www.mayoclinic.com/health/atrial-septal-defect/DS00628

PROGNOSIS

- ASD closure in asymptomatic or minimally symptomatic adults reduces morbidity but not mortality (9).
- ASD closure before age 25 years in symptomatic adults reduces morbidity and likely also mortality.
- ASD repair deferred until after adolescence may not decrease long-term risk of future atrial arrhythmias.
- Up to 50% mortality by age 50 years in untreated symptomatic patients with large defects

COMPLICATIONS

- Unrepaired: congestive heart failure, stroke, pulmonary hypertension/Eisenmenger syndrome, atrial arrhythmias, increased infection risk (pulmonary, cerebral abscess, infective endocarditis)
- Surgically repaired: late-onset arrhythmias 10–20 years after surgery (5%), perioperative atrial tachyarrhythmias in 10–13% of patients
- Device closure: device embolization (1%), cardiac perforation, thrombus formation, endocarditis, supraventricular arrhythmias

REFERENCES

1. Warnes CA, Williams RG, Bashore TM, et al. ACC/AHA 2008 guidelines for the management of adults with congenital heart disease. *J Am Coll Cardiol*. 2008;52(23):e143–e263.
2. Geva T, Martins JD, Wald RM. Atrial septal defects. *Lancet*. 2014;383(9932):1921–1932.
3. McMahon CJ, Feltes TF, Fraley JK, et al. Natural history of growth of secundum atrial septal defects and implications for transcatheter closure. *Heart*. 2002;87(3):256–259.
4. Hanslik A, Pospisil U, Salzer-Muhar U, et al. Predictors of spontaneous closure of isolated secundum atrial septal defect in children: a longitudinal study. *Pediatrics*. 2006;118(4):1560–1565.
5. Nishimura RA, Carabello BA, Faxon DP, et al. ACC/AHA 2008 guideline update on valvular heart disease: focused update on infective endocarditis. *Circulation*. 2008;118(8):887–896.
6. Wilson W, Taubert KA, Gewitz M, et al. Prevention of infective endocarditis: guidelines from the American Heart Association: a guideline from the American Heart Association Rheumatic Fever, Endocarditis, and Kawasaki Disease Committee, Council on Cardiovascular Disease in the Young, and the Council on Clinical Cardiology, Council on Cardiovascular Surgery and Anesthesia, and the Quality of Care and Outcomes Research Interdisciplinary Working Group. *Circulation*. 2007;116(15):1736–1754.
7. Holzer R, Hijazi ZM. Interventional approach to congenital heart disease. *Curr Opin Cardiol*. 2004;19(2):84–90.
8. Crandall M, Daoud E, Daniels C, et al. Percutaneous radiofrequency catheter ablation for atrial fibrillation prior to atrial septal defect closure. *J Cardiovasc Electrophysiol*. 2012:23(1):102–104.
9. Attie F, Rosas M, Granados N, et al. Surgical treatment for secundum atrial septal defects in patients >40 years old. A randomized clinical trial. *J Am Coll Cardiol*. 2001;38(7):2035–2042.

SEE ALSO

Aortic Valvular Stenosis; Coarctation of the Aorta; Patent Ductus Arteriosus; Pulmonary Valve Stenosis; Tetralogy of Fallot; Ventricular Septal Defect

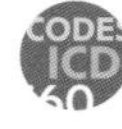

CODES

ICD10

- Q21.1 Atrial septal defect
- Q21.2 Atrioventricular septal defect

CLINICAL PEARLS

- ASD is often missed due to subtle clinical presentation.
- Ideally, hemodynamically significant ASDs should be closed in early childhood, although some benefit from closure is present in older patients.
- Many ASDs can be treated by catheter-directed percutaneous closure rather than open-heart surgery.
- Routine endocarditis prophylaxis is not recommended for unrepaired ASDs.
- Generally, symptomatic and hemodynamically significant ASDs are repaired; management of asymptomatic small ASDs is debated.
- Patent foramen ovales, unlike large ASDs, are very common and generally require no treatment in asymptomatic individuals.

ATTENTION DEFICIT/HYPERACTIVITY DISORDER, ADULT

Wynne S. Morgan, MD

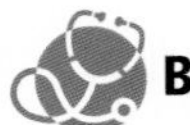

BASICS

- Adult attention deficit hyperactivity disorder (adult ADHD) is a psychiatric condition resulting in inattention and/or hyperactivity or impulsivity. It is associated with low self-esteem and challenges in interpersonal relationships, often impacting work environments.
- Adult ADHD has been shown to affect a significant portion of the adult population; >30% of patients diagnosed with this disorder as a child will meet criteria for this disorder into adulthood, and many more will have symptoms related to the disorder (1).
- Young adults aging out of pediatric services and into adult services often lose access to ADHD medications in the transition period, leaving them at risk for disruption in their daily functioning.

DESCRIPTION

- ADHD is one of the most common pediatric disorders that also affects patients into adulthood who have symptoms as a child.
- Symptoms include difficulty concentrating, impulsivity, and hyperactivity/overactivity.
- The 3 main types of ADHD are the following: (i) Primary symptoms include hyperactivity-impulsivity; (ii) primary symptoms include inattentiveness; and (iii) combined symptoms of inattention and hyperactivity
- Cost to society in 2010 U.S. dollars estimated to be $105–194 billion, with most of this cost from productivity and income losses, with "spillover" costs paid by families ranging from $33 to $43 billion (1)[A].

EPIDEMIOLOGY

Prevalence

General population prevalence for adult ADHD 2.5–4.4%, but population prevalence declines with age (2)[A],(3)[B].

Genetics

ADHD has substantial heritability, 1st-degree biologic relatives with ADHD are found more often in patients with ADHD. Some genes have been correlated with ADHD, although not necessary or sufficient causal factors (4)[A].

RISK FACTORS

History of childhood and adolescent ADHD diagnosis, particularly symptoms of hyperactivity and/or impulsivity, persisting into adulthood. ADHD is more frequent in males than females (3)[B].

COMMONLY ASSOCIATED CONDITIONS

- Substance use and substance abuse disorders
- Mood disorders
- Anxiety disorders
- Intellectual disabilities
- Obsessive-compulsive disorder (OCD)
- Tic disorders

DIAGNOSIS

- Diagnosis is made from patient's history and detailing patient's current level of functioning in at least two different settings (i.e., work & home).
- It is particularly important to gather history of patient's childhood and school performance. ADHD symptoms should be present before age 12 years. If no diagnosis or concern for ADHD as a child, it is unlikely to be diagnosed as an adult.
- *DSM-5* criteria are used for adults as well as children.

HISTORY

- History of childhood ADHD symptoms before age 12 years
- *DSM-5* criteria include ≥5 hyperactivity/impulsivity symptoms and/or ≥5 inattentive symptoms. These symptoms must be present for ≥6 months.
- Symptoms must result in maladaptive behavior that impairs the patient's function.
- There also must be some impairment in ≥2 settings, such as work and home.
- Clear evidence must exist of impairment of function in work, home life, and education secondary to these symptoms of inattention/hyperactivity.
- These symptoms must happen outside an episode of psychosis, mood disorder, or related to autistic spectrum disorder and may not be better explained by another *DSM* diagnosis.
- CAGE and substance abuse questions will help identify substance abuse issues but will not determine if the substance abuse is the primary diagnosis or if the patient has this in addition to adult ADHD.
- History of cardiac disease and family history of cardiac disease and sudden death should be documented.
- History of lead exposure or other toxins
- History of thyroid disease

PHYSICAL EXAM

- Physical exam is the key to rule out other medical conditions.
- Exam should focus on the thyroid and neurologic exam. Examine the body for any sequelae of substance abuse.
- BP and baseline weight are also important to record and monitor when considering starting medication treatment.

DIFFERENTIAL DIAGNOSIS

Hearing impairment; hyperthyroid/hypothyroid; sleep deprivation; sleep apnea; phenylketonuria; OCD; lead toxicity; substance abuse (5)[A]

DIAGNOSTIC TESTS & INTERPRETATION

- Adult ADHD screening tools: There are retrospective tools like the Childhood Symptom Scale and the Wender Utah Rating Scale; also current symptom scales, such as the Adult ADHD Rating Scale IV, Adult Self Report Scale Symptom Checklist, and the Connor Adult Rating Scale. These scales can take 5–20 minutes to complete.
- Provider/patient screening checklist
  - http://help4adhd.org/documents/AdultADHDSelfReportScale-ASRS-v1-1.pdf
  - http://webdoc.nyumc.org/nyumc_d6/files/psych_adhd_screener.pdf
- ECG with concerns for cardiac disease in patient or family history
- Record baseline blood pressure, pulse, and BMI.

Initial Tests (lab, imaging)

- Thyroid-stimulating hormone (TSH)
- Liver function test monitoring (with atomoxetine)
- Rapid plasma reagin (RPR) or VDRL (Venereal Disease Research Laboratory) test
- Serum lead levels (pending history)

Follow-Up Tests & Special Considerations

- A history of childhood behaviors is helpful to make the diagnosis, but adult patients often don't accurately recall childhood symptomology.
- Consider speaking with patient's parents or obtaining old school records and a developmental history as well as any family history of ADHD, substance abuse, or tic disorder to ensure accurate diagnosis.
- Caution stimulant use in pregnancy as significant risk for low fetal birth weight and preterm birth. Risks and benefits must be discussed with family (6)[B].
- Caution use of stimulants in adult patients with cardiac history.

ALERT

Mood disorders, generalized anxiety disorders, and substance abuse can also co-occur with adult ADHD; treating both the ADHD and comorbid condition will provide the greatest prognosis for the patient.

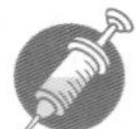

TREATMENT

- Most of the research and medication trials have been performed in children.
- There are more data showing stimulants and nonstimulants that are used in children are also effective in adults (5,6)[A].

ALERT

Stimulant medication prescriptions risk inducing dependency, substance abuse, and diversion. Perform pill counts and urine drug testing, as well as screening for signs of prescription drug abuse. Misuse of amphetamines may cause sudden death and serious cardiovascular adverse events.

GENERAL MEASURES

When prescribing stimulant medications for adults with ADHD, watch for misuse, abuse, and diversion of prescription medications. When substance abuse is not present, stimulants are 1st-line treatment for ADHD and highly efficacious. There are multiple formulations of stimulants, and patients may require multiple trials of different preparations for effective response.

MEDICATION

- Psychotropic medications play a large part in the treatment of ADHD symptoms. Medications should be titrated slowly to effective dose to avoid side effects.
- Stimulants are more effective than antidepressants or nonstimulants, but up to 30% discontinue medications because of side effects.
- Stimulants can be divided into two different classes: Methylphenidate and amphetamine come in both short-acting and long-acting preparations.
- Antidepressants studied for ADHD include bupropion, which has been shown to have a medium effect compared with stimulants (7)[A].

First Line

- Stimulants: methylphenidate (Concerta, Ritalin), dexmethylphenidate (Focalin), dextroamphetamine/amphetamine (Adderall), dextroamphetamine (Dexedrine), lisdexamfetamine (Vyvanse)
  - Methylphenidate preparations are available in short-acting, intermediate-acting, long-acting, and patch formulations.
  - Ritalin LA may be used for patient's naive to stimulants. It can be started at 20 mg daily and dose titrated by 10 mg increments weekly to symptoms response. Max dose of 60 mg
  - Concerta ER is another option in adults up to 65 years of age. Starting dose of 18 mg and adjust in increments of 18 mg weekly until symptoms improve. Max dose 72 mg/day. Concerta also has an oral osmotic release to decrease abuse potential.
  - Amphetamines also come in immediate-release preparations and sustained release preparations.
  - Dextroamphetamine is commonly used with a half-life of 4–6 hours with an initial dose of 5 mg. Caution: Immediate-release preparations have high abuse potential.
  - Dextroamphetamine/amphetamine (Adderall) is a 75%/25% mix that also comes in an extended-release form.
  - Lisdexamfetamine (Vyvanse) is an extended-release stimulant that is a prodrug requiring metabolization to active component, dextroamphetamine.
  - Common side effects of stimulants include hypertension (HTN), tachycardia, insomnia, weight loss, stomach upset, increased anxiety/irritability, or worsening of tics (8)[A].
- Nonstimulants: Atomoxetine (Strattera) has been shown effective in adults with ADHD when compared to placebo (9)[B]. It may be given as a single dose or split dose and has low abuse potential, making it a better choice over a stimulant medication for patients with substance abuse history. Onset of effect may take up to 4 weeks. Atomoxetine may require dose adjustments with strong inhibitors of cytochrome P2D6 (e.g., Paxil or Prozac). Also, there are rare cases of liver damage associated with these medications. Monitor for increased suicidal thinking.
- Antidepressants: best used for those at risk or have history of substance abuse disorder
  - Bupropion (Wellbutrin) is an antidepressant effective in adults with ADHD symptoms (8)[A].

ISSUES FOR REFERRAL

Patients with comorbid conditions may need specialist evaluation to diagnose and treat, and to manage complex ADHD symptomatology cases. Cardiology consult may be considered using stimulants in patients with known cardiac issues. May consider referral to perinatal psychiatry when treating pregnant women with ADHD

ADDITIONAL THERAPIES

Cognitive-behavioral therapy can be useful in conjunction with medication to help patient modify and cope with symptoms.

COMPLEMENTARY & ALTERNATIVE MEDICINE

No data effective

ONGOING CARE

Often times, young adults transitioning from pediatrics to adult care will discontinue their ADHD medication, leading to issues with school, work, and personal life and also makes them at greater risk of substance abuse and criminal activities.

FOLLOW-UP RECOMMENDATIONS

- Close follow-up of medication as dose is titrated
- Continue to monitor for medication side effects.
- Repeat screening checklists to quantify benefit of interventions as needed.
- Reinforce behavioral change (e.g., self-initiated, through cognitive-behavioral therapy), which is the cornerstone of long-term management.

REFERENCES

1. Doshi JA, Hodgkins P, Kahle J, et al. Economic impact of childhood and adult attention-deficit/hyperactivity disorder in the United States. *J Am Acad Child Adolesc Psychiatry*. 2012;51(10):990–1002.
2. Simon V, Czobor P, Bálint S, et al: Prevalence and correlates of adult attention-deficit hyperactivity disorder: a meta-analysis. *Br J Psychiatry*. 2009;194(3):204–211.
3. Kessler RC, Adler L, Barkley R, et al. The prevalence and correlates of adult ADHD in the United States: results from the National Comorbidity Survey Replication. *Am J Psychiatry*. 2006;163(4):716–723.
4. Gatt JM, Burton KL, Williams LM, et al. Specific and common genes implicated across major mental disorders: a review of meta-analysis studies. *J Psychiatr Res*. 2015;60C:1–13.
5. Castells X, Ramos-Quiroga JA, Bosch R, et al. Amphetamines for attention deficit hyperactivity disorder (ADHD) in adults. *Cochrane Database Syst Rev*. 2011;(6):CD007813.
6. Epstein T, Patsopoulos NA, Weiser M. Immediate-release methylphenidate for attention deficit hyperactivity disorder (ADHD) in adults. *Cochrane Database Syst Rev*. 2014;9:CD005041.
7. Verbeeck W, Tuinier S, Bekkering GE. Antidepressants in the treatment of adult attention-deficit hyperactivity disorder: a systematic review. *Adv Ther*. 2009;26(2):170–184.
8. Maneeton N, Maneeton B, Srisurapanont M, et al. Bupropion for adults with attention-deficit hyperactivity disorder: meta-analysis of randomized, placebo-controlled trials. *Psychiatry Clin Neurosci*. 2011;65(7):611–617.
9. Asherson P, Bushe C, Saylor K, et al. Efficacy of atomoxetine in adults with attention deficit hyperactivity disorder: an integrated analysis of the complete database of multicenter placebo-controlled trials. *J Psychopharmacol*. 2014;28(9):837–846.

ADDITIONAL READING

- American Psychiatric Association. *Diagnostic and Statistical Manual of Mental Disorders*. 5th ed. Arlington, VA: American Psychiatric Association; 2013.
- Bader A, Adesman A. Complementary and alternative therapies for children and adolescents with ADHD. *Curr Opin Pediatr*. 2012;24(6):760–769.
- Mongia M, Hechtman L. Cognitive behavior therapy for adults with attention-deficit/hyperactivity disorder: a review of recent randomized controlled trials. *Curr Psychiatry Rep*. 2012;14(5):561–567.
- Post RE, Kurlansik SL. Diagnosis and management of adult attention-deficit/hyperactivity disorder. *Am Fam Physician*. 2012;85(9):890–896.
- U.S. Food and Drug Administration. Ritalin (FDA approval). http://www.accessdata.fda.gov/drugsatfda_docs/label/2013/010187s077lbl.pdf. Accessed 2014.

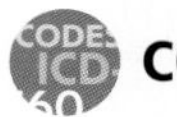

CODES

ICD10

- F90.9 Attention-deficit hyperactivity disorder, unspecified type
- F90.0 Attn-defct hyperactivity disorder, predom inattentive type
- F90.1 Attn-defct hyperactivity disorder, predom hyperactive type

CLINICAL PEARLS

- Adult ADHD results in inattention, hyperactivity, and impulsive behavior; it is associated with low self-esteem and challenges in interpersonal relationships, including work environments.
- Psychotropic medications plus cognitive-behavioral treatments are the cornerstone of management.
- Substance abuse is a common comorbidity; recommend use nonstimulant medication management in those at risk.

ATTENTION DEFICIT/HYPERACTIVITY DISORDER, PEDIATRIC

Laura Novak, MD • Suman Vellanki, MD

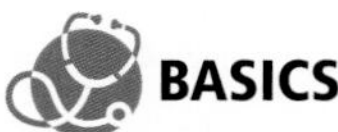

BASICS

DESCRIPTION

- Attention deficit hyperactivity disorder (ADHD) is a neurodevelopmental problem that manifests in early childhood characterized by distractibility, impulsivity, hyperactivity, and/or inattention.
- 3 subsets: predominantly hyperactivity-impulsive (ADHD-HI), predominantly inattentive (ADHD-I), or combined (ADHD-C)
- System(s) affected: nervous
- Synonym(s): attention deficit disorder; hyperactivity

EPIDEMIOLOGY

- Predominant age: onset <12 years; lasts into adolescence and adulthood; 50% meet diagnostic criteria by age 4 years
- Predominant sex: m > f (2:1); predominantly inattentive type may be more common in girls

Prevalence

- Varies from 2–18% depending on diagnostic criteria and the population studied
- 42% increase from estimated prevalence in 2003 according to 2011 National Survey of Children's Health

ETIOLOGY AND PATHOPHYSIOLOGY

Not definitive; imbalance of catecholamine metabolism in cerebral cortex appears to play a primary role

Genetics

Familial pattern

RISK FACTORS

- Family history
- Medical causes (affecting brain development)
- Environmental causes (toxins such as lead, fetal alcohol, and nutritional deficiencies)

GENERAL PREVENTION

- Children are at risk for abuse, depression, and isolation.
- Parents need regular support and advice.
- Parents should establish contact with teacher each school year.

COMMONLY ASSOCIATED CONDITIONS

- Depression (in up to 1/3 of cases and more common in inattentive and combined subtypes)
- Oppositional defiant disorder (more common in combined and hyperactive-impulsive subtypes)
- Conduct disorder
- Anxiety disorder
- Learning disabilities

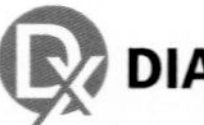

DIAGNOSIS

- American Academy of Pediatrics (AAP) guidelines recommend *DSM-5* criteria to establish diagnosis.
- Children undergoing extreme stress (divorce, illness, homelessness, abuse) may demonstrate ADHD behaviors secondary to stress (1). This can be assessed using the American Academy of Child and Adolescent Psychiatry (AACAP) screening tool.
- If diagnostic behaviors are noted in only 1 setting, explore the stressors in that setting.
- The diagnostic behaviors are more noticeable in tasks that require concentration or boredom tolerance than in free play or office situations.
- Response to stimulant medication cannot be used to confirm or refute the diagnosis of ADHD.
- *DSM-5* criteria: For children <17 years, ≥6 inattention criteria and/or ≥6 hyperactivity/impulsivity criteria. Symptoms must occur often, be present before age of 12 years, for >6 months, be noticed in 2 settings (e.g., home and school), and be excessive for development level of child (1)[A].
- Inattention
  - Careless mistakes in tasks; difficulty sustaining attention or in organizing tasks; does not seem to listen, follow through, or finish tasks; avoids tasks that require sustained mental effort; loses things; forgetful in daily activities
- Hyperactivity/impulsivity
  - Fidgets; difficulty remaining seated; runs/climbs excessively or inappropriately; difficulty playing quietly; acts as if "driven by a motor" or seeming to always be "on the go"; talks excessively; blurts out answers before question is complete; has difficulty waiting turn; interrupts others

HISTORY

- Birth and development history
- Psychosocial evaluation of home environment
- School performance history and school absences
- Psychiatric history or comorbid disorder(s)

PHYSICAL EXAM

- Baseline weight for future monitoring
- Focus on soft neurologic signs, such as tics, clumsiness, mixed handedness
- Assess hearing and vision

DIFFERENTIAL DIAGNOSIS

- Activity level appropriate for age
- Language or communication disorders
- Hearing/vision disorder
- Dysfunctional family situation
- Learning disability (e.g., dyslexia)
- Autism spectrum disorders
- Oppositional/defiant disorder or conduct disorder
- Tourette syndrome: motor and verbal tics
- Absence seizures (inattentive-type ADHD only)
- Lead poisoning
- Sequelae of central nervous system infection/trauma
- Medication reaction (decongestant, antihistamine, theophylline, phenobarbital)

DIAGNOSTIC TESTS & INTERPRETATION

- Behavior rating scales (e.g., Connors) should be completed by parents, caregivers, and teachers. They are repeated after therapy is started to gauge differences (*DSM-5* criteria can be used in place of a rating scale).
- ADHD toolkit with forms is available from http://www.nichq.org/adhd.html and includes Vanderbilt Assessment Scales
- Testing for learning disability (e.g., dyslexia) through the school may be needed.

Initial Tests (lab, imaging)

Lead level if high risk

Diagnostic Procedures/Other

EEG not needed unless symptoms are highly suggestive of seizure disorder (e.g., absence seizures).

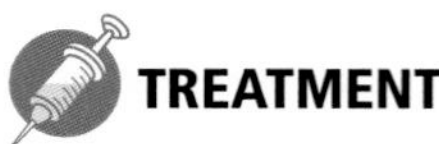

TREATMENT

GENERAL MEASURES

- Parent/school/patient education
- Work closely with teacher.
- Behavioral therapy/environmental changes

MEDICATION

First Line

2011 AAP guideline recommends stimulant medications as first-line treatment (2)[A], (3)[A]. Medications should be used as an adjunct to behavioral interventions for preschool children (4 through 5 years) (3)[B]. A 2nd type of stimulant should be tried if the 1st treatment fails.

- *Stimulant*:
  - Dexmethylphenidate
    - Focalin: initial: 2.5 mg BID; Increase total daily by 2.5–5 mg weekly up to maximum dose of 20 mg/day
    - Focalin XR: initial: 5 mg in AM; increase daily dose by 5 mg weekly up to maximum dose of 30 mg/day
  - Methylphenidate
    - Short-acting→ Ritalin, Methylin, Methylin oral: initial 5 mg BID before breakfast and lunch; increase by 5–10 mg weekly to maximum dose of 60 mg/day (2 or 3 divided doses)
    - Intermediate-acting→ Ritalin SR: 20 mg once in AM; increase by 10 mg weekly up to 40–60 mg; Metadate ER: 10 mg BID; increase by 10 mg weekly to 40–60 mg
    - Long-acting→ Metadate CD: 20 mg in AM; increase by 10–20 mg weekly to 40–60 mg; Quillivant XR: 20 mg in AM; increase 10–20 mg weekly until 40–60 mg; Ritalin LA: 10–20 mg in AM; increase 10 mg weekly until 40–60 mg; Concerta: 18–36 mg in AM; increase by 18 mg weekly until 54–72 mg; Daytrana transdermal patch: 10 mg patch on (hip area) 2 hours before effect is needed; patch removed 9 hours after application; increase to next higher patch weekly until 30 mg patch if needed
  - Dextroamphetamine
    - Dexedrine spansule (long-acting): 5 mg BID; increase by 5 mg weekly to maximum dose of 40 mg daily
  - Dextroamphetamine and amphetamine (mixed salts)
    - Short-acting: Adderall: 5 mg daily or BID; increase by 5–10 mg weekly to a maximum dose of 40 mg daily divided into 1–3 doses
    - Long-acting: Adderall XR: 5–10 mg in AM; increase by 5–10 mg weekly until maximum dose of 30 mg/day
  - Lisdexamfetamine
    - Vyvanse: 30 mg in AM; increase by 10–20 mg weekly up to a maximum of 70 mg/day

ALERT
The FDA recommends that a personal or family history of congenital heart disease or sudden death be screened with an ECG and possible cardiology consultation before beginning stimulant medication.

- Precautions:
  - If not responding, check compliance and consider another diagnosis.
  - Some children experience withdrawal (tearfulness, agitation) after a missed dose or when medication wears off. A small, short-acting dose at 4 PM may help to prevent this.
  - Stimulants are drugs of abuse and should be monitored carefully.
  - Drug holidays are not recommended.
- Common adverse effects:
  - Anorexia, GI effects, headache, and insomnia
- Signicant possible interactions: may increase levels of anticonvulsants, SSRIs, tricyclics, and warfarin

Pregnancy Considerations
Medications are Category C: caution in pregnancy

Second Line
Nonstimulant:

- Atomoxetine (Strattera):
  - Children/adolescents ≤70 kg: 0.5 mg/kg/day initial; increase after a minimum of 3 days to target dose of 1.2 mg/kg/day; maximum of 1.4 mg/kg/day
  - Children/adolescents >70 kg: 40 mg daily; increase after minimum of 3 days to target dose of 80 mg/day; dose may be increased to maximum of 100 mg/day after additional 2–4 weeks
- Clonidine extended-release
  - Kapvay: 0.1 mg once daily at bedtime; increase by 0.1 mg weekly; doses should be taken twice daily with equal or higher split dosage given at HS; maximum of 0.4 mg/day; taper when discontinued
- Guanfacine extended-release
  - Intuniv: 1 mg daily; increase by 1 mg weekly until 1 to 4 mg daily; taper when discontinued

ALERT
- Atomoxetine carries a "black box" warning regarding potential exacerbation of suicidality (similar to SSRIs). Close follow-up recommended.
  - Associated with hepatic injury in a small number of cases; check liver enzymes if symptoms develop.
    - Interacts with paroxetine (Paxil), fluoxetine (Prozac), and quinidine
    - Extended-release guanfacine and extended-release clonidine and other nonstimulant drugs (e.g., tricyclic antidepressants, SSRIs): have mixed efficacy and high side effects. Consider consultation.

ISSUES FOR REFERRAL
Should be considered for children <6 years for psychological or medical complications, developmental disorder or intellectual disability, or poor response to medication.

ADDITIONAL THERAPIES
- Medication alone or combined with behavioral therapy produced better results than therapy alone.
- For preschool-aged children (4–5 years), prescribe evidence-based parent- and/or teacher-administered behavior therapy as the first line of treatment.

COMPLEMENTARY & ALTERNATIVE MEDICINE
- Surveys have shown that parents of children with ADHD use herbals and complementary treatments frequently (20–60%).
- Omega-3 fatty acids (found in fish oil and some supplements) showed improvement in rating scales in 2 double-blind, placebo-controlled studies of 116 and 130 patients (4).

ONGOING CARE

FOLLOW-UP RECOMMENDATIONS

Patient Monitoring
- Parent/teacher rating scales
- Office visits to monitor side effects and efficacy: End points are improved grades, improved rating scales, acceptable family interactions, and improved peer interactions.
- Monitor growth (especially weight) and BP.

DIET
- "Insufficient evidence to suggest that dietary interventions reduce the symptoms of ADHD (4)."
- The AAP recommends that "For a child without a medical, emotional, or environmental etiology of ADHD behaviors, a trial of a preservative-free food coloring–free diet is a reasonable intervention" (4).

PATIENT EDUCATION
- Excellent reference: http://www.parentsmedguide.org
- Key points for parents:
  - Behavioral interventions may help; find things child is good at and emphasize these; reinforce good behavior; give one task at a time; stop behavior with quiet discipline; coordinate homework with teachers; have set schedule.
- Support groups:
  - Children and Adults with Attention Deficit Disorder (CHADD): http://www.chadd.org
  - Attention Deficit Disorder Warehouse: http://www.addwarehouse.com
  - National Information Center for Children and Youth with Disabilities: http://www.nichcy.org

PROGNOSIS
- May last into adulthood; hyperactivity may become easier to control with age.
- Relative deficits in academic and social functioning may persist into late adolescence/adulthood.
- Encourage career choices that allow autonomy and mobility.

COMPLICATIONS
- Untreated ADHD can lead to failing in school, parental abuse, social isolation, and poor self-esteem.
- Some children experience withdrawal after a missed dose or when medication wears off.
- Monitor growth with stimulant use. If appetite is poor, eat before the medication is given and after it wears off.
- Increased risk of substance abuse is controversial and may be related to comorbid conditions (conduct disorder).
- 2–4 times increase in automobile accidents and injuries; decreases with medication

REFERENCES

1. American Psychiatric Association. *Diagnostic and Statistical Manual of Mental Disorders*. 5th ed. Washington, DC: American Psychiatric Association; 2013.
2. Rader R, McCauley L, Callen EC. Current strategies in the diagnosis and treatment of childhood attention-deficit/hyperactivity disorder. *Am Fam Physician*. 2009;79(8):657–665.
3. Subcommittee on Attention-Deficit/Hyperactivity Disorder; Steering Committee on Quality Improvement and Management; Wolraich M, Brown L, Brown RT, et al. ADHD: clinical practice guideline for the diagnosis, evaluation, and treatment of attention-deficit/hyperactivity disorder in children and adolescents. *Pediatrics*. 2011;128(5): 1007–1022.
4. Sinn N. Nutritional and dietary influences on attention deficit hyperactivity disorder. *Nutr Rev*. 2008;66(10):558–568.

ADDITIONAL READING

- Laforett DR, Murray DW, Kollins SH. Psychosocial treatments for preschool-aged children with attention-deficit hyperactivity disorder. *Dev Disabil Res Rev*. 2008;14(4):300–310.
- Larson K, Russ SA, Kahn RS, et al. Patterns of comorbidity, functioning, and service use for US children with ADHD, 2007. *Pediatrics*. 2011;127(3):462–470.
- Millichap JG, Yee MM. The diet factor in attention-deficit/hyperactivity disorder. *Pediatrics*. 2012;129(2):330–337.
- Weber W, Newmark S. Complementary and alternative medical therapies for attention-deficit/hyperactivity disorder and autism. *Pediatr Clin North Am*. 2007;54(6):983–1006; xii.

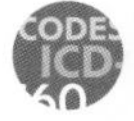

CODES

ICD10
- F90.9 Attention-deficit hyperactivity disorder, unspecified type
- F90.0 Attn-defct hyperactivity disorder, predom inattentive type
- F90.1 Attn-defct hyperactivity disorder, predom hyperactive type

CLINICAL PEARLS

- Children undergoing extreme stress (divorce, illness, homelessness, abuse) may demonstrate ADHD behaviors secondary to stress.
- 50% of children with ADHD have a parent with ADHD.
- AAP recommends the use of stimulant medications as the first-line treatment.

AUTISM SPECTRUM DISORDERS

Macario C. Corpuz, MD, MBA, FAAFP • Jennifer Luo Powell, DO

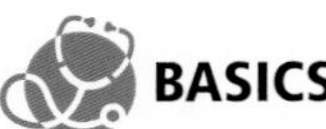

BASICS

DESCRIPTION

Group of neurodevelopmental disorders of early childhood: DSM-5 has included autism spectrum disorders (ASDs) to include autistic disorder, childhood disintegrative disorder, Asperger disorder, pervasive developmental disorder not otherwise specified (PDD-NOS); and now, it also encompasses early infantile autism, childhood autism, Kanner autism, high-functioning autism, and atypical autism (1)[A].

- 2 symptom clusters
  - Social/communication
    - Impairment of effective social skills and absent or impaired communication skills
  - Fixed interests/repetitive behaviors
    - Repetitive and/or stereotyped behaviors and interests, especially in inanimate objects (2)[A]
- Severity levels
  - Level 1: requiring support
  - Level 2: requiring substantial support
  - Level 3: requiring very substantial support
- Important to distinguish autism disorder from social (pragmatic) communication disorder. Separate DSM-5 criteria for individuals with social communication deficits but do not meet autism-spectrum criteria.

EPIDEMIOLOGY

- Predominant age: onset in early childhood
- Predominant sex: male > female (5:1)

Pediatric Considerations

Symptom onset seen in children <3 years of age (except for childhood disintegrative disorder)

Prevalence

- Estimated 1/100–1/500 children
- Among 6–17 years–aged children within the United States, in 2011–2012, there is found to be a 2% (1 in 50) parent-reported prevalence compared to 1.16% (1 in 86) as reported in 2007.

ETIOLOGY AND PATHOPHYSIOLOGY

- No single cause has been identified.
- General consensus: A genetic abnormality leads to altered neurologic development.
- No scientific evidence relating vaccines, such as vaccines for measles, mumps, or rubella (MMR), or thimerosal causing ASDs (3)[C]
- Pathophysiology is incompletely understood.

Genetics

- High concordance in monozygotic twins
- Increased recurrence risk (2–18%) in subsequent siblings

RISK FACTORS

Siblings of affected children have a 5-times greater risk of developing autism. Prevalence ranging from 2 to 8%

GENERAL PREVENTION

- Early screening for early treatment means a better prognosis.
- Some ASDs are caused by genetic or chromosomal disorders.
- Economic costs
  - An additional $17,000–21,000 is an estimated cost for raising an ASD child (4)[B].
  - Medical costs in 2005 were estimated to be 6× more, totaling $10,709 per child.
  - Intensive behavioral interventions costs range $40,000–$60,000 (5)[C].

COMMONLY ASSOCIATED CONDITIONS

- Mental retardation, ADHD, anxiety, depression, or obsessive behavior
- Phenylketonuria (PKU), tuberous sclerosis, fragile X syndrome, Angelman syndrome, and fetal alcohol syndrome (rare)
- Seizures (increased risk if severe mental retardation)
- Maternal use of selective serotonin reuptake inhibitors (SSRIs) during pregnancy

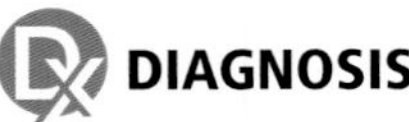

DIAGNOSIS

HISTORY

- Impairment in social interaction
  - Impairment in nonverbal behaviors such as eye-to-eye gaze, facial expression
  - Unable to develop peer relationships
  - Does not smile nor share emotions
  - Loss of social or emotional reciprocity
- Communication impairment
  - Delay or lack of development in language skills
  - Inability to initiate or sustain conversation
  - Stereotyped and repetitive use of language
  - Preoccupation with parts of toys or body parts
- Repetitive and stereotyped patterns of behavior
  - Excessively lines up toys or other objects
  - Unusually attached to 1 particular toy or object
  - Repetitive odd movements (toe walking, hand flapping)
  - Adherence to specific routines or rituals
- Prenatal, neonatal, and developmental history
- Seizure disorder
- Family history of autism, genetic disorders, learning disabilities, psychiatric illness, neurologic disorders, genetic disorders, or mental retardation
- Commonly associated with sleep disorders

PHYSICAL EXAM

- Macrocephaly in 25%; head circumference growth peaks at age 6 months and begins to decline by 1 year.
- Dysmorphic features consistent with genetic disorder (fragile X syndrome)
- Hypotonia occurs in autism but should prompt imaging.
- Wood lamp skin exam to rule out tuberous sclerosis

DIFFERENTIAL DIAGNOSIS

Other mental and CNS disorders

- Obsessive-compulsive disorder
- Elective mutism
- Language disorder/hearing impairment
- Intellectual disability/global developmental delay
- Stereotyped movement disorder
- Severe early deprivation/reactive attachment disorder
- Anxiety disorder
- Social communication disorder
- Developmental language disorder

DIAGNOSTIC TESTS & INTERPRETATION

- Checklist for Autism in Toddlers (CHAT) to screen for ASDs at 18 months of age. (To order: http://www.autism.org.uk/working-with/health/screening-and-diagnosis/checklist-for-autism-in-toddlers-chat.aspx)
- The Pervasive Developmental Disorders Screening Test-II (PDDST-II) to screen for ASDs beginning at 18 months
- Modified Checklist for Autism in Toddlers (M-CHAT) to screen for ASDs at 16–30 months
- Social Communication Questionnaire (SCQ) (formerly Autism Screening Questionnaire)—used with children age 4+ years—the gold standard diagnostic interview used in research studies

Initial Tests (lab, imaging)

- Lead and PKU screening
- Karyotype and DNA analysis (fragile X, PKU, tuberous sclerosis, and others)
- Metabolic testing if signs of
  - Lethargy, limited endurance, unusual habits, hypotonia, recurrent vomiting and dehydration, developmental regression, or specific food intolerance
- MRI is useful only if focal neurologic symptoms.

Follow-Up Tests & Special Considerations

- Hearing tests: audiometry and brainstem auditory evoked response (BAERS)
- Comprehensive speech and language evaluation
- Evaluation by multidisciplinary team: includes a psychiatrist, neurologist, psychologist, speech therapist, and other autism specialists
- Intellectual level needs to be established and monitored, as it is one of the best measures of prognosis.
- Test used to follow autism are the following:
  - Autism Behavior Checklist (ABC)
  - Gilliam Autism Rating Scale (GARS)
  - Childhood Autism Rating Scale (CARS)
  - Autism Diagnosis Interview-Revised (ADI-R)
  - Autism Diagnostic Observation Schedule-Generic (ADOS-G) Imaging

Diagnostic Procedures/Other

EEG if history of seizures or spells

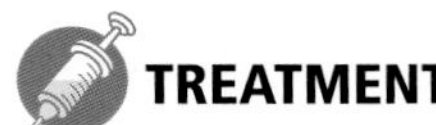

TREATMENT

GENERAL MEASURES

- Comprehensive structured educational programming of a sustained and intensive design, most commonly applied behavioral analysis therapy
- Core features of a successful education program
  - High staff–student ratio 1:2, or less
  - Individualized programming
  - Specialized teacher training with ongoing evaluation of teachers and programs
  - 25 hours a week minimum of specialized services
  - A structured routine environment that emphasizes attention, imitation, communication, socialization, and play interactions (6)[C]
  - Functional analysis of behavioral problems
  - Transition planning and involvement of the family
- Currently no cure for ASDs. Early diagnosis and initiation of multidisciplinary intervention help enhance functioning in later life.
- Early intensive behavioral intervention (EIBI) involving treatment for 20–40 hours per week is a well-established treatments for ASD.
- School-based special education for older children
- Some evidence indicates social skills groups can improve social competence for some children and adolescents with ASD.
- Find alternative methods of communication: sign language; picture exchange communication system

MEDICATION

- Autism behavior issues should be managed with maximal behavioral management prior to medication.
- Medication directed at managing symptoms

First Line

- No true 1st-line medical therapy; medications used to treat targeted symptoms
- Stimulants (such as methylphenidate): efficacious in treating concomitant symptoms of ADHD such as impulsiveness, hyperactivity, and inattention; however, the magnitude of response is less than in typically developing children, and adverse effects are more frequent.
- SSRIs have limited evidence for autism. It has shown help in reducing ritualistic behavior and improving mood and language skills. Initial choice for anxiety and depressive mood (7)[B]
- Risperidone has shown short-term efficacy for treatment for irritability, repetitious behaviors, and social withdrawal. Aripiprazole has shown efficacy for treating short-term irritability, hyperactivity, and repetitive movements (8)[B].
- Melatonin used for patients with concomitant sleep disorders

Second Line

- **Vitamin B_6** and magnesium: inconclusive evidence in improving behavior, speech, and language of children with ASD (9)[C]
- Tricyclic antidepressants have limited and conflicting evidence of effect (10)[B].

ISSUES FOR REFERRAL

- Refer early to
  - Early learning for evaluation of behavior and language, genetic counseling, and audiology
- Consider referrals to psychiatry, ophthalmology, otolaryngology, neurology, and nutrition (11).
- Refer family members to parent support groups and respite programs.

COMPLEMENTARY & ALTERNATIVE MEDICINE

- Parent-mediated early intervention for young children with autism spectrum has sufficient evidence of benefit in child outcomes related to language understanding and severity of autism characteristics (12)[B].
- Music therapy has been shown to improve communication skills in autistic patients; however, more research is needed (13)[C].
- "Theory of mind," or related skills, can be taught to ASD patients, but further research is needed (14)[C].
- No evidence to support use of auditory integration therapy or other sound therapies as an effective treatment for ASD (15)[B]
- No evidence to support acupuncture for treatment of ASD (6)[C]
- IV secretin has shown no evidence of efficacy and is not currently recommended as a treatment for ASD (16)[C].

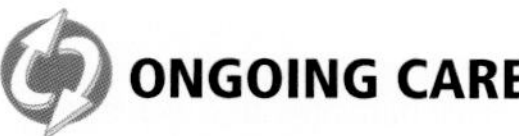

ONGOING CARE

FOLLOW-UP RECOMMENDATIONS

Patient Monitoring

- Constant monitoring by caregivers
- Reevaluation every 6–12 months by physician for seizures, sleep and nutritional problems, and prescribed medical management
- Intellectual and language testing every 2 years in childhood

DIET

- Gluten- and casein-free diets: Current evidence for efficacy is poor (17)[C].
- Omega-3 fatty acids supplementation has not been found to improve outcomes (18)[C].

PROGNOSIS

- Beginning treatment at a young age (2–4 years) results in better outcomes.
- Prognosis is closely related to initial intellectual abilities, with only 20% functioning above the mentally retarded level.
- Communicative language development before 5 years is also associated with a better outcome.
- The general expected course is for a lifelong need for supervised structured care.

COMPLICATIONS

- Increasing incidents of seizure disorders in up to 1 in 4 children
- Increased risk for physical and sexual abuse
- With pica, increased risk of lead poisoning
- Limited variety of food consumed due to dietary obsessions
- Increased risk for GI symptoms, including weight abnormalities and abnormal stool patterns

REFERENCES

1. Wingate M, Mulvihill B, Kirby RS, et al. Prevalence of autism spectrum disorders—Autism and Developmental Disabilities Monitoring Network, 14 sites, United States, 2008. *MMWR Surveill Summ*. 2012;61(3):1–19.
2. Blumberg SJ, Bramlett MD, Kogan MD, et al. Changes in prevalence of parent-reported autism spectrum disorder in school-aged U.S. children: 2007 to 2011–2012. *Natl Health Stat Report*. 2013;(65):1–11.
3. Demicheli V, Rivetti A, Debalini MG, et al. Vaccines for measles, mumps and rubella in children. *Cochrane Database Syst Rev*. 2012;2:CD004407.
4. Lavelle TA, Weinstein MC, Newhouse JP, et al. Economic burden of childhood autism spectrum disorders. *Pediatrics*. 2014;133(3):e520–e529.
5. Shimabukuro TT, Grosse SD, Rice C. Medical expenditures for children with an autism spectrum disorder in a privately insured population. *J Autism Dev Disord*. 2008;38(3):546–552.
6. Cheuk DK, Wong V, Chen WX. Acupuncture for autism spectrum disorders (ASD). *Cochrane Database Syst Rev*. 2011;(9):CD007849.
7. Williams K, Wheeler DM, Silove N, et al. Selective serotonin reuptake inhibitors (SSRIs) for autism spectrum disorders (ASD). *Cochrane Database Syst Rev*. 2013;8:CD004677.
8. Ching H, Pringsheim T. Aripiprazole for autism spectrum disorders (ASD). *Cochrane Database Syst Rev*. 2012;5:CD009043.
9. Nye C, Brice A. Combined vitamin B6-magnesium treatment in autism spectrum disorder. *Cochrane Database Syst Rev*. 2005;(4):CD003497.
10. Hurwitz R, Blackmore R, Hazell P, et al. Tricyclic antidepressants for autism spectrum disorders (ASD) in children and adolescents. *Cochrane Database Syst Rev*. 2012;3:CD008372.
11. Reichow B, Steiner AM, Volkmar F. Social skills groups for people aged 6 to 21 with autism spectrum disorders (ASD). *Cochrane Database Syst Rev*. 2012;7:CD008511.
12. Oono IP, Honey EJ, McConachie H. Parent-mediated early intervention for young children with autism spectrum disorders (ASD). *Cochrane Database Syst Rev*. 2013;4:CD009774.
13. Geretsegger M, Elefant C, Mössler KA, et al. Music therapy for people with autism spectrum disorder. *Cochrane Database Syst Rev*. 2014;6:CD004381.
14. Fletcher-Watson S, McConnell F, Manola E, et al. Interventions based on the Theory of Mind cognitive model for autism spectrum disorder (ASD). *Cochrane Database Syst Rev*. 2014;3: CD008785.
15. Sinha Y, Silove N, Hayen A, et al. Auditory integration training and other sound therapies for autism spectrum disorders (ASD). *Cochrane Database Syst Rev*. 2011;(12):CD003681.
16. Williams K, Wray JA, Wheeler DM. Intravenous secretin for autism spectrum disorders (ASD). *Cochrane Database Syst Rev*. 2012;4:CD003495.
17. Millward C, Ferriter M, Calver S, et al. Gluten- and casein-free diets for autistic spectrum disorder. *Cochrane Database Syst Rev*. 2013;(2) CD003498.
18. James S, Montgomery P, Williams K. Omega-3 fatty acids supplementation for autism spectrum disorders (ASD). *Cochrane Database Syst Rev*. 2011;(11):CD007992.

ADDITIONAL READING

- Reichow B, Barton EE, Boyd BA, et al. Early intensive behavioral intervention (EIBI) for young children with autism spectrum disorders (ASD). *Cochrane Database Syst Rev*. 2012;10:CD009260.
- Vriend JL, Corkum PV, Moon EC, et al. Behavioral interventions for sleep problems in children with autism spectrum disorders: current findings and future directions. *J Pediatr Psychol*. 2011;36(9):1017–1029.

SEE ALSO

Algorithm: Intellectual Disability

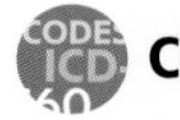

CODES

ICD10

- F84.0 Autistic disorder
- F84.5 Asperger's syndrome
- F84.3 Other childhood disintegrative disorder

CLINICAL PEARLS

ALARM mnemonic from the American Academy of Pediatrics (AAP)

- **A**SD is prevalent (screen ALL children between 18 and 24 months).
- **L**isten to parents when they feel something is wrong.
- **A**ct early: Screen all children who fall behind in language and social developmental milestones (use early learning to help with evaluation).
- **R**efer to multidisciplinary teams (speech and language evaluation, genetic screening, social support groups).
- **M**onitor support for patient and families.

BACK PAIN, LOW

Millicent King Channell, DO, MA, FAAO

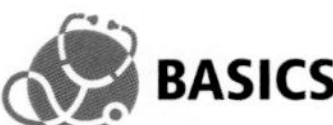

BASICS

DESCRIPTION

- Low back pain (LBP) is extremely common and includes a wide range of symptoms involving the lumbosacral spine and pelvic girdle.
- LBP can be characterized by duration or associated symptoms.
- **Duration** (1)[A]
  - Acute (<6 weeks)
  - Subacute (>6 weeks but <3 months)
  - Chronic (>3 months)
- **Associated symptoms** (1)[A]
  - Localized/nonspecific "mechanical" low back pain
  - Back pain with lower extremity symptoms
  - Systemic and visceral symptoms
- A specific cause is not found for most patients with low back pain. Most cases resolve 4–6 weeks after onset.
- It is important to rule out "red" flag symptoms that indicate the need for immediate intervention.
- System(s) affected: musculoskeletal, neurologic
- Synonym(s): lumbago, lumbar sprain/strain, low back syndrome

EPIDEMIOLOGY

Incidence

- 1-year incidence: 6–15% (1)[A]
- LBP is one of the most common primary care complaints (1)[A].

Prevalence

- Lifetime prevalence: 84% (1)[A]
- Global point prevalence: 9% (1)[A]
- Predominant sex: male = female
- Age: The highest incidence is in the 3rd decade (20–29 years), overall prevalence increases with age until age 65 years and then declines (1)[A].

ETIOLOGY AND PATHOPHYSIOLOGY

A clear etiology is not found in most patients. Age-related degenerative changes of the lumbosacral spine, and atrophy of supporting musculature may contribute (2)[A].

RISK FACTORS

- Age (1)[A]
- Activity (lifting, sudden twisting, bending) (1)[A]
- Obesity (1)[A]
- Sedentary lifestyle (1)[A]
- Physically strenuous work (1)[A]
- Psychosocial factors such as anxiety, depression, and stress (1)[A]
- Smoking (1)[A]

GENERAL PREVENTION

- Maintain normal weight (1)[A].
- Maintain physical fitness and activity (1)[A].
- Stress reduction (1)[A]
- Proper lifting technique
- Good posture
- Smoking cessation
- USPSTF states there is insufficient evidence to recommend for or against preventive intervention in adults.

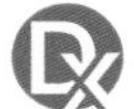

DIAGNOSIS

HISTORY

- Onset of pain (sudden or gradual) (1)[A]
- Pain from spinal structures (musculature, ligaments, facet joints, and disks) can refer to the thigh region but rarely below the knee (1)[A].
- Sacroiliac pain often refers to the thigh and can also radiate below the knee (1)[A].
- Irritation, impingement, or compression of lumbar nerve roots often results in more leg pain than back pain (1)[A].
- Pain from the L1–L3 nerve roots radiates to the hip and/or thigh, whereas pain from the L4–S1 nerve roots radiates below the knee.
- **Red flags**
  - Recent trauma
  - Neurologic deficits
    - Bowel/bladder incontinence or bladder retention
    - Saddle anesthesia
    - Weakness, falls
  - Night pain, sweats, fever, weight loss
  - Age >70 years with or without trauma
  - Age >50 years with minor trauma
  - History of cancer
  - Osteoporosis
  - Immunosuppression, prolonged glucocorticoid use
- **Yellow flags** predicting poor long-term prognosis
  - Lack of social support
  - Unsupportive work environment
  - Depression and/or anxiety
  - Abuse of alcohol or other substances
  - History of physical or sexual abuse
- Pain can be provoked with motion: flexion–extension, side-bending rotation, sitting, standing, and lifting. Pain often relieved with rest.
- Radicular pain may radiate to buttocks, thighs and lower legs.

PHYSICAL EXAM

- Observe gait, position on examination table, and facial expressions.
- Test lumbar spine range of motion.
- Evaluate for point tenderness or muscle spasm.
- Neurologic examination
  - Visual examination: signs of muscle atrophy
  - Test reflexes, strength, pulses, sensation
  - Straight leg test
  - FABER test (flexion, abduction and external rotation)

DIFFERENTIAL DIAGNOSIS

- Localized/nonspecific "mechanical" low back pain (87%) (1)[A]
  - Lumbar strain/sprain (70%)
  - Disc/facet degeneration (10%)
  - Osteoporotic compression fracture (4%)
  - Spondylolisthesis (2%)
  - Severe scoliosis, kyphosis,
  - Asymmetric transitional vertebrae (<1%)
  - Traumatic fracture (<1%)
- Back pain with lower extremity symptoms (7%) (1)[A]
  - Disc herniation (4%)
  - Spinal stenosis (3%)
- Systemic and visceral symptoms (1)[A]
  - Neoplasia (0.7%)
    - Multiple myeloma
    - Metastatic carcinoma
    - Lymphoma/leukemia
    - Spinal cord tumors
    - Retroperitoneal tumors
  - Infection (0.01%)
    - Osteomyelitis
    - Septic discitis
    - Paraspinous abscess
    - Epidural abscess
    - Shingles
  - Inflammatory disease (0.03%)
    - Ankylosing spondylitis
    - Psoriatic spondylitis
    - Reactive arthritis
    - Inflammatory bowel disease
  - Visceral disease (0.05%)
    - Prostatitis
    - Endometriosis
    - Chronic pelvic inflammatory disease
    - Nephrolithiasis
    - Pyelonephritis
    - Perinephric abscess
    - Aortic aneurysm
    - Pancreatitis
    - Cholecystitis
    - Penetrating ulcer
  - Other
    - Osteochondrosis
    - Paget disease

DIAGNOSTIC TESTS & INTERPRETATION

Initial Tests (lab, imaging)

- Imaging studies are unnecessary during the first 6 weeks if no red flag signs or symptoms.
  - X-ray of the lumbar spine (1,3,4)[A]
    - Not recommended for initial presentation or without red flags including trauma. Defer plain films for 6 weeks unless there is a high risk of disease.
    - Useful for bony etiology such as suspected fracture
  - MRI of the lumbar spine (1,3,4)[A]
    - If patient presents with neurologic deficits, fails to improve within 6 weeks of conservative treatment, or if there is a strong suspicion of cancer or cauda equina syndrome
    - Useful for suspected herniated disc, nerve root compression, or metastatic disease
  - CT scan of the lumbar spine (1,3,4)[A]
    - Appropriate alternative to MRI for patient with pacemaker, metallic hardware, or other contra-indication to MRI

- Labs are unnecessary with initial presentation if no related red flags, signs, or symptoms present (1,3,4)[A].
- If infection or bone marrow neoplasm is suspected, consider (1,3,4)[A]
  - Complete blood count with differential (CBC)
  - Erythrocyte sedimentation rate (ESR)
  - C-reactive protein level (CRP)

Diagnostic Procedures/Other

- Neurosurgical consult for acute neurologic deficits or suspected cauda equina syndrome (1,4)[A]
- Epidural injections provide short-term relief of persistent pain associated with herniated disc (1,4)[A].
- There is no significant evidence to support intradisc steroid injections, facet joint injections, medial branch blocks, and radiofrequency denervation (1,4)[A].

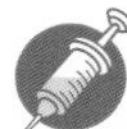

TREATMENT

- The primary goal is to provide supportive care and allow return to functional activity. Patients should be aware of alarm symptoms that should prompt a return visit to their physician.

First Line

- Patient education (4)[A]
  - Patients should be reassured that pain is usually self-limited; treatment should aim to relieve pain and improve function.
  - Encouraging activity as tolerated leads to quicker recovery.
- Medications (1,3,5)[A]
  - Acetaminophen 325–650 mg PO q4–6h PRN pain (max 4 g/day)
  - NSAIDs
    - Ibuprofen 400–600 mg PO 3–4 times daily (max 3,200 mg/day)
    - Naproxen 250–500 mg PO q12h (max 1,500 mg/day)
- Manual medicine (4)[A]
  - Osteopathic manipulative treatments (4)[A] myofascial, counter-strain, bilateral ligamentous techniques, as well as muscle energy, if tolerated

Second Line

- Second-line therapy for moderate to severe pain (1,3,5)[A]
  - Cyclobenzaprine 5–10 mg PO up to TID PRN (max 30 mg/day)
  - Tizanidine 2 mg PO up to TID PRN
  - Hydrocodone 2.5–10 mg PO q4–6h PRN pain; use of hydrocodone or other opioids for low back pain is based on clinical judgment.
- Alternate methods (1,3)[A]
  - Epidural corticosteroid injections in patients with documented radicular symptoms caused by herniated disc
- Antidepressants (1,3,5)[A]
  - Tricyclic antidepressants (amitriptyline, nortriptyline, desipramine) have been shown in randomized trials to provide a small pain reduction in patients. No clear evidence that SSRIs are more effective than placebo in cases of chronic LBP.

COMPLEMENTARY & ALTERNATIVE MEDICINE

- Acupuncture is superior to no treatment, but evidence is mixed regarding the effectiveness of acupuncture over other treatment modalities (1,3,4)[A].
- Yoga can be helpful in chronic low back pain (1,3,4)[A].

ONGOING CARE

FOLLOW-UP RECOMMENDATIONS

- Regular exercise (3,6)[A]
- Patient education regarding chronicity, recurrence, and red flags (3,6)[A]

Patient Monitoring

- Reassurance is key. Follow up within 2–4 weeks of initial presentation to monitor progress:
  - Assess severity and quality of pain as well as range of motion and other historical features.
- Reevaluate for possible underlying organic causes for pain if patients fail to improve.

COMPLICATIONS

- Regular NSAID use can increase risk of gastrointestinal toxicity and nephrotoxicity (1,4)[A].
- Acetaminophen has potential hepatotoxicity (1,4)[A].
- Centrally acting skeletal muscle relaxants and opioid agonist risk sedation, confusion, dependence, and abuse (1,4)[A].

REFERENCES

1. Golob AL, Wipf JE. Low back pain. *Med Clin North Am*. 2014;98(3):405–428.
2. Duffy RL. Low back pain: an approach to diagnosis and management. *Prim Care*. 2010;37(4):729–741, vi.
3. Chaparro LE, Furlan AD, Deshpande A, et al. Opioids compared with placebo or other treatments for chronic low back pain: an update of the Cochrane Review. *Spine (Phila Pa 1976)*. 2014;39(7):556–563.
4. Casazza BA. Diagnosis and treatment of acute low back pain. *Am Fam Physician*. 201215;85(4):343–350.
5. Lee TJ. Pharmacologic treatment for low back pain: one component of pain care. *Phys Med Rehabil Clin N Am*. 2010;21(4):793–800.
6. Savigny P, Watson P, Underwood M; Guideline Development Group. Early management of persistent non-specific low back pain: summary of NICE guidance. *BMJ*. 2009;338:b1805.

ADDITIONAL READING

- Chou R, Huffman LH; American Pain Society; American College of Physicians. Medications for acute and chronic low back pain: a review of the evidence for an American Pain Society/American College of Physicians clinical practice guideline. *Ann Intern Med*. 2007;147(7):505–514.
- Dahm KT, Brurberg KG, Jamtvedt G, et al. Advice to rest in bed versus advice to stay active for acute low-back pain and sciatica. *Cochrane Database Syst Rev*. 2010;(6):CD007612.
- de Leon-Casasola OA. Opioids for chronic pain: new evidence, new strategies, safe prescribing. *Am J Med*. 2013;126(3)(Suppl 1):S3–S11.
- Engers A, Jellema P, Wensing M, et al. Individual patient education for low back pain. *Cochrane Database Syst Rev*. 2011;(1):CD004057.
- Falco FJ, Manchikanti L, Datta S, et al. An update of the effectiveness of therapeutic lumbar facet joint interventions. *Pain Physician*. 2012;15(6):E909–E953.
- Flynn TW, Smith B, Chou R. Appropriate use of diagnostic imaging in low back pain: a reminder that unnecessary imaging may do as much harm as good. *J Orthop Sports Phys Ther*. 2011;41(11):838–846.
- Gleason JM, Slezak JM, Jung H, et al. Regular nonsteroidal anti-inflammatory drug use and erectile dysfunction. *J Urol*. 2011;1854(4):1388–1393.
- Henschke N, Ostelo RW, van Tulder MW, et al. Behavioural treatment for chronic low-back pain. *Cochrane Database Syst Rev*. 2010;(7):CD002014.
- Hutchinson AJ, Ball S, Andrews JC, et al. The effectiveness of acupuncture in treating chronic non-specific low back pain: a systematic review of the literature. *J Orthop Surg Res*. 2012;7:36.
- Kuijpers T, van Middelkoop M, Rubinstein SM, et al. A systematic review on the effectiveness of pharmacological interventions for chronic non-specific low-back pain. *Eur Spine J*. 2011;20(1):40–50.
- Srinivas SV, Deyo RA, Berger ZD. Application of "less is more" to low back pain. *Arch Intern Med*. 2012;172(13):1016–1020.
- Urquhart DM, Hoving JL, Assendelft WW, et al. Antidepressants for non-specific low back pain. *Cochrane Database Syst Rev*. 2010;(1):CD001703.
- Walker BF, French SD, Grant W, et al. A Cochrane review of combined chiropractic interventions for low-back pain. *Spine*. 2011;36(3):230–242.
- Waterman BR, Belmont PJ, Shoenfeld AJ. Low back pain in the United States: incidence and risk factors for presentation in the emergency setting. *Spine J*. 2012;12(1):63–70.
- Wegner I, Widyahening IS, van Tulder MW, et al. Traction for low-back pain with or without sciatica. *Cochrane Database Syst Rev*. 2013;8:CD003010.

SEE ALSO

- Lumbar (Intervertebral) Disc Disorders
- Algorithm: Low Back Pain, Acute

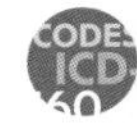

CODES

ICD10

- M54.5 Low back pain
- G89.29 Other chronic pain

CLINICAL PEARLS

- Low back pain is one of the most common complaint seen in primary care. Most patients do not have an identifiable cause of pain, and most cases resolve within 4–12 weeks of onset.
- Review red flag symptoms that may indicate neurologic compromise, infection, or cancer.
- Labs and imaging studies are unnecessary for most cases of back pain if no red flag symptoms are present.

BACTERIURIA, ASYMPTOMATIC

Mony Fraer, MD, FACP, FASN • Kantima Phisitkul, MD

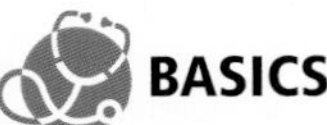

BASICS

DESCRIPTION

Asymptomatic bacteriuria (ASB) is diagnosed when significant bacteriuria is not accompanied by signs and symptoms referable to urinary tract infection (UTI).

EPIDEMIOLOGY

Incidence

- General population: 3.5%
- Pregnancy: 7–10%
- Older women: 16–18%

Prevalence

- Variable, increased with age, female gender, sexual activity, and presence of genitourinary (GU) abnormalities
- Pregnancy: 2–10%
- Short- and long-term indwelling catheter 9–23% and 100%, respectively
- Long-term care residents in women 25–50% and men 15–40%

ETIOLOGY AND PATHOPHYSIOLOGY

- Microbiology is similar to that of other UTI, with bacteria originating from periurethral area, vagina, or gut.
- Organisms are less virulent in ASB than those causing UTI.
- The most common organism in pregnancy is *Escherichia coli*. Other common organisms are *Klebsiella pneumonia*, *Proteus mirabilis*, *Staphylococcus aureus*, group B *Streptococcus* (GBS), and *Enterococcus*.

Genetics

Genetic variations that reduce toll-like receptor-4 function (TLR4) have been associated with ASB by lowering innate immune response and delaying bacterial clearance.

RISK FACTORS

- Older age
- Female gender
- Sexual activity, use of diaphragm with spermicide
- GU abnormalities: neurogenic bladder, urinary retention, urinary catheter use (indwelling, intermittent, or condom catheter)
- Institutionalized residents
- Diabetes mellitus
- Immunocompromised status
- Spinal cord injuries or functional impairment
- Hemodialysis

COMMONLY ASSOCIATED CONDITIONS

Depends on the risk factors

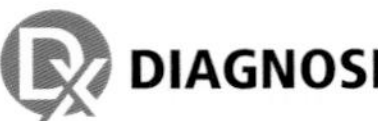

DIAGNOSIS

HISTORY

- Asymptomatic
- Negative symptoms referable to UTI such as fever, acute dysuria (<1 week), new or worsening urinary urgency/frequency/incontinence, or acute gross hematuria

PHYSICAL EXAM

- Afebrile
- No suprapubic and costovertebral angle tenderness

DIFFERENTIAL DIAGNOSIS

- UTI
- Contaminated urine specimen

DIAGNOSTIC TESTS & INTERPRETATION

Initial Tests (lab, imaging)

- Urinalysis (UA): pyuria (common)
- Screening urine culture in asymptomatic patients is indicated in only two conditions:
  - Pregnancy: screening between 12 and 16 weeks' gestation or at first prenatal visit if later (1)[A]
  - Prior to transurethral resection of prostate (TURP) (1)[A] or any urologic interventions when mucosal bleeding is anticipated (1)[C]
- Screening for ASB in men and nonpregnant women is not recommended.

Follow-Up Tests & Special Considerations

- Noncontaminated urine specimen should be used for urine culture.
- In pregnancy, periodic screening urine culture should be done after ASB treatment (1)[A] but not required in GBS bacteriuria (2,3)[C].

Test Interpretation

- Per Infectious Disease Society of America
  - Significant bacteriuria is defined based on type of urine specimen, sex, and the amount of bacteria.
  - By midstream, clean catch specimen
    - Male: >100,000 CFU/mL of single bacteria species
    - Female: the same criteria as male but needs 2 positive consecutive specimens
  - By catheterized specimen
  - Male and female: >100 CFU/mL of 1 bacterial species. Required 1-time collection only
- Patient with significant bacteriuria with or without pyuria and without symptoms referable to UTI should be diagnosed as ASB.

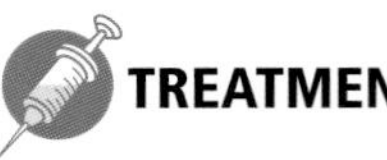

TREATMENT

GENERAL MEASURES

ALERT

- Antibiotic treatment of ASB is indicated in two conditions;
  - Pregnancy (1)[A]
    - Rationale: Treatment has been shown to significantly reduce the incidence of acute pyelonephritis and low birth weight.
  - Prior to urologic procedure particularly TURP (1)[A]
    - Rationale: Antibiotic treatment can effectively prevent postprocedure bacteremia and sepsis.
- Treatment of ASB in other conditions (nonpregnant women, diabetic women, indwelling catheter, patients with spinal cord injury, or the elderly living in the community) does not provide any known clinical benefit, does not reduce the risk of symptomatic infection nor improvement in morbidity or mortality. Indeed, it increases health care cost, adverse drug side effects, development of resistant organisms, and reinfection rate (1,4).
- Inadequate evidence to guide management in nonurologic procedure and solid organ transplant (1,4)

MEDICATION

First Line

- Pregnancy
  - Intrapartum antibiotic prophylaxis with intravenous penicillin or clindamycin (penicillin allergy) is recommended for women with GBS bacteriuria occurring at any stage of pregnancy and of any colony count to prevent GBS disease in the newborn (2)[C].
  - No consensus on choice of antibiotics and duration of treatment in pregnancy, however, the cure rate is higher for the 4–7 days of treatment than 1-day treatment (1)[A].
  - Choice of antibiotics should be guided by bacterial pathogen, local resistance rate, adverse effects, and comorbidities of patients (5).
  - Common oral antibiotics that have been used
    - Nitrofurantoin 100 mg BID × 5 days (low level of resistance, may cause hemolysis in glucose-6-phosphate dehydrogenase deficiency)
    - Amoxicillin/clavulanate 500/125 BID × 5–7 days
    - Cefuroxime 250 mg BID × 5 days
    - Cephalexin 500 mg BID × 5 days
    - Fosfomycin 3 g × 1 single dose (not effective when glomerular filtration rate is less than 30 mL/min, may be used in highly resistant bacteria such as methicillin-resistant *Staphylococcus aureus* [MRSA], vancomycin-resistant enterococci [VRE], and extended-spectrum beta-lactamase [ESBL]-producing organism bacteria) (6)
  - Avoid trimethoprim in 1st trimester and sulfa after 32 weeks' gestation.
  - Contraindicated: fluoroquinolones (FDA-C), tetracyclines (FDA-D)
- Prior to urologic interventions
  - Initiate antibiotic the night before or immediately before the procedure (1)[A].
  - Antibiotic should be continued until the indwelling catheter is removed postprocedure (1)[B].

ONGOING CARE

FOLLOW-UP RECOMMENDATIONS

No consensus on screening frequency of ASB in pregnancy, but monthly screening of urine culture after ASB treatment is recommended except GBS (1,2).

Patient Monitoring

Development of any signs/symptoms of UTI should warrant antibiotic treatment.

DIET

Daily cranberry juice may reduce the frequency of ASB during pregnancy, but it has not been confirmed in large study (see "Additional Reading").

PATIENT EDUCATION

Patient should seek medical attention when UTI symptoms develop.

COMPLICATIONS

- Late pregnancy pyelonephritis occurs in 20–35% of women with untreated bacteriuria (20–30-fold higher than women with negative initial screening urine cultures or in whom bacteriuria was treated). Pyelonephritis is associated with premature delivery and worse fetal outcomes (infant with group B streptococcal infections, low–birth weight infant). Antimicrobial treatment will decrease the risk of subsequent pyelonephritis from 20–35% to 1–4% and the risk of having a low–birth weight baby from 15 to 5%.
- If bacteriuria remains untreated in patients who undergo traumatic urologic procedures, up to 60% develop bacteremia after the procedure and 5–10% progress to severe sepsis/septic shock.

REFERENCES

1. Nicolle LE, Bradley S, Colgan R, et al. Infectious Diseases Society of America guidelines for the diagnosis and treatment of asymptomatic bacteriuria in adults. *Clin Infect Dis*. 2005;40(5):643–654.
2. Zolotor AJ, Carlough MC. Update on prenatal care. *Am Fam Physician*. 2014;89(3):199–208.
3. Nicolle LE. Asymptomatic bacteriuria. *Curr Opin Infect Dis*. 2014;27(1):90–96.
4. Trautner BW, Grigoryan L. Approach to a positive urine culture in a patient without urinary symptoms. *Infect Dis Clin North Am*. 2014;28(1):15–31.
5. Mody L, Juthani-Mehta M. Urinary tract infections in older women: a clinical review. *JAMA*. 2014; 311(8):844–854.
6. Keating GM. Fosfomycin trometamol: a review of its use as a single-dose oral treatment for patients with acute lower urinary tract infections and pregnant women with asymptomatic bacteriuria. *Drugs*. 2013;73(17):1951–1966.

ADDITIONAL READING

- Ragnarsdóttir B, Svanborg C. Susceptibility to acute pyelonephritis or asymptomatic bacteriuria: host-pathogen interaction in urinary tract infections. *Pediatr Nephrol*. 2012;27(11):2017–2029.
- Wing DA, Rumney PJ, Preslicka CW. Daily cranberry juice for the prevention of asymptomatic bacteriuria in pregnancy: a randomized, controlled pilot study. *J Urol*. 2008;180(4):1367–1372.

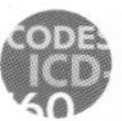

CODES

ICD10

- N39.0 Urinary tract infection, site not specified
- B96.20 Unsp Escherichia coli as the cause of diseases classd elswhr

CLINICAL PEARLS

- ASB is common, benign, and not harmful in most patients.
- Pyuria is common in ASB and not an indication for antimicrobial treatment on its own.
- Antibiotic treatment is indicated for ASB in pregnancy and patients who require urologic procedure in which mucosal bleeding is anticipated.
- Treatment of ASB in other conditions does not decrease the frequency of UTI or improve other outcome.
- Overtreatment of ASB may result in negative consequences such as antimicrobial resistance, adverse drug reaction, and unnecessary cost.

BALANITIS, PHIMOSIS, AND PARAPHIMOSIS

James P. Miller, MD

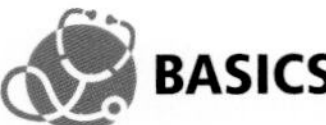

BASICS

DESCRIPTION

- Balanitis:
  - An inflammation of the glans penis
  - Posthitis is an inflammation of the foreskin.
  - Balanitis xerotica obliterans (BXO) is lichen sclerosus of the glans penis (uncommon).
- Phimosis and paraphimosis:
  - Phimosis: tightness of the distal penile foreskin that prevents it from being drawn back from over the glans
  - Paraphimosis: constriction by foreskin of an uncircumcised penis, preventing the foreskin from returning to its position over the glans; occurs after the retracted foreskin becomes swollen and engorged; a urologic emergency
- System(s) affected: renal/urologic; reproductive; skin/exocrine

ALERT

- Recurrent infection and irritations (condom catheters) can lead to phimosis.
- Recurrent balanitis, either chemical or infectious, can lead to an acquired phimosis.
- Inappropriate forced reduction of a physiologic foreskin can lead to chronic scarring and acquired phimosis. Unfortunately, many times done due to instructions from health care providers.

EPIDEMIOLOGY

- Balanitis: predominant age: adult; predominant gender: male only
- Phimosis/paraphimosis: predominant age: infancy and adolescence; unusual in adults; risk returns in geriatrics; predominant sex: male only

Incidence

Balanitis: will affect 3–11% of males

Prevalence

Phimosis: in the United States: 8% of boys age 6 years and 1% of men >16 years of age (1)

ETIOLOGY AND PATHOPHYSIOLOGY

- Balanitis:
  - Allergic reaction (condom latex, contraceptive jelly)
  - Infections (*Candida albicans*, *Borrelia vincentii*, streptococci, *Trichomonas,* HPV)
  - Fixed-drug eruption (sulfa, tetracycline)
  - Plasma cell infiltration (Zoon balanitis)
  - Autodigestion by activated pancreatic transplant exocrine enzymes
- Phimosis:
  - Physiologic: present at birth; resolves spontaneously during the first 2–3 years of life through nocturnal erections, which slowly dilate the phimotic ring
  - Acquired: recurrent inflammation, trauma, or infections of the foreskin
- Paraphimosis:
  - Often iatrogenically or inadvertently induced by the foreskin not being pulled back over the glans after voiding, cleaning, cystoscopy, or catheter insertion

Geriatric Considerations

Condom catheters can predispose to balanitis.

Pediatric Considerations

Oral antibiotics predispose male infants to *Candida balanitis*. Inappropriate care of physiologic phimosis can lead to acquired phimosis by repeated forced reduction of the foreskin.

RISK FACTORS

- Balanitis:
  - Presence of foreskin
  - Morbid obesity
  - Poor hygiene
  - Diabetes; probably most common
  - Nursing home environment
  - Condom catheters
  - Chemical irritants
  - Edematous conditions: CHF, nephrosis
- Phimosis:
  - Poor hygiene
  - Diabetes by repeated balanitis
  - Frequent diaper rash in infants
  - Recurrent posthitis
- Paraphimosis:
  - Presence of foreskin
  - Inexperienced health care provider (leaving foreskin retracted after catheter placement)
  - Poor education about care of the foreskin

GENERAL PREVENTION

- Balanitis:
  - Proper hygiene and avoidance of allergens
  - Circumcision
- Phimosis/paraphimosis:
  - If the patient is uncircumcised, appropriate hygiene and care of the foreskin are necessary to prevent phimosis and paraphimosis.

DIAGNOSIS

HISTORY

- Balanitis:
  - Pain
  - Drainage
  - Dysuria
  - Odor
  - Ballooning of foreskin with voiding
  - Redness
- Phimosis:
  - Painful erections
  - Recurrent balanitis
  - Foreskin balloons when voiding
  - Inability to retract foreskin at appropriate age
- Paraphimosis:
  - Uncircumcised
  - Pain
  - Drainage
  - Voiding difficulty

PHYSICAL EXAM

- Balanitis:
  - Erythema
  - Edema
  - Discharge
  - Ulceration
  - Plaque
- Phimosis
  - Foreskin will not retract.
  - Secondary balanitis
  - Physiologis phimosis—preputial orifice appears normal and healthy.
  - Pathologic phimosis—preputial orifice has fine white fibrous ring of scar.
- Paraphimosis
  - Edema of prepuce and glans
  - Drainage
  - Ulceration

DIFFERENTIAL DIAGNOSIS

- Balanitis:
  - Leukoplakia
  - Lichen planus
  - Psoriasis
  - Reiter syndrome
  - Lichen sclerosus et atrophicus
  - Erythroplasia of Queyrat
  - BXO: atrophic changes at end of foreskin; can form band that prevents retraction
- Phimosis/paraphimosis:
  - Penile lymphedema, which can be related to insect bites, trauma, or allergic reactions
  - Penile tourniquet syndrome: foreign body around penis, most commonly hair
  - Anasarca

DIAGNOSTIC TESTS & INTERPRETATION

Initial Tests (lab, imaging)

- Microbiology culture
- Wet mount
- Serology for syphilis
- Serum glucose; ESR (if concerns about Reiter syndrome)
- STD testing
- HIV testing
- Gram stain

Diagnostic Procedures/Other

Biopsy, if persistent

Pathologic Findings

Plasma cells infiltration with Zoon balanitis

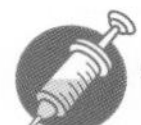

TREATMENT

GENERAL MEASURES

- Consider circumcision for recurrent balanitis and paraphimosis.
- Warm compresses or sitz baths
- Local hygiene

MEDICATION

- Balanitis:
  - Antifungal:
    - Clotrimazole (Lotrimin) 1% BID
    - Nystatin (Mycostatin) BID–QID
    - Fluconazole: 150 mg PO single dose
- Antibacterial:
  - Bacitracin QID
  - Neomycin–polymyxin B–bacitracin (Neosporin) QID
  - If cellulitis, cephalosporin or sulfa drug PO or parenteral:
    - Dermatitis: topical steroids QID
    - Zoon balanitis: topical steroids QID
- Phimosis:
  - 0.05% fluticasone propionate daily for 4–8 weeks with gradual traction placed on foreskin (2)[B]
  - 1% pimecrolimus BID for 4–6 weeks. Not for use in children <2 years (3)[C].
- Paraphimosis:
  - Manual reduction, if possible (should be done with the patient sedated). Place the middle and index fingers of both hands on the engorged skin proximal to the glans. Place both thumbs on glans and, with gentle pressure, push on the glans and pull on the foreskin to attempt reduction. If unsuccessful, a dorsal slit will be necessary, with eventual circumcision after the edema resolves.
  - Osmotic agents: granulated sugar placed on edematous tissue for several hours to reduce edema
  - Puncture technique: Multiple punctures of foreskin with a 21-gauge needle will allow edematous fluid to escape and thus allow reduction.
  - Dorsal slit; done by surgeon or urologist
- BXO:
  - 0.05% betamethasone BID
  - 0.1% tacrolimus BID

ISSUES FOR REFERRAL

Recurrent infections or development of meatal stenosis

SURGERY/OTHER PROCEDURES

- Balanitis and phimosis: Consider circumcision as preventive measure.
- For paraphimosis:
  - Represents a true surgical emergency to avoid necrosis of glans
  - Dorsal slit with delayed circumcision, if reduction is not possible
  - Operative exploration if the possibility of penile tourniquet syndrome cannot be eliminated. Hair removal cream can be applied if a hair is thought to be the cause of the tourniquet.

INPATIENT CONSIDERATIONS

Admission Criteria

- Uncontrolled diabetes
- Sepsis

Nursing

Appropriate hygiene if condom catheters are used

Discharge Criteria

Resolution of problem

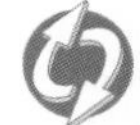

ONGOING CARE

FOLLOW-UP RECOMMENDATIONS

Patient Monitoring

Balanitis:

- Every 1–2 weeks until etiology has been established
- Persistent balanitis may require biopsy to rule out malignancy or BXO.
- Evaluation for resolution of phimosis

DIET

Weight reduction, if obese

PATIENT EDUCATION

- Need for appropriate hygiene
- Appropriate foreskin care
- Avoidance of known allergens
- No sexual activity for 2–3 weeks after circumcision

PROGNOSIS

Should resolve with appropriate treatment

COMPLICATIONS

- Meatal stenosis
- Premalignant changes from chronic irritation
- UTIs
- Acquired phimosis
- Unreducible paraphimosis can lead to gangrene.
- Posthitis (inflammation of the prepuce)

REFERENCES

1. Oster J. Further fate of the foreskin. Incidence of preputial adhesions, phimosis, and smegma among Danish schoolboys. *Arch Dis Child*. 1968; 43(228):200–203.
2. Zavras N, Christianakis E, Mpourikas D, et al. Conservative treatment of phimosis with fluticasone proprionate 0.05%: a clinical study in 1185 boys. *J Pediatr Urol*. 2009;5(3):181–185.
3. Georgala S, Gregoriou S, Georgala C, et al. Pimecrolimus 1% cream in non-specific inflammatory recurrent balanitis. *Dermatology*. 2007;215(3):209–212.

ADDITIONAL READING

- Kiss A, Csontai A, Pirót L, et al. The response of balanitis xerotica obliterans to local steroid application compared with placebo in children. *J Urol*. 2001;165(1):219–220.
- Palmer LS, Palmer JS. The efficacy of topical betamethasone for treating phimosis: a comparison of two treatment regimens. *Urology*. 2008;72(1): 68–71.
- Pandher BS, Rustin MH, Kaisary AV. Treatment of balanitis xerotica obliterans with topical tacrolimus. *J Urol*. 2003;170(3):923.
- Stary A, Soeltz-Szoets J, Ziegler C, et al. Comparison of the efficacy and safety of oral fluconazole and topical clotrimazole in patients with candida balanitis. *Genitourin Med*. 1996;72(2):98–102.

SEE ALSO

Reiter Syndrome

CODES

ICD10

- N48.1 Balanitis
- N47.1 Phimosis
- N47.2 Paraphimosis

CLINICAL PEARLS

- Balanitis is an inflammation of the glans penis. Posthitis is an inflammation of the foreskin. BXO is lichen sclerosus of the glans penis.
- With recurrent infections and a plaque, a biopsy should be done to rule out BXO or malignancy.
- If there is a true phimosis that interferes with appropriate hygiene, treat the phimosis with steroids or circumcision to help with hygiene.

BAROTRAUMA OF THE MIDDLE EAR, SINUSES, AND LUNG

Robert A. Baldor, MD, FAAFP

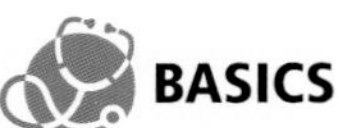

BASICS

DESCRIPTION

- Barotrauma is tissue damage resulting from the direct effects of pressure. Extreme changes or imbalances between ambient pressure and pressure within an enclosed body cavity can cause physical damage to tissue lining the cavity.
- Body cavities at greatest risk for barotrauma
  - Middle ear (otic barotrauma)
  - Paranasal sinuses (sinus barotrauma)
  - Lungs (pulmonary barotrauma)
- Dental barotrauma
  - Dental work can create small pockets of air, which can damage teeth in scuba divers or aviators during pressure change.
- Synonym(s): dysbarism; aerotitis; otitic barotrauma; middle ear barotrauma

ALERT

- Dizziness and sensorineural hearing loss warrant immediate ENT referral for inner ear involvement.
- Valsalva maneuver can spread nasopharyngeal infection into the middle ear.

EPIDEMIOLOGY

Incidence

- Pulmonary barotrauma is the 2nd leading cause of death among divers.
- Pulmonary barotrauma affects 3% of mechanically ventilated patients.
- Otic barotrauma is common in air travel.

Pediatric Considerations

- Children have difficulty opening the eustachian tube and commonly develop upper respiratory infections. This combination results in higher risk for otic and sinus barotraumas with smaller pressure changes than adults.
- Mechanical ventilation of neonates is associated with barotrauma and contributes to bronchopulmonary dysplasia.

ALERT

Increased nasal congestion in pregnancy increases risk of barotitis media (barotrauma of the middle ear).

ETIOLOGY AND PATHOPHYSIOLOGY

- Boyle law states that the volume of a gas varies inversely with pressure if temperature is held constant. When gas is trapped in a confined space, such as the middle ear, paranasal sinus, or lungs, a sudden decrease in ambient pressure causes expansion of the gas within the cavity.
- Otalgia (earache) and hearing loss occur as a result of stretching and deformation of the tympanic membrane.
- Sudden pressure differentials between middle and inner ear may lead to rupture of the round or oval window. This can create a labyrinthine fistula, which consequently can allow leakage of perilymph. Damage to inner ear may be permanent.
- When the transalveolar pressure disrupts the structural integrity of the alveolus, the alveolar wall can rupture, leading to interstitial emphysema, pneumothorax, or pneumomediastinum.
- Otic and sinus barotrauma:
  - Associated with rapid or extreme changes in environmental pressure: air travel, mountain climbing, scuba diving
    - Nasal congestion or eustachian tube dysfunction increases risk of damage.
    - Failure of eustachian tube to equilibrate pressure may distort the tympanic membrane, causing discomfort or rupture.
    - Rupture of round or oval membrane may cause inner ear barotrauma, vertigo, and sensorineural hearing loss.
- Pulmonary barotrauma
  - Iatrogenic complication of mechanical ventilation or complication of scuba diving.

RISK FACTORS

- Otic or sinus
  - High-risk activities
    - Scuba diving, especially with rapid ascent or breath-holding
    - Airplane flight; sky diving; high-altitude travel
    - High-impact sports: boxing, soccer, water skiing
  - Recurrent upper respiratory infections
  - Nasal congestion or allergic rhinitis
  - Eustachian tube dysfunction
  - Blast exposure
  - The most common complication of hyperbaric oxygen treatment is middle ear barotrauma, which can lead to permanent hearing loss and vertigo.
  - Pregnancy (associated nasal congestion)
  - Anatomic obstruction in the nasopharynx
    - Deviated nasal septum
    - Nasal polyps
    - Congenital anomalies, including cleft palate
  - Previous history of ear trauma
- Pulmonary
  - Iatrogenic:
    - Mechanical ventilation, especially in the presence of asthma, chronic interstitial lung disease, acute respiratory distress syndrome
    - Hyperbaric oxygen therapy
  - Scuba diving or other underwater activities
  - Air travel with preexisting pulmonary pathology

GENERAL PREVENTION

- Pulmonary barotrauma
  - Cautious use of mechanical ventilation and hyperbaric oxygen therapy
  - Avoid breath holding during ascent while scuba diving.
- Otic barotrauma
  - Avoid altitude changes or scuba diving with eustachian tube dysfunction.
  - Treat upper respiratory congestion.
- Equilibration of pressure: Valsalva maneuver, yawning, swallowing, drinking, or chewing gum

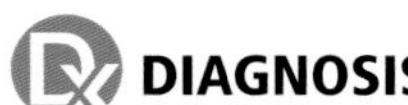

DIAGNOSIS

HISTORY

- History of high-risk activity
- Otic (middle ear) barotrauma:
  - Otalgia, sensation of fullness or pressure in the ear
  - Hearing loss
  - Vertigo
  - Transient facial paralysis
  - Otorrhea
- All patients with middle ear barotrauma should be evaluated for inner ear barotrauma:
  - Hearing loss
  - Tinnitus
  - Vertigo
  - Disorientation
- Sinus barotrauma
  - Facial pain, sensation of fullness or pressure
- Pulmonary barotrauma: Ask about scuba diving, mechanical ventilation, air travel with preexisting lung disease:
  - Chest pain, dyspnea

PHYSICAL EXAM

- Otic barotrauma
  - Otoscopic exam: otorrhea, pneumotoscopy
  - Assess balance and hearing.
  - Palpate eustachian tube for tenderness.
- Otic (middle ear) barotrauma
  - Conductive hearing loss with Weber and Rinne tests
  - Transient facial paralysis
- All patients with middle ear barotrauma should be evaluated for inner ear barotrauma:
  - Sensorineural hearing loss with Weber and Rinne tests
- Sinus barotrauma
  - Facial tenderness
- Pulmonary barotrauma
  - Hypoxia, hypotension
  - Auscultation, percussion
  - Assessment of respiratory distress

DIFFERENTIAL DIAGNOSIS

- Acute and chronic otitis media
- Otitis externa
- Temporomandibular joint syndrome
- Pulmonary: pulmonary embolism; complications of mechanical ventilation

DIAGNOSTIC TESTS & INTERPRETATION

Initial Tests (lab, imaging)

- Otic or sinus
  - CT to rule out nasopharyngeal tumor or chronic sinus disease, if suspected
- Pulmonary
  - Chest radiograph
  - Chest CT if CXR not informative
  - Arterial blood gases (ABG)
- Other: ultrasound

Diagnostic Procedures/Other

- Otic barotrauma
  - Tympanometry
  - Audiometry: conductive (middle ear) versus sensorineural (inner ear) hearing loss
  - Surgical exploration to rule out inner ear involvement, if suspected
- Pulmonary barotrauma: chest tube insertion, if clincally indicated, for pneumothorax

Test Interpretation

- Tympanic membrane (TM) retraction or bulging
  - Teed 0: no visible damage
  - Teed 1: congestion around umbo
  - Teed 2: congestion of entire TM
  - Teed 3: hemorrhage into middle ear
  - Teed 4: extensive middle ear hemorrhage; TM may rupture.
  - Teed 5: entire middle ear filled with deoxygenated blood
- Inner ear involvement with rupture of the round or oval windows, perilymphatic fistula, and leakage of perilymph into the middle ear
- Pulmonary barotrauma
  - Alveolar rupture may progress to interstitial emphysema, pneumoperitoneum, and pneumothorax.

- Petechial hemorrhages in area covered by diver's mask, as well as subconjunctival hemorrhages

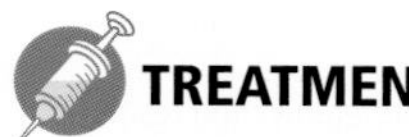

TREATMENT

GENERAL MEASURES

- Prevention/avoidance is best: Avoid flying or diving when risk factors are present.
- Autoinflate the eustachian tube during pressure changes 1[B].
  - Valsalva during ascent and descent in air travel
  - Infants: breastfeeding, pacifier use or bottle feed
  - ≥4 years: chewing gum
  - ≥8 years: blowing up a balloon
  - Adults: chewing gum, swallowing, or yawning
- The nasal balloon is effective for prevention 1[B].
- Pressure-equalizing earplugs are not recommended in air travel and do not prevent ear barotrauma 2[B].
- For inner ear barotrauma
  - Bed rest with head elevated to avoid leakage of perilymph
  - Tympanotomy and repair of round or oval window may be necessary.
  - Sudden or progressive sensorineural hearing loss accompanied by dizziness following barotrauma should prompt consideration of a perilymph fistula. Early surgical exploration is recommended to improve hearing and vestibular symptoms 3[C].
- Treatment of pneumothorax
  - Removal of air from pleural space (chest tube; Heimlich valve)
- Correct iatrogenic cause (e.g., adjustment of mechanical ventilation).

MEDICATION

- Treat predisposing conditions (e.g., upper respiratory congestion prior to air travel):
  - Oral decongestants
  - Nasal decongestants
  - Antihistamines
- Antibiotics are not indicated for middle ear effusion secondary to barotrauma.
- HBO therapy is the treatment of choice for patients with inner ear decompression sickness but is contraindicated in patients with inner ear barotrauma 4[B].
- Analgesics for pain control
- Tinnitus can be treated with high-dose steroids if given within 3 weeks of onset 5[C].

ISSUES FOR REFERRAL

- Refer to otolaryngology if inner ear is exposed, perilymphatic fistula is present, or sensorineural hearing loss experienced.
- Consultation with a hyperbaric specialist if recompression is required
- Chest tube placement

SURGERY/OTHER PROCEDURES

- If necessary, myringotomy or tympanoplasty
- Tympanotomy and repair of round or oval window may be necessary for inner ear barotrauma.
- Tube thoracostomy for persistent pneumothorax

INPATIENT CONSIDERATIONS

Admission Criteria/Initial Stabilization

- Patients with complicating emergencies (e.g., incapacitating pain requiring myringotomy, large tympanic perforation requiring tympanoplasty)
- Inner ear barotrauma with hearing loss
- Management of pneumothorax

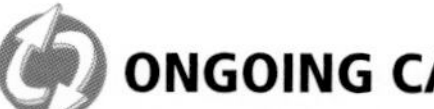

ONGOING CARE

FOLLOW-UP RECOMMENDATIONS

- No flying or diving until complete resolution of all signs and symptoms and Valsalva maneuver succeeds in equalizing pressure
- Complete bed rest for inner ear barotrauma
- No high-risk activities or air travel until pneumothorax is completely resolved.

Patient Monitoring

- Repeat physical examination until symptoms clear.
- Audiograms and tympanometry if tympanic rupture

PATIENT EDUCATION

- Demonstrate proper Valsalva maneuver.
- Appropriately treat sinus infections.
- American Academy of Pediatrics travel safety tips: http://www.aap.org
- Divers Alert Network of Duke University Medical Center information line: (919) 684-2948

PROGNOSIS

- Mild barotitis media may resolve spontaneously.
- Tympanic rupture takes weeks to months for healing.
- Hearing loss may be permanent in barotitis externa.
- Prognosis of pulmonary barotrauma depends on the extent of underlying pathology.

COMPLICATIONS

- Permanent hearing loss
- Ruptured tympanic membrane
- Chronic tinnitus, vertigo
- Fluid exudate in middle ear
- Perilymphatic fistula
- Sensorineural hearing loss

REFERENCES

1. Stangerup SE, Klokker M, Vesterhauge S, et al. Point prevalence of barotitis and its prevention and treatment with nasal balloon inflation: A prospective, controlled study. *Otol Neurotol*. 2004;25(2):89–94.
2. Klokker M, Vesterhauge S, Jansen EC. Pressure-equalizing earplugs do not prevent barotrauma on descent from 8000 ft cabin altitude. *Aviat Space Environ Med*. 2005;76(11):1079–1082.
3. Park GY, Byun H, Moon IJ. Effects of early surgical exploration in suspected barotraumatic perilymph fistulas. *Clin Exp Otorhinolaryngol*. 2012;5(2):74–80.
4. Klingmann C. Treatment of acute cochleovestibular damage after diving. *HNO*. 2004;52(10):891–896.
5. Duplessis C, Hoffer M. Tinnitus in an active duty navy diver: A review of inner ear barotrauma, tinnitus, and its treatment. *Undersea Hyperbaric Med*. 2006;33(4):223–230.

SEE ALSO

Algorithm: Ear Pain

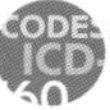

CODES

ICD10

- T70.0XXA Otitic barotrauma, initial encounter
- T70.1XXA Sinus barotrauma, initial encounter
- T70.29XA Other effects of high altitude, initial encounter

CLINICAL PEARLS

- Small children can equalize eustachian tube pressure by breastfeeding or sucking on bottles or pacifiers. Crying also serves as autoinflation.
- Pulmonary barotrauma is the 2nd leading cause of death among divers.
- Otic barotrauma is common in air travel, especially among flight personnel.
- Pulmonary barotrauma is noted in 3% of mechanically ventilated patients.
- Sudden or progressive sensorineural hearing loss accompanied by dizziness following barotrauma suggests a perilymphatic fistula. Early surgical exploration is recommended to preserve hearing and vestibular functions.

BARRETT ESOPHAGUS

Jonathan T. Lin, MD • Harlan G. Rich, MD, FACP, AGAF

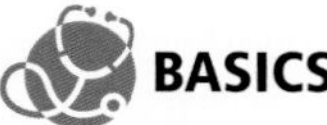

BASICS

DESCRIPTION

- Metaplasia of the distal esophageal mucosa from the normal stratified squamous epithelium to abnormal columnar (intestinalized) epithelium, likely as a consequence of chronic GERD
- Predisposes to the development of adenocarcinoma of the esophagus

EPIDEMIOLOGY

- Predominant age: >50 years
- May occur in children (rare <5 years)

Incidence

- 10–15% of patients undergoing endoscopy for evaluation of reflux symptoms (1)
- Esophageal adenocarcinoma incidence is one of the fastest rising malignancies in the United States (1,2):
  - From 1975 to 2001, nearly a 6-fold increase from 4 to 23 cases per million person-years
  - Attributed to changes in smoking and obesity rather than reclassification or overdiagnosis

Prevalence

- Difficult to ascertain because of different populations studied, varying definitions used, and common nature of asymptomatic cases
- As many as 1.5–2.0 million adults in the United States (extrapolated from a 1.6% prevalence in Swedish general population) (1)

ETIOLOGY AND PATHOPHYSIOLOGY

- Chronic gastric reflux injures the esophageal mucosa, triggering the development of columnar metaplasia. Bile acids in reflux felt to induce differentiation in gastroesophageal junction (GEJ) cells.
- Columnar cells in the esophagus have higher malignant potential than squamous cells. Activation of CDX2 gene and overexpression of HER2/neu (ERBB2) oncogene promotes carcinogenesis.
- Elevated levels of COX-2, a mediator of inflammation and regulator of epithelial cell growth, have been associated with Barrett esophagus (2).
- Classic progression: normal epithelium → esophagitis → metaplasia (Barrett esophagus) → dysplasia (low- or high-grade) → adenocarcinoma

Genetics

- Familial predisposition to GERD and Barrett esophagus has been described, along with multiple genetic markers.
- Acquired genetic changes lead to adenocarcinoma and are being investigated for use as biomarkers for risk stratification and early detection.

RISK FACTORS

- Chronic reflux (>5 years)
- Hiatal hernia
- Age >50 years
- Male gender
- White ethnicity—incidence in white males is much higher than white women and African American men
- Smoking history
- Intra-abdominal obesity
- Family history with at least 1 1st-degree relative with Barrett esophagus or esophageal adenocarcinoma

GENERAL PREVENTION

Weight loss, smoking cessation, dietary intake of fruits and vegetables, and wine consumption may decrease risk of both Barrett esophagus and lower progression to esophageal cancer (3)[C].

COMMONLY ASSOCIATED CONDITIONS

GERD, obesity, hiatal hernia

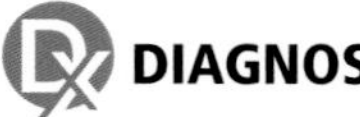

DIAGNOSIS

HISTORY

- Assess underlying risk factors
- GERD symptoms common: heartburn, regurgitation, or dysphagia
- Less common symptoms include chest pain, odynophagia, chronic cough, water brash, globus sensation, laryngitis, or wheezing.
- Symptoms suggestive of complicated GERD or cancer: weight loss, anorexia, dysphagia, odynophagia, hematemesis, or melena

ALERT

Up to 25% of patients with Barrett esophagus are asymptomatic (2).

PHYSICAL EXAM

No abnormal findings on physical exam are specific for Barrett esophagus. A general physical examination including vital signs, oral examination, cardiopulmonary examination, abdominal examination, and search for lymphadenopathy should be performed.

DIFFERENTIAL DIAGNOSIS

- Erosive esophagitis
- GERD

DIAGNOSTIC TESTS & INTERPRETATION

Endoscopy with multiple biopsies for histologic examination are required to diagnose Barrett esophagus.

- Gastric fundic-type epithelium may be found on pathology but does not have clear malignant potential and may reflect sampling error.
- Specialized intestinal metaplasia at the GEJ: cancer risk difficult to assess with varying definitions of GEJ landmarks

ALERT

Screening for Barrett esophagus in the general population with GERD is **not** recommended because of the lack of demonstrated impact on mortality. The 2011 American Gastroenterological Association (AGA) guidelines suggest individualized screening for patients with multiple risk factors (3)[C].

Initial Tests (lab, imaging)

None:

- *Helicobacter pylori* testing is not indicated. Meta-analyses show an inverse relationship between *H. pylori* infections and Barrett esophagus, which may be related to decreased acid production (4)[C].
- No biomarkers currently effective for diagnosis; many are under investigation for risk stratification (1,3)[B].

Diagnostic Procedures/Other

- Endoscopy: visual identification of columnar epithelium (reddish, velvety appearance) replacing the squamous lining of the distal esophagus
  - Extent of disease may be characterized:
    - Long-segment (≥3 cm) versus short-segment (<3 cm)
    - Prague C (circumference) and M (maximum extent) criteria
  - White light endoscopy (preferably high resolution) remains the standard of diagnosis.
    - Advanced imaging techniques, such as narrow band imaging (NBI) and confocal laser endomicroscopy, may help identify dysplasia but are still preliminary (1)[A].
- Systematic biopsies from endoscopy showing columnar epithelium confirm the diagnosis:
  - Seattle protocol: 4-quadrant biopsies at regular intervals with additional biopsies of visible mucosal irregularities
    - More time-consuming but higher diagnostic yield than random biopsies (3)[A]
- Capsule endoscopy is still under development and currently has poor sensitivity compared with conventional endoscopy (5)[B].

Test Interpretation

Specialized intestinal metaplasia (also called specialized columnar epithelium) is diagnostic:

- Dysplasia (and grade) should be confirmed by an expert pathologist before treatment (3,5)[B].
- Cardia-type columnar epithelium may predispose to malignancy but with an unclear magnitude of risk; the AGA currently recommends against including this type of epithelium in the definition of Barrett esophagus (3)[B].

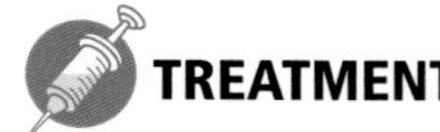

TREATMENT

ALERT

Neither suppression of gastric acid production via high-dose proton pump inhibitors (PPIs) nor reduction in esophageal acid exposure via antireflux surgery induces regression of Barrett esophagus. These therapies may decrease cancer risk.

MEDICATION

- The goal of medical therapy is to control GERD to reduce esophagitis.
- Therapy usually does **not** result in reversal of Barrett esophagus but may decrease risk of progression to cancer (1,2)[A],(5,6)[B].

First Line

Unlike the stepwise management of GERD without evidence of Barrett esophagus, patients with Barrett esophagus and GERD symptoms should be treated initially with a once-daily PPI:

- PPIs should be dosed 30 minutes before a meal (ideally, the 1st meal of the day).

ALERT

PPI therapy should be titrated to symptoms; pH monitoring is **not** recommended (1,2)[C].

- Chemoprevention of neoplastic progression is under active investigation.
- Case-controlled studies have shown that aspirin and NSAIDs may prevent progression to esophageal cancer due to the inhibition of COX-2:
  - Administration of the COX-2 selective inhibitor celecoxib was not shown to affect progression of Barrett dysplasia to adenocarcinoma (2)[A].
  - The use of aspirin and a PPI for chemoprevention of esophageal cancer is being investigated (1–3).

B

- Low-dose aspirin may be considered in patients with Barrett esophagus who also have risk factors for cardiovascular disease (2)[C].
- Statins, alone or in combination with aspirin or NSAIDs, appear to be effective in chemoprevention but are not yet generally recommended (3)[B],(7)[A].

Second Line

If once-daily PPI does not control symptoms, twice-daily dosing is recommended (5)[A].

ISSUES FOR REFERRAL

- PPI therapy should be initiated prior to endoscopy to reduce reactive esophagitis/atypia, which may be confused with low-grade dysplasia on biopsy (5)[C].
- Patients considering esophagectomy should be referred to a high-volume institution.

ADDITIONAL THERAPIES

- Low-grade dysplasia: Treatment is controversial.
  - Endoscopic eradication may prevent progression to high-grade dysplasia or esophageal adenocarcinoma (3)[B],(8)[A].
- High-grade dysplasia, without or with very limited submucosal invasion (stage T1SM1 or lower by endoscopic ultrasound): Endoscopic eradication therapy is recommended (1,2,5)[B]:
  - Photodynamic therapy (PDT): eradication rate 77–100% but with strictures in ~40%
  - Radiofrequency ablation (RFA): eradication rate 54–90%, comparable efficacy to PDT, fewer adverse effects
  - Endoscopic mucosal resection (EMR): eradication rate 86–100%, excision to submucosa, allows staging, preferred for visible irregularities
  - Combination therapy:
    - EMR may be coupled with RFA or PDT to attempt to eliminate all Barrett epithelium.
    - Focal EMR combined with RFA of other areas is considered the most effective eradication therapy (3)[B].
- Cryotherapy and other ablative procedures: Additional studies are still required before they can be recommended.

ALERT

Endoscopic eradication therapy is **not** recommended for Barrett esophagus in the absence of dysplasia, but surveillance should be continued.

SURGERY/OTHER PROCEDURES

Antireflux surgery such as fundoplication may control GERD symptoms but not convincingly shown to reverse Barrett esophagus, decrease risk of cancer, or be more effective than medical therapy (1,2)[A],(5)[B].

ALERT

Available data suggest that antireflux surgery does **not** decrease risk of esophageal cancer.

- Esophagectomy is definitive and should be offered as an alternative to endoscopic eradication therapy for high-grade dysplasia (1,3)[B]:
  - Preferred for patients with evidence of submucosal invasion (stage T1SM2 or higher)
  - Added benefit of lymph nodes removal
  - Mortality rate: <5% in patients with high-grade dysplasia who are otherwise healthy
  - Serious postoperative complications: 30–50%
  - Ideally should be performed by an experienced surgeon in a high-volume medical center (2,3)[A]

COMPLEMENTARY & ALTERNATIVE MEDICINE

A prospective study of 339 men and women with Barrett esophagus found those taking either a multivitamin, vitamin C, or vitamin E once a day were less likely to develop esophageal adenocarcinoma (9)[B].

Geriatric Considerations

If the patient is a poor operative candidate for endoscopic eradication therapy or esophagectomy, surveillance or no treatment may be preferable.

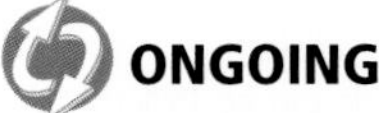

ONGOING CARE

FOLLOW-UP RECOMMENDATIONS

- Surveillance (to detect high-grade dysplasia or early carcinoma) remains controversial but is recommended in patients with histologically confirmed Barrett.
- Surveillance intervals depend on the grade of dysplasia, 2011 AGA guidelines for surveillance intervals in Barrett esophagus (3)[C]
- No dysplasia: 3–5 years
- Low-grade dysplasia: 6–12 months
- High-grade dysplasia without eradication therapy: 3 months

ALERT

- Adherence to recommended surveillance protocols may improve rates of dysplasia and cancer detection.
- Surveillance should continue even if the patient has had endoscopic ablation therapy, antireflux surgery, or esophagectomy.

DIET

Patients should avoid foods that can trigger reflux: caffeine, alcohol, chocolate, peppermint, carbonated drinks, garlic, onions, spicy foods, fatty foods, citrus, and tomato-based products.

PATIENT EDUCATION

- Lifestyle modifications:
  - Smoking cessation
  - Weight loss
  - Avoiding supine position after eating
  - Avoiding tight-fitting clothes
  - Head of bed elevation
- *No evidence that treating GERD will reverse Barrett esophagus or prevent esophageal cancer.*

PROGNOSIS

Annual incidence of esophageal cancer in patients with Barrett esophagus is ≤0.33% per year (2,3)[B]:

- Low-grade dysplasia: may be transient; cancer risk 0.5–0.6% per year
- High-grade dysplasia: cancer risk 5–7% per year

COMPLICATIONS

Same as GERD: stricture, bleeding, ulceration

REFERENCES

1. Sharma P. Clinical practice. Barrett's esophagus. *N Engl J Med*. 2009;361(26):2548–2556.
2. Spechler SJ, Sharma P, Souza RF, et al. American Gastroenterological Association technical review on the management of Barrett's esophagus. *Gastroenterology*. 2011;140(3):e18–e52; quiz e13.
3. American Gastroenterological Association, Spechler SJ, Sharma P, Souza RF, et al. American Gastroenterological Association medical position statement on the management of Barrett's esophagus. *Gastroenterology*. 2011;140(3):1084–1091.
4. Fischbach LA, Nordenstedt H, Kramer JR, et al. The association between Barrett's esophagus and Helicobacter pylori infection: a meta-analysis. *Helicobacter*. 2012;17(3):163–175.
5. Wang KK, Sampliner RE; Practice Parameters Committee of the American College of Gastroenterology. Updated guidelines 2008 for the diagnosis, surveillance and therapy of Barrett's esophagus. *Am J Gastroenterol*. 2008;103(3):788–797.
6. Singh S, Garg SK, Singh PP, et al. Acid-suppressive medications and risk of oesophageal adenocarcinoma in patients with Barrett's oesophagus: a systematic review and meta-analysis. *Gut*. 2014;63(8):1229–1237.
7. Kastelein F, Spaander MC, Biermann K, et al; Probar-study Group. Nonsteroidal anti-inflammatory drugs and statins have chemopreventative effects in patients with Barrett's esophagus. *Gastroenterology*. 2011;141(6):2000–2008; quiz e13–e14.
8. Phoa KN, van Vilsteren FG, Weusten BL, et al. Radiofrequency ablation vs endoscopic surveillance for patients with Barrett esophagus and low-grade dysplasia: a randomized clinical trial. *JAMA*. 2014;311(12):1209–1217.
9. Dong LM, Kristal AR, Peters U, et al. Dietary supplement use and risk of neoplastic progression in esophageal adenocarcinoma: a prospective study. *Nutr Cancer*. 2008;60(1):39–48.

ADDITIONAL READING

- Dunbar KB, Spechler SJ. Controversies in Barrett esophagus. *Mayo Clin Proc*. 2014;89(7):973–984.
- Zimmerman TG. Common questions about Barrett esophagus. *Am Fam Physician*. 2014;89(2):92–98.

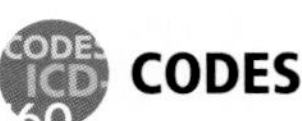

CODES

ICD10

- K22.70 Barrett's esophagus without dysplasia
- K22.719 Barrett's esophagus with dysplasia, unspecified
- K22.710 Barrett's esophagus with low grade dysplasia

CLINICAL PEARLS

- The incidence of esophageal carcinoma is rising faster than any other major malignancy. Barrett esophagus is a known precursor.
- Highest incidence is among white males >50 years.
- Endoscopic eradication therapy is the preferred treatment for high-grade dysplasia with or without submucosal invasion.
- Esophagectomy offers definitive therapy: Consider all patients with high-grade dysplasia; preferred for patients with submucosal invasion.
- Promising areas of research include the use of biomarkers for risk stratification, chemoprevention of neoplastic progression, capsule endoscopy for screening and use of vitamins and antioxidants.

BASAL CELL CARCINOMA

Frank J. Domino, MD

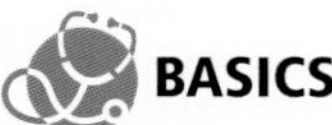

BASICS

DESCRIPTION

Basal cell carcinoma (BCC) is the most common cancer, originating from the basal cell layer of the skin appendages.

- Rarely metastasizes but capable of local tissue destruction

Geriatric Considerations

- Greater frequency in geriatric patients (ages 55–75 years have 100× incidence compared with those aged <20 years)
- The incidence is rapidly increasing in those 20–40 years of age.

Pediatric Considerations

Rare in children, but childhood sun exposure is important in adult disease.

EPIDEMIOLOGY

Worldwide, the most common form of cancer

Incidence

- Incidence in the United States: 1 million cases per year; increasing about 10% each year
- Predominant age: generally >40 years; incidence increasing in younger populations
- Predominant sex: male > female (although incidence is increasing in females)
- Lifetime risk of white North Americans: 30%

ETIOLOGY AND PATHOPHYSIOLOGY

- UV-induced inflammation and cyclooxygenase activation in skin
- Mutation of *PTCH1* (patched homolog 1), a tumor-suppressor gene that inhibits the hedgehog signaling pathway
- Mutation of the *SMO* (smoothened homolog) gene, which is also involved in the hedgehog signaling pathway
- UV-induced mutations of the *TP53* (tumor protein 53), a tumor-suppressor gene
- Activation of *BCL2*, an antiapoptosis proto-oncogene

Genetics

Several genetic conditions increase the risk of developing BCC:

- Albinism (recessive alleles)
- Xeroderma pigmentosum (autosomal recessive)
- Bazex syndrome (rare, X-linked dominant)
- Nevoid BCC syndrome/Gorlin syndrome (rare, autosomal dominant)
- Cytochrome P-450 CYP2D6 and glutathione S-transferase detoxifying enzyme gene mutations (especially in truncal BCC, marked by clusters of BCCs and a younger age of onset)

RISK FACTORS

- Chronic sun exposure (UV radiation)
- Most common in the following phenotypes
  - Light complexion: skin type I (burns but does not tan) and skin type II (usually burns, sometimes tans)
  - Red or blond hair
  - Blue or green eyes
- Tendency to sunburn
- Male sex, although increasing risk in women due to lifestyle changes, such as tanning beds
- History of nonmelanoma skin cancer
  - After initial diagnosis of skin cancer, 35% risk of new nonmelanoma skin cancer at 3 years and 50% at 5 years
- Family history of skin cancer
- 3–4 decades after chronic arsenic exposure
- 2 decades after therapeutic radiation
- Chronic immunosuppression: transplant recipients (10× higher incidence), patients with HIV or lymphomas

GENERAL PREVENTION

- Use broad-spectrum sunscreens of at least SPF 30 daily and reapply after swimming or sweating.
- Avoid overexposure to the sun by seeking shade between 10 AM and 4 PM and wearing wide-brimmed hats and long-sleeved shirts.
- Avoid tanning and sunburns (including tanning salons).

COMMONLY ASSOCIATED CONDITIONS

- Cosmetic disfigurement because head and neck most often affected
- Loss of vision with orbital involvement
- Loss of nerve function due to perineural spread or extensive and deep invasion
- Ulcerating neoplasms are prone to infections.

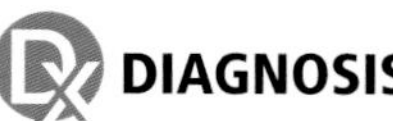

DIAGNOSIS

HISTORY

Exposure to risk factors, family history

PHYSICAL EXAM

- 80% on face and neck, 20% on trunk and lower limbs (mostly women)
- Nodular: most common (60%); presents as pinkish, pearly papule, plaque, or nodule often with telangiectatic vessels, ulceration, and a rolled periphery usually on face
  - Pigmented: presents as a translucent papule with "floating pigment"; more commonly seen in darker skin types
- Superficial: 30%; light red, scaly papule or plaque with atrophic center, ringed by translucent micropapules, usually on trunk or extremities; more common in men
- Morpheaform: 5–10%; firm, smooth, flesh-colored, scar-like papule or plaque with ill-defined borders

DIFFERENTIAL DIAGNOSIS

- Sebaceous hyperplasia
- Epidermal inclusion cyst
- Intradermal nevi (pigmented and nonpigmented)
- Molluscum contagiosum
- Squamous cell carcinoma (SCC)
- Nummular dermatitis
- Psoriasis
- Melanoma (pigmented lesions)
- Atypical fibroxanthoma
- Rare adnexal neoplasms

DIAGNOSTIC TESTS & INTERPRETATION

Diagnostic Procedures/Other

- Clinical diagnosis and histologic subtype are confirmed through skin biopsy and pathologic examination.
- Shave biopsy is typically sufficient; however, punch biopsy is more useful to assess depth of tumor and perineural invasion.
- If a genetic disorder is suspected, additional tests may be needed to confirm it.

Test Interpretation

- Nodular BCC
  - Extending from the epidermis are nodular aggregates of basaloid cells.
  - Tumor cells are uniform; rarely have mitotic figures; large, oval, hyperchromatic nuclei with little cytoplasm, surrounded by a peripheral palisade
  - Early lesions are usually connected to the epidermis, unlike late lesions.
  - Increased mucin in dermal stroma
    - Cleft formation (retraction artifact) common between BCC "nests" and stroma due to mucin shrinkage during fixation and staining
- Superficial BCC
  - Appear as buds of basaloid cells attached to undersurface of epidermis
  - Peripheral palisading
- Morpheaform BCC
  - Thin cords and strands of basaloid cells, embedded in dense, fibrous, scar-like stroma
  - Less peripheral palisading and retraction, greater subclinical involvement
- Infiltrating BCC
  - Like morpheaform BCC but no scar-like stroma and thicker, more spiky, irregular strands
  - Less peripheral palisading and retraction, greater subclinical involvement
- Micronodular BCC
  - Small, nodular aggregates of tumor cells
  - Less retraction artifact and higher subclinical involvement than nodular BCC

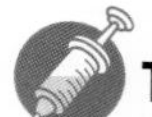

TREATMENT

MEDICATION

- May be especially useful in those who cannot tolerate surgical procedures and in those who refuse to have surgery
- 5-fluorouracil cream inhibits thymidylate synthetase, interrupting DNA synthesis for superficial lesions in low-risk areas; primary treatment only 5% applied BID for 3–10 weeks.
- Imiquimod (Aldara) cream approved for treatment of low-risk superficial BCC; daily dosing for 6–12 weeks; 90% histologic cure

ADDITIONAL THERAPIES

- Radiation therapy
  - Useful for patients who cannot or will not undergo surgery
  - Used following surgery, particularly if margins of tumor were not cleared
  - Cure rate is ~90%.
  - Tumors that recur in areas previously treated with radiation are harder to treat, and the area is more difficult to reconstruct.
- Photodynamic therapy (PDT)
  - 5-aminolevulinic acid, a photosensitizer, is activated by specific wavelengths of light, creating singlet oxygen radicals that destroy local tissue (no damage to surrounding or deep tissues) (1)[B].
  - Useful in areas where tissue preservation is cosmetically or functionally important

SURGERY/OTHER PROCEDURES

- Generally first choice; specific treatment selection varies with extent and location of lesion as well as tumor border demarcation (2)[A].
- High-risk areas
  - Inner canthus, nasolabial sulcus, philtrum, preauricular area, retroauricular sulcus, lip, temple
- Curettage and electrodesiccation
  - If nodular lesion <1 cm, in low-risk area, not deeply invasive
- Excision
  - Useful for lesions in high-risk areas
  - Not as dependent on lesion size
- Cryosurgery
  - Reserved for small lesions in low-risk areas
  - May want pre- and posttreatment biopsies
- Mohs surgery
  - Preferred microsurgically controlled surgical treatment for lesions in high-risk areas, recurrent lesions, and lesions exhibiting an aggressive growth pattern
  - Requires referral to appropriately trained dermatologic surgeon

INPATIENT CONSIDERATIONS

Outpatient, unless extensive lesion

ONGOING CARE

FOLLOW-UP RECOMMENDATIONS

- Avoid sun exposure.
- Oral retinoids may prevent the development of new BCCs in patients with Gorlin syndrome, renal transplant recipients, and patients with severe actinic damage.

Patient Monitoring

- Every month for 3 months, then twice yearly for 5 years; yearly thereafter
- Increased risk of other skin cancers

PATIENT EDUCATION

- Teach patient-appropriate sun-avoidance techniques, sunscreens, and so forth.
- Monthly skin self-exam
- Educate patients concerning adequate vitamin D intake.

PROGNOSIS

- Proper treatment yields 90–95% cure.
- Most recurrences happen within 5 years.
- Development of new BCCs: Patients (36%) will develop a new lesion within 5 years.

COMPLICATIONS

- Local recurrence and spread
- Usually, recurrences will appear within 5 years.
- Metastasis: rare (<0.1%), but metastatic disease usually fatal within 8 months

REFERENCES

1. Soler AM, Angell-Petersen E, Warloe T, et al. Photodynamic therapy of superficial basal cell carcinoma with 5-aminolevulinic acid with dimethylsulfoxide and ethylenediaminetetraacetic acid: a comparison of two light sources. *Photochem Photobiol*. 2000;71(6):724–729.
2. Bath-Hextall FJ, Bong J, Perkins W, et al. Interventions for basal cell carcinoma of the skin. *Cochrane Database Syst Rev*. 2003;(2):CD003412.

ADDITIONAL READING

- Friedman GD, Tekawa IS. Association of basal cell skin cancers with other cancers (United States). *Cancer Causes Control*. 2000;11(10):891–897.
- Wong CS, Strange RC, Lear JT. Basal cell carcinoma. *BMJ*. 2003;327(7418):794–798.

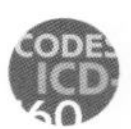

CODES

ICD10

- C44.91 Basal cell carcinoma of skin, unspecified
- C44.31 Basal cell carcinoma of skin of other and unspecified parts of face
- C44.41 Basal cell carcinoma of skin of scalp and neck

CLINICAL PEARLS

- Nodular: pearly papule, plaque, or nodule often with telangiectatic vessels, ulceration, and a rolled periphery, usually on face
- Pigmented: presents as a translucent papule with "floating pigment"; more commonly seen in darker skin types
- Superficial: Scaly papule or plaque with atrophic center, ringed by translucent micropapules, usually on trunk or extremities; more common in men
- Morpheaform: firm, smooth, flesh-colored, scar-like papule or plaque with ill-defined borders
- Use diagnostic keys above to differentiate between BCC and cutaneous SCC. SCC arises from actinic keratosis in 60% of cases and generally presents as an asymptomatic hyperkeratotic lesion. If unsure, biopsy or refer to a specialist.
- Some hyperpigmented BCCs may appear similar to melanoma. Remember the ABCDEs of melanoma recognition: **A**symmetry, **B**order irregularities, **C**olor variability, **D**iameter >6 mm, **E**nlargement. If unsure, refer to a specialist.
- The USPSTF concludes insufficient evidence and recommends for or against routine total body skin exams for melanoma, BCC, or SCC. Exams should be based on risk factors, including exposure and family and prior medical history. All patients should receive education about risks and self-exam.

BED BUGS

Fawn Winkelman, DO

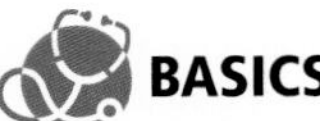

BASICS

DESCRIPTION

- Nocturnal obligate blood parasites that take refuge on furniture and bedding
- 5–7 mm oval, reddish brown, flat, wingless

EPIDEMIOLOGY

Incidence

- According to the 2013 "Bugs Without Borders" survey, bed bug infestations are increasing and continue to remain the most difficult pest to treat, more difficult than cockroaches, termites, and ants (1)[B].
- Resurgence is due to the use of less toxic, less persistent insecticides as well as increased travel, use of secondhand furniture, and a high turnover rate of residents in hotels.

Prevalence

- Infestations are increasing across the United States.
- Sharp increase in prevalence, as only 11% of survey respondents reported bed bug calls more than 10 years ago.
- Bed bug encounters have become more common in public places (schools, hospitals, hotels/motels, aircrafts) than in previous years, increasing by 10–30% (2)[B].

ETIOLOGY AND PATHOPHYSIOLOGY

- Insect family Cimicidae
- 3 species that bite humans: *Cimex lectularius*, *Cimex hemipterus*, and *Leptocimex boueti* (2)[B]
- Most prevalent species is *C. lectularius* (2)[B]
- Found in tropical or temperate climates
- Hide in crevices of mattresses, box springs, headboards, and baseboards
- Infestations occur in hotels/motels, hospitals, cinemas, transportation vehicles, aircrafts, and homes.
- Reactions range from an absent or minimal response to a more typical reaction presenting as pruritic, erythematous macules and papules or a less common urticarial and anaphylactic response.
- Skin reactions are due to host immunologic response to the parasite salivary proteins.
- Papular urticarial reactions are mediated via immunoglobulin (Ig) G antibody response to salivary proteins (3)[B].
- Bullous reactions are caused by an IgE-mediated hypersensitivity to nitrophorin, the substance that transports nitric oxide in bed bug saliva (3)[B].
- Bed bugs locate warmth and carbon dioxide production, which allows them to migrate to humans (4).

GENERAL PREVENTION

- Bed bug monitors and traps can be purchased which contain carbon dioxide as well as heat to attract and trap the bugs but can be cost prohibitive (5)[B].
- Avoidance of bed bugs: vacuum regularly, reduce clutter, seal cracks in walls, inspect luggage and clothing
- Launder all bedding and cloth items in 130°F (50°C) or hotter for 2 hours or 20°F (−5°C) or cooler for 5 days
- If present in the home, eradication is essential via professional extermination. Some pest control companies have employed pest control canines to detect live bed bugs and eggs based on pheromones from the bed bugs but are expensive and generate false positives and negatives depending on the training of the dog (5)[B].

RISK FACTORS

- Immunologically weak or compromised
- Recent travel
- High turnover environment
- Secondhand furniture in home

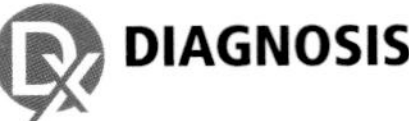

DIAGNOSIS

HISTORY

- Recent travel
- Blood specks on sheets
- Bed bug sighting
- New skin lesions in the morning
- Intense pruritus, pain, or burning

PHYSICAL EXAM

- Characteristic lesions are erythematous pruritic papules in an irregular linear pattern.
- Found on body surfaces exposed during sleeping such as face, neck, arms, legs, and shoulders
- May appear hours to days after being bitten
- Patients are usually asymptomatic but may be anaphylactic and present with papular urticaria, diffuse urticaria, and/or bullous lesions.

DIFFERENTIAL DIAGNOSIS

- Urticaria
- Insect or spider bite
- Scabies
- Dermatitis herpetiformis

DIAGNOSTIC TESTS & INTERPRETATION

Initial Tests (lab, imaging)

- Skin scraping with mineral oil preparation
- Skin biopsy

Test Interpretation

- Skin scraping is negative with mineral oil, which helps to exclude scabies.
- Skin biopsy shows nonspecific perivascular eosinophilic infiltrate consistent with arthropod bite reaction.

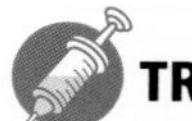

TREATMENT

GENERAL MEASURES

- Self-limited and resolves within 1–2 weeks
- Treat symptomatically
- Avoidance of the bed bugs by inspection
- Prevention by laundering bedding and cloth

MEDICATION

First Line

- Disease is self-limited; treat symptoms
- Oral antihistamines (i.e., diphenhydramine, hydroxyzine)
- Topical antipruritics (i.e., pramoxine/calamine ointment or doxepin cream)
- Topical low to midpotency corticosteroids for 2 weeks (i.e., hydrocortisone, triamcinolone)
- Systemic corticosteroids (severe cases)

ADDITIONAL THERAPIES

- If secondarily infected, use topical or oral antibiotics against *Staphylococcus* and *Streptococcus* spp. (i.e., cephalexin, tetracycline, doxycycline, clindamycin, topical mupirocin).
- Epinephrine for anaphylaxis
- Professional extermination may be necessary.

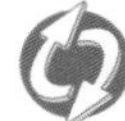

ONGOING CARE

FOLLOW-UP RECOMMENDATIONS

- Not necessary as disease is self-limited
- Recommended in extreme cases or if anaphylaxis ensues

PATIENT EDUCATION

- Avoid scratching to prevent superinfection.
- Inspect bedding, furniture, and luggage regularly.
- CDC: www.cdc.gov/parasites/bedbugs/
- EPA: www.epa.gov/bedbugs/

COMPLICATIONS

- Bed bug dermatitis, allergic reactions, asthma exacerbations, anaphylaxis
- Significant psychological distress (insomnia, depression, anxiety, delusional parasitosis) (3)
- Secondary bacterial infections
- Transmission of blood-borne diseases (rare)

REFERENCES

1. Studdiford JS, Conniff KM, Trayes KP, et al. Bedbug infestation. *Am Fam Physician*. 2012;86(7):653–658.
2. Kolb A, Needham GR, Neyman KM, et al. Bedbugs. *Dermatol Ther*. 2009:22(4):347–352.
3. Goddard J, deShazo R. Bedbugs (*Cimex lectularius*) and clinical consequences of their bites. *JAMA*. 2009;301(13):1358–1366.
4. Williams K, Willis MS. Bedbugs in the 21st century: the reemergence of an old foe. *Lab Medicine*. 2012;43:141–148.
5. Vaidyanathan R, Feldlaufer MF. Bed bug detection: current technologies and future directions. *Am J Trop Med Hyg*.2013;88(4):619–625.

ADDITIONAL READING

Thomas I, Kihiczak GG, Schwartz RA. Bedbug bites: a review. *Int J Dermatol*. 2004;43(6):430–433.

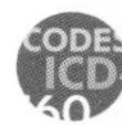

CODES

ICD10

- S00.96XA Insect bite (nonvenomous) of unspecified part of head, initial encounter
- S10.96XA Insect bite of unspecified part of neck, initial encounter
- S40.269A Insect bite (nonvenomous) of unspecified shoulder, initial encounter

CLINICAL PEARLS

- 90% of infestations occur within 3 feet of beds.
- Wash bedding/clothing regularly in hot water.
- Vacuum carpet daily or steam clean daily.
- Inspect furniture, bedding, and luggage regularly.
- Use professional services if necessary.
- Patient education and vigilance is paramount for bed bug prevention and avoidance.

BEHAVIORAL PROBLEMS, PEDIATRIC

William G. Elder, PhD

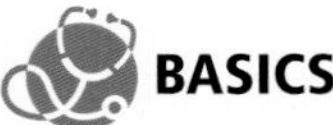

BASICS

DESCRIPTION

Behavior that disrupts at least 1 area of psychosocial functioning. Commonly reported behavioral problems are as follows:

- Noncompliance: active or passive refusal to do as requested by parent or other authority figure
- Temper tantrums: loss of internal control provoked by overtiredness, physical discomfort, or fear that leads to crying, whining, breath-holding, or in extreme cases, acts of aggression
- Sleep problems: sleep patterns that are distressing to caregivers or child; difficulty going to sleep or staying asleep at night, nightmares, and night terrors
- Nocturnal enuresis: enuresis that occurs only at night in children >5 years of age with no medical problems
  - Primary: children who have never been dry at night
  - Secondary: children dry at night for at least 6 months
- Functional encopresis: repeated involuntary fecal soiling that is not caused by organic defect or illness
- Problem eating: "picky eating," difficult mealtime behaviors
- Normative sexual behaviors: developmentally appropriate behaviors in children in the absence of abuse
- Thumb sucking: An innate reflex that is self-soothing. May be protective against sudden infant death. If persists past eruption of primary teeth, can affect teeth alignment and mouth shape.

EPIDEMIOLOGY

- Noncompliance: May manifest as children develop autonomy; males have a modestly greater likelihood of being noncompliant. Decreases with age.
- Temper tantrums: 70% of 18–24-month-old children; 7% of 3–5-year-old children; in children with severe tantrums, 52% have other behavioral/emotional problems (1).
- Sleep problems
  - Night waking in 25–50% of infants 6–12 months; bedtime refusal in 10–30% of toddlers
  - Nightmares in 10–30% of preschoolers; peaks between ages 6 and 10 years
  - Night terrors in 1–6.5% early childhood; peaks between ages 4 and 12 years
  - Sleepwalking frequently in 3–5%; peaks between ages 5 and 8 years (2)
- Nocturnal enuresis
  - At least 20% of children in the 1st grade wet the bed occasionally; 4% wet ≥2 times per week.
  - At 10 years of age, 9% in boys, 3% in girls (3)
- Functional encopresis
  - Rare before age 3 years, most common in 5–10-year-olds; more common in boys (4)
- Problem eating
  - Prevalence peaks at 50% at 24 months of age; no relation to sex/ethnicity/income (5)
- Normative sexual behaviors
  - Rare in infancy, except hand to genital contact
  - Increased in 3–5-year-olds; less observed in >5-year-olds because more covert (6)
- Thumb sucking: decreases with age; most children spontaneously stop between 2 and 4 years.

COMMONLY ASSOCIATED CONDITIONS

- Noncompliance: if exceeds what seems normative, rule out depression, compulsive patterns, adjustment disorder, inappropriate discipline
- Temper tantrums: difficult child temperament, stress
- Sleep problems: often with inconsistent bedtime routine or sleep schedule, stimulating bedtime environment; can be associated with hyperactive behavior, poor impulse control, and poor attention in young children (2)
- Enuresis: secondary often with medical problems, especially constipation, and frequent behavior problems, especially ADHD
- Functional encopresis: enuresis, UTIs, ADHD
- Normative sexual behaviors: family stressors such as separation or divorce (6)

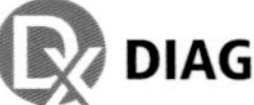

DIAGNOSIS

HISTORY

- Noncompliance: complete history from caregivers and teachers, if applicable; direct observation of child or child–caregiver interaction
  - Criteria: is problematic for at least some adults, leading to difficult interactions for at least 6 months
  - Reduces child's ability to take part in structured activities
  - Creates stressful relationships with compliant children
  - Disrupts academic progress; places child at risk for physical injury
- Temper tantrums: history, with focus on development, family functioning, or violence; may consist of stiffening limbs and arching back, dropping to the floor, shouting, screaming, crying, pushing/pulling, stamping, hitting, kicking, throwing, or running away (1)
- Sleep disorders: screening questions about sleep during well-child visit, such as the BEARS screen (Bedtime problems, Excessive daytime sleepiness, Awakenings during the night, Regularity and duration of sleep, and Snoring); bedtime routine (2)[C]
- Nocturnal enuresis: severity, onset, and duration; daytime wetting or any associated genitourinary symptoms; family history of enuresis; medical and psychosocial history; constipation; child and caregiver's motivation for treatment (7)[C]
- Problem eating: review of child's diet, growth curves, nutritional needs, and caregiver's response to behavior (5)[C]
- Normative sexual behaviors: When was behavior first noticed? Any recent changes or stressors in family? Behavior solitary or with another; if with another, what age? Changes in frequency or nature of behaviors; occurs at home, daycare, school? Is behavior disruptive, intrusive, or coercive? (6) (See "Child Sexual Behavior Inventory" in the following discussion).

PHYSICAL EXAM

- Nocturnal enuresis
  - Physical exam of abdomen for enlarged bladder, kidneys, or fecal masses; rectal exam if history of constipation; back for spinal dysraphism seen in dimpling or hair tufts
  - Neurologic exam: focus on lower extremities
  - Genital urinary exam
    - Males: meatal stenosis, hypospadias, epispadias, phimosis
    - Females: vulvitis, vaginitis, labial adhesions, ureterocele at introitus; wide vaginal orifice with scar or healed laceration may be evidence of abuse.
- Functional encopresis
  - Height and weight; abdominal exam for masses or tenderness; rectal exam for tone, size of rectal vault, fecal impaction, masses, fissures, hemorrhoids; back for signs of spinal dysraphism seen in dimpling or hair tufts (4)

DIAGNOSTIC TESTS & INTERPRETATION

Initial Tests (lab, imaging)

- For nocturnal enuresis: urinalysis (dipstick test OK); if abnormal, consider urine culture
  - For secondary enuresis: serum glucose, creatinine, thyrotropin (8)[C]
  - Urinary tract imaging and urodynamic studies if significant daytime symptoms with history or diagnosis of UTI or history of structural renal abnormalities (8)[C]
- For functional encopresis: tests for hypothyroidism or celiac disease if poor growth or family history; urinalysis and culture if enuresis or features of UTI (4)
  - Spine imaging if evidence of spinal dysraphism or if both encopresis and daytime enuresis; barium enema if suspect Hirschsprung disease

Follow-Up Tests & Special Considerations

Sleep disorders: Sleep studies may be performed in children if there is a history of snoring and daytime ADHD–type symptoms (2).

Diagnostic Procedures/Other

- Pediatric symptom checklist: www.brightfutures.org/mentalhealth/pdf/professionals/ped_symptom_chklst.pdf
- National Initiative for Children's Healthcare Quality (NICHQ) Vanderbilt Assessment (ADHD screen): www.myadhd.com/vanderbiltparent6175.html
- Child Sexual Behavior Inventory. Completed by female caregiver to assist with differentiation of normative versus abnormal behaviors particularly those related to sexual abuse: www.nctsnet.org/content/child-sexual-behavior-inventory-csbi

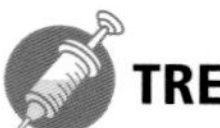

TREATMENT

- General: Educate caregiver about specific behavioral problem.
- Noncompliance: In the case of extreme child disobedience, consider parent training programs. Child may need to be formally screened for ADHD, obsessive-compulsive disorder (OCD), oppositional defiant disorder (ODD), or conduct disorder (CD).
- Temper tantrums: Remind caregiver this is a normal aspect of childhood.
  - If tantrum is set off by external factors, such as hunger or overtiredness, then correct.
  - Other methods for dealing with a tantrum include one of the following:
    - Ignore the tantrum; remove the child and place him or her in time-out (1 minute for each year of age); hold/restrain child until calmed down; provide child with clear, firm, and consistent instructions as well as enough time to obey.

- Sleep problems: Intervention consists largely of education of the caregiver who may need a roadmap for dealing with this difficult and distressing problem. Developmental stages; environmental factors and cues; caregiver emotions and reactions; and child fears, stress, and habits are all important factors in sleep onset and maintenance that should be explored and explained to caregiver.
- Specific recommendations may also consist of other interventions including the following (2)[A]:
  - Graduated extinction: Caregiver ignores cries/tantrums for specified period. Can check at a fixed time or increasing intervals.
  - "Fading": Gradual decrease in direct contact with the child as child falls asleep; goal is for caregiver to exit the room and allow child to fall asleep independently.
  - Consider the "5S Intervention" for settling problems in toddlers (used to comfort infants in nurseries): swaddling, sucking, shushing, stomach/side position, and swinging.
  - If fearful, preferred routines or inert sprays or glitter spread by the child (while avoiding the eyes) may help the child feel more secure.
- Nocturnal enuresis
  - Bedwetting alarm: 1st-line therapy for caregivers who can overcome objection of having their sleep disturbed; about 2/3 of children respond while using the alarm; if enuresis recurs after use, it will often resolve with a 2nd trial (7)[A].
  - Decrease fluids an hour before bedtime.
  - Little evidence from clinical trials but good empirical evidence for behavioral training, including positive reinforcement (small reward for each dry night) or responsibility training (if developmentally able, child is responsible for changing or washing sheets), encouraging daily bowel movements, and frequent bladder emptying during the day
- Functional encopresis
  - First disimpaction: PO with polyethylene glycol solution or mineral oil; if unsuccessful, manual, mineral oil enemas
  - Maintenance therapy
    - Medical: osmotics, such as polyethylene glycol, fiber, lactulose; stimulants, such as senna or bisacodyl
  - Behavior modification: toileting after meals for 10 minutes 2–3 times a day, star charts and rewards (4)[C]
- Problem eating
  - Avoid punishment, prodding, or rewards. Offer a variety of healthy foods at every meal; limit milk to 24 oz/day and decrease juice (5)[C].
- Normative sexual behavior: No treatment needed; caregivers may need encouragement not to punish or admonish child and to use gentle distraction to redirect behavior when in public setting.
- Thumb sucking: Recommendations to caregivers include praising children when not sucking their thumb, offer alternatives that are soothing (e.g., stuffed toys), provide reminders or negative reinforcement in the form of a bandage around or bitters on the thumb (5)[C].

MEDICATION

Most pediatric behavioral issues respond well to nonpharmacologic therapy:

- Sleep disorders
  - For certain delayed sleep-onset disorders, after behavioral methods are exhausted, melatonin 0.5–10 mg PO can be tried while behavior modification is continued. Sleep latency is likely to be reduced, but not total time asleep. However, this is not approved by the FDA for children. Daytime exposure to bright or sun light should be assured before treatment.
- Nocturnal enuresis
  - Desmopressin can decrease urine output to reduce enuresis episodes. Not before age 6 years; begin with 0.2 mg tablet nightly 1 hour before bedtime; titrate to 0.6 mg (8)[B]. However, use is questionable because its effects do not persist post treatment (9)[A]. Intranasal formulations can cause severe hyponatremia, resulting in seizures and death in children. Behavioral interventions should be 1st-line treatment (7)[C].

ISSUES FOR REFERRAL

- A patient who exhibits self-injurious behaviors, slow recovery time from tantrums, more tantrums in the home than outside the home, or more aggressive behaviors toward others may require referral to a child psychologist or psychiatrist.
- A child with loud nightly snoring, with observed apnea spells, daytime excessive sleeping, and neurobehavioral signs such as mood changes, ADHD-like symptoms, or academic problems, should be referred for sleep studies (2).
- With enuresis and obstructive sleep apnea symptoms, refer for sleep studies because surgical correction of airway obstruction often improves or cures enuresis and daytime wetting (8).
- Must distinguish sexual behavior problems: Developmentally inappropriate behaviors—greater frequency or much earlier age than expected—becomes a preoccupation, recurs after adult intervention/corrective efforts. If abuse not suspected, consider referral to a child psychologist. If abuse is suspected, must report to child protective services (6).
- If disimpaction by either manual or medical methods is unsuccessful, consult gastroenterology or general surgery. Patients who show no improvement after 6 months of maintenance medical therapy should be referred to gastroenterology (4).
- Thumb sucking resistant to behavioral intervention and threatening oral development may be evaluated by a pediatric dentist for use of habit breaking dental appliances.

ONGOING CARE

DIET

Nutrition is very important in behavioral issues. Avoiding high-sugar foods and caffeine and providing balanced meals has been shown to decrease aggressive and noncompliant behaviors in children.

PATIENT EDUCATION

- See *Parent Training Programs: Insight for Practitioners* at: www.cdc.gov/violenceprevention/pdf/Parent_Training_Brief-a.pdf
- *The Happiest Baby Guide to Great Sleep: Simple Solutions for Kids from Birth to 5 Years*. Harvey Karp, MD New York, HarperCollins Publishers 2012, 384 pp.
- Products
  - www.bedwettingstore.com

REFERENCES

1. Potegal M, Davidson RJ. Temper tantrums in young children: 1. Behavioral composition. *J Dev Behav Pediatr*. 2003;24(3):140–147.
2. Bhargava S. Diagnosis and management of common sleep problems in children. *Pediatr Rev*. 2011;32(3):91–98.
3. Robson WL. Clinical practice. Evaluation and management of enuresis. *N Engl J Med*. 2009;360(14):1429–1436.
4. Har AF, Croffie JM. Encopresis. *Pediatr Rev*. 2010;31(9):368–374; quiz 374.
5. Tseng AG, Biagioli FE. Counseling on early childhood concerns: sleep issues, thumb sucking, picky eating, and school readiness. *Am Fam Physician*. 2009;80(2):139–142.
6. Kellogg ND. Sexual behaviors in children: evaluation and management. *Am Fam Physician*. 2010;82(10):1233–1238.
7. Vande-Walle J, Rittig S. Practical consensus guidelines for management of enuresis. *Eur J Pediatr*. 2012;171(6):971–983.
8. Ramakrishnan K. Evaluation and treatment of enuresis. *Am Fam Physician*. 2008;78(4):489–496.
9. Glazener CMA, Evans JHC. Desmopressin for nocturnal enuresis in children. *Cochrane Database Syst Rev*. 2002;(3):CD002112.

ADDITIONAL READING

- Gringras P. When to use drugs to help sleep. *Arch Dis Child*. 2008;93(11):976–981.
- Gringras P, Gamble C. Melatonin for sleep problems in children with neurodevelopmental disorders: randomised double masked placebo controlled trial. *BMJ*. 2012;345.
- Miller JW. Screening children for developmental behavioral problems: principles for the practitioner. *Prim Care*. 2007;34(2):177–201.
- Strachan E, Staples B. Masturbation. *Pediatr Rev*. 2012;33(4):190–191.
- Zahrt DM, Melzer-Lange MD. Aggressive behavior in children and adolescents. *Pediatr Rev*. 2011;32(8):325–332.

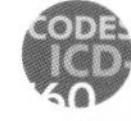

CODES

ICD10

- F98.9 Unspecified behavioral and emotional disorders with onset usually occurring in childhood and adolescence
- F91.1 Conduct disorder, childhood-onset type
- F91.2 Conduct disorder, adolescent-onset type

CLINICAL PEARLS

- Well-child visits provide opportunities for systematic screening for these common conditions.
- Parental education, including a review of age-appropriate discipline, is a key component of treatment.

BELL PALSY

Robert A. Baldor, MD, FAAFP

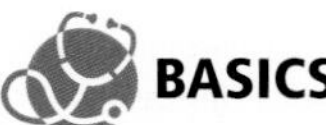

BASICS

DESCRIPTION

A peripheral lower motor neuron facial palsy, usually unilateral, which arises secondary to inflammation and subsequent swelling and compression of cranial nerve VII (facial) and the associated vasa nervorum

EPIDEMIOLOGY

- Affects 0.02% of the population annually
- Predominant sex: male = female
- Median age of onset is 40 years but affects all ages
- Accounts for 60–75% of all cases of unilateral facial paralysis
- Occurs with equal frequency on the left and right sides of the face
- Most patients recover, but as many as 30% are left with facial disfigurement and pain.

Incidence

- 20–30 cases per 100,000 people in the United States per year
- Lowest in children ≤10 years of age; highest in adults ≥70 years of age
- Higher among pregnant women

Prevalence

Affects 40,000 Americans every year

ETIOLOGY AND PATHOPHYSIOLOGY

- Results from damage to the facial cranial nerve (VII)
- Inflammation of cranial nerve VII causes swelling and subsequent compression of both the nerve and the associated vasa nervorum.
- May arise secondary to reactivation of latent herpesvirus (herpes simplex virus [HSV] type 1 and herpes zoster virus) in cranial nerve ganglia or due to ischemia from arteriosclerosis associated with diabetes mellitus

Genetics

May be associated with a genetic predisposition, but it remains unclear which factors are inherited

RISK FACTORS

- Pregnancy
- Diabetes mellitus
- Age >30 years
- Exposure to cold temperatures
- Upper respiratory infection (e.g., coryza, influenza)

COMMONLY ASSOCIATED CONDITIONS

- HSV
- Lyme disease
- Diabetes mellitus
- Hypertension
- Herpes zoster virus
- Ramsay-Hunt syndrome
- Sjögren syndrome
- Sarcoidosis
- Eclampsia
- Amyloidosis

DIAGNOSIS

HISTORY

- Time course of the illness (rapid onset)
- Predisposing factors: recent viral infection, trauma, new medications, hypertension, diabetes mellitus
- Presence of hyperacusis or history of recurrent Bell palsy (both associated with poor prognosis)
- Any associated rash (suggestive of herpes zoster, Lyme disease, or sarcoid)
- Weakness on affected side of face, often sudden in onset
- Pain in or behind the ear in 50% of cases, which may precede the palsy in 25% of cases (1)[C]
- Subjective numbness on the ipsilateral side of the face
- Alteration of taste on the ipsilateral anterior 2/3 of the tongue (chorda tympani branch of the facial nerve)
- Hyperacusis (nerve to the stapedius muscle)
- Decreased tear production

PHYSICAL EXAM

- Neurologic
  - Determine if the weakness is caused by a problem in either the central or peripheral nervous systems.
  - Flaccid paralysis of muscles on the affected side, *including the forehead*
    - Impaired ability to raise the ipsilateral eyebrow
    - Impaired closure of the ipsilateral eye
    - Impaired ability to smile, grin, or purse the lips
    - Bell phenomenon: upward diversion of the eye with attempted closure of the lid
  - Patients may complain of numbness, but no deficit is present on sensory testing.
  - Examine for involvement of other cranial nerves.
- Head, ears, eyes, nose, and throat
  - Carefully examine to exclude a space occupying lesion
  - Perform pneumatic otoscopic exam.
- Skin: Examine for erythema migrans (Lyme disease) and vesicular rash (herpes zoster virus).

DIFFERENTIAL DIAGNOSIS

Etiologies include the following:

- Infectious
  - Acute or chronic otitis media
  - Malignant otitis externa
  - Osteomyelitis of the skull base
- Cerebrovascular
  - Brainstem stroke involving anteroinferior cerebellar artery
  - Aneurysm involving carotid, vertebral, or basilar arteries
- Neoplastic (Onset of palsy is usually slow and progressive and accompanied by additional cranial nerve deficits and/or headache.) (2)[C]
  - Tumors of the parotid gland
  - Cholesteatoma
  - Skull base tumor
  - Carcinomatous meningitis
  - Leukemic meningitis
- Traumatic
  - Temporal bone fracture
  - Mandibular bone fracture
- Other
  - Multiple sclerosis
  - Myasthenia gravis (should be considered in cases of recurrent or bilateral facial palsy)
  - Guillain-Barré syndrome (may also present with bilateral facial palsy)
  - Sjögren syndrome
  - Sarcoidosis
  - Amyloidosis
  - Melkersson-Rosenthal syndrome
  - Mononeuritis or polyneuritis

DIAGNOSTIC TESTS & INTERPRETATION

Initial Tests (lab, imaging)

- Blood glucose level (if diabetes a consideration)
- Lyme titer ELISA and Western blot for immunoglobulin (Ig) M, IgG for *Borrelia burgdorferi*
- ESR
- Consider CBC.
- Consider rapid plasma reagin test.
- Consider HIV test.
- In appropriate clinical circumstances, consider titers for varicella-zoster virus, cytomegalovirus, rubella, hepatitis A, hepatitis B, and hepatitis C.

Follow-Up Tests & Special Considerations

- CSF analysis
  - CSF protein is elevated in 1/3 of cases.
  - CSF cells show mild elevation in 10% of cases with a mononuclear cell predominance.
  - Not routinely indicated
- Salivary polymerase chain reaction for HSV1 or herpes zoster virus (largely reserved for research purposes)
- Facial radiographs
  - In the setting of trauma, evaluate for fracture.
- IV contrast–enhanced head CT
  - Evaluate for fracture.
  - Evaluate for stroke, if stroke is in the differential.
- IV contrast–enhanced brain MRI (1)[A]
  - Evaluate for central pontine, temporal bone, and parotid neoplasms.
  - Not routinely indicated

Diagnostic Procedures/Other

- Electromyograph: Nerve conduction on affected and nonaffected sides can be compared to determine the extent of nerve injury, especially if there is dense palsy or no recovery after several weeks.
- Electroneurography: Evoked potentials of affected and nonaffected sides can be compared.

Test Interpretation

Invasive diagnostic procedures are not indicated because biopsy could further damage cranial nerve XII.

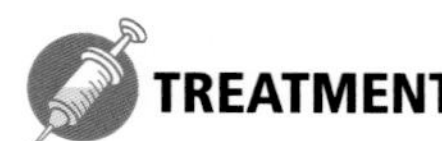

TREATMENT

GENERAL MEASURES

- Artificial tears should be used to lubricate the cornea.
- The ipsilateral eye should be patched and taped shut at night to avoid drying and infection.

MEDICATION

- Corticosteroids decrease inflammation and limit nerve damage, thereby reducing the number of patients with residual facial weakness (3,4)[A].
- Routine use of antiviral medication is not recommended. Antiviral agents targeting herpes simplex, when administered concurrently with corticosteroids, may further reduce the risk of unfavorable outcomes in patients with a dense Bell palsy (5,6)[A]:
  - Antivirals alone are less likely to produce full recovery than corticosteroids (3)[A].
  - A combination of valacyclovir and steroids provides only minimal added benefit over steroid use alone (7)[B].
- Corticosteroids
  - Prednisolone: total of 500 mg over 10 days, 25 mg PO BID
    - Treatment with prednisolone within 48 hours of palsy onset has shown higher complete recovery rates and less synkinesis compared with no prednisolone (8)[B].
    - Antivirals in combination with corticosteroids
      - Valacyclovir: 1,000 mg TID × 7 days plus prednisolone 60 mg/day × 5 days; then tapered by 10 mg/day for total treatment length of 10 days (7)[B]
- Contraindications
  - Documented hypersensitivity
  - Preexisting infections, including tuberculosis (TB) and systemic mycosis
- Precautions: use with discretion in pregnant patients and those with peptic ulcer disease and diabetes
- Significant possible interactions: measles-mumps-rubella, oral polio virus vaccine, and other live vaccines

Pregnancy Considerations

Steroids should be used cautiously during pregnancy; consult with an obstetrician.

ISSUES FOR REFERRAL

Patients may need to be referred to an ear, nose, and throat specialist or a neurologist.

ADDITIONAL THERAPIES

- Physical therapy: no evidence of significant benefit or harm, but facial exercises may reduce time to recover and/or sequelae (9,10)[C]
- Electrostimulation and mirror biofeedback rehabilitation have limited evidence of effect (11,12)[C].
- Acupuncture with strong stimulation has shown some therapeutic promise (12)[C].

SURGERY/OTHER PROCEDURES

- Surgical treatment of Bell palsy remains controversial and is reserved for intractable cases (13)[A].
- There is insufficient evidence to decide whether surgical intervention is beneficial or harmful in the management of Bell palsy (9)[B].
- In those cases where surgical intervention is performed, cranial nerve XII is surgically decompressed at the entrance to the meatal foramen where the labyrinthine segment and geniculate ganglion reside (1)[A].
- Decompression surgery should not be performed >14 days after the onset of paralysis because severe degeneration of the facial nerve is likely irreversible after 2–3 weeks (1)[A].

ONGOING CARE

FOLLOW-UP RECOMMENDATIONS

Patient Monitoring

- Patients should start steroid treatment immediately and be followed for 12 months.
- Patients who do not recover complete facial nerve function should be referred to an ophthalmologist for tarsorrhaphy.

PATIENT EDUCATION

American Academy of Family Physicians: www.aafp.org/afp/2007/1001/p1004.html

PROGNOSIS

- Most patients achieve complete spontaneous recovery within 2 weeks. More than 80% recover within 3 months.
- 85% of untreated patients will experience the first signs of recovery within 3 weeks of onset.
- 16% are left with a partial palsy, motor synkinesis, and autonomic synkinesis.
- 5% experience severe sequelae, and a small number of patients experience permanent facial weakness and dysfunction.
- Poor prognostic factors include the following:
  - Age >60 years
  - Complete facial weakness
  - Hypertension
  - Ramsay-Hunt syndrome
- The Sunnybrook and House-Brackmann facial grading systems are clinical prognostic models that identify Bell palsy patients at risk for nonrecovery at 12 months.
- Treatment with prednisolone or no prednisolone and the Sunnybrook score are significant factors for predicting nonrecovery at 1 month (14)[C].

COMPLICATIONS

- Corneal abrasion or ulceration
- Steroid-induced psychological disturbances; avascular necrosis of the hips, knees, and/or shoulders
- Steroid use can unmask subclinical infection (e.g., TB).

REFERENCES

1. Gilden DH. Clinical practice. Bell's palsy. *N Engl J Med*. 2004;351(13):1323–1331.
2. Holland NJ, Weiner GM. Recent developments in Bell's palsy. *BMJ*. 2004;329(7465):553–557.
3. Gronseth GS, Paduqa R; American Academy of Neurology. Evidence-based guideline update: steroids and antivirals for Bell palsy: report of the Guideline Development Subcommittee of the American Academy of Neurology. *Neurology*. 2012;79(22):2209–2213.
4. Salinas RA, Alvarez G, Daly F, et al. Corticosteroids for Bell's palsy (idiopathic facial paralysis). *Cochrane Database Syst Rev*. 2010;(3):CD001942.
5. Lockhart P, Daly F, Pitkethly M, et al. Antiviral treatment for Bell's palsy (idiopathic facial paralysis). *Cochrane Database Syst Rev*. 2009;(4):CD001869.
6. Thaera GM, Wellik KE, Barrs DM, et al. Are corticosteroid and antiviral treatments effective for bell palsy? A critically appraised topic. *Neurologist*. 2010;16(12):138–140.
7. Worster A, Keim SM, Sahsi R, et al. Do either corticosteroids or antiviral agents reduce the risk of long-term facial paresis in patients with new-onset Bell's palsy? *J Emerg Med*. 2010;38(4):518–523.
8. Madhok V, Falk G, Fahey T. Prescribe prednisolone alone for Bell's palsy diagnosed within 72 hours of symptom onset. *BMJ*. 2009;338:b255.
9. Axelsson S, Berg T, Jonsson L, et al. Prednisolone in Bell's palsy related to treatment start and age. *Otol Neurotol*. 2011;32(1):141–146.
10. Teixeira LJ, Valbuza JS, Prado GF. Physical therapy for Bell's palsy (idiopathic facial paralysis). *Cochrane Database Syst Rev*. 2011;(12):CD006283.
11. Alakram P, Puckree T. Effects of electrical stimulation on House-Brackmann scores in early Bell's palsy. *Physiother Theory Pract*. 2010;26(3):160–166.
12. Xu SB, Huang B, Zhang C. Effectiveness of strengthened stimulation during acupuncture for the treatment of Bell palsy: a randomized control trial. *CMAJ*. 2013;185(6):473–479.
13. McAllister K, Walker D, Donnan PT, et al. Surgical interventions for the early management of Bell's palsy. *Cochrane Database Syst Rev*. 2011;(2):CD007468.
14. Marsk E, Bylund N, Jonsson L. Prediction of nonrecovery in Bell's palsy using Sunnybrook grading. *Laryngoscope*. 2012;122(4):901–906.

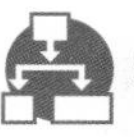

SEE ALSO

Amyloidosis; Diabetes Mellitus, Type 1; Diabetes Mellitus, Type 2; Herpes Simplex; Herpes Zoster (Shingles); Lyme Disease; Melkersson-Rosenthal Syndrome; Ramsay-Hunt Syndrome; Sarcoidosis; Sjögren Syndrome

CODES

ICD10

G51.0 Bell's palsy

CLINICAL PEARLS

- Initiate steroids immediately following the onset of symptoms.
- Look closely at the voluntary movement on the upper part of the face on the affected side; in Bell palsy, all of the muscles are involved (weak or paralyzed), whereas in a stroke, the upper muscles are spared (because of bilateral innervation).
- Protect the affected eye with lubrication and taping.
- In areas with endemic Lyme disease, Bell palsy should be considered to be Lyme disease until proven otherwise.

BIPOLAR I DISORDER

Laurie A. Carrier, MD

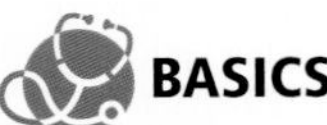

BASICS

DESCRIPTION

- Bipolar I (BP-I) is a mood disorder characterized by at least 1 manic or mixed episode, often alternating with episodes of major depression, that causes marked impairment and/or hospitalization.
- Symptoms are not caused by a substance (e.g., drug), a general medical condition, or a medication.

Geriatric Considerations

New onset in older patients (>50 years of age) requires a workup for organic or chemically induced pathology.

Pediatric Considerations

There is overlap with symptoms of attention deficit hyperactivity disorder (ADHD) and oppositional defiant disorder (ODD). Children and adolescents experience more rapid cycling and mixed states. Depression often presents as irritable mood.

Pregnancy Considerations

- Potential teratogenic effects of commonly used medications (e.g., lithium, valproic acid)
- Symptoms may be exacerbated in the postpartum period.

EPIDEMIOLOGY

- Onset usually between 15 and 30 years of age
- More common in single and divorced persons
- Less common in college graduates
- Increased incidence in higher socioeconomic groups

Prevalence

- 1.0–1.6% lifetime prevalence
- Equal among men and women (manic episodes more common in men; depressive episodes more common in women)
- Equal among races; however, clinicians tend to misdiagnose schizophrenia in African Americans with BP-I.

ETIOLOGY AND PATHOPHYSIOLOGY

Genetic predisposition and major life stressors can trigger initial and subsequent episodes:

- Dysregulation of biogenic amines or neurotransmitters (particularly serotonin, norepinephrine, and dopamine)
- MRI findings suggest abnormalities in prefrontal cortical areas, striatum, and amygdala that predate illness onset (1)[C].

Genetics

- Monozygotic twin concordance 40–70%
- Dizygotic twin concordance 5–25%
- 50% have at least 1 parent with a mood disorder
- 1st-degree relatives are 7× more likely to develop BP-I than the general population.

RISK FACTORS

Genetics, major life stressors (especially loss of parent or spouse), or substance abuse

GENERAL PREVENTION

Treatment adherence and education can help to prevent relapses.

COMMONLY ASSOCIATED CONDITIONS

Substance abuse (60%), ADHD, anxiety disorders, and eating disorders

DIAGNOSIS

- The diagnosis of BP-I requires at least 1 manic or mixed episode (simultaneous mania and depression). Although a depressive episode is not necessary for the diagnosis, 80–90% of people with BP-I also experience depression.
- Manic episode, *DSM-5* criteria (2):
  - Distinct period of abnormally and persistently elevated, expansive, or irritable mood lasting at least 1 week (or any duration if hospitalization is necessary)
  - During the period of mood disturbance, 3 or more of the "DIG FAST" symptoms must persist (4 if the mood is only irritable) and must be present to a significant degree:
    - Distractibility
    - Insomnia, decreased need for sleep
    - Grandiosity or inflated self-esteem
    - Flight of ideas or racing thoughts
    - Agitation or increase in goal-directed activity
    - Speech pressured/more talkative than usual
    - Taking risks: excessive involvement in pleasurable activities that have a high potential for painful consequences (e.g., financial or sexual)
  - Mixed episode: Criteria are met for both a manic and major depressive episode nearly every day during at least a 1-week period, and the mood disturbance causes significant impairment in functioning.
  - Signs and symptoms more likely in bipolar than in unipolar depression: agitation/restlessness, suicidal ideation/planning, increased frequency of depressive episodes, melancholia, psychomotor retardation, younger age of onset, hyperphagia, hypersomnia, family history of bipolar disorder, subsyndromal hypomanic symptoms (particularly increased goal-directed activity) (3)[B].

HISTORY

- Collateral information makes diagnostics more complete and is often necessary for a clear history.
- History: safety concerns (e.g., Suicidal/homicidal ideation? Safety plan? Psychosis present?), physical well-being (e.g., Number of hours of sleep? Appetite? Substance abuse?), personal history (e.g., Told life of the party? Talkative? Speeding? Spending sprees or donations? Credit card or gambling debt? Promiscuous? Other risk-taking behavior? Legal trouble? Religious infatuation?)

PHYSICAL EXAM

- Mental status exam in acute mania:
  - General appearance: bright clothing, excessive makeup, disorganized or discombobulated, psychomotor agitation
  - Speech: pressured, difficult to interrupt
  - Mood/affect: euphoria, irritability/expansive, labile
  - Thought process: flight of ideas (streams of thought occur to patient at rapid rate), easily distracted
  - Thought content: grandiosity, paranoia, hyperreligious
  - Perceptual abnormalities: 3/4 of manic patients experience delusions, grandiose or paranoid
  - Suicidal/homicidal ideation: Irritability or delusions may lead to aggression toward self or others; suicidal ideation is common with mixed episode.
  - Insight/judgment: poor/impaired
- See "Bipolar II Disorder" for an example of a mental status exam in depression.
- With mixed episodes, patients may exhibit a combination of manic and depressive mental states.

DIFFERENTIAL DIAGNOSIS

- Other psychiatric considerations: unipolar depression ± psychotic features, schizophrenia, schizoaffective disorder, personality disorders (particularly antisocial, borderline, histrionic, and narcissistic), ADD ± hyperactivity, substance-induced mood disorder
- Medical considerations: epilepsy (e.g., temporal lobe), brain tumor, infection (e.g., AIDS, syphilis), stroke, endocrine (e.g., thyroid) disease, multiple sclerosis
- In children, consider ADHD and ODD.

DIAGNOSTIC TESTS & INTERPRETATION

- BP-I is a clinical diagnosis.
- The Mood Disorder Questionnaire is a self-assessment screen for bipolar disorders (sensitivity 73%, specificity 90%) (4).
- Patient Health Questionnaire-9 helps to determine the presence and severity of a depressive episode.

Initial Tests (lab, imaging)

- TSH, CBC, BMP, LFTs, ANA, RPR, HIV, ESR
- Drug/alcohol screen with each presentation
- Dementia workup if new onset in seniors
- Consider brain imaging (CT, MRI) with initial onset of mania to rule out organic cause (e.g., tumor, infection, or stroke), especially with onset in elderly and if psychosis is present.

Diagnostic Procedures/Other

Consider EEG if presentation suggests temporal lobe epilepsy (hyperreligiosity, hypergraphia).

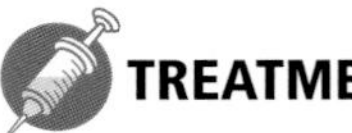

TREATMENT

- Ensure safety.
- Psychotherapy (e.g., cognitive-behavioral therapy, social rhythm therapy)
- Stress reduction
- Patient and family education

GENERAL MEASURES

- Psychotherapy (e.g., cognitive-behavioral therapy, social rhythm, interpersonal) in conjunction with medications
- Regular exercise, a healthy diet, and sobriety have been shown to help prevent worsening of symptoms.

MEDICATION

First Line

- Treatment may consist of 1–4 mood stabilizers or other psychotropic medications. When combining these agents, add different classes (e.g., an atypical antipsychotic and/or an antiseizure medication and/or lithium).
- Lithium (Lithobid, Eskalith, generic): dosing: 600–1,200 mg/day divided BID–QID; start 600–900 mg/day divided BID–TID, titrate based on blood levels. *Warning:* Caution in kidney and heart disease; use can lead to diabetes insipidus or thyroid disease. Caution with diuretics or ACE inhibitors; dehydration can lead to toxicity (seizures, encephalopathy, arrhythmias). Pregnancy Category D (Ebstein anomaly). *Monitor:* Check ECG >40 years, TSH, BUN, creatine, electrolytes at baseline and every

6 months; check level 5–7 days after initiation or dose change, then every 2 weeks × 3, then every 3 months (goal: 0.8–1.2 mmol/L).
- Antiseizure medications
  - Divalproex sodium, valproic acid (Depakote, Depakene, generic): dosing: start 250–500 mg BID–TID; maximum 60 mg/kg/day. *Black box warnings:* hepatotoxicity, pancreatitis, thrombocytopenia, pregnancy Category D. *Monitor:* CBC, LFTs at baseline and every 6 months; check level 5 days after initiation and dose changes (goal: 50–125 μg/mL).
  - Carbamazepine (Equetro, Tegretol, generic): dosing: 800–1,200 mg/day PO divided BID–QID; start 100–200 mg PO BID and titrate to lowest effective dose. *Warning:* Do not use with TCA or within 14 days of an MAOI. Caution in kidney/heart disease; risk of aplastic anemia/agranulocytosis, enzyme inducer; pregnancy Category D. *Monitor:* CBC, LFTs at baseline and every 3–6 months; check level 4–5 days after initiation and dose changes (goal: 4–12 μg/mL).
  - Lamotrigine (Lamictal, generic): dosing: 200 mg/day; start 25 mg/day × 2 weeks, then 50 mg/day × 2 weeks, then 100 mg/day × 1 week, then 150 mg/day. (*Note:* Use different dosing if adjunct to valproate). *Warning:* Titrate slowly (risk of Stevens-Johnson syndrome); caution with kidney/liver/heart disease; pregnancy Category C
  - Oxcarbazepine (Trileptal), gabapentin (Neurontin), and topiramate (Topamax) are also used in BP-I, but are not approved by the FDA.
- Atypical antipsychotics
  - Side effects: orthostatic hypotension, metabolic side effects (glucose and lipid dysregulation, weight gain), tardive dyskinesia, neuroleptic malignant syndrome (NMS), prolactinemia (except Abilify), increased risk of death in elderly with dementia-related psychosis, pregnancy Category C
  - Monitor: LFTs, lipids, glucose at baseline, 3 months, and annually; check for extrapyramidal symptoms (EPS) with Abnormal Involuntary Movement Scale (AIMS) and assess weight (with abdominal circumference) at baseline, at 4, 8, and 12 weeks, and then every 3–6 months; monitor for orthostatic hypotension 3–5 days after starting or changing dose.
  - Risperidone (Risperdal, Risperdal Consta, generic): dosing: 1–6 mg/day divided QD–QID IM preparation available (q2wk)
  - Olanzapine (Zyprexa, Zydis, generic): dosing: 5–20 mg/day; most likely to cause metabolic side effects (weight gain, diabetes)
  - Symbyax (olanzapine + fluoxetine): dosing: 6/25 mg/day
  - Quetiapine (Seroquel, Seroquel XR, generic): dosing: In mania, 200–400 mg BID; in bipolar depression, 50–300 mg qhs. XR dosing 50–400 mg qhs.
  - Aripiprazole (Abilify): dosing: 15–30 mg/day; less likely to cause metabolic side effects
  - Ziprasidone (Geodon): dosing: 40–80 mg BID; less likely to cause metabolic side effects. *Caution:* QTc prolongation (>500 ms) has been associated with use (0.06%). Consider ECG at baseline.
  - Asenapine (Saphris): dosing: 5–10 mg BID; comes in sublingual tab

Second Line
- Antidepressants (in addition to mood stabilizers) have mixed evidence to support use.
- Benzodiazepines (for acute agitation with mania, associated anxiety)
- Sleep medications

ISSUES FOR REFERRAL
- Depends on comfort level of the doctor, stability of patient
- Patients benefit from a multidisciplinary team, including a primary care physician, psychiatrist, and therapist.

ADDITIONAL THERAPIES
- Electroconvulsive therapy can be helpful in acute mania and depression.
- Light therapy for seasonal component to depressive episodes (use with caution because it can precipitate manic episode)
- Modest evidence supports transcranial magnetic stimulation, vagus nerve stimulation, ketamine infusion, sleep deprivation, and hormone therapy (e.g., thyroid) in bipolar depression.

INPATIENT CONSIDERATIONS
Admit if dangerous to self or others.

Admission Criteria/Initial Stabilization
To admit involuntarily, the patient must have a psychiatric diagnosis (e.g., BP-I) and present a danger to self or others or the mental disease must be inhibiting the person from obtaining basic needs (e.g., food, clothing).

Nursing
Alert staff to potentially dangerous or agitated patients. Acute suicidal threats need continuous observation.

Discharge Criteria
Determined by safety

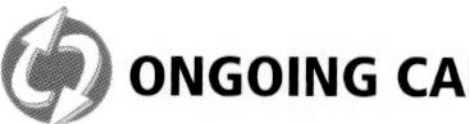

ONGOING CARE

FOLLOW-UP RECOMMENDATIONS
- Regularly scheduled visits support adherence with treatment.
- Frequent communication among primary care doctor, psychiatrist, and therapist

Patient Monitoring
Mood charts are helpful to monitor symptoms.

PATIENT EDUCATION
- National Alliance on Mental Illness (NAMI): www.nami.org/
- National Institutes of Mental Health (NIMH): www.nimh.nih.gov

PROGNOSIS
- Frequency and severity of episodes are related to medication adherence, consistency with therapy, quality of sleep, and support systems (5)[B].
- 40–50% of patients experience another manic episode within 2 years of 1st episode.
- 25–50% attempt suicide, and 15% die by suicide.
- Substance abuse, unemployment, psychosis, depression, and male gender are associated with a worse prognosis.

REFERENCES

1. Fornito A, Yücel M, Wood SJ, et al. Anterior cingulate cortex abnormalities associated with a first psychotic episode in bipolar disorder. *Br J Psychiatry*. 2009;194(5):426–433.
2. American Psychiatric Association. *Diagnostic and Statistical Manual of Mental Disorders*. 5th ed. Arlington, VA: American Psychiatric Association; 2013.
3. Perlis RH, Brown E, Baker RW, et al. Clinical features of bipolar depression versus major depressive disorder in large multicenter trials. *Am J Psychiatry*. 2006;163(2):225–231.
4. Hirshfeld RM. Validation of the mood disorder questionnaire. *Bipolar Depression Bulletin*. 2004.
5. Depp CA, Moore DJ, Patterson TL, et al. Psychosocial interventions and medication adherence in bipolar disorder. *Dialogues Clin Neurosci*. 2008;10(2):239–250.

ADDITIONAL READING

- Agency for Healthcare Research and Quality. Antipsychotic medicines for treating schizophrenia and bipolar disorder: a review of the research for adults and caregivers. In: *Comparative Effectiveness Review Summary Guides for Consumers*. Rockville, MD: Agency for Healthcare Research and Quality; 2013.
- American Psychiatric Association. Practice guideline for the treatment of patients with bipolar disorder (revision). *Am J Psychiatry*. 2002;159(4)(Suppl):1–50.
- Licht RW. A new balance in bipolar I disorder. *Lancet*. 2010;375(9712):350–352.

SEE ALSO
Algorithm: Depressive Episode, Major

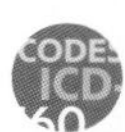

CODES

ICD10
- F31.9 Bipolar disorder, unspecified
- F31.10 Bipolar disorder, current episode manic without psychotic features, unspecified
- F31.30 Bipolar disord, crnt epsd depress, mild or mod severt, unsp

CLINICAL PEARLS
- Bipolar I is characterized by at least 1 manic or mixed episode, often alternating with episodes of major depression, that causes marked impairment.
- 25–50% of BP-I patients attempt suicide, and 15% die by suicide.
- There is no way to prevent the onset of BP-I, but treatment adherence and education can help to prevent further episodes.
- Goal of treatment is to decrease the intensity, length, and number of episodes as well as greater mood stability between episodes.

BIPOLAR II DISORDER

Laurie A. Carrier, MD

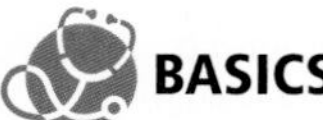

BASICS

DESCRIPTION

Bipolar II (BP-II) is a mood disorder characterized by at least 1 episode of major depression and at least 1 episode of hypomania, a milder form of mania.

Geriatric Considerations

New onset in older patients (>50 years) requires a workup for organic or chemically induced pathology.

Pediatric Considerations

- Large overlap with symptoms of attention deficit hyperactivity disorder (ADHD) and oppositional defiant disorder (ODD)
- Depression often presents as irritable mood.

Pregnancy Considerations

- Counsel women of childbearing age about potentially teratogenic effects of commonly used medications (e.g., lithium, valproic acid).
- Symptoms may be exacerbated in the postpartum period.

EPIDEMIOLOGY

More common in women

Prevalence

0.5–1.1% lifetime prevalence

ETIOLOGY AND PATHOPHYSIOLOGY

- Dysregulation of biogenic amines or neurotransmitters (particularly serotonin, norepinephrine, and dopamine)
- Genetics
- Major life stressors (especially loss of parent or spouse)

Genetics

Heritability estimate: >77%

GENERAL PREVENTION

No way to prevent the onset of BP-II, but treatment adherence and education can help to prevent further episodes

COMMONLY ASSOCIATED CONDITIONS

Substance abuse or dependence, ADHD, anxiety disorders, and eating disorders

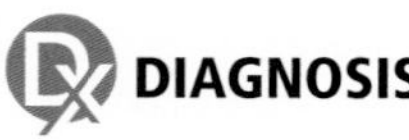

DIAGNOSIS

- *DSM-5* criteria: Patient must experience at least 1 hypomanic episode and at least 1 major depressive episode. The symptoms have caused *some* distress or impairment in social, occupational, or other areas of functioning. There can be no history of full manic or mixed episodes 1[C].
- Hypomania is a distinct period of persistently elevated, expansive, or irritable mood, different from usual nondepressed mood, lasting at least 4 days:
  - The episode must include at least 3 of the "DIG FAST" symptoms below (4 if the mood is only irritable):
    - Distractibility
    - Insomnia, decreased need for sleep
    - Grandiosity or inflated self-esteem
    - Flight of ideas or racing thoughts
    - Agitation or increase in goal-directed activity (socially, at work or school, or sexually)
    - Speech pressured/more talkative than usual
    - Taking risks: excessive involvement in pleasurable activities that have high potential for painful consequences (e.g., sexual or financial)
- The symptoms are not severe enough to cause *marked* impairment in functioning or hospitalization, and there is no associated psychosis as with BP-I.
- Major depression
  - Depressed mood or diminished interest and 4 or more of the "SIG E CAPS" symptoms are present during the same 2-week period:
    - **S**leep disturbance (e.g., trouble falling asleep, early morning awakening)
    - **I**nterest: loss or anhedonia
    - **G**uilt (or feelings of worthlessness)
    - **E**nergy, loss of
    - **C**oncentration, loss of
    - **A**ppetite changes, increase or decrease
    - **P**sychomotor changes (retardation or agitation)
    - **S**uicidal/homicidal thoughts
  - BP-II with rapid cycling is diagnosed when a patient experiences at least 4 episodes of a mood disturbance in a 12-month period (either major depression or hypomania).
- Signs, symptoms, and history seen more often in BP-II than in unipolar depression:
  - Agitation, hyperphagia, hypersomnia, melancholia, psychomotor retardation, suicidal ideation/planning, increased frequency of depressive episodes, younger age of onset, family history of bipolar disorder, subsyndromal hypomanic symptoms (e.g., overactivity) (2)[C]
- Note: If symptoms have *ever* met criteria for a full manic episode or hospitalization was necessary secondary to manic/mixed symptoms or psychosis was present, then the diagnosis changes to BP-I.

HISTORY

Collateral information makes diagnostics more complete and is often necessary for a clear history.

PHYSICAL EXAM

- Mental status exam in hypomania
  - General appearance: usually appropriately dressed, with psychomotor agitation
  - Speech: may be pressured, talkative, difficult to interrupt
  - Mood/affect: euphoria, irritability/congruent, or expansive
  - Thought process: may be easily distracted, difficulty concentrating on 1 task
  - Thought content: usually positive, with "big" plans
  - Perceptual abnormalities: none
  - Suicidal/homicidal ideation: low incidence of homicidal or suicidal ideation
  - Insight/judgment: usually stable/may be impaired by their distractibility
- Mental status exam in acute depression
  - General appearance: unkempt, psychomotor retardation, poor eye contact
  - Speech: low, soft, monotone
  - Mood/affect: sad, depressed/congruent, flat
  - Thought process: ruminating thoughts, generalized slowing
  - Thought content: preoccupied with negative or nihilistic ideas
  - Perceptual abnormalities: 15% of depressed patients experience hallucinations or delusions.
  - Suicidal/homicidal ideation: Suicidal ideation is very common.
  - Insight/judgment: often impaired

DIFFERENTIAL DIAGNOSIS

- Other psychiatric considerations
  - BP-I disorder, unipolar depression, personality disorders (particularly borderline, antisocial, and narcissistic), ADD with hyperactivity, substance-induced mood disorder
- Medical considerations
  - Epilepsy (e.g., temporal lobe), brain tumor, infection (e.g., AIDS, syphilis), stroke, endocrine (e.g., thyroid disease), multiple sclerosis
- In children, consider ADHD and ODD.

DIAGNOSTIC TESTS & INTERPRETATION

- BP-II is a clinical diagnosis.
- Mood Disorder Questionnaire, self-assessment screen for BP, sensitivity 73%, specificity 90% (3)[B]
- Hypomania Checklist-32 distinguishes between BP-II and unipolar depression (sensitivity 80%, specificity 51%) (4)[B].
- Patient Health Questionnaire-9 helps to determine the presence and severity of depression.

Initial Tests (lab, imaging)

- Rule out organic causes of mood disorder during initial episode.
- Drug/alcohol screen is prudent with each presentation.
- Dementia workup if new onset in seniors
- With initial presentation: Consider CBC, chem 7, TSH, LFTs, ANA, RPR, HIV, and ESR.
- Consider brain imaging (CT, MRI) with initial onset of hypomania to rule out organic cause, especially with onset in the elderly.

TREATMENT

- Ensure safety
- Medication management
- Psychotherapy (e.g., cognitive-behavioral therapy [CBT], social rhythm therapy, interpersonal therapy)
- Stress reduction
- Patient and family education

GENERAL MEASURES

- Psychotherapy (e.g., CBT, social rhythm, interpersonal, family focused) in conjunction with medications is the key.
- Regular exercise, a healthy diet, and sobriety have been shown to help prevent worsening of symptoms.

MEDICATION

- Less research has been conducted on the appropriate treatment of BP-II, but current consensus is to treat with the same medications as BP-I.
- Antidepressant medications must be used with caution during depressive episodes, as they may precipitate hypomanic episodes (less common than with BP-I).

First Line

- American Psychological Association guidelines state lithium or lamotrigine as first-line treatment for bipolar depression (5)[C].
- Treatment may be a combination of 1–4 different agents. When combining mood stabilizers, consider adding different classes (e.g., an atypical antipsychotic and/or an antiseizure medication and/or lithium).
- Lithium (Lithobid, Eskalith, generic): dosing 600–1,200 mg/day divided BID–QID, titrate based on blood levels:
  - Caution in kidney or heart disease; use can lead to diabetes insipidus, thyroid disease; caution in sodium-depleted patients (diuretics, ACE inhibitors); dehydration can lead to toxicity, which may cause seizures, encephalopathic syndrome, arrhythmias, pregnancy Category D (Ebstein anomaly with 1st-trimester use).
  - Monitor electrocardiogram in patients >40 years, TSH, BUN, creatinine, electrolytes at baseline and q6mo; check level 5–7 days after initiation or dose change, then q1–2wk × 3, then q3mo (goal: 0.8–1.2 mmol/L).
- Anticonvulsants
  - Valproic acid, divalproex sodium: dosing: Start 250–500 mg BID–TID, max 60 mg/kg/day. *Warning*: hepatotoxicity, pancreatitis, thrombocytopenia, pregnancy Category D (neural tube defects). *Monitor*: CBC, LFTs at baseline and q6mo; check valproic acid level 5 days after initiation and dose changes (goal: 50–125 μm/mL).
  - Carbamazepine: dosing: 800–1,200 mg/day PO divided BID–QID, start 100–200 mg PO BID and titrate to lowest effective dose. Do not use with tricyclic antidepressants or within 14 days of monoamine oxidase inhibitor; caution with kidney or heart disease, may cause aplastic anemia/agranulocytosis, pregnancy Category D. Monitor: CBC, LFTs at baseline and q3–6mo; check level 4–5 days after initiation and dose changes (goal: 4–12 μm/mL).
  - Lamotrigine: dosing: 200 mg/day start 25 mg × 2 weeks, then 50 mg × 2 weeks, then 100 mg × 1 week. (Note: Different dosing if adjunct to valproate.) Selected warnings: Titrate slowly (risk of Stevens-Johnson syndrome); caution with kidney, liver, or heart impairment; pregnancy Category C. Monitor: Patient to monitor for rash.
  - Oxcarbazepine, gabapentin, and topiramate are also used in bipolar depression but are not FDA approved.
- Atypical antipsychotics (AAs)
  - Side effects of AAs: orthostatic hypotension, negative metabolic side effects (effect glucose and lipid regulation, weight gain), tardive dyskinesia, neuroleptic malignant syndrome, prolactinemia (except Abilify), increased risk of mortality in elderly with dementia-related psychosis, pregnancy Category C
  - Monitor: LFTs, lipids, glucose at baseline, 3 months, and annually; check for extrapyramidal symptoms with Abnormal Involuntary Movement Scale (AIMS) and assess weight (with abdominal circumference) at baseline, then 4, 8, and 12 weeks, then q3–6mo; monitor for orthostatic hypotension 3–5 days after starting or changing dose.
  - Aripiprazole: dosing: 15 mg/day, max 30 mg/day, less likely to cause metabolic side effects
  - Olanzapine: dosing: 5–20 mg/day, most likely AA to cause metabolic side effects (weight gain, diabetes mellitus)
  - Symbyax (olanzapine + fluoxetine): dosing: 6/25 mg/day, FDA approved for bipolar depression
  - Quetiapine: dosing: hypomania 200–400 mg BID; depression: 50–300 mg qhs
  - Risperidone: dosing: 1–6 mg/day every day–BID; generic and q2wk IM preparations available
  - Ziprasidone: dosing: 40–80 mg BID. Less likely to cause metabolic side effects. *Warning*: QTc prolongation (>500 ms) has been associated with use (0.06%); consider ECG at baseline.
  - Asenapine (Saphris): dosing: 5–10 mg BID; comes in sublingual tab, FDA approved for acute and maintenance treatment

Second Line

- Antidepressants (in addition to mood stabilizers) have better data in BP-II than BP-I.
- Benzodiazepines (for acute agitation, anxiety)
- Sleep medications

ISSUES FOR REFERRAL

Patients benefit from care by a multidisciplinary team, including a primary care physician, therapist, and psychiatrist.

ADDITIONAL THERAPIES

- Electroconvulsive therapy with severe depression (may precipitate hypomania)
- Light therapy if there is a seasonal component to depressive episodes (may precipitate hypomania)
- Modest evidence exists to support transcranial magnetic stimulation, vagal nerve stimulation, ketamine infusion, sleep deprivation, and hormone therapy (e.g., thyroid) in bipolar depression.

INPATIENT CONSIDERATIONS

If hypomanic symptoms are severe enough to necessitate hospitalization, the patient automatically meets criteria for mania and BP-I.

Admission Criteria/Initial Stabilization

To admit patients (>18 years) to a psychiatric unit involuntarily, they must have a psychiatric diagnosis (e.g., major depression) and present a danger to themselves or others, or their mental disease must be inhibiting them from providing their basic needs (e.g., food, clothing, shelter).

Nursing

Acute suicidal threats need closer observation.

Discharge Criteria

Determined by safety

ONGOING CARE

FOLLOW-UP RECOMMENDATIONS

- Regularly scheduled visits support treatment adherence.
- Frequent communication between primary care doctor, psychiatrist, and therapist ensures comprehensive care.

Patient Monitoring

Mood charts are helpful adjuncts to care.

PATIENT EDUCATION

- Support groups for patients and families are recommended.
- National Alliance on Mental Illness: http://www.nami.org/

PROGNOSIS

- Frequency and severity of problematic episodes are related to medication adherence, consistency with psychotherapy, sleep, support systems, regularity of daily activities, and social history.
- Substance abuse, unemployment, persistent depression, and male gender are associated with a worse prognosis.
- Although data are limited, evidence indicates that patients with BP-II may be at greater risk of both attempting and completing suicide than with BP-I and unipolar depression.

REFERENCES

1. American Psychiatric Association. *Diagnostic and Statistical Manual of Mental Disorders*. 5th ed. Arlington, VA: American Psychiatric Association; 2013.
2. Perlis RH, Brown E, Baker RW, et al. Clinical features of bipolar depression versus major depressive disorder in large multicenter trials. *Am J Psychiatry*. 2006;163(2):225–231.
3. Hirshfeld RM. Validation of the mood disorder questionnaire. *Bipolar Depression Bulletin*. 2004.
4. Angst J, Adolfsson R, Benazzi F, et al. The HCL-32: towards a self-assessment tool for hypomanic symptoms in outpatients. *J Affect Disord*. 2005;88(2):217–233.
5. American Psychiatric Association. Practice guideline for the treatment of patients with bipolar disorder (revision). *Am J Psychiatry*. 2002;159(4 Suppl):1–50.

ADDITIONAL READING

- Benazzi F. A prediction rule for diagnosing hypomania. *Prog Neuropsychopharmacol Biol Psychiatry*. 2009;33(2):317–322.
- Benazzi F. Bipolar disorder—focus on bipolar II disorder and mixed depression. *Lancet*. 2007;369(9565):935–945.
- Licht RW. A new BALANCE in bipolar I disorder. *Lancet*. 2010;375(9712):350–352.

SEE ALSO

Algorithm: Depressive Episode, Major

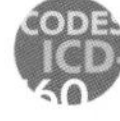

CODES

ICD10

F31.81 Bipolar II disorder

CLINICAL PEARLS

- BP-II is characterized by at least 1 episode of major depression and 1 episode of hypomania.
- Patients are often resistant to treatment during a hypomanic episode, as they enjoy the elevated mood and productivity.
- Evidence indicates that patients with BP-II may be at greater risk of both attempting and completing suicide than with BP-I and unipolar depression.

BITES, ANIMAL AND HUMAN

Kathryn Samai, PharmD, BCPS • Brian James Kimbrell, MD, FACS

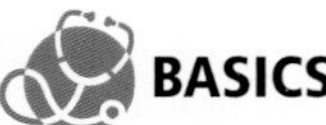

BASICS

DESCRIPTION

- Animal bites to humans from dogs (60–90%), cats (5–20%), rodents (2–3%), humans (2–3%), and rarely other animals, including snakes
- System(s) affected: potentially any

Pediatric Considerations

Young children are more likely to sustain bites and have bites that include the face, upper extremity, or trunk.

EPIDEMIOLOGY

- Predominant age: all ages but children > adults
- Predominant gender: dog bites, male > female; cat bites, female > male

Incidence

- 2–5 million animal bites per year in the United States
- Account for 1% of all emergency room visits
- 1–2% will require hospital admission, and 10–20 victims will die from bites annually (1).

ETIOLOGY AND PATHOPHYSIOLOGY

- Most dog bite wounds are from a domestic pet known to the victim.
- 89% of cat bites are provoked.
- Males, pit bull terriers, and German shepherds are most commonly associated with dog bites (2).
- Human bites are often the result of 1 person striking another in the mouth with a clenched fist.
- Bites can also occur incidentally in the case of paronychia due to nail biting, or thumb sucking, or "love nips" to the face, breasts, or genital areas.
- Animal bites can cause tears, punctures, scratches, avulsions, or crush injuries.
- Contamination of wound with flora from the mouth of the biting animal or from the broken skin of the victim can lead to infection.

RISK FACTORS

- Male dogs and older dogs are more likely to bite.
- Clenched-fist human bites are frequently associated with the use of alcohol.
- Patients presenting >8 hours following the bite are at greater risk of infection.

GENERAL PREVENTION

- Instruct children and adults about animal hazards and strongly enforce animal control laws.
- Educate dog owners.

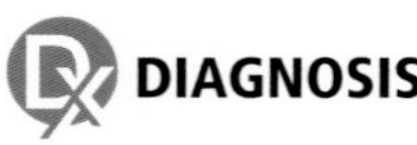

DIAGNOSIS

HISTORY

- Obtain detailed history of the incident (provoked or unprovoked).
- Type of animal
- Vaccine status
- Site of the bite
- Geographic setting

PHYSICAL EXAM

- Dog bites (60–90% of bites)
  - Hands and face most common site of injury in adults and children, respectively
  - More likely to have associated crush injury
- Cat bites (5–20% of bites)
  - Predominantly involve the hands, followed by lower extremities, face, and trunk
- Human bites (2–3% of bites)
  - Intentional bite: semicircular or oval area of erythema and bruising, with or without break in skin
  - Clenched-fist injury: small wounds over the metacarpophalangeal joints from striking the fist against another's teeth
- Signs of wound infection include fever, erythema, swelling, tenderness, purulent drainage, and lymphangitis.

ALERT

Cat bites (often puncture wounds) are twice as likely to cause infection as dog bites, with higher risks of osteomyelitis, tenosynovitis, and septic arthritis.

Pediatric Considerations

If human bite mark on child has intercanine distance >3 cm, bite probably came from an adult and should raise concerns about child abuse.

DIAGNOSTIC TESTS & INTERPRETATION

Initial Tests (lab, imaging)

- Drainage from infected wounds should be Gram-stained and cultured (3)[A].
  - If wound fails to heal, perform cultures for atypical pathogens (fungi, *Nocardia*, and mycobacteria) and ask lab to keep bacterial cultures for 7–10 days (some pathogens are slow-growing).
- 85% of bite wounds will yield a positive culture, with an average of 5 pathogens.
- Aerobic and anaerobic blood cultures should be obtained before starting antibiotics if bacteremia suspected (e.g., fever or chills).
- Previous antibiotic therapy may alter culture results.

ALERT

If bite wound is near a bone or joint, a plain radiograph is needed to check for bone injury and to use for comparison later if osteomyelitis is subsequently suspected (3)[B].

- Radiographs are needed to check for fractures in clenched-fist injuries.

Follow-Up Tests & Special Considerations

Subsequent suspicion of osteomyelitis warrants comparison of plain radiograph or MRI. Severe skull bites warrant a CT scan and ultrasound can be useful for detection of abscess.

Diagnostic Procedures/Other

Surgical exploration may be needed to ascertain extent of injuries or to drain deep infections (such as tendon sheath infections), especially in serious hand wounds.

Test Interpretation

- Dog bites (4,5)
  - *Pasteurella* species is present in 50% of bites.
  - Also found: viridans streptococci, *Staphylococcus aureus*, *Staphylococcus intermedius*, *Bacteroides*, *Capnocytophaga canimorsus*, *Fusobacterium*
- Cat bites (5)
  - *Pasteurella* species is present in 75% of bites.
  - Also found: *Streptococcus* spp. (including *Streptococcus pyogenes*), *Staphylococcus* spp. (including methicillin-resistant *Staphylococcus aureus* [MRSA]), *Fusobacterium* spp., *Bacteroides* spp., *Porphyromonas* spp., *Moraxella* spp.
- Human bites
  - *Streptococcus* spp., *Staphylococcus aureus*, *Eikenella corrodens* (29%), and various anaerobic bacteria (e.g., *Fusobacterium*, *Peptostreptococcus*, *Prevotella*, and *Porphyromonas* spp.)
  - Although rare, case reports have suggested transmission of viruses such as hepatitis, HIV, and herpes simplex.
- Reptile bites
  - If from a venomous snake, use antivenom. Bacteria: *Pseudomonas aeruginosa*, *Proteus* spp., *Salmonella*, *Bacteroides fragilis*, and *Clostridium* spp.
- Rodent bites
  - *Streptobacillus moniliformis* or *Spirillum minor*, which causes rat-bite fever
- Monkey bites
  - All monkey bites can transmit rabies, and bites of a macaque monkey may transmit herpes B virus, which is potentially fatal. Providers should contact CDC and administer an antiviral, such as valacyclovir, active against herpes B virus.

ALERT

Asplenic patients and those with underlying hepatic disease are at risk of bacteremia and fatal sepsis after dog bites infected with *Capnocytophaga canimorsus* (gram-negative rod).

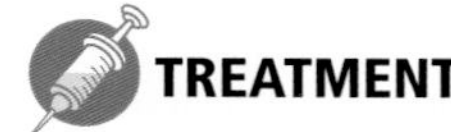

TREATMENT

GENERAL MEASURES

- Elevation of the injured extremity to prevent swelling
- Contact the local health department regarding the prevalence of rabies in the species of animal involved (highest in bats).
- Snake bite: If venomous, patient needs rapid transport to facility capable of definitive evaluation. If envenomation has occurred, patient should receive antivenom. Be sure patient is stable for transport; consider measuring and/or treating coagulation and renal status along with any anaphylactic reactions before transport.

MEDICATION

- Consider need for antirabies therapy: rabies immunoglobulin and human diploid cell rabies vaccine for those bitten by wild animals (in the United States, primary vector is bat bite), rabid pets, or unvaccinated pets or if animal cannot be quarantined for 10 days.
- Tetanus toxoid for those previously immunized but >10 years since their last dose (3)[C]; tetanus immunoglobulin and tetanus vaccination in patients without a full primary series of immunizations

- A patient negative for anti-HBs and bitten by an HBsAg-positive individual should receive both hepatitis B immunoglobulin (HBIG) and hepatitis B vaccine.
- HIV postexposure prophylaxis is generally not recommended for human bites, given the extremely low risk for transmission.
- Preemptive antibiotics are only recommended for human bites and high-risk wounds (deep puncture, crush injury, venous or lymphatic compromise, hands or near joint, face or genital area, immunocompromised hosts, requiring surgical repair, asplenic, advanced liver, edema).
- For preemptive and for empiric treatment of established infection, amoxicillin and clavulanate is first-line (3)[B],(6)
  - Adults: 875 mg PO BID
  - Children: <3 months: 30 mg/kg/day PO q12h; ≥3 months and <40 kg: 45 mg/kg/day q12h; >40 kg, use adult dosing
    - Adverse reaction: Amoxicillin and clavulanate should be given with food to decrease GI side effects.
    - Precautions: Dose antibiotics by body weight and renal function.
    - Significant possible interactions: Antibiotics may decrease efficacy of oral contraceptives.
  - Duration of therapy: preemptive, 3–5 days; treatment of cellulitis/skin abscess, 5–10 days; bacteremia, 10–14 days
    - Adults: clindamycin (300–450 mg PO TID) *plus* either
    - Trimethoprim-sulfamethoxazole (TMP-SMX; 1 DS tablet PO BID–TID) *or*
    - Ciprofloxacin (500 mg PO BID) for 7–21 days
    - Children: clindamycin (5–10 mg/kg IV [to a maximum of 600 mg] followed by 10–30 mg/kg/day in 3–4 divided doses to a maximum of 300 mg per dose) *plus*
    - TMP-SMX (8–10 mg/kg/day of trimethoprim) in 2 divided doses
- Avoid 1st-generation cephalosporins (e.g., cephalexin), penicillinase-resistant penicillins (e.g., dicloxacillin), macrolides (e.g., erythromycin), and clindamycin (when not administered with another agent) as they lack activity against *Pasteurella multocida* (dog/cat bites) and *E. corrodens* (human bites).

Pregnancy Considerations

- Penicillin-allergic pregnant women
  - Azithromycin 250–500 mg PO every day
- Observe closely and note potential increased risk of failure.

ALERT

Consider community-acquired MRSA as possible pathogen (from human skin or colonized pet). If high suspicion, doxycycline or TMP-SMX provide good coverage (7).

ISSUES FOR REFERRAL

- Deep wounds to the hand and face should be referred to a hand surgeon or plastic surgeon, respectively.
- Bites from primates or unusual species of animals should be referred to infectious disease specialist.

SURGERY/OTHER PROCEDURES

- Copious irrigation of the wound with normal saline via a catheter tip is needed to reduce risk of infection.
- Devitalized tissue needs débridement.
- Débridement of puncture wounds is not advised.
- Primary closure can be considered if the wound is clean after irrigation and bite is <12 hours old and in bites to the face (cosmesis).
- Infected wounds and those at risk of infection (cat bites, human bites, bites to the hand, crush injuries, presentation >12 hours from injury) should be left open (8).
- Delayed primary closure in 3–5 days is an option for infected wounds.
- Splint hand if it is injured.
- Large, gaping wounds should be reapproximated with widely spaced sutures or Steri-Strips.

INPATIENT CONSIDERATIONS

Admission Criteria/Initial Stabilization

Patients with deep or severe wound infections, systemic infections requiring IV antibiotics, those requiring surgery, and the immunocompromised require ABCs for associated trauma or severe infection and IV antibiotic therapy

- Adults: ampicillin and sulbactam 3 g IV q6h *or* piperacillin and tazobactam 3.375 g IV q6h (3). Alternative: ciprofloxacin 400 mg IV q12h *or* levofloxacin 500 mg IV every day with metronidazole 500 mg IV q8h (3)
- Children: ampicillin and sulbactam 200 mg/kg/day IV given in 4 divided doses to maximum of 3 g per dose

Discharge Criteria

Pending clinical improvement

ONGOING CARE

FOLLOW-UP RECOMMENDATIONS

Patient Monitoring

- Patient should be rechecked in 24–48 hours if not infected at time of 1st encounter.
- Daily follow-up is warranted for infections.
- Subsequent revisions of empiric antibiotic therapy should be based on culture results and clinical response.

PATIENT EDUCATION

- Educate parents at well-child checks about how to avoid animal bites.
- AAFP: http://familydoctor.org/familydoctor/en/prevention-wellness/staying-healthy/pets-animals/dog-bites-how-to-teach-your-children-to-be-safe.html
- CDC: http://www.cdc.gov/HomeandRecreationalSafety/Dog-Bites/index.html

PROGNOSIS

Wounds should steadily improve and close over by 7–10 days.

COMPLICATIONS

- Septic arthritis
- Osteomyelitis
- Extensive soft tissue injuries with scarring
- Hemorrhage
- Gas gangrene
- Sepsis
- Meningitis
- Endocarditis
- Posttraumatic stress disorder
- Death

REFERENCES

1. Goldstein EJ. New horizons in the bacteriology, antimicrobial susceptibility and therapy of animal bite wounds. *J Med Microbiol*. 1998;47(2):95–97.
2. Wiley JF II. Mammalian bites. Review of evaluation and management. *Clin Pediatr (Phila)*. 1990;29(5):283–287.
3. Stevens DL, Bisno AL, Chambers HF, et al. Practice guidelines for the diagnosis and management of skin and soft tissue infections: 2014 update by the Infectious Disease Society of America. *Clin Infect Dis*. 2014;59(2):e10–e52.
4. Bini JK, Cohn SM, Acosta SM, et al. Mortality, mauling, and maiming by vicious dogs. *Ann Surg*. 2011;253(4):791–797.
5. Abrahamian FM, Goldstein EJ. Microbiology of animal bite wound infections. *Clin Microbiol Rev*. 2011;24(2):231–246.
6. Medeiros I, Saconato H. Antibiotic prophylaxis for mammalian bites. *Cochrane Database Syst Rev*. 2001;(2):CD001738.
7. Oehler RL, Velez AP, Mizrachi M, et al. Bite-related and septic syndromes caused by cats and dogs. *Lancet Infect Dis*. 2009;9(7):439–447.
8. Benson LS, Edwards SL, Schiff AP, et al. Dog and cat bites to the hand: treatment and cost assessment. *J Hand Surg Am*. 2006;31(3):468–473.

ADDITIONAL READING

- Okonkwo U, Changulani M, Moonot P. Animal bites: practical tips for effective management. *J Emerg Nurs*. 2008;34(3):225–226.
- Rittner AV, Fitzpatrick K, Corfield A. Best evidence topic report. Are antibiotics indicated following human bites? *Emerg Med J*. 2005;22(9):654.

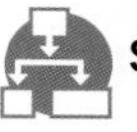

SEE ALSO

Cellulitis; Rabies; Snake Envenomations; *Bartonella* Infections

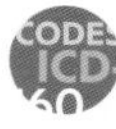

CODES

ICD10

- S61.459A Open bite of unspecified hand, initial encounter
- S01.85XA Open bite of other part of head, initial encounter
- S20.97XA Other superficial bite of unspecified parts of thorax, initial encounter

CLINICAL PEARLS

- Wound cleansing, débridement, and culture are essential. Most wounds should be left open.
- Prophylaxis is recommended for human bites and high-risk wounds.
- Consider rabies and tetanus vaccination.
- Antibiotic and duration of therapy should be adjusted based on culture results and clinical improvement.
- Patients bitten by animals or humans require close follow-up to monitor for infection.

BLADDER CANCER

Margaret E. Thompson, MD

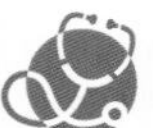

BASICS

DESCRIPTION

- Primary malignant neoplasms arising in the urinary bladder
- Most common type is transitional cell carcinoma (90%)
- Other types include adenocarcinoma, small cell carcinoma, and squamous cell carcinoma.
- Rhabdomyosarcoma of the bladder may occur in children.

EPIDEMIOLOGY

Incidence

- Increases with age (median age at diagnosis is 73 years) (1)
- More common in Caucasians than in Asians or African Americans
- Male > female (4:1), but in smokers, risk is 1:1
- 36.2/100,000 men per year (1)
- 8.8/100,000 women per year (1)
- 20.5/100,000 men and women per year (1)

Prevalence

In 2011, 571,518 cases in the United States (1)

ETIOLOGY AND PATHOPHYSIOLOGY

Unknown, other than related to risk factors:

- 70–80% is superficial (in lamina propria or mucosa):
  - Usually highly differentiated with long survival
  - Initial event seems to be activation of an oncogene on chromosome 9 in superficial cancers.
- 20% of tumors are invasive (deeper than lamina propria) at presentation:
  - Tend to be high grade with worse prognosis
  - Associated with other chromosome deletions

Genetics

Hereditary transmission is unlikely, although transitional cell carcinoma pathophysiology is related to oncogenes.

RISK FACTORS

- Smoking is the single greatest risk factor (increases risk 4-fold) and increases risk equally for men and women (2).
- Use of pioglitazone for more than 1 year may be associated with an increased risk of bladder cancer. The risk seems to increase with duration of therapy and may also be present with other thiazolidinediones.
- Other risk factors:
  - Occupational carcinogens in dye, rubber, paint, plastics, metal, carbon black dust, and automotive exhaust
  - Schistosomiasis in Mediterranean (squamous cell) cancer
  - Arsenic in well water
  - History of pelvic irradiation
  - Chronic lower UTI
  - Chronic indwelling urinary catheter
  - Cyclophosphamide exposure
  - High-fat diet
  - Coffee consumption associated with reduced risk (RR 0.83; 95% CI, 0.73–0.94) (3)

ALERT

Any patient who smokes and presents with microscopic or gross hematuria or irritative voiding symptoms such as urgency and frequency not clearly due to UTI should be evaluated by cystoscopy for the presence of a bladder neoplasm.

GENERAL PREVENTION

- Avoid smoking and other risk factors.
- Counseling of individuals with occupational exposure
- The U.S. Preventive Services Task Force has concluded that there is insufficient evidence to determine the balance between risk and harm of screening for bladder cancer.

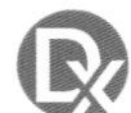

DIAGNOSIS

HISTORY

- Painless hematuria is most common symptom.
- Urinary symptoms (frequency, urgency)
- Abdominal or pelvic pain in advanced disease
- Exposures (see "Risk Factors")

PHYSICAL EXAM

Normal in early cases, pelvic or abdominal mass in advanced disease, wasting in systemic disease

DIFFERENTIAL DIAGNOSIS

- Other urinary tract neoplasms
- UTI
- Prostatism
- Bladder instability
- Interstitial cystitis
- Urolithiasis
- Interstitial nephritis
- Papillary urothelial hyperplasia

DIAGNOSTIC TESTS & INTERPRETATION

Initial Tests (lab, imaging)

- Urinalysis is the initial test in patients presenting with gross hematuria or urinary symptoms such as frequency, urgency, and dysuria.
- Urine cytology (consult your local lab for volume needed and proper fixative/handling)
- Cystoscopy with biopsy is the gold standard for at-risk patients with painless hematuria.
- Macroscopic hematuria (55% sensitivity, positive predictive value [PPV] 0.22 for urologic cancer) (4)[C]

Follow-Up Tests & Special Considerations

- Urine cytology: 54% sensitivity overall (lower in less advanced tumors), 94% specific (5)[A]
- Other urine markers (of little clinical benefit):
  - Nuclear matrix protein-22 (NMP22): 67% sensitive, 78% specific (5)[A]
  - Bladder tumor–associated antigen stat: 70% sensitive, 75% specific (5)[A]
  - Fluorescence in situ hybridization assay (FISH): 69% sensitive, 78% specific (PPV 27.1, negative predictive value 95.3) for all tumors, more sensitive and specific for higher grade (6)[B]
  - *FGFR3* mutation has high specificity (99.9%) but low sensitivity (34.5%); PPV 95.2% (7)[A].
- *Bottom line: None of the urine markers is sensitive enough to rule out bladder cancer on its own.*
- Liver function tests, alkaline phosphatase if metastasis suspected
- Done for staging and to evaluate extent of disease but not for diagnosis itself:
  - CT urogram replacing IVP to image upper tracts if there is suspicion of disease there
  - Diffusion-weighted MRI and multidimensional CT scan are undergoing study for use in diagnosis and staging of bladder tumors.
  - For invasive disease, metastatic workup should include chest x-ray.
  - Bone scan should be performed if the patient has bone pain or if alkaline phosphatase is elevated.
- Urologic CT scan (abdomen, pelvis, with and without contrast) or MRI (40–98% accurate), with MRI slightly more accurate, is recommended if metastasis is suspected (8)[B].
- Regular cystoscopy (initiated at 3 months postprocedure) is indicated after transurethral resection of superficial tumor (TURBT) and intravesical chemotherapy for superficial bladder cancers.

Diagnostic Procedures/Other

- Cystoscopy with biopsy is the gold standard for diagnosis, but one study showed that 33% of patients had residual tumor after TURBT (8)[B].
- Using photodynamic diagnosis (PDD; employing a photosensitizing agent in the bladder that is taken up by tumor cells and visualized using a particular wavelength of light, which is changed to a different wavelength by the photosensitizing agent) has been shown to increase detection and identification of cancerous superficial tumors when compared with plain white light cystoscopy. A recent meta-analysis shows that this increases the likelihood of total resection (9)[A].

Test Interpretation

- Characterized as superficial or invasive
- 70–80% present as superficial lesion.
- Superficial lesions
  - Carcinoma in situ: flat lesion, high grade
  - Ta: noninvasive papillary carcinoma
  - T1: extends into submucosa, lamina propria
- Invasive cancer
  - T2: invasion into muscle
    - pT2a: invasion into superficial muscle
    - pT2b: invasion into deep muscle
  - T3: invasion into perivesical fat
    - pT3a: microscopic
    - pT3b: macroscopic
  - T4: invasion into adjacent organs
    - aT4a: invades prostate, uterus, or vagina
    - aT4b: invades abdominal or pelvic wall
- N1–N3: invades lymph nodes
- M: metastasis to bone or soft tissue

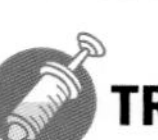

TREATMENT

For superficial bladder cancer, the treatment is generally removal via cystoscopic surgery (see earlier discussion re: PDD). For muscle-invasive cancer, a radical cystectomy is preferred.

MEDICATION

First Line

- A recent meta-analysis demonstrated neoadjuvant chemotherapy using platinum-based combination chemotherapy (with ≥1 of doxorubicin/epirubicin, methotrexate, or vinblastine), but not platinum alone, confers a significant survival advantage in patients with invasive bladder cancer, with an increase in survival at 5 years from 45% (without neoadjuvant treatment) to 50% (with treatment) (combined hazard ratio 0.86; 95% CI, 0.77–0.95) (10)[A].
- Intravesical bacillus Calmette-Guérin (BCG) after TURBT in high-grade lesions has been shown to decrease recurrence in Ta and T1 tumors (11)[A].

Second Line

- Chemotherapy is the 1st-line treatment for metastatic bladder cancer:
  - Methotrexate-vinblastine-doxorubicin-cisplatin (MVAC) is the preferred regimen.
- A recent review showed that gemcitabine plus cisplatin may be better tolerated and result in equivalent survival to MVAC, making it a possible 1st choice in metastatic bladder cancer.

ISSUES FOR REFERRAL

Patients with microscopic or gross hematuria not otherwise explained or resolving should be referred to a urologist for cystoscopy.

ADDITIONAL THERAPIES

Radiotherapy:

- In the United States, used for patients with muscle-invasive cancer who are not surgical candidates
- Preoperative (radical cystectomy) radiotherapy also an option
- Treatment of choice for muscle-invasive cancer in some European and Canadian centers:
  - 65–70 Gy over 6–7 weeks is standard.

SURGERY/OTHER PROCEDURES

- Surgery is definitive therapy for superficial and invasive cancer:
  - Superficial cancer: TURBT sometimes followed by intravesical therapy
- Invasive cancer
  - Radical cystectomy for invasive disease that is confined to the bladder is more effective than radical radiotherapy. There is insufficient evidence to recommend one form of urinary diversion over another (12).

INPATIENT CONSIDERATIONS

Admission Criteria/Initial Stabilization

Need for surgery or intensive therapy

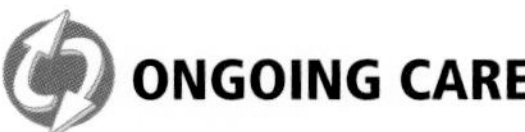

ONGOING CARE

FOLLOW-UP RECOMMENDATIONS

- Superficial cancers
  - Urine cytology alone has not been shown to be sufficient for follow-up.
  - Cystoscopy every 3 months for 18–24 months, every 6 months for the next 2 years, then annually
- Follow-up for invasive cancers depends on the approach to treatment.
- Patients treated with BCG require lifelong follow-up.

DIET

Continue adequate fluid intake.

PATIENT EDUCATION

Smoking cessation

PROGNOSIS

- 5-year relative survival rates (1)
  - Overall survival: 77.4%
    - In situ: 96.2%
    - Localized: 69.2%
    - Regional metastasis: 33.7%
    - Distant metastasis: 5.5%
- Superficial bladder cancer
  - BCG treatment prevents recurrence versus TURBT alone; difference 30%, NNT 3.3
  - BCG prevents progression versus TURBT alone, difference 8%
- Invasive cancer
  - T2 disease: Radical cystectomy results in 60–75% 5-year survival.
  - T3 or T4 disease: Radical cystectomy results in 20–40% 5-year survival.
  - Neoadjuvant chemotherapy with cystectomy has led to varying degrees of increased survival.
  - Radiation with chemotherapy has led to varying degrees of increased survival.
- Metastatic cancer:
  - MVAC resulted in mean survival of 12.5 months.

COMPLICATIONS

- Superficial bladder cancer
  - Local symptoms
    - Dysuria, frequency, nocturia, pain, passing debris in urine
    - Bacterial cystitis
    - Perforation
  - General symptoms
    - Flulike symptoms
    - Systemic infection
- Invasive cancer
  - Symptoms related to definitive treatment, including incontinence, bleeding
  - Patients with neobladder at risk for azotemia and metabolic acidosis

REFERENCES

1. National Cancer Institute. SEER stat fact sheets: bladder cancer. http://seer.cancer.gov/statfacts/html/urinb.html. Accessed July 2, 2014.
2. Freedman N, Silverman DT, Hollenbeck AR, et al. Association between smoking and risk of bladder cancer among men and women. *JAMA*. 2011;306(7):737–745.
3. Yu X, Bao Z, Zou J, et al. Coffee consumption and risk of cancers: a meta-analysis of cohort studies. *BMC Cancer*. 2011;11:96. doi:10.1186/1471-2407-11-96.
4. Buntinx F, Wauters H. The diagnostic value of macroscopic haematuria in diagnosing urological cancers: a meta-analysis. *Fam Pract*. 1997;14(1):63–68.
5. Glas AS, Roos D, Deutekom M, et al. Tumor markers in the diagnosis of primary bladder cancer. A systematic review. *J Urol*. 2003;169(6):1975–1982.
6. Sarosdy MF, Kahn PR, Ziffer MD, et al. Use of a multitarget fluorescence in situ hybridization assay to diagnose bladder cancer in patients with hematuria. *J Urol*. 2006;176(1):44–47.
7. Karnes RJ, Fernandez CA, Shuber AP. A noninvasive mulitanalyte urine-based diagnostic assay for urothelial cancer of the bladder in the evalatuion of hematuria. *Mayo Clin Proc*. 2012;87(9):835–342.
8. Kirkali Z, Chan T, Manoharan M, et al. Bladder cancer: epidemiology, staging and grading, and diagnosis. *Urology*. 2005;66(6)(Suppl 1):4–34.
9. Mowatt G, N'Dow J, Vale L, et al. Photodynamic diagnosis of bladder cancer compared with white light cystoscopy: systematic review and meta-analysis. *Int J Technol Assess Health Care*. 2011;27(1):3–10.
10. Advanced Bladder Cancer Meta-analysis Collaboration. Neoadjuvant chemotherapy for advanced bladder cancer (Cochrane Review). In: Cochrane Library, Issue 2, 2012. Chichester, UK: John Wiley and Sons, Ltd.
11. Shelley M, Court JB, Kynaston H, et al. Intravesical bacillus Calmette-Guerin in Ta and T1 bladder cancer (Cochrane Review). In: Cochrane Library, Issue 3, 2010. Chichester, UK: John Wiley and Sons, Ltd.
12. Cody JD, Nabi G, Dublin N, et al. Urinary diversion and bladder reconstruction/replacement using intestinal segments for intractable incontinence or following cystectomy. *Cochrane Database Syst Rev*. 2012;2:CD003306.

ADDITIONAL READING

- Msaouel P, Koutsilieris M. Diagnostic value of circulating tumor cell detection in bladder and urothelial cancer: systematic review and meta-analysis. *BMC Cancer*. 2011;11:336.
- Sharma S, Ksheersagar P, Sharma P. Diagnosis and treatment of bladder cancer. *Am Fam Physician*. 2009;80(7):717–723.
- Zhu Z, Shen Z, Lu Y, et al. Increased risk of bladder cancer with pioglitazone therapy in patients with diabetes: a meta-analysis. *Diabetes Res Clin Pract*. 2012;98(1):159–163.

SEE ALSO

- Hematuria
- Algorithm: Hematuria

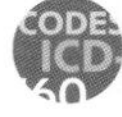

CODES

ICD10

- C67.9 Malignant neoplasm of bladder, unspecified
- C67.4 Malignant neoplasm of posterior wall of bladder
- C67.3 Malignant neoplasm of anterior wall of bladder

CLINICAL PEARLS

- Painless hematuria in smokers should be evaluated with cystoscopy.
- Be aware of potential link between pioglitazone treatment and risk for bladder cancer.
- The U.S. Preventive Services Task Force recommends against routine screening for bladder cancer.

BLADDER INJURY

Greg Murphy, MD • Joseph R. Wagner, MD

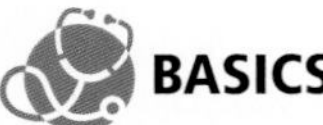

BASICS

DESCRIPTION

- The bladder is well protected deep within the bony pelvis.
- Bladder injury is caused by trauma, iatrogenic surgical complication, or spontaneous rupture.
  - The mechanism of traumatic injury is characterized as blunt or penetrating.
- Bladder injury can be classified as a contusion or rupture.
  - Rupture is classified as intraperitoneal or extraperitoneal.
- Bladder injury is often associated with other traumatic injuries, most commonly pelvic fracture.

EPIDEMIOLOGY

Incidence

- 1.6% of blunt abdominal trauma cases have an associated bladder injury (1)[C].
  - 80% of bladder injuries are associated with pelvic fracture.
  - 10% of pelvic fractures are associated with bladder injury.
  - 90% of bladder injuries due to blunt trauma are caused by motor vehicle collision (MVC).
- 15–40% of bladder rupture from penetrating trauma (2)[B].
  - 85% secondary to gunshot wounds (GSW), 15% from stab wounds
- Bladder ruptures: 55% extraperitoneal, 40% intraperitoneal, and 5% combined (1)[C]
- The bladder is the most common organ damaged during pelvic surgery (1)[C].
  - Obstetric injuries and gynecologic surgery are the most common causes of iatrogenic bladder injury.

ETIOLOGY AND PATHOPHYSIOLOGY

- Bladder contusion (1)[C]
  - Damage to bladder mucosa or muscularis without full thickness injury, usually presenting with gross hematuria but no extravasation on cystogram
- Blunt bladder trauma is associated with rapid deceleration (1)[C].
  - The bladder is well protected within the bony pelvis. It takes a significant amount of blunt force to cause a rupture.
  - MVC, fall, or crush mechanism are most common.
  - Fracture of the bony pelvis tears fascial attachments to the bladder, causing rupture.
  - Bone fragments can directly lacerate the bladder, although this is less common.
  - A blow to abdomen with a full bladder can lead to a rise in intravesical pressure and rupture at the dome with or without associated pelvic fracture.
- Penetrating bladder injuries (1)[C]
  - GSW or stab injury to bladder
  - Iatrogenic surgical injury
    - Complication of open, laparoscopic, or robotic surgeries as well as cystoscopic procedure
- Spontaneous rupture (1)[C]
  - Patients may have neurologic disease, bladder outlet obstruction, or prior urologic surgery.

Pediatric Considerations

Lower rates of bladder injury in children with blunt trauma and pelvic fracture (1)[C]

RISK FACTORS

- Rapid deceleration injury
- Pelvic fracture
- Penetrating trauma to the pelvis
- Prior pelvic surgery
- Prior pelvic radiation

GENERAL PREVENTION

- Seat belts
- Void prior to driving

COMMONLY ASSOCIATED CONDITIONS

80–94% blunt bladder trauma associated with injuries to other structures

- Pelvic fracture is the most common associated injury.
- Urethral injury occurs in 15% of cases of bladder rupture (1)[C].

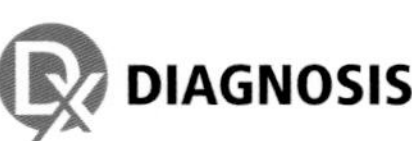

DIAGNOSIS

HISTORY

- Determine mechanism of injury: trauma (blunt or penetrating), surgery, or spontaneous.
- Gross hematuria and pelvic fracture (1,3)[B]
- Urinary retention (1,4)[C]
- Inability to void or oliguria (1,4)[C]
- Suprapubic pain (1,4)[C]
- Abdominal distention (1,4)[C]

PHYSICAL EXAM

- Abdominal exam: Assess for suprapubic tenderness, peritoneal signs, distention, bruising, laceration, or scars (4)[C].
- Genitourinary exam: Assess for blood at the meatus, gross hematuria, ecchymosis, or hematoma (4)[C].
- Rectal exam: high riding prostate—assess for concomitant urethral injury (4)[C].
- Catheterization to evaluate for gross hematuria (4)[C]
  - If blood is seen at the meatus or a catheter cannot be easily passed, evaluate for a urethral injury with a retrograde urethrogram.
- Intraoperative finding with iatrogenic surgical injury to the bladder (1)[C]
  - Gross hematuria
  - Pneumaturia (air in the catheter) during laparoscopic or robotic procedure

DIFFERENTIAL DIAGNOSIS

Other urologic injury: urethral, ureteral, or renal injury causing gross hematuria

DIAGNOSTIC TESTS & INTERPRETATION

Initial Tests (lab, imaging)

- Urinalysis may demonstrate microscopic hematuria.
- Basic metabolic panel: Elevated BUN/creatinine may be seen secondary to peritoneal absorption of urine after intraperitoneal ruptures (4)[C].
- Hemoglobin/hematocrit and PT/PTT: Evaluate in patients with gross hematuria.
- Cystogram (1,3,4)[B]
  - Technique: Fill the bladder with a minimum of 300 mL of contrast or until discomfort. Need precontrast, full bladder, and postcontrast imaging with two views.
  - Contusion: normal or distortion of bladder wall without extravasation
  - Extraperitoneal perforation: flame-shaped perivesical contrast; teardrop deformity seen with compression from pelvic hematoma
  - Intraperitoneal perforation: Contrast outlines bowel loops.
- CT cystogram: Bladder needs to be filled in a retrograde fashion similar to a cystogram. Dilute contrast should be used. Only 1 view is required with a full bladder. Unacceptably high rate of false-negative studies if the catheter is clamped and IV contrast is allowed to fill the bladder in an antegrade fashion (1,3,4)[B].
- Absolute indication for a cystogram: blunt trauma, pelvic fracture, and gross hematuria (1,3,4)[B]
- Relative indication for a cystogram: blunt trauma, pelvic fracture, and microscopic hematuria or gross hematuria and a high index of suspicion (1,3,4)[C]
- Ultrasound is not an adequate study to diagnose or rule out bladder rupture (1)[C].
- Penetrating trauma usually requires operative exploration. Gross hematuria in the setting of penetrating trauma warrants either emergent exploration or a cystogram if the patient is clinically stable (1)[C].

Follow-Up Tests & Special Considerations

Oliguric/anuric patient with ascites and risk factors needs to be ruled out for an intraperitoneal bladder rupture (1,3,4)[C].

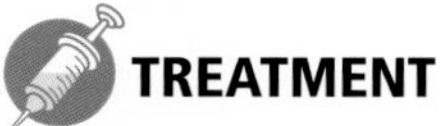

TREATMENT

GENERAL MEASURES

- Place a catheter to drain the bladder.
- Control pain.
- Short course of prophylactic antibiotics
- Obtain appropriate labs and imaging studies.
- See surgery section for details

MEDICATION

First Line

- 3 days of prophylactic antibiotics to cover common uropathogens recommended (i.e., ciprofloxacin 500 mg PO BID)
- Opioids as needed for pain control
- Anticholinergics/antispasmodics for bladder spasms (i.e., oxybutynin 5 mg PO TID PRN for bladder spasms)

ISSUES FOR REFERRAL

Whenever possible, urology should be consulted for all patients with bladder injury.

SURGERY/OTHER PROCEDURES

- Contusion: observation or catheter drainage until hematuria resolves (1)[C]
- Extraperitoneal bladder perforation (1,3)[C]
  - Can be managed with catheter drainage alone for 10–14 days if otherwise uncomplicated; large-bore catheters preferred for adequate drainage (20–22F)
  - Indications for operative repair:
    - Bladder neck injury
    - Concomitant vaginal or rectal injury (concern for fistula formation)
    - Bone fragments present in bladder wall (concern for poor healing)
    - Orthopedic hardware required to fix pelvic fracture (concern for urine infecting hardware)
    - Exploratory laparotomy for other associated injuries
  - Surgical approach: exploratory laparotomy. Open the bladder and repair defect intravesically with 1–2 layer closure of absorbable suture. Do not attempt to repair extravesically as a hematoma under tamponade may be released, causing serious bleeding.
- Intraperitoneal bladder perforation or penetrating injury (1,3,4)[B]
  - Requires urgent operative repair
  - Débridement of devitalized tissue
  - Need to rule out concomitant ureteral injury either by passage of ureteral catheters or efflux of urine/methylene blue from the ureteral orifice
  - 2 layer water-tight closure with absorbable suture
  - Foley catheter should be left to drainage for 10–14 days.
  - Suprapubic tube placement can be considered if concern for inadequate urethral catheter drainage but is otherwise not required (3,5)[B].
  - Consider leaving an intra-abdominal drain to control and test for a postoperative urine leak.

INPATIENT CONSIDERATIONS

Admission Criteria/Initial Stabilization

- Trauma evaluation
- Hemodynamic stabilization and resuscitation
- All traumatic bladder injuries will require inpatient monitoring of hemodynamics, hematocrit, electrolytes, and renal function.

IV Fluids

Isotonic fluids for resuscitation

Nursing

- Ensure the catheter is draining.
- Irrigate clots as needed.
- Avoid continuous bladder irrigation if possible.

Discharge Criteria

- Pain is controlled.
- Patient able to void or catheter is draining with minimal hematuria.
- Patient can manage all injuries at home and activities of daily living.

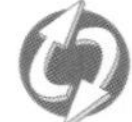

ONGOING CARE

FOLLOW-UP RECOMMENDATIONS

Patients with bladder perforation should undergo a cystogram prior to catheter removal around 10–14 days to rule out a persistent leak (3)[C].

DIET

No restrictions

PROGNOSIS

The goal is for patients to store urine and void volitionally to completion without complaint. If there is no associated neurologic injury, this is typically accomplished.

COMPLICATIONS

- Urinary tract infection
- Urine leak
- Abscess
- Fistula
- Bladder calculi
- Death (usually from other associated injuries)

REFERENCES

1. Gomez RG, Cabellos L, Coburn M, et al. Consensus statement on bladder injuries. *BJU Int*. 2004;94(1):27–32.
2. Pereira BM, de Campos CC, Calderan TR, et al. Bladder injuries after external trauma: 20 year experience report in a population-based cross-sectional view. *World J Urol*. 2013;31(4):913–917.
3. Morey AF, Brandes S, Dugi DD III, et al. Urotrauma: AUA guideline. *J Urol*. 2014;192(2):327–335.
4. Morey AF, Iverson AJ, Swan A, et al. Bladder rupture after blunt trauma: guidelines for diagnostic imaging. *J Trauma*. 2001;51(4):683–636.
5. Parry NG, Rozycki GS, Feliciano DV, et al. Traumatic rupture of the urinary bladder: is the suprapubic tube necessary? *J Trauma*. 2003;54(3):431–436.

ADDITIONAL READING

Morey AF, Dugi DD III. Genital and lower urinary tract trauma. In: Wein AJ, Kavoussi AC, Novick AW, et al, eds. *Campbell-Walsh Urology*. 10th ed. Philadelphia: Elsevier Saunders; 2012.

SEE ALSO

Hematuria

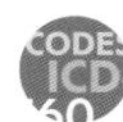

CODES

ICD10

- S37.20XA Unspecified injury of bladder, initial encounter
- S37.29XA Other injury of bladder, initial encounter
- S37.22XA Contusion of bladder, initial encounter

CLINICAL PEARLS

- Bladder injuries are usually associated with blunt trauma and pelvic fracture.
- Gross hematuria is the most common presenting sign.
- A cystogram needs to be performed when a bladder injury is suspected.
- Bladder contusions and uncomplicated extraperitoneal injuries can be managed with catheter drainage alone.
- Intraperitoneal bladder perforations or complicated extraperitoneal injuries require urgent operative intervention.
- Catheter drainage is required until bladder is healed, usually around 10–14 days.
- A cystogram should be obtained prior to catheter removal to evaluate for a leak.
- Persistent leaks are most often managed conservatively with prolonged catheter drainage.

BLEPHARITIS

Robert A. Baldor, MD, FAAFP

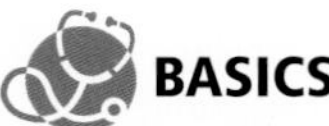

BASICS

DESCRIPTION

- An inflammatory reaction of the eyelid margin
  - Usually occurs as seborrheic or staphylococcal blepharitis
  - Multiple types may coexist.
  - Itchiness, redness, flaking, and crusting of the eyelids
  - Categorization
    - Based on the length of disease process: acute or chronic
    - Anatomic location of disease: anterior (e.g., staphylococcal and seborrheic blepharitis), posterior (e.g., meibomian gland dysfunction), parasitic, or mixed
- System(s) affected: skin/exocrine
- Synonym(s): granulated eyelids

EPIDEMIOLOGY

Incidence

- Very common
- All ethnic groups
- Predominant age: adult
- Predominant sex: male = female

RISK FACTORS

- Seborrheic dermatitis
- Contact dermatitis
- Herpes simplex dermatitis
- Varicella-zoster dermatitis
- Acne rosacea
- Diabetes mellitus
- Immunocompromised state (e.g., AIDS, chemotherapy)
- Isotretinoin use
- Dry eye syndromes

ETIOLOGY AND PATHOPHYSIOLOGY

- Seborrheic
  - Accelerated shedding of skin cells with associated sebaceous gland dysfunction
  - *Malassezia furfur* (formerly *Pityrosporum ovale*)
- Staphylococcal
  - Superinfection of Zeis glands of lid margin and meibomian glands posterior to lashes with *Staphylococcus aureus*
  - Usually part of mixed blepharitis
- Meibomian gland dysfunction: obstruction and inflammation of the meibomian glands; associated with acne rosacea, acne vulgaris, and oral retinoid therapy
- Other types of blepharitis:
  - Ulcerative blepharitis: more severe blepharitis with small marginal ulceration and destruction of the hair follicles
  - Contact dermatitis/blepharitis:
    - Develops from type IV hypersensitivity; common causes include ocular medications, topical anesthetics, antivirals, and cosmetics
    - May occur with secondary *Staphylococcus* infection
  - Eczematoid blepharitis
    - Caused by type I hypersensitivity reaction to exotoxins and antigens from local flora
    - Strong association with eczema, asthma
    - Staphylococcal infection common
  - Angular blepharitis: often caused by *Staphylococcus* or *Moraxella* infection
- The exact etiopathogenesis is unknown.
- Suspected to be multifactorial
  - Chronic low-grade infections of the ocular surface with bacteria
  - Infestations with certain parasites such as the mite *Demodex*
  - Inflammatory skin conditions such as atopy and seborrhea

COMMONLY ASSOCIATED CONDITIONS

See "Risk Factors" and "Differential Diagnosis."

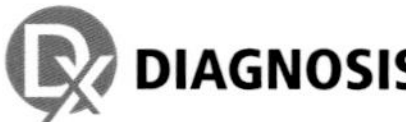

DIAGNOSIS

HISTORY

- Duration of symptoms
- Unilateral or bilateral presentation
- Note any exacerbating conditions (e.g., smoke, allergens, wind, contact lenses).
- Symptoms related to systemic diseases
- Current and recent medication use
- Recent exposure to infected individuals
- Frequently reported in all types of blepharitis
  - Burning
  - Itching
  - Eyelid erythema
  - Conjunctival infection (red eyes)
  - Lacrimation, tearing
  - Tear deficiency
  - Foreign body sensation
  - Photophobia (light sensitivity)
  - Impaired vision

PHYSICAL EXAM

- Test of visual acuity
- External exam (skin and eyelids)
  - Staphylococcal
    - Recurrent stye (external or internal hordeolum)
    - Missing, broken, or misdirected eyelashes (trichiasis)
    - Eyelid deposits: matted, hard scales; collarettes (ringlike formation around the lash shaft)
    - Ulcerations at base of eyelashes (rare)
    - Eyelid scarring may occur.
  - Seborrheic blepharitis
    - Eyelid deposits: dry flakes; oily or greasy secretions on lid margins and/or lashes
    - Associated dandruff of scalp, eyebrows
  - Meibomian gland dysfunction
    - Eyelash misdirection may occur with long-standing disease.
    - Eyelid deposits: fatty deposits; may be foamy
    - Eyelid margin thickening
    - Plugged meibomian gland orifices
    - Chalazion (sometimes multiple)
    - Eyelid scarring with long-term disease
    - Association with ocular rosacea
  - Mixed blepharitis: Signs and symptoms of >1 type of blepharitis may be present.

DIFFERENTIAL DIAGNOSIS

Masquerade syndrome (1)

- Persistent inflammation and thickening of eyelid margin may indicate squamous cell, basal cell, or sebaceous cell carcinoma masquerading as blepharitis. These carcinomas also may mimic styes or chalazia.
- Sebaceous carcinoma of the eyelid has a 22% fatality rate. Up to 1/2 of these potentially fatal sebaceous cell carcinomas may resemble benign inflammatory diseases, particularly chalazia and chronic blepharoconjunctivitis.
- Consider masquerade syndrome in all cases of recurrent, persistent, or atypical chalazion; chronic unilateral unresponsive blepharoconjunctivitis; diffuse or nodular tumors of the eyelid; orbital mass developing after removal of an eyelid or caruncular tumor; and any tumor developing in a person with a history of ocular radiotherapy.

DIAGNOSTIC TESTS & INTERPRETATION

Follow-Up Tests & Special Considerations

- Cultures in atypical blepharitis
- Biopsy in atypical cases for carcinoma
- Slit-lamp biomicroscopy
  - Examine tear film, eyelid margins, eyelashes, tarsal and bulbar conjunctivae, and cornea.
  - Reveals loss of lashes (madarosis), whitening of the lashes (poliosis), trichiasis, crusting, eyelid margin ulcers, and lid irregularities

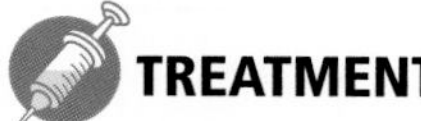

TREATMENT

GENERAL MEASURES

- Promote proper eyelid hygiene (2,3)[C]
  - Apply warm compresses for several minutes once a day to soften adherent encrustations.
  - The eyelid margins then are scrubbed gently with eyelid cleanser or diluted baby shampoo twice a day to remove adherent material and clean the meibomian gland orifices (4)[C].
- Brief, gentle massage of the eyelids can help to express meibomian secretions in patients with meibomian gland dysfunction (2)[C].
- Discontinue soft contact lenses use during an acute case of blepharitis (3)[B].

MEDICATION

First Line

- According to Cochrane 2012, topical antibiotics provided some symptomatic relief and were effective in eradicating bacteria from the eyelid margin for anterior blepharitis. Lid hygiene may provide symptomatic relief for anterior and posterior blepharitis. The effectiveness of other treatments for blepharitis, such as topical steroids and PO antibiotics, was inconclusive (5)[A].
- No strong evidence supports any of the treatments in terms of curing chronic blepharitis (5)[A].
- Topical treatment to lid, if *Staphylococcus* likely:
  - Bacitracin ointment: 500 μg/g or (2nd choice)
  - Erythromycin: 0.5% ophthalmic ointment
    - Apply with a cotton-tipped applicator.
    - The frequency and duration of treatment are guided by the severity (2)[C].
      - Topical corticosteroids (short term) may be useful for eyelid or ocular surface inflammation. The minimum effective dose should be used; long-term use should be avoided if possible.
- For patients with meibomian gland dysfunction inadequately controlled with eyelid hygiene, consider doxycycline 100 mg/day or tetracycline 1,000 mg/day in divided doses, tapered after clinical improvement (2–4 weeks) to doxycycline 50 mg/day or tetracycline 250–500 mg/day (2)[C].
- Because aqueous tear deficiency is common in blepharitis, use twice-daily artificial tears in addition to eyelid hygiene and medications.
- Contraindications: allergy to medication; tetracyclines are not for use in pregnancy, nursing women, or children <8 years of age.
- Precautions: Tetracyclines may cause photosensitivity; sunscreen is recommended. Corticosteroids may increase intraocular pressure and risk of cataract.

Second Line

- Topical fluoroquinolones (e.g., gatifloxacin 0.3%, levofloxacin 0.5%, or moxifloxacin 0.5%) may be helpful for persistent or recurrent staphylococcal blepharitis or for those patients who prefer a solution.
- Seborrheic blepharitis may respond to antifungal agents, such as a short course of itraconazole (6)[C].

ISSUES FOR REFERRAL

Chronic recurrent blepharitis requires referral to an ophthalmologist for evaluation whether patient should continue soft lens use.

ADDITIONAL THERAPIES

Various commercial products are marketed to consumers and prescribed to patients; however, there is no substantial evidence of effectiveness (5)[A].

ONGOING CARE

FOLLOW-UP RECOMMENDATIONS

Patient Monitoring

- Patients should schedule a return visit if their condition worsens despite treatment.
- Return visit intervals for patients with severe disease vary.
- If corticosteroid is prescribed, reevaluate within a few weeks to measure intraocular pressure and determine response to therapy.

PATIENT EDUCATION

- "Blepharitis Fact Sheet" from the American Academy of Ophthalmology
- Advise patient that blepharitis is a chronic condition likely to recur if eyelid hygiene is not maintained after antibiotic treatment is discontinued.

PROGNOSIS

- Symptoms frequently can be lessened but rarely are eliminated.
- Long-term eyelid hygiene is required for control.

COMPLICATIONS

- Stye and chalazion
- Scarring of eyelid margin
- Corneal infection
- Superficial keratopathy
- Corneal neovascularization and ulceration
- Ectropion/entropion

REFERENCES

1. Tsai T, O'Brien JM. Masquerade syndromes: malignancies mimicking inflammation in the eye. *Int Ophthalmol Clin*. 2002;42(1):115–131.
2. American Academy of Ophthalmology Cornea/External Disease Panel, Preferred Practice Patterns Committee. *Preferred Practice Pattern: Blepharitis*. San Francisco, CA: American Academy of Ophthalmology; 2003.
3. Eyelid hygiene for blepharitis. *Insight*. 2011;36(1):24.
4. McCulley JP, Shine WE. Changing concepts in the diagnosis and management of blepharitis. *Cornea*. 2000;19(5):650–658.
5. Lindsley K, Matsumura S, Hatef E. Interventions for chronic blepharitis. *Cochrane Database Syst Rev*. 2012;5:CD005556.
6. Ninomiya J, Nakabayashi A, Higuchi R, et al. A case of seborrheic blepharitis: treatment with itraconazole. *Nihon Ishinkin Gakkai Zasshi*. 2002;43(3):189–191.

SEE ALSO

Lacrimal Disorders (Dry Eye Syndrome)

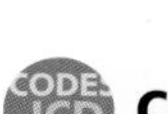

CODES

ICD10

- H01.009 Unspecified blepharitis unspecified eye, unspecified eyelid
- H01.019 Ulcerative blepharitis unspecified eye, unspecified eyelid
- L21.8 Other seborrheic dermatitis

CLINICAL PEARLS

- Blepharitis is often a chronic condition; symptoms frequently can be lessened but rarely are eliminated.
- Promote proper eyelid hygiene.
- Bacitracin ophthalmic ointment is the 1st-line treatment if *Staphylococcus* is suspected.

BORDERLINE PERSONALITY DISORDER

Daniel E. Melville, MD • William G. Elder, PhD

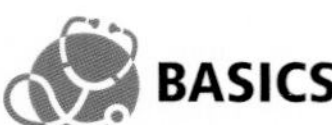

BASICS

DESCRIPTION

Beginning no later than adolescence or early adulthood, borderline personality disorder (BPD) is a consistent and pervasive pattern of labile affect and sense of self, impulsivity, and volatile interpersonal relationships (1).

- Common behaviors and variations
  - Self-mutilation: pinching, scratching, cutting
  - Suicide: ideation, history of attempts, plans
  - Splitting: idealizing then devaluing others
  - Presentation of helplessness or victimization
  - High use of emergency department and resultant inpatient hospitalizations for psychiatric treatment (2)
  - BPD patients are frequent users of primary care (3).
- High rate of associated mental disorders
- Typically display little insight into behavior

Geriatric Considerations

Illness (both acute and chronic) may exacerbate BPD and may lead to intense feelings of fear and helplessness.

Pediatric Considerations

Diagnosis is rarely made in children. Axis I disorders and general medical conditions are more probable.

Pregnancy Considerations

Physical, emotional, and social concerns may transiently mimic symptoms of BPD; consider delay in diagnosis until pregnancy completed. Pregnancy may also induce stress or increased fears, resulting in escalation of borderline behaviors.

EPIDEMIOLOGY

Predominant age: onset no later than adolescence or early adulthood (may go undiagnosed for years)

Prevalence

- General population: 0.5–5.9% of United States population (3)
- Estimated lifetime prevalence: 10–13% (3)
- 10% of all psychiatric outpatients and between 15% and 25% of patients in psychiatry inpatient settings have BPD (3).
- 20–30% of patients in primary care outpatient settings have a personality disorder.

ETIOLOGY AND PATHOPHYSIOLOGY

Undetermined but generally accepted that psychiatric disorders are due to a combination of the following:

- Hereditary temperamental traits
- Environment (i.e., history of childhood sexual and/or physical abuse, history of childhood neglect, ongoing conflict in home)
- Stress is theorized to exert damaging effects on the brain, specifically the hippocampus (3,4).
- Neurobiologic research of BPD continues to increase the understanding of the etiology:
  - Abnormalities of the frontolimbic circuitry in relation to poor emotional stability (3)
  - Potential alterations in the sensitivity of opioid receptors and/or deficiencies with endogenous opioids (5)
  - Heightened activity in brain circuits involved in the experience of negative emotions and reduced activation that normally suppresses negative emotion once it is generated (6)

Genetics

1st-degree relatives are at greater risk for this disorder (undetermined if due to genetic or psychosocial factors).

RISK FACTORS

- Genetic factors contribute; however, no specific genes have yet been identified as causative (3).
- Childhood sexual and/or physical abuse and neglect
- Disrupted family life
- Physical illness and external social factors may exacerbate borderline personality behaviors.

GENERAL PREVENTION

- Tends to be a multigenerational problem
- Children, caregivers, and significant others should have some time and activities away from the borderline individual, which may protect them.

COMMONLY ASSOCIATED CONDITIONS

Other psychiatric disorders include the following:

- Co-occurring personality disorders, frequent
- Mood disorders, common
- Anxiety disorders, common
- Substance-related disorders, common
- Eating disorders, common
- Posttraumatic stress disorder, common
- BPD does not appear to be independently associated with increased risk of violence.

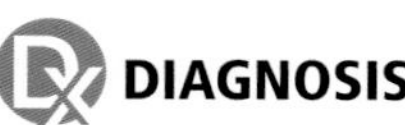

DIAGNOSIS

- The comprehensive evaluation should focus on the following (7,8)[B]:
  - Comorbid conditions
  - Functional impairments
  - Adaptive/maladaptive coping styles
  - Psychosocial stressors
  - Patient strengths; needs/goals
- Initial assessment should focus on determining treatment setting (7,8)[B]:
  - Establish treatment agreement with patient, and outline treatment goals.
  - Assess suicide ideation and self-harm behavior.
  - Assess for psychosis.
  - Hospitalization is necessary if patient presents a threat of harm to self or others.

HISTORY

- Clinic visits for problems that do not have biologic findings
- Conflicts with medical staff members
- Idealizing or unexplained anger at physician
- History of unrealistic expectations of physician (e.g., "I know you can take care of me." "You're the best, unlike my last provider.")
- Obtain collateral information (i.e., from family, partner) about patient behaviors.

PHYSICAL EXAM

- BPD patients should have a thorough physical examination to help lower suspicion of organic disease, (especially thyroid disease) (1,3).
- Often, physical examination reveals no gross abnormalities, other than related to scarring from self-mutilation.

DIFFERENTIAL DIAGNOSIS

- Mood disorders
  - Look at baseline behaviors when considering BPD versus mood disorder.
  - BPD symptoms increase the likelihood of misdiagnosing bipolar disorder.
  - In particular, disruptive mood dysregulation disorder, a new diagnosis appearing in *DSM-5* and characterized by severe recurrent temper outbursts manifesting verbally or behaviorally and grossly out of proportion to the situation, may appear quite similar to the acting out and intense emotions seen in BPD. Look for other symptoms characteristic of BPD to differentiate (1).
- Psychotic disorder
  - With BPD, typically only occurs under intense stress and is characterized as "micropsychotic"
- Other PD
  - Thoughts, feelings, and behavior will differentiate BPD from other PDs.
- General medical condition (GMC)
  - Traits may emerge due to the effect of a GMC on the CNS.
- Substance use

DIAGNOSTIC TESTS & INTERPRETATION

- Consider age of onset. To meet criteria for BPD, borderline pattern will be present from adolescence or early adulthood.
- Formal psychological testing
- Rule out personality change due to a GMC (1)[C]:
  - Traits may emerge due to the effect of a GMC on the CNS.
- Rule out symptoms related to substance use.
- If symptoms begin later than early adulthood or are related to trauma (e.g., after a head injury), a GMC, or substance use, then consider other diagnoses.

DIAGNOSTIC PROCEDURES/OTHER

According to *DSM-5* criteria, patient must meet at least 5 of the following criteria (1)[C]:

- Attempt to avoid abandonment
- Volatile interpersonal relationships
- Identity disturbance
- Impulsive behavior
  - In ≥2 areas
  - Impulsive behavior is self-damaging.
- Suicidal or self-mutilating behavior
- Mood instability
- Feeling empty
- Is unable to control anger, or finds it difficult
- Paranoid or dissociative when under stress
- With advent of *DSM-5*, an alternative model is being promulgated that may come to define the diagnosis as impairments in personality functioning AND the presence of pathologic traits. Attention to these features may ultimately enhance provider understanding, diagnosis, and treatment of patients with personality dysfunction.
  - Criteria regarding personality functioning refer to impairments of self-functioning (i.e., identity or self-direction) AND interpersonal functioning (i.e., empathy or intimacy).
    - Criteria regarding personality functioning refer to impairments of self-functioning (i.e., identity or self-direction) AND interpersonal functioning (i.e., empathy or intimacy).
    - Pathologic personality traits refer to characteristics in the domains of negative affectivity (i.e., emotional liability, anxiousness, separation insecurity, deppresivity); disinhibition (i.e., impulsivity, risk taking); OR antagonism (1).

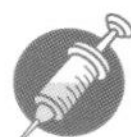

TREATMENT

- Outpatient psychotherapy for BPD is the preferred treatment (3,7,8)[B].
  - Dialectical behavior therapy (DBT) combines cognitive-behavioral techniques for emotional regulation and reality-testing with concepts of distress tolerance, acceptance, and self-awareness.
    - Following a dialectal process, therapists are tough-minded allies who validate feelings and are unconditionally accepting while also reminding patients to accept their dire level of emotional dysfunction and to apply better alternative behaviors.
    - DBT may be done individually and in groups.
- Consider transference-focused psychotherapy.
- Patient may need to be placed on suicide watch.
- Brief inpatient hospitalizations are ineffective in changing Axis II disorder behaviors.
  - Hospitalizations should be limited and of short duration to adjust medications, implement psychotherapy for crisis intervention, and to stabilize patients from psychosocial stressors.
- Extended inpatient hospitalization should be considered for the following reasons (7,8)[B]:
  - Persistent/severe suicidal ideation or risk to others
  - Comorbid substance use and/or nonadherence to outpatient or partial hospitalization treatments
  - Comorbid Axis I disorders that may increase threat to life for the patient (i.e., eating disorders, mood disorders)

GENERAL MEASURES

Focus on patient management rather than on "fixing" behaviors:

- Schedule consistent appointment follow-ups to relieve patient anxiety.
- Meet with and rely on treatment team to avoid splitting of team by patient and to provide opportunity to discuss patient issues.
- Treatment is usually most effective when both medications and psychotherapy are used simultaneously.

MEDICATION

- Although no specific medications are approved by the FDA to treat BPD, American Psychiatric Association (APA) guidelines recommend pharmacotherapy to manage symptoms (3)[A],(7,8)[B].
- Treat Axis I disorders (7,8)[B].
- Consider high rate of self-harm and suicidal behavior when prescribing (3)[A].
- APA guideline recommendations (7,8)[B]
  - Affective dysregulation: mood stabilizers, selective serotonin reuptake inhibitor (SSRIs), and monoamine oxidase inhibitors (MAOIs)
  - Impulsive-behavioral control: SSRIs and mood stabilizers
  - Cognitive-perceptual symptoms: antipsychotics
- With more neurobiologic causes considered in relation to BPD, there is more emphasis on mood stabilizers and atypical antipsychotics, but research is uncertain and inconclusive (9)[B].
- Antipsychotics have short-lived benefit and offer no value other than transient treatment of cognitive perceptual symptoms (9)[B].

ISSUES FOR REFERRAL

- If hospitalized, consider for suicide risk, mood or anxiety disorders, or substance-related disorders.
- Urgency for scheduled follow-up depends on community resources (e.g., outpatient day programs for suicidal patients, substance abuse programs) .
  - With increased risk for self-harm or self-defeating behaviors and low community resources, the patient can/will have increased need for frequent visits.

ADDITIONAL THERAPIES

Consider referring patient for specialty mental health behavioral services, including partial hospital therapy.

COMPLEMENTARY & ALTERNATIVE MEDICINE

Omega-3 fatty acid dietary supplementation has shown beneficial effects (3)[B].

INPATIENT CONSIDERATIONS

Admission Criteria/Initial Stabilization

Admit for inpatient services immediately in presence of psychosis or threat of injury to self or others; include police, as necessary, for safety measures.

- Assess suicidal ideation.
- Consider trial of antipsychotic medications for psychosis.

Nursing

Nurses can be instrumental in managing and calling patients, potentially relieving patient stress.

Discharge Criteria

- Patient should not present risk of harm to self or others and have a safety plan.
- Follow-up should be scheduled with a mental health specialist and primary care provider.

ONGOING CARE

FOLLOW-UP RECOMMENDATIONS

- Schedule visits that are short, more frequent, and focused to relieve patients' anxiety about relationships with their physician/provider and to help reduce risk of provider burnout.
- Maintain open lines of communication with mental health professionals providing psychological support.
- Emphasize importance of healthy lifestyle modifications (i.e., exercise, rest, diet).

Patient Monitoring

Monitor for suicidal or other self-harm behaviors.

PATIENT EDUCATION

Include patients in the diagnosis so they can make sense of their disease process and participate in the treatment strategy (7,8,10)[C].

PROGNOSIS

- Borderline behaviors may decrease with age and over time.
- Patients in treatment improve at a rate of seven times compared with following natural course (11).
- Treatment is complex and takes time.
- Medical focus includes patient management and caring for medical and Axis I disorders.

REFERENCES

1. American Psychiatric Association. *Diagnostic and Statistical Manual of Mental Disorders*. 5th ed. Arlington, VA: American Psychiatric Association; 2013.
2. Foti ME, Geller J, Guy LS, et al. Borderline personality disorder: considerations for inclusion in the Massachusetts parity list of "biologically-based" disorders. *Psychiatr Q*. 2011;82(2):95–112.
3. Leichsenring F, Leibing E, Kruse J, et al. Borderline personality disorder. *Lancet*. 2011;377(9759): 74–84.
4. Ruocco AC, Amirthavasagam S, Zakzanis KK. Amygdala and hippocampal volume reductions as candidate endophenotypes for borderline personality disorder: a meta-analysis of magnetic resonance imaging studies. *Psychiatry Res*. 2012;201(3):245–252.
5. Bandelow B, Schmahl C, Falkai P, et al. Borderline personality disorder: a dysregulation of the endogenous opioid system? *Psychol Rev*. 2010;117(2):623–636.
6. Ruocco A, Amirthavasagam S, Choi-Kain LW, et al. Neural correlates of negative emotionality in borderline personality disorder: an activation-likelihood-estimation meta-analysis. *Biol Psychiatry*. 2013;73(2):153.
7. American Psychiatric Association. *Practice Guideline for the Treatment of Patients With Borderline Personality Disorder*. Arlington, VA: American Psychiatric Association; 2001.
8. Oldham JA. *Guideline Watch: Practice Guideline for the Treatment of Patients With Borderline Personality Disorder*. Arlington, VA: American Psychiatric Association; 2005.
9. Feurino L III, Silk KR. State of the art in the pharmacologic treatment of borderline personality disorder. *Curr Psychiatry Rep*. 2011;13(1):69–75.
10. Sanislow CA, Marcus KL, Reagan EM. Long-term outcomes in borderline psychopathology: old assumptions, current findings, and new directions. *Curr Psychiatry Rep*. 2012;14(1):54–61.
11. Elder W, Walsh E. Personality disoders. In South-Paul J, Matheny S, Lewis E, eds. *Current Diagnosis & Treatment: Family Medicine*. New York, NY: McGraw-Hill; 2011.

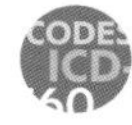

CODES

ICD10

F60.3 Borderline personality disorder

CLINICAL PEARLS

- View BPD as a chronic condition with waxing and waning features. It is important to adjust medications/treatments as clinically appropriate when symptoms change.
- If there are problems with the patient disrespecting the physician or support staff, clear guidelines should be established with the treatment team and then with the patient.
- When considering terminating care, the patient may improve if empathetically confronted about certain behaviors and is given clear guidelines on how to behave in the clinic. It is the patient's job to follow the guidelines, and it is you and your team's job to enforce the guidelines. Designate a case management nurse or well-trained support staff person who can be the primary contact person for the patient.
- Have an agenda when you visit with BPD patients. Be cordial—they deserve the same professionalism that any patient gets. Have and identify 1–2 issues to be discussed per clinic visit. Frequently scheduled visits can help with this.
- Regularly scheduled psychotherapy treatment helps physician performance by becoming the "home" for mental health treatment, leaving the physician to focus on the patient's immediate medical issues.

BRAIN INJURY, TRAUMATIC

Elise Taylor Nissen, MD • Ashley K. Christiani, MD

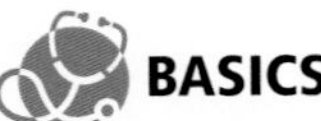

BASICS

DESCRIPTION

- Traumatic brain injury (TBI) is defined as an alteration in brain function, or other evidence of brain pathology, caused by an external force.
- System(s) affected: neurologic; psychiatric; cardiovascular; endocrine/metabolic; gastrointestinal
- Synonym(s): head injury, concussion

EPIDEMIOLOGY

Incidence

- 2.2 million ED visits and 280,000 hospitalizations/year
- 50,000 deaths/year; ~30% of all injury-related deaths
- Incidence in males twice that of females with 4-fold risk fatal trauma

Prevalence

- Predominant age: 0–4 years, 15–19 years, and >65 years
- Predominant gender: male > female (2:1)

ETIOLOGY AND PATHOPHYSIOLOGY

- Falls (40%)
- Motor vehicle accidents (14%)
- Assault (10%)
- Child abuse (24% of TBI age 2 years and younger)
- Recreational activities (21% of pediatric TBI peak seasons spring/summer; peak ages 10–14 years)
- Primary insult: direct mechanical damage
- Secondary insult: actuation of complex cellular and molecular cascades that promote cerebral edema, ischemia, and apoptotic cell death

RISK FACTORS

Alcohol and drug use, prior/recurrent head injury, contact sports, seizure disorder, ADHD, male sex, luteal phase of female menstrual cycle

Geriatric Considerations

Subdural hematomas are common after a fall or blow in elderly; symptoms may be subtle and not present until days after trauma.

GENERAL PREVENTION

- Safety education
- Seat belts; bicycle and motorcycle helmets
- Protective headgear for contact sports

Pediatric Considerations

Child abuse: Consider if dropped or fell <4 feet (e.g., off bed, couch) and significant injury present or any retinal hemorrhages.

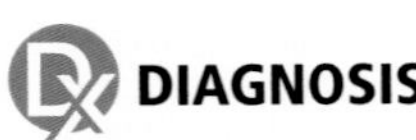

DIAGNOSIS

HISTORY

- Loss of consciousness (LOC)
- Headache
- Vomiting
- Amnesia
- Epidural hemorrhage from blunt trauma: 30% with a "lucid interval" (initial LOC followed by recovery of consciousness, then LOC recurs and persists)

PHYSICAL EXAM

- Neurologic and cognitive testing important
- Repeat neurologic exams every 30 minutes until 2 hours after GCS reaches 15, then hourly for 4 hours, then every 2 hours.
- Evidence of increased intracranial pressure (ICP) (elevated BP, decreased pulse rate, or slow/irregular breathing [Cushing triad]—only 30% have all 3)
- Decorticate or decerebrate posturing
- Signs of basilar skull fracture: raccoon eyes, Battle sign, hemotympanum, CSF rhinorrhea or otorrhea

DIFFERENTIAL DIAGNOSIS

Other causes of altered mental status (e.g., toxicologic, infectious, metabolic, vascular)

DIAGNOSTIC TESTS & INTERPRETATION

Initial Tests (lab, imaging)

- Mild TBI and concussions cognitive screening tests
  - Sports Concussion Assessment Tool V3 (SCAT3)
  - Child SCAT3
  - Concussion Recognition Tool (CRT)
  - Standardized Assessment of Concussion (SAC)
  - King-Devick Test
  - Balance Error Scoring System (BESS)
- Evaluate for coagulopathy.
- Type and screen for possible surgical intervention.
- Perform drug and alcohol screening.
- CT, noncontrast, is study of choice to review bone windows, tissue windows, and subdural space.
- NEXUS II study demonstrated that if all 8 clinical criteria are absent, there is a low likelihood of significant TBI:
  - Evidence of significant skull fracture (depressed, basilar, or diastatic)
  - Altered level of alertness
  - Neurologic deficit
  - Persistent vomiting
  - Presence of scalp hematoma
  - Abnormal behavior
  - Coagulopathy
  - Age >65 years

Follow-Up Tests & Special Considerations

Blast-related TBI: much higher rates of postconcussive syndrome, PTSD, depression, and chronic pain. Chronic impairment is strongly correlated with psychological factors. Return to battlefield guidelines similar to return to play in sports (see "General Measures") (1)[A]

Pediatric Considerations

Skull radiographs are not indicated unless abuse is suspected, in which case they can detect fractures not seen under CT. No return to activity until they are asymptomatic, and return to school should precede return to sport/physical activity (2)[A].

Diagnostic Procedures/Other

- CSF rhinorrhea
  - Contains glucose; nasal mucus does not.
  - Check for the double-halo sign: If nasal discharge contains CSF and blood, two rings appear when placed on filter paper—a central ring followed by a paler ring.
- Placement of ICP monitor, when indicated

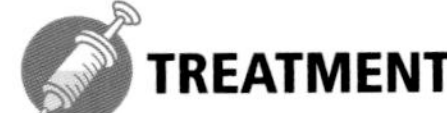

TREATMENT

GENERAL MEASURES

- Acute management depends on injury severity. Most patients need no interventions.
- Immediate goal: Determine who needs further therapy, imaging studies (CT), and hospitalization to prevent further injury.
- For the mildly injured patient:
  - Early education is beneficial for recovery (3)[A]
  - **Return to play (RTP)**
    - Never RTP on same day.
    - Strict guidelines for graduated return to cognitive and physical activity when there are no evident signs or symptoms (physical, cognitive, emotional, or behavioral) on neuropsychological and clinical evaluation (2)[A]
- For the moderate to severely injured patient
  - Avoid hypotension or hypoxia. Head injury causes increased ICP secondary to edema, and cerebral perfusion pressure (CPP) should be maintained between 60 and 70 mm Hg (4)[A].
  - 30-degree head elevation decreases ICP and improves CPP.
  - Hyperventilation (hypocapnia)
    - Use should be limited to patients with impending herniation while preparing for definitive treatment or intraoperatively. Risk of worsening cerebral ischemia and organ damage (4,5,6)[A]
    - Addition of tromethamine can offset deleterious effects and lead to better outcomes (6)[A].
  - Mild systematic hypothermia lowers ICP but leads to increased rates of pneumonia. Selective brain cooling may also decrease ICP with improved outcomes at 2 years post injury (6)[A].
- Seizure prophylaxis
  - Does not change morbidity or mortality. Consider phenytoin or levetiracetam for 1 week post injury or longer for patients with early seizures, dural-penetrating injuries, multiple contusions, and/or subdural hematomas requiring evacuation (7)[A].

MEDICATION

First Line

- Pain
  - Morphine: 1–2 mg IV PRN, with caution, because can depress mental status, further altering serial neurologic evaluations

ALERT

Bolus doses increase ICP and decrease CPP (8)[A].

- Increased ICP
  - Hypertonic saline: 2 mL/kg IV decreases ICP without adverse hemodynamic status; preferred agent (4,8)[A]
  - Mannitol: 0.25–2 g/kg (0.25–1 g/kg in children) given over 30–60 minutes in patients with adequate renal function. Prophylactic use is associated with worse outcomes (8)[A].
- Sedation
  - Propofol: preferred due to short duration of action. Avoid high doses to prevent propofol infusion syndrome. When combined with morphine, it can also effectively decrease ICP and decrease use of other meds (8)[A].
  - Midazolam: similar sedating effect to propofol but may cause hypotension (8)[A]
- Seizures
  - Phenytoin (Dilantin): 15 mg/kg IV (1 mg/kg/min IV, not to exceed 50 mg/min). Stop infusion if QT interval increases by >50%.

ALERT

Avoid corticosteroid use, as it increases mortality rates and risk of developing late seizures (8)[A]. Avoid barbiturates due to risk of hypotension (8)[A].

ISSUES FOR REFERRAL

Consult neurosurgery for:

- All penetrating head trauma
- All abnormal head CTs

ADDITIONAL THERAPIES

Emerging therapies with limited but promising evidence: coma arousal therapy: amantadine, zolpidem, and levodopa/carbidopa; postcoma therapy: bromocriptine; prophylactic therapy: Progesterone may be protective against secondary insult.

SURGERY/OTHER PROCEDURES

- Early evacuation of trauma-related intracranial hematoma decreases mortality especially with GCS <6 and CT evidence of hematoma, cerebral swelling, or herniation (9)[A].
- Decompressive craniectomy reduces ICP especially when a large bone flap is removed. ONLY for adults and ONLY with GCS >6 (6)[A].
- Hyperbaric oxygen temporarily lowers ICP and improves mortality, but evidence is conflicting about outcomes at 6–12 months post injury (6)[A]. The combination of hyperbaric and normobaric hyperoxia reduces ICP and improves overall morbidity/mortality (10)[B].
- CSF drainage reduces ICP but has not been demonstrated to have long-term benefit (6)[A].
- CSF leakage often resolves in 24 hours with bed rest, but if not, may require surgical repair (4)[A].

COMPLEMENTARY & ALTERNATIVE MEDICINE

- Insufficient evidence for use of acupuncture, but it may improve overall functional outcome (11)[A].
- Music therapy in conjunction with multimodal stimulation improves awareness in comatose TBI patients (9)[B].

INPATIENT CONSIDERATIONS

Admission Criteria/Initial Stabilization

- Abnormal GCS or CT
- Clinical evidence of basilar skull fracture
- Persistent neurologic deficits (e.g., confusion, somnolence)
- Patient with no competent adult at home for observation
- Possibly admit: LOC, amnesia, patients on anticoagulants with negative CT
- ABCs take priority over head injury.
- C-spine immobilization should be considered in all head trauma.

IV Fluids

Use normal saline for resuscitation fluid.

Discharge Criteria

Normal CT with return to normal mental status and responsible adult to observe patient at home (see "Patient Monitoring")

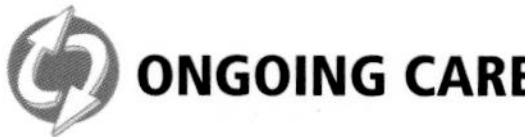

ONGOING CARE

FOLLOW-UP RECOMMENDATIONS

- Schedule regular follow-up within a week to determine return to activities.
- Rehabilitation indicated following a significant acute injury. Set realistic goals.
- For patients on anticoagulants, net benefit to restarting therapy after discharge despite increased bleeding risk.

Patient Monitoring

Patient should be discharged to the care of a competent adult with clear instructions on signs and symptoms that warrant immediate evaluation (e.g., changing mental status, worsening headache, focal findings, or any signs of distress). Patients should be monitored but not awakened from sleep.

DIET

As tolerated

PATIENT EDUCATION

Proper counseling, symptomatic management, and gradual return to normal activities are essential.

PROGNOSIS

- Gradual improvement may continue for years.
- 30–50% of severe head injuries may be fatal.
- Predicting outcome is difficult; many with even minor to moderate injuries have moderate to severe disability at 1 year, whereas prolonged coma may be followed by satisfactory outcome.
- Patients may have new onset seizures over 2 years following trauma.
- Poor prognostic factors: low GCS on admission, nonreactive pupils, old age, comorbidity, midline shift

COMPLICATIONS

- Chronic subdural hematoma, which may follow even "mild" head injury, especially in the elderly; often presents with headache and decreased mentation
- Delayed hematomas and hydrocephalus
- Emotional disturbances and psychiatric disorders resulting from head injury may be refractory to treatment
- Seizures: seen in 50% of penetrating head injuries, 20% of severe closed head injuries, and $<5\%$ of head injuries overall. Hematomas increase risk of epilepsy.
- Postconcussion syndrome can follow mild head injury without LOC and includes headaches, dizziness, fatigue, and subtle cognitive or affective changes.
- Second-impact syndrome occurs when the CNS loses autoregulation. An individual with a minor head injury is returned to a contact sport and, following even minor trauma (e.g., whiplash), the patient loses consciousness and may quickly herniate, with a 50% mortality. A similar syndrome of malignant edema can occur in children with even a single injury.
- Increased risk for Alzheimer disease, Parkinson disease, and other brain disorders whose prevalence increases with age

REFERENCES

1. Rosenfeld JV, McFarlane AC, Bragge P, et al. Blast-related traumatic brain injury. *Lancet Neurol*. 2013;12(9):882–893.
2. McCrory P, Meeuwisse WH, Aubry M, et al. Consensus statement on concussion in sport: the 4th International Conference on Concussion in Sport held in Zurich, November 2012. *Br J Sports Med*. 2013;47(5):250–258.
3. Nygren-de Boussard C, Holm LW, Cancelliere C, et al. Nonsurgical interventions after mild traumatic brain injury: a systematic review. *Arch Phys Med Rehabil*. 2014;95(3)(Suppl):S257–S264.
4. Tsang KKT, Whitfield PC. Traumatic brain injury: review of current management strategies. *Br J Oral Maxillofac Surg*. 2012;50(4):298–308.
5. Curley G, Kavanagh BP, Laffey JG. Hypocapnia and the injured brain: more harm than benefit. *Crit Care Med*. 2010;38(5):1348–1359.
6. Meyer MJ, Megyesi J, Meythaler J, et al. Acute management of acquired brain injury part I: an evidence-based review of non-pharmacological interventions. *Brain Inj*. 2010;24(5):694–705.
7. Agrawal A, Timothy J, Pandit L, et al. Post-traumatic epilepsy: an overview. *Clin Neurol Neurosurg*. 2006;108(5):433–439.
8. Meyer MJ, Megyesi J, Meythaler J, et al. Acute management of acquired brain injury part II: an evidence-based review of pharmacological interventions. *Brain Inj*. 2010;24(5):706–721.
9. Kim YJ. The impact of time to surgery on outcomes in patients with traumatic brain injury: a literature review. *Int Emerg Nurs*. 2014;22(4):214–219.
10. Rockswold SB, Rockswold GL, Zaun DA, et al. A prospective, randomized phase II clinical trial to evaluate the effect of combined hyperbaric and normobaric hyperoxia on cerebral metabolism, intracranial pressure, oxygen toxicity, and clinical outcome in severe traumatic brain injury. *J Neurosurg*. 2013;118(6):1317–1328.
11. Wong V, Cheuk DKL, Lee S, et al. Acupuncture for acute management and rehabilitation of traumatic brain injury. *Cochrane Database Syst Rev*. 2013;3:CD007700.

ADDITIONAL READING

Carroll LJ, Cassidy JD, Cancelliere C, et al. Systematic review of the prognosis after mild traumatic brain injury in adults: cognitive, psychiatric, and mortality outcomes: results of the International Collaboration on Mild Traumatic Brain Injury Prognosis. *Arch Phys Med Rehabil*. 2014;95(3)(Suppl 2): S152– S173.

SEE ALSO

Brain Injury—Post Acute Care Issues; Postconcussion Syndrome (Mild Traumatic Brain Injury); Seizure Disorders

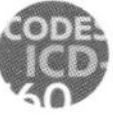

CODES

ICD10

- S06.9X0A Unsp intracranial injury w/o loss of consciousness, init
- S06.5X0A Traum subdr hem w/o loss of consciousness, init
- S06.6X0A Traum subrac hem w/o loss of consciousness, init

CLINICAL PEARLS

- TBI involves two distinct phases: the primary mechanical insult and secondary dysregulation of the cerebrovascular system with cerebral edema, ischemia, and cell-mediated death.
- Indications for imaging include evidence of skull fracture, altered consciousness, neurologic deficit, persistent vomiting, scalp hematoma, abnormal behavior, coagulopathy, age >65 years.
- Strict criteria exist for patients to return to normal sport activity following head injury to avoid the second-impact syndrome, which has 50% mortality.

BREAST ABSCESS

Shumaila Athar, MD • Tamara McGregor, MD

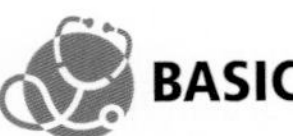

BASICS

DESCRIPTION

- Collection of pus (usually localized) within breast parenchyma
- Can be associated with lactation or fistulous tracts secondary to squamous epithelial neoplasm or duct occlusion
- System(s) affected: skin/exocrine
- Synonym(s): mammary abscess; peripheral breast abscess; subareolar abscess; puerperal abscess

Pregnancy Considerations

Most commonly associated with postpartum lactation

EPIDEMIOLOGY

- Predominant age
  - Puerperal abscess: lactational
  - Subareolar abscess: postmenopausal
- Predominant sex: female
- Higher incidence in African American women

Incidence

- 0.1–0.5% of breastfeeding women
- Puerperal abscess rare after first 6 weeks of lactation

ETIOLOGY AND PATHOPHYSIOLOGY

- Delayed treatment of mastitis
- Puerperal abscesses: blocked lactiferous duct
- Subareolar abscess: squamous epithelial neoplasm with keratin plugs or ductal extension with associated inflammation
- Peripheral abscess: stasis of the duct leading to microbial accumulation and secondary abscess formation
- Microbiology
  - Most common cause
    - *Staphylococcus aureus*
  - Less common causes
    - *Streptococcus pyogenes*
    - *Escherichia coli*
    - *Bacteroides*
    - *Corynebacterium*
    - *Pseudomonas*
    - *Proteus*
- Methicillin-resistant *Staphylococcus aureus* (MRSA) is an increasingly important pathogen in postpartum women; risk factors for postpartum *S. aureus* (SA) breast abscess have not changed with rise in community-associated MRSA.

RISK FACTORS

- Puerperal mastitis
  - 5–11% go on to abscess:
    - Most often due to inadequate or incomplete therapy
  - Risk factors (stasis):
    - Infrequent or missed feeds
    - Poor latch
    - Damage or irritation of the nipple
    - Illness in mother or baby
    - Rapid weaning
    - Blocked nipple or duct
    - Maternal stress or fatigue (1)
    - Maternal malnutrition
- General factors
  - Smoking
  - Diabetes
  - Rheumatoid arthritis
  - Obesity
- Medically induced factors
  - Steroids
  - Silicone/paraffin implant
  - Lumpectomy with radiation
- Nipple retraction
- Nipple piercing (mastitis) (2)
- Higher recurrence rate if multiorganism abscess

GENERAL PREVENTION

- Early treatment of mastitis with milk expression and cold compresses
- Early treatment with antibiotics

COMMONLY ASSOCIATED CONDITIONS

Lactation

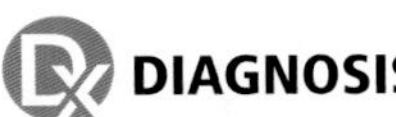

DIAGNOSIS

HISTORY

- Tender breast lump, usually unilateral
- Breastfeeding
- Postmenopausal
- Tender breast lump, fluctuant, usually unilateral
- Systemic malaise (usually less than with mastitis)

PHYSICAL EXAM

- Fever, tachycardia
- Erythema of overlying skin
- Tenderness, fluctuance on palpation
- Draining pus
- Local edema
- Nipple and skin retraction
- Regional lymphadenopathy

DIFFERENTIAL DIAGNOSIS

- Carcinoma (inflammatory or primary squamous cell)
- Engorgement
- Galactocele
- Tuberculosis (may be associated with HIV infection)
- Sarcoid
- Granulomatous disease
- Syphilis
- Foreign body reactions (e.g., to silicone and paraffin)
- Mammary duct ectasia

DIAGNOSTIC TESTS & INTERPRETATION

- CBC (leukocytosis)
- Elevated ESR
- Culture and sensitivity of abscess fluid or expressed breast milk to identify pathogen (usually staphylococci or streptococci)
- MRSA is an increasingly important pathogen in both lactational and nonlactational abscesses.
- Other bacteria:
  - Nonlactational abscess and recurrent abscesses associated with anaerobic bacteria
    - *E. coli*, *Proteus*; mixed bacteria less common
- Ultrasound (US) helps identify fluid collection within breast tissue.
- Mammogram

Diagnostic Procedures/Other

Aspiration of abscess for culture (not accurate to exclude carcinoma)

Test Interpretation

- Squamous metaplasia of the ducts
- Intraductal hyperplasia
- Epithelial overgrowth
- Fat necrosis
- Duct ectasia

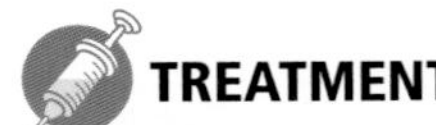

TREATMENT

GENERAL MEASURES

- Cold compresses for pain control
- *Important to continue to breastfeed or express milk* to drain the affected breast

B

MEDICATION

Combination of antibiotics and drainage for cure:

- Culture midstream sample of milk for mastitis.
- Culture abscess fluid for breast abscess.

- There is insufficient evidence regarding the effectiveness of antibiotic therapies for lactational mastitis alone (3)[A].

First Line

- NSAIDs for analgesia and/or antipyresis

- Dicloxacillin 500 mg QID for 10–14 days (4)[A]

- If no response in 24–48 hours, switch to cephalexin 500 mg QID for 10–14 days.
  - Or amoxicillin-clavulanate (Augmentin) 250–500 mg TID
- Clindamycin 300 mg QID if anaerobes are suspected
- If MRSA is a concern, TMP-SMZ DS 1–2 PO BID for 10–14 days. Clindamycin 300 mg PO QID as alternative
- *Contraindications*: antibiotic allergy
- In severe infections, vancomycin as an inpatient may be necessary.
  - Dose (30 mg/kg) IV in 2 divided doses every 24 hours may be necessary until culture results are available.
  - A 3rd-generation or a combination of a beta-lactam and beta-lactamase agent may need to be added as well.
- Subareolar abscess may need addition of metronidazole for anaerobic coverage.
  - Dose: 500 mg PO TID for 7–14 days
- Percutaneous intracavitary urokinase irrigation has been used to treat large abscesses in nonlactating women (5)[C].

SURGERY/OTHER PROCEDURES

- Aspiration under US guidance (5,6)[B],(7)[C]

- Serial aspirations under US may be necessary (q2–3d) if patients fail to respond (8)[C].

- Needle aspiration alone (without antibiotics) may be effective for small breast abscesses (9)[A].

- If aspiration and antibiotics fail, incision and drainage should be considered to remove loculations.
- Biopsy nonpuerperal abscesses to rule out carcinoma.
- Open all fistulous tracts, especially in nonlactating abscesses.

- US-guided aspiration of breast abscess with judicious use of antibiotics is superior to incision and drainage (10)[A].

COMPLEMENTARY & ALTERNATIVE MEDICINE

- Lecithin supplementation may help in some women.

- Acupuncture may help with breast engorgement, and possibly with breast abscess prevention (11)[A].

INPATIENT CONSIDERATIONS

Admission Criteria/Initial Stabilization

Outpatient, unless systemically immunocompromised or septic

ONGOING CARE

FOLLOW-UP RECOMMENDATIONS

Patient Monitoring

Ensure resolution to exclude carcinoma.

PATIENT EDUCATION

- Wound care
- Continue with breastfeeding or pumping (if breastfeeding is not possible due to location of abscess) to prevent engorgement. Milk can be discarded in some cases.

PROGNOSIS

- Complete healing expected in 8–10 days
- Subareolar abscesses frequently recur, even after incision and drainage (I&D) and antibiotics; may require surgical removal of ducts

COMPLICATIONS

- Fistula: mammary duct or milk fistula
- Poor cosmetic outcome

REFERENCES

1. Branch-Ellinman W, Golen TH, Nielsen KR, et al. Risk factors for *Staphylococcus aureus* postpartum breast abscess. *Clin Infect Dis*. 2012;54(1):71–77.
2. Gollapalli V, Liao J, Dudkavic A, et al. Risk factors for development and recurrence of primary breast abscess. *J Am Coll Surg*. 2010;211(1):41–48.
3. Jahanfar S, Ng CJ, Teng CL. Antibiotics for mastitis in breastfeeding women. *Cochrane Database Syst Rev*. 2013;2:CD005458.
4. Cusack L, Brennan M. Lactational mastitis and breast abscess—diagnosis and management in general practice. *Aust Fam Physician*. 2011;40(12):976–979.
5. Schwarz RJ, Shrestha R. Needle aspiration of breast abscesses. *Am J Surgery*. 2001;182(2):117–119.
6. Dener C, Inan A. Breast abscesses in lactating women. *World J Surg*. 2003;27(2):130–133.
7. Christensen AF, Al-Suliman N, Nielsen KR, et al. Ultrasound-guided drainage of breast abscesses: results in 151 patients. *Br J Radiol*. 2005;78(297):186–188.
8. Elder EE, Brennan M. Nonsurgical management should be first-line therapy for breast abscess. *World J Surg*. 2010;34(9):2257–2258.
9. Thirumalaikumar S, Kommu S. Best evidence topic reports. Aspiration of breast abscesses. *Emerg Med J*. 2004;21:333–334.
10. Naeem M, Rahimnajjad MK, Rahimnajjad NA, et al. Comparison of incision and drainage against needle aspiration for treatment of breast abscess. *Am Surg*. 2012;78(11):1224–1227.
11. Mangesi L, Dowswell T. Treatments for breast engorgement during lactation. *Cochrane Database Syst Rev*. 2010;(9):CD006946.

ADDITIONAL READING

- Berná-Serna JD, Berná-Mestre JD, Galindo PJ, et al. Use of urokinase in percutaneous drainage of large breast abscesses. *J Ultrasound Med*. 2009;28(4):449–454.
- Dabbas N, Chand M, Pallett A, et al. Have the organisms that cause breast abscess changed with time?—implications for appropriate antibiotic usage in primary and secondary care. *Breast J*. 2010;16(4):412–415.
- Rizzo M, Gabram S, Staley C, et al. Management of breast abscesses in nonlactating women. *Am Surg*. 2010;76(3):292–295.
- Trop I, Dugas A, David J, et al. Breast abscesses: evidence-based algorithms for diagnosis, management, and follow-up. *Radiographics*. 2011;31(6):1683–1699.

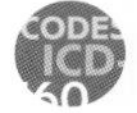

CODES

ICD10

- N61 Inflammatory disorders of breast
- O91.13 Abscess of breast associated with lactation
- O91.12 Abscess of breast associated with the puerperium

CLINICAL PEARLS

- Risk factors for mastitis are those that result in milk stasis (infrequent feeds, missing feeds). 5–11% of cases of puerperal mastitis go on to abscess (most often due to inadequate therapy for mastitis).
- Abscesses not associated with lactation should be treated with antibiotics that cover anaerobic bacteria.
- Treatment of choice for most breast abscesses is the combination of antibiotics and aspiration.
- US-guided aspiration of breast abscess is preferred to incision and drainage in most cases.
- Cointinuing to empty the breast (feeding, pumping or expression of breast milk) is recommended during the presence of lactation-associated breast infection.

BREAST CANCER

Bethany Gentilesco, MD • Aaron Kofman, MD • Komal Talati, MD

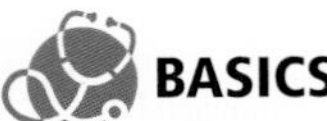

BASICS

DESCRIPTION

- Malignant tumor originating from breast epithelial cells, glandular cells, or connective tissue (rare)
- Types: ductal carcinoma in situ (DCIS—a precursor to invasive disease), invasive infiltrating ductal carcinoma, invasive lobular carcinoma, inflammatory breast cancer, Paget disease of the nipple, phyllodes tumor, angiosarcoma

EPIDEMIOLOGY

Incidence

- 122 cases per 100,000 women per year, 2005–2009
- New invasive cancer 2013 (est.): women: 232,340
- New in situ cancer 2013 (est.): 64,640 (85% DCIS)
- Breast cancer (BC) deaths 2013 (est.): 39,620; lifetime risk BC: 1 in 8 (12.2%); lifetime risk BC death (2007–2009): 2.76% (1 in 36)
- Most common malignancy in United States women, second only to lung cancer (CA) as cause of CA death

Prevalence

Over 2.8 million women with a history of BC in the United States (2013 est.) (1)[A]

ETIOLOGY AND PATHOPHYSIOLOGY

- Genetic mutations, such as *BRCA1* and *BRCA2*, can cause hereditary breast and ovarian cancer. These genes function as tumor suppressor genes, and a mutation leads to cell cycle progression and limitations in DNA repair.
- Mutations in estrogen/progesterone receptors through genetic changes can cause BC by inducing cyclin D1 and *c-myc* expression downstream, leading to cell cycle progression.
- ~1/3 of BCs do not express estrogen receptor (ER) mutations; however, many of these tumors may display cross-talk with ER and epidermal growth factors receptors (EGFR).

Genetics

- Criteria for additional risk evaluation/gene testing in *affected individual* (2)[A]
  - BC at age ≤50 years
  - BC at any age and ≥1 family member with BC ≤50 years of age or ovarian/fallopian tube/primary peritoneal CA any age or ≥2 family members with BC or pancreatic CA any age or population at increased risk (e.g., Ashkenazi Jew with BC or ovarian CA at any age)
  - Triple-negative BC (ER-, PR-, HER2-)
  - 2 BC primaries in single patient
  - Ovarian/fallopian tube/primary peritoneal CA
  - 1+ family member with BC and CA of thyroid, adrenal cortex, endometrium, pancreas, CNS, diffuse gastric, aggressive prostate (Gleason >7), leukemia, lymphoma, sarcoma, dermatologic manifestations and/or macrocephaly, GI hamartomas
  - Male BC
  - Known BC *susceptibility gene* mutation in family
- Criteria for additional risk evaluation/gene testing in *unaffected BC individual*
  - 1st- or 2nd-degree relative with BC ≤45 years of age
  - ≥2 breast primaries in one individual or ≥1 ovarian/fallopian tube/primary peritoneal CA from same side of family or ≥2 w/ breast primaries on same side of family
  - 1+ family member with BC and CA of thyroid, adrenal cortex, endometrium, pancreas, CNS, diffuse gastric, aggressive prostate (Gleason >7), leukemia, lymphoma, sarcoma, dermatologic manifestations, and/or macrocephaly, GI hamartomas
  - Ashkenazi Jewish with breast/ovary cancer at any age
  - Male BC
  - Known BC *susceptibility gene* mutation in family
- *BRCA1* and *BRCA2*
- Other genes: *ATM*, *BARD1*, *BRIP*, *CDH1*, *PTEN*, *STK11*, *CHEK2*, *p53*, *ERBB2*, *DIRAS3*, *NBN*, *RAD50*, *RAD51*
- Cowden syndrome (*PTEN*): autosomal dominant, BC, hamartomas of skin, intestine, oral mucosa (trichilemmoma), microencephaly, endometrial CA, nonmedullary thyroid CA, benign thyroid lesions
- Li-Fraumeni syndrome (*TP53*): autosomal dominant, BC and CA in CNS, leukemia, sarcoma, osteosarcoma, adrenal cortex
- Ataxia-telangiectasia (*ATM*): autosomal recessive, ataxia, telangiectasia, lymphoma, leukemia, CA of breast, stomach, ovary
- Peutz-Jeghers (*STK11*): autosomal dominance; hamartomatous polyps of GI tract, mucocutaneous melanin in lips, buccal mucosa, fingers, toes; CA in GI, lung, breast, uterus, ovary

RISK FACTORS

- Female, race (e.g., Ashkenazi Jewish), family history (FH), genetics, nulliparity or older age at first live birth, early menarche, delayed menopause, increasing age, personal history of BC or ovarian cancer, prolonged hormone replacement therapy, obesity/high body mass index, heavy alcohol intake, physical inactivity, mammographic breast density, active oral contraceptive use (disappears once discontinued)
- Benign/at-risk breast disease: atypical hyperplasia (ductal/lobular); lobular carcinoma in situ (LCIS) increases risk for bilateral BC
- Prior chest radiation (lymphoma), DES (diethylstilbestrol) exposure
- Number of prior breast biopsies of different lesions
- Men less at risk for BC but at increased risk with Klinefelter syndrome, testicular pathology, FH, or *BRCA2* mutations
- Prior radiation therapy (RT) between ages 10 years and 30 years
- Strong FH of hereditary breast and/or ovarian CA OR genetic predisposition (*high risk*)
  - Women: CBE 6–12 months starting at age 30 years; mammogram and MRI annually or individualized to earliest age of onset in family; at age 30 years: semiannual transvaginal US
- Risk-modifying agents
  - Premenopausal: Consider tamoxifen if history of LCIS, DCIS, or atypical ductal or lobular hyperplasia or if Gail modeling finds >1.66% over 5 years.
  - Postmenopausal: aromatase inhibitors or selective ER modulator, raloxifene. Tamoxifen use dependent on comorbid conditions, uterus status, and age. Discuss risk-reducing mastectomy and salpingo-oophorectomy (limited to *BRCA1* or *BRCA2*) done after age 35 years or after childbearing.
- Men: CBE 6–12 months starting at age 35 years; baseline mammogram at age 40 years; annual mammogram if gynecomastia or parenchymal/glandular breast

GENERAL PREVENTION

General population screening (normal risk)

- Breastfeeding, regular exercise, lean body weight
- Risk assessment tool: http://www.cancer.gov/bcrisktool/
- Clinical breast examination (CBE) if age 25–39 years: every 1–3 years (controversial; no evidence CBE improves outcomes but may decrease patient anxiety); age ≥40 years: every year
- Mammography: USPSTF recommends every other year starting at age 50 years; NCCN recommends every other year starting at age 40 years.

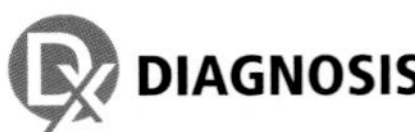

DIAGNOSIS

PHYSICAL EXAM

- Visualize breasts with patient sitting for skin dimpling, peau d'orange, asymmetry.
- Palpation of breast and regional lymph node exam: supraclavicular, infraclavicular, axillary

DIFFERENTIAL DIAGNOSIS

- Benign breast disease: fibrocystic disease, fibroadenoma, intraductal papilloma (bloody nipple discharge), duct ectasia, cyst, sclerosing adenosis, fat necrosis (s/p breast trauma)
- Infection: abscess, cellulitis, mastitis

DIAGNOSTIC TESTS & INTERPRETATION

Initial Tests (lab, imaging)

- Mammography BI-RADS: Breast Imaging–Reporting and Data System is a quality assurance (QA) method published by the American Radiology Society.
- BI-RADS interpretation: 0: incomplete (need additional imaging); 1: negative; 2: benign; 3: probably benign; 4: suspicious; 5: highly suggestive of malignancy; 6: known biopsy—proven malignancy
- All newly diagnosed BC: history and physical, CBC, LFTs, ALP, pathology review, ER/PR and HER2 status determination, genetic counseling if high risk, fertility counseling if indicated
- Clinical sign
  - Palpable mass ≥30 years: Obtain screening mammogram, which may be followed by diagnostic mammogram.
    - If BI-RADS 1–3, then get ultrasound ± biopsy.
    - If BI-RADS 4–6, then get core needle biopsy ± surgical excision.
  - Palpable mass <30 years: Obtain ultrasound ± mammogram ± biopsy; if low clinical suspicion, observe for 1–2 menstrual cycles for resolution.
  - Spontaneous, reproducible nipple discharge: Obtain mammogram, ± ultrasound.
    - If BI-RADS 1–3, then get ductogram or MRI.
    - If BI-RADS 4–5, then surgical excision
  - Asymmetric thickening/nodularity ≥30 years: Obtain mammogram + ultrasound ± biopsy.
  - Asymmetric thickening/nodularity <30 years: Obtain ultrasound ± mammogram ± biopsy.
  - Skin changes, peau d'orange: Obtain mammogram ± ultrasound ± biopsy.

Follow-Up Tests & Special Considerations

- Early disease (clinical stage I and IIB)
  - Consider additional studies only if signs and symptoms warrant.

- Advanced disease (stage IIIA or higher)
  - Chest diagnostic CT, abdominal ± pelvis CT, FDG positron emission tomography (PET)/CT scan, bone scan or sodium fluoride PET/CT if FDG-PET/CT indeterminate
  - Most common metastasis: lungs, liver, bone, brain
  - Bone scan: localized pain, elevated alkaline phosphate
  - Abdominal ± pelvis CT: abdominal symptoms, elevated alkaline phosphate, abnormal LFTs
  - Chest imaging: pulmonary symptoms
  - MRI: CNS/spinal cord symptoms

Diagnostic Procedures/Other

- Primary tumor: Fine-needle aspiration, ultrasound-guided core needle biopsy, stereotactic-guided core needle biopsy ± wire localization, sentinel lymph node, surgical excision, sentinel lymph node biopsy, post biopsy may get inflammatory changes/hematoma.
- Genomic assay on formalin-fixed tissue for select +ER, −HER2, node negative tumor to assess chemotherapy responsiveness

Test Interpretation

- Ductal/lobular/other: tumor size, inflammatory component, invasive/noninvasive, margins, nodal involvement
- Nodal micrometastases: increased risk of disease recurrence
- ER, PR, HER2 assay

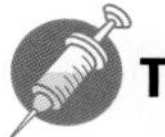

TREATMENT

MEDICATION

- Secondary prevention
  - ASA use at least once per week may be associated with as much as a 50% reduction in death from BC (see "Additional Reading")
  - Chemoprevention/hormone therapy for patients ages ≥35 years
    - Risk reduction for ER-positive tumors
- Hormone therapy for ER-positive tumors
  - Tamoxifen: premenopausal at diagnosis: 5-year treatment and consider for additional 5 years; avoid during lactation, pregnancy, or in patients with history of deep venous thrombosis/pulmonary embolism; routine CYP2D6 (tamoxifen metabolizing enzyme) testing not recommended; use strong CYP2D6-inhibiting medications with caution in conjunction with tamoxifen
  - Aromatase inhibitors: postmenopausal women, 5-year treatment following tamoxifen for 4.5–6 years, or tamoxifen for up to 10 years
  - Ovarian ablation or suppression with luteinizing hormone–releasing hormone agonists: premenopausal women
  - Anti-HER2/neu antibody (e.g., trastuzumab) in select HER2/neu-positive patients
  - Monitor cardiac toxicity via ECG, especially with anthracycline.
- Neoadjuvant chemotherapy (preop): Premenopausal women should be counseled on potential effect of chemotherapy on fertility, refer to fertility expert.
  - Locally advanced, inoperable advanced BC (stage III)
  - Early operable BC for breast conservation surgery
  - Triple negative BC
- Cytotoxic therapy: anthracyclines, taxanes, alkylating agents, antimetabolites
  - Higher risk patients with nonmetastatic operable tumors
  - Patients with high risk of recurrence after local treatment (serial/parallel [s/p] surgery ± radiation)
  - Online tool to estimate recurrence risk and benefits of adjuvant chemotherapy (http://www.adjuvantonline.com/online.jsp)
  - Dose-dense chemotherapy demonstrates overall survival advantage in early BC (3)[A].
- Advanced disease
  - Hormone therapy
  - Cytotoxic therapy
  - Bisphosphonates to decrease skeletal complications
  - Antivascular endothelial growth factor antibody
  - Anti-HER2/neu antibody in select HER2/neu-positive patients
- Metastatic disease
  - Monitoring metastatic disease: system assessment, physical examination, performance status, weight, LFT/CBC, CT scan/chest/abdomen/pelvis, bone scan, PET/CT, tumor markers

SURGERY/OTHER PROCEDURES

Secondary prevention

- Risk-reducing mastectomy and bilateral salpingo-oophorectomy for breast and ovary CA syndromes
- Breast-conserving partial mastectomy/lumpectomy, if possible
- Negative margins; tumor usually <5 cm
- No prior breast radiation, relative contraindication: connective tissue disease (lupus, scleroderma)
- Modified radical mastectomy
- Large tumors; multicentric disease; young women with known *BRCA*; consider immediate or delayed reconstruction
- RT should be initiated without delay:
- After breast-conserving therapy (BCT), stage I, IIA, IIB treatable with BCT + radiation
- Postmastectomy in select high-risk patients; palliation of metastatic disease; cord compression
- Pregnancy (treatment varies on trimester)
- Surgical: mastectomy or breast conservation: mastectomy preferred due to limitations of radiation during pregnancy
- Sentinel lymph node biopsy: safe to use with lymphoscintigraphy
- Chemotherapy: appropriate in 2nd and 3rd trimesters, trastuzumab contraindicated
- RT: Avoid until after delivery.

INPATIENT CONSIDERATIONS

Discharge Criteria

Postmastectomy

- Complications: seroma, phantom breast syndrome, cellulitis, chest wall/axilla/arm pain, long thoracic nerve damage leading to winged scapula sign
- Lymphedema; avoid having BP taken on side of surgery

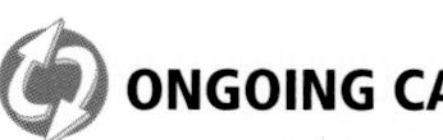

ONGOING CARE

FOLLOW-UP RECOMMENDATIONS

- Every 4–6 months × 5 years, then annually
- No evidence to support the use of routine CBC, LFTs, "tumor markers," bone scan, CXR, liver ultrasound, CT scans, MRI, PET
- Mammogram/imaging 1 year after initial mammogram but 6–12 months postradiation, then annually
- Annual gynecologic exam for women on tamoxifen; bone mineral density at baseline and follow-up for women on aromatase inhibitors or with ovarian failure secondary to treatment

PROGNOSIS

Stage	5-year Relative Survival Rate
0	100%
I	100%
II	93%
III	72%
IV	22%

(4)[A]

COMPLICATIONS

- Hypercalcemia, metastatic disease, lymphedema
- Emotional issues, especially depression and body-image alteration

REFERENCES

1. American Cancer Society. Cancer facts & figures 2013. Available at http://www.cancer.org. Accessed June 8, 2014.
2. National Comprehensive Cancer Network. NCCN guidelines: breast and/or ovarian cancer genetic assessment (Version1. 2012) © 2012. Breast Cancer National Comprehensive Cancer Network, Inc. Available at http://www.nccn.org. Accessed June 8, 2014.
3. Lyman GH, Barron RL, Natoli JL, et al. Systematic review of efficacy of dose-dense versus non-dose-dense chemotherapy in breast cancer, non-Hodgkin lymphoma, and non-small cell lung cancer. *Crit Rev Oncol Hematol*. 2012;81(3):296–308.
4. American Cancer Society. Breast cancer survival by stage. Available at www.cancer.org. Accessed June 8, 2014.

ADDITIONAL READING

- Holmes MD, Chen WY, Li L, et al. Aspirin intake and survival after breast cancer. *J Clin Oncol*. 2010;28(9):1467–1472.
- Rothwell PM, Wilson M, Price JF, et al. Effect of daily aspirin on risk of cancer metastasis: a study of incident cancers during randomized controlled trials. *Lancet*. 2012;379(9826):1591–1601.

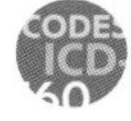

CODES

ICD10

- C50.919 Malignant neoplasm of unsp site of unspecified female breast
- D05.90 Unspecified type of carcinoma in situ of unspecified breast
- Z12.31 Encntr screen mammogram for malignant neoplasm of breast

CLINICAL PEARLS

- BC is most common malignancy in women in the United States, with lifetime risk of 1 in 8.
- High alcohol use, high body mass index (BMI), and physical inactivity are modifiable risk factors.
- Pursue/refer all abnormal breast physical examination/imaging findings.
- If patient ≥30 years of age with palpable mass, obtain mammogram, if <30 years of age obtain ultrasound.
- Normal mammography does not exclude possibility of CA with a palpable mass.

BREASTFEEDING

Zaiba Jetpuri, DO, MBA

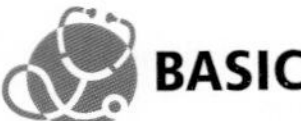

BASICS

- Breastfeeding is the natural process of feeding infant human milk directly from the breast.
- Breast milk is the preferred nutritional source for all newborns and infants.
- The American Academy of Pediatrics (AAP), the American Academy of Family Physicians (AAFP), WHO, and other medical organizations recommend exclusive breastfeeding for 6 months, with continuation of breastfeeding for ≥1 year as desired by mother and infant (1)[A].

DESCRIPTION

- Maternal benefits (as compared with mothers who do not breastfeed) include the following (2):
  - Decreased postpartum bleeding (due to oxytocin release)
  - Association of decreased risk of postpartum depression
  - Associated postpartum weight loss
  - Decreased risk of breast cancer
  - Association of decreased risk of ovarian cancer
  - Decreased risk of type 2 diabetes
  - Increased bonding
  - Convenience and economic savings
- Infant benefits (as compared with children who are formula-fed) include the following (1,2):
  - Ideal food: easily digestible, nutrients well absorbed, less constipation
  - Lower rates of virtually all infections via maternal antibody protection
    - Fewer respiratory and GI infections
    - Decreased incidence of otitis media
    - Decreased risk of bacterial meningitis and sepsis
    - Decreased incidence of necrotizing enterocolitis
  - Decreased incidence of obesity and type 1 and 2 diabetes
  - Decreased incidence of allergies and atopic dermatitis in childhood
  - Decreased risk of developing celiac disease and inflammatory bowel disease
  - Decreased risk of childhood leukemia
  - Decreased risk of sudden infant death syndrome (SIDS) and decreased mortality
  - Higher intelligence scores and better neurodevelopmental outcomes
  - Increased attachment between mother and baby

EPIDEMIOLOGY

Incidence

- According to the most recent breastfeeding scorecard, United States breastfeeding rates are on the rise. Based on the CDC, in 2014: any breastfeeding: 79.2.0% (however, differs among different sociodemographic and culture) (3)
- Breastfeeding at 6 months: 49.4%
- Breastfeeding at 12 months: 26.7%
- Exclusive breastfeeding at 3 months: 40.7%
- Exclusive breastfeeding at 6 months: 18.8%

ETIOLOGY AND PATHOPHYSIOLOGY

The overarching mechanism of milk production is based on supply and demand.

- Stimulation of areola causes secretion of oxytocin.
- Oxytocin is responsible for let-down reflex when milk is ejected into milk ducts (4).
- Sucking stimulates secretion of prolactin, which triggers milk production.
- Endocrine/metabolic: Thyroid dysfunction may cause delayed lactation or decreased milk.

GENERAL PREVENTION

- Most vaccinations can be given to breastfeeding mothers. The CDC recommends that the diphtheria-tetanus-acellular pertussis, hepatitis B, inactivated influenza virus (as opposed to live attenuated), measles-mumps-rubella (MMR), and inactivated polio and varicella vaccines can be given. The CDC recommends avoiding the yellow fever or smallpox vaccine in breastfeeding mothers (5).
- The inactivated influenza virus is preferred to the live attenuated virus in women with infants' age 6–23 months, regardless of whether these infants are being breastfed (5).

DIAGNOSIS

PHYSICAL EXAM

Examine breasts, ideally during pregnancy, looking for scars, lumps, or inverted nipples.

ALERT

A breast lump should be followed to complete resolution or worked up if present and not just attributed to changes from lactation.

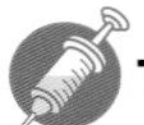

TREATMENT

GENERAL MEASURES

- Breastfeeding initiation
  - Initiate breastfeeding immediately after birth, ideally placing the infant on mother's chest skin-to-skin IN FIRST HOUR (1,6)[A].
  - Get mother in a comfortable position, usually sitting or reclining with the baby's head in crook of her arm.
  - Baby's belly and mother's belly should face each other or touch ("belly to belly"). Initiate the rooting reflex by tickling baby's lips with nipple or finger. As baby's mouth opens wide, mother guides her nipple to back of her baby's mouth while pulling the baby closer. This will ensure that the baby's gums are sucking on the areola, not the nipple.
  - Feed every 2–3 hours, 10–15 minutes/side
  - Rooming-in to encourage on-demand feeding
  - Observation of a nursing session by an experienced physician, nurse, or lactation consultant
  - Avoid supplementation with formula or water.
- Contraindications
  - Contraindications to breastfeeding are few (WHO) (1).
    - Maternal HIV (in industrialized world) or human T-cell leukemia virus (HTLV) infection
    - Active untreated tuberculosis
    - Active herpes simplex virus (HSV) lesions on the breast*
    - Substances of abuse and some medications that will pass into human milk
    - Infants with galactosemia or maple syrup urine disease should not be fed with breast milk. Infants with phenylketonuria may be fed breast milk under close observation.
    - Mothers who develop varicella 5 days before through 2 days after delivery*
    - Mothers acutely infected with influenza H1N1 until afebrile*
    - Maternal hepatitis is NOT a contraindication.

*Expressed milk can be used.

ISSUES FOR REFERRAL

- Refer to trained physician, nurse, or lactation consultant for inpatient and/or outpatient teaching.
- Frequent follow-up if having problems with latching, sore nipples, or inadequate milk production.

COMPLEMENTARY & ALTERNATIVE MEDICINE

Galactagogues (7)[C]

- Metoclopramide, oxytocin, fenugreek, and milk thistle have mixed results in improving milk production but efficacy and safety data are lacking in literature.

ONGOING CARE

FOLLOW-UP RECOMMENDATIONS

See mother and baby within a few days of hospital discharge, especially if 1st-time breastfeeding.

- Risk factors for suboptimal initiation
  - Breast surgery, especially reduction surgery, prior to pregnancy may disrupt breast milk production in the future.
  - Severe postpartum hemorrhage may lead to Sheehan syndrome, which is associated with difficulty breastfeeding due to poor milk production.
  - Parity
  - Delivery mode and duration of labor
  - Use of non–breast milk fluids or pacifiers
  - Maternal infection
  - Culture

Patient Monitoring

- Monitor infant's weight and output closely.
- Supplementation with infant formula recommended only if infant has lost ≥7% of birth weight or shows signs of dehydration such as decreased urine output.
- Supplementation without persistent breast stimulation with frequent feedings or breast pump use will decrease milk production and decrease breastfeeding success.

DIET

- For mothers:
  - Drink plenty of fluids: 8 glasses of liquid a day.
  - Breastfeeding mothers require ~500 more calories a day than prepregnancy needs (1).
  - Gassy foods, such as cabbage, may cause baby to have colic.
  - Limit caffeine to 300 mg/day.
  - Alcohol should be avoided. 1–2 drinks/week of alcohol may be okay, but mothers should avoid nursing 2–3 hours after a drink. <2% of alcohol is passed to baby via breast milk.
- Continue prenatal vitamin supplements.
- For infants:
  - In 2008, the AAP increased its recommended daily intake of vitamin D in infants from 200 to 400 IU. For exclusively breastfed babies, this will require taking a vitamin supplement, such as Poly-Vi-Sol or Vi-Daylin vitamin drops, 0.5 mL/day, beginning in the 1st few days of life (1).

B

- In 2010, the AAP recommended adding supplementation for breastfed infants with oral iron 1 mg/kg/day beginning at age 4 months.
  - Preterm infants fed human milk should receive an iron supplement of 2 mg/kg/day by 1 month of age, and this should be continued until the infant is weaned to iron-fortified formula or begins eating complementary foods that supply the 2 mg/kg of iron.
  - Fluoride supplement is unnecessary until 6 months of age (1).

PATIENT EDUCATION

- Primary care–initiated interventions to promote breastfeeding have been shown to be successful with respect to child and maternal health outcomes.
  - U.S. Preventive Services Task Force (USPSTF) recommends structured breastfeeding education and behavioral counseling programs to promote breastfeeding.
    - Regular promotion of the advantages of breastfeeding/risks of not breastfeeding (6)[A]
    - Emphasize importance of exclusive breastfeeding for first 4 weeks of life to allow adequate buildup of sufficient milk supply.
- Milk usually comes in about postpartum day 3.
- Frequent nursing (feedings 8–12/24 hours)
- Baby should have ~6 wet diapers/day and 3–4 bowel movements/day.
- Signs of adequate nursing
  - Hard breasts become soft after feeding.
  - Baby satisfied; appropriate weight gain (average 1 oz/day in first few months)
- Weaning
  - Solid food may be introduced at 6 months.
  - For mothers going to work, start switching the baby to breast milk feeding (or formula feeding) during hours mother will be gone about a week ahead of time.
- Family planning
  - Lactational amenorrhea method (LAM): Breastfeeding may be used as effective birth control option if (i) infant is <6 months old, (ii) infant is exclusively breastfeeding, and (iii) mother is amenorrheic.
  - Other options include barrier methods, implants, Depo-Provera, PO contraception, and intrauterine devices (IUDs). ACOG recommends that progesterone-only pills be used 2–3 weeks postpartum, and that Depo-Provera, IUDs, combined OCPs, and Implanon can be used 6 weeks postpartum. However, ACOG recommends delaying use of combined OCPs until after 6 weeks postpartum when lactation is well established.

COMPLICATIONS

- Breast milk jaundice should be considered if jaundice persists for >1 week in an otherwise healthy, well-hydrated newborn. It peaks at 10–14 days.
- Plugged duct
  - Mother is well except for sore lump in 1 or both breasts without fever.
  - Use moist, hot packs on lump prior to, and during, nursing; more frequent nursing on affected side.
- Mastitis (see topic "Mastitis")
  - Sore lump in 1 or both breasts plus fever and/or redness on skin overlying lump
  - Use moist, hot packs on lump prior to, and during, nursing.
  - Antibiotics covering for *Staphylococcus aureus* (most common organism)
  - Other possible sources of fever should be ruled out, that is, endometritis and pyelonephritis.
  - Mother should get increased rest; use acetaminophen (Tylenol) PRN.
  - Fever should resolve within 48 hours or consider changing antibiotics. Lump should resolve. If it continues, an abscess may be present, requiring surgical drainage.
- Milk supply inadequate
  - Check infant weight gain.
  - Review signs of adequate supply; technique, frequency, and duration of nursing.
  - Check to see if mother has been supplementing with formula, thereby decreasing her own milk production.
- Sore nipples
  - Check technique and improve latch-on.
  - Baby should be taken off the breast by breaking the suction with a finger in the mouth.
  - Air-dry nipples after each nursing and/or coat with expressed breast milk.
  - Use lanolin cream to help healing.
  - Do not wash nipples with soap and water.
  - Check for signs of thrush in baby and on mother's nipple. If affected, treat both.
  - Check for evidence of ankyloglossia (tongue tie) in the infant. Correction of ankyloglossia leads to decreased nipple soreness and improved breastfeeding.
- Flat or inverted nipples
  - When stimulated, inverted nipples will retract inward, flat nipples remain flat; check for this on initial prenatal physical.
  - Nipple shells, a doughnut-shaped insert, can be worn inside the bra during the last month of pregnancy to force the nipple gently through the center opening of the shell.
- Engorgement
  - Develops after milk first comes in (day 3 or 4 postpartum), resolves within a day or 2
  - Signs are warm, hard, sore breasts.
    - To resolve, offer baby more frequent nursing; breastfeed long enough to empty breasts.

REFERENCES

1. American Academy of Pediatrics, Section on Breastfeeding. Breastfeeding and the use of human milk. *Pediatrics*. 2012;129(3):e827–e841.
2. Ip S, Chung M, Raman G, et al. *Breastfeeding and Maternal and Infant Health Outcomes in Developed Countries*. Rockville, MD: Agency for Health Care Research and Quality; 2007.
3. Centers for Disease Control and Prevention. *Breastfeeding Report Card—United States 2014*. Atlanta: GA: Center for Disease Control and Prevention; 2014. http://www.cdc.gov/breastfeeding/pdf/2014breastfeedingreportcard.pdf. Accessed 2014.
4. Sinusas K, Gagliardi A. Initial management of breastfeeding. *Am Fam Physician*. 2001;64(6): 981–988.
5. Centers for Disease Control and Prevention. *Breastfeeding Vaccinations*. Atlanta, GA: Center for Disease Control and Prevention; 2010. http://www.cdc.gov/breastfeeding/recommendations/vaccinations.htm. Accessed 2014.
6. American College of Obstetricians and Gynecologists Women's Health Care Physicians; Committee on Health Care for Underserved Women. Committee opinion no. 570: breastfeeding in underserved women: increasing initiation and continuation of breastfeeding. *Obstet Gynecol*. 2013;122(2, Pt 1): 423–428.
7. Foranish AB, Yancey AM, Barnes KN, et al. The use of galactogogues in the breastfeeding mother. *Ann Pharmacother*. 2012;46(10):1392–1404.

ADDITIONAL READING

- American Academy of Pediatrics, American College of Obstetricians and Gynecologists. *Breastfeeding Handbook for Physicians*. Elk Grove Village, IL: American Academy of Pediatrics; 2006.
- Casey CF, Slawson DC, Neal LR. Vitamin D supplementation in infants, children, and adolescents. *Am Fam Physician*. 2010;81(6):745–748.
- Wagner CL, Greer FR, American Academy of Pediatrics Section on Breastfeeding, American Academy of Pediatrics Committee on Nutrition. Prevention of rickets and vitamin D deficiency in infants, children, and adolescents. *Pediatrics*. 2008;122(5):1142–1152.
- Websites/Books:
  - La Leche League at www.llli.org
  - World Health Organization. *Protecting, Promoting and Supporting Breastfeeding: The Special Role of Maternity Services. A Joint World Health Organization/United Nations Children's Fund (WHO/UNICEF) Statement*. Geneva, Switzerland: World Health Organization; 1989. http://www.unicef.org/newsline/tenstps.htm. Accessed 2014.
  - The Academy of Breastfeeding Medicine. A worldwide organization of physicians dedicated to the promotion, protection, and support of breastfeeding and human lactation. www.bfmed.org. Accessed 2014.

CODES

ICD10

Z39.1 Encounter for care and examination of lactating mother

CLINICAL PEARLS

- Breast milk is the optimal food for infants, with myriad health benefits for mothers and children.
- USPSTF recommends regular, structured education during pregnancy to promote breastfeeding.
- Vitamin D and iron supplementation should begin at birth and 4 months of age, respectively, for exclusively breastfed infants.

BRONCHIECTASIS

Sumera R. Ahmad, MD • Scott E. Kopec, MD

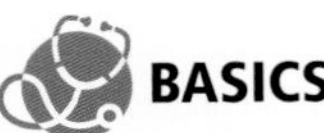

BASICS

DESCRIPTION

- Bronchiectasis is an irreversible dilatation of ≥1 airways accompanied by recurrent transmural bronchial infection/inflammation and chronic mucopurulent sputum production.
- Generally classified into cystic fibrosis (CF) and noncystic fibrosis (non-CF) bronchiectasis.

EPIDEMIOLOGY

- Predominant age: Most commonly presents in 6th decade of life.
- Predominant sex: female > male

Incidence

Incidence has decreased in the United States for 2 reasons:

- Widespread childhood vaccination against pertussis
- Effective treatment of childhood respiratory infections with antibiotics

Prevalence

- Prevalence in adult U.S. population estimated to be >110,000 affected individuals
- Internationally, prevalence increases with age from 4.2/100,000 persons aged 18–34 years to 271.8/100,000 among those aged 75 years and older (1).

ETIOLOGY AND PATHOPHYSIOLOGY

- CF bronchiectasis: bronchiectasis due to CF
- Non-CF bronchiectasis
  - Most cases are idiopathic.
  - Most commonly associated with non-CF bronchiectasis is childhood infection.
- Vicious circle hypothesis: Transmural infection, generally by bacterial organisms, causes inflammation and obstruction of airways. Damaged airways and dysfunctional cilia foster bacterial colonization, which leads to further inflammation and obstruction.

RISK FACTORS

- Nontuberculous mycobacterial infection is both a cause and a complication of non-CF bronchiectasis.
- Severe respiratory infection in childhood (measles, adenovirus, influenza, pertussis, or bronchiolitis)
- Systemic diseases (e.g., rheumatoid arthritis and inflammatory bowel disease)
- Chronic rhinosinusitis
- Recurrent pneumonia
- Aspirated foreign body
- Immunodeficiency
- Congenital abnormalities

GENERAL PREVENTION

- Routine immunizations against pertussis, measles, *Haemophilus influenza* type B, influenza, and pneumococcal pneumonia
- Genetic counseling if congenital condition is etiology
- Smoking cessation

COMMONLY ASSOCIATED CONDITIONS

- Mucociliary clearance defects
  - Primary ciliary dyskinesia
  - Young syndrome (secondary ciliary dyskinesia)
  - Kartagener syndrome
- Other congenital conditions
  - α1-Antitrypsin deficiency
  - Marfan syndrome
  - Cartilage deficiency (Williams-Campbell syndrome)
- Chronic obstructive pulmonary disease
- Pulmonary fibrosis, causing traction bronchiectasis
- Postinfectious conditions
  - Bacteria (*H. influenzae* and *Pseudomonas aeruginosa*)
  - Mycobacterial infections (tuberculosis [TB] and *Mycobacterium avium* complex [MAC])
  - Whooping cough
  - *Aspergillus* species
  - Viral (HIV, adenovirus, measles, influenza virus)
- Immunodeficient conditions
  - Primary: hypogammaglobulinemia
  - Secondary: allergic bronchopulmonary aspergillosis [ABPA], posttransplantation
- Sequelae of toxic inhalation or aspiration (e.g., chlorine, luminal foreign body)
- Rheumatic/chronic inflammatory conditions
  - Rheumatoid arthritis
  - Sjögren syndrome
  - Systemic lupus erythematosus
  - Inflammatory bowel disease
- Miscellaneous
  - Yellow nail syndrome

DIAGNOSIS

- Typical symptoms include chronic productive cough, wheezing, and dyspnea.
- Symptoms are often accompanied by repeated respiratory infections (2).
- Once diagnosed, investigate etiology.

HISTORY

- Any predisposing factors (congenital, infectious, and/or exposure-related)
- Immunization history

PHYSICAL EXAM

Symptoms are commonly present for many years and include the following:

- Chronic cough (90%)
- Sputum: may be copious and purulent (90%)
- Rhinosinusitis (60–70%)
- Fatigue: may be a dominant symptom (70%)
- Dyspnea (75%)
- Chest pain: May be pleuritic (20–30%)
- Hemoptysis (20–30%)
- Wheezing (20%)
- Bibasilar crackles (60%)
- Rhonchi (44%)
- Digital clubbing (3%)

DIFFERENTIAL DIAGNOSIS

- CF
- Chronic obstructive pulmonary disease
- Asthma
- Chronic bronchitis
- Pulmonary TB
- ABPA

DIAGNOSTIC TESTS & INTERPRETATION

- Spirometry
  - Moderate airflow obstruction and hyperresponsive airways
  - Forced expiratory volume in the 1st second of expiration (FEV_1): <80% predicted and FEV_1/FVC <0.7
- Special tests
  - Ciliary biopsy by electron microscopy
- Sputum culture
  - *H. influenzae*, nontypeable form (42%)
  - *P. aeruginosa* (18%)
  - Cultures may also be positive for *Streptococcus pneumoniae, Moraxella catarrhalis*, MAC, and *Aspergillus*.
  - Of all isolates, 30–40% will show no growth.
- Special tests
  - Sweat test for CF
  - Purified protein derivative (PPD) test for TB
  - Skin test for *Aspergillus*
  - HIV
  - Serum immunoglobulins to test for humoral immunodeficiency
  - Protein electrophoresis to test for α1-antitrypsin deficiency
  - Barium swallow to look for abnormalities of deglutition, achalasia, esophageal hypomotility
  - pH probe to characterize reflux
  - Screening tests for rheumatologic diseases
- Chest radiograph
  - Nonspecific; increased lung markings or may appear normal
- Chest computed tomography (CT)
  - Noncontrast high-resolution chest CT is the most important diagnostic tool.
  - Bronchi are dilated and do not taper, resulting in "tram track sign"; parallel opacities seen on scan.
  - Varicose constrictions and balloon cysts may be seen.
  - For focal bronchiectasis, rule out endobronchial obstruction.
  - For exclusively upper lobe bronchiectasis, consider CF and ABPA.

Diagnostic Procedures/Other

- Bronchoscopy may be used to obtain cultures and evacuate sputum.
- Bronchoscopy for hemoptysis
- Bronchoscopy may be useful to rule out airway obstructing lesions with focal bronchiectasis.

Test Interpretation

Bronchoscopy findings include the following:

- Dilatation of airways and purulent secretions
- Thickened bronchial walls with necrosis of bronchial mucosa
- Peribronchial scarring

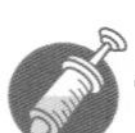

TREATMENT

- Treat underlying conditions.
- Recognize an acute exacerbation with 4 out of 9 criteria (3)
  - Change in sputum production
  - Increased dyspnea
  - Increased cough
  - Fever
  - Increased wheezing
  - Malaise, fatigue, lethargy
  - Reduced pulmonary function
  - Radiographic changes
  - Changes in chest sounds
- Non-CF bronchiectasis: Determine cause of exacerbations; promote good bronchopulmonary hygiene via daily airway clearance.
- Consider surgical resection of damaged lung for focal disease that is refractory to medical management.
- Medical management: Reduce morbidity by controlling symptoms and preventing disease progression.
- Patients with non-CF bronchiectasis may not respond to CF treatment regimens in the same way as patients with CF do.

GENERAL MEASURES

- Maintain hydration (nebulized hypertonic saline, 3% or 7% may be used to help increase mucus clearance) (4)[A].
- Noninvasive positive-pressure ventilation

MEDICATION

- Insufficient evidence exists to support efficacy of short-course antibiotics in adults and children with bronchiectasis (5)[A].
- Frequent exacerbations may be treated with prolonged and aerosolized antibiotics (2)[A].
- Role of mucolytics, anti-inflammatory agents, and bronchodilators is still unclear (2)[A].

First Line

- Antibiotics
  - Potentially useful in acute exacerbations
  - Chronic therapy decreases sputum volume and purulence, but it does not diminish the frequency of exacerbations (6)[A].
  - Patients may require twice the usual dose and longer treatment for 14 days (7)[C].
  - Sputum culture and sensitivity should direct therapy; antibiotic selection is complicated by a wide range of pathogens and resistant organisms.
  - Should be administered IV in cases of severe infection
    - Augmentin: 500 mg PO q8–12h Pediatric: Base dosing on amoxicillin content.
    - Trimethoprim (TMP)/sulfamethoxazole (SMX) : 160 mg TMP/800 mg SMX PO q12h Pediatric: ≥2 months, 8 mg/kg TMP and 40 mg/kg SMX PO/24 hours, administered in 2 divided doses q12h
    - Doxycycline and cefaclor given PO are also effective.
    - Nebulized aminoglycosides (tobramycin): 300 mg by aerosol BID (8)[B]
    - Ciprofloxacin: 750 mg PO q12h for adults for susceptible strain of *Pseudomonas*
    - Macrolides: appear to have immunomodulatory benefits
- Chronic use of azithromycin as an oral macrolide in non-CF bronchiectasis has been shown to reduce exacerbations. Needs caution with respect to cardiovascular deaths, where it is a QTc-prolonging medication (9).
- Bronchodilators
  - Chronic use of β2-agonists (e.g., albuterol) reverses airflow obstruction.
- Inhaled corticosteroids
  - Insufficient evidence exists to recommend use of inhaled steroids with stable bronchiectasis (10)[A].
  - A therapeutic trial of inhaled steroids may be justified in adults with difficult-to-control symptoms (10)[A].
  - Decrease sputum and tend to improve lung function
    - Fluticasone propionate: 110–220 μg inhaled BID
  - Potential synergistic effect of long-acting β2-agonists with inhaled corticosteroids, allowing for lower steroid dose (11):
    - Budesonide 160 μg/Formoterol 4.5 μg 2 puffs inhaled BID

Second Line

Other broad-spectrum antimicrobials, including those with antipseudomonal coverage

ADDITIONAL THERAPIES

Sputum clearance techniques, including physiotherapy (percussion and postural drainage) and pulmonary rehabilitation (improves exercise tolerance)

SURGERY/OTHER PROCEDURES

- Surgery if area of bronchiectasis is localized and symptoms remain intolerable despite medical therapy or if disease is life threatening (2)[A].
- Surgery effectively improves symptoms in 80% of these cases.

INPATIENT CONSIDERATIONS

Admission Criteria/Initial Stabilization

Bronchiectasis can present as life-threatening massive hemoptysis. In this situation, in addition to airway protection and resuscitation, bronchial artery embolization or surgical intervention is necessary to control bleeding.

ONGOING CARE

Long-term outpatient treatment recommendations for bronchiectasis in children (12)[B]:

- Children with CF- and non–CF-related bronchiectasis should be treated by comprehensive interdisciplinary chronic disease management programs.
- Pathogen-directed aerosolized tobramycin treatment should be used long-term on a regular basis to improve the course of CF-related bronchiectasis.
- PO macrolide antibiotic use long-term (up to 6 months) improves lung function among children with CF-related bronchiectasis.
- Long-term antibiotic use (PO or aerosolized) in children with non–CF-related bronchiectasis has not been studied enough to warrant routine use.
- Hypertonic saline administered by inhalation used long-term (48 weeks) improves lung function and is safer when used with pretreatment bronchodilator therapy among children who have CF.
- Nebulized dornase improves multiple pulmonary outcomes of children who have CF and is indicated for long-term use.
- Risks for long-term oral corticosteroid use outweigh pulmonary benefits in the treatment of CF-related bronchiectasis.
- High-dose ibuprofen therapy reduces the rate of decline among children with mild CF-related bronchiectasis and is indicated for long-term use.
- Mucolytic agents, airway hydrating treatments, anti-inflammatory therapy, chest physical therapy (CPT), and bronchodilator therapy have not been studied sufficiently long-term in children with non–CF-related bronchiectasis to merit their routine use.

FOLLOW-UP RECOMMENDATIONS

Regular exercise is recommended.

Patient Monitoring

- Serial spirometry, every 2–5 years, to monitor the course of the disease
- Chest CTs to monitor progression of disease may be indicated with some conditions such as bronchiectasis with MAC infections.
- Routine microbiological sputum analysis

PATIENT EDUCATION

http://www.lungusa.org

PROGNOSIS

- Mortality rate (death due directly to bronchiectasis) is 13%.
- *Pseudomonas* infection is associated with poorer prognosis.

COMPLICATIONS

- Hemoptysis
- Recurrent pulmonary infections
- Pulmonary hypertension
- Cor pulmonale
- Lung abscess

REFERENCES

1. Pappalettera M, Aliberti S, Castellotti P, et al. Bronchiectasis: an update. *Clin Respir J*. 2009; 3(3):126–134.
2. ten Hacken NH, Wijkstra PJ, Kerstjens HA. Treatment of bronchiectasis in adults. *BMJ*. 2007;335(7629):1089–1093.
3. O'Donnell AE, Barker AF, Ilowite JS, et al. Treatment of idiopathic bronchiectasis with aerosolized human recombinant DNase 1. rhDNase Study Group. *Chest*. 1998;113(5):1329–1334.
4. Kellett F, Robert NM. Nebulised 7% hypertonic saline improves lung function and quality of life in bronchiectasis. *Resp Med*. 2011;105(12): 1831–1835.
5. Wurzel D, Marchant JM, Yerkovich ST, et al. Short courses of antibiotics for children and adults with bronchiectasis. *Cochrane Database Sys Rev*. 2011;(6):CD008695.
6. Evans DJ, Bara AI, Greenstone M. Prolonged antibiotics for purulent bronchiectasis. *Cochrane Database Sys Rev*. 2003;(4):CD001392.
7. Pasteur MC Bilton D, Hill AT, et al. British Thoracic Society guideline for non-CF bronchoectasis. *Thorax*. 2010;65(Suppl 1):i1–i58.
8. Lobue PA. Inhaled tobramycin: not just for cystic fibrosis anymore? *Chest*. 2005;127(4):1098–1101.
9. Wong C, Jayaram L, Karalus N, et al. Azithromycin for exacerbations of non-cystic fibrosis bronchiectasis (EMBRACE): a randomized, double-blind, placebo- controlled trial. *Lancet*. 2012;380(9842):660–667.
10. Kapur N, Bell S, Kolbe J. Inhaled steroids for bronchiectasis. *Cochrane Database Sys Rev*. 2009;(1):CD000996.
11. Martinez-Garcia MA, Soler-Cataluña JJ, Catalan-Serra P, et al. Clinical efficacy and safety of budesonide-formoterol in non-cystic fibrosis bronchiectasis. *Chest*. 2012;141(2):461–468.
12. Redding GJ. Bronchiectasis in children. *Pediatr Clin North Am*. 2009;56(1):157–171.

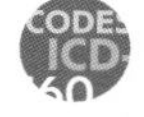

CODES

ICD10

- J47.9 Bronchiectasis, uncomplicated
- J47.1 Bronchiectasis with (acute) exacerbation
- J47.0 Bronchiectasis with acute lower respiratory infection

CLINICAL PEARLS

- Symptoms of bronchiectasis include chronic productive cough, wheezing, and dyspnea, often accompanied by repeated respiratory infections.
- A chest x-ray has poor sensitivity and specificity for the diagnosis; a noncontrast high-resolution chest CT is the most important diagnostic tool.
- Current practice guidelines recommend treating acute exacerbations with a 14-day course of antibiotics. Frequent exacerbations may be treated with prolonged and aerosolized antibiotics.

BRONCHIOLITIS

Dennis E. Hughes, DO, FAAFP, FACEP

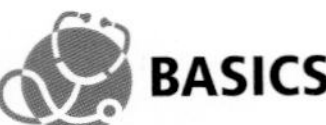

BASICS

DESCRIPTION

- Inflammation and obstruction of small airways and reactive airways generally affecting infants and young children—upper respiratory infection (URI) prodrome followed by increased respiratory effort and wheezing
- Usual course: insidious, acute, progressive
- Leading cause of hospitalizations in infants and children in most Western countries
- Predominant age: newborn–2 years (peak age <6 months). Neonates are not protected despite transfer of maternal antibody.
- Predominant sex: male > female

EPIDEMIOLOGY

Incidence

- 21% in North America
- May be seasonal (October–May in the Northern Hemisphere) and often occurs in epidemics
- 18.8% (90,000 annually) of all pediatric hospitalizations (excluding live births) in children <2 years
- Incidence increasing since 1980 (with concomitant increase in relative rate of hospitalization from 2002 to 2007)

ETIOLOGY AND PATHOPHYSIOLOGY

RSV accounts for 70–85% of all cases (children younger than 12 months of age), but rhinovirus, parainfluenza virus, adenovirus, influenza virus, *Mycoplasma pneumoniae*, and *Chlamydophila pneumoniae* have all been implicated:

- Infection results in necrosis and lysis of epithelial cells and subsequent release of inflammatory mediators.
- Edema and mucus secretion, which combined with accumulating necrotic debris and loss of cilia clearance, results in airflow obstruction.
- Ventilation–perfusion mismatching resulting in hypoxia.
- Air trapping is caused by dynamic airways narrowing during expiration, which increases work of breathing.
- Bronchospasm appears to play little or no role.

RISK FACTORS

- Secondhand cigarette smoke
- Low birth weight, premature birth
- Immunodeficiency
- Formula feeding (little or no breastfeeding)
- Contact with infected person (primary mode of spread)
- Children in daycare environment
- Congenital cardiopulmonary disease
- Majority have no underlying condition.

GENERAL PREVENTION

- Handwashing
- Contact isolation of infected babies
- Persons with colds should keep contact with infants to a minimum.
- Palivizumab (Synagis), a monoclonal product, administered monthly, October–May, 15 mg/kg IM; used for RSV prevention ONLY in high-risk patients
- High-risk considerations for use:
  - 32–35 weeks' gestation and <3 months of age at the start of RSV season with at least one risk factor: either attending daycare or with a sibling <5 years at home
  - 28–32 weeks' gestation and age <6 months
  - <28 weeks' gestation and age <12 months
  - Younger than 2 years of age with cyanotic or other complicated congenital heart disease
  - Younger than 2 years of age with congential airway or neuromuscular disorders
  - Once begun, continue through end of season regardless of age attained (1)[A].

Pediatric Considerations

Prior infection does not seem to confer subsequent immunity.

COMMONLY ASSOCIATED CONDITIONS

- Upper respiratory congestion
- Conjunctivitis
- Pharyngitis
- Otitis media
- Diarrhea

DIAGNOSIS

History and physical examination should be the basis for the diagnosis of bronchiolitis.

HISTORY

- Irritability
- Anorexia
- Fever
- Noisy breathing (due to rhinorrhea)
- Cough
- Grunting
- Cyanosis
- Apnea
- Vomiting

PHYSICAL EXAM

- Tachypnea
- Retractions
- Rhinorrhea
- Wheezing
- Upper respiratory findings: pharyngitis, conjunctivitis, otitis

DIFFERENTIAL DIAGNOSIS

- Other pulmonary infections such as pertussis, croup, or bacterial pneumonia
- Aspiration
- Vascular ring
- Foreign body
- Asthma
- Heart failure
- Gastroesophageal reflux
- Cystic fibrosis

DIAGNOSTIC TESTS & INTERPRETATION

Laboratory and other ancillary testing (including chest x-ray) not required

Initial Tests (lab, imaging)

- Arterial oxygen saturation by pulse oximetry (<94% significant)
- Rapid respiratory viral antigen testing (not necessary during RSV season because the disease is managed symptomatically but may be useful for epidemiologic, hospital cohorting, or in the very young to reduce unnecessary other workup.
- The American Association of Pediatrics (AAP) does not recommend routine RSV testing in infants and children with bronchiolitis:
  - Sensitivity 87–91%; specificity 96–100%
- Chest x-ray findings:
  - Increased anteroposterior diameter
  - Flattened diaphragm
  - Air trapping
  - Patchy infiltrates
  - Focal atelectasis: right upper lobe common
  - Peribronchial cuffing

TREATMENT

Mainstay of therapy is supportive to include upper airway suctioning, prevention of significant and prolonged hypoxia, and dehydration. The other interventions noted have historically varying effect on the course of the illness despite numerous studies.

MEDICATION

First Line

- Humidified oxygen for hypoxia only
- Nebulized hypertonic saline (3%) to reduce mucus plugging and mobilize airway secretions (2)[A]
- Epinephrine aerosols (0.5 mL of 2.25% solution in 3 mL NS): Some studies support short-term improvement in outpatient settings.
- Corticosteroids:
  - Oral dexamethasone (1 mg/kg loading dose, then 0.6 mg/kg daily for 5 days) especially for those with asthma risk (3)[B]
  - Nebulized dexamethasone (2–4 mg in 3 mL NS) may have anecdotal benefit; studies show mixed results.

B

Second Line

- Nebulized albuterol (0.15 mg/kg/dose) is often tried for acute symptoms; a trial of therapy may be reasonable in the presence of a suspected bronchospastic component (or with a family history of asthma).
- Antibiotics only if secondary bacterial infection present (rare)
- Positive-pressure ventilation (PPV) in the form of continuous positive airway pressure (CPAP) can be used in cases of respiratory failure. There is limited clinical evidence other than observational studies (4).
- High-flow nasal cannula oxygen widely used in various settings to improve oxygen saturation with resultant reduction in end-tidal CO_2 ($ETCO_2$) and respiratory rate, but overall effectiveness remains unproven to date (4).

ADDITIONAL THERAPIES

- Ribavirin (palivizumab) for patients at high risk (for prophylaxis per CDC/AAP guidelines) (1)[A]
- Heliox therapy (70% helium and 30% oxygen) may be of benefit early in moderate to severe bronchiolitis to reduce degree of respiratory distress, but Cochrane review found little evidence of sustained benefit at 24 hours (5)[A].

INPATIENT CONSIDERATIONS

Bronchiolitis can be associated with apnea in children <6 weeks of age.

Admission Criteria/Initial Stabilization

- Respiratory rate >45/min with respiratory distress or apnea
- Hypoxia is common so clinical criteria are more helpful (pulse oximetry <94% used by many as cutoff).
- Ill or toxic appearance
- Underlying heart condition, respiratory condition, or immune suppression
- High risk for apnea (age <30 days, preterm birth [<37 weeks])
- Dehydrated or unable to feed
- Uncertain home care
- Use of Respiratory Distress Assessment Instrument may aid in determining admission. The five best predictors of admission: Age, respiratory rate, heart rate, oxygen saturation, and duration of symptoms were recently incorporated into a scoring instrument.
- Supplemental oxygen for pulse oximetry <94% on room air if clinically indicated. AAP recommends O_2 saturation >90% if infant otherwise well.

IV-Fluids

Indicated only if tachypnea precludes oral feeding. Weight-based maintenance rate plus insensible losses.

Discharge Criteria

Normal respiratory rate and no oxygen requirement. Recent small studies suggest that after a period of observation, children can be safely discharged on home oxygen.

ONGOING CARE

FOLLOW-UP RECOMMENDATIONS

Patient Monitoring

- Hospitalization is usually required only if oxygen is a requirement or unable to feed/drink.
- For a hospitalized patient, monitor as needed depending on the severity of the infection.
- If the patient is receiving home care, follow daily by telephone for 2–4 days; the patient may need frequent office visits.

PATIENT EDUCATION

- American Academy of Pediatrics: http://www.aap.org
- American Academy of Family Physicians: http://www.familydoctor.org

PROGNOSIS

- Recovery time is variable. 40% can have symptoms at 14 days and 10% at 4 weeks.
- Mortality statistics differ but probably <1%.
- High-risk infants (bronchopulmonary dysplasia, congenital heart disease) may have a prolonged course.

COMPLICATIONS

- Bacterial superinfection
- Bronchiolitis obliterans
- Apnea
- Respiratory failure
- Death
- Increased incidence of development of reactive airway disease (asthma)

REFERENCES

1. Pickering LK, Kimberlin DW, Long SS, eds. *Red Book: 2012 Report of the Committee on Infectious Diseases*. 29th ed. Elk Grove Village, IL: American Academy of Pediatrics; 2012.
2. Zhang L, Medoza-Sassi RA, Wainwright C, et al. Nebulized saline solution for acute bronchiolitis in infants. *Cochrane Database Syst Rev*. 2013,7:CDC006458.
3. Alansari K, Sakran M, Davidson BL, et al. Oral dexamethasone for bronchiolitis: a randomized trial. *Pediatrics*. 2013;132(4),810–816.
4. Øymar K, Skjerven HO, Mikalsen IB. Acute bronchiolitis in infants, a review. *Scand J Trauma Resuc Emerg Med*. 2014,22:23.
5. Liet JM, Ducruet T, Gupta V, et al. Heliox inhalation therapy for bronchiolitis in infants. *Cochrane Database Syst Rev*. 2010;(4):CD006915.

ADDITIONAL READING

- Beggs S, Wong Z, Kaul S, et al. High flow nasal cannula therapy for infants with bronchilotis. *Cochrane Database Syst Rev*. 2014,1:CDC009609.
- Fernandes RM, Bialy LM, Vandermeer B, et al. Glucocorticoids for acute viral bronchiolitis in infants and young children. *Cochrane Database Syst Rev*. 2013;6:CD004878.
- García CG, Bhore R, Soriano-Fallas A, et al. Risk factors in children hospitalized with RSV bronchiolitis versus non-RSV bronchiolitis. *Pediatrics*. 2010;126(6):e1453–1460.
- Zorc JJ, Hall CB. Bronchiolitis: recent evidence on diagnosis and management. *Pediatrics*. 2010;125(2):342–349.

CODES

ICD10

- J21.9 Acute bronchiolitis, unspecified
- J21.0 Acute bronchiolitis due to respiratory syncytial virus
- J21.8 Acute bronchiolitis due to other specified organisms

CLINICAL PEARLS

- Bronchiolitis is the leading cause of hospitalizations in infants and children—especially <3 months of age.
- Diagnosis is a clinical one.
- Antibiotics are not helpful in most cases.
- Nebulized hypertonic saline may be of most benefit.
- Parental education of expected course of illness is most important—especially potential duration.

BRONCHIOLITIS OBLITERANS AND ORGANIZING PNEUMONIA

Jason Cohn, DO, MS • Amit Bhojwani, DO • Edward Scheiner, DO

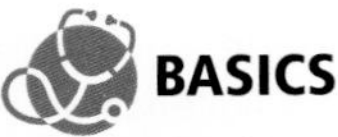

BASICS

DESCRIPTION

- A primary (cryptogenic) or secondary process of the lungs characterized by granulation-like tissue involving the distal airways and alveoli
- Bronchiolitis obliterans and organizing pneumonia (BOOP) is a restrictive problem that is completely reversible.
- A specific reaction of lung tissue to a variety of injuries
- It may occur as patchy infiltrates, or it may be nodular or secondary to another lung disease.
- May also appear to be a migrating process
- May have a gradual or sudden onset
- Lungs show a pattern of multiple patchy pneumonia, which are seen on the chest x-ray (CXR) as patchy alveolar or ground glass opacifications, with or without interstitial infiltrates; there may be air bronchograms as well.
- Most cases will respond to corticosteroids, which may have to be given for a year or more.
- Synonym(s): intraluminal fibrosis of distal airways; idiopathic BOOP; cryptogenic organizing pneumonia; obliterative bronchiolitis

Geriatric Considerations

More common than originally thought and may be sudden and very severe

Pediatric Considerations

- Rare but has been reported after viral pneumonia (adenovirus influenza)
- Characteristics include delayed recovery, persistent cough, crackles, or wheezing after pneumonia.
- Laboratory findings generally not helpful
- Imaging shows: ventilation perfusion ratio–matched defects; high-resolution CT, bronchiectasis, bronchogram, pruned tree appearance
- Diagnosis is confirmed by biopsy.

EPIDEMIOLOGY

- Incidence/prevalence in the United States: estimated at 0.01% but may be underdiagnosed
- Predominant age: Reported cases range age 0–70 years; most commonly seen in ages 40–60s

Prevalence

Unknown

ETIOLOGY AND PATHOPHYSIOLOGY

Idiopathic: a complex response to a variety of injuries such as toxic inhalation, postmycoplasma, viral and bacterial infection, aspiration, immunologic factors, drugs

Genetics

No known genetic component

RISK FACTORS

- AIDS
- Immunocompromised patients, including transplant recipients
- Smoking

GENERAL PREVENTION

Except for prevention of relapse, none known

COMMONLY ASSOCIATED CONDITIONS

- Drug-induced pneumonitis
  - Paraquat poisoning
  - Amiodarone toxicity
  - Acebutolol toxicity
  - Amphotericin B
- Beta blockers
  - Bleomycin
  - Carbamazepine
  - Cephalosporins
  - Gold
  - Minocycline
  - Nitrofurantoin
  - Phenytoin
  - Sulfamethoxypyridazine
  - Sulfasalazine
  - Ticlopidine
- Antineoplastic agents
  - Freebase cocaine pulmonary toxicity
  - Overdose of L-tryptophan
- Infections
  - Chronic infectious pneumonia
  - Malaria
  - *Chlamydia*
  - *Legionella*
  - *Mycoplasma*
  - *Pneumocystis*
  - *Cryptococcus*
- Immunocompromised (bone marrow, lung, renal transplantation)
- Malignancy: colon, breast, lymphoma
- Bronchial obstruction (lack of mucociliary clearance), that is, lung cancer
- Connective tissue diseases
  - BOOP itself is an autoimmune connective tissue disorder, so autoimmune connective tissue disorders confer a higher risk of acquiring the disease.
- Rheumatoid arthritis
  - Sjögren syndrome
  - Polymyositis
  - Scleroderma
  - Essential mixed cryoglobulinemia
  - Wegener granulomatosis
- Miscellaneous
  - Cystic fibrosis
  - Bronchopulmonary dysplasia
  - Renal failure
  - Congestive heart failure (CHF)
  - Adult respiratory distress syndrome
- Idiopathic pulmonary fibrosis
  - Chronic eosinophilic pneumonia
  - Hypersensitivity pneumonitis
  - Histiocytosis X
  - Sarcoidosis
  - Pneumoconioses
- Radiation pneumonitis

DIAGNOSIS

Think of the possibility in patients presenting with

- Flulike illness that lasts 4–10 weeks or longer. Most have been treated with antibiotics without success.
- Fatigue, fever, and weight loss
- Dry cough
- Dyspnea may be severe.
- Bilateral crackles

HISTORY

- Fatigue
- Malaise
- Fever/chills
- Weight loss
- Dry cough
- Dyspnea may be severe.

PHYSICAL EXAM

- Hypoxia
- Cyanosis
- Respiratory distress
- Bilateral crackles and/or
- Wheezing
- Dry cough
- Shortness of breath
- Rarely: hemoptysis, respiratory distress

DIFFERENTIAL DIAGNOSIS

- Usual interstitial pneumonitis
- Noninfectious diseases
- Tuberculosis
- Sarcoidosis
- Histoplasmosis
- Berylliosis
- Goodpasture syndrome
- Neoplasm
- Polyarteritis nodosa
- Systemic lupus erythematosus
- Wegener granulomatosis
- Sjögren syndrome
- Chronic eosinophilic pneumonia
- Cryptogenic bronchiolitis

DIAGNOSTIC TESTS & INTERPRETATION

- May have normal or nonspecific laboratory findings
- Leukocytosis with a normal differential
- Elevated ESR
- Eosinophilia
- Anemia
- If secondary to autoimmune process, may have elevated levels of antinuclear antibodies (ANA), rheumatoid factor (RF), anti-SSA/Ro, anti-SSB/La, anti-Jo, etc.
- Negative cultures
- Negative serology for *Mycoplasma*, *Coxiella*, *Legionella*, psittacosis, and fungus
- Negative viral studies
- CXR: often appears more normal than the physical examination
  - CXR may show bilateral patchy alveolar opacities (typical pattern), often in the middle or upper lung area, a ground glass pattern that may have air bronchograms.
  - CXR can also reveal a solitary focal nodule or mass known as a focal pattern (1)[B].
- Throughout the disease, new infiltrates may appear or may seem to migrate.
- Effusions and cavitary lesions are rare on x-ray.
- Patients with linear opacities at lung bases may have a poorer prognosis.
- CT scans more accurately define the distribution and extent of the patchy alveolar opacities with areas of hyperlucency. Findings are commonly described as a "reversed halo sign" or "Atoll sign," a focal round area of ground glass attenuation; however, this is a nonspecific finding (2,3)[A].
- Up to 90% of CT scans may show airspace consolidation with air bronchograms.
- Pulmonary function shows a restrictive/obstructive pattern.
- Flow-volume loop shows terminal airway obstruction.
- The involved area may seem to migrate.
- Ventilation–perfusion ratio scan: matched patchy defects

Diagnostic Procedures/Other

- In one study, open lung biopsy established the correct diagnosis in 1/3 of patients (4)[B].
- Transbronchial biopsy has yielded a correct diagnosis in 2/3 of cases (4,5)[B].
- It may be wise to use a trial of steroids as a diagnostic trial, although not all would agree.
- If a diagnostic trial is successful, be prepared to treat the patient for at least 1 year.
- Bronchoalveolar lavage (BAL) fluid in patients with BOOP have shown larger amounts of natural killer cells, natural killer T-like cells, Fas and tumor necrosis factor receptor expression indicating cytotoxicity and local inflammation (5,6)[C]. In one specific study, the most frequent BAL profile was mixed alveolitis with lymphocytic predominance, a CD4/CD8 index of 0.4, and foamy macrophages, which was shown to be specific (88.8%) but not sensitive (4)[C].

Test Interpretation

- Intraluminal fibrosis of distal airspaces is the major pathologic feature.
- Fibroblasts and plugs of inflammatory cells and loose connective tissue fill these distal airways, known as Masson bodies.
- Inflammatory cells are mainly lymphocytes and plasma cells.
- Interstitial fibrosis is present.
- Plugs of edematous granulation tissue in the terminal and respiratory bronchioles and alveolar ducts do not cause permanent damage.

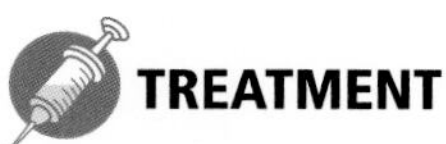

TREATMENT

Inpatient care may be required.

GENERAL MEASURES

- Monitor blood gases or pulse oximetry.
- Oxygen, as necessary

MEDICATION

First Line

Prednisone

- 1 mg/kg (up to 60 mg/day) for 1–3 months, then 40 mg/day for 3 months, then 10–20 mg/day for up to 1 year
- May consider a 6-month-only taper or alternate day dosing for 1 year to limit steroid exposure
- Increase length of taper for patients on long-term therapy to avoid precipitating addisonian crisis.
- Treatment may be needed for ≥1 year.
- In one study, the best response to corticosteroid therapy was seen in individuals younger than 35 years of age, nonsmokers, and with morphologic features (large bronchial plugs, mild inflammatory reaction) and immunohistochemical markers (presence of collagen IV, absence of collagen III, CD-68-positive cells and positive VEGF) (7)[B].
- Contraindications: Refer to the manufacturer's literature.
- Precautions: Be aware of the patient's Mantoux status and history of peptic ulcer disease. Long-term steroid treatment is associated with significant adverse effects, including Cushing syndrome, fluid retention, osteoporosis, hyperkalemia, and poor wound healing.

Pediatric Considerations

Prednisone: 1 mg/kg q24h for 1 month, followed by weaning over several months

Second Line

- Steroids other than prednisone may be used.
- Prescribe antimicrobials if the original infection is persistent. The proper choice depends on the pathogen.
- Anecdotal use of inhaled triamcinolone and cyclophosphamide has been reported.
- Macrolide antibiotics have also been used for their anti-inflammatory properties; however, not employed in most cases (4)[C]

ISSUES FOR REFERRAL

Patients should be followed by a pulmonologist.

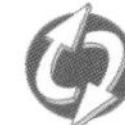

ONGOING CARE

FOLLOW-UP RECOMMENDATIONS

Patient Monitoring

- Frequent visits, weekly at first
- Prednisone must be continued because of the chance of relapse.
- Monitor the lung disease and the side effects of prednisone therapy:
  - Annual Mantoux/purified protein derivative
  - Monthly CBC
  - Funduscopic examination every 3–6 months
  - Serial dual energy x-ray absorptiometry (DEXA) scans for osteoporosis
- Smoking cessation is encouraged. Advice and information about smoking cessation interventions should be provided (i.e., counseling, nicotine replacement, medications, etc.).

DIET

No special diet

PATIENT EDUCATION

- Compliance: Emphasize the need to continue prednisone because of the chance of a relapse.
- Recurrence in up to 1/3 who do not complete full steroid treatment.

PROGNOSIS

Typically complete recovery, but individual case management is mandatory.

COMPLICATIONS

- Bronchiectasis
- Most people recover completely without permanent sequelae if full course of steroids completed.
- Death occurs in up to 7% but usually in individuals who are elderly or have preexisting comorbid conditions.

REFERENCES

1. Cottin V, Cordier JF. Cryptogenic organizing pneumonia. *Semin Respir Crit Care Med*. 2012;33(5):462–475.
2. Marchiori E, Zanetti G, Hochhegger B, et al. Reversed halo sign on computed tomography: state-of-the-art review. *Lung*. 2012;190(4):389–394.
3. Marchiori E, Irion KL, Zanetti G, et al. Atoll sign or reversed halo sign? Which term should be used? *Thorax*. 2011;66(11):1009–1010.
4. Drakopanagiotakis F, Paschalaki K, Abu-Hijleh M, et al. Cryptogenic and secondary organizing pneumonia: clinical presentation, radiographic findings, treatment response, and prognosis. *Chest*. 2011;139(4):893–900.
5. Jara-Palomares L, Gomez-Izquierdo L, Gonzalez-Vergara D, et al. Utility of high-resolution computed tomography and BAL in cryptogenic organizing pneumonia. *Respir Med*. 2010;104(11):1706–1711.
6. Papakosta D, Manika K, Gounari E, et al. Bronchoalveolar lavage fluid and blood natural killer and natural killer T-like cells in cryptogenic organizing pneumonia. *Respirology*. 2014;19(5):748–754.
7. Ye Q, Dai H, Sarria R, et al. Increased expression of tumor necrosis factor receptors in cryptogenic organizing pneumonia. *Respir Med*. 2011;105(2):292–297.

ADDITIONAL READING

- Cordier JF, Loire R, Brune J. Idiopathic bronchiolitis obliterans organizing pneumonia. Definition of characteristic clinical profiles in a series of 16 patients. *Chest*. 1989;96(5):999–1004.
- Drakopanagiotakis F, Polychronopoulos V, Judson MA. Organizing pneumonia. *Am J Med Sci*. 2008;335(1):34–39.
- Limper AH. Chemotherapy-induced lung disease. *Clin Chest Med*. 2004;25(1):53–64.
- Moonnumakal SP, Fan LL. Bronchiolitis obliterans in children. *Curr Opin Pediatr*. 2008;20(3):272–278.
- Müller NL, Staples CA, Miller RR. Bronchiolitis obliterans organizing pneumonia: CT features in 14 patients. *AJR Am J Roentgenol*. 1990;154(5):983–987.
- Ruth-Sahd LA, White KA. Bronchiolitis obliterans organizing pneumonia. *Dimens Crit Care Nurs*. 2009;28(5):204–208.
- Schlesinger C, Koss MN. The organizing pneumonias: an update and review. *Curr Opin Pulm Med*. 2005;11(5):422–430.
- White KA, Ruth-Sahd LA. Bronchiolitis obliterans organizing pneumonia. *Crit Care Nurse*. 2007;27(3):53–66; quiz 67.

SEE ALSO

Sjögren Syndrome

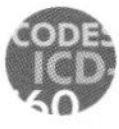

CODES

ICD10

- J84.89 Other specified interstitial pulmonary diseases
- J44.9 Chronic obstructive pulmonary disease, unspecified

CLINICAL PEARLS

- BOOP is a restrictive problem that is completely reversible.
- Major risk factors for BOOP include immunosuppression and smoking.
- When diagnosing BOOP, one should perform an autoimmune workup.
- The classic CT finding of BOOP is the "reversed halo sign" also known as "Atoll sign."
- BOOP treatment is a prolonged course of corticosteroids.

BRONCHITIS, ACUTE

Alan Cropp, MD, FCCP • Ghazaleh Bigdeli, MD, FCCP

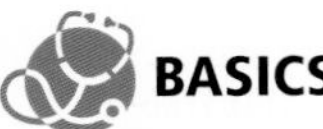

BASICS

DESCRIPTION

- Inflammation of trachea, bronchi, and bronchioles resulting from a respiratory tract infection or chemical irritant (1)
- Cough, the predominant symptom, may last as long as 3 weeks (2,3).
- Generally self-limited, with complete healing and full return of function (2)
- Most infections are viral if no underlying cardiopulmonary disease is present (2).
- Synonym(s): tracheobronchitis

Geriatric Considerations

Can be serious, particularly if part of influenza, with underlying COPD or CHF (3)

Pediatric Considerations

- Usually occurs in association with other conditions of upper and lower respiratory tract (trachea usually involved) (4)
- If repeated attacks occur, child should be evaluated for anomalies of the respiratory tract, immune deficiencies, or for chronic asthma.
- When acute bronchitis is caused by RSV, it may be fatal.
- Antitussive medication not indicated in patients younger than age 6 years (2).

EPIDEMIOLOGY

- Predominant age: all ages
- Predominant gender: male = female

Incidence

- ~5% of adults per year (5)
- Common cause of infection in children (4)

Prevalence

Results in 10–12 million office visits per year

ETIOLOGY AND PATHOPHYSIOLOGY

- Viral infections such as adenovirus, influenza A and B, parainfluenza virus, coxsackie virus, RSV, rhinovirus, coronavirus (types 1–3), herpes simplex virus (2)
- Bacterial infections, such as *Chlamydia pneumoniae* TWAR agent, *Mycoplasma*, *Bordetella pertussis*, *Haemophilus influenzae*, *Streptococcus pneumoniae*, *Moraxella catarrhalis*, and *Mycobacterium tuberculosis* (2)
- Secondary bacterial infection as part of an acute upper respiratory infection
- Possibly fungal infections
- Chemical irritants
- Acute bronchitis causes an injury to the epithelial surfaces, resulting in an increase in mucous production and thickening of the bronchiole wall (1).

Genetics

No known genetic pattern

RISK FACTORS

- Infants
- Elderly
- Air pollutants
- Smoking
- Secondhand smoke
- Environmental changes
- Chronic bronchopulmonary diseases
- Chronic sinusitis
- Tracheostomy
- Bronchopulmonary allergy
- Hypertrophied tonsils and adenoids in children
- Immunosuppression
  - Immunoglobulin deficiency
  - HIV infection
  - Alcoholism
- Gastroesophageal reflux disease (GERD)

GENERAL PREVENTION

- Avoid smoking and secondhand smoke.
- Control underlying risk factors (i.e., asthma, sinusitis, and reflux).
- Avoid exposure, especially daycare.
- Pneumovax, influenza immunization

COMMONLY ASSOCIATED CONDITIONS

- Allergic rhinitis
- Sinusitis
- Pharyngitis
- Epiglottitis (rare but can be rapidly fatal)
- Coryza
- Croup
- Influenza
- Pneumonia
- Asthma
- COPD/emphysema
- GERD

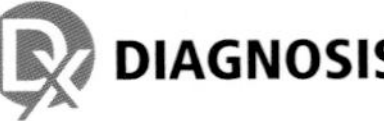

DIAGNOSIS

HISTORY

- Sudden onset of cough and no evidence of pneumonia, asthma, exacerbation of COPD, or the common cold (3)
- Cough is initially dry and nonproductive, then productive; later, mucopurulent sputum, which may indicate secondary infection
- Dyspnea, wheeze, fever, and fatigue may occur.
- Possible contact with others who have respiratory infections (1)

PHYSICAL EXAM

- Fever
- Tachypnea
- Pharynx injected
- Rales, rhonchi, wheezing
- No evidence of pulmonary consolidation

DIFFERENTIAL DIAGNOSIS

- Common cold
- Acute sinusitis
- Bronchopneumonia
- Influenza
- Bacterial tracheitis
- Bronchiectasis
- Asthma
- Reactive airways dysfunction syndrome (RADS)
- Allergy
- Eosinophilic pneumonitis
- Aspiration
- Retained foreign body
- Inhalation injury
- Cystic fibrosis
- Bronchogenic carcinoma
- Heart failure
- GERD

DIAGNOSTIC TESTS & INTERPRETATION

Initial Tests (lab, imaging)

- None normally needed; diagnosis is based on history and physical exam showing no postnasal drip or rales (1,3).
- For a complicated picture, consider the following:
  - WBC with differential
  - Sputum culture/sensitivity if CXR is abnormal (3)
  - Influenza titers (if appropriate for time of year) (1)
  - Viral panel
- No testing needed unless concerned about pneumonia
- CXR
  - Lungs normal, if uncomplicated
  - Helps to rule out other diseases (pneumonia) or complications

Follow-Up Tests & Special Considerations

- Arterial blood gases: hypoxemia (rarely)
- Pulmonary function tests (seldom needed during acute stages): increased residual volume, decreased maximal expiratory rate (2)

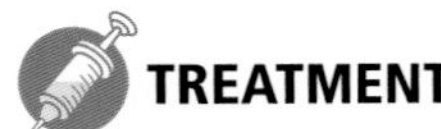

TREATMENT

GENERAL MEASURES

- Rest
- Stop smoking or avoid smoke.
- Steam inhalations
- Vaporizers
- Adequate hydration
- Antitussives
- Antibiotics are usually not recommended (1,3,6)[A].
- Treat associated illnesses (e.g., GERD).

MEDICATION

ALERT

Antibiotics are not recommended (1,3,6)[A] unless a treatable pathogen has been identified or significant comorbidities are present. This should be explained to patients who likely expect an antibiotic to be prescribed (3)[B].

First Line

- Supportive; increased fluids (cough results in increased fluid loss)
- Antipyretic analgesic such as aspirin, acetaminophen, or ibuprofen
- Decongestants if accompanied by sinus condition
- Cough suppressant for troublesome cough (not with COPD); honey, benzonatate (Tessalon), guaifenesin with codeine or dextromethorphan. Not indicated in children younger than age 6 years (2)[C]
- Mucolytic agents are not recommended (3)[B].
- Inhaled β-agonist (e.g., albuterol) or in combination with high-dose inhaled corticosteroids for cough with bronchospasm (2)[B]
- If influenza is highly suspected and symptom onset is <48 hours: oseltamivir (Tamiflu) or zanamivir (Relenza) (2)[B].
- Antibiotics ONLY if a treatable cause (i.e., pertussis) is identified (2)[A]
  - Clarithromycin (Biaxin): 500 mg q12h or azithromycin (Zithromax) Z-pack for atypical or pertussis infection (1)[A]
  - In patients with acute bronchitis of a suspected bacterial cause, azithromycin tends to be more effective in terms of lower incidence of treatment failure and adverse events than amoxicillin or amoxicillin-clavulanic acid (7)[B].
    - Doxycycline: 100 mg/day × 10 days if *Moraxella*, *Chlamydia*, or *Mycoplasma* suspected
    - Quinolone for more serious infections or other antibiotic failure or in elderly or patients with multiple comorbidities
- Contraindication(s): Doxycycline and quinolones should not be used during pregnancy or in children.
- Precautions:
  - Multiple antibiotics have the potential to interfere with the effectiveness of PO contraceptives.
  - Antibiotic use can be associated with *Clostridium difficile* infections.
  - Cough and cold preparations should not be used in children <6 years (2)[B].

Second Line

Other antibiotics if indicated by sputum culture

ISSUES FOR REFERRAL

- Complications such as pneumonia or respiratory failure
- Comorbidities such as COPD
- Cough lasting >3 months

ADDITIONAL THERAPIES

- Antipyretic for fever (e.g., acetaminophen, aspirin, or ibuprofen)
- Inhaled β-agonist (e.g., albuterol) or in combination with high dose inhaled corticosteroids for cough with bronchospasm (2)[B]
- Oral corticosteroids probably not indicated (2)[C]

COMPLEMENTARY & ALTERNATIVE MEDICINE

Throat lozenges for pharyngitis

INPATIENT CONSIDERATIONS

Admission Criteria/Initial Stabilization

- Hypoxia
- Severe bronchospasm
- Exacerbation of underlying disease
- Outpatient, unless elderly or complicated by severe underlying disease
- May require supplemental oxygen in selected patients
- Bronchodilators if patient is bronchospastic

IV Fluids

May be helpful if patient is dehydrated

Nursing

- Ensure patient comfort and monitor for signs of deterioration, especially if underlying lung disease exists.
- May need to follow oxygen saturation in patients with underlying lung disease

Discharge Criteria

Improvement in symptoms and comorbidities

ONGOING CARE

FOLLOW-UP RECOMMENDATIONS

- Usually a self-limited disease not requiring follow-up
- Cough may linger for several weeks.
- In children, if recurrent, need to consider other diagnoses, such as asthma (6)

PATIENT MONITORING

- Oximetry until no longer hypoxemic
- Recheck for chronicity.

DIET

Increased fluids (3–4 L/day) while febrile

PATIENT EDUCATION

- For patient education materials favorably reviewed on this topic, contact the American Lung Association: 1740 Broadway, New York, NY 10019 (212) 315-8700; www.lungusa.org.
- American Academy of Family Physicians: www.familydoctor.org

PROGNOSIS

- Usual: complete resolution
- Can be serious in the elderly or debilitated
- Cough may persist for several weeks after an initial improvement.
- Postbronchitic reactive airways disease (rare)
- Bronchiolitis obliterans and organizing pneumonia (rare)

COMPLICATIONS

- Superinfection such as bronchopneumonia
- Bronchiectasis
- Hemoptysis
- Acute respiratory failure
- Chronic cough

REFERENCES

1. Wenzel RP, Fowler AA. Clinical practice. Acute bronchitis. *N Engl J Med*. 2006;355(20):2125–2130.
2. Albert RH. Diagnosis and treatment of acute bronchitis. *Am Fam Physician*. 2010;82(11):1345–1350.
3. Braman SS. Chronic cough due to acute bronchitis: ACCP evidence-based clinical practice guidelines. *Chest*. 2006;129(1)(Suppl):95S–103S.
4. Fleming DM, Elliot AJ. The management of acute bronchitis in children. *Expert Opin Pharmacother*. 2007;8(4):415–426.
5. Llor L, Moragas A, Bayona C, et al. Efficacy of anti-inflammatory or antibiotic treatment in patients with non-complicated acute bronchitis and discolored sputum: randomized placebo controlled trial. *BMJ*. 2013;347:f5762.
6. Gonzales R, Anderer T, McCulloch C, et al. A cluster randomized trial of decision support for reducing antibiotic use in acute bronchitis. *JAMA Intern Med*. 2013;173(4): 267–273.
7. Panpanich R, Lerttrakarnnon P, Laopaiboon M. Azithromycin for acute lower respiratory tract infections. *Cochrane Database Syst Rev*. 2008;(1):CD001954.

SEE ALSO

- Asthma; Chronic Obstructive Pulmonary Disease and Emphysema
- Algorithm: Cough, Chronic

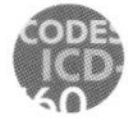

CODES

ICD10

- J20.9 Acute bronchitis, unspecified
- J68.0 Bronchitis and pneumonitis due to chemicals, gases, fumes and vapors
- B97.0 Adenovirus as the cause of diseases classified elsewhere

CLINICAL PEARLS

- Acute bronchitis is a common and generally self-limited disease.
- It usually does not require treatment with antibiotics. This needs to be explained to patients who expect antibiotics to be prescribed.
- Cough may linger for several weeks.
- Recurrent or seasonal episodes may suggest another disease process, such as asthma.

BULIMIA NERVOSA

Umer Farooq, MD, MBBS • Najm Hasan Siddiqui, MD

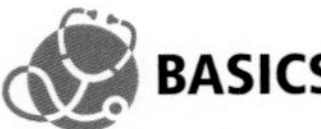

BASICS

DESCRIPTION
- A pattern of discrete periods of uncontrolled eating (within 2-hour period), followed by compensatory behaviors (at least 1 time per week for 3 months)
- *DSM-V* classifies bulimia nervosa as:
  - Mild: 1–3 episodes of compensatory behaviors
  - Moderate: 4–7 episodes of compensatory behaviors
  - Severe: 8–13 episodes of compensatory behaviors
  - Extreme: 14 or more episodes of compensatory behaviors
- System(s) affected: oropharyngeal; endocrine/metabolic; gastrointestinal; dermatologic; cardiovascular; nervous

EPIDEMIOLOGY
- Predominant age: adolescents and young adults
- Mean age of onset: 18–21 years
- Predominant sex: female > male (10–20:1)

Incidence
28.8 women, 0.8 men per 100,000 per year

Prevalence
- More prevalent than anorexia nervosa
- 1–3% in women age 16–35 years
- 0.5% in young men (higher among gay and bisexual men)

ETIOLOGY AND PATHOPHYSIOLOGY
- Combination of biologic, psychological, environmental, and social factors. Unique contribution of any specific factor remains unclear.
- Strong evidence of serotonergic dysregulation in bulimia nervosa
- Substantial literature shows genetic evidence for bulimia nervosa (1)[B].

RISK FACTORS
- Female gender
- History of obesity and dieting
- Body dissatisfaction
- Critical comments by family or others about weight, body shape, or eating
- Severe life stressor
- Low self-esteem
- Perceived pressure to be thin
- Perfectionist or obsessive thinking
- Poor impulse control, alcohol misuse
- Environment stressing high achievement, physical fitness (e.g., armed forces, ballet, cheerleading, gymnastics, or modeling)
- Family history of substance abuse, affective disorders, eating disorder, or obesity
- Type 1 diabetes
- Sexual abuse is not causally related to bulimia.

GENERAL PREVENTION
- Prevention programs can reduce risk factors and future onset of eating disorders (2)[A].
- Target adolescents and young women ≥15 years
- Realistic and healthy weight management strategies and attitudes
- Decrease body dissatisfaction and promote self-esteem.
- Reduce focus on thin as ideal.
- Decrease anxiety/depressive symptoms and improve stress management.

COMMONLY ASSOCIATED CONDITIONS
- Major depression and dysthymia
- Anxiety disorders
- Substance abuse/dependence
- Bipolar disorder
- Obsessive-compulsive disorder
- Borderline personality disorder

DIAGNOSIS

HISTORY
- Patients unlikely to self-identify binge eating or purging behaviors; corroborate with parent/relative
- Unhappiness and/or preoccupation with weight and diet attempts
- Pattern of restricting diet, binge eating, and compensatory behaviors:
  - Binge is context specific (usually within 2-hour period, they will eat what would be an unusually large amount for most people)
  - Vomiting (often with little effort)
  - Vigorous aerobic exercise
  - Distress/shame related to loss of control
- Depressed mood and self-depreciation following the binges
- Relief following the purges
- Other possible signs and symptoms:
  - Requesting weight loss help and mildly underweight to overweight
  - Diet pill, diuretic, laxative, ipecac, and thyroid medication use/abuse
  - Menstrual disturbance
  - Fatigue and lethargy
  - Abdominal pain, bloating, constipation, diarrhea, rectal prolapse
  - Sore throat
  - Thermal tooth sensitivity
  - Frequent fluctuations in weight
  - Omission/underdosing insulin in diabetes patients

PHYSICAL EXAM
- Often normal
- Bradycardia
- Eroded tooth enamel
- Perimylolysis
- Cheilosis
- Gingivitis
- Sialadenosis
- Asymptomatic, noninflammatory parotid gland enlargement
- Epigastric tenderness to palpation
- Calluses, abrasions, bruising on hand, thumb (Russell sign)
- Peripheral edema

DIFFERENTIAL DIAGNOSIS
- Anorexia, binge eating/purging type
- Major depressive disorder
- Anxiety disorders
- Malabsorption
- Addison disease
- Celiac disease
- Diabetes mellitus
- Hyperthyroidism, hypothyroidism
- Hyperpituitarism
- Hypothalamic brain tumor
- Kleine-Levin syndrome
- Body dysmorphic disorder
- Borderline personality disorder

DIAGNOSTIC TESTS & INTERPRETATION
All lab results may be within normal limits and are not necessary for diagnosis.
- Psychological self-report screening tests may be helpful, but diagnosis is based on meeting the *DSM-IV-TR* criteria:
  - Eating Disorder Inventory
  - Eating Disorder Screen for Primary Care

Initial Tests (lab, imaging)
- Blood work
  - Hypokalemia, hypochloremia
  - Hypomagnesemia, hyponatremia, hypocalcemia, hypophosphatemia
  - Serum amylase levels
  - Alkalosis
  - Elevated BUN
  - Hypoglycemia
- Urinalysis
  - Increased urine specific gravity

Diagnostic Procedures/Other
Electrocardiogram
- Bradycardia or arrhythmias
- Conduction defects
- Depressed ST segment due to hypokalemia

Test Interpretation
- Esophagitis
- Acute pancreatitis
- Cardiomyopathy and muscle weakness due to ipecac abuse
- Melanosis coli
- Cathartic colon syndrome
- Delayed or arrested skeletal growth
- Stress fracture
- Irreversible dental erosions
- Osteopenia/osteoporosis

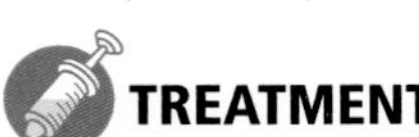

TREATMENT

- Cognitive-behavioral therapy (CBT) should be considered as first-line treatment (3,4)[A].
- Guided self-help therapies may be effective.
- Interpersonal therapies and group therapies have been found to be helpful.

GENERAL MEASURES
- Psychotherapies should be employed as first-line treatments.
- Multidisciplinary team:
  - Primary care physician, behavioral health provider, nutritionist
- Build trust; increase motivation for change
- Assess psychological and nutritional status
- Consider evidence-based self-help program

- CBT for bulimia nervosa (3,4)[A]:
  - 16–20 50-minute appointments
  - Involve patient in establishing goals.
  - Self-monitoring of food intake, frequency of binges/purges, related antecedents, consequences, thoughts, and emotions
  - Self-monitoring of weight once per week
  - Educate about ineffectiveness of purging for weight control and adverse outcomes
  - Establish prescribed eating plan to develop regular eating habits and realistic weight goal
  - Gradually introduce feared foods into diet
  - Problem-solve how to cope with triggers
  - Decrease ruminations about calories, weight, and purging
  - Challenge fear of loss of control
  - Establish relapse prevention plan
  - Gradual laxative withdrawal
- Interpersonal therapy:
  - May act more slowly than CBT
- Transdiagnostic CBT
- Dialectical behavior therapy
- Family therapy for adolescents
- Nutritional education, relaxation techniques
- Educate patient to brush teeth and use baking soda to rinse mouth after vomiting.

MEDICATION

First Line

- Selective serotonin reuptake inhibitors (SSRIs) (5)[A],(6)[B], particularly fluoxetine (Prozac) titrated to 60 mg/day, are effective in reducing symptoms with relatively few side effects. Higher doses than standard doses for depression are often needed:
  - Combination of medication and CBT has been shown to have added benefit over medication or therapy alone.
- To prevent relapse, maintain antidepressant at full therapeutic dose for at least 1 year.
- Avoid bupropion: contraindicated due to its association with seizures in patients who purge
- Precautions:
  - Serious toxicity following overdose is common.
  - Patients may vomit medications.

Second Line

- Select different SSRI.
- Tricyclic antidepressants (imipramine, nortriptyline)
- Ondansetron (Zofran) 4–8 mg TID between meals can help prevent vomiting.
- Psyllium (Metamucil) preparations, 1 tbs QHS with glass of water, can prevent constipation during laxative withdrawal.

ISSUES FOR REFERRAL

- Patients with bulimia require a multidisciplinary team, including a primary care physician, behavioral health provider, and a nutritionist. Important part of treatment is to arrange mental health therapist for psychotherapy.
- Binge eating disorder: Lisdexamfetamin dimesylate (Vyvnase) was approved in 2015; dosing: titrate from 30–70 mg q AM.

ADDITIONAL THERAPIES

Most patients can be treated as outpatients.

COMPLEMENTARY & ALTERNATIVE MEDICINE

Bright light therapy may help.

INPATIENT CONSIDERATIONS

- If possible, admit to a specialized eating disorders unit.
- Supervised meals and bathroom privileges
- Monitor weight and physical activity.
- Monitor electrolytes.
- Gradually shift control to patients as they demonstrate improvement.

Admission Criteria/Initial Stabilization

Hospitalize if severe malnutrition, dehydration, electrolyte disturbances, cardiac dysrhythmia, uncontrolled binging and purging, psychiatric emergency (threat to self/others), or if outpatient treatment failed.

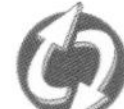

ONGOING CARE

FOLLOW-UP RECOMMENDATIONS

Patient Monitoring

- Binge–purge activity, including antecedents and consequences
- Level of exercise activity
- Self-esteem, comfort with body and self
- Ruminations and depressive symptoms
- Repeat any abnormal lab values weekly or monthly until stable.

DIET

- Balanced diet, normal eating pattern
- Reintroduce feared foods.

PATIENT EDUCATION

- Astrachan-Fletcher E, Maslar M. *The Dialectical Behavior Therapy Skills Workbook for Bulimia: Using DBT to Break the Cycle and Regain Cntrol of Your Life*. Oakland, CA: New Harbinger; 2009.
- http://www.mayoclinic.org/diseases-conditions/bulimia/basics/definition/con-20033050
- http://www.nami.org/helpline/bulimia.htm

PROGNOSIS

- After effective CBT:
  - In the short term, 50% of treated individuals do not meet criteria for diagnosis.
  - In the long term (2–10 years), 70% may be asymptomatic.
  - Symptomatic individuals may demonstrate remissions, relapses, subclinical, or other eating disorder–related behaviors.
- Untreated
  - Likely to remain chronic/relapsing problem
- Greater weight fluctuations, other impulsive behaviors, childhood obesity, low self-esteem, family history of alcohol abuse, psychiatric comorbidity, and personality disorder diagnoses (e.g., avoidant personality disorder) may predict poor prognosis.
- Mortality rate: 0.4%

COMPLICATIONS

- Drug and alcohol abuse
- Osteopenia/osteoporosis
- Stress fracture
- Gastric dilatation
- Boerhaave syndrome
- Mallory-Weiss tears
- Pseudo-Bartter syndrome
- Spontaneous pneumomediastinum
- Potassium depletion, cardiac arrhythmia, cardiac arrest
- Suicide

Pregnancy Considerations

Maternal and fetal problems if pregnant:

- Binging/purging behaviors may persist, increase, or decrease with pregnancy.
- Increased risk for preterm delivery, operative delivery, and infants with low birth weight should be managed as high risk.

REFERENCES

1. Raevuori A. Genetic etiology of eating disorders, *Duodecim*. 2013;129(20):2126–2132.
2. Stice E, Shaw H, Marti CN. A meta-analytic review of eating disorder prevention programs: encouraging findings. *Annu Rev Clin Psychol*. 2007;3:207–231.
3. Hay PP, Bacaltchuk J, Stefano S, et al. Psychological treatments for bulimia nervosa and binging. *Cochrane Database Syst Rev*. 2009;(4):CD000562.
4. Shapiro JR, Berkman ND, Brownley KA, et al. Bulimia nervosa treatment: a systematic review of randomized controlled trials. *Int J Eat Disord*. 2007;40(4):321–336.
5. Bacaltchuk J, Hay P, Trefiglio R. Antidepressants versus psychological treatments and their combination for bulimia nervosa. *Cochrane Database Sys Rev*. 2001;(4):CD003385.
6. Bellini M, Merli M. current drug treatment of patients with bulimia nervosa and binge-eating disorder: selective serotonin reuptake inhibitors versus mood stabilizers. *Int J Psychiatry Clin Pract*. 2004;8(4):235–243.

ADDITIONAL READING

- American Psychiatric Association. *Practice Guideline for the Treatment of Patients with Eating Disorders*. 3rd ed. Washington, DC: American Psychiatric Association. http:www.psych.org. Accessed 2014.
- National Institute for Clinical Excellence. *Eating Disorders: Core Interventions in the Treatment of Anorexia Nervosa, Bulimia Nervosa, and Related Eating Disorders*. NICE Clinical Guideline no. 9. London, United Kingdom: National Institute for Clinical Excellence; 2004. http://www.nice.org.uk. Accessed 2014.

SEE ALSO

- Anorexia Nervosa; Hyperkalemia; Laxative Abuse; Salivary Gland Tumors
- Algorithm: Weight Loss

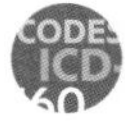

CODES

ICD10

F50.2 Bulimia nervosa

CLINICAL PEARLS

- Asking "Are you satisfied with your eating patterns?" and/or "Do you worry that you have lost control over how much you eat?" may help to screen for an eating problem.
- Weight is not severely lowered as in anorexia nervosa.
- Consider using a stepped-care approach. Start with a guided self-help program using instructional aids; next, begin CBT (e.g., 16–20 sessions over 4–5 months).
- SSRIs, particularly fluoxetine (60 mg daily), may be helpful as a 1st step or as an adjunctive treatment with CBT.

BUNION (HALLUX VALGUS)

Jennifer G. Chang, MD, Maj, USAF, MC

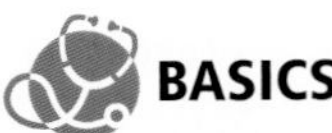

BASICS

DESCRIPTION

- Lateral deviation of the great toe. Hallux valgus derives from the Latin for "big toe askew"; also commonly known as a bunion
- This lateral deviation with medial deviation of the 1st metatarsal leads to a medial prominence of the 1st metatarsophalangeal (MTP) joint and a potentially painful and/or debilitating deformity.
- Progressive subluxation of the 1st MTP joint is common.
- System(s) affected: musculoskeletal/skin

EPIDEMIOLOGY

- Predominant age: more common in adults
  - Estimated 23% in adults aged 18–65 years
  - Estimated 35.7% in elderly >65 years
- Predominant sex: female > male by ~2:1

Prevalence

- Prevalence increases with age particularly in females.
- Juvenile hallux valgus
  - More common in girls (>80% of cases)
- Commonly bilateral
- Pain is not usually the presenting symptom.

ETIOLOGY AND PATHOPHYSIOLOGY

Multifactorial. Contributing factors include the following:

- Valgus deviation of the hallux promotes varus position of the first metatarsal.
- Medial MTP joint capsule stretches and attenuates while the lateral capsule contracts.
- Metatarsal head moves medially, causing the sesamoid bones to a lateral position.
- Extensor hallucis longus deviates laterally.
- Lateral and plantar migration of abductor hallucis moves the great toe into plantar flexion and pronation laterally.
- Medial collateral ligament stretches and eventually ruptures due to this deviation, decreasing stability and causing progressive subluxation of the 1st MTP joint.

RISK FACTORS

- Familial predisposition
- Abnormal biomechanics (i.e., flexible flat feet)
- Joint laxity
- Pronation of hindfoot
- Achilles tendon contracture
- Pes planus (fallen arches)
- Metatarsus primus varus
- Amputation of 2nd toe
- Inflammatory joint disease
- Neuromuscular disorders
- Improper footwear, narrow toe box

GENERAL PREVENTION

Although the condition is known to be familial, proper foot wear may decrease the progression of the disease.

COMMONLY ASSOCIATED CONDITIONS

- Medial bursitis of the 1st MTP joint (most common)
- Hammertoe deformity of the 2nd phalanx
- Plantar callus
- Metatarsalgia
- Degeneration of 1st metatarsal head cartilage
- Pronated feet
- Ankle equinus
- Onychocryptosis (Ingrown toenail)
- Entrapment of the medial dorsal cutaneous nerve
- Synovitis of the MTP joint

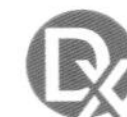

DIAGNOSIS

- Based on clinical exam
- Radiographs are used for staging

HISTORY

- Painful MTP joint (most common symptom in adults)
- Abnormal position of great toe
- Enlargement of the MTP joint medially (patients complain of a "bump")
- Shoes don't fit properly
- Pain on ambulation
- Skin irritation, blistering, callus formation at 1st MTP

PHYSICAL EXAM

- Observe gait; may be antalgic due to pain
- Increased distal metatarsal articular angle (DMAA)
- Medial prominence at the MTP joint
- Inflammation and ulceration at the MTP joint medially
- Skin changes: inflammation, blistering, callus formation
- Great toe over- or underriding the 2nd toe
- Examine the entire first ray for the following:
  - 1st MTP range of motion
  - 1st tarsometatarsal mobility
  - Neurovascular integrity
  - Degenerative osteoarthritis

DIFFERENTIAL DIAGNOSIS

- Trauma
  - Turf toe
  - Sesamoiditis
  - Stress fracture
- Infection
  - Osteomyelitis
  - Septic arthritis
- Joint disorder
  - Osteoarthritis
  - Rheumatoid arthritis
  - Pseudogout
  - Gout
- Tendon disorder
  - Tendinosis
  - Tenosynovitis
  - Tendon rupture
- Other
  - Bursitis
  - Ganglia
  - Foreign body granuloma

DIAGNOSTIC TESTS & INTERPRETATION

- Weight-bearing AP and lateral radiographs (sesamoid view optional) to assess for the following:
  - Joint congruency and degenerative changes
  - Lateral sesamoid bone displacement (1)[A]
  - Rounded 1st MT head (1)[A]
  - Longer 1st metatarsal (1)[A]
- Radiographic parameters:
  - Hallux valgus angle: Long axis of the 1st MT and proximal phalanx is normally <15 degrees.
  - Intermetatarsal angle: Between long axis of 1st and 2nd MT is normally <9 degrees.
  - DMAA: Between 1st MT long axis and line through base of distal articular cap is normally <15 degrees.
  - Hallux valgus interphalangeus: Between long axis of distal phalanx and proximal phalanx is normally <10 degrees.

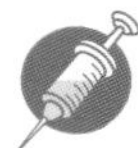

TREATMENT

- Primary indication for treatment is pain.
- There are conservative and surgical approaches.
- Surgical treatment is generally more effective in improving pain; surgery has attendant risks.

GENERAL MEASURES

Several nonoperative treatment options may improve symptoms and delay the progression of hallux valgus deformity, although high-quality evidence is limited:

- Proper fitting footwear: low-heeled, wide-toe shoes to decrease stress on MTP joint (i.e., wide toe box)
- Orthoses: Shoe inserts to correct foot alignment (pes planus and overpronation). Improving gait may prevent bunion formation and reduce pressure on the MTP.
- Night splinting: In theory, splinting stabilizes and balances soft tissue structures around the MTP. Limited evidence shows improvement in degree of angulation in mild hallux valgus.
- Manual and manipulative therapy (MMT): stretches contracted soft tissue
- Foot exercises and stretching to improve intrinsic foot muscle strength and increase range of motion
- Pads/spacers: Pads can decrease friction on the MTP joint. Placement of a toe spacer in the 1st interdigital space can straighten the hallux and may reduce pain (2)[C].

MEDICATION

- Topical and PO medications (NSAIDs) can be used to relieve pain and swelling. Other topical options include capsaicin cream.
- Corticosteroid injections improve the pain associated with bunions.

ADDITIONAL THERAPIES

Custom orthoses are a safe intervention that may decrease pain at 6 and 12 months compared with no treatment; however, this improvement is less than that seen with surgical intervention (3)[B].

SURGERY/OTHER PROCEDURES

- Surgery is indicated if patient has severe pain, dysfunction, or symptoms that do not abate with conservative therapy.
- Surgery is more beneficial than conservative therapy for patients with severe symptoms (3)[B]:
  - >150 different surgical techniques to treat hallux valgus; however, none has been proven to be superior, and no universally accepted standard exists for selecting 1 procedure over another.
  - Choice of surgical technique depends on the severity of disease, the HA and IM angles, congruency and subluxation of the MTP joint, patient-specific factors, and the pathologic element the surgeon determines needs correcting. Examples include the following:
    - Arthrodesis: fusion of the 1st MTP joint; reserved for severe and/or recurrent hallux valgus
    - Arthroplasty: removing the joint or replacing it with a prosthesis
    - Exostectomy/bunionectomy: removing the medial bony prominence of the MTP joint
    - Soft tissue realignment: alters the function of surrounding ligaments and tendons; used for minor, flexible deformities
    - Osteotomy and realignment: can correct large deformities, but evidence of long-term outcome is lacking (4)[C]
    - Mini-tight rope procedure: use of a Fiberwire to correct the misalignment of the deformity; reportedly allows for faster recovery and earlier weight bearing (5)[C]
- Surgery can decrease pain and increase foot alignment in patients. However, some may have little to no improvement in symptoms despite interventions.
- Establishing realistic expectations prior to surgery may improve patient satisfaction (6)[C].
- In pediatric patients, surgery should generally be delayed until skeletal maturity (7)[C].

COMPLEMENTARY & ALTERNATIVE MEDICINE

Marigold ointment may reduce pain and soft tissue swelling over an 8-week period (8)[C].

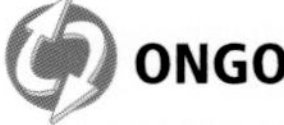

ONGOING CARE

FOLLOW-UP RECOMMENDATIONS

- Postoperative treatment may include physical therapy, physiotherapy, use of supportive shoe, continuous passive motion, or manual manipulation.
- Time until full weight bearing depends on the surgical procedure. Patients should follow instructions based on individual procedure

PROGNOSIS

Patient outcome varies depending on biomechanical factors, severity of the deformity, and treatment modality used. The radiologic HA angle is a predictor of surgical correction; patients with an HA angle <37 degrees have a higher chance of having the deformity successfully corrected with surgery compared with patients with an HA angle >37 degrees (9)[C].

COMPLICATIONS

- Risks associated with surgery include infection, lack of improvement in pain, and poor cosmetic result.
- Additional risks vary with the type of surgical procedure.
- Other complications may include the following:
  - Early swelling
  - Hallux varus
  - Recurrence of bunion
  - Decreased sensation over the 1st metatarsal or phalanx

REFERENCES

1. Nix SE, Vicenzino BT, Collins NJ, et al. Characteristics of foot structure and footwear associated with hallux valgus: a systematic review. *Osteoarthritis and Cartilage*. 2012;20(10):1059–1074.
2. Tehraninasr A, Saeedi H, Forogh B, et al. Effects of insole with toe-separator and night splint on patients with painful hallux valgus: a comparative study. *Prosthet Ortho Int*. 2008;32(1):78–83.
3. Torkki M, Malmivaara A, Seitsalo S, et al. Surgery vs. orthosis vs. watchful for hallux valgus: a randomized controlled trial. *JAMA*. 2001;285(19):2474–2480.
4. Choi JH, Zide JR, Coleman SC, et al. Prospective study of treatment of adult primary hallux valgus with scarf osteotomy and soft tissue realignment. *Foot Ankle Int*. 2013;34(5):684–690.
5. Holmes GB, Hsu AR. Correction of intermetatarsal angle in hallux valgus using small suture button device. *Foot Ankle Int*. 2013;34(4):543–549.
6. Dux K, Smith N, Rottier FJ. Outcome after metatarsal osteotomy for hallux valgus: a study of postoperative foot function using revised foot function index short form. *J Foot Ankle Surg*. 2013;52(4):422–425.
7. Chell J, Dhar S. Pediatric hallux valgus. *Foot Ankle Clin*. 2014;19(2):235–243.
8. Khan MT. The podiatric treatment of hallux abductor valgus and its associated condition, bunion, with Tagetes patula. *J Pharm Pharmacol*. 1996;48(7):768–770.
9. Deenik AR, de Visser E, Louwerens JW, et al. Hallux valgus angle as main predictor for correction of hallux valgus. *BMC Musculoskelet Disord*. 2008;9:70.

ADDITIONAL READING

- Glasoe WM, Nuckley DJ, Ludewig PM, et al. Hallux valgus and the first metatarsal arch segment: a theoretical biomechanical perspective. *Phys Ther*. 2010;90(1):110–120.
- Mafulli NI, Longo UG, Marinozzi AN, et al. Hallux valgus: effectiveness and safety of minimally invasive surgery. A systematic review. *Brit Med Bull*. 2010;97:149–167.
- Nix S. Prevalence of hallux valgus in the general population: a systemic review and meta-analysis. *J Foot Ankle Res*. 2010;3:21.
- Perera AM, Mason L, Stephens MM. The pathogenesis of hallux valgus. *J Bone Joint Surg Am*. 2011;93(17):1650–1661.
- Schuh R, Hofstaetter SG, Adams SB, et al. Rehabilitation after hallux valgus surgery: importance of physical therapy to restore weight bearing of the first day during the stance phase. *Phys Ther*. 2009;89(9):934–945.
- Smith SE, Landorf KB, Butterworth PA, et al. Scarf versus chevron osteotomy for the correction of 1–2 intermetatarsal angle in hallux valgus: a systematic review and meta-analysis. *J Foot Ankle Surg*. 2012;51(4):437–444.
- Trnka HJ, Krenn S, Schuh R. Minimally invasive hallux valgus surgery: a critical review of the evidence. *Int Orthop*. 2013;37(9):1731–1735.

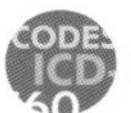

CODES

ICD10

- M20.10 Hallux valgus (acquired), unspecified foot
- M20.11 Hallux valgus (acquired), right foot
- M20.12 Hallux valgus (acquired), left foot

CLINICAL PEARLS

- Avoiding footwear with high heels, pointed toe boxes, or inadequate toe space may reduce development or progression of bunions.
- Surgery generally results in superior outcomes for pain relief in appropriately selected patients.
- No single surgical method has shown to be superior for long-term pain relief.
- Establishing realistic expectations prior to surgery may improve patient satisfaction.

BURNS

James R. Yon, MD • Edward James Kruse, DO

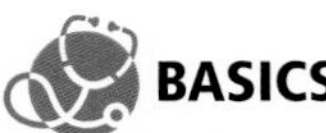

BASICS

DESCRIPTION

- Tissue injuries caused by application of heat, chemicals, electricity, or irradiation
- Extent of injury (depth of burn) is result of intensity and duration of exposure.
  - 1st degree involves superficial layers of epidermis
  - 2nd degree involves varying amounts of epidermis (with blister formation) and part of the dermis
  - 3rd degree involves destruction of all skin elements (full thickness) with coagulation of subdermal plexus
- System(s) affected: endocrine/metabolic, pulmonary, skin/exocrine

Geriatric Considerations

- Prognosis is poorer for severe burns.
- Patients >60 years of age account for 11% of burns.

Pediatric Considerations

Consider child abuse or neglect when dealing with hot water burns in children; abuse accounts for 15% of pediatric burns. Special concerns are sharply demarcated wounds, immersion injuries, and suspect stories. Involve child welfare services early.

EPIDEMIOLOGY

- Predominant age: 30 years; 13% infants; 11% >60 years of age
- Predominant gender: males account for 70%

Incidence

Per year in the United States

- 1.2–2 million burns; 700,000 emergency room visits; 45,000–50,000 hospitalizations; 3,900 deaths owing to burn-related complications
- In children: 250,000 burns; 15,000 hospitalizations; 1,100 deaths
- Estimated total cost of $2 billion annually for burn care
- House fires cause 75% of deaths.
- Burn deaths decreasing nationally due to improved prevention and treatment
- Increase in burns from the illegal production of methamphetamines. Patients can present with a combination of chemical burn, thermal burn, and explosion injury.

ETIOLOGY AND PATHOPHYSIOLOGY

- Open flame and hot liquid are the most common causes of burns (heat usually ≥45°C): flame burns more common in adults; scald burns more common in children.
- Caustic chemicals or acids (may show little signs or symptoms for the first few days)
- Electricity (may have significant injury with very little damage to overlying skin)
- Excess sun exposure

RISK FACTORS

- Water heaters set too high
- Workplace exposure to chemicals, electricity, or irradiation
- Young children and older adults with thin skin are more susceptible to injury
- Carelessness with burning cigarettes: related to 18% of fatal fires in 2006
- Inadequate or faulty electrical wiring
- Lack of smoke detectors: Lacking or nonfunctioning smoke alarms are implicated in 63% of residential fires.
- Arson: cause of 27% of fires that resulted in fatalities in 2006

GENERAL PREVENTION

Home safety education should be a key mechanism for injury prevention.

- Families educated on home safety were more likely to have safe hot water temperatures.
- Safety education results in more families having functioning smoke alarms and increased use of fireguards.
- There is no evidence that home safety education results in increasing the chance of possessing a fire extinguisher.
- Home safety education did not improve the odds of keeping hot drinks or food out of reach of children and did not increase the safe storage of matches.
- There is a lack of evidence that home safety education (with or without the provision of safety equipment) results in a reduction of thermal injuries.

COMMONLY ASSOCIATED CONDITIONS

Smoke inhalation syndrome

- May involve thermal burn to respiratory mucosa (e.g., trachea, bronchi) as well as carbon monoxide inhalation
- Occurs within 72 hours of burn
- Should be suspected in all burns occurring in an enclosed space or exposure to explosions

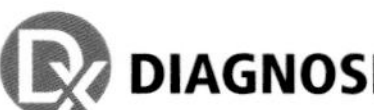

DIAGNOSIS

HISTORY

- History of source of burn
- In children or elderly: Check for consistency between the history and the burn's physical characteristics.

PHYSICAL EXAM

- 1st degree
  - Erythema of involved tissue
  - Skin blanches with pressure
  - Skin may be tender
- 2nd degree
  - Skin is red and blistered.
  - Skin is very tender.
- 3rd degree
  - Burned skin is tough and leathery.
  - Skin nontender
- Rule of 9s (1)[C]
  - Each upper extremity: adult and child 9%
  - Each lower extremity: adult 18%; child 14%
  - Anterior trunk: adult and child 18%
  - Posterior trunk: adult and child 18%
  - Head and neck: adult 10%; child 18%
- Quick estimate: The surface area of the patient's hand (palmar surface plus fingers) is 1% of the body surface area (BSA).
- Careful documentation of extent of burn and the estimated depth of burn
- Check for any signs suggestive of potential airway involvement: singed nasal hair, facial burns, carbonaceous sputum, progressive hoarseness, inflamed oropharynx, circumferential burns around the neck, tachypnea

DIAGNOSTIC TESTS & INTERPRETATION

- Children: glucose (hypoglycemia may occur in children because of limited glycogen storage)
- Smoke inhalation: arterial blood gas, carboxyhemoglobin
- Electrical burns: ECG, urine myoglobin, creatine kinase isoenzymes

Initial Tests (lab, imaging)

- Hematocrit
- Type and cross
- Electrolytes, including BUN and creatinine
- Urinalysis
- Chest radiograph
- Xenon scan useful in suspected smoke inhalation

Diagnostic Procedures/Other

Bronchoscopy may be necessary in smoke inhalation to evaluate lower respiratory tract (2)[A].

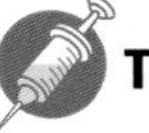

TREATMENT

- Prehospital care (1)[C]
  - Remove the patient from the source of burn
  - Extinguish and remove all burning clothing
  - Room-temperature water may be poured onto burn but only in the first 15 minutes following burn exposure.
  - Wrap patient to prevent hypothermia.
  - All patients to receive 100% oxygen via face mask
- Hospitalization for all serious burns
  - 2nd-degree burns >10% of BSA
  - Any 3rd-degree burn
  - Burns of hands, feet, face, or perineum
  - Electrical or lightning burns
  - Inhalation injury
  - Chemical burns
  - Circumferential burn
- Transfer to burn center for (3)[C]
  - 2nd- and 3rd-degree burns >10% of BSA in patients <10 years and >50 years of age
  - 2nd-degree burns >20% of BSA and full-thickness burns >5% BSA in any age range
  - 3rd-degree burns in any age group
  - Burns of hands, feet, face, or perineum
  - Electrical or lightning burns
  - Inhalation injury
  - Chemical burns
  - Circumferential burn
  - Burns in patients with additional trauma (fractures, etc.) in which the burn is the more severe injury. Otherwise, send to trauma center for stabilization.
  - Burn injuries in patients with preexisting medical conditions that could affect management, mortality, or recovery

GENERAL MEASURES

- Based on depth of burns and accurate estimate of total BSA involved (rule of 9s)
- Tetanus prophylaxis (if not current)
- Remove all rings, watches, and other items from injured extremities to avoid tourniquet effect.
- Remove clothing and cover all burned areas with dry sheets.
- Flush area of chemical burn (for ~2 hours).
- For all major burns, use 100% oxygen administration; consider early intubation.
- Do not apply ice to burn site.
- Nasogastric tube (high risk of paralytic ileus)
- Foley catheter
- Analgesia
- ECG monitoring in first 24 hours following electrical burn

- Whirlpool hydrotherapy followed by silver sulfadiazine (Silvadene) occlusive dressings in severe burns
- Daily or BID cleansing with dressing changes
- Burn fluid resuscitation (1)[C]
  - Calculate fluid resuscitation from time of burn, not from time treatment begins.
  - 2–4 mL lactated Ringer × body weight (kg) × % BSA burn (1/2 given in first 8 hours, in second 8 hours, and in third 8 hours); in children, this is given in addition to maintenance fluids and is adjusted according to urine output and vital signs. Protocol-based resuscitation leads to superior outcomes.
  - Colloid solutions are not recommended during the first 12–24 hours of resuscitation (1)[C],(4)[A].
  - Other: Use of biologic membranes or skin substitutes may be indicated for burn coverage.
- Inhalation injury
  - Intubation, ventilation with positive end-expiratory pressure assistance
  - Hyperbaric oxygen treatment may be useful in patients with carbon monoxide levels >25%, patients with coma, focal neurologic deficit, ischemic ECG changes, and pregnant patients (1)[C].

MEDICATION

First Line

- IV morphine or hydromorphone (Dilaudid) for severe pain
- Oral analgesics, such as acetaminophen (Tylenol) with codeine, acetaminophen with oxycodone (Percocet), or acetaminophen with hydrocodone (Lortab) for moderate pain
- Silver sulfadiazine (Silvadene): Apply topically to burn site (can cause leukopenia). Do not use in sulfa-allergic patients, women who are pregnant/breastfeeding, or infants younger than 2 months)
- Neosporin or bacitracin ointment: Apply to facial burns.
- Mupirocin: has potent inhibitory activity against methicillin-resistant *Staphylococcus aureus* (MRSA) (5)[B]
- Acticote A.B. (a dressing consisting of 2 sheets of high-density polyethylene mesh coated with nanocrystalline silver) has a more controlled, prolonged release of silver, allowing less frequent dressing changes (5)[B].
- Electrical burn with myoglobinuria will require alkalinization of urine and mannitol.
- Consider H2 blockers (e.g., famotidine) or proton-pump inhibitors (e.g., lansoprazole, pantoprazole) for stress ulcer prophylaxis in severely burned patients.
- Tetanus toxoid/tetanus immunoglobulin
- There is no clear indication for prophylactic systemic antibiotics (5)[B].
- Use of negative pressure wound therapy may result in a low-protease environment with higher levels of angiogenic factor (vascular endothelial growth factor [VEGF]) during wound healing, leading to more chaotic, hyperkeratinized, thickened epidermis when compared with a standard hydrocolloid dressing (6)[C].

Second Line

- Mafenide (Sulfamylon) for full-thickness burn, best against *Pseudomonas* (*Caution:* metabolic acidosis, painful)
- Silver nitrate 0.5% (messy, leeches electrolytes from burn, causes water toxicity)
- Povidone–iodine (Betadine) may result in iodine absorption from burn and "tan eschar," makes débridement more difficult
- Travase (enzymatic debridement)

SURGERY/OTHER PROCEDURES

- Escharotomy may be necessary in constricting circumferential burns of extremities or chest due to compartment syndrome.
- Tangential excision with split-thickness skin grafts
- Early excision of burns results in a significant reduction in mortality (excluding patients with inhalational injury) and a significant decrease in hospital length of stay (7)[B].
- Various dressings (e.g., biosynthetic, biologic) are available to help reduce number of dressing changes and promote healing.

ONGOING CARE

FOLLOW-UP RECOMMENDATIONS

Early mobilization is the goal.

DIET

- High-protein, high-calorie diet when bowel function resumes
- Nasogastric tube feedings may be required in early postburn period.
- Total parenteral nutrition if NPO expected for >5 days
- Early initiation of enteral nutrition in first 24 hours of admission results in shorter intensive care unit (ICU) stay and lower wound infection rates

PATIENT EDUCATION

- Use of sunscreen: Skin grafts or newly epithelialized skin is highly sensitive to sun exposure and thermal extremes.
- Prevent access to electrical cords/outlets.
- Isolate household chemicals.
- Use low-temperature setting for water heater (below 54°C).
- Household smoke detectors with special emphasis on maintenance
- Family/household evacuation plan
- Proper storage and use of flammable substances
- Burn management: www.aafp.org/afp/20001101/2029ph.html
- Burn prevention: www.aafp.org/afp/20001101/2032ph.html

PROGNOSIS

- 1st-degree burn: complete resolution
- 2nd-degree burn: epithelialization in 10–14 days (deep 2nd-degree burns probably will require skin graft)
- 3rd-degree burn: no potential for re-epithelialization; skin graft required
- Length of hospital stay and need for ICU care depend on extent of burn, smoke inhalation, comorbidities, and age.
- A 50% survival rate can be expected with a 62% burn in patients aged 0–14 years, 63% burn in patients aged 15–40 years, 38% burn in patients aged 40–65 years, and 25% burn in patients >65 years of age (1)[C].
- 90% of survivors can be expected to return to an occupation comparable to their preburn employment.

COMPLICATIONS

- Gastroduodenal ulceration (Curling ulcer)
- Marjolin ulcer: malignant squamous cell carcinoma developing in old burn site
- Signs of infection: discoloration, green fat, edema, eschar separation, and conversion of 2nd-degree to 3rd-degree wound
- Biopsy best way to diagnose wound infection.
- Burn wound sepsis: most commonly *S. aureus* (including MRSA), vancomycin-resistant enterococci, and gram-negative organisms (5)[B].
- Pneumonia
- Decreased mobility with possibility of future flexion contractures
- Hypertrophic scarring common with burns

REFERENCES

1. Teague H, Sweneki SA, Tang A. The burned patient: assessment, diagnosis, and management in the ED. *Trauma Reports*. 2005;6:1–12.
2. Dries DJ, Endorf FW. Inhalation injury: epidemiology, pathology, treatment strategies. *Scand J Trauma Resusc Emerg Med*. 2013;21:31.
3. Bezuhly M, Fish JS. Acute burn care. *Plast Reconstr Surg*. 2012;130(2):349E–358E.
4. Perel P, Roberts I, Ker K. Colloids versus crystalloids for fluid resuscitation in critically ill patients. *Cochrane Database Syst Rev*. 2013;(2):CD000567.
5. Church D, Elsayed S, Reid O, et al. Burn wound infections. *Clin Microbiol Rev*. 2006;19(2):403–434.
6. Caulfield RH, Tyler MP, Austyn JM, et al. The relationship between protease/anti-protease profile, angiogenesis and re-epithelialisation in acute burn wounds. *Burns*. 2008;34(4):474–486.
7. Ong YS, Samuel M, Song C. Meta-analysis of early excision of burns. *Burns*. 2006;32(2):145–150.

ADDITIONAL READING

Endorf FW, Ahrenholz D. Burn management. *Curr Opin Crit Care*. 2011;17(6):601–605.

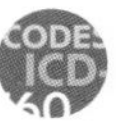

CODES

ICD10

- T30.0 Burn of unspecified body region, unspecified degree
- T30.4 Corrosion of unspecified body region, unspecified degree

CLINICAL PEARLS

- 1st degree: erythema of involved tissue; skin blanches with pressure. Skin may be tender.
- 2nd degree: Skin is red and blistered. Skin is very tender.
- 3rd degree: Burned skin is tough and leathery. Skin is not tender.

BURSITIS

Jeff Wang, MD, MPH • J. Herbert Stevenson, MD

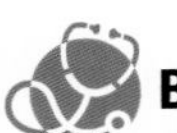

BASICS

DESCRIPTION

- Bursae are synovial fluid-filled sacs found in areas subject to friction, such as when tendons pass over bony prominences.
- Although there are at least 78 different sites where bursae are found, the most common sites of clinical bursitis are the following:
  - Subdeltoid/subacromial
  - Olecranon ("student's elbow")
  - Prepatellar ("housemaid's knee")
  - Infrapatellar ("clergyman's knee")
  - Trochanteric
  - Radiohumeral
  - Ischial ("weaver's bottom")
  - Pes anserinus
  - Retrocalcaneal
- Bursae serve a lubricating function, allowing for musculotendinous units to glide over bony prominences.
- Bursae are lined with synovial membrane and play a role in synovial fluid mechanics.
- System(s) affected: musculoskeletal

Pediatric Considerations

Bursitis is less common in children.

EPIDEMIOLOGY

Predominant age

- 15–50 years (most common in skeletally mature)
- Traumatic bursitis is more likely in patients <35 years of age.

Incidence

- Bursitis: 32/1,000 per year (1)[B]
- Approximately 1 in 31; 3.2% or 8.7 million people in the United States impacted annually (1)[B]
- Trochanteric pain: 1.8/1,000 per year (2)[B]

ETIOLOGY AND PATHOPHYSIOLOGY

- Trauma: acute or chronic
- Repetitive movement: Upper extremity bursitis, in particular, is usually the result of repetitive microtrauma.
- Infections: most commonly *Staphylococcus aureus*
- Systemic disease: rheumatoid disease, tuberculosis, pancreatitis, lupus
- Crystal deposition: gout and pseudogout

RISK FACTORS

- Individuals who engage in repetitive motion and/or vigorous training
- Prolonged pressure on particular bursae (e.g., "clergyman's knee" and "student's elbow")
- Sudden increase in level of activity
- Leg length discrepancy and Trendelenburg gait increase risk for trochanteric bursitis.
- Anabolic steroid use increases risk of bursitis due to increased training, estrogen suppression causing increased inflammation, and muscle stiffness.

GENERAL PREVENTION

- Appropriate warmup and cool-down maneuvers
- Frequent breaks between repetitive activities
- Use of protective gear (e.g., knee pads)
- Maintain fitness and general health.

COMMONLY ASSOCIATED CONDITIONS

- Tendinitis
- Sprains, strains
- Associated stress fractures
- Muscular tightness and physical deconditioning

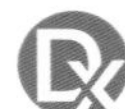

DIAGNOSIS

HISTORY

- Pain in the affected region, usually gradual in onset; can be rapid if due to trauma.
- Decreased ROM or stiffness of the affected region
- Recent changes in recreational or occupational physical activity
- History of prior injury
- Subacromial bursitis: repetitive overhead activities, pain with overhead activity
- Trochanteric bursitis: recent increase in running or lower extremity exercise
- Prepatellar bursitis: fall on patella, prolonged kneeling or running
- Olecranon bursitis: leaning on elbows, trauma, decreased ROM at the elbow
- Radiohumeral bursitis: repetitive forearm pronation (medial epicondylitis/golfer's elbow) or supination (lateral epicondylitis/tennis elbow) and pain with opening jars, wringing out hair or opening doors

PHYSICAL EXAM

- Pain and point tenderness of affected area
- Decreased ROM of affected region (particularly shoulder)
- Erythema
- Swelling
- Crepitus
- Point tenderness

DIFFERENTIAL DIAGNOSIS

- Septic arthritis; Lyme disease
- Osteoarthritis
- Gout, pseudogout
- Rheumatic disorders
- Tendinitis, strains, and sprains
- Fractures and contusions
- Cellulitis

DIAGNOSTIC TESTS & INTERPRETATION

Consider ECG (if left shoulder pain suggests cardiac pain).

Initial Tests (lab, imaging)

- The diagnosis of bursitis is typically clinical.
- The following tests help in differentiating soft tissue disease from rheumatic and connective tissue disease (but are not necessary for routine bursitis diagnosis):
  - CBC with differential
  - ESR
  - Serum protein electrophoresis
  - Rheumatoid factor
  - Anti-CCP
  - ANA
  - Joint fluid analysis
- Calcific deposits may be seen on plain radiograph.
- MRI may help if diagnosis is unclear.
- US useful for direct visualization and to guide injection (3)[B]

Diagnostic Procedures/Other

- Aspiration
  - Fluid analysis, Gram stain, cell count, culture, and examination for presence of crystals
  - White blood cell (WBC) 2,000–5,000/μL implies inflammatory cause; >5,000/μL implies infectious cause. Noninflammatory fluid contains <2,000 WBCs/μL.
  - If the Gram stain and culture indicate infection, treat with appropriate antibiotics.

Test Interpretation

- Acutely (early inflammation), bursa is distended with watery or mucoid fluid.
- Infection: purulent fluid on aspiration
- Chronic bursitis
  - Bursal wall is thickened, and inner surface is shaggy and trabeculated.
  - Bursal space is filled with granular, brown, inspissated blood with gritty, calcific precipitations.

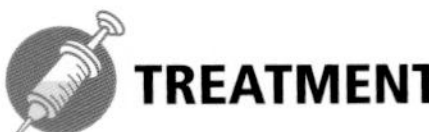

TREATMENT

Outpatient; refer only difficult cases.

GENERAL MEASURES

- Goal is to reduce pain and irritation and prevent recurrence.
- Conservative therapy consists of rest, ice, and local care; elevation; and gentle compression (often referred to as PRICE therapy [protection-rest-ice-compression-elevation]).
- Compression
- Bursa aspiration (particularly if suspicion for infection)
- Corticosteroid injection if infectious etiology ruled out
- Treat any underlying infection.
- Treat underlying causes such as overtraining, poor body mechanics, repetitive trauma, or tight or deconditioned muscles.
- For prepatellar bursitis resulting from trauma, have patient wear knee pads during prolonged kneeling.

MEDICATION

First Line

- NSAIDs or aspirin (4)[C]
- Antibiotic therapy if infection present; cover for staph and strep species (most common)

Second Line

- Injectable corticosteroids once infectious etiology ruled out (2,4)[C],(5)[B]
- Systemic steroids provide limited short-term benefit (6)[B].
- Local corticosteroid injection may be used in the management of prepatellar and olecranon bursitis; however, steroid injection into the retrocalcaneal bursa may adversely affect the biomechanical properties of the Achilles tendon (7)[C].
- US guidance for bursa injections increases anatomic accuracy and effectiveness of therapy.

ADDITIONAL THERAPIES

- For trochanteric bursitis, low-energy shock wave therapy (SWT) may be superior to other nonoperative modalities (8)[A].
- Platelet-rich plasma (PRP) injections are increasingly used to treat bursitis (9)[C].
- Physical therapy to correct biomechanical abnormalities and strengthen surrounding musculature

SURGERY/OTHER PROCEDURES

- Surgical excision in severe cases unresponsive to conservative treatments
- Outpatient arthroscopic bursectomy under local anaesthesia is an effective procedure for the treatment of posttraumatic prepatellar bursitis after failed conservative treatments.

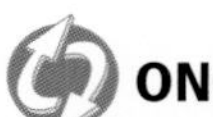

ONGOING CARE

FOLLOW-UP RECOMMENDATIONS

Rest and elevation of affected extremity

Patient Monitoring

- Discontinue NSAIDs as soon as possible to avoid side effects.
- Some patients may require repeated injections (usually no more than 3) of a corticosteroid and lidocaine (2,3)[C].

DIET

Consider dietary changes if bursitis is directly related to obesity/crystalline deposition.

PROGNOSIS

- Most bouts of bursitis heal uneventfully.
- Repetitive bouts may lead to chronic bursitis, necessitating repeated joint/bursal aspirations or (rarely) surgical excision of involved bursa.
- Although multiple aspirations may not be curative, they can provide significant symptom relief while awaiting a more definitive treatment (i.e., surgery).

COMPLICATIONS

- Septic bursitis may extend to nearby joint.
- Acute bursitis leading to chronic pain, limitation of motion, and dysfunction

REFERENCES

1. Centers for Disease Control and Prevention. National health interview survey. http://www.cdc.gov/nchs/nhis.htm. Accessed 2014.
2. Williams BS, Cohen SP. Greater trochanteric pain syndrome: a review of anatomy, diagnosis and treatment. *Anesth Analg*. 2009;108(5):1662–1670.
3. Finlay K, Friedman L. Ultrasonography of the lower extremity. *Orthop Clin North Am*. 2006;37(3):245–275, v.
4. Tallia AH, Cardone DA. Diagnostic and therapeutic injection of the shoulder region. *Am Fam Physician*. 2003;67(6):1271–1278.
5. Gasparre G, Fusaro I, Galletti S, et al. Effectiveness of ultrasound-guided injections combined with shoulder exercises in the treatment of subacromial adhesive bursitis. *Musculoskelet Surg*. 2012;96(Suppl 1):S57–S61.
6. Buchbinder R, Hoving JL, Green S, et al. Short course prednisolone for adhesive capsulitis (frozen shoulder or stiff painful shoulder): a randomised, double blind, placebo controlled trial. *Ann Rheum Dis*. 2004;63(11):1460–1469.
7. Aaron DL, Patel A, Kayiaros S, et al. Four common types of bursitis: diagnosis and management. *J Am Acad Orthop Surg*. 2011;19(6):359–367.
8. Lustenberger DP, Ng VY, Best TM, et al. Efficacy of treatment of trochanteric bursitis: a systematic review. *Clin J Sport Med*. 2011;21(5):447–453.
9. Hsu WK, Mishra A, Rodeo SR, et al. Platelet-rich plasma in orthopaedic applications: evidence-based recommendations for treatment. *J Am Acad Orthop Surg*. 2013;21(12):739–748.

ADDITIONAL READING

- Cardone DA, Tallia AF. Diagnostic and therapeutic injection of the hip and knee. *Am Fam Physician*. 2003;67(10):2147–2152.
- Hsieh LF, Hsu WC, Lin YJ, et al. Is ultrasound-guided injection more effective in chronic subacromial bursitis? *Med Sci Sports Exerc*. 2013;45(12):2205–2213.
- McFarland EG, Gill HS, Laporte DM, et al. Miscellaneous conditions about the elbow in athletes. *Clin Sports Med*. 2004;23(4):743–763, xi–xii.
- Wiegerinck JI, Kok AC, van Dijk CN. Surgical treatment of chronic retrocalcaneal bursitis. *Arthroscopy*. 2012;28(2):283–293.

SEE ALSO

- Tendinitis
- Video: Olecranon Bursitis Aspiration

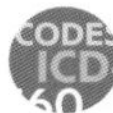

CODES

ICD10

- M71.9 Bursopathy, unspecified
- M75.50 Bursitis of unspecified shoulder
- M70.20 Olecranon bursitis, unspecified elbow

CLINICAL PEARLS

- PRICE for conservative therapy
  - Protect (protective gear or padding)
  - Rest affected area.
  - Ice inflamed bursa.
  - Compress (with Ace wrap or neoprene sleeve)
  - Elevate joint.
- Treat underlying cause of the bursitis. Rehabilitation to restore biomechanics and strengthen surrounding musculature helps to prevent recurrence.

BURSITIS, PES ANSERINE

Jennifer Schwartz, MD

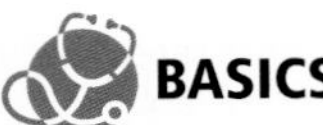

BASICS

DESCRIPTION

- The pes anserinus ("goosefoot") is the combined insertion of the sartorius, gracilis, and semitendinosus ("SGT"-from medial to lateral) tendons on the anteromedial tibia.
- The pes anserine muscles help flex the knee and resist valgus stress.
- The pes anserine bursa lies deep to the SGT tendons and superficial to the tibial attachment of the medial collateral ligament.
- *Pes anserine syndrome* is due to irritation of the bursa and/or tendons in this area.

EPIDEMIOLOGY

Incidence

Pes anserine bursa inflammation is detected in up to 2.5% of MRI studies on patients who are symptomatic (1). The overall incidence is likely higher.

ETIOLOGY AND PATHOPHYSIOLOGY

Pes anserine bursitis occurs secondary to the following:

- Overuse injury
- Excessive valgus and rotary stresses
- Mechanical forces and degenerative changes
- Direct trauma

RISK FACTORS

- Obesity
- Female
- Pes planus
- Genu valgum
- Knee joint laxity/ligamentous injury
- Long distance running, hill running; change in mileage
- Swimming ("breaststroker's knee")
- Cycling
- Sports with side-to-side (cutting) activity (soccer, basketball, racquet sports).

COMMONLY ASSOCIATED CONDITIONS

- Osteoarthritis (OA)
  - Knee pain due to osteoarthritis is often associated with pes bursitis, both of which may need condition-specific treatment (1)[C].
  - Higher grades of OA associated with a thicker pes bursa and a larger area of bursitis (2,3)[C]
- Valgus knee deformity
- Obesity
- Diabetes mellitus (questionable association)

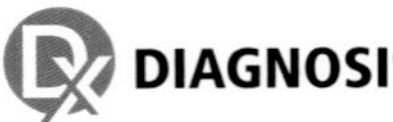

DIAGNOSIS

HISTORY

- Medial knee pain is the most common complaint.
- Changes in training regimen or mileage often accompany knee pain.
- Pain is located 4–6 cm distal to the medial joint line on the anteromedial aspect of the tibia.
- Pain exacerbated by knee flexion:
  - Going up or down stairs
  - Getting out of a chair

PHYSICAL EXAM

- Common findings
  - Tenderness to palpation at the pes anserine insertion
    - 30% of asymptomatic patients also have tenderness to deep palpation in this area.
  - Pain worsens with flexion of the knee against resistance.
  - Localized swelling of the pes anserine insertion
- Findings that suggest an alternative diagnosis: joint effusion, tenderness directly over the joint line, erythema or warmth, locking of the knee, systemic signs such as fever or pain with passive knee movement

DIFFERENTIAL DIAGNOSIS

- Medial collateral ligament injury
- Medial meniscal injury
- Medial plica syndrome
- Medial compartment osteoarthritis
- Semimembranosus bursitis
- Popliteal/meniscal cyst
- Tibial stress fracture
- Septic arthritis

DIAGNOSTIC TESTS & INTERPRETATION

Initial Tests (lab, imaging)

- Primarily a clinical diagnosis
- Lab work not indicated unless infection is suspected, in which CBC, ESR, C-reactive protein, and analysis if joint fluid aspirate are indicated.
- Imaging is not indicated unless there is concern for bony injury/fracture, ligamentous injury, or meniscal tear.

Follow-Up Tests & Special Considerations

- Ultrasound (US)
  - Can demonstrate focal edema within the pes anserine bursa but has poor correlation with clinical findings
  - Many patients clinically diagnosed with pes anserine bursitis have no morphologic changes of the pes anserine complex on US (4)[C].
- MRI: can demonstrate inflammation of the bursa, delineate the pes anserine bursa from other structures and rule out other etiologies
- T2W axial images best (5)[C]
  - No large studies exist to evaluate the correlation between clinical diagnosis of pes anserine bursitis and radiographic evidence of pes anserine pathology on MRI.
  - May see fluid in the pes bursa on MRI in 5% of asymptomatic patients (6)[C]

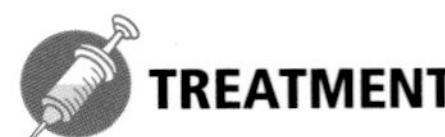

TREATMENT

Pes anserine bursitis is often self-limited. Therefore, conservative therapy is the most common treatment approach:

- Relative rest, activity modification to encourage avoiding offending movements (especially knee flexion)
- Ice
- Physical therapy
- NSAIDs
- Corticosteroid injection
- Weight loss

MEDICATION

First Line

NSAIDs, such as ibuprofen, (800 mg PO TID) or naproxen (500 mg PO BID) are often used as 1st-line therapy.

Second Line

- Corticosteroid injection combined with local anesthetic has been shown to provide relief in many patients (7)[C].
  - The injection is usually performed at the point of maximal tenderness: The area is prepared with standard aseptic practices.
  - ~2 mL of anesthetic (i.e., 1% lidocaine) and 1 mL of steroid (i.e., 40 mg of methylprednisolone) is injected into the bursa using a small (e.g., 25-gauge 1-inch needle).

- Insert needle perpendicular to the skin until bone is felt and then withdraw slightly before injecting.
- Care should be taken to avoid injecting directly into the tendon (8)[C].

- US-guided injection appears to be superior to blind injection (9)[C].
- Platelet rich plasma injections also shown to provide pain relief (10)[C].
- Injection of steroid and anesthetic allows for pain relief, which can hasten physical therapy and rehabilitative efforts.

ADDITIONAL THERAPIES

Physical therapy

- Hamstring and achilles stretching
- Quadriceps strengthening—particularly of the vastus medialis (terminal 30 degrees of knee extension)
- Adductor strengthening

SURGERY/OTHER PROCEDURES

- No role for surgery in routine isolated cases
- Drainage or removal of bursa may be used in severe/refractory cases.

ONGOING CARE

Home exercise program focusing on flexibility and strengthening

DIET

Consider dietary changes as part of a comprehensive weight-loss program if obesity is a contributing factor.

PROGNOSIS

Most cases of pes anserine syndrome respond to conservative therapy. Recurrence is common, and multiple treatments may be required.

REFERENCES

1. Rennie WJ, Saifuddin A. Pes anserine bursitis: incidence in symptomatic knees and clinical presentation. *Skeletal Radiol*. 2005;34(7):395–398.
2. Toktas H, Dundar U, Adar S, et al. Ultrasonographic assessment of pes anserinus tendon and pes anserinus tendinitis bursitis syndrome in patients with knee osteoarthritis. *Mod Rheumatol*. 2014;19:1–6.
3. Uysal F, Akbal A, Gokmen E, et al. Prevalance of pes anserine bursitis in symptomatic osteoarthritis patients: an ultrasonographic prospective study [published online ahead of print May 6, 2014]. *Clin Rheumatol*.
4. Helfenstein M, Kuromoto J. Anserine syndrome [in English, Portuguese]. *Rev Bras Reumatol*. 2010;50(3):313–327.
5. Chatra, P. Bursae around the knee joints. *Indian J Radiol Imaging*. 2012(22):27–30.
6. Rennie WJ, Saifuddin A. Pes anserine bursitis: incidence in symptomatic knees and clinical presentation. *Skeletal Radiol*. 2005;34(7):395–398.
7. Yoon HS, Kim SE, Suh YR, et al. Correlation between ultrasonographic findings and the response to corticosteroid injection in pes anserinus tendinobursitis syndrome in knee osteoarthritis patients. *J Korean Med Sci*. 2005;20(1):109–112.
8. Stephens MB, Beutler AI, O'Connor FG. Musculoskeletal injections: a review of the evidence. *Am Fam Physician*. 2008;78(8):971–976.
9. Finnoff JT, Nutz DJ, Henning PT, et al. Accuracy of ultrasound-guided versus unguided pes anserinus bursa injections. *PM R*. 2010;2(8):732–739.
10. Rowicki K, Płomiński J, Bachta A. Evaluation of the effectiveness of platelet rich plasma in treatment of chronic pes anserinus pain syndrome. *Ortop Traumatol Rehabil*. 2014;16(3):307–318.

ADDITIONAL READING

- Alvarez-Nemegyei J. Risk factors for pes anserine tendinitis/bursitis syndrome: a case control study. *J Clin Rheumatol*. 2007;13(2):63–65.
- Wittich CM, Ficalora RD, Mason TG, et al. Musculoskeletal injection. *Mayo Clin Proc*. 2009;84(9):831–836; quiz 837.

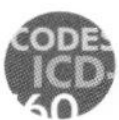

CODES

ICD10

- M71.569 Other bursitis, not elsewhere classified, unspecified knee
- M65.869 Other synovitis and tenosynovitis, unspecified lower leg
- M76.899 Oth enthesopathies of unspecified lower limb, excluding foot

CLINICAL PEARLS

- Consider pes anserine syndrome in patients presenting with medial knee pain.
- Occurs relatively commonly in athletes and in older, obese patients with osteoarthritis
- Physical examination reveals tenderness over the insertion of the pes anserine tendon on the medial aspect of the tibia 4–6 cm distal to the joint line.
  - Patients without pes anserine syndrome may have tenderness to palpation in this area, so it is important to correlate the entire clinical picture.
- Consider pes anserine syndrome in patients who have persistent symptoms associated with medial-sided osteoarthritis. A local steroid/anesthetic injection may help differentiate the two conditions and provide pain relief.

CANDIDIASIS, MUCOCUTANEOUS

Hugh J. Silk, MD, MPH • Sheila O. Stille, DMD

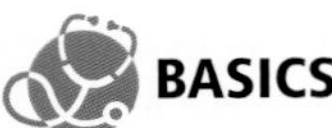

BASICS

DESCRIPTION

- Heterogeneous mucocutaneous disorder caused by infection with various *Candida* spp.
- Characterized by superficial infection of the skin, mucous membranes, and nails
- Due to impaired cell-mediated immunity against *Candida* species; can be transient or chronic
- >20 *Candida* species cause infection in humans. *Candida albicans is most common.*
- Affected systems include the following:
  - Gastrointestinal
    - Oropharyngeal candidiasis: mouth, pharynx
    - Angular cheilitis: corner of the mouth
    - Esophageal candidiasis
    - GI candidiasis: gastritis and/or ulcers, associated with thrush; alimental or perianal
  - Non-GI
    - Candida vulvovaginitis: vaginal mucosa and/or vulvar skin
    - Candidal balanitis: glans of the penis
    - Candidal paronychia: nail bed or nail folds
    - Folliculitis
    - Interdigital candidiasis: webs of the digits
    - Candidal diaper dermatitis and intertrigo (skin folds of groin)
- Synonym(s): monilia; thrush; yeast; intertrigo

ALERT
Vaginal antifungal creams and suppositories can weaken condoms and diaphragms.

Pregnancy Considerations

- Vaginal candidiasis is common during pregnancy due to hormonal changes.
- Treatment during pregnancy should be extended by several days when using topical agents.
- Vaginal yeast infection at birth can increase the risk of thrush to the newborn but is of no overall harm to baby.

EPIDEMIOLOGY

- Common in the United States; particularly with immunodeficiency and/or uncontrolled diabetes
- Age considerations
  - Infants and seniors: thrush and cutaneous infections (infant diaper rash)
  - Women of childbearing age: vaginitis
  - Prepubertal or postmenopausal: yeast vaginitis
  - Predominant sex: female > male

Incidence

Unknown—relatively high prevalence of mucocutaneous candidiasis with low incidence of complications in immunocompetent patients

Prevalence

Candida species are normal flora of oral cavity, pharynx, esophagus, and GI tract present in >70% U.S. population.

ETIOLOGY AND PATHOPHYSIOLOGY

C. albicans (responsible for 80–92% vulvovaginal and 70–80% oral isolates)

Genetics

Chronic mucocutaneous candidiasis is a heterogeneous, genetic syndrome with infection of skin, nails, hair, and mucous membranes; typically presents in infancy.

RISK FACTORS

- Immunosuppression
- Antibacterial therapy (broad-spectrum antibiotics)
- Douches, chemical irritants, and concurrent vaginitides alter vaginal pH and predispose to yeast vaginitis
- Denture wear
- Birth control pills
- Hyperglycemia; diabetes
- Uncircumcised men at higher risk for balanitis

GENERAL PREVENTION

- Judicious medication use—antibiotics and steroids in particular; rinse mouth after inhaled steroid use (1)[A].
- Avoid douching. Treat other vaginal infections.
- Minimize moisture (wear cotton underwear; frequent diaper changes).
- Clean dentures often; use well-fitting dentures, and remove during sleep.
- Glycemic control in diabetic patients
- Preventive regimens during cancer treatments (2)[A]
- Fluconazole prophylaxis against oral candidiasis in HIV-infected adults (3)[A]

COMMONLY ASSOCIATED CONDITIONS

- HIV
- Leukopenias
- Diabetes mellitus
- Cancer and other immunosuppressive conditions

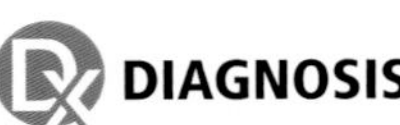

DIAGNOSIS

HISTORY

- Infants/children
  - Oral: adherent white patches on oral mucosae or on the tongue
  - Perineal: erythematous rash with characteristic satellite lesions; painful if eroding skin layers. 40–75% of diaper rashes lasting >3 days are *C. albicans* (4,5)[A].
  - Angular cheilitis: painful fissures
- Adults
  - Vulvovaginal lesions; thin to thick, whitish, discharge; pruritus; burning
- Immunocompromised hosts
  - Oral: white, raised, painless, distinct patches; red, slightly raised patches
  - Esophagitis: dysphagia, odynophagia, retrosternal pain; usually concomitant thrush
  - GI symptoms: abdominal pain
  - Balanitis: erythema, erosions, scaling; dysuria
  - Folliculitis: follicular pustules
  - Interdigital: redness, itchiness at base of fingers and/or toes, possible maceration

PHYSICAL EXAM

- Infants/children
  - Oral: white, raised, distinct patches within the mouth; wiping off reveals red base
  - Perineal: erythematous maculopapular rash with satellite pustules or papules
  - Angular cheilitis: tender fissures in mouth corners, often cracked and bleeding
- Adults
  - Vulvovaginal: thick, whitish, cottage cheese–like discharge; vagina or perineum erythema
- Immunocompromised hosts
  - Oral: white, raised, nontender, distinct patches; red, slightly raised patches; thick, dark-brownish coating; deep fissures
  - Esophagitis: Often, oral thrush is visible.
  - Balanitis: erythema, linear erosions, scaling
  - Folliculitis: follicular pustules
  - Interdigital: redness, excoriations at base of fingers and/or toes, often maceration

DIFFERENTIAL DIAGNOSIS

- For oral candidiasis
  - Leukoplakia
  - Lichen planus
  - Geographic tongue
  - Herpes simplex
  - Erythema multiforme
  - Pemphigus
- Baby formula or breast milk can mimic thrush—easier to wipe away than thrush
- Hairy leukoplakia: does not rub off; lateral tongue
- Angular cheilitis from vitamin B or iron deficiency, staphylococcal infection, or edentulous overclosure
- Bacterial vaginosis and *Trichomonas vaginalis* tend to have more odor, itch, and a different discharge.

DIAGNOSTIC TESTS & INTERPRETATION

Initial Tests (lab, imaging)

- KOH slide preparation: mycelia (hyphae) or pseudomycelia (pseudohyphae) yeast forms; few WBC
- pH paper <4 (normal = 4.5–5.5)
- Barium swallow: cobblestone appearance, fistulas, or dilatation (denervation)

Diagnostic Procedures/Other

- If 1st-line treatment fails, perform culture for type and sensitivity, alternative infection.
- Esophagitis may require endoscopy with biopsy.
- Biopsy if suspicious for cancer.
- HIV seropositivity plus thrush with dysphagia relieved by antifungal diagnostic for *Candida* esophagitis.

Test Interpretation

Biopsy: epithelial parakeratosis with polymorphonuclear leukocytes in superficial layers; periodic acid–Schiff staining reveals presence of candidal hyphae.

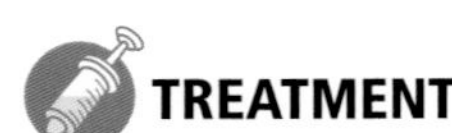

TREATMENT

GENERAL MEASURES

Screen immunodeficient patients.

MEDICATION

First Line

- Vaginal (choose 1)
  - Miconazole (Monistat) 2% cream: 1 applicator or 200 mg (1 suppository), intravaginally qhs for 7 days
  - Clotrimazole (Gyne-Lotrimin, Mycelex): intravaginal tablets (100 mg qhs for 7 days; 200 mg qhs for 3 days; 500 mg daily for 1 day) or 2% cream (1 applicator qhs for 3 days)
  - Fluconazole 150 mg PO single dose

- Oropharyngeal
  - Mild disease
    - Clotrimazole (Mycelex): oral 10 mg troche; 20 minutes 5 times daily for 7–14 days or
    - Nystatin suspension: 100,000 U/mL swish and swallow 400,000–600,000 U 4×/day or
    - Nystatin pastilles: 200,000 U each, QID daily for 7–14 days (6)[B],(7)[A]
    - Denture wearers
      - Nystatin ointment: 100,000 U/g under denture and corners of mouth for 3 weeks
      - Remove dentures at night; clean 2× weekly with diluted (1:20) bleach.
      - Moderate to severe disease
    - Fluconazole: 200 mg load then 100–200 mg (peds: 3 mg/kg) daily for 7–14 days
- Esophagitis
  - Fluconazole: 400 mg load then 200–400 mg/day for 14–21 days
  - Itraconazole (Sporanox)
    - Oral solution: 200 mg daily for 14–21 days

Pregnancy Considerations

2% Miconazole cream, intravaginally, for 7 days in uncomplicated candidiasis. Systemic amphotericin B for invasive candidiasis in pregnancy.

Second Line

- Vaginal
  - Terconazole (Terazol): Recurrent cases: 0.4% cream (1 applicator qhs for 7 days of induction therapy); 0.8% cream/80-mg suppositories (1 applicator or 1 suppository qhs for 3 days)
  - Prophylaxis: Fluconazole, 150 mg once per week for 6 months to prevent recurrence
    - In HIV patients: Concerns with this regimen include emergence of drug resistance (8)[A].
- Oropharyngeal
  - Clotrimazole troches 10 mg 5 times daily
  - Nystatin oral suspension (100,000 U/mL)
    - Infants: 0.5 mL in each cheek QID for 10 days
    - Children: 5–10 mL QID for 10 days
    - Adults: Swish and swallow 5–10 mL QID for 14 days; prophylaxis—same dosage 2–5×/day.
  - Fluconazole: 100 mg/day for 7–14 days (load immunocompromised patient with 200 mg)
  - Itraconazole (Sporanox) suspension: 200 mg (20 mL) daily; swish-swallow for 7–14 days
  - Miconazole oral gel (20 mg/mL): QID, swish and swallow
  - Amphotericin B (Fungizone) oral suspension (100 mg/mL): 1 mL QID daily, swish and swallow; use between meals
- Esophagitis
  - Amphotericin B (variable dosing) IV dose of 0.3–0.7 mg/kg daily; an echinocandin should be used for patients who cannot tolerate oral therapy.
- Continue treatments for 2 days after infection gone:
  - Contraindications
    - Ketoconazole, itraconazole, or nystatin (if swallowed): severe hepatotoxicity
    - Amphotericin B: can cause nephrotoxicity
  - Precautions
    - Miconazole: can potentiate the effect of warfarin but drug of choice in pregnancy
    - Fluconazole: renal excretion; rare hepatotoxicity; resistance frequent
    - Itraconazole: Doubling the dosage results in ~3-fold increase in itraconazole plasma concentrations.
- Possible interactions (rarely seen with creams, lotions, or suppositories)
  - Fluconazole
    - Rifampin: decreased fluconazole concentrations
    - Tolbutamide: decreased concentrations
    - Warfarin, phenytoin, cyclosporine: altered metabolism; check levels.
  - Itraconazole: potent CYP 3A4 inhibitor. Carefully assess all coadministered medications.

ISSUES FOR REFERRAL

- Patients without obvious reasons for recurrent superficial candidal infections
- GI candidiasis

ADDITIONAL THERAPIES

- For infants with thrush: Boil pacifiers and bottle nipples; assess mother's breasts/nipples for candida infections as well.
- For denture-related candidiasis, disinfection of the denture (using soak solution of benzoic acid, 0.12% chlorhexidine gluconate, 1:20 NaOCl or alkalize proteases), in addition to oral antifungal therapy

COMPLEMENTARY & ALTERNATIVE MEDICINE

Probiotics: *Lactobacillus* and *Bifidobacterium* may inhibit *Candida* spp.

INPATIENT CONSIDERATIONS

Nursing

Elderly patients should be properly trained in oral hygiene. Protocols for brushing, proper denture care, and moistening the oral cavity reduce oral candidiasis.

ONGOING CARE

FOLLOW-UP RECOMMENDATIONS

Patient Monitoring

Immunocompromised persons benefit from regular symptom evaluation and screening.

DIET

Active-culture yogurt or other live lactobacillus may decrease colonization; indeterminate evidence.

PATIENT EDUCATION

- Advise patients at risk for recurrence about antibacterial therapy overgrowth.
- "Azole" medications are pregnancy Category C.

PROGNOSIS

- Immunocompetent: benign course, excellent prognosis
- For immunosuppressed persons, *Candida* may become an AIDS-defining illness and cause morbidity.

COMPLICATIONS

In immunosuppressed, complications depend on the severity. In HIV infection, moderate immunosuppression (e.g., CD4 200–500 cells/mm^3) may be associated with chronic candidiasis. In severe immunosuppression (e.g., CD4 <100 cells/mm^3), thrush may lead to esophagitis or systemic infection.

REFERENCES

1. Yang IA, Clarke MS, Sim EH, et al. Inhaled corticosteroids for stable chronic obstructive pulmonary disease. *Cochrane Database Syst Rev*. 2012;(7):CD002991.
2. Glenny AM, Gibson F, Auld E, et al. The development of evidence-based guidelines on mouth care for children, teenagers and young adults treated for caner. *Eur J Cancer*. 2010;46(8):1399–1412.
3. Pienaar ED, Young T, Holmes H. Interventions for the prevention and management of oropharyngeal candidiasis associated with HIV infection in adults and children. *Cochrane Database Syst Rev*. 2010;(11):CD003940.
4. Nield LS, Kamat D. Prevention, diagnosis, and management of diaper dermatitis. *Clin Pediatr*. 2007;46(6):480–486.
5. Williams DW, Jordan RP, Wei XQ, et al. Interactions of *Candida albicans* with host epithelial surfaces. *J Oral Microbiol*. 2013;5.
6. Pappas PG, Kauffman CA, Andes D, et al. Clinical practice guidelines for the management of candidiasis: 2009 update by the Infectious Diseases Society of America. *Clin Infect Dis*. 2009;48(5):503–535.
7. Martins N, Ferreira IC, Barros L, et al. Candidiasis: predisposing factors, prevention, diagnosis and alternative treatment. *Mycopathologia*. 2014;177(5–6):223–240.
8. Ray A, Ray S, George AT, et al. Interventions for prevention and treatment of vulvovaginal candidiasis in women with HIV infection. *Cochrane Database Syst Rev*. 2011;(8):CD008739.

ADDITIONAL READING

- Nyirjesy P, Sobel JD. Genital mycotic infections in patients with diabetes. *Postgrad Med*. 2013;125(3):33–46.
- Strus M, Kucharska A, Kukla G, et al. The in vitro activity of vaginal *Lactobacillus* with probiotic properties against *Candida*. *Infect Dis Obstet Gynecol*. 2005;13(2):69–75.
- Terai H, Shimahara M. Tongue pain: burning mouth syndrome vs Candida-associated lesion. *Oral Dis*. 2007;13(4):440–442.

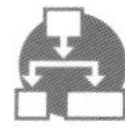

SEE ALSO

Candidiasis, Invasive; Candidiasis, Mucocutaneous; HIV/AIDS

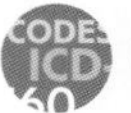

CODES

ICD10

- B37.9 Candidiasis, unspecified
- B37.0 Candidal stomatitis
- B37.49 Other urogenital candidiasis

CLINICAL PEARLS

- Candidiasis is generally a clinical diagnosis with or without KOH scrapings. Rarely, a culture of skin scrapings or even a biopsy is needed to identify resistant strains.
- Person-to-person transmission is rare. Rarely, *Candida* vaginitis may be sexually transmitted.
- If tongue pain continues after treatment, consider burning mouth syndrome. Biopsy if concern for cancer.
- Oral antifungal medications are hepatically metabolized and may have serious side effects.

CARDIAC ARREST

Brent J. Levy, MD • Ryan R. Knapp, MD, MS

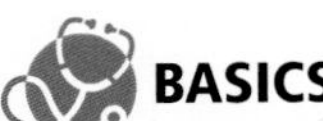

BASICS

DESCRIPTION

- The absence of effective mechanical cardiac activity
- This section is not a substitute for an American Heart Association (AHA)-approved Advanced Cardiac Life Support (ACLS) course and is intended only as a quick reference.
- Synonym(s): "Code" or "Code Blue" in many institutions

Geriatric Considerations

This condition has a low rate of survival and a poor long-term outcome. Discuss Do Not Resuscitate (DNR) orders with patients at risk.

Pediatric Considerations

Bradycardia is linked to hypoxia. Bradycardia is the most common initial form of cardiac arrest in children and is often the response to hypoxia. Adequate oxygenation and ventilation are critical.

Pregnancy Considerations

- Displace the uterus to the left, either manually or by placing a rolled towel under the right hip. If the patient cannot be resuscitated within 5–15 minutes, consider an emergency C-section to relieve uterine obstruction and increase blood return to the heart. This may also be done to save the fetus if the fetus has reached gestational age of viability.
- Consider amniotic fluid embolism or eclampsia-related seizures as precipitating factors.

EPIDEMIOLOGY

- Predominant age: Risk increases with age.
- Predominant sex: male > female

Incidence

0.5–1.5/1,000 persons per year

ETIOLOGY AND PATHOPHYSIOLOGY

- Asystole (confirm in 2 leads)
- Ventricular fibrillation (VF)
- Pulseless ventricular tachycardia (VT)
- Pulseless electrical activity (PEA)
- Consider possible reversible causes (6 Hs and 5 Ts):
  - Hypoxia, hypovolemia, hyper- and hypokalemia, [H^+] (acidosis), hypothermia, hypoglycemia
  - Cardiac tamponade, tension pneumothorax, thrombosis (pulmonary embolism, myocardial infarction [MI]), toxins (medications and overdoses), trauma

RISK FACTORS

- Male gender
- Advanced age
- Hypercholesterolemia
- Hypertension (HTN)
- Cigarette smoking
- Family history of atherosclerosis
- Diabetes
- Cardiomyopathy
- Prolonged QT

COMMONLY ASSOCIATED CONDITIONS

- Coronary artery disease/acute coronary syndrome (ACS) (cardiac arrest may be presenting symptom)
- Valvular heart disease
- HTN
- Pulmonary embolism

DIAGNOSIS

- Loss of consciousness secondary to CNS hypoperfusion
- Absence of pulses in large arteries
- Apnea or agonal breathing
- Cyanosis or pallor

HISTORY

- Witnessed versus unwitnessed
- Approximate downtime
- Initial resuscitation efforts and response
- History or risk factors
- Associated trauma
- DNR/Do Not Intubate (DNI) status

PHYSICAL EXAM

- Check for pulses.
- Check lungs (i.e., Did patient have respiratory decline prior to cardiac decline?).
- Check for signs suggesting possible reversible causes:
  - Check for dialysis shunt: Patients on dialysis are at increased risk for an electrolyte imbalance that can cause arrest (especially hyperkalemia).
  - Check pupils: may indicate drug overdose (cannot interpret if patient has received atropine).
  - Check for obvious signs of trauma.

DIAGNOSTIC TESTS & INTERPRETATION

Laboratory results have limited value during initial resuscitation.

Initial Tests (lab, imaging)

- Fingerstick glucose
- Arterial blood gas (ABG)/venous blood gas (VBG)
- Chemistry and/or electrolyte panel
- Blood type and cross, if indicated
- Cardiac enzymes (troponin, creatine kinase [CK], CK-MB)
- CBC with platelets
- Drug levels, if indicated (toxicology screen, acetaminophen/aspirin levels, history of specific medication (e.g., digoxin, antiepileptics)
- Consider
  - RUSH (Rapid Ultrasound in SHock) exam to evaluate "the pump, tank, and pipes" to guide resuscitation (1)[C]
  - Perform emergency echocardiogram for pericardial effusion, assessment of cardiac motion, and presence of intraventricular clot.
  - Chest x-ray for endotracheal tube (ET) placement, pneumothorax
  - Once stabilized, consider a CT scan of the brain.

Diagnostic Procedures/Other

- Obtain access
  - Peripheral IV as close to central circulation as possible (preferred)
  - Intraosseous (IO) if no venous access
  - Consider central venous access if unable to achieve alternative access; femoral approach preferred to minimize interruptions in CPR
  - Many medications may be administered by ET if access is otherwise unobtainable (double dose and flush with saline).
- Airway management/intubation
- Needle decompression/chest tube for pneumothorax
- Pericardiocentesis for cardiac tamponade
- ECG

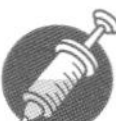

TREATMENT

- C-A-B (circulation, airway, breathing). Use compressions 1st, then check airway and breathing.
- Prompt initiation of high-quality CPR, particularly chest compressions (at least 100 per minute, depth 2 inches in adults, allowing recoil after each compression), and immediate defibrillation (in witnessed VF and pulseless VT but not in PEA) are 1st priority (2)[A]:
  - In unwitnessed arrest, complete 2 minutes of CPR before attempting defibrillation (3)[A].
  - Capnography should be used to evaluate the efficacy of chest compressions (2)[A].
  - Avoid excessive ventilation (2)[A].
- Establishing IV access, intubation, and medications are 2nd priority.
- Continue CPR for 1–2 minutes following the return of a potentially perfusing rhythm before stopping for a pulse check, except for witnessed arrest with a prompt return of rhythm following defibrillation.
- Patients with a return of spontaneous circulation (ROSC) should have an ECG and be strongly considered for primary coronary intervention. If not available in your facility, then consider transfer to a hospital with this capacity. Early 12-lead ECG may not demonstrate MI, but this may develop late. Intervention should not be delayed in the appropriate setting.

GENERAL MEASURES

- Perform CPR: 100/min, allowing for chest wall recoil, with minimal interruptions (4)[B]
- Sequence should be as follows:
  - CPR
  - Rhythm check
  - Resume CPR
  - Shock/medicines (charge defibrillator and administer drugs during CPR)
  - Continue CPR (after shocking) for 5 cycles before rechecking rhythm (repeat as needed) (4)[B].
- In VF/pulseless VT, 1 shock should be delivered, then continue sequence above (4)[B]:
  - Monophasic automatic external defibrillators (AEDs) initial and subsequent shocks at 360 J
  - Biphasic AEDs
    - 150–200 J for biphasic truncated exponential waveform
    - 120 J for rectilinear biphasic waveform
    - If not specified on the biphasic defibrillator, use default of 200 J.
  - Subsequent shocks should be the same or higher energy.
  - Pediatric manual defibrillation energy should be initial dose of 2 J/kg for the 1st attempt, followed by 4 J/kg for the next attempt. Increase energy with subsequent attempts but do not exceed 10 J/kg or maximum adult dose.
- Consider possible causes of VT/VF, including hypoxia, hyperkalemia, hypokalemia, preexisting acidosis, drug overdose, and hypothermia.
- Administer 100% oxygen by bag-valve mask or ET.
- IV and IO are the preferred methods of medication administration, followed by ET.
- Start IV lines as close to the heart as possible. Large-bore peripheral lines can deliver fluid more quickly than a triple-lumen catheter.

- Use an end-tidal CO_2 (ET-CO_2) monitor to assess gas exchange, if available. Capnography is the test of choice to assess ET placement, as esophageal intubation will produce a very low ET-CO_2 and requires proper reintubation (2). The use of sodium bicarbonate will increase ET-CO_2 levels.
- Consider a termination of efforts if no reversible underlying cause is found. Consider patient's age, comorbid conditions, and length of downtime to help guide decision making.

MEDICATION

First Line

- Vascular access for medications: IV or IO
- Consider medications after initiation of CPR and defibrillation attempt; medications should be administered during CPR as soon as possible following a rhythm check.
- Epinephrine: 1 mg IV q3–5min or vasopressin 40 U IV single dose (4)[B] (can be used once in lieu of the 1st or 2nd dose of epinephrine in VT or VF but not in PEA):
  - Vasopressin is not recommended in children.
  - Pediatric dose of epinephrine: 0.01 mg/kg
- Magnesium sulfate: 1–2 g diluted in 10 mL D_5W IV push in suspected torsades de pointes (4)[B]:
  - Magnesium is relatively contraindicated in renal failure, but given the consequences of not correcting this rhythm, contraindication is only relative in this setting.
- Antiarrhythmics:
  - Consider if VT/VF is unresponsive to 2–3 shocks and the 1st dose of vasopressor.
  - Amiodarone is the drug preferred by the AHA. Dosing: 300 mg IV push followed by 2nd dose of 150 mg IV (4)[B].
  - Amiodarone for perfusing tachyarrhythmias: 150 mg over 10 minutes; repeat as needed followed by a maintenance infusion of 1 mg/min for the first 6 hours.
  - Lidocaine: Initial dose, 1–1.5 mg/kg IV; a repeat loading dose of 1–1.5 mg/kg can be given at 5–10-minute intervals if VT/VF persist to maximum dose of 3 mg/kg, then followed by drip if perfusing rhythm is recovered.
- Endotracheal medications (NAVEL): naloxone, atropine, vasopressin (and Valium), epinephrine, or lidocaine. Each may be placed in 5–10 mL of normal saline or sterile water and given by ET followed by bagging. Dosage should be 2–2.5× recommended IV dose. IV or IO is preferred.

Second Line

- Dopamine: 2–10 mcg/kg/min IV for bradycardia
- Procainamide: 30 mg/min IV in refractory VF/VT (maximum dose: 17 mg/kg) is permissible. However, because the time to a useful level by infusion is so long, it is unlikely to be of benefit in cardiac arrest but may be useful in perfusing tachycardias (4)[C].
- Calcium: may be useful in hyperkalemia, ionized hypokalemia secondary multiple transfusions, and Ca^+ channel blocker toxicity; otherwise, no clear benefit is shown.
- High-dose epinephrine: No survival benefit is seen with a high dose (0.1 mg/kg), but it should be considered in exceptional situations, such as β-blocker or calcium channel blocker overdoses.
- Bicarbonate: Generally ineffective in sudden cardiac arrest; 1 mEq/kg IV only in known preexisting bicarbonate-responsive acidosis, hyperkalemia, or to correct widened QRS complex in known responsive overdoses (i.e., tricyclics). Also may be considered in patients with prolonged or unknown downtime (4)[C].

ISSUES FOR REFERRAL

- Consider communication with the medical examiner's office.
- Consider communication with an organ/tissue bank.

ADDITIONAL THERAPIES

Therapeutic hypothermia after resuscitation (to 32–34°C within 6 hours of collapse for 12–24 hours) should be performed if possible. The greatest benefit is seen in VF as initial rhythm and short downtime (<25 minutes), but it should be considered with any patient who has ROSC and coma state (5). New evidence suggests that a strategy of targeted temperature management (temperature <36°C) confers the same benefits as hypothermia for out-of-hospital arrests (6).

INPATIENT CONSIDERATIONS

Admission Criteria/Initial Stabilization

- Decreasing the emergency medical services (EMS) response interval increases survival (4)[A].
- The home use of AEDs does not improve survival (7).

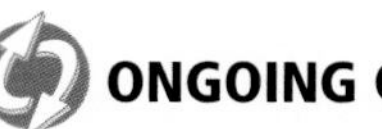

ONGOING CARE

FOLLOW-UP RECOMMENDATIONS

Patient Monitoring

- Admit to ICU or coronary care unit (CCU) on continuous monitoring.
- Consider electroencephalogram (EEG) to assess for nonconvulsive status epilepticus.

PROGNOSIS

- The outcome is related to underlying disease, age, duration of arrest, and other factors.
- The outcome is poor with the following indicators:
  - >4 minutes to CPR or >8 minutes to ACLS
  - Arrest occurs out of hospital
  - Resuscitation effort >30 minutes
- ~17% survive in-hospital arrest
- ~1–10% survive to leave the hospital in out-of-hospital arrest, varying by geographic region.
- ~10–15% of those with VF survive.
- If the arrest is out of hospital without a return of vital signs from advanced life support (ALS) prehospital care, the patient is unlikely to respond to emergency department (ED) resuscitation efforts.
- If the patient has an ROSC with coma, strongly consider induced hypothermia to improve the neurologic outcome (number needed to treat in VF = 6).

COMPLICATIONS

- Significant neurologic, hepatic, renal, or cardiac ischemic injury or multiorgan systems failure
- Rib fractures, hemopneumothorax, abdominal organ injury from CPR

REFERENCES

1. Perera P, Mailhot T, Riley D, et al. The RUSH exam: Rapid Ultrasound in SHock in the evaluation of the critically ill. *Emerg Med Clin North Am*. 2010;28(1):29–56, vii.
2. Neumar RW, Otto CW, Link MS, et al. Part 8: adult advanced cardiovascular life support: 2010 American Heart Association Guidelines for Cardiopulmonary Resuscitation and Emergency Cardiovascular Care. *Circulation*. 2010;122(18 Suppl 3):S729–S767.
3. Stiell IG, Nichol G, Leroux BG, et al. Early versus later rhythm analysis in patients with out-of-hospital cardiac arrest. *N Engl J Med*. 2011;365(9):787–797.
4. Hypothermia after Cardiac Arrest Study Group. Mild therapeutic hypothermia to improve the neurologic outcome after cardiac arrest. *N Engl J Med*. 2002;346(8):549–556.
5. Testori C, Sterz F, Behringer W, et al. Mild therapeutic hypothermia is associated with favourable outcome in patients after cardiac arrest with non-shockable rhythms. *Resuscitation*. 2011;82(9):1162–1167.
6. Nielsen N, Wetterslev J, Cronberg T, et al. Targeted temperature management at 33°C versus 36°C after cardiac arrest. *N Engl J Med*. 2013;369(23):2197–2206.
7. Bardy GH, Lee KL, Mark DB, et al. Home use of automated external defibrillators for sudden cardiac arrest. *N Engl J Med*. 2008;358(17):1793–1804.

ADDITIONAL READING

- Holzer M. Targeted temperature management for comatose survivors of cardiac arrest. *N Engl J Med*. 2010;363(13):1256–1264.
- Wik L, Hansen TB, Fylling F, et al. Delaying defibrillation to give basic cardiopulmonary resuscitation to patients with out-of-hospital ventricular fibrillation: a randomized trial. *JAMA*. 2003;289(11):1389–1395.

SEE ALSO

Algorithm: Coronary Syndrome, Acute

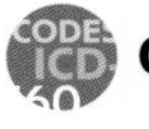

CODES

ICD10

- I46.9 Cardiac arrest, cause unspecified
- I46.2 Cardiac arrest due to underlying cardiac condition
- I46.8 Cardiac arrest due to other underlying condition

CLINICAL PEARLS

- C-A-B replaces ABCs for the priority of approach to a patient with a suspected cardiac arrest.
- Prompt initiation of CPR, particularly chest compressions (push hard, push fast, and don't interrupt!), and immediate defibrillation (in witnessed VF and pulseless VT but not in PEA) are 1st priority.
- For an unwitnessed arrest, complete 2 minutes of CPR before attempting defibrillation.
- Epinephrine is the 1st drug to give in any case requiring CPR: IO and endotracheal routes are preferred if peripheral access is not attainable. Central line may be considered if unable to achieve access and if performed femoral approach is preferred.
- Therapeutic hypothermia has significantly improved neurologic outcomes in cardiac arrest and should be initiated as soon as possible in any patient with ROSC and coma state.

CARDIOMYOPATHY, END STAGE

Timothy P. Fitzgibbons, MD, PhD • Theo E. Meyer, MD, DPhil

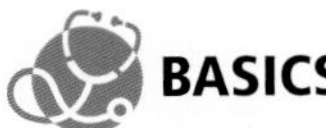

BASICS

DESCRIPTION

- Cardiomyopathy encompasses a large group of diseases of the myocardium that commonly result in mechanical pump dysfunction. The current classification scheme attempts to differentiate between myocardial diseases confined to the myocardium (primary) and those due to systemic disorders (secondary). Specific causes of myocardial dysfunction due to other cardiovascular disorders are considered a third, separate category (1).
- Classification of cardiomyopathy
  - Primary
    - Genetic
    - Hypertrophic cardiomyopathy (HCM)
    - Arrhythmogenic right ventricular cardiomyopathy/dysplasia (ARVC/D)
    - Left ventricular (LV) noncompaction (LVNC)
    - Glycogen storage (Danon type, PRKAG2)
    - Conduction defects
    - Mitochondrial myopathies
    - Ion channel disorders: long QT syndrome, Brugada, short QT syndrome, catecholaminergic ventricular tachycardia (CVPT), Asian SUNDS
    - Mixed
    - Dilated cardiomyopathy (DCM) (genetic or nongenetic)
    - Restrictive
    - Acquired
    - Myocarditis, stress cardiomyopathy, peripartum, tachycardia-induced, infants of type 1 diabetic mothers
  - Secondary (see list below)
  - Specific
    - Ischemic
    - Valvular
    - Hypertensive
    - Congenital heart disease
- Patients with end-stage cardiomyopathy have stage D heart failure or severe symptoms at rest refractory to standard medical therapy.
- System(s) affected: cardiovascular; renal

Pediatric Considerations

Etiology: idiopathic, viral, congenital heart disease, and familial

Pregnancy Considerations

May occur in women postpartum

EPIDEMIOLOGY

Predominant age: Ischemic cardiomyopathy is the most common etiology; predominantly in patients aged >50 years. Consider uncommon causes in young.

Incidence

- 60,000 patients <65 years die each year from end-stage heart disease.
- 35,000–70,000 people might benefit from cardiac transplant or chronic support.

Prevalence

Most rapidly growing form of heart disease

ETIOLOGY AND PATHOPHYSIOLOGY

The most frequent causes are in bold:

- Ischemic heart disease: most common etiology; up to 66% of patients
- Hypertension
- Valvular heart disease
- Primary genetic causes
- Congenital heart disease
- Peripartum/postpartum
- Endocrine
  - Diabetes mellitus
  - Hyperthyroidism
  - Hypothyroidism
  - Hyperparathyroidism
  - Pheochromocytoma
  - Acromegaly
- Nutritional deficiencies
  - Beriberi, pellagra, scurvy, selenium, carnitine, kwashiorkor
- Autoimmune/collagen
  - Systemic lupus erythematosus
  - Dermatomyositis
  - Rheumatoid arthritis
  - Scleroderma
  - Polyarteritis nodosa
- Infectious causes
  - Viral (e.g., HIV, coxsackievirus, adenovirus)
  - Bacterial and mycobacterial (e.g., diphtheria, rheumatic fever)
  - Parasitic (e.g., toxoplasmosis, *Trypanosoma cruzi*)
- Infiltrative (2)
  - Amyloidosis
  - Gaucher disease
  - Hurler disease
  - Hunter disease
  - Fabry disease
- Storage
  - Hemochromatosis
  - Fabry disease
  - Glycogen storage disease (type II, Pompe)
  - Niemann-Pick disease
- Neuromuscular/neurologic
  - Duchenne and Emery-Dreifuss muscular dystrophies
  - Friedreich ataxia
  - Myotonic dystrophy
  - Neurofibromatosis
  - Tuberous sclerosis
- Toxic
  - Alcohol
  - Drugs and chemotherapy: anthracyclines, cyclophosphamide, Herceptin
  - Radiation
  - Heavy metal, chemical agents
- Inflammatory (granulomatous):
  - Sarcoidosis
- Idiopathic
- Endomyocardial
  - Endomyocardial fibrosis
  - Hypereosinophilic syndrome (Loeffler endocarditis)

Genetics

Autosomal dominant HCM is the most common form of primary genetic cardiomyopathy (1/500 in the general population). Genetic causes of DCM are less common, accounting for 1/3 cases, with mostly autosomal dominant inheritance. LNC and ARVC are also inherited in an autosomal dominant fashion in addition to LQTS and other ion-channel disorders.

RISK FACTORS

- Hypertension
- Hyperlipidemia
- Obesity
- Coronary artery diease
- Diabetes mellitus
- Smoking
- Physical inactivity
- Excessive alcohol intake
- Dietary sodium
- Obstructive sleep apnea
- Chemotherapy

GENERAL PREVENTION

Reduce salt and water intake; home BP and daily weight measurement

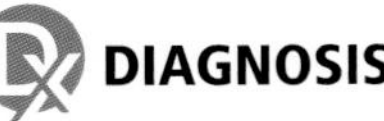

DIAGNOSIS

HISTORY

- Dyspnea at rest or with exertion
- Paroxysmal nocturnal dyspnea
- Orthopnea
- Postprandial dyspnea
- Right upper quadrant pain or bloating
- Midabdominal pain
- Fatigue
- Syncope
- Edema

PHYSICAL EXAM

- Tachypnea
- Cheyne-Stokes breathing
- Low pulse pressure
- Cool extremities
- Jugular venous distention
- Bibasilar rales
- Tachycardia
- Displaced point of maximal impulse (PMI)
- S_3 gallop
- Blowing systolic murmur
- Hepatosplenomegaly
- Ascites
- Edema

DIFFERENTIAL DIAGNOSIS

- Severe pulmonary disease
- Primary pulmonary hypertension
- Recurrent pulmonary embolism
- Constrictive pericarditis
- Some advanced forms of malignancy
- Anemia

DIAGNOSTIC TESTS & INTERPRETATION

- ECG: LV hypertrophy, interventricular conduction delay, atrial fibrillation, evidence of prior Q-wave infarction
- Hyponatremia
- Prerenal azotemia
- Anemia
- Mild elevation in troponin
- Elevated B-type natriuretic peptide (BNP) or pro-BNP
- Mild hyperbilirubinemia
- Elevated liver function tests
- Elevated uric acid

Initial Tests (lab, imaging)

- ECG
- Chest radiograph
  - Cardiomegaly
  - Increased vascular markings to the upper lobes
  - Pleural effusions may or may not be present.

- Echocardiography
  - In dilated cardiomyopathy, 4-chamber enlargement and global hypokinesis are present.
  - In hypertrophic cardiomyopathy, severe LV hypertrophy is present.
  - Segmental contraction abnormalities of the LV are indicative of previous localized myocardial infarction.
- Cardiac MRI
  - May be useful to characterize certain nonischemic cardiomyopathies
- Myocardial stress perfusion imaging (MPI)
  - Recommended in those with new-onset LV dysfunction or when ischemia is suspected

Diagnostic Procedures/Other

Cardiac catheterization

- Helpful to rule out ischemic heart disease
- Characterize hemodynamic severity
- Pulmonary artery catheters may be reasonable in patients with refractory heart failure to help guide management.

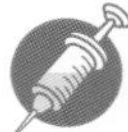

TREATMENT

See "Heart Failure, Chronic" for detailed treatment protocols.

GENERAL MEASURES

- Reduction of filling pressures
- Treatment of electrolyte disturbances

MEDICATION

First Line

- Systolic failure syndromes
  - ACE inhibitors: All considered equally effective; initiate at low doses and titrate as tolerated to target doses (3)[A].
  - Loop diuretics
    - May need to be given IV initially and then orally as patient stabilizes
  - Furosemide, 40–120 mg/day or TID (3)[A]
  - β-Blockers
    - Use with caution in acutely decompensated or low–cardiac output states.
    - Initiate with low doses and titrate as tolerated.
  - Metoprolol succinate, 12.5–200 mg/day; carvedilol, 3.125–25 mg BID; or bisoprolol, 1.25–10 mg/day (3)[A]
  - Patients with New York Heart Association (NYHA) II–IV heart failure, ejection fraction (EF) <35%, on standard therapy: aldosterone antagonists: spironolactone or eplerenone (3)[A]
  - Digoxin, 0.125–0.25 mg/day for symptomatic patients on standard therapy (3)[B]
  - Combination hydralazine/isosorbide dinitrate is 1st-line treatment in African American patients with class III–IV symptoms already on standard therapy and for all patients with reduced EF and symptoms incompletely responsive to ACE inhibitor and β-blocker (3)[A].
    - Contraindications
  - β-Blockers: low cardiac output, 2nd- or 3rd-degree heart block
  - Avoid use of diltiazem and verapamil in patients with systolic dysfunction.
  - Aldosterone antagonists: oliguria, anuria, renal dysfunction
  - Loop diuretics: hypokalemia, hypomagnesemia
  - ACE inhibitors: pregnancy, angioedema
- Precautions
  - In patients with chronic kidney disease, digoxin dosage should be $\leq$0.125 mg/day and drug levels followed carefully to avoid toxicity.
  - Closely monitor electrolytes.
  - ACE inhibitors: Initiate with care if BP is low. Begin with low-dose captopril, such as 6.25 mg TID.
  - β-Blockers: Avoid in patients with evidence of poor tissue perfusion; they may further depress systolic function.
  - Milrinone, dobutamine: long-term use associated with increased mortality
- Medications TO AVOID
  - NSAIDs
  - Glitazones
  - Cilostazol

Second Line

- Angiotensin receptor blockers as an alternative to ACE inhibitors
- Inotropic therapy (e.g., dobutamine or milrinone) for cardiogenic shock and support prior to surgery or cardiac transplantation (3)[B]
- Continuous inotrope infusion may be considered in stage D outpatients for symptom control in those who are not eligible for transplantation or mechanical circulatory support (3)[B].

ISSUES FOR REFERRAL

Management by a heart failure team improves outcomes and facilitates early transplant referral.

ADDITIONAL THERAPIES

- Prophylactic implantable cardioverter defibrillator (ICD) should be considered for patients with a left ventricular ejection fraction (LVEF) <35% and mild to moderate symptoms (3)[A].
- Cardiac resynchronization therapy (CRT) is recommended and should be considered for patients in sinus rhythm with a QRS >150 msec, LVEF <35%, in FC I–III and ambulatory FC IV patients (3)[A].
- Patients with severe, refractory heart failure with no reasonable expectation of improvement should not be considered for an ICD.
- Consideration of an LV assist device as "permanent" or destination therapy or cardiac transplantation is reasonable in selected stage D patients.

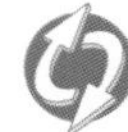

ONGOING CARE

DIET

Low-fat, low-salt, fluid restriction

PROGNOSIS

~20–40% of patients in NYHA functional class IV die within 1 year. With a transplant, 1-year survival is as high as 94%.

COMPLICATIONS

Worsening congestive heart failure syncope, renal failure, arrhythmias, or sudden death

REFERENCES

1. Maron BJ, Towbin JA, Thiene G, et al. Contemporary definitions and classification of the cardiomyopathies: an American Heart Association Scientific Statement from the Council on Clinical Cardiology, Heart Failure and Transplantation Committee; Quality of Care and Outcomes Research and Functional Genomics and Translational Biology Interdisciplinary Working Groups; and Council on Epidemiology and Prevention. *Circulation*. 2006;113(14):1807–1816.
2. Seward JB, Casaclang-Verzosa G. Infiltrative cardiovascular diseases: cardiomyopathies that look alike. *J Am Coll Cardiol*. 2010;55(27):1769–1779.
3. Yancy CW, Jessup M, Bozkurt B, et al. 2013 ACCF/AHA guideline for the management of heart failure: a report of the American College of Cardiology Foundation/American Heart Association Task Force on Practice Guidelines. *Circulation*. 2013;128:1–375.

SEE ALSO

Alcohol Abuse and Dependence; Alcohol Withdrawal; Amyloidosis; Congestive Heart Failure; Diabetes Mellitus, Type 1; Diabetes Mellitus, Type 2; Hypertension, Essential; Hypothyroidism, Adult; Idiopathic Hypertrophic Subaortic Stenosis; Protein Energy Malnutrition; Rheumatic Fever; Sarcoidosis

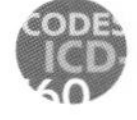

CODES

ICD10

- I42.9 Cardiomyopathy, unspecified
- I42.2 Other hypertrophic cardiomyopathy
- I42.1 Obstructive hypertrophic cardiomyopathy

CLINICAL PEARLS

- Cardiomyopathy represents the end-stage of a large number of disease processes involving the heart muscle.
- Ischemic, hypertensive, postviral, familial, alcoholic, and incessant tachycardia-induced are the most common cardiomyopathy varieties seen in the United States.
- Core therapy for heart failure applies: salt restriction, diuretics, ACE inhibitors, β-blockers, digoxin, and electrical treatments, such as cardiac resynchronization and implantable defibrillators, as appropriate.

CAROTID STENOSIS

Edlira Yzeiraj, DO, MS • Maria M. Plummer, MD

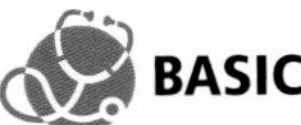

BASICS

Carotid stenosis may be caused by atherosclerosis, intimal fibroplasia, vasculitis, adventitial cysts, or vascular tumors; atherosclerosis is the most common etiology.

DESCRIPTION

- Narrowing of carotid artery lumen is typically due to atherosclerotic changes in the vessel wall. Atherosclerotic plaques are responsible for 90% of extracranial carotid lesions and up to 30% of all ischemic strokes.
- A "hemodynamically significant" carotid stenosis produces a drop in pressure, reduction in flow, or both and corresponds approximately to a 60% diameter-reducing stenosis (1).
- Carotid lesions are classified by the following:
  - Symptom status
    - Asymptomatic: tend to be homogenous and stable
    - Symptomatic (stroke, transient cerebral ischemic event): tend to be heterogeneous and unstable
  - Degree of stenosis
    - High grade: 80–99% stenosis
    - Moderate grade: 50–79% stenosis
    - Low grade: <50% stenosis

EPIDEMIOLOGY

More common in men and with increasing age (see "Risk Factors")

Incidence

Unclear (asymptomatic patients often go undiagnosed)

Prevalence

- Moderate stenosis (2)
  - Age <50 years: men 0.2%, women 0%
  - Age >80 years: men 7.5%, women 5%
- Severe stenosis (2)
  - Age <50 years: men 0.1%, women 0%
  - Age >80 years: men 3.1%, women 0.9%

ETIOLOGY AND PATHOPHYSIOLOGY

- Atherosclerosis begins during adolescence, consistently at carotid bifurcation. The carotid bulb has unique blood flow dynamics. Hemodynamic disturbances cause endothelial injury and dysfunction. Plaque formation in vessel wall results, and stenosis then ensues.
- Initial cause not well understood, but certain risk factors are frequently present (see "Risk Factors"). Tensile stress on the vessel wall, turbulence, and arterial wall shear stress seem to be involved.

Genetics

- Increased incidence among family members
- Genetically linked factors
  - Diabetes mellitus (DM), race, hypertension (HTN), family history, obesity
  - In a recent single nucleotide polymorphism study, the following genes were strongly associated with worse carotid plaque: *TNFSF4*, *PPARA*, *TLR4*, *ITGA2*, and *HABP2*.

RISK FACTORS

- Nonmodifiable factors: advanced age, male sex, family history, cardiac disease, congenital arteriopathies (1)
- Modifiable factors: smoking, diet, dyslipidemia, physical inactivity, obesity, HTN, DM

GENERAL PREVENTION

- Antihypertensive treatment to maintain BP <140/90 mm Hg (systolic BP of 150 mm Hg is target in elderly)
- Smoking cessation to reduce the risk of atherosclerosis progression and stroke
- Lipid control: regression of carotid atherosclerotic lesions seen with statin therapy

COMMONLY ASSOCIATED CONDITIONS

- Transient ischemic attack (TIA)/stroke
- Coronary artery disease (CAD)/myocardial infarction (MI)
- Peripheral vascular disease (PVD)
- HTN
- DM
- Hyperlipidemia

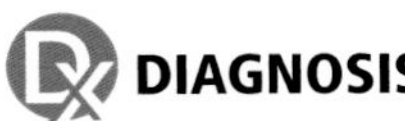

DIAGNOSIS

Screening for carotid stenosis is not recommended. However, in the setting of symptoms suggestive of stroke or TIA, workup for this condition may be indicated.

HISTORY

- Identification of modifiable and nonmodifiable comorbidities (see "Risk Factors")
- History of cerebral ischemic event
- Stroke, TIA, amaurosis fugax (monocular blindness), aphasia
- Coronary artery disease/MI
- Peripheral arterial disease
- Review of systems, with focus on risk factors for
  - Cardiovascular disease
  - Stroke (HTN and arrhythmia)

PHYSICAL EXAM

- Lateralizing neurologic deficits: contralateral motor and/or sensory deficit
- Amaurosis fugax: ipsilateral transient visual obscuration from retinal ischemia
- Visual field defect
- Dysarthria and, in the case of dominant (usually left) hemisphere involvement, aphasia
- Carotid bruit (low sensitivity and specificity)

DIFFERENTIAL DIAGNOSIS

- Aortic valve stenosis
- Aortic arch atherosclerosis
- Arrhythmia with cardiogenic embolization
- Migraine
- Brain tumor
- Metabolic disturbances
- Functional/psychological deficit
- Seizure

DIAGNOSTIC TESTS & INTERPRETATION

Initial Tests (lab, imaging)

Workup for suspected TIA/stroke may include the following:

- CBC with differential
- Basic metabolic panel
- ESR (if temporal arteritis a consideration)
- Glucose/glycated hemoglobin (HbA1c)
- Fasting lipid profile
- Duplex ultrasound (US) identifies ≥50% stenosis, with 98% sensitivity and 88% specificity. Doppler US determines degree of stenosis by assessing velocity of blood flow through stenotic vessel. Although findings should be confirmed by angiogram (MR or CT), US is increasingly used to screen prior to surgical assessment.

Follow-Up Tests & Special Considerations

- Proceed to imaging if there is suggestion of stenosis from history or physical exam.
- Other noninvasive imaging techniques can add detail to duplex results:
  - CT angiography
    - 88% sensitivity and 100% specificity
    - Requires contrast load with risk for subsequent renal morbidity
  - MR angiography
    - 95% sensitivity and 90% specificity
    - Evaluates cerebral circulation (extracranial and intracranial) as well as aortic arch and common carotid artery
    - The presence of unstable plaque can be determined if the following characteristics are seen:
      - Presence of thin/ruptured fibrous cap
      - Presence of lipid-rich necrotic core
    - Tends to overestimate degree of stenosis

Diagnostic Procedures/Other

Cerebral (catheter) angiography is the traditional gold standard for diagnosis:

- Delineates anatomy pertaining to aortic arch and proximal vessels
- However, procedure is invasive and has multiple risks:
  - Contrast-induced renal dysfunction (1–5% complication rate)
  - Thromboembolic-related complications (1–2.6% complication rate) and neurologic complications
  - Should be used only when other tests are not conclusive

Test Interpretation

- Stenosis consistently occurs at carotid bifurcation, with plaque formation most often at proximal internal carotid artery:
  - Plaque is thickest at the carotid bifurcation.
  - Plaque occupies the intima and inner media and avoids outer media and adventitia.
- Plaque histology
  - Homogenous (stable) plaques seldom hemorrhage or ulcerate:
    - Fatty streak and fibrous tissue deposition
    - Diffuse intimal thickening
  - Heterogenous (unstable) plaques may hemorrhage or ulcerate:
    - Presence of lipid-laden macrophages, necrotic debris, cholesterol crystals
    - Ulcerated plaques
  - Soft and gelatinous clots with platelets, fibrin, and red and white blood cells

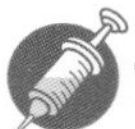

TREATMENT

Smoking cessation, BP control, use of antiplatelet medication, and statin medication are the primary treatments for both asymptomatic and symptomatic carotid stenosis.

GENERAL MEASURES

- Lifestyle modifications: dietary control and weight loss, exercise of 30 min/day at least 5 days/week.
- Patients should be advised to quit smoking and offered smoking cessation intervention to reduce the risk of atherosclerotic progression and stroke.
- Control of HTN with antihypertensive agents to maintain BP <140/90 (3)[A]

MEDICATION

- Antihypertensive treatment (<140/90 mm Hg)
- Diet and exercise are useful adjuncts to therapy (3).
  - Statin initiation is recommended (3)[A] to reduce LDL cholesterol <100 mg/dL; choose moderate- to high-intensity statin therapy for anti-inflammatory benefit.
- Aspirin: 75–325 mg/day (3)[A]
- If patient has sustained ischemic stroke or TIA, antiplatelet therapy with
  - Aspirin alone (75–325 mg/day) (3)[A] *or*
  - Clopidogrel alone (75 mg/day) (3)[A], *or*
  - Aspirin plus extended-release dipyridamole (25 and 200 mg BID, respectively) (3)[A]

ISSUES FOR REFERRAL

- For acute symptomatic stroke, order imaging and contact neurology.
- For known carotid stenosis, some suggest duplex imaging every 6 months if stenosis is >50% and patient is a surgical candidate.

SURGERY/OTHER PROCEDURES

- Symptomatic carotid stenosis
  - Carotid endarterectomy (CEA) is recommended in symptomatic patients with a carotid stenosis of 70–99% without near-occlusion. Benefit in patients with carotid near-occlusion is uncertain in the long term (4)[A].
  - CEA is recommended for patients with a life expectancy of at least 5 years. The anticipated rate of perioperative stroke or mortality must be <6% (3)[A].
  - Treatment with aspirin (81–325 mg/day) is recommended for all patients who are having CEA. Aspirin should be started prior to surgery and continued for at least 3 months postsurgery but may be continued indefinitely (5)[B].
  - Carotid artery stenting (CAS) provides similar long-term outcomes as CEA (6)[A]. Age should be considered when planning a carotid intervention.
    - CAS has an increased risk of adverse cerebrovascular events in the elderly compared to the young but similar mortality risk. CEA is associated with similar neurologic outcomes in the elderly and young, at the expense of increased mortality (7)[A].
    - CAS is suggested in select patients with neck anatomy unfavorable for arterial surgery and those with comorbid conditions that greatly increase the risk of anesthesia and surgery (3)[A].
- Asymptomatic patients
  - Some recommend CEA for asymptomatic men who have 60–99% stenosis, have a life expectancy of at least 5 years, and the perioperative risk of stroke and death is <3% (6)[B]. There is no evidence supporting CEA for the treatment of asymptomatic women and meta-analysis of the asymptomatic carotid stenosis (ACAS) and asymptomatic carotid surgery trial (ACST) data showed no benefit (8)[A].
  - The advantage of surgical compared with medical therapy has decreased with contemporary medical management. It is not possible to make an evidence-based recommendation for or against surgical therapy with current literature (9)[A].

INPATIENT CONSIDERATIONS

Admission Criteria/Initial Stabilization

Any patient with presentation of acute symptomatic carotid stenosis should be hospitalized for further diagnostic workup and appropriate therapy.

Rapid evaluation for symptoms compatible with TIA should be obtained in the emergency department (ED) or inpatient setting.

Discharge Criteria

24–48 hours post-CEA, if ambulating, taking adequate PO intake, and neurologically intact

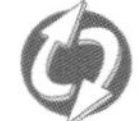

ONGOING CARE

FOLLOW-UP RECOMMENDATIONS

Patient Monitoring

After CEA, overnight in postanesthesia care unit or step-down

- Duplex at 2–6 weeks postop
- Duplex every 6–12 months
- Reoperative CEA or CAS is reasonable if there is rapidly progressive restenosis (3)[A].

DIET

Low-fat, low-cholesterol, low-salt diet at discharge

PATIENT EDUCATION

- Signs and symptoms of TIA/stroke
  - Lateralizing neurologic deficits, monocular blindness, aphasia
- Diet and lifestyle modification

COMPLICATIONS

- Untreated: TIA/Stroke (risk of ipsilateral stroke approximately 1.68% per year [9])
- Postoperative (s/p CEA)
  - Perioperative (within 30 days)
    - Stroke/death, cranial nerve injury, hemorrhage, hemodynamic instability, MI
  - Late (>30 days postop)
    - Recurrent stenosis, false aneurysm at surgical site

REFERENCES

1. Goldstein LB, Bushnell CD, Adams RJ, et al. Guidelines for the primary prevention of stroke: a guideline for healthcare professionals from the American Heart Association/American Stroke Association. *Stroke*. 2011;42(2):517–584.
2. de Weerd M, Greving JP, Hedblad B, et al. Prevalence of asymptomatic carotid artery stenosis in the general population: an individual participant data meta-analysis. *Stroke*. 2010;41(6):1294–1297.
3. Brott TG, Halperin JL, Abbara S, et al. 2011 ASA/ACCF/AHA/AANN/AANS/ACR/ASNR/CNS/SAIP/SCAI/SIR/SNIS/SVM/SVS guideline on the management of patients with extracranial carotid and vertebral artery disease: executive summary. *J Am Coll Cardiol*. 2011;57(8):1002–1044.
4. Rerkasem K, Rothwell PM. Carotid endarterectomy for symptomatic carotid stenosis. *Cochrane Database Syst Rev*. 2011;(4):CD001081.
5. Chaturvedi S, Bruno A, Feasby T. Carotid endarterectomy—an evidenced–based review: report of the Therapeutics and Technology Assessment Subcommittee of the American Academy of Neurology. *Neurology*. 2005 65(6):794–801.
6. Bonati LH, Lyrer P, Ederle J, et al. Percutaneous transluminal balloon angioplasty and stenting for carotid artery stenosis. *Cochrane Database Syst Rev*. 2012;(9):CD000515.
7. Antoniou GA, Georgiadis GS, Georgakarakos EI, et al. Meta-analysis and meta-regression analysis of outcomes of carotid endarterectomy and stenting in the elderly. *JAMA Surg*. 2013;148(12):1140–52.
8. Rothwell PM, Goldstein LB. Carotid endarterectomy for asymptomatic carotid stenosis: asymptomatic carotid surgery trial. *Stroke*. 2004;35(10):2425– 2427.
9. Raman G, Moorthy D, Hadar N, et al. Management strategies for asymptomatic carotid stenosis: a systematic review and meta-analysis. *Ann Intern Med*. 2013;158(9):676–685.

ADDITIONAL READING

- Lovrencic-Huzjan A, Rundek T, Katsnelson M. Recommendations for management of patients with carotid stenosis. *Stroke Res Treat*. 2012;2012:175869.
- Paraskevas KI, Mikhailidis DP, Veith FJ. Comparison of the five 2011 guidelines treatment of carotid stenosis. *J Vasc Surg*. 2012;55(5):1504–1508.
- Roger VL, Go AS, Lloyd-Jones DM, et al. Heart disease and stroke statistics—2012 update: a report from the American Heart Association. *Circulation*. 2012;125(1):2–e220.

SEE ALSO

Algorithms: Transient Ischemic Attack; Stroke; Hypercholesterolemia

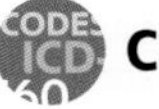

CODES

ICD10

- I65.29 Occlusion and stenosis of unspecified carotid artery
- I65.21 Occlusion and stenosis of right carotid artery
- I65.22 Occlusion and stenosis of left carotid artery

CLINICAL PEARLS

- Atherosclerosis is responsible for 90% of all cases of carotid artery stenosis.
- Duplex US is the best initial imaging modality.
- Antiplatelet therapy and aggressive treatment of vascular risk factors are the mainstays of medical therapy.
- Compared with CEA, CAS increases the risk of any stroke and decreases the risk of MI. For every 1,000 patients opting for stenting rather than endarterectomy, 19 more patients would have strokes and 10 fewer would have MIs.

CARPAL TUNNEL SYNDROME

Philip Aurigemma, MD • Marci D. Jones, MD

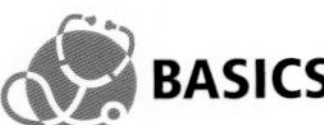

BASICS

DESCRIPTION

- Carpal tunnel syndrome (CTS) is a symptomatic compression neuropathy of the median nerve.
- Increased pressure within the carpal tunnel leads to compression of the median nerve and characteristic of motor-sensory findings.
- The dorsal element of the carpal tunnel is composed of the carpal bones. The transverse carpal ligament defines the palmar boundary:
  - The carpal tunnel contains nine flexor tendons in addition to the median nerve.
- Symptoms most commonly affect the dominant hand, but >50% of patients will experience bilateral symptoms.
- System(s) affected: musculoskeletal, nervous

ALERT

Pregnancy: increased incidence during pregnancy (up to 20–45%) of patients

EPIDEMIOLOGY

- Predominant age: 40–60 years
- Predominant sex: female > male (3:1–10:1)

Incidence

- 2 peaks: Late 50s in women and again in late 70s where gender ratio is more equal
- Incidence up to 276/100,000 has been reported.
- Incidence increases with age.

Prevalence

- 9.2% in women and 6% in men. 50 cases per 1,000 subjects per year in United States (1)[C]
- Diabetic prevalence rate of 14% (without neuropathy) and 30% (with diabetic neuropathy)
- Rising prevalence may be the result of increasing lifespan and increasing prevalence of diabetes.

ETIOLOGY AND PATHOPHYSIOLOGY

- Combination of mechanical trauma, inflammation, increased pressure, and ischemic injury to the median nerve within the carpal tunnel
- Acute CTS caused by rapid and sustained pressure in carpal tunnel, usually secondary to trauma, may require urgent surgical decompression.
- Chronic CTS divided into four categories (1)[C]:
  - Idiopathic: combination of edema and fibrous hypertrophy without inflammation
  - Anatomic: persistent median artery, ganglion cyst, infection, space-occupying lesion within carpal tunnel
  - Systemic: associated with medical conditions such as obesity, diabetes, hypothyroidism, rheumatoid arthritis, amyloidosis, scleroderma, renal failure as well as drug toxicity
  - Exertional: attributed to repetitive use of wrists and digits, repeated palmar impact, and use of vibratory tools. Repetitive use has not been objectively shown as a cause of CTS.

Genetics

Unknown; however, a familial type has been reported.

RISK FACTORS

- Prolonged postures in extremes of wrist ranges of motion and repetitive exposure to vibration
- Conditions that alter the fluid balance in the body including pregnancy, menopause, obesity, renal failure, hypothyroidism, congestive heart failure (CHF), and oral contraceptive use
- Neuropathic factors, such as diabetes, alcoholism, vitamin deficiency, or exposure to toxins, can play a role in eliciting CTS symptoms.
- No universal agreement that CTS is job related.

GENERAL PREVENTION

There is no known prevention for CTS. It is recommended to take a break once an hour when doing repetitive work involving hands.

COMMONLY ASSOCIATED CONDITIONS

- Diabetes
- Obesity
- Pregnancy
- Hypothyroidism
- Hyperparathyroidism, hypocalcemia
- Other miscellaneous associations include the following:
  - Acromegaly
  - Lupus erythematosus
  - Leukemia
  - Pyogenic infections
  - Sarcoidosis
  - Primary amyloidosis
  - Paget disease
  - Hormone replacement therapy

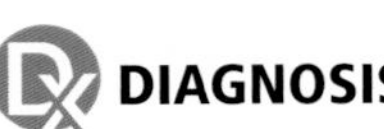

DIAGNOSIS

HISTORY

- Patients report nocturnal pain, numbness, and tingling in the thumb, index, long, and radial 1/2 of the ring fingers; patients may not localize and describe the entire hand as being affected.
- Hand weakness during tasks as opening jars is often noted early in the disorder.
- Atypical presentation involves paresthesias in radial digits, with pain radiating proximally along median nerve to elbow and sometimes the shoulder (1)[C].
- Symptoms characteristically are relieved by shaking or rubbing the hands.
- During waking hours, symptoms occur when driving, talking on the phone, and occasionally when using the hands for repetitive maneuvers.
- Presence of predisposing factors, such as diabetes, obesity, acromegaly, pregnancy

PHYSICAL EXAM

- Positive Tinel sign: Tapping over the palmar surface of the wrist proximal to the carpal tunnel may produce an electric sensation perceived by the patient (50% sensitivity; 77% specificity) along the distribution of the median nerve.
- Positive Phalen sign: Holding the wrist in a flexed position for 60 seconds may precipitate paresthesias (68% sensitivity; 73% specificity).
- Durkan compression test: Direct compression of median nerve at carpal tunnel for 30 seconds can also elicit symptoms (87% sensitivity; 90% specificity) (1)[C].
- Wasting of the thenar muscles is a late sign.
- Loss of 2-point discrimination

DIFFERENTIAL DIAGNOSIS

- Cervical spondylosis (carpal tunnel may also occur with cervical spine disease; "double crush")
- Generalized peripheral neuropathy
- Brachial plexus lesion, in particular upper trunk
- CNS disorders (multiple sclerosis, small cerebral infarction)
- Thoracic outlet syndrome
- Pronator syndrome
- Anterior interosseous syndrome
- Disorders affecting the musculoskeletal system in the region of the wrist, including the following:
  - Trauma or distal radius fracture
  - Degenerative joint disease
  - Rheumatoid arthritis
  - Ganglion cyst
- Scleroderma

DIAGNOSTIC TESTS & INTERPRETATION

No laboratory test is diagnostic.

- Normal serum thyrotropin (thyroid-stimulating hormone [TSH]) and normal serum glucose may be helpful in excluding secondary conditions associated with CTS.

Initial Tests (lab, imaging)

- Special tests
  - Electrodiagnostic studies
    - Sensitivity 85%; specificity 95%
    - Nerve conduction studies compare latency and amplitude of median nerve segment across the carpal tunnel to another nerve segment such as the radial or ulnar nerve.
    - Prolonged distal latency of the median motor and/or sensory fibers may be seen. Axon loss is suggested when amplitudes are decreased.
    - The most sensitive indicator is the median sensory distal latency, which is prolonged in CTS. Further, the sensory nerve action potential may be reduced or unobtainable.
    - Electromyographic changes are indicative of more long-standing or severe nerve dysfunction.
- Stimulation of the ulnar nerve should also take place to exclude generalized polyneuropathy.
- Standard radiographs of the wrist to evaluate bony anatomy and degenerative joint disease
- Special radiographic views of the carpal tunnel are of limited use.
- Magnetic resonance imaging and ultrasound are of limited benefit in diagnosis of CTS.

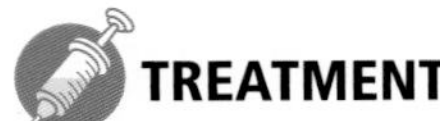

TREATMENT

GENERAL MEASURES

- Splinting of the wrist in a neutral position while sleeping may provide significant symptom relief:
  - Limited evidence indicates that splints worn at night are more effective than no treatment in the short term. Insufficient evidence to recommend 1 splint design or wearing regimen over any others (2)[A].
- Splinting (sometimes prolonged) typically allows symptoms to resolve.
- Corticosteroid injections are effective for up to 3 months compared with placebo (3)[A].
- Outcomes at 1 year show no benefit for local steroid injections compared to placebo (3)[A].

MEDICATION

First Line

NSAIDs, such as ibuprofen or naproxen sodium, are commonly used. There is insufficient evidence to determine the efficacy of this approach:

- Contraindications: GI intolerance
- Precautions: GI side effects of NSAIDs may preclude their use in selected patients.

Second Line

- Local steroid injection: Methylprednisolone injections are more effective than systemic steroids or placebo at 1 and 3 months and more effective than splinting at 6 months (4)[A].
- Response to injections can help confirm diagnosis of CTS and predict a better response to surgery.
- Possible side effects include reduction of collagen and proteoglycan synthesis, limiting tenocytes, and reducing mechanical strength of tendon, leading to further degeneration.
- Oral steroids may provide a short-term improvement (2–8 weeks) in symptoms.
- The long-term risks of even a short course of steroids should be balanced with the limited potential benefit of symptom improvement.

ISSUES FOR REFERRAL

Most surgeons do not perform operative release of the carpal tunnel without preoperative electrodiagnostic studies.

SURGERY/OTHER PROCEDURES

- Surgical decompression of the carpal tunnel by completely dividing the transverse carpal ligament provides symptom relief in >95% of patients.
- Surgical decompression is an outpatient procedure performed under local or regional anesthesia.
- Healing of the incision generally takes 2 weeks; an additional 2 weeks of recuperation may be required before the hand can be used for tasks requiring strength.
- Long-term results of open carpal tunnel release are excellent, with patients experiencing consistent pain relief over 10–15 years (5)[B].
- Recent randomized, controlled studies indicate that surgery leads to better functional improvements at 1 year compared with nonoperative management.
- Open versus endoscopic surgical procedures produce similar outcomes at 1 year. The approach should be based on surgeon and patient preference.
- Endoscopic carpal tunnel release likely has lower rates of minor complications and allows a faster return to work (6)[A].
- Therapeutic ultrasound, exercise, and mobilization interventions have limited benefit compared with other nonsurgical interventions. Poor quality evidence shows ultrasound may be more effective than placebo (7,8)[A].

COMPLEMENTARY & ALTERNATIVE MEDICINE

No trial data support the use of vitamin B_6 in the prevention or treatment of CTS.

INPATIENT CONSIDERATIONS

Admission Criteria/Initial Stabilization

Outpatient

ONGOING CARE

FOLLOW-UP RECOMMENDATIONS

Patient Monitoring

- Patients treated nonoperatively (splinting, injections) require follow-up over 4–12 weeks to ensure adequate progress.
- There is only limited, low-quality evidence to suggest that rehabilitation exercises such as wrist immobilization, ice therapy, and multimodal hand rehabilitation are beneficial.
- 7–20% of patients treated surgically may experience recurrence.

PATIENT EDUCATION

- Free online and printable patient information from the American Society for Surgery of the Hand: http://www.assh.org/Public/HandConditions/Pages/CarpalTunnelSyndrome.aspx
- Carpal Tunnel Syndrome Foundation. For patient education materials favorably reviewed on this topic, contact: American Academy of Family Physicians Foundation, P.O. Box 8418, Kansas City, MO 64114 (800) 274-2237, Ext. 4400.

PROGNOSIS

- Patients with severe CTS may not recover completely even after surgical release. Although paresthesias and weakness may persist, night symptoms generally resolve.
- Untreated, more severe cases of CTS can lead to numbness and weakness in the hand, with atrophy of the thenar muscles and permanent loss of median nerve function.

COMPLICATIONS

- Postoperative infection (rare)
- Injury to the median nerve or its recurrent (motor) branch

REFERENCES

1. Cranford CS, Ho JY, Kalainov DM, et al. Carpal tunnel syndrome. *J Am Acad Orthop Surg*. 2007;15(9):537–548.
2. Page MJ, Massy-Westropp N, O'Connor D, et al. Splinting for carpal tunnel syndrome. *Cochrane Database Syst Rev*. 2012;(7):CD010003.
3. Atroshi I, Flondell M, Hofer M, et al. Methylprednisolone injections for the carpal tunnel syndrome: a randomized, placebo-controlled trial. *Ann Intern Med*. 2013;159(5):309–317.
4. Marshall S, Tardif G, Ashworth N. Local corticosteroid injection for carpal tunnel syndrome. *Cochrane Database Syst Rev*. 2007;(2):CD001554. 17443508.
5. Louie DL, Earp BE, Collins JE, et al. Outcomes of open carpal tunnel release at a minimum of ten years. *J Bone Joint Surg*. 2013;95(12):1067–1073.
6. Vasiliadis HS, Georgoulas P, Shrier I, et al. Endoscopic release for carpal tunnel syndrome. *Cochrane Database Syst Rev*. 2014;(1):CD008265.
7. Page MJ, O'Connor D, Pitt V, et al. Exercise and mobilisation interventions for carpal tunnel syndrome. *Cochrane Database Syst Rev*. 2012;(6):CD009899.
8. Page MJ, O'Connor D, Pitt V, et al. Therapeutic ultrasound for carpal tunnel syndrome. *Cochrane Database Syst Rev*. 2013;(3):CD009601.

ADDITIONAL READING

- Fowler JR, Gaughan JP, Ilyas AM. The sensitivity and specificity of ultrasound for the diagnosis of carpal tunnel syndrome: a meta-analysis. *Clin Orthop Relat Res*. 2011;469(4):1089–1094.
- Graham B. Nonsurgical treatment of carpal tunnel syndrome. *J Hand Surg Am*. 2009;34(3):531–534.
- Huisstede BM, Hoogvliet P, Randsdorp MS, et al. Carpal tunnel syndrome. Part I: effectiveness of nonsurgical treatments—a systematic review. *Arch Phys Med Rehabil*. 2010;91(7):981–1004.
- Peters S, Page MJ, Coppieters MW, et al. Rehabilitation following carpal tunnel release. *Cochrane Database Syst Rev*. 2013;(6):CD004158.
- Shi Q, MacDermid JC. Is surgical intervention more effective than non-surgical treatment for carpal tunnel syndrome? A systematic review. *J Orthop Surg Res*. 2011;6:17.
- Tai TW, Wu CY, Su FC, et al. Ultrasonography for diagnosing carpal tunnel syndrome: a meta-analysis of diagnostic test accuracy. *Ultrasound Med Biol*. 2012;38(7):1121–1128.

SEE ALSO

- Arthritis, Rheumatoid; Hypoparathyroidism; Scleroderma; Systemic Lupus Erythematosus (SLE)
- Algorithms: Carpal Tunnel Syndrome; Pain in Upper Extremity

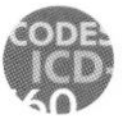

CODES

ICD10

- G56.00 Carpal tunnel syndrome, unspecified upper limb
- G56.01 Carpal tunnel syndrome, right upper limb
- G56.02 Carpal tunnel syndrome, left upper limb

CLINICAL PEARLS

- The altered sensation (tingling or prickling) in CTS is characteristically confined to the thumb, index, long, and radial 1/2 of the ring fingers.
- Thenar atrophy is a late finding, indicating severe disease.
- Durkan (carpal compression) test is superior to Tinels sign (tapping on median nerve over carpal tunnel) and Phalen maneuver (holding wrists in flexion) for the clinical diagnosis of CTS.
- Steroid injections offer short-term relief, but clinical outcomes at 1 year are no different than placebo.

CATARACT

Yasir Ahmed, MD • Ingrid U. Scott, MD, MPH

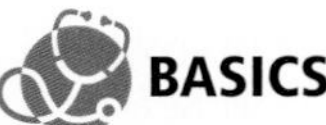

BASICS

DESCRIPTION

- A cataract is any opacity or discoloration of the lens, localized or generalized; the term is usually reserved for changes that affect visual acuity (1,2).
- Etymology: from Latin *catarractes*, for "waterfall"; named after foamy appearance of opacity
- Leading cause of blindness worldwide, estimated 20 million people (1,2)
- Types include the following:
  - Age related: 90% of total
  - Metabolic (diabetes via accelerated sorbitol pathway, hypocalcemia, Wilson disease)
  - Congenital (1/250 newborns; 10–38% of childhood blindness)
  - Systemic disease associated (myotonic dystrophy, atopic dermatitis)
  - Secondary to associated eye disease, so-called complicated (e.g., uveitis associated with juvenile rheumatoid arthritis or sarcoid, tumor such as melanoma or retinoblastoma)
  - Traumatic (e.g., heat, electric shock, radiation, concussion, perforating eye injuries, intraocular foreign body)
  - Toxic/nutritional (e.g., corticosteroids)
- Morphologic classification:
  - Nuclear: exaggeration of normal aging changes of *central* lens nucleus, often associated with myopia due to increased refractive index of lens (some elderly patients consequently may be able to read again *without spectacles*, so-called second sight of the aged)
  - Cortical: outer portion of lens; may involve anterior, posterior, or equatorial cortex; radial, spoke-like opacities
  - Subcapsular: Posterior subcapsular cataract has more profound effect on vision than nuclear or cortical cataract; patients particularly troubled under conditions of miosis; near vision frequently impaired more than distance vision.
- System(s) affected: nervous

Geriatric Considerations

Some degree of cataract formation is expected in all people >70 years of age.

Pediatric Considerations

See "Cataract, Pediatric"; may present as leukocoria.

Pregnancy Considerations

See "Congenital Cataract" (i.e., medications, metabolic dysfunction, intrauterine infection, and malnutrition).

EPIDEMIOLOGY

Incidence

- ~48% of the 37 million cases of blindness worldwide result from cataracts (1,2).
- Leading cause of treatable blindness and vision loss in developing countries (1,2)
- Predominant age: depends on type of cataract
- Predominant sex: male > female

Prevalence

- Cataract type and prevalence highly variable based on population demographic
- An estimated 50% of people 65–74 years of age and 70% of people >75 years of age have age-related cataract.

ETIOLOGY AND PATHOPHYSIOLOGY

- Age-related cataract:
  - Continual addition of layers of lens fibers throughout life creates hard, dehydrated lens nucleus that impairs vision (nuclear cataract).
  - Aging alters biochemical and osmotic balance required for lens clarity; outer lens layers hydrate and become opaque, adversely affecting vision.
- Congenital:
  - Usually unknown etiology
  - Drugs (corticosteroids in 1st trimester, sulfonamides)
  - Metabolic (diabetes in mother, galactosemia in fetus)
  - Intrauterine infection during 1st trimester (e.g., rubella, herpes, mumps)
  - Maternal malnutrition
- Other cataract types:
  - Common feature is a biochemical/osmotic imbalance that disrupts lens clarity.
  - Local changes in lens protein distribution lead to light scattering (lens opacity).

Genetics

- Congenital (e.g., chromosomal disorders [Down syndrome])
- Genetics of age-related cataract not yet established but likely multifactorial contribution

RISK FACTORS

- Aging
- Cigarette smoking
- Ultraviolet (UV) sunlight exposure
- Diabetes
- Prolonged high-dose steroids
- Positive family history
- Alcohol

GENERAL PREVENTION

- Use of UV protective glasses
- Avoidance of tobacco products
- Effective control of diabetes
- Care with high-dose, long-term steroid use (systemic therapy > inhaled treatment)
- Protective methods using pharmaceutical intervention (e.g., antioxidants, acetylsalicylic acid [ASA], hormone replacement therapy [HRT]) show no proven benefit to date.

COMMONLY ASSOCIATED CONDITIONS

- Diabetes (especially with poor glucose control)
- Myotonic dystrophy (90% of patients develop visually innocuous change in 3rd decade; becomes disabling in 5th decade)
- Atopic dermatitis (AD) (10% of patients with severe AD develop cataracts in 2nd–4th decades, often bilateral)
- Neurofibromatosis type 2
- Associated ocular disease or "secondary cataract" (e.g., chronic anterior uveitis, acute [or repetitive] angle–closure glaucoma or high myopia)
- Drug induced (e.g., steroids, chlorpromazine)
- Trauma

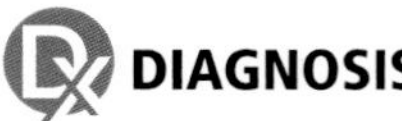

DIAGNOSIS

HISTORY

- Age-related cataract:
  - Decreased visual acuity, blurred vision, distortion, or "ghosting" of images (1,2)
  - Problems with visual acuity in any lighting condition
  - Falls or accidents; injuries (e.g., hip fracture)
- Congenital: often asymptomatic, leukocoria, parents notice child's visual inattention or strabismus
- Other types of cataract:
  - May also present with decreased visual acuity
  - Appropriate clinical history or signs to help with diagnosis

PHYSICAL EXAM

- Visual acuity assessment for all cataracts
- Age-related cataract: lens opacity on eye examination
- Congenital:
  - Lens opacity present at birth or within 3 months of birth
  - Leukocoria (white pupil), strabismus, nystagmus, signs of associated syndrome (as with Down or rubella syndrome)
  - *Note:* must always rule out ocular tumor; early diagnosis and treatment of retinoblastoma may be lifesaving
- Other types of cataract: may present with decreased visual acuity associated with characteristic physical findings (e.g., metabolic, trauma)

DIFFERENTIAL DIAGNOSIS

- An opaque-appearing eye may be due to opacities of the cornea (e.g., scarring, edema, calcification), lens opacities, tumor, or retinal detachment. Biomicroscopic examination (slit lamp) or careful ophthalmoscopic exam should provide diagnosis.
- In the elderly, visual impairment is often due to multiple factors such as cataract and macular degeneration, both contributing to visual loss.

- Age-related cataract is significant if symptoms and ophthalmic exam support cataract as a major cause of vision impairment.
- Congenital lens opacity in the absence of other ocular pathology may cause severe amblyopia.
- *Note:* Cataract *does not* produce a relative afferent pupillary reaction defect. Abnormal pupillary reactions mandate further evaluation for other pathology.

DIAGNOSTIC TESTS & INTERPRETATION

- Visual quality assessment: Glare testing, contrast sensitivity sometimes indicated.
- Retinal/macular function assessment: potential acuity meter testing
- Workup of underlying process

Test Interpretation

Consistent with lens changes found in the type of cataract; however, diagnosis is made by clinical examination.

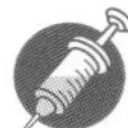

TREATMENT

- Outpatient (usually)
- ~1.64 million cataract extractions in the United States yearly (3,4)

GENERAL MEASURES

Eye protection from UV light

MEDICATION

There are currently no medications to prevent or slow the progression of cataracts.

ISSUES FOR REFERRAL

If patient has cataract and symptoms do not seem to support recommended surgery, a second opinion by another ophthalmologist may be indicated.

SURGERY/OTHER PROCEDURES

- Age-related cataract:
  - Surgical removal is indicated if visual impairment–producing symptoms are distressing to the patient, interfering with lifestyle or occupation, or posing a risk for fall or injury (3,4)[A].
  - Because significant cataract may develop gradually, the patient may not be aware of how it has changed his or her lifestyle. Physician may note a significant cataract, and patient reports "no problems." Thus, evaluation requires effective physician–patient exchange of information.
  - Surgical technique: Cataract extraction via small incisions, followed by implantation of a prosthetic intraocular lens; lenses have power calculated based on size of the eye and curvature of cornea usually to correct for distance vision; surgery performed on one (worse) eye, with contralateral surgery only after recovery and if deemed necessary; generally takes <1 hour depending on surgical technique
  - Anesthesia: usually regional injection or topical with sedation and monitoring of vital signs
  - Preoperative evaluation: by the primary care physician:
    - Patients on anticoagulants may need to be temporarily discontinued 1–2 weeks before surgery if possible (but not always necessary; thus, need to discuss with ophthalmologist).
    - Patients who have ever taken an α-blocker such as tamsulosin (Flomax) should alert their ophthalmologist (increased risk of intraoperative floppy iris syndrome [IFIS] even in patients who no longer use these drugs).
  - Postoperative care: usually protective eye shield as directed, topical antibiotic, NSAIDs, and steroid ophthalmic medications; avoid lifting or bending over for a few weeks
- Congenital cataract:
  - Treatment is surgical removal of cataract. Newborns may require surgery within days to reduce risk of severe amblyopia. Use of lens implants is controversial because the eyes are growing.
  - Postoperative care: long-term patching program for good eye to combat amblyopia; refractive correction of operative eye, with multiple repeat examinations; challenging for physician and parents

ONGOING CARE

FOLLOW-UP RECOMMENDATIONS

Patient Monitoring

- As cataract progresses, an ophthalmologist may change spectacle correction to maintain vision. When this is no longer successful and interferes with patient's activities of daily living, surgery is indicated.
- Following surgery, spectacle correction may be required to maximize near and/or far visual acuity. Refraction is usually prescribed several weeks after surgery.

PATIENT EDUCATION

Medline Plus on cataracts at: www.nlm.nih.gov/medlineplus/cataract.html

PROGNOSIS

- Ocular prognosis good after cataract removal if no prior or coexisting ocular disease: 94.3% of otherwise healthy eyes achieve best corrected visual acuity of 20/40 or better. Success rates are lower with comorbidities such as diabetes and glaucoma (5).
- In congenital cataracts, prognosis often is poorer because of the high risk of amblyopia.

COMPLICATIONS

- Vary widely from delay in visual recovery or protracted visual discomfort to blindness and loss of eye
- Nearly all reported complications occur rarely (<2% of eyes) except for posterior capsule opacification (14.7–42.7% of eyes, usually treated with Nd-YAG laser capsulotomy in office with a rate of 4–25.3%) (6,7)[B].

REFERENCES

1. Asbell PA, Dualan I, Mindel J, et al. Age-related cataract. *Lancet*. 2005;365(9459):599–609.
2. Abraham AG, Condon NG, West Gower E. The new epidemiology of cataract. *Ophthalmol Clin North Am*. 2006;19(4):415–425.
3. Riaz Y, Mehta JS, Wormald R, et al. Surgical interventions for age-related cataract. *Cochrane Database Syst Rev*. 2006;(4):CD001323.
4. Fedorowicz Z, Lawrence D, Gutierrez P. Day care versus in-patient surgery for age-related cataract. *Cochrane Database Syst Rev*. 2005;(1):CD004242.
5. Biber JM, Sandoval HP, Trivedi RH, et al. Comparison of the incidence and visual significance of posterior capsule opacification between multifocal spherical, monofocal spherical, and monofocal aspheric intraocular lenses. *J Cataract Refract Surg*. 2009;35(7):1234–1238.
6. Findl O, Buehl W, Bauer P, et al. Interventions for preventing posterior capsule opacification. *Cochrane Database Syst Rev*. 2010;(2):CD003738.
7. Lundström M, Barry P, Henry Y, et al. Visual outcome of cataract surgery; study from the European Registry of Quality Outcomes for Cataract and Refractive Surgery. *J Cataract Refract Surg*. 2013;39(5):679.

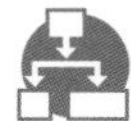

SEE ALSO

- Algorithm: Cataracts
- Floppy Iris Syndrome

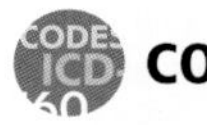

CODES

ICD10

- H26.9 Unspecified cataract
- H25.9 Unspecified age-related cataract
- Q12.0 Congenital cataract

CLINICAL PEARLS

- Cataracts are the leading cause of blindness worldwide; 90% are age related.
- Primary indication for cataract surgery is visual impairment leading to significant lifestyle changes for the patient.
- For congenital cataracts, must always rule out ocular tumor because early diagnosis and treatment of retinoblastoma may be lifesaving.
- Before prescribing an α-blocker for an older adult with hypertension or a prostate or urinary retention problem, consider whether the patient has cataracts (due to increased risk of IFIS).

CELIAC DISEASE

Suma Chennubhotla, MD • Amaninderapal S. Ghotra, MD • Thomas L. Abell, MD

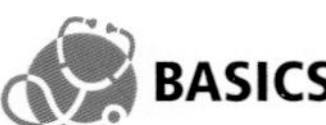

BASICS

DESCRIPTION

- An autoimmune condition characterized by an immune-mediated reaction to dietary gluten (found in wheat, barley, rye). Primarily affects the small intestine in genetically predisposed individuals.
- NOT a food allergy
- Celiac presentations
  - Typical
    - Diarrheal illness characterized by villous atrophy with symptoms of malabsorption (steatorrhea, weight loss, vitamin deficiencies, anemia). Symptoms resolve with a gluten-free diet.
  - Atypical
    - Minor GI symptoms, with a myriad of extraintestinal manifestations (e.g., anemia, dental enamel defects, neurologic symptoms, infertility)
  - Asymptomatic (silent) disease
    - Found when screening 1st-degree relatives
  - Latent
    - Positive laboratory tests and genetics, without signs/symptoms
- System(s) affected: gastrointestinal
- Synonym(s): celiac sprue; gluten enteropathy

EPIDEMIOLOGY

Incidence

- Disease primarily of individuals of Northern European ancestry
- Predominant sex: female > male (3:2)

Prevalence

- ~1/133–160 persons in the United States; an estimated 3 million Americans have celiac disease (1).
- Prevalence is increasing worldwide.

ETIOLOGY AND PATHOPHYSIOLOGY

Sensitivity to gluten, specifically gliadin fraction. Tissue transglutaminase modification of protein leads to immunologic cross-reactivity, inflammation, and tissue damage (villous atrophy) with subsequent malabsorption.

Genetics

Homogenicity for *HLA-DQ2* increases the risk of celiac disease and enteropathy-associated T-cell lymphoma.

RISK FACTORS

- 1st-degree relatives: 5–10% incidence (2)
- Monozygotic twins: 70% incidence
- 25% in family member with an autoimmune disease

GENERAL PREVENTION

Avoid gluten-containing products (wheat, barley, rye, and possibly oat products).

COMMONLY ASSOCIATED CONDITIONS

- *Dermatitis herpetiformis*: strong association with celiac disease; (3) 85% of patients have celiac disease. All patients should follow gluten-free diet.
- Secondary lactase deficiency
- Osteopenia
- Thyroid disease: Hashimoto thyroiditis
- Diabetes, type 1: 3–10% of patients have celiac disease.
- Elevated AST and ALT (with no direct cause)
- Hyposplenism
- Recurrent fetal loss/infertility
- Irritable bowel syndrome (IBS)
- Restless leg syndrome
- GI lymphoma and adenocarcinoma: Celiac disease is associated with increased risk for adenocarcinoma and lymphoma of the small bowel.
  - Particular increase in prevalence of T-cell non-Hodgkin lymphoma (4)
  - The risk of lymphoproliferative malignancies in celiac disease is dependent on small intestinal histopathology.
  - There appears to be little to no increased risk in latent celiac disease (seropositive but normal biopsy) (5)[A].
- Migraine (more prevalent in patients with celiac disease) (6)
- Addison disease, Turner syndrome, Raynaud syndrome
- Autoimmune disorders: systemic lupus erythematosus (SLE), rheumatoid arthritis (RA), scleroderma, Sjögren syndrome

Pregnancy Considerations

- Celiac disease may be an underappreciated cause of male and female infertility.
- Consider celiac disease in pregnant women with severe anemia.

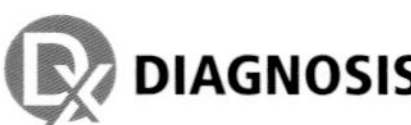

DIAGNOSIS

HISTORY

- Diarrhea, cramping, gas pains
- Steatorrhea (fatty stools)
- Muscle cramps
- Iron deficiency anemia
- Nervousness, depression
- Weight loss
- Failure to thrive (slowing velocity of weight gain)
- Weakness, fatigue
- Flatulence (can be explosive)
- Abdominal pain, nausea, vomiting
- Recurrent aphthous stomatitis
- Abdominal distention
- Delayed puberty
- Tingling numbness in hands, feet
- Bone or joint pain
- Migraines

Pediatric Considerations

Failure to thrive and delayed growth with short stature may be early manifestations. Some children may outgrow wheat intolerance after prolonged gluten-free diets but should watch for signs of recurrence in middle age.

PHYSICAL EXAM

Often normal but look for

- Oropharynx: aphthous stomatitis
- Skin: *Dermatitis herpetiformis* (excoriations, symmetric erythematous papules and blisters on elbows, knees, buttocks, and back)
- Abdomen: distention

DIFFERENTIAL DIAGNOSIS

- Short bowel syndrome
- Dyspepsia, gastroesophageal reflux disease (GERD)
- Pancreatic insufficiency
- Crohn disease
- Whipple disease
- Hypogammaglobulinemia
- Tropical sprue
- Lymphoma
- HIV/AIDS
- Acute enteritis
- Giardiasis
- Eosinophilic gastroenteritis
- Pancreatic disease

DIAGNOSTIC TESTS & INTERPRETATION

Initial Tests (lab, imaging)

In general, diagnosis should not be made based on serology alone. Patients with symptoms highly suggestive of celiac disease or those with positive serologies should undergo endoscopy for biopsy. Tissue biopsy is the gold standard for diagnosis.

- IgA antiendomysial antibodies (IgA anti-EmA)
- IgA antitissue transglutaminase (IgA- anti-TTG)
- Total serum IgA

ALERT

Positive IgA anti-EMA and IgA TTG have high sensitivity and specificity (sensitivity, 90–98%; specificity, 98%) when on normal (non–gluten-free) diet for at least 4 weeks.

- IgA-deficient patients have false-negative IgA anti-endomysial and IgA antitransglutaminase antibodies.
- Selective IgA deficiency is 10–15× more prevalent in patients with celiac disease.
  - This can delay diagnosis due to "negative" IgA anti-EMA testing.
- The TTG antibody test is the preferred test (over the deamidated gliadin peptide [DGP] antibody) (7,8,9)[A].

- Assessment of symptoms, risk, predisposition, then antibody tests (anti-TTG antibody is gold standard)

Follow-Up Tests & Special Considerations

- If patient is IgA deficient OR if IgA EMA and IgA anti-TTG are negative, follow up blood tests.
  - Anti-DGP (DGP–IgA and IgG)
    - Sensitivity, 94%; specificity, 99% (similar to anti-TTG) (9)
- Antigliadin antibody (AgA–IgG and IgA)
  - Not considered sufficiently sensitive/specific for adults

Pediatric Considerations

- Consider evaluation for premature osteoporosis.
- Antigliadin antibody (AgA–IgG and IgA) may be used for children age <2 years because TTG and EMA antibodies may be absent.
- Anti-DGP test is sensitive in this group.
- 72-hour fecal fat showing >7% fat malabsorption
- Elevated liver function test (LFT) results
- d-Xylose test showing malabsorption
- Decreased calcium; cholesterol; vitamin A, C, D, and B_{12} (rare); folate, iron (common); total protein; hemoglobin (common)
- Increased prothrombin time (PT)
- Decreased neutral fats

Diagnostic Procedures/Other

- *Endoscopy with multiple diagnostic biopsies of the duodenal mucosa with repeat endoscopy and normal biopsy on a gluten-free diet is necessary before a firm diagnosis can be made* (2).

- Although endoscopy with small bowel biopsy is the gold standard for confirmation, recent studies suggest that video capsule endoscopy is a promising alternative, particularly when antibody screening and the clinical picture are consistent with celiac disease, even if duodenal biopsies are nondiagnostic (10)[A].

Test Interpretation

Small bowel biopsy

- Flattened villi/villous atrophy, hyperplasia and lengthening of crypts, infiltration of plasma cells, and intraepithelial lymphocytosis in lamina propria

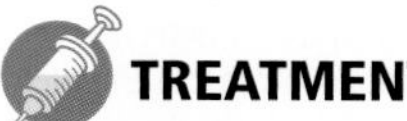

TREATMENT

GENERAL MEASURES

- Removal of gluten from the diet
  - Rice, corn, and soybean flour are safe, palatable substitutes.
- Levels of IgA antigliadin normalize with gluten abstinence.
- LIFELONG abstinence is required; immune response to gluten will recur with resumption of gluten consumption.

MEDICATION

First Line

Usually no medications: gluten-free diet is the treatment.

Second Line

- In refractory disease, consider
  - Steroids (prednisone, 40–60 mg/day PO in cases of refractory sprue)
  - Azathioprine (immunosuppressants should be used with caution; use may lead to lymphoma in celiac disease)
  - Cyclosporine
  - Infliximab
  - Cladribine
- Patients may develop nutritional deficiencies depending on the severity of the disease.

Third Line

There are currently numerous ongoing clinical trials testing the efficacy of intraluminally acting agents such as lactobacilli to gluten endopeptidases, inhibitors of transepithelial gliaden uptake, immunomodulation, and even vaccination (11). Results of these studies are largely pending and awaiting further validation at this time.

ISSUES FOR REFERRAL

- Additional nutritional support
- Refractory disease

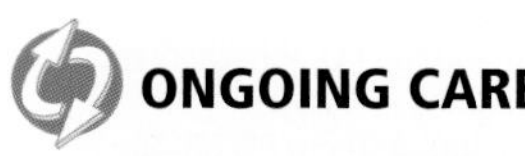

ONGOING CARE

FOLLOW-UP RECOMMENDATIONS

- Consultation with registered dietitian
- Screen for osteoporosis and treat accordingly.

Patient Monitoring

- Repeat EGD in 1 year on a gluten-free diet to document normalization of villi.
- Increased intraepithelial lymphocytes may persist for up to 5 years after initial diagnosis, in some cases may persist indefinitely even with symptom resolution.
- Follow anti-TTG IgA or deaminated antigliadin antibodies as a measure of response/compliance with diet (vs. antigliadin IgA or IgG).

DIET

- Removal of gluten: wheat, rye, barley, and those with gluten additives
- This can be a challenging diet (especially learning sources of "hidden" gluten) and should be coordinated with a skilled registered dietitian.

PATIENT EDUCATION

- Discuss how to recognize gluten in various products.
- Highlight potential complications and outcomes of failing to follow a gluten-free diet.

PROGNOSIS

- Good prognosis with correct diagnosis and adherence to gluten-free diet
- Patients should feel better within 7 days of dietary modification.
- Symptoms usually disappear in 4–6 weeks.
- It is unknown whether strict dietary adherence decreases cancer risk.

COMPLICATIONS

- Malignancy: $<$10% of patients (50% of whom develop small bowel lymphoma)
- Refractory sprue
  - May respond to prednisone 40–60 mg/day PO
  - Refractory sprue unresponsive to corticosteroid therapy suggests adult-onset autoimmune enteropathy or cryptic T-cell lymphoma. In this circumstance, screening for antienterocyte autoantibodies and scrutiny of the small intestine, including retroperitoneal lymph node biopsy with full-thickness small bowel biopsy, may be needed.
- Chronic ulcerative jejunoileitis
  - Associated with multiple ulcers, intestinal bleeding, strictures, perforation, obstruction, and peritonitis
  - 7% mortality
- Osteoporosis secondary to decreased vitamin D and calcium absorption
- Dehydration
- Electrolyte depletion
- Refractory cases may need total parenteral nutrition.

REFERENCES

1. Biagi F, Klersy C, Balduzzi D, et al. Are we not over-estimating the prevalence of coeliac disease in the general population? *Ann Med*. 2010;42(8):557–561.
2. Rubio-Tapia A, Hill I, Kelly C, et al. ACG Clinical guidelines: diagnosis and management of celiac disease. *Am J Gastroenterol*. 2013;108(5): 656–676.
3. Bolotin D, Petronic-Rosic V. Dermatitis herpetiformis. Part II. Diagnosis, management, and prognosis. *J Am Acad Dermatol*. 2011;64(6):1027–1033.
4. Tio M, Cox MR, Eslick GD. Meta-analysis: coeliac disease and the risk of all-cause mortality, any malignancy and lymphoid malignancy. *Aliment Pharmacol Ther*. 2012;35(5):540–551.
5. Elfström P, Granath F, Ekström Smedby K, et al. Risk of lymphoproliferative malignancy in relation to small intestinal histopathology among patients with celiac disease. *J Natl Cancer Inst*. 2011;103(5):436–444.
6. Dimitrova AK, Ungaro RC, Lebwohl B, et al. Prevalence of migraine in patients with celiac disease and inflammatory bowel disease. *Headache*. 2012;53(2):344–355.
7. Lewis NR, Scott BB. Meta-analysis: deamidated gliadin peptide antibody and tissue transglutaminase antibody compared as screening tests for coeliac disease. *Aliment Pharmacol Ther*. 2010;31(1):73–81.
8. van der Windt DA, Jellema P, Mulder CJ, et al. Diagnostic testing for celiac disease among patients with abdominal symptoms: a systematic review. *JAMA*. 2010;303(17):1738–1746.
9. Sugai E, Vázquez H, Nachman F, et al. Accuracy of testing for antibodies to synthetic gliadin-related peptides in celiac disease. *Clin Gastroenterol Hepatol*. 2006;4(9):1112–1117.
10. Rokkas T, Niv Y. The role of video capsule endoscopy in the diagnosis of celiac disease: a meta-analysis. *Eur J Gastroenterol Hepatol*. 2012;84(3):303–308.
11. Crowe, S. Management of celiac disease: beyond the gluten-free diet. *Gastroenterology*. 2014;146(7):1594–1596.

C

ADDITIONAL READING

- AGA Institute. AGA Institute Medical Position Statement on the Diagnosis and Management of Celiac Disease. *Gastroenterology*. 2006;131(6):1977–1980.
- Celiac Disease Foundation. Guidelines for a Gluten-Free Lifestyle. 3rd ed. Studio City, CA: Celiac Disease Foundation; 2002. http://www.celiac.org. Accessed 2014.
- Celiac Sprue Association (CSA): http://www.csaceliacs.org. Accessed 2014.
- Giersiepen K, Lelgemann M, Stuhldreher N, et al. Accuracy of diagnostic antibody tests for coeliac disease in children: summary of an evidence report. *J Pediatr Gastroenterol Nutr*. 2012;54(2):229–241.
- Gluten Intolerance Group (GIG). http://www.gluten.net. Accessed 2014.
- Green PHR, Jones R. *Celiac Disease: A Hidden Epidemic*. New York, NY: HarperCollins; 2006.
- Prince HE. Evaluation of the INOVA diagnostics enzyme-linked immunosorbent assay kits for measuring serum immunoglobulin G (IgG) and IgA to deamidated gliadin peptides. *Clin Vaccine Immunol*. 2006;13(1):150–151.
- Celiac Disease Foundation. Quick start gluten-free diet guide for celiac disease and non-celiac gluten sensitivity. http://celiac.org/wp-content/uploads/2013/12/quick-start-guide.pdf. Accessed 2014.
- Rozenberg O, Lerner A, Pacht A, et al. A novel algorithm for the diagnosis of celiac disease and a comprehensive review of celiac disease diagnostics. *Clin Rev Allergy Immunol*. 2012;42(3):331–341.

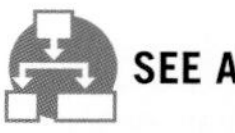

SEE ALSO

Algorithms: Diarrhea, Chronic; Malabsorption Syndrome

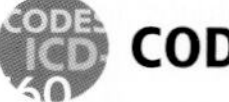

CODES

ICD10

K90.0 Celiac disease

CLINICAL PEARLS

- Test for celiac disease in patients with presumed IBS or *Dermatitis herpetiformis*.
- Test IgA levels along with IgA anti-EMA and anti-TTG antibodies.
- Positive serology alone is not sufficient to ascertain diagnosis; endoscopic biopsy is the gold standard for diagnosis.
- Definitive treatment is a gluten-free diet. Patient symptoms should improve within 7 days if fully compliant with gluten-free diet.

CELLULITIS

Jowhara Al-Qahtani, MD • Amer Homsi, MD • Bakr Nour, MD, PhD, FACS

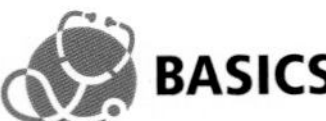

BASICS

DESCRIPTION

- An acute bacterial skin and skin structure infection (ABSSI) of the dermis and subcutaneous tissue; commonly characterized by pain, erythema, warmth, and swelling
  - Periorbital cellulitis: bacterial infection of the eyelid and surrounding tissues (anterior compartment)
  - Orbital cellulitis: infection of the eye posterior to the septum; sinusitis is the most common risk factor.
  - Facial cellulitis: preceded by upper respiratory infection or otitis media
  - Buccal cellulitis: infection of cheek in children associated with bacteremia (common before *Haemophilus influenzae* type B vaccine)
  - Peritonsillar cellulitis: common in children associated with fever, sore throat, and "hot potato" speech
  - Abdominal wall cellulitis: common in morbidly obese
  - Perianal cellulitis: sharply demarcated, bright, perianal erythema
  - Necrotizing cellulitis: gas-producing bacteria in the lower extremities; common in diabetics
- System(s) affected: skin/exocrine

EPIDEMIOLOGY

Predominant sex: male = female (common in elderly and adults, except perianal cellulitis which is common in children)

Incidence

200/100,000 patient/years

Prevalence

The exact prevalence is uncertain as this disease is very common and not reportable. It affects all age groups and all races; however, certain types of cellulitis/microorganisms occur in certain populations. Recent studies showed that prevalence of community-acquired methicillin resistant *Staphylococcus aureus* [CA-MRSA] has increased in athletes in contact sports (i.e., wrestling).

ETIOLOGY AND PATHOPHYSIOLOGY

Cellulitis is caused by bacterial penetration through a break in the skin. Hyaluronidase mediates subcutaneous (SC) spread.

- Microbiology
  - β-Hemolytic streptococci (groups A, B, C, G, and F), *S. aureus*, including MRSA and gram-negative aerobic bacilli (accounts for 27 and 51%, respectively)
  - *S. aureus*: periorbital and orbital cellulitis and IV drug users
  - *Pseudomonas aeruginosa*: diabetics and other immunocompromised patients
  - *Aeromonas hydrophila* and *Vibrio vulnificus:* cellulitis caused by waterborne pathogens
  - *H. influenzae:* buccal cellulitis
  - Clostridia and non–spore-forming anaerobes: necrotizing cellulitis (crepitant/gangrenous)
  - *Streptococcus agalactiae*: cellulitis following lymph node dissection
  - *Pasteurella multocida* and *Capnocytophaga canimorsus*: cellulitis preceded by bites
  - *Streptococcus iniae*: immunocompromised hosts
  - Rare causes: mycobacterium, fungal (mucormycosis, aspergillosis, syphilis)

Genetics

No genetic pattern

RISK FACTORS

- Disruption to skin barrier: trauma, infection, insect bites, and injection drug use
- Inflammation: eczema or radiation therapy
- Edema due to venous insufficiency, and lymphatic obstruction due to surgical procedures
- Increased risk factor: elderly, diabetes, hypertension, obesity
- Recurrent cellulitis: immunocompromised, diabetes, hypertension, cancer, peripheral arterial or venous diseases, chronic kidney disease, dialysis, IV or SC drug use

GENERAL PREVENTION

- Maintain good skin hygiene.
- Wear support stockings to decrease edema.
- Maintain tight glycemic control and proper foot care for diabetics.

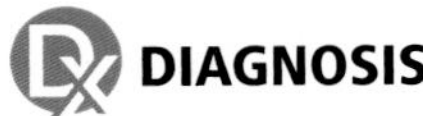

DIAGNOSIS

Mostly clinical diagnosis; high index of suspicion

HISTORY

- Previous trauma, surgery, animal/human bites, dermatitis, fungal infection; all may serve as a portal of entry for bacterial pathogens.
- Patient will often complain of pain, itching, and/or burning.
- Fever, chills, and malaise

PHYSICAL EXAM

- Localized pain and tenderness to touch with notable erythema, induration, swelling, and warmth
- Peau d'orange appearance
- Regional lymphadenopathy of the face, periorbital region, neck, or extremities
- Purulent drainage from abscesses
- Orbital cellulitis: proptosis, globe displacement, limitation of ocular movements, vision loss, diplopia
- Facial cellulitis: malaise, anorexia, vomiting, pruritus, burning, anterior neck swelling

DIFFERENTIAL DIAGNOSIS

Toxic shock syndrome, venous stasis dermatitis (commonly mistaken as cellulitis), bursitis, acute dermatitis or intertrigo, herpes zoster or herpetic whitlow, deep vein thrombosis or thrombophlebitis, acute gout or pseudogout, necrotizing fasciitis or myositis, gas gangrene, osteomyelitis, erythema chronicum migrans or malignancy, drug reaction, sunburn, or insect stings

DIAGNOSTIC TESTS & INTERPRETATION

Initial Tests (lab, imaging)

- For signs of systemic disease (fever, heart rate >100 bpm, or systolic blood pressure <90 mm Hg): blood cultures, CPK, CRP. Consider serum lactate levels.
- WBC has 84.5% specificity and 43.0% sensitivity, whereas CRP had a sensitivity of 67.1% and specificity of 94.8% (PPV 94.65 and NPV 67.9%).
- Aspirates from point of maximum inflammation yield 45% positive culture compared with 5% from leading edge.
- Blood cultures: Pathogens isolated in <5% of patients. Blood cultures in children are more likely to show a contaminant than true positive.
- CREST guidelines recommend wound swabs on open cellulitis wound.
- Plain radiographs, CT, or MRI useful if osteomyelitis, fracture, necrotizing fasciitis, or retained foreign body is suspected or underlying abscess
- Gallium[67] scintillography is helpful for detecting cellulitis superimposed on recently increasing chronic lymphedema of a limb.

Diagnostic Procedures/Other

Lumbar puncture should be considered for children with *H. influenzae* type B or if with meningeal signs and facial cellulitis.

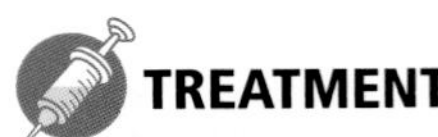

TREATMENT

GENERAL MEASURES

- Immobilization and elevation of the involved limb to reduce swelling
- Sterile saline dressings or cool aluminum acetate compresses for pain relief
- Edema: compression stocking, pneumatic pumps, and diuretic therapy
- Steroids (prednisone 0.5 mg/kg/day for 5–8 days) if partial response to antibiotics in hemorrhagic or bullous cellulitis
- Mark the area of cellulitis to monitor its progress and assist the efficacy of the antibiotics regimen.
- Tetanus immunization if needed

MEDICATION

First Line

- Treatment should be modified as indicated in the setting of known pathogens, underlying conditions such as diseases, or certain exposure like animal bites.
- Antibiotics selection relies on clinical presentation of purulent versus nonpurulent:
  - Nonpurulent cellulitis
    - With nonpurulent drainage, treatment should be targeted toward β-hemolytic streptococci and methicillin-sensitive *S. aureus* (MSSA).
    - Outpatient: Cover for β-hemolytic streptococci and MSSA; treatment duration of 5–10 days
      - Oral: for mild cellulitis
        - Cephalexin 500 mg PO q6h; children: 25–50 mg/kg/day in 3–4 doses
        - Dicloxacillin 500 mg PO q6h; children: 25–50 mg/kg/day in 4 doses
        - Clindamycin 300–450 mg PO q6–8h; children: 20–30 mg/kg/day in 4 doses
      - IV: for rapidly progressing cellulitis
        - Cefazolin 1–2 g IV q8h; children: 100 mg/kg/day IV in 2–4 divided doses
        - Oxacillin 2 g IV q4h; children: 150–200 mg/kg/day IV in 4–6 doses
        - Nafcillin 2 g IV q4h; children: 150–200 mg/kg/day IV in 4–6 doses
        - Clindamycin 600–900 mg IV q8h; children: 25–40 mg/kg/day IV in 3–4 doses

- Purulent cellulitis (probable CA-MRSA
  - Culture should be taken of all purulent wounds and followed up in 48 hours.
  - If suspected CA-MRSA is a concern, management entails incision and drainage of abscess and empiric antibiotic therapy followed by culture-based therapy (5–10 days); duration should be individualized to patient outcome 1[B]:
    - Oral
      - Clindamycin 300–450 mg PO; children: 40 mg/kg/day in 3–4 doses
      - Trimethoprim-sulfamethoxazole (TMP-SMZ) 1 DS tab PO BID; children: dose based on TMP at 8–12 mg/kg/day divided in 2 doses
      - Doxycycline 100 mg PO BID; children >8 years of age: ≤45 kg: 4 mg/kg/day divided in 2 doses; >45 kg: 100 mg PO BID
      - Minocycline 200 mg PO once, then 100 mg PO BID; children >8 years old: 4 mg/kg PO once, then 4 mg/kg PO BID
      - Linezolid 600 mg PO BID; children <12 years: 10 mg/kg/dose (max 600 mg/dose) PO TID; ≥12 years: 600 mg PO BID
      - Tedizolid 200 mg PO once daily; children: dosing not established
    - IV
      - Vancomycin 15–20 mg/kg/dose IV every 8–12 hours
      - Daptomycin 4 mg/kg/dose IV once daily; if bacteremia is present or suspected: 6 mg/kg IV once daily
      - Linezolid 600 mg IV BID
      - Tedizolid 200 mg IV once daily
      - Ceftaroline 600 mg IV q12h
      - Tigecycline 100 mg IV once, thereafter 50 mg IV q12h
- Necrotizing cellulitis: clostridial and anaerobic, requires broad-spectrum coverage: ampicillin-sulbactam 1.5–3.0 g q6–8h IV or piperacillin-tazobactam 3.37 g q6–8h IV plus ciprofloxacin 400 mg q12h IV plus clindamycin 600–900 mg q8h IV
- In patients with recurrent infection underlying predisposing conditions, previous episode of proven MRSA infection, or systemic toxicity. Patients should be educated on personal hygiene and proper wound care. Use agents with activity against MRSA as outlined earlier.
- Freshwater exposure: penicillinase-resistant: penicillin plus gentamicin or fluoroquinolone; in salt water exposure: doxycycline 200 mg IV in 2 divided doses
- Bites: The combination of amoxicillin and clavulanic acid has been shown to be effective in treating human bites and dog bites. Ticarcillin and clavulanic acid or the combination of a 3rd-generation cephalosporin (i.e., ceftriaxone) plus metronidazole will provide adequate parenteral therapy for animal or human bites. If allergic to penicillin, use fluoroquinolone plus metronidazole.
- Facial cellulitis in adults: ceftriaxone IV
- Diabetic foot infection: ampicillin/sulbactam or imipenem/cilastatin or meropenem; alternative: combinations of targeting anaerobes as well as gram-positive and gram-negative aerobes
- Severe infection, toxicity, immunocompromised patients, or worsening infection despite empirical therapy. Patient should be admitted, and empiric antibiotic therapy covering MRSA as listed earlier should be started immediately.
- Recurrent streptococcal cellulitis: penicillin 250 mg BID, or if penicillin-allergic, use erythromycin 250 mg BID

Pediatric Considerations

Avoid doxycycline in children ≥8 years old and during pregnancy.

Second Line

Mild infection

- Penicillin allergy: erythromycin 500 mg PO q6h
- Cephalexin remains a cost-effective therapy for outpatient management of cellulitis at current estimated MRSA levels.

SURGERY/OTHER PROCEDURES

- Débridement for gas and purulent matter
- Intubation or tracheotomy may be needed for cellulitis of the head or neck.

INPATIENT CONSIDERATIONS

Admission Criteria/Initial Stabilization

- Severe infection, suspicion of deeper or rapidly spreading infection, tissue necrosis, or severe pain
- Marked systemic toxicity or worsening symptoms that do not resolve after 24–48 hours of therapy
- Patients with underlying risk factors or severe comorbidities

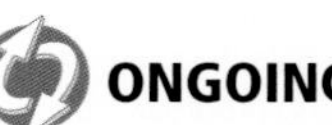

ONGOING CARE

FOLLOW-UP RECOMMENDATIONS

Patient Monitoring

- Repeat blood count if patient is toxic.
- Repeat lumbar puncture in case of meningitis.
- Consider prophylaxis of deep vein thrombosis.
- Cutaneous inflammation may worsen in first 24 hours due to release of bacterial antigens. Symptomatic improvement usually occurs in 24–48 hours, but visible improvement may take up to 72 hours.

DIET

Strict glucose control in diabetics

PATIENT EDUCATION

Practice good skin hygiene, especially with minor cuts, and report skin changes early.

PROGNOSIS

With adequate antibiotic treatment, prognosis is good.

- New study showed that low dose of penicillin for prophalyxis in patients with recurrent cellulitis has decreased the cellulitis attacks; however, it recurred once prophylaxis stopped (2)[A].

COMPLICATIONS

- Local abscess or bacteremia
- Superinfection with gram-negative organisms
- Lymphangitis, especially if recurrent
- Thrombophlebitis or venous thrombosis
- Bacterial meningitis
- Gangrenous disorder

REFERENCES

1. Champion A, Goodwin TA, Brolinson P, et al. Prevalence and characterization of methicillin-resistant. *Ann Clin Microbiol Antimicrob*. 2014;13(1):33.
2. Thomas KS, Crook AM, Nunn AJ, et al. Penicillin to prevent recurrent leg cellulitis. *N Engl J Med*. 2013;368(18):1695–1703.

C

ADDITIONAL READING

- Brook I. Management of human and animal bite wounds: an overview. *Adv Skin Wound Care*. 2005;18(4):197–203.
- Gunderson CG. Cellulitis: definition, etiology, and clinical features. *Am J Med*. 2011;124(12): 1113–1122.
- Hepburn MJ, Dooley DP, Skidmore PJ, et al. Comparison of short-course (5 days) and standard (10 days) treatment for uncomplicated cellulitis. *Arch Intern Med*. 2004;164(15):1669–1674.
- Kilburn SA, Featherstone P, Higgins B, et al. Interventions for cellulitis and erysipelas. *Cochrane Database Syst Rev*. 2010;(6):CD004299.
- Liu C, Bayer A, Cosgrove SE, et al. Clinical practice guidelines by the Infectious Diseases Society of America for the treatment of methicillin-resistant *Staphylococcus aureus* infections in adults and children. *Clin Infect Dis*. 2011;52:1–38.
- Phoenix G, Das S, Joshi M. Diagnosis and management of cellulitis. *BMJ*. 2012;345:e4955.
- Quirke M, O'Sullivan R, McCabe A, et al. Are two penicillins better than one? A systematic review of oral flucloxacillin and penicillin V versus oral flucloxacillin alone for the emergency department treatment of cellulitis. *Eur J Emerg Med*. 2013;21(3):170–174.
- Stevens DL, Bisno AL, Chambers HF, et al. Practice guidelines for the diagnosis and management of skin and soft-tissue infections. *Clin Infect Dis*. 2005;41(10):1373–1406.
- Swartz MN. Cellulitis. *N Engl J Med*. 2004;350(9):904.

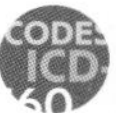

CODES

ICD10

- L03.90 Cellulitis, unspecified
- H05.019 Cellulitis of unspecified orbit
- L03.211 Cellulitis of face

CLINICAL PEARLS

- *S. aureus* and group A *Streptococcus* cause most cases of cellulitis.
- Consider MRSA if cellulitis is not responding to antibiotics in the 1st 48 hours.
- Rapid expansion of infected area with red/purple discoloration and severe pain may suggest necrotizing fasciitis, requiring urgent surgical evaluation.

CELLULITIS, ORBITAL

Fozia Akhtar Ali, MD • Rachel Myers, MD

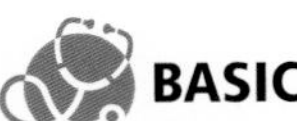

BASICS

DESCRIPTION

- Acute infection of orbital contents posterior to orbital septum. Retro-orbital cellulitis is infection posterior to the globe. Periorbital (preseptal) cellulitis is anterior to the septum; distinguishing location determines the appropriate treatment (1).
- Synonym(s): postseptal cellulitis

ALERT

- Differentiating orbital from preseptal cellulitis is the critical diagnostic step.
- Diplopia, proptosis, vision loss, and fever suggest orbital involvement.
- Contrast CT is imaging method of choice.
- Treat with immediate IV antibiotics; ophthalmology referral; monitor frequently for vision loss, cavernous sinus thrombosis, abscess, and meningitis.
- Intraorbital foreign body (FB) may cause delayed orbital cellulitis.
- Metastatic tumors and autoimmune inflammation may masquerade as orbital cellulitis in rare cases.

EPIDEMIOLOGY

- More common in winter due to increased incidence of sinusitis
- No difference in frequency between genders in adults.
- More common in children; mean age of surgical cases: 10.1 years; medical pediatric cases: 6.1 years
- *Haemophilus influenzae* type b (Hib): most common organism prior to Haemophilus influenzae type b (Hib) vaccine

Incidence

Orbital cellulitis has declined since Hib vaccine was introduced in 1985. In 2000, incidence per 100,000 in California was 3.5 in whites, 6.1 in blacks, and 3.2 in Hispanics, compared to 6.5 in whites, 10.2 in blacks, and 5.5 in Hispanics in 1990.

ETIOLOGY AND PATHOPHYSIOLOGY

- Sinusitis is major risk factor.
- Cellulitis in closed bony orbit causes proptosis, globe displacement, orbital apex syndrome, optic nerve compression, and vision loss.
- Orbital abscess (medial wall most common), meningitis, and cavernous sinus fibrosis may occur.
- Cultures in adults often grow multiple organisms, but >1/3 of cases have no pathogen recovered (2).
- Most common organisms (3,4)[C]
  - *Staphylococcus aureus*, *Streptococcus pneumoniae*, *Streptococcus anginosus*
- Less common organisms/precursor causes the following:
  - *Moraxella catarrhalis*, *H. influenzae*, group A β-hemolytic *Streptococcus*, *Pseudomonas aeruginosa*, anaerobes, phycomycosis (mucormycosis), aspergillosis, *Mycobacterium tuberculosis*, *Mycobacterium avium complex*, trichinosis, Echinococcus
- Since routine vaccination, *Hib* is no longer leading cause of orbital cellulitis (3,4)[B].

Genetics

No known genetic predisposition

RISK FACTORS

- Sinusitis present in 80–90% of cases (3)[C]
- Orbital trauma, retained orbital FB, ophthalmic surgery
- Dental, periorbital, skin, or intracranial infection; acute dacryocystitis and acute dacryoadenitis

GENERAL PREVENTION

- Appropriate treatment of bacterial sinusitis
- Proper wound care and perioperative monitoring of orbital surgery and trauma
- Routine Hib vaccination
- High index of suspicion in febrile patients presenting with eyelid and conjunctival erythema

COMMONLY ASSOCIATED CONDITIONS

- >80% cases have contiguous sinusitis.
- Trauma and intraorbital FB
- Preseptal cellulitis
- Orbital apex syndrome, vision loss, abscess, meningitis, or cavernous sinus thrombosis
- Neutropenia and asthma are associated with orbital cellulitis, but the relationship is unclear.

DIAGNOSIS

- Clinical signs help to distinguish periorbital from orbital cellulitis. Periorbital infection causes erythema, induration, and tenderness of the periorbital tissues, and patients rarely show signs of systemic illness.
- Orbital cellulitis may have not only the same signs and symptoms but also results in proptosis, conjunctival edema, ophthalmoplegia (pain with ocular movement), or decreased visual acuity (5).
- New evidence-based staging in cases resulting from acute sinusitis (3)[A]
  - Stage I: no abscess
  - Stage II a, b, c: small, large, or extending medial subperiosteal abscess
  - Stage III: orbital abscess
- Chandler staging is less widely used due to availability of imaging but remains widely accepted: (6)[C]
  - Stage I: periorbital cellulitis (considered different entity)
  - Stage II: orbital lining edema, chemosis, proptosis, limitation of extraocular movement, fever
  - Stage III: includes stage II with subperiosteal abscess and occasional vision loss
  - Stage IV: orbital abscess, ophthalmoplegia with vision loss
  - Stage V: extension to cavernous sinus, subdural space, meninges, or brain (3,5)

HISTORY

- History of surgery, trauma, sinus or upper respiratory infection, dental infection
- Malaise, fever, stiff neck, mental status changes
- Systemic immunosuppression or diabetes
- Signs of orbital cellulitis include the following:
  - Proptosis, double vision, vision loss (or decreased field of vision), pain with eye movement, decreased color vision

ALERT

- Ophthalmoplegia, mental status changes, contralateral cranial nerve palsy, or bilateral orbital cellulitis may indicate CNS involvement.
- MRSA orbital cellulitis may present without associated upper respiratory infection.

PHYSICAL EXAM

- Vital signs
  - Visual assessment (with glasses if required)
  - Lid exam and palpation of the orbit
  - Pupillary reflex for afferent pupillary defect
  - Extraocular movements; assessing pain with eye movement
  - Red desaturation: Patient views red object with 1 eye and compares to the other; reduced red color may indicate optic nerve involvement.
  - Confrontation visual field testing

DIFFERENTIAL DIAGNOSIS

- Preseptal cellulitis
  - Eyelid erythema with or without conjunctival erythema, afebrile, no pain on eye movement, no diplopia, normal eye exam (7)
- Idiopathic orbital inflammatory disease (orbital pseudotumor) (3)[C]
  - Afebrile, normal WBCs; can be acute, may have pain, responds to steroids
- Orbital FB
- Arteriovenous fistula (carotid-cavernous fistula)
  - Spontaneous or due to trauma; bruit may be present.
- Cavernous sinus thrombosis
  - Signs of orbital cellulitis with cranial nerve 3, 4, 5, and 6 findings; often bilateral and acute (7)
- Acute thyroid orbitopathy
  - Afebrile; possible signs of thyroid disease
- Orbital tumor
  - Acute rhabdomyosarcoma in children; acute lymphoblastic leukemia, or metastatic
- Trauma, insect bite, ruptured dermoid cyst (6)

DIAGNOSTIC TESTS & INTERPRETATION

- CBC with differential, C-reactive protein, ESR
- Cultures of eye secretions or nasopharyngeal aspirates often contaminated by normal flora but may identify antibiotic-resistant organisms.
- Cultures from orbital and sinus abscesses more often yield positive results but should be limited to cases where invasive procedures are indicated. Cultures from sinus aspirates and abscesses may grow multiple organisms.
- Blood cultures should be obtained prior to initiation of antibiotic therapy.

Initial Tests (lab, imaging)

CT scan of orbits and sinuses with axial and coronal views, with and without contrast, is diagnostic modality of choice. US and MRI are alternatives (8)[B].

- Contrast CT is most widely used for evaluating orbital cellulitis. Consider CT imaging if concern for Chandler stage III or IV disease (8)[B].
  - Thin section (2 mm) CT, coronal and axial views with bone windows to differentiate periorbital from orbital cellulitis, confirm extension into orbit, detect coexisting sinus disease, and identify orbital or subperiosteal abscesses.
  - Deviation of medial rectus indicates intraorbital involvement.

- MRI offers superior resolution of soft tissue infections for identification of cavernous sinus thrombosis but is less effective for bone imaging.
- US is used to rule out orbital myositis, locate FBs or abscesses, and follow progression of drained abscess.

Follow-Up Tests & Special Considerations
- A full septic evaluation with lumbar puncture should be considered before antibiotic administration in toxic patients or if meningitis is suspected (6)[C].
- Frequent eye exam and vitals q4h is essential for early diagnosis and treatment of associated conditions, such as meningitis or abscess.
- Consult ophthalmology for slit lamp and dilated funduscopic exam; exophthalmometry measurement for proptosis, color vision, and automated visual field

Diagnostic Procedures/Other
Consult otolaryngology if surgical management of sinus involvement is necessary.

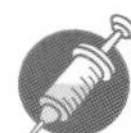

TREATMENT

Patients with orbital cellulitis should be admitted for careful monitoring of ocular status and treatment with broad-spectrum antibiotics covering gram-positive/-negative and anaerobic organisms (2).

MEDICATION
- Empiric antibiotic therapy to cover pathogens associated with acute sinusitis (*Streptococcus pneumoniae*, *H. influenzae*, *M. catarrhalis*, *Streptococcus pyogenes*), as well as for *Staphylococcus aureus*, *Streptococcus anginosus*, and anaerobes
- Modify IV antibiotic treatment when microbiologic sensitivities are available. Duration of IV therapy is usually a week, with additional PO therapy depending on clinical response.
- PO antibiotic therapy for 2–3 weeks or longer (3–6 weeks) is recommended for patients with severe sinusitis and bony destruction.

First Line
- Ampicillin/sulbactam (Unasyn) or ceftriaxone plus metronidazole or clindamycin if anaerobic infection is suspected (2).
  - Ampicillin/sulbactam: 3 g IV q6h for adult; 200–300 mg/kg/day divided q6h for children
  - Ceftriaxone: 1–2 g IV q12h for adults or 100 mg/kg/day divided BID in children with maximum 4 g/day
  - Clindamycin: 600 mg IV q8h for adults; 20–40 mg/kg/day IV q6–8h for children (9)
  - Metronidazole: 500 mg IV q8 h for adult; 30–35 mg/kg/day divided q8h for children
- In severe, culture-proven or suspected MRSA infection, vancomycin remains parenteral drug of choice.
  - Vancomycin: 1 g IV q12h for adults; 40 mg/kg/day IV divided q8–12h, max daily dose 2 g for children (2)

ADDITIONAL THERAPIES
- Steroid use is controversial but may be recommended for orbital cellulitis secondary to sinusitis (3)[C].
- PO steroids as an adjunct to IV antibiotic therapy for orbital cellulitis may hasten resolution of inflammation (10)[C].
- Topical erythromycin or nonmedicated ophthalmic ointment protects the eye from exposure in cases with severe proptosis.
- PO antibiotics for ≥2 weeks are traditionally recommended following IV treatment.
- Children may be treated with amoxicillin/clavulanate 20–40 mg/kg/day divided TID or in adults 250–500 mg TID. Cefaclor may be used 20–40 mg/kg/day, divided TID in children or 250–500 mg TID in adults

ISSUES FOR REFERRAL
Consultation with ophthalmology, ID, ENT for orbital cellulitis and neurology/neurosurgery if intracranial spread is suspected

SURGERY/OTHER PROCEDURES
- IV antibiotic therapy is preferred initial therapy.
- Surgical intervention warranted for visual loss, complete ophthalmoplegia, or well-defined large abscess (>10 mm) on presentation or no clinical improvement after 24 hours of antibiotic therapy.
- Trauma cases may need débridement or FB removal.
- Orbital abscess may need surgical drainage, and treatment of choice for brain abscess is surgical drainage with 4–8 weeks of antibiotics.
- Surgical interventions may include external ethmoidectomy, endoscopic ethmoidectomy, uncinectomy, antrostomy, and subperiosteal drainage.

INPATIENT CONSIDERATIONS
Patients with orbital cellulitis should be admitted for IV antibiotics and serial eye exams to evaluate progression of infection or involvement of optic nerve.
- Follow temperature, WBC, visual acuity, pupillary reflex, ocular motility, and proptosis.
- Repeat CT, surgical intervention, lumbar puncture may be required for worsening orbital cellulitis cases.

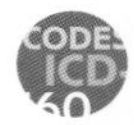

ONGOING CARE

FOLLOW-UP RECOMMENDATIONS

Patient Monitoring
Serial visual acuity testing and slit lamp exams

ALERT
Bedside exam q4h is indicated, as complications can develop rapidly.

PATIENT EDUCATION
- Maintain proper hand washing and good skin hygiene.
- Avoid skin or lid trauma.

COMPLICATIONS
- Vision loss, CNS involvement, and death
- Permanent vision loss
  - Corneal exposure
  - Optic neuritis
  - Endophthalmitis
  - Septic uveitis or retinitis
  - Exudative retinal detachment
  - Retinal artery or vein occlusions
  - Globe rupture
  - Orbital compartment syndrome
- CNS complications
  - Intracranial abscess, meningitis, cavernous sinus thrombosis (4)[B]

REFERENCES

1. Pasternak A, Irish B. Ophthalmologic infections in primary care. *Clin Fam Pract*. 2004;6(1):19–33.
2. Seltz LB, Smith J, Durairaj VD, et al. Microbiology and antibiotic management of orbital cellulitis. *Pediatrics*. 2011;127(3):e566–e572.
3. Chadha NK. An evidence-based staging system for orbital infections from acute rhinosinusitis. *Laryngoscope*. 2012;122(Suppl 4):S95–S96.
4. Hauser A, Fogarasi S. Periorbital and orbital cellulitis. *Pediatr Rev*. 2010;31(6):242–249.
5. Distinguishing periorbital from orbital cellulitis. *Am Fam Physician*. 2003;67(6):1349–1353.
6. Kloek CE, Rubin PA. Role of inflammation in orbital cellulitis. *Int Ophthalmol Clin*. 2006;46(2):57–68.
7. Papier A, Tuttle DJ, Mahar TJ. Differential diagnosis of the swollen red eyelid. *Am Fam Physician*. 2007;76(12):1815–1824.
8. Rudloe TF, Harper MB, Prabhu SP, et al. Acute periorbital infections: who needs emergent imaging? *Pediatrics*. 2010;125(4):e719–e726.
9. Bedwell J, Bauman NM. Management of pediatric orbital cellulitis and abscess. *Curr Opin Otolaryngol Head Neck Surg*. 2011;19(6):467–473.
10. Pushker N,Tejwani LK, Bajaj MS, et al. Role of oral corticosteroids in orbital cellulitis. *Am J Ophthalmol*. 2013;156(1):178–183.e1.

CODES

ICD10
- H05.019 Cellulitis of unspecified orbit
- H05.011 Cellulitis of right orbit
- H05.012 Cellulitis of left orbit

CLINICAL PEARLS
- Most orbital cellulitis cases result from sinusitis.
- MRSA orbital cellulitis may present without associated upper respiratory infection.
- Older age (>10 years) and diplopia may predict need for surgical intervention in children.
- Patients with orbital cellulitis should be admitted for visual monitoring and IV antibiotic therapy.
- Ophthalmoplegia, mental status changes, contralateral cranial nerve palsy, or bilateral orbital cellulitis may herald intracranial involvement.
- CT of orbits and sinuses with axial and coronal views with and without contrast is diagnostic modality of choice for suspected cases of orbital cellulitis.

CELLULITIS, PERIORBITAL

Fozia Akhtar Ali, MD

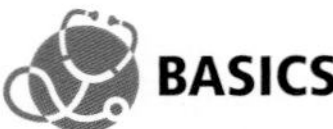

BASICS

DESCRIPTION

- An acute bacterial infection of the skin and SC tissue anterior to the orbital septum; does not involve orbital structures (globe, fat, and ocular muscles)
- Synonym(s): preseptal cellulitis

ALERT

It is important to distinguish periorbital cellulitis from orbital cellulitis, which is a potentially life-threatening condition. *Orbital cellulitis is posterior to the orbital septum; symptoms include restricted eye movement, pain with eye movement, proptosis, and vision changes.*

EPIDEMIOLOGY

- Occurs more commonly in children; mean age 21 months
- 3 times more common than orbital cellulitis (1)[C]

Incidence

Increased incidence in the winter months (due to increased number of cases of sinusitis) (1)[C]

ETIOLOGY AND PATHOPHYSIOLOGY

- The anatomy of the eyelid distinguishes preseptal from orbital cellulitis:
  - The orbital septum is a sheet of connective tissue extending from the orbital bones to the margins of the upper and lower eyelids; it acts as a barrier to infection deep in the orbital structures.
  - Infection of tissues anterior to the orbital septum is periorbital (preseptal) cellulitis.
  - Infection deep to the orbital septum is orbital (postseptal) cellulitis.
- Periorbital cellulitis classically arises from a contiguous infection of soft tissues of the face.
  - Sinusitis (via lamina papyracea) extension
  - Local trauma
  - Insect or animal bites
  - Foreign bodies
  - Dental abscess extension
  - Hematogenous seeding
- Common organisms (1)[C]
  - *Staphylococcus aureus,* typically MSSA (although increasing incidence of MRSA)
  - *Staphylococcus epidermidis*
  - *Streptococcus pyogenes*
- Atypical organisms
  - *Acinetobacter* sp.
  - *Nocardia brasiliensis*
  - *Bacillus anthracis*
  - *Pseudomonas aeruginosa*
  - *Neisseria gonorrhoeae*
  - *Proteus* sp.
  - *Pasteurella multocida*
  - *Mycobacterium tuberculosis*
  - *Trichophyton* sp. (ringworm)
- Since the introduction of the *Hib* vaccine, the incidence of *Haemophilus influenzae* has decreased; however, this organism should still be suspected in unimmunized or partially immunized patients.

Genetics

No known genetic predisposition.

RISK FACTORS

- Contiguous spread from upper respiratory infection
- Sinusitis
- Local skin trauma/puncture wound
- Insect bite
- Bacteremia

GENERAL PREVENTION

- Avoid dermatologic trauma around the eyes.
- Avoid swimming in fresh or salt water, particularly with facial skin abrasions.
- Routine vaccination: *H. influenzae* type B and *Streptococcus pneumoniae* in particular

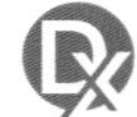

DIAGNOSIS

HISTORY

- Induration, erythema, warmth, and/or tenderness of periorbital soft tissue, usually with normal vision and eye movements
- Chemosis (conjunctival swelling), proptosis; pain with extraocular eye movements can occur in severe cases of periorbital cellulitis, although these symptoms are more common with orbital cellulitis.
- Fever (although not necessary for diagnosis)

ALERT

Pain with eye movement (ophthalmoplegia) and conjunctival swelling raise the suspicion for orbital cellulitis.

PHYSICAL EXAM

- Vital signs and general appearance (Patients with orbital cellulitis often appear systemically ill.)
- Thorough inspection of the eye and surrounding structures—lids, lashes, conjunctiva, and skin
- Erythema, swelling, and tenderness of lids without orbital congestion
  - Violaceous discoloration of eyelid is more commonly associated with *H. influenzae*.
- Evaluate for any skin break.
- Look for vesicles to rule out herpetic infection.
- Inspect nasal vaults and palpate sinuses for signs of acute sinusitis.
- Examine oral cavity for dental abscesses.
- Test ocular motility and visual acuity.

DIFFERENTIAL DIAGNOSIS

- Orbital cellulitis
  - Orbital cellulitis may have the same signs and symptoms as periorbital cellulitis, with more extensive proptosis, chemosis, ophthalmoplegia, decreased visual acuity, or fever.
- Abscess
- Dacryocystitis
- Hordeolum (stye)
- Allergic inflammation
- Orbital or periorbital trauma
- Idiopathic inflammation from orbital pseudotumor
- Orbital myositis
- Rapidly progressive tumors
  - Rhabdomyosarcoma
  - Retinoblastoma
  - Lymphoma
- Leukemia

DIAGNOSTIC TESTS & INTERPRETATION

Initial Tests (lab, imaging)

- CBC with differential
- Blood cultures (low yield) (2)[C]
- Wound culture of purulent drainage (if available)
- If suspicious for orbital involvement, consider imaging studies.
- Imaging is indicated in individuals who exhibit marked eyelid swelling, fever, and leukocytosis or those who fail to improve on appropriate antibiotics in 24–48 hours.
- CT can be used to evaluate the extent of infection and detect orbital inflammation or abscess (3)[B]:
  - The classic sign of orbital cellulitis on CT scan is bulging of the medial rectus.
  - CT should be performed with contrast, thin sections (2 mm), coronal, and axial views with bone windows.

Follow-Up Tests & Special Considerations

- Children with periorbital or orbital cellulitis often have underlying sinusitis.
- If the child is febrile, <15 months old, and appears toxic, blood cultures should be performed and lumbar puncture considered.

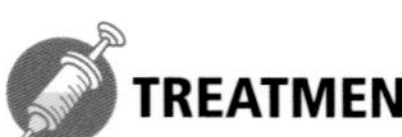

TREATMENT

MEDICATION

- Empiric antibiotic treatment regimens are based on coverage of the most likely organisms (*Staphylococcus* and *Streptococcus*) (3)[C].
- Pay attention to local prevalence and characteristics of MRSA to determine therapy.
- No evidence that IV antibiotics are more effective than PO in reducing recovery time or preventing secondary complications in the management of simple periorbital cellulitis (1)[C]
- No evidence for steroid use

C

First Line

- Uncomplicated posttraumatic
  - Usually due to skin flora, including *Staphylococcus* and *Streptococcus*
  - Cephalexin 500 mg PO q6h or dicloxacillin 500 mg PO q6h
  - Clindamycin 300 mg PO TID, doxycycline 100 mg PO BID, or trimethoprim-sulfamethoxazole (TMP-SMX) 1–2 DS tablets PO every 12 hours if MRSA is suspected
- Extension from sinusitis
  - Amoxicillin-clavulanate 875 mg PO BID
  - 3rd-generation cephalosporin (e.g., cefdinir 300 mg PO BID)
- Dental abscess
  - Amoxicillin-clavulanate 875 mg PO BID or clindamycin 300 mg PO TID
- Bacteremic cellulitis
  - May be associated with meningitis
  - Ceftriaxone 1 g IV q24h plus vancomycin 15 mg/kg/dose IV q8–12h or clindamycin 600–900 mg IV q8h to cover MRSA
- Duration of therapy should be 7–10 days:
  - If symptoms do not improve within 24 hours, IV antibiotic therapy is indicated.

ISSUES FOR REFERRAL

Consult otolaryngologists and ophthalmologists when there is concern of orbital cellulitis or when 1st-line treatment has failed (4).

SURGERY/OTHER PROCEDURES

- Usually not indicated in uncomplicated cases
- If there is an abscess or potential compromise of critical structures, such as the brain or eye, seen on imaging, orbital surgery is indicated.
- Diplopia is the strongest clinical predictor of surgery.

INPATIENT CONSIDERATIONS

Mild cases in adults and children >1 year of age can be managed on an outpatient basis, provided the patient is stable and without systemic signs of toxicity.

Admission Criteria/Initial Stabilization

Consider hospitalization and IV antibiotics:

- Children <1 year of age (4,5)[C]
- Patients not immunized against *S. pneumoniae* or *H. influenzae*
- If no signs of clinical improvement are apparent after 24 hours of antibiotic therapy
- Cases with high suspicion of orbital cellulitis (eyelid swelling with reduced vision, diplopia, abnormal light reflexes, or proptosis)

Discharge Criteria

- No strict guidelines indicate when to switch therapy from parenteral to PO agents.
- Generally, switch to PO therapy after the patient is afebrile and the skin findings have begun to resolve (typically 2–3 days).
- Therapy is typically for 10–14 days for orbital cellulitis or complicated periorbital cellulitis.

ONGOING CARE

FOLLOW-UP RECOMMENDATIONS

Patient Monitoring

Follow for signs of orbital involvement, including decreased visual acuity or painful/limited ocular motility.

PATIENT EDUCATION

- Maintain good skin hygiene.
- Avoid skin trauma.
- Report early skin changes to health care professional.

PROGNOSIS

- With timely treatment, patients do well.
- 10-day course of antibiotic treatment generally is sufficient.
- Recurrent periorbital cellulitis is a clinical entity in which a patient has ≥3 periorbital infections in the span of 1 year with at least 1 month of convalescence; must be differentiated from treatment failure due to antibiotic resistance (1)[C]

COMPLICATIONS

- Orbital cellulitis
- Abscess formation
- Scarring
- Delay in diagnosis and adequate treatment may result in serious complications, including blindness.

REFERENCES

1. Hauser A, Fogarasi S. Periorbital and orbital cellulitis. *Pediatr Rev*. 2010;31(6):242–249.
2. Baring DE, Hilmi OJ. An evidence based review of periorbital cellulitis. *Clin Otolaryngol*. 2011;36(1):57–64.
3. Beech T, Robinson A, McDermott AL, et al. Paediatric periorbital cellulitis and its management. *Rhinology*. 2007;45(1):47–49.
4. Upile NS, Munir N, Leong SC, et al. Who should manage acute periorbital cellulitis in children? *Int J Pediatr Otorhinolaryngol*. 2012;76(8):1073–1077.
5. Georgakopoulos CD, Eliopoulou MI, Stasinos S, et al. Periorbital and orbital cellulitis: a 10-year review of hospitalized children. *Eur J Ophthalmol*. 2010;20(6):1066–1072.

ADDITIONAL READING

- Chaudhry IA, Shamsi FA, Elzaridi E, et al. Inpatient preseptal cellulitis: experience from a tertiary eye care centre. *Br J Ophthalmol*. 2008;92(10):1337–1341. doi:10.1136/bjo.2007.128975.
- Goldstein SM, Shelsta HN. Community-acquired methicillin-resistant *Staphylococcus aureus* periorbital cellulitis: a problem here to stay. *Ophthal Plast Reconstr Surg*. 2009;25(1):77.
- Mahalingam-Dhingra A, Lander L, Preciado DA, et al. Orbital and periorbital infections: a national perspective. *Arch Otolaryngol Head Neck Surg*. 2011;137(8):769–773.
- Yeilding RH, O'Day DM, Li C, et al. Periorbital infections after Dermabond closure of traumatic lacerations in three children. *JAAPOS*. 2012;16(1):168–172.

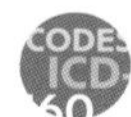

CODES

ICD10

- H05.019 Cellulitis of unspecified orbit
- H05.013 Cellulitis of bilateral orbits
- H05.011 Cellulitis of right orbit

CLINICAL PEARLS

- Periorbital (preseptal) and orbital (postseptal) cellulitis occur most commonly in children.
- It is critical to differentiate between periorbital cellulitis and orbital cellulitis; the latter is more dangerous and can be life threatening.
- CT scan of the patient's sinuses and orbits can be used to differentiate periorbital cellulitis from orbital cellulitis.
- Early detection and treatment of periorbital cellulitis is important to prevent complications.
- The 2 most important predisposing factors for periorbital cellulitis are upper respiratory infections and eyelid trauma; sinusitis is more typically associated with orbital cellulitis (5)[C].

CEREBRAL PALSY

Christina Mezzone, DO, MS • Michael J. Terzella, DO

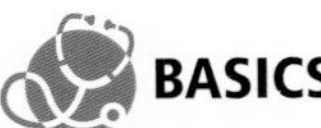

BASICS

DESCRIPTION

Cerebral palsy (CP) is a group of clinical syndromes characterized by motor and postural dysfunction due to permanent and nonprogressive disruptions in the developing fetal brain. Motor impairment resulting in activity limitation is necessary for this diagnosis. CP is classified by the nature of the movement disorder and its functional severity. Individuals with this disorder are affected with secondary musculoskeletal and neurologic problems (intellectual, sensory, speech and language impairment, and seizures).

EPIDEMIOLOGY

Incidence

- Overall, 1.5–2.5/1,000 live births
- Incidence increases as gestational age (GA) at birth decreases:
  - 146/1,000 for GA of 22–27 weeks
  - 62/1,000 for GA of 28–31 weeks
  - 7/1,000 for GA of 32–36 weeks
  - 1/1,000 for GA of 37+ weeks

Prevalence

3–4/1,000 of the population

ETIOLOGY AND PATHOPHYSIOLOGY

- Multifactorial; CP results from static injury or lesions in the developing brain, occurring prenatally, perinatally, or postnatally.
- Neuropathology linked to GA at time of brain insult
- Cytokines, free radicals, and inflammatory response are likely contributing factors.
- Etiology is most likely multifactorial and depends on timing of brain insult: prenatally, perinatally, or postnatally (see "Risk Factors").
- Spastic CP is most common, usually related to premature birth, with either periventricular leukomalacia or germinal matrix hemorrhage.
- Dystonic or athetotic CP, often resulting from kernicterus, is now rare due to improved management of hyperbilirubinemia.

Genetics

There are reports of associations between CP and candidate genes: thrombophilic, cytokines, and apolipoprotein E.

RISK FACTORS

- Prenatal: congenital anomalies, multiple gestation, in utero stroke, intrauterine infection (cytomegalovirus [CMV], varicella), intrauterine growth retardation (IUGR), clinical and histologic chorioamnionitis, antepartum bleeding, maternal factors (cognitive impairment, seizure disorders, hyperthyroidism), abnormal fetal position (e.g., breech)
- Perinatal: preterm birth, low birth weight, periventricular leukomalacia, perinatal hypoxia/asphyxia, intracranial hemorrhage/intraventricular hemorrhage, neonatal seizure or stroke, hyperbilirubinemia
- Postnatal: traumatic brain injury or stroke, sepsis, meningitis, encephalitis, asphyxia, and progressive hydrocephalus

GENERAL PREVENTION

- Treating mothers with magnesium sulfate during preterm delivery is neuroprotective for fetus. Effect on term fetus is unknown.
- Improved management of hyperbilirubinemia with decrease in kernicterus has greatly reduced dyskinetic CP.
- Prevention or reduction of chorioamnionitis and premature births

COMMONLY ASSOCIATED CONDITIONS

- Seizure disorder (22–40%)
- Intellectual impairment (23–44%)
- Behavioral problems
- Speech and language impairment (42–81%)
  - May have an impact on expressive and/or receptive language
  - May be nonverbal
- Sensory impairments
  - Hearing deficits
  - Visual (62–71%): poor visual acuity, strabismus (50%), or hemianopsia
- Feeding impairment, swallowing dysfunction, and aspiration: when severe, may require gastrostomy feedings
- Poor dentition, excessive drooling
- GI conditions: constipation (59%), vomiting (22%), gastroesophageal reflux
- Decreased linear growth and weight abnormalities (under- and overweight)
- Osteopenia
- Bowel and bladder incontinence
- Orthopedic: contractures, hip subluxation/dislocation, scoliosis (60%)

DIAGNOSIS

- A clinical diagnosis including
  - Delayed motor milestones
  - Abnormal tone
  - Abnormal neurologic exam suggesting a cerebral etiology for motor dysfunction
  - Absence of regression (not losing function)
  - Absence of underlying syndromes or alternative explanation for etiology
- Although the pathologic lesion is static, clinical presentation may change as the infant grows and develops.
- Accurate early diagnosis remains difficult. Neurologic abnormalities observed in the first 1–2 years of life may resolve; be cautious of diagnosing CP before age 2 years.
- Serial exams are often required for a definitive diagnosis.

HISTORY

- Presentation: concerns over movements or delayed motor development
- Ask about
  - Prenatal, perinatal, and postnatal risk factors
  - Neurobehavioral signs
    - Poor feeding/frequent vomiting
    - Irritability
  - Timing of motor milestones: Delay in milestones is not sensitive or specific until after 6 months of age.
  - Abnormal spontaneous general movements
  - Asymmetry of movements such as early hand preference
- Regression of motor skills does not occur with CP.

PHYSICAL EXAM

- Assess for more than one type of neurologic impairment:
  - Spasticity: increased tone/reflexes/clonus
  - Dyskinesia: abnormal movements
  - Hypotonia: decreased tone
  - Ataxia: abnormal balance/coordination
- Areas of exam
  - Tone: may be increased or decreased
  - Trunk and head control: often poor but may be advanced due to high tone
  - Reduced strength and motor control
  - Persistence of primitive reflexes
  - Asymmetry of movement or reflexes
  - Decreased joint range of motion and contractures
  - Brisk deep tendon reflexes
  - Clonus
  - Delayed motor milestones: serial exams most effective
  - Gait abnormalities: scissoring, toe-walking
- CP is classified by the following:
  - Muscle tone or movement disorder
    - Spasticity
      - Unilateral: hemiplegic
      - Bilateral: diplegic (lower extremity [LE] > upper extremity [UE] involvement) or quadriplegic (UE ≥ LE involvement)
    - Dystonia: hypertonia and reduced movement
    - Choreoathetosis: irregular spasmodic involuntary movements of the limbs or facial muscles
    - Ataxia: loss of orderly muscular coordination
  - Motor function severity
    - The Gross Motor Function Classification System (GMFCS) scores I–IV
      - Score of I: ambulates without limitation
      - Score of II: ambulates without assistive devices but some limitation
      - Score of III: ambulates with assistive mobility devices
      - Score of IV: self-mobility limited, but technology can help
      - Score of V: self-mobility severely limited, even with technology
    - The Manual Ability Classification System (MACS) can be used to assess upper extremity and fine motor function.

DIFFERENTIAL DIAGNOSIS

Benign congenital hypotonia, brachial plexus injury, familial spastic paraplegia, dopa-responsive dystonia, transient toe-walking, muscular dystrophy, metabolic disorders (e.g., glutaric aciduria type 1), mitochondrial disorders, genetic disorders (e.g., Rett syndrome)

DIAGNOSTIC TESTS & INTERPRETATION

CP is a clinical diagnosis based on history, physical, and risk factors. Laboratory testing is not needed to make diagnosis but can help exclude other etiologies.

- Testing for metabolic and genetic syndromes (1)[C]
  - Not routinely obtained in the evaluation for CP
  - Considered if no specific etiology is identified by neuroimaging or there are atypical features in clinical presentation.
  - Detection of certain brain malformations may warrant genetic or metabolic testing to identify syndromes.
- Screening for coagulopathies: Diagnostic testing for coagulopathies should be considered in children with hemiplegic CP with cerebral infarction identified on neuroimaging (1)[C].

Initial Tests (lab, imaging)

- Neuroimaging is not essential, but it is recommended in children with CP for whom the etiology has not been established (1)[C].
- MRI is preferred for determining etiology and timing of a brain insult (1)[C].

- Abnormalities in 80–90% of patients: brain malformation, cerebral infarction, intraventricular or other intracranial hemorrhage, periventricular leukomalacia, ventricular enlargement, or other CSF space abnormalities

Diagnostic Procedures/Other

- The Communication Function Classification System has recently been developed as another means of assessing function.
- Screening for comorbid conditions: developmental delay/intellectual impairment, vision/hearing impairments, speech and language disorders, feeding/swallowing dysfunction, or seizures
- Electroencephalograms (EEGs) should only be obtained if there is a history of suspected seizures.

Test Interpretation

Perinatal brain injury may include the following:

- White matter damage
  - Most common in premature infants
  - Periventricular leukomalacia: gliosis with or without focal necrosis with resulting cysts and scarring. May be multiple lesions of various ages. Necrosis can lead to cysts/scarring.
  - Germinal matrix hemorrhage: may lead to intraventricular hemorrhage
- Gray matter damage: more common in term infants; cortical infarcts, focal neuronal damage, myelination abnormalities

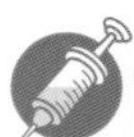

TREATMENT

Focuses on control of symptoms; treatments reduce spasticity to prevent painful contractures, manage comorbid conditions, and optimize functionality and quality of life.

GENERAL MEASURES

- Early intervention programs for preterm infants influences motor and cognitive outcomes (2)[A].
- Referral to early intervention for children ages 0–3 years is essential.
- Various therapy modalities enhance functioning:
  - Physical therapy to improve posture stability and gait, motor strength and control, and prevent contractures
  - Occupational therapy to increase functional activities of daily living and other fine motor skills
  - Speech therapy for verbal and nonverbal speech and to aid in feeding
- Equipment optimizes participation in activities:
  - Orthotic splinting (ankle–foot orthosis) maintains functional positioning and prevents contractures.
  - Spinal bracing (body jacket) may slow down scoliosis.
  - Augmentative communication with pictures, switches, or computer systems for nonverbal individuals
  - Therapeutic and functional electrical stimulation decreases activity limitation in gait.
  - Use of adaptive equipment such as crutches, walkers, gait trainers, and wheelchairs for mobility and standers for weight bearing

MEDICATION

First Line

- Diazepam (3)[A]
  - Short-term treatment for generalized spasticity; insufficient evidence on motor function
  - A γ-aminobutyric acid-A ($GABA_A$) agonist that facilitates CNS) inhibition at spinal and supraspinal levels to reduce spasticity
  - Adverse effects: ataxia and drowsiness
  - Adult dose: 2–12 mg/dose PO q6–12h
  - Pediatric dose (<12 years and <15 kg): <8.5 kg: 0.5–1 mg HS; 8.5–15 kg: 1–2 mg HS; children 5–16 years of age and ≥15 kg: 1.25 mg TID
- Botulinum toxin type A (3)[A]
  - Injected directly into muscles of interest for localized spasticity; insufficient evidence on motor function
  - Higher functional benefit when combined with occupational therapy
  - Acts at neuromuscular junction to inhibit the release of acetylcholine to reduce tone
  - Lasts for 12–16 weeks following injection

Second Line

- Baclofen (3)[A]
  - $GABA_B$ agonist, facilitates presynaptic inhibition of mono- and polysynaptic reflexes
  - Adverse effects: drowsiness and sedation
  - Abrupt withdrawal symptoms: spasticity, hallucinations, seizures, confusion, hyperthermia
  - Adults: Initial dose is 5 mg TID; increase dosage every 3 days to an average maintenance dose of 20 mg TID 80 mg/day maximum.
  - Pediatric dose (>2 years): initial 10–15 mg/day. Titrate to effective dose (maximum 40 mg/day). <8 years old: 60 mg/day maximum. >8 years old: 60 mg/day maximum
- Intrathecal baclofen (baclofen pump) (4)[A]
  - Continuous intrathecal route allows greater maximal response with smaller dosage to reduce spasticity.
  - May help ambulatory individuals with gait but no improvement seen in nonambulatory patients.
  - Adverse effects: infection, catheter malfunction, CSF leakage

ADDITIONAL THERAPIES

- Multidisciplinary care including ophthalmology; neurology; orthopedics; physiatry along with physical, occupational, and speech therapists
- A primary care "medical home" that coordinates medical and community services, provides support for the patient and the patient's family

SURGERY/OTHER PROCEDURES

- Dorsal root rhizotomy selectively cuts dorsal rootlets from L1–S2. Best for patients with normal intelligence with spastic diplegia. Decreases spasticity in lower limbs when done in conjunction with physiotherapy but associated with adverse effects. Evidence is lacking as to long-term outcomes.
- Surgical treatment of joint dislocations/subluxation, scoliosis management, tendon lengthening, gastrostomy

COMPLEMENTARY & ALTERNATIVE MEDICINE

- Hyperbaric oxygen is controversial and not recommended in those who do not suffer hypoxic ischemic encephalopathy (5)[A].
- Therapeutic horse riding or hippotherapy improves postural control and balance.
- Aquatherapy improves gross motor function in patients with various motor severities (6)[B].

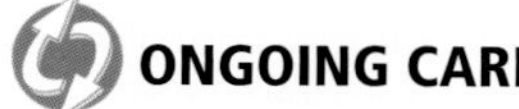

ONGOING CARE

PROGNOSIS

Reduced lifespan strongly associated with level of functional impairment and intellectual disability

REFERENCES

1. Ashwal S, Russman BS, Blasco PA, et al. Practice parameter: diagnostic assessment of the child with cerebral palsy: report of the Quality Standards Subcommittee of the American Academy of Neurology and the Practice Committee of the Child Neurology Society. *Neurology*. 2004;62(6):851–863.
2. Spittle A, Orton J, Anderson P, et al. Early developmental intervention programmes post-hospital discharge to prevent motor and cognitive impairments in preterm infants. *Cochrane Database Syst Rev*. 2012;(12):CD005495.
3. Quality Standards Subcommittee of the American Academy of Neurology and the Practice Committee of the Child Neurology Society; Delgado MR, Hirtz D, Aisen M, et al. Practice parameter: pharmacologic treatment of spasticity in children and adolescents with cerebral palsy (an evidence-based review): report of the Quality Standards Subcommittee of the American Academy of Neurology and the Practice Committee of the Child Neurology Society. *Neurology*. 2010;74(4):336–343.
4. Pin TW, McCartney L, Lewis J, et al. Use of intrathecal baclofen therapy in ambulant children and adolescents with spasticity and dystonia of cerebral origin: a systematic review. *Dev Med Child Neurol*. 2011;53(10):885–895.
5. Lacey DJ, Stolfi A, Pilati LE. Effects of hyperbaric oxygen on motor function in children with cerebral palsy. *Ann Neurol*. 2012;72(5):695–703.
6. Lai CJ, Liu WY, Yang TF, et al. Pediatric aquatic therapy on motor function and enjoyment in children diagnosed with cerebral palsy of various motor severities [published online ahead of print June 5, 2014]. *J Child Neurol*.

ADDITIONAL READING

- Himpens E, Van den Broeck C, Oostra A, et al. Prevalence, type, distribution, and severity of cerebral palsy in relation to gestational age: a meta-analytic review. *Dev Med Child Neurol*. 2008;50(5):334–340.
- Nguyen TM, Crowther CA, Wilkinson D, et al. Magnesium sulphate for women at term for neuroprotection of the fetus. *Cochrane Database Syst Rev*. 2013;(2):CD009395.
- O'Shea TM. Diagnosis, treatment, and prevention of cerebral palsy. *Clin Obstet Gynecol*. 2008;51(4):816–828.

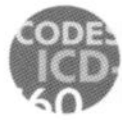

CODES

ICD10

- G80.9 Cerebral palsy, unspecified
- G80.1 Spastic diplegic cerebral palsy
- G80.2 Spastic hemiplegic cerebral palsy

CLINICAL PEARLS

- Management should focus on maximizing functioning and quality of life using multidisciplinary team approach.
- Regression of motor skills does not occur with CP.

CERVICAL HYPEREXTENSION INJURIES

Shane L. Larson, MD • Derek G. Zickgraf, DO

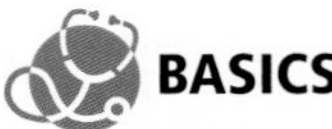

BASICS

DESCRIPTION

- Variety of injuries involving the neck that typically result from a rapid, forceful, backward motion
- May involve the following:
  - Injury to vertebral and paravertebral structures: fractures, dislocations, ligamentous tears, and disc disruption/subluxation
  - Spinal cord injury: traumatic central cord syndrome (CCS) secondary to cord compression or vascular insult
  - Blunt cerebrovascular injury (BCVI): vertebral artery or carotid artery dissection
  - Soft tissue injury around cervical spine: cervical strain/sprain

EPIDEMIOLOGY

- Predominant age: trauma and sports injuries more common in young adults (average age 29.4 years); however, CCS mostly seen in older population (average age 53 years)
- Predominant sex: male > female

Incidence

In the United States

- Cervical fractures: 2–5/100 blunt trauma patients
- CCS: 3.6/100,000 people/year
- BCVI: estimated 1/1,000 of hospitalized trauma patients; incidence increased with cervical spine or thoracic injury.
- Cervical strain: 3–4/1,000 people/year

ETIOLOGY AND PATHOPHYSIOLOGY

Blunt trauma due to motor vehicle accidents, sports injuries, falls, and assaults

RISK FACTORS

- Fractures: osteoporosis, conditions predisposing to spinal rigidity such as ankylosing spondylitis or other spondyloarthropathies
- CCS: Preexisting spinal stenosis is present in >50% of cases, which may be the following:
  - Acquired: prior trauma, spondylosis
  - Congenital: Klippel-Feil syndrome (congenital fusion of any 2 cervical vertebra) with cervical stenosis

GENERAL PREVENTION

Seat belts, use of proper safety equipment, rule changes, and technique-coaching emphasis in sports activities can potentially prevent or minimize injury.

COMMONLY ASSOCIATED CONDITIONS

Closed head injuries (mild TBI, cerebral contusions, intracranial hemorrhage), facial fractures, other spinal injury, soft tissue trauma

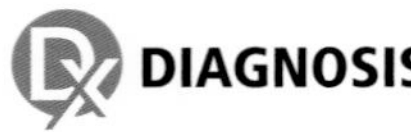

DIAGNOSIS

HISTORY

Usually acute presentation with mechanism of cervical hyperextension (see "Etiology") and complaints of neck pain, stiffness, or headaches ± neurologic symptoms

PHYSICAL EXAM

- External signs of trauma on the head and neck such as abrasions, lacerations, or contusions are clues to mechanism.
- Presence, severity, and location of neck tenderness often helps localize involved structure(s):
  - Posterior midline, bony tenderness concerning for fracture
  - Paraspinal or lateral soft tissue tenderness suggests muscular/ligamentous injury.
  - Anterior tenderness concerning for vascular injury
- Carotid bruit suggests carotid dissection.
- Neurologic exam: Paresthesias, weakness suggests spinal cord injury or stroke secondary to BCVI:
  - CCS often presents as the following:
    - Distal > proximal symptom distribution, upper extremity > lower extremity
    - Extremity weakness/paralysis predominates.
    - Variable sensory changes below level of lesion (including paresthesias and dysesthesia)
    - Bladder/bowel incontinence may occur.

DIFFERENTIAL DIAGNOSIS

- Acute or chronic disc pathology (including herniation or internal disruption)
- Osteoarthritis
- Cervical radiculopathy
- For CCS
  - Bell cruciate palsy
  - Bilateral brachial plexus injuries
  - Carotid or vertebral artery dissection

DIAGNOSTIC TESTS & INTERPRETATION

Initial Tests (lab, imaging)

- Low-risk patients can be cleared clinically (without imaging) using either the Canadian C-spine Rule (CCR) or the National Emergency X-Ray Utilization Study (NEXUS) criteria (1)[B]:
  - CCR: Clinically clear a stable, adult patient with no history of cervical spine disease/surgery if all of the following conditions are met:
    - Glasgow Coma Scale (GCS) ≥15
    - Nonintoxicated patients without a distracting injury
    - No dangerous mechanism or extremity paresthesias
    - Age <65 years
    - At least 1 "low-risk factor" (i.e., simple rear-end motor vehicle accident [MVA], ambulation at the accident scene, no midline cervical tenderness, delayed onset of neck pain, or sitting position at the time of exam)
  - NEXUS: Clinically clear if all of the following are met:
    - No alteration of mental status or intoxication
    - No focal/neuro deficits
    - No distracting injury
    - No posterior, midline C-spine tenderness
  - Reported sensitivity/specificity: CCR (99.4%/45.1%), NEXUS (90.7%/36.8%)
- In patients with high-risk mechanism or any concerning historical/physical exam elements, imaging should strongly be considered. Choose from the following options based on the suspected injury and level of clinical suspicion:
  - Plain radiographs: recommended by some in patients who cannot be cleared clinically but still are in low-suspicion category: sensitivity for C-spine injury as low as 39%
    - Static: lateral, anteroposterior (AP), and odontoid views; in addition to bony abnormalities, may show prevertebral soft tissue swelling
    - Dynamic: flexion/extension; only if asymptomatic and no neurologic deficits or mental impairment, poor identification of ligamentous injury, limited diagnostic value (2)[A]
  - CT: axial CT from occiput to T1 with coronal and sagittal reconstructions; has replaced plain radiography as the test of choice for cases with moderate to high clinical suspicion of C-spine injury, given high sensitivity (90–100%)
  - MRI: test of choice in CCS with direct visualization of traumatic cord lesions (edema or hematomyelia), soft tissue compressing cord, and/or stenosis of canal. Detects ligamentous injury and abnormalities of intervertebral discs and soft tissues. MRI is poor with fractures due to false-positive results from nonspecific findings. Some authors suggest MRI is required to screen for occult injury in obtunded patients with a negative CT scan; however, this recommendation is controversial with limited evidence.
  - CT angiography: visualization of cervical and cerebral vascular structures to detect BCVI, with reported sensitivity approaching 100% when a ≥16-slice CT scanner is used. MR angiography is an alternative modality, although reported sensitivities of 47–50% limit its use, and it may have limited accessibility in some hospital settings.

Test Interpretation

- Vertebral fractures: See "General Measures."
- CCS: currently thought to be due to axonal disruption within the white matter of the lateral column, particularly the corticospinal tracts
- BCVI: intimal disruption, leading to thrombosis and embolization
- Acute cervical strain/sprain: Models based on animal, cadaver, and postmortem studies show myofascial tearing, edema, and inflammation, but facet joint capsular pain may also play a role.

Geriatric Considerations

- Degenerative changes of the C-spine may be confused with acute traumatic change, and osteopenia may limit visualization of fractures, particularly on x-ray; CT imaging differentiates the two.
- Degenerative disease and osteopenia increases the risk of upper cervical spine injuries despite low-velocity trauma (3)[B].

Pediatric Considerations

Consider spinal cord injury without radiographic abnormality (SCIWORA): high incidence at <9 years and accounts for up to 50% of all pediatric cervical spine injuries. MRI may help detect the injury.

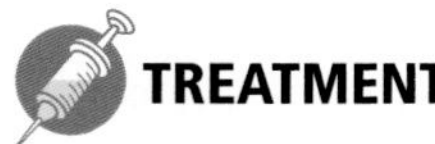

TREATMENT

GENERAL MEASURES

- Fractures
  - Stability determined by imaging; decompression and stabilization are indicated in the following:
    - Incomplete spinal cord injuries with spinal canal compromise
    - Clinical deterioration or failure to improve despite conservative management
  - Hangman's fracture: traumatic spondylolisthesis of C2 with bilateral fractures through C2 pedicles, often with anterior subluxation of C2 over C3; can be unstable
    - Managed with halo vest immobilization for 12 weeks until repeated flexion/extension films normalize
  - Odontoid fractures: treated according to type
    - I: through apex; usually stable; external immobilization with a cervical collar (less often halo vest) for up to 12 weeks

    - II: most common, at base of dens, usually unstable; nonunion rates of up to 67% with halo immobilization alone, especially with dens displacement >6 mm or age >50 years
    - III: through C2 body, usually stable; immobilization in halo or cervical collar for 12–20 weeks
  - Hyperextension teardrop fractures
    - If stable, rigid collar or cervicothoracic brace for 8–14 weeks
    - If unstable, halo brace for up to 3 months
- CCS: neck immobilization with cervical collar, physical therapy/occupational therapy (PT/OT)
- Cervical strain: No evidence of different outcomes with active (PT) versus passive (immobilization, rest) treatment but may use soft cervical collar for up to 10 days for symptomatic relief, then mobilization and activity as tolerated.
- Lack of clear effective treatments in current medical literature in absence of fracture (4)[B]

MEDICATION

- Fractures: pain control as needed with opiate analgesics
- CCS: Within 8 hours of injury, consider methylprednisolone 30 mg/kg IV over 15 minutes, then continuous infusion 5.4 mg/kg/h IV for 23 hours. Further improvement in motor function recovery may be seen if infusion is continued for 48 hours, especially if initial bolus administration is delayed by 3–8 hours after injury (5)[A].
- BCVI: Anticoagulation with IV heparin, followed by warfarin therapy for 3–6 months, then long-term antiplatelet therapy is common practice. However, an antiplatelet agent is used as the sole initial therapy in patients with contraindications to anticoagulation. To date, no randomized controlled trials compare the efficacy of antiplatelets versus anticoagulant therapy, so evidence-based recommendations are unavailable.
- Cervical strain: muscle relaxants, acetaminophen/NSAIDs ± opiate analgesics are commonly used.

ISSUES FOR REFERRAL

- When cervical spine injury is suspected, the patient should be immobilized and sent to the ED for evaluation.
- Emergent consultation from a spinal surgeon (orthopedics or neurosurgery) is indicated if there is any concern for unstable fracture or spinal cord injury.

SURGERY/OTHER PROCEDURES

- Fractures
  - Hangman fracture: Consider surgical fixation for excessive angulation or subluxation, disruption of intervertebral disc space, or failure to obtain alignment with external orthosis.
  - Odontoid fractures
    - Type II: Early surgical stabilization recommended in setting of age >50 years, dens displacement >5 mm, and specific fracture patterns.
    - Type III: Surgical intervention often reserved for cases of nonunion/malunion after trial of external immobilization.
  - Hyperextension teardrop fractures: Consider surgical repair if unstable with neurologic deficit.
- CCS: Surgical decompression/fixation indicated in setting of unstable injury, herniated disc, or when neurologic function deteriorates.
- BCVI: Surgical and/or angiographic intervention may be required if there is evidence of pseudoaneurysm, total occlusion, or transection of the vessel.

INPATIENT CONSIDERATIONS

Admission Criteria/Initial Stabilization

- Varies by injury; clinical judgment, imaging findings, concomitant injuries, and need for operative intervention
- Advanced Trauma Life Support protocol with backboard and collar

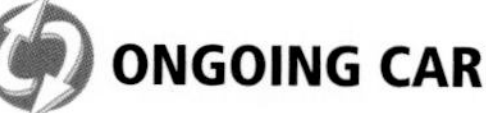

ONGOING CARE

FOLLOW-UP RECOMMENDATIONS

Patient Monitoring

Patients with known injuries will often be followed with serial imaging under the care of a specialist (i.e., a spinal surgeon, neurologist, and/or physiatrist).

PATIENT EDUCATION

For patient instruction on prevention: ThinkFirst Foundation: http://www.thinkfirst.org

PROGNOSIS

- Overall, the most important prognostic factor is the patient's presenting neurologic status.
- Fractures
  - Hangman's fracture: 93–100% fusion rate after 8–14 weeks external immobilization
  - Odontoid fracture, fusion rate by type: type I ~100% with external immobilization alone; type III, 85% with external immobilization, 100% with surgical fixation
- BCVI: With early diagnosis and initiation of antithrombotic therapy, patients may have fewer neurologic sequelae.
- CCS
  - Spontaneous recovery of motor function in >50% of cases over several weeks, with younger patients more likely to regain function
  - Leg, bowel, and bladder functions return first, followed by upper extremities.
- Cervical strain: Up to 50% of patients continue to have neck pain at 1 year:
  - Prognostic factors for development of late whiplash syndrome (>6 months of symptoms affecting normal activity) include increased initial pain intensity, pain-related disability, and cold hyperalgesia.

COMPLICATIONS

- Fractures: instability or malunion/nonunion necessitating 2nd operation, reactions, and infection related to orthosis
- BCVI: embolic ischemic events and pseudoaneurysm formation

REFERENCES

1. Stiell IG, Clement CM, McKnight RD, et al. The Canadian C-spine rule versus the NEXUS low-risk criteria in patients with trauma. *N Engl J Med.* 2003;349(26):2510–2518.
2. Sierink JC, van Lieshout WA, Beenen LF, et al. Systematic review of flexion/extension radiography of the cervical spine in trauma patients. *Eur J Radiol.* 2013;82(6):974–981.
3. Watanabe M, Sakai D, Yamamoto Y, et al. Upper cervical spine injuries: age-specific clinical features. *J Orthop Sci.* 2010;15(4):485–492.
4. Verhagen AP, Scholten-Peeters GG, van Wijngaarden S, et al. Conservative treatments for whiplash. *Cochrane Database Syst Rev.* 2007;(2):CD003338.
5. Bracken MB. Steroids for acute spinal cord injury. *Cochrane Database Syst Rev.* 2012;1:CD001046.

ADDITIONAL READING

- Chinnock P, Roberts I. Gangliosides for acute spinal cord injury. *Cochrane Database Syst Rev.* 2005;(2):CD004444.
- Franz RW, Willette PA, Wood MJ, et al. A systematic review and meta-analysis of diagnostic screening criteria for blunt cerebrovascular injuries. *J Am Coll Surg.* 2012;214(3):313–327.
- Kwan I, Bunn F, Roberts I. Spinal immobilisation for trauma patients. *Cochrane Database Syst Rev.* 2001;(2):CD002803.
- Liu BC, Ivers R, Norton R, et al. Helmets for preventing injury in motorcycle riders. *Cochrane Database Syst Rev.* 2008;(1):CD004333.
- Shears E, Armitstead CP. Surgical versus conservative management for odontoid fractures. *Cochrane Database Syst Rev.* 2008;(4):CD005078.

SEE ALSO

Algorithm: Cervical Hyperextension Injury

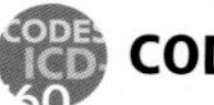

CODES

ICD10

- S13.4XXA Sprain of ligaments of cervical spine, initial encounter
- S13.101A Dislocation of unspecified cervical vertebrae, init encntr
- S14.109A Unsp injury at unsp level of cervical spinal cord, init

CLINICAL PEARLS

- Follow NEXUS or Canadian Cervical Spine rules on every patient with potential neck injury to determine imaging needs, but they do not supercede clinical judgment!
- Inquire about preexisting cervical spine conditions, especially in the elderly, as they may increase risk of injury or change radiographic interpretation.
- Suspect spinal cord injury until exam and imaging suggest otherwise.
- Consider BCVI when neurologic deficits are inconsistent with level of known injury or significant mechanism exists.

CERVICAL MALIGNANCY

Benjamin P. Brown, MD • Meaghan Tenney, MD

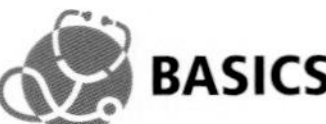

BASICS

DESCRIPTION
- Invasive cancer of the uterine cervix
- Commonly involves the vagina, parametria, and pelvic side walls
- Invasion of bladder, rectum, and other pelvic sites in advanced disease

EPIDEMIOLOGY

Incidence
- Worldwide, cervical cancer is the 3rd most common malignancy among women.
- There is a higher incidence of cervical cancer in developing countries, contributing >80% of reported cases annually.
- In the developed world, it is the 10th most common malignancy among women. In the United States, it is the 3rd most common gynecologic cancer.
- The disease has a bimodal distribution, with the highest risk among women age 40–59 years and >70.

Prevalence
- In 2014, the American Cancer Society (ACS) estimated there were 12,360 new cases in the United States, with 4,020 deaths from the malignancy.
- African Americans and women in lower socioeconomic groups have the highest age-standardized cervical cancer death rates.
- Hispanic and Latina women have the highest incidence of the malignancy.

ETIOLOGY AND PATHOPHYSIOLOGY
- Arises from preexisting dysplastic lesions, usually following persistent human papillomavirus (HPV) infection
- Pattern of local growth may be exophytic or endophytic.
- Lymphatic spread, typically through cervical lymphatic drainage
- Local tumor extension involving the bladder, ureters, rectum, and distant metastasis from hematogenous spread (Halstedian growth)
- Epidemiologic and experimental evidence supports HPV strains 16 and 18 as etiologic agents in ~70% of cervical cancers.
- Association with E6 and E7 oncogenic proteins responsible for malignant cell transformation by inactivation of p53 and Rb tumor suppressor genes
- Slow progression from dysplasia to invasive cancer allows sufficient time for effective screening and treatment of preinvasive disease.

Genetics
Not an inherited disease, except in very rare cases of Peutz-Jeghers syndrome

RISK FACTORS
- Causative agent in the majority of cases is persistent HPV infection.
- Other risk factors include the following:
  - Lack of regular Pap smears
  - Early coitarche
  - Multiple sexual partners
  - Unprotected sex
  - A history of sexually transmitted diseases (STDs)
  - Low socioeconomic status
  - High parity
  - Cigarette smoking
  - Immunosuppression
  - Diethylstilbestrol (DES) exposure in utero

GENERAL PREVENTION
- Patient education regarding safer sex, decreasing number of sexual partners
- Smoking cessation
- HPV vaccines
  - Gardasil vaccine: Quadrivalent vaccine containing proteins from HPV strains 6, 11, 16, and 18. FDA approved in females and in males (for prevention of genital warts and anal cancer)
  - Cervarix vaccine: Bivalent vaccine against oncogenic HPV strains 16 and 18.
  - Neither vaccine yet conclusively shown to prevent cancer.
  - Recommended age of vaccination is 11–12 years (prior to coitarche), but Gardasil is approved from 9 to 26 years and Cervarix from 10 to 25 years.
- Regular Pap smears and pelvic exams at appropriate intervals. In patients with no history of abnormal Paps, current guidelines from the American College of Obstetricians and Gynecologists (ACOG) are as follows:
  - Cytology alone every 3 years between 21 and 30 years
  - Cytology plus HPV testing every 5 years after 30 years (1)[C]
- The International Federation of Gynecology and Obstetrics (FIGO) recommends visual inspection with acetic acid (VIA) or Lugol iodine (VILI) as reasonable alternatives to Pap smear screening in resource-poor settings. A 3–5-year screening interval is currently recommended (2)[C].
- Despite HPV vaccination, cervical cancer screening will remain the main preventive measure for both vaccinated and nonvaccinated women.

COMMONLY ASSOCIATED CONDITIONS
- Condyloma acuminata
- Preinvasive/invasive lesions of the vulva and vagina

DIAGNOSIS

HISTORY
- May be asymptomatic
- Most common symptom is vaginal bleeding, often postcoital.
- Other gynecologic symptoms include intermenstrual or postmenopausal bleeding and vaginal discharge.
- Other less common symptoms include low back pain with radiation down posterior leg, lower extremity edema, vesicovaginal and rectovaginal fistula, and urinary symptoms.

PHYSICAL EXAM
- Disease is staged clinically not surgically.
- Thorough internal and external pelvic exam is needed to look for lesions:
  - Many patients have a normal exam, especially with microinvasive disease.
  - Lesions may be exophytic, endophytic, polypoid, papillary, ulcerative, or necrotic.
  - Watery, purulent, or bloody discharge
- Bimanual and rectovaginal examination for uterine size, vaginal wall, rectovaginal septum, parametrial, uterosacral, and pelvic sidewall involvement
- Enlarged supraclavicular or inguinal lymphadenopathy, lower extremity edema, ascites, or decreased breath sounds with lung auscultation may indicate metastases or advanced stage disease.

DIFFERENTIAL DIAGNOSIS
- Marked cervicitis and erosion
- Glandular hyperplasia
- Sexually transmitted infection
- Cervical condyloma, leiomyoma, or polyp
- Metastasis from endometrial carcinoma or gestational trophoblastic neoplasia

DIAGNOSTIC TESTS & INTERPRETATION

Initial Tests (lab, imaging)
- Biopsy of gross lesions and colposcopically directed biopsies are the definitive means of diagnosis.
- CBC may show anemia.
- Urinalysis may show hematuria.
- In advanced disease, BUN, creatinine, and liver function tests (LFTs) may be helpful.
- Initially, a CT scan of the chest, abdomen, and pelvis and/or a positron emission tomography (PET) scan.
- Apart from chest x-ray (CXR) and intravenous pyelogram (IVP), imaging does not alter tumor stage.
- MRI may be helpful in evaluating parametrial involvement in patients who are surgical candidates or for radiation treatment planning.

Follow-Up Tests & Special Considerations
Prompt multidisciplinary plan of care

DIAGNOSTIC PROCEDURES/OTHER
- Exam under anesthesia may help in determining clinical stage and disease extent and determine if patient is a surgical candidate.
- Endocervical curettage and cervical conization as indicated to determine depth of invasion and presence of lymphovascular involvement
- Cystoscopy to evaluate bladder invasion
- Proctoscopy for invasion into rectum

Test Interpretation
- Majority of cases (80%) are invasive squamous cell types usually arising from the ectocervix.
- Adenocarcinomas comprise 10–15% of cervical cancer arising from endocervical mucus-producing glandular cells. Often, no exophytic lesion but a "bulky" "barrel-shaped" cervix present on exam.
- Other cell types that may be present include rare mixed cell types, neuroendocrine tumors, sarcomas, lymphomas, and melanomas.

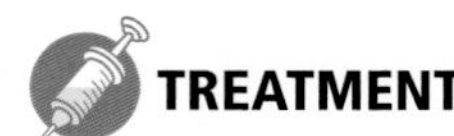

TREATMENT

GENERAL MEASURES
Improve nutritional state, correct any anemia, and treat any vaginal and/or pelvic infections.

MEDICATION
- Chemoradiation with cisplatin-containing regimen has superior survival rates over pelvic and extended-field radiation alone (3)[A].
- Neoadjuvant chemotherapy may improve survival for early and locally advanced tumors, but more data are needed (4)[A].
- Adjuvant chemotherapy after chemoradiation may improve progression-free survival in patients who receive primary chemoradiation for stages IIB–IVA tumors. The OUTBACK trial will further investigate these findings (http://www.clinicaltrials.gov).

- The addition of bevacizumab to standard combination chemotherapy (cisplatin/topotecan or cisplatin/paclitaxel) for recurrent, persistent, or metastatic disease has been shown to improve overall survival (5)[A].

ISSUES FOR REFERRAL

Multidisciplinary management of patients as needed and in a timely fashion

ADDITIONAL THERAPIES

- Chemoradiation (without surgery) is the first-line therapy for tumors stage IIB and higher (gross lesions with obvious parametrial involvement) and for most bulky stage IB2 tumors (6)[A].
- Combination of external beam pelvic radiation and brachytherapy is usually employed.
- If para-aortic lymph node metastases are suspected, extended-field radiation or lymph node dissection prior to radiation therapy may be performed.

SURGERY/OTHER PROCEDURES

- Surgical management is an option for patients with early-stage tumors.
- Removal of precursor lesions (cervical intraepithelial neoplasia [CIN]) by loop electrosurgical excision procedure (LEEP), cold knife conization, laser ablation, or cryotherapy
- Stage IA1 (lesions with <3-mm invasion from basement membrane) without lymphovascular space invasion: option of conization or simple extrafascial hysterectomy (6)[A]
- Stage IA2 (lesions with >3-mm but <5-mm invasion from basement membrane): option of radical hysterectomy with lymph node dissection or radiation, depending on clinical setting (6)[A]
- Stages IA2–IB1: Fertility-sparing radical trachelectomy may be considered in selected patients (6)[A].
- Stages IB1–IIA (gross lesions without obvious parametrial involvement): option of radical hysterectomy with lymph node sampling or primary chemoradiation with brachytherapy and teletherapy, depending on clinical setting (6)[A]
- Stage IVA (lesions limited to central metastasis to the bladder and/or rectum): Primary pelvic exenteration may be feasible (6)[A].
- Stage IVB disease is treated with goal of palliation. Early referral to palliative care should be made (6)[A],(7)[C].

Pregnancy Considerations

- Management is guided by consideration of stage of lesion, gestational age, and maternal assessment of risks and benefits from treatment.
- Abnormal cytology is best followed up by colposcopy with directed biopsies.
- CIN1 or less: postpartum follow-up
- CIN2–3: management per established guidelines
- Microinvasive carcinoma: conization or trachelectomy. If depth of invasion ≤3 mm, follow up at the 6-week postpartum visit
- Invasive carcinoma: definitive therapy, with timing determined by maternal preference, stage of disease, and gestational age

INPATIENT CONSIDERATIONS

Admission Criteria/Initial Stabilization

- Signs of active bleeding
- Urinary symptoms
- Dehydration
- Complications from surgery, chemotherapy, or radiation
- Active vaginal bleeding can be controlled with timely vaginal packing and radiation therapy.
- Recognition of ureteral blockage, hydronephrosis, urosepsis, and timely intervention

Discharge Criteria

Discharge criteria based on multidisciplinary assessment

ONGOING CARE

FOLLOW-UP RECOMMENDATIONS

Patient Monitoring

- With completion of definitive therapy and based on individual risk factors, patients are evaluated with physical/pelvic examinations:
  - Every 3–6 months for 2 years
  - Every 6–12 months until the 5th year
  - Yearly thereafter (8)[C]
- Pap smears may be performed yearly but have a low sensitivity for detecting recurrence (8)[C].
- CT and PET scan are useful in locating metastases when recurrence is suspected (8)[C].
- Signs of recurrence include vaginal bleeding, unexplained weight loss, leg edema, and pelvic or thigh pain.

PATIENT EDUCATION

Patient education material available through the ACOG at http://www.acog.org, the Society of Gynecologic Oncology at http://www.sgo.org, the Foundation for Women's Cancer at http://www.foundationforwomenscancer.org, the American Cancer Society at http://www.cancer.org, and the National Cancer Institute at http://www.cancer.gov.

PROGNOSIS

Stage	5-yr Survival (%)
1	76–98
2	66–73
3	40–42
4	9–22

COMPLICATIONS

- Loss of ovarian function from radiotherapy or indication for bilateral oophorectomy
- Hemorrhage
- Pelvic infection
- Genitourinary fistula
- Bladder dysfunction
- Sexual dysfunction
- Ureteral obstruction with renal failure
- Bowel obstruction
- Pulmonary embolism
- Lower extremity lymphedema

REFERENCES

1. Committee on Practice Bulletins—Gynecology. ACOG Practice Bulletin Number 131: screening for cervical cancer. *Obstet Gynecol*. 2012;120(5):1222–1238.
2. International Federation of Obstetrics and Gynecology. Global guidance for cervical cancer prevention and control. http://www.rho.org/files/FIGO_cervical_cancer_guidelines_2009.pdf. Accessed 2014.
3. Chemoradiotherapy for Cervical Cancer Meta-analysis Collaboration (CCCMAC). Reducing uncertainties about the effects of chemoradiotherapy for cervical cancer: individual patient data meta-analysis. *Cochrane Database Syst Rev*. 2010;(1):CD008285.
4. Rydzewska L, Tierney J, Vale CL, et al. Neoadjuvant chemotherapy plus surgery versus surgery for cervical cancer. *Cochrane Database Syst Rev*. 2012;(12):CD007406.
5. Tewari KS, Sill MW, Long HJ III, et al. Improved survival with bevacizumab in advanced cervical cancer. *N Engl J Med*. 2014;370(8):734–743.
6. National Comprehensive Cancer Network. NCCN Clinical Practice Guidelines in Oncology: cervical cancer. http://www.nccn.org/professionals/physician_gls/pdf/cervical.pdf. Accessed 2014.
7. Smith TJ, Temin S, Alesi ER, et al. American Society of Clinical Oncology provisional clinical opinion: the integration of palliative care into standard oncology care. *J Clin Oncol*. 2012;30(8):880–887.
8. Salani R, Backes FJ, Fung MF, et al. Posttreatment surveillance and diagnosis of recurrence in women with gynecologic malignancies: Society of Gynecologic Oncologists recommendations. *Am J Obstet Gynecol*. 2011;204:466–478.

ADDITIONAL READING

- American Society for Colposcopy and Cervical Pathology (ASCCP). Algorithms: updated consensus guidelines for managing abnormal cervical cancer screening tests and cancer precursors. http://www.asccp.org/Portals/9/docs/Algorithms%207.30.13.pdf. Accessed 2014.
- Martin-Hirsch PP, Paraskevaidis E, Bryant A, et al. Surgery for cervical intraepithelial neoplasia. *Cochrane Database Syst Rev*. 2013;(12):CD001318.
- Scarinci IC, Garcia FA, Kobetz E, et al. Cervical cancer prevention: new tools and old barriers. *Cancer*. 2010;116(11):2531–2542.

SEE ALSO

Abnormal Pap and Cervical Dysplasia

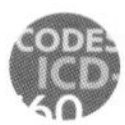

CODES

ICD10

- C53.9 Malignant neoplasm of cervix uteri, unspecified
- C53.0 Malignant neoplasm of endocervix
- C53.1 Malignant neoplasm of exocervix

CLINICAL PEARLS

- Worldwide, cervical cancer is the 3rd most common malignancy among women. Improving access to screening is likely to have the greatest impact in reduction of burden of disease.
- Women with cervical cancer may be asymptomatic and have a normal physical exam.
- Surgical management is an option for patients with early-stage tumors.
- Chemoradiation is the first-line therapy for higher stage tumors.

CERVICITIS, ECTROPION, AND TRUE EROSION

Ileana Bembenek, MD • Chris Wheelock, MD

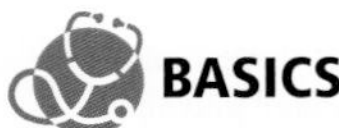

BASICS

DESCRIPTION

Cervicitis represents any acute or chronic cervical inflammatory changes; etiology may be infectious or noninfectious.

- Ectropion is the eversion of the endocervix, exposing the columnar cells to the vaginal environment. More common in adolescents and pregnancy and often confused for cervicitis.
- True erosion occurs with the loss of overlying cervical epithelium due to trauma (e.g., forceful insertion of vaginal speculum in patient with atrophic mucosa).
- System(s) affected: reproductive

Geriatric Considerations

- Chronic cervicitis in postmenopausal women may be related to low levels of estrogen.
- Infectious cervicitis should not be overlooked in geriatric patients because many remain sexually active.

Pregnancy Considerations

All pregnant women should be screened for infectious cervicitis by *screening for chlamydia and gonorrhea* to protect the health of mothers and infants (1).

Pediatric Considerations

Infectious cervicitis in children should lead to an investigation of possible sexual abuse.

EPIDEMIOLOGY

Incidence

- Cervicitis: most commonly due to infectious etiologies, including, but not limited to the following:
  - Chlamydia: 1,422.976 cases were reported to the CDC in 2012, 69% of reported cases occurring among 15–24-year-olds (1).
  - Gonorrhea: second most commonly reported notifiable disease after chlamydia in the United States; 334,826 cases reported to the CDC in 2012 and a 4.1% increase since 2011 (1)
  - Other infectious etiology: HSV and *Trichomonas*; however not routinely reported to CDC. Per CDC (2), trend data for *Trichomonas* are limited to estimates of initial physician office visits from the National Disease and Therapeutic Index (NDTI), which showed 219,000 initial visits in 2012, up from the 168,000 visits in 2011 (2).
  - *Mycoplasma genitalium:* increasingly recognized as a common sexually transmitted pathogen among high-risk, sexually active women (3)
- Ectropion: typically related to higher levels of estrogen; ectropion is common among adolescents, women using oral contraceptive pills OCPs, and pregnant women.
- True erosion: can be seen in women who have undergone cervical trauma

ETIOLOGY AND PATHOPHYSIOLOGY

- Cervicitis: Often, no specific etiology is identified.
  - Infectious: *Chlamydia trachomatis, Neisseria gonorrhoeae,* most commonly identified—affect the columnar epithelium of the endocervix; *Trichomonas vaginalis* and herpes simplex virus (HSV; especially primary infections of HSV-2) affect the squamous epithelium; mycoplasmas (e.g., *M. genitalium*) are becoming increasingly recognized as causative organism.
  - Noninfectious: physical or chemical irritation (e.g., douching, latex exposure, contraceptive creams, or vaginal foreign bodies such as tampons, cervical caps), radiation therapy, inflammatory diseases, malignancy
- Ectropion
  - Hormonal changes with puberty, oral contraceptive use, or pregnancy
  - Resulting from cervical laceration during childbirth
- True erosion: injury to atrophic epithelium; estrogen-deficient states such as menopause

RISK FACTORS

- Infectious cervicitis (4)
  - Multiple sexual partners
  - New sexual partner
  - Younger than 25 years old (adolescence and young adulthood)
  - Unprotected sex or sporadic use of condoms
  - History of sexually transmitted infection (STI)
  - Smoking
  - Other reproductive tract infections: vaginitis, pelvic inflammatory disease (PID)
- Noninfectious cervicitis
  - Foreign objects: pessary, diaphragm, cervical cap, etc.
- Ectropion: adolescence, pregnancy, use of OCP
- True erosion: estrogen deficiency, trauma from foreign body

GENERAL PREVENTION

- STIs (chlamydia, gonorrhea, trichomoniasis)

Follow CDC-recommended screening measures (5)[A]:

- Annual screening for *C. trachomatis* infection of all sexually active nonpregnant young women ≤25 years and all older nonpregnant women at increased risk. Screen all pregnant women (1) and repeat test in 3–6 months (5).
- Annual screening for *N. gonorrhoeae* among all at-risk sexually active women (new or multiple partners, from communities with high prevalence). Screen among pregnant women at risk early in pregnancy and repeat in 3–6 months (6).
- At least annual screening of trichomoniasis among HIV-positive women
- Treat sexual partners of infected women.
- Advise use of condoms and safer sexual practices.

- Estrogen deficiency: estrogen replacement therapy

DIAGNOSIS

HISTORY

- May be asymptomatic (6,7); vaginal discharge
- Dyspareunia
- Lower abdominal pain/pelvic pain
- Postcoital or intermenstrual bleeding/spotting (7)

PHYSICAL EXAM

- Cervicitis: most evident is mucopurulent/purulent discharge from cervix and cervical friability (6,7)
- Other symptoms: erythema, ulceration (HSV), punctate hemorrhage ("strawberry" cervix appearance in trichomoniasis). Consider coexistence with PID with cervical motion tenderness on bimanual exam (6).
- Ectropion: Cervix appears red due to the color of the columnar epithelium.
- True erosion: vaginal bleeding, sharply defined ulcers of cervix

DIFFERENTIAL DIAGNOSIS

- Cervical dysplasia
- Carcinoma of the cervix
- Bacterial vaginosis (discharge is noninflammatory)

DIAGNOSTIC TESTS & INTERPRETATION

- Nucleic acid amplification tests (NAATs) is the recommended test by CDC for *C. trachomatis/ N. gonorrhoeae* detection (8)[A].

- Vaginal swab is the optimal specimen; endocervical specimen may be used if speculum exam performed.
- First-catch urine may detect 10% fewer infections than vaginal or endocervical swabs.
- NAAT is also the most sensitive test for *M. genitalium*, although testing for this is not widely available. Cultures may be used when evaluating a potential *N. gonorrhoeae* treatment failure (8).
- Vaginal wet mount for *T. vaginalis*
  - Culture, antigen assays, and nucleic acid amplification tests should be considered in cases where microscopy is unavailable or inconclusive. Sensitivity for microscopy is low (~50%).
  - Pap smears should not be used to diagnose trichomoniasis.
- If ulcerations are present, culture for HSV.

Diagnostic Procedures/Other

Colposcopy may be helpful in cases of chronic inflammation, with biopsy of suspicious areas.

Test Interpretation

- Cervicitis: acute and chronic inflammatory changes, presence of infective organisms
- Ectropion: none/squamous metaplasia
- True erosion: sharply defined ulcer borders, loss of epithelium

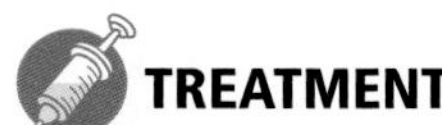

TREATMENT

MEDICATION

First Line

- If infectious cervicitis suspected, treat without awaiting culture results: ceftriaxone 250 mg single dose IM, followed by either azithromycin 1 g single dose or doxycycline 100 mg PO BID × 7 days. Option of ceftriaxone and azithromycin removes patient-compliance factor because they are 1-time doses.
- Chlamydia: for nonpregnant women, azithromycin 1 g PO single dose or doxycycline 100 mg BID PO × 7 days; for pregnant women, azithromycin 1 g single dose or erythromycin base 500 mg QID PO × 7 days or erythromycin ethylsuccinate 800 mg QID × 7 days
- Gonorrhea: Due to increased resistance to antibiotics, the CDC currently recommends ceftriaxone 250 mg single dose IM, followed by either azithromycin 1 g PO single dose or doxycycline 100 mg PO BID × 7 days regardless of the chlamydial coinfection status.

- Trichomoniasis: metronidazole 2 g PO single dose or 500 mg PO BID × 7 days. A single oral dose of 2 g of tinidazole is also effective (6)[A].

- *M. genitalium*: azithromycin 1 g PO as a single dose or 500 mg PO once followed by 250 mg PO daily × 4 days
- Ectropion: none, unless patient is extremely symptomatic with copious discharge. In that case, acid-buffered vaginal jelly can be used to decrease discharge. Cautery can be used but generally is considered overly invasive.

- True erosion: conjugated estrogen cream applied vaginally daily for 1–2 weeks, followed by maintenance dosing twice weekly or oral hormone replacement therapy (HRT)
- Contraindications:
  - Metronidazole: Older references state that metronidazole is relatively contraindicated during 1st trimester of pregnancy. More recent meta-analyses suggest absence of teratogenicity.
  - Doxycycline: pregnancy or lactation
  - Estrogen: See extended list of contraindications to estrogen use in standard texts.
- Precautions:
  - Metronidazole and tinidazole: Avoid alcohol and breastfeeding during treatment and 24 hours after completion of treatment with metronidazole and 72 hours after completion of treatment with tinidazole (6)[A].
  - Doxycycline: possible fetal harm if used during pregnancy; staining of the infant's teeth if used during breastfeeding; allergy; photosensitization
  - Erythromycin: nausea or vomiting
  - Estrogens: history of estrogen-dependent neoplasms; history of thromboembolic diseases. See extended list of contraindications to estrogen therapy in standard texts.
- Significant possible interactions:
  - Metronidazole: ethanol
  - Doxycycline: dairy products, iron preparations, warfarin, and oral contraceptives (advise use of alternative contraceptive method)
  - Erythromycin: theophylline (elevated theophylline level)
  - Estrogen: N/A

Pregnancy Considerations
Doxycycline should be avoided in pregnancy.

Second Line
- Chlamydia
  - Levofloxacin 500 mg PO daily × 7 days
  - Ofloxacin 300 mg PO BID × 7 days 6[A]
- Gonorrhea: If an injectable cephalosporin is not an option, oral cephalosporin therapy with azithromycin or doxycycline can be considered as 2nd-line therapy:
  - Cefixime: 400 mg PO single dose is an acceptable alternative to ceftriaxone, (however, necessitates that the patient return in 1 week for a test of cure) plus azithromycin 1 g single dose or doxycycline 100 mg PO BID × 7 days (9)[A].
  - In the case of a true penicillin allergy, alternative regimens include the following:
    - Azithromycin: 2 g PO as a single dose; however, due to evidence of increasing resistance to macrolides, use should be limited. Return 1 week after treatment for a test of cure at the infected anatomic site.
    - CDC no longer recommends fluoroquinolones for treatment of gonorrhea, since 2007, due to emergence of fluoroquinolone-resistant *N. gonorrhoeae* in United States (9)[A].
    - *M. genitalium*: moxifloxacin 400 mg PO daily × 7–10 days (10)[C] in patients with persistent *M. Genitalium* despite azithromycin treatment, although studies are limited
- Estrogen deficiency: A number of estrogen vaginal preparations are available commercially.

Pregnancy Considerations
Quinolones are also contraindicated in pregnancy.

SURGERY/OTHER PROCEDURES
- Chronic cervicitis with negative cultures that does not respond to empirical medical treatment may be treated with cryosurgery, electrocautery, or loop excision.
- Adverse effects of cautery or cryosurgery can include cervical stenosis, which may affect fertility.

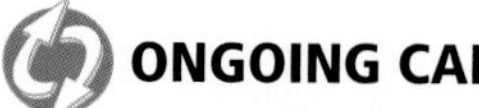

ONGOING CARE

FOLLOW-UP RECOMMENDATIONS

Patient Monitoring
- Test of cure for *C. trachomatis* is recommended in pregnant patients to document eradication of infection; perform at least 3 weeks following treatment.
- Reinfection with gonorrhea and chlamydia is common; repeat screening should be performed routinely for all patients 3–4 months following treatment (6)[A].
- Estrogen deficiency: Reexamine in 1 month to confirm healing.

ALERT

For *C. trachomatis*, the test of cure with nucleic acid amplification tests should not be done <3 weeks after treatment because of false-positive results due to dead organisms. For gonorrhea, however, the test of cure should be done at the infected anatomic site 1 week after treatment. The test of cure ideally should be performed with NAAT or culture.

PATIENT EDUCATION
If the etiology of cervicitis is a confirmed STI, the patient's sex partners within the preceding 60 days must be evaluated for *N. gonorrhoeae* or *C. trachomatis* and treated accordingly. Patient should abstain from sexual intercourse for 7 days after a single-dose regimen or after completion of a 7-day regimen to avoid reinfection.

PROGNOSIS
- Cervicitis: excellent after bacterial infection is eradicated
- Ectropion: spontaneous regression postpartum and with cessation of use of oral contraceptives
- True erosion: spontaneous healing

COMPLICATIONS
- Cervicitis due to *C. trachomatis* or *N. gonorrhoeae* carries an 8–10% risk of developing subsequent PID. Adolescents should be screened at least once yearly because they are a high-risk group for reinfection with sexually transmitted organisms.
- *M. genitalium* may be associated with PID.
- Women positive for HIV with cervicitis have an increased risk of viral shedding and transmission to sexual partners.

REFERENCES

1. Centers for Disease Control and Prevention. Reported STDs in the United States: 2012 national data for chlamydia, gonorrhea and syphilis; CDC fact sheet. http://www.cdc.gov/nchhstp/newsroom/docs/STD-Trends-508.pdf. Accessed 2014.
2. Centers for Disease Control and Prevention. 2012 sexually transmitted diseases surveillance: Table 45. Selected STDs and complications—initial visits to physicians' offices, National Disease and Therapeutic Index, United States, 1966-2012. http://www.cdc.gov/std/stats12/tables/45.htm. Accessed 2014.
3. Manhart LE, Mycoplasma genitalium: an emergent sexually transmitted disease? *Infect Dis Clin North Am*. 2013;27(4):779–792.
4. Centers for Disease Control and Prevention. 2011 sexually transmitted diseases surveillance. http://www.cdc.gov/std/stats11/toc.htm. Accessed April 4, 2014.
5. Centers for Disease Control and Prevention; National Center for HIV/AIDS, Viral Hepatitis, STD, and TB Prevention (United States). Incidence, prevalence, and cost of sexually transmitted infections in the United States. http://www.cdc.gov/std/stats/sti-estimates-fact-sheet-feb-2013.pdf. Accessed 2014.
6. Workowski Ka, Berman S; Centers For Disease Control and Prevention. Sexually transmitted disease guidelines, 2010. *MMWR Recomm Rep*. 2010;59(RR-12):1–110.
7. Workowski K. In the clinic. Chlamydia and gonorrhea. *Ann Intern Med*. 2013;158(3):ITC2-1.
8. Centers for Disease Control and Prevention. Recommendations for the laboratory-based detection of *Chlamydia trachomatis* and *Neisseria gonorrhoeae*—2014. *MMWR Recomm Rep*. 2014:63(RR-02):1–19.
9. Centers For Disease Control and Prevention. Update to CDC's sexually transmitted diseases treatment guidelines, 2010: oral cephalosporins no longer a recommended treatment for gonococcal infections. *MMWR Morb Mortal Wkly Rep*. 2012;61(31):590–594.
10. Manhart LE, Broad JM, Golden MR. *Mycoplasma genitalium*: should we treat and how? *Clin Infect Dis*. 2011;53(Suppl 3):S129–142.

ADDITIONAL READING

- Cazanave C, Manhart LE, Bébéar C. *Mycoplasma genitalium*, an emerging sexually transmitted pathogen. *Med Mal Infect*. 2012;42(9):381–392.
- Cook RL, Hutchison SL, Østergaard L, et al. Systematic review: noninvasive testing for *Chlamydia trachomatis* and *Neisseria gonorrhoeae*. *Ann Intern Med*. 2005;142(11):914–925.
- Gülmezoglu AM, Azhar M. Interventions for trichomoniasis in pregnancy. *Cochrane Database Syst Rev*. 2011;(5):CD000220.
- Haggerty CL, Taylor BD. *Mycoplasma genitalium*: an emerging cause of pelvic inflammatory disease. *Infect Dis Obstet Gynecol*. 2011;2011:959816.
- Johnson LF, Lewis DA. The effect of genital tract infections on HIV-1 shedding in the genital tract: a systematic review and meta-analysis. *Sex Transm Dis*. 2008;35(11):946–959.
- Sutton M, Sternberg M, Koumans EH, et al. The prevalence of *Trichomonas vaginalis* infection among reproductive-age women in the United States, 2001–2004. *Clin Infect Dis*. 2007;45(10):1319–1326.
- U.S. Preventive Services Task Force. Screening for chlamydial infection: U.S. Preventive Services Task Force recommendation statement. *Ann Intern Med*. 2007;147(2):128–134.
- Wilson JF. In the clinic. Vaginitis and cervicitis. *Ann Intern Med*. 2009;151:ITC3-1–ITC3-15; quiz ITC3-16.

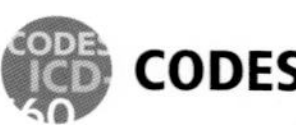

CODES

ICD10
- N72 Inflammatory disease of cervix uteri
- N86 Erosion and ectropion of cervix uteri

CLINICAL PEARLS
- If infectious cervicitis is suspected, treatment of choice is ceftriaxone 250 mg IM plus azithromycin 1 g PO × 1 dose. Do not wait for test results.
- Sexual partner(s) need to be treated.
- Positive results for *N. gonorrhoeae* or chlamydia should be reported to local or state health department.

CHANCROID

Jeffery T. Kirchner, DO, FAAFP, AAHIVS

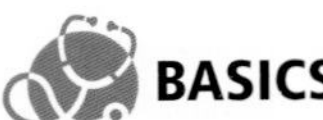

BASICS

DESCRIPTION

- A sexually transmitted infection characterized by painful genital ulcerations and inflammatory inguinal adenopathy
- Uncommon in the United States, present worldwide
- Chancroid is endemic in developing countries, especially sub-Saharan Africa, and is a cofactor for HIV transmission.
- Synonyms: soft chancre; ulcus molle

EPIDEMIOLOGY

Incidence

- <50 cases reported to CDC in 2004–2012 (1)
- Actual numbers are considered higher due to lack of testing and underreporting.

Prevalence

- Endemic in developing countries; annual estimated global prevalence of 4–6 million; actual prevalence is unknown due to lack of testing.
- More common in
  - Sub-Saharan Africa
  - Southeast Asia
  - Latin America

ETIOLOGY AND PATHOPHYSIOLOGY

- *Haemophilus ducreyi* enters through abraded skin during sexual activity and attaches to susceptible cells.
- Cytotoxin is secreted, which may play a role in epithelial injury and ulcer formation.
- The bacterium contains a fimbria-like protein (flp) operon that encodes proteins that contribute to adherence and pathogenesis.
- Dendritic cells and natural killer cells respond to *H. ducreyi*, and this innate host response determines bacterial clearance versus disease progression.

H. ducreyi (gram-negative rod) thought to be strictly a human pathogen. Following exposure, a local tissue reaction generates an erythematous papule that progresses to a pustule in 4–7 days. Central ulceration and necrosis follow, leading to the clinical chancre.

RISK FACTORS

- Multiple sexual partners
- Uncircumcised men
- Other genital ulcerative diseases (syphilis, herpes simplex)
- HIV

GENERAL PREVENTION

Condom use should be demonstrated and promoted.

COMMONLY ASSOCIATED CONDITIONS

- Syphilis: concurrent in 10% of patients
- Herpes simplex virus (HSV) or HIV infection

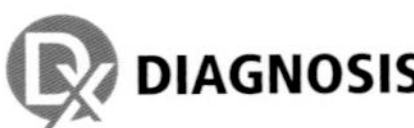

DIAGNOSIS

HISTORY

- Exposure to infected individual
- Local manifestations (lack of systemic symptoms); dysuria, chancre (painful); inguinal lymph node swelling
- Women can be asymptomatic carriers, making diagnosis more challenging.

PHYSICAL EXAM

- Tender erythematous genital papule that progresses into a pustule that erodes into an ulcer:
  - Infected persons commonly have 1–3 ulcers.
- Typical ulcer is 1–2 cm, but size is variable.
- Ulcers are painful, with erythematous base and ragged edges, which are sometimes undermined:
  - Common sites for ulcers in men include the penile shaft, glans, and meatus.
  - Common sites for ulcers in women include labia, introitus, and perianal areas.
- Inguinal lymphadenitis with abscess (bubo) formation occurs in ~50% of men. Less common in women
- Buboes arise 1–2 weeks after ulceration and are typically painful.
- Buboes may spontaneously rupture if the primary disease is untreated.
- Atypical presentations include folliculitis and foreskin abscess.

DIFFERENTIAL DIAGNOSIS

- Syphilis (*Treponema pallidum*)
- Genital herpes (HSV-1 and -2)
- Lymphogranuloma venereum (*Chlamydia trachomatis*)
- Granuloma inguinale (*Klebsiella granulomatis*)
- Drug eruption; Behçet disease

DIAGNOSTIC TESTS & INTERPRETATION

CDC criteria for presumptive diagnosis

- Definite: Isolation of *H. ducreyi* from a lesion
- Probable: clinical findings, including one or more painful genital ulcers and regional adenopathy, *plus* negative dark field exam, negative serologic test for syphilis, negative cultures for HSV, or a clinical presentation not typical for HSV (2)

Initial Tests (lab, imaging)

- "School of fish" pattern on Gram stain, with organisms clumped in long parallel strands
- Serologic testing for antibody to *H. ducreyi* with ELISA (although may not be diagnostic of acute infection) (3)
- Culture of the organism on Mueller-Hinton agar with incorporated vancomycin, but sensitivity is <80%.
- Multiplex polymerase chain reaction (PCR) has sensitivity of 95–98% but no FDA-approved tests in the United States; available from some commercial labs

Follow-Up Tests & Special Considerations

- All patients should be tested for syphilis and HIV.
- Test of cure is not recommended.

Diagnostic Procedures/Other

Gram stain and culture of exudate

- Aspiration of inguinal bubo (lymph node); can also obtain culture material from base of cleansed ulcer
- PCR testing of ulcer exudate for *H. ducreyi* DNA
- Dark-field examination of exudate to rule out *T. pallidum* infection
- Culture or PCR testing for HSV

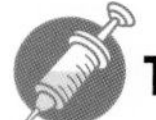

TREATMENT

GENERAL MEASURES

- Outpatient treatment
- Saline or Burrow solution to soak ulcers
- Aspiration of buboes if >5 cm; approached through adjacent skin. Also consider incision and drainage for larger lesions.

ALERT

HIV may affect treatment response.

MEDICATION

First Line

- Azithromycin: 1 g PO single dose, *or*
- Ceftriaxone 250 mg IM single dose (4,5)[A]

Second Line

- Ciprofloxacin 500 mg PO BID for 3 days
- Erythromycin base 500 mg QID for 7 days
- Contraindications
  - Allergy to the medication
  - Ciprofloxacin during pregnancy and lactation and in patients <18 years

ONGOING CARE

FOLLOW-UP RECOMMENDATIONS

Patient Monitoring

- Avoid sexual activity until ulcers are resolved.
- Clinical improvement usually occurs within 48 hours.
- Patients should be reexamined 3–7 days after initiation of therapy and followed closely until all clinical signs of infection are resolved.
- Baseline HIV and syphilis serology, repeat 3–6 months post treatment.

PATIENT EDUCATION

- Counseling on safe sexual practices and condom use
- Local wound care
- Treat sexual partners
- HIV and syphilis testing

PROGNOSIS

- Full clinical resolution with appropriate treatment
- Failure to respond may be due to
  - Incorrect diagnosis
  - Coinfection with syphilis
  - Coinfection with HIV
  - Medication nonadherence
  - Resistant *H. ducreyi*
- 5% relapse after treatment

COMPLICATIONS

- Phimosis
- Balanoposthitis
- Rupture of buboes with fistula formation and scarring

REFERENCES

1. Adams DA, Jajosky RA, Ajani U, et al; Centers for Disease Control and Prevention. Summary of notifiable diseases—United States, 2012. *MMWR Morb Mortal Wkly Rep*. 2014;61(53):1–121.
2. Lewis DA, Ison CA. Chancroid. *Sex Transm Infect*. 2006;82(Suppl 4):iv19–iv20.
3. Alfa M. The laboratory diagnosis of *Haemophilus ducreyi*. *Can J Infect Dis Med Microbiol*. 2005;16(1):31–34.
4. Centers for Disease Control and Prevention. Sexually transmitted diseases treatment guidelines—2010. *MMWR Morb Mortal Wkly Rep*. 2010;59(19):19–20.
5. Kemp M, Christensen JJ, Lautenschlager S, et al. European guideline for the management of chancroid, 2011. *Int J STD AIDS*. 2011;22(5):241–244.

ADDITIONAL READING

- Cone MM, Whitlow CB. Sexually transmitted and anorectal infectious diseases. *Gastroenterol Clin North Am*. 2013;42(4):877–892.
- Janowicz DM, Li W, Bauer ME. Host-pathogen interplay of *Haemophilus ducreyi*. *Curr Opin Infect Dis*. 2010;23(1):64–69.
- Janowicz DM, Ofner S, Katz BP, et al. Experimental infection of human volunteers with *Haemophilus ducreyi*: fifteen years of clinical data and experience. *J Infect Dis*. 2009;199(11):1671–1679.
- Markle W, Conti T, Kad M. Sexually transmitted disease. *Prim Care*. 2013;40(3):557–587.
- Mutua FM, Mimunya JM, Wiysonge CS. Genital ulcer disease treatment for reducing sexual acquisition of HIV. *Cochrane Database Syst Rev*. 2012;8:CD007933.
- Roett MA, Mayor MT, Uduhiri KA. Diagnosis and management of genital ulcers. *Am Fam Physician*. 2012;85(3):254–262.

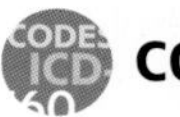

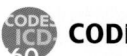

CODES

ICD10

A57 Chancroid

CLINICAL PEARLS

- Chancroid is characterized by genital papules that progress to pustules that open, producing painful ulcers. It is rare in the United States.
- Treatment of choice is a single dose of azithromycin.
- Treat sexual partners (from prior 3 months) even in the absence of signs or symptoms of disease.
- All patients should be tested for syphilis and HIV.

CHICKENPOX (VARICELLA ZOSTER)

Kay A. Bauman, MD, MPH

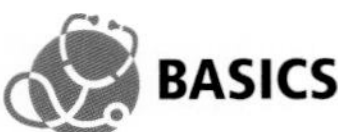

BASICS

DESCRIPTION

- Common, highly contagious generalized exanthem characterized by crops of pruritic vesicles on the skin and mucous membranes caused by exposure to varicella-zoster virus (VZV)
- VZV is spread by respiratory (airborne) droplets and direct contact with vesicles.
- VZV establishes latency in the dorsal root ganglia; reactivation results in zoster (shingles).
- Outbreaks tend to occur late winter to early spring in temperate climates.
- Usual incubation period is 14–16 days (range, 10–21). Patients are infectious from ~48 hours before appearance of vesicles until the final lesions have crusted. Historically, most people acquired chickenpox during childhood and developed lifelong immunity. Varicella is now part of recommended primary vaccination schedule
- System(s) affected: nervous, skin/exocrine
- Synonym(s): varicella

EPIDEMIOLOGY

- Predominant age: peak incidence in preschoolers to 9 years but may occur at any age
- Predominant gender: male = female

Incidence

- Decreasing incidence since vaccination became routine; estimated 3.5 million cases annually prior to vaccine, with an incidence of 8–9% in children age 1–9 years
- Reported U.S. varicella cases : 1991, 147,076; 2011, 14,513; provisionally reported for 2012, 13,447 cases (1–3)
- Prior to vaccine, ~100 deaths/year were reported in the United States; in 2012, 3 reported deaths (2)
- U.S. rates: 1994, prior to vaccine: 135.8/100,000 persons; 2012: 4.3/100,000 persons
- Rates of varicella in the United States dropped after vaccine introduction until mid-2000s when they plateaued; 2nd dose of vaccine was recommended in 2006, and rates have declined again since.
- In developing countries, varicella continues to cause a severe disease burden with complications, hospitalizations, and deaths.

ETIOLOGY AND PATHOPHYSIOLOGY

- Skin lesions identical histologically to those of herpes simplex virus
- In fatal cases, intranuclear inclusions are found in vascular endothelium and most organs.
- VZV is a double-stranded DNA virus of the α-Herpesviridae subfamily.
- Humans are primary disease reservoir.

RISK FACTORS

- No history of varicella infection or prior immunization
- Immunocompromised patients (especially children with leukemia/lymphoma in remission or receiving high-dose corticosteroids)
- Pregnancy

Geriatric Considerations

- Infection more severe in adults than in children
- Reactivation of latent infection causes zoster (shingles).
- Herpes zoster vaccine, a live attenuated vaccine licensed in 2006, is recommended as a single dose for all persons ≥60 years regardless of prior clinical history of shingles or chickenpox (http://www.cdc.gov/vaccines/vpd-vac/shingles/hcp-vaccination.htm).
- Most common cause of death: primary viral pneumonia

Pediatric Considerations

- Neonates born to mothers who develop chickenpox from 5 days before to 2 days after delivery are at risk for serious disease and should receive varicella-zoster immune globulin (VZIG).
- Newborns are at highest risk for severe disease during the 1st month of life, especially if mother is sero-negative.
- Delivery prior to 28 weeks increases risk.
- Varicella bullosa is seen mainly in children younger than 2 years. Lesions appear as bullae instead of vesicles. The clinical course is similar.
- Most common cause of death: septic complications and encephalitis
- Avoid aspirin/acetylsalicylic acid in children because of link to Reye syndrome.

Pregnancy Considerations

- 25% risk of transplacental infection after maternal infection
- Congenital malformations are seen in 2% of patients when the fetus is infected during the 1st or 2nd trimesters, characterized by limb atrophy and scarring of the skin of the extremities and occasional CNS and eye manifestations.
- Morbidity (e.g., pneumonia) is increased in women infected during pregnancy.

GENERAL PREVENTION

- Susceptible (immunologically naive) individuals exposed to varicella are at risk to develop disease and are also potentially infectious for 21 days.
- Isolate hospitalized patients.
- When indicated, passive immunization with IM VZIG should be given within 96 hours (but can be as long as up to 10 days) after exposure (4).
  - VZIG is recommended for people exposed to chickenpox or shingles who are immunocompromised, newborns of mothers with onset of chickenpox <5 days before delivery or <2 days after delivery, premature infants (<28 weeks) exposed in neonatal period either whose mothers are not immune, or babies who weigh <1,000 g regardless of maternal immunity (4).
- Active immunization after exposure has been shown to prevent or reduce the severity of varicella if given within 72 hours postexposure.
- Active immunization: varicella virus vaccine (Varivax): live attenuated vaccine approved by FDA in 1995 for pediatric immunization and recommended by ACIP for immunization of healthy patients ≥12 months who have not had chickenpox
  - 12 months–12 years: initial dose 0.5 mL SC at age 12–15 months; 2nd dose age 4–6 years. Prelicensure studies showed efficacy rates: 70–90% against any disease and 95% against severe disease 7–10 years after vaccination. Other studies showed 100% efficacy at 1 year and 98% at 2 years after vaccination. Moreover, single dose is 85–94% effective in preventing severe disease. The 2-dose regimen is 96–98% effective. Breakthrough disease generally has <50 lesions, shorter duration of illness, and lower incidence of fever (5)[A].
  - ≥13 years: two 0.5 mL SC doses 4–8 weeks apart, seroconversion rates 78–82% after 1 dose, 99% after 2 doses. Adults have efficacy rates in the lower end of this range.
  - 2009 U.S. estimate: 90% 2-dose vaccine coverage for children ages 19–35 months
  - Vaccine side effects are pain and redness at vaccine site. 1 in 10 develop fever. 1 in 25 will develop a mild varicella-like rash up to 1 month after vaccination.
  - Vaccine contraindications (6)
    - Severe allergic reaction (e.g., anaphylaxis) to a previous dose or vaccine component
    - Severe immunodeficiency (e.g., severely immunocompromised HIV patients, on chemotherapy, congenital immunodeficiency, or long-term immunosuppressive therapy)
    - Pregnancy
- MMRV vaccine, which combines the measles, mumps, and rubella vaccine with varicella, is equally effective. There are rare reports of an increased risk of febrile seizures 5–12 days after vaccination in 1/2,300–2,600 patients (7)[A].
- May be considered for a subset of HIV-positive children in CDC class I with CD4 >25%
  - Vaccine recipients who develop a rash should avoid contact with immunocompromised people, pregnant women who have never had chickenpox, and their newborns.
  - Children needing catch-up vaccination need at least 3 months between doses 1 and 2.

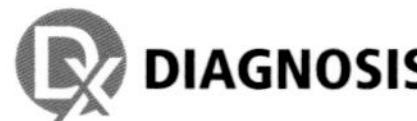

DIAGNOSIS

HISTORY

- Prodromal symptoms: fever, malaise, anorexia, mild headache
- Malaise, muscle aches, arthralgias, and headache more common in adults
- Subclinical in ~4% of cases

PHYSICAL EXAM

- Characteristic rash: crops of vesicles on erythematous bases ("dewdrops on a rose petal")
- Lesions erupt in successive crops.
- Progress from macule to papule to vesicle, then begin to crust
- Pruritic rash is present in various stages of development.
- Lesions may be present on mucous membranes, both oral and vaginal.

DIFFERENTIAL DIAGNOSIS

- Herpes simplex: herpes zoster
- Smallpox
- Impetigo

- Coxsackievirus infection
- Scabies
- Dermatitis herpetiformis
- Drug rash
- Rickettsial pox infection

DIAGNOSTIC TESTS & INTERPRETATION

The diagnosis of chickenpox is based primarily on clinical grounds. Other testing is generally used for complicated cases and epidemiologic studies

Initial Tests (lab, imaging)

- Leukocyte count may be normal, low, or mildly increased.
- Marked leukocytosis suggests secondary infection.
- Multinucleated giant cells visible on Tzanck smear from scrapings of vesicles
- Isolated virus from human tissue culture

Follow-Up Tests & Special Considerations

- Serologies can show response to acute infection (IgM) or prior infection (IgG).
- Visualization of the virus by electron microscopy, tissue culture (costly), and various methods of acute and convalescent sera collection: latex agglutination (most available), enzyme immunoassay, indirect immunofluorescence antibody, fluorescent antibody to membrane assay, or polymerase chain reaction (PCR) assay, which can detect wild from vaccine viral strains
- Vaccine-modified cases can be more difficult to diagnose; consider PCR testing of skin lesions (8)[B].

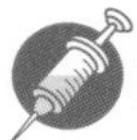

TREATMENT

Outpatient, except for complicating emergencies

GENERAL MEASURES

- Supportive/symptomatic treatment
- Antihistamines and/or oatmeal baths, as needed, for itch
- Acetaminophen and/or ibuprofen, as needed for pain and fever
- Nail clipping in children can help prevent scarring or secondary infection from itching.

MEDICATION

First Line

- Supportive: antipyretics for fever; avoid aspirin in children
- Local and/or systemic antipruritic agents for itching
- VZIG available for passive immunization for
- Immunocompromised patients, newborn infants whose mothers have signs and symptoms of varicella around the time of delivery, premature infants born at 28 weeks or more whose mothers do not have evidence of immunity to varicella, and premature infants less than 28 weeks' gestation or who weigh <1,000 g regardless of mothers' evidence of immunity. VZIG should be given within 96 hours after exposure to be most beneficial (9).
- Acyclovir: decreases duration of fever and shortens time of viral shedding; recommended for adolescents, adults, and high-risk patients; most beneficial if initiated early in the disease (≤24 hours)
  - 2–16-year-old patients: 20 mg/kg/dose (max 800 mg/dose) QID for 5 days
  - Adults: 800 mg 5 times daily for 5 days
- Contraindications
  - Hypersensitivity to the drug
- Precautions
  - Possible renal insufficiency with acyclovir
  - Concurrent administration of probenecid increases half-life; increased effects with zidovudine (e.g., drowsiness, lethargy)

Second Line

- Famciclovir: 500 mg TID for 7–10 days (adults)
- Valacyclovir: 1 g TID for 7–10 days (adults)

ONGOING CARE

FOLLOW-UP RECOMMENDATIONS

Patient Monitoring

- Usually none needed in mild cases. If complications occur, intensive supportive care may be required.
- Activity as tolerated. Children may return to school when lesions have scabbed.

DIET

No special diet

PATIENT EDUCATION

- In the healthy child, chickenpox is rarely serious and recovery is complete.
- Native chickenpox typically confers lifelong immunity.
- Second attack rare, but subclinical infection can occur; happens occasionally after vaccination in children
- Infection becomes latent and may recur years later as herpes zoster in adults (and sometimes in children).
- Fatalities rarely occur from complications.

COMPLICATIONS

- Although only 2% of cases are reported after 2nd decade, 35% of deaths occur in this age group.
- Secondary bacterial infection: cellulitis, abscess, erysipelas, sepsis, septic arthritis/osteomyelitis, or staphylococcal pyomyositis
- Pneumonia: 20–30% of adults with chickenpox have lung involvement; 1/400 is hospitalized.
- Encephalitis (the most common CNS complication)
- Meningitis
- Reye syndrome
- Purpura
- Thrombocytopenia
- Glomerulonephritis
- Arthritis
- Hepatitis

REFERENCES

1. Centers for Disease Control and Prevention. MMWR: summary of notifiable diseases. http://www.cdc.gov/mmwr/mmwr_nd/. Accessed 2014.
2. Provisional cases of notifiable diseases. *MMWR*. 2013;62:670.
3. Center for Disease Control and Prevention. *MMWR*. 2013;61:731.
4. Centers for Disease Control and Prevention. FDA approval of an extended period for administering VariZIG for postexposure prophylaxis of varicella. *MMWR Morb Mortal Wkly Rep*. 2012;61(12):212.
5. Marin M, Güris D, Chaves SS, et al. Prevention of varicella: recommendations of the Advisory Committee on Immunization Practices (ACIP). *MMWR Recomm Rep*. 2007;56(RR-4):1–40.
6. National Center for Immunization and Respiratory Diseases. General recommendations on immunization—recommendations of the Advisory Committee on Immunization Practices (ACIP). *MMWR Recomm Rep*. 2011;60(2):1–64.
7. Marin M, Broder KR, Temte JL, et al. Use of combination measles, mumps, rubella, and varicella vaccine: recommendations of the Advisory Committee on Immunization Practices (ACIP). *MMWR Recomm Rep*. 2010;59(RR-3):1–12.
8. Leung J, Harpaz R, Baughman AL, et al. Evaluation of laboratory methods for diagnosis of varicella. *Clin Infect Dis*. 2010;51(1):23–32.
9. Centers for Disease Control and Prevention. Updated recommendations for use of VariZig—United States, 2013. *MMWR Morb Mortal Wkly Rep*. 2013;62(28):574–576

ADDITIONAL READING

- Centers for Disease Control and Prevention. Summary of notifiable diseases, United States—1991. *MMWR Morb Mortal Wkly Rep*. 1992;40(53):1–63.
- Centers for Disease Control and Prevention. Varicella-related deaths—United States, January 2003-June 2004. *MMWR Morb Mortal Wkly Rep*. 2005;54(11):272–274.
- Galea SA, Sweet A, Beninger P, et al. The safety profile of varicella vaccine: a 10-year review. *J Infect Dis*. 2008;197(Suppl 2):S165–S169.

SEE ALSO

Herpes Zoster

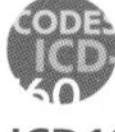

CODES

ICD10

- B01.9 Varicella without complication
- B02.9 Zoster without complications
- P35.8 Other congenital viral diseases

CLINICAL PEARLS

- Infection is more likely to produce serious illness in adults than in children.
- Introduction of the varicella vaccine has reduced morbidity and mortality. Currently, 2 doses of vaccine are recommended.
- Herpes zoster vaccine (Zostavax) is recommended for persons ≥60 years of age to prevent shingles (zoster).

CHILD ABUSE

Karen Hulbert, MD

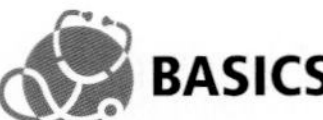

BASICS

DESCRIPTION
- Types of abuse: neglect (most common and highest mortality), physical abuse, emotional/psychological abuse, sexual abuse
- System(s) affected: gastrointestinal (GI), endocrine/metabolic, musculoskeletal, nervous, renal, reproductive, skin/exocrine, psychiatric
- Synonym(s): suspected nonaccidental trauma; child maltreatment; child neglect

EPIDEMIOLOGY

Incidence
- The National Incidence Study (NIS) estimates the incidence of neglect in the United States using estimates from child protective services (CPS) statistics and other sources. Most recent *NIS-4* (published 2010) looked at data from 2004 to 2009.
- Using the stringent "harm standard" definition, >1.25 million children experience maltreatment (1 in 58).
- Using the "endangerment standard," 3 million children experienced maltreatment (1 child in 25) (1).

Prevalence
- In 2012, a nationally estimated 3.2 million children received either an investigation or alternative CPS response (2).
- There was a nationally estimated 686,000 victims of abuse and neglect, resulting in a rate of 9.2 victims per 1,000 children in the population.
- More than one quarter of victims were younger than 3 years. 20% were in the age group 3–5 years.
- The greatest percentage of children were neglected (78.3%) compared to 18.3% suffering physical abuse and 9.3% suffering sexual abuse.
- Professionals submitted three-fifths of reports.

RISK FACTORS
- All ages; male = female:
  - Risk of physical abuse increases with age.
  - Risk of fatal abuse more common in those <2 years
  - Physical abuse 2.1× higher among children with disabilities (2)
- Poverty, drug abuse, lower educational status, parental history of abuse, mentally ill parent/maternal depression, poor support network, and domestic violence:
  - Child abuse 4.9× more likely in family with spouse abuse (3)
  - Children in households with unrelated adults, 50× more likely to die of inflicted injuries (3)
  - Adults who were abused as children are at higher risk of becoming abusers than those not abused.

GENERAL PREVENTION
- Know your patients and document their family situations; have increased suspicion to screen for risk factors at prenatal, postnatal, and pediatric visits.
- Physicians can educate parents on range of normal behaviors to expect in infants and children:
  - Anticipatory guidance on ways to handle crying infants; methods of discipline for toddlers
- Train first responders—teachers, childcare workers—to look for signs of abuse.
- Some studies suggest developing screening tools to identify high-risk families early and offer interventions such as early childhood home visitation programs.

COMMONLY ASSOCIATED CONDITIONS
- Failure to thrive
- Prematurity
- Developmental deficits
- Poor school performance
- Poor social skills
- Low self-esteem, depression

DIAGNOSIS

- Relatively minor injuries, frenulum tears, or bruising in precruising infants, may be the first indication of child physical abuse; these minor, suspicious injuries have been termed "sentinel injuries" (4)[B].
- In a retrospective study of infants who were definitely abused, 27.5% had a sentinel injury (80% had a bruise), and in 41.9% of those cases, the parent reported that a medical provider was aware of the injury (4)[B].

- Documentation:
  - The medical record is an important piece of evidence for investigation and litigation (5)[C].
  - Critical elements include the following (5)[C]:
    - Brief statement of child's disclosure or caregiver's explanation, including any alternate explanations offered
    - Time the incident occurred and date/time of disclosure
    - Whether witnesses were present
    - Developmental abilities of child
    - Objective medical findings
    - Interpretation of the findings
- DO NOT use terms such as "rule out," "R/O," and "alleged." They may cause ambiguity; clearly state physician opinion (5)[C].
- Documentation should include disposition of patient, and record any report made to CPS (5)[C].

HISTORY
- History of a sentinel injury should prompt consideration of abuse; it may be the first and only abusive injury; there may be escalating and repeated violence instead of a single event of momentary loss of control (4)[B].

- Use nonjudgmental, open-ended questions (ask: who, what, when, and where; NEVER why).
- Use quotes whenever possible.
- Document past medical and developmental history, child's temperament, and interactions among family members.
- Suggestive of intentional trauma:
  - No explanation or vague explanation (3)[C]
  - Important detail of explanation changes dramatically (3)[C].
  - Explanation is inconsistent with pattern, age, or severity (3)[C].
  - Explanation is inconsistent with child's physical or developmental abilities (3)[C].
  - Different witnesses provide markedly different history (3)[C].
  - Considerable delay in seeking treatment
- Nonspecific symptoms of abuse:
  - Behavior changes; self-destructive behavior
  - Anxiety and/or depression
  - Sleep disturbances, night terrors
  - School problems

PHYSICAL EXAM
- Explain what the exam will involve and why procedures are needed.
- Examine child in a comfortable setting.
- Allow child to choose who will be in the room.
- Use appropriate positions to examine the anal and genital areas of children.
- General assessment for signs of physical abuse, neglect, and self-injurious behaviors
- Thorough physical exam:
  - Skin, head, eyes, ears, nose, and mouth
  - Chest/abdomen
  - Genital (consider exam under sedation) or refer to emergency department (ED)
  - Extremities, with focus on inner arms and legs
  - Growth data
- Maintain high index of suspicion for occult head, chest, and abdominal trauma.
- Physical abuse:
  - Skin markings (e.g., lacerations, burns, ecchymoses, linear/shaped contusions, bites)
  - Immersion injuries with clearly distinguished outlines (e.g., from boiling water)
  - Oral trauma (e.g., torn frenulum, loose teeth)
  - Ear trauma (e.g., signs of ear pulling)
  - Eye trauma (e.g., hyphema, hemorrhage)
  - Head/abdominal blunt trauma
  - Fractures
- Sexual abuse:
  - Unexplained penile, vaginal, hymenal, perianal, or anal injuries/bleeding/discharge
  - Pregnancy or STIs
  - Sperm is a definitive finding of child abuse.
- Neglect:
  - Child may be low weight for height, unclean, or unkempt.
  - Rashes
  - Fearful or too trusting
  - Clinging to or avoiding caregiver
  - Flat or balding occiput
  - Abnormal development or growth parameters
- Measurements, photographs, and careful descriptions are critical for accurate diagnosis.
- Collaboration with specialist and child abuse assessment team (3)[C]

DIFFERENTIAL DIAGNOSIS
- Physical trauma:
  - Accidental injury; toxic ingestion
  - Bleeding disorders (e.g., classic hemophilia)
  - Metabolic or congenital conditions
  - Conditions with skin manifestations (e.g., Mongolian spots, Henoch-Schönlein purpura, meningococcemia, erythema multiforme, hypersensitivity, car seat burns, staphylococcal scalded skin syndrome, chickenpox, impetigo)
  - Cultural practices (e.g., cupping, coining)
- Neglect:
  - Endocrinopathies (e.g., diabetes mellitus)
  - Constitutional
  - GI (clefts, malabsorption, irritable bowel)
  - Seizure disorder
  - Sudden infant death syndrome (SIDS)
- Skeletal trauma:
  - Obstetrical trauma
  - Nutritional (scurvy, rickets)
  - Infection (congenital syphilis, osteomyelitis)
  - Osteogenesis imperfecta

C

DIAGNOSTIC TESTS & INTERPRETATION

Initial Tests (lab, imaging)

- Directed by history and physical exam:
  - Urinalysis (e.g., abdominal/flank/back/genital trauma), urine DNA probe for STIs
  - Complete blood chemistry. Consideration of coagulation studies and platelet count (e.g., rule out bleeding disorder, abdominal trauma) as appropriate.
  - Electrolytes, creatinine, BUN, glucose
  - Liver and pancreatic function tests (e.g., abdominal trauma)
  - Guaiac stool (abdominal trauma)
- In cases of suspected neglect:
  - Stool exam, calorie count, purified protein derivative and anergy panel, sweat test, lead and zinc levels
- In cases of suspected sexual abuse:
  - STI testing: gonorrhea, chlamydia, *Trichomonas*; also consider HIV, herpes simplex virus (HSV), hepatitis panel, syphilis
  - Serum pregnancy test
- A skeletal survey for abusive fractures, especially if <6 months. Obtain follow-up survey even if initial is negative in cases with significant concern (6)[B].
- In one retrospective analysis, 79% of detected cases of abuse had healing fractures due to victims being abused on >1 occasion (6)[B].
- All children with fractures and children with suspicious injuries <2 years:
  - Skeletal survey: X-rays include two views of each extremity; skull, anteroposterior (AP) and lateral; spine, AP and lateral; chest x-ray; and/or rib (posterior), abdomen, pelvis, hands, and feet.
  - Consider bone scan for acute rib fractures and subtle long bone fractures.
- Intracranial and extracranial injury:
  - CT scan of head
  - Consider MRI of head/neck for better dating of injuries, looking at subtle findings, intercerebral edema, or hemorrhage.
- Intra-abdominal injuries:
  - CT scan of abdomen

Follow-Up Tests & Special Considerations

- Bruising is a common presenting feature:
  - Bruising in babies who are not independently mobile is very uncommon (<1%).
- Patterns suggestive of abuse:
  - Bruises seen away from bony prominences
  - Bruises to face, back, abdomen, arms, buttocks, ears, hands
  - Multiple bruises in clusters or uniform shape
  - Patterned injuries (such as bite marks or the imprint of an object like a belt or cord) should be considered inflicted until proven otherwise.
- Red flags (3)[B]:
  - History that is inconsistent with the injury
  - No explanation offered for the injury or injury blamed on sibling or another child
  - History that is inconsistent with the child's developmental level

Diagnostic Procedures/Surgery

Sexual abuse:

- Consider photocolposcopy.
- <72 hours from time of abuse: Collect samples for the forensic laboratory (contact authorities for appropriate protocol).

Test Interpretation

- Spiral fractures in nonambulatory patients (children who are not walking or cruising should not have bruising or fractures from "falls")
- Chip or bucket-handle fractures
- Epiphyseal/metaphyseal rib fractures in infants
- Rupture of liver/spleen in abdominal blunt trauma
- Retinal hemorrhages in shaken baby syndrome
- Recent literature notes a greater risk of abuse with skull and femur fractures, unexplained injuries, and a delay in seeking care (6)[C].

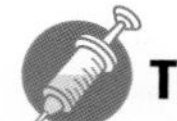

TREATMENT

GENERAL MEASURES

Test for STIs before treatment.

MEDICATION

First Line

Antibiotics as indicated for STIs

Second Line

Consider antidepressants if needed.

ALERT

Emergency contraception reduces rate of pregnancy after sexual assault:

- Levonorgestrel: single dose of 1.5 mg or two 0.75 mg doses taken together or 12 hours apart. Take as soon as possible; effective up to 72 hours (7)[A].
- Ulipristal (Ella) 30 mg single dose as soon as possible; effective up to 120 hours (7)[A]

ISSUES FOR REFERRAL

- Consider managing in ED to collect forensic specimens and maintain chain of evidence.
- Mandatory reporting to child protective authorities

INPATIENT CONSIDERATIONS

Admission Criteria/Initial Stabilization

- Moderate to severe injuries or unstable
- Acute psychological trauma
- If safety of child outside the hospital cannot be guaranteed

Discharge Criteria

- Child should be sent to another relative or into foster care if the suspected abuser lives with the child.
- Counseling for individual and family
- After initial evaluation, consider referral to sexual assault center.

ONGOING CARE

FOLLOW-UP RECOMMENDATIONS

As clinically indicated

Patient Monitoring

- Refer to the state protective services.
- Monitor injury healing over time.
- Follow-up assessment for STIs that may not present acutely (e.g., HPV)

PROGNOSIS

Without intervention, child abuse is often a chronic and escalating phenomenon.

COMPLICATIONS

Growing evidence that sexual, physical, and emotional abuse in childhood are risk factors for poorer adult mental and physical health.

REFERENCES

1. Sedlak AJ, Mettenburg J, Basena M, et al. *Fourth National Incidence Study of Child Abuse and Neglect (NIS-4): Report to Congress, Executive Summary.* Washington, DC: U.S. Department of Health and Human Services, Administration for Children and Families; 2010.
2. U.S. Department of Health and Human Services, Administration for Children and Families, Administration on Children, Youth and Families, Children's Bureau. Child maltreatment 2012. http://www.acf.hhs.gov/sites/default/files/cb/cm2012.pdf. Accessed 2014.
3. Kellogg N; American Academy of Pediatrics Committee on Child Abuse and Neglect. The evaluation of child physical abuse. *Pediatrics.* 2007;119(6):1232–1241.
4. Sheets LK, Leach ME, Koszewski AM, et al. Sentinel injuries in infants evaluated for child physical abuse. *Pediatrics.* 2013;131(4):701–707.
5. Jackson AM, Rucker A, Hinds T, et al. Let the record speak: medicolegal documentation in cases of child maltreatment. *Clin Ped Emerg Med.* 2006;7(3):181–185.
6. Preer G, Sorrentino D, Newton AW. Child abuse pediatrics: prevention, evaluation, and treatment. *Curr Opin Pediatr.* 2012;24(2):266–273.
7. Bosworth M, Olusola P, Low S. An update of emergency contraception. *Am Fam Physician.* 2014;89(7):545–550.

ADDITIONAL READING

- Harris T. Bruises in children: normal or child abuse? *J Pediatr Health Care.* 2010;24(4):216–221.
- van Rijn RR, Sieswerda-Hoogendoorn T. Educational paper: imaging child abuse: the bare bones. *Eur J Pediatr.* 2012:171(2):215–224.

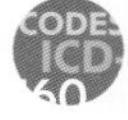

CODES

ICD10

- T74.12XA Child physical abuse, confirmed, initial encounter
- T74.32XA Child psychological abuse, confirmed, initial encounter
- T74.22XA Child sexual abuse, confirmed, initial encounter

CLINICAL PEARLS

- When a bruise is present, it should be considered as potentially sentinel for physical abuse if no plausible explanation is given (4)[B].
- High index of suspicion is important for prevention and recognition of abuse.
- Neglect is the most common and lethal form of abuse and should be aggressively reported.
- Detailed exam with documentation is key.
- Mandated reporting is required for suspected child abuse and neglect; the physician does not have to prove abuse before reporting.
- Child Abuse Hotline by state: http://www.childwelfare.gov/responding/reporting.cfm

CHLAMYDIA INFECTION (SEXUALLY TRANSMITTED)

Casandra Cashman, MD

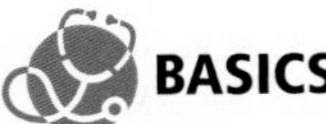

BASICS

DESCRIPTION

- *Chlamydia trachomatis* is an intracellular membrane-bound prokaryotic organism. Chlamydia is from Greek word for "cloak."
- Chlamydia is the most common bacterial sexually transmitted infection (STI) in the United States (1)[A].
- Transmitted through vaginal, anal, or oral sex; transmitted vertically during vaginal delivery
- Majority of cases are asymptomatic, especially in females. Untreated disease can lead to pelvic inflammatory disease (PID), ectopic pregnancy, and infertility.
- System(s) affected: reproductive

Pregnancy Considerations

Perinatal acquisition may result in neonatal pneumonia and/or conjunctivitis.

EPIDEMIOLOGY

Incidence

- Mandatory reporting started in 1985; steady increase in incidence since
- 1.42 million *reported* cases in 2012 increasing incidence reflects broader screening, improved testing, and better reporting (as opposed to a large increase in disease burden).
- Swedish new variant chlamydia (nvCT) first reported in 2006; often produces false-negative tests; largely confined to Nordic countries.

Prevalence

- 458/100,000 people in the United States in 2012
- Populations most affected: young females, particularly those in ethnic minority groups
- Peak incidence: age 18–20 years
- Predominant sex: females > males. Females have >2.5× higher reported incidence and prevalence than males. This likely reflects increased testing in females. Increasing use of urine screening may increase identification in males.
- Infection rates >7× higher in blacks than whites. Rates are higher in larger urban areas.
- Highest male prevalence in heterosexual adolescents
- Estimated to affect ~2% of young sexually active individuals in the United States

ETIOLOGY AND PATHOPHYSIOLOGY

C. trachomatis serotypes D–K associated with genital tract infections. Chlamydia is an obligate intracellular organism. Chlamydia has biphasic life cycle. Extracellularly exists as elementary body (EB) which are metabolically inactive and infectious. Once taken up by host cell (typically columnar epithelium of the genital tract), the EB prevents lysosomal phagocytosis and transforms to reticulate body (RB) which requires energy from host cell to synthesize RNA, DNA, and proteins. After taking up host cell residence, EB are released and are capable of infecting neighboring cells or spreading the infection through sexual contact.

RISK FACTORS

Risk correlates with the following:

- Number of lifetime sexual partners and number of concurrent sexual partners
- No use of barrier contraception during intercourse
- Younger age (highest in females 15–19 years, males 20–24 years)
- Black/Hispanic/Native American and Alaskan Native ethnicity

GENERAL PREVENTION

- Populations with prevalence >5% should be screened at least annually (1)[A].
- Screening recommended if new or >1 sex partner in past 6 months; attending an adolescent clinic, family-planning clinic, STD or abortion clinic, or attending a jail or other detention center clinic. Screen if rectal pain, discharge or tenesmus, testicular pain; test all individuals with urethral or cervical discharge.
- All sexually active women ≤25 years of age should be screened at least yearly. Repeat testing in ~3 months is recommended for those who screen positive because reinfection rate is high regardless of whether the sexual partner is treated (2)[A].
- Screening sexually active men ≤25 years of age should be strongly considered, particularly in high-risk populations.
- Annual screening is recommended for men who have sex with men.
- Nucleic acid amplification test (NAAT) is the preferred screening test in all circumstances except child sexual abuse involving boys or rectal/oropharyngeal testing in prepubescent girls. For these situations, culture and susceptibility testing is preferred (3)[A].
- Acceptable to screen women for chlamydia on same day as intrauterine device insertion (4)[B]

COMMONLY ASSOCIATED CONDITIONS

- Females
  - PID: ~10% develop PID within 12 months if untreated.
  - Infertility, ectopic pregnancy
  - Chronic pelvic pain
  - Urethral syndrome (dysuria, frequency, and pyuria in the absence of infection)
  - Arthritis (less common)
  - Spontaneous abortion
- Males
  - Epididymitis and nongonococcal urethritis
  - Reiter syndrome (HLA-B27)
  - Proctitis
- Neonates
  - Inclusion conjunctivitis (occurs in ~40% of exposed neonates)
  - Otitis media
  - Pneumonia
  - Pharyngitis
- Diseases caused by other chlamydial species
  - Lymphogranuloma venereum (LGV): *C. trachomatis* serotypes L1–L3
  - Trachoma: *C. trachomatis* serotypes A–C

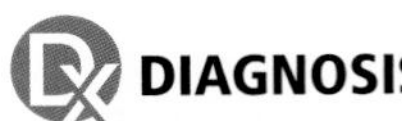

DIAGNOSIS

Many patients are asymptomatic.

Pregnancy Considerations

- Test all patients at first prenatal visit.
- Test of cure 3 weeks after treatment for all pregnant patients
- Repeat test in 3rd trimester (2)[A].

HISTORY

- Complete sexual history, including number of sex partners lifetime and past year, prior history of STIs, use of barrier protection, exchange of money or drugs for sex, oral or anal receptive intercourse, and partner fidelity
- In females, the most common symptoms are the following:
  - Mucopurulent vaginal discharge, dysuria (urethral syndrome), bartholinitis, abdominopelvic pain (endometritis, salpingitis/PID), right upper quadrant pain (Fitz-Hugh-Curtis perihepatitis syndrome)
- In males, the most common symptoms are the following:
  - Dysuria, urethral discharge (urethritis), scrotal pain (epididymitis), rectal pain or discharge (proctitis), acute arthritis (Reiter syndrome)

PHYSICAL EXAM

- Men and women: external genitalia (rash? lesions?), urethra (discharge? dysuria?), inguinal lymph nodes, pharynx, and perianal area, if history indicates
- In addition, for women: cervix (discharge, motion tenderness), uterus, ovaries, adnexa
- LGV (*C. trachomatis* serovars L1, L2, or L3): Primary lesion is a small papule that may ulcerate at the site of transmission after an incubation period of 3–30 days. May manifest as unilateral tender lymphadenopathy. With rectal transmission, LGV causes an invasive proctocolitis.

DIFFERENTIAL DIAGNOSIS

- *Neisseria gonorrhoeae*: urethritis, proctitis, epididymitis, cervicitis, PID, Bartholin abscess
- *Mycoplasma* or *Ureaplasma urealyticum*: urethritis, epididymitis, Reiter disease, PID
- *C. trachomatis* (serotypes L1–L3): LGV, proctitis
- Trichomoniasis

DIAGNOSTIC TESTS & INTERPRETATION

Initial Tests (lab, imaging)

- *Test of choice is NAAT*: sensitivity >95%; specificity >99%
- Urine equally sensitive to cervical swab
- Patient self-collected vaginal swabs also effective.
- Lab tests may remain positive for as long as 3 weeks after successful treatment.
- Test for concurrent STIs, including gonorrhea, HIV, syphilis; perform cervical cancer (PAP) screening if clinically appropriate.

Follow-Up Tests & Special Considerations

See "Patient Monitoring."

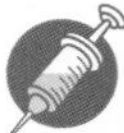

TREATMENT

GENERAL MEASURES

- Offer patients with known or suspected chlamydia testing for gonorrhea, HIV (after counseling and consent), and possibly syphilis. Also, ensure females are up to date with cervical cancer screening.
- Consider treating gonorrhea empirically.
- All partners (most recent partner and all partners within the past 60 days) should be tested and treated empirically, if possible.

MEDICATION

First Line

- http://www.cdc.gov/std/treatment/2010/chlamydial-infections.htm
- Treatment of chlamydial urethritis, cervicitis (including sexual partners of infected persons)
- Azithromycin 1 g PO single dose *or*
- Doxycycline 100 mg PO BID × 7 days
- 1st-line PID treatment (outpatient)
  - Ceftriaxone 250 mg IM × 1 *PLUS* doxycycline 100 mg PO × 14 days with or without metronidazole 500 mg PO BID × 14 days *or*
  - Cefoxitin 2 g IM × 1 with probenecid 1 g PO × 1 *PLUS* doxycycline 100 mg PO × 14 days with or without metronidazole 500 mg PO BID × 14 days
- Azithromycin and ceftriaxone may be given simultaneously in the office to treat both chlamydia and gonorrhea. This reduces patient nonadherence (2)[A].
- Asymptomatic rectal chlamydia can be treated with doxycycline 100 mg BID × 7 days. Azithromycin 1 g × 1 is slightly less effective but can also be used, especially if compliance or medication availability is an issue (5,6)[A].

ALERT

Use azithromycin with caution in patients with known QT prolongation, hypokalemia, hypomagnesemia, bradycardia, or who are currently treated with antiarrythmics.

Pregnancy Considerations

- Tetracyclines (doxycycline) and quinolones (ofloxacin, levofloxacin) are contraindicated in pregnant women.
- Consider the following:
  - Azithromycin 1 g PO *OR*
  - Amoxicillin 500 mg PO TID × 7 days (2)[A] *OR*
  - Erythromycin base 500 mg PO QID × 7 days

ALERT

Tetracyclines and quinolones are contraindicated in young children:

- <45 kg: erythromycin base or ethinyl succinate 500 mg/kg/day PO QID × 14 days
- >45 kg but <8 years: azithromycin 1 g PO × 1 day
- >8 years: adult regimen
- Rule out sexual abuse in children with chlamydial infections.

Second Line

For chlamydial urethritis/cervicitis

- Erythromycin base 500 mg PO QID × 7 days *OR* erythromycin ethylsuccinate 800 mg PO QID × 7 days
- Levofloxacin 500 mg PO daily × 7 days *or* ofloxacin 300 mg PO BID × 7 days

ADDITIONAL THERAPIES

Patient delivered partner therapy (PDPT) or expedited partner therapy (EPT): provide medications or prescriptions to take to sexual partners of persons infected with STIs without clinical assessment

- EPT is more effective than traditional partner referral in reducing recurrence rates.
- www.cdc.gov/std/ept/legal/default.htm

INPATIENT CONSIDERATIONS

Patients falling into the following categories are recommended for inpatient treatment of PID: pregnancy, lack of response or intolerance to oral medicines, suspicion of poor compliance, severe clinical illness, pelvic abscess, and possible need for surgical intervention.

Admission Criteria/Initial Stabilization

Outpatient treatment, unless patient is moderately or severely ill

ONGOING CARE

FOLLOW-UP RECOMMENDATIONS

Patient and all partners should abstain from sexual contact until at least 7 days after completing treatment.

Patient Monitoring

- Test of cure: not routinely recommended, except in pregnancy
- Sexual partners should be treated.

PATIENT EDUCATION

- Counseling regarding safe sexual practices, use of barrier protection, and delay of initiation of sexual activity
- Patient and partner should both finish entire course of antibiotics.

PROGNOSIS

Prognosis is good following therapy.

COMPLICATIONS

- Both sexes: Chlamydial infection enhances transmission of and susceptibility to HIV.
- Females: tubal infertility (most common cause of acquired infertility), tubal (ectopic) pregnancy, chronic pelvic pain
  - Annual screening of sexually active women would prevent 61% of chlamydia-related PID.
- Males: transient oligospermia and postepididymitis urethral stricture (rare)

REFERENCES

1. Centers for Disease Control and Prevention. 2012 Sexually transmitted disease surveillance. http://www.cdc.gov/std/stats12/chlamydia.htm. Accessed 2014.
2. Workowski KA, Berman S; Centers for Disease Control and Prevention. Sexually transmitted diseases treatment guidelines, 2010. *MMWR Recomm Rep*. 2010;59(RR-12):1–110.
3. Centers for Disease Control and Prevention. Recommendations for the laboratory-based detection of *Chlamydia trachomatis* and *Neisseria gonorrhoeae*—2014. http://www.cdc.gov/std/laboratory/2014/labrec/default.htm. Accessed 2014.
4. Sufrin CB, Postlethwaite D, Armstrong MA, et al. *Neisseria gonorrhea* and *Chlamydia trachomatis* screening at intrauterine device insertion and pelvic inflammatory disease. *Obstet Gynecol*. 2012;120(6):1314–1321.
5. Elgalib A, Alexander S, Tong CY, et al. Seven days of doxycycline is an effective treatment for asymptomatic rectal *Chlamydia trachomatis* infection. *Int J STD AIDS*. 2011;22(8):474–477.
6. Drummond F, Ryder N, Wand H, et al. Is azithromycin adequate treatment for asymptomatic rectal chlamydia? *Int J STD AIDS*. 2011;22(8):478–480.

C

ADDITIONAL READING

- Baud D, Goy G, Jaton K, et al. Role of *Chlamydia trachomatis* in miscarriage. *Emerg Infect Dis*. 2011;17(9):1630–1635.
- Price MJ, Ades AE, De Angelis D, et al. Risk of pelvic inflammatory disease following *Chlamydia trachomatis* infection: analysis of prospective studies with a multistate model. *Am J Epidemiol*. 2013;178(3):484–492.
- Ray WA, Murray KT, Hall K, et al. Azithromycin and the risk of cardiovascular death. *N Engl J Med*. 2012;366(20):1881–1890.
- Unemo M, Clarke IN. The Swedish new variant of *Chlamydia trachomatis*. *Curr Opin Infect Dis*. 2011;24(1):62–69.
- Won H, Ramachandran P, Steece R, et al. Is there evidence of the new variant *Chlamydia trachomatis* in the United States? *Sex Transm Dis*. 2013;40(5):352–353.

SEE ALSO

Cervicitis, Ectropion, and True Erosion; Epididymitis; Gonococcal Infections; HIV/AIDS; Pelvic Inflammatory Disease; Syphilis; Urethritis

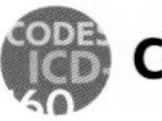

CODES

ICD10

- A56.8 Sexually transmitted chlamydial infection of other sites
- A56.01 Chlamydial cystitis and urethritis
- A56.02 Chlamydial vulvovaginitis

CLINICAL PEARLS

- *C. trachomatis* is common in young sexually active individuals. Screening is recommended annually in sexually active women 25 years of age and younger.
- To prevent recurrence, treat patients and their partners concurrently.
- Test of cure is recommended for pregnant patients at 3 weeks. Pregnant women diagnosed in the 1st trimester should have a second test of cure 3 months after treatment.

CHLAMYDOPHILA PNEUMONIAE

Fozia Akhtar Ali, MD • Teny Anna Philip, MD

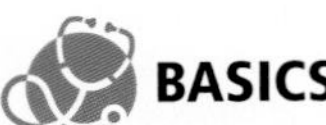

BASICS

DESCRIPTION

- Chlamydophila pneumoniae (formerly known as Chlamydia pneumoniae) is an obligate intracellular gram-negative bacterium causing atypical pneumonia or bronchitis in adolescents and young adults (1).
- Causes a more severe persistent latent infection in older adults
- Humans are the only known reservoir.

EPIDEMIOLOGY

- Responsible for 10–20% of community-acquired pneumonia (CAP) among adults, 2nd to mycoplasma in cases of atypical pneumonia (1)
- Epidemiologic studies suggest 4-year peaks.
- The incubation period is ~3–4 weeks.
- Most infected persons are asymptomatic.
- Typically presents as mild upper respiratory infection (URI). Bronchitis and pneumonia may follow in 1–4 weeks.
- Primary infection more common in ages 7–40 years; reinfection pneumonia more common in elderly
- Serologic evidence of previous infection is found in 50% of adults and 75% of elderly.
- Male > female (60–90%); possibly due to smoking

Incidence

Outbreaks have occurred among military recruits, university students, and nursing home residents, with incidence highest in elderly.

Prevalence

- 300,000 cases per year in the United States
- 10–20% of CAP cases among adults

ETIOLOGY AND PATHOPHYSIOLOGY

- The elementary body is the infectious form.
  - Metabolically inactive with rigid cell wall allows survival outside the host cell for a limited time.
- The elementary body infects the host cell by receptor-mediated endocytosis and becomes a reticulate body (2).
- Reticulate bodies divide intracellularly, forming intracytoplasmic inclusions that divide and release chlamydial antigens. This elicits a host immune response that leads to mucus production in the nasal passages, sinuses, bronchial tree, and alveoli, along with nasopharyngeal and airway inflammation and bronchospasm.
- After 48–72 hours, the reticulate bodies become elementary bodies and are released by cell lysis.

RISK FACTORS

Close quarters such as classrooms, military barracks, shelters, and nursing homes

GENERAL PREVENTION

- Transmission is by respiratory droplets. Hand washing and avoiding exposure to infected persons are key preventive steps.
- Incidence high among military recruits during basic training; weekly azithromycin prophylaxis reduced cases by 58%.

COMMONLY ASSOCIATED CONDITIONS

- Chronic obstructive pulmonary disease
- Asthma
- HIV infection
- Cystic fibrosis
- Diabetes mellitus

DIAGNOSIS

HISTORY

- Illness varies in clinical severity from mild and self-limited URI to fulminant pneumonia.
- Onset is typically gradual.
- Sore throat and hoarseness may precede cough by a week or more, leading to biphasic constellation of symptoms (uncommon in *Legionella*, less common with *Mycoplasma*, *Streptococcus pneumoniae*, and *Haemophilus influenzae*).
- Dry cough
- Low-grade fever (usually early in illness)
- Chills
- Rhinitis
- Headache
- Malaise
- Myalgias
- Sinus congestion
- Nausea
- Altered mental status; elderly patients are less likely to exhibit respiratory symptoms with pneumonia and may present with altered mental status or history of falls.

PHYSICAL EXAM

- General appearance usually nontoxic
- Fever
- Tachypnea
- Tachycardia
- Crackles or wheezing
- Bronchial breath sounds
- Percussion dullness and egophony less sensitive but more specific for pneumonia
- Pharyngeal erythema without exudate

DIFFERENTIAL DIAGNOSIS

- Other causes of atypical pneumonia, including *Mycoplasma pneumoniae* and *Legionella pneumophila*
- Other bacterial causes of pneumonia, including *S. pneumoniae*, *H. influenzae*, *Moraxella catarrhalis*, and *Staphylococcus aureus*
- Respiratory viruses: adenovirus, influenza A, influenza B, parainfluenza virus, and respiratory syncytial virus
- Endemic fungal pathogens: coccidioidomycosis, histoplasmosis
- Opportunistic fungal pathogens: *Candida* species, *Aspergillus* species, *Mucor* species, *Cryptococcus neoformans*
- Other: psittacosis, Q fever, TB, tularemia
- Conditions that mimic CAP: acute respiratory disease syndrome, idiopathic pulmonary fibrosis, neoplasm, pulmonary embolus, sarcoidosis, congestive heart failure

DIAGNOSTIC TESTS & INTERPRETATION

Initial Tests (lab, imaging)

- Most commonly used test and practical test of choice is the microimmunofluorescence (MIF) test.
  - Sensitivity of 50–90% if using paired sera
  - IgM 1:16 or higher
  - IgG 1:512 or higher
  - IgM may not be detectable early in the disease.
- White blood count is usually normal.
- Alkaline phosphate levels may be elevated. Blood cultures are recommended if patient is toxic and requires ICU admission; otherwise less helpful.
- Culture with oropharyngeal swab is the gold standard diagnostic method (not widely available).
  - Specificity 100%; sensitivity 50–70% (3)
  - Specimen should be kept cool and transported in specific media.
  - Most easily cultured using HL or HEp2 cells (4)
- PCR from pharyngeal swab or bronchioalveolar lavage specimen (30–95% sensitivity, >95% specificity) (4); during an outbreak, one study showed PCR was less sensitive (68% vs. 79%) but more specific (93% vs. 86%) than MIF IgM (5).
- Complement fixation for *Chlamydia* is available but cannot distinguish *C. pneumoniae* from *Chlamydophila psittaci*.
- Chest x-ray (CXR) (6)[A]
- No characteristic radiograph findings
- CXR most commonly shows a single subsegmental infiltrate that is mainly located in the lower lobes.
- Extensive consolidation is rare, although cases of acute respiratory distress syndrome (ARDS) have been reported.
- Pleural effusion seen in 20–25% of cases
- Histologically, intra-alveolar inflammation with mild interstitial reaction is characteristic of chlamydial pneumonias. Alveolar lining cells contain intracytoplasmic inclusions.

Diagnostic Procedures/Other

Although serology is 95% specific, definitive diagnosis requires a positive culture or PCR testing.

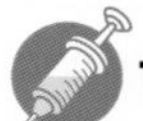

TREATMENT

MEDICATION

An advantage in clinical efficacy or mortality by empiric coverage of atypical pathogens in patients with CAP has not been shown (7)[A].

First Line

- Doxycycline: 100 mg PO BID for 10–14 days (may use IV in inpatient setting) *OR*
- Tetracycline: 500 mg PO QID for 10–14 days *OR*
- Azithromycin: 500 mg on day 1, then 250 mg on days 2–5 *OR*
- Clarithromycin: 500 mg q12h for 10–14 days
  - Tetracyclines not for use during pregnancy or in children <8 years
  - Tetracyclines may cause photosensitivity; sunscreen is recommended.

Second Line

Alternative drugs

- Levofloxacin: 250–500 mg/day (PO or IV) or other respiratory fluoroquinolones have good bioavailability and the convenience of once-daily dosing but are recommended for use only when patients have failed treatment with a 1st-line drug, have had recent antibiotics, significant comorbidities, or have allergies to 1st-line medications.

Pregnancy Considerations

Avoid tetracyclines in pregnant women.

INPATIENT CONSIDERATIONS

- Usually outpatient care. Those with severe pneumonia or coexisting illness may require hospitalization.
- Pneumonia severity index can help predict morbidity and need for hospitalization in context of clinical judgment (6).

Admission Criteria/Initial Stabilization

Infection in debilitated or hospitalized patients can be severe; ventilatory support for respiratory failure

Discharge Criteria

Reversal of respiratory distress, tolerating PO medications, otherwise stable medically, and clinically stable for discharge

ONGOING CARE

FOLLOW-UP RECOMMENDATIONS

Patient Monitoring

- Monitor patients weekly until well.
- Follow-up CXR can document resolution.
- Reinfection is possible.

PROGNOSIS

- Pneumonia is more likely to be life-threatening in older adults and patients with other underlying pulmonary disease (e.g., asthma, chronic obstructive pulmonary disease [COPD]) or the immune compromise (e.g., diabetes), with an overall 0.5–29% mortality rate.
- Death usually from secondary infection or underlying comorbidity

COMPLICATIONS

- Reactive airway disease
- Erythema nodosum
- Otitis media
- Endocarditis
- Pericarditis or myocarditis
- Meningoencephalitis
- Possible association with atherosclerotic disease: *C. pneumoniae* has been cultured from atherosclerotic plaque in patients with coronary artery disease and stroke. Treatment for *C. pneumoniae* has not been shown to affect cardiovascular mortality.
- *C. pneumoniae* infection is associated with an increased risk for lung cancer (8).

REFERENCES

1. Blasi F, Tarsia P, Aliberti S. *Chlamydophila pneumoniae*. *Clin Microbiol Infect*. 2009;15(1):29–35.
2. Thibodeau KP, Viera AJ. Atypical pathogens and challenges in community-acquired pneumonia. *Am Fam Physician*. 2004;69(7):1699–1706.
3. Kumar S, Hammerschlag MR. Acute respiratory infection due to *Chlamydia pneumoniae*: current status of diagnostic methods. *Clin Infect Dis*. 2007;44(4):568–576.
4. Burillo A, Bouza E. *Chlamydophila pneumoniae*. *Infect Dis Clin North Am*. 2010;24(1):61–71.
5. Hvidsten D, Halvorsen DS, Berdal BP, et al. *Chlamydophila pneumoniae* diagnostics: importance of methodology in relation to timing of sampling. *Clin Microbiol Infect*. 2009;15(1):42–49.
6. Lutfiyya MN, Henley E, Chang LF, et al. Diagnosis and treatment of community-acquired pneumonia. *Am Fam Physician*. 2006;73(3):442–450.
7. Shefet D, Robenshtock E, Paul M, et al. Empiric antibiotic coverage of atypical pathogens for community acquired pneumonia in hospitalized adults. *Cochrane Database Sys Rev*. 2005;1:CD004418.
8. Zhan P, Suo LJ, Qian Q, et al. *Chlamydia pneumoniae* infection and lung cancer risk: a meta-analysis. *Eur J Cancer*. 2011;47(5):742–747.

C

ADDITIONAL READING

- Centers for Disease Control and Prevention. Chlamydophila pneumoniae infection. http://www.cdc.gov/pneumonia/atypical/chlamydophila.html. Accessed 2014.
- Conklin L, Adjemian J, Loo J, et al. Investigation of a *Chlamydia pneumoniae* outbreak in a federal correctional facility in Texas. *Clin Infect Dis*. 2013;57(5):639–647.

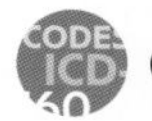

CODES

ICD10

- J16.0 Chlamydial pneumonia
- A70 Chlamydia psittaci infections

CLINICAL PEARLS

- Consider *C. pneumoniae* in young patients who look fine but present clinically with pneumonia.
- Formal diagnosis of *C. pneumoniae* is difficult. Culture is the gold standard. Serodiagnosis is used for acute infection.
- Tetracyclines or macrolides are initial drugs of choice.

CHOLELITHIASIS

Hongyi Cui, MD, PhD, FACS, FICS

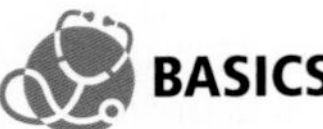

BASICS

DESCRIPTION

- Cholelithiasis is the presence of cholesterol, pigment, or mixed stones (calculi) formed within the gallbladder.
- Synonym(s): gallstones

Pediatric Considerations

- Uncommon at <10 years
- Most gallstones in the pediatric population are pigment stones associated with blood dyscrasias.

EPIDEMIOLOGY

Incidence

- Increased in Native Americans and Hispanics
- Increases with age by 1–3% per year; peaks at 7th decade; 2% of the U.S. population develops gallstones annually.

Prevalence

- Population: 8–10% of the United States; 20% of those >65 years of age
- Predominant sex: female > male (2–3:1)

ETIOLOGY AND PATHOPHYSIOLOGY

Gallstone formation is a complex process mediated by genetic, metabolic, immune, and environmental factors. Gallbladder sludge (a mixture of cholesterol crystals, calcium bilirubinate granules, and mucin gel matrix) serves as the nidus for gallstone formation.

- Production of bile supersaturated with cholesterol (cholesterol stones) from excess cholesterol secretion precipitates as microcrystals that aggregate and expand. Stone formation enhanced by biliary stasis or impaired gallbladder motility.
- Decrease in bile content of either phospholipid (lecithin) or decreased bile salt secretion
- Generation of excess unconjugated bilirubin in patients with hemolytic diseases; passage of excess bile salt into the colon with subsequent absorption of excess unconjugated bilirubin in patients with inflammatory bowel disease (IBD) or after distal ileal resection (black or pigment stones)
- Hydrolysis of conjugated bilirubin or phospholipid by bacteria in patients with biliary tract infection or stricture (brown stones or primary bile duct stones; rare in the Western world and common in Asia)

RISK FACTORS

- Age (peak in 60–70s)
- Female gender, pregnancy, multiparity, obesity, and metabolic syndrome
- Caucasian, Hispanic, or Native American descent
- High-fat diet rich in cholesterol
- Cholestasis or impaired gallbladder motility in association with prolonged fasting, long-term total parenteral nutrition (TPN), and rapid weight loss
- Hereditary (p.D19H variant for the hepatocanalicular cholesterol transporter ABCG5/ABG8)
- Short gut syndrome, terminal ileal resection, inflammatory bowel disease
- Hemolytic disorders (hereditary spherocytosis; sickle cell anemia, etc.); cirrhosis (black/pigment stones)
- Medications (birth control pills, estrogen replacement therapy at high doses, and long-term corticosteroid or cytostatic therapy)
- Viral hepatitis, biliary tract infection and stricture (promotes intraductal formation of pigment stones)

GENERAL PREVENTION

- Ursodiol (Actigall) taken during rapid weight loss prevents gallstone formation.
- Regular exercise and dietary modification may reduce the incidence of gallstone formation.
- Lipid-lowering drugs (statins) may prevent cholesterol stone formation by reducing bile cholesterol saturation.

COMMONLY ASSOCIATED CONDITIONS

90% of people with gallbladder carcinoma have gallstones.

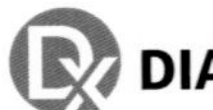

DIAGNOSIS

HISTORY

- Mostly asymptomatic (80%): 2% become symptomatic each year. Over their lifetime, <1/2 of patients with gallstones develop symptoms.
- Episodic right upper quadrant or epigastric pain lasting >15 minutes and sometimes radiating to the back (biliary colic), usually postprandially; pain sometimes awakens the patient from sleep; most patients develop recurrent symptoms after first episode of biliary colic.
- Nausea, vomiting; indigestion or bloating sensation; fatty food intolerance

PHYSICAL EXAM

- Physical exam is *usually normal* in patients with cholelithiasis without acute attack.
- Epigastric and/or right upper quadrant tenderness (Murphy sign) is traditional physical finding—associated with cholecystitis
- Charcot triad: fever, jaundice, right upper quadrant pain
- Reynold pentad: fever, jaundice, right upper quadrant pain, hemodynamic instability, mental status changes; classically associated with ascending cholangitis
- Flank and periumbilical ecchymoses (Cullen sign and Grey-Turner sign) in patients with acute hemorrhagic pancreatitis
- Courvoisier sign: palpable mass in the right upper quadrant in patient with obstructive jaundice most commonly due to tumors within the biliary tree or pancreas

DIFFERENTIAL DIAGNOSIS

- Peptic ulcer diseases and gastritis
- Hepatitis
- Pancreatitis
- Cholangitis
- Gallbladder cancer
- Gallbladder polyps
- Acalculous cholecystitis
- Biliary dyskinesia
- Choledocholithiasis

DIAGNOSTIC TESTS & INTERPRETATION

No lab study is specific for cholelithiasis.

Initial Tests (lab, imaging)

- Leukocytosis and elevated C-reactive protein level are associated with acute calculus cholecystitis.
- US (best technique) can detect gallstones in 97–98% of patients.
- Thickening of the gallbladder wall (≥5 mm), pericholecystic fluid, and direct tenderness when the probe is pushed against the gallbladder (sonographic Murphy sign) are associated with acute cholecystitis.

Follow-Up Tests & Special Considerations

- CT scan (no advantage over US except in detecting distal common bile duct stones)
- MR cholangiopancreatography (MRCP) is reserved for cases of suspected common bile duct stones due to high cost. MRCP is recommended as a secondary imaging study if ultrasounography does not clearly demonstrate acute cholecystitis or gallstones (1)[C].
- Endoscopic US has been shown to be as sensitive as endoscopic retrograde cholangiopancreatography (ERCP) for detection of common bile duct stones in patients with gallstone pancreatitis.
- Hepatobiliary iminodiacetic acid (HIDA) scan is useful in diagnosing acute cholecystitis secondary to cystic duct obstruction. It is also useful in differentiating acalculous cholecystitis from other causes of abdominal pain. False-positive results can arise from fasting status, insufficient resistance of the sphincter of Oddi, and gallbladder agenesis.
- Cholecystokinin (CCK)-HIDA is specifically used to diagnose gallbladder dysmotility (biliary dyskinesia).
- 10–30% of gallstones are radiopaque calcium or pigment-containing gallstones and are more likely to be visible on plain x-ray. A "porcelain gallbladder" is a calcified gallbladder, visible by x-ray; associated with gallbladder cancer.

Test Interpretation

- Pure cholesterol stones have a white or slightly yellow color.
- Pigment stones may be black or brown. Black stones contain polymerized calcium bilirubinate, most often secondary to cirrhosis or hemolysis; these almost always form in the gallbladder.
- Brown stones are associated with biliary tract infection, caused by bile stasis, and as such may form either in the bile ducts or gallbladder.

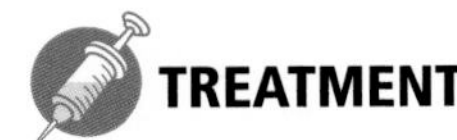

TREATMENT

GENERAL MEASURES

- Treat only symptomatic gallstones.
- Attempt conservative therapy during pregnancy. Surgery preferred in the 2nd trimester if necessary.
- Prophylactic cholecystectomy for patients with calcified (porcelain) gallbladder (risk for gallbladder cancer), patients with large stones (>3 cm), patients with sickle cell disease, patients planning an organ transplant, and patients with recurrent pancreatitis due to microlithiasis
- In morbidly obese patients, simultaneous cholecystectomy may be performed in combination with bariatric procedures (2) to reduce subsequent stone-related comorbidities.

Geriatric Considerations

Gallstones are more common in the elderly. Age alone should not alter the therapy plan.

MEDICATION

First Line

- Analgesics for pain relief
  - A recent meta-analysis shows NSAIDs are the 1st-choice treatments as they control pain with the same efficacy as opioids (2)[A].
  - Opioids may be considered for patients who cannot tolerate or fail to respond to NSAIDs.
- Antibiotics for patients with acute cholecystitis
- Prophylactic antibiotics in low-risk patients do not prevent infections during laparoscopic cholecystectomy (3,4)[A].

ISSUES FOR REFERRAL

Patients with retained or recurrent bile duct stones following cholecystectomy should be referred for ERCP.

SURGERY/OTHER PROCEDURES

- Surgery should be considered for patients who have symptomatic cholelithiasis or gallstone-related complications (cholecystitis) or in asymptomatic patients with immune suppression, calcified gallbladder, or family history of gallbladder cancer. Open or laparoscopic cholecystectomy (LC) has similar mortality and complication rates. LC offers less pain and quicker recovery. In well-selected patients, single-incision LC (SILC) and robotic LC are novel methods for the treatment of symptomatic cholelithiasis. SILC has not been shown to be superior to conventional multiport LC in terms of pain and risk of complications (5)[A]. Natural orifice transluminal endoscopic surgery (NOTES) is still in investigational stage. Surgery-related complications include common bile duct injury (0.5%), right hepatic duct/artery injury, retained stones, cystic duct or duct of Luschka leak, biloma formation, or bile duct stricture in the long term.
  - Conversion to open procedure is based on clinical picture and judgment of the operating surgeon. Factors that increase the risk of conversion to open cholecystectomy include male gender, previous upper abdominal surgery, thickened gallbladder wall, and acute cholecystitis.
  - In 10–15% of patients with symptomatic cholelithiasis, common bile duct (CBD) stones are detected during LC by intraoperative cholangiogram (IOC). CBD stone(s) can be removed by laparoscopic CBD exploration or postoperative ERCP.
  - IOC helps delineate bile duct anatomy when dissection is difficult. Routine use of IOC is debatable but may be associated with earlier recognition and/or decreased incidence of bile duct injury.
- Percutaneous cholecystostomy (PC) is used in high-risk patients with cholecystitis or gallbladder empyema. PC may also be used in patients with symptoms of cholecystitis for >72 hours in which altered anatomy might significantly increase the surgical risk. Interval cholecystectomy is advisable.

INPATIENT CONSIDERATIONS

For patients with symptomatic cholelithiasis, laparoscopic cholecystectomy is typically an outpatient procedure. For patients with complications (i.e., cholecystitis, cholangitis, pancreatitis), inpatient care is necessary.

Admission Criteria/Initial Stabilization

- Acute phase: NPO, IV fluids, and antibiotics
- Adequate pain control with narcotics and/or NSAIDs

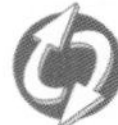

ONGOING CARE

FOLLOW-UP RECOMMENDATIONS

Patient Monitoring

- Follow for signs of symptomatic cholelithiasis
- Patients on oral dissolution agents should be followed with serial liver enzyme, serum cholesterol, and imaging studies.

DIET

A low-fat diet may be helpful.

PATIENT EDUCATION

- Change in lifestyle (e.g., regular exercise) and dietary modification (low-fat diet and reduction of total caloric intake) may reduce gallstone-related hospitalizations.
- Patients with asymptomatic gallstones should be educated about the typical symptoms of biliary colic and gallstone-related complications.

PROGNOSIS

- <1/2 of patients with gallstones become symptomatic.
- Cholecystectomy: mortality <0.5% elective, 3–5% emergency; morbidity <10% elective, 30–40% emergency
- ~10–15% of the patients will have associated choledocholithiasis.
- After cholecystectomy, stones may recur within the biliary tree.

COMPLICATIONS

- Acute cholecystitis (90–95% secondary to gallstones)
- Gallstone pancreatitis
- Common bile duct stones with obstructive jaundice and acute cholangitis
- Biliary-enteric fistula and gallstone ileus; Bouveret syndrome is a variant of gallstone ileus where the gallstone lodges in the duodenum or pylorus causing a gastric outlet obstruction.
- Gallbladder cancer
- Mirizzi syndrome (extrinsic bile duct obstruction caused by gallstones lodged in gallbladder or cystic duct)

REFERENCES

1. American College of Radiology. ACR appropriateness criteria: right upper quadrant pain. http://www.acr.org/~/media/ACR/Documents/AppCriteria/Diagnostic/RightUpperQuadrantPain.pdf. Accessed 2014.
2. Colli A, Conte D, Valle SD, et al. Meta-analysis: nonsteroidal anti-inflammatory drugs in biliary colic. *Aliment Pharmacol Ther*. 2012;35(12):1370–1378.
3. Sanabria A. Dominguez LC, Valdivieso E, et al. Antibiotic prophylaxis for patients undergoing elective laparoscopic cholecystectomy. *Cochrane Database Syst Rev*. 2010;(12):CD005265.
4. Zhou H, Zhang J, Wang Q, et al. Meta-analysis: Antibiotic prophylaxis in elective laparoscopic cholecystectomy. *Aliment Pharmacol Ther*. 2009;29(10):1086–1095.
5. Gurusamy KS, Vaughan J, Rossi M, et al. Fewer-than-four-port versus four ports for laparoscopic cholecystectomy. *Cochrane Database Syst Rev*. 2014;2:CD007109.

ADDITIONAL READING

- Brown LM, Rogers SJ, Cello JP, et al. Cost-effective treatments of patients with symptomatic cholelithiasis and possible common bile duct stones. *J Am Coll Surg*. 2011;212(6):1049–1060.
- Connor S, Garden OJ. Bile duct injury in the era of laparoscopic cholecystectomy. *Br J Surg*. 2006;93(2):158–168.
- Gurusamy KS, Samraj K. Cholecystectomy versus no cholecystectomy in patients with silent gallstones. *Cochrane Database Syst Rev*. 2007;(1):CD006230.
- Keus F, Gooszen HG, van Laarhoven CJ, et al. Open, small-incision, or laparoscopic cholecystectomy for patients with symptomatic cholecystolithiasis. An overview of Cochrane Hepato-Biliary Group reviews. *Cochrane Database Syst Rev*. 2010;(1):CD008318.
- Society for Surgery of the Alimentary Tract. SSAT patient care guidelines. Treatment of gallstone and gallbladder disease. *J Gastrointest Surg*. 2007;11(9):1222–1224.
- Uy MC, Talingdan-Te MC, Espinosa WZ, et al. Ursodeoxycholic acid in the prevention of gallstone formation after bariatric surgery: a meta-analysis. *Obes Surg*. 2008;18(12):1532–1538.
- Zehetner J, Pelipad D, Darehzereshki A, et al. Single-access laparoscopic cholecystectomy versus classic laparoscopic cholecystectomy: a systematic review and meta-analysis of randomized controlled trials. *Surg Laparosc Endosc Percutan Tech*. 2013;23(3):235–243.

SEE ALSO

Cholangitis, Acute; Choledocholithiasis

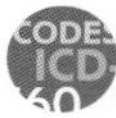

CODES

ICD10

- K80.20 Calculus of gallbladder w/o cholecystitis w/o obstruction
- K80.21 Calculus of gallbladder w/o cholecystitis with obstruction
- K80.01 Calculus of gallbladder w acute cholecystitis w obstruction

CLINICAL PEARLS

- Most patients with gallstones are asymptomatic.
- Laparoscopic cholecystectomy is the preferred procedure for symptomatic cholelithiasis; lithotripsy and oral dissolution therapy may be considered in rare circumstances.
- Acute acalculous cholecystitis is associated with bile stasis and gallbladder ischemia.
- Prophylactic cholecystectomy is not indicated in patients with diabetes and asymptomatic gallstones.
- Transabdominal ultrasound is the preferred imaging modality for diagnosis of cholelithiasis (sensitivity, 97%; specificity, 95%).
- Consider gallstones in patients complaining of "gas pains" after bariatric surgery adjusting to a new diet.

CHRONIC FATIGUE SYNDROME

Anthony F. Valdini, MD, MS, FACP, FAAFP

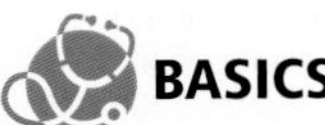

BASICS

DESCRIPTION

- A condition characterized by profound mental and physical exhaustion, with at least 6 months presence of multiple systemic and neuropsychiatric symptoms, and at least 4 of 8 associated conditions are required per CDC definition:
  - Impaired memory
  - Sore throat
  - Tender lymph nodes
  - Persistent muscle or joint pain
  - New headaches
  - Nonrefreshing sleep
  - Postexertional malaise >24 hours
- Must have a new or definite onset (not lifelong)
- Fatigue is not relieved by rest and results in >50% reduction in previous activities (occupational, educational, social, and personal). Other potential medical causes must be ruled out (1).
- Exclusions: See "History."

EPIDEMIOLOGY

- Predominant age: 20–50 years
- Predominant sex: male < female
- All socioeconomic groups
- Various, and at times contradictory, associations between ethnicity and incidence have been reported. Higher rates found in ethnic minorities (Native Americans and African Americans) compared with white populations based on a population study. Service-based studies (tertiary care) have reported higher rates among whites or no association between incidence and ethnicity (2).

Prevalence

Estimates vary widely and depend on case definition and population studied, but a reasonable estimate using a strict case definition is 100 cases per 100,000 population. Community-based studies have reported prevalence rates of 0.23 and 0.42%.

ETIOLOGY AND PATHOPHYSIOLOGY

- Unknown and likely multifactorial
  - Possible interaction between genetic predisposition, environmental factors, an initiating stressor, and perpetuating factors
- Physiologic or environmental stressor could be precipitant.
- Many patients with chronic fatigue recall significant stressors (e.g., major medical procedure, loss of a loved one, loss of employment) in months before symptoms began.
- Systems hypothesized to contribute to altered physiology include the following:
  - Neuroendocrine (e.g., diminished cortisol response to increased corticotropin concentrations)
  - Immune (e.g., increased C-reactive protein and β-2 microglobulin)
  - Neuromuscular (e.g., dysfunction of oxidative metabolism)
  - Autonomic (Orthostatic hypotension is reported in a proportion of chronic fatigue syndrome [CFS] sufferers.)
  - Serotonergic (e.g., hyperserotonergic mechanisms or upregulation of serotonin receptors)

Genetics

Higher concordance among monozygotic twins compared with dizygotic twins

RISK FACTORS

Possible predisposing factors include the following:

- Personality characteristics (neuroticism and introversion)
- Lifestyle
  - Childhood inactivity or overactivity
  - Inactivity in adulthood after infectious mononucleosis
  - Familial predisposition
  - Comorbid mood disorders of depression and anxiety
- Long-standing medical conditions in childhood
- Childhood trauma (emotional, physical, sexual abuse) (4)
- Prolonged idiopathic chronic fatigue
- Postinfectious fatigue and CFS have followed: mononucleosis, Ross River virus, *Coxiella burnetii*, and *Guardia lamblia*

COMMONLY ASSOCIATED CONDITIONS

Common comorbidities include the following:

- Fibromyalgia (more common in women)
- Irritable bowel syndrome
- Temporomandibular joint disorder
- Anxiety disorders
- Major depression
- Posttraumatic stress disorder (including physical and/or sexual past abuse)
- Domestic violence
- Attention-deficit hyperactivity disorder (ADHD)
- Postural orthostatic tachycardia syndrome (POTS)

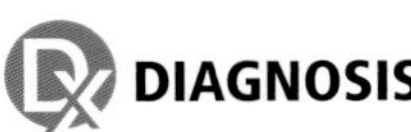

DIAGNOSIS

HISTORY

- Discrete onset
- Profound mental and physical exhaustion
- At least 6 months presence of multiple systemic and neuropsychiatric symptoms
- Significantly interferes with daily activites/work
- At least 4 of 8 associated conditions per CDC definition:
  - Impaired memory, sore throat, tender lymph nodes, persistent muscle or joint pain, new headaches, nonrefreshing sleep, postexertional malaise
- Exclusion criteria
  - <2 years after recovery of substance/alcohol abuse
  - Any past or current dx of anorexia nervosa or bulimia, dementia, schizophrenia, or bipolar disease
  - BMI ≥45
  - Malignancy
  - Previously diagnosed medical condition, unresolved clinically (e.g., hepatitis B or C)

PHYSICAL EXAM

Complete physical exam to rule out other medical causes for symptoms. Note: Tender adenopathy is one of the defining criteria.

ALERT

Detailed mental status examination (or referral to psychiatrist) to rule out other primary etiologies or comorbidities

DIFFERENTIAL DIAGNOSIS

- Idiopathic chronic fatigue (i.e., fatigue of unknown cause for >6 months without meeting criteria for CFS)
- Psychiatric disorders
  - Major depression
  - Somatization disorder
- Physiologic fatigue (inadequate or disrupted sleep, menopause)
- Pregnancy until 3 months postpartum
- Insomnia: primary (no clear etiology) versus secondary (e.g., due to anxiety, depression, environmental factors, poor sleep hygiene)
- Other known or defined systemic disease
- Endocrine disorder (hypothyroidism, Addison disease, Cushing syndrome, diabetes mellitus)
- Localized infection (e.g., occult abscess)
- Chronic or subacute bacterial disease (e.g., endocarditis)
- Lyme disease
- Fungal disease (e.g., histoplasmosis, coccidioidomycosis)
- Parasitic disease (e.g., amebiasis, giardiasis, helminth infestation)
- HIV or related disease
- Iatrogenic (e.g., medication side effects)
- Toxic agent exposure
- Morbid obesity, BMI >40
- Malignancy
- Autoimmune disease
- Chronic inflammatory disease (sarcoidosis, Wegener granulomatosis)
- Neuromuscular disease (multiple sclerosis, myasthenia gravis)

DIAGNOSTIC TESTS & INTERPRETATION

- No single diagnostic test available and finding an abnormal result is not always the same as discovering the cause of fatigue. Be prepared to renew the search for the cause if the problem is treated and the patient remains fatigued.

Initial Tests (lab, imaging)

- Standard laboratory tests are recommended to rule out other causes for symptoms:
  - Chemistry panel
  - CBC
  - Urinalysis
  - Thyroid-stimulating hormone (TSH)
  - ESR or C-reactive protein
  - Liver function
  - Screen for drugs of abuse
  - Age/gender-appropriate cancer screening
- Additional studies, if clinical findings are suggestive or patient at risk:
  - Antinuclear antibodies and rheumatoid factor (if elevated ESR)
  - Creatine kinase
  - Tuberculin skin test
  - Serum cortisol
  - HIV
  - Venereal Disease Research Laboratory or rapid plasma reagin
  - Lyme serology
  - IgA tissue transglutaminase
- No applicable imaging tests available; however, EEG and/or MRI may be useful if patient has CNS symptoms; polysomnography, if patient is sleepy (4).

Follow-Up Tests & Special Considerations

- Assess for comorbid psychiatric disorders.
- Assess for personality and psychosocial factors and maladaptive coping styles.
- In patients with sleep disturbance, polysomnography may reveal a treatable comorbid disease.

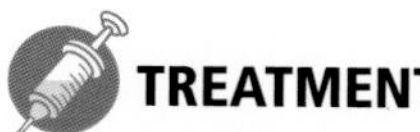

TREATMENT

Focus on changes in lifestyle and insight, with a goal to avoid complicating treatments (e.g., addicting medications, invasive testing) or interventions that support secondary gain.

GENERAL MEASURES

ALERT

Treatment cornerstones include *both* cognitive-behavioral therapy (CBT) and graded exercise therapy. Medication is of little value. 2 treatments have been shown effective, often used in combination (5)[A]:

- Individual CBT: challenge fatigue-related cognition; plan social and occupational rehabilitation.
- Graded exercise therapy (GET): Track amount of exercise patient can do without exacerbating symptoms and gradually increase intensity and duration. Both involve a careful balance between activity and rest (6)[A]. Fear of movement and avoidance of physical activity are common in CFS.
- Patients learn how to gradually increase activity in a way that will not exacerbate their illness. Vigorous exercise can trigger relapse, perhaps related to immune dysregulation.
- Improves functional capacity and diminishes sense of fatigue
- GET is more effective with educational interventions using telephone reminders.
- Duration of illness does not predict treatment outcome; aggressive combined care indicated for all.

MEDICATION

- No established pharmacologic treatment recommendations
- Studies have been conducted with antidepressants, immunoglobulins, hydrocortisone, and modafinil. None has shown clear benefit.
- Agomelatine, an antidepressant with agonist activity at melatonin receptors, is promising in early studies (7)[C].
- If insomnia is present, use of nonaddicting sleep aids (hydroxyzine, trazodone, doxepin, etc.) may improve outcomes.

ISSUES FOR REFERRAL

- Psychiatrist to assist in managing comorbid disorders if needed
- Rehabilitative medicine

COMPLEMENTARY & ALTERNATIVE MEDICINE

- Insufficient to recommend any complementary and alternative medicine option for all (8)
- Social support groups have not proven to be effective.

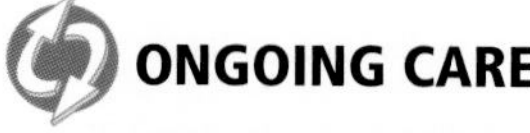

ONGOING CARE

FOLLOW-UP RECOMMENDATIONS

- Gradual increase in physical exercise with scheduled rest periods.
- Avoid extended periods of rest.

Patient Monitoring

Although no consensus exists, periodic reevaluation is appropriate for support, relief of symptoms, and assessment for other possible causes of symptoms.

DIET

- No diet has been shown to be effective for treatment of CFS.
- A BMI of 40 has been associated with fatigue in general, and BMI ≥45 is a CFS exclusion.
- Whether weight loss improves symptoms in obese CFS patients has yet to be tested.

PATIENT EDUCATION

- Patient education is an important part of treatment of CFS, such as education on the benefits of cognitive therapies, lifestyle changes, and pharmacologic therapy directed at specific-associated symptoms.
- Chronic Fatigue and Immune Dysfunction Syndrome Association of America: http://www.cfids.org
- CDC, Chronic Fatigue Syndrome: http://www.cdc.gov/cfs/

PROGNOSIS

- Fluctuating course is common.
- Generally, improvement is slow, with a course of months to years.
- An estimated 5% fully recover.
- Patients with poor social adjustment, a strong belief in an organic etiology, financial secondary gain, or age >50 years are less likely to improve (9).

COMPLICATIONS

- Depression
- Unemployment: Although studies document improvement with treatment, <1/3 of patients in trials return to work.
- The U.S. Social Security Administration lists CFS as a bona fide form of disability.
- Receipt of government payments (secondary gain) has been associated with treatment nonresponse.
- Polypharmacy
- Chronic immune activation or an infection associated with CFS may play a role in an increased risk for non-Hodgkins lymphoma in elderly (>80 years) CFS patients.

REFERENCES

1. Baker R, Shaw EJ. Diagnosis and management of chronic fatigue syndrome or myalgic encephalomyelitis (or encephalopathy): summary of NICE guidance. *BMJ*. 2007;335(7617):446–448.
2. Dinos S, Khoshaba B, Ashby D, et al. A systematic review of chronic fatigue, its syndromes and ethnicity: prevalence, severity, co-morbidity and coping. *Int J Epidemiol*. 2009;38(6):1554–1570.
3. Lievesley K, Rimes KA, Chalder T. A review of the predisposing, precipitating and perpetuating factors in chronic fatigue syndrome in children and adolescents. *Clin Psychol Rev*. 2014;34(3):233–248.
4. Duffy FH, McAnulty GB, McCreary MC, et al. EEG spectral coherence data distinguish chronic fatigue syndrome patients from healthy controls and depressed patients—a case control study. *BMC Neurol*. 2011;11:82.
5. White PD, Goldsmith KA, Johnson AL, et al. Comparison of adaptive pacing therapy, cognitive behaviour therapy, graded exercise therapy, and specialist medical care for chronic fatigue syndrome (PACE): a randomised trial. *Lancet*. 2011;377(9768):823–836.
6. Nijs J, Paul L, Wallman K. Chronic fatigue syndrome: an approach combining self-management with graded exercise to avoid exacerbations. *J Rehabil Med*. 2008;40(4):241–247.
7. Pardini M, Cordano C, Benassi F, et al. Agomelatine but not melatonin improves fatigue perception: a longitudinal proof-of-concept study. *Euro Neuropsychopharmacol*. 2014;24(6):939–944.
8. Adams D, Wu T, Yang X, et al. Traditional Chinese medicinal herbs for the treatment of idiopathic chronic fatigue and chronic fatigue syndrome. *Cochrane Database Syst Rev*. 2009;(4):CD006348.
9. Cairns R, Hotopf M. A systematic review describing the prognosis of chronic fatigue syndrome. *Occup Med*. 2005;55(1):20–31.

ADDITIONAL READING

- Centers for Disease Control and Prevention. Diagnosis and management of chronice fatigue syndrome, CDC course for clinicians. http://www.cdc.gov/cfs/education/diagnosis/idex.html. Accessed 2014.
- Freeman R, Wieling W, Axelrod FB, et al. Consensus statement on the definition of orthostatic hypotension, neutrally mediated syncope and the postural tachycardia syndrome. *Clin Auton Res*. 2011;21(2):69–72.
- Social Security Administration. Providing medical evidence to the social security administration for individuals with chronic fatigue syndrome—fact sheet. https://www.socialsecurity.gov/disability/professionals/cfs-pub063.htm. Accessed 2014.

SEE ALSO

Algorithm: Fatigue

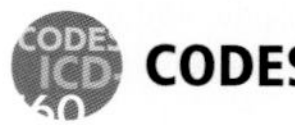

CODES

ICD10

R53.82 Chronic fatigue, unspecified

CLINICAL PEARLS

- CFS and depression can be comorbid. However, to differentiate between the 2, sore throat, tender lymph nodes, and postexercise fatigue are much more characteristic of CFS.
- No universal pharmacologic agents (e.g., antidepressants, immune modulators) have been shown to be consistently effective.
- ~70% of patients show improvement with CBT, compared to 55% with GET; in many cases, these 2 treatments can be undertaken in combination.
- There are many more patients with idiopathic chronic fatigue than true CFS. To diagnose CFS, CDC criteria need to be met; standardized instruments (SF-36, symptom index and Multidimentional Fatigue Inventory [MFI]) have been shown to be of use in the empirical diagnosis of CFS and may be helpful for following patients' progress.

CHRONIC KIDNEY DISEASE

Urooj Najm, MBBS • Najm Hasan Siddiqui, MD

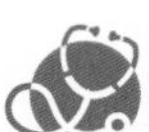

BASICS

Chronic kidney disease (CKD) is defined as structural or functional abnormalities of the kidney for ≥3 months, as determined by either pathologic abnormalities or markers of damage—including abnormalities in blood or urine tests, histology, imaging studies, or history of kidney transplant—*or a* GFR <60 mL/min/1.73 m² for ≥3 months.

DESCRIPTION

- In 2012, Kidney Disease Improving Global Outcome (KDIGO) classified CKD in 6 categories by GFR estimation:
  - G1: Kidney damage with normal or increased GFR ≥90 mL/min/1.73 m²
  - G2: Mild ↓ GFR 60–89 mL/min/1.73 m²
  - G3a: Mild to moderate ↓ GFR 45–59 mL/min/1.73 m²
  - G3b: Moderate to severe ↓ GFR 30–44 mL/min/1.73 m²
  - G4: Severe ↓ GFR 15–29 mL/min/1.73 m²
  - G5: Kidney failure: GFR <15 mL/min/1.73 m² or dialysis
- CKD per albumin-to-creatinine ratio (ACR) category:
  - A1: Normal to mildly increased: <30 mg/g or <3 mg/mmol
  - A2: Moderately increased: 30–300 mg/g or 3–30 mg/mmol (formerly called microalbuminiuria)
  - A3: Severely increased: >300 mg/g or >30 mg/mmol (formerly called macroalbuminuria)
- System(s) affected: renal/urinary, cardiovascular, skeletal, endocrine, metabolic, hematologic, lymphatic, immune, neurologic
- Synonym(s): chronic renal failure; chronic renal insufficiency

Geriatric Considerations

GFR normally decreases with age, despite normal creatinine (Cr). Adjust renally cleared drugs for GFR in the elderly.

Pediatric Considerations

CKD definition is not applicable for children <2 years because of lower GFR even when corrected for body surface area. Calculated GFR based on serum Cr is used in this age group.

Pregnancy Considerations

- Renal function in CKD may deteriorate during pregnancy. Cr >1.5 and hypertension (HTN) are major risk factors for worsening renal function.
- Increased risk of premature labor, preeclampsia, and/or fetal loss
- ACE inhibitors and angiotensin receptor blockers (ARBs) are contraindicated due to teratogenicity. Use diuretics with caution.

EPIDEMIOLOGY

- Majority of people with CKD in stages 1–3
- African Americans are 3.6 × more likely to develop chronic kidney disease than Caucasians.
- Predominant sex: similar in both sexes; however, incidence rate of end-stage renal disease (ESRD) is 1.6 × higher in males than females.

Incidence

Estimated annual incidence of 1,700/1 million population

Prevalence

Overall prevalence of CKD is 14.2%. Unadjusted prevalence/incidence rates of ESRD (stage 5) are 1,752 and 362.4/1 million, respectively. Numbers do not reflect the burden of earlier stages of CKD (stages 1–4), which are estimated to affect 13.1% of the population nationwide, or 26.3 million in the United States.

ETIOLOGY AND PATHOPHYSIOLOGY

Progressive destruction of kidney nephrons; GFR will drop gradually, and plasma Cr values will approximately double, with 50% reduction in GFR and 75% loss of functioning nephrons mass. Hyperkalemia usually develops when GFR falls to <20–25 mL/min. Anemia develops from decreased renal synthesis of erythropoietin:

- Renal parenchymal/glomerular
  - Nephritic: hematuria, RBC casts, HTN, variable proteinuria
    - Focal proliferative: IgA nephropathy, systemic lupus erythematosus (SLE), Henoch-Schönlein purpura, Alport syndrome, proliferative glomerulonephritis, crescentic glomerulonephritis
    - Diffuse proliferative: membranoproliferative glomerulonephritis, SLE, cryoglobulinemia, rapidly progressive glomerulonephritis (RPGN), Goodpasture syndrome
  - Nephrotic: proteinuria (>3.5 g/day), hypoalbuminemia, hyperlipidemia, and edema
    - Minimal change disease, membranous nephropathy, focal segmental glomerulosclerosis
    - Amyloidosis, diabetic nephropathy
- Vascular: HTN, thrombotic microangiopathies, vasculitis (Wegener), scleroderma
- Interstitial-tubular: infections, obstruction, toxins, allergic interstitial nephritis, multiple myeloma, connective tissue disease, cystic disease
- Postrenal: obstruction (benign prostatic hyperplasia), neoplasm, neurogenic bladder

Genetics

- Alport syndrome, Fabry disease, sickle cell anemia, SLE, and autosomal dominant polycystic kidney disease can lead to CKD.
- Polymorphisms in gene that encodes for podocyte nonmuscle myosin IIA are more common in African Americans than Caucasians and appear to increase risk for nondiabetic ESRD

RISK FACTORS

- Type 1 or 2 diabetes mellitus (DM); most common
- Age >60 years
- Cardiovascular disease (e.g., HTN [common], renal artery stenosis, atheroemboli)
- Previous kidney transplant
- Urinary tract obstruction (e.g., benign prostatic hyperplasia)
- Autoimmune disease, vasculitis/connective tissue disorder
- Family history of CKD
- Nephrotoxic drugs (lithium, salicylate, high-dose or chronic NSAIDs, sulfa)
- Congenital anomalies, obstructive uropathy, renal aplasia/hypoplasia/dysplasia, reflux nephropathy
- Hyperlipidemia
- Low income/education/ethnic minority status
- Obesity/smoking/heroin use
- Chronic infection (hepatitis B, hepatitis C, HIV)

GENERAL PREVENTION

- Treat reversible causes: hypovolemia, infections, diuretics, drugs (NSAIDs, aminoglycosides, IV contrast).
- Treat risk factors: DM, HTN, hyperlipidemia, smoking, and obesity; adjust medication doses to prevent renal toxicity.

COMMONLY ASSOCIATED CONDITIONS

HTN, DM, cardiovascular disease

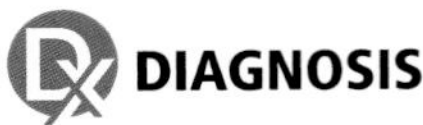

DIAGNOSIS

HISTORY

Patients with CKD stages 1–3 are usually asymptomatic; can present with

- Oliguria, nocturia, polyuria, hematuria, change in urinary frequency
- Bone disease
- Edema, HTN, dyspnea
- Fatigue, depression, weakness
- Pruritus, ecchymosis
- Metallic taste in mouth, anorexia, nausea, vomiting
- Hyperlipidemia, claudication, restless legs
- Erectile dysfunction, decrease libido, amenorrhea

PHYSICAL EXAM

- Volume status (pallor, BP/orthostatic; edema; jugular venous distention; weight)
- Skin: sallow complexion, uremic frost
- Ammonia-like odor (uremic fetor)
- Cardiovascular: assess for murmurs, bruits, pericarditis.
- Chest: pleural effusion
- Rectal: enlarged prostate
- CNS: asterixis, confusion, seizures, coma, peripheral neuropathy

DIAGNOSTIC TESTS & INTERPRETATION

Initial Tests (lab, imaging)

- GFR can be estimated by multiple equations (freely available in medical calculators) including MDRD equation:
  - GFR (mL/min/1.73 m²) = 175 × [(serum Cr μmol/1/88.4)$^{-1.154}$] × [age (years)$^{-0.203}$] × 0.742 for females *or* 1.21 for African American
  - Often used as estimate in electronic health records
- Cr clearance (CrCl) can be calculated using Cockroft-Gault formula:
  - CrCl (male) = [(140 − age) × weight(kg)/(serum Cr × 72)]
  - CrCl (female) = CrCl (male) × 0.85
  - Formula used for determining cut points for renally adjusted medications
- Urine analysis
  - Urine microscopy: WBC casts in pyelonephritis, RBC casts in glomerulonephritis/vasculitis, dysmorphic RBCs
  - Urine electrolytes: sodium, Cr, urea (if on loop diuretics)
  - Proteinuria/albuminuria
    - 24-hour urine collection: >30–300 mg/24 hr (20–200 μg/min) is microalbuminuria and >300 mg/24 hr (>200 μg/min) is macroalbuminuria.
    - Albumin/Cr ratio (ACR): See "Description"
- Hematology: normochromic, normocytic anemia; increased bleeding time
- Chemistry
  - Elevated BUN, Cr, hyperkalemia, metabolic acidosis
  - Increased parathyroid hormone, decreased 25-(OH) vitamin D, hypocalcemia, hyperphosphatemia
  - Hyperlipidemia, decreased albumin

ALERT

Drugs that may alter lab result:

- Cimetidine: inhibits Cr tubular secretion
- Trimethoprim: inhibits Cr and K^+ secretion and may cause/worsen hyperkalemia
- Cefoxitin and flucytosine: increases serum Cr
- Diltiazem and verapamil (like ACE/ARBs) have significant antiproteinuric effects in patients with CKD.
- Ultrasound (initial test of choice): small, echogenic kidneys; may see obstruction (e.g., hydronephrosis); cysts; kidneys may be enlarged with HIV and diabetic nephropathy
- Doppler ultrasound to assess for renovascular disease, thrombosis
- Noncontrast CT scan: obstruction, calculi, cysts, neoplasm, renal artery stenosis
- MRI/MRA: Avoid gadolinium because of the risk of nephrogenic systemic fibrosis.
- Renal arteriogram for renal artery stenosis can be therapeutic (angioplasty or stenting).
- Renal scan to screen for differential function between kidneys
- Retrograde pyelogram: if strong suspicion for obstruction despite negative finding on ultrasound

Follow-Up Tests & Special Considerations

- Serology: antinuclear antibody (ANA); double-stranded DNA, antineutrophil cytoplasmic antibody; complements (C3, C4, CH50); anti-glomerular basement membrane (GBM) antibodies; hepatitis B, C; and HIV screening
- Serum and urine immunoelectrophoresis

Diagnostic Procedures/Other

Biopsy: hematuria, proteinuria, acute/progressive renal failure, nephritic or nephrotic syndrome

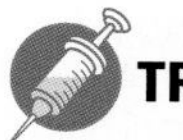

TREATMENT

GENERAL MEASURES

- Lowering salt intake to <2 g/day of sodium in adults, unless contraindicated (1)[C]
- Minimize radiocontrast exposure; prehydrate; *N*-acetylcysteine use is controversial. Avoid nephrotoxins (NSAIDs, aminoglycosides, etc.).
- Renal replacement: Prepare for dialysis or transplant when GFR <30 mL/min/1.73 m^2.
- Vaccines: pneumococcal, influenza.
- Encourage smoking cessation, encourage weight loss (if applicable), and limit alcohol consumption

MEDICATION

- HTN: Goal is BP <130/80 mm Hg (in nonhemodialysis patients) and <140/90 mm Hg (in patients on hemodialysis) in the nephrology literature, but more recent analysis based on outcomes suggests a universal BP target of <140/90 mm Hg (2).
- Antihypertensive agents should be selected based on the type of CKD and presence of cardiovascular disease.
- Long-acting (once daily) agents should be prescribed preferentially and given at bedtime.
- ACE inhibitors (drugs of choice) or ARBs for BP control and antiproteinuric effect
  - Potential for hyperkalemia
  - Can tolerate up to 30% rise in serum Cr unless hyperkalemia develops
  - If goal not reached, add diuretic; thiazides are recommended for GFR ≥30 mL/min/1.73 m^2; loop diuretics are recommended for GFR <30 mL/min/1.73 m^2), followed by diltiazem or verapamil or a β-blocker.
- Secondary hyperparathyroidism
  - Cinacalcet, paricalcitol (decrease PTH levels)
- Recommended serum phosphate maintenance levels for CKD patients:

Stage	mg/day	mmol/L
Normal range *may vary by institution*	2.5–4.5	0.81–1.45
Stage 3 and 4 CKD (not on dialysis)	2.7–4.6	0.87–1.49
Stage 5 and ALL stages on dialysis	3.5–5.5	1.13–1.78

  - Stages 3–5 CKD (not on dialysis): Restrict dietary phosphate to 800–1,000 mg/day:
    - Calcium-containing phosphate binders (with meals): calcium carbonate, calcium acetate (risk of hypercalcemia)
    - Non–calcium phosphate binders (with meals): sevelamer, lanthanum
    - Vitamin D: inactive vitamin D 25 (ergocalciferol or cholecalciferol), calcitriol (active vitamin D 1,25 [OH]): Vitamin D may increase absorption of phosphate by intestines and should not be started until serum phosphate concentration is controlled.
  - Anemia: ferrous sulfate, erythropoietin-stimulating agents (ESAs): Before starting ESAs, nonrenal causes of anemia/iron stores should be checked. Start when Hgb <10 g/dL; goal range 10–11 g/dL, not to exceed 11.5 g/dL
  - Hyperlipidemia: Statins with low-density lipoprotein (LDL) goal is similar to coronary heart disease patients (LDL <70–100).
  - Glycemic control: Target HbA1c 7.0%, but it should be individualized based on life expectancy of patient, risk for adverse events related to glucose control, and patient preference (1). Tighter control may slow progression of microalbuminuria but may not reduce progression to ESRD and death in patients with type 2 diabetes. Use of metformin is not advised with serum Cr ≥1.5 mg/dL in males and ≥1.4 mg/dL in females because of possible risk of lactic acidosis.
  - Metabolic acidosis: Start treatment when bicarb <20 mEq/L; goal 23-29 mEq/L
    - Sodium bicarbonate: daily dose of 0.5–1 mEq/kg/day *or* sodium citrate (should be avoided in patients taking aluminum-containing antacid)

ISSUES FOR REFERRAL

- Nephrology consult: GFR <15: immediate
- GFR 15–29: urgent
- GFR 30–59: nonurgent referral
- GFR 60–89: not required unless with comorbidities

SURGERY/OTHER PROCEDURES

Placement of dialysis access or transplantation

INPATIENT CONSIDERATIONS

Admission Criteria/Initial Stabilization

Uremia: nausea/vomiting, fluid overload, pericarditis, uremic encephalopathy, resistant HTN, hyperkalemia, metabolic acidosis, hyperphosphatemia

ONGOING CARE

DIET

Nutrition consult for CKD diet: Protein restriction in early CKD is controversial but may be beneficial in ESRD; restricted intake of phosphates; sodium and water restriction to avoid volume overload; potassium restriction if hyperkalemic

PATIENT EDUCATION

National Kidney Federation patient Web site at: www.kidney.org/patients

PROGNOSIS

Patients with CKD gradually progress to ESRD, with bad prognoses. 5-year survival rate for U.S. patients on dialysis is ~35%.

COMPLICATIONS

HTN, anemia, secondary hyperparathyroidism, renal osteodystrophy, sleep disturbances, infections, malnutrition, electrolyte imbalances, platelet dysfunction/bleeding, pseudogout, gout, metabolic calcification, sexual dysfunction

REFERENCES

1. Mancia G, Fagard R, Narkiewicz K, et al. 2013 ESH/ESC guidelines for the management of arterial hypertension: the Task Force for the Management of Arterial Hypertension of the European Society of Hypertension (ESH) and of the European Society of Cardiology (ESH). *J Hypertens.* 2013;31(7):1281–1357.
2. Kidney Disease: Improving Global Outcomes (KDIGO) CKD Work Group. KDIGO 2012 clinical practice guideline for the evaluation and management of chronic kidney disease. *Kidney Inter Suppl.* 2013;3:1–150. www.kdigo.org/clinical_practice_guidelines/pdf/CKD/KDIGO_2012_CKD_GL.pdf. Accessed 2014.

SEE ALSO

- Hydronephrosis; Nephrotic Syndrome; Polycystic Kidney Disease; Proteinuria
- Algorithm: Anuria or Oliguria

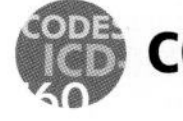

CODES

ICD10

- N18.9 Chronic kidney disease, unspecified
- Q63.9 Congenital malformation of kidney, unspecified
- N18.3 Chronic kidney disease, stage 3 (moderate)

CLINICAL PEARLS

- Maintaining BP <140/90 mm Hg is imperative (in patients not on dialysis).
- Avoid nephrotoxins including ACE/ARB in acute kidney injury (AKI) with or without CKD.
- CKD is a CHD risk equivalent.

CHRONIC OBSTRUCTIVE PULMONARY DISEASE AND EMPHYSEMA

Alan Cropp, MD, FCCP • Bryon Veynovich, DO

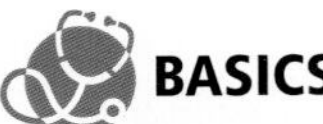

BASICS

DESCRIPTION

- Chronic obstructive pulmonary disease (COPD) usually describes a mixture of chronic bronchitis and emphysema. It is characterized by airflow limitation that is not fully reversible, inflammation, and is progressive (1,2).
- Chronic bronchitis is defined clinically by increased mucus production and recurrent cough present on most days for at least 3 months per year during at least 2 consecutive years.
- Emphysema, the destruction of interalveolar septa, occurs in the distal or terminal airways and involves both airways and lung parenchyma.

EPIDEMIOLOGY

Incidence

Affects more than 5% of adults in the Unites States and is the 12th leading cause of morbidity (1)

Prevalence

- 3rd leading cause of death in the Unites States (1)
- Projected to be the 3rd leading cause of death globally by 2020 (2)

ETIOLOGY AND PATHOPHYSIOLOGY

Cigarette and/or cannabis smoking, air pollution (including indoor), antiprotease deficiency (α_1-antitrypsin), occupational exposure (firefighters), infection (viral), occupational pollutants (cadmium, silica)

- Impaired gas (carbon dioxide and oxygen) exchange
- Chronic bronchitis: airway obstruction (3)
- Emphysema: destruction of lung parenchyma

Genetics

- Chronic bronchitis is not a genetic disorder.
- Antiprotease deficiency (due to α_1-antitrypsin deficiency) is an inherited, rare disorder due to 2 autosomal codominant alleles.

RISK FACTORS

- Smoking; passive smoking, especially adults whose parents smoked; cannabis use (1 joint is equivalent to 2.5–5 cigarettes) (1–3)
- Severe pneumonia early in life including viral (4)
- Aging
- Lower level of education and poverty (4)
- Airway hyperactivity
- Indoor pollution (open fire for cooking or heating) (4)
- Occupational organic or inorganic dusts (4)

GENERAL PREVENTION

- Avoidance of smoking is the most important preventive measure.
- Early detection through pulmonary function tests (PFTs) in high-risk patients may be useful in preserving remaining lung function.

COMMONLY ASSOCIATED CONDITIONS

- Pulmonary: lung cancer, chronic respiratory failure, acute bronchitis, sleep apnea, pulmonary hypertension
- Cardiac: coronary artery disease, arrhythmia
- Ear, nose, and throat (ENT): chronic sinusitis, laryngeal carcinoma
- Miscellaneous: malnutrition, osteoporosis, muscle dysfunction, depression

DIAGNOSIS

HISTORY

- Discuss patient's habits with regard to tobacco
- Consider indoor pollution (coal furnace) (4)
- Review possible causes of exacerbation (e.g., recent infection) and history of cough, sputum, dyspnea
- Chronic bronchitis: cough, sputum production, frequent infections, intermittent dyspnea, wheeze, hemoptysis, morning headache, pedal edema
- Emphysema: minimal cough, scant sputum, dyspnea, weight loss, occasional infections

PHYSICAL EXAM

- Rarely diagnostic for COPD (2)
- Chronic bronchitis: cyanosis, wheezing, weight gain, diminished breath sounds, distant heart sounds
- Emphysema: barrel chest, minimal wheezing, accessory muscle use, pursed lip breathing, cyanosis slight or absent, breath sounds diminished

DIFFERENTIAL DIAGNOSIS

- Asthma (including occupational)
- Bronchiectasis
- Lung cancer
- Acute viral infection
- Normal aging of lungs
- Chronic pulmonary embolism
- Sleep apnea
- Primary alveolar hypoventilation
- Chronic sinusitis
- Reactive airways dysfunction syndrome (RADS)
- Congestive heart failure (CHF)
- Bronchiolitis obliterans
- Gastroesophageal reflux disease
- Cystic fibrosis

DIAGNOSTIC TESTS & INTERPRETATION

Spirometry (the most reliable/objective measurement of airflow obstruction) (1–3)[A]

Initial Tests (lab, imaging)

- Chronic bronchitis
  - Arterial blood gases (ABGs) may show hypercapnia and hypoxia.
  - Hemoglobin may be increased.
- Emphysema
  - Normal serum hemoglobin or polycythemia
  - Normal partial pressure of arterial carbon dioxide ($PaCO_2$) on ABGs unless forced expiratory volume in 1 second (FEV_1) <1 L, in which case it can be elevated
  - Mild hypoxia
- Spirometry (1–3)
- Chronic bronchitis CXR: increased bronchovascular markings and cardiomegaly
- Emphysema CXR: small heart, hyperinflation, flat diaphragms, and possibly bullous changes
- CT may show emphysema, air trapping, or bronchial wall thickening (5).

Follow-Up Tests & Special Considerations

- Consider checking continuous overnight oximetry in selected patients.
- α_1-Antitrypsin screening for those with COPD age younger than 45 years or have a blood relative with this disease
- Chest CT may show diffuse bullous changes or upper lobe predominance. Also, small lung nodules may be identified (6)[B].

Diagnostic Procedures/Other

- PFTs (1,2)[A]
  - Not indicated during acute exacerbation (3)
  - Decreased FEV_1 and resulting reduction in FEV_1:FVC (forced vital capacity) ratio
  - Poor or absent reversibility to bronchodilator
  - Normal or reduced FVC
  - Normal or increased total lung capacity
  - Increased residual volume and functional residual capacity
  - Diffusing capacity is normal or reduced.
- Staging: Global Initiative for Obstructive Lung Disease (GOLD) criteria (3)
  - Mild COPD: FEV_1 ≥80% predicted
  - Moderate COPD: FEV_1 between 50% and 80% predicted
  - Severe COPD: FEV_1 between 30% and 50% predicted
  - Very severe COPD: FEV_1 <30% predicted or FEV_1 <50% predicted plus chronic respiratory failure

Test Interpretation

- Chronic bronchitis: bronchial mucous gland enlargement, increased number of secretory cells in surface epithelium, thickened small airways from edema and inflammation, smooth muscle hyperplasia, mucus plugging, bacterial colonization of airways
- Emphysema: entire lung affected, bronchi usually clear of secretions, anthracotic pigment, alveoli enlarged with loss of septa, cartilage atrophy, bullae

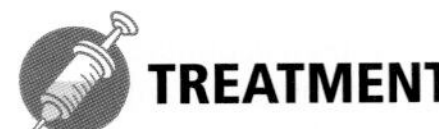

TREATMENT

GENERAL MEASURES

- Smoking cessation: This is the most important intervention to decrease risk (1,2)[A].
- Aggressive treatment of infections (3)[B]
- Treat any reversible bronchospasm.
- Home oxygen: may improve survival; should be initiated partial pressure of arterial oxygen (PaO_2) ≤55 mm Hg or pulse oximetry trends ≤88% (1)[A]
- Influenza and pneumococcal immunizations (2)[B]
- Tiotropium (Spiriva) may slow disease progression (5)[B].

MEDICATION

Medications help reduce symptoms and exacerbations (1).

First Line

- All patients should have a short-acting β-agonist (albuterol) to use as a rescue drug (1).
- Anticholinergics (2)[A]
  - Ipratropium (Atrovent), tiotropium (Spiriva), aclidinium bromide (Turdoza) *AND/OR*
- Long-acting β-agonists
  - Salmeterol (Serevent), formoterol (Foradil), 1 inhalation q12h; or arformoterol (Brovana), formoterol (Perforomist), nebulized q12h (1,2)[A]

ALERT

Acute exacerbation: Use oxygen, inhaled β-agonists, inhaled anticholinergic agents, and oral or IV corticosteroids prednisone (up to 1 mg/kg/day commonly 40 mg/day for 5 days) (7)[A]. Antibiotics should be given for those with moderate/severe exacerbations showing clinical signs of bacterial infection (increased sputum volume, increased sputum purulence); optimal antibiotic therapy has not been determined (3)[B].

Second Line

- Trial of inhaled corticosteroids for moderate or severe disease (2)[A]
  - May initiate earlier if suggestion of asthmatic component to disease

- Systemic corticosteroids; prednisone (Deltasone) can be given orally 7.5–15 mg/day in selected patients.
- Long-term monotherapy with steroids (oral or inhaled) is not recommended (2,3)[A].
- Among patients with COPD, inhaled corticosteroid is associated with an increased risk of serious pneumonia (3).

- Theophylline if other long-term treatment is unavailable or unaffordable: 400 mg/day; increase by 100–200 mg in 1–2 weeks, if necessary (2)[B]
  - Reduce dosage in patients with impaired renal or liver function, age older than 55 years, or CHF
  - Monitor serum level. Therapeutic range is 8–13 μg/mL.
  - Low-dose theophylline may help inflammatory component (5)[B].
- Combination of inhaled corticosteroid, long-acting β-agonist, and anticholinergic indicated for severe disease (2)[A]
- Mucolytic agents may improve secretions but do not improve outcomes.
- Phosphodiesterase-4 inhibitor (PDE4) inhibitor (roflumilast) in severe chronic bronchitis may reduce exacerbations (2)[B].
- α_1-antitrypsin, if deficient: 60 mg/kg/week to maintain level >80 mg/dL
- Precautions
  - Sympathomimetics: Excessive use may be dangerous. May need to reduce dosage or use levalbuterol (Xopenex) in patients with cardiovascular disease, hypertension (HTN), hyperthyroidism, diabetes, or convulsive disorders.
  - Anticholinergics: narrow-angle glaucoma, benign prostatic hyperplasia, bladder neck obstruction
  - Corticosteroids: weight gain, diabetes, adrenal suppression, osteoporosis, infection (pneumonia)
- Sympathomimetics may be aerosolized.
- Anticholinergics: Ipratropium (Atrovent) may be aerosolized or combined with albuterol (Combivent Respimat).

ISSUES FOR REFERRAL

Severe exacerbation, frequent hospitalizations, age younger than 40 years, rapid progression, weight loss, severe disease, or surgical evaluation

ADDITIONAL THERAPIES

- Adequate hydration and pulmonary hygiene
- Consider postural drainage, flutter valve, or other devices to assist mucus clearance.
- Pulmonary rehabilitation (1–3)[A]
- Intermittent, noninvasive ventilation may help in severe chronic respiratory failure.
- Short course of antibiotics (5–10 days) for acute exacerbations (2)[B]
- Immunizations
- Supplemental oxygen if indicated

SURGERY/OTHER PROCEDURES

- Lung reduction surgery (selected cases)
- Lung transplantation (selected cases)

INPATIENT CONSIDERATIONS

Admission Criteria/Initial Stabilization

- Outpatient treatment is usually adequate.
- Exacerbation with acute decompensation (hypoxemia, hypercarbia)
- Serious comorbidities (i.e., decompensated CHF)
- Systemic steroids have been shown to reduce recovery time and improve hypoxia (2,7)[A].
- Supplemental oxygen and short-acting bronchodilators should be given (3).

ALERT

- If not already in place, have patient delineate an **a**dvance **d**irective, and if they have one, review patient's preferences.
- www.agingwithdignity.org, www.putitinwriting.org
- Progressive nature of disease and severity of treatment methods (ventilation, etc.) make revisiting patient preferences beneficial.
- Acute respiratory failure may require ICU and invasive or noninvasive (NIV) ventilation (2)[A].
- Systemic steroids (prednisone 40 mg/day for 5 days or equivalent) have been shown to reduce recovery time and improve hypoxia (7)[A].
- A short course of antibiotics for change in sputum volume, purulence, and increased dyspnea (2,3)[B]

Nursing

Teach proper inhaler use.

Discharge Criteria

- Ability to ambulate (3)
- Patient should have adequate gas exchange (3).
- Hypoxia can be treated with home oxygen (may only be temporary) (2)[A].
- Inhaled short-acting β-agonist therapy no more frequently than q4h (3)
- Ability to eat and sleep without interruption caused by dyspnea (3)

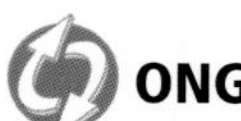

ONGOING CARE

FOLLOW-UP RECOMMENDATIONS

- May taper or stop oral steroids as outpatient
- If pneumonia caused exacerbation, need to follow CXR or chest CT until clear or stable
- Pulmonary rehabilitation for exertional dyspnea (1)[A]

PATIENT MONITORING

- Severe or unstable patients should be seen monthly. When stable, see every 6 months.
- Check theophylline level with dose adjustment, then check every 6–12 months.
- With use of home oxygen, check ABGs yearly or with change in condition. Frequently monitor saturation (pulse oximetry).
- Some patients only desaturate at night, thus only need nocturnal oxygen.
- Travel at high altitude with supplemental oxygen if necessary.
- Discuss advance directive and health care proxy.

DIET

A high-protein diet is suggested. Decreased carbohydrates may benefit those with hypercarbia.

PATIENT EDUCATION

American Lung Association: www.lung.org/lung-disease/copd/

PROGNOSIS

- Patient's age and postbronchodilator FEV_1 are the most important predictors of prognosis.
- Supplemental O_2, when indicated, is shown to increase survival (may only need at night) (1)[A].
- Smoking cessation improves prognosis—consider E-cigarettes (2).
- Malnutrition, cor pulmonale, hypercapnia, and pulse >100 indicate a poor prognosis.

COMPLICATIONS

- Malnutrition, poor sleep quality, infections, secondary polycythemia
- Acute or chronic respiratory failure, bullous lung disease, pneumothorax
- Arrhythmias, cor pulmonale, pulmonary HTN

C

REFERENCES

1. Amir Q, Wilt T, Weinberger S, et al. Diagnosis and management of stable chronic obstructive pulmonary disease: a clinical practice guideline update from the American College of Physician, American College of Chest Physicians, American Thoracic Society, and European Respiratory Society. *Ann Intern Med*. 2011;155(3):179–191.
2. Vestbo J, Hurd S, Agusti A, et al. Global strategy for the diagnosis, management, and prevention of chronic obstructive pulmonary disease: GOLD executive summary. *Am J Respir Crit Care Med*. 2013;187(4):347–365.
3. Global Initiative for Chronic Obstructive Lung Disease. Global strategy for the diagnosis, management, and prevention of COPD. Revised 2013. http://www.goldcopd.org/guidelines-global-strategy-for-diagnosis-management.html. Accessed 2014.
4. Lamprecht B, McBurnie M, Vollmer W, et al. COPD in never smokers: results from the population-based burden of obstructive lung disease study. *Chest*. 2011;139(4):752–763.
5. Csikesz N, Gartman E. New developments in the assessment of COPD: early diagnosis is key. *Int J of Chron Obstruct Pulmon Dis*. 2014;9:277–286.
6. Detterbeck F, Mazzone P, Naidich D, et al. Screening for lung cancer: diagnosis and management of lung cancer, 3rd ed: American College of Chest Physicians evidence-based guidelines. *Chest*. 2013;143(5)(Suppl):e78S–e92S.
7. Leuppi J, Schuetz P, Bingisser R, et al. Short-term vs conventional glucocorticoid therapy in acute exacerbations of chronic obstructive pulmonary disease: the REDUCE randomized clinical trial. *JAMA*. 2013;309(21):2223–2231.

SEE ALSO

- Bronchitis, Acute
- Algorithms: Clubbing; Cyanosis

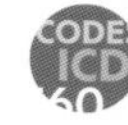

CODES

ICD10

- J44.9 Chronic obstructive pulmonary disease, unspecified
- J43.9 Emphysema, unspecified
- J42 Unspecified chronic bronchitis

CLINICAL PEARLS

- Consider screening PFTs on any high-risk patient.
- Overnight oximetry if daytime SaO_2 is borderline
- Influenza/pneumococcal vaccines should be current.
- Advance directive before patient is seriously ill
- Consider chest CT for patients age 55–74 years plus a 30 pack-year smoking history for lung cancer screening.

CHRONIC PAIN MANAGEMENT: AN EVIDENCE-BASED APPROACH

Jennifer Reidy, MD, MS, FAAHPM

BASICS

- Chronic pain is pain persisting beyond the time of normal tissue healing, usually >3 months.
- Over time, neuroplastic changes in the CNS transform pain into a chronic disease itself. Pain levels can exceed observed pathology on exam or imaging.
- Pain experience is inherently related to emotional, psychological, and cognitive factors.
- An epidemic of undertreated pain coexists with an epidemic of prescription drug abuse in the United States.
- Use a system-based practice to safely and effectively prescribe opioids when indicated for chronic nonmalignant pain.

EPIDEMIOLOGY

Incidence

Incidence is rising, but exact rate is unclear. The annual economic cost of chronic pain in the United States is estimated at $560–635 billion (1)[B].

Prevalence

In the United States, an estimated 100 million adults live with chronic pain—more than the total affected by heart disease, cancer, and diabetes combined (1)[B].

Chronic pain accounts for 20% of outpatient visits and 12% of all prescriptions (2)[B].

ETIOLOGY AND PATHOPHYSIOLOGY

- With intense, repeated, or prolonged stimulation of damaged or inflamed tissues, the threshold for activating primary afferent pain fibers is lowered, the frequency of firing is higher, and there is increased response to noxious and/or normal stimuli (peripheral and central sensitization). The amygdala, prefrontal cortex, and cortex are thought to relay emotions and thoughts that create the pain experience and these areas may undergo structural and functional changes with chronic pain.
- Many patients have an identifiable etiology (most commonly musculoskeletal problems or headache), but pain levels can be worse than observable tissue injury. A significant percentage of patients have no obvious cause of chronic pain.

Genetics

Current research suggests genetic polymorphism in opioid receptors, which may affect patient's response and/or side effects to individual opioids.

RISK FACTORS

- Traumatic: motor vehicle accidents, repetitive motion injuries, sports injuries, work-related injuries, and falls
- Postsurgical: any surgery but especially back surgeries, amputations and thoracotomies
- Medical conditions: See "Commonly Associated Conditions" later.
- Psychiatric comorbidities: substance abuse, depression, posttraumatic stress disorder (PTSD), personality disorders
- Aging: increased incidence with age but should not be considered a "normal" part of aging

GENERAL PREVENTION

- Avoidance of work-related injuries through the use of ergonomically correct workplace design
- Exercise and physical therapy to help prevent work-related low back pain
- Varicella vaccine and rapid treatment of shingles to lower risk of postherpetic neuralgia
- Tight glycemic control for diabetic patients, alcohol cessation for alcoholics, smoking cessation

COMMONLY ASSOCIATED CONDITIONS

Any chronic disease and/or its treatment can cause chronic pain, including diabetes, cardiovascular disease, HIV, progressive neurologic conditions, lung disease, cirrhosis, autoimmune disease, cancer, renal failure, depression, and mental illness.

DIAGNOSIS

Chronic pain can be divided into 2 general categories:

- Nociceptive pain (2 types)
  - Somatic: skin, bone, soft tissue disease; described as well localized, sharp, stabbing, aching
  - Visceral: visceral inflammation/injury; described as poorly localized, dull, aching; may refer to sites remote from lesion
- Neuropathic pain: damaged peripheral or central nerves; described as burning, tingling, and/or numbness
  - Sympathetically mediated pain: Peripheral nerve injury can cause severe burning pain, swelling of the affected limb, and focal changes in sweat production and skin appearance. Example: complex regional pain syndrome.

HISTORY

- Obtain pain history: location, onset, intensity, duration, quality, temporal pattern, exacerbators, alleviators, prior treatments
- Assess and document how pain affects patient's functioning and quality of life and what they expect from treatment.
- Screen for personal or family history of substance abuse (including tobacco addiction), mental health conditions, domestic violence, or sexual abuse.
- Use standardized tools: Pain severity—Brief Pain Inventory (short form); mood—Patient Health Questionnaire-9 (PHQ-9); substance abuse—Screener and Opioid Assessment for Patients with Pain (SOAPP), multiple versions
- Use this screening to risk stratify patients for risks of chronic opioid therapy and increased monitoring; a positive screen does not automatically exclude patients from opioid therapy.

PHYSICAL EXAM

Exam is guided by history and should include functional and mental assessments.

DIFFERENTIAL DIAGNOSIS

- The causes of pain are numerous, and clinic presentations are protean, depending on the individual patient.
- There is a spectrum of aberrant drug-taking behaviors, and differential diagnosis includes
  - Inadequate analgesia ("pseudoaddiction"), disease progression, opioid-resistant pain, opioid-induced hyperalgesia, addiction, opioid tolerance, self-medication of nonpain symptoms, criminal intent (diversion)

DIAGNOSTIC TESTS & INTERPRETATION

Testing is based on differential diagnosis of pain syndrome to elucidate etiology.

Initial Tests (lab, imaging)

If substance abuse suspected, order urine drug screen. Most tests are immunoassays, which usually detect morphine and heroin but often not other opioids. Laboratory-based chromatography/spectrometry can identify specific drugs. Clinicians should be aware of uses and limitations of local laboratory testing (http://www.aafp.org/afp/2010/0301/p635.html).

Follow-Up Tests & Special Considerations

- If patient is taking chronic opioid therapy, order random urine drug screens as part of the "universal precautions" approach (see "Ongoing Care").
- Urine drug screen: Order qualitative analysis for drugs of abuse and quantitative analysis for the drug you are prescribing.

Diagnostic Procedures/Other

- Consider interventional pain clinic for complicated joint injections and nerve root blocks, which can be diagnostic.
- If complex regional pain syndrome is suspected, a sympathetic block can be diagnostic and possibly prevent chronic pain.

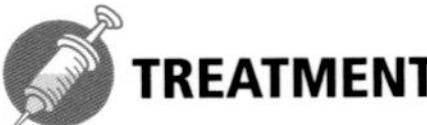

TREATMENT

- Goals of treatment are pain relief and restoring function, while balancing risks and benefits of therapies.
- Intradisciplinary teams offer most effective approach to chronic pain, including its physical, emotional, and psychological aspects. These teams may include the patient, family, primary care doctor, nurse, pain management specialist, pharmacist, psychologist, psychiatrist, physical and occupational therapists, physiatrist, complementary medicine practitioners, social worker, and (if needed) addiction medicine specialist (3)[B].
- Treatment should always include nonpharmacologic therapies such as exercise, cognitive-behavioral therapy (CBT), patient and family education, yoga, massage, relaxation techniques, support groups, meditation, and acupuncture.

GENERAL MEASURES

Keep a pain and function diary to record pain and activity levels and how much medication is taken.

MEDICATION

- Always begin with exercise, physical therapy, CBT and self-management skills before or with pain medications. Use sequential time-limited trials of medications, starting at low doses and gradually increasing until either effect or dose-limiting side effects are reached. Rational polypharmacy may be indicated (such as an opioid + neuropathic agent).
- For mild to moderate chronic pain
  - Acetaminophen: daily dose not to exceed total 4 g in healthy adults and 2 g in the elderly or those with hepatic disease or active or past history of alcohol use

- NSAIDs: COX-2 selective inhibitors should be used with caution because of cardiac risks, but may have less gastric risk. If high cardiac risk consider nonselective COX inhibitor (such as naproxen) with or without gastric prophylaxis (depending on ulcer risk).
- "Weak" opioids, including tramadol. Caution: Opioid analgesic combinations can lead to serious acetaminophen or NSAID toxicities if patients exceed safely prescribed doses.
- Topical agents: NSAIDs, lidocaine (gel less expensive than patch), ketamine, capsaicin

- For neuropathic pain
  - Classes of medications include: (i) tricyclic antidepressants (desipramine and nortriptyline have fewer side effects); (ii) serotonin-norepinephrine reuptake inhibitor (SNRI) antidepressants (duloxetine); (iii) anticonvulsants (alpha 2-delta ligands, gabapentin, and pregabalin); (iii) opioids, including tramadol. Example: combination of nortriptyline + gabapentin.
  - See "Neuropathic Pain" topic.
- For moderate to severe chronic pain
  - Strong opioids, including morphine, oxycodone, hydromorphone, oxymorphone, fentanyl. Check opioid equianalgesic tables for dosing by route of administration.
  - No evidence supports any of these strong opioids as superior or having improved side effect profile.
  - In patients with chronic back pain, opioids may be efficacious for short-term use, but long-term benefits and side effects are unclear; in addition, aberrant medication-taking behaviors range from 5% to 24%.
    - Morphine should be avoided in patients with significant renal insufficiency.
    - Methadone should only be prescribed by experienced providers. The only opioid that also acts as *N*-methyl-d-aspartate receptor antagonist, methadone has many drug interactions and can contribute to potentially fatal cardiac arrhythmias.
  - Once stable dose of opioids is established, change to sustained-release formulations if pain constant or very frequent. Short-acting formulations are only for breakthrough or episodic pain.
  - Common side effects: constipation: Senna should be prescribed at time opioids are started; also nausea, sedation, mental status changes, and pruritus

ALERT

Patients on chronic opioid therapy must agree to monitoring. Clinicians should use universal precautions and systems-based practice, including written agreements, random urine drug screens, pill/patch counts, and other measures (see "Ongoing Care") (4,5)[B].

SURGERY/OTHER PROCEDURES

Consider interventional procedures, including joint injections, nerve blocks, spinal cord stimulation, and intrathecal medication among others, as needed.

COMPLEMENTARY & ALTERNATIVE MEDICINE

- Acupuncture: efficacy in chronic neck and back pain and fibromyalgia
- Exercise: efficacy in low back pain and fibromyalgia
- Improved mood and coping skills, decreased disability with CBT
- Mind–body interventions: yoga, tai chi, hypnosis, progressive muscle relaxation, meditation

ONGOING CARE

FOLLOW-UP RECOMMENDATIONS

Patient Monitoring

- It can be difficult to identify appropriate pain relief–seeking behavior from inappropriate drug-seeking, but consistent patient–clinician relationships over time can often discern the difference.
- Always maintain a risk–benefit stance and avoid judging a patient.
- Assess and document benefits, pain levels, functioning, and quality of life. In general, patients successfully taking opioids for pain become more engaged (better relationships and productive work).
- At each visit, assess and document harm, using universal precautions approach. This system-based practice includes the following:
  - Informed consent for opioid therapy
  - Written or electronic agreement between patient and clinician
  - 1 prescribing clinician (or designee) and 1 pharmacy
  - No after-hours prescriptions or early refills
  - Mandatory police reports for medication thefts
  - Random urine drug tests, pill/patch counts
  - Requirements for patient to continue with physical therapy, counseling, psychiatric medications, or other necessary treatments
  - Participate in state's prescription drug monitoring program: See www.pmpalliance.org.
  - Taper and discontinue medications (10% dose reduction per week) if patient does not benefit, if side effects outweigh benefits, or if medications are abused or diverted. If addiction is suspected, always offer treatment for substance abuse (4,5)[B].

PATIENT EDUCATION

American Chronic Pain Association: http://theacpa.org

COMPLICATIONS

- Rate of addiction in chronic pain patients is unclear (3–19% in published literature), but it may reflect rate in the general population.
- Definitions
  - Addiction: chronic biopsychologic disease characterized by impaired control over drug use, compulsive use, and continued use despite harm
  - Physical dependence: withdrawal syndrome produced by abrupt cessation or rapid dose reduction; is not addiction but a physiologic phenomenon
  - Tolerance: state of adaptation when a drug induces changes that diminish its effects over time
  - Diversion: selling drugs or giving them to persons other than for whom they are prescribed

ALERT

Caution: From 1999 to 2007, the rate of unintentional overdose death increased by 124%, largely due to prescription opioid overdoses (especially methadone). In 2011, prescription narcotic overdose was the leading cause of accidental death in the United States (http://www.cdc.gov/homeandrecreationalsafety/overdose/facts.html) (6)[B].

REFERENCES

1. Institute of Medicine, Committee on Advancing Pain Research, Care and Education. *Relieving Pain in America: A Blueprint for Transforming Prevention, Care, Education and Research*. Washington, DC: The National Academies Press; 2011.
2. Alford DP, Krebs EE, Chen IA, et al. Update in pain medicine. *J Gen Intern Med*. 2010;25(11):1222–1226.
3. Dobscha SK, Corson K, Perrin NA, et al. Collaborative care for chronic pain in primary care: a cluster randomized trial. *JAMA*. 2009;301(12):1242–1252.
4. American Society of Anesthesiologists Task Force on Chronic Pain Management, American Society of Regional Anesthesia and Pain Medicine. Practice guidelines for chronic pain management: an updated report by the American Society of Anesthesiologists Task Force on Chronic Pain Management and the American Society of Regional Anesthesia and Pain Medicine. *Anesthesiology*. 2010;112(4):810–833.
5. Manchikanti L, Abdi S, Atluri S, et al. American Society of Interventional Pain Physicians (ASIPP) guidelines for responsible opiod prescribing in chronic non-cancer pain: Part 2—guidance. *Pain Physician*. 2012;15(Suppl 3):S67–S116.
6. Bohnert AS, Valenstein M, Bair MJ, et al. Association between opioid prescribing patterns and opioid overdose-related deaths. *JAMA*. 2011;305(13):1315–1321.

ADDITIONAL READING

- Federation of State Medical Boards of the United States, Inc. Model policy for the use of controlled substances for the treatment of pain www.painpolicy.wisc.edu/sites/www.painpolicy.wisc.edu/files/model04.pdf. Accessed 2014.
- Washington State Agency Medical Director's Group. Interagency guideline on opioid dosing for chronic non-cancer pain: an educational aid to improve care and safety with opioid therapy. www.agencymeddirectors.wa.gov

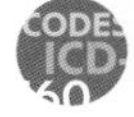

CODES

ICD10

- G89.29 Other chronic pain
- G89.21 Chronic pain due to trauma
- G89.28 Other chronic postprocedural pain

CLINICAL PEARLS

- Start with the presumption that the patient's pain is *real*, even if pathophysiologic evidence for it cannot be found.
- Emphasize that being pain-free may not be possible but that better function and quality of life can be shared goals.
- Use a multidisciplinary approach with nonpharmacologic therapies, exercise, patient self-management strategies, and thoughtful medication use with clear goals, expectations, and documentation of care plan.
- Use universal precautions and systems-based practice to safely and effectively prescribe opioids for chronic pain.

CIRRHOSIS OF THE LIVER

Urooj Najm, MBBS • Najm Hasan Siddiqui, MD

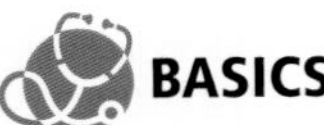

BASICS

DESCRIPTION
A chronic hepatocellular disease involving inflammation, necrosis, and fibrosis potentially leading to liver failure and/or cancer.

EPIDEMIOLOGY
- Predominant age: 40–50 years old
- Predominant sex: male > female; more women get cirrhosis from alcohol abuse.
- 9th leading cause of death among U.S. adults

ETIOLOGY AND PATHOPHYSIOLOGY
- Chronic hepatitis C (26%)
- Alcohol abuse (21%)
- Hepatitis C with alcoholic liver disease (15%)
- Nonalcoholic steatohepatitis/obesity (~10%)
- Hepatitis B plus hepatitis D infection (15%)
- Other: hemochromatosis; autoimmune hepatitis; primary biliary cirrhosis; secondary biliary cirrhosis; primary sclerosing cholangitis; Wilson disease; α_1-antitrypsin deficiency; granulomatous disease (e.g., sarcoidosis); drug-induced liver disease (e.g., methotrexate, α-methyldopa, amiodarone); venous outflow obstruction (e.g., Budd-Chiari syndrome, veno-occlusive disease); chronic right-sided heart failure; tricuspid regurgitation; and rare genetic, metabolic, and infectious causes

Genetics
Hemochromatosis, Wilson disease, and α_1-antitrypsin deficiency in adults are associated with cirrhosis.

RISK FACTORS
Alcohol abuse; intravenous drug abuse; obesity; blood transfusion

GENERAL PREVENTION
- Mitigate risk factors (e.g., alcohol abuse); *>80% of chronic liver disease is preventable.*
- Limit alcohol consumption; advise weight loss in overweight or obese patients.
  - Elevated BMI and alcohol with additive link to liver disease (1)

COMMONLY ASSOCIATED CONDITIONS
Diabetes, alcoholism, drug abuse, depression, obesity

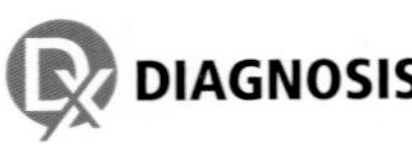

DIAGNOSIS

HISTORY
- Review risk factors (alcohol abuse, viral hepatitis; family history of primary liver cancer, other liver disease, or autoimmune disease)
- Symptoms
  - Fatigue, malaise, weakness
  - Anorexia, weight loss (gain if ascites/edema)
  - Right upper abdominal pain
  - Absent/Irregular menses
  - Diminished libido, erectile dysfunction
  - Tea-colored urine, clay-colored stools
  - Edema, abdominal swelling/bloating
  - Bruising, bleeding, hematemesis, hematochezia, melena, pruritus
  - Night blindness

PHYSICAL EXAM
Physical exam may be normal until end-stage disease:
- Skin changes: spider angiomata, palmar erythema, jaundice, scleral icterus, ecchymoses, caput medusa, hyperpigmentation
- Hepatomegaly (small, fibrotic liver in end-stage disease)
- Splenomegaly (if portal hypertension)
- Central obesity
- Abdominal fluid wave, shifting dullness (ascites)
- Gynecomastia
- Dupuytren contractures
- Pretibial, presacral pitting edema and clubbing (especially in hepatopulmonary syndrome)
- Asterixis; mental status changes
- Muscle wasting, weakness

DIFFERENTIAL DIAGNOSIS
Steatohepatitis, other causes of portal hypertension (e.g., portal vein thrombosis, lymphoma), metastatic or multifocal cancer in the liver, vascular congestion (e.g., cardiac cirrhosis), acute alcoholic hepatitis

DIAGNOSTIC TESTS & INTERPRETATION

Initial Tests (lab, imaging)
- Aspartate aminotransferase/alanine aminotransferase (AST/ALT): mildly elevated; typically AST > ALT; enzymes normalize as cirrhosis progresses.
- Elevated alkaline phosphatase (ALP), gamma-glutamyl transpeptidase (GGT), and total/direct bilirubin indicates cholestasis.
- Anemia from hemolysis, folate deficiency, and splenomegaly
- Decreased platelet count from portal hypertension with splenomegaly
- Impaired synthetic liver function
  - Low albumin and cholesterol
  - Prolonged prothrombin (PT), international normalized ratio (INR), partial thromboplastin time (PTT). Vitamin K–dependent clotting factors
- Progressive cirrhosis
  - Elevated ammonia level; BUN, sodium, and potassium
- α-Fetoprotein level at diagnosis to screen for hepatocellular carcinoma (HCC)
- Abdominal ultrasound q6–12 months to screen for hepatocellular carcinoma
- Doppler ultrasound of hepatic/portal veins
- MRI best follow-up test for HCC if α-fetoprotein elevated and/or liver mass found on ultrasound
- Noninvasive modalities, such as elastography, are being researched as an alternative to liver biopsy (2).

Follow-Up Tests & Special Considerations
To determine specific etiology, consider the following:
- Hepatitis serologies (particularly B and C)
- Serum ethanol and GGT if alcohol abuse suspected
- Antimitochondrial antibody to screen for primary biliary cirrhosis
- Anti–smooth muscle and antinuclear antibodies to screen for chronic active (autoimmune) hepatitis. Iron saturation (>50%) and ferritin (markedly increased) to screen for hemochromatosis; if abnormal, check hemochromatosis (HFE) genetics/mutation analysis.
- α_1-Antitrypsin phenotype screen
- Ceruloplasmin level to screen for Wilson disease; if low, check copper excretion (serum copper plus 24-hour urine copper).

Diagnostic Procedures/Other
- Liver biopsy: percutaneous if INR <1.5 and no ascites; otherwise, transjugular
- Liver–spleen scan to diagnose portal hypertension if biopsy cannot be performed
- Endoscopy if portal hypertension; rule out esophageal varices/portal hypertensive gastropathy (3)[C].

Test Interpretation
- Fibrous bands and regenerative nodules are classic features of cirrhosis on biopsy.
- Other histologic findings vary with etiology
  - Alcoholic liver disease: steatosis, polymorphonuclear (PMN) leukocyte infiltrate, ballooning degeneration of hepatocytes, Mallory bodies, giant mitochondria
  - Chronic hepatitis B and C: periportal lymphocytic inflammation
  - Nonalcoholic steatohepatitis (NASH): identical to alcoholic liver disease and confirmed by history. Steatosis may be absent in advanced disease ("burned-out NASH")
  - Biliary cirrhosis: PMN infiltrate in wall of bile ducts, inflammation increased in portal spaces, progressive loss of bile ducts in portal spaces.
  - Hemochromatosis: intrahepatic iron stores increased (iron stain or weighted biopsy tissue)
  - α_1-Antitrypsin deficiency: positive periodic acid–Schiff (PAS) bodies in hepatocytes

TREATMENT

Outpatient care except for major GI bleeding, altered mental status, sepsis/infection, rapidly progressing hepatic decompensation, and renal failure

GENERAL MEASURES
- Patients *must* abstain from alcohol, drugs, hepatotoxic medications, and hepatotoxic herbs.
- Immunize for pneumococcus, hepatitis A/B, and influenza.
- NASH: weight reduction, exercise, optimal control of lipids/glucose

MEDICATION

First Line
Treat the underlying cause first (*note prescribing precautions in decompensated cirrhosis*):
- Hepatitis C: Goal of treatment is to eradicate hepatitis C virus (HCV) RNA in serum ≥6 months after completing antiviral treatment. Combination therapy of pegylated interferon (PEG-IFN) with ribavirin is the standard of care for most genotypes.
- Hepatitis B: Goal of treatment is to achieve HBeAg seroconversion. Adefovir 10 mg PO daily, entecavir 0.5–1 mg PO daily, telbivudine 600 mg PO daily, or lamivudine 100 mg PO daily for minimum of 1 year, or continue for at least 6 months after HBeAg seroconversion; alternatively, peginterferon-α 2a, 180 μg SC weekly for 48 weeks. Lamivudine is no longer recommended as first-line agent due to high rates of resistance.
- Biliary cirrhosis: ursodeoxycholic acid (ursodiol) 13–15 mg/kg PO divided BID–QID with food, indefinitely (4)[A]; bile acid sequestrants (BAS) are first-line therapy for pruritus: cholestyramine 4–8 g PO BID; antihistamines; rifampicin 150–300 mg BID or PO opiate antagonists such as naltrexone 50 mg/day can be used for pruritus if ursodiol is ineffective.

- Wilson disease: initial treatment with penicillamine 1,000–1,500 mg/day PO BID–QID or trientine 750–1,500 mg/day PO BID–TID on empty stomach. Trientine (Syprine) is better tolerated. After 1 year, zinc acetate 150 mg/day PO BID–TID for maintenance. Zinc is a drug of choice for presymptomatic, pregnant, and pediatric populations.
- Autoimmune (chronic active) hepatitis: prednisone 30–60 mg/day initially, maintenance 5–20 mg/day with or without azathioprine (Imuran) 0.5–1 mg/kg; adjust to keep transaminase levels normal. The combination regime is preferred. Maintenance therapy can be discontinued after at least 24 months of treatment and continued normal AST and ALT.
- Esophageal varices: propranolol 40–160 mg or nadolol 40 mg daily to lower portal pressure by 20 mm Hg, systolic pressure to 90–100 mm Hg, and pulse rate by 25% (3)[A].
- Ascites/edema: low-sodium (<2 g/day) diet and spironolactone 100–400 mg/day with or without furosemide 40–160 mg/day PO; torsemide may substitute for furosemide.
- Encephalopathy: lactulose 15–45 mL BID, titrate to induce 3 loose bowel movements daily. Combination therapy with rifaximin (550 mg PO BID) is superior to prevent recurrent hepatic encephalopathy (5)[B].
- Pruritus: ursodiol, cholestyramine, and antihistamines (e.g., hydroxyzine)
- Renal insufficiency: Stop diuretics and nephrotoxic drugs, normalize electrolytes, and hospitalize for plasma expansion or dialysis.
- Prophylactic antibiotics for invasive procedures, GI bleeding, or history of spontaneous bacterial peritonitis (3)[A]
- Proton pump inhibitor for esophageal varices requiring banding or portal hypertensive gastropathy (6)[A]
- Recombinant factor VIIa to correct bleeding shows no survival benefit (7).

ISSUES FOR REFERRAL

Liver transplant evaluation at first onset of complications (ascites, variceal bleeding, encephalopathy), jaundice, or liver lesion suggestive of hepatocellular carcinoma and/or when evidence of hepatic dysfunction develops (Child-Turcotte-Pugh >7 and Model for End-stage Liver Disease [MELD] >10).

SURGERY/OTHER PROCEDURES

- Varices: endoscopic ligation, typically 4–6 treatments (if acute bleed, use pre-esophagogastroduodenoscopy [EGD] octreotide as vasoconstrictor); transjugular intrahepatic shunt (TIPS) second-line or salvage therapy for acute bleed (3)
- Ascites: if tense, therapeutic paracentesis every 2 weeks PRN; caution if pedal edema absent
- Fulminant hepatic failure: liver transplantation
- Hepatocellular carcinoma: curable if small with radiofrequency ablation or resection and transplant

COMPLEMENTARY & ALTERNATIVE MEDICINE

- Zinc sulfate 220 mg BID may improve dysgeusia and appetite. Adjunct for hepatic encephalopathy.
- Milk thistle (silymarin) may lower transaminases and improve symptoms.
- Danshen and huang qi injections may promote improvement; further studies needed (8)[B].
- Hepatotoxicity and drug interactions are common with many herbal medications (9).

INPATIENT CONSIDERATIONS

Admission Criteria/Initial Stabilization

Major GI bleeding, altered mental status, sepsis/infection, rapidly progressing hepatic decompensation, renal failure

ONGOING CARE

FOLLOW-UP RECOMMENDATIONS

Regular conditioning may help fatigue.

Patient Monitoring

- Once stable, monitor liver enzymes, platelets, and PT q6–12 months.
- Patients older than 55 years old with chronic hepatitis B or C, elevated INR, or low platelets are at highest risk for HCC. Check α-fetoprotein and liver ultrasound q6–12 months for screening in patients with cirrhosis (7,10)[C].
- Endoscopy at diagnosis and every 3 years in compensated and every 1 year in decompensated cirrhotic patients to screen for varices (3)[C]

DIET

- Protein (1–1.5 g/kg body weight), high fiber, daily multivitamin (without iron), and sodium (<2 g/day, essential if ascites/edema)
- A high-protein diet may precipitate encephalopathy, but protein restriction is no longer recommended (7).
- Coffee consumption has a graded and inverse association with liver cancer (11)[A].

PATIENT EDUCATION

- Educate about when to seek emergency care (e.g., hematemesis, altered mental status).
- Maintain sobriety/recovery/smoking cessation (includes no cannabis).
- Update all required immunizations and educate about hepatitis C transmission precautions.

PROGNOSIS

- At diagnosis of cirrhosis, expect 5–20 years of asymptomatic disease.
- At onset of complications, death typically within 5 years if no transplant
  - 5% per year develop HCC
  - 50% of cirrhotics develop ascites over 10 years; 50% 5-year survival once ascites develops
  - Acute variceal bleeding is the most common fatal complication; 30% mortality
  - Median survival after complications (ascites, variceal bleeding, encephalopathy) is 1.5 years (7).
  - With transplant, 85% survive 1 year; after transplant, ~5% annual mortality
- <25% of eligible patients receive a transplant because of donor organ shortage.

COMPLICATIONS

Ascites; edema; infections; encephalopathy; GI bleeding; esophageal varices, gastropathy, colopathy; hepatorenal syndrome; hepatopulmonary syndrome; hepatocellular carcinoma; fulminant hepatic failure; complications after transplant (e.g., surgical, rejection, infections)

REFERENCES

1. Hart CL, Morrison DS, Batty GD, et al. Effect of body mass index and alcohol consumption on liver disease: analysis of data from two prospective cohort studies. *BMJ*. 2010;340:c1240.
2. Tsochatzis EA, Gurusamy KS, Ntaoula S, et al. Elastography for the diagnosis of severity of fibrosis in chronic liver disease: a meta-analysis of diagnostic accuracy. *J Hepatol*. 2011;54(4):650–659.
3. Garcia-Tsao G, Sanyal AJ, Grace ND, et al. Prevention and management of gastroesophageal varices and variceal hemorrhage in cirrhosis. *Hepatology*. 2007;46(3):922–938.
4. Lindor KD, Gershwin ME, Poupon R, et al. Primary biliary cirrhosis. *Hepatology*. 2009;50(1):291–308.
5. Sharma BC, Sharma P, Lunia MK, et al. A randomized, double-blind, controlled trial comparing rifaximin plus lactulose with lactulose alone in treatment of overt hepatic encephalopathy. *Am J Gastroenterol*. 2013;108(9):1458–1463.
6. Leontiadis GI, Sharma VK, Howden CW. Proton pump inhibitor therapy for peptic ulcer bleeding: cochrane collaboration meta-analysis of randomized controlled trials. *Mayo Clin Proc*. 2007;82(3):286–296.
7. Garcia-Tsao G. Managing the complications of cirrhosis, hepatitis annual update 2008, clinical care options: hepatitis. http://clinicaloptions.com/Hepatitis/Annual%20Updates/2008%20Annual%20Update.aspx. Accessed 2014.
8. Zhu C, Cao H, Zhou X, et al. Meta-analysis of the clinical value of danshen injection and huangqi injection in liver cirrhosis. *Evid Based Complement Alternat Med*. 2013;2013:842824.
9. Verma S, Thuluvath PJ. Complementary and alternative medicine in hepatology: review of the evidence of efficacy. *Clin Gastroenterol Hepatol*. 2007;5(4):408–416.
10. Yang JD, Roberts LR. Hepatocellular carcinoma: a global view. *Nat Rev Gastroenterol Hepatol*. 2010;7(8):448–458.
11. Bravi F, Bosetti C, Tavani A, et al. Coffee reduces risk for hepatocellular carcinoma: an updated meta-analysis. *Clin Gastroenterol Hepatol*. 2013;11(11):1413–1421.

ADDITIONAL READING

- Chou R, Wasson N. Blood tests to diagnose fibrosis or cirrhosis in patients with chronic hepatitis C virus infection: a systematic review. *Ann Intern Med*. 2013;158(11):807–820.
- Nierhoff J, Chávez Ortiz AA, Herrmann E, et al. The efficiency of acoustic radiation force impulse imaging for the staging of liver fibrosis: a meta-analysis. *Eur Radiol*. 2013;23(11):3040–3053.

SEE ALSO

Algorithm: Cirrhosis

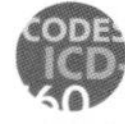

CODES

ICD10

- K74.60 Unspecified cirrhosis of liver
- K70.30 Alcoholic cirrhosis of liver without ascites
- K74.69 Other cirrhosis of liver

CLINICAL PEARLS

- 80% of chronic liver disease that leads to cirrhosis is preventable (primarily alcoholic).
- Check abdominal ultrasound every 6 months for early detection of hepatocellular carcinoma.
- Update necessary immunizations and focus on treatment of underlying cause of cirrhosis (hepatitis C; alcohol abuse, etc.).

CLOSTRIDIUM DIFFICILE INFECTION

Samuel Luke Brown, DO • Scott W. Rodi, MD, MPH, FACEP

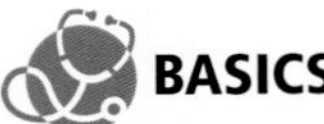

BASICS

DESCRIPTION

- *Clostridium difficile* is a gram-positive, spore-forming anaerobic bacillus that releases toxins to produce clinical disease.
- Infection caused by *C. difficile* is usually linked to broad-spectrum antibiotic use, hospitalization, and age.
- Severity of infection can range from diarrhea to colitis to perforation to death.
- System(s) affected: gastrointestinal
- Synonyms(s): *C. difficile*–associated disease or diarrhea (CDAD); *C. difficile* colitis; antibiotic-associated diarrhea; *C. difficile*

EPIDEMIOLOGY

Incidence

- *C. difficile* infection is among the most common causes of hospital-acquired infection along with methicillin-resistant Staphylococcus aureus and vancomycin-resistant enterococcus (1).
- Rates of complications associated with *C. difficile* such as treatment failure and recurrence are increasing (1).

Prevalence

- *C. difficile* causes ~25% of all cases of antibiotic-associated diarrhea.
- Community-acquired *C. difficile* infection is increasing, which may make prevalence much higher than previously thought.
- *C. difficile* is present as a commensurate organism in 2–5% of the adult U.S. population.

ETIOLOGY AND PATHOPHYSIOLOGY

- *C. difficile* are motile bacteria existing in vegetative and spore forms. *C. difficile* spores can survive for months even in harsh conditions.
- *C. difficile* can thrive in the colon and cause infection if the normal flora is disrupted.
- Host factors, such as the presence of antibodies to *C. difficile* toxins, reduce severity and prevent recurrences of infection.
- *C. difficile* produces toxins that mediate disease:
  - Toxins A (enterotoxin) and B (cytotoxin) attract neutrophils and monocytes and degrade colonic epithelial cells, causing colitis, pseudomembrane colitis, and watery diarrhea.
- BI/NAP1/027 strain of *C. difficile* has been shown to produce more virulent characteristics.
- Binary toxin produces a virulent form of disease (different from toxin A or B); this may result in increased rates of colectomies and mortality.
- Spread by fecal–oral contact. Once ingested, spores are acid-resistant (pass through stomach) and take up residence in the colon on exposure to bile acids.
- *C. difficile* can produce heat-resistant spores that are not killed by routine cleaning or alcohol-based hand sanitizers.

Genetics

No known genetic factors

RISK FACTORS

- Host risk factors
  - Age >65 years
  - Hospitalization or stay in long-term health care facility. The length of stay is directly correlated with the risk.
  - Comorbidities, including inflammatory bowel disease, immunosuppression, tube feeding, chronic liver disease, and end-stage renal disease
  - Previous *C. difficile* infection
- Recurrence from prior infection
  - Recurrence rates are shown to be 15–35%. Patients who have 1 recurrence are 45% more likely to have a 2nd recurrence, and patients with 2nd recurrences have up to a 65% chance of 3rd recurrence.
- Factors disrupting normal colonic microbiota
  - Exposure to almost all antibiotics is associated with *C. difficile* infection (this includes perioperative prophylaxis). Fluoroquinolones, cephalosporins, and clindamycin are most commonly implicated (alter normal intestinal flora).
  - Use of antacids, especially proton pump inhibitors (PPIs)
- Community-acquired *C. difficile* infections may affect patients without risk factors (younger, no recent antibiotic exposure).

Geriatric Considerations

C. difficile is the most common cause of acute diarrheal illness in long-term care facilities. Elderly patients also commonly have multiple other risk factors (comorbid disease, antibiotic exposure, medication use).

Pediatric Considerations

Neonates have a higher rate of *C. difficile* colonization (25–80%) but are generally less symptomatic than adults (possibly due to immature toxin receptors).

GENERAL PREVENTION

- A comprehensive infection control program decreases the incidence of *C. difficile* infection.
- 2010 Society for Healthcare Epidemiology of America (SHEA)/Infectious Diseases Society of America (IDS) guidelines
  - Measures for health care workers, patients, and visitors:
    - Contact precautions, including gloves and gowns, on entry to room
    - Hand hygiene with soap and water before and after patient interaction
    - Accommodate patients with *C. difficile* infection in private rooms, if possible.
  - Environmental cleaning and disinfection
    - Disinfection with hypochlorite solution or other spore-killing solutions
    - Identification and reduction of environmental sources of *C. difficile,* including the use of nondisposable rectal thermometers
  - Antimicrobial use restrictions
    - Minimize the frequency and duration of antibiotic therapy.

COMMONLY ASSOCIATED CONDITIONS

Pseudomembranous colitis, toxic megacolon, sepsis, colonic perforation

DIAGNOSIS

HISTORY

- Identify known risk factors such as recent antibiotic use (especially broad-spectrum fluoroquinolones and cephalosporins)
- Diarrhea (defined as >3 stools in 24 hours) that is watery, foul-smelling, and sometimes bloody (1)
- Fever (<10%), anorexia, nausea
- Recent hospitalization or stay at nursing facility

PHYSICAL EXAM

There is a wide range of physical exam findings, ranging from mild abdominal pain to peritoneal findings and shock:

- Mild or moderate disease: mild lower abdominal pain, often cramping pain
- Severe disease: fever, nausea/vomiting, dehydration
- Severe, complicated disease: shock, peritonitis, ileus

DIFFERENTIAL DIAGNOSIS

- Antibiotic-associated diarrhea
- inflammatory bowel disease
- Enteric infections
- Food poisoning

DIAGNOSTIC TESTS & INTERPRETATION

- SHEA/IDSA guidelines
  - Mild or moderate disease: leukocytosis with white blood cell (WBC) count <15,000 cells/μL and a serum creatinine level <1.5× the premorbid level
  - Severe, uncomplicated disease: leukocytosis with a WBC count >15,000 cells/μL or a serum creatinine level >1.5× the premorbid level
  - Severe, complicated disease: Markers of severe infection include hypotension, sepsis, markedly elevated WBC count, and bandemia.
    - Other signs seen on imaging include obstruction, perforation, toxic megacolon, and colonic wall thickening.
- Current recommendations are for 2-step testing using a sensitive initial screening test followed by a more specific confirmatory test if positive.
- General approach: Screen with the *C. difficile* common antigen test; if positive, confirm with either enzyme immunoassay test or cell cytotoxic assay.

Initial Tests (lab, imaging)

- Screening: *C. difficile* common antigen test: Tests for glutamate dehydrogenase (GDH), found in both toxic and nontoxic strains of *C. difficile* (sensitivity, 85–95%; specificity, 89–99%).
- Confirmatory: enzyme immunoassay for toxins (A/B or A); rapid results, inexpensive, easy to use (sensitivity 63–94%)
- Confirmatory: cell cytotoxicity assay; 24–48 hours for results; labor-intensive (sensitivity 67–100%)
- Stool culture is the most sensitive test; however, non–toxin-producing strains also detected. Generally, used to evaluate epidemiology.
- Polymerase chain reaction (PCR)–based testing is becoming the preferred test for *C. difficile* (1).
- Repeat testing during the same episode of diarrhea is discouraged because stool carriage persists for 3–6 weeks after successful treatment (2).

Diagnostic Procedures/Other

- Endoscopy can be used to evaluate for pseudomembranes and exclude other conditions:
  - Although not all patients with *C. difficile* infection have pseudomembranes, their presence is pathognomonic for *C. difficile*.
- Flexible sigmoidoscopy may miss 15–20% of pseudomembranes that may be more proximal in the colon.
- Colonoscopy evaluates the entire colon: used when diagnosis is in doubt or severity demands rapid diagnosis.
- Plain films may show thumbprinting and colonic distension.
- CT radiography may show mucosal wall thickening, thickened colonic wall, and pericolonic inflammation.

Test Interpretation
Pseudomembranes consist of inflammatory and cellular debris that forms visible exudates that can obscure the underlying mucosa. These exudates have a yellow to grayish color.

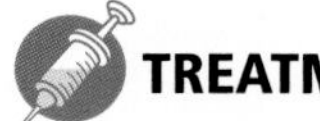

TREATMENT

GENERAL MEASURES
- Avoid antimotility agents and opiates.
- Avoid indiscriminate use of antibiotics.
- PPIs, associated with a 42% increased risk of recurrence if used concurrently with treatment for *C. difficile* colitis
- Discontinue offending antibiotic, if possible.

MEDICATION
First Line
- Mild or moderate infection
  - Metronidazole is the drug of choice for mild to moderate *C. difficile* infection due to low cost and to minimize the emergence of vancomycin-resistant organisms:
    - 500 mg PO TID for 10–14 days
    - If patient is unable to take oral medications, then intravenous (IV) metronidazole or intraluminal vancomycin can be used.
- Severe infection
  - Vancomycin is 1st-line therapy in patients with severe or fulminant *C. difficile* infection:
    - 125 mg PO QID for 10–14 days
    - Vancomycin retention enema if unable to take PO or there is evidence of poor gastrointestinal motility
- Severe, complicated infection
  - Vancomycin: 500 mg PO QID *AND* metronidazole 500 mg PO TID
- 1st recurrence
  - Treat the same as 1st episode.
- 2nd recurrence
  - Vancomycin taper and/or pulse: vancomycin 125 mg PO QID for 10–14 days, then 125 mg PO BID for 7 days, then 125 mg PO once daily for 7 days, then 125 mg PO every 2–3 days for 2–8 weeks:
    - The pulse dosing every 2–3 days allows spores to germinate and then be killed.

ALERT
When using vancomycin for treatment of *C. difficile* infection, oral or rectal formulations must be used. IV formulations are not excreted into the colonic lumen.

Second Line
- Vancomycin: indicated for patients who cannot tolerate or have failed metronidazole therapy and for those who are pregnant
- Fidaxomicin is another option 200 mg PO BID. Similar cure rates to vancomycin and lower recurrence rates:
- Fidaxomicin rapidly kills *C. difficile*, whereas vancomycin inhibits growth. Fidaxomicin has a narrow antimicrobial spectrum and helps preserve normal anaerobic flora.
- Fecal transplant is an effective treatment, especially for virulent 027 strain and recurrent infections. Stool is biologically active and contains a mixture of living organisms that can help restore normal recipient gut microbiota. Recipient gut flora have been transformed in as few as 3 days following fecal transplantation (3).
- A recent meta-analysis of 11 studies showed a cure rate of 89% with no adverse events in over 500 patients (1).
- Donors are carefully screened. Donor stool is homogenized in water and infused via nasogastric tube or colonoscopy.

SURGERY/OTHER PROCEDURES
If *C. difficile* infection progresses to toxic megacolon, peritonitis, or sepsis, consult specialty services such as surgery, critical care, and/or infectious diseases.

COMPLEMENTARY AND ALTERNATIVE MEDICINE
- Adjunctive therapy with intravenous immunoglobulin (IVIG) has shown initial promise, but more data are required before routine clinical use (2).
- Probiotics may play a role in prevention. Probiotics have an (strain-specific) inhibitory effect on *C. difficile*.
- Other treatment options under investigation include the following:
  - New antibiotics (Rifalazil, Tolevamer, and Ramoplanin)
  - Monoclonal antibodies to directly modulate the effects of toxins
  - Vaccine form of *C. difficile* antitoxin antibody

INPATIENT CONSIDERATIONS
Admission Criteria/Initial Stabilization
- Hypovolemia
- Inability to keep up with enteric losses
- Hematochezia
- Electrolyte disturbances

IV Fluids
To maintain volume status

Discharge Criteria
- Improved diarrhea severity and frequency
- Tolerating oral diet and medications
- Do not repeat testing for toxins, as they may shed for weeks following an acute infection.

ONGOING CARE

FOLLOW-UP RECOMMENDATIONS
Many patients can be treated as outpatients.

Patient Monitoring
- Relapses of colitis occur in 15–30%.
- Relapses typically occur 2–10 days after discontinuing antibiotics.

DIET
Regular diet

PATIENT EDUCATION
Educate patients about *C. difficile* transmission, the importance of hand washing, and the appropriate use of antibiotics.

ALERT
Alcohol-based hand sanitizers are not effective against *C. difficile*. Wash with soap and water.

PROGNOSIS
- Most patients improve with conservative management and oral antibiotics.
- 1–3% of patients develop severe colitis requiring emergency colectomy.

REFERENCES

1. Khanna S, Pardi DS. *Clostridium difficile* infection: management strategies for a difficult disease. *Therap Adv Gastroenterol*. 2014;7(2):72–86.
2. Oldfield EC IV, Oldfield EC III, Johnson DA. Clinical update for the diagnosis and treatment of *Clostridium difficile* infection. *World J Gastrointest Pharmacol Ther*. 2014;5(1):1–26.
3. Shankar V, Hamilton MJ, Khoruts A, et al. Species and genus level resolution analysis of gut microbiota in *Clostridium difficile* patients following fecal microbiota transplantation. *Microbiome*. 2014;2:13.

ADDITIONAL READING

- Cohen SH, Gerding DN, Johnson S, et al. Clinical practice guidelines for *Clostridium difficile* infection in adults: 2010 update by the Society for Healthcare Epidemiology of America (SHEA) and the Infectious Diseases Society of America (IDSA). *Infect Control Hosp Epidemiol*. 2010;31(5):431–455.
- Kassam Z, Lee CH, Yuan Y, et al. Fecal microbiota transplantation for *Clostridium difficile* infection: systematic review and meta-analysis. *Am J Gastroenterol*. 2013;108(4):500–508.
- McCollum DL, Rodriguez JM. Detection, treatment, and prevention of *Clostridium difficile* infection. *Clin Gastroenterol Hepatol*. 2012;10(6):581–592.

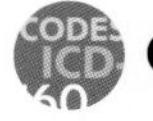

CODES

ICD10
A04.7 Enterocolitis due to Clostridium difficile

CLINICAL PEARLS
- *C. difficile* is spread by fecal–oral contact.
- Alcohol-based hand sanitizers are ineffective against *C. difficile*. Wash hands with soap and water.
- Testing and treatment of asymptomatic patients is not recommended.
- Patients may shed organism or toxin for weeks after treatment. Repeat toxin assays are not helpful.

COLIC, INFANTILE

Daniel T. Lee, MD, MA • Arthur Ohannessian, MD

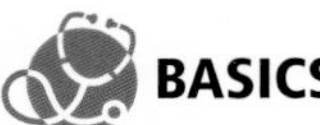

BASICS

DESCRIPTION

- Colic is defined as excessive crying in an otherwise healthy baby.
- A commonly used criteria is the Wessel criteria or the Rule of Three: crying lasts for:
  - >3 hours a day
  - >3 days a week
  - Persists >3 weeks
- Many clinicians no longer use the criterion of persistence for >3 weeks because few parents or clinicians will wait that long before evaluation or intervention.
- Some clinicians feel that colic represents the extreme end of the spectrum of normal crying, whereas most feel that colic is a distinct clinical entity.

EPIDEMIOLOGY

Incidence

- Predominant age: between 2 weeks and 4 months of age
- Predominant sex: male = female

Prevalence

- Probably between 10% and 25% of infants
- Range is somewhere between 8% and 40% of infants.

Pediatric Considerations

This is a problem during infancy.

ETIOLOGY AND PATHOPHYSIOLOGY

The cause is unknown. Factors that may play a role include the following:

- Infant gastroesophageal reflux disease
- Allergy to cow's milk, soy milk, or breast milk protein
- Fruit juice intolerance
- Swallowing air during the process of crying, feeding, or sucking
- Overfeeding or feeding too quickly; underfeeding also has been proposed
- Inadequate burping after feeding
- Family tension
- Parental anxiety, depression, and/or fatigue
- Parent–infant interaction mismatch
- Baby's inability to console himself or herself when dealing with stimuli
- Increased gut hormone motilin, causing hyperperistalsis
- Functional lactose overload (i.e., breast milk that has a lower lipid content can have faster transit time in the intestine, leading to more lactose fermentation in the gut and hence gas and distension) (1)[C]
- Tobacco smoke exposure

RISK FACTORS

- Physiologic predisposition in infant but no definitive risk factors have been established. However, emerging data suggest maternal smoking or exposure to nicotine replacement therapy during pregnancy is associated with higher incidence of infantile colic (2)[B].
- Infants with a maternal history of migraine headaches are twice as likely to have colic (3)[B].

GENERAL PREVENTION

Colic is generally not preventable.

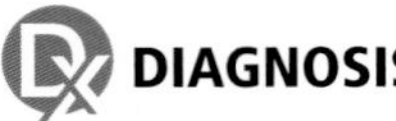

DIAGNOSIS

HISTORY

- Evaluation for Wessel criteria: crying lasts for >3 hours per day, >3 days per week, and persists >3 weeks.
- The colicky episodes may have a clear beginning and end.
- The crying is generally spontaneous, without preceding events triggering the episodes.
- The crying is typically different from normal crying. Colicky crying may be louder, more turbulent, variable in pitch, and appear more like screaming.
- The infant may be difficult to soothe or console regardless of how the parents try to help.
- The infant acts normally when not colicky.
- Assess the support system of caregivers and families, including coping skills.

PHYSICAL EXAM

- A comprehensive physical exam is normal.
- Because excessive crying may be a risk factor for shaken baby syndrome or other forms of child abuse (4)[B], be sure to examine the child carefully for signs of shaken baby syndrome or other types of child abuse.

DIFFERENTIAL DIAGNOSIS

Any organic cause for excessive or qualitatively different crying in infants such as:

- Infections (e.g., meningitis, sepsis, otitis media, or UTI)
- GI issues such as gastroesophageal reflux, intussusception, lactose intolerance, constipation, anal fissure, or strangulated hernia
- Trauma, which includes foreign bodies, corneal abrasion, occult fracture, digit or penile hair tourniquet syndrome, or child abuse

DIAGNOSTIC TESTS & INTERPRETATION

Diagnostic Procedures/Other

A thorough history and physical exam should be performed to rule out other causes. Otherwise, no diagnostic procedures or imaging is indicated.

TREATMENT

GENERAL MEASURES

- Soothe by holding and rocking the baby.
- Use a pacifier.
- Use of gentle rhythmic motion (e.g., strollers, infant swings, car rides).
- Place near white noise (e.g., vacuum cleaner, clothes dryer, white noise machine).
- Crib vibrators or car-ride simulators have not proven to be helpful (5)[B].
- Increased carrying or use of infant carrier has not been shown to improve colic (5)[B].
- Burping does not significantly lower colic events and can cause significant increase in regurgitation episodes (6)[B].
- Employ the 5Ss (need to be done concurrently):
  - Swaddling: tight wrapping with blanket; may be especially beneficial in infants <8 weeks old (7)[B]
  - Side: laying baby on side
  - Shushing: loud white noise
  - Swinging: rhythmic, jiggly motion
  - Sucking: sucking on anything (e.g., nipple, finger, pacifier)

MEDICATION

- Dicyclomine (Bentyl) has been proven beneficial, but the potential serious adverse effects (apnea, seizures, and syncope) have precluded its use. Furthermore, the manufacturer has made the medication contraindicated for infants <6 months (8)[B].
- Simethicone has not been shown to be beneficial (8)[B].

ISSUES FOR REFERRAL

Excessive vomiting, poor weight gain, recurrent respiratory diseases, or bloody stools should prompt referral to a specialist.

COMPLEMENTARY & ALTERNATIVE MEDICINE

- Recent data from a large randomized controlled study involving nine neonatal units in Italy found that prophylactic use of *Lactobacillus reuteri* was beneficial. At 3 months of age, the mean duration of crying time (38 vs. 71 minutes; $P < .01$), the mean number of regurgitations per day (2.9 vs. 4.6; $P < .01$), and the mean number of evacuations per day (4.2 vs. 3.6; $P < .01$) for the *L. reuteri* 17938 and placebo groups, respectively, were significantly different (9)[A].
- However, the effect of *L. reuteri* has not been as robust in infants already diagnosed with colic. A placebo-controlled study of 50 infants given *L. reuteri* had significantly reduced median daily crying times throughout the study (370–35 min/day vs. 300–90 min/day in placebo group). However, weight gain, stooling frequency, and incidence of regurgitation were similar in both groups (10)[B].
- *L. reuteri* is available as over-the-counter drops, but it is not regulated by the FDA.
  - A 2013 systematic review found probiotics effective for breastfed infants but not formula-fed infants.
- Herbal teas and supplements may help but are not recommended because of limited, inconclusive evidence. Examples:
  - One study concluded that herbal teas containing mixtures of chamomile, vervain, licorice, fennel, and balm-mint used up to TID may be beneficial (4)[C]. However, the study used high dosages, raising clinical concerns that this therapy may impair needed milk consumption in infants and be impractical to administer. In addition, preparations used in the study may not be commercially available in the United States.
  - A second double-blind, randomized trial of 0.1% fennel seed oil emulsion versus placebo demonstrated a decrease in colic symptoms according to the Wessel criteria. However, this preparation of fennel seed oil is not commercially available in the United States, and the long-term health effects are unknown (11)[B].

- A home-based intervention focusing on reducing infant stimulation and synchronizing infant sleep–wake cycles with the environment, as well as parental support, has been shown to be effective (12)[B].
- Use of music may help (13)[C],(14)[C].
- Chiropractic treatment has shown no benefit over placebo.
- Infant massage has not been shown to be helpful.

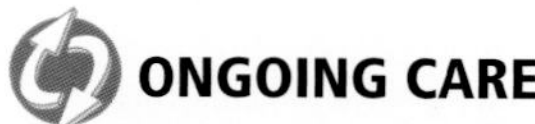

ONGOING CARE

FOLLOW-UP RECOMMENDATIONS

Frequent outpatient visits as needed for parental reassurance, education, and monitoring and to ensure the health of the infant and parents

Patient Monitoring

Follow for proper feeding, growth, and development.

DIET

- If breastfeeding:
  - Continue breastfeeding. Switching to formula probably will not help.
  - Possible therapeutic benefit from eliminating milk products, eggs, wheat, and/or nuts from the diet of breastfeeding mothers (5)[B].
  - Along with eliminating the preceding foods from the maternal diet, removing soy, nuts, and fish may be beneficial.
- If formula feeding:
  - Feeding the infant in a vertical position using a curved bottle or bottle with collapsible bag may help to reduce air swallowing.
  - If no intervention or dietary change has improved the situation, consider a 1-week trial of hypoallergenic formulas such as whey hydrolysate (e.g., Good Start) or casein hydrolysate (e.g., Alimentum, Nutramigen, Pregestimil) (5)[B],(8)[C].
  - The American Academy of Pediatrics concluded that there is no proven role for soy formula in the treatment of colic (15)[C].
  - Adding fiber to formula also has not been shown to be helpful (5,13)[B].
- Supplementing with sucrose solution may be helpful, but the effect may be short lived (<1 hour) (5,8)[B].
- Despite the proposed mechanism of functional lactose overload, use of lactase enzymes in formula or breast milk or given directly to the infant has no therapeutic benefit (5)[B].

PATIENT EDUCATION

- Reassure parents that colic is not the result of bad parenting, and advise parents about having proper rest breaks, adequate sleep, and help in caring for the infant.
- Explain the spectrum of crying behavior.
- Avoid overfeeding or underfeeding.
- Instruct in better feeding techniques such as improved bottles (low air, curved) and sufficient burping after feeding.
- Colic information at American Family Physician: www.aafp.org/afp/2004/0815/p741.html

PROGNOSIS

- Usually subsides by 3–6 months of age, often on its own
- Despite apparent abdominal pain, colicky infants eat well and gain weight normally.
- A handful of studies indicate temper tantrums may be more common among formerly colicky infants as studied in toddlers up to 4 years old (16)[C],(17)[C].
- Colic has no bearing on the baby's intelligence or future development.

COMPLICATIONS

- Colic is self-limiting and does not result in lasting effects to infant or maternal mental health (18)[C].
- However, case-control studies have shown an increased incidence of diagnosing childhood migraine headaches in patients with a history of colic during infancy (19)[B].

REFERENCES

1. Douglas P, Hill P. Managing infants who cry excessively in the first few months of life. *BMJ*. 2011;343:d7772.
2. Milidou I, Henriksen TB, Jensen MS, et al. Nicotine replacement therapy during pregnancy and infantile colic in the offspring. *Pediatrics*. 2012;129(3):e652–658.
3. Romanello S, Spiri D, Marcuzzi E, et al. Association between childhood migraine and history of infantile colic. *JAMA*. 2013;309(15):1607–12.
4. Reijneveld SA, van der Wal MF, Brugman E, et al. Infant crying and abuse. *Lancet*. 2004;364(9442):1340–1342.
5. Garrison MM, Christakis DA. A systematic review of treatments for infant colic. *Pediatrics*. 2000;106(1, Pt 2):184–190.
6. Kaur R, Bharti B, Saini SK. A randomized controlled trial of burping for the prevention of colic and regurgitation in healthy infants. *Child Care Health Dev*. 2015;41(1):52–56.
7. van Sleuwen BE, L'hoir MP, Engelberts AC, et al. Comparison of behavior modification with and without swaddling as interventions for excessive crying. *J Pediatr*. 2006;149(4):512–517.
8. Wade S, Kilgour T. Extracts from "clinical evidence": infantile colic. *BMJ*. 2001;323(7310):437–440.
9. Indrio F, Di Mauro A, Riezzo G, et al. Prophylactic use of a probiotic in the prevention of colic, regurgitation, and functional constipation: a randomized clinical trial. *JAMA Pediatr*. 2014;168(3):228–33.
10. Savino F, Cordisco L, Tarasco V, et al. Lactobacillus reuteri DSM 17938 in infantile colic: a randomized double-blind placebo-controlled trial. *Pediatrics*. 2010;126(3):e526–e533.
11. Alexandrovich I, Rakovitskaya O, Kolmo E, et al. The effect of fennel (*Foeniculum vulgare*) seed oil emulsion in infantile colic: a randomized, placebo-controlled study. *Altern Ther Health Med*. 2003;9(4):58–61.
12. Keefe MR, Lobo ML, Froese-Fretz A, et al. Effectiveness of an intervention for colic. *Clin Pediatr (Phila)*. 2006;45(2):123–133.
13. Clemons RM. Issues in newborn care. *Prim Care*. 2000;27(1):251–267.
14. McCollough M, Sharieff GQ. Common complaints in the first 30 days of life. *Emerg Med Clin North Am*. 2002;20(1):27–48.
15. O'Connor NR. Infant formula. *Am Fam Physician*. 2009;79(7):565–570.
16. Canivet C, Jakobsson I, Hagander B, et al. Infantile colic. Follow-up at four years of age: still more "emotional." *Acta Paediatr*. 2000;89(1):13–17.
17. Rautava P, Lehtonen L, Helenius H, et al. Infantile colic: child and family three years later. *Pediatrics*. 1995;96(1, Pt 1):43–47.
18. Clifford TJ, Campbell MK, Speechley KN, et al. Sequelae of infant colic: evidence of transient infant distress and absence of lasting effects on maternal mental health. *Arch Pediatr Adolesc Med*. 2002;156(12):1183–1188.
19. Gelfand AA, Thomas KC, Goadsby PJ. Before the headache: infant colic as an early life expression of migraine. *Neurology*. 2012;79(13):1392–1396.

ADDITIONAL READING

- Anabrees J, Indrio F, Paes B, et al. Probiotics for infantile colic: a systematic review. *BMC Pediatr*. 2013;13:186.
- Hill DJ, Roy N, Heine RG, et al. Effect of a low-allergen maternal diet on colic among breastfed infants: a randomized, controlled trial. *Pediatrics*. 2005;116(5):e709–e715.
- Savino F, Pelle E, Palumeri E, et al. Lactobacillus reuteri (American Type Culture Collection Strain 55730) versus simethicone in the treatment of infantile colic: a prospective randomized study. *Pediatrics*. 2007;119(1):e124–e130.

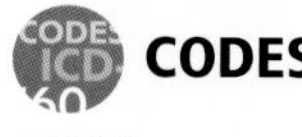

CODES

ICD10

R10.83 Colic

CLINICAL PEARLS

- Colic is defined as excessive crying in an otherwise healthy baby.
- Excessive crying may be a risk factor for shaken baby syndrome or other forms of child abuse.
- Usually subsides spontaneously by 3–6 months of age
- Provide advice, support, and reassurance to parents.
- Prevent caregiver burnout by advising parents to get proper rest breaks, sleep, and help in caring for the infant.

COLITIS, ISCHEMIC

Pia Prakash, MD • Ben P. Alencherry, MD • Marie L. Borum, MD, EdD, MPH

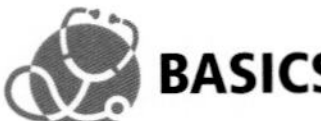

BASICS

Ischemic colitis (IC) results from decreased blood flow to the colon with resultant inflammation and tissue damage.

DESCRIPTION

- More common in the elderly but can affect patients of all ages
- Patients can present with the following:
  - *Nonacute IC* from a chronic process with irreversible ischemic injury
  - *Acute process* with self-limited transient mucosal ischemia
- IC is self-limited and reversible in 80% of patients:
  - 20% of patients progress to full-thickness necrosis and require surgical intervention.
- Most commonly, ischemia is related to nonocclusive reduction in blood flow:
  - Occlusive events can occur but are less common.
- Presentation varies, but patients with acute IC present with localized abdominal pain and tenderness. Frequent loose, bloody stools may be seen within 12–24 hours of onset.
- Laboratory and radiographic findings are nonspecific and must be correlated closely with clinical presentation.
- Colonoscopy is the gold standard for diagnosis of IC.
- In the absence of complications, most patients recover with supportive care including IV fluids, bowel rest, and monitoring for clinical decompensation.

EPIDEMIOLOGY

- Men and women at equal risk
- Patients with inflammatory bowel disease or COPD have an increased risk.
- Seen in 1 of every 100 endoscopies

Geriatric Considerations

Rare in patients <60 years. Average age of diagnosis is 70 years.

Incidence

- 4.5–44 cases per 100,000 in the general population
- 1 of every 2,000 hospital admissions
- True incidence may be underestimated due to nonspecific clinical manifestations.

Prevalence

19 cases per 100,000 in the general population

ETIOLOGY AND PATHOPHYSIOLOGY

- Results from reduction in blood flow to the colon, compromising ability to meet metabolic demands
- Most commonly, an acute, self-limited process
- The colon is perfused by both the superior and inferior mesenteric arteries (SMAs and IMAs) and branches of the internal iliac arteries. With extensive collateral circulation, occlusion of branches of the SMA or IMA rarely leads to ischemic consequences.
- Watershed areas of the colon (splenic flexure and rectosigmoid junction) are most susceptible to ischemic damage. Blood is carried by narrow branches of the SMA and IMA to these areas, putting them at increased risk for ischemia. The splenic flexure is supplied by the terminal branches of the SMA, and the rectosigmoid junction is supplied by the terminal branches of the IMA.
- Left colon more commonly affected than the right.
- The rectum is often spared because of additional blood supply from the internal iliac arteries.
- Poor perfusion may result from systemic etiologies, local vascular compromise, and anatomic or functional changes in the colon itself. An occlusion of large vessels is usually not identified.
  - Hypoperfusion from shock
  - Embolic occlusion of mesenteric vessels
  - Hypercoagulable states
  - Sickle cell disease
  - Arterial thrombosis
  - Venous thrombosis
  - Vasculitis
  - Mechanical colonic obstruction (e.g., tumor, adhesions, hernia, volvulus, prolapse, diverticulitis)
  - Surgical complications (e.g., related to abdominal aortic aneurism repair)
  - Trauma
  - Medications (intestinally active vasoconstrictive substances, medications that induce hypotension and thus hypoperfusion)
  - Cocaine abuse
  - Aortic dissection
  - Strenuous physical activity (e.g., long-distance running)
- Acute IC is largely self-limited and often resolves without long-term complications.
- Repeated episodes of ischemia and inflammation may result in chronic colonic ischemia, possible stricture formation, recurrent bacteremia, and sepsis. These patients may have unresolving areas of colitis and require segmental colonic resection.

RISK FACTORS

- Age >60 years (90% of patients)
- Hypertension
- Diabetes mellitus
- Rheumatologic disorders/vasculitis
- Cerebrovascular disease
- Ischemic heart disease
- Recent abdominal surgery
- Constipation-inducing medications
- History of vascular surgery
- Hypoalbuminemia
- Hemodialysis
- Smoking
- Hypercoagulable state

DIAGNOSIS

- Diagnosis is based on history, risk factors, and physical examination (1)[A].
- Laboratory values and radiographic findings are usually nonspecific (1)[A].
- Colonoscopy is diagnostic (1)[A].

HISTORY

- Symptoms vary, depending on severity (2)[A].
- Sudden-onset, mild to moderate abdominal pain with tenderness over the affected segment of bowel (1)[A]
- Sudden urge to defecate followed by passage of either bright red or maroon stool (2)[A]
- Lower GI bleeding is rarely heavy (1)[A].
- Loose, bloody bowel movements may occur, typically within 12–24 hours of abdominal pain onset (2)[A].

PHYSICAL EXAM

- Individual signs and symptoms are poorly predictive of IC (3)[A].
- Vital signs: hypotension
- Tenderness to palpation over the involved segment of bowel (2)[A]
- Abdominal distention with vomiting due to an associated ileus (1)[A]
- In the uncommon setting of transmural ischemia, patients may develop peritoneal signs such as rebound and guarding (4)[A].

DIFFERENTIAL DIAGNOSIS

- Infectious colitis (4)[A]
- Inflammatory bowel disease (ulcerative colitis, Crohn disease) (4)[A]
- Colon cancer (4)[A]
- Diverticulitis (4)[A]
- Pseudomembranous colitis (3)[A]

DIAGNOSTIC TESTS & INTERPRETATION

- Depends on the clinical presentation, extensiveness of colonic involvement, depth of mural involvement, and the acuteness of onset (1)[A]
- CT scan used as initial diagnostic test when patients present with nonspecific abdominal pain (3)[A]
- Colonoscopy is the most sensitive diagnostic test (1)[A].
- Radiographic tests and laboratory values are nonspecific (3)[A].

Initial Tests (lab, imaging)

- The following lab markers of ischemia are not specific to IC and are more common in severe ischemia (3)[A]:
  - CBC (leukocytosis) (3)[A]
  - BMP; ABG (signs of metabolic acidosis) (3)[A]
  - Lactate (3)[A]
  - CPK (3)[A]
  - Alkaline phosphatase (3)[A]
  - Lactate dehydrogenase (LDH) (3)[A]
  - Amylase (3)[A]
- Abdominal plain film should be obtained:
  - In 20% of patients, signs of IC such as thumbprinting and mural thickening may be present (4)[A].
  - Necessary to rule out bowel perforation and pneumoperitoneum (4)[A]
- No role for routine mesenteric angiography (1)[A]
- Abdominal CT scan with contrast should also be obtained in suspected IC (1)[A]:
  - Common CT findings include hyperdense mucosa, submucosal edema, mesenteric inflammation, and moderate continuous circumferential thickening of colonic wall (1)[A].
  - Pneumatosis, pneumoperitoneum, and free peritoneal fluid may also be seen, suggesting advanced ischemia (1)[A].

Follow-Up Tests & Special Considerations

- Stool cultures, fecal leukocytes, stool ova, and parasites to rule out infectious etiologies (3)[A]
- Patients undergoing aortic surgery should have postoperative colonoscopy within 2–3 days to look for signs of IC (2)[A].

- Cardiac workup including electrocardiogram, Holter monitoring, or transthoracic echocardiogram to exclude cardiac-originating embolism should be considered (3)[A].

Diagnostic Procedures/Other

- Colonoscopy is gold standard; sigmoidoscopy may also be used: (1)[A]
  - Visualization of cyanotic hemorrhagic tissue and edematous mucosa suggests ischemia (2)[A].
  - Segmental distribution (watershed), hemorrhagic nodules, and rectal sparing (2)[A]
  - "Colon single-stripe sign" refers to a single line of erythema, associated with a 75% histopathologic yield (2)[A].
  - Routine biopsy no longer advised, as results are typically nonspecific (1)[A].
- In cases of isolated right colon ischemia, noninvasive vascular imaging studies are recommended due to possible acute superior mesenteric artery occlusion (2)[A].

Test Interpretation

- Fulminant gangrenous IC seen in 15% of cases. Requires surgical intervention (1)[A]
- Acute transient IC seen in 85% of cases requires clinical evaluation for further workup (1)[A].
- Biopsied specimens reveal mucosal infarction and ghost cells, which show normal cellular outlines but lack intracellular contents (1)[A].

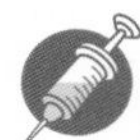

TREATMENT

- Treatment depends on disease severity (1)[A].
- Continuous monitoring of clinical status, including vital signs and serial abdominal exams (4)[A]
- In the absence of colonic necrosis or perforation, most patients respond to supportive care (2)[A]:
  - Bowel rest (2)[A]
  - IV fluids to maintain hemodynamic stability (2)[A]
  - In ill patients, broad-spectrum antibiotics to cover aerobic and anaerobic bacteria to avoid bacterial translocation secondary to colonic mucosal damage (2)[A]
    - Ciprofloxacin
    - Metronidazole
  - Avoid intestinally active vasoconstrictive medications (2)[A].
  - Avoid systemic corticosteroids, which may worsen ischemic damage and increase risk of perforation (1)[A].
  - If ileus is present, place nasogastric tube (1)[A].
- If radiographic abnormalities are present, serial abdominal x-rays may be helpful to follow improvement (2)[A].
- If signs of clinical deterioration are present despite supportive care, including increased abdominal pain, peritoneal signs, persistent diarrhea, bleeding, or sepsis, consider surgery (1)[A].

MEDICATION

- Broad-spectrum antibiotics (i.e., metronidazole, ciprofloxacin) (2)[A]
- If cardiac workup reveals CHF or cardiac arrhythmias, appropriate medical treatment should be initiated (2)[A].

ADDITIONAL THERAPIES

Stem cell implantation in ischemic colonic wall in a rat model enhanced tissue healing by promoting angiogenesis (5)[B].

SURGERY/OTHER PROCEDURES

- 20% of patients require surgical intervention (6)[A].
- Evidence of pneumatosis intestinalis, portal vein air, or free peritoneal air are other indications for immediate surgery prior to endoscopic confirmation of IC (1)[A].
- Surgery may be indicated for patients with the following:
  - Peritoneal signs, increased abdominal tenderness, new-onset shock, lactic acidosis, or acute renal failure (1)[A]
  - Diarrhea, lower GI bleeding, or exudative colitis persisting past 14 days (1)[A]
- Most common surgical intervention is colectomy with end ileostomy (3)[A].
  - Cholecystectomy may prevent resuscitation-related acute acalculous cholecystitis, which in a postoperative patient may have severe consequences (1)[A].

ONGOING CARE

DIET

- Bowel rest until symptoms resolve
- Parenteral nutrition for patients needing prolonged bowel rest who have contraindications to surgery

PROGNOSIS

- In most patients, symptoms of IC resolve within 24–48 hours.
- Radiographic or endoscopic resolution is seen within 2 weeks.
- Right-sided IC appears to be the most significant predictor of outcome. Patients with right-sided IC have a 2-fold greater mortality and a 5-fold increased morbidity.
- Secondary prevention of cardiovascular risk factors minimizes recurrence.

COMPLICATIONS

20–30% of patients develop chronic IC, with persistent diarrhea or stricture formation requiring surgical intervention.

REFERENCES

1. Moszkowicz D, Mariani A, Trésallet C, et al. Ischemic colitis: the ABCs of diagnosis and surgical management. *J Visc Surg*. 2013;150(1):19–28.
2. Feuerstadt P, Brandt LJ. Colon ischemia: recent insights and advances. *Curr Gastroenterol Rep*. 2010;12(5):383–390.
3. Theodoropoulou A, Koutroubakis IE. Ischemic colitis: clinical practice in diagnosis and treatment. *World J Gastroenterol*. 2008;14(48):7302–7308.
4. Sun MY, Maykel JA. Ischemic colitis. *Clin Colon Rectal Surg*. 2007;20(1):5–12.
5. Joo HH, Jo HJ, Jung TD, et al. Adipose-derived stem cells on the healing of ischemic colitis: a therapeutic effect by angiogenesis. *Int J Colorectal Dis*. 2012;27(11):1437–1443.
6. Tortora A, Purchiaroni F, Scarpellini E, et al. Colitides. *Eur Rev Med Pharmacol Sci*. 2012;16(13): 1795–1805.

ADDITIONAL READING

- Huguier M, Barrier A, Boelle PY, et al. Ischemic colitis. *Am J Surg*. 2006;192(5):679–684.
- Iacobellis F, Berritto D, Somma F, et al. Magnetic resonance imaging: a new tool for diagnosis of acute ischemic colitis? *World J Gastroenterol*. 2012;18(13):1496–1501.
- O'Neill S, Yalamarthi S. Systematic review of the management of ischaemic colitis. *Colorectal Dis*. 2012;14(11):e751–e763. doi:10.1111/j.1463-1318.2012.03171.x.
- Paterno F, McGillicuddy EA, Schuster KM, et al. Ischemic colitis: risk factors for eventual surgery. *Am J Surg*. 2010;200(5):646–650.

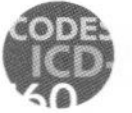

CODES

ICD10

- K55.9 Vascular disorder of intestine, unspecified
- K55.0 Acute vascular disorders of intestine
- K55.1 Chronic vascular disorders of intestine

CLINICAL PEARLS

- Suspect IC in patients with multiple risk factors who present with abdominal pain and loose bloody stools.
- Colonoscopy is the diagnostic gold standard.
- Most often, IC is self-limited, responding well to conservative management with IV fluids, bowel rest, and empiric broad-spectrum antibiotics.
- Peritoneal signs or lack of clinical improvement suggests more extensive ischemia, requiring surgical intervention.
- Right-sided IC is associated with higher morbidity and mortality.

COLONIC POLYPS

Stephen D. Cagle, Jr., MD, Capt, USAF, MC • Brandon Q. Jones, MD

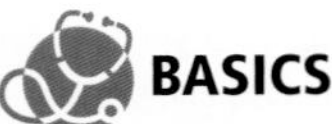

BASICS

DESCRIPTION

- Colonic polyps are (typically) benign, intraluminal outgrowths arising from the epithelium of the colon and rectum:
  - Potential for malignant transformation necessitates ongoing monitoring (see "Colorectal Malignancy").
- Polyps are also seen in children and adolescents.
  - Juvenile polyp: named for histology (not patient age)
  - Polyps seen in children and adolescence typically include those associated with familial adenomatous polyposis (FAP), attenuated familial adenomatous polyposis and MUTYH-associated polyposis syndromes which tend to be adenomatous polyps.

EPIDEMIOLOGY

Higher risk in

- Men
- Industrialized countries
- Older age

Incidence

- ~5% of the U.S. population
- ~20% of middle-aged and older adults
- 50% seen in ≥50 years

Prevalence

Average prevalence: ~25% in patients <40 years and up to 55% by age 80 years

ETIOLOGY AND PATHOPHYSIOLOGY

- Several types of colonic polyps in adults:
  - Adenomas: represent ~10% of polyps; may become malignant
    - Villous adenomas (10%). Typically occur in the rectum, are nonpedunculated, and have larger surface area (with greater potential for malignant transformation)
    - Tubular (75%). Most common of the adenomas. Can be found anywhere in the colon.
    - Tubulovillous (15%)
    - Sessile serrated (SSA). Have both adenomatous and hyperplastic features. Also have malignant potential.
- Hyperplastic polyps: most common type, representing up to 90% of all colonic polyps; rarely malignant (only malignant in setting of hyperplastic polyposis syndrome)
- Inflammatory polyps: no malignant potential; often found in association with underlying colitis
- Hamartomatous polyps—contain a mixture of normal tissues

Genetics

- May occur in the setting of genetic syndromes associated with specific gene mutations
- Polyposis syndromes: FAP; hereditary nonpolyposis colorectal cancer—also known as Lynch syndrome; Gardner syndrome; Peutz-Jeghers syndrome; Coden disease; familial juvenile polyposis, hyperplastic polyposis, serrated polyposis syndrome

RISK FACTORS

- Advancing age
- Male
- Abdominal obesity
- Family history of intestinal polyposis, polyps, or colorectal cancer (CRC)
- Inflammatory bowel disease
- Current cigarette smoking
- Excessive alcohol intake: >8 drinks a week (1)
- Sedentary lifestyle

GENERAL PREVENTION

- Diet: High-fiber diet has been a controversial risk modifier; however, there is no evidence to support increasing dietary fiber has any effect on incidence or recurrence of adenomatous polyps (2)[A].
- Avoid smoking.
- Limit alcohol intake.
- Calcium supplement: reduces colorectal adenoma recurrence (2)[A]
- Aspirin reduces the recurrence of sporadic adenomatous polyps after 1–3 years and promote regression of colorectal adenomas in FAP (3)[A].
- Patients on statins are 30% less likely to develop CRC; need more trial data before routinely recommending statins for primary prevention (2)[B].

COMMONLY ASSOCIATED CONDITIONS

Associated with several hereditary disorders

- FAP
- Peutz-Jeghers syndrome
- Gardner syndrome
- hereditary nonpolyposis colorectal cancer

ALERT
Patients who present with painless rectal bleeding should be evaluated for colon polyps.

DIAGNOSIS

HISTORY

- Many patients are asymptomatic. Assess for risk factors (social and occupational history; family history)
- Hematochezia (Painless rectal bleeding is a common presentation in adults and children.)
- Melena
- Diarrhea or constipation
- Anemia
- Fatigue
- Abdominal pain

PHYSICAL EXAM

- Usually normal
- Rectal lesions occasionally noted on digital rectal examination.

DIAGNOSTIC TESTS & INTERPRETATION

Initial Tests (lab, imaging)

- CBC: anemia
- Electrolyte abnormalities: in villous adenoma with hypersecretory syndrome

Diagnostic Procedures/Other

- Tests that detect polyps and colon cancer
  - Colonoscopy: gold standard (2)[B]
    - Polypectomy is often performed during the procedure, allowing screening and treatment of polyps to be performed at a single visit.
  - CT colonography may be a more suitable initial test than optical colonoscopy and can accurately detect polyps >10 mm (2)[B].
  - Sigmoidoscopy every 5 years combined with fecal occult blood test (FOBT) every 1–3 years (2)[C]
  - Chromoscopy: Studies are examining narrow-band imaging for histologic differentiation between adenomatous and hyperplastic polyps and is used in conjunction with standard colonoscopy (4)[A].
    - Chromoscopy enhances the detection of neoplastic lesions in the colon and the rectum that could be missed with conventional colonoscopy.
    - Cap-assisted colonoscopy increased detection of polyps, with better success of cecal intubation compared with standard colonoscopy.
  - Air-contrast barium enema
    - Misses small lesions
- Tests that detect colon cancer
  - FOBT
    - Higher false-positive rate
    - Decreases mortality by 16% (2)[A]
    - Recommend yearly FOBT screening if used as single screening modality (2)[A]
  - Fecal DNA testing
  - Fecal immunochemical test (FIT): Better at detecting advanced adenomatous polyps over traditional FOBT. Patients are more likely to undergo a FIT screen than colonoscopy screen (2)[A].
    - If used as single screening modality, annual screening is recommended (2)[C].

ALERT
Identification of any polyp with potentially malignant appearance merits histopathologic evaluation.

Test Interpretation

- Villous adenoma
  - Gross: velvety, multiple-frond projections
  - Micro: Glands proliferate in fingerlike projections and malignant degenerations.

- Tubular adenoma
  - Gross: smooth, firm, pink surface; microlobulated; fissures; pedunculated
  - Glands proliferate in tubular fashion, nuclei elongated, and hyperchromatic.
- Juvenile polyp

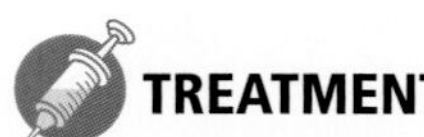

TREATMENT

SURGERY/OTHER PROCEDURES

- Endoscopic polypectomy: Major risks include perforation and bleeding (2)[A].
- Colonic resection: for multiple intestinal polyps associated with FAP (5)[A]

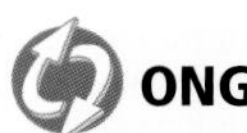

ONGOING CARE

FOLLOW-UP RECOMMENDATIONS

Follow-up recommendations are based on polyp type, size, and number.

Patient Monitoring

Offer CRC screening for average-risk patients beginning at age 50 years, earlier for at-risk patients:

- Most guidelines recommend to stop screening if life expectancy is <10 years (2)[A].

DIET

There is insufficient evidence to support dietary supplementation or modification in the primary or secondary prevention of colonic polyps (2,6)[A].

PROGNOSIS

- Polypectomy prevents villous adenoma from progressing to colon cancer if completely resected.
- 50% of postpolypectomy patients have a recurrence within 7.6 years and should, therefore, be followed at recommended intervals.
- Adenomatous polyps may undergo malignant transformation if not removed.
- Multiple polyps increase the risk of developing CRC.

COMPLICATIONS

Perforation with colonoscopy is rare.

REFERENCES

1. Anderson JC, Alpern Z, Sethi G, et al. Prevalence and risk of colorectal neoplasia in consumers of alcohol in a screening population. *Am J Gastroenterol*. 2005;100(9):2049–2055.
2. Wilkins T, Reynolds PL. Colorectal cancer: a summary of the evidence for screening and prevention. *Am Fam Physician*. 2008;78(12):1385–1392.
3. Asano TK, McLeod RS. Nonsteroidal anti-inflammatory drugs (NSAID) and aspirin for preventing colorectal adenomas and carcinomas. *Cochrane Database Syst Rev*. 2010;(2):CD004079.
4. Brown SR, Baraza W, Hurlstone P. Chromoscopy versus conventional endoscopy for the detection of polyps in the colon and rectum. *Cochrane Database Syst Rev*. 2007;(4):CD006439.
5. Durno CA. Colonic polyps in children and adolescents. *Can J Gastroenterol*. 2007;21(4):233–239.
6. Asano TK, McLeod RS. Dietary fibre for the prevention of colorectal adenomas and carcinomas. *Cochrane Database Syst Rev*. 2002;(2):CD003430.

ADDITIONAL READING

- Brown SR, Baraza W. Chromoscopy versus conventional endoscopy for the detection of polyps in the colon and rectum. *Cochrane Database Syst Rev*. 2010;(10):CD006439.
- Elwood PC, Gallagher AM, Duthie GG, et al. Aspirin, salicylates, and cancer. *Lancet*. 2009;373(9671):1301–1309.
- Kim DH, Pickhardt PJ, Taylor AJ, et al. CT colonography versus colonoscopy for the detection of advanced neoplasia. *N Engl J Med*. 2007;357(14):1403–1412.
- Larsen IK, Grotmol T, Almendingen K, et al. Lifestyle as a predictor for colonic neoplasia in asymptomatic individuals. *BMC Gastroenterol*. 2006;6:5.
- Levi Z, Birkenfeld S, Vilkin A, et al. A higher detection rate for colorectal cancer and advanced adenomatous polyp for screening with immunochemical fecal occult blood test than guaiac fecal occult blood test, despite lower compliance rate. A prospective, controlled, feasibility study. *Int J Cancer*. 2011;128(10):2415–2424.
- Pickhardt PJ, Hassan C, Halligan S, et al. Colorectal cancer: CT colonography and colonoscopy for detection—systematic review and meta-analysis. *Radiology*. 2011;259(2):393–405.
- Quintero E, Castells A, Bujanda L, et al. Colonoscopy versus fecal immunochemical testing in colorectal-cancer screening. *N Engl J Med*. 2012;366(8):697–706.
- Rastogi A, Pondugula K, Bansal A, et al. Recognition of surface mucosal and vascular patterns of colon polyps by using narrow-band imaging: interobserver and intraobserver agreement and prediction of polyp histology. *Gastrointest Endosc*. 2009;69(3 Pt 2):716–722.
- Weingarten MA, Zalmanovici A, Yaphe J. Dietary calcium supplementation for preventing colorectal cancer and adenomatous polyps. *Cochrane Database Syst Rev*. 2008;(1):CD003548.
- Westwood DA, Alexakis N, Connor SJ. Transparent cap-assisted colonoscopy versus standard adult colonoscopy: a systematic review and meta-analysis. *Dis Colon Rectum*. 2012;55(2):218–225.
- Yood MU, Oliveria S, Boyer JG, et al. Colon polyp recurrence in a managed care population. *Arch Intern Med*. 2003;163(4):422–426.
- Zijta FM, Bipat S, Stoker J. Magnetic resonance (MR) colonography in the detection of colorectal lesions: a systematic review of prospective studies. *Eur Radiol*. 2010;20(5):1031–1046.

SEE ALSO

Algorithm: Bleeding, Upper GI

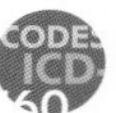

CODES

ICD10

- K63.5 Polyp of colon
- D12.6 Benign neoplasm of colon, unspecified
- D12.5 Benign neoplasm of sigmoid colon

CLINICAL PEARLS

- Villous adenomatous polyps are the "villains" (most likely to become malignant).
- Hyperplastic polyps are rarely cancerous.
- Up to 50% of patients who have polyps removed will have recurrent polyps.
- Aspirin reduces the recurrence of sporadic adenomatous polyps after 1–3 years.

COLORECTAL CANCER

Stephen Scott, MD, MPH

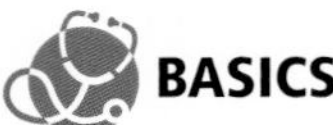

BASICS

DESCRIPTION

- Colorectal cancer (CRC) denotes a neoplasm that develops in the colon or rectum.
- CRC is the 2nd leading cause of cancer deaths and is the 3rd most common cancer in men and women in the United States.
- Screening for CRC reduces the incidence of and mortality from CRC.

EPIDEMIOLOGY

Incidence

96,830 new cases of colon cancer; 40,000 new cases of rectal cancer; and 50,310 deaths from colon and rectal cancer combined were estimated in the United States in 2014 (1).

Prevalence

- The lifetime risk for developing CRC in the United States is about 1 in 21 (4.8%).
- Incidence and death rates have been declining due to improved screening, prevention, and treatment.

ETIOLOGY AND PATHOPHYSIOLOGY

- Progression from the 1st abnormal cells to the appearance of CRC usually occurs over 10–15 years; a disease characteristic that contributes to the effectiveness of prevention.
- High-risk polyp findings include multiple polyps, villous polyps, and larger polyps; hyperplastic polyps are less likely to evolve into CRC.
- Multiple genetic and environmental factors have been linked to the development of CRC.

Genetics

- There does not seem to be a single genetic pathway to CRC.
- <10% of CRC cases are linked to an inherited gene:
  - APC, a tumor suppressor gene, is altered in FAP.
  - Genes encoding DNA mismatch repair (MMR) enzymes are implicated in hereditary nonpolyposis colon cancer (HNPCC): MLH1, MSH2, MSH6, PMS1, PMS2, and others.
  - STK11, a tumor suppressor gene, is altered in Peutz-Jeghers syndrome.
- Sporadic cases of CRC have been linked to oncogenes: kras, c-myc, src, HER2/neu, and others.

RISK FACTORS

- Age: >90% of people diagnosed with CRC are >50 years of age.
- Personal history of colorectal polyps
  - Risks increase with multiple polyps, villous polyps, and larger polyps.
- Personal history of cancer
  - Rectal cancer has a higher incidence of local recurrence than proximal cancers (20–30% vs. 2–4%).
- History of inflammatory bowel disease
  - Prevalence of CRC in ulcerative colitis and Crohn disease is ~3%, with a cumulative risk of CRC of 2% at 10 years, 8% at 20 years, and 18% at 30 years.
- Family history of CRC
  - Having a single 1st-degree relative with a history of CRC increases risk 1.7-fold.
  - Risk is more than double for those who have a history of CRC or polyps in:
    - Any 1st-degree relative <60 years of age
    - ≥2 1st-degree relatives, regardless of age
- Inherited syndromes
  - HNPCC also called Lynch syndrome.
    - Often develops at younger age (Average age at diagnosis of CRC is 44 years.)
    - Lifetime risk of CRC is 52–69%.
    - Accounts for ~2% of all CRCs
  - Familial adenomatous polyposis (FAP)
    - Affected individuals develop hundreds to thousands of polyps in colon and rectum
    - CRC usually present by age 40 years.
    - Accounts for <1% of CRCs
  - Peutz-Jeghers syndrome
    - Individuals may have freckles (mouth, hands, feet) and large polyps in GI tract.
    - Greatly increased risk for CRC and cancers
- Race and ethnicity
  - African Americans have highest CRC incidence and mortality rates in the United States.
  - Several different gene mutations have been identified among Ashkenazi Jews.
- Miscellaneous
  - Patients with obesity, diabetes, acromegaly, smoking, and alcohol use are at increased risk.

GENERAL PREVENTION

- Diets high in fruits and vegetables have been linked with decreased risk; those high in red and processed meats may increase CRC risk.
- Some studies suggest that vitamin D, calcium, folate, and fiber may lower CRC risk; more research is needed to understand how diet affects risks of CRC.
- People who are physically inactive are at higher risk for CRC.
- Long-term smokers are more likely than nonsmokers to develop and die from CRC.
- CRC has been linked to heavy alcohol consumption; may be related to low folate intake or absorption
- NSAIDs may reduce risk in some groups; experts do not recommend NSAID use as a cancer prevention strategy in people at average risk for CRC.
- Colon cancer screening is one of the most powerful tools in preventing colon cancer.

ALERT

The U.S. Preventive Services Task Force (USPSTF) strongly recommends that clinicians screen men and women between the ages of 50 and 75 years for CRC using fecal occult blood testing, sigmoidoscopy, or colonoscopy (2).

- American Cancer Society recommendations for screening include the following (3):
  - fecal occult blood testing annually
  - Fecal immunochemical test (FIT) annually
  - Flexible sigmoidoscopy every 5 years
  - Colonoscopy every 10 years
  - CT colonography every 5 years (colonoscopy completed if positive)*
  - Double-contrast barium enema every 5 years*
  - Stool DNA test (sDNA) (non–FDA-approved; studies of next generation tests are ongoing)*

  *The USPSTF does <u>not</u> recommend barium enema as a screening test and concludes the evidence is insufficient to assess the benefits and harms of CT colonography and stool DNA testing as screening modalities for CRC.

- Screening in high-risk groups
  - People with a personal history of polyps need more frequent colonoscopy screening, depending on risk (i.e., 1 or 2 <1 cm polyps with low-grade dysplasia is deemed low risk and may warrant repeat colonoscopy in 5–10 years; decision is influenced by family history, age, quality of initial colonoscopy, and patient comorbidities).
  - People who have a family history of CRC or adenomatous polyps before age 60 years should begin colonoscopy at age 40 or 10 years younger than the age of relative at cancer diagnosis, whichever is earlier.
  - People with inflammatory bowel disease should have regular surveillance colonoscopy with biopsies to detect dysplasia; guidelines for timing and location vary by professional society but generally indicate starting surveillance by ~8 years of onset of disease followed by surveillance every 1–2 years.
  - Genetic testing may be appropriate for individuals with a strong family history of CRC or polyps:
    - Family members of a person affected by HNPCC should start colonoscopy surveillance as early as age 20 years.
    - Individuals with suspected FAP should have yearly flexible sigmoidoscopy beginning at age 10–12 years; those who test positive for the gene linked to FAP may consider colectomy.

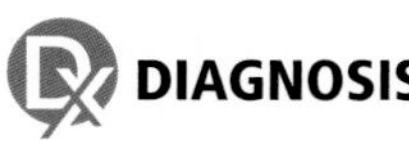

DIAGNOSIS

HISTORY

- Many patients with CRC are asymptomatic.
- Common presenting symptoms and signs in symptomatic patients include the following:
  - Abdominal pain or cramping
  - Change in bowel habits (constipation, diarrhea, narrowing of stool)
  - Rectal bleeding, dark stools, or blood in stool
  - Weakness or fatigue
  - Anemia
  - Weight loss
- Other presentations may include symptoms due to the presence of metastatic lesions (lymph nodes, liver, lung, peritoneum), fever of unknown origin, and *Streptococcus bovis* or *Clostridium septicum* sepsis.

PHYSICAL EXAM

- Weight loss
- Signs of anemia (i.e., conjunctival pallor)
- Palpable abdominal mass

DIFFERENTIAL DIAGNOSIS

- >95% of CRCs are adenocarcinomas.
- Other colonic tumors include carcinoid tumors, lymphomas, and Kaposi sarcoma in HIV.
- Many conditions can mimic CRC, including other cancers, hemorrhoids, inflammatory bowel disease, infection, and extrinsic masses (i.e., cysts, abscesses).

DIAGNOSTIC TESTS & INTERPRETATION

Initial Tests (lab, imaging)

- CBC (to evaluate anemia)
- Liver function (CRC may spread to the liver)
- Colonoscopy
- CT colography if colonoscopy incomplete

Follow-Up Tests & Special Considerations

- Carcinoembryonic antigen (CEA) should be obtained preoperatively to assist with follow-up screening.
- CT to evaluate presence of metastatic disease
- Chest x-ray to evaluate presence of chest metastases
- Endoscopic ultrasound (EUS) may be used to evaluate the extent of rectal cancers; endorectal MRI may also provide further detail.
- Intraoperative US may be used to evaluate solid organs (e.g., the liver) after tumor resection.
- Positron emission tomography (PET) may be used in some cases to detect metastatic disease.

Diagnostic Procedures/Other

- Biopsy is usually performed (most often during colonoscopy) if CRC is suspected.
- CT needle-guided biopsy may be needed to evaluate a suspected tumor or metastasis.

Test Interpretation

The American Joint Committee on Cancer (AJCC) TNM staging is preferred:

- Stage 0: limited to the mucosa (carcinoma in situ or intramucosal carcinoma (Tis, N0, M0)
- Stage I: invades mucosa (T1) or muscularis propria (T2); no invasion of lymph nodes or distant sites (T1, N0, M0 or T2, N0, M0)
- Stage IIA: invades pericolorectal tissues; no lymph nodes or distant sites (T3, N0, M0)
- Stage IIB: penetrates to surface of visceral peritoneum; no lymph nodes or distant sites (T4a, N0, M0)
- Stage IIC: directly invades or adherent to other organs or structures (T4b, N0, M0)
- Stage IIIA: invades submucosa or muscularis propria with spread to 1–3 lymph nodes; no distant sites (T1, N1, M0 or T2, N1, M0)
- Stage IIIB: invades pericolorectal tissues or surface of visceral peritoneum + spread to 1–3 lymph nodes; no distant sites (T3, N1, M0, or T4a, N1, M0)
- Stage IIIC: invades pericolorectal tissues or peritoneum or other organs and to ≥4 nearby lymph nodes; no distant sites (any T3 or T4, N2, M0)
- Stage IVA: any level of invasion with spread to one organ or site (any T, any N, M1a)
- Stage IVB: any level of invasion with spread to more than 1 organ or site or peritoneum (any T, any N, M1b)

TREATMENT

MEDICATION

- **Surgical resection is the primary treatment for CRC, as noted in the following texts.** Adjuvant chemotherapy is most clearly beneficial for stage III (node-positive) disease, in which improvements of ~30% may be achieved in both disease recurrence and overall survival, compared with nontreated controls. Chemotherapeutic regimens for metastatic disease may extend overall survival from 6 months to ~2 years (4)[B].

First Line

Combination chemotherapy is common and may include oxaliplatin, irinotecan, fluorouracil, leucovorin, and capecitabine.

Geriatric Considerations

Elderly patients tend to tolerate CRC chemotherapy and should be considered for treatment.

Second Line

Targeted therapies may be used alongside 1st-line agents or alone if 1st-line agents are ineffective:

- Bevacizumab (Avastin) is a monoclonal antibody that targets vascular endothelial growth factor (VEGF); inhibits angiogenesis
- Cetuximab (Erbitux) and panitumumab (Vectibix) are monoclonal antibodies that target epidermal growth factor receptor (EGFR).
- Aflibercept and regorafenib are newer agents with actions on VEGF.

SURGERY/OTHER PROCEDURES

- Surgery is the primary treatment for localized CRC:
  - May involve segmental resection, hemicolectomy, or colectomy, as well as resection of nodes, depending on size and invasion
  - Laparoscopic-assisted colectomy is an emerging option for earlier stage tumors.
  - Surgery for rectal cancer may include local transanal, low anterior, or abdominoperineal resection or pelvic exenteration.
- Radiation therapy is most often used for peritoneal or rectal cancers; it may also be used to relieve symptoms.

COMPLEMENTARY & ALTERNATIVE MEDICINE

- May serve as an adjunct to treatment for CRC
- 70–75% of cancer survivors report using at least 1 type of complementary and alternative medicine (CAM), and almost all report that the alternative therapy improved well-being.

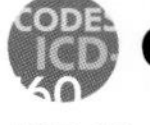

ONGOING CARE

FOLLOW-UP RECOMMENDATIONS

Patient Monitoring

- People with a personal history of proximal cancer (nonrectal) should have follow-up colonoscopy in 1 year and, if normal, in 3 and 5 years subsequently.
- CEA and/or CA 19-9 are used to detect recurrence in people treated for CRC. (Note: CEA levels may be elevated in ulcerative colitis, nonmalignant GI tumors, liver disease, lung disease, and in smokers.)

PATIENT EDUCATION

- NIH: Colorectal Cancer: http://www.nlm.nih.gov/medlineplus/colorectalcancer.html
- AAFP: Colorectal Cancer: http://familydoctor.org/familydoctor/en/diseases-conditions/colorectal-cancer.html

PROGNOSIS

5-year relative survival rate is determined by stage (adjusted for patients dying of other diseases): stage I: 93%; stage II: 72–85%; stage III: 44–83%; stage IV: 8%.

COMPLICATIONS

- Colorectal surgery: pain, deep vein thrombosis, anastomotic leaks, infection, scarring, bowel obstruction
- Chemotherapy: hair loss, nausea, vomiting, bruising, fatigue, increased risk for infections
- Radiation therapy: skin irritation, nausea, rectal pain, incontinence, bladder irritation, fatigue, and sexual problems

REFERENCES

1. Siegel R, Ma J, Zou Z, et al. Cancer statistics, 2014. *CA Cancer J Clin*. 2014;64(1):9–29.
2. U.S. Preventive Services Task Force. Colorectal cancer: screening. http://www.uspreventiveservicestaskforce.org/uspstf08/colocancer/colors.htm. Accessed July 9, 2014.
3. American Cancer Society. Guidelines for the early detection of cancer. http://www.cancer.org/healthy/findcancerearly/cancerscreeningguidelines/american-cancer-society-guidelines-for-the-early-detection-of-cancer. Accessed July 9, 2014.
4. Brenner H, Kloor M, Pox CP. Colorectal cancer. *Lancet*. 2014;383(9927):1490–1502.

ADDITIONAL READING

- Benson AB III, Venook AP, Bekaii-Saab T, et al. Colon cancer, version 3.2014. *J Natl Compr Canc Netw*. 2014;12(7):1028–1059.
- National Institutes of Health, National Cancer Institute. Colon cancer treatment (PDQ®). http://www.cancer.gov/cancertopics/pdq/treatment/colon/Patient. Accessed 2014.
- National Institutes of Health, National Cancer Institute. Colon and rectal cancer. http://www.cancer.gov/cancertopics/types/colon-and-rectal. Accessed 2014.

CODES

ICD10

- C19 Malignant neoplasm of rectosigmoid junction
- C18.9 Malignant neoplasm of colon, unspecified
- C20 Malignant neoplasm of rectum

CLINICAL PEARLS

- The USPSTF recommends screening beginning at age 50 years and notes that evidence supports fecal occult blood testing (yearly), sigmoidoscopy, or colonoscopy (every 10 years).
- High-risk polyp findings include multiple polyps, villous polyps, and larger polyps; hyperplastic polyps are less likely to become cancerous.
- 10% of cases of CRC occur in people <50 years of age. People who have a family history of CRC without other risks (i.e., polyposis syndrome) should begin colonoscopy at age 40 years or 10 years younger than the age of relative at cancer diagnosis, whichever is earlier.
- Iron deficiency anemia in the elderly should prompt a search for CRC and should not be attributed to normal aging.

COMPLEMENTARY AND ALTERNATIVE MEDICINE

Paul Crawford, MD

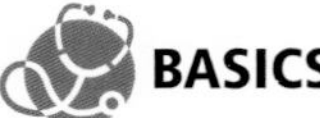

BASICS

- Complementary and alternative medicine (CAM) are medical and health care systems, practices, and products not presently considered part of conventional medicine.
- The National Center for Health Statistics (NCHS) 2012 survey (1) reports nonvitamin, nonmineral dietary supplements, chiropractic or osteopathic manipulation, yoga, and massage therapy were most common complementary health approaches used.
- Medical professionals who incorporate CAM into their medical practice will often refer to their health care model as "integrative medicine."

DESCRIPTION

- Definitions and additional terms
  - *Complementary medicine* is used with conventional medicine to address a health concern. For example, massage plus physical therapy to address low back pain, or medication plus osteopathic manipulation to address recurrent headaches.
  - *Alternative medicine* is used in place of conventional medicine to promote healing of conditions that cannot be explained by the conventional biomedical model or for which the effectiveness of therapy is not yet established by clinical research.
  - *Integrative medicine* is the combination of allopathic medicine with CAM and may be provided to the patient by a single licensed medical professional trained in CAM or by a group of diverse health care providers.
  - *Holistic* is a descriptive term for a practitioner's approach to patient care. A holistic practitioner assesses the emotional, spiritual, mental, and physical state of wellness of the client, then works to provide comprehensive care. A holistic practice may include practitioners of different disciplines to best address all aspects of wellness or illness.
- *Biologically based therapies*: diets, herbals, vitamins, supplements, flower essences
- *Manipulative and body-based methods*
  - Massage therapy is the manipulation of the body's soft tissues, whereby the licensed practitioner uses knowledge of anatomy and physiology to restore function, promote relaxation, and relieve pain. There are several different types of massage.
  - Osteopathic manipulative medicine focuses on the musculoskeletal system. It includes indirect techniques (e.g., muscle energy, myofascial release, osteopathy in the cranial field, and strain–counterstrain approach), as well as direct action techniques (high-velocity thrusts).
  - Craniosacral therapy is a gentle manual treatment focusing on the release of bony and fascial restrictions in the craniosacral system (cranium, sacrum, spinal cord, meninges, CSF).
  - Chiropractic therapy focuses on the musculoskeletal and nervous systems and how imbalances in these systems can affect general health. It is used to treat back pain, neck pain, and joint pain. Doctors of Chiropractic (DCs) complete 4–5 years of intensive training in anatomy, physiology, and manipulation.
- *Mind–body medicine*
  - Meditation is a practice of detachment in which a person sits quietly, generally focusing on the breath, while releasing all thoughts from the mind with the intention to center the self, restore balance, and enhance well-being. Mindfulness meditation involves making oneself aware of the most immediate of activities in order to gain control over actions and anxiety.
  - Spiritual practices; for example, prayer
  - Yoga is an exercise of mindfulness, meditation, strength, and balance. It is composed of *asanas* (postures) and *pranayamas* (focused breathing).
  - Aromatherapy uses highly concentrated plant extracts to stimulate healing processes. These aromatic oils are rubbed on the skin, aerosolized, or used in compresses.
  - Relaxation techniques include breathing exercises, progressive muscle relaxation, and guided imagery.
  - *Tai chi* and *qi gong* are Chinese exercise systems that combine meditation, regulated breathing, and flowing dance-like movements to enhance and balance *chi* (*qi*), or life force energy.
- *Alternative medical systems*
  - Traditional Chinese medicine incorporates Chinese herbs and acupuncture. Acupuncture is the practice of regulating *chi* by inserting hair-thin needles at specific points along meridian pathways of the body. *Chi* movement is responsible for animating and protecting the body; relieving pain; and regulating blood, oxygen, and nourishment to every cell.
  - Ayurvedic medicine originated in India and is one of the world's oldest medical systems. It uses healing modalities and herbs to integrate and balance the body, mind, and spirit.
  - Homeopathy is a system of therapy based on the concept that very dilute quantities of an offending agent can stimulate the body's own immune system to produce a reaction against this offense, thereby healing itself. In general, homeopathic remedies are considered safe and unlikely to cause serious adverse reactions. Only 3 states license homeopaths.
  - Naturopathy is based on providing natural and minimally invasive options for prevention and treatment of disease. Treatment regimens can include herbs, vitamins, supplements, dietary counseling, homeopathic remedies, manipulative therapies, acupuncture, and hydrotherapy. 4-year doctoral training programs are available; however, only 20 states/territories have licensing laws for naturopathic practitioners.
- *Energy therapies*
  - *Reiki*, which means "source energy," is a healing practice from Japan. Laying hands lightly on the patient or holding the hands just above the body, the *reiki* practitioner facilitates spiritual and physical healing by stimulating a patient's life force energy.
- Common reasons patients choose CAM
  - Additive therapy to address aspects not provided for in conventional medical treatment
  - Conventional medicine has been unsuccessful in fully addressing ailment.
  - Preventive health care
  - Desire for a holistic and natural approach to well-being
  - Preference for noninvasive treatment options
  - Concern about side effects of medication
  - Desire for spiritual support to be incorporated into healing practice
  - Cultural or familial belief system may be more aligned with "natural" solutions not provided for or supported by the standard allopathic model of health care

EPIDEMIOLOGY

- All ages use CAM, but it is most prevalent among adults aged 30–69 years.
- Gender ratio: female > male
- College graduates and residents from western states are more likely to use CAM.
- Cancer survivors are more likely than the general population to use CAM.
- 6 most used CAM therapies based on the NCHS 2012 survey. These CAM therapies were used by the indicated percentage of survey participants:
  - Nonvitamin, nonmineral dietary supplements (17.9%)
  - Chiropractic and osteopathic manipulation (8.5%)
  - Yoga (8.4%)
  - Massage (6.8%)
  - Meditation (4.1%)
  - Special diets (3.0%).

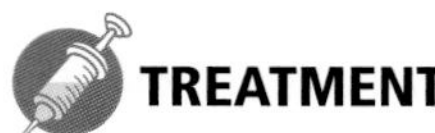

TREATMENT

- Variable evidence supports both safety and efficacy of
  - *Meditation* for lowering BP (2)[C]
  - *Acupuncture* for chronic low back pain (3)[B]
  - *Acupuncture* to improve fertility (4)[C]
  - *Spinal manipulative therapy* for prophylactic treatment of headaches
  - Ginger for nausea, including that associated with chemotherapy
  - *Manipulation*, *massage*, and mobilization for acute low back and posterior neck pain
  - *Massage therapy* to promote weight gain in preterm infants
  - *Massage* (30 minutes × 3) during labor shortens the second stage and reduces pain (5)[A].
  - *Acupuncture* for chemotherapy-induced nausea and vomiting
  - *Tai chi* for improving balance and decreasing the risk of and fear of falling in elderly
  - *Mind–body techniques* for migraines, chronic pain, and insomnia
  - *Homeopathic remedy* for the treatment of chemotherapy-induced stomatitis in children
  - Riboflavin for migraine prophylaxis
  - Horse chestnut seed extract to improve lower leg venous tone, pain, and edema
  - Glucosamine for osteoarthritis and knee pain
  - *Yoga and meditation* appear to improve endothelial function in patients with CAD and can have potential beneficial effects on depressive disorders.
  - *Yoga* throughout pregnancy shortens labor by 140–190 minutes.

– *Exercise* in both preconception and early pregnancy reduces chance of gestational diabetes mellitus (6)[A].
– *Breast stimulation* in late pregnancy increases successful induction of labor (NNT 3.2) and reduces postpartum hemorrhage (NNT 19) (7)[A].
– Oral probiotics in preterm infants to decrease necrotizing enterocolitis and reduce mortality (8)[A].
– Oral probiotics to prevent URIs in children and influenza in the elderly (9,10)[A]
– Oral probiotics to shorten the duration of acute and antibiotic-associated diarrhea and as prophylaxis for traveler's diarrhea (10),(11)[A],(12,13)
– Vitamin D 800 IU/day may reduce falls and fractures in the elderly (14)[A].
– *Acupuncture* for recurrent headache

- Evidence supports safety, but evidence regarding efficacy is inconclusive:
  – *Homeopathy* for induction and augmentation of labor
  – Chondroitin sulfate is ineffective for osteoarthritis.
  – *Sterile water injections* do not reduce pain in labor.
  – Omega-3 fatty acids may reduce inflammation and anxiety in young healthy adults.
  – *Dietary fat reduction* for certain types of cancer
  – *Mind–body techniques* for metastatic cancer
  – *Copper and magnetic bracelets* for pain
  – *Vitamin D levels* >30 ng/mL correlate with lower risk of some cancers. Adequate vitamin D intake may decrease atopy and asthma symptoms.
- Evidence supports efficacy, but evidence regarding safety is inconclusive:
  – St. John's wort extract for short-term treatment of depression in adults
  – Licorice for gastritis
- Evidence indicates serious risk:
  – Black cohosh, blue cohosh, and evening primrose oil are unsafe to induce labor.
  – Delay in seeking medical care or replacement of curative conventional treatment
  – Use of toxic herbs or substances
  – Known herb–drug interactions

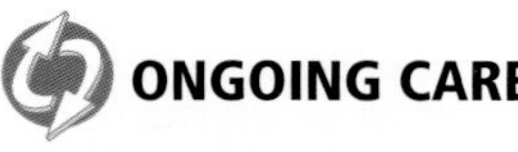

ONGOING CARE

PATIENT EDUCATION

The National Center for Complementary and Alternative Medicine (nccam.nih.gov)

COMPLICATIONS

ALERT

Ginkgo and St. John's wort account for most herb–drug interactions described in the medical literature.

- Herbs with possible adverse effects
  – Serious adverse events from herbal remedies remain uncommon.
  – Some ethnic medicines, as those prescribed by practitioners of Ayurveda or traditional Chinese medicine, may intentionally contain heavy metals or other toxic substances. These are usually listed by their pharmacopeial names, for example, Qian Dan = lead oxide.
  – Bitter orange (*Citrus sinensis*): sympathomimetic; increases heart rate (HR), BP
  – California poppy (*Eschscholzia californica*): may cause respiratory depression, drowsiness; contains opioids
  – Cascara sagrada (*Frangula purshiana*): depletes serum potassium
  – Chaparral (*Larrea tridentata*): hepatotoxic
  – Ephedra (*Ephedra* spp.): sympathomimetic; increases HR, BP; insomnia, gastric distress
  – Ginkgo (*Ginkgo biloba*): extravasation, increased bleeding time
  – Guarana (*Paullinia cupana*): tachycardia, hypertension; contains caffeine
  – Kava (*Piper methysticum*): decreases use of niacin; possibly hepatotoxic
  – Licorice (*Glycyrrhiza* spp.): Long-term use depletes serum potassium.
  – Lily of the valley (*Convallaria majalis*): contains cardiac glycosides
  – Poke root (*Phytolacca species*): strong gastric irritant, may cause sedation
  – Senna (*Cassia* senna): depletes serum potassium
  – Snakeroot (*Aristolochia* spp.): nephrotoxic
  – St. John's wort (*Hypericum perforatum*): numerous drug interactions; induces CYP(3a4) pathway, speeding metabolism of many drugs
  – Wormwood (*Artemisia absinthium*): elevates serotonin level, may raise BP
  – Yohimbe (*Pausinystalia yohimbe*): elevates BP

Geriatric Considerations

Gingko biloba commonly interacts with Coumadin.

Pediatric Considerations

ALERT

Iron is a leading cause of accidental poisoning in children <6 years of age. Minerals (i.e., potassium, calcium, magnesium, zinc, copper, and selenium) may cause toxicity.

- Vitamin A is most common cause of hypervitaminosis.
- Beta-carotene may have a limited potential for overdose.

REFERENCES

1. Peregoy JA, Clarke TC, Jones LI, et al. *Regional variation in use of complementary health approaches by U.S. adults. NCHS data brief, no 146*. Hyattsville, MD: National Center for Health Statistics; 2014.
2. Anderson JW, Liu C, Kryscio RJ. Blood pressure response to transcendental meditation: a meta-analysis. *Am J Hypertens*. 2008;21(3):310–316.
3. Manheimer E, White A, Berman B, et al. Meta-analysis: acupuncture for low back pain. *Ann Intern Med*. 2005;142(8):651–663.
4. Park JJ, Kang M, Shin S, et al. Unexplained infertility treated with acupuncture and herbal medicine in Korea. *J Altern Complement Med*. 2010;16(2):193–198.
5. Mortazavi SH, Khaki S, Moradi R, et al. Effects of massage therapy and presence of attendant on pain, anxiety and satisfaction during labor. *Arch Gynecol Obstet*. 2012;286(1):19–23.
6. Tobias DK, Zhang C, van Dam RM, et al. Physical activity before and during pregnancy and risk of gestational diabetes mellitus: a meta-analysis. *Diabetes Care*. 2011;34(1):223–229.
7. Kavanagh J, Kelly AJ, Thomas J. Breast stimulation for cervical ripening and induction of labour. *Cochrane Database Syst Rev*. 2005;(3):CD003392.
8. Alfaleh K, Anabrees J, Bassler D, et al. Probiotics for prevention of necrotizing enterocolitis in preterm infants. *Cochrane Database Syst Rev*. 2011;(3):CD005496.
9. Guillemard E, Tondu F, Lacoin F, et al. Consumption of a fermented dairy product containing the probiotic Lactobacillus casei DN-114001 reduces the duration of respiratory infections in the elderly in a randomised controlled trial. *Br J Nutr*. 2010;103(1):58–68.
10. Hojsak I, Snovak N, Abdović S, et al. Lactobacillus GG in the prevention of gastrointestinal and respiratory tract infections in children who attend day care centers: a randomized, double-blind, placebo-controlled trial. *Clin Nutr*. 2010;29(3):312–316.
11. Johnston BC, Supina AL, Ospina M, et al. Probiotics for the prevention of pediatric antibiotic-associated diarrhea. *Cochrane Database Syst Rev*. 2007;(2):CD004827.
12. Hickson M, D'Souza AL, Muthu N, et al. Use of probiotic Lactobacillus preparation to prevent diarrhoea associated with antibiotics: randomised double blind placebo controlled trial. *BMJ*. 2007;335(7610):80.
13. McFarland LV. Meta-analysis of probiotics for the prevention of traveler's diarrhea. *Travel Med Infect Dis*. 2007;5(2):97–105.
14. Makariou S, Liberopoulos EN, Elisaf M, et al. Novel roles of vitamin D in disease: what is new in 2011? *Eur J Intern Med*. 2011;22(4):355–362.

CLINICAL PEARLS

- Oral probiotics reduce respiratory and diarrheal infections and reduce mortality in preterm infants.
- Acupuncture is effective for back pain, headaches, and infertility.
- Yoga and breast stimulation shorten labor.
- Ginkgo and St. John's wort account for most herb–drug interactions described in the medical literature.

COMPLEX REGIONAL PAIN SYNDROME

Dennis E. Hughes, DO, FAAFP, FACEP

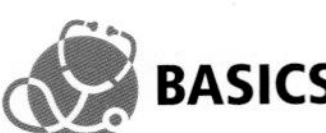

BASICS

DESCRIPTION

- Complex regional pain syndrome (CRPS) is a pain syndrome that is seemingly disproportionate in time or degree to any known trauma or lesion.
  - Type I: no nerve injury (reflex sympathetic dystrophy [RSD])
  - Type II: associated with a demonstrable nerve injury (causalgia)
- Synonym(s): traumatic erythromelalgia; Weir Mitchell causalgia; causalgia; reflex sympathetic dystrophy; posttraumatic neuralgia; sympathetically maintained pain

EPIDEMIOLOGY

- Incidence of 5.46/100,000 and prevalence of 20.57/1000,000 in United States
- Peak age 50–70 years
- Predominant gender: female > male (3:1, 60–81%)
- Recent studies found 3.8% occurrence after wrist fracture and 7% occurrence after ankle fracture (1)
- Extremely rare in children

ETIOLOGY AND PATHOPHYSIOLOGY

- Poorly understood activation of abnormal sympathetic reflex that lowers pain threshold.
  - Increased excitability of nociceptive neurons in the spinal cord; "central sensitization"
  - Exaggerated responses to normally nonpainful stimuli (hyperalgesia, allodynia)
- Other than known nerve injury (type II or causalgia), no known definitive pathogenesis

Genetics

No known genetic pattern

RISK FACTORS

- Minor or severe trauma (upper extremity fracture noted in 44%)
- Surgery (particularly carpal tunnel release)
- Lacerations
- Burns
- Frostbite
- Casting/immobilization after extremity injury
- Penetrating injury
- Polymyalgia rheumatica
- Myocardial infarction (MI)
- Cerebral vascular accident

GENERAL PREVENTION

- Early mobilization after fracture, stroke, and MI has proven benefit in reducing incidence of CRPS.
- 1 study of wrist fractures found that addition of 500 mg/day of vitamin C lowered rates of CRPS.
- There is evidence that limiting use of tourniquets, liberal regional anesthetic use, and ensuring adequate perioperative analgesia can reduce the incidence of CRPS-I.

COMMONLY ASSOCIATED CONDITIONS

- Serious injury to bone and soft tissue
- Herpes zoster
- Postherpetic neuralgia results from partial or complete damage to afferent nerve pathways.
- Pain occurs in dermatomes as a sequela of herpes zoster.

DIAGNOSIS

Unprovoked pain is the hallmark of the condition, and the diagnosis of CRPS is excluded by the existence of conditions that would otherwise account for the degree of symptoms. Clinical diagnostic criteria (2):

HISTORY

- Continuing pain which is disproportionate to any inciting event.
- One reported symptom in 3 of the 4 following categories:
  - Sensory: hyperalgesia and/or allodynia
  - Vasomotor: skin, temperature, color asymmetry
  - Sudomotor/edema: edema, sweating changes, or sweating asymmetry
  - Motor/trophic: decreased range of motion or motor dysfunction and/or trophic changes (hair, nail, skin)

PHYSICAL EXAM

At least one sign at evaluation in 2 of the following:

- Sensory: hyperalgesia (to pinprick) or allodynia (to light touch, pressure, or joint movement)
- Vasomotor: evidence of temperature, skin, color asymmetry
- Sudomotor/edema: evidence of edema or sweating changes or asymmetry
- Motor/trophic: decreased range of motion, motor dysfunction, or trophic changes in hair, nails, skin

DIFFERENTIAL DIAGNOSIS

- Infection
- Hypertrophic scar
- Bone fragments
- Neuroma
- CNS tumor or syrinx
- Deep vein thrombosis or thrombophlebitis
- Thoracic outlet syndrome

DIAGNOSTIC TESTS & INTERPRETATION

Initial Tests (lab, imaging)

- CBC
- Erythrocyte sedimentation rate (ESR)
- Plain radiographs may show patchy demineralization within 3–6 weeks of onset of CRPS and more pronounced than would be see from disuse alone.
- 3-phase bone scanning has varying sensitivity but is most accurate for support of the diagnosis when there is diffuse activity (especially on phase 3).
- Bone density

Diagnostic Procedures/Other

- Electromyelography (EMG) shows nerve injury with type II CRPS.
- Sudomotor function testing (resting sweat testing, resting skin temperature, quantitative sudomotor axon reflex testing; all related to increased autonomic activity of the affected limb)

Test Interpretation

- Partial or complete damage to afferent nerve pathways and probably reorganized central pain pathways
- Nerves most commonly involved are median and sciatic.
- Atrophy in affected muscles
- Incomplete nerve plexus lesion

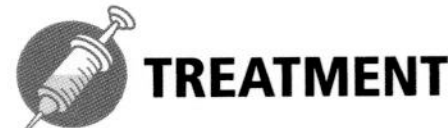

TREATMENT

GENERAL MEASURES

Discourage maladaptive behaviors (pain medication seeking, secondary gain). Principal of functional restoration is a stepwise and multidisciplinary approach.

MEDICATION

First Line

- NSAIDS recommended early in course but mixed support in literature
- The following have literature support of either limited or suggestive benefit in treatment of CRPS-I:
  - Corticosteroids (prednisone 30 mg/day × 2–12 weeks with taper) are the only class of drugs that have direct clinical trial support early in the course.
  - Gabapentin 600–1,800 mg/day for 8 weeks following diagnosis
  - 50% DMSO cream applied to affected extremity up to 5 times daily
  - N-acetylcysteine 600 mg TID
  - Bisphosphonates (alendronate) at 40 mg/day (however, optimal dose uncertain)
  - Nifedipine 20 mg/day showed benefit early in the course of the condition.

- Although many have advocated the use of tricyclic antidepressants in the treatment of CRPS, there is no credible evidence of improvement of pain. They may be helpful in controlling depressive symptoms that develop with disease progression (2).

Second Line

A number of small randomized controlled trials, clinical research, and observational studies show significant reduction in symptoms with the use of short courses (~1 week) of IV (and topical) ketamine (3)[B]; limited by toxicity at effective doses.

ISSUES FOR REFERRAL

- After 2 months of the illness, psychological evaluation generally is indicated to identify and treat any comorbid conditions.
- Identifying local resources and early referral for expert management give increased likelihood of long-term success in controlling condition.

ADDITIONAL THERAPIES

Type I

- Physical and occupational therapy (beneficial to the overall prognosis for recovery)
  - Should be started early
  - "Mirror therapy" has shown good results.
- Transcutaneous nerve stimulation
- Psychotherapy

SURGERY/OTHER PROCEDURES

- Type II responds more favorably to nerve-directed treatment
  - Sympathetic blocks
  - Cervicothoracic or lumbar sympathectomies have little data to support their use and should be used judici1ously and after all other therapies have failed (4)[A].
- Anesthetic blockade (chemical or surgical) of sympathetic nerve function
  - Transient relief suggests that chemical or surgical sympathectomy will be helpful.
  - Little in the way of quality clinical trials exist to support local sympathetic blockage as the gold standard of therapy.
- IV regional sympathetic block with guanethidine or reserpine by pain specialist or anesthetist
- Transcutaneous electric nerve stimulation (controversial)
- Inject myofascial painful trigger points
- Spinal cord stimulation (quality of life improved only with implanted system)
- Intrathecal analgesia
- Amputation as a last resort in severe cases, with patients reporting improved quality of life

COMPLEMENTARY & ALTERNATIVE MEDICINE

- Vitamin C (500 mg/day) may help to prevent CRPS in those with wrist fracture.
- Briskly rub the affected part several times per day
- Acupuncture
- Hypnosis can be suggested
- Relaxation training (alternate muscle relaxing and contracting)
- Biofeedback

INPATIENT CONSIDERATIONS

Admission Criteria/Initial Stabilization

Only for proposed surgical therapy

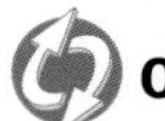

ONGOING CARE

FOLLOW-UP RECOMMENDATIONS

Weekly, to monitor progress and initiate additional modalities as needed

PATIENT EDUCATION

- Stress need to remain active physically
- Instruct carefully about any prescribed medications
- Reflex Sympathetic Dystrophy Syndrome Association, www.rsds.org, 203-877-3790
- American RSD Hope Group, www.rsdhope.org, 207-583-4589

PROGNOSIS

Most improve with early treatment, but symptoms may be lifelong if there is limited response to initial treatments.

COMPLICATIONS

- Depression
- Disability
- Opioid dependence

REFERENCES

1. Fukushima FB, Bezerra DM, Villas Boas PJF, et al. Complex regional pain syndrome. *BMJ*. 2014;348:g3683.
2. Harden RN, Oaklander AL, Burton AW, etal. Complex regional pain syndrome: practical diagnostic and treatment guidelines, 4th edition. *Pain Med*. 2013;14(2):180–229.
3. Azari P, Lindsay DR, Briones D, et al. Efficacy and safety of ketamine in patients with complex regional pain syndrome: a systematic review. *CNS Drugs*. 2012;26(3):215–228.
4. Straube S, Derry S, Moore RA, et al. Cervico-thoracic or lumbar sympathectomy for neuropathic pain and complex regional pain syndrome. *Cochrane Database Syst Rev*. 2013;9:CD002918.

C

ADDITIONAL READING

- Ezendam D, Bongers RM, Jannink MJ, et al. Systematic review of the effectiveness of mirror therapy in upper extremity function. *Disabil Rehabil*. 2009;31(26):2135–2149.
- Goebel A. Complex regional pain syndrome in adults. *Rheumatology*. 2011;50(10):1739–1750.
- Perez RS, Zollinger PE, Dijkstra PU, et al. Evidence based guidelines for complex regional pain syndrome type I. *BMC Neurol*. 2010;10:20.
- Tran De QH, Duong S, Bertini P, et al. Treatment of complex regional pain syndrome: a review of the evidence. *Can J Anaesth*. 2010;57(2):149–166.

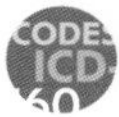

CODES

ICD10

- G90.50 Complex regional pain syndrome I, unspecified
- G90.519 Complex regional pain syndrome I of unspecified upper limb
- G90.529 Complex regional pain syndrome I of unspecified lower limb

CLINICAL PEARLS

- A pain syndrome disproportioned to injury
- Pain control and early mobility are the key to recovery.
- Avoid use of opiate analgesics.
- Use a multidisciplinary approach.

CONCUSSION (MILD TRAUMATIC BRAIN INJURY)

Nathan Cardoos, MD • J. Herbert Stevenson, MD

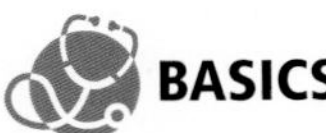

BASICS

DESCRIPTION

- Concussion (or mild traumatic brain injury [mTBI]) is defined as a complex pathophysiologic process affecting the brain, induced by traumatic biomechanical forces. This can be caused by a direct blow to the head or indirectly anywhere on the body where impulsive force is then transmitted to the head.
- Concussion may or may not involve loss of consciousness; headache, dizziness, and confusion are identified as the most common complaints. There is currently no widely accepted classification system for concussions.

Pediatric Considerations

Resolution of symptoms and return to neurocognitive baseline often take longer in pediatric and adolescent athletes (<18 years) (1)[B].

EPIDEMIOLOGY

- The CDC estimates 1.6–3.8 million concussions every year, although many go unreported.
- >1 million ER visits every year are due to TBIs (falls, MVAs, assault, sports, other); >1/2 of these visits are by children aged 5–18 years.
- High school and college athlete concussion rates have increased in the past 30 years, likely in part due to increased reporting.
- American football is associated with the highest number of TBIs.
- Concussions occur more often in games than practices.
- Female athletes have more reported concussions than male athletes in similar sports and more frequently suffer cognitive impairment.

Incidence

- The most common cause of TBI in the elderly (>65 years of age) is falls.
- Up to 1/3 of all sports-related concussions may go unreported or undiagnosed (2)[B].
- Sports (numbers per 1,000 athlete exposures, defined as one athlete playing in one game or practice) (3)[B]
  - Football: college 0.61 (0.39 in practice, 3.02 in games), high school 0.47 (0.21 in practice, 1.55 in games)
  - Basketball (college): males 0.16; females 0.22
  - Ice hockey (college): males 0.41, females 0.91
  - Lacrosse (college): males 0.26, females 0.25
  - Soccer: males 0.49, high school males 0.22, college females 0.63, high school females 0.36
  - Skiing and snowboarding: 0.005 and 0.004, respectively. Snowboarders have a higher incidence of severe brain injuries than skiers.

ETIOLOGY AND PATHOPHYSIOLOGY

- Direct or indirect injury to the head
  - Falls
  - Sports-related injuries
  - Motor vehicle accidents
  - Assaults
- Identifiable metabolic changes include alterations in intra-/extracellular potassium, calcium, and glutamate with subsequent neuron dysfunction. Microtearing of cerebral blood vessels and a relative decrease in cerebral blood flow also occurs. An increased requirement for glucose by the brain, coupled with decreased blood flow, may result in cellular dysfunction and increased susceptibility to subsequent brain insults. Other biochemical changes are currently being studied.
- Structural abnormalities of the brain are typically absent based on imaging studies.

RISK FACTORS

- Patients at high risk for falls: elderly, intoxication
- History of previous concussion
- Contact sports (particularly football): activities such as bicycling, cheerleading, skiing, and snowboarding; organized sports > leisure physical activity
- There are no reported incidences of concussion associated with heading a soccer ball in a 6-year study (4)[B].

GENERAL PREVENTION

- Educate athletes, coaches, parents, and officials about signs and symptoms of concussions.
- Preparticipation exams to identify risk factors in athletes
- Strength and conditioning (athletes and elderly)
- Rule enforcement in sports (e.g., penalties for spearing or head-to-head contact) and teaching athletes correct sports-specific techniques
- Protective equipment, such as helmets and mouth guards, decrease injuries but have not been shown to decrease concussion rates.

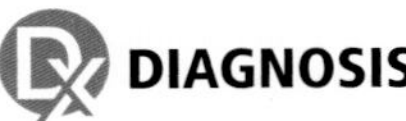

DIAGNOSIS

HISTORY

- Cognitive signs and symptoms
  - Confusion
  - Posttraumatic amnesia
  - Retrograde amnesia
  - Loss of consciousness (LOC, occurs in <10%)
  - Disorientation
  - Feeling "in a fog," "zoned out"
  - Inability to focus (i.e., difficulty at work or school)
  - Delayed verbal and motor responses
  - Slurred/incoherent speech
  - Excessive drowsiness
- Physical signs and symptoms
  - Headache (most common symptom)
  - Fatigue
  - Disequilibrium, dizziness
  - Visual disturbances
  - Phonophobia
  - Nausea
- Emotional signs and symptoms
  - Emotional lability
  - Irritability
  - Personality changes
- Sleep disturbance

PHYSICAL EXAM

Variable and dependent on acuteness of assessment, degree of injury:

- ABCs
- Evaluate for C-spine stability and possible serious head injury.
- Assess for focal neurologic signs and symptoms.
- Thorough neurologic exam, including
  - State of alertness and orientation
  - Cranial nerves
  - 3- or 5-word recall at 5 minutes
  - Concentration/attention (serial 3s or 7s)
  - Cerebellar function (finger-to-nose, gait assessment) and postural stability assessment (Romberg test, single leg balance)
  - Deep tendon reflexes
  - Extremity strength

DIFFERENTIAL DIAGNOSIS

- Subdural hematoma
- Epidural hematoma
- Cerebral contusion
- Facial or skull fracture
- Seizure

DIAGNOSTIC TESTS & INTERPRETATION

- Serial cognitive and neurologic evaluations should be done by an experienced health care provider. Other assessment tools, such as the sport concussion assessment tool (SCAT3), can also be used. However, if baseline testing has not been done, assessment tools may not be helpful because a perfect baseline score cannot be assumed, particularly in adolescents.
- SCAT3 testing is appropriate for patients >13 years of age. The Child-SCAT3 was developed for children 5–12 years of age (5).
- The gold standard is a thorough evaluation and individualized treatment by a trained physician. Studies have not yet validated computerized testing as either improving outcomes or being cost effective.

Initial Tests (lab, imaging)

- C-spine x-rays for midline cervical tenderness, abnormal neurologic findings, or dangerous mechanism. Structural neuroimaging is usually normal in the setting of concussion.
- CT head or MRI is indicated with loss of consciousness, amnesia, focal neurologic deficit, age >65 years, coagulopathy, GCS score <15, seizure, evidence of skull fracture, persistent vomiting, or overall worsening symptoms.
- Various clinical decision rules for imaging exist including the NEXUS and Canadian CT head and C-spine rules.

Diagnostic Procedures/Other

- Monitoring for several hours after injury is paramount, as signs and symptoms may worsen.
- EEG testing is not commonly used; however, in studies, electrophysiologic abnormalities have been identified in concussed athletes for days after injury.

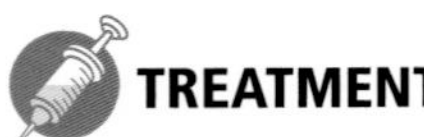

TREATMENT

GENERAL MEASURES

- There are no specific treatments for concussion. Physical and cognitive rest are the most important factors in initial management.
- Sunglasses, ear plugs if needed
- Consider no texting, video games, school, work, play, exercise, or sexual activity until symptoms begin to improve.
- A graded, individualized return to play plan can be initiated after complete resolution of all signs and symptoms (see "Follow-Up Recommendations").

MEDICATION

- Ibuprofen or acetaminophen may be used for headache once structural brain injury ruled out; limit use to a few days to reduce risk for rebound headache
- Prolonged symptoms such as sleep disturbance, depression, or anxiety may benefit from appropriate pharmacologic treatment for symptom relief (i.e., SSRIs, amitriptyline, etc.).

ISSUES FOR REFERRAL
- Most concussions can be managed by primary care physicians; referral to a specialist is not mandatory.
- Patients with prolonged signs and symptoms of concussion, or who have suffered recurrent concussions, should be referred to a sports medicine physician or neurologist for management and clearance prior to returning to sports activities.

SURGERY/OTHER PROCEDURES
Not indicated, unless signs of more severe TBI are present with increased intracranial pressure or large bleeding

INPATIENT CONSIDERATIONS
Admission Criteria/Initial Stabilization
- ABCs take priority over head injury and concussion.
- C-spine immobilization should be considered in all head trauma, especially for GCS <15, neck pain or tenderness, or focal neurologic deficit.
- Admit for progressive neurologic symptoms, including deterioration of mental status, seizures, and focal neurologic signs, or when no competent adult at home.

DISCHARGE CRITERIA
- Improving mental status at or near baseline
- Competent adult at home for patient observation

ONGOING CARE

FOLLOW-UP RECOMMENDATIONS
- Any athlete with a suspected concussion should not be allowed to return to play on the same day.
- Return to play guidelines: Decisions for athletes should be individualized, graded, and not made without follow-up evaluation(s). This includes the following:
  - Complete rest until symptom-free
  - Gradual reintroduction of activity as long as symptom-free. Each step should generally be done 24 hours apart (6)[C]:
    - Light aerobic exercise
    - Sports-specific exercise
    - Noncontact training drills
    - Full-contact training
    - Game play
- If any signs or symptoms recur (i.e., exertional headache, visual disturbance, or disequilibrium), stop all activity until again asymptomatic for 24 hours. Restart return to play protocol at last step that the patient was asymptomatic.
- For student athletes, the period of time away from class and homework should be individualized and symptom-based.
- Athletes at high risk for prolonged recovery include pediatric athletes and athletes with mood disorders, learning disabilities, or migraine headaches. These athletes should have a slower return to play progression and may require more intensive evaluation (formal neuropsychologic, balance, symptom testing).
- Athletes with multiple concussions should have slower return to play and may benefit from sports medicine consultation or neurology referral.

Patient Monitoring
- Written instructions regarding postconcussion management should be given to a competent adult, describing signs to watch for and when to bring the patient back for further evaluation.
- Have a follow-up plan prior to discharge to home, ideally to be seen within a few days.
- Instruct patients and families regarding postconcussive signs and symptoms.
- Ensure adequate cognitive and physical rest and symptom-free return to school, work, and sports-related activities.
- Some states now require specific training in order to provide medical clearance for return to sport after concussion.

DIET
As tolerated

COMPLICATIONS
- Delayed hematomas, including subdural hematomas, can present minutes to hours after initial injury, necessitating serial neurologic checks and close observation.
- Second-impact syndrome describes rare but life-threatening cerebral edema that occurs after repeated head injury, before the brain has had adequate time to completely recover (highest susceptibility within first 7–10 days of initial concussion). The etiology is thought to be due to loss of regulation of either cerebral circulation or glucose metabolism in the concussed brain.
- Recovery can be prolonged or complicated by concussion history, age (youths need more time to heal than adults), and preexisting conditions (migraines, depression, ADHD, anxiety, learning disabilities).
- Postconcussion syndrome occurs when symptoms of concussion, such as headache, fatigue, memory changes, or emotional lability, are persistent and last at least 1–3 months or longer.
- Chronic traumatic encephalopathy (CTE) with chronic cognitive, mood, and potential Parkinson-type symptoms is a distinct neurodegenerative disease that may be related to repeated concussions, although causality has not been proven.

REFERENCES

1. Zuckerman SL, Odom M, Lee YM, et al. Sport-related concussion and age: number of days to neurocognitive baseline. *Neurosurgery*. 2012;71(2):E558.
2. Meehan WP III, Mannix RC, O'Brien MJ, et al. The prevalence of undiagnosed concussions in athletes. *Clin J Sport Med*. 2013;23(5):339–342.
3. Daneshvar DH, Nowinski CJ, McKee AC, et al. The epidemiology of sport-related concussion. *Clin Sports Med*. 2011;30(1):1–17, vii.
4. Fuller CW, Junge A, Dvorak J. A six year prospective study of the incidence and causes of head and neck injuries in international football. *Br J Sports Med*. 2005;39(Suppl 1):i3–i9.
5. Guskiewicz KM, Register-Mihalik J, McCrory P, et al. Evidence-based approach to revising the SCAT2: introducing the SCAT3. *Br J Sports Med*. 2013;47(5):289–293.
6. McCrory P, Meeuwisse W, Aubry M, et al. Consensus statement on concussion in sport: the 4th International Conference on Concussion in Sport held in Zurich, November 2012. *Br J Sports Med*. 2013;47(5):250–258.

ADDITIONAL READING

- Almasi SJ, Wilson JJ. An update on the diagnosis and management of concussion. *WMJ*. 2012;111(1):21–27; quiz 28.
- Grady MF. Concussion in the adolescent athlete. *Curr Probl Pediatr Adolesc Health Care*. 2010;40(7):154–169.
- Guskiewicz KM, Marshall SW, Bailes J, et al. Association between recurrent concussion and late-life cognitive impairment in retired professional football players. *Neurosurgery*. 2005;57(4):719–726; discussion 719–726.
- Halstead ME, Walter KD; Council on Sports Medicine and Fitness. American Academy of Pediatrics. Clinical report—sport-related concussion in children and adolescents. *Pediatrics*. 2010;126(3):597–615.
- Herring SA, Kibler WB, Putukian M, et al. Team Physician Consensus Statement: 2013 update. *Med Sci Sports Exerc*. 2013;45(8):1618–1622.
- Jinguji TM, Bompadre V, Harmon KG, et al. Sport Concussion Assessment Tool-2: baseline values for high school athletes. *Br J Sports Med*. 2012;46(5):365–370.
- Khurana VG, Kaye AH. An overview of concussion in sport. *J Clin Neurosci*. 2012;19(1):1–11.
- Valovich McLeod TC, Bay RC, Lam KC, et al. Representative baseline values on the Sport Concussion Assessment Tool 2 (SCAT2) in adolescent athletes vary by gender, grade, and concussion history. *Am J Sports Med*. 2012;40(4):927–933.

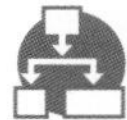

SEE ALSO
Brain Injury, Traumatic; Postconcussion Syndrome (Mild Traumatic Brain Injury); Seizure Disorders

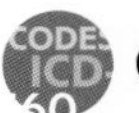

CODES

ICD10
- S06.0X0A Concussion without loss of consciousness, initial encounter
- S06.9X0A Unsp intracranial injury w/o loss of consciousness, init
- S06.0X9A Concussion w loss of consciousness of unsp duration, init

CLINICAL PEARLS
- Concussions occur from direct or indirect force to the head; loss of consciousness is not required.
- Any athlete with a suspected concussion should not be allowed to return to play on the same day.
- Monitor for several hours after concussion; frequent waking from sleep is controversial, and sleep deprivation can make symptoms worse.
- Complete cognitive and physical rest are paramount to the initial management of concussion.
- Complete resolution of concussion symptoms most often spontaneously occurs within 7–10 days. Pediatric and adolescent populations, those with certain medical conditions, and those with a previous history of concussion may take more time to fully recover.
- An individualized, graded return to play plan can be initiated after complete resolution of signs and symptoms of concussion. If symptoms recur during any step of the plan, the athlete should postpone activity until asymptomatic for 24 hours.

CONDYLOMATA ACUMINATA

Tayseer Husain Chowdhry, MD, MA • Edward James Kruse, DO

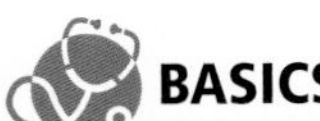

BASICS

DESCRIPTION

- Condylomata acuminata are soft, skin-colored, fleshy lesions (commonly called genital warts) that are caused by human papillomavirus (HPV):
  - Warts appear singly or in groups (a single wart is a "condyloma"; multiple warts are "condylomas" or "condylomata"); small or large; typically appear on the anogenital skin (penis, scrotum, introitus, vulva, perianal area); and may occur in the anogenital tract (vagina, cervix, rectum, urethra, anus); also conjunctival, nasal, oral, and laryngeal warts
- System(s) affected: skin/exocrine, reproductive, occasionally respiratory
- HIV considerations:
  - Treatment for external genital warts should not be different for HIV-infected persons (1).
  - May have larger or more numerous warts (1)
  - May not respond as well as immunocompetent persons to therapy (1)

Pediatric Considerations

- Consider sexual abuse if seen in children, although children can be infected by other means (e.g., transfer from wart on another child's hand or prolonged latency period) (2).
- American Academy of Pediatrics recommends all school-aged children who present with lesions be evaluated for abuse and screened for other STDs (2).

Pregnancy Considerations

- Warts often grow larger during pregnancy and regress spontaneously after delivery.
- Virus does not cross the placenta. Treatment during pregnancy is somewhat controversial. Cesarean section is not absolutely indicated for maternal condylomata (3)[A].
- Cervical infection has been found to be a risk factor for preterm birth (3)[A].
- Few documented cases of laryngeal papillomas due to HPV transmission at the time of delivery. Although rare, the condition is life-threatening (4).
- HPV vaccination is contraindicated in pregnancy.
- The safety of imiquimod, sinecatechins, podophyllin, and podofilox during pregnancy has not been established (3)[C].

EPIDEMIOLOGY

- HPV types 6 and 11 associated with 90% of condylomata acuminata. Types 16, 18, 31, 33, and 35 may be found in warts and may be associated with high-grade intraepithelial dysplasia in immunocompromised states such as HIV.
- Highly contagious; incubation period may be from 1 to 8 months. Initial infections may very well go unrecognized, so a "new" outbreak may be a relapse of an infection acquired years prior.
- Predominant age: 15–30 years
- Predominant sex: male = female
- Most infections are transient and clear spontaneously within 2 years.

Incidence

- One study population demonstrated that from 2007 to 2010, with the introduction of HPV vaccines, the incidence of genital warts decreased 35% (from 0.94% per year to 0.61% per year) in females < 21 years, and decreased 19% in males <21.
- Increased size and number of warts in immunocompromised patients

Prevalence

- Most common viral sexually transmitted infection (STI) in the United States. Most sexually active men and women will have acquired a genital HPV infection, usually asymptomatic, at some time.
- Peak prevalence in ages 17–33 years
- 10–20% of sexually active women may be actively infected with HPV. Studies in men suggest a similar prevalence.
- Pregnancy and immunosuppression favor recurrence and increased growth of lesions.

ETIOLOGY AND PATHOPHYSIOLOGY

HPV is a circular, double-stranded DNA molecule. There are >120 HPV subtypes. HPV types that cause genital warts do not cause anogenital cancers.

RISK FACTORS

- Usually acquired by sexual activity
  - Young adults and adolescents
  - Multiple sexual partners; short interval between meeting new sex partner and first intercourse
  - Not using condoms
  - Young age of commencing sexual activity
  - History of other STI
- Immunosuppression (particularly HIV)

GENERAL PREVENTION

- Sexual abstinence or monogamy
- Quadrivalent HPV vaccine available against genital warts and cervical cancer. This vaccine is targeted to adolescents before the period of their greatest risk for exposure to HPV. The vaccine does not treat previous infections:
  - Immunity has been documented to last at least 5 years after HPV vaccination.
  - The HPV quadrivalent vaccine (Gardasil) protects against the 2 most common HPV serotypes (types 6 and 11, which cause most anogenital warts) and the 2 most cancer-promoting types (16 and 18) (5).
  - Quadrivalent vaccine is indicated for females and males ages 9–26 years: Vaccine is administered IM; 3 doses at 0, 2, and 6 months to achieve optimal seroconversion (6).
  - Vaccine efficacy for preventing external genital warts is related to age of administration of 1st dose: 76% if aged <20 years, 93% if < 14.
- Bivalent HPV vaccine is available but does not cover the HPV types that cause most condyloma lesions (Cervarix) (5).
- Quadrivalent vaccine has been proven effective in prevention of external lesions in males 16–26 years of age (5).
- Use of condoms is partially effective, although warts may be easily spread by lesions not covered by a condom (e.g., 40% of infected men have scrotal warts).
- Abstinence until treatment completed

COMMONLY ASSOCIATED CONDITIONS

- >90% of cervical cancer associated with HPV types 16, 18, 31, 33, and 35
- 60% of oropharyngeal and anogenital squamous cell carcinomas are associated with HPV.
- STIs (e.g., gonorrhea, syphilis, chlamydia), AIDS

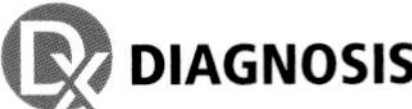

DIAGNOSIS

HISTORY

- Explore sexual history, contraception use, and other lifestyle issues.
- Most warts are asymptomatic but may cause
  - Pruritus, burning, redness, pain, bleeding
  - Vaginal discharge
  - Large warts may cause obstructive symptoms in the anus (with defecation) or vaginal canal (with intercourse or childbirth).

PHYSICAL EXAM

- Lesions often have a typical rough, warty appearance with multiple fingerlike projections but may be soft, sessile, and smooth.
- Large lesions are cauliflower-like and may grow to >10 cm.
- Most common sites: penis, vaginal introitus, and perianal region
- May be seen anywhere on the anogenital epithelium or in the anogenital tract
- Warts often occur in clusters.
- Bleeding or irritation of the lesions may be noted.

DIFFERENTIAL DIAGNOSIS

- Condylomata lata (flat warts of syphilis)
- Lichen planus
- Normal sebaceous glands
- Seborrheic keratosis
- Molluscum contagiosum
- Keratomas, micropapillomatosis
- Scabies
- Crohn disease
- Skin tags
- Melanocytic nevi
- Vulvar intraepithelial neoplasia
- Squamous cell carcinoma

DIAGNOSTIC TESTS & INTERPRETATION

- Diagnosis is usually clinical, made by unaided visual examination of the lesions.
- Biopsy
- Acetowhitening test: Subclinical lesions can be visualized by wrapping the penis with gauze soaked with 5% acetic acid (vinegar) for 5 minutes. Using a 10× hand lens or colposcope, warts appear as tiny white papules. A shiny white appearance of the skin represents foci of epithelial hyperplasia (subclinical infection), but because of low specificity, the CDC recommends against routine use of this test to screen for HPV mucosal infection.

Initial Tests (lab, imaging)

- Usually not required for diagnosis
- Serologic tests for syphilis may be helpful to rule out condylomata lata.
- Other testing for STIs
- Pap smear may be indicated.

Follow-Up Tests & Special Considerations

Because squamous cell carcinoma may resemble or coexist with condylomata, biopsy may be considered for lesions refractory to therapy.

Diagnostic Procedures/Other

- Biopsy with highly specialized identification techniques, such as HPV DNA detected through polymerase chain reaction, is rarely useful.

- Colposcopy, antroscopy, anoscopy, and urethroscopy may be required to detect anogenital tract lesions.
- Screening men who have sex with men (MSM) with anal Pap smears is controversial.

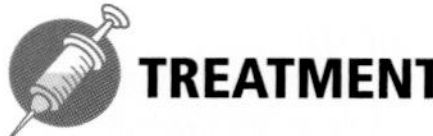

TREATMENT

GENERAL MEASURES

- May resolve spontaneously
- Change therapy if no improvement after 3 treatments, no complete clearance after 6 treatments, or therapy's duration or dosage exceeds manufacturer's recommendations.
- Appropriate screening/counseling of partners

MEDICATION

First Line

- No single therapy for genital warts is ideal for all patients or clearly superior to other therapies.
- Recommendations for external genital warts, patient-applied:
  - Podofilox (Condylox): antimitotic action; apply 0.5% solution or gel to warts twice daily (allowing to dry) for 3 consecutive days at home followed by 4 days of no therapy; may repeat up to 4 total cycles; maximum of 0.5 mL/day or area less than 10 cm^2 (3)[A],(7)
  - Imiquimod (Aldara): immune enhancer; self-treatment with a 5% cream applied once daily at bedtime 3 times weekly until warts resolve for up to 16 weeks. Wash off with soap and water 6–10 hours after application. Imiquimod has been noted to weaken condoms and diaphragms; therefore, patients should refrain from sexual contact while the cream is on the skin (3)[A],(8).
  - Sinecatechins (Veregen): immune enhancer and antioxidant, extract from green tea; apply a 0.5-cm strand of ointment 3 times daily for up to 16 weeks. Do not wash off after use (3)[A].
- Recommendations for external genital warts, provider-applied:
  - Cryotherapy: liquid nitrogen applied to warts for two 10-second bursts with thawing in between; usually requires 2–3 weekly sessions (3)[A]
  - Podophyllin 10–25% in tincture of benzoin. Apply directly to warts, air-dry in office before coming into contact with clothes. Wash off in 1–4 hours. Repeat every 7 days in office until gone (3)[A],(7).
  - Trichloroacetic acid (TCA): 80% solution. Apply only to warts; powder/talc to remove unreacted acid. Repeat in office at weekly intervals; ideal for isolated lesions in pregnancy (3)[A]
- Recommendations for exophytic cervical warts: biopsy to exclude high-grade squamous intraepithelial lesion (SIL) (3)[A]
- Recommendations for vaginal warts: cryotherapy or TCA or bichloracetic acid (BCA) 80–90% (3)[A]
- Recommendations for urethral meatus warts: cryotherapy or podophyllin 10–25% in compound tincture of benzoin (3)[A]
- Recommendations for anal warts: cryotherapy, TCA or BCA 80–90%, or surgery; specialty consultation for intra-anal warts (3)[A]

Pregnancy Considerations

Cryotherapy, surgery, or TCA. Medications contraindicated in pregnancy: podophyllin, podophyllotoxin, sinecatechins, interferon, and imiquimod (3)[C]

Second Line

Intralesional interferon, photodynamic therapy, topical cidofovir (3)[A]

SURGERY/OTHER PROCEDURES

- Larger warts may require surgical excision, laser treatment, or electrocoagulation (including infrared therapy):
  - Precaution: Laser treatment may create smoke plumes that contain HPV. CDC recommendation is for the use of a smoke evacuator no less than 2 inches from the surgical site. Masks are recommended, N95 the most efficacious.
- Intraurethral, external (penile and perianal), anal, and oral lesions can be treated with fulgurating CO_2 laser. Oral or external penile/perianal lesions can also be treated with electrocautery or surgery.

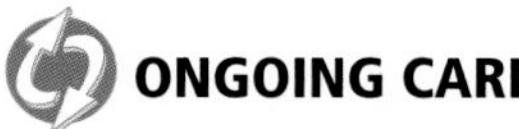

ONGOING CARE

FOLLOW-UP RECOMMENDATIONS

No restrictions, except for sexual contact

Patient Monitoring

- Patients should be seen every 1–2 weeks until lesions resolve.
- Patients should follow up 3 months after completion of treatment.
- Persistent warts require biopsy.
- Sexual partners require monitoring.

PATIENT EDUCATION

- Provide information on HPV, STI prevention, and condom use.
- Explain to patients that it is difficult to know how or when a person acquired an HPV infection; a diagnosis in 1 partner does not prove sexual infidelity in the other partner.
- Emphasize the need for women to follow recommendations for regular Pap smears.

PROGNOSIS

- Asymptomatic infection persists indefinitely.
- Treatment has not clearly been shown to decrease transmissible infectivity.
- Warts may clear with treatment or resolve spontaneously, but recurrences are frequent, particularly in the first 3 months, and may necessitate repeated treatments.

COMPLICATIONS

- Cervical dysplasia (probably does not occur with type 6 or 11, which cause most warts)
- Malignant change: Progression of condylomata to cancer rarely, if ever, occurs, although squamous cell carcinoma may coexist in larger warts.
- Urethral, vaginal, or anal obstruction from treatment
- The prevalence of high-grade dysplasia and cancer in anal canal is higher in HIV-positive than in HIV-negative patients, probably because of increased HPV activity.

REFERENCES

1. Gormley RH, Kovarik CL. Human papillomavirus-related genital disease in the immunocompromised host: part II. *J Am Acad Dermatol*. 2012;66(6):883.e1–883.e17; quiz 899–900.
2. Unger ER, Fajman NN, Maloney EM, et al. Anogenital human papillomavirus in sexually abused and nonabused children: a multicenter study. *Pediatrics*. 2011;128(3):e658–e665.
3. Workowski KA, Berman S; Centers for Disease Control and Prevention (CDC). Sexually transmitted diseases treatment guidelines, 2010. *MMWR Recomm Rep*. 2010;59(RR-12):1–110.
4. Gerein V, Schmandt S, Babkina N, et al. Human papilloma virus (HPV)-associated gynecological alteration in mothers of children with recurrent respiratory papillomatosis during long-term observation. *Cancer Detect Prev*. 2007;31(4):276–281.
5. Centers for Disease Control and Prevention. FDA licensure of bivalent human papillomavivaccine (HPV2, Cervarix) for use in females and updated HPV vaccination recommendations from the Advisory Committee on Immunization Practices (ACIP). MMWR Morb Mortal Wkly Rep. 2010;59(20):626–629
6. Centers for Disease Control and Prevention. Recommendations on the use of quadrivalent human papillomavirus vaccine in males—Advisory Committee on Immunization Practices (ACIP), 2011. *MMWR Morb Mortal Wkly Rep*. 2011;60(50):1705–1708.
7. Stockfleth E, Beti H, Orasan R, et al. Topical Polyphenon E in the treatment of external genital and perianal warts: a randomized controlled trial. *Br J Dermatol*. 2008;158(6):1329–1338.
8. Gotovtseva EP, Kapadia AS, Smolensky MH, et al. Optimal frequency of imiquimod (aldara) 5% cream for the treatment of external genital warts in immunocompetent adults: a meta-analysis. *Sex Transm Dis*. 2008;35(4):346–351.

ADDITIONAL READING

- Bauer HM, Wright G, Chow J. Evidence of human papillomavirus vaccine effectiveness in reducing genital warts: an analysis of California public family planning administrative claims data, 2007–2010. *Am J Public Health*. 2012;102(5):833–835.
- Giuliano AR, Palefsky JM, Goldstone S, et al. Efficacy of quadrivalent HPV vaccine against HPV infection and disease in males. *N Engl J Med*. 2011;364(5):401–411.
- Gormley RH, Kovarik CL. Human papillomavirus-related genital disease in the immunocompromised host: part I. *J Am Acad Dermatol*. 2012;66(6):867.e1–867.e14; quiz 881–882.

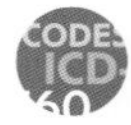

CODES

ICD10

A63.0 Anogenital (venereal) warts

CLINICAL PEARLS

- Condylomata acuminata are soft, skin-colored, fleshy lesions caused by HPV subtypes 6, 11, 16, 18, 31, 33, and 35.
- Quadrivalent HPV vaccine addresses the 2 most common HPV serotypes to be contracted in warts types 6 and 11 and the 2 most cancer-promoting types in 16 and 18 (Gardasil).
- Vaccine: 0.5 mL IM first dose and at months 2 and 6
- The majority of sexually active men and women will have acquired a genital HPV infection, usually asymptomatic, at some time.
- No single therapy for genital warts is ideal for all patients or clearly superior to other therapies.
- Quadrivalent HPV vaccine is effective in preventing HPV infection, particularly if administered prior to the onset of engaging in sexual activity. Gardasil is approved and recommended for use in males and females aged 9–26 years.

CONSTIPATION

Robert A. Baldor, MD, FAAFP • Mark B. Stephens, MD, MS, FAAFP, CAPT, MC, USN

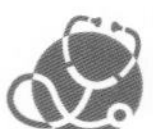

BASICS

- A group of syndromes with similar findings that include unsatisfactory defecation characterized by infrequent stools, difficult stool passage, or both
- Characteristics include <3 bowel movements a week, hard stools, excessive straining, prolonged time spent on the toilet, a sense of incomplete evacuation, and abdominal discomfort/bloating.

DESCRIPTION

- System(s) affected: gastrointestinal (GI)
- Synonym(s): obstipation

Geriatric Considerations

Colorectal neoplasms may be associated with constipation as individuals age; new-onset constipation after age 50 years is a "red flag."

Pediatric Considerations

Consider Hirschsprung disease (absence of colonic ganglion cells): 25% of all newborn intestinal obstructions, milder cases diagnosed in older children with chronic constipation, abdominal distension, decreased growth. 5:1 male-to-female ratio; associated with inherited conditions such as Down syndrome

EPIDEMIOLOGY

- More pronounced in children and elderly
- Predominant sex: female > male (2:1)
- Nonwhites > whites

Incidence

- 5 million office visits annually
- 100,000 hospitalizations

Prevalence

~15% of population affected

ETIOLOGY AND PATHOPHYSIOLOGY

- As food leaves the stomach, the ileocecal valve relaxes (gastroileal reflex) and chyme enters the colon (1–2 L/day) from the small intestine. In the colon, sodium is actively absorbed in exchange for potassium and bicarbonate. Water follows because of the osmotic gradient. Peristaltic contractions move chyme through the colon into the rectum. Chyme is converted into feces (200–250 mL).
- Normal transit time is 4 hours to reach the cecum and 12 hours to reach the pelvic colon.
- Defecation reflexively follows once stool reaches the rectal vault. This reflex can be inhibited by voluntarily contracting the external sphincter or facilitated by straining to contract the abdominal muscles while voluntarily relaxing the anal sphincter. Rectal distention initiates the defecation reflex. The urge to defecate occurs as rectal pressures increase. Distention of the stomach by food also initiates rectal contractions and a desire to defecate.
- Primary constipation
  - Slow colonic transit time (13%)
  - Pelvic floor/anal sphincter dysfunction (25%)
  - Functional: normal transit time and sphincter function, subjective symptoms (bloating, abdominal discomfort, perceived difficulty defecating, presence of hard stools) (69%)
- Secondary constipation
  - Irritable bowel syndrome (IBS)
  - Endocrine dysfunction (diabetes mellitus, hypothyroid)
  - Metabolic disorder (increased calcium, decreased potassium)
  - Mechanical (obstruction, rectocele)
  - Pregnancy
  - Neurologic disorders (Hirschsprung, multiple sclerosis, spinal cord injuries)
- Medication effect
  - Anticholinergic effects (antidepressants, narcotics, antipsychotics)
  - Antacids (calcium, aluminum)
  - Calcium channel blockers

Genetics

Unknown but may be familial

RISK FACTORS

- Extremes of life (very young and very old)
- Polypharmacy
- Sedentary lifestyle or condition
- Improper diet and inadequate fluid intake

GENERAL PREVENTION

High-fiber diet, adequate fluids, exercise, and training to "obey the urge" to defecate

COMMONLY ASSOCIATED CONDITIONS

- General debilitation (disease or aging)
- Dehydration
- Hypothyroidism
- Hypokalemia
- Hypercalcemia

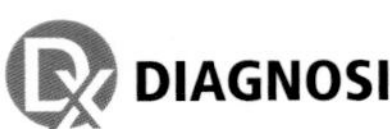

DIAGNOSIS

ALERT

Red flags:

- New onset after age of 50 years
- Hematochezia/melena
- Unintentional weight loss
- Anemia
- Neurologic defects

HISTORY

Rome III criteria (1)[C]:

- At least 2 of the following for 12 weeks in the previous 6 months:
  - <3 stools/week
  - Straining at least a 1/4 of the time
  - Hard stools at least 1/4 of time
  - Need for manual assist at least 1/4 of time
  - Sense of incomplete evacuation at least 1/4 of time
  - Sense of anorectal blockade at least 1/4 of time
- Loose stools rarely seen without use of laxatives.

PHYSICAL EXAM

- Vital signs, height, weight
- Digital rectal exam (masses, pain, stool, fissures, hemorrhoids, anal tone)
- Abdominal/gynecologic exam (masses, pain)
- Neurologic exam

DIFFERENTIAL DIAGNOSIS

- Congenital
  - Hirschsprung disease/syndrome
  - Hypoganglionosis
  - Congenital dilation of the colon
  - Small left colon syndrome

DIAGNOSTIC TESTS & INTERPRETATION

Primarily a clinical diagnosis

Initial Tests (lab, imaging)

CBC, glucose, TSH, calcium, and creatinine routinely and sigmoid/colonoscopy if red flags are present

Follow-Up Tests & Special Considerations

- If condition is refractory, pursue further testing:
  - Colonoscopy
  - Barium enema to look for obstruction and/or megarectum, megacolon, or Hirschsprung disease
- Additional testing
  - Measure colonic transit time by ingesting radiopaque (Sitz-Mark) markers.
  - Plain abdominal film obtained 5 days later (120 hours): Retention >20% markers indicates slow transit.
  - Markers seen exclusively in distal colon/rectum suggests defecatory disorder.

Diagnostic Procedures/Other

Consider referral in refractory cases to evaluate:

- Balloon expulsion
- Defecography using a barium paste
- Anorectal manometry with a rectal catheter

Test Interpretation

- Most cases are functional.
- Paucity or absence of intramural enteric ganglia in certain cases of congenital or acquired megacolon
- Neuromuscular abnormalities in certain cases of pseudo-obstruction

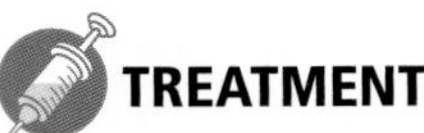

TREATMENT

Address immediate concerns:

- Bloating/discomfort/straining: osmotic agents
- Postoperative, after childbirth, hemorrhoids, fissures: stool softener to aid defecation
- If impacted: manual disimpaction, then treat the chronic underlying condition

GENERAL MEASURES

- Attempt to eliminate medications that may cause or worsen constipation.
- Increase fluid intake.
- Increase fiber in diet.
- Enemas if other methods fail

MEDICATION

In patients with no known secondary causes of constipation, conservative nonpharmacologic treatment is recommended:

- Regular exercise
- Increased fluid intake
- Bowel habit training

First Line

Bulking agents (must be accompanied by adequate amounts of liquid to be useful):

- Hydrophilic colloids (bulk-forming agents)
  - Psyllium (Konsyl, Metamucil, Perdiem Fiber): 1 tbsp in 8-oz liquid PO daily up to TID
  - Methylcellulose (Citrucel): 1 tbsp in 8-oz liquid PO daily up to TID
  - Polycarbophil (Mitrolan, FiberCon): 2 caplets with 8-oz liquid PO up to QID

- Stool softeners
  - Docusate sodium (Colace): 100 mg PO TID
- Osmotic laxatives
  - Polyethylene glycol (PEG) (MiraLax) 17 g/day PO dissolved in 4–8 oz of beverage (current evidence shows PEG to be superior to lactulose) (2)[B]
  - Lactulose (Chronulac): 15–60 mL PO QHS (flatulence, bloating, cramping)
  - Sorbitol: 15–60 mL PO QHS (as effective as lactulose)
  - Magnesium salts (milk of magnesia); 15–30 mL PO once daily; avoid in renal insufficiency

Second Line

- Stimulants (irritate bowel, causing muscle contraction; usually combined with a softener; work in 8–12 hours):
  - Senna/docusate (Senokot-S, Ex-lax, Peri-Colace): 1–2 tablets or 15–30 mL PO at bedtime
  - Bisacodyl (Dulcolax, Correctol): 1–3 tablets PO daily
- Lubricants (soften stool and facilitate passage of the feces by its lubricating oily effects):
  - Mineral oil (15–45 mL/day)
  - Short-term use only. Can bind fat-soluble vitamins, with the potential for deficiencies; may similarly decrease absorption of some drugs
  - Avoid in those at risk for aspiration (lipoid pneumonia)
- Suppositories
  - Osmotic: sodium phosphate
  - Lubricant: glycerin
  - Stimulatory: Bisacodyl
  - Enemas: saline (Fleet enema)
- Lubiprostone (Amitiza): a selective chloride channel activator; 24 μg PO BID:
  - Avoid in pregnancy and breastfeeding
- Linaclotide (Linzess): guanylate cyclase-C agonist; dose: 145 μg PO once daily; adult use only
- Methylnaltrexone (Relistor): a peripherally acting μ-opioid receptor (PAM-OR) antagonist; dose: 38–<62 kg: 8 mg; 62–114 kg: 12 mg SC every other day PRN:
  - Indicated for short-term (<4 months) palliative care use for opioid-induced constipation
  - Side effects: abdominal pain and flatulence
- Prokinetic agents (partial 5-HT4 agonists) have been withdrawn due to cardiac side effects; only available via IND protocols: tegaserod (Zelnorm), cisapride (Propulsid)
- Other agents not approved by the FDA:
  - Misoprostol (Cytotec): a prostaglandin that increases colonic motility
  - Colchicine: neurogenic stimulation to increase colonic motility

ADDITIONAL THERAPIES

Other nonpharmacologic therapies include the following:

- Biofeedback therapy
- Behavior therapy
- Electric stimulation

SURGERY/OTHER PROCEDURES

Surgery rarely indicated

INPATIENT CONSIDERATIONS

Toxic megacolon

Nursing

Manual disimpaction occasionally required in chronic refractory cases

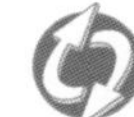

ONGOING-CARE

FOLLOW-UP RECOMMENDATIONS

Encourage exercise and physical activity.

Patient Monitoring

If what seems to be simple, functional constipation persists, further investigate for a possible organic cause.

DIET

Increase fiber, but bloating and gas can be problematic:

- Gradually increase intake to 25 g/day over a 6-week period.
- Insoluble, less fermentable fiber, like wheat bran, tends to be better tolerated.
- Bran (hard outer layer of cereal grains)
- Vegetables and fruits
- Whole grain foods
- Encourage liberal intake of fluids.

PATIENT EDUCATION

- Occasional mild constipation is normal.
- Instruction in consistent bowel training; the best time to move bowels is in the morning, after eating breakfast, when the normal bowel transit and defecation reflexes are typically functioning to move the bowels.

PROGNOSIS

- Occasional constipation responsive to simple measures is harmless.
- Habitual constipation can be a lifelong nuisance.
- Patients with neurologic compromise can suffer from ill effects such as obstipation, impaction, and toxic megacolon.
- No evidence for laxative dependence
- No evidence for harm from stimulant use; melanosis coli may develop, but it is a benign condition.

COMPLICATIONS

- Volvulus
- Toxic megacolon
- Acquired megacolon: in severe, long-standing cases
- Fluid and electrolyte depletion: laxative abuse
- Rectal ulceration (stercoral ulcer) related to recurrent fecal impaction
- Anal fissures

REFERENCES

1. Bove A, Pucciani F, Bellini M, et al. Consensus statement AIGO/SICCR: diagnosis and treatment of chronic constipation and obstructed defecation (part I: diagnosis). *World J Gastroenterol*. 2012;18(14):1555–1564.
2. Lee-Robichaud H, Thomas K, Morgan J, et al. Lactulose versus polyethylene glycol for chronic constipation. *Cochrane Database Syst Rev*. 2010;7:CD007570.

ADDITIONAL READING

- American College of Gastroenterology Chronic Constipation Task Force. An evidence-based approach to the management of chronic constipation in North America. *Am J Gastroenterol*. 2005;(100)(Suppl 1):S1–S4.
- Basilisco G, Coletta M. Chronic constipation: a critical review. *Dig Liver Dis*. 2013;45(11):886–893. doi:10.1016/j.dld.2013.03.016.
- Locke GR III, Pemberton JH, Phillips SF. American Gastroenterological Association Medical Position Statement: guidelines on constipation. *Gastroenterology*. 2000;119(6):1761–1766.
- Longstreth GF, Thompson WG, Chey WD, et al. Functional bowel disorders. *Gastroenterology*. 2006;130(5):1480–1491.
- Müller-Lissner SA, Kamm MA, Scarpignato C, et al. Myths and misconceptions about chronic constipation. *Am J Gastroenterol*. 2005;100(1):232–242.
- Roarty TP, Weber F, Soykan I, et al. Misoprostol in the treatment of chronic refractory constipation: results of a long-term open label trial. *Aliment Pharmacol Ther*. 1997;11(6):1059–1066.
- van Dijk M, Benninga MA, Grootenhuis MA, et al. Chronic childhood constipation: a review of the literature and the introduction of a protocolized behavioral intervention program. *Patient Educ Couns*. 2007;67(1–2):63–77.
- Verne GN, Davis RH, Robinson ME, et al. Treatment of chronic constipation with colchicine: randomized, double-blind, placebo-controlled, crossover trial. *Am J Gastroenterol*. 2003;98(5):1112–1116.
- Spinzi G, Amato A, Imperiali G, et al. Constipation in the elderly: management strategies. *Drugs Aging*. 2009;26(6):469–474.

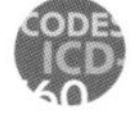

CODES

ICD10

- K59.00 Constipation, unspecified
- K59.01 Slow transit constipation
- K59.09 Other constipation

CLINICAL PEARLS

- Constipation can be characterized as unsatisfactory defecation, with infrequent stools, difficult stool passage, or both for 3 months.
- Functional constipation (normal transit time and sphincter function) is most common.
- Workup is necessary for red flags: onset >50 years, hematochezia/melena, unintentional weight loss, anemia, neurologic defects.
- Osmotic agents (polyethylene glycol [PEG]) have most evidence to support clinical effectiveness.

CONTRACEPTION

Ronya L. Green, MD, MPH

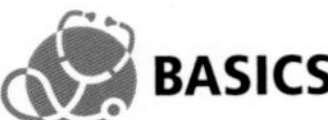

BASICS

DESCRIPTION

- To control the timing of pregnancy and prevent unintended pregnancies
- Contraception is selected based on patient preference, effectiveness, STD prevention, side effects, and contraindications.
- Contraception options are divided into 2 major categories: hormonal and nonhormonal.
- The most effective methods of contraception are vasectomy, female sterilization, and the long-acting reversible contraceptive (LARC) methods, including the intrauterine devices and progesterone implant.

EPIDEMIOLOGY

Incidence

- The estimated prevalence of contraception use among reproductive age women is 63% worldwide and 77% in the United States (1).
- However, 50% of all pregnancies in the United States are unintended. 50% of these occur in women using a form of reversible contraception. 50% of all unintended pregnancies in the United States result in termination.
- The most frequently used forms of contraception in the United States (in order of prevalence) are oral contraceptive pills (OCPs), female sterilization, male condom, male sterilization, and depot injectables. Despite their proven safety, effectiveness, and cost-effectiveness, LARC methods (intrauterine devices [IUDs] and the subdermal implant) are underused in the United States.

RISK FACTORS

- Unintended pregnancy: women ages 18–24 years and 35–44 years, unmarried/cohabitating women, women with less than a college education, minority women, pregnancy ambivalence (1)
- Contraception nonuse: being dissatisfied with one's method of contraception, behavioral errors or mistakes, and side effects

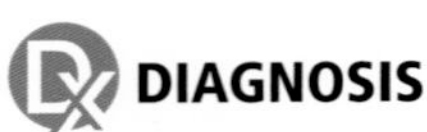

DIAGNOSIS

HISTORY

Review contraindications for selected methods.

- Contraindications to estrogen-containing hormonal contraception (2)[A]
  - History of coronary artery disease (CAD) or multiple risk factors (age >55 years, smoking, high BP, diabetes mellitus)
  - History of deep vein thrombosis (DVT)/pulmonary embolism (PE) or personal history of cerebrovascular accident (CVA)
  - History of migraines at age >35 years or migraine at any age with aura
  - Current or past breast cancer, active liver disease, or hepatic tumor
  - Pregnancy, unexplained abnormal uterine bleeding without further investigation
  - Relative contraindication to estrogen-containing hormonal contraception: smokers >35 years
  - Women with a history of uncontrolled hypertension, hyperlipidemia, and peripheral vascular disease who also take combined estrogen/progestin pills (COCs) are at increased CVA risk (3).
- Contraindications to IUDs: pregnancy, active uterine infection, malignancy in the uterus or cervix, an inability to place or retain the device, unexplained abnormal bleeding, and adverse reaction to product ingredients

DIAGNOSTIC TESTS & INTERPRETATION

- A negative pregnancy test (urine or serum) is advised prior to initiating contraception (2)[A].
- Testing for gonorrhea and chlamydia may be performed but is not required prior to IUD insertion. In high-risk populations, active infection should be ruled out prior to IUD insertion.
- In family history of thrombophilia, testing can be considered before initiation of estrogen-containing contraception, especially if specific defect is known (e.g., factor V Leiden or prothrombin 20210 mutation). In absence of known specific defect, current genetic testing not likely to be useful for patient in context of contraception.

Follow-Up Tests & Special Considerations

Routine 2–3-month follow-up after initiation of all methods of contraception to assess patient tolerance and acceptability of contraceptive method. BP check within 3 months of initiation in patients on combined OCPs due to the rare occurrence of hypertension in this population is often advised.

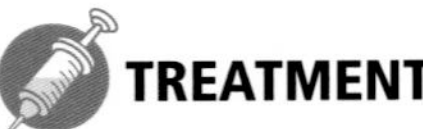

TREATMENT

GENERAL MEASURES

Nondrug methods

- Barrier methods: condoms (benefit: reduces risk of STIs), diaphragm (needs fitting), cervical cap (3 sizes, may cause vaginal irritation)
- Fertility awareness methods: calendar method, cervical mucus method, temperature method. These methods are low cost but generally not as effective as most other methods.
- Withdrawal method: Male partner withdraws from vagina before ejaculation. Failure occurs if withdrawal is not timed accurately or if the pre-ejaculatory fluid contains sperm.
- Lactational amenorrhea method: Breastfeeding is effective contraception only if (i) the infant is <6 months old, (ii) the infant is exclusively breastfeeding, and (iii) the mother has not resumed her regular menses.
- Abstinence

MEDICATION

- OCPs
  - COCs should be used for nonbreastfeeding patients without a contraindication to estrogen-containing contraception (see above):
    - Pills may be started at any time after pregnancy has been ruled out. Some providers prefer a "Sunday start" because they feel this is less confusing for patients. 1 study found better compliance at 3 months among patients assigned to start pills the day they were prescribed ("Quick start").
    - All COCs contain the same type of estrogen (ethinyl estradiol). COCs differ in the level of estrogen (range of 20–50 μg) and the type of progestin. Newer progestogens are less androgenic but may have increased rate of venous thromboembolism (VTE).
    - Patient response to any 1 type of COC is unpredictable. A starting pill is one that is inexpensive (generic); contains an average amount of estrogen (30–35 μg); and contains a well-studied, lower androgenicity progestin. Portia or Loestrin 1.5/30 are reasonable starting pills.
    - Patients should be instructed to take the pill every day and use backup birth control for the first 2 weeks after the initiation of pills. If a pill is missed, she should take 2 pills the following day. If 2 pills are missed, she should take 3 pills the following day and use a backup method for 7 days. If ≥3 pills are missed, the patient should be instructed to restart a new pack and use a backup for 2 weeks.
    - Most pills have a 21/7 regimen (21 active days and 7 placebo). Some new preparations have 24/4 combinations. It is reasonable for patients to skip the placebo pills and begin a new pack immediately on the active pill so as to avoid a period (continuous dosing). A withdrawal bleed 4 times a year reduces unplanned ("breakthrough") bleeding.
    - The most common side effects include nausea, bloating, headaches, and mastalgia. These symptoms tend to decrease over time. Nausea can be reduced by taking the pill at nighttime. Women who experience headaches can be counseled that these usually decrease over time.
  - Breastfeeding women desiring oral contraceptive medications should be prescribed progestin-only pills (e.g., Micronor), especially for the first months. Patients should be instructed to take these pills at the same time every day.
- Weekly hormonal patch (Ortho-Evra): The "patch" contains 20 μg ethinyl estradiol and 150 μg norelgestromin. It is applied transdermally and changed weekly. Produces higher serum estrogen levels than oral 20 μg pill and may be associated with a slightly increased risk of blood clot. Patch may cause local skin irritation. Not as reliable in women >90 kg
- Vaginal contraceptive ring (NuvaRing): a flexible polymer ring containing 15 μg ethinyl estradiol and 120 μg etonogestrel; inserted into vagina for 3 weeks/cycle (also may be used for continuous cycling for 4 weeks and replaced immediately with a fresh ring [off label])
- Medroxyprogesterone (Depo-Provera), also known as depot-medroxyprogesterone acetate (DMPA): 150 mg IM *or* 104 mg/0.65 mL SC, both are given every 3 months. Contraceptive levels of hormone persist for up to 4 months (2–4-week margin of safety). Major side effects include irregular bleeding and weight gain. Potential for decreased bone mineral density (BMD) if used for >2 years, so recommend that women take 1,300 mg of calcium and 400 IU of vitamin D when using DMPA. No evidence for increased fracture risk related to this method, and BMD recovers quickly on discontinuation.
- IUDs: These are highly effective, LARC methods with few side effects. 5-year failure rates are approximately 0.5%. IUD may be inserted anytime pregnancy is ruled out. May also be inserted immediately postpartum (within 10 minutes of removal of placenta) as well as postabortion. IUDs are commonly used in adolescents and other nulliparous women. 3 types of IUDs are currently available in the United States (4).
  - ParaGard (Copper T): interferes with sperm transport and ova fertilization; approved for up to 10 years but likely remains effective for longer. May increase menstrual blood loss. Also effective as postcoital contraceptive up to 5 days from intercourse

 - Mirena (Levonorgestrel intrauterine system): a T-shaped IUD that releases 20 μg/dose of levonorgestrel (very low serum levels). Approved for use up to 5 years; has been used off label for up to 7 years. Safe and effective for use in adolescents and nulliparous women. Side effects include irregular menstrual spotting for the first 3–6 months that usually resolves after 6 months of use. Some will not have menses after 1 year, although others may have continuing irregular spotting for years.
 - Skyla (Levonorgestrel intrauterine system): very similar to Mirena but releases lower hormone dose (14 μg/dose of levonorgestrel), is slightly smaller, and lasts 3 years. Smaller insertion tube might make this an easier IUD for nulliparous women. More bleeding days than Mirena
- Etonogestrel implant (Nexplanon): a small, single, plastic rod that is implanted into the superficial SC tissue of the upper arm and provides continuous contraception via progestin hormone. This prevents ovulation and thickens cervical mucus to halt fertilization. Effective for up to 3 years. The device may be inserted only by trained and certified providers. Menstrual irregularities are common the first 6–12 months (and beyond); some will not have menses after 1 year, although others may have continuing irregular spotting for years.
- Spermicides: All contain nonoxynol-9; may alter vaginal flora and mucosal barrier.
- Sponge (Today Sponge): Soft foam disk contains nonoxynol-9. Moisten with water before use; effective for 24 hours; must leave in for 6 hours after use; less effective in women who have given birth.
- Emergency contraception: Start within 72 hours for maximum effectiveness, but evidence supports up to 120 hours (5)[A]:
 - Levonorgestrel: 1.5 mg taken as 2 0.75-mg tablets (Plan B) or one 1.5-mg tablet (Plan B 1-Step). Less nausea and slightly more effective than the "Yuzpe regimen" (see below): available over the counter but may be less expensive for many women if prescribed
 - Estradiol/levonorgestrel (Preven, Ovral, Ogestrel): "Yuzpe regimen" 50 μg/0.25 mg, 2 tablets q12h (4 tablets total). Other OCs may be used as long as the dose of estrogen component ≥100 μg/dose. *Note*: Antinausea medication (e.g., Phenergan) should be given 1–2 hours before the doses.
 - Copper-bearing IUD (Paragard): Insert up to 5 days after intercourse; >99% effective in preventing pregnancy and continues to provide contraception for up to 10 years.
 - Ulipristal acetate (Ella): 30 mg × 1 dose; approved by FDA in 2010. Selective progesterone modulator, approved for use up to 5 days following unprotected intercourse.

Pediatric Considerations

Levonorgestrel is recommended for adolescent and teen girls who need emergency contraception. It may be purchased over the counter for women ages 17 years and older and men ages 18 years and older. A prescription is required for women younger than age 17 years. The medication is unavailable to men younger than.

SURGERY/OTHER PROCEDURES

Permanent sterilization. Female: tubal ligation or Essure (fallopian tube inserts placed hysteroscopically). Essure requires confirmation with hysterosalpingogram 3 months after procedure. Male: vasectomy. Male sterilization less complicated than female

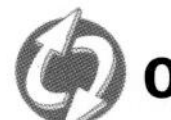

ONGOING CARE

FOLLOW-UP RECOMMENDATIONS

Patient Monitoring

- Pelvic exam, Pap smear, and STI testing, per guidelines
- Check for IUD strings 1 month after insertion. Spontaneous expulsion rate highest in 1st month. The patient should monitor presence of the string monthly following menses.

DIET

Some herbals, such as St. John' wort, may alter estrogen levels, reducing efficacy or causing breakthrough bleeding.

PATIENT EDUCATION

- Condoms: Water-based lubricants (inside and outside) reduce the risk of breakage. Withdraw penis before it becomes flaccid. New condom is required for each sex act. Male condoms available in both latex and nonlatex (if allergic to latex).
- IUD: Check string periodically.
- Diaphragm: Refit after childbirth or if weight changes by >10%. Before inserting, 1 tbs of water-soluble spermicidal jelly or cream should be placed in the dome. Leave in at least 6 hours after coitus. If coitus is repeated <6 hours, insert another teaspoon of spermicidal jelly into the vagina without removing the diaphragm.
- OCP: Pill should be taken at approximately the same time each day. If a pill is missed, see above instructions.
- Emergency contraception prevents pregnancy via several proposed mechanisms, including inhibition of sperm motility, alterations in tubal transport, unfavorable uterine receptivity, and/or fertilization inhibition. Emergency contraception does not affect an established pregnancy: 1-888-NOT-2-LATE or http://www.planbonestep.com/

COMPLICATIONS

- Hormonal contraceptives, serious: stroke, thromboembolism, hypertension, myocardial infarction
- Hormonal contraceptives, minor: nausea and vomiting: Take after eating. Breakthrough bleeding: usually self-limiting after 3 months; if persists, change pill. Amenorrhea: Pregnancy must be ruled out. Cyclic weight gain: Use smallest dose of estrogen available. Breast tenderness: rare with low-dose pill. Depression: rare with low-dose pill. Chloasma: Stop pill or cover with makeup. Acne or hirsutism: Change to a less-androgenic progesterone. Cholestatic jaundice: Stop pill; do not restart. Weight gain throughout cycle: Use triphasic pill to minimize dose of progesterone or use newer progesterone.
- Hormonal contraceptive users have an overall 5-fold increased risk of venous thrombosis compared to nonusers. This risk is comparable to the 4-fold increased risk of venous thrombosis during pregnancy (6)[B].
- Injectable contraceptive (Depo-Provera): irregular bleeding: No treatment needed; NSAID may help. Weight gain: average of 5 lb/year of use. Amenorrhea: common after 1 year of use. Possible ↑ bone resorption and ↓ BMD but rapid recovery following discontinuation. FDA recommends BMD for use >2 years and to consider periodic estrogen.
- Progesterone implant: irregular bleeding: Counsel patients extensively prior to insertion.
- Sponge and diaphragm: associated with toxic shock syndrome (rare)
- IUD: Pelvic inflammatory disease (PID) or salpingitis: Device removal is not necessary for mild PID treated as outpatient. For infections requiring hospitalization: Remove device. For heavy bleeding and cramps: trial of combined oral contraceptives, consider removing device. Although absolute risk less than without IUD, pregnancy, when it occurs, is more likely to be ectopic (5)[B].

REFERENCES

1. Blumenthal PD, Voedisch A, Gemzell-Danielsson K. Strategies to prevent unintended pregnancy: increasing use of long-acting reversible contraception. *Hum Reprod Update*. 2011;17(1):121–137.
2. For Centers for Disease Control and Prevention. United States Medical Eligibility Criteria (USMEC) for Contraceptive Use - Reproductive Health, see http://www.cdc.gov/reproductivehealth/unintendedpregnancy/USMEC.htm
3. Fehr AD, Mounsey A, Yates JE, et al. FPIN's clinical inquiries. Cardiovascular risks of combined oral contraceptive use. *Am Fam Physician*. 2012;86(12):1–2.
4. Shimoni N. Intrauterine contraceptives: a review of uses, side effects, and candidates. *Semin Reprod Med*. 2010;28(2):118–125.
5. Cheng L, Gülmezoglu AM, Piaggio G, et al. Interventions for emergency contraception. *Cochrane Database Syst Rev*. 2008;(3):CD001324.
6. Van Hylckama Vlieg A, Helmerhorst FM, Vandenbroucke JP, et al. The venous thrombotic risk of oral contraceptives, effects of oestrogen dose and progestogen type: results of the MEGA case-control study. *BMJ*. 2009;339:b2921.

ADDITIONAL READING

- Centers for Disease Control and Prevention. U.S. Medical Eligibility Criteria for Contraceptive Use, 2010. *MMWR Recomm Rep*. 2010;59(RR-4):1–86. http://www.cdc.gov/mmwr/pdf/rr/rr59e0528.pdf. Accessed 2014.
- Excellent chart comparing contraceptive methods: ARHP Method Match at http://www.arhp.org/methodmatch

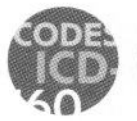

CODES

ICD10

- Z30.9 Encounter for contraceptive management, unspecified
- Z30.41 Encounter for surveillance of contraceptive pills
- Z30.431 Encounter for routine checking of intrauterine contracep dev

CLINICAL PEARLS

- Hormonal and IUD contraceptives may be initiated immediately ("Quick start") if the likelihood of preexisting pregnancy is low.
- Clearly established noncontraceptive benefits of OCPs include reduction in ovarian cancer, endometrial cancer, ectopic pregnancies, and PID; dysmenorrhea and anemia; functional ovarian cysts. Also, a regular menstrual cycle; improvement in acne. LARC methods provide high efficacy and convenience for patients.

COR PULMONALE

Parag Goyal, MD • Sergey G. Gurevich, MD • James M. Horowitz, MD, FACC

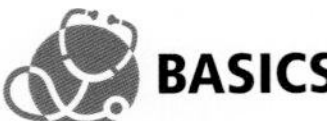

BASICS

DESCRIPTION

- Enlargement and subsequent dysfunction and failure of the right ventricle (RV) in the presence of pulmonary hypertension secondary to abnormalities of the pulmonary system, including disorders of the lung parenchyma, pulmonary circulation, chest wall, and ventilatory mechanisms.
- For the purposes of this review, pulmonary arterial hypertension (WHO Group I) will not be considered as a cause of cor pulmonale.
- May occur in acute or chronic setting
  - Acute: rapid increase of pulmonary arterial pressure resulting in RV overload, dysfunction, and potential cardiovascular collapse
  - Chronic: progressive hypertrophy and dilation of the RV over months to years, leading to dysfunction, and potentially failure

EPIDEMIOLOGY

- ~6–7% of all types of adult heart disease in United States
- Estimated 10–30% of heart failure admissions in the United States are the result of cor pulmonale, most commonly related to chronic obstructive pulmonary disease (COPD).

Incidence

Difficult to assess: Best estimate is 1/10,000–3/10,000/year.

Prevalence

Difficult to assess: Best estimate is 2/1,000–6/1,000.

ETIOLOGY AND PATHOPHYSIOLOGY

- Acute: A sudden event, such as large pulmonary embolism (PE), increases resistance to blood flow in the pulmonary vasculature, causing a quick and significant increase of pressure proximally. The RV is unable to overcome this pressure, leading to low RV cardiac output, which ultimately leads to low left ventricle (LV) cardiac output. Increased RV pressures in conjunction with a low cardiac output may cause coronary ischemia, further impairing cardiac output and potentially causing complete cardiovascular collapse.
- Chronic: A disorder of the pulmonary system causing chronic hypoxia leads to vasoconstriction of the pulmonary vasculature. Over time, the pulmonary vasculature hypertrophies and the intrinsic vasodilatory mechanisms (mediated by nitric oxide) become dysregulated, leading to increases in pulmonary vasculature resistance. The resulting pulmonary hypertension (WHO Group III) transmits increased pressures and volumes to the thin-walled low-pressure RV, causing maladaptive remodeling (concentric hypertrophy, followed by eccentric dilation frequently with associated tricuspid regurgitation) and subsequent impairment in RV systolic and diastolic function.
- Pulmonary disorders
  - Lung parenchymal disease: COPD (most common), interstitial lung disease
  - Pulmonary circulation: Thromboembolic disease (associated with pulmonary hypertension WHO Group IV)
  - Chest wall: severe obesity, kyphoscoliosis
  - Ventilation: obstructive sleep apnea and obesity hypoventilatory syndrome, neuromuscular diseases such as Guillain-Barré syndrome, muscular dystrophy, myasthenia gravis, spinal cord injuries)
- LV failure is not considered a cause of cor pulmonale.

RISK FACTORS

- Acute cor pulmonale (most commonly caused by PE)
  - Risk factors associated with PE:
    - Vessel injury
    - Stasis
    - Hypercoagulable states
- Chronic cor pulmonale (most commonly caused by underlying pulmonary disorder)
  - Risk factors associated with pulmonary disorders
    - Tobacco use (COPD)
    - Occupational exposures (interstitial lung disease)
    - Hypercoagulable state (chronic thromboembolic disease)
    - Obesity, age (chest wall abnormalities)

GENERAL PREVENTION

Management of underlying pulmonary disorder, including aggressive correction of hypoxia and acidosis, which may contribute to worsening pulmonary hypertension

COMMONLY ASSOCIATED CONDITIONS

Pulmonary hypertension, defined as the presence of a resting mean pulmonary artery pressure (PAP) >25 mm Hg

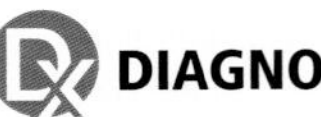

DIAGNOSIS

HISTORY

- Dyspnea is most common symptom, though nonspecific; may be present at rest, with exertion, or occur as paroxysmal nocturnal dyspnea
- Other pulmonary symptoms: pleuritic chest pain, cough, hemoptysis
- General heart failure symptoms: fatigue, lethargy, syncope, exertional angina less likely
- Right-sided heart failure symptoms: anorexia, early satiety, right upper quadrant discomfort from hepatic congestion, lower extremity edema
- Hoarseness secondary to compression of the left recurrent laryngeal nerve by enlarged pulmonary vessels
- Cardiovascular collapse, shock, and/or cardiac arrest may occur in acute or advanced chronic setting.

PHYSICAL EXAM

- Peripheral edema is the most common sign of right-sided heart failure, although it is nonspecific.
- General: pallor, diaphoresis, cyanosis, tachypnea
- Neck: jugular venous distension, with prominent *a*-wave
- Lungs: tachypnea, wheezing
- Heart
  - Increased intensity of pulmonic component of second heart sound (P_2)
  - Splitting of S_2 over the cardiac apex with inspiration
  - Audible right-sided S_3 or S_4
  - Jugular venous pressure JVP, with prominent v-wave
  - RV heave
  - Pansystolic murmur heard best at right midsternal border increasing with inspiration, consistent with tricuspid regurgitation (typically a late sign)
  - Early diastolic murmur heard best at left upper sternal border, consistent with pulmonary regurgitation
- Abdomen: hepatomegaly
- Extremities: clubbing, bilateral lower extremity edema, also signs of deep vein thrombosis (DVT) such as tenderness or unilateral swelling

DIFFERENTIAL DIAGNOSIS

Other causes of right-sided failure:

- Left-sided heart failure (WHO Group II)
- WHO Groups I and V pulmonary hypertension
- Right-sided cardiomyopathy

DIAGNOSTIC TESTS & INTERPRETATION

- 2D echocardiogram
  - Initial diagnostic test of choice
  - Elevated pulmonary artery pressure (limited in the absence of tricuspid regurgitation)
  - Right ventricular hypertrophy
  - Bulging of the interventricular septum into the left ventricle with systole
  - Flattening of the interventricular or interatrial septum
  - Dilation and hypokinesis of the right ventricle
  - Tricuspid regurgitation
  - Dilation of the right atrium
  - Acute thromboembolic pulmonary disease as evidenced by right ventricular hypokinesis with sparing of the apex (McConnell sign)
  - Echocardiography can over- or underestimate the PAP depending on image quality or operator. PAP should therefore be verified by catheter.
- MRI
  - If echocardiography is inconclusive or as a substitute
  - Most accurate modality for diagnosing emphysema and interstitial lung disease
  - Can assess pressures, size, function, myocardial mass, and viability
  - Despite being superior to echocardiogram, diagnosis of cor pulmonale still requires assessment via catheterization.
- Right heart catheterization
  - Gold standard for diagnosis of cor pulmonale
  - Elevated central venous pressure (CVP)
  - Mean pulmonary artery pressure >25 mm Hg at rest
  - Absence of left heart failure (pulmonary capillary wedge pressure <15 mm Hg)

Initial Tests (lab, imaging)

- CBC may show signs of polycythemia due to chronic hypoxia.
- Basic metabolic panel (BMP) may demonstrate elevated creatinine secondary to poor cardiac output.
- Liver function tests (LFTs) may be elevated due to hepatic congestion secondary to RV failure.

- Brain natriuretic peptide (BNP) and cardiac troponin can be elevated secondary to right ventricular strain.
- D-dimer may be positive as evidence of underlying thromboembolic pulmonary disease.
- Arterial blood gas may show hypercapnea due to COPD.
- ECG often shows signs of right-sided enlargement
  - Right axis deviation
  - An R/S wave ratio greater than 1 in V_1
  - Right ventricular hypertrophy (R wave in V_1 and V_2 with S waves in V_5 and V_6)
  - Right atrial enlargement as evidenced by P pulmonale (increased amplitude of P wave in lead II)
  - Incomplete or complete right bundle branch block
  - $S_1S_2S_3$ pattern, or $S_1Q_3T_3$, inverted pattern
- Chest x-ray
  - Cardiomegaly
  - Enlargement of the central pulmonary arteries and reduced size of peripheral vessels (oligemia)
  - Reduced retrosternal space due to right ventricular enlargement on lateral views
  - Enlargement of the right atrium resulting in prominence of the right heart border
  - Evidence of COPD, interstitial lung disease (ILD), and structural disease (i.e., kyphosis)
  - Evidence of pulmonary embolism (Westermark sign and Hampton hump)
- Spiral CT scan of chest
  - Diagnosis of acute pulmonary embolism
  - Diagnosis of COPD and ILD
- Ventilation/perfusion scan (V/Q)
  - High specificity and sensitivity for acute and chronic thromboembolic disease
  - May be used for diagnosis of acute thromboembolic disease if contraindication to chest spiral CT
  - May be preferred to chest spiral CT for diagnosis of chronic thromboembolic pulmonary disease, given higher sensitivity (can detect peripheral pulmonary emboli otherwise missed by spiral CT)
  - Diagnosis of chronic thromboembolic disease may warrant confirmation by pulmonary angiography.
- Pulmonary angiography
  - Gold standard in diagnosis of chronic thromboembolic pulmonary disease
- Polysomnography
  - Gold standard for diagnosis of obstructive sleep apnea (OSA)
- Pulmonary function tests (PFTs)
  - Impaired diffusion capacity
  - Obstructive and restrictive ventilatory defects (ILD, structural abnormalities, and COPD)

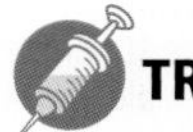

TREATMENT

Reduce symptoms and improve quality of life and survival. Reduce disease burden via oxygenation, preservation of cardiac function, and attenuation of pulmonary hypertension.

GENERAL MEASURES

- Treat underlying disease (1)[A].
  - For underlying pulmonary disease, bronchodilators and/or steroids may be beneficial.
  - For underlying chronic thromboembolic disease, anticoagulation may be indicated.
- Supportive therapy as necessary
  - Continuous positive airway pressure/bilevel positive airway pressure may be used for hypoxia/sleep disorders.
  - Ventilation using positive-pressure masks, negative-pressure body suits, or mechanical ventilation is suggested for patients with neuromuscular disease.
  - Phlebotomy may be indicated for severe polycythemia (hematocrit $>55\%$).

MEDICATION

- Oxygen (2)[A]
  - Long-term continuous oxygen therapy improves the survival of hypoxemic patients with COPD and cor pulmonale.
  - All patients with pulmonary hypertension whose PaO_2 is consistently <55 mm Hg or saturation ≤88% at rest, during sleep, or with ambulation should be prescribed oxygen to keep O_2 >92 mm Hg.
- Preservation of cardiac function (3)[B]
  - Inotropes: dobutamine and milrinone may improve cardiac output; should be reserved for hemodynamically unstable patients
  - Diuretics: decrease RV filling pressures; also reduces peripheral edema secondary to RHF
    - Excessive volume depletion should be avoided.
    - Monitor closely for metabolic alkalosis, as this may suppress ventilatory drive and contribute to hypoxia.
- Ameliorate pulmonary hypertension (3)
  - Treatment of underlying disease is hallmark of treatment.
  - When refractory to traditional medical treatment, advanced therapies may be beneficial, though evidence is lacking.
    - If "vasoreactive," calcium channel blockers (nifedipine, diltiazem, amlodipine) may be used; verapamil should be avoided.
    - Other advanced therapies include phosphodiesterase inhibitors (sildenafil, tadalafil), endothelin receptor antagonists (bosentan, ambrisentan), prostanoids (iloprost, treprostinil, epoprostenol), and/or nitric oxide.

ISSUES FOR REFERRAL

Patients with cor pulmonale should be referred to a specialized center for expert consultation.

SURGERY/OTHER PROCEDURES

- Endarterctomy for chronic thromboembolic disease (WHO Group IV)
- Moderate to severe disease refractory to medication may require lung and/or heart transplantation.

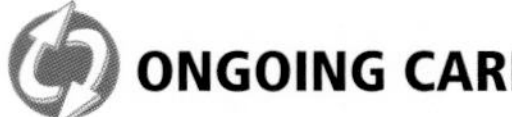

ONGOING CARE

DIET

Salt and fluid restriction

PATIENT EDUCATION

- Smoking cessation and avoidance of exposure to secondary smoke is strongly recommended.
- Exertional activity should be limited.
- Pregnancy should be avoided.

PROGNOSIS

- Patients with cor pulmonale resulting from COPD have a greater likelihood of dying than do similar patients with COPD alone.
- Pulmonary arterial pressure is a reliable indicator of prognosis; higher pressure is associated with a worse prognosis.
- In patients with COPD and mild disease (PAP 20–35 mm Hg), 5-year survival is 50%.

REFERENCES

1. McLaughlin VV, Archer SL, Badesch DB, et al. ACCF/AHA 2009 expert consensus document on pulmonary hypertension a report of the American College of Cardiology Foundation Task Force on Expert Consensus Documents and the American Heart Association developed in collaboration with the American College of Chest Physicians; American Thoracic Society, Inc.; and the Pulmonary Hypertension Association. *J Am Coll Cardiol.* 2009;53(17):1573–1619.
2. Naeije R. Pulmonary hypertension and right heart failure in chronic obstructive pulmonary disease. *Proc Am Thorac Soc.* 2005;2(1):20–22.
3. Price LC, Wort SJ, Finney SJ, et al. Pulmonary vascular and right ventricular dysfunction in adult critical care: current and emerging options for management: a systematic literature review. *Crit Care.* 2010;14(5):R169.

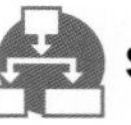

SEE ALSO

Chronic Obstructive Pulmonary Disease and Emphysema; Congestive Heart Failure; Pulmonary Arterial Hypertension; Pulmonary Embolism

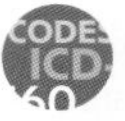

CODES

ICD10

- I27.81 Cor pulmonale (chronic)
- I26.09 Other pulmonary embolism with acute cor pulmonale

CLINICAL PEARLS

- Treatment of cor pulmonale requires treatment of an underlying disease.
- Continuous, long-term oxygen therapy improves life expectancy and quality of life in cor pulmonale.
- Referral of patients with cor pulmonale to a specialized center is strongly recommended.

CORNEAL ABRASION AND ULCERATION

John N. Dorsch, MD

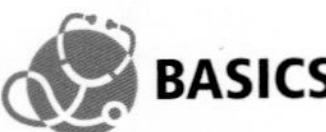

BASICS

DESCRIPTION

- Corneal abrasions result from scratching, denuding, abrading, or cutting of the epithelial layer of the cornea. They are usually traumatic and accidental but can occur spontaneously as well.
- Corneal ulcers usually represent an infection deeper in the cornea by bacteria, viruses, or fungi as a result of breakdown in the protective epithelial barrier.
- Both corneal abrasions and ulcerations can result in scarring, which may impair vision.
- Both lesions can occur centrally or marginally.

EPIDEMIOLOGY

Incidence

- Corneal abrasion is the most common ophthalmologic visit to the emergency department and is a commonly seen problem in urgent care:
  - 64% of cases are caused by direct minor trauma to eye.
  - 12% of cases are due to contact lens–related problems.
- Ulceration is also common in the United States.

ETIOLOGY AND PATHOPHYSIOLOGY

- Corneal abrasions most commonly result from accidental trauma (e.g., fingernail scratch, makeup brush):
  - Dirt, sand, sawdust, or other foreign body gets caught under eyelid.
- Corneal ulcers result from presence of an entryway to the external eye through dry eye; burns; abrasion; contact lenses; inappropriate use of topical anesthetics, antibiotics, or antiviral drops; immunosuppressant drugs; diabetes; or immunodeficiency. Causes of ulcerations include the following:
  - Infection with gram-positive organisms ~29–53% (*Staphylococcus aureus* and coagulase-negative *Streptococcus* are common ones)
  - Infection with gram-negative organisms ~47–50% (*Pseudomonas* being most common, followed by *Serratia marcescens*, *Proteus mirabilis*, and gram-negative enteric bacilli)

ALERT

Patients with contact lenses may have colonization of the cornea with *Pseudomonas* and other gram-negative bacteria and should be treated with ophthalmic quinolones or aminoglycosides to prevent corneal ulceration and infection (1)[A].

- Viral infections, especially herpes
- Fungal infections (*Candida*, *Aspergillus*, *Fusarium*, *Acanthamoeba*) in agricultural workers or associated with ocular corticosteroid use
- Autoimmune disorders, such as rheumatoid arthritis (RA), systemic lupus erythematosus (SLE), and scleroderma, are the usual cause of peripheral ulcerative keratitis.
- Vitamin A deficiency may cause corneal necrosis or keratomalacia.

RISK FACTORS

- Any abrasive injury
- Foreign body in eye
- Contact lenses (especially soft lenses and extended-wear lenses)
- Blepharitis
- Dry eye syndrome
- Entropion (with lashes scratching cornea)
- Chronic topical steroid use
- Abuse of topical anesthetics
- Autoimmune disorders
- Vitamin A deficiency
- Chronic corneal exposure (e.g., Bell palsy, exophthalmos)
- Recent eye surgery
- Immunosuppression and trigeminal nerve abnormalities
- Flash burn (welding burn or prolonged gazing directly at bright sunlight; symptoms often begin several hours after exposure)

GENERAL PREVENTION

- Eye protection to avoid injury during work, crafts, and sports
- Proper contact lens handling
  - Do not sleep while wearing contact lens.
- Artificial tears for those with inability to blink or known dry eyes
- Lenses to block UV rays (e.g., welding helmets)

COMMONLY ASSOCIATED CONDITIONS

- Chronic ulcerations may be associated with neurotrophic keratitis due to lack of 5th nerve innervation of the cornea. Individuals with thyroid disease, diabetes, or immunosuppressive conditions are particularly at risk.
- Any cause of fat malabsorption may be associated with vitamin A deficiency.

DIAGNOSIS

HISTORY

- Sudden onset of eye pain, photophobia, tearing, foreign body sensation, blurring of vision, and/or conjunctival injection
- Abrasions and ulcerations are usually unilateral.
- History remarkable for contact lens use, dry eyes, rubbing eye, history of trauma from foreign body, or chemical burn
- History of connective tissue disorder

PHYSICAL EXAM

- Visual acuity may be decreased if abrasion or ulcer is centrally located.
- Conjunctival injection
- Increased lacrimation on affected side
- Photophobia
- Blepharospasm
- Lesion seen on slit-lamp exam and area of damage shows fluorescein uptake; staining seen using Wood's lamp or cobalt blue slit lamp:
  - "Dendritic" staining pattern with fluorescein indicative of viral keratitis
- Examine for foreign body under eyelids or in cornea ("rust ring")

DIFFERENTIAL DIAGNOSIS

- Foreign body in eye
- Unilateral iritis
- Acute or chronic glaucoma
- Keratitis
- Scleritis with corneal melting
- Herpes simplex or zoster
- Bilateral or true idiopathic lesions may suggest basement membrane dystrophy.

DIAGNOSTIC TESTS & INTERPRETATION

Initial Tests (lab, imaging)

- Culture ulcer and contact lens, if applicable.
- Pretreatment with topical antibiotics may alter culture results.

Diagnostic Procedures/Other

Scrapings of the corneal ulcer for culture and sensitivity ideally should be obtained before beginning local antibiotics. The sample should be plated directly onto the culture medium.

Test Interpretation

Scrapings for Gram and Giemsa stain may demonstrate bacteria, yeast, or intranuclear inclusions that may aid in the diagnosis.

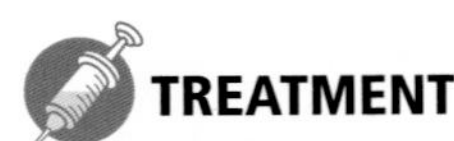

TREATMENT

GENERAL MEASURES

- Simple corneal abrasions <4 mm in diameter can be managed by primary care physicians. See indications for referral in the following text.
- All patients with corneal ulceration should be referred immediately to an ophthalmologist. Corneal cultures should be obtained before starting antibiotics. If immediate referral is not possible, it is reasonable to start antibiotics without delay.

- Flash burns from welding or prolonged exposure to sunlight may be treated like corneal abrasions (2)[C].
- Topical ophthalmic steroids should be avoided: may delay healing of corneal abrasions (3)[C]. Use of topical anesthetics outside of clinical settings should be avoided: may develop corneal toxicity with prolonged use (4)[A]

MEDICATION

First Line

- Eye patching does not reduce pain or speed the healing process (5)[A].
- Topical NSAIDs have been proven to reduce eye pain (5)[A].
  - Ophthalmic NSAIDs: Diclofenac 0.1% QID helps relieve moderate pain:
    - Alternatives include ketorolac 0.5% and bromfenac 0.09%.
    - Caution: Ophthalmic NSAIDs may rarely cause corneal melting and perforation.
- Ophthalmic antibiotics may help prevent further infection and ulceration of corneal abrasions (2)[C].
- Some ophthalmic antibiotics include ciprofloxacin 0.3%, ofloxacin 0.3%, gentamicin 0.3%, erythromycin 0.5%, polymyxin B/trimethoprim (Polytrim), and tobramycin 0.3%:
  - Ointment preparations may be more soothing to the eye than solutions.
  - Topical antibiotics should be continued until eye pain is resolved.
  - Chloramphenicol should be avoided due to high risk of toxicity and Stevens-Johnson syndrome.
- Large corneal abrasions (>4 mm) or very painful abrasions should be treated with combination of topical antibiotic and topical NSAID.
- Reevaluate in 24 hours. If improving, no need for further follow-up (2)[C].
- Fungal keratitis is treated with a protracted course of topical antifungal agents (by ophthalmologist).
- Herpetic keratitis should be referred promptly to ophthalmologist and treated initially with trifluridine:
  - Vidarabine and acyclovir are alternatives.

Second Line

- Oral analgesic medication (hydrocodone and other opioids) if topical analgesia not adequate
- Supplemental topical cycloplegics (i.e., homatropine 5% and cyclopentolate 1%) have not been found to be beneficial in relieving pain in corneal abrasion (6)[B].

ISSUES FOR REFERRAL

- Consultation with an ophthalmologist is recommended for all ulcers to help determine appropriate therapy. Moreover, ulcers need corneal cultures to be taken directly onto culture media.
- Also refer to ophthalmologist if there is history of the following:
  - Significant ocular trauma
  - Corneal infection is suspected (including viral keratitis)
  - Recurrent or nonhealing abrasion is encountered despite standard treatment
  - Severe ocular pain not explained by apparent pathology (e.g., traumatic iritis)

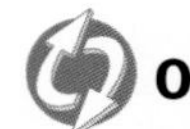

ONGOING CARE

FOLLOW-UP RECOMMENDATIONS

Patient Monitoring

- Contact lens wearer should be monitored daily with slit lamp for signs of secondary infection.
- Minor abrasion should be reevaluated only if it becomes more painful (2)[C].
- Large abrasion (>4 mm) should be reevaluated in 24 hours, and if improving, no need to follow further unless symptoms worsen again (2)[C].

PATIENT EDUCATION

Prevention of abrasions and proper handling of contact lenses can prevent recurrence of corneal ulcers.

PROGNOSIS

- Corneal abrasions and ulcerations should improve daily and heal with appropriate therapy.
- If healing does not occur within 24–48 hours or the lesion extends, obtain an ophthalmology consultation.

COMPLICATIONS

- Recurrence
- Scarring of the cornea
- Loss of vision
- Corneal perforation

REFERENCES

1. Dargin JM, Lowenstein RA. The painful eye. *Emerg Med Clin North Am*. 2008;26(1):199–216, viii.
2. Fraser S. Corneal abrasion. *Clin Ophthalmol*. 2010;4:387–390.
3. Tomas-Barberan S, Fagerholm P. Influence of topical treatment on epithelial wound healing and pain in the early postoperative period following photorefractive keratectomy. *Acta Ophthalmol Scand*. 1999;77(2):135–138.
4. Duffin RM, Olson RJ. Tetracaine toxicity. *Ann Ophthalmol*. 1984;16(9):836, 838.
5. Turner A, Rabiu M. Patching for corneal abrasion. *Cochrane Database Syst Rev*. 2006;(2):CD004764.
6. Carley F, Carley S. Towards evidence based emergency medicine: best BETs from the Manchester Royal Infirmary. Mydriatics in corneal abrasion. *Emerg Med J*. 2001;18(4):273.

ADDITIONAL READING

- Ehlers JP, Shah CP, Fenton GL. *The Wills Eye Manual: Office and Emergency Room Diagnosis and Treatment of Eye Disease*. Baltimore: Lippincott Williams & Wilkins; 2008.
- Vemuganti GK, Murthy SI, Das S. Update on pathologic diagnosis of corneal infections and inflammations. *Middle East Afr J Ophthalmol*. 2011;18(4):277–284.
- Watson SL, Barker NH. Interventions for recurrent corneal erosions. *Cochrane Database Syst Rev*. 2007;(4):CD001861, revised in *Cochrane Database Syst Rev*. 2012;9:CD001861.
- Wilhelmus KR. Therapeutic interventions for herpes simplex virus epithelial keratitis. *Cochrane Database Syst Rev*. 2008;(1):CD002898.
- Wipperman JL, Dorsch JN. Evaluation and management of corneal abrasions. *Am Fam Physician*. 2013;87(2):114–120.
- Wirbelauer C. Management of the red eye for the primary care physician. *Am J Med*. 2006;119(4):302–306.

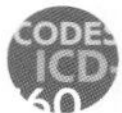

CODES

ICD10

- S05.00XA Inj conjunctiva and corneal abrasion w/o fb, unsp eye, init
- H16.009 Unspecified corneal ulcer, unspecified eye
- H16.049 Marginal corneal ulcer, unspecified eye

CLINICAL PEARLS

- Contact lens use should be discontinued until corneal abrasion or ulcer is healed and pain is fully resolved.
- Eye patching is not recommended.
- Prescribe topical and/or oral analgesic medication for symptom relief and consider ophthalmic antibiotics.
- Prompt referral to an ophthalmologist should be made with suspicion of an ulcer, recurrence of abrasion, retained foreign body, viral keratitis, significant visual loss, or lack of improvement despite therapy.

CORNS AND CALLUSES

Neil J. Feldman, DPM, FACFAS

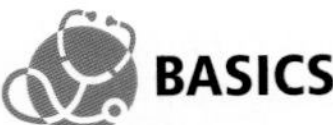

BASICS

DESCRIPTION

- A callus (tyloma) is a diffuse area of hyperkeratosis, usually without a distinct border.
  - Typically the result of exposure to repetitive forces, including friction and mechanical pressure; tend to occur on the palms of hands and soles of feet (1).
- A corn (heloma) is a circumscribed hyperkeratotic lesion with a central conical core of keratin that causes pain and inflammation. The conical core in a corn is a thickening of the stratum corneum.
- Hard corn or heloma durum (more common): more often on toe surfaces, especially 5th toe (proximal interphalangeal [PIP]) joint
- Soft corn (heloma molle): commonly in the interdigital space (1)
- Digital corns are also known as clavi.
- Intractable plantar keratosis is usually located under a metatarsal head (1st and 5th most common), is typically more difficult to resolve, and often is resistant to usual conservative treatments.

EPIDEMIOLOGY

Corns and calluses have the largest prevalence of all foot disorders.

Incidence

Incidence of corns and calluses increases with age. Less common in pediatric patients. Women affected more often than men. Blacks report corns and calluses 30% more often than whites.

Prevalence

- 9.2 million Americans
- ~38/1,000 people affected

ETIOLOGY AND PATHOPHYSIOLOGY

Increased activity of keratinocytes in superficial layer of skin leading to hyperkeratosis. This is a normal response to excess friction, pressure, or stress.

- Calluses typically arise from repetitive friction, motion, or pressure to skin.
- Soft corns arise from increased moisture from perspiration leading to skin maceration, along with mechanical irritation, especially between toes.
- Hard corns are an extreme form of callus with a keratin-based core. Often found on the digital surfaces and commonly linked to bony protrusions, causing skin to rub against shoe surfaces.

Genetics

No true genetic basis identified because most corns and calluses are due to mechanical stressors on the foot/hands.

RISK FACTORS

- Extrinsic factors producing pressure, friction, and local stress
  - Ill-fitting shoes
  - Not using socks, gloves
  - Manual labor
  - Walking barefoot
  - Activities that increase stress applied to skin of hands or feet (running, walking, sports)
- Intrinsic factors
  - Bony prominences: bunions, hammertoes
- Enlarged bursa or abnormal foot function/structure: hammertoe, claw toe, or mallet toe deformity

GENERAL PREVENTION

External irritation is by far the most common cause of calluses and corns. General measures to reduce friction on the skin are recommended to reduce incidence of callus formation. Examples include wearing shoes that fit well and using socks and gloves.

Geriatric Considerations

In elderly patients, especially those with neurologic or vascular compromise, skin breakdown from calluses/corns may lead to increased risk of infection/ulceration. 30% of foot ulcers in the elderly arise from eroded hyperkeratosis. Regular foot exams are emphasized for these patients as well as diabetic patients (2).

COMMONLY ASSOCIATED CONDITIONS

- Foot ulcers, especially in diabetic patients or patients with neuropathy or vascular compromise
- Infection: look for warning signs of
  - Increasing size or redness
  - Puslike drainage
  - Increased pain/swelling
  - Fever
  - Change in color of fingers or toes
- Signs of gangrene

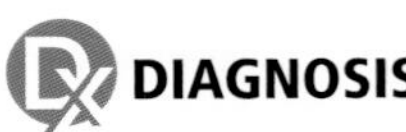

DIAGNOSIS

- Most commonly a clinical diagnosis based on visualization of the lesion
- Examination of footwear may also provide clues.

HISTORY

- Careful history can usually pinpoint cause.
- Ask about neurologic and vascular history and diabetes. These may be risk factors for progression of corns/calluses to frank ulcerations and infection.

PHYSICAL EXAM

- Calluses
  - Thickening of skin without distinct borders
  - Often on feet, hands; especially over palms of hands, soles of feet
  - Colors from white to gray-yellow, brown, red
  - May be painless or tender
  - May throb or burn
- Corns
  - Hard corns: commonly on dorsum of toes or dorsum of 5th PIP joint
    - Varied texture: dry, waxy, transparent to a hornlike mass
    - Distinct borders
    - More common on feet
    - Often painful
  - Soft corns
    - Often between toes, especially between 4th and 5th digits at the base of the webspace
    - Often yellowed, macerated appearance
    - Often extremely painful

DIFFERENTIAL DIAGNOSIS

- Plantar warts (typically a loss of skin lines within the wart) which are viral in nature
- Porokeratoses (blocked sweat gland)
- Underlying ulceration of skin, with or without infection (rule out especially with diabetic patients)

DIAGNOSTIC TESTS & INTERPRETATION

Initial Tests (lab, imaging)

- Radiographs may be warranted if no external cause found. Look for abnormalities in foot structure, bone spurs.
- Use of metallic radiographic marker and weight-bearing films often highlight the relationship between the callus and bony prominence.

Diagnostic Procedures/Other

Biopsy with microscopic evaluation in rare cases

Test Interpretation

Abnormal accumulation of keratin in epidermis, stratum corneum

TREATMENT

GENERAL MEASURES

- Débridement of affected tissue and use of protective padding
- Low-heeled shoes; soft upper with deep and wide toebox
- Extra-width shoes for 5th-toe corns
- Avoidance of activities that contribute to painful lesions
- Prefabricated or custom orthotics

MEDICATION

- Most therapy for corns and calluses can be done as self-care in the home (1).
- Use bandages, soft foam padding, or silicone sleeve over the affected area to decrease friction on the skin and promote healing with digital clavi.
- Use socks or gloves regularly.
- Use lotion/moisturizers for dry calluses and corns.
- Keratolytic agents, such as urea or ammonium lactate, can be applied safely.
- Use sandpaper discs or pumice stones over hard, thickened areas of skin.

Geriatric Considerations

Use of salicylic acid corn plasters can cause skin breakdown and ulceration in patients with thin, atrophic skin; diabetes; and those with vascular compromise. The skin surrounding the callus will often turn white and can become quite painful.

ISSUES FOR REFERRAL

- May benefit from referral to podiatrist if use of topical agents and shoe changes are ineffective
- Abnormalities in foot structure may require surgical treatment.
- Diabetic, vascular, and neuropathic patients may benefit from referral to podiatrist for regular foot exams to prevent infection or ulceration.

SURGERY/OTHER PROCEDURES

- Surgical treatment to areas of protruding bone where corns and calluses form
- Rebalancing of foot pressure through functional foot orthotics
- Shaving or cutting off hardened area of skin using a chisel or 15-blade scalpel. For corns, remove keratin core and place pad over area during healing.

COMPLEMENTARY AND ALTERNATIVE MEDICINE

- Many over-the-counter topical ointments and lotions are available for calluses (Keralac, CalleX, urea, Lac-Hydrin). Do not use on broken skin.
- Epsom salt soaks for 5 minutes at a time

INPATIENT CONSIDERATIONS

Admission Criteria/Initial Stabilization

- Admission usually not necessary, unless progression to ulcerated lesion with signs of severe infection, gangrene
- May require aggressive débridement in operating room should an abscess or deep-space infection be suspected. The deep-space infection is where an abscess can penetrate into tendon sheaths and/or deep compartments within the foot or hand, potentially leading to rapid sepsis.

Nursing

Wound care, dressing changes for infected lesions

ONGOING CARE

PATIENT EDUCATION

- General information. http://www.mayoclinic.org/diseases-conditions/corns-and-calluses/basics/definition/con-20014462
- American Podiatric Medical Association: http://www.apma.org

PROGNOSIS

Complete cure is possible once factors causing pressure or injury are eliminated.

COMPLICATIONS

Ulceration, infection

REFERENCES

1. Freeman DB. Corns and calluses resulting from mechanical hyperkeratosis. *Am Fam Physician*. 2002;65(11):2277–2280.
2. Pinzur MS, Slovenkai MP, Trepman E, et al. Guidelines for diabetic foot care: recommendations endorsed by the Diabetes Committee of the American Orthopaedic Foot and Ankle Society. *Foot Ankle Int*. 2005;26(1):113–119.

ADDITIONAL READING

Theodosat A. Skin diseases of the lower extremities in the elderly. *Dermatol Clin*. 2004;22(1):13–21.

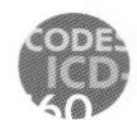

CODES

ICD10

L84 Corns and callosities

CLINICAL PEARLS

Most therapy for corns and calluses can be done as self-care in the home using padding over the affected area to decrease friction or pressure. However, if simple home care is not helpful, then removal of the lesions is often immediately curative.

C

CORONARY ARTERY DISEASE AND STABLE ANGINA

Daniel J. Stein, MD, MPH • Stephen K. Lane, MD, FAAFP

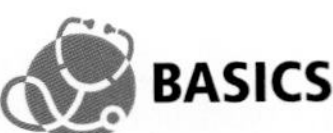

BASICS

DESCRIPTION

- Predictable (consistent) and reproducible chest discomfort occurring in a consistent pattern at a certain level of exertion or emotional stress and relieved with rest or sublingual nitroglycerin
- Definitions:
  - Typical angina: a sense of choking, pressure, or heaviness deep to the precordium, frequently radiating to the jaw, arms, or epigastrium; usually brought on by exertion or anxiety and relieved by rest. Discomfort may be described with a clenched fist over the sternum (Levine sign).
  - Atypical angina: nonclassical symptoms and signs such as absence of substernal localization and character, exertional trigger, or relief with nitroglycerin or rest
  - Anginal equivalent: Patients with angina may present without chest discomfort but with nonspecific symptoms such as dyspnea, diaphoresis, fatigue, belching, nausea, light-headedness, or indigestion.
  - Unstable angina: anginal symptoms that are new or are changed in character to become more frequent, more severe, or both. It is considered an acute coronary syndrome in the same continuum as non–ST-segment elevation myocardial infarction (NSTEMI) but without troponin leak.
- Low-risk unstable angina (age <70 years, exertional pain lasting <20 minutes, pain not rapidly accelerating, normal or unchanged ECG, no elevation of cardiac markers) may be treated similarly to stable ischemic heart disease.
- Canadian Cardiovascular Society grading of chronic stable angina severity:
  - Class 1: Ordinary physical activity does not cause angina; angina with strenuous or rapid or prolonged exertion
  - Class 2: slight limitation of ordinary activity (walking rapidly or >2 blocks, climbing >1 flight of stairs, emotional stress)
  - Class 3: marked limitation of ordinary physical activity
  - Class 4: inability to carry on any physical activity without discomfort. Angina may occur at rest.
- System(s) affected: cardiovascular

Geriatric Considerations

Elderly patients may present with atypical anginal symptoms. Maintain a high degree of suspicion during evaluation. They may also be very sensitive to the side effects of medications.

EPIDEMIOLOGY

- Most common in middle-age and older men, postmenopausal women
- Predominant sex: male > female

Incidence

~785,000 new cases of stable angina occur yearly in patients aged ≥45.

Prevalence

17 million with coronary heart disease and nearly 10 million with angina pectoris (1)

ETIOLOGY AND PATHOPHYSIOLOGY

- Anginal symptoms occur during times of myocardial ischemia caused by a mismatch between coronary perfusion and myocardial oxygen demand.
- Atherosclerotic narrowing of the coronary arteries is the most common pathology, with symptoms arising from stenosis of >70% in epicardial coronary arteries or >50% stenosis of the left main artery.
- Angina may occur in those with significant aortic stenosis, pulmonary hypertension, or hypertrophic cardiomyopathy, even with normal coronary arteries due to high demand.
- Sensory nerves from the heart travel up the sympathetic chain and enter the spinal cord at levels C7–T4, causing diffuse referred pain/discomfort in the associated dermatomes.

RISK FACTORS

Risk factors for coronary artery disease (CAD) include the following:

- Family history of premature CAD in 1st-degree relatives (in male, relatives <55 years; in female, relatives <65 years)
- Personal history of obesity, hyperlipidemia, hypertension, smoking, diabetes mellitus, male gender, increased age, sedentary lifestyle

GENERAL PREVENTION

- Smoking cessation
- Low-fat (increasingly controversial)/low-cholesterol diet and statin medication if indicated by current Adult Treatment Panel (ATP) guidelines or a risk-based approach
- Regular aerobic exercise program and weight loss (goal BMI <25 kg/m^2)
- BP control (goal <140/90 mm Hg)
- Diabetic management

COMMONLY ASSOCIATED CONDITIONS

Hypercholesterolemia, peripheral vascular disease, hypertension, obesity, diabetes mellitus

DIAGNOSIS

HISTORY

- Predictable and reproducible anginal symptoms lasting 3–15 minutes brought on by exertion, emotional stress, meals, cold air, or smoking; symptoms relieved by rest or nitrates. Careful history is important in eliciting symptoms of angina.
- Dyspnea on exertion may present as the only symptom. Atypical symptoms are more likely in women, elderly, and diabetic patients.
- May present with symptoms similar to gastric reflux or GI upset (indigestion, nausea, diaphoresis)
- Underlying history of heart disease or valvular disease; assess risk factors.
- Family history of myocardial infarction (MI), CAD, sudden death

PHYSICAL EXAM

- Normal physical exam/vital signs does not exclude diagnosis of angina.
- Cardiac exam may reveal dysrhythmias, heart murmurs indicative of valvular disease, signs of ventricular hypertrophy, gallops, or signs of congestive heart failure.
- Vascular exam may show signs of peripheral vascular disease (diminished pulses, bruits, abdominal aneurysm).

DIFFERENTIAL DIAGNOSIS

- Vascular: aortic dissection, pericarditis, myocardial infarction
- Pulmonary: pleuritis, pulmonary embolism
- Gastroesophageal: gastric reflux, esophageal spasm, gastric/duodenal ulcer
- Musculoskeletal: costochondritis, arthritis, muscle strain
- Other: anxiety, psychosomatic, cocaine abuse

DIAGNOSTIC TESTS & INTERPRETATION

Initial Tests (lab, imaging)

- CBC (evaluate for anemia, infectious cause)
- Fasting lipid profile—dyslipidemia associated with increased cardiovascular risk
- Diabetic evaluation if not previously diagnosed
- Basic metabolic panel to rule out electrolyte abnormalities and assess renal function
- Cardiac enzymes for prolonged acute chest pain
- ECG
  - Should be routinely obtained unless there is an noncardiac cause of the chest pain (1)[B]
  - May show evidence of prior MI
  - Frequently unremarkable between angina episodes; may show signs of myocardial ischemia during symptomatic episodes
  - Bundle branch block, Wolff-Parkinson-White syndrome, or intraventricular conduction delay may make stress ECG interpretation unreliable.
- Chest x-ray may exclude other causes of chest pain.

Follow-Up Tests & Special Considerations

Further diagnostic testing is most useful in patients at intermediate risk and consists of the following:

- Stress testing is helpful for patients with a less classic presentation because of either atypical symptoms or atypical demographics:
  - Exercise testing for those who can physically exercise (≥5 metabolic equivalents [METS]) (1)[A]
    - Standard exercise ECG for those with normal baseline ECG
    - Exercise stress testing with echo or perfusion imaging for those with abnormal baseline ECG or in premenopausal women
  - In patients who cannot tolerate exercise, pharmacologic stress testing is a good alternative (1)[B].
- Coronary angiography is the gold standard for confirmation and delineation of coronary disease and direction of interventional therapy or surgery.
- Consider echocardiogram if valvular disease or hypertrophic cardiomyopathy is suspected. Routine assessment for patients with normal ECG and no exam findings or history of MI is unlikely to contribute to management (1)[C].
- CT coronary angiography or MRI angiography can be considered as a supplement to stress testing in patients with (1)[C]:
  - Need for better anatomic definition of disease
  - Continued symptoms with negative stress testing
  - Inconclusive testing
  - Unable to undergo stress testing

Diagnostic Procedures/Other

- Assessment of infarction risk with stress test, angiography, or cross-sectional imaging (as above) should be considered in patients at high risk.
- Goal is to detect possible high risk coronary lesions, where intervention would improve long-term mortality. The definition of who is at high-risk is not well defined (1).
- Similar to the diagnostic workup, exercise testing with ECG or nuclear/echo imaging is preferred in those able to exercise and pharmacologic stress for those unable to do so (1)[B].

- Echocardiogram should be obtained in patients with murmur (not previously imaged), signs of previous MI, concern for heart failure, or complex arrhythmias (1)[B]; can be considered in patients with hypertension or diabetes and abnormal ECG (1)[C]

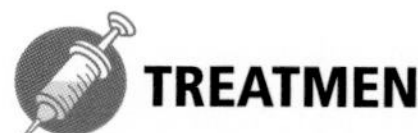

TREATMENT

GENERAL MEASURES

Lifestyle modifications are very important:

- BP control goal: <140/90 mm HG for most
- Smoking cessation goal: complete cessation, no exposure to secondhand smoke
- Physical activity goal: 30–60 minutes of moderate aerobic activity, at least 5 days/week and preferably 7 days/week
- Weight management goal: BMI 18.5–24.9 kg/m^2; waist circumference <35 inches (women) or <40 inches (men)
- Lipid management (see "Medication")
- Glycemic control in diabetics: individualize based on life expectancy, risk for adverse events related to glucose control, and patient preference

MEDICATION

First Line

- Anti-ischemic (antianginal) medications
  - β-Blockers decrease heart rate, BP, and myocardial contractility (decreased demand).
  - Metoprolol (25–200 mg daily [succinate] or divided BID [tartrate]). Carvedilol can also be considered starting at 3.125 mg BID with maximum dosing of 25–50 mg BID.
  - Adjust doses according to clinical response. Aim to maintain resting heart rate of 50–60 bpm.
  - Improves mortality in patients with congestive heart failure (CHF) or a history of MI only
- Calcium channel blockers (CCBs) cause arterial vasodilation, decrease myocardial oxygen demand, and improve coronary blood flow. They have similar effectiveness to β-blockers and are used as replacement (if β-blocker nontolerated) or supplementation (continued symptoms despite β-blocker). Only long-acting CCBs should be used:
  - Dihydropyridine CCBs such as nifedipine (30–90 mg/day), amlodipine (5–10 mg/day), or felodipine (2.5–10 mg/day) cause more vasodilation.
  - Nondihydropyridine CCBs such as diltiazem (120–480 mg/day) or verapamil (120–480 mg/day).
  - Amlodipine is preferred in patients with low ejection fraction.
  - Side effects include constipation and peripheral edema. The nondihydropyridine CCBs may also cause bradycardia and heart block and precipitate heart failure in those with severe systolic dysfunction.
  - Nitrates dilate systemic veins and arteries (including coronary vessels) and cause decreased preload; at higher doses, decreases BP and thus decreases afterload and increases myocardial flow:
    - Sublingual nitroglycerin 0.4 mg. For acute anginal episodes. Repeat 2–3 times over a 10–15-minute period; if no relief, immediate medical attention must be sought.
    - Long-acting nitrates: should be used with a drug-free interval of 8–12 hours to prevent tolerance. Side effects such as headaches and hypotension tend to clear with continued usage.
- Treatment of atherosclerosis is indicated with the following three agent classes unless patient-specific contraindications exist:
  - Antiplatelet therapy in all patients: Standard therapy is 75–162 mg of aspirin daily (1)[A]:
    - Clopidogrel (75 mg/day) may be used in patients with contraindications to aspirin.
    - Combination of aspirin and clopidogrel is indicated after stent placement.
  - Statins (e.g., atorvastatin) for hypercholesterolemia
    - Most effective medication for secondary prevention in those with CAD; decrease incidence of symptomatic CAD and reduce MI/death from MI
    - Current ATP guidelines support high-intensity statin (e.g., atorvastatin 40–80 mg daily, rosuvastatin 20–40 mg daily) in those ≤75 years old; those >75 years or with intolerance should receive moderate-intensity statin (2)[A].
    - Side effects may include myalgias. May rarely cause myositis or rhabdomyolysis. Monitor labs with any changes in medication doses.
  - ACE inhibitors have been shown to reduce both cardiovascular death and MI.
    - Indicated in patients with CAD or other vascular disease, particularly in those with diabetes or left ventricular (LV) systolic dysfunction (1)[A]
    - Angiotensin receptor blockers may be used in patients intolerant of ACE inhibitors.
    - Other antihypertensives should be used as appropriate according to current guidelines such as JNC 8 (3).

Second Line

Ranolazine (500–1,000 mg BID) decreases ischemia-associated calcium overload. Does not affect heart rate or BP. Use as adjunctive therapy in those who are still symptomatic on optimal doses of β-blockers, nitrates, or amlodipine. Side effects may include nausea, constipation, dizziness, and headache.

SURGERY/OTHER PROCEDURES

Revascularization should be considered when noninvasive testing suggests a high-risk lesion. It can also be considered if optimal medication management is inadequate in controlling symptoms.

- Percutaneous coronary intervention (PCI), balloon angioplasty, and/or stent placement (with drug eluting or bare metal stent). Although patients may become symptom-free faster, PCI does not decrease mortality or MI compared with optimal medical management in those with stable angina.
- Coronary artery bypass grafting (CABG)
- For refractory angina: spinal cord stimulation, enhanced external counterpulsation, myocardial laser revascularization therapy

COMPLEMENTARY & ALTERNATIVE MEDICINE

Relaxation/stress reduction therapy may help reduce anginal episodes.

INPATIENT CONSIDERATIONS

Admission Criteria/Initial Stabilization

Inpatient evaluation for any patient with changes in angina symptoms, as this is classified as unstable angina in the continuum of acute coronary syndromes

Discharge Criteria

Without myonecrosis, discharge may be considered after appropriate risk stratification has been determined.

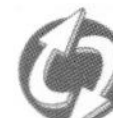

ONGOING CARE

FOLLOW-UP RECOMMENDATIONS

Lifestyle modifications should be aggressively stressed at every visit.

Patient Monitoring

Frequent follow-up after initial event: every 4–6 months in 1st year, then 1–2 × per year

DIET

Reduced intake of saturated fat and cholesterol, especially trans fatty acids (1)[B]

PROGNOSIS

Variable; depends on severity of symptoms, extent of CAD, and LV function

COMPLICATIONS

Unstable angina or MI, arrhythmia, cardiac arrest, heart failure

REFERENCES

1. Fihn SD, Gardin JM, Abrams J, et al. 2012 ACCF/AHA/ACP/AATS/PCNA/SCAI/STS guideline for the diagnosis and management of patients with stable ischemic heart disease. *J Am Coll Cardiol*. 2012;60(24):2564–2603.
2. Stone NJ, Robinston JG, Lichtenstein AH, et al. 2013 ACC/AHA guideline on the treatment of blood cholesterol to reduce atherosclerotic cardiovascular risk in adults. *Circulation*. 2014;129(25)(Suppl 2):S1–S45.
3. James PA, Oparil S, Carter BL, et al. 2014 Evidence-based guideline for the management of high blood pressure in adults: report from the panel members appointed to the Eighth Joint National Committee (JNC 8). *JAMA*. 2014;311(5):507–520.

SEE ALSO

Algorithms: Chest Pain/Acute Coronary Syndrome

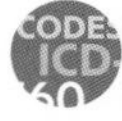

CODES

ICD10

- I25.119 Athscl heart disease of native cor art w unsp ang pctrs
- I25.111 Athscl heart disease of native cor art w ang pctrs w spasm
- I25.118 Athscl heart disease of native cor art w oth ang pctrs

CLINICAL PEARLS

- Maximize antianginal therapy: Combine β-blockers, CCBs, and nitrates in those still symptomatic with monotherapy.
- Lifestyle changes and optimal medical therapy must be emphasized to control complicating factors that trigger ischemia and to prevent progression of the atherosclerotic process.

C

COSTOCHONDRITIS

Smriti Ohri, MD • Scott A. Fields, MD, MHA

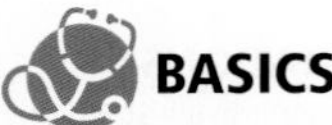

BASICS

DESCRIPTION

- Anterior chest wall pain associated with pain and tenderness of the costochondral and costosternal regions
- System(s) affected: musculoskeletal
- Synonym(s): costosternal syndrome; parasternal chondrodynia; anterior chest wall syndrome; chondrocostal junction syndrome

Pediatric Considerations

Pay special attention to psychogenic chest pain in children who perceive family discord.

EPIDEMIOLOGY

- Predominant age: 20–40 years
- Predominant gender: female

Incidence

~30% of patients presenting to emergency room with chest pain; 15–20% of teenagers with chest pain may have costochondritis.

ETIOLOGY AND PATHOPHYSIOLOGY

- Not fully understood
- Trauma
- Overuse

RISK FACTORS

- Unusual physical activity or overuse
- Recent trauma (including motor vehicle accident, domestic violence) or new activity
- Recent upper respiratory infection (URI)

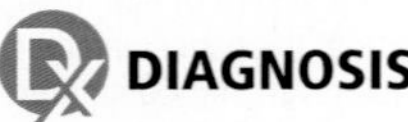

DIAGNOSIS

- Insidious onset
- Pain is usually sharp, achy, or pressurelike, sometimes pleuritic
- Pain involves multiple locations, the 2nd–5th costal cartilages most often involved.
- Pain is most often unilateral.
- Pain is exacerbated by upper body movements and exertional activities.
- Pain is reproduced by palpation of the affected cartilage segments.
- Chest tightness is often associated with the pain.
- Redness and warmth at sites of tenderness

HISTORY

- A complete and thorough history is mandatory for the diagnosis, with special emphasis on cardiac risk factor evaluation.
- Social history: careful screening and evaluation for domestic violence and substance abuse

PHYSICAL EXAM

- A physical exam to exclude more serious conditions that may present with chest pain is necessary for the diagnosis.
- Tenderness elicited over the costochondral junctions is necessary to establish the diagnosis but does not completely exclude other causes of chest pain.
- If swelling of the costal cartilage is involved, this may be termed as Tietze syndrome.
- Movement of upper extremity of the same side may reproduce the pain (1).
- Palpation of epigastric region to evaluate for gastroesophageal reflux disease (GERD) and deep palpation in right upper quadrant of abdomen to evaluate gallbladder

Geriatric Considerations

Often presents with multiple problems capable of causing chest pain, making a thorough history and physical exam imperative

DIFFERENTIAL DIAGNOSIS

- Cardiac
  - Coronary artery disease (CAD)
  - Cardiac contusion from trauma
  - Aortic aneurysm
  - Mitral valve prolapse
  - Pericarditis
  - Myocarditis
- GI
  - Gastroesophageal reflux
  - Peptic esophagitis
  - Esophageal spasm
- Musculoskeletal
  - Fibromyalgia
  - Slipping rib syndrome
  - Costovertebral arthritis
  - Painful xiphoid syndrome
  - Rib trauma with swelling
  - Ankylosing spondylitis
  - Precordial catch syndrome
- Psychogenic
  - Anxiety disorder
  - Panic attacks
  - Hyperventilation
- Respiratory
  - Asthma
  - Pulmonary embolism
  - Pneumonia
  - Chronic cough
  - Pneumothorax
- Other
  - Domestic violence and abuse
  - Herpes zoster
  - Spinal tumor
  - Metastatic cancer
  - Substance abuse (cocaine)

DIAGNOSTIC TESTS & INTERPRETATION

- The diagnosis of costochondritis is primarily based on a thorough history and physical exam.
- Laboratory exams should be used to exclude other differential diagnosis.
- ESR is inconsistently elevated.

Initial Tests (lab, imaging)

No imaging is indicated for the diagnosis of costochondritis; chest x-ray and rib films are often normal.

Diagnostic Procedures/Other

- None indicated for the diagnosis of costochondritis.
- Consider ECG in patients age >35 years, those with history or risk of CAD (2)[C].
- Also consider chest x-ray in patients with cardiopulmonary symptoms (2)[C].
- Consider spiral CT for pulmonary embolism and D-dimer if history or risk factors are present.

Test Interpretation

Costochondral joint inflammation

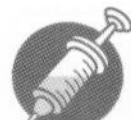

TREATMENT

Reassurance of benign nature of condition and potential for long, slow recovery from pain

GENERAL MEASURES

- Patient reassurance, rest, and heat (or ice massage, whichever makes the patient feel better) (3,4)[C]
- Stretching exercises (5)
- Minimizing activities that provoke the symptoms (e.g., reducing the frequency or intensity of exercise or work activities) (3)[C],(4)[C]

MEDICATION

Pain relief with NSAIDs (ibuprofen, naproxen, or diclofenac); acetaminophen or other analgesics may be considered in noninflammatory disorders (3,4)[C].

Use of skeletal muscle relaxants may be beneficial if associated muscle spasm.

ISSUES FOR REFERRAL

Consider referral to physical therapy or osteopathy. Refractory cases of costochondritis can be treated with local injections of combined lidocaine (Xylocaine)/corticosteroid into costochondral areas if severe; however, this is rarely necessary (3,4,6)[C].

COMPLEMENTARY & ALTERNATIVE MEDICINE

Limited data on use of manipulation or ice massage but may be safely tried if patient interested

INPATIENT CONSIDERATIONS

Admission Criteria/Initial Stabilization

Only indicated if differential diagnosis is unclear and cardiac or other more serious etiology of chest pain is being considered

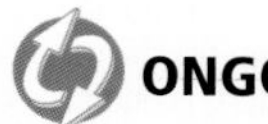

ONGOING CARE

FOLLOW-UP RECOMMENDATIONS

Follow up within 1 week if diagnosis is unclear or symptoms do not abate with conservative treatment.

PATIENT EDUCATION

- Educate the patient in regard to the self-limited (although potentially recurrent) nature of the illness.
- Instruct patient on proper physical activity regimens to avoid overuse syndromes.
- Stress importance of avoiding sudden, significant changes in activity.

PROGNOSIS

- Self-limited illness lasts for weeks to months but usually abates by 1 year, although sometimes chronic especially in adolescents.
- Often recurs

COMPLICATIONS

Incomplete attention to differential diagnosis or overly aggressive interventions to ensure a more life-threatening diagnosis is not missed.

REFERENCES

1. Fam AG. Approach to musculoskeletal chest wall pain. *Prim Care*. 1988;15(4):767–782.
2. Miller CD, Lindsell CJ, Khandelwal S, et al. Is the initial diagnostic impression of "noncardiac chest pain" adequate to exclude cardiac disease? *Ann Emerg Med*. 2004;44(6):565–574.
3. How J, Volz G, Doe S, et al. The causes of musculoskeletal chest pain in patients admitted to hospital with suspected myocardial infarction. *Eur J Intern Med*. 2005;16(6):432–436.
4. Spalding L, Reay E, Kelly C. Cause and outcome of atypical chest pain in patients admitted to hospital. *J R Soc Med*. 2003;96(3):122–125.
5. Rovetta G, Sessarego P, Monteforte P. Stretching exercises for costochondritis pain. *G Ital Med Lav Ergon*. 2009;31(2):169–171.
6. Aspegren D, Hyde T, Miller M. Conservative treatment of a female collegiate volleyball player with costochondritis. *J Manipulative Physiol Ther*. 2007;30(4):321–325.

ADDITIONAL READING

- Cayley WE Jr. Diagnosing the cause of chest pain. *Am Fam Physician*. 2005;72(10):2012–2021.
- Freeston J, Karim Z, Lindsay K, et al. Can early diagnosis and management of costochondritis reduce acute chest pain admissions? *J Rheumatol*. 2004;31(11):2269–2271.
- Proulx AM, Zryd TW. Costochondritis: diagnosis and treatment. *Am Fam Physician*. 2009;80(6):617–620.
- Verdon F, Herzig L, Burnand B, et al. Chest pain in daily practice: occurrence, causes and management. *Swiss Med Wkly*. 2008;138(23–24):340–347.

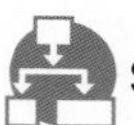

SEE ALSO

Algorithm: Chest Pain/Acute Coronary Syndrome

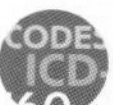

CODES

ICD10

M94.0 Chondrocostal junction syndrome [Tietze]

CLINICAL PEARLS

- A very common disorder, accounting for perhaps 30% of all cases of chest pain
- Educate the patient in regard to the self-limited (although potentially recurrent) nature of the illness. Instruct patient on proper physical activity regimens to avoid overuse syndromes. Also stress importance of avoiding sudden, significant changes in activity.
- Consider an anxiety disorder as a contributor to all cases of persistent chest pain whether musculoskeletal or cardiac.

COUNSELING TYPES

William T. Garrison, PhD

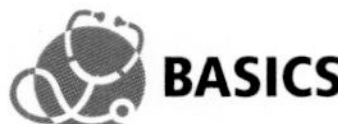

BASICS

DESCRIPTION

- Psychotherapeutic and counseling interventions play an important role in the management of chronic and acute-onset diseases and disorders. They are typically the primary initial mode of evaluation and/or treatment for most mild to moderate psychiatric disorders that reach criteria using the *DSM-5* (1) or *ICD-10* (2) diagnostic classification systems. It should be noted that the *DSM* system has recently been revised with significant changes in several disorder categories and their criteria. Treatment and successful control of either medical or psychological conditions require some form of professional counseling experience. Best outcomes occur when they are employed by a skilled practitioner. However, psychotherapy differs from generic counseling, which can take many forms and is delivered commonly in nonmedical settings, with mixed results.
- Counseling approaches are usually tailored to the specific presenting problem or issue and serve educational and emotional support functions. Typically, such counseling in medical settings will be time limited and problem focused and often not intended to lead to major medical symptom relief or major behavioral changes.
- The goals of psychotherapy range from increasing individual psychological insight and motivation for change to reduction of interpersonal conflict in the marriage or family, reduction of chronic or acute emotional suffering, and reversal of dysfunctional or habitual behaviors. There are several general types of psychotherapy, starting with individual, marital, or family approaches. In addition, a number of psychological theories guide various methods and treatment philosophies. The following is a brief overview of commonly used psychotherapeutic and counseling methods.
- Psychodynamic therapy: Unconscious conflict manifests as patient's symptoms/problem behaviors:
  - Short-term (4–6 months) and long-term (≥1 year)
  - Focus is on increasing insight of underlying conflict or processes to initiate symptomatic change.
  - Therapist actively helps patient identify patterns of behavior stemming from existence of an unconscious conflict or motivations that may not be accurately perceived.
- Cognitive-behavioral therapy (CBT): Patterns of thoughts and behaviors can lead to development and/or maintenance of symptoms. Thought patterns may not accurately reflect reality and may lead to psychological distress:
  - Therapy aims at modifying thought patterns by increasing cognitive flexibility and changing dysfunctional behavioral patterns.
  - Encourages patient self-monitoring of symptoms and the precursors or results of maladaptive behavior
  - Uses therapist-assisted challenges to patient's basic beliefs/assumptions
  - May use *exposure*, a procedure derived from basic learning theories, which encourages gradual steps toward change.
  - Can be offered in group or individual formats
  - Therapist's role is suggestive and supportive.
- Dialectical behavior therapy (DBT): Techniques such as social skills training, mindfulness, and problem solving are used to modulate impulse control and affect management:
  - Derivative of CBT
  - Originally used in treatment of patients with self-destructive behaviors (e.g., cutting, suicide attempts)
  - Seeks to change rigid patterns of cognitions and behaviors that have been maladaptive
  - Uses both individual and group treatment modalities
  - Therapist takes an active role in interpretation and support.
- Interpersonal psychotherapy: Interpersonal relationships in a patient's life are linked to symptoms. Therapy seeks to alleviate symptoms and improve social adjustment through exploration of patient's relationships and experiences. Focus is on one of four potential problem areas:
  - Grief
  - Interpersonal role disputes
  - Role transitions
  - Interpersonal deficits: Therapist works with the patient in resolving the problematic interpersonal issues to facilitate change in symptoms.
- Family therapy: focuses on the family as a unit of intervention
  - Uses psychoeducation to increase patient's and family's insight
  - Teaches communication and problem-solving skills
- Motivational interviewing: focuses on motivation as a key to successful change process
  - Short term and problem focused
  - Focuses on identifying discrepancies between goals and behavior
  - "5 A's" model is a brief counseling framework developed specifically for physicians to effect behavioral change in patients:
    - Assess for a problem.
    - Advise making a change.
    - Agree on action to be taken.
    - Assist with self-care support to make the change.
    - Arrange follow-up to support the change.
- Counseling (heterogeneous treatment)
  - Often focuses on situational factors maintaining symptoms
  - Often encourages the use of community resources
- Behavioral therapy: relatively nontheoretical approach to behavioral change or symptom reduction/eradication through application of principles of stimulus and response

Pediatric Considerations

- Important distinctions are made between psychotherapy and counseling for children/teens compared to adults/couples.
- The focus of evaluation must include attention to parent and family processes and factors. Interventions typically include interactions and sessions with parents as well as collateral work with teachers and other school personnel.
- Younger children will often be evaluated and diagnosed through behavioral descriptions provided by parents and other adults who know them well as well as through direct observation and/or play techniques. Children of all ages should be screened using behavioral checklists that are norm referenced for age.
- Any child or teenager who requests counseling should be interviewed initially by the primary care provider and referred appropriately. Most referrals will be in response to parental request, however.
- Psychotherapeutic interventions with the strongest empirical basis with children include behavior therapy/modification, CBT, and family/parenting therapy. Play therapy has the least empirical support, and insight-oriented therapies appear to be more effective with older children (>11 years).
- There is controversy regarding the efficacy of psychopharmacologic treatment in preadolescents, although clear benefits have been demonstrated in some studies. Treatment guidelines for mild to moderate depressed mood and/or anxiety disorders typically recommend pediatric CBT initially, and studies have typically supported this approach in preteen and milder cases.

EPIDEMIOLOGY

- ~18.8 million adults suffer from clinical depression, and 20 million suffer from a diagnosable anxiety disorder.
- One in four Americans report seeking some form of mental health treatment in their adult life. This includes generic counseling in nonmedical settings such as work, clergy, or school settings and also includes visits to primary care providers. It is estimated that between 3.5% and 5% of adults in the United States actually participate in formal mental health psychotherapy annually.
- Public health experts report that the majority of those adults with diagnosable psychiatric disorders, however, do not receive professional mental health services. This is due to multiple factors, including failure to identify, noncompliance with psychiatric referral, regional shortages of providers, economic barriers, and excessive time duration from referral to available service.
- A large study conducted between 1987 and 1997 concluded that the percentage of adults in psychotherapy remained relatively stable over that decade, the use of psychopharmacology doubled, and older adults (aged 55–64 years) increasingly sought psychotherapy services. In that same study, it was found that psychotherapy duration (number of sessions) decreased substantially and about 1/3 of psychotherapy patients only attended one or two sessions.

RISK FACTORS

The need for psychotherapy or counseling services is directly and indirectly associated with a host of socioeconomic and biogenetic factors, including the general effects of poverty, family or marital dysfunction; life stressors; medical diseases or conditions; and individual biologic predisposition to mental health disorders.

GENERAL PREVENTION

It is generally assumed that early identification and intervention of child and adolescent psychopathology increases the likelihood of reducing the risk for adult psychopathology, but this has not been sufficiently validated in all categories of psychological disorders. Data support such claims in disorders such as childhood ADHD, anxiety disorders, and habit disorders of childhood, however.

TREATMENT

GENERAL MEASURES

There is evidence of a "dose effect" in psychotherapy outcomes research, with some investigators suggesting that 6–8 sessions are necessary to yield positive initial effects and upward of 15–20 sessions for longer term, sustainable therapeutic effects. This dose effect may not be applicable to counseling services with primarily informational or emotional/supportive functions. Also, long-term therapy should be evaluated at 6–12-month intervals to determine efficacy.

MEDICATION

- Psychotherapy is most likely to be accompanied by use of pharmaceutical adjuncts in moderate to severe cases of psychological dysfunction that do not respond to other therapies or in cases of extremely poor quality of life or high risk. The most common examples are in cases of clinical depression or anxiety that clearly incapacitates the patient or significantly reduces his or her quality of life. Patients at risk for suicide or who represent a danger to others are also candidates for acute psychopharmacotherapy. Studies suggest that verbal and behaviorally oriented therapies can add efficacy to medication treatment in both depression and anxiety.
- There is controversy in the research field regarding the efficacy of medication alone versus psychotherapy alone versus combined treatments. The most recent consensus has been that combined treatments in moderate to severe psychological dysfunction are most likely to render positive short-term results and increase the likelihood that such effects can be sustained over time.

ADDITIONAL THERAPIES

- Anxiety disorders
  - Panic disorder with and without agoraphobia: CBT, psychodynamic therapy
  - Generalized anxiety disorder: CBT
  - Obsessive-compulsive disorder: CBT
  - Posttraumatic stress disorder: CBT
  - Specific phobia: CBT
  - Social phobia: CBT
- Mood disorders
  - Unipolar depression: CBT, interpersonal therapy, psychodynamic therapy
  - Bipolar disorder: family therapy, interpersonal therapy, CBT
  - Schizophrenia: psychodynamic therapy, family therapy, CBT
- Eating disorders
  - Binge eating disorder: CBT, interpersonal therapy
  - Bulimia nervosa: CBT, interpersonal therapy
- Personality disorders
  - Borderline: DBT, CBT
- Substance-use disorders
  - Alcohol: counseling, CBT, motivational interviewing
  - Cocaine: CBT, counseling
  - Heroin: CBT, counseling
  - Smoking: 5 A's
- Somatoform disorders
  - Hypochondriasis: CBT
  - Body dysmorphic disorder: CBT

COMPLEMENTARY & ALTERNATIVE MEDICINE

A host of nonempirically based psychological and nutritional therapies can be found outside of mainstream medicine and psychological science. Very little or no evidence exists to support such experimental therapies, but all have the considerable power of the placebo effect fueling their anecdotal supports or claims. Placebo effects are also thought to be powerfully enhanced by the use of ingested or applied substances that create real physiologic, although not therapeutic, changes in the patient. If it makes them feel different, they are more likely to believe it helps.

REFERENCES

1. American Psychiatric Association. *Diagnostic and Statistical Manual of Mental Disorders*. 5th ed. Arlington, VA: American Psychiatric Association; 2013.
2. World Health Organization. *The ICD-10 Classification of Mental and Behavioural Disorders: Clinical Descriptions and Diagnostic Guidelines*. Geneva, Switzerland: World Health Organization; 1992.

ADDITIONAL READING

- Bortolotti B, Menchetti M, Bellini F, et al. Psychological interventions for major depression in primary care: a meta-analytic review of randomized controlled trials. *Gen Hosp Psychiatry*. 2008;30(4):293–302.
- Eddy KT, Dutra L, Bradley R, et al. A multidimensional meta-analysis of psychotherapy and pharmacotherapy for obsessive-compulsive disorder. *Clin Psychol Rev*. 2004;24(8):1011–1030.
- Furukawa TA, Watanabe N, Churchill R. Combined psychotherapy plus antidepressants for panic disorder with or without agoraphobia. *Cochrane Database Syst Rev*. 2007;(1):CD004364.
- Hunot V, Churchill R, Silva de Lima M, et al. Psychological therapies for generalised anxiety disorder. *Cochrane Database Syst Rev*. 2007;(1):CD001848.

C

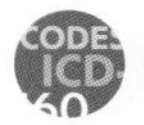

CODES

ICD10

- Z71.9 Counseling, unspecified
- Z71.89 Other specified counseling
- Z63.9 Problem related to primary support group, unspecified

CLINICAL PEARLS

- Combined medication and psychotherapeutic treatments in moderate to severe psychological dysfunction are most likely to render positive short-term results and increase the likelihood such effects can be sustained over time. Relapse is common over time and/or as treatments are discontinued. Children <10 years may benefit significantly from counseling or psychotherapy alone for symptom relief. Older children and those with more severe symptoms typically require psychopharmacologic options in concert with counseling or verbal therapy approaches.
- There is evidence of a "dose effect" in psychotherapy outcomes research, with some investigators suggesting that 6–8 sessions are necessary to yield positive initial effects and upward of 15–20 sessions for longer term, sustainable therapeutic effects. This dose effect may not be applicable to counseling services with primarily informational or emotional/supportive functions. Because many patients cease attendance to psychotherapy sessions after one or a few sessions, most interventions of this type cannot be accurately evaluated by the referring provider. Long-term therapy should also be evaluated for effectiveness at regular periods.

CROHN DISEASE

Eric Ji-Yuan Mao, MD • Samir A. Shah, MD, FACG, FASGE, AGAF

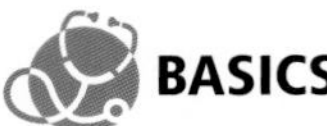

BASICS

DESCRIPTION

Crohn disease (CD) is a chronic, relapsing inflammatory GI tract disorder, most commonly involving the terminal ileum (80%).

- Hallmark features
  - Transmural inflammation, which can result in fibrosis, stricture formation, and fissures leading to sinus tracts, abscesses, or fistulas
  - Noncaseating granulomas (30%), crypt abscesses
  - Skip lesions: patchy, segmental distribution of disease; lesions may affect multiple bowel segments, interspersed with areas of normal mucosa; disease can also be continuous, potentially mimicking ulcerative colitis (UC)
  - Diverse presentations: ileocolitis (50%); isolated colitis (20%) are most common. In cases of isolated colitis, 10% involve the rectum and 33% involve the anorectal area.
- Early disease
  - Ulcerations: focal lesions with surrounding edema, resembling aphthous ulcers
  - Perianal disease (pain, anal fissures, perirectal abscess) may precede intestinal disease.
  - May present as wasting illness or anorexia
- Developed disease
  - Mucosal cobblestoning; luminal stenosis; creeping fat; fissures between mucosal folds, result in strictures/adhesions and/or fistulae

EPIDEMIOLOGY

Incidence

- In North America, 8–13 cases/100,000 adults; incidence is rising in North America and Western Europe.
- Bimodal age distribution: Predominant age is 15–25 years, with a 2nd smaller peak at 50–70 years.
- Women slightly more affected than men; increased incidence among patients in northern climates
- Increased risk in whites versus non-whites: 2–5×
- Increased risk in Ashkenazi Jews: 3–5×

Prevalence

United States adults: 100–200 cases/100,000

ETIOLOGY AND PATHOPHYSIOLOGY

- General: Clinical manifestations result from activation of inflammatory cells, whose by-products produce nonspecific tissue injury.
- Mechanism of diarrhea: excess fluid secretion and impaired fluid absorption; bile salt malabsorption in inflamed ileum, with subsequent steatorrhea; bacterial overgrowth
- Multifactorial: Genetic, environmental triggers, and immunologic abnormalities result in inflammation and tissue injury in the genetically predisposed.

Genetics

Of CD patients, 15% have a 1st-degree relative with inflammatory bowel disease (IBD); 1st-degree relative of an IBD patient has 3–30× increased risk of developing IBD by age 28 years. At least 163 different genes associated with IBD.

- Mutations in susceptibility loci
  - Ileal CD: IBD1 gene (chromosome 16)
  - Early-onset CD (age <15 years): mutations in 5q31-33 (IBD5), 21q22, and 20q13
  - North American white men with CD: 30% have HLA-DR7 and DQ4.
  - Extraintestinal manifestations of CD: mutations in HLA-A2, HLA-DR1, HLA-DQw5
  - Others: IL-10, IL-23 receptors; ATG16L1; IRGM
- Genetic syndromes associated with IBD: Turner and Hermansky-Pudlak syndromes, glycogen storage disease type 1b

RISK FACTORS

- Environmental factors
  - Cigarette smoking doubles the risk of developing CD; cessation may reduce frequency of flares, relapse after surgery.
  - Dietary factors: higher incidence if diet high in refined sugars, protein (meat, fish)
  - *Salmonella* or *Campylobacter* increase risk of developing IBD
  - *Clostridium difficile* infection may trigger flare of IBD and make treatment more difficult.
- Immunologic abnormalities: not clear if IBD immune response is directed against self-antigens of intestinal epithelium or foreign, bacterial antigens.
  - Tumor necrosis factor (TNF): upregulation of inflammatory Th1 cytokines
  - Tissue inflammation may result from increased secretion of cytokine IL-17, by Th17 subset of CD4+ T cells.

COMMONLY ASSOCIATED CONDITIONS

- Extraintestinal manifestations
  - Arthritis (20%): seronegative, primarily involving large joints; axial arthritis or ankylosing spondylitis (AS) and sacroiliitis (SI).
  - Skin disorders (10%): erythema nodosum, pyoderma gangrenosum, psoriasis
  - Ocular disease (5%): uveitis, iritis, episcleritis
  - Kidney stones: calcium oxalate stones (from steatorrhea and diarrhea) or uric acid stones (from dehydration and metabolic acidosis)
  - Fat-soluble vitamin deficiency (A, D, E, K), B_{12}
  - Osteopenia and osteoporosis; hypocalcemia
  - Hypercoagulability: venous thromboembolism prophylaxis essential in hospitalized patients
  - Gallstones: cholesterol stones resulting from impaired bile acid reabsorption
  - Primary sclerosing cholangitis (5%): more common in men with UC; asymptomatic, elevated alkaline phosphatase as marker
  - Autoimmune hemolytic anemia
- Conditions correlated with increased disease activity
  - Peripheral arthropathy (but not SI and AS)
  - Episcleritis (but not uveitis)
  - Oral aphthous ulcers and erythema nodosum
  - SI, AS, and uveitis are associated with HLA-B27.
- Other significant complications: GI bleed, toxic megacolon, bowel perforation/peritonitis, malignancy, sclerosing cholangitis; rectovaginal fistula

DIAGNOSIS

HISTORY

Hallmarks: fatigue, fever, weight loss, prolonged diarrhea; perianal disease, crampy abdominal pain, with or without gross bleeding. Children may present with failure to thrive.

- Factors exacerbating CD: concurrent infection, smoking, NSAIDs, and possibly stress

PHYSICAL EXAM

Presentation varies with location of disease

- General: signs of sepsis/disease activity (fever, tachycardia, hypotension) or wasting/malnutrition
- Abdominal: focal or diffuse tenderness, distension, rebound/guarding; rectal bleeding
- Perianal: fistulae, fissures
- Skin: erythema nodosum; psoriasis

DIFFERENTIAL DIAGNOSIS

- Acute, severe abdominal pain: perforated viscus, pancreatitis, appendicitis, diverticulitis, bowel obstruction, kidney stones, ovarian torsion
- Chronic diarrhea with crampy pain (colitis-like): UC, radiation colitis, infection, drugs, ischemia, microscopic colitis, IBD, celiac disease, malignancy (lymphoma, carcinoma), carcinoid
- Wasting illness: malabsorption, malignancy, psychiatric illness

DIAGNOSTIC TESTS & INTERPRETATION

Initial Tests (lab, imaging)

- CBC; chem 10; LFTs; ESR/C-reactive protein (CRP); serum iron, vitamin B_{12}, vitamin D-25 OH
- If diarrhea, stool specimen for routine culture, fecal leukocytes, *C. difficile*, and ova and parasites
- In hospitalized patients with severe flare-ups, KUB to rule out toxic megacolon
- Colon: colonoscopy with ileoscopy provides the greatest diagnostic sensitivity and specificity.
- Small bowel: sensitivity of CT or magnetic resonance enterography (MRE) better than small bowel follow through. MRE has no radiation exposure (important in younger patients). Capsule endoscopy allows small bowel visualization but no biopsy (1)[A].
  - Signs of small bowel disease: narrowed lumen with nodularity and/or string sign; cobblestone appearance, fistula and abscess formation, bowel loop separation (transmural inflammation)
- Gastroduodenal: upper GI endoscopy
  - Signs of gastroduodenal disease: antral narrowing and segmental duodenal stricturing; inflammatory mucosal disease on endoscopy
- Perirectal complications: optimal results from combination of endoscopic ultrasound (EUS) or MRI, with exam under anesthesia (EUA)
- Contraindications to endoscopy: perforated viscus, recent myocardial infarction, severe diverticulitis, toxic megacolon, or inability to undergo appropriate bowel preparation. In most cases, unprepared limited sigmoidoscopy allows adequate visualization to assess severity, extent, and aspirate stool for *C. difficile*, obtain biopsies to assess histologic severity, exclude other disorders (e.g., cytomegalovirus)

Follow-Up Tests & Special Considerations

Evidence of complications

- Stricture: obstructive signs: nausea, vomiting, pain, weight loss, diarrhea, or inability to pass gas or feces
- Abscess/phlegmon: localized abdominal peritonitis with fever and abdominal pain; diffuse peritonitis suggests intestinal perforation or abscess rupture (may be masked by steroids, narcotics)
- Fistulae (33–50% of patients, after 10 and 20 years of disease, respectively)
  - Enteroenteric: asymptomatic or a palpable, commonly indolent abdominal mass
  - Enterovesical: pneumaturia, recurrent polymicrobial UTI
  - Retroperitoneal: psoas abscess, ureteral obstruction
  - Enterovaginal: vaginal passage of gas or feces; clear, nonfeculent drainage from ileal fistula may be misdiagnosed as primary vaginal infection.

Diagnostic Procedures/Other

How to distinguish CD from UC

- CD: small bowel disease, rectal sparing; skip lesions; granulomas, perianal disease, and/or fistulae; no gross bleeding: RLQ pain more common
  - Commercially available antibody tests (overall 70% sensitive): anti-*Saccharomyces cerevisiae* antibody (ASCA), Cbir-1, OmpC, I2
- UC: diffuse, continuous involving the rectum; loss of normal vascularity, friable tissue; perinuclear antineutrophil cytoplasmic antibody (pANCA); LLQ pain; typically only affects colon; rectal bleeding common

ALERT

CD can mimic UC with continuous, not intermittent involvement; 10–15% of cases are difficult to differentiate; diagnosed as IBD undetermined (IBD-U).

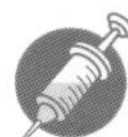

TREATMENT

- Assessment of disease severity: Crohn Disease Activity Index (CDAI)
  - Asymptomatic remission (CDAI <150)
  - Mild to moderate CD: ambulatory patients able to tolerate PO intake without dehydration, obstruction, or >10% weight loss. No abdominal tenderness, toxicity, or mass (CDAI 150–220).
  - Moderate to severe CD: patients who have failed initial treatment or who continue to have mild symptoms such as fever, weight loss, and abdominal pain (CDAI 220–450)
  - Severe: persistent symptoms despite outpatient therapy with glucocorticoids and/or biologics, or fulminant disease (peritonitis, cachexia, intestinal obstruction, abscess) (CDAI >450)
- General strategies
  - Step-up approach: Begin treatment with milder therapy (5-ASA, antibiotics) followed by more aggressive agents (steroids, immunomodulators, anti-TNF agents), as needed.
  - Top-down approach: early management with immunomodulators and/or anti-TNF agents before patients receive steroids, become steroid-dependent, or require surgery

GENERAL MEASURES

Additional therapies depend on location of disease.

- Oral lesions: triamcinolone acetonide in benzocaine and carboxymethyl cellulose or topical sucralfate for aphthous ulcers, cheilitis, and/or granulomatous sialadenitis
- Gastroduodenal CD: no clinical trials, although slow-release mesalamine may be beneficial, as it is partially released in proximal small bowel. Case reports note success of anti-TNF therapies. Symptomatic relief possible from proton pump inhibitors, H_2-receptor blockers, and/or sucralfate.
- Ileitis: supplementation of fat-soluble vitamins, as well as iron, B_{12}, and/or folate, and calcium to prevent bone loss.
- Treatment toxicity: pancreatitis, bone marrow toxicity, lymphoma, nonmelanoma skin cancer, infections (TB, histoplasmosis, others), malignancy

MEDICATION

First Line

- Asymptomatic patients: observation
- Mild CD
  - Mesalamine preferred for ileitis (2)[C]. For ileocolitis, sulfasalazine (2–4 g/day) or mesalamine (2)[C], (3)[C].
  - Antibiotics use is also controversial.
  - Glucocorticoid therapy: controlled ileal release budesonide (9 mg/day for 8–16 weeks, then discontinued over 2–4-week taper) for distal ileum and/or right colon involvement (2)[A], (3)[A]
  - Consider adjunctive therapy: antidiarrheals (loperamide); bile acid-binding resin (cholestyramine 4–12 g/day); probiotics (selected species either alone or in combination may prevent recurrent intestinal inflammation and reduce symptoms in acute CD).
  - Induction: controversial: slow-release oral 5-ASA agent (1.6–4.8 g/day). Evidence does not support this approach, but clinical practice suggests that some patients respond; therefore, it is commonly used as 1st-line therapy (2)[C].
  - Maintenance: 5-ASA is not recommended (3)[C]. Controlled ileal release budesonide, 6 mg/day, effective for maintenance for up to 6 months (2)[A].
- Moderate to severe CD
  - Induction: prednisone 40–60 mg/day (2)[A] or controlled-release budesonide (for isolated, moderate ileitis) or anti-TNF agents as initial induction agent or for lack of response to corticosteroid or immunomodulator (2)[A],(3)[A] (see below)
  - Maintenance: little role for mesalamine. If steroids required for induction, then use immunomodulator (2,3)[B] or biologic (anti-TNF agent) (2)[A],(3)[B] for maintenance. Except for budesonide, do not use steroids for maintenance (1)[A].
- Severe disease: immunomodulators, anti-TNF agents ± steroids
  - Azathioprine or 6-mercaptopurine: thiopurine methyltransferase (TPMT) and LFTs prior to initiation. Check CBC and LFTs every 2–3 months.
  - Methotrexate: effective for steroid-dependent and steroid-refractory CD (2)[B]
    - Folic acid 1 mg/day; follow LFTs
  - Anti-TNF therapies: active disease, fistulae, steroid sparing, some extraintestinal disease. Infliximab, adalimumab, certolizumab pegol
    - Prior to initiation of anti-TNF therapy: Check for evidence of TB, HBV infection.
    - Avoid live vaccines.
    - Monitoring: Consider anti-drug Ab levels to assess for immunogenicity. Serum concentrations of anti-TNF agents may also correlate with disease activity (4)[B].
- Combination therapy
  - Azathioprine + infliximab more effective than either alone in patients not previously treated with either (5)[A].
  - Rare: hepatosplenic T-cell lymphoma (fatal)
- Anti-adhesion molecules: prevent inflammatory cells from entering GI tract
  - Vedolizumab: gut-specific, can be used in anti-TNF failures or anti-TNF naive patients as induction and maintenance (6)[A]; given IV, no risk of progressive multifocal leukoencephalopathy (PML); FDA approved May 2014
  - Natalizumab: non-gut-specific, PML risk (1/1000). Can minimize risk by testing for John Cunningham (JC) virus antibody. However, can avoid risk of PML now that vedolizumab is available.

ADDITIONAL THERAPIES

Complications

- Peritonitis: bowel rest and antibiotic therapy (7–10 days parenteral antibiotics, followed by 2–4 week course of PO ciprofloxacin and metronidazole); surgery, as indicated
  - Consider holding steroids, which mask sepsis.
- Abscess: antibiotics, percutaneous drainage, or surgery with resection of affected segments
- Small bowel obstruction: IV hydration, nasogastric (NG) suction, total parenteral nutrition (TPN) for malnutrition, with resolution typically in 24–48 hours. Surgery for nonresponders

ONGOING CARE

FOLLOW-UP RECOMMENDATIONS

Patient Monitoring

Vaccinations in CD

- Check titers; avoid live vaccines (MMR, varicella, zoster) in patients on immunosuppressive therapy (steroids, 6MP, AZA, MTX, or anti-TNF).
- Regardless of immunosuppression: HPV, influenza, pneumococcal, meningococcal, hepatitis A, B; Tdap.

PATIENT EDUCATION

Crohn and Colitis Foundation of America (800) 343-3637; www.ccfa.org

REFERENCES

1. Baumgart DC, Sandborn WJ. Crohn's disease. *Lancet*. 2012;380(9853):1590–1605.
2. Lichtenstein GR, Hanauer SB, Sandborn WJ. Management of Crohn's disease in adults. *Am J Gastroenterol*. 2009;104(2):465–483.
3. Talley NJ, Abreu MT, Achkar JP, et al. An evidence-based systematic review on medical therapies for inflammatory bowel disease. *Am J Gastroenterol*. 2011;106(Suppl 1):S2–S25.
4. Ben-Horin S, Yavzori M, Katz L, et al. The immunogenic part of infliximab is the F(ab')2, but measuring antibodies to the intact infliximab molecule is more clinically useful. *Gut*. 2011;60(1):41–48.
5. Colombel JF, Sandborn WJ, Reinisch W, et al. Infliximab, azathioprine, or combination therapy for Crohn's disease. *N Engl J Med*. 2010;362(1):1383–1395.
6. Sandborn W, Feagan BG, Rutgeerts P, et al. Vedolizumab as induction and maintenance therapy for Crohn's disease. *N Engl J Med*. 2013;369(8):711–721.

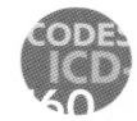

CODES

ICD10

- K50.919 Crohn's disease, unspecified, with unspecified complications
- K50.00 Crohn's disease of small intestine without complications
- K50.10 Crohn's disease of large intestine without complications

CLINICAL PEARLS

- The incidence of CD has risen over the past four decades.
- Magnetic resonance enterography allows assessment of luminal and extraluminal CD without radiation exposure.
- Assess for TB and HBV infection prior to initiating anti-TNF therapy.
- Cigarette smoking doubles the risk of developing CD; cessation may reduce frequency of flares and need for surgery.
- Test for *C. difficile* infection when evaluating diarrhea in all CD patients.
- Hospitalized CD patients require deep vein thrombosis prophylaxis.

CROUP (LARYNGOTRACHEOBRONCHITIS)

Garreth C. Debiegun, MD, FACEP

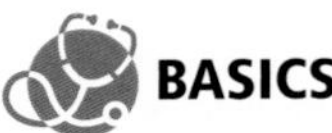

BASICS

DESCRIPTION

- Croup is a subacute viral illness characterized by upper airway symptoms such as barking cough, stridor, and fever. "Croup" is used to refer to viral laryngotracheitis or laryngotracheobronchitis (LTB), although it is sometimes used for LTB with pneumonitis, bacterial tracheitis, or spasmodic croup.
- Most common cause of upper airway obstruction or stridor in children
- Spasmodic croup: noninfectious form with sudden resolution
  - No fever or radiographic changes
  - Initially treated as croup
  - Usually self-limiting and resolves with mist therapy at home
  - Often recurs on same night or in 2–3 nights
- System(s) affected: pulmonary and respiratory
- Synonym(s): infectious croup; viral croup

EPIDEMIOLOGY

- Predominant age
  - Common among children 7 months–3 years
  - Most common during the 2nd year of life
  - Rare among those >6 years
- Predominant sex: male > female (1.5:1)
- Timing
  - Possible during any time of year but is most common in autumn and winter (with parainfluenza 1 and respiratory syncytial virus [RSV])

Incidence

- 6 cases per year per 100 children <6 years old
- 1.5–6% of cases require hospitalization.
- 2–6% of those require intubation.
- Decreasing incidence in the United States and Canada

ETIOLOGY AND PATHOPHYSIOLOGY

- Subglottic region/larynx is entirely encircled by the cricoid cartilage.
- Inflammatory edema and subglottic mucus production decrease airway radius.
- Small children have small airways with more compliant walls.
- Negative-pressure inspiration pulls airway walls closer together.
- Small decrease in airway radius causes significant increase in resistance (Poiseuille law: resistance proportional to 1/radius^4).
- Usually viruses that initially infect oropharyngeal mucosa and then migrate inferiorly
- Parainfluenza virus
  - Most common pathogen: 75% of cases
  - Type 1 is most common, causing 18% of all cases of croup.
  - Types 2, 3, and 4 are also common.
  - Type 3 may cause a particularly severe illness.
- Other viruses: RSV, paramyxovirus, influenza virus type A or B, adenovirus, rhinovirus, enteroviruses (coxsackie and echo), reovirus, measles virus where vaccination not common, and metapneumovirus
- *Haemophilus influenzae* type B now rare with routine immunization
- May have bacterial cause: *Mycoplasma pneumoniae* has been reported.

RISK FACTORS

- History of croup
- Recurrent upper respiratory infections
- Atopic disease increases the risk of spasmodic croup.

COMMONLY ASSOCIATED CONDITIONS

If recurrent (>2 episodes in a year) or during first 90 days of life, consider host factors.

- Underlying anatomic abnormality (e.g., subglottic stenosis)
  - In 1 study, found to be present in 59% children with recurrent croup
- Paradoxical vocal cord dysfunction
- Gastroesophageal reflux disease
- Neonatal intubation

DIAGNOSIS

- Most children who present with acute onset of barky cough, stridor, and chest wall indrawing have croup.
- Croup is a clinical diagnosis; lab tests and imaging serve only ancillary purposes.
- Classic "seal-like" barking, spasmodic cough
- May have biphasic stridor
- Low-grade to moderate fever
- Upper respiratory infection prodrome lasting 1–7 days
- Severity usually is determined by clinical observation for signs of respiratory effort: nasal flaring, retractions, tripoding, sniffing position, abdominal breathing, and tachypnea. Later symptoms: hypoxia/cyanosis or fatigue
- Westley croup scale (≤2 mild; 3–7 moderate; ≥8 severe), most useful for research purposes
  - Level of consciousness: normal, including sleep = 0; disoriented = 5
  - Cyanosis: none = 0; with agitation = 4; at rest = 5
  - Stridor: none = 0; with agitation = 1; at rest = 2
  - Air entry: normal = 0; decreased = 1; markedly decreased = 2
  - Retractions: none = 0; mild = 1; moderate = 2; severe = 2
- No change in stridor with positioning
- Nontender larynx
- Inflamed subglottic region with normal-appearing supraglottic region
- Differentiate from epiglottitis: nontoxic appearing, normal voice, no drooling, is coughing (1)

HISTORY

- 2–3 days of nonspecific prodromal syndrome with low-grade fever, coryza, and rhinorrhea
- Onset and recurrence at night when child is sleeping
- Symptoms often resolve en route to the hospital as the child is exposed to cool night air.
- Lack of prodrome indicates spasmodic croup.

PHYSICAL EXAM

- Pulse oximetry often is normal because there is no disturbance of alveolar gas exchange.
- Overall appearance: Is the child comfortable or struggling?
- Work of breathing: labored or comfortable?
- Sound of breathing and voice: hoarse, stridor, inspiratory wheezing, short sentences?
- Observed/subjective tidal volume: sufficient for child's size?

DIFFERENTIAL DIAGNOSIS

- Epiglottitis: currently rare
- Foreign body aspiration
- Subglottic stenosis (congenital or acquired)
- Bacterial tracheitis
- Simple upper respiratory infection
- Retropharyngeal or peritonsillar abscess
- Trauma
- Allergic reaction (acute angioneurotic edema)
- Airway anomalies (e.g., tracheo-/laryngomalacia)
- Other anatomic obstructions: subglottic hemangioma, subglottic cyst

DIAGNOSTIC TESTS & INTERPRETATION

- No laboratory abnormality is diagnostic.
- WBCs may be low, normal, or elevated.
- Lymphocytosis is expected but not required.
- Rapid antigen or viral culture tests are available in some centers.
  - Guide isolation precautions, not management

Initial Tests (lab, imaging)

- Posteroanterior and lateral neck films show funnel-shaped subglottic region with normal epiglottis: "steeple," "hourglass," or "pencil point" sign (present in 40–60% of children with LTB).
- CT may be more sensitive for defining obstruction in a confusing clinical picture.
- Patient should be monitored during imaging; airway obstruction may occur rapidly.

Test Interpretation

- Inflammatory reaction of respiratory mucosa
- Loss of epithelial cells
- Thick mucoid secretions

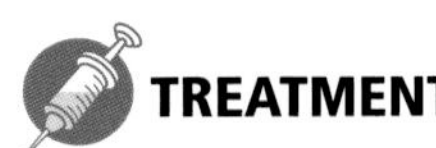

TREATMENT

GENERAL MEASURES

- Minimize lab tests, imaging, and procedures that upset the child; agitation worsens tachypnea and can be more detrimental than accepting a clinical diagnosis.
- ECG monitoring and pulse oximetry
  - Frequent checks are more sensitive to worsening disease than is pulse oximetry.

MEDICATION

First Line

- Well established in the literature; cornerstones of treatment are immediate nebulized epinephrine and dexamethasone.
- Racemic or L-epinephrine (equal efficacy and side effect profiles; L-epinephrine is used for most other hospital purposes and is less expensive.) (2)[A]
  - Reserved for more severe cases with stridor at rest
  - Racemic epinephrine: 0.05 mL/kg/dose (max, 0.5 mL) of 2.25% solution nebulized in normal saline to total volume of 3 mL
  - L-epinephrine: 0.5 mL/kg/dose (max, 5 mL) of a 1:1,000 dilution nebulized
  - Onset in 1–5 minutes, duration of 2 hours
  - Repeat as necessary if side effects are tolerated.
  - Observe child for 2 hours to ensure no recurrence after epinephrine wears off.
- Corticosteroids
  - Dexamethasone (least expensive, easiest), 0.15–0.6 mg/kg; higher doses have been traditional care, but studies have shown 0.15 mg/kg has equal efficacy (3)[B]. Single dose; IV/IM/PO has proven equal efficacy.

– Randomized controlled trials show this begins to improve symptoms within 30 minutes (4)[A]; full effect by 4 hours
– Other steroids (betamethasone, budesonide (5)[A], prednisolone) are beneficial, there may be minimal superiority of dexamethasone, also dexamethasone carries benefit of single-dose administration (6,7)[A].

- Heliox: a helium–oxygen mixture
  – Smaller, lower mass helium molecule (compared with nitrogen) theoretically maintains laminar flow in narrower airways and serves as bridge therapy to steroids.
  – Minimum of 60% helium must be used; 70% is preferable; 79% if patient has no oxygen requirement.
  – Limited data; a Cochrane review found no benefit in mild cases but likely benefit in moderate to severe croup as a bridge to steroid effect (8)[A].
- Antibiotics not indicated in this viral illness
  – Antecedent or subsequent bacterial infection is possible but uncommon.
- Oxygen as needed
- Humidified air shows no clinical benefit.

Second Line

Oseltamivir for influenza A

SURGERY/OTHER PROCEDURES

- Intubation rarely is required; tube 0.5–1 mm smaller than normal.
  – After trial of medical management, intubation is for fatigue caused by work of breathing or beginning total obstruction; not secondary to low oxygen saturation.
  – Extubate in 3–5 days when there is an appropriate air leak around the endotracheal tube.
- Tracheotomy: rarely; maintenance 3–7 days

COMPLEMENTARY & ALTERNATIVE MEDICINE

- Although proven no benefit in hospital, may be helpful at home. Do not use high-temperature misters (e.g., teakettles) because of a risk of burns. A hot shower running in a bathroom is a good steam generator.
- Some children respond well to cold, dry air.
- Probiotics may decrease the incidence of upper respiratory tract infections (9)[A].

INPATIENT CONSIDERATIONS

Admission Criteria/Initial Stabilization

Minor cases need no visit to a hospital or primary care physician (PCP).

- Outpatient care in mild cases
- Admit patients who do not respond to therapy or have recurrent stridor at rest after epinephrine wears off. Also admit those who have oxygen requirement, pneumonia, or congestive heart failure.
- In most cases, observation in the ED after medical management is sufficient.

Discharge Criteria

- >2 hours since last epinephrine
- No stridor at rest, no difficulty breathing
- Child able to tolerate liquids PO
- No underlying medical condition
- Caretakers able to assess changes to clinical picture and reaccess medical care

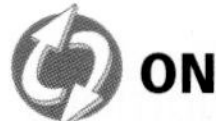

ONGOING CARE

FOLLOW-UP RECOMMENDATIONS

Patient Monitoring

Most patients will be seen in an ED or PCP office setting.

DIET

- NPO and IV fluids for severe cases
- Frequent small feedings with increased fluids for mild cases

PATIENT EDUCATION

- Must keep the patient quiet; crying may exacerbate symptoms.
- Educate parents about when to seek emergency care if mild cases progress.
- Provide emotional support and reassurance for the patient.

PROGNOSIS

- Up to 1/3 of patients will have a recurrence.
- Recovery is usually full and without lasting effects.
- If multiple recurrences, consider referral to ENT specialist to evaluate for possible anatomic etiology.

COMPLICATIONS

- Rare
- Subglottic stenosis in intubated patients
- Bacterial tracheitis
- Cardiopulmonary arrest
- Pneumonia

REFERENCES

1. Tibballs J, Watson T. Symptoms and signs differentiating croup and epiglottitis. *J Paediatr Child Health*. 2011;47(3):77–82.
2. Bjornson C, Russell KF, Vandermeer B, et al. Nebulized epinephrine for croup in children. *Cochrane Database Syst Rev*. 2013;10:CD006619.
3. Dobrovoljac M, Geelhoed GC. 27 years of croup: an update highlighting the effectiveness of 0.15 mg/kg of dexamethasone. *Emerg Med Australas*. 2009;21(4):309–314.
4. Dobrovoljac, Geelhoed GC. How fast does oral dexamethasone work in mild to moderately severe croup? A randomized double-blinded clinical trial. *Emerg Med Australas*. 2012;24(1):79–85.
5. Cetinkaya F, Tüfekçi BS, Kutluk G. A comparison of nebulized budesonide, and intramuscular, and oral dexamethasone for treatment of croup. *Int J Pediatr Otorhinolaryngol*. 2004;68(4):453–456.
6. Russell KF, Liang Y, O'Gorman K, et al. Glucocorticoids for croup. *Cochrane Database Syst Rev*. 2011;(1):CD001955.
7. Garbutt JM, Conlon B, Sterkel R, et al. The comparative effectiveness of prednisolone and dexamethasone for children with croup: a community-based randomized trial. *Clin Pediatrics (Phila)*. 2013;52(11):1014–1021.
8. Moraa I, Sturman N, McGuire T, et al. Heliox for croup in children. *Cochrane Database Syst Rev*. 2013;12:CD006822.
9. Hao Q, Lu Z, Dong BR, et al. Probiotics for preventing acute upper respiratory tract infections. *Cochrane Database Syst Rev*. 2011;(9):CD006895.

ADDITIONAL READING

- Bjornson CL, Johnson DW. Croup. *Lancet*. 2008;371(9609):329–339.
- Cherry JD. Clinical practice. Croup. *N Engl J Med*. 2008;358(4):384–391.

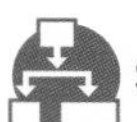

SEE ALSO

Bronchiolitis; Tracheitis, Bacterial

CODES

ICD10

- J05.0 Acute obstructive laryngitis [croup]
- J20.9 Acute bronchitis, unspecified
- J38.5 Laryngeal spasm

CLINICAL PEARLS

- Parainfluenza virus is the most common pathogen but caused by many viruses.
- Nebulized epinephrine only for stridor at rest
- Dexamethasone 0.6 mg/kg PO × 1
- Lateral neck films show funnel-shaped subglottic region with normal epiglottis: "steeple," "hourglass," or "pencil point" sign (present in 40–60% of children with LTB).

CRYPTORCHIDISM

Pamela Ellsworth, MD

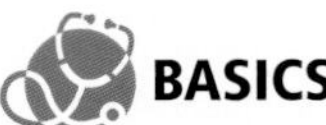

BASICS

DESCRIPTION

- Incomplete or improper descent of 1 or both testicles; also called *undescended testes* (1)
- Normally, descent is in the 7th–8th month of gestation. The cryptorchid testis may be palpable or nonpalpable.
- Types of cryptorchidism:
  - Abdominal: located inside the internal ring
  - Canalicular: located between the internal and external rings
  - Ectopic: located outside the normal path of testicular descent from abdominal cavity to scrotum; may be ectopic to perineum, femoral canal, superficial inguinal pouch (most common), suprapubic area, or opposite hemiscrotum
  - Retractile: fully descended testis that moves freely between the scrotum and the groin.
  - Iatrogenic: Previously descended testis becomes undescended secondary to scar tissue after inguinal surgery, such as an inguinal hernia repair or hydrocelectomy.
  - Also may be referred to as *palpable* versus *nonpalpable* (1)
- System(s) affected: reproductive
- Synonym(s): undescended testes (UDT)

EPIDEMIOLOGY

Incidence

- Predominant age: premature newborns
- Predominant sex: male only

Prevalence

- In the United States, cryptorchidism occurs in 1–3% of full-term and 15–30% of premature newborn males (2).
- Spontaneous testicular descent occurs by age 1–3 months in 50–70% of full-term males with cryptorchidism.
- Descent at 6–9 months of age is rare (3).

ETIOLOGY AND PATHOPHYSIOLOGY

- Not fully known
- May involve alterations in
  - Mechanical factors (gubernaculum, length of vas deferens and testicular vessels, groin anatomy, epididymis, cremasteric muscles, and abdominal pressure), hormonal factors (gonadotropin, testosterone, dihydrotestosterone, and müllerian-inhibiting substance), and neural factors (ilioinguinal nerve and genitofemoral nerve)
  - Major regulators of testicular descent from intra-abdominal location into the bottom of the scrotum are the Leydig cell–derived hormones, testosterone, and insulin-like growth factor 3 (IGF-3).
  - Mutations in the gene for IGF-3 and in the androgen receptor gene have been evaluated as possible causes of cryptorchidism as well as chromosomal alterations (1).
  - Environmental factors acting as endocrine disruptors of testicular descent also may contribute to the etiology of cryptorchidism (4).
- Risk of ascent may be as high as 32% in retractile testis (5).

Genetics

Occurrence of UDT in siblings, as well as fathers, suggests a genetic etiology.

RISK FACTORS

- Family history of cryptorchidism: highest risk if brother had UDT, followed by uncle then father (6)
- Low birth weight, prematurity, and small for gestational age are associated with a substantial increase in incidence of cryptorchidism (1). Retractile testes are at increased risk for ascent (5).

COMMONLY ASSOCIATED CONDITIONS

- Inguinal hernia/hydrocele
- Abnormalities of vas deferens and epididymis
- Intersex abnormalities
- Hypogonadotropic hypogonadism
- Germinal cell aplasia
- Prune-belly syndrome
- Meningomyelocele
- Hypospadias
- Wilms' tumor
- Prader-Willi syndrome
- Kallmann syndrome
- Cystic fibrosis

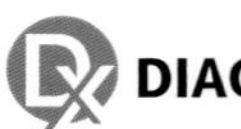

DIAGNOSIS

HISTORY

- ≥1 testicles in a site other than the scrotum
- May be an isolated defect or associated with other congenital anomalies

PHYSICAL EXAM

- Performed with warm hands, with child in sitting, standing, and squatting position
- A Valsalva maneuver and applied pressure to lower abdomen may help to identify the testes, especially a gliding testis.
- Failure to palpate a testis after repeated exams suggests an intra-abdominal or atrophic testis.
- An enlarged contralateral testis in the presence of a nonpalpable testis suggests testicular atrophy/absence.
- Testes should be palpated for quality and position at each recommended well-child visit (1)[B].

DIFFERENTIAL DIAGNOSIS

- Retractile testis (hypermobile testis) a normally descended testis that ascends into the inguinal canal because of an active cremasteric reflex (more common in males 4–6 years of age)
- Atrophic testis: may occur as a result of neonatal torsion
- Vanished testis may be the result of a lack of development or in utero torsion.

DIAGNOSTIC TESTS & INTERPRETATION

Initial Tests (lab, imaging)

- In phenotypic male newborn with bilateral, nonpalpable UDTs, hormone levels are helpful to determine whether the testes are present and should be evaluated for possible disorder of sexual development (1)[A].
  - Luteinizing hormone (LH)
  - Follicle-stimulating hormone (FSH)
  - Müllerian-inhibiting substance (MIS)
  - Testosterone
  - Serum electrolytes
  - Karyotype
- If bilateral nonpalpable testes and presenting >3 months of age, obtain a human chorionic gonadotropin (hCG) stimulation test to determine presence or absence of testicular tissue (hCG 2,000 IU/day × 3 days, and check testosterone before and after stimulation) as well as gonadotropins—to say testes are absent—need negative stimulation test and elevated gonadotropins (7).
- Ultrasound or other imaging modalities should not be performed in the evaluation of boys with cryptorchidism prior to referral to a specialist, as they are rarely needed in decision making (1)[B].

Follow-Up Tests & Special Considerations

- In newborns and children <6 months of age, periodic examination to determine if testis is palpable and descended prior to considering further intervention (1)
- In the absence of spontaneous testicular descent by 6 months of age (gestational age adjusted), infant should be referred to appropriate specialist and should perform surgery within 1 year (1,8)[B].
- In children with retractile testes, examination should be performed at least yearly to rule out subsequent ascent (1)[B].

Diagnostic Procedures/Other

Laparoscopy is useful in a child with nonpalpable cryptorchidism to confirm testicular absence or presence accurately and to determine the feasibility of performing a standard orchidopexy.

Test Interpretation

- Higher incidence of carcinoma in UDT and alterations in spermatogenesis (9)
- Histologic changes occur by 1.5 years of age and include smaller seminiferous tubules, fewer spermatogonia, and more peritubular tissue (9,10).

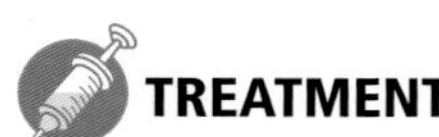

TREATMENT

GENERAL MEASURES

- Rule out retractile testis.
- Appropriate health care: outpatient until surgery performed
- Administration of chorionic gonadotropin may cause testicular descent in some boys. Reports of efficacy are inconsistent American Urological Association (AUA) guidelines on cryptorchidism do not recommend use of hormonal therapy to induce testicular descent due to low response rate and lack of evidence for long-term efficacy (1).

MEDICATION

Medical therapy is not indicated in the United States per the AUA guidelines on cryptorchidism 2014 (1).

ISSUES FOR REFERRAL

- ≥1 testes not descended by 6 months age (1)[B]
- Bilateral nonpalpable UDTs (1)
- Newly diagnosed cryptorchidism after 6 months of age (1)[B]

SURGERY/OTHER PROCEDURES

- Reasons to consider: avoids torsion, averts trauma, decreases but does not eliminate risk of malignancy, and prevents further alterations in spermatogenesis

- In the absence of spontaneous testicular descent by 6 months of age (gestational age-adjusted), surgery should be performed within 1 year (1)[B].
- Prepubertal orchidopexy decreases risk of testicular cancer and results in 2- to 6-fold reduction in relative risk compared to postpubertal orchidopexy (1,11–13).
- Laparoscopy/abdominal exploration is performed first if testis is nonpalpable (14).
- If palpable, an inguinal approach is usually performed. If low-lying, a single-incision scrotal approach can also be considered but may increase the risk of hernia (15,16).

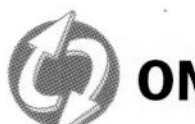

ONGOING CARE

FOLLOW-UP RECOMMENDATIONS

- Initial follow-up within 1 month of surgery and periodically thereafter to assess testicular size/growth.
- Patients with retractile testes should be examined at least annually to monitor for secondary ascent until testis is no longer retractile (1)[B].

Patient Monitoring

- Patients should be followed after surgery to evaluate testicular growth.
- Testicular tumors occur mainly during or after puberty; thus, these children should be taught self-examination when they are older.

DIET

No restrictions

PATIENT EDUCATION

Discuss with parents about causes, available treatments, and possible effects on patient's reproductive potential and also increased risk for testicular cancer and need for regular self-examination.

PROGNOSIS

- Disorder is usually corrected with medical or surgical therapy; however, there are possible lifelong consequences.
- If testicle is absent or orchiectomy is required, may consider placement of testicular prosthesis
- Early orchidopexy may decrease risk of testicular damage and risk of malignancy.

COMPLICATIONS

- Progressive failure of spermatogenesis, if left untreated; even with orchidopexy, the fertility rate is still reduced, especially with bilateral UDTs.
- Spermatogenesis is related to the duration of cryptorchidism and the location of the testis (17).
- Formerly, bilaterally cryptorchid men have a greater decrease in fertility compared with unilateral cryptorchid male and the general male population (1,18–22).
- Abnormalities also have been identified in the contralateral descended testis, although less severe.

REFERENCES

1. Kolon TF, Herndon CDA, Baker LA, et al. Cryptorchidism. AUA Guideines. www.auanet.org/education/guidelines/cryptorchidism.cfm. Accessed 2014.
2. Sijstermans K, Hack WW, Meijer RW, et al. The frequency of undescended testis from birth to adulthood: a review. *Int J Androl*. 2008;31(1):1–11.
3. Berkowitz GS, Lapinski RH, Dolgin SE, et al. Prevalence and natural history of cryptorchidism. *Pediatrics*. 1993;92(1):44–49.
4. Main KM, Skakkebaek NE, Toppari J. Cryptorchidism as part of the testicular dysgenesis syndrome: the environmental connection. *Endocr Dev*. 2009;14:167–173.
5. Agarwal PK, Diaz M, Elder JS. Retractile testis—is it really a normal variant. *J Urol*. 2006;175(4):1496–1499.
6. Elert A, Jahn K, Heidenreich A, et al. Population-based investigation of familial undescended testis and its association with other urogenital anomalies. *J Ped Urol*. 2005;1(6):403–407.
7. Docimo SG, Silver RI, Cromie W. The undescended testicle: diagnosis and management. *Amer Fam Physician*. 2000;62(9):2037–2044.
8. Surgical Advisory Panel. Referral to pediatric surgical specialists. *Pediatrics*. 2014;133(2):350–356.
9. Cortes D, Thorup JM, Visfeldt J. Cryptorchidism: aspects of fertility and neoplasms. A study including data of 1,335 consecutive boys who underwent testicular biopsy simultaneously with surgery for cryptorchidism. *Horm Res*. 2001;55(1):21–27.
10. Park KH, Lee JH, Han JJ, et al. Histological evidences suggest recommending orchiopexy within the first year of life for children with unilateral inguinal cryptorchid testis. *Int J Urol*. 2007;14(7): 616–621.
11. Wood HM, Elder JS. Cryptorchidism and testicular cancer: separating fact from fiction. *J Urol*. 2009;181(2):452–461.
12. Walsh TJ, Dall'Era MA, Croughan MS, et al. Prepubertal orchiopexy for cryptorchidism may be associated with lower risk of testicular cancer. *J Urol*. 2007;1784, Pt 1:1440–1446.
13. Pettersson A, Richiardi L, Nordenskjold A, et al. Age at surgery for undescended testis and risk of testicular cancer. *N Engl J Med*. 2007;356(18):1835–1841.
14. Patil KK, Green JS, Duffy PG. Laparoscopy for impalpable testis. *BJU Int*. 2005;95(5):704–708.
15. Al-Mandil M, Khoury AE, El-Hout Y, et al. Potential complications with the prescrotal approach for the palpable undescended testis? A comparison of single prescrotal incision to the traditional inguinal approach. *J Urol*. 2008;180(2):686–689.
16. Na SW, Kim SO, Hwang EC, et al. Single scrotal incision orchiopexy for children with palpable low-lying undescended testis: early outcome of a prospective randomized controlled study. *Korean J Urol*. 2011;52(9):637–641.
17. Wilkerson ML, Bartone FF, Fox L, et al. Fertility potential: a comparion of intra-abdominal and intracanalicular testes by age groups in children. *Horm Res*. 2001;55(1):18–20.
18. Bremholm Rasmussen T, Ingerslev HJ, Hostrup H. Bilateral spontaneous descent of the testis after the age of 10: subsequent effects on fertility. *Br J Surg*. 1988;75(8):820–823.
19. Gilhooly PE, Meyers F, Lattimer JK. Fertility prospects for children with cryptorchidism. *Am J Dis Child*. 1984;138(10):940–943.
20. Fallon B, Kennedy TJ. Long-term follow-up of fertility in cryptorchid patients. *Urology*. 1985;25(5):502–504.
21. Gracia J, Sánchez Zalabardo J, Sánchez Garcia J, et al. Clinical, physical, sperm and hormonal data in 251 adults operated on for cryptorchidism in childhood. *BJU Int*. 2000;85(9):1100–1103.
22. Trsinar B, Muravec UR. Fertility potential after unilateral and bilateral orchidopexy for cryptorchidism. *World J Urol*. 2009;27(4):513–519.

C

ADDITIONAL READING

- Barthold JS. Undescended testis: current theories of etiology. *Curr Opin Urol*. 2008;18(4):395–400.
- Barthold JS, Gonzalez R. The epidemiology of congential cryptorchidism, testicular ascent and orchidopexy. *J Urol*. 2003;170(6):2396–2401.
- Cortes D. Cryptorchidism—aspects of pathogenesis, histology and treatment. *Scan J Nephrol Suppl*. 1998;196:1–54.
- Foresta C, Zuccarello D, Garolla A, et al. Role of hormones, genes, and environment in human cryptorchidism. *Endocr Rev*. 2008;29(5):560–580.
- Hutson JM, Balic A, Nation T, et al. Cryptorchidism. *Semin Pediatr Surg*. 2010;19(3):215–224.
- Kollin C, Hesser U, Ritzen EM, et al. Testicular growth from birth to two years of age, and the effect of orchidopexy at 9 months of age: a randomized, controlled study. *Acta Paediatr*. 2006;95(3):318–324.
- Lee PA. Fertility after cryptorchidism: epidemiology and other outcome studies. *Urology*. 2005;66(2):427–431.

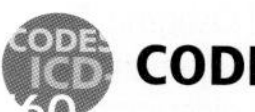

CODES

ICD10

- Q53.9 Undescended testicle, unspecified
- Q53.10 Unspecified undescended testicle, unilateral
- Q53.20 Undescended testicle, unspecified, bilateral

CLINICAL PEARLS

- If testicular descent does not occur by 6 months of age, it is unlikely to occur. Therefore, refer patients to a specialist if a testis has not descended by 6 months of age.
- Children with bilateral, nonpalpable UDTs require laboratory evaluation to determine if viable testicular tissue is present and to rule out disorder of sexual differentiation.
- Radiologic imaging has no role in the initial evaluation of cryptorchidism.
- The risk of infertility is increased with bilateral UDTs.

CUBITAL TUNNEL SYNDROME AND OTHER ULNAR NEUROPATHIES

James Winger, MD

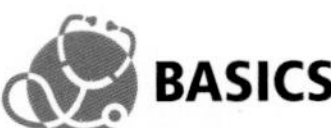

BASICS

DESCRIPTION

- Compression of the ulnar nerve on the medial aspect of the elbow where it enters the cubital tunnel results in cubital tunnel syndrome (CuTS); often resulting in elbow pain, loss of grip strength, and paresthesias of the forearm, wrist, and 4th and 5th fingers.
- Synonym(s): ulnar neuropathy
- Compression of the ulnar nerve at the wrist results in ulnar tunnel syndrome (UTS).

EPIDEMIOLOGY

- Predominant sex: male > female (3–8× more common)
- Elbow is most common site of compression of ulnar nerve resulting in cubital tunnel syndrome.
  - Less common sites of entrapment include the following:
    - Arcade of Struthers
    - Medial intermuscular septum
    - Medial epicondyle
    - Deep flexor pronator aponeurosis (1)
- CuTS is 2nd to carpal tunnel syndrome as the most common nerve compression of upper extremity (2).

ETIOLOGY AND PATHOPHYSIOLOGY

- The ulnar nerve is the terminal branch of the medial cord of the brachial plexus; it is composed of portions of the C8 and T1 nerve roots.
- The ulnar nerve becomes more superficial as it enters the ulnar sulcus near the medial epicondyle. The nerve runs posterior to the medial epicondyle and medial to the olecranon to enter the cubital tunnel (2).
- The cubital tunnel is a fibro-osseous canal. The roof is defined by the arcuate ligament of Osborne. The floor consists of the medial collateral ligament of the elbow, the joint capsule, and the olecranon.
- Elbow flexion increases distance from medial epicondyle to olecranon 5 mm for every 45 degrees of flexion.
- Elbow flexion places stress on medial (ulnar) collateral ligament, overlying retinaculum, and ulnar nerve.
- Shape of cubital tunnel changes from circular to ovoid and loses 2.5 mm of height with elbow flexion.
- Loss of height of cubital tunnel with elbow flexion decreases tunnel volume by 55%, doubling intraneural pressure on the ulnar nerve.
- Maximal pressure on the ulnar nerve in cubital tunnel is created by shoulder abduction, elbow flexion, and wrist extension.
- Elbow flexion decreases volume of cubital tunnel, causing compression of ulnar nerve.
- Compression of ulnar nerve causes pain at medial aspect of elbow and symptoms of the forearm and hand.
- Caused by constricting fascial bands, subluxation of ulnar nerve over medial epicondyle, cubitus valgus, bony spurs, hypertrophied synovium, tumors, ganglia, or direct compression of ulnar nerve as it crosses cubital tunnel
- Compression by ganglia, anomalous musculature, carpal bone fracture, or direct hypothenar pressure results in ulnar tunnel syndrome (3).

RISK FACTORS

- Patients who sleep or position themselves with their elbows bent, their arms overhead
- Patients with occupations demanding prolonged time with elbows bent (4)[A]
- Athletes in throwing sports, racquet sports, weightlifting, skiing, and cycling
- Preexisting polyneuropathy
- Patients on hemodialysis
- Patients in dependent position (surgery, ICU)

GENERAL PREVENTION

- Avoid long periods of elbow flexion, pressure on elbows or anterior ulnar aspect of the wrist
- Sleep with elbows straight; avoid sleeping with arms overhead.
- Keep proper posture when working at a desk.

COMMONLY ASSOCIATED CONDITIONS

- Ulnar nerve subluxation
- Ulnar collateral ligament laxity
- Osteoarthritis of elbow joint
- Carpal tunnel syndrome

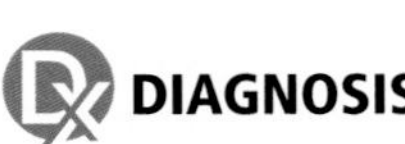

DIAGNOSIS

HISTORY

- Nocturnal elbow pain
- Medial elbow pain
- Paresthesias along medial forearm, wrist, and 4th and 5th digits
- Paresthesias may be intermittent at first and then become more constant.
- History of trauma over the area
- Repetitive elbow flexion and extension activities (e.g., hammering)
- Overhead throwing athlete with repetitive elbow motion
- Chronic symptoms: loss of grip strength and loss of fine motor skills in hand

PHYSICAL EXAM

- Inspect carrying angle of both elbows.
- Palpate medial epicondyle and cubital tunnel for areas of tenderness or ulnar nerve subluxation.
- Assess elbow range of motion.
- Positive Hoffman-Tinel test (CuTS) (percussion at ulnar nerve reproduces symptoms) (3)
- Pain on palpation over ulnar nerve
- Atrophy of intrinsic hand muscles
- Loss of sensation of 5th digit and medial 4th digit
- Wasting of hypothenar muscles and flexion contracture of 4th and 5th digits (ulnar claw)
- Wartenberg sign is clawing or abduction of the 5th digit with extension.
- Assess ability to cross 2nd and 3rd digits.
- Evaluate grip and pinch strength for weakness
- Froment sign is hyperflexion of the interphalangeal joint of the thumb while trying to secure a sheet of paper between the thumb and 1st finger as the examiner pulls the paper away (3).
- Assess vibration and light touch sensation.
- Scratch-collapse test: Patient faces examiner with arms adducted, elbows flexed, hands outstretched, and wrist in neutral position. The examiner gently pushes against both forearms, asking the patient to maintain steady resistance. The examiner scratches the skin overlying the potentially compressed ulnar nerve. The test is positive if the patient decreases resistance. Sensitivity for the scratch collapse was 69% compared with 54% and 46% for Tinel test and elbow flexion-compression test, respectively. Tinel test; however, had the highest negative predictive value (98%) of all tests for cubital tunnel (5).
- Compression prior to or within Guyon canal produces intrinsic muscle weakness and dorsolateral sensation loss (6).
- Intact sensation to dorsolateral hand implies nerve compromise distal to the takeoff of the dorsal sensory branch.
- Sensory loss to dorsolateral hand without hypothenar and interosseous weakness implies compression of superficial branch of ulnar nerve.

DIFFERENTIAL DIAGNOSIS

- C8–T1 radiculopathy
- Thoracic outlet syndrome
- Carpal tunnel syndrome
- Medial epicondylosis
- Ulnar collateral ligament injury
- Pancoast syndrome
- Metabolic disorders creating peripheral neuropathies
- Multiple sclerosis and other myelopathies

DIAGNOSTIC TESTS & INTERPRETATION

McGowan grades quantify the degree of physical exam findings and are specific for cubital tunnel syndrome.

- McGowan grade I: no wasting or weakness of intrinsic muscles, feeling of clumsiness in affected hand, mild paresthesias in ulnar nerve distribution
- McGowan grade II: intermediate lesions with weak interossei and muscle wasting
- McGowan grade III: severe lesions with paralysis of interossei and a marked weakness of the hand

Initial Tests (lab, imaging)

Initial approach

- X-ray may reveal osteophyte impingement of cubital tunnel or hamulus fracture in the wrist. Radiographs may also show signs of instability, deformity from old trauma, or presence of a supracondylar process (which can cause median nerve compression). Include anteroposterior (AP), lateral, and cubital tunnel views (1).
- Cubital tunnel view: Elbow is maximally flexed and x-ray beam is shot as an AP view of the distal humerus.

Follow-Up Tests & Special Considerations

- Chest x-ray if patient has history of smoking and ulnar nerve symptoms (to exclude Pancoast tumor)
- MRI shows inflammation and irritation of ulnar nerve.
- High-resolution ultrasound

Diagnostic Procedures/Other

- 1 mL lidocaine and 20–40 mg methylprednisolone injected into ulnar groove, parallel to ulnar nerve for CuTS (7)
- Electromyogram with nerve conduction studies (EMG/NCS) is not essential when diagnosis is obvious on clinical exam. Use to determine the efficacy of conservative treatment or when the diagnosis is unclear.

Test Interpretation

Delayed conduction of solely the ulnar nerve on an EMG/NCS implies a likely compressive neuropathy. Subjective improvement after diagnostic injection indicates anatomic site of compression at injection site.

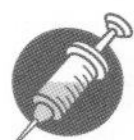

TREATMENT

- Mild cubital tunnel syndrome can often be treated without surgery. Consider surgery if no change after 3 months.
- If provocative causes can be identified and avoided, some recovery is likely.
- Patients with constant symptoms and/or muscle atrophy typically require surgical intervention (1)[C].
- If UTS is caused by direct compression, activity modification has shown to be effective (8)[C].
- Conservative treatment is initial approach if no motor weakness (3,9)[C].

GENERAL MEASURES

- Activity modification
- Avoid aggravating activities
- Avoid prolonged elbow flexion
- Avoid prolonged pressure/compression of ulnar nerve at elbow or wrist.
- Ice for symptom relief
- Splint or brace while sleeping to keep affected elbow in extension and take pressure off cubital tunnel (e.g., wrap towel around elbow and hold in place with tape; use a small size soft knee splint placed backward on the elbow, tie a scarf around waist then around wrist).
- For cyclists with UTS, frequent hand repositioning on handlebars is recommended.
- Physical therapy (nerve mobilization techniques and forearm and wrist stretching)
- Workplace/ergonomic modifications (e.g., correct posture, avoid long periods with elbows bent)
- Otherwise activity, as tolerated

MEDICATION

First Line

NSAIDs and activity modification to limit elbow flexion or hypothenar pressure; corticosteroid injection into the cubital tunnel (7)[B].

ISSUES FOR REFERRAL

CuTS: Failure of 3–6 months of conservative treatment, loss of grip strength, flexion contracture of 4th and 5th digits, and positive EMG for motor conduction delay merit surgical consultation (9)[C].

UTS: organic compressive lesion, motor deficit, failure of conservative treatment or dysesthesia greater than 36 hours after wrist fracture (3)[C]

ADDITIONAL THERAPIES

Hand therapy and custom-splint prescription

COMPLEMENTARY & ALTERNATIVE MEDICINE

Vitamin B_6 (100 mg/day) not effective in randomized trials

SURGERY/OTHER PROCEDURES

- Goal of surgery in CuTS is to create more space for the ulnar nerve (9).
- Many surgical treatments exist for the treatment of cubital tunnel syndrome. Comparative studies have shown some short-term advantages to one or another technique, but overall results between the treatments have essentially been equivalent. The choice of surgical procedure is based on multiple factors, and a single surgical approach cannot be applied to all clinical situations (10)[A].

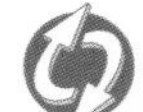

ONGOING CARE

FOLLOW-UP RECOMMENDATIONS

Patient Monitoring

- In severe cases, the nerve damage may be permanent.
- Patients with symptoms lasting >6 months have a worse prognosis.

DIET

No restrictions

PATIENT EDUCATION

- Use correct posture; avoid putting pressure on elbows, and place padding under elbows.
- Inability to fully extend affected fingers is a sign of severe ulnar nerve damage. Patients with this level of irritation usually do not recover, even with surgery.

PROGNOSIS

- Both conservative and surgical methods result in good to excellent results in 85–90% of cases.
- For McGowan grade III: Anterior IM transposition has best outcome (9)[C].

COMPLICATIONS

Anterior transposition and simple decompression may be complicated by recurrent subluxation of the ulnar nerve.

REFERENCES

1. Hariri S, McAdams TR. Nerve injuries about the elbow. *Clin Sports Med*. 2010;29(4):655–675.
2. Palmer BA, Hughes TB. Cubital tunnel syndrome. *J Hand Surg Am*. 2010;35(1):153–163.
3. Chen SH, Tsai TM. Ulnar tunnel syndrome. *J Hand Surg Am*. 2014;39(3):571–579.
4. van Rijn RM, Huisstede BM, Koes BW, et al. Associations between work-related factors and specific disorders at the elbow: a systematic literature review. *Rheumatology (Oxford)*. 2009;48(5):528–536.
5. Anderton M, Webb M. Cubital tunnel syndrome. *Br J Hosp Med (Lond)*. 2010;71(11):M167–M169.
6. Cheng CJ, Mackinnon-Patterson B, Beck JL, et al. Scratch collapse test for evaluation of carpal and cubital tunnel syndrome. *J Hand Surg Am*. 2008;33(9):1518–1524.
7. Rampen AJ, Wirtz PW, Tavy DL, et al. Ultrasound-guided steroid injection to treat mild ulnar neuropathy at the elbow. *Muscle Nerve*. 2011;44(1):128–130.
8. Murata K, Shih JT, Tsai TM. Causes of ulnar tunnel syndrome: a retrospective study of 31 subjects. *J Hand Surg Am*. 2003;28(4):647–651.
9. Mowlavi A, Andrews K, Lille S, et al. The management of cubital tunnel syndrome: a meta-analysis of clinical studies. *Plast Reconstr Surg*. 2000;106(2):327–334.
10. Mitsionis GI, Manoudis GN, Paschos NK, et al. Comparative study of surgical treatment of ulnar nerve compression at the elbow. *J Shoulder Elbow Surg*. 2010;19(4):513–519.

ADDITIONAL READING

- Assmus H, Antoniadis G, Bischoff C, et al. Cubital tunnel syndrome—a review and management guidelines. *Cent Eur Neurosurg*. 2011;72(2):90–98.
- Shi Q, MacDermid J, Grewal R, et al. Predictors of functional outcome change 18 months after anterior ulnar nerve transposition. *Arch Phys Med Rehabil*. 2012;93(2):307–312.
- Shi Q, MacDermid JC, Santaguida PL, et al. Predictors of surgical outcomes following anterior transposition of ulnar nerve for cubital tunnel syndrome: a systematic review. *J Hand Surg Am*. 2011;36(12):1996–2001.e1–e6.

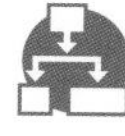

SEE ALSO

Epicondylitis

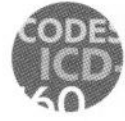

CODES

ICD10

- G56.20 Lesion of ulnar nerve, unspecified upper limb
- G56.22 Lesion of ulnar nerve, left upper limb
- G56.21 Lesion of ulnar nerve, right upper limb

CLINICAL PEARLS

- Elbow flexion decreases depth of cubital tunnel, compressing the ulnar nerve, and contributing to cubital tunnel syndrome.
- Sleeping with the elbow bent and arm overhead can exacerbate symptoms.
- Improper posture when working at a desk can exacerbate symptoms.
- Conservative treatment consists of ice, rest, hand therapy, splint fabrication, and activity modifications for 3 months in selected patients.
- Both conservative and surgical methods result in good to excellent results most of the time.

CUSHING DISEASE AND CUSHING SYNDROME

Linda Paniagua, MD • Geetha Gopalakrishnan, MD

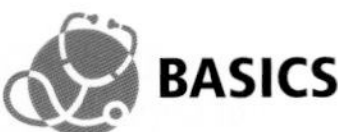

BASICS

DESCRIPTION

- Clinical abnormalities associated with chronic exposure to excessive amounts of cortisol (the major adrenocorticoid)
- Cushing syndrome is defined as excessive corticosteroid exposure from exogenous sources (medications) or endogenous sources (pituitary, adrenal, pulmonary, etc.) or tumor. Exogenous intake of steroids is the primary cause of Cushing syndrome.
- Cushing disease is defined as glucocorticoid excess due to excessive adrenocorticotropic hormone (ACTH) secretion from a pituitary tumor, the most common cause of primary Cushing syndrome.
- System(s) affected: endocrine/metabolic; musculoskeletal; skin/exocrine; cardiovascular; neuropsychiatric

Pediatric Considerations

- Rare in infancy and childhood
- Cushing disease accounts for approximately 75% of all cases of Cushing syndrome in children >7 years.
- In children <7 years, adrenal causes of Cushing syndrome (adenoma, carcinoma, or bilateral hyperplasia) are more common.
- Most common presenting symptom is lack of growth consistent with the weight gain.

Pregnancy Considerations

- Pregnancy may exacerbate disease.
- Cortisol levels increase in normal pregnancy states.

EPIDEMIOLOGY

Incidence

Uncommon: 0.7–2.4/1 million per year (1)

Prevalence

2–5% prevalence reported in difficult-to-control diabetics with obesity and hypertension (HTN)

ETIOLOGY AND PATHOPHYSIOLOGY

- Syndrome: excessive corticosteroid exposure from exogenous sources (medications) or endogenous sources (pituitary, adrenal, pulmonary, etc.) or tumor
- Disease: pituitary tumor causing excess ACTH (corticotropin)
- General population
  - Exogenous glucocorticoids
  - Endogenous ACTH–dependent hypercortisolism: 80–85%
    - ACTH-secreting pituitary tumor: 75%
    - Ectopic ACTH production (e.g., small cell carcinoma of lung, bronchial carcinoid): 20%
  - Endogenous ACTH–independent hypercortisolism: 15–20%
    - Adrenal adenoma
    - Adrenal carcinoma
    - Macronodular or micronodular hyperplasia
- Pediatric/adolescent (1)
  - Adrenal hyperplasia secondary to McCune-Albright: mean age 1.2 years
  - Adrenocortical tumors: mean age 4.5 years
  - Ectopic ACTH syndrome: mean age 10.1 years
  - Primary pigmented nodular adrenocortical disease: mean age 13.0 years
  - Cushing disease: mean age 14.1 years
- Pregnancy (2)
  - Pituitary-dependent Cushing syndrome: 33%
  - Adrenal causes: 40–50%
  - ACTH-independent adrenal hyperplasia: 3%

Genetics

- Multiple endocrine neoplasia
- Carney complex (an inherited multiple neoplasia syndrome)
- McCune-Albright syndrome (mutation of *GNAS1* gene)
- Familial isolated pituitary adenomas (mutations in the aryl hydrocarbon receptor–interacting protein gene)

RISK FACTORS

- Prevalent sex: female > male (3:1) (3)
- Most often occurs between the ages of 25 and 40 years
- Prolonged use of corticosteroids

GENERAL PREVENTION

Avoid corticosteroid exposure, when possible.

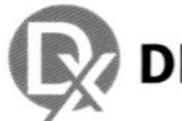

DIAGNOSIS

HISTORY

- Weight gain: 95%
- Decreased libido: 90%
- Menstrual irregularity: 80%
- Depression/emotional lability: 50–80%
- Easy bruising: 65%
- Diabetes or glucose intolerance: 60%

PHYSICAL EXAM

- Obesity (usually central): 95%
- Facial plethora: 90%
- Moon face (facial adiposity): 90%
- Thin skin: 85%
- Hypertension: 75%
- Skeletal growth retardation in children (epiphyseal plates remain open): 70–80%
- Hirsutism: 75%
- Proximal muscle weakness: 60%
- Purple striae on the skin
- Increased adipose tissue in neck and trunk
- Acne

DIFFERENTIAL DIAGNOSIS

- Obesity
- Diabetes mellitus
- HTN
- Metabolic syndrome X
- Polycystic ovarian disease
- Pseudo-Cushing (e.g., alcoholism, physical stress, severe major depression)

DIAGNOSTIC TESTS & INTERPRETATION

Initial Tests (lab, imaging)

- Recent guidelines (4)[C]
  - The 2008 Endocrine Society guidelines recommend against widespread testing for Cushing syndrome except in patients with the following:
    - Adrenal incidentaloma
    - Multiple progressive features suggestive of Cushing syndrome
    - Unusual features for their age such as osteoporosis and HTN
    - Abnormal growth (children)
- Late-night salivary cortisol, 24-hour urinary free cortisol, or low-dose dexamethasone suppression testing
  - Elevated late-night salivary cortisol: Obtain at least two measurements. Cortisol secretion is highest in the morning and lowest between 11 PM and midnight. The nadir of serum cortisol is maintained in pseudo-Cushing (e.g., obesity, alcoholism, depression) but not in Cushing syndrome. Sensitivity and specificity are >90–95% (5,6)[B].
  - 24-hour urinary free cortisol level: Obtain ≥2 samples to rule out intermittent hypercortisolism if results are normal and suspicion is high. Also measure 24-hour urinary creatinine excretion to verify adequacy of collection. Results may be falsely low if glomerular filtration rate <30 mL/min. Overall sensitivity and specificity varies, 90–97% and 85–96%, respectively (5)[B]. Avoid drinking excessive amounts of water due to risk of false-positive values. False-positive values can be seen in the presence of pseudo-Cushing states.
  - Low-dose dexamethasone suppression testing: Dexamethasone 1 mg is given between 11 PM and midnight, and fasting plasma cortisol is measured between 8 and 9 AM the following morning. A serum cortisol level below 1.89 μg/dL excludes Cushing syndrome, but specificity is limited. The presence of pseudo-Cushing states (depression, obesity, etc.), hepatic or renal disease, or any drug that induces cytochrome P-450 enzymes may cause a false result.
- High-dose dexamethasone suppression test may be useful when baseline ACTH levels are indeterminate:
  - 8 mg overnight dexamethasone suppression test: 8 mg of oral dexamethasone is given at 11 PM, with measurement of an 8-AM cortisol level the next day. A baseline 8-AM cortisol measurement is also obtained the morning prior to ingesting dexamethasone. Suppression of serum cortisol level to <50% of baseline is suggestive of a pituitary source of ACTH rather than ectopic ACTH or primary adrenal disease. Sensitivity and specificity are 95% and 100%, respectively (7)[B].
- If the initial results are positive or if clinical suspicion is high, perform additional studies to confirm diagnosis. Other tests to consider include the following:
  - Awake midnight plasma cortisol: Obtain samples on 3 consecutive nights. A late-evening serum cortisol >7.5 μg/dL has a sensitivity of 96% and specificity of 100% (8)[B]. Persistently elevated serum cortisol implies Cushing syndrome; nadir of serum cortisol is maintained in obese patients but not in Cushing.
  - Corticotropin-releasing hormone (CRH) after dexamethasone: used to distinguish Cushing syndrome from pseudo-Cushing syndrome. Dexamethasone 0.5 mg is given q6h for 48 hours starting at noon. CRH (1 μg/kg) is given 2 hours after the last dose of dexamethasone. Plasma cortisol is >1.4 μg/dL 15 minutes after CRH in patients with Cushing syndrome but not in those with pseudo-Cushing (9)[B].
- Pituitary MRI scan if pituitary tumor is suspected
- Abdominal CT scan if adrenal disease is suspected
- Chest CT scan if ectopic ACTH secretion is suspected
- Octreotide scintigraphy to look for occult ACTH-secreting tumor
- Dual energy x-ray absorptiometry to evaluate for osteoporosis

ALERT
- Antiepileptic drugs, progesterone, oral contraceptives (withdraw estrogen-containing drugs 6 weeks before testing), rifampin, and spironolactone may cause a false-positive dexamethasone suppression test.
- Pregnancy (4)[C]: Urine free cortisol is recommended instead of dexamethasone testing in the initial evaluation of pregnant women. Only urine free cortisol in the 2nd or 3rd trimester >3× the upper limit of normal can be taken to indicate Cushing syndrome.
- Epilepsy (4)[C]: Best to use measured cortisol from saliva and urine instead of serum cortisol after dexamethasone. No data to guide length of time needed after withdrawal of such medication to allow dexamethasone metabolism to return to normal; such medication change may not be clinically possible.

Follow-Up Tests & Special Considerations
- Once the diagnosis of Cushing syndrome is confirmed, localization is the next step:
  - ACTH level: elevated in ACTH-dependent Cushing syndrome (e.g., pituitary and ectopic tumor) and low in ACTH-independent Cushing syndrome (e.g., adrenal tumors and exogenous glucocorticoids)
  - High-dose dexamethasone suppression testing: used to distinguish between an ACTH-secreting pituitary tumor and ectopic ACTH-secreting tumors. 0.5 mg dexamethasone is given q6h for eight doses, with serum cortisol measured at 2 and 6 hours after last dose (sensitivity 79%, specificity 74%) (7)[B].
- Diagnosis of Cushing syndrome is complicated by the nonspecificity and high prevalence of clinical symptoms in patients without the disorder and involves a variety of tests of variable sensitivity and specificity. Efficient screening and confirmatory procedures are essential before considering therapy.

Diagnostic Procedures/Other
Diagnostic procedure depends on clinical judgment. Inferior petrosal sinus sampling with CRH stimulation can be considered if ACTH-dependent tumor is suspected but not localized.

Test Interpretation
- Thyroid function suppressed
- HTN
- Dyslipidemia
- Polycystic ovarian syndrome/hyperandrogenism
- Oligomenorrhea/hypogonadism
- Myopathy/cutaneous wasting
- Neuropsychiatric problems
- Ipsilateral adrenal gland hyperplasia and contralateral adrenal gland atrophy
- Hypercoagulable state
- Osteoporosis
- Nephrolithiasis
- Growth hormone reduced

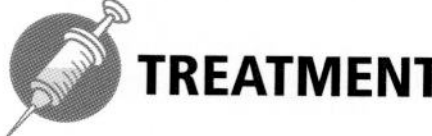

TREATMENT

MEDICATION
- Drugs usually not effective for primary long-term treatment; used in preparation for surgery or as adjunctive treatment after surgery, pituitary radiotherapy, or both
- Metyrapone, ketoconazole, and mitotane all lower cortisol by directly inhibiting synthesis and secretion in the adrenal gland. Replacement glucocorticoid therapy often required. As initial treatment, remission rates up to 85% (10,11)[C]
- Mifepristone is a potent antagonist of the glucocorticoid and progesterone receptors. It is FDA approved to control hyperglycemia in adults with endogenous Cushing syndrome who have type 2 diabetes or glucose intolerance secondary to hypercortisolism that has not responded to (or who are not candidates for) surgery.

SURGERY/OTHER PROCEDURES
- Tumor-specific surgery
  - Transsphenoidal surgery for Cushing disease (remission rate: 60–80%)
  - Resection of the ACTH-producing ectopic tumor
  - Adrenal surgery
    - For unilateral adrenal adenomas, laparoscopic surgery is the treatment of choice.
    - For nodular hyperplasia, bilateral adrenalectomy is usually recommended.
    - For patients with Cushing disease, bilateral laparoscopic adrenalectomy can be considered if the patient has persistent disease even after pituitary surgery and radiotherapy.
- Pituitary radiotherapy can be used to treat persistent hypercortisolism after transsphenoidal surgery.
- Benefits of surgery have not been definitively established for mild or intermittent hypercortisolism.

ONGOING CARE

PATIENT EDUCATION
- Teaching regarding diet and monitoring daily weight, early treatment of infections, emotional lability
- National Adrenal Disease Foundation. Great Neck, NY 11021; 516-407-4992

PROGNOSIS
- Guardedly favorable prognosis with surgery for Cushing disease; generally chronic course with cyclic exacerbations and rare remissions
- Better prognosis following surgery for benign adrenal tumors; long-term recurrence rate is 20%.
- Poor with small cell carcinoma of the lung producing ectopic hormone; neuroendocrine tumors (bronchial carcinoid) have much better prognosis.

COMPLICATIONS
- Osteoporosis
- Increased susceptibility to infections
- Metastases of malignant tumors
- Increased cardiovascular risk even after treatment
- Lifelong glucocorticoid dependence following treatment with bilateral adrenalectomy
- Nelson syndrome (pituitary tumor) after treatment with bilateral adrenalectomy (can occur in 8–38% of patients)

REFERENCES

1. Storr HL, Chan LF, Grossman AB, et al. Pediatric Cushing's syndrome: epidemiology, investigation and therapeutic advances. *Trends Endocrinol Metab*. 2007;18(4):167–174.
2. Lindsay JR, Nieman LK. Adrenal disorders in pregnancy. *Endocrinol Metab Clin North Am*. 2006;35(1):1–20, v.
3. Newell-Price J, Bertagna X, Grossman AB, et al. Cushing's syndrome. *Lancet*. 2006;367(9522):1605–1617.
4. Nieman LK, Biller BM, Findling JW, et al. The diagnosis of Cushing's syndrome: an Endocrine Society clinical practice guideline. *J Clin Endocrinol Metab*. 2008;93(5):1526–1540.
5. Putignano P, Toja P, Dubini A, et al. Midnight salivary cortisol versus urinary free and midnight serum cortisol as screening tests for Cushing's syndrome. *J Clin Endocrinol Metabol*. 2003;88(9):4153–4157.
6. Yaneva M, Mosnier-Pudar H, Dugué MA, et al. Midnight salivary cortisol for the initial diagnosis of Cushing's syndrome of various causes. *J Clin Endocrinol Metab*. 2004;89(7):3345–3351.
7. Aytug S, Laws ER, Vance ML. Assessment of the utility of the high-dose dexamethasone suppression test in confirming the diagnosis of Cushing disease. *Endocr Pract*. 2012;18(2):152–157.
8. Isidori AM, Kaltsas GA, Pozza C, et al. The ectopic adrenocorticotropin syndrome: clinical features, diagnosis, management and long-term follow-up. *J Clin Endocrinol Metabol*. 2006;91(2):371–377.
9. Yanovski JA, Cutler GB, Chrousos GP, et al. Corticotropin-releasing hormone stimulation following low-dose dexamethasone administration. A new test to distinguish Cushing's syndrome from pseudo-Cushing's states. *JAMA*. 1993;269(17):2232–2238.
10. Findling JW, Raff H. Cushing's syndrome: important issues in diagnosis and management. *J Clin Endocrinol Metab*. 2006;91(10):3746–3753.
11. Nieman LK, Ilias I. Evaluation and treatment of Cushing's syndrome. *Am J Med*. 2005;118(12):1340–1346.

SEE ALSO

Algorithm: Cushing Syndrome

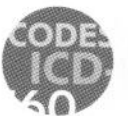

CODES

ICD10
- E24.9 Cushing's syndrome, unspecified
- E24.0 Pituitary-dependent Cushing's disease
- E24.2 Drug-induced Cushing's syndrome

CLINICAL PEARLS
- Cushing disease is due to excessive ACTH secretion from a pituitary tumor, resulting in corticosteroid excess.
- Cushing syndrome is due to excessive corticosteroid exposure from exogenous sources (medications) or endogenous sources (pituitary, adrenal, pulmonary, etc.) or tumor.
- Depression, alcoholism, medications, eating disorders, and other conditions can cause mild clinical and laboratory findings similar to those in Cushing syndrome (pseudo-Cushing syndrome).

CUTANEOUS DRUG REACTIONS

Angela M. Riegel, DO

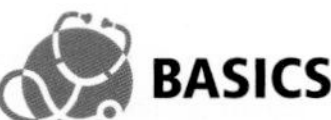

BASICS

DESCRIPTION

- An adverse cutaneous reaction in response to administration of a drug. Skin reactions are the most common adverse drug reactions.
- Severity can range from mild eruptions that resolve after the removal of the inciting agent to severe skin damage with multiorgan involvement.
- Morbilliform/simple exanthem (75–95%) and urticarial (5–6%) eruptions are most common, but multiple morphologic types may occur.
- System(s) affected: skin/mucosa/exocrine, hematologic/lymphatic/immunologic

EPIDEMIOLOGY

- All ages affected
- Predominant sex: female > male
- Special consideration in the geriatric population who are on multiple medications: increased likelihood of severe cutaneous and systemic reactions; also consider in the pediatric group: difficult to distinguish from viral exanthems

Incidence

In the United States, prevalence of 2–3% in hospitalized patients; estimated 1/1,000 hospitalized patients has had a severe cutaneous reaction.

ETIOLOGY AND PATHOPHYSIOLOGY

- Predictable adverse reactions are due to overdose, side effect, or drug interaction.
- Unpredictable reactions include intolerance, drug idiosyncrasy secondary to abnormality in metabolism, or immune reaction. >700 drugs are known to cause a dermatologic reaction:
  - Immunologically mediated reaction: immunoglobulin (Ig) E–mediated reaction (type I hypersensitivity), cytotoxic/IgG/IgM induced (type II), immune complex reactions (type III), and delayed-type hypersensitivity (type IV) with T cells, eosinophils, neutrophils, and monocytes
  - Acneiform: OCPs, corticosteroids, iodinated compounds, hydantoins, lithium
  - Erythema multiforme/Stevens-Johnson syndrome (SJS)/toxic epidermal necrolysis (TEN): sulfonamides, penicillins, barbiturates, hydantoins, anticonvulsants, NSAIDs, cephalosporins, tetracycline, terbinafine
  - Fixed drug eruptions: NSAIDS, sulfonamides, tetracycline, barbiturates, salicylates, OCPs
  - Lichenoid: thiazides, NSAIDS, gold, ACE inhibitors, proton pump inhibitors, antimalarials, sildenafil
  - Photosensitivity: doxycycline, thiazides, sulfonylureas, quinolones, sulfonamides, NSAIDs
  - Hypersensitivity vasculitis: hydralazine, penicillins, cephalosporins, thiazides, gold, sulfonamides, NSAIDs,
  - Drug rash with eosinophilia and systemic symptoms (DRESS) syndrome: anticonvulsants, sulfonamides, dapsone, minocycline, allopurinol
  - Acute generalized exanthematous pustulosis (AGEP): penicillins, cephalosporins, macrolides, calcium channel blockers, antimalarials, carbamazepine, acetaminophen, terbinafine, nystatin, vancomycin
  - Sweet syndrome (acute febrile neutrophilic dermatosis): sulfa drugs, granulocyte colony-stimulating factor (G-CSF), granulocyte-macrophage colony-stimulating factor (GM-CSF), diazepam, minocycline, nitrofurantoin
  - Serum sickness-like reaction: penicillins, TMP-SMX, propranolol, bupropion, minocycline
  - Morbilliform/urticarial/exfoliative erythroderma: numerous medications, including penicillins, cephalosporins, sulfonamides, tetracyclines, ibuprofen, naproxen, allopurinol, acetylsalicylic acid, radiocontrast media (1)[A]

Genetics

Genetics may play a role, as certain HLA antigens have been associated with increased predisposition to specific drug eruptions:

- HLA-B*5801, HLA-B*5701 and HLA-B*1502 have been linked to allopurinol-induced and carbamazepine-induced SJS/TEN, respectively.
- HLA class I antigens, such as HLA-A2, HLA-B12 and HLA-B22, have been linked to TEN and fixed drug eruptions, respectively.

RISK FACTORS

Previous drug reaction, multiple medications, concurrent infections, immunocompromised, disorders of metabolism, and certain genetic HLA haplotypes

GENERAL PREVENTION

Always ask patients about prior adverse drug events. Be aware of medications with higher incidence of reactions as well as drug cross-reactions.

DIAGNOSIS

HISTORY

- New medications within the preceding 6 weeks: all oral, parenteral, and topical agents, including over the counter drugs, vitamins, and herbal remedies
- Consider other etiologies: bacterial infections, viral exanthems, or underlying skin disease including cutaneous lymphoma

PHYSICAL EXAM

May present as a number of different eruption types, including, but not limited to the following:

- Morbilliform eruptions (exanthems)
  - Most frequent cutaneous reaction (75–95%); difficult to distinguish from viral exanthem; often secondary to antibiotic
  - Starts on trunk as pruritic red macules and papules and extends to extremities in confluent fashion, sparing face, palms, soles, and mucous membranes
  - Onset 7–21 days after drug initiation (2)[C]
- Urticaria
  - Pruritic erythematous wheals distributed anywhere on the body, including mucous membranes; may progress to angioedema, appearing as nonpitting edema without erythema or margins
  - Individual lesions fade within 24 hours, but new lesions may develop (2).
- Acneiform eruptions
  - Folliculocentric, monomorphous pustules typically involving the face, chest, and back distinguished from acne vulgaris by absence of comedones grossly and microscopically
  - Often become secondarily infected (2)[C]
- Fixed drug eruptions
  - Single/multiple, round, sharply demarcated, violaceous plaques with gray center that leave postinflammatory hyperpigmentation; occur on skin or mucous membrane.
  - Appear shortly after drug exposure and recur in identical location after reexposure; some patients have a refractory period during which the drug fails to activate lesions.
  - Onset usually 48 hours after ingestion of drug (2)
- AGEP
  - Multiple sterile pinhead-sized nonfollicular pustules on erythematous background with desquamation after 7–10 days
  - Involves intertriginous areas, but can be generalized and involve the face
  - Appears similar to pustular psoriasis, but AGEP has fever and marked leukocytosis with neutrophilia and/or eosinophilia (2)[C]
- DRESS syndrome
  - Classic triad of fever, exanthem, and internal organ involvement with possible pharyngitis and lymphadenopathy
  - Can lead to exfoliative dermatitis, often accompanied by facial edema
  - Internal organ involvement: 80% hepatic, 40% renal, 33% pulmonary, and cardiac lab tests show elevated liver transaminases and eosinophilia.
  - Onset 2–8 weeks after drug exposure; may develop 3 months or later into therapy (3)[B]
- Erythema multiforme
  - Most commonly associated with herpes simplex virus and other viral/bacterial etiologies; less likely secondary to drug exposure
  - 3-zone target lesions and raised atypical 2-zone targets with localized erythema
  - Lesions predominant on distal extremities including on acral surface with limited mucosal involvement; <10% epidermal detachment (4)[B]
- SJS/TEN
  - Classification and distinction between SJS and TEN determined by affected body surface area (BSA)
    - SJS: <10% BSA; SJS-TEN overlap: 10–30% BSA; TEN: >30% BSA
  - Unlike erythema multiforme, strong association with preceding drug exposure as opposed to infection except in children where infection is more common (e.g., mycoplasma)
  - Onset 1–3 weeks after starting offending agent: Flat atypical 2-zone target lesions and erythematous macules that are truncal and generalized with mucosal involvement
  - May develop confluent areas of bullae, erosions, and necrosis; significant risk for infection and sepsis
  - SJS: 5–15% mortality; TEN: 30% mortality (5)[C],(6)[A]
- Lichenoid eruptions
  - Flat-topped, violaceous, pruritic papules on extensor surfaces and involving oral mucosa
  - Reticular pattern: lesions heal with hyperpigmentation
  - Chronic lesions: persist for weeks/months after drug discontinued (2)
- Photosensitivity reaction
  - Phototoxic reactions within 24 hours of light exposure with exaggerated sunburn reaction; confined to sun-exposed areas
  - Photoallergic reactions: caused by UVA exposure; more pruritic than painful; can involve non–sun-exposed areas

- Hypersensitivity vasculitis
  - Petechiae/palpable purpura and/or maculopapular rash concentrated on lower extremities and dependent areas
  - Biopsy shows neutrophils around an arteriole or venule
  - Possible renal, joint, and CNS involvement with fever, myalgias, arthritis, and abdominal pain (2)
- Sweet syndrome
  - Fever, neutrophilia, tender edematous violaceous papules, plaques, or nodules, with or without pustules/vesicles that spontaneously resolve
  - May have oral ulcers or ocular manifestations, such as conjunctivitis
  - Classically seen in young women after a mild respiratory illness, but 7–56% associated with malignancy and pregnancy
- Serum sickness–like reaction
  - Fever, nonspecific cutaneous eruption with possible bullous lesions, arthralgias
  - Onset 7–14 days
- Exfoliative dermatitis/erythroderma
  - Generalized erythema with exfoliation and/or fine desquamation over 90% of body surface
  - Difficult to distinguish between drug, primary cutaneous lymphoma, or inflammatory etiology
  - Lymphadenopathy, hepatosplenomegaly, leukocytosis, eosinophilia, or anemia may be present.
  - Increased risk of secondary infection and insensible fluid and temperature loss with hemodynamic instability

DIFFERENTIAL DIAGNOSIS

- Viral exanthem: presence of fever, lymphocytosis, and other systemic findings may help in the differential
- Primary dermatosis: Correlation of drug withdrawal to rash resolution may clarify diagnosis; skin biopsy is helpful.
- Bacterial infection: Cultures of pustules may distinguish primary infection from AGEP and acneiform eruptions.

DIAGNOSTIC TESTS & INTERPRETATION

Initial Tests (lab, imaging)

A minimum number of tests are useful in evaluating for internal organ involvement. CBC with differential; significant eosinophilia may be seen in DRESS and other drug-induced allergic reactions. LFT, urinalysis, and serum creatinine; chest x-ray if suspected vasculitis

Diagnostic Procedures/Other

- Special tests depend on suspected mechanism:
  - Type I: skin/intradermal testing, radioallergosorbent (RAST)
  - Type II: direct/indirect Coombs test
  - Type III: ESR, C-reactive protein, ANA, antihistone antibody, tissue biopsy for immunofluorescence studies
  - Type IV: patch testing, lymphocyte proliferation assay (investigational)
  - Anaphylaxis/nonimmunologic mast and basophil cell reaction: serum tryptase levels
- Cultures useful in excluding infectious etiology; skin biopsy is nonspecific but useful in characterizing an eruption and excluding primary skin pathologies.
- Develop a timeline documenting the onset and duration of all drugs, dosages, and onset of cutaneous eruption (1)[A].

Test Interpretation

- Nonspecific histologic findings are superficial epidermal and dermal infiltrates composed variably of lymphocytes, neutrophils, and eosinophils.
- SJS/TEN: partial or full-thickness necrosis of the epidermis, necrotic keratinocytes, vacuolization leading to subepidermal blister at basal membrane zone

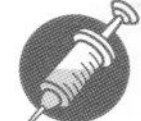

TREATMENT

GENERAL MEASURES

- Monitor for signs of impending cardiovascular collapse: Anaphylactic reactions, DRESS, SJS/TEN, extensive bullous reactions, and generalized erythroderma may require inpatient treatment.
- Do not rechallenge with drugs causing urticaria, bullae, angioedema, DRESS, anaphylaxis, or erythema multiforme.

MEDICATION

- Withdrawal of offending drug. Depending on the type of eruption, symptomatic treatment may be useful, but most require no additional therapy except cessation of offending agent.
- Anaphylaxis or widespread urticaria: epinephrine 0.2–0.5 mg (1:1000 [1 mg/mL] solution) SC every 5–15 min; prednisone may be given to prevent recurrence.
- Acute urticaria (<6 weeks) and chronic urticaria (>6 weeks): 2nd-generation antihistamines (preferred): cetirizine 10–20 mg daily, loratadine 10–20 mg daily, fexofenadine 180 mg daily, levocetirizine 5–10 mg daily. 1st-generation antihistamines: diphenhydramine 10–25 mg QHS, hydroxyzine 10–25 mg TID, doxepin 10–50 mg QHS H_2 antagonists: cimetidine 400 mg BID, ranitidine 150 mg BID
- Anaphylaxis, severe urticaria: prednisone PO 1 mg/kg in tapering doses
- Erythema multiforme
  - Treatment is generally supportive with management of suspected underlying infection.
  - Herpes simplex virus (HSV)–associated: prophylaxis with acyclovir 400 mg BID, valacyclovir 500–1,000 mg/day, or famciclovir 250 mg BID
  - "Magic mouthwash" BID or TID is helpful for mucosal erosions. Consider ophthalmology consult for severe ocular involvement (4)[B].
- SJS/TEN: Treatment is supportive. Consult with a dermatologist and ophthalmologist. Systemic corticosteroid use remains controversial. Consider IVIG 2–3 g/kg for severe disease. In pediatric TEN patients, low-dose IVIG (0.05–0.1 g/kg/day) was effective. Varied success rates reported with use of anti–tumor necrosis factor-α agents, cyclosporine, cyclophosphamide, and plasmapheresis (5)[C],(6)[A].
- DRESS: prompt removal of offending drug and supportive measures; high-potency topical steroids for rash; systemic steroids with severe organ involvement; prednisone 0.5–2 mg/kg/day with prolonged taper 8–12 weeks (3)[B].

ONGOING CARE

FOLLOW-UP RECOMMENDATIONS

Patient Monitoring

- For urticarial, bullous, DRESS, or erythema multiforme spectrum lesions, close follow-up is needed.
- Patients with anaphylaxis/angioedema should be given EpiPen for secondary prevention and a Med Alert bracelet; label the patient's medical record with the agent and reaction.
- If the patient needs to take the inciting drug (e.g., antibiotic) in the future, induction of drug tolerance or graded challenge procedures may be necessary.

PROGNOSIS

- Eruptions generally begin fading within days after removing offending agent. With morbilliform eruptions, eruption may spread distally even when agent is removed, resolving over time.
- Anaphylaxis, angioedema, DRESS, and bullous reactions are potentially fatal.

COMPLICATIONS

Anaphylaxis, bone marrow suppression, hepatitis (dapsone, hydantoin), renal failure, and pulmonary and thyroid toxicity

REFERENCES

1. Joint Task Force on Practice Parameters, American Academy of Allergy, Asthma and Immunology, American College of Allergy, Asthma and Immunology, et al. Drug allergy: an updated practice parameter. *Ann Allergy Asthma Immunol*. 2010;105(4):259–273.
2. Ahmed A, Pritchard S, Reichenberg J. A review of cutaneous drug eruptions. *Clin Geriatr Med*. 2013;29(2):527–545.
3. Chen YC, Chiu HC, Chu CY. Drug reaction with eosinophilia and systemic symptoms: a retrospective study of 60 cases. *Arch Dermatol*. 2010;146(12):1373–1379.
4. Wetter DA, Davis MD. Recurrent erythema multiforme: clinical characteristics, etiologic associations, and treatment in a series of 48 patients at Mayo Clinic, 2000–2007. *J Am Acad Dermatol*. 2010;62(1):45.
5. Mockenhaupt M. Stevens-Johnson syndrome and toxic epidermal necrolysis: clinical patterns, diagnostic considerations, etiology, and therapeutic management. *Semin Cutan Med Surg*. 2014;33(1):10–16.
6. Schneck J, Fagot JP, Sekula P, et al. Effects of treatments on the mortality of Stevens-Johnson syndrome and toxic epidermal necrolysis: a retrospective study on patients included in the prospective EuroSCAR study. *J Am Acad Dermatol*. 2008;58(1):33–40.

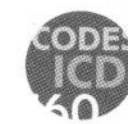

CODES

ICD10

- L27.1 Loc skin eruption due to drugs and meds taken internally
- L50.0 Allergic urticaria
- R21 Rash and other nonspecific skin eruption

CLINICAL PEARLS

- Virtually, any drug can cause a rash; antibiotics are the most common culprits that cause cutaneous drug reactions.
- Focus on drug history with new suspicious skin eruptions.
- Usually self-limited after withdrawal of offending agent
- Symptoms such as tongue swelling/angioedema, skin necrosis, blisters, high fever, dyspnea, and mucous membrane erosions signify more severe drug reactions.

CYBERBULLYING

Elizabeth Janopaul-Naylor, MD • Edward Feller, MD, FACP, FACG

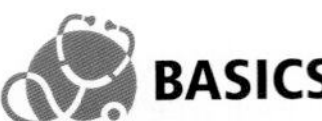

BASICS

DESCRIPTION

- Bullying: repetitive intentional behavior to harm based on imbalance of power
- Cyberbullying: behavior via electronic or digital media that communicates hostile or aggressive messages intended to harm or discomfort others
  - Includes threats, rumors, harassment, sexually explicit or embarrassing images, impersonation carried out through social media, e-mail, online forums, or instant messaging services
  - Can occur between similar and different ages; can occur between strangers and known persons. (¾ of victims report knowing their bully; similarly, ¼ of bullies report NOT knowing their victim)
- Computer and phone ubiquity allow continuous online access; victimization occurs anywhere, anytime. Increase in accessibility and internet use has drawn attention to cyberbullying, which has similarly grown in popularity:
  - Teens using the Internet (93%); owning a cell phone (75%)
- Popular media focuses on high-profile cases, but minor, common episodes are pervasive and corrosive and may have more significant effects on the mental health of victims. Minor incidents may precede major bullying incidents and take an additive toll on emotional health.
- Compared with traditional bullying, cyberbullying is anonymous, opportunistic, free from supervision, and easily accessible. Power differential may be absent.
- Large overlap between traditional bullies and victims and cyberbullies and victims; but youth not engaged in traditional bullying may participate due to limited consequences, lack of perceived harm to victims due to the ability to use a false name, or assume someone else's on-screen identity.
- Intervention is difficult because cyberbullying occurs in spaces not monitored by school staff or supervisory adults in nonschool settings.
- Infrequently reported, usually to a friend (30%), parent (<10%), rarely to school personnel (<5%). Cyberbullying creates a permanent record that can cause lasting emotional and social harm.
- Types of cyberbullying:
  - Like traditional bullying, cyberbullying can be direct, where an individual contacts his or her victim, or indirect, where the bully uses technology to spread rumors, for example.
  - Direct: text, call, instant message, e-mail
  - Indirect: commenting on public Web site, posting pictures/videos to public forum
  - The most common social media site used is Facebook, which is also the leading medium for cyberbullying. Twitter, YouTube, and MySpace are other popularly used cites commonly used for cyberbullying.
  - The most common venue for cyberbullying is through instant messaging.
  - Anonymity can facilitate disinhibition, for example, allowing students to post inappropriate evaluations of teachers on Web sites such as ratemyteacher.com.
  - Commonly, a pediatric or early adult issues; but cyberbullying can occur at any age or any locale, such as the workplace. Adult-on-child cyberbullying is uncommon.
  - Microepidemics can occur in schools or sports teams. Multiple bullies—a contagion of peer-group bullying—piling on a single victim or group.

EPIDEMIOLOGY

Incidence

1-year incidence ~15% for high school students and a 2-month incidence of 18% for middle school students.

Prevalence

- Cyberbullying is pervasive; globally, between 20 and 40% of adolescents report cyber victimization (2).
- As many as one-half of all middle and high schoolers report being targeted; one-third cyberbullied others.
- 60% of cyberbullying victims were also bullying victims; one-third of bullying victims were also cyberbullying victims; one-half of all middle and high schoolers report being targeted; one-third cyberbullied others (1,2).
- Bullying behavior is thought to peak in middle school.
- Due to the openness of the internet, much bullying is witnessed by third parties. A study of undergraduates showed that over half of respondents reported being an observer of cyberbullying (3).

RISK FACTORS

- For bully victims:
  - Frequent Internet or social media use
  - Previous offline harassment
  - More likely to have psychosomatic, emotional, or peer problems or social anxiety
  - More likely to come from families with structures other than 2 biologic parents
  - Female, correlation with depression and cyber victimization
  - Males are more likely to stand up to their bully than females.
  - Targets may be youth perceived as different due to physical or mental disability, race/ethnicity, socioeconomic class, gender expression, or sexual preference.
    - Lesbian, gay, bisexual, or transgender (LGBT) students experience more frequent electronic harassment than peers (4)[B].
    - Being bullied for sexual orientation has a higher association with depression and suicidality than bullying for other reasons.
- For cyberbullies:
  - Males are three times more likely to cyberbully (5)[B].
  - Hyperactivity, conduct disorder
  - Frequent smoking, alcohol
  - Not feeling safe at school
  - Low prosocial behavior (limited empathy)
  - Engagement in relational aggression (spreading rumors, exclusion)
  - Poor emotional bond with caregiver
  - Previous victims of traditional bullying
  - Younger children may unintentionally bully, viewing the Internet similarly to a video game, where there are no consequences.
  - Intend online content as jokes
  - Youth who are both cyber victims and cyberbullies have higher rates of severe psychiatric illness (6)[B].

GENERAL PREVENTION

Recommendations to parents/guardians:

- Communicate with children about online use.
  - Discuss positive and negative aspects of social media and Internet usage.
  - Learn about technologies children use.
- Teach children that jokes may be difficult to interpret when not in person. When they poke fun or criticize, they may unwittingly offend.
- Encourage children to report witnessing cyberbullying as well as resisting the pressure to reinforce bullying when others are reinforcing.
- Form an online-use plan with children:
  - Reduce time online or on social media sites.
  - Negotiate policies that fit desires and needs of both parents and children.
- Check privacy settings and supervise online activities:
  - Understand limitations of software monitoring to assess Internet use.

ALERT

- Recommendations to physicians:
  - Screening for cyberbullying should be included in adolescent mental health assessment: "Have you ever received, sent, or seen messages on the Internet that might be seen as bullying?"
- Recommendations to schools and communities:
  - Open periodic discussions with youth and parents/guardians about online use and cyberbullying.
  - Multimodality, long-term, school-wide interventions against bullying have been shown to be effective in decreasing rates of cyberbullying.
  - Vigilance and intervention during after-school and extracurricular activities
  - Some bullying behaviors may represent delinquent or criminal offenses:
    - Of 48 states with antibullying legislation, the majority have specific provisions addressing cyberbullying (7).

COMMONLY ASSOCIATED CONDITIONS

- Traditional bullying
- Behavioral health consequences
- Internet addiction (8)
- Cyber immersion: use of cyber technology and Internet as a central element of daily life, communication, and relationships
- Bullied victims are more likely to bring guns to school and engage in school violence (9). Half of adolescents expressing shooting threats online had prepared to carry out threats (10).
- Victims of cyberbullying via phone may report more safety concerns than victims of Internet bullying.
- Cyberbullying victims report more depressive symptoms, whereas cyberbullies report more problems with substance use.

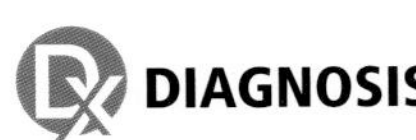

DIAGNOSIS

HISTORY

Unique technology-associated characteristics (11)[C]:

- Avoiding computers, cell phones, and other devices
- Stress receiving e-mail, instant message, or text
- Avoiding conversations about computer use
- Emotional or peer problems; not feeling safe at school; fear of a particular person
- Poor academic performance

- Physical complaints: headache, abdominal pain, difficulty sleeping
- Withdrawal from family, friends; reluctance to attend school and social events
- See "Risk Factors"

PHYSICAL EXAM

Signs consistent with depression: flattened affect, fatigue

DIFFERENTIAL DIAGNOSIS

- Traditional bullying: physical abuse, sexual or verbal harassment
- Child abuse or neglect
- Depression
- Conduct disorder
- Malingering, prevarication
- Cyberbullying as a feature of underlying psychiatric illnesses

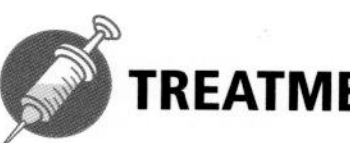

TREATMENT

GENERAL MEASURES

- Community-based approach: Parents, teachers, and school officials should be aware of communications technology used by youth. Learn how technology is used and new trends in positive and negative social communications.
- Encourage cyberbullying reporting to parents, teachers, and other supervising adults.
- School-wide programs addressing traditional bullying may also be effective in cyberbullying.
- Prepare parents to discuss online safety.
- In traditional bullying, mediation between bully and victim may be counterproductive as mediation is only successful if both parties have equal power and incentive to end conflict, which is inherently not true in bullying situations; less evidence is available for cyberbullying.
- Gather information about the methods and context of cyberbullying:
  - Duration: establish timeline, previous history as victim or bully.
  - When and where does the bullying occur?
  - How does bullying occur? Mediums of online communication, traditional bullying
  - Content: Review printouts, text messages, and so forth; look for themes.
  - Relationship between victim and bully: power differential, age differences, previous conflicts
  - Check for external and internal consistency, malingering.
  - Bullies may view behavior as joking or not malicious.
  - Identify other participants because cyberbullying may occur with multiple offenders or onlookers.

ISSUES FOR REFERRAL

- Psychiatric sequelae such as depression, anxiety
- Suicidality or homicidal ideation should be referred urgently for psychiatric care.
- Any online sexual solicitations of minors by adults should be reported to law enforcement.
- Severe cases of cyberbullying may require referral for legal and criminal input.

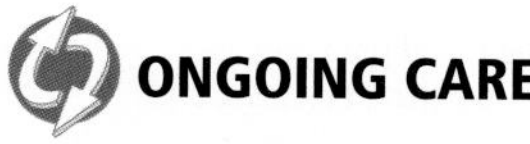

ONGOING CARE

FOLLOW-UP RECOMMENDATIONS

- Screen for cyberbullying at medical visits.
- Discuss efficacy of online privacy measures.
- Screen for traditional forms of bullying.
- Consider referral for ongoing psychiatric sequelae.

Patient Monitoring

- Screen for depression, substance and alcohol abuse, suicidality, and homicidal ideation.
- Monitor technology use.
- Effective coping measures (12)[A]:
  - Removing self from Web sites
  - Avoiding Internet use
  - Informing school or adult
- Ineffective coping measures:
  - Bullying the bully
  - Pretending to ignore the bully
  - Drug use

PATIENT EDUCATION

- Directed toward youth and parents
- See "General Measures"
- Efforts must be multidimensional, repeated, and involve school and health care personnel and community-wide involvement.
- http://www.stopbullying.gov/cyberbullying/
- http://kidshealth.org/parent/positive/talk/cyberbullying.html
- http://www.commonsensemedia.org/cyberbullying

PROGNOSIS

- Varies widely; lack of long-term demographic studies
- Bullying and cyberbullying may have chronic social, psychological, and medical sequelae that may not be evident during episodes.

COMPLICATIONS

- Linked with depression and suicidality. Highest rates of suicidal ideation are associated with victims of both traditional and cyberbullying. In a study of middle schoolers, males with depressive-like symptoms were more than eight times as likely to have experienced cyber victimization.
- Popular media has portrayed high rates of suicide directly caused by cyberbullying, but data are unclear whether there exists a statistical link between cyberbullying and completed suicide (13)[A].
- Decreased self-esteem, poor interpersonal relationships, loneliness, and often drop in grades
- Victims of cyberbullying and traditional bullying show high rates of depressive symptoms and suicidality.
- Cyber victims may in fact have worse depression symptoms due to increased sense of isolation.
- Long-term data for cyberbullies and victims do not exist, but traditional bullies have a much higher future incarceration rate.
- Both cyberbullies and victims have increased rates of aggression.
- Legal complications:
  - Some Web sites are exploring installation of automatic bullying monitoring. Many sites such as Facebook and YouTube have current settings for users to report inappropriate content.
  - Many states have clauses pertaining to electronic communication in their stalking and harassment laws. Jurisdictions now have cybercrime units.
  - A question facing courts is how far to pursue cases and if this infringes on free speech.

REFERENCES

1. Schneider SK, O'Donnell L, Stueve A, et al. Cyberbullying, school bullying, and psychological distress: a regional census of high school students. *Am J Public Health*. 2012;102(1):171–177.
2. Tokunaga RS. Following you home from school: a critical review and synthesis of research on cyberbullying victimization. *Computers in Human Behavior*. 2010;26(3):277–287.
3. Carter MA. Third party observers witnessing cyber bullying on social media sites. *Procedia-Soc Behav Sci*. 2013;84:1296–1309.
4. Patrick DL, Bell JF, Huang JY, et al. Bullying and quality of life in youths perceived as gay, lesbian, or bisexual in Washingtom State, 2010. *Am J Public Health*. 2013;103(7):1255–1261.
5. Bauman S, Toomey RB, Walker JL. Associations among bullying, cyberbullying, and suicide in high school students. *J Adolesc*. 2013;36(2):341–350.
6. Sourander A, Klomek AB, Ikonen M, et al. Psychosocial risk factors associated with cyberbullying among adolescents. *Arch Gen Psychiatry*. 2010;67(7):720–728.
7. Freeman BW, Thompson C, Jacques C. Forensic aspects and assessment of school bullying. *Psychiatr Clin North Am*. 2012;35(4):877–900.
8. Englander EK. Spinning our wheels: improving our ability to respond to bullying and cyberbullying. *Child Adolesc Psychiatr Clin N Am*. 2012;21(1):43–55.
9. Suzuki K, Asaga R, Sourander A, et al. Cyberbullying and adolescent mental health. *Int J Adolesc Med Health*. 2012;24(1):27–35.
10. Lindberg N, Oksanen A, Sailas, E, et al. Adolescents expressing school massacre threats online: something to be extremely worried about? *Child Adolesc Psychiatry Ment Health*. 2012;6(1):39.
11. Donnerstein E. Internet bullying. *Pediatr Clin North Am*. 2012;59:623–633.
12. Jacobs NC, Dehue F, Völlink T, et al. Determinants of adolescents' ineffective and improved coping with cyberbullying: a Delphi study. *J Adolesc*. 2014;37(4):373–385.
13. Messias E, Kindrick K, Castro J. School bullying, cyberbullying, or both: correlates of teen suicidality in the 2011 CDC Youth Risk Behavior Survey. *Compr Psychiatry*. 2014;55(5):1063–1068.

ADDITIONAL READING

- Bostic JQ, Brunt CC. Cornered: an approach to school bullying and cyberbullying, and forensic implications. *Child Adolesc Clin N Am*. 2011;20(3):447–465.
- Moreno MA, Kolb J. Social networking sites and adolescent health. *Pediatr Clin North Am*. 2012;59(3):601–612.
- Olweus D. School bullying: development and some important challenges. *Annu Rev Clin Psychol*. 2013;9:751–780.

CLINICAL PEARLS

- Cyberbullying is anonymous, occurs anywhere anytime, may leave a permanent record, and occurs without witnesses so more difficult to protect against; parents are unaware of extent.
- Cyberbullying can profoundly affect mental health.
- Rarely reported to adults; daily microaggressions may have cumulative effects not perceived by parents, guardians, or school officials.
- Students viewed as different due to disability, socioeconomic status, gender identity, sexual orientation, race, or ethnicity are more likely to be cyberbullied.
- Prevention requires awareness of this common issue and sustainable, community-wide interventions.

CYSTIC FIBROSIS

Emily Forbes, DO • Reem Abu-Sbaih, DO

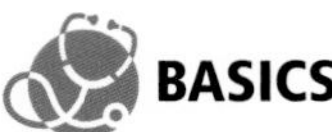

BASICS

DESCRIPTION

- Cystic fibrosis (CF) is an autosomal recessive genetic condition that most prominently affects the lungs and pancreas.
- The GI, endocrine, and reproductive systems as well as the liver, sinuses, and skin can all be involved.
- Initially a pediatric disease, CF has become a chronic pediatric and adult medical condition as improvements in medical care have led to a dramatic increase in long-term survival.

EPIDEMIOLOGY

CF is the most common lethal inherited disease in Caucasians and is found in every racial group.

Incidence

Number of infants born with CF in relation to the total number of live births in the United States

- 1 in 3,000 Caucasians
- 1 in 4,000–10,000 Latin Americans
- 1 in 15,000–20,000 African Americans
- Uncommon in Africa and Asia, with reported frequency in Japan of 1 in 350,000 (1)[A]

Prevalence

- 30,000 patients with CF living in the United States
- ~1,000 new diagnoses are made annually.

ETIOLOGY AND PATHOPHYSIOLOGY

- Abnormal CFTR function leads to abnormally viscous secretions that alter organ function.
- The lungs: obstruction, infection, and inflammation negatively affect lung growth, structure, and function
  - Decreased mucociliary clearance
  - Infection is accompanied by an intense neutrophilic response.
  - Degradation of supporting tissues causes bronchiectasis and eventual failure.

Genetics

CFTR gene (cystic fibrosis transmembrane conductance regulator): >1,500 mutations exist that can cause phenotypic CF, all of which are recessively inherited. Most common is loss of the phenylalanine residue at 508th position (deltaF508), which accounts for 8.7% of affected alleles in the CF population in the United States. *G551D* mutation accounts for 4.3% of affected alleles (2)[A].

RISK FACTORS

CF is a single-gene disorder. The severity of the phenotype can be affected by the specific *CFTR* mutation (most predictive of pancreatic disease), other modifier genes (*CFTM1* for meconium ileus), gastroesophageal reflux disease (GERD), severe respiratory virus infection, and environmental factors such as tobacco smoke exposure.

GENERAL PREVENTION

- American Congress of Obstetricians and Gynecologists (ACOG) recommends genetic analysis for all North American couples planning a pregnancy, with appropriate counseling to identified carriers and genetic analysis of siblings of known CF patients.
- Newborn screening for CF is offered throughout the United States. Identification of affected newborns has resulted in a reduction of new cases.
- Amelioration of complications of CF can be accomplished through early diagnosis (by newborn screening) followed by referral to an accredited regional CF center.

COMMONLY ASSOCIATED CONDITIONS

- Upper respiratory
  - Rhinosinusitis is seen in up to 100% of patients with CF.
  - Nasal polyps are seen in up to 86% of patients.
- The GI tract
  - Pancreatic exocrine insufficiency (85–90%) (1)[A]
  - Malabsorption of fat, protein, and fat-soluble vitamins (A, D, E, and K)
  - Hepatobiliary disease (10.8%)
    - Focal biliary cirrhosis
    - Cholelithiasis
  - Meconium ileus at birth (10–15%) (1)[A]
  - Distal intestinal obstruction syndrome (DIOS): intestinal blockage that typically occurs in older children and adults (5.1%) (2)[A]
  - GERD (30.5%) (2)[A]
- Endocrine
  - CF-related diabetes (CFRD)
    - May present as steady decline in weight, lung function, or increased frequency of exacerbation
    - Leading comorbid complication (30.5% in patients age <18 years)
    - Result of progressive insulin deficiency
    - Early screening and treatment may improve reduced survival found in CFRD.
  - Bone mineral disease (14.8%) (2)[A]
  - Joint disease (2.9%) (2)[A]
  - Hypogonadism
    - Frequent low testosterone levels in men
    - Menstrual irregularities are common.
- Reproductive organs
  - Congenital bilateral absence of the vas deferens: obstructive azoospermia in 98% of males
- Depression (12%) (2)[A]

Pregnancy Considerations

- Pulmonary disease may worsen during pregnancy.
- Originally considered too dangerous for women with CF, successful pregnancies occur more frequently. In 2012, 249 women with CF became pregnant (2)[A].
- Advances in fertility treatments now allow men with CF to father children (2)[A].

DIAGNOSIS

- Median age at diagnosis: 4 months (2)[A]
- General (any age)
  - Family history
  - Chronic/recurrent respiratory symptoms, including airway obstruction and infections
  - Persistent infiltrates on chest x-rays (CXRs)
  - Hypochloremic metabolic acidosis
- Neonatal
  - Meconium ileus
  - Prolonged jaundice
- Infancy
  - Failure to thrive
  - Chronic diarrhea
  - Anasarca/hypoproteinemia
  - Pseudotumor cerebri (vitamin A deficiency)
  - Hemolytic anemia (vitamin E deficiency)
- Childhood
  - Recurrent endobronchial infection
  - Bronchiectasis
  - Recurrent sinusitis
  - Steatorrhea
  - Poor growth
  - DIOS
  - Allergic bronchopulmonary aspergillosis
- Adolescence and adulthood
  - Recurrent endobronchial infection
  - Bronchiectasis
  - Allergic bronchopulmonary aspergillosis
  - Chronic sinusitis
  - Hemoptysis
  - Pancreatitis
  - Portal hypertension
  - Azoospermia
  - Delayed puberty

HISTORY

Suspect with failure to thrive, steatorrhea, and recurrent respiratory problems

PHYSICAL EXAM

- Respiratory
  - Rhonchi and/or crackles
  - Hyperresonance on percussion
  - Nasal polyps
- GI: Hepatosplenomegaly when cirrhosis present.
- Other: digital clubbing, growth retardation, and pubertal delay

DIFFERENTIAL DIAGNOSIS

- Pulmonary
  - Difficult-to-manage asthma
  - Chronic bronchitis
  - Recurrent pneumonia
  - Chronic/recurrent sinusitis
  - Primary ciliary dyskinesia
- GI
  - Celiac disease
  - Protein-losing enteropathy
  - Pancreatitis of unknown etiology
  - Shwachman-Diamond syndrome

DIAGNOSTIC TESTS & INTERPRETATION

Initial Tests (lab, imaging)

- Newborn screening (~61% of new cases) tests blood levels of immunoreactive trypsin (IRT) (2)[A].
- Sweat test (gold standard)
  - Sweat chloride
    - >60 mmol/L is positive for CF.
    - <40 mmol/L is normal.
- CFTR mutation analysis
  - Limited panel testing: Allele-specific polymerase chain reaction (PCR) identifies >90% of mutations; finite chance of false-negative finding. Full-sequence testing is more costly and time-consuming.
- CXR
  - Hyperinflation early in disease
  - Bronchial thickening and plugging
  - Nodular densities, patchy atelectasis, and confluent infiltrates
  - Bronchiectasis

Follow-up Tests & Special Considerations

- Sputum culture (common CF organisms)
- Pulmonary function tests (PFTs)

- 72-hour fecal fat
- Stool elastase
- Oral glucose tolerance test (OGTT) annually after age 10 years
- Head CT: Abnormal sinus CT findings are nearly universal in CF and may include mucosal thickening, intraluminal sinus polyps, and sinus effusions. Many children with CF never develop aerated frontal sinuses.
- Chest CT (not routine): Useful when unusual findings noted on CXR

Diagnostic Procedures/Other

- Flexible bronchoscopy
- Bronchoalveolar lavage

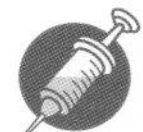

TREATMENT

GENERAL MEASURES

- Annual influenza vaccination for all CF patients age >6 months
- Palivizumab for prophylaxis of respiratory syncytial virus (RSV) in infants with CF <2 years (3)[A]
- Avoidance of smoke

MEDICATION

- Pulmonary
  - Antibiotics, oral
    - *Staphylococcus aureus*: Bactrim or cephalexin
    - *Pseudomonas aeruginosa*: fluoroquinolones
    - Azithromycin (anti-inflammatory properties)
  - Antibiotics, inhaled
    - **TOBI** (tobramycin): for *P. aeruginosa*, nebulizer twice daily for 28 days; stop for 28 days then resume use (4)[A]
    - Colistin (more commonly used in Europe)
    - Cayston (aerosolized aztreonam) (4)[A]
  - Antibiotics, IV
    - *S. aureus*: Zosyn or nafcillin
    - Methicillin-resistant *S. aureus* (MRSA): vancomycin or linezolid
    - *P. aeruginosa*: Zosyn or ceftazidime plus aminoglycoside (tobramycin)
    - *Burkholderia cepacia*: ≥3 drugs based on synergy studies
  - Inhalation therapy
    - β-agonist in conjunction with chest physiotherapy
    - Recombinant human DNAse (Dornase alpha) (4)[A]
    - Hypertonic saline (4)[A]
  - Anti-inflammatory agents
    - Oral steroids (useful in setting of ABPA)
    - Ibuprofen (high dose)
  - CFTR modulation therapy
    - Ivacaftor (VX770): A small-molecule CFTR potentiator shown to improve lung function and improve risk of pulmonary exacerbations in patients 6 years and older with at least 1 copy of *G551D* mutation (4)[A].
- GI
  - Pancreatic enzymes (87.3%) (2)[A]
    - Use in pancreatic-insufficient patients.
  - Fat-soluble vitamin supplementation (A, D, E, and K)
  - Liver disease (cholestasis)
    - Ursodeoxycholic acid

ISSUES FOR REFERRAL

All patients should be followed in a CF center (accredited sites are listed at www.cff.org).

ADDITIONAL THERAPIES

- Airway clearance techniques (5)[A]
- Routine chest physiotherapy with postural drainage is critical in prevention of pulmonary exacerbations
  - VEST (airway clearance system)
- Endocrine
  - CFRD: Insulin is the primary therapy, and dietary restrictions should be avoided (6)[A].
  - CF-related bone disease: Consider bisphosphonate therapy.

SURGERY/OTHER PROCEDURES

- Lung transplantation reserved for patients with limited life expectancy (forced expiratory volume in 1 second [FEV_1] <30% predicted)
  - 205 patients with CF underwent lung transplantation during 2012 (2)[A].
  - 5-year posttransplant survival is up to 62%.
- Liver transplantation is reserved for progressive liver failure ± portal hypertension with GI bleeding; 19 patients received liver transplantation in 2012 (2)[A].
- Nasal polypectomy in 4.5% of CF patients (2)[A]

INPATIENT CONSIDERATIONS

Admission Criteria/Initial Stabilization

- Pulmonary exacerbation (most common reason for admission)
  - Increased cough, sputum production, and decreased pulmonary function
  - Change in lung examination (rales, retractions, tachypnea)
  - New abnormalities on CXR
  - Decreased energy level and appetite and weight loss
  - Fever, leukocytosis, elevation of acute-phase reactants
- Bowel obstruction (due to DIOS, previously known as meconium ileus equivalent [MIE])
- Pancreatitis (in pancreatic-sufficient patients)
- Nasal cannula oxygen when the patient is hypoxemic (SaO_2 <90%)

IV Fluids

- Increased salt loss increases risk of hyponatremic hypochloremic dehydration.
- Cautious use of IV fluids with worsening lung disease

Nursing

Nursing assignments should involve only 1 CF patient per nurse for isolation purposes.

ONGOING CARE

FOLLOW-UP RECOMMENDATIONS

- Upon discharge for a pulmonary exacerbation, follow-up with CF provider within 2–4 weeks
- Routine clinic visits every 3 months, with airway cultures and pulmonary function testing
- Annual comprehensive nutritional evaluation
- Annual OGTT after 10 years of age
- Bone densitometry after age 18 years

DIET

High-calorie, high-fat diet with added salt

PATIENT EDUCATION

Cystic Fibrosis Foundation: www.cff.org

PROGNOSIS

- Most recent median survival is 41.1years, as of 2012 CF Foundation Patient Registry (2)[A].
- Progression of lung disease usually determines length of survival.

C

REFERENCES

1. O'Sullivan BP, Freedman SD. Cystic fibrosis. *Lancet*. 2009;373(9678):1891–1904.
2. Cystic Fibrosis Foundation Patient Registry. *Annual Data Report*. Bethesda, MD: Cystic Fibrosis Foundation; 2012.
3. Cystic Fibrosis Foundation; Borowitz D, Robinson KA, Rosenfeld M, et al. Cystic Fibrosis Foundation evidence-based guidelines for management of infants with cystic fibrosis. *J Pediatr*. 2009; 155(6 Suppl): S73–S93.
4. Mogayzel PJ Jr, Naureckas ET, Robinson KA, et al. Cystic fibrosis pulmonary guidelines: chronic medications for maintenance of lung health. *Am J Respir Crit Care Med*. 2013;187(7):680–689.
5. Flume PA, Robinson KA, O'Sullivan BP, et al. Cystic fibrosis pulmonary guidelines: airway clearance therapies. *Respir Care*. 2009;54(4):522–537.
6. Moran A, Brunzell C, Cohen RC, et al. Clinical care guidelines for cystic fibrosis-related diabetes: a position statement of the American Diabetes Association and a clinical practice guideline of the Cystic Fibrosis Foundation, endorsed by the Pediatric Endocrine Society. *Diabetes Care*. 2010;33(12):2697–2708.

ADDITIONAL READING

- Conwell LS, Chang AB. Bisphosphonates for osteoporosis in people with cystic fibrosis. *Cochrane Database Syst Rev*. 2014;(3):CD002010.
- Oomen KP, April MM. Sinonasal manifestations in cystic fibrosis. *Int J Otolaryngol*. 2012;2012:789572.
- Ramsey BW, Davies J, McElvaney NG, et al. A CFTR potentiator in patients with cystic fibrosis and the G551D mutation. *N Engl J Med*. 2011;365(18): 1663–1672.

CODES

ICD10

- E84.9 Cystic fibrosis, unspecified
- E84.11 Meconium ileus in cystic fibrosis
- E84.0 Cystic fibrosis with pulmonary manifestations

CLINICAL PEARLS

- CF must be considered in *any* child with chronic diarrhea, especially if associated with poor growth or failure to thrive.
- All children with nasal polyps, digital clubbing, or bronchiectasis should be evaluated.
- Children with CF may present with generalized edema due to protein/calorie malnutrition.
- A rapid decline in pulmonary function suggests the acquisition of resistant organisms (e.g., *B. cepacia*), CF-related diabetes, allergic bronchopulmonary aspergillosis (ABPA), or GERD.

CYTOMEGALOVIRUS (CMV) INCLUSION DISEASE

Nick Singh, MD • Christina Kelly, MD, FAAFP

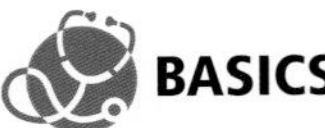

BASICS

Cytomegalovirus (CMV) is ubiquitous and commonly infects people of all ages, ethnic and socioeconomic groups, and geographic areas.

- Although most CMV infections are asymptomatic or cause mild disease, the virus can cause serious disease in neonates and immunocompromised people.
- Because of its ubiquity, it is often difficult to define the role of CMV in a disease process.

DESCRIPTION

- CMV is a DNA virus in the *Herpesvirus* family, also known as HHV-5. It is a member of the β-herpesvirus subfamily, which also includes HHV-6 and HHV-7.
- Primary infection: often asymptomatic; may remain latent for prolonged periods if not immunocompromised
- Wide spectrum of disorders ranging from asymptomatic subclinical infection to a mononucleosis syndrome in healthy patients to disseminated disease in immunocompromised hosts and fulminant disease in neonates
- Severe disease can result from primary infection of the fetus and newborn or reactivation in setting of immunocompromise or organ transplantation.
- Name derives from large intranuclear inclusions ("owl's eye") in infected cells.
- Not highly contagious
  - Spread via close contact with persons shedding virus from saliva, urine, blood, breast milk, feces, semen, or organ transplantation
  - Any organ can be affected.
- Categories of CMV infections:
  - Congenital
  - Perinatal
  - Acute infection in a normal host
  - Latent infection
  - Infection in immunocompromised hosts: solid organ transplant; bone marrow transplant; AIDS patients
- System(s) affected: ophthalmic; pulmonary; GI; neurologic; renal; skin/exocrine, hepatic, cardiac
- Synonym(s): giant cell inclusion disease; CID CMV, HHV-5

Pregnancy Considerations

- CMV infection in pregnancy may cause broad range of illness in the newborn, ranging from asymptomatic infection to severe disease or even death.
- Infection may occur in utero, intrapartum, or postnatally.
- Preexisting maternal CMV seropositivity substantially decreases (but does not eliminate) fetal infection.

Pediatric Considerations

Breastfeeding can transmit virus to high-risk preterm infants. However, there is low risk of symptomatic disease and no evidence of long-term sequelae from transmission via breastfeeding. Currently, there are no recommendations for avoidance or treated breast milk.

EPIDEMIOLOGY

Incidence

- Common, but frequently asymptomatic
- <2–3 cases of end-organ disease per 100 person-years in HIV patients
- CMV infection is more prevalent in populations at higher risk for HIV infection (IV drug users, 75%; homosexual males, 90%).
- CMV reactivation frequently occurs in immunocompromised hosts (organ transplant recipients and HIV patients).
- Predominant age: all ages, peaks at <3 months, 16–40 years, and 40–75 years
- Predominant sex: male > female

Prevalence

- Occurs worldwide; higher prevalence in underdeveloped countries
- 40–100% of the general U.S. population is seropositive from prior exposure during childhood or early adulthood.
- 20% of children in the United States are seropositive before reaching puberty.
- Most common perinatally transmitted infection: 0.2–2.2% of births in the United States

ETIOLOGY AND PATHOPHYSIOLOGY

- Primary infection. Virus infects epithelial cells, macrophages, and T cells causing coalescence (protects from antibody). Intact host cell–mediated immunity required to attack CMV infection.
- Reinfection with different CMV strains
- Reactivation of latent virus in patients who are immunosuppressed

RISK FACTORS

- HIV infection with specific risks, including the following:
  - CD4 count <50 cells/μL
  - Absence of treatment with or failure to respond to ART
  - Previous opportunistic infections
  - HIV viral load >100,000
- Organ transplantation
- Blood transfusion
- Immunocompromise
- Living in closed population, daycare, nursing home, military barracks, correctional facilities
- Corticosteroid therapy
- Maternal infection during pregnancy (neonatal disease)
- Low socioeconomic status
- Critically ill immunocompetent adults in ICU settings (up to 1/3 develop CMV, primarily between days 4 and 12 after admission)
- Inflammatory bowel disease

GENERAL PREVENTION

- Hand washing/personal hygiene
- Avoid immunosuppression; maintain CD4 count >100 cells/mm^3 in HIV patients.
- Highly active antiretroviral therapy (HAART) is the best method of prevention for high-risk HIV patients.
- Primary prophylaxis is not recommended.
- Chronic maintenance therapy for secondary prophylaxis in HIV patients (1,2)[A]
- Options include the following:
  - Parenteral or PO ganciclovir
  - Parenteral foscarnet
  - Combined parenteral ganciclovir and foscarnet
  - Parenteral cidofovir
  - Ganciclovir via intraocular implant or repetitive intravitreous injection of fomivirsen
- CMV antibody+, HIV+ children who are severely immunosuppressed require PO ganciclovir 1,000 mg TID.
- Antiviral suppression of CMV reactivation in CMV+ transplant recipients or recipients of CMV+ organs:
  - Solid organ transplant: prophylactic or preemptive treatment with PO ganciclovir, valganciclovir
  - Bone marrow transplant: IV ganciclovir
- CMV immunoglobulins decrease rate of severe disease after liver transplant and decrease incidence of disease after renal transplant.

COMMONLY ASSOCIATED CONDITIONS

AIDS, corticosteroid therapy, transplantation, or immunosuppression

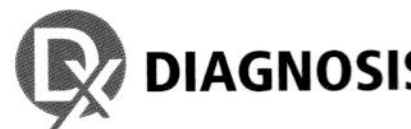

DIAGNOSIS

HISTORY

- Congenital
  - ~1% (0.2–2.5%) of newborns are congenitally infected with CMV.
  - Most infected newborns appear normal and are asymptomatic.
  - As many as 15% develop progressive hearing loss, which is most often unilateral.
  - ~5–15% of congenitally infected newborns are symptomatic at birth (small size for gestational age, hepatosplenomegaly, petechial or purpuric rash, and jaundice).
- Perinatal: exposure to CMV in maternal cervicovaginal secretions, breast milk, or from blood product transfusions; often asymptomatic
- Acute infection in a normal host: Symptomatic infection commonly presents with acute mononucleosis syndrome.
- Latent infection: Higher IgG titers may contribute to development of atherosclerotic disease.
- Infection in bone marrow and solid organ transplant patients:
  - Heart transplant: early myocarditis followed by late atherosclerosis
  - Lung and bone marrow transplant: interstitial pneumonia
  - Liver transplant: hepatitis and colitis
  - Kidney transplant: graft loss
- AIDS: most commonly CMV retinitis; then colitis, followed by esophagitis and neurologic disease
- Infections in other immunocompromised patients: Pulmonary, GI, or renal disease

PHYSICAL EXAM

- Congenital
  - Asymptomatic cytomegaloviremia
  - Symptomatic: small for gestational age, purpura/petechiae, jaundice, hepatosplenomegaly, chorioretinitis, microcephaly, intracranial calcifications, hearing impairment
  - 90% have late complications: sensorineural hearing loss in 14%; 3–5% moderate to severe
  - Mental retardation, chorioretinitis, optic atrophy, seizures, learning disabilities
- Acquired: acute infection in a normal host
  - Usually asymptomatic
  - Mononucleosis syndrome: fever, malaise, sore throat, headache, antibiotic rash
  - Less common: exudative pharyngitis, splenomegaly, cervical adenopathy, rash

- Infections in AIDS patients:
  - Retinitis: usually unilateral, floaters, scotomata, peripheral field defects. Diagnosis is made when characteristic retinal changes are noted by ophthalmologist on funduscopic exam.
  - Colitis: fever, weight loss, anorexia, abdominal pain, diarrhea, malaise; hemorrhage or perforation rare but serious
  - Esophagitis: fever, odynophagia, nausea, abdominal discomfort
  - Pneumonitis: dyspnea with or without exertion, nonproductive cough, hypoxemia
  - Neurologic disease: dementia, lethargy, confusion, fever, focal neurologic signs
- Infections in transplant recipients:
  - Persistent fever (most common)
  - Bone marrow transplant: interstitial pneumonia
  - Liver transplant: hepatitis
  - Kidney transplant: CMV syndrome (fever, leucopenia, atypical lymphocytes, hepatomegaly, myalgia, arthralgia)

DIFFERENTIAL DIAGNOSIS

- Congenital: toxoplasmosis, rubella, syphilis, hepatitis B
- Early infancy: chlamydia, human respiratory syncytial virus
- Acquired in immunocompetent: Epstein-Barr virus (EBV) mononucleosis, viral hepatitis
- Acquired immunocompromised: other viral, bacterial, fungal opportunistic infections

DIAGNOSTIC TESTS & INTERPRETATION

Initial Tests (lab, imaging)

- Congenital (3)[C]
  - Isolation of the virus in urine or saliva collected within the first 3 weeks of life
  - Direct hyperbilirubinemia >3 mg/dL
  - Thrombocytopenia (<75,000/mL)
  - Elevated liver transaminases
- Acute infection in a normal host:
  - Elevated liver transaminases in 92%, rarely to >5× normal
  - Anemia; thrombocytopenia
  - Positive cold agglutinins
  - Lymphocytosis with >10% atypical
  - Negative heterophil antibody test (rules out Epstein-Barr virus mononucleosis)
  - Positive CMV IgM antibodies; may not peak until 4–7 weeks after acute infection
  - CMV IgG should increase 4-fold during acute infection.
- Immunocompromised
  - Viremia: PCR, antigen assays (pp65 lower matrix protein in leukocytes), blood culture; although viremia can be present without CMV disease
  - Serum CMV antibodies not useful; can be falsely negative due to immunosuppression
  - Neurologic disease: CMV detected in CSF or brain tissue clinches diagnosis; enhanced by PCR analysis
  - Recovery of virus from tissue in symptomatic patient (GI or pulmonary tissue) indicates infection, although 1–6 weeks are required for distinctive cytopathic events to occur.
  - Quantitative DNA polymerase chain reaction (PCR) can be used for diagnosis and to monitor therapy.
- Head CT or MRI: periventricular enhancement (CMV neurologic disease in neonate)
- Chest x-ray: interstitial infiltrates (CMV pneumonitis)

Diagnostic Procedures/Other

- Bronchoscopy: CMV inclusion bodies in lung tissue in context of pulmonary infiltrates (pneumonitis)
- GI endoscopy: mucosal ulcerations and colitis, esophagitis on biopsy

Test Interpretation

Giant cells with basophilic inclusion bodies

TREATMENT

MEDICATION

First Line

- Congenital disease: ganciclovir 5 mg/kg IV q12h for 6 weeks
- Pediatric disseminated disease: IV ganciclovir
- CMV mononucleosis/asymptomatic viremia: no treatment
- Retinitis: Effective treatments include the following and should be chosen in consultation with an ID specialist:
  - PO valganciclovir (for peripheral lesions)
  - IV ganciclovir
  - IV ganciclovir followed by PO valganciclovir
  - IV foscarnet
  - IV cidofovir
  - Ganciclovir intraocular implant with PO *or* IV valganciclovir
  - Treat until CD4 >100 for 3–6 months.
- Colitis or esophagitis: Treat 21–42 days or until symptom resolution: IV ganciclovir *or PO* valganciclovir
- IV foscarnet
- Neurologic disease: prompt treatment with IV ganciclovir *and* IV foscarnet. Pneumonitis: IV ganciclovir *or* IV foscarnet
- CMV disease in transplant patients: IV ganciclovir for 2–4 weeks

Second Line

- Adult CMV retinitis: fomivirsen
- Pediatric disseminated disease: foscarnet 60 mg/kg q8h for 14–21 days, combination ganciclovir and foscarnet CMV disease in transplant patients: valganciclovir
- CMV in bone marrow transplant patients
  - Prophylaxis: valacyclovir
  - Preemptive: foscarnet

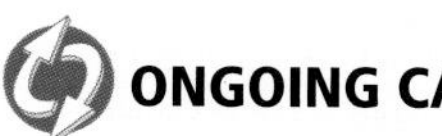

ONGOING CARE

FOLLOW-UP RECOMMENDATIONS

Patient Monitoring

- CMV urine culture at birth for all HIV-infected or exposed with annual testing in CMV seronegative/HIV+ children
- Patients with CD4 counts <50 should have ophthalmologic screening every 3–6 months.
- Patients on therapy should be followed for neutropenia, anemia, and thrombocytopenia.

PROGNOSIS

Severe disease with primary infection in newborns and reactivation in immunocompromised

COMPLICATIONS

- Congenital: hearing loss, mental retardation, optic atrophy, seizures, learning disabilities
- Colitis: hemorrhage and perforation

REFERENCES

1. Guidelines for the prevention and treatment of opportunistic infections in HIV-infected adults and adolescents: recommendations from the CDC, the NIH, and IDSA. http://aidsinfo.nih.gov/contentfiles/lvguidelines/adult_oi.pdf. Accessed December 10, 2014.
2. Mofenson LM, Oleske J, Serchuck L, et al. Treating opportunistic infections among HIV-exposed and infected children: recommendations from CDC, the National Institutes of Health, and the Infectious Diseases Society of America. *MMWR Recomm Rep*. 2004;53(RR-14):1–92.
3. Kotton CN. CMV: prevention, diagnosis and therapy. *Am J Transplant*. 2013;13(Suppl 3):24–40.

ADDITIONAL READING

- Cascio A, Iaria C, Ruggeri P, et al. Cytomegalovirus pneumonia in patients with inflammatory bowel disease: a systematic review. *Int J Infect Dis*. 2012;16(7):e474–e479.
- Grosse SD, Ross DS, Dollard SC. Congenital cytomegalovirus (CMV) infection as a cause of permanent bilateral hearing loss: a quantitative assessment. *J Clin Virol*. 2008;41(2):57–62.
- Kadambari S, Williams EJ, Luck S, et al. Evidence based management guidelines for the detection and treatment of congenital CMV. *Early Hum Dev*. 2011;87(11):723–728.
- Kurath S, Halwachs-Baumann G, Müller W, et al. Transmission of cytomegalovirus via breast milk to the prematurely born infant: a systematic review. *Clin Microbiol Infect*. 2010;16(8):1172–1178.
- Osawa R, Singh N. Cytomegalovirus infection in critically ill patients: a systematic review. *Crit Care*. 2009;13(3):R68.
- Razonable RR, Emery VC; 11th Annual Meeting of the IHMF (International Herpes Management Forum). Management of CMV infection and disease in transplant patients. 27–29 February 2004. *Herpes*. 2004;11(3):77–86.
- Salzberger B, Hartmann P, Hanses F, et al. Incidence and prognosis of CMV disease in HIV-infected patients before and after introduction of combination antiretroviral therapy. *Infection*. 2005;33(5–6):345–349.
- Taylor GH. Cytomegalovirus. *Am Fam Physician*. 2003;67(3):519–524.

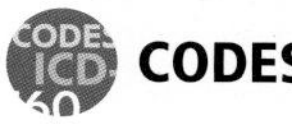

CODES

ICD10

- B25.9 Cytomegaloviral disease, unspecified
- P35.1 Congenital cytomegalovirus infection
- B25.8 Other cytomegaloviral diseases

CLINICAL PEARLS

- CMV mononucleosis syndrome has less cervical adenopathy and/or splenomegaly than EBV mono in adults.
- CMV is a major cause of sensorineural hearing loss in young children.
- Up to 80% of adults worldwide have antibodies to CMV.

DE QUERVAIN TENOSYNOVITIS

Alexandra Sophocles, MD • J. Herbert Stevenson, MD

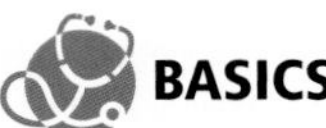

BASICS

DESCRIPTION

- First identified in 1895, de Quervain tenosynovitis is a painful condition due to tendon sheath stenosis in the first dorsal compartment of the radial aspect of the wrist.
- Caused by repetitive motion of the extensor pollicis brevis (EPB) and abductor pollicis longus (APL) over the radial styloid with irritation of the surrounding tendon sheath

EPIDEMIOLOGY

The predominant age range is 30–50 years and women are affected much more often than men (1).

Incidence

- The overall incidence of de Quervain tenosynovitis is 0.9/1,000 person-years (1).
- For patients age >40 years, the incidence is 1.4/1,000 person-years compared with 0.6/1,000 person-years for those younger than 20 years.
- Women have an incidence rate ratio of 2.8/1,000 person-years compared with 0.6/1,000 person-years in men.
- The incidence ratio rate of de Quervain tenosynovitis is 1.3/1,000 person-years in blacks and 0.8 in whites.

ETIOLOGY AND PATHOPHYSIOLOGY

- Repetitive motions of the wrist and/or thumb result in microtrauma and thickening of the tendons (EPB, APL) and surrounding tendon sheath.
- This thickening causes pain with movements of the thumb and wrist, as EPB and APL movement is resisted as they glide over the radial styloid.

RISK FACTORS

- Women age 30–50 years
- Pregnancy (primarily 3rd trimester and postpartum)
- African American race
- Systemic diseases (e.g., rheumatoid arthritis)
- Participation in activities that include repetitive motion or forceful grasping with thumb and wrist deviation such as golf, fly fishing, racquet sports, rowing, or bicycling
- Repetitive movements with the hand/thumb requiring forceful grasping with wrist involving ulnar/radial deviation; seen in dental hygienists, musicians, carpenters, assembly workers, and machine operators

GENERAL PREVENTION

Avoid overuse or repetitive movements of the wrist and/or thumb associated with forceful grasping and ulnar/radial deviation.

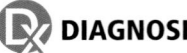

DIAGNOSIS

HISTORY

- Often involves repetitive motion activity or overuse of wrist or thumb.
- Patients may complain of gradual worsening pain along the radial aspect of the thumb and wrist with certain movements, such as ulnar deviation of the wrist.
- Pregnancy
- Sports, leisure, and occupational history
- Rarely, associated with trauma

PHYSICAL EXAM

- Pain is present over the radial styloid, which may be exacerbated when patients move the thumb or make a fist.
- Crepitus with movement of the thumb
- Swelling over the radial styloid and base of the thumb
- Decreased range of motion of the thumb
- Pain over the 1st dorsal compartment on resisted thumb abduction or extension
- Tenderness may extend proximally or distally along the tendons with palpation or stress.

DIFFERENTIAL DIAGNOSIS

- Scaphoid fracture
- Scapholunate ligament tear
- Dorsal wrist ganglion
- Osteoarthritis of the 1st carpometacarpal joint
- Flexor carpi radialis tendonitis
- Infectious tenosynovitis
- Tendonitis of the wrist extensors
- Intersection syndrome
- Trigger thumb

DIAGNOSTIC TESTS & INTERPRETATION

- Finkelstein test: The examiner grasps the affected thumb and deviates the hand sharply in the ulnar direction. A positive test occurs when there is pain along the distal radius.
- Eickhoff test: Patient's grasp a flexed thumb and the examiner deviates the wrist in an ulnar direction.
- Finkelstein test is more sensitive for determining tenosynovitis of the APL and EPB tendons (2)[A].

Initial Tests (lab, imaging)

- This disease is primarily a clinical diagnosis. Radiographs of the wrist may be obtained to rule out other pathology, such as carpometacarpal (CMC) arthritis, if the diagnosis is in question.
- MRI is the test of choice to rule out coexisting soft tissue injury or wrist joint pathology.

Follow-Up Tests & Special Considerations

Ultrasound is helpful to detect anatomic variations in the 1st dorsal extensor compartment of the wrist and for targeting corticosteroid injections which may improve outcomes (3),(4)[C],(5)[B].

Test Interpretation

Inflamed and thickened retinacular sheath of the tendon

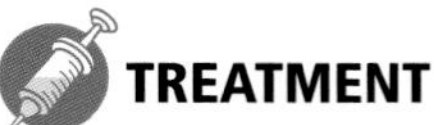

TREATMENT

- Most cases of de Quervain syndrome are self-limited.
- Rest and NSAIDs (2)[A]
- Ice (15–20 minutes 5–6 times a day)
- Immobilization with a thumb spica splint (2)[A]
- Corticosteroid injection (preferably ultrasound guided) (6)[A]
- Surgery (if conservative measures fail >6 months) (7,8)[A]

GENERAL MEASURES

- If full relief is not achieved, a corticosteroid injection of the tendon sheath can improve symptoms.
- Anatomic variation, including 2 tendon sheaths in the 1st compartment or the EPB tendon traveling in a separate compartment may complicate treatment. Ultrasound can distinguish these variants and improve anatomic accuracy of injections (3),(9)[B],(10,11).
- Surgical release may be indicated after 3–6 months of conservative treatment if symptoms persist. Surgery is highly efficacious with low complication rate (7,8)[A].

MEDICATION

First Line

Splinting, rest, and NSAIDs

Second Line

- Corticosteroid injection of the tendon sheath has shown significant cure rates. An 83% success rate after single injection has been reported. Additional injections are sometimes required (6)[A].
- Corticosteroid injection plus immobilization is more effective than immobilization alone (5)[B].
- A 4-point injection technique may be preferred to 1- and 2-point injection techniques in high-resistance training athletes (12)[B].
- Percutaneous tenotomy and/or injection of platelet-rich plasma are newer techniques that are showing promise for treatment of de Quervain tenosynovitis.

ISSUES FOR REFERRAL

Referral to a hand surgeon is indicated if there is no improvement with conservative therapy.

ADDITIONAL THERAPIES

- Hand therapy, along with iontophoresis/phonophoresis, may help improve outcomes in persistent cases.
- Patients may use thumb-stretching exercises as part of their rehabilitation.

SURGERY/OTHER PROCEDURES

- Indicated for patients who have failed conservative treatment.
- Endoscopic release may provide earlier relief, fewer superficial radial nerve complications, and greater scar satisfaction, compared with open release (5)[B].

INPATIENT CONSIDERATIONS

Admission Criteria/Initial Stabilization

Hospitalization for care associated with surgical treatment

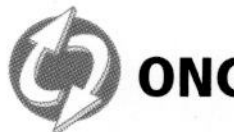

ONGOING CARE

FOLLOW-UP RECOMMENDATIONS

- Additional corticosteroid injection may be performed at 4–6 weeks if symptoms persist.
- Avoid repetitive motions and activities that cause pain.

DIET

As tolerated

PATIENT EDUCATION

Modification of activities eliciting pain, such as repetitive movement of the wrist/thumb and forceful grasping

PROGNOSIS

Prognosis is extremely good with conservative treatment. Complete resolution can take up to 1 year. 95% success rates have been shown with conservative therapy over 1 year. Up to 1/3 of patients will have recurrence (6)[A].

COMPLICATIONS

- Most complications are secondary to treatment. This includes GI, renal, and hepatic injury secondary to NSAID use.
- Nerve damage may occur during surgery (13)[B].
- Hypopigmentation, fat atrophy, bleeding, infection, and tendon rupture have been reported as potential adverse events from corticosteroid injection. Ultrasound guidance reduces the rate of complications (14)[B].
- If not appropriately treated, thumb flexibility may be lost due to fibrosis.

REFERENCES

1. Wolf JM, Sturdivant RX, Owens BD. Incidence of de Quervain's tenosynovitis in a young, active population. *J Hand Surg Am*. 2009;34(1):112–115.
2. Huisstede BM, Coert JH, Friden J, et al. Consensus on a multidisciplinary treatment guideline for de Quervain disease: results from the European HANDGUIDE study. *Phys Ther*. 2014;94(8):1095–1110.
3. Choi SJ, Ahn JH, Lee YJ, et al. De Quervain disease: US identification of anatomic variations in the first extensor compartment with an emphasis on subcompartmentalization. *Radiology*. 2011;260(2):480–486.
4. Di Sante L, Martino M, Manganiello I, et al. Ultrasound-guided corticosteroid injection for the treatment of de Quervain's tenosynovitis. *Am J Phys Med Rehabil*. 2013;92(7):637–638.
5. Kang HJ, Koh IH, Jang JW, et al. Endoscopic versus open release in patients with de Quervain's tenosynovitis: a randomised trial. *Bone Joint J*. 2013;95-B(7):947–951.
6. Ashraf MO, Devadoss VG. Systematic review and meta-analysis on steroid injection therapy for de Quervain's tenosynovitis in adults. *Eur J Orthop Surg Traumatol*. 2014;24(2):149–157.
7. Ilyas AM, Ast M, Schaffer AA, et al. De Quervain tenosynovitis of the wrist. *J Am Acad Orthop Surg*. 2007;15(12):757–764.
8. Ilyas AM. Nonsurgical treatment for de Quervain's tenosynovitis. *J Hand Surg Am*. 2009;34(5):928–929.
9. Kume K, Amano K, Yamada S, et al. In de Quervain's with a separate EPB compartment, ultrasound-guided steroid injection is more effective than a clinical injection technique: a prospective open-label study. *J Hand Surg Eur Vol*. 2012;37(6):523–527.
10. Kwon BC, Choi SJ, Koh SH, et al. Sonographic identification of the intracompartmental septum in de Quervain's disease. *Clin Orthop Relat Res*. 2010;468(8):2129–2134.
11. Rousset P, Vuillemin-Bodaghi V, Laredo JD, et al. Anatomic variations in the first extensor compartment of the wrist: accuracy of US. *Radiology*. 2010;257(2):427–433.
12. Pagonis T, Ditsios K, Toli P, et al. Improved corticosteroid treatment of recalcitrant de Quervain's tenosynovitis with a novel 4-point injection technique. *Am J Sports Med*. 2011;39(2):398–403.
13. Scheller A, Schuh R, Hönle W, et al. Long-term results of surgical release of de Quervain's stenosing tenosynovitis. *Int Orthop*. 2009;33(5):1301–1303.
14. Jeyapalan K, Choudhary S. Ultrasound-guided injection of triamcinolone and bupivacaine in the management of De Quervain's disease. *Skeletal Radiol*. 2008;38(11):1099–1103.

ADDITIONAL READING

Peters-Veluthamaningal C, van der Windt DA, Winters JC, et al. Corticosteroid injection for de Quervain's tenosynovitis. *Cochrane Database Syst Rev*. 2009;(3):CD005616.

SEE ALSO

Algorithm: Pain in Upper Extremity

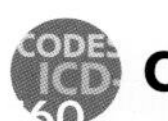

CODES

ICD10

M65.4 Radial styloid tenosynovitis [de Quervain]

CLINICAL PEARLS

- De Quervain tenosynovitis is thickening of the tendon sheath that surrounds the EPB and the APL in the first dorsal compartment of the wrist leading to pain with certain movements of the thumb.
- Repetitive movements of the wrist and thumb and activities that require forceful grasping are the most common causes of de Quervain tenosynovitis.
- Initial treatment includes rest, thumb immobilization, and NSAIDs. Corticosteroid injections are helpful and have lower complication rates if done under ultrasound guidance.

DEEP VEIN THROMBOPHLEBITIS

Denisse V. Tafur, MD • Alfonso Tafur, MD, MS, RPVI

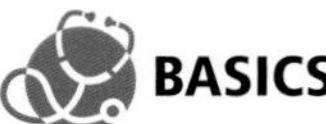

BASICS

DESCRIPTION
- Development of blood clot within the deep veins, usually accompanied by inflammation of the vessel wall
- Major clinical consequences are embolization (usually to the lung) and postphlebitic syndrome.
- System(s) affected: cardiovascular

EPIDEMIOLOGY
- Age and gender adjusted incidence of venous thromboembolism (VTE) is 100× higher in the hospital than in the community.
- Of patients with VTE, 1/3 die within 30 days, 20% will have sudden death due to pulmonary embolism (PE). The 28-day DVT fatality rate is 9%.

Incidence
- In the United States, VTE occurs for the 1st time in 100/100,000/year.
- ~2/3 of the new VTE cases are DVT alone.
- Higher incidence among Caucasians and African Americans relative to Hispanics and Asians
- Complicates ~1/1,000 pregnancies

Prevalence
Variable; depends on medical condition or procedure
- 22–52% of the patients with PE have DVT.
- 25% of patients with superficial venous thrombosis (1)[B]
- Present in 11% of patients with acquired brain injury entering to neurorehabilitation

ETIOLOGY AND PATHOPHYSIOLOGY
Factors involved may include venous stasis, endothelial injury, and abnormalities of coagulation.

Genetics
- Factor V Leiden is found in 5% of the population and in 20% of all VTE events. It is the most common thrombophilia. Homozygosity is found in 1/5,000 persons. It increases the risk of VTE 3–8-fold in heterozygous carriers and 50–80-fold in homozygous.
- Prothrombin 20210A is found in 3% of Caucasians. Increases the risk of thrombosis ~3-fold.

RISK FACTORS
- Acquired: age, previous thrombosis, immobilization, major surgery, orthopedic surgery, malignancy, oral contraceptives, hormonal replacement therapy, antiphospholipid syndrome, polycythemia vera, paroxysmal nocturnal hemoglobinuria, pregnancy/puerperium, diabetes who developed VTE
- Inherited: antithrombin deficiency, protein C deficiency, protein S deficiency, factor V Leiden R506Q, prothrombin G20210A, dysfibrinogenemia
- Mixed/unknown: hyperhomocysteinemia, high levels of factor VIII, high levels of factor IX, high levels of thrombin activatable fibrinolysis inhibitor (TAFI), high levels of factor XI

GENERAL PREVENTION
- Mechanical thromboprophylaxis is recommended in patients with high bleeding risk and as adjunct to anticoagulant-based thromboprophylaxis.
- Compression stockings have conflicting data on postthrombotic syndrome prevention (2)[B].
- For acutely ill and for critically ill hospitalized patients at increased risk of thrombosis, low-molecular-weight heparin [LMWH], low-dose unfractionated heparin [LDUH], or fondaparinux are recommended (3)[C].
- For surgical patients, the use of a prediction score for VTE is strongly recommended. If the risk is moderate or higher, LMWH is preferred.
- Rivaroxaban and apixaban are approved in United States for surgical DVT prevention.
- For most patients, prolonged prophylaxis is not recommended.

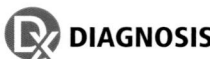

DIAGNOSIS

Modified Wells criteria
- Active cancer +1 point. Calf swelling >3 +1 point. Collateral superficial veins +1 point. Pitting edema +1 point. Previous documented DVT +1 point. Swelling of entire leg +1 point. Localized pain along distribution of deep venous system +1 point. Paralysis, paresis, or recent cast immobilization of lower extremities +1 point. Recently bedridden >3 days or major surgery requiring regional or general anesthetic in past 4 weeks +1 point. Alternative diagnosis at least as likely −2 points
  - Interpretation: Score 0–1 DVT unlikely. Score ≥2: moderate to high probability.

HISTORY
- Establish pretest probability based on Wells criteria.
- Classify as "provoked" or "idiopathic." Determine the presence of risk factors, including family history.
- Clinical assessment of bleeding risk: bleeding with previous history of anticoagulation, history of liver disease, recent interventions, history of GI bleed

PHYSICAL EXAM
- Physical exam is only 30% accurate for DVT.
- Resistance to dorsiflexion of the foot (Homan sign) is unreliable.
- Swelling of collateral veins. Massive edema with cyanosis is a medical emergency (phlegmasia cerulea dolens, rare).
- Thoracic outlet maneuvers in upper extremity DVT
- Attention to signs of possible malignancy

DIFFERENTIAL DIAGNOSIS
Cellulitis, fracture, ruptured synovial cyst (Baker cyst), lymphedema, muscle strain/tear, extrinsic compression of vein (e.g., by tumor/enlarged lymph nodes), compartment syndrome, localized allergic reaction

DIAGNOSTIC TESTS & INTERPRETATION

Initial Tests (lab, imaging)
- D-dimer (sensitive but not specific; has a high negative predictive value [NPV])
- Patients with a prior DVT and those with malignancy have a high rate of VTE, which decreases the NPV of Wells prediction rule (4).
- CBC, platelet count, activated partial thromboplastin time (aPTT), prothrombin time (PT)/INR
- In young patients with idiopathic/recurrent VTE, consider thrombophilia testing.
- Compression ultrasound (CUS): noninvasive; sensitive and specific for popliteal, femoral thrombi but has poor ability to detect calf vein thrombi
- Contrast venography: gold standard, is technically difficult, risk of morbidity
- Impedance plethysmography: as accurate as duplex US, less operator dependent but poor at detecting calf vein thrombi; not widely available
- MR venography: as accurate as contrast venography; may be useful for patients with contraindications to IV contrast
- ^{125}I-fibrinogen scan: detects only active clot formation; very good at detecting ongoing calf thrombi; takes 4 hours for results
- In patients with suspected DVT, the choice of diagnostic test process should be guided by the assessment of the pretest probability.
  - Low pretest probability: D-dimer, proximal CUS
  - Moderate pretest probability: D-dimer, proximal CUS, whole leg US
  - High pretest probability: proximal CUS, whole leg US
  - If negative, no further testing is recommended. If positive
    - Low pretest probability, then CUS
    - Moderate pretest probability, then proximal CUS/whole leg US
    - CUS: if positive, treat DVT; if negative
  - Low pretest probability, no further testing
  - Moderate pretest probability, repeat proximal CUS in 1 week

Follow-Up Tests & Special Considerations
Risk of an underlying malignancy is more likely if recurrent VTE, risk 3.2 (95% CI 2.0–4.8). Unprovoked VTE, 4.6× higher (vs. secondary); upper extremity DVT, not catheter associated; odds ratio (OR) 1.8, abdominal DVT; OR 2.2, (5) bilateral lower extremity DVT, OR 2.1 (5)

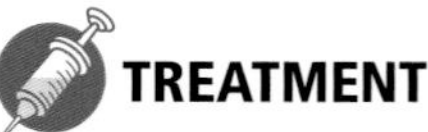

TREATMENT

MEDICATION
All proximal DVTs should receive treatment. Consider starting therapy even before confirmation in patients with high pretest probability.

First Line
- Unfractionated heparin (UFH)
  - IV drip: initial dose of 80 U/kg or 5,000 U followed by continuous infusion of 18 U/kg/hr. Target an aPTT ratio >1.5. The aPTT prolongation should correspond to a 0.3–0.7 anti-Xa level.
  - SC UFH: monitored: 17,500 U or 250 U/kg BID with aPTT adjustment to an equivalent to 0.3–0.7 anti-Xa. Alternatively, fixed dose: 333 U/kg followed by BID dose 250 U/kg.
- Enoxaparin (Lovenox): 1 mg/kg/dose SC q12h or 1.5 mg/kg/dose/day
- Dalteparin (Fragmin): 200 U/kg SC q24h
- Fondaparinux (Arixtra): 5 mg (body weight <50 kg), 7.5 mg (body weight = 50–100 kg), or 10 mg (body weight >100 kg) SC once daily
- Rivaroxaban (Xarelto): 15 mg PO twice daily with food for the first 3 weeks.
- Apixaban (Eliquis): 10 mg PO twice daily for 1 week followed by 2.5–5 mg PO twice daily
- Maintenance therapy
  - Warfarin (Coumadin): 5 mg/day for 3 days, then adjust to a target INR of 2–3; overlap with injectable anticoagulant for minimum of 5 days and 2 consecutive therapeutic INRs

- Rivaroxaban (Xarelto): 20 mg PO once daily with food after the first 3 weeks
- Apixaban (Eliquis): 2.5–5 mg PO twice daily after the first 1 week
- Dabigatran (Pradaxa): 150 mg PO twice daily (CrCl >30 mL/min) after 5–10 days of parenteral anticoagulant

- Adverse effects
  - Heparin or LMWH: bleeding, edema, injection site irritation, skin eruptions, hematoma, thrombocytopenia
  - Fondaparinux: bleeding, injection site irritation, rash, fever, anemia
  - Warfarin: bleeding, skin necrosis, teratogenicity
- Contraindications
  - Heparin or LMWH: bleeding, heparin hypersensitivity, heparin-induced thrombocytopenia (HIT), idiopathic thrombocytopenic purpura (ITP)
  - Fondaparinux: bleeding, thrombocytopenia
  - Warfarin: current bleeding, alcoholism, preeclampsia, pregnancy, surgery

Second Line

Heparin can be given by intermittent SC self-injection.

Pregnancy Considerations

- Warfarin (Coumadin) is a teratogen; treat with full-dose heparin initially, followed by SC heparin starting at 15,000 U q12h.
- Warfarin is safe with breastfeeding.
- LMWH, dalteparin, and fondaparinux are pregnancy Category B.

ADDITIONAL THERAPIES

Edoxaban after initial treatment with heparin is noninferior to warfarin and has less bleeding complications (6)[B].

SURGERY/OTHER PROCEDURES

- In selected patients with proximal DVT (iliofemoral DVT, <2 weeks of symptoms, good functional status, >1 year of life expectancy), consider catheter-directed thrombolysis/open thrombectomy.
- When anticoagulants have failed or are contraindicated, filtering devices are recommended.

INPATIENT CONSIDERATIONS

Admission Criteria/Initial Stabilization

Admission for respiratory distress, proximal VTE, candidate for thrombolysis, active bleeding, renal failure, phlegmasia cerulea dolens, history of HIT

Nursing

Limb elevation

Discharge Criteria

Medically stable and properly anticoagulated; overlap of anticoagulation and warfarin monitoring may be done as an outpatient.

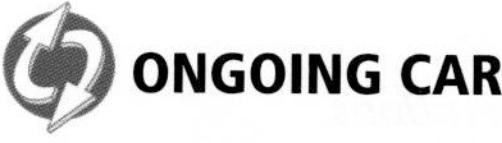

ONGOING CARE

FOLLOW-UP RECOMMENDATIONS

- Gradual resumption of normal activity, with avoidance of prolonged immobility
- Duration of warfarin treatment after DVT
  - 3 months for treatment of a DVT secondary to a reversible risk factor
  - Patients with unprovoked DVT can be considered for prolonged secondary prophylaxis
    - In patients who have completed 3 months of anticoagulation after an unprovoked VTE, a positive D-dimer 1 month after discontinuation of therapy correlates with the risk of VTE recurrence (7)[A].

Patient Monitoring

- Monitor platelet count while on heparin, LMWH, fondaparinux.
- An anti-Xa activity level may help guide LMWH titration of therapy, but it is not usually needed.
- Investigate significant bleeding (e.g., hematuria or GI hemorrhage) because anticoagulant therapy may unmask a preexisting lesion (e.g., cancer, peptic ulcer disease, or arteriovenous malformation).

PATIENT EDUCATION

- Patients should wear compression stockings post-DVT.
- Dietary habits should be discussed when warfarin is initiated to ensure that intake of vitamin K–rich foods is monitored.

PROGNOSIS

- 20% of untreated proximal (e.g., above the calf) DVTs progress to pulmonary emboli, and 10–20% of those are fatal; with anticoagulant therapy, mortality is decreased 5–10-fold.
- DVT confined to the infrapopliteal veins has a small risk of embolization but can propagate into the proximal system.

COMPLICATIONS

PE (fatal in 10–20%), arterial embolism (paradoxical embolization) with arteriovenous (AV) shunting, chronic venous insufficiency, postphlebitic syndrome (pain and swelling in affected limb without new clot formation), treatment-induced hemorrhage, soft tissue ischemia associated with massive clot and high venous pressures; phlegmasia cerulea dolens (rare but a surgical emergency)

REFERENCES

1. Decousus H, Quéré I, Presles E, et al. Superficial venous thrombosis and venous thromboembolism: a large, prospective epidemiologic study. *Ann Intern Med*. 2010;152(4):218–224.
2. Kahn S, Shapiro S, Wells P, et al. Compression stockings to prevent post-thrombotic syndrome: a randomised placebo-controlled trial. *Lancet*. 2013;383(9920):880–888.
3. Holbrook A, Schulman S, Witt DM, et al. Evidence-based management of anticoagulant therapy: antithrombotic therapy and prevention of thrombosis, 9th ed: American College of Chest Physicians evidence-based clinical practice guidelines. *Chest*. 2012;141(2)(Suppl):e152S–e184S.
4. Geersing GJ, Zuithoff NP, Kearon C, et al. Exclusion of deep vein thrombosis using the Wells rule in clinically important subgroups: individual patient data meta-analysis. *BMJ*. 2014;348:g1340.
5. Tafur AJ, Kalsi H, Wysokinski WE, et al. The association of active cancer with venous thromboembolism location: a population-based study. *Mayo Clin Proc*. 2011;86(1):25–30.
6. Büller HR, Décousus H, Grosso MA, et al; Hokusai VTE Investigators. Edoxaban versus warfarin for the treatment of symptomatic venous thromboembolism. *N Engl J Med*. 2013:369(15):1406–1415.
7. Palareti G, Cosmi B, Legnani C, et al. D-dimer testing to determine the duration of anticoagulation therapy. *N Engl J Med*. 2006;355(17):1780–1789.

ADDITIONAL READING

- Agnelli G, Buller H, Cohen A, et al. Oral apixaban for the treatment of acute venous thromboembolism. *N Eng J Med*. 2013;369(9):799–808.
- Bauersachs R, Berkowitz SD, Brenner B, et al; EINSTEIN Investigators. Oral rivaroxaban for symptomatic venous thromboembolism. *N Eng J Med*. 2010;363(26):2499–2510.
- Kyrle PA, Rosendaal FR, Eichinger S. Risk assessment for recurrent venous thrombosis. *Lancet*. 2010;376(9757):2032–2039.
- Lyman GH, Khorana A, Kuderer N, et al. Venous thromboembolism prophylaxis and treatment in patients with cancer: American Society of Clinical Oncology clinical practice guideline update. *J Clin Oncol*. 2013;31(17):2189–2204.
- Prins M, Lensing A, Bauersachs R, et al. Oral rivaroxaban versus standard therapy for the treatment of symptomatic venous thromboembolism: a pooled analysis of the EINSTEIN-DVT and PE randomized studies. *Thromb J*. 2013;11(1):21.

SEE ALSO

Antithrombin Deficiency; Factor V Leiden; Protein C Deficiency; Protein S Deficiency; Prothrombin 20210 (Mutation); Pulmonary Embolism

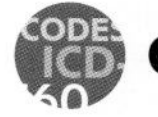

CODES

ICD10

- I80.209 Phlbts and thombophlb of unsp deep vessels of unsp low extrm
- I80.299 Phlebitis and thombophlb of deep vessels of unsp low extrm
- I80.10 Phlebitis and thrombophlebitis of unspecified femoral vein

CLINICAL PEARLS

- Many cases are asymptomatic and are diagnosed after embolization.
- Of the patients with superficial thrombophlebitis, 25% will have DVT at presentation.
- Heparin and warfarin should overlap for a minimum of 5 days to achieve target INR.
- The current American Society of Clinical Oncology guidelines acknowledge the value of primary prophylaxis in selected patients with active cancer receiving outpatient chemotherapy.

D

DEHYDRATION

Jerin Mathew, MD • Mony Fraer, MD, FACP, FASN

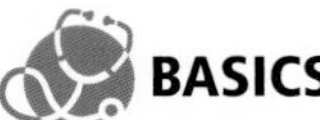

BASICS

DESCRIPTION

- Dehydration is a state of negative fluid balance; strictly defined as free water deficiency
- The 2 types of dehydration
  - Water loss
  - Salt and water loss (combination of dehydration and hypovolemia)

EPIDEMIOLOGY

- Cause of 10% of all pediatric hospitalizations in the United States
- Gastroenteritis, 1 of its leading causes, accounts to 13/1,000 children <5 years of age annually in the United States.

Incidence

- More than a half-million hospital admissions annually in the United States for dehydration
- Of hospitalized older persons, 7.8% have the diagnosis of dehydration (1).
- Worldwide, ~3–5 billion cases of acute gastroenteritis occur each year in children <5 years of age, resulting in nearly 2 million deaths.

ETIOLOGY AND PATHOPHYSIOLOGY

- Negative fluid balance occurs when ongoing fluid losses exceed fluid intake.
- Fluid losses can be insensible (sweat, respiration), obligate (urine, stool), or abnormal (diarrhea, vomiting, osmotic diuresis in diabetic ketoacidosis).
- Negative fluid balance can ultimately lead to severe intravascular volume depletion (hypovolemia) and ultimately end-organ damage from inadequate perfusion.
- The elderly are at increased risk as kidney function, urine concentration, thirst sensation, aldosterone secretion, release of vasopressin, and renin activity are all significantly lowered with age.
- Decreased intake
- Increased output: vomiting, diarrheal illnesses, sweating, frequent urination
- Third spacing of fluids: effusions, ascites, capillary leaks from burns or sepsis

Genetics

Some underlying causes of dehydration have a genetic component (diabetes), whereas others do not (gastroenteritis).

RISK FACTORS

- Children <5 years of age at highest risk
- Elderly
- Decreased cognition
- Lack of access to water such as in critically sick intubated patients

GENERAL PREVENTION

- Patient/parent education on the early signs of dehydration
- Observing universal precautions (including hand hygiene)

Geriatric Considerations

A systematic approach in assessing risk factors is necessary for early prevention and management of dehydration in the elderly, especially those in long-term care facilities.

COMMONLY ASSOCIATED CONDITIONS

- Hypo-/hypernatremia
- Hypokalemia
- Hypovolemic shock
- Renal failure

DIAGNOSIS

Calculate % dehydration = (preillness weight – illness weight) / preillness weight × 100. Supplement this along with the ongoing fluid loss.

- Weight loss: <5%, 10%, or >15%
- Mental status
- Head: sunken anterior fontanelle (for infants)
- Eyes: sunken, ± tear production
- Mucous membranes: tacky, dry, or parched
- Capillary refill: ranges from brisk to >3 seconds

DIFFERENTIAL DIAGNOSIS

- Decreased intake: ineffective breastfeeding, inadequate thirst response, anorexia, malabsorption, metabolic disorder, obtunded state
- Excessive losses: gastroenteritis, diarrhea, febrile illness, diabetic ketoacidosis, hyperglycemia, hyperosmolar hyperglycemic state, diabetes insipidus, intestinal obstruction, sepsis

Clinical Finding (2)	Mild	Moderate	Severe
Dehydration: children	5–10%	10–15%	>15%
Dehydration: adults	3–5%	5–10%	>10%
General condition: infants	Thirsty, alert, restless	Lethargic/drowsy	Limp, cold, cyanotic extremities, may be comatose
General condition: older children	Thirsty, alert, restless	Alert, postural dizziness	Apprehensive, cold, cyanotic extremities, muscle cramps
Quality of radial pulse	Normal	Thready/weak	Feeble or impalpable
Quality of respiration	Normal	Deep	Deep and rapid/tachypnea
BP	Normal	Normal to low	Low (shock)
Skin turgor	Normal skin turgor	Reduced skin turgor, cool skin	Skin tenting, cool, mottled, acrocyanotic skin
Eyes	Normal	Sunken	Very sunken
Tears	Present	Absent	Absent
Mucous membranes	Moist	Dry	Very dry
Urine output	Normal	Reduced	None passed in many hours
Anterior fontanelle	Normal	Sunken	Markedly sunken

HISTORY

- Fever
- Intake (including description and amount)
- Diarrhea (including duration, frequency, consistency, ± mucus/blood)
- Vomiting (including duration, frequency, consistency, ± bilious/nonbilious)
- Urination pattern
- Sick contacts
- Medication history (e.g., diuretics, laxatives)

PHYSICAL EXAM

- The most useful individual signs for identifying dehydration in children are prolonged capillary refill time, abnormal skin turgor, and abnormal respiratory pattern (3).
- Vitals: pulse, BP, temperature
- Orthostatic vital signs: Take BP and heart rate (HR) while supine, sitting, and standing.
  - Systolic BP decrease by 20, diastolic BP decrease by 10, or HR increase by 20 highly suggestive of hypovolemia (4)

DIAGNOSTIC TESTS & INTERPRETATION

Initial Tests (lab, imaging)

- For mild dehydration: generally not necessary
- For moderate to severe dehydration
  - Blood work, including electrolytes, BUN, creatinine, and glucose
  - Urinalysis (specific gravity, hematuria, glucosuria)
- Imaging does not play a role in the diagnosis of dehydration, unless diagnosis of the specific medical condition causing the dehydration requires imaging.
- In adults, there is evidence to support the use of inferior vena cava collapsibility as a surrogate marker for volume status.

Pediatric Considerations

Infants and the elderly may not concentrate urine maximally, so a nonelevated specific gravity should *not* be reassuring.

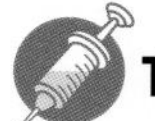

TREATMENT

MEDICATION

First Line

- Oral rehydration is 1st-line treatment in dehydrated children. If this is unsuccessful, use IV rehydration. If IV unobtainable, nasogastric (NG) rehydration can be considered (5).
- Oral rehydration is 1st-line treatment in dehydrated adults as long as they can tolerate fluids. Have a lower threshold for IV rehydration if needed.
- If the patient is experiencing excessive vomiting, consider using an antiemetic.
- Ondansetron (PO/IV) may be effective in decreasing the rate of vomiting, improving the success rate of oral hydration, preventing the need for IV hydration, and preventing the need for hospital admission (6,7).
- Other antiemetics can be used.

Second Line

- Loperamide may reduce the duration of diarrhea compared with placebo in children with mild to moderate dehydration (2 randomized controlled trials [RCTs] yes, 1 RCT no).
- In children ages 3–12 years with mild diarrhea and minimal dehydration, loperamide decreases diarrhea duration and frequency when used with oral rehydration.

Pediatric Considerations

Given a higher risk for serious adverse events, loperamide is not indicated for children <3 years of age with acute diarrhea.

ISSUES FOR REFERRAL

- For severe dehydration, critical care referral and ICU-level care may be warranted.
- Surgical consultation for acute abdominal issues

SURGERY/OTHER PROCEDURES

For specific underlying causes of dehydration, such as intestinal obstruction or appendicitis

INPATIENT CONSIDERATIONS

Admission Criteria/Initial Stabilization

- Intractable vomiting/diarrhea
- Electrolyte abnormalities
- Hemodynamic instability
- Inability to tolerate oral rehydration therapy (ORT)
- Stabilize ABCs.
- If mild dehydration, try ORT.
- If excessive vomiting/severe dehydration with shock, start IV access and IV fluids immediately.

IV Fluids

- Stage I
  - For moderate to severe dehydration in children: isotonic saline or Ringer lactate solution bolus of 10–20 mL/kg; may repeat up to 60 mL/kg; if still hemodynamically unstable, consider colloid replacement (blood, albumin, fresh frozen plasma) and address other causes for shock.
  - For moderate to severe hypovolemia in adults: isotonic saline or Ringer lactate 20 mL/kg/hr until normal state of consciousness returns/vital signs stabilize. Also consider colloid replacement if continued fluids required beyond 3 L.
- Stage II: Replace fluid deficit along with maintenance over 48 hours. Fluid deficit = preillness weight − illness weight.
- An alternative IV treatment option for moderate (10%) dehydration in children
  - Bolus with NS/LR at 20 mL/kg for 1 hour
  - Replete fluid deficit with D5 1/2 NS + 20 mEq KCl/L at 10 mL/kg for 8 hours (hours 2–9)
  - Replete 1.5 × maintenance fluids with D5 1/4 NS + 20 mEq/L of KCl for 16 hours (hours 10–24)
- An alternative to IV fluids is hypodermoclysis, the SC infusion of fluids into the body.
  - Indications: hydration of patients with mild to moderate dehydration who do not tolerate oral intake because of cognitive impairment, severe dysphagia, advanced terminal illness, or intractable vomiting. It is also indicated to prevent dehydration, especially in frail elderly residents living in long-term care settings who reject the oral route for any reason; useful technique for patients with difficult IV access.
  - Contraindications: severe dehydration or shock, patients with coagulopathy or receiving full anticoagulation, patients with severe generalized edema (anasarca) or congestive heart failure, and those with fluid overload (8).

Nursing

Strict intake and outputs: oral and IV intake and output of urine and stool, which may include weighing wet diapers

Discharge Criteria

- Intake > output
- Underlying etiology treated and improving

ONGOING CARE

FOLLOW-UP RECOMMENDATIONS

Activity as tolerated

- If mild to moderate dehydration, the patient may be mobile without restrictions, although watch for orthostasis/falls.
- If moderate to severe dehydration, bed rest.

Patient Monitoring

Ongoing surveillance for recurrence

DIET

- Bland food such as a BRAT diet (bananas, rice, apples, toast)
- If diarrhea, avoid dairy for 48 hours after symptoms resolve. One review of weak RCTs and 3 of 5 subsequent RCTs found that lactose-free feeds reduced the duration of diarrhea in children with mild to severe dehydration, compared with lactose-containing feeds. However, 2 subsequent RCTs found no difference between lactose-free and lactose-containing feeds in duration of diarrhea.
- Small frequent sips of room-temperature liquids
- For children, Pedialyte (liquid or popsicles)
- Continue breastfeeding ad lib.

PATIENT EDUCATION

- Patients should go to the nearest emergency facility or call 911 if they or their child feels faint or dizzy when rising from a sitting or lying position, becomes lethargic and/or confused, or complains of a rapid heart rate.
- Patients should call their physician if they are unable to keep down any fluids, vomiting has been going on >24 hours in an adult or >12 hours in a child, diarrhea has lasted >2 days in an adult/child, or an infant/child is much less active than usual or is very irritable.
- Patient information on dehydration: www.mayoclinic.com/health/dehydration/DS00561
- Additional patient information: http://familydoctor.org/online/famdocen/home/children/parents/common/stomach/196.html

PROGNOSIS

Self-limited if treated early; potentially fatal

COMPLICATIONS

- Seizures
- Renal failure
- Cardiovascular arrest

REFERENCES

1. Thomas DR, Cote TR, Lawhorne L, et al. Understanding clinical dehydration and its treatment. *J Am Med Dir Assoc.* 2008;9(5):292–301.
2. Gorelick MH, Shaw KN, Murphy KO. Validity and reliability of clinical signs in the diagnosis of dehydration in children. *Pediatrics.* 1997;99(5):E6.
3. Steiner MJ, DeWalt DA, Byerley JS. Is this child dehydrated? *JAMA.* 2004;291(44):2746–2754.
4. Lanier JB, Mote MB, Clay EC. Evaluation and management of orthostatic hypotension. *Am Fam Physician.* 2011;84(5):527–536.
5. Rouhani S, Meloney L, Ahn R, et al. Alternative rehydration methods: a systematic review and lessons for resource-limited care. *Pediatrics.* 2011;127(3):e748–e757.
6. Colletti JE, Brown KM, Sharieff GQ, et al. The management of children with gastroenteritis and dehydration in the emergency department. *J Emerg Med.* 2010;38(5):686–698.
7. Carter B, Fedorowicz Z. Antiemetic treatment for acute gastroenteritis in children: an updated Cochrane systematic review with meta-analysis and mixed treatment comparison in a Bayesian framework. *BMJ Open.* 2012;2(4):e000622.
8. Lopez JH, Reyes-Ortiz CA. Subcutaneous hydration by hypodermoclysis. *Rev Clin Gerontol.* 2010;20:105–113.

SEE ALSO

Oral Rehydration

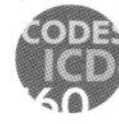

CODES

ICD10

- E86.0 Dehydration
- E87.1 Hypo-osmolality and hyponatremia
- E86.1 Hypovolemia

CLINICAL PEARLS

- Dehydration is the result of a negative fluid balance and is a common cause of hospitalization in both children and the elderly.
- Begin by assessing the level of dehydration and determining the underlying cause.
- Treatment is directed at restoring fluid balance via oral rehydration (1st-line) therapy or IV fluids and treating underlying causes.

DELAYED SLEEP-WAKE PHASE DISORDER (DSWPD)

Adam J. Sorscher, MD

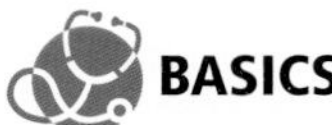

BASICS

DESCRIPTION

- Circadian rhythm sleep disorders (CRSDs) are a family of conditions that occur when an individual's preferred timing of sleep is not synchronized to commitments to job, school, family, or social engagements. In CRSDs, intrinsic sleep is normal (i.e., there is no sleep fragmenting condition such as obstructive sleep apnea or periodic limb movement disorder). However, when forced by obligations to attempt sleep at nonpreferred times, individuals with CRSDs complain of both sleep-initiation insomnia and excessive sleepiness in wake time. These symptoms resolve entirely if the individual is allowed to sleep at his or her preferred time.
- Delayed sleep-wake phase disorder (DSWPD) is marked by a stable but persistent inability to initiate sleep at a desired time. Individuals are typically unable to initiate sleep until 2–6 hours later than societal norms (typically after 2 AM), and this frequently results in insufficient sleep/sleepiness in the day that follows.

EPIDEMIOLOGY

DSWPD is the most common circadian rhythm disorder seen by referral in sleep medicine clinics.

Prevalence

DSWPD has an estimated prevalence of 0.1–0.2% in the general population. It is most common in adolescents, with a prevalence of 7–16%.

ETIOLOGY AND PATHOPHYSIOLOGY

In all mammals, an oscillating signal from the suprachiasmatic nucleus (SCN) in the anterior hypothalamus establishes circadian rhythms, including the propensity to be awake or asleep. The average period of this signal in humans is 24.2 hours. Certain factors, most significantly light, can shift the timing of the circadian rhythm and thereby synchronize it to the shorter environmental cycle day by day. DSWPD and other circadian rhythm disorders occur when the circadian rhythm is not adequately synchronized to the shorter 24-hour environmental cycle, creating a mismatch between them. Some theories to account for inadequate synchronization are that it occurs in individuals who have an abnormally long circadian period (>25 hours) or whose circadian clock does not properly respond to synchronizing agents such as light (1).

- Release of melatonin from the pineal gland in the evening initiates a cascade of events that usually triggers sleep behavior several hours later. Studies suggest that the timing of melatonin release within the circadian cycle is delayed by 40–120 minutes in late adolescence compared with prepuberty. This suggests that the tendency for teenagers to delay sleep onset is largely a genetically programmed developmental phenomenon.
- DSWPD is the result of biologic, behavioral, and psychosocial factors. The relative contributions of genetically predetermined endogenous factors (the shifting of the circadian phase just described) versus voluntary behaviors that delay bedtime are not fully delineated.

Genetics

Emerging evidence indicates a genetic component to DSWPD—a positive family history is reported in approximately 40% of individuals. In one familial case report, DSWPD was shown to occur in an autosomal dominant inheritance pattern. Polymorphisms in circadian rhythm genes such as *hPer3* and *clock* among individuals with DSWPD constitute evidence of a genetic component to the disorder (2).

RISK FACTORS

DSWPD primarily affects adolescents and young adults who have a biologic tendency to delay the onset of sleep yet often need to be up early for school/work responsibilities. Children with autism spectrum disorders frequently have disturbed circadian rhythm cycles.

GENERAL PREVENTION

In DSWPD (and all CRSDs), careful attention to sleep hygiene is necessary to establish and maintain a desired sleep schedule. The most important behavioral practices needed to prevent an undesirably late fall-asleep time are as follows:

- Maintain a regular sleep/wake schedule 7 days/week.
- Avoid napping.
- Minimize caffeine and stimulants.
- Avoid stimulating activities in the late evening, such as computer, TV, and social interactions. A 30-minute "wind-down" time prior to bedtime in which homework, socializing, and electronic devices are off-limits is helpful.
- Adolescents who sleep ad lib on the weekends (sometimes into the afternoon) often find that they have especially great difficulty initiating sleep on Sunday night and, thus, get the week off to a bad start; to prevent this, they should be advised to arise at a similar time on weekends as on the school/work mornings.

DIAGNOSIS

HISTORY

- People with DSWPD report both sleep initiation insomnia and excessive sleepiness in the daytime. They struggle to awaken for school/work in the morning.
- Careful questioning should explore for competing/comorbid causes of insomnia (poor sleep hygiene, significant mental health disorders, restless legs syndrome, medical conditions/medication side effects, and substance abuse disorders) and for competing/comorbid causes of hypersomnolence (symptoms of narcolepsy and obstructive sleep apnea, voluntary insufficient sleep, medical conditions/medication side effects, and substance abuse disorders).
- Individuals with psychophysiologic insomnia (psychologically conditioned arousal when attempting to initiate sleep) do not usually experience genuine hypersomnolence in the daytime despite short sleep times overnight, but instead complain of fatigue.
- People with DSWPD will have no complaint about sleep/wakefulness and their sleep will be of normal duration when they are able to sleep at their preferred time (e.g., they do not have sleep/wakefulness issues when on summer vacation from school).

PHYSICAL EXAM

Explore for features of sleep apnea, a competing cause of hypersomnolence: obesity/large neck circumference; hypertension, crowded oropharynx

DIFFERENTIAL DIAGNOSIS

DSWPD and other CRSDs are unique in that they are marked by the twin complaints of insomnia when attempting to sleep *and* hypersomnolence in the wake period. Other sleep disorders cause either insomnia or hypersomnolence but not both. DSWPD and other CRSDs resolve entirely if the individual is allowed to sleep at his or her preferred time.

DIAGNOSTIC TESTS & INTERPRETATION

- Diagnosis of DSWPD is made primarily by thorough history taking.
- Sleep logs completed over 3 weeks time graphically reveal fall-asleep times that are consistently 3–6 hours later than societal norms and much later wake-up times (not infrequently in the afternoon) on days off from school/work (3)[B].
- Wrist actigraphy (using a wristwatch-like device with an accelerometer), undertaken for 3 weeks, also provides an accurate display of sleep and wake timing but is currently not reimbursable and is not needed if the individual can complete sleep logs (3)[B].
- Testing in the sleep lab is not indicated unless a suspicion exists of comorbid intrinsic disorders of sleep, such as sleep apnea, narcolepsy, or parasomnias (unusual behaviors arising out of sleep) (3)[A].

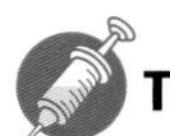

TREATMENT

- The goal of treatment in DSWPD is to help the individual consistently initiate sleep at an earlier time. The principal therapies that advance sleep onset are light and melatonin (factors that shift the circadian rhythm are called zeitgebers). Comparatively, light is much more potent than melatonin in its phase-shifting ability. The phase-shifting effects of light and melatonin depend on the timing at which they are provided as depicted in the phase-response curve (see online version). Key points: Light will advance sleep onset to an earlier time if provided after the body's temperature nadir that occurs ~2/3 through the habitual sleep phase and for several hours thereafter. Proper timing is critical because exposure to light in the evening or *before* the temperature nadir (i.e., in the initial 2/3 of the sleep period) will have the opposite effect—it will further delay sleep onset. For melatonin, the most potent phase-advancing effect occurs if it is provided in the evening, 5–6 hours before an individual's usual sleep onset time.

- Use the following rules to guide prescribing of light in order to advance sleep phase (3)[B]:
  - No single rule exists for intensity, duration, or wavelength for light therapy. Most protocols employ a 2,500–10,000 lux full-spectrum light box, set 2–3 feet from the individual for 30–120 minutes. A common prescription is 10,000 lux box for 30 minutes upon awakening in the morning. Retailers of full-spectrum light boxes abound on the Internet. Sunlight, when present in the morning in warm-weather seasons, is equally effective.
  - Prescribe exposure to full-spectrum light immediately upon awakening. (Note: Although the phase-advancing effect of light is actually greatest if it is provided *immediately* after the body temperature nadir that occurs ~2/3 through the sleep period, the strategy of waiting until the habitual waking time is preferred for these reasons: [i] it acknowledges that it is onerous for the individual to wake up artificially early for light therapy and [ii] it minimizes the risk of unintentionally providing light *before* the temperature nadir, which further delays the sleep phase.)
  - Light exposure in the evening has the effect of delaying sleep phase and worsening DSWPD. Instruct individuals to limit light exposure in the evening (consider using sunglasses or curtailing outdoors activities in warm-weather months).
  - Contraindications to phototherapy include retinopathy, photosensitivity, and bipolar disorder.

MEDICATION

- Prescribe melatonin to be taken 5–6 hours before the habitual (usual) fall-asleep time, *not* at bedtime. Melatonin in minute doses is as effective as higher doses in producing phase-shift; therefore, use the lowest dose available—usually 1 or 3 mg (3)[B].
- Once earlier sleep onset and wake-up occurs, adjust the timing of therapies every 3–5 days—continue to use light directly upon awakening; provide melatonin earlier and earlier in the evening corresponding to 5–6 hours before the newly observed fall-asleep time.

ALERT

Melatonin has a weak sedating effect, and individuals should be counseled not to drive/operate dangerous machines after taking the medication. Other side effects include headache and unusual taste in mouth.

ISSUES FOR REFERRAL

- Referral for evaluation and testing at a sleep clinic is not necessary in most cases of DSWPD. The chief indications for referral are suspicion of the following comorbid disorders:
  - Obstructive sleep apnea: indicated by loud snoring, obesity/large neck, witnessed apneas, and history of hypertension
  - Narcolepsy: indicated by severe levels of daytime sleepiness, despite adequate sleep quantity, and sometimes accompanied by cataplexy (bouts of sudden muscular weakness triggered by strong emotions)
  - Parasomnias: undesirable experiential/behavioral phenomena that arise out of sleep, such as dangerous sleepwalking or dream-enactment behavior
- In addition, many individuals with the complaint of insomnia/sleepiness have comorbid mental health disorders, primarily depression and possibly substance abuse. Referral for mental health disorders/substance abuse treatment is indicated if these are present.

ADDITIONAL THERAPIES

- Chronotherapy is an older strategy in which the individual is instructed to delay sleep and wake times by 2–3 hours every 2–3 days, shifting the sleep cycle across the 24-hour day, until the individual reaches a desired bedtime. Carried out over several weeks, this protocol is extremely disruptive to daytime schedules and also has not been demonstrated to be effective. It is seldom used (4).
- Some early reports suggest that vitamin B_{12} has circadian phase-shifting properties. This finding has not been confirmed in subsequent investigations, and presently, no evidence seen of benefit to the use of this supplement in CRSDs (3)[B].
- Use of sedative-hypnotic medications to treat the insomnia component and stimulant medications to treat daytime sleepiness has not been shown to be effective in the context of DSWPD (3)[C].

ONGOING CARE

Remind patients to practice healthy sleep behaviors (see "General Prevention") if they wish to maintain an earlier sleep/wake pattern.

PATIENT EDUCATION

http://www.aafp.org/afp/1999/0401/p1918.html

REFERENCES

1. Wyatt JK, Stepanski EJ, Kirkby J. Circadian phase in delayed sleep phase syndrome: predictors and temporal stability across multiple assessments. *Sleep*. 2006;29(8):1075–1080.
2. Ebisawa T, Uchiyama M, Kajimura N, et al. Association of structural polymorphisms in the human period3 gene with delayed sleep phase syndrome. *EMBO Rep*. 2001;2(4):342–346.
3. Morgenthaler TI, Lee-Chiong T, Alessi C, et al. Practice parameters for the clinical evaluation and treatment of circadian rhythm sleep disorders. An American Academy of Sleep Medicine report. *Sleep*. 2007;30(11):1445–1459.
4. Sack RL, Auckley D, Auger RR, et al. Circadian rhythm sleep disorders: part II, advanced sleep phase disorder, delayed sleep phase disorder, free-running disorder, and irregular sleep-wake rhythm. An American Academy of Sleep Medicine review. *Sleep*. 2007;30(11):1484–1501.

ADDITIONAL READING

- Barion A, Zee PC. A clinical approach to circadian rhythm sleep disorders. *Sleep Med*. 2007;8(6): 566–577.
- Kanathur N, Harrington J, Lee-Chiong T Jr, et al. Circadian rhythm sleep disorders. *Clin Chest Med*. 2010;31(2):319–325.
- Kripke DF, Rex KM, Ancoli-Israel S, et al. Delayed sleep phase cases and controls. *J Circadian Rhythms*. 2008;6:6.
- Wilson SJ, Nutt DJ, Alford C, et al. British Association for Psychopharmacology consensus statement on evidence-based treatment of insomnia, parasomnias and circadian rhythm disorders. *J Psychopharmacol*. 2010;24(11):1577–1601.

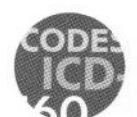

CODES

ICD10

G47.21 Circadian rhythm sleep disorder, delayed sleep phase type

CLINICAL PEARLS

- The tendency to become "night-owlish" with adolescence is, to a large extent, a biologically programmed phenomenon, not strictly a behavioral choice. Enlightened public policy would recognize this and allow for later start times for high schools.
- DSWPD can be diagnosed with careful history-taking and sleep logs; referral for formal sleep studies is usually not indicated.
- Use of light and melatonin can shift habitual sleep onset and offset time by their action on the human circadian rhythm.
- To maintain a desirable sleep phase, individuals with DSWPD usually need to maintain meticulous attention to sleep hygiene, including a regular sleep/wake schedule 7 days/week, to avoid lapsing into a delayed phase pattern.

DELIRIUM

Jonathan M. Flacker, MD, AGSF • Katrina A. Booth, MD

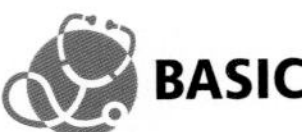

BASICS

DESCRIPTION

- A neurologic complication of illness and/or medication(s), especially common in older patients, manifested by new confusion and impaired attention
- A medical emergency requiring immediate evaluation to decrease morbidity and mortality
- System(s) affected: nervous
- Synonym(s): acute confusional state, altered mental status, organic brain syndrome, acute mental status change

EPIDEMIOLOGY

- Predominant age: older persons
- Predominant sex: male = female

Incidence

- >50% in older ICU patients
- 11–51% in postoperative patients
- 10–40% in hospitalized older patients

Prevalence

- 8–17% in older ER patients
- 14% in older postacute care patients

ETIOLOGY AND PATHOPHYSIOLOGY

- Multifactorial: believed to result from a decline in physiologic reserves with aging, resulting in a vulnerability to new stressors.
- Neuropathophysiology is not clearly defined; cholinergic deficiency, dopamine excess, and neuroinflammation are leading hypotheses.
- Often interaction between predisposing and precipitating risk factors
- With more predisposing factors (i.e., frail patients), fewer precipitating factors needed to cause delirium.
- If few predisposing factors (e.g., very robust patients), more precipitating factors needed to cause delirium.
- Multicomponent approach addressing contributing factors can reduce incidence and complications.

RISK FACTORS

- Predisposing risk factors (1)
  - Advanced age, >70 years
  - Prior cognitive impairment
  - Functional impairment
  - Dehydration; high BUN:creatinine ratio
  - History of alcohol abuse
  - Malnutrition
  - Hearing or vision impairment
- Precipitating risk factors
  - Severe illness in any organ system(s)
  - Presence of a urinary catheter
  - >3 medications
  - Specific medications, especially benzodiazepines, opioids (meperidine), and anticholinergics (diphenhydramine)
  - Pain
  - Any iatrogenic event
  - Surgery
  - Restraints
  - Sleep deprivation

GENERAL PREVENTION

Follow treatment approach.

COMMONLY ASSOCIATED CONDITIONS

Multiple but most common are the following:

- New medicine or medicine changes
- Infections (especially lung and urine but consider meningitis as well)
- Toxic-metabolic (especially low sodium, elevated calcium, renal failure, and hepatic failure)
- Heart attack
- Stroke
- Alcohol or drug withdrawal
- Preexisting cognitive impairment increases risk

DIAGNOSIS

- DSM-5 diagnostic criteria include the following (2):
  - Disturbance in attention and awareness
  - Change in cognition not due to dementia
  - Onset over short (hours to days) period and fluctuates during course of day
  - Evidence from history, exam, or lab that disturbance is caused by physiologic consequence of medical condition, intoxicating substance, medication use, or more than one cause

- The confusion assessment method (CAM) is the most well-validated and tested tool and has been adapted for ICU setting in adults (CAM-ICU) and children (pediatric CAM-ICU [pCAM-ICU]) (3)[B].

ALERT

- Key diagnostic features of the CAM
  - Acute change in mental status that fluctuates
  - Abnormal attention and either disorganized thinking or altered level of consciousness
- Any of the following nondiagnostic symptoms may be present
  - Short- and long-term memory problems
  - Sleep–wake cycle disturbances
  - Hallucinations and/or delusions
  - Emotional lability
  - Tremors and asterixis
- Subtypes based on level of consciousness
  - Hyperactive delirium (15%): Patients are loud, agitated, and disruptive.
  - Hypoactive delirium (20%): quietly confused; sleepy, may sit and not eat, drink, or move
  - Mixed delirium (50%): features of both hyperactive and hypoactive delirium
  - Normal consciousness delirium (15%): still displays disorganized thinking, along with acute onset, inattention, and fluctuation

HISTORY

- Time course of mental status changes
- Recent medication changes
- Symptoms of infection
- New neurologic signs

PHYSICAL EXAM

- Comprehensive cardiorespiratory exam is essential.
- Focal neurologic signs are usually absent.
- Formal Mini-Mental State Exam is not diagnostic but is helpful as a structured interview and followed serially over time.
- GI/GU exam for constipation/urinary retention

DIFFERENTIAL DIAGNOSIS

- Depression (slow onset, disturbance of mood, normal level of consciousness, fluctuates weeks to months)
- Dementia (insidious onset, memory problems, normal level of consciousness, fluctuates days to weeks)
- Psychosis (rarely sudden onset in older adults)

DIAGNOSTIC TESTS & INTERPRETATION

Initial Tests (lab, imaging)

- Guided by history and physical exam
  - CBC
  - Electrolytes, BUN, and creatinine
  - Urinalysis, urine culture
  - Medication levels (digoxin, theophylline, antiepileptics where applicable)
- Chest radiograph for most
- ECG as necessary
- Other if indicated by history and exam

Follow-Up Tests & Special Considerations

- If lab tests listed above do not indicate a precipitator of delirium, consider
  - Arterial blood gases
  - Troponin
  - Toxicology screen
  - Liver panel
  - Thyroid-stimulating hormone
- Noncontrast-enhanced head CT scan if
  - Unclear diagnosis
  - Recent fall
  - Receiving anticoagulants
  - New focal neurologic signs
  - Need to rule out increased intracranial pressure before lumbar puncture

Diagnostic Procedures/Other

- Lumbar puncture (rarely necessary)
  - Perform if clinical suspicion of a CNS bleed or infection is high.
- EEG (rarely necessary)
  - Consider after above evaluation if cause remains unclear or suspicion of seizure activity.

TREATMENT

- The best treatment is prevention (4)[A].

- Principles: maintain safety, identify causes, and manage symptoms.
- Stabilize vital signs if needed.
- Ensure immediate evaluation. Addressing 6 risk factors (i.e., cognitive impairment, sleep deprivation, dehydration, immobility, vision impairment, and hearing impairment) in at-risk hospitalized patients can reduce the incidence of delirium by 33%.

GENERAL MEASURES

- Postoperative patients should be monitored and treated for
  - Myocardial infarction/ischemia
  - Pulmonary complications/pneumonia
  - Pulmonary embolism
  - Urinary or stool retention (attempt catheter removal by postoperative day 2)
- Anesthesia route (general vs. epidural) does not affect the risk of delirium.

- ICU sedation-avoidance of benzodiazepines may reduce risk (5)[B]. Multifactorial treatment: identify

contributing factors and provide preemptive care to avoid iatrogenic problems, with special attention to
- CNS oxygen delivery (attempt to attain the following)
  - $SaO_2 > 90\%$ with goal of $SaO_2 > 95\%$
  - Systolic BP <2/3 of baseline or >90 mm Hg
  - Hematocrit >30%
- Fluid/electrolyte balance
  - Sodium, potassium, and glucose normal (glucose <300 mg/dL in diabetics)
  - Treat fluid overload or dehydration.
- Treat pain
  - Schedule acetaminophen (650 mg QID) if daily pain
  - Opioids alone (morphine) or in combination (oxycodone, hydrocodone) may be used for break-through pain if acetaminophen is ineffective.

ALERT
- Avoid meperidine (Demerol).
- Eliminate unnecessary medications.
  - Investigate new symptoms as potential medication side effects.
- Regulate bowel/bladder function.
  - Bowel movement at least every 48 hours
  - Screen for urinary retention.
- Prevent major hospital-acquired problems.
  - 6-inch-thick foam mattress overlay or a pressure-reducing mattress
  - Avoid urinary catheter.
  - Incentive spirometry, if bed-bound
  - Venous thromboembolism (VTE) prophylaxis if bed-fast
  - Early mobilization
  - Environmental stimulation
    - Glasses and hearing aids
    - Clock and calendar
    - Soft lighting
    - Radio, tapes, and television, if desired
  - Sleep
    - Quiet environment
    - Soft music
    - Therapeutic massage
- Restraints increase risk of falls/injury
  - Use only in the most difficult-to-manage patients, as briefly as possible

MEDICATION
- Nonpharmacologic approaches are preferred for initial treatment, but medication may be needed for behavioral management, especially in the ICU setting (6)[C].
- Medications treat only the symptoms and do not address the underlying cause.
- No medication is FDA approved for delirium.

First Line
- Antipsychotics
  - Haloperidol (Haldol): initially, 0.25–0.5 mg PO/IM/IV; reevaluate and potentially redose hourly. Critical care guidelines do not support use of antipsychotics for prevention of ICU delirium [5].
  - Quetiapine (Seroquel) 12.5–25 mg PO BID
  - Risperidone (Risperdal) 0.25–0.5 mg/day PO
- Benzodiazepines should be avoided except in alcohol withdrawal.
  - Lorazepam (Ativan): initially, 0.25–0.5 mg PO/IM/IV q6–8h; may need to adjust to effect (caution in patients with impaired liver function)
- Contraindications: Avoid typical antipsychotics in patients with parkinsonism or Parkinson disease.
- Precautions: Typical antipsychotics may cause extrapyramidal effects; benzodiazepines may cause delirium. Both increase fall risk. Antipsychotics may prolong the QTc interval.

Second Line
- Olanzapine (Zyprexa) 2.5–5.0 mg/day PO
- Multiple trials demonstrate adverse events with cholinesterase inhibitors in the management of delirium; evidence does not support their use.

ISSUES FOR REFERRAL
Geriatric, psychiatric, or neurologic consultation is helpful if delirium is not easily explainable after full evaluation. Interprofessional team approach is best.

ADDITIONAL THERAPIES
Early mobilization critical
- Out of bed on hospital day 2 (or postoperative day 1) if no contraindications
- Out of bed several hours daily if able
- Daily therapy if not ambulating independently
- Daily therapy if not functionally independent

INPATIENT CONSIDERATIONS
General measures described earlier are also applicable to delirium prevention.

Admission Criteria/Initial Stabilization
New delirium is a medical emergency and requires admission, except in the setting of palliative home care.

IV Fluids
As needed for dehydration

Nursing
- Screen for development of delirium.
- Institute skin care program for patients with established incontinence.
- Turning regimen if at risk of pressure ulcers
- Maintain mobility.
- Maintain day/night orientation.
- Encourage family presence.

Discharge Criteria
- Resolution of precipitating factor(s)
- Safe discharge site if still delirious

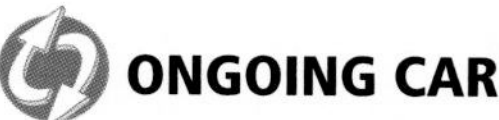

ONGOING CARE

FOLLOW-UP RECOMMENDATIONS
- If delirium at discharge, will usually be followed in postacute facility
- If no delirium at discharge, follow-up with primary care physician in 1–2 weeks.

Patient Monitoring
- Evaluate and assess mental status daily.
- Depends on specific conditions present

DIET
- Liberalize diet to increase oral intake.
- Nutritional supplements (1–3 cans/day) if intake poor
- Consider temporary nasogastric tube if unable to eat and bowels working.

PROGNOSIS
- May take weeks/months to fully resolve
- Usually improves with treatment of underlying condition(s) but may become chronic
- Delirium complicating medical illness significantly increases a person's chance of dying even up to 1 year later.

COMPLICATIONS
- Falls
- Pressure ulcers
- Malnutrition
- Functional decline
- Future cognitive dysfunction
- Death

REFERENCES

1. Inouye SK, Westendorp RG, Saczynski JS. Delirium in elderly people. *Lancet*. 2014;383(9920):911–922.
2. American Psychiatric Association. *Diagnostic and Statistical Manual of Mental Disorders*. 5th ed. Arlington, VA: American Psychiatric Association; 2013.
3. van Eijk MM, van Marum RJ, Klijn IA, et al. Comparison of delirium assessment tools in a mixed intensive care unit. *Crit Care Med*. 2009;37:1881–1885.
4. Reston JT, Schoelles KM. In-facility delirium prevention programs as a patient safety strategy: a systematic review. *Ann Intern Med*. 2013:158 (5, Pt 2):375–380.
5. Kalabalik J, Brunetti L, El-Srougy R. Intensive care unit delirium: a review of the literature. *J Pharm Pract*. 2014;27(2):195–207.
6. Barr J, Fraser GL, Puntillo K, et al. Clinical practice guidelines for the management of pain, agitation, and delirium in adult patients in the intensive care unit. *Crit Care Med*. 2013;41(1):263–306.

ADDITIONAL READING

- Inouye SK, Bogardus ST Jr, Charpentier PA, et al. A multicomponent intervention to prevent delirium in hospitalized older adults. *N Engl J Med*. 1999;340(9):669–676.
- Jones RN, Fong TG, Metzger E, et al. Aging, brain disease, and reserve: implications for delirium. *Am J Geriatr Psychiatry*. 2010;18(2):117–127.
- National Clinical Guideline Centre. Delirium: Diagnosis, Prevention, and Management. London, United Kingdom: National Clinical Guideline Centre; 2010.
- Quinlan N, Marcantonio ER, Inouye SK, et al. Vulnerability: the crossroads of frailty and delirium. *J Am Geriatr Soc*. 2011;59(Suppl 2):S262–S268.

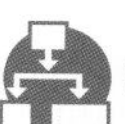

SEE ALSO

- Dementia; Depression; Substance Use Disorders
- Algorithm: Delirium

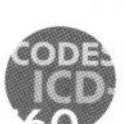

CODES

ICD10
- R41.0 Disorientation, unspecified
- F19.931 Oth psychoactive substance use, unsp w withdrawal delirium
- F10.231 Alcohol dependence with withdrawal delirium

CLINICAL PEARLS
- The CAM criteria for delirium are acute onset of fluctuating mental status, inattention, and either disorganized thinking or altered level of consciousness.
- Hypoactive subtype of delirium can easily be missed.
- Addressing 6 risk factors (i.e., cognitive impairment, sleep deprivation, dehydration, immobility, vision impairment, and hearing impairment) in hospitalized patients can reduce the incidence of delirium by 33%.
- Delirium may not resolve as soon as the treatable contributors resolve; may take weeks or months.
- Avoid diphenhydramine and benzodiazepines in older patients. Nonpharmacologic measures are preferable as a sleep aid; if needed, trazodone (25–50 mg at bedtime) is a reasonable alternative.

DEMENTIA

Umer Farooq, MD, MBBS • Najm Hasan Siddiqui, MD

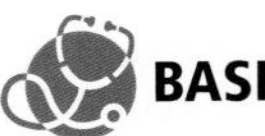

BASICS

DESCRIPTION

- DSM-5 classifies dementias under neurocognitive disorders (major and mild).
- Evidence of cognitive decline from previous level of performance in one of cognitive domains (attention, executive function, learning, and memory). The cognitive deficits interfere significantly with ADLs (for major only) and do not occur exclusively in the context of delirium.
- DSM-5 specifies the cause of neurocognitive decline secondary to the following:
  - Alzheimer dementia (AD)
    - Progressive cognitive decline; most common older than age 65 years
  - Vascular dementia (VaD)
    - Usually correlated with a cerebrovascular event and/or cerebrovascular disease
    - Stepwise deterioration with periods of clinical plateaus
  - Lewy body dementia
    - Fluctuating cognition associated with parkinsonism, hallucinations and delusions, gait difficulties, and falls
  - Frontotemporal dementia
    - Language difficulties, personality changes, and behavioral disturbances
  - Creutzfeldt-Jakob disease (CJD)
    - Very rare; rapid onset
  - HIV dementia
  - Substance/medication use

EPIDEMIOLOGY

Prevalence

- In patients age ≥71 years
  - AD: 70%
  - VaD: 17%
  - Other: 13%
- Estimated 5.4 million Americans had AD in 2010
  - 5 million >65 years of age; 200,000 <65 years
  - Prevalence expected to double by 2030

ETIOLOGY AND PATHOPHYSIOLOGY

- AD: Unknown but involves β-amyloid protein accumulation and/or neurofibrillary tangles (NFTs), synaptic dysfunction, neurodegeneration, and eventual neuronal loss: Age, genetics, systemic disease, behaviors (smoking), and other host factors may influence the response to amyloid-β and/or the pace of progression toward the clinical manifestations of AD.
- VaD: cerebral atherosclerosis/emboli with clinical/subclinical infarcts

Genetics

- AD: Positive family history in 50%, but 90% AD is sporadic: *APOE4* increases risk but full role unclear
- Familial/autosomal dominant AD accounts for <5% AD: amyloid precursor protein (APP), presenilin-1 (PSEN-1), and presenilin-2 (PSEN-2)

RISK FACTORS

- Age; sex: female > male
- Genetic predisposition
- Hypertension: AD; VaD
- Hypercholesterolemia: AD; VaD
- Diabetes: VaD
- Cigarette smoking: VaD
- Endocrine/metabolic abnormalities: hypothyroidism, Cushing syndrome; thiamine and vitamin B_{12} deficiency
- Chronic alcoholism, other drugs
- Lower educational status
- Head injury early in life
- Sedentary lifestyle

GENERAL PREVENTION

- Treat reversible causes of dementia, such as drug induced, alcohol induced, and vitamin deficiencies.
- Treat hypertension, hypercholesterolemia, and diabetes.
- No evidence for statins (or any other specific medication) to prevent onset of dementia (1)[A]
- BP control and low-dose aspirin may prevent or lessen cognitive decline in VaD.

COMMONLY ASSOCIATED CONDITIONS

- Anxiety and depression
- Psychosis (delusions; delusions of persecution are common)
- Delirium
- Behavioral disturbances (agitation, aggression)
- Sleep disturbances

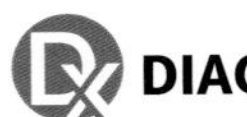

DIAGNOSIS

HISTORY

Probable diagnosis AD: (2)[B]

- Age between 40 and 90 years (usually >65 years)
- Progressive cognitive decline of insidious onset
- No disturbances of consciousness
- Deficits in areas of cognition
- No other explainable cause of symptoms
- Specifically rule out thyroid disease, vitamin deficiency (B_{12}), grief reaction, and depression
- Supportive factors: family history of dementia

PHYSICAL EXAM

- Often normal physical
- No disturbances of consciousness
- Cognitive decline demonstrated by standardized instruments, including the following:
  - Mini-Mental State Exam
  - MOCA (Montreal Cognitive Assessment Test)
  - ADAS-Cog
  - Clock draw test
  - Use caution in relying solely on cognition scores, especially in those with learning difficulty, language barriers, or similar limitations

DIFFERENTIAL DIAGNOSIS

- Major depression
- Medication side effect
- Chronic alcohol use
- Delirium
- Subdural hematoma
- Normal pressure hydrocephalus
- Brain tumor
- Thyroid disease
- Parkinson disease
- Vitamin B_{12} deficiency
- Toxins (aromatic hydrocarbons, solvents, heavy metals, marijuana, opiates, sedative-hypnotics)

DIAGNOSTIC TESTS & INTERPRETATION

Initial Tests (lab, imaging)

- Used to rule out causes
  - CBC, comprehensive metabolic profile
  - Thyroid-stimulating hormone
  - Vitamin B_{12} level
- Select patients
  - HIV, rapid plasma regain (RPR)
  - Erythrocyte sedimentation rate (ESR)
  - Folate
  - Heavy metal and toxicology screen
- Research studies with cerebrospinal fluid (CSF) biomarkers in patient with confirmed AD have shown decreased A beta (1–42) and increased tau and p-tau levels, which are specific features of AD, and CSF tau proteins are increased in CJD (3)[A].
- Neuroimaging (CT/MRI of brain): cerebral atrophy
  - Early age of onset (<65 years), rapid progression, focal neurologic deficits, cerebrovascular disease risk, or atypical symptoms: neuroimaging (MRI/CT) to rule out other causes
  - Important findings
    - AD: diffuse cerebral atrophy starting in association areas, hippocampus, amygdala
    - VaD: old infarcts, including lacunar

Diagnostic Procedures/Other

PET scan not routinely recommended; has been approved to differentiate between Alzheimer disease and frontotemporal dementia

Test Interpretation

AD

- Neurofibrillary tangles: abnormally phosphorylated tau protein
- Senile plaques: amyloid precursor protein derivatives
- Microvascular amyloid

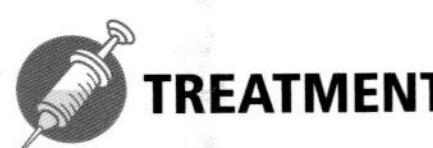

TREATMENT

GENERAL MEASURES

- Daily schedules and written directions
- Emphasis on nutrition, personal hygiene, accident-proofing the home, safety issues, sleep hygiene, and supervision
- Socialization (adult daycare)
- Sensory stimulation (display of clocks and calendars) in the early to middle stages
- Discussion with the family concerning support and advance directives

MEDICATION

Cognitive dysfunction

- Medications for AD (4)[A] show a small, statistically significant improvement in some cognitive measures, but it remains unclear if the improvement is clinically significant.
- Cognitive dysfunction, mild
  - Cholinesterase inhibitors: donepezil (Aricept), 5–10 mg/day; rivastigmine (Exelon), 1.5–6 mg BID, transdermal system 4.6 mg/24 hours and 9.5 mg/24 hours; galantamine (Razadyne), 4–12 mg BID, extended release 8–24 mg/day
    - Adverse events: nausea, vomiting, diarrhea, anorexia, nightmares, bradycardia/syncope

- Galantamine warning: associated with mortality in patients with mild cognitive impairment in clinical trial
- Start drug with lowest acquisition cost; also consider adverse event profile, adherence, medical comorbidity, drug interactions, and dosing profiles.

- Cognitive dysfunction, moderate to severe
  - Cholinesterase inhibitors *OR*
  - Memantine (Namenda), 5–20 mg/day
    - Adverse events: dizziness, confusion, headache, constipation
    - *OR* combination cholinesterase inhibitor and memantine
- Commonly associated conditions
  - Psychosis and agitation/aggressive behavior:
    - Look for precipitating factors (infection, pain, depression, medications).
    - Nonpharmacologic therapies (behavioral interventions, music therapy, etc.) are preferred as first-line treatment.
    - Mood stabilizers (valproic acid, carbamazepine) have been used although evidence is lacking.
    - For moderate/severe symptoms; antipsychotics: Initiate low doses, risperidone 0.25–1 mg/day; olanzapine 1.25–5 mg/day; quetiapine 12.5–50 mg/day; aripiprazole 5 mg/day; ziprasidone 20 mg/day.
    - Atypical antipsychotics associated with a better side effect profile: quetiapine and aripiprazole often first line due to decreased extrapyramidal side effect

ALERT
Black box warning on antipsychotics due to increased mortality in elderly with dementia

- Depression and insomnia
  - Depression:
    - Selective serotonin reuptake inhibitors (SSRIs): Initiate low doses, citalopram (Celexa) 10 mg/day; escitalopram (Lexapro) 5 mg/day; sertraline (Zoloft) 25 mg/day.
    - Adverse events: nausea, vomiting, agitation, parkinsonian effects, sexual dysfunction, hyponatremia
    - Venlafaxine, mirtazapine, and bupropion are also useful.
  - Sleep disturbances:
    - Low-dose antidepressants (e.g., Remeron) have significant sedative properties at 7.5 or 15 mg.
    - Trazodone 25–100 mg is frequently used because of better side effect profile
    - Zolpidem 5–10 mg; zaleplon 5–10 mg
  - Psychosis and agitation/aggressive behavior:
    - Some data for SSRIs
    - Benzodiazepines if agitation with anxiety; in elderly, use PRN

Geriatric Considerations
Initiate pharmacotherapy at low doses and titrate slowly up if necessary.

- Benzodiazepine are potentially inappropriate for older adults, yet their use persists.

ALERT
Benzodiazepine use is associated with increased fall risk (5)[B].

- Watch decreased renal function and hepatic metabolism.

ISSUES FOR REFERRAL
Neuropsychiatric evaluation particularly helpful in early stages or mild cognitive impairment

ADDITIONAL THERAPIES
Behavioral modification

- Socialization, such as adult daycare, to prevent isolation and depression
- Sleep hygiene program as alternative to pharmaceuticals for sleep disturbance
- Scheduled toileting to prevent incontinence

COMPLEMENTARY & ALTERNATIVE MEDICINE
- Vitamin E is no longer recommended due to lack of evidence.
- Ginkgo biloba is not recommended due to lack of evidence.
- NSAIDs, selegiline, and estrogen lack efficacy and safety data.

INPATIENT CONSIDERATIONS
Admission Criteria/Initial Stabilization
- Worsening physical health issues
- Psychiatry admission may be required because of safety concerns (self-harm/harm to others), self-neglect, aggressive behaviors, or other behavioral issues

ONGOING CARE

FOLLOW-UP RECOMMENDATIONS
Patient Monitoring
- Progression of cognitive impairment by use of standardized tool (e.g., MMSE, ADAS-Cog)
- Development of behavioral problems: sleep, depression, psychosis
- Adverse events of pharmacotherapy
- Nutritional status
- Caregiver evaluation of stress
- Evaluate issues that may affect quality of life.

PATIENT EDUCATION
- Safety concerns
- Long-term issues: management of finances, medical decision making, possible placement when appropriate; legal guardianship, if necessary, to avoid capacity and competency issues
- Advance directives
- National Institute on Aging. About Alzheimer's disease: other dementias. http://www.nia.nih.gov/alzheimers/topics/other-dementias

PROGNOSIS
- AD: usually steady progression leading to profound cognitive impairment:
  - Average survival of AD is about 8 years.
- VaD: incrementally worsening dementia, but cognitive improvement is unlikely
- Secondary dementias: Treatment of the underlying condition may lead to improvement. Commonly seen with normal pressure hydrocephalus, hypothyroidism, and brain tumors.

COMPLICATIONS
- Wandering
- Delirium
- Sundowner syndrome: It is frequently common in older people (who are sedated) and also in people who have dementia (adverse reaction to small dose of psychoactive substances).
- Falls with injury
  - Hip fracture
  - Head trauma/hematomas
- Neglect and abuse
- Caregiver burnout

REFERENCES

1. McGuinness B, Craig D, Bullock R, et al. Statins for the prevention of dementia. *Cochrane Database Syst Rev*. 2009;(2):CD003160.
2. Blass DM, Rabins PV. In the clinic. Dementia. *Ann Intern Med*. 2008;148(7):ITC4-1–ITC4-16.
3. van Harten AC, Kester MI, Visser PJ, et al. Tau and p-tau as CSF biomarkers in dementia: a meta-analysis. *Clin Chem Lab Med*. 2011;49(3):353–366.
4. Birks J. Cholinesterase inhibitors for Alzheimer's disease. *Cochrane Database Syst Rev*. 2006;(1):CD005593.
5. Softic A, Beganlic A, Pranjic N, et al. The influence of the use of benzodiazepines in the frequency falls in the elderly. *Med Arch*. 2013;67(4):256–259.

ADDITIONAL READING

- Rabins PV, Blacker D, Rovner BW, et al; APA Work Group on Alzheimer's Disease and Other Dementias. American Psychiatric Association practice guideline for the treatment of patients with Alzheimer's disease and other dementias. Second edition. *Am J Psychiatry*. 2007;164(Suppl 12):5–56.
- Lyketsos CG, Colenda CC, Beck C. Position statement of the American Association for Geriatric Psychiatry regarding principles of care for patients with dementia resulting from Alzheimer disease. *Am J Geriatr Psychiatry*. 2006;14(7):561–572.
- National Collaborating Centre for Mental Health. *Dementia: The NICE-SCIE Guideline on Supporting People with Dementia and Their Carers in Health and Social Care*. London, United Kingdom: British Psychological Society, Royal College of Psychiatrists; 2007. (National clinical practice guideline number 42). http://www.nice.org.uk/nicemedia/live/10998/30320/30320/pdf. Accessed 2014.

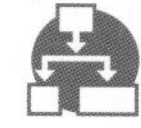

SEE ALSO

Algorithm: Dementia

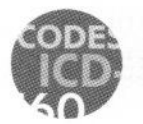

CODES

ICD10
- F03 Unspecified dementia
- G30.9 Alzheimer's disease, unspecified
- F01.50 Vascular dementia without behavioral disturbance

CLINICAL PEARLS

- Medications for AD show a small, statistically significant improvement in some cognitive measures, but it remains unclear if the improvement is clinically significant.
- Do not forget the role of adult protective services in case of elderly abuse.
- A particular concern in nursing homes relates to the use of physical restraints and antipsychotic medication, which are regulated by Omnibus Reconciliation Act of 1987.

DEMENTIA, VASCULAR

Birju B. Patel, MD, FACP, AGSF • N. Wilson Holland, MD, FACP, AGSF

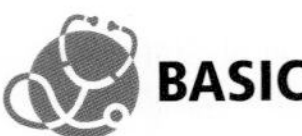

BASICS

Vascular dementia is a heterogeneous disorder caused by the sequel of cerebrovascular disease that manifests in cognitive impairment affecting memory, thinking, language, behavior, and judgment.

DESCRIPTION

- Vascular dementia (previously known as multi-infarct dementia) was first mentioned by Thomas Willis in 1672. Later, it was further described in the late 19th century by Binswanger and Alzheimer as a separate entity from dementia paralytica caused by neurosyphilis. This concept has evolved tremendously since the advent of neuroimaging modalities (1).
- Synonym(s): vascular cognitive impairment (VCI); vascular cognitive disorder (VCD); arteriosclerotic dementia; poststroke dementia; senile dementia due to hardening of the arteries; Binswanger disease. *Diagnostic and Statistical Manual of Mental Disorders* (*DSM-5*) categorizes vascular dementia as mild or major VCD (2).

EPIDEMIOLOGY

Second most common cause of dementia after Alzheimer dementia in the elderly

Incidence

About 6–12 cases/1,000/person age >70 years

Prevalence

- ~1.2–4.2% in those age >65 years
- 14–32% prevalence of dementia after a stroke

ETIOLOGY AND PATHOPHYSIOLOGY

Upon autopsy of those with dementia, many have significant vascular pathology present, but this is not necessarily correlated clinically with vascular dementia. No set pathologic criteria exist for the diagnosis of vascular dementia such as those that exist for Alzheimer dementia. Pathology includes the following:

- Large vessel disease: cognitive impairment that follows a stroke
- Small vessel disease: includes white matter changes (leukoaraiosis), subcortical infarcts, and incomplete infarction. This is usually the most common cause of multi-infarct dementia.
- Subcortical ischemic vascular disease: due to small vessel involvement within cerebral white matter, brain stem, and basal ganglia. Lacunar infarcts and deep white matter changes are typically included in this category.
- Noninfarct ischemic changes and atrophy
- Transient ischemic attack (TIA)/stroke
- Vascular, demographic, genetic factors
- Vascular disease (i.e., hypertension [HTN], peripheral vascular disease [PVD], atrial fibrillation, hyperlipidemia, diabetes) (3)

Genetics

- Cerebral autosomal dominant arteriopathy with subcortical infarcts (CADASIL) is caused by a mutation in the *NOTCH3* gene on chromosome 19 that results in leukoencephalopathy and subcortical infarcts. This is clinically manifested in recurrent strokes and associated cognitive decline.
- Apolipoprotein E gene type: Those with ApoE4 subtypes are at higher risk of developing both vascular and Alzheimer dementia.
- Amyloid precursor protein (APP) gene: leads to a form of vascular dementia called heritable cerebral hemorrhage with amyloidosis (4,5)

RISK FACTORS

- Age
- Previous stroke
- Smoking
- Diabetes
- HTN
- Atrial fibrillation
- PVD
- Hyperlipidemia
- Metabolic syndrome
- Coronary atherosclerotic heart disease (6)

GENERAL PREVENTION

- Optimization and aggressive treatment of vascular risk factors, such as HTN, diabetes, and hyperlipidemia
- HTN is the single most modifiable risk factor and treatment for it must be optimized.
- Lifestyle modification: weight loss, physical activity, smoking cessation
- Medication management for vascular risk reduction: aspirin usage, statin therapy for hyperlipidemia, antihypertensive therapy (7)[B]

COMMONLY ASSOCIATED CONDITIONS

- CADASIL
- Cerebral amyloid angiopathy (CAA): accumulation of amyloid in cerebral vasculature resulting in infarctions and hemorrhages

DIAGNOSIS

Differentiation between Alzheimer dementia and vascular dementia can be difficult, and significant overlap is seen in the clinical presentation of these two dementias. The diagnosis of vascular dementia is a clinical diagnosis.

HISTORY

- Gradual, stepwise progression is typical.
- Ask about onset and progression of cognitive impairment and the specific cognitive domains involved.
- Ask about vascular risk factors and previous attempts to control these risk factors.
- Ask about medication compliance.
- Ask about urinary incontinence and gait disturbances. Abnormal gait and falls are strong predictors of development of vascular dementia, particularly unsteady, frontal, and hemiparetic types of gait.
- Look for early symptoms, including difficulty performing cognitive tasks, memory, mood, and assessment of instrumental activities of daily living (IADLs).
- Past history may include TIAs, cerebrovascular accidents (CVAs), coronary atherosclerotic heart disease, atrial fibrillation, hyperlipidemia, and/or PVD.

PHYSICAL EXAM

- Screen for HTN. Average daily BP and not office BP is associated with progression of cerebrovascular disease and cognitive decline in the elderly.
- Focal neurologic deficits may be present.
- Gait assessment is important, especially looking at gait initiation, gait speed, and balance (8)[C],(9)[B].
- Check for carotid bruits as well as abdominal bruits and assess for presence of PVD.
- Check body mass index and waist circumference.
- Do a thorough cardiac evaluation that includes looking for arrhythmias (i.e., atrial fibrillation).

DIFFERENTIAL DIAGNOSIS

- Alzheimer dementia
- Depression
- Drug intoxication
- CNS tumors
- Hypothyroidism
- Vitamin B_{12} deficiency

DIAGNOSTIC TESTS & INTERPRETATION

- Cognitive testing, such as Mini-Mental Status Exam (MMSE), Saint Louis University Mental Status (SLUMS), and Montreal Cognitive Assessment (MOCA), provides more definitive information in terms of cognitive deficits, especially executive function, which may be lost earlier in vascular dementia.
- Neuropsychological testing may also be beneficial, especially in evaluating multiple cognitive domains and their specific involvements and deficits.

Initial Tests (lab, imaging)

As appropriate, consider: CBC, comprehensive metabolic profile, lipid panel, thyroid function, hemoglobin A1C, and vitamin B_{12}.

- Imaging is used in conjunction with history and physical examination to support a clinical diagnosis of vascular dementia.
- Cognitive deficits observed clinically do not always have to correlate with findings found on neuroimaging studies.
- MRI is best in terms of evaluation of subtle subcortical deficits.
- White matter changes and specific location of these changes can be associated with executive dysfunction and episodic memory impairment (10)[C].

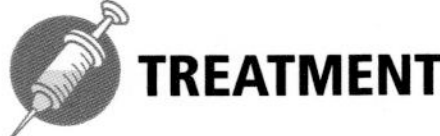

TREATMENT

Prevention is the real key to treatment:

- Control of risk factors, including HTN, hyperlipidemia, and diabetes
- Avoidance of tobacco and smoking cessation
- Healthy, low-cholesterol diet

MEDICATION

- Acetylcholinesterase inhibitors may be used but are of limited benefit in vascular dementia (11)[A].
- Clinical evidence for use of memantine is limited with the clinical benefit likely modest.
- Controlling BP with any antihypertensive medications, treatment of dyslipidemia (e.g., statins), and treatment of diabetes are very important.

- Nicardipine has been studied and has been found to have some neuroprotective effects for vascular dementia (12)[B].
- Selective serotonin receptor inhibitors (SSRIs) may be of benefit for agitation and psychosis in vascular dementia (13)[A].

ADDITIONAL THERAPIES

- Limit alcohol drink intake to ≤1/day in women and 2/day in men.
- Heavy sustained alcohol use contributes to HTN.
- Aspirin and/or clopidogrel may be useful in some cases.

SURGERY/OTHER PROCEDURES

Carotid endarterectomy/stenting should be considered if evidence of significant internal carotid artery stenosis (i.e., >70–80%).

COMPLEMENTARY & ALTERNATIVE MEDICINE

Ginkgo biloba should be avoided due to increased risk of bleeding, especially in CAA.

INPATIENT CONSIDERATIONS

- Remain sensitive to functional assessment and avoidance of pressure ulcers after CVAs.
- Avoid Foley catheter usage unless absolutely necessary due to increased risk of infection.

Nursing

- Nonpharmacologic approaches to behavior management should be attempted prior to medication usage.
- Providing optimal sensory input to patients with cognitive impairment is important during hospitalizations to avoid delirium and confusion. Patients should be given frequent cues to keep them oriented to place and time. They should be informed of any changes in the daily schedule of activities and evaluations. Family and caregivers should be encouraged to be with patients with dementia as much as possible to further help them from becoming confused during hospitalization. Recreational, physical, occupational, and music therapy can be beneficial during hospitalization in avoiding delirium and preventing functional decline.
- Particular emphasis has to be placed on screening for, and optimizing, the mood of the patient. Depression is very common in older patients, especially those who have had strokes and have become hospitalized. Depression in itself can present as "pseudodementia" with worsening confusion during hospitalization and is a treatable condition.

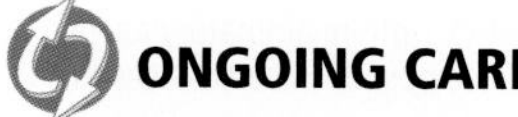

ONGOING CARE

Vascular dementia is a condition that should be followed with multiple visits in the office setting with goals of optimizing cardiovascular risk profiles for patients. Future planning and advanced directives should be addressed early. Family and caregiver evaluation and burden should also be evaluated.

FOLLOW-UP RECOMMENDATIONS

Perform regular follow-up with a primary care provider or geriatrician for risk factor modification and education on importance of regular physical and mental exercises as tolerated.

Patient Monitoring

Appropriate evaluation and diagnosis of this condition, need for future planning, optimizing vascular risk factors, lifestyle modification counseling, therapeutic interventions

DIET

- The American Heart Association diet and dietary approaches to stop hypertension (DASH) diet is recommended for optimal BP and cardiovascular risk factor control.
- Low-fat, decreased concentrated sweets and carbohydrates, especially in those with metabolic syndrome

PATIENT EDUCATION

- Lifestyle modification is important in vascular risk reduction (smoking cessation, exercise counseling, dietary counseling, weight-loss counseling).
- Optimizing vascular risk factors via medications (i.e., HTN, diabetes, atrial fibrillation, PVD, heart disease)
- Avoiding smoking, including secondhand smoke
- Home BP monitoring and glucometer testing of blood sugars if HTN, impaired glucose tolerance, and/or diabetes is present.

PROGNOSIS

- Lost cognitive abilities that persist after initial recovery of deficits from stroke do not usually return. Some individuals can have intermittent periods of self-reported improvement in cognitive function.
- Risk factors for progression of cognitive and functional impairment poststroke include age, prestroke cognitive abilities, depression, polypharmacy, and decreased cerebral perfusion during acute stroke.

COMPLICATIONS

- Physical disability from stroke
- Severe cognitive impairment
- Death

REFERENCES

1. OBrien RJ. Vascular dementia: atherosclerosis, cognition and Alzheimer disease. *Curr Alzheimer Res*. 2011;8(4):341–344.
2. Sachdev P, Kalaria R, O'Brien J, et al. Diagnostic criteria for vascular cognitive disorders: a VASCOG statement. *Alzheimer Dis Assoc Disord*. 2014;28(3):206–218.
3. Arvanitakis Z, Leurgans SE, Barnes LL, et al. Microinfarct pathology, dementia, and cognitive systems. *Stroke*. 2011;42(3)722–727.
4. Russell MB. Genetics of dementia. *Acta Neurol Scand Suppl*. 2010 ;(190):58–61.
5. Kalimo H, Ruchoux MM, Viitanen M, et al. CADASIL: a common form of hereditary arteriopathy causing brain infarcts and dementia. *Brain Pathol*. 2002;12(3):371–384.
6. Gorelick PB, Scuteri A, Black SE, et al. Vascular contributions to cognitive impairment and dementia: a statement for healthcare professionals from the American Heart Association/American Stroke Association. *Stroke*. 2011;42(9):2672–2713.
7. White WB, Wolfson L, Wakefield DB, et al. Average daily blood pressure, not office blood pressure, is associated with progression of cerebrovascular disease and cognitive decline in older people. *Circulation*. 2011;124(21):2312–2319.
8. Montero-Odasso M, Verghese J, Beauchet O, et al. Gait and cognition: a complementary approach to understanding brain function and the risk of falling. *J Am Geriatr Soc*. 2012;60(11):2127–2136.
9. Verghese J, Lipton RB, Hall CB, et al. Abnormality of gait as a predictor of non-Alzheimer's dementia. *N Engl J Med*. 2002;347(22):1761–1768.
10. Smith EE, Salat DH, Jeng J, et al. Correlations between MRI white matter lesion location and executive function and episodic memory. *Neurology*. 2011;76(17):1492–1499.
11. Kavirajan H, Schneider LS. Efficacy and adverse effects of cholinesterase inhibitors and memantine in vascular dementia: a meta-analysis of randomised controlled trials. *Lancet Neurol*. 2007;6(9):782–792.
12. Amenta F, Lanari A, Mignini F, et al. Nicardipine use in cerebrovascular disease: a review of controlled clinical studies. *J Neurol Sci*. 2009;283 (1–2):219–223.
13. Seitz DP, Adunuri N, Gill SS, et al. Antidepressants for agitation and psychosis in dementia. *Cochrane Database Syst Rev*. 2011;(2):CD008191.

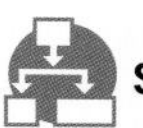

SEE ALSO

Alzheimer Disease; Depression; Mild Cognitive Impairment

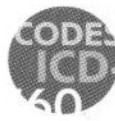

CODES

ICD10

- F01.50 Vascular dementia without behavioral disturbance
- F01.51 Vascular dementia with behavioral disturbance

CLINICAL PEARLS

- Executive dysfunction and gait abnormalities are often seen early and are more pronounced in vascular dementia as opposed to Alzheimer dementia.
- Memory is relatively preserved in vascular dementia when compared with Alzheimer dementia in the early stages of this disease.
- Stepwise progression, as opposed to progressive decline in Alzheimer dementia, is typical.
- Considerable overlap exists between vascular dementia and Alzheimer dementia in clinical practice and classification into one of these categories is often difficult.

DENTAL INFECTION

Hugh J. Silk, MD, MPH • Sheila O. Stille, DMD

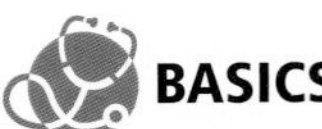

BASICS

DESCRIPTION

- Very painful area ± swelling in the head and neck region arising from the teeth and supporting structures; if left untreated, can lead to serious and potentially life-threatening illnesses
- Assume any head and neck infection or swelling to be odontogenic in origin until proven otherwise.

EPIDEMIOLOGY

Incidence

- Caries (aka tooth decay or cavity) is a contagious bacterial infection that causes demineralization and destruction of the hard tissues of the teeth (enamel, dentin, and cementum).
- Transmitted vertically from caregivers
- Completely preventable disease with good oral hygiene and diet
- The introduction of fluoride has dramatically decreased dental caries.

Prevalence

- >25% of 2–5-year-olds have caries (1)[A].
- Percentage of children 6–19 years with untreated dental caries: 16.2% (2005–2008) (2)[A]
- 92% of adults 20–64 years have had dental caries; 23% have untreated dental caries (2005–2008) (2)[A].
- 25% of children 5–17 years account for 80% of caries in the United States.
- 5% of adults age 20–64 years have no teeth.

ETIOLOGY AND PATHOPHYSIOLOGY

Caries or trauma can lead to pulpal death, which in turn leads to infection of pulp and/or abscess of adjacent tissues via direct or hematogenous bacterial colonization.

- *Streptococcus mutans* vertically transmitted to newly dentate infants from caregivers
- Acidic secretions from *S. mutans* are implicated in early caries.
- Often polymicrobial mix of strict anaerobes and facultative anaerobes in dental abscess
- Anaerobes, including *peptostreptococci*, *Bacteroides*, *Prevotella*, and *Fusobacterium*, have been implicated. *Lactobacilli* not seen in healthy subjects but seen in those with rampant caries (3)[B].

RISK FACTORS

- Low socioeconomic status
- Parent and/or sibling with history of caries or existing untreated dental caries
- Previous caries
- Poor access to dental and health care
- Fear of dentist
- Poor oral hygiene
- Poor nutrition, including high level of sugary foods and drinks
- Trauma to the teeth or jaws
- Inadequate access to and use of fluoride
- Gingival recession (increased risk of root caries)
- Physical and mental disabilities
- Decreased salivary flow (e.g., use of anticholinergic medications, immunologic diseases, radiation therapy to head and neck)

GENERAL PREVENTION

- Prevent caries and contagious bacterial infection (*S. mutans*).
- Majority of dental problems can be avoided through flossing; brushing with fluoride toothpaste, systemic fluoride (fluoridated bottled water; fluoride supplements for high-risk patients in nonfluoridated areas), and fluoride varnish for moderate- to high-risk patients; and regular dental cleanings (4)[B].
- Consider prevention of transmission of *S. mutans* from mother to infant by improving mother's dental care and decreasing mother's bacterial load through proper dental care, chlorhexidine gluconate rinses, and use of xylitol products. Avoid smoking, which is linked to severe periodontal disease (5)[A].
- Good control of systemic diseases (e.g., diabetes)
- Fluoride varnish provided by primary care providers twice per year (4)[B]

COMMONLY ASSOCIATED CONDITIONS

- Rampant caries throughout dentition, faulty restorations, extractions, and multiple missing teeth
- Periapical abscesses associated with necrotic teeth
- Periodontal abscesses
- Soft tissue cellulitis
- Periodontitis (deep inflammation ± infection of gingiva and ligaments)

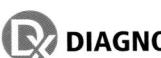

DIAGNOSIS

HISTORY

- Pain at infected site or referred pain to ears, jaw, cheek, neck, or sinuses. Unexplained headaches.
- Sensitivity to hot or cold stimuli
- Unprovoked, intermittent, or constant throb along nerve pathway
- Pain on biting or chewing
- Trismus (inability to open mouth)
- Bleeding or purulent drainage from gingival tissues
- When severe infection (systemic)
  - Fever
  - Difficulty breathing or swallowing
  - Mental status changes
- Children <4 years with stiff neck, sore throat, and dysphagia should be worked up for retropharyngeal abscess secondary to primary molar infection.

PHYSICAL EXAM

- Gingival edema and erythema
- Cheek (extraoral swelling) or intraoral swelling
- Presence of fluctuant mass
- Suppuration of gingival margin or from tooth
- Submandibular or cervical lymphadenopathy on side of complaint
- Severe (systemic) infection may present with dysphagia, fever, and signs of airway compromise.

DIFFERENTIAL DIAGNOSIS

- Bacterial or viral throat infection
- Pericoronitis (inflamed ± infection of gum flap over mandibular last molar, typically 3rd molars)
- Otitis media
- Sinusitis
- Viral (HSV1, herpangina, hand-foot-mouth disease) or aphthous stomatitis
- Temporomandibular joint (TMJ) dysfunction (myofascial pain or internal derangement of TMJ)
- Parotitis
- Cyst
- Jaw pain can be anginal equivalent, especially in women, and especially lower left portion of the jaw.

DIAGNOSTIC TESTS & INTERPRETATION

Initial Tests (lab, imaging)

- No initial labs needed, unless patient looks acutely ill
- If acutely ill
  - Consider CBC with differential.
  - Culture and sensitivity; if abscess present, aspirate pus and culture for aerobes and anaerobes (3)[A].
  - Multiple organisms involved, most likely anaerobic gram-negative rods and anaerobic gram-positive cocci (4)[B]
- Individual dental films of suspected teeth, including root apices; test with palpation, percussion, and cold test to diagnose correct tooth
- Panoramic film of the teeth and jaw for evaluation of the extent of infection

Follow-Up Tests & Special Considerations

- Panoramic radiograph on patients with trismus
- In large facial swellings extending below inferior border of mandible or into infraorbital space (eye closing), CT scan can be used to determine the extent and density of the swelling, locating the abscess within the soft tissue and bone. This aids in determining treatment course and planning need for and location of external drainage by oral and maxillofacial surgeon or ENT.

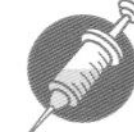

TREATMENT

- Place patient on appropriate antibiotic, if indicated (if systemic). Pain without swelling does not warrant antibiotic use.
- If localized infection, incision and drainage may be warranted.
- Appropriate pain control: Anti-inflammatory agents are 1st line; short-course opioids in some cases (6)[A].
- Refer to dentist as soon as possible for definitive treatment: root canal or extraction or gum therapy (7)[B]
- If infection is severe (systemic symptoms), consider hospitalization with IV antibiotics until stabilized. Patient may need intraoral or extraoral incision and drainage of abscess as well.

GENERAL MEASURES

- Ibuprofen 600–800 mg (peds: 10 mg/kg) q6h *or* acetaminophen 650–1,000 mg (peds: 10–15 mg/kg) q4–6h PRN for pain
- For more severe pain, consider acetaminophen or ibuprofen + short course of opioids.
- Can consider local anesthetic nerve block with long-acting anesthetic (bupivacaine) as adjunct; avoid penetrating infection with needle to avoid tracking infection.

MEDICATION

First Line

- Amoxicillin: 500 mg TID for 7–10 days; in children, 40–60 mg/kg/day divided TID
- If penicillin-allergic, use clindamycin 300 mg PO TID for 7 days (8)[B].

Second Line

If long-standing infection or previously treated infection that does not respond to 1st-line treatment

- Clindamycin: 300 mg PO TID for 7–10 days
- Amoxicillin/clavulanic acid (500 mg/125 mg), 1 tablet PO TID for 7 days (8)[B]
- If severe infection, consider IV antibiotics (ampicillin-sulbactam, cefoxitin, cefotetan)
- Consider double coverage with metronidazole 500 mg PO TID for 7 days for better bone penetration and good anaerobic coverage. Do not use metronidazole alone. Will increase development of resistant strains; can be used with amoxicillin or clindamycin (8)[B]

ISSUES FOR REFERRAL

A dentist should be consulted and follow-up definitive care appointment should be secured prior to discharge from medical office, emergency room, or hospital unit.

SURGERY/OTHER PROCEDURES

- Incision and drainage of abscess should be performed if abscess is large and fluctuant.
- Root canal or extraction should be performed as definitive treatment.

INPATIENT CONSIDERATIONS

Admission Criteria/Initial Stabilization

Criteria for hospital admission include swelling involving deep spaces of the neck, floor of the mouth, or infraorbital region; unstable vital signs; fever; chills; confusion or delirium; or evidence of invasive infection or cellulitis.

- Secure airway, if compromised, with either endotracheal intubation or tracheotomy.
- IV fluid resuscitation with normal saline may be indicated in acutely ill patients.

Nursing

- Ensure good oral hygiene.
- Rinse or swab mouth with chlorhexidine gluconate BID.
- Use warm saltwater rinses several times per day to encourage drainage, especially after incision and drainage. In conjunction, use ice packs on outside of face to decrease swelling and help encourage drainage into mouth.

DISCHARGE CRITERIA

Discharge patient if

- Airway not compromised
- Abscess and sepsis eliminated
- Able to take PO intake and ambulate

ONGOING CARE

Educate patient in need for proper oral hygiene, need for follow-up dental care, and need for routine dental care and stress medical complications that can and have occurred due to lack of dental care.

FOLLOW-UP RECOMMENDATIONS

- Follow-up with dentist within 24 hours.
- Ensure adequate PO intake, including protein.

DIET

- Maintain a healthful diet; bacteria thrive on refined sugar and starch.
- Avoid sugary foods that stick between the teeth.
- Avoid continuous sugary/carbonated drinks throughout day; encourage water as beverage of choice between meals.

Pediatric Considerations

In children, limit the frequency of sugary drinks and advise against sleeping with a bottle to decrease the chance of dental caries.

PATIENT EDUCATION

- Manage dental disease, comprehensively—caries and periodontal disease need to be controlled.
- Minimally, biannual dental visits after disease control
- Nutritional education
  - Limit the frequency of sugar/carbonated drinks and sugary or sticky foods.
- In young children, avoid sleeping with a bottle to decrease the chance of dental caries.
- Brush twice daily and floss daily.
- Caretakers should tend to their personal oral hygiene ± chlorhexidine gluconate rinses in 1st 3 years of the child's life to decrease the risk of transmission of the caries-causing microorganisms.

PROGNOSIS

Prognosis is excellent with proper treatment.

COMPLICATIONS

- Ludwig angina
- Retropharyngeal and mediastinal infection
- Osteomyelitis
- Endocarditis
- Submental infection
- Submandibular infection
- Can cause unstable diabetes in diabetics/worsen preexisting heart disease
- Brain abscess/death

REFERENCES

1. Centers for Disease Control and Prevention. Chronic disease prevention and health promotion. Oral health: preventing cavities, gum disease, tooth loss, and oral cancers at a glance 2011. http://www.cdc.gov/chronicdisease/resources/publications/aag/doh.htm. Accessed 2014.
2. National Center for Health Statistics. Health, United States, 2011: with special feature on socioeconomic status and health. Table 76. Hyattsville, MD: National Center for Health Statistics; 2012. http://www.cdc.gov/nchs/data/hus/hus11.pdf/. Accessed 2014.
3. Robertson D, Smith AJ. The microbiology of the acute dental abscess. *J Med Microbiol*. 2009; 58(Pt 2):155–162.
4. Marinho VC, Higgins JP, Logan S, et al. Topical fluoride (toothpastes, mouth rinses, gels or varnishes) for preventing dental caries in children and adolescents. *Cochrane Database Syst Rev*. 2007;(4):CD002782.
5. Mickenautsch S, Yengopal V. Anticariogenic effect of xylitol versus fluoride—a quantitative systematic review of clinical trials. *Int Dent J*. 2012;62(1):6–20.
6. Ong CK, Seymour RA. An evidence-based update of the use of analgesics in dentistry. *Periodontol*. 2008;46(1):143–164.
7. Douglass AB, Douglass JM. Common dental emergencies. *Am Fam Physician*. 2003;67:511–516.
8. Flynn TR. What are the antibiotics of choice for odontogenic infections, and how long should the treatment course last? *Oral Maxillofac Surg Clin North Am*. 2011; 23(4):519–536.

ADDITIONAL READING

- Clark MB, Douglass AB, Maier R, et al. *Smiles for Life: A National Oral Health Curriculum*. 3rd ed. Leawood, Kansas: Society of Teaachers of Family Medicine; 2010. http://www.smilesforlifeoralhealth.com/buildcontent.aspx?tut=555&pagekey=62948&cbreceipt=0. Accessed 2014.
- Lockhart PB, ed. *Oral Medicine and Medically Complex Patients*. 6th ed. New York, NY: Elsevier; 2013.
- U.S. Preventive Services Task Force. Dental caries in children from birth through age 5 years: screening. AHRQ Publication No. 12-05170-EF-2. http://www.uspreventiveservicestaskforce.org/Page/Document/RecommendationStatementFinal/dental-caries-in-children-from-birth-through-age-5-years-screening. Accessed 2014.

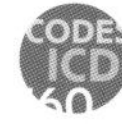

CODES

ICD10

- K02.9 Dental caries, unspecified
- K04.7 Periapical abscess without sinus
- K12.2 Cellulitis and abscess of mouth

CLINICAL PEARLS

- Do not ignore toothache pain.
- Treat patients with facial swelling aggressively, as infections can spread quickly, leading to significant morbidity or death.
- Promote prevention (oral hygiene, fluoride, dental visits) to avoid infections.

DEPRESSION

Rachel Bramson, MD • Michael L. Brown, MD • Suzanne Shurtz, MLIS, AHIP

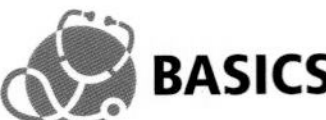

BASICS

DESCRIPTION
- A primary mood disorder characterized by a sustained depressed mood and/or decreased interest in things that used to give pleasure (anhedonia), which represents a change from previous functioning.
- Variants: (1) major depressive disorder (MDD), (2) dysthymic disorder, and (3) depressive disorder not otherwise specified (NOS). (Last two disorders have slightly different diagnostic criteria but are still treated as below.)

EPIDEMIOLOGY
Incidence
In United States, 6.9% 18 years of age or older in past year

Prevalence
- 16.2% lifetime risk of having major depressive disorder
- Patients can relapse; risk decreases with longer remission period but increases in patients with severe episodes, episodes at a younger age, and multiple episodes.
- Predominant age
  - Low risk before early teens but highest prevalence in teens and young adults
- Predominant gender
  - Females > males (2:1)

ETIOLOGY AND PATHOPHYSIOLOGY
Complex etiology with 2 major models in the literature
- *Monoamine-deficiency hypothesis*: symptoms related to decreased levels of norepinephrine (dullness and lethargy) and serotonin (irritability, hostility, and suicidal ideation) in multiple regions of the brain; other neurotransmitters involved include dopamine, acetylcholine, γ-aminobutyric acid (GABA), glutamate.
- *Stress/hypothalamic-pituitary-adrenal axis*: Abnormalities in cortisol response lead to depression; elevated cortisol levels can be associated with depression, but cortisol tests are not indicated for diagnosis.
- Other areas of research interest: inflammatory processes and abnormal circadian rhythms; impaired synthesis/metabolism of neurotransmitters
- Environmental factors and learned behavior may affect neurotransmitters and/or have an independent influence on depression.

Genetics
Multiple gene loci place a person at increased risk when faced with environmental stressor; twin studies suggest 37% concordance (1).

RISK FACTORS
- Female > male (2:1)
- Severity of 1st episode
- Persistent sleep disturbances
- Presence of chronic disease(s), recent myocardial infarction (MI), cardiovascular accident (CVA)
- Strong family history (depression, bipolar, suicide, substance abuse), spouse with depression
- Substance abuse and dependence, domestic abuse/violence
- Losses, stressors, unemployment
- Single, divorced, or unhappily married

COMMONLY ASSOCIATED CONDITIONS
- Bipolar disorder, cyclothymic disorder, grief reaction, anxiety disorders, somatoform disorders, schizophrenia/schizoaffective disorders
- Medical comorbidity
- Substance abuse

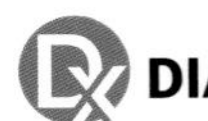

DIAGNOSIS

HISTORY
DSM-5 requires all of the following criteria for MDD:
- Criterion A: ≥5 of the following symptoms present nearly every day during the same 2-week period, with at least 1 of the 5 being either depressed mood or loss of interest or pleasure:
  - Depressed mood most of the day by subjective report or observation from other people
  - Diminished interest or pleasure in all activities most of the day by subjective report or observation from other people
  - Decreased or increased appetite or significant weight loss without dieting
  - Insomnia or hypersomnia
  - Fatigue or energy loss
  - Restlessness, irritability, or withdrawal observable by others
  - Worthlessness, excessive/inappropriate guilty feelings
  - Diminished thinking/concentration, poor memory, indecisiveness
  - Recurrent thoughts of death, suicidal ideations, and may or may not have a specific plan
- Criterion B: symptoms cause significant social, occupational, or functional distress or impairment
- Criterion C: symptoms not attributable to substance effects or other medical conditions

Geriatric Considerations
- Difficult to diagnose due to medical comorbidity
- Can present with memory difficulties as chief complaint; treatment reverses memory difficulty
- Can be the initial presentation of irreversible dementia
- Geriatric Depression Scale (GDS 15) improves rate of diagnosis in primary care setting (2,3)[A].

Pediatric Considerations
- Can present as irritable or angry rather than sad or dejected
- Failure to make expected weight gains can substitute weight loss symptom above.
- A sudden and remarkable drop in grades can indicate difficulty concentrating.
- Can present with separation anxiety

PHYSICAL EXAM
Complete physical with focus on endocrine, cardiac, neurologic, and psychiatric (affect, attention, cognition, memory); look for evidence of contributing medical or neurologic disorder

DIFFERENTIAL DIAGNOSIS
- Psychiatric: depressed phase of bipolar disorder—inquire if prior mania, family or personal history of bipolar disorder, prior agitation or excitement with antidepressant medication. If positive, monitor carefully for mood elevation or destabilization, adjustment disorder, and bereavement.
- Neurologic or degenerative CNS diseases, dementias
- Medical comorbidity: adrenal disease, thyroid disorders, diabetes, metabolic abnormalities (hypercalcemia), liver/renal failure, malignancy, chronic fatigue syndrome, fibromyalgia, lupus
- Nutritional: pernicious anemia, pellagra
- Medications/substances: abuse, side effects, overdose, intoxication, dependence, withdrawal

DIAGNOSTIC TESTS & INTERPRETATION
- A clinical diagnosis made by eliciting personal, family, social, and psychosocial factors
- The Patient Health Questionnaire (PHQ-9) is a brief screening test valid for diagnosis of major depressive disorder in primary care settings (3)[A].
- Other validated standard rating scales include the following: Beck Depression Inventory, Zung, GDS 15, and so forth. Rating scales are also useful to track response to treatment over time (3)[A].
- Rule out hypothyroidism, anemia, and metabolic disorders with TSH, CBC, and comprehensive metabolic panel (CMP).
- Order urine drug screen if symptoms suggest intoxication.

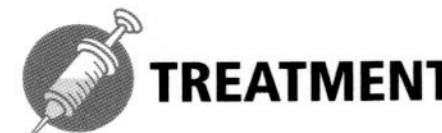

TREATMENT

American Psychiatric Association (APA) 2010 guidelines recommend phasic approach: acute phase (first 3 months), continuation phase (4–9 months), and maintenance (9 months until discontinuation) (4)[A].
- Acute phase
  - Full evaluation, including risk to self and others, with selection of appropriate treatment setting (hospitalization for those at risk of harm to self or others, or so incapacitated as to be unable to take care of themselves and/or who have no support system to assist with treatment)
  - Goal should be symptom remission, with intervention based on clinical picture, including patient's preference, availability of services
  - For mild to moderate depression, psychotherapies (individual, interpersonal or cognitive-behavioral therapy [CBT]) and/or medication are recommended.
  - For refractory/severe depression, medication is indicated.
  - For patients not responding to medication alone, CBT should be initiated.
  - Continue to increase dosage q3–4wk until symptoms in remission. Full medication effect is complete in 4–6 weeks. Augmentation with 2nd medication may be necessary.
  - See within 2–4 weeks of starting medication and q2wk until improvement, then monthly to monitor medication changes.
  - ≥6 visits recommended for monitoring (younger patients, those at high suicide risk, see within 1st week, and follow frequently).
- Continuation/maintenance phase
  - Regular visits to monitor for signs of relapse, q3–6mo if stable; depression rating scales should be used.
  - Once remission achieved, dosage should be continued for at least 6–9 months to reduce relapse; CBT is also effective in reducing relapse (visits typically q2wk).

– If/when drug discontinuation is considered, medications should be tapered gradually (weeks to months).
- Primary care considerations
  – Refer immediately for active suicidal ideations, psychosis, severe agitation, severe self-neglect, and significant risk of self-harm.
  – Caution with personal or family history of bipolar disorder: antidepressants can precipitate mania.
  – Refer to psychiatry for failed response to medication trials, suspected bipolar disorder, more persistent suicidal thoughts, and self-neglect.

MEDICATION

- Effectiveness of medications is comparable between/within classes; selection should be based on provider familiarity and patient characteristics/preferences (5)[A].
- Selective serotonin reuptake inhibitors (SSRIs) and tricyclic antidepressants (TCAs) are effective, but TCAs are 2nd-line due to side effects and lethality in overdose. Tolerability is much poorer than newer antidepressants.
- First-line SSRIs (starting dose; usual dose)
  – Fluoxetine (Prozac): 20 mg/day; 20–60 mg/day
  – Sertraline (Zoloft): 50 mg/day; 50–200 mg/day
  – Paroxetine (Paxil): 10 mg/day; 20–50 mg/day
  – Paroxetine CR (Paxil CR): 12.5 mg/day; 25–62.5 mg/day
  – Citalopram (Celexa): 20 mg/day; 20–40 mg/day (higher doses not advised; EKG monitoring for doses >40 mg/day due to increased risk of QTc prolongation)
  – Escitalopram (Lexapro): 10 mg/day; 10–20 mg/day
  – Precautions: abrupt discontinuation may result in withdrawal symptoms (i.e., dizziness, nausea, headache, paresthesia)
  – Fluoxetine, paroxetine may raise serum levels of other drugs; escitalopram, sertraline have minimal to no drug interactions.
  – Common side effects: sexual dysfunction (20%), nausea, GI upset, dizziness, insomnia; headache: typically resolve in the 1st week
  – Less common side effects: drowsiness, weight gain, emotional blunting, dry mouth
  – Lower starting doses for elderly, adolescents, those with comorbid conditions, panic disorder, significant anxiety or hepatic conditions
- Others (starting dose; usual dose)
  – Venlafaxine (Effexor, Effexor XR): 37.5 mg/day; 75–225 mg/day
  – Bupropion XL (Wellbutrin XL): 150 mg/day; 150–300 mg/day (precautions: powers seizure threshold at doses >450 mg/day)
  – Duloxetine (Cymbalta): 30 mg/day; 30–60 mg/day
  – Desvenlafaxine (Pristiq): 50 mg/day
  – Vilazodone: start 10 mg/day; usual target 40 mg/day
  – Vortioxetine: start 5 mg/day; target dose 20 mg/day
  – Levomilnacipran: start 20 mg/day; target dose 40–120 mg/day

Second Line

- TCAs (starting dose; usual dose)
  – Amitriptyline (Elavil): 25–50 mg/day; 100–300 mg/day
  – Nortriptyline (Pamelor): 25 mg/day; 50–150 mg/day
  – Doxepin (Prudoxin, Zonalon): 25–50 mg/day; 100–300 mg/day
  – Imipramine (Tofranil, Tofranil-PM): 25–50 mg/day; 100–300 mg/day
  – Desipramine (Norpramin): 25–50 mg/day; 100–300 mg/day
  – Precautions: advanced age, glaucoma, benign prostate hyperplasia, hyperthyroidism, cardiovascular disease, liver disease, monamine oxidase inhibitor (MAOI) treatment, potential for fatal overdose, arrhythmia, worsening glycemic control, SSRIs recommended for patients with diabetes (4)[A]
  – Common side effects: dry mouth, blurred vision, constipation, urinary retention, tachycardia, confusion/delirium, elderly particularly susceptible
- α_2-Antagonists (sedating) (starting dose; usual dose)
  – Mirtazapine (Remeron): 15 mg/day; 15–45 mg/day
- Atypical antipsychotics
  – Adjunctive treatment: aripiprazole or quetiapine
  – Treatment-resistant depression (TRD): olanzapine
  – Significant side effects: dyslipidemia, hypertriglyceridemia, glucose dysregulation, diabetes mellitus, hyperprolactinemia, tardive dyskinesia, neuroleptic malignant syndrome, QTc prolongation (6)[A]
  – Recommended for depression with psychotic features; consult with psychiatry and consider carefully before starting (4)[A].
- Significant potential interactions
  – TCAs: amphetamines, barbiturates, clonidine, epinephrine, ethanol, norepinephrine
  – ALL ANTIDEPRESSANTS: allow 14-day washout period before starting MAOIs
  – MAOIs: not recommended in primary care. Significant drug and food interactions limit use.

ALERT

- Black box warning: increased risk of suicidality in children, adolescents, and young adults up to age 25 years who are treated with antidepressants. Although this has not been extended to adults, suicide risk assessments are warranted for all patients.
- Serotonin syndrome—a rare but potentially lethal complication from rapid increase in dose or new addition of medication with serotonergic effects

Pregnancy Considerations

SSRIs: fluoxetine, sertraline, and bupropion considered safe in pregnancy (paroxetine Category D; other SSRIs Category C).

ADDITIONAL THERAPIES

- Electroconvulsive therapy (ECT) for refractory cases
- Repetitive transcranial magnetic stimulation (rTMS) may be helpful for TRD (6)[A].

COMPLEMENTARY & ALTERNATIVE MEDICINE

Used in mild depression but *not* regulated by FDA nor recommended by APA

- Hypericum perforatum (St. John's wort): multiple drug interactions; not safe in pregnancy.
- Data do not support S-adenosyl methionine (SAM-e) or acupuncture.

INPATIENT CONSIDERATIONS

Admission Criteria/Initial Stabilization

Inpatient care is indicated for severe depression, patients at risk of suicide/homicide, and for comorbid conditions.

Discharge Criteria

Depressive symptoms abating, no longer suicidal, appropriate outpatient follow-up in place

ONGOING CARE

PATIENT EDUCATION

- Depression is a common medical illness, not a character defect.
- Emphasize the need for long-term treatment and follow-up, which includes lifestyle changes.
- Exercise, good sleep hygiene, good nutrition, and decreased use of tobacco and alcohol are recommended. The optimal regimen is one the patient prefers and will adhere to.

PROGNOSIS

- 70% show significant improvement.
- Of patients with a single depressive episode, 50% will relapse over their lifetime.

COMPLICATIONS

- Suicide
- Lower quality of life

D

REFERENCES

1. Flint J, Kendler KS. The genetics of major depression. *Neuron*. 2014;81(3):484–503.
2. Mitchell AJ, Bird V, Rizzo M, et al. Diagnostic validity and added value of the Geriatric Depression Scale for depression in primary care: a meta-analysis of GDS30 and GDS15. *J Affect Disord*. 2010;125(1–3):10–17.
3. Deneke DE, Schultz H, Fluent TE. Screening for depression in the primary care population. *Prim Care*. 2014;41(2):399–420.
4. American Psychiatric Association. Practice guidelines for the treatment of patients with major depressive disorder. http://www.psychiatryonline.com/pracGuide/pracGuideTopic_7.aspx. Accessed 2014.
5. Arroll B, Elley CR, Fishman T, et al. Antidepressants versus placebo for depression in primary care. *Cochrane Database Syst Rev*. 2009;(3):CD007954.
6. McIntyre RS, Filteau MJ, Martin L, et al. Treatment-resistant depression: definitions, review of the evidence, and algorithmic approach. *J Affect Disord*. 2014;156:1–7.

ADDITIONAL READING

- American Psychiatric Association. *Diagnostic and Statistical Manual of Mental Disorders*. 5th ed. Arlington, VA: American Psychiatric Association; 2013.
- Patient Health Questionnaire (PHQ) Screeners: http://www.phqscreeners.com/overview.aspx?Screener=03_GAD-7.

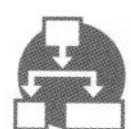

SEE ALSO

Algorithms: Depressed Mood Associated with Medical Illness; Depressive Episode, Major

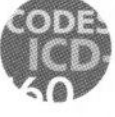

CODES

ICD10

- F32.9 Major depressive disorder, single episode, unspecified
- F33.9 Major depressive disorder, recurrent, unspecified
- F34.1 Dysthymic disorder

CLINICAL PEARLS

- Therapeutic alliance is important to treatment success.
- Given the high recurrence rates, long-term treatment is often necessary.

DEPRESSION, ADOLESCENT

Kenia Mansilla-Rivera, MD

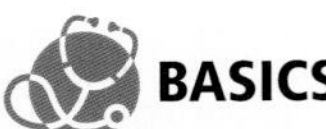

BASICS

DESCRIPTION

- *DSM-5* depressive disorders include disruptive mood dysregulations disorder (DMDD), major depressive disorder (MDD), dysthymia, premenstrual dysphoric disorder, substance/medication-induced depressive disorder, and other nonspecific depression (1). This chapter focuses on MDD.
- MDD is a primary mood disorder characterized by sadness and/or irritable mood with impairment of functioning, abnormal psychological development, and a loss of self-worth, energy, and interest in typically pleasurable activities.
- DMDD is characterized by a chronic, severe persistent irritability with frequent temper outbursts in response to frustration.
- Dysthymic disorder is differentiated from major depression by less intense symptoms that are more persistent, lasting at least 1 year.
- Treatment-resistant depression is a failure of treatment with 2 antidepressants administered in adequate dosage for at least 6 weeks.
- Adolescents with depression are likely to suffer broad functional impairment across social, academic, family, and occupational domains, along with a high incidence of relapse and a high risk for substance abuse and other psychiatric comorbidity.

EPIDEMIOLOGY

Incidence

During adolescence, 1–6%; many do not receive appropriate care.

Prevalence

- MDD: 6–12% of adolescents; twice as common in females (2)
- DMDD: 2–5%; more prominent in males (1)

ETIOLOGY AND PATHOPHYSIOLOGY

- Unclear; low levels of neurotransmitters (serotonin, norepinephrine) may produce symptoms; decreased functioning of the dopamine system also contributes
- External factors may affect neurotransmitters independently.

Genetics

A 76% concordance rate is found in monozygotic twins reared together and a 67% concordance rate among those reared apart, along with a 19% concordance rate in dizygotic twins reared together.

RISK FACTORS

- Increased 3–6× if 1st-degree relative has a major affective disorder; 3–4× in offspring of parents with depression
- Prior depressive episodes
- History of low self-esteem, anxiety disorders, attention deficit hyperactivity disorder (ADHD), and/or learning disabilities
- Hormonal changes during puberty
- Female gender
- Low socioeconomic status
- General stressors: adverse life events, difficulties with peers, loss of a loved one, academic difficulties, abuse, chronic illness, and tobacco abuse

GENERAL PREVENTION

Insufficient evidence for universal depression prevention programs (psychological and social) (3)[B]. There is evidence that participation in sports (specifically team sports) is associated with improved psychological and social health (4); however, no evidence of significant benefit to prevent episodes of depression by exercise (5)[B].

- Some evidence indicates that child and adolescent mental health can be improved by successfully treating maternal depression (6).
- Agency for Healthcare Research and Quality (AHRQ) recommends the screening of adolescents (12–18 years of age) for major depressive disorder when systems are in place to ensure accurate diagnosis, psychotherapy (cognitive-behavioral or interpersonal), and follow-up (7).

COMMONLY ASSOCIATED CONDITIONS

- Eating disorders (especially bulimia)
- Alcohol and substance abuse
- Anxiety and somatization disorders
- Behavioral disorders (i.e., ADHD, oppositional-defiant disorder, conduct disorder)
- Learning disorders
- Headaches

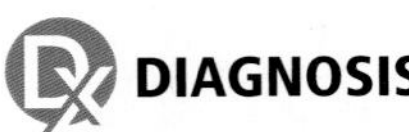

DIAGNOSIS

HISTORY

- Adolescents may present with medically unexplained somatic complaints (fatigue, irritability, headache).
- Based on *DSM-5* criteria, ≥5 of the following symptoms have been present during the same 2-week period and represent a change from previous functioning: At least 1 of the symptoms is either depressed mood or loss of interest or pleasure (1):
  - Criterion A
    - Depressed mood most of the day, nearly every day by either subjective report or observation by others (feelings of sadness, emptiness, hopelessness; in children, can be irritability)
    - Markedly diminished interest or pleasure in all activities most of the day, nearly every day
    - Significant weight loss when not dieting or weight gain (>5% body weight in 1 month)
    - Insomnia or hypersomnia
    - Psychomotor agitation or retardation nearly every day
    - Fatigue or loss of energy
    - Feelings of worthlessness or excessive or inappropriate feelings of guilt nearly every day
    - Diminished ability to think or concentrate, or indecisiveness, nearly every day
    - Recurrent thoughts of death, recurrent suicidal ideation, or attempt
  - Criterion B. Symptoms cause clinically significant distress or impairment in social, occupational, or other important areas of functioning.
  - Criterion C. Episode is not attributable to substances effects or other medical conditions.
  - Criterion D. Episode is not better explained by a schizoaffective, schizophreniform, or delusional disorder.
  - Criterion E. There has never been a manic or hypomanic episode.

PHYSICAL EXAM

- Psychomotor retardation/agitation may be present.
- Clinicians should carefully assess patients for signs of self-injury (wrist lacerations) or abuse.

DIFFERENTIAL DIAGNOSIS

- Normal bereavement
- Substance-induced mood disorder
- Bipolar disorder
- Mood disorder secondary to a medical condition (thyroid, anemia, vitamin deficiency, diabetes)
- Organic CNS diseases
- Malignancy
- Infectious mononucleosis or other viral diseases
- ADHD, posttraumatic stress disorder (PTSD), eating disorders, and anxiety disorders
- Sleep disorder

DIAGNOSTIC TESTS & INTERPRETATION

Initial Tests (lab, imaging)

May be used to rule out other diagnoses (i.e., CBC, TSH, glucose, mono spot, and urine drug)

Follow-Up Tests & Special Considerations

None with sufficient sensitivity/specificity for diagnosis

Diagnostic Procedures/Other

- Depression is primarily diagnosed after a formal interview, with supporting information from caregivers and teachers.
- Standardized tests are useful as screening tools and to monitor response to treatment but should not be used as the sole basis for diagnosis:
  - Beck Depression Inventory (BDI): 12–18 years (2)
  - Child Depression Inventory (CDI): ages 7–17 years
  - Reynolds Adolescent Depression Scale (RADS): teenagers in grades 7–12
  - Mood and Feelings Questionnaire (MFQ) (6)
  - Patient Health Questionnaire-9 (PHQ-9): ages 13–17 with ideal cut point of 11 or higher (instead of 10 used for adults) (8)
- The USPSTF concludes that the current evidence is insufficient to assess the balance of benefits and harms of screening for suicide risk in adolescents in a primary care setting (9).

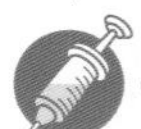

TREATMENT

- Psychotherapy, active support, and monitoring is recommended for mild cases (3)[B].
- In moderate to severe cases, starting medication with/without psychotherapy is recommended (3)[A].

GENERAL MEASURES

- Evidence for the effectiveness of cognitive-behavioral therapy (CBT) alone is mixed but may be effective for mild to moderate depression and useful adjunct to SSRIs, although overall there is limited evidence for long-term benefit (2,6)[A]. Goal is to alter thoughts and behaviors to increase coping and communication skills, problem solving, to regulate emotions, improve mood, and decrease negative thinking.
- Interpersonal psychotherapy (IPT) has been shown to be effective for adolescent depression. The treatment targets interpersonal problems to improve both interpersonal functioning and mood (6).
- Regular exercise may help reduce depressive symptoms (4,5)[B].

MEDICATION

First Line

- Fluoxetine: FDA approved for depression in age >8 years. Starting dose 10 mg/day; may increase after 1 week. Effective dose 20–40 mg/day. The most studied SSRI and with the most favorable effectiveness and safety data (2,10,11)
- Escitalopram: Starting dose 10 mg/day. Effective dose 10–20 mg/day. May increase after 3 weeks. FDA approved for depression age >12 years (2,11,12)
- Citalopram: Starting dose 20 mg/day. May increase up to 20 mg after 2 weeks. FDA approved for depression in age >12 years (2,11)
- Sertraline: Starting dose 25 mg/day (6–12 years old); 50 mg (13–17 years old). Effective dose 50–200 mg/day. May titrate every 1 week. FDA approved for depression in age >12 years (2,11)
- Monitor for suicidal thoughts and behavior, given the possible increased risk while taking any antidepressant. Some studies have shown increases in the rate of adolescent suicide following the FDA black box warning, although is controversial (2,10,13)[C].

Second Line

Other antidepressants (less studied, but reasonable if failed 2 SSRIs):

- Venlafaxine: 37.5–75 mg/day (consider if comorbid anxiety/if failed 2 SSRIs)
- Desvenlafaxine: 50 mg/day
- Bupropion: 37.5–400 mg/day (consider if comorbid ADHD)
- Duloxetine: 20–60 mg/day (although no randomized controlled trials in minors)
- Mirtazapine has shown recently positive outcomes in efficacy and safety (11).

Pediatric Considerations

- Tricyclic antidepressants (TCAs) have not been proven to be effective in adolescents and should NOT be used (11).
- Paroxetine (SSRI): Avoid use due to short half-life, associated withdrawal symptoms, and higher association with suicidal ideation.

ISSUES FOR REFERRAL

Pediatric depression is often managed by primary care providers: Refer to a child psychiatrist for severe, recurrent, or treatment-resistant depression or if the patient has comorbidities (13).

COMPLEMENTARY & ALTERNATIVE MEDICINE

No evidence supports the use of St. John's wort or acupuncture.

INPATIENT CONSIDERATIONS

Admission Criteria/Initial Stabilization

If severely depressed, psychotic, suicidal, or homicidal, 1-on-1 supervision may be needed.

ONGOING CARE

Treatment for at least 6 months reduced the likelihood of suicide attempts, compared with treatment for <8 weeks (12,13).

FOLLOW-UP RECOMMENDATIONS

- Systematic and regular tracking of goals and outcomes from treatment should be performed, including assessment of depressive symptoms and functioning in home, school, and peer settings (13).
- Diagnosis and initial treatment should be reassessed if no improvement is noted after 6–8 weeks of treatment (13).

Patient Monitoring

- Once started on antidepressants, patients are seen weekly for 1st month, biweekly for the 2nd month, and at least 12-week intervals thereafter. Monitor for suicidal thoughts/behavior, particularly in the first 2 months after initiation or dose increase. Monitor for signs of antidepressant-induced mania, especially between 1st and 4th weeks (12).
- Length of medication treatment:
  - 1st episode: minimum 6–9 months followed by a slow taper over 6–8 weeks (risk of discontinuation syndrome highest with paroxetine)
  - 2nd episode: at least 1 year
  - 3rd episode: 1–3 years
  - >3 episodes: lifelong
- Adverse effects (e.g., nausea, headaches, behavioral activation) occur in up to 93% treated with SSRIs and occur earlier than therapeutic response. Routine monitoring and discussion of possible side effects is critical for those treated with antidepressants. Although it is rare, serotonin syndrome can occur with multiple medications or high doses of SSRIs (12).

PATIENT EDUCATION

Educate patients and parents about mental health and the fact that depression is a medical illness, not a character defect.

PROGNOSIS

- If left untreated, major depressive episode in adolescents typically lasts 7–9 months, with 90% resolving within 2 years.
- Recurrence is 40% by 2 years and 50–70% by 5 years.
- Persistent and severe depression in adulthood is more likely with an earlier onset of disease (6).
- Patients with family conflict, drug and alcohol use, and anxiety disorders are less likely to achieve remission (14).
- Psychological depression prevention programs were effective in preventing recurrent episodes of illness (1).

COMPLICATIONS

- Treatment-induced mania, aggression, or lack of improvement in symptoms
- School failure/refusal
- Suicide

REFERENCES

1. American Psychiatric Association. *Diagnostic and Statistical Manual of Mental Disorders*. 5th ed. Arlington, VA: American Psychiatric Association; 2013.
2. Clark MS, Jansen KL, Cloy A. Treatment of childhood and adolescent depression. *Am Fam Physician*. 2012;86(5):442–448.
3. Merry SN, Hetrick SE, Cox GR, et al. Psychological and educational interventions for preventing depression in children and adolescents. *Cochrane Database Syst Rev*. 2011;(12):CD003380.
4. Eime RM, Young JA, Harvey JT, et al. A systematic review of the psychological and social benefits of participation in sport for children and adolescents: informing development of a conceptual model of health through sport. *Int J Beh Nutr Phys Act*. 2013;10:98.
5. Larun L, Nordheim LV, Ekeland E, et al. Exercise in prevention and treatment of anxiety and depression among children and young people. *Cochrane Database Syst Rev*. 2006;(3):CD004691.
6. Thapar A, Ollishaw S, Potter R, et al. Managing and preventing depression in adolescents. *BMJ*. 2010;340:c209.
7. U.S. Preventive Services Task Force. Screening and treatment for major depressive disorder in children and adolescents: US Preventive Services Task Force Recommendation Statement. *Pediatrics*. 2009;123(4):1223–1228.
8. Richardson LP, McCAuley E, Grossman DC, et al. Evaluation of the Patient Health Questionnaire-9 item for detecting major depression among adolescents. *Pediatrics*. 2010;126(6):1117–1123.
9. LeFevre ML; U.S. Preventive Services Task Force. Screening for suicide risk in adolescents, adults, and older adults in primary care: U.S. Preventive Services Task Force recommendation statement. *Ann Intern Med*. 2014;160(10):719–727.
10. Hetrick SE, McKenzie JE, Cox GR, et al. Newer generation antidepressants for depressive disorders in children and adolescents. *Cochrane Database Syst Rev*. 2012;11:CD004851.
11. Ma D, Zhang Z, Zhang X, et al. Comparative efficacy, acceptability, and safety of medicinal, cognitive-behavioral therapy, and placebo treatments for acute major depressive disorder in children and adolescents: a multiple-treatments meta-analysis. *Curr Med Res Opin*. 2014;30(6):971–995.
12. Smiga SM, Elliott GR. Psychopharmacology of depression in children and adolescents. *Pediatr Clin North Am*. 2011;58(1):155–171.
13. Cheung AH, Kozloff N, Sacks D. Pediatric depression: an evidence-based update on treatment interventions. *Curr Psychiatry Rep*. 2013;15(8):381.
14. Emslie GJ. Treatment of resistant depression in adolescents (TORDIA): week 24 outcomes. *Am J Psychiatry*. 2010;167(7):782–791.

ADDITIONAL READING

Cheung AH, Zuckerbrot RA, Jensen PS, et al. Guidelines for Adolescent Depression in Primary Care (GLAD-PC): II. Treatment and ongoing management. *Pediatrics*. 2007;120(5):e1313–e1326.

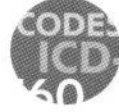

CODES

ICD10

- F32.9 Major depressive disorder, single episode, unspecified
- F33.9 Major depressive disorder, recurrent, unspecified
- F33.8 Other recurrent depressive disorders

CLINICAL PEARLS

- Adolescent depression is underdiagnosed and often presents with irritability and anhedonia.
- Fluoxetine and escitalopram are the most studied FDA approved for treatment of adolescent depression.
- Citalopram, sertraline, and mirtazapine are also FDA approved antidepressants.
- CBT combined with fluoxetine is efficacious for adolescents with major depression.
- Paroxetine and TCAs should not be used to treat adolescent depression.
- Referral to a child psychiatrist is appropriate for complex cases or treatment-resistant depression.
- Monitor all adolescents with depression for suicidality, especially during the 1st month of treatment with an antidepressant.

D

DEPRESSION, GERIATRIC

Robert A. Baldor, MD, FAAFP

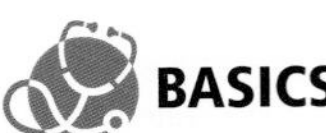

BASICS

DESCRIPTION

- Depression is a primary mood disorder characterized by a depressed mood and/or a markedly decreased interest or pleasure in normally enjoyable activities for at least 2 weeks and causing significant distress or impairment in daily functioning.
- It is not considered a part of normal aging.

EPIDEMIOLOGY

Prevalence rates among the elderly vary, largely depending on the specific diagnostic instruments used and their current health and/or home environment:

- 1–3% of community-dwelling elderly
- 7.5% seen in primary care clinics
- 10–21% of hospitalized elderly patients
- 12–27% of nursing home residents

ETIOLOGY AND PATHOPHYSIOLOGY

- Significant gaps exist in the understanding of the underlying pathophysiology.
- Ongoing research has identified several possible mechanisms, including the following:
  - Monoamine transmission and associated transcriptional and translational activity
  - Epigenetic mechanisms and resilience factors
  - Neurotrophins, neurogenesis, neuroimmune systems, and neuroendocrine systems
- Depression appears to be a complex interaction between heritable and environmental factors.

RISK FACTORS

- General
  - Chronic physical health condition(s)
  - History of mental health problems
  - Death of a loved one
  - Caregiving
  - Social isolation
  - Lack/loss of social support
  - Significant loss of independence
  - Uncontrolled pain
  - Insomnia/sleep disturbance
- Prevalence of depression in medical illness
  - Stroke (22–50%)
  - Cancer (18–50%)
  - Myocardial infarction (15–45%)
  - Parkinson disease (10–39%)
  - Rheumatoid arthritis (13%)
  - Diabetes mellitus (5–11%)
  - Alzheimer dementia (5–15%)
- Suicide
  - Suicide is the 11th leading cause of death in the United States for all ages.
  - Suicide rates are higher for Americans age >65 years compared with the general population (~15/100,000 people).
  - Suicide rates are highest for males aged >75 years (rate 38.5/100,000).

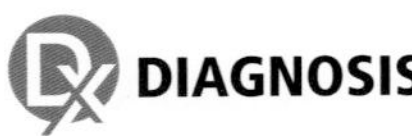

DIAGNOSIS

HISTORY

- Depressed mood most of the day, nearly every day, and/or loss of interest/pleasure in life for at least 2 weeks
- Other common symptoms include the following:
  - Feeling hopeless, helpless, or worthless
  - Insomnia and loss of appetite/weight (alternatively, hypersomnia with increased appetite/weight in atypical depression)
  - Fatigue and loss of energy
  - Somatic symptoms (headaches, chronic pain)
  - Neglect of personal responsibility or care
  - Psychomotor retardation or agitation
  - Diminished concentration, indecisiveness
  - Thoughts of death or suicide
- Screening with "SIGECAPS"
  - **S**leep: changes in sleep habits from baseline, including excessive sleep, early waking, or inability to fall asleep
  - **I**nterest: loss of interest in previously enjoyable activities
  - **G**uilt: guilt that may or may not focus on a specific problem or circumstance
  - **E**nergy: perceived lack of energy
  - **C**oncentration: inability to concentrate on specific tasks
  - **A**ppetite: increase/decrease in appetite
  - **P**sychomotor: restlessness and agitation or the perception that everyday activities are too strenuous to manage
  - **S**uicidality: desire to end life or hurt oneself, harmful thoughts directed internally or thoughts of homicidality

PHYSICAL EXAM

Mental status exam

DIFFERENTIAL DIAGNOSIS

Concurrent medical conditions, cognitive disorders, and medications may produce neurovegetative symptoms that may mimic depression:

- Medical conditions: hypothyroidism, vitamin B_{12} deficiency, liver or renal failure, cancers, stroke
- Medication-induced: interferon-α, β_2-blockers, isotretinoin
- Dementia and neurodegenerative disorders
- Delirium
- Psychiatric disorders: bipolar disorder, dysthymic disorder, anxiety disorders, substance abuse–related mood disorders, psychotic disorders

DIAGNOSTIC TESTS & INTERPRETATION

Initial Tests (lab, imaging)

Initial laboratory evaluation is done primarily to rule out potential medical factors that could be causing symptoms.

- Thyroid-stimulating hormone (TSH)
- CBC with differential
- Comprehensive metabolic panel, including liver function
- Urine drug screen
- Vitamin B_{12}

Follow-Up Tests & Special Considerations

Additional testing for possible confounding medical and cognitive disorders, as warranted

Diagnostic Procedures/Other

Validated screening tools and rating scales:

- Geriatric Depression Scale: 15- or 30-point scales
- Patient Health Questionnaire (PHQ-2 or PHQ-9)
- Hamilton Depression Rating Scale
- Beck Depression Inventory
- Cornell Scale for Depression in Dementia 1H

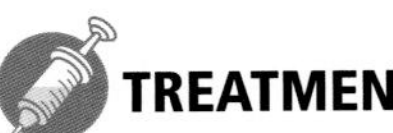

TREATMENT

Although response alone, usually interpreted as a 50% reduction in symptoms, can be clinically meaningful, the goal is to treat patients to the point of remission (i.e., essentially the absence of depressive symptoms).

GENERAL MEASURES

Psychotherapy: Studies do show some benefit in depressed elderly patients (1)[B]:

- Cognitive-behavioral therapy
- Problem-solving therapy
- Interpersonal therapy
- Psychodynamic psychotherapy

MEDICATION

- Typically more conservative initial dosing and titration of antidepressants in the elderly, starting with 1/2 of the usual initiation dose and increasing within a couple of weeks, if tolerated
- Continue titrating dose every 2–4 weeks, as appropriate. It is important to reach an adequate treatment dose.

First Line

- SSRIs have been found to be effective in treating depression in the elderly (2)[A].
- No single SSRI clearly outperforms others in the class; choice of medication often reflects side effect profile or practitioner familiarity:
  - Citalopram: Start at 10 mg/day. Treatment range 10–20 mg/day.
  - Sertraline: Start at 25 mg/day. Treatment range 50–200 mg/day.
  - Escitalopram: Start at 5–10 mg/day. Treatment range 10–20 mg/day.
  - Fluoxetine: Start at 10 mg/day. Treatment range 20–60 mg/day.
  - Paroxetine: Start at 10 mg/day. Treatment range 20–40 mg/day.
- SSRIs should not be used concomitantly with monoamine oxidase inhibitors (MAOIs).

Second Line

- Atypical antidepressants: more effective than placebo in treatment of depression in the elderly, although additional studies are needed to better delineate patient factors that determine response (3)[A]:
  - Bupropion (immediate, sustained/twice a day, and extended/once daily available): Start at 100 mg/day. Increase dose in 3–4 days. Treatment range 200–300 mg/day. Avoid in patients with elevated seizure risk.
  - Venlafaxine (immediate- and extended-release available): Start at 37.5 mg/day extended-release and titrate weekly. Treatment range 75–225 mg/day. May be associated with elevated BP at higher doses.
  - Duloxetine: Start at 30 mg/day. Treatment range 30–60 mg/day. Also may be associated with elevated BP.
  - Mirtazapine: Start at 7.5–15/day mg nightly. Treatment range 15–45 mg/day; can produce problems with weight gain, sedation, and cognitive dysfunction
  - Desvenlafaxine: 50 mg/day in AM; higher doses do not confer additional benefit; 50 mg every other day if CrCl <30 mL/min
  - Vilazodone: Start at 10 mg/day with food. Treatment range 20–40 mg/day; can produce diarrhea and nausea
- For patients who have not responded to initial SSRI trial:
  - Switch to a different SSRI medication, switch to an atypical antidepressant, or augment initial antidepressant with bupropion (4)[A].

ISSUES FOR REFERRAL

Depression with suicidal ideation, psychotic depression, bipolar disorder, comorbid substance abuse issues, severe or refractory illness

ADDITIONAL THERAPIES

- Tricyclic antidepressants (TCAs) have been shown to be effective in treating depression in the elderly. However, they are difficult for elderly patients to tolerate due to side effect profile and are potentially lethal in overdose, limiting their use as initial treatment agents (2)[A].
- Although not FDA approved, buspirone, lithium, or triiodothyronine are sometimes used off-label to augment a primary antidepressant (4)[B].
- MAOIs also appear more effective than placebo in the treatment of depression in the elderly. They are not used frequently in clinical practice due to potential side effects and necessary dietary restrictions (2)[A].
- Evidence for benefit of antidepressants in the treatment of depression in patients with dementia is equivocal. Consideration should be made for a limited trial with follow-up for improvement and side effects or use only in patients with severe symptoms (5)[A].
- Electroconvulsive therapy (ECT): has been shown to produce remission of depressive symptoms in the elderly. It should be considered as an initial option for patients with severe or psychotic depression (6)[B].
- Exercise: may be beneficial for depression in the elderly population (7)[A]

COMPLEMENTARY & ALTERNATIVE MEDICINE

- Acupuncture: equally beneficial as counseling (8)[B]
- St. John's wort may have minimal benefit (9)[A].
- Tryptophan and hydroxytryptophan: 150–300 mg/day; possible efficacy, additional investigation required (10)[B]

INPATIENT CONSIDERATIONS

Inpatient care indicated for imminent safety risk (e.g., acutely suicidal patients) or for those patients unable to care adequately for themselves due to depression

ONGOING CARE

FOLLOW-UP RECOMMENDATIONS

Due to the delay of benefit following initiation of antidepressant therapy (2–4 weeks), it is necessary to ensure open communication with the patient to prevent premature discontinuation of therapy. An adequate explanation of potential side effects with instructions to call the office before discontinuing therapy is imperative.

Patient Monitoring

- A patient with severe depression who exhibits suicidality may require admission to an appropriate facility.
- Monitor for worsening anxiety symptoms or increase in suicidality.

DIET

No dietary restrictions are necessary, except for patients taking MAOIs, which necessitates dietary restriction of foods high in tyramine.

PATIENT EDUCATION

- Depression is a treatable illness.
- Medications may need to be taken for at least 2–4 weeks before any beneficial effect is noted.
- Depression is often a recurring illness.
- National Suicide Prevention Lifeline at 1-800-273-TALK (8255) is a free, 24-hour hotline available to anyone in suicidal crisis or emotional distress. Calls will be routed to the nearest crisis center.

PROGNOSIS

- Treatment outcomes in the elderly may be worse than in the general population, possibly mediated by physical comorbidities and other factors.
- Depending on the population studied and specific clinical measures used, estimates vary for initial clinical response and remission (between 30% and 70%).

COMPLICATIONS

- Impairment in social, occupational, or interpersonal functioning
- Difficulty performing activities of daily living and self-care
- Increase in medical services utilization and increased costs of care
- Suicide

REFERENCES

1. Wilson KC, Mottram PG, Vassilas CA. Psychotherapeutic treatments for older depressed people. *Cochrane Database Syst Rev*. 2008;(1):CD004853.
2. Wilson K, Mottram P, Sivanranthan A, et al. Antidepressant versus placebo for depressed elderly. *Cochrane Database Syst Rev*. 2001;(2):CD000561.
3. Nelson JC, Delucchi K, Schneider LS. Efficacy of second generation antidepressants in late-life depression: a meta-analysis of the evidence. *Am J Geriatr Psychiatry*. 2008;16(7):558–567.
4. Ruhé HG, Huyser J, Swinkels JA, et al. Switching antidepressants after a first selective serotonin reuptake inhibitor in major depressive disorder: a systematic review. *J Clin Psychiatry*. 2006;67(12):1836–1855.
5. Nelson JC, Devanand DP. A systematic review and meta-analysis of placebo-controlled antidepressant studies in people with depression and dementia. *J Am Geriatr Soc*. 2011;59(4):577–585.
6. Van der Wurff FB, Stek ML, Hoogendijk WL, et al. Electroconvulsive therapy for the depressed elderly. *Cochrane Database Syst Rev*. 2003;(2):CD003593.
7. Blake H, Mo P, Malik S, et al. How effective are physical activity interventions for alleviating depressive symptoms in older people? A systematic review. *Clin Rehabil*. 2009;23(10):873–887.
8. MacPherson H, Richmond S, Bland M, et al. Acupuncture and counselling for depression in primary care: a randomised controlled trial. *PLoS Med*. 2013;10(9):e1001518.
9. Linde K, Mulrow CD, Berner M, et al. St. John's wort for depression. *Cochrane Database Syst Rev*. 2005;(2):CD000448.
10. Shaw K, Turner J, DelMar C. Tryptophan and 5-hydroxytryptophan for depression. *Cochrane Database Syst Rev*. 2002;(1):CD003198.

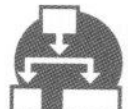

SEE ALSO

Algorithms: Depressed Mood Associated with Medical Illness; Depressive Episode, Major

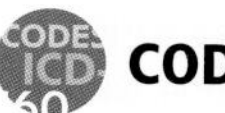

CODES

ICD10

- F32.9 Major depressive disorder, single episode, unspecified
- F03 Unspecified dementia
- F43.21 Adjustment disorder with depressed mood

CLINICAL PEARLS

- Depression is not a normal part of aging.
- Depression in the elderly may be difficult to diagnose precisely due to medical and cognitive comorbidities.
- Depression may present primarily with cognitive dysfunction. Cognitive function may improve with treatment of the depression.
- A multidisciplinary approach to the treatment of depression is often most efficacious.
- SSRIs are considered 1st-line therapy for safety and tolerability. A full remission may take upward of 12 weeks of treatment. Long-term treatment may be needed to prevent recurrence.

DEPRESSION, POSTPARTUM

Isheeta Zalpuri, MD • Nancy Byatt, DO, MBA, FAPM

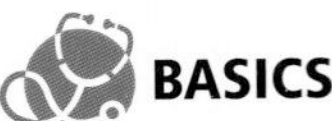

BASICS

DESCRIPTION

- Major depressive disorder (MDD) that recurs or has its onset in the postpartum period. May also occur in mothers adopting a baby or in fathers
- Postpartum depression (PPD) is similar to non-pregnancy depression (sleep disorders, anhedonia, psychomotor changes, etc.); it has its onset within the first 12 weeks postpartum.
- Different than postpartum "blues" (sadness and emotional lability) which is experienced by 30–70% of women and has an onset and resolution within first 10 days postpartum

EPIDEMIOLOGY

Incidence

14.5% of women have a new episode of major or minor depression during postpartum period (1).

Prevalence

As many as 19.2% women suffer from depression in postpartum period (1).

ETIOLOGY AND PATHOPHYSIOLOGY

- May be related to sensitivity in hormonal fluctuations, including estrogen; progesterone; and other gonadal hormones as well as neuroactive steroids; cytokines; hypothalamic–pituitary–adrenal (HPA) axis hormones; altered fatty acid, oxytocin, and arginine vasopressin levels; and genetic and epigenetic factors
- Multifactorial including biologic–genetic predisposition in terms of neurobiologic deficit, destabilizing effects of hormone withdrawal at birth, inflammation, and psychosocial stressors

RISK FACTORS

- Previous episodes of PPD
- History of MDD
- MDD during pregnancy
- Anxiety during pregnancy
- History of premenstrual dysphoria
- Family history of depression
- Unwanted pregnancy
- Socioeconomic stress
- Low self-esteem
- Young maternal age
- Alcohol abuse
- Marital conflict
- Multiple births
- African Americans and Hispanics may have higher rates of PPD.
- Preterm and low birth weight baby
- Postpartum pain, sleep disturbance, and fatigue
- Recent immigrant status
- Increased stressful life events
- History of childhood sexual abuse
- Decision to decrease antidepressants during pregnancy
- Intimate partner violence (2)

GENERAL PREVENTION

- Universal screening during pregnancy to allow for detection and treatment
- Screening using Edinburgh Postnatal Depression Scale during the postpartum year: http://www.testandcalc.com/etc/tests/edin.asp
- For women with depression, continuation of antidepressants during pregnancy may prevent PPD.
- Postnatal visits, psychotherapy, and/or psychoeducation for high-risk women
- Depression care manager who provides education, routine telephone contact, and follow-up to engage women in treatment

COMMONLY ASSOCIATED CONDITIONS

- Bipolar mood disorder
- Depressive disorder not otherwise specified
- Dysthymic disorder
- Cyclothymic disorder
- MDD

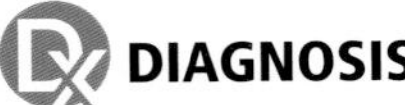

DIAGNOSIS

HISTORY

- Increased/decreased sleep
- Decreased interest in formerly compelling or pleasurable activities
- Guilt, low self-esteem
- Decreased energy
- Decreased concentration
- Increased/decreased appetite
- Psychomotor agitation or retardation
- Suicidal ideation

DIFFERENTIAL DIAGNOSIS

- Baby blues: not a psychiatric disorder; mood lability resolves within days
- Postpartum psychosis: a psychiatric emergency
- Postpartum anxiety/panic disorder
- Postpartum obsessive-compulsive disorder
- Hypothyroidism
- Postpartum thyroiditis: can occur in up to 5.7% of patients in the United States and can present as depression (3)

DIAGNOSTIC TESTS & INTERPRETATION

Initial Tests (lab, imaging)

Thyroid-stimulating hormone (TSH)

Diagnostic Procedures/Other

- Edinburgh Postnatal Depression Scale is the primary screening tool.
- Beck, Hamilton, and Zung depression inventories may provide information about the severity of the depression and suicidal risks.
- Edinburgh Postnatal Depression Scale (Partner Version): to be completed by mother's partner to obtain his/her view of mother's depression

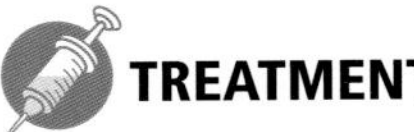

TREATMENT

GENERAL MEASURES

- Outpatient individual psychotherapy in combination with pharmacotherapy
- Support/psychotherapy groups may be helpful.
- Assess suicidal ideation.
- Assess homicidal ideation and thoughts of harming baby. Thoughts of harming baby require immediate hospitalization.
- Visiting nurse services can provide direct observations of the mother regarding safety concerns and mother–child bonding.
- Peer support

MEDICATION

First Line

- For nonbreastfeeding women, selection of antidepressants is similar to nonpostpartum patients.
- Selective serotonin reuptake inhibitors (SSRIs) are generally effective and safe:
  - Fluoxetine (Prozac): 20–80 mg/day PO (most activating of all SSRIs)
  - Sertraline (Zoloft): 50–200 mg/day PO (mildly sedating)
  - Paroxetine (Paxil): 20–60 mg/day PO (sedating)
  - Citalopram (Celexa): 20–40 mg/day PO (FDA recommendation)
  - Escitalopram (Lexapro): 10–20 mg/day PO
- Tricyclic antidepressants (TCAs) are effective and less expensive yet also are lethal in overdose and have unfavorable side effects:
  - Avoid TCAs in mothers with a history of suicidal ideation.
- Bupropion (Wellbutrin): 150–450 mg/day PO in patients with depression plus psychomotor retardation and hypersomnia and with weight gain. Bupropion is less likely to cause weight gain or sexual dysfunction and is highly activating.
- Mirtazapine (Remeron): 15–45 mg/day PO at bedtime; may assist with sleep restoration and weight gain; no sexual dysfunction
- Serotonin–norepinephrine reuptake inhibitors (SNRIs)
  - Venlafaxine (Effexor XR): A dual-action antidepressant that blocks the reuptake of serotonin in doses of up to 150 mg/day and then blocks the reuptake of norepinephrine in doses of 150–450 mg/day PO.
  - Duloxetine (Cymbalta): more balanced serotonin/norepinephrine reuptake throughout dosing; 40–60 mg/day PO (doses >60 mg have not been demonstrated to be more effective)
  - Desvenlafaxine (Pristiq): 50 mg/day PO
- Bipolar disorder requires treatment with mood stabilizer.
- Among breastfeeding mothers
  - Weigh potential efficacy of treatment with antidepressant, prior treatment history, risks of exposure to infant, and negative effects of untreated PPD on child development.
  - All antidepressants are excreted in breast milk but are generally compatible with lactation.
  - Paroxetine and sertraline have lower translactal passage.
  - SSRIs and nortriptyline have a better safety profile.
  - Translactal passage is greater with fluoxetine and citalopram (4)[B].
  - Start with low doses and increase slowly. Monitor infant for adverse side effects.
  - Continuing an efficacious medication is preferred over switching antidepressants to avoid exposing mother and infant to the risks of untreated PPD (4)[B].
  - Breastfeeding women need additional education and support regarding the risks and benefits of use of antidepressants during breastfeeding.
  - Discussions of the treatment options must be held with the patient and her partner. These include the patient's personal psychiatric history and previous response to treatment, the risks

of no treatment or undertreatment, available data about the safety of medications during breastfeeding, and her individual expectations and treatment preferences (4)[B].

– For further information: *Medications and Mother's Milk* by Thomas Hale, PhD.

Second Line

Consider switching to a different antidepressant or augmentation if patient has a partial response electroconvulsive therapy (ECT). This is an option for depressed postpartum women who do not respond to antidepressant medications, have severe or psychotic symptoms, cannot tolerate antidepressant medications, are actively engaged in suicidal self-destructive behaviors, or have a previous history of response to ECT (5)[B].

ISSUES FOR REFERRAL

- Obtain psychiatric consultation for patients with psychotic symptoms.
- Immediate hospitalization is mandatory if delusions or hallucinations are present.
- Hospitalization is indicated if mother's ability to care for self and/or infant is significantly compromised.

ADDITIONAL THERAPIES

- Psychoeducation, including providing reading material for the patient and family
- Psychotherapy: Interpersonal psychotherapy, cognitive behavioral therapy, and psychodynamic psychotherapy have shown to be effective (5)[B].

COMPLEMENTARY & ALTERNATIVE MEDICINE

- Breastfeeding is effective in reducing stress and protecting maternal mood.
- Infant massage, infant sleep intervention, exercise, and bright light therapy may be beneficial (5)[B].

INPATIENT CONSIDERATIONS

ALERT

Obtain psychiatric consultation for patients with psychotic symptoms. If delusions or hallucinations are present, immediate hospitalization is mandatory. The psychotic mother should *not* be left alone with the baby.

Admission Criteria/Initial Stabilization

Presence of suicidal or homicidal ideation and/or psychotic symptoms and/or thoughts of harming baby and/or inability to care for self or infant, severe weight loss

Discharge Criteria

- Absence of suicidal or homicidal ideation and/or psychotic symptoms and/or thoughts of harming baby
- Mother must be able to care for self and infant.

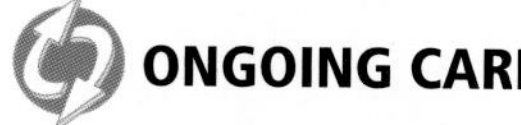

ONGOING CARE

FOLLOW-UP RECOMMENDATIONS

Patient Monitoring

- Collaborative care approach, including primary care visits and case manager follow-ups
- Consultation with the infant's doctor, particularly if mother is breastfeeding while taking psychotropic medications

DIET

- Good nutrition and hydration, especially when breastfeeding
- Mixed evidence to support the addition of multivitamin with minerals and omega-3 fatty acids

PATIENT EDUCATION

- *This Isn't What I Expected: Overcoming Postpartum Depression*, by Karen R. Kleinman and Valerie Davis Radkin
- *Down Came the Rain: My Journey Through Postpartum Depression*, by Brooke Shields, 2005
- *Behind the Smile: My Journey Out of Postpartum Depression*, by Marie Osmond, Marcie Wilkie, and Judith Morre, 2001
- *A Medication Guide for Breastfeeding Moms*, by Thomas Hale and Ghia Mcafee, 2008
- Web resources
  - Postpartum support international: http://www.postpartum.net
  - http://www.4women.gov
  - La Leche League: http://www.lalecheleague.org
  - http://toxnet.nlm.nih.gov
  - www.mededppd.org
  - www.womensmentalhealth.org
  - www.motherrisk.org
  - www.step-ppd.com

PROGNOSIS

- Treatment of maternal depression to remission has been shown to have a positive impact on children's mental health.
- Some patients, particularly those with undertreated or undiagnosed depression, may develop chronic depression requiring long-term treatment.
- Untreated maternal depression is linked to impaired cognitive and language development delay in infants and children (6).
- Postpartum psychosis is associated with tragic outcomes such as maternal suicide and infanticide.

COMPLICATIONS

- Suicide
- Self-injurious behavior
- Psychosis
- Neglect of baby
- Harm to the baby

REFERENCES

1. Gavin NI, Gaynes BN, Lohr KN, et al. Perinatal depression: a systematic review of prevalence and incidence. *Obstet Gynecol*. 2005;106(5, Pt 1):1071–1083.
2. Cerulli C, Talbot NL, Tang W, et al. Co-occurring intimate partner violence and mental health diagnoses in perinatal women. *J Womens Health (Larchmt)*. 2011;20(12):1797–1803.
3. Nicholson WK, Robinson KA, Smallridge RC, et al. Prevalence of postpartum thyroid dysfunction: a quantitative review. *Thyroid*. 2006;16(6):573–582.
4. Pearlstein T, Howard M, Salisbury A, et al. Postpartum depression. *Am J Obstet Gynecol*. 2009;200(4):357–364.
5. Fitelson E, Kim S, Baker AS, et al. Treatment of postpartum depression: clinical, psychological and pharmacological options. *Int J Womens Health*. 2010;3:1–14.
6. Kingston D, Tough S, Whitfield H. Prenatal and postpartum maternal psychological distress and infant development: a systematic review. *Child Psychiatry Hum Dev*. 2012;43(5):683–714.

ADDITIONAL READING

- Edinburgh Postnatal Depression Scale. http://www.testandcalc.com/etc/tests/edin.asp
- Gjerdingen D, Katon W, Rich DE. Stepped care treatment of postpartum depression: a primary care-based management model. *Womens Health Issues*. 2008;18(1):44–52.
- Harrington AR, Greene-Harrington CC. Healthy Start screens for depression among urban pregnant, postpartum and interconceptional women. *J Natl Med Assoc*. 2007;99(3):226–231.
- Hirst KP, Moutier CY. Postpartum major depression. *Am Fam Physician*. 2010;82(8):926–933.
- Howard LM, Boath E, Henshaw C. Antidepressant prevention of postnatal depression. *PLoS Med*. 2006;3(10):e389.
- Kendall-Tackett K. A new paradigm for depression in new mothers: the central role of inflammation and how breastfeeding and anti-inflammatory treatments protect maternal mental health. *Int Breastfeed J*. 2007;2:6.
- Musters C, McDonald E, Jones I. Management of postnatal depression. *BMJ*. 2008;337:a736.
- Ng RC, Hirata CK, Yeung W, et al. Pharmacologic treatment for postpartum depression: a systematic review. *Pharmacotherapy*. 2010;30(9):928–941.
- Sit DK, Wisner KL. Identification of postpartum depression. *Clin Obstet Gynecol*. 2009;52(3):456–468.
- Tammentie T, Tarkka MT, Astedt-Kurki P, et al. Family dynamics and postnatal depression. *J Psychiatr Ment Health Nurs*. 2004;11(2):141–149.

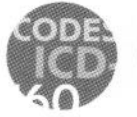

CODES

ICD10

F53 Puerperal psychosis

CLINICAL PEARLS

- PPD is a common, debilitating medical condition that impairs a mother's ability to function and interact with her infant and family.
- Universal screening for PPD is recommended during the 3rd trimester and at regular intervals during the postpartum period.
- Early diagnosis and treatment are vital, as untreated PPD can lead to developmental difficulties for the infant and prolonged disability and suffering for the mother.
- Breastfeeding is recommended for maternal and child health. Several medication options for treating depression in mothers are safe for breastfeeding infants.
- Treatment with antidepressants should be individualized for breastfeeding mothers (4)[B].

DEPRESSION, TREATMENT RESISTANT

Michelle Magid, MD • Roger Lowell McRoberts, III, MD

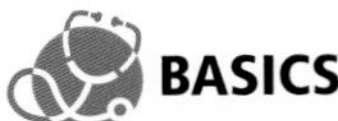

BASICS

DESCRIPTION

- Major depressive disorder (MDD) that has failed to respond to ≥2 adequate trials of antidepressant therapy in ≥2 different classes (1)
- Antidepressant therapy must be given for 6 weeks at standard doses before being considered a failure.

EPIDEMIOLOGY

- Depression affects >18 million people in the United States and >340 million people worldwide.
- 16% lifetime risk of MDD (2,3). Approximately 1/3 of patients with MDD will develop treatment-resistant depression (3,4).

ETIOLOGY AND PATHOPHYSIOLOGY

- Unclear. Low levels of neurotransmitters (serotonin, norepinephrine, dopamine) have been indicated.
- Serotonin has been linked to irritability, hostility, and suicidal ideation.
- Norepinephrine has been linked to low energy.
- Dopamine may play a role in low motivation and depression with psychotic features.
- Environmental stressors such as abuse and neglect may affect neurotransmission.

Genetics

Limited studies have shown that a genetic abnormality in the serotonin transporter gene (5-HTTLPR) may increase risk for treatment-resistant depression.

RISK FACTORS

- Severity of disease
- Mislabeling patients with depression who are bipolar
- Comorbid medical disease (including chronic pain)
- Comorbid personality disorder
- Comorbid anxiety disorder
- Comorbid substance abuse
- Familial predisposition to poor response to antidepressants

GENERAL PREVENTION

- Medication adherence in combination with psychotherapy
- Maintenance electroconvulsive therapy (ECT) may prevent relapse.

COMMONLY ASSOCIATED CONDITIONS

- Suicide
- Bipolar disorder
- Substance abuse
- Anxiety disorders
- Dysthymia
- Eating disorders
- Somatic symptom disorders

DIAGNOSIS

HISTORY

- Symptoms are the same as in MDD. However, patients do not respond to standard form of treatment. Severity and duration are extreme.
- Especially important to screen for suicidality in treatment-resistant depression
- Screening with SIGECAPS
  - Sleep: too much or too little
  - Interest: failure to enjoy activities
  - Guilt: excessive and uncontrollable
  - Energy: poor energy
  - Concentration: inability to focus on tasks
  - Appetite: too much or too little
  - Psychomotor changes: restlessness/agitation or slowing/lethargy
  - Suicidality: desire to end life

PHYSICAL EXAM

Mental status exam may reveal poor hygiene, poor eye contact, blunted affect, tearfulness, weight loss or gain, psychomotor retardation, or agitation.

DIFFERENTIAL DIAGNOSIS

- Bipolar disorder
- Dysthymia
- Dementia
- Early-stage Parkinson disease
- Personality disorder
- Medical illness such as malignancy, thyroid disease, HIV
- Substance abuse

DIAGNOSTIC TESTS & INTERPRETATION

Initial Tests (lab, imaging)

- Used to rule out medical factors that could be causing/contributing to treatment resistance
  - CBC
  - Complete metabolic profile, including liver tests, calcium, and glucose
  - Urine drug screen
  - Thyroid-stimulating hormone (TSH)
  - Vitamin D level (25-OH vitamin D)
  - Testosterone
- CT or MRI of the brain if neurologic disease, tumor, or dementia is suspected

Follow-Up Tests & Special Considerations

Delirium and dementia may often look like depression.

Diagnostic Procedures/Other

- Depression is a clinical diagnosis.
- Validated depression rating scales to assist
  - Beck Depression Inventory
  - Hamilton Rating Scale for Depression
  - Patient Health Questionnaire 9 (PHQ-9)

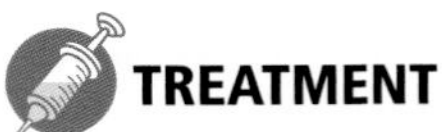

TREATMENT

MEDICATION

First Line

- Please see "Depression" topic. When those fail, augmentation and combination strategies are as follows:
  - Antidepressants in combination
    - Citalopram (Start 20 mg/day. Max dose 40 mg/day) + bupropion (start 100 mg BID; max dose 450 mg total) (4,5)[B]
    - Tricyclic antidepressants (TCAs) and selective serotonin reuptake inhibitors (SSRIs) may be used in combination. Proceed with caution due to risk of serotonin syndrome. Citalopram (start 20 mg/day; max dose 40 mg/day) + nortriptyline (start 50 mg at bedtime; max dose 150 mg at bedtime)
  - Antidepressants + antipsychotics
    - Citalopram (start 20 mg/day; max dose 40 mg/day) + aripiprazole (2–5 mg/day, different mechanism of action at higher doses) *OR* + risperidone (start 0.5–1 mg at bedtime; max dose 6 mg/day) *OR* + quetiapine (start 25 mg at bedtime; titrate to 100–300 mg at bedtime. Maximum dose 600 mg/day) (6,7)[A]
  - Antidepressant + lithium
    - TCA: nortriptyline (start 50 mg at bedtime; max dose 150 mg at bedtime) + lithium (start 300 mg at bedtime; max dose 900 mg BID) (1,6,8)[A]
    - SSRI: citalopram (start 20 mg/day; max dose 40 mg QD) + lithium (start 300 mg at bedtime; max dose 900 mg BID) (1,4,6)[B]
  - Antidepressant + thyroid supplementation
    - Citalopram (start 20 mg/day; max dose 40 mg/day) + triiodothyronine (T_3) (12.5–50 μg/day) (4,9)[B]
- In above combinations, citalopram (Celexa) can be replaced with other SSRIs such as fluoxetine (Prozac) 20–80 mg/day, sertraline (Zoloft) 50–200 mg/day, and escitalopram (Lexapro) 10–20 mg/day or with serotonin–norepinephrine reuptake inhibitors (SNRIs) duloxetine (Cymbalta) 30–120 mg/day or venlafaxine XR (Effexor XR) 75–225 mg/day.
- Maximum doses for medication in treatment-resistant cases may be higher than in treatment-responsive cases.

Second Line

Monamine oxidase inhibitor (MAOI)

- Tranylcypromine (Parnate): Start 10 mg BID, increase 10 mg/day every 1–3 weeks; max dose 60 mg/day
- Selegiline transdermal (Emsam patch): Apply 6-mg patch daily, increase 3 mg/day; max dose 12 mg/day

- Side-effect profile (e.g., hypertensive crisis), drug–drug interactions, and dietary restrictions make MAOIs less appealing. Patch version does not require dietary restrictions at lower doses.
- High risk of serotonin syndrome, if combined with another antidepressant; 2-week washout period is advised.

ISSUES FOR REFERRAL
Treatment-resistant depression should be managed in consultation with a psychiatrist.

ADDITIONAL THERAPIES
- First line
  - ECT: safe and effective treatment for treatment-resistant and life-threatening depression, with a 60–90% success rate (10,11)[A]:
    - Known to rapidly relieve suicidality, psychotic depression, and catatonia
    - Controversy due to cognitive side effects during the treatment
    - 3 types of lead placements
      - Bitemporal: rapid and effective. Usually need 6–10 treatments at 1.5× seizure threshold
      - Right unilateral: may be slightly less rapid but fewer cognitive side effects. Usually need 8–12 treatments at 6× seizure threshold
      - Bifrontal: newer technique that may offer similar speed to bitemporal, with slightly improved side-effect profile
- Second line
  - Deep brain stimulation (DBS): surgical implantation of intracranial electrodes, connected to an impulse generator implanted in the chest wall (12,13)[C]:
    - Reserved for those who have failed medications, psychotherapy, and ECT
    - Preliminary data are promising, showing 40–70% response rate and 35% remission rate, but further trials are warranted.
  - Transcranial magnetic stimulation (TCMS): noninvasive brain stimulation technique that is generally safe. A few case reports on efficacy in treatment-resistant depression but thus far is only FDA approved for less severe forms of the illness (8,13)[C].
  - Vagus nerve stimulation (VNS): surgical implantation of electrodes onto left vagus nerve. Its use in treatment-resistant depression has become limited in recent years (13)[C].
  - Ketamine—not FDA approved, but evidence of rapid improvement in mood and suicidal thinking in most participants, although the literature is limited. In addition, the effects of ketamine appear temporary, disappearing after days to weeks (8,14)[C].

INPATIENT CONSIDERATIONS
Admission Criteria/Initial Stabilization
Inpatient care is indicated for severely depressed, psychotic, catatonic, or suicidal patients.

Discharge Criteria
Symptoms improving, no longer suicidal, psychosocial stressors addressed

ONGOING CARE

FOLLOW-UP RECOMMENDATIONS
- Frequent visits (i.e., every month)
- During follow-up, evaluate side effects, dosage, and effectiveness of medication as well as need for referral to ECT.
- Patients who have responded to ECT may need maintenance treatments (q3–12wk) to prevent relapse.
- Combination of lithium/nortriptyline after ECT appears to be as effective as maintenance ECT in reducing relapse.

DIET
Patients on MAOIs need dietary restriction.

PATIENT EDUCATION
- Educate patients that depression is a medical illness, not a character defect.
- Review signs and symptoms of worsening depression and when patient needs to come in for further evaluation.
- Discuss safety plan to address suicidal thoughts.

PROGNOSIS
With medication adherence, close follow-up, improved social support, and psychotherapy, prognosis improves.

COMPLICATIONS
- Suicide
- Disability
- Poor quality of life

REFERENCES

1. Keller MB. Issues in treatment-resistant depression. *J Clin Psychiatry*. 2005;66(Suppl 8):5–12.
2. Kessler RC, Berglund P, Demler O, et al. The epidemiology of major depressive disorder: results from the National Comorbidity Survey Replication. *JAMA*. 2003;289(23):3095–3105.
3. Olchanski N, McInnis Myers M, Halseth M, et al. The economic burden of treatment-resistant depression. *Clinical Ther*. 2013;35(4):512–522.
4. Rush AJ. Acute and longer-term outcomes in depressed patients who require one or several treatment steps: a STAR*D report. *Am J Psychiatry*. 2006;163(11):1905–1917.
5. Trivedi MH, Fava M, Wisniewski SR, et al. Medication augmentation after the failure of SSRIs for depression. *N Engl J Med*. 2006;354(12):1243–1252.
6. Hicks P, Hicks XP, Meyer H, et al. How to best manage treatment-resistant depression? *J Fam Pract*. 2010;59(9);490–497.
7. Maglione M, Maher AR, Hu J-H, et al. *Off-Label Use of Atypical Antipsychotics: An Update*. Rockville, MD: Agency for Healthcare Research and Quality; 2011. Report No. 11-EHC087-EF. AHRQ Comparative Effectiveness Reviews.
8. Holtzheimer PE. Advances in the management of treatment-resistant depression. *FOCUS*. 2010;8(4):488–500.
9. Nierenberg AA, Fava M, Trivedi MH, et al. A comparison of lithium and T3 augmentation following two failed medication treatments for depression: a STAR*D report. *Am J Psychiatry*. 2006;163(9):1519–1530.
10. American Psychiatric Association. Practice guideline for the treatment of patients with major depressive disorder, third edition. *Am J Psychiatry*. 2010;167(10):1–118. http://psychiatryonline.org/data/Books/prac/PG_Depression3rdEd.pdf. Accessed 2014.
11. Weiner RD. *The Practice of Electroconvulsive Therapy: Recommendations for Treatment, Training, and Privileging: A Task Force Report of the American Psychiatric Association*. 2nd ed. Washington DC: American Psychiatric Association; 2001:5–25.
12. Morishita T, Fayad SM, Higuchi MA, et al. Deep brain stimulation for treatment-resistant depression: systematic review of clinical outcomes. *Neurotherapeutics*. 2014;11(3):475–84.
13. Holtzheimer PE, Mayberg HS. Deep brain stimulation for treatment-resistant depression. *Am J Psychiatry*. 2010;167(12):1437–1444.
14. Caddy C, Giaroli G, White TP, et al. Ketamine as the prototype glutamatergic antidepressant: pharmacodynamics actions, and a systematic review and meta-analysis of efficacy. *Ther Adv Psychopharmacol*. 2013;4(2):75–99.

ADDITIONAL READING

- Kasper S. Treatment-resistant depression: a challenge for future research. *Acta Neuropsychiatr*. 2014;26(3):131–133.
- Vieta E, Colom F. Therapeutic options in treatment-resistant depression. *Ann Med*. 2011;43(7):512–530.

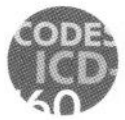

CODES

ICD10
- F32.9 Major depressive disorder, single episode, unspecified
- F33.9 Major depressive disorder, recurrent, unspecified

CLINICAL PEARLS
- Treatment-resistant depression is common, affecting 1/3 of those with MDD.
- Combination and augmentation strategies with antidepressants, antipsychotics, and mood stabilizers can be helpful.
- ECT should be considered in severe and life-threatening cases.

DERMATITIS HERPETIFORMIS

Cindy England Owen, MD • Jewell V. Gaulding, MD

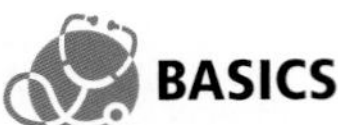

BASICS

DESCRIPTION

- Dermatitis herpetiformis (DH) is a chronic, polymorphous, intensely pruritic, erythematous papulovesicular eruption with symmetrical distribution primarily involving extensor skin surfaces of the elbows, knees, buttocks, back, and scalp.
- DH is a multifactorial disease with genetic, environmental, and immunologic influences.
- DH is distinguished from other bullous diseases by characteristic histologic and immunologic findings, as well as associated gluten-sensitive enteropathy (GSE).
- System(s) affected: skin
- Synonym(s): Duhring disease

EPIDEMIOLOGY

- Occurs most frequently in those of Northern European origin
- Rare in persons of Asian or African American origin
- Predominant age: most common in 4th decade but may present at any age
- Predominant sex: male > female (1.5:1 in the United States, 2:1 worldwide) (1)

Incidence

1/100,000 persons per year in the United States

Prevalence

11/100,000 persons in the U.S. population; as high as 39/100,000 persons worldwide

ETIOLOGY AND PATHOPHYSIOLOGY

- Evidence suggests that epidermal transglutaminase (eTG) 3, a keratinocyte enzyme involved in cell envelope formation and maintenance, is the autoantigen in DH.
- eTG is highly homologous with tissue transglutaminase (tTG), which is the antigenic target in celiac disease and GSE.
- The initiating event for DH is presumed to be the interaction of wheat peptides with tTGs, which results in the formation of an autoantigen with high affinity for particular class II major histocompatibility complex (MHC) molecules.
- Presentation of the autoantigen leads to activation of T cells and the humoral immune system.
- IgA antibodies against tTG cross-react with eTG and result in IgA-eTG immune complexes that are deposited in the papillary dermis. Subsequent activation of complement and recruitment of neutrophils to the area result in inflammation and microabscesses.
- Skin eruption may be delayed 5–6 weeks after exposure to gluten.
- Gluten applied directly to the skin does not result in the eruption, whereas gluten taken by mouth or rectum does. This implies necessary processing by the GI system.
- Thought to be immune complex–mediated disease

Genetics

- High association with human leukocyte antigen DQ2 (95%), with remaining patients being positive for DQ8, DR4, or DR3 (2)
- Strong association with combination of alleles DQA1*0501 and DQB1*0201/0202, DRB1*03 and DRB1*05/07, *or* DQA1*0301 and DQB1*0302 (2)

RISK FACTORS

- GSE: >90% of those with DH will have GSE, which may be asymptomatic.
- Family history of DH or celiac disease

GENERAL PREVENTION

Gluten-free diet (GFD) results in improvement of DH and reduces dependence on medical therapy. GFD also may reduce the risk of lymphomas associated with DH.

COMMONLY ASSOCIATED CONDITIONS

- Gluten-sensitive enteropathy, gluten ataxia
- Gastric atrophy, hypochlorhydria, pernicious anemia
- GI lymphoma, non-Hodgkin lymphoma
- Hypothyroidism, hyperthyroidism, thyroid nodules, thyroid cancer
- Down syndrome, Turner syndrome
- IgA nephropathy
- Autoimmune disorders, including systemic lupus erythematosus, dermatomyositis, Sjögren syndrome, rheumatoid arthritis, sarcoidosis, Raynaud phenomenon, insulin-dependent diabetes mellitus, myasthenia gravis, Addison disease, vitiligo, alopecia areata, primary biliary cirrhosis, and psoriasis

DIAGNOSIS

Diagnosis of DH involves a clinicopathologic correlation among clinical presentation, histologic and direct immunofluorescence evaluation, serology, and response to therapy or dietary restriction.

HISTORY

- Waxing and waning, intensely pruritic eruption with papules and tiny vesicles
- Eruption may worsen with gluten intake.
- GI symptoms may be absent or may not be reported until prompted.

PHYSICAL EXAM

- Polymorphic presentation with symmetric, grouped, erythematous papules and vesicles
- May primarily present with erosions, excoriations, lichenification, hypopigmentation, and/or hyperpigmentation secondary to scratching and healing of old lesions
- Areas involved include extensor surfaces of elbows (90%), knees (30%), shoulders, buttocks, and sacrum. The scalp is also frequently affected. Oral lesions are rare (1,2).
- In children, purpura may be visible on digits and palmoplantar surfaces.
- Adults with associated enteropathy are most often asymptomatic, with ~20% experiencing steatorrhea and <10% with findings of bloating, diarrhea, or malabsorption (3).
- Children with associated enteropathy may present with abdominal pain, diarrhea, iron deficiency, and reduced growth rate (4).

DIFFERENTIAL DIAGNOSIS

- In adults (4)
  - Bullous pemphigoid: linear deposition of C3 and IgG at the basement membrane zone
  - Linear IgA disease: homogeneous and linear deposition of IgA at the basement membrane zone, absence of GSE
  - Nodular prurigo
  - Urticaria: wheals, angioedema, dermal edema
  - Erythema multiforme
- In children (4)
  - Atopic dermatitis: face and flexural areas
  - Scabies: interdigital areas, axillae, genital region
  - Papular urticaria: dermal edema
  - Impetigo

DIAGNOSTIC TESTS & INTERPRETATION

Initial Tests (lab, imaging)

- Serum IgA tTG antibodies: Detection of tTG antibodies was noted to be up to 95% sensitive and >90% specific for DH in patients on unrestricted diets.
- Serum IgA eTG antibodies: Antibodies to eTG, the primary autoantigen in DH, were shown to be more sensitive than antibodies to tTG in the diagnosis of patients with DH on unrestricted diets (95% vs. 79%).
- Serum IgA endomysial antibodies: have a sensitivity between 50% and 100% and a specificity close to 100% in patients on unrestricted diets (4)

Follow-Up Tests & Special Considerations

Serologic assessment of anti-tTG and anti-eTG correlate with intestinal involvement of disease and in conjunction with antiendomysial antibodies (EMA) may be useful in monitoring major deviations from GFD (4,5).

Diagnostic Procedures/Other

The "gold standard" for diagnosing DH is a skin biopsy of perilesional skin evaluated via direct immunofluorescence, which demonstrates granular IgA deposited in dermal papillae and/or basement membrane (5,6).

Test Interpretation

- Direct immunofluorescence of perilesional skin reveals a granular pattern of IgA deposition in the dermal papillae (4).
- Histopathology of lesion with routine staining reveals neutrophilic microabscesses in the tips of the dermal papillae and may show subepidermal blistering (2).

TREATMENT

MEDICATION

- Disease control is achieved with dietary modification and medication.
- Medication is useful for immediate symptom management but should be used as an adjunct to dietary modification (6).
- A GFD is necessary for long-term management of underlying gluten sensitivity.

First Line

- Dapsone is approved by the FDA for use in DH and is the most widely used medication (2)[A]. Adult doses begin with 25–50 mg/day, which result in improvement of symptoms within 24–48 hours. Use minimum effective dose with slow titration based on patient response and tolerability. Average maintenance dose is 1 mg/kg/day (50–150 mg/day). Minor outbreaks on the face and scalp are common even with treatment. Not ideal for long-term use in DH.
- Dapsone works by inhibiting neutrophil recruitment and IL-8 release, inhibiting the respiratory burst of neutrophils, and protecting cells from neutrophil-mediated injury, thereby suppressing the skin reaction. It has no role in preventing IgA deposition or mitigating the immune reaction in the gut (2).

- Precautions
  - Common side effects include nausea, vomiting, headache, dizziness, weakness, and hemolysis.
  - A drop in hemoglobin of 1–2 g is characteristic with dapsone 100 mg/day.
  - G6PD deficiency increases severity of hemolytic stress. Dapsone should be avoided, if possible, in those who are G6PD-deficient.
  - Dose-related methemoglobinemia may occur with doses >100 mg/day. Cimetidine may reduce the severity of this side effect.
  - Risk of distal motor neuropathy

ALERT

- Monitor for potentially fatal dapsone-induced sulfone syndrome: fever, jaundice and hepatic necrosis, exfoliative dermatitis, lymphadenopathy, methemoglobinemia, and hemolytic anemia.
- Can occur 48 hours or 6 months after treatment, most often 5 weeks after initiation

Pediatric Considerations

- <2 years: dosing not established
- >2 years: 0.5–1.0 mg/kg/day

Pregnancy Considerations

- Category C: Safety during pregnancy is not established.
- Secreted in breast milk and will produce hemolytic anemia in infants
- Adherence to a strict GFD 6–12 months before conception should be considered with the hope of eliminating need for dapsone during pregnancy.

Second Line

Sulfapyridine (1–2 g/day) is FDA approved for use in DH and is thought to be the active metabolite in sulfasalazine (2–4 g/day) and sulfamethoxypyridazine (0.25–1.5 g/day) (7). Common side effects include nausea, vomiting, and anorexia. Enteric-coated form may reduce side effects. Other side effects include hypersensitivity reactions, hemolytic anemia, proteinuria, and crystalluria (4,7).

ISSUES FOR REFERRAL

Over time, interdisciplinary treatment may involve a dermatologist, gastroenterologist, and registered dietician. Genetic counseling and testing should be considered on diagnosis (6).

ADDITIONAL THERAPIES

GFD

- Average of 2 years is often necessary for diet to completely eliminate skin eruptions, and lesions usually recur within 12 weeks of gluten reintroduction (4).
- Fundamentals of the GFD (8)
  - Grains that should be avoided: wheat (includes spelt, kamut, semolina, and triticale), rye, and barley (including malt)
  - Safe grains (gluten-free): rice, amaranth, buckwheat, corn, millet, quinoa, sorghum, teff (an Ethiopian cereal grain), and oats
  - Sources of gluten-free starches that can be used as flour alternatives
    - Cereal grains: amaranth, buckwheat, corn, millet, quinoa, sorghum, teff, rice (white, brown, wild, basmati, jasmine), and montina
    - Tubers: arrowroot, jicama, taro, potato, and tapioca
    - Legumes: chickpeas, lentils, kidney beans, navy beans, pea beans, peanuts, and soybeans
    - Nuts: almonds, walnuts, chestnuts, hazelnuts, and cashews
    - Seeds: sunflower, flax, and pumpkin

ONGOING CARE

FOLLOW-UP RECOMMENDATIONS

Patient Monitoring

If treating with dapsone, check a baseline CBC with differential, renal function test, liver function tests, and urinalysis and then follow safety monitoring protocol. If WBC count falls below 4,000 cells/mm^3 discontinue therapy. Screening for commonly associated autoimmune conditions is also indicated (6).

DIET

- 87% of patients showed complete remission of skin manifestations after 18 months of a GFD.
- Improvement in cutaneous disease and normalization of small bowel mucosa result from strict compliance with a GFD.

PATIENT EDUCATION

- Patients on dapsone should be made aware of potential hemolytic anemia and the signs associated with methemoglobinemia.
- American Academy of Dermatology, 930 N. Meacham Road, P.O. Box 4014, Schaumberg, IL 60168-4014; (708) 330-0230
- The University of Chicago Celiac Disease Center, 5841 S. Maryland Ave., Mail Code 4069, Chicago, IL 60637; (773) 702-7593; www.celiacdisease.net or www.cureceliacdisease.org
- Gluten Intolerance Group of North America, 31214-124 Ave. SE, Auburn, WA 98092; (206) 246-6652; fax (206) 246-6531; www.gluten.net
- The Celiac Disease Foundation, 13251 Ventura Blvd., #1, Studio City, CA 9160; (818) 990-2354; fax (818) 990-2379

PROGNOSIS

- Lifelong disease with favorable prognosis
- 10–15 year survival rates do not seem to differ from general population (6).
- Remission in 10–15% (9)
- Skin disease responds readily to dapsone. Occasional new lesions (2–3/week) are to be expected and are not an indication for altering daily dosage.
- Strict adherence to a GFD improves clinical symptoms and decreases dapsone requirement. GFD is the only sustainable method of eliminating cutaneous and GI disease.
- Risk of lymphoma may be decreased in those who maintain a GFD.

COMPLICATIONS

- Malnutrition, weight loss, nutritional deficiencies (folate, B_{12}, iron)
- Abdominal pain, dyspepsia
- Osteoporosis, dental abnormalities
- Autoimmune diseases
- Lymphomas

REFERENCES

1. Bolotin D, Petronic-Rosic V. Dermatitis herpetiformis. Part I. Epidemiology, pathogenesis, and clinical presentation. *J Am Acad Dermatol*. 2011;64(6):1017–1024; quiz 1025–1026.
2. Kárpáti S. An exception within the group of autoimmune blistering diseases: dermatitis herpetiformis, the gluten-sensitive dermopathy. *Immunol Allergy Clin North Am*. 2012;32(2):255–262, vi.
3. Cardones AR, Hall RP III. Management of dermatitis herpetiformis. *Immunol Allergy Clin North Am*. 2012;32(2):275–281.
4. Caproni M, Antiga E, Melani L, et al. Guidelines for the diagnosis and treatment of dermatitis herpetiformis. *J Eur Acad Dermatol Venereol*. 2009;23(6):633–638.
5. Kárpáti S. Dermatitis herpetiformis. *Clin Dermatol*. 2012;30(1):56–59.
6. Bolotin D, Petronic-Rosic V. Dermatitis herpetiformis. Part II. Diagnosis, management, and prognosis. *J Am Acad Dermatol*. 2011;64(6):1027–1033; quiz 1033–1034.
7. Cardones AR, Hall RP III. Pathophysiology of dermatitis herpetiformis: a model for cutaneous manifestations of gastrointestinal inflammation. *Immunol Allergy Clin North Am*. 2012;32(2):263–274.
8. Green PH, Cellier C. Celiac disease. *N Engl J Med*. 2007;357(17):1731–1743.
9. Paek SY, Steinberg SM, Katz SI. Remission in dermatitis herpetiformis: a cohort study. *Arch Dermatol*. 2011;147(3):301–305.

ADDITIONAL READING

- Bonciolini V, Bonciani D, Verdelli A, et al. Newly described clinical and immunopathological feature of dermatitis herpetiformis. *Clin Dev Immunol*. 2012;2012:967974. doi:10.1155/2012/967974.
- Karell K, Korponay-Szabo I, Szalai Z, et al. Genetic dissection between coeliac disease and dermatitis herpetiformis in sib pairs. *Ann Hum Genet*. 2002;66(Pt 5–6):387–392.
- Nicolas ME, Krause PK, Gibson LE, et al. Dermatitis herpetiformis. *Int J Dermatol*. 2003;42:588–600.

SEE ALSO

- Celiac Disease
- Algorithm: Rash, Focal

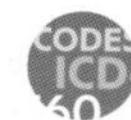

CODES

ICD10

L13.0 Dermatitis herpetiformis

CLINICAL PEARLS

- DH is a chronic, intensely pruritic, papulovesicular eruption primarily involving extensor skin surfaces.
- Strong association with gluten-sensitive enteropathy
- Skin biopsy with direct immunofluorescence demonstrating granular IgA deposits in the dermal papillae is pathognomonic.
- Serologic levels of IgA transglutaminase aid in diagnosis and monitoring of deviations from GFD.
- Mainstay of treatment is a gluten-free diet with dapsone.

DERMATITIS, ATOPIC

Dennis E. Hughes, DO, FAAFP, FACEP

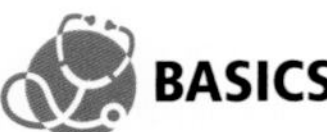

BASICS

DESCRIPTION

- A chronic, relapsing, pruritic eczematous condition affecting characteristic sites
- Early onset cases have coexisting allergen sensitization more often than late onset.
- Clinical phenotypical presentation highly variable, suggesting multifactorial pathophysiology.

EPIDEMIOLOGY

- 45% of all cases begin in the first 6 months of life with 95% onset prior to age 5 years.
- 70% of affected children will have a spontaneous remission before adolescence.
- Incidence on the rise for the past 3 decades in industrialized countries; overall, affects ~15% of children at some time (United States).
- Also, may have late-onset dermatitis in adults or relapse of childhood condition—primarily hand eczema
- Asians and blacks affected more often than whites
- 60% if one parent affected; rises to 80% if both parents affected

ETIOLOGY AND PATHOPHYSIOLOGY

- Two main hypothesis: immunologic with unbalanced immune response and/or skin barrier dysfunction (1)
- Alteration in stratum corneum results in transepidermal water loss and defect in barrier function.
- Epidermal adhesion is reduced either as a result of (a) genetic mutation resulting in altered epidermal proteins or (b) defect in immune regulation causing an altered inflammatory response.
- Interleukin-31 (IL-31) upregulation is thought to be a major factor in pruritus mediated by cytokines and neuropeptides rather than histamine excess.

Genetics

- Recent discovery of association between atopic dermatitis (AD) and mutation in the filaggrin gene (on chromosome 1), which codes for a skin barrier protein (2)
- Both epidermal and immune coding likely involved

RISK FACTORS

- "Itch–scratch cycle" (stimulates histamine release)
- Skin infections
- Emotional stress
- Irritating clothes and chemicals
- Excessively hot or cold climate
- Food allergy in children (in some cases)
- Exposure to tobacco smoke
- Family history of atopy
  - Asthma
  - Allergic rhinitis

COMMONLY ASSOCIATED CONDITIONS

- Food sensitivity/allergy in many cases
- Asthma
- Allergic rhinitis
- Hyper-IgE syndrome (Job syndrome)
  - AD
  - Elevated IgE
  - Recurrent pyodermas
  - Decreased chemotaxis of mononuclear cells

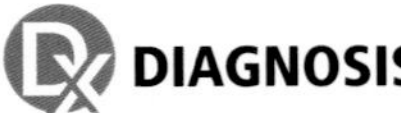

DIAGNOSIS

HISTORY

Presence of major symptoms, including relapsing of condition, family history, typical distribution, and morphology necessary to make diagnosis of AD

PHYSICAL EXAM

- Distribution of lesions
  - Infants: trunk, face, and flexural surfaces; diaper-sparing
  - Children: antecubital and popliteal fossae
  - Adults: hands, feet, face, neck, upper chest, and genital areas
- Morphology of lesions
  - Infants: erythema and papules; may develop oozing, crusting vesicles
  - Children and adults: Lichenification and scaling are typical with chronic eczema as a result of persistent scratching and rubbing (lichenification rare in infants).
- Associated signs
  - Facial erythema, mild to moderate
  - Perioral pallor
  - Infraorbital fold (Dennie sign/Morgan line)
  - Dry skin
  - Increased palmar linear markings
  - Pityriasis alba (hypopigmented asymptomatic areas on face and shoulders)
  - Keratosis pilaris

DIFFERENTIAL DIAGNOSIS

- Photosensitivity rashes
- Contact dermatitis (especially if only the face is involved)
- Scabies
- Seborrheic dermatitis (especially in infants)
- Psoriasis or lichen simplex chronicus if only localized disease is present in adults
- Rare conditions of infancy
  - Histiocytosis X
  - Wiskott-Aldrich syndrome
  - Ataxia-telangiectasia syndrome
- Ichthyosis vulgaris

DIAGNOSTIC TESTS & INTERPRETATION

Initial Tests (lab, imaging)

- No test is diagnostic.
- Serum IgE levels are elevated in as many as 80% of affected individuals, but test is not routinely ordered.
- Eosinophilia tends to correlate with disease severity.
- Scoring atopic dermatitis (SCORAD) is scoring system for AD comprising scores for area, intensity, and subjective symptoms.

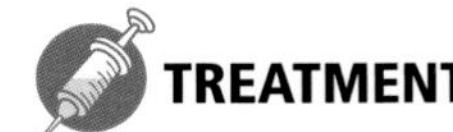

TREATMENT

GENERAL MEASURES

- Minimize flare-ups and control the duration and intensity of flare-up.
- Avoid agents that may cause irritation (e.g., wool, perfumes).
- Minimize sweating.
- Lukewarm (not hot) bathing
- Minimize use of soap (superfatted soaps best).
- Sun exposure may be helpful.
- Humidify the house.
- Avoid excessive contact with water.
- Avoid lotions that contain alcohol.
- If very resistant to treatment, search for a coexisting contact dermatitis.

Pediatric Considerations

Chronic potent fluorinated corticosteroid use may cause striae, hypopigmentation, or atrophy, especially in children.

MEDICATION

First Line

- Frequent systemic lubrication with thick emollient creams (e.g., Eucerin, Vaseline) over moist skin is the mainstay of treatment before any other intervention is considered (1),(3)[A].
- Infants and children: 0.5–1% topical hydrocortisone creams or ointments (use the "fingertip unit [FTU]" dosing) (1)

- Adults: higher potency topical corticosteroids in areas other than face and skin folds
- Short-course, higher potency corticosteroids for flares; then return to the lowest potency (creams preferred) that will control dermatitis.
- Antihistamines for pruritus (e.g., hydroxyzine 10–25 mg at bedtime and as needed)

Second Line

- Topical immunomodulators (tacrolimus or pimecrolimus) for episodic use for children >2 years. There is a black box warning from the FDA regarding potential cancer risk.
- Plastic occlusion in combination with topical medication to promote absorption
- For severe AD, consider systemic steroids × 1–2 weeks (e.g., prednisone 2 mg/kg/day PO [maximum 80 mg/d] initially, tapered over 7–14 days).
- Topical tricyclic doxepin, as a 5% cream may decrease pruritus
- Modified Goeckerman regimen (tar and ultraviolet light)
- Low-dose methotrexate established as effective treatment in adults, and recent review suggests safe for children and adolescents (4)[B]

ISSUES FOR REFERRAL

- Ophthalmology evaluation for persistent vernal conjunctivitis
- If using topical steroids around eyes for extended periods, ophthalmology follow-up for cataract evaluation

ADDITIONAL THERAPIES

- Methods to reduce house mite allergens (micropore filters on heating, ventilation, and air-conditioning systems; impermeable mattress covers)
- Behavioral relaxation therapy to reduce scratching
- Bleach baths may reduce staph colonization, but definitive evidence for benefit in the condition is lacking. Recommend 1/2 cup of standard 6% household bleach for a full tub of water, and soak for 5–10 minutes, blotting skin dry upon leaving the bath.

COMPLEMENTARY & ALTERNATIVE MEDICINE

- Evening primrose oil (includes high content of fatty acids)
  - May decrease prostaglandin synthesis
  - May promote conversion of linoleic acid to omega-6 fatty acid
- Probiotics may reduce the severity of the condition, thus reducing medication use.

ONGOING CARE

FOLLOW-UP RECOMMENDATIONS

Patient Monitoring

Evaluate to ensure that secondary bacterial or fungal infection does not develop as a result of disruption of the skin barrier. Most patients with AD are colonized by *Staphylococcus*. There is little evidence for the routine use of antimicrobial interventions to reduce skin bacteria, but treatment of clinical infection with coverage for *Staphylococcus* is recommended.

DIET

- Trials of elimination may find certain "triggers" in some patients.
- Breastfeeding in conjunction with maternal hypoallergenic diets may decrease the severity in some infants.

PATIENT EDUCATION

- http://www.aad.org/skin-conditions/dermatology-a-to-z/atopic-dermatitis
- National Eczema Association: www.nationaleczema.org

PROGNOSIS

- Chronic disease
- Declines with increasing age
- 90% of patients have spontaneous resolution by puberty.
- Localized eczema (e.g., chronic hand or foot dermatitis, eyelid dermatitis, or lichen simplex chronicus) may continue in some adults.

COMPLICATIONS

- Cataracts are more common in patients with AD.
- Skin infections (usually *Staphylococcus aureus*); sometimes subclinical
- Eczema herpeticum
  - Generalized vesiculopustular eruption caused by infection with herpes simplex or vaccinia virus
  - Causes acute illness requiring hospitalization
- Atrophy and/or striae if fluorinated corticosteroids are used on face or skin folds
- Systemic absorption may occur if large areas of skin are treated, particularly if high-potency medications and occlusion are combined.

REFERENCES

1. Thomsen SF. Atopic dermatitis: natural history, diagnosis, and treatment. *ISRN Allergy*. 2014;2014:354250.
2. Wollenberg A, Seba A, Antal AS. Immunological and molecular targets of atopic dermatitis treatment. *Br J Dermatol*. 2014;170(Suppl 1):7–11.
3. Silverberg JI. Atopic Dermatitis: an evidence-based treatment update. *Am J Clin Dermatol*. 2014;15(3):149–164.
4. Deo M, Yung A, Hill S, et al. Methotrexate for treatment of atopic dermatitis in children and adolescents. *Int J Dermatol*. 2014;53(8):1037–1041.

D

ADDITIONAL READING

- Bieber T. Atopic dermatitis. *N Engl J Med*. 2008;358(14):1483–1494.
- Boguniewicz M, Leung DY. Recent insights into atopic dermatitis and implications for management of infectious complications. *J Allergy Clin Immunol*. 2010;125(1):1–17.
- Catherine Mack Correa M, Nebus J. Management of patients with atopic dermatitis: the role of emollient therapy. *Dermatol Res Pract*. 2012;2012:836931.

SEE ALSO

Algorithm: Rash, Focal

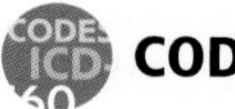

CODES

ICD10

- L20.9 Atopic dermatitis, unspecified
- L20.89 Other atopic dermatitis

CLINICAL PEARLS

- Institute early and proactive treatment to reduce inflammation.
- Monitor for secondary bacterial infection.
- Frequent systemic lubrication with thick emollient creams (e.g., Eucerin, Vaseline) over moist skin is the mainstay of treatment before any other intervention is considered.
- Use the lowest potency topical steroid that controls symptoms.

DERMATITIS, CONTACT

Aamir Siddiqi, MD

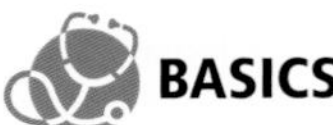

BASICS

DESCRIPTION

- A cutaneous reaction to an external substance
- Primary irritant dermatitis is due to direct injury of the skin. It affects individuals exposed to specific irritants and generally produces discomfort immediately after exposure (1).
- Allergic contact dermatitis (ACD) affects only individuals previously sensitized to a substance. It represents a delayed hypersensitivity reaction, requiring several hours for the cascade of cellular immunity to be completed to manifest itself (2).
- System(s) affected: skin/exocrine
- Synonym(s): dermatitis venenata

EPIDEMIOLOGY

Common

Incidence

Occupational contact dermatitis:
20.5/100,000 workers/year in one Australian study

Prevalence

- Contact dermatitis represents >90% of all occupational skin disorders.
- Predominant sex: male = female
  - Variations due to differences in exposure to offending agents, as well as normal cutaneous variations between males and females (eccrine and sebaceous gland function and hair distribution)

Geriatric Considerations

Increased incidence of irritant dermatitis secondary to skin dryness

Pediatric Considerations

Increased incidence of positive patch testing due to better delayed hypersensitivity reactions (3)

ETIOLOGY AND PATHOPHYSIOLOGY

Hypersensitivity reaction to a substance generating cellular immunity response (4)

- Plants
  - Urushiol (allergen): poison ivy, poison oak, poison sumac
  - Primary contact: plant (roots/stems/leaves)
  - Secondary contact: clothes/fingernails (not blister fluid)
- Chemicals
  - Nickel: jewelry, zippers, hooks, and watches
  - Potassium dichromate: tanning agent in leather
  - Paraphenylenediamine: hair dyes, fur dyes, and industrial chemicals
  - Turpentine: cleaning agents, polishes, and waxes
  - Soaps and detergents
- Topical medicines
  - Neomycin: topical antibiotics
  - Thimerosal (Merthiolate): preservative in topical medications
  - Anesthetics: benzocaine
  - Parabens: preservative in topical medications
  - Formalin: cosmetics, shampoos, and nail enamel

Genetics

Increased frequency of ACD in families with allergies

RISK FACTORS

- Occupation
- Hobbies
- Travel
- Cosmetics
- Jewelry

GENERAL PREVENTION

- Avoid causative agents.
- Use of protective gloves (with cotton lining) may be helpful.

DIAGNOSIS

HISTORY

- Itchy rash
- Assess for prior exposure to irritating substance.

PHYSICAL EXAM

- Acute
  - Papules, vesicles, bullae with surrounding erythema
  - Crusting and oozing
  - Pruritus
- Chronic
  - Erythematous base
  - Thickening with lichenification
  - Scaling
  - Fissuring
- Distribution
  - Where epidermis is thinner (eyelids, genitalia)
  - Areas of contact with offending agent (e.g., nail polish)
  - Palms and soles relatively more resistant, although hand dermatitis is common.
  - Deeper skin folds spared
  - Linear arrays of lesions
  - Lesions with sharp borders and sharp angles are pathognomonic.
- Well-demarcated area with a papulovesicular rash

DIFFERENTIAL DIAGNOSIS

- Based on clinical impression
  - Appearance, periodicity, and localization
- Groups of vesicles
  - Herpes simplex
- Diffuse bullous or vesicular lesions
  - Bullous pemphigoid
- Photodistribution
  - Phototoxic/allergic reaction to systemic allergen
- Eyelids
  - Seborrheic dermatitis
- Scaly eczematous lesions
  - Atopic dermatitis
  - Nummular eczema
  - Lichen simplex chronicus
  - Stasis dermatitis
  - Xerosis

DIAGNOSTIC TESTS & INTERPRETATION

Diagnostic Procedures/Other

Consider patch tests for suspected allergic trigger (systemic corticosteroids or recent, aggressive use of topical steroids may alter results).

Test Interpretation

- Intercellular edema
- Bullae

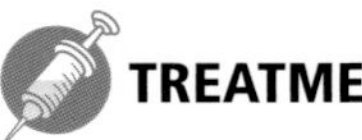

TREATMENT

GENERAL MEASURES

- Remove offending agent:
  - Avoidance
  - Work modification
  - Protective clothing
  - Barrier creams, especially high-lipid content moisturizing creams (e.g., Keri lotion, petrolatum, coconut oil)
- Topical soaks with cool tap water, Burow solution (1:40 dilution), saline (1 tsp/pt water), or silver nitrate solution
- Lukewarm water baths
- Aveeno oatmeal baths
- Emollients (white petrolatum, Eucerin)

MEDICATION

First Line

- Topical medications (5)
  - Lotion of zinc oxide, talc, menthol 0.15% (Gold Bond), phenol 0.5%
  - Corticosteroids for ACD as well as irritant dermatitis
    - High-potency steroids: fluocinonide (Lidex) 0.05% gel, cream, or ointment TID–QID
    - Use high-potency steroids only for a short time, then switch to low- or medium-potency steroid cream or ointment.
    - Caution regarding face/skin folds: Use lower potency steroids, and avoid prolonged usage. Switch to lower potency topical steroid once the acute phase is resolved.
- Calamine lotion for symptomatic relief
- Topical antibiotics for secondary infection (bacitracin, erythromycin)
- Systemic
  - Antihistamine
    - Hydroxyzine: 25–50 mg PO QID, especially useful for itching
    - Diphenhydramine: 25–50 mg PO QID
    - Cetirizine: 10 mg PO BID–TID
- Corticosteroids
  - Prednisone: Taper starting at 60–80 mg/day PO, over 10–14 days.
  - Used for moderate to severe cases
  - May use burst dose of steroids for up to 5 days
- Antibiotics for secondary skin infections
  - Dicloxacillin: 250–500 mg PO QID for 7–10 days
  - Amoxicillin-clavulanate (Augmentin): 500 mg PO BID for 7–10 days
  - Erythromycin: 250 mg PO QID in penicillin-allergic patients
  - Trimethoprim-sulfamethoxazole (Bactrim DS): 160 mg/800 mg (1 tab) PO BID for 7–10 days (suspected resistant *Staphylococcus aureus*)
- Precautions
  - Antihistamines may cause drowsiness.
  - Prolonged use of potent topical steroids may cause local skin effects (atrophy, stria, telangiectasia).
  - Use tapering dose of oral steroids if using >5 days.

Second Line

Other topical or systemic antibiotics, depending on organisms and sensitivity

Pregnancy Considerations

Usual caution with medications.

ISSUES FOR REFERRAL

May need referral to a dermatologist or allergist if refractory to conventional treatment

COMPLEMENTARY & ALTERNATIVE MEDICINE

The use of complementary and alternative treatment is a supplement and not an alternative to conventional treatment.

Admission Criteria/Initial Stabilization

Rarely needs hospital admission

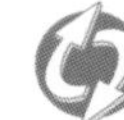

ONGOING CARE

FOLLOW-UP RECOMMENDATIONS

Stay active, but avoid overheating.

Patient Monitoring

- As necessary for recurrence
- Patch testing for etiology after resolved

DIET

No special diet

PATIENT EDUCATION

- Avoidance of irritating substance
- Cleaning of secondary sources (nails, clothes)
- Fallacy of blister fluid spreading disease

PROGNOSIS

- Self-limited
- Benign

COMPLICATIONS

- Generalized eruption secondary to autosensitization
- Secondary bacterial infection

REFERENCES

1. Ale IS, Maibacht HA. Diagnostic approach in allergic and irritant contact dermatitis. *Expert Rev Clin Immunol*. 2010;6(2):291–310.
2. Tan CH, Rasool S, Johnston GA. Contact dermatitis: allergic and irritant. *Clin Dermatol*. 2014;32(1):116–124.
3. Admani S, Jacob SE. Allergic contact dermatitis in children: review of the past decade. *Curr Allergy Asthma Rep*. 2014;14(4):421.
4. Martin SF. Contact dermatitis: from pathomechanisms to immunotoxicology. *Exp Dermatol*. 2012;21(5):382–389.
5. Usatine RP, Riojas M. Diagnosis and management of contact dermatitis. *Am Fam Physician*. 2010;82(3):249–255.

SEE ALSO

Algorithm: Rash, Focal

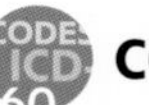

CODES

ICD10

- L25.9 Unspecified contact dermatitis, unspecified cause
- L23.9 Allergic contact dermatitis, unspecified cause
- L25.5 Unspecified contact dermatitis due to plants, except food

CLINICAL PEARLS

- Anyone exposed to irritants or allergic substances is predisposed to contact dermatitis, especially in occupations that have high exposure to chemicals.
- The most common allergens causing contact dermatitis are plants of the *Toxicodendron* genus (poison ivy, poison oak, poison sumac).
- The usual treatment for contact dermatitis is avoidance of the allergen or irritating substance and temporary use of topical steroids.
- A contact dermatitis eruption presents in a nondermatomal geographic fashion due to the skin being in contact with an external source.

DERMATITIS, DIAPER

Dennis E. Hughes, DO, FAAFP, FACEP

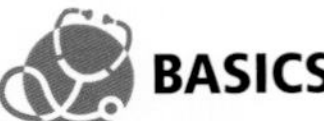

BASICS

DESCRIPTION

- Diaper dermatitis is a rash occurring under the covered area of a diaper. It is usually initially a contact dermatitis.
- System(s) affected: skin/exocrine
- Synonym(s): diaper rash; nappy rash; napkin dermatitis.

Geriatric Considerations

Incontinence is a significant cofactor.

EPIDEMIOLOGY

Incidence

- The most common dermatitis found in infancy
- Peak incidence: 7–12 months of age, then decreases
- Lower incidence reported in breastfed babies due to lower pH, urease, protease, and lipase activity.

Prevalence

Prevalence has been variably reported from 4–35% in the first 2 years of life.

ETIOLOGY AND PATHOPHYSIOLOGY

- Immature infant skin with histologic, biochemical, functional differences compared to mature skin (1)
- Wet skin is central in the development of diaper dermatitis, as prolonged contact with urine or feces results in susceptibility to chemical, enzymatic, and physical injury; wet skin is also penetrated more easily.
- Fecal proteases and lipases are irritants.
- Superhydrase urease enzyme found in the stratum corneum liberates ammonia from cutaneous bacteria.
- Fecal lipase and protease activity is increased by acceleration of GI transit; thus, a higher incidence of irritant diaper dermatitis is observed in babies who have had diarrhea in the previous 48 hours.
- Once the skin is compromised, secondary infection by *Candida albicans* is common. 40–75% of diaper rashes that last >3 days are colonized with *C. albicans*.
- Bacteria may play a role in diaper dermatitis through reduction of fecal pH and resulting activation of enzymes.
- Allergy is exceedingly rare as a cause in infants.

RISK FACTORS

- Infrequent diaper changes
- Improper laundering (cloth diapers)
- Family history of dermatitis
- Hot, humid weather
- Recent treatment with oral antibiotics
- Diarrhea (>3 stools per day increases risk)
- Dye allergy
- Eczema may increase risk.

GENERAL PREVENTION

Attention to hygiene during bouts of diarrhea

COMMONLY ASSOCIATED CONDITIONS

- Contact (allergic or irritant) dermatitis
- Seborrheic dermatitis
- Psoriasis
- Candidiasis
- Atopic dermatitis

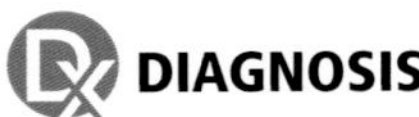

DIAGNOSIS

HISTORY

- Onset, duration, and change in the nature of the rash
- Presence of rashes outside the diaper area
- Associated scratching or crying
- Contact with infants with a similar rash
- Recent illness, diarrhea, or antibiotic use
- Fever
- Pustular drainage
- Lymphangitis

PHYSICAL EXAM

- Mild forms consist of shiny erythema ± scale.
- Margins are not always evident.
- Moderate cases have areas of papules, vesicles, and small superficial erosions.
- It can progress to well-demarcated ulcerated nodules that measure ≥1 cm in diameter.
- It is found on the prominent parts of the buttocks, medial thighs, mons pubis, and scrotum.
- Skin folds are spared or involved last.
- *Tidemark dermatitis* refers to the bandlike form of erythema of irritated diaper margins.
- Diaper dermatitis can cause an id reaction (autoeczematous) outside the diaper area.

DIFFERENTIAL DIAGNOSIS

- Contact dermatitis
- Seborrheic dermatitis
- Candidiasis
- Atopic dermatitis
- Scabies
- Acrodermatitis enteropathica
- Letterer-Siwe disease
- Congenital syphilis
- Child abuse
- Streptococcal infection
- Kawasaki disease
- Biotin deficiency
- Psoriasis
- HIV infection

DIAGNOSTIC TESTS & INTERPRETATION

Initial Tests (lab, imaging)

Rarely needed

Follow-Up Tests & Special Considerations

- Consider a culture of lesions or a potassium hydroxide (KOH) preparation.
- The finding of anemia in association with hepatosplenomegaly and the appropriate rash may suggest a diagnosis of Langerhans cell histiocytosis or congenital syphilis.
- Finding mites, ova, or feces on a mineral oil preparation of a burrow scraping can confirm the diagnosis of scabies.

Test Interpretation

- Biopsy is rare.
- Histology may reveal acute, subacute, or chronic spongiotic dermatitis.

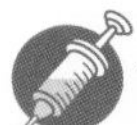

TREATMENT

Prevention is the key to treatment of this condition.

GENERAL MEASURES

- Expose the buttocks to air as much as possible.
- Use mild slightly acidic cleanser with water; no rubbing and pat dry.
- Avoid impermeable waterproof pants during treatment (day or night); they keep the skin wet and subject to rash or infection.
- Change diapers frequently, even at night, if the rash is extensive.
- Superabsorbable diapers are beneficial, as they wick urine away from skin and still allow air to permeate (2,3)[C].
- Discontinue using baby lotion, powder, ointment, or baby oil (except zinc oxide).
- Use of appropriately formulated baby wipes (fragrance-free) is safe and as effective as water.
- Apply zinc oxide ointment or other barrier cream to the rash at the earliest sign and BID or TID (e.g., Desitin or Balmex). Thereafter, apply to clean, thoroughly dried skin (3)[C].
- Cornstarch can reduce friction. Talc powders that do not enhance the growth of yeast can provide protection against frictional injury in diaper dermatitis, but do not form a continuous lipid barrier layer over the skin and obstruct the skin pores. These treatments are not recommended.

MEDICATION

First Line

- For a pure contact dermatitis, a low-potency topical steroid (hydrocortisone 0.5–1% TID for 3–5 days) and removal of the offending agent (urine, feces) should suffice.
- If candidiasis is suspected or diaper rash persists, use an antifungal such as miconazole nitrate 2% cream, miconazole powder, econazole (Spectazole), clotrimazole (Lotrimin), or ketoconazole (Nizoral) cream at each diaper change.
- If inflammation is prominent, consider a very low-potency steroid cream such as hydrocortisone 0.5–1% TID along with an antifungal cream ± a combination product such as clioquinol–hydrocortisone (Vioform–hydrocortisone) cream.
- If a secondary bacterial infection is suspected, use an antistaphylococcal oral antibiotic or mupirocin (Bactroban) ointment topically.
- Precautions: Avoid high- or moderate-potency steroids often found in combination steroid antifungal mixtures—these should never be used in the diaper area.

Second Line

Sucralfate paste for resistant cases

ISSUES FOR REFERRAL

Consider if a systemic disease such as Langerhans cell histiocytosis, acrodermatitis enteropathica, or HIV infection is suspected

INPATIENT CONSIDERATIONS

Admission Criteria/Initial Stabilization

- Febrile neonates
- Recalcitrant rash suggestive of immunodeficiency
- Toxic-appearing infants

Nursing

Assist first-time parents with hygiene education.

ONGOING CARE

FOLLOW-UP RECOMMENDATIONS

Patient Monitoring

Recheck weekly until clear; then at times of recurrence.

PATIENT EDUCATION

Patient education is vital to the treatment and prevention of recurrent cases.

PROGNOSIS

- Quick, complete clearing with appropriate treatment
- Secondary candidal infections may last a few weeks after treatment is begun.

COMPLICATIONS

- Secondary bacterial infection (consider community-acquired methicillin-resistant *Staphylococcus aureus* [MRSA] in pustular dermatitis that does not respond to normal therapy)
- Rare complication is inoculation with group A β-hemolytic *Streptococcus* resulting in necrotizing fasciitis.
- Secondary yeast infection

REFERENCES

1. Stamatas GN, Tierney NK. Diaper dermatitis: etiology, manifestations, prevention, and management. *Pediatr Dermatol*. 2014;31(1):1–7.
2. Erasala GN, Romain C, Merlay I. Diaper area and disposable diapers. *Curr Probl Dermatol*. 2011;40:83–89.
3. Humphrey S, Bergman JN, Au S. Practical management strategies for diaper dermatitis. *Skin Therapy Lett*. 2006:11(7):1–6.

ADDITIONAL READING

Serdaroglu S, Ustunbas TK. Diaper dermatitis (napkin dermatitis, nappy rash). *J Turk Acad Dermatol*. 2010;4(4):04401r.

SEE ALSO

Algorithm: Rash, Focal

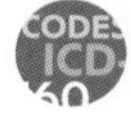

CODES

ICD10

- L22 Diaper dermatitis
- B37.2 Candidiasis of skin and nail

CLINICAL PEARLS

- Hygiene is the main preventative measure.
- Look for secondary infection in persistent cases.

D

DERMATITIS, SEBORRHEIC

Juan Qiu, MD, PhD

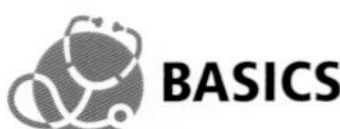

BASICS

DESCRIPTION

Chronic, superficial, recurrent inflammatory rash affecting sebum-rich, hairy regions of the body, especially scalp, eyebrows, and face

EPIDEMIOLOGY

Incidence

- Predominant age: infancy, adolescence, and adulthood
- Predominant sex: male > female

Prevalence

Seborrheic dermatitis: 3–5%

ETIOLOGY AND PATHOPHYSIOLOGY

- Skin surface yeasts *Malassezia* (formerly *Plasmodium ovale*) may be a contributing factor (1,2).
- The mite *Demodex folliculorum* may have a direct/indirect role (3).
- Genetic and environmental factors: Flares are common with stress/illness.
- Parallels increased sebaceous gland activity in infancy and adolescence or as a result of some acnegenic drugs
- Seborrheic dermatitis is more common in immunosuppressed patients, suggesting that immune mechanisms are implicated in the pathogenesis of the disease, although the mechanisms are not well defined (1).

Genetics

Positive family history; no genetic marker identified to date

RISK FACTORS

- Parkinson disease
- AIDS (disease severity correlated with progression of immune deficiency)
- Emotional stress
- Medications may flare/induce seborrheic dermatitis: auranofin, aurothioglucose, buspirone, chlorpromazine, cimetidine, ethionamide, gold, griseofulvin, haloperidol, interferon-α, lithium, methoxsalen, methyldopa, phenothiazine, psoralen, stanozolol, thiothixene, trioxsalen (2)

GENERAL PREVENTION

Seborrheic skin should be washed more often than usual.

COMMONLY ASSOCIATED CONDITIONS

- Parkinson disease
- AIDS

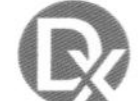

DIAGNOSIS

Diagnosis of seborrheic dermatitis usually can be made by history and physical exam.

HISTORY

- Intermittent active phases manifest with burning, scaling, and itching, alternating with inactive periods; activity is increased in winter and early spring, with remissions commonly occurring in summer.
- Infants
  - Cradle cap: greasy scaling of scalp, sometimes with associated mild erythema
  - Diaper and/or axillary rash
  - Age at onset typically ~1 month
  - Usually resolves by 8–12 months
- Adults
  - Red, greasy, scaling rash in most locations consisting of patches and plaques with indistinct margins
  - Red, smooth, glazed appearance in skin folds
  - Minimal pruritus
  - Chronic waxing and waning course
  - Bilateral and symmetric
  - Most commonly located in hairy skin areas: scalp and scalp margins, eyebrows and eyelid margins, nasolabial folds, ears and retroauricular folds, presternal area, middle to upper back, buttock crease, inguinal area, genitals, and armpits

PHYSICAL EXAM

- Scalp appearance varies from mild, patchy scaling to widespread, thick, adherent crusts. Plaques are rare.
- Seborrheic dermatitis can spread onto the forehead, the posterior part of the neck, and the postauricular skin, as in psoriasis.
- Skin lesions manifest as brawny or greasy scaling over red, inflamed skin.
- Hypopigmentation is seen in African Americans.
- Infectious eczematoid dermatitis, with oozing and crusting, suggests secondary infection.
- Seborrheic blepharitis may occur independently.

DIFFERENTIAL DIAGNOSIS

- Atopic dermatitis: Distinction may be difficult in infants.
- Psoriasis
  - Usually knees, elbows, and nails are involved.
  - Scalp psoriasis will be more sharply demarcated than seborrhea, with crusted, infiltrated plaques rather than mild scaling and erythema.
- *Candida*
- Tinea cruris/capitis: Suspect these when usual medications fail/hair loss occurs.
- Eczema of auricle/otitis externa
- Rosacea
- Discoid lupus erythematosus: Skin biopsy will be beneficial.
- Histiocytosis X: may appear as seborrheic-type eruption
- Dandruff: scalp only, noninflammatory

DIAGNOSTIC TESTS & INTERPRETATION

Diagnostic Procedures/Other

Consider biopsy if:

- Usual therapies fail
- Petechiae noted
- Histiocytosis X suspected
- Fungal cultures in refractory cases or when pustules and alopecia are present.

Test Interpretation

Nonspecific changes

- Hyperkeratosis, acanthosis, accentuated rete ridges, focal spongiosis, and parakeratosis are characteristic.
- Parakeratotic scale around hair follicles and mild superficial inflammatory lymphocytic infiltrate

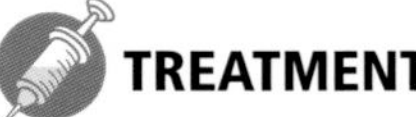

TREATMENT

GENERAL MEASURES

- Increase frequency of shampooing.
- Sunlight in moderate doses may be helpful.
- Cradle cap
  - Frequent shampooing with a mild, nonmedicated shampoo
  - Remove thick scale by applying warm mineral oil, then wash off 1 hour later with a mild soap and a soft-bristle toothbrush or terrycloth washcloth.
- Adults: Wash all affected areas with antiseborrheic shampoos. Start with over-the-counter products (selenium sulfide) and increase to more potent preparations (containing coal tar, sulfur, or salicylic acid) if no improvement is noted.
- For dense scalp scaling, 10% liquor carbonic detergens in Nivea oil may be used at bedtime, covering the head with a shower cap. This should be done nightly for 1–3 weeks.

MEDICATION

First Line

- Cradle cap: Use a coal tar shampoo or ketoconazole (Nizoral) shampoo if the nonmedicated shampoo is ineffective.
- Adults
  - Topical antifungal agents
    - Ketoconazole or miconazole 2% shampoo twice a week for clearance, then once a week or every other week for maintenance (1,4–6)[A]
    - Ketoconazole (Nizoral) and sertaconazole 2% cream may be used to clear scales in other areas (1,4–6)[A].
    - Ciclopirox 1% shampoo twice weekly (1)[A]
  - Topical corticosteroids
    - Begin with 1% hydrocortisone and advance to more potent (fluorinated) steroid preparations, as needed (1,4–6)[A].
      - Avoid continuous use of the more potent steroids to reduce the risk of skin atrophy, hypopigmentation, or systemic absorption (esp. in infants and children).
      - Precautions: Fluorinated corticosteroids and higher concentrations of hydrocortisone (e.g., 2.5%) may cause atrophy or striae if used on the face or on skin folds.
  - Other topical agents
    - Coal tar 1% shampoo twice a week
    - Selenium sulfide 2.5% shampoo twice a week (1,4–6)[A]
    - Zinc pyrithione shampoo twice a week
    - Lithium succinate ointment twice a week
- Once controlled, washing with zinc soaps or selenium lotion with periodic use of steroid cream may help to maintain remission.

Second Line

- Calcineurin inhibitors
  - Pimecrolimus 1% cream BID (7)[B]
  - Tacrolimus 0.1% ointment BID (1,4–6)[A]
- Systemic antifungal therapy
  - Data are limited.
  - For moderate to severe seborrheic dermatitis
    - Ketoconazole: 200 mg/day (8)[A]
    - Itraconazole: 200 mg/day (8)[A]
    - Daily regimen for 1–2 months followed by twice-weekly dosing for chronic treatment
    - Monitor potential hepatotoxic effects.
- Low-molecular-weight hyaluronic acid
  - Hyaluronic acid sodium salt gel 0.2% BID (9)[B]

ISSUES FOR REFERRAL

No response to 1st-line therapy and concerns regarding systemic illness (e.g., HIV)

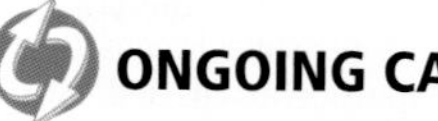

ONGOING CARE

FOLLOW-UP RECOMMENDATIONS

Patient Monitoring

Every 2–12 weeks, as necessary, depending on disease severity and degree of patient sophistication

PATIENT EDUCATION

http://familydoctor.org/familydoctor/en/diseases-conditions/seborrheic-dermatitis/treatment.html

PROGNOSIS

- In infants, seborrheic dermatitis usually remits after 6–8 months.
- In adults, seborrheic dermatitis is usually chronic and unpredictable, with exacerbations and remissions. Disease is usually easily controlled with shampoos and topical steroids.

COMPLICATIONS

- Skin atrophy/striae is possible from fluorinated corticosteroids, especially if used on the face.
- Glaucoma can result from use of fluorinated steroids around the eyes.
- Photosensitivity is caused occasionally by tars.
- Herpes keratitis is a rare complication of herpes simplex: Instruct patient to stop eyelid steroids if herpes simplex develops.

REFERENCES

1. Dessinioti C, Katsambas A. Seborrheic dermatitis: etiology, risk factors, and treatment: facts and controversies. *Clin Dermatol*. 2013:31(4):343–351.
2. Hay RJ. Malassezia, dandruff and seborrhoeic dermatitis: an overview. *Br J Dermatol*. 2011; 165(Suppl 2):2–8.
3. Karincaoglu Y, Tepe B, Kalayci B, et al. Is *Demodex folliculorum* an aetiological factor in seborrhoeic dermatitis? *Clin Exp Dermatol*. 2009;34(8): e516–e520.
4. Shin H, Kwon OS, Won CH, et al. Clinical efficacies of topical agents for the treatment of seborrheic dermatitis of the scalp: a comparative study. *J Dermatol*. 2009;36(3):131–137.
5. Stefanaki I, Katsambas A. Therapeutic update on seborrheic dermatitis. *Skin Therapy Lett*. 2010;15(5):1–4.
6. Kastarinen H, Oksanen T, Okokon EO, et al. Topical anti-inflammatory agents for seborrheic dermatitis of the face or scalp. *Cochrane Database Syst Rev*. 2014;(5):CD009446.
7. Kim GK, Rosso JD. Topical pimecrolimus 1% cream in the treatment of seborrheic dermatitis. *J Clin Aesthet Dermatol*. 2013;6(2):29–34.
8. Gupta AK, Richarson M, Paquet M. Systematic review of oral treatments for seborrheic dermatitis. *J Eur Acad Dermatol Venereol*. 2014:28(1): 16–26.
9. Schlesinger T, Rowland Powell C. Efficacy and safty of a low molecular weight hyaluronic acid topical gel in the treatment of facial seborrheic dermatitis final report. *J Clin Aesthet Dermatol*. 2014:7(5):15–18.

ADDITIONAL READING

- Bikowski J. Facial seborrheic dermatitis: a report on current status and therapeutic horizons. *J Drugs Dermatol*. 2009;8(2):125–133.
- Darabi K, Hostetler SG, Bechtel MA, et al. The role of Malassezia in atopic dermatitis affecting the head and neck of adults. *J Am Acad Dermatol*. 2009;60(1):125–136.
- Johnson BA, Nunley JR. Treatment of seborrheic dermatitis. *Am Fam Physician*. 2000;61(9):2703–2710, 2713–2714.
- Naldi L, Rebora A. Clinical practice. Seborrheic dermatitis. *N Engl J Med*. 2009;360(4):387–396.
- Shemer A, Kaplan B, Nathansohn N, et al. Treatment of moderate to severe facial seborrheic dermatitis with itraconazole: an open non-comparative study. *Isr Med Assoc J*. 2008;10(6):417–418.

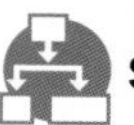

SEE ALSO

Algorithm: Rash, Focal

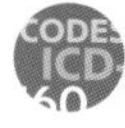

CODES

ICD10

- L21.9 Seborrheic dermatitis, unspecified
- L21.1 Seborrheic infantile dermatitis
- L21.0 Seborrhea capitis

CLINICAL PEARLS

- Search for an underlying systemic disease in a patient who is unresponsive to usual therapy.
- In adults, seborrheic dermatitis is usually chronic and unpredictable, with exacerbations and remissions. Disease is usually easily controlled with shampoos and topical steroids.

DERMATITIS, STASIS

Joseph A. Florence, MD • Fereshteh Gerayli, MD, FAAFP

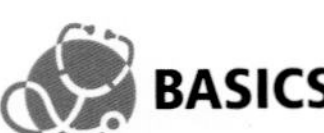

BASICS

DESCRIPTION

- Chronic, eczematous, erythema, scaling, and noninflammatory edema of the lower extremities accompanied by cycle of scratching, excoriations, weeping, crusting, and inflammation in patients with chronic venous insufficiency due to impaired circulation and other factors (nutritional edema)
- Clinical skin manifestation of chronic venous insufficiency usually appears late in the disease.
- May present as a solitary lesion
- System(s) affected: skin/exocrine
- Synonym(s): gravitational eczema; varicose eczema; venous dermatitis

EPIDEMIOLOGY

Prevalence

- In the United States: common in patients age older than 50 years (6–7%)
- Predominant age: adult, geriatric
- Predominant sex: female > male

Geriatric Considerations

Common in this age group

- Estimated to affect 15–20 million patients age older than 50 years in the United States

ETIOLOGY AND PATHOPHYSIOLOGY

- Incompetence of perforating veins causing blood to backflow to the superficial venous system leading to venous hypertension (HTN) and cutaneous inflammation
- Deposition of fibrin around capillaries
- Microvascular abnormalities
- Ischemia
- Continuous presence of edema in ankles, usually present because of venous valve incompetency (varicose veins)
- Weakness of venous walls in lower extremities
- Trauma to edematous, eczematized skin
- Itch may be caused by inflammatory mediators (from mast cells, monocytes, macrophages, or neutrophils) liberated in the microcirculation and endothelium.
- Abnormal leukocyte–endothelium interaction is proposed to be a major factor.
- A cascade of biochemical events leads to ulceration.

Genetics

Familial link probable

RISK FACTORS

- Atopy
- Superimposition of itch–scratch cycle
- Trauma
- Previous deep vein thrombosis (DVT)
- Previous pregnancy
- Prolonged medical illness
- Obesity
- Secondary infection
- Low-protein diet
- Old age
- Genetic propensity
- Chronic edema
- Tight garments that constrict the thigh
- Vein stripping
- Vein harvesting for coronary artery bypass graft surgery
- Previous cellulitis

GENERAL PREVENTION

- Use compression stockings to avoid recurrence of edema and to mobilize the interstitial lymphatic fluid from the region of stasis dermatitis and also following DVT.
- Topical lubricants twice a day to prevent fissuring and itching

COMMONLY ASSOCIATED CONDITIONS

- Varicose veins
- Venous insufficiency
- Other eczematous disease
- Hyperhomocysteinemia
- Venous HTN

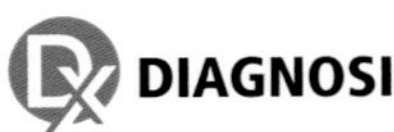

DIAGNOSIS

HISTORY

- Itching, pain, and burning may precede skin signs, which are aggravated during evening hours.
- Insidious onset
- Usually bilateral
- Description may include aching/heavy legs.
- Erythema, scaling, edema of lower extremities
- Noninflammatory edema preceded the skin eruption and ulceration.
- Edema initially develops around the ankle.

PHYSICAL EXAM

- Evaluation of the lower extremities characteristically reveals
  - Bilateral scaly, eczematous patches; papules; and/or plaques
  - Violaceous (sometimes brown), erythematous-colored lesions due to deoxygenation of venous blood (postinflammatory hyperpigmentation and hemosiderin deposition within the cutaneous tissue)
- Distribution: medial aspect of ankle, with frequent extension onto the foot and lower leg
- Brawny induration
- Stasis ulcers (frequently accompany stasis dermatitis) secondary to cuts, bruises, and excoriations to the weakened skin around the ankle
- Excoriations
- Weeping, crusting, inflammation of the skin
- Varicosities are often associated with ulcers.
- Clinical inspection reveals swelling and warmth.
- Skin changes are more common in the lower 1/3 of the extremity and medially.
- Early signs include prominent superficial veins and pitting ankle edema.
- May present as a solitary lesion mimicking a neoplasm

DIFFERENTIAL DIAGNOSIS

- Other eczematous diseases
  - Atopic dermatitis
  - Uremic dermatitis
  - Contact dermatitis (due to topical agents used to self-treat)
  - Neurodermatitis
  - Arterial insufficiency
  - Sickle cell disease causing skin ulceration
  - Cellulitis
  - Erysipelas
- Tinea dermatophyte infection
- Pretibial myxedema
- Nummular eczema
- Lichen simplex chronicus
- Xerosis
- Asteatotic eczema
- Amyopathic dermatomyositis

DIAGNOSTIC TESTS & INTERPRETATION

Initial Tests (lab, imaging)

Duplex ultrasound imaging is helpful in diagnosis.

Diagnostic Procedures/Other

Rule out arterial insufficiency (check peripheral pulses); ankle-brachial pressure index (ABPI or ABI).

Check for diabetes.

Test Interpretation

- ABPI <0.8 is suggestive of arterial insufficiency.
- ABPI can be falsely elevated in diabetic patients and others with distal small vessel calcifications.
- Arterial duplex ultrasound and angiography are the gold standards.

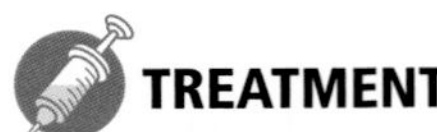

TREATMENT

GENERAL MEASURES

- Primary role of treatment is to reverse effects of venous HTN; appropriate health care
- Outpatient
  - Reduce edema
    - Leg elevation: heels higher than knees; knees higher than hips
    - Compression therapy: elastic bandage wraps: ace bandages or Unna paste boot (zinc gelatin) or compression stockings (Jobst or nonfitted type)
    - Graduated elastic compression of at least 30–40 mm Hg at the ankle improves ulcer healing rate (1)[A].
    - No specific type of topical dressing (hydrocolloid vs. simple nonadherent dressing) superior to another when used with compression therapy. Maintain moist wound environment.
    - Multilayer or bilayer compression bandages—more effective than nonelastic or short stretch bandages for severe cases
    - High compression is contraindicated in arterial insufficiency
    - Pneumatic compression devices
  - Treat infection: Debride the ulcer base of necrotic tissue.
- Improvement of lipodermatosclerosis
  - Activity
    - Avoid standing still.
    - Stay active and exercise regularly.
    - Elevate foot of bed unless contraindicated.
- Inpatient, for endovascular radiofrequency ablation, vein stripping, sclerotherapy, or skin grafts
  - Venous ulcer treatment includes autolytic, biologic, chemical, mechanical, and surgical.
    - Autolytic: hydrogels, alginates, hydrocolloids, foams, and films
    - Biologic: Topical application of granulocyte macrophage colony-stimulating factor promotes healing of ulcers.
    - Chemical: enzyme debriding agents
    - Mechanical: wet to dry dressings, hydrotherapy, and irrigation
    - Surgical: modifying cause of venous HTN (by venous ligation, valvuloplasty, and endoscopic perforator vein surgery); treat ulcer by graft.

MEDICATION

First Line

- Pentoxifylline 400 mg TID is effective in treating venous leg ulcer (2)[A].
- Enteric-coated aspirin (at least 300 mg) daily improves venous ulcer healing (3)[B].
- Use of antibiotics topically or systemically is controversial, as stasis ulcer may not be infected.
- In light of increasing bacterial resistance to antibiotics, current guidelines recommend the use of antibacterial preparations only for clinical infection (cellulitis, increased pain, warmth, malodorous exudate) not for bacterial colonization (4)[A].
- If secondary infection, treat with PO antibiotics for *Staphylococcus* or *Streptococcus* organisms (e.g., dicloxacillin 250 mg QID, cephalexin250 mg QID or 500 mg BID, or levofloxacin 250 mg daily).
- Current evidence does not support the routine use of honey- or silver-based products.
- There is no reliable evidence in the effectiveness of topical preparations such as povidone-iodine, peroxide-based preparations, mupirocin, and chlorhexidine (4)[A].
- Uncomplicated stasis dermatitis can be treated with short courses of topical steroids (5)[B] (topical triamcinolone 0.1% cream/ointment TID or betamethasone valerate 0.1% cream/ointment/solution TID).
- Topical antipruritic: pramoxine, camphor, menthol, and doxepin
- Topical anesthetic (e.g., lidocaine/prilocaine) may reduce ulcer pain.
- Systemic steroids for severe cases
- Insufficient evidence exists to either support or refute the routine use of silver sulfadiazine (SSD) for ambulatory patients with either partial-thickness burns or stasis dermatitis ulcers to decrease mortality, prevent infection, or augment wound healing.

Second Line

- Consider antibiotics on basis of culture results of exudate from infected ulcer craters.
- Lubricants when dermatitis is quiescent
- Chronic stasis dermatitis can be treated with topical emollients (e.g., white petroleum, lanolin, etc.).
- Antipruritic medications (e.g., diphenhydramine, cetirizine hydrochloride, desloratadine)

ISSUES FOR REFERRAL

Consider referral for the following:

- Nonhealing ulcer
- Arterial insufficiency
- Uncertain diagnosis
- Rheumatoid arthritis
- Patch testing to evaluate for contact dermatitis
- Associated disease (e.g., symptomatic varicose veins)

ADDITIONAL THERAPIES

If the patient is on amlodipine therapy, consider discontinuing amlodipine.

SURGERY/OTHER PROCEDURES

Sclerotherapy and surgery may be required for associated disease.

ONGOING CARE

FOLLOW-UP RECOMMENDATIONS

Patient Monitoring

If Unna boot compression is used: Cut off and reapply boot once a week. Unna boots reduce edema by compression and prevent scratching.

Regular use of high compression stockings reduces chance of recurrent venous ulcer (6)[A].

DIET

Lose weight, if overweight.

PATIENT EDUCATION

- Encourage staying active to keep circulation and leg muscles in good condition. Walking is ideal.
- Keep legs elevated while sitting or lying.
- Do not wear girdles, garters, or pantyhose with tight elastic tops.
- Do not scratch.
- Avoid leg injury.
- Elevate foot of bed with 2–4-inch blocks.
- Apply compression stockings prior to getting out of bed when less edema is present. Regular use of high compression stockings may prevent recurrence of venous ulcers.

PROGNOSIS

- Chronic course with intermittent exacerbations and remissions
- The healing process for ulceration is often prolonged and may take months.

COMPLICATIONS

- Sensations of itching, pain, and burning have negative impact on the quality of life.
- Secondary bacterial infection
- DVT
- Bleeding at dermatitis sites
- Squamous cell carcinoma in edges of long-standing stasis ulcers
- Scarring, which in turn leads to further compromise to blood flow and increased likelihood of minor trauma

REFERENCES

1. O'Meara S, Cullum N, Nelson EA, et al. Compression for venous leg ulcers. *Cochrane Database Syst Rev*. 2012;11:CD000265.
2. Jull A, Waters J, Arroll B. Pentoxifylline for treatment of venous leg ulcers: a systematic review. *Lancet*. 2002;359(9317):1550–1554.
3. Layton AM, Ibbotson SH, Davies JA, et al. Randomised trial of oral aspirin for chronic venous leg ulcers. *Lancet*. 1994;344(8916):164–165.
4. O'Meara S, Al-Kurdi D, Ovington LG, et al. Antibiotics and antiseptics for venous leg ulcers. *Cochrane Database Syst Rev*. 2014;1:CD003557.
5. Weiss SC, Nguyen J, Chon S, et al. A randomized controlled clinical trial assessing the effect of betamethasone valerate 0.12% foam on the short-term treatment of stasis dermatitis. *J Drugs Dermatol*. 2005;4(3):339–345.
6. Nelson EA, Bell-Syer SE. Compression for preventing recurrence of venous ulcers. *Cochrane Database Syst Rev*. 2012;8:CD002303.
7. Palfreyman SJ, Nelson EA, Lochiel R, et al. WITHDRAWN: dressings for healing venous leg ulcers. *Cochrane Database Syst Rev*. 2014;5:CD001103.

ADDITIONAL READING

- Coleridge-Smith PD. Leg ulcer treatment. *J Vasc Surg*. 2009;49(3):804–808.
- Coleridge-Smith P, Labropoulos N, Partsch H, et al. Duplex ultrasound investigation of the veins in chronic venous disease of the lower limbs—UIP consensus document. Part I. Basic principles. *Eur J Vasc Endovasc Surg*. 2006;31(1):83–92.
- Collins L, Seraj S. Diagnosis and treatment of venous ulcers. *Am Fam Physician*. 2010;81(8):989–996.
- Partsch H, Flour M, Smith PC; International Compression Club. Indications for compression therapy in venous and lymphatic disease consensus based on experimental data and scientific evidence. Under the auspices of the IUP. *Int Angiol*. 2008;27(3):193–219.
- Sippel K, Mayer D, Ballmer B, et al. Evidence that venous hypertension causes stasis dermatitis. *Phlebology*. 2011;26(8):361–365.

SEE ALSO

- Varicose veins
- Algorithm: rash, focal

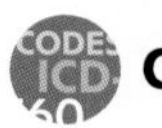

CODES

ICD10

- I83.10 Varicose veins of unsp lower extremity with inflammation
- I83.11 Varicose veins of right lower extremity with inflammation
- I83.12 Varicose veins of left lower extremity with inflammation

CLINICAL PEARLS

- Treatment of edema associated with stasis dermatitis via elevation and/or compression stockings is essential for optimal results.
- No difference in healing rate of venous stasis ulcers by use of hydrocolloid dressing versus simple nonadherent dressing when used beneath compression. Decision about the dressing should be based on local cost and patient or physician's preferences (7)[A].
- Mild topical corticosteroids reduce inflammation and itching; however, these may potentiate infection; high-potency topical corticosteroids should be avoided due to increased risk of atrophy and ulceration.

DIABETES MELLITUS, TYPE 1

Sani Mathew Roy, MD • Vibin Roy, MD

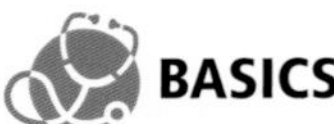

BASICS

DESCRIPTION

- Type 1 diabetes mellitus (T1DM) is a chronic disease caused by pancreatic insufficiency (deficiency) of insulin production.
- Results in hyperglycemia and end-organ complications (e.g., accelerated atherosclerosis, neuropathy, nephropathy, and retinopathy)
- Features include the following:
  - Patients are insulinopenic and require insulin.
  - Polyphagia, polydipsia, and polyuria
  - Ketosis
  - Usually rapid onset
  - Body habitus: normal or thin physique
- System(s) affected: endocrine/metabolic

Pregnancy Considerations

- Hyperglycemia increases the incidence of congenital malformations. Tight control of blood sugar prior to conception (goal A1C <7%) is important (1).
- Women with microalbuminuria during the 1st trimester are at increased risk for preeclampsia and preterm delivery.
- A safe pregnancy is possible with vaginal delivery of a term baby. Close monitoring of blood sugar during labor is important.
- Many drugs used to treat diabetic complications are relatively/absolutely contraindicated in pregnancy.

EPIDEMIOLOGY

- Age of onset peaks between 5 and 7 years of age and again around puberty. Rapid decline in incidence after adolescence
- Slightly more common in males than females
- Overall incidence is increasing worldwide.
- More cases are diagnosed in the autumn and winter than in spring and summer.

Incidence

- 18/100,000 per year in the United States (0–60/100,000 worldwide) (2)
- Average lifetime prevalence risk of T1DM in the general population is 0.4%.
- Racial predilection for whites
- African Americans have lowest overall incidence.

Pediatric Considerations

- Although onset is usually before the age of 19 years, T1DM can occur for the 1st time in patients who are well into their 30s.
- Young children are more likely to present in diabetic ketoacidosis (DKA) due to atypical presentation and because they may not express thirst or obtain fluids as readily as older children or adults.

ETIOLOGY AND PATHOPHYSIOLOGY

- Genetic predisposition is thought to exist.
- Alteration in immunologic integrity, placing the β cell at special risk for inflammatory damage
- Autoantibodies present in >90% of patients at presentation: glutamic acid decarboxylase (GAD), insulinoma-associated autoantigen 2 (IA2A), zinc transporter 8 (ZnT8A), and insulin (IAA) (2)
- Associated environmental triggers (none have been verified):
  - Vitamin D deficiency
  - Infant feeding practices (short-term breastfeeding, early exposure to complex proteins)
  - Viruses (e.g., enteroviruses, retroviruses)
  - Environmental toxins
- Various epigenetic modifications of gene expression (DNA methylation, histone modifications, and microRNA dysregulation) have been noted, further suggesting a role between genetics and environment in the development of T1DM (3).

Genetics

- T1DM is a polygenic disorder with 40+ loci known to affect susceptibility to the disease (2).
- Genes located on major histocompatibility complex (MHC) on chromosome 6 provide about half of the genetic susceptibility leading to T1DM risk (2).
- HLA class II shows the strongest association with T1DM risk, but class I MHCs also affect risk (2).

RISK FACTORS

- Certain human leukocyte antigen (HLA) types, MHC classes, and autoantibodies (2)
- Increased susceptibility to T1DM is inheritable (3):
  - Only 10–15% of newly diagnosed T1DM patients have a positive family history of T1DM.
  - Among autoimmune conditions, T1DM has the highest concordance rates in monozygotic twins.
  - Average prevalence risk of T1DM in children of patients with T1DM is ~6%.
  - Relative risk for siblings of patients with T1DM is about 15.
- See environmental triggers above (2).

COMMONLY ASSOCIATED CONDITIONS

- Autoimmune diseases, such as celiac disease vitamin B_{12} deficiency, and hypothyroidism
- T1DM can also be seen as part of autoimmune polyendocrine syndromes.

DIAGNOSIS

DIFFERENTIAL DIAGNOSIS

- Benign renal glycosuria
- Glucose intolerance
- Type 2 diabetes
- Consider monogenic diabetes if
  - Diabetes diagnosed before 6 months of age
  - Strong family history of diabetes without classic features of type 2 diabetes
  - Mild fasting hyperglycemia
  - Nonobese diabetic child with negative autoantibodies
- Secondary diabetes
  - Pancreatic disease (chronic pancreatitis, cystic fibrosis, hereditary hemochromatosis)
  - Endocrine-associated diabetes: acromegaly, Cushing syndrome, pheochromocytoma, glucagonoma, neuroendocrine tumors
  - Drug- or chemical-induced glucose intolerance: glucocorticosteroids, HIV protease inhibitors, atypical antipsychotics, tacrolimus, cyclosporine
- Acute poisonings (Salicylate poisoning can cause hyperglycemia and glycosuria and may mimic DKA.)

DIAGNOSTIC TESTS & INTERPRETATION

Initial Tests (lab, imaging)

- Criteria for the diagnosis of diabetes (1)[C]:
  - Fasting glucose >126 mg/dL (7.0 mmol/L) *or*
  - Random of >200 mg/dL (11.1 mmol/L) in a patient with classic symptoms of hyperglycemia *or*
  - Oral glucose tolerance test; plasma glucose ≥200 mg/dL 2 hours after a glucose load of 1.75 g/kg (max dose 75 g) *or*
  - Glycated hemoglobin (HbA1c) level ≥6.5%
- Other tests to consider:
  - Serum electrolytes, especially in sicker patients who may have ketoacidosis
  - Urinalysis for glucose, ketones, and microalbuminuria
  - Pancreatic autoantibodies
    - Islet cell, IAA, GAD, IA2A, and ZnT8A
  - CBC (WBC count and hemoglobin may be elevated)
- C-peptide insulin level if needed to differentiate from type 2 diabetes

Test Interpretation

Inflammatory changes, lymphocytic infiltration around the islets of Langerhans, or islet cell loss

HISTORY

- Polyuria and polydipsia (4)[C]
  - Polyuria may present as nocturia, bedwetting, or incontinence in a previously continent child.
  - Polyuria may be difficult to appreciate in diaper-clad children.
- Weight loss 10–30%
  - Often almost devoid of body fat at diagnosis due to hypovolemia and increased catabolism
- Prolonged or recurrent candidal infection, usually in the diaper area
- Increased fatigue, lethargy, muscle cramps
- Abdominal discomfort, nausea
- Vision changes, such as blurriness
- Altered school or work performance

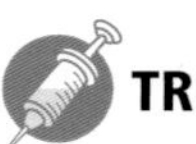

TREATMENT

GENERAL MEASURES

- Overall control of carbohydrate metabolism for the very young child (1)[B]:
  - Normoglycemia (adjusted for age): strive for blood glucose levels in range of 80–150 mg/dL (4.4–8.3 mmol/L) at all times (80–120 mg/dL in older patients)
  - Very tight control might be dangerous in young children due to risk of repeated hypoglycemia.
  - HbA1c target levels:
    - Children <6 years: <8.5%
    - Children 6–12 years: <8.0%
    - Adolescents 13–19 years: <7.5% (<7.0% if achieved without excessive hypoglycemia)
    - Adults: <7.0%
- Normal growth and development and overall good health (asymptomatic) (4)[C]:
  - Reach optimal height for genetic potential
  - Appropriate and timely pubertal maturation
  - Coping psychosocial development: normal school or work attendance and performance; normal goals/career plans. Screen children ≥10 years of age annually for depression

- Prevent acute complications, including the following:
  - Hypoglycemic insulin reactions
  - Ketoacidosis
- Delay or prevent chronic end-organ complications.

MEDICATION

- All type 1 diabetes patients will require some form of insulin supplementation.
- Types of insulin (1)[C]:
  - Long-acting insulin analogues: insulin glargine (Lantus) and insulin detemir (Levemir). These should not be mixed with other insulins in the same syringe.
  - Intermediate-acting insulin (NPH)—Humulin N or Novolin N—can be mixed with other insulins.
  - Short-acting (regular) insulin: Novolin R or Humulin R
  - Very rapid-acting insulin analogues: insulin lispro (Humalog), insulin aspart (Novolog), and insulin glulisine (Apidra)

First Line

- Flexible intensive insulin therapy is the gold standard.
- Multiple dose insulin (MDI) or continuous subcutaneous insulin infusion (CSII) have equal efficacy (1)[B].
- Total initial dose is 0.2–0.4 U/kg/day for insulin-naïve patients (will often need 0.6–0.7 U/kg/day).
- 40–60% of total dose given as basal insulin, with the rest as bolus insulin
- MDI regimen (5)[C]:
  - Basal, long-acting insulin once or twice a day
  - Prandial, short-acting insulin based on number of carbohydrate portions (e.g., 1:10, meaning 1 U of insulin for every 10 g of carbohydrate to be eaten)
  - Correctional short-acting mealtime insulin based on premeal blood glucose level (subtract target blood glucose level and divided by sensitivity factor)
  - Administration of the mealtime insulin before a meal may be more efficacious than during or after the meal.
- CSII regimen:
  - May use regular insulin or rapid-acting insulin analogues
  - Basal insulin is infused continuously at a preset rate, and bolus doses are given with meals as above.

Second Line

- Twice-daily injections with NPH along with regular or rapid-acting insulin
- Not physiologic, but lower cost and fewer injections may improve adherence in the less motivated patient.
- Premixed insulin available as NPH/regular (Novolin or Humulin 70/30) or NPH/rapid-acting insulin (e.g., Novolog 75/25 Mix or Humulin 75/25 Mix) (5)[C]
- Pancreatic transplantation is usually reserved for patients with end-stage renal failure, who may receive kidney-pancreatic transplants at the same time.
- Oral hypoglycemics not indicated in type 1 diabetes (except in obese patients, who may have a combination of type 1 and type 2): Metformin (Glucophage)

INPATIENT CONSIDERATIONS

Newly diagnosed type 1 diabetics may require hospitalization during initiation of insulin therapy.

ONGOING CARE

FOLLOW-UP RECOMMENDATIONS

- Normal; full participation in sports activities
- Regular aerobic exercise is recommended.

Patient Monitoring

- BP monitoring at every office visit. If elevated, consider an ACE inhibitor (such as Vasotec [enalapril]) or an angiotensin receptor blocker; avoid in pregnancy (1)[C]
- Monitor height, weight, and sexual maturation (in children) (5)[C].
- Daily home blood glucose monitoring with home blood glucose meter: Blood tests should be done at least 4–6 times daily (more frequently in pump patients) for optimal monitoring.
- Quarterly measurement of HbA1c
- Annual screenings (1)[C]:
  - Microalbuminuria for earliest signs of possible nephropathy
  - Ophthalmology exam (after 3–5 years of diabetes, also depending on glycemic control); annually thereafter
  - Annual lipid profile, thyroid levels, blood chemistries, CBC
  - Annual influenza vaccine in patients ≥6 months of age
  - Pneumococcal polysaccharide vaccine to all patients ≥2 years
  - Hepatitis B vaccination to unvaccinated adults aged 19–59 years

DIET

- American Diabetic Association diet: http://www.diabetes.org/food-and-fitness/food/
- Carbohydrate counting using insulin-to-carbohydrate ratio with all meals and snacks; allows patient flexibility in eating and ability to eat almost anything

PROGNOSIS

- Initial remission or honeymoon phase with decreased insulin needs and easier control, usually 3–6 months
- Current prognosis for reduced life expectancy:
  - Increasing longevity and quality of life with careful blood glucose monitoring, improvement in insulin delivery regimens, and appropriate glycemic control

COMPLICATIONS

- Microvascular disease (retinopathy, nephropathy, neuropathy)
- Hyperlipidemia
- Macrovascular disease (coronary and cerebral artery disease)
- Chronic foot ulcers/amputations
- Hypoglycemia
- DKA
- Excessive weight gain
- Increased risk for preeclampsia and preterm delivery
- Driving mishaps
- Psychological problems of chronic disease

REFERENCES

1. American Diabetes Association. Standards of medical care in diabetes. *Diabetes Care*. 2013;36(Suppl 1):S11–S65.
2. Atkinson MA, Eisenbarth GS, Michels AW. Type 1 diabetes. *Lancet*. 2014;383(9911):69–82.
3. Stankov K, Benc D, Draskovic D. Genetic and epigenetic factors in etiology of diabetes mellitus type 1. *Pediatrics*. 2013;132(6):1112–1122.
4. Silverstein J, Klingensmith G, Copeland K, et al. Care of children and adolescents with type 1 diabetes: a statement of the American Diabetes Association. *Diabetes Care*. 2005;28(1):186–212.
5. Mooradian AD, Bernbaum M, Albert SG. Narrative review: a rational approach to starting insulin therapy. *Ann Intern Med*. 2006;145(2):125–134.

ADDITIONAL READING

- Cox DJ, Ford D, Gonder-Frederick L, et al. Driving mishaps among individuals with type 1 diabetes: a prospective study. *Diabetes Care*. 2009;32(12):2177–2180.
- Gillett MJ. International Expert Committee report on the role of the A1c assay in the diagnosis of diabetes: Diabetes Care 2009;32(7):1327–1334. *Clin Biochem Rev*. 2009;30(4):197–200.
- Husebye ES, Anderson MS. Autoimmune polyendocrine syndromes: clues to type 1 diabetes pathogenesis. *Immunity*. 2010;32(4):479–487.

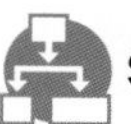

SEE ALSO

Diabetes Mellitus, Type 2; Diabetic Ketoacidosis

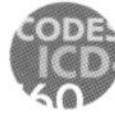

CODES

ICD10

- E10.9 Type 1 diabetes mellitus without complications
- E10.8 Type 1 diabetes mellitus with unspecified complications
- E10.69 Type 1 diabetes mellitus with other specified complication

CLINICAL PEARLS

- Polyuria may present as nocturia, bedwetting, or incontinence in a previously continent child.
- Young children are more likely to present in DKA because they may not express thirst or obtain fluids as readily as older children or adults.
- Onset usually before the age of 19 years, but type 1 diabetes can present in patients who are well into their 30s.

DIABETES MELLITUS, TYPE 2

Swathi A.N. Rao, MD • Sathya S. Krishnasamy, MD

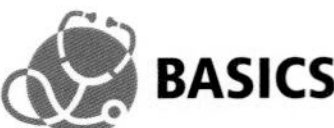

BASICS

DESCRIPTION

- Diabetes mellitus (DM) type 2 can manifest as nonketotic hyperglycemia and is due to a progressive insulin secretory defect in the setting of insulin resistance.
- Significant contributing factor to blindness, renal failure, and lower limb amputations

Geriatric Considerations

Monitor elderly for hypoglycemia; adjust doses for renal/hepatic dysfunction and cognitive function.

Pediatric Considerations

Incidence is increasing and parallels weight gain.

Pregnancy Considerations

First-line drug is insulin (class B) but may consider glyburide after the 1st trimester. Metformin may be continued through 1st trimester (class B) (1).

EPIDEMIOLOGY

Incidence

1.7 million new diagnoses/year in 2012

Prevalence

- In 2012, 29.1 million Americans or 9.3% of the population had DM; men and women equally affected
- 7.6% of non-Hispanic Caucasians, 12.8% of Hispanics, 13.2% of non-Hispanic African Americans, 9% of Asian Americans, and 15.9% of Native Americans

ETIOLOGY AND PATHOPHYSIOLOGY

- Peripheral insulin resistance
- Defective insulin secretion
- Increased gluconeogenesis
- Genetic factors: monogenic (e.g., *PPAR*γ and insulin gene mutations) and polygenic
- Obesity
- Hemochromatosis
- Drug- or chemical-induced (e.g., glucocorticoids, highly active antiretroviral therapy [HAART], atypical antipsychotics, posttransplant immunosuppressants)

Genetics

50% concordance in monozygotic twins

RISK FACTORS

- Family history: 1st-degree relative
- Gestational diabetes or history of baby with birth weight ≥4 kg (9 lb)
- Polycystic ovary syndrome (PCOS)
- Obesity (body mass index [BMI] ≥25 kg/m^2) and visceral adiposity
- Hypertriglyceridemia or low high-density lipoprotein (HDL)
- Ethnicity: African American, Latino, Native American, Asian, and Pacific Islander
- Impaired fasting glucose (IFG)/impaired glucose tolerance (IGT)
- Sedentary lifestyle
- Genetic factors

GENERAL PREVENTION

Weight loss of 5–10% body weight, exercise 150 min/week, and decrease in fat and caloric intake. Follow USDA dietary recommendation of 14 g fiber/1,000 kcal; metformin or TZDs in high-risk prediabetics with cardiovascular risk factors (1)[A]

COMMONLY ASSOCIATED CONDITIONS

Hypertension, hyperlipidemia, metabolic syndrome, fatty liver disease, infertility, PCOS, acanthosis nigricans (2)

DIAGNOSIS

HISTORY

Polyuria, polydipsia, polyphagia, weight loss, weakness, fatigue, blurry vision, and frequent infections

PHYSICAL EXAM

BMI, funduscopic exam, oral exam, cardiopulmonary exam, abdominal exam for hepatomegaly, focused neurologic exam, and diabetic foot exam

DIFFERENTIAL DIAGNOSIS

- Type 1 DM
- Cushing syndrome, acromegaly, and glucagonoma

DIAGNOSTIC TESTS & INTERPRETATION

Initial Tests (lab, imaging)

Criteria for diagnosis (2)[A]

- HbA1c ≥6.5% is diagnostic.
- Hyperglycemic crisis + random plasma glucose ≥200 mg/dL (11.1 mmol/L) *or*
- Fasting plasma glucose (FPG) ≥126 mg/dL (7.0 mmol/L) on 2 occasions *or*
- 2-hour plasma glucose ≥200 mg/dL (11.1 mmol/L) during oral glucose tolerance test (OGTT) with 75-g glucose load
- If equivocal, repeat testing.

Follow-Up Tests & Special Considerations

Screen patients with history of gestational diabetes for persistent diabetes/prediabetes 6–12 weeks postpartum with OGTT and at least every 3 years thereafter.

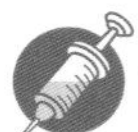

TREATMENT

- Use patient-centered approach (individualized).
- A1C targets
  - A1C <7.0: for those with a long life expectancy and no cardiovascular disease (CVD) who have had DM for a short duration and no history of hypoglycemia
  - A1C 8.0–8.5%: for those with a limited life expectancy, advanced micro- or macrovascular complications, extensive comorbidities, and a history of hypoglycemia or long-standing DM in whom the general goal is difficult to attain
- FPG goal is <110 mg/dL (5.5 mmol/L) and 2-hour postprandial goal is <140 mg/dL (American Association of Clinical Endocrinologists guidelines 2011):
  - Use drugs from different classes to achieve adequate control and limit side effects.
  - Consider the addition of insulin if FPG is not controlled by oral agents (1,2)[A].

GENERAL MEASURES

- Diabetic foot exam at every visit
- Nephropathy: annual urine microalbumin-to-creatinine ratio
- Retinopathy: annual diabetic eye exam
- If DM TI or T2 and 40–75 years old, begin a statin—moderate intensity for low-risk and high-intensity statin if greater than or equal to 7.5% ASCVD risk (3)[A]. Low-dose aspirin for all adults with CVD risk unless contraindicated.
- Hypertension: goal BP <140/80 mm Hg (SBP <130 preferred if tolerated)
- Angiotensin-converting enzyme (ACE) inhibitor/angiotensin receptor blocker: 1st-line hypertension drug. If contraindicated, consider calcium channel blocker.
- Vaccination recommendation (CDC) update: hepatitis B to unvaccinated adults age 19–59 years
- Limit protein intake to 0.8–1 g/kg body weight/day for diabetics with early stages of chronic kidney disease (CKD).
- Limit protein intake to 1 g/kg body weight/day for diabetic patients with advanced CKD.

PATIENT EDUCATION

- Diabetes self-management education and support by certified diabetes educator
- Nutritional therapy by a registered dietician
- Lifestyle modifications with pharmacotherapy delays prediabetes progression to diabetes (1,2)[A].

MEDICATION

First Line

- Biguanides
  - Metformin (Glucophage, Fortamet, Riomet, Glumetza): preferred 1st medication because it promotes weight loss and improves insulin resistance. Dosage: 500–2,000 mg in divided doses or ER 1,000–2,000 mg every evening. Maximum effective dose 2,000 mg/day.
  - Avoid metformin and combination drugs containing metformin in renal insufficiency, prior to radiocontrast agent use, surgery, and severe acute illnesses (e.g., liver disease, cardiogenic shock, pancreatitis, hypoxia) due to increased risk of lactic acidosis.
  - Caution with acute heart failure, alcohol abuse, elderly
  - Associated with GI side effects, vitamin B_{12} deficiency
- Dipeptidyl peptidase-4 inhibitors
  - Considered to be weight neutral with minimal risk for hypoglycemia; dose adjustments in renal function decline with exception of linagliptin
  - Sitagliptin (Januvia): 100 mg/day
  - Saxagliptin (Onglyza): 2.5 mg/day, maximum 5 mg/day
  - Linagliptin (Tradjenta): 5 mg/day
  - Alogliptin (Nesina) 25 mg/day
- Sulfonylureas
  - Caution with renal or liver disease, sulfa allergy, creatinine clearance <50 mL/min, pregnancy
  - Glipizide (Glucotrol): 2.5–40 mg/day. Dosage >10 mg/day given BID 30 minutes before meals
  - Glipizide extended-release: 5–20 mg/day
  - Glyburide (DiaBeta, Glynase, Micronase): 1.25–20 mg/day, Glynase 0.75–12 mg/day
  - Glimepiride (Amaryl): 1–8 mg/day
- Thiazolidinediones:
  - Obtain baseline liver function tests; if abnormal, use with caution; routine monitoring of liver function tests not recommended in those without liver disease. Contraindicated in patients with NYHA Class III or IV heart failure.
  - Pioglitazone (Actos): 15–45 mg/day. Concerns for increased risk of bladder cancer in a 5-year study, 10-year study results to be published
  - Rosiglitazone (Avandia): 4–8 mg/day

- Numerous combination products are commercially available.
  - Linagliptin/metformin (Jentadueto): 2.5/500 mg PO BID, maximum 2.5/1,000 mg PO BID
- Alogliptin + metformin significant interactions
  - Drugs that may potentiate effects of sulfonylureas: salicylates, clofibrate, warfarin (Coumadin), ethanol, and ACE inhibitors
  - Thiazides can cause IGT.
  - Fluoroquinolones have been associated with either severe hypo-/hyperglycemia.
  - Drug binders, such as cholestyramine resin, should be taken at least 2 hours apart from α-glucosidase inhibitors.

Second Line

- Insulin: rapid (aspart, lispro, glulisine), short (regular insulin), intermediate (neutral protamine hagedorn), long-acting (glargine, detemir)
  - May be used in combination with certain oral agents
  - Long-acting insulins have lower risk of hypoglycemia than short-acting insulin.
  - Insulin detemir (Levemir) or insulin glargine (Lantus): 10 units (or 0.1–0.2 units/kg) once daily in the evening or 2 divided doses; added to oral agents. Onset of action 1 hour. No peak. Duration of action 16–23 hours.
  - Combination basal/bolus insulin may be used (0.5–2 U/kg/day) after failure or oral agents.
  - Human insulin inhalation powder (Afrezza). Given as a single inhalation before a meal, in combination with long-acting insulin; contraindicated in chronic lung disease; can cause edema when given with TZDs (4)[B]
  - Concentrated human regular insulin (U-500) Eli Lilly: used for extreme insulin resistance (5)[B]
  - Consider insulin pump therapy and V-Go in select patients.
- Amylinomimetic
  - Pramlintide (Symlin): 60–120 μg SC before every major meal
  - Prandial insulins (short-acting/rapid-acting) should be reduced by 50% if pramlintide is initiated to avoid hypoglycemia.
  - Avoid anticholinergics that slow intestinal absorption of nutrients.
- GLP-1 (glucagonlike peptide-1) receptor agonist (incretins) (6)[B]
  - Exenatide (Byetta): 5–10 μg SC BID within 60 minutes before meals and at least 6 hours apart
  - Liraglutide (Victoza): 0.6 mg/day SC for 1 week, then increase to 1.2, maximum 1.8 mg/day. Less expensive and better tolerated than exenatide; should not be used in patients with personal history/family history of medullary thyroid cancer or multiple endocrine neoplasia (MEN) type 2 (black box warning).
  - Albiglutide (Tanzeum): 30–50 mg SC q week in a single-dose pen
  - Dulaglutide 0.75–1.5 mg weekly exenetide extended-release) (Bydureon): 2 mg/wk
  - Associated increased risk of acute pancreatitis with GLP-1 agonists and DPP4 inhibitors and caution with use in CKD ≥stage 4 (6)[B]. GLP-1 analogs and Symlin require insulin adjustment and may exacerbate gastroparesis.
- α-Glucosidase inhibitors
  - Acarbose (Precose): 25–100 mg TID
  - Miglitol (Glyset): 25–100 mg TID
  - Take at beginning of meals to decrease postprandial hyperglycemia.
  - Poor patient compliance due to GI symptoms
  - Avoid in renal insufficiency and bowel diseases.
- Meglitinides
  - Repaglinide (Prandin): 0.5–4 mg before meals; may be useful in patients with sulfa allergy or renal impairment
- Diphenylalanine derivatives
  - Nateglinide (Starlix): 60–120 mg before meals TID
- Bile acid sequestrants
  - Colesevelam: 3.75 g/day or 1.875 g BID
- Dopamine-2 agonists
  - Bromocriptine mesylate (Cycloset): 0.8–1.6 mg/day within 2 hours of awakening
  - Alters hypothalamic regulation of metabolism, reduces hepatic gluconeogenesis (7)[B]
  - May cause dizziness, nausea, fatigue, rhinitis
- SGLT2 Inhibitors
  - Inhibits glucose reabsorption by sodium glucose cotransporter-2 inhibition
  - Canagliflozin (Invokana) 100–300 mg single dose before breakfast; adjust dose with renal function decline
  - Dapagliflozin (Farxiga) 5–10 mg daily; avoid use if eGFR <60
  - Empagliflozin (Jardiance) 10–25 mg daily; avoid use if eGFR <45
  - May cause hypotension, genital mycotic infections, UTI, impairment of renal function

SURGERY/OTHER PROCEDURES

For patients with BMI >35 years, consider bariatric surgery (8)[B].

COMPLEMENTARY & ALTERNATIVE MEDICINE

Cinnamon may improve glycemic control, with improvements in A1C and FBG (9)[B].

ONGOING CARE

FOLLOW-UP RECOMMENDATIONS

Patient Monitoring

- Frequency of office visits at physician's discretion. Telemedicine and mobile communications on the rise. Home blood glucose monitoring with glucose testing kits is helpful with treatment titration.
- Monitor glucose, HbA1c, BP, body weight, lipid profile, and renal and liver function (10)[A].
- A1c twice a year for patients with well-controlled blood glucose and quarterly for patients with hyperglycemia or recent changes in therapy
- Consider continuous glucose monitoring as clinically indicated.

PROGNOSIS

There is evidence that intensive glycemic control in newly diagnosed diabetics may reduce long-term CVD rates.

COMPLICATIONS

- Emergencies: hyperosmolar coma, diabetic ketoacidosis (DKA), Charcot joints
- CVD: coronary artery disease, peripheral vascular disease, stroke
- Microvascular: peripheral neuropathy, proliferative retinopathy, nephropathy, erectile dysfunction, and CKD
- Ophthalmic: blindness, cataracts, glaucoma, retinopathy
- GI: nonalcoholic fatty liver disease, gastroparesis, diarrhea
- Neurologic: autonomic dysfunction
- Foot ulcers and soft tissue infections

REFERENCES

1. American Diabetes Association. Standards of medical care in diabetes—2014. *Diabetes Care*. 2014;37(Suppl 1):S14–S80.
2. Blonde L. Current antihyperglycemic treatment guidelines and algorithms for patients with type 2 diabetes mellitus. *Am J Med*. 2010;123(3 Suppl):S12–S18.
3. Handelsman Y, Mechanick JI, Blonde L, et al. American Association of Clinical Endocrinologists Medical Guidelines for Clinical Practice for developing a diabetes mellitus comprehensive care plan. *Endocr Pract*. 2011;17(Suppl 2):1–53.
4. MannKind Corporation Endocrinologic and Metabolic Drug Advisory Committee. AFREZZA® (insulin human [rDNA origin]) inhalation powder: an ultra-rapid acting insulin treatment to improve glycemic control in adult patients with diabetes mellitus. http://www.fda.gov/downloads/advisorycommittees/committeesmeetingmaterials/drugs/endocrinologicandmetabolicdrugsadvisorycommittee/ucm390865. Accessed 2014.
5. Boldo A, Comi RJ. Clinical experience with U500 insulin: risks and benefits. *Endocr Pract*. 2012;18(1):56–61.
6. Fakhoury WK, Lereun C, Wright D. A meta-analysis of placebo-controlled clinical trials assessing the efficacy and safety of incretin-based medications in patients with type 2 diabetes. *Pharmacology*. 2010;86(1):44–57.
7. Defronzo RA. Bromocriptine: a sympatholytic, d2-dopamine agonist for the treatment of type 2 diabetes. *Diabetes Care*. 2011;34(4):789–794.
8. Schauer PR, Kashyap SR, Wolski K, et al. Bariatric surgery versus intensive medical therapy in obese patients with diabetes. *N Engl J Med*. 2012;366(17):1567–1576.
9. Akilen R, Tsiami A, Devendra D, et al. Cinnamon in glycaemic control: systematic review and meta analysis. *Clin Nutr*. 2012;31(5):609–715.
10. Stone NJ, Robinson JG, Lichtenstein AH, et al. 2013 ACC/AHA guideline on the treatment of blood cholesterol to reduce atherosclerotic cardiovascular risk in adults: a report of the American College of Cardiology/American Heart Association Task Force on Practice Guidelines. *Circulation*. 2014;129(25 Suppl 2):S1–S45.

SEE ALSO

- Diabetes Mellitus, Type 1; Diabetic Ketoacidosis (DKA); Hypertension, Essential
- Algorithm: Diabetes Mellitus, Type 2

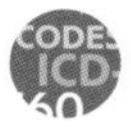

CODES

ICD10

- E11.9 Type 2 diabetes mellitus without complications
- E11.319 Type 2 diabetes mellitus with unspecified diabetic retinopathy without macular edema
- E11.21 Type 2 diabetes mellitus with diabetic nephropathy

CLINICAL PEARLS

Target A1C <7.0 for those with a long life expectancy and no CVD, who have had DM for a short duration and no history of hypoglycemia.

D

DIABETIC KETOACIDOSIS

Charmiane Lieu, MD • Melanie J. Lippmann, MD

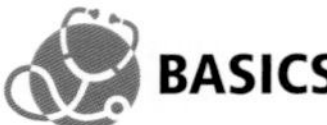

BASICS

DESCRIPTION

- A true medical emergency secondary to severe insulin deficiency and characterized by hyperglycemia, ketosis, and metabolic acidosis
- System(s) affected: endocrine/metabolic

EPIDEMIOLOGY

Incidence

- In the United States: 46 episodes/10,000 diabetics; 2/100 patient-years of type 1 diabetes mellitus (DM) (1)
- Predominant age: 19–44 years (56%) and 45–65 years (24%); only 18% are younger than 20 years.

ETIOLOGY AND PATHOPHYSIOLOGY

A deficiency of insulin, exacerbated by an increase in counterregulatory hormones (e.g., catecholamines, cortisol, glucagon, and growth hormone) leading to a hyperglycemic crisis, osmotic diuresis, and metabolic acidosis and ketosis

- Noncompliance/insufficient insulin: 25%
- Infection: 30–40%
- 1st presentation of DM: 10–20%
- Myocardial infarction (MI): 5–7%
- No cause identified: 10–30%
- Cerebrovascular accident (CVA)
- Medications (corticosteroids, thiazides, SSRI, sympathomimetics)
- Drugs (cocaine)
- Trauma
- Surgery
- Emotional stress
- Pregnancy

RISK FACTORS

- Type 1 > type 2 DM
- Younger patients at higher risk

GENERAL PREVENTION

- Close monitoring of glucose during periods of stress, infection, and trauma
- Careful insulin control and monitoring of the blood glucose level
- "Sick day" management instructions

COMMONLY ASSOCIATED CONDITIONS

Complications of chronic DM such as nephropathy, neuropathy, and retinopathy

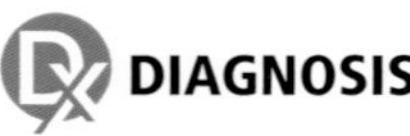

DIAGNOSIS

HISTORY

- Recent illness
- Changes in diet or medications
- Missed insulin doses/noncompliance
- Polyuria, nocturia
- Polydipsia, polyphagia
- Generalized weakness
- Malaise, lethargy
- Anorexia or increased appetite
- Nausea, vomiting
- Abdominal pain
- Decreased perspiration
- Fever

PHYSICAL EXAM

- Hypotension
- Tachycardia
- Hypothermia or fever
- Tachypnea, Kussmaul respirations
- Fruity odor to breath (acetone smell)
- Decreased reflexes
- Abdominal tenderness, decreased bowel sounds
- Dry mucous membranes, poor skin turgor
- Decreased perspiration
- Altered mental status
- Coma

DIFFERENTIAL DIAGNOSIS

- Hyperosmolar hyperglycemic crisis
- Alcoholic ketoacidosis
- Starvation ketosis
- Toxic ingestions (e.g., salicylates)
- Lactic acidosis
- Acute hypoglycemic coma
- Uremia/chronic renal failure

DIAGNOSTIC TESTS & INTERPRETATION

- ECG
  - Usually shows sinus tachycardia
  - Changes consistent with electrolyte abnormalities
  - Ischemia/MI as a precipitating factor
- Urine and blood cultures
- Consider lumbar puncture (meningitis).
- Chest x-ray to rule out possible infectious etiology

Initial Tests (lab, imaging)

ALERT

- Diagnostic criteria (1)[C]:
  - Hyperglycemia (glucose usually 250–800 mg/dL)
  - HCO_3 (usually $\leq$18 mEq/L)
  - Metabolic acidosis on arterial blood gases (pH <7.3)
  - Anion gap = serum sodium − (serum chloride + bicarbonate), > 10 mmol
- Other pertinent labs:
  - Serum ketosis: Check β-hydroxybutyrate (β-HB) instead of ketones to evaluate ketosis (2)[B]. β-HB is the predominant ketone produced and is preferred over serum ketones. β-HB >3 mg/dL is abnormal and should be decreased to <1.5 mg/dL within 12–24h (3)[B].
  - Urine ketosis (urinalysis [UA]) may only identify acetoacetate and not β-HB.
  - Glycosuria
  - Hyperamylasemia, hyperlipasemia
  - Hypertriglyceridemia/hypercholesterolemia
  - Increased creatinine and BUN: Markedly increased serum ketones may cross-react and cause a falsely high serum creatinine.
  - Pseudohyponatremia: Hyperglycemia or hypertriglyceridemia may cause an artificially low sodium concentration. The measured sodium is suppressed by 1.6 mg/dL for every 100 mg/dL of glucose over normal.
  - Decreased calculated total body K^+: Severe acidosis gives an artificially high K^+ level.
  - Increased serum osmolality (mOsm/kg)= [2 × serum Na (mEq/L) + glucose (mg/dL)/18 + BUN (mg/dL)/2.8]; if calculated osmolality <320 mOsm/kg, consider other etiologies than diabetic ketoacidosis (DKA).
  - Elevated base deficit
  - A1C helps determine history of diabetic control

- CBC, electrolytes, BUN, creatinine
- Serum β-HB or ketones
- Arterial blood gases (ABGs); venous blood gases (VBGs) may also be used (VBG pH correlates with 0.03 lower than ABG pH)
- Chest x-ray to rule out pulmonary infection
- Head CT scan if suspected CVA or cerebral edema
- If necessary, cardiac enzymes and blood cultures

Diagnostic Procedures/Other

Only if surgical problem is the underlying precipitant (e.g., appendicitis)

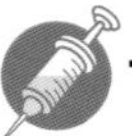

TREATMENT

- Oxygen and airway management, as needed
- Establish IV access.
- Cardiac monitoring
- Start isotonic crystalloid solution (0.9% saline).
- Fingerstick glucose testing
- Empirical naloxone if altered mental status

GENERAL MEASURES

- All but mild cases require inpatient management; severe DKA requires an ICU setting.
- Goals
  - Fluid resuscitation
  - Insulin therapy
  - Resolution of anion gap acidosis
  - Correction of electrolytes
- Attempt to find precipitating cause (i.e., source of infection).
- Laboratory testing during management:
  - Serum glucose q1–2h until stable
  - Electrolytes, phosphorus, and venous pH q2–6h as needed

MEDICATION

First Line

- Insulin (1)[C]
  - Bolus 0.1 U/kg IV then continuous infusion at 0.1 U/kg/hr
  - If without bolus, 0.14 U/kg/hr continuous infusion (4)
  - When glucose 200 mg/dL, reduce infusion to 0.02–0.05 U/kg/hr IV or give rapid-acting insulin at 0.1 U/kg SC q2h; goal glucose is 150–200 mg/dL.
  - Overlap and continue IV insulin infusion for 1–2 hours after SC insulin is initiated.
- IV fluids: Start with 0.9% NaCl bolus, calculate corrected sodium; if serum Na^+ is high, consider 0.45% NaCl to replace free fluid loss or when adding potassium replacement.
  - When glucose is 200 mg/dL, change to 5% dextrose with 0.45% NaCl at 150–250 mL/hr.
- Potassium: falsely elevated due to acidosis; when K^+ $\leq$5.2 mg/dL and if urine output is adequate, start replacement with 20–30 mEq/L of K^+ in 1 L IV fluids (1).
  - Hold insulin if K^+ $\leq$3.3 mg/dL; give IV potassium 20–30 mEq/hr with fluids until >3.3 mg/dL to prevent cardiac arrhythmia (class III).
  - For each 0.1 unit of pH, serum K^+ will change by ~0.6 mEq in opposite direction.
- Phosphorus: Routine replacement may lead to hypocalcemia; if very low (<1.0), give 20–30 mEq/L of K-Phos in fluids.

- Sodium bicarbonate: no demonstrable benefit with a pH >7.0 (2,5)[B]; rehydration usually leads to resolution of acidosis. Guidelines recommend its use with pH <6.9 or in patients with life-threatening hyperkalemia; however, there is evidence that it may increase cerebral edema especially in children (6)[A].
- Magnesium: If Mg ≤1.8 mg/dL and the patient is symptomatic, consider replacement.
- Precautions
  - If the patient is on an insulin pump, it should be stopped.
  - If glucose does not fall by 10% in 1st hour, give regular insulin 0.14 U/kg IV bolus, then continuous infusion at previous rate.
  - If using bicarbonate, add 100 mmol or 2 ampules of sodium bicarbonate to 400 mL isotonic solution with 20 mEq KCL over 200 mL/hr for 2 hours until venous pH is >7.0, then stop infusion (1).

Second Line

Insulin, SC or IM: Load with 0.3 U/kg SC, followed by 0.1 U/kg/hr. Space dosing to q2h once glucose <250 mg/dL. In uncomplicated DKA, may be safe and cost effective (7)[B].

Pediatric Considerations

- Children with moderate to severe DKA should be transferred to the nearest pediatric critical care hospital.
- Cerebral edema is a rare complication (~1%) but has mortality of 20–50%:
  - Diagnostic criteria exist for diagnosis; CT may rule out alternative diagnoses (8).
  - Treat with IV bolus of mannitol 1 g/kg in 20% solution, reduce IV fluid rate, and consider hypertonic 3% saline (9).

Geriatric Considerations

Must be careful with impaired renal function or congestive heart failure when correcting fluid and electrolyte abnormalities

Pregnancy Considerations

- Pregnancy itself is diabetogenic. It also results in a compensated respiratory alkalosis (HCO_3 19–20 mEq/L) with theoretically reduced buffering capacity. Therefore, pregnant patients are more susceptible to DKA.
- Euglycemic DKA
- Increased risk of preeclampsia and fetal death
- β-Tocolytics and corticosteroids can trigger DKA.
- Perinatal death: 9–35%

INPATIENT CONSIDERATIONS

Admission Criteria/Initial Stabilization

ADA admission guidelines: blood glucose >250 mg/dL; pH <7.3; HCO_3 ≤15 mEq/L; ketones in urine; ICU setting for severe DKA (10)

IV Fluids

- 1–1.5 L over the 1st hour, then, if serum corrected Na is high or normal, give 0.45% NaCl at 250–500 mL/hr depending on hydration state.
- Switch to 5% dextrose in 0.45% saline at maintenance rate when serum glucose <200 mg/dL. Maintain blood glucose between 150–250 mg/dL. Overly rapid correction of fluid balance may precipitate cerebral edema (2)[C]. If the blood glucose level is falling too rapidly, consider using a 10% dextrose solution instead.

Pediatric Considerations

Bolus 10–20 mL/kg initially; 4-hour fluid total should be <50 mL/kg to reduce chance of cerebral edema.

Discharge Criteria

Discharge when DKA has resolved: anion gap <12, glucose <200 mg/dL; pH >7.3; bicarbonate >18 mEq/L; additionally, patients must be tolerating PO intake and able to resume home medication regimen. Underlying precipitant (e.g., infection) must be identified and treated.

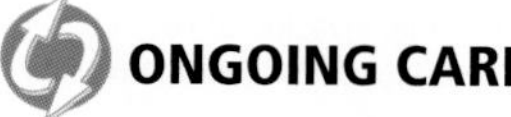

ONGOING CARE

FOLLOW-UP RECOMMENDATIONS

Bed rest

Patient Monitoring

- Monitor mental status, vital signs, and urine output q30–60min until improved, then q2–4h.
- Monitor blood sugar q1h until <200 mg/dL, then q2–6h.
- Monitor electrolytes, BUN, venous pH, and creatinine q2–4h.

DIET

- NPO initially
- Advance to preketotic diet when nausea and vomiting are controlled.
- Avoid foods with high glycemic index (e.g., soft drinks, fruit juice, white bread, etc.).

PROGNOSIS

- 16% of all diabetes-related fatalities
- Death 1–2%
- In children younger than 10 years of age, DKA causes 70% of diabetes-related fatalities.

COMPLICATIONS

- Cerebral edema (most common cause of death in children)
- Pulmonary edema
- Vascular thrombosis
- Hypokalemia
- Hypophosphatemia
- Cardiac dysrhythmia
- MI
- Acute gastric dilatation
- Late hypoglycemia (secondary to treatment)
- Erosive gastritis
- Infection, mucormycosis
- Respiratory distress

REFERENCES

1. Kitabchi AE, Umpierrez GE, Miles JM, et al. Hyperglycemic crises in adult patients with diabetes. *Diabetes Care*. 2009;32(7):1335–1343.
2. Agus MS, Wolfsdorf JI. Diabetic ketoacidosis in children. *Pediatr Clin North Am*. 2005;52(4):1147–1163, ix.
3. Trachtenbarg DE. Diabetic ketoacidosis. *Am Fam Physician*. 2005;71(9):1705–1714.
4. Kitabchi AE, Murphy MB, Spencer J, et al. Is a priming dose of insulin necessary in a low-dose insulin protocol for the treatment of diabetic ketoacidosis? *Diabetes Care*. 2008;31(11):2081–2085.
5. Kitabchi AE, Umpierrez GE, Murphy MB, et al. Hyperglycemic crises in diabetes. *Diabetes Care*. 2004;27(Suppl 1):S94–S102.
6. Chua HR, Schneider A, Bellomo R. Bicarbonate in diabetic ketoacidosis—a systematic review. *Ann Intensive Care*. 2011;1(1):23.
7. Umpierrez GE, Latif K, Stoever J, et al. Efficacy of subcutaneous insulin lispro versus continuous intravenous regular insulin for the treatment of patients with diabetic ketoacidosis. *Am J Med*. 2004;117(5):291–296.
8. Watts E. How can cerebral edema during treatment of diabetic ketoacidosis be avoided? *Pediatr Diabetes*. 2014:15(4);271–276.
9. Brown TB. Cerebral oedema in childhood diabetic ketoacidosis: is treatment a factor? *Emerg Med J*. 2004;21(2):141–144.
10. American Diabetes Association. Hospital admission guidelines for diabetes. *Diabetes Care*. 2004;27(Suppl 1):S103.

D

ADDITIONAL READING

- Agus MS, Wolfsdorf JI. Diabetic ketoacidosis in children. *Pediatr Clin North Am*. 2005;52(4):1147–1163, ix.
- American Diabetes Association. Standards of medical care in diabetes—2013. *Diabetes Care*. 2013;36(Suppl 1):S11–S66.
- Carroll MA, Yeomans ER. Diabetic ketoacidosis in pregnancy. *Crit Care Med*. 2005;33(Suppl 10):S347–S353.
- Chua HR, Schneider A, Bellomo R. Bicarbonate in diabetic ketoacidosis—a systematic review. *Ann Intensive Care*. 2011;1(1):23.
- Sheikh-Ali M, Karon BS, Basu A, et al. Can serum beta-hydroxybutyrate be used to diagnose diabetic ketoacidosis? *Diabetes Care*. 2008;31(4):643–647.

SEE ALSO

Diabetes Mellitus, Type 1

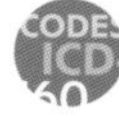

CODES

ICD10

- E10.10 Type 1 diabetes mellitus with ketoacidosis without coma
- E13.10 Oth diabetes mellitus with ketoacidosis without coma
- E10.11 Type 1 diabetes mellitus with ketoacidosis with coma

CLINICAL PEARLS

- Admit if blood glucose >250 mg/dL, pH <7.3, HCO_3 ≤15 mEq/L, and ketones in urine.
- Potassium is falsely elevated due to acidosis; start replacement when K^+ ≤5.2 mg/dL and urine output is adequate.

DIARRHEA, ACUTE

Pia Prakash, MD • Abdullah A. Al-Shahrani, MBBS • Marie L. Borum, MD, EdD, MPH

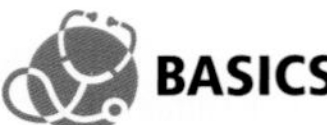

BASICS

DESCRIPTION

- Acute diarrhea is an abnormal increase in stool water content, volume, or frequency (≥3 in 24 hours) for <14 days duration.
- Acute viral diarrhea (50–70%)
  - Most common
  - Usually occurs for 1–3 days
  - Typically self-limited
- Bacterial diarrhea (15–20%)
  - Develops 6–24 hours after ingestion of contaminated food
  - Suspect when concurrent illness in others who have shared potentially contaminated food.
  - Suspect *Clostridium difficile* in patients with recent antibiotic use or hospitalization.
- Protozoal infections (10–15%)
  - Prolonged, watery diarrhea in areas with contaminated water supply
  - Consider if diarrhea lasts >7 days.
- Traveler's diarrhea typically begins 3–7 days after arrival in foreign location; rapid onset

EPIDEMIOLOGY

- In developing countries, acute diarrhea is more common in children. No age predilection in developed countries
- Acute diarrhea accounts for >128,000 U.S. hospital admissions and approximately 1.5 million worldwide deaths annually (1).

Prevalence

- 7th leading cause of death worldwide (1)
- Affects 11% of the general population
- In developing countries, acute diarrhea is most common in children aged <5 years.
- Rotavirus and adenovirus common in children aged <2 years
- In developing world, acute diarrhea is largely due to contaminated food and water supply.

ETIOLOGY AND PATHOPHYSIOLOGY

- Bacterial
  - *Escherichia coli*
  - *Salmonella*
  - *Shigella*
  - *Campylobacter jejuni*
  - *Vibrio parahaemolyticus*
  - *Vibrio cholerae*
  - *Yersinia enterocolitica*
  - *Clostridium difficile*
  - *Staphylococcus aureus*
  - *Bacillus cereus*
  - *Clostridium perfringens*
  - *Listeria monocytogenes*
- Viral
  - Rotavirus and norovirus (most common)
  - Adenovirus
  - Astrovirus
  - Cytomegalovirus (CMV) (HIV, immunocompromised)
- Protozoal
  - *Giardia lamblia*
  - *Entamoeba histolytica*
  - *Cryptosporidium*
  - *Isospora belli*
  - *Cyclospora*
  - *Microspora*
- Pathophysiology (2)
  - Noninflammatory: increased intestinal secretions without disruption of intestinal mucosa
  - Inflammatory: disrupts intestinal mucosal integrity, with subsequent tissue invasion/damage
- Viral diarrhea: changes in small intestine cell morphology that include villous shortening, increased number of crypt cells, and increased cellularity of the lamina propria
- Bacterial diarrhea: Bacterial invasion of colonic wall leads to mucosal hyperemia, edema, and leukocytic infiltration.

RISK FACTORS

- Travel to developing countries
- Immunocompromised host
- Antibiotic use
- Proton pump inhibitor (PPI) use
- Daycare attendance
- Nursing home residence
- Pregnancy (12-fold increase for *listeriosis)* (2)

GENERAL PREVENTION

- Frequent hand washing
- Proper food and water precautions, particularly during foreign travel—"boil it, peel it, cook it, or forget it."
- Avoid undercooked meats.
- Probiotics have not been shown to prevent traveler's diarrhea (3).
- Rotavirus vaccine (for infants) (4)
- Typhoid fever and cholera vaccine (for endemic areas) (5,6)

COMMONLY ASSOCIATED CONDITIONS

- Inflammatory bowel disease
- Medications
- Ileal resection
- Gastrectomy
- Hyperthyroidism
- Diabetes mellitus
- Immunocompromise (HIV, malignancy, chemotherapy)

DIAGNOSIS

HISTORY

- Duration of symptoms <14 days
- Historical clues for dehydration: orthostatic hypotension, dizziness, increased thirst, decreased urinary output, or altered mental status
- Description of stool—characteristics and output
  - Frequency
  - Quantity
  - Presence of mucus, blood, or fat
  - Consistency
  - Floating (7)[A]
- Weight loss
- Associated symptoms: change in appetite, abdominal pain or bloating, nausea/vomiting, or fever
- Recent hospitalization or antibiotic use
- Travel history
- Ingestion of
  - Raw or undercooked meat
  - Raw seafood
  - Unpasteurized milk
- Sick contacts (7)[A]
- Immunocompromise or pregnancy
- Daycare attendance
- Nursing home residence
- *Giardia* associated with abdominal cramping and pale, greasy stools; fatigue, weight loss

PHYSICAL EXAM

- General: fever, volume status
- Cardiovascular: tachycardia, orthostatic hypotension
- Abdominal: bowel sounds, abdominal distention, abdominal tenderness, masses, hepatomegaly
- Rectal: stool with blood or mucus, tenderness

Geriatric Considerations

Watery diarrhea with chronic constipation may be caused by fecal impaction or obstructing neoplasm.

DIFFERENTIAL DIAGNOSIS

- Inflammatory bowel disease
- Malabsorption
- Medications (cholinergic agents, magnesium-containing antacids, chemotherapy)
- Pseudomembranous colitis secondary to antibiotic use
- Diverticulitis
- Spastic (irritable) colon
- Fecal impaction
- Ischemic colitis
- Endocrinopathies
- Neoplasia

DIAGNOSTIC TESTS & INTERPRETATION

Initial Tests (lab, imaging)

- CBC
  - Leukocytosis may indicate infectious diarrhea.
  - Anemia from blood loss
  - Eosinophilia associated with extraintestinal migration phase of parasitic infection
- Serum electrolytes
- BUN, creatinine may be elevated secondary to volume depletion.
- Nonanion gap metabolic acidosis
- Stool sample
  - Occult blood present in inflammatory bowel disease, bowel ischemia, and certain bacterial infections
  - Fecal leukocytes
  - Stool ova and parasites
  - Stool culture
    - For bloody diarrhea, consider *Salmonella*, *Shigella*, *Campylobacter*, *E. coli* 0157:H7, *Y. enterocolitica*, *E. histolytica*.
  - *C. difficile* toxin (especially important if recent hospitalization or antibiotic use) (7)[B]
  - *Giardia* ELISA >90% sensitive in at-risk population
  - Abdominal radiographs (flat plate and upright) indicated with severe abdominal pain or if there is concern for obstruction
  - Abdominal CT scan is preferred if both intra-abdominal and intestinal disease are included in the differential diagnosis.

Diagnostic Procedures/Other

- Sigmoidoscopy or colonoscopy should be considered in patients with persistent diarrhea, when there is no clear diagnosis after routine blood and stool tests, and if empiric or supportive therapy is ineffective.
- Colonoscopy should be considered in patients with HIV to evaluate for CMV colitis.
- Colonoscopy helps to distinguish infectious diarrhea from inflammatory bowel disease.

TREATMENT

GENERAL MEASURES

- Oral rehydration and electrolyte management are key elements in successful treatment of patients with acute diarrhea (8)[A].
- Diet, as tolerated. If the gut works, use it.
- IV fluids if patient cannot tolerate oral rehydration or present with severe dehydration

MEDICATION

First Line

- Empiric antibiotics (fluoroquinolones or macrolides) should be considered in patients with signs and symptoms of systemic infection and severe cases of traveler's diarrhea as suggested by the following (9):
  - Fever
  - Bloody diarrhea
  - Presence of fecal leukocytes
  - Immunocompromised host
  - Signs of volume depletion
  - Symptoms >1 week
- Tailor antibiotic regimen according to stool culture results (10):
  - *Giardia*: metronidazole, tinidazole
  - *E. histolytica*: metronidazole
  - *Shigella*: ciprofloxacin or azithromycin
  - *Campylobacter*: azithromycin or erythromycin
  - *C. difficile*: metronidazole, PO vancomycin, or fidaxomicin
  - Traveler's diarrhea: patients without fever or dysentery: rifamixin or ciprofloxacin. Patients with fever or dysentery: azithromycin
- General considerations
  - Antibiotics are not recommended in *Salmonella* infections unless caused by *Salmonella typhosa*, or if the patient is febrile or immunocompromised.
  - Antibiotics should be avoided in patients with *E. coli* 0157:H7 due to increased risk of hemolytic-uremic syndrome.
  - Antibiotics are not indicated in foodborne toxigenic diarrhea.
  - Antimotility agents (e.g., loperamide) should generally be avoided in patients suspected of having infectious diarrhea (especially, *E. coli* 0157:H7) or antibiotic-associated colitis.
  - Antimotility agents may, however, speed recovery from traveler's diarrhea when used in combination with an antibiotic (11)[A].
- Significant medication interactions
  - Salicylate absorption from bismuth subsalicylate can cause toxicity in patients already taking aspirin-containing compounds and may alter anticoagulation control in patients taking Coumadin.
  - Avoid alcoholic beverages with metronidazole due to the possibility of a disulfiram reaction.

COMPLEMENTARY & ALTERNATIVE MEDICINE

- In patients with antibiotic-associated diarrhea, administration of a probiotic at levels above 10^{10}/g may be of use (3)[A].
- The use of probiotics is controversial in the treatment of acute diarrhea. Probiotics should be avoided in immunocompromised patients (3,12)[A].
- Zinc supplementation can decrease diarrhea-related morbidity and mortality (13)[A].

INPATIENT CONSIDERATIONS

Admission Criteria/Initial Stabilization

Outpatient management, except for patients who are severely ill with signs of volume depletion

ONGOING CARE

DIET

- Early refeeding is encouraged. Regular diets are just as effective as restricted diets.
- The traditional bananas, rice, applesauce, toast diet (BRAT diet) has little evidence-based support, despite heavy clinical use, and may result in suboptimal nutrition.
- During periods of active diarrhea, coffee, alcohol, dairy products, fruits, vegetables, red meats, and heavily seasoned foods may exacerbate symptoms.

PATIENT EDUCATION

See guidelines in "Prevention" section.

PROGNOSIS

Acute diarrhea is rarely life-threatening if adequate hydration is maintained and causative agent can be identified.

COMPLICATIONS

- Volume depletion
- Sepsis
- Shock
- Anemia
- Hemolytic uremic syndrome with *E. coli* 0157:H7
- Guillain-Barré syndrome with *C. jejuni*
- Reactive arthritis with *Salmonella*, *Shigella*, *and Yersinia*
- Functional bowel disorders (e.g., postinfectious irritable bowel syndrome [PI-IBS])

REFERENCES

1. World Health Organization. The top 10 causes of death in the world 2000-2012 fact sheet. http://www.who.int/mediacentre/factsheets/fs310/en/.
2. Barr W, Smith A. Acute diarrhea. *Am Fam Physician*. 2014;89(3):180–189.
3. Ritchie ML, Romanuk TN. A meta-analysis of probiotic efficacy for gastrointestinal diseases. *PLoS One*. 2012;7(4):e34938.
4. Soares-Weiser K, MacLehose H, Bergman H, et al. Vaccines for preventing rotavirus diarrhoea: vaccines in use. *Cochrane Database Syst Rev*. 2012;11:CD008521.
5. Anwar E, Goldberg E, Fraser A, et al. Vaccines for preventing typhoid fever. *Cochrane Database of Syst Rev*. 2014;1:CD001261.
6. Sinclair D, Abba K, Zaman K, et al. Oral vaccines for preventing cholera. *Cochrane Database Syst* Rev. 2011;3: CD008603.
7. Pawlowski SW, Warren CA, Guerrant R. Diagnosis and treatment of acute or persistent diarrhea. *Gastroenterology*. 2009;136(6):1874–1886.
8. DuPont HL. Clinical practice. Bacterial diarrhea. *N Engl J Med*. 2009;361(16):1560–1569.
9. Dryden MS, Gabb RJ, Wright SK. Empirical treatment of severe acute community-acquired gastroenteritis with ciprofloxacin. *Clin Infect Dis*. 1996;22(6):1019–1025.
10. DuPont HL. Acute infectious diarrhea in immunocompetent adults. *N Engl J Med*. 2014;370(16):1532–1540.
11. Riddle MS, Arnold S, Tribble DR. Effect of adjunctive loperamide in combination with antibiotics on treatment outcomes in traveler's diarrhea: a systematic review and meta-analysis. *Clin Infect Dis*. 2008;47(8):1007–1014.
12. Goldenberg JZ, Ma SS, Saxton JD, et al. Probiotics for the prevention of Clostridium difficile-associated diarrhea in adults and children. *Cochrane Database Syst Rev*. 2013;5:CD006095.
13. Walker CL, Black RE. Zinc for the treatment of diarrhoea: effect on diarrhoea morbidity, mortality and incidence of future episodes. *Int J Epidemiol*. 2010;39(Suppl 1):i63–i69.

D

ADDITIONAL READING

- Chen CC, Kong MS, Lai MW, et al. Probiotics have clinical, microbiologic, and immunologic efficacy in acute infectious diarrhea. *Pediatr Infect Dis J*. 2010;29(2):135–138.
- DuPont HL. Systematic review: the epidemiology and clinical features of travellers' diarrhoea. *Aliment Pharmacol Ther*. 2009;30(3):187–196.
- Johnston BC, Ma SS, Goldenberg JZ, et al. Probiotics for the prevention of *Clostridium difficile*-associated diarrhea: a systematic review and meta-analysis. *Ann Intern Med*. 2012;157(12):878–888.
- Koo HL, DuPont HL. Rifaximin: a unique gastrointestinal-selective antibiotic for enteric diseases. *Curr Opin Gastroenterol*. 2010;26(1):17–25.
- McFarland LV. Evidence-based review of probiotics for antibiotic-associated diarrhea and Clostridium difficile infections. *Anaerobe*. 2009;15(6):274–280.
- McFarland LV. Meta-analysis of probiotics for the prevention of traveler's diarrhea. *Travel Med Infect Dis*. 2007;5(2):97–105.

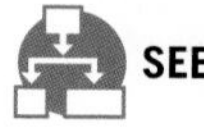

SEE ALSO

Botulism; Cholera; Food Poisoning, Bacterial

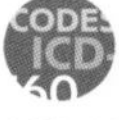

CODES

ICD10

- R19.7 Diarrhea, unspecified
- A09 Infectious gastroenteritis and colitis, unspecified
- A08.4 Viral intestinal infection, unspecified

CLINICAL PEARLS

- Viruses, especially norovirus, are the most common causes of acute diarrheal illness in the United States.
- Oral rehydration and correction of electrolyte imbalances are the most important in the treatment of acute diarrhea.
- Routine stool culture is not recommended, unless the patient presents with bloody diarrhea, fever >38.5°C, severe dehydration, signs of inflammatory disease, persistent symptoms >3–7 days, or immunosuppression.
- Empiric antibiotics should be started in patients who are severely ill or immunocompromised.

DIARRHEA, CHRONIC

Neha Jakhete, MD • M Aung S. Myint, DO • Marie L. Borum, MD, EdD, MPH

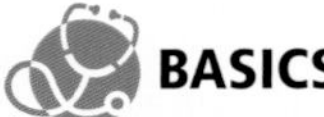

BASICS

DESCRIPTION

- Chronic diarrhea is an increase in frequency of defecation or decrease in stool consistency (typically >3 loose stools per day) for >4 weeks (1–3):
  - Etiologies include osmotic, secretory, malabsorptive, inflammatory, and hypermotility
  - Infectious etiologies are possible but less common in a chronic setting.
- System(s) affected: gastrointestinal (GI)

EPIDEMIOLOGY

Prevalence

Variable depending on etiology, but overall ~3–5% of the U.S. population is affected (3).

ETIOLOGY AND PATHOPHYSIOLOGY

In most cases, chronic diarrhea is the result of disturbances in the intestinal luminal water and electrolyte balance. This varies depending on etiology.

- Osmotic (fecal osmotic gap >125 mOsm/kg) (2,3)
  - Carbohydrate malabsorption
    - Disaccharides including lactose
    - Monosaccharides including fructose
    - Polyols including sorbitol, xylotil, sucralose and saccharin (common sugar substitutes)
    - These substances cannot be metabolized, thus creating an osmotic gradient.
  - Substances including magnesium, phosphate, sulfate
- Secretory (fecal osmotic gap <50 mOsm/kg) (2,3)
  - Stimulant laxative ingestion
  - Postcholecystectomy
    - Leads to excessive bile salts in intestinal lumen causing cholerheic diarrhea; often resolves in 6–12 months
  - Ileal bile acid malabsorption
    - Ileal resection of <100 cm leads to cholerheic diarrhea due to excessive presentation of bile salts to colon.
  - Disordered motility
    - Postvagotomy
    - Diabetic autonomic neuropathy
    - Hyperthyroidism
  - Neuroendocrine tumors
    - VIPoma
    - Gastrinoma
    - Somatostatinoma
    - Carcinoid syndrome
  - Metastatic medullary carcinoma of the thyroid
  - Systemic mastocytosis
  - Protein-losing enteropathy
- Malabsorption (2,3)
  - Whipple disease
  - Giardiasis
  - Celiac disease
  - Short bowel syndrome
    - Ileal resection of >100 cm leads to insufficient bile salt concentrations in the duodenum for optimal fat absorption, leading to fat and fat-soluble vitamin malabsorption.
  - Small intestinal bacterial overgrowth
  - Pancreatic exocrine insufficiency (CF, chronic pancreatitis)
  - Inadequate bile acid production/secretion
- Inflammatory (2,3)
  - Ulcerative colitis
  - Crohn disease
  - Microscopic colitis (lymphocytic or collagenous)
  - Vasculitis
  - Radiation enterocolitis
  - Eosinophilic enterocolitis
- Hypermotility (normal fecal osmotic gap) (1–3)
  - Irritable bowel syndrome (IBS)
  - Functional diarrhea
- Drugs: NSAIDs, colchicine, metformin, digoxin, SSRIs (3)
- Herbal products: St. John's wort, echinacea, garlic, saw palmetto, ginseng, cranberry extract, aloe vera
- Infectious (2,3)
  - Bacterial: *Clostridium difficile*, *Mycobacterium avium intracellulare*
  - Viral: cytomegalovirus
  - Parasitic: *Giardia lamblia*, *Cryptosporidium*, *Isospora*
  - Helminthic: *Strongyloides*

Genetics

- Celiac disease is associated with HLA-DQ2 and HLA-DQ8 haplotypes on major histocompatibility complex (MHC) class II antigen-presenting cells (4).
- IBD is polygenic, and genome-wide association studies demonstrate new polymorphisms (5).
- Cystic fibrosis (CF) is caused by a mutation in the CF transmembrane conductance regulator (CFTR), resulting in abnormal exocrine gland secretions.
- Familial diarrhea syndrome is linked to a missense mutation in GUCY2C resulting in hyperactivation of CFTR (6).

RISK FACTORS

- Osmotic
  - Excessive ingestion of nonabsorbable carbohydrates
  - Lactose intolerance
  - Celiac disease
- Secretory
  - Extensive small bowel resection/ileal surgery
  - History of neuroendocrine disease
  - History of stimulant laxative abuse
  - Dysmotility syndromes
- Malabsorptive
  - CF
  - Chronic alcohol abuse
  - Chronic pancreatitis/pancreatic insufficiency
  - Celiac disease
  - Medications (e.g., orlistat, acarbose)
- Inflammatory
  - Inflammatory bowel disease (IBD)
  - NSAID use
  - Thoracoabdominal radiation
  - HIV/AIDS
  - Antibiotic use
  - Immunosuppressant therapy
- Hypermotility
  - Psychosocial stress
  - Preceding infection
- Genetic predisposition

ALERT

Diabetes mellitus and history of cholecystectomy can cause both secretory and osmotic diarrhea.

GENERAL PREVENTION

- Variable depending on etiology of the diarrhea
- Treat the underlying disorder.

COMMONLY ASSOCIATED CONDITIONS

- Extraintestinal manifestations of IBD include arthralgias, aphthous stomatitis, uveitis/episcleritis, erythema nodosum, pyoderma gangrenosum, perianal fistulas, rectal fissures, ankylosing spondylitis, and primary sclerosing cholangitis.
- Celiac disease is associated with dermatitis herpetiformis.
- A significant number of patients with IBS have psychiatric comorbidities.

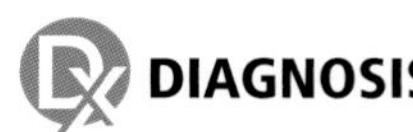

DIAGNOSIS

HISTORY

- Detailed history of symptoms, including the following (1–3):
  - Onset
  - Pattern and frequency
  - Stool volume and quality (including presence of blood or mucus)
  - Presence of nocturnal symptoms
  - Travel history
  - Antibiotic exposure
  - Dietary habits
  - Current medications
  - Family history
- Evaluate for aggravating or alleviating factors, including changes with oral intake or improvement with selective food avoidance (e.g., dairy products).
- Evaluate for recent unintentional weight loss.
- Complete review of systems, including rashes, arthritis, ocular problems, heat intolerance, polyuria/polydipsia, headache, fever, flushing, alcohol intake
- Evaluate for IBS or functional diarrhea by Rome III criteria (3):
  - IBS: recurrent abdominal pain or discomfort at least 3 days/month in last 3 months. ≥2 of the following criteria must be met:
    - Improvement with defecation
    - Onset associated with change in frequency of stool
    - Onset associated with change in form of stool
  - Functional diarrhea: loose or watery stools ≥75% of the time without pain for >3 months (symptoms >6 months)

PHYSICAL EXAM

- General: assess for volume depletion, nutritional status, recent weight loss (2,3)
- Skin: flushing (carcinoid), erythema nodosum (IBD), pyoderma gangrenosum (IBD), ecchymoses (vitamin K deficiency), dermatitis herpetiformis (celiac disease) (1–3)
- HEENT: iritis/uveitis (IBD)
- Neck: goiter (hyperthyroid), lymphadenopathy (Whipple disease)
- Cardiovascular: tachycardia (hyperthyroid)
- Pulmonary: wheezing (carcinoid)
- Abdomen: hyperactive bowel sounds (IBD), abdominal distention (IBD/IBS), diffuse tenderness (IBD/IBS)
- Anorectal: anorectal fistulas (IBD), anal fissures (IBD)
- Extremities: arthritis (IBD)
- Neurologic: tremor (hyperthyroid)

DIFFERENTIAL DIAGNOSIS

See above.

DIAGNOSTIC TESTS & INTERPRETATION

Initial Tests (lab, imaging)

- Blood: CBC with differential, electrolytes (Mg, P, Ca), total protein, albumin, thyroid-stimulating hormone (TSH), free T_4, erythrocyte sedimentation rate, iron studies (2,3)
- Stool: WBCs, culture, ova and parasites, *Giardia* stool antigen, *C. difficile* toxin, stool electrolytes (fecal osmotic gap), fecal occult blood, qualitative fecal fat (Sudan stain) (2,3).

- Plain film of the abdomen to evaluate for obstruction, toxic megacolon, bowel ischemia (1)
- CT to rule out chronic pancreatitis if abnormal pancreatic enzymes or evidence of malabsorption (1,2)

Follow-Up Tests & Special Considerations

- Celiac disease: antiendomysial antibody IgA, antitissue transglutaminase (TTG) IgA, antigliadin (AGA) IgA, serum IgA (10% of celiac patients have IgA deficiency that may result in false-negative results) (4)[A]
- Chronic pancreatic insufficiency: fecal elastase (2)[A]
- Protein-losing enteropathy: fecal α_1 antitrypsin (2)[A]
- Carbohydrate malabsorption: fecal pH (3)[A]
- Small bowel overgrowth: hydrogen breath test
- Prior history of hospitalization or antibiotics: *C. difficile* toxin (3)[A]
- HIV ELISA, special stains for *Isospora* and *Cryptosporidium* (2)[A]
- Allergy testing (2)[C]
- Neuroendocrine tumor
  - Serum: chromogranin A, VIP, gastrin (1,3)
  - Urine: 5-HIAA, histamine (1,3)

Diagnostic Procedures/Other

- Colonoscopy with ileal intubation and biopsies: to diagnose IBD, microscopic colitis, CMV colitis, and colorectal neoplasia (7)[A]
- Flexible sigmoidoscopy: especially if pregnant, with comorbidities, or if left-sided symptoms predominate (tenesmus and urgency) (7)[A]
- Esophagogastroduodenoscopy (EGD) with small bowel biopsies if malabsorption suspected:
  - Celiac, *Giardia* infection, Crohn disease, eosinophilic gastroenteropathy, Whipple disease, intestinal amyloid, pancreatic insufficiency (7)[A]
- Capsule endoscopy if further evaluation of small bowel is needed (7)[C]
- Upper GI series with small bowel follow-through
- CT or magnetic resonance (MR) enterography (1,2)

Test Interpretation

- Celiac disease: Marsh classification:
  - Intraepithelial lymphocytosis, crypt hyperplasia, villous atrophy (4)
- Crohn disease: cobblestoning, linear ulcerations, skip lesions, noncaseating granulomas
- Ulcerative colitis: crypt abscesses, superficial inflammation
- Lymphocytic colitis: increased intraepithelial infiltration of lymphocytes, increased inflammatory cells within the lamina propria, normal mucosal architecture (8)
- Melanosis coli suggests laxative abuse (2).

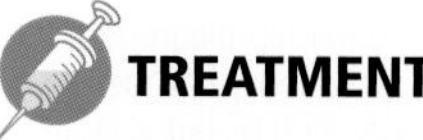

TREATMENT

GENERAL MEASURES

- Volume resuscitation if depleted (2)[A]
- Electrolyte replacement if indicated (2)[A]
- If the patient is stable, therapy is generally outpatient.

MEDICATION

First Line

- Based on underlying cause:
  - Lactose intolerance: lactose-free diet (9)[A]
  - Cholecystectomy or ileal resection: cholestyramine or colestipol (10)[A]
  - Diabetes: aggressive diabetes management and glucose control
  - Hyperthyroidism: methimazole, propylthiouracil (PTU), thyroid ablation
  - *C. difficile*: vancomycin PO or metronidazole (Flagyl) or fidaxomicin (newer therapy)
  - *G. lamblia*: metronidazole or nitazoxanide (2)[A]
  - Whipple disease: ceftriaxone IV for 14 days then Bactrim DS PO for 1–2 years (11)[A]
  - Small intestinal bacterial overgrowth: rifaximin, fluoroquinolones, metronidazole, penicillins (12)[A]
  - Pancreatic insufficiency: pancreatic enzyme replacement (1)[A]
  - HIV/AIDS: antiretroviral therapy
  - Microscopic colitis: budesonide, mesalamine, Pepto-Bismol (8)[A]
  - IBD: 5-aminosalicylic acid (5-ASA), corticosteroids (short-term only), antibiotics (short-term only), immunomodulators (6-mercaptopurine [6-MP], azathioprine, methotrexate), anti-TNF therapy (infliximab, adalimumab, certolizumab) (5)[A]
  - Neuroendocrine tumor: octreotide (2,13)[A]
  - Celiac disease: gluten-free diet (wheat/barley/rye avoidance) (4)[A]
  - IBS diarrhea predominant: antidiarrheals (14)[A]
- Symptom relief:
  - Loperamide (Imodium)
  - Diphenoxylate-atropine (Lomotil) (2)[A]

SURGERY/OTHER PROCEDURES

- Resection of neuroendocrine tumors (13)[A]
- Intestinal resection for medically refractory IBD

COMPLEMENTARY AND ALTERNATIVE MEDICINE

Many homeopathic and naturopathic formulations are available to treat diarrhea; however, most have not been evaluated by the FDA.

ONGOING CARE

DIET

Abstain from gluten-containing foods, nonabsorbable carbohydrates, lactose-containing products, and food allergens depending of etiology of diarrhea.

PATIENT EDUCATION

- Reassure patient of wide variation in what is accepted as "normal" bowel habits.
- Restrict colon stimulants.
- Dietary changes as appropriate
- Specific education based on underlying etiology

PROGNOSIS

Depends on etiology

COMPLICATIONS

- Fluid and electrolyte abnormalities (1,3)
- Malnutrition (1)
- Anemia (1,3)
- Malignancy (colon cancer in IBD, small bowel cancer in celiac disease and Crohn disease, lymphoma with IBD therapies) (5)
- Infection with immunomodulator, biologic, and corticosteroid therapies for IBD (5)

REFERENCES

1. Schiller LR. Definitions, pathophysiology, and evaluation of chronic diarrhea. *Best Pract Res Clin Gastroenterol*. 2012;26(5):551–562.
2. Fine KD, Schiller LR. AGA technical review on the evaluation and management of chronic diarrhea. *Gastroenterology*. 1999;116(6):1464–1486.
3. Juckett G, Trivedi R. Evaluation of chronic diarrhea. *Am Fam Physician*. 2011;84(10):1119–1126.
4. Rubio-Tapia A, Hill ID, Kelly CP, et al. ACG clinical guidelines: diagnosis and management of celiac disease. *Am J Gastroenterol*. 2013;108(5):656–676.
5. Talley NJ, Abreu MT, Achkar JP, et al. An evidence-based systematic review on medical therapies for inflammatory bowel disease. *Am J Gastroenterol*. 2011;106(Suppl 1):S2–S25.
6. Fiskerstrand T, Arshad N, Haukanes BI, et al. Familial diarrhea syndrome caused by an activating GUCY2C mutation. *N Engl J Med*. 2012;366(17):1586–1595.
7. American Society for Gastrointestinal Endoscopy Standards of Practice Committee, Shen B, Khan K, Ikenberry SO, et al. The role of endoscopy in the management of patients with diarrhea. *Gastrointest Endosc*. 2010;71(6):887–892.
8. Temmerman F, Baert F. Collagenous and lymphocytic colitis: systematic review and update of the literature. *Dig Dis*. 2009;27(Suppl 1):137–145.
9. Shaukat A, Levitt M, Taylor BC, et al. Systematic review: effective management strategies for lactose intolerance. *Ann Intern Med*. 2010;152(12):797–803.
10. Wilcox C, Turner J, Green J. Systematic review: the management of chronic diarrhea due to bile acid malabsorption. *Aliment Pharmacol Ther*. 2014;39(9):923–939.
11. Fenollar F, Puéchal X, Raoult D. Whipple's disease. *N Engl J Med*. 2007;356(1):55–66.
12. Fan X, Sellin JH. Review article: small intestinal bacterial overgrowth, bile acid malabsorption and gluten intolerance as possible causes of chronic watery diarrhea. *Aliment Pharmacol Ther*. 2009;29(10):1069–1077.
13. Sidéris L, Dubé P, Rinke A. Antitumor effects of somatostatin analogs in neuroendocrine tumors. *The Oncologist*. 2012;17(6):747–755.
14. Grundmann O, Yoon SL. Irritable bowel syndrome: epidemiology, diagnosis and treatment: an update for health-care practitioners. *J Gastroenterol Hepatol*. 2010;25(4):691–699.

SEE ALSO

Algorithm: Diarrhea, Chronic

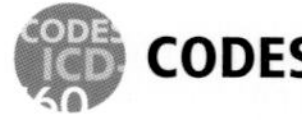

CODES

ICD10

K52.9 Noninfective gastroenteritis and colitis, unspecified

CLINICAL PEARLS

- In patients with chronic diarrhea, consider IBS, IBD, malabsorption syndromes (such as lactose intolerance), celiac disease, and chronic infections (particularly in patients who are immunocompromised).
- A thorough medical history guides the appropriate workup.
- Consider over-the-counter medications and herbal products as potential causative agents.

DIFFUSE INTERSTITIAL LUNG DISEASE

Jacqueline L. Olin, MS, PharmD, BCPS, CPP, CDE, FASHP • Brian Hertz, MD • J. Andrew Woods, PharmD, BCPS

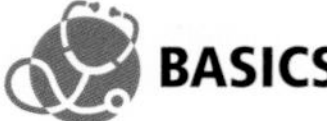

BASICS

DESCRIPTION

- Interstitial lung diseases (ILDs) represent a diverse group of chronic progressive lung diseases associated with alveolar inflammation and/or potentially irreversible pulmonary fibrosis.
- >200 individual diseases may present with similar characteristics, making ILD difficult to classify.
- A classification scheme proposed by the American Thoracic Society and European Respiratory Society includes these subtypes:
  - Known causes (environmental, occupational, or drug-associated disease)
  - Systemic disorders (e.g., sarcoidosis, Wegener granulomatosis, collagen vascular disease)
  - Rare lung diseases (e.g., pulmonary histiocytosis, lymphangioleiomyomatosis)
  - Idiopathic interstitial pneumonias (IIPs)
- Based on clinical, radiologic, and histologic features, IIPs are further subclassified into the following diagnoses (1):
  - Major IIPs, including Idiopathic pulmonary fibrosis (IPF), nonspecific interstitial pneumonia (NSIP), respiratory bronchiolitis–associated ILD (cryptogenic organizing pneumonia [COP], etc.)
  - Rare IIPs
  - Unclassifiable IIPs
- Classification of IIPs and relationships between the subtypes are difficult to classify due to mixed patterns of injury (1).

Pediatric Considerations

ILD in infants and children represents a heterogeneous group of respiratory disorders. Diseases result from a variety of processes involving genetic factors and inflammatory or fibrotic responses, and these processes are distinct from those that cause ILD in adults (2). Some diseases result from developmental disorders and growth abnormalities in infancy (2,3). After common causes are excluded, referral of infants to a subspecialist is recommended (2).

EPIDEMIOLOGY

Incidence

- Exact incidence is difficult to determine because of differences in case definitions and procedures used in diagnosis.
- Ranges cited for incidence of IPF: 4.6–10.7/100,000 (4) and pediatric ILD of 1.32/1,000,000 (3)

Prevalence

- Exact prevalence is difficult to determine because of differences in case definitions and procedures used in diagnosis.
- Ranges cited for prevalence of IPF: 2–29 cases/100,000 in the general population (4) and pediatric ILD of 3.6/1 million (3)

ETIOLOGY AND PATHOPHYSIOLOGY

- Alveolar inflammation may progress into irreversible fibrosis.
- Varying degrees of ventilatory dysfunction occur among the ILD subtypes.
- ILD associated with collagen vascular disease and systemic connective disorders can manifest involvement of skin, joints, muscular, and ocular systems.

Some types of ILD are associated with specific exposures:

- Medications (amiodarone, antibiotics [especially nitrofurantoin], chemotherapy agents, gold, illicit drugs)
- Inorganic dusts (silicates, asbestos, talc, mica, coal dust, graphite)
- Organic dusts (moldy hay, inhalation of fungi, bacteria, animal proteins)
- Metals (tin, aluminum, cobalt, iron, barium)
- Gases, fumes, vapors, aerosols

Genetics

Some subtypes of ILD may be associated with specific predisposing genes and environmental exposures; however, the role of genetic factors is unknown.

RISK FACTORS

- Environmental or occupational exposure to inorganic or organic dusts
- 66–75% of patients with ILD have a history of smoking.
- Due to diversity of diseases, age is not a reliable predictor of pathology:
  - Most patients with connective tissue disease–related pathology and inherited subtypes present between ages 20 and 40 years.
  - Median age of patients with IPF is 66 years. Studies of clinical predictors of survival including age, ethnicity, and smoking status have been inconsistent (5).

GENERAL PREVENTION

Avoiding environmental/occupational exposure to organic or inorganic dust and smoking cessation may reduce incidence or improve clinical course in patients with established ILD.

COMMONLY ASSOCIATED CONDITIONS

Many systemic disorders and primary diseases are associated with ILD. A partial list includes the following:

- Collagen vascular disease
- Sarcoidosis
- Amyloidosis
- Goodpasture syndrome
- Churg-Strauss syndrome
- Wegener granulomatosis

DIAGNOSIS

- Diagnosis should be based on clinical, radiologic, and histologic data.
- A multidisciplinary consensus is recommended for diagnosis because even among experts, diagnostic criteria are subject to interpretation.
- Accurate diagnosis is imperative, as treatment choices and prognosis can vary with pathogenesis.
- Diagnosis of IPF requires exclusion of other known ILD causes, the presence of a UIP pattern on high-resolution computed tomography (HRCT), and/or surgical lung biopsy pattern (4).

HISTORY

- Symptoms may include progressive exertional dyspnea and nonproductive cough.
- Patients may also present with hemoptysis or fatigue.
- Obtaining a history of illness duration (acute vs. chronic), potential environmental/occupational exposures, travel, medical conditions (including systemic diseases), and medication reconciliation is important in assessing the cause of the ILD.
- Some cases of lung disease may occur weeks to years after discontinuation of an offending agent (e.g., carmustine).

PHYSICAL EXAM

Physical findings are usually nonspecific. Some common features includes the following:

- Crackles (typically present on auscultation of lung bases on posterior axillary line)
- Rales
- Inspiratory "squeaks"
- Clubbing of the digits and cyanosis in advanced disease

DIFFERENTIAL DIAGNOSIS

- Acute pulmonary edema
- Diffuse hemorrhage
- Atypical pneumonia
- Diffuse bronchoalveolar cell carcinoma or lymphatic spread of tumor

DIAGNOSTIC TESTS & INTERPRETATION

Initial Tests (lab, imaging)

- O_2 saturation
- Peak expiratory flow rate
- CBC with differential, comprehensive metabolic profile
- CRP or sedimentation rate
- Chest x-ray (CXR): most commonly reticular pattern, less commonly nodular or mixed patterns

Follow-Up Tests & Special Considerations

HRCT of the chest is the most useful tool for distinguishing among ILD subclasses, especially if normal CXRs:

- If indicated, arterial blood gas (ABG), hypersensitivity pneumonitis panel, plasma ACE inhibitor concentration (sarcoidosis)
- If a systemic disorder is suspected, consider antinuclear antibody (ANA), rheumatoid factor (RF), erythrocyte sedimentation rate (ESR), and antineutrophil cytoplasmic antibodies (ANCA).

Diagnostic Procedures/Other

- Pulmonary function testing (PFT; spirometry, lung volumes, carbon monoxide diffusing capacity)
  - Commonly demonstrates a restrictive defect (decreased vital capacity and total lung capacity)
  - Forced vital capacity (FVC) has been shown to decline 100–200 mL/year in the placebo arm of IPF patients in clinical trials (5).
- Bronchoscopy
  - Bronchoalveolar lavage (BAL) cellular analysis studies may be useful in distinguishing subtypes (including sarcoidosis, hypersensitivity pneumonitis, cancer). If performed, the BAL target site should be chosen based on the HRCT finding (6).
  - Bronchoscopic transbronchial lung biopsy may help diagnose sarcoidosis and, on occasion, is sufficiently supportive of other ILD diagnoses.
- Thoracoscopic surgery for lung biopsy has the greatest diagnostic specificity for ILDs but is less frequently used given improved specificity of HRCT. May be indicated if a diagnosis cannot be determined from transbronchial biopsy or HRCT

Test Interpretation

- Diagnostic classifications of IIPs are based on histopathologic patterns seen on lung biopsy.
- Major histologies include an inflammation and fibrotic and granulomatous patterns.
- Characteristic changes on HRCT may help to distinguish between the following subtypes:
  - Reticulonodular, ground glass opacities, and, in later stages, honeycombing may be seen.
  - Associated hilar and mediastinal adenopathy are characteristic of stage I and II sarcoidosis.

- No specific test is the gold standard, which emphasizes the importance of a multidisciplinary consensus for diagnosis with clinical, radiologic, and pathologic findings.

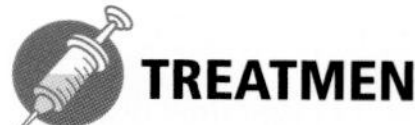

TREATMENT

- Evidence does not support the routine use of any specific therapy for ILD in general, and especially IPF (4).
- No survival benefit of home oxygen use in ILD (7)[A].
- Small prospective trials with co-trimoxazole, thalidomide, and/or sildenafil have shown improvement in some quality of life parameters.
- Corticosteroids have a role in some ILD subtypes (8)[A].
- Current evidence does not clearly support routine use of noncorticosteroid anti-inflammatory agents for IPF, including cyclosporine, azathioprine, colchicines, cyclophosphamide, cytokines, bosentan, etanercept, methotrexate, or interferon.
- Clinical trials have indicated that anticoagulation (warfarin) and endothelin receptor antagonists (ambrisentan, bosentan) are ineffective, potentially harmful, and therefore not recommended in the treatment of IPF.

GENERAL MEASURES

- Avoid/minimize offending environmental/occupational exposures/medications.
- Smoking cessation
- Supplemental oxygen, if indicated

MEDICATION

First Line

- Corticosteroids are most effective for certain ILDs, especially exacerbations of sarcoidosis, NSIP, COP, and hypersensitivity pneumonitis. However, response rates have been variable across and within subtypes. The optimal dose and duration of therapy are unknown.
- Common starting dose of prednisone is 0.5–1 mg/kg/day for 4–12 weeks, with potential up-titration to 0.5 mg/kg based on patient response.

Second Line

- Some 2nd-line agents have been used for IPF alone or in combination with steroids, with varied success rates:
  - Interim analysis of a multicenter, three-arm trial comparing combination therapy (prednisone, azathioprine, *N*-acetylcysteine [NAC]), NAC alone, and placebo revealed that combination therapy was associated with increased mortality, hospitalization, and adverse events compared with placebo. The combination arm was terminated (9)[A]. With respect to preservation of FVC, rate of acute exacerbation and death, NAC monotherapy offers no significant benefit in comparison to placebo (10)[A].
  - Pirfenidone, an orally active antifibroblast agent available outside the United States has demonstrated a favorable risk-to-benefit profile in 3 randomized, placebo-controlled trials of IPF patients with mild-to-moderate impairment of lung function. The ASCEND trial demonstrated that use of pirfenidone led to a significant reduction in rate of decline in FVC compared with placebo. (11)[A].
  - Nintedanib (BIBF 1120) a tyrosine kinase inhibitor has been evaluated in patients with IPF. Treatment resulted in a significant reduction in the annual rate of decline in FVC and fewer acute exacerbations. Nintedanib was most frequently associated with diarrhea (12)[A].
- Several 2nd-line agents have been used in Wegener granulomatosis:
  - Cyclophosphamide is commonly used in treatment of Wegener granulomatosis. It is given 1.5–2 mg/kg/day PO for 3–6 months.
  - Methotrexate has been used in treatment of mild Wegener granulomatosis in combination with corticosteroids. A studied dosing regimen consisted of an initial methotrexate dose of 0.3 mg/kg (maximum dose of 15 mg) once weekly, with 2.5 mg titration each week (maximum dose of 25 mg/week).
  - Other 2nd-line agents that have been studied include mycophenolate, mofetil, and rituximab.

SURGERY/OTHER PROCEDURES

Single- or double-lung transplantation may be a treatment of last resort. Some ILDs associated with systemic disease may recur in the recipient lung.

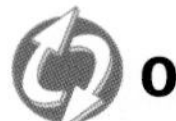

ONGOING CARE

FOLLOW-UP RECOMMENDATIONS

Follow-up testing should include PFTs, cardiopulmonary stress test, pulse oximetry, and CXR.

PATIENT EDUCATION

National Heart, Lung, and Blood Institute: www.nhlbi.nih.gov/health/dci/Diseases/ipf/ipf_whatis.html

PROGNOSIS

IPF confers the worst prognosis (median survival of 2.5–3 years) (5). A clinical prediction model to estimate the risk of death from ILD has been described (13). Other subtypes, including hypersensitivity pneumonitis, nonspecific interstitial pneumonia, and cryptogenic organizing pneumonia, have a good prognosis.

COMPLICATIONS

- Cor pulmonale
- Pneumothorax
- Progressive respiratory failure

REFERENCES

1. Travis, WD, Costabel U, Hansell DM, et al. An official American Thoracic Society/European Respiratory Society statement: update of the international multidisciplinary classification of the idiopathic interstitial pneumonias. *Am J Respir Crit Care Med*. 2013;188(6):733–748.
2. Kurland G, Deterding RR, Hagood JS, et al. An official American Thoracic Society clinical practice guideline: classification, evaluation, and management of childhood interstitial lung disease in infancy. *Am J Respir Crit Care Med*. 2013;188(3):376–394.
3. Cazzato S, di Palmo E, Ragazzo V, et al. Interstitial lung disease in children. *Early Hum Dev*. 2013; 89(Suppl 3): S39–S43.
4. Raghu G, Collard HR, Egan JJ, et al. An official ATS/ERS/JRS/ALAT statement: idiopathic pulmonary fibrosis: evidence-based guidelines for diagnosis and management. *Am J Respir Crit Care Med*. 2011;183(6):788–824.
5. Ley B, Collard HR, King TE, et al. Clinical course and prediction of survival in idiopathic pulmonary fibrosis. *Am J Respir Crit Care Med*. 2011;183(4):431–440.
6. Meyer KC, Raghu G, Baughman RP, et al. An official American Thoracic Society clinical practice guideline: the clinical utility of bronchoalveolar lavage cellular analysis in interstitial lung disease. *Am J Respir Crit Care Med*. 2012;185(9):1004–1014.
7. Crockett A, Cranston JM, Antic N. Domiciliary oxygen for interstitial lung disease. *Cochrane Database Syst Rev*. 2010;(3):CD002883.
8. Richeldi L, Davies HR, Ferrara G, et al. Corticosteroids for idiopathic pulmonary fibrosis. *Cochrane Database Syst Rev*. 2009;(3):CD002880.
9. Idiopathic Pulmonary Fibrosis Clinical Research Network, Raghu G, Anstrom KJ, et al. Prednisone, azathioprine, and N-acetylcysteine for pulmonary fibrosis. *N Engl J Med*. 2012;366(21):1968–1977.
10. Idiopathic Pulmonary Fibrosis Clinical Research Network, Martinez FJ, de Andrade JA, et al. Randomized trial of acetylcysteine in idiopathic pulmonary fibrosis. *N Engl J Med*. 2014; 370(22): 2093–2101.
11. King TE, Bradford WZ, Castro-Bernardini S, et al. A phase 3 trial of pirfenidone in patients with idiopathic pulmonary fibrosis. *N Engl J Med*. 2014; 370(22):2083–2092.
12. Richeldi L, du Bois RM, Raghu G, et al. Efficacy and safety of nintedanib in idiopathic pulmonary fibrosis. *N Engl J Med*. 2014;370(22): 2071–2082.
13. Ryerson CJ, Vittinghoff E, Ley B, et al. Predicting survival across chronic interstitial lung disease: the ILD-GAP model. *Chest*. 2014;145(4):723–728.

ADDITIONAL READING

- King TE Jr, Brown KK, Raghu G, et al. BUILD-3: a randomized, controlled trial of bosentan in idiopathic pulmonary fibrosis. *Am J Respir Crit Care Med*. 2011;184(1):92–99.
- Noth I, Anstrom KJ, Calvert SB, et al. A placebo-controlled randomized trial of warfarin in idiopathic pulmonary fibrosis. *Am J Respir Crit Care Med*. 2012;186(1):88–95.
- Raghu G, Behr J, Brown JJ, et al. Treatment of idiopathic pulmonary fibrosis with ambrisentan: a parallel, randomized trial. *Ann Intern Med*. 2013;158(9):641–649.
- Spagnolo P, Del Giovane C, Luppi F, et al. Non-steroid agents for idiopathic pulmonary fibrosis. *Cochrane Database Syst Rev*. 2010;(9):CD003134.

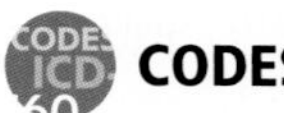

CODES

ICD10

- J84.9 Interstitial pulmonary disease, unspecified
- J84.10 Pulmonary fibrosis, unspecified
- J84.111 Idiopathic interstitial pneumonia, not otherwise specified

CLINICAL PEARLS

- ILD differs from chronic obstructive pulmonary disease (COPD); anatomically, ILD involves the lung parenchyma (i.e., alveoli) and COPD involves both airways and alveoli.
- In some cases, avoiding or minimizing offending environmental/occupational exposures, medications, and smoking may alter disease severity.

DISSEMINATED INTRAVASCULAR COAGULATION

Jan Cerny, MD, PhD, FACP • Mary L. Lopresti, DO

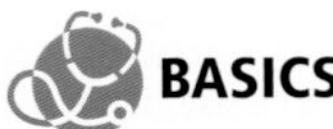

BASICS

DESCRIPTION

- Disseminated intravascular coagulation (DIC) is an acquired syndrome characterized by diffuse activation of intravascular coagulation. It can originate from and cause damage to the microvasculature, which, if sufficiently severe, can produce organ dysfunction.
- Occurs as a complication of pregnancy (e.g., abruptio placentae, fetus retention, amniotic fluid embolism), infection (especially gram-negative), malignancy (uncontrolled, metastatic tumor or leukemia), trauma, and other severe illnesses
- System(s) affected: Hematologic/lymphatic/immunologic
- Synonym(s): consumptive coagulopathy

EPIDEMIOLOGY

Incidence

Present in 1% of hospitalized patients (1)

Prevalence

- Predominant age: none
- Predominant sex: male = female

ETIOLOGY AND PATHOPHYSIOLOGY

- Systemic formation of fibrin is the result of the simultaneous coexistence of (2):
  - Increased thrombin generation via tissue factor-/factor VII-mediated pathway
  - Suppression of the physiologic anticoagulant pathways
    - Antithrombin due to consumption, degradation, and impaired synthesis
    - Proteins C and S due to decreased levels of thrombomodulin (TM)
  - Impaired fibrinolysis (early on)
    - Sustained increase in plasminogen activator inhibitor, type 1
- Increased fibrinolysis (late during the process) leads to bleeding.

Causes can be classified as acute or chronic, systemic or localized:

- Sepsis/severe infection (any microorganism)
- Trauma (polytrauma, neurotrauma)
- Obstetric complications (amniotic fluid embolism, abruptio placentae, hemorrhage, acute fatty liver of pregnancy, fetal demise, hemolysis, elevated liver function, and low platelets [HELLP] syndrome, preeclampsia)
- Solid tumors and leukemias (especially acute promyelocytic leukemia)
- Vascular disorders, such as Kasabach-Merritt syndrome, large vascular aneurysms, and thrombosis
- Organ destruction (severe pancreatitis, severe liver failure)
- Severe toxic or immunologic reactions
  - Snake bite
  - Recreational drugs
  - Transfusion reactions
  - Transplant rejection
  - Thermal injury
- Infant and adult respiratory distress syndrome
- Neonatal purpura fulminans

RISK FACTORS

See "Etiology and Pathophysiology."

GENERAL PREVENTION

Aggressive interventions aimed at early treatment of the underlying clinical conditions

COMMONLY ASSOCIATED CONDITIONS

Thromboembolic phenomena are associated with venous thrombosis, thrombotic vegetations on the aortic heart valve, arterial emboli, and neonatal purpura fulminans (homozygous protein C or protein S deficiency).

Pediatric Considerations

Neonatal purpura fulminans is associated with DIC and protein C or protein S deficiency (homozygous).

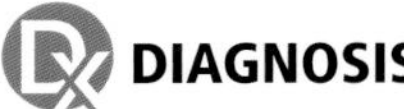

DIAGNOSIS

Symptoms and signs are related to the underlying disease process and DIC.

HISTORY

Symptoms of microvascular thrombosis (e.g., renal failure) as well as diffuse bleeding

PHYSICAL EXAM

- Bleeding manifestations
  - Skin (petechiae, purpura, ecchymosis, generalized oozing from venipuncture sites and wounds)
  - Renal (hematuria)
  - GI (mucous membranes and intestinal bleeding)
  - Neurologic (hemorrhagic infarction, massive intracerebral bleeding)
  - Respiratory (epistaxis, pulmonary hemorrhage)
- Microvascular thrombosis
  - Skin (skin infarction, digital gangrene)
  - GI (mucosal ulcerations, bowel infarction)
  - Renal (oliguria, anuria, uremia)
  - Pulmonary (hypoxemia, acute respiratory distress syndrome)
  - Neurologic (convulsions, delirium, coma, multifocal cortical infarction)

DIFFERENTIAL DIAGNOSIS

- Fulminant liver failure or massive hepatic necrosis
- Vitamin K deficiency
- Thrombotic thrombocytopenic purpura
- Hemolytic-uremic syndrome
- Heparin-induced thrombocytopenia
- Primary fibrinolysis
- HELLP syndrome in pregnancy

DIAGNOSTIC TESTS & INTERPRETATION

No single laboratory test is sensitive and specific enough to allow a definitive diagnosis of DIC.

Initial Tests (lab, imaging)

- CBC with different prothrombin time (PT)/INR, partial thromboplastin time (PTT), fibrinogen, fibrin degradation product (FDP), D-dimer, antithrombin III
- Thrombocytopenia (3)
- Increased PTT
- Increased PT
- Decreased fibrinogen (serial levels)
- Increased FDP
- Positive D-dimer
- Decreased antithrombin III, decreased protein C
- Other labs that may have prognostic significance
  - Decreased Adams-13
  - Increase soluble TM, plasminogen activator inhibitor-1 (PAI-1), von Willebrand factor peptide
  - Decrease des-R-prothrombin activation peptide fragment 2 (4)
- Microangiopathic hemolytic anemia (schistocytes, increased lactate dehydrogenase levels, low hemoglobin)

ALERT

Diagnostic algorithm for overt DIC (International Society on Thrombosis and Haemostasis) (5):

- Assess if underlying disease is known to be associated with DIC:
  - YES: Proceed with this algorithm.
  - NO: Do not use this algorithm.
- Order global coagulation tests (PT, PTT, fibrinogen, soluble fibrin monomers, or FDPs).
- Score global coagulation test results:
  - Platelet count (>100 = 0, <100 = 1, <50 = 2)
  - Elevated fibrin-related markers (no increase = 0, moderate increase = 2, strong increase = 3)
  - Prolonged PT (<3 seconds = 0, >3 but <6 seconds = 1, >6 seconds = 2)
  - Fibrinogen level (>1 g/L = 0, <1 g/L = 1)
- Calculate score:
  - If ≥5: compatible with DIC, repeat scoring daily. If <5: suggestive of nonovert DIC, repeat in 1–2 days

Follow-Up Tests & Special Considerations

Frequent follow-up of initially abnormal laboratory tests to see effect of therapeutic interventions

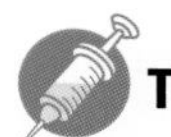

TREATMENT

Heterogeneity of the underlying disorders and the clinical presentations makes the therapeutic approach to DIC difficult:

- Appropriate health care: inpatient and intensive care unit (ICU) (depending on underlying condition)
- Treat underlying condition (e.g., evacuation of uterus in abruptio placentae; broad-spectrum antibiotics for gram-negative sepsis).
- Do not treat abnormal lab parameters. Supportive care with transfusions in patients who are bleeding, going for surgery, or at high risk of bleeding:
  - Fresh frozen plasma
  - Platelet concentrates
  - Cryoprecipitate or fibrinogen concentrates
  - Anticoagulants remain very controversial. Therapeutic heparin may be considered in cases where thrombosis dominates. Deep venous thrombosis prophylaxis is recommended in patients who are not bleeding.
- Restoration of anticoagulant pathways
  - Recombinant human-activated protein C once had a level of evidence for use only in selected high-risk patients in ICU setting. The drug was, however, removed from the market in 2012 (6).
  - Activated factor VII, antithrombin, and recombinant human TM-α use remains controversial. Investigation is ongoing.
  - Antifibrinolytic treatment is generally not recommended but may be considered in those with severe bleeding and marked hyperfibrinolytic state (i.e., trauma, acute promyelocytic leukemia, cavernous hemangioma).

MEDICATION

Broad-spectrum antibiotics for sepsis

SURGERY/OTHER PROCEDURES

Surgical treatment or procedures should be considered, especially if they are treating the underlying condition (e.g., evacuation of uterus in abruptio placentae; some trauma or bleeding situations).

INPATIENT CONSIDERATIONS

Admission Criteria/Initial Stabilization

Usually dictated by severity of underlying condition. Some cases can be managed in a standard ward, but ICU care is typical.

- Treat underlying disorder.
- Frequent monitoring of clinical and laboratory response

Discharge Criteria

Once clinical and laboratory criteria are significantly improved and underlying reason for DIC is under control

ONGOING CARE

FOLLOW-UP RECOMMENDATIONS

Patient Monitoring

- Monitor closely until much improved.
- Serial platelet count, coagulation tests, and fibrinogen levels to see effect of therapeutic interventions

PROGNOSIS

- Related to the severity of cause
- Decreased antithrombin level is a poor prognostic factor in DIC.

COMPLICATIONS

- Acute renal failure
- Shock
- Cardiac tamponade
- Hemothorax
- Intracerebral hematoma
- Various thrombotic complications, including myocardial infarction, stroke, gangrene, and loss of digits

REFERENCES

1. Matsuda T. Clinical Aspects of DIC—disseminated intravascular coagulation. *Pol J Pharmacol*. 1996; 48(1):73–75.
2. Franchini M, Lippi G, Manzato F. Recent acquisitions in the pathophysiology, diagnosis and treatment of disseminated intravascular coagulation. *Thromb J*. 2006;4:4.
3. Levi M, van der Poll T. Disseminated intravascular coagulation: a review for the internist. *Intern Emerg Med*. 2013;8(1):23–32.
4. Chung S, Kim JE, Kim HK, et al. Serum des-R prothrombin activation peptide fragment 2: a novel prognostic marker for disseminated intravascular coagulation. *Thromb Res*. 2013;131(6):547–553.
5. Voves C, Wuillemin WA, Zeerleder S. International Society on Thrombosis and Haemostasis score for overt disseminated intravascular coagulation predicts organ dysfunction and fatality in sepsis patients. *Blood Coagul Fibrinolysis*. 2006;17(6):445–451.
6. Vincent JL, Bernard GR, Beale R, et al. Drotrecogin alfa (activated) treatment in severe sepsis from the global open-label trial ENHANCE: further evidence for survival and safety and implications for early treatment. *Crit Care Med*. 2005;33(10):2266–2277.

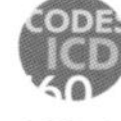

CODES

ICD10

- D65 Disseminated intravascular coagulation
- P60 Disseminated intravascular coagulation of newborn
- O46.009 Antepartum hemorrhage w coag defect, unsp, unsp trimester

CLINICAL PEARLS

- Treat underlying condition(s); transfusions represent supportive measures.
- Transfusions are not indicated in patients with abnormal laboratory parameters without clinical bleeding.

D

DIVERTICULAR DISEASE

David M. Hardy, MD • Steven B. Holsten, Jr., MD, FACS

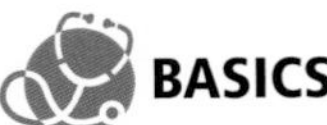

BASICS

DESCRIPTION

Diverticular disease includes asymptomatic diverticulosis, symptomatic uncomplicated diverticulitis, symptomatic complicated diverticulitis, and diverticular bleeding.

- Diverticulum (single) or diverticula (multiple) outpouchings of colonic mucosa and submucosa through weakened muscle layers in the colonic wall:
  - Diverticulosis is less common in vegetarians and more common in cultures with low-fiber diets.
  - Most diverticula occur on the left side of the colon; Asian populations have more right-sided disease.
  - Prevalence of diverticulosis and the number of diverticula increase with age.
- Diverticular bleeding: occurs in 3–5% of patients with diverticular disease:
  - Accounts for >40% of lower GI bleeds and 30% of cases of hematochezia in general
  - Bleeding is more common if right sided.
- Symptomatic uncomplicated diverticular disease: recurrent abdominal pain attributed to diverticula in the absence of macroscopically overt colitis or diverticulitis (1)
- Uncomplicated diverticulitis: diverticular inflammation and/or infection without systemic sequelae, affects 10–25% of patients with diverticulosis
- Complicated diverticulitis inflammation/infection with secondary abscess formation, bowel obstruction or perforation, peritonitis, fistula, or stricture formation
- System(s) affected: entire GI tract except the rectum

EPIDEMIOLOGY

Incidence

- Diverticulosis <5% in general population, diverticulitis 1–2% in the United States (1)
- Yearly mortality rate: 2.5/100,000

Prevalence

- Increased from 61.8 to 75.5/100,000 persons from 1998 to 2005, large increase in incidence for patients <45 years old, largely due to changes in diet
- Male = female overall. More common in men <65 years of age and more common in women >65 years.

ETIOLOGY AND PATHOPHYSIOLOGY

Diverticula form where intestinal blood flow (vasa recta) penetrate the colonic mucosa. This results in decreased resistance to intraluminal pressure. Diverticulitis occurs when there is diverticular inflammation, infection and/or perforation.

- Age-related degeneration of mucosal wall; increased intraluminal pressure from dense, fiber-depleted stools, and abnormal colonic motility contribute to diverticular disease.
- Thinning of the vasa recta over the neck of the diverticula increases susceptibility to bleeding.
- Diverticulitis occurs when local inflammation and infection contribute to tissue necrosis with risk for mucosal micro- or macroperforation.
- Most right-sided diverticula are true diverticula (all layers of the colonic wall).
- Most left-sided diverticula are pseudodiverticula (outpouchings of the mucosa and submucosa only).
- Surgical and autopsy studies show mycosis, a constellation of thickened circular muscle (pseudohypertrophy due to increased elastin in the taeniae), short taeniae, and luminal narrowing.
- Diverticulitis: inflammation with lymphocytic infiltrate, ulceration, mucin depletion necrosis, Paneth cell metaplasia, and cryptitis
- Alterations in intestinal microbiota contribute to chronic inflammation (1,2).
- Diverticular disease and irritable bowel syndrome (IBS) may be on the same disease continuum.

Genetics

- No known genetic pattern
- Asian and African populations have lower prevalence but develop diverticular disease with adoption of a Western lifestyle.

RISK FACTORS

- Age >40 years
- Low-fiber diet
- Sedentary lifestyle, obesity
- Previous diverticulitis. Risk for diverticulitis rises with the number of diverticula
- Smoking increases the risk of perforation (1).
- NSAIDs, steroids, and opiate analgesics increase risk for diverticular bleeding. Calcium channel blockers and statins appear to protect against diverticular bleeding.

GENERAL PREVENTION

High-fiber diet or nonabsorbable fiber (psyllium) (>30 g/day of fiber)

COMMONLY ASSOCIATED CONDITIONS

Connective tissue diseases, colon cancer, and inflammatory bowel disease

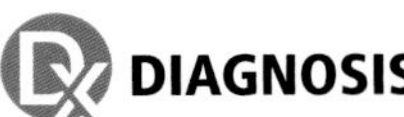

DIAGNOSIS

HISTORY

- Diverticulosis
  - 80–85% of patients are asymptomatic. Of the 15–20% with symptoms, 1–2% will need hospitalization and 0.5% will need surgery.
  - Abdominal pain: dull, colicky, mostly in left lower quadrant (LLQ). Pain can be exacerbated by eating and alleviated following bowel movement or passage of flatus.
  - Diarrhea or constipation
- Diverticulitis: uncomplicated (75%) and complicated (25%)
  - Abdominal pain: acute onset, typically in LLQ
  - Fever and/or chills
  - Anorexia, nausea (20–62%), or vomiting
  - Constipation (50%) or diarrhea (25–35%)
  - Dysuria and urinary frequency suggest bladder or ureteral irritation due to bowel inflammation.
  - Pneumaturia, fecaluria can occur if colovesical fistula develops.
- Diverticular hemorrhage
  - Melena, hematochezia
  - Painless rectal bleeding
- Immunocompromised patients may not present with fever or leukocytosis but are at higher risk for perforation and abscess formation (2).

PHYSICAL EXAM

- Diverticulosis
  - Exam may be completely normal.
  - May have intermittent distension or tympany
  - No signs of peritoneal inflammation
- Diverticulitis
  - Abdominal tenderness usually localized to the LLQ
  - Rebound tenderness, involuntary guarding, or rigidity (suggests peritoneal inflammation or potential bowel perforation)
  - Palpable mass in LLQ (20%) that is tender, firm, or fixed
  - Abdominal distension and tympany
  - Bowel sounds hypoactive or could be high-pitched and intermittent if obstruction ensues.
  - Rectal exam may reveal tenderness or mass.
  - Colovaginal, colovesical, and perirectal fistulae may be the initial manifestation (rarely).

DIFFERENTIAL DIAGNOSIS

IBS, lactose intolerance, carcinoma, inflammatory bowel disease, fecal impaction, incarcerated hernia, gallbladder disease, angiodysplasia, colitis, acute appendicitis, ectopic pregnancy

DIAGNOSTIC TESTS & INTERPRETATION

Initial Tests (lab, imaging)

- WBC normal in diverticulosis and up to 45% of cases of diverticulitis. As diverticulitis worsens, WBC typically elevated with left shift.
- Hemoglobin normal (unless bleeding)
- ESR elevated in diverticulitis
- Urinalysis (UA) may show microscopic pyuria or hematuria
- Urine culture: usually normal. Persistent infection suspicious for colovesical fistula
- Blood cultures positive in systemic cases of diverticulitis with bowel perforation and hematogenous spread
- Diverticulosis
  - Asymptomatic diverticulosis is a common incidental finding on routine colonoscopy.
- Diverticulitis
  - Plain films of the abdomen (acute abdominal series—supine and upright) assess for air under the diaphragm (bowel perforation) and signs of bowel obstruction (dilated loops of bowel)
  - CT scan with IV, oral, and rectal contrast to stage disease and map medical versus surgical treatment plan (3)[A]
  - Ultrasound (US) is effective for acutely identifying diverticulitis.
  - Barium enema is not recommended due to risk of peritoneal extravasation.
- Diverticular bleeding/hematochezia
  - Endoscopy is the test of choice for the evaluation of GI bleeding (4).
  - Angiography if massive bleeding obscures endoscopy or when endoscopy cannot visualize a source (4).

Follow-Up Tests & Special Considerations

Once episodes of acute diverticulitis have resolved, colonoscopy to exclude any associated malignancies, strictures, or inflammatory bowel disease (3).

Diagnostic Procedures/Other

- For evaluation of hematochezia in suspected diverticular hemorrhage
  - Place nasogastric (NG) tube for NG lavage to exclude upper GI sources of bleeding (4).
  - 99mTc-pertechnetate–labeled RBC scan can be used before angiography (more sensitive than angiography) with follow-up angiography to localize a bleeding source (not studied in a comparison trial) (4).

- For diverticulitis, gallium- or indium-labeled leukocytes to localize abscess (rarely used)

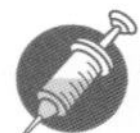

TREATMENT

GENERAL MEASURES

- Diverticulosis: outpatient therapy with fiber supplementation and/or bulking agents (psyllium) to soften stools
- Outpatient diverticulitis: pain, tenderness, leukocytosis, but no toxicity or peritoneal signs; use oral broad-spectrum antibiotics. 1–2% of subjects require hospitalization for toxicity, septicemia, peritonitis, or failure of symptoms to resolve. Up to 30% of patients may require surgery at 1st episode of diverticulitis. Recurrent bouts of diverticulitis increase requirement for surgical intervention.
- Patients who appear septic or hemodynamically unstable require hospitalization, bowel rest, and broad-spectrum antibiotic therapy until symptoms improve.
- Symptomatic improvement is expected within 2–3 days. Antibiotics should be continued for a 7–10 day course of therapy.
- 80% of diverticular bleeding resolve spontaneously (4).

MEDICATION

First Line

- Diverticulosis
  - High-fiber intake is recommended (preferably >20–30 g/day) (3)[A].
- Symptomatic uncomplicated diverticular disease: cyclical rifaximin or continuous mesalamine (3)[B]
- Uncomplicated diverticulitis
  - Oral antibiotics for outpatient treatment of mild disease: cover for anaerobes and gram-negative rods with
    - A fluoroquinolone (ciprofloxacin 750 mg BID or levofloxacin 750 QD) *plus* metronidazole 500 mg QID (may use clindamycin if metronidazole intolerant) *or*
    - Trimethoprim/sulfamethoxazole DS BID *plus* metronidazole 500 QID
    - Treat for 7–10 days
  - The routine use of antibiotics in uncomplicated diverticulitis is controversial (5)[A].
  - Inpatient: Use IV antibiotics:
    - Monotherapy with a β-lactam/β-lactamase inhibitor: piperacillin/tazobactam (3,375 g IV QID) or ampicillin/sulbactam or ertapenem
    - Penicillin-allergic patient: Quinolone (levofloxacin 750 mg IV QD plus metronidazole (500 mg IV QID)
    - Unresponsive or severe disease: imipenem or meropenem
  - Recurrences of acute diverticulitis may be decreased by using mesalamine ± rifaximin (6)[A] or probiotics.
- Diverticular bleeding
  - Consider vasopressin 0.2–0.3 units/min through selective intra-arterial catheter.
- Precautions
  - Avoid morphine and other opiates that may increase intraluminal pressure or promote ileus.
  - Increased fiber intake is not recommended in the acute management of diverticulitis.

Second Line

- Outpatient: amoxicillin/clavulanate monotherapy (1,000/62.5) two tablets BID (contraindicated in patients with clearance less than 30 mL/min) or moxifloxacin (400 mg PO QD) *plus* metronidazole (500 mg QID)
- Severely ill inpatients: ampicillin + metronidazole + a quinolone *or* ampicillin + metronidazole + an aminoglycoside

ISSUES FOR REFERRAL

Patients with complicated diverticulitis manifesting with hemodynamic instability or failure to respond to initial IV antibiotic therapy should have appropriate surgical and critical care/infectious disease consultations.

SURGERY/OTHER PROCEDURES

- Indication for emergent surgery: peritonitis, uncontrolled sepsis, visceral perforation, colonic obstruction, or acute deterioration
- Decision for elective resection in nonemergent or recurrent cases of diverticulitis is made on a case-by-case basis (3)[B]:
  - After 1st episode, there is a 33% chance of recurrence. After a second episode, there is a 66% chance of further recurrence.
  - Most complications occur during first bout of diverticulitis.
  - Emergent surgery carries a much higher risk of morbidity/mortality.
  - Recommendations for elective surgery recommendations should be based on severity of complications (not solely on number of recurrences).
  - Elective resection is typically advised after recovery from a complicated diverticulitis treated nonoperatively (3)[B].
  - Age: Younger patients more likely to have recurrence.
  - Immunocompromised patients: more likely to present with acute complicated diverticulitis, fail medical management, and have complications from elective surgery
- Large abscesses (>4 cm) can be drained with radiographic guidance and managed nonoperatively (3).
- In diverticular hemorrhage, if >4 units of RBC transfused, then 60% chance of requiring surgical intervention (4).

COMPLEMENTARY & ALTERNATIVE MEDICINE

Probiotics such as *Lactobacillus casei* and *Escherichia coli* Nissle 1917 have been used with mixed success to prevent recurrence.

INPATIENT CONSIDERATIONS

Admission Criteria/Initial Stabilization

- Admit for toxicity, septicemia, and/or peritonitis
- IV fluids, analgesics, antibiotics, NG suction

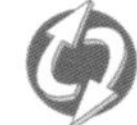

ONGOING CARE

DIET

- NPO during acute diverticulitis; advance diet as tolerated as bowel function returns
- Patients with known diverticulosis or a history of diverticulitis should consume a high-fiber diet (>30 g/day) to prevent recurrence (7).
- Nuts and popcorn do not increase risk for diverticulosis or diverticular complications (8).

PROGNOSIS

- Typically good with early detection and prompt treatment of complications
- Risk for recurrence increases with each subsequent bout of diverticulitis.
- Rebleeding occurs in up to 6%.
- Diverticulitis recurs more often in younger patients, but severity is similar to elderly.

COMPLICATIONS

Hemorrhage, perforation, peritonitis, obstruction, abscess, or fistula

REFERENCES

1. Strate LL, Modi R, Cohen E, et al. Diverticular disease as a chronic illness: evolving epidemiologic and clinical insights. *Am J Gastroenterol*. 2012;107(10):1486–1493.
2. Sheth AA, Longo W, Floch MH. Diverticular disease and diverticulitis. *Am J Gastroenterol*. 2008;103(6):1550–1556.
3. Rafferty J, Shellito P, Hyman NH, et al. Practice parameters for sigmoid diverticulitis. *Dis Colon Rectum*. 2006;49(7):939–944.
4. Zuccaro G. Management of the adult patient with acute lower gastrointestinal bleeding. American College of Gastroenterology. Practice Parameters Committee. *Am J Gastroenterol*. 1998;93(8):1202–1208.
5. Shabanzadeh DM, Wille-Jørgensen P. Antibiotics for uncomplicated diverticulitis. *Cochrane Database Syst Rev*. 2012;(11):CD009092.
6. Gatta L, Vakil N, Vaira D, et al. Efficacy of 5-ASA in the treatment of colonic diverticular disease. *J Clin Gastroenterol*. 2010;44(2):113–119.
7. Ravikoff JE, Korzenik JR. Presentations the role of fiber in diverticular disease. *J Clin Gastroenterol*. 2011;45:S7–S11.
8. Strate LL, Liu YL, Syngal S, et al. Nut, corn, and popcorn consumption and the incidence of diverticular disease. *JAMA*. 2008;300(8):907–914.

ADDITIONAL READING

- Boynton W, Flock M. New strategies for the management of diverticular disease: insights for the clinician. *Therap Adv Gastroenterol*. 2013;6(3):205–213.
- Katz LH, Guy DD, Lahat A, et al. Diverticulitis in the young is not more aggressive than in the elderly, but it tends to recur more often: systematic review and meta-analysis. *J Gastroenterol Hepatol*. 2013;28(8):1274–1281.
- Templeton AW, Strate LL. Updates in diverticular disease. *Curr Gastroenterol Rep*. 2013;15(8):339.

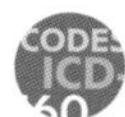

CODES

ICD10

- K57.90 Dvrtclos of intest, part unsp, w/o perf or abscess w/o bleed
- K57.30 Dvrtclos of lg int w/o perforation or abscess w/o bleeding
- K57.92 Diverticulitis of intestine, part unspecified, without perforation or abscess without bleeding

CLINICAL PEARLS

- Diverticular disease affects 15% of individuals by the 5th decade of life and increases to 70% by the 9th decade.
- Patients with known diverticular disease should eat a high-fiber diet (30 g/day).
- IBS and diverticular disease often coexist. IBS does not cause diverticular disease and vice versa.

DOMESTIC VIOLENCE

Rhonda A. Faulkner, PhD • Mary Segraves Lindholm, MD

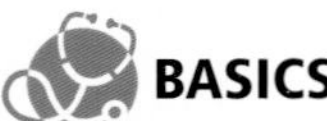

BASICS

DESCRIPTION

- Domestic violence (DV) is behavior in any relationship that is used to gain or maintain power and control over an intimate partner.
- May include physical, sexual, and/or emotional abuse, economic or psychological actions, or threats of actions that influence another person
- Although women are at greater risk of experiencing DV, it occurs among patients of any race, age, sexual orientation, religion, gender, socioeconomic background, and education level.
- Synonym(s): intimate partner violence (IPV); spousal abuse; family violence

EPIDEMIOLOGY

Incidence

8% in the United States; women are more likely to report partner violence than men.

Prevalence

- DV occurs in 1 of 4 American families. Nearly 5.3 million incidents of DV occur each year among U.S. women aged ≥18 and 3.2 million incidents among men.
- DV results in nearly 2 million injuries and up to 4,000 deaths annually in the United States.
- 30% of women and 22% of men have experienced physical, sexual, or psychological IPV during their lifetime in the United States.
- 14–35% of adult female patients in emergency departments report experiencing DV within the past year.
- Costs of DV are estimated to exceed $5.8 billion annually, of which $4.1 billion are for direct medical and mental health services.
- DV survivors have a 1.6–2.3-fold increase in health care use compared with the nonabused population.

Geriatric Considerations

- 4–6% of elderly are abused, with ~2 million elderly persons experiencing abuse and/or neglect each year. In 90% of cases, the perpetrator is a family member.
- Elder abuse is any form of mistreatment that results in harm or loss to an older person; may include physical, sexual, emotional, financial abuse, and/or neglect.

Pediatric Considerations

- >3 million children aged 3–17 years are at risk of witnessing acts of DV.
- ~1 million abused children are identified in the United States each year.
- Children living in violent homes are at increased risk of physical, sexual, and/or emotional abuse; anxiety and depression; decreased self-esteem; emotional, behavioral, social, and/or physical disturbances; and lifelong poor health.

Pregnancy Considerations

DV occurs during 7–20% of pregnancies. Women with unintended pregnancy are at 3× greater risk of DV. 25% of abused women report exacerbation of abuse during pregnancy. There is a positive correlation between DV and postpartum depression.

RISK FACTORS

- Patient/victim risk factors
  - Substance abuse
  - Poverty/financial stressors/unemployment
  - Recent loss of social support
  - Family disruption and lifecycle changes
  - History of abusive relationships or witness to abuse as child
  - Mental or physical disability in family
  - Social isolation
  - Pregnancy
- Abuser risk factors
  - Substance abuse (e.g., heavy drinking)
  - Young age
  - Unemployment
  - Low academic achievement
  - Witnessing or experiencing violence as child
  - Depression
  - Personality disorders
- Relational risk factors
  - Marital conflict
  - Marital instability
  - Economic stress
  - Traditional gender role norms
  - Poor family functioning

Geriatric Considerations

Factors associated with the abuse of older adults include increasing age, nonwhite race, low-income status, functional impairment, cognitive disability, substance use, poor emotional state, low self-esteem, cohabitation, and lack of social support.

Pediatric Considerations

Factors associated with child abuse or neglect include low-income status, low maternal education, nonwhite race, large family size, young maternal age, single-parent household, parental psychiatric disturbances, and presence of a stepfather.

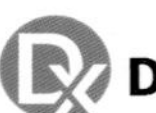

DIAGNOSIS

- DV is often underdiagnosed, with only 10–12% of physicians conducting routine screening.
- Although prevalence of DV in primary care settings is 7–50%, <15% are screened.
- Pregnancy increases risk.
- Barriers to screening: time constraints, discomfort with the subject, fear of offending the patient, and lack of perceived skills and resources to manage DV
- Abused patients may refuse to disclose abuse for many reasons, which includes the following:
  - Not feeling emotionally ready to admit the reality of the situation
  - Shame and self-blame
  - Feelings of failure if abuse is admitted
  - Fear of rejection by the physician
  - Fear of retribution from abuser
  - Belief that abuse will not happen again
  - Belief that no alternatives or available resources exist

HISTORY

- Physicians should introduce the subject of DV in a general way (i.e., "I routinely ask all patients about domestic violence. Have you ever been in a relationship where you were afraid?").
- How to screen
  - Screen patient alone, without partner or others present.
  - Ask screening questions in patient's primary language; do not use children or other family members as interpreters.
- Partner violence screen (sensitivity 35–71%; specificity 80–94%)
  - "Have you ever been hit, kicked, punched, or otherwise, hurt by someone within the past year? If so, by whom?"
  - "Do you feel safe in your current relationship?"
  - "Is there a partner from a previous relationship who is making you feel unsafe now?"
- CDC-recommended RADAR system
  - **R:** Routinely screen every patient; make screening a part of everyday practice in prenatal, postnatal, routine gynecologic visits, and annual health screenings.
  - **A:** Ask questions directly, kindly, and be nonjudgmental.
  - **D:** Document findings in the patient's chart using the patient's own words, with details. Use body maps and photographs as necessary.
  - **A:** Assess the patient's safety and see if the patient has a safety plan.
  - **R:** Review options for dealing with DV with the patient and provide referrals.
- SAFE questions
  - **S**tress/safety: "Do you feel safe in your relationship?"
  - **A**fraid/abused: "Have you ever been in a relationship where you were threatened, hurt, or afraid?"
  - **F**riends/family: "Are your friends or family aware that you have been hurt? Could you tell them, and would they be able to give you support?"
  - **E**mergency plan: "Do you have a safe place to go and the resources you need in an emergency?"
- "How often does your partner: physically hurt you? insult or talk down to you? threaten you with harm? scream or curse at you?"
- Assess pregnancy difficulties such as poor/late prenatal care, low-birth-weight babies, and perinatal deaths
- Pelvic and abdominal pain, chronic without demonstrable pathology
- Headaches, back pain
- Gynecologic disorders
- Sexually transmitted infections (STIs) including HIV/AIDS
- Depression, suicidal ideation, anxiety, fatigue
- Substance abuse
- Eating disorders
- Overuse of health services/frequent emergency room visits
- Noncompliance

PHYSICAL EXAM

- Clinical presentation/psychological signs and symptoms
  - Delay in seeking treatment
  - Inconsistent explanation of injuries
  - Reluctance to undress
  - Signs of battered woman syndrome and/or posttraumatic stress disorder (PTSD) (flat affect/avoidance of eye contact, evasiveness, heightened startle response, sleep disturbance, traumatic flashbacks)
  - Depression, anxiety, chronic fatigue, substance abuse
  - Suspicious partner accompaniment at appointment; overly solicitous partner and/or refusal to leave exam room
- Physical signs and symptoms
  - Tympanic membrane rupture
  - Rectal or genital injury (centrally located injuries with bathing-suit pattern of distribution—concealable by clothing)

- Head and neck injuries (site of 50% of abusive injuries)
- Facial scrapes, loose or broken tooth, bruises, cuts, or fractures to face or body
- Knife wounds, cigarette burns, bite marks, welts with outline of weapon (such as belt buckle)
- Broken bones
- Defensive posture injuries
- Injuries inconsistent with the explanation given
- Injuries in various stages of healing

DIAGNOSTIC TESTS & INTERPRETATION

- The U.S. Preventive Services Task Force (USPSTF) in 2013 issued guidelines recommending that clinicians screen all women of childbearing age (14–46 years old) for DV and provide or refer women to intervention services when appropriate (1)[B].
- Other recommendations
  - American College of Physicians (ACP) recommends routine screening for DV for all women in primary care settings at periodic intervals and when women present for emergency care with traumatic injuries.
  - The American Medical Association (AMA) recommends that all patients be routinely screened for DV with inquiry into history of family violence.
  - The World Health Organization (WHO) recommends against DV screening or routine inquiry about exposure to DV; however, they recommend asking about exposure to DV when assessing conditions that may be caused or complicated by abuse (2)[B].
  - U.S. Surgeon General and American Association of Family Practitioners recommend that physicians consider the possibility of DV as a cause of illness and injury.
  - The Partner Violence Screen is a 3-question screening tool with a high specificity.
  - There is no evidence of harm in screening for DV.

Pediatric Considerations

American Academy of Pediatrics (AAP) and AMA recommend that physicians remain alert for signs and symptoms of child physical and sexual abuse in the routine exam.

Pregnancy Considerations

American Congress of Obstetrics and Gynecologists (ACOG) and AMA guidelines on DV recommend that physicians routinely assess all pregnant women for DV. ACOG recommends periodic screening throughout obstetric care (at the first prenatal visit, at least once per trimester, at the postpartum checkup).

Initial Tests (lab, imaging)

Liver function tests (LFTs), amylase, lipase if abdominal trauma is suspected

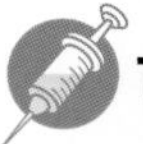

TREATMENT

- Treatment includes initial diagnosis; ongoing medical care; emotional support, counseling, and patient education regarding the DV cycle; referrals to community and supportive services as needed.
- On diagnosis, use the SOS-DoC intervention:
- **S:** Offer *S*upport and assess *S*afety:
  - Support: "You are not to blame. I am sorry this is happening to you. There is no excuse for DV."
  - Remind patient of your commitment to confidential communication.
  - Safety: Listen and respond to safety issues for the patient: "Do you feel safe going home?"; "Are your children safe?"
- **O:** Discuss *O*ptions, including safety planning and follow-up:
  - Provide information about DV and help when needed. Make referrals to local resources:
    - "Do you need or want to access a safety shelter or DV service agency?"
    - "Do you want police intervention and if so, would you like me to call the police so they can make a report with you?"
    - Offer numbers to local resources and National DV Hotline: 1-800-799-SAFE (open 24/7; can provide physicians in every state with information on local resources).
- **S:** Validate patient's *S*trengths:
  - "It took courage for you to talk with me today. You have shown great strength in very difficult circumstances."
- **Do:** *D*ocument *o*bservations, assessment, and plans:
  - Use patient's own words regarding injury and abuse.
  - Legibly document injuries: Use a body map.
  - If possible, take instant photographs of patient's injuries if given patient consent.
  - Make patient safety plan. Prepare patient to get away in an emergency:
    - Encourage patient to keep the following items in a safe place: keys (house and car); important papers (Social Security card, birth certificates, photo ID/driver's license, passport, green card); cash, food stamps, credit cards; medication for self and children; children's immunization records; important phone numbers/addresses (friends, family, local shelters); personal care items (e.g., extra glasses).
    - Encourage patient to arrange a signal with someone to let that person know when she or he needs help.
- **C:** Offer *C*ontinuity:
  - Offer a follow-up appointment and assess barriers to access.

GENERAL MEASURES

- Reporting child and elder abuse to protective services is mandatory in most states. Several states have laws requiring mandatory reporting of IPV.
- Contact the local DV program to find out about laws and community resources before they are needed.
- Display resource materials (National DV Hotline: 1-800-799-SAFE) in the office, all exam rooms, and restrooms.

ADDITIONAL THERAPIES

- National DV Hotline: 1-800-799-SAFE (7233)
- Post in all exam rooms posters in both English and Spanish; available at www.thehotline.org/resources/resource-download-center/

ONGOING CARE

FOLLOW-UP RECOMMENDATIONS

- Schedule prompt follow-up appointment.
- Inquire about what has happened since last visit.
- Review medical records and ask about past episodes to convey concern for the patient and a willingness to address this health issue openly.
- DV often requires multiple interventions over time before it is resolved.

PATIENT EDUCATION

- Counsel patients about nonviolent ways to resolve conflict.
- Educate patients about the cycle of violence.
- Counsel parents about developmentally appropriate ways to discipline their children.
- Educate parents about the negative consequences of arguments on children and each other.
- National Coalition Against Domestic Violence: www.ncadv.org
- CDC: www.cdc.gov/violenceprevention

PROGNOSIS

Most DV perpetrators do not voluntarily seek therapy unless pressured by partners or upon legal mandate. Current evidence is insufficient on effectiveness of therapy for perpetrators.

D

REFERENCES

1. U.S. Preventive Services Task Force. *Screening for Intimate Partner Violence and Abuse of Elderly and Vulnerable Adults*. Rockville, MD: Agency for Healthcare Research and Quality; 2013.
2. Feder G, Wathen CN, MacMillan HL. An evidence-based response to intimate partner violence. *JAMA*. 2013;310(5):479–480.

ADDITIONAL READING

- Cronholm PF, Fogarty CT, Ambuel B, et al. Intimate partner violence. *Am Fam Physician*. 2011;83(10):1165–1172.
- Rhodes KV, Kothari CL, Ditcher M, et al. Intimate partner violence identification and response: time for a change in strategy. *J Gen Intern Med*. 2011;26(8):294–899.
- Walton MA, Murray R, Cunningham RM, et al. Correlates of intimate partner violence among men and women in an inner city emergency department. *J Addict Dis*. 2009;28(4):366–381.
- Wu Q, Chen HL, Xu XJ. Violence as a risk factor for postpartum depression in mothers: a meta-analysis. *Arch Womens Ment Health*. 2012;15(2):107–114.

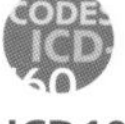

CODES

ICD10

- T74.91XA Unspecified adult maltreatment, confirmed, initial encounter
- T74.11XA Adult physical abuse, confirmed, initial encounter
- T74.31XA Adult psychological abuse, confirmed, initial encounter

CLINICAL PEARLS

- Display resource materials in the office (e.g., posting abuse awareness posters/National DV Hotline, 1-800-799-SAFE, in both English and Spanish, in all exam rooms and restrooms).
- Given the high prevalence of DV and the lack of harm and potential benefits of screening, routine screening is recommended.
- For those who screen positive, offer resources, reassure confidentiality, and provide close follow-up.

DOWN SYNDROME

Michele Roberts, MD, PhD • Brian G. Skotko, MD, MPP

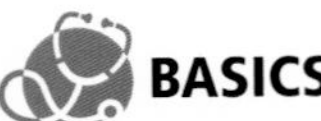

BASICS

DESCRIPTION

- Down syndrome (DS) is a congenital condition associated with intellectual disability and an increased risk of multisystem medical problems
- System(s) affected: neurologic (100%), cardiac (40–50%), GI (8–12%)
- Etiology: presence of all or part of an extra chromosome 21
- Synonym(s): trisomy 21

Pediatric Considerations

Murmur may not be present at birth. Delay in recognition of heart condition may lead to irreversible pulmonary hypertension.

Geriatric Considerations

- Life expectancy has increased to ~60 years.
- Age-related health issues occur at earlier age than in the general population.
- Communication difficulties may interfere with prompt recognition of some medical issues.

Pregnancy Considerations

- American Congress of Obstetricians and Gynecologists (ACOG) recommends all pregnant women be offered traditional prenatal screening and diagnostic testing for DS.
  - Maternal prenatal screening may be performed in the 1st or 2nd trimester.
  - Prenatal diagnosis includes chorionic villus sampling or amniocentesis.
- ACOG and the Society for Maternal-Fetal Medicine (SMFM) recommend noninvasive prenatal screening (NIPS) for "high-risk" women.
- Most, but not all, men with DS are believed to be infertile.
- Most women with DS are subfertile but can conceive children with and without DS.

EPIDEMIOLOGY

Incidence

In the United States, 1 per 830 live births, ~4,700 births/year (1)

Prevalence

~250,000 persons in the United States

ETIOLOGY AND PATHOPHYSIOLOGY

- Trisomy 21: 95% of DS, an extra chromosome 21 is found in all cells due to nondisjunction, usually in maternal meiosis.
- Translocation DS: 3–4% of DS, extra chromosome 21q material is translocated to another chromosome (usually 13, 14, or 21); ~25% have parental origin.
- Mosaic trisomy 21: 1–2% of DS, manifestations may be milder.

Genetics

- Online Mendelian Inheritance in Man (OMIM) 190685
- Inheritance: most commonly sporadic nondisjunction resulting in trisomy 21
- Chance of having another child with DS is
  - 1% (or age risk, whichever is greater) after conceiving a pregnancy with nondisjunction trisomy 21
  - 10–15% for mothers/sisters and 3–5% for fathers/brothers who carry balanced translocation with chromosome 21
  - 100% if the parental balanced translocation is 21:21 (45,t[21:21])
  - Unclear after child with mosaic DS but ~1%

RISK FACTORS

- DS believed to occur in all races with equal frequency.
- Chance of having an infant with DS increases with mother's age.
- Relatively more infants with DS are born to younger mothers because younger women are more likely to become pregnant.
- Prenatal diagnosis of DS is more common in older women, and a high percentage of such pregnancies are electively terminated.

GENERAL PREVENTION

- No prevention for nondisjunction trisomy 21
- Preimplantation diagnosis with in vitro fertilization (IVF), prenatal diagnosis and termination, and adoption are current options for expectant parents who do not wish to raise a child with DS.

COMMONLY ASSOCIATED CONDITIONS

- Cardiac
  - Congenital heart defects (40–50%)
- GI/growth
  - Feeding problems are common in infancy.
  - Structural defects (~12%)
  - Gastroesophageal reflux
  - Constipation
  - Celiac disease (~5%)
- Pulmonary
  - Tracheal stenosis/tracheoesophageal fistula
  - Pulmonary hypertension
  - Obstructive sleep apnea (50–75%)
- Genitourinary
  - Cryptorchidism, hypospadias
- Hematologic/neoplastic
  - Transient myeloproliferative disorder (~10%): generally resolves spontaneously; can be preleukemic (acute megakaryoblastic leukemia [AMKL]) in 20–30%
  - Leukemia (AMKL or acute lymphoblastic leukemia [ALL]) in 0.5–1%
  - Decreased risk of most solid tumors; increased risk of germ cell tumors
- Endocrine
  - Hypothyroidism: congenital or acquired (4–18%)
  - Diabetes
- Skeletal
  - Atlantoaxial instability (15%): 2% symptomatic
  - Short stature is common.
  - Scoliosis (some cases have adult onset)
  - Hip problems (1–4%)
- Immune/rheumatologic
  - Abnormal immune function with increased rate of respiratory infections
  - Increased risk of autoimmune disorders, including Hashimoto thyroiditis, celiac disease, and alopecia
- Neurologic
  - Intellectual ability ranging from near-normal to severe disability. Average is moderate intellectual disability.
  - Autism spectrum disorder (<18%); autism (<6%)
  - Seizures: (8%), typically occurring <1 year of age or >30 years of age
  - Alzheimer disease: at least 40% at age 40 years develop signs of dementia; percentage increases with age
- Psychiatric
  - Attention deficit hyperactivity disorder (ADHD), obsessive-compulsive disorder (OCD), oppositional-defiant disorder, and autism spectrum disorder increased frequency in children.
  - Generalized depression and anxiety with increased frequency in young adults/adults
- Sensory
  - Hearing loss (75%): mostly conductive due to high frequency of asymptomatic middle ear effusion; otitis media (50–70%)
  - Visual impairment (60%): mostly strabismus (refractive errors, 15%), nystagmus, cataracts (15%)
- Dermatologic
  - Xerosis, eczema, palmoplantar hyperkeratosis, atopic or seborrheic dermatitis, onychomycosis, syringomas, furunculosis/folliculitis

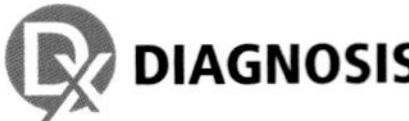

DIAGNOSIS

HISTORY

~85% of mothers of infants with DS learn of the diagnosis postnatally, although this is changing with the availability of noninvasive prenatal testing.

PHYSICAL EXAM

- Typical growth curves should be used (2).
- Infants and children
  - Brachycephaly (100%)
  - Hypotonia (80%)
  - Small ears, often low set and simplified
  - Up-slanting palpebral fissure (90%)
  - Epicanthic folds (90%)
  - Brushfield spots
  - Depressed nasal bridge
  - Short neck, often with increased nuchal folds
  - Single palmar crease, single flexion crease on 5th finger
  - Increased space between toes 1 and 2, 5th finger clinodactyly, brachydactyly

DIAGNOSTIC TESTS & INTERPRETATION

Initial Tests (lab, imaging)

- Maternal prenatal screening includes the following:
  - 1st trimester: combined screen (maternal age, β-human chorionic gonadotropin [β-hCG], pregnancy-associated plasma protein A, and nuchal translucency)
  - 2nd trimester: quad screen (α-fetoprotein, β-hCG, estriol, inhibin-A)
  - Sequential screen (combined screen in 1st trimester, if abnormal, obtain amniocentesis *or* await 2nd trimester quad screening)
  - Integrated screen (combined screening in 1st trimester plus quad screen in 2nd trimester)
  - NIPS with cell-free DNA (beginning at 10 weeks' gestation)
- Prenatal diagnosis includes the following:
  - Chorionic villus sampling: 1st trimester, ~99% accurate, ~1% miscarriage
  - Amniocentesis: 2nd trimester, ~99% accurate, ~0.25% miscarriage rate

- Postnatal diagnosis
  - Fluorescence in situ hybridization (FISH) can be performed at time of clinical suspicion, but karyotype should always be done to differentiate type of DS.
  - Parental (and adult-aged sibling) chromosome study is indicated only if translocation DS found in child.
- Echo, with or without murmur (2)
- CBC with differential (to look for transient myeloproliferative disorder) (2)
- Thyroid-stimulating hormone (TSH) (2)
- Audiogram (2)
- Ophthalmologic exam (look for red reflex) (2)
- Swallowing study for those with feeding difficulties (2)

Follow-Up Tests & Special Considerations

- After delivering a prenatal diagnosis, the physician should offer "Understanding a Down Syndrome Diagnosis" (www.lettercase.org) (3).
- If the diagnosis is postnatal, the mother and her partner should be informed of the diagnosis promptly by a physician (preferably the obstetrician and pediatrician or family physician), on the basis of clinical observations and before the karyotype is available, but with consideration of extenuating circumstances (e.g., mother's medical condition). The spouse/partner and infant should be present unless this would cause undue delay. The meeting should be private. Refer to the baby by name (4).
- In the postnatal setting, the physician should be knowledgeable on the subject of DS and should conduct a discussion with content that is current, respectful, balanced, informative, and realistic, but not overly pessimistic, concentrating on what is relevant to the first year of life (4,5).
- Cardiac follow-up, as indicated (2).

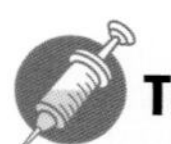

TREATMENT

GENERAL MEASURES

Genetic evaluation and counseling

ISSUES FOR REFERRAL

- Infant stimulation programs (early intervention) (6)[A]
- Lactation consultant
- Physical/occupational/speech therapy (6)[A]
- Inclusion programs can be successful.
- Pediatric cardiologist, if indicated.
- DS specialty clinics can improve medical outcomes (7)[B].

SURGERY/OTHER PROCEDURES

Repair of congenital anomalies is appropriate. Plastic surgery for facial features is not recommended.

COMPLEMENTARY & ALTERNATIVE MEDICINE

- There is no evidence to support the use of antioxidant or folinic acid supplements in children with DS.
- Craniosacral manipulation is dangerous due to potential atlantoaxial instability.
- Sicca is illegal in United States, potentially dangerous, and without any evidence of benefit.
- Piracetam is much publicized, without scientific evidence of benefit.

INPATIENT CONSIDERATIONS

Discharge Criteria

If the social situation indicates adoption: the National Down Syndrome Adoption Network (NDSAN) (www.ndsan.org), national registry of families seeking to adopt a child with DS.

ONGOING CARE

FOLLOW-UP RECOMMENDATIONS

Patient Monitoring

The American Academy of Pediatrics recommends ongoing assessment and review, at least annually, the following surveillance (2)[C]:

- Vision: Assess for strabismus, cataracts, and nystagmus by ophthalmologist by 6 months, annually between ages 1 and 5 years; every 2 years ages 5–13 years; every 3 years ages 13–21 years.
- Hearing: neonatal screen with auditory brainstem response (ABR) or otoacoustic emissions (OAE), then audiogram every 6 months until age 3 years, then annually
- Thyroid: initial newborn screen. Repeat TSH at 6 months, 12 months, and then annually.
- Screening for celiac disease (total IgA and tissue transglutaminase [TTG]-IgA) annually, if symptomatic
- 3-view cervical spine films if patient symptomatic, beginning at 3–5 years of age
- Hemoglobin annually to screen for iron deficiency anemia
- Echocardiogram for all newborns, regardless of murmur. Repeat in teens if with murmur or fatigue.

DIET

- No special diet, but caloric needs are lower in adolescents/adults with DS than their peers.
- Obesity is prevalent at all ages.
- No scientific evidence supports megavitamin therapy or dietary supplements.

PATIENT EDUCATION

- National Down Syndrome Congress 800-232-NDSC; www.ndsccenter.org
- National Down Syndrome Society 800-221-4602; www.ndss.org
- The Down Syndrome Research and Treatment Foundation provides information on the latest research for people with DS: www.dsrtf.org
- www.lettercase.org provides peer-reviewed booklet for parents who have received a prenatal diagnosis of DS and have not yet made a decision about their pregnancy.
- http://Downsyndromepregnancy.org provides a free downloadable book for expectant mothers who have decided to continue their pregnancies after a prenatal diagnosis of DS.
- www.downsyndromediagnosis.org

PROGNOSIS

- Associated congenital anomalies are the immediate concern during the newborn period.
- 99% of young adults/adults with DS report being happy with their lives.
- Life expectancy ~60 years

REFERENCES

1. Parker SE, Mai CT, Canfield MA, et al. Updated national birth prevalence estimates for selected birth defects in the United States, 2004–2006. *Birth Defects Res A Clin Mol Teratol*. 2010;88(12):1008–1016.
2. Bull MJ; Committee on Genetics. Health supervision for children with Down syndrome. *Pediatrics*. 2011;128(2):393–406.
3. Skotko BG, Kishnani PS, Capone GT; Down Syndrome Diagnosis Study Group. Prenatal diagnosis of Down syndrome: how best to deliver the news. *Am J Med Genet A*. 2009;149A(11):2361–2367.
4. Sheets KB, Crissman BG, Feist CD, et al. Practice guidelines for communicating a prenatal or postnatal diagnosis of Down syndrome: recommendations of the national society of genetic counselors. *J Genet Couns*. 2011;20(5):432–441.
5. Skotko BG, Capone GT, Kishnani PS, et al. Postnatal diagnosis of Down syndrome: synthesis of the evidence on how best to deliver the news. *Pediatrics*. 2009;124(4):e751–e758.
6. Blauw-Hospers CH, Hadders-Algra M. A systematic review of the effects of early intervention on motor development. *Dev Med Child Neurol*. 2005;47(6):421–432.
7. Skotko BG, Davidson EJ, Weintraub GS. Contributions of a specialty clinic for children and adolescents with Down syndrome. *Am J Med Genet A*. 2013;161A(3):430–437.

ADDITIONAL READING

National Center for Prenatal and Postnatal Down Syndrome Resources. Lexington, KY: University of Kentucky's Human Development Institute; 2012. http://www.downsyndromediagnosis.org. Accessed 2014.

SEE ALSO

Algorithm: Mental Retardation

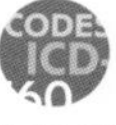

CODES

ICD10

- Q90.9 Down syndrome, unspecified
- Q90.1 Trisomy 21, mosaicism (mitotic nondisjunction)
- Q90.0 Trisomy 21, nonmosaicism (meiotic nondisjunction)

CLINICAL PEARLS

- 99% of young adults/adults with DS report being happy with their lives.
- DS specialty clinics can improve medical outcomes.

D

DRUG ABUSE, PRESCRIPTION

Edward Han, PharmD • Matthew A. Silva, PharmD, RPh, BCPS • Jeffrey Baxter, MD

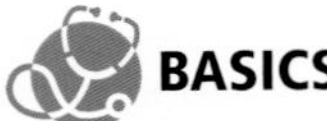

BASICS

DESCRIPTION

- Prescription drug abuse behaviors exist on a continuum and may include the following:
  - Using medication for nonmedical reasons such as to get high or enhance performance
  - Using medication for medical reasons other than what the prescriber intended
  - Using medication for any reason by someone other than the person for whom the medication was originally prescribed
- Commonly abused prescription medications include opioid analgesics (morphine, oxycodone, hydrocodone, oxymorphone, hydromorphone, fentanyl, methadone, buprenorphine), stimulants (amphetamine, methylphenidate), benzodiazepines (alprazolam, clonazepam), and barbiturates (secobarbital, amobarbital).
- *Diversion* is a term used to describe the rerouting of medications from prescriptions or other legitimate supplies for recreational use or criminal activity, such as selling prescription medication for personal profit.

EPIDEMIOLOGY

- In 2010, 49.6% of the 2.5 million drug-related ED visits attributed to drug misuse and abuse were due to pharmaceuticals (1.24 million) (1).
- A 2010 study found 62% of college students diverted ADHD medicine and 35% diverted prescription analgesics (1).
- Prescription opioids are the 2nd most commonly used class to initiate illicit drug use (1.9 million) (2).

Incidence

- Predominant sex: males > females (2)
- Predominant age: highest among adults 18–25 years, then adolescents and teens 12–17 years, followed by adults ≥26 years (2)
- >20% of the 3.1 million persons who were 1st-time substance abusers in 2011 used prescription medications nonmedically (2).
- The average age of persons with the 1st reported instance of nonmedical prescription drug use is 22.4 years (2).

Prevalence

- The number of persons with nonmedical opioid dependence increased from 936,000 in 2002 to 1.4 million in 2011 (2).
- Lifetime prevalence of prescription drug abuse is highest for opioids, benzodiazepines, and stimulants.

ETIOLOGY AND PATHOPHYSIOLOGY

- Prescription medications are now perceived by young adults to be more socially acceptable than other illicit drugs.
- Pharmacokinetics, compound purity, government approval, and extensive media advertising, along with personal or family experiences with prescription medication, contribute to perceived advantages of prescription drug misuse over street drugs and other illicit substances.

Genetics

Variant alleles affecting the expression and function of opioid, dopamine, acetylcholine, serotonin, and GABA may explain susceptibility to all forms of prescription and nonprescription drug abuse behaviors.

RISK FACTORS

- Sociodemographic, psychosocial, pain- and drug-related factors
- Genetics and environment; family history

GENERAL PREVENTION

- Educate and raise awareness about the dangers of misuse and abuse of prescription drugs. Focus on individuals, then families, then communities.
- Educate and reinforce safe practices in evaluating patients and prescribing medications. Use office based peer-to-peer education and follow-up with pharmacies when abuse behaviors are suspected.
- Develop or adopt a standard practice agreement for prescribing and monitoring controlled substances with abuse potential (3–5).
- Prescription monitoring plans (PMP) show fair evidence in reducing doctor shopping but have not reliably shown reductions in ED visits for drug overdose and prescription drug-abuse–related deaths (3).
- Avoid prescribing benzodiazepines and hypnotics to elderly (6).
- Avoid using benzodiazepines >2–4 weeks.
- Minimize controlled substances when patients have a personal or family history of substance abuse or psychiatric disorders (7).
- Limit or avoid prescribing controlled medications on 1st visit and until a relationship can be established.
- Take a thorough history, contact family members and past prescribers, and perform observed urine drug screens. Stop prescribing prescription analgesics for chronic pain when they are not working, if a patient is unable to take medications as prescribed, or if there are problems related to opioid and nonopioid analgesics. Identify and treat underlying substance abuse problems and involve behavioral health providers when possible.

COMMONLY ASSOCIATED CONDITIONS

- Benzodiazepines: withdrawal syndromes/delirium, psychosis, anxiety, sleep driving, blackout states, cognitive impairment, impaired driving while awake; increased fall risk and mortality in elderly patients
- Amphetamines: hypertension, tachyarrhythmias, myocardial ischemia, seizures, hypothermia, psychosis, hallucinations, paranoia, anxiety
- Opioids: respiratory depression and death with overdose, low testosterone, and sexual dysfunction with chronic abuse. Methadone is associated with QT-prolongation, which increases risk for torsades de pointes.

DIAGNOSIS

Screening: "How many times in the past year have you used an illegal drug or used a prescription medication for nonmedical reasons?"; primary care setting sensitivity of 100% and specificity of ~75% (8)[C]

HISTORY

Consider aberrant behaviors found when taking a history. Patient may ask for dose escalations and early refills ("spilled the bottle, pharmacist shorted me . . . etc."), has strong preference for one drug, targets appointments at end of day and after hours, and shows hostile/threatening behavior or overly flattering behavior.

DIAGNOSTIC TESTS & INTERPRETATION

- Urine drug screens are recommended to identify patients who are noncompliant or abusing prescription drugs despite limited evidence of reliability and accuracy (3,9)[C].
- Urine drug screen (UDS): Order an expanded panel to detect commonly used opioids (ask specifically for semisynthetics [hydrocodone, hydromorphone, oxycodone] and synthetics [methadone, fentanyl, propoxyphene, meperidine]) along with tramadol, and buprenorphine.
- Clonazepam and lorazepam rarely show up as benzodiazepines in routine UDS and should be ordered specifically.

Initial Tests (lab, imaging)

- Interpretation: Results are positive if drugs that are not prescribed are present; positive in presence of illicit drugs (marijuana, cocaine); can be negative for prescribed drug (suspect diversion)
- Be suspicious if patient refuses test.
- OxyContin will only be positive for oxycodone.
- Hydrocodone will be positive for hydrocodone and hydromorphone.
- Codeine will be positive for codeine plus morphine.
- Heroin will be positive for morphine.
- Thus, if UDS is positive for morphine, it could mean that a patient took morphine, codeine, heroin, or hydrocodone.

Diagnostic Procedures/Other

CAGE (Cut down, Anger at being questioned about use, Guilt about prior use, Eye-opener use early in day) or AUDIT (alcohol use disorders identification test) to assess current alcohol use. DAST (drug abuse screening test) helps determine patient's involvement with drugs over the past year. Details: http://counsellingresource.com/lib/quizzes/drug-testing/drug-abuse/. SOAPP (Screener and Opioid Assessment for Patients with Pain), ORT (Opioid Risk Tool), and DIRE (Diagnosis, Intractability, Risk, Efficacy) are tools used to assess risk of opioid misuse (10)[C].

Test Interpretation

See "History."

TREATMENT

- Whenever there is evidence of prescription opioid abuse, the controlled substance should be tapered to begin discontinuing drug therapy (3)[C].
- Benzodiazepines cannot be stopped abruptly for risk of seizures and death. A Cochrane Review supported a gradual benzodiazepine withdrawal over 10 weeks (11)[A].
- Amphetamines can be stopped abruptly without risk of severe withdrawal or death.
- The general approach to treatment includes inpatient, residential, or outpatient detoxification as required; counseling and intensive counseling as needed; and ongoing medication-assisted treatment.

GENERAL MEASURES

Alcoholics Anonymous/Narcotics Anonymous is helpful, as are Alanon/Alateen for family members. Nonjudgmental interactions and cognitive-behavioral therapy focused on motivational interviewing, goal-setting, and brief interventions help manage anxiety, insomnia, and denial and improve willingness to change.

MEDICATION

- Opioid detoxification programs use clonidine (12)[A], buprenorphine (12,13)[A], or methadone (14)[A] under the direction of an addiction specialist. Buprenorphine is as effective as methadone but safer (15)[A]. Both buprenorphine and methadone are more effective than clonidine for detoxification.
- Buprenorphine and methadone have been found to be similarly effective when used in long-term opioid maintenance therapy. Long-term therapy supervised by an addiction specialist is preferable to short-term detoxification.
- Subutex (buprenorphine) lacks naloxone and is prone to diversion and abuse because patients can crush, snort, or shoot to get high. Suboxone (buprenorphine and naloxone) discourages abuse and diversion because naloxone displaces buprenorphine binding to opioid receptors. Newer Suboxone sublingual film is preferred as the dosage form is difficult to adulterate.
- There is neither support for using or converting to long half-life benzodiazepines before beginning a slow, gradual 10-week benzodiazepine taper, although diazepam is often preferred, nor are there any benefits shown using propranolol, buspirone, progesterone, hydroxyzine, or dothiepin to manage withdrawal symptoms. Carbamazepine may be useful in patients who were dependent on ≥20 mg diazepam equivalents daily, and antidepressants may be helpful for depression and anxiety linked to benzodiazepine withdrawal.
- Atomoxetine and bupropion SR can also be helpful in managing ADHD symptoms in select patients.

ISSUES FOR REFERRAL

Refer to chemical dependency groups/addiction specialists/pain management and psychiatry/psychology when patients have polysubstance abuse and to treat underlying mood and anxiety disorders, PTSD, and ADHD. See related topic "Substance Abuse Disorders."

COMPLEMENTARY AND ALTERNATIVE MEDICINE

Acupuncture, yoga, meditation, or martial arts may aid in anxiety management and stress reduction.

INPATIENT CONSIDERATIONS

Admission Criteria/Initial Stabilization

Indications for inpatient detoxification are concomitant alcohol and benzodiazepine dependence (increased risk of seizures), mental confusion/delirium, history of seizures, psychosis, active suicidal ideation, serious comorbid medical issues, and absence of social support.

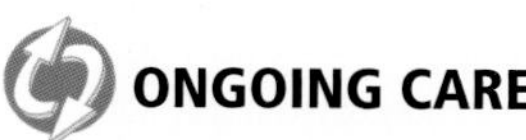

ONGOING CARE

PATIENT EDUCATION

- Advise patients receiving controlled medication to keep them hidden and inaccessible to others. Inform patients that giving their medication to others may result in legal charges. Warn about potential addiction when starting controlled substances and about withdrawal symptoms when a medication is stopped abruptly. Warn of the dangers of respiratory depression and death when opioids are mixed with benzodiazepines. Advise patients on controlled substances; avoid all alcohol and any illicit drugs.
- Tell patient to come to you if he or she begins to need medication in increasing amounts, uses it to feel high or overcome stress, or spends a lot of time craving it and thinking about the next dose. Emphasize that you will create a mutual plan to stop the medication and try something new. Inform spouse/family members when family dynamics are an important behavioral component.

REFERENCES

1. Substance Abuse and Mental Health Services Administration. *Drug Abuse Warning Network, 2011: National Estimates of Drug-Related Emergency Department Visits*. Rockville, MD: Substance Abuse and Mental Health Services Administration; 2013. HHS Publication No. (SMA) 13-4760, DAWN Series D-39.
2. Substance Abuse and Mental Health Services Administration. *Results from the 2011 National Survey on Drug Use and Health: Summary of National Findings* Rockville, MD: Substance Abuse and Mental Health Services Administration; 2012. HHS Publication No. (SMA) 12-4713.
3. Manchikanti L, Abdi S, Atluri S, et al. American Society of Interventional Pain Physicians (ASIPP) guidelines for responsible opioid prescribing in chronic non-cancer pain: part I–evidence assessment. *Pain Physician*. 2012;15(3)(Suppl):S1–S65.
4. Hariharan J, Lamb GC, Neuner JM. Long-term opioid contract use for chronic pain management in primary care practice. A five year experience. *J Gen Intern Med*. 2007;22(4):485–490.
5. Starrels JL, Becker WC, Alford DP, et al. Systematic review: treatment agreements and urine drug testing to reduce opioid misuse in patients with chronic pain. *Ann Intern Med*. 2010;152(11):712–720.
6. American Geriatrics Society 2012 Beers Criteria Update Expert Panel. American Geriatrics Society updated Beers Criteria for potentially inappropriate medication use in older adults. *J Am Geriatr Soc*. 2012;60(4):616–631.
7. Miotto K, Kaufman A, Kong A, et al. Managing co-occurring substance use and pain disorders. *Psychiatr Clin North Am*. 2012;35(2):393–409.
8. Smith PC, Schmidt SM, Allensworth-Davies D, et al. A single-question screening test for drug use in primary care. *Arch Intern Med*. 2010;170(13):1155–1160.
9. Manchikanti L, Abdi S, Atluri S, et al. American Society of Interventional Pain Physicians (ASIPP) guidelines for responsible opioid prescribing in chronic non-cancer pain: part 2–guidance. *Pain Physician*. 2012;15(3)(Suppl):S67–S116.
10. Chou R, Fanciullo GJ, Fine PG, et al. Clinical guidelines for the use of chronic opioid therapy in chronic noncancer pain. *J Pain*. 2009;10(2):113–130.
11. Denis C, Fatséas M, Lavie E, et al. Pharmacological interventions for benzodiazepine mono-dependence management in outpatient settings. *Cochrane Database Syst Rev*. 2006;(3):CD005194.
12. Gowing L, Ali R, White JM, et al. Buprenorphine for the management of opioid withdrawal. *Cochrane Database Syst Rev*. 2009;(3):CD002025.
13. Maremmani I, Gerra G. Buprenorphine-based regimens and methadone for the medical management of opioid dependence: selecting the appropriate drug for treatment. *Am J Addictions*. 2010;19(6):557–568.
14. Mattick RP, Breen C, Kimber J, et al. Methadone maintenance therapy versus no opioid replacement therapy for opioid dependence. *Cochrane Database Syst Rev*. 2009;(3):CD002209.
15. Mattick RP, Breen C, Kimber J, et al. Buprenorphine maintenance versus placebo or methadone maintenance for opioid dependence. *Cochrane Database Syst Rev*. 2008;(2):CD002207.

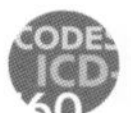

CODES

ICD10

- F19.10 Other psychoactive substance abuse, uncomplicated
- F11.10 Opioid abuse, uncomplicated
- F15.10 Other stimulant abuse, uncomplicated

CLINICAL PEARLS

- Education and prescription monitoring programs are important for preventing prescription drug abuse.
- Use a standardized office practice agreement when prescribing controlled substances.
- Screening: "How many times in the past year have you used an illegal drug or prescription medication for nonmedical reasons?"
- Avoid prescribing controlled substances and nonbenzodiazepine hypnotics to patients at risk for substance abuse or with an Axis 1 or Axis 2 diagnosis.
- Discontinue prescription opioid analgesics if pain or functionality does not improve and if there's evidence of prescription or illicit drug abuse (i.e., positive UDS, driving while intoxicated [DWI], accidental or intentional overdose, early refills).
- Limit benzodiazepine use to 2–4 weeks.
- Do frequent, observed UDS.
- Addiction is a potentially fatal disease.

DUCTAL CARCINOMA IN SITU

Bradley M. Turner, MD, MPH, MHA • David G. Hicks, MD

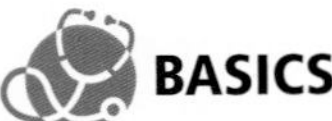

BASICS

DESCRIPTION

- Ductal carcinoma in situ (DCIS) is a heterogeneous group of lesions that have in common the presence of a clonal proliferation of neoplastic epithelial cells confined to ducts and lobules.
- Considered premalignant lesions—the neoplastic epithelial cells do not extend beyond the basement membrane and thus are not invasive (pure DCIS).
- Classification is subjective; however, typically considered as either low-, intermediate-, or high-grade based on architectural features and growth patterns (comedo, solid, cribriform, clinging, papillary, and micropapillary), nuclear grade (1, 2, or 3), and the absence/presence of necrosis.
- Mortality from DCIS with subsequent progression to invasive carcinoma is low regardless of histologic type or type of treatment.

EPIDEMIOLOGY

Incidence

- Estimated 65,000 new diagnoses of DCIS in 2013.
- DCIS accounts for approximately 80–85% of in situ breast carcinomas (lobular carcinoma in situ [LCIS] accounts for approximately 15–20%).
- Overall, incidence has increased in the United States between 1983 and 2003 with the introduction of mammographic screening—more stable over the last several years.
- Declining incidence in women >50 years of age over the last several years.
- Continued increased incidence in women <50 years of age over the last several years.
- Represents ~25% of all new invasive breast cancers—an estimated 58,168 new cases in 2014
- Rate of DCIS is comparable among women of different ethnicities.

ETIOLOGY AND PATHOPHYSIOLOGY

- A non-obligate precursor to invasive breast cancer
- Presumed to be the final step prior to invasive breast carcinoma, part of a poorly understood spectrum of polyclonal (hyperplasia) and clonal (atypical ductal hyperplasia [ADH]) epithelial proliferative lesions
- Either low- or high-grade DCIS has the potential for subsequent invasion into the surrounding stroma; however, the changes necessary for transition to invasive carcinoma are poorly understood.
- Molecular evidence suggests that low- and high-grade DCIS are genetically distinct lesions, with high-grade DCIS associated with more aggressive disease.

Genetics

- Low-grade DCIS typically shows diffuse and strong expression of estrogen receptor (ER) and progesterone receptor (PR), without HER2 protein overexpression or amplification.
- High-grade DCIS not consistently ER+ or PR+; frequent HER2 protein overexpression and amplification; commonly associated with p53 gene mutations
- HER2 overexpression is even more frequent in high-grade DCIS compared to invasive carcinoma.
- *BRCA1* and *BRCA2* associations observed
- If patients are high risk, consider genetic counseling after diagnosis of DCIS.

RISK FACTORS

- Similar to invasive breast cancer, although not as strongly associated
- Female gender, older age nulliparity, late age at first birth, late age at menopause, family history of a first-degree relative with breast cancer, prior breast biopsies, long-term use of postmenopausal hormone replacement therapy, elevated body mass index in postmenopausal women not taking hormone replacement, high mammographic breast density.
- Association with smoking, lactation, early menarche, increased alcohol consumption, and oral contraceptive use are less clear.

GENERAL PREVENTION

- Recent observational studies have created some controversy, suggesting that screening may result in an increase in overdiagnosis with little or no reduction in the incidence of advanced cancers.
- General screening guidelines have been suggested for women with an average risk of breast carcinoma.
- Women with increased risk should have more aggressive screening (risk assessment tool available at http://www.cancer.gov/bcrisktool/Default.aspx).
- General screening guidelines—U.S. Preventive Services Task Force (USPSTF)
  - USPSTF recommendations based on outcome data
    - Biennial mammography for women aged 50–74 years
    - Avoid routine screening mammography in women aged 40–49 years of age. The decision to start biennial mammographic screening before age 50 years should be individualized, based on patient's values regarding specific benefits or harms.
    - Discourage teaching breast self-exam (BSE).
    - Insufficient evidence to assess the value of clinical breast exam (CBE) in women after age 40 years. If this service is offered, the patient should understand this uncertainty.
    - Insufficient evidence to assess the benefit or harm of digital mammography or MRI over film mammography. If this service is offered, the patient should understand this uncertainty.
- General screening guidelines—National Comprehensive Cancer Network (NCCN)
  - NCCN recommends that women should be familiar with their breast; promptly report changes to their health care provider; and that periodic, consistent BSE may facilitate breast self-awareness.
  - For asymptomatic patients with negative physical exam
    - Ages 25–39 years: breast awareness, CBE every 1–3 years
    - Age 40 years and older: breast awareness, annual CBE, annual screening mammography
- Clinicians should use judgment when applying screening guidelines.
- Mammography screening should be individualized.
- If no intervention would occur based on screening findings, patient should not undergo screening.
- Risk reduction
  - Assess for familial/genetic and other elements that contribute to an increase risk of breast cancer.
  - Lifestyle modifications: Limit alcohol intake to <1 drink/day, exercise, maintain healthy diet, and weight control.
  - Risk reduction surgery supported for carefully selected women at high risk of breast cancer who desire this intervention.
  - Risk reduction agents (i.e., tamoxifen) are recommended in certain high-risk women ≥35 years of age.

DIAGNOSIS

HISTORY

- Most DCIS is now diagnosed by screening mammography (presence of microcalcifications in approximately 72%); patients may be asymptomatic with nonpalpable mass (12%) (1,2)[A].
- More advanced lesions may present with a palpable mass, spontaneous nipple discharge, or Paget disease (1,3)[A].

PHYSICAL EXAM

- CBE with inspection of breasts with patient in upright and supine position, evaluating for asymmetry, spontaneous discharge, skin changes (peau d'orange, erythema, scaling), nipple retraction/excoriation (Paget disease).
- Palpation of all breast quadrants with patient in upright and supine position and lymph node examination (axillary, supraclavicular, and internal mammary nodes).

- Positive clinical findings: Refer for consideration of diagnostic imaging and/or surgical evaluation, unless <30 years of age with a low clinical suspicion (observe 1–2 menstrual cycles; if positive clinical findings persist, refer for imaging) (3)[A].

DIFFERENTIAL DIAGNOSIS

Usual ductal hyperplasia, flat epithelial atypia, ADH, LCIS, microinvasive carcinoma (1)[A].

DIAGNOSTIC TESTS & INTERPRETATION

Initial Tests (lab, imaging)

- Mammography Breast Imaging Reporting and Data System (BI-RADS) developed by the American College of Radiology is used for uniform reporting of mammography results.
- BI-RADS interpretation: **Category 0:** incomplete and needs additional imaging; **Category 1:** negative; **Category 2:** benign finding; **Category 3:** probably benign finding; **Category 4:** suspicious abnormality; **Category 5:** highly suggestive of malignancy; **Category 6:** known biopsy-proven malignancy
- Similar BI-RADS interpretations for diagnostic ultrasound (US)
- Screening BI-RADS category 0: diagnostic workup with consideration for diagnostic imaging
- Screening BI-RADS categories 1 and 2: screening recommendations.
- Screening BI-RADS category 3: diagnostic imaging at 6 months, then every 6–12 months for 2–3 years; consider biopsy if patient anxious or follow-up uncertain.
- Screening BI-RADS categories 4 and 5: diagnostic imaging with follow-up
- Screening BI-RADS category 6: technically not a "screening" category other than to assess a known cancer that might need additional evaluation. NCCN guidelines for breast cancer should be followed.

- DCIS is commonly seen on imaging as clustered microcalcifications (2)[A].

- Diagnostic imaging will result in consideration for tissue biopsy.

Follow-Up Tests & Special Considerations

- US not recommended for screening (3)[A].
- The sensitivity of breast MRI screening is higher than mammography but has lower specificity resulting in a greater number of false positives (2,3)[A].

- Screening with MRI is only recommended in certain women: *BRCA* mutation, first-degree relative of *BRCA* carrier, ≥20% lifetime risk of breast cancer, radiation to chest between the ages of 10 and 30 years, presence of Li-Fraumeni, Cowden, or Bannayan-Riley-Ruvalcaba syndrome in patient or first-degree relative (3)[A].
- Screening with MRI is not recommended in women with <15% lifetime risk of breast cancer.
- MRI can also complement mammography in the diagnostic setting, particularly in patients with skin changes (3)[A].
- Although MRI and US are complementary diagnostic methods to mammography, US is less sensitive in detecting most microcalcifications and MRI does not typically detect microcalcifications at all (2,3)[A].
- Pathology
  - Tissue necessary for diagnosis: typically core needle (CN) or vacuum-assisted (VA) biopsy (mammographic/stereotactic, US or MRI guided). Open surgical biopsy in patients not amenable to CN or VA biopsy.
  - Fine-needle aspiration (FNA) is not adequate for specific diagnosis of DCIS; however, it can suggest the presence of neoplastic cells.
- Histologic classification
  - Traditionally classified by architectural pattern (comedo, solid, cribriform, clinging, papillary, and micropapillary), morphology, nuclear grade, and the presence of necrosis (1,2).
  - Grade is more important for prognosis, risk for progression, and local recurrence.
  - Ductal intraepithelial neoplasia (DIN) is an alternative histologic classification using size as a discriminatory factor to separate low-grade DCIS from ADH (2,4)[C].
- Presence of necrosis is often used to classify DCIS.
- Comedo necrosis (necrosis filling central portion of involved duct), typically seen in high-grade DCIS.
- Varying degrees of necrosis in other types of DCIS.
- Determination of ER and PR status (1)[A].
- Studies show unclear or weak evidence of HER2 status as a prognostic indicator in DCIS (5)[A].

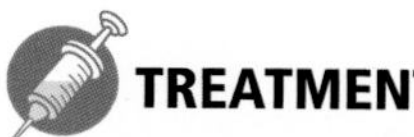

TREATMENT

SURGERY/OTHER PROCEDURES

- Surgery is the primary treatment option. Options for surgery are based on risk of recurrence, anatomic location, extent of disease, and the ability to achieve "negative" margins (5)[A].
- Positive margins are considered "ink on tumor" (6)[A].
- Negative margins controversial with DCIS (5)[C]
- Margins <1 mm considered inadequate (1,5)[A]
- Totality of evidence may not support distinguishing between margins of "no ink on tumor" and margins of <1 mm (6)[C].
- Margins <1 mm at the breast fibroglandular boundary (chest wall or skin) do not mandate surgical excision but may be an indication for higher boost dose radiation in patients opting for breast conservation (5)[A].
- Surgical options include the following:
  - **Breast conservation (lumpectomy) with or without whole breast radiation therapy** (5)[A]
    - Radiation decreases recurrence rates by about 50 % (2,7,8)[A].
    - ∼50% of recurrences are pure DCIS; ∼50% are invasive cancer (1,5)[A].
    - Recurrence generally requires mastectomy with consideration for systemic treatment (2)[C].
  - **Mastectomy with or without sentinel node biopsy ± breast reconstruction** (5)[A]
    - Mastectomy provides maximum local control.
    - Recurrence type similar to lumpectomy
    - Recurrence should be treated with wide local excision, chest wall radiation, and consideration for systemic treatment (5)[A].
    - Long-term cause-specific survival seems to be equivalent to lumpectomy with whole breast radiation (5)[A].
- Secondary chemoprevention following breast-conserving surgery for ER + DCIS
  - Tamoxifen for 5 years (5)[A]
  - Considered in lumpectomy patients with or without whole breast radiation (5)[A]
  - Benefit of trastuzumab in patients with ER-negative/HER2-positive disease is unclear (1,9)[C].

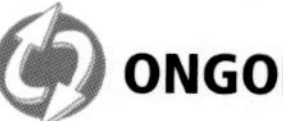

ONGOING CARE

FOLLOW-UP RECOMMENDATIONS

- History and physical exam every 6 months for first 5 years, then annually
- Mammography 6–12 months after whole breast radiation, then every 12 months

PROGNOSIS

- Good prognosis: 10-year breast cancer–specific survival rates of >95%; overall mortality after diagnosis of treated pure DCIS generally >98%
- Risk of local recurrence after mastectomy generally reported as 1–2% (higher in some studies)
- Higher risk of local recurrences after breast-conserving therapy in younger age (particularly before age 40 years), larger tumor size, high nuclear grade, comedo necrosis, and close/positive margin status (DCIS volume related)
- ER+ tumors associated with lower recurrence risk

REFERENCES

1. Siziopikou KP. Ductal carcinoma in situ of the breast: current conceptys and future directions. *Arch Pathol Lab Med*. 2013;137(4):462–466.
2. Lee RJ, Vallow LA, McLaughlin SA, et al. Ductal carcinoma in situ of the breast. *Int J Surg Oncol*. 2012;2012:1–12.
3. NCCN clinical practice guidelines in oncology: breast cancer screening and diagnosis (Version 1.2014) 2014. National Comprehensive Cancer Network Web site. http://www.nccn.org. Accessed on June 16, 2013.
4. Tavassoli FA. Breast pathology: rationale for adopting the ductal intraepithelial (DIN) classification. *Nat Clin Pract Oncol*. 2005;2(3):116–117.
5. NCCN clinical practice guidelines in oncology: breast cancer (Version 3.2014) 2014. National Comprehensive Cancer Network Web site. http://www.nccn.org. Accessed on June 16, 2014.
6. Moran MS, Schnitt S, Giuliano AE, et al. Society of Surgical Oncology-American Society for Radiation Oncology concensus guideline on margins for breast-conserving surgery with whole-breast irradiation in stages I and II invasive breast cancer. *J Clin Oncol*. 2014;32(14):1507–1515.
7. Donker M, Litiére S, Werutsky G, et al. Breast conserving treatment with or without radiotherapy in ductal carcinoma in situ: 15-year recurrence rates and outcome after a recurrence, from the EORTC 10853 randomized phase III trial. *J Clin Oncol*. 2013;31(32):4054–4059.
8. Goodwin A, Parker S, Ghersi D, et al. Post-operative radiotherapy for ductal carcinoma in situ of the breast. *Cochrane Database Syst Rev*. 2013;(11):CD000563.
9. Carraro D, Elias E, Andrade V. Ductal carcinoma in situ of the breast: morphological and molecular features implicated in progression. *Biosci Rep*. 2014;34(1):19–28.

ADDITIONAL READING

- Gøtzxche PC, Jørgensen KJ. Screening for breast cancer with mammography. *Cochrane Database Syst Rev*. 2013;(6):CD001877.
- Kerlikowske K. Epidemiology of ductal carcinoma in situ. *J Natl Cancer Inst Monogr*. 2010;2010(41):139–141.
- Lim YJ, Kim K, Chie EK, et al. Treatment outcome of ductal carcinoma in situ patients treated with postoperative radiation therapy. *Radiat Oncol J*. 2014;32(1):1–6.
- Owen D, Tyldesley S, Alexander C, et al. Outcomes in patients treated with mastectomy for ductal carcinoma in situ. *Int J Radiat Oncol Biol Phys*. 2013;85(3):e129–e134.
- Punglia RS, Schnitt SJ, Weeks JC. Treatment of ductal carcinoma in situ after excision: would a prophylactic paradigm be more appropriate? *J Natl Cancer Inst*. 2013;105(20):1527–1533.
- Siegel R, Ma J, Zou Z, et al. Cancer statistics, 2014. *CA Cancer J Clin*. 2014;64(1):9–29.
- US Preventive Services Task Force. Screening for breast cancer: U.S. Preventative Services Task Force recommendation statement. *Ann Intern Med*. 2009;151(10):716–726.
- Wehner P, Lagios MD, Silverstein MJ. DCIS treated with excision alone using the National Comprehensive Cancer Network (NCCN) guidelines. *Ann Surg Oncol*. 2012;20(10):3175–3179.
- Wilkinson JB, Vicini F, Shah C, et al. Twenty-year outcomes after breast-conserving surgery and definitive radiotherapy for mammographically detected ductal carcinoma in situ. *Ann Surg Oncol*. 2012;19(12):3785–3791.

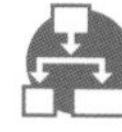

SEE ALSO

- Breast Cancer

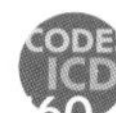

CODES

ICD10

- D05.10 Intraductal carcinoma in situ of unspecified breast
- D05.11 Intraductal carcinoma in situ of right breast
- D05.12 Intraductal carcinoma in situ of left breast

CLINICAL PEARLS

- DCIS is a heterogeneous group of noninvasive neoplastic lesions arising from the breast ductal epithelial cells.
- The incidence of DCIS has continued to increase in women <50 years of age, with a more stable incidence in women >50 years of age.
- The goal of DCIS treatment is to prevent invasive breast cancer.
- Current standard of care is breast-conserving therapy with consideration for postoperative whole breast radiation therapy and/or postsurgical tamoxifen therapy, unless otherwise contraindicated.
- With appropriate therapy, the overall prognosis of pure DCIS is good.

DUMPING SYNDROME

Hongyi Cui, MD, PhD, FACS, FICS

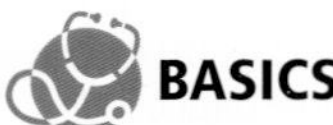

BASICS

DESCRIPTION

GI and vasomotor symptoms resulting from rapid gastric emptying and delivery of large amounts of hyperosmolar content into the small intestine

- Usually occurs following gastric and esophageal surgery (gastrectomy, vagotomy, pyloroplasty, esophagectomy, Nissen fundoplication, or gastric bypass procedures).

EPIDEMIOLOGY

- Overall, ~10% of patients following gastric surgery and up to 50% of patients who undergo esophagectomy develop dumping symptoms.
- Predominant age: middle age to elderly
- Predominant sex: female > male

Incidence

- In the United States, 0.9% of patients undergoing proximal gastric vagotomy without any drainage procedure; 10–22% truncal vagotomy and drainage
  - After partial gastrectomy, 14–20% of patients develop symptoms of dumping.
- Prominent feature after bariatric surgery:
  - >70% of gastric bypass patients experience varying degrees of dumping symptoms.
  - Regarded as a beneficial feature of gastric bypass surgery because patients learn to avoid calorie-rich foods and eat small meals

ETIOLOGY AND PATHOPHYSIOLOGY

The pathogenesis of dumping syndrome is multifactorial.

- Alterations in the storage function of the stomach and/or the pyloric emptying mechanism lead to rapid delivery of hyperosmolar material into the intestine. Fluid shifts from the intravascular compartment into the bowel lumen lead to rapid small bowel distention and an increased frequency of bowel contractions (early dumping).
- Supraphysiologic release of GI peptides/vasoactive mediators lead to paradoxical vasodilation in a relatively volume-contracted state.
- Reactive hypoglycemia secondary to hyperinsulinemia caused by high concentration of carbohydrates in the proximal small intestine and rapid absorption of glucose (late dumping)
- Pancreatic islet cell hyperplasia, rather than late dumping, is thought to be the underlying mechanism for hyperinsulinemic hypoglycemia with nesidioblastosis after gastric bypass. These patients do not respond to treatment for dumping syndrome, and the confirmation of this rare condition is difficult.

RISK FACTORS

Gastric surgery is the main risk factor. The severity of dumping syndrome is proportional to the rate of gastric emptying following different surgical procedures:

- Bariatric surgery (i.e., Roux-en-Y gastric bypass)
  - Laparoscopic sleeve gastrectomy (LSG) for morbid obesity is also associated with symptoms of dumping syndrome.
- Gastric drainage procedures (e.g., pyloroplasty)
- Partial gastrectomy
- Total gastrectomy: Pouch formation has less dumping and heartburn.
- Esophagectomy
- Antiulcer surgery (e.g., vagotomy)
- Antireflux surgery (e.g., Nissen fundoplication, especially in pediatric patients)

GENERAL PREVENTION

- Dietary modifications (frequent, small, dry meals that contain limited amount of refined carbohydrates; restrict fluids to between meals; avoid milk products and increase protein/fat intake; supplement dietary fiber)
- Postural changes (supine for 30 minutes after meals)
- New bariatric surgical techniques may reduce postoperative dumping syndrome.

COMMONLY ASSOCIATED CONDITIONS

- Peptic ulcer disease
- Reactive hypoglycemia
- Gastrectomy/vagotomy/pyloroplasty
- Esophagectomy
- Post-Nissen fundoplication (pediatric reflux)
- After gastric bypass or sleeve gastrectomy procedure for morbid obesity

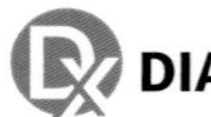

DIAGNOSIS

A suggestive symptom profile in a patient who has undergone gastric (including bariatric) or esophageal surgery.

HISTORY

- History of gastric or esophageal surgery
- Early dumping symptoms include GI and vasomotor symptoms.
- Late dumping includes systemic and vasomotor symptoms.
- GI symptoms (early dumping)
  - Cramping abdominal pain
  - Diarrhea (postprandial)
  - Borborygmi
  - Bloating or epigastric fullness
  - Nausea/vomiting
- Systemic/vasomotor symptoms (early and late dumping)
  - Palpitations
  - Diaphoresis
  - Faintness, fatigue, and headache
  - Flushing
  - Light-headedness and desire to lie down
  - Confusion and syncope
  - Malnutrition and weight loss

PHYSICAL EXAM

- Diagnosis is based primarily on typical symptoms in patients with history of gastric procedures.
- A diagnostic scoring system is available (1):
  - A score index >7 is suggestive of dumping syndrome.
  - The score also helps assess response to therapy.

Sigstad's Scoring System:	
Shock	+5
Fainting, syncope, unconscious	+4
Desire to lie or sit down	+4
Breathlessness, dyspnea	+3
Weakness, exhaustion	+3
Sleepiness, drowsiness, apathy	+3
Palpitation	+3
Dizziness	+2
Restlessness	+2
Headaches	+1
Feeling of warmth, sweating, pallor, clammy	+1
Nausea	+1
Abdominal fullness	+1
Borborygmus	+1
Eructation	−1
Vomiting	−1

- No physical signs are specific for dumping syndrome.

DIFFERENTIAL DIAGNOSIS

- Afferent loop syndromes
- Bile acid reflux after surgery
- Bowel obstruction
- Celiac disease
- Gastroenteric fistula
- Cholecystitis
- Inflammatory bowel disease
- Hypoglycemia
- Pancreatic insufficiency

DIAGNOSTIC TESTS & INTERPRETATION

Dumping syndrome is a clinical diagnosis based on typical symptoms in patients who have undergone gastric surgery.

Initial Tests (lab, imaging)

- Postprandial hypoglycemia
- Anemia
- Hypoalbuminemia
- Upper GI series: barium rapidly emptying from stomach (barium fluoroscopy)
- Nuclear medicine gastric emptying study (radionuclide scintigraphy)
- Endoscopy (to define anatomy and exclude mechanical obstruction)

Diagnostic Procedures/Other

- Oral glucose challenge test (i.e., oral intake of 50 g of glucose following 10-hour fasting) can elicit typical signs and symptoms in patients with dumping syndrome. A rise in heart rate by ≥10 beats/minute in the 1st hour is the best predictor for dumping syndrome.
- Hydrogen breath test after oral ingestion of glucose

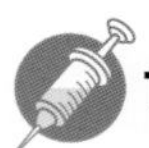

TREATMENT

- *Dietary modification is the mainstay of treatment*
- Medical therapy is effective in patients with incapacitating symptoms who fail dietary modifications.
- Remedial surgery is only considered in patients who are refractory to medical management.

GENERAL MEASURES

Most patients can be managed conservatively with dietary modification and medical treatment. Only a small percentage of patients ultimately require surgical intervention.

MEDICATION

First Line

- Octreotide (Sandostatin, 50 μg SC BID–TID) relieves dumping symptoms by delaying gastric emptying and inhibiting the release of GI hormones. Expensive.
  - Patients may have increased steatorrhea during octreotide treatment, and pancreatic enzyme supplement is effective in relieving this symptom.
  - Gallstone formation, steatorrhea, and diarrhea are side effects associated with octreotide.
- Late dumping symptoms can be ameliorated by the α-glucosidase inhibitor acarbose (100–200 mg PO TID), which lowers blood glucose by delaying GI absorption of carbohydrates.
  - Acarbose therapy is associated with bloating diarrhea due to bacterial fermentation of unabsorbed carbohydrate in the intestine.
- Pectin/Guar gum (ingestion of up to 15 g with each meal) is effective by delaying glucose absorption and prolonging small bowel transit time.

Second Line

Anticholinergics: generally not helpful

ADDITIONAL THERAPIES

- Continuous trophic enteral feeding via a jejunostomy has been reported to be an effective approach in patient who are refractory to other treatments.
- Individual psychotherapy with behavior modification and (in selected cases) hypnotherapy
- Adjuncts: group therapy, expressive art therapy, occupational and recreational therapy when not associated with dissociative amnesia or fugue

SURGERY/OTHER PROCEDURES

- Remedial surgery is indicated only if dietary and medical management unsuccessful and symptoms debilitating. The results are variable and unpredictable. A proper selection of the surgical intervention is very important. Most patients with dumping syndrome due to gastric bypass report that symptoms improve over time (>2 years).
- Surgical options include Roux-en-Y conversion (from Billroth I and II), pyloric reconstruction (for patients who have severe dumping following pyloroplasty), reversed jejunal segment (for patients who failed Roux-en-Y reconstruction), and conversion of Billroth II to Billroth I anastomosis.
- Patients with refractory dumping symptoms after loop gastrojejunostomy may benefit from simple takedown of the anastomosis; conversion to Roux-en-Y gastrojejunostomy is reasonable for patients with disabling dumping after distal gastrectomy. Other procedures have had limited success.
- The syndrome of hyperinsulinemic hypoglycemia with nesidioblastosis (a hyperplasia of islet cells) after Roux-en-Y gastric bypass (>1–2 years postop) can usually be managed with low-carbohydrate diet and α-glucosidase inhibitors.
- For selected patients with medical refractory hyperinsulinemic hypoglycemia after Roux-en-Y gastric bypass (RYGB), laparoscopic reversal of RYGB to normal anatomy or modified sleeve gastrectomy is an option (2)[B].

ONGOING CARE

FOLLOW-UP RECOMMENDATIONS

Lying supine for 30 minutes after eating or when symptoms occur may reduce the chance of syncope.

Patient Monitoring

Follow to be sure of adequate nutrition.

DIET

Mainstay of treatment for dumping syndrome:

- Low-carbohydrate, high-protein diet
- Add dietary fiber.
- Milk or milk products should be avoided.
- Frequent small meals with minimal liquid. Drink liquids between meals (rather than with meals).
- Avoid hyperosmolar liquids.

PATIENT EDUCATION

National Digestive Diseases Information Clearinghouse, Box NDDIC, Bethesda, MD 20892, (301) 468-6344, digestive.niddk.nih.gov

PROGNOSIS

Favorable

COMPLICATIONS

- Hypoglycemia
- Malnutrition and weight loss
- Electrolyte disturbances, including hypokalemia

REFERENCES

1. Sigstad H. A Clinical Diagnostic Index in the diagnosis of the dumping syndrome. Changes in plasma volume and blood sugar after a test meal. *Acta Med Scand*. 1970;188(6):479–486.
2. Campos GM, Ziemelis M, Paparodis R, et al. Laparoscopic reversal of Roux-en-Y gastric bypass: technique and utility for treatment of endocrine complications. *Surg Obes Relat Dis*. 2014;10(1):36–43.

ADDITIONAL READING

- Banerjee A, Ding Y, Mikami DJ, et al. The role of dumping syndrome in weight loss after gastric bypass surgery. *Surg Endosc*. 2013;27(5):1573–1578.
- Bouras EP, Scolapio JS. Gastric motility disorders: management that optimizes nutritional status. *J Clin Gastroenterol*. 2004;38(7):549–557.
- Dikic S, Randjelovic T, Dragojevic S, et al. Early dumping syndrome and reflux esophagitis prevention with pouch reconstruction. *J Surg Res*. 2012;175(1):56–61.
- Gertler R, Rosenberg R, Feith M, et al. Pouch vs. no pouch following total gastrectomy: meta-analysis and systematic review. *Am J Gastroenterol*. 2009;104(11):2838–2851.
- Gonzalez-Sánchez JA, Corujo-Vázquez O, Sahai-Hernández M. Bariatric surgery patients: reasons to visit emergency department after surgery. *Bol Asoc Med P R*. 2007;99(4):279–283.
- Penning C, Vecht J, Masclee AA. Efficacy of depot long-acting release octreotide therapy in severe dumping syndrome. *Aliment Pharmacol Ther*. 2005;22(10):963–969.
- Tack J, Arts J, Caenepeel P. Pathophysiology, diagnosis and management of postoperative dumping syndrome. *Nat Rev Gastroenterol Hepatol*. 2009;6(10):583–590.
- Tzovaras G, Papamargaritis D, Sioka E, et al. Symptoms suggestive of dumping syndrome after provocation in patients after laparoscopic sleeve gastrectomy. *Obes Surg*. 2012;22(1):23–28.
- Ukleja A. Dumping syndrome: pathophysiology and treatment. *Nutr Clin Pract*. 2005;20(5):517–525.

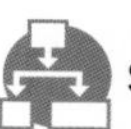

SEE ALSO

- Diarrhea, Chronic; Hypoglycemia, Nondiabetic; Peptic Ulcer Disease
- Algorithm: Diarrhea, Chronic

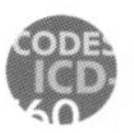

CODES

ICD10

K91.1 Postgastric surgery syndromes

CLINICAL PEARLS

- Dumping syndrome is the most common cause for emergency room presentation after bariatric surgery.
- An increase in heart rate of 10 bpm is noted after glucose challenge (50 g PO glucose) in patients with dumping syndrome.
- Vagotomy affects gastric emptying through increased gastric tone and decreased receptive relaxation.
- Dietary modification is the mainstay of treatment for dumping syndrome.

D

DUPUYTREN CONTRACTURE

Jeffrey F. Minteer, MD

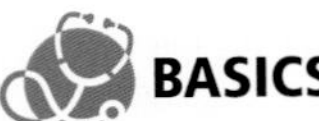

BASICS

DESCRIPTION

- Palmar fibromatosis; caused by progressive fibrous proliferation and tightening of the fascia of the palms, resulting in flexion deformities and loss of function
- Not the same as "trigger finger," which is caused by thickening of the distal flexor tendon
- Similar change may rarely occur in plantar fascia; it usually appears simultaneously.
- System(s) affected: musculoskeletal
- Synonyms: morbus Dupuytren; Dupuytren disease; "Celtic hand"

EPIDEMIOLOGY

Prevalence

- 4% in the United States
- Norway: 30% of males >60 years; Spain: 19% of males >60 years
- More common in Caucasians of Scandinavian or Northern European ancestry

ETIOLOGY AND PATHOPHYSIOLOGY

Unknown; possibly a T-cell–mediated autoimmune disorder. Disease occurs in three stages:

- Proliferative phase: proliferation of myofibroblasts with nodule development on palmar surface
- Involutional stage: spread along palmar fascia to fingers with cord development
- Residual phase: spread into fingers with cord tightening and contracture formation

Genetics

- Autosomal dominant with incomplete penetrance:
  - Siblings with 3-fold risk
- 68% of male relatives of affected patients develop disease at some time.

RISK FACTORS

- Smoking (mean 16 pack-years, odds ratio 2.8)
- Increasing age
- Male/Caucasian; male > female (1.7:1)
- Workers exposed to vibration—risk doubled with weekly exposure (1)
- Diabetes mellitus (affected, increases with time, usually mild; middle and ring finger involved)
- Epilepsy
- Chronic illness (e.g., pulmonary tuberculosis, liver disease, HIV)
- Hypercholesterolemia
- Alcohol consumption

GENERAL PREVENTION

Avoid risk factors, especially in those with a strong family history.

COMMONLY ASSOCIATED CONDITIONS

- Alcoholism
- Epilepsy
- Diabetes mellitus
- Chronic lung disease
- Occupational hand trauma (vibration)
- Hypercholesterolemia
- Carpal tunnel syndrome; Peyronie disease

DIAGNOSIS

HISTORY

- Caucasian male aged 50–60 years
- Family history
- Mild pain early:
  - Begins in palm then spread to digits
- Unilateral or bilateral (50%)
- Right hand more frequent
- Ring finger more frequent
- Ulnar digits more affected than radial digits
- Flexion contracture of metacarpophalangeal (MCP) before proximal interphalangeal (PIP) joint

PHYSICAL EXAM

- Painless plaques or nodules in palmar fascia
- Cordlike band in the palmar fascia
- Skin adheres to fascia and becomes puckered.
- Nodules can be palpated under the skin.
- Reduced flexibility of MCP and PIP joints
- No sign of inflammation
- Web space contractures
- Ectopic Dupuytren can involve plantar (Ledderhose—10%) and penile (Peyronie—2%) fascia:
  - Knuckle pads over PIP:
    - Garrod nodes commonly associated with severe disease.
- Disease stages:
  - Early: skin pits (can also be seen in nevoid basal cell cancer and palmar keratosis)
- Intermediate: nodules and cords. Nerves and vessels can be entwined in cords.
  - Late: contractures

DIFFERENTIAL DIAGNOSIS

- Tendon abnormalities
- Camptodactyly: early teens; tight fascial bands on ulnar side of small finger
- Diabetic cheiroarthropathy: all 4 fingers
- Volkmann ischemic contracture

DIAGNOSTIC TESTS & INTERPRETATION

Diagnostic Procedures/Other

MRI can assess cellularity of lesions that correlate with higher recurrence after surgery.

Test Interpretation

- Myofibroblasts predominate.
- Nodules: Lumps fixed to skin hypercellular masses.
- Cords: organized collagen type III arranged parallel and hypocellular
- 1st stage (proliferative): increased myofibroblasts
- 2nd stage (residual): dense fibroblast network
- 3rd stage (involutional): Myofibroblasts disappear.

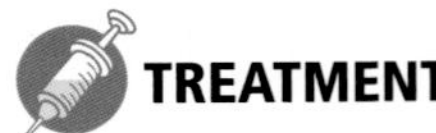

TREATMENT

GENERAL MEASURES

- Physiotherapy alone is ineffective:
  - Intermittent splinting is unlikely to be effective.
  - Continuous splinting may be helpful pre- and postoperatively.
- Isolated involvement of palmar fascia can be followed conservatively.
- MCP joint involvement can be followed conservatively if flexion contracture is <30 degrees.

MEDICATION

First Line

- Steroid injection for acute tender nodule, painful knuckle pad
- Clostridial collagenase injections (FDA approved 2010):
  - Degrades collagen to allow manual rupture of diseased cord
  - Best for isolated cord of MCP joint 77% and PIP 40%
  - Recurrence rate at 8 years; 67% in MCP joints but less severe than initial contracture (2)[B]
  - Complications: edema, pain
  - Can do 2 cords concurrently
  - Can be effective for recurrence postsurgery

Second Line

- Topical high-potency steroids: case report of improvement with clobetasol 0.05% BID and at bedtime for 2–4 weeks
- Surgery for contracture >30%

ISSUES FOR REFERRAL

- Any involvement of PIP joints
- MCP joints contracted >30 degrees
- Positive Hueston tabletop test: When the palm is placed on a flat surface, the digits cannot be simultaneously placed fully on the same surface as the palm because of flexion contractures.

ADDITIONAL THERAPIES

- Continuous elongation (atraumatic elongation using an external device, typically on 4th and 5th digits) is useful to prepare a severely contracted PIP joint for surgery.
  - The digit can frequently be completely extended; will relapse if surgery is not performed.
- Prophylactic external beam radiation: 87% either no progression or improvement at 12 months; concern about local effects in a benign disease
- Intraoperative 5-fluorouracil ineffective
- Percutaneous and needle fasciotomy:
  - Best for MCP joint
  - Recurrence common
  - Not indicated in severe or recurrent disease

SURGERY/OTHER PROCEDURES

- Selective fascial ray release/partial fasciectomy (3)[B]:
  - Studies pending to compare collagenase injection with limited fasciectomy or percutaneous needle fasciotomy (recurrence 84% vs. 21% in limited fasciectomy) (4).
  - Night extension orthosis in combination with standard hand therapy no different maintaining finger extension than hand therapy alone in the 3 months following surgical release (5)[C].
- Indications:
  - Any involvement of the PIP joints
  - MCP joints contracted at least 30 degrees
  - Positive Hueston tabletop test
- May require skin grafts for wound closure with severe cutaneous shrinkage. Reports of clinical regression with continuous passive skeletal traction in extension and under a skin graft. Skin tears in 11% using collagenase.
- 80% have full range of movement with early surgery.
- Amputation of 5th digit if severe and deforming
- MCP joints respond better to surgery than PIP joints, especially if contracted >45 degrees.
- Percutaneous needle aponeurotomy: Elderly with comorbid conditions may do better when used for MCP joints; has higher rate of recurrence.

ONGOING CARE

FOLLOW-UP RECOMMENDATIONS

Patient Monitoring

Regular follow-up by physician every 6 months–1 year

PATIENT EDUCATION

- Avoid risk factors, especially in those with a strong family history.
- Mild disease: Passively stretch digits twice a day and avoid recurrent gripping of tools.

PROGNOSIS

- Unpredictable but usually slowly progressive
- 10% may regress spontaneously.
- Dupuytren diathesis predicts aggressive course. Features include ethnicity (Nordic), family history, bilateral lesions outside of palm, age <50 years—all factors with 71% risk of recurrence compared to baseline 23% without any risk factors.
- Prognosis better for MCP versus PIP joint after surgery and collagenase injection.

COMPLICATIONS

- Reflex sympathetic dystrophy postsurgery
- Postoperative recurrence or extension in 46–80%
- Postoperative hand edema and skin necrosis
- Digital infarction

REFERENCES

1. Descatha A, Jauffret P, Chastang JF, et al. Should we consider Dupuytren's contracture as work-related? A review and meta-analysis of an old debate. *BMC Musculoskelet Disord*. 2011;12:96.
2. Watt AJ, Curtin CM, Hentz VR, et al. Collagenase injection as nonsurgical treatment of Dupuytren's disease: 8-year follow-up. *J Hand Surg Am*. 2010;35(4):534–539, 539.e1.
3. van Rijssen AL, Werker PM. Treatment of Dupuytren's contracture: an overview of options [in Dutch]. *Ned Tijdschr Geneeskd*. 2009;153:A129.
4. Stanbury SJ, Hammert WC. Dupuytren contracture. *J Hand Surg Am*. 2011;36(12):2038–2040.
5. Collis J, Collocott S, Hing W, et al. The effect of night extension orthoses following surgical release of Dupuytren contracture: a single-center, randomized, controlled trial. *J Hand Surg Am*. 2013;38(7):1285.e2–1294.e2.
6. Rayan GM. Clinical presentation and types of Dupuytren's disease. *Hand Clin*. 1999;15(1):87–96, vii.

ADDITIONAL READING

- Ball C, Pratt AL, Nanchahal J. Optimal functional outcome measures for assessing treatment for Dupuytren's disease: a systematic review and recommendations for future practice. *BMC Musculoskelet Disord*. 2013;14:131.
- Black E, Blazar P. Dupuytren disease: an evolving understanding of an age-old disease. *J Am Acad Orthop Surg*. 2011;19(12):746–757.
- Rayan GM. Dupuytren disease: anatomy, pathology, presentation, and treatment. *J Bone Joint Surg Am*. 2007;89(1):189–198.
- Sweet S, Blackmore S. Surgical and therapy update on the management of Dupuytren's disease. *J Hand Ther*. 2014;27(2):77–84.

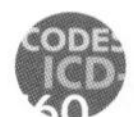

CODES

ICD10

M72.0 Palmar fascial fibromatosis [Dupuytren]

CLINICAL PEARLS

- Dupuytren contracture is a fixed flexion deformity of (most commonly) the 4th and 5th digits due to palmar fibrosis. 90% of cases are progressive.
- Refer patients with involvement of the PIP joints or MCP involvement with contractures of >30 degrees.
- Both surgical and enzymatic fasciotomy have high rate of recurrence (6).

DYSHIDROSIS

Cara Marshall, MD

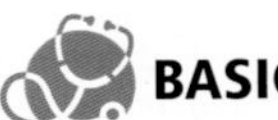

BASICS

DESCRIPTION

- A skin rash (dermatitis) within the "dyshidrosis" family. Literature supports the presence of several different classes within the family dyshidrosis but no general agreement about a strict definition of these classes.
- Dyshidrotic eczema
  - Common, chronic, or recurrent; nonerythematous; symmetric vesicular eruption primarily of the palms, soles, and interdigital areas
  - Associated with burning, itching, and pain
- Pompholyx (from Greek "bubble")
  - Rare condition characterized by abrupt onset of large bullae.
  - Sometimes used interchangeably with dyshidrotic eczema (small vesicles). Some believe these to be discrete entities.
- Lamellar dyshidrosis
  - Fine, spreading exfoliation of the superficial epidermis in the same distribution as described above.
- System(s) affected: dermatologic, exocrine, immunologic
- Synonym(s): cheiropompholyx, keratolysis exfoliativa, vesicular palmoplantar eczema, desquamation of interdigital spaces, palmar pompholyx reaction, acute and recurrent hand dermatitis (1)

EPIDEMIOLOGY

Incidence

- Mean age of onset is 40 years and younger
- Male = female
- Comprises 5–20% of hand eczema cases

Prevalence

20 cases/100,000 populations

ETIOLOGY AND PATHOPHYSIOLOGY

- Exact mechanism unknown; thought to be multifactorial
- Dermatopathology: spongiosis with intraepidermal vesicles
- Despite the name, sweat glands are not altered/affected (2).
- Vesicles remain intact due to thickness of stratum corneum of palmar/plantar skin (1).
- Exact cause not known.
- Aggravating factors (debated)
  - Hyperhidrosis (in 40% of patients with the condition)
  - Climate: hot/cold weather; humidity
  - Contact sensitivity (in 30–67% of patients with the condition) (2)
  - Nickel, cobalt, and chromate sensitivity (may include implanted orthopedic or orthodontic metals) (1)
  - Irritating compounds and solutions
  - Stress
  - Dermatophyte infection (present in 10% of patients with the condition) (2)
  - Prolonged wear of occlusive gloves
  - IV immunoglobulin therapy
  - Smoking

Genetics

- Atopy: 50% of patients with dyshidrotic eczema have atopic dermatitis (1).
- Rare autosomal dominant form of pompholyx found in Chinese population maps to chromosome 18q22.1–18q22.3 (2).

RISK FACTORS

- Many risk factors are disputed in the literature, with none being consistently associated.
- Atopy
- Other dermatologic conditions
  - Atopic dermatitis (early in life)
  - Contact dermatitis (later in life)
  - Dermatophytosis
- Sensitivity to
  - Foods
  - Drugs: neomycin, quinolones, acetaminophen, and oral contraceptives
  - Contact and dietary: nickel (more common in young women), chromate (more common in men), and cobalt (1)
  - Smoking in males

GENERAL PREVENTION

- Control emotional stress.
- Avoid excessive sweating.
- Avoid exposure to irritants.
- Avoid diet high in metal salts (chromium, cobalt, nickel).
- Avoid smoking.

COMMONLY ASSOCIATED CONDITIONS

- Atopic dermatitis
- Allergic contact dermatitis
- Parkinson disease
- HIV (2)

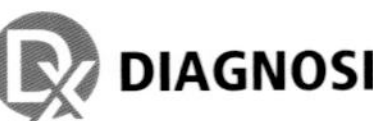

DIAGNOSIS

HISTORY

- Episodes of pruritic rash
- Recent emotional stress
- Familial or personal history of atopy
- Exposure to allergens or irritants (3)
  - Occupational, dietary, or household
  - Cosmetic and personal hygiene products
  - Vesicular eruption typically occurs 24 hours after allergen challenge (1).
- Costume jewelry use
- IV immunoglobulin therapy
- HIV
- Smoking

PHYSICAL EXAM

- Symmetric distribution on the palms and soles; also may affect the dorsal aspects of hands and feet
- Lesions may not heal completely between flares (1).
- Early findings
  - 1–2 mm, clear, nonerythematous, deep-seated vesicles
- Late findings
  - Unroofed vesicles with inflamed bases
  - Desquamation
  - Peeling, rings of scale, or lichenification common

DIFFERENTIAL DIAGNOSIS

- Vesicular tinea pedis/manuum
- Vesicular id reaction
- Contact dermatitis (allergic or irritant)
- Scabies
- Chronic vesicular hand dermatitis
- Drug reaction
- Dermatophytid
- Bullous disorders: dyshidrosiform bullous pemphigoid, pemphigus, bullous impetigo, epidermolysis bullosa
- Pustular psoriasis
- Acrodermatitis continua
- Erythema multiforme
- Herpes infection
- Pityriasis rubra pilaris
- Vesicular mycosis fungoides

DIAGNOSTIC TESTS & INTERPRETATION

Follow-Up Tests & Special Considerations

- Skin culture in suspected secondary infection (most commonly, *Staphylococcus aureus*) (4)
- Consider antibiotics based on culture results and severity of symptoms.

Diagnostic Procedures/Other

- Diagnosis is based on clinical exam.
- Potassium hydroxide (KOH) wet mount (if concerned about dermatophyte infection)
- Patch test (if suspecting allergic cause)

Test Interpretation

- Fine, 1–2-mm spongiotic vesicles intraepidermally with little to no inflammatory change
- No eccrine glandular involvement
- Thickened stratum corneum

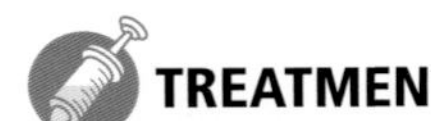

TREATMENT

GENERAL MEASURES

- Avoid possible causative factors: stress, direct skin contact with irritants, nickel, occlusive gloves, household cleaning products, smoking, sweating
- Use moisturizers/emollients for symptomatic relief and to maintain effective skin barrier.
- Skin care
  - Wear shoes with leather rather than rubber soles (e.g., sneakers).
  - Wear socks and gloves made of cotton and change frequently.
  - Wash infrequently, carefully dry, then apply emollient.
  - Avoid direct contact with fresh fruit (5)[C].

MEDICATION

First Line

- Mild cases: topical steroids (high potency) (2)[B]
  - Considered cornerstone of therapy but limited published evidence
- Moderate to severe cases
  - Ultrahigh-potency topical steroids with occlusion over treated area (4)[B]
  - Prednisone 40–100 mg/day tapered after blister formation ceases (2)[B]
  - Psoralens plus ultraviolet (UV)-A therapy (PUVA), either systemic/topical *or* immersion in psoralens (2)[B]
- Recurrent cases (4)[B]
  - Systemic steroids at onset of itching prodrome
  - Prednisone 60 mg PO × 3–4 days

Second Line

- Topical calcineurin inhibitors (mitigate the long-term risks of topical steroid use)
  - Topical tacrolimus (6)[B]
  - Topical pimecrolimus (6)[B]
  - May not be as effective on plantar surface
- Other therapies (typically with dermatology consultation)
  - Oral cyclosporine (4)[B]
  - Injections of botulinum toxin type A (BTXA) (6)[B]
    - Newer topical forms of BTXA currently being developed show promise.
    - Painful, requires nerve block
  - Systemic alitretinoin (teratogenic) (5)[B]
  - Topical bexarotene (a teratogenic retinoid X receptor agonist approved for use in cutaneous T-cell lymphoma) (6)[B]
  - Methotrexate (6)[C]
  - Azathioprine (1)[C]
  - Disulfiram or sodium cromoglycate in nickel-allergic patients (1)[C]
  - Mycophenolate mofetil (2)[C]
  - Tapwater iontophoresis (2)[C]

ISSUES FOR REFERRAL

- Allergist (if allergen testing required)
- Psychologist (if stress modification needed)

ADDITIONAL THERAPIES

- Radiation therapy (1)[C]
- UV-free phototherapy (5)[C]
- Treat underlying dermatophytosis (1).

COMPLEMENTARY & ALTERNATIVE MEDICINE

- Topical treatments to minimize pruritus (not curative) (4)[C]: Burow solution (aluminum acetate) or vinegar compress
- Exposure to sunlight as maintenance therapy, 12 minutes every other day, 10–15 exposures (5)[C]
- Dandelion juice (avoid in atopic patients) (6)[C]

ONGOING CARE

FOLLOW-UP RECOMMENDATIONS

Patient Monitoring

- Dyshidrotic Eczema Area and Severity Index (DASI) (1)
- Parameters used in the DASI score
  - Number of vesicles per square centimeter
  - Erythema
  - Desquamation
  - Severity of itching
  - Surface area affected
- Grading: mild (0–15), moderate (16–30), severe (31–60)
- Monitor BP and glucose in patients receiving systemic corticosteroids.
- Monitor for adverse effects of medications.

DIET

- Consider diet low in metal salts if there is history of nickel sensitivity (4)[B].
- Updated recommendations for low-cobalt diet are available (1).

PATIENT EDUCATION

- Instructions on self-care, complications, and avoidance of triggers/aggravating factors
- PubMed Health: Dyshidrotic Eczema at: http://www.ncbi.nlm.nih.gov/pubmedhealth/PMH0001835/

PROGNOSIS

- Condition is benign.
- Usually heals without scarring.
- Lesions may spontaneously resolve.
- Recurrence is common.

COMPLICATIONS

- Secondary bacterial infections (*S. aureus* most common)
- Dystrophic nail changes
- Fissures
- Skin tightening/discomfort
- Psychological distress

REFERENCES

1. Veien NK. Acute and recurrent vesicular hand dermatitis. *Dermatol Clin*. 2009;27(3):337–353.
2. Wollina U. Pompholyx: a review of clinical features, differential diagnosis, and management. *Am J Clin Dermatol*. 2010;11(5):305–314.
3. Guillet MH, Wierzbicka E, Guillet S, et al. A 3-year causative study of pompholyx in 120 patients. *Arch Dermatol*. 2007;143(12):1504–1508.
4. Lofgren SM, Warshaw EM. Dyshidrosis: epidemiology, clinical characteristics, and therapy. *Dermatitis*. 2006;17(4):165–181.
5. Letic M. Use of sunlight to treat dyshidrotic eczema. *JAMA Dermatol*. 2013;149(5):634–635.
6. Wollina U. Pompholyx: what's new? *Expert Opin Investig Drugs*. 2008;17(6):897–904.

ADDITIONAL READING

- Chen J, Liang YH, Zhou FS, et al. The gene for a rare autosomal dominant form of pompholyx maps to chromosome 18q22.1–18q22.3. *J Invest Dermatol*. 2006;126(2):300–304.
- Molin S, Diepgen TL, Ruzicka T, et al. Diagnosing chronic hand eczema by an algorithm: a tool for classification in clinical practice. *Clin Exp Dermatol*. 2011;36(6):595–601.
- Schuttelaar ML, Coenraads PJ, Huizinga J, et al. Increase in vesicular hand eczema after house dust mite inhalation provocation: a double-blind, placebo-controlled, cross-over study. *Contact Dermatitis*. 2013;68(2):76–85.
- Stuckert J, Nedorost S. Low-cobalt diet for dyshidrotic eczema patients. *Contact Dermatitis*. 2008;59(6):361–365.
- Sumila M, Notter M, Itin P, et al. Long-term results of radiotherapy in patients with chronic palmo-plantar eczema or psoriasis. *Strahlenther Onkol*. 2008;184(4):218–223.
- Thiers BH. What's new in dermatologic therapy. *Dermatol Ther*. 2008;21(2):142–149.
- Tzaneva S, Kittler H, Thallinger C, et al. Oral vs. bath PUVA using 8-methoxypsoralen for chronic palmoplantar eczema. *Photodermatol Photoimmunol Photomed*. 2009;25(2):101–105.

SEE ALSO

Algorithm: Rash, Focal

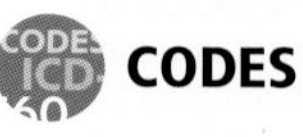

CODES

ICD10

L30.1 Dyshidrosis [pompholyx]

CLINICAL PEARLS

- Dyshidrosis is a transient, recurrent vesicular eruption most commonly of the palms, soles, and interdigital areas.
- Etiology and pathophysiology are unknown but are most likely related to a combination of genetic and environmental factors.
- Best prevention is effective skin care and limiting exposure to irritating agents.
- Treatments are based on disease severity; preferred treatments include topical steroids, oral steroids, and calcineurin inhibitors.
- Condition is benign and usually heals spontaneously and without scarring. Medical treatment decreases healing time and risk for progression to secondary bacterial infection.

D

DYSMENORRHEA

Kristen A. Reineke-Piper, MD • LaShell LaBounty, DO

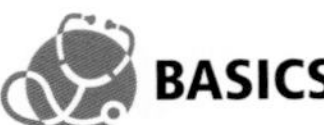

BASICS

DESCRIPTION

- Pelvic pain occurring at/around time of menses; a leading cause of absenteeism for women <30 years old
- Primary dysmenorrhea: without pathologic physical findings
- Secondary dysmenorrhea: often more severe, having a secondary pathologic (structural) cause
- Severity based on activity impairment
  - Mild: painful, rarely limits daily function or requires analgesics
  - Moderate: daily activity affected, rare absenteeism, requires analgesics
  - Severe: daily activity affected, likelihood absenteeism, limited benefit from analgesics
- System affected: reproductive
- Synonym(s): menstrual cramps

EPIDEMIOLOGY

- Predominant age
  - Primary: teens to early 20s
  - Secondary: 20s–30s
- Predominant sex: women only

Prevalence

- Up to 95% of menstruating females have experienced primary dysmenorrhea
- Up to 42% lose days of school/work monthly due to dysmenorrhea

ETIOLOGY AND PATHOPHYSIOLOGY

- Primary: Elevated production of prostaglandins (PGF2α) through indirect hormonal control (stimulation of production by estrogen), which causes hypercontractility and increased uterine muscle tone with vasoconstriction and resultant uterine ischemia. Ischemia results in type C pain neuron stimulation through buildup of anaerobic metabolites.
- Secondary
  - Endometriosis (up to 10%)
  - Congenital abnormalities of uterine/vaginal anatomy
  - Cervical stenosis
  - Pelvic infection
  - Adenomyosis
  - Ovarian cysts
  - Pelvic tumors, especially leiomyomata (fibroids) and uterine polyps

Genetics

Not well studied

RISK FACTORS

- Primary
  - Cigarette smoking
  - Alcohol use
  - Weight loss
  - Early menarche (age <12 years)
  - Age <30 years
  - Irregular/heavy menstrual flow
  - Non-use of oral contraceptives
  - Sexual abuse
  - Psychological symptoms (depression, anxiety, etc.)
- Secondary (10%)
  - Pelvic infection
  - Use of intrauterine device (IUD)
  - Structural pelvic malformations
  - Family history endometriosis in first-degree relative

GENERAL PREVENTION

- Primary: choose a diet low in animal fats.
- Secondary: reduce risk of sexually transmitted infections (STIs)

Pediatric Considerations

Onset with 1st menses raises probability of genital tract anatomic abnormality (i.e., transverse vaginal septum, imperforate or minimally perforated hymen, uterine anomalies).

COMMONLY ASSOCIATED CONDITIONS

- Irregular/heavy menstrual periods
- Longer menstrual cycle length/duration of bleeding
- Endometriosis

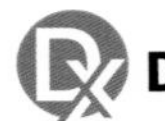

DIAGNOSIS

Based on characteristic history of cramping pain felt in suprapubic/lower back occurring at or near onset of menstrual flow lasting for 8–72 hours (1).

HISTORY

- Onset once ovulatory cycles are established in adolescents; 2 years after menarche on average
- Patients may have associated diarrhea, headache, fatigue, or pain radiating into the inner thighs.
- Recurrence at or just before the onset of the menstrual flow
  - Pelvic pain occurring between menstrual periods is not likely to be dysmenorrhea.
  - Present with most menstrual periods (cyclic)
- Relief associated with the following:
  - Continued bleeding for the usual duration
  - Use of analgesics, especially NSAIDs
  - Orgasm
  - Local heat application
- Response to NSAIDs helps confirm diagnosis.

PHYSICAL EXAM

- Primary: Physical exam typically is normal. Examine to rule out secondary dysmenorrhea.
- Secondary: Evaluate for cervical discharge, uterine enlargement, tenderness, irregularity, or fixation.

DIFFERENTIAL DIAGNOSIS

- Primary: History is characteristic.
- Secondary
  - Pelvic/genital infection
  - Complication of pregnancy
  - Missed/incomplete abortion
  - Ectopic pregnancy
  - Uterine/ovarian neoplasm
  - Endometriosis
  - UTI
  - Complication with IUD use

DIAGNOSTIC TESTS & INTERPRETATION

Initial Tests (lab, imaging)

- Pregnancy test
- Urine testing for infection
- Gonorrhea/chlamydia cervical testing, especially in women age <25 years and in high prevalence areas.
- Primary: Consider pelvic ultrasound to rule out secondary abnormalities if history is not characteristic or suspected abnormality on exam.
- Secondary: Ultrasound/laparoscopy to define anatomy for severe/refractory cases. MRI may be useful as second-line noninvasive imaging if ultrasound is nondiagnostic and torsion, deep endometriosis, or adenomyosis suspected.

Follow-Up Tests & Special Considerations

Counsel regarding appropriate preventive measures for STI and pregnancy.

Diagnostic Procedures/Other

Laparoscopy is rarely needed.

Test Interpretation

- Primary: none
- Secondary: Specific anatomic abnormalities may be noted (see "Differential Diagnosis").

Pregnancy Considerations

Consider ectopic pregnancy when pelvic pain occurs with vaginal bleeding.

TREATMENT

- Reassure the patient that treatment success is very likely with adherence to recommendations.
- Relief may require the use of several treatment modalities at the same time.

GENERAL MEASURES

- Exercise and local heat are noninvasive general measures to relieve pain.
- High-frequency transcutaneous electrical nerve stimulation (TENS) has been found to be beneficial. There is conflicting evidence for low-frequency TENS.
- Secondary dysmenorrhea: Treatment of infections; suppression of endometrium if endometriosis suspected; remove IUD if contributing factor.

MEDICATION

First Line

- NSAIDs: No NSAID has been found to be superior over others. In theory, COX-2 inhibitors are more selective for the endometrium, although they have not been FDA approved for use in primary dysmenorrhea. Medication should be taken on scheduled dosing 1–2 days prior to onset of menses and continued for 2–3 days (1,2)[A]
  - Ibuprofen 400 mg q8h
  - Naproxen sodium 500 mg BID
  - Celecoxib 400mg ×1, then 200mg q12h
- Hormonal contraceptives: recommended for primary dysmenorrhea in women desiring contraception (1)[B]. Continuous rather than cyclic dosing may initially be more effective at reducing pain; however, may have similar benefit after 6 months (3)[B]. Estrogen-containing contraceptives are recommended first-line for secondary dysmenorrhea due to endometriosis, although progestin-only methods have also been shown to be beneficial (1)[B].
- Levonorgestrel IUDs can decrease primary dysmenorrhea (4)[B].

- Potential contraindications to NSAIDs and combined oral contraceptives (COCs)
  - Platelet disorders
  - Gastric ulceration or gastritis
  - Thromboembolic disorders
  - Vascular disease
  - Migraine with aura
- Precautions
  - GI irritation
  - Lactation

  - Coagulation disorders
  - Impaired renal function
  - Heart failure
  - Liver dysfunction
- Significant possible interactions
  - Coumadin-type anticoagulants
  - Aspirin with other NSAIDs

Second Line

- Local heat can help relieve pain and may be as effective as NSAIDs (1)[B].
- Exercise may have beneficial effects in relieving pain (5)[B].
- β_2-adrenoceptor agonists have not definitively been shown to relieve pain in dysmenorrhea (6)[B].
- Behavioral interventions, such as relaxation exercises, may help alleviate pain in primary dysmenorrhea.

SURGERY/OTHER PROCEDURES

Laparoscopic uterosacral nerve ablation has been shown to relieve pain at >12 months postoperatively.

COMPLEMENTARY & ALTERNATIVE MEDICINE

- Spinal manipulation has not been shown to be effective in treating pain (7)[A].
- Chinese herbal medicine shows promising evidence of decreasing pain, but more evidence is needed.
- Acupuncture treatments have been shown to decrease pain in dysmenorrhea, but further randomized, well-designed studies are needed (1,8)[B].
- Acupoint stimulation, particularly noninvasive stimulation (acupressure), can relieve pain (9)[B].
- Aromatherapy abdominal massage performed daily for 10 minutes, 7 days prior to onset of menses can decrease primary dysmenorrhea (10)[B].
- Further research needed to determine benefit and safety for use of oral fennel, extracorporeal magnetic innervation, vitamin K1 injection into the spleen-6 acupuncture point, use of high frequency vibratory stimulation tampon, and vaginal sildenafil.

INPATIENT CONSIDERATIONS

Both primary and secondary dysmenorrhea are usually managed in the outpatient setting.

Admission Criteria/Initial Stabilization

- Primary: outpatient care
- Secondary: usually outpatient care

ONGOING CARE

FOLLOW-UP RECOMMENDATIONS

Normal

DIET

- Vitamin B_1 100 mg daily, omega-3 fatty acid (1)[B], and fish oil supplementation may be beneficial (11)[B].
- Magnesium has been shown to be useful, but the correct dosage has not been determined.
- Insufficient evidence to show usefulness of zinc and vitamin E at this time
- Low-fat vegetarian diet can be helpful in some patients.

PATIENT EDUCATION

Reassure the patient that primary dysmenorrhea is treatable with use of NSAIDs, COCs, or local heat and that it will usually abate with age and parity.

PROGNOSIS

- Primary: reduced with age and parity
- Secondary: likely to require therapy based on underlying cause

COMPLICATIONS

- Primary: anxiety and/or depression
- Secondary: infertility from underlying pathology

REFERENCES

1. Osaynde AS, Mehulic S. Diagnosis and initial management of dysmenorrhea. *Am Fam Physician*. 2014;89(5):341–346.
2. Lethaby A, Duckitt K, Farquhar C. Non-steroidal anti-inflammatory drugs for heavy menstrual bleeding. *Cochrane Database Syst Rev*. 2013;(1):CD0004000.
3. Dmitrovic R, Kunselman AR, Legro RS. Continuous compared with cyclic oral contraceptives for the treatment of primary dysmenorrhea: a randomized controlled trial. *Obstet Gynecol*. 2012;119(6):1143–1150.
4. Bayer LL, Hillard PJ. Use of levonorgestrel intrauterine system for medical indications in adolescents. *J Adolesc Health*. 2013;52(Suppl 4) S54–S58.
5. Brown J, Brown S. Exercise for dysmenorrhoea. *Cochrane Database Syst Rev*. 2010;(2):CD004142.
6. Fedorowicz Z, Nasser M, Jagannath VA, et al. Beta2-adrenoceptor agonists for dysmenorrhoea. *Cochrane Database Syst Rev*. 2012;(5):CD008585.
7. Kannan P, Claydon LS. Some physiotherapy treatments may relieve menstrual pain in women with primary dysmenorrhea: a systematic review. *J Physiother*. 2014;60(1):13–21.
8. Reyes-Campos MD, Diaz-Toral LG, Verdin-Teran SL, et al. Acupuncture as an adjunct treatment for primary dysmenorrhea: a comparative study. *Med Acupunct*. 2013;25(4):291–294.
9. Chen MN, Chien LW, Liu CF. Acupuncture or acupressure at the Sanyinjiao (SP6) Acupoint for the treatment of primary dysmenorrhea: a meta-analysis. *Evid Based Complement Alternat Med*. 2013;2013:493038.
10. Marzouk TMF, El-Nemer AMR, Baraka HN. The effect of aromatherapy abdominal massage on alleviating menstrual pain in nursing students: a prospective randomized cross-over study. *Evid Based Complement Alternat Med*. 2013;2013:742421.
11. Hansen SO, Knudsen UB. Endometriosis, dysmenorrhoea and diet. *Eur J Obstet Gynecol Reprod Biol*. 2013;169(2):162–171.

ADDITIONAL READING

- Akin MD, Weingand KW, Hengehold DA, et al. Continuous low-level topical heat in the treatment of dysmenorrhea. *Obstet Gynecol*. 2001;97(3):343–349.
- Allen LM, Lam AC. Premenstrual syndrome and dysmenorrhea in adolescents. *Adolesc Med State Art Rev*. 2012;23(1):139–163.
- Altunyurt S, Göl M, Altunyurt S, et al. Primary dysmenorrhea and uterine blood flow: a color Doppler study. *J Reprod Med*. 2005;50(4):251–255.
- Cho SH, Hwang EW. Acupuncture for primary dysmenorrhoea: a systematic review. *BJOG*. 2010;117(5):509–521.
- Dawood MY. Primary dysmenorrhea: advances in pathogenesis and management. *Obstet Gynecol*. 2006;108(2):428–441.
- Eby G. Zinc treatment prevents dysmenorrhea. *Med Hypoth*. 2007;69(2):297–301.
- Khan KS, Champaneria R, Latthe PM. How effective are non-drug, non-surgical treatments for primary dysmenorrhoea? *BMJ*. 2012;344:e3011.
- Latthe P, Mignini L, Gray R, et al. Factors predisposing women to chronic pelvic pain: systematic review. *BMJ*. 2006;332(7544):749–755.
- Polat A, Celik H, Gurates B, et al. Prevalence of primary dysmenorrhea in young adult female university students. *Arch Gynecol Obstet*. 2009;279(4):527–532.
- Proctor M, Farquhar C. Diagnosis and management of dysmenorrhea. *BMJ*. 2006:332(7550):1134–1138.
- Proctor ML, Murphy PA. Herbal and dietary therapies for primary and secondary dysmenorrhoea. *Cochrane Database Syst Rev*. 2001;(3):CD002124.
- Weissman AM, Hartz AJ, Hansen MD, et al. The natural history of primary dysmenorrhoea: a longitudinal study. *BJOG*. 2004;111(4):345–352.
- Willman EA, Collins WP, Clayton SG. Studies in the involvement of prostaglandins in uterine symptomatology and pathology. *Br J Obstet Gynaecol*. 1976;83(5):337–341.
- Ylikorkala O, Dawood MY. New concepts in dysmenorrhea. *Am J Obstet Gynecol*. 1978;130(7):833–847.
- Zahradnik HP, Hanjalic-Beck A, Groth K. Non-steroidal anti-inflammatory drugs and hormonal contraceptives for pain relief from dysmenorrhea: a review. *Contraception*. 2010;81(3):185–196.
- Zannoni L, Giorgi M, Spagnolo E, et al. Dysmenorrhea, absenteeism from school, and symptoms suspicious for endometriosis in adolescents. *J Pediatr Adolesc Gynecol*. 2014;27(5):258–256.
- Zhu X, Proctor M, Bensoussan A, et al. Chinese herbal medicine for primary dysmenorrhoea. *Cochrane Database Syst Rev*. 2008;(2):CD005288.

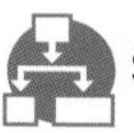

SEE ALSO

- Endometriosis
- Dyspareunia
- Menorrhagia
- Premenstrual Syndrome (PMS) and Premenstrual Dysphoric Disorder (PMDD)
- Algorithm: Pelvic Pain

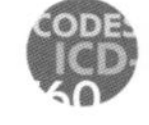

CODES

ICD10

- N94.6 Dysmenorrhea, unspecified
- N94.4 Primary dysmenorrhea
- N94.5 Secondary dysmenorrhea

CLINICAL PEARLS

- Dysmenorrhea is a leading cause of absenteeism for women age <30 years.
- In women who desire contraception, hormonal contraceptives are preferred treatment.
- All NSAIDs studied have been found to be equally effective in the relief of dysmenorrhea and should be initiated 1–2 days prior to onset of menses with scheduled dosing.

DYSPAREUNIA

Scott T. Henderson, MD

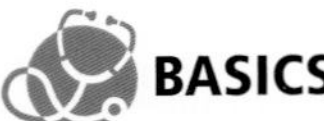

BASICS

DESCRIPTION

- Recurrent and persistent genital pain associated with sexual activity, which is not exclusively due to lack of lubrication or vaginismus.
- May be the result of organic, emotional, or psychogenic causes
  - Primary: present throughout one's sexual history
  - Secondary: arising from some specific event or condition (e.g., menopause, drugs)
  - Superficial: pain at, or near, the introitus or vaginal barrel associated with penetration
  - Deep: pain after penetration located at the cervix or lower abdominal area
  - Complete: present under all circumstances
  - Situational: occurring selectively with specific situations
- System(s) affected: reproductive

EPIDEMIOLOGY

- Predominant age: all ages
- Predominant sex: female > male

Incidence

>50% of all sexually active women will report dyspareunia at some time.

Geriatric Considerations

Incidence increases dramatically in postmenopausal women primarily because of vaginal atrophy.

Prevalence

- Most sexually active women will experience dyspareunia at some time in their lives.
  - ~15% (4–40%) of adult women will have dyspareunia on a few occasions during a year.
  - ~1–2% of women will have painful intercourse on a more-than-occasional basis.
- Male prevalence is ~1%.

ETIOLOGY AND PATHOPHYSIOLOGY

- Disorders of vaginal outlet
  - Adhesions
  - Clitoral irritation
  - Episiotomy scars
  - Fissures
  - Hymeneal ring abnormalities
  - Inadequate lubrication
  - Infections
  - Lichen planus
  - Lichen sclerosus
  - Postmenopausal atrophy
  - Trauma
  - Vulvar papillomatosis
  - Vulvar vestibulitis/vulvodynia
- Disorders of vagina
  - Abnormality of vault owing to surgery or radiation
  - Congenital malformations
  - Inadequate lubrication
  - Infections
  - Inflammatory or allergic response to foreign substance
  - Masses or tumors
  - Pelvic relaxation resulting in rectocele, uterine prolapse, or cystocele
- Disorders of pelvic structures
  - Endometriosis
  - Levator ani myalgia/spasm
  - Malignant or benign tumors of the uterus
  - Ovarian pathology
  - Pelvic adhesions
  - Pelvic inflammatory disease (PID)
  - Pelvic venous congestion
  - Prior pelvic fracture
- Disorders of the GI tract
  - Constipation
  - Crohn disease
  - Diverticular disease
  - Fistulas
  - Hemorrhoids
  - Inflammatory bowel disease
- Disorders of the urinary tract
  - Interstitial cystitis
  - Ureteral or vesical lesions
- Chronic disease
  - Behçet syndrome
  - Diabetes
  - Sjögren syndrome
- Male
  - Cancer of penis
  - Genital muscle spasm
  - Infection or irritation of penile skin
  - Infection of seminal vesicles
  - Lichen sclerosus
  - Musculoskeletal disorders of pelvis and lower back
  - Penile anatomy disorders
  - Phimosis
  - Prostate infections and enlargement
  - Testicular disease
  - Torsion of spermatic cord
  - Urethritis
- Psychological disorders
  - Anxiety
  - Conversion reactions
  - Depression
  - Fear
  - Hostility toward partner
  - Phobic reactions
  - Psychological trauma

RISK FACTORS

- Fatigue
- Stress
- Depression
- Diabetes
- Estrogen deficiency
  - Menopause
  - Lactation
- Previous PID
- Vaginal surgery
- Alcohol/marijuana consumption
- Medication side effects (antihistamines, tamoxifen, bromocriptine, low-estrogen oral contraceptives, depo-medroxyprogesterone, desipramine)

Pregnancy Considerations

Pregnancy is a potent influence on sexuality; dyspareunia is common.

COMMONLY ASSOCIATED CONDITIONS

Vaginismus

Pregnancy Considerations

Episiotomies do not have a protective effect (1)[A].

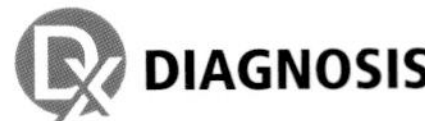

DIAGNOSIS

HISTORY

- Identify pain characteristics:
  - Onset
  - Duration
  - Location: entry versus deep, single versus multiple sites, positional
  - Intensity/quality: varying degrees of pelvic/genital pressure, aching, tearing, and/or burning
  - Pattern (precipitating or aggravating factors): when pain occurs (at entry, during, or after intercourse)
  - Relief measures: Avoid intercourse, change positions, and have intercourse only at certain times of the month.
- Include menstrual, obstetric, reproductive, sexual, domestic violence, and rape histories with medical and psychosocial history.

PHYSICAL EXAM

- A complete exam, including a focused pelvic exam, to identify pathology and provide patient education
- Because examination often reproduces the pain, examiner should be cautious and sensitive to patient's anxiety. Exam must include inspection and palpation of vulva and vaginal areas, palpation of the uterine and adnexal structures, and a rectovaginal exam. Sensory mapping with a cotton-tipped applicator to identify sensitive and painful areas.
- Inspect and palpate urethra and base of the bladder.

DIFFERENTIAL DIAGNOSIS
Vaginismus

DIAGNOSTIC TESTS & INTERPRETATION
Initial Tests (lab, imaging)
Based on history and exam findings
- Wet mount
- Gonorrhea and chlamydia cultures
- Herpes culture
- Urinalysis and urine culture
- Pap smear

Follow-Up Tests & Special Considerations
- Serum estradiol if vulvodynia or atrophic vaginitis.
- Voiding cystourethrogram if urinary tract involvement
- GI contrast studies if GI symptoms.
- Ultrasound and CT scan are of limited value; perform if clinically indicated.

Diagnostic Procedures/Other
Based on history and exam findings
- Colposcopy and biopsy if vaginal/vulvar lesions
- Laparoscopy if complex deep-penetration pain
- Cystoscopy if urinary tract involvement
- Endoscopy if GI involvement

Test Interpretation
Depends on etiology

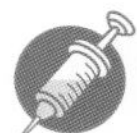

TREATMENT
- Potential relationships exists between primary dyspareunia and vaginismus, low libido, and arousal disorders.
- Endocrine factors, such as primary amenorrhea, might reduce the biologic basis of sexual response.
- If pain prevents penetration, severe vaginismus may be present.

GENERAL MEASURES
- Educate the patient and partner regarding the nature of the problem. Reassure both there are solutions to the problem.
- Initiate specific treatment when initial evaluation identifies an organic cause.
- Once organic causes are ruled out, treatment is a multidimensional and multidisciplinary approach (2)[C].
  - Individual behavioral therapy
    - Indicated to help the patient deal with intrapersonal issues and assess the role of the partner
  - Couple behavioral therapy
    - Indicated to help resolve interpersonal problems
    - May involve short-term structured intervention or sexual counseling
    - Designed to desensitize systemically uncomfortable sexual responses and intercourse through a series of interventions over a period of weeks
    - Interventions range from muscle relaxation and mutual body massage to sexual fantasies and erotic massage.

MEDICATION
First Line
Depends on the etiology
- Antibiotics, antifungals, or antivirals, as indicated, for infection
- Vaginal moisturizers and lubricants for dryness
- Analgesics and topical anesthetics for pain
- Topical estrogen for vaginal and vulvar atrophy
- Neuropathic pain associated with vulvar vestibulitis/vulvodynia may respond to tricyclic antidepressants (amitriptyline or nortriptyline) or gabapentin.

Second Line
Ospemifene for moderate to severe symptoms due to menopause-related vulvar and vaginal atrophy

ISSUES FOR REFERRAL
Referral for long-term therapy may be necessary.

ADDITIONAL THERAPIES
Physical therapy for pelvic floor muscle pain

SURGERY/OTHER PROCEDURES
- Laparoscopic excision of endometriotic lesions has shown benefit (3)[C].
- Surgical vestibulectomy can be considered if medical measures fail with vulvar vestibulitis (4)[B].

COMPLEMENTARY & ALTERNATIVE MEDICINE
- Sitz baths may relieve painful inflammation.
- Perineal massage
- Antioxidants may improve symptoms associated with endometriosis.

ONGOING CARE

FOLLOW-UP RECOMMENDATIONS
Patient Monitoring
- Outpatient follow-up depends on therapy.
- Every 6–12 months once resolved

DIET
A high-fiber diet may help if constipation is a contributing cause.

PATIENT EDUCATION
- Boston Women's Health Book Collective. *Our Bodies, Ourselves: A New Edition for a New Era*. New York, NY: Simon & Schuster; 2005.
- Kegel exercise information
- Provide couples with information about sexual arousal techniques.

PROGNOSIS
Depends on underlying cause but most patients will respond to treatment.

REFERENCES

1. Carroli G, Mignini L. Episiotomy for vaginal birth. *Cochrane Database Syst Rev*. 2009;(1):CD000081.
2. Crowley T, Richardson D, Goldmeier D; Bashh Special Interest Group for Sexual Dysfunction. Recommendations for the management of vaginismus: BASHH Special Interest Group for Sexual Dysfunction. *Int J STD AIDS*. 2006;17(1):14–18.
3. Ferrero S, Abbamonte LH, Giordano M, et al. Deep dyspareunia and sex life after laparoscopic excision of endometriosis. *Hum Reprod*. 2007;22(4):1142–1148.
4. Steege JF, Zolnoun DA. Evaluation and treatment of dyspareunia. *Obstet Gynecol*. 2009;113(5):1124–1136.

ADDITIONAL READING

- Boardman LA, Stockdale CK. Sexual pain. *Clin Obstet Gynecol*. 2009;52(4):682–690.
- Frank JE, Mistretta P, Will J. Diagnosis and treatment of female sexual dysfunction. *Am Fam Physician*. 2008;77(5):635–642.
- Sung SC, Jeng CJ, Lin YC. Sexual health care for women with dyspareunia. *Taiwan J Obstet Gynecol*. 2011;50(3):268–274.

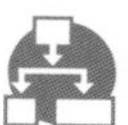

SEE ALSO

- Balanitis; Endometriosis; Pelvic Inflammatory Disease (PID); Sexual Dysfunction in Women; Vaginismus; Vulvovaginitis, Estrogen Deficient; Vulvovaginitis, Prepubescent
- Algorithms: Dyspareunia; Discharge, Vaginal

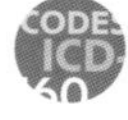

CODES

ICD10
- N94.1 Dyspareunia
- F52.6 Dyspareunia not due to a substance or known physiol cond

CLINICAL PEARLS
- Careful history to determine if patient feels pain before, during, or after intercourse will help identify cause.
  - Pain before intercourse suggests a phobic attitude toward penetration and/or the presence of vestibulitis.
  - Pain during intercourse combined with the location of the pain is most predictive of the causes of pain.
  - Introital pain after intercourse suggests vestibulitis in women of childbearing age, hypertonic pelvic floor, or vulvovaginal dystrophia.
- Potential relationship exists between primary dyspareunia and vaginismus, low libido, and arousal disorders.
- Episiotomy does not offer any benefit in the prevention of dyspareunia; a mediolateral episiotomy in fact may cause more future discomfort.

D

DYSPEPSIA, FUNCTIONAL

Kristina G. Burgers, MD • Matthew W. Short, MD

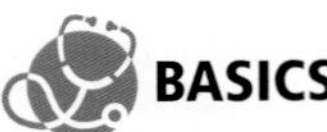

BASICS

DESCRIPTION

- A condition defined as the presence of bothersome postprandial fullness, early satiety, or epigastric pain/burning in the absence of causative structural disease (to include upper endoscopy) for the preceding 3 months with initial symptom onset at least 6 months prior to diagnosis (Rome III criteria)
- Rome III criteria divide patients into two subtypes:
  - Postprandial distress syndrome
  - Epigastric pain syndrome
- System(s) affected: GI
- Synonym(s): idiopathic dyspepsia; nonulcer dyspepsia; nonorganic dyspepsia; postprandial distress syndrome; epigastric pain syndrome

EPIDEMIOLOGY

Incidence

- Unknown
- Accounts for 70% of patients with dyspepsia
- Accounts for ~5% of primary care visits

Prevalence

- 15–30% prevalence in developed countries (3–10% when strict Rome III criteria are used)
- Predominant age: adults, but can be seen in children
- Predominant gender: female > male

ETIOLOGY AND PATHOPHYSIOLOGY

Unknown, but proposed mechanisms or associations include gastric motility disorders, visceral hypersensitivity to pain, *Helicobacter pylori* infection, alteration in upper GI microbiome, medications, anxiety, and depression

Genetics

Possible link to G-protein β-3 subunit 825 CC genotype and serotonin transport genes

Pediatric Considerations

Be alert for family system dysfunction.

Pregnancy Considerations

Pregnancy may exacerbate symptoms.

Geriatric Considerations

Patients older than age 55 years with new-onset dyspepsia should have an upper endoscopy.

RISK FACTORS

- Other functional disorders
- Anxiety/depression psychosocial factors: divorce, unemployment
- Smoking

GENERAL PREVENTION

Avoid foods and habits known to exacerbate symptoms.

COMMONLY ASSOCIATED CONDITIONS

Other functional bowel disorders

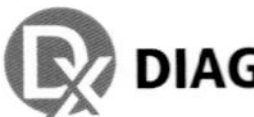

DIAGNOSIS

HISTORY

- Postprandial fullness (1)[B]
- Early satiety (1)[B]
- Epigastric pain (1)[B]
- Epigastric burning (1)[B]

- Symptoms for 3 months (1)[C]
- Inquire about warning signs that necessitate a more aggressive workup to include endoscopy (2)[C]:
  - Unintended weight loss
  - Progressive dysphagia
  - Persistent vomiting
  - GI bleeding
  - Family Hx of cancer
  - Older than age 55 years

PHYSICAL EXAM

Physical exam help to rule out other disorders:

- Document weight status (3)
- Examine for other signs of systemic illness (3)
  - Murphy sign for cholelithiasis
  - Rebound and guarding for ulcer perforation
  - Palpation during muscle contraction for abdominal wall pain
  - Jaundice
  - Thyromegaly

DIFFERENTIAL DIAGNOSIS

- Peptic ulcer disease
- Gastroesophageal reflux disease
- Cholecystitis
- Gastric or esophageal cancer
- Esophageal spasm
- Malabsorption syndromes
- Celiac disease
- Pancreatic cancer
- Pancreatitis
- Inflammatory bowel disease
- Carbohydrate malabsorption
- Gastroparesis
- Ischemic bowel disease
- Intestinal parasites
- Irritable bowel syndrome
- Ischemic heart disease
- Diabetes mellitus
- Thyroid disease
- Connective tissue disorders
- Conversion disorder
- Medication effects

DIAGNOSTIC TESTS & INTERPRETATION

Initial Tests (lab, imaging)

- Functional dyspepsia is a diagnosis of exclusion. Labs should be ordered based on clinical suspicion for underlying organic disease (3)[C].
- CBC (if anemia or infection suspected)
- LFT (if hepatobiliary disease suspected

- Test for *H. pylori* (stool antigen or urea breath test) in areas of high *H. pylori* prevalence (4)[A].

- Order upper endoscopy for patients >55 years or those with alarm symptoms (weight loss, signs of blood loss, dysphagia, concern for cancer) (3)[C].
- Perform upper endoscopy if patient does not respond to gastric acid suppression trial (3)[C].

Diagnostic Procedures/Other

Esophageal manometry or gastric accommodation studies are rarely needed (3)[C].

Test Interpretation

None (by definition a functional disorder)

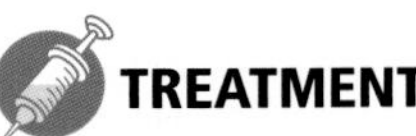

TREATMENT

GENERAL MEASURES

- Few treatment options are proven to be effective (5).
- Reassurance and physician support are helpful (3)[C].
- Treatment is based on presumed etiologies.
- Discontinue offending medications (3)[C].

MEDICATION

First Line

- Treat *H. pylori* if confirmed on testing (4)[A].
- Trial of once-daily proton pump inhibitor (PPI) medication (e.g., omeprazole 20 mg PO QD) or H2RA (e.g., ranitidine 150mg BID) for up to 8 weeks in patients without alarm symptoms (5)[A]

Second Line

- Trial of low-dose tricyclic antidepressant (TCA) medication if no response to PPIs (amitriptyline 10 mg or trazodone 25 mg at bedtime); consider increasing to double dose after a few days. Caution in elderly due to side effects (5,6)[A].
- Consider a 1-month trial of prokinetic medication (metoclopramide) or buspirone if no response to TCA (5,6)[B]. Caution with metoclopramide in elderly due to side effects of tardive dyskinesia and parkinsonian symptoms.

ADDITIONAL THERAPIES

- Stress reduction (5,6)[A]
  - Relaxation techniques
  - Physical exercise
  - Reflux precautions where applicable
- Psychological therapy effective in some patients (6)[A]
  - Cognitive-behavioral therapy
  - Hypnotherapy
  - Psychotherapy

COMPLEMENTARY & ALTERNATIVE MEDICINE

- Alternative approaches need further study.
  - Peppermint oil +/− caraway oil
  - Probiotics have theoretical benefit but only one controlled trial (5)[B].
  - Iberogast: mixture of 9 plant extracts (3)[B]

ONGOING CARE

FOLLOW-UP RECOMMENDATIONS

Patient Monitoring

- Provide ongoing support and reassurance.
- Refer for upper endoscopy for persistent symptoms.

DIET

- Limited data to support dietary modification
- Consider limiting fatty foods (5,6)[C].
- Avoid foods that exacerbate symptoms: wheat and cow milk proteins, peppers or spices, coffee and tea, and alcohol (5,6)[C].

PATIENT EDUCATION

Reassurance and stress reduction techniques

PROGNOSIS

Long-term/chronic symptoms with symptom-free periods

COMPLICATIONS

Iatrogenic, from evaluation to rule out serious pathology

REFERENCES

1. Tack J, Talley NJ. Functional dyspepsia—symptoms, definitions and validity of the Rome III criteria. *Nat Rev Gastroenterol Hepatol*. 2013;10(3):134–141.
2. Loyd R, McClellan D. Update on the evaluation and management of functional dyspepsia. *Am Fam Phys*. 2011;83(5):547–552.
3. Oustamanolakis P, Tack J. Dyspepsia: organic versus functional. *J Clin Gastroenterol*. 2012;46(3):175–190.
4. Zhao B, Zhao J, Cheng W, et al. Efficacy of *Helicobacter pylori* eradication therapy on functional dyspepsia: a meta-analysis of randomized controlled studies with 12-month follow-up. *J Clin Gastroenterol*. 2014;48(3):241–247.
5. Stein B, Everhart KK, Lacy BE. Treatment of functional dyspepsia and gastroparesis. *Curr Treat Options Gastroenterol*. 2014;12(4):385–397. doi:10.1007/s11938-014-0028-5.
6. Vanheel H, Tack J. Therapeutic options for functional dyspepsia. *Dig Dis*. 2014;32(3):230–234. doi:10.1159/000358111.

ADDITIONAL READING

- Amini M, Ghamar Chehreh ME, Khedmat H, et al. Famotidine in the treatment of functional dyspepsia: a randomized double-blind, placebo-controlled trial. *J Egypt Public Health Assoc*. 2012;87(1–2):29–33.
- Ford A, Moayyedi P. Dyspepsia. *Curr Opin Gastroenterol*. 2013;29(6):662–668. doi:10.1097/MOG.0b013e328365d45d.
- Ganesh M, Nurko S. Functional dyspepsia in children. *Pediatr Ann*. 2014;43(4):e101–e105. doi:10.3928/00904481-20140325-12.
- Graham D, Rugge M. Clinical practice: diagnosis and evaluation of dyspepsia. *J Clin Gastroenterol*. 2010;44(3):167–172.
- Kaminski A, Kamper A, Thaler K, et al. Antidepressants for the treatment of abdominal pain-related functional gastrointestinal disorders in children and adolescents. *Cochrane Database Syst Rev*. 2011;(7):CD008013. doi: 10.1002/14651858.CD008013.pub2
- Lacy BE, Talley NJ, Locke GR 3rd, et al. Review article: current treatment options and management of functional dyspepsia. *Aliment Pharmacol Ther*. 2012;36(1):3–15.
- Lan L, Zeng F, Liu GJ, et al. Acupuncture for functional dyspepsia. *Cochrane Database Syst Rev*. 2014;10:CD008487. doi: 10.1002/14651858.CD008487.pub2.
- Overland MK. Dyspepsia. *Med Clin North Am*. 2014;98(3):549–564. doi: 10.1016/j.mcna.2014.01.007.
- Tack J, Masaoka T, Janssen P, et al. Functional dyspepsia. *Curr Opin Gastroenterol*. 2011;27(6):549–557.
- Tack J, Talley N, Camilleri M, et al. Functional gastroduodenal disorders. *Gastroenterology*. 2006;130(5):1466–1479. doi:10.1053/j.gastro.2005.11.059.

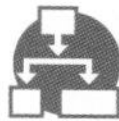

SEE ALSO

- Dyspepsia; Endoscopic-Negative Reflux Disease; Gastritis; Irritable Bowel Syndrome
- Algorithms: Dyspepsia; Epigastric Pain; Esophageal Regurgitation

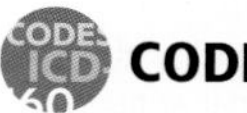

CODES

ICD10

K30 Functional dyspepsia

CLINICAL PEARLS

- When no organic cause for dyspepsia is found, it is considered functional or idiopathic.
- Consider empiric treatment with acid suppression as 1st-line therapy.
- Treat *H. pylori* if present.
- Extensive diagnostic testing is not recommended unless alarm symptoms are present.

DYSPHAGIA

Felix B. Chang, MD, DABMA, ABIHM

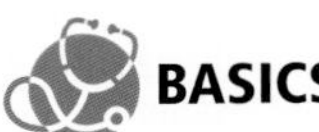

BASICS

Difficulty transmitting the alimentary bolus from the mouth to the stomach

DESCRIPTION

- Oropharyngeal: difficulty transferring food bolus from oropharynx to proximal esophagus
- Esophageal dysphagia: difficulty moving food bolus through esophagus

EPIDEMIOLOGY

10% of individuals >50 years of age

Prevalence

- Common primary care complaint
- Impaired swallowing common in nursing home residents 29–32%

ETIOLOGY AND PATHOPHYSIOLOGY

- Oropharyngeal (transfer dysphagia):
  - *Mechanical causes*: pharyngeal and laryngeal cancer, acute epiglottitis, carotid body tumor, pharyngitis, tonsillitis, strep throat, lymphoid hyperplasia of lingual tonsil, lateral pharyngeal pouch, hypopharyngeal diverticulum
- Esophageal:
  - *Esophageal mechanical lesions*: carcinomas, esophageal diverticula, esophageal webs, Schatzki ring, structures (peptic, chemical, trauma, radiation), foreign body
  - *Extrinsic mechanical lesions*: peritonsillar abscess, thyroid disorders, tumors, mediastinal compression, vascular compression (enlarged left atrium, aberrant subclavius, aortic aneurysm), osteoarthritis cervical spine, adenopathy, esophageal duplication cyst
- Neuromuscular: achalasia, diffuse esophageal spasm, hypertensive lower esophageal sphincter, scleroderma, nutcracker esophagus, CVA, Alzheimer disease, Huntington chorea, Parkinson disease, multiple sclerosis, skeletal muscle disease (polymyositis, dermatomyositis), neuromuscular junction disease (myasthenia gravis, Eaton-Lambert syndrome, botulism), hyper-hypothyroidism, Guillain-Barré syndrome, systemic lupus erythematous, acute lymphoblastic leukemia, amyloidosis, diabetic neuropathy, brainstem tumors, Chagas disease
- Infection: diphtheria, chronic meningitis, tertiary syphilis, Lyme disease, rabies, poliomyelitis, CMV, esophagitis (*Candida*, herpetic)

RISK FACTORS

- Children: hereditary and/or congenital malformations
- Adults: age >50 years. Elderly: GERD, stroke, COPD, chronic pain
- Smoking, excess alcohol intake, obesity
- Medications: quinine, potassium chloride, vitamin C, tetracycline, Bactrim, clindamycin, NSAIDs, procainamide, anticholinergics, bisphosphates
- Neurologic events or diseases: CVA, myasthenia gravis, multiple sclerosis, Parkinson disease, amyotrophic lateral sclerosis (ALS), Huntington chorea
- HIV patients with CD4 cell count <100 cells/mm^3
- Trauma or irradiation of head, neck, and chest; mechanical lesions
- Extrinsic mechanical lesions: lung, thyroid tumors, lymphoma, metastasis
- Iron deficiency
- Anterior cervical spine surgery (up to 71% first 2 weeks postop; 12–14% 1 year postop)

GENERAL PREVENTION

- Correct poorly fitting dentures in older patients.
- Educate patients on prolonged chewing and drinking large volumes of water to accompany meals.
- Diet consisting of liquids and soft foods
- Avoid drinking alcohol with meals.
- Prophylactic swallowing exercises in patients with head and neck cancer undergoing chemoradiation

COMMONLY ASSOCIATED CONDITIONS

Peptic structure, esophageal webs and rings, carcinoma; history of stroke, dementia, pneumonia

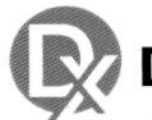

DIAGNOSIS

HISTORY

- Dysphagia to both solids and liquids from the onset is likely an esophageal motility disorder.
- Oropharyngeal dysphagia presents as difficulty in initiating the swallowing process.
- Dysphagia for solids that later progresses to involve liquids is more likely to reflect mechanical obstruction.
- Progressive dysphagia is usually caused by cancer or a peptic stricture, whereas intermittent dysphagia is most often related to a lower esophageal ring.
- Inquire about heartburn, weight loss, hematemesis, coffee ground emesis, anemia, regurgitation of food particles, and respiratory symptoms.
- Is there regurgitation, aspiration, or drooling immediately after swallowing?
  - May represent oropharyngeal dysphagia
- Does the food bolus feel stuck?
  - Upper sternum or back of throat may represent oropharyngeal dysphagia, whereas sensation over the lower sternum is typical of esophageal dysphagia.
- Is odynophagia present?
  - May represent inflammation, achalasia, diffuse esophageal spasm, esophagitis, pharyngitis, pill-induced esophagitis, cancer
- Globus sensation?
  - Indicates cricopharyngeal or laryngeal disorders
- History of sour taste in the back of the throat or history of chronic heartburn?
  - GERD
- Inquire about alcohol and/or tobacco use.
- Are there associated symptoms such as weight loss or chest pain?
  - Double aortic arch, right aortic arch with retroesophageal left subclavian artery and left ligamentum arteriosum
  - Anticholinergics, antihistamines, and some antihypertensives can decrease salivary production.
- Halitosis: Rule out diverticulitis.
- Connective tissue disorder?
- Changes in speech, hoarseness, weak cough, dysphonia? Rule out neuromuscular dysfunction.

PHYSICAL EXAM

- General: vital signs
- Skin:
  - Telangiectasia, sclerodactyly, calcinosis (r/o autoimmune), Reynaud phenomenon, sclerodactyly may be found in CREST syndrome or systemic scleroderma; stigmata of alcohol abuse (palmar erythema; telangiectasia)
- Head, eye, ear, nose, throat (HEENT):
  - Oropharyngeal:
    - Pharyngeal erythema/edema, tonsillitis, pharyngeal ulcers or thrush, odynophagia (bacterial, viral, fungal infections)
    - Tongue fasciculations (ALS)
  - Neck:
    - Neck masses, lymphadenopathy, neck tenderness, goiter
    - Neck tenderness: acute thyroiditis
- Neurologic:
  - Cranial nerve exam:
    - Sensory testing of cranial nerves V, IX, and X
    - Motor examination of cranial nerves V, VII, X, XI, and XII
  - CNS, mental status exam, strength testing, Horner syndrome, ataxia, cogwheel rigidity (CVA, dementia, Parkinson disease, Alzheimer disease)
    - Eye position, extraocular motility: stroke
  - Informal bedside swallowing evaluation:
    - Observe level of consciousness, postural control-upright position, oral hygiene, mobilization of oral secretions.

DIFFERENTIAL DIAGNOSIS

See "Etiology and Pathophysiology."

DIAGNOSTIC TESTS & INTERPRETATION

Adults:

- Barium swallow
- Fiberoptic endoscopic examination of swallowing (FEES)
- Gastroesophageal endoscopy
- Barium cine/video esophagogram
- Ambulatory 24-hour pH testing

- Esophageal manometry
- Videofluoroscopic swallowing study (VFSS): oropharyngeal dysphagia

Initial Tests (lab, imaging)

- Guided by specific diagnostic considerations (1)[C]
  - CBC (infection and inflammation)
  - Serum protein and albumin levels for nutritional assessment
  - Thyroid function studies to detect dysphagia associated with hypothyroidism or hyperthyroidism, cobalamin levels
  - Antiacetylcholine antibodies in selected patients
- Barium swallow: Detects mild strictures, evaluation of stenosis

Follow-Up Tests & Special Considerations

- CT scan of chest
- MRI of brain and cervical spine
- Videofluoroscopic swallowing function study (VSFS) (lips, tongue, palate, pharynx, larynx, proximal esophagus)
- No significant difference regarding the diagnostic efficacy of fiberoptic endoscopic evaluation of swallowing compared to videofluoroscopy (2)[C].

Diagnostic Procedures/Other

Endoscopy with biopsy; esophageal manometry; esophageal pH monitoring

Test Interpretation

- Squamous cell or adenocarcinoma
- Barrett metaplasia
- Fibrous tissue of a ring, web, or stricture
- Loss of smooth muscle (scleroderma)

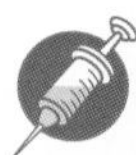

TREATMENT

GENERAL MEASURES

Exclude cardiac disease. Ensure airway and pulmonary function. Assess nutritional status. Speech therapy evaluation is helpful.

MEDICATION

First Line

- For esophageal spasms: calcium channel blockers: nifedipine 10–30 mg TID; imipramine 50 mg at bedtime; sildenafil 50 mg/day PRN
- For esophagitis:
  - Antacids: Tums, Mylanta, Maalox
  - H_2 blockers: cimetidine, ranitidine, nizatidine, famotidine
  - Proton pump inhibitors: omeprazole, lansoprazole, rabeprazole, esomeprazole, pantoprazole
  - Prokinetic agents: metoclopramide, erythromycin (rarely used due to contraindications)
- Precautions: may need to use liquid forms of medications because patients might have difficulty swallowing pills

ISSUES FOR REFERRAL

- Gastroenterology: endoscopy, refractory
- Surgery: dilation, esophageal myotomy, biopsy

ADDITIONAL THERAPIES

Speech therapy for swallowing assessment, dietary and positioning recommendations, and muscle-strengthening exercise; no eating at bedtime; remaining upright after eating

SURGERY/OTHER PROCEDURES

- Esophageal dilatation (pneumatic or bougie)
- Esophageal stent; laser for cancer palliation (2)[A]
- Treatment for underlying problem (e.g., thyroid goiter, vascular ring, esophageal atresia)
- Nd:YAG laser incision of lower esophageal rings refractory to dilation
- Photodynamic therapy (cancer) (3)[C]
- Cricopharyngeal myotomy (for oropharyngeal dysphagia)
- Surgery for Zenker diverticulum, refractory strictures, or myotomy (for achalasia)
- Percutaneous gastrostomy (PEG) decreases risk of dysphagia when compared with nasogastric tube.

COMPLEMENTARY & ALTERNATIVE MEDICINE

- Acupuncture for neurogenic dysphagia
- Electroacupuncture combined with dilating granule in the treatment of GERD
- Botulinum toxin insufficient evidence

INPATIENT CONSIDERATIONS

Admission Criteria/Initial Stabilization

- Complete or partial esophageal obstruction with malnutrition or hypovolemia/dehydration
- Comorbid conditions complicating etiology of dysphagia
- Enteral feeding requirement
- Outpatient for conditions where patient is able to maintain nutrition and has little risk of complications
- Hospitalization may be required for adults when dysphagia is associated with total or near-total obstruction of esophageal lumen.
- Endoscopy and/or esophageal dilation; surgery diagnostic or therapeutic

IV Fluids

For dehydrated, hypovolemic patients and patients with impaired consciousness

Discharge Criteria

Tolerating adequate diet without nausea/pain

ONGOING CARE

DIET

See "General Prevention."

PATIENT EDUCATION

Dietary modification, no eating at bedtime, remaining upright after eating, smoking cessation

PROGNOSIS

Vary with specific diagnosis

COMPLICATIONS

- Oropharyngeal: pneumonia, lung abscess, aspiration, airway obstruction
- Malnutrition and dehydration

REFERENCES

1. Al-Hussaini A, Latif EH, Singh V. 12-minute consultation: an evidence-based approach to the management of dysphagia. *Clin Otolaryngol*. 2013;38(3):237–243. doi:10.1111/coa.12116.
2. American Society for Gastrointestinal Endoscopy Standards of Practice Committee, Pasha SF, Acosta RD, et al. The role of endoscopy in the evaluation and management of dysphagia. *Gastrointest Endosc*. 2014;79(2):191–201.
3. Dai Y, Li C, Xie Y, et al. Interventions for dysphagia in oesophageal cancer. *Cochrane Database Syst Rev*. 2014;10:CD005048. doi:10.1002/14651858.CD005048.pub4.

ADDITIONAL READING

- American College of Radiology. *ACR appropriateness Criteria*. https://acsearch.acr.org/docs/69471/Narrative/ Accessed 2014.
- Anderson U, Beck A, Kjaersgaard A, et al. Systematic review and evidence based recommendations on texture modified foods and thickened fluids for adults with oropharyngeal dysphagia. *E-SPEN Journal*. 2013;(8):e127–e134. doi:10.1016/j.clnme.2013.05.
- Cho SK, Lu Y, Lee DH. Dysphagia following anterior cervical spinal surgery: a systematic review. *Bone Joint J*. 2013;95-B(7):868–873. doi:10.1302/0301-620X.95B7.31029.
- Geeganage C, Beavan J, Ellender S, et al. Interventions for dysphagia and nutritional support in acute and subacute stroke. *Cochrane Database Syst Rev*. 2012;10:CD000323. doi:10.1002/14651858.CD000323.pub2.
- Regan J, Murphy A, Chiang M, et al. Botulinum toxin for upper oesophageal sphincter dysfunction in neurological swallowing disorders. *Cochrane Database Syst Rev*. 2014;5:CD009968. doi:10.1002/14651858.CD009968.pub2.

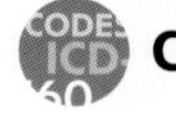

CODES

ICD10

- R13.10 Dysphagia, unspecified
- R13.12 Dysphagia, oropharyngeal phase
- R13.14 Dysphagia, pharyngoesophageal phase

CLINICAL PEARLS

- Weight loss is usually associated with malignancy or achalasia.
- Dysphagia is common after stroke and increases risk of aspiration pneumonia.
- Self-expanded metal stent is safe, effective, and quicker in palliating dysphagia compared to others modalities.

DYSPLASTIC NEVUS SYNDROME

Andrew Kim, MD • Dori Goldberg, MD

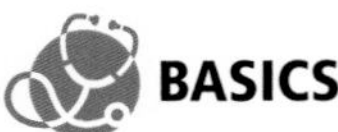

BASICS

Dysplastic nevus syndrome (DNS), also known as atypical mole syndrome (AMS), is a sporadic or hereditary disorder resulting in numerous clinically atypical nevi and an increased risk for developing malignant melanoma.

DESCRIPTION

- Condition resulting in elevated total body nevi count, including clinically atypical nevi
  - Usually >50, although often >100
  - Larger number in hereditary DNS versus sporadic dysplastic nevi (DN) (as few as <10 in sporadic, although high numbers also possible)
- Increased risk of melanoma (1)
  - Up to 90% occurrence by age 80 years in certain high-risk individuals
  - Earlier onset than sporadic melanoma cases
  - Most arise out of healthy skin as opposed to a preexisting atypical nevus
  - Higher risk for appearance at unusual sites (e.g., scalp)
- DNS terminology often used interchangeably with AMS, familial atypical multiple mole melanoma (FAMMM) syndrome, and B-K mole syndrome
- Median age of diagnosis for melanoma is 10–20 years earlier than the general population, with documented cases of melanoma as early as in the early teens and 20s (2).
- Melanomas in the setting of DNS are most often superficial spreading or nodular type.

EPIDEMIOLOGY

Incidence

Uncertain due to phenotype variability and limited data but ~10% of melanoma cases are diagnosed as familial.

Prevalence

At least 32,000 cases in the United States per National Institutes of Health (NIH) calculations (3)

ETIOLOGY AND PATHOPHYSIOLOGY

CDKN2A (cyclin-dependent kinase inhibitor 2A) mutations have been observed in kindreds with familial DNS and multiple melanomas. The *CDKN2A* gene on 9p21 encodes for the proteins p16 and p14. The p16 binds to CDK4 and 6 and is a negative cell-cycle regulator via inhibition of the CDK-cyclin D interaction needed for cell-cycle progression from G_1 to S. Similarly, p14 functions by stabilizing the tumor-suppressor protein p53 in the G_1 phase of the cell cycle.

- Unclear for sporadic cases, although somatic p16 inactivation noted in 40% of familial melanoma
- Familial cases of germline *CDKN2A* mutations considered to be transmitted genetically in an autosomal dominant fashion.

Genetics

- Autosomal dominant inheritance in hereditary cases but variable expressivity and incomplete penetrance
- *CDKN2A* mutation observed in 25–40% of hereditary cases

RISK FACTORS

Family history DN, DNS, and/or melanoma

GENERAL PREVENTION

- No currently available prevention strategies
- Treatment is directed toward secondary prevention of melanoma complications with routine skin exams, biopsy of suspect lesions, and environmental risk mitigation (e.g., sun protection and sun avoidance).
- Experimental early detection protocols for pancreatic cancer in use with some high-risk individuals

COMMONLY ASSOCIATED CONDITIONS

- Malignant melanoma, including ocular melanoma
- Ocular nevi
- Pancreatic cancer in *CDKN2A* mutation

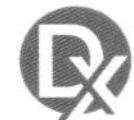

DIAGNOSIS

DNS is a clinical diagnosis with various classifications schemes proposed in the past. Although not widely accepted, diagnostic criteria as defined by the NIH require the 3 features of (i) malignant melanoma in ≥1 1st- or 2nd-degree relatives; (ii) numerous melanocytic nevi (frequently >50), some of which are clinically atypical; and (iii) nevi that have certain histologic features on pathologic examination (4).

HISTORY

- Changing lesions: bleeding, scaling, size, texture, nonhealing, hyper- or hypopigmentation
- Prior skin biopsies
- Prior melanoma
- Pancreatic cancer
- In 1st- or 2nd-degree relatives
  - DNS
  - Melanoma
  - Pancreatic cancer

PHYSICAL EXAM

- ABCDE mnemonic for pigmented lesions: Asymmetry, Border irregularity, Color variegation, Diameter >6 mm, and Evolving lesion
  - Melanoma typically with several characteristics of ABCDEs on gross exam (DN often defined as ≥5 mm + at least 2 other features)
  - Difficult differentiating DN from melanoma using these criteria
- "Ugly duckling sign" (5)
- Melanoma screening strategy of identifying atypical nevi straying from the predominant nevus pattern when numerous atypical nevi present.
- Most common features of DN on dermatoscopy magnification per the pattern analysis method include the following (6):
  - Atypical pigment network
  - Irregular/peripheral depigmentation areas
  - Irregular distribution of brown globules
  - Pigmentation with central heterogeneity and abrupt termination
- Some dermatoscopic features more suggestive of melanoma include the following (6):
  - Depigmented areas
  - Whitish veil
  - Homogenous areas distributed irregularly, in multiple areas, or >25% of total lesion
  - ≥4 colors

DIFFERENTIAL DIAGNOSIS

- Acquired melanocytic nevi
- Sporadic atypical nevi
- Melanoma
- Seborrheic keratosis
- Dermatofibroma
- Lentigo
- Pigmented actinic keratosis

DIAGNOSTIC TESTS & INTERPRETATION

Initial Tests (lab, imaging)

Genetic testing is available for *CDKN2A* mutations, but it is not recommended outside of research studies as the results cannot be adequately used for management or surveillance (7)[C].

- When the total nevus count is high and individually following each nevus impractical, total-body photography may aid in the evaluation of evolving nevi as well as in documenting new nevi (8)[C].
- Further exam of nevi with a dermatoscope may help in distinguishing between benign and malignant pigmented lesions.

Diagnostic Procedures/Other

- Biopsy is recommended of any new lesion where melanoma cannot be excluded or for any existing evolving lesion concerning for melanoma.
- Preferred method entails full-thickness biopsy of the entire lesion with a narrow 2-mm margin of normal skin by excisional, incisional, or punch biopsy (8)[C].
  - Excisional biopsy provides the most accurate diagnosis and should be performed when possible.
  - Take care to provide a sufficiently deep sample down to the fat to allow assessment of the depth of any melanomas.
  - Scoop shave biopsy including a sufficient lateral and deep margin can also be used, but care must be taken to not transect the deep margin.

Test Interpretation

DN: Possible features include melanocyte proliferation in the dermoepidermal junction, bridging of rete ridges by melanocytic nests, dermal fibrosis, and interstitial lymphocytic inflammation.

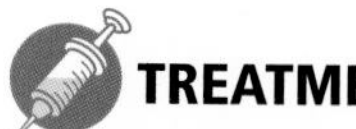

TREATMENT

MEDICATION

No medications are available at this time to treat atypical nevi.

ISSUES FOR REFERRAL

- Referral to a dermatologist for routine skin exam
- Consider referral to a specialty pigmented lesion clinic.
- Ophthalmologic exams for ocular nevi/melanoma screening
- Oncology or specialized genetics study group involvement if strong family predisposition to pancreatic cancer
- Possible cosmetic surgery consultation for cosmetically poor excision outcomes

ADDITIONAL THERAPIES

- Topical chemo- and immunotherapies therapies have been unsuccessfully attempted to treat atypical nevi.
- Laser treatment should be avoided because it is both unsafe and ineffective for melanocytic nevi.

SURGERY/OTHER PROCEDURES

Surgical excision of all atypical nevi is not recommended as most melanomas in DNS appear de novo on healthy skin and the procedure leads to both poor cosmetic outcomes and a false sense of security. Lesions suspicious for melanoma should be biopsied or removed surgically.

ONGOING CARE

FOLLOW-UP RECOMMENDATIONS

Close follow-up with a dermatologist and sun avoidance/protection is highly advised.

Patient Monitoring

- Total body skin exam (including nails, scalp, genital area, and oral mucosa) every 3–6 months initially, starting at puberty; may be reduced to annually once nevi are stable.
- Dermatoscopic evaluation for suspect lesions
- Ocular exam for those with familial DNS
- Excision of suspect lesions
- Total body photography at baseline
- Monthly self-exams of skin
- Sun avoidance and sun protection

PATIENT EDUCATION

- Teach patients the "ABCDE" mnemonic + ugly duckling sign for assessing nevi and identifying potential melanomas.
- Encourage sun protection/minimization of sun exposure.
- Educate on sun avoidance, proper application of sunscreen, use of protective clothing (e.g., hats), and avoidance of tanning booths.
- Provide instruction on skin self-exam techniques.
- A sample listing of patient-centric review sources on this topic are as follows:
  - American Academy of Dermatology (http://www.aad.org/dermatology-a-to-z/diseases-and-treatments/m---p/moles/who-gets-types)
  - Skin Cancer Foundation (http://www.skincancer.org/skin-cancer-information/dysplastic-nevi)
  - Melanoma Research Foundation (http://www.melanoma.org/learn-more/melanoma-101/what-melanoma)

PROGNOSIS

- Multiple classification schemes have been developed over the years to delineate risk of melanoma in patients with DNS. Individuals with a family history of melanoma are at greatest risk. A classification system developed by Rigel is simply and readily applied in the clinical setting. Points are assigned based on incidence of melanoma, with 1 point given for a personal history with melanoma, and 2 points for each family member with melanoma (modified nuclear family consisting of 1st-degree relatives + grandparents and uncles/aunts) and stratified as follows (9):
  - Score = 0, Rigel group 0, 6% 25-year accumulated risk for melanoma
  - Score = 1, Rigel group 1, 10% risk
  - Score = 2, Rigel group 2, 15% risk
  - Score ≥3, Rigel group 3, 50% risk
- The *CDKN2A* mutation has also been associated with a 60–90% risk of melanoma by age 80 years and a 17% risk for pancreatic cancer by age 75 years.

COMPLICATIONS

- Malignant melanoma
- Poor cosmetic outcomes from biopsy

REFERENCES

1. Newton JA, Bataille V, Griffiths K, et al. How common is the atypical mole syndrome phenotype in apparently sporadic melanoma? *J Am Acad Dermatol*. 1993;29(6):989–996.
2. Silva JH, Sá BC, Avila AL, et al. Atypical mole syndrome and dysplastic nevi: identification of populations at risk for developing melanoma—review article. *Clinics (Sao Paulo)*. 2011;66(3):493–499.
3. Mize DE, Bishop M, Reese E, et al. Familial atypical multiple mole melanoma syndrome. In: Riegert-Johnson DL, Boardman LA, Hefferon T, et al, eds. *Cancer Syndromes*. Bethesda, MD: National Center for Biotechnology Information; 2009.
4. NIH Consensus conference. Diagnosis and treatment of early melanoma. *JAMA*. 1992;268(10):1314–1319.
5. Grob JJ, Bonerandi JJ. The 'ugly duckling' sign: identification of the common characteristics of nevi in an individual as a basis for melanoma screening. *Arch Dermatol*. 1998;134(1):103–104.
6. Salopek TG, Kopf AW, Stefanato CM, et al. Differentiation of atypical moles (dysplastic nevi) from early melanomas by dermoscopy. *Dermatol Clin*. 2001;19(2):337–345.
7. Kefford R, Bishop JN, Tucker M, et al. Genetic testing for melanoma. *Lancet Oncol*. 2002;3(11):653–654.
8. Duffy K, Grossman D. The dysplastic nevus: from historical perspective to management in the modern era: part I. Historical, histologic, and clinical aspects. *J Am Acad Dermatol*. 2012;67(1):1.e1–e16; quiz 17–18.
9. Rigel DS, Rivers JK, Friedman RJ, et al. Risk gradient for malignant melanoma in individuals with dysplastic naevi. *Lancet*. 1988;1(8581):352–353.

D

ADDITIONAL READING

- Czajkowski R, Placek W, Drewa G, et al. FAMMM syndrome: pathogenesis and management. *Dermatol Surg*. 2004;30(2, Pt 2):291–296.
- Farber MJ, Heilman ER, Friedman RJ. Dysplastic nevi. *Dermatol Clin*. 2012;30(3):389–404.
- Friedman RJ, Farber MJ, Warycha MA, et al. The "dysplastic" nevus. *Clin Dermatol*. 2009;27(1):103–115.
- Moloney FJ, Guitera P, Coates E, et al. Detection of primary melanoma in individuals at extreme high risk: a prospective 5-year follow-up study [published online ahead of print June 25, 2014]. *JAMA Dermatol*. doi:10.1001/jamadermatol.2014.514.
- Naeyaert JM, Brochez L. Clinical practice. Dysplastic nevi. *N Engl J Med*. 2003;349(23):2233–2240.
- Robson ME, Storm CD, Weitzel J, et al. American Society of Clinical Oncology policy statement update: genetic and genomic testing for cancer susceptibility. *J Clin Oncol*. 2010;28(5):893–901.
- Slade J, Marghoob AA, Salopek TG, et al. Atypical mole syndrome: risk factor for cutaneous malignant melanoma and implications for management. *J Am Acad Dermatol*. 1995;32(3):479–494.

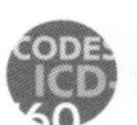

CODES

ICD10

- D23.9 Other benign neoplasm of skin, unspecified
- D23.4 Other benign neoplasm of skin of scalp and neck

CLINICAL PEARLS

- Melanoma in DNS tends to arise from healthy skin despite a large number of atypical nevi.
- ~20% of individuals with familial DNS will develop pancreatic cancer by age 75 years.
- Patients with DNS tend to produce neoplasms in unusual sites such as the scalp, eyes, and double sun-protected areas (e.g., gluteal folds).
- ~10% of melanomas are featureless on dermatoscopy.

ECTOPIC PREGNANCY

Ryan J. Callery, MD

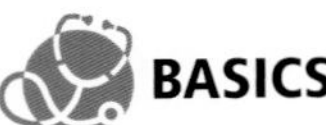

BASICS

DESCRIPTION

Ectopic: pregnancy implanted outside the confines of the uterine cavity. Subtypes include the following:

- Tubal: pregnancy implanted in any portion of the fallopian tube
- Abdominal: pregnancy implanted intra-abdominally, most commonly after tubal abortion or rupture of tubal ectopic pregnancy
- Heterotopic: pregnancy implanted intrauterine and a separate pregnancy implanted outside uterine cavity
- Ovarian: implantation of pregnancy in ovarian tissue
- Cervical: implantation of pregnancy in cervix
- Intraligamentary: implantation of pregnancy within the broad ligament

EPIDEMIOLOGY

Incidence

- 108,800 cases in 1992 in the United States, according to CDC census (most recent data available) meaning that 1.5–2.0% of all pregnancies were ectopic. The true incidence is difficult to estimate because many patients are treated in the outpatient setting.
- In the United States, ectopic pregnancy is the leading cause of 1st trimester maternal deaths and accounts for 6% of all pregnancy-related deaths.
- Heterotopic pregnancy, although rare (1:30,000), occurs with greater frequency in women undergoing in vitro fertilization (IVF) (1/1,000).

Prevalence

~33% recurrence rate if prior ectopic pregnancy

ETIOLOGY AND PATHOPHYSIOLOGY

- 97% of ectopic pregnancies occur in the fallopian tube, of which, 55% in the ampullary portion of the tube, 25% in the isthmus, and 17% in the fimbria.
- Of the remaining 3%, most are ovarian, cervical, abdominal pregnancies, or heterotopic.
- For a tubal pregnancy, impaired movement of the fertilized ovum to the uterine cavity due to dysfunction of the tubal cilia, scarring, or narrowing of the tubal lumen
- Other locations are rare but may occur from reimplantation of an aborted tubal pregnancy or from uterine structural abnormalities (mainly cervical pregnancy).

RISK FACTORS

- History of pelvic inflammatory disease (PID), endometritis, or current gonorrhea/chlamydia infection
- Previous ectopic pregnancy
- History of tubal surgery (~33% of pregnancies after tubal ligation will be ectopic)
- Pelvic adhesive disease (infection or prior surgery)
- Use of an IUD: Overall chance of pregnancy of any type with an IUD is low; however, there is an increased likelihood of ectopic location if pregnancy occurs.

ALERT

- IUDs reduce absolute risk of ectopic pregnancy.
- Use of assisted reproductive technologies
- Diethylstilbestrol exposure in utero (DES was last used in 1972)
- Tobacco use
- Patients with disorders that affect ciliary motility may be at increased risk (e.g., endometriosis, Kartagener).

GENERAL PREVENTION

- Reliable contraception or abstinence
- Screening and treatment of STIs (i.e., gonorrhea, chlamydia) that can cause PID and tubal scarring

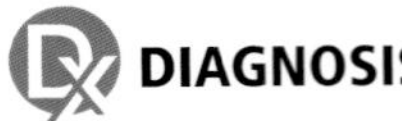

DIAGNOSIS

HISTORY

In >50% of presenting cases, patients have sudden-onset abdominal pain coupled with cessation of/or irregular menses. Other common symptoms include nausea and/or vomiting, vaginal bleeding, and pain referred to the shoulder (from hemoperitoneum).

PHYSICAL EXAM

- Abdominal tenderness ± rebound tenderness
- Vaginal bleeding
- Palpable mass on pelvic exam (adnexal or cul-de-sac fullness)
- Cervical motion tenderness
- In cervical cases, an hourglass-shaped cervix might be noted.
- In cases of rupture and significant intraperitoneal bleeding, signs of shock such as pallor, tachycardia, and hypotension may be present.

DIFFERENTIAL DIAGNOSIS

- Missed, threatened, inevitable, or completed abortion
- Gestational trophoblastic neoplasia ("molar pregnancy")
- Appendicitis
- Salpingitis, PID
- Ruptured corpus luteum or hemorrhagic cyst
- Ovarian tumor, benign or malignant
- Ovarian torsion
- Cervical polyp, cancer, trauma, or cervicitis

DIAGNOSTIC TESTS & INTERPRETATION

Initial Tests (lab, imaging)

- Human chorionic gonadotropin (hCG): Serial quantitative serum levels normally increase by at least 53% every 48 hours: Abnormal rise should prompt workup for gestational abnormalities. Clinical impression of acute abdomen/intraperitoneal bleeding concurrent with a positive hCG level is indicative of ectopic pregnancy until proven otherwise (1).
- CBC and ABO type and antibody screen
- Serum progesterone level (>20 mg/mL associated with lower risk of ectopic pregnancy). In women with pain and/or bleeding who have an inconclusive US, serum progesterone level <3.2 ng/mL ruled out a viable pregnancy in 99.2% of women (2).
- Under investigation: evaluation of serum progesterone levels in conjunction with vascular endothelial growth factor, inhibin A, and activin A using an algorithm. This diagnosed patients with ectopic pregnancy with 99% accuracy (3).
- Transvaginal US (TVUS) is the gold standard for diagnosis:
  - Failure to visualize a normal intrauterine gestational sac when serum hCG is above the discriminatory level (>1,500–2,000 IU/L) suggests an abnormal pregnancy (4).
  - Recent studies show an hCG level of 3,500 IU/L to be associated with a 99% probability of detecting a normal intrauterine gestational sac in clinical practice (5).
  - These values are not valid for multiple gestations.
- MRI is also useful, but costly, and rarely used if TVUS is available.

Diagnostic Procedures/Other

- In the setting of an undesired pregnancy, sampling of the uterine cavity with endometrial biopsy or D&C can identify the presence/absence of intrauterine chorionic villi. When an intrauterine pregnancy (IUP) has been evacuated by curettage, hCG levels should drop by 15% the next day (6).
- Historically, culdocentesis was performed to confirm suspected hemoperitoneum prior to surgical management. Currently, TVUS quantification of pelvic fluid is sufficient.

Test Interpretation

Products of conception (POC; especially chorionic villi) outside the uterine cavity

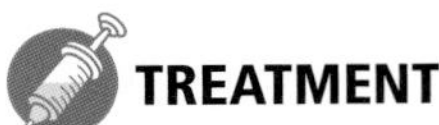

TREATMENT

MEDICATION

- Methotrexate (MTX): treatment for unruptured tubal pregnancy or for remaining POCs after laparoscopic salpingostomy. MTX inhibits DNA synthesis via folic acid antagonism by inactivating dihydrofolate reductase. Most effective when pregnancy is <3 cm diameter, hCG <5,000 mIU/mL, and no fetal heart movement is seen. Success rate is 88% if hCG <1,000, 71% if hCG <2,000:
  - Dosage:
    - Single: IM methotrexate: 50 mg/m^2 of body surface area; may repeat once (preferred method) if <15% decline in hCG by day 7
    - Two-dose: methotrexate 50 mg/m^2 of body surface area once and then repeated on day 4; if <15% decline in hCG on day 7, may repeat dose on days 7 and 11
    - Multidose: methotrexate 1 mg/kg IM/IV every other day, with leucovorin 0.1 mg/kg IM in between. Maximum 4 doses; course may be repeated 7 days after last dose if necessary.
  - Contraindications:
    - Hemodynamic instability or any evidence of rupture
    - Moderate to severe anemia
    - Severe hepatic or renal dysfunction
    - Immunodeficiency
  - Relative contraindications:
    - Fetal heart rate seen
    - Large gestational sac
    - Noncompliance or limited access to hospital or transportation
    - High hCG count >5,000
- Precautions: immunologic, hematologic, renal, GI, hepatic, and pulmonary disease, or interacting medications
- Pretreatment testing: serum hCG, CBC, liver and renal function tests, blood type, and screen
- Patient counseling: During therapy, refrain from use of alcohol, aspirin, NSAIDs, and folate supplements (decreases efficacy of MTX); avoid excessive sun exposure:
  - Adherence to scheduled follow-up appointments is critical.
  - Increased abdominal pain may occur during treatment; however, severe pain, nausea, vomiting, bleeding, dizziness, or light-headedness may indicate treatment failure and require urgent evaluation.

- Rupture of ectopic pregnancy during MTX treatment ranges from 7% to 14%.
- Side effects include stomatitis, conjunctivitis, abdominal cramping, and rarely neutropenia, pneumonitis, or alopecia (7–9).

ISSUES FOR REFERRAL

Refer to a gynecologist for surgical care.

ADDITIONAL THERAPIES

- Physician or patient may elect for surgical treatment as primary method, then post-op hCG should guide need for MTX.
- After evidence of medical failure or tubal rupture, surgery is necessary.
- Surgery may either be salpingostomy (with preservation of tube) or salpingectomy (tubal removal). Abdominal entry is typically laparoscopic.
- Treatment of cervical, ovarian, abdominal, or other ectopic pregnancy is complicated and requires immediate specialist referral.
- Follow all patients treated medically to an hCG of 0 to ensure no need for surgical intervention.
- Offer anti-D Rh prophylaxis at a dose of 50 μg to all Rh-negative women who have a surgical procedure to manage an ectopic pregnancy.
- Expectant management to allow for spontaneous resolution of ectopic pregnancy is acceptable in asymptomatic patients with no evidence of rupture or hemodynamic instability coupled with an appropriately low hCG (<200 mU/mL) and no extrauterine mass suggestive of ectopic. Ruptured tubal pregnancies may occur even with extremely low hCG levels (<100 mU/mL) (10).

SURGERY/OTHER PROCEDURES

- Indications include ruptured ectopic pregnancy, inability to comply with medical follow-up, previous tubal ligation, known tubal disease, current heterotopic pregnancy, desire for permanent sterilization at time of diagnosis.
- Laparoscopy is 1st-line surgical management.
- Salpingostomy preferred in patients who wish to maintain fertility particularly if contralateral tube is damaged/absent:
  - No difference in recurrence rate compared to salpingectomy (11).
  - Persistent trophoblastic tissue with salpingostomy remains in the fallopian tube in 4–15% of cases.
- Salpingectomy indicated for uncontrolled bleeding, recurrent ectopic pregnancy, severely damaged tube, large gestational sac, or patient desire for sterilization.

INPATIENT CONSIDERATIONS

Admission Criteria/Initial Stabilization

- Fails criteria for methotrexate management, suspicion of rupture, orthostatic, shock, and severe abdominal pain requiring IV narcotics
- Inpatient observation in the setting of an uncertain diagnosis, particularly with an unreliable patient, may be appropriate.

Surgical emergency:

- Two IV access lines should be placed immediately if suspicion of rupture; aggressive resuscitation as needed
- Blood product transfusion if necessary en route to OR.
- In cases of shock, pressors and cardiac support may be necessary.

IV Fluids

- Unnecessary for a stable ectopic pregnancy being medically treated
- Critical for a surgical patient who is bleeding

Nursing

Strict input/output, hourly vitals, orthostatics if mobile, frequent abdominal exams, serial hematocrit, pad counts if heavy vaginal bleeding

Discharge Criteria

Afebrile, abdominal pain resolving or resolved, diagnosis established, surgical treatment, and recovery complete

ONGOING CARE

FOLLOW-UP RECOMMENDATIONS

Patient Monitoring

- Serial serum quantitative hCG until level drops to zero
  - After methotrexate administration, a strict monitoring protocol should be followed (8).
  - Following salpingostomy, weekly levels are appropriate.
  - Following salpingectomy, further follow-up may be unnecessary.
- Pelvic US for persistent or recurrent masses
- Pain control: brief course of opioids usually necessary
- Liver and renal function tests following methotrexate administration if repeat dosing is required
- Delay of subsequent pregnancy for at least 3 months after treatment with methotrexate due to teratogenicity (folate deficiency)

DIET

- During treatment, avoid foods and vitamins high in folate (leafy greens, liver, edamame) due to interaction with methotrexate efficacy.
- Maintain excellent hydration.

PATIENT EDUCATION

- Signs and symptoms of ectopic pregnancy should be reviewed.
- Patients should be encouraged to plan subsequent pregnancies and seek early medical care on discovery of future pregnancies.

PROGNOSIS

- Chronic ectopic pregnancies are rare and treated with surgical removal of the fallopian tube.
- Future fertility depends on fertility prior to ectopic pregnancy and degree of tubal compromise.
- ~66% of women with a history of ectopic pregnancy will have a future IUP if they are able to conceive.
- If infertility persists beyond 12 months, the fallopian tubes should be evaluated.

COMPLICATIONS

- Hemorrhage and hypovolemic shock
- Persistent trophoblastic tissue after medical or surgical management
- Infection
- Infertility
- Blood transfusions with associated infections/transfusion reaction
- Disseminated intravascular coagulation in the setting of massive hemorrhage

REFERENCES

1. Barnhart KT, Sammel MD, Rinaudo PF, et al. Symptomatic patients with an early viable intrauterine pregnancy: hCG curves redefined. *Obstet Gynecol*. 2004;104(1):50–55.
2. Verhaegen J, Gallos ID, van Mello NM, et al. Accuracy of single progesterone test to predict early pregnancy outcome in women with pain or bleeding: meta-analysis of cohort studies. *BMJ*. 2012;345:e6077.
3. Rausch ME, Sammel MD, Takacs P, et al. Development of a multiple marker test for ectopic pregnancy. *Obstet Gynecol*. 2011;117(3):573–582.
4. Barnhart K, Mennuti MT, Benjamin I, et al. Prompt diagnosis of ectopic pregnancy in an emergency department setting. *Obstet Gynecol*. 1994;84(6):1010–1015.
5. Connolly A, Ryan DH, Stuebe AM, et al. Reevaluation of discriminatory and threshold levels for serum β-hcg in early pregnancy. *Obstet Gynecol*. 2013;121(1):65–70.
6. Seeber BE, Barnhart KT. Suspected ectopic pregnancy. *Obstet Gynecol*. 2006;107(2, Pt 1):399–413.
7. Bachman EA, Barnhart KT. Medical management of ectopic pregnancy: a comparison of regimens. *Clin Obstet Gynecol*. 2012;55(2):440–447.
8. Practice Committee of the American Society for Reproductive Medicine. Medical treatment of ectopic pregnancy. *Fertil Steril*. 2006;86(5)(Suppl 1):S96–S102.
9. Menon S, Colins J, Barnhart KT. Establishing a human chorionic gonadotropin cutoff to guide methotrexate treatment of ectopic pregnancy: a systematic review. *Fertil Steril*. 2007;87(3):481–484.
10. American College of Obstetricians and Gynecologists. ACOG Practice Bulletin No. 94: medical management of ectopic pregnancy. *Obstet Gynecol*. 2008;111(6):1479–1485.
11. Mol F, van Mello NM, Strandell A, et al. Salpingotomy versus salpingectomy in women with tubal pregnancy (ESEP study): an open-label, multicentre, randomised controlled trial. *Lancet*. 2014;383(9927):1483–1489.

ADDITIONAL READING

Hajenius PJ, Mol F, Mol BW, et al. Interventions for tubal ectopic pregnancy. *Cochrane Database Syst Rev*. 2007;(1):CD000324.

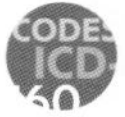

CODES

ICD10

- O00.9 Ectopic pregnancy, unspecified
- O00.1 Tubal pregnancy
- O00.0 Abdominal pregnancy

CLINICAL PEARLS

- 97% of ectopic pregnancies occur in the fallopian tube.
- Diagnosis requires high clinical suspicion in the setting of abdominal pain and a positive pregnancy test.

EJACULATORY DISORDERS

Payam Sazegar, MD

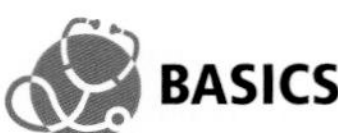

BASICS

DESCRIPTION

- Premature ejaculation (PE): inability to control ejaculatory reflex resulting in ejaculation sooner than desired; most common type of sexual dysfunction affecting all age groups
  - Defined as an ejaculation that always or nearly always occurs prior to or within 1 minute of penetration, an inability to ejaculate on or nearly all penetrations, and with negative personal consequences (1,2).
  - Natural biologic response is to ejaculate within 2–5 minutes after vaginal penetration.
  - Ejaculatory control is an acquired behavior that increases with experience.
- Delayed ejaculation (DE): prolonged time to ejaculate (>30 minutes) despite desire, stimulation, and erection
- Aspermia (lack of sperm in the ejaculate)
  - Anejaculation (AE): lack of emission or contractions of bulbospongiosus muscle
  - Retrograde ejaculation (RE): partial or complete ejaculation of semen into the bladder
  - Obstruction: ejaculatory duct obstruction or urethral obstruction
- Painful ejaculation: genital or perineal pain during or after ejaculation
- Ejaculatory anhedonia: normal ejaculation lacking orgasm or pleasure
- Hematospermia: presence of blood in the ejaculate
- Ejaculatory duct obstruction
- Synonym(s): rapid ejaculation; retarded ejaculation; inhibited orgasm in males; ejaculatory dysfunction

EPIDEMIOLOGY

Prevalence

- PE is common. Reported prevalence in U.S. males ranges from 20 to 30% depending definition.
- DE is reported in 5–8% of men age 18–59 years, but <3% experience the problem for >6 months.
- Predominant age: all sexually mature age groups
- Predominant sex: male only

ETIOLOGY AND PATHOPHYSIOLOGY

Male sexual response are as follows:

- Erection mediated by parasympathetic nervous system
- Normal ejaculation consists of 3 phases:
  - Emission phase: Semen is deposited into urethra by contraction of prostate, seminal vesicles, and vas deferens; under autonomic sympathetic control
  - Ejaculation phase: Semen is forcibly propelled out of urethra by rhythmic contractions of bulbospongiosus and ischiocavernosus muscles. This is mediated by the somatic nervous system on the motor branches of the pudendal nerve. Bladder neck contracture induced by α-adrenergic receptors ensures anterograde ejaculation.
  - Orgasm: the pleasurable sensation associated with ejaculation (cerebral cortex); smooth muscle contraction of accessory sexual organs; release of pressure in posterior urethra
- PE has many theoretical causes:
  - Penile hypersensitivity
  - 5-hydroxytryptamine (5-HT)-receptor sensitivity
  - Sexual inexperience
  - High level of sexual arousal and/or long interval since last ejaculation
  - Fear of sexually transmitted infections (STIs)
  - Anxiety or guilty feelings about sex
  - Lack of privacy
  - Interpersonal maladaptation (e.g., marital problems, unresponsiveness of partner)
- DE
  - Rarely due to underlying painful disorder (e.g., prostatitis, seminal vesiculitis)
  - Psychogenic
  - Sexual performance anxiety and other psychosocial factors
  - Medications may impair ejaculation (e.g., MAOIs, SSRIs, α- and β-blockers, thiazides, antipsychotics, tricyclic and quadricyclic antidepressants, NSAIDs, opiates, alcohol).
- Never any ejaculate
  - Congenital structural disorder (müllerian duct cyst, wolffian abnormality)
  - Acquired (radical prostatectomy, postinfectious, posttraumatic, T10–T12 neuropathy)
- AE
  - Retroperitoneal lymph node (LN) dissection
  - Spinal cord injury or other (traumatic) sympathetic nerve injury
  - Medications (α- and β-blockers, benzodiazepines, SSRIs, MAOIs, TCAs, antipsychotics, aminocaproic acid
  - Diabetes mellitus (DM) (neuropathy)
  - Radical prostatectomy
- RE
  - Transurethral resection of the prostate (25%) or other prostate resection procedures
  - Surgery on the neck of the bladder
  - Extensive pelvic surgery
  - Retroperitoneal LN dissection for testicular cancer (also may produce failure of emission)
  - Neurologic disorders (multiple sclerosis [MS], DM)
  - Medications (α-blockers, in particular tamsulosin, ganglion blockers, antipsychotics)
  - Urethral stricture (may be posttraumatic)
- Painful ejaculation
  - Infection or inflammation (orchitis, epididymitis, prostatitis, urethritis)
  - Ejaculatory duct obstruction
  - Seminal vesicle calculi
  - Obstruction of the vas deferens
  - Psychological/functional
- Ejaculatory anhedonia
  - Medications
  - Psychological
  - Hormonal imbalances
  - Decreased libido
- Hematospermia (often unable to find cause)
  - Inflammation/infection
  - Calculi: bladder, seminal vesicle, prostate, urethra
  - Trauma to genital area (cycling, constipation)
  - Obstruction
  - Cyst
  - Tumor (prostate cancer [1–3% present with hematospermia])
  - Arteriovenous malformations
  - Iatrogenic
  - Hypertension

COMMONLY ASSOCIATED CONDITIONS

- Neurologic disorders (e.g., MS)
- DM
- Prostatitis
- Ejaculatory duct obstruction
- Urethral stricture
- Psychological disorders
- Endocrinopathies
- Relationship/interpersonal difficulties

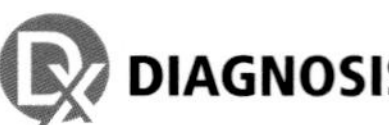

DIAGNOSIS

- Ejaculation occurs before individual wishes (PE).
- Ejaculation does not occur following normal stimulation (including masturbation).

HISTORY

- Detailed sexual history, which includes the following:
  - Time frame of the problem
  - Quality of patient's sexual response
  - Sense of ejaculatory control and sexual distress
  - Overall assessment of the relationship
  - Ask specific questions as patients often reluctant to discuss openly
- Detailed history of recent and current medications
- History of past trauma or recent infections
- Past surgical history with particular attention to genitourinary (GU) surgeries
- Supplements and alternative therapies tried
- Many men do not distinguish initially between problems related to erection and ejaculation.
- Some men have unrealistic expectations of ejaculatory response and frequency.
- Include the sexual partner in the interview, especially if the patient expresses a belief that he is not meeting his partner's needs.
- In review of systems, elicit any evidence of testosterone deficiency or prolactin excess especially if anhedonia present.

PHYSICAL EXAM

- Check vitals. Look for focal neurologic signs (MS, spinal cord injury) and psychiatric disorders.
- Thorough GU exam, which includes the following:
  - Size and texture of testes and epididymis
  - Verification of the presence of the vas deferens
  - Location and patency of urethral meatus
  - Digital rectal examination to evaluate prostate consistency and size and possible midline lesions

DIAGNOSTIC TESTS & INTERPRETATION

- Laboratory test results may be normal.
- Fasting glucose or HgbA1c to rule out diabetes
- Postorgasmic urinalysis will confirm RE. Semen fructose level, sperm count, and viscosity can be measured. Patient may complain of cloudy urine.
- AE will have fructose negative, sperm negative, nonviscous postorgasmic urinalysis.
- In painful ejaculation, urinalysis and urine culture

- If prostate cancer is considered, check prostate-specific antigen (PSA).
- In anhedonia, consider checking testosterone, prolactin, glucose, and thyroid levels.
- In hematospermia, painful ejaculation, or if ejaculatory duct obstruction is considered, transrectal ultrasound (TRUS) may be helpful.
- TRUS-guided seminal vesicle aspiration; if ejaculatory duct obstruction is present, then the aspirate will contain sperm.
- If suspicious of anatomic abnormality, can get scrotal US and/or MRI.

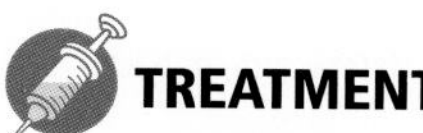

TREATMENT

GENERAL MEASURES

- Identifying any medical cause (even if not reversible) helps patient accept condition.
- Improve partner communication.
- Psychological counseling for patient and partner
- Reduce performance pressure through reassurance.
- Use of a variety of resources may be necessary (e.g., psychiatrist, psychologist, sex therapist, vascular surgeon, urologist, endocrinologist, neurologist).
- PE
  - Use sensate focus therapy (gradual progression of nonsexual contact to sexual contact)
  - Quiet vagina: female partner stops moving just prior to ejaculation
  - Techniques to learn ejaculatory control (e.g., coronal squeeze technique [squeezing the glans penis until ejaculatory urge ceases] or start-and-stop technique [cessation of penile stimulation when ejaculation approaches and resumption of stimulation when ejaculatory feeling ends]) (3)[B]
- DE
  - Change to antidepressant less likely to cause DE (fluvoxamine, nefazodone).
- AE/RE
  - Discontinue offending medication(s).
  - Diabetic control
  - If urethral obstruction is present, refer to urologist.
  - RE may be helped if intercourse occurs when bladder is full.
  - Consider penile vibratory stimulation (effective in spinal cord injuries >T10) or electroejaculation (place on monitor if lesions above T6 because autonomic dysreflexia may result) to collect sperm in AE cases.
- Painful ejaculation
  - Counseling may be beneficial.
  - If seminal vesicle stones are possible, refer to urologist.
- Hematospermia
  - Often resolves spontaneously, without known cause
  - May try empiric antibiotic, but little evidence to support
  - If persistent or high degree of suspicion for abnormality, refer to urologist

MEDICATION

- PE
  - Treating underlying erectile dysfunction (if identified) with PDE5 inhibitors
  - First line
  - Topical anesthetic gel applied (2.5% prilocaine ± 2.5% lidocaine [EMLA]) 2.5 g under a condom for 30 minutes prior to intercourse (4,5)[A]
  - Daily dosing of clomipramine 12.5–50 mg, sertraline 25–200 mg, fluoxetine 5–20 mg, or paroxetine 10–40 mg can delay ejaculation within 1–3 weeks of starting (4)[A].
  - Dapoxetine, a short-acting SSRI, used "on demand" 30–60 mg 1–2 hours prior to sexual activity (2,4)[A]
  - Tramadol 25–50 mg used on demand 2 hours before sex; effective in many studies (6)[A]
  - Some other on-demand options include clomipramine 20–40 mg 4–24 hours before intercourse, sertraline 50 mg 4–8 hours before intercourse, and paroxetine 20 mg 3–4 hours before intercourse (2)[A].
  - Second line: behavioral/sex therapy, pelvic floor muscle therapy (3)[B]
- DE (limited options)
- Patients who must continue SSRIs may respond to bupropion, buspirone (1)[B], or PDE-5 inhibitors (1)[C] before intercourse.
  - Sex therapy, self-stimulation therapies (1)[B]
  - Some evidence that amantadine or cyproheptadine may be helpful (2)[B]
- AE/RE
  - α-Agonists and antihistamines can be helpful but are not approved by the FDA.
  - First line
    - Pseudoephedrine 60 mg PO daily to QID (7)[A]
    - Imipramine 25–75 mg PO BID (7)[A]
  - Second line: For RE, can try postejaculation bladder harvest of sperm (if fertility desired). For AE, can try midodrine, penile vibratory stimulation, or electroejaculation (7)[B].
- Painful ejaculation
  - Treat underlying infection/inflammatory process.
  - α-Blockers may have some benefit.

ISSUES FOR REFERRAL

The following conditions, when suspected, should be referred to a urologist:

- Ejaculatory duct obstruction
- Seminal vesicle or prostatic stones
- Urethral obstruction
- Vas deferens obstruction
- Calculi
- Persistent or severe hematospermia

SURGERY/OTHER PROCEDURES

Surgical treatment of ejaculatory duct obstruction:

- Transurethral resection of the ejaculatory ducts

ONGOING CARE

PATIENT EDUCATION

See "General Measures."

PROGNOSIS

Often improves with therapy and counseling

COMPLICATIONS

Psychological impact on some males: signs of severe inadequacy, self-doubt, additional anxiety, and guilt

REFERENCES

1. Rowland D, McMahon CG, Abdo C, et al. Disorders of orgasm and ejaculation in men. *J Sex Med*. 2010;7(4):1668–1686.
2. McMahon CG, Jannini E, Waldinger M, et al. Standard operating procedures in the disorders of orgasm and ejaculation. *J Sex Med*. 2013;10(1): 204–229.
3. Melnik T, Althof S, Atallah AN, et al. Psychosocial interventions for premature ejaculation. *Cochrane Database Syst Rev*. 2011;(8):CD008195.
4. Porst H. An overview of pharmacotherapy in premature ejaculation. *J Sex Med*. 2011;8(Suppl 4): 335–341.
5. Wyllie MG, Powell JA. The role of local anaesthetics in premature ejaculation. *BJU Int*. 2012;110(11, Pt C): E943–E948.
6. Wong BLK, Malde S. The use of tramadol "on-demand" for premature ejaculation: a systematic review. *Urology*. 2013;81(1):98–103.
7. Barazani Y, Stahl PJ, Nagler HM, et al. Management of ejaculatory disorders in infertile men. *Asian J Androl*. 2012;14(4):525–529.

E

ADDITIONAL READING

- Fode M, Krogh-Jespersen S, Brackett NL, et al. Male sexual dysfunction and infertility associated with neurological disorders. *Asian J Androl*. 2012; 14(1):61–68.
- Giuliano F, Clement P. Pharmacology for the treatment of premature ejaculation. *Pharmacol Rev*. 2012;64(3):621–644.
- Jefferys A, Siassakos D, Wardle P. The management of retrograde ejaculation: a systematic review and update. *Fertil Steril*. 2012;97(2):306–312.
- Siegel AL. Pelvic floor muscle training in males: practical applications. *Urology*. 2014;84(1):1–7.

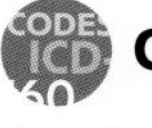

CODES

ICD10

- F52.4 Premature ejaculation
- N53.11 Retarded ejaculation
- N53.14 Retrograde ejaculation

CLINICAL PEARLS

- If erectile dysfunction is contributing to ejaculatory difficulty, management of erectile dysfunction should precede attempted management of ejaculatory disorders.
- Medications should always be thoroughly reviewed, as they may be the primary cause of ejaculatory disorders.
- PE and DE generally have both psychogenic and physical causes, whereas AE and RE are due to organic neurogenic/autonomic dysfunction.
- A multidisciplinary approach, including the primary care physician, urologists, psychologists, and other appropriate health care professionals, is essential to the proper treatment of ejaculatory disorders.

ELDER ABUSE

Nitin Budhwar, MD

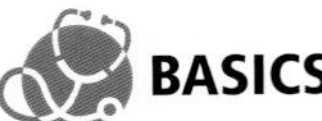

BASICS

DESCRIPTION

- The National Center of Elder Abuse divides abuse in to 3 categories (older than age 60 years) (1)[A]
  - **Domestic:** abuse from someone who has a special relationship with the elderly individual (spouse, child, friend, or in-home caregiver) that occurs in the home of the elderly or caregiver.
  - **Institutional:** occurs in the setting of a facility that is responsible for caring for the elderly, such as a nursing home or long-term care facility.
  - **Self-neglect:** The behavior of the elderly individual leads to harm.
- Types of abuse in estimated order of occurrence
  - Self-neglect (estimated 50%): The most common form of abuse (2)[C].
  - Financial
  - Neglect
  - Emotional
  - Physical
  - Sexual
  - Taken advantage of misinformation and unregulated online pharmaceutical, financial companies, etc., that specifically target the elderly leading to deleterious outcomes (3)[C].

EPIDEMIOLOGY

Incidence

Estimate is that as many as 1:10 have been victims of abuse, placing a conservative number at 50,000 cases per year. Majority of whom are believed to be women (4)[A].

Prevalence

A recent national survey measuring prevalence of abuse in individuals of at least 60 years of age and older found that 11.9% of the surveyed population suffered some form of abuse.

- 5.2% encountered financial mistreatment by family members.
- 5.1% suffered potential neglect.
- 4.6% encountered emotional mistreatment, mostly by humiliation or verbal abuse.
- 1.6% encountered physical mistreatment, mostly through battery.
- 0.6% sexually mistreated, mostly through forced intercourse

ETIOLOGY AND PATHOPHYSIOLOGY

The etiology of elder abuse is a complex biopsychosocial combination of increased dependence on the caregiver by the abuser in a suboptimal environment with poor behavioral coping methods, which is compounded by increased stress.

Genetics

Not contributory

RISK FACTORS

- The victim
  - Advanced age
  - Dementia or other cognitive impairment
  - Female gender
  - Disability in caring for himself or herself
  - Depression
  - Social isolation
  - Stress: health, financial, or situational
- The abuser
  - Mental illness
  - Financial dependency
  - Substance abuse
  - History of violence
  - Other antisocial behavior (5)[C]

GENERAL PREVENTION

- Improve patient social contact and support.
- Identify and correct potential risk factors for elder abuse:
  - Home visit to identify for potential risks of fall hazards and barriers to ambulation that could lead to fractures and functional decline that could leave the individual vulnerable to abuse
  - Evaluate for assist devices that help the patient independently complete his or her activities of daily living (ADLs) and prevent caregiver dependence.
  - Screen for depression using validated tools such as the Geriatric Depression Scale.
  - Early identification and treatment of cognitive impairment
- Identify caregiver stress and burden; refer to community programs that aid with emotional assistance.
- Advance life directives planning, including identifying possible caregivers; choosing a medical power of attorney (MPOA), estate, and will planning; and so forth.

COMMONLY ASSOCIATED CONDITIONS

Most commonly associated conditions with elder abuse are also identified as risk factors, social isolation, increased dependence for ADL/instrumental activities of daily living (IADLs), depression, cognitive impairment, and aggressive behavior (5)[C],(6)[B].

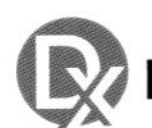

DIAGNOSIS

A high index of suspicion when risk factors are present is important; types of abuse should be kept in mind as some types might not be obvious. It can be difficult to diagnose elder abuse in a single clinic visit, so it is important to get social services involved and to consider doing home visits when abuse is suspected (5)[C].

HISTORY

It is important to take a detailed history with focus on the living arrangements, degree of functionality, who the caregivers are, and other risk factors listed above.

PHYSICAL EXAM

- It is important to objectively document positive and negative findings in your physical exam and to be very detailed because it can be admissible in court if abuse is suspected.
- Vital signs: check weight and assess for progressive loss in weight; BP can be an indicator of dehydration that could be secondary to neglect.
- General overall appearance
  - Wasting or cachexia
  - Poor hygiene, unkempt clothing
  - If the patient is bedbound, it is important to assess the integrity of the mattress and sheets. Look for excessive skin flakes, hair, or urine-soiled mattresses.
- Oral exam
  - Assess for poor dentition, oral ulcers, or abscesses.
- Skin exam
  - Most bruises from elder abuse are large (>5 cm) and located on the face, lateral arm, or back.
  - Bite marks
  - It is important to check for pressure ulcers on the bony prominences of the patient, elbows, sacrum, heels, and scapula.
- Mental/psychiatric
  - Withdrawn, anxious, fearful, blunted
- Genital/rectal exam if sexual abuse is suspected (4)[A].

DIFFERENTIAL DIAGNOSIS

- Advanced dementia can present with individuals appearing withdrawn, and they are often malnourished.
- Elderly with advanced dementia of Alzheimer type or Lewy body dementia can present with delusions of persecution and aggression that can be confused for elder abuse.
- Patients with Parkinson disease often fall and may exhibit fractures and bruises on a frequent basis that may mimic recurrent physical abuse.
- Coagulopathy seen in patients in advanced malignancy with bone marrow suppression or invasion and those on chronic antiplatelet therapy can appear with bruising that can be easily confused with elder abuse.
- Wasting from malignancy, infections, chronic disease
- Thyroid disorder can present with altered mental status (AMS), depression, or anxiety.
- Chronic lung disease can present with decreased weight.
- Delirium from acute electrolyte disturbances, infectious etiology, or cardiovascular compromise can all present similar to elder abuse.
- Impaired financial status can also be confused with self-neglect.

DIAGNOSTIC TESTS & INTERPRETATION

The following workup is recommended.

- Nutritional assessment: iron, vitamin B_{12}, folate, thiamine, albumin, prealbumin, CBC, liver function tests (LFTs), electrolytes
- Malignancy workup, as per current guidelines
- If bruising is noted, check for coagulopathies (e.g., platelets, bleeding times, PT/INR, and PTT.
- If cognitive impairment is observed, check thyroid-stimulating hormone, vitamin B_{12} level; consider syphilis and HIV testing if indicated.
- Assessment of infection: may include urinalysis and culture, chest radiograph, blood count, and cultures

- Radiographic imaging of areas below soft tissue injury is indicated if there is evidence of infection (osteomyelitis) at a pressure ulcer site or bruising of a limb (fracture).
- If physical abuse is suspected and cognitive impairment present, then cranial imaging to look for hemorrhage (e.g., subdural) is indicated using CT scan or MRI.

Diagnostic Procedures/Other

- Pulse test: Check BP and pulse in presence and absence of suspected abuser. Elevation of either in the presence of the suspected abuser should raise suspicion. Useful in patients with dementia or other condition that makes history-taking difficult.
- Folstein Mini-Mental State Examination (MMSE), Montreal Cognitive Assessment (MOCA), or other validated tools to assess for cognitive impairment if suspected
- Geriatric Depression Screen if suspected
- Documentation: Practitioners may make statements of "suspected mistreatment" but should avoid making definitive diagnosis of abuse in their initial assessment, unless it is very obvious.

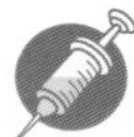

TREATMENT

Most states require all health care providers to report suspected elder abuse to a local agency such as the Adult Protective Services (http://www.nccafv.org/state_elder_abuse_hotlines.htm).

MEDICATION

None

INPATIENT CONSIDERATIONS

Admission Criteria/Initial Stabilization

- Victims of elder abuse should be admitted to the hospital if there are no safe discharge alternatives.
- Management of uncontrolled chronic conditions due to neglect (i.e., wound care from ulcers or infections)
- Cases of suspected abuse *must be reported* to the state's Adult Protective Services agency or a designated alternative (e.g., if patient resides in nursing home, then report to that state's regulatory entity). Social services may help. If physical harm has occurred, consider reporting to local law enforcement for investigation.
- Hospital security may need to be notified if restricted visitor access to a patient is required, and the patient's name may be hidden from the public hospital census.
- If the patient is a victim of elder abuse, he or she must be relocated to a safer alternative and may need admission for sequelae caused by the abuse.

Discharge Criteria

Victims should not be discharged to a potentially abusive environment. Alternatives to discharge to the unsafe environment may include the following:

- Friend or family member
- Nursing home
- Personal care home
- Assisted living facility
- Local victims' rescue or sheltering program if available

ONGOING CARE

FOLLOW-UP RECOMMENDATIONS

Victims of abuse should not be discharged without adequate follow-up including:

- Primary care physician visit within 1 week
- Follow-up with Adult Protective Services or other agency; a home visit should be scheduled prior to discharge if the patient is going back home.
- Home Health Agency for assessment of safety (physical therapy)
- Follow-up with appropriate mental health care

Patient Monitoring

The patient should have frequent visits and be followed through the appropriate agencies to reduce continuation of abuse and to identify recurring abuse.

PATIENT EDUCATION

- For Elder Abuse Resources in your state, you can go to the National Center of Elder Abuse at www.ncea.aoa.gov.
- Or your local representative by calling 1-800-677-1166

PROGNOSIS

Elder abuse and self-neglect are associated with an overall increased risk in mortality (7)[B].

COMPLICATIONS

Complications of elder abuse can lead to worsening depression, increased mortality, and overall poor quality of life.

REFERENCES

1. National Center on Elder Abuse. *Elder Abuse Prevalence and Incidence*. Washington, DC: National Center on Elder Abuse; 2005.
2. Mosqueda L, Dong X. Elder abuse and self-neglect: "I don't care anything about going to the doctor, to be honest. . ." *JAMA*. 2011;306(5):532–540.
3. Liang BA, Lovett KM, Mackey TK. Elder abuse. *J Am Geriatr Soc*. 2012;60(2):398–400.
4. Committee Opinion No. 568: elder abuse and women's health. *Obstet Gynecol*. 2013;122(1):187–191.
5. Halphen JM, Varas GM, Sadowsky JM. Recognizing and reporting elder abuse and neglect. *Geriatrics*. 2009;64(7):13–18.
6. Acierno R, Hernandez MA, Amstadter AB, et al. Prevalence and correlates of emotional, physical, sexual, and financial abuse and potential neglect in the United States: the National Elder Mistreatment Study. *Am J Public Health*. 2010;100(2):292–297.
7. Dong X, Simon M, Mendes de Leon C, et al. Elder self-neglect and abuse and mortality risk in a community-dwelling population. *JAMA*. 2009;302(5):517–526.

ADDITIONAL READING

- Burnett J, Dyer CB, Halphen JM, et al. Four subtypes of self-neglect in older adults: results of a latent class analysis. *J Am Geriatr Soc*. 2014;62(6):1127–1132.
- Cooper C, Katona C, Finne-Soveri H, et al. Indicators of elder abuse: a crossnational comparison of psychiatric morbidity and other determinants in the Ad-HOC study. *Am J Geriatr Psychiatry*. 2006;14(6):489–497.
- Lachs MS, Pillemer K. Elder abuse. *Lancet*. 364(9441):1263–1272.
- Lachs MS, Williams CS, O'Brien S, et al. Adult protective service use and nursing home placement. *Gerontologist*. 2002;42(6):734–739.
- Lachs MS, Williams CS, O'Brien S, et al. The mortality of elder mistreatment. *JAMA*. 1998;280(5):428–432.
- Widera E, Steenpass V, Marson D, et al. Finances in the older patient with cognitive impairment: "He didn't want me to take over." *JAMA*. 2011;305(7):698–706.
- Wiglesworth A, Austin R, Corona M, et al. Bruising as a marker of physical elder abuse. *J Am Geriatr Soc*. 2009;57(7):1191–1196.
- Wiglesworth A, Mosqueda L, Mulnard R, et al. Screening for abuse and neglect of people with dementia. *J Am Geriatr Soc*. 2010;58(3):493–500.

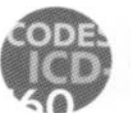

CODES

ICD10

- T74.11XA Adult physical abuse, confirmed, initial encounter
- T74.21XA Adult sexual abuse, confirmed, initial encounter
- T74.01XA Adult neglect or abandonment, confirmed, initial encounter

CLINICAL PEARLS

- Elder abuse, or elder mistreatment, is a condition in which the physical, psychological, or financial well-being of an older adult is infringed upon through intentional acts or lack of action, even if harm is not intended.
- It is important to identify vulnerable individuals through proper evaluation of potential risk factors for abuse (social isolation, depression, cognitive impairment, disability requiring assistance, and financial dependence by the caregiver).
- Correction of risk factors is important to reduce the incidence of elder abuse (strengthen the patients' social support, treat depression, provide the patient with assist devices, screen for cognitive impairment with a trial of medication if possible, and identify caregiver burn out).
- Clearly document your physical exam with only specific objective findings.
- Contact Adult Protective Services or your local resources if elder abuse is suspected; it is unlawful not to report suspected elder abuse.

ENCEPHALITIS, VIRAL

Aditya Chandrasekhar, MD, MPH • Sarah H. Cheeseman, MD

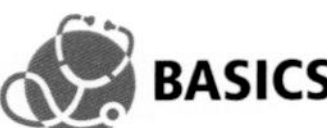

BASICS

DESCRIPTION

- Inflammatory process of the brain associated with clinical evidence of neurologic dysfunction
- System(s) affected: nervous
- Synonym(s): meningoencephalitis

EPIDEMIOLOGY

Incidence

3.5–7.4/100,000 persons/year

Prevalence

- Seasonal variation (e.g., arboviruses, enteroviruses)
- Nonseasonal: most others (e.g., herpes simplex virus [HSV])
- Vaccines have altered prevalence and seasonality (e.g., mumps and measles were common in winter before routine immunization).

ETIOLOGY AND PATHOPHYSIOLOGY

- Most common entry site is through the respiratory or GI tract, followed by hematogenous spread.
- Rarer modes of entry include neurotropic spread (e.g., rabies).
- Specific cell lines may be infected and are associated with specific symptom complexes:
  - Neurons: associated with seizures
  - Oligodendroglia: may cause demyelination alone, cortical infection, or reactive parenchymal swelling; altered levels of consciousness
  - Brainstem neurons: coma, respiratory failure
  - Microglia, macrophages: neurologic dysfunction
- Pathologic changes seen with postinfectious and postvaccinal encephalomyelitis include perivascular mononuclear infiltrates.
- Most commonly identified etiologies in the United States are HSV, West Nile virus (WNV), and enteroviruses.
- Despite extensive evaluations, the etiologic agent is frequently not identified in cases of viral meningitis.

RISK FACTORS

- Age: increased incidence in infants and elderly
- Contact with animals or insect vectors
- Impaired immune status
- Occupation (e.g., lab or animal care workers)
- Recreational activities (e.g., camping, hunting)
- Transfusion and transplantation
- Travel to endemic areas
- Recent vaccinations/unvaccinated status

GENERAL PREVENTION

- Use of mosquito repellants (DEET, Picaridin) and appropriate clothing to prevent arthropod bites
- Avoidance and prompt removal of ticks
- Elimination of mosquito breeding sources
- Vaccination (e.g., mumps, measles, polio, rabies, Japanese encephalitis)

COMMONLY ASSOCIATED CONDITIONS

- Seizures
- Hyperthermia
- Increased intracranial pressure (ICP)
- Inappropriate antidiuretic hormone (ADH) secretion

DIAGNOSIS

- Major and minor diagnostic criteria proposed in 2014 for probable and confirmed encephalitis of presumed infectious or autoimmune etiology
- Epidemiologic risk factor assessment in all patients with encephalitis.
- Consider acute disseminated encephalomyelitis (ADEM) in patients with history of recent infectious illness or vaccination (1)[B].

HISTORY

- The classic encephalitis triad includes the following:
  - Fever
  - Headache
  - Altered mental status
- Focal neurologic deficits correlate with areas affected by individual viruses (e.g., personality changes with frontal lobe involvement or speech deficits with temporal lobe involvement in HSV)
- Assess travel, animal exposure, occupation, and vaccination status
- General medical history to include use of immunosuppressive medications (e.g., steroids), diabetes, HIV, autoimmune disease

PHYSICAL EXAM

- General signs:
  - Fever
  - Rash
  - Parotitis
- Neurologic findings:
  - Altered level of consciousness
  - Acute cognitive dysfunction
  - Behavioral changes
  - Neck stiffness
  - Focal neurologic signs
  - Cranial nerve palsies
  - Paresthesias
- Other:
  - Loss of temperature or vasomotor control

DIFFERENTIAL DIAGNOSIS

- Autoimmune (e.g., anti-NMDA)
- Meningitis
- Intracranial space-occupying lesions
- Nonviral encephalitis (e.g., rickettsia, *Borrelia burgdorferi, Mycoplasma pneumoniae)*
- Noninfectious encephalopathies (e.g., poisoning)
- Infectious encephalopathies (e.g., progressive multifocal leukoencephalopathy)
- Infectious endocarditis with CNS involvement
- Vasculitis
- Paraneoplastic syndromes
- Postinfectious encephalitis
- Postimmunization encephalitis
- ADEM

DIAGNOSTIC TESTS & INTERPRETATION

- Recommended general diagnostic studies (outside CNS) for all patients suspected of having encephalitis:
  - Blood cultures (1)[B]
  - Serum samples: at presentation; store for future studies
  - HIV testing (2)[C]
- Additional studies based on risk factors and clinical findings:
  - Nucleic acid amplification tests (polymerase chain reaction [PCR]) (e.g., HSV PCR)
  - Cultures of stool, nasopharynx, sputum (1)[B]
  - Skin scrapings of active vesicles (direct fluorescent antibody [DFA] testing to identify viral antigen)
  - Tissue biopsies with culture, antigen detection, nucleic acid amplification testing, and histology (1)[A]
  - Serologic testing: IgM and IgG antibodies (test of choice for WNV)
  - Serum cryptococcal antigen testing
  - Acute and convalescent phase serum (helpful for the retrospective diagnosis of a specific pathogen) (1)[B]
  - Serum IgG antibodies in patients where encephalitis may be due to reactivation of a previously acquired infection (e.g., toxoplasmosis in HIV).
  - Serum monospot test (Epstein-Barr virus (EBV) encephalitis)

Initial Tests (lab, imaging)

- Lumbar puncture (unless specific contraindication) (1)[A]
  - CSF pleocytosis (10–2,000 cells/mm^3). Mononuclear cells usually predominate. Finding of CSF eosinophils may suggest helminthes (can also be seen with other pathogens).
  - CSF glucose normal or mildly depressed
  - CSF protein usually mild or moderately increased
  - Direct examination of CSF fluid with Gram stain for bacteria and acid-fast stain for *Mycobacteria*
  - CSF culture for bacteria, mycobacteria, fungi, amoeba, and viruses
  - CSF viral culture not routinely recommended
  - CSF nucleic acid amplification tests (e.g., PCR); herpes simplex PCR should be performed on all specimens, and if negative, consider repeat in 3–7 days for those with compatible clinical syndrome or temporal lobe findings on neuroimaging (1)[A].
  - Enterovirus PCR based on clinical suspicion and season
  - CSF testing for cryptococcal antigen is superior to India ink preparations.
- In up to 10% of cases, CSF findings are normal.
- MRI is imaging modality of choice and should be obtained in all cases, unless contraindicated (or diagnosis is already certain) (2).
- MRI is most sensitive for HSV encephalitis when T2-weighted and fluid attenuated inversion recovery (FLAIR) images show temporal lobe and limbic involvement.
- Diffusion-weighted imaging is superior to conventional MRI in encephalitis caused by HSV, enterovirus, and WNV.
- CT, with and without contrast enhancement, is less sensitive and used if MRI is not an option (1)[B].

Follow-Up Tests & Special Considerations
- PCR may be negative early on; repeat in 3–7 days if symptoms persist and suspicion is high.
- Follow-up imaging is generally not necessary.

Diagnostic Procedures/Other
- CSF culture is not routinely used to diagnose encephalitis.
- Electroencephalogram (EEG) is typically nondiagnostic but may be useful in early herpes simplex encephalitis and, less commonly, in other herpes viruses (varicella-zoster virus [VZV], EBV, human herpesvirus 6 [HHV6]).
- Brain biopsy: *rarely used and not routinely recommended*; consider if unknown etiology and condition is deteriorating despite treatment with acyclovir (1)[B]

Test Interpretation
- Prominent inflammatory reaction in meninges and in a perivascular distribution
- Swelling and degenerative changes

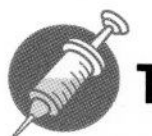

TREATMENT

- Many patients will require intensive care.
- In general, empiric therapy with acyclovir is appropriate in most cases of suspected encephalitis while waiting on formal diagnosis (1)[A].
- Combine with therapy for bacterial, rickettsial, or ehrlichia infection based on clinical suspicion, risk factors, and epidemiology.
- Once an etiologic agent has been identified, change to pathogen-specific therapy.

GENERAL MEASURES
- Supportive therapy
- Monitoring for drug-related toxicities

MEDICATION
- No specific drug therapy is available for most types of viral encephalitis.
- HSV is the most important exception: acyclovir 10 mg/kg IV q8h in adults with normal renal function
- Acyclovir is also effective against VZV encephalitis.
- Foscarnet IV 60–90 mg/kg/dose every 8–12 hours and ganciclovir IV 5 mg/kg/dose every 12 hours are effective against cytomegalovirus (CMV) or acyclovir-resistant HSV.
- Appropriate antiviral therapy (i.e., oseltamivir PO, 75 mg every 12 hours) should be started for suspected influenza infection (3)[C].
- Doxycycline PO/IV 100 mg every 12 hours should be added to an empiric regimen when clinical setting suggests rickettsial or ehrlichia infection (1)[A].
- Use of corticosteroids in viral encephalitis continues to remain controversial and is not currently recommended as standard of practice but is important for antibody-mediated encephalitis, such as anti-NMDA disease (4)[A].

ISSUES FOR REFERRAL
- Monitoring and management of ICP
- Evaluation and treatment of seizures
- Multidisciplinary teams often provide care.

ADDITIONAL THERAPIES
- There is limited data for most adjunctive therapies; in general, should not use without consulting infectious diseases specialists (e.g., interferon-α or IVIG in WNV encephalitis)
- Rabies encephalitis has been treated using induced coma with the Milwaukee protocol.

SURGERY/OTHER PROCEDURES
- No surgical treatment routinely indicated
- Central line placement, intubation, and other procedures as needed for support

INPATIENT CONSIDERATIONS
- Admit suspected cases for evaluation, supportive care, and treatment. Many require intensive care.
- Standard isolation precautions

Admission Criteria/Initial Stabilization
All suspected cases of encephalitis warrant admission:
- Protect airway and provide supplemental oxygen as needed:
  - Intubation and mechanical ventilatory support in severe cases
- Assess and manage circulatory status, fluids, glucose, and electrolytes.

IV Fluids
Assess for syndrome of inappropriate ADH hypersecretion.

Nursing
- Isolation, when indicated (e.g., rabies, influenza)
- Precautions for seizure and altered mental status
- Routine nursing care for skin care, patient comfort, monitoring, and family support
- Educate families about the importance of vaccination.

Discharge Criteria
Patients may be discharged when symptoms have resolved and hospital care is no longer needed.

ONGOING CARE

FOLLOW-UP RECOMMENDATIONS
- Postencephalitis sequelae are primarily neurologic, and follow-up should be guided by patient's condition (e.g., anticonvulsants for seizures).
- Physical therapy may be necessary.

PATIENT EDUCATION
- DEET-containing mosquito repellants and tick removal
- Avoid outdoor activities during periods of peak mosquito activity.
- Use protective clothing.
- Adequate vector control and environmental sanitation
- Vaccination
- Prompt treatment of animal bites or bat exposure

PROGNOSIS
- Often difficult to predict. Anticipate slow, but complete, recovery from deficits in most cases.
- Outcomes worse in elderly and infants
- Some viruses have high mortality (rabies, herpes B virus, untreated HSV, eastern equine encephalitis), than others (West Nile virus, enteroviruses).

COMPLICATIONS
Vary with age, etiologic agent, and clinical course

REFERENCES

1. Tunkel AR, Glaser CA, Bloch KC, et al. The management of encephalitis: clinical practice guidelines by the Infectious Diseases Society of America. *Clin Infect Dis*. 2008;47(3):303–327.
2. Solomon T, Michael BD, Smith PE, et al. Management of suspected viral encephalitis in adults—Association of British Neurologists and British Infection Association National Guidelines. *J Infect*. 2012;64(4):347–373.
3. Centers for Disease Control and Prevention. Neurologic complications associated with novel influenza A (H1N1) virus infection in children—Dallas, Texas, May 2009. *MMWR Morb Mortal Wkly Rep*. 2009;58(28):773–778.
4. Ramos-Estebanez C, Lizarraga KJ, Merenda A. A systematic review on the role of adjunctive corticosteroids in herpes simplex virus encephalitis: is timing critical for safety and efficacy? *Antivir Ther*. 2014;19(2):133–139.

ADDITIONAL READING

Venkatesan A, Tunkel AR, Bloch KC, et al. Case definitions, diagnostic algorithms, and priorities in encephalitis: consensus statement of the international encephalitis consortium. *Clin Infect Dis*. 2013;57(8):1114–1128.

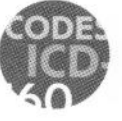

CODES

ICD10
- A86 Unspecified viral encephalitis
- A85.2 Arthropod-borne viral encephalitis, unspecified
- A84.9 Tick-borne viral encephalitis, unspecified

CLINICAL PEARLS

- All patients with suspected encephalitis must have MRI and CSF analysis, unless otherwise contraindicated.
- Reinforce the importance of protective clothing, vector control, and vaccination to prevent viral disease.
- Empiric treatment with acyclovir is warranted in cases of suspected viral encephalitis pending identification of the causative organism. Most patients require hospitalization and supportive care.

ENCOPRESIS

Jay Fong, MD • William T. Garrison, PhD

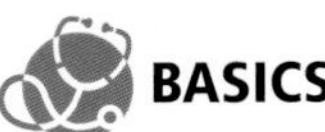

BASICS

DESCRIPTION

- Voluntary or involuntary fecal soilage by a child 4–18 years of age who was (typically) previously toilet-trained
  - Age may be chronologic or developmental.
  - Absence of underlying organic process
  - At least 1 event per month for 3 months
  - Classified into functional constipation (retentive encopresis) and functional nonretentive fecal incontinence (FNRFI); both cause fecal incontinence. There is no constipation in FNRFI. *Functional constipation is more common*.
- System(s) affected: GI; psychological
- Synonyms(s): fecal incontinence, soiling

EPIDEMIOLOGY

Incidence

Predominant sex: male > female (4–6:1). Constipation accounts for 3% of general pediatric referrals; up to 84% of constipated children have fecal incontinence at some point.

Prevalence

Occurs in 1–3% of children 4 years of age

ETIOLOGY AND PATHOPHYSIOLOGY

- In 90% of cases, encopresis develops as a consequence of chronic constipation, with resulting overflow incontinence, which typically is termed *retentive encopresis*. The other 10% are caused by specific organic etiologies.
- Chronic constipation due to irregular and incomplete evacuation results in progressive rectal distension and stretching of both the internal and external anal sphincters.
- As a child habituates to chronic rectal distension, they may no longer sense the normal urge to defecate. Eventually, soft or liquid stool leaks around the retained fecal mass.
- Many children voluntarily withhold stool in response to the urge to defecate for fear of pain or due to a preoccupation with not interrupting social activities.
- Psychological
  - Stool withholding, fear, anxiety
  - Difficulty with toilet training, including unusual anxiety or conflict with parent
  - Resistance to using public toilet facilities, such as school bathrooms or outdoor toilets
  - Known association with sexual abuse in boys; likely similar association in girls
  - Developmental delay
- Anatomic
  - Rectal distension and desensitization
  - Anal fissure or painful defecation
  - Muscle hypotonia
  - Slow intestinal motility
  - Hirschsprung disease
  - Cystic fibrosis
  - Spinal cord defects (e.g., spina bifida)
  - Congenital anorectal malformations
  - Anal stenosis
  - Anterior displacement of the anus
  - Postoperative stricture of anus or rectum
  - Pelvic mass
  - Neurofibromatosis
- Dietary or metabolic
  - Inadequate dietary fiber
  - Excessive protein or milk intake
  - Inadequate water intake
  - Hypothyroidism
  - Hypercalcemia
  - Hypokalemia
  - Diabetes insipidus; diabetes mellitus
  - Food allergy
  - Gluten enteropathy
- Medication side effects

Genetics

None known; although incidence may be higher in children with family history of constipation.

RISK FACTORS

- Male gender
- Constipation
- Very low birth weight
- Painful defecation
- Difficulty with bowel training, including social pressure related to early daycare placement
- Organic/anatomic causes
- Anxiety and depression
- Insufficient fluid or fiber intake
- Refusal to use public restrooms
- Attention deficit

GENERAL PREVENTION

Family education: Avoid toilet training prior to readiness, optimize fluid and fiber intake.

COMMONLY ASSOCIATED CONDITIONS

- Constipation, Hirschsprung disease
- Cerebral palsy, cystic fibrosis
- Developmental and behavioral diagnoses, urinary incontinence

DIAGNOSIS

HISTORY

- Look for signs/symptoms of constipation:
  - Hard, large-caliber stools
  - <3 defecations/week
  - Pain or discomfort with stool passage, withholding of stool
  - Blood on stool or in diaper/toilet bowl
  - Decreased appetite
  - Abdominal pain that improves with stool passage
  - Hiding while defecating before child is toilet-trained; avoiding use of the toilet
  - Diet low in fiber or fluids, high in dairy
  - No stool passed within first 48 hours of life.
  - Pasty stool found on underclothes
  - Recurrent UTIs
- Abrupt onset after age 5 years more likely to be associated with psychological trauma.
- Overlap with attention deficit disorder (ADD) common in children >5 years
- Medications, such as opiates, phenobarbital, and tricyclic antidepressants (TCAs)
- Family history of constipation

PHYSICAL EXAM

- Neurologic exam of lower extremities and perineal area, with attention to S1–S4 distribution, perineal sensation, cremasteric reflex, and anal sphincter tone
- Genital examination and digital rectal exam: Assess for anal fissures, sphincter tone, rectal distension/impaction, presence of occult or visible blood.
- Abdominal exam: Assess bowel sounds, percussion note (tympany), presence of abdominal distension; palpate for stool (most common in left lower quadrant).

DIAGNOSTIC TESTS & INTERPRETATION

Most cases of encopresis can be diagnosed by history and physical examination and do not require extensive lab work.

Initial Tests (lab, imaging)

- Done to rule out organic causes when conventional treatment fails
- UA/urine culture: UTI/glucosuria
- Thyroid function tests: hypothyroidism
- Electrolyte panel, including calcium, may show hypokalemia, hypercalcemia, or hyperglycemia.
- Abdominal plain films if impaction is suspected and not detected by abdominal or rectal exam.

Follow-Up Tests & Special Considerations

Failure to pass meconium within 48 hours of birth, failure to thrive, bloody diarrhea, or bilious vomiting in a neonate should be promptly evaluated to exclude aganglionic megacolon. Constipation and diarrhea, rash, failure to thrive, or recurrent pneumonia should prompt evaluation for cystic fibrosis. Patients with abdominal distension or ileus should be evaluated for possible obstruction.

Diagnostic Procedures/Other

Manometric studies may be useful in patients who have constipation that does not respond to treatment.

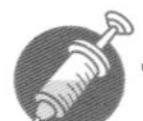

TREATMENT

GENERAL MEASURES

- Anticipatory guidance relative to toilet training beginning at 18 months, with special attention to when children should reduce reliance on diapers or pull-ups during the daytime hours.
- Eliminate impaction prior to initiating maintenance therapy.
- Avoid frequent and repeated rectal exams, enemas, and suppositories, especially in infants.
- Once stools are regular in frequency, child should sit on toilet BID at the same time each day for 10–15 minutes and for 10–15 minutes after meals. Incorporate positive reinforcement for successful bowel movements.

MEDICATION

- Remove impaction and start maintenance treatment.
- No randomized, controlled studies have compared methods of disimpaction: can use oral agents, enemas, and rectal suppositories; oral agents are least traumatic. Glycerin suppositories best option for infants

First Line

- Disimpaction with polyethylene glycol (PEG)
  - Give 17 g (240 mL) water or juice: 1–1.5 g/kg/day × 3 days for disimpaction.
  - 0.4–0.8 g/kg/day for maintenance
- Disimpaction with mineral oil for child >1 year also effective; give 15–30 mL/year of age to max 240 mL.
  - Maintenance: 1–3 mL/kg/day or divided BID
  - May mix with orange juice to make palatable; *avoid in infants to avoid aspiration and lipoid pneumonia*.
- Other maintenance regimens include the following:
  - Milk of magnesia (MOM) 400 mg (5 mL): 1–2 mL/kg/day BID
  - Lactulose 10 g (15 mL): 1–3 mL/kg/day divided BID
  - Senna syrup 8.8 g sennoside (5 mL): age 2–6 years: 2.5–7.5 mL/day divided BID; age 6–12 years: 5–15 mL/day divided BID
  - Bisacodyl suppository 10 mg: 0.5–1 suppository once or twice per day

ISSUES FOR REFERRAL

If symptoms do not improve after 6 months of good compliance with a multifactorial treatment model, refer to pediatric gastroenterologist for recommendations and further evaluation.

ADDITIONAL THERAPIES

Behavioral treatment and counseling

COMPLEMENTARY & ALTERNATIVE MEDICINE

- Children with volitional stool holding who receive behavioral treatment in addition to medications are more likely to have resolution of encopresis at 3 and 6 months than children receiving medication alone (1)[A].
- No evidence that biofeedback training adds benefit to conventional treatment for functional fecal incontinence in children (2)[A]
- Behavioral interventions plus laxative therapy (rather than laxative therapy alone) improves continence in children with functional fecal incontinence associated with constipation (1)[B].

SURGERY/OTHER PROCEDURES

If ongoing constipation is refractory to a combination of medical and behavioral therapy, consider anorectal manometry to evaluate for internal anal sphincter achalasia (or ultrashort-segment Hirschsprung disease). If present, this condition can be treated successfully in most patients with an internal sphincter myectomy.

INPATIENT CONSIDERATIONS

Admission Criteria/Initial Stabilization

- Continued soiling and recurrent impaction on outpatient medical therapy, whether from lack of medication efficacy or patient medication nonadherence
- Decreased intake leading to malnutrition or dehydration
- Recalcitrant vomiting or concern for obstruction
- Hospital admission and abdominal films may be necessary to ensure complete removal of impaction. This may include direct gastric administration of balanced electrolyte–polyethylene glycol solutions if the patient cannot tolerate by mouth. Serial abdominal films and observation of the rectal effluent can help to determine treatment adequacy.

IV Fluids

IV fluids if the patient is dehydrated and having difficulty tolerating oral hydration

Nursing

Nursing to document stool output and character

Discharge Criteria

- Stools that are looser in consistency and clearer in appearance are a successful inpatient end point.
- Abdominal radiographs showing less fecal loading (compared with a pretreatment radiograph) with improving serial abdominal exams

ONGOING CARE

FOLLOW-UP RECOMMENDATIONS

Patient Monitoring

- Continue maintenance treatment from 6 months to 2 years.
- Visits every 4–10 weeks for support and to ensure compliance; more often with oppositional or anxious children
- Provider availability (telephone or virtual visits) to adjust doses and to provide continued encouragement to caregivers
- Treat recurrences of impaction promptly.
- Emphasize compliance with medication and self-initiation of regular bathroom visits.
- Children who do not progress using a well-designed behavior plan should be referred for more in-depth mental health evaluation and counseling.

DIET

Adequate fluid and fiber intake (2)[A]; trial of decrease or avoid cow's milk products. Avoid excessive consumption of bananas, rice, apples, and gelatin.

PATIENT EDUCATION

- Demystify the defecation process.
- Carefully explain the treatment plan including medications and dietary changes.
- Avoid punishment for inadvertent soiling.
- In children >4 years of age, explain to parents how overreliance on diapers and pull-ups, while convenient, can prolong the problem.
- Always attempt to use positive reinforcement for successful toilet sits and medication compliance.
- If positive approach is unsuccessful, consider removing daily desired privileges (e.g., TV, video games, time with friends) for noncompliance with behavioral plan. Some children respond better to use of a token economy (chips or tickets to earn privileges) to promote desired behavior.

PROGNOSIS

- Many children exhibit a good response and have a high relapse rate due to noncompliance by parents and/or child.
- From 30 to 50% of children may still have encopresis after 5 years of treatment.
- Children with psychosocial or emotional problems that preceded the encopresis are more recalcitrant to treatment.

COMPLICATIONS

- Colitis due to excessive enema/suppository
- Perianal dermatitis
- Anal fissure

REFERENCES

1. Brazzelli M, Griffiths PV, Cody JD, et al. Behavioural and cognitive interventions with or without other treatments for the management of faecal incontinence in children. *Cochrane Database Syst Rev*. 2011;7(12):CD002240.
2. Tabbers MM, Dilorenzo C, Berger MY, et al. Evaluation and treatment of functional constipation in infants and children: evidence-based recommendations from ESPGHAN and NASPGHAN. *J Pediatr Gastroenterol Nutr*. 2014;58(2):258–274.

ADDITIONAL READING

- Borowitz SM, Cox DJ, Tam A, et al. Precipitants of constipation during early childhood. *J Am Board Fam Pract*. 2003;16(3):213–218.
- Constipation Guideline Committee of the North American Society for Pediatric Gastroenterology, Hepatology and Nutrition. Evaluation and treatment of constipation in infants and children: recommendations of the North American Society for Pediatric Gastroenterology, Hepatology and Nutrition. *J Pediatr Gastroenterol Nutr*. 2006;43(3):e1–e13.
- Levitt M, Peña A. Update on pediatric faecal incontinence. *Eur J Pediatr Surg*. 2009;19(1):1–9.
- Loening-Baucke V, Pashankar DS. A randomized, prospective, comparison study of polyethylene glycol 3350 without electrolytes and milk of magnesia for children with constipation and fecal incontinence. *Pediatrics*. 2006;118(2):528–535.

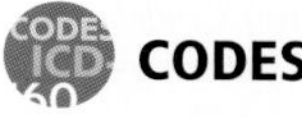

CODES

ICD10

- R15.9 Full incontinence of feces
- R15.1 Fecal smearing
- F98.1 Encopresis not due to a substance or known physiol condition

CLINICAL PEARLS

- 90% of encopresis results from chronic constipation.
- Address toddler constipation early by decreasing excessive milk intake, increasing fruits/vegetables intake, and ensuring adequate fluid and fiber intake.
- Disimpact before initiating maintenance therapy.

ENDOCARDITIS, INFECTIVE

Mariya Milko, DO • Theodore B. Flaum, DO, FACOFP

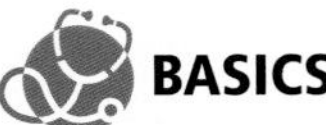

BASICS

DESCRIPTION

- An infection of the valvular (primarily) and mural (rarely) endocardium
- System(s) affected: cardiovascular, endocrine/metabolic, hematologic/lymphatic, immunologic, pulmonary, renal/urologic, skin/exocrine, neurologic
- Synonym(s): bacterial endocarditis; subacute bacterial endocarditis (SBE); acute bacterial endocarditis (ABE)

EPIDEMIOLOGY

Incidence

- In industrialized countries: 3–9/100,000
- 1.5–3.0% incidence 1 year after prosthetic valve replacement; at 5 years, the incidence is 3–6%
- Increasing incidence of cardiovascular device-related infections, due to higher frequency of implantable devices, especially in the elderly

ETIOLOGY AND PATHOPHYSIOLOGY

- ABE: *Staphylococcus aureus*; *Streptococcus* groups A, B, C, G; *Streptococcus pneumoniae*; *Staphylococcus lugdunensis*; *Enterococcus* spp. (gram-positive); *Haemophilus influenzae* or *parainfluenzae*; *Neisseria gonorrhoeae* (gram-negative)
- SBE: α-Hemolytic streptococci (viridans group strep), *Streptococcus bovis*, *Enterococcus* spp., *Staphylococcus aureus*, *Staphylococcus epidermidis* (gram-positive); HACEK organisms: *Haemophilus aphrophilus* or *paraphrophilus*, *Actinobacillus (aggregatibacter) actinomycetemcomitans*, *Cardiobacterium hominis*, *Eikenella corrodens*, *Kingella kingae*
- Endocarditis in IV drug abusers (tricuspid valve): *Staphylococcus aureus*, *Enterococcus* spp. (gram-positive); *Pseudomonas aeruginosa*, *Burkholderia cepacia*, other bacilli (gram-negative); *Candida* spp.
- Early prosthetic-valve endocarditis (<60 days after valve implantation): *Staphylococcus aureus*, *Staphylococcus epidermidis* (gram-positive); gram-negative bacilli; fungi: *Candida* spp., *Aspergillus* spp.
- Late prosthetic valve endocarditis (>60 days after valve implantation): α-Hemolytic streptococci, *Enterococcus* spp., *S. epidermidis* (gram-positive); *Candida* spp., *Aspergillus* spp.
- Culture-negative endocarditis: 10% of cases; *Bartonella quintana* (homeless); *Brucella* spp., fungi, *Coxiella burnetii* (Q fever), *Chlamydia trachomatis*, *Chlamydophila psittaci*, HACEK organisms; abiotrophia (formerly B_6-deficient streptococci); use of antibiotics prior to blood cultures
- Device-related endocarditis: coagulase-negative staphylococci or *S. aureus*

RISK FACTORS

- Injection drug use, IV catheterization, certain malignancies (colon cancer)
- High-risk conditions
  - Prosthetic cardiac valve, implantable devices (pacemaker, automatic implantable cardioverter defibrillator [AICD]), total parenteral nutrition
  - Previous infective endocarditis (IE)
  - Congenital heart disease (CHD): unrepaired cyanotic CHD, including palliative shunts and conduits; repaired CHD with prosthetic device during the first 6 months; repaired CHD with residual defects at or near prosthetic site; cardiac transplant with valvulopathy (1)[B]

GENERAL PREVENTION

- Maintain good oral hygiene.
- Antibiotic prophylaxis is only recommended for high-risk cardiac conditions (1)[B]—prosthetic heart valve, history of endocarditis, transplant with abnormal valvular function, CHD (see "Risk Factors").
- *Procedures requiring prophylaxis*
  - Oral/upper respiratory tract: any manipulation of gingival tissue or periapical region of teeth or perforation of the oral mucosa (1)[B], invasive respiratory procedures involving incision, or biopsy of the respiratory mucosa, use amoxicillin 2 g PO (if penicillin allergic, clindamycin 600 mg PO) 30–60 minutes before procedure or ampicillin 2 g IV/IM. For penicillin-allergic patients use clindamycin 600 mg IV, *or* cephalexin 2 g PO, *or* azithromycin/clarithromycin 500 mg PO, *or* cefazolin/ceftriaxone 1 g IV/IM 30 minutes before procedure. For pediatric doses, use amoxicillin 50 mg/kg PO (max 2 g), cephalexin 50 mg/kg PO (max 2 g), clindamycin 20 mg/kg PO (max 600 mg), and ampicillin or ceftriaxone 50 mg/kg (maximum 1 g) IM/IV.
  - GI/GU: Only consider coverage for enterococcus (with penicillin, ampicillin, piperacillin, or vancomycin) for patients with an established infection undergoing procedures (1)[B].
  - Cardiac valvular surgery or placement of prosthetic intracardiac/intravascular materials: perioperative cefazolin 1–2 g IV 30 minutes preop, or vancomycin 15 mg/kg (maximum 1 g) 60 minutes preop in the penicillin-allergic patient (1)[B]
  - Skin: incision and drainage of infected tissue; use agents active against skin pathogens (e.g., cefazolin 1–2 g IV q8h or vancomycin 15 mg/kg q12h; max 1 g) if penicillin-allergic or if methicillin-resistant *Staphylococcus aureus* (MRSA) suspected.

DIAGNOSIS

- Modified Duke Criteria for Diagnosis of IE (2)[B] (definite: 2 major criteria, or 1 major and 3 minor criteria, or 5 minor criteria; possible: 1 major and 1 minor criteria, or 3 minor criteria)
- Major clinical criteria
  - Positive blood culture: isolation of typical microorganism for IE from 2 separate blood cultures *or* persistently positive blood culture
  - Single positive blood culture for *C. burnetii* or anti–phase-1 IgG antibody titer >1:800
  - Positive echocardiogram: presence of vegetation, abscess, or new partial dehiscence of prosthetic valve; must be performed rapidly if IE is suspected
  - New valvular regurgitation (change in preexisting murmur not sufficient)
- Minor criteria
  - Predisposing heart condition or IV drug use
  - Fever ≥38.0°C (100.4°F)
  - Vascular phenomena: major arterial emboli, septic pulmonary infarcts, mycotic aneurysm, intracranial hemorrhage, conjunctival hemorrhage, Janeway lesions
  - Immunologic phenomena: glomerulonephritis, Osler nodes, Roth spots, rheumatoid factor (RF)
  - Microbiologic evidence: positive blood culture, but not a major criterion (excluding single positive cultures for coagulase-negative staphylococci and organisms that do not cause endocarditis) or serologic evidence of infection likely to cause IE

HISTORY

- Fever (>38°C), chills, cough, dyspnea, orthopnea; especially in subacute endocarditis: night sweats, weight loss, fatigue
- Predisposition to IE (see "Risk Factors")
- Symptoms of transient ischemic attack, cerebrovascular accident (CVA), or myocardial infarction (MI) on presentation

PHYSICAL EXAM

- Most patients with IE have new murmur or change in existing murmur; signs of heart failure (rales, edema) if valve function compromised
- Peripheral stigmata of IE: splinter hemorrhages in fingernail beds, Osler nodes on fleshy portions of extremities, "Roth spot" retinal hemorrhages, Janeway lesions (cutaneous evidence of septic emboli), palatal or conjunctival petechiae, splenomegaly, hematuria (due to emboli or glomerulonephritis)
- Neurologic findings consistent with CVA, such as visual loss, motors weakness, and aphasia

DIFFERENTIAL DIAGNOSIS

Fever of unknown origin, infected central venous catheter, marantic endocarditis, connective tissue diseases, intra-abdominal infections, rheumatic fever, salmonellosis, brucellosis, malignancy, tuberculosis, atrial myxoma, septic thrombophlebitis

DIAGNOSTIC TESTS & INTERPRETATION

- 3 sets of blood cultures drawn >2 hours apart *before administration of antibiotics*
- Leukocytosis common in acute endocarditis
- Anemia, decreased C3, C4, CH50, and RF in subacute endocarditis
- ESR, C-reactive protein (CRP)
- Hematuria, microscopic or macroscopic
- Consider serologies for *Chlamydia*, Q fever, and *Bartonella* in "culture-negative" endocarditis.
- Transthoracic or transesophageal echocardiogram (TTE/TEE) should be performed as soon as IE is suspected.
- CT scan may help locate embolic abscesses (e.g., splenic abscess).
- Vegetations are composed of platelets, fibrin, and colonies of microorganisms. Destruction of valvular endocardium, perforation of valve leaflets, rupture of chordae tendineae, abscesses of myocardium, rupture of sinus of Valsalva, and pericarditis may occur.
- Emboli, abscesses, and/or infarction may be found in any organ.
- Immune-complex glomerulonephritis

TREATMENT

MEDICATION

First Line

- Initial empirical treatment: should be started after 3 sets of blood cultures have been drawn while waiting for a causative organism to be identified
  - Native valves: Ampicillin-sulbactam 12 g/day IV divided into 4 doses with gentamicin 3 mg/kg/day IV/IM in 2 or 3 doses. If penicillin allergic, use vancomycin 30 mg/kg/day IV in 2 doses with

gentamicin 3 mg/kg/day IV/IM in 2 or 3 doses and ciprofloxacin 1,000 mg/day PO or 800 mg/day IV, both in 2 doses (3)[A].
  - Prosthetic valves: Vancomycin 30 mg/kg/day IV in 2 doses with gentamicin 3 mg/kg/day IV/IM in 2 or 3 doses and rifampin 1,200 mg/day PO in 2 doses, if <12 months postsurgery. If >12 months, use native valve regimen (3)[A].
- Penicillin-susceptible viridans group streptococci or *S. bovis*
  - Native valve: penicillin G 12–18 million U/day IV continuously or in 4–6 doses *or* ceftriaxone 2 g/day IV/IM in 1 dose, both for 4 weeks (2)[B]
  - Prosthetic valve: penicillin G 24 million U/day IV continuously or 4–6 doses for 6 weeks *or* ceftriaxone 2 g/day IV/IM in 1 dose ± gentamicin 3 mg/kg IV/IM q24h for 2 weeks (peak gentamicin level 3 μg/mL and trough <1 μg/mL) (2)[B]
- Penicillin-resistant viridans group streptococci or *S. bovis*
  - Native valve: penicillin G 24 million U/day IV, either continuously or in 6 equally divided doses *or* ceftriaxone 2 g/day IV/IM in 1 dose for 4 weeks + gentamicin 3 mg/kg IV/IM q24h for 2 weeks (peak gentamicin level 3 μg/mL and trough <1 μg/mL) (2)[B]
  - Prosthetic valve: Regimen is equivalent, but length of therapy is 6 weeks for all antibiotics.
- *Staphylococcus*
  - Native valve: oxacillin or nafcillin 2 g IV q4h for 4–6 weeks. Use of gentamicin 3 mg/kg q8h IV/IM for the first 3–5 days does not improve survival and increases the chance of nephrotoxicity. For oxacillin-resistant strains, use vancomycin 15 mg/kg/day IV q12h for 6 weeks for goal trough of 15–20 μg/mL (2)[B].
  - Prosthetic valve: oxacillin or nafcillin 12 g/day IV in 6 doses + rifampin 300 mg IV/PO q8h, for 6 weeks, + gentamicin 3 mg/kg q8h IV/IM for first 2 weeks (peak gentamicin level 3 μg/mL and trough <1 μg/mL). For oxacillin-resistant strains, use vancomycin 15 mg/kg IV q12h, + rifampin 300 mg IV/PO q8h, both for 6 weeks, + gentamicin 3 mg/kg/day IV/IM in 2–3 doses for the first 2 weeks (peak gentamicin level 3 μg/mL and trough <1 μg/mL) (2)[B].
- Penicillin-sensitive *Enterococcus*, native or prosthetic valve: ampicillin 12 g IV divided q4h *or* penicillin G 18–30 million U/day IV continuously or in 6 doses plus gentamicin 3 mg/kg IV q8h for 4–6 weeks (peak gentamicin level 3 μg/mL and trough <1 μg/mL) (2)[B]. Consider expert consultation for penicillin-resistant enterococci.
- *HACEK* organisms: Ceftriaxone 2 g IM or IV q24h for 4 weeks (2)[B] *or* ampicillin-sulbactam 12 g IV divided q4h for 4 weeks *or* ciprofloxacin 1 g/day PO or 800 mg/day IV in 2 equally divided doses for 4 weeks
  - Cardiac device-related endocarditis: Whole device removal is recommended for all patients with lead infection, followed by antibiotic therapy based on organism susceptibility (4)[B].
- Precautions: In patients with renal impairment, dosage adjustment should be made for penicillin G, gentamicin, cefazolin, ampicillin, ampicillin/sulbactam, ciprofloxacin, and vancomycin. Rapid infusion of vancomycin <1 hour may cause "red-man syndrome" due to histamine release, not an allergic reaction. Treat with antihistamines and decrease infusion rate.
- Interactions: Vancomycin + gentamicin increases renal toxicity. Rifampin increases the requirement for Coumadin and oral hypoglycemic agents.

Second Line

For patients allergic to penicillin:

  - Penicillin-susceptible or resistant viridans group streptococci or *S. bovis*: vancomycin 30 mg/kg (not to exceed 2 g/day) IV for 4 weeks (6 weeks for prosthetic valve endocarditis) for goal trough of 15–20 μg/mL (2)[B]
  - *Enterococcus*, native or prosthetic valve: Desensitization to penicillin should be considered. Vancomycin 15 mg/kg (usual dose, 1 g) IV q12h, + gentamicin or streptomycin (peak gentamicin level 3 μg/mL and trough <1 μg/mL) for 4–6 weeks (6 weeks for prosthetic valve endocarditis) (2)[B]
  - *Staphylococcus* of native valve: cefazolin 2 g IV q8h (not to be used in patients with immediate-type hypersensitivity to penicillin) for 4–6 weeks *or* vancomycin 30 mg/kg (usual dose, 1 g) IV q12h for a goal trough of 15–20 μg/mL, for 6 weeks (2)[B]

SURGERY/OTHER PROCEDURES

Surgical therapy is required in 50% of IE cases. Indications for surgery include the following (3)[A]:

- Heart failure due to involvement of aortic or mitral valve
  - Prevention of embolism: aortic or mitral valve vegetations >10 mm with prior embolic episodes; isolated very large vegetation >15 mm; in patients with major ischemic stroke, surgery is delayed for at least 4 weeks, if possible (5)[C].
- Uncontrolled infection: persistent fever and positive cultures >7–10 days; infection caused by fungi or resistant organism; presence of abscess, fistula, false aneurysm, or enlarging vegetations
- Early prosthetic valve IE

ONGOING CARE

FOLLOW-UP RECOMMENDATIONS

Patient Monitoring

- Check gentamicin peak (~3 μg/mL) and trough (<1 μg/mL) levels if used for >5 days and with renal dysfunction. Perform twice-weekly BUN and serum creatinine while on gentamicin. Consider audiometry baseline and follow-up during long-term aminoglycoside therapy.
- Check vancomycin trough (15–20 μg/mL) levels in all patients (usually prior to 4th dose) (3)[B].
- Baseline ECG, and monitor ECG for conduction disturbances/MI in initial weeks of therapy
- TTE at the conclusion of therapy
- Blood cultures q48h until negative

PROGNOSIS

Late complications contribute to the poor prognosis of IE. The main complications are heart failure, reinfection, and cerebral emboli. 10-year survival is 60–90% (6)[A].

COMPLICATIONS

- Cerebral complications are the most frequent and severe, occurring in 15–20% of patients (1)[A].
- Emboli: arterial (e.g., MI, mesenteric, splenic, cerebral infarction), infectious (e.g., abscesses of heart, lung, brain, meninges, bone, pericardium)
  - Neurologic events are the most frequent complications in patients with IE requiring ICU admission. Ischemic stroke is the presenting symptom of IE in 20% of cases (6)[A].
- Inflammatory/immune disorders (e.g., arthritis, myositis, glomerulonephritis)
- Other complications: congestive heart failure (CHF), ruptured valve cusp, sinus of valsalva aneurysm, arrhythmia, and mycotic aneurysms

REFERENCES

1. Wilson W. Prevention of infective endocarditis: guidelines from the American Heart Association: a Guideline from the American Heart Association Rheumatic Fever, Endocarditis, and Kawasaki Disease Committee, Council on Cardiovascular Disease in the Young, and the Council on Clinical Cardiology, Council on Cardiovascular Surgery and Anesthesia, and the Quality of Care and Outcomes Research Interdisciplinary Working Group. *Circulation*. 2007;116(15):1736–1754.
2. Baddour LM, Wilson WR, Bayer AS, et al. Infective endocarditis: diagnosis, antimicrobial therapy, and management of complications: a statement for healthcare professionals from the Committee on Rheumatic Fever, Endocarditis, and Kawasaki Disease, Council on Cardiovascular Disease in the Young, and the Councils on Clinical Cardiology, Stroke, and Cardiovascular Surgery and Anesthesia, American Heart Association: endorsed by the Infectious Diseases Society of America. *Circulation*. 2005;111(23):e394–e434.
3. Habib G, Hoen B, Tornos P, et al. Guidelines on the prevention, diagnosis, and treatment of infective endocarditis (new version 2009): the Task Force on the Prevention, Diagnosis, and Treatment of Infective Endocarditis of the European Society of Cardiology (ESC). Endorsed by the European Society of Clinical Microbiology and Infectious Diseases (ESCMID) and the International Society of Chemotherapy (ISC) for infection and cancer. *Eur Heart J*. 2009;30(19):2369–2413.
4. Baddour LM, Epstein AE, Erickson CC, et al. Update on cardiovascular implantable electronic device infections and their management: a scientific statement from the American Heart Association. *Circulation*. 2010;121(3):458–477.
5. Byrne JG, Rezai K, Sanchez JA, et al. Surgical management of endocarditis: the society of thoracic surgeons clinical practice guideline. *Ann Thorac Surg*. 2011;91(6):2012–2019.
6. Sonneville R, Mirabel M, Hajage D, et al. Neurologic complications and outcomes of infective endocarditis in critically ill patients: the ENDOcardite en REAnimation prospective multicenter study. *Crit Care Med*. 2011;39(6):1474–1481.

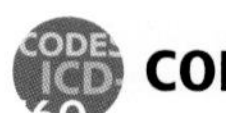

CODES

ICD10

- I33.0 Acute and subacute infective endocarditis
- I39 Endocarditis and heart valve disord in dis classd elswhr
- A54.83 Gonococcal heart infection

CLINICAL PEARLS

- Antibiotic prophylaxis is recommended for patients with artificial heart valves, history of IE, CHDs, and cardiac transplants with valvulopathy.
- TEE/TTE and blood cultures are the mainstays in diagnosis of IE.
- Most common organisms involved in IE include viridians *Streptococcus* spp. and *Staphylococcus*.

ENDOMETRIAL CANCER AND UTERINE SARCOMA

Radhika Sharma, MD • Michael P. Hopkins, MD, MEd

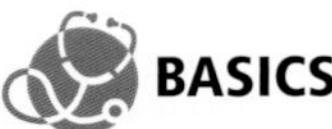

BASICS

DESCRIPTION

- Endometrial cancer: malignancy of the endometrial lining of the uterus
  - 2 types
    - I: estrogen dependent, grade1 or grade 2, better prognosis, endometrioid histology
    - II: estrogen independent, higher grade, more aggressive, include grade 3 endometrioid and nonendometrioid: serous, clear cell, mucinous, poor prognosis (1)[A]
- Cell types: adenocarcinoma, adenosquamous (malignant squamous elements), clear cell, and papillary serous
- Sarcomas: malignancy of the uterine mesenchyme and mixed tumors
  - Mixed müllerian sarcoma (carcinosarcoma): Heterologous sarcoma elements are not native to the müllerian system (e.g., cartilage or bone); homologous sarcoma elements are native to the müllerian system (40–50% prevalence of all sarcomas).
  - Leiomyosarcoma develops in the myometrium, characterized by cellular atypic mitoses and coagulative necrosis (30% prevalence of all sarcomas).
  - Endometrial stromal sarcoma develops from the stromal component of the endometrium (15% prevalence of all sarcomas).
  - Poorer prognosis (2)[C]
- Predominant age
  - Endometrial cancer: Most patients are postmenopausal:
    - Average age of diagnosis: 61years old
- Sarcomas: age 40–69 years (2)[C]
- 68% uterine cancers confined to primary site at time of diagnosis (1)[A]
- System(s) affected: reproductive
- Synonym(s): uterine cancer; endometrial cancer; corpus cancer

Pregnancy Considerations

This malignancy is not associated with pregnancy.

EPIDEMIOLOGY

Incidence

- Endometrial cancer is the most common gynecologic malignancy; 4th most common cancer in women and 8th leading cause of cancer-related death in women worldwide.
- In the United States, it is estimated that endometrial cancer will account for 49,560 new cases and 8,190 deaths in 2014 (2)[C].

Prevalence

500,000 women in the United States

ETIOLOGY AND PATHOPHYSIOLOGY

Continuous estrogen stimulation unopposed by progesterone

- Endometrial: unopposed estrogen
  - Estrogen replacement therapy without concomitant progesterone increases the risk. Addition of progesterone decreases risk to that of general population.
- Sarcomas: etiology unknown

Genetics

- Endometrial: Lynch syndrome (hereditary nonpolyposis colorectal cancer)
- Sarcoma: African American, higher incidence of leiomyosarcoma, childhood retinoblastoma survivors

RISK FACTORS

- Early menarche/late menopause
- Nulliparity
- Personal or family history of colon or reproductive system cancer
- Obesity
- Diabetes mellitus
- Hypertension
- Polycystic ovarian syndrome
- Estrogen-secreting tumor
- Endometrial hyperplasia
- Unopposed estrogens
- Tamoxifen use
- Increasing age

GENERAL PREVENTION

- In young women who are obese or anovulatory, the risk of endometrial cancer can be reduced by taking oral contraceptive pills, permanently losing weight, or taking cyclic progesterone to prevent unopposed estrogen's effects on the uterus (3)[A].
- Estrogen replacement therapy should always include progesterone unless the woman has had a hysterectomy (3)[A].
- Cigarette smoking has been associated with a lower risk of endometrial cancer; however, it is not recommended secondary to its many health risks.

COMMONLY ASSOCIATED CONDITIONS

- Endometrial hyperplasia: 1–25% will progress to endometrial adenocarcinoma:
  - Simple without atypia
  - Complex without atypia
  - Simple with atypia
  - Complex with atypia
    - 43% with complex hyperplasia with atypia have concurrent endometrial cancer.
- Endometrial cancer patients should be screened regularly for breast and colon cancer because of an increased risk of these cancers.
- Patients who have breast or colon cancer are at increased risk for endometrial cancer.
- Granulosa cell tumors of the ovary produce estrogen; these patients will have an increased risk of endometrial cancer.

DIAGNOSIS

HISTORY

- Endometrial cancer
  - Postmenopausal bleeding is the most frequent sign. Any spotting or abnormal discharge mandates evaluation.
  - Premenopausal patients with history of anovulation and heavy, irregular, or prolonged periods that fail multiple medical managements mandate evaluation.
- Sarcoma
  - Mixed müllerian sarcoma: bleeding and prolapsing tissue, pain (2)[C]
  - Leiomyosarcoma: pelvic pain, pressure, uterine mass, abnormal bleeding

PHYSICAL EXAM

Pelvic exam: enlarged, fixed

DIFFERENTIAL DIAGNOSIS

- Atypical complex hyperplasia: a premalignant lesion of the endometrium
- Cervical cancer
- Ovarian cancer invading the uterus
- Endometriosis
- Adenomyosis
- Leiomyoma

DIAGNOSTIC TESTS & INTERPRETATION

Initial Tests (lab, imaging)

- Liver and renal function tests
- Transvaginal ultrasound usually shows increased endometrial thickness (>4 mm in postmenopausal patients or in patients with irregular or heavy periods if >35 years of age) (1)[A].
- Levels of cancer antigen 125 (CA-125) may be elevated when intra-abdominal disease is present (1)[A].
- Chest x-ray (CXR): Most common site of metastases is the lungs.
- Mammogram and colonoscopy: Endometrial cancer is associated with breast and colon cancer.

Follow-Up Tests & Special Considerations

- A biopsy of a pregnant uterus can produce tissue that looks hyperplastic or premalignant.
- Pap smear is rarely positive.
- CT scan, bone scan, liver and spleen scan: not part of the routine evaluation but may be needed if metastasis is suspected
- MRI has been reported to show the depth of myometrial penetration accurately but is not always cost-effective (4)[A].

Diagnostic Procedures/Other

- Office endometrial biopsy (90% accurate): If negative with high suspicion for cancer, a dilation and curettage (D&C) is necessary. Endometrial stromal sarcoma and leiomyosarcoma rarely are diagnosed preoperatively. Any patient with history of irregular, heavy, or prolonged periods should undergo endometrial biopsy prior to endometrial ablation procedures.
- Fractional D&C is 99% accurate except in cases of sarcoma.
- Hysteroscopy, which may be associated with higher risk of positive washings/cytology, is controversial (4,5)[A].

Test Interpretation

- Federation of Gynecology and Obstetrics Staging System: revised 2009
  - Stage I (confined to corpus uteri)
    - A: no or <1/2 myometrial invasion
    - B: invasion ≥1/2 the myometrium
  - Stage II: Tumor invades cervical stroma but does not extend beyond the uterus.
  - Stage III: local and/or regional spread
    - A: uterine serosal and/or adnexal invasion
    - B: vaginal and/or parametrial involvement
    - C: metastases to pelvic and/or para-aortic lymph nodes
    - IIIC1: +pelvic nodes
    - IIIC2: +para-aortic lymph nodes positive pelvic lymph nodes

- Stage IV: Tumor invades bladder and/or bowel mucosa and/or distant metastases:
  - A: Tumor invades bladder and/or bowel mucosa.
  - B: distant metastases, including intra-abdominal metastases and/or inguinal lymph nodes (1)[A]
- Uterine sarcoma criteria for diagnosis: mitotic index, cellular atypia, and areas of coagulative necrosis separated from tumor (6)[C]

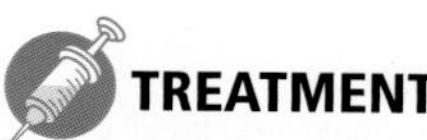

TREATMENT

GENERAL MEASURES

- Main treatment for uterine cancer is surgery.
- Radiation is used to prevent tumor recurrence at the vaginal cuff.

MEDICATION

First Line

- Endometrial
  - Chemotherapy for advanced or recurrent disease incurable with surgery and radiation
    - Doxorubicin + cisplatin + paclitaxel
    - Paclitaxel + carboplatin
- Hormonal therapy
  - Medroxyprogesterone acetate: for recurrence or metastases
  - Megestrol (Megace) 160 mg/day for at least 2 months for women with premalignant lesions, atypical complex hyperplasia, or well-differentiated endometrial cancer in patients desiring fertility. Follow with D&C to determine cancer resolution.
  - Levonorgestrel-containing intrauterine device: as mentioned earlier for patients who desire future fertility (3,7,8)[A]
- Sarcoma
  - Chemotherapy
    - Doxorubicin as single agent or in combination (6)[A]
- Hormonal
  - Tamoxifen or aromatase inhibitors; not fully studied
  - Progesterones (3)[A]

Second Line

Ondansetron (Zofran), dronabinol (Marinol), metoclopramide (Reglan), and others to control nausea from chemotherapy

ADDITIONAL THERAPIES

Radiation therapy

- Nonoperative candidates: radiation therapy alone
- Low risk: no adjuvant radiation therapy
- Intermediate risk: Consider adjuvant vaginal brachytherapy; reduces local recurrences but has no effect on overall survival
- High risk: chemotherapy and radiation therapy in some cases (4,5)[A]

SURGERY/OTHER PROCEDURES

Surgical staging

- Extrafascial hysterectomy and bilateral salpingo-oophorectomy
- Cytologic washings
- Pelvic and para-aortic lymph node dissection
- Omental sampling, as indicated
- Optimal tumor debulking (1)[A]

Geriatric Considerations

Older (and obese) patients may be at high risk for surgery. Alternative radiation therapy can be considered.

INPATIENT CONSIDERATIONS

Admission Criteria/Initial Stabilization

- Excessive vaginal bleeding
- Preoperative stabilization

Nursing

Routine; ensure postoperative pain is controlled.

Discharge Criteria

Postsurgical criteria: pain controlled, tolerating diet, ambulating, and voiding

ONGOING CARE

FOLLOW-UP RECOMMENDATIONS

Speculum and rectovaginal exam every 3–4 months for 2–3 years, then every 6 months for 3 years, and then annually for life

Patient Monitoring

Annual CXR

DIET

As tolerated and according to comorbidities

PATIENT EDUCATION

After surgery:

- No intercourse for ~6 weeks
- No lifting >10–15 lb
- No driving until pain free
- Do not expect resumption of full activity for 6 weeks.

PROGNOSIS

5-year survival rates

- Uterine adenocarcinoma

Stage	Survival (%)
IA	88
IB	75
II	69
IIIA	58
IIIB	50
IIIC	47
IVA	17
IVB	15

- Uterine sarcoma

Stage	Survival (%)
I	70
II	45
III	30
IV	15

(3,4)[A]

COMPLICATIONS

- Surgical: excessive bleeding, wound infection, lymphedema, deep vein thrombosis (DVT), and damage to the urinary or intestinal systems
- Radiation: diarrhea, ileus, bowel obstruction or fistula, radiation cystitis, proctitis, vaginal stenosis, DVT
- Chemotherapy: per the drug given

REFERENCES

1. Creasman W. Revised FIGO staging for carcinoma of the endometrium. *Int J Gynaecol Obstet*. 2009;105(2):109.
2. American College of Obstetricians and Gynecologists. ACOG practice bulletin, clinical management guidelines for obstetrician-gynecologists, number 65, August 2005: management of endometrial cancer. *Obstet Gynecol*. 2005;106(2):413–425.
3. Polyzos NP, Pavlidis N, Paraskevaidis E, et al. Randomized evidence on chemotherapy and hormonal therapy regimens for advanced endometrial cancer: an overview of survival data. *Eur J Cancer*. 2006;42(3):319–326.
4. Humber C, Tierney J, Symonds P, et al. Chemotherapy for advanced, recurrent or metastatic endometrial carcinoma. *Cochrane Database Syst Rev*. 2005;(4):CD003915.
5. Einhorn N, Tropé C, Ridderheim M, et al. A systematic overview of radiation therapy effects in uterine cancer (corpus uteri). *Acta Oncol*. 2003;42(5–6):557–561.
6. Gadducci A, Cosio S, Romanini A, et al. The management of patients with uterine sarcoma: a debated clinical challenge. *Crit Rev Oncol Hematol*. 2008;65(2):129–142.
7. Bramwell VH, Anderson D, Charette ML; Sarcoma Disease Site Group. Doxorubicin-based chemotherapy for the palliative treatment of adult patients with locally advanced or metastatic soft tissue sarcoma. *Cochrane Database Syst Rev*. 2003;(3):CD003293.
8. Fleming GF, Brunetto VL, Cella D, et al. Phase III trial of doxorubicin plus cisplatin with or without paclitaxel plus filgrastim in advanced endometrial carcinoma: a Gynecologic Oncology Group study. *J Clin Oncol*. 2004;22(11):2159–2166.

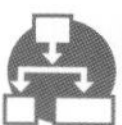

SEE ALSO

- Cervical Malignancy
- Algorithm: Pelvic Pain

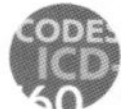

CODES

ICD10

- C54.1 Malignant neoplasm of endometrium
- C55 Malignant neoplasm of uterus, part unspecified
- C54.2 Malignant neoplasm of myometrium

CLINICAL PEARLS

- Most common presenting symptom is abnormal uterine bleeding.
- Any patient with history of irregular, heavy, or prolonged periods should undergo endometrial biopsy.
- Primary cause is unopposed estrogen.
- Endometrial thickness on transvaginal ultrasound of <5 mm makes endometrial cancer very unlikely.
- Primary treatment is with surgery, with possible chemotherapy ± radiation.

ENDOMETRIOSIS

Katherine L. Ball, MD • Jeanne Cawse-Lucas, MD

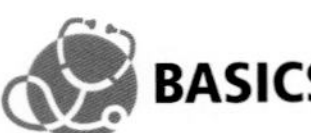

BASICS

DESCRIPTION

- Endometriosis is a common gynecologic condition affecting women of reproductive age, often recurring and persisting into early menopause (1). Generally associated with pelvic pain and infertility
- Thought to be estrogen-dependent implants of endometrial glands and stroma found outside the uterus
  - Pelvic sites: peritoneal surfaces (bladder, cul-de-sac, pelvic walls, ligaments, and fallopian tubes), vagina, cervix, lymph nodes, ovaries, bowel
  - Distant sites: abdominal wall, spleen, gallbladder, stomach, nasal mucosa, spinal canal, lungs, breasts, diaphragm, pleura, pericardium
- Staged according to the American Society for Reproductive Medicine surgical scoring system
  - Based on disease severity: size, depth, location, and characteristics of endometrial implants and adhesions
  - Stage I (minimal) to IV (severe)
- System(s) affected: reproductive
- Synonym(s): endometriosis externa

ALERT

Staging is useful in therapeutic planning but does not correlate with pain severity or predict response to treatment for symptoms or infertility.

EPIDEMIOLOGY

Prevalence

- Predominant sex: female only
- Affects 0.5–5% of fertile women
- Found in 30–50% of infertile women (2)
- Found in 50–60% of women and adolescent women with pelvic pain
- Difficult to assess true prevalence as some women are asymptomatic
- Estimated to affect 10% of reproductive-age women (3)

Pediatric Considerations

Endometriosis may begin with puberty as endometrial implants are dependent on ovarian hormones. This can lead to debilitating pelvic pain and severe dysmenorrhea associated with missed school, social, and family activities.

Pregnancy Considerations

Infertility is significantly associated with endometriosis. However, pelvic endometriosis generally improves during pregnancy.

Geriatric Considerations

Although menopause often results in a resolution of symptoms, pelvic endometriosis may extend into menopause and is exacerbated by hormone replacement therapy (HRT).

ETIOLOGY AND PATHOPHYSIOLOGY

- Not fully understood; generally thought that abnormal endometrial tissue implants and proliferates, causing chronic peritoneal inflammation
- Theories include the following:
  - **Sampson theory:** Retrograde menstruation results in peritoneal implantation and disease. Affected women have an immune dysfunction that prevents clearing of implants.
  - **Halban theory:** Distant disease probably caused by hematogenous/lymphatic dissemination or metaplastic transformation.
  - **Coelomic metaplasia:** Coelomic epithelium remains undifferentiated in the peritoneal cavity and differentiates to form functioning endometrium.
- Endometrial-associated infertility is multifactorial:
  - Pelvic inflammation
  - Anatomic disruption of pelvic structures (involvement of the fallopian tube may cause isthmic tubal obstruction)
  - Proliferation and activation of peritoneal macrophages (may predispose to gamete phagocytosis)
  - Alteration in eutopic endometrium

Genetics

Genetic predisposition is common.

RISK FACTORS

- Diethylstilbestrol exposure in utero
- Low birth weight
- Obstruction of menstrual flow (müllerian anomalies)
- Prolonged exposure to endogenous estrogen
  - Early menarche
  - Short menstrual cycles
  - Late menopause
  - Delayed childbearing
  - Obesity
- Hereditary/genetic predisposition
- Exposure to endocrine-disrupting chemicals
- Increased dietary intake of red meat and trans fats

GENERAL PREVENTION

- No evidence for prevention at this time
- Some factors are considered protective:
  - Fruits, green vegetables, n-3 long-chain fatty acids
  - Multiple pregnancies
  - Prolonged lactation
- Early diagnosis and treatment might help prevent the possible sequelae.

COMMONLY ASSOCIATED CONDITIONS

Associated with increased risk of autoimmune diseases and some epithelial ovarian cancers

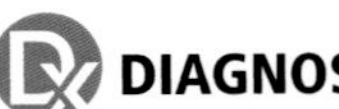

DIAGNOSIS

- Diagnosis can be challenging as symptoms overlap with many other gynecologic and nongynecologic conditions.
- Collect a complete medical history.
- Perform a complete physical exam, including a pelvic/rectovaginal exam.

HISTORY

- Dysmenorrhea (50–90% of cases)
- Dyspareunia
- Chronic pelvic pain (≥6 months) that worsens with time and activity
  - Intermittent/continuous
  - Dull/throbbing/sharp
- Premenstrual spotting
- Dyschezia, painful defecation, hematochezia
- Cyclic nausea, abdominal distention, and early satiety
- Hematuria
- Infertility
- Spontaneous abortion (theoretical)
- History of pelvic pain, infertility, and hysterectomy in 1st- or 2nd-degree relative

PHYSICAL EXAM

- Focal pain/tenderness on pelvic exam (associated with endometriosis in 66% of patients) (4)
- Pelvic mass
- Immobile pelvic organs (frozen pelvis)
- Rectovaginal exam revealing uterosacral nodules, beading, or tenderness

DIFFERENTIAL DIAGNOSIS

Differential diagnosis of pelvic pain includes all causes of acute abdomen and:

- Complications of intrauterine/ectopic pregnancy
- Pelvic adhesions
- Acute salpingitis/pelvic inflammatory disease
- Ruptured ovarian cyst
- Uterine leiomyomas
- Adenomyosis
- Irritable bowel syndrome
- Inflammatory bowel disease
- Intussusception
- UTI/cystitis
- Interstitial cystitis
- Malignancies
- Depression
- History of sexual abuse
- Myofascial pain

DIAGNOSTIC TESTS & INTERPRETATION

Initial Tests (lab, imaging)

- Labs are not useful in diagnosis.
- CA-125 levels may be elevated but are not recommended (poor sensitivity and specificity) and may be falsely elevated due to peritoneal irritation.
- Routine imaging is not recommended.
- If history and physical exam reveal adnexal pain or tenderness with/without fullness on pelvic exam
  - Transvaginal ultrasound (US) and MRI are equally effective in detecting ovarian endometriomas: sensitivity, 80–90%; specificity, 60–98% for both (4).
  - US is preferred (less costly).
  - Both modalities are poor in detecting peritoneal implants and adhesions.

Diagnostic Procedures/Other

Definitive diagnosis is made with visualization of lesions during laparoscopy or laparotomy.

Test Interpretation

- Red and blue-black lesions described as "powder-burns," adhesions, and "chocolate cysts"
- Endometrial glands and stroma on histologic analysis of biopsied lesions

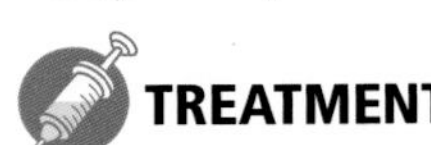

TREATMENT

GENERAL MEASURES

Endometriosis should be considered a chronic disease with the goal of optimizing medical management to avoid repeat surgical procedures.

MEDICATION

Medications may be helpful in treating symptoms of pain and dysmenorrhea, but symptoms frequently recur.

First Line

Empirical medical treatment is indicated for symptom management but has not been shown to improve fertility (4):

- NSAIDs initiated at the beginning or just before menses. Evidence is inconclusive on effectiveness (5)[B].
- Cyclic combined oral contraceptive pills (OCPs) suppress ovulation.

Second Line

- Continuous combined OCPs. Switch from cyclic to continuous OCPs for 3–6 months if symptoms persist or if there is chronic, noncyclic pelvic pain.
- Progestins: induce endometrial decidualization and atrophy
  - Levonorgestrel intrauterine device (IUD) (Mirena) found to decrease recurrence of painful menstruation (although not FDA approved for this indication) (6)[A]
- Medroxyprogesterone acetate 150 mg IM or 104 mg SC every 3 months. Prolonged use may lead to loss of bone mineral density of uncertain clinical significance. Gonadotropin-releasing hormone (GnRH) agonists: inhibit pituitary gonadotropin synthesis and induce a hypoestrogenic state (3)[A]: initial treatment continued for up to 6 months
  - Leuprolide acetate (Depo-Lupron) 3.75 mg IM each month or 11.25 mg IM every 3 months (gluteal)
  - Nafarelin (Synarel) intranasal 1 spray (200 mcg) in 1 nostril each morning and the other nostril each evening (start between days 2 and 4 of menstrual cycle)
  - Goserelin (Zoladex) implant 3.6 mg SC in upper abdominal wall every 28 days
- GnRH agonists should be given with estrogen-progestogen add-back therapy to minimize effects of hypoestrogenism (most importantly, reduced bone mineral density):
  - Norethindrone acetate 5 mg PO once daily
  - Conjugated equine estrogen 0.635 mg PO once daily
- Danazol: effective but second or third line due to androgenic side effects (7)[A]
- Aromatase inhibitors (anastrozole and letrozole) reduce local estrogen production and endometriotic growth. Risk with long-term use is reduction in bone mineral density.
- Anti-TNFα: have not been found to alleviate pain associated with endometriosis (8)

ALERT

Calcium (1,000–1,500 mg/day) with vitamin D 1,000–2,000 IU daily is recommended when using GnRH agonists to prevent calcium loss.

ISSUES FOR REFERRAL

- Refer early to a board-certified reproductive endocrinologist or gynecologist with expertise in infertility if the patient has difficulty conceiving.
- Other indications for referral to a gynecologist include the following:
  - Need for definitive diagnosis (failure to respond to a conservative first-line therapy)
  - Chronic pelvic pain
  - Adolescent with severe dysmenorrhea/dyspareunia

ADDITIONAL THERAPIES

Regular exercise and counseling for pain-management strategies (avoidance of narcotics is ideal)

SURGERY/OTHER PROCEDURES

Surgery (laparoscopy or laparotomy) is both diagnostic and therapeutic (first line or when conservative measures fail):

- Peritoneal endometriosis: laser ablation/excision/fulguration
- Ovarian endometriosis (endometriomas) >3 cm: ablation, excision, drainage
- Lysis of adhesions (LOA)
- Hysterectomy with bilateral salpingo-oophorectomy for debilitating symptoms refractory to other medical or surgical treatments:
  - Relieves pain in 80–90%, but pain recurs in 10% within 1–2 years after surgery.
  - Postoperative HRT should include estrogen and progestogen.
- Interruption of nerve pathways: Laparoscopic ablations and presacral neurectomy improve dysmenorrhea.
- Fertility procedures: Ablation of lesions with LOA is recommended to treat infertility in stages I–II disease:
  - Spontaneous conception should be attempted for 1 year prior to assisted reproduction techniques.
  - Disease does not endanger in vitro fertilization (IVF) pregnancies.

ALERT

Surgery for endometriomas may decrease ovarian reserve in advanced disease.

COMPLEMENTARY & ALTERNATIVE MEDICINE

- Physical therapy (4)[C]
- Postsurgical use of Chinese herbal medicine (oral and enema administration) is more effective than danazol at improving dysmenorrhea and reducing size of adnexal masses and has fewer side effects (9)[B].
- Acupuncture may be more effective than danazol to decrease pain, irregular menstruation, back pain, and perineal swelling (4)[C]. Also found to be more effective than Chinese herbal medicine (10)[B].
- Osteopathic manipulation

ONGOING CARE

FOLLOW-UP RECOMMENDATIONS

Routine gynecologic care

Patient Monitoring

Symptomatic and asymptomatic pelvic masses: http://www.acog.org

PROGNOSIS

- Excellent, especially if diagnosis and treatment plans are initiated early in disease course
- Poor for recovery of fertility if the disease has progressed to stage III/IV

COMPLICATIONS

Possible sequelae include chronic pelvic pain, repetitive surgical intervention, costs, and infertility.

REFERENCES

1. Brown J, Farquhar C. Endometrosis: an overview of Cochrane Reviews. *Cochrane Database Syst Rev.* 2014;(3):CD009590.
2. Ozkan S, Murk W, Arici A. Endometriosis and infertility: epidemiology and evidence-based treatments. *Ann N Y Acad Sci.* 2008;1127:92–100.
3. Brown J, Pan A, Hart RJ, et al. Gonadotrophin-releasing hormone analogues for pain associated with endometriosis. *Cochrane Database Syst Rev.* 2010;(12):CD008475.
4. Giudice LC. Clinical practice. Endometriosis. *N Engl J Med.* 2010;362(25):2389–2398.
5. Allen C, Hopewell S, Prentice A, et al. Nonsteroidal anti-inflammatory drugs for pain in women with endometriosis. *Cochrane Database Syst Rev.* 2009;(2):CD004753.
6. Abou-Setta AM, Houston B, Al-Inany HG, et al. Levonorgestrel-releasing intrauterine device (LNG-IUD) for symptomatic endometriosis following surgery. *Cochrane Database Syst Rev.* 2013;(1):CD005072.
7. Selak V, Farquhar C, Prentice A, et al. Danazol for pelvic pain associated with endometriosis. *Cochrane Database Syst Rev.* 2007;(4):CD000068.
8. Lu D, Song H, Shi G. Anti-TNF-α treatment for pelvic pain associated with endometriosis. *Cochrane Database Syst Rev.* 2013;(3):CD008088.
9. Flower A, Liu JP, Lewith G, et al. Chinese herbal medicine for endometriosis. *Cochrane Database Syst Rev.* 2012;(5):CD006568.
10. Zhu X, Hamilton KD, McNicol ED. Acupuncture for pain in endometriosis. *Cochrane Database Syst Rev.* 2011;(9):CD007864.

E

ADDITIONAL READING

- Davis L, Kennedy SS, Moore J, et al. Modern combined oral contraceptives for pain associated with endometriosis. *Cochrane Database Syst Rev.* 2007;(3):CD001019.
- de Ziegler D, Borghese B, Chapron C, et al. Endometriosis and infertility: pathophysiology and management. *Lancet.* 2010;376(9742):730–738.
- Härkki P, Tiitinen A, Ylikorkala O, et al. Endometriosis and assisted reproduction techniques. *Ann N Y Acad Sci.* 2010;1205:207–213.
- Hughes E, Brown J, Collins JJ, et al. Ovulation suppression for endometriosis. *Cochrane Database Syst Rev.* 2007;(3):CD000155.
- Jacobson TZ, Duffy JM, Barlow D, et al. Laparoscopic surgery for pelvic pain associated with endometriosis. *Cochrane Database Syst Rev.* 2009;(4):CD001300.
- Practice Committee of American Society for Reproductive Medicine. Treatment of pelvic pain associated with endometriosis. *Fertil Steril.* 2008;90(5 Suppl):S260–S269.

SEE ALSO

Algorithm: Pelvic Pain

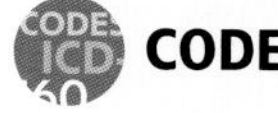

CODES

ICD10

- N80.2 Endometriosis of fallopian tube
- N80.3 Endometriosis of pelvic peritoneum
- N80.9 Endometriosis, unspecified

CLINICAL PEARLS

- Severe dysmenorrhea and dyspareunia are never normal. Failure to respond to NSAIDs and/or OCPs warrants further investigation.
- A rectovaginal exam can be useful in patients suspected of having endometriosis.

ENDOMETRITIS AND OTHER POSTPARTUM INFECTIONS

Justin P. Lavin, Jr., MD, FACOG • Jacoby D. Spittler, DO • Danielle Taylor, DO, MS

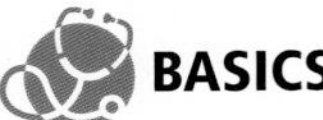

BASICS

DESCRIPTION

- Endometritis (infection of the endometrium) is the most common postpartum infection.
- Bacterial infection of genital tract, usually within the 1st week after delivery, can occur as late as 1–6 weeks postpartum.
- Less common are postpartum infections of the myometrium and parametrial tissues, vaginal and cervical infections, perineal cellulitis, pelvic cellulitis, septic pelvic vein thrombophlebitis, and parametrial phlegmon.
- System(s) affected: reproductive
- Synonym(s): postpartum infection; endometritis; endoparametritis; endomyometritis; myometritis; endomyoparametritis; metritis; metritis with pelvic cellulitis

EPIDEMIOLOGY

Incidence

- Predominant age: women of childbearing years
- Predominant sex: female only

Prevalence

- Occurs after 1–3% of all births
- 10 times more likely following cesarean section
  - 2–15% of infections occur prior to labor
  - 30–35% occur after labor in absence of appropriate antibiotic prophylaxis
  - 2–15% after labor with prophylaxis
  - 5th leading cause of maternal mortality, accounting for 11% of maternal deaths

ETIOLOGY AND PATHOPHYSIOLOGY

- Endometritis is more common in labors complicated by chorioamnionitis.
- Other infections follow trauma to the perineum, vagina, cervix, and uterus.
- Postpartum infections are almost always polymicrobial and involve organisms that have ascended from the lower genital tract:
  - Aerobic isolates in 70%: *Streptococcus faecalis, Streptococcus agalactiae, Streptococcus viridans, Staphylococcus aureus, Escherichia coli*
  - Anaerobic isolates in 80%: *Peptococcus* sp., *Peptostreptococcus* sp., *Clostridium* sp., *Bacteroides bivius, Bacteroides fragilis, Fusobacterium* sp.
- Other genital mycoplasmata
- Herpes simplex virus and cytomegalovirus should be considered, particularly in immunocompromised patients who fail to improve on appropriate antibiotics.
- Superficial layer of infected necrotic tissue in microscopic sections of uterine lining
- Thrombosis of any pelvic vein, including vena cava
- Phlegmon on leaves of the broad ligament

RISK FACTORS

- Cesarean delivery is primary risk factor.
- Chorioamnionitis
- Bacterial vaginosis
- Group B streptococcal colonization of genital tract
- HIV infection
- Prolonged labor
- Prolonged rupture of membranes
- Multiple vaginal examinations
- Internal fetal monitoring during labor
- Operative vaginal delivery
- Manual extraction of the placenta
- Low socioeconomic status
- Obesity
- Anemia
- Care in a teaching hospital

GENERAL PREVENTION

- Vaginal delivery
  - Avoid unnecessary vaginal examinations.
  - Treat chorioamnionitis during labor.
  - Avoid manual placental extraction, retained placental fragments, or membranes.
  - Antibiotic prophylaxis for 3rd- and 4th-degree laceration (1)[B]
  - Use of aseptic technique during operative vaginal delivery
  - No data to support antibiotic prophylaxis for operative vaginal delivery (2)[A]
- Cesarean delivery
  - Preoperative preparation using a paint and scrub technique with a 10% povidone-iodine scrub and topical solution decreases puerperal infection by up to 38% (3)[B].
  - Prophylactic antibiotics before both emergency and scheduled cesarean deliveries prior to skin incision reduces the prevalence of postpartum infection (4)[A],(5,6)[B].
    - Antibiotics should be administered within 1 hour of the surgery start time (6)[B].
    - Appropriate administration of antibiotics results in a 40% reduction in postpartum maternal infections without any increase in neonatal infectious outcomes (6)[B].
  - Extending the spectrum of coverage to include both a cephalosporin and a macrolide may further decrease infection risk (7)[A],(8)[B].
  - Vaginal preparation with povidone-iodine solution immediately before cesarean delivery reduces the risk of postoperative endometritis (9)[A].
  - Weight-based antibiotic dosage helps ensure appropriate tissue concentrations prior to skin incision (10).

COMMONLY ASSOCIATED CONDITIONS

- Chorioamnionitis
- Wound infection

DIAGNOSIS

HISTORY

- History of cesarean delivery or chorioamnionitis
- Fever and chills
- Malaise
- Headache
- Anorexia
- Abdominal pain
- Heavy vaginal bleeding or foul smelling vaginal discharge

PHYSICAL EXAM

- Oral temperature >38.7°C (101.6°F) in first 24 hours postpartum or >38°C (100.4°F) in 2 of first 10 days postpartum (excluding first 24 hours)
- Tachycardia
- Uterine tenderness on exam
- Other localized abdominopelvic tenderness on exam
- Purulent or malodorous lochia
- Heavy vaginal bleeding
- Ileus
- Group A or B streptococcal bacteremia may have no localizing signs.

DIFFERENTIAL DIAGNOSIS

- UTI
- Viral syndrome
- Dehydration
- Pneumonia
- Wound infection
- Thrombophlebitis
- Thyroid storm
- Mastitis
- Appendicitis
- Drug/medication-related fever

DIAGNOSTIC TESTS & INTERPRETATION

Initial Tests (lab, imaging)

- CBC: Interpret with care because *physiologic leukocytosis may be as high as 20,000 WBCs*.
- 2 sets of blood cultures (especially if sepsis is suspected)
- Note: Diagnosis is usually made based on clinical grounds. Potential testing includes the following:
  - Genital tract cultures and rapid test for group B streptococci (may be done during labor)
  - Amniotic fluid Gram stain: usually polymicrobial
  - Uterine tissue cultures: Prep the cervix with Betadine and use a shielded specimen collector or Pipelle; difficult to obtain without contamination
- If patient is not responsive to antibiotics in 24–48 hours:
  - Ultrasound for retained products of conception, pelvic abscess, or mass
  - CT or MRI looking for pelvic vein thrombophlebitis, abscess, or deep-seated wound infection

Diagnostic Procedures/Other

Paracentesis/culdocentesis with culture rarely necessary

Test Interpretation

>5 neutrophils per high-power field in superficial endometrium; ≥1 plasma cell in endometrial stroma

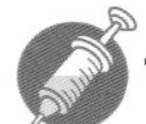

TREATMENT

MEDICATION

First Line

- Clindamycin 900 mg IV q8h + gentamicin 5 mg/kg IV q24h (11)[A]
- Potential side effects include nephrotoxicity, ototoxicity, pseudomembranous colitis, or diarrhea (in up to 6%).

Second Line

- Ampicillin-sulbactam 3 g IV q6h (12)[A]
- Metronidazole 500 mg q8–12h + penicillin 5 million units q6h, *or*
- Ampicillin 2 g q6h + gentamicin 5 mg/kg q24h (11)[A]
- Cefoxitin 2 g IV q6h. Add ampicillin 2 g IV q6h, if clinical failure after 48 hours
- Cefotetan 2 g IV q12h. Add ampicillin 2 g IV q6h, if clinical failure after 48 hours (11)[A]

- Note: Base therapy on cultures, sensitivities, and clinical response.
- Contraindications:
  - Drug allergy
  - Renal failure (aminoglycosides)
  - Avoid sulfa, tetracyclines, and fluoroquinolones before delivery and if breastfeeding. Metronidazole is relatively contraindicated if breastfeeding; however, consider clinical scenario.
- Precautions:
  - Clindamycin and other antibiotics occasionally cause pseudomembranous colitis.
  - Antibiotic-associated diarrhea (*Clostridium difficile*)
- Significant possible interactions: Refer to the manufacturer's literature for each drug.
- Note: Consider adding a macrolide antibiotic (for chlamydia coverage) for infections occurring after 48 hours.
- Note: Heparin typically indicated for septic pelvic vein thrombophlebitis; requires 10 days of full anticoagulation

SURGERY/OTHER PROCEDURES

- Curettage of retained products of conception
- Surgery to drain an abscess
- Surgery to decompress the bowel
- Surgical drainage of a phlegmon is not advised unless it is suppurative.

INPATIENT CONSIDERATIONS

Admission Criteria/Initial Stabilization

- Inpatient care for postpartum infections
- Most infections (94%) occur after hospital discharge.
- IV antibiotics and close observation for severe infections
- Open and drain infected wounds.
- Optimize fluid status.

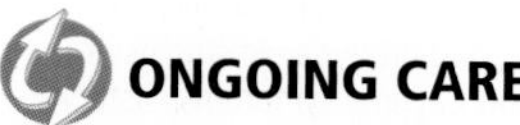

ONGOING CARE

FOLLOW-UP RECOMMENDATIONS

Patient Monitoring

- Individualize according to severity
- IV antibiotics can be stopped when the patient is afebrile for 24–48 hours.
- Oral antibiotics on discharge are not necessary, except in cases of bacteremia; then continue oral antibiotics to complete a 7-day course.

DIET

As tolerated, although may be limited by ileus

PATIENT EDUCATION

- Advise patient to contact physician with fever >38°C (100.4°F) postpartum, heavy vaginal bleeding, foul-smelling lochia, or other symptoms of infection.
- Information available at http://www.healthline.com/yodocontent/pregnancy/infections-postpartum-endometritis.html

PROGNOSIS

- With supportive therapy and appropriate antibiotics, most patients improve relatively quickly and recover without complication.
- If no improvement occurs on antibiotics, consider retained placental fragments or membranes, abscess, wound infection, hematoma, cellulitis, phlegmon, or septic pelvic vein thrombosis.

COMPLICATIONS

- Resistant organisms
- Peritonitis
- Pelvic abscess
- Septic pelvic thrombophlebitis
- Ovarian vein thrombosis
- Sepsis
- Death

REFERENCES

1. Duggal N, Mercado C, Daniels K, et al. Antibiotic prophylaxis for prevention of postpartum perineal wound complications: a randomized controlled trial. *Obstet Gynecol*. 2008;111(6):1268–1273.
2. Liabsuetrakul T. Antibiotic prophylaxis for operative vaginal delivery. *Cochrane Database Sys Rev*. 2009;(1):CD004455
3. Weed S, Bastek JA, Sammel MD, et al. Comparing postcesarean infectious complication rates using two different skin preparations. *Obstet Gynecol*. 2011;117(5):1123–1129.
4. Smaill FM, Gyte GM. Antibiotic prophylaxis versus no prophylaxis for preventing infection after cesarean section. *Cochrane Database Sys Rev*. 2010;(1):CD007482.
5. Dinsmoor MJ, Gilbert S, Landon MB, et al. Perioperative antibiotic prophylaxis for nonlaboring cesarean delivery. Eunice Kennedy Shriver National Institute of Child Health and Human Development Maternal-Fetal Medicine Units Network. *Obstet Gynecol*. 2009;114(4):752–756.
6. American College of Obstetricians and Gynecologist. ACOG practice bulletin no. 120: use of prophylactic antibiotics in labor and delivery. *Obstet Gynecol*. 2011;117(6):1472–1483.
7. Costantine MM, Rahman M, Ghulmiyah L, et al. Timing of perioperative antibiotics for cesarean delivery: a metaanalysis. *Am J Obstet Gynecol*. 2008;199(3):301.e1–301.e6.
8. Tita AT, Owen J, Stamm AM, et al. Impact of extended-spectrum antibiotic prophylaxis on incidence of postcesarean surgical wound infection. *Am J Obstet Gynecol*. 2008;199(3):303.e1–303.e3.
9. Haas DM, Morgan S, Contreras K. Vaginal preparation with antiseptic solution before cesarean section for preventing postoperative infections. *Cochrane Database Syst Rev*. 2013;1:CD007892.
10. Pevzner L, Swank M, Krepel C, et al. Effects of maternal obesity on tissue concentrations of prophylactic cefazolin during cesarean delivery. *Obstet Gynecol*. 2011;117(4):877–882.
11. French LM, Smaill F. Antibiotic regimens for endometritis after delivery. *Cochrane Database Sys Rev*. 2009;(1):CD001067.
12. McGregor JA, Crombleholme W, Newton E, et al. Randomized comparison of ampicillin-sulbactam to cefoxitin and doxycycline or clindamycin and gentamicin in the treatment of pelvic inflammatory disease or endometritis. *Am J Obstet Gynecol*. 1994;83:998–1004.

ADDITIONAL READING

- Baaqeel H, Baaqeel R. Timing of administration of prophylactic antibiotics for caesarean section: a systematic review and meta-analysis. *BJOG*. 2013;120(6):661–669.
- Bianco A, Roccia S, Nobile CG, et al. Postdischarge surveillance following delivery: the incidence of infections and associated factors. *Am J Infect Control*. 2013;41(6):549–553.
- Maharaj D. Puerperal pyrexia: a review. Part I. *Obstet Gynecol Surv*. 2007;62(6):393–399.
- Maharaj D. Puerperal pyrexia: a review. Part II. *Obstet Gynecol Surv*. 2007;62(6):400–406.
- Srinivas SK, Fager C, Lorch SA. Variations in postdelivery infection and thrombosis by hospital teaching status. *Am J Obstet Gynecol*. 2013;209(6):567.e1–567.e7.
- Sun J, Ding M, Liu J, et al. Prophylactic administration of cefazolin prior to skin incision versus antibiotics at cord clamping in preventing postcesarean infectious morbidity: a systematic review and meta-analysis of randomized controlled trials. *Gynecol Obstet Invest*. 2013;75(3):175–178.

SEE ALSO

Algorithm: Pelvic Pain

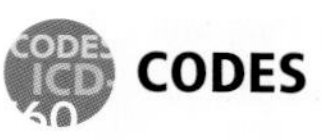

CODES

ICD10

- O86.12 Endometritis following delivery
- O86.4 Pyrexia of unknown origin following delivery
- O86.13 Vaginitis following delivery

CLINICAL PEARLS

- Postpartum endometritis follows 1–3% of all births.
- Infections are typically polymicrobial and involve organisms ascending from the lower genital tract.
- Evidence supports antibiotic prophylaxis prior to skin incision for all cesarean deliveries but not for operative vaginal deliveries.
- Recommended treatment of endometritis is clindamycin 900 mg IV q8h and gentamicin 5 mg/kg q24h until the patient is afebrile for 24–48 hours.
- Antibiotics can be stopped completely when the patient has been afebrile for 24–48 hours, except in cases of documented bacteremia, which require a 7-day course of therapy.

ENURESIS

Melanie J.S. Malec, MD

BASICS

DESCRIPTION

- Nocturnal enuresis (NE): repeated spontaneous voiding of urine during sleep after the anticipated age of bladder control (age 5 years)
- Daytime incontinence: uncontrollable leakage of urine while awake
- Bladder dysfunction: NE with daytime symptoms
- Classification
  - Primary NE: 1% of adult population; 80% of all cases; child/adult who has never established urinary continence on consecutive nights for a period of ≥6 months
  - Secondary NE: 20% of cases; resumption of enuresis after at least 6 months of urinary continence
- Also categorized as follows:
  - Monosymptomatic NE (uncomplicated): bed wetting without lower urinary tract (LUT) symptoms other than nocturia and no history of bladder dysfunction
  - Nonmonosymptomatic NE: bed wetting with LUT symptoms such as frequency, urgency, daytime wetting, hesitancy, straining, weak or intermittent stream, posturination dribbling, lower abdominal or genital discomfort, sensation of incomplete emptying
  - Daytime LUT condition: bed wetting with LUT daytime symptoms

ALERT

Adult-onset NE with absent daytime incontinence is a serious symptom; complete urologic evaluation and therapy are warranted.

- System(s) affected: nervous; renal/urologic
- Synonym(s): bed wetting; sleep enuresis; nocturnal incontinence; primary NE

EPIDEMIOLOGY

Incidence

- Depends on family history
- Spontaneous resolution: 15% per year, 99% children are dry by age 15 years.

Prevalence

- Very common. Affects 5–7 million children in the United States
- 40% of 3-year-olds; 10% of 6-year-olds; 3% of 12-year-olds; 1% of adults
- Male > female (3:1)
- Nocturnal > day (3:1)

Geriatric Considerations

Infrequent; often associated with daytime incontinence (formerly referred to as diurnal enuresis)

ETIOLOGY AND PATHOPHYSIOLOGY

- A disorder of sleep arousal, a low nocturnal bladder capacity, and nocturnal polyuria are the 3 factors that interrelate to cause NE (1)[C].
- Both functional and organic causes (below); many theories, none absolutely confirmed
- Detrusor instability
- Deficiency of arginine vasopressin (AVP); decreased nocturnal AVP or decreased AVP stimulation secondary to an empty bladder (bladder distension stimulates AVP)
- Maturational delay of CNS
- Severe NE with some evidence of interaction between bladder overactivity and brain arousability: association with children with severe NE and frequent cortical arousals in sleep
- Organic urologic causes in 1–4% of enuresis in children: UTI, occult spina bifida, ectopic ureter, lazy bladder syndrome, irritable bladder with wide bladder neck, posterior urethral valves
- Organic nonurologic causes: epilepsy, diabetes mellitus, food allergies, obstructive sleep apnea, chronic renal failure, hyperthyroidism, pinworm infection, sickle cell disease
- NE occurs in all stages of sleep.

Genetics

Most commonly, NE is an autosomal-dominant inheritance pattern with high penetrance (90%).

- 1/3 of all cases are sporadic.
- 75% of children with enuresis have a 1st-degree relative with the condition.
- Higher rates in monozygotic versus dizygotic twins (68% vs. 36%)
- If both parents had NE, risk in child is 77%; 44% if 1 parent affected. Parental age of resolution often predicts when child's enuresis should resolve.

RISK FACTORS

- Family history
- Stressors (emotional, environmental) common in secondary enuresis (e.g., divorce, death)
- Constipation
- Encopresis
- Organic disease: 1% of monosymptomatic NE (e.g., urologic and nonurologic causes)
- Psychological disorders
  - Comorbid disorders are highest with secondary NE: depression, anxiety, social phobias, conduct disorder, hyperkinetic syndrome, internalizing disorders
  - Association with ADHD; more pronounced in ages 9–12 years
  - Abuse; 11% sexually abused girls
- Altered mental status or impaired mobility

GENERAL PREVENTION

No known measures

COMMONLY ASSOCIATED CONDITIONS

- Obstructive sleep apnea syndrome; ↑ atrial natriuretic factor → inhibits renin-angiotensin-aldosterone pathway → ↑ diuresis
- Constipation (1/3 of patients with NE)
- Behavioral problems (specifically ADHD)

DIAGNOSIS

HISTORY

- Age of onset, duration, severity
- LUT tract symptoms
- Constipation and encopresis (15% with comorbid encopresis)
- Daily intake patterns
- Voiding and elimination patterns (voiding diary)
- Psychosocial history
- Family history of enuresis
- Investigation and previous treatment history

PHYSICAL EXAM

- ENT: evaluation for adenotonsillar hypertrophy
- Abdomen: enlarged bladder, kidneys, fecal masses, or impaction
- Back: Look for dimpling or tufts of hair on sacrum.
- Genital urinary exam
  - Males: meatal stenosis, hypospadias, epispadias, phimosis
  - Females: vulvitis, vaginitis, labial adhesions, ureterocele at introitus; evidence of abuse
- Rectal exam: tone and constipation
- Neurologic exam, especially lower extremities

DIFFERENTIAL DIAGNOSIS

- Primary NE
  - Delayed physiologic urinary control
  - UTI (both)
  - Spina bifida occulta
  - Obstructive sleep apnea (both)
  - Idiopathic detrusor instability
  - Previously unrecognized myelopathy or neuropathy (e.g., multiple sclerosis, tethered cord, epilepsy)
  - Anatomic urinary tract abnormality (e.g., ectopic ureter)
- Secondary NE
  - Bladder outlet obstruction
  - Neurologic disease, neurogenic bladder (e.g., spinal cord injury)

DIAGNOSTIC TESTS & INTERPRETATION

Initial Tests (lab, imaging)

- Only obligatory test in children is urinalysis
- Urinalysis and urine culture: UTI, pyuria, hematuria, proteinuria, glycosuria, and poor concentrating ability (low specific gravity) may suggest organic etiology, especially in adults.
- Urinary tract imaging is usually not necessary.
- If abnormal clinical findings or adult onset: renal and bladder US
- IV pyelogram, voiding cystourethrogram (VCUG) or retrograde pyelogram as indicated
- Spine radiographs for spina bifida occulta

Follow-Up Tests & Special Considerations

- Secondary enuresis: serum glucose, BUN, creatinine, thyroid-stimulating hormone (TSH), urine C/S
- In children, imaging and urodynamic studies are helpful for significant daytime symptoms, history of UTIs, suspected structural abnormalities, and in refractory cases.

Diagnostic Procedures/Other

Urodynamic studies may be beneficial in adults and nonmonosymptomatic NE.

Test Interpretation

- Dysfunctional voiding
- Detrusor instability and/or reduced bladder capacity most common findings

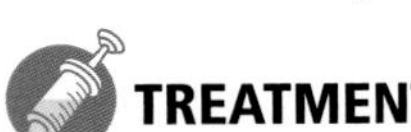

TREATMENT

- Prior to either alarm or pharmacologic treatment, supportive treatment measures should be attempted.
  - Counseling and information provision such as explanation of the 3 pathophysiologic factors
  - Review of eating and drinking habits, with emphasis on normal drinking patterns during daytime hours and reduction of intake in the hours prior to sleep.
  - Positive reinforcement of the child should also be encouraged.
- If supportive measures have no success, combined therapy (e.g., enuresis alarm, bladder training, motivational therapy, and pelvic floor muscle training) is more effective than each component alone or than pharmacotherapy (2)[A].

GENERAL MEASURES

- Use nonpharmacologic approaches as first line before prescribing medications (3)[A].
- Simple behavioral interventions (e.g., scheduled wakening, positive reinforcement, bladder training, diet changes) are effective.
- Enuresis alarms (bells or buzzers)
  - 66–70% success rate; must be used nightly for 3–4 months; offers cure; significant parental involvement; disruption of sleep for entire family
  - In children, number needed to treat (NNT) = 2 (4)[A].
- See "Patient Education" for options.

MEDICATION

First Line

- Desmopressin (DDAVP): synthetic analogue of vasopressin that decreases nocturnal urine output (5)[A]
  - Adults only: 20 μg (2 sprays) intranasally at bedtime
  - FDA recommends against use in children due to reports of severe hyponatremia resulting in seizures and deaths in children using intranasal formulations of desmopressin.
  - Oral DDAVP: dose dependent: begin at 0.2 mg tablet taken at bedtime on empty stomach; may titrate to 0.6 mg
    - Maximally effective in 1 hour; cleared within 9 hours
    - Trial nightly for 6 months, then stop for 2 weeks for test of dryness
    - Suspend dose in children who experience acute condition affecting fluid/electrolyte balances (fever, vomiting, diarrhea, vigorous exercise).
  - 10–70% success; safe even when used for >12 months; high relapse rate after discontinuation without a structured withdrawal program
  - In children, NNT = 6 (6)[A].
- Anticholinergics
  - Oxybutynin (Ditropan, Ditropan XL, Oxytrol patch): anticholinergic; smooth muscle relaxant, antispasmodic; may increase functional bladder capacity and aids in timed voiding
    - Ditropan: adults and children >5 years of age: 5 mg PO TID–QID; children 1–5 years of age: 0.02 mg/kg/dose BID–QID (syrup 5 mg/5 mL)
    - Ditropan XL: adults: 5 mg/day PO; increase to 30 mg/day PO (5-, 10-mg tabs)
    - Oxytrol patch: 1 patch every 3–4 days (3.9 mg/patch) (periodic trials off the medication, that is, weekends or weeks at a time, will help determine efficacy and resolution of primary disturbance)
    - Ditropan: 5–10 mg at night; 30–50% success; 50% relapse after stopped
  - Tolterodine (Detrol, Detrol LA): anticholinergic; fewer side effects than Ditropan
    - Detrol: 1–2 mg PO BID
    - Detrol LA: 2–4 mg/day

Pediatric Considerations

FDA recommends against using intranasal formulations of desmopressin in children due to reports of severe hyponatremia resulting in seizures and deaths (7,8)[A].

Second Line

- Imipramine (Tofranil): tricyclic antidepressant, anticholinergic effects; increases bladder capacity, antispasmodic properties
  - Primarily in adults; use in children is reserved for resistant cases
  - Dose: adults, 25–75 mg and children >6 years, 10–25 mg PO at bedtime; increase by 10–25 mg at 1–2-week intervals; treat for 2–3 months; then taper
  - 25–30% success when used >3 months.
  - Pretreatment ECG recommended identifying underlying rhythm disorders.
- Precautions
  - Oxybutynin: glaucoma, myasthenia gravis, GI or genitourinary obstruction, ulcerative colitis, megacolon; use a decreased dose in the elderly.
  - Tolterodine: urinary retention, gastric retention, or uncontrolled narrow-angle glaucoma; significant drug interactions with CYP2D6, CYP3A3/4 substrates
  - DDAVP: Avoid in patients at risk for electrolyte changes or fluid retention (congestive heart failure [CHF], renal insufficiency).
  - Imipramine: Do not use with monoamine oxidase inhibitors (MAOIs), hypotension, and arrhythmias; low toxic therapeutic ratio.
- Combination therapy with DDAVP and oxybutynin has better results than individual use.
- Prostaglandin inhibitors (e.g., indomethacin) have been studied; may increase bladder capacity; not as effective as DDAVP and ↑ adverse effects.

ALERT

Imipramine: Cardiotoxicity and death with overdose have been described.

ISSUES FOR REFERRAL

- Primary NE: persistent enuresis despite nonpharmacologic and pharmacologic therapies
- Diurnal incontinence or nonmonosymptomatic enuresis with voiding dysfunction or underlying medical condition

ADDITIONAL THERAPIES

Individual psychotherapy, crisis intervention, and family therapy

SURGERY/OTHER PROCEDURES

Only for surgically correctable causes (e.g., tethered cord, ectopic ureter, benign prostatic hypertrophy, obstructive sleep apnea)

COMPLEMENTARY & ALTERNATIVE MEDICINE

Acupuncture and hypnosis are other treatments offered; few data support their use (9,10)[B].

ONGOING CARE

FOLLOW-UP RECOMMENDATIONS

Patient Monitoring

Follow patient until condition resolves. Monitor therapy.

DIET

- Limit fluid and caffeine intake 2 hours prior to bedtime.
- Limit dairy products 4 hours prior to bedtime (decrease osmotic diuresis).

PATIENT EDUCATION

Web resources for alarms and supplies

- www.bedwettingstore.com/index.htm; www.dri-sleeper.com; www.enurad.com; www.nitetrain-r.com; www.sleepydryalarm.com; www.wetstop.com; www.pottypager.com/

PROGNOSIS

In children, NE is usually self-limiting; 1% will persist as adult; evaluate for organic causes.

COMPLICATIONS

UTI, perineal excoriation, psychological disturbance (especially in children)

REFERENCES

1. Robson WL. Current management of nocturnal enuresis. *Curr Opin Urol*. 2008;18(4):425–430.
2. Zaffanello M, Giacomello L, Brugnara M, et al. Therapeutic options in childhood nocturnal enuresis. *Minerva Urol Nefrol*. 2007;59(2):199–205.
3. Robson WL. Clinical practice. Evaluation and management of enuresis. *N Engl J Med*. 2009;360(14):1429–1436.
4. Glazener CM, Evans JH, Peto RE. Alarm interventions for nocturnal enuresis in children. *Cochrane Database Syst Rev*. 2005;(2):CD002911.
5. Vande Walle J, Stockner M, Raes A, et al. Desmopressin 30 years in clinical use: a safety review. *Curr Drug Saf*. 2007;2(3):232–238.
6. Glazener CM, Evans JH. Desmopressin for nocturnal enuresis in children. *Cochrane Database Syst Rev*. 2002;(3):CD002112.
7. Graham KM, Levy JB. Enuresis. *Pediatr Rev*. 2009;30(5):165–172; quiz 173.
8. U.S. Food and Drug Administration. Desmopressin acetate (marketed as DDAVP nasal spray, DDAVP rhinal tube, DDAVP, DDVP, Minirin, and stimate nasal spray. http://www.accessdata.fda.gov/scripts/cder/drugsatfda/index.cfm?fuseaction=Search.SearchAction&SearchTerm=desmopressin&SearchType=BasicSearch. Updated June 20, 2013.
9. Neveus T, Eggert P, Evans J, et al. Evaluation of and treatment for monosymptomatic enuresis: a standardization document from the International Children's Continence Society. *J Urol*. 2010;183(2):441–447.
10. Libonate J, Evans S, Tsao JC. Efficacy of acupuncture for health conditions in children: a review. *ScientificWorldJournal*. 2008;8:670–682.

ADDITIONAL READING

Vande Walle J, Rittig S, Bauer S, et al. Practical consensus guidelines for the management of enuresis. *Eur J Pediatr*. 2012;171(6):971–983.

SEE ALSO

- Incontinence, Urinary Adult Female; Incontinence, Urinary Adult Male
- Algorithm: Enuresis

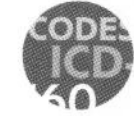

CODES

ICD10

- N39.44 Nocturnal enuresis
- R32 Unspecified urinary incontinence
- F98.0 Enuresis not due to a substance or known physiol condition

CLINICAL PEARLS

- Diagnosis is usually made based on history, physical examination, and urinalysis.
- If the condition is not distressing to child and caretakers, treatment is unnecessary.
- Dryness is possible for most children.

EOSINOPHILIC ESOPHAGITIS

Benjamin Hyatt, MD

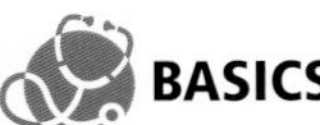

BASICS

Eosinophilic esophagitis (EoE) is a chronic, immune-mediated, inflammatory esophageal disease characterized clinically in adults by dysphagia, food impaction, and heartburn and in children with non-specific abdominal complaints, abdominal pain, and failure to thrive. Histologically, EoE is characterized by eosinophilic predominate inflammation (1)[A].

EPIDEMIOLOGY

All ages, most common in 20s–30s; male > female, 3:1

Incidence

Incidence in general population is 0.03% (2)[A].

- Incidence in those with gastroesophageal reflux disease (GERD)/dysphagia symptoms: 2.8% (2)[A]

Prevalence

Gradually increasing, perhaps due to better case finding, understanding of EoE in multiple clinical guises; 45–55/100,000

- Increased prevalence in those with celiac disease.

ETIOLOGY AND PATHOPHYSIOLOGY

- Believed to be an atopic inflammatory disease, whose pathogenesis is an aberrant immune response to antigenic stimulation
- Like eczema and asthma, T-helper 2 (T_H2) lymphoctyes play a role, as do mixed IgE and non–IgE-mediated allergic responses to food and environmental allergens.
- Although not well understood, the pathophysiology of EoE is postulated to be due to increased recruitment and activation of eosinophils in the esophagus. Eosinophil chemoattractants include eotaxin-3, IL-5, and IL-13.

Genetics

- EoE susceptibility may be caused by polymorphisms in thymic stromal lymphopoietin protein (TSLP) (2)[A].
- Potential new subphenotype of EoE (may also overlap with GERD): proton pump inhibitor (PPI)–responsive esophageal eosinophilia, where PPIs may act to decrease the inflammatory response in EoE (2)[A]

RISK FACTORS

- >50% with EoE have personal history of atopy/allergic disorders, such as asthma, hay fever, or eczema (1)[A].
- High rate of associated food antigen allergies/anaphylaxis

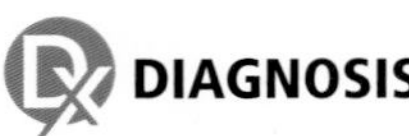

DIAGNOSIS

There are no pathognomonic findings for EoE. A definitive diagnosis is made by esophageal endoscopy and biopsy.

HISTORY

- Solid food dysphagia and food impaction are the most common symptoms and are usually present for 3–4 years prior to the diagnosis.
- Patients may also have reflux symptoms. Often, the diagnosis is entertained after patients fail a trial of antireflux medications. Other common complaints include nausea or vomiting, regurgitation, chest pain, upper abdominal pain, or decreased appetite.
- Patients may also have a history of food or environmental allergies, as well as asthma or atopic conditions (e.g., dermatitis).

PHYSICAL EXAM

No specific physical exam findings are associated with the diagnosis. However, signs and symptoms of allergies or asthma with symptoms of ongoing dysphagia or GERD-like symptoms should raise suspicion; some patients will have signs indicating weight loss or malnutrition.

DIFFERENTIAL DIAGNOSIS

- GERD
  - Associated with EoE; diseases may coexist in individual patients.
- PPI-responsive esophageal eosinophilia (PPI-REE)
  - Characteristics of PPI-REE
    - Shows classic EoE symptoms
    - Diagnosis of GERD has been excluded.
    - Responds to PPIs clinically and histologically
- Secondary causes of esophageal eosinophilia including celiac disease, Crohn esophagitis, infection, vasculitis, PPIs, achalasia, connective tissue disease, eosinophilic gastrointestinal diseases
- Functional dyspepsia
- Congenital rings
- Esophageal carcinoma
- Esophageal motility disorders

DIAGNOSTIC TESTS & INTERPRETATION

- To exclude PPI-REE, patients with suspected EoE should be given a 2-month course of PPI followed by endoscopy with biopsies.
- Solid food dysphagia is an indication for esophagogastroduodenoscopy (EGD), as are other concerning or "red-flag" symptoms, many of which occur in patients with EoE; they include the following:
  - Odynophagia
  - wWeight loss
  - Early satiety or vomiting
  - Aspiration/wheezing or cough
  - GI bleeding
  - Unexplained iron deficiency anemia
  - Male >45 years with long-standing symptoms
- GERD patients who show no symptomatic improvement after 8–12 weeks of a PPI should also be considered for EGD and biopsy.
- Serum IgE levels are elevated in 70% of patients.
- Peripheral eosinophilia occurs in 10–50% of patients.

Follow-Up Tests & Special Considerations

Testing for asthma and IgE-mediated food/inhalant allergies, if clinically relevant, can help manage coexisting atopic conditions:

- Serum IgE, skin prick test, or atopy patch test

Diagnostic Procedures/Other

EGD: 17% of biopsy-proven cases of EoE had an endoscopically normal exam (3)[A].

- Endoscopic findings: esophageal rings (tracheálization), strictures, white plaques or exudates, linear furrows, narrow-caliber esophagus, and pallor or decreased vasculature
- Esophageal biopsies are required for diagnosis; 2–4 biopsies from both proximal and distal esophagus. At initial diagnosis, biopsies should be obtained from antrum and/or duodenum to rule out other causes of esophageal eosinophilia in all children and adults with gastric or small intestinal symptoms or endoscopic abnormalities (1)[A].
  - Biopsy specimen: Pathologic findings may include surface layering of eosinophils, eosinophilic microabscesses, subepithelial lamina propria fibrosis, or basal cell hyperplasia.

- Barium contrast radiography
  - Can help to identify anatomic abnormalities in EoE but has a low sensitivity for diagnosis
  - May be an alternative to repeated endoscopies in previously treated patients who have changing symptoms
- pH monitoring: may be helpful in differentiating EoE from GERD

- Consensus American Gastroenterologic Association guidelines for diagnosis of EoE (1)[A]
  - Clinical symptoms of esophageal dysfunction
  - ≥15 eosinophils in 1 high-power field on biopsy
  - Mucosal eosinophilia is isolated to esophagus and persists after PPI use.
  - Secondary causes of esophageal eosinophilia are excluded.

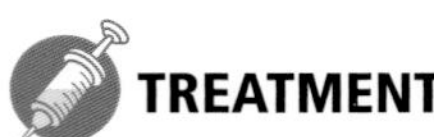

TREATMENT

Endpoints of therapy of EoE include improvements in clinical symptoms and esophageal eosinophilic inflammation. Defining evidence-based endpoints in EoE is still an area of active research (1)[A].

MEDICATION

First Line

- Corticosteroids
  - Topical steroids (swallowed, not inhaled) are 1st-line pharmacologic treatment:
    - Initial dosing for treatment of EoE: Swallowed fluticasone dose in adults is 880–1,760 mcg/day in a divided dose and in children is determined based on age or weight. Swallowed budesonide

dose in adults is 2 mg/day, typically in divided doses; in children determined based on age or weight. Initial duration of treatment is 8 weeks. Medication should be discontinued if patient develops side effects or other intolerances. Patients have relapsed after withdrawal of the medication. Inhaled topical steroid trials are ongoing.

- Systemic steroids: Prednisone can be helpful if topical steroids are not effective or for patients who require a more rapid improvement to symptoms, such as those with refractory dysphagia and in patients who are hospitalized. Long-term toxicity limits use (1)[A].
- Diet
  - Dietary elimination is considered initial therapy in both children and adults.
  - 3 dietary regimens have been shown to be effective in treatment of EoE: 1) Elemental amino acid–based diet, 2) elimination diet based on various food allergy tests, and 3) 6-food elimination diet of the most common food groups known to trigger EoE: wheat, soy, cow's milk, eggs, nuts, and seafood. All 3 methods have been shown to be effective in children for both clinical and histologic improvement, with the elemental diet being most effective:
    - In children, success rates of 77–98% have been reported for clinical and histologic remission using an elemental amino acid formula. A retrospective chart review comparing the 3 diets showed that the elemental diet was superior, with 96% remission (4)[B]. Yet this treatment has not gained popularity because of its high cost, impaired quality of life, and overall practicality.
  - In adults, a recent study indicates food allergy plays an important role in EoE and single food elimination diet (SFED) is an effective therapy (5)[B]:
    - Gonsalves et al. evaluated SFED in adult patients with EoE and demonstrated clinical, endoscopic, and histologic improvement. Symptoms improved in 94% of patients. Reintroduction of eliminated food caused reactivation of EoE with wheat (60%) and cow's milk (50%) as the leading causative agents. Skin-prick allergy testing was only 13% predictive in identifying food triggers.

Second Line

- Endoscopic esophageal dilation
  - May be used effectively in symptomatic patients with strictures that are resistant to medical or dietary treatments and initially in patients with severe and symptomatic esophageal stenosis (1)[A]
  - A systematic review showed that 92% of patients treated with dilation had improvement in dysphagia symptoms for up to 1–2 years.
  - Patients should be informed of the risks of esophageal dilation. The most common risk being postprocedure chest pain, which occurs in 75% of patients. The perforation rate for dilation is 0.3%, contrary to early reports which showed higher rates of perforation. Bleeding requiring endoscopic intervention or blood products is very rare, with only 1 occurence reported to date (1,6)[A].

ISSUES FOR REFERRAL

Refer to an allergist and/or nutritionist to help identify/manage allergic disorders and diet regimens.

ADDITIONAL THERAPIES

Other pharmacologic therapies

- Montelukast, mepolizumab (IL-5 monoclonal antibody), acid suppression therapy, purine analogues, anti-TNF therapy. Biologic agents have been well tolerated with low adverse effects (AEs), yet no studies have shown prolonged symptomatic relief (1)[A].
- Antihistamines: Case studies showed no benefit.

ONGOING CARE

FOLLOW-UP RECOMMENDATIONS

- EoE is a chronic disease with symptom recurrence after discontinuing treatment the rule rather than the exception. Prevention of progression of esophageal dysfunction is primary. Maintenance therapy with swallowed topical corticosteroid therapy and/or dietary restriction should be considered in all patients after clinicopathologic remission indefinitely or PRN (1)[A]. This is not yet standardized; only 1 RCT maintenance study has been done using low-dose budesonide (0.25 mg BID) versus placebo after remission for 50 weeks. Those maintained on budesonide had modest reduction in eosinophilia and fewer symptom recurrence, but there was still significant recurrence (7)[A]. As such, ongoing therapy needs to be tailored to individual patient cases.
- Patient should be counseled on the high likelihood of symptom recurrence after discontinuing treatment.

Patient Monitoring

- No guidelines yet established. It is reasonable to order periodic endoscopy based on symptoms or after completing a recent therapeutic regimen.
- There is no evidence to date of esophageal malignancy or hypereosinophilic syndromes associated with EoE.
- Esophageal candidiasis is a common side effect of chronic corticosteroid therapy.

PROGNOSIS

EoE does not seem to affect life expectancy. Quality of life is affected to some extent due to the chronic nature of the disease, difficulty in adhering to a restrictive diet, etc. Nutritional status can be maintained with appropriate care and diligence.

COMPLICATIONS

- Food impaction
- Esophageal stricture/ring/narrowing
- Nutritional deficiencies
- Subglottic stenosis or laryngeal edema is very rare.

REFERENCES

1. Dellon ES, Gonsalves N, Hirano I, et al. ACG Clinical Guidelines: evidenced based approach to diagnosis and management of esophageal eosinophilia and eosinophilic esophagitis (EoE). *Am J Gastroenterol*. 2013;108(5):679–692.
2. Liacouras CA, Furuta GT, Hirano I, et al. Eosinophilic esophagitis: updated consensus recommendations for children and adults. *J Allergy Clin Immunol*. 2011;128(1):3.e6–20.e6.
3. Kim HP, Vance RB, Shaheen NJ, et al. The prevalence and diagnostic utility of endoscopic features of eosinophilic esophagitis: a meta-analysis. *Clin Gastroenterol Hepatol*. 2012;10(9):988.e5–996.e5.
4. Henderson CJ, Abonia JP, King EC, et al. Comparative dietary therapy effectiveness in remission of pediatric eosinophilic esophagitis. *J Allergy Clin Immunol*. 2012;129(6):1570–1578.
5. Gonsalves N, Yang GY, Doerfler B, et al. Elimination diet effectively treats eosinophilic esophagitis in adults; food reintroduction identifies causative factors. *Gastroenterology*. 2012;142(7):1451.e1–1459.e1.
6. Bohm ME, Richter JE. Review article: oesophageal dilation in adults with eosinophilic oesophagitis. *Aliment Pharmacol Ther*. 2011;33(7):748–757.
7. Straumann A, Conus S, Degen L, et al. Long-term budesonide maintenance treatment is partially effective for patients with eosinophilic esophagitis. *Clin Gastroenterol Hepatol*. 2011;9(5):400.e1–409.e1.

ADDITIONAL READING

- Dellon ES, Jensen ET, Martin CF, et al. Prevalence of eosinophilic esophagitits in the United States. *Clin Gastroenterol Hepatol*. 2014;12(4):589.e1–596.e1.
- Stewart MJ, Shaffer E, Urbanski SJ. The association between celiac disease and eosinophilic esophagitis in children and adults. *BMC Gastroenterol*. 2013;13:96.

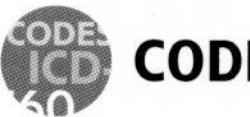

CODES

ICD10

K20.0 Eosinophilic esophagitis

CLINICAL PEARLS

- Food impaction or recurrent solid food dysphagia in a young, adult male: Think EoE.
- EoE commonly mimics disorders like GERD and PPI-REE.
- A PPI trial is now required prior to the diagnosis of EoE.
- Remember "red flags" in patients with empiric GERD: dysphagia, odynophagia, weight loss, early satiety or vomiting, aspiration/wheezing/cough, GI bleeding, unexplained iron deficiency anemia, age >50 years. Each "red flag" justifies EGD.

E

EPICONDYLITIS

Kevin Heaton, DO, CAQSM

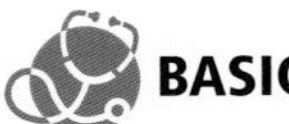

BASICS

DESCRIPTION

- Tendinopathy of the elbow characterized by pain and tenderness at the origins of the wrist flexors/extensors at the humeral epicondyles
- May be acute (traumatic) or chronic (overuse)
- 2 types
  - Medial epicondylitis or "golfer's elbow"
    - Involves the wrist flexors and pronators, which originate at the medial epicondyle
  - Lateral epicondylitis or "tennis elbow"
    - Involves the wrist extensors and supinators, which originate at the lateral epicondyle
- May be caused by many different athletic or occupational activities
- Common in carpenters, plumbers, gardeners, and athletes
- Usually involves epicondyles of the dominant arm
- Lateral epicondylitis is more common.

EPIDEMIOLOGY

- Predominant age: >40 years
- Predominant sex: male = female

Incidence

- Common overuse injury
- Lateral > medial
- Estimated between 1% and 3%

Prevalence

- Lateral epicondylitis: 1.3%
- Medial epicondylitis: 0.4%

ETIOLOGY AND PATHOPHYSIOLOGY

- Acute (tendonitis)
  - Inflammatory response to injury
- Chronic (tendinosis)
  - Overuse injury
  - Tendon degeneration, fibroblast proliferation, microvascular proliferation, lack of inflammatory response
- Repetitive wrist motions
- Tool/racquet gripping
- Shaking hands
- Sudden maximal muscle contraction
- Direct blow

RISK FACTORS

- Repetitive wrist motions
  - Flexion/pronation: medial
  - Extension/supination: lateral
- Smoking
- Obesity
- Upper extremity forceful activities

GENERAL PREVENTION

- Limit overuse of the wrist flexors, extensors, pronators, and supinators.
- Use proper techniques when working or playing racquet sports.
- Use lighter tools and smaller grips.

DIAGNOSIS

HISTORY

- Occupational activities
- Sport participation
- Direct trauma
- Duration and location of symptoms
- Prior treatments or medication use
- Pain with gripping
- Sensation of mild forearm weakness

PHYSICAL EXAM

- Localized pain just distal to the affected epicondyle
- Increased pain with wrist flexion/pronation (medial)
- Increased pain with wrist extension/supination (lateral)
- Medial epicondylitis
  - Tenderness at origin of wrist flexor tendons
  - Increased pain with resisted wrist flexion and pronation
  - Normal elbow range of motion
  - Increased pain with gripping
- Lateral epicondylitis
  - Tenderness at origin of wrist extensors
  - Increased pain with resisted wrist extension/supination
  - Normal elbow range of motion
  - Increased pain with gripping

DIFFERENTIAL DIAGNOSIS

- Elbow osteoarthritis
- Epicondylar fractures
- Posterior interosseous nerve entrapment (lateral)
- Ulnar neuropathy (medial)
- Synovitis
- Medial collateral ligament injury
- Referred pain from shoulder or neck

DIAGNOSTIC TESTS & INTERPRETATION

Initial Tests (lab, imaging)

No imaging is required for initial evaluation and treatment of a classic overuse injury.

Follow-Up Tests & Special Considerations

- Anterior-posterior/lateral radiographs if decreased range of motion, trauma, or no improvement with initial conservative therapy. Assess for fractures or signs of arthritis.
- For recalcitrant cases
  - Musculoskeletal ultrasound (US) reveals abnormal tendon appearance (e.g., tendon thickening, partial tear at tendon origin, calcifications) and neovascularity if color flow Doppler is used. US can also be used to guide steroid or other anesthetic injections.
  - MRI can show intermediate or high T2 signal intensity within the common flexor or extensor tendon or the presence of peritendinous soft tissue edema.

Diagnostic Procedures/Other

Infiltration of local anesthetic with subsequent resolution of symptoms can help support the diagnosis if clinically in doubt.

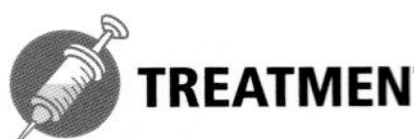

TREATMENT

GENERAL MEASURES

Initial treatment consists of activity modification, counterforce bracing, oral or topical NSAIDs, ice, and physical therapy:

- Observation: If left untreated, symptoms typically last between 6 months and 2 years. For patients with good function and minimal pain, conservative management using a "wait and see" approach may be considered based on patient preference.
- Activity modification, relative rest, and correction of faulty biomechanics
- Counterforce bracing with a forearm strap is easy and inexpensive. Systematic reviews are inconclusive about overall efficacy, but initial bracing may help to improve the ability to perform daily activities in the first 6 weeks.
- Nighttime wrist splinting can also be effective. Consider for repetitive daily activities if counterforce bracing fails.
- Frequent ice application after activities
- Physical therapy
  - Begin once acute pain is resolved. Infiltration of local anesthetic can help reduce pain to allow for physical therapy
  - Eccentric strength training regimen and stretching program
  - US therapy
  - Corticosteroid iontophoresis
  - Dry needling

MEDICATION

First Line

- Topical NSAIDs: Low-quality evidence suggests topical NSAIDS are significantly more effective than placebo with respect to pain and number needed to treat to benefit (7) in the short term (up to 4 weeks) with minimal adverse effects (1)[A].
- Oral NSAIDs: Unclear efficacy with respect to pain and function, but may offer short-term pain relief. Associated with adverse GI effects (1)[A].

Second Line

Corticosteroid injections: Short-term (≤8 weeks) reduction in pain. No benefits found for intermediate or long-term outcomes (2)[A].

ISSUES FOR REFERRAL

Failure of conservative therapy

ADDITIONAL THERAPIES

- Platelet-rich plasma (PRP) injections
  - Involves the injection of a concentrated portion of the patient's platelet-rich plasma. The localized injection leads to a local inflammatory response causing the platelets to degranulate, releasing growth factors, which then stimulates the physiologic healing cascade.
  - Treatment of patients with chronic lateral epicondylitis with PRP significantly reduces pain and increases function, exceeding the effect of corticosteroid injection even after a follow-up of 2 years (3)[B].
- US-guided percutaneous needle tenotomy
  - Involves the injection of a local anesthetic followed by US-guided tendon fenestration, calcification fragmentation and aspiration, and abrading the underlying bone. The procedure is thought to break apart scar tissue and stimulate an inflammatory and healing response.
- Prolotherapy
  - Involves the injection of a dextrose solution into and around the tendon attachment. This stimulates a localized inflammatory response, leading to increased blood supply to the area, which increases the flow of nutrients and healing mediators to stimulate tendon healing.
- Glyceryl trinitrate (GTN) transdermal patch
  - Nitric oxide (NO) is a small free radical generated by 3 isoenzymes called nitric oxide synthases. NO is expressed by fibroblasts and is postulated to aid in collagen synthesis. Topical application of glyceryl trinitrate theoretically improves healing by this mechanism. 1/4 of a 5-mg/24-hour GTN transdermal patch is applied once daily for up to 24 weeks.
  - Significant decreases in pain are seen at 3 weeks and 6 months compared to placebo patch (4)[B].
- Botulinum toxin A for chronic lateral epicondylitis
  - Injections into the forearm extensor muscles (60 units) can be performed in the outpatient setting.

SURGERY/OTHER PROCEDURES

- Elbow surgery may be indicated in the following refractory cases:
  - Fair evidence for treatment (5)[B]
  - Involves débridement and release of the involved tendons
  - Can be performed open or arthroscopically
- Denervation of the lateral humeral epicondyle
  - Transection of the posterior cutaneous nerve of the forearm with implantation into the triceps may help with chronic symptoms and pain.

COMPLEMENTARY AND ALTERNATIVE MEDICINE

Acupuncture: effective for short-term pain relief for lateral epicondyle pain

ONGOING CARE

PROGNOSIS

Good: Majority resolve with conservative care.

REFERENCES

1. Pattanittum P, Turner T, Green S, et al. Non-steroidal anti-inflammatory drugs (NSAIDs) for treating lateral elbow pain in adults. *Cochrane Database of Syst* Rev. 2013;5:CD003686.
2. Krogh TP, Bartels EM, Ellingsen T, et al. Comparative effectiveness of injection therapies in lateral epicondylitis: a systematic review and network meta-analysis of randomized controlled trials. *Am J Sports Med*. 2013;41(6):1435–1446.
3. Gosens T, Peerbooms JC, van Laar W, et al. Ongoing positive effect of platelet-rich plasma versus corticosteroid injection in lateral epidondylitis: a double-blind randomized controlled trial with 2-year follow-up. *Am J Sports Med*. 2011;39(6):1200–1208.
4. Ozden R, Uruç V, Doğramaci Y, et al. Management of tennis elbow with topical glyceryl trinitrate. *Acta Orthop Traumatol Turc*. 2014;48(2):175–180.
5. Yeoh KM, King GJ, Faber KJ, et al. Evidence-based indications for elbow arthroscopy. *Arthroscopy*. 2012;28(2):272–282.

ADDITIONAL READING

- Cullinane FL, Boocock MG, Trevelyan FC. Is eccentric exercise an effective treatment for lateral epicondylitis? A systematic review. *Clin Rehabil*. 2014;28(1):3–19.
- Dingemanse R, Randsdorp M, Koes BW, et al. Evidence for the effectiveness of electrophysical modalities for treatment of medial and lateral epicondylitis: a systematic review. *Br J Sports Med*. 2013;48(12):957–965.
- Green S, Buchbinder R, Barnsley L, et al. Acupuncture for lateral elbow pain. *Cochrane Database Syst Rev*. 2002;(1):CD003527.
- Kalichman L, Bannuru RR, Severin M, et al. Injection of botulinum toxin for treatment of chronic lateral epicondylitis: systematic review and meta-analysis. *Semin Arthritis Rheum*. 2011;40(6):532–538.
- McShane JM, Shah VN, Nazarian LN. Sonographically guided percutaneous needle tenotomy for treatment of common extensor tendinosis in the elbow: is a corticosteroid necessary? *J Ultrasound Med*. 2008;27(8):1137–1144.
- Rose NE, Forman SK, Dellon AL. Denervation of the lateral humeral epicondyle for treatment of chronic lateral epicondylitis. *J Hand Surg Am*. 2013;38(2):344–349.

SEE ALSO

Algorithm: Pain in Upper Extremity

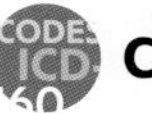

CODES

ICD10

- M77.00 Medial epicondylitis, unspecified elbow
- M77.10 Lateral epicondylitis, unspecified elbow
- M77.01 Medial epicondylitis, right elbow

CLINICAL PEARLS

- Tendon injury (acute or chronic) characterized by pain and tenderness at the tendinous origins of the wrist flexors/extensors on the epicondyles of the humerus
- Medial epicondylitis or golfer's elbow involves wrist flexors and pronators at the medial epicondyle.
- Lateral epicondylitis or tennis elbow involves wrist extensors and supinators at the lateral epicondyle.
- Left untreated, symptoms typically last between 6 months and 2 years.
- Most patients improve using conservative treatment with bracing, actvitity modification, and physical therapy.

EPIDIDYMITIS

Katherine Vlasica, DO

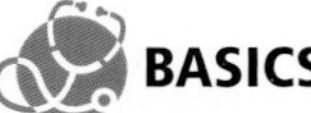

BASICS

- Acute epididymitis: pain for <6 weeks
- Chronic epididymitis: pain for >3 months

DESCRIPTION

- Inflammation (infectious or noninfectious) of epididymis resulting in scrotal pain and swelling, induration of the posterior epididymis, and eventual scrotal wall edema, involvement of the adjacent testicle, and hydrocele formation
- Classification: infectious (bacterial, viral, fungal, parasitic) versus sterile (chemical, traumatic, autoimmune, idiopathic, industrial, noninfectious, vasoepididymal reflux syndrome, vasal reflux syndrome); chronic versus acute
- System(s) affected: reproductive
- Synonym(s): epididymo-orchitis

EPIDEMIOLOGY

- Predominant age: usually younger, sexually active men or older men with UTIs; in older men, usually secondary to bladder outlet obstruction
- Predominant sex: male only

Pediatric Considerations

In prepubertal boys: Epididymitis is found to be the most common cause of acute scrotum—more common than testicular torsion.

Incidence

- Common (600,000 cases annually in the United States) (1)
- 1 in 1,000 males per year

Prevalence

Common

ETIOLOGY AND PATHOPHYSIOLOGY

- Infectious epididymitis
  - Retrograde passage of urine or urinary bacteria from the prostate or urethra to the epididymis via the ejaculatory ducts and the vas deferens; rarely, hematogenous spread
  - Causative organism is identified in 80% of patients and varies according to patient age.
- Sterile epididymitis
  - Can develop as a sequelae of strenuous exercise with a full bladder when urine is pushed through internal urethral sphincter (located at proximal end of prostatic urethra)
  - Reflux of urine through orifice of ejaculatory ducts at verumontanum may occur with history of urethritis/prostatitis, as inflammation may produce rigidity in musculature surrounding orifice to ejaculatory ducts, holding them open.
  - Exposure of epididymis to foreign fluid may produce inflammatory reaction within 24 hours.
- <35 years and sexually active
  - Usually *Chlamydia trachomatis* or *Neisseria gonorrhoeae*
  - Look for serous urethral discharge (chlamydia) or purulent discharge (gonorrhea)
  - With anal intercourse, likely *Escherichia coli* or *Haemophilus influenzae*
- >35 years
  - Coliform bacteria usually, but sometimes *Staphylococcus aureus* or *Staphylococcus epidermidis*
  - In elderly men, often with distal urinary tract obstruction, benign prostatic hyperplasia (BPH), UTI, or catheterization
  - Tuberculosis, if sterile pyuria and nodularity of vas deferens (hematogenous spread)
  - Sterile urine reflux after transurethral prostatectomy
  - Granulomatous reaction following BCG intravesical therapy for bladder cancer
- Prepubertal boys
  - Usually coliform bacteria
  - Evaluate for underlying congenital abnormalities, such as vesicoureteral reflux, ectopic ureter, or anorectal malformation (rectourethral fistula).
- Amiodarone may cause noninfectious epididymitis; resolves with decreasing drug dosage
- Syphilis, blastomycosis, coccidioidomycosis, and cryptococcosis are rare causes, but brucellosis can be a common cause in endemic areas.

RISK FACTORS

- UTI, prostatitis
- Indwelling urethral catheter
- Urethral instrumentation or transurethral surgery
- Urethral or meatal stricture
- Transrectal prostate biopsy
- Prostate brachytherapy (seeds) for prostate cancer
- Anal intercourse
- High-risk sexual activity
- Strenuous physical activity
- Prolonged sedentary periods
- Bladder obstruction (benign prostatic hyperplasia, prostate cancer)
- HIV-immunosuppressed patient
- Severe Behçet disease
- Presence of foreskin
- Constipation
- Sterile epididymitis
  - Increased intra-abdominal pressure (due to frequent physical strain)
    - Military recruits, especially who begin physically unprepared
    - Laborers; restaurant kitchen workers
    - Full bladder during intense physical exertion

GENERAL PREVENTION

- Vasectomy or vasoligation during transurethral surgery
- Safer sexual practices
- Mumps vaccination
- Antibiotic prophylaxis for urethral manipulation
- Early treatment of prostatitis/BPH
- Avoid vigorous rectal exam with acute prostatitis.
- Sterile epididymitis
- Emptying the bladder prior to physical exertion
- Physically conditioning the body prior to engaging in regular intense physical exertion
- Treat constipation.

COMMONLY ASSOCIATED CONDITIONS

- Prostatitis/urethritis/orchitis
- Hemospermia
- Constipation
- UTI

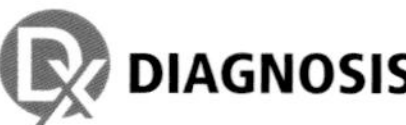

DIAGNOSIS

- Scrotal pain, sometimes radiating to the groin region, may begin acutely over several hours.
- Urethral discharge or symptoms of UTI, such as frequency of urination, dysuria, cloudy urine, or hematuria
- Initially, only the posterior-lying epididymis, usually the lowermost tail section, is very tender and indurated; will eventually progress to involvement of body and head of epididymis
- Elevation of the testes/epididymis reduces the discomfort (Prehn sign).
- Entire hemiscrotum becomes swollen and red; the testis becomes indistinguishable from the epididymis; the scrotal wall becomes thick and indurated; and reactive hydrocele may occur.
- Sterile epididymitis
  - Unilateral scrotal pain and swelling preceded by several hours of intense physical exertion. Patient may recall full bladder prior to exertion.
  - No symptoms of infection

Pediatric Considerations

- In prepubertal patients, may be postinfectious inflammatory condition; treat with anti-inflammatories, analgesics, and usually no antibiotics.
- Bacteremia from *H. influenzae* infection may produce acute epididymitis.
- In adolescent males, particularly age >13 years, must rule out testicular torsion
- History not helpful in distinguishing epididymitis from testicular torsion

Geriatric Considerations

Diabetics with sensory neuropathy may have no pain despite severe infection/abscess.

PHYSICAL EXAM

- The tail of the epididymis is larger in comparison with the contralateral side.
- Epididymis is markedly tender to palpation.
- Absence of a cremasteric reflex should raise suspicion for testicular torsion.

DIFFERENTIAL DIAGNOSIS

- Epididymal congestion following vasectomy
- Testicular torsion
- Torsion of testicular appendages
- Orchitis
- Testicular malignancy
- Testicular trauma
- Epididymal cyst
- Inguinal hernia
- Urethritis
- Spermatocele
- Hydrocele
- Hematocele
- Varicocele
- Epididymal adenomatoid tumor
- Epididymal rhabdomyosarcoma
- Vasculitis (Henoch-Schönlein purpura)

DIAGNOSTIC TESTS & INTERPRETATION

Initial Tests (lab, imaging)

- Urinalysis and urine culture, preferably on first-void urine
- GC/chlamydia testing (urethral swab or urine testing)
- Gram stain urethral discharge

- CRP >24 mg/L suggestive of epididymitis (2).
- Urinalysis clear and culture-negative suggest sterile epididymitis.
- If testicular torsion cannot be excluded (especially in children), Doppler ultrasound is test of choice (1).
- In adult men, Doppler ultrasound: sensitivity and specificity of 100% in evaluation of acute scrotum (3)

Pediatric Considerations

Further radiographic imaging in children should be done to rule out anatomic abnormalities.

Diagnostic Procedures/Other

This is a clinical diagnosis.

Test Interpretation

- Epididymis
  - Surrounding tissue fibrosis and scarring
  - Interstitial, nonspecific acute infiltration, edema, congestion, PMNs, and lymphocytes
  - Fine inflammatory adhesions
  - Can progress to abscess or necrosis
- Vas deferens
  - Possible fibrosis of this structure

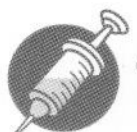

TREATMENT

- Bed rest or restriction on activity
- Athletic scrotal supporter
- Scrotal elevation
- Ice pack/warm compress
- If chemical epididymitis
  - No strenuous physical activity and avoidance of any Valsalva maneuvers for several weeks
  - Empty bladder prior to strenuous exercises.

GENERAL MEASURES

Spermatic cord block with local anesthesia in severe cases

MEDICATION

First Line

- <35 years, or suspected STD etiology: doxycycline 100 mg PO BID for 10 days **PLUS** ceftriaxone 250 mg IM × 1. Refer sexual partner(s) for evaluation and treatment if contact within 60 days of the onset of symptoms (4).
- ≥35 years, with suspected enteric organism
  - Levofloxacin (Levaquin) 500 mg/day PO for 10 days (4) OR
  - Ofloxacin 300 mg PO BID for 10 days
- Men who are at risk for both STD and enteric organism (i.e., men who have sex with men who report insertive anal intercourse): ceftriaxone 250 mg IM × 1 plus fluoroquinolone
- Analgesia (infectious and chemical epididymitis)
  - NSAIDs (e.g., naproxen or ibuprofen) for mild to moderate pain
  - Consider corticosteroid if patient cannot tolerate NSAID.
  - Acetaminophen-codeine or acetaminophen-oxycodone for moderate to severe pain
- Septic or toxic patient
  - 3rd-generation cephalosporin or aminoglycoside
- For Beçhet, sarcoid, Henoch-Schönlein purpura
  - Corticosteroids, such as methylprednisolone, 40 mg/day recommended

Second Line

- Trimethoprim-sulfamethoxazole (Bactrim, Septra) double-strength PO BID for 10–14 days; increasing bacterial resistance may limit effectiveness.
- Add rifampin (rifampicin) or vancomycin, as required.

ISSUES FOR REFERRAL

- If suspicion is high for testicular torsion or cancer, consult a urologist.
- Epididymitis in prepubertal boys requires a urology referral due to high incidence of associated urogenital abnormalities.
- If medical management fails, should be referred to urologist to rule out anatomic abnormality or chemical epididymitis

SURGERY/OTHER PROCEDURES

- Vasostomy to drain infected material if severe or refractory case
- Scrotal exploration if unable clinically to distinguish between epididymitis or testicular torsion
- Drainage of abscesses, epididymectomy (acute suppurative), or epididymo-orchiectomy in severe cases refractory to antibiotics
- Surgery to correct underlying anatomic abnormality or obstruction

INPATIENT CONSIDERATIONS

Admission Criteria/Initial Stabilization

- Intractable pain
- Sepsis
- Abscess
- Persistent vomiting
- Scheduled surgery
- Purulent drainage
- Most cases can be managed with outpatient care.

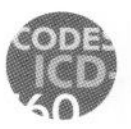

ONGOING CARE

FOLLOW-UP RECOMMENDATIONS

Patient Monitoring

- Office visits until all signs of infection have cleared
- In chemical epididymitis, follow up in 4 weeks to assess efficacy of NSAIDs and lifestyle changes.

DIET

If constipation is contributing to chemical epididymitis, consider a high-fiber diet.

PATIENT EDUCATION

- Stress completing course of antibiotics, even when asymptomatic.
- Early recognition and treatment of UTI or prostatitis
- Safer sexual practices
- If chemical epididymitis, then educate on noninfectious etiology and proper lifestyle changes.

PROGNOSIS

- Pain improves within 1–3 days, but induration may take several weeks/months to completely resolve.
- If bilateral involvement, sterility may result.
- In chemical epididymitis, symptoms usually resolve in <1 week.

COMPLICATIONS

- Recurrent epididymitis
- Infertility
- Oligospermia
- Testicular necrosis or atrophy
- Secondary abscess formation
- Fournier gangrene (necrotizing synergistic infection)

REFERENCES

1. Trojian TH, Lishnak TS, Heiman D. Epididymitis and orchitis: an overview. *Am Fam Physician*. 2009; 79(7):583–587.
2. Crawford P, Crop JA. Evaluation of scrotal masses. *Am Fam Physician*. 2014;89(9):723–727.
3. Rizvi SA, Ahmad I, Siddiqui MA, et al. Role of color Doppler ultrasonography in evaluation of scrotal swellings: pattern of disease in 120 patients with review of literature. *Urol J*. 2011;8(1):60–65.
4. http://www.cdc.gov/std/treatment/2010/default.htm. Accessed 2014.

ADDITIONAL READING

- Akinci E, Bodur H, Cevik MA, et al. A complication of brucellosis: epididymoorchitis. *Int J Infect Dis*. 2006;10(2):171–177.
- Bennett RT, Gill B, Kogan SJ. Epididymitis in children: the circumcision factor? *J Urol*. 1998;160(5): 1842–1844.
- Somekh E, Gorenstein A, Serour F. Acute epididymitis in boys: evidence of a post-infectious etiology. *J Urol*. 2004;171(1):391–394.
- Tracy CR, Steers WD, Costabile R. Diagnosis and management of epididymitis. *Urol Clin North Am*. 2008;35(1):101–108; vii.
- Wolin LH. On the etiology of epididymitis. *J Urol*. 1971;105(4):531–533.

CODES

ICD10

- N45.1 Epididymitis
- N45.3 Epididymo-orchitis
- N45.4 Abscess of epididymis or testis

CLINICAL PEARLS

- With epididymitis, the pain is gradual in onset and the tenderness is mostly posterior to the testis. With testicular torsion, the symptoms are quite rapid in onset, the testis will be higher in the scrotum and may have a transverse lie, and the cremasteric reflex will be absent. The absence of leukocytes on urine analysis and decreased blood flow on scrotal ultrasound with Doppler will suggest torsion.
- Prostatic massage is contraindicated in epididymitis because the risk for worsening local infection and potential for sepsis are increased with acute prostatitis.
- Chemical epididymitis is a clinical diagnosis of exclusion, and infectious causes are much more common; but certain occupations, such as soldiers and laborers, must be considered.

E

EPISCLERITIS

Sean M. Oser, MD, MPH • Tamara K. Oser, MD

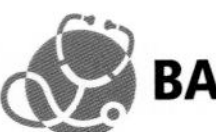

BASICS

- Episcleritis is localized inflammation of the vascular connective tissue superficial to the sclera.
- Usually a self-limited condition, typically resolving within 3 weeks.
- Most cases resolve without treatment.
- Topical lubricants and/or topical corticosteroid treatment may relieve symptoms while awaiting spontaneous resolution.

DESCRIPTION

- Edema and injection confined to the episcleral tissue
- 2 types
  - Simple (diffuse scleral involvement—more common)
  - Nodular (focal area[s] of involvement—less common)

EPIDEMIOLOGY

Slight female predominance (~60–65%)

Incidence

- May occur at any age
- Peak incidence in 40s–50s
- Community incidence not well known (~20–50 cases/100,000 person-years)

Prevalence

Not historically well known; a recent community study found a prevalence of 53 cases/100,000 persons.

ETIOLOGY AND PATHOPHYSIOLOGY

Etiology: usually idiopathic but other causes may be found (either nonimmune or immune)

Pathophysiology

- Nonimmune (e.g., dry eye syndrome, with histology showing widespread vasodilation, edema, lymphocytic infiltration)
- Immune (systemic vasculitis or rheumatologic disease)

COMMONLY ASSOCIATED CONDITIONS

- Usually not associated with another condition
- Less commonly associated conditions include the following:
  - Rheumatoid arthritis
  - Vasculitis
  - Inflammatory bowel disease
  - Ankylosing spondylitis
  - Systemic lupus erythematosus
  - Gout
  - Herpes zoster
  - Hypersensitivity disorders
    - Rosacea
    - Contact dermatitis
    - Penicillin sensitivity
    - Erythema multiforme

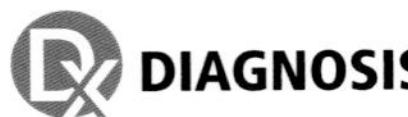

DIAGNOSIS

Episcleritis is a clinical diagnosis (1,2)[C].

HISTORY

- History should elicit potential causative factors, recurrence, or associated systemic disease (2)[C].
- Pain is often absent; when present, it is usually mild and localized to the eye (1–3)[C].
- Mild tearing may be present (2)[C].

PHYSICAL EXAM

- Check visual acuity; decreased vision is very unusual with episcleritis, and its presence should raise suspicion for another condition such as scleritis (1–3)[C].
- Focal hyperemia (2,4)[C]
- Pupils equal and reactive (2)[C]
- Superficial episcleral vascular dilation (1,2)[C]
- Episcleral edema (1,2)[C]
  - Diffuse in simple episcleritis
  - Focal in nodular episcleritis
- Tenderness over involved area may be present (2)[C] but is usually absent (3,4)[C].
- Superficial episcleral vascular hyperemia blanches with topical phenylephrine (1,4)[C].

ALERT

Recurrent episodes, difficulty confirming the diagnosis, or worsening symptoms require prompt ophthalmology referral (2)[C].

DIFFERENTIAL DIAGNOSIS

- Scleritis
- Bacterial conjunctivitis
- Viral conjunctivitis
- Herpes (ulcerative) keratitis
- Superficial keratitis
- Increased intraocular pressure (ocular hypertension)

DIAGNOSTIC TESTS & INTERPRETATION

Most patients with episcleritis do not require any further lab work or diagnostic studies (5)[C].

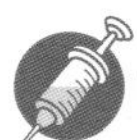

TREATMENT

MEDICATION

Treatment for episcleritis typically consists of symptomatic relief. The goal is to suppress the inflammation, which will, in turn, relieve the discomfort or pain. In most cases, treatment is not needed.

First Line

Topical lubricants such as artificial tears are typically used for initial management of symptomatic episcleritis (2)[C].

Second Line

- Topical corticosteroids are useful when discomfort is not sufficiently controlled by conservative measures (2,5,6)[C].
  - Fluorometholone 0.1% drops 4 times daily; if not effective may increase frequency
  - Prednisolone 0.5–1% eye drops
- Refractory episcleritis may be treated with oral NSAIDs, typically indomethacin 25 mg 3 or 4 times daily (5)[C].

ISSUES FOR REFERRAL

Recurrent episodes, uncertain diagnosis, and/or worsening symptoms should prompt ophthalmology referral. Rarely, episcleritis may progress to scleritis, in which case ophthalmology referral is also recommended.

ADDITIONAL THERAPIES

- Topical NSAIDs have not been shown to have a significant benefit over artificial tears (7)[B].
- When episcleritis results from viral infection, appropriate antiviral therapy is indicated (6)[C].

ONGOING CARE

FOLLOW-UP RECOMMENDATIONS

Episcleritis is usually self-limited (up to 21 days) and does not typically require follow-up.

PROGNOSIS

- Most patients have no ocular complications.
- Prognosis for episcleritis is excellent, with most patients making a full recovery.

COMPLICATIONS

Associated complications are rare, even at tertiary care referral centers, where referral bias likely overestimates their community incidence. When complications do occur, they tend not to be severe.

- Anterior uveitis may occur in 4–16% of cases (1,5,6)[C].
- Decreased vision may occur in 0–4% of cases (1,5,6)[C].
- Ocular hypertension has been in reported in 0–3.5% of cases (1,5,6)[C].

REFERENCES

1. Sainz de la Maza M, Molina N, Gonzalez-Gonzalez LA, et al. Clinical characteristics of a large cohort of patients with scleritis and episcleritis. *Ophthalmology*. 2012;119(1):43–50.
2. Cronau H, Kankanala RR, Mauger T. Diagnosis and management of red eye in primary care. *Am Fam Physician*. 2010;81(2):137–144.
3. Garrity JA. Ocular manifestations of small-vessel vasculitis. *Cleve Clin J Med*. 2012;79(Suppl 3): S31–S33.
4. Galor A, Thorne JE. Scleritis and peripheral ulcerative keratitis. *Rheum Dis Clin North Am*. 2007;33(4):835–854.
5. Jabs DA, Mudun A, Dunn JP, et al. Episcleritis and scleritis: clinical features and treatment results. *Am J Ophthalmol*. 2000;130(4):469–476.
6. Berchicci L, Miserocchi E, Di Nicola M, et al. Clinical features of patients with episcleritis and scleritis in an Italian tertiary care referral center. *Eur J Ophthalmol*. 2014;24(3):293–298.
7. Williams CP, Browning AC, Sleep TJ, et al. A randomized, double-blind trial of topical ketorolac vs artificial tears for the treatment of episcleritis. *Eye (Lond)*. 2005;19(7):739–742.

ADDITIONAL READING

- Homayounfar G, Nardone N, Borkar DS, et al. Incidence of scleritis and episcleritis: results from the Pacific Ocular Inflammation Study. *Am J Ophthalmol*. 2013;156(4):752–758.
- Honik G, Wong IG, Gritz DC. Incidence and prevalence of episcleritis and scleritis in Northern California. *Cornea*. 2013;32(12):1562–1566.

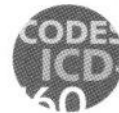

CODES

ICD10

- H15.109 Unspecified episcleritis, unspecified eye
- H15.101 Unspecified episcleritis, right eye
- H15.102 Unspecified episcleritis, left eye

CLINICAL PEARLS

- Episcleritis typically is a benign, self-limited disorder.
- Is often not painful and presents without decrease in visual acuity
- Although treatment is often not needed, when employed, the goal is symptomatic relief while awaiting spontaneous resolution.
- Associated complications are uncommon and not severe but may include anterior uveitis, decreased vision, and ocular hypertension.
- Episcleritis can be an early presentation of scleritis, which is more severe. Accurate diagnosis of episcleritis is important.

E

ERECTILE DYSFUNCTION

Michael C. Barros, PharmD, BCPS, BCACP • Neela Bhajandas, PharmD • Paul N. Williams, MD

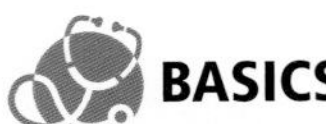

BASICS

DESCRIPTION

- Erectile dysfunction (ED): the consistent or recurrent inability to acquire or sustain an erection of sufficient rigidity and duration for sexual intercourse
- In the past, ED was assumed to be a symptom of the aging process in men, but it can result from concurrent medical conditions of the patient or from medications that patients may be taking to treat those conditions.
- Sexual problems are frequent among older men and have a detrimental effect on their quality of life but are infrequently discussed with their physicians (1).
- Synonym(s): impotence

ALERT
When ED occurs in a younger man, it is associated with a significantly increased risk of future cardiac events (2).

EPIDEMIOLOGY

Incidence

It is estimated that >600,000 new cases of ED will be diagnosed annually in the United States, although this may be an underestimation of the true incidence, as ED is vastly underreported.

Prevalence

Overall prevalence for ED:

- 52% in men age 40–70 years
- Age-related increase ranging from 12.4% in men age 40–49 years up to 46.6% in men age 50–69 years

ETIOLOGY AND PATHOPHYSIOLOGY

- ED is a neurovascular event.
  - With stimulation, there is release of nitrous oxide, which increases production of guanosine 3′,5′-cyclic monophosphate (cGMP).
  - This leads to relaxation of cavernous smooth muscle, leading to increased blood flow to penis.
  - As cavernosal sinusoids distend with blood, there is passive compression of subtunical veins, which decreases venous outflow, and this leads to an erection.
- Alterations in any of these events leads to ED.
- ED may result from problems with systems required for normal penile erection.
  - Vascular: diseases that compromise blood flow
    - Peripheral vascular disease, arteriosclerosis, essential hypertension
  - Neurologic: diseases that impair nerve conduction to brain or penile vasculature
    - Spinal cord injury, stroke, diabetes
  - Endocrine: diseases associated with changes in testosterone, luteinizing hormone, prolactin levels
  - Psychological: patients suffering from malaise, depression, performance anxiety
- Social habits such as smoking or excessive alcohol intake
- Medications may cause ED.
- Structural injury or trauma (bicycling accident)

Genetics

Rarely related to chromosomal disorders

RISK FACTORS

- Advancing age
- Cardiovascular disease
- Diabetes mellitus
- Metabolic syndrome
- Cigarette smoking
- Urologic surgery, radiation, trauma/injury to pelvic area or spinal cord
- Medications that induce ED
- Central neurologic and endocrinologic conditions
- Substance abuse
- Psychological conditions: stress, anxiety, or depression

GENERAL PREVENTION

The 2 best ways to prevent ED are by the following:

- Making healthy lifestyle choices by exercising regularly, eating well-balanced meals, limiting alcohol, and avoiding smoking
- Treating existing health problems and working with your patients to manage diabetes, heart disease, and other chronic problems

ALERT
Aging alone is not a cause.

COMMONLY ASSOCIATED CONDITIONS

- Cardiovascular disease:
  - Men with ED have a greater likelihood of having angina, myocardial infarction, stroke, transient ischemic attack, congestive heart failure, or cardiac arrhythmia compared to men without ED (3).
- Diabetes
- Psychiatric disorders

DIAGNOSIS

Inability to achieve or maintain erection satisfactory for intercourse

HISTORY

- Identify concurrent medical illnesses or surgical procedures, history of trauma, and a list of current medications (e.g., antihypertensive meds)
- Psychosocial history: smoking, ethanol intake, recreational drug use, anxiety and depression, satisfaction with current relationship
- Presence or absence of morning erections
- Speed of onset and duration of symptoms
- Relationship of symptoms to libido
- Detailed sexual history important to rule out premature ejaculation, as this is frequently confused with ED

PHYSICAL EXAM

- Signs and symptoms of hypogonadism: gynecomastia, small testicles, decreased body hair
- Penile plaques (Peyronie disease)
- Detailed examination of the cardiovascular, neurologic, and genitourinary systems
  - Blood pressure
  - Check femoral and lower extremity pulses to assess vascular supply to genitals.
  - Check anal sphincter tone and genital reflexes, including cremasterics and bulbocavernosus.

DIFFERENTIAL DIAGNOSIS

- Premature ejaculation
- Decreased libido
- Anorgasmia
- Sudden versus chronic ED

DIAGNOSTIC TESTS & INTERPRETATION

Vascular and/or neurologic assessment, and monitoring of nocturnal erections may be indicated in selected patients but not for routine workup (4)[C].

Initial Tests (lab, imaging)

- Fasting serum glucose level, lipid panel, TSH, and morning total testosterone level (3)[C]
- Doppler, angiogram, and cavernosogram are available radiologic modalities but not recommended in routine practice for the diagnosis of ED (4)[C].

Follow-Up Tests & Special Considerations

Other hormonal tests, such as prolactin, should only be ordered when there is suspicion for a specific endocrinopathy.

Diagnostic Procedures/Other

Questionnaires can be offered to assess the severity of ED, including the International Index of Erectile Function (IEFF) and its validated and more easily administered abridged version, the Sexual Health Inventory for Men (SHIM) (4)[C].

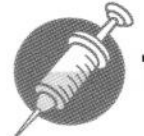

TREATMENT

- Lifestyle modifications and managing medications contributing to ED is 1st-line therapy for ED (5)[C]. Use least invasive therapy first; reserve more invasive therapies for nonresponders.
- Phosphodiesterase type 5 (PDE-5) inhibitor choice should be based on patient's preference (cost, ease of use, and adverse effects).

GENERAL MEASURES

- Psychotherapy alone or in combination with psychoactive drugs may be helpful in men whose ED is related to depression or anxiety.
- Weight loss and increased physical activity for obese men with ED

MEDICATION

First Line

Phosphodiesterase type 5 (PDE-5) inhibitors are effective in the treatment of ED in many men, including those with diabetes mellitus and spinal cord injury and sexual dysfunction associated with antidepressants (3)[A]. There is insufficient evidence to support the superiority of 1 agent over the others (5)[A]:

- Sildenafil (Viagra): usual daily dose: 50–100 mg within at least 60 minutes of sexual intercourse
- Vardenafil (Levitra): usual daily dose 5–20 mg within at least 60 minutes of sexual intercourse
- Vardenafil (Staxyn): ODT: usual dose 10 mg within 60 minutes of sexual intercourse

- Tadalafil (Cialis): usual daily dose 5–20 mg within at least 30 minutes of sexual intercourse or 2.5 mg once daily without regard to sexual activity
  - Adverse effects of PDE-5 inhibitors: headache, facial flushing, dyspepsia, nasal congestion, dizziness, hypotension, increased sensitivity to light (sildenafil and vardenafil), vision changes, lower back pain (tadalafil), and priapism (with excessive doses)
  - Sildenafil and vardenafil should be taken on an empty stomach for maximum effectiveness.

Geriatric Considerations

Use doses at the lower end of the dosing range for elderly patients.

- Sildenafil 25 mg daily
- Vardenafil 5 mg daily

Second Line

Intraurethral and intracavernosal injectables are 2nd-line therapies shown to be effective and should be administered based on patient preference (3)[B]. Intraurethral suppositories are a less invasive treatment option than intracavernosal injections; however, they are not as effective (5)[C]. Alprostadil, also known as prostaglandin E1, causes smooth muscle relaxation of the arterial blood vessels and sinusoidal tissues in the corpora:

- Intraurethral alprostadil (Muse):
  - Urethral suppository: 125-, 250-, 500-, and 1,000-μg pellets. Administer 5–50 minutes before intercourse. No more than 2 doses in 24 hours are recommended.
- Intracavernosal alprostadil (available in 2 formulations):
  - Alprostadil (Caverject): usual dose: 10–20 μg, with max dose of 60 μg. Injection should be made at right angles into one of the lateral surfaces of the proximal third of the penis using a 0.5-inch 27- or 30-gauge needle. Do not use >3 times a week or more than once in 24 hours.
  - Alprostadil may also be combined with papaverine (Bimix) plus phentolamine (Tri-Mix).

ALERT

- Initial trial dose of 2nd-line agents should be administered under supervision of a specialist or primary care physician with expertise in these therapies.
- Patient should notify physician if erection lasts >4 hours for immediate attention.
- Vacuum pump devices are a noninvasive 2nd-line option and are available over the counter. Do not use vacuum devices in men with sickle cell anemia or blood dyscrasias.
- Testosterone supplementation in men with hypogonadism improves ED and libido (3)[B]. Available formulations include injectable depots, transdermal patches and gels, SC pellets, and oral therapy.
- Contraindications:
  - Nitroglycerin (or other nitrates) and phosphodiesterase inhibitors: potential for severe, potentially fatal hypotension
  - Precautions/side effects:
    - Testosterone: *precautions*: Exogenous testosterone reduces sperm count and thus do not use in patients wishing to keep fertility; *side effects*: acne, sodium retention
    - Intraurethral suppository: local penile pain, urethral bleeding, dizziness, and dysuria
    - Intracavernosal injection: penile pain, edema and hematoma, palpable nodules or plaques, and priapism
    - Sildenafil: hypotension (caution for patients on nitrates)
    - PDE-5 inhibitors: Use caution with congenital prolonged QT syndrome, class Ia or II antiarrhythmics, nitroglycerin, α-blockers (e.g., terazosin, tamsulosin), retinal disease, unstable cardiac disease, liver and renal failure.
    - Significant possible interactions
    - PDE-5 inhibitor concentration is affected by CYP3A4 inhibitors (e.g., erythromycin, indinavir, ketoconazole, ritonavir, amiodarone, cimetidine, clarithromycin, delavirdine, diltiazem, fluoxetine, fluvoxamine, grapefruit juice, itraconazole, nefazodone, nevirapine, ritonavir, saquinavir, and verapamil). Serum concentrations and/or toxicity may be increased. Lower starting doses should be used in these patients.
    - PDE-5 inhibitor concentration may be reduced by rifampin and phenytoin.

ADDITIONAL THERAPIES

Behavioral therapy: Couples therapy aimed at improving relationship difficulties found that men who received this therapy plus sildenafil had more successful intercourse than those who received only sildenafil (6)[A].

SURGERY/OTHER PROCEDURES

Penile prosthesis should be reserved for patients who have failed or are ineligible 1st- or 2nd-line therapies.

COMPLEMENTARY & ALTERNATIVE MEDICINE

Trazodone, yohimbine, and herbal therapies are not recommended for the treatment of ED, as they have not proven to be efficacious.

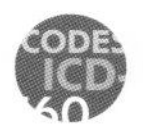

ONGOING CARE

FOLLOW-UP RECOMMENDATIONS

Patient Monitoring

Treatment should be assessed at baseline and after the patient has completed at least 1–3 weeks of a specific treatment: Monitor the quality and quantity of penile erections, and monitor the level of satisfaction patient achieves.

DIET

Diet and exercise recommended to achieve a normal body mass index; limit alcohol

PROGNOSIS

- All commercially available PDE-5 inhibitors are equally effective. In the presence of sexual stimulation, they are 55–80% effective.
  - Lower success rates with diabetes mellitus and radical prostatectomy patients who suffer from ED
- Overall effectiveness is 70–90% for intracavernosal alprostadil and 43–60% for intraurethral alprostadil (4)[B].
- Penile prostheses are associated with an 85–90% patient satisfaction rate (4)[C].

REFERENCES

1. Lindau ST, Schumm LP, Laumann EO, et al. A study of sexuality and health among older adults in the United States. *N Engl J Med*. 2007;357(8):762–774.
2. Inman BA, Sauver JL, Jacobson DJ, et al. A population-based, longitudinal study of erectile dysfunction and future coronary artery disease. *Mayo Clin Proc*. 2009;84(2):108–113.
3. Heidelbaugh JJ. Management of erectile dysfunction. *Am Fam Physician*. 2010;81(3):305–312.
4. McVary KT. Clinical practice. Erectile dysfunction. *N Engl J Med*. 2007;357(24):2472–2481.
5. The American Urological Association. Guideline on the management of erectile dysfunction: Diagnosis and treatment recommendations. Reviewed and Validity Confirmed in 2011. http://www.auanet.org/education/guidelines/erectile-dysfunction.cfm. Accessed 2015.
6. Melnik T, Soares BGO, Nasselo AG. Psychosocial interventions for erectile dysfunction. *Cochrane Database Syst Rev*. 2007;(3):CD004825.

CODES

ICD10

- N52.9 Male erectile dysfunction, unspecified
- N52.1 Erectile dysfunction due to diseases classified elsewhere
- F52.21 Male erectile disorder

CLINICAL PEARLS

- Nitrates should be withheld for 24 hours after sildenafil or vardenafil administration and for 48 hours after use of tadalafil. PDE-5 inhibitors are contraindicated in patients taking concurrent nitrates of any form (regular or intermittent nitrate therapy), as it can lead to severe hypotension and syncope.
- Reserve surgical treatment for patients who do not respond to drug treatment.
- The use of PDE-5 inhibitors with alpha-adrenergic antagonists may increase the risk of hypotension. Tamsulosin is the least likely to cause orthostatic hypotension.
- ED serves as a predictor for future cardiovascular events; thus, these patients should be followed vigilantly.

ERYSIPELAS

Fozia Akhtar Ali, MD • Mary Anne de la Cruz Estacio, DO

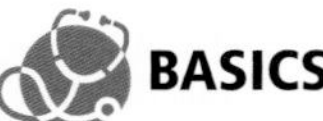

BASICS

DESCRIPTION

- Distinct form of cellulitis notable for acute, well-demarcated, superficial bacterial skin infection with lymphatic involvement almost always caused by *Streptococcus pyogenes*
- Usually acute, but a chronic recurrent form also exists (1)
- Nonpurulent
- System(s) affected: skin, exocrine
- Synonym(s): St. Anthony's fire

EPIDEMIOLOGY

- Predominant age: infants, children, and adults >40 years
- Greatest in elderly (>75 years)
- No gender/racial predilection
- Affects all races

Incidence

- Erysipelas occurs in ~1/1,000 persons/year (2).
- Incidence on the rise since the 1980s (3)

Prevalence

Unknown

ETIOLOGY AND PATHOPHYSIOLOGY

- Group A streptococci induce inflammation and activation of the contact system, a proinflammatory pathway with antithrombotic activity, releasing proteinases and proinflammatory cytokines.
- The generation of antibacterial peptides and the release of bradykinin, a proinflammatory peptide, increase vascular permeability and induce fever and pain.
- The M proteins from the group A streptococcal cell wall interact with neutrophils, leading to the secretion of heparin-binding protein, an inflammatory mediator that also induces vascular leakage.
- This cascade of reactions leads to the symptoms seen in erysipelas: fever, pain, erythema, and edema.
- Group A β-hemolytic streptococci primarily; commonly *S. pyogenes*, occasionally, other streptococcus groups C/G
- Rarely, group B streptococci/*Staphylococcus aureus* may be involved.

RISK FACTORS

- Disruption in the skin barrier (surgical incisions, insect bites, eczematous lesions, local trauma, abrasions, dermatophytic infections, intravenous drug user [IVDU])
- Chronic diseases (diabetes, malnutrition, nephrotic syndrome, heart failure)
- Immunocompromised (HIV)/debilitated
- Fissured skin (especially at the nose and ears)
- Toe-web intertrigo and lymphedema (2)
- Leg ulcers/stasis dermatitis
- Venous/lymphatic insufficiency (saphenectomy, varicose veins of leg, phlebitis, radiotherapy, mastectomy, lymphadenectomy)
- Alcohol abuse
- Morbid obesity
- Recent streptococcal pharyngitis
- Varicella

GENERAL PREVENTION

- Good skin hygiene
- It is recommended that predisposing medical conditions, such as tinea pedis and stasis dermatitis, be appropriately managed first.
- Men who shave within 5 days of facial erysipelas are more likely to have a recurrence.
- With recurrences, search for other possible sources of streptococcal infection (e.g., tonsils, sinuses).
- Compression stockings should be encouraged for patients with lower extremity edema.
- Consider suppressive prophylactic antibiotic therapy, such as penicillin, in patients with >2 episodes in a 12-month period.

Pediatric Considerations

Group B Streptococcus may be a cause of erysipelas in neonates/infants.

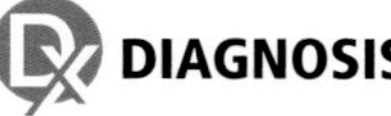

DIAGNOSIS

Prodromal symptoms before the skin eruption of erysipelas may include the following:

- Moderate- to high-grade fever
- Chills
- Headache
- Malaise
- Anorexia, usually in the 1st 48 hours (4)[B]
- Vomiting
- Arthralgias

ALERT

It is important to differentiate erysipelas from a methicillin-resistant *S. aureus* (MRSA) infection, which usually presents with an indurated center, significant pain, and later evidence of abscess formation.

PHYSICAL EXAM

- Vital signs: moderate- to high-grade fever with resultant tachycardia. Hypotension may occur.
- The presence of a fever in erysipelas can be considered a differentiating factor from other skin infections.
- Headache and vomiting may be prominent.
- Acute onset of intense erythema; well-demarcated painful plaque (5)
- Peau d'orange appearance
- Milian's ear sign distinguishing for erysipelas
- Vesicles and bullae may form but are not uniformly present.
- Desquamation may occur later.
- Lymphangitis
- Location
  - Lower extremity 70–80% of cases
  - Face involvement is less common (5–20%), especially nose and ears.
  - Chronic form usually recurs at site of the previous infection and may recur years after initial episode.
- Patients on systemic steroids may be more difficult to diagnose because signs and symptoms of the infection may be masked by anti-inflammatory action of the steroids.
- Systemic toxicity resolves rapidly with treatment; skin lesions desquamate on days 5–10 but usually heal without scarring.
- In geriatric patients, facial involvement presents in a butterfly pattern. Pustules characteristically absent and regional lymphadenopathy with lymphangitic streaking is seen.

Pediatric Considerations

- Abdominal involvement more common in infants, especially around umbilical stump
- Face, scalp, and leg involvement common in older children due to the excoriations of anterior rhinitis sicca allowing an easy port of entry

Geriatric Considerations

- Fever may not be as prominent.
- Face and lower extremity are the most common areas.
- High-output cardiac failure may occur in debilitated patients with underlying cardiac disease.
- More susceptible to complications

DIFFERENTIAL DIAGNOSIS

- Cellulitis (margins are less clear)
- Necrotizing fasciitis (systemic illness and more pain)
- Skin abscess (feel for area of fluctuance)
- DVT (need to rule out if clinically suspected)
- Acute gout (check patient history)
- Insect bite (check patient history)
- Dermatophytes
- Impetigo (blistered/crusted appearance; superficial)
- Ecthyma (ulcerative impetigo)
- Herpes zoster (dermatomal distribution)
- Erythema annulare centrifugum (raised pink-red ring/bulls-eye marks)
- Contact dermatitis (no fever, pruritic, not painful)
- Giant cell urticaria (transient, wheal-appearance, severe itching)
- Angioneurotic edema (no fever)
- Scarlet fever (widespread rash with indistinct borders and without edema; rash is most common early in skin folds; develops generalized "sandpaper" feeling as it progresses)
- Toxic shock syndrome (diffuse erythema with evidence of multiorgan involvement)
- Lupus (of the face; less fever, positive antinuclear antibodies)
- Polychondritis (common site is the ear)
- Other bacterial infections to consider:
  - Meat, shellfish, fish, and poultry workers: *Erysipelothrix rhusiopathiae* (known as erysipeloid)
  - Human bite: *Eikenella corrodens*
  - Cat/dog bite: *Pasteurella multocida/Capnocytophaga canimorsus*
  - Salt water exposure: *Vibrio vulnificus*
  - Fresh/brackish water exposure: *Aeromonas hydrophila*

DIAGNOSTIC TESTS & INTERPRETATION

Reserve diagnostic tests for severely ill, toxic patients, or those who are immunosuppressed.

Initial Tests (lab, imaging)

- Leukocytosis
- Blood culture (<5% positive)
- Elevated erythrocyte sedimentation rate (ESR) and C-reactive protein (CRP)
- Streptococci may be cultured from exudate/noninvolved sites.

Test Interpretation

Biopsy is not needed. However, skin findings would show

- Dermal and epidermal edema, extending into the SC tissues
- Peau d'orange appearance caused by edema in the superficial tissue surrounding the hair follicles
- Vasodilation and enlarged lymphatics
- Mixed interstitial infiltrate mainly consisting of neutrophils and mononuclear cells
- Endothelial cell swelling

- Gram-positive cocci in lymphatics and tissue with rare invasion of local blood vessels
- Fibrotic thickening of lymphatic vessel walls with possible luminal occlusion may be seen in recurrent erysipelas.

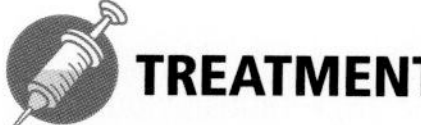

TREATMENT

GENERAL MEASURES

- Symptomatic treatment of myalgias and fever
- Adequate fluid intake
- Local treatment with cold compresses
- Elevation of affected extremity
- Appropriate therapy for any underlying predisposing condition

MEDICATION

- Antibiotics cure 50–100% of infections, but we don't know which regimen is most successful.
- We don't know whether antibiotics are as effective when given orally or intravenously.
- A 5-day course of antibiotics may be as effective as a 10-day course at curing (6)[A]

First Line

- Adults
  - Extremities, nondiabetic
    - Primary
      - Penicillin G: 1–2 million U IV q6h *or* cefazolin 1 g IV q8h
    - Alternative (if penicillin allergic)
      - Vancomycin 15 mg/kg IV q12h
      - When afebrile **Pen VK** 500 mg PO QID ac and hs
  - Total 10 days diabetics
    - Early-mild:
      - Trimethoprim-sulfamethoxazole (TMP-SMX)-DS: 1–2 tablets PO BID and penicillin VK 500 mg PO QID *or* cephalexin 500 mg PO QID
  - Severe disease
    - IMP or MER or ERTA IV and linezolid 600 mg IV/PO BID *or* vancomycin IV or daptomycin 4 mg/kg IV q24h
  - Facial
    - Primary
      - Vancomycin: 15 mg/kg (actual wt) IV q8–12h with target trough 15–20
    - Alternative
      - Daptomycin 4 mg/kg IV q24h or linezolid 600 mg IV q12h
- Children
  - Penicillin G
    - 0–7 days, <2,000 g: 50,000 U/kg q12h
    - 8–28 days, <2,000 g: 50,000 U/kg q8h
    - 0–7 days, >2,000 g = 50,000 U/kg q8h
    - 8–28 days, >2,000 g = 50,000 U/kg q6h
    - >28 days: 100,000–300,000 U/kg/day divided
  - Cefazolin
  - 0–7 days, <2,000 g: 25 mg/kg q12h
  - 8–28 days, <2,000 g: 25 mg/kg q12h
  - 0–7 days, >2,000 g = 25 mg/kg q12h
  - 8–28 days, > 2,000 g = 25 mg/kg q8h
  - >28 days: 25 mg/kg q8h
- No reported group A streptococci resistance to β-lactam antibiotics
- In chronic recurrent infections, prophylactic treatment after the acute infection resolves:
  - Penicillin G benzathine: 1.2 million U IM q4wk *or* penicillin VK 500 mg PO BID or azithromycin 250 mg PO QD
- If staphylococcal infection is suspected or patient is acutely ill, consider a β-lactamase-stable antibiotic.
- Consider community-acquired MRSA and, depending on regional sensitivity, may treat MRSA with TMP-SMX DS 1 tablet PO BID or vancomycin 1 g IV q12h or doxycycline 100 mg PO BID

ISSUES FOR REFERRAL

Recurrent infection, treatment failure

ADDITIONAL THERAPIES

Some patients may notice a deepening of erythema after initiating antimicrobial therapy. This may be due to the destruction of pathogens that release enzymes, increasing local inflammation. In this case, treatment with corticosteroids in addition to antimicrobials can mildly reduce healing time and antibiotic duration in patients with erysipelas. Consider prednisolone 30 mg/day with taper over 8 days (7).

INPATIENT CONSIDERATIONS

Admission Criteria/Initial Stabilization

- Patient with systemic toxicity
- Patient with high-risk factors (e.g., elderly, lymphedema, postsplenectomy, diabetes)
- Failed outpatient care

IV Fluids

IV therapy if systemic toxicity/unable to tolerate PO

Discharge Criteria

No evidence of systemic toxicity with resolution of erythema and swelling

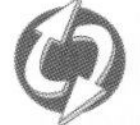

ONGOING CARE

FOLLOW-UP RECOMMENDATIONS

Bed rest with elevation of extremity during acute infection, then activity as tolerated

Patient Monitoring

Patients should be treated until all symptoms and skin manifestations have resolved.

PATIENT EDUCATION

Stress importance of completing prescribed medication regimen.

PROGNOSIS

- Patients should recover fully if adequately treated.
- May experience deepening of erythema after initiation of antibiotics
- Most respond to therapy after 24–48 hours.
- Mortality is <1% in patients receiving appropriate treatment.
- Bullae formation suggests longer disease course and often indicates a concomitant *S. aureus* infection that may require antibiotic coverage for MRSA.
- Chronic edema/scarring may result from chronic recurrent cases.
- Rarely, obstructive lymphadenitis may result from chronic recurrent cases.

COMPLICATIONS

- Recurrent infection
- Abscess (suggests staphylococcal infection)
- Necrotizing fasciitis
- Lymphedema (most prominent risk factor for recurrence) (8)
- Bacteremia, which may lead to sepsis
- Pneumonia (due to sepsis/toxin-producing organism)
- Meningitis (due to sepsis/toxin-producing organism)
- Embolism
- Gangrene
- Bursitis, septic arthritis, tendinitis, or osteitis

REFERENCES

1. Gabillot-Carré M, Roujeau JC. Acute bacterial skin infections and cellulitis. *Curr Opin Infect Dis.* 2007;20(2):118–123.
2. Bernard P. Management of common bacterial infections of the skin. *Curr Opin Infect Dis.* 2008;21(2):122–128.
3. Celestin R, Brown J, Kihiczak G, et al. Erysipelas: a common potentially dangerous infection. *Acta Dermatovenerol Alp Pannonica Adriat.* 2007;16(3):123–127.
4. Stevens DL. Practice guidelines for the diagnosis and management of skin and soft-tissue infections. *Clin Infect Dis.* 2005;41(10):1373–1406.
5. Breen JO. Skin and soft tissue infections in immunocompetent patients. *Am Fam Physician.* 2010;81(7):893–899.
6. Morris AD. Cellulitis and erysipelas. *BMJ Clin Evid.* 2008;1:1708.
7. Bergkvist PI, Sjöbeck K. Antibiotic and prednisolone therapy of erysipelas: a randomized, double blind, placebo-controlled study. *Scand J Infect Dis.* 1997;29(4):377–382.
8. Inghammar M, Rasmussen M, Linder A. Recurrent erysipelas—risk factors and clinical presentation. *BMC Infect Dis.* 2014;14:270.

ADDITIONAL READING

Gilbert D, Chambers HF, Eliopoulos GM, eds. *The Sanford Guide to Antimicrobial Therapy.* Sperryville, VA: Sanford Guides; 2014.

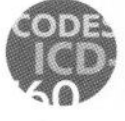

CODES

ICD10

A46 Erysipelas

CLINICAL PEARLS

- Athlete's foot is the most common portal of entry.
- Erysipelas is distinguished from cellulitis by its sharp, shiny, fiery-red, raised border.
- In recurrent cases, search for other possible source of streptococcal infection (e.g., tonsils, sinuses, intertrigo).
- Most erysipelas infections now occur on the legs rather than the face.

ERYTHEMA MULTIFORME

Cindy England Owen, MD

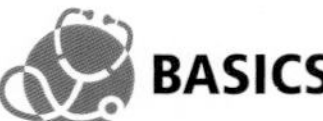

BASICS

- Erythema multiforme (EM) is an acute, self-limited hypersensitivity reaction.
  - Mostly (~90% of cases) triggered by infectious agents (up to 50% by herpes simplex virus [HSV]-1 or -2) or, less commonly, by drugs (1)
  - Involving the skin and the mucous membrane, most commonly the mouth (60–70% of all patients with EM have oral lesions)
  - Skin lesions include raised typical target or "iris" lesions or raised atypical lesions predominantly involving the extremities; flat, atypical lesions and macules with or without blisters are more suggestive of Stevens-Johnson (SJS) or toxic epidermal necrolysis (TEN).
- Currently, there are no universal diagnostic criteria for EM. It was previously considered a spectrum of disease, consisting of EM, EM major, SJS, and TEN; however, a growing consensus believes EM is a condition distinct from SJS and TEN due to the differences in clinical presentation, histopathologic features, patient demographics, possible etiology and pathogenesis, and treatment plan.

DESCRIPTION

- 2 subtypes, erythema multiforme minor (EMm) and erythema multiforme major (EMM), with the former involving none or 1 mucous membrane, and the latter involving at least 2 mucous membrane sites
- Recurrent EM is defined as >3 attacks but has a mean number of 6 attacks (range 2–24) per year and a mean duration of 6–9.5 years (range 2–36) (2,3).

EPIDEMIOLOGY

Incidence

Annual U.S. incidence is estimated at 0.01–1% (1).

Prevalence

- Peak incidence in 20s and 40s; rare <3 years and >50 years of age
- Male > Female (3:2–2:1)

ETIOLOGY AND PATHOPHYSIOLOGY

- The exact pathophysiology of EM is unknown.
- Possible immunologically mediated lymphocytic reaction to an infectious agent or a drug at the dermal–epidermal junction
- HSV-triggered EM seems to involve CD4$^+$ T-cell infiltration and associated IFN-γ activation.
- Drug-triggered EM (<10% of cases) involves CD8$^+$ T-cells and associated TNF-α activation.
- Most cases appear to be due to a preceding infection (~90% of cases), especially HSV and *Mycoplasma pneumoniae* (2,4).
- Viral infections, particularly HSV (up to 50% of cases); also Epstein-Barr, coxsackie, echovirus, varicella, mumps, poliovirus, hepatitis C, cytomegalovirus, HIV, molluscum contagiosum virus (2,4)
- Bacterial infections, particularly *M. pneumoniae;* other reported bacterial infections include *Treponema pallidum* and *Gardnerella vaginalis* (2,4).
- Fungal infection, including *Histoplasma capsulatum* and *Coccidioides immitis* (2,4)
- Medications, including sulfonamides, penicillins, anticonvulsants (carbamazepine, phenytoin, phenylbutazone, phenothiazines, barbiturates), hydantoins, NSAIDs, oral contraceptives, and statins. Other sparsely reported medications include cimetidine, salicylic acid, angiotensin receptor blockers, metformin, bupropion, ciprofloxacin, sorafenib, gemfibrozil, risperidone, paclitaxel, metoprolol, tumor necrosis factor (TNF) inhibitors (adalimumab, etanercept, infliximab), and methotrexate (2,4,5)
- Vaccines: tetanus/diphtheria, bacillus Calmette-Guérin, oral polio, hepatitis B, human papillomavirus, H1N1 influenza
- Occupational exposures: herbicides (alachlor and butachlor), iodoacetonitrile
- Protozoan infections
- Radiation therapy
- Premenstrual hormone changes
- Sarcoidosis
- Cannabis-induced EM-like drug eruption
- Rowell syndrome: lupus erythematosus (specifically, chronic cutaneous LE) with EM-like lesions

Genetics

Strong association with HLA-DQ3 in herpes-related cases (6); possible association in recurrent cases with HLA-B15, -B35, -A33, -DR53, DQB1*0301, and DQW3 (7)

RISK FACTORS

Previous history of EM

GENERAL PREVENTION

- Known or suspected etiologic agents should be avoided.
- Acyclovir or valacyclovir may help prevent herpes-related recurrent EM.

COMMONLY ASSOCIATED CONDITIONS

See "Etiology and Pathophysiology" earlier.

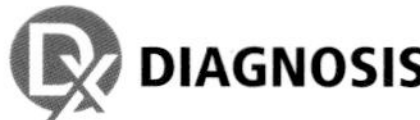

DIAGNOSIS

Clinical

HISTORY

- Absent or mild prodromal symptoms
- Preceding HSV infection (up to 50% of cases) 10–15 days before the skin eruptions
- Rash involving the skin and sometimes the mucous membrane, most commonly the mouth

PHYSICAL EXAM

- Pleomorphic skin eruption with a mixture of papules of various sizes and target lesions
  - Typical target lesions: raised and cyanotic center, edematous light intermediate ring and bright erythematous border (3 zones)
  - Raised atypical target lesions: 2 zones only (center and intermediate ring) with poorly defined border
  - Symmetrically distributed eruption, mainly on the palms, soles, dorsum of the hands, and extensor surface of the extremities and the face
- Mucosal involvement
  - Minimal involvement in EM minor; if present, most commonly involves the mouth (usually cutaneous or mucosal lips)
  - At least 2 mucosal sites involved in EM major, including eyes (conjunctivitis, keratitis); mouth (stomatitis, cheilitis, characteristic blood-stained crusted erosions on lips); and probable trachea, bronchi, GI tract, or genital tract (balanitis and vulvitis)
  - Multiple papules and vesicles, superficial irregular erosions, shallow painful ulcers with erythematous margin

DIFFERENTIAL DIAGNOSIS

- SJS
  - Generalized distribution of lesions; concentrated on the trunk
  - Absence of raised typical target lesions
  - Atypical flat target lesions or macules with coalescence of lesions
  - Blisters and skin detachment <10% of the total body surface area
  - Usually with systemic complications (i.e., CNS, lung, GI system, kidney); 1–5% mortality rate
  - Presence of high fever (>38.5°C) more likely with SJS than EM
  - More likely to have mucosal involvement at ≥2 sites, lymphadenopathy, high C-reactive protein levels (>10 mg/dL), and hepatic dysfunction
- TEN
  - Full-thickness skin necrosis and skin detachment >30% of the total body surface area
  - 10–30% mortality rate
  - Otherwise similar to SJS
- Urticaria
- Pemphigus vulgaris
- Pemphigoid
- Paraneoplastic pemphigoid
- Mucocutaneous lymph node syndrome
- Erythema annulare centrifugum
- Acute hemorrhagic edema of infancy
- Subacute cutaneous lupus erythematosus
- Necrotizing vasculitis
- Drug eruptions
- Contact dermatitis
- Pityriasis rosea
- HSV
- Secondary syphilis
- Tinea corporis
- Dermatitis herpetiformis
- Herpes gestationis
- Septicemia
- Serum sickness
- Viral exanthem
- Rocky Mountain spotted fever
- Meningococcemia
- Lichen planus
- Behçet syndrome
- Recurrent aphthous ulcers
- Herpetic gingivostomatitis
- Granuloma annulare

DIAGNOSTIC TESTS & INTERPRETATION

- No lab test is indicated to make the diagnosis of EM.
- Skin biopsy of lesional and perilesional tissue in equivocal conditions
- Direct and indirect immunofluorescence (DIF and IIF) to differentiate EM from other vesiculobullous diseases. DIF is detected on a biopsy of perilesional skin, and IIF is detected from a blood sample.
- HSV tests in recurrent EM (serologic tests, swab culture, or tests using skin biopsy sample to check HSV antigens or DNA in keratinocytes by direct immunofluorescence [DFA] or polymerase chain reaction [PCR])
- Antibody staining to IFN-γ and TNF-α to differentiate HSV- from drug-associated EM
- Elevated *M. pneumoniae* antibody titer in *M. pneumoniae*–associated EM

Initial Tests (lab, imaging)

No imaging studies are indicated in most cases unless there is suspicion for *M. pneumoniae*.

Follow-Up Tests & Special Considerations

Chest x-ray may be necessary if an underlying pulmonary infection (*M. pneumoniae*) is suspected.

Test Interpretation

- Vacuolar interface dermatitis with CD4^{+} T lymphocytes and histiocytes in papillary dermis and the dermal–epidermal junction
- Superficial perivascular lymphocytic inflammation
- Satellite cell necrosis
- Necrotic keratinocytes mainly in the basal layer
- Papillary dermal edema

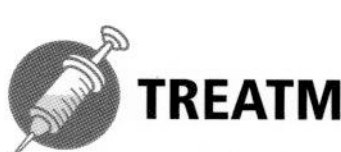

TREATMENT

GENERAL MEASURES

- Meticulous wound care and Burow solution or Domeboro solution dressings for severe cases with epidermal detachment followed by Vaseline gauze and curlex.
- Mouth washes with warm saline or a solution of diphenhydramine, lidocaine (Xylocaine), and Kaopectate for oral lesions to provide symptomatic relief and oral hygiene and to facilitate oral intake

MEDICATION

First Line

- Treatment of any underlying or causative disease
- Withdrawal of any drugs that might be the cause
- Symptomatic treatment with oral antihistamines and topical corticosteroids for mild cases; mouthwashes or topical steroid gels for oral disease
- Early treatment with acyclovir may lessen the number and duration of cutaneous lesions for patients with coexisting or recent HSV infection (2)[B].
  - Acyclovir for adults: 200 mg, 5× a day for 7–10 days in the onset of EM
  - For pediatric patients: 10 mg/kg/dose TID for 7–10 days
- Recurrent EM: oral acyclovir (400 mg BID), even if HSV infection has not been confirmed
- Valacyclovir (Valtrex, 500–1,000 mg/day) and famciclovir (Famvir, 125–250 mg/day) may be tried: Reduce dosage once the patient is recurrence-free for 4 months and eventually discontinue (8)[B].

Second Line

- Recurrent EM cases nonresponsive to antiviral therapy: dapsone (100–150 mg/day), azathioprine (Imuran, 100–150 mg/day), thalidomide (100–200 mg/day), tacrolimus (0.1% ointment daily), mycophenolate mofetil (CellCept 1000–1500 mg twice daily), hydroxychloroquine (400 mg/day), colchicine ($<$1.2 mg/day) (2,9,10)[B]
- Cyclosporine given intermittently (4 mg/kg/day for a week) may also be used for recurrent EM (10)[B].
- Systemic steroid use is controversial: may decrease the patient's resistance to HSV and increase EM eruptions

INPATIENT CONSIDERATIONS

Admission Criteria/Initial Stabilization

- Care at home
- Hospitalization needed for fluid and electrolyte management in patient with severe mucous membrane involvement, impaired oral intake, and dehydration
- IV antibiotics if secondary infection develops

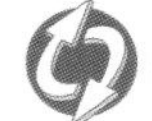

ONGOING CARE

FOLLOW-UP RECOMMENDATIONS

Patient Monitoring

- The disease is self-limiting.
- Complications are rare, with no mortality.

DIET

As tolerated, with increased fluid intake

PATIENT EDUCATION

- The disease is self-limiting. However, the recurrence risk may be 30%.
- Antiviral therapy with acyclovir may reduce the duration and frequency of outbreaks.
- Avoid any identified etiologic agents.

PROGNOSIS

- Rash evolves over 1–2 weeks and subsequently resolves within 2–6 weeks, generally without scarring or sequelae.
- Following resolution, there may be some postinflammatory hyper- or hypopigmentation.

COMPLICATIONS

Secondary infection

REFERENCES

1. Huff JC, Weston WL, Tonnesen MG. Erythema multiforme: a critical review of characteristics, diagnostic criteria, and causes. *J Am Acad Dermatol*. 1983;8(6):763.
2. Wetter DA, Davis MD. Recurrent erythema multiforme: clinical characteristics, etiologic associations, and treatment in a series of 48 patients at Mayo Clinic, 2000 to 2007. *J Am Acad Dermatol*. 2010;62(1):45–53.
3. Schofield JK, Tatnall FM, Leigh IM. Recurrent erythema multiforme: clinical features and treatment in a large series of patients. *Br J Dermatol*. 1993;128(5):542.
4. Huff JC, Weston WL, Tonnesen MG. Erythema multiforme: a critical review of characteristics, diagnostic criteria, and causes. *J Am Acad Dermatol*. 1983;8(6):763.
5. Assier H, Bastuji-Garin S, Revuz J, et al. Erythema multiforme with mucous membrane involvement and Stevens-Johnson syndrome are clinically different disorders with distinct causes. *Arch Dermatol*. 1995;131(5):539.
6. Khalil I, Lepage V, Douay C, et al. HLA DQB1*0301 allele is involved in the susceptibility to erythema multiforme. *J Invest Dermatol*. 1991;97(4):697.
7. Schofield JK, Tatnall FM, Brown J, et al. Recurrent erythema multiforme: tissue typing in a large series of patients. *Br J Dermatol*. 1994;131(4):532.
8. Tatnall FM, Schofield JK, Leigh IM. A double-blind placebo-controlled trial of continuous acyclovir in recurrent erythema multiforme. *Br J Dermatol*. 1995;132(2):267.
9. Chen M, Doherty SD, Hsu S, et al. Innovative uses of thalidomide. *Dermatol Clin*. 2010;28(3):577–586.
10. Bakis S, Zagarella S. Intermittent oral cyclosporine for recurrent herpes simplex virus associated erythema multiforme. *Australas J Dermatol*. 2005;46(1):18.

E

ADDITIONAL READING

American Academy of Allergy, Asthma and Immunology; American College of Allergy, Asthma and Immunology; Joint Council of Allergy, Asthma and Immunology. Drug allergy: an updated practice parameter. *Ann Allergy Asthma Immunol*. 2010;105(4):259.e78–273.e78.

SEE ALSO

Cutaneous Drug Reactions; Dermatitis Herpetiformis; Herpes Gestationalis; Stevens-Johnson Syndrome; Toxic Epidermic Necrotisis; Urticaria

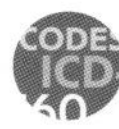

CODES

ICD10

- L51.9 Erythema multiforme, unspecified
- L51.8 Other erythema multiforme
- L51.0 Nonbullous erythema multiforme

CLINICAL PEARLS

- EM is diagnosed clinically by careful review of the history, thorough detailed physical exam, and by excluding other similar disorders. No lab tests are required for the diagnosis.
- Typical lesions are characteristic target or "iris" lesions but can include raised atypical (2-zone) targets.
- Lesions are symmetrically distributed on palms, soles, dorsum of the hands, and extensor surfaces of extremities and face. The oral mucosa is the most affected mucosal region in EM.
- Management of EM involves determining the etiology when possible. The first step is to treat the suspected infection or discontinue the causative drug.
- Complications are rare. Most cases are self-limited. However, the recurrence risk may be as high as 30%.
- Recurrent cases often are secondary to HSV infection. Antiviral therapy may be beneficial.

ERYTHEMA NODOSUM

Amy L. Lee, MD

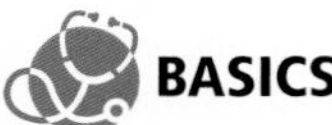

BASICS

DESCRIPTION

- A delayed-type hypersensitivity reaction to various possible antigens, or an autoimmune reaction, presenting as a panniculitis that affects subcutaneous (SC) fat
- Clinical pattern of multiple, bilateral, erythematous, tender SC nodules that undergo a characteristic pattern of color changes, similar to that seen in bruises. Unlike erythema induratum, the lesions of erythema nodosum (EN) do not typically ulcerate.
- Occurs most commonly on the shins, less commonly on the thighs, forearms, trunk, head, or neck
- May be accompanied by fever and arthralgias
- Often idiopathic but may be associated with a number of clinical entities
- Usually remits spontaneously in weeks to months without scarring or atrophy
- Synonym(s): dermatitis contusiformis

Pregnancy Considerations

May have repeat outbreaks during pregnancy

Pediatric Considerations

Rare pediatric variant has lesions only on palms or soles, often unilateral.

EPIDEMIOLOGY

Incidence

- 1–5/100,000/year
- Predominant age: 20–30 years
- Predominant sex: female > male (3:1)

Prevalence

Varies geographically depending on the prevalence of disorders associated with EN

ETIOLOGY AND PATHOPHYSIOLOGY

- Idiopathic: 33–60%
- Bacterial: 44%. Streptococcal infections (most common cause in children), tuberculosis, leprosy, tularemia, gonorrhea, *Yersinia enterocolitica*, *Campylobacter*, *Salmonella*, *Shigella*
- Sarcoidosis: 11–25%
- Drugs: sulfonamides, amoxicillin, oral contraceptives, bromides, azathioprine, vemurafenib
- Pregnancy, progesterone injection during 1st trimester as part of assisted reproductive therapy
- Fungal: dermatophytes, coccidioidomycosis, histoplasmosis, blastomycosis
- Viral/chlamydial: infectious mononucleosis, lymphogranuloma venereum, paravaccinia, HIV
- Enteropathies: ulcerative colitis, Crohn disease, Behçet disease, celiac disease, diverticulitis
- Malignancies: lymphoma/leukemia, sarcoma, myelodysplastic syndrome, after radiation therapy
- Sweet syndrome

RISK FACTORS

See "Etiology and Pathophysiology."

COMMONLY ASSOCIATED CONDITIONS

See "Etiology and Pathophysiology."

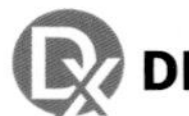

DIAGNOSIS

HISTORY

- Increasingly tender and aching nodules on the legs, usually over the shins
- Fever, malaise, chills, fatigue
- Eruptions often preceded by symptoms of pharyngitis or upper respiratory infection
- Headache
- Arthralgias

PHYSICAL EXAM

- Initially warm, tender, brightly erythematous nodules, often raised, on anterior shins; lesions become bluish and fluctuant, gradually fading to resemble a bruise.
- May occur on any area with SC fat
- Diameter usually 2–6 cm but may rarely be larger

DIFFERENTIAL DIAGNOSIS

- Nodular vasculitis or erythema induratum (warm ulcerating calf nodules)
- Superficial thrombophlebitis
- Cellulitis
- Septic emboli
- Weber-Christian disease (violaceous, scarring nodules)
- Lupus panniculitis
- Cutaneous polyarteritis nodosa
- Sarcoidal granulomas
- Cutaneous T-cell lymphoma
- Erythema nodosum leprosum (clinically similar to EN but shows vasculitis on histopathology)
- Vasculitis

DIAGNOSTIC TESTS & INTERPRETATION

Diagnosis is made clinically, with support of testing.

- ESR or C-reactive protein (CRP): may be elevated or normal (1)[C]
- CBC: mild leukocytosis (1)[C]
- Urine pregnancy test in women (1)[C]
- Throat culture, antistreptolysin O titer (1)[C]
- Blood and/or stool culture, stool ova and parasites (O&P)
- Tuberculin skin testing (1)[C]
- Drugs that may alter lab results: Prior antibiotics may affect cultures.

Initial Tests (lab, imaging)

CXR for hilar adenopathy or infiltrates related to sarcoidosis or tuberculosis (1)[C]

Diagnostic Procedures/Other

Deep-incisional skin biopsy including SC fat; rarely necessary except in atypical cases with ulceration, duration >12 weeks (2)[C]

Test Interpretation

- Septal panniculitis without vasculitis
- Neutrophilic infiltrate in septa of fat tissue early in course
- Actinic radial (Miescher) granulomas, consisting of collections of histocytes around a central stellate cleft, may be seen.
- Fibrosis, paraseptal granulation tissue, lymphocytes, and multinucleated giant cells predominate late in course.

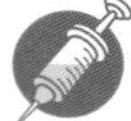

TREATMENT

- Medication more effective for acute than chronic disease
- Condition usually self-limited
- All medications listed as treatment for erythema nodosum are off-label uses of the medications. There are no FDA-approved medications for EN.

GENERAL MEASURES

- Mild compression bandages and leg elevation may reduce pain. (Wet dressings, hot soaks, and topical medications are not useful.)
- Discontinue potentially causative drugs.
- Treat underlying disease.

MEDICATION

First Line

- NSAIDs
  - Ibuprofen 400 mg PO q4–6h (not to exceed 3,200 mg/day)
  - Indomethacin 25–50 mg PO TID
  - Naproxen (Naprosyn) 250–500 mg PO BID
- Precautions
  - GI upset/bleeding
  - Fluid retention
  - Renal insufficiency
  - Dose reduction in elderly, especially those with renal disease, diabetes, or heart failure
  - May mask fever
  - NSAIDs can increase cardiovascular (CV) risk.
- Significant possible interactions
  - May blunt antihypertensive effects of diuretics and β-blockers
  - NSAIDs can elevate plasma lithium levels.
  - NSAIDs can cause significant elevation and prolongation of methotrexate levels.

Second Line

- Potassium iodide 400–900 mg/day divided BID or TID × 3–4 weeks (for persistent lesions); need to monitor for hypothyroidism with prolonged use; pregnancy class D (3)[B]
- Corticosteroids for severe, refractory cases in which an infectious workup is negative. Prednisone 1 mg/kg/day for 1–2 weeks often helps resolve the lesions. Potential side effects include hyperglycemia, hypertension, weight gain, worsening gastroesophageal reflux disease (GERD), mood changes, bone loss, osteonecrosis, myopathy.
- For EN related to Behçet disease, colchicine 0.6–1.2 mg BID. Potential side effects include GI upset and diarrhea (4)[B].
- Some case reports of treating refractory EN successfully with minocycline (5)[C] and hydroxychloroquine (6)[C].

COMPLEMENTARY & ALTERNATIVE MEDICINE

Vitamin B_{12} replacement. A single case report of resolution of lesions with B_{12} replacement in a patient who had B_{12} deficiency and EN (7)[C].

INPATIENT CONSIDERATIONS

Admission Criteria/Initial Stabilization

Occasionally, admission may be needed for the antecedent illness (e.g., tuberculosis).

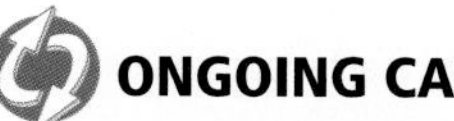

ONGOING CARE

FOLLOW-UP RECOMMENDATIONS

- Keep legs elevated.
- Elastic wraps or support stockings may be helpful when patients are ambulating.

Patient Monitoring

Monthly follow-up or as dictated by underlying disorder

DIET

No restrictions

PATIENT EDUCATION

- Lesions will resolve over a few weeks to months
- Scarring is unlikely.
- Joint aches and pains may persist.
- <20% recur

PROGNOSIS

- Individual lesions resolve generally within 2 weeks.
- Total time course of 6–12 weeks but may vary with underlying disease.
- Joint aches and pains may persist for years.
- Lesions do not scar.
- Recurrences in 12–14% of patients: Occurs over variable periods, averaging several years; seen most often in sarcoid, streptococcal infection, pregnancy, and oral contraceptive use.

COMPLICATIONS

- Vary according to underlying disease
- None expected from lesions of erythema nodosum

REFERENCES

1. Cribier B, Caille A, Heid E, et al. Erythema nodosum and associated diseases. A study of 129 cases. *Int J Dermatol*. 1998;37(9):667–672.
2. Requena L, Yus ES. Erythema nodosum. *Dermatol Clin*. 2008;26(4):425–438.
3. Horio T, Imamura S, Danno K, et al. Potassium Iodide in the treatment of erythema nodosum and nodular vasculitis. *Arch Dermatol*. 1981;117(1):29–31.
4. Yurdakul S, Mat C, Tüzün Y, et al. A double-blind trial of colchicine in Behçet's syndrome. *Arthritis Rheum*. 2001;44(11):2686–2692.
5. Davis MD. Response of recalcitrant erythema nodosum to tetracyclines. *J Am Acad Dermatol*. 2011;64(6):1211–1212.
6. Alloway JA, Franks LK. Hydroxychloroquine in the treatment of chronic erythema nodosum. *Br J Dermatol*. 1995;132(4):661–662.
7. Volkov I, Rudoy I, Press Y. Successful treatment of chronic erythema nodosum with vitamin B12. *J Am Board Fam Pract*. 2005;18(6):567–569. 16322421.

ADDITIONAL READING

- Bartyik K, Várkonyi A, Kirschner A, et al. Erythema nodosum in association with celiac disease. *Pediatr Dermatol*. 2004;21(3):227–230.
- Chong TA, Hansra NK, Ruben BS, et al. Diverticulitis: an inciting factor in erythema nodosum. *J Am Acad Dermatol*. 2012;67(1):e60–e62.
- Harris T, Henderson MC. Concurrent Sweet's syndrome and erythema nodosum. *J Gen Intern Med*. 2011;26(2):214–215.
- Jeon HC, Choi M, Paik SH, et al. A case of assisted reproductive therapy-induced erythema nodosum. *Ann Dermatol*. 2011;23(3):362–364.
- Schwartz RA, Nervi SJ. Erythema nodosum: a sign of systemic disease. *Am Fam Physician*. 2007;75(5):695–700.
- Then C, Langer A, Adam C, et al. Erythema nodosum associated with myelodysplastic syndrome: a case report. *Onkologie*. 2011;34(3):126–128.

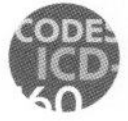

CODES

ICD10

- L52 Erythema nodosum
- A18.4 Tuberculosis of skin and subcutaneous tissue

CLINICAL PEARLS

- Lesions of EN appear to be erythematous patches, but when palpated, their underlying nodularity is appreciated.
- Evaluation for a concerning underlying etiology is necessary in EN, but most cases are idiopathic.
- EN in the setting of hilar adenopathy may be seen with multiple etiologies and does not exclusively indicate sarcoidosis.
- In patients with a history of Hodgkin lymphoma, EN may be an early sign of recurrence.

ESOPHAGEAL VARICES

Avani Sinha, MD • Edward Feller, MD, FACP, FACG

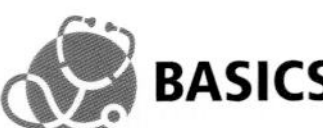

BASICS

DESCRIPTION

- Dilated distal esophageal veins connecting the portal and systemic circulations
- Results from portal hypertension (most commonly due to cirrhosis of the liver), resistance to portal blood flow, and increased portal venous blood inflow
- Superficial location of distal esophageal veins makes them susceptible to rupture.
- Esophageal variceal rupture is the most common fatal complication of cirrhosis; severity of liver disease correlates with presence of varices and risk of bleeding.

EPIDEMIOLOGY

Incidence

- At the time of diagnosis, 30% of patients with cirrhosis have varices. This increases to 90% after 10 years (1).
- 1-year rate of first variceal bleeding is 5% for small varices, 15% for large varices.

Pediatric Considerations

Portal hypertension is a common complication of chronic liver disease in children. No clear guidelines for screening, endoscopy, or pharmacologic treatment (2)

Prevalence

- 50% of patients with esophageal varices will have a bleeding episode at some point during their lifetime.
- Bleeding from esophageal varices is associated with 15–20% mortality in the first 6 weeks following the bleeding episode.
- Predominant gender: male > female

ETIOLOGY AND PATHOPHYSIOLOGY

- Fibrous tissue and regenerative nodules associated with cirrhosis lead to splanchnic arteriolar vasodilatation, increased portal inflow, and increased resistance to outflow resulting in portal hypertension. Increased production of endothelin-1 and decreased production of nitrous oxide causes intrahepatic vasoconstriction and further reductions in flow (1).
- Portal hypertension: defined as a pressure gradient >10 mm Hg between the portal vein and inferior vena cava. Collateral vessels (varices) form to decompress portal circulation.
- Cirrhotic portal hypertension
  - >90% of cases
  - Alcohol and hepatitis C are the most common causes. Less common are hemochromatosis, hepatitis B, and nonalcoholic fatty liver disease such as biliary and autoimmune cirrhosis.
- Noncirrhotic portal hypertension
  - Extrahepatic portal or splenic vein thrombosis from umbilical vein infection, trauma, chronic pancreatitis, thrombotic disease, polycythemia
  - Malignant invasion of liver sinusoids/portal vein in lymphoma, leukemia, hepatocellular, or other carcinomas.
  - Metabolic disease altering liver sinusoids: amyloidosis, Gaucher disease, Budd-Chiari syndrome, veno-occlusive disease

Genetics

Cirrhosis is rarely hereditary.

RISK FACTORS

- Cirrhosis: alcohol abuse, viral hepatitis, autoimmune inflammation, hemochromatosis, Wilson disease, primary biliary cirrhosis, primary sclerosing cholangitis, nonalcoholic fatty liver disease, or medications
- In cirrhotic patients, thrombocytopenia and splenomegaly, correlated with portal hypertension, are independent predictors of esophageal varices.
- Noncirrhotic portal hypertension

GENERAL PREVENTION

- Prevention of underlying causes of cirrhosis: alcohol abuse, hepatitis B vaccine, needle hygiene, or detox in IV drug use (IVDU) to avoid hepatitis C exposure; specific screening and therapy for hepatitis B and C, hemochromatosis (3)
- See "Treatment" section for prevention of 1st and 2nd bleeds.

COMMONLY ASSOCIATED CONDITIONS

- Portal hypertensive gastropathy; varices in stomach, duodenum, colon, rectum (causes massive bleeding, unlike hemorrhoids); rarely at umbilicus (caput medusa) or ostomy sites
- Isolated gastric varices can occur due to splenic vein thrombosis/stenosis from hypercoagulability/contiguous inflammation (most commonly, chronic pancreatitis). Tumors can compress/infiltrate the splenic vein leading to pressure increase in short gastric veins. Signs of portal hypertension may be absent (4).
- Other complications of cirrhosis: hepatic encephalopathy, ascites, hepatorenal syndrome, spontaneous bacterial peritonitis, hepatocellular carcinoma

DIAGNOSIS

- First indication of varices often associated with GI bleeding episode: painless hematemesis, hematochezia, and/or melena
- Occult bleeding (anemia): uncommon

HISTORY

- Underlying history of cirrhosis/liver disease. Variceal bleed can be initial presentation of previously undiagnosed cirrhosis.
- Painless hematemesis, melena, or hematochezia
- Rapid upper GI bleed can present as rectal bleeding.

PHYSICAL EXAM

- Assess hemodynamic stability: hypotension/tachycardia (active bleeding).
- Assess airway integrity.
- Small, hard liver; hepatomegaly possible
- Splenomegaly, ascites
- Visible abdominal periumbilical collateral circulation (caput medusae)
- Peripheral stigmata of alcoholism: spider angiomata on chest/back, palmar erythema, testicular atrophy, gynecomastia
- Anal varices (which collapse with digital pressure, whereas hemorrhoids do not)
- Hepatic encephalopathy; asterixis
- Blood on rectal exam

DIFFERENTIAL DIAGNOSIS

- Upper GI bleeding: 10–30% due to varices
  - In patients with known varices, as many as 50% bleed from nonvariceal sources.
  - Peptic ulcer disease; gastritis
  - Gastric/esophageal malignancy
  - Congestive gastropathy of portal hypertension
  - Arteriovenous malformation
  - Mallory-Weiss tears
  - Aortoenteric fistula
  - Hemoptysis; nosebleed
- Lower GI bleeding
  - Rectal varices; hemorrhoids
  - Colonic neoplasia
  - Diverticulosis/arteriovenous malformation
  - Rapidly bleeding upper GI site
- Continued/recurrent bleeding risk: actively bleeding/large varix, high Childs-Pugh severity score, infection, renal failure

DIAGNOSTIC TESTS & INTERPRETATION

Initial Tests (lab, imaging)

- Anemia from blood loss; hemoglobin may be normal in cases of active bleeding; may require 6–24 hours to equilibrate; other causes of anemia are common in cirrhotics.
- Thrombocytopenia: most sensitive and specific lab parameter—indicates portal hypertension, large esophageal varices
- Abnormal aspartate aminotransferase (AST), alanine aminotransferase (ALT), alkaline phosphatase, bilirubin, prolonged PT, or low albumin reflects cirrhosis (6).
- BUN, creatinine
- Esophagogastroduodenoscopy (7)[A]
  - Can identify actively bleeding varices as well as large varices and stigmata of recent bleeding
  - Can treat active bleeding with esophageal band ligation (preferred to sclerotherapy); prevent rebleeding; can detect gastric varices, portal hypertensive gastropathy; diagnose alternative bleeding site, such as ulcer
  - Can also identify and treat nonbleeding varices appearing as protruding submucosal veins in the distal third of the esophagus.

Diagnostic Procedures/Other

- Hepatic vein pressure gradient (HVPG) > 10 mm Hg: significant portal hypertension (normal: 1–5 mm Hg) (5)[A]. Non-invasive alternatives to HVPG (e.g., measure of spleen stiffness) are not sufficiently accurate.
- Video capsule endoscopy screening: In early trials, has lower sensitivity and specificity for detection; not able to treat varices; may be an alternative for those unwilling to undergo screening endoscopy
- Doppler sonography (second line): demonstrates patency, diameter, and flow in portal and splenic veins, and intra-abdominal collaterals; very sensitive for gastric varices; and to document patency after ligation or transjugular intrahepatic portosystemic shunt (TIPS)

- MRI (second line, not routine): demonstrates large vascular channels in abdomen, mediastinum; demonstrates patency of intrahepatic portal vein and splenic vein
  - Venous-phase celiac arteriography: demonstrates portal vein and collaterals; diagnoses hepatic vein occlusion
  - Portal pressure measurement using retrograde catheter in hepatic vein

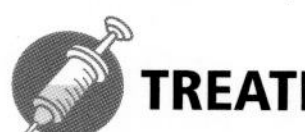

TREATMENT

GENERAL MEASURES

- Treat underlying comorbidities related to cirrhosis.
- Variceal bleeding is often complicated by hepatic encephalopathy and infection.
- Active bleeding (7)[A]
  - IV access, hemodynamic resuscitation.
  - Type and cross-match packed RBCs. Overtransfusion increases portal pressure and increases rebleeding risk.
  - Treat coagulopathy as necessary. Fresh frozen plasma may increase blood volume and increase rebleeding risk.
  - Avoid sedation, monitor mental status, and avoid nephrotoxic drugs and β-blockers acutely.
  - Thiamine replacement as indicated, monitor blood glucose, risk for alcohol withdrawal and delirium tremens
  - IV octreotide to lower portal venous pressure as adjuvant to endoscopic management. IV bolus of 50 μg followed by drip of 50 μg/hour.
  - Terlipressin (alternative): 2 mg q4h IV for 24–48 hours, then 1 mg q4h
  - Urgent upper endoscopy for diagnosis and treatment
    - Variceal band ligation/sclerotherapy for any bleeding varices. Also for nonbleeding medium-to-large varices to decrease bleeding risk
    - Variceal band ligation is preferred, fewer complications and more rapid cessation of bleeding.
- Repeat ligation/sclerosant for rebleeding.
- If endoscopic treatment fails to stop bleeding, consider per oral placement of Sengstaken-Blakemore-type tube to stabilize patient for TIPS.
- As many as two-thirds of patients with variceal bleeding develop an infection. Antibiotic prophylaxis for spontaneous peritonitis with oral norfloxacin 400 mg or IV ceftriaxone 1 g every 12 hours for up to a week.
- In active bleeding, avoid β-blockers, which decrease BP and blunt the physiologic increase in heart rate during acute hemorrhage.
- Preventing recurrence of acute bleeding
  - Vasoconstrictors: terlipressin, octreotide (reduce portal pressure)
  - Endoscopic band ligation (EBL): if bleeding recurs/portal pressure measurement shows portal pressure remains >12 mm Hg
  - TIPS: Second-line therapy if above methods fail; TIPS decreases portal pressure by creating communication between hepatic vein and an intrahepatic portal vein branch.

MEDICATION

Primary prevention of variceal bleeding

- Endoscopy: assesses variceal size, presence of red wale sign (longitudinal variceal reddish streak that suggests either a recent bleed or a pending bleed) to determine risk stratification.
  - Endoscopy every 2–3 years if cirrhosis but no varices; every 1–2 years if small varices and not receiving β-blockers

First Line

- (Not actively bleeding). Nonselective β-blockers reduce portal pressure and decrease risk of first bleed from 25% to 15% in primary prophylaxis. Used in cirrhosis with small varices and increased hemorrhage risk, as well as cirrhosis + medium-to-large varices (8)[A]
  - Propranolol: 40 mg BID increase until heart rate decreased by 25% from baseline
  - Nadolol 80 mg daily; increase as above
  - Contraindications: severe asthma
- Chronic prevention of rebleeding (secondary prevention): Nonselective β-blockers and EBL reduce the rate of rebleeding to a similar extent, but β-blockers reduce mortality, whereas ligation does not.

Second Line

Obliteration of varices with esophageal banding for those intolerant of medication prophylaxis

- During ligation: proton pump inhibitors, such as lansoprazole 30 mg/day, until varices obliterated

ISSUES FOR REFERRAL

Primarily, those associated with endoscopy, liver transplantation, interventional radiology for TIPS procedure; refer for liver transplantation in appropriate (eligible) patients.

ADDITIONAL THERAPIES

Patients should receive pneumococcal vaccine and hepatitis A/B virus (HAV/HBV) vaccine.

SURGERY/OTHER PROCEDURES

- Esophageal transection: in rare cases of uncontrollable, exsanguinating bleeding
- Liver transplantation: referral after diagnosis

INPATIENT CONSIDERATIONS

Admission Criteria/Initial Stabilization

Inpatient for acute bleeding and hemodynamic stabilization and therapeutic endoscopy. ICU care often most appropriate initially.

Discharge Criteria

Cessation of bleeding, stability of comorbidities, complications

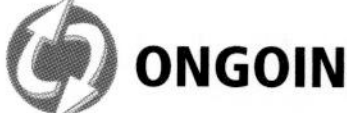

ONGOING CARE

FOLLOW-UP RECOMMENDATIONS

Patient Monitoring

- Close monitoring of vital signs
- Endoscopic variceal ligation, repeated every 1–4 weeks until varices eradicated
- If TIPS, repeat endoscopy if clinically bleeding.
- Post-TIPS follow-up: Doppler sonogram every 6 months to assess shunt patency
- Endoscopic screening in patients with known cirrhosis every 2–3 years; yearly in patients with decompensated cirrhosis

PATIENT EDUCATION

National Digestive Information Clearinghouse, (digestive.niddk.nih.gov/) or American Liver Foundation, (www.liverfoundation.org)

PROGNOSIS

- Depends on underlying comorbidities
- In patients with cirrhosis, 1-year survival is 50% for those surviving 2 weeks following a variceal bleed
- Prognosis in noncirrhotic portal fibrosis is better than for patients with cirrhosis.

COMPLICATIONS

- Formation of gastric varices or varices in other uncommon locations may occur after eradication of esophageal varices.
- Esophageal varices can recur.
- Hepatic encephalopathy, renal dysfunction, hepatorenal syndrome
- Infections are common after banding/ligation of varices.

REFERENCES

1. Asrani SK, Kamath PS. Natural history of cirrhosis. *Curr Gastroenterol Rep*. 2013;15(2):8–13.
2. D'Antiga L. Medical management of esophageal varices and portal hypertension in children. *Semin Pediatr Surg*. 2012;21(3):211–218.
3. Simonetto DA, Shah VH, Kamath PS. Primary prophylaxis of variceal bleeding. *Clin Liver Dis*. 2014; 18(2):335–345.
4. Irani S, Kowdley K, Kozarek R. Gastric varices: an updated review of management. *J Clin Gastroenterol*. 2011;45(2):133–148.
5. de Franchis R, Dell'Era A. Invasive and noninvasive methods to diagnose portal hypertension and esophageal varices. *Clin Liver Dis*. 2014;18:293–302.
6. Woreta TA, Alqahtani SA. Evaluation of abnormal liver tests. *Med Clin North Am*. 2014;98(1):1–16.
7. Herrera JL. Management of acute variceal bleeding. *Clin Liver Dis*. 2014;18(2):347–357.
8. Albillos A, Tejedor M. Secondary prophylaxis for esophageal variceal bleeding. *Clin Liver Dis*. 2014;18(2):359–370.

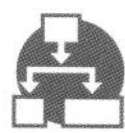

SEE ALSO

Cirrhosis of the Liver; Portal Hypertension

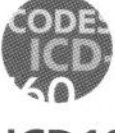

CODES

ICD10

- I85.00 Esophageal varices without bleeding
- I85.01 Esophageal varices with bleeding
- I85.10 Secondary esophageal varices without bleeding

CLINICAL PEARLS

- In acute bleeding, avoid β-blockers, which decrease BP and blunt the physiologic increase in heart rate.
- In acute bleeding, overtransfusion can elevate portal pressure and increases bleeding risk.
- Thrombocytopenia: sensitive marker of increased portal pressure, large esophageal varices
- During bleeding, consider antibiotic prophylaxis for spontaneous peritonitis and other infections with IV ciprofloxacin or oral norfloxacin for 7–10 days.
- Upper GI bleeds, with brisk variceal bleeding, can present with painless rectal bleeding.

E

ESSENTIAL TREMOR SYNDROME

Jonathon M. Firnhaber, MD

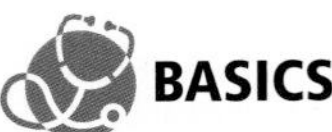

BASICS

DESCRIPTION

- A postural (occurring with voluntary maintenance of a position against gravity) or kinetic (occurring during voluntary movement) flexion–extension tremor that is slow and rhythmic and primarily affects the hands and forearms, head, and voice with a frequency of 4–12 Hz
- Older patients tend to have lower frequency tremors, whereas younger patients exhibit frequencies in the higher range.
- May be familial, sporadic, or associated with other movement disorders
- Can begin at any age but the incidence and prevalence increase with age
- The tremor can be exacerbated by emotional or physical stresses, fatigue, and caffeine.
- System(s) affected: neurologic, musculoskeletal, ear/nose/throat (ENT) (voice)

EPIDEMIOLOGY

Essential tremor is the most common pathologic tremor in humans.

Incidence

- Can occur at any age but bimodal peaks exist in the 2nd and 6th decades.
- Incidence rises significantly after age 49 years.

Prevalence

The overall prevalence for essential tremor has been estimated between 0.4 and 0.9% but is increased in older (65 years) patients to 4.6% and in advanced age (95 years) up to 22% (1)[B].

ETIOLOGY AND PATHOPHYSIOLOGY

- Suspected to originate from an abnormal oscillation within thalamocortical and cerebello-olivary loops, as lesions in these areas tend to reduce essential tremor.
- Essential tremor is not a homogenous disorder; many patients have other motor manifestations and nonmotor features, including cognitive and psychiatric symptoms.

Genetics

- Positive family history in 50–70% of patients; autosomal dominant inheritance is demonstrated in many families, but twin studies suggest that environmental factors are also involved.
- A link to genetic loci exists on chromosomes 2p22–25, 3q13, and 6p23. In addition, a Ser9Gly variant in the dopamine D_3 receptor gene on 3q13 has been suggested as a risk factor.

COMMONLY ASSOCIATED CONDITIONS

- Can be present in 10% of patients with Parkinson disease (PD); characteristics of PD that distinguish it from essential tremor include 3–5-Hz resting tremor; accompanying rigidity, bradykinesia, or postural instability; and no change with alcohol consumption.
- Patients with essential tremor have a 4% risk of developing PD. Although action tremors may precede PD, they will be diagnosed as essential tremor as long as the bradykinesia and rigidity of PD are not yet present (1)[B].
- Resting tremor, typically of the arm, may be seen in up to 20–30% of patients with essential tremor. Although action tremor is the hallmark feature of essential tremor, it is commonly found in patients with PD as well.

DIAGNOSIS

HISTORY

- Core criteria for diagnosis
  - Bilateral (less likely unilateral) action (postural or kinetic) tremor of the hands and forearms that is most commonly asymmetric
  - Absence of other neurologic signs, with the exception of cogwheel phenomenon
  - May have isolated head tremor with no signs of dystonia
- Secondary criteria include long duration (>3 years), positive family history, and beneficial response to alcohol (2)[C].

PHYSICAL EXAM

- Tremor can affect upper limbs (~95% of patients).
- Less commonly, the tremor affects head (~34%), lower limbs (~30%), voice (~12%), tongue (~7%), face (~5%), and trunk (~5%).

DIFFERENTIAL DIAGNOSIS

- PD
- Wilson disease
- Hyperthyroidism
- Multiple sclerosis
- Dystonic tremor
- Cerebellar tremor
- Asterixis
- Psychogenic tremor
- Orthostatic tremor
- Drug-induced or enhanced physiologic tremor (amiodarone, cimetidine, lamotrigine, itraconazole, valproic acid, SSRIs, steroids, lithium, cyclosporine, β-adrenergic agonists, ephedrine, theophylline, tricyclic antidepressants [TCAs], antipsychotics) (3)[B].

DIAGNOSTIC TESTS & INTERPRETATION

Initial Tests (lab, imaging)

- No specific biologic marker or diagnostic test is available.
- Ceruloplasmin and serum copper to rule out Wilson disease
- Thyroid-stimulating hormone to rule out thyroid dysfunction
- Serum electrolytes, BUN, creatinine
- Brain MRI usually is not necessary or indicated unless Wilson disease is found or exam findings imply central lesion.

Diagnostic Procedures/Other

- Accelerometry evaluates tremor frequency and amplitude; more than 95% of PD cases exhibit frequencies in the 4–6-Hz range, and 95% of essential tremor cases exhibit frequencies in the 5–8-Hz range.
- Surface electromyography is less helpful in distinguishing essential tremor from PD.

Test Interpretation

Posture-related tremor

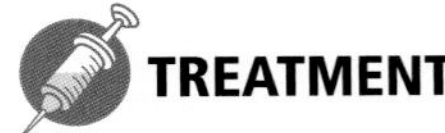

TREATMENT

MEDICATION

Pharmacologic treatment should be considered when tremor interferes with activities of daily living (ADLs) or causes psychological distress.

First Line

- Propranolol 60–320 mg/day in divided doses or in long-acting formulation reduces limb tremor magnitude by ~50%, and almost 70% of patients experience improvement in clinical rating scales. There is insufficient evidence to recommend propranolol for vocal tremor. Single doses of propranolol, taken before social situations that are likely to exacerbate tremor, are useful for some patients.
- Primidone 25 mg at bedtime, gradually titrated to 150–300 mg at bedtime, improves tremor amplitude by 40–50%. Maximum dose is 750 mg/day, with doses >250 mg/day typically divided to BID or TID. Low-dose therapy (<250 mg/day) is just as effective as high-dose (750 mg/day) therapy.
- Propranolol and primidone have similar efficacy when used as initial therapy for limb tremor; both carry a level A recommendation (4)[A].
- 30–50% of patients will not respond to either propranolol or primidone.

Second Line

- Topiramate at a mean dose of 292 mg/day demonstrated significantly greater reduction in tremor rating scale (TRS) compared with placebo (7.7 vs. 0.08; $p < .005$; baseline TRS = 37.0) in a small study combining results of 3 double-blind, randomized, controlled trials following a common protocol. Use is limited by dropout rates as high as 40% due to appetite suppression, weight loss, paresthesias, and concentration difficulties (5)[B].
- Gabapentin up to 400 mg TID
- Sotalol, nadolol, and atenolol are alternative β-blockers; each has less evidence than propranolol to support use.
- Clonazepam and alprazolam should be used with caution because of abuse potential.
- Clozapine has shown efficacy at doses of 6–75 mg/day but is recommended only for refractory cases of limb tremor because of a 1% risk of agranulocytosis. The American Academy of Neurology (AAN) indicates that insufficient evidence exists to support or refute the efficacy of clozapine for chronic use (4)[A].
- Memantine, in a pilot study using doses up to 40 mg/day, showed significant benefit in a small subset of the study group. Adverse events at this dose included dizziness, somnolence, and poor energy (6)[B].
- Levetiracetam and 3,4-diaminopyridine are probably ineffective at reducing limb tremor and should not be considered according to the AAN (4)[A].
- Other medications that have been evaluated for treatment of essential tremor, with limited data to support their use, include acetazolamide, clonidine, flunarizine, methazolamide, nimodipine, olanzapine, phenobarbital, pregabalin, quetiapine, sodium oxybate, and zonisamide (4)[A].
- Alcohol may provide transient improvement in symptoms, but its brief duration of action, subsequent rebound, and associated risk of developing alcohol addiction make it an inappropriate treatment.
- Botulinum toxin A injections should be offered as a treatment option for cervical dystonia (level A recommendation from AAN) and may be offered for blepharospasm, focal upper extremity dystonia, adductor laryngeal dystonia, and upper extremity essential tremor. Limited data support its use for head and voice tremor (7)[B].

ISSUES FOR REFERRAL

Referral to a neurologist can help to differentiate those with dystonia, neuropathic tremor, PD, or drug-induced tremor.

SURGERY/OTHER PROCEDURES

- Deep brain stimulation provides a magnitude of benefit that is superior to all available medications and may be used to treat medically refractory limb tremor; it has fewer adverse effects than thalamotomy (8)[B].
- Bilateral thalamic stimulation is effective in reducing tremor and functional disability; however, dysarthria is a possible complication.
- Unilateral thalamotomy may be used to treat limb tremor that is refractory to medical management.
- Bilateral thalamotomy is not recommended because of adverse side effects.

ONGOING CARE

DIET

Avoid caffeine.

PROGNOSIS

Tremor tends to worsen with age, increasing in amplitude.

REFERENCES

1. Elias WJ, Shah BB. Tremor. *JAMA*. 2014;311(9):948–954.
2. Bain P, Brin M, Deuschl G, et al. Criteria for the diagnosis of essential tremor. *Neurology*. 2000;54(11 Suppl 4):S7.
3. Zeuner KE, Deuschl G. An update on tremors. *Curr Opin Neurol*. 2012;25(4):475–482.
4. Zesiewicz TA, Elble RJ, Louis ED, et al. Evidence-based guideline update: treatment of essential tremor: report of the Quality Standards subcommittee of the American Academy of Neurology. *Neurology*. 2011;77(19):1752–1755.
5. Connor GS, Edwards K, Tarsy D. Topiramate in essential tremor: findings from double-blind, placebo-controlled, crossover trials. *Clin Neuropharmacol*. 2008;31(2):97–103.
6. Handforth A, Bordelon Y, Frucht SJ, et al. A pilot efficacy and tolerability trial of memantine for essential tremor. *Clin Neuropharm*. 2010;33(5):223–226.
7. Simpson DM, Blitzer A, Brashear A, et al; Therapeutics and Technology Assessment Subcommittee of the American Academy of Neurology. Assessment: botulinum neurotoxin for the treatment of movement disorders (an evidence-based review): report of the Therapeutics and Technology Assessment Subcommittee of the American Academy of Neurology. *Neurology*. 2008;70(19):1699–1706.
8. Flora ED, Perera CL, Cameron AL, et al. Deep brain stimulation for essential tremor: a systematic review. *Mov Disord*. 2010;25(11):1550–1559.

ADDITIONAL READING

- Buijink AW, Contarino MF, Koelman JH, et al. How to tackle tremor—systematic review of the literature and diagnostic work-up. *Front Neurol*. 2012;3:146.
- Deuschl G, Raethjen J, Hellriegel H, et al. Treatment of patients with essential tremor. *Lancet Neurol*. 2011;10(2):148–161.
- Sullivan KL, Hauser RA, Zesiewicz TA. Essential tremor: epidemiology, diagnosis, and treatment. *Neurologist*. 2004;10(5):250–258.
- Thenganatt MA, Louis ED. Distinguishing essential tremor from Parkinson's disease: bedside tests and laboratory evaluations. *Expert Rev Neurother*. 2012;12(6):687–696.

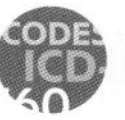

CODES

ICD10

G25.0 Essential tremor

CLINICAL PEARLS

- Core criteria for diagnosis of essential tremor include bilateral action (intention) tremor of the hands, forearm, and/or head without resting component.
- Beneficial response to alcohol and positive family history help to differentiate essential tremor from PD (PD is characterized by tremor at rest, bradykinesia, and rigidity, and it does not improve with alcohol use).
- 10% of patients with PD will have both resting tremors of PD and essential (intention) tremors.
- Wilson disease, thyroid disease, and medication effect should be ruled out.
- Brain MRI is usually not necessary or indicated.
- First-line treatments include propranolol and primidone.

EUSTACHIAN TUBE DYSFUNCTION

Adam W. Kowalski, MD • Vernon Wheeler, MD, FAAFP

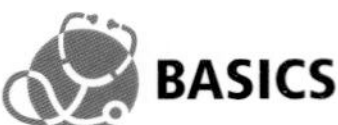

BASICS

DESCRIPTION

- Eustachian tube dysfunction (ETD) represents a spectrum of disorders involving an impairment in the functional valve of the eustachian tube of the middle ear.
- ETD can be classified as *patulous dysfunction*, in which the eustachian tube is excessively open, or *dilatory dysfunction*, in which there is failure of the tubes to dilate appropriately.
- Pathophysiology is thought to be related to pressure dysregulation, impaired protection secondary to reflux of irritating material into the middle ear, or impaired clearance by the mucociliary system.
- May occur in the setting of pressure changes (e.g., scuba diving or air travel) or acute upper airway inflammation (e.g., allergic or infectious rhinosinusitis)
- Chronic ETD may lead to a retracted tympanic membrane, recurrent serous effusion, recurrent otitis media (OM), adhesive OM, chronic mastoiditis, or cholesteatoma.
- System(s) affected: auditory
- Synonym(s): auditory tube dysfunction; eustachian tube disorder; blocked eustachian tube; patulous eustachian tube

ALERT

- Sudden single-sided deafness (SSNHL) can be misdiagnosed as ETD.
- A simple 512-Hz tuning fork test lateralizes to the opposite ear in sudden sensorineural hearing loss and to the affected ear in ETD with conductive hearing loss
- Any sudden sensorineural hearing loss is a medical emergency and should be referred to an otolaryngologist immediately.

EPIDEMIOLOGY

- Most common in children <5 years of age
- Usually decreases with age

Incidence

70% of children by age 7 years have experienced ETD.

Prevalence

- Males > females
- Highest prevalence among Native Americans, Inuits, Australian Aborigines, Hispanics, Africans

ETIOLOGY AND PATHOPHYSIOLOGY

- Under normal circumstances, the eustachian tube (ET) is closed but can open to release a small amount of air to equalize pressure between the middle ear and the surrounding atmosphere.
- ETD is failure of the ET, palate, nasal cavities, and nasopharynx to regulate middle ear and mastoid pressure.
- ET functions
  - Ventilation/regulation of middle ear pressure
  - Protection from nasopharyngeal secretions
  - Drainage of middle ear fluid
  - ET is closed at rest and opens with yawning, swallowing, and chewing.
- Cycle of dysfunction: Structural or functional obstruction of the ET compromises 3 functions:
  - Negative pressure develops in middle ear.
  - Serous exudate is drawn from the middle ear by negative pressure or refluxed into the middle ear if the ET opens momentarily.
  - Infection of static fluid causes edema and release of inflammatory mediators, which exacerbates cycle of inflammation and obstruction.
- In children, a horizontal and shorter ET predisposes to difficulties with ventilation and drainage.
- Adenoid hypertrophy can block the torus tubarius (proximal opening of the ET).
- In adults, paradoxical closing with swallowing has been noted in a majority of affected patients.

Genetics

Twin studies show a genetic component. Specific genetic cause is still undefined.

RISK FACTORS

- Adult and pediatric
  - Allergic rhinitis, tobacco exposure, GERD, chronic sinusitis, adenoid hypertrophy or nasopharyngeal mass, neuromuscular disease, altered immunity
- Pediatric
  - In addition to the earlier mentioned, prematurity and low birth weight, young age, daycare, crowded living conditions, low socioeconomic status, prone sleeping position, prolonged bottle use, craniofacial abnormalities (e.g., cleft palate, Down syndrome)

Pregnancy Considerations

ETD may be exacerbated by rhinitis of pregnancy; symptoms resolve postpartum.

GENERAL PREVENTION

- Control sources of upper airway inflammation: allergies, infectious rhinosinusitis, GERD
- Autoinsufflation of middle ear (i.e., blow gently against pinched nostril and closed mouth)
- Avoid atmospheric pressure changes (e.g., plane flight, scuba diving) in the setting of acute allergy exacerbation or URI.
- Avoid exposure to environmental irritants: tobacco smoke and pollutants.

COMMONLY ASSOCIATED CONDITIONS

- Hearing loss
- OM: acute, chronic, and serous
- Chronic mastoiditis
- Cholesteatoma
- Allergic rhinitis
- Chronic sinusitis/URI
- Adenoid hypertrophy
- GERD
- Cleft palate
- Down syndrome
- Obesity
- Nasopharyngeal carcinoma or other tumor

DIAGNOSIS

HISTORY

- Symptoms of ear pain, fullness, "plugging," hearing loss, tinnitus, popping or snapping noises, and vertigo are commonly seen with ETD.
- ETDQ-7 is a disease-specific symptom score for adult patients with ETD that has shown promise in small studies. Questions are answered based on the presence and intensity of symptoms in the past 1 month. Severity of each symptom is rated on an ascending scale of 1–7, with 1 indicating no problem and 7 indicating severe problems. A total score cutoff point >14.5 categorizes the patient as having the diagnosis of ETD (1)[B].
  - Pressure in ears in past 1 month?
  - Pain in ears in past 1 month?
  - A feeling that ears are clogged or "under water"?
  - Ear symptoms when you have cold or sinusitis?
  - Crackling or popping sounds in the ears?
  - Ringing in ears?
  - A feeling that your hearing is muffled?
- Other historical elements
  - Unilateral or bilateral. Adults presenting with persistent unilateral symptoms should be evaluated for nasopharyngeal process (tumor).
  - History of previous ear infections, surgeries, head trauma, recent flying or diving
  - Voice change (hypo- or hypernasal voice, consider NP mass or palatal dysfunction)
  - Differentiate patulous dysfunction, in which patient's own voice and breath sounds are amplified (autophony), from dilatory dysfunction, in which patient complains more of ear pain, "plugged" ear, hearing loss, and tinnitus.

PHYSICAL EXAM

- Pneumatic otoscopy: retracted tympanic membrane, effusion, decreased drum movement
- Toynbee maneuver: view changes of the drum while patient autoinsufflates against closed lips and pinched nostrils; may show various degrees of retraction
  - Entire drum may be retracted and "lateralize" with insufflation.
  - Posterosuperior quadrant (pars flaccida) may form a retraction pocket.
- Tuning fork tests: 512-Hz fork placed on the forehead lateralizes to affected ear (Weber test); the fork will be louder behind the ear on the mastoid than in front of the ear (bone conduction > air conduction, Rinne test) in conductive hearing loss.
- Nasopharyngoscopy: adenoid hypertrophy or nasopharyngeal mass
- Anterior rhinoscopy: deviated nasal septum, polyps, mucosal hypertrophy, turbinate hypertrophy

DIFFERENTIAL DIAGNOSIS

- SSNHL (a medical emergency)
- Tympanic membrane perforation
- Barotrauma
- Temporomandibular joint disorder
- Ménière disease
- Superior semicircular canal dehiscence

DIAGNOSTIC TESTS & INTERPRETATION

Initial Tests (lab, imaging)

- Radiologic studies are not performed routinely if clinical signs/symptoms suggest ETD.
- CT scan (not necessary) may show changes related to OM or middle ear/mastoid opacification.
- Functional MRI might determine cause of ETD (in recalcitrant cases), as the ET opening can be visualized during Valsalva.

Diagnostic Procedures/Other

- Audiogram may show conductive hearing loss.
- Tympanometry: type B or C tympanograms indicate fluid or retraction, respectively. Negative middle ear peak pressures seen even with normal (type A) tympanograms.

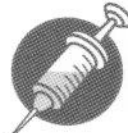

TREATMENT

- Due to limited high-quality evidence, it is difficult to recommend any one treatment option/intervention as superior (2).
- Generally, principle of treatment is to reduce cycle of infection/inflammation.
- Tympanostomy tubes ± adenoidectomy when indicated for recurrent ear infections or severe progressive retractions

MEDICATION

- Few data support pharmacologic treatments such as decongestants, nasal steroids, or antihistamines for ETD.
- Medication options are for treatment of comorbid conditions.
- Decongestants, topical, oral
  - Avoid prolonged use (>3 days); can cause rhinitis medicamentosa
  - Decongestants are most useful for acute ETD related to a resolving URI.
  - Decongestants are not typically used for relief of chronic ETD in children.
    - Phenylephrine: adults and children ≥12 years of age, 1 (10 mg) tablet q4h PRN; children 6–11 years of age, 5 mg q4h PRN; children 4–5 years of age, 2.5 mg q4h PRN
    - Pseudoephedrine: adults, 60 mg q4–6h PRN; children 6–12 years of age, 30 mg q4–6h PRN; children 4–5 years of age, 15 mg q4–6h PRN
    - Oxymetazoline: adults and children ≥6 years of age, 1–2 sprays each nostril q12h PRN. Limit use to ≤3 days.
    - Phenylephrine: adults, 1–2 sprays each nostril q4h PRN. Limit use to ≤3 days.
- Nasal steroids (may be beneficial for those with allergic rhinitis) (3)[A]
  - Beclomethasone (Beconase, Vancenase): adults and children ≥12 years of age, 1–2 sprays each nostril BID; children 6–11 years of age, 1 spray each nostril BID. Not recommended for children <6 years of age.
  - Budesonide (Rhinocort): adults and children ≥6 years of age, 1 spray each nostril daily
  - Ciclesonide (Omnaris) (a prodrug activated on nasal mucosa): adults and children ≥6 years of age, 2 sprays each nostril daily
  - Flunisolide (Nasarel, Nasalide): adults and children ≥6 years of age, 2 sprays each nostril BID
  - Fluticasone furoate (Veramyst): adults and children ≥12 years of age, 2 sprays each nostril daily; children 2–11 years of age, 1 spray each nostril daily
  - Fluticasone propionate (Flonase): adults 1–2 sprays each nostril daily; children ≥4 years of age, 1 spray each nostril daily
  - Mometasone (Nasonex): adults and children ≥12 years of age, 2 sprays each nostril daily; children 2–12 years of age, 1 spray each nostril daily.
  - Triamcinolone (Nasocort): adults and children ≥6 years of age, 1–2 sprays each nostril daily; children 2–5 years of age, 1 spray each nostril daily
- 2nd-generation H_1 antihistamines (may be beneficial for those with ETD and chronic rhinitis)
  - Cetirizine (Zyrtec) (tablets, chewable tablets, liquid): adults and children ≥6 years of age, 5–10 mg/day PO; children 12 months to 5 years of age: 2.5 mg/day PO; may increase to BID; children 6–<12 months of age: 2.5 mg/day PO
  - Desloratadine (Clarinex) (tablets, Redi-tabs, liquid): adults and children ≥12 years of age, 5 mg/day PO; children 6–11 years of age, 2.5 mg/day PO; children 12 months to 5 years of age, 1.25 mg/day PO; children 6–11 months of age, 1 mg/day PO
  - Fexofenadine (Allegra) (tablets, Redi-tabs, liquid): adults and children ≥12 years of age, 60 mg PO BID or 180 mg/day PO; children 2–11 years of age, 30 mg PO BID
  - Levocetirizine (Xyzal) (tablets, liquid): adults and children ≥12 years of age, 2.5–5 mg PO every evening; children 6–11 years of age, 2.5 mg PO every evening; children 6 months to 5 years of age, 1.25 mg PO every evening
- Antihistamine nasal sprays (may be beneficial for those with ETD and chronic rhinitis)
  - Azelastine (Astepro or Astelin): adults and children ≥12 years of age, 1–2 sprays each nostril BID; children 6–11 years of age, 1 spray each nostril BID
  - Olopatadine (Patanase): adults and children ≥12 years of age, 2 sprays each nostril BID; children 6–11 years of age, 1 spray each nostril BID

SURGERY/OTHER PROCEDURES

- Myringotomy and pressure equalization tube placement to ventilate middle ear, relieve pressure, and prevent sequelae of chronically retracted drum
- Patients with ETD during pressure changes may benefit from minimally invasive laser eustachian tuboplasty.
- New studies are emerging regarding balloon tubuloplasty but to date are very limited in terms of efficacy, safety, and long-term outcomes (4,5).
- Adenoidectomy if hypertrophied tissue is present.
  - In children, 1st set of tubes are typically placed alone. Adenoidectomy is performed with 2nd set of tubes if problems recur.
  - Some advocate adenoidectomy even in absence of excess tissue; reduces frequency and number of subsequent tubes

ONGOING CARE

FOLLOW-UP RECOMMENDATIONS

- Monitor pressure equalization tubes every 6–8 months in children and every 6–12 months in adults.
- Monitor tympanic membrane retraction pocket for progression every 6–12 months to allow for early intervention for progression in hearing loss, obvious ossicular erosion, or cholesteatoma.

DIET

In newborns, breastfeeding has been associated with lower incidence of ETD and OM.

PROGNOSIS

If symptoms of ETD persist beyond age 7 years, patient is more likely to have long-term problems and require regular monitoring.

COMPLICATIONS

Morbidity related to hearing compromise or associated sequela of chronic ear infections

REFERENCES

1. McCoul ED, Anand VK, Christos PJ. Validating the clinical assessment of eustachian tube dysfunction: the Eustachian Tube Dysfunction Questionnaire (ETDQ-7). *Laryngoscope*. 2012;122(5):1137–1141.
2. Norman G, Llewellyn A, Harden M, et al. Eustachian tube dysfunction: a health technology assessment. *Clin Otolaryngol*. 2014;(39):6–21.
3. Simpson SA, Lewis R, van der Voort J, et al. Oral or topical nasal steroids for hearing loss associated with otitis media with effusion in children. *Cochrane Database Syst Rev*. 2011;(5):CD001935.
4. Gurtler N, Husner A, Flurin H. Balloon dilation of the Eustachian tube: early outcome analysis. *Otol Neurotol*. 2015;36(3):437–443.
5. Bluestone CD. Balloon dilation of the eustachian tube is indeed a "gizmo" until future research proves safety and efficacy. *Otolaryngol Head Neck Surg*. 2014;151(3):374.

E

ADDITIONAL READING

- Bluestone CD. Studies in otitis media: Children's Hospital of Pittsburgh-University of Pittsburgh progress report–2004. *Laryngoscope*. 2004;114(11 Pt 3 Suppl 105):1–26.
- Gluth MB, McDonald DR, Weaver AL, et al. Management of eustachian tube dysfunction with nasal steroid spray: a prospective, randomized, placebo-controlled trial. *Arch Otolaryngol Head Neck Surg*. 2011;137(5):449–455. doi:10.1001/archoto.2011.56.
- Jumah MD, Jumah M, Pazen D, et al. Laser Eustachian tuboplasty: efficiency evaluation in the pressure chamber. *Otol Neurotol*. 2012;33(3):406–412.
- Seibert JW, Danner CJ. Eustachian tube dysfunction and the middle ear. *Otolaryngol Clin North Am*. 2006;39(6):1221–1235.

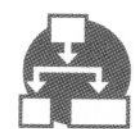

SEE ALSO

Algorithm: Ear Pain

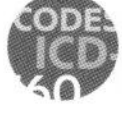

CODES

ICD10

- H69.90 Unspecified Eustachian tube disorder, unspecified ear
- H69.00 Patulous Eustachian tube, unspecified ear
- H68.109 Unspecified obstruction of Eustachian tube, unspecified ear

CLINICAL PEARLS

- ETD can be acute or chronic. Treatment is based on the underlying etiology.
- SSNHL (medical emergency) can be misdiagnosed as ETD and should always be ruled out, especially in patients with unilateral symptoms.

FACTOR V LEIDEN

Laura Howe, MD • Samuel B. Carli, MD

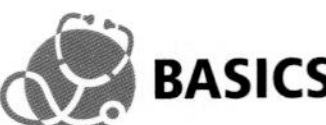

BASICS

DESCRIPTION

- Factor V Leiden is a genetic mutation in the coagulation pathway that results in the most common thrombophilic disease.
- System(s) affected: cardiovascular, gastrointestinal, hemo-/lymphatic/immunologic, nervous, pulmonary, reproductive
- Synonym(s): factor V Leiden thrombophilia; factor V Leiden mutation, hereditary APC resistance

Pediatric Considerations

Increased thrombosis risk in patients with factor V Leiden

Pregnancy Considerations

Recurrent late pregnancy loss is a possible complication.

EPIDEMIOLOGY

- Predominant age: Thrombosis typically occurs after the second decade.
- Predominant sex: male = female

Prevalence

Most common in Caucasians: Studies estimate ~5–8% occurrence in Caucasians, with Asian Americans affected the least at ~0.45%.

ETIOLOGY AND PATHOPHYSIOLOGY

- In the "checks and balances" of the coagulation pathway, the clotting cascade and ultimately thrombin, will create activated protein C (APC) in an effort to establish a negative feedback loop.
- APC and its cofactor, protein S, lead to inactivation of factors V and VIII.
- Point mutation causing substitution of arginine for glutamine in location 506 of factor V gene, rendering it less susceptible to inactivation by activated protein C (APC).
- This, in turn, reduces the anticoagulant role of factor V and increases the *procoagulant* role of activated factor V, as there is now 20-fold slower degradation of activated factor V Leiden.

RISK FACTORS

- Risk for venous thromboembolism (VTE) is ~7-fold in heterozygous and ~80-fold in homozygous factor V Leiden individuals, compared with individuals without the mutation (1).
- Having non-O blood type (A, B, or AB) can increase the risk VTE in both heterozygotes and homozygotes by 2- to 4-fold.
- Increased estrogen states may cause an acquired resistance to APC, thus
  - Oral contraceptives in homozygotes may increase the risk 100-fold; in heterozygotes, 35-fold.
  - The increased risk is halved when the patient uses desogestrel-containing oral contraceptives.
- Hormone replacement therapy (HRT) and selective estrogen receptor modulators (SERMs) both increase the risk of thrombosis; in patients with factor V Leiden, that risk is increased substantially.
- Pregnancy and *homozygous* factor V Leiden increase the risk of thrombosis 7–16-fold during pregnancy and the puerperium. Other complications of pregnancy may be increased in patients with factor V Leiden.
- Data are conflicting with regard to risk for recurrent VTE for patients with factor V Leiden but trend toward an increased risk (2,3).

GENERAL PREVENTION

ALERT

Patients with factor V Leiden without thrombosis do not require prophylactic anticoagulation.

COMMONLY ASSOCIATED CONDITIONS

Venous thrombosis

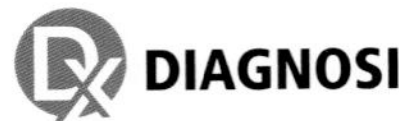

DIAGNOSIS

HISTORY

- Previous thrombosis
- Family history of thrombosis

PHYSICAL EXAM

- Family history of factor V Leiden mutation
- Findings suggestive of VTE, which can include deep venous thrombosis (DVT), pulmonary embolus (PE), and cerebral vein thrombosis: 10–26% of patients with VTE are carriers of the factor V Leiden mutation.
- Thrombosis in unusual locations, such as the sagittal sinus, mesentery, and portal systems, is less common in patients with factor V Leiden than in patients with deficiency of protein C or S.
- Obstetric complications and venous thrombosis are increased in patients with factor V Leiden and especially in those taking oral contraceptives.
- There is a weak, however significant, association between procoagulant states (including factor V Leiden) and coronary events in younger patients (4).

DIFFERENTIAL DIAGNOSIS

- Protein C deficiency
- Protein S deficiency
- Antithrombin deficiency
- Other causes of activated protein C resistance (e.g., antiphospholipid antibodies)
- Dysfibrinogenemia
- Dysplasminogenemia
- Homocystinemia
- Prothrombin 20210 mutation
- Elevated factor VIII levels

DIAGNOSTIC TESTS & INTERPRETATION

Initial Tests (lab, imaging)

- For evaluation of a new clot in patient at risk: CBC with peripheral smear, PT/INR, aPTT, thrombin time, lupus anticoagulant, antiphospholipid antibodies, factor VIII, anticardiolipin antibody, anti-β2 glycoprotein I antibody, activated protein C resistance, protein S antigen and resistance, antithrombin III assay, fibrinogen, factor V Leiden, prothrombin G20210A
- Genetic test: DNA-based test for factor V mutation; will be unaffected by anticoagulation and other drugs
- Functional test: plasma-based coagulation assay using factor V–deficient plasma to which patient plasma is added along with purified activated protein C. The relative prolongation of the activated partial thromboplastin time (aPTT) is used to assay for the defect. Heparin, direct thrombin inhibitors, and factor Xa inhibitor may cause false-negative results.
- Extremity US for DVT
- V/Q scan of spiral CT for PE

Follow-Up Tests & Special Considerations

- US may not show DVT acutely; repeat in 5–7days if strong suspicion.
- V/Q scan may be difficult to interpret in patients with other lung disease.

Diagnostic Procedures/Other

Magnetic resonance angiography (MRA), venography, or arteriography to detect thrombosis

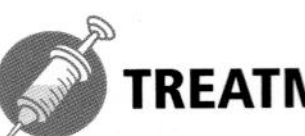

TREATMENT

Indicated if thrombotic event

GENERAL MEASURES

- Like general VTE treatment, patients with factor V Leiden and a 1st thrombosis should be anticoagulated initially with heparin or LMWH and warfarin for at least 3 months.
- Treatment with low-molecular-weight heparin (LMWH) is recommended over unfractionated heparin, unless the patient has severe renal failure (5)[A].
- Treat as outpatient, if possible (5)[A].
- Initiate warfarin with LMWH on the 1st treatment day and discontinue LMWH after minimum of 5 days and when INR >2 for 2 consecutive days (5)[A].
- Patients should be maintained on warfarin with an INR of 2–3 for at least 3 months (5)[A].
- For those patients with recurrence, the risks and benefits of indefinite anticoagulation need to be assessed.

MEDICATION

First Line

- LMWH:
  - Enoxaparin (Lovenox): 1 mg/kg SC BID, start warfarin simultaneously, continue enoxaparin for minimum of 5 days and until INR is >2 for 2 consecutive days, at which time enoxaparin can be stopped.
  - Fondaparinux (Arixtra): 5 mg (body weight <50 kg), 7.5 mg (body weight 50–100 kg), or 10 mg (body weight >100 kg) SC daily
  - Tinzaparin (Innohep): 175 anti-Xa IU/kg SC daily for minimum of 5 days and patient is adequately anticoagulated with warfarin (INR of at least 2 for 2 consecutive days)
  - Dalteparin (Fragmin): 200 IU/kg SC daily
- Oral anticoagulant
  - Warfarin (Coumadin) PO with dose adjusted to an INR of 2–3 (3)[A].
- Contraindications
  - Active bleeding precludes anticoagulation.
  - Risk of bleeding is a relative contraindication to long-term anticoagulation.
  - Warfarin is contraindicated in patients with history of warfarin skin necrosis (5)[A].
  - Warfarin is contraindicated in pregnancy.
- Precautions
  - Observe patient for signs of embolization, further thrombosis, or bleeding.
  - Avoid IM injections. Periodically check stool and urine for occult blood; monitor CBCs, including platelets.
  - Heparin: thrombocytopenia and/or paradoxic thrombosis with thrombocytopenia
  - Warfarin: necrotic skin lesions (typically breasts, thighs, or buttocks)
  - LMWH: Adjust dosage in renal insufficiency. May also need dose adjustment in pregnancy

- Significant possible interactions
  - Agents that intensify the response to oral anticoagulants: alcohol, allopurinol, amiodarone, anabolic steroids, androgens, many antimicrobials, cimetidine, chloral hydrate, disulfiram, all NSAIDs, sulfinpyrazone, tamoxifen, thyroid hormone, vitamin E, ranitidine, salicylates, acetaminophen
  - Agents that diminish the response to anticoagulants: aminoglutethimide, antacids, barbiturates, carbamazepine, cholestyramine, diuretics, griseofulvin, rifampin, oral contraceptives

Second Line

- Heparin 80 mg/kg IV bolus followed by 18 g/kg/h continuous infusion
- Adjust dose depending on aPTT.
- In patients requiring large daily doses of heparin, measure an anti-Xa level for dose guidance.
- Alternatively, for outpatients, weight-adjusted subcutaneous unfractionated heparin with 333 U/kg first, then 250 U/kg, without monitoring (5)[A]
- Consider deficiency of antithrombin as a co-mutation in patients with significant elevated heparin requirements.

ISSUES FOR REFERRAL

- Recurrent thrombosis on anticoagulation
- Difficulty anticoagulating
- Genetic counseling

SURGERY/OTHER PROCEDURES

- Anticoagulation must be held for surgical interventions.
- For most patients with DVT, recommendations are against routine use of vena cava filter in addition to anticoagulation except when there is contraindication for anticoagulation (5)[A].
- Thrombectomy may be necessary in some cases.

IN-PATIENT CONSIDERATIONS

Admission Criteria/Initial Stabilization

Complicated thrombosis, such as PE

Nursing

- Teach LMWH and warfarin use.
- See above for drug interactions.

Discharge Criteria

Stable on anticoagulation

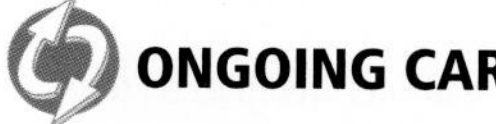

ONGOING CARE

FOLLOW-UP RECOMMENDATIONS

Patient Monitoring

Warfarin use requires periodic (~monthly after initial stabilization) INR measurements, with a goal of 2–3 (5)[A].

DIET

- No restrictions
- Large amounts of foods rich in vitamin K may interfere with anticoagulation with warfarin.

PATIENT EDUCATION

- Patients should be educated about the following
  - Use of oral anticoagulant therapy
  - Avoidance of NSAIDs while on warfarin
- The role of family screening is unclear, as most patients with this mutation do not have thrombosis. In a patient with a family history of factor V Leiden, consider screening during pregnancy or if considering oral contraceptive use.

PROGNOSIS

- Most patients heterozygous for factor V Leiden do not have thrombosis.
- Homozygotes have about a 50% lifetime incidence of thrombosis.
- Recurrence rates after a 1st thrombosis are not clear, with some investigators finding rates as high as 5% and others finding rates similar to the general population.
- Despite the increased risk for thrombosis, factor V Leiden does not increase overall mortality.

COMPLICATIONS

- Recurrent thrombosis
- Bleeding on anticoagulation

REFERENCES

1. Rosendaal FR, Koster T, Vandenbroucke JP, et al. High risk of thrombosis in patients homozygous for factor V Leiden (activated protein C resistance). *Blood*. 1995;85(6):1504–1508.
2. Lijfering WM, Middeldorp S, Veeger NJ, et al. Risk of recurrent venous thrombosis in homozygous carriers and double heterozygous carriers of factor V Leiden and prothrombin G20210A. *Circulation*. 2010;121(15):1706–1712.
3. Ho WK, Hankey GJ, Quinlan DJ, et al. Risk of recurrent venous thromboembolism in patients with common thrombophilia: a systematic review. *Arch Intern Med*. 2006;166(7):729–736.
4. Ye Z, Liu EH, Higgins JP, et al. Seven haemostatic gene polymorphisms in coronary disease: meta-analysis of 66,155 cases and 91,307 controls. *Lancet*. 2006;367(9511):651–658.
5. Guyatt GH, Akl EA, Crowther M, et al. Executive summary: antithrombotic therapy and prevention of thrombosis, 9th ed: American College of Chest Physicians evidence-based clinical practice Guidelines. *Chest*. 2012;141(Suppl 2):7S–47S.

ADDITIONAL READING

Seligsohn U, Lubetsky A. Genetic susceptibility to venous thrombosis. *N Engl J Med*. 2001;344(16):1222–1231.

SEE ALSO

Deep Vein Thrombophlebitis (DVT)

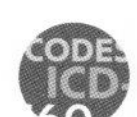

CODES

ICD10

D68.51 Activated protein C resistance

CLINICAL PEARLS

- Extremely rare in Asian and African populations
- Asymptomatic patients with factor V Leiden do not need anticoagulation.
- For pregnant women homozygous for factor V Leiden but no prior history of VTE, postpartum prophylaxis with prophylactic or intermediate-dose LMWH or vitamin K antagonists with target INR 2–3 for 6 weeks is recommended. Antepartum prophylaxis is added if there is positive family of VTE.

FAILURE TO THRIVE

Durr-e-Shahwaar Sayed, DO • Uzma Malik, MD

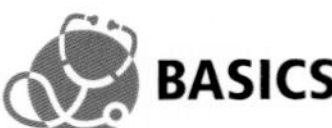

BASICS

DESCRIPTION

- Failure to thrive (FTT) is not a diagnosis but a sign of inadequate nutrition in young children manifested by a failure of physical growth, usually affecting weight. In severe cases, decreased length and/or head circumference may develop.
- Various parameters are used to define FTT, but in clinical practice, it is commonly defined as either weight for age that falls below the 5th percentile on more than 1 occasion or weight that drops 2 or more major percentile lines on standard growth charts.
- A combination of anthropometric criteria rather than one criterion should be used to identify children at risk of FTT (1)[C].

Pediatric Considerations

- Children with genetic syndromes, intrauterine growth restriction (IUGR), or prematurity follow different growth curves.
- 25% of children will decrease their weight or height crossing ≥2 major percentile lines in the first 2 years of life. These children are failing to reach their genetic potential or demonstrating constitutional growth delay (slow growth with a bone age < chronologic age). After shifting down, these infants grow at a normal rate along their new percentile and do not have FTT.

EPIDEMIOLOGY

Incidence

- Predominant age: 6–12 months; 80% <18 months
- Predominant sex: male = female

Prevalence

- As many as 10% of children seen in primary care have signs of growth failure.
- 1–5% of pediatric inpatient admissions are for FTT.
- Occurs more frequently in children living in poverty (1).

ETIOLOGY AND PATHOPHYSIOLOGY

- Mismatch between caloric intake and caloric expenditure
- Often grouped into 4 major categories:
  - Inadequate caloric intake (most frequent)
  - Inadequate caloric absorption
  - Excessive caloric expenditure
  - Defective utilization
- Traditionally, FTT was classified as organic or nonorganic, but most cases are multifactorial.
- FTT often begins with a specific event and may lead to persistent difficulties.
- Causes of FTT can be grouped by pathophysiology (including examples):
  - Inadequate intake: breastfeeding difficulty, incorrect formula preparation, poor transition to food (6–12 months), poor feeding habits (e.g., excessive juice, restrictive diets), mechanical problems (e.g., oromotor dysfunction, congenital anomalies, GERD, CNS or PNS anomalies), oral aversion, poverty, neglect, poor parent–child interaction
  - Inadequate absorption: necrotizing enterocolitis, short gut syndrome, biliary atresia, liver disease, cystic fibrosis, celiac disease, milk protein allergy, vitamin/mineral deficiency
  - Increased expenditure: hyperthyroidism, congenital/chronic cardiopulmonary disease, HIV, immunodeficiencies, malignancy, renal disease
  - Defective utilization: metabolic disorders, congenital infections (TORCH: toxoplasmosis, other agents, rubella, cytomegalovirus, herpes simplex)

Genetics

Multiple genetic disorders can cause FTT.

RISK FACTORS

- Psychosocial risks
  - Poverty, parent(s) with mental health disorder or cognitive impairment, poor parenting skills or hypervigilant parents, families with unique health/nutritional beliefs, physical or emotional abuse, substance abuse, and social isolation
- Medical risks
  - Intrauterine exposures, history of IUGR (symmetric or asymmetric), congenital abnormalities, oromotor dysfunction, premature or sick newborn, infant with physical deformity, acute or chronic medical conditions, developmental delay, lead poisoning, anemia

Pregnancy Considerations

FTT is linked to intrauterine exposures, IUGR, and prematurity.

GENERAL PREVENTION

- Educate parents on normal feeding and parenting skills.
- Access to supplemental feeding programs (WIC)

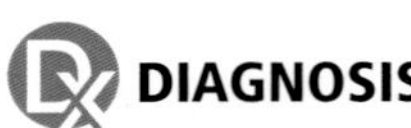

DIAGNOSIS

HISTORY

- Prenatal and developmental history
- Past medical history: acute/chronic disease affecting caloric intake, digestion, absorption, or causing increased energy need or defective utilization
- Medication history, including complementary and alternative medications
- Family history: stature of parents and growth trajectories of siblings, chronic diseases, genetic disorders, developmental delay
- Diet history from birth: breastfeeding or formula feeding; timing and introduction of solids; who feeds the child, when, and how often; placement of child during feeds; amounts consumed/caloric intake; beverages consumed; snacking; vomiting or stooling associated with feeds; oral aversions or unusual behaviors during feeding
- Social history: family composition, socioeconomic status, child-rearing beliefs, stressors, parental depression, parental substance abuse, caretaker personal history of abuse/neglect
- Review of systems: anorexia, activity level, mental status, fevers, dysphagia, vomiting, gastroesophageal reflux, stooling pattern/consistency, dysuria, urinary frequency

PHYSICAL EXAM

- Accurate measurement of height, weight, and head circumference on National Center for Health Statistics (NCHS) growth charts (www.cdc.gov/growthcharts) (2).
- The World Health Organization (WHO) growth charts may be more appropriate for breastfed infants (www.who.int/childgrowth/standards/en/)
- Growth charts exist for many other syndromes/conditions such as Down syndrome, Turner syndrome, and the premature infant.
- Exam should assess for the following:
  - Signs of dehydration or severe malnutrition are as follows:
    - Severity of malnutrition estimated via Gomez classification: compare current weight for age with expected weight for age (50th percentile): severe, <60% of expected; moderate, 61–75%; mild, 76–90%
  - Underlying medical disease
  - Dysmorphic features
  - Mental status (alert, responsive to stimuli)
  - Any signs of physical abuse and/or neglect
- Observe interaction with caregivers and feeding techniques, specifically bonding and social/psychological cues.

DIFFERENTIAL DIAGNOSIS

Differentiate based on growth patterns

- FTT classically presents as low weight for age, normal linear growth, normocephalic *or* low weight for age, followed by decreased linear growth *or* low weight for age, leading to decreased linear growth and decreased head circumference (without neurologic signs).
  - In this situation, consider differential diagnosis as outlined in "Etiology and Pathophysiology."
- If low linear growth with normal weight for length *or* low linear growth and proportionately low weight and decreased head circumference:
  - Consider genetic potential (constitutional short stature or growth delay), genetic syndromes, teratogens, endocrine disorders
- If microcephaly with prominent neurologic signs, with poor growth secondary to presumed neurologic disorder:
  - Consider TORCH infections, genetic syndromes, teratogens, brain injury (i.e., hypoxic/ischemic)

DIAGNOSTIC TESTS & INTERPRETATION

- Labs useful only in ~1% of cases and are generally not recommended (1)[C].
- A period of addressing nutritional causes is preferable prior to extensive labs and other workup.

Initial Tests (lab, imaging)

Labs should be ordered based on history and physical exam findings and the age of the patient.

- Tests often considered in initial evaluation:
  - CBC, ESR
  - Electrolytes, BUN/creatinine, liver function tests
  - Urinalysis and urine culture
  - Lead level
- Other tests as dictated by the history and exam:
  - TSH, amylase/lipase, serum zinc level, iron studies, karyotype, genetic testing, sweat chloride test, stool for ova and parasite or fat/reducing substances, guaiac, α-1-antitrypsin and elastase, radioallergosorbent test for IgE food allergies, tissue transglutaminase and total IgA (celiac sprue), P-ANCA and anti-*Saccharomyces cerevisiae* antibodies for inflammatory bowel disease [IBD]), TB test, HIV, ELISA, hepatitis A and B, other infections

Follow-Up Tests & Special Considerations

- Prospective 3-day food diary for accurate record of caloric intake should be obtained.
- Home visit by a clinician to observe infant feeding, interaction of caretakers, and home environment (3)
- Observe breastfeeding and/or formula preparation to ensure adequacy and offer instruction.

- Additional indicated evaluations may be performed by dietitians, occupational, physical and speech therapists, social workers, developmental specialists, psychiatrists, psychologists, visiting nurses, lactation consultants, and/or child protection services.
- Can consider
  - Skeletal survey if suspicion of physical abuse
  - Bone age if possible endocrine disorder
  - Swallowing studies, small bowel follow-through if possible oromotor dysfunction, GERD, structural abnormalities
  - Brain imaging if microcephalic and/or neurologic findings on examination

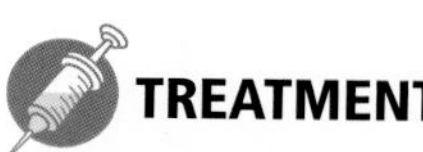

TREATMENT

GENERAL MEASURES

- Treat underlying conditions.
- Caregiver and infant interaction should be evaluated in infants and children with FTT.
- The goal is to improve nutrition to allow catch-up growth (weight gain 2–3 times > average for age).
- Calculate energy needs based on recommended energy intake for age, increased by 50%.
  - Recommended energy intake (use *expected*, not actual weight, to calculate needs)
    - 0–1 month: 120 kcal/kg/day
    - 1–2 months: 115 kcal/kg/day
    - 2–3 months: 105 kcal/kg/day
    - 3–6 months: 95 kcal/kg/day
    - 6 months to 3 years: 90 kcal/kg/day (4)[C]
- Alternatively, may calculate caloric requirements for infants to achieve catch-up growth
  - kcal/kg/day required = RDA for age (kcal/kg) × Ideal weight for height/Actual weight, where ideal weight for height is the median weight for the patient's height
- Try various strategies to increase caloric intake, such as the following:
  - Optimize breastfeeding support, consider supplementation
  - Higher calorie formulas
  - Addition of rice cereal or fats to current foods
  - Limit intake of milk to 24–32 oz/day.
  - Avoid juice and soda.
  - Vitamin and/or nutritional supplements
  - Assist with social and family problems (women, infants, and children [WIC], food stamps, and other transitional assistance).
- Rapid high-calorie intake can cause diarrhea, malabsorption, hypokalemia, and hypophosphatemia. Therefore, increasing formulas more than 24 kcal/oz is not recommended.
- The target energy intake should be slowly increased to goal over 5–7 days.
- Catch-up growth should be seen in 2–7 days.
- Accelerated growth should be continued for 4–9 months to restore weight and height.

MEDICATION

Use only for identified underlying conditions

ISSUES FOR REFERRAL

- Refer as indicated for underlying conditions.
- Multidisciplinary care is beneficial (1)[A]. Specialized multidisciplinary clinics may be of benefit for children with complicated situations, failure to respond to initial treatment, or when the PCP does not have access to specialized services such as nutrition, psychology, PT/OT, and speech therapy (2).

ADDITIONAL THERAPIES

In severe cases, nasogastric tube feedings or gastrostomy may be considered.

INPATIENT CONSIDERATIONS

Most cases of FTT can be managed as outpatients.

Admission Criteria/Initial Stabilization

Hospitalization should be considered if

- Outpatient management fails.
- There is evidence of severe dehydration or malnutrition.
- There are signs of abuse or neglect.
- There are concerns that the psychosocial situation presents harm to child.
- During catch-up growth, some children will develop nutritional recovery syndrome:
  - Symptoms include sweating, increased body temperature, hepatomegaly (increased glycogen deposits), widening of cranial sutures (brain growth > bone growth), increased periods of sleep, fidgetiness, and mild hyperactivity.
- There may also be an initial period of malabsorption with resultant diarrhea.

Discharge Criteria

Catch-up growth should be seen in 2–7 days. If this is not seen, reevaluation of causes is needed.

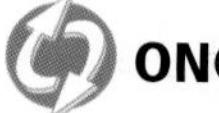

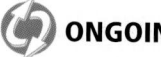

ONGOING CARE

FOLLOW-UP RECOMMENDATIONS

- If specific disease identified, follow-up as indicated.
- Close long-term follow-up with frequent visits is important to create and maintain a healthy, supportive environment (3).
- Children with history of FTT are at increased risk of recurrent FTT, and growth should be monitored closely (1,4).
- If the family fails to comply, child protection authorities must be notified.

DIET

Nutritional requirements for a "normal" child:

- Infant
  - 120 kcal/kg/day, decreased to 95 kcal/kg/day at 6 months; if breastfed, ensure appropriate frequency and duration of feeding.
  - Between 6 and 12 months, continue breast milk and/or formula, but pureed foods should be consumed several times a day during this period.
- Toddler
  - 3 meals plus 2 nutritional snacks, 16–32 oz milk/day; avoid juice and soda, and feed in a social environment.
  - Do not restrict fat and cholesterol in children <2 years.
- Rate of weight gain expected for age:
  - 0–3 months: 26–31 g/day
  - 3–6 months: 17–18 g/day
  - 6–9 months: 12–13 g/day
  - 9–12 months: 9 g/day
  - 1–3 years: 7–9 g/day

PATIENT EDUCATION

- Counsel parents regarding the need to avoid "food battles," which worsen the problem.
- Educate parents regarding infant social and physiologic cues, formula/food preparation, proper feeding techniques, and importance of relaxed and social mealtimes.
- When environmental deprivation is identified, educating in a nonpunitive way is essential.
- "Failure to thrive: What this means for your child," available from AAFP at: www.aafp.org/afp/2011/0401/p837.html
- WIC provides grants to states for supplemental foods, health care referrals, and nutrition education for low-income pregnant, breastfeeding, and non-breastfeeding postpartum women and to infants and children up to age 5 years at nutritional risk: www.fns.usda.gov/wic/

PROGNOSIS

- Many children with FTT show adequate improvement in dietary intake with intervention.
- Some studies looking at children with FTT have demonstrated an association with later problems with cognitive development, behavioral issues, and growth, but there is no consensus on these long-term outcomes or their clinical significance (1).
- Children with FTT are at increased risk for future undernutrition, overnutrition, and eating disorders.

REFERENCES

1. Cole SZ, Lanham JS. Failure to thrive: an update. *Am Fam Physician*. 2011;83(7):829–834.
2. Grissom M. Disorders of childhood growth and development: failure to thrive versus short stature. *FP Essent*. 2013;410:11–19.
3. Shields B, Wacogne I, Wright CM, et al. Weight faltering and failure to thrive in infancy and early childhood. *BMJ*. 2012;345:e5931.
4. Krugman SD, Dubowitz H. Failure to thrive. *Am Fam Physician*. 2003;68(5):879–884.

ADDITIONAL READING

- Atalay A, McCord M. Characteristics of failure to thrive in a referral population: implications for treatment. *Clin Pediatr (Phila)*. 2012;51(3):219–225.
- Jaffe AC. Failure to thrive: current clinical concepts. *Pediatr Rev*. 2011;32(3):100–107.

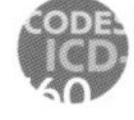

CODES

ICD10

- R62.51 Failure to thrive (child)
- P92.6 Failure to thrive in newborn

CLINICAL PEARLS

- FTT is a sign of inadequate nutrition.
- Underlying medical and/or social issues are generally suggested by history and physical exam, and extensive laboratory or imaging tests are rarely needed.
- A multidisciplinary team approach to diagnosis and treatment is critical to help children with FTT and their families.
- Prompt diagnosis and intervention is important to decrease the risk of adverse effects

F

FECAL IMPACTION

Pia Prakash, MD • Abdullah A. Al-Shahrani, MBBS • Marie L. Borum, MD, EdD, MPH

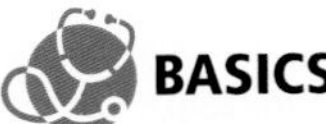

BASICS

DESCRIPTION

Incomplete evacuation of feces leading to the formation of a large, firm, immovable mass of stool in the rectum or distal sigmoid colon with resultant partial or complete obstruction

EPIDEMIOLOGY

Incidence

Incidence increases with age

- Predominant age: >70 years

Geriatric Considerations

42% of patients in a geriatric ward with fecal impaction (1)

Prevalence

- 60% of patients with fecal impaction have a history of chronic constipation (2).
- In North America, the prevalence of constipation among the general population is 2–27%.
- Constipation is more common in females, nonwhites, and people from low socioeconomic class (3).
- 78% of all children with encopresis have fecal impaction (4).
- In children, encopresis is 3× more common in boys than girls (4).

ETIOLOGY AND PATHOPHYSIOLOGY

- Age-related degenerative changes of the enteric nervous system, colonic hypomotility, and age-related anatomic changes of the lower GI tract contribute to delayed gut transit time and decreased stool water content.
- The rectosigmoid colon dilates to accommodate fecal material, which is not pliable enough to pass through the anal canal (5).
- Impacted stool may exist as a single mass (stercolith) or as a composite of small, rounded fecal particles (scybalum).
- Poor diet
  - Inadequate fiber, water, and caloric intake
- Medication side effect (6,7)
  - Stimulant laxatives
  - Opiate analgesics
  - Anticholinergics
  - Diuretics
  - Calcium channel blockers
  - Aluminum (sucralfate, antacids)
  - Iron
  - NSAIDs
- Neurogenic disorders
  - Hirschsprung disease
  - Chagas disease
  - Autonomic neuropathy
  - Multiple sclerosis
  - Spinal cord injury (13%) (8)
  - Cauda equina
  - Parkinson disease
- Metabolic derangements
  - Hypothyroidism
  - Hyperparathyroidism
  - Diabetes mellitus
- Electrolyte disturbances
  - Hypokalemia
  - Hypercalcemia
  - Hypermagnesemia
- Anatomic
  - Anorectal stenosis
  - Neoplasm
  - Megarectum
  - Painful rectal conditions inhibiting voluntary defecation (anal fissure, hemorrhoids, fistulas)
- Psychological
  - Depression
  - Anxiety
  - Anorexia nervosa
- Immobility (1% of hospitalized patients) (9)
- Pelvic floor dysfunction or dyssynergia
- Irritable bowel syndrome, constipation predominant
- Idiopathic
- Withholding behavior (most common cause in children) (10)

Genetics

Fecal impaction of the cecum (cystic fibrosis)

RISK FACTORS

- Institutionalization
- Constipation
- Psychogenic illness
- Immobility, inactivity
- Pica
- Chronic renal failure
- Urinary incontinence
- Cognitive decline, disability
- Heavy metal ingestion or exposure
- Poor toileting habits
- Excessive seed consumption (common in Middle East cultures), leading to rectal seed bezoars
- Medication (opioids in particular)

Pediatric Considerations

Habitual neglect of defecation urge may promote impaction.

GENERAL PREVENTION

- Maintain adequate hydration.
- Maintain high-fiber diet (11)[C].
- Regular exercise and ambulation (11)[B]
- Establish regular toilet time leveraging gastrocolic reflex to promote defecation after meals (11)[C].
- Psyllium (12)[B]
- Periodic enemas, if indicated
- Periodic polyethylene glycol powder (MiraLAX) (12)[A]
- Lactulose (12)[A]

DIAGNOSIS

HISTORY

- Abdominal pain and bloating
- Constipation
- Rectal discomfort
- Fecal incontinence, paradoxical (overflow) diarrhea
- Nausea, vomiting, anorexia
- General malaise
- Agitation and confusion in elderly
- Urinary frequency
- Urinary incontinence
- Straining

PHYSICAL EXAM

May be unremarkable

- Vital signs
  - Tachycardia
  - Tachypnea
  - Low-grade fever
- General
  - Agitated
  - Confused
  - Poor hydration status
- Abdominal
  - Distention
  - Palpable, tubular mass in lower quadrant
- Rectal
  - Copious amount of stool in rectal vault. If impaction is in sigmoid colon, rectal exam will be nondiagnostic.
  - Hard stool
  - Anal fissures
  - Hemorrhoids
  - Loss of sphincter tone

DIFFERENTIAL DIAGNOSIS

- Colitis
- Diverticulitis
- Appendicitis
- Colorectal cancer

DIAGNOSTIC TESTS & INTERPRETATION

Initial Tests (lab, imaging)

- Laboratory tests are often unremarkable. If obtained, the following are possible:
  - Leukocytosis
  - Hyponatremia
  - Hypokalemia
  - Hypercalcemia
  - Hypermagnesemia
  - Hypothyroidism
  - Stool may be positive for occult blood.
- Plain abdominal radiography may reveal stool or signs of obstruction, including dilated colon or small bowel, and air-fluid levels.
- CT scan may show a localized fecal material with a diameter that is greater than or equal to the colon diameter (13).

Geriatric Considerations

Attempts to identify underlying cause should be carried out in all patients. Thyroid and electrolyte disturbances are common in elderly patients presenting with impaction.

Follow-Up Tests & Special Considerations

Pediatrics

- Celiac antibodies (antigliadin and antiendomysial)
- Lead levels

Diagnostic Procedures/Other

Sigmoidoscopy may be used to clarify the nature of a rectosigmoid mass.

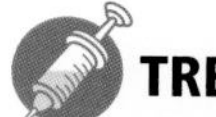

TREATMENT

GENERAL MEASURES

- Treatment centers on removal of the impaction and prevention of future recurrence.
- Manual disimpaction and extraction of fecal mass is often required.
- For stool located higher in the rectum, a rigid proctoscope may be used to disimpact stool or to pass enema solution to soften stool (7).

MEDICATION

First Line

- Enemas to soften stool and stimulate defecation
  - Mineral oil enema or warm water enema to aid passage of stool
- Osmotic laxatives, such as polyethylene glycol solutions and magnesium citrate, may soften stool.
- Enemas and polyethylene glycol are equally effective in treating fecal impaction in children. However, enemas have a faster relief (14).
- Precautions
  - Use of osmotic laxatives is contraindicated with bowel obstruction (7).
  - Use magnesium citrate with caution in patients with renal insufficiency.
  - Lactulose may result in colonic distension due to bacterial fermentation.
  - Avoid soap, hot water, and hydrogen peroxide enemas as they may result in rectal mucosal irritation.

SURGERY/OTHER PROCEDURES

- Neostigmine combined with glycopyrrolate for patients with spinal cord injury (8), and severe impaction must be used in ICU setting.
- Surgery may be necessary with intestinal perforation.
- After disimpaction, colonoscopy or barium enema can be considered to evaluate for anatomic abnormalities contributing to impaction (15).

COMPLEMENTARY & ALTERNATIVE MEDICINE

Biofeedback improves constipation in patients with dyssynergic defecation, which may decrease incidence of impaction.

INPATIENT CONSIDERATIONS

Admission Criteria/Initial Stabilization

- Disimpaction is usually performed in outpatient setting.
- Hospitalization is necessary if several attempts at outpatient management have failed.
- Signs and symptoms of obstruction, intestinal perforation, or peritonitis
- Hemodynamic instability or poor hydration status

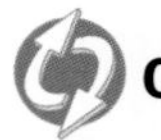

ONGOING CARE

FOLLOW-UP RECOMMENDATIONS

Patient Monitoring

Attempt at maintaining >3 bowel movements/week

DIET

High fiber (30 g/day) with adequate hydration (minimum 2 L/day). Fermentable (soluble) fiber sources: psyllium seed husk, oat bran, barley, soybeans, chia, broccoli, almonds, avocados, plums, berries, pears, apples.

PATIENT EDUCATION

- Increased activity
- Comprehensive program, including use of osmotic laxatives, bulking agents, behavioral changes, dietary changes
- Effective education with regard to constipation is crucial in changing chronic behavior patterns.
- Regular toileting using gastrocolic reflex
- Attempt defecation when urge for bowel movement is sensed.
- Maintain a good hydration status.

PROGNOSIS

- Reimpaction is likely if program is not followed.
- Prognosis is poor if complicated by intestinal perforation or peritonitis.
- Mortality with impaction and obstruction is highest in the very young and the very old (up to 16%).

COMPLICATIONS

- Intestinal obstruction
- Urinary tract obstruction
- Recurrent UTIs
- Spontaneous perforation of colon
- Incarcerated hernia
- Volvulus
- Megacolon
- Rectal prolapse
- Rectovaginal fistula
- Dystocia in pregnancy
- Peritonitis (16)
- Colonic volvulus (16)
- Sepsis with perforation

REFERENCES

1. Read NW, Abouzekry L, Read MG, et al. Anorectal function in elderly patients with fecal impaction. *Gastroenterology*. 1985;89(5):959–966.
2. Maurer CA, Renzulli P, Mazzucchelli L, et al. Use of accurate diagnostic criteria may increase incidence of stercoral perforation of the colon. *Dis Colon Rectum*. 2000;43(7):991–998.
3. Higgins PD, Johanson JF. Epidemiology of constipation in North America: a systematic review. *Am J Gastroenterol*. 2004;99(4):750–759.
4. Constipation Guideline Committee of the North American Society for Pediatric Gastroenterology, Hepatology and Nutrition. Evaluation and treatment of constipation in infants and children: recommendations of the North American society for pediatric gastroenterology, hepatology and nutrition. *J Pediatr Gastroenterol Nutr*. 2006;43(3):e1–e13.
5. McCrea GL, Miaskowski C, Stotts NA, et al. Pathophysiology of constipation in the older adult. *World J Gastroenterol*. 2008;14(17):2631–2638.
6. Leung L, Riutta T, Kotecha J, et al. Chronic constipation: an evidence-based review. *J Am Board Fam Med*. 2011;24(4):436–451.
7. Araghizadeh F. Fecal impaction. *Clin Colon Rectal Surg*. 2005;18(2):116–119.
8. Ebert E. Gastrointestinal involvement in spinal cord injury: a clinical perspective. *J Gastrointestin Liver Dis*. 2012;21(1):75–82.
9. Fargo MV, Latimer KM. Evaluation and management of common anorectal conditions. *Am Fam Physician*. 2012;85(6):624–630.
10. Benninga MA, Voskuijl WP, Taminiau JA. Childhood constipation: is there new light in the tunnel? *J Pediatr Gastroenterol Nutr*. 2004;39(5):448–464.
11. Hsieh C. Treatment of constipation in older adults. *Am Fam Physician*. 2005;72(11):2277–2284.
12. Brandt LJ, Prather CM, Quigley EM, et al. Systematic review on the management of chronic constipation in North America. *Am J Gastroenterol*. 2005;100(Suppl 1):S5–S22.
13. Kumar P, Pearce O, Higginson A. Imaging manifestations of faecal impaction and stercoral perforation. *Clin Radiol*. 2011;66(1):83–88. doi:10.1016/j.crad.2010.08.002.
14. Miller MK, Dowd MD, Friesen CA, et al. A randomized trial of enema versus polyethylene glycol 3350 for fecal disimpaction in children presenting to an emergency department. *Pediatr Emerg Care*. 2012;28(2):115–119.
15. Rao SS, Seaton K, Miller M, et al. Randomized controlled trial of biofeedback, sham feedback, and standard therapy for dyssynergic defecation. *Clin Gastroenterol Hepatol*. 2007;5(3):331–338.
16. Halawi HM, Maasri KA, Mourad FH, et al. Faecal impaction: in-hospital complications and their predictors in a retrospective study on 130 patients. *Colorectal Dis*. 2012;14(2):231–236.

F

ADDITIONAL READING

Enck RE. An overview of constipation and newer therapies. *Am J Hosp Palliat Care*. 2009;26(3): 157–158.

SEE ALSO

Constipation; Diarrhea, Chronic; Encopresis

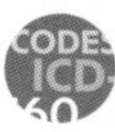

CODES

ICD10

- K56.41 Fecal impaction
- K59.00 Constipation, unspecified
- R15.9 Full incontinence of feces

CLINICAL PEARLS

- Constipation and resulting fecal impaction are often seen in elderly and hospitalized patients.
- When treating chronic pain patients with opioid preparations, be sure to supplement with stool softeners or osmotic laxatives.
- Prevent recurrent fecal impaction with increased fiber intake, adequate hydration, exercise, osmotic laxatives, and bulking agents.

FEMALE ATHLETE TRIAD

David A. Ross, MD • Rahul Kapur, MD, CAQSM

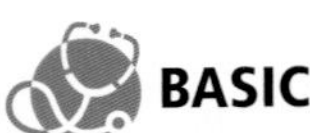

BASICS

Syndrome of 3 interrelated clinical entities: low energy availability (EA) (with or without disordered eating [DE]), menstrual dysfunction (MD), and low bone mineral density (BMD) (1).

DESCRIPTION

- Female athlete triad first described in 1992: Athletes may meet criteria for only 1 or 2 parts of the triad.
- Prevention and early intervention are essential to prevent progression to serious clinical end points of eating disorders, amenorrhea, and osteoporosis.
- 2014 Female Athlete Triad Coalition Consensus Statement supports the 2007 American College of Sports Medicine (ACSM) Position Stand (1):
  - Each component of the triad represents a spectrum ranging from health to dysfunction.
  - Energy availability is fundamental to the propagation of the triad.
  - Full recovery is not possible without correction of low energy availability.
- Energy availability (EA)
  - Dietary energy intake minus exercise energy expenditure. Considered to be the core component of the triad.
  - Represents the amount of dietary energy remaining for bodily functions after correcting for exercise training
  - Low EA results in reduced capacity for cellular maintenance, thermoregulation, and growth.
  - Low EA serves a causal role in the induction of exercise-associated menstrual disturbances.
  - Low EA occurs either intentionally or inadvertently. Examples include increasing training disproportionately to energy intake; disordered eating; and reducing energy intake by restricting, fasting, binging, and purging or by using diet pills, laxatives, diuretics, or enemas. Only some athletes meet the diagnostic criteria from *Diagnostic and Statistical Manual of Mental Disorders* 5th edition (*DSM-5*) for clinical eating disorders.
- Menstrual dysfunction (MD)
  - Low EA alters the hypothalamic-pituitary axis, resulting in decreased estrogen levels.
  - MD is a spectrum ranging from eumenorrhea to amenorrhea.
  - MD includes athletes who have low estrogen levels but still experience menstruation.
  - Energy deficit results in menstrual dysfunction at ~30 kcal/kg lean body mass per day.
  - MD includes luteal suppression (shortened luteal phase, prolonged follicular phase, and decreased estradiol level), anovulation, oligomenorrhea (menstrual cycle >35 days), and primary and secondary hypothalamic amenorrhea.
  - Primary amenorrhea, although less common, can occur in young athletes. Secondary amenorrhea is defined as the absence of menstrual cycles for >3 months after menarche established.
  - Although hypothalamic suppression is the most common cause of secondary amenorrhea in these athletes, other causes must be ruled out.
- BMD
  - Ranges from optimal bone health to osteoporosis
  - Bone health encompasses bone strength as well as bone quality. Current technology allows for the measurement of bone density but not quality. Therefore, two athletes with the same BMD may have very different bone fracture histories.
    - ACSM Position Stand recommends using the International Society of Clinical Densitometry (ISCD) guidelines for BMD, which refers to *Z*-scores below −2.0
    - Because most athletes have a higher BMD than nonathletes, ACSM recommends further workup for any athlete with a *Z*-score <−1, even in the absence of fracture.
  - Endothelial dysfunction
    - Emerging evidence that the female athlete triad is associated with endothelial dysfunction. Reduced levels of estrogen directly reduces vasodilation. Athletic amenorrhea is associated with reduced brachial artery flow-mediated dilation, which has a 95% positive predictive value for coronary endothelial dysfunction. Consequences include decreased blood flow to muscles during exercise and accelerated atherosclerosis. In the future, this clinical syndrome may be considered a tetrad (2).

EPIDEMIOLOGY

Prevalence

- Overall prevalence: 0–16% of female athletes (3). Prevalence of 2 criteria varies: MD + BMD 0–8% (n = 460), MD + LE 18% (n = 80), and BMD + LE 4% (n = 80) (3)
- Disordered eating higher than general population (3)
- Menstrual dysfunction: Prevalence of secondary amenorrhea is as high as 60% in female athletes compared to 2–5% in the general population (3).
- Bone health: Using the World Health Organization (WHO) criteria for low BMD, prevalence ofosteopenia (T-score between −1 and −2) ranges from 0 to 40% in female athletes, as compared to ~12% in the general population (3).

ETIOLOGY AND PATHOPHYSIOLOGY

- Low EA causes disruption in the hypothalamic-pituitary-ovarian axis, decreasing pulsatile gonadotropin-releasing hormone (GnRH) release (4).
- Low GnRH levels decrease luteinizing hormone (LH) and follicle-stimulating hormone (FSH) levels, decreasing estrogen production with resultant menstrual dysfunction.
- Estrogen deficiency negatively affects bone density. A chronic state of malnutrition reduces the rate of bone formation and increases the rate of bone resorption. Changes in bone metabolism occur within 5 days of reductions in EA.

RISK FACTORS

- History of menstrual irregularities and amenorrhea, history of stress fractures and recurrent or non-healing injuries, history of critical comments about eating or weight from parent or coach, history of depression, history of dieting, personality factors including perfectionism and/or obsessiveness, overtraining, and inappropriate coaching behaviors (1).
- Lean physique, sports with an aesthetic component (ballet, figure skating, gymnastics, distance running, diving, and swimming), or sports with weight classifications (martial arts and wrestling). Frequent weigh-ins, consequences for weight gain, and win-at-all-cost attitude all increase risk of developing triad (5).
- A lack of family or social support, intense training hours, social isolation, or entering a new environment (boarding school or college); an athlete with comorbid psychological conditions (anxiety, depression, and/or obsessive-compulsive disorder)

GENERAL PREVENTION

- Education of athletes (middle school through college), coaches, trainers, parents, and physicians. Young athletes are extremely impressionable and may turn negative comments and unhealthy advice into maladaptive eating and exercising habits.
- General screening during preparticipation exam (PPE) and annual physicals is endorsed by AAP, AAFP, ACSM, AAOSM, and AMSSM (5).
- Female Athlete Triad Coalition has 11-question screening to use during PPE.
- Athletes presenting with "red flag" conditions such as fractures, weight changes, fatigue, amenorrhea, bradycardia, orthostatic hypotension, syncope, arrhythmia, electrolyte abnormalities, or depression should be screened.

COMMONLY ASSOCIATED CONDITIONS

- Anorexia nervosa, bulimia nervosa, avoidant or restrictive food intake disorder, and other psychological disorders, including low self-esteem, depression, and anxiety (4)
- Low BMD predisposes athletes to stress fractures and may not be fully reversible. This may lead to a higher rate of fractures after menopause.

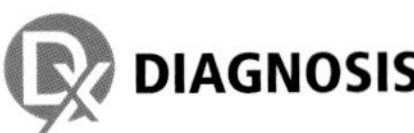

DIAGNOSIS

The female athlete triad is a clinical diagnosis based primarily on patient history. Screening for the female athlete triad should occur at annual sports physicals or during routine exams and acute visits if there are any concerning complaints or evident components of the triad (1,4)[A].

HISTORY

Assess menstrual history (including oral contraceptive use), fracture history, and symptoms of depression. Assess dietary practices, eating behaviors, and history of weight changes. Dietary intake logs and a nutritional assessment by a sports dietitian can be helpful. Assess body image, fear of weight gain, fluctuations in weight, history of disordered eating, and use of laxatives, diet pills, or enemas.

PHYSICAL EXAM

- Height, weight, body mass index (BMI) <17.5% kg/m^2 or less than 85% of expected body weight in adolescents (1)[A]
- Common findings in patients at risk for the triad include bradycardia, orthostatic hypotension, hypothermia, cold or cyanotic extremities, lanugo, parotid gland enlargement or tenderness, epigastric tenderness, eroded tooth enamel, and knuckle or hand calluses (Russell sign).
- Patients with amenorrhea should undergo a pelvic exam to verify the presence of a uterus and evaluate for outflow tract abnormalities. Vaginal atrophy may be present if the patient is hypoestrogenic.

DIFFERENTIAL DIAGNOSIS

Screen for anorexia nervosa, bulimia nervosa, avoidant/restrictive food intake disorder, and rumination disorder using the *DSM-5* criteria. Rule out the following in amenorrheic patients:

- Pregnancy
- Endocrine abnormalities: thyroid dysfunction, Cushing syndrome
- Hypothalamic dysfunction: psychological stress-induced amenorrhea, medication-induced amenorrhea, Kallmann syndrome
- Pituitary dysfunction: prolactinoma, Sheehan syndrome, sarcoidosis, empty sella syndrome
- Ovarian dysfunction: polycystic ovarian syndrome, premature ovarian failure, menopause, gonadal dysgenesis, Turner syndrome, ovarian neoplasm, autoimmune disease
- Uterine dysfunction: Asherman syndrome, absence of uterus

DIAGNOSTIC TESTS & INTERPRETATION

Initial Tests (lab, imaging)

- Basic metabolic panel, magnesium, phosphorus, albumin, CBC with differential, ESR, thyroid-stimulating hormone (TSH), calcium, 25-OH vitamin D, and urinalysis (1,5)
- Evaluation for secondary amenorrhea includes urine hCG, FSH, LH, prolactin, and TSH.
- Pelvic ultrasound in patients with hyperandrogenism to confirm polycystic ovaries or rule out virilizing ovarian tumors
- ECG to rule out prolonged QT interval

Follow-Up Tests & Special Considerations

- BMD testing by dual-energy x-ray absorptiometry (DEXA) is based on a risk stratification model (1). Risk factors include disordered eating, eating disorders >6 months, hypoestrogenism, amenorrhea, oligomenorrhea, and/or in patients with a history of stress fractures or fractures from minimal impact.
- In patients with persistent components of the triad, ISCD 2013 guidelines indicate reevaluation by the same DEXA machine is recommended every 1–2 years.

TREATMENT

- The goal is to optimize nutritional status by establishing healthy eating behaviors and treating any associated maladaptive behavioral disorders. (1,3)[A].
- A multidisciplinary team including a physician (or other health care provider), registered dietitian, and a mental health provider is important. Build open lines of communication with coaches, trainers, and family.
- A positive EA of >30 kcal/kg of fat-free muscle mass/day is sufficient to restore menses (4)[A].
- Physically active females should strive for an EA of >45 kcal/kg of fat-free muscle mass/day (1)[A].

MEDICATION

First Line

- Increasing EA through nutritional intervention is the best strategy for normalizing gonadotropin pulsatility and release. The use of combination oral contraceptive pills (cOCPs), hormone replacement therapy (HRT), and/or bisphosphonates has not been clearly shown to increase BMD or aid in the restoration of normal menstrual cycling. cOCPs or transdermal estradiol with cyclic progesterone can be considered in patients with particularly low BMD *Z*-scores and fracture histories who do not respond to 1 year of nonpharmacologic management.
- cOCP or transdermal estradiol can also be given to minimize further bone loss in patients >16 years and <21 years who, despite adequate nutrition and body weight gain, continue to have decreasing BMD and functional hypothalamic amenorrhea.
- Calcium and vitamin D supplementation to maintain serum levels within 32–50 mg/mL is recommended (1)[A].

INPATIENT CONSIDERATIONS

Patients with eating disorders should be evaluated for potentially life-threatening conditions requiring hospital admission, including bradycardia, severe orthostatic hypotension, significant electrolyte imbalances, hypothermia, arrhythmias, or prolonged QT interval.

ONGOING CARE

- Patients with components of the triad should have regular follow-up with a multidisciplinary treatment team (5)[A].
- Cognitive-behavioral therapy (CBT) is effective for exercising women with ED and may be more beneficial than nutritional counseling alone in women with disordered eating behavior.
- "Clearance and Return to Play (RTP) Guidelines by Medical Risk Stratification" are helpful in determining when to safely allow an athlete to return to competition. More research is needed in order to validate this model (1)[A].
- To continue training and competing, athletes with eating disorders must agree to the following stipulations as part of a behavioral contract: to comply with all treatment strategies; to be closely monitored by health care providers; to place treatment goals over training goals; and to modify the type, duration, and intensity of training or competition as necessary.

PATIENT EDUCATION

All young female patients should be counseled on the importance of proper nutrition, calcium, and vitamin D intake and the benefits of regular weight-bearing exercise. Patients presenting with ≥1 components of the triad should be educated about the short- and long-term effects of low BMD (1,3)[A].

PROGNOSIS

- The short- and long-term prognosis for patients with female athlete triad depends on time to diagnosis and response to treatment.
- It is estimated that amenorrheic women will lose 2–3% of bone mass per year without intervention.
- With early diagnosis and treatment using a multidisciplinary team, prognosis for patients with the female athlete triad is good. Patients regain normal menstrual cycling and fertility and increase BMD.
- Because the triad often occurs within the age window of optimal bone strengthening, patients with a prolonged disease course may suffer from complications of decreased BMD throughout their adolescent and adult life.
- Patients with disordered eating behaviors often require long-term therapy to manage their disease.

REFERENCES

1. DeSouza MJ, Nattiv A, Joy E, et al. 2014 Female Athlete Triad Coalition consensus statement on treatment and return to play of the female athlete triad: 1st International Conference held in San Francisco, CA, May 2012, and 2nd International Conference held in Indianapolis, IN, May 2013. *Clin J Sport Med*. 2014;24(2):96–119.
2. Lanser EM, Zach KN, Hoch AZ, et al. The female athlete triad and endothelial dysfunction. *PM R*. 2011;3(5):458–465.
3. Barrack MT, Ackerman KE, Gibbs JC. Update on the female athlete triad. *Curr Rev Musculoskeletal Med*. 2013;6(2):195–204.
4. Hoch AZ, Temme KE. Recognition and rehabilitation of the female athlete triad/tetrad: a multidisciplinary approach. *Curr Sports Med Rep*. 2013;12(3):190–199.
5. Deimel JF, Dunlap BJ. The female athlete triad. *Clin Sports Med*. 2012;31(2):247–254.

ADDITIONAL READING

Nattiv A, Loucks AB, Manore MM, et al. American College of Sports Medicine position stand. The female athlete triad. *Med Sci Sports Exerc*. 2007;39(10):1867–1882.

SEE ALSO

Algorithms: Amenorrhea, Primary (Absence of Menarche by Age 16); Amenorrhea, Secondary; Weight Loss

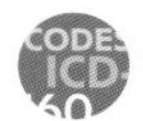

CODES

ICD10

- F50.9 Eating disorder, unspecified
- N91.2 Amenorrhea, unspecified
- M81.8 Other osteoporosis without current pathological fracture

CLINICAL PEARLS

- The female athlete triad consists of pathology in 3 clinical areas: low EA (with or without DE), menstrual dysfunction, and BMD. Athletes may exhibit varying degrees of dysfunction in any of these three areas.
- Screening at-risk women is critical to early diagnosis and intervention.
- Early intervention by a multidisciplinary team, including physicians, registered dietitians, mental health professionals, coaches, trainers, and parents, is the most successful strategy to minimize further bone loss, recover BMD, and regain normal menstrual function.
- Current guidelines recommend screening for abnormal BMD using DEXA studies for patients with disordered eating, eating disorders >6 months, hypoestrogenism, amenorrhea, oligomenorrhea, and/or in patients with a history of stress fractures or fractures from minimal impact.

FEVER OF UNKNOWN ORIGIN (FUO)

Scott T. Henderson, MD

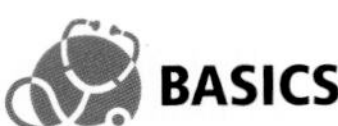

BASICS

DESCRIPTION

- Classic definition
  - Fever >38.3°C on several occasions
  - Fever duration at least 3 weeks
  - Uncertain diagnosis after 1 week of study in the hospital
- Modifications to FUO definition have evolved over time. In-hospital evaluation has been eliminated as well as shortening the time of undiagnosed fever.
- Some expand the definition to include nosocomial, neutropenic, and shorter duration HIV-associated fevers.

EPIDEMIOLOGY

Incidence

Incidence unclear

ETIOLOGY AND PATHOPHYSIOLOGY

- >200 causes; each with prevalence of ≤5%
- *Most commonly an atypical presentation of a common condition*
- Infection
  - Abdominal or pelvic abscesses
  - Amebic hepatitis
  - Catheter infections
  - Cytomegalovirus
  - Dental abscesses
  - Endocarditis/pericarditis
  - HIV (advanced stage)
  - Mycobacterial infection (often with advanced HIV)
  - Osteomyelitis
  - Renal
  - Sinusitis
  - Wound infections
  - Other miscellaneous infections
- Neoplasms
  - Atrial myxoma
  - Colorectal cancer
  - Hepatoma
  - Lymphoma
  - Leukemia
  - Solid tumors (renal cell carcinoma)
- Noninfectious inflammatory disease
  - Connective tissue diseases
    - Adult Still disease
    - Rheumatoid arthritis
    - Systemic lupus erythematosus
  - Granulomatous disease
    - Crohn disease
    - Sarcoidosis
  - Vasculitis syndromes
    - Giant cell arteritis
    - Polymyalgia rheumatica
- Other causes
  - Alcoholic hepatitis
  - Cerebrovascular accident
  - Cirrhosis
  - Drug fever/medication induced
    - Allopurinol, captopril, carbamazepine, cephalosporins, cimetidine, clofibrate, erythromycin, heparin, hydralazine, hydrochlorothiazide, isoniazid, meperidine, methyldopa, nifedipine, nitrofurantoin, penicillin, phenytoin, procainamide, quinidine, sulfonamides
  - Endocrinologic diseases
  - Factitious/fraudulent fever
  - Occupational causes
  - Periodic fever
  - Pulmonary emboli/deep vein thrombosis
  - Thermoregulatory disorders
- In up to 20% of cases, the cause of the fever will not be identified despite thorough workup.

RISK FACTORS

- Recent travel
- Exposure to biologic or chemical agents
- HIV-infection (particularly in advanced stages)
- Elderly
- Drug abuse
- Immigrants
- Young female health care workers (consider factitious fever)

Geriatric Considerations

Acute leukemia, Hodgkin lymphoma, intra-abdominal infections, tuberculosis (TB), and temporal arteritis are more common causes in elderly. Infections account for over half of cases. Collagen vascular diseases are 2nd most common etiology in older patients.

Pediatric Considerations

- ~50% of FUO in published pediatric case series are infectious; collagen vascular disease, malignancy also common (1)[A].
- Inflammatory bowel is a common cause in older children and adolescents.

DIAGNOSIS

HISTORY

- Important symptoms associated with fever
  - Common constitutional symptoms
    - Chills, night sweats, myalgias, weight loss with an intact appetite (infectious)
    - Arthralgias, myalgias, fatigue (inflammatory)
    - Fatigue, night sweats, weight loss with loss of appetite (neoplasms)
- Past medical history should explore previously treated chronic infections, abdominal diseases, transfusion history, malignancy, psychiatric illness, and recent hospitalization.
- Past surgical history should include specific information about type of surgery performed, postoperative complications, and any indwelling foreign materials.
- Obtain a comprehensive list of all medications, including over-the-counter and herbal remedies.
- Family history, such as periodic fever syndromes and recent febrile illnesses in family members to which the patient may have been exposed

ALERT

Care should be taken to obtain a thorough travel history, psychosocial history, occupational history, sexual history, and any history of drug use/abuse.

PHYSICAL EXAM

- Physical exam with high diagnostic yield
  - Funduscopic exam for choroid tubercles or Roth spots
  - Temporal artery tenderness
  - Oral-mucosal lesions
  - Auscultation for bruits and murmurs
  - Abdominal palpation for organomegaly
  - Rectal examination
  - Testicular examination
  - Lymph node examination
  - Skin and nail bed exam for clubbing, nodules, lesions, and erosions
  - Focal neurologic signs
  - Bony tenderness or joint effusion
  - Serial exams are often helpful for evolving physical signs associated with FUO (e.g., lesions associated with endocarditis).

DIFFERENTIAL DIAGNOSIS

See "Etiology and Pathophysiology"

DIAGNOSTIC TESTS & INTERPRETATION

Initial Tests (lab, imaging)

- CBC
- Peripheral blood smear
- LFTs
- C-reactive protein, ESR
- HIV testing
- Blood cultures (not to exceed 6 sets)
- Urinalysis and urine culture
- Chest x-ray
- CT or MRI of abdomen and pelvis (with directed biopsy, if indicated) (2)[C].

Follow-Up Tests & Special Considerations

- Rheumatoid factor and antinuclear antibody test
- Serologic tests: Epstein-Barr, hepatitis, syphilis, Lyme disease, Q fever, cytomegalovirus, amebiasis, coccidioidomycosis
- Serum ferritin
- Serum protein electrophoresis
- Sputum and urine cultures for TB
- Thyroid function tests
- Tuberculin skin test
  - May not be helpful if anergic or acute infection
  - If test negative, repeat in 2 weeks
  - If indicated, consider an interferon gamma release assay (IGRA) test
- Technetium-based scan, if infectious process or tumor suspected (2)[B]
- FDG-PET/CT scan if infectious process, inflammatory process, or tumor suspected; PET scans have a high negative predictive value and good sensitivity (but may have false positives) (3)[A].

- Ultrasound of abdomen and pelvis (plus directed biopsy, if indicated) if renal obstruction or gallbladder/biliary tree pathology suspected
- Echocardiogram if cardiac valve lesions (endocarditis), atrial myxomas, or pericardial effusion suspected
- Lower extremity Doppler if deep vein thrombosis/pulmonary embolism suspected
- CT scan of chest if pulmonary emboli suspected
- Indium-labeled leukocyte scanning if inflammatory process or occult abscess suspected
- Bone scan if osteomyelitis or metastatic disease suspected

Diagnostic Procedures/Other

- Liver biopsy if granulomatous disease suspected (2)[C]
- Temporal artery biopsy, particularly in the elderly
- Lymph node, muscle, or skin biopsy, if clinically indicated
- Bone marrow biopsy with histologic examination
- Spinal tap, if clinically indicated

Test Interpretation

Depends on etiology

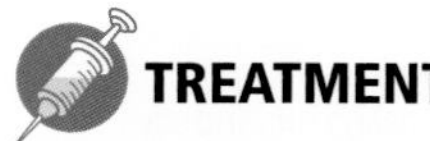

TREATMENT

GENERAL MEASURES

- Treatment depends on the specific etiology, which should be determined before initiating therapy if at all possible
- Therapeutic trials are a last resort and should be as specific as possible based on available clinical evidence. Such "shotgun" approaches are condemned because they obscure the clinical picture, have untoward effects, and do not solve the problem (2)[C].

MEDICATION

First Line

- First-line drugs depend on the diagnosis.
- Evidence does not support isolated treatment of fever (4)[C].

Second Line

If the patient has localizing symptoms associated with the fever or continues to decline, consider a therapeutic trial:

- Antibiotic trial based on patient's history
- Antituberculous therapy if there is a high risk for TB pending definitive culture results
- Steroid trial based on patient's history (once occult malignancy is ruled out)

ALERT

If a steroid trial is initiated, patient may have a relapse after treatment or if certain conditions (e.g., TB) have been undiagnosed.

ADDITIONAL THERAPIES

Febrile patients have increased caloric and fluid demands.

SURGERY/OTHER PROCEDURES

The need for exploratory laparotomy has been largely eliminated with the advent of more sophisticated tests and imaging modalities.

INPATIENT CONSIDERATIONS

Admission Criteria/Initial Stabilization

- Reserved for the ill and debilitated
- Consider if factitious fever has been ruled out or an invasive procedure is indicated

ONGOING CARE

FOLLOW-UP RECOMMENDATIONS

Patient Monitoring

If the etiology of the fever remains unknown, it is helpful to repeat the history and physical exam along with screening lab studies.

DIET

No specific dietary recommendations have been shown to ameliorate undiagnosed fever.

PATIENT EDUCATION

Maintain an open line of communication between physician and patient/family as the workup progresses:

- The extended time required in establishing a diagnosis can be frustrating.

PROGNOSIS

- Depends on etiology and age
  - Patients with HIV have the highest mortality.
- 1-year survival rates (reflecting deaths due to all causes)

Age	Survival
$<$35 years	91%
35–64 years	82%
$>$64 years	67%

COMPLICATIONS

Dependent on etiology

Pregnancy Considerations

Fever increases the risk of neural tube defects in pregnancy and can also trigger preterm labor.

REFERENCES

1. Chow A, Robinson JL. Fever of unknown origin in children: a systematic review. *World J Pediatr*. 2011;7(1):5–10.
2. Mourad O, Palda V, Detsky AS. A comprehensive evidence-based approach to fever of unknown origin. *Arch Intern Med*. 2003;163(5):545–551.
3. Hao R, Yuan L, Kan Y, et al. Diagnostic performance of 18F-FDG PET/CT in patients with fever of unknown origin: a meta-analysis. *Nucl Med Commun*. 2013;34(7):682–688.
4. Plaisance KI, Mackowiak PA. Antipyretic therapy: physiologic rationale, diagnostic implications, and clinical consequences. *Arch Intern Med*. 2000;160(4):449–456.

ADDITIONAL READING

- Ben-Baruch S, Canaani J, Braunstein R, et al. Predictive parameters for a diagnostic bone marrow biopsy specimen in the work-up of fever of unknown origin. *Mayo Clin Proc*. 2012;87(2):136–142.
- Hayakawa K, Ramasamy B, Chandrasekar PH. Fever of unknown origin: an evidence-based review. *Am J Med Sci*. 2012;344(4):307–316.
- Hersch EC, Oh RC. Prolonged febrile illness and fever of unknown origin in adults. *Am Fam Physician*. 2014;90(2):91–96.
- Varghese GM, Trowbridge P, Doherty T. Investigating and managing pyrexia of unknown origin in adults. *BMJ*. 2010;341:C5470.

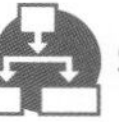

SEE ALSO

- Arthritis, Juvenile Idiopathic; Colorectal Cancer; Cytomegalovirus Inclusion Disease; Endocarditis, Infective; Hepatoma; HIV Infection and AIDS; Leukemia; Lupus Erythematosus, Discoid; Osteomyelitis; Polyarteritis Nodosa; Polymyalgia Rheumatica; Pulmonary Embolism; Rheumatic Fever; Sinusitis; Stroke, Acute; Temporal Arteritis
- Algorithms: Fever, Acute; Fever in the First 3 Months of Life; Fever of Unknown Origin

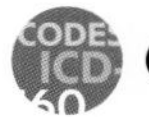

CODES

ICD10

R50.9 Fever, unspecified

CLINICAL PEARLS

- A sequential approach to FUO based on a careful history, physical examination, and targeted testing/imaging typically leads to a rational diagnosis or rules out common causes of FUO in most cases.
- Avoid a "shotgun" approach to diagnosis treatment; use empiric therapy only in carefully defined circumstances.
- FUO cases that defy precise diagnosis after intensive investigation and prolonged observation generally carry a favorable prognosis.
- In many cases, FUO in older persons may represent atypical presentations of common diseases.

FIBROCYSTIC CHANGES OF THE BREAST

Katherine M. Callaghan, MD

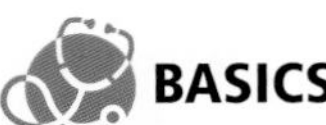

BASICS

DESCRIPTION

- Fibrocystic changes (FCC) of the breast is a generalized term for a heterogeneous group of changes affecting the stromal and glandular tissues of the breast.
- It is the most common of all benign breast conditions.
- Commonly presents as mastalgia, engorgement, increased breast nodularity, and/or cysts
  - Mastalgia (breast pain) is usually in upper outer quadrants of breast, bilateral, and may radiate to shoulders or upper arms.
  - Localized pain may occur with a rapidly enlarging cyst.
  - Nodules are usually small (2–10 mm), diffuse, and bilateral, with a rubbery consistency.
  - Cysts are more common in women in their 40s.
  - Larger cysts may have consistency of a water-filled balloon.
- Symptoms are most prominent in premenstrual (luteal) phase.
- System(s) affected: endocrine/metabolic, reproductive
- Synonym(s): fibrocystic breast disease; mammary dysplasia; chronic cystic mastitis

EPIDEMIOLOGY

Most common in women of reproductive years; occasionally seen after menopause with hormone replacement

Incidence

Unknown but very frequent

Prevalence

50–60% of women without breast disease are found to have this pattern of fibrous change and cyst formation.

ETIOLOGY AND PATHOPHYSIOLOGY

- Estrogen likely a causative factor for many
- May be the result of an exaggerated response of breast tissue to cycling hormones or a subtle imbalance in the ratio of estrogen to progesterone
- Cystic disease is caused by dilation of ducts and acini, proliferation and metaplasia of epithelial lining, and multiplication of ducts and acini, resulting in obstruction of the terminal ductal lobular unit.

RISK FACTORS

- The effect of consumption of methylxanthine-containing substances (e.g., coffee, tea, cola, and chocolate) has not been found to be a contributing factor.
- Diet high in fruits and vegetables and high parity independently decrease risk of FCC.
- Diet high in saturated fats may increase risk of FCC.

COMMONLY ASSOCIATED CONDITIONS

FCC found clinically confers no increased risk of breast cancer.

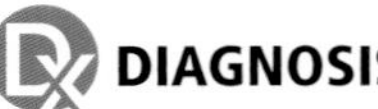

DIAGNOSIS

HISTORY

- May present in 3 overlapping, indistinct stages:
  - Mastoplasia (breast enlargement) and mastalgia which may subside after menses; common in women in their 20s
  - Adenosis: appearance of multiple small breast nodules; common in women in their 30s
  - Cystic phase: tender cysts, usually small, but up to 5 cm in diameter; common in women in their 40s
- Obtain personal history of breast biopsy and family history of breast disease (benign or malignant).

PHYSICAL EXAM

- With patient first upright, then supine, turn rotated on to contralateral hip, evaluate all breast tissue from sternum to midaxillary line, from clavicle to mammary ridge.
- Using fingertip, proceed in a linear fashion from top of sternum past breast tissue using 3 different depths of pressure at each palpation. Continue superiorly again to clavicle in a "lawn mower" fashion.
- Quantitate size, consistency, mobility, location, and skin changes.
- Findings in FCC may include the following:
  - Smooth, tense, or fluctuant masses
  - Bilateral masses
  - Breast thickening
  - Nipple discharge
- Palpate for axillary lymph nodes.

DIFFERENTIAL DIAGNOSIS

- Pain
  - Mastitis
  - Costochondritis
  - Pectoralis muscle strain
  - Neuralgia
  - Breast cancer
  - Angina pectoris
  - Gastroesophageal reflux (GERD)
  - Superficial phlebitis of the thoracoepigastric vein (Mondor disease)
- Masses
  - Breast cancer
  - Sebaceous cyst
  - Fibroadenoma
  - Lipoma
  - Fat necrosis
- Skin changes
  - Breast cancer (peau d'orange: thickened skin similar to peel of an orange)
  - Eczema

DIAGNOSTIC TESTS & INTERPRETATION

- Evaluation should focus on excluding breast cancer.
- Testing may be conducted based on a level of clinical suspicion.

Initial Tests (lab, imaging)

- Ultrasound (US): Signs of malignancy include irregular mass, clustered masses, calcifications, architectural distortion, and dilated duct; US is useful for differentiating cystic from solid lesions.
- Mammography may reveal mass or dense tissue $\pm$ calcifications.

Follow-Up Tests & Special Considerations

- Mammogram may be normal in presence of malignancy and difficult to interpret in women $<$35 years of age due to dense breast tissue; US may be more helpful, particularly in the presence of a palpable mass.
- MRI is indicated in patients with *BRCA1* or *BRCA2* mutation or in any woman with $\geq$25% lifetime risk for breast cancer (1).

Diagnostic Procedures/Other

- Fine-needle aspiration (FNA) and biopsy
  - Allows differentiation of cystic and solid lesions
  - Aspirate may be straw-colored, dark brown, or green.
  - Cells sent for cytology can reveal cancer with high accuracy.
  - Low morbidity
- If mass disappears, no further evaluation is necessary (including cytologic evaluation of aspirated fluid).

Test Interpretation
Certain histologic changes in the setting of fibrocystic change confer an increased risk for breast cancer:
- Atypia: relative risk of 4.24
- Proliferative changes without atypia: relative risk of 1.88
- Nonproliferative changes: relative risk of 1.27 (2)

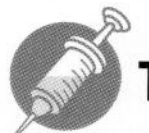

TREATMENT

- After ruling out malignancy by means of examination, and/or imaging and diagnostic procedures, FCC may not require treatment and often resolves with time.
- Cool compresses, avoiding trauma, and around-the-clock wearing of a well-fitting, supportive brassiere may be useful for symptom relief.

MEDICATION
First Line
For cyclic pain and swelling: NSAIDs
- Ibuprofen 400 mg QID/PRN
- Naproxen 500 mg BID/PRN

Second Line
- Oral contraceptives may be useful in modulating symptoms or in preventing the development of new changes.
- For severe pain, consider the following (3,4):
  - Danazol (Danocrine) 100–400 mg/day divided in 2 doses × 4–6 months
  - Bromocriptine 1.25–2.5 mg BID × 3 months
  - Tamoxifen 10 mg/day × 3–6 months
  - These medications are not without serious side effects and thorough counseling is required. Consultation with a breast specialist may be considered.

ISSUES FOR REFERRAL
- If discrete palpable lesion in a woman ≥35 years: US, then refer to a surgeon.
- If discrete palpable lesion in a woman >35 years: Diagnostic mammography ± US, then refer to surgeon.

SURGERY/OTHER PROCEDURES
Breast cyst aspiration can be both diagnostic and therapeutic.

COMPLEMENTARY & ALTERNATIVE MEDICINE
Evidence supporting evening primrose oil, vitamin E, or pyridoxine as treatment for the discomforts of FCC is insufficient to draw conclusions about effectiveness (5).

ONGOING CARE

FOLLOW-UP RECOMMENDATIONS
Condition is benign, chronic, and recurrent.

Patient Monitoring
- The patient needs to be assessed with clinical examination, radiologic studies, and sometimes biopsy to be certain a lump is not malignant.
- Follow-up times are variable, depending on the clinical situation.
- US is useful to differentiate cysts from solid lesions and in evaluating women <35 years of age for FCC but is not useful for screening.
- Screening mammograms should be obtained after age 40–50 years. Refer to the USPSTF, ACOG, or ACS recommendations for screening schedules.
- Aspiration cytology is useful to differentiate cysts from solid lesions. The sensitivity and specificity of cyst aspirate cytology for cancer diagnosis depends on the skill of the clinician and cytopathologist and may be as high as 98%.
- When physical examination, mammography, and FNA are used in combination, detection rates for breast cancer range from 93 to 100%.

DIET
There is insufficient evidence that changes in diet (e.g., caffeine intake) affect symptoms of FCC. Individual patient response will vary.

PATIENT EDUCATION
- Patient information on fibrocystic breasts from the Mayo Foundation for Medical Education and Research: www.mayoclinic.com/health/fibrocystic-breasts/DS01070
- Information on breast cancer prevention from the National Cancer Institute: www.cancer.gov
- Information on fibrocystic breasts from the American Cancer Society: www.cancer.org/Healthy/FindCancerEarly/WomensHealth/Non-CancerousBreastConditions/non-cancerous-breast-conditions-fibrocystic-changes

REFERENCES

1. Morris EA. Diagnostic breast MR imaging: current status and future directions. *Magn Reson Imaging Clin North Am*. 2010;18(1):57–74.
2. Hartmann LC, Sellers TA, Frost MH, et al. Benign breast disease and the risk of breast cancer. *N Engl J Med*. 2005;353(3):229–237.
3. Srivastava A, Mansel RE, Arvind N, et al. Evidence-based management of mastalgia: a meta-analysis of randomised trials. *Breast*. 2007;16(5):503–512.
4. Mousavi SR, Mousavi SM, Samsami M, et al. Comparison of tamoxifen with danazol in the management of fibrocystic disease. *Int J Med Med Sci*. 2011;2:329–331.
5. Horner NK, Lampe JW. Potential mechanisms of diet therapy for fibrocystic breast conditions show inadequate evidence of effectiveness. *J Am Diet Assoc*. 2000;100(11):1368–1380.

ADDITIONAL READING

- Amin AL, Purdy AC, Mattingly JD, et al. Benign breast disease. *Surg Clin North Am*. 2013;93(2):299–308.
- Griffin JL, Pearlman MD. Breast cancer screening in women at average risk and high risk. *Obstet Gynecol*. 2010;116(6):1410–1421.
- Meisner AL, Fekrazad MH, Royce ME. Breast disease: benign and malignant. *Med Clin North Am*. 2008;92(5):1115–1141.
- Rinaldi P, Ierardi C, Costantini M, et al. Cystic breast lesions: sonographic findings and clinical management. *J Ultrasound Med*. 2010;29(11):1617–1626.
- Santen RJ, Mansel R. Benign breast disorders. *N Engl J Med*. 2005;353(3):275–285.
- Saslow D, Boetes C, Burke W, et al. American Cancer Society guidelines for breast screening with MRI as an adjunct to mammography. *CA J Clin*. 2007;57(2):75–89.

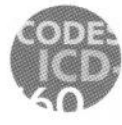

CODES

ICD10
- N60.19 Diffuse cystic mastopathy of unspecified breast
- N60.09 Solitary cyst of unspecified breast
- N60.29 Fibroadenosis of unspecified breast

CLINICAL PEARLS

- Fibrocystic breast change is a common finding in reproductive-aged women and generally does not confer an increased cancer risk.
- Symptoms can be managed expectantly with NSAIDs or oral contraceptives.
- Palpable breast lesions should be evaluated as clinically indicated.

FIBROMYALGIA

F. Stuart Leeds, MS, MD

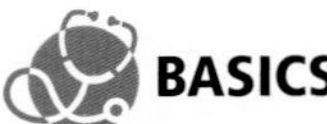

BASICS

DESCRIPTION

- Chronic, widespread noninflammatory musculoskeletal pain syndrome with multisystem manifestations. Although the specific pathophysiology has not been elucidated, it is generally thought to be a disorder of altered central pain regulation.
- Synonym(s): FMS; fibrositis, fibromyositis; "psychogenic rheumatism" (archaic and inaccurate)

EPIDEMIOLOGY

Incidence

- Predominant sex: female > male ($\sim$90% are females)
- Predominant age range: 20–65 years

Prevalence

2–5% of adult U.S. population (1)

ETIOLOGY AND PATHOPHYSIOLOGY

Idiopathic but appears to be a primary disorder of central pain processing, termed central sensitization (2); decrease in blood flow to the thalamus and caudate nucleus

- Afferent augmentation of peripheral nociceptive stimuli
- Alterations in neuroendocrine, neuromodulation, neurotransmitter, neurotransporter, biochemical, and neuroreceptor function/physiology
- Sleep abnormalities—alpha-wave intrusion (3)
- Inflammation is not a feature of fibromyalgia.
- May be triggered or exacerbated by a situational stressor, physical injury, or illness

Genetics

- Genetics
  - High familial aggregation
  - Inheritance is unknown but likely polygenic
  - Odds ratio may be as high as 8.5 for a 1st-degree relative of a familial proband (4).
  - Commonly comorbid with mood or anxiety disorders in families
- Environmental
  - Physical trauma or injury or severe illness
  - Stressors (e.g., work, family, life events, and abuse)
  - Some studies report correlations to certain infections (e.g., Lyme disease and hepatitis C).

RISK FACTORS

- Female gender
- Poor functional status
- Negative/stressful life events
- Low socioeconomic status

GENERAL PREVENTION

No specific prevention known

COMMONLY ASSOCIATED CONDITIONS

- Fibromyalgia presents as the "fibromyalgia syndrome," with widespread pain and regional/functional manifestations. It may occur concomitant to other rheumatologic or neurologic disorders.
- Obesity is frequently present and is associated with increased severity of symptoms (5).

DIAGNOSIS

- Per the 2010 revised ACR criteria (1)
  - Based on Widespread Pain Index (WPI) and Symptom Score (SS)
    - Must have ($\text{WPI} \geq 7 + \text{SS} \geq 5$) or ($\text{WPI} \geq 3$ and $\text{SS} \geq 9$); *and*
    - Symptoms for >3 months; *and*
    - No other explanation for these symptoms
- Per the original 1990 ACR criteria, still used by many clinicians: a) pain in all 4 quadrants, b) axial (neck/spine) involvement, c) tender points (TPs) –11+/18; a questionnaire tool to facilitate WPI/SS patient scoring and diagnosis may be found at: ***www.fmnetnews.com/docs/NewFibroCriteriaSurvey.pdf***
- This tool assesses the following:
  - WPI counts the number of sites of regional pain occurring over past week (**score 0–19**):
    - Above the waist
      - Jaw, right and left
      - Neck
      - Shoulder girdle, right and left
      - Upper back
      - Upper arm, right and left
      - Lower arm, right and left
      - Chest
      - Abdomen
      - Lower back
    - Below the waist
      - Hip (buttock, trochanter), right and left
      - Upper leg, right and left
      - Lower leg, right and left
      - The SS scale score is the sum of two parts.
      - Part (1) grades the 3 key symptoms on a 0–3 scale, giving a score of 0–9: **fatigue**, **waking unrefreshed**, and **cognitive symptoms**
      - Part (2) counts 40+ associated symptoms, giving a 0–3 score corresponding to **none**, **few**, **moderate**, **or many** symptoms.
      - Part (1) and (2) are added together to give a total SS of **0–12**.
  - The Visual Analogue Scale Fibromyalgia Impact Questionnaire (VASFIQ) (6) is recommended for initial and serial assessment of patient's functional status. It may be found at: ***http://www.ncbi.nlm.nih.gov/pmc/articles/PMC3383533/figure/fig1-1759720X11416863/***

HISTORY

- Universal symptoms include the following
  - Chronic widespread pain ≥3 months: bilateral limbs and in the axial skeleton
  - Generalized fatigue and sleep disturbances
- Often present
  - Mood disorders, including depression, anxiety, and panic symptoms
  - Cognitive impairment: qualitatively different from that seen in isolated mood disorders ("fibrofog") (7)
  - Headaches: typically, tension and migraine types
  - Other regional pain syndromes, such as irritable bowel syndrome, chronic pelvic pain, vulvodynia, and interstitial cystitis
  - Paresthesias, often "nonanatomic"
  - Exercise intolerance, dyspnea, and palpitations
  - Sexual dysfunction
  - Ocular dryness
  - "Multiple chemical sensitivity" and an increased tendency to report drug reactions
  - Impaired social/occupational functioning
  - Symptoms can wax and wane on a day-to-day basis, varying in quality, intensity, and location.

PHYSICAL EXAM

- Classic fibromyalgia TPs: 9 symmetric pairs (5 anterior, 4 posterior) located at anterior sternocleidomastoids, upper mid trapezius, medial 2nd intercostals space, lateral epicondyles, medial fat pad of knees, and, posteriorly, at occipital insertions, upper medial scapular insertions, upper outer quadrants of gluteals, and posterior greater trochanters. The presence of 11+/18 TPs carries a sensitivity of 88.4% and specificity 81.1% for the disease (1). These are distinct from the "trigger points" found in myofascial pain syndrome.
- Generalized hyperalgesia and allodynia
- Joints examined for swelling, tenderness, erythema, decreased range of motion, crepitus, and cystic or mass lesions—all typically absent in isolated fibromyalgia
- Document absence of inflammatory musculoskeletal disease features (e.g., no synovitis, enthesopathy, dermatologic/ocular findings)
- Neurologic exam: typically unremarkable

DIFFERENTIAL DIAGNOSIS

- RA, SLE, sarcoidosis, and other inflammatory connective tissue disorders
- Diffuse/advanced OA
- Seronegative spondyloarthropathies (AS, psoriatic arthritis, etc.)
- Polymyalgia rheumatica
- Inherited myopathies
- Drug-induced and endocrine myopathies
- Viral/postviral polyarthralgia
- Anemia and iron deficiency
- Electrolyte disturbances: Mg, Na, K, Ca
- Obstructive sleep apnea
- Osteomalacia/vitamin D deficiency
- Opioid-induced hyperalgesia
- Hypothyroidism
- Multiple sclerosis
- Lyme disease
- Hepatitis B and C (chronic)
- Inclusion-body myositis
- Spinal stenosis/neuropathies
- Peripheral vascular disease
- Somatoform disorder
- Overlap syndromes
  - Chronic fatigue syndrome/chronic fatigue immune dysfunction syndrome
  - Myofascial pain syndrome (more anatomically localized than fibromyalgia, but they may co-occur)

DIAGNOSTIC TESTS & INTERPRETATION

Initial Tests (lab, imaging)

- CBC with differential, ESR or CRP, CPK, TSH, comprehensive metabolic profile; consider 25-OH vitamin D, Mg, B_{12}, folate, and urine drug screen.
- ANA, RF, and other rheumatologic labs unnecessary, unless there is evidence of an inflammatory connective tissue disorder.
- Imaging not indicated, except to exclude other diagnoses.

Diagnostic Procedures/Other

- Sleep studies may be indicated to rule out obstructive sleep apnea or narcolepsy.
- Consider psychiatric or neuropsychiatric evaluation for mood disorders and cognitive disturbances.

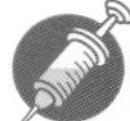

TREATMENT

According to the HHS National Guideline Summary (8), evidence-based interventions include the following:

- Nonpharmacologic
  - Educate the patient about the diagnosis, signs, symptoms, and treatment options (8)[A].
  - Provide Internet education resources.
    - www.fmaware.org
    - www.nfra.net
    - www.fmnetnews.com
  - Use the Fibromyalgia Impact Questionnaire (VAS-FIQ) for initial assessment and interval evaluation during treatment (8)[A].
  - Cognitive-behavioral therapy: improves mood, energy, pain, and functional status (8)[A]
  - Aerobic exercise: moderately intense, with gradual progression to avoid symptom exacerbation (9)[A]
  - Weight loss may augment the benefits of exercise.
  - Strength/resistance training—mild to moderate (9)[A]
- Pharmacologic
  - The 3 FDA-approved drugs are duloxetine, milnacipran, and pregabalin; others are used off-label.

MEDICATION

First Line

- Amitriptyline: 10–50 mg PO at bedtime to treat pain, fatigue, and sleep disturbances (10)[A]
- Duloxetine: initially 30 mg/day × 1 week, then increase to 60 mg/day as tolerated. Taper if discontinued (10)[A].
- Milnacipran day 1: 12.5 mg/day; days 2–3, *begin dividing doses*: 12.5 mg BID; days 4–7: 25 mg BID; after day 7: 50 mg BID; max dose 100–200 mg BID. Taper if discontinued (10)[A].
- Pregabalin: Start with 75 mg BID, titrate over 1 week to 150 BID; max dose 450 mg/day divided BID–TID (11)[A].
- Cyclobenzaprine 5 mg HS; titrate up to 10 mg BID–TID (8)[B].

Second Line

- Gabapentin start at 300 mg HS, titrate to 1,200–2,400 mg/day divided BID–TID (8)[B].
- Fluoxetine 10–80 mg/day PO (higher doses may be more effective). Taper if discontinued (8)[B].
- Paroxetine CR 12.5–62.5 mg/day. Taper if discontinued (8)[B].
- Tramadol 50–100 mg q6h; likely more effective in combination with acetaminophen (8)[C]
- Medications likely to be *ineffective* include NSAIDs, opioids, benzodiazepines, magnesium, guaifenesin, thyroxine, corticosteroids, DHEA, melatonin, calcitonin (8)[C].
- Several investigational agents show some promise of benefit, including pramipexole (12), naltrexone, quetiapine, sodium oxybate (3), and nabilone.
- Cholecalciferol may be beneficial in patients with low 25-OH vitamin D levels (13).

ISSUES FOR REFERRAL

In the case of unclear diagnosis or poor response to therapy, may refer to rheumatology, neurology, and/or pain management.

COMPLEMENTARY & ALTERNATIVE MEDICINE

- Acupuncture, biofeedback, hypnotherapy (8)[B]
- Balneotherapy (mineral-rich baths): hot or cold, with or without massage (8)[B]
- Treatments likely to be *ineffective*: chiropractic treatment, massage, electrotherapy, ultrasound, trigger point injections (8)[A]
- Yoga, tai chi, and qi gong—improve sleep, fatigue, and quality of life but may not decrease pain (14)
- Limited double-blind trials have shown effectiveness of supplementation with 5-HTP (may not be safe), S-adenosyl methionine, and acetyl-L-carnitine.
- Transcranial direct current stimulation and repetitive transcranial magnetic stimulation may be considered for those with inadequate symptom relief using other therapies (15).

ONGOING CARE

FOLLOW-UP RECOMMENDATIONS

Patient Monitoring

- For efficacy of therapy at 2–4-week intervals
- Patient follow-up required if intolerant to exercise; reduce intensity and duration until tolerated.

DIET

No proven efficacy of any specific diet. A nutrient-rich, varied diet with avoidance of processed foods is generally recommended. Caloric or carbohydrate restriction may be helpful in obese patients.

PROGNOSIS

- 50% partial remission after 2–3 years of therapy (16)
- Typically has fluctuating, chronic course
- Poorer outcome with
  - Longer illness duration, more severe symptoms, depression, advanced age, lack of social support

REFERENCES

1. Wolfe F, Häuser W. Fibromyalgia diagnosis and diagnostic criteria. *Ann Med*. 2011;43(7):495–502.
2. Smith HS, Harris R, Clauw D. Fibromyalgia: an afferent processing disorder leading to a complex pain generalized syndrome. *Pain Physician*. 2011;14(2):E217–E245.
3. Russell IJ, Holman AJ, Swick TJ, et al. Sodium oxybate reduces pain, fatigue, and sleep disturbance and improves functionality in fibromyalgia: results from a 14-week,randomized, double-blind, placebo-controlled study. *Pain*. 2011;152(5):1007–1017.
4. Arnold LM, Hudson JI, Hess EV, et al. Family study of fibromyalgia. *Arthritis Rheum*. 2004;50(3):944–952.
5. Okifuji A, Donaldson GW, Barck L, et al. Relationship between fibromyalgia and obesity in pain, function, mood, and sleep. *J Pain*. 2010;11(12):1329–1337.
6. Boomershine CS, Emir B, Wang Y, et al. Simplifying fibromyalgia assessment: the VASFIQ Brief Symptom Scale. *Ther Adv Musculoskelet Dis*. 2011;3(5): 215–226.
7. Glass JM. Cognitive dysfunction in fibromyalgia and chronic fatigue syndrome: new trends and future directions. *Curr Rheumatol Rep*. 2006;8(6):425–429.
8. National Guideline Clearinghouse. Guideline summary NGC-7367: management of fibromyalgia syndrome in adults. http://f.i-md.com/medinfo/material/8d0/4eb2854244ae46d1d13648d0/4eb2855d44ae46d1d13648d3.pdf. Accessed 2014.
9. Häuser W, Klose P, Langhorst J, et al. Efficacy of different types of aerobic exercise in fibromyalgia syndrome: a systematic review and meta-analysis of randomised controlled trials. *Arthritis Res Ther*. 2010;12(3):R79.
10. Häuser W, Petzke F, Üçeyler N, et al. Comparative efficacy and acceptability of amitriptyline, duloxetine and milnacipran in fibromyalgia syndrome: a systematic review with meta-analysis. *Rheumatology (Oxford)*. 2011;50(3):532–543.
11. Häuser W, Walitt B, Fitzcharles MA, et al. Review of pharmacological therapies in fibromyalgia syndrome. *Arthritis Res Ther*. 2014;16(1):201.
12. Holman AJ, Myers RR. A randomized, double-blind, placebo-controlled trial of pramipexole, a dopamine agonist, in patients with fibromyalgia receiving concomitant medications. *Arthritis Rheum*. 2005;52(8):2495–2505.
13. Wepner F, Scheuer R, Schuetz-Wieser B, et al. Effects of vitamin D on patients with fibromyalgia syndrome: a randomized placebo-controlled trial. *Pain*. 2014;155(2):261–268.
14. Langhorst J, Klose P, Dobos GJ, et al. Efficacy and safety of meditative movement therapies in fibromyalgia syndrome: a systematic review and meta-analysis of randomized controlled trials. *Rheumatol Int*. 2013;33(1):193–207.
15. Marlow NM, Bonilha HS, Short EB. Efficacy of transcranial direct current stimulation and repetitive transcranial magnetic stimulation for treating fibromyalgia syndrome: a systematic review. *Pain Pract*. 2012;13(2):131–145.
16. Forseth KO, Førre O, Gran JT. A 5.5 year prospective study of self-reported musculoskeletal pain and of fibromyalgia in a female population: significance and natural history. *Clin Rheumatol*. 1999;18(2):114–121.

ADDITIONAL READING

- Hassett AL, Williams DA. Non-pharmacological treatment of chronic widespread musculoskeletal pain. *Best Pract Res Clin Rheumatol*. 2011;25(2):299–309.
- Häuser W, Bernardy K, Arnold B, et al. Efficacy of multicomponent treatment in fibromyalgia syndrome: a meta-analysis of randomized controlled clinical trials. *Arthritis Rheum*. 2009;61(2):216–224.

SEE ALSO

Algorithm: Fatigue

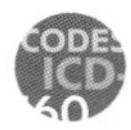

CODES

ICD10

M79.7 Fibromyalgia

CLINICAL PEARLS

- Suspect fibromyalgia when a patient describes severe symptoms of chronic pain, fatigue, and multiple regional complaints in the *absence* of laboratory or physical exam findings.
- Use rigorous ACR criteria to make the diagnosis.
- Fibromyalgia is not a somatoform disorder and is not merely a manifestation of depression or anxiety, although, as with all chronic pain syndromes, it is frequently associated with mood disturbances.
- The pathophysiology is still unclear, but the disease is currently believed to be a disorder of pain regulation, known as "central sensitization." Best outcomes occur in patients who understand their illness and are willing to actively engage in a multimodal treatment plan, including exercise, medication, CBT, and lifestyle modifications.

F

FOLLICULITIS

Joseph R. Adams, DO • Miles C. Layton, DO, MAJ, MC, USA • Samuel N. Sigoloff, DO, CPT, MC, USA

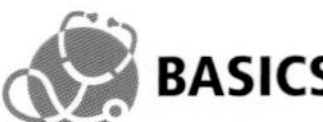

BASICS

DESCRIPTION

- Inflammation of a follicle, usually a hair follicle, caused by infection, physical injury (traction), or chemical irritation (1)
- Can occur anywhere on the body that hair is found
- Most frequent symptom is pruritus.
- Painless or tender pustules, vesicles or pink/red papulopustules up to 5 mm in size
- Most commonly infectious in etiology:
  - *Staphylococcus aureus* bacteria (most common)
  - *Pseudomonas aeruginosa* infects areas of the body exposed to poorly chlorinated hot tubs, pools, or contaminated water.
  - *Aeromonas hydrophila* with recreational water exposure
  - Fungal (dermatophytic, *Pityrosporum*, *Candida*)
  - Viral (VZV, HSV)
  - Parasitic (*Demodex* spp. mites, schistosomes)
- Noninfectious types
  - Acneiform folliculitis
  - Actinic superficial folliculitis
  - Acne vulgaris
  - Keloidal folliculitis
  - Folliculitis decalvans
  - Perioral dermatitis
  - Rosacea
  - Fox-Fordyce disease
  - Pruritus folliculitis of pregnancy
  - Eosinophilic pustular folliculitis (3 variants: Ofuji disease in patients of Asian descent, HIV-positive/immunocompromised, infantile)
  - Toxic erythema of the newborn
  - Eosinophilic folliculitis (seen in HIV-positive/immunocompromised)
  - Follicular mucinosis
- Skin disorders may produce a follicular eruption that includes the following:
  - Pseudofolliculitis: similar in appearance; occurs after shaving; affects the face, scalp, pubis, and legs. Pseudofolliculitis barbae, or razor bumps, occurs frequently in black men.
  - Atopic dermatitis
  - Follicular psoriasis

EPIDEMIOLOGY

Affects persons of all ages, gender, and race

ETIOLOGY AND PATHOPHYSIOLOGY

Predisposing factors to folliculitis

- Chronic staphylococcal carrier
- Diabetes mellitus
- Malnutrition
- Pruritic skin disease (e.g., scabies, eczema, etc.)
- Exposure to poorly chlorinated swimming pools/hot tubs or water contaminated with *P. aeruginosa*, *A. hydrophila*, or schistosomes
- Occlusive corticosteroid use (for multiple hours)
- Bacteria
  - Superficial or deep
  - Most frequently due to *S. aureus* (increasing number of MRSA cases)
  - Also due to *Streptococcus* species, *Pseudomonas* (following exposure to water contaminated with the species), or *Proteus*
  - May progress to furunculosis (painful pustular nodule with central necrosis that leaves a permanent scar after healing)
- Fungal
  - Dermatophytic (tinea capitis, corporis, pedis)
  - *Pityrosporum (Pityrosporum orbiculare)* commonly affecting teenagers and men, predominantly on upper chest and back.
  - *Candida albicans*, although rare, has been reported with broad-spectrum antibiotic use, glucocorticoid use, immunosuppression, and in those who abuse heroin, resulting in candidemia that leads to pustules and nodules in hair-bearing areas.
- Viral
  - Herpes simplex virus
  - May be due to molluscum contagiosum, usually a sign of immunosuppression
- Parasitic
  - *Demodex* spp. mites (most commonly *Demodex folliculorum*)
  - Schistosomes (swimmer's itch)
- Acneiform type commonly drug-induced (systemic and topical corticosteroids, lithium, isoniazid, rifampin), EGFR inhibitors
- Severe vitamin C deficiency
- Actinic superficial type occurs within 24–48 hours of exposure to the sun, resulting in multiple follicular pustules on the shoulders, trunk, and arms.
- Acne vulgaris
- Keloidal folliculitis is a chronic condition affecting mostly black patients; involves the neck and occipital scalp, resulting in hypertrophic scars and hair loss; usually secondary to folliculitis barbae from shaving
- Folliculitis decalvans is a chronic folliculitis that leads to progressive scarring and alopecia of the scalp.
- Rosacea consists of papules, pustules, and/or telangiectasias of the face; individuals are genetically predisposed. *Helicobacter pylori* and *D. folliculorum* have also been implicated.
- Perioral dermatitis seen most commonly in children and young women; restricted to the perioral region as well as the lower eyelids. May be due to cosmetics, hyperandrogenemia, or use of fluorinated topical corticosteroids
  - Typically spares vermillion border
- Fox-Fordyce disease affects the skin containing apocrine sweat glands (i.e., axillae), resulting in chronic pruritic, annular, follicular papules.
- Eosinophilic pustular folliculitis (EPF) has 3 variants: classic (Ofuji disease), associated with HIV infection, and infantile.
- Toxic erythema of the newborn is a self-limiting pustular eruption usually appearing during the first 3–4 days of life and subsequently fading in the following 2 weeks.
- Malassezia infections in adult males with lesions on trunk (2)[B]

RISK FACTORS

- Hair removal (shaving, plucking, waxing, epilating agents)
- Other pruritic skin conditions: eczema, scabies
- Occlusive dressing or clothing
- Personal carrier or contact with methicillin-resistant *Staphylococcus aureus* (MRSA)-infected persons
- Diabetes mellitus
- Immunosuppression (medications, chemotherapy, HIV)
- Use of hot tubs or saunas
- Use of EGFR inhibitors
- Chronic antibiotic use (Gram [−] folliculitis)

GENERAL PREVENTION

- Good hygiene practices
  - Wash hands frequently.
  - Antimicrobial soap
  - Wash towels, clothes, and linens frequently with hot water to avoid reinfection.
- Good hair removal practices
  - Exfoliate beforehand.
  - Use witch hazel, alcohol, or Tend Skin afterward.
  - Shave in direction of hair growth; use moisturizer/warm water.
  - Decrease frequency of shaving.
  - Use clippers primarily or single blade razors if straight shaving is desired.

COMMONLY ASSOCIATED CONDITIONS

- Impetigo
- Furunculosis
- Scabies
- Acne
- Follicular psoriasis
- Eczema

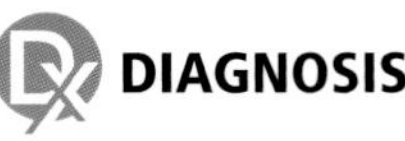

DIAGNOSIS

HISTORY

- Recent use of hot tubs, swimming pools, topical corticosteroids, certain hair styling and shaving practices, antibiotics or systemic steroids
- HIV status
- History of STDs (specifically syphilis)
- MRSA exposures/carrier status
- Ask about home and work environment (risk/exposure potential).
- *Pityrosporum* folliculitis occurs more often in warm, moist climates.
- Inquire about the timeline in which the lesions have occurred, including previous similar episodes.

PHYSICAL EXAM

- Characteristic lesions are 1–5-mm–wide vesicles, pustules, or papulopustules with surrounding erythema.
- Rash occurs on hair-bearing skin, especially the face (beard), proximal limbs, scalp, and pubis.
- Pseudomonal folliculitis appears as a widespread rash, mainly on the trunk and limbs.
- In pseudofolliculitis, the growing hair curls around and penetrates the skin at shaved areas.

DIFFERENTIAL DIAGNOSIS

- Acne vulgaris/acneiform eruptions
- Arthropod bite
- Contact dermatitis
- Cutaneous candidiasis
- Milia
- Atopic dermatitis
- Follicular psoriasis
- Hidradenitis suppurativa

DIAGNOSTIC TESTS & INTERPRETATION

Initial Tests (lab, imaging)

- Diagnosis usually made clinically, taking risk factors, history, and location of lesion into account.
- Culture and Gram stain of the pustule by scraping the pustule with a no. 15 blade and not directly swabbing the skin to identify infectious agent and sensitivities to antibiotics
- KOH preparation as well as Wood lamp fluorescence to identify *Candida* or yeast

- Tzanck smear where suspicion of herpetic simplex viral folliculitis is high

Follow-Up Tests & Special Considerations
- If risk factors or clinical suspicion exist, consider serologies for HIV or syphilis.
- If recurrent, consider HIV testing and A1C/fasting blood sugar testing to evaluate for diabetes.
- Punch biopsy may be considered if lesions persist despite treatment (3)[C].

Test Interpretation
- Treat positive bacterial culture according to sensitivities.
- Positive HIV serology: Follow up with CD4 count and punch biopsy to rule out eosinophilic folliculitis.
- Eosinophilic folliculitis: Collect eosinophils within superficial follicle (4)[B].

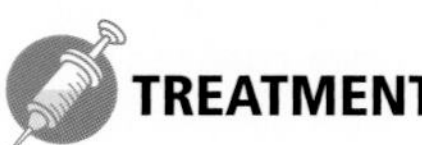

TREATMENT

GENERAL MEASURES
- Lesions usually resolve spontaneously.
- Avoid shaving and waxing affected areas (5)[C].
- Warm compresses may be applied TID.
- Systemic antibiotics are typically unnecessary.
- Topical mupirocin may be used in presumed *S. aureus* infection.
- Topical antifungals for fungal folliculitis (2)[B]
- Preventive measures are keys to avoidance of recurrence:
  - Antibacterial soaps (Dial soap, chlorhexidine, or benzyl peroxide wash when showering/bathing)
  - Bleach baths (1/2 cup of 6% bleach per standard bathtub and soak for 5–15 minutes followed by water rinse 1–2 times a week)
  - Keep skin intact; daily skin care with noncomedogenic moisturizers; avoid scratching.
  - Clean shaving instruments daily or use disposable razor, disposing after 1 use.
  - Change washcloths, towels, and sheets daily.

MEDICATION
Antiseptic and supportive care is usually enough. Systemic antibiotics may be used with questionable efficacy.

First Line
- Staphylococcal folliculitis
  - Mupirocin ointment applied TID for 10 days
  - Cephalosporin (cephalexin): 250–500 mg PO QID for 7–10 days
  - Dicloxacillin: 250–500mg PO QID for 7–10 days
- For MRSA:
  - Bactrim DS: 1–2 tablets (160 mg/800 mg) BID PO for 5–10 days
  - Clindamycin: 300 mg PO TID for 10–14 days
  - Minocycline: 200 mg PO initially then 100 mg BID for 5–10 days
  - Doxycycline: 50–100 mg PO BID for 5–10 days
- Pseudomonal folliculitis
  - Topical dilute acetic acid baths
  - Ciprofloxacin: 500–750 mg PO BID for 7–14 days only if patient is immunocompromised or lesions are persistent
- Eosinophilic folliculitis/eosinophilic pustular folliculitis
  - HAART treatment for HIV-positive–related causes
  - Topical corticosteroids: betamethasone 0.1% BID for 3–24 weeks *or*
  - Antihistamines (hydroxyzine, cetirizine) *or*
  - Tacrolimus: topically BID for 3–24 weeks *or*
  - Isotretinoin: 0.5 mg/kg/day PO for 4–8 weeks *or*
  - Itraconazole or metronidazole
- Fungal folliculitis
  - Topical antifungals: ketoconazole 2% cream or shampoo or selenium sulfide shampoo daily *or*
  - Econazole cream applied to affected area BID for 2–3 weeks
    - Systemic antifungals for relapses fluconazole (100–200 mg/day for 3 weeks) *or* itraconazole (200 mg/day for 1–3 weeks)
    - Griseofulvin (tinea capitis in children; 10–20 mg/kg/day for 6 weeks minimum)
- Parasitic folliculitis
  - 5% permethrin: Apply to affected area, leave on for 8 hours and wash off.
  - Ivermectin: 200 μg/kg × 1 followed by topical permethrin
- Herpetic folliculitis
  - Valacyclovir: 500 mg PO TID for 5–10 days *or*
  - Famciclovir: 500 mg PO TID for 5–10 days *or*
  - Acyclovir: 200 mg PO 5× daily for 5–10 days

ISSUES FOR REFERRAL
Unusual or persistent cases should be biopsied and then referred to dermatology.

ADDITIONAL THERAPIES
Public Health Measures
- Outbreaks of culture-positive *Pseudomonas* hot tub folliculitis should be reported so that source identification can be determined and superchlorination (14 parts/million) can occur.

SURGERY/OTHER PROCEDURES
Incision and drainage is unlikely to be necessary and typically not preferred due to potential for scar formation.

ONGOING CARE

FOLLOW-UP RECOMMENDATIONS
Patient Monitoring
- Resistant cases should be followed every 2 weeks until cleared.
- 1 return visit in 2 weeks if symptoms abate

DIET
For obese patients, weight reduction will decrease skin-on-skin friction.

PATIENT EDUCATION
Avoid shaving in involved areas.

PROGNOSIS
- Usually resolves with treatment; however, *S. aureus* carriers may experience recurrences.
- Mupirocin nasal treatment for carrier status and for family/household members might be helpful.
- Resistant or severe cases may warrant testing for diabetes mellitus or immunodeficiency (HIV) (3)[C].

COMPLICATIONS
- Primary complication is recurrent folliculitis.
- Extensive scarring with hyperpigmentation
- Progression to furunculosis or abscesses

REFERENCES

1. Breitkopf T, Leung G, Yu M, et al. The basic science of hair biology: what are the causal mechanisms for the disordered hair follicle. *Dermatol Clin*. 2013;31(1):1–19.
2. Song HS, Kim SK, Kim YC. Comparison between Malassezia folliculitis and Non-Malassezia folliculitis. *Ann Dermatol*. 2014;26(5):598–602.
3. Tilley DH, Satter EK, Kakimoto CV, et al. Disseminated verrucous varicella zoster with exclusive follicular involvement. *Arch Dermatol*. 2012;148(3):405–407.
4. Annam V, Yelikar BR, Inamadar AC, et al. Clinicopathological study of itchy folliculitis in HIV-infected patients. *Indian J Dermatol Venereol Leprol*. 2010;76(3):259–262.
5. Khanna N. Post waxing folliculitis: a clinicopathological evaluation. *Int J Dermatol*. 2014;53(7):849–854.

ADDITIONAL READING

- Bachet JB, Peuvrel L, Bachmeyer C, et al. Folliculitis induced by EGFR inhibitors, preventive and curative efficacy of tetracyclines in the management and incidence rates according to the type of EGFR inhibitor administered: a systematic literature review. *Oncologist*. 2012;17(4):555–568.
- Böer A, Herder N, Winter K, et al. Herpes folliculitis: clinical, histopathological, and molecular pathologic observations. *Br J Dermatol*. 2006;154(4):743–746.
- Brooke RCC, Griffiths CEM. Folliculitis decalvans. *Clin Exp Dermatol*. 2001;26(1):120–122.
- Ellis E, Scheinfeld N. Eosinophilic pustular folliculitis: a comprehensive review of treatment options. *Am J Clin Dermatol*. 2004;5(3):189–197.
- Fiorillo L, Zucker M, Sawyer D, et al. The *Pseudomonas* hot-foot syndrome. *N Engl J Med*. 2001;345(5):335–338.
- Fridkin SK, Hageman JC, Morrison M, et al. Methicillin-resistant *Staphylococcus aureus* disease in three communities. *N Engl J Med*. 2005;352(14):1436–1444.
- James WD. Clinical practice. Acne. *N Engl J Med*. 2005;352(14):1463–1472.
- Luelmo-Aguilar J, Santandreu MS. Folliculitis: recognition and management. *Am J Clin Dermatol*. 2004;5(5):301–310.
- Nervi SJ, Schwartz RA, Dmochowski M. Eosinophilic pustular folliculitis: a 40 year retrospect. *J Am Acad Dermatol*. 2006;55(2):285–289.

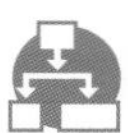

SEE ALSO

Algorithm: Rash, Focal

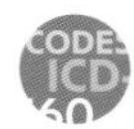

CODES

ICD10
- L73.9 Follicular disorder, unspecified
- L66.2 Folliculitis decalvans
- L73.8 Other specified follicular disorders

CLINICAL PEARLS

- Folliculitis lesions are typically 1–5 mm clusters of pruritic erythematous papules and pustules.
- Most commonly due to *S. aureus*. If community has increased incidence of MRSA, consider anti-MRSA treatment.
  - It is extremely important to educate patients on proper hygiene and skin care techniques in order to prevent chronic or recurrent cases.

F

FOOD ALLERGY

Stanley Fineman, MD

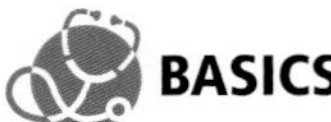

BASICS

DESCRIPTION

- Hypersensitivity reaction caused by certain foods
- System(s) affected: gastrointestinal, hemic/lymphatic/immunologic, pulmonary, skin/exocrine
- Synonym(s): allergic bowel disease; dietary protein sensitivity syndrome

EPIDEMIOLOGY

- Predominant age: all ages but more common in infants and children
- Predominant sex: male > female (2:1)

Incidence

Prospective studies indicate ~2.5% of infants experience hypersensitivity reactions to cow's milk in their 1st year of life (1)[B].

Prevalence

- The true prevalence of IgE-mediated food allergy when assessed by double-blind, placebo-controlled food challenge is 3% (2)[B].
- The self-reported prevalence of food allergy is 12% in children and 13% in adults (2)[B].
- In young children, the most common food allergies are cow's milk (2.5%), egg (1.3%), peanut (0.8%), and wheat (0.4%) (3)[B].
- Adults tend to have allergies to shellfish (2%), peanut (0.6%), tree nuts (0.5%), and fish (0.4%).
- In general, only 3–4% of children >4 years of age have persisting food allergy; it is frequently a transient phenomenon (4)[B].
- 20% of children with peanut protein allergy may outgrow their sensitivity by school age.

ETIOLOGY AND PATHOPHYSIOLOGY

Allergic response triggered by immunologic mechanisms, such as the classic IgE-allergic response or nonimmunologic-mediated mechanisms

- Any food or ingested substance can cause allergic reactions:
  - Most commonly implicated foods include cow's milk, egg whites, wheat, soy, peanuts, fish, tree nuts (walnut and pecan), and shellfish.
- Several food dyes and additives may elicit non–IgE-mediated allergic-like reactions.

Genetics

In family members with a history of food hypersensitivity, the probability of food allergy in subsequent siblings may be as high as 50%.

RISK FACTORS

- Persons with allergic or atopic predisposition have increased risk of hypersensitivity reaction to food.
- Family history of food hypersensitivity

GENERAL PREVENTION

- Avoidance of offending food
- In patients at risk for anaphylaxis, epinephrine autoinjectors should be readily available.

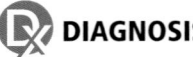

DIAGNOSIS

PHYSICAL EXAM

- GI (system usually affected)
  - More common: nausea, vomiting, diarrhea, abdominal pain, occult bleeding, flatulence, and bloating
  - Less common: malabsorption, protein-losing enteropathy, eosinophilic-enteritis, colitis
- Dermatologic
  - More common: urticaria/angioedema, atopic dermatitis, pallor, or flushing
  - Less common: contact rashes
- Respiratory
  - More common: allergic rhinitis, asthma and bronchospasm, cough, serous otitis media
  - Less common: pulmonary infiltrates (Heiner syndrome), pulmonary hemosiderosis
- Neurologic
  - Less common: migraine headaches
- Other symptoms
  - Systemic anaphylaxis, vasculitis

DIFFERENTIAL DIAGNOSIS

- A careful history is necessary to document a temporal relationship with the manifestations of suspected food hypersensitivity.
- GI, dermatologic, respiratory, neurologic, or other systemic manifestations may mimic a variety of clinical entities.

DIAGNOSTIC TESTS & INTERPRETATION

Initial Tests (lab, imaging)

- Eosinophilia in blood or tissue suggests atopy.
- Epicutaneous (prick or puncture) allergy skin tests are used to document IgE-mediated immunologic hypersensitivity and can be done using commercially available extracts (variable sensitivities) or fresh-food skin testing.
- Patient history has a greater sensitivity than skin testing or serum IgG.
- Skin testing using the suspect food is helpful. If positive on skin test, an oral challenge may aid in diagnosis. The overall correlation between commercially available allergy skin testing and oral food challenge is 60% but increases to 90% when fresh-food skin testing is done (i.e., a positive skin test correlates with a positive challenge to a particular food)
  - Skin testing has a high sensitivity (low false-negative rate) *but* a low specificity (high false-positive rate) so *only* skin test against antigens found on history (5)[B]
- Food-specific IgE assays (radioallergosorbent [RAST] and fluorescent enzyme immunoassay [FEI]) detect specific IgE antibodies to offending foods and are less sensitive to skin testing
  - In certain laboratories, the ImmunoCap food-specific IgE was almost as accurate as a skin test in predicting positive oral challenges.
  - Using a serum assay alone to diagnose food allergy has been shown to result in misdiagnosis of true clinical food allergic sensitivity, particularly in children with atopic dermatitis. Do not test using a panel but rather for specific IgE to foods based on patient history.
- Periodic monitoring of the peanut-specific IgE levels every 2 years may be helpful. If the level of peanut-specific IgE falls to <0.5 kU/L, then a cautious oral challenge under the supervision of an allergist may be considered. A fresh-food skin test with peanut protein should be considered prior to the oral challenge (6)[B].
- Patch testing for foods for determining delayed-sensitivity immunologic reactions, in patients with eosinophilic esophagitis and atopic dermatitis, is considered of marginal benefit (7)[B].
- Widespread allergy skin testing or serum IgE tests are *not* recommended because of their poor predictive value without a clinical correlating history (3)[B].
- Leukocyte histamine release and assays for circulating immune complexes are predominantly research procedures and are of limited use in clinical practices:
  - Assays for IgG and IgG 4 subclass antibodies are commercially available.
  - No convincing data suggest that these tests are reliable for the diagnosis of food allergy (4)[B].
- The provocative injection and sublingual provocative tests are highly controversial and have been proven useless for diagnosis of food allergy.
- The leukocytotoxic assay is an unproven diagnostic procedure and is not useful for the diagnosis of allergy (7)[B].
- Other unproven diagnostic procedures that are not recommended include provocative neutralization, lymphocyte stimulation, hair analysis, and applied kinesiology (3)[B].

Diagnostic Procedures/Other

Elimination and challenge test is the best procedure for confirming food allergy:

- The suspected food is eliminated from the diet for 1–2 weeks.
- The patient's symptoms are monitored. If they disappear or substantially improve, an oral challenge with the suspected food should be performed under medical supervision.
- Optimally, this challenge should be performed in a double-blind, placebo-controlled manner.
- Patients with history of anaphylaxis should not have an oral challenge unless lack of IgE sensitivity can be documented.
- Most allergic reactions will occur within 30 minutes to 2 hours after challenge, although late reactions have also been described that may occur from 12 to 24 hours.

Test Interpretation

Pathologic findings are not common in food allergies; however, inflammatory changes can sometimes be seen in the GI tract. The diagnosis of eosinophilic esophagitis is defined by the finding of >15–20 eosinophils per high-power field on esophageal biopsy (8)[C].

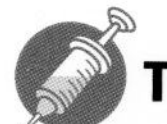

TREATMENT

GENERAL MEASURES

- Avoiding the offending food is the most effective mode of treatment for patients with food allergies.
- Those patients with exquisite and severe allergy hypersensitivity to a food should be more cautious in their avoidance of that food. They should carry epinephrine for self-administration in the event that the offending food is ingested unknowingly and a subsequent immediate reaction develops.
- Immunotherapy or hyposensitization with food extracts by various routes, including SC immunotherapy or sublingual neutralization, are not recommended. Research studies are in progress, but immunotherapy is considered experimental at this time.

MEDICATION

- Patients with significant type 1, IgE-mediated hypersensitivity should have epinephrine for autoinjection available in case of accidental ingestion and resulting severe anaphylactic reaction.
- After receiving epinephrine for a systemic anaphylactic reaction to a food, the patient should be monitored in a medical facility because 15–25% of patients may require >1 dose of epinephrine.
- Symptomatic treatment for milder reactions (e.g., antihistamine)
- The use of cromolyn has been suggested but is not recommended for use in most patients with food allergy.

COMPLEMENTARY & ALTERNATIVE MEDICINE

There are reports of benefit using various Chinese herbal medicines in laboratory animals with induced food allergy. Benefits have not been reported in humans at this time.

ONGOING CARE

FOLLOW-UP RECOMMENDATIONS

Patient Monitoring

As needed

DIET

- As determined by tests and clinical evaluation
- Strict avoidance of offending food

PATIENT EDUCATION

- Patients should be counseled by a dietitian to maintain a nutritionally sound diet despite avoiding those foods to which the patient is sensitive.
- Patient support: Food Allergy Research & Education, Inc.: 7925 Jones Branch Drive Suite 1100 McLean, VA 22102 Toll-Free: 800-929-4040; Web site www.foodallergy.org
- Other information available at www.aanma.org, www.acaai.org, and www.aaaai.org

PROGNOSIS

- Most infants will outgrow their food hypersensitivity by 2–4 years:
  - It may be possible to reintroduce the offending food cautiously into the diet (particularly helpful when the food is one that is difficult to avoid). It is critical that a specific IgE to the offending food is checked, optimally by fresh-food allergy skin test, and is negative prior to an oral challenge.
  - 20% of young children with peanut allergy experience resolution by the age of 5 years.
  - 42% of children with egg allergy and 48% of children with milk allergy develop clinical tolerance and lose their sensitivity over time (3)[B].
- Adults with food hypersensitivity (particularly to milk, fish, shellfish, or nuts) tend to maintain their allergy for many years (3)[B].

COMPLICATIONS

- Anaphylaxis
- Angioedema
- Bronchial asthma
- Enterocolitis
- Eosinophilic esophagitis
- Eczematoid lesions

REFERENCES

1. Bernstein IL, Li JT, Bernstein DI, et al. Allergy diagnostic testing: an updated practice parameter. *Ann Allergy Asthma Immunol*. 2008;100(3)(Suppl 3):S1–S148.
2. Rona RJ, Keil T, Summers C, et al. The prevalence of food allergy: a meta-analysis. *J Allergy Clin Immunol*. 2007;120(3):638–646.
3. Boyce JA, Assa'ad A, Burks AW, et al. Guidelines for the diagnosis and management of food allergy in the United States: summary of the NIAID-Sponsored Expert Panel Report. *J Allergy Clin Immunol*. 2010;126(6):1105–1118.
4. Burks AW, Tang M, Sicherer S, et al. ICON: food allergy. *J Allergy Clin Immunol*. 2012;129(4):906–920.
5. Chafen JJ, Newberry SJ, Riedl MA, et al. Diagnosing and managing common food allergies: a systematic review. *JAMA*. 2010;303(18):1848–1856.
6. Fleischer DM, Bock SA, Spears GC, et al. Oral food challenges in children with a diagnosis of food allergy. *J Pediatr*. 2011;158(4):578–583.e1.
7. Spergel JM, Brown-Whitehorn T, Beausoleil JL, et al. Predictive values for skin prick test and atopy patch test for eosinophilic esophagitis. *J Allergy Clin Immunol*. 2007;119(2):509–511.
8. Furuta GT, Liacouras CA, Collins MH, et al. Eosinophilic esophagitis in children and adult: a systematic review and consensus recommendations for diagnosis and treatment. *Gastroenterology*. 2007;133(4):1342–1363.

ADDITIONAL READING

- American College of Allergy, Asthma, & Immunology. Food allergy: a practice parameter. *Ann Allergy Asthma Immunol*. 2006;96(3)(Suppl 2):S1–S68.
- Høst A, Halken S. A prospective study of cow milk allergy in Danish infants during the first 3 years of life. Clinical course in relation to clinical and immunological type of hypersensitivity reaction. *Allergy*. 1990;45(8):587–596.
- Maloney JM, Rudengren M, Ahlstedt S, et al. The use of serum-specific IgE measurements for the diagnosis of peanut, tree nut, and seed allergy. *J Allergy Clin Immunol*. 2008;122(1):145–151.

SEE ALSO

Anaphylaxis; Celiac Disease; Irritable Bowel Syndrome

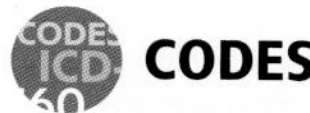

CODES

ICD10

- T78.1XXA Oth adverse food reactions, not elsewhere classified, init
- T78.00XA Anaphylactic reaction due to unspecified food, init encntr
- L27.2 Dermatitis due to ingested food

CLINICAL PEARLS

- Recent studies suggest that up to 20% of children with peanut allergy may outgrow their sensitivity:
  - Periodic monitoring of the peanut-specific IgE levels every 2 years may be helpful. If the level of peanut-specific IgE falls to <0.5 kU/L, then a cautious oral challenge under the supervision of an allergist may be considered. A fresh-food skin test with peanut protein should be considered prior to the oral challenge.
- Oral itching following ingestion of fresh fruit may be a warning of risk for anaphylaxis but may also represent oral allergy syndrome
  - This syndrome is the result of cross-reacting proteins in pollens (e.g., patients sensitive to birch tree pollen frequently have cross-reactivity to fresh apples and pears. Cooked fruits are usually tolerated).
- Current evidence does not support a major role for maternal dietary restrictions during pregnancy or lactation in the prevention of atopic disease in infants. It is generally recommended to exclusively breastfeed for the first 6 months of life, particularly when there is a family history of atopy and food allergy. Although solid foods should not be introduced before 4–6 months of age, there is no convincing evidence that delaying their introduction beyond this period has a significant protective effect on the development of allergies.

FOOD POISONING, BACTERIAL

Amy Okpaku, DO

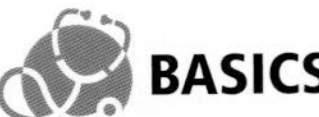

BASICS

DESCRIPTION

- Food poisoning (also known as foodborne infection) is an illness resulting from the consumption of contaminated food (1,2).
- Most cases are due to noroviruses, approximately 50% in the United States (1).
- The illness may be produced by bacterial infection or by toxins produced by the bacteria (1,2).
- The most commonly recognized bacterial foodborne infections acquired in the United States are the following: *Salmonella*, *Campylobacter*, and *Clostridium perfringens*. In traveler's diarrhea, *Escherichia coli* enters this group (1,2).

EPIDEMIOLOGY

Incidence

- In the United States, an estimated 48 million cases of foodborne poisoning annually (most due to viral etiology), resulting in 128,000 hospitalizations and 3,000 deaths. ~1 of 6 Americans will have an episode (2).
- >1/2 of waterborne bacterial food poisoning in the United States occurs in water not intended for drinking—untreated or inadequately treated ground water.

ETIOLOGY AND PATHOPHYSIOLOGY

- Short incubation period (1–6 hours): likely preformed toxin–induced
  - *Bacillus cereus*
    - Food sources: improperly cooked rice/fried rice and red meats
    - Causes sudden onset of severe nausea and vomiting. Diarrhea may be present.
  - *Staphylococcus aureus*
    - Food sources: nonrefrigerated or improperly refrigerated meats and potato and egg salads
    - Causes sudden onset of severe nausea and vomiting. Abdominal cramps and fever may be present.
- Medium incubation period (8–16 hours)
  - *Bacillus cereus* (toxin)
    - Food sources: meat, stew gravy, vanilla sauce
    - Causes watery diarrhea, abdominal cramps, nausea
  - *C. perfringens*
    - Food sources: dry/precooked meats and poultry
    - Causes watery diarrhea, nausea, abdominal cramps
- Long incubation period (>16 hours)
  - Toxin-producing organisms
    - *Clostridium botulinum*: Source is commercially canned or improperly home-canned foods. Causes vomiting, diarrhea, slurred speech, diplopia, dysphagia, and descending muscle weakness/flaccid paralysis
    - Enterohemorrhagic *E. coli* (e.g., 0157:H7): Food sources are undercooked beef, especially hamburger, unpasteurized milk, raw fruits and vegetables, and contaminated water. Causes severe diarrhea that often becomes bloody, abdominal pain, vomiting. More common in children <4 years of age
    - Enterotoxigenic *E. coli*: Food sources are foods or water contaminated by human feces. Causes watery diarrhea, abdominal cramps, and vomiting
    - *Vibrio cholerae*: Food sources are contaminated water, fish, and shellfish, especially food sold by street vendors. Causes profuse watery diarrhea and vomiting, which can lead to severe dehydration and death within hours
  - Invasive organisms: often bloody stool and fever
    - *Salmonella*: Food sources are contaminated eggs, poultry, unpasteurized milk or juice, cheese, contaminated raw fruits and vegetables, and contaminated peanut butter. Causes watery diarrhea, fever, abdominal cramps, vomiting
    - *Campylobacter jejuni*: Food sources are raw and undercooked poultry, unpasteurized milk, and contaminated meats. Causes diarrhea (may be bloody), cramps, vomiting, fever
    - *Shigella*: Food sources are food or water contaminated by human fecal material. Causes abdominal cramps, fever, diarrhea
    - *Vibrio parahaemolyticus*: Food source is raw shellfish. Causes nausea, vomiting, diarrhea, abdominal pain
    - *Vibrio vulnificus*: Food source is undercooked and raw seafood; wounds exposed to sea water. Causes vomiting, diarrhea, abdominal pain, bacteremia, wound infections. Can be fatal in patients with liver disease or those who are immunocompromised
    - *Yersinia enterocolitica* and *Y. pseudotuberculosis*: Food sources are undercooked pork, unpasteurized milk, tofu, contaminated water. Causes appendicitis-like symptoms: abdominal pain, fever, diarrhea, vomiting; occurs primarily in older children and younger adults.
    - *Listeria*: Sources include unpasteurized/contaminated milk, soft cheese, and processed/delicatessen meats. Causes nausea, vomiting, fever, watery diarrhea

RISK FACTORS

- Travel to developing countries
- Improper food storage/handling
- Cross-contamination during preparation of food
- Weakened immune system, pregnancy, very young, elderly, and those with chronic diseases
- Underlying GI disorders
- Patients taking antacids, H_2 blockers, and proton pump inhibitors

GENERAL PREVENTION

- When preparing food at home
  - Clean
    - Wash hands, cutting boards, and surfaces before food preparation and after preparing each food item.
    - Wash fresh produce thoroughly before eating.
  - Separate
    - Keep raw meat, poultry, fish, and their juices away from other food that will not be cooked (e.g., salad).
    - Place cooked meat on a clean platter.
  - Cook: Thoroughly cook meat to the following internal temperature
    - Fresh beef, veal, pork, and lamb: 145°F
    - Ground meats and egg dishes: 160°F
    - Poultry: 165°F. Cook chicken eggs thoroughly until the yolk is firm.
  - Chill
    - Refrigerate leftovers within 2–3 hours in clean, shallow, and covered containers. If the temperature is >90°F, refrigerate within 1 hour.
- When traveling to underdeveloped countries
  - Eat only freshly prepared foods.
  - Avoid beverages diluted with nonpotable water, such as ice and milk.
  - Avoid food washed in nonpotable water, such as salads.
  - Other risky foods include raw or undercooked meat and seafood, unpeeled raw fruits, and vegetables.
  - In developing nations: "Boil it, Cook it, Peel it, or Forget it."
  - Bottled, carbonated, and boiled beverages are generally safe to drink.
- Bismuth subsalicylate (Pepto-Bismol), two 262-mg tablets QID has been shown to protect travelers to developing countries ~60% of the time. However, it is not recommended for persons taking anticoagulants or other salicylates.

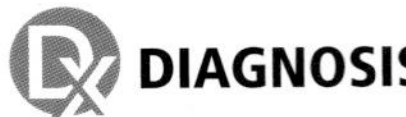

DIAGNOSIS

HISTORY

- The definition of diarrhea is >3 or more unformed stools daily (1).
- Suspect bacterial food poisoning when multiple persons have rapid onset of symptoms after eating the same meal; have high fever, blood, or mucus in stool; severe abdominal pain or neurologic involvement; or recent traveling in a foreign country.
- Any of the following should prompt further evaluation and possible supportive treatment: high fever (≥101.5°F), blood in the stools, prolonged vomiting, signs of dehydration (decrease in urination, a dry mouth and throat, and feeling dizzy when standing up), and diarrheal illness that lasts >3 days (1).
- Suspect *Clostridium difficile* colitis if with recent prolonged antibiotic use or recurrent *C. difficile* infection in repeated episodes (1,3).

PHYSICAL EXAM

- Focus on signs of dehydration: skin turgor, mucous membranes, and orthostatic changes.
- Abdominal exam: distension with tenderness (suggestive of bowel obstruction). Auscultation may demonstrate increased bowel sound in obstruction or decreased bowel sounds with an ileus.
- Neurologic: weakness, paresthesias, diplopia

DIFFERENTIAL DIAGNOSIS

- Infectious gastroenteritis of any kind (i.e., viral)
- *C. difficile* colitis
- Inflammatory bowel disease
- Appendicitis and other acute abdominal surgical processes
- Hepatitis
- Malabsorption

DIAGNOSTIC TESTS & INTERPRETATION

Initial Tests (lab, imaging)

- Culture of stool and sensitivity, fecal leukocytes, and Hemoccult testing; consider ova and parasites if dehydration, history of foreign travel, or symptoms lasting >2 weeks (1)[C]
- CBC, BMP for severe cases with dehydration, inpatient, and nursing home exposure (1)[C]

- Flexible sigmoidoscopy and colonoscopy are reserved for severe cases or when pathogen is suspected in setting of negative stool cultures (1).
- Abdominal CT may be helpful when intra-abdominal pathology or bowel disease are in the differential (1).

Follow-Up Tests & Special Considerations
Epidemiologic investigation may be warranted.

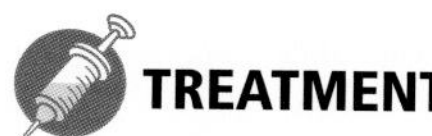

TREATMENT

Most cases of food poisoning are self-limiting and do not require medication.

MEDICATION

First Line

- Children, the elderly, and pregnant patients with signs of mild diarrhea should be started on oral rehydration solution to prevent dehydration (2)[C].
- Oral rehydration options can be purchased or mixed simply from common home ingredients: 6 tsp sugar and 1/2 tsp salt in 1 L of clean, potable water (2)[B].
- Travelers may consider empiric treatment for diarrhea with a single dose of ciprofloxacin 750 mg together with loperamide (see "Additional Treatment") (2)[A].

Second Line

For severe cases of food poisoning (up to 8% have bacteremia) or if the patient has a prosthetic valve, the following medications are recommended.

- *B. cereus* (2)
  - Supportive care only
- *Campylobacter jejuni* (1,2)
  - Mild: supportive care only
  - Severe: children: azithromycin 10 mg/kg/day for 3 days
  - Severe: adults: azithromycin 500 mg/day for 3 days or ciprofloxacin 500mg BID for 5 days
- *Clostridium botulinum*
  - Supportive care. Antitoxin can be helpful if administered early in the course of the illness.
- *Clostridium perfringens*
  - Supportive care only
- *Clostridium difficile* (1,2,4)
  - Mild disease: metronidazole 500 mg TID for 10 days
  - Severe disease: vancomycin 125 mg PO QID for 10 days, fidaxomicin 200 mg BID × 10 days
  - Severe disease, complicated (hypotension/shock, ileus, megacolon): vancomycin 500 mg PO QID plus metronidazole 500 mg IV every 8 hours
  - Discontinue offending antibiotic if applicable.
- Enterohemorrhagic *E. coli* (e.g., 0157:H7) (1)
  - Supportive care only. Closely monitor renal function, hemoglobin, and platelets. Infection associated with hemolytic uremic syndrome (HUS). Antibiotics may increase this risk.
- Enterotoxigenic *E. coli* (common cause of traveler's diarrhea) (1,2)
  - Generally self-limited. Antibiotics shorten course of illness.
  - Children: azithromycin 10 mg/kg/day for 3 days or ceftriaxone 50 mg/kg/day for 3 days
  - Adults: ciprofloxacin 500 mg BID for 3 days or azithromycin 1 g × single dose. Rifaximin is rising as an alternative.
- *Salmonella* (1,2,5)
  - No therapy in mild disease.
  - Moderate ciprofloxacin 500 mg BID × 10–14 days, levofloxacin 500 mg daily × 10 days or TMP/SMX DS 160/800 mg twice per day for 5–7 days
  - Severe diarrhea, immunocompromised, systemic signs, positive blood cultures, IV ceftriaxone 1–2 g daily for 7–10 days
- *Shigella* (1,2)
  - Ciprofloxacin 500 mg twice per day for 3 days, or 2-g single dose; alternative options: azithromycin 500 mg twice per day for 3 days, TMP/SMX DS 160/800 mg twice per day for 5 days, or ceftriaxone 1–2 g/day for 5 days
- *S. aureus* (1)
  - Supportive care only
- Noncholeraic *Vibrio* (1)
  - Ciprofloxacin 750 mg once daily for 3 days or azithromycin 500 mg once daily for 3 days
- *Vibrio cholera* (1)
  - Children: erythromycin 30 mg/kg/day given TID for 3 days or azithromycin 10 mg/kg/day for 3 days
  - Adults: doxycycline 300 mg 1-time dose in most cases or tetracycline 500 mg QID for 3 days or erythromycin 250 mg TID for 3 days or azithromycin 500 mg/day for 3 days
- *Yersinia* (2)
  - Usually supportive care only
  - Quinolones or 3rd-generation cephalosporin if severe

ADDITIONAL THERAPIES

- Loperamide 4 mg initially, then 2 mg after each loose stool to a maximum of 16 mg in a 24-hour period may be used *unless* high fever, bloody diarrhea, and/or severe abdominal pain present (signs of enteroinvasion). Among travelers with mild–moderate diarrhea and cramping, a single dose of ciprofloxacin 750 mg together with loperamide may eliminate the diarrhea (2)[A]. If symptoms persist after 24 hours, treat with antibiotics for an additional 1–2 days (2).
- Bismuth subsalicylate (Pepto-Bismol) may be combined with loperamide and is more effective than either alone (2)[B].
- Probiotics (i.e., *Lactobacillus* sp.) have been shown to reduce severity and sometimes duration by 24 hours. May also decrease likelihood of antibiotic-associated diarrhea (1,2,6).
- Diligent hand washing during course will decrease spread (2)[A].

ONGOING CARE

DIET

- Avoid food while nausea is present, but drink plenty of fluids in frequent sips.
- As the nausea subsides, drink adequate fluids; add in bland, low-fat meals; and rest. Avoid alcohol, coffee, nicotine, and spicy foods.
- Nursing infants should continue to be breastfed on demand, and infants and older children should be offered their usual food.

PROGNOSIS

Most infections are self-limited and will resolve over the course of 4–5 days.

COMPLICATIONS

- Dehydration
- HUS (3–5% *E. coli* 0157:H7)
- Guillain-Barré syndrome after *Campylobacter* enteritis
- Reiter syndrome after *Salmonella* enteritis
- *Clostridium difficile* colitis after antibiotic use
- Postinfectious irritable bowel

REFERENCES

1. DuPont HL. Acute infectious diarrhea in immunocompetent adults. *N Engl J Med*. 2014;370(16):1532–1540.
2. Barr W, Smith A. Acute diarrhea. *Am Fam Physician*. 2014;89(3):180–189.
3. Debast SB, Bauer MP, Kuijper EJ. European Society of Clinical Microbiology and Infectious Diseases: update of the treatment guidance document for *Clostridium difficile* infection. *Clin Microbiol Infect*. 2014;20(Suppl 2):1–26.
4. Slimings C, Riley TV. Antibiotics and hospital-acquired *Clostridium difficile* infection: update of systematic review and meta-analysis. *J Antimicrob Chemother*. 2014;69(4):881–891.
5. Onwuezobe IA, Oshun PO, Odigwe CC. Antimicrobials for treating symptomatic non-typhoidal *Salmonella* infection. *Cochrane Database Syst Rev*. 2012;11:CD001167.
6. Kligler B, Cohrssen A. Probiotics. *Am Fam Physician*. 2008;78(9):1073–1078.

ADDITIONAL READING

- Allen SJ, Martinez EG, Gregorio GV, et al. Probiotics for treating acute infectious diarrhoea. *Cochrane Database Syst Rev*. 2010;(11):CD003048.
- Ang JY, Mathur A. Traveler's diarrhea: updates for pediatricians. *Pediatr Ann*. 2008;37(12):814–820.
- *Trends in Foodborne Illness in the United States, 2012*. Atlanta, GA: Centers for Disease Control and Prevention; 2013.

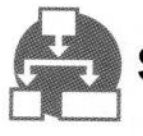

SEE ALSO

Appendicitis, Acute; Botulism; Brucellosis; Dehydration; Diarrhea, Acute; Guillain-Barré Syndrome; Hypokalemia; Intestinal Parasites; Salmonella Infection; Typhoid Fever

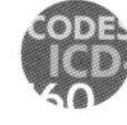

CODES

ICD10

- A05.9 Bacterial foodborne intoxication, unspecified
- A02.0 Salmonella enteritis
- A04.5 Campylobacter enteritis

CLINICAL PEARLS

- Consider bacterial food poisoning when multiple people present after ingesting the same food with fevers and blood/mucus in stool or have recently returned from a developing nation.
- In developing nations: "Boil it, Cook it, Peel it, or Forget it."
- Consider culture and antibiotics in a prolonged febrile state with blood/mucus in stool, septicemic states, and traveler's diarrhea.
- With signs of enteroinvasion (high prolonged fever, bloody diarrhea, severe pain, septicemia) consider withholding antispasmodics (e.g., Imodium)

F

FRAGILE X SYNDROME

Thomas J. Hansen, MD

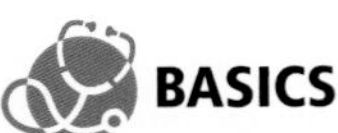

BASICS

DESCRIPTION

- Fragile X syndrome (FXS) is the most common inherited form of mental retardation (also referred to as mental impairment) and is one of the leading known causes of autism (1).
- Among the genetic causes of mental impairment, FXS is the 2nd most common cause following Down syndrome.
- In addition to mental impairment, FXS is characterized by a group of symptoms that may include specific physical features, distinctive behavior patterns, defective speech and language, seizure disorder, and cognitive deficits (2).
- Synonym(s): marker X syndrome; Martin-Bell syndrome; Escalante syndrome

EPIDEMIOLOGY

- Although this condition is seen in both sexes, males are usually more severely affected than females.
- Affected males almost always have mental impairment, mostly of moderate severity.
- Only 1/3–1/2 of affected females have mental impairment, usually in the mild to moderate range (2).

Prevalence

- FXS with full mutation is seen in 1:4,000 males and 1:8,000 females (3).
- FXS with premutation is seen in 1:800 males and 1:200 females (2).

Genetics

- This is an X-linked dominant disorder with variable penetrance.
- The syndrome is caused by an abnormal expansion of cytosine-guanine-guanine (CGG) on the fragile X mental retardation 1 (*FMR1*) gene. *FMR1* normally synthesizes the fragile X protein (FMRP), but mutations in *FMR1* lead to a lack of FMRP synthesis, which is important for normal brain development (4).
- The number of CGG repeats in the *FMR1* gene are classified as follows:
  - Full mutation (>200 CGG repeats)
  - Premutation (~6–200 CGG repeats)
- Most males with full mutation have mental impairment in addition to some form of the physical and behavioral features.
- Males with premutation have normal intelligence but have an increased risk for tremor-ataxia syndrome between age 50 and 60 years.
- Females with full mutation have a ~50% chance of having mental impairment in addition to some form of physical and behavioral features.
- Females with premutation have normal intelligence but have a 20% risk for premature ovarian failure.
- Because a male has only 1 X chromosome, it is never passed on to his son. He will pass the affected chromosome to all of his daughters.
- An affected female has a 50% chance of passing her affected chromosome to all of her children.

COMMONLY ASSOCIATED CONDITIONS

- Autistic spectrum disorder (3)
- Connective tissue manifestations, including flat feet and inguinal hernias (3)
- Mitral valve prolapse (develops during adolescence and adulthood) (3)
- Recurrent otitis media and sinusitis in childhood (3)
- Seizure disorder (15–20% for boys and 5% for girls) (4)
- Social phobias and other anxiety disorders (4)

DIAGNOSIS

HISTORY

- Family history of mental impairment, particularly with multiple male relatives
- Family history of premature ovarian failure or fragile X-related tremor ataxia syndrome
- Delay of ≥1 developmental milestones, especially when there is mental impairment in the family (2)
- After the 1st year of life, delay in speech and language along with impaired fine motor skills

Pediatric Considerations

Average age at the time of diagnosis is 8 years, reflecting the subtlety of features in young children (2).

PHYSICAL EXAM

- Physical characteristics become more prominent with advancing age (5).
- Birth–1 month
  - Examine for orthopedic abnormalities, especially congenital hip dysplasia and clubfoot.
  - Evaluate occipitofrontal circumference, which may be increased.
  - Monitor for feeding difficulties and gastroesophageal reflux (GERD).
- 1 month–1 year
  - Monitor for hypotonia that frequently results in mild motor delay.
  - Monitor for irritability secondary to sensory problems.
  - Evaluate for feeding problems and the presence of vomiting secondary to GERD.
- 1–5 years
  - Perform an ophthalmologic evaluation to check for strabismus and refractory errors.
  - Monitor for ptosis and nystagmus.
  - Evaluate for orthopedic problems related to connective tissue dysplasia such as pes planus, hypermobile joints, and scoliosis.
  - Examine for inguinal hernias.
  - Monitor for recurrent otitis media, conductive hearing loss, and recurrent sinusitis.
  - Monitor for language delay.
  - Monitor for emotional and behavioral status closely, especially tantrums and hyperactivity, and signs of autism.
- 5–12 years
  - Evaluate for macroorchidism and hernias in boys and precocious puberty in females.
  - Monitor for the child's developmental status.
  - Assess for hyperactivity, obsessive-compulsive behaviors, and anxiety.
  - Assess for cognitive impairments.
- 13–21 years
  - Assess for seizures, especially atypical seizures.
  - Monitor for cardiac murmur or click.
- Adulthood
  - Assess for mitral valve prolapse.
  - Evaluate for premature menopause (up to 20% before age 40 years).
  - Assess for fragile X–associated tremor/ataxia syndrome as patients approach the age of 50 years.

DIFFERENTIAL DIAGNOSIS

- Pervasive developmental disorder
- Learning disability
- Autism
- Attention deficit hyperactivity disorder (ADHD)
- Other causes of mental impairment

DIAGNOSTIC TESTS & INTERPRETATION

Diagnosis of FXS is made by DNA-based molecular tests, such as Southern blot test and polymerase chain reaction (PCR), to isolate the *FMR1* gene mutation. Indications for testing include the following (1):

- Patients with a family history of mental impairment or FXS
- Any child with developmental delay of uncertain etiology or autism
- Individual with mental impairment of unknown etiology
- Women with premature ovarian failure of unknown cause
- Individuals with late-onset intentional tremor or ataxia, especially with a family history of movement disorders, FXS, or undiagnosed mental impairment
- Prenatal testing is offered only if maternal premutation or full mutation is present.
  - Chorionic villus sampling or amniocentesis is used for prenatal diagnosis.
  - Preimplantation genetic diagnosis may be another option for women with a premutation FXS; however, there are several limitations to this approach.

Initial Tests (lab, imaging)

Newborn screening for FXS is not routine at present (6)[B].

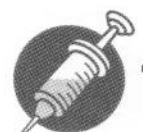

TREATMENT

- Treatment is usually supportive and includes the use of stimulants, selective serotonin reuptake inhibitors (SSRIs), atypical antipsychotics, and α-agonists; treatment is individualized according to symptoms.
- However, there currently is no robust evidence to support recommendations on pharmacologic treatments in patients with FXS in general or in those with an additional diagnosis of ADHD or autism (7).

MEDICATION

Depending on the clinical presentation, pharmacotherapy may include the following (8)[B]:

- Atypical antipsychotics
- SSRIs
- Antiepileptics
- Methylphenidate
- Dextroamphetamines
- Clonidine
- Guanfacine

Second Line

Impossible to draw conclusions about the effect of folic acid on FXS patients due to the low quality of current evidence (9)

ISSUES FOR REFERRAL

- The proband and family should be referred for genetic counseling and tested for the *FMR1* gene.
- Also see "Additional Therapies" section.

ADDITIONAL THERAPIES

Nonpharmacologic therapies are of tremendous value (10)[B] and include the following:

- Behavior therapy
- Speech and language therapy
- Psychotherapy and counseling
- Occupational and physical therapy
- Social skill training, support group
- Special education and preschool intervention programs (10)

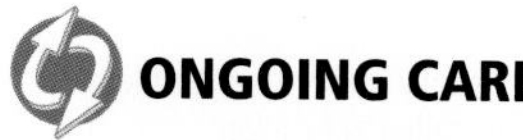

ONGOING CARE

PATIENT EDUCATION

- In young females with FXS who are planning for future pregnancies, review the reproductive options such as egg donation, prenatal diagnosis, adoption, and preimplantation genetic diagnosis.
- Useful Web sites
  - The National Fragile X Foundation (www.fragilex.org)
  - FRAXA research foundation (http://www.fraxa.org)
  - Gene tests (www.genetests.org, www.geneclinics.org)
  - American College of Medical Genetics (www.acmg.net)
  - Dolan DNA learning center: your genes, your health (www.ygyh.org)
  - National Institute of Child Health and Human Development (www.nichd.nih.gov)

PROGNOSIS

- Patients with FXS have a normal lifespan.
- About 20–33% of women carrying a premutation for FXS are at increased risk for premature ovarian failure.
- 1/3 of males and, to a lesser extent, females carrying the premutation are at increased risk for late-onset (>50 years) progressive neurodegenerative disorder. It is characterized by intentional tremor and ataxia, called fragile X-associated tremor/ataxia syndrome (FXTAS). Other associated findings include parkinsonism, autonomic dysfunction, peripheral neuropathy, and dementia.

REFERENCES

1. Santoro MR, Bray SM, Warren ST. Molecular mechanisms of fragile X syndrome: a twenty-year perspective. *Annu Rev Pathol*. 2012;7:219–245.
2. Wattendorf DJ, Muenke M. Diagnosis and management of fragile X syndrome. *Am Fam Physician*. 2005;72(1):111–113.
3. Visootsak J, Warren ST, Anido A, et al. Fragile X syndrome: an update and review for the primary pediatrician. *Clin Pediatr (Phila)*. 2005;44(5):371–381.
4. Tsiouris JA, Brown WT. Neuropsychiatric symptoms of fragile X syndrome: pathophysiology and pharmacotherapy. *CNS Drugs*. 2004;18(11):687–703.
5. Hersh JH, Saul RA; Committee on Genetics. Health supervision for children with fragile X syndrome. *Pediatrics*. 2011;127(5):994–1006.
6. Bailey DB Jr, Skinner D, Davis AM, et al. Ethical, legal, and social concerns about expanded newborn screening: fragile X syndrome as a prototype for emerging issues. *Pediatrics*. 2008;121(3):e693–e704.
7. Rueda JR, Ballesteros J, Tejada MI. Systematic review of pharmacological treatments in fragile X syndrome. *BMC Neurol*. 2009;9:53.
8. Hagerman RJ, Berry-Kravis E, Kaufmann WE, et al. Advances in the treatment of fragile X syndrome. *Pediatrics*. 2009;123(1):378–390.
9. Rueda JR, Ballesteros J, Guillen V, et al. Folic acid for fragile X syndrome. *Cochrane Database Syst Rev*. 2011;(5):CD008476.
10. Solomon M, Hessl D, Chiu S, et al. A genetic etiology of pervasive developmental disorder guides treatment. *Am J Psychiatry*. 2007;164(4):575–580.

ADDITIONAL READING

- American College of Obstetricians and Gynecologists Committee on Genetics. ACOG committee opinion. No. 338: screening for fragile X syndrome. *Obstet Gynecol*. 2006;107(6):1483–1485.
- Cornish KM, Gray KM, Rinehart NJ. Fragile X syndrome and associated disorders. *Adv Child Dev Behav*. 2010;39:211–235.
- McConkie-Rosell A, Finucane B, Cronister A, et al. Genetic counseling for fragile x syndrome: updated recommendations of the national society of genetic counselors. *J Genet Couns*. 2005;14(4):249–270.
- McLennan Y, Polussa J, Tassone F, et al. Fragile x syndrome. *Curr Genomics*. 2011;12(3):216–224.
- Orr HT, Zoghbi HY. Trinucleotide repeat disorders. *Annu Rev Neurosci*. 2007;30:575–621.

F

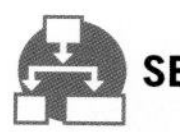

SEE ALSO

Algorithm: Mental Retardation

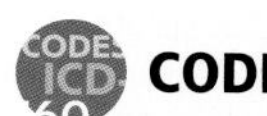

CODES

ICD10

Q99.2 Fragile X chromosome

CLINICAL PEARLS

- FXS is the most common inherited form of mental retardation.
- FXS is an X-linked dominant disorder with variable penetrance. Therefore, although this condition is seen in both sexes, males are usually more severely affected than females.
- Newborn screening for FXS is not routine.
- The average age at the time of diagnosis is 8 years.

FURUNCULOSIS

Zoltan Trizna, MD, PhD

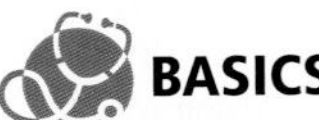

BASICS

DESCRIPTION

- Acute bacterial abscess of a hair follicle (often *Staphylococcus aureus*)
- System(s) affected: skin/exocrine
- Synonym(s): boils

EPIDEMIOLOGY

Incidence

- Predominant age
  - Adolescents and young adults
  - Clusters have been reported in teenagers living in crowded quarters, within families, or in high school athletes.
- Predominant sex: male = female

Prevalence

Exact data are not available.

ETIOLOGY AND PATHOPHYSIOLOGY

- Infection spreads away from hair follicle into surrounding dermis.
- Pathogenic strain of *S. aureus* (usually); most cases in United States are now due to community-acquired methicillin-resistant *S. aureus* (CA-MRSA), whereas methicillin-sensitive *S. aureus* (MSSA) is most common elsewhere (1).

Genetics

Unknown

RISK FACTORS

- Carriage of pathogenic strain of *Staphylococcus* sp. in nares, skin, axilla, and perineum
- Rarely, polymorphonuclear leukocyte defect or hyperimmunoglobulin E–*Staphylococcus* sp. abscess syndrome
- Diabetes mellitus, malnutrition, alcoholism, obesity, atopic dermatitis
- Primary immunodeficiency disease and AIDS (common variable immunodeficiency, chronic granulomatous disease, Chediak-Higashi syndrome, C3 deficiency, C3 hypercatabolism, transient hypogammaglobulinemia of infancy, immunodeficiency with thymoma, Wiskott-Aldrich syndrome)
- Secondary immunodeficiency (e.g., leukemia, leukopenia, neutropenia, therapeutic immunosuppression)
- Medication impairing neutrophil function (e.g., omeprazole)
- The most important independent predictor of recurrence is a positive family history.

GENERAL PREVENTION

Patient education regarding self-care (see "General Measures"); treatment and prevention are interrelated.

COMMONLY ASSOCIATED CONDITIONS

- Usually normal immune system
- Diabetes mellitus
- Polymorphonuclear leukocyte defect (rare)
- Hyperimmunoglobulin E–*Staphylococcus* sp. abscess syndrome (rare)
- See "Risk Factors."

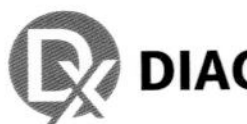

DIAGNOSIS

HISTORY

- Located on hair-bearing sites, especially areas prone to friction or repeated minor traumas (e.g., underneath belt, anterior aspects of thighs, nape, buttocks).
- No initial fever or systemic symptoms
- The folliculocentric nodule may enlarge, become painful, and develop into an abscess (frequently with spontaneous drainage).

PHYSICAL EXAM

- Painful erythematous papules/nodules (1–5 cm) with central pustules
- Tender, red, perifollicular swelling, terminating in discharge of pus and necrotic plug
- Lesions may be solitary or clustered.

DIFFERENTIAL DIAGNOSIS

- Folliculitis
- Pseudofolliculitis
- Carbuncles
- Ruptured epidermal cyst
- Myiasis (larva of botfly/tumbu fly)
- Hidradenitis suppurativa
- Atypical bacterial or fungal infections

DIAGNOSTIC TESTS & INTERPRETATION

Initial Tests (lab, imaging)

Obtain culture if with multiple abscesses marked by surrounding inflammation, cellulitis, systemic symptoms such as fever, or if immunocompromised.

Follow-Up Tests & Special Considerations

- Immunoglobulin levels in rare (e.g., recurrent or otherwise inexplicable) cases
- If culture grows gram-negative bacteria or fungus, consider polymorphonuclear neutrophil leukocyte functional defect.

Test Interpretation

Histopathology (although a biopsy is rarely needed)

- Perifollicular necrosis containing fibrinoid material and neutrophils
- At deep end of necrotic plug, in SC tissue, is a large abscess with a Gram stain positive for small collections of *S. aureus*.

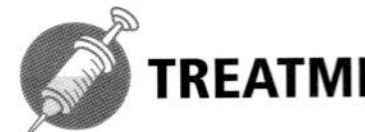

TREATMENT

GENERAL MEASURES

- Moist, warm compresses (provide comfort, encourage localization/pointing/drainage) 30 minutes QID
- If pointing or large, incise and drain: consider packing if large or incompletely drained.
- Routine culture is not necessary for localized abscess in nondiabetic patients with normal immune system.
- Sanitary practices: change towels, washcloths, and sheets daily; clean shaving instruments; avoid nose picking; change wound dressings frequently; do not share items of personal hygiene (2)[B].

MEDICATION

First Line

- Systemic antibiotics usually *unnecessary*, unless extensive surrounding cellulitis or fever
- If suspecting MRSA, see "Second Line."

- If multiple abscesses, lesions with marked surrounding inflammation, cellulitis, systemic symptoms such as fever, or if immunocompromised: place on antibiotics therapy directed at *S. aureus* × 10–14 days.
  - Dicloxacillin (Dynapen, Pathocil) 500 mg PO QID *or* cephalexin 500 mg PO QID *or* clindamycin 300 mg TID, if penicillin-allergic

Second Line

- Resistant strains of *S. aureus* (MRSA): clindamycin 300 mg q6h or doxycycline 100 mg q12h or trimethoprim-sulfamethoxazole (TMP-SMX DS) 1 tab q8–12h or minocycline 100 mg q12h
- If known or suspected impaired neutrophil function (e.g., impaired chemotaxis, phagocytosis, superoxide generation), add vitamin C 1,000 mg/day × 4–6 weeks (prevents oxidation of neutrophils).
- If antibiotic regimens fail:
  - May try PO pentoxifylline 400 mg TID × 2–6 months
  - Contraindications: recent cerebral and/or retinal hemorrhage; intolerance to methylxanthines (e.g., caffeine, theophylline); allergy to the particular drug selected
  - Precautions: prolonged prothrombin time (PT) and/or bleeding; if on warfarin, frequent monitoring of PT

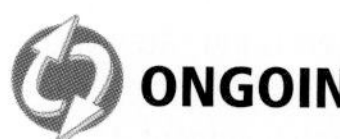

ONGOING CARE

FOLLOW-UP RECOMMENDATIONS

Patient Monitoring

Instruct patient to see physician if compresses are unsuccessful.

DIET

Unrestricted

PROGNOSIS

- Self-limited: usually drains pus spontaneously and will heal with or without scarring within several days.
- Recurrent/chronic: may last for months or years
- If recurrent, usually related to chronic skin carriage of staphylococci (nares or on skin). Treatment goals are to decrease or eliminate pathogenic strain *or* suppress pathogenic strain.
  - Culture nares, skin, axilla, and perineum (culture nares of family members).
  - Mupirocin 2%: apply to both nares BID × 5 days each month
  - Culture anterior nares every 3 months; if failure, retreat with mupirocin or consider clindamycin 150 mg/day × 3 months.
- Especially in recurrent cases, wash entire body and fingernails (with nailbrush) daily for 1–3 weeks with povidone-iodine (Betadine), chlorhexidine (Hibiclens), or hexachlorophene (pHisoHex soap), although all can cause dry skin.

COMPLICATIONS

- Scarring
- Bacteremia
- Seeding (e.g., septal/valve defect, arthritic joint)

REFERENCES

1. Demos M, McLeod MP, Nouri K. Recurrent furunculosis: a review of the literature. *Br J Dermatol*. 2012;167(4):725–732.
2. Fritz SA, Camins BC, Eisenstein KA, et al. Effectiveness of measures to eradicate *Staphylococcus aureus* carriage in patients with community-associated skin and soft-tissue infections: a randomized trial. *Infect Control Hosp Epidemiol*. 2011;32(9):872–880.

ADDITIONAL READING

- El-Gilany AH, Fathy H. Risk factors of recurrent furunculosis. *Dermatol Online J*. 2009;15(1):16.
- McConeghy KW, Mikolich DJ, LaPlante KL, et al. Agents for the decolonization of methicillin-resistant *Staphylococcus aureus*. *Pharmacotherapy*. 2009;29(3):263–280.
- Rivera AM, Boucher HW. Current concepts in antimicrobial therapy against select gram-positive organisms: methicillin-resistant *Staphylococcus aureus*, penicillin-resistant pneumococci, and vancomycin-resistant enterococci. *Mayo Clin Proc*. 2011;86(12):1230–1243.
- Wahba-Yahav AV. Intractable chronic furunculosis: prevention of recurrences with pentoxifylline. *Acta Derm Venereol*. 1992;72(6):461–462.
- Winthropp KL. An outbreak of mycobacterium furunculosis associated with footbaths at a nail salon. *N Engl J Med*. 2002;346(18):1366–1371.

SEE ALSO

Folliculitis; Hidradenitis Suppurativa

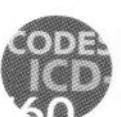

CODES

ICD10

- L02.92 Furuncle, unspecified
- L02.12 Furuncle of neck
- L02.429 Furuncle of limb, unspecified

CLINICAL PEARLS

- Pathogens may be different in different localities. Keep up-to-date with the locality-specific epidemiology.
- If few, furuncles/furunculosis do not need antibiotic treatment. If systemic symptoms (e.g., fever), cellulitis, or multiple lesions occur, oral antibiotic therapy is used.
- Other treatments for MRSA include linezolid PO or IV and IV vancomycin.
- Folliculitis, furunculosis, and carbuncles are parts of a spectrum of pyodermas.
- Other causative organisms include aerobic (e.g., *Escherichia coli, Pseudomonas aeruginosa,* and *Streptococcus faecalis*), anaerobic (e.g., *Bacteroides, Lactobacillus, Peptobacillius*, and *Peptostreptococcus*), and *Mycobacteria*.
- Decolonization (treatment of the nares with topical antibiotic) is only recommended if the colonization was confirmed by cultures because resistance is common and treatment is of uncertain efficacy.

GALACTORRHEA

Katherine M. Callaghan, MD

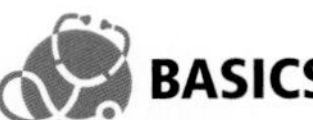

BASICS

DESCRIPTION

- Milky nipple discharge not associated with gestation or present >1 year after weaning. Galactorrhea does not include serous, purulent, or bloody nipple discharge.
- System(s) affected: endocrine/metabolic, nervous, reproductive
- Synonym(s): disordered lactation; nipple discharge

Pregnancy Considerations

Most cases of galactorrhea during pregnancy are physiologic.

EPIDEMIOLOGY

- Predominant age: 15–50 years (reproductive age)
- Predominant sex: female > male (rare, e.g., in patients with multiple endocrine neoplasia type 1 [MEN1], the most common anterior pituitary tumors are prolactinomas)

Incidence

Common

Prevalence

6.8% of women referred to physicians with a breast complaint have nipple discharge.

ETIOLOGY AND PATHOPHYSIOLOGY

Disorders of lactation are associated with elevated prolactin levels, either from overproduction or loss of inhibitory regulation by dopamine.

- Nipple stimulation
- Pituitary gland overproduction
  - Prolactinoma
- Loss of dopamine via hypothalamic dysregulation
  - Craniopharyngiomas
  - Meningiomas or other tumors
  - Sarcoid
  - Irradiation
  - Vascular insult
  - Stalk disruption
  - Traumatic injury
- Medications that suppress dopamine (1):
  - Typical and atypical antipsychotics
  - SSRIs
  - Tricyclic antidepressants
  - Cimetidine
  - Ranitidine
  - Reserpine
  - α-Methyldopa
  - Verapamil
  - Estrogens
  - Isoniazid
  - Opioids
  - Stimulants
  - Neuroleptics
  - Metoclopramide
  - Domperidone
  - Protease inhibitors
- Chest wall injury
  - Zoster, surgical or other trauma
- Postoperative condition, especially oophorectomy
- Renal failure
- Other causes:
  - Primary hypothyroidism
  - Cirrhosis
  - Cushing disease
  - Ectopic prolactin secretion
  - Renal failure
  - Sarcoid
  - Lupus
  - Multiple sclerosis
  - Polycystic ovary syndrome
- Idiopathic
  - Normal prolactin levels

GENERAL PREVENTION

- Frequent nipple stimulation can cause galactorrhea.
- Avoid medications that can suppress dopamine.

COMMONLY ASSOCIATED CONDITIONS

See "Etiology and Pathophysiology."

DIAGNOSIS

- Findings vary with causes.
- Look for signs/symptoms of associated conditions:
  - Adrenal insufficiency
  - Acromegaly
  - Hypothyroidism
  - Chest wall conditions

HISTORY

- Usually bilateral milky nipple discharge; may be spontaneous or induced by stimulation
- Determine possibility of pregnancy or recent discontinuation of lactation.
- Signs of hypogonadism from hyperprolactinemia:
  - Oligomenorrhea, amenorrhea
  - Inadequate luteal phase, anovulation, infertility
  - Decreased libido (especially in affected males)
- Mass effects from pituitary enlargement:
  - Headache, cranial neuropathies
  - Bitemporal hemianopsia, amaurosis, scotomata

PHYSICAL EXAM

Breast examination should be performed with attention to the presence of spontaneous or induced nipple discharge.

DIFFERENTIAL DIAGNOSIS

- Pregnancy-induced lactation or recent weaning
- Nonmilky nipple discharge
  - Intraductal papilloma
  - Fibrocystic disease
- Purulent breast discharge
  - Mastitis
  - Breast abscess
  - Impetigo
  - Eczema
- Bloody breast discharge: Consider malignancy (Paget disease, breast cancer).

DIAGNOSTIC TESTS & INTERPRETATION

Perform formal visual field testing if pituitary adenoma suspected.

Initial Tests (lab, imaging)

- Prolactin level, thyroid-stimulating hormone, pregnancy test, liver, and renal functions
- Drugs that may alter lab results: medications that can cause hyperprolactinemia
- Situations that may alter lab results:
  - Lab evaluation of prolactin may be falsely elevated by a recent breast examination.
  - Vigorous exercise
  - Sexual activity
  - High-carbohydrate diet
  - Consider repeating the test under different circumstances if the value is borderline (30–40) elevated.
- Prolactin levels may fluctuate. Elevated prolactin levels should be confirmed with at least 1 additional level drawn in a fasting, nonexercised state, with no breast stimulation (2)[C].
- Prolactin levels >250 ng/mL are highly suggestive of a pituitary adenoma (3)[C].
- If a breast mass is palpated in the setting of nipple discharge, evaluation of that mass is indicated with mammogram and/or ultrasound.
- Pituitary MRI with gadolinium enhancement if the serum prolactin level is significantly elevated (>200 ng/mL) or if a pituitary tumor is otherwise suspected.

Follow-Up Tests & Special Considerations

- Consider evaluation of follicle-stimulating hormone and luteinizing hormone if amenorrheic.
- Consider evaluation of growth hormone levels if acromegaly suspected.
- Measure adrenal steroids if signs of Cushing disease present.

Diagnostic Procedures/Other

If diagnosis is in question, confirm by microscopic evaluation that nipple secretions are lipoid.

Test Interpretation

None unless pituitary resection required

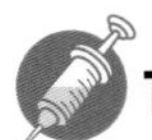

TREATMENT

- Avoid excess nipple stimulation.
- Idiopathic galactorrhea (normal prolactin levels) does not require treatment.
- Discontinue causative medications, if possible.
- Treat to manage symptoms, reduce patient anxiety, and restore fertility.
- Treat tumors >10 mm (even if asymptomatic) to reduce pituitary tumor size or prevent progression to avoid neurologic sequelae.
- If microadenoma, watchful waiting can be appropriate, because 95% do not enlarge.

MEDICATION

- Dopamine agonists work to reduce prolactin levels and shrink tumor size. Therapy is suppressive, not curative (4)[C].
- Treatment is discontinued when tumor size has reduced or regressed completely or after pregnancy has been achieved.
- Cabergoline (Dostinex)
  - Start at 0.25 mg PO twice weekly and increase by 0.25 mg monthly until prolactin levels normalize. Usual dose ranges from 0.25 to 1.00 mg PO once or twice weekly.
  - More effective and better tolerated than bromocriptine (5)[A]
  - Convenient dosing
- Although cabergoline has been associated with valvular heart disease in patients treated for Parkinson disease, the lower doses used in treatment of prolactinomas have not been adequately studied (6)[C].
- Bromocriptine
  - Start at 1.25 mg/day PO with food and increase weekly by 1.25 mg/day until therapeutic response achieved (usually 2.5–15 mg/day, divided once daily/TID).
  - More expensive and more frequent dosing, however, most providers have experience with this effective drug.
  - Long-term treatment can cause woody fibrosis of the pituitary gland.
- Contraindications are similar for all and include the following:
  - Uncontrolled hypertension
  - Sensitivity to ergot alkaloids
- Precautions:
  - Nausea, vomiting, and drowsiness are common.
  - Orthostasis, light-headedness, or syncope
  - Hypertension, seizures, acute psychosis, and digital vasospasm are rare.
- Significant possible interactions:
  - Phenothiazines, butyrophenones, other drugs listed under "Etiology and Pathophysiology"

SURGERY/OTHER PROCEDURES

- Surgery
  - Macroadenomas need surgery if (a) medical management does not halt growth, (b) neurologic symptoms persist, (c) size >10 mm, or (d) patient cannot tolerate medications. Also considered in young patients with microadenomas to avoid long-term medical therapy
  - Transsphenoidal pituitary resection
  - 50% recurrence after surgery
- Radiotherapy
  - Radiation is an alternate tumor therapy for macroprolactinomas not responsive to other modes of treatment:
    - 20–30% success rate
    - 50% risk of panhypopituitarism after radiation
    - Risk of optic nerve damage, hypopituitarism, neurologic dysfunction, and increased risk for stroke and secondary brain tumors

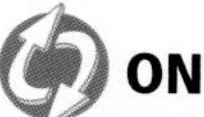

ONGOING CARE

FOLLOW-UP RECOMMENDATIONS

- Outpatient care unless pituitary resection required
- Bromocriptine patients need adequate hydration.
- Dopamine agonist therapy should be discontinued in pregnancy.

Patient Monitoring

- Varies with cause
- Check prolactin levels every 6 weeks until normalized, then every 6–12 months.
- Monitor visual fields and/or MRI at least yearly until stable.

DIET

No restrictions

PATIENT EDUCATION

- Warn about symptoms of mass enlargement in pituitary.
- Discuss treatment rationale, risks of treating, and expectant management.
- Patient education material available from American Family Physician: www.aafp.org/afp/20040801/553ph.html

PROGNOSIS

- Depends on underlying cause
- Symptoms can recur after discontinuation of a dopamine agonist.
- Surgery can have 50% recurrence.
- Prolactinomas <10 mm can resolve spontaneously.

COMPLICATIONS

- If enlarging pituitary adenoma, risk of permanent visual field loss
- Panhypopituitarism can complicate radiation or surgical therapy.
- Osteoporosis if amenorrhea persists without estrogen replacement.

REFERENCES

1. Molitch ME. Drugs and prolactin. *Pituitary*. 2008;11(2):209–218.
2. Huang W, Molitch ME. Evaluation and management of galactorrhea. *Am Fam Physician*. 2012;85(11):1073–1080.
3. Melmed S, Casanueva FF, Hoffman AR, et al. Diagnosis and treatment of hyperprolactinemia: an Endocrine Society clinical practice guideline. *J Clin Endocrinol Metab*. 2011;96(2):273–288.
4. Majumdar A, Mangal NS. Hyperprolactinemia. *J Hum Reprod Sci*. 2013;6(3):168–175.
5. Wang AT, Mullan RJ, Lane MA, et al. Treatment of hyperprolactinemia: a systematic review and meta-analysis. *Syst Rev*. 2012;1:33.
6. Córdoba-Soriano JG, Lamas-Oliveira C, Hidalgo-Olivares VM, et al. Valvular heart disease in hyperprolactinemic patients treated with low doses of cabergoline. *Rev Esp Cardiol*. 2013;66(5):410–412.

ADDITIONAL READING

- Mancini T, Casanueva FF, Giustina A. Hyperprolactinemia and prolactinomas. *Endocrinol Metab Clin North Am*. 2008;37(1):67–99.
- Schlechte JA. Long-term management of prolactinomas. *J Clin Endocrinol Metab*. 2007;92(8):2861–2865.

SEE ALSO

Hyperprolactinemia

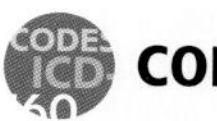

CODES

ICD10

N64.3 Galactorrhea not associated with childbirth

CLINICAL PEARLS

- Galactorrhea is a common disorder, affecting up to 50% of reproductive-age women.
- Common causes include idiopathic, from excess nipple stimulation, dopamine-suppressing medications, or pituitary prolactinoma.
- Most cases may be adequately evaluated by thyroid-stimulating hormone, prolactin, and human chorionic gonadotropin measurement, with additional testing as suggested by the presence of other symptoms or signs.
- Lab evaluation of prolactin may be falsely elevated due to recent sexual activity, breast examination, exercise, or a high-carbohydrate diet. Repeat any borderline elevation before continuing evaluation or initiating treatment.
- Evaluate prolactin >200 ng/mL (or suspicion of pituitary macroadenoma) with a gadolinium-enhanced MRI.

GAMBLING ADDICTION

Rebecca Collins, DO, MPH, FAAFP

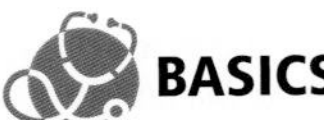

BASICS

DESCRIPTION

Gambling is the act of placing something of value at risk in the hopes of gaining something of greater value. Pathologic gambling (PG) and problem gambling affect up to 15 million Americans with the number of those affected increasing, especially in young people. The essential feature of gambling disorder is persistent and recurrent maladaptive gambling behavior that disrupts personal, family, and/or vocational pursuits. Individuals with gambling disorder have high rates of comorbidity with other mental disorders (substance use, depression, anxiety, and personality disorders). There is debate as to whether gambling addiction is an impulse-control disorder or a non substance abuse–related disorder.

EPIDEMIOLOGY

- Predominant sex: male > female, though gap narrowing
- Rates of pathologic and problem gambling are higher in adolescents and middle-age persons than older adults.
- The younger a person starts gambling, the more likely he or she is to become a pathologic gambler.

Prevalence

- Lifetime gambling disorder prevalence is 0.4–1% in the U.S. adults.
  - Males 0.6%, females 0.2%
  - African American 0.9%, Caucasian 0.4%, Hispanic 0.3%
- Living in closer proximity to a casino increases prevalence.

GENERAL PREVENTION

- Focus on treatment; patient education; and awareness of risk factors, associated conditions, and warning signs of pathologic or problematic gambling behaviors.
- Primary prevention using educational programs that target at-risk youth and adults

ETIOLOGY AND PATHOPHYSIOLOGY

- *DSM 5* characterizes gambling disorder as a non–substance related and addictive disorder, however there is debate whether it is an impulse-control disorder or possibly both.
- Impulse control: changes in serotonin metabolites in pathologic gamblers and patients with impulse-control disorders
- Substance abuse: similarities found between pathologic gambling and substance use (tolerance, withdrawal, anticipatory craving, relapses)
- The brains of pathologic gamblers may have some predisposition to illness. Functional MRI studies indicate that the ventromedial prefrontal cortex is less activated when gambling stimuli are presented to pathologic gamblers.
- Abnormalities in the neurotransmitters serotonin, norepinephrine, dopamine, and glutamate may be implicated in PG.
  - Norepinephrine: Low levels seem to help a patient avoid gambling, whereas high levels may lead to poor decision making.
  - Serotonin: involved in impulse control by helping a patient weigh the risks of gambling
  - Dopamine: High levels in the nucleus accumbens while gambling lead to a pleasurable rush. May induce reversible PG in Parkinson patients who take dopamine agonists.
- Medicine classes for each category have been used to treat.

Genetics

- *SLC6A4* serotonin transporter gene has been associated with PG in males but not females.
- Dopamine receptor genes *DRD1*, *DRD2*, *DRD3*, and *DRD4* have been correlated with pathologic gambling.
- More prevalent among 1st-degree relatives of alcoholics than among general population.

RISK FACTORS

- Some types of gambling present a greater risk to cause PG than other types: pull tabs, casino gambling, bingo, and card games outside a casino
- Being involved with several gaming modalities is related to PG and suggests that the gambler is very captivated with risking money for excitement as opposed to risking money for social pleasure or for an interest in sports.
- Lower socioeconomic status
- Adults in mental health treatment
- Substance abuse (nicotine, alcohol, inhalants, marijuana)
- Positive family history
- Antisocial personality disorder, depressive and bipolar disorders, other substance abuse disorders (especially alcohol)

COMMONLY ASSOCIATED CONDITIONS

- Poor nutrition
- Stress-related medical conditions (e.g., peptic ulcer disease [PUD], hypertension, migraine, palpitations)
- Suicidal ideation and attempts
- Substance abuse disorder (especially alcohol)
- Attention-deficit/hyperactivity disorder
- Bipolar disorder and other mood disorders
- Impulse-control disorders
- Personality disorders
- Incarceration
- Financial problems (e.g., previous bankruptcy)

DIAGNOSIS

DSM 5 criteria for gambling disorder (1):

- Persistent and recurrent gambling behavior leading to significant impairment or distress as indicated by ≥4 of the following in a 12-month period, AND gambling behavior is not better explained by a manic episode:
  - Often preoccupied with gambling
  - Need to gamble with increasing amounts of money to achieve the desired excitement
  - Repeated unsuccessful efforts to control, cut back, or stop gambling
  - Restless or irritable when attempting to cut down or stop gambling
  - Often gambles when feeling distressed (e.g., helpless, guilty, anxious, depressed)
  - After losing money gambling, often returns another day to get even ("chasing" one's loses)
  - Lies to conceal the extent of involvement with gambling
  - Has jeopardized or lost a significant relationship, job, or educational or career opportunity because of gambling
  - Relies on others to provide money to relieve a desperate financial situation caused by gambling ("bailout" behavior)
- Specifiers:
  - Episodic: meets diagnostic criteria at more than one time point with symptoms subsiding for at least several months
  - Persistent: continuous symptoms for multiple years
  - Early remission: After criteria met previously, none met for ≥3 months but <12 months.
  - Sustained remission: After criteria met previously, no criteria met for ≥12 months.
  - Current severity: mild (4–5 criteria), moderate (6–7 criteria), or severe (8–9 criteria)

HISTORY

- Preoccupation with gambling and chasing losses are most frequently endorsed criteria.
- Those with moderate to severe forms of disorder are usually the individuals who present for treatment.
- May have distortions in thinking (e.g., denial, superstitions, sense of power and control over outcome of chance events)
- Preoccupation with money; belief that money is cause and solution to their problems
- Personality characteristics: impulsivity, competitive, energetic, restless OR depressed, lonely, helpless, guilty
- 50% of patients in treatment for PG have suicidal ideation, 17% have suicide attempts.
- Symptoms can develop anytime from adolescence through older adulthood.
- Amounts of money wagered is not in themselves indicative of gambling disorder (some individuals can wager thousands of dollars per month and not have a problem, some may wager much smaller amounts but experience substantial gambling-related difficulties).
- Loss of important relationships with family or friends
- Absenteeism or poor work/school performance
- Poor general health; high use of medical services
- Unexplained new financial problems
- New participation in illegal or dishonest money-making endeavors or activities
- Disruptions in personal life or career
- Patient may ask his or her family and friends to pay off his or her debts ("bailing them out").

DIFFERENTIAL DIAGNOSIS

- Social gambling
- Professional gambling
- Bipolar disorder, manic episode
- Personality disorder
- Other medical conditions (patients on dopaminergic medications, e.g., Parkinson)

DIAGNOSTIC TESTS & INTERPRETATION

- South Oaks Gambling Screen (SOGS):
  - Most extensively used and validated screening tool
  - 20-question screen for PG
  - Score of 3–4 suggests problem gambling.
  - Score of ≥5 indicates probable PG.
  - Criticized as having high false-positive rate and being too lengthy to administer

- Gamblers Anonymous 20 questions:
  - Easily obtainable from Gamblers Anonymous Web site
  - Scores of >7 are indicative of problem/PG.
- Lie/Bet method: "Have you ever had to lie to people important to you about how much you gambled?" "Have you ever felt a need to bet more money?":
  - A patient who answers at least one question with a "Yes" suggests further investigation needed to see if criteria are met for PG.
  - This test has been shown to have >85% specificity and >95% sensitivity.

Initial Tests (lab, imaging)

None usually indicated

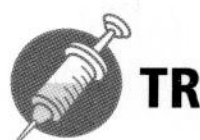

TREATMENT

To treat PG, treat comorbidities first. The usual comorbid disorders are substance abuse, bipolar disorder, ADHD, and other impulse-control disorders. Nonpharmacologic therapies are more effective than pharmacologic therapies. Some data suggest that gambling abstinence is not necessary for treatment; patients can still exhibit controlled gambling.

GENERAL MEASURES

- Get a sense of the patient's readiness for change.
- Provide intervention/patient education. Although there are no FDA-approved drug treatments for PG, make clinically based medication recommendations.
- Screen for and treat comorbid conditions.
- Provide referrals:
  - Addiction psychiatrist/counselor
  - Gamblers Anonymous
  - Consumer credit organizations
  - Bankruptcy lawyers
  - Gam-Anon for family members

MEDICATION

- There are no FDA-approved medicines for gambling addiction; pharmacotherapy most effective when directed toward patient's comorbid psychiatric condition (2)[A].
- SSRIs:
  - Currently seen as beneficial for treating comorbid impulse-control disorders, although their efficacy has been under question for PG
  - All studies with SSRIs limited due to small size, short follow-up, conflicting outcomes, and in some cases study design; confirmation for some positive findings need larger randomized controlled trials with extended follow-up before recommendations for use can be made
- Opiate antagonists have the ability to decrease dopamine release in the dopamine reward pathway. Naltrexone and nalmefene have been reported to cause improvements on gambling symptom assessment scores (3,4)[B].

ADDITIONAL THERAPIES

- Cognitive-behavioral therapy (CBT):
  - The main effective interventions for PG are psychoeducation, cognitive restructuring, problem solving, social skills training, and relapse prevention. Studies indicated that CBT resulted in significant improvement as short-term therapy.
  - CBT may be done in several formats: individual, group, brief group, and dual diagnosis. All these formats have been shown to be effective. Group therapy is favored because patients are often extroverted. Couple or family therapy also may be used.
- Gamblers Anonymous:
  - A 12-step program similar to Alcoholics Anonymous for a person suffering from a gambling addiction
  - Dropout rate is high if this is the only means of therapy.
  - Patients may deny need to attend in the first place, and for that reason, Gamblers Anonymous may not be appropriate for patients who are in the precontemplation stage.
- Motivational enhancement therapy (MET):
  - Provides nonargumentative exploration of patient's stage of change
  - Patient receives positive reinforcement from clinician.
  - Motivational enhancement strategies support self-efficacy.
  - Improves patient rapport; aids in removing barriers to treatment
  - In one study, MET alone did not show any improvement, but MET and CBT together improved outcome measures.
- Because of increased suicide rates, patients may need to be hospitalized acutely for safety and to prevent gambling.
- Because patients are at increased risk from mental and physical illness, they benefit from relaxation exercises to reduce stress, identify triggers, substitute gambling with other activities, and a complete physical and lab work with nutrition evaluation.

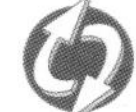

ONGOING CARE

FOLLOW-UP RECOMMENDATIONS

Patients seeking treatment for gambling addiction should be followed routinely to monitor the response to treatment, tolerance to medications, and relapse.

PATIENT EDUCATION

- Gamblers Anonymous:
  - www.gamblersanonymous.org
  - National hotline 1-888-GA-HELPS (888-424-3577)
- Gam-Anon: support group for spouses, family, or close friends: www.gam-anon.org
- Responsible Gambling Council: www.responsiblegambling.org
- Humphrey H. *This must be hell: A look at pathological gambling*. Bloomington, IN: iUniverse; 2000.
- Lee B. *Born to lose: Memoirs of a compulsive gambler*. Center City, MN: Hazelden; 2005.

PROGNOSIS

- Patients with gambling addiction can be treated, but many relapse.
- 36–39% of patients did not experience any gambling-related problems according to one study, and only 7–12% sought formal treatment or Gamblers Anonymous meetings.
- Roughly 1/3 of patients who have a gambling addiction recover without any intervention.

REFERENCES

1. American Psychiatric Association. *Diagnostic and Statistical Manual of Mental Disorders*. 5th ed. Arlington, VA: American Psychiatric Association; 2013:585–589.
2. Dell'Osso B, Allen A, Hollander E. Comorbidity issues in the pharmacological treatment of pathological gambling: a critical review. *Clin Pract Epidemiol Ment Health*. 2005;1:21.
3. Kim SW, Grant JE, Adson DE, et al. Double-blind naltrexone and placebo comparison study in the treatment of pathological gambling. *Biol Psychiatry*. 2001;49(11):914.
4. Grant JE, Potenza MN, Hollander E, et al. Multicenter investigation of the opioid antagonist nalmefene in the treatment of pathological gambling. *Am J Psychiatry*. 2006;163(2):303–312.

ADDITIONAL READING

- Chou K, Afifi TO. Disordered (pathologic or problem) gambling and axis I psychiatric disorders: results from the National Epidemiologic Survey on Alcohol and Related Conditions. *Am J Epidemiol*. 2011; 173(11):1289–1297.
- Leung KS, Cottler LB. Treatment of pathological gambling. *Curr Opin Psychiatry*. 2009;22(1):69–74.
- Nussbaum D, Honarmand K, Govoni R, et al. An eight component decision-making model for problem gambling: a systems approach to stimulate integrative research. *J Gambl Stud*. 2011;27(4): 523–563.
- Okuda M, Balan I, Petry NM, et al. Cognitive-behavioral therapy for pathological gambling: cultural considerations. *Am J Psychiatry*. 2009;166(12): 1325–1330.
- Potenza MN. Review. The neurobiology of pathological gambling and drug addiction: an overview and new findings. *Philos Trans R Soc Lond B Biol Sci*. 2008;363(1507):3181–3189.
- Potenza MN, Fiellin DA, Heninger GR, et al. Gambling: an addictive behavior with health and primary care implications. *J Gen Intern Med*. 2002;17(9):721–732.
- Rossow I, Molde H. Chasing the criteria: comparing SOGS-RA and the Lie/Bet screen to assess prevalence of problem gambling and "at-risk" gambling among adolescents. *J Gambling Issues*. 2006; 18:57–71.

CODES

ICD10

- F63.0 Pathological gambling
- Z72.6 Gambling and betting

CLINICAL PEARLS

- Several brief screening strategies can be used to identify PG, including the SOGS, the Gamblers Anonymous 20 questions, and the Lie/Bet method.
- To treat PG, first treat comorbidities such as substance abuse, bipolar disorder, ADHD, and other mental health/substance abuse disorders.
- Nonpharmacologic therapies are more effective than pharmacologic therapies. There is no FDA-approved therapy for PG.
- Patients seeking treatment for gambling addiction should be followed routinely by physicians and counselors to monitor the response to treatment, tolerance to medications, and possibility of relapse.

GANGLION CYST

Mary Segraves Lindholm, MD

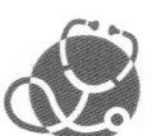

BASICS

- Ganglions are common benign tumors that are not related to nerve tissue (as implied incorrectly by the name).
- Can be located throughout the body, usually adjacent to or within joints and tendons, mostly on wrist, foot, and ankle
- Because pathology does not show an epithelial lining, it is not a true cyst.
- Average size is 3 cm.
- Most are asymptomatic except for changing size, but local nerve compression can result in pain or activity limitation.
- Synonym: synovial cyst; myxoid cyst; Gideon disease; Bible bump

EPIDEMIOLOGY

- Can affect all age groups but unusual in children
- Most common in young adults and 3× more common in women
- Common in dorsal wrist, radial wrist, and dorsum of the distal interphalangeal (DIP) joint (referred to as a mucous cyst)
- Mucous cysts are usually seen in older patients.
- 60–70% of hand and wrist ganglion cysts are in dorsal wrist; 15–20% are at the volar wrist (1).

Prevalence

- Prevalence of wrist ganglia in patients presenting with wrist pain is as high as 19%.
- Prevalence of ganglia in patients with a palpable mass in the wrist is as high as 27%.
- Reported prevalence in ankles is 5.6%.

ETIOLOGY AND PATHOPHYSIOLOGY

Pathogenesis is unclear. Several theories include the following:

- Mucoid degeneration of connective tissue results in formation of hyaluronic acid, leading to cystic space formation.
- Herniation of synovial lining creates a one-way valve. Hypothesis supported by dye studies that show communication of fluid from the wrist joint into the cyst but not from the cyst to the joint. Lack of epithelial lining of cyst wall argues against this hypothesis.
- A rent in the joint capsule or tendon sheath allows synovial fluid to leak into surrounding tissue. Local irritation leads to production of a pseudocapsule and ganglion (explains lack of epithelial lining).
- Recurrent stress and microtrauma at the synovial–capsular interface may stimulate mucin production by mesenchymal cells or fibroblasts.
- May be associated with trauma, but most patients do recall inciting traumatic event.

Genetics

No specific genetic links have been found.

RISK FACTORS

- Female > male
- Osteoarthritis for mucoid cysts
- No known occupational risk factors

COMMONLY ASSOCIATED CONDITIONS

Mucous cysts are usually associated with some level of osteoarthritis of DIP joint.

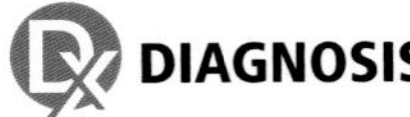

DIAGNOSIS

- Usually made on basis of history and physical examination
- Patients usually present when there is pain, increased size, interference with activities, or weakness.

HISTORY

- Patients usually present with asymptomatic mass that has been present for months or years.
- Variable: in size; most commonly of hands, wrists, and fingers
- Mostly asymptomatic but can be associated with pain and limitations in activity

PHYSICAL EXAM

- Mass
  - Compressible
  - Subcutaneous
  - Transilluminating
  - Slightly mobile
  - Without overlying skin changes
- Extension or flexion of wrist can cause pain through nerve compression.
- Small ganglions may only be palpable in full wrist flexion or extension.
- Occult ganglions are not palpable but can be quite painful.

DIFFERENTIAL DIAGNOSIS

- Giant cell tumor, lipoma, sarcoma
- Hamartoma, interosseous neuroma
- Tenosynovitis

DIAGNOSTIC TESTS & INTERPRETATION

Unless diagnosis is unclear, most ganglions do not require imaging for confirmation.

Initial Tests (lab, imaging)

- Most are apparent clinically and do not need imaging.
- Plain films can exclude bony pathology.
- Other options
  - US
  - MRI
  - Bone scintigraphy, arthroscopy
- US and MRI have similar rates of sensitivity and specificity. US is less expensive than MRI but more operator-dependent.
- Scintigraphy is less specific and not useful.
- Arthroscopy is used for both diagnostic and therapeutic purposes and should be considered when initial workup is nondiagnostic and conservative treatment is not effective.

Test Interpretation

- Gross pathologic evaluation shows that cysts are often multilobulated.
- Microscopic exam reveals a relatively acellular outer wall with several layers of randomly oriented collagen fibers and mesenchymal cells in the collagen fibers.
- Viscous fluid contains glucosamine, albumin, globulin, and hyaluronic acid.
- Ganglions are histopathologically identical regardless of anatomic location.

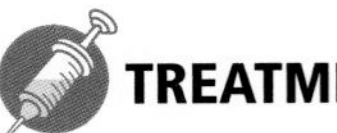

TREATMENT

Four primary treatment options

- Reassurance and observation: Ganglia are not likely to be malignant or to cause damage.
  - 33% dorsal ganglions and 45% volar ganglions resolve spontaneously by 6 years; up to 80% of ganglion in children resolve (2)[B].
- Closed rupture: historically done by hitting cyst with a book
  - Results in initial decreased clinical symptoms by 22–66%, recurrence is common.
- Aspiration: can be done in the office under local anesthesia with a 16-gauge needle at base of cyst
  - Studies demonstrate mixed results on aspirations; evidence supporting injecting steroids into ganglion cyst after aspiration is weak; splinting after the procedure may help cure rate. Recurrence may be as high as 80% after a single aspiration. This can be reduced to 20% with multiple aspirations.
  - Aspirations with US guidance allow direct visualization of the ganglion.
  - Volar gangliа should not be aspirated without US guidance due to risk of damage to neurovascular structures.
  - Mucous cysts can be aspirated, but recurrence is >50% and pain may not resolve if due to underlying osteoarthritis.
- Surgical excision
  - 1/3 of patients presenting with ganglion cyst elect for surgical intervention (2)[B].

MEDICATION

First Line

- Evidence for steroid injection after aspiration is mixed.
- No other medications have been shown to be effective.

SURGERY/OTHER PROCEDURES

- 6-year study comparing blind aspiration to surgery to watchful waiting found
  - Recurrence rates: 58% after aspiration, 39% after surgery, and 58% in untreated patients
  - Patient satisfaction: 81% aspiration, 83% surgery, and 53% with simple reassurance
  - No significant difference seen in pain, weakness, or stiffness between groups
  - Significant reduction in pain was seen in all groups.
  - Neither aspiration nor surgical excision provides a clear long-term benefit over simple observation. The primary benefit of surgery is early resolution of the appearance of the ganglia (3)[B].
- Bottom line
  - Surgical excision yields less risk of recurrence but similar rates of pain, weakness, and stiffness as aspiration or reassurance.
  - Patient satisfaction is higher with excision or aspiration; however, longer time out of work is seen with excision compared with aspiration and reassurance.
- Two methods
  - Arthroscopic and open excision: After 1 year, ~10% had recurrence; no significant difference in surgical approaches (4)[B].

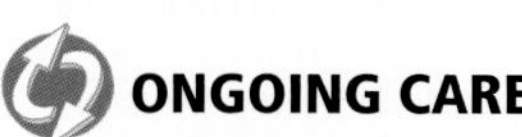

ONGOING CARE

May require supervised hand therapy after surgical repair to aid in pain reduction and improve stiffness and function

FOLLOW-UP RECOMMENDATIONS

- Hand/occupational therapy may be helpful if ganglion symptoms persist despite rest.
- Improved resolution rates with multiple aspirations
- Splinting is often used after surgical repair and follow-up with hand therapy for residual symptoms.

PROGNOSIS

- Generally very good
- Up to 50% will resolve with watchful waiting.
- Higher rate of resolution in children

COMPLICATIONS

- Risk of recurrence is present regardless of treatment; no specific recommendations to minimize this risk.
- Risks of surgical excision include the following:
  - Residual pain
  - Poor cosmesis
  - Neuropathy
  - Stiffness and instability of the wrist, especially scapholunate ligament instability; also may require open excision if arthroscopic treatment fails to resolve symptoms

REFERENCES

1. Thommasen HV, Johnston S, Thommasen A. Management of the occasional wrist ganglion. *Can J Rural Med*. 2006;11(1):51–53.
2. Dias J, Buch K. Palmar wrist ganglion: does intervention improve outcome? A prospective study of the natural history and patient-reported treatment outcomes. *J Hand Surg [Br]*. 2003;28(2):172–176.
3. Dias JJ, Dhukaram V, Kumar P. The natural history of untreated dorsal wrist ganglia and patient reported outcome 6 years after intervention. *J Hand Surg Eur*. 2007;32(5):502–508.
4. Kang L, Akelman E, Weiss AP. Arthroscopic versus open dorsal ganglion excision: a prospective, randomized comparison of rates of recurrence and of residual pain. *J Hand Surg [Am]*. 2008;33(4):471–475.

ADDITIONAL READING

- Kang HJ, Koh IH, Kim JS, et al. Coexisting intraarticular disorders are unrelated to outcomes after arthroscopic resection of dorsal wrist ganglions *Clin Orthop Relat Res*. 2013;471(7):2212–2218.
- Lee SW, Kim SG, Oh-Park M. Ganglion cyst of radiocapitellar joint mimicking lateral epicondylitis: role of ultrasonography. *Am J Phys Med Rehabil*. 2013;92(5):459–460.
- Wong AS, Jebson PJ, Murray PM, et al. The use of routine wrist radiography is not useful in the evaluation of patients with a ganglion cyst of the wrist. *Hand*. 2007;2(3):117–119.

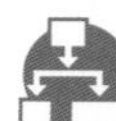

SEE ALSO

Algorithm: Pain in Upper Extremity

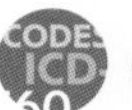

CODES

ICD10

- M67.40 Ganglion, unspecified site
- M67.48 Ganglion, other site
- M67.439 Ganglion, unspecified wrist

CLINICAL PEARLS

- Ganglion cysts are the most wrist masses and are technically not true cysts.
- Diagnosis is based on history and physical examination.
- Treatment options include observation, aspiration, and excision. Long-term outcomes are generally similar with all three approaches.
- Volar wrist ganglia should not be aspirated without US guidance due to the risk of damage to neurovascular structures from blind aspiration.

GASTRIC CANCER

Scott T. Henderson, MD

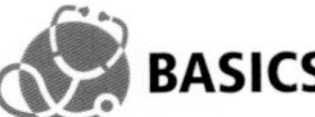

BASICS

DESCRIPTION
- Malignant neoplasm occuring anywhere in the stomach
- Infiltration to lymph nodes, omentum, lungs, and liver is rapid.
- Uncommon in U.S. natives
- Synonym(s): linitis plastica ("leather bottle stomach")

Pediatric Considerations
Rare

Pregnancy Considerations
- Rarely diagnosed during pregnancy
- Prognosis is poor.

EPIDEMIOLOGY
- Predominant age: >55 years (2/3 >65 years)
- Predominant gender: male > female (1.7:1)
- Incidence is decreasing globally but in worldwide is still the 3rd leading cause of cancer death.

Incidence
- 5.9/100,000 males (North America)
- 2.5/100,000 females (North America)
- 21,130 new cases per year (United States)

ETIOLOGY AND PATHOPHYSIOLOGY
Unknown

Genetics
- More common in people with blood group A
- 2–4 times more common in 1st-degree relatives
- 1–3% of gastric cancers are associated with inherited gastric cancer predisposition syndromes (hereditary diffuse gastric cancer [*CDH1*] gene).
- Amplification or overexpression of the HER2 protein is associated with some gastric cancers.

RISK FACTORS
- *Helicobacter pylori* infection is primary risk in 65–80%.
- Smoking/tobacco abuse is second leading risk factor.
- Diet rich in additives (e.g., smoked, pickled, or salted foods; highly spiced foods). Nitrates and nitrites have been implicated.
- Atrophic gastritis/intestinal metaplasia
- Pernicious anemia
- Preexisting diabetes mellitus
- Overweight and obesity: strength of association increases with increasing body mass index (BMI).
- Familial polyposis
- Barrett esophagus
- Patients in lower socioeconomic status have higher risk of gastric cancer.
- Low consumption of fruits and vegetables
- Ethnicity: Hispanic, Japanese, Chilean, Costa Rican
  - Migrants from high-incidence areas (e.g., Iceland, Chile, or Japan) to low-incidence areas maintain an increased risk, whereas their offspring have an occurrence rate that corresponds to that of the new location.

GENERAL PREVENTION
- Avoid tobacco, have a regular exercise, maintain optimal body weight, and pay attention to dietary intake.
  - Diets that include 5–20 servings of both fruits and vegetables each week reduce the risk of gastric malignancy by ~50%.
- Insufficient data to recommend routine gastric cancer screening
- Screening may be of benefit in high-prevalence areas to identify and eradicate *H. pylori*.

COMMONLY ASSOCIATED CONDITIONS
- Giant hypertrophic gastritis (Ménétrier disease)
- Intestinal metaplasia
- Atrophic gastritis
- *H. pylori* infection

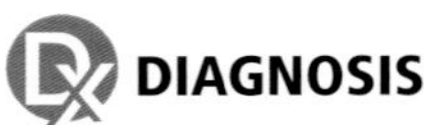

DIAGNOSIS

ALERT
Symptoms often present late in the course.

HISTORY
- Assess history of risk factors (tobacco use; *H.* pylori infection, dietary history; family history)
- Anorexia/weight loss (70–80%)
- Early satiety
- Heartburn, nausea and vomiting
- Change in bowel habits
- Chronic noncolicky abdominal pain (especially in epigastrium)
  - Postprandial fullness to severe steady pain
  - Unrelieved by antacids
  - Exacerbated by food
  - Relieved by fasting
- GI bleeding (10%)
- Dysphagia (rare)

PHYSICAL EXAM
- Abdominal palpation for masses and/or ascites
- Palpation for lymph nodes
  - Left supraclavicular node (Virchow)
  - Sister Mary Joseph nodule at umbilicus
- Assess for jaundice

DIFFERENTIAL DIAGNOSIS
- Angiodysplasia of the colon
- Carcinoma of body or tail of the pancreas
- Carcinoma of the colon
- Crohn disease
- Eosinophilic gastroenteritis
- Functional dyspepsia
- Gastric lymphoma
- GI sarcoidosis
- Peptic ulcer with or without hemorrhage
- Small intestinal lymphoma

DIAGNOSTIC TESTS & INTERPRETATION

Initial Tests (lab, imaging)
- CBC and platelet count:
  - Hemoglobin <12 g/dL (1.86 mmol/L)
  - Hematocrit <35 (0.35)
- Serum chemistry analysis
  - Albumin <3 g/dL
- Coagulation studies
- *H. pylori* testing
- Stool guaiac
- Upper endoscopy is the diagnostic test of choice. Allows for direct visualization, biopsy, and cytology:
  - Minimum of 6 biopsies should be done to confirm a diagnosis of malignancy (1)[C].
- CT scan of chest, abdomen, and pelvis with contrast and gastric distension are done for staging (1)[C].

Follow-Up Tests & Special Considerations
- Pentagastrin test (stomach pH <6)
  - Pernicious anemia may cause a false-positive pentagastrin test.
- Consider pelvic ultrasound (US) in females.

Diagnostic Procedures/Other
- Endoscopic US is most accurate preoperative staging tool to identify proximal and distal extent of tumor (2)[C].
- Laparoscopy may be useful in select patients for staging (3)[C].

Test Interpretation
- Adenocarcinomas: 90% (intestinal [well-differentiated] and diffuse [undifferentiated/linitis plastica])
- Gastric lymphomas, sarcomas, other rare types: 10%

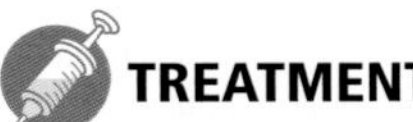

TREATMENT

GENERAL MEASURES
- Multidisciplinary treatment is needed.
- Surgical excision of the tumor is the only potentially curative option:
  - Extent of lymph node resection is controversial.
  - Endoscopic mucosal resection for early gastric mucosal cancers (≤2 cm in size, histologically differentiated, and nonulcerated) and high-grade dysplasia may be curative (2)[B].
  - Patients with advanced (incurable) disease should discuss surgical reduction, which offers the best form of palliation and improves the likelihood of benefit if chemotherapy and/or radiation therapy is administered.

- Adjuvant chemotherapy may provide benefit compared to surgery alone (4)[A].
- Patients with inoperable, locally advanced disease should be offered chemotherapy and reassessed for surgery if response is favorable (2)[A].
- Patients with stage IV disease should be offered chemotherapy, which improves survival compared with the best supportive care (2)[A].

- Radiation therapy
  - Used in combination with surgery and/or chemotherapy
  - Little benefit when used alone because of the radiation resistance of gastric tumors
  - Has role in palliation of pain, reducing risk of bleeding, and mitigating obstruction

MEDICATION

First Line

Combination chemotherapy improves survival compared to single-agent 5-FU (4)[A]:

- Higherst survival achieved with regimens containing a fluoroporyrimidine (5-FU), anthracyclines, and a platinum compound (cisplatin).
- In this category, epirubicin, cisplatin, and continuous-infusion 5-FU are tolerated best.

Second Line

- Ondansetron (Zofran), dronabinol (Marinol), metoclopramide (Reglan), and others for nausea control
- Pain control with opioids

ISSUES FOR REFERRAL

Refer to a high-volume surgery-oncology center

ADDITIONAL THERAPIES

- Trastuzumab in combination with cisplatin or 5-FU should be considered in patients with HER2-positive tumors (1)[A].

- The neoadjuvant use of radiotherapy is not recommended outside clinical trials.

SURGERY/OTHER PROCEDURES

- Radical subtotal gastrectomy with gastrojejunostomy or gastroduodenostomy is the usual treatment:
  - Removal of a large part of the stomach along with the greater and lesser omentum en bloc
  - Splenectomy or distal pancreatectomy done in certain situations
  - Excision of direct tumor extensions at the time of surgery
- Total gastrectomy is indicated only if necessary to remove the local lesion.
- Local excision, endoscopic laser therapy, or electrocautery for palliation of incurable lesion by resection of bleeding area or area of obstruction

COMPLEMENTARY & ALTERNATIVE MEDICINE

Commonly used but with little supportive evidence

INPATIENT CONSIDERATIONS

Admission Criteria/Initial Stabilization

- Inpatient care typical but depends on stage at time of diagnosis
- Most follow-up treatment is outpatient.

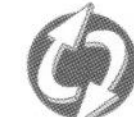

ONGOING CARE

FOLLOW-UP RECOMMENDATIONS

Symptom-driven follow-up visits to monitor disease state, assess treatments, monitor for recurrence/metastasis, and assess nutritional status (2)[B].

Patient Monitoring

Monitor vitamin B_{12} and iron levels following surgical resection; supplement if needed.

DIET

- Maximize preoperative nutritional state.
- All patients undergoing surgery should be considered for early postoperative nutritional support:
  - Enteral route preferred
  - Consider placement of jejunostomy feeding tube.

PATIENT EDUCATION

- Contact local American Cancer Society: http://www.cancer.org
- Cancer Research Institute Helpbook: What to Do If Cancer Strikes. FDR Station, Box 5199, New York, NY 10150-5199

PROGNOSIS

- Because most lesions do not produce symptoms until late in course, gastric carcinomas are usually advanced at the time of diagnosis.
- Overall 5-year relative survival rate is 24% (if local disease 61%, regional spread 24%, distant spread 3%).
- Early detection of gastric cancers usually occurs when performing screening endoscopy in endemic areas or as an otherwise incidental finding.
- Primary gastric lymphoma is more treatable than gastric adenocarcinoma
  - 5-year survival rate is 40–60% with subtotal gastrectomy followed by combination chemotherapy.

COMPLICATIONS

- Early lymphatic spread
- Aggressive metastatic disease (especially hepatic, cerebral, peritoneum, and pulmonary)
- Anemia (especially pernicious)
- Pyloric stenosis
- Dumping syndrome may occur following gastric surgery.

REFERENCES

1. Allum WH, Blazeby JM, Griffin SM, et al. Guidelines for the management of oesophageal and gastric cancer. *Gut*. 2011;60(11):1449–1472.
2. Okines A, Verheij M, Allum W, et al. Gastric cancer: ESMO Clinical Practice Guidelines for diagnosis, treatment and follow-up. *Ann Oncol*. 2010;21(Suppl 5):v50–v54.
3. Sarela AI, Lefkowitz R, Brennan MF, et al. Selection of patients with gastric adenocarcinoma for laparoscopic staging. *Am J Surg*. 2006;191(1):134–138.
4. Wagner AD, Unverzagt S, Grothe W, et al. Chemotherapy for advanced gastric cancer. *Cochrane Database Syst Rev*. 2010;(3):CD004064.

ADDITIONAL READING

- Chen WW, Wang F, Xu RH. Platinum-based versus non-platinum-based chemotherapy as first line treatment of inoperable, advanced gastric adenocarcinoma: a meta-analysis. *PLoS One*. 2013;8(7):e68974.
- Choi IJ. Current evidence of effects of *Helicobacter pylori* eradication on prevention of gastric cancer. *Korean J Intern Med*. 2013;28(5):525–537.
- Karpeh MS Jr. Palliative treatment and the role of surgical resection in gastric cancer. *Dig Surg*. 2013;30(2):174–180.
- Khushalani N. Cancer of the esophagus and stomach. *Mayo Clin Proc*. 2008;83(6):712–722.

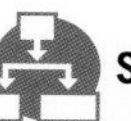

SEE ALSO

Multiple Endocrine Neoplasia (MEN) Syndromes

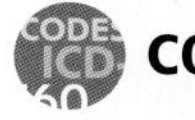

CODES

ICD10

- C16.9 Malignant neoplasm of stomach, unspecified
- C16.8 Malignant neoplasm of overlapping sites of stomach
- C16.2 Malignant neoplasm of body of stomach

CLINICAL PEARLS

- Consider gastric malignancy in patients presenting with epigastric pain and early satiety.
- Accurate preoperative staging is necessary to enhance survival. Endoscopic US is the most accurate preoperative staging tool.
- Treatment generally combines surgery, chemotherapy, and radiation therapy.

GASTRITIS

Miles C. Layton, DO, MAJ, MC, USA • Matthew W. Short, MD

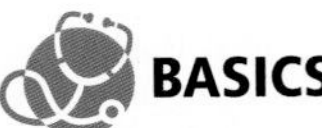

BASICS

DESCRIPTION

- Inflammatory reaction in the gastric mucosa
- Patchy erythema of gastric mucosa
  - A common endoscopic finding; usually insignificant
- Erosive gastritis
  - A reaction to mucosal injury by a noxious chemical agent (especially NSAIDs or alcohol)
- Reflux gastritis
  - A reaction to protracted reflux exposure to bile and pancreatic juice, usually associated with a defective pylorus
  - Typically limited to the prepyloric antrum
- Hemorrhagic gastritis (stress ulceration)
  - A reaction to hemodynamic disorder (e.g., hypovolemia or hypoxia [as in shock])
  - Also common in ICUs
  - Seen after severe burns and severe physical trauma
  - Seen rarely with dabigatran, the 1st oral thrombin inhibitor
- Infectious gastritis
  - Commonly associated with *Helicobacter pylori* (possibly causative, maybe opportunistic)
  - Viral infection, usually as a component of systemic infection, is common.
  - Significant infection by other specific microbes is rare.
  - 2/3 world population colonized with *H. pylori*
- Atrophic gastritis
  - Frequent, in varying degrees, in the elderly
  - Primarily from long-standing *H. pylori* infections
  - May be caused by prolonged PPI use
  - Major risk factor for onset of gastric cancer
  - Associated with primary (pernicious) anemia
  - Autoimmune disease
  - Patches of lymphoid follicles noted in chronic gastritis, along with plasma cells and macrophages; antibodies to parietal cells and intrinsic factor
- Synonym(s): erosive gastritis; reflux gastritis; hemorrhagic gastritis; acute gastritis

Geriatric Considerations

Persons age >60 years often harbor *H. pylori* infection.

Pediatric Considerations

Gastritis rarely occurs in infants or children.

EPIDEMIOLOGY

- Predominant age: all ages
- Predominant sex: male = female

ETIOLOGY AND PATHOPHYSIOLOGY

- Noxious agents cause a breakdown in the gastric mucosal barrier, leaving the epithelial cells unprotected.
- Infection: *H. pylori* (most common cause), *Staphylococcus aureus* exotoxins, and viral infection
- Alcohol
- Aspirin and other NSAIDs
- Bile reflux
- Pancreatic enzyme reflux
- Portal hypertensive (HTN) gastropathy
- Emotional stress

Genetics

Unknown, but observational studies show that 10% of a given population is never colonized with *H. pylori*, regardless of exposure. Genetic variations in *TLR1* may help explain some of this observed variation in individual risk for *H. pylori* infection.

RISK FACTORS

- Age >60 years
- Exposure to potentially noxious drugs or chemical agents, including alcohol or NSAIDs
- Hypovolemia, hypoxia (shock), burns, head injury, complicated postoperative course
- Autoimmune diseases (thyroid and diabetes mellitus 1)
- Family history of *H. pylori* and/or gastric cancer
- Stress (hypovolemia or hypoxia)
- Tobacco use
- Radiation
- Ischemia
- Pernicious anemia
- Gastric mucosal atrophy

GENERAL PREVENTION

- Avoid injurious drugs or chemical agents.
- Patients with hypovolemia or hypoxia (especially patients confined to an intensive care ward) should receive prophylactic antacid therapy.
- In ICU patients (particularly burn and trauma), H_2 receptor antagonists, prostaglandins, or sucralfate used for gastric mucosal protection
- Consider testing for *H. pylori* (and eradicating if present) in patients facing long-term NSAID therapy.

COMMONLY ASSOCIATED CONDITIONS

- Gastric or duodenal peptic ulcer
- Primary (pernicious) anemia—atrophic gastritis
- Portal HTN, hepatic failure
- Gastric lymphoma linked to lymphoid follicles

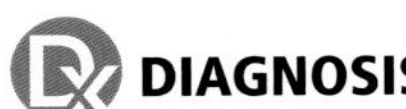

DIAGNOSIS

HISTORY

- Nondescript epigastric distress, often aggravated by eating, often severe, burning
- Anorexia
- Nausea, with or without vomiting
- Significant bleeding is unusual except in hemorrhagic gastritis.
- Hiccups
- Bloating or abdominal fullness

PHYSICAL EXAM

- Mild epigastric tenderness but may have normal abdominal exam
- May have heme-positive stool
- Stool may be black in color.
- Examine for stigmata of chronic alcohol abuse.

DIFFERENTIAL DIAGNOSIS

- Functional GI disorder
- Peptic ulcer disease
- Viral gastroenteritis
- Pancreatic disease
- Gastric cancer (elderly)
- Cholecystitis
- Pancreatic disease (inflammation vs. tumor)

DIAGNOSTIC TESTS & INTERPRETATION

Initial Tests (lab, imaging)

- Usually unremarkable
- CBC to evaluate for blood loss/anemia
- ^{13}C-urea breath test for *H. pylori*
  - 95% specificity and sensitivity
- Serologic test available for *H. pylori*, serum IgG (office and clinical laboratory):
  - Inexpensive
  - 85% sensitivity 79% specificity
  - Cannot be used to assess eradication
- Stool analysis for fecal *H. pylori* antigen
  - 95% specificity and sensitivity
- Gastric acid analysis may be abnormal but is not a reliable indicator of gastritis.
- Low serum pepsinogen I (PG I) relative to PG II is associated with fundal intestinal metaplasia
- Drugs that may alter lab results: Antibiotics or PPIs may affect urea breath test for *H. pylori*.
  - Hold PPIs for 2 weeks, H_2 receptor antagonists for 24 hours, and antibiotics for 4 weeks prior to stool or breath tests (1,2)[C].

Follow-Up Tests & Special Considerations

Endoscopy for *H. pylori*

- Culture
- Polymerase chain reaction (PCR)
- Histology
- Rapid urease testing

Diagnostic Procedures/Other

- Gastroscopy with biopsy allows for a precise diagnosis and is a 1st-line diagnostic tool in
  - Age >55 years with new-onset signs and symptoms
  - Weight loss, persistent vomiting, or GI bleed (1)[C]
- Biopsies (multiple) in both body and antrum recommended if there is a poor response to the initial treatment (3)[C],(4)[B]. *Patient must discontinue PPIs for 2 weeks prior to endoscopy to improve accuracy of result*

Test Interpretation

Acute or chronic inflammatory infiltrate in gastric mucosa, often with distortion or erosion of adjacent epithelium. Presence of *H. pylori* may be confirmed.

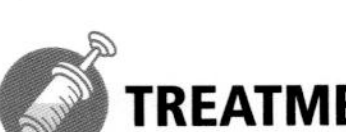

TREATMENT

GENERAL MEASURES

- Treatment of *H. pylori* gastritis is required to relieve symptoms.
- Parenteral fluid and electrolyte supplements required if oral intake is compromised.
- Consider discontinuing NSAIDs.
- Encourage alcohol and smoking cessation.
- Endoscopy indicated for patients not responsive to treatment

MEDICATION

First Line

- Antacids: best given in liquid form, 30 mL 1 hour after meals and at bedtime; useful mainly as an emollient
- H_2 receptor antagonists (e.g., cimetidine [Tagamet]): oral cimetidine 300 mg q6h (or ranitidine [Zantac] or famotidine [Pepcid] or nizatidine [Axid]); not shown to be clearly superior to antacids
- Sucralfate (Carafate): 1 g q4–6h on an empty stomach; rationale uncertain but empirically helpful
- Prostaglandins (misoprostol [Cytotec]): can help allay gastric mucosal injury; suggested dosage 100–200 μg QID
- PPIs can be used if there is no response to antacids or H_2 receptor blockers.
- *H. pylori* eradication
  - Clarithromycin triple therapy (CTT)
    - A short-course therapy (10–14 days) of amoxicillin 1 g BID, standard dose PPI BID (omeprazole 20 mg BID, etc), and clarithromycin 500 mg BID (1,2,5)[A].
    - 70–85% eradication
    - Optimal treatment regimens continue to be debated and tested.
    - IF PCN ALLERGIC: Substitute amoxicillin with metronidazole 500 mg BID.
  - Bismuth quadruple therapy (BQT)
    - PPI (omeprazole 20 mg) BID plus bismuth (Pepto-Bismol) 30 mL liquid or 2 tablets QID plus metronidazole 250 mg QID plus tetracycline 500 mg QID for 10–14 days (1,2,5,6)[A].
    - 75–90% eradication
    - Use as initial therapy in areas of high clarithromycin resistance (>15%)
    - Consider in penicillin-allergic patients
- Consider sequential antibiotic therapy with standard dose PPI (i.e., omeprazole 20 mg) and amoxicillin 1 g BID for 5 days followed by clarithromycin 500 mg and tinidazole 500 mg PO BID with standard dose PPI (omeprazole 20 mg) BID for 5 days. Some studies show it works just as well or better than triple therapy (1,2)[B],(5)[A].
- With treatment failure, use a different regimen, avoiding clarithromycin (unless resistance testing confirms susceptibility):
  - Bismuth quadruple therapy for 7–14 days (1,2,5)[A].
  - Consider levofloxacin 250 mg BID, amoxicillin 1 g BID, and standard dose PPI BID for 14 days in those who fail two attempts (1,2,5)[A].
- Contraindications: hypersensitivity to the drug(s)
- Precautions:
  - If bismuth is prescribed, warn the patient about the side effect of stool becoming black.
  - Refer to the manufacturer's profile of each drug.
- Significant possible interactions: Refer to the manufacturer's profile of each drug.

INPATIENT CONSIDERATIONS

Gastritis may occur in ICU patients.

Admission Criteria/Initial Stabilization

Outpatient, except for severe hemorrhagic gastritis

ONGOING CARE

FOLLOW-UP RECOMMENDATIONS

Usually no restrictions.

- For *H. pylori*, confirm eradication in patients with
  - Gastric ulcer
  - Persistent dyspepsia despite treatment
  - *H. pylori*–associated mucosa-associated lymphoid tissue (MALT) lymphoma
  - History of resection of early gastric cancer

PATIENT MONITORING

- Gastroscopy should be repeated after 6 weeks if gastritis was severe or if patient has a poor symptomatic response to treatment.
- Surveillance gastroscopy every 3–5 years in patients with atrophic gastritis in both the antrum and body, within 1 year for patients with low-grade dysplasia, and immediately (with extensive biopsy sampling) followed by surveillance at 6 and 12 months in patients with high-grade dysplasia (4)[B].

DIET

Restrictions, if any, depend on symptom severity (e.g., bland, light, soft foods); avoid caffeine and spicy foods as well as alcohol.

PATIENT EDUCATION

- Smoking cessation
- Dietary changes
- Relaxation therapy

PROGNOSIS

- Most cases clear spontaneously when the cause has been identified and treated.
- Recurrence of *H. pylori* infection requires a repeated course of treatment.

COMPLICATIONS

- Bleeding from extensive mucosal erosion or ulceration
- Clearing *H. pylori* before chronic gastritis develops may prevent development of gastric cancer.

REFERENCES

1. McColl KE. Clinical practice. *Helicobacter pylori* infection. *N Engl J Med*. 2010;362(17):1597–1604.
2. Chey WD, Wong BC; Practice Parameters Committee of the American College of Gastroenterology. Management of *Helicobacter pylori* infection. *Am J Gastroenterol*. 2007;102(8):1808–1825.
3. Hirota WK, Zuckerman MJ, Adler DG, et al. ASGE guideline: the role of endoscopy in the surveillance of premalignant conditions of the upper GI tract. *Gastrointestinal Endoscopy*. 2006;63(4):570–580.
4. Dinis-Ribeiro M, Areia M, de Vries AC, et al. Management of precancerous conditions and lesions in the stomach (MAPS): guideline from the European Society of Gastrointestinal Endoscopy (ESGE), European *Helicobacter* Study Group (EHSG), European Society of Pathology (ESP), and the Sociedade Portuguesa de Endoscopia Digestiva (SPED). *Endoscopy*. 2012;44(1):74–94.
5. Malfertheiner P, Megraud F, O'Morain CA, et al. Management of *Helicobacter pylori* infection—the Maastricht IV/Florence Consensus report. *Gut*. 2012; 61(5):646–664.
6. Venerito M, Krieger T, Ecker T, et al. Meta-analysis of bismuth quadruple therapy versus clarithromycin triple therapy for empiric primary treatment of *Helicobacter pylori* infection. *Digestion*. 2013;88(1):33–45.

ADDITIONAL READING

- El-Zimaity H, Serra S, Szentgyorgyi E, et al. Gastric biopsies: the gap between evidence-based medicine and daily practice in the management of gastric *Helicobacter pylori* infection. *Can J Gastroenterol*. 2013;27(10):e25–e30.
- Eslami L, Nasseri-Moghaddam S. Meta-analyses: does long-term PPI use increase the risk of gastric premalignant lesions? *Arch Iran Med*. 2013;16(8):449–458.
- Gisbert JP. Rescue therapy for *Helicobacter pylori* infection 2012. *Gastroenterol Res Pract*. 2012;2012:974594.
- Graham DY, Rimbara E. Understanding and appreciating sequential therapy for *Helicobacter pylori* eradication. *J Clin Gastroenterol*. 2011;45(4):309–313.
- Lanza FL, Chan FK, Quigley EM, et al. Guidelines for prevention of NSAID-related ulcer complications. *Am J Gastroenterol*. 2009;104(3):728–738.
- Mayerle J, den Hoed CM, Schurmann C, et al. Identification of genetic loci associated with *Helicobacter pylori* serologic status. *JAMA*. 2013;309(18): 1912–1920.
- Nazareno J, Driman DK, Adams P. Is *Helicobacter pylori* being treated appropriately? A study of inpatients and outpatients in a tertiary care centre. *Can J Gastroenterol*. 2007;21(5):285–288.
- Rugge M, Pennelli G, Pilozzi E, et al. Gastritis: the histology report. *Dig Liver Dis*. 2011;43(Suppl 4):S373–S384.

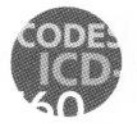

CODES

ICD10

- K29.70 Gastritis, unspecified, without bleeding
- K29.71 Gastritis, unspecified, with bleeding
- K29.00 Acute gastritis without bleeding

CLINICAL PEARLS

- *H. pylori* is the most common cause of gastritis.
- >50% of adult patients are colonized with *H. pylori*.
- *H. pylori* antibodies decline in the year after treatment and should not be used to determine eradication. *H. pylori* antibody titers rise significantly with reinfection.
- *H. pylori* stool antigen tests can be used before and after therapy to assess for eradication and reinfection.
- Several rescue therapies may be necessary to eradicate *H. pylori*.
- Discontinue PPIs 2 weeks prior to endoscopy to improve diagnostic accuracy in cases of suspected gastritis.

GASTROESOPHAGEAL REFLUX DISEASE

Angela Lye, PharmD • Eric F. Hussar, MD

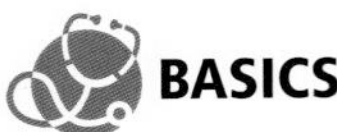

BASICS

DESCRIPTION

Reflux of stomach contents causing episodes of troublesome symptoms that adversely affect quality of life at least twice per week

EPIDEMIOLOGY

Incidence

Incidence: 5 per 1,000 person-years

Prevalence

- Prevalence of gastroesophageal reflux disease (GERD): 18–28% in the United States
- As many as 40% of U.S. adults report symptoms of reflux disease.
- Nonerosive reflux disease: 50–85% of GERD patients
- Barrett esophagus (metaplasia): ~10% of patients
- Prevalence of Barrett esophagus: 2–5% in the United States
- 50% of infants have reflux at 4 months; declines to 5–10% by 12 months of age

ETIOLOGY AND PATHOPHYSIOLOGY

- Associated with defective lower esophageal sphincter (LES) pressure
- Most commonly due to inappropriate LES relaxation
  - Foods that relax LES include high fat content, spicy foods and acidic foods, coffee
  - Nicotine, alcohol
  - Medications (anticholinergic, smooth muscle relaxants—calcium channel blockers, nitrates)
- Other contributing factors:
  - Pregnancy (progestational hormones decrease LES pressure)
  - Ineffective peristalsis
  - Alteration in mucosal resistance
  - Hiatal hernia
  - Scleroderma
  - Delayed gastric emptying
  - Positional: Recumbent or forward bending postures exacerbate reflux symptoms

Genetics

Gene polymorphism associated with GERD has been identified.

RISK FACTORS

- Obesity
- Hiatal hernia
- Scleroderma
- Alcohol use
- Smoking
- Pregnancy

GENERAL PREVENTION

- Avoid triggering foods and beverages.
- Tobacco cessation
- Avoid meals before bedtime.
- Elevate head of bed.
- Avoid lying down after meals.
- Infants: Use car seat for 2–3 hours after meals; thickened feedings

COMMONLY ASSOCIATED CONDITIONS

- Nonerosive esophagitis
- Erosive esophagitis
- Extraesophageal reflux: aspiration, chronic cough, laryngitis, vocal cord granuloma, sinusitis, otitis media
- Halitosis
- Hiatal hernia: Acid pocket (zone of high acidity in the proximal stomach after a meal) above the diaphragm in patients with hiatal hernia is a risk factor (1)[B].
- Peptic stricture: 10% of patients with GERD
- Barrett esophagus
- Esophageal adenocarcinoma

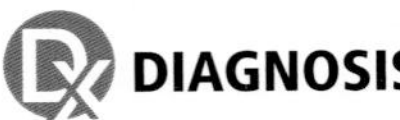

DIAGNOSIS

- Typical symptoms: acid regurgitation, heartburn
- Atypical symptoms: epigastric fullness/pressure/pain, dyspepsia, nausea, bloating, belching
- Extraesophageal signs and symptoms: chronic cough, bronchospasm, wheezing, hoarseness, sore throat, asthma, laryngitis, dental erosions

HISTORY

- Heartburn: retrosternal burning
- Regurgitation; sour or acid taste in mouth ("water brash")
- Symptoms worse with bending or recumbency
- Extraesophageal symptoms (cough; wheezing; hoarseness)
- Diet, alcohol, smoking
- Diagnosis often solely based on history

PHYSICAL EXAM

Typically unremarkable

- Evaluate BMI.
- Rare epigastric tenderness or palpable epigastric mass
- Look for stigmata of chronic systemic disease or alcohol use.

DIFFERENTIAL DIAGNOSIS

- Infectious esophagitis (*Candida*, herpes, HIV, cytomegalovirus)
- Chemical esophagitis
- Pill-induced esophagitis
- Radiation injury
- Crohn disease
- Angina
- Esophageal stricture or anatomic defect (ring, sling)
- Esophageal adenocarcinoma
- Achalasia
- Scleroderma
- Peptic ulcer disease

DIAGNOSTIC TESTS & INTERPRETATION

- Treat empirically if there are no red flags (dysphagia odynophagia, weight loss, early satiety, anemia, new onset, male >50 years) to suggest serious disease.

Initial Tests (lab, imaging)

Check for anemia (bleeding esophageal erosions or poor B_{12} absorption on proton pump inhibitor (PPI).

Diagnostic Procedures/Other

- Upper endoscopy
  - Not required initially if patient has typical GERD symptoms
  - Recommended if there are alarm symptoms such as dysphagia, bleeding, anemia, weight loss, recurrent vomiting, or if patient is unresponsive to 4–8 weeks of maximal PPI treatment
  - Confirms mucosal injury; erosive esophagitis, Barrett esophagus; visually directed biopsy if suspicious for adenocarcinoma
  - ~50–70% of patients with heartburn have negative endoscopy findings (nonerosive or endoscopy—negative reflux disease).
- Savary-Miller classification
  - For grading esophagitis based on endoscopy
    - Grade I: ≥1 nonconfluent reddish spots, with or without exudate
    - Grade II: erosive and exudative lesions in the distal esophagus; may be confluent but not circumferential
    - Grade III: circumferential erosions in the distal esophagus
    - Grade IV: chronic complications such as deep ulcers, stenosis, or scarring with Barrett metaplasia
- Ambulatory reflux monitoring
  - Used preoperatively for nonerosive disease. Also for refractory GERD symptoms or if GERD diagnosis is in question
  - Used to correlate symptoms with reflux, document abnormal acid exposure and the frequency of reflux
- Barium swallow
  - Not used for GERD diagnosis. Used to evaluate complaints of dysphagia (outline anatomic abnormalities)
- Esophageal manometry
  - Records pressure of LES and effectiveness of peristalsis
    - Not recommended for primary GERD diagnosis; used for preoperative surgical evaluation

Test Interpretation

- Acute inflammation (especially eosinophils)
- Epithelial basal zone hyperplasia seen in 85%
- Barrett epithelial change: Gastric columnar epithelium replaces squamous epithelium in distal esophagus (metaplasia).

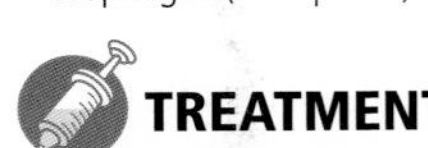

TREATMENT

GENERAL MEASURES

Lifestyle changes are 1st-line intervention:

- Elevate head of bed.
- Avoid meals 2–3 hours before bedtime.
- Avoid stooping, bending.
- Avoid tight-fitting garments.
- Avoid medications that relax LES (anticholinergic drugs; calcium channel blockers).
- Weight loss
- Tobacco cessation
- Avoid alcohol.
- Moderate consumption of patient-specific food triggers (global elimination of all reflux-causing foods is not necessary or beneficial)
- Stepped therapy
  - Phase I: lifestyle and diet modifications, antacids plus H_2 blockers or PPIs
  - Phase II: If symptoms persist, consider endoscopic evaluation.
  - Phase III: If symptoms still persist, consider surgical options.

MEDICATION

First Line

- H_2 blockers in equipotent oral doses (e.g., cimetidine 800 mg BID or 400 mg QID, ranitidine 150 mg BID, famotidine 20 mg BID, or nizatidine 150 mg BID)
  - Renally dosed

- PPIs: Irreversibly bind proton pump (H^+/K^+ ATPase), effective onset within 4 days. Omeprazole 20–40 mg/day, lansoprazole 15–30 mg/day, dexlansoprazole 30 mg/day, pantoprazole 40 mg/day, rabeprazole 20 mg/day, esomeprazole 40 mg/day
  - No major differences in efficacy among PPIs (2)[A]
  - Dose 30–60 minutes before meals with the exception of dexlansoprazole (3)[A].
- Nonerosive esophagitis: PPI therapy superior to H_2 blocker and prokinetics (4)[A]
- Erosive esophagitis: 8 weeks of PPI effective in 90%
  - PPI more effective than H_2 blocker for healing erosive esophagitis (2)[A]
  - Rabeprazole better than omeprazole for symptomatic relief, but no significant difference in endoscopic changes of erosive GERD for treatment up to 8 weeks (5)[A]

Pediatric Considerations

Antacids or liquid H_2 blockers and omeprazole are available. Reflux typically resolves spontaneously in young children.

Second Line

- Antacids or barrier agents (sucralfate 1 g PO QID 1 hour before meals and at bedtime for 4–8 weeks) may relieve breakthrough symptoms.
- Prokinetics: metoclopramide 5–10 mg before meals
- Baclofen as add-on therapy with a PPI
- Precautions
  - Blood dyscrasias and anemia with PPIs and H_2 blockers
  - Metoclopramide is a dopamine blocker; risk of dystonia and tardive dyskinesia
  - Tachyphylaxis may occur with H_2 blockers.
  - B_{12} and iron absorption and calcium absorption compromised on PPI
- Significant possible interactions
  - PPIs and H_2 blockers: multiple cytochrome P450 drug interactions; that is, warfarin, phenytoin, antifungals, digoxin

SURGERY/OTHER PROCEDURES

Laparoscopic fundoplication (wrapping gastric fundus around distal esophagus) increases pressure gradient between stomach and esophagus. Indicated if

- Patient desires to discontinue medical therapy, has unacceptable side effects associated with medical therapy, has a large hiatal hernia, has esophagitis refractory to medical therapy, or has refractory symptoms (3)[A].
- Rule out esophageal dysmotility prior to surgery. If motility problem identified, consider a partial (270 degrees, Toupet) wrap rather than a full 360 degrees wrap.
- Best surgical response seen in patients with typical symptoms who respond well to PPI therapy
- If it is estimated that a patient will require >10 years of PPI treatment, surgery may be more cost-effective.
- Bariatric surgery can be considered for patients with comorbid obesity. Gastric bypass preferred (3)[A]

Pediatric Considerations

Surgery for severe symptoms (apnea, choking, persistent vomiting)

ONGOING CARE

FOLLOW-UP RECOMMENDATIONS

Patient Monitoring

- Follow symptoms over time.
- Repeat endoscopy at 4–8 weeks if there is a poor symptomatic response to medical therapy, especially in older patients.
- Endoscopic surveillance every 2–3 years in patients with Barrett esophagus to screen for malignant transformation (in patients who would opt for treatment if cancer is detected)

DIET

Avoid foods that trigger or worsen symptoms.

PATIENT EDUCATION

- Lifestyle and dietary modifications: eat small meals; avoid lying down soon after meals; elevate head of bed; weight loss, smoking cessation, avoid alcohol and caffeine

PROGNOSIS

- Symptoms and esophageal inflammation often return promptly when treatment is withdrawn. To prevent relapse of symptoms, continue antisecretory therapy (in addition to lifestyle and dietary modifications):
  - PPI maintenance therapy likely improves quality of life better than H_2 blocker maintenance.
  - Full-dose PPIs more effective than half-dose for maintenance (2)[A].
  - In erosive esophagitis, daily maintenance therapy with PPI prevents relapse; intermittent PPI therapy not as effective (6)[A]
- Medical and surgical therapy are equally effective for symptom reduction (2)[A].
- Antireflux surgery
  - 90–94% symptom response. Patients with persistent symptoms should have repeat anatomic evaluation (endoscopy or esophagram).
  - Some surgically treated patients eventually require medical therapy.
- Regression of Barrett epithelium does not routinely occur despite aggressive medical or surgical therapy.

COMPLICATIONS

- Peptic stricture: 10–15%
- Barrett esophagus: 10%
  - Adenocarcinoma cancer develops at an annual rate of 0.5%.
  - Primary treatment for Barrett esophagus with high-grade dysplasia is endoscopic radiofrequency ablation (7)[B].
- Extraesophageal symptoms: hoarseness, aspiration, (including pneumonia)
- Bleeding due to mucosal injury
- Noncardiac chest pain

Geriatric Considerations

Complications more likely (e.g., aspiration pneumonia)

REFERENCES

1. Beaumont H, Bennink RJ, de Jong J, et al. The position of the acid pocket as a major risk factor for acidic reflux in healthy subjects and patients with GORD. *Gut*. 2010;59(4):441–451.
2. Agency for Healthcare Research and Quality. Comparing effectiveness of management strategies for gastroesophageal reflux disease. An update to the 2005 report. http://effectivehealthcare.ahrq.gov/index.cfm/search-for-guides-reviews-and-reports/?productid=781&pageaction=displayproduct. Accessed September 22, 2014.
3. Katz PO, Gerson LB, Vela MF. Guidelines for the diagnosis and management of gastroesophageal reflux disease. *Am J Gastroenterol*. 2013;108(10):308–328.
4. van Pinxteren B, Sigterman KE, Bonis P, et al. Short-term treatment with proton pump inhibitors, H2-receptor antagonists and prokinetics for gastro-oesophageal reflux disease-like symptoms and endoscopy negative reflux disease. *Cochrane Database Syst Rev*. 2010;(11):CD002095.
5. Xia XM, Wang H. Gastroesophageal reflux disease relief in patients treated with rabeprazole 20 mg versus omeprazole 20 mg: a meta-analysis. *Gastroenterol Res Pract*. 2013;2013:327571.
6. Zacny J, Zamakhshary M, Sketris I, et al. Systematic review: the efficacy of intermittent and on-demand therapy with histamine H2-receptor antagonists or proton pump inhibitors for gastro-oesophageal reflux disease patients. *Aliment Pharmacol Ther*. 2005;21(11):1299–1312.
7. Hur C, Choi SE, Rubenstein JH, et al. The cost effectiveness of radiofrequency ablation for Barrett's esophagus. *Gastroenterology*. 2012;143(3):567–575.

G

ADDITIONAL READING

- Badillo R, Francis D. Diagnosis and treatment of gastroesophageal reflux disease. *World J Gastrointest Pharmacol Ther*. 2014;5(3):105–112.
- Martigne L, Delaage PH, Thomas-Delecourt F, et al. Prevalence and management of gastroesophageal reflux disease in children and adolescents: a nationwide cross-sectional observational study. *Eur J Pediatr*. 2012;171(12):1767–1773.

SEE ALSO

Algorithms: Dyspepsia; Epigastric Pain

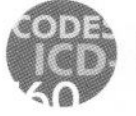

CODES

ICD10

- K21.9 Gastro-esophageal reflux disease without esophagitis
- K21.0 Gastro-esophageal reflux disease with esophagitis

CLINICAL PEARLS

- Treatment with PPI does not alter Barrett-related epithelial change or inhibit neoplastic progression.
- Most cases of GERD can be diagnosed based on medical history alone.
- Empiric treatment with H_2 blockers or PPI leads to symptomatic relief in most cases. Persistent symptoms should be evaluated with endoscopy.

GENITO-PELVIC PAIN/PENETRATION DISORDER (VAGINISMUS)

Adriana C. Linares, MD, MPH, DrPH

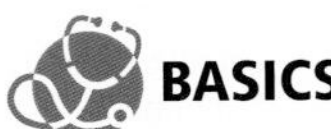

BASICS

Genito-pelvic pain/penetration disorder is the name of the conditions formally known as vaginismus and dyspareunia. It has overlapping elements of hypertonic pelvic floor muscles (recurrent or persistent involuntary contractions), pain, and avoidance of sexual intercourse leading to difficulty in vaginal penetration.

DESCRIPTION

- Persistent or recurrent difficulties for 6 months or more with at least 1 of the following:
  - Inability to have vaginal intercourse/penetration on at least 50% of attempts
  - Marked genito-pelvic pain during at least 50% of vaginal intercourse/penetration attempts
  - Marked fear of vaginal intercourse/penetration or of genito-pelvic pain during intercourse/penetration on at least 50% of vaginal intercourse/penetration attempts
  - Marked tensing or tightening of the pelvic floor muscles during attempted vaginal intercourse/ penetration on at least 50% of occasions
- The disturbance causes marked distress or interpersonal difficulty.
- Specify if with a general medical condition (e.g., lichen sclerosis, endometriosis) (1)

Pregnancy Considerations

- Pregnancy can occur in patients with genito-pelvic pain/penetration disorder when ejaculation occurs on the perineum.
- Vaginismus may be an independent risk factor for cesarean delivery.

EPIDEMIOLOGY

Incidence

The incidence of vaginismus is thought to be about 1–17% per year worldwide.

Prevalence

- True prevalence is unknown due to limited data/ reporting.
- Population-based studies report prevalence rates of 0.5–30%.
- Affects women in all age groups
- Approximately 15% of women in North America report recurrent pain during intercourse.

ETIOLOGY AND PATHOPHYSIOLOGY

Most often multifactorial in both primary and secondary vaginismus:

- Primary
  - Psychological and psychosocial issues
    - Negative messages about sex and sexual relations in upbringing may cause phobic reaction.
    - Poor body image and limited understanding of genital area
    - History of sexual trauma
  - Abnormalities of the hymen
- Secondary
  - Vaginal infection
  - Inflammatory dermatitis
  - Surgical or postdelivery scarring
  - Endometriosis
  - Inadequate vaginal lubrication
  - Pelvic radiation
  - Estrogen deficiency
  - Conditioned response to pain from physical issues previously listed

RISK FACTORS

- Although the exact role in the condition is unclear, many women report a history of abuse or sexual trauma.
- Often associated with other sexual dysfunctions

COMMONLY ASSOCIATED CONDITIONS

- Marital stress, family dysfunction
- Anxiety
- Vulvodynia/vestibulodynia

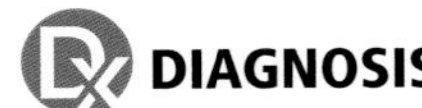

DIAGNOSIS

DSM-5 has combined vaginismus and dyspareunia in a condition called genito-pelvic pain/penetration disorder.

HISTORY

- Complete medical history
- Full psychosocial and sexual history, including the following
  - Relationship difficulty
  - Inability to allow vaginal entry for different purposes:
    - Sexual (penis, digit, object)
    - Hygiene (tampon use)
    - Health care (pelvic examination)
  - Infertility
  - Past traumatic experiences
  - Religious beliefs
  - Views on sexuality

PHYSICAL EXAM

- Pelvic examination is necessary to exclude structural abnormalities or organic pathology.
- Educating the patient about the examination and giving her control over the progression of the examination is essential, as genital/pelvic examination may induce varying degrees of anxiety in patients.
- Referral to a gynecologist, family physician, or other provider specializing in the treatment of sexual disorders may be appropriate.
- Lamont classification system aids in the assessment of severity:
  - 1st degree: perineal and levator spasm relieved with reassurance
  - 2nd degree: perineal spasm maintained throughout the pelvic exam
  - 3rd degree: levator spasm and elevation of buttocks
  - 4th degree: levator and perineal spasm and elevation with adduction and retreat

DIFFERENTIAL DIAGNOSIS

- Vaginal infection
- Vulvodynia/vestibulodynia
- Vulvovaginal atrophy
- Urogenital structural abnormalities
- Interstitial cystitis

DIAGNOSTIC TESTS & INTERPRETATION

No laboratory tests indicated. When diagnosing of this disorder has been conducted, five factors should be considered:

- Partner factors
- Relationship factors
- Individual vulnerability factors
- Cultural/religious factors
- Medical factors

Test Interpretation

Not available, may be needed to check for secondary causes

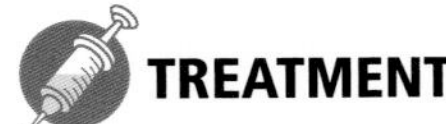

TREATMENT

- Genito-pelvic pain penetration disorder may be successfully treated (2)[B]

- Outpatient care is appropriate.
- Treatment of physical conditions, if present, is 1st line (see "Secondary" under "Etiology and Pathophysiology").
- Role for pelvic floor physical therapy and myofascial release

- Some evidence suggests that cognitive-behavioral therapy may be effective, including desensitization techniques, such as gradual exposure, aimed at decreasing avoidance behavior and fear of vaginal penetration (3)[A].
- Based on a Cochrane review, a clinically relevant effect of systematic desensitization cannot be ruled out (2)[A].
- Evidence suggests that Masters and Johnson sex therapy may be effective (4)[B].
  - Involves Kegel exercises to increase control over perineal muscles
  - Stepwise vaginal desensitization exercises:
    - With vaginal dilators that the patient inserts and controls
    - With woman's own finger(s) to promote sexual self-awareness
    - Advancement to partner's fingers with patient's control
    - Coitus after achieving largest vaginal dilator or 3 fingers; important to begin with sensate-focused exercises/sensual caressing without necessarily a demand for coitus
    - Female superior at first; passive (nonthrusting); female directed
    - Later, thrusting may be allowed.
- Topical anesthetic with desensitization exercises may be considered.
- Patient education is an essential component of treatment (see "Patient Education" section).

MEDICATION

Botulinum neurotoxin type A injections may improve vaginismus in patients who do not respond to standard cognitive-behavioral and medical treatment for vaginismus:

- Dosage: 20, 50, and 100–400 U of botulinum toxin type A injected in the levator ani muscle have been shown to improve vaginismus.

ISSUES FOR REFERRAL

For diagnosis and treatment recommendations, the following resources may be consulted:

- Obstetrics/gynecology
- Pelvic floor physical therapy
- Psychiatry
- Sex therapy
- Hypnotherapy

SURGERY/OTHER PROCEDURES

Contraindicated

COMPLEMENTARY & ALTERNATIVE MEDICINE

- Biofeedback
- Functional electrical stimulation

ONGOING CARE

FOLLOW-UP RECOMMENDATIONS

Desensitization techniques of gentle, progressive, patient-controlled vaginal dilation

Patient Monitoring

General preventive health care

DIET

No special diet

PATIENT EDUCATION

- Education about pelvic anatomy, nature of vaginal spasms, normal adult sexual function
- Handheld mirror can help the woman to learn visually to tighten and loosen perineal muscles.
- Important to teach the partner that spasms are not under conscious control and are not a reflection on the relationship or a woman's feelings about her partner
- Instruction in techniques for vaginal dilation
- Resources:
  - American College of Obstetricians & Gynecologists (ACOG), 409 12th St., SW, Washington, DC 20024-2188; 800-762-ACOG. http://www.acog.org
  - Valins L. *When a Woman's Body Says No to Sex: Understanding and Overcoming Vaginismus*. New York, NY: Penguin; 1992.

PROGNOSIS

Favorable, with early recognition of the condition and initiation of treatment

REFERENCES

1. American Psychiatric Association. *Diagnostic Statistical Manual of Mental Disorders*. 5th ed. Arlington, VA. American Psychiatric Association; 2013.
2. Melnik T, Hawton K, McGuire H. Interventions for vaginismus. *Cochrane Database Syst Rev*. 2012;(12):CD001760.
3. Ter Kuile MM, Both S, van Lankveld JJ. Cognitive behavioral therapy for sexual dysfunctions in women. *Psychiatr Clin North Am*. 2010;33(3):595–610.
4. Pereira VM, Arias-Carrión O, Machado S, et al. Sex therapy for female sex dysfunction. *Int Arc Med*. 2013;6(1):37.

ADDITIONAL READING

- Basson R, Wierman ME, van Lankveld J. Summary of the recommendations on sexual dysfunctions in women. *J Sex Med*. 2010;7(1, Pt 2):314–326.
- Crowley T, Goldmeier D, Hiller J. Diagnosing and managing vaginismus. *BMJ*. 2009;338:b2284.
- Jeng CJ, Wang LR, Chou CS, et al. Management and outcome of primary vaginismus. *J Sex Marital Ther*. 2006;32(5):379–387.
- Pacik PT. Understanding and treating vaginismus: a multimodal approach. *Int Urogynecol J*. 2014;25(12):1613–1620.
- Pacik PT. Vaginismus: review of current concepts and treatment using botox injections, bupivacaine injections, and progressive dilation with the patient under anesthesia. *Aesthetic Plast Surg*. 2011;35(6):1160–1164.
- Reissing ED, Binik Y, Khalifé S, et al. Etiological correlates of vaginismus: sexual and physical abuse, sexual knowledge, sexual self-schema, and relationship adjustment. *J Sex Marital Ther*. 2003;29(1):47–59.
- Simons JS, Carey MP. Prevalence of sexual dysfunctions: results from a decade of research. *Arch Sex Behav*. 2001;30(2):177–219.
- ter Kuile MM, van Lankveld JJ, de Groot E, et al. Cognitive-behavioral therapy for women with lifelong vaginismus: process and prognostic factors. *Behav Res Ther*. 2007;45(2):359–373.

SEE ALSO

Dyspareunia; Sexual Dysfunction in Women

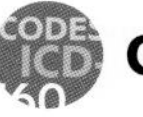

CODES

ICD10

- N94.2 Vaginismus
- F52.5 Vaginismus not due to a substance or known physiol condition
- N94.1 Dyspareunia

CLINICAL PEARLS

- In a patient with suspected genito-pelvic pain penetration disorder, a complete medical history, including a comprehensive psychosocial and sexual history, and a patient-centric, patient-controlled educational pelvic exam should be conducted.
- This condition can be treated effectively.
- Cognitive-behavioral therapy may be effective for the treatment of this condition.
- Botox injection therapy is in the experimental stages but looks promising for the treatment of vaginismus. Bupivacaine and dilation under general anesthesia has also been tried as a treatment for vaginismus.

GIARDIASIS

Kristyn T. Fagerberg, MD

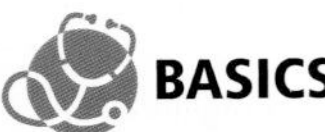

BASICS

DESCRIPTION

- Intestinal infection caused by the protozoan parasite *Giardia lamblia*:
  - *G. lamblia* is also called *G. duodenalis* and *G. intestinalis*.
- Infection results from ingestion of the cysts, which excyst into trophozoites:
  - Trophozoites colonize the small intestine and cause symptoms.
  - Cycle is continued when the trophozoites encyst in the small intestine and subsequently transmitted through water, food, or hands contaminated by feces of infected person.
- Most infections result from fecal–oral transmission or ingestion of contaminated water (e.g., swimming).
- Less commonly, giardiasis is the result of contaminated food.

EPIDEMIOLOGY

- Predominant age:
  - All ages but most common in early childhood ages 1–9 years and adults 35–44 years
- Predominant gender:
  - male > female (slightly)
- There is minimal seasonal variability; however, a slight increase in cases is noted in summer months.

Pediatric Considerations

Common in early childhood

Prevalence

- 5% of patients with stools submitted for ova and parasite exams
- >19,000 cases/year in reportable US states:
  - Giardia is not reportable in Indiana, Kentucky, Mississippi, North Carolina, and Texas.

ETIOLOGY AND PATHOPHYSIOLOGY

Giardia trophozoites colonize the surface of the proximal small intestine: The mechanism by which they cause diarrhea is unknown.

Genetics

No known genetic risk factors

RISK FACTORS

- Daycare centers
- Anal intercourse
- Wilderness camping
- Travel to developing countries
- Children adopted from developing countries
- Public swimming pools
- Pets with giardia infection/diarrhea

GENERAL PREVENTION

- Hand hygiene
- Water purification when camping and when traveling to developing countries
- Properly cook all foods.

COMMONLY ASSOCIATED CONDITIONS

Hypogammaglobulinemia and possibly IgA deficiency: diarrhea more severe and prolonged in these patients

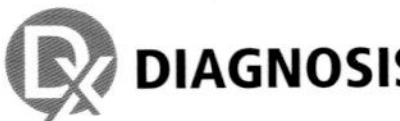

DIAGNOSIS

HISTORY

- 25–50% of infected persons are symptomatic.
- Symptoms usually appear 1–2 weeks after an exposure.
- Chronic diarrhea (lasting >5–7 days and frequently weeks)
- Abdominal bloating
- Flatulence
- Loose, greasy, foul-smelling stools that tend to float
- Weight loss
- Nausea
- Lactose intolerance

PHYSICAL EXAM

- Typically normal vital signs
- Nonspecific; abdominal exam; may have bloating tenderness or increased bowel sounds

DIFFERENTIAL DIAGNOSIS

- Infectious causes include cryptosporidiosis, isosporiasis, and cyclosporiasis.
- Other causes of malabsorption include celiac sprue, tropical sprue, bacterial overgrowth syndromes, and Crohn ileitis.
- Suspect irritable bowel if diarrhea is not accompanied by weight loss.

DIAGNOSTIC TESTS & INTERPRETATION

Initial Tests (lab, imaging)

- Stool for ova and parasites:
  - Repeated 3× on separate days
  - Cysts seen in fixed or fresh stools and, occasionally, trophozoites are found in fresh diarrheal stools.
- Fluorescent antibody (FA) and ELISA fecal tests:
  - *A single FA or ELISA is at least as sensitive as 3 stools for ova and parasites* (1,2)[B].
- Polymerase chain reaction (PCR) techniques are more sensitive than microscopy but have not been widely adopted due to high cost.

Follow-Up Tests & Special Considerations

String test (Enterotest):

- A gelatin capsule on a string is swallowed and left in the duodenum for several hours or overnight.
- The end of the string is then visualized microscopically.

Diagnostic Procedures/Other

Esophagogastroduodenoscopy (EGD) with biopsy and sample of small intestinal fluid

Test Interpretation

Intestinal biopsy shows flattened, mild lymphocytic infiltration and trophozoites on the surface.

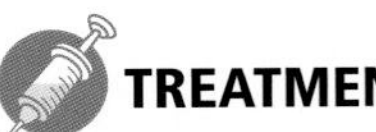

TREATMENT

Outpatient for mild cases; inpatient if symptoms are severe enough to cause dehydration warranting parenteral fluid replacement

GENERAL MEASURES

- Medical therapy for all infected individuals
- Fluid replacement if dehydrated

MEDICATION

First Line

- Metronidazole (Flagyl): 250 mg PO TID for 5–7 days (2)[B]
- Tinidazole: 2 g PO single dose (50 mg/kg up to 2 g for children)
- Albendazole: 400 mg/day PO for 5 days:
  - Albendazole has comparable effectiveness to metronidazole with fewer side effects and low cost
- Precautions:
  - Theoretical risk of carcinogenesis with metronidazole
- Significant possible interactions: occasional disulfiram reaction with metronidazole or tinidazole

Pregnancy Considerations

Medications to treat giardiasis are relatively contraindicated during pregnancy; consider appropriate consultation with infectious disease or maternal-fetal medicine specialist.

Second Line

- Furazolidone: 8 mg/kg/day TID for 10 days (slightly less effective but commonly used in pediatrics because it is well tolerated); not available in United States
- Paromomycin (Humatin): a nonabsorbable aminoglycoside that is probably less effective but commonly recommended in pregnancy because of theoretical risk of teratogenicity of other agents
- Quinacrine: 100 mg TID for 5–7 days; was the treatment of choice for giardiasis but has been withdrawn from the U.S. market

- Nitazoxanide suspension was approved by the FDA in 2003 for treatment of giardiasis in children age 1–11 years. Children age 1–4 years receive 100 mg BID and age 5–11 years receive 200 mg BID for 3 days.
- 2 other nitroimidazole antibiotics, omidazole and secnidazole, are effective against *Giardia* but are not available in the United States.

ADDITIONAL THERAPIES

- Lactose intolerance may follow *Giardia* infection and be a cause of persistent diarrhea post treatment.
- There have been anecdotal reports of herbal products containing *Mentha crispa* being effective in the treatment of *Giardia*. However, when studied, it was shown to be only 47.8% effective when compared to 84% for secnidazole (a metronidazole analog).
- A recent study showed tetrahydrolipstatin (Orlistat) had activity against *Giardia* and may be investigated as a potential treatment option in the future for patients who are resistant to metronidazole (3)[C].

ONGOING CARE

FOLLOW-UP RECOMMENDATIONS

Patient Monitoring

Symptoms, weight, stool exams if patients fail to improve

DIET

Good nutrition, low lactose, low fat, monitor for dehydration

PATIENT EDUCATION

- Hand washing may be more important than water purification to prevent transmission in outdoor recreationalists.
- CDC Facts about *Giardia* and Swimming Pools: www.cdc.gov/healthywater/pdf/swimming/resources/giardia-factsheet.pdf:
  - Don't swim when you have diarrhea.
  - Wash hands with soap after changing diapers before you return to the pool.
  - Avoid ingestion of pool, lake, or river water.
  - Use chlorine to kill giardia in water used for recreational activities.

PROGNOSIS

- Untreated giardiasis lasts for weeks.
- Patients usually (90%) respond to treatment within a few days:
  - Most nonresponders or relapses respond to a 2nd course with the same or a different agent.

COMPLICATIONS

Malabsorption, reactive arthritis, and weight loss

ALERT
Notifiable disease

REFERENCES

1. L Alexander C, Niebel M, Jones B. The rapid detection of *Cryptosporidium* and *Giardia* species in clinical stools using the Quik Chek immunoassay *Parasitol Int*. 2013;62(6):552–553.
2. Granados CE, Reveiz L, Uribe LG, et al. Drugs for treating giardiasis. *Cochrane Database Syst Rev*. 2012;12:CD007787.
3. Hahn J, Seeber F, Kolodziej H, et al. High sensitivity of *Giardia duodenalis* to tetrahydolipstatin (orlistat) in vitro. *PLoS One*. 2013;8(8):e71597. doi:10.1371/journal.pone.0071597.

ADDITIONAL READING

- Almirall P, Escobedo AA, Ayala I, et al. Mebendazole compared with secnidazole in the treatment of adult giardiasis: a randomised, no-inferiority, open clinical trial. *J Parasitol Res*. 2011;2011:636857.
- Cañete R, Rodríguez P, Mesa L, et al. Albendazole versus metronidazole in the treatment of adult giardiasis: a randomized, double-blind, clinical trial. *Curr Med Res Opin*. 2012;28(1):149–154.
- Fallah M, Rabiee S, Moshtaghi AA. Comparison between efficacy of a single dose of tinidazole with a 7-day standard dose course of metronidazole in giardiasis. *Pak J Med Sci*. 2007;23:43–46.
- Haque R, Roy S, Siddique A, et al. Multiplex real-time PCR assay for detection of *Entamoeba histolytica, Giardia intestinalis,* and *Cryptosporidium* spp. *Am J Trop Med Hyg*. 2007;76(4):713–717.
- Lal A, Hales S, French N, et al. Seasonality in human zoonotic enteric diseases: a systematic review. *PLoS ONE*. 2012;7(4):e31883.
- Shields JM, Gleim ER, Beach MJ. Prevalence of *Cryptosporidium* spp. and *Giardia intestinalis* in swimming pools, Atlanta, Georgia. *Emerg Infect Dis*. 2008;14(6):948–950.
- Solaymani-Mohammadi S, Genkinger JM, Loffredo CA, et al. A meta-analysis of the effectiveness of albendazole compared with metronidazole as treatments for infections with *Giardia duodenalis*. *PLoS Negl Trop Dis*. 2010;4(5):e682.
- Teles NS, Fechine FV, Viana FA, et al. Evaluation of the therapeutic efficacy of *Mentha crispa* in the treatment of giardiasis. *Contemp Clin Trials*. 2011;32(6):809–813.
- Yoder JS, Harral C, Beach MJ, et al. Giardiasis surveillance—United States, 2006–2008. *MMWR Surveill Summ*. 2010;59(6):15–25.

SEE ALSO

Algorithm: Diarrhea, Chronic

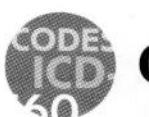

CODES

ICD10

A07.1 Giardiasis [lambliasis]

CLINICAL PEARLS

- Daycare facilities and public swimming pools are common sources of *Giardia* (don't assume camping or travel is required).
- Treatment with metronidazole is often poorly tolerated but has higher cure rates.
- Most treatment failures respond to a 2nd course of antibiotics (whether or not you switch drugs).
- A single FA or ELISA is at least as sensitive as 3 stool samples for ova and parasites.

GILBERT DISEASE

Robert A. Marlow, MD, MA

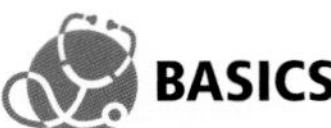

BASICS

DESCRIPTION

Mild chronic or intermittent unconjugated hyperbilirubinemia (not due to hemolysis) with otherwise normal liver function (1)

Pediatric Considerations

Rare for the disorder to be diagnosed before puberty (2)

Pregnancy Considerations

The relative fasting that may occur with morning sickness can elevate bilirubin level.

EPIDEMIOLOGY

- Predominant age: present from birth but most often presents in the 2nd or 3rd decade of life; heterozygous for single abnormal gene (3)
- Predominant sex: male > female (2–7:1)

Prevalence

Prevalence in the United States: ~7% of the population (4); ~1 in 3 of those affected are not aware that they have the disorder.

ETIOLOGY AND PATHOPHYSIOLOGY

The hyperbilirubinemia results from impaired hepatic bilirubin clearance (~30% of normal). Hepatic bilirubin conjugation (glucuronidation) is reduced, although this is likely not the only defect (3).

Genetics

A gene defect resulting in reduced bilirubin uridine diphosphate–glucuronosyltransferase-1 appears to be necessary but not sufficient for Gilbert syndrome (5).

RISK FACTORS

Male gender

COMMONLY ASSOCIATED CONDITIONS

Gilbert disease may be part of a spectrum of hereditary disorders that includes types I and II Crigler-Najjar syndrome.

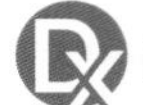

DIAGNOSIS

HISTORY

No significant symptoms, although a variety of nonspecific symptoms have been described. An episode of nonpruritic jaundice can be triggered by stressors such as fasting, dehydration, infections, physical exertion, lack of sleep, and surgery. Some medications may also trigger episodes of jaundice, such as drugs that inhibit glucuronyl transferase, such as gemfibrozil and the protease inhibitors atazanavir and indinavir. Any symptoms present during an episode of jaundice, including fatigue, are caused by the triggering factor and are not directly a result of the Gilbert disease (6).

PHYSICAL EXAM

No abnormal physical findings other than occasional mild jaundice that can be precipitated by the abovementioned triggers (fasting, dehydration, infections, physical exertion, lack of sleep, and surgery).

DIFFERENTIAL DIAGNOSIS

- Hemolysis
- Ineffective erythropoiesis (megaloblastic anemias, certain porphyrias, thalassemia major, sideroblastic anemia, severe lead poisoning, congenital dyserythropoietic anemias)
- Cirrhosis
- Chronic persistent hepatitis
- Pancreatitis
- Biliary tract disease

DIAGNOSTIC TESTS & INTERPRETATION

Initial Tests (lab, imaging)

- Bilirubin: Elevated but <6 mg/dL (103 μmol/L) and usually <3 mg/dL (51 μmol/L), virtually all unconjugated (indirect), with conjugated bilirubin within the normal range and/or <20% of the total bilirubin (6).
- CBC with peripheral smear is normal.
- Reticulocyte count is normal.
- Liver function tests (LFTs) (aspartate aminotransferase [AST], alanine transaminase [ALT], alkaline phosphatase, and gamma-glutamyl transpeptidase [GGT]) are normal.
- Fasting and postprandial serum bile acids are normal.
- Up to 60% of patients have clinically insignificant mild hemolysis that frequently can only be detected with sophisticated red cell survival studies.
- Drugs that may alter lab results: Bilirubin level may be raised by nicotinic acid and lowered by phenobarbital.
- Disorders that may alter lab results: Bilirubin levels increase during fasting and may increase during a febrile illness.

Diagnostic Procedures/Other

ALERT

A liver biopsy is not usually needed to exclude other diagnoses (4).

- Some clinicians recommend confirming the diagnosis by reducing daily caloric intake to 400 kcal for 48 hours, which results in a 2–3-fold increase in unconjugated bilirubin, but other clinicians consider this impractical and nonspecific for Gilbert disease.
- After 12 hours of fasting, an increase of total bilirubin to >1.9 mg/dL 2 hours after an oral dose of rifampin 900 mg distinguishes patients with Gilbert disease with a sensitivity of 100% and a specificity of 100% (7).

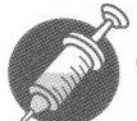

TREATMENT

- Outpatient
- The most important treatment is to make a positive diagnosis of Gilbert disease to reassure the patient and prevent further unnecessary procedures.

ONGOING CARE

FOLLOW-UP RECOMMENDATIONS

Patient Monitoring

If history, physical exam, and laboratory tests are normal, see the patient on 2–3 further occasions during the ensuing 12–18 months. If the patient develops no symptoms, reticulocytosis, or new liver function abnormalities, make the diagnosis of Gilbert disease.

PATIENT EDUCATION

Reassure the patient that the condition is benign with no known sequelae.

PROGNOSIS

- The disorder is benign with an excellent prognosis.
- There is some preliminary evidence that patients with Gilbert disease may have a lower incidence of cardiovascular disease (8,9). Elevated levels of bilirubin may exert an antioxidation effect (9).
- Patients with Gilbert syndrome are able to serve as donors for right lobe of liver for transplantation (10).

COMPLICATIONS

No known complications

REFERENCES

1. Bosma PJ. Inherited disorders of bilirubin metabolism. *J Hepatol*. 2003;38(1):107–117.
2. Fretzayas A, Moustaki M, Liapi O, et al. Gilbert syndrome. *Eur J Pediatr*. 2012;171(1):11–15.
3. Strassburg CP. Pharmacogenetics of Gilbert's syndrome. *Pharmacogenomics*. 2008;9(6):703–715.
4. Radu P, Atsmon J. Gilbert's syndrome—clinical and pharmacological implications. *Isr Med Assoc J*. 2001;3(8):593–598.
5. Bosma PJ, Chowdhury JR, Bakker C, et al. The genetic basis of the reduced expression of bilirubin UDP-glucuronosyltransferase 1 in Gilbert's syndrome. *N Engl J Med*. 1995;333(18):1171–1175.
6. Claridge LC, Armstrong MJ, Booth C, et al. Gilbert's syndrome. *BMJ*. 2011;342:d2293.
7. Murthy GD, Byron D, Shoemaker D, et al. The utility of rifampin in diagnosing Gilbert's syndrome. *Am J Gastroenterol*. 2001;96(4):1150–1154.
8. Inoguchi T, Sasaki S, Kobayashi K, et al. Relationship between Gilbert syndrome and prevalence of vascular complications in patients with diabetes. *JAMA*. 2007;298(12):1398–1400.
9. Bulmer AC, Blanchfield JT, Toth I, et al. Improved resistance to serum oxidation in Gilbert's syndrome: a mechanism for cardiovascular protection. *Atherosclerosis*. 2008;199(2):390–396.
10. Demirbas T, Piskin T, Dayangac M, et al. Right-lobe liver transplant from donors with Gilbert syndrome. *Exp Clin Transplant*. 2012;10(1):39–42.

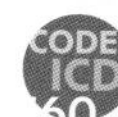

CODES

ICD10

- E80.4 Gilbert syndrome
- E80.6 Other disorders of bilirubin metabolism

CLINICAL PEARLS

- Gilbert disease: a mild chronic or intermittent unconjugated hyperbilirubinemia (not due to hemolysis) with otherwise normal liver function
- The hyperbilirubinemia results from impaired hepatic bilirubin clearance (30% of normal). Hepatic bilirubin conjugation (glucuronidation) is reduced, although this is likely not the only defect.
- The most important reason to make the diagnosis of Gilbert disease is to reassure the patient that this is a benign condition with no known sequelae and to prevent unnecessary procedures.
- To diagnose Gilbert disease: History, physical exam, and laboratory tests (LFTs, reticulocytosis, etc.) are normal on visits every 6 months over 18 months.
- A liver biopsy is not usually needed to rule out other liver diseases. The diagnosis can be confirmed by otherwise normal LFTs, no evidence of hemolysis, and the response to fasting or a dose of rifampin.
- The etiology of Gilbert disease can result when the patient has a gene defect resulting in reduced conjugation of bilirubin. The gene defect is necessary but not sufficient to produce Gilbert disease.

GINGIVITIS

Hugh J. Silk, MD, MPH • Sheila O. Stille, DMD • Alliam Regan, MD

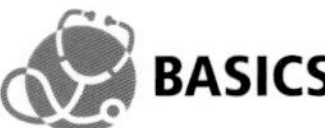

BASICS

DESCRIPTION

Gingivitis is a reversible form of inflammation of the gingiva. It is a mild form of periodontal disease. Classification includes the following:

- Plaque-induced
- Not plaque-induced (bacterial, viral, or fungal; e.g., acute necrotizing gingivitis, Vincent disease ["trench mouth"], denture-related)
- Modified by systemic factors (e.g., pregnancy, puberty, HIV, diabetes, smoking, leukemia)
- Modified by medications (calcium channel blockers, antipsychotics, antiepileptics, antirejection medications, hormones)
- Modified by malnutrition (vitamin deficiencies)
- System(s) affected: gastrointestinal; ears, nose, throat; dental
- Synonym(s): mild periodontal disease; gum disease

Geriatric Considerations

More frequent in this age group (due more to additive effects than to increased susceptibility)

Pediatric Considerations

Mild cases common in children (most common form of pediatric periodontal disease) and usually require no specific interventions other than improved oral hygiene

Pregnancy Considerations

- Very common in pregnant women; hormonal effect
- Self-limited

EPIDEMIOLOGY

- Predominant age: teenagers and young adults. Periodontitis, the outcome of chronic gingivitis, >35 years (but as young as 5 years of age)
- Predominant sex: slightly more males than female
- Prevalence ~50% of children
- ~90% of adolescents and adult population
- ~30–75% of pregnant women

ETIOLOGY AND PATHOPHYSIOLOGY

Inflammation of gingiva. This can progress to deeper, destructive inflammation. If involving supporting bone, will be periodontitis, not gingivitis.

- Usually noncontagious
- Inadequate plaque removal
- Blood dyscrasias (pregnancy)
- Oral contraceptives
- Allergic reactions
- Nutritional deficiencies
- Vasoconstriction (nicotine, methamphetamine)
- Endocrine/hormonal variations
  - Pregnancy
  - Menses
  - Menarche
- Chronic debilitating disease
- Vincent disease
  - Synergistic infection with fusiform bacillus (*Fusobacterium* spp.) and spirochete (*Borrelia vincentii*)
- Pathology
  - Acute or chronic inflammation
  - Hyperemic capillaries
  - Polymorphonuclear infiltration
  - Papillary projections in subepithelial tissue
  - Fibroblasts

Genetics

Possible genetic link (up to 30% of population). Rare condition called hereditary gingival fibromatosis associated with hirsutism.

RISK FACTORS

- Poor dental hygiene/plaque formation
- Pregnancy
- Uncontrolled diabetes mellitus
- Malocclusion or dental crowding
- Smoking
- Mouth breathing
- Xerostomia
- Faulty dental restoration
- HIV-positive; AIDS
- Stress
- Hospitalization (1)[A]
- Vitamin C deficiency; coenzyme Q10 deficiency
- Dental appliances (dentures, braces)
- Eruption of primary or secondary teeth
- Necrotizing ulcerative gingivitis
  - Stress
  - Lack of sleep
  - Malnutrition
  - Viral illness
  - Typically teens and young adults
- Bronchial asthma and other respiratory diseases (2,3)[B]
- Rheumatoid arthritis (4)[B]

GENERAL PREVENTION

- Good oral hygiene
  - Adults
    - Regular twice-daily brushing with fluoride toothpaste and increased benefit of using circular oscillating electric brush rather than regular brush or sonic/vibration (5,6)[A]
    - Daily "high-quality" flossing (studies show that flossing only helps when it is done correctly) (7)[A]
    - Chlorhexidine with oral hygiene better than other oral rinse agents (8,9)[A]
      - Use in acute phase sparingly (10)[B]
  - Pediatrics
    - Regular twice-daily brushing with fluoride toothpaste under parental supervision until full manual dexterity (~8 years of age)
    - Regular flossing if no spaces between teeth
- Cleaning by a dentist or hygienist every 6 months or more frequently, if indicated
- Mouth rinse with essential oils (menthol, thymol, eucalyptol; e.g., Listerine) combined with brushing reduces gingivitis more than brushing alone (11)[B].
  - Caution: Long-term use of alcohol-based mouth rinse may be associated with an increased risk of oral cancer (12)[B].

COMMONLY ASSOCIATED CONDITIONS

- Periodontitis
- Glossitis
- Pedunculated growths (pyogenic granulomata)

DIAGNOSIS

HISTORY

- Gum erythema, swelling, and edema
- Gums are tender when touched but otherwise painless.
- Bleeding of gums when brushing, flossing, or eating
- Inquire about HIV risk, pregnancy, nutritional deficiencies, diabetes, and other risk factors as indicated (see "Risk Factors").
- Smoking history
- Oral hygiene, dental visit history

PHYSICAL EXAM

- Normal gums should appear pink, firm, stippled, and scalloped.
- Gingivitis—gum swelling and edema (usually painless, except to touch)
- Gum erythema: bright red or red-purple appearance
- Bleeding with manipulation of gums
- Change of normal gum contours
- Plaque and calculus (not easily removed)
- Edema of interdental papillae
- HIV gingivitis
  - Also called linear gingival erythema
  - Narrow band of bright red inflamed gum surrounding neck of tooth
  - Painful
  - Bleeds easily
  - Rapid destruction of gingival tissue and can progress to periodontitis with destruction of underlying support tissues (periodontal ligament, supporting alveolar bone)
- Vincent disease
  - Ulcers
  - Fever
  - Malaise
  - Regional lymphadenopathy
  - Pain
  - Mouth odor

DIFFERENTIAL DIAGNOSIS

- Periodontitis (deeper inflammation, causing destruction to connective tissue, ligaments, and alveolar bone)
- Glossitis
- Desquamative gingivitis (painful, persistent, usually middle-aged women)
- Pericoronitis (gum flap traps food and plaque over partially erupted third molar), common in adolescence
- Gingival ulcers (aphthous, herpetic, malignancy, TB, syphilis)
- Specific forms of gingivitis: See "Description," including acute necrotizing ulcerative gingivitis (Vincent disease) and HIV gingivitis (linear gingival erythema).

DIAGNOSTIC TESTS & INTERPRETATION

Initial Tests (lab, imaging)

- No tests usually needed
- Possible smear or culture to identify causative agent (HIV gingivitis includes gram-negative anaerobes, enteric strains, and *Candida*)
- Labs for contributing conditions (HIV, pregnancy, diabetes, nutritional deficiencies)

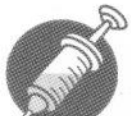

TREATMENT

GENERAL MEASURES

- Stop any contributing medications.
- Remove irritating factors (plaque, calculus, faulty dental restorations, or partial dentures).
- Good oral hygiene (see "General Prevention")
- Regular dental checkups (for scaling and polishing if plaque and/or tartar are present)
- Smoking cessation
- Warm saline rinses BID
- Special care needs patients: use of tray-applied 10% carbamide peroxide gels (13)[C]

MEDICATION

First Line

- Chlorhexidine rinses or varnishes may be used (14)[B].
- Mouth rinses with essential oils (EOMW) may be equally effective to chlorhexidine for reduction of gingival inflammation (while EOMW is not as effective for plaque control) (15)[A].
- Both chlorhexidine and EOMW rinses are as clinically effective as oral prophylaxis and oral hygiene instruction at 6-month recall (16)[B].

- Antibiotics indicated only for acute necrotizing ulcerative gingivitis (Vincent disease)
- Antibiotics
  - Penicillin V: pediatric dose, 25–50 mg/kg/day divided q6h; adult dose, 250–500 mg q6h, *OR*
  - Metronidazole: pediatric dose, 30 mg/kg/day PO/IV divided q6h; maximum 4 g/day; adult dose, 500 mg BID or TID for 10 days *OR*
  - Amoxicillin/clavulanic acid: pediatric dose, 30 mg/kg/day PO divided q12h; info: use 125 mg/31.25 mg/5 mL susp; adult dose, 875 mg/125 mg PO BID for 10 days
  - Erythromycin: pediatric dose 30–40 mg/kg/day divided q6h; adult dose, 250 mg q6h
  - Doxycycline: adult dose, 100 mg BID 1st day, then QD × 10 days
- Topical corticosteroids
  - Triamcinolone 0.1% in Orabase (spray or ointment), applied locally TID, QID
    - Contraindications
      - Allergy to specific medication
- Precautions
  - Erythromycin frequently causes GI issues.

Second Line

- Acetaminophen or ibuprofen for any pain (rare)
- Other antibiotics or antifungal rinses or systemics according to culture or smear
- Decapinol oral rinse (surfactant that acts as a physical barrier, making it harder for bacteria to stick to tooth and mucosal surfaces) to reduce bacteria (not recommended for pregnant women or children <12 years); should be used in conjunction with other oral hygiene practices when those practices alone are not enough

ISSUES FOR REFERRAL

- Dental referral for cleanings and further treatment, as needed
- If gingivitis becomes periodontitis, deep root scaling, planning, and antibiotics may be indicated.

SURGERY/OTHER PROCEDURES

- Debridement for acute necrotizing gingivitis
- Minor surgery may be necessary to correct tissue overgrowth for gingivitis caused by medicines.

COMPLEMENTARY & ALTERNATIVE MEDICINE

- Bilberry: potentially helpful in reducing inflammation and stabilizing collagen tissue
- Coenzyme Q10: topically, to restore coenzyme Q10 deficiency
- Replace any other deficiencies (e.g., vitamin C).

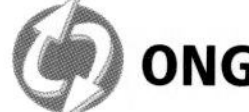

ONGOING CARE

FOLLOW-UP RECOMMENDATIONS

- Outpatient
- No restrictions

Patient Monitoring

Until clear; dental follow-up for continued cleanings and secondary prevention

DIET

- Well-balanced diet that includes fruits, vegetables, vitamin C; avoid sugary snacks and drinks, which contribute to plaque formation
- Soft foods during flare, if significant inflammation/ bleeding

PATIENT EDUCATION

- Good oral hygiene, including twice-daily brushing with circular oscillating electric brush, fluoridated toothpaste, and daily flossing; regular dental visits
- Printable and viewable patient information available under "gum diseases" from the American Dental Association at http://www.mouthhealthy.org and the American Academy of Periodontology under "patient resources" at http://www.perio.org.

PROGNOSIS

- Usual course: acute, relapsing, intermittent; chronic
- Prognosis: generally favorable, responds well to appropriate treatment
- Left untreated, may progress to periodontitis (controversial), which is a major cause of tooth loss

COMPLICATIONS

Severe periodontal disease (which is associated with heart disease, diabetes, and preterm birth)

REFERENCES

1. Terezakis E, Needleman I, Kumar N, et al. The impact of hospitalization on oral health: a systematic review. *J Clin Periodontol*. 2011;38(7):628–636.
2. Mehta A, Sequeira PS, Sahoo RC, et al. Is bronchial asthma a risk factor for gingival diseases? A control study. *N Y State Dent J*. 2009;75(1):44–46.
3. Widmer RP. Oral health of children with respiratory diseases. *Paediatr Respir Rev*. 2010;11(4):226–232.
4. Nilsson M, Kopp S. Gingivitis and periodontitis are related to repeated high levels of circulating tumor necrosis factor-alpha in patients with rheumatoid arthritis. *J Periodontol*. 2008;79(9):1689–1696.
5. Robinson PG, Deacon SA, Deery C, et al. Manual versus powered toothbrushing for oral health. *Cochrane Database Syst Rev*. 2005;(2):CD002281.
6. Klukowska M, Grender JM, Conde E, et al. A 12-week clinical comparison of an oscillating-rotating power brush versus a marketed sonic brush with self-adjusting technology in reducing plaque and gingivitis. *J Clin Dent*. 2013;24(2): 55–61.
7. Sambunjak D, Nickerson JW, Poklepovic T, et al. Flossing for the management of periodontal diseases and dental caries in adults. *Cochrane Database Syst Rev*. 2011;(12):CD008829.
8. Van Strydonck DA, Slot DE, Van der Velden U, et al. Effect of a chlorhexidine mouthrinse on plaque, gingival inflammation and staining in gingivitis patients: a systematic review. *J Clin Periodontol*. 2012;39(11):1042–1055.
9. Babu JP, Garcia-Godoy F. In vitro comparison of commercial oral rinses on bacterial adhesion and their detachment from biofilm formed on hydroxyapatite disks. *Oral Health Prev Dent*. 2014;12(4):365–371.
10. Eliot MN, Michaud DS, Langevin SM, et al. Periodontal disease and mouthwash use are risk factors for head and neck squamous cell carcinoma. *Cancer Causes Control*. 2013;24(7):1315–1322.
11. Stoeken JE, Paraskevas S, van der Weijden GA. The long-term effect of a mouthrinse containing essential oils on dental plaque and gingivitis: a systematic review. *J Periodontol*. 2007;78(7):1218–1228.
12. McCullough M, Farah CS. The role of alcohol in oral carcinogenesis with particular reference to alcohol-containing mouthwashes. *Aust Dent J*. 2008;53(4):302–305.
13. Lazarchik DA, Haywood VB. Use of tray-applied 10 percent carbamide peroxide gels for improving oral health in patients with special-care needs. *J Am Dent Assoc*. 2010;141(6):639–646.
14. Puig-Silla M, Montiel-Company JM, Almerich Silla JM. Use of chlorhexidine varnishes in preventing and treating periodontal disease. A review of the literature. *Med Oral Patol Oral Cir Bucal*. 2008;13(4):E257–E260.
15. Van Leeuwen MP, Slot DE, Van der Weijden GA. Essential oils compared to chlorhexidine with respect to plaque and parameters of gingival inflammation: a systematic review. *J Periodontol*. 2011;82(2):174–194.
16. Osso D, Kanani N. Antiseptic mouth rinses: an update on comparative effectiveness, risks and recommendations. *J Dent Hyg*. 2013;87(1): 10–18.

ADDITIONAL READING

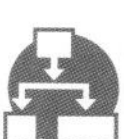

SEE ALSO

- Dental Infection; Glossitis
- Algorithm: Bleeding Gums

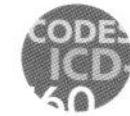

CODES

ICD10

- K05.10 Chronic gingivitis, plaque induced
- K05.11 Chronic gingivitis, non-plaque induced
- K05.00 Acute gingivitis, plaque induced

CLINICAL PEARLS

- Gingivitis may be prevented and treated with regular dental cleanings, good oral hygiene, and use of certain mouth rinses including chlorhexidine.
- Untreated, gingivitis may progress to periodontitis, a possible contributor to systemic inflammation and its consequences (e.g., coronary artery disease and uncontrolled diabetes).
- New-onset or difficult-to-treat gingivitis, consider differential of etiology: pregnancy, HIV, diabetes, medications, and vitamin deficiencies.

G

GLAUCOMA, PRIMARY CLOSED-ANGLE

Ryan B. Feeney, PharmD • Michael C. Barros, PharmD, BCPS, BCACP • Paul N. Williams, MD

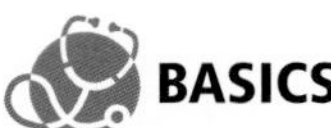

BASICS

DESCRIPTION

- Acute-angle closure (the term *glaucoma* is added when glaucomatous optic neuropathy is present)
  - At least 2 of the following symptoms: ocular pain, nausea/vomiting, intermittent blurred vision with halos, *plus*
  - At least 3 of the following signs: intraocular pressure (IOP) >21 mm Hg, conjunctival injection, corneal epithelial edema, mid-dilated nonreactive pupil, shallower chamber in the presence of occlusion
- Primary-angle closure (the term *glaucoma* is added when glaucomatous optic neuropathy is present)
  - Occludable drainage angle *plus* signs that the peripheral iris has obstructed the trabecular meshwork (e.g., elevated IOP, lens opacities)
- Chronic angle-closure glaucoma: refers to an eye with permanent closure of areas of the anterior chamber angle by peripheral anterior synechiae

Geriatric Considerations

Increased risk with age and prior history of cataract, hyperopia, and/or uveitis

Pregnancy Considerations

Medications used may cross the placenta and be excreted into breast milk.

EPIDEMIOLOGY

- Leading cause of blindness is glaucoma of this type.
- Age >40 years
- Female > male
- Inuit and Asian > African and European
- Most common form of glaucoma worldwide but only 10% of glaucoma in the United States

Prevalence

Acute-angle closure glaucoma occurs in 1 in 1,000 Caucasians; 1 in 100 Asians; and 2–4 in 100 Eskimos (lifetime).

ETIOLOGY AND PATHOPHYSIOLOGY

- Peripheral iris apposition to the trabecular meshwork obstructs the outflow of aqueous humor through the trabecular meshwork, which causes elevation in IOP.
- The underlying mechanism is anterior lens displacement or other anatomic abnormality, leading to pupillary block in which aqueous humor egress through the pupil is limited. This causes pressure to build posterior to the iris, leading to anterior iris displacement.
- Predisposing ocular anatomy

Genetics

Polygenic inheritance: 1st-degree relatives have a 2–5% lifetime risk.

RISK FACTORS

- Hyperopia
- Age >40 years
- Shallow anterior chamber
- Female gender
- Family history of angle closure
- Asian or Inuit descent
- Pseudoexfoliation
- Short axial length
- Thick crystalline lens
- Medications that may induce angle-closure glaucoma:
  - Angiotensin-converting enzyme (ACE) inhibitors (rare), adrenergic agonists (albuterol), anticholinergics, antihistamines, antidepressants including selective serotonin reuptake inhibitors (SSRIs) and tricyclic antidepressants (TCAs), cholinergic agents (pilocarpine), noncatecholamine adrenergic agonists, sulfa-based drugs, topiramate, warfarin (rare)

GENERAL PREVENTION

- Routine eye exam with gonioscopy for high-risk populations
- U.S. Preventive Services Task Force: insufficient evidence to recommend for or against screening adults for glaucoma

COMMONLY ASSOCIATED CONDITIONS

- Cataract
- Hyperopia
- Microphthalmos
- Systemic hypertension

DIAGNOSIS

HISTORY

- Patient's previous medical and ophthalmologic history
- Family history of glaucoma
- Obtain history of prescription, over-the-counter, and herbal medications
- Precipitating factors (dim light, medicines)
- Review of symptoms
- Acute
  - Severe unilateral ocular pain
  - Blurred vision
  - Lacrimation
  - Photophobia
  - Halos around lights/objects
  - Frontal, ipsilateral, headache
  - Nausea and vomiting
- Chronic
  - May have subacute symptoms (intermittent subacute attacks)
  - Compromised peripheral, then central vision
  - Usually asymptomatic until advanced vision loss has occurred

PHYSICAL EXAM

- Includes, but is not limited to, the following in the undilated eye (1)[C]
  - Visual acuity
  - Visual field testing and ocular motility
  - Pupil size and reactivity (mid-dilated, minimally reactive)
  - External examination
  - Undilated fundus exam (congestion, cupping, atrophy of optic nerve)
  - Slit-lamp biomicroscopy (anterior segments)
  - Tonometry (determination of IOP)
  - Gonioscopy (visualization of the angle)
- Acute
  - Elevated IOP (40–80 mm Hg)
  - Corneal microcystic edema (haze)
  - Lid edema, conjunctival hyperemia, and circumcorneal injection (ciliary flush)
  - Fixed mid-dilated pupil (often oval) and firm globe
  - Shallow anterior chamber, often with inflammatory reaction (cell and flare)
  - Blepharospasm (severe cases)
  - Pain with eye movement
  - Closed angle by gonioscopy
- Chronic
  - Multiple peripheral anterior synechiae
  - Normal or elevated IOP
  - Increased cup-to-disc ratio or excavation of disc
  - Glaucoma flecks (lens) and iris atrophy (previous acute attacks)

DIFFERENTIAL DIAGNOSIS

- Acute orbital compartment syndrome
- Traumatic hyphema
- Conjunctivitis, episcleritis
- Corneal abrasion
- Glaucoma, malignant or neovascular
- Herpes zoster ophthalmicus
- Iritis and uveitis
- Orbital/periorbital infection
- Plateau iris syndrome
- Vitreous or subconjunctival hemorrhage
- Tight necktie, causing increased IOP
- Lens-induced angle closure

DIAGNOSTIC TESTS & INTERPRETATION

Initial Tests (lab, imaging)

Ultrasound (US) biomicroscopy

Diagnostic Procedures/Other

Careful ophthalmic examination, including gonioscopy and tonometry (1–3)[C]

Test Interpretation

- Corneal stromal and epithelial edema
- Endothelial cell loss (guttata)
- Iris stromal necrosis
- Anterior subcapsular cataract (*glaukomflecken*)
- Optic disc congestion, cupping, excavation
- Optic nerve atrophy

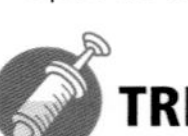

TREATMENT

Goals of treatment:

- Reverse or prevent angle-closure process
- Control IOP
- Prevent damage to the optic nerve

GENERAL MEASURES

- For acute form:
  - Manage nausea and pain
  - Immediate ophthalmology consultation
- Ocular goals of therapy through medical and surgical treatment:
  - Reduce IOP to <35 mm Hg or by >25% of presenting IOP (4)[B]

MEDICATION

- Acute angle-closure glaucoma is managed with PO glycerin (50%) for a rapid decrease in IOP; after the cornea clears, a peripheral iridotomy is done.
- Initiate medical therapy first, using some or all of the following (1)[C],(4)[B]:
  - Systemic carbonic anhydrase inhibitors (CAIs):
    - Acetazolamide (Diamox): 500 mg IV/PO; may repeat with 250 mg in 2–4 hours to a maximum of 1 g/day:
      - When used acutely, give with a topical β-blocker and topical steroid, such as prednisolone (Predsol) 0.5% solution, followed by further topical therapy to achieve IOP goals.
      - Methazolamide (Neptazane): 50–100 mg PO 2–3 BID to TID

- Topical CAIs:
  - Dorzolamide (Trusopt) 2% eyedrops: 1 drop in affected eye(s) TID
  - Brinzolamide (Azopt) 1% suspension: 1 drop in affected eye(s) TID:
    - Contraindications/precautions: sulfa allergy (risk of cross-sensitivity)
- β-Blockers:
  (requires weeks to stabilize IOP)
  - Timolol (Timoptic) 0.25–0.5% solution: 1 drop in affected eye(s) BID
  - Timolol (Istalol) 0.5% solution: 1 drop daily in the morning
  - Timolol (Timolol GFS, Timoptic-XE) 0.25–0.5% gel-forming solution: 1 drop daily
  - Levobunolol (Betagan) 0.25–0.5% solution: 1 drop in affected eye(s) 1–2 times daily
  - Betaxolol (Betoptic) 0.5% solution: 1–2 drops in affected eye(s) BID
  - Carteolol 1% solution: 1 drop in affected eye(s) BID
  - Metipranolol (OptiPranolol) 0.3% solution: 1 drop in affected eye(s) BID:
    - Contraindications/precautions: decompensated heart failure, sinus bradycardia, heart block, severe COPD/asthma; increased risk of bradycardia or heart block with digoxin, verapamil, diltiazem, or clonidine; effect on IOP may be lessened in patients taking oral β-blockers
- α_2-Agonists: (used as adjunct therapy)
  - Apraclonidine (Iopidine) 0.5% solution: 1–2 drops in affected eye(s) TID
  - Brimonidine (Alphagan P) 0.1–0.2% solution: 1 drop in affected eye(s) TID:
    - Contraindications/precautions: MAO inhibitor therapy, CNS depression
- Prostaglandin analogs: (↑ dose or frequency may ↓ effect)
  - Latanoprost (Xalatan) 0.005% solution, travoprost (Travatan Z) 0.004% solution, bimatoprost (Lumigan) 0.01% solution, tafluprost (Zioptan) 0.0015% solution: 1 drop in affected eye(s) nightly:
    - Precautions: irreversible changes to iris, eyelid and eyelash pigmentation, eyelash growth, itching, redness, edema
      - Bimatoprost (Latisse) 0.03% topical solution: indicated for hypotrichosis of the eyelashes
- Direct cholinergic agonists:
  - Pilocarpine (IsoptoCarpine) (1%, 2%, 4% solution): 1–2 drops up to 6 times daily; per ophthalmologist
  - Carbachol (IsoptoCarbachol) 3% solution: 1–2 drops up to TID
- Cholinesterase inhibitor:
  - Echothiophate iodide (Phospholine Iodide) 0.125% solution: 1 drop BID:
    - Precautions: may worsen the condition due to anterior rotation of the lens–iris diaphragm, impaired night vision
- Combination products:
  - Timolol-Dorzolamide (Cosopt) 0.5/2% solution: 1 drop in affected eye(s) BID
  - Timolol-Brimonidine (Combigan) 0.5/0.2% solution: 1 drop in affected eye(s) BID
  - Brinzolamide-Brimonidine (Simbrinza**)** 1/0.2% solution: 1 drop in affected eye(s) TID
- Miscellaneous product:
  - Unoprostone (Rescula) 0.15% solution: 1 drop in affected eye(s) BID
    - Mechanism unknown: may effect big potassium (BK) and ClC-2 chloride channels

ADDITIONAL THERAPIES

Keep patient supine.

SURGERY/OTHER PROCEDURES

- Acute (1,5)[B]
  - Laser peripheral iridotomy per ophthalmology (1,5)[B]
  - Perform surgical iridectomy if laser is not possible.
- Chronic
  - Goniosynechialysis
  - Phacoemulsification

INPATIENT CONSIDERATIONS

Admission Criteria/Initial Stabilization

- Patient requires metabolic ± electrolyte and volume status monitoring (with osmotic agents).
- Maintain ophthalmology follow-up.

ONGOING CARE

FOLLOW-UP RECOMMENDATIONS

Schedule an immediate ophthalmologic follow-up.

Patient Monitoring

- Postsurgical follow-up
- Fellow eye evaluation
- Chronic monitoring post–acute attack per ophthalmology

PATIENT EDUCATION

- Advise patient to seek emergency medical attention if experiencing a change in visual acuity, blurred vision, eye pain, or headache.
- If narrow angles but no peripheral iridotomy performed: Avoid decongestants, motion sickness medications, adrenergic agents, antipsychotics, antidepressants, and anticholinergic agents.
- Correct eyedrop administration technique, including the following:
  - Remove contact lenses before administration and wait 15 minutes before reinserting.
  - Allow at least 5 minutes between administration of multiple ophthalmic products.
- Patients with significant visual impairment should be referred to vision rehab and social services.
- Patient education materials:
  - Glaucoma Research Foundation: http://www.glaucoma.org
  - National Eye Institute: http://www.nei.nih.gov
  - Glaucoma handout from American Academy of Family Physicians
  - Handout on using glaucoma eyedrops in *Am Fam Physician* 1999;59(7):1882

PROGNOSIS

- With timely treatment, most patients do not have permanent vision loss.
- Prognosis depends on ethnicity, underlying eye disease, and time-to-treatment.

COMPLICATIONS

- Chronic corneal edema
- Corneal fibrosis and vascularization
- Iris atrophy
- Cataract
- Optic atrophy
- Malignant glaucoma
- Central retinal artery/vein occlusion
- Permanent decrease in visual acuity
- Repeat episode
- Fellow eye attack

REFERENCES

1. American Academy of Ophthalmology. *Primary Angle Closure Preferred Practice Pattern*. San Francisco, CA: American Academy of Ophthalmology; 2010. http://www.aao.org. Accessed 2014.
2. Asrani S, Sarunic M, Santiago C, et al. Detailed visualization of the anterior segment using Fourier-domain optical coherence tomography. *Arch Ophthalmol*. 2008;126(6):765–771.
3. Barkana Y, Dorairaj SK, Gerber Y, et al. Agreement between gonioscopy and ultrasound biomicroscopy in detecting iridotrabecular apposition. *Arch Ophthalmol*. 2007;125(10):1331–1335.
4. Choong YF, Irfan S, Menage MJ. Acute angle closure glaucoma: an evaluation of a protocol for acute treatment. *Eye*. 1999;13(Pt 5):613–616.
5. Saw SM, Gazzard G, Friedman DS. Interventions for angle-closure glaucoma: an evidence-based update. *Ophthalmology*. 2003;110(10):1869–1878; quiz 1878–1879, 1930.

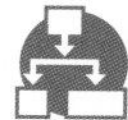

SEE ALSO

Glaucoma, Primary Open-Angle

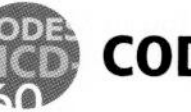

CODES

ICD10

- H40.20X0 Unsp primary angle-closure glaucoma, stage unspecified
- H40.219 Acute angle-closure glaucoma, unspecified eye
- H40.2290 Chronic angle-closure glaucoma, unsp eye, stage unspecified

CLINICAL PEARLS

- Examiner can determine if patient is hyperopic by observing the magnification of the patient's face through his or her glasses (myopic lenses minify).
- A careful history may reveal similar episodes of angle closure that resolved spontaneously.
- Miotics are ineffective in the setting of high IOP (due to iris sphincter ischemia) and potentially can worsen angle closure by causing anterior rotation of the lens–iris diaphragm.
- Latanoprost, a prostaglandin analog, has recently become available generically. This agent has shown greater reductions in IOP compared to β-blockers and CAIs. Although all of these agents can still be used as 1st-line treatment, an increase in the use of prostaglandin analogs may be seen in the future as other agents in this class become generically available and the cost of their therapy becomes comparable with these other agents. Generic latanoprosta availability provides the option of once-daily medication administration, helping to improve patient adherence.

GLAUCOMA, PRIMARY OPEN-ANGLE

Richard W. Allinson, MD

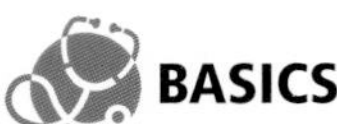

BASICS

DESCRIPTION

- Primary open-angle glaucoma (POAG) is an optic neuropathy resulting in visual field loss frequently associated with increased intraocular pressure (IOP).
- Normal IOP is 10–22 mm Hg. However, glaucomatous optic nerve damage also can occur with normal IOP and as a secondary manifestation of other disorders such as corticosteroid-induced glaucoma.
- System(s) affected: nervous
- Synonym(s): chronic open-angle glaucoma

Pregnancy Considerations

Prostaglandins should be avoided during pregnancy in the treatment of POAG.

EPIDEMIOLOGY

Incidence

- Predominant age: usually >40 years
- Increases with age
- Predominant gender: male = female

Prevalence

Prevalence in persons >40 years of age is ~1.8%.

Geriatric Considerations

Increasing prevalence with increasing age

ETIOLOGY AND PATHOPHYSIOLOGY

- Abnormal aqueous outflow resulting in increased IOP
- Normally, aqueous is produced by the ciliary epithelium of the ciliary body and is secreted into the posterior chamber of the eye.
- Aqueous then flows through the pupil and enters the anterior chamber to be drained by the trabecular meshwork in the iridocorneal angle of the eye into the Schlemm canal and into the venous system of the episclera.
- 5–10% of the total aqueous outflow leaves via the uveoscleral pathway.
- Impaired aqueous outflow through the trabecular meshwork
  - Increased resistance within the aqueous drainage system

Genetics

A family history of glaucoma increases the risk for developing glaucoma.

RISK FACTORS

- Increased IOP
- Myopia
- Diabetes mellitus (DM)
- African American
- Elderly
- Hypothyroidism
- Positive family history
- Central corneal thickness <550 μm
- Larger vertical cup-to-disc ratio (CDR)
- Larger horizontal CDR
- CDR asymmetry
- Disc hemorrhage
- Prolonged use of topical, periocular, inhaled, or systemic corticosteroids
- Obstructive sleep apnea
- Hypertension (1)[B]
- Corneal hysteresis (CH) (2)[B]
  - A measure of the viscoelastic damping of the cornea
  - Lower CH associated with faster rates of visual field loss

GENERAL PREVENTION

Possible reduced risk of open-angle glaucoma with long-term use of oral statins among persons with hyperlipidemia

COMMONLY ASSOCIATED CONDITIONS

DM

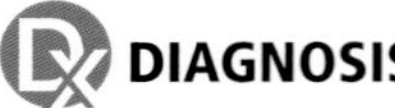

DIAGNOSIS

HISTORY

Painless, slowly progressive visual loss; patients are generally unaware of the visual loss until late in the disease. Central visual acuity remains unaffected until late in the disease.

PHYSICAL EXAM

- Visual acuity and visual field assessment
- Ophthalmoscopy to assess optic nerve for glaucomatous damage
- Increased IOP
- CDR >0.5: Normal eyes show a characteristic configuration for disc rim thickness of inferior ≥superior ≥nasal ≥temporal (ISNT rule).
- Earliest visual field defects are paracentral scotomas and peripheral nasal steps.

DIFFERENTIAL DIAGNOSIS

- Normal-tension glaucoma
- Optic nerve pits
- Anterior ischemic optic neuropathy
- Compressive lesions of the optic nerve or chiasm
- Posthemorrhagic (shock optic neuropathy)

DIAGNOSTIC TESTS & INTERPRETATION

Initial Tests (lab, imaging)

Optical coherence tomography can be useful in the detection of glaucoma by measuring the thickness of the retinal nerve fiber layer (RNFL).

- RNFL is thinner in patients with glaucoma.
- RNFL tends to be thinner with older age, in Caucasians, greater axial length, and smaller optic disc area.

Diagnostic Procedures/Other

- Visual field testing: perimetry
  - A multifocal intraocular lens may reduce visual sensitivity on standard automated perimetry.
- Tonometry to measure IOP

Test Interpretation

- Atrophy and cupping of optic nerve
- Loss of retinal ganglion cells and their axons produces defects in the RNFL.

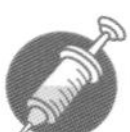

TREATMENT

GENERAL MEASURES

- Early Manifest Glaucoma Trial
  - Early treatment delays progression.
  - The magnitude of initial IOP reduction influences disease progression (3)[A].
- Ocular Hypertension Treatment Study
  - Patients who only had increased IOP in the range of 24–32 mm Hg were treated with topical ocular hypotensive medication.
  - Treatment produced ~20% reduction in IOP.
  - At 5 years, treatment reduced the incidence of POAG by >50%: 9.5% in the observation group versus 4.4% in the medication-treated group (4)[A].
- The Advanced Glaucoma Intervention Study
  - Eyes were randomized to laser trabeculoplasty or filtering surgery when medical therapy failed.
  - In follow-up, if IOP was always <18 mm Hg, visual fields tended to stabilize. When IOP was >17 mm Hg, more than 1/2 the time, patients tended to have worsening of visual fields (5)[A].
  - Whites did better with trabeculectomy first, whereas African Americans did better with argon laser trabeculoplasty as the initial procedure.
- Collaborative Initial Glaucoma Treatment Study
  - Both initial medical and surgical (trabeculectomy) treatment achieved significant IOP reduction, and both had little visual field loss over time (6)[A].
  - There was a 5-year risk of endophthalmitis of 1.1% after trabeculectomy (7)[A].

MEDICATION

- >1 medication, with different mechanisms of action, may be needed.
- When ≥3 medications are required, compliance is difficult, and surgery may be needed. Ocular hypotensive agent categories
  - β-adrenergic antagonists (nonselective and selective): decrease aqueous formation; best when used as add-on therapy: timolol 0.25% (initial) −0.5% 1 drop in affected eye q12h; gel-forming solution (0.35% or 0.5%) 1 drop affected eye once daily; betaxolol 0.5% 1 drop affected eye twice daily
  - Parasympathomimetics (miotic), including cholinergic (direct-acting) and anticholinesterase agents (indirect-acting parasympathomimetic): increase aqueous outflow
    - Pilocarpine 1–4%: 1 drop in affected eye BID–QID (cholinergic)
- Carbonic anhydrase inhibitors (oral, topical): decrease aqueous formation
  - Acetazolamide: 250 mg PO 1–4 times per day
  - Dorzolamide 2%: 1 drop TID
  - Brinzolamide 1%: 1 drop TID
- Adrenergic agonists (nonselective and selective α_2-adrenergic agonists)
  - Epinephrine 0.5–2%: 1 drop BID and Propine (dipivefrin) 0.1% 1 drop BID are both nonselective agents that increase aqueous outflow through the trabecular meshwork and increase uveoscleral outflow.
  - Brimonidine tartrate 0.1%: 1 drop TID (α_2-adrenergic agonist) decreases aqueous formation and increases uveoscleral outflow.
- Prostaglandin analogues: enhance uveoscleral outflow and increase aqueous outflow through the trabecular meshwork: latanoprost 0.005% 1 drop at bedtime; travoprost 0.004% 1 drop at bedtime
- Hyperosmotic agents: increase blood osmolality, drawing water from the vitreous cavity
  - Mannitol 20% solution: administered IV at 2 g/kg of body weight
  - Glycerin 50% solution: administered PO; dosage is usually 4–7 oz.
- Contraindications/precautions
  - Nonselective β-adrenergic antagonists: Avoid in asthma, chronic obstructive pulmonary disease (COPD), 2nd- and 3rd-degree atrioventricular (A-V) block, and decompensated heart failure. Betaxolol is a selective β-adrenergic antagonist and is safer in pulmonary disease.

- Parasympathomimetics (miotic): Indirect-acting parasympathomimetic agents increase risk of ocular and systemic side effects and are used rarely.
- Carbonic anhydrase inhibitors
  - Do not use with sulfa drug allergies.
  - Do not use with cirrhosis because of the risk of hepatic encephalopathy.
- Adrenergic agonists: Caution recommended when using brimonidine and monoamine oxidase (MAO) inhibitor or tricyclic antidepressant (TCA) and in patients with vascular insufficiency. Brimonidine can cause excessive sleepiness and lethargy in children.
- Prostaglandin analogues: caution with uveitis and avoided during pregnancy
- Hyperosmotic agents
  - Glycerin can produce hyperglycemia or ketoacidosis in diabetic patients.
  - Can cause congestive heart failure
  - Do not use in patients with anuria.
- Precautions
  - β-adrenergic antagonists: caution with obstructive pulmonary disease, heart failure, and DM
  - Parasympathomimetics (miotic): cause pupillary constriction and may cause decreased vision in patients with a cataract; may cause eye pain or myopia due to increased accommodation. All miotics break down the blood–aqueous barrier and may induce chronic iridocyclitis.
  - Adrenergic agonists (e.g., brimonidine): caution with vascular insufficiency
  - Contact lens wearers: Many products contain benzalkonium chloride; remove contact lens prior to administration and wait 15 minutes before reinsertion.
  - Prostaglandin analogues may cause increased pigmentation of the iris and periorbital tissue (eyelid).
    - Increased pigmentation and growth of eyelashes
    - Should be used with caution in active intraocular inflammation (iritis/uveitis)
    - Caution is also advised in eyes with risk factors for herpes simplex, iritis, and cystoid macular edema.
    - Macular edema may be a complication associated with treatment.
- Hyperosmotic agents: caution in diabetics; dehydrated patients; and those with cardiac, renal, and hepatic disease
- Significant possible interactions: β-adrenergic antagonists: caution in patients taking calcium antagonists because of possible A-V conduction disturbances, left ventricular failure, or hypotension
- Parasympathomimetics (miotic): Indirect-acting parasympathomimetic agents, anticholinesterase eye drops, can reduce serum pseudocholinesterase levels. If succinylcholine is used for induction of general anesthesia, prolonged apnea may result.

SURGERY/OTHER PROCEDURES

- Argon laser trabeculoplasty (ALT)
  - Can be applied up to 180 degrees of the trabecular meshwork
  - Improves aqueous outflow
  - The Glaucoma Laser Trial Research Group showed in newly diagnosed, previously untreated patients with POAG that ALT was as effective as topical glaucoma medication within the first 2 years of follow-up.
  - Usually reserved for patients needing better IOP control while taking topical glaucoma drops
- Selective laser trabeculoplasty (SLT)
  - 532-nm Nd:YAG laser
  - Appears to be as effective as ALT in lowering IOP
- Trabeculectomy (glaucoma filtering surgery)
  - Usually reserved for patients needing better IOP control after maximal medical therapy and who may have previously undergone an ALT
  - Mitomycin C can be applied at the time of surgery to increase the chances of a surgical success.
  - Subconjunctival bevacizumab may be a beneficial adjunctive therapy for reducing late surgical failure after trabeculectomy.
- Shunt (tube) surgery
  - For example, Molteno and Ahmed devices
  - Generally reserved for difficult glaucoma cases in which conventional filtering surgery has failed or is likely to fail
- Tube Versus Trabeculectomy (TVT) Study
  - After 5 years of follow-up, both procedures were associated with similar IOP reduction and the number of glaucoma medications needed (8)[A].
- Ciliary body ablation: indicated to lower IOP in patients with poor visual potential or those who are poor candidates for filtering or shunt procedures
- Canaloplasty can control IOP in patients with POAG. Canaloplasty involves the placement of a microcatheter circumferentially through Schlemm canal, viscodilation of the canal, and placement of a nylon tensioning suture.
- Cataract extraction can decrease IOP in patients with ocular hypertension (9)[A].

ONGOING CARE

FOLLOW-UP RECOMMENDATIONS

Patient Monitoring

- Monitor vision and IOP every 3–6 months.
- Visual field testing every 6–18 months
- Optic nerve evaluation every 3–18 months, depending on POAG control
- A worsening of the mean deviation by 2 dB on the Humphrey field analyzer and confirmed by a single test after 6 months had a 72% probability of progression.
- The IOP response to ocular hypotensive agents tends to be reduced in persons with thicker corneas.

PATIENT EDUCATION

POAG is a silent robber of vision, and patients may not appreciate the significance of their disease until much of their visual field is lost.

PROGNOSIS

- With standard glaucoma therapy, the rate of visual field loss in POAG is slow.
- Patients still may lose vision and develop blindness, even when treated appropriately.
- The rate of legal blindness from POAG over a follow-up of 22 years is 19%.
- The rate of progression of visual field loss increases with older age.

COMPLICATIONS

Blindness

REFERENCES

1. Zhao D, Cho J, Kim MH, et al. The association of blood pressure and primary open-angle glaucoma: a meta-analysis. *Am J Ophthalmol*. 2014;158(3):615–627.
2. Medeiros FA, Meira-Freitas D, Lisboa R, et al. Corneal hysteresis as a risk factor for glaucoma progression: a prospective longitudinal study. *Ophthalmology*. 2013;120(8):1533–1540.
3. Heijl A, Leske MC, Bengtsson B, et al; Early Manifest Glaucoma Trial Group. Reduction of intraocular pressure and glaucoma progression: results from the Early Manifest Glaucoma Trial. *Arch Ophthalmol*. 2002;120(10):1268–1279.
4. Kass MA, Heuer DK, Higginbotham EJ, et al. The Ocular Hypertension Treatment Study: a randomized trial determines that topical ocular hypotensive medication delays or prevents the onset of primary open-angle glaucoma. *Arch Ophthalmol*. 2002;120(6):701–713; discussion 829–830.
5. The Advanced Glaucoma Intervention Study (AGIS): 7. The relationship between control of intraocular pressure and visual field deterioration. The AGIS investigators. *Am J Ophthalmol*. 2000;130(4):429–440.
6. Lichter PR, Musch DC, Gillespie BW; CIGTS Study Group. Interim clinical outcomes in the Collaborative Initial Glaucoma Treatment Study comparing initial treatment randomized to medications or surgery. *Ophthalmology*. 2001;108(11):1943–1953.
7. Zahid S, Musch DC, Nizol LM, et al. Risk of endophthalmitis and other long-term complications of trabeculectomy in the Collaborative Initial Glaucoma Treatment Study (CIGTS). *Am J Ophthalmol*. 2013;155(4):674–680.
8. Gedde SJ, Schiffman JC, Feuer WJ, et al. Treatment outcomes in the Tube Versus Trabeculectomy (TVT) Study after five years of follow-up. *Am J Ophthalmol*. 2012;153(5):789–803.
9. Mansberger SL, Gordon MO, Jampel H, et al. Reduction in intraocular pressure after cataract extraction: the Ocular Hypertension Treatment Study. *Ophthalmology*. 2012;119(9):1826–1831.

ADDITIONAL READING

- Aychoua N, Junoy Montolio FG, Jansonius NM. Influence of multifocal intraocular lenses on standard automated perimetry test results. *JAMA Ophthalmol*. 2013;131(4):481–485.
- Lin CC, Hu CC, Ho JD, et al. Obstructive sleep apnea and increased risk of glaucoma: a population-based matched-cohort study. *Ophthalmology*. 2013;120(8):1559–1564.

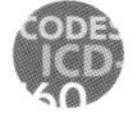

CODES

ICD10

- H40.11X0 Primary open-angle glaucoma, stage unspecified
- H40.11X1 Primary open-angle glaucoma, mild stage
- H40.11X2 Primary open-angle glaucoma, moderate stage

CLINICAL PEARLS

- Topical or systemic steroids can cause the IOP to increase.
- Pain is not a frequent symptom of POAG.
- Painless, slowly progressive visual loss; patients generally are unaware of the visual loss until late in the disease. Central visual acuity remains unaffected until late in the disease.
- Patients still may lose vision and develop blindness, even when treated appropriately.

GLOMERULONEPHRITIS, ACUTE

Jonathan T. Lin, MD • Michael J. Ross, MD

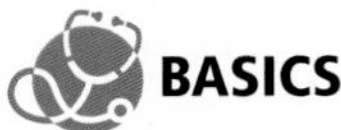

BASICS

DESCRIPTION

- Acute glomerulonephritis (GN) is an inflammatory process involving the glomerulus of the kidney, resulting in a clinical syndrome consisting of hematuria, proteinuria, and renal insufficiency, often in association with hypertension and edema.
- Acute GN may be caused by primary glomerular disease or secondary to systemic disease:
  - Postinfectious GN
  - IgA nephropathy/Henoch-Schönlein purpura (HSP)
  - Antiglomerular basement membrane disease (anti-GBM disease)
  - Antineutrophil cytoplasmic antibody (ANCA)–associated GN
  - Membranoproliferative GN (MPGN)
  - Lupus nephritis
  - Cryoglobulin-associated GN
- Clinical severity ranges from asymptomatic microscopic or gross hematuria to a rapid loss of kidney function over days to weeks, termed rapidly progressive GN (RPGN).

ALERT

Urgent investigation and treatment are required to avoid irreversible loss of kidney function.

EPIDEMIOLOGY

- Postinfectious GN
  - Most commonly follows group A β-hemolytic *Streptococcus* infection but can occur as a result of other bacterial infections or less commonly in the setting of viral or parasitic infections
  - Accounts for 80% of acute GN in children
  - May also occur in the setting of infective endocarditis
- IgA nephropathy
  - Most common form of primary acute GN
  - Occurs mainly in the 2nd and 3rd decades
  - Male > female (2:1)
  - Incidence differs geographically: Asia > United States
  - HSP typically childhood illness, usually <10 years old
- Anti-GBM disease
  - A notable cause of the pulmonary–renal syndrome known as Goodpasture disease
  - Peak distribution in 3rd and 6th decades
- ANCA-associated GN
  - Often has a relapsing and remitting course
  - Four disease presentations:
    - Granulomatosis with polyangiitis (GPA, formerly Wegener granulomatosis)
    - Microscopic polyangiitis (MPA)
    - Isolated Pauci-immune GN—when isolated to kidneys
    - Churg-Strauss disease—GN relatively common but renal involvement rarely severe
  - Older patients are more commonly affected, although this GN can affect any age group.
- MPGN
  - May be primary or secondary
  - May present in the setting of a systemic viral (hepatitis B or hepatitis C) or rheumatologic illness
  - Classification by immunofluorescence: immune complex mediated or complement mediated (dense deposit disease [DDD] and C3 glomerulonephritis [C3GN])
  - Classification by electron microscopy: MPGN types I–III
- Lupus nephritis
  - 30–70% of systemic lupus patients will have renal involvement.
- Cryoglobulin-associated vasculitis
  - 80% of cases are associated with hepatitis C infection.

ETIOLOGY AND PATHOPHYSIOLOGY

- In general, an immunologic mechanism triggers inflammation and proliferation of glomerular tissue.
- Postinfectious GN: immune complex disease with host immune reaction to nephritogenic strains of streptococci as a trigger
- IgA nephropathy: relates to an abnormal glycosylation of IgA
- Anti-GBM disease: caused by autoantibodies that target type IV collagen of basement membranes
- ANCA-associated GN: Autoantibodies against neutrophil granules are involved in the pathogenesis.
- MPGN: An immune or genetic etiology is presumed, which triggers renal deposits and inflammation.
- Lupus nephritis: an immune complex–mediated glomerular disease
- Cryoglobulin-associated GN: An immune etiology is presumed but not clearly defined.

Genetics

Genetic factors are likely to play a role in susceptibility to many of the acute GNs, although these have not been sufficiently defined to be clinically useful in most circumstances.

RISK FACTORS

- Epidemics of nephritogenic strains of streptococci are triggers for postinfectious GN.
- Hepatic cirrhosis, celiac disease, and HIV infection place patients at risk for IgA nephropathy.
- Anti-GBM disease has been associated with influenza A infection and inhaled hydrocarbon solvent exposure.
- ANCA-associated GN is increased in settings where there is increased silica exposure (i.e., earthquakes and farming).
- Infection with hepatitis B or C is known to be associated with MPGN.
- Infection with hepatitis C is a risk factor for developing cryoglobulinemic GN.
- Mutations in alternate complement pathway genes are associated with complement-mediated MPGN.

GENERAL PREVENTION

Early detection is paramount.

DIAGNOSIS

HISTORY

- Patients may report cola- or tea-colored urine and decreased urine volume.
- Edema occurs in many patients, typically face and lower extremities.
- Shortness of breath may occur with significant fluid overload.
- Generalized malaise
- Timing
  - Postinfectious GN typically occurs 1–3 weeks after pharyngitis or 2–6 weeks after skin infection.
  - IgA nephropathy may present within several days after an acute infection.
- Patients may also present with complaints more specific to the associated disease:
  - Joint pain or rash in lupus nephritis
  - Hemoptysis in anti-GBM disease
  - Sinusitis, pulmonary infiltrates, arthralgias in ANCA-associated GN
  - Abdominal or joint pain and purpura in IgA–Henoch-Schönlein purpura
  - Purpura and skin vasculitis in cryoglobulinemia-associated GN

PHYSICAL EXAM

- A complete physical exam may discover clues to systemic disease as a potential cause.
- Sinus disease: ANCA-associated GN, most commonly GPA
- Pharyngitis or impetigo: postinfectious GN or IgA nephropathy
- Pulmonary hemorrhage (pulmonary–renal syndrome): anti-GBM disease/Goodpasture, ANCA-associated GN, HSP, cryoglobulinemia, or lupus nephritis
- Hepatomegaly or liver tenderness could point to cryoglobulinemia-associated GN or IgA nephropathy.
- Purpura may point to ANCA-associated GN or HSP/IgA nephropathy.

DIFFERENTIAL DIAGNOSIS

Non-glomerular hematuria: trauma, prostate diseases, urologic cancer, or renal stone disease

DIAGNOSTIC TESTS & INTERPRETATION

Initial Tests (lab, imaging)

- Urinalysis with examination of sediment: Dysmorphic RBCs or RBC casts on urine microscopy indicate glomerular hematuria and strongly suggest the diagnosis of an acute GN. Pyuria and white blood cell casts may also be present.
- Electrolytes, BUN, creatinine, CBC
- Antistreptolysin O titer, Streptozyme: often positive in poststreptococcal GN
- Complement levels (C3, C4)
  - C3 complement levels are low in postinfectious GN.
  - C3 and C4 are abnormal in lupus nephritis and MPGN.
  - C4 can be low in cryoglobulinemia.
- Proteinuria: 24-hour collection or random urine protein/creatinine ratio
  - Typically mild to moderate proteinuria, sometimes nephrotic range
- Antinuclear antibody (ANA) to rule out lupus nephritis
- ANCA antibody screen: MPO and PR3 antibodies
- Anti-GBM antibody

- Hepatitis B surface antigen and antibody
- Hepatitis C antibody
- HIV testing
- A chest x-ray may be useful in the setting of hemoptysis or a suspected infiltrate on exam.

Test Interpretation

Renal biopsy:

- If clinical picture is consistent with postinfectious GN in a child, a biopsy may not be required.
- If there is clinical suspicion for other causes of acute GN, renal biopsy should be done.
- Light microscopy
  - Diffuse hypercellularity suggests a proliferative disease such as IgA nephropathy, lupus nephritis, or postinfectious GN.
  - Presence of crescents correlates with RPGN and disease severity.
- Immunofluorescence
  - Isolated IgA staining is pathognomonic for IgA nephropathy, with the absence of immune complex staining suggesting ANCA-associated GN.
  - Pattern of IgG, IgM, C3, and C4 staining may also aid in characterizing the GN.
  - Lupus nephritis typically positive for all immunoglobulins and complements ("full house")
- Electron microscopy: The location of immunoglobulin deposits is useful in pointing to a particular diagnosis.

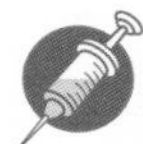

TREATMENT

Supportive in postinfectious GN

MEDICATION

First Line

- Hypertension
  - Diuretics are useful for management of salt retention and edema.
  - Calcium channel blockers
  - Avoid angiotensin-converting enzyme inhibitors (ACE-I) or angiotensin receptor blockers (ARBs) if acute renal dysfunction is present.
- Peripheral edema: Loop diuretics are often required due to the degree of edema.
- Pulmonary edema: oxygen and diuretic

Second Line

- Each of the glomerular diseases often requires a specific treatment plan based on renal biopsy results; therefore, a nephrologist is often guiding care at this point.
- Empiric pulse methylprednisolone prior to kidney biopsy may be indicated in cases of RPGN (1)[C].
- Crescents on renal biopsy may be an indication for steroids in postinfectious GN and in other cases are often an indication for potent immunosuppressive medications in addition to steroids (2)[C].
- Steroids plus either cyclophosphamide, rituximab, or mycophenolate may be used to treat ANCA-associated renal disease and proliferative forms of lupus nephritis (2–6)[A].
- Plasmapheresis may also be considered in some cases for RPGN or anti-GBM disease or ANCA-associated renal disease with diffuse pulmonary hemorrhage (2)[C],(4,7)[A].
- Dialysis may be needed for uremia, hyperkalemia refractory to medical management, intractable acidosis, and diuretic-resistant pulmonary edema.
- IgA nephropathy: ACE-Is or ARBs recommended for patients with proteinuria (1,2)[C]

ISSUES FOR REFERRAL

Consultation with a nephrologist is usually required to assist with renal biopsy to confirm diagnosis and assist with management.

INPATIENT CONSIDERATIONS

Admission Criteria/Initial Stabilization

Consider admission for patients with no urine output, rapidly deteriorating renal function, significant hypertension, and suspicion of pulmonary hemorrhage or fluid overload that is compromising heart or respiratory function.

Discharge Criteria

Hemodynamically stable patients without complications may be managed as outpatients.

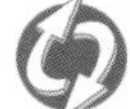

ONGOING CARE

FOLLOW-UP RECOMMENDATIONS

Patient Monitoring

Depends on type of GN:

- Regular BP checks and urinalysis to detect recurrence, assessment of renal function to detect acute or follow chronic renal disease as a result of the primary event, and regular clinical assessment to detect suspicious symptoms that may herald a recurrence (i.e., rash, joint complaint, hemoptysis)
- Periodic reassessment of serology tests to detect asymptomatic individuals

DIET

- No-added-salt diet and fluid restriction until edema and hypertension clear
- Avoid high-potassium foods if significant renal dysfunction is present.

PATIENT EDUCATION

- National Kidney Foundation, 30 E. 33rd Street, Suite 1100, New York, NY 10016; 212-889-2210
- Web site: http://vsearch.nlm.nih.gov/vivisimo/cgi-bin/query-meta?v%3Aproject=medlineplus&query=glomerulonephritis&x=48&y=10 (search under the individual disease)

PROGNOSIS

- In general, the prognosis depends on the cause of the GN.
- The GN may be self-limited (as often is the case in postinfectious GN) or part of a chronic disease that makes the possibility of recurrence of acute disease likely, with the potential for progressive loss of renal function over time.

COMPLICATIONS

- Hypertensive retinopathy and encephalopathy
- Rapidly progressive GN
- Microscopic hematuria may persist for years.
- Chronic kidney disease
- Nephrotic syndrome (~10%)

REFERENCES

1. Chadban SJ, Atkins RC. Glomerulonephritis. *Lancet*. 2005;365(9473):1797–1806.
2. Beck L, Bomback AS, Choi MJ, et al. KDOQI US commentary on the 2012 KDIGO clinical practice guideline for glomerulonephritis. *Am J Kidney Dis*. 2013;62(3):403–41. doi:10.1053/j.ajkd.2013.06.002.
3. Hahn BH, McMahon MA, Wilkinson A, et al; American College of Rheumatology. American College of Rheumatology guidelines for screening, treatment, and management of lupus nephritis. *Arthritis Care Res (Hoboken)*. 2012;64(6):797–808. doi:10.1002/acr.21664.
4. Walters G, Willis NS, Craig JC. Interventions for renal vasculitis in adults. *Cochrane Database Syst Rev*. 2008;(3):CD003232. doi:10.1002/14651858.CD003232.pub2.
5. Stone JH, Merkel PA, Spiera R, et al. Rituximab versus cyclophosphamide for ANCA-associated vasculitis. *N Engl J Med*. 2010;363(3):221–232. doi:10.1056/NEJMoa0909905.
6. Bomback AS, Appel GB. Updates on the treatment of lupus nephritis. *J Am Soc Nephrol*. 2010;21(12):2028–35. doi:10.1681/ASN.2010050472.
7. Jayne DR, Gaskin G, Rasmussen N, et al; European Vasculitis Study Group. Randomized trial of plasma exchange or high-dosage methylprednisolone as adjunctive therapy for severe renal vasculitis. *J Am Soc Nephrol*. 2007;18(7):2180–2188.

SEE ALSO

- Hyperkalemia; Hypertensive Emergencies; Renal Failure, Acute
- IgA Nephropathy
- Glomerulonephritis, Poststreptococcal
- Algorithm: Hematuria

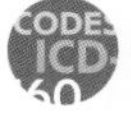

CODES

ICD10

- N00.9 Acute nephritic syndrome with unsp morphologic changes
- N00.2 Acute nephritic syndrome w diffuse membranous glomrlneph
- N00.8 Acute nephritic syndrome with other morphologic changes

CLINICAL PEARLS

- Dysmorphic RBCs and RBC casts are a key component of the urinalysis in GN.
- Postinfectious GN in children is typically a self-limited disease.
- Searching for other organ involvement is useful in establishing a definitive diagnosis.
- With discovery of a GN, monitor the initial renal function labs frequently to identify a rapidly progressive GN.

GLOMERULONEPHRITIS, POSTINFECTIOUS

Kelly H. Beers, DO • Theodore B. Flaum, DO, FACOFP

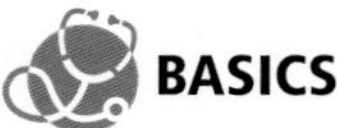

BASICS

DESCRIPTION

Postinfectious glomerulonephritis (PIGN) is an immune complex disease preceded by nonrenal infection with certain strains of bacteria, most commonly *Streptococcus* and *Staphylococcus*. The most common form of PIGN, poststreptococcal glomerulonephritis (PSGN), predominantly affects children. The clinical presentation varies from asymptomatic to the acute nephritic syndrome, characterized by gross hematuria, proteinuria, edema, hypertension (HTN), and acute kidney injury.

EPIDEMIOLOGY

A global decline in incidence, especially in developed countries, is attributed to better hygiene and a decreased incidence of streptococcal skin infections. Of cases, 97% occur in developing countries. PSGN is primarily a pediatric disease, but a recent increase has been seen in nonstreptococcal GN in adults.

Incidence

- Pediatrics: 24.3 cases/100,000 persons per year in developing countries, 6 cases/100,000 persons per year in developed countries
- Adults: 2 cases/100,000 persons/year in developing countries, 0.3 cases/100,000 persons/year in developed countries. Global burden of 68,000 cases per year.
- Globally, 34% of cases are now seen in adults.
- Male > female (2:1) (1)

ETIOLOGY AND PATHOPHYSIOLOGY

- Glomerular immune complex disease induced by specific nephritogenic strains of bacteria:
  - Group A β-hemolytic *Streptococcus* (GAS)
  - Staphylococcus (predominantly *Staphylococcus aureus*; more commonly methicillin-resistant *S. aureus* [MRSA], occasionally coagulase-negative *Staphylococcus*)
  - Gram-negative bacteria including *Escherichia coli*, *Yersinia*, *Pseudomonas*, and *Haemophilus* (1)
- Proposed mechanisms for the glomerular injury (2):
  - Deposition of circulating immune complexes with streptococcal or staphylococcal antigens—these complexes can be detected in patients with streptococcal- or staphylococcal-related GN but do not correlate to disease activity (3).
  - In situ immune complex formation from deposition of antigens within the glomerular basement membrane (GBM) and subsequent antibody binding
  - In situ glomerular immune complex formation promoted by antibodies to streptococcal or staphylococcal antigens
  - Alteration of normal renal antigen leading to molecular mimicry that elicits an autoimmune response
- Glomerular immune complex causing complement activation and inflammation:
  - Nephritis-associated plasmin receptor (NAPlr): activates plasmin, contributes to activation of the alternative complement pathway
  - Streptococcal pyrogenic exotoxin B (SPE B): binds plasmin and acts as a protease; promotes the release of inflammatory mediators
- Activation of the alternative complement pathway causes initial glomerular injury as evidenced by C3 deposition and decreased levels of serum C3. The lectin pathway of complement activation has also been recently implicated in glomerular injury (4).

RISK FACTORS

- Children 5–12 years of age
- Older patients (>65 years of age) (1):
  - Diabetics
  - Patients with immunocompromising comorbid conditions
  - Alcohol abuse

GENERAL PREVENTION

- Early antibiotic treatment for streptococcal and staphylococcal infections, when indicated, although efficacy in preventing GN is uncertain
- Improved hygiene
- Prophylactic penicillin treatment to be used in closed communities and household contacts of index cases in areas where PIGN is prevalent

COMMONLY ASSOCIATED CONDITIONS

Streptococcal infection, staphylococcal infection

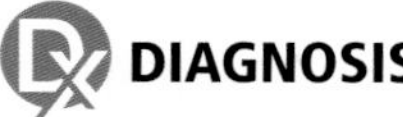

DIAGNOSIS

HISTORY

- Patients present with acute nephritic syndrome, characterized by sudden onset of hematuria associated with edema and HTN 1–2 weeks after an infection.
- A triad of edema, hematuria, and HTN is classic.
- PIGN in children usually follows GAS skin/throat infection.
- The latent period between GAS infection and PIGN depends on the site of infection: 1–3 weeks following GAS pharyngitis and 3–6 weeks following GAS skin infection.
- Adult PIGN most commonly follows staphylococcal infections (3× more common than streptococcal infections) of the upper respiratory tract, skin, heart, lung, bone, or urinary tract. Studies show 7–16% of cases of adult PIGN have no preceding evidence of infection and, in 24–59%, the offending microorganism cannot be identified (5)[A].

PHYSICAL EXAM

- Edema: present in ~2 of 3 adult patients due to sodium and water retention; less common in pediatric patients
- Gross hematuria: present in 25–60% of patients. Urine described as "tea-colored" or "cola-colored."
- HTN: present in 80–90% of patients and varies from mild to severe; secondary to fluid retention Hypertensive encephalopathy is an uncommon but serious complication.
- Microscopic hematuria: subclinical cases of PIGN
- Respiratory distress: due to pulmonary edema (rare)

DIFFERENTIAL DIAGNOSIS

The diagnosis of PIGN is generally by history once the diagnosis of acute nephritis is made, with documentation of a recent infection, with nephritis beginning to resolve 1–2 weeks after presentation. However, with progressive disease >2 weeks, persistent hematuria/HTN >4–6 weeks, or no adequate documentation of a GAS or other infection, the differential diagnosis of GN needs to be considered and renal biopsy ordered:

- Membranoproliferative glomerulonephritis (MPGN): The presentation of MPGN may be indistinguishable initially with hematuria, HTN, proteinuria, and hypocomplementemia after an upper respiratory infection. However, patients with MPGN continue to have persistent nephritis and hypocomplementemia beyond 4–6 weeks and possibly also have a further elevation in serum creatinine. Patients with PIGN tend to have resolution of their disease and a return of normal C3 and CH50 levels within 2–4 weeks.
- Secondary causes of GN: Lupus nephritis and Henoch-Schönlein purpura nephritis have features similar to PIGN. Extrarenal manifestations and laboratory tests for these underlying systemic diseases help differentiate them from PIGN. Hypocomplementemia is not characteristic of Henoch-Schönlein purpura and the hypocomplementemia that occurs in lupus nephritis is with reductions in both C3 and C4, whereas C4 levels are normal in PIGN.
- IgA nephropathy often presents after an upper respiratory infection. It can be distinguished from PIGN based on a shorter time frame between the upper respiratory illness and hematuria, as well as history of gross hematuria, as PIGN recurrence is rare. IgA nephropathy is a chronic illness and will recur. Patients with IgA nephropathy have normal C3/C4 levels. Note: IgA-dominant PIGN is a newly recognized form of PIGN occurring in poststaphylococcal GN. This differs from primary IgA nephropathy in that these patients do not have a history of renal disease (1)[A].
- Pauci-immune crescentic GN: In elderly patients with severe renal failure and active urine sediment, this is much more common, so antineutrophil cytoplasmic antibody (ANCA) testing should be done (1)[A].

DIAGNOSTIC TESTS & INTERPRETATION

Initial Tests (lab, imaging)

Urinalysis shows hematuria. Can be with/without RBC casts and pyuria. Proteinuria present, but nephrotic range proteinuria is uncommon in children (more likely in adults).

Follow-Up Tests & Special Considerations

- Culture: PSGN usually presents weeks after a GAS infection; only ~25% of patients will have either a positive throat or skin culture.
- Complement: 90% of pediatric patients (slightly fewer adult patients) will have depressed C3 and CH50 levels in the first 2 weeks of the disease, whereas C2 and C4 levels remain normal. C3 and CH50 levels return to normal within 4–8 weeks after presentation.

- Creatinine: Elevated to the point of renal insufficiency in 25–83% of cases, more commonly in adults (83%) (4)[A]
- Serology: Elevated titers of antibodies support evidence of a recent GAS infection. Streptozyme test measuring antistreptolysin O (ASO), antihyaluronidase (AHase), antistreptokinase (ASKase), anti–nicotinamide-adenine dinucleotidase (anti-NAD), and anti-DNAse B antibodies: Positive in >95% of patients with PSGN due to pharyngitis and 80% with skin infections. In pharyngeal infection, ASO, anti-DNAse B, anti-NAD, and AHase titers elevated. In skin infection, only the anti-DNAse and AHase titers are typically elevated.

Diagnostic Procedures/Other

Renal biopsy is rarely done in children. Recommended in most adults to confirm the diagnosis and rule out other glomerulopathies with similar clinical presentations that require immunosuppressive treatment.

Test Interpretation

- Light microscopy: diffuse proliferative glomerulonephritis with prominent endocapillary proliferation and numerous neutrophils within the capillary lumen. Deposits may also be found in the mesangium ("starry sky"). Severity of involvement varies and correlates with clinical findings. Crescent formation is uncommon and is associated with a poor prognosis.
- Immunofluorescence microscopy: Deposits of C3 and IgG distributed in a diffuse granular pattern.
- Electron microscopy: dome-shaped subepithelial electron-dense deposits that are referred to as "humps." These deposits are immune complexes and they correspond to the deposits of IgG and C3 found on immunofluorescence. Rate of clearance of these deposits affects recovery time.
- Renal biopsy: usually not performed in most patients to confirm the diagnosis of PIGN as clinical history is highly suggestive and resolution of PIGN typically begins within 1 week of presentation. A biopsy is done when other glomerular disorders are being considered, such as in the case of persistently low C3 levels beyond 6 weeks for possible diagnosis of MPGN, recurrent episodes of hematuria suggestive of IgA nephropathy, or a progressive increase in serum creatinine not characteristic of PIGN.

TREATMENT

MEDICATION

- No specific therapy exists for PIGN, and no randomized controlled trials indicate that aggressive immunosuppressive therapy has a beneficial effect in patients with rapidly progressive crescentic disease. Despite this, patients with >30% crescents on renal biopsy are often treated with steroids (4)[A].
- Older patients often require hospitalization to prevent and treat complications of heart failure (HF) from volume overload (1).
- Management is supportive, with focus on treating the clinical manifestations of PIGN. These include HTN and pulmonary edema:
  - General measures include salt and water restriction and loop diuretics.
  - Calcium channel blockers/angiotensin-converting enzyme (ACE) inhibitors may be used in cases of severe HTN (4)[A].
- Patients with evidence of persistent bacterial infection should be given a course of antibiotic therapy.

SURGERY/OTHER PROCEDURES

Acute dialysis is required in approximately 50% of elderly patients (1).

ONGOING CARE

FOLLOW-UP RECOMMENDATIONS

Patient Monitoring

- Repeat urinalysis to check for clearance of hematuria and/or proteinuria.
- Consider other diagnosis if no improvement within 2 weeks.
- Recurrence is rare.

DIET

Renal diet if requiring instances of dialysis

PROGNOSIS

- Most children with PIGN have an excellent outcome, with >90% of cases achieving full recovery of renal function.
- Elderly patients, especially adults, develop HTN, recurrent proteinuria, and renal insufficiency long after the initial illness. Adults with multiple comorbid factors have the worst prognosis and highest incidence of chronic renal injury following PIGN (1).
- Complete remission in adult PIGN is only 26–56%. This has declined since the 1990s, suggesting prognosis is worsening (5).
- The presence of diabetes, higher creatinine levels, and more severe glomerular disease (e.g., crescents) on biopsy are all risk factors for developing end-stage renal disease (1).

REFERENCES

1. Nasr SH, Radhakrishnan J, D'Agati VD. Bacterial infection-related glomerulonephritis in adults. *Kidney Int*. 2013;83(5):792–803.
2. Nadasdy T, Hebert LA. Infection-related glomerulonephritis: understanding mechanisms. *Semin Nephrol*. 2011;31(4):369–375.
3. Uchida T, Oda T, Watanabe A, et al. Clinical and histologic resolution of poststreptococcal glomerulonephritis with large subendothelial deposits and kidney failure. *Am J Kidney Dis*. 2011;58(1):113–117.
4. Ramdani B, Zamd M, Hachim K, et al. Acute postinfectious glomerulonephritis [in French]. *Nephrol Ther*. 2012;8(4):247–258.
5. Wen YK. Clinicopathological study of infection-associated glomerulonephritis in adults. *Int Urol Nephrol*. 2010;42(2):477–485.

ADDITIONAL READING

- Eison TM, Ault BH, Jones DP, et al. Post-streptococcal acute glomerulonephritis in children: clinical features and pathogenesis. *Pediatr Nephrol*. 2011;26(2):165–180.
- Nasr SH, Fidler ME, Valeri AM, et al. Postinfectious glomerulonephritis in the elderly. *J Am Soc Nephrol*. 2011;22(1):187–195.
- Nast CC. Infection-related glomerulonephritis: changing demographics and outcomes. *Adv Chronic Kidney Dis*. 2012;19(2):68–75.
- Rodriguez-Iturbe B, Musser JM. The current state of poststreptococcal glomerulonephritis. *J Am Soc Nephrol*. 2008;19(10):1855–1864.
- Singh GR. Glomerulonephritis and managing the risks of chronic renal disease. *Pediatr Clin North Am*. 2009;56(6):1363–1382.

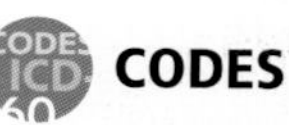

CODES

ICD10

- N05.9 Unsp nephritic syndrome with unspecified morphologic changes
- N00.9 Acute nephritic syndrome with unsp morphologic changes

CLINICAL PEARLS

- PIGN is an immune complex disease occurring after infection with certain strains of bacteria, most commonly group A *Streptococcus pyogenes*.
- The clinical presentation varies from asymptomatic to the acute nephritic syndrome, characterized by gross hematuria, proteinuria, edema, HTN, and acute kidney injury.
- Treatment is primarily supportive and includes treating HTN and edema, along with antibiotics for any ongoing bacterial infection.
- Persistent nephritis and low C3 levels for >2 weeks should prompt evaluation for other causes of GN, such as MPGN or systemic lupus erythematosus nephritis.

GLUCOSE INTOLERANCE

Kristina McGraw, DO • Jennifer Lee, DO

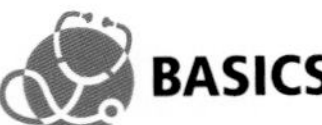

BASICS

DESCRIPTION

- Glucose intolerance is chronic condition defined as blood glucose higher than considered normal yet does not meet criteria levels for diabetes.
- Individuals with impaired fasting glucose (IFG) and/or impaired glucose intolerance (IGT) have been referred to as having prediabetes:
  - IFG: 100–125 mg/dL
  - IGT: 140–199 mg/dL 2 hours after ingestion of 75 g oral glucose load.
  - Hemoglobin A1c as a screening test 5.7–6.4% (1)

EPIDEMIOLOGY

- As of 2010, it is estimated that 1 of every 3 U.S. adults ≥20 years of age have prediabetes (2).
- An estimated 86 million people in the United States are living with prediabetes.
- Only 11% of people with prediabetes are aware of their condition (3).
- Prediabetes has a 37% prevalence among adults >20 years old and 51% of adults 65 years and older in the United States (4).

Incidence

- 15–30% of people with prediabetes will develop type 2 diabetes within 5 years.
- Prospective studies indicate that A1c range of 5.5–6.0% have a 5-year cumulative incidence from 9 to 25% for developing diabetes (2).
- Highest incidence in American Indians/Alaska Natives, non-Hispanic blacks, and Hispanics (2)

ETIOLOGY AND PATHOPHYSIOLOGY

Insulin resistance and progressive insulin secretary defect (5)

RISK FACTORS

- Body mass index (BMI) ≥25: overweight
- Obesity and metabolic syndrome
- 10-fold risk increase for future diabetes in A1c ranges 5.7–6.4%.
- History of gestational diabetes (GDM)
- Sedentary lifestyle
- Glucocorticoids and antipsychotic use

GENERAL PREVENTION

- Lifestyle modification with weight reduction and increased physical activity
- A decrease in excess body fat provides the greatest risk reduction.
- Medical therapy: weight loss medications
  - Phentermine
  - Orlistat
  - Locaserin
  - Phentermine topiramate ER
- Surgical therapy (BMI ≥35)
  - Lap band
  - Gastric sleeve
  - Gastric bypass
- Patients with other cardiovascular risk factors (e.g., dyslipidemia, hypertension, obesity, tobacco use) should receive appropriate counseling to modify diet and exercise.

Pregnancy Considerations

- Screening for diabetes in pregnancy is based on risk factor analysis:
  - High risk: 1st prenatal visit
  - Average risk: 24–28 weeks' gestation
- Women with GDM should be screened for diabetes 6–12 weeks postpartum (6).

COMMONLY ASSOCIATED CONDITIONS

- Obesity (abdominal and visceral obesity)
- Dyslipidemia with high triglycerides (TG)
- Metabolic syndrome
- PCOS
- GDM
- Low HDL
- HTN
- Congenital diseases (Down, Turner, Klinefelter, and Wolfram syndromes)

DIAGNOSIS

Who to screen

- BMI ≥25kg/m^2
- Age >45 years
- 1st-degree relative with diabetes
- Low HDL <35 mg/dL
- High TG >250 mg/dL
- HTN: BP >140/90 mm Hg or on treatment
- Hx of GDM
- Physical inactivity
- Hx of cardiovascular disease
- Ethnic group at increased risk (non-Hispanic black, Native American, Hispanics, Asian American, Pacific Islander)
- HgbA1c ≥5.7%, IGT, or IFG on previous testing
- PCOS
- Conditions associated with insulin resistance such as severe obesity or acanthosis nigricans

HISTORY

- No clear symptoms
- Polyuria
- Polydipsia
- Weight loss
- Blurred vision
- Polyphagia

PHYSICAL EXAM

- General physical exam
- BMI assessment

DIFFERENTIAL DIAGNOSIS

- Type A insulin resistance
- Leprechaunism
- Rabson-Mendenhall syndrome
- Lipoatrophic diabetes
- Pancreatitis
- Cystic fibrosis
- Hemachromatosis
- Acromegaly
- Cushing syndrome
- Glucagonoma
- Pheochromocytoma
- Hyperthyroidism
- Somatostatinoma
- Aldosteronoma
- Drug-induced hyperglycemia
  - Thiazide diuretics (high doses)
  - Beta-blockers
  - Corticosteroids (including inhaled corticosteroids)
  - Thyroid hormone
  - Alpha interferon
  - Pentamidine
  - Protease inhibitors
  - Atypical antipsychotics

DIAGNOSTIC TESTS & INTERPRETATION

Initial Tests (lab, imaging)

- Fasting glucose
- 2-hour OGTT
- HbA1c
- Repeat screen at least at 3-year intervals with normal results or sooner depending on risk status (5).

Follow-Up Tests & Special Considerations

- Fasting lipid profile
- Creatinine and GFR
- Urinalysis
- Microalbumin-to-creatinine ratio
- Thyroid-stimulating hormone with free T_4

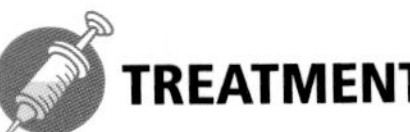

TREATMENT

- Lifestyle aimed at increasing physical activity and weight loss prevents or delays the development of diabetes in people with IGT [A] and IFG (6)[C].
- Exercise and lifestyle:
  - At least 150 minute/week of moderate-intensity aerobic exercise and/or at least 90 minute/week of vigorous aerobic exercise
  - Resistance exercise improves insulin sensitivity to the same extent as aerobic exercise; resistance training 3 ×/week is recommended for those with type 2 diabetes
  - Smoking cessation
- Follow up counseling (6)[B]
- Diabetes prevention programs are cost effective (6)[B].
  - Diabetes prevention program (participants <60 years of age, BMI ≥35 kg/m^2, women with a history of gestational diabetes) showed that loss of weight through diet and exercise reduces risk of developing diabetes by 58% and demonstrated that lifestyle modification decreases risk of diabetes more than metformin.
- Because of its effectiveness, low cost, and long-term safety, the ADA recommends consideration of metformin for prevention of diabetes in individuals with IGT [A], IFG [C], or an A1c 5.7–6.4% [C], especially for those with BMI >35kg/m^2, aged <60 years, and women with history of GDM [A].

- Dietary recommendations:
  - Either low-carbohydrate, low-fat calorie-restricted, or Mediterranean diets may be effective.
  - Diets high in fiber-rich foods such as vegetables, fruits, whole grains, seeds, and nuts plus white meat sources are protective against type 2 diabetes (7).
  - Restrict beverages containing simple sugars, as they increase risk of diabetes (7).
  - Intake of polyunsaturated fatty acid (PUFA) may improve glycemic control; however, data is inconsistent regarding PUFA and other types of fatty acids (7).
  - Individuals who have prediabetes or diabetes should receive individualized MNT (medical nutrition therapy) as needed to achieve treatment goals, preferably provided by a registered dietitian familiar with the components of diabetes MNT (6).

MEDICATION

First line

Metformin (drug of choice) 500 mg BID or 850 mg daily may reduce incidence of new-onset diabetes and BMI (level 2); contraindicated with Cr >1.5 in males and >1.4 in females because it increases risk of lactic acidosis (6).

Second line

Acarbose: started as 50 mg PO once daily and titrated to 100 mg PO TID may reduce incidence of diabetes; GI upset is common (7).

ISSUES FOR REFERRAL

- Nutritionist
- Diabetes educator/registered dietitian upon diagnosis
- Exercise physiologist
- Lifestyle coaching

ADDITIONAL THERAPIES

- Weight loss of 5–10% improves glycemic control, increases insulin sensitivity, improves lipids, and lowers BP.
- Alternative/botanical therapy:
  - Fenugeek, Bitter melon, and cinnamon have reduced hyperglycemia and improved insulin sensitivity in studies by Deng (8) and Graf et al. (9).

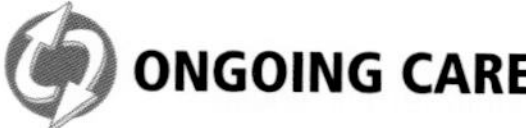

ONGOING CARE

FOLLOW-UP RECOMMENDATIONS

Patient Monitoring

- Consider self-monitoring of blood glucose.
- At least annual monitoring for development of diabetes with HbA1c, 2-hour OGTT, or fasting glucose
- BP should be routinely measured.
- Annual testing for lipid abnormalities and microalbuminuria (for detection and therapy modification of incipient diabetic nephropathy)

DIET

- Monitor carbohydrate intake.
- Macronutrient distribution should be based on individual assessment of eating patterns, preferences, and metabolic goals.
- Consider Mediterranean diet.
- Maximize low glycemic index foods.
- Low-fat (<25%) intake: Saturated fat intake should be <7% of total calories.
- Minimize *trans* fat intake.
- Low-sodium intake <2,300 mg/day
- High-fiber (~50 g/day; 14 g/1,000 kcal) and whole-grain intake
- Drink ample quantities of water, minimum of 64 oz of water daily, and strictly avoid sugar-sweetened beverages.
- Moderate alcohol intake: 1 drink/day for women; 2 drinks/day for men

PROGNOSIS

- Individuals with IFG and/or IGT have high risk for the future development of diabetes.
- Prediabetes increases the risk of developing type 2 diabetes, heart disease, and stroke.
- The potential impact of interventions to reduce mortality or the incidence of cardiovascular disease has not been demonstrated to date.
- 20–70% of individuals with prediabetes who do not lose weight, change their dietary habits, and/or engage in moderate physical activity will progress to type 2 diabetes within 3–6 years (7).
- HbA1c >6.5% at age 12–39 years associated with increased risk of death before age 55 years compared with HbA1c <5.7%

COMPLICATIONS

- Cardiovascular disease
- PAD
- Stroke: 2–4 times higher risk
- Ketoacidosis
- Sexual dysfunction
- Gastroparesis
- Nephropathy and potential for renal failure
- Retinopathy and potential for loss of vision
- Peripheral and autonomic neuropathy

REFERENCES

1. Nathan DM, Davidson MB, DeFronzo RA, et al. Impaired fasting glucose and impaired glucose tolerance: implications for care. *Diabetes Care*. 2007;30(3):753.
2. Centers for Disease Control and Prevention. *National Diabetes Statistics Report: Estimates of Diabetes and Its Burden in the United States, 2014*. Atlanta, GA: U.S. Department of Health and Human Services; 2014.
3. Centers for Disease Control and Prevention. Awareness of prediabetes—United States, 2005–2010. *MMWR Morb Mortal Weekly Rep*. 2013:62(11): 209–212.
4. Centers for Disease Control and Prevention. Prediabetes facts. http://www.cdc.gov/diabetes/pub/statsreport14/prediabetes-infographic.pdf. Accessed 2014.
5. American Diabetes Association. Diagnosis and classification of diabetes mellitus. Position Statement. *Diabetes Care*. 2014;37(Suppl 1):S81–S90.
6. American Diabetes Association. Standards of medical care in diabetes —2014. *Diabetes Care*. 2014;37(Suppl 1):S14–S79.
7. Stull AJ. Lifestyle approaches and glucose intolerance [published online ahead of print October 14, 2014]. *Am J Lifestyle Med*. doi:10.1177/1559827614554186.
8. Deng R. A review of the hypoglycemia effects of five commonly used herbal food supplements. *Recent Pat Food Nutr Agric*. 2012;4(1):50–60.
9. Graf BL, Raskin I, Cefalu WT, et al. Plant-derived therapeutics for the treatment of metabolic syndrome. *Curr Opin Investig Drugs*. 2010;11(10):1107–1115.

ADDITIONAL READING

- Maruthur NM, Ma Y, Delahanty LM, et al. Early response to preventive strategies in the Diabetes Prevention Program. *J Gen Intern Med*. 2013;28(12):1629–1636.
- Ramachandran A, Riddle MC, Kabali C, et al. Relationship between A1C and fasting plasma glucose in dysglycemia or type 2 diabetes: an analysis of baseline data from the ORIGIN trial. *Diabetes Care*. 2012;35(4):749–753.

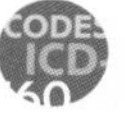

CODES

ICD10

- E74.39 Other disorders of intestinal carbohydrate absorption
- R73.09 Other abnormal glucose
- R73.01 Impaired fasting glucose

CLINICAL PEARLS

- Lifestyle optimization is essential for all patients with prediabetes.
- Research shows that you can lower your risk for type 2 diabetes by 58% by losing 7% of your body weight (or 15 lb if you weigh 200 lb).
- Exercising moderately (such as brisk walking) 30 minutes a day, 5 days a week
- Consider concurrent cardiovascular risks and further workup as indicated clinically.
- Patient education and lifestyle reinforcement should be emphasized in all clinical encounters.

GONOCOCCAL INFECTIONS

Julissa Mendoza, MD • Stephen J. Conner, MD

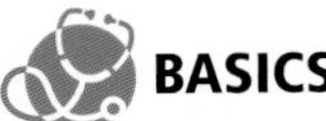

BASICS

DESCRIPTION

Gonorrhea is a sexually or vertically transmitted bacterial infection caused by *Neisseria gonorrhoeae*:

- *N. gonorrhoeae* is a fastidious gram-negative intracellular diplococcus (1)[A].
- Can present as conjunctival, pharyngeal, urogenital or anorectal infections. Urogenital infections are most common (1)[A].
- Hematogenous dissemination may also occur leading to fever, skin lesions, arthralgias, purulent or sterile arthritis, tenosynovitis, endocarditis, or (rarely) meningitis (1)[A].
- Asymptomatic carrier state can occur in both sexes.
- In newborns, gonococcal ophthalmia neonatorum, a purulent conjunctivitis, may occur after vaginal delivery by an infected mother, potentially leading to blindness if not treated promptly (1,2)[A].
- System(s) affected: cardiovascular, musculoskeletal, nervous, reproductive, skin/exocrine
- Synonym(s): gonococcal infection (GC); clap

EPIDEMIOLOGY

- Predominant age: 15–24 years (1,2)[A]
- Predominant sex: women 105/100,000 versus men 92/100,000 (2)[A]

Incidence

CDC Statistics: 2012: 334,826 reported cases (107.5/100,000 U.S. population) (2)[A]

Prevalence

As a treatable disease, incidence and prevalence of diagnosed disease are approximately equal. The true prevalence is higher due to the asymptomatic nature of the disease (2)[A]:

- Rates peaked in mid-1970s and fell 74% over the next 20 years with national control program (2)[A].
- Highest rate: women aged 20–24 years (578.5/100,000) followed by women aged 15–19 years (521.2/100,000) (2)[A]
- Blacks (462.0/100,000) have higher reported rates of infections than whites (31.0/100,000) (2)[A].
- The southern regions of the United States have higher reported rates. Highest reported state rate is Mississippi (230.8/100,000) (2)[A].

ETIOLOGY AND PATHOPHYSIOLOGY

Infection requires 4 steps: (i) mucosal attachment. Bacterial proteins bind to receptors on host cells; (ii) local penetration/invasion; (iii) local proliferation; (iv) inflammatory response or dissemination *N. gonorrhoeae* (gonococcus). *N. gonorrhoeae* spreads most commonly during sexual relations.

Genetics

Congenital deficiency of late components of complement cascade (C7,8,9) are prone to develop dissemination of local gonococcal infections.

RISK FACTORS

- History of previous gonorrhea infection or other STIs
- Sexual exposure to an infected individual without barrier protection (condom)
- New/multiple sexual partners
- Inconsistent condom use
- Commercial sex work or drug use
- Infants: infected mother
- Children: sexual abuse by infected individual
- Autoinoculation (finger to eye)

GENERAL PREVENTION

- Condoms offer partial protection but must be used for oral, anal, and vaginal intercourse to be effective.
- Treat sexual contacts; consider expedited partner therapy (EPT) (2,3)[A]

COMMONLY ASSOCIATED CONDITIONS

Other STIs: *Chlamydia*, syphilis, HIV, hepatitis B, herpes (2–4)[A]

DIAGNOSIS

HISTORY

- Sexual history
  - Number of partners and age of onset of sexual activity; STI history
  - New/recent change in sexual partner
  - Contact with commercial sex workers
  - Condom use
  - Menses and possibility of pregnancy
- *10% males and 20–40% of women are asymptomatic (2)[A].*
- If symptomatic, explore the onset, context, duration, timing, severity, and associated symptoms:
  - Symptoms typically appear within 1–14 days after exposure (when present) (1)[A].
- Ocular symptoms: discharge, itch, redness (1)[A]
- Pharyngeal symptoms: asymptomatic infection (98%), sore throat (1)[A]
- GI symptoms: acute diarrhea (1)[A]
- Urinary symptoms: urinary frequency, urgency, dysuria (1)[A]
- Urethral symptoms: copious urethral discharge (1,2)[A]
  - Males: scant to copious purulent urethral discharge (82%), dysuria (53%), testicular pain (1%), asymptomatic infection (10%), proctitis
  - Females: asymptomatic cervical infection (20%), endocervical discharge (96%), vaginal discharge, Bartholin gland abscess, dysmenorrhea, menometrorrhagia, abdominal pain/tenderness, dyspareunia, cervical motion tenderness, rebound, infertility, chronic pelvic pain
- Either sex, for receptive anal intercourse: rectal discharge, tenesmus, rectal burning, asymptomatic
- Disseminated syndromes (1,2)[A]
  - Fever, chills, malaise, skin rash, arthralgia
  - Endocarditis: high fevers
  - Meningitis: meningeal signs, headache, skin lesions, fever, altered mental status

PHYSICAL EXAM

- General: fever, chills (1)[A]
- Ocular: purulent discharge, conjunctivitis, chemosis, eyelid edema, corneal ulceration (1)[A]
- Pharyngeal infection: exudative pharyngitis (<1%) (1)[A]
- GI: acute diarrhea, hyperactive bowel sounds (1)[A]
- Genitourinary (GU) (1)[A]
  - Males: scant to copious purulent urethral discharge (82%), testicular tenderness (1%), asymptomatic infection (10%), proctitis
  - Females: asymptomatic cervical infection (20%), endocervical discharge (96%), Bartholin gland abscess, abdominal pain/tenderness, cervical motion tenderness, rebound tenderness
- Either sex, for receptive anal intercourse: rectal discharge; may appear normal (1)[A]
- Disseminated syndromes (1)[A]:
  - Fever, chills, malaise, tenosynovitis, maculopapular-pustular rash, polyarthralgia—typically large joints (knee, wrist, ankle), purulent arthritis
  - Endocarditis: rapid cardiac valve destruction, heart murmurs, high fevers
  - Meningitis: meningeal signs, headache, skin lesions, fever, altered mental status

DIFFERENTIAL DIAGNOSIS

Chlamydia trachomatis, UTIs, other vaginitis, or urethritis (bacterial, viral, or parasitic)

DIAGNOSTIC TESTS & INTERPRETATION

Initial Tests (lab, imaging)

- The CDC recommends nucleic acid amplification (NAAT) as the most sensitive and specific test for *N. gonorrhoeae* (2)[A]. Other options include the following:
  - Genital culture
  - Add pharyngeal culture in adolescents.
  - Gram stain (recommended for urethritis)
  - Urethral smear, sensitivity in symptomatic male: ≥95%. Sensitivity of endocervical smear in infected woman: 40–60%. Specificity: 100%
- DNA probes and polymerase chain reaction (PCR) sensitivity: 92–99% dependent on population. Specificity: >97%; can replace culture
- Sensitivity of blood culture in disseminated disease: 50%. Sensitivity of joint fluid culture in septic arthritis: 50%
- Screen for additional STIs, especially chlamydia, syphilis, and HIV
- Imaging is not generally recommended.

Follow-Up Tests & Special Considerations

- Test of cure not generally recommended (1–3)[A].
- Follow-up testing may be considered in cases of recurrent infection and/or in areas where significant antibiotic resistance exists (2,3)[A].
- Pelvic ultrasound or CT scan may demonstrate thick, dilated fallopian tubes or abscess formation.

Diagnostic Procedures/Other

Culdocentesis may demonstrate free purulent exudate and provide material for Gram staining and culture. Gram-staining material from unroofed skin lesions may show typical organisms.

Test Interpretation

- Gram-negative intracellular diplococci
- Nonpathologic gram-negative diplococci may be found in extragenital locations. For this reason, Gram stain of pharyngeal or rectal swabs is not recommended.

TREATMENT

GENERAL MEASURES

- STI counseling and condom use
- In children and adolescents, suspect sexual abuse.

MEDICATION

- *N. gonorrhoeae* multidrug antimicrobial resistance continues to increase: *CDC recommends dual therapy for all uncomplicated GC infections in U.S. adults and adolescents* (both to treat for concomitant chlamydia and to increase efficacy against drug-resistant strains) (2–4)[A].
- Quinolones are not recommended since 2007 (2–4)[A].
- *If treatment fails, check culture and sensitivities, and report to CDC through local health authorities* (2–4)[A].
- Treat routinely with regimen that is also effective against uncomplicated genital chlamydial infection (2–4)[A].

First Line

- Uncomplicated urogenital, anorectal, and pharyngeal gonorrheal infection (2,3)[A]
  - Ceftriaxone 250 mg IM in a single dose
  - *PLUS* treatment for chlamydia (azithromycin 1 g PO single dose or doxycycline 100 mg PO BID for 7 days)
- Pharyngitis: ceftriaxone 250 mg IM once PLUS treatment for chlamydia (azithromycin 1 g PO single dose or doxycycline 100 mg PO BID for 7 days) (1–3)[A]
- Conjunctivitis: ceftriaxone, 1 g IM single dose (1–3)[A]
- Pelvic inflammatory disease (PID): Parenteral and oral treatments are equivalent for mild to moderate severity PID. If using IV therapy, switch to PO within 24–48 hours of clinical improvement (1–3)[A].
  - Cefotetan 2 g IV q12r OR cefoxitin 2 g IV q6h + doxycycline 100 mg PO or IV q12h OR
  - Clindamycin 900 mg IV q8h + gentamicin loading dose IV or IM (2 mg/kg of body weight), followed by a maintenance dose (1.5 mg/kg) q8h. Daily dosing (3–5 mg/kg) can be substituted.
  - Preferred "oral" regimen includes the following:
    - Ceftriaxone 250 mg IM once + doxycycline, 100 mg PO b.i.d. for 14 days
    - With or without metronidazole, 500 mg PO b.i.d. for 14 days
- Disseminated infection in adults (1–3)[A]
  - Ceftriaxone 1 g IM or IV q24h until 24–48 hours after improvement begins, then switch to cefixime 400 mg PO b.i.d. to complete at least 1 week of antibiotic treatment. *Also treat for chlamydial infection.*
- Meningitis and endocarditis (1–3)[A]
  - Ceftriaxone 1–2 g IV q12h 10–14 days for meningitis; 4 weeks for endocarditis
- *Contraindications:* Doxycycline *is contraindicated in pregnancy and young children.*

Pediatric Considerations

- Children >45 kg same dosing as adults (1–3)[A]
- Children <45 kg: uncomplicated urethral, cervical, rectal or pharyngeal gonococcal infections (1–3)[A]
  - Ceftriaxone 125 mg IM in single dose
  - Disseminated infections: ceftriaxone 50 mg/kg IV or IM daily (max dose 1 g) in single dose; bacteremia: 7 days; meningitis: 10–14 days; endocarditis: 4 weeks
- Ophthalmic neonatorum prophylaxis: single application of erythromycin 0.5% ophthalmic ointment to each eye immediately after delivery (1–3)[A]
- Neonatal conjunctivitis: ceftriaxone 25–50 mg/kg IV or IM in a single dose (not to exceed 125 mg) (1–3)[A]
- *Conjunctival exudates should be cultured for definitive diagnosis* (1–3)[A].
- Scalp abscesses (from scalp electrodes) (1–3)[A]
  - Ceftriaxone 25–50 mg/kg/day IV or IM in a single daily dose for 7 days, with duration of 10–14 days if meningitis is documented.
- Asymptomatic infants born to mothers with untreated gonorrhea (1–3)[A]
  - Ceftriaxone 25–50 mg/kg IV or IM, not to exceed 125 mg in a single dose

Pregnancy Considerations

Pregnant women should be treated with cephalosporin or recommended alternate (1–4)[A].

- Azithromycin 2 g orally in single dose for women intolerant to cephalosporin
- Treat with azithromycin or amoxicillin for presumed *C. trachomatis* coinfection.
- Women with 1st-trimester gonococcal infection should be retested within 3–6 months.
- High-risk uninfected pregnant women should be retested during the 3rd trimester.

Second Line

- Due to antimicrobial resistance, combination therapy using 2 agents with different mechanisms of action improves treatment efficacy and decreases resistance to cephalosporins (1–3)[A].
  - Use of a 2nd antimicrobial (azithromycin as a single 1-g oral dose or doxycycline 100 mg orally twice daily for 7 days) is recommended for use with ceftriaxone (1–3)[A].
  - Azithromycin as 2nd antimicrobial is preferred to doxycycline because of convenience and compliance of single-dose therapy as well as higher resistance with tetracyclines (1–3)[A].
- For additional treatment options, see CDC STD treatment guidelines: http://www.cdc.gov/std/treatment/2010/gonococcal-infections.htm

INPATIENT CONSIDERATIONS

Admission Criteria/Initial Stabilization

- Hematogenously disseminated infection
- Pneumonia or eye infection in infants
- PID: if unable to take oral medications, significant tubo-ovarian abscess, or patient is pregnant

ONGOING CARE

FOLLOW-UP RECOMMENDATIONS

Patient Monitoring

U.S. Preventive Services Task Force (USPSTF) (4)[A]

- Screen all sexually active women, including those who are pregnant if they are at increased risk of infection (*young or have other individual/population risk factor*) **Grade B recommendation**
- Insufficient evidence to recommend for or against screening men at increased risk of infection **Grade I recommendation**
- No routine screening in men and women who are low risk for infection **Grade D recommendation**
- Insufficient evidence to recommend for or against screening in pregnant women who are not at increased risk for infection **Grade I recommendation**
- Prophylactic ocular topical medication for *all* newborns **Grade A recommendation**
- Gonorrhea is a reportable disease (3,4)[A].
  - *Providers must contact both the state health department and the CDC.*

PATIENT EDUCATION

- Counseling concerning risk reduction, condom use, future fertility, and full STI testing
- Encourage patient to notify partners (from past 60 days); consider EPT.

PROGNOSIS

With adequate early therapy, complete cure with return to normal function is the rule.

COMPLICATIONS

- Infertility
- Urethral stricture
- Corneal scarring
- Destruction of joint articular surfaces
- Cardiac valvular damage

Pediatric Considerations

Vertical transmission to newborn infants is a significant risk among patients with gonococcal infection at the time of delivery (1,2)[A].

REFERENCES

1. Mayor MT, Roett MA, Uduhiri KA. Diagnosis and management of gonococcal infections. *Am Fam Physician*. 2012;86(10):931–938.
2. Centers for Disease Control and Prevention. 2010 sexually transmitted diseases treatment guidelines: gonococcal infections. http://www.cdc.gov/std/treatment/2010/gonococcal-infections.htm. Accessed 2014.
3. Centers for Disease Control and Prevention. Update to CDC's sexually transmitted diseases treatment guidelines, 2010: oral cephalosporins no longer a recommended treatment for gonococcal infections. *MMWR Morb Mortal Wkly Rep*. 2012;61(31):590–594.
4. U.S. Preventive Services Task Force. Gonorrhea: screening. http://www.uspreventiveservicestaskforce.org/uspstf05/gonorrhea/gonup.pdf. Accessed 2014.

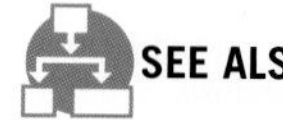

SEE ALSO

Chlamydial Sexually Transmitted Diseases; HIV/AIDS; Pelvic Inflammatory Disease; Syphilis

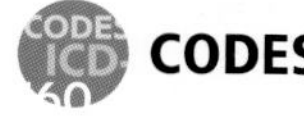

CODES

ICD10

- A54.9 Gonococcal infection, unspecified
- A54.31 Gonococcal conjunctivitis
- A54.03 Gonococcal cervicitis, unspecified

CLINICAL PEARLS

- Due to rising treatment recommendations for uncomplicated gonorrhea, should include 2 drugs, one of which is effective against chlamydia.
- Patients testing positive for gonorrhea should generally be screened for chlamydia, syphilis, HIV, and hepatitis.

GOUT

Ryan B. Feeney, PharmD • Michael C. Barros, PharmD, BCPS, BCACP • Paul N. Williams, MD

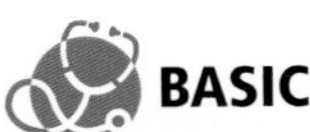

BASICS

DESCRIPTION

- Gout is an inflammatory arthritis related to a hyperuricemia (serum uric acid [SUA] level >6.8 mg/dL) (1).
- Acute gouty arthritis can affect ≥1 joints; the 1st metatarsophalangeal joint is most commonly involved at presentation (podagra).
- Although hyperuricemia is necessary for the development of gout, it is not the only determining factor.
- Characterized by deposition of monosodium urate (MSU) crystals that accumulate in joints and soft tissues, resulting in acute and chronic arthritis, soft-tissue masses called tophi, urate nephropathy, and uric acid nephrolithiasis
- After an initial flare, a 2nd flare occurs in ~60% of patients within 1 year and 78% within 2 years of the initial attack (2).
- Management involves treating acute attacks and preventing recurrent disease by long-term reduction of SUA levels through pharmacology and lifestyle adjustments.

EPIDEMIOLOGY

Incidence

Annual incidence of gout (3):

- Uric acid 7–8.9 mg/dL is 0.5%.
- Uric acid >9 mg/dL is 4.5%.

Prevalence

- Increasing prevalence over the past decades (3)
- 2007–2008 prevalence of gout in the United States (3):
  - Men 5.8% (6.1 million)
  - Women 2.0% (2.2 million)
- 2008 prevalence of hyperuricemia in the United States (3):
  - Men 21.2% (SUA >7.0 mg/dL)
  - Women 21.6% (SUA >5.7 mg/dL)

ETIOLOGY AND PATHOPHYSIOLOGY

- Hyperuricemia results from urate overproduction, underexcretion, or often a combination of the 2.
- Gout occurs when MSU, a product of purine metabolism, precipitates out of solution and accumulates in joints and soft tissues.
- Transient changes in urate solubility caused by local temperature decrease, trauma, or acidosis may lead to an acute gouty attack.
- Urate crystals that precipitate trigger an immune response.
- Left untreated, this crystal deposition leads to permanent joint damage and tophus formation.

Genetics

- Phosphoribosyl pyrophosphate (PRPP) deficiency and hypoxanthine-guanine-phosphoribosyltransferase (HGPRT) deficiency (Lesch-Nyan syndrome) are inherited enzyme defects associated with overproduction of uric acid.
- Polymorphisms in the URAT1 and SLC 2A9 (GLUT9) renal transporters are hereditary enzyme defects resulting in primary underexcretion of uric acid.

RISK FACTORS

- Age >40 years
- Male gender
- Increased purine uptake (meats and seafood)
- Alcohol intake (especially beer)
- High fructose intake
- Obesity
- Hyperuricemia
- Congestive heart failure
- Coronary artery disease
- Dyslipidemia
- Renal disease
- Organ transplant
- Hypertension
- Hyperinsulinemia
- Metabolic syndrome
- Diabetes mellitus
- Urate-elevating medications:
  - Thiazide diuretics: ethambutol
  - Loop diuretics (less of a risk vs. thiazides)
  - Niacin
  - Calcineurin inhibitors (cyclosporine and tacrolimus)
  - Acetylsalicylic acid (*not* recommended in high doses)

GENERAL PREVENTION

- Maintain optimal weight.
- Regular exercise
- Diet modification (purine rich foods)
- Reduce alcohol consumption (beer and liquor).
- Maintain fluid intake and avoid dehydration.

COMMONLY ASSOCIATED CONDITIONS

- Hypertension
- Dyslipidemia
- Nontraumatic joint disorders
- Heart disease
- Urinary tract disease
- Diabetes mellitus
- Metabolic syndrome
- Obesity
- Renal disease

DIAGNOSIS

HISTORY

- Classic presentation of acute gouty arthritis:
  - Intense pain and tenderness in the 1st metatarsophalangeal joint (podagra)
  - Can occur in the midtarsal, ankle, or knee joints
  - Joint may be swollen, warm, and red
  - Often awakes patients from sleep due to an intolerance to contact with clothing or bed sheets
  - There is a rapid onset of intense pain, often beginning in the early morning and progressing rapidly over 12–24 hours.
  - In the absence of treatment, flares can last up to 10 days.
- Fever can be seen.
- SC or intraosseous nodules, referred to as tophi
- Pain with urination secondary to uric acid renal stones

PHYSICAL EXAM

- Examine suspected joint(s) for tenderness, swelling, and range of motion (ROM).
- Assess for presence of firm nodules known as tophi.
- In patients with chronic gout, tophi can frequently be found in the helix of the ear, over the olacrenon process, or on the Achilles tendon.
- Patients with untreated chronic gout can have evidence of joint inflammation and deformity.

DIFFERENTIAL DIAGNOSIS

Acute bursitis, tendonitis, septic arthritis, pseudogout (calcium pyrophosphate deposition disease), cellulitis, osteoarthritis

DIAGNOSTIC TESTS & INTERPRETATION

- SUA (may be normal during an acute flare)
- CBC (can see elevation of WBC during an acute gout flare)
- Synovial fluid analysis: urate crystals (negatively birefringent under polarizing microscopy), cell count (WBC usually 2,000–50,000/mm^3); culture to rule out infection. Some guidelines suggest that gout can be diagnosed clinically without synovial fluid analysis.
- Screen for uric acid overproduction 24-hour urinary uric acid in those patients with gout onset before the age of 25 years or a history of urolithiasis (1)[C].
- Radiograph is normal early in disease but can reveal
  - Swelling in acute gout
  - Periarticular erosions with periosteum overgrowth in chronic gout
- Urate kidney stones are radiolucent and thus invisible on radiograph.

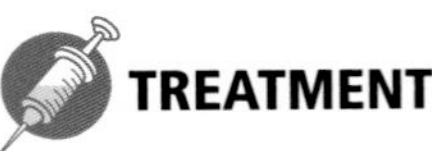

TREATMENT

GENERAL MEASURES

Topical ice as needed (4)[B]

MEDICATION

- Acute treatment
  - General principles:
    - Acute gouty arthritis attacks should be treated with pharmacologic therapy (4)[C].
    - Pharmacologic treatment should be initiated within 24 hours of acute gout attack onset (4)[C].
    - Ongoing pharmacologic urate-lowering therapy should not be interrupted during an acute gout attack (4)[C].
    - Choice of agent is based on severity of pain and the number of joints involved (4).
  - Mild/moderate gout severity (≤6 of 10 on visual analog pain scale, particularly for an attack involving only 1 or a few small joints or 1–2 large joints)
    - NSAIDs
      - Naproxen (Naprosyn, Anaprox, Aleve): 750 mg followed by 250 mg q8h for 5–8 days (4)[A]
      - Indomethacin (Indocin): 50–150 mg/day for 2–7 days (4)[A]
      - Sulindac (Clinoril): 200 mg BID for 7–10 days (4)[A]
      - Celecoxib (Celebrex)
      - Not FDA approved but can be considered in selected patients with contraindications or intolerance to NSAIDs (4)[B].
        - Dose at 800 mg once followed by 400 mg on day 1, then 400 mg BID for 1 week (4)[B]
    - Corticosteroids
      - Those with an acute flare involving 1–2 large joints can consider intra-articular corticosteroids; can consider using PO corticosteroids in combination.
      - For other acute flares, use PO corticosteroids:
        - Prednisone (Sterapred): 0.5 mg/kg/day for 5–10 days followed by discontinuation (4)[A] or alternately 2–5 days at full dose followed by tapering for 7–10 days and then discontinuing (4)[C]

- Methylprednisolone (Medrol) dose pack (4)[C]
- Triamcinolone acetonide (Trivaris): 60 mg IM single dose followed by oral corticosteroids (4)[C]
- Colchicine (Colcrys)
  - Used for gout attacks where the onset was <36 hours prior to treatment initiation (4)[A]
  - Begin a loading dose of 1.2 mg followed by 0.6 mg 1 hour later, followed by 0.6 mg once or twice daily 12 hours later, until the gout attack resolves (4)[C].
  - Dose reduction recommended in moderate to severe kidney disease and in those on inhibitors of cytochrome P450 3A4 and P-glycoprotein (clarithromycin, erythromycin, cyclosporine, and disulfiram) (4).
- Severe gout (≥7 of 10 on visual analog pain scale, involving ≥4 joints with arthritis involving >1 region, or involving 3 separate large joints)
  - Initial combination therapy is an option and includes the use of full doses of the following (4)[C]:
    - Colchicine and NSAIDs
    - PO corticosteroids and colchicine
    - Intra-articular steroids with all other modalities
- For patients not responding to initial pharmacologic monotherapy, add a 2nd agent (4)[C].

• Chronic treatment
- Indications for pharmacologic urate-lowering therapy include any patient with
  - Tophus or tophi by clinical exam or imaging study (1)[A]
  - Frequent attacks of acute gouty arthritis (≥2 attacks/year) (1)[A]
  - Chronic kidney disease (CKD) stage 2 or worse (1)[C]
  - Past urolithiasis (1)[C]
- Treat to the serum urate:
  - Minimum serum urate target is <6 mg/dL (1)[A].
  - Serum urate target may need to be <5 mg/dL to improve gout signs and symptoms (1)[B].
- Urate-lowering agents can be prescribed during an acute attack provided that effective anti-inflammatory prophylaxis has been initiated prior to urate lowering-therapy (1)[C].
- Anti-inflammatory prophylaxis required when initiating urate-lowering therapy include the following:
  - 1st line
    - Low-dose colchicine: 0.6 mg once or twice daily (4)[A]
    - Low-dose NSAIDs with proton pump inhibitor where indicated: naproxen 250 mg PO BID (4)[C]
  - 2nd line: Use of colchicine and NSAIDs both are not tolerated, contraindicated, or ineffective:
    - Low-dose prednisone or prednisolone at ≤10 mg/day (4)[C]
  - Treatment duration for the greater of
    - At least 6 months (4)[A] *or*
    - 3 months after achieving serum urate appropriate for the patient with no tophi on exam (4)[B] or for 6 months after achieving serum urate appropriate for the patient with ≥1 tophi on exam (4)[C]
- Pharmacologic urate-lowering agents:
  - Allopurinol (Zyloprim): xanthine oxidase inhibitor (1)[A]
    - Starting dose should be no higher than 100 mg/day (1)[B].
    - Starting dose should be 50 mg/day in stage 4 CKD or worse
    - Gradually titrate the dose upward q2–5wk to appropriate maximum dose (1)[C].
    - Dose can be >300 mg/day, even with renal impairment, as long as accompanied by patient education and monitoring for drug toxicity; maximum FDA-approved dosage is 800 mg/day (1)[B].
    - Regularly monitor for allopurinol hypersensitivity syndrome (AHS), pruritus, rash, elevated hepatic transaminases, and eosinophilia.
    - Screening for the HLA-B*5801 allele for AHS should be performed in those of Korean descent with stage 3 CKD or worse and Han Chinese or Thai descent irrespective of renal function (1)[A].
  - Febuxostat (Uloric): selective xanthine oxidase inhibitor (1)[A]
    - No renal or hepatic adjustments needed for mild-to-moderate hepatic or renal impairment
    - Starting dose 40 mg/day; may be titrated to 80 mg/day
    - In select instances, may dose up to 120 mg/day (not FDA approved) (1)[A]
  - Probenecid: uricosuric agent (1)[B]
    - Alternative 1st-line urate-lowering therapy; use if at least 1 xanthine oxidase inhibitor is contraindicated or not tolerated (1)[B]
    - May be used in addition to allopurinol or febuxostat if serum urate target not achieved
    - Multiple drug interactions exist as well as risk of urolithiasis with this agent.
    - Not recommended if creatinine clearance (CrCl) is <50 or with patient history of urolithiasis (1)[C].
    - Starting dose is 250 mg BID; gradually titrate to 2,000 mg/day

• Other treatment
- Acute treatment: adrenocorticotropic hormone (ACTH): 25–40 IU SC (4)[A]; especially in those NPO
- Pegloticase in select severe instances (1)

SURGERY/OTHER PROCEDURES

Large tophi that are infected or interfering with joint motion may need to be surgically removed.

ONGOING CARE

FOLLOW-UP RECOMMENDATIONS

Patient Monitoring

- SUA q2–5wk while titrating urate-lowering treatment to goal (1)[C]
- Regularly monitor CBC, renal function, liver function test, and urinalysis.

DIET

- General lack of evidence regarding specific recommendations, although the American College of Rheumatology has outlined the following (1)[C]:
- General measures:
  - Weight loss for obese patients
  - Healthy overall diet
  - Exercise
  - Smoking cessation
  - Stay well hydrated
- Avoid
  - Organ meats high in purine content (sweetbreads, liver, kidney) (1)[A]
  - High-fructose corn syrup–sweetened sodas, other beverages, or foods
  - Alcohol overuse (>2 servings per day for men and >1 serving per day for women) (1)[A]
  - Any alcohol use in gout during periods of frequent gout attacks or advanced gout under poor control
- Limit
  - Serving sizes of beef, lamb, pork, and seafood with high purine content such as sardines and shellfish (1)[B]
  - Servings of naturally sweetened fruit juices
  - Table sugar and sweetened beverages and desserts
  - Table salt, including in sauces and gravies
  - Alcohol (particularly beer) in all gout patients (1)[B]
- Encourage
  - Low-fat or nonfat dairy products
  - Vegetables

PATIENT EDUCATION

- Dietary and lifestyle modifications (1)[B]
- Patient instructions on initiating treatment on signs and symptoms of an acute gout attack without the need to consult health care provider for each attack (1)[B]
- Discussion that gout is caused by excess uric acid and that effective urate-lowering therapy is essential treatment (1)[B]

PROGNOSIS

Gout can usually be successfully managed with proper treatment.

COMPLICATIONS

- AHS
- Increased susceptibility to infection
- Urate nephropathy
- Renal stones

G

REFERENCES

1. Khanna D, Fitzgerald JD, Khanna PP, et al. 2012 American College of Rheumatology guidelines for management of gout. Part 1: systematic nonpharmacologic and pharmacologic therapeutic approaches to hyperuricemia. *Arthritis Care Res.* 2012;64(10):1431–1446.
2. Doghramji PP. Managing your patient with gout: a review of treatment options. *Postgrad Med.* 2011;123(3):56–71.
3. Zhu Y, Pandya BJ, Choi HK. Prevalence of gout and hyperuricemia in the US general population: the National Health and Nutrition Examination Survey 2007–2008. *Arthritis Rheum.* 2012;63(10): 3136–3141.
4. Khanna D, Khanna PP, Fitzgerald JD, et al. 2012 American College of Rheumatology guidelines for management of gout. Part 2: therapy and antiinflammatory prophylaxis of acute gouty arthritis. *Arthritis Care Res.* 2012;64(10):1447–1461.

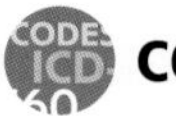

CODES

ICD10

- M10.9 Gout, unspecified
- M10.00 Idiopathic gout, unspecified site
- M10.30 Gout due to renal impairment, unspecified site

CLINICAL PEARLS

- MSU crystals found in synovial fluid aspirate are pathognomonic for gout.
- Acute gout and sepsis can coexist.
- Asymptomatic hyperuricemia does not require treatment.
- Losartan possesses uricosuric properties, therefore it may be an excellent agent if patient is hypertensive.

GRANULOMA ANNULARE

Jeremy Golding, MD, FAAFP

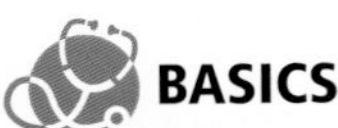

BASICS

DESCRIPTION

A benign skin condition characterized by grouped papules, which typically occur in an annular pattern. 5 variants have been described, the most common of which is localized granuloma annulare (GA). The other types are generalized, patch type, SC (deep dermal), and perforating.

EPIDEMIOLOGY

Incidence

- GA is not common, although its occurrence in the general population is unknown.
- Predominant sex: female > male (2:1)
- Most lesions resolve in 2–24 months but may last up to 5–10 years. 2/3 of patients are <30 years, and the age distribution varies by type, as follows:
  - Localized: children and adults <30 years
  - Generalized: bimodal: children <10 years and adults 30–60 years
  - Patch type: adults >30 years
  - SC: children 2–10 years
  - Perforating: typically children but also young adults

Prevalence

Among cases of GA, the approximate distribution is as follows:

- Localized: 75%
- Generalized: 10–15%
- Patch type: <5%
- SC: <5%
- Perforating: <5% (perhaps higher in Hawaii)

ETIOLOGY AND PATHOPHYSIOLOGY

The cause of GA remains unknown, although it is hypothesized to be a delayed-type hypersensitivity to an unknown antigen.

Genetics

There is some evidence for a possible hereditary component.

RISK FACTORS

No definite risk factors have been identified. There is weak evidence for possible associations with diabetes mellitus; TB; HIV, EBV, and other viral infections; interferon-α therapy; trauma; insect bites; borreliosis; and malignancies (most commonly lymphoma).

GENERAL PREVENTION

There are no established strategies for preventing GA.

COMMONLY ASSOCIATED CONDITIONS

A recent case-control study found that those patients with granuloma annulare were more likely to have dyslipidemia, with the strongest association seen in patients with generalized subtype.

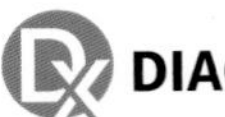

DIAGNOSIS

HISTORY

Cutaneous lesions of GA are generally asymptomatic. They may persist for months or years; longer duration is more often seen in the generalized subtype. They typically resolve spontaneously, and they may recur.

PHYSICAL EXAM

- Localized: small (1–2 mm) papules arranged in a ring, which may enlarge from 5 mm to 5 cm. Color may range from skin-colored to red. The most common locations are the dorsal aspects of the distal extremities.
- Generalized: similar to localized but a higher number of lesions (>10), which are more diffuse distribution, often larger, and typically persist longer
- Patch type: erythematous macules and patches distributed symmetrically on the extremities and trunk. The typical annular configuration may not be present.
- SC: firm, nontender, SC nodule, which tends to grow rapidly. Usually solitary but may occur in groups. Most common location is lower extremities, especially pretibial; other sites include upper extremities, scalp, and buttocks.
- Perforating: Papules may be up to 4 mm and display umbilication, crusting, or scale. Lesions are often generalized and may occur anywhere.

DIFFERENTIAL DIAGNOSIS

- Localized: tinea corporis, annular lichen planus, necrobiosis lipoidica, pityriasis rosea, erythema migrans of Lyme disease, leprosy
- Generalized: sarcoidosis, lichen planus, cutaneous metastases, mycosis fungoides
- Patch type: erythema migrans
- SC: rheumatoid nodule
- Perforating: molluscum contagiosum, sarcoidosis, insect bites

DIAGNOSTIC TESTS & INTERPRETATION

Initial Tests (lab, imaging)

- Diagnosis is typically established by the history and physical, so lab investigations are rarely needed. Skin scraping/KOH test may be useful for excluding a fungal process.
- Consideration could be given to testing for dyslipidemia.
- Rarely indicated but may occasionally be useful in the workup of suspected SC subtype

Diagnostic Procedures/Other

Skin punch biopsy is useful to confirm the diagnosis and designate subtype. Immunohistochemical streptavidin-biotin-horseradish peroxidase (HRP) analysis for CD68/KP-1, which is a marker for histiocytic differentiation, may aid in the diagnosis.

Test Interpretation

Dermal granulomatous infiltrate demonstrating foci of degenerative collagen associated with palisading around an anuclear dermis with mucin deposition. Histologic variants include interstitial (histiocytic infiltrate between collagen fibers), classic (palisading dermal granulomas), and epithelioid (tuberculoid and sarcoidal granulomas).

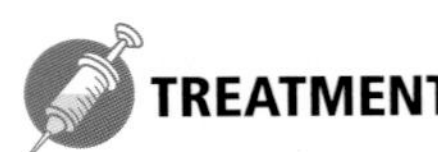

TREATMENT

GENERAL MEASURES

GA is a self-limited, asymptomatic condition that is likely to regress spontaneously. The clinician's primary role after diagnosis is to educate the patient regarding the anticipated natural history and to provide reassurance.

MEDICATION

- No strong evidence supports therapeutic intervention for GA. Reassurance with observation may be adequate treatment for localized, asymptomatic disease.
- The trauma induced by biopsy alone can cause involution of the lesions through an unknown mechanism.
- The following therapies have been tried with variable success, and the possible benefit of treatment must be weighed against the significant toxicities of these treatments.

First Line

Corticosteroids (1)

- High-potency topical, with or without occlusion
- Intralesional triamcinolone: 2.5–5 mg/mL

Second Line

- Methotrexate: 15 mg IM weekly (2)
- Rifampin: 600 mg, ofloxacin 400 mg, with minocycline 100 mg once daily (3)
- Pimecrolimus 1% cream BID
- Isotretinoin: 0.5–0.75 mg/kg/day
- Dapsone: 100 mg/day
- Chloroquine: 3 mg/kg/day
- Hydroxychloroquine: 3–6 mg/kg/day
- Cyclosporine: 3–4 mg/kg/day
- Niacinamide: 500 mg TID
- TNF-α inhibitors, such as infliximab 5 mg/kg IV weeks 0, 2, and 6 and monthly thereafter × 10 months or adalimumab 80 mg SC × 1 for the 1st week then 40 SC × 1 for weeks 2–4

ADDITIONAL THERAPIES

- Fractional thermolysis (Er:YAG fractionated laser)
- Psoralen ultraviolet A (PUVA)
- Cryotherapy
- Surgical excision for SC GA

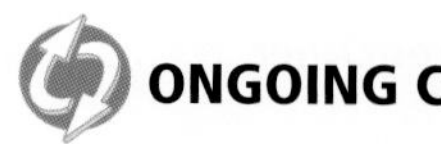

ONGOING CARE

FOLLOW-UP RECOMMENDATIONS

Routine follow-up is not required unless treatment is initiated. Then follow-up may be important to monitor for possible adverse effects associated with treatment. Referral to a dermatologist is prudent in cases of generalized GA and in those cases that persist despite conservative therapy.

PATIENT EDUCATION

The patient should be educated that GA is a benign, self-limited condition that may persist a long time, resolve, and/or recur.

PROGNOSIS

>50% of cases resolve spontaneously within 2 months–2 years, although recurrence—typically at the original site—is common (>40%). Patients <39 years have been shown to have a shorter duration of illness.

COMPLICATIONS

Complications of treatment are much more likely than complications from GA.

REFERENCES

1. Cyr PR. Diagnosis and management of granuloma annulare. *Am Fam Physician*. 2006;74(10):1729–1734.
2. Plotner AN, Mutasim DF. Successful treatment of disseminated granuloma annulare with methotrexate. *Br J Dermatol*. 2010;163(5):1123–1124.
3. Marcus DV, Mahmoud BH, Hamzavi IH. Granuloma annulare treated with rifampin, ofloxacin, and minocycline combination therapy. *Arch Dermatol*. 2009;145(7):787–789.

ADDITIONAL READING

- Browne F, Turner D, Goulden V. Psoralen and ultraviolet A in the treatment of granuloma annulare. *Photodermatol Photoimmuno Photomed*. 2011;27(2):81–84.
- Duarte AF, Mota A. Generalized granuloma annulare—response to doxycycline. *J Eur Acad Dermat and Vener*. 2009;23(1):84–85.
- Liu A, Hexsel CL, Moy RL, et al. Granuloma annulare successfully treated using fractional photothermolysis with a 1,550-nm erbium-doped yttrium aluminum garnet fractionated laser. *Dermatol Surg*. 2011;37(5):712–715.
- Mazzatenta C, Ghilardi A, Grazzini M. Treatment of disseminated granuloma annulare with allopurinol: case report. *Dermatol Therapy*. 2010;23(Suppl 1):S24–S27.
- Misago N, Narisawa Y. Subcutaneous granuloma annulare with overlying localized granuloma annulare. *J Dermatol*. 2010;37(8):755–757.
- Plotner AN, Mutasim DF. Successful treatment of disseminated granuloma annulare with methotrexate. *Br J Dermatol*. 2010;163(5):1123–1124.
- Shanmuga SC, Rai R, Laila A, et al. Generalized granuloma annulare with tuberculoid granulomas: a rare histopathologic variant. *Indian J Dermatol Venereol Leprol*. 2010;76(1):73–75.
- Werchau S, Enk A, Hartmann M. Generalized interstitial granuloma annulare—response to adalimumab. *Int J Dermatol*. 2010;49(4):457–460.
- Wu W, Robinson-Bostom L, Kokkotou E. Dyslipidemia in granuloma annulare: a case-control study. *Arch Dermatol*. 2012;148(10):1131–1136.

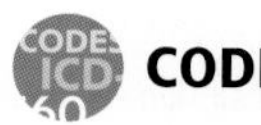

CODES

ICD10

L92.0 Granuloma annulare

CLINICAL PEARLS

- This condition is benign.
- In cases of suspected tinea that lack scaling, consider GA.
- Consider lipid testing, especially in those with generalized subtype.

GRANULOMA, PYOGENIC

Eddie Needham, MD, FAAFP

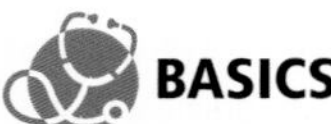

BASICS

DESCRIPTION

- Pyogenic granulomas (PG) are benign, acquired, solitary vascular proliferations that occur most often on the head and neck, the lips and oral cavity, the trunk, and the extremities (1).
- They are friable and tend to bleed easily due to the vascular nature of the lesion.
- Smooth, red to purple, sessile or pedunculated, grow rapidly over several weeks
- Synonym(s): Given that PG are neither pyogenic nor granulomatous, another term is lobular capillary hemangioma.

EPIDEMIOLOGY

The peak incidence of PG are the 2nd and 3rd decades of life. (2)

Incidence

- In children, PG accounts for <1% of all skin lesions.
- 42% of all cases occur by age 5 years (2).
- 2% of pregnant women in the United States develop a PG by 5 months' pregnancy (3).

Prevalence

Relatively common condition

ETIOLOGY AND PATHOPHYSIOLOGY

- Thought to be an aberrant healing response to minor trauma in many cases
- May be related to hormonal changes in pregnancy
- Not caused by bacterial infection but associated with capillary proliferation
- Not considered a hemangioma or neoplasm
- Associated with acute and chronic trauma, peripheral nerve injury, inflammatory systemic diseases, infection, drugs (systemic steroids, protease inhibitors, retinoids, epidermal growth factor receptor inhibitors)

RISK FACTORS

- Pregnancy
- Trauma
- Intraoral trauma or surgery
- Inflammatory systemic diseases

GENERAL PREVENTION

Good oral hygiene may be helpful.

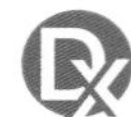

DIAGNOSIS

HISTORY

- Solitary lesion that develops rapidly from days to weeks after minor trauma
- Tends to bleed easily
- Grows early in pregnancy and partially regresses postpartum

PHYSICAL EXAM

- Most commonly located at head, neck, and upper extremities, especially in children
- Among oral lesions, gingiva is the most common location.
- Usually a bright red, friable papule. Can also be purple, yellow, or brown
- Moist and sometimes scaly-appearing surface
- Usually <1 cm but ranges from a few millimeters to 2–3 cm in diameter
- Giant lesions may occur on areas such as the foot (rare).
- Soft; pedunculated or sessile
- Solitary red papule, grows rapidly, forming a stalk, may bleed and ulcerate.
- On diascopy, red structureless areas surrounded by a white collarette intersected by white lines
- Erythematous, soft compressible papule with serosanguineous crusting and sharp demarcation

DIFFERENTIAL DIAGNOSIS

- Benign lesions
  - Cherry/infantile hemangioma (4)
  - Fibrous papule (1,4)
  - Bacillary angiomatosis, from by *Bartonella* (1)
- Malignant lesions
  - Basal cell carcinoma (1)
  - Squamous cell carcinoma (1)
  - Amelanotic melanoma (1)
  - Kaposi sarcoma (1)
  - Cutaneous metastases (1)

DIAGNOSTIC TESTS & INTERPRETATION

Initial Tests (lab, imaging)

No labs are necessary for the diagnosis.

Diagnostic Procedures/Other

- Excisional/shave biopsy
- Send for pathology.

Test Interpretation

Microscopic examination reveals

- Small, endothelial-lined vascular spaces
- Loose/dense connective tissue stroma
- Acute and chronic inflammatory cells

- *No true granuloma formation*
- Abundant mitotic activity
- Resembles granulation tissue in an edematous matrix, showing immature capillaries with interspersed tissue

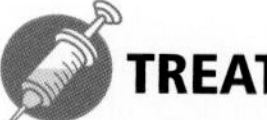

TREATMENT

When feasible, surgical excision is best to yield material for histopathologic analysis (1,5).

MEDICATION

- Cryotherapy with liquid nitrogen (recur 2%) (6)[B]
- Laser (recur 5%) (6)[B]
- Topical imiquimod (recur 0%) (6)[B]
- Silver nitrate (recur 15%) (6)[A]
- Topical 1.5% phenol solution may be used for periungual lesion (6)[B].
- Perform excision for bx if recurrent.

SURGERY/OTHER PROCEDURES

- Excisional biopsy should be tried in all situations, if possible, to ensure a proper diagnosis (i.e., not missing malignancies such as amelanotic melanoma or basal cell carcinoma) (recur 2–3%) (6)[B]. For smaller lesions in noncosmetically sensitive areas, surgical excision with simple closure gives the best result with least recurrence (6)[B].
- Liquid nitrogen may be nonsurgical option with the lowest recurrence rate (recur 2%) (6)[B].
- Shave excision with cautery may be optimal treatment for a lesion on fingertips (recur 7–9%) (6)[B].
- Electrosurgery: electrodesiccation and curettage (recur 7–9%) (6)[B]
- Excision must be adequate to avoid recurrence. Even a small fragment of tissue left behind may lead to recurrence.

ONGOING CARE

PATIENT EDUCATION

Patient should avoid trauma to area following excision.

PROGNOSIS

- Some lesions spontaneously resolve on their own (usually within 6 months).
- Complete resolution is expected with adequate excision.

COMPLICATIONS

Recurrence: After removal or destruction of solitary lesion, multiple satellite lesions can form around original treatment site.

REFERENCES

1. Lin RL, Janniger CK. Pyogenic granuloma. *Cutis*. 2004;74(4):229–233.
2. Harris MN, Desai R, Chuang TY, et al. Lobular capillary hemangiomas: an epidemiologic report, with emphasis on cutaneous lesions. *J Am Acad Dermatol*. 2000;42(6):1012–1016.
3. Kroumpouzos G, Cohen LM. Dermatoses of pregnancy. *J Am Acad Dermatol*. 2001;45(1):1–19.
4. Pagliai KA, Cohen BA. Pyogenic granuloma in children. *Pediatr Dermatol*. 2004;21(1):10–13.
5. Gilmore A, Kelsberg G, Safranek S. Clinical inquiries. What's the best treatment for pyogenic granuloma? *J Fam Pract*. 2010;59(1):40–42.
6. Lee J, Sinno H, Tahiri Y, et al. Treatment options for cutaneous pyogenic granulomas: a review. *J Plast Reconstr Aesthet Surg*. 2011;64(9):1216–1220.

ADDITIONAL READING

- Greene AK. Management of hemangiomas and other vascular tumors. *Clin Plast Surg*. 2011;38(1):45–63.
- Losa Iglesias ME, Becerro de Bengoa Vallejo RB. Topical phenol as a conservative treatment for periungual pyogenic granuloma. *Dermatol Surg*. 2010;36(5):675–678.
- Piraccini BM, Bellavista S, Misciali C, et al. Periungual and subungual pyogenic granuloma. *Br J Dermatol*. 2010;163(5):941–953.
- Zalaudek I, Kreusch J, Giacomel J, et al. How to diagnose nonpigmented skin tumors: a review of vascular structures seen with dermoscopy: part II. Nonmelanocytic skin tumors. *J Am Acad Dermatol*. 2010;63(3):377–386.

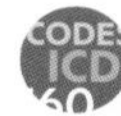

CODES

ICD10

- L98.0 Pyogenic granuloma
- K06.8 Oth disrd of gingiva and edentulous alveolar ridge
- K13.4 Granuloma and granuloma-like lesions of oral mucosa

CLINICAL PEARLS

- Benign, acquired, usually rapidly growing, solitary vascular proliferation that involves exposed areas, such as distal extremities and face, as well as in the oral cavity
- Excision must be adequate to avoid recurrence.
- Excisional biopsy recommended to ensure proper diagnosis (and to not miss a malignant lesion)
- Excision with primary closure or excision with cautery should be the 1st choice for treatment in most lesions.

GRAVES DISEASE

Mohita Patel, MD • Nora Gimpel, MD

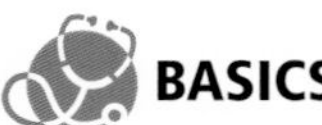

BASICS

DESCRIPTION

Autoimmune disease in which thyroid-stimulating antibodies cause increased thyroid function; most common cause of hyperthyroidism. Classic findings are goiter, ophthalmopathy (orbitopathy), and occasionally dermopathy (pretibial or localized myxedema).

EPIDEMIOLOGY

Prevalence

- Overall prevalence of hyperthyroidism in United States: ~2% for women and 0.2% for men
- More common in white and Hispanic populations in comparison to the black population
- Graves disease accounts for 60–80% of all cases of hyperthyroidism.
- Hyperthyroidism occurs in 0.2% of pregnancies, of which 95% is due to Graves disease.
- Predominant age: 30–40 years
- Synonym(s): Basedow disease

ETIOLOGY AND PATHOPHYSIOLOGY

- Excessive production of TSH receptor antibodies from B cells primarily within the thyroid, likely due to genetic clonal lack of suppressor T cells
- Binding of these antibodies to TSH receptors in the thyroid activates the receptor, stimulating thyroid hormone synthesis and secretion as well as thyroid growth (leading to goiter).
- Binding to similar antigen in retro-orbital connective tissue causes ocular symptoms.

Genetics

Higher risk with personal or family history of any autoimmune disease, especially Hashimoto thyroiditis

RISK FACTORS

- Female gender
- Postpartum period
- Stressful life events
- Medications: iodine, amiodarone, lithium, highly active antiretroviral (HAART); rarely, immune-modulating medications (e.g., interferon therapy)
- Smoking (higher risk of developing ophthalmopathy)

GENERAL PREVENTION

Screening thyroid-stimulating hormone (TSH) in asymptomatic patients is not recommended. No data conclusively show that treatment of subclinical thyroid dysfunction improves quality of life or clinical outcome measures.

COMMONLY ASSOCIATED CONDITIONS

- Mitral valve prolapse
- Type 1 diabetes mellitus
- Addison disease, hypokalemic periodic paralysis
- Vitiligo, alopecia areata
- Other autoimmune disorders (myasthenia gravis, celiac disease)

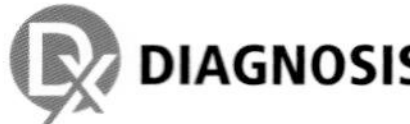

DIAGNOSIS

Hyperthyroid patients appear hypermetabolic with increased adrenergic tone.

HISTORY

- Tachycardia, palpitations
- Tremor, restlessness
- Hyperactivity, anxiety, emotional lability, insomnia
- Sweating, heat intolerance
- Pruritus, skin changes
- Weight loss with increased appetite
- Fatigue, dyspnea (due to muscle weakness)
- Oligo-/amenorrhea (women), loss of libido, erectile dysfunction (men), gynecomastia
- Loose, frequent stools
- Blurred vision or diplopia, lacrimation, photophobia, gritty sensation in eyes (ocular dryness), retro-orbital discomfort, painful eye movement, loss of color vision or visual acuity
- Worsening of chronic medical conditions (anxiety, bipolar disorder, glucose intolerance, heart failure, or angina)

Geriatric Considerations

Elderly patients may not display classic symptoms; may present with atrial fibrillation, weight loss, or shortness of breath (1)[B]

PHYSICAL EXAM

- Ophthalmologic (present in 50% of cases): grittiness/discomfort in the eyes, retrobulbar pressure/pain, lid lag/retraction, proptosis, ophthalmoplegia; papilledema and loss of color vision may signify optic neuropathy
- Thyroid: enlarged (goiter), nontender, and without nodules; possible bruit (increased blood flow)
- Integumentary: fine hair, warm skin, onycholysis, palmar erythema, possible pretibial myxedema (orange peel appearance), possible hyperpigmented plaques (dermopathy)
- Cardiac: resting tachycardia, hyperdynamic circulation, possible atrial fibrillation
- Extremities: fine tremor, hyperreflexia, proximal myopathy; rarely, soft tissue edema of extremities and clubbing of digits (acropachy)

DIFFERENTIAL DIAGNOSIS

- Toxic multinodular goiter (multiple hormone-producing nodules)
- Toxic adenoma (single hormone-producing nodule)
- Thyroiditis (hormone leakage)
  - Subacute, usually postviral (thyroid will be tender)
  - Lymphocytic, including postpartum
  - Hashimoto thyroiditis (antithyroperoxidase [TPO] antibodies may stimulate TSH receptors)
- Iatrogenic (treatment-induced)
  - Iodine-induced (dietary, radiographic contrast, or medications)
  - Amiodarone
  - Thyroid hormone overreplacement (accidental or intentional)
- Tumor
  - Pituitary adenoma producing TSH
  - Human chorionic gonadotropin (hCG)-producing tumors (stimulate TSH receptors)
  - Extraglandular thyroid hormone production (e.g., struma ovarii or metastatic thyroid cancer)

DIAGNOSTIC TESTS & INTERPRETATION

Initial Tests (lab, imaging)

- TSH is initial test: suppressed (low or undetectable) TSH confirms hyperthyroidism.
- Free T_4 level will be high in Graves disease.
- After confirming suppressed TSH and high T_4, perform radioactive iodine uptake (RAIU) and scan. Patients with Graves disease will have diffuse, elevated RAIU (vs. localized/nodular elevated uptake in adenoma and multinodular goiter, and decreased uptake in thyroiditis or exogenous thyroid hormone).

Pregnancy Considerations

Increase in serum T_4-binding globulin concentration and initial stimulation of TSH by hCG results in a total T_4 and T_3 rise during first ½ of pregnancy. The TSH level is decreased throughout pregnancy and should be compared to the trimester-specific ranges for pregnancy. Measurement of thyrotropin receptor antibody (TRAb) is positive in 95% of patients with Graves and should be used if diagnosis is unclear in pregnancy (2)[B].

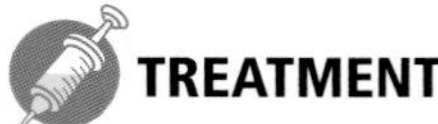

TREATMENT

MEDICATION

Goal is to correct hypermetabolic state with the fewest side effects and lowest incidence of posttreatment hypothyroidism.

First Line

- β-blockers provide prompt control of adrenergic symptoms; start while workup is in progress. Long-acting propranolol is used most commonly and titrated to symptom control (40–320 mg/day). Calcium channel blockers are an alternative in patients who cannot take β-blockers (3)[C].
- Radioactive iodine (RAI)
  - Concentrates in the thyroid gland and destroys thyroid tissue
  - Treatment of choice in the United States for Graves disease (4)[C]
  - High cure rate with single treatment, especially with high-dose regimen
  - Risks: side effects (neck soreness, flushing, decreased taste); worsening ophthalmopathy (15% incidence, higher in smokers); posttreatment hypothyroidism (80% incidence, not dosage-dependent); radiation thyroiditis (1% incidence); need to adhere to safety precautions until radiation is eliminated from the body
  - May worsen Graves orbitopathy (GO): Symptoms are usually mild and transient in those patients with no or mild ophthalmopathy; however, treatment for patients with moderate to severe GO is still guided by expert opinion pending further study (5)[C].
  - Pretreatment with antithyroid medication should be considered in patients with severe disease and the elderly to reduce risk of posttreatment transient hyperthyroidism and posttreatment radiation thyroiditis as well as quicker return to normal thyroid function. Controversy remains regarding whether pretreatment results in treatment failure, and no definitive data support use (6)[C].
  - May be repeated in as soon as 3 months but usually after 6 months if not euthyroid

Pregnancy Considerations

RAI is contraindicated in pregnancy and during breastfeeding:

- Antithyroid drugs: methimazole (MMI) and propylthiouracil (PTU)
  - Compete with the thyroid for iodine, thereby decreasing the synthesis of thyroid hormone; PTU blocks peripheral conversion of T_4 to T_3.
  - Treatment of choice for children and for adults who refuse radioactive iodine
  - May use as pretreatment for older or cardiac patients before radioactive iodine or surgery

– MMI is usually first choice due to lower cost and once-daily dosing; additionally, the risk of hepatocellular inflammation and severe liver damage (0.1%) with PTU make it second line to MMI for most patients (7)[C].
– No improvement in remission rates noted with higher dose MMI; lowest effective dose should be used (8)[B].
– Minor side effects (<5% incidence): controlled by switching from 1 agent to another: rash, fever, arthralgias, GI side effects
– Major side effects necessitating change in treatment: polyarthritis (1–2%), agranulocytosis (<0.5%), and cholestasis/jaundice (rare)
– Discontinue treatment after 1 year if patient is euthyroid and thyroid-stimulating antibody level is undetectable.
– 60% remission rate with 2 years of treatment (standard regimen); newer studies suggest no increased benefit to treatment beyond 18 months (4,9)[B].
– Relapse rates up to 50% in patients who respond initially; higher rates if smoker, large goiter, or positive thyroid-stimulating antibodies at end of treatment.

Pregnancy Considerations
PTU is preferred in 1st trimester of pregnancy due to teratogenic effects of MMI. Switch to MMI in 2nd and 3rd trimesters due to risk of PTU-induced hepatotoxicity (10,11)[C].

Second Line
Plasmapheresis is under investigation as a treatment option (3)[C], as is rituximab (immune modulator) for thyroid eye disease (12)[C] and possibly dermatopathy (13)[C].

ISSUES FOR REFERRAL
- Endocrinologist for radioactive iodine therapy; if patient is pregnant or breastfeeding
- Graves ophthalmopathy
- Surgery if failed drug therapy or refusing RAI; obstruction or cosmesis

ADDITIONAL THERAPIES
- Symptom control may be achieved with iodides, which block conversion of T_4 to T_3 and inhibit TSH release. Use for pregnant patients who do not tolerate antithyroid medication or in conjunction with antithyroid medications. Should not be used long term (may cause paradoxical increase in TSH release) or in combination with radioactive iodine.
- For corneal protection: tinted glasses when outdoors, artificial tears, patching/taping the lids at night
- For orbitopathy: Mild cases can be treated with lubricants, nocturnal ointments, botulinum toxin injection for upper lid retraction, and smoking cessation (14)[C]. Moderate to severe cases should be treated with pulse-dose IV glucocorticoid if no contraindications (15)[C]. Alternative is PO steroid (prednisone 60–80 mg/day for 2–4 weeks, then taper off).
- For dermopathy, medium- to high-potency topical corticosteroid

SURGERY/OTHER PROCEDURES
Total thyroidectomy (TT) is the procedure of choice (4)[C] and offers a better chance of cure than a bilateralsubtotal thyroidectomy (preserves some thyroid function but has a less predictable outcome) (16)[C].

COMPLEMENTARY & ALTERNATIVE MEDICINE
Nutritional supplementation with L-carnitine may act as an antagonist of thyroid hormone and reduce hyperthyroid symptoms as well as decrease bone demineralization.

INPATIENT CONSIDERATIONS
Indications for hospital admission:
- Thyroid storm (rare but life-threatening complication): Admit to ICU.
- Ophthalmopathy with visual impairment: severe cardiac symptoms (heart failure, rapid atrial fibrillation, angina)

ONGOING CARE

FOLLOW-UP RECOMMENDATIONS
Patient Monitoring
- Monitoring is for resolution of hyperthyroidism and for development of hypothyroidism.
- Check TSH and T_4 levels every 1–2 months for first 6 months after treatment, then every 3 months for a year, then every 6–12 months thereafter. For patients on treatment with PTU and MMI, CBC, check anti-TSH receptor antibodies at 12 months of treatment to determine possibility of discontinuing medication.

Pregnancy Considerations
Postpartum exacerbation of hyperthyroidism is common for women not currently under treatment, so TSH and symptoms should be monitored.

PATIENT EDUCATION
Adherence to both follow-up surveillance and medication regimens is the most important way to achieve a good outcome and promote lifelong health.

PROGNOSIS
- Generally good with treatment
- May have irreversible ocular, cardiac, and psychiatric consequences
- Increased morbidity and mortality due to osteoporosis, atherosclerotic disease, insulin resistance and obesity, and endothelial cell dysfunction (thromboembolic risk)

COMPLICATIONS
Hypothyroidism is most common consequence of treatment (25–80%, depending on treatment modality). Patients should be monitored annually, even if asymptomatic.

REFERENCES

1. Bartalena L. The dilemma of how to manage Graves' hyperthyroidism in patients with associated orbitopathy. *J Clin Endocrinol Metab*. 2011;96(2):592–599.
2. Bahn Chair RS, Burch HB, Cooper DS, et al. Hyperthyroidism and other causes of thyrotoxicosis: management guidelines of the American Thyroid Association and American Association of Clinical Endocrinologists. *Thyroid*. 2011;21(6):593–646.
3. Reid JR, Wheeler SF. Hyperthyroidism: diagnosis and treatment. *Am Fam Physician*. 2005;72(4):623–630.
4. Benker G, Reinwein D, Kahaly G, et al. Is there a methimazole dose effect on remission rate in Graves' disease? Results from a long-term prospective study. The European Multicentre Trial Group of the Treatment of Hyperthyroidism with Antithyroid Drugs. *Clin Endocrinol*. 1998;49(4):451–457.
5. Boelaert K, Torlinska B, Holder RL, et al. Older subjects with hyperthyroidism present with a paucity of symptoms and signs: a large cross-sectional study. *J Clin Endocrinol Metab*. 2010;95(6):2715–2726.
6. Cooper DS, Rivkees SA. Putting propylthiouracil in perspective. *J Clin Endocrinol Metab*. 2009;94(6):1881–1882.
7. Hegedüs L, Smith TJ, Douglas RS, et al. Targeted biological therapies for Graves' disease and thyroid-associated ophthalmopathy. Focus on B-cell depletion with Rituximab. *Clin Endocrinol (Oxf)*. 2011;74(1):1–8.
8. Helfand M; U.S. Preventive Services Task Force. Screening for subclinical thyroid dysfunction in nonpregnant adults: a summary of the evidence for the U.S. Preventive Services Task Force. *Ann Intern Med*. 2004;140(2):128–141.
9. Maugendre D, Gatel A, Campion L, et al. Antithyroid drugs and Graves' disease—prospective randomized assessment of long-term treatment. *Clin Endocrinol*. 2004;50(1):127–132.
10. Mitchell AL, Gan EH, Morris M, et al. The effect of B cell depletion therapy on anti-TSH receptor antibodies and clinical outcome in glucocorticoid-refractory Graves' orbitopathy. *Clin Endocrinol*. 2013;79(3):437–442.
11. Oszukowska L, Knapska-Kucharska M, Lewiński A. Effects of drugs on the efficacy of radioiodine (131I) therapy in hyperthyroid patients. *Arch Med Sci*. 2010;6(1):4–10.
12. Stagnaro-Green A, Abalovich M, Alexander E, et al. Guidelines of the American Thyroid Association for the diagnosis and management of thyroid disease during pregnancy and postpartum. *Thyroid*. 2011;21(10):1081–1125.
13. Yoshihara A, Noh J, Yamaguchi T, et al. Treatment of Graves' disease with antithyroid drugs in the first trimester of pregnancy and the prevalence of congenital malformation. *J Clin Endocrinol Metab*. 2012;97(7):2396–2403.
14. Melcescu E, Horton WB, Kim D, et al. Graves orbitopathy: update on diagnosis and therapy. *South Med J*. 2014;107(1):34–43.
15. Zang S, Ponto KA, Kahaly GJ. Clinical review: intravenous glucocorticoids for Graves' orbitopathy: efficacy and morbidity. *J Clin Endocrinol Metab*. 2011;96(2):320–332.
16. Feroci F, Rettori M, Borrelli A, et al. A systematic review and meta-analysis of total thyroidectomy versus bilateral subtotal thyroidectomy for Graves' disease. *Surgery*. 2014;155(3):529–540.

SEE ALSO

See also topics: Anxiety; Cardiac Arrhythmias; Weight Loss

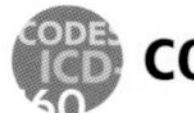

CODES

ICD10
- E05.00 Thyrotoxicosis w diffuse goiter w/o thyrotoxic crisis
- E05.01 Thyrotoxicosis w diffuse goiter w thyrotoxic crisis or storm

CLINICAL PEARLS

Thyroid hormone controls metabolic rate and affects many organ systems. Hyperthyroid patients appear hypermetabolic, with symptoms and signs of increased adrenergic tone.

G

GROWTH HORMONE DEFICIENCY

Abigail Weil Hoffman, MD • Rod Pellenberg, MD • Edward James Kruse, DO

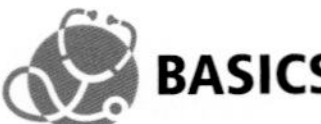

BASICS

DESCRIPTION

- Insufficient production of growth hormone (GH) in adults or children caused by problems arising in the pituitary gland
- GH is produced by somatotroph cells of the anterior pituitary gland, which is stimulated by growth hormone–releasing hormone (GHRH) and inhibited by somatostatin from the hypothalamus.
- GH, also called *somatotropin*, is a polypeptide hormone that stimulates growth and cell reproduction.
- Hypopituitarism is GH deficiency (GHD) plus a deficiency in at least 1 other anterior pituitary hormone.
- Panhypopituitarism is a deficiency in all the hormones produced in the pituitary gland.
- System(s) affected: endocrine, musculoskeletal, psychological
- Synonym(s) and keywords: hypopituitarism; familial short stature; short height; growth pattern; pituitary dwarfism; acquired GHD; isolated GHD; congenital GHD; panhypopituitarism

EPIDEMIOLOGY

Incidence

- Most common cause of GHD in children is idiopathic.
- Most common cause of GHD in adults is a pituitary adenoma or treatment of the adenoma with surgery or radiotherapy:
  - 76% of patients with GHD had a pituitary tumor.
  - 13% had an extrapituitary tumor.
  - 8% idiopathic cause
  - 1% had sarcoidosis.
  - 0.5% had Sheehan syndrome.

Prevalence

- In children, isolated GHD is reported to affect 1 in 5,000.
- Adult-onset idiopathic GHD is extremely rare.

ETIOLOGY AND PATHOPHYSIOLOGY

- GHD is caused by a genetic or acquired absence or decline in production of GH.
- Hypothalamus secretes GHRH, which stimulates the pituitary to secrete GH.
- Somatostatin is secreted by the hypothalamus to inhibit GH secretion.
- When GH pulses are secreted into the blood, then insulin-like growth factor (IGF)-1 is released.
- GHD may result from disruption of the GH axis—in the higher brain, the hypothalamus, or the pituitary gland (1)[C].
- Congenital
  - Genetic (see "Genetics")
  - Structural brain defects
    - Agenesis of corpus callosum
    - Septo-optic dysplasia
    - Empty sella syndrome
    - Encephalocele
    - Hydrocephalus
    - Arachnoid cyst
  - Associated midline facial defects
    - Single central incisor
    - Cleft lip/palate
- Acquired
  - Trauma
  - CNS infection
  - Tumors of hypothalamus or pituitary
    - Pituitary adenoma
    - Craniopharyngioma
    - Rathke cleft cyst
    - Glioma/astrocytoma
    - Germinoma
    - Metastatic tumor
  - Infiltrative/granulomatous disease
    - Sarcoidosis
    - Tuberculosis
    - Langerhans cell histiocytosis
    - Hypophysitis
  - Cranial irradiation
  - Idiopathic
  - Pituitary infarction
  - Surgical
  - Hemochromatosis (rare)

Genetics

A variety of congenital genetic causes of GHD:

- Transcription factor defects (POU1F1/PIT-1, PROP-1, LHX3/4, HESX-1, and PITX-2)
- GHRH-receptor gene defects
- GH secretagogue receptor gene defects
- GH receptor/postreceptor defects
- Prader-Willi syndrome
- Deletion and mutation of GH-1

COMMONLY ASSOCIATED CONDITIONS

- Macroadenoma
- Sarcoidosis
- Sheehan syndrome

DIAGNOSIS

HISTORY

- Children
  - Poor height velocity, slower muscular development, and delayed gross motor milestones, such as standing, walking, and jumping
  - Clinical questions
    - Birth weight and length
    - Previous growth points
    - Nutritional history
    - General health of child
    - Height of parents
    - Timing of puberty in parents
- Adults: Always consider evaluation in patients with structural hypothalamic/pituitary disease, surgery or radiation to hypothalamic/pituitary region, head traumatic brain injury, or a subarachnoid hemorrhage and evidence of other pituitary disorders:
  - Fatigue
  - Muscle weakness
  - Depression
  - Social withdrawal
  - Poor memory
  - Loss of strength and/or stamina
  - Reduced physical performance

PHYSICAL EXAM

- Children with GHD
  - Most common presentation is short stature and drop off in height, then weight, then head circumference on the growth curve:
    - Strong suspicion if >2.5 *SD* below mean (corresponds to <0.5 percentile) for height (for chronologic, age, sex, and background) and/or height velocity >2 *SD* below mean (corresponds to approximately <3rd percentile) (2)[C]
  - Newborns may present with hypoglycemia, prolonged jaundice, or micropenis.
  - Children with severe GHD have maxillary hypoplasia and forehead prominence.
  - Accurately measure height and weight.
  - Assess pubertal status using Tanner staging system.
- Adults
  - Decreased lean body mass
  - Increased fat mass, particularly in the abdominal region
  - Poor bone density
  - Reduced physical performance: loss of strength, stamina, and muscle
  - Reduced quality of life: poor memory, social withdrawal, and depression
  - Abnormal labs
    - Dyslipidemia
    - Increased insulin resistance
    - Glucose intolerance

DIFFERENTIAL DIAGNOSIS

- Adrenal insufficiency
- Hypothyroidism
- Turner syndrome
- Renal failure
- Small size for gestational age in newborns
- Prader-Willi syndrome
- Idiopathic short stature
- Noonan syndrome
- Russell-Silver syndrome
- Down syndrome

DIAGNOSTIC TESTS & INTERPRETATION

Initial Tests (lab, imaging)

- Thyroid-stimulating hormone (TSH): Hypothyroidism should be excluded, and thyroxine should be adequately replaced prior to testing for GHD.
- Serum electrolytes (low bicarbonate levels may indicate renal tubular acidosis)
- CBC
- ESR
- Karyotype (in females to rule out Turner syndrome)
- Radiograph of hand and wrist to determine skeletal age in children
- GHD is effectively excluded in children with normal bone age and height velocity.

Follow-Up Tests & Special Considerations

- If labs above are normal and growth curve shows short stature and drop off in height, then weight, then head circumference, consider IGF-1 and insulin-like growth factor–binding protein (IGFBP-3) (both decreased in GHD).

- IGF-1 is a good screening test for GHD in younger, lean patients (<40 years; BMI <25 kg/m^2) with evidence of hypopituitarism; however, a normal IGF-1 does not rule out GHD at any age.
- Multiple blood sample testing for GH levels: Testing for GHD by random measurement of GH in a single blood sample is not beneficial because GH is nearly undetectable for most of the day.
- Brain MRI to evaluate for a pituitary tumor

Diagnostic Procedures/Other

Stimulatory tests should be done after abnormal levels of IGF-1 or IGFBP-3 are obtained and if they are not explainable by malnutrition:

- Insulin tolerance test (ITT) is considered the gold standard in adults by American Association of Clinical Endocrinologists (AACEs). It is recommended to perform ITT under careful medical management in an experienced endocrine unit and is contraindicated for several clinical conditions including history of seizures or ischemic heart disease (3)[C].
- GHRH-arginine and GHRH + GH releasing peptide-2 (GHRP-2) are most common, although not widely available.
- Alternative provocative tests: Give a dose of an agent that in a normal person causes a surge in the release of GH: Common agents used include arginine, clonidine, glucagons, insulin, levodopa, and propranolol (3)[C].
- After agent is given, GH serum levels are drawn q15min for a total of 60 minutes.

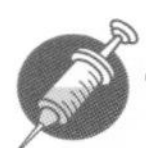

TREATMENT

MEDICATION

- GHD is treated with GH replacement.
- The goal of replacement therapy is to correct the metabolic, functional, and psychological abnormalities associated with GHD.
- Recombinant human growth hormone (rhGH) was first approved for childhood GHD in 1985.
- The recommended rhGH dose for children in the United States is 0.175–0.35 mg/kg/wk, with 0.3 mg/kg/wk being most commonly used. Stepwise increase during pubertal stages has been shown to improve growth velocity. It has also been shown that pulsatile administration is more effective than 3 times weekly.
- The rhGH therapy for adults with GHD offers significant clinical benefits in body composition, including skeletal integrity, lipids, quality of life, and exercise capacity. The dosing plans have evolved from weight-based to individualized dose-titration strategies based on age, gender, estrogen status, IGF-1 levels, appropriate clinical response, and avoidance of side effects (4)[C].
- Several GH-releasing peptides (GHRPs) or nonpeptide analogs are to be evaluated in children and adults. It is too early to evaluate their long-term safety and efficacy.
- Treatment is expensive, costing as much as $10,000–40,000 per year.

ISSUES FOR REFERRAL

Patients with GHD would benefit from a referral to an endocrinologist.

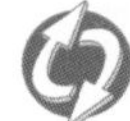

ONGOING CARE

FOLLOW-UP RECOMMENDATIONS

- Children: Follow-up with a pediatric endocrinologist. Most endocrinologist will monitor growth and adjust dose every 3–6 months.
- Childhood onset GHD, the need for continuation of GH replacement should be evaluated following completion of statural growth (usually <20 years).
- Adults: Follow-up with an endocrinologist is recommended. Consider monitoring every 1–2 months during dose titration, then every 6 months. Assess clinical status, side effects, IGF-1 levels. Check fasting lipids and glucose annually. Consider dual-energy x-ray absorptiometry (DEXA) scan for prolonged treatments (>2 years) to quantify changes in body composition and assess bone density (5)[C].

DIET

No restrictions

PROGNOSIS

- Determined by response to GH replacement therapy; is generally favorable
- GH treatment is meant for replacement therapy with expectations of growth at a normal rate.
- 5 independent predictors of pubertal growth:
  - Gender
  - Age at onset of puberty
  - Age at end of growth
  - Dose of GH at onset of puberty
  - Deviation of target height from height at onset of puberty

COMPLICATIONS

- In children:
  - Slipped capital femoral epiphysis
  - Scoliosis
- In adults and children:
  - Premature cardiovascular disease
  - Osteoporosis
  - Psychiatric disturbances
  - Insulin resistance
  - Metabolic effects (monitor thyroid and adrenal functions)
  - Antibodies to GH
  - Cancer: lymphoma, colon, tumor recurrence
  - Fluid retention: pseudotumor cerebri, carpal tunnel syndrome, pancreatitis, and edema

REFERENCES

1. Fukuda I, Hizuka N, Muraoka T, et al. Adult growth hormone deficiency: current concepts. *Neurol Med Chir (Tokyo)*. 2014;54(8):599–605.
2. Miller BS. rhGH safety and efficacy update. Adv *Pediatr*. 2011;58(1):207–241.
3. Molich ME, Clemmons DR, Malozowski S, et al. Evaluation and treatment of adult growth hormone deficiency: an Endocrine Society Clinical Practice Guideline. *J Clin Endocrinol Metab*. 2006;91(5):1621–1634.
4. Molitch ME, Clemmons DR, Malozowski S, et al. Evaluation and treatment of adult growth hormone deficiency: an Endocrine Society Clinical Practice Guideline. *J Clin Endocrinol Metab*. 2011;96(6):1587–1609.
5. Ho KK; 2007 GH Deficiency Consensus Workshop Participants. Consensus guidelines for the diagnosis and treatment of adults with GH deficiency II: a statement of the GH Research Society in association with the European Society for Pediatric Endocrinology, Lawson Wilkins Society, European Society of Endocrinology, Japan Endocrine Society, and Endocrine Society of Australia. *Eur J Endocrinol*. 2007;157(6):695–700.

ADDITIONAL READING

- Binder G. Growth hormone deficiency: new approaches to the diagnosis. *Pediatr Endocrinol Rev*. 2011;9(Suppl 1):535–537.
- Cook DM, Yuen KC, Biller BM, et al. American Association of Clinical Endocrinologists medical guidelines for clinical practice for growth hormone use in growth hormone-deficient adults and transition patients—2009 update. *Endocr Pract*. 2009;15(Suppl 2):1–29.
- Kirk J. Indications for growth hormone therapy in children. *Arch Dis Child*. 2012;97(1):63–68.
- Richmond EJ, Rogol AD. Growth hormone deficiency in children. *Pituitary*. 2008;11(2):115–120.

SEE ALSO

Pituitary Adenoma

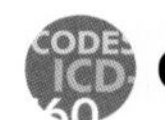

CODES

ICD10

E23.0 Hypopituitarism

CLINICAL PEARLS

- Most common cause of GHD in children is idiopathic.
- Most common cause of GHD in adults is pituitary adenoma.
- Most common presentation of childhood GHD is short stature and poor growth velocity.
- Patients taking replacement GH therapy should have regular monitoring for both adverse effects and physiologic benefits in addition to IGF-1 levels.

G

GUILLAIN-BARRÉ SYNDROME

David Anthony, MD, MSc

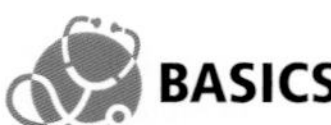

BASICS

DESCRIPTION

- A group of acquired autoimmune disorders causing acute peripheral neuropathy and ascending paralysis
- Subtypes classified by pattern of neural injury:
  - Acute inflammatory demyelinating polyradiculoneuropathy (AIDP)
    - Accounts for ~95% of cases in Europe and North America
    - Progressive limb weakness with areflexia
  - *Acute motor axonal neuropathy* (*AMAN*): Pure motor neuropathy accounts for about 5% of cases in Europe and North America but 30–47% of cases in China, Japan, and Central and South America
  - *Acute motor-sensory axonal neuropathy* (*AMSAN*): Combined motor–sensory neuropathy; poor prognosis
  - *Miller Fisher Syndrome* (*MFS*): *Opthalmoplegia with ataxia and areflexia; antibodies to GQ1b present in 90% of patients with MFS*
- In Guillain-Barré syndrome (GBS), symptoms progress for up to 4 weeks. This distinguishes it from subacute and chronic inflammatory demyelinating polyradiculoneuropathy (CIDP), in which the onset phase lasts 4–8 weeks or >8 weeks, respectively.
- Synonym(s): GBS, acute inflammatory demyelinating polyneuropathy; Landry-Guillain-Barré-Strohl syndrome; acute inflammatory polyneuropathy; idiopathic polyneuritis; acute autoimmune neuropathy; Landry ascending paralysis

ALERT

25–30% of patients have respiratory paralysis. Rapidly progressive forms may cause quadriplegia and a need for mechanical ventilation within 48 hours.

ALERT

Absent reflexes are a red flag for GBS in patients with rapidly progressive limb weakness.

ALERT

A history of weakness preceded by respiratory or GI infection suggests GBS.

EPIDEMIOLOGY

Incidence

- In the United States: 1.8/100,000 (0.8/100,000 in children <18 years of age; 3.2/100,000 in adults >60 years of age)

Prevalence

- In the US: 3–10/100,000
- Male > female (1.5:1)

ETIOLOGY AND PATHOPHYSIOLOGY

- Autoimmune disorder targeted against myelin and/or gangliosides in peripheral nerve tissue causing destruction of peripheral nerves in susceptible individuals
- The pathogenesis is felt to involve molecular mimicry (i.e., invoking an immune response to antigenic targets that are coincidentally shared by infectious organisms and host peripheral nerve tissue).

Genetics

Host factors appear to play a role in GBS, but no clear genetic risk factors have been identified.

RISK FACTORS

- Of patients with GBS, 2/3 have history of a preceding GI (especially *Campylobacter jejuni*), respiratory (especially influenza), or sinus infection.
- Incidence increases with age.
- Males have 1.8 times the risk of females.

COMMONLY ASSOCIATED CONDITIONS

- 2/3 of cases associated with antecedent bacterial or viral infection, usually of the respiratory or GI tract
  - *C. jejuni*: The most common precipitant of GBS, seen in 21–32% of cases:
    - Associated with axonal degeneration, slower recovery, more severe residual disability
  - Cytomegalovirus (CMV): Primary CMV infection precedes 10–22% of cases.
  - Also associated with *Mycoplasma pneumoniae* (5%), influenza, Epstein-Barr virus (EBV), varicella zoster virus, and HIV infections
- Influenza vaccinations
  - Based on 1992–1994 data, inactivated seasonal flu vaccines are associated with a very small increase in the risk of GBS equivalent to about 1 case/million vaccines above background incidence. A steady decline seen in the number of cases of GBS associated with influenza vaccine in the United States between 1993 and 1994 (0.17 per 100,000) and 2002 and 2003 (0.04 per 100,000).
  - Influenza A (H1N1) 2009 monovalent inactivated vaccines were the largest mass vaccination initiative in recent U.S. history and closely studied for adverse effects. A small increased risk of GBS was associated was noted (incidence rate ratio 2:35, 95% CI 1.42–4,01, p = 0.0003). This finding translated to about 1.6 cases of GBS per million people vaccinated. *The benefits of pandemic vaccines outweigh the risks*.
  - By comparison, the attributable risk of GBS following influenza vaccine was 1.03 cases per million doses compared to 17.3 cases of GBS per million episodes of influenza.
  - *Of historical note*: Increased incidence during 1976 U. S. National Immunization Program against swine-origin influenza A H1N1 subtype A/NJ/76; vaccine-attributable risk 8.8 per million recipients

DIAGNOSIS

HISTORY

- AIDP presents as an acute neuropathy, defined as progressive onset of limb weakness that reaches its worst within 4 weeks; 73% of patients reach a nadir of clinical function at 1 week.
- 2/3 of patients have an antecedent, respiratory illness or gastroenteritis, within the prior 6 weeks.
- Earliest symptoms are pain, numbness, paresthesias, or limb weakness. Numbness and paresthesias affect the extremities and spread proximally.
- Pain is present in most patients, commonly in the back and lower extremities; pain may be severe
- A purely sensory syndrome (without weakness) excludes GBS.

PHYSICAL EXAM

Diagnostic criteria for typical GBS

- Features required for diagnosis
  - Progressive weakness of >1 limb
  - Areflexia
  - Paresthesias with only mild changes in objective sensory function (e.g., pinprick)
  - Progression to nadir between 12 hours and 28 days
- Features strongly supporting diagnosis
  - Relative symmetry
  - Antecedent infection
  - Mild sensory symptoms or signs
  - Cranial nerve involvement, especially bilateral weakness of facial muscles
  - Recovery beginning within 4 weeks after progression ceases
  - Autonomic dysfunction
  - Absence of fever at onset

DIFFERENTIAL DIAGNOSIS

Differential diagnosis of acute flaccid paralysis

- Brain: basilar artery stroke, brain stem encephalitis
- Spinal cord: transverse myelitis, cord compression
- Motor neuron: poliomyelitis
- Peripheral neuropathy other than GBS: vasculitis, critical illness polyneuropathy, infectious (e.g., diphtheria, Lyme disease), CIDP, acute intermittent porphyria
- Neuromuscular junction: myasthenia gravis, Eaton-Lambert, botulism, toxins (e.g., heavy metals, inhalant abuse, organophosphates)
- Muscle: electrolyte disturbance (hypokalemia, hypophosphatemia), inflammatory myopathy, critical illness myopathy, acute rhabdomyolysis, trichonosis, periodic paralysis
- Psychological cause of weakness

DIAGNOSTIC TESTS & INTERPRETATION

Initial Tests (lab, imaging)

- Studies to establish the diagnosis:
  - Nerve conduction study: *The most useful confirmatory test*; conduction velocities abnormal in 85% of patients with demyelination, even early in the disease. If nondiagnostic, repeat after 1–2 weeks.
    - Repeat study 3–8 weeks later correctly classifies the subtype of GBS (1)[B].
  - CSF: increase in CSF protein (>0.55 g/L) without pleocytosis (i.e., albuminocytologic dissociation). Elevated protein present in ~80% of patients but often normal within the first 48 hours of symptom onset:
    - CSF should be analyzed before treatment with IVIG, which can also cause aseptic meningitis.
- Studies related to finding underlying cause:
  - Stool culture and serology for *C. jejuni*
  - Acute and convalescent serology for CMV, EBV, and *Mycoplasma pneumoniae*
  - Anti-GQ1b antibodies in Miller Fisher variant
- Imaging is not generally required as the diagnosis can be established by clinical criteria, CSF analysis, and nerve conduction studies.

Follow-Up Tests & Special Considerations

If indicated, labs targeted at specific differential diagnoses.

Diagnostic Procedures/Other

Sural nerve biopsy not indicated unless necessary to rule out vasculitis or amyloidosis.

TREATMENT

GENERAL MEASURES

Pain: Both gabapentin and carbamazepine have been shown to decrease opiate requirements in patients with GBS. One is not preferred over the other (2)[A].

MEDICATION

First Line

- Plasma exchange (PE)
  - Compared with supportive treatment, patients treated with PE are quicker to recover walking, have less requirement for artificial ventilation, have a shorter duration of artificial ventilation, recover full muscle strength more quickly, and have fewer severe sequelae at 1 year (3)[A].
  - In mild GBS, 2 sessions of PE are superior to none. In moderate GBS, 4 sessions are superior to 2. In severe GBS, 6 sessions are not significantly better than 4 (3)[A].
  - PE most beneficial if started within 7 days of disease onset but still helpful until up to 30 days (3)[A].
  - Value of PE in children <12 years is not known.
- IVIG 0.4 g/kg/day for 5 days
  - In severe disease, IVIG started within 2 weeks of onset hastens recovery as much as PE (4)[A].
  - In children, IVIG likely hastens recovery compared with supportive care alone (4)[A].
  - IVIG and PE are equally effective and associated with similar rates of adverse events. IVIG may be preferred due to ease of administration (4)[A].
  - Treatment with IVIG after PE does not confer additional benefit when compared with either treatment alone (4)[A].

Second Line

Corticosteroids have not been shown to be beneficial. Steroids do not significantly hasten recovery from GBS or affect the long-term outcome (5)[A].

COMPLEMENTARY & ALTERNATIVE MEDICINE

A small trial showed that the Chinese herbal medicine Tripterygium polyglycoside hastened recovery significantly more than corticosteroids, but additional confirmatory studies are needed (6)[A].

INPATIENT CONSIDERATIONS

Admission Criteria/Initial Stabilization

- Admit patients suspected of having GBS.
- Mildly affected patients who remain capable of walking unaided and are stable for >2 weeks are unlikely to experience disease progression and may be managed as outpatients.
- 25–30% of patients will require mechanical ventilation, yet classic signs of respiratory distress occur too late to serve as guidelines for management. Serial measurement of vital capacity (VC) and static inspiratory and expiratory pressures (PI_{max} and PE_{max}) are the most useful parameters for evaluating respiratory compromise.
- Predictors of respiratory failure include rapid disease progression (≥3 days between onset of weakness and hospital admission), the presence of facial and/or bulbar weakness, VC <20 mL/kg, VC decrease >30%, and Medical Research Council (MRC) sum score indicating muscle weakness.
- Monitor closely for complications of autonomic dysfunction (e.g., hemodynamic instability, urinary retention, ileus).

Nursing

- Prevent complications of immobilization with graduated compression stockings and SC heparin.
- Respiratory care, aspiration precautions, pulmonary toilet and frequent turning
- Monitor bowel and bladder function for urinary retention and ileus.

ONGOING CARE

FOLLOW-UP RECOMMENDATIONS

Patient Monitoring

- Pulmonary function testing (vital capacity, respiratory frequency) q2–6h in the progressive phase and q6–12h in the plateau phase
- Monitor bulbar weakness and ability to handle airway secretions.
- Telemetry in patients with severe disease

PATIENT EDUCATION

Emphasize expectation for significant recovery and explain phases of illness

PROGNOSIS

- If untreated, 3 phases of illness
  - Initial progression phase up to 4 weeks; highest risk of death and complication
  - Variable plateau phase
  - Recovery phase (weeks–months): return of proximal then distal strength
- Recent mortality estimate of 3% at 6 months and 4% at 1 year. Older patients and those with severe disease have highest risk of mortality (7)[B].
- ~80% of patients achieve functional recovery within 6–12 months. Recovery is maximal at 18 months past onset.
- Up to 20% of patients have residual disability at 1 year. This includes neurologic sequelae such as bilateral footdrop, intrinsic hand muscle wasting, sensory ataxia, and dysesthesia.
- Factors associated with poor functional outcome include age >60 years, rapid disease progression, severe disease indicated by GBS disability score or MRC sum score, preceding diarrhea, positive *C. jejuni* or CMV serology, axonal degeneration, and need for mechanical ventilation.

REFERENCES

1. Shahrizaila N, Goh KJ, Abdullah S, et al. Two sets of nerve conduction studes may suffice in reaching a reliable electrodiagnosis in Guillain-Barré syndrome. *Clin Neurophysiol*. 2013;124(7)1456–1459.
2. Liu J, Wang LN, McNicol ED. Pharmacological treatment for pain in Guillain-Barré syndrome. *Cochrane Database Syst Rev*. 2013;(10):CD009950.
3. Raphaël JC, Chevret S, Hughes RA, et al. Plasma exchange for Guillain-Barré syndrome. *Cochrane Database Syst Rev*. 2002;(2):CD001798.
4. Hughes RA, Swan AV, van Doorn PA. Intravenous immunoglobulin for Guillain-Barré syndrome. *Cochrane Database Syst Rev*. 2012;(7):CD002063.
5. Hughes RAC, van Doorn PA. Corticosteroids for Guillain-Barré syndrome. *Cochrane Database Syst Rev*. 2012,(8):CD001446.
6. Hughes RAC, Pritchard J, Hadden RDM. Pharmacological treatment other than corticosteroids, intravenous immunoglobulin and plasma exchange for Guillain-Barré syndrome. *Cochrane Database Syst Rev*. 2013;(2):CD008630.
7. van den Berg B, Bunschoten C, van Doorn PA, et al. Mortality in Guillain-Barré syndrome. *Neurology*. 2013;80(18):1650–1654.

ADDITIONAL READING

- Kwong JC, Vasa PP, Campitelli MA, et al. Risk of Guillain-Barré syndrome after seasonal influenza vaccination and influenza health-care encounters: a self-controlled study. *Lancet Infect Dis*. 2013; 13(9):769–776.
- Pandey CK, Raza M, Tripathi M, et al. The comparative evaluation of gabapentin and carbamazepine for pain management in Guillain-Barré syndrome patients in the intensive care unit. *Anesth Analg*. 2005;101(1):220–225.
- Rinaldi S. Update on Guillain-Barré syndrome. *J Peripher Nerv Syst*. 2013;18(2):99-112.
- Salmon DA, Proschan M, Forshee R, et al. Association between Guillain-Barré syndrome and influenza A (H1N1) 2009 monovalent inactivated vaccines in the USA: a meta-analysis. *Lancet*. 2013;381(9876):1461–1468.
- Sejvar JJ, Baughman AL, Wise M, et al. Population incidence of Guillain-Barré syndrome: a systematic review and meta-analysis. *Neuroepidemiology*. 2011;36(2):123–133.
- Walgaard C, Lingsma HF, Ruts L, et al. Prediction of respiratory insufficiency in Guillain-Barré syndrome. *Ann Neurol*. 2010;67(6):781–787.

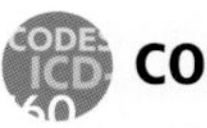

CODES

ICD10

G61.0 Guillain-Barre syndrome

CLINICAL PEARLS

- Suspect GBS in cases of ascending flaccid paralysis with antecedent history of viral respiratory illness or gastroenteritis.
- Natural history of uncomplicated GBS is for slow spontaneous recovery. Treatment with IVIG or PE speeds rate of recovery and reduces disability.
- Most useful diagnostic tests are nerve conductions studies and lumbar puncture.
- If GBS is suspected, evaluate vital capacity and inspiratory force for signs of respiratory compromise.
- Risk of GBS following influenza infection 40–70× greater than risk following seasonal influenza vaccine.

GYNECOMASTIA

Christine Clarice Zacharia, MD, MS • Geetha Gopalakrishnan, MD

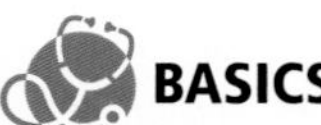

BASICS

DESCRIPTION

- Benign glandular proliferation of male breast tissue
- Increase in estrogens relative to androgens leads to the development of gynecomastia
- Gynecomastia can be transient and represent the normal physiologic changes that occur in utero or in adolescence. However, gynecomastia presenting or persisting in adulthood is typically pathologic in nature.

EPIDEMIOLOGY

- 60–90% of infants have transient gynecomastia (1).
- 48–64% of pubertal males have mild transient gynecomastia (onset at 10–12 years of age and resolution by age 18 years in most individuals) (1).
- 24–65% of men between 50–80 years of age report gynecomastia (2).

ETIOLOGY AND PATHOPHYSIOLOGY

Increase in estrogen activity relative to androgen activity leads to the development of gynecomastia (3). Estrogen stimulates ductal cell hyperplasia, facilitates ductal branching and lengthening, increases vascularity, and results in the proliferation of periductal fibroblasts. These changes occur within 12 months and are followed by fibrosis in the later stages of gynecomastia. Multiple factors can alter the estrogen to androgen ratio and precipitate gynecomastia:

- Decrease in androgen production
- Increase in estrogen production
- Increase in peripheral conversion to estrogen
- Inhibition of the androgen receptor
- Increase in the level of sex hormone–binding globulin (SHBG) or the affinity of androgens to SHBG (decreases free or bioavailable testosterone)
- Displacement of estrogen relative to testosterone from SHBG due to medications

RISK FACTORS

Gynecomastia can be physiologic or pathologic in nature.

- Physiologic gynecomastia presents in infants and adolescent boys and resolves spontaneously.
  - Neonatal gynecomastia: The placenta converts dehydroepiandrosterone (DHEA) and dehydroepiandrosterone sulfate (DHEA-S) to estrone and estradiol resulting in transient gynecomastia.
  - Adolescent gynecomastia: Transient increases in estradiol levels at the onset of puberty leads to gynecomastia.
- Pathologic gynecomastia refers to persistent or adult-onset gynecomastia. Multiple medications and medical conditions can alter the estrogen to androgen ratio and precipitate gynecomastia. However, 25% of cases are idiopathic in nature.
  - Medications: spironolactone, calcium channel blockers, proton pump inhibitors, cimetidine, efavirenz, ketoconazole, phenytoin, cytotoxic drugs, antidepressants, antiandrogen, estrogen, gonadotropin-releasing hormone (GnRH) agonists, 5-alpha rductase inhibitors, growth hormone (4,5)

ALERT

Illicit drugs (likely most common cause): marijuana, heroin, methadone, alcohol, amphetamines

- Primary or secondary hypogonadism
- Testicular tumor: germ cell (secrete human chorionic gonadotropin or hCG), Leydig cell (secrete estrogen), Sertoli cell (excessive aromatization to estrogens)
- Adrenal tumors (secrete DHEA-S and estrogens)
- Ectopic hCG tumors (hepatoblastoma, gastric tumors, renal cell carcinomas)
- Prolactinemia: leads to secondary hypogonadism and gynecomastia. Prolactin can stimulate milk production in breast tissue.
- Hyperthyroidism
- Cirrhosis
- Renal disease or dialysis
- Malnutrition/starvation
- Androgen insensitivity syndromes (defect in the androgen receptor)
- True hermaphroditism (both testicular and ovarian tissue present)
- Aromatase excess syndrome (increased peripheral conversion of androgens to estrogen)
- Idiopathic: most likely secondary to age-associated decline in free testosterone and adipose tissue–mediated aromatase activity

Pediatric Considerations

Transient gynecomastia is seen in neonates or pubertal boys. Typically resolves within 6–24 months.

Geriatric Considerations

Age-associated decline in testosterone production and increase in SHBG production leads to low free testosterone levels in the elderly population. Furthermore, the increased ratio of fat mass to lean mass noted with aging leads to adipose tissue—mediated peripheral conversion of androgens to estrogen. Both factors contribute to the development of idiopathic gynecomastia in the elderly. Medications also play a significant role in the development of gynecomastia in this population.

COMMONLY ASSOCIATED CONDITIONS

- Peutz-Jeghers syndrome—autosomal dominant disorder associated with Sertoli cell tumors, benign hamartomatous polyps, and mucocutaneous hyperpigmentation
- Carney complex—autosomal dominant disorder associated with Sertoli cell tumors, myxoma, hyperpigmentation of the skin (lentiginosis), and endocrine disorders like Cushing syndrome
- Prostate carcinoma—treatment with estrogen and antiandrogen leads to gynecomastia in 50% of patients.
- Klinefelter syndrome—congenital abnormality leads to primary hypogonadism and gynecomastia. These patients are at risk for breast cancer and need regular breast exams.

DIAGNOSIS

HISTORY

- Inquire about duration of breast growth, increase in breast tissue size, associated breast pain and discharge.
- If suspicious of hypogonadism, ask about erectile dysfunction, muscle mass, and decreased shaving frequency and libido.
- Obtain a complete medical history including headache, loss of vision, loss of appetite, weight loss, malignancy, thyroid disorders, liver disease, renal disease, and genetic abnormalities.
- Obtain a family history including Carney complex and Peutz-Jeghers syndrome.
- Review medication list extensively and inquire about the use of illicit substances.

PHYSICAL EXAM

- Careful breast exam to evaluate characteristics:
  - Firm, concentric glandular tissue beneath the nipple and areola palpable by pinching the thumb and forefinger together from either side of the breast toward the nipple
  - May involve one or both breasts
  - Usually asymptomatic but may be painful or tender if it is of recent onset
  - Off center, hard, fixed mass is concerning for malignancy while palpation of subareolar fat is more consistent with pseudogynecomastia
  - Breast discharge should raise concern for malignancy or prolactinemia. In the latter, the discharge is typically clear or milky.
- Thyroid exam (evaluate for diffuse enlargement and palpable nodules and check extremities for tremor and brisk reflexes)
- Abdominal exam (evaluate for masses and liver size)
- Gentiourinary exam (evaluate for testicular size, hair pattern, and presence of ovary or uterus)
- Visual field exam (evaluate for peripheral fileld defect)

DIFFERENTIAL DIAGNOSIS

- Pseudogynecomastia—fat deposition without glandular proliferation often seen in obesity
- Breast cancer—on exam the lesion is typically unilateral; firm; eccentric to the nipple; and associated with skin dimpling, nipple retraction/discharge, and lymphadenopathy
- Lipomas
- Sebaceous cyst
- Dermoid cyst
- Mastitis
- Hematoma
- Hamartoma

DIAGNOSTIC TESTS & INTERPRETATION

- Laboratory and radiologic investigations should be tailored to fit history and physical exam findings.
- Idiopathic gynecomastia is a diagnosis of exclusion and therefore, laboratory tests to rule out medical conditions associated with gynecomastia is recommended.

Initial Tests (lab, imaging)

- Luteinizing hormone (LH)—elevated in primary hypogonadism and decreased in secondary hypogonadism (6)[C]
- Morning total and free testosterone—decreased testosterone level in hypogonadism (6)[C]
- Human chorionic gonadotropin (hCG)—elevated in germ cell tumors and ectopic hCG tumors (6)[C]
- Estradiol—elevated in leydig cell tumors, Sertoli cell tumors, adrenal tumors, and with increased aromatase activity (6)[C]
- Urine for drugs of abuse (UDA)
- Other tests to consider include creatinine, liver function test, thyroid function tests, and prolactin.

Follow-Up Tests & Special Considerations

Consider imaging studies based on laboratory findings.

- Testicular ultrasound (testicular tumor)
- Chest x-ray (CXR) and abdominal CT/MRI (extragonadal germ cell tumor, ectopic hCG tumor, and adrenal tumor)
- MRI of pituitary (pituitary tumor)

Diagnostic Procedures/Other

Based on physical exam findings, consider biopsy of breast mass to rule out malignancy (i.e., off center, hard, fixed, discharge).

Test Interpretation

- **Elevated hCG:** Check testicular ultrasound. If positive for a mass, likely a testicular germ cell tumor. If the ultrasound is negative, consider extragonadal germ cell tumor or hCG-secreting neoplasm and order a CXR and CT abdomen (6)[C].
- **Elevated LH:** if in relation to low testosterone, likely primary hypogonadism. If elevated in relation to high testosterone, check thyroid-stimulating hormone (TSH) and free thyroxine (FT4). If FT4 elevated and TSH is suppressed, likely hyperthyroidism; if TSH and FT4 are normal, likely androgen resistance (6)[C]
- **Normal or decreased LH in relation to low testosterone:** Check prolactin level. If prolactin is elevated, likely due to a prolactin-secreting pituitary tumor; if normal, likely due to secondary hypogonadism (6)[C]
- **Normal or decreased LH in relation to increased estradiol:** Check testicular ultrasound. If positive for a mass, likely Leydig or Sertoli cell tumor. If negative for mass, check CT abdomen to evaluate the adrenals. If mass is present, possible adrenal neoplasm versus adenoma; if no mass is detected, then likely due to increased aromatase activity in extraglandular tissue (6)[C]
- hCG, LH, testosterone, and estradiol are normal: likely idiopathic or medication/drug-induced gynecomastia (6)[C]

TREATMENT

GENERAL MEASURES

- Gynecomastia usually regresses spontaneously within 6 months of onset. This is true even for adult males. Therefore, patients can be monitored for the first 6 months and treatment considered if gynecomastia persists.
- The histologic changes early in the disease process can be reversed with medical therapy. However, with the development of fibrotic tissue, surgery is typically required. Typically, 1–2 years after the onset of gynecomastia, fibrotic changes can be seen and medical intervention is less effective (7)[C].
- Neonatal and pubertal gynecomastia spontaneously resolves within 6–24 months. Persistent pubertal gynecomastia (>24 months) occurs in 8% of pubertal boys. In adult males, 75% of gynecomastia is secondary to persistent pubertal gynecomastia, medications, and idiopathic conditions. Only 25% is related to an underlying medical condition.
- All illicit drug use and offending medications should be stopped if appropriate and patients monitored for clinical improvement.
- Underlying medical conditions need to be treated (i.e., testosterone replacement for hypogonadal men, dopamine agonist for prolactinoma, appropriate treatment for thyrotoxicosis, and tumor resection).
- Medical and surgical therapy to reduce gynecomastia should be considered in patients with significant physical or psychological discomfort.

MEDICATION

- There are no FDA-approved medications for the treatment of gynecomastia but clinical trials involving selective estrogen receptor modulators and aromatase inhibitors demonstrate partial regression and symptom relief (i.e., breast tenderness).
  - Selective estrogen receptor modulators (SERMs): Clinical trials of both tamoxifen (10–20 mg/day) and raloxifene (60 mg/day) showed partial reduction in pubertal gynecomastia in 90% of study participants after 3–9 months but 40% of patients in both treatment groups were not satisfied with the final results and underwent surgical removal (7)[B]. Tamoxifen has also been shown to reduce breast tenderness and prevent the development of gynecomastia in prostate cancer patients on androgen deprivation therapy. Therefore, SERMs (particularly tamoxifen) can be considered in men with 6–12 months of severe, painful gynecomastia symptoms.
  - Aromatase inhibitors block peripheral conversion of androgens to estrogens. In clinical trials, anastrozole (1 mg daily) has shown mixed results with one study reporting reduced breast volume in pubertal males and others not reporting a benefit. In prostate cancer patients, anastrozole prevented the development of gynecomastia in patients undergoing androgen deprivation therapy (8,9)[B].

ISSUES FOR REFERRAL

- Refer patients to an endocrinologist if abnormally elevated hormone levels are confirmed.
- If patients have refractory gynecomastia despite medical therapy and have prolonged gynecomastia characterized by the late fibrotic stage or symptoms concerning for breast cancer, referral to a surgeon would be appropriate.

ADDITIONAL THERAPIES

In clinical trials, prophylactic radiotherapy (10–15 Gy in one fraction over 3 days) prevented the development of gynecomastia in prostate cancer patients on androgen deprivation therapy. Higher doses (20 Gy in five fractions) improved pain symptoms in the same population. More studies are needed to evaluate the use of radiation therapy in other populations.

SURGERY/OTHER PROCEDURES

Surgery to remove breast tissue is recommended if:

- Gynecomastia does not regress within 12 months either spontaneously or after medical therapy
- Significant discomfort (i.e., pain, tenderness)
- Causes embarrassment or anxiety
- Biopsy suspicious for malignancy

Patient Monitoring

- Every 3–6 months for 24 months; consider medical therapy (i.e., tamoxifen) if severe, painful symptoms persist after 6–12 months and surgery after 12–24 months. In individuals with asymptomatic or mild disease, routine yearly breast and physical exam is recommended.
- Patients with Klinefelter syndrome are at increased risk of breast cancer and should have routine breast exams done.

PATIENT EDUCATION

Patients should be encouraged to do periodic breast examination and to alert their clinical provider if a nodule is palpated in the breast or axilla, skin discoloration occurs, or nipple discharge develops.

PROGNOSIS

- Good in physiologic cases, as they often regress spontaneously within 3–6 months (6)
- Majority of patients experience regression once underlying disorder is treated or offending agents are eliminated (6).
- In patients who undergo surgery, majority are satisfied with the postop cosmetic appearance (10).

REFERENCES

1. Bembo SA, Carlson HE. Gynecomastia: its features, and when and how to treat it. *Cleve Clin J Med*. 2004;71(6):511–517.
2. Cuhaci N, Polat SB, Evranos B, et al. Gynecomastia: clinical evaluation and management. *Indian J Endocrinol Metab*. 2014;18(2):150–158.
3. Boccardo F, Rubagotti A, Battaglia M, et al. Evaluation of tamoxifen and anastrozole in the prevention of gynecomastia and breast pain induced by bicalutamide monotherapy of prostate cancer. *J Clin Oncol*. 2005;23(4):808–815.
4. Bowman JD, Kim H, Bustamante JJ. Drug induced gynecomastia. *Pharmacotherapy*. 2012;32(12):1123–1140.
5. Jover F, Cuadrado JM, Roig P, et al. Efavirinez-associated gynecomastia: report of five cases and review of the literature. *Breast J*. 2004;10(3):244–246.
6. Braunstein GD. Clinical practice. Gynecomastia. *N Eng J Med*. 2007;357(12):1229–1237.
7. Lawrence SE, Faught KA, Vethamuthu J, et al. Beneficial effects of raloxifene and tamoxifen in the treatment of pubertal gynecomastia. *J Pediatr*. 2004;145(1):71–76.
8. Mauras N, Bishop K, Merinbaum D, et al. Pharmacokinetics and pharmacodynamics of anastrozole in pubertal boys with recent-onset gynecomastia. *J Clin Endocrinol Metab*. 2009;94(8):2975–2978.
9. Plourde PV, Reiter EO, Jou HC, et al. Safety and efficacy of anastrazole for the treatment of pubertal gynecomastia: a randomized, double-blind, placebo-controlled trial. *J Clin Endocrinol Metab*. 2004;89(9):4428–4433.
10. Gioffrè F, Alfio AR, Famà F, et al. Evaluation of complications and long-term results after surgery for gynecomastia [in Italian]. *Chir Ital*. 2004;56(1):113–116.

ADDITIONAL READING

Eckman A, Dobs A. Drug-induced gynecomastia. *Expert Opin Drug Saf*. 2008;7(6):691–702.

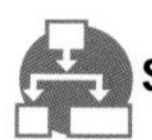

SEE ALSO

Algorithm: Gynecomastia

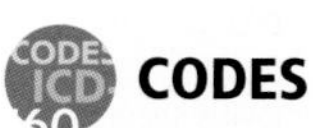

CODES

ICD10

N62 Hypertrophy of breast

CLINICAL PEARLS

- Gynecomastia can be transient and represents the normal physiologic changes in neonates or adolescents. However, gynecomastia presenting or persisting in adulthood is typically pathologic in nature.
- Thorough history and physical exam should be performed on all patients and offending medications eliminated.
- Lab and radiologic studies should be conducted to rule out medical conditions associated with gynecomastia including thyrotoxicosis, prolactinemia, hypogonadism, testicular tumors, adrenal tumors, and ectopic hCG tumors. Treatment should be tailored to exam findings.
- ~25% of gynecomastia is idiopathic in nature and treatment should focus on symptom control.
- Clinical trials of SERMs, aromatase inhibitors, and radiation therapy seem promising. Surgery is the treatment of choice for refractory gynecomastia.

G

HAMMER TOES

Leslie Lemanek, MD • Mary DiGiulio, DO

BASICS

Hammer toes are deformities of digits 2–5 ("lesser" digits).

DESCRIPTION

- Plantar flexion deformity of the proximal interphalangeal (PIP) joint with varying degrees of hyperextension of the metatarsophalangeal (MTP) and distal interphalangeal (DIP) joints occurring primarily in sagittal plane (1)
- Can be flexible, semirigid, or fixed
  - Flexible: passively correctable to neutral position
  - Semirigid: partially correctable to neutral position
  - Fixed: not correctable to neutral position without intervention

EPIDEMIOLOGY

Most common deformity of lesser digits, typically affecting only one or two toes:

- 2nd toe most commonly involved

Incidence

- Undefined
- Increases with age, duration of deformity (from flexible to rigid)

Prevalence

- Predominant sex: female > male (2)
  - Female predominance from 2.5:1 to 9:1, depending on age group
- Can range from 1 to 20% of population studied
- Blacks more often affected than whites (2)

ETIOLOGY AND PATHOPHYSIOLOGY

- Can be congenital or acquired
- Biomechanical dysfunction results in loss of function of extensor digitorum longus (EDL) tendon at PIP joint and the flexor digitorum longus (FDL) tendon at the MTP joint; the intrinsic muscles sublux dorsally as the MTP hyperextends. This results in plantar flexion of the PIP joint and hyperextension of the MTP joint (2).
- Specific pathomechanics vary by etiology:
  - Toe length discrepancy or narrow footwear toe box induces PIP joint flexion by forcing digit to accommodate shoe.
    - May also lead to MTP joint synovitis secondary to overuse, with elongation of plantar plate and MTP joint hyperextension
  - Rheumatoid arthritis (RA) causes MTP joint destruction and resultant subluxation.
  - Any condition that compromises intra-articular and periarticular tissues, such as 2nd ray longer than 1st, inflammatory joint disease, improper fitting shoes, and trauma (1)
  - Damage to joint capsule, collateral ligaments, or synovia leads to unstable PIP joint or MTP joint.

Genetics

- Significant heritability rates of 49–90% (3)
- Specific genetic markers not identified

RISK FACTORS

- Pes cavus and planus
- Hallux valgus
- Metatarsus adductus
- Ankle equinus
- Neuromuscular disease (rare)
- Trauma
- Improperly fitted shoes (narrow toe box) and/or tight hosiery
- Abnormal metatarsal and/or digit length
- Inflammatory joint disease (e.g., RA)
- Connective tissue disease
- Diabetes mellitus

GENERAL PREVENTION

- No documented means of prevention
- Use of pressure-dispersive foot wear helps reduce pain.
- Foot orthoses modulate biomechanical dysfunction and muscular imbalance, preventing progression (2).
- Control of predisposing factors (e.g., inflammatory joint disease) may also slow progression.

COMMONLY ASSOCIATED CONDITIONS

- Hallux valgus
- Cavus foot
- Metatarsus adductus
- Dorsal callus

DIAGNOSIS

History and physical exam typically sufficient for diagnosis of hammer toes. Additional testing are available to exclude other conditions.

HISTORY

- Location, duration, severity, and rate of progression of foot deformity (4)[C]
- Type, location, duration of pain
  - Patients often relate sensation of lump on plantar aspect of MTP joint.
- Degree of functional impairment
- Factors that improve and exacerbate the condition
- Type of footwear and hosiery worn
- Peripheral neurologic symptoms
- Any prior treatment rendered

PHYSICAL EXAM

- Note MTP joint hyperextension, PIP joint flexion, and DIP joint extension.
- Observe any adjacent toe deformities (e.g., hallux valgus, flexion contractures).
- Assess degree of flexibility and reducibility of deformity in both weight-bearing and non–weight-bearing positions (2)[C].
- Note any hyperkeratosis over the joint, ulcers, clavi (dorsal PIP joint, metatarsal head), adventitious bursa, erythema, or skin breakdown (2).
- Palpate for pain over dorsal aspect of PIP joint or MTP joint.
- Drawer test of MTP joint
- Palpate web spaces to exclude interdigital neuroma.
- Neurovascular evaluation (e.g., pulses, sensation, muscle bulk)

DIFFERENTIAL DIAGNOSIS

- Hammer toe: hyperextension of the MTP and DIP joints and plantar flexion of the PIP joint
- Claw toe: dorsiflexion of MTP joint and plantar flexion of the DIP joint
- Mallet toe: fixed or flexible deformity of the DIP joint of the toe
- Overlapping 5th toe
- Interdigital neuroma
- Plantar plate rupture
- Nonspecific synovitis of MTP joint
- Exostosis
- Arthritis (e.g., rheumatoid, psoriatic)
- Fracture

DIAGNOSTIC TESTS & INTERPRETATION

Initial Tests (lab, imaging)

- Not required unless clinically indicated to rule out suspected metabolic or inflammatory arthropathies (2)[C]: rheumatoid factor, antinuclear antibodies (ANA), HLA-B27 serologies for inflammatory disease
- Weight-bearing x-rays of affected foot in anterior–posterior (AP), lateral, and oblique views (2)[C]:
  - AP view superior for assessing MTP subluxation or dislocation
  - Lateral view best for evaluation of hammer toe

Follow-Up Tests & Special Considerations

MRI or bone scan if osteomyelitis is suspected

Diagnostic Procedures/Other

- Nerve conduction studies or EMG if neurologic disorder is suspected
- Doppler or plethysmography if impaired circulation and surgery is considered
- Computerized weight-bearing pressure testing is indicated only in setting of neuromuscular deficiencies of toes.

Test Interpretation

Histologic evaluation typically not necessary before treatment

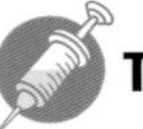

TREATMENT

- Goal of treatment is to reduce or relieve symptoms and help patients return to their normal activity level.
- Management includes surgical and nonsurgical interventions.
- Mild cases may not require treatment.

GENERAL MEASURES

Nonsurgical (conservative) treatment includes

- Shoe modifications (wider and/or deeper toe box) may be used to accommodate the deformity and decrease the pressure over osseous prominences. Avoid high-heeled shoes (2)[C].
- Toe sleeve or orthodigital padding of the hammer toe prominence (5)[C]
- Hammer toe–straightening orthotics or taping to reduce flexible deformities

- Débridement of hyperkeratotic lesions can reduce symptoms. Topical keratolytics may be helpful (2)[C].
- Shoe orthotics mitigate abnormal biomechanics.
- Physical therapy for stretching and strengthening of the toes may help to preserve flexibility.

MEDICATION

Indicated if adequate pain relief is achievable nonsurgically or patient is poor surgical candidate

First Line

NSAIDs may be helpful in managing symptoms of pain as well as soft tissue and joint inflammation.

Second Line

Anti-inflammatory (cortisone) injections if local inflammation or bursitis exists (1)[C]

ISSUES FOR REFERRAL

If nonsurgical (conservative) treatment is unsuccessful and/or impractical or patient has combined deformity of MTP joint, PIP joint, and/or DIP joint, then patient may be referred to an orthopedic surgeon or surgical podiatrist.

SURGERY/OTHER PROCEDURES

- Surgical procedures for the correction of hammer toes depend on the degree and flexibility of the contracture(s) and related abnormalities.
- Surgical interventions for *flexible* hammer toes include (1,5,6)[C]
  - PIP joint arthroplasty (most common)
  - Flexor tendon lengthening/flexor tenotomy
  - Extensor tendon lengthening/tenotomy/MTP joint capsulotomy
  - Flexor to extensor tendon transfer
  - Exostosectomy
  - Implant arthroplasty
- Surgical interventions for semirigid/rigid hammer toes include (1,5)[C]
  - PIP joint resection arthroplasty or arthrodesis
  - Girdlestone-Taylor flexor-to-extensor transfer
  - Metatarsal shortening (Weil osteotomy)
  - Exostosectomy
  - Diaphysectomy of the proximal phalanx (less common)
  - Middle phalangectomy (less common)
  - Soft tissue releases/lengthening
- Procedures may be performed as isolated operations or in conjunction with other procedures.
- Contraindications for surgery: active infection, inadequate vascular supply, and desire for cosmesis alone

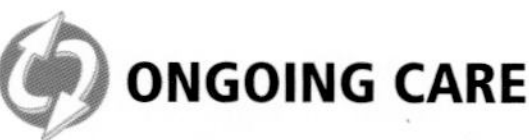

ONGOING CARE

FOLLOW-UP RECOMMENDATIONS

- Radiographs should be taken immediately following surgery or at the first postoperative visit. Subsequent x-rays may be taken as needed.
- Full weight bearing in a postoperative (surgical) shoe or other device is indicated based on the procedure(s) performed and the individual patient.
- Elevate the foot to minimize swelling.
- Return to regular shoe wear after pain is controlled, swelling has subsided, and wounds have healed.
- Role and efficacy of postoperative physical therapy (3 × a week for 2–3 weeks) unclear

Patient Monitoring

In the absence of complications, the patient should be seen initially within the first week following the procedure(s). Frequency of subsequent visits is determined based on the procedure(s) performed and the postoperative course.

PATIENT EDUCATION

- Patients should be aware of mild to moderate swelling and plantar foot discomfort that may persist for many (1–6) months after surgery and may limit footwear options until resolved.
- MTP joint and PIP joint may remain stiff for extended periods of time.
- "Molding" of the operative toe (assuming the contours of adjacent toes) is common.
- Encourage patients to wear shoes of adequate size with rounded or squared toe box.

PROGNOSIS

- Nonoperative (conservative) treatment usually alleviates pain; however, the deformity may progress despite diligent care.
- Surgical treatment of flexible hammer toe deformity reliably corrects the deformity and alleviates pain. Recurrence and progression are common, especially if the patient continues to wear ill-fitting shoes.
- Surgical treatment of fixed hammer toe deformity provides reliable deformity correction and pain relief. Recurrence is uncommon.

COMPLICATIONS

- Common complications specific to digital surgery include but are not limited to
  - Persistent edema
  - Recurrence of deformity
  - Residual pain
  - Excessive stiffness
  - Metatarsalgia
- Less common complications include
  - Numbness (e.g., digital nerve palsy)
  - Flail toe
  - Symptomatic osseous regrowth
  - Malposition of toe
  - Malunion/nonunion
  - Infection
  - Vascular impairment (e.g., toe ischemia, gangrene)

REFERENCES

1. Academy of Ambulatory Foot and Ankle Surgery. *Hammertoe Syndrome*. Philadelphia: Academy of Ambulatory Foot and Ankle Surgery; 2003.
2. Clinical Practice Guideline Forefoot Disorders Panel, Thomas JL, Blitch EL IV, et al. Diagnosis and treatment of forefoot disorders. Section 1: digital deformities. *J Foot Ankle Surg*. 2009;48(2):230–238.
3. Hannan MT, Menz HB, Jordan JM, et al. High heritability of hallux valgus and lesser toe deformities in adult men and women. *Arthritis Care Res (Hoboken)*. 2013;65(9):1515–1521.
4. Schrier JC, Verheyen CC, Louwerens JW. Definitions of hammer toe and claw toe: an evaluation of the literature. *J Am Podiatr Med Assoc*. 2009;99(3):194–197.
5. Smith BW, Coughlin MJ. Disorders of the lesser toes. *Sports Med Arthrosc*. 2009;17(3):167–174.
6. Kwon JY, De Asla RJ. The use of flexor to extensor transfers for the correction of the flexible hammer toe deformity. *Foot Ankle Clin*. 2011;16(4):573–582.

ADDITIONAL READING

- Miller JM, Blacklidge DK, Ferdowsian V, et al. Chevron arthrodesis of the interphalangeal joint for hammertoe correction. *J Foot Ankle Surg*. 2010;49(2):194–196.
- O'Kane C, Kilmartin T. Review of proximal interphalangeal joint excisional arthroplasty for the correction of second hammer toe deformity in 100 cases. *Foot Ankle Int*. 2005;26(4):320–325.
- Pietrzak WS, Lessek TP, Perns SV. A bioabsorbable fixation implant for use in proximal interphalangeal joint (hammer toe) arthrodesis: biomechanical testing in a synthetic bone substrate. *J Foot Ankle Surg*. 2006;45(5):288–294.
- Shirzad K, Kiesau CD, DeOrio JK, et al. Lesser toe deformities. *J Am Acad Orthop Surg*. 2011;19(8):505–514.

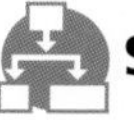

SEE ALSO

Algorithm: Foot Pain

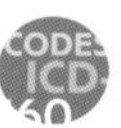

CODES

ICD10

- M20.40 Other hammer toe(s) (acquired), unspecified foot
- M20.41 Other hammer toe(s) (acquired), right foot
- M20.42 Other hammer toe(s) (acquired), left foot

CLINICAL PEARLS

- Hammer toe is plantar flexion deformity of PIP joint.
- Patients complain of pain at the PIP or MTP joint.
- Initial management of hammer toe deformity is conservative. Consider surgery if pain persists or the deformity worsens.
- Properly fitting footwear helps minimize recurrence. Patients should be aware of mild to moderate swelling and plantar foot discomfort that may persist for many (1–6) months after surgery and may limit footwear options until resolved.

HAND-FOOT-AND-MOUTH DISEASE

Chris Wheelock, MD

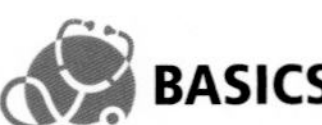

BASICS

DESCRIPTION

- Common acute viral illness affecting mostly children
- Characterized by vesicles on the buccal mucosa and tongue and peripherally distributed small, tender cutaneous lesions on the hands, feet, buttocks, and (less commonly) genitalia
- Group A coxsackieviruses are the most common causative agent (1).
- Synonym(s): herpangina

EPIDEMIOLOGY

- Self-limiting illness resolves in 7–10 days
- Moderately contagious
- Infection is spread by direct contact with nasal discharge, saliva, blister fluid, or stool.
- Infected individuals are most contagious during the 1st week of the illness.
- The viruses that cause hand-foot-and-mouth disease (HFM) can persist for weeks after symptoms have resolved, most commonly in stool, allowing transmission following resolution of symptoms.
- The incubation period is 3–5 days (2).

Incidence

- Children <10 years of age are most commonly affected.
- Can occur as isolated cases, outbreaks, or epidemics
- Occurs worldwide
- Mother to fetus transmission is possible.
- Most large outbreaks occur in Southeast Asia.

ETIOLOGY AND PATHOPHYSIOLOGY

Transmission by the fecal–oral route or contact with skin lesions or oral secretions

- Most commonly coxsackievirus A16
- Also coxsackieviruses A5, A7, A9, A10, B2, B5, and Enterovirus 71 (3)

GENERAL PREVENTION

- Hand washing, especially around food handling or stooling/diaper changes (4)[B]
- Exclusion of children from group settings during the first few days of the illness in the setting of open lesions in the mouth or on the skin may reduce the spread of infection (2)[C].
- Hand hygiene measures are effective in reducing transmission (4,5).
- Pregnant woman should avoid contact with infected individuals.

DIAGNOSIS

HISTORY

- Rash on hands and feet
- Sore throat
- Painful mouth lesions
- 1-day prodrome of fever, anorexia, malaise, abdominal pain, upper respiratory symptoms
- Fever may last 3–4 days.
- Often history of sick contacts

PHYSICAL EXAM

- Tender vesicles or ulcers on buccal mucosa, sides of tongue, and palate
- Begin as small red papules and evolve into vesicles and then ulcerations
- May persist for up to 1 week
- Cutaneous vesicles 3–5 mm in diameter start as maculopapular eruptions, occur typically on dorsal aspect of fingers and toes.
- May also occur on the palms, soles, buttocks, and groin
- Adults are less likely to have cutaneous findings.

DIFFERENTIAL DIAGNOSIS

- Herpes simplex
- Herpes zoster
- Scarlet fever
- Roseola infantum
- Fifth disease
- Other enteroviral infections
- Kawasaki disease
- Viral pharyngitis
- Erythema multiforme
- Varicella (6)

DIAGNOSTIC TESTS & INTERPRETATION

Typically clinically diagnosed

Initial Tests (lab, imaging)

Culture for responsible virus (virus isolation) can be obtained from oral lesions, cutaneous vesicles, nasopharyngeal swabs, stool, and CSF, although not typically performed. PCR of throat swabs and vesicle fluid is the most efficient test if enterovirus 71 is suspected (7).

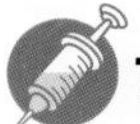

TREATMENT

- Symptomatic
- Avoid spicy or acidic foods to limit oral pain.
- Numbing sprays or cautious use of viscous lidocaine can be used for oral pain.
- IV fluids may be required in more severe cases of dehydration.

MEDICATION

- Symptomatic care using acetaminophen or ibuprofen for pain from oral ulcers or fever
- Soothing mouthwashes can be compounded by the pharmacy containing equal amounts of viscous lidocaine, diphenhydramine, and Maalox. Instruct to swish and spit (caution in young children due to risk of lidocaine toxicity).

Pediatric Considerations

Avoid aspirin use in treating febrile illness in children.

INPATIENT CONSIDERATIONS

- Patients with CNS manifestations may require hospitalization.
- Admit those with dehydration unable to maintain adequate oral hydration.

ONGOING CARE

DIET

- Encourage cold liquids (e.g., milk products, popsicles) to prevent dehydration.
- Avoid acidic, salty, and spicy foods, as they will increase pain.

COMPLICATIONS

- Dehydration most common due to painful oral ulcerations
- Rarely, aseptic meningitis or other neurologic complications
- Concomitant CNS disease may occur when HFM syndrome is caused by Enterovirus 71. In Southeast Asia, this results in a mortality rate of 3 deaths per 10,000 cases.
- Cardiopulmonary complications include myocarditis, pneumonitis, and pulmonary edema.
- Fever >3 days and lethargy are associated with CSF pleocytosis.
- Usually resolves in 7–10 days without complications

REFERENCES

1. Frydenberg A, Starr M. Hand, foot and mouth disease. *Aust Fam Physician*. 2003;32(8):594–595.
2. Centers for Disease Control and Prevention. Notes from the field: severe hand, foot, and mouth disease associated with coxsackievirus A6–Alabama, Connecticut, California, and Nevada, November 2011-February 2012. *MMWR Morb Mortal Wkly Rep*. 2012;61(12):213–214.
3. Richardson M, Elliman D, Maguire H, et al. Evidence base of incubation periods, periods of infectiousness and exclusion policies for control of communicable diseases in schools and preschools. *Pediatr infect Dis J*. 2001;20(4):380–391.
4. Ruan F, Yang T, Ma H, et al. Risk factors for hand, foot, and mouth disease and herpangina and the preventive effect of hand-washing. *Pediatrics*. 2011;127(4):e898–e904.
5. Ma E, Wong S, Wong C, et al. Effects of public health interventions in reducing transmission of hand, foot, and mouth disease. *Pediatr Infect Dis J*. 2011;30(5):432–435.
6. Quail G. The painful mouth. *Aust Fam Physician*. 2008;37(11):935–938.
7. Ooi MH, Wong SC, Lewthwaite P, et al. Clinical features, diagnosis, and management of enterovirus 71. *Lancet Neurol*. 2010;9(11):1097–1105.

ADDITIONAL READING

- Chang LY, Tsao KC, Hsia SH, et al. Transmission and clinical features of enterovirus 71 infections in household contacts in Taiwan. *JAMA*. 2004;291(2):222–227.
- Scott LA, Stone MS. Viral exanthems. *Dermatol Online J*. 2003;9(3):4.

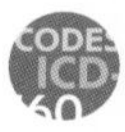

CODES

ICD10

- B08.4 Enteroviral vesicular stomatitis with exanthem
- B34.1 Enterovirus infection, unspecified
- B08.5 Enteroviral vesicular pharyngitis

CLINICAL PEARLS

- Most common May–October
- Children <5 years of age tend to have worse symptoms than older children.
- Hand-foot-and-mouth disease is the most common cause of mouth sores in pediatric patients.
- Usually self-limiting, resolving in 7–10 days
- Careful hand washing to limit spread

HEADACHE, CLUSTER

Jeffrey Phillips, MD

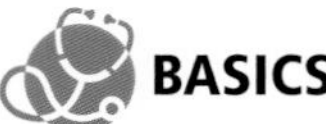

BASICS

DESCRIPTION

- Primary headache disorder
- Multiple attacks of unilateral, excruciating, sharp, searing, or piercing pain. Typically localized in the periorbital area and temple accompanied by signs of ipsilateral autonomic features.
- Autonomic symptoms: parasympathetic hyperactivity signs (ipsilateral lacrimation, eye redness, nasal congestion) and sympathetic hypoactivity (ipsilateral ptosis and miosis)
- Patients often pace, rubbing their heads to try to alleviate the pain.
- Symptoms usually remain on the same side during a single cluster attack.
- Individual attacks last 15–180 minutes if untreated and occur from once every other day to 8 times per day.
- Attacks usually occur in series (cluster periods) lasting for weeks or months separated by remission periods usually lasting months or years. However, about 10–15% of patients have chronic symptoms without remissions.

EPIDEMIOLOGY

Incidence

1-year incidence: 53/100,000

Prevalence

- Lifetime prevalence 124/100,000 (~0.1%)
- Predominant sex: male > female (4.3:1)
- Mean age of onset: between 29.6 and 35.7 years
- Episodic/chronic ratio 6:1

ETIOLOGY AND PATHOPHYSIOLOGY

- Complex and incompletely understood
- Proposed mechanisms include the following:
  - Activation of posterior hypothalamus may trigger an attack, causing activation of the trigeminal nerve, leading to intense pain symptoms.
  - Autonomic symptoms: activation of craniofacial parasympathetic nerve fibers secondary to pathologic activation of trigemino-autonomic brainstem reflex

Genetics

- Usually sporadic: autosomal dominant in 5% of cases, autosomal recessive or multifactorial in other families
- Evidence varies: 1st-degree relatives carry 5–8-fold; 2nd degree 1–3-fold increased relative risk of disease

RISK FACTORS

- Male gender
- Age (70% onset before age 30 years)
- Cigarette smoking
- Family history of cluster headache (CH)
- Head trauma
- Alcohol induces attacks during a cluster but not during remission.
- Small amounts of vasodilators (e.g., alcohol, nitroglycerin, sildenafil)
- Strong odors

COMMONLY ASSOCIATED CONDITIONS

- Depression (24%)
- Increased risk of suicide secondary to the extreme nature of the pain
- Medication overuse headache
- Asthma (9%)
- History of migraine, frequently in female patients
- Sleep apnea (14%)
- Increased prevalence of cardiac right-to-left shunt and patent foramen ovale (relationship unclear)

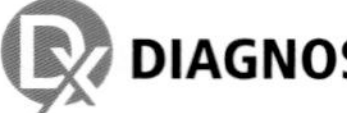

DIAGNOSIS

- Diagnosis is clinical.
- *International Classification of Headache Disorders* (2nd edition) criteria: at least 5 attacks of severe or very severe unilateral orbital, supraorbital, or temporal pain lasting 15–180 minutes if untreated
- At least 1 of the following:
  - Ipsilateral
    - Conjunctival injection and/or lacrimation
    - Nasal congestion and/or rhinorrhea
    - Eyelid edema
    - Forehead and facial sweating
    - Miosis and/or ptosis
  - Sense of restlessness or agitation
- Attack frequency: 1 every other day to 8 per day
- Episodic CH: at least 2 cluster periods lasting 7 days–1 year, separated by a pain-free interval of >1 month (80–90% of cases)
- Chronic CH: cluster-free interval of <1 month in a ≥12-month period

HISTORY

- Episodic periods of headache described as excruciating, unilateral, sharp, searing, or piercing pain, typically localized in the periorbital area
- Eye redness, tearing, nasal discharge, sweating
- Timing of headaches often circadian in nature

PHYSICAL EXAM

- Usually patients seen between attacks
- Acute distress, crying, screaming, restless, and/or agitated during attacks
- Ipsilateral lacrimation, injected conjunctivae, ptosis, and miosis
- Nasal stuffiness or rhinorrhea
- Bradycardia or tachycardia

DIFFERENTIAL DIAGNOSIS

- Paroxysmal hemicrania, short-lasting unilateral neuralgiform headache attacks with conjunctival injection and tearing (SUNCT).
- Hemicrania continua, hypnic headaches, trigeminal and other facial neuralgias, migraine, temporal arteritis, herpes zoster
- Secondary CH
  - Vertebral or carotid artery dissection, brain arteriovenous malformations, intracranial artery aneurysms
  - Pituitary tumors
  - Nasopharyngeal carcinoma
  - Maxillary sinus foreign body/sinusitis
  - Cavernous hemangioma
  - Meningiomas/carcinomas/metastases

DIAGNOSTIC TESTS & INTERPRETATION

- Diagnosis is primarily clinical.
- Diagnosis is often delayed (>40% report 5-year delay in diagnosis)
- Consider neuroimaging (MRI/CT head and vascular imaging of brain):
  - Abnormal neurologic exam
  - Suspect secondary CH

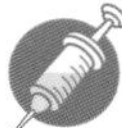

TREATMENT

Many of the medications discussed in the following section are used off-label in the treatment of CH.

GENERAL MEASURES

- Avoid major changes in sleep habits.
- Stop smoking.
- Avoid use of alcohol during cluster period.
- Avoid extreme changes in altitude due to changes in oxygen levels.
- Avoid exposure to chemical agents/solvents.

MEDICATION

- Avoid pain therapy, especially narcotic analgesics, for acute attacks.
- Goal is abortion of acute attack and prophylaxis for expected duration of the cluster.
- Assess cardiovascular risk before instituting a vasoactive drug, such as triptans or ergot derivatives.

First Line

For acute attacks:

- Oxygen
  - 100% at 6–12 L/min for 15 minutes via nonrebreathing mask provides relief within 15 minutes (1)[A].
  - Avoid in severe chronic obstructive pulmonary disease (COPD) as might affect hypoxic respiratory drive.
- Sumatriptan (Imitrex)
  - 6 mg SC, max 12 mg/24 hr with at least 1 hour between injections is most effective medication for acute attacks. NNT (needed to treat) 2.4 for headache relief in 15 minutes. Sumatriptan nasal spray: 20 mg. May repeat in 2 hours, max dose 40 mg/24 hr. NNT 3.2 for headache relief at 30 minutes (2)[A].
- Zolmitriptan
  - Nasal spray: 5- and 10-mg dosage both effective. May repeat in 2 hours, max 10 mg/24 hr. NNT 12 and 4.9 for headache relief in 15 minutes for 5 and 10 mg, respectively. Zolmitriptan tablet: 5- and 10-mg dosage both effective. May repeat in 2 hours, max dose 10 mg/24 hr. NNT 6.7 and 4.5 for headache relief in 30 minutes for 5 and 10 mg, respectively (2)[A].

ALERT

Triptans are contraindicated in ischemic cardiac disease, stroke, uncontrolled hypertension, prinzmetal angina, basilar migraine, hemiplegic migraine, ischemic bowel disease, and peripheral vascular disease.

- Prophylaxis: used at start of cluster period to prevent and shorten further attacks. Start as soon as possible:
  - Verapamil
    - Can start at 240 mg/day and increase by 40–80 mg every 10–14 days. Short- or long-acting equivalent. Most patients respond to daily dose of 200–480 mg but up to 960 mg/day may be needed. NNT = 1.2 (3)[A]
    - ECG monitoring for doses/increments >480 mg/day required because of risk of bradycardia (q3m used as a guideline)
    - Similar efficacy to lithium, but fewer adverse effects and faster onset make it the preferred choice.

Second Line

- Acute attack
  - Lidocaine/cocaine: 10 mg (1 mL) of lidocaine or 40–50 mg of 10% cocaine intranasal. No well well-controlled randomized controlled trials (RCTs) done. Most common side effects are nasal congestion, unpleasant taste (4)[B].
  - Octreotide: SC 100 μg. Can be considered in patients when triptans are contraindicated. Main side effect is GI upset (5)[A].
  - Ergotamine/dihydroergotamine (DHE): original treatments for CH. Now rarely used because of significant side effects. No controlled trials done. Still used for transitional prophylaxis (see below).
- Prophylaxis
  - Lithium: Start 300 mg b.i.d., titrate to therapeutic range of 0.8–1.1 mEq/L. Most patients benefit from 600 to 1,200 mg/day. Widely used without formal evidence of efficacy. Retrospective case series show that lithium led to >50% reduction in attack frequency within 2 weeks in 77% of the patients with episodic CH. Must monitor levels, liver, renal, and thyroid function. Caution with nephrotoxic drugs, diuretics. Inferior to verapamil (6)[B]
  - Melatonin: 10 mg in the evening showed reduction in headache frequency versus placebo in small RCT. No side effects were reported.
  - Antiepileptics: topiramate, sodium valproate, gabapentin: Open studies showed reduction of cluster duration and frequency of headache, but RCT did not show superiority to placebo. Significant adverse effects
  - Civamide: 100 μL of 0.025% into each nostril daily. Only studied in episodic CH in 1 trial of 28 patients. Not available in the United States. Most common side effects were nasal burning, lacrimation, pharyngitis, and rhinorrhea.
  - Capsaicin: 0.025% ipsilateral nostril for 7 days shows benefit in small RCT.
  - Methysergide: No studies available to confirm efficacy. Has serious adverse effects, including pulmonary and retroperitoneal fibrosis. Cannot be given with triptans and ergots
  - Pizotifen: Modest benefit limited by fatigue and weight gain

ADDITIONAL THERAPIES

Transitional preventive treatment:

- Used until longer term preventive treatment becomes effective. Longer term maintenance agents are started concurrently:
  - Steroids: Several open studies suggested benefit, but no rigorous trials to prove efficacy. Studies support at least 40 mg/day (up to 80 mg/day) prednisone with a 10–30-day taper provides benefit to 60–90% patients. Adverse effects for short-term use: insomnia, psychosis, hyponatremia, edema, hyperglycemia, peptic ulcer

ALERT

Ergots are contraindicated in patients with cardiovascular disease and cannot be used with triptans.

Pregnancy Considerations

Collaboration between headache specialist, obstetrician, and pediatrician strongly encouraged. Patient should be informed of treatment benefits and risks as well as drug's potential teratogenic effect. For abortive treatment, oxygen is most appropriate 1st-line therapy. Nasal lidocaine (pregnancy Category B) can be used as 2nd-line therapy. As preventive therapy, verapamil (pregnancy Category C) and steroids (pregnancy Category C) remain the preferred options. Use of SC or intranasal sumatriptan (pregnancy Category C) should be limited as much as possible. Avoid ergotamines (pregnancy Category X).

ISSUES FOR REFERRAL

Consider a neurology or headache center referral for refractory or complicated patients.

SURGERY/OTHER PROCEDURES

- Surgery may be considered only for patients who are refractory to, or have contraindications to, medical therapy.
- Various techniques focus on stimulation or ablation of segments of trigeminal nerve root and sphenopalatine ganglion. Other techniques are aimed at decreasing pain and inflammation surrounding the greater occipital nerve.
- Greater occipital nerve steroid injection: A retrospective analysis showed ~80% of patients with partial or complete response. Effect lasted 3.5 weeks; 21 mg of betamethasone and 2 mL of 2% lidocaine were used. One class I RCT showed benefit within 72 hours in 85% of lidocaine/betamethasone group compared with none in lidocaine/saline group. Cortivazol injection reduced severity and frequency of headache compared with placebo in an RCT (7)[A].
- No evidence for Botox or hyperbaric oxygen treatment.
- Neurostimulation
  - Occipital nerve stimulation (ONS) was shown to reduce severity and attack frequency in chronic CH patients.
  - Deep brain stimulation (DBS) of the posterior inferior hypothalamus shows moderate therapeutic effect.

INPATIENT CONSIDERATIONS

Suicidal ideation, unwilling to contract for safety

ONGOING CARE

FOLLOW-UP RECOMMENDATIONS

Patient Monitoring

- Anticipate cluster bouts and initiate early prophylaxis.
- Monitor for depression.
- Watch for adverse medication response and side effects, such as unmasking of underlying cardiovascular disorder when using medications to treat CH.

PROGNOSIS

- Unpredictable course. With aging, attack frequency often decreases.
- Poor prognosis associated with older age of onset, male gender, disease duration of >20 years for episodic form
- Possibility of transformation of episodic cluster to chronic cluster and occasionally chronic cluster to episodic cluster

COMPLICATIONS

- Depression and suicide
- Side effects of medication, including unmasking of coronary artery disease
- Potential for drug abuse/misuse

REFERENCES

1. Cohen AS, Burns B, Goadsby PJ, et al. High-flow oxygen for treatment of cluster headache: a randomized trial. *JAMA*. 2009;302(22):2451–2457.
2. Law S, Derry S, Moore RA. Triptans for acute cluster headache. *Cochrane Database Syst Rev*. 2010;(4):CD008042.
3. Leone M, D'Amico D, Frediani F, et al. Verapamil in the prophylaxis of episodic cluster headache: a double-blind study versus placebo. *Neurology*. 2000;54(6):1382–1385.
4. Costa A, Pucci E, Antonaci F, et al. The effect of intranasal cocaine and lidocaine on nitroglycerin-induced attacks in cluster headache. *Cephalalgia*. 2000;20(2):85–91.
5. Matharu MS, Levy MJ, Meeran K, et al. Subcutaneous octreotide in cluster headache: randomized placebo-controlled double-blind crossover study. *Ann Neurol*. 2004;56(4):488–494.
6. Stochino ME, Deidda A, Asuni C, et al. Evaluation of lithium response in episodic cluster headache: a retrospective case series. *Headache*. 2012;52(7):1171–1175.
7. Leroux E, Valade D, Taifas I, et al. Suboccipital steroid injections for transitional treatment of patients with more than two cluster headache attacks per day: a randomised, double-blind, placebo-controlled trial. *Lancet Neurol*. 2011;10(10): 891–897.

ADDITIONAL READING

- Ashkenazi A, Schwedt T. Cluster headache—acute and prophylactic therapy. *Headache*. 2011;51(2):272–286.
- Beck E, Sieber WJ, Trejo R. Management of cluster headache. *Am Fam Phyician*. 2005;71(4):717–724.
- Fontaine D, Lanteri-Minet M, Ouchchane L, et al. Anatomical location of effective deep brain stimulation electrodes in chronic cluster headache. *Brain*. 2010;133(Pt 4):1214–1223.
- Hainer BL, Matheson EM. Approach to acute headache in adults. *Am Fam Physician*. 2013;87(10):682–687.
- International Headache Society: http://www.ihs-headache.org
- Nagy AJ, Gandhi S, Bhola R, et al. Intravenous dihydroergotamine for inpatient management of refractory primary headaches. *Neurology*. 2011;77(20):1827–1832.

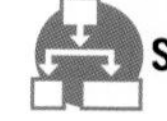

SEE ALSO

Algorithm: Headache, Chronic

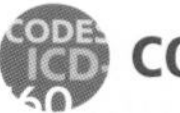

CODES

ICD10

- G44.009 Cluster headache syndrome, unspecified, not intractable
- G44.019 Episodic cluster headache, not intractable
- G44.029 Chronic cluster headache, not intractable

CLINICAL PEARLS

- CHs are rare but disabling. Patients are often agitated and restless during the attack.
- Oxygen and triptans, not narcotics, are 1st-line therapy for acute attacks.
- Abortive, transitional, and prophylaxic treatment must all be considered.

HEADACHE, MIGRAINE

Jay H. Levin, MD • Michelle L. Mellion, MD

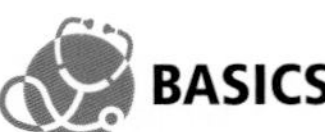

BASICS

DESCRIPTION

Recurrent headache disorder manifesting in attacks lasting 4–72 hours. Typical characteristics of the headache are unilateral location, pulsating quality, moderate or severe intensity, aggravation by routine physical activity, and association with nausea and/or photophobia and phonophobia (1). Most frequent subtypes of migraine are the following:

- Without aura (common migraine): defining >80% of attacks, often associated with nausea, vomiting, photophobia, and/or phonophobia
- With aura (classic migraine): visual or other types of fully reversible neurologic phenomenon lasting 5–60 minutes
- Chronic (transformed) migraine: chronic headache pattern evolving from episodic migraine. Migraine-like attacks are superimposed on a daily or near-daily headache pattern (e.g., tension headaches), >15 headache days/month for at least 3 months.
- Medication overuse headache: headache occurring 10 or more days per month for more than 3 months as a consequence of regular overuse of an acute or symptomatic headache medication.
- With brainstem aura (basilar migraine): brainstem symptoms such as dysarthria, vertigo, tinnitus, or ataxia, which are fully reversible and lasting 5–60 minutes.
- Hemiplegic migraine: aura consisting of fully reversible hemiplegia and/or hemiparesis
- Recurrent painful ophthalmoplegic neuropathy (ophthalmoplegic migraine): neuralgia accompanied by paresis of an ocular cranial nerve with ipsilateral headache
- Retinal: repeated attacks of monocular visual disturbance, including scintillations, scotomata, or blindness, associated with migraine headache
- Menstrual-related (moliminal) migraine: associated with onset of menstrual period
- Status migrainosus: debilitating migraine that lasts >72 hours
- Migrainous infarction: one or more migraine aura symptoms associated with an ischemic brain lesion in the appropriate territory demonstrated by neuroimaging

EPIDEMIOLOGY

Female > male (3:1)

Prevalence

- Affects >28 million Americans
- Adults: women 18%; men 6%

ETIOLOGY AND PATHOPHYSIOLOGY

- No longer believed to be primarily vascular in etiology; rather, cortical spreading depolarization/depression
- Trigeminovascular hypothesis: hyperexcitable trigeminal sensory neurons in brainstem are stimulated and release neuropeptides, such as substance P and calcitonin gene–related peptide (CGRP), leading to vasodilation and neurogenic inflammation.

Genetics

- >80% of patients have a positive family history.
- Familial hemiplegic migraine has been shown to be linked to both chromosomes 1, 2, and 19 (1).

RISK FACTORS

- Family history of migraine
- Female gender
- Stress
- Menstrual cycle, hormones
- Sleep pattern disruption
- Diet: skipped meals (40–56%), alcohol (29–35%), chocolate (19–22%), cheese (9–18%), caffeine overuse (14%), monosodium glutamate (MSG) (12%), and artificial sweeteners (e.g., aspartame, sucralose)
- Medications: estrogens, vasodilators

GENERAL PREVENTION

- Avoid precipitants of attacks.
- Biofeedback, education, and psychological intervention
- Preventative therapy if attacks frequent, interfere with lifestyle, or are not controlled by acute interventions
- Lifestyle modifications are the cornerstone of migraine prevention: sleep hygiene, stress management, healthy diet, and regular aerobic exercise.

COMMONLY ASSOCIATED CONDITIONS

- Depression, psychiatric disorders
- Sleep disturbance (e.g., sleep apnea)
- Cerebral vascular disease
- Peripheral vascular disease
- Seizure disorders
- Irritable bowel syndrome
- Obesity
- Patent foramen ovale (PFO)

DIAGNOSIS

A thorough history and neurologic examination are usually all that is necessary to make the diagnosis. Migraine is a clinical diagnosis.

HISTORY

- Screening mnemonic "POUND": **P**ulsating, duration of 4–72 h**O**urs, **U**nilateral, **N**ausea, **D**isabling
  - Likelihood ratio (LR) = 24 for migraine diagnosis if 4 of 5 criteria present
  - LR = 0.41 for migraine diagnosis if ≤2 criteria present (2)
    - Headache usually begins with mild pain that escalates into a unilateral (30–40% bilateral) throbbing (40% nonthrobbing) pain lasting 4–72 hours.
    - Intensified by movement and associated with systemic manifestations: nausea (87%), vomiting (56%), diarrhea (16%), photophobia (82%), phonophobia (78%), muscle tenderness (65%), lightheadedness (72%), and vertigo (33%)
    - May be preceded by aura
  - Visual disruptions are most common, including scotoma, hemianopsia, fortification spectra, geometric visual patterns, and occasionally hallucinations.
  - Somatosensory disruption in face or arms
  - Speech difficulties
    - Obtain adequate headache profile: total number of headaches/month; number of days/month whereby headaches limit daily activities; and frequency and amount of all headache medications used.
    - Identify possible triggers (e.g., stress, sleep disturbance, food, caffeine, alcohol).

PHYSICAL EXAM

A full neurologic exam should be performed; abnormalities consistent with other causes to severe headaches MIGHT include the following:

- Gait abnormalities and other new cerebellar findings
- Loss of gross and/or fine motor function
- Altered mental status including possible hallucinations (visual, auditory, olfactory)
- Short-term memory loss

DIFFERENTIAL DIAGNOSIS

- Other primary headache syndromes
- If focal neurologic signs/symptoms are present, consider transient ischemic attack (TIA) or stroke.
- Secondary headaches: tumor, infection, vascular pathology, prescription or illicit drug use
- Drug-seeking patients
- Psychiatric disease
- Rarely, atypical forms of epilepsy

DIAGNOSTIC TESTS & INTERPRETATION

Neuroimaging is appropriate ONLY with suspicious symptomatology and/or an abnormality on physical examination (3). Other red flags include the following:

- New onset in patient >50 years of age
- Change in established headache pattern
- Atypical pattern or unremitting/progressive neurologic symptoms
- Prolonged or bizarre aura

Pregnancy Considerations

- Migraine frequency may decrease in 2nd and 3rd trimesters.
- Nonpharmacologic methods are mainstay of treatment (see in the following text).
- No treatment drug has FDA approval during pregnancy.
  - Acetaminophen, short-acting opioids, and antiemetics (e.g., prochlorperazine) can be considered for acute headaches during pregnancy.
  - Ergotamines are contraindicated.
  - Avoid herbal remedies.
  - Early data for sumatriptan and naratriptan suggest no increase in birth defects.
  - Sumatriptan by injection is ideal for breastfeeding women with disabling migraines.
  - Propranolol is safe and effective for migraine prevention during pregnancy/lactation.

TREATMENT

GENERAL MEASURES

- Most patients manage attacks with self-care.
- Cold compresses to area of pain
- Withdrawal from stressful surroundings
- Sleep is desirable.

MEDICATION

- **First-line abortive treatments**
  - Mild to moderate attacks
    - NSAIDs, such as ibuprofen, naproxen, and diclofenac are generally inexpensive and effective in up to 60% of cases.
    - Aspirin 500 mg–acetaminophen 500 mg–caffeine 130 mg (AAC) combination (e.g., Excedrin Migraine) is an inexpensive, nonprescription, and FDA-approved treatment for acute migraine.
  - Moderate to severe attacks:
    - Triptans are preferred when OTC agents fail for mild/moderate attacks *OR* as initial treatment for moderate to severe attacks:
    - All triptans have similar effectiveness and tolerability, but some patients may respond better to one triptan over another.

- Early intervention with triptans during the aura, prior to onset of pain, may prevent headache 89% of the time.
- Common adverse drug reactions include chest pressure, flushing, weakness, dizziness, feeling of warmth, and paresthesia.
  - Suggested initial doses (refer to individual labeling for more detailed dosing instructions)
  - Sumatriptan 100 mg PO; 6 mg SQ; 20 mg intranasal
  - SQ route quickest onset followed by intranasal then PO
  - Eletriptan 40 mg PO
  - Rizatriptan 10 mg PO
  - Zolmitriptan 2.5 mg PO; 5 mg intranasal
  - Naratriptan 2.5 mg PO
  - Frovatriptan 2.5 mg PO
    - 44–77% of patients taking triptans report complete pain relief within 2 hours.
    - Frovatriptan and naratriptan have slowest onset, however, least likely to cause adverse effects
- Combination triptan and NSAID: supatriptan 85 mg/naproxen 500 mg PO at onset of HA
- Antiemetics: Consider antinausea medications that antagonize dopamine receptors:
  - Metoclopramide, prochlorperazine
  - IV dexamethasone: Use as adjunctive emergency therapy; 10–25 mg single dose (4)[A].
- Contraindications to treatments
  - Avoid 5-HT-1 agonists (triptans) and ergots in coronary artery disease, peripheral vascular disease, uncontrolled hypertension, and complicated migraine (e.g., brainstem or hemiplegic migraine).
  - Triptans should not be used with ergot derivative, MAOI, or other triptans.
  - Avoid opioids or butalbital in addiction-prone patients and patients with frequent migraines.
- Precautions
  - Frequent use of acute-treatment drugs may lead to increase in migraine patterns and medication overuse headache.

- **Second-line abortive treatment**
  - Paracetamol (acetaminophen 1,000 mg) or aspirin (975 mg) plus the addition of a dopamine antagonist (e.g., metoclopramide 10 mg) may be as effective as PO sumatriptan 100 mg for acute migraine headache
  - Ergotamines (e.g., dihydroergotamine SC, Migranal intranasal): drug of choice in status migrainosus and nonpregnant patients but limited use due to side effects and replaced by triptans
  - Opiate use is controversial.
    - Opiates may contribute to medication overuse or chronic daily headache with use as few as 8 days per month (5).
- **First-line preventative treatment**
  - Lifestyle modifications: sleep hygiene, stress management, healthy diet, regular aerobic exercise, and medication use
  - ~38% of migraineurs need preventative therapy, but only 3–13% use it (6). Trial and error is needed to determine optimal therapy.
  - Consider starting preventative treatment when:
    - Quality of life is severely impaired
    - ≥2 attacks/month
    - Migraine attacks do not respond to acute drug treatment
    - Frequent, very long, or uncomfortable auras occur
  - For prevention of *episodic migraine*, effective treatments include valproate, topiramate, propranolol, timolol, and (off-label) metoprolol (6)[A].
    - Topiramate 50–100 mg BID or low-dose amitriptyline 25–75 mg daily are considered 1st-line migraine preventative treatments (7)[A].
    - Venlafaxine XR is probably effective (6)[B]. Calcium channel blockers (e.g., verapamil) are effective for some patients. Other antidepressants and antihypertensives lack definitive data.
    - NSAIDs, such as fenoprofen, ibuprofen, ketoprofen, and naproxen, are probably effective for migraine prevention but pose a risk for medication overuse headache (8)[B].
  - For treatment of *chronic migraine*, FDA has approved botulinum toxin A (Botox), as it significantly reduced the frequency of headache days in chronic migraineurs.

ISSUES FOR REFERRAL

- Obscure diagnosis, concomitant medical conditions, significant psychopathology
- Unresponsive to usual treatment
- Analgesic-dependent headache patterns

COMPLEMENTARY & ALTERNATIVE MEDICINE

- Butterbur (*Petasites hybridus*; Petadolex): 50–75 mg BID (8)[A]
- Riboflavin (vitamin B_2): 400 mg/day (8)[B]
- Magnesium: 400 mg/day (8)[B]
- MIG-99 (feverfew): 6.25 mg TID (8)[B]
- Histamine SC: 1–10 ng twice weekly (8)[B]

INPATIENT CONSIDERATIONS

Admission Criteria/Initial Stabilization

Consider if diagnosis not clear; status migrainosus; may need to exclude intracranial bleeds, TIA, stroke; monitor vital signs and patient comfort.

IV Fluids

Fluids are a necessary part of inpatient management. Keeping patients hydrated and on antiemetics around the clock may be helpful.

Discharge Criteria

Judgment based on patient's overall clinical status and patient's ability to tolerate PO medications

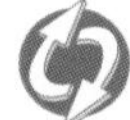

ONGOING CARE

FOLLOW-UP RECOMMENDATIONS

- Early intervention is key at the onset of an attack.
- Preventative treatment should aim to decrease frequency and severity of acute attacks, make acute treatments more efficacious, and minimize adverse drug reactions.

Patient Monitoring

- Monitor frequency of attacks, pain behaviors, and medication usage via headache diary.
- Encourage lifestyle modifications. Counsel patients and manage expectations.

PATIENT EDUCATION

Educate patients about migraine triggers.

PROGNOSIS

- With increasing age, there may be a reduction in severity, frequency, and disability of attacks.
- Most attacks subside within 72 hours.

COMPLICATIONS

- Status migrainosus (>72 hours)
- Cerebral ischemic events (rare)
- Iatrogenic effects of treatment

REFERENCES

1. Headache Classification Committee of the International Headache Society. The International Classification of Headache Disorders, 3rd edition (beta version). *Cephalalgia*. 2013;33(9):629–808.
2. Detsky ME, McDonald DR, Baerlocher MO, et al. Does this patient with headache have a migraine or need neuroimaging? *JAMA*. 2006;296(10):1274–1283.
3. Loder E, Weizenbaum E, Frishberg B, et al. Choosing wisely in headache medicine: the American Headache Society's list of five things physicians and patients should question. *Headache*. 2013;53(10):1651–1659.
4. Gilmore B, Michael M. Treatment of acute migraine headache. *Am Fam Physician*. 2011;83(3):271–280.
5. Taylor FR, Kaniecki RG. Symptomatic treatment of migraine: when to use NSAIDs, triptans, or opiates. *Curr Treat Options Neurol*. 2011;13(1):15–27.
6. Silberstein SD, Holland S, Freitag F, et al. Evidence-based guideline update: pharmacologic treatment for episodic migraine prevention in adults: report of the Quality Standards Subcommittee of the American Academy of Neurology and the American Headache Society. *Neurology*. 2012;78(17):1337–1345.
7. Fenstermacher N, Levin M, Ward T. Pharmacological prevention of migraine. *BMJ*. 2011;342:d583.
8. Holland S, Silberstein SD, Freitag F, et al. Evidence-based guideline update: NSAIDs and other complementary treatments for episodic migraine prevention in adults: report of the Quality Standards Subcommittee of the American Academy of Neurology and the American Headache Society. *Neurology*. 2012;78(17):1346–1353.

SEE ALSO

Algorithm: Headache, Chronic

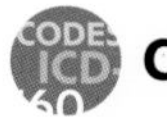

CODES

ICD10

- G43.909 Migraine, unsp, not intractable, without status migrainosus
- G43.109 Migraine with aura, not intractable, w/o status migrainosus
- G43.409 Hemiplegic migraine, not intractable, w/o status migrainosus

CLINICAL PEARLS

- Migraine is a chronic headache disorder of unclear etiology often characterized by unilateral, throbbing headaches that may be associated with additional neurologic symptoms.
- Accurate diagnosis of migraine is crucial.
- Consider nonspecific analgesics for milder attacks; migraine-specific treatments (triptans) for more severe attacks. Avoid opiates when possible. In frequent migraineurs, consider preventative treatments.

HEADACHE, TENSION

Kaelen C. Dunican, PharmD • Brandi Hoag, DO

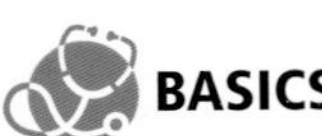

BASICS

DESCRIPTION

- Typically characterized by bilateral mild to moderate pain and pressure; may be associated with pericranial tenderness at the base of the occiput
- 2 types:
  - Episodic tension–type headache (ETTH) divided into
    - Infrequent: <1 day per month
    - Frequent: ≥1 but <15 days per month
  - Chronic tension–type headache (CTTH): ≥15 days per month for >3 months
- Synonym(s): muscle contraction headache; stress headache

EPIDEMIOLOGY

Most common type of primary headache

Prevalence

- Global prevalence in adults is 42% (1).
- Lifetime prevalence is 79%.
- More prevalent among women
- Prevalence of CTTH is 3%.
- Prevalence of ETTH decreases with age, whereas the prevalence of CTTH increases with age.

ETIOLOGY AND PATHOPHYSIOLOGY

- Debatable: peripheral and/or central mechanisms
- Activation of peripheral nociceptors leads to muscle tenderness in ETTH.
- Central sensitization is associated with CTTH:
  - Nitric oxide may play an important role in central sensitization.
  - Debatable: low-platelet serotonin
- Peripheral: may provoke the central mechanism leading from ETTH to CTTH
- Stress is the most frequently reported precipitating factor.

Genetics

An increased genetic risk has been suggested by studies, particularly for CTTH.

RISK FACTORS

Associated with triggers/precipitating factors

- Stress (mental or physical)
- Change in sleep regimen
- Skipping meals
- Certain foods (caffeine, alcohol, chocolate)
- Dehydration
- Physical exertion
- Environmental factors (sun glare, odors, smoke, noise, lighting)
- Poor or sustained posture
- Female hormonal changes
- Medications (e.g., nitrates, SSRIs, antihypertensives)
- Overuse of abortive headache medication

GENERAL PREVENTION

- Identify and avoid triggers/precipitating factors.
- Minimize emotional stress.
- Encourage relaxation techniques:
  - Biofeedback, relaxation therapy, and physical therapy
  - Consider counseling/psychotherapy.

COMMONLY ASSOCIATED CONDITIONS

- 83% of patients with migraine headaches also suffer from tension-type headaches.
- Debatable: increased prevalence of comorbid anxiety and depression

DIAGNOSIS

HISTORY

Obtain a thorough headache history to rule out other headache disorders, including severity, symptoms, onset, location and radiation of pain; quality of pain; concurrent medical conditions and medications; and recent trauma or other procedures.

Diagnosis is based on clinical symptoms.

- Diagnostic criteria provided by the International Headache Society:
  - Headache lasting 30 minutes–7 days
  - At least 2 of the following:
    - Bilateral location
    - Pressing/tightening (nonpulsating) quality
    - Mild or moderate intensity
    - Not aggravated by routine physical activity
  - Not associated with nausea or vomiting (chronic type may be associated with nausea)
  - No more than 1 of the following: photophobia or phonophobia
- Headache not due to another disorder
- Fronto-occipital or generalized pain (dull, pressing, or bandlike)
- Associated symptoms:
  - Fatigue
  - Irritability
  - Difficulty concentrating
  - Muscular tightness; tenderness; or stiffness in neck, occipital, and frontal regions

PHYSICAL EXAM

- General physical exam: vital signs, funduscopic and cardiovascular assessment, palpation of the head and neck
- Neurologic exam: mental status, pupillary responses, motor-strength testing, deep tendon reflexes, sensation, cerebellar function, gait testing, signs of meningeal irritation

DIFFERENTIAL DIAGNOSIS

- Migraine headache
- Cluster headache
- Head trauma
- Subarachnoid hemorrhage
- Subdural hematoma
- Unruptured vascular malformation
- Ischemic cerebrovascular disease
- Temporal arteritis
- Arterial hypertension (HTN)
- Cerebral venous thrombosis
- Benign intracranial HTN
- Intracranial neoplasm, infection, or meningitis
- Low CSF pressure
- Medication (nonprescription analgesic dependency, nitrates)
- Caffeine dependency
- Metabolic disorders (hypoxia, hypercapnia, hypoglycemia)
- Toxic effects from drugs or fumes
- Temporomandibular joint syndrome
- Eyes: glaucoma, refractive errors
- Sinusitis or middle ear infection
- Cervical spondylosis
- Severe anemia or polycythemia
- Uremia and hepatic disorders
- Paget disease of bone

DIAGNOSTIC TESTS & INTERPRETATION

Labs and neuroimaging (CT or MRI) are only necessary when a secondary cause is suspected:

- Atypical pattern of headache (does not fit specific category such as migraine, cluster, or tension)
- Rapid increase in frequency (2)[C]
- Focal neurologic findings
- New onset after age 40 years
- Sudden onset or worsening with exertion CT scan, with and without contrast, is as sensitive as MRI and is the test of choice.
- Use MRI when lesions of the posterior fossa or an aneurysm is suspected.

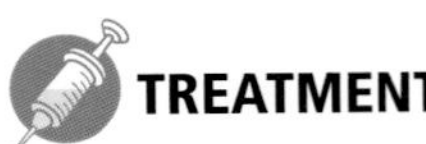

TREATMENT

- NSAIDs, acetaminophen (APAP), and aspirin (ASA) are effective for short-term pain relief of ETTH (3,4)[B].
- Amitriptyline should be considered first line for prophylaxis of CTTH (3,4)[B].

GENERAL MEASURES

Relief measures: relaxation routines; rest in quiet, dark room; hot bath or shower; massage of back of neck and temples

MEDICATION

Choice of simple analgesic is based on patient-specific parameters:

- NSAIDs may be more effective than APAP for ETTH (3)[C]:
  - Ibuprofen and naproxen may be preferred due to better GI tolerability.
- APAP should be considered for patients taking warfarin, unable to tolerate NSAIDs, or allergic to ASA or NSAIDs.

First Line

- For acute attack (ETTH): NSAIDs, APAP, or ASA:
  - NSAIDs:
    - Ibuprofen (Motrin, Advil): 400–800 mg; may repeat q8h PRN (max 3.2 g/day)
    - Naproxen (Naprosyn): 375–500 mg or naproxen sodium (Aleve, Anaprox) 440–550 mg; may repeat q8–12h PRN (max 1,250 mg naproxen base/d)
    - Ketoprofen (Orudis): 12.5–50 mg; may repeat q6–8h PRN (max 300 mg/day)
    - Diclofenac (Voltaren, Cataflam): 50–100 mg; may repeat q8h PRN (max 150 mg/day)
    - Contraindications: ASA or NSAID allergy or bronchospasm, renal disease, bleeding disorders, increased risk of cardiovascular events (myocardial infarction [MI], stroke, new onset, or worsening of HTN)
    - Drug interactions: antihypertensives, anticoagulants, antiplatelet drugs, ASA, lithium, methotrexate
    - Adverse effects: epigastric distress, peptic ulcer
  - APAP (Tylenol): 1,000 mg; may repeat q6h PRN (max 4 g/day):
    - Adverse effects (rare): rash, pancytopenia, liver damage
    - Precaution: hepatic impairment, consumption of ≥3/day alcoholic beverages

- Aspirin: 500–1,000 mg; may repeat q6h PRN (max 4 g/day):
  - Contraindication: ASA or NSAID allergy or bronchospasm, bleeding disorders
  - Drug interactions: anticoagulants, antiplatelet drugs, ACE inhibitors, β-blockers, corticosteroids, NSAIDs, sulfonylureas
  - Adverse effects: GI irritation/bleeding, thrombocytopenia
- Prophylaxis for CTTH: tricyclic antidepressants (TCAs) (amitriptyline [Elavil]) 10–75 mg/day:
  - Not FDA approved for CTTH
  - Contraindications: acute recovery phase of MI, use of monamine oxidase inhibitors (MAOIs) within 14 days
  - Drug interactions: clonidine, MAOIs, quinolone antibiotics, SSRIs, sympathomimetics, azole antifungals, valproic acid
  - Adverse effects: drowsiness, dry mouth, tachycardia, heart block, blurred vision, urinary retention, seizure

Second Line

- For acute attack (ETTH):
  - Caffeine combinations: 130 mg caffeine with 500 mg APAP and/or 500 mg ASA q6h PRN (3)[C]
  - Narcotic analgesics (rarely indicated; consider secondary causes of headache or secondary gain such as drug-seeking behavior for personal use or diversion/sale)
  - Ketorolac: 60 mg IM, single dose
- For CTTH prophylaxis:
  - Mirtazapine: 15–30 mg/day (not FDA approved for CTTH) (3,4)[B]
  - Venlafaxine XR (Effexor XR): 37.5–300 mg/day (not FDA approved for CTTH) (3,4)[B]

ALERT

Use of abortive agents >2 days/week may lead to *medication-overuse headaches*; must withdraw acute treatment to diagnose.

Pediatric Considerations

ASA and antidepressants are contraindicated.

ADDITIONAL THERAPIES

- The combination of stress management therapy and a TCA (amitriptyline) may be most effective for CTTH.
- Maprotiline: 75 mg/day (not FDA approved for CTTH) (3)[C]
- Topiramate: 100 mg/day (limited clinical evidence for prevention of CTTH; not FDA approved for CTTH)
- Alternative TCAs (although limited evidence of benefit, all are widely used for prophylaxis) (5)[B]
  - Desipramine (Norpramin): 50–100 mg/day
  - Imipramine (Tofranil): 50–100 mg/day
  - Nortriptyline (Pamelor): 25–50 mg/day
  - Protriptyline (Vivactil): 25 mg/day
- Drugs with conflicting clinical evidence for CTTH (not FDA approved for CTTH):
  - Tizanidine: 2–6 mg TID
  - Memantine: 20–40 mg/day
- Botulinum toxin type A is not likely to be effective for ETTH or CTTH (6)[A).

COMPLEMENTARY & ALTERNATIVE MEDICINE

- Electromyographic (EMG) biofeedback may be effective and is enhanced when combined with relaxation therapy (3,7)[C].
- Cognitive-behavioral therapy may be helpful (3,7)[C].
- Physical therapy, including positioning, ergonomic instruction, massage, transcutaneous electrical nerve simulation, and application of heat/cold may help.
- Alternative agents (not FDA approved for TTH)
  - Tiger Balm or peppermint oil applied topically to the forehead may be effective for ETTH.
  - Limited evidence for use of acupuncture and physical therapy (7)[B]
- Chiropractic spinal manipulation cannot be recommended for the management of ETTH; recommendations cannot be made for CTTH (8)[B].

INPATIENT CONSIDERATIONS

Admission Criteria/Initial Stabilization

Outpatient treatment

ONGOING CARE

FOLLOW-UP RECOMMENDATIONS

- Regulate sleep schedule.
- Regular exercise

DIET

- Identify and avoid dietary triggers.
- Regulate meal schedule.

PATIENT EDUCATION

For additional information, contact:

- National Headache Foundation: http://www.headaches.org
- American Council for Headache Education: http://www.achenet.org

PROGNOSIS

- Usually follows a chronic course when life stressors are not changed
- Most cases are intermittent.

COMPLICATIONS

- Lost days of work and productivity (more with CTTH)
- Cost to health system
- Dependence/addiction to narcotic analgesics
- GI bleeding from NSAID use

REFERENCES

1. Ferrante T, Manzoni GC, Russo M, et al. Prevalence of tension-type headache in adult general population: the PACE study and review of the literature. *Neurol Sci*. 2013;34(Suppl 1):S17–S138.
2. Freitag F. Managing and treating tension-type headache. *Med Clin North Am*. 2013;97(2): 281–292.
3. Bendtsen L, Jensen R. Treating tension-type headache—an expert opinion. *Expert Opin Pharmacother*. 2011;12(7):1099–1109.
4. Bendtsen L, Evers S, Linde M, et al. EFNS guideline on the treatment of tension-type headache—report of an EFNS task force. *Eur J Neurol*. 2010;17(11):1318–1325.
5. Verhagen AP, Damen L, Berger MY, et al. Lack of benefit for prophylactic drugs of tension-type headache in adults: a systematic review. *Fam Pract*. 2010;27(2):151–165.
6. Jackson JL, Kuriyama A, Hayashino Y. Botulinum toxin A for prophylactic treatment of migraine and tension headaches in adults: a meta-analysis. *JAMA*. 2012;307(16):1736–1745.
7. Sun-Edelstein C, Mauskop A. Complementary and alternative approaches to the treatment of tension-type headache. *Curr Pain Headache Rep*. 2012;16(6):539–544.
8. Bryans R, Descarreaux M, Duranleau M, et al. Evidence-based guidelines for the chiropractic treatment of adults with headache. *J Manipulative Physiol Ther*. 2011;34(5):274–289.

SEE ALSO

Algorithm: Headache, Chronic

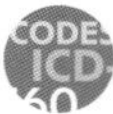

CODES

ICD10

- G44.209 Tension-type headache, unspecified, not intractable
- G44.219 Episodic tension-type headache, not intractable
- G44.229 Chronic tension-type headache, not intractable

CLINICAL PEARLS

- Tension-type headache may be difficult to distinguish from migraine without aura. A tension-type headache is typically described as bilateral, mild to moderate, dull pain, whereas a migraine is typically pulsating; unilateral; and associated with nausea, vomiting, and photophobia or phonophobia.
- Evidence suggests that NSAIDs may be more effective than APAP for ETTH. Consider APAP for patients who cannot tolerate, or have a contraindication, to NSAIDs. Initial dose of APAP should be 1,000 mg (500 mg may not be as effective).
- CTTH is difficult to treat, and these patients are more likely to develop medication-overuse headache. Clinical evidence supports the use of amitriptyline + stress-management therapy for CTTH.
- Medication-overuse headaches must be avoided by limiting use of abortive agents to no more than 2 days/week.
- A headache diary may be useful to identify triggers, response to treatment, and medication-overuse headaches.

HEARING LOSS

Robert A. Baldor, MD, FAAFP

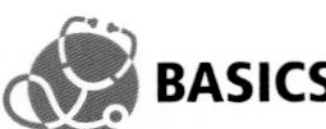

BASICS

DESCRIPTION
- Decrease in the ability to comprehend sound. It can be partial, complete, unilateral, or bilateral.
- Types of hearing loss include conductive hearing loss (CHL or air–bone gap), sensorineural hearing loss (SNHL), or mixed hearing loss.
- System(s) affected: auditory; external and middle ear (CHL) or inner ear (SNHL)

EPIDEMIOLOGY
- All ages affected; common in children (CHL) and elderly (SNHL)
- Predominant sex: male = female

Incidence
- 3/10 people >60 years of age
- At least 1.4 million children (≤18 years of age)

Prevalence
Hearing loss has decreased from 12.2% (1992) to 8.1% (2000) in men and 7% (1992) to 4.2% (2000) in women.

Geriatric Considerations
- ~50% of people age >85 years have hearing loss.
- Hearing aids are underused.
- Loss of communication is a source of emotional stress and a physical risk for the elderly.

Pediatric Considerations
- Congenital hearing loss
  - 1–3/1,000 infants have hearing loss.
  - Mandatory newborn screening (otoacoustic emission [OAE] and auditory brainstem response [ABR] testing are ideal)
- Audiologic testing after major intracranial infection (meningitis)

Pregnancy Considerations
Otosclerosis can worsen during pregnancy.

ETIOLOGY AND PATHOPHYSIOLOGY
- CHL: Hearing loss can result from middle ear effusion, obstruction of canal (cerumen/foreign body, osteomas/exostoses, cholesteatoma, tumor), loss of continuity (ossicular discontinuity), stiffening of the components (myringosclerosis, tympanosclerosis, and otosclerosis), and loss of the pressure differential across the tympanic membrane (TM) (perforation).
- SNHL: damage along the pathway from oval window, cochlea, auditory nerve, and brainstem. Examples include vascular/metabolic insult, mass effect, infection and inflammation, and acoustic trauma.
  - Noise-induced hearing loss is caused by acoustic insult that affects outer hair cells in the organ of Corti, causing them to be less stiff. Over time, severe damage occurs with fusion and loss of stereocilia. Eventually may progress to inner hair cells and auditory nerve as well
- Large vestibular aqueduct or superior canal dehiscence: Third mobile window shunts acoustic energy away from cochlea.

Genetics
- Connexin 26 (13q11–12): most common cause of nonsyndromic genetic hearing loss
- Mitochondrial disorders (may predispose to aminoglycoside ototoxicity)
- Otosclerosis: familial
- Most common congenital syndromes:
  - Hemifacial microsomia
  - Stickler syndrome
  - Congenital cytomegalovirus
  - Usher syndrome
  - Branchio-oto-renal syndrome
  - Pendred syndrome
  - CHARGE association
  - Neurofibromatosis type 2
  - Waardenburg syndrome

RISK FACTORS
- Conductive
  - Chronic sinusitis; allergy
  - Cigarette smoking
  - Sleep apnea with continuous positive airway pressure (CPAP) use
  - Adenoid hypertrophy; nasopharyngeal mass
  - Eustachian tube dysfunction
  - Neuromuscular disease
  - Family history/heredity
  - Prematurity and low birth weight
  - Craniofacial abnormalities (e.g., cleft palate, Down syndrome)
  - Third mobile window (superior canal dehiscence or large vestibular aqueduct)
- Sensorineural
  - Aging/older age
  - Loud noise/acoustic trauma
  - Dizziness/vertigo: especially Ménière disease or history of labyrinthitis
  - Medications (aminoglycosides, loop diuretics, quinine, aspirin, chemotherapeutic agents)
  - Bacterial meningitis
  - Head trauma
  - Atherosclerosis
  - Vestibular schwannoma/skull base neoplasm
  - Previous ear surgery
- Sensorineural, pediatric specific
  - Postnatal asphyxia
  - Mechanical ventilation lasting ≥5 days
  - In utero infections (TORCH syndrome; toxoplasmosis; other agents, rubella, cytomegalovirus, herpes simplex)
  - Toxemia of pregnancy
  - Maternal diabetes
  - Rh incompatibility
  - Prematurity or birth weight <1,500 g
  - Hyperbilirubinemia; exchange transfusions
  - Anomalous temporal bone (Mondini or large vestibular aqueduct)
  - Infectious diseases: chickenpox, measles, encephalitis, influenza, mumps

GENERAL PREVENTION
- Limit noise exposure; use hearing protection.
- Avoid ear canal instrumentation (e.g., cotton swabs).
- Limit ototoxic medications.

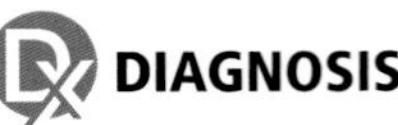

DIAGNOSIS

HISTORY
- Social problems and comments from friends and family members are often the 1st presentation of presbycusis, as patients are often not aware of the degree of hearing loss they experience and how it affects their life. Onset is gradual.
- Difficulty hearing
  - Rapid versus gradual decline: Rapid loss (<3 days) is a medical emergency. If suspicious of a sudden SNHL, urgently refer to ENT.
  - Difficulty with discrimination of sounds, hearing in crowds or turning up the volume of television sets
  - Frequently having to ask speakers to repeat
  - Friends/family complain of hearing loss
- Tinnitus, bilateral, or unilateral
- Otalgia
- Otorrhea, clear or purulent
- Dizziness or vertigo
- Ear fullness
- Autophony (hearing own voice louder or echoing)
- Depression or anxiety
- History of ear infections or ear surgeries
- History of trauma or noise exposure
- Family history of hearing loss
- History of recent viral infection
- Nasal obstruction
- Frequent epistaxis

PHYSICAL EXAM
- A simple 512-Hz tuning fork test lateralizes to unaffected ear in sudden SNHL (emergency) and lateralizes to the affected ear in CHL (not an emergency).
- Whispering screen: A whisper heard from ~2 feet away is a good screen for intact hearing. Patients with SNHL have difficulty with this because their hearing loss is usually in the high frequency range.
- 512-Hz tuning fork tests:
  - Sensorineural loss
    - Placed on the forehead: lateralizes to nonaffected ear (Weber test)
    - Base of tuning fork placed on the mastoid and then fork end placed next to ear; heard louder next to ear (Rinne test)
  - Conductive loss
    - Placed on the forehead or teeth lateralizes to affected or symptomatic ear
    - Placed on the mastoid and then next to ear; heard louder behind the ear on the side of conductive deficit
- Otoscopy: Assess for deformity, canal patency, and otorrhea; TM integrity/retraction/mobility with insufflation; canal; or middle ear mass.
- Facial symmetry
- Cranial nerve exam
- Nasopharyngoscopy: adenoid hypertrophy or nasopharyngeal mass (mandatory in adult patient with new unilateral serous effusion)
- Pediatric: Survey for syndromic anomalies.

DIFFERENTIAL DIAGNOSIS

- Conductive
  - Cerumen impaction/foreign body
  - Perforation of TM
  - Middle ear fluid (serous otitis media)
  - Acute otitis media/adhesive otitis media
  - Ossicular erosion (infection, cholesteatoma)
  - Myringosclerosis/tympanosclerosis
  - Temporal bone fracture
  - Otosclerosis
  - Glomus tumor
- Sensorineural
  - Presbycusis (hearing loss related to aging)
  - Noise-induced (recreational, occupational)
  - Ménière disease
  - Ototoxicity (aspirin, aminoglycosides)
  - Viral labyrinthitis
  - Cerebellopontine angle tumor
  - Large vestibular aqueduct syndrome
  - Syndromic hearing loss
  - Congenital cochlear malformation
  - Syphilis
  - Cytomegalovirus; rubella
  - Temporal bone fracture
  - Metabolic (hyper-/hypothyroid)
  - Paget disease
  - Perilymphatic (inner ear) fistula

DIAGNOSTIC TESTS & INTERPRETATION

Often labs are not needed. If indicated

- Pendred syndrome (goiter, mental retardation + SNHL): perchlorate test, thyroid function tests
- Alport syndrome (nephritis + SNHL): urinalysis, renal function tests
- Jervell and Lange-Nielsen syndrome (syncope, family history of sudden death + profound SNHL): ECG
- Any pediatric patient with SNHL: Consider genetic testing for connexin 26, mitochondrial studies.
- TORCH screening (congenital infection)
- Rapid plasma reagin (RPR) or Venereal Disease Research Laboratory (VDRL) confirmed by fluorescent treponemal antibody absorption (FTA-ABS)
- Lyme titer in endemic areas
- Antinuclear antibodies and sedimentation rate as a screen for autoimmune disease
- Fine-cut CT temporal bones without contrast may help in the evaluation of CHL.
- MRI of brain and brainstem with gadolinium to evaluate SNHL in congenital, early onset, and asymmetric hearing loss

Diagnostic Procedures/Other

- Audiometry: pure tone (air and bone), speech testing, and impedance (middle ear pressure) testing
- Tympanometry: Type B or C tympanograms indicate fluid or retraction, respectively. Negative middle ear peak pressures seen even with normal (type A) tympanograms.
- Other tests:
  - Auditory brainstem response
  - OAEs: "echo" of the cochlea
  - Behavioral (visual reinforcement) audiometry; used in children 6 months–5 years
- Myringotomy and tubes can be considered for persistent fluid with hearing loss.

Test Interpretation

Varies depending on etiology

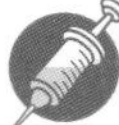

TREATMENT

Hearing rehabilitation:

- Personal amplifiers, situation-specific amplification (e.g., amplified phone), or personal hearing aids can be considered for any individual who has significant communication difficulties due to hearing loss.
- Cochlear implants for patients with bilateral severe to profound hearing loss who no longer derive benefit from hearing aids

MEDICATION

- Depends on cause
- Any sudden SNHL (usually unilateral) is a medical emergency; obtain a hearing testing and start steroid therapy.
- Treatment should begin ASAP, ideally within 1–2 weeks of onset with high-dose oral steroids: 1 mg/kg or 60–100 mg/day prednisone or 12–16 mg/day dexamethasone for 7–14 days, followed by a taper: For patients who cannot tolerate systematic steroids, intratympanic steroids are equally effective (1)[A].
  - Clinical practical guidelines for sudden hearing loss include the following (2)[C]:
    - Distinguishing SNHL from CHL; testing for bilateral sudden hearing loss in patients with unilateral sudden hearing loss; obtaining an MRI, auditory brainstem response or audiometric follow-up to evaluate for retrocochlear pathology; offer intratympanic steroid perfusion for refractory cases after initial management fails to treat idiopathic SNHL (ISSNHL) and follow-up within 6 month of diagnosis.
    - May offer corticosteroids as initial therapy to patients with ISSNHL and hyperbaric oxygen within 3 months of ISSNHL diagnosis
    - Recommended against prescribing antivirals, thrombolytics, vasodilators, vasoactive substances, or antioxidants to patients with ISSNHL
    - Also recommended against routine laboratory tests in patients with ISSNHL

ISSUES FOR REFERRAL

- Audiology: If hearing loss is suspected, refer to audiology for formal evaluation. Audiologists also provide hearing aid options and maintenance.
- Genetics: if congenital syndrome or familial hearing loss is suspected
- Speech therapist: if speech delay or speech impediment is present
- Endocrinology: Pendred syndrome, other associated endocrine disorder (hypo-/hyperthyroidism)
- Cardiology: Jervell and Lange-Nielsen syndrome
- Ophthalmology: Usher syndrome
- Neurotology and neurosurgery: cerebellopontine angle (CPA) lesion, intracranial complication of middle ear disease

SURGERY/OTHER PROCEDURES

- CHL often has surgical options for repair.
  - Tympanostomy and tube placement
  - Tympanoplasty
  - Mastoidectomy
  - Ossicular chain reconstruction
  - Stapedectomy/stapedotomy
  - Canaloplasty
- Those with profound bilateral SNHL may qualify for cochlear implantation.

ONGOING CARE

FOLLOW-UP RECOMMENDATIONS

Patient Monitoring

Audiogram and clinical exam are primary means of monitoring patient. Patients with hearing-assist devices benefit from audiology involvement.

DIET

Salt restriction to 2 g/day is helpful for patients with Ménière disease.

PATIENT EDUCATION

National Institute on Deafness and Other Communication Disorders: www.nidcd.nih.gov/health/hearing/

PROGNOSIS

SNHL is usually permanent and may be progressive. However, amplification devices (e.g., hearing aids) may help improve functionality.

COMPLICATIONS

Acute middle ear problems may become chronic (perforations, cholesteatoma).

REFERENCES

1. Spear SA, Schwartz SR. Intratympanic steroids for sudden sensorineural hearing loss: a systematic review. *Otolaryngol Head Neck Surg*. 2011;145(4):534–543.
2. Stachler RJ, Chandrasekhar SS, Archer SM, et al. Clinical practice guideline: sudden hearing loss. *Otolaryngol Head Neck Surg*. 2012;146(3)(Suppl):S1–S35.

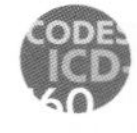

CODES

ICD10

- H91.90 Unspecified hearing loss, unspecified ear
- H90.2 Conductive hearing loss, unspecified
- H90.5 Unspecified sensorineural hearing loss

CLINICAL PEARLS

- In sudden hearing loss, if a 512-Hz tuning fork test (Weber test) lateralizes to the *unaffected ear*, suspect sensorineural causes (emergent evaluation needed), but if it lateralizes to the *affected* ear, the diagnosis is CHL (not an emergency).
- ~50% of people age >85 years have hearing loss, encourage screening and treatment, especially in patients with early dementia.

H

HEART FAILURE, ACUTELY DECOMPENSATED

Jeremy Golding, MD, FAAFP

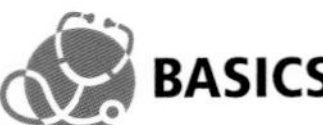

BASICS

DESCRIPTION

Acute decompensated heart failure (ADHF) is a heterogeneous syndrome of acute impairment in cardiac pump function resulting in inefficient perfusion to bodily tissues. This may be due to structural or functional cardiac disorders and may represent a new diagnosis or worsening of preexisting chronic HF.

EPIDEMIOLOGY

Incidence

- Medicare spends more to diagnose and treat HF than any other medical condition. In 2009, the total cost of HF approached $37 billion. In the United States, there are 670,000 new cases annually. HF is the primary cause of >55,000 deaths each year and a contributing factor in >280,000 deaths.
- 1 million admissions/year; 30% incident ADHF; 70% decompensated chronic HF
- About ½ of people who have HF die within 5 years of diagnosis.

Prevalence

- ~5.8 million people in the United States carry an HF diagnosis; <1% in those <50 years of age, increasing to 10% of those >70 years of age
- Primarily a disease of the elderly; 75% of hospital admissions for HF are in persons >65 years of age.

ETIOLOGY AND PATHOPHYSIOLOGY

- Two physiologic components explain most of the clinical findings of ADHF.
  - Systolic dysfunction: an *inotropic* abnormality, often due to myocardial infarction (MI) or dilated or ischemic cardiomyopathy, resulting in diminished systolic emptying (ejection fraction <45%)
  - Diastolic dysfunction: a *compliance* abnormality, often due to hypertensive cardiomyopathy, in which the ventricular relaxation is impaired (ejection fraction >45%)
- Common causes of ADHF
  - Exacerbation of chronic HF caused by dietary or medication nonadherence, infection, or any of the following as cause of new HF or exacerbation
  - Coronary artery disease (CAD), MI (especially new-onset ADHF)
  - Arrhythmia (afib or tachyarrhythmias, high-grade heart block)
  - Valvular and vascular abnormalities: aortic stenosis or regurgitation, rheumatic heart disease (mitral and aortic valvular disease)
  - Severe hypertension (both systemic and pulmonary)
  - High-output states: hyperthyroidism, anemia
  - Medications: cardiac depressants (β-blocker overdose), chemotherapeutic agents
  - Other (infiltrative disease, Chagas disease, pericardial disease, postpartum cardiomyopathy, wet beriberi, sepsis)

Genetics

Familial cardiomyopathy predisposes to development of HF (rare).

RISK FACTORS

- History of chronic HF
- CAD and MI
- Hypertension (HTN), systemic or pulmonary
- Valvular heart disease
- Diabetes mellitus
- Cardiotoxic medications
- Renal insufficiency and renal failure
- Arrhythmia
- Infection

GENERAL PREVENTION

Control BP and other risk factors. Thiazide diuretics and ACE inhibitors are superior to other agents in preventing development of HF. Treat cardiovascular disease.

COMMONLY ASSOCIATED CONDITIONS

- Dysrhythmia followed by pump failure is the leading cause of death in ADHF. Most patients have >5 comorbid medical conditions (especially CAD, chronic kidney disease, and diabetes) and take >5 medications.
- Cardiogenic shock
- Hyponatremia and altered mental status, especially in the elderly

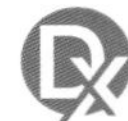

DIAGNOSIS

Clinical diagnosis, no gold standard; ED diagnosis of ADHF is incorrect 10–20%.

HISTORY

- History of HF
- Dyspnea on exertion: *cardinal sign of left-sided HF*. Deteriorating exercise capacity: easy fatigue, general weakness, possibly chest pain/discomfort if acute coronary syndrome (ACS) is present
- Nocturnal nonproductive cough, orthopnea, and paroxysmal nocturnal dyspnea; sometimes frothy or pink sputum
- Wheezing, especially nocturnal, in absence of history of asthma or infection (cardiac asthma)
- Edema, abdominal bloating (ascites), or anasarca; cyanosis

PHYSICAL EXAM

- S_3 and/or jugular venous distension most useful positive finding, although no vital sign/PE finding has sensitivity >70%
- Peripheral edema, cool extremities, edema, cyanosis, hepatomegaly, hepatojugular reflex, hypotension, laterally displaced apical impulse
- Lung exam: rales (crackles) and sometimes wheezing, Cheyne-Stokes respirations

DIFFERENTIAL DIAGNOSIS

Pulmonary embolism, exertional asthma, acute MI, cardiac ischemia with angina, chronic obstructive pulmonary disease (COPD), constrictive pericarditis, pneumonia, tamponade, tension pneumothorax, high-output states: anemia, sepsis, hyperthyroidism

DIAGNOSTIC TESTS & INTERPRETATION

- Laboratory data are adjunctive and indicative of complications.
- Perform ECG to evaluate for ACS.

Initial Tests (lab, imaging)

- Cardiac troponins (to evaluate for ACS)
- B-type natriuretic peptide (BNP) and/or N-type pro-BNP (BT-BNP) may be helpful in (1)[A].
  - ED setting to help differentiate the cause of dyspnea. BNP <100 essentially rules out HF as a cause of dyspnea with negative predictive value (NPV) of ~99%. Most dyspneic patients with ADHF have BNP >400. Elevation in BNP is not able to differentiate systolic versus nonsystolic HF adequately.
  - BNP may be higher in obesity or if renal disease is present. BNP and N-type pro-BNP have been shown to have similar specificities and sensitivities in identifying ADHF.
  - BNP values of 100–400 are more problematic, as they may indicate HF or may be due to conditions such as pulmonary embolism, renal failure, ACS, and pulmonary HTN.
  - Patients may have BNP elevated due to HF, but acute dyspnea may be from another cause (pneumonia or pulmonary embolism).
  - Other lab findings in early and mild to moderately severe ADHF include respiratory alkalosis, mild azotemia, and dilutional hyponatremia (poor prognosis).
  - Chest x-ray (CXR) (changes lag clinical symptoms by up to 6 hours): increased heart size, vascular redistribution (cephalization) with "butterfly" pattern of pulmonary edema, interstitial and alveolar edema, Kerley B lines, pleural effusions
  - Bedside cardiac US (available in the ED) to assess pump function (identify systolic vs. diastolic dysfunction, tamponade, valvular abnormalities, etc.)

Follow-Up Tests & Special Considerations

Please see "Chronic Heart Failure" topic.

Diagnostic Procedures/Other

Determining ejection fraction (EF) is critical to proper diagnosis and management: Formal echocardiographic study is most useful single test to determine EF and valvular abnormalities; may be repeated if change suspected in underlying cardiac status. Pulmonary artery catheterization may be performed to guide therapy in severe cases with cardiogenic shock.

Test Interpretation

Cardiac pathology depends on the etiology of HF. Please refer to "Chronic Heart Failure" topic.

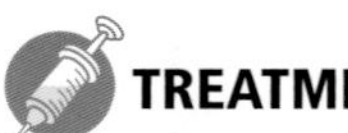

TREATMENT

Approach is to improve symptoms, hemodynamics, and renal function and to minimize myocardial damage and hospital length of stay. See "Chronic Heart Failure" chapter as well.

MEDICATION

ALERT

Many medications have been shown to improve hemodynamics and symptoms in ADHF but do not decrease mortality. Diuretics are used initially in fluid overload acute HF, with nitrates added if needed. Nitrates are primary therapy in ischemic acute HF (flash pulmonary edema) and hypertensive ADHF, with diuretics secondary. Once acute HF is stabilized, an ACE inhibitor or β-blocker should be started. Instruct patients not to use NSAIDs. Avoid use of diltiazem and verapamil in patients with systolic dysfunction.

First Line

- Loop diuretics initially for fluid-overloaded ADHF in hemodynamically stable patients (contraindicated if SBP <90 mm Hg, severe hyponatremia, acidosis) (2)[A]; be cautious of electrolyte abnormalities if kidney disease is present. Avoid if possible diagnosis of pneumonia. Continuous infusion is not better

than bolus, and high dose is not significantly better than low dose.
- Furosemide (Lasix): 40 mg IV
- If on Lasix chronically, initial IV dose should be equal or exceed chronic oral daily dose (max 180 mg). Monitor for appropriate urine output.
- Metolazone (Zaroxolyn): 2.5–20 mg/day PO, more useful if reduced creatinine clearance

- Thiazides in combination with loop diuretics may be useful if resistant to diuresis (HCTZ 25 mg PO). Thiazides and spironolactone or eplerenone (25–50 mg PO) may be used in combination with loop diuretics if excessive volume overload.
- Vasodilators: first line in addition to diuretics if severe HTN or acute pulmonary edema; don't use if SBP <90 mm Hg, history of aortic stenosis, or phosphodiesterase inhibitor use
  - IV nitroglycerin may be of short-term benefit to decrease preload, afterload, and systemic resistance (IV 10–20 μg/min)
  - IV nitroprusside: Administer with caution, infusion rate 5–10 μg/min. Consider an arterial line.
- Morphine: IV boluses 2.5–5 mg IV helps with chest pain and restlessness. Monitor respirations.

Second Line

- Tolvaptan (an oral vasopressin antagonist), in addition to normal treatment (including diuretics), may improve dyspnea and decrease body weight at 24 hours but confers no survival or morbidity benefit.
- Inotropes: Consider adding if signs of hypoperfusion and in patients with dilated cardiomyopathy. Withdraw as soon as hemodynamic parameters improve, as these may increase short- and medium-term mortality.
  - Phosphodiesterase inhibitors (milrinone, enoximone) decrease pulmonary resistance; may be used for patients on β-blockers but may increase medium-term mortality in CAD patients
  - Dobutamine infusion requires close BP monitoring; avoid in cardiogenic shock or with tachyarrhythmias
  - Low-dose dopamine infusion may be considered.
  - Levosimendan (calcium sensitizer) improves hemodynamic parameters but not survival compared to placebo while improving hemodynamic parameters and survival compared to dobutamine.
- Nesiritide, a BNP analog, is not recommended for most hospitalized patients with ADHF; higher rates of hypotension, no benefit on death or rehospitalization rates

ADDITIONAL THERAPIES

- Oxygen: Begin treatment early; ideally, arterial oxygen saturation >92% (90% if COPD). For acute cardiogenic pulmonary edema, noninvasive ventilation (BiPAP, CPAP) decreases early mortality compared to standard therapy.
- No significant difference between continuous positive airway pressure (CPAP) and noninvasive positive pressure ventilation (NIPPV). If possible, avoid mechanical ventilation for patients with right HF (3)[A].
- Treat anemia with transfusion: conservative trigger Hgb <8; target Hgb 10.
- For patients with new-onset arrhythmias, consider pacing and/or antiarrhythmics.
- For patients in severe cardiogenic shock, consider intra-aortic balloon pump or percutaneous or surgically implanted ventricular assist devices (VADs).
- Please refer to "Chronic Heart Failure" for maintenance treatments.

SURGERY/OTHER PROCEDURES

- Heart valve surgery if defective heart valve is responsible
- PCI/CABG for patients with CAD/MI if applicable
- Cardiac transplantation considered in patients <55 years of age and without other disqualifying medical problems who are developing chronic decompensated HF unresponsive to other therapeutic maneuvers and who are considered to have a life expectancy of >1 year

INPATIENT CONSIDERATIONS

Postdischarge appointment, left ventricular EF assessment, and start on ACEi (or ARB) and β-blocker if left ventricular systolic dysfunction present

Admission Criteria/Initial Stabilization

See earlier discussion.

- Acute change in HF, with pulmonary edema accompanied by decreased oxygenation, change in mental status, with acute renal insufficiency, or significant hyponatremia
- Consider observation unit stay for hemodynamically stable ED patients assuming preexisting HF and the following:
  - No acute interventions needed for comorbid condition
  - SBP >120 mm Hg, BUN <40, creatinine <3.0, absence of elevated troponins/ischemic ECG changes
  - Respiratory rate <32 breaths/min without needing noninvasive ventilation
  - No actively titrated vasoactive IV infusions
  - Partial improvement in vital signs and/or increased urine output with initial treatment
  - Clinical impression that patient could be discharged in the next 24 hours and rapid outpatient follow-up is available.

IV Fluids

Restrict fluids if possible. Avoid sodium-containing fluids unless necessary to urgently correct hyponatremia.

Discharge Criteria

Subjective improvement, resting heart rate (HR) <100 bpm, systolic BP >80 mm Hg, HF outpatient education performed

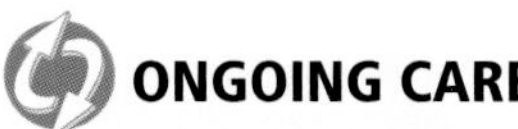

ONGOING CARE

FOLLOW-UP RECOMMENDATIONS

Critical patient education performed at all outpatient and inpatient physician visits. Please see "Chronic Heart Failure" topic.

Patient Monitoring

Rapid office follow-up after hospitalization and home health monitoring by specially trained nurses have both been shown to decrease frequency of hospitalizations.

DIET

Reduce sodium (2 g); maintain cardiac or diabetic diet if these comorbidities are present.

PATIENT EDUCATION

- Definition and etiology: Understand the cause of HF and why symptoms occur.
- Prognosis: Understand important prognostic factors and make realistic decisions.
- Symptom monitoring and self-care: Recognize signs/symptoms, record daily weight, know how and when to contact a healthcare provider; may increase diuretic dose with >1 kg in a day or >2 kg weight gain in 5 days or dyspnea/contact health care provider
- Pharmacologic treatment: Understand indications, dosing, effects, and side effects of drugs.
- Adherence: Understand the importance of maintaining the treatment plan.
- Alcohol, smoking, and drugs: Modest intake/abstinence is recommended in patients with alcohol-induced cardiomyopathy. Otherwise, normal alcohol guidelines apply. Smoking and illicit drug cessation.
- Exercise: Understand the benefits of exercise, perform regularly, be comfortable about physical activity.

PROGNOSIS

- The ADHERE risk tree stratifies ADHF patients for inpatient mortality using systolic blood pressure, BUN, and creatinine.
- S_3 on physical exam correlates with poor prognosis.
- After diagnosis, 1-year survival ~75%, 5-year survival <50%, 10-year <25%

COMPLICATIONS

Sudden death (arrhythmic), acute pulmonary edema, hyponatremia, death

REFERENCES

1. Worster A, Balion CM, Hill SA, et al. Diagnostic accuracy of BNP and NT-proBNP in patients presenting to acute care settings with dyspnea: a systematic review. *Clin Biochem*. 2008;41(4–5):250–259.
2. Felker GM, Lee KL, Bull DA, et al. Diuretic strategies in patients with acute decompensated heart failure. *N Engl J Med*. 2011;364(9):797–805.
3. Mariani J, Macchia A, Belziti C, et al. Noninvasive ventilation in acute cardiogenic pulmonary edema: a meta-analysis of randomized controlled trials. *J Card Fail*. 2011;17(10):850–859.

ADDITIONAL READING

- Centers for Disease Control and Prevention. Heart failure fact sheet. http://www.cdc.gov/dhdsp/data_statistics/fact_sheets/docs/fs_heart_failure.pdf. Accessed 2014.
- Delaney A, Bradford C, McCaffrey J, et al. Levosimendan for the treatment of acute severe heart failure: a meta-analysis of randomised controlled trials. *Int J Cardiol*. 2010;138(3):281–289.
- Konstam MA, Gheorghiade M, Burnett JC Jr, et al. Effects of oral tolvaptan in patients hospitalized for worsening heart failure: the EVEREST Outcome Trial. *JAMA*. 2007;297(12):1319–1331.
- McMurray JJV, Adamopoulos S, Anker SD, et al. ESC guidelines for the diagnosis and treatment of acute and chronic heart failure 2012: the Task Force for the Diagnosis and Treatment of Acute and Chronic Heart Failure 2012 of the European Society of Cardiology. Developed in collaboration with the Heart Failure Association (HFA) of the ESC. *Eur Heart J*. 2012;33(14):1787–1847.
- O'Connor CM, Starling RC, Hernandez AF, et al. Effect of nesiritide in patients with acute decompensated heart failure. *N Engl J Med*. 2011;365(1):32–43.

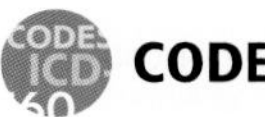

CODES

ICD10

I50.9 Heart failure, unspecified

CLINICAL PEARLS

- BNP is overused diagnostically and is best reserved for situations in which diagnosis of ADHF is unclear.
- Look for underlying cause of each episode of ADHF.
- IV diuretics are used initially in fluid-overload acute HF, with nitrates added if needed. Nitrates are primary therapy in ischemic acute HF.

HEART FAILURE, CHRONIC

Jeffrey Shih, MD • David DeNofrio, MD

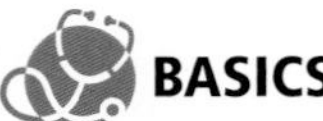

BASICS

DESCRIPTION

- Heart failure (HF) is the condition resulting from inability of the heart to fill and/or pump blood sufficiently to meet tissue metabolic needs. Alternatively, HF may occur when adequate cardiac output can be achieved only at the expense of elevated filling pressures. It is the principal complication of heart disease.
- HF is the preferred term over congestive heart failure (CHF) because patients are not always congested (fluid overloaded).
- HF may involve the left heart, the right heart, or be biventricular. The New York Heart Association (NYHA) Classification is a subjective grading scale used for classifying patients with HF: NYHA I: asymptomatic; NYHA II: symptomatic with moderate exertion; NYHA III: symptomatic with mild exertion and may limit activities of daily living; NYHA IV: symptomatic at rest. For acute HF see "Heart Failure (CHF), Acutely Decompensated."

EPIDEMIOLOGY

The annual direct and indirect cost of HF in the United States is ~$34.4 billion.

Incidence

In the United States, 550,000 new cases diagnosed annually with >250,000 deaths per year.

Prevalence

- ~5.7 million people in the United States have HF; <1% in those age <50 years, increasing to 10% of those age >80 years
- Primarily a disease of the elderly; 75% of hospital admissions for HF are for persons >65 years of age.

ETIOLOGY AND PATHOPHYSIOLOGY

2 physiologic components explain most of the clinical findings of HF and result in classifications of patients in 4 general categories:

- HF with reduced ejection fraction (HFrEF) or systolic HF: an *inotropic* abnormality, often due to myocardial infarction (MI) or dilated cardiomyopathy, resulting in diminished systolic emptying (ejection fraction [EF] ≤40%).
- HF with preserved ejection fraction (HFpEF) or diastolic HF: a *compliance* abnormality, often due to hypertensive cardiomyopathy, in which the ventricular relaxation is impaired (EF ≥50%)
- Borderline HFpEF (EF 41–49%): mild systolic dysfunction but clinically behaves like HFpEF
- Improved HFpEF (EF >40%): previously HFrEF but with improvement in systolic function
- Patients with systolic dysfunction may also have diastolic dysfunction.
- Most common etiologies: coronary artery disease (CAD)/MI and hypertension (HTN)
- Myocarditis and cardiomyopathy (CM): alcoholic, viral, long-standing HTN, drugs (e.g., chemotherapeutic agents), muscular dystrophy, infiltrative (e.g., amyloidosis, sarcoidosis), postpartum state, infectious (e.g., Chagas disease, HIV), hypertrophic CM (HCM), inherited familial dilated CM, left ventricular noncompaction
- Valvular and vascular abnormalities: any valvular stenosis or regurgitation, rheumatic heart; renal artery stenosis, usually bilateral, may cause recurrent "flash" pulmonary edema, especially in setting of severe chronic HTN
- Chronic lung disease and pulmonary HTN (cor pulmonale)
- Iatrogenic volume overload (requires extreme overload in patients with normal hearts and kidneys)
- Arrhythmias (atrial fibrillation and other tachyarrhythmias, high-grade heart block)
- Miscellaneous: high-output states: hyperthyroidism, anemia; cardiac depressants (β-blocker overdose), stress-induced
- Idiopathic: 20–50% of idiopathic dilated cardiomyopathies are familial.
- HF is progressive—manifested by the remodeling (altered heart geometry) process

Genetics

Multiple genetic abnormalities responsible for a variety of phenotypes have been identified (HCM, arrhythmogenic right ventricular [RV] dysplasia, left ventricular [LV] noncompaction, dilated CM). Consider genetic screening 1st-degree relatives of HCM and arrhythmogenic RV dysplasia.

RISK FACTORS

For development of HF: CAD/MI, HTN (80% of cases of HF in the United States caused by either CAD or HTN), valvular heart disease, diabetes mellitus, cardiotoxic medications (e.g., anthracyclines, tyrosine-kinase inhibitors, TNF-α inhibitors), obesity, older age

GENERAL PREVENTION

Control HTN and other risk factors. Thiazide diuretics and angiotensin-converting enzyme inhibitors (ACE-I) are superior to other agents in preventing development of HF.

COMMONLY ASSOCIATED CONDITIONS

Sudden cardiac death and progressive pump failure are the leading causes of death. Most patients have >5 comorbid medical conditions and take >5 medications.

DIAGNOSIS

HISTORY

- Dyspnea on exertion: *cardinal sign of left HF*. Deteriorating exercise capacity: easy fatigue, general weakness
- Nocturnal nonproductive cough, orthopnea, and paroxysmal nocturnal dyspnea; sometimes frothy or pink sputum. Wheezing, especially nocturnal, in absence of history of asthma or infection (cardiac asthma); Cheyne-Stokes respirations
- Anorexia and/or fullness or dull pain in right upper quadrant (hepatic congestion). Nausea and poor appetite may indicate advanced HF.

PHYSICAL EXAM

- Increased filling pressures: rales (crackles) and sometimes wheezing, peripheral edema, S_3 gallop, hepatomegaly, jugular venous distension, hepatojugular reflux, ascites
- Remodeling: enlarged or displaced point of maximal impulse
- Poor cardiac output: hypotension, pulsus alternans, tachycardia, narrow pulse pressure, cool extremities, cyanosis

DIFFERENTIAL DIAGNOSIS

Simple dependent edema, pulmonary embolism, exertional asthma, cardiac ischemia, asthma/COPD, constrictive pericarditis, nephrotic syndrome, cirrhosis, venous occlusive disease with subsequent peripheral edema, high-output states: anemia, sepsis, hyperthyroidism, lymphedema, tamponade

DIAGNOSTIC TESTS & INTERPRETATION

Diagnosis should be primarily clinical, with laboratory data as adjunctive and indicative of complications.

Initial Tests (lab, imaging)

- β-type natriuretic peptide (BNP) and N-type pro-BNP (NT-BNP) helpful in the acute setting to differentiate the cause of dyspnea (BNP <100 essentially rules out HF; most dyspneic patients with HF have a BNP >400) (1)[A]. Other, non-HF conditions, such as pulmonary embolism, renal failure, and acute coronary syndromes, may cause elevated BNP. Obesity may lower BNP levels. The use of BNP-guided therapy in chronic HF and acutely decompensated HF is not well-established.
- Lab findings include respiratory alkalosis, mild azotemia, decreased ESR, proteinuria (usually <1 g/24 hr), elevated creatinine (cardiorenal syndrome), dilutional hyponatremia (poor prognosis), hyperuricemia, and hyperbilirubinemia.
- Chest x-ray (changes lag clinical symptoms by up to 6 hours): increased heart size, vascular redistribution (cephalization) with "butterfly" pattern of pulmonary edema, interstitial and alveolar edema, Kerley B lines, and pleural effusions. Findings of pulmonary edema may be absent in long-standing HF.

Diagnostic Procedures/Other

Determination of left ventricular ejection fraction (LVEF) is critical to proper diagnosis and management:

- Echocardiogram is the most useful test to determine LVEF, RV function, diastolic dysfunction, ventricular size, wall thickness, and valvular abnormalities. May be repeated if change suspected in underlying cardiac status
- Nuclear imaging to estimate ventricular sizes, assess for ischemia or infarction and systolic function
- Cardiac MRI can be considered in select circumstances: suspicion of cardiac sarcoidosis, arrhythmogenic RV CM, acute myocarditis, amyloidosis, and hemochromatosis. It is also useful for differentiating restrictive CM and constrictive pericarditis.
- Cardiac catheterization is important for excluding CAD as an etiology in the setting of risk factors.
- Endomyocardial biopsy should not be performed routinely, only in special circumstances (e.g., suspected giant cell myocarditis) that may change therapy (1)[C].

Test Interpretation

Cardiac pathology depends on underlying etiology.

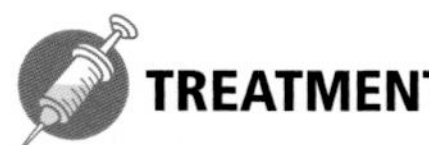

TREATMENT

GENERAL MEASURES

Correct and treat risk factors for HF. The treatment of chronic HF is focused on improving hemodynamics, relieving symptoms, and blocking the neurohormonal response to hopefully improve survival.

MEDICATION

Diuretics are used initially in fluid overload acute HF. The addition of ACE-I and aldosterone antagonists can be added at any time. Once acute HF is stabilized, a β-blocker should be started. Avoid nonsteroidal anti-inflammatory drugs (NSAIDs), which markedly worsen HF. Avoid use of diltiazem and verapamil in patients with systolic dysfunction as they may increase mortality and have negative inotropic effects.

First Line

- ACE-I: used to decrease afterload. Shown to increase survival, improve symptoms and overall exercise capacity in patients in all NYHA classifications; benefit greatest for patients with systolic dysfunction and post-MI. Number needed to treat (NNT) ~25 per year for mortality. All ACE-I considered equally effective. Initiate at low doses and titrate as tolerated to target doses.
- Angiotensin receptor blockers (ARBs) are indicated for those who are intolerant to ACE-I. They are probably slightly less effective than ACE-I. Avoid combination of ACE-I and ARB.
- β-blockers: used in systolic or diastolic HF (Note: initiate in hemodynamically stable/compensated patients at low dose and titrate upward slowly); NNT = 25 for mortality. Mortality decreased in systolic HF. Evidence for titration to heart rate rather than specific dose (1)[A].
  - Carvedilol: 3.125 mg PO BID to a target of 25 mg PO BID; metoprolol succinate extended release: 12.5 mg/day PO to a target of 200 mg/day PO or bisoprolol 1.25–10 mg once daily (currently not FDA approved for the treatment of HF).
- Diuretics are helpful to manage volume overload/ reduce preload.
  - Furosemide (Lasix): 20–320 mg/day IV/IM/PO divided dose; bumetanide (Bumex): 0.5 mg–10 mg/ day IV/PO divided; torsemide (Demadex): 10–200 mg/day PO divided (1)[C].
  - Metolazone (Zaroxolyn): 2.5–20 mg/day PO divided dose; hydrochlorothiazide: 12.5–100 mg/day PO divided; chlorothiazide (Diuril): 250–2,000 mg/ day IV/PO divided.
  - Spironolactone, eplerenone (improve mortality when added to standard therapy in NYHA class II-IV + EF<35%): spironolactone 12.5–25 mg/ day PO; maximum 50 mg/day PO; eplerenone 25–50 mg/day. Caution regarding hyperkalemia and chronic kidney disease (CKD) (1)[A].
- Digoxin reduces symptoms but has not clearly shown any positive effect on mortality: In patients with preserved renal function (creatinine clearance >50 mL/min), the recommended dose is 0.125 mg/ day. Levels lower than used for atrial fibrillation are effective and safer (1)[B].
- The combination of hydralazine (75 mg/day divided BID or TID) and isosorbide dinitrate (40 mg QID) is effective for African Americans (1)[A] or if unable to take ACE-I or an ARB (1)[B].
- Anticoagulation is not recommended in patients with HFrEF unless there are other indications such as atrial fibrillation, cardioembolism, or intracardiac thrombus (1,2)[A].
- In diastolic HF, no medical therapy has improved survival (1,3)[A]. ARBs and spironolactone can be used to potentially reduce hospitalizations (1,4)[B].

ADDITIONAL THERAPIES

Device therapy including implantable cardioverter defibrillators (ICD) and cardiac resynchronization (CRT) shown to improve outcomes

- CRT is recommended for patients in sinus rhythm with a QRS width ≥150 ms due to left bundle branch block (LBBB) and LVEF ≤35% and persistent mild to moderate HF (NYHA II–III) despite optimal medical therapy. CRT may be considered for ambulatory NYHA class IV patients in sinus rhythm with a QRS width ≥150 ms, LBBB, and LVEF ≤35% (1)[A].
- CRT may be considered for patients with LVEF ≤35%, sinus rhythm, QRS width ≥150 ms, non-LBBB pattern, and NYHA III or ambulatory NYHA IV symptoms (1)[A].
- CRT may also be considered for patients with a QRS width between 120 and 150 ms, LBBB, LVEF ≤35%, and persistent mild to severe HF (NYHA II–IV) despite optimal medical therapy (1)[B].
- ICDs are recommended for primary prevention in patients with *non-ischemic* CM and *ischemic* CM who are at least 40 days post-MI; LVEF ≤35%, NYHA class II or III HF (1)[A], or LVEF ≤30%, NYHA I HF (1)[B]; and on optimal medical therapy and >1 year estimated survival. Generally not indicated in American Heart Association (AHA) stage D (end-stage) HF
- CRT is recommended in patients with reduced LVEF and chronic RV pacing or with bradyarrhythmias and an anticipated need for a pacemaker (5)[A].

SURGERY/OTHER PROCEDURES

- Heart valve surgery if defective heart valve is responsible; mitral valve repair especially helpful if mitral regurgitation is the primary issue and not functional.
- Advanced therapies such as cardiac transplantation and LV assist device (LVAD) implantation can be considered in patients with HF refractory to conventional medical/device therapies without other disqualifying medical and psychosocial conditions. Cardiac transplantation is generally considered for patients ≤70 years old with a predicted 1-year survival worse than that afforded by transplantation. Indications for LVAD implantation are generally similar to cardiac transplantation but are evolving.

INPATIENT CONSIDERATIONS

Admission Criteria/Initial Stabilization

- Sublingual nitroglycerin is rapid-onset and reduces preload. Oxygen for symptoms. Diuretics to reduce preload. See "Heart Failure, Acutely Decompensated."
- Admit patients with hemodynamic/respiratory compromise, hypoxia/hypoxemia, change in mental status, acute renal insufficiency, significant volume overload, and significant electrolyte abnormalities (e.g., hyponatremia).

Discharge Criteria

Subjective improvement, euvolemia on clinical assessment, resting heart rate (HR) <100 bpm, systolic BP >80 mm Hg, HF outpatient education performed

ONGOING CARE

FOLLOW-UP RECOMMENDATIONS

Critical patient education performed at all outpatient and inpatient physician visits: "MAWDS"

- **M**edications: Take every day; don't skip.
- **A**ctivity: A little every day; don't overdo.
- **W**eight: Daily. If gain >2 lb in a day or 5 lb above ideal, CALL.
- **D**iet: Eat low salt, heart healthy diet and limit fluids and alcohol.
- **S**ymptoms: Know the signs of worsening HF (cough, weight gain, worsening or rest dyspnea, swelling) and call the doctor early! Quit smoking, if a smoker!

Patient Monitoring

Rapid office follow-up (1–2 weeks) after hospitalization and home health monitoring by specially trained nurses have both been shown to decrease frequency of hospitalizations. Readmissions remain problematic.

DIET

Reduce sodium load (<1.5–2 g/day).

PATIENT EDUCATION

AHA: www.americanheart.org

PROGNOSIS

After diagnosis: 1-year survival ~75%, 5-year survival <50%, and 10 year <25%

COMPLICATIONS

Sudden death (arrhythmic), acute pulmonary edema, death, progressive pump failure

REFERENCES

1. Yancy C, Jessup M, Bozkurt B, et al. 2013 ACCF/AHA guideline for the management of heart failure: a report of the American College of Cardiology Foundation/ American Heart Association task force on practice guidelines. *J Am Coll Cardiol*. 2013;62(16):e147–e239.
2. Homma S, Thompson JLP, Pullicino PM, et al. Warfarin and aspirin in patients with heart failure and sinus rhythm. *N Engl J Med*. 2012;366(20):1859–1869.
3. Massie BM, Carson PE, McMurray JJ, et al. Irbesartan in patients with heart failure and preserved ejection fraction. *N Engl J Med*. 2008;359(23): 2456–2467.
4. Pitt B, Pfeffer MA, Assmann SF, et al; TOPCAT Investigators. Spironolactone for heart failure with preserved ejection fraction. *N Engl J Med*. 2014; 370(15):1383–1392.
5. Curtis AB, Worley SJ, Adamson PB, et al. Biventricular pacing for atrioventricular block and systolic dysfunction. *N Engl J Med*. 2013;368(17):1585–1593.

ADDITIONAL READING

- Al-Majed NS, McAlister FA, Bakal JA, et al. Meta-analysis: cardiac resynchronization therapy for patients with less symptomatic heart failure. *Ann Intern Med*. 2011;154(6):401–412.
- Felker GM, Lee KL, Bull DA, et al. Diuretic strategies in patients with acute decompensated heart failure. *N Engl J Med*. 2011;364(9):797–805.
- Nohria A, Lewis E, Stevenson LW. Medical management of advanced heart failure. *JAMA*. 2002;287(5): 628–640.
- Stevenson WG, Hernandez AF, Carson PE, et al. Indications for cardiac resynchronization therapy: 2011 update from the Heart Failure Society of America Guideline Committee. *J Card Fail*. 2012;18(2):94–106.
- Zannad F, McMurray JJ, Krum H, et al. Eplerenone in patients with systolic heart failure and mild symptoms. *N Engl J Med*. 2011;364(1):11–21.

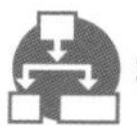

SEE ALSO

- Heart Failure (CHF), Acutely Decompensated
- Algorithms: Congestive Heart Failure

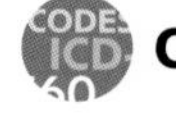

CODES

ICD10

- I50.9 Heart failure, unspecified
- I50.1 Left ventricular failure
- I50.22 Chronic systolic (congestive) heart failure

CLINICAL PEARLS

- Have patients weigh themselves daily and report weight gains of >2 lb in a day or 5 lb above dry weight.
- β-Blockers, ACE-I, and aldosterone antagonists are the core medications for management of chronic HF.
- Consider referral for biventricular pacing in patients with bundle branch block and ICD in those with low EF.
- Refer to an HF specialist if frequently hospitalized.

HEAT EXHAUSTION AND HEAT STROKE

Brian Frank, MD • Scott A. Fields, MD, MHA

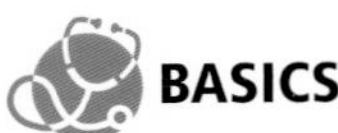

BASICS

DESCRIPTION

- A continuum of increasingly severe heat illnesses caused by dehydration, electrolyte losses, and failure of the body's thermoregulatory mechanisms
  - Heat exhaustion is an acute heat injury with hyperthermia owing to dehydration.
  - Heat stroke is extreme hyperthermia with thermoregulatory failure and profound CNS dysfunction (1).
- System(s) affected: endocrine/metabolic; nervous
- Synonym(s): heat illness; heat injury; hyperthermia; heat collapse; heat prostration

Geriatric Considerations

Elderly persons are more susceptible.

Pediatric Considerations

Children are more susceptible.

Pregnancy Considerations

Pregnant women may be more susceptible to volume depletion with heat stress.

EPIDEMIOLOGY

- Predominant age: more likely in children or elderly
- Predominant sex: male = female

Incidence

Depends on intensity of heat; estimate of 20/100,000 persons per season (1)

Prevalence

- Depends on predisposing conditions in combination with environmental factors
- Roughly 600 deaths/year in the United States (2)

ETIOLOGY AND PATHOPHYSIOLOGY

- Direct cellular toxicity of heat, imbalance between inflammatory and anti-inflammatory cytokines, and vascular endothelial damage causing end-organ dysfunction
- Interplay between failure of heat-dissipating mechanisms, an overwhelming heat stress, and an exaggerated acute-phase inflammatory response (3)

RISK FACTORS

- Poor acclimatization to heat or poor physical conditioning
- Salt or water depletion
- Obesity
- Acute febrile or GI illnesses
- Chronic illnesses: uncontrolled diabetes mellitus or hypertension, cardiac disease
- Alcohol and other substance abuse
- High heat and humidity, poor air circulation in environment
- Heavy, restrictive clothing (4,5)
- Nutritional supplementation that includes ephedra (6)

GENERAL PREVENTION

- The most important factor in preventing heat stress is adequate fluid replacement.
- Allow acclimatization to hot weather through proper conditioning and activity modification.
- Dress appropriately with loose-fitting, open-weaved, light-colored clothing.
- Avoid dehydration by consuming a proper amount of fluids during activity or exercise: 8 oz fluid intake for every 15 minutes of moderate exercise.
- Never leave children unattended in cars during hot weather.
- Try to gain access to air-conditioned environments during hot weather (7).

PROGNOSIS

- The prognosis is good when mental function is not altered and when serum enzymes are not elevated; recovery is within 24–48 hours in most cases.
- The mortality rate for heat stroke (10–80%) is directly related to the duration and intensity of hyperthermia, as well as to the speed and effectiveness of diagnosis and treatment (1).

COMPLICATIONS

- May involve failure of any major organ system
- Cardiac arrhythmias or infarction
- Pulmonary edema, acute respiratory distress syndrome
- Coma, seizures
- Acute renal failure
- Rhabdomyolysis
- Disseminated intravascular coagulopathy (DIC)
- Hepatocellular necrosis

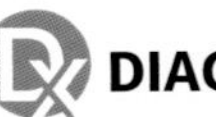

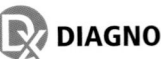

DIAGNOSIS

- Heat exhaustion: Symptoms are milder than in heat stroke, with no severe CNS derangements:
  - Fatigue and lethargy
  - Weakness
  - Dizziness
  - Nausea, vomiting
  - Myalgias
  - Headache
  - Profuse sweating
  - Tachycardia
  - Hypotension
  - Lack of coordination
  - Agitation
  - Intense thirst
  - Hyperventilation
  - Paresthesias
  - Core temperature elevated but <103°F (<39.4°C)
- Heat stroke: divided into 2 categories, classic and exertional:
  - Classic: caused by environmental exposure, primarily in elderly or chronically ill patients, and may develop gradually over days
    - Delirium
    - Confusion
    - Coma
    - Core temperature >104°F (>40°C)
    - Hot, flushed, dry skin
  - Exertional: typically younger, very active patients; rapid onset
    - Exhaustion
    - Confusion, disorientation
    - Delirium
    - Coma
    - Hot, flushed skin, typically with sweating
    - Core temperature >105°F (>40.5°C) (1,8)

DIFFERENTIAL DIAGNOSIS

- Other causes of elevated temperature, dehydration, or circulatory collapse
- Febrile illnesses, sepsis
- Drug-induced fluid loss
- Cardiac arrhythmia or infarction
- Acute cocaine intoxication
- Neuroleptic malignant syndrome
- Malignant hyperthermia (an autosomally inherited disorder of skeletal and cardiac muscle in which patients have abnormal muscle metabolism on exposure to halothane or skeletal muscle reactants)

DIAGNOSTIC TESTS & INTERPRETATION

Used primarily to detect end-organ damage

Initial Tests (lab, imaging)

- Electrolytes, urinalysis
- Creatinine, BUN
- Liver enzymes, muscle enzymes (creatine phosphokinase)
- CBC
- Increased urine-specific gravity
- Results of these studies may indicate hypernatremia, hyperchloremia, and hemoconcentration.
- Drugs that may alter lab results: diuretics

Diagnostic Procedures/Other

Rectal temperature monitoring (do not rely on oral temp) (9)[A]

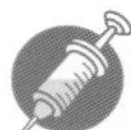

TREATMENT

GENERAL MEASURES

- Fluid and electrolyte replacement with normal saline gradually; avoid hypotonic fluids (7)[C].
- Consider CVP monitoring.
- Body immersion in ice water (1,8)[C]
- Evaporative cooling: spraying water over the patient and facilitating evaporation and convection with the use of fans (1,8)[C]
- Immersing the hands and forearms in cold water (1,8)[C]
- Use of ice or cold packs on the neck, groin, and axillae (10)[C]
- No clear superiority of any one method (8).

MEDICATION

First Line

No medications are required in the initial management. Use isotonic saline solution to rehydrate (1,7)[C].

Second Line

- Consider immunomodulators such as corticosteroids (8)[C].
- Iced gastric, bladder, or peritoneal lavage (1,8)[C]
- In DIC, consider appropriate replacement therapy.

INPATIENT CONSIDERATIONS

Admission Criteria/Initial Stabilization

- Emergency treatment; best in a hospital setting
- Rapid cooling: Remove clothing, wet patient down, and apply ice packs.

ONGOING CARE

FOLLOW-UP RECOMMENDATIONS

Rest with legs elevated (1,8)[C].

Patient Monitoring

- Rectal temperature monitoring: Cooling may be discontinued when the core temperature drops to 102°F (38.9°C) and stabilizes.
- Heat stroke patients may require airway management, hemodynamic monitoring, and careful fluid and electrolyte administration and monitoring.
- Consider CVP monitoring.

DIET

- Cool or cold clear liquids only (noncarbonated)
- Avoid caffeine.
- Unrestricted sodium

PATIENT EDUCATION

- The key to prevention is proper hydration.
- Stress the importance of proper conditioning and acclimatization.
- Instruct patients to recognize heat stress signs and symptoms.
- Maintain as much skin exposure as possible in hot, humid conditions while using proper sun-block protection.

REFERENCES

1. Yeo TP. Heat stroke: a comprehensive review. *AACN Clin Issues*. 2004;15(2):280–293.
2. Xu J. QuickStats: Number of heat-related deaths, by sex—National Vital Statistics System, United States, 1999–2010. http://www.cdc.gov/mmwr. Accessed 2014.
3. Bouchama A, Knochel JP. Heat Stroke. *N Engl J Med*. 2002;346(25):1978–1988.
4. Cleary M. Predisposing risk factors on susceptibility to exertional heat illness: clinical decision-making considerations. *J Sport Rehabilitation*. 2007;16(3): 204–214.
5. Muldoon S, Bunger R, Deuster P, et al. Identification of risk factors for exertional heat illness: a brief commentary on genetic testing. *J Sport Rehabilitation*. 2007;16(3):222–226.
6. Charaton F. Ephedra supplement may have contributed to sportsman's death. *Br Med J*. 2003; 326(7387):464.
7. Glazer JL. Management of heatstroke and heat exhaustion. *Am Fam Physician*. 2005;71(11): 2133–2140.
8. Bouchama A, Dehbi M, Chaves-Carballo E. Cooling and hemodynamic management in heatstroke: practical recommendations. *Crit Care*. 2007;11(3):R54.
9. Mazerolle S, Ganio M, Casa DJ, et al. Is oral temperature an accurate measurement of deep body temperature? A systematic review. *J Athl Train*. 2014;46(5):566–573.
10. Gaffin SL, Gardner JW, Flinn SD. Cooling methods for heatstroke victims. *Ann Intern Med*. 2000; 132(8):678.

ADDITIONAL READING

- American College of Sports Medicine, Armstrong LE, Casa DJ, et al. American College of Sports Medicine position stand. Exertional heat illness during training and competition. *Med Sci Sports Exerc*. 2007;39(3):556–572.
- Smith JE. Cooling methods used in the treatment of exertional heat illness. *Br J Sports Med*. 2005;39(8): 503–507; discussion 507.

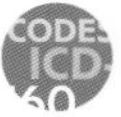

CODES

ICD10

- T67.5XXA Heat exhaustion, unspecified, initial encounter
- T67.0XXA Heatstroke and sunstroke, initial encounter
- T67.3XXA Heat exhaustion, anhydrotic, initial encounter

CLINICAL PEARLS

- The diagnosis of heat stroke relies on both hyperthermia and CNS dysfunction (e.g., irritability, ataxia, confusion, seizures, or coma).
- Start the cooling process immediately when heat exhaustion or heat stroke is recognized, beginning with wetting the skin with a cool mist and giving oral rehydration solutions containing saline, if the patient is alert and oriented.
- Do not rely on oral temperature.

HEMATURIA

Tracy O. Middleton, DO

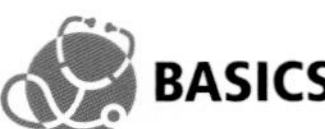

BASICS

DESCRIPTION

- Gross (visible) or microscopic (nonvisible) blood in the urine
- Symptomatic or asymptomatic

EPIDEMIOLOGY

Prevalence

- Microscopic hematuria in school-aged children: 0.5–2%
- Microscopic hematuria in asymptomatic adults varies from 0.19 to 31%, depending on population studied (1).

ETIOLOGY AND PATHOPHYSIOLOGY

- Trauma
  - Exercise-induced (resolves with rest)
  - Abdominal trauma or pelvic fracture with renal, bladder, or ureteral injury
  - Iatrogenic from abdominal or pelvic surgery; chronic indwelling catheters
  - Foreign body, physical/sexual abuse
- Neoplasms
  - Urologic malignancies
  - Benign tumors
  - Endometriosis of the urinary tract (suspect in females with cyclic hematuria)
- Inflammatory causes
  - UTI: most common cause of hematuria in adults
  - Renal diseases: radiation nephritis and cystitis, acute/chronic tubulointerstitial nephritis (due to drugs, infections, systemic disease)
  - Glomerular disease
    - Goodpasture syndrome (antiglomerular basement membrane disease; autoimmune; associated pulmonary hemorrhage)
    - IgA nephropathy
    - Lupus nephritis
    - Henoch-Schönlein purpura
    - Membranoproliferative, poststreptococcal, or rapidly progressive glomerulonephritis (GN)
    - Wegener granulomatosis
  - Endocarditis/visceral abscesses
  - Other infections: schistosomiasis, TB, syphilis
- Metabolic causes
  - Stones (85% have hematuria)
    - Hypercalciuria: a common cause of both gross and microscopic hematuria in children
    - Hyperuricosuria
- Congenital/familial causes
  - Cystic disease: polycystic, solitary renal cyst
  - Benign familial hematuria or thin basement membrane nephropathy (autosomal dominant)
  - Alport syndrome (X-linked in 85%; hematuria, proteinuria, hearing loss, corneal abnormalities)
  - Fabry disease (X-linked recessive inborn error of metabolism; vascular kidney disease)
  - Nail-patella syndrome (autosomal dominant; nail and patella hypoplasia; hematuria in 33%)
  - Renal tubular acidosis type 1 (autosomal dominant or autoimmune)
- Hematologic causes
  - Bleeding dyscrasias (e.g., hemophilia)
  - Sickle cell anemia/trait (renal papillary necrosis)
- Vascular causes
  - Hemangioma
  - Arteriovenous malformations (rare)
  - Nutcracker syndrome: compression of left renal vein and subsequent renal parenchymal congestion
  - Renal artery/vein thrombosis
  - Arterial emboli to kidney
- Chemical causes
  - Aminoglycosides, cyclosporine, analgesics, oral contraceptives, Chinese herbs
- Obstruction
  - Strictures or posterior urethral valves
  - Hydronephrosis from any cause
  - Benign prostatic hyperplasia: Rule out other causes of hematuria.
- Other causes: loin pain hematuria (most often in young women on oral contraceptives)

RISK FACTORS

- Smoking
- Occupational exposures (dyes, rubber, or tire manufacturing)
- Analgesic abuse (e.g., phenacetin)
- Medications (e.g., cyclophosphamide)
- Pelvic irradiation
- Chronic infection, especially with calculi
- Recent upper respiratory tract infection
- Positive family history of renal diseases (stones, GN)
- Underlying primary renal disorder
- Chronic indwelling foreign body

DIAGNOSIS

HISTORY

Considerations

- Burning, urgency, frequency: UTI
- Dark cola-colored urine: glomerular origin
- Clots: extraglomerular bleeding
- Arthritis/arthralgias/rash: lupus, vasculitis, Henoch-Schönlein purpura
- Flank pain: stones, infarction, pyelonephritis
- Recent upper respiratory infection (URI): poststreptococcal GN, membranoproliferative GN
- Concurrent URI: IgA nephropathy
- Excessive vitamin use: stones
- Marathon runner: traumatic, rhabdomyolysis
- Travel: schistosomiasis, TB
- Painless hematuria and/or weight loss: malignancy
- Family history: Alport disease (hereditary nephritis), sickle cell, polycystic, IgA nephropathy, thin basement membrane disease

PHYSICAL EXAM

Considerations

- Elevated BP, edema, and weight gain: glomerular disease
- Fever: infection
- Palpable kidney: neoplasm, polycystic
- Genitalia: Look for meatal erosion, lesions.

DIAGNOSTIC TESTS & INTERPRETATION

- A hematuria risk index may assist in stratifying patients at risk for urothelial malignancies who require more intensive testing. High-risk indicators are gross hematuria, age >50 years, male gender, and smoking (2)[B].
- American Urological Association (AUA) suggests upper urinary tract imaging in all adults with unexplained hematuria (3)[C].

Initial Tests (lab, imaging)

- Urine dipstick (sensitivity 91–100%; specificity 65–99%)
  - False negatives are rare but can be caused by high-dose vitamin C.
  - False positives (35%): oxidizers (povidone, bacterial peroxidases, bleach), myoglobin, alkaline urine (>9), semen, food coloring, food (beets, blackberries, rhubarb, paprika) (1,4)
  - Phenazopyridine may discolor the dipstick, making interpretation difficult.
- Microscopic urinalysis should always be done to confirm dipstick findings and quantify RBCs.
  - AUA defines clinically significant microscopic hematuria as ≥3 RBCs/HPF on a properly collected urinary specimen when there is not an obvious benign cause (3)[C].
  - Positive dipstick but a negative microscopic exam should be followed by 3 repeat tests. If any 1 is positive, proceed with a workup (3)[C].
  - Exclude factitious or nonurinary causes, such as menstruation, mild trauma, exercise, poor collection technique, or chemical/drug causes, through cessation of activity/cause and a repeat urinalysis in 48 hours (1)[C].
- Voided urine cytology
  - No longer recommended by AUA for routine evaluation of hematuria (3)[C]
  - Some still consider cytology in those with risk factors for urinary malignancy (1)[C].
- Renal function tests (eGFR, BUN, creatinine) to differentiate intrinsic renal disease and to evaluate for risks for imaging contrast dye or certain medications
  - Indicators of renal disease are significant (>500 mg/day) proteinuria, red cell casts (pathognomonic of glomerular disease), dysmorphic RBCs, and increased creatinine (3)[C].
- Urine culture if suspected infection/pyuria (1)[C]
- PT/INR for patients on warfarin or suspected of abusing warfarin
- Multidetector CT urography (MDCTU); sensitivity 91–100%, specificity 94–97% (1)[C]
  - The initial imaging of choice in nonpregnant adults with unexplained hematuria (1)[C],(4,5)[B]
  - Highly specific and relatively sensitive for the diagnosis of urinary tract neoplasms, especially when >1 cm (5)[B]
  - Higher radiation dose; weigh risk of disease versus risk of radiation exposure.
  - Does not obviate the need for cystoscopy, particularly in high-risk patients (5)[B]
  - Presence of calculi on noncontrast does not exclude another diagnosis or need for contrast phase.
  - Visualization of ureters is discontinuous.
  - Less cost-efficient
- CT
  - Perform unenhanced helical CT for suspected stone disease in children if US is negative (6)[C].
  - Perform CT abdomen and pelvis with contrast in children with traumatic hematuria (6)[C].
- Renal ultrasound
  - Best for differentiating cystic from solid masses
  - Sensitive for hydronephrosis
  - No radiation or iodinated contrast exposure

- Cost-efficient
- Poor sensitivity for renal masses <3 cm
- Main disadvantage is inability to thoroughly evaluate the urothelium for transitional cell cancer.
- Magnetic resonance urography (MRU)
  - High sensitivity/specificity for renal parenchyma; less useful for collecting system or stones
  - Can be used in patients with contraindications to MDCTU (3)[C]
- IV urography (IVU)
  - Limited sensitivity for small renal masses and for differentiating cystic from solid masses
  - Addition of US or CT often necessary to evaluate renal parenchyma
  - Potential reactions to IV iodine contrast media
- MRI
  - Similar to CT in sensitivity for renal masses
  - No radiation exposure
  - Least cost-efficient
  - Limited ability to reliably detect urinary tract calcifications
  - Can be combined with retrograde pyelogram (RPG) for patients who cannot tolerate MDCTU or MRU (3)[C]

Diagnostic Procedures/Other

- Flexible cystoscopy
  - Best for evaluation of bladder pathology, especially small urothelial lesions; negative predictive value for bladder tumors is 99% (1)[C].
  - AUA recommends all patients with hematuria who are ≥35 years of age and all patients with risk factors for bladder cancer regardless of age to receive cystoscopy (3)[C].
- Renal biopsy
  - Not routine but may be necessary to diagnose GN or in the face of increasing renal insufficiency
- RPG
  - Reserved for patients in which findings on MDCTU are equivocal or in addition to US or noncontrast studies in patients who are contraindicated for contrast or MRI (3)[C]
  - Sensitive for small lesions of supravesicular collecting system
  - Requires cystoscopy
- Ureteroscopy/pyeloscopy
  - For visualization of suspected supravesical collecting system lesions
  - Biopsy, excision, fulguration, or extraction of lesions/stones possible
  - Requires anesthesia
  - Requires cystoscopy
  - Risk of injury to collecting system

Follow-Up Tests & Special Considerations

- Other tests depend on suspected etiology: STD testing, antineutrophil cytoplasmic antibody (ANCA), C3, C4, antistreptolysin O (ASO) titer, hemoglobin electrophoresis (7)[C].
- Insufficient evidence to recommend routine use of urinary tumor markers
- Malignancies are detected in up to 5% of patients with microscopic hematuria and up to 40% of patients with gross hematuria (1)[C].

Pregnancy Considerations

Renal US is initial imaging choice for pregnant patients. MRU or RPG combined with either MRI or US are alternatives (3)[C].

Pediatric Considerations

- Consider GN, Wilms tumor, child abuse
- Isolated asymptomatic microscopic hematuria may not need full workup; these patients rarely need cystoscopy; observe for development of hypertension, gross hematuria, or proteinuria (7)[C].
- Gross or symptomatic hematuria needs a full workup.
  - If eumorphic RBCs, consider US (rule out stones, congenital abnormalities) and urinary Ca:Cr ratio. Urine Ca:Cr ratio >0.2 is suggestive of hypercalciuria in children >6 years of age (7)[C].
- If dysmorphic RBCs, consider renal consult.
- Renal US identifies most congenital and malignant conditions; CT is reserved for cases of suspected trauma (with contrast) or stones (without contrast) (6,7)[C].

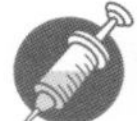

TREATMENT

MEDICATION

None indicated for undiagnosed hematuria

ISSUES FOR REFERRAL

Prompt nephrology referral for proteinuria, red cell casts, and elevated serum creatinine (3)[C].

SURGERY/OTHER PROCEDURES

Gross hematuria: Clots may require continuous bladder irrigation with a large-bore Foley catheter (2- or 3-way catheter may be helpful) to prevent clot retention.

ONGOING CARE

FOLLOW-UP RECOMMENDATIONS

Patient Monitoring

Some experts still recommend periodic urinalysis; recent literature suggests that, after thorough initial negative investigations (imaging, cystoscopy), no follow-up is indicated for the asymptomatic patient with microscopic hematuria unless symptoms or frank hematuria develop. AUA recommends annual urinalyses in these patients, until 2 consecutive are negative and the consideration for a repeat workup at 3–5 years if hematuria is persistent (1,3)[C].

DIET

Increased fluids for stones or clots and decreased soda intake for stone prevention

PROGNOSIS

- Generally excellent for common causes of hematuria
- Poorer for malignant tumors and certain types of nephritis

- Persistent asymptomatic microscopic hematuria is associated with an increased risk of end-stage renal disease in patients aged 16–25 years (8)[B].

REFERENCES

1. Sharp VJ, Barnes KT, Erickson BA. Assessment of asymptomatic microscopic hematuria in adults. *Am Fam Physician*. 2013;88(11):747–754.
2. Loo RK, Lieberman SF, Slezak JM, et al. Stratifying risk of urinary tract malignant tumors in patients with asymptomatic microscopic hematuria. *Mayo Clin Proc*. 2013;88(2):129–138.
3. Davis R, Jones JS, Barocas DA, et al. Diagnosis, evaluation and follow-up of asymptomatic microhematuria (AMH) in adults: AUA guideline. *J Urol*. 2012;188(6)(Suppl):2473–2481.
4. Choyke PL. Radiologic evaluation of hematuria: guidelines from the American College of Radiology's appropriateness criteria. *Am Fam Physician*. 2008;78(3):347–352.
5. Sudakoff GS, Dunn DP, Guralnick ML, et al. Multidetector computerized tomography urography as the primary imaging modality for detecting urinary tract neoplasms in patients with asymptomatic hematuria. *J Urol*. 2008;179(3):862–867.
6. Dillman JR, Coley BD, Karmazyn B, et al. *Expert Panel on Pediatric Imaging. ACR Appropriateness Criteria® Hematuria—Child*. Reston, VA: American College of Radiology; 2012. http://www.guideline.gove/content.aspx?id=43874. Accessed 2014.
7. Massengill SF. Hematuria. *Pediatr Rev*. 2008;29(10):342–348.

SEE ALSO

Algorithm: Hematuria

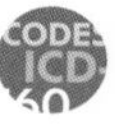

CODES

ICD10

- R31.9 Hematuria, unspecified
- R31.1 Benign essential microscopic hematuria
- R31.0 Gross hematuria

CLINICAL PEARLS

- Screening asymptomatic patients for microscopic hematuria is an "I" recommendation from the USPSTF (1)[B].

- Asymptomatic hematuria and hematuria persisting after treatment of UTIs must be evaluated.
- Patients with bladder cancer can have intermittent microscopic hematuria; a thorough evaluation in high-risk patients is needed after just 1 episode.
- Routine use of anticoagulants should not cause hematuria unless there is an underlying urologic abnormality (1)[C].
- Signs of underlying renal disease indicate the need for a nephrologic workup, but a urologic evaluation is still needed in the presence of persistent hematuria (3)[C].

HEMOCHROMATOSIS

Robert A. Marlow, MD, MA

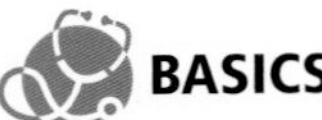

BASICS

DESCRIPTION

Hemochromatosis is a hereditary disorder in which the small intestine absorbs excessive iron (1,2).

- Early clinical features include arthralgia, fatigue, and decreased libido.
- Late effects include cirrhosis of the liver, diabetes, hypermelanotic pigmentation of the skin, and heart failure.
- Because there is no mechanism to excrete excess iron, the excess is stored in muscle and in organs, including the liver, pancreas, and heart, eventually resulting in severe damage to the affected organs.
- Liver damage ultimately may result in hepatocellular carcinoma.
- System(s) affected: endocrine/metabolic
- Synonym(s): bronze diabetes; Troisier-Hanot-Chauffard syndrome

EPIDEMIOLOGY

Incidence

- Predominant age: Metabolic abnormality is congenital, but symptoms usually present in the 5th and 6th decades.
- Predominant sex: gene frequency: male = female (8:1), although clinical signs are more frequent in men (3)

Prevalence

- 3/1,000 people (heterozygote frequency, 1/10) (4)
- The most common genetic abnormality in the United States

Pediatric Considerations

Rarely, iron overload may occur as early as 2 years of age. The disorder can be diagnosed before iron overload is clinically apparent.

ETIOLOGY AND PATHOPHYSIOLOGY

- Type 1 hemochromatosis is caused by mutations in the *HFE* gene, type 2 by mutations in either the *HFE2* gene or *HAMP* gene, type 3 by mutations in the *TFR2* gene, and type 4 by mutations in the *SLC40A1* gene. The cause of neonatal hemochromatosis is unknown.
- The mechanism for increased iron absorption in the face of excessive iron stores is not clear. Iron metabolism appears normal in this disease except for a higher level of circulating iron.
- Iron overload may be caused by thalassemia, sideroblastic anemia, liver disease, excess iron intake, or chronic transfusion.

Genetics

- Genetically heterogeneous disorder of iron overload; types 1, 2, and 3 are autosomal recessive; type 4 is autosomal dominant. Neonatal hemochromatosis is rare.
- Penetrance is incomplete; expressivity is variable.
- Factors contributing to variable expressivity include different mutations in the same gene, mitigating or exacerbating genes, and environmental factors.

RISK FACTORS

- The disease is a genetic disorder.
- Affected individuals should not ingest iron supplements, eat raw shellfish, or eat large quantities of iron-rich food, such as red meat.
- Alcohol increases the absorption of iron. (As many as 41% of patients with symptomatic disease are alcoholic.)
- Loss of blood, such as that which occurs during menstruation and pregnancy, delays the onset of symptoms.

GENERAL PREVENTION

- Family members of affected individuals should be screened.
- Pregnant women with the disorder should avoid iron supplements.

ALERT

Screening of population is *not* recommended because the vast majority of those with homozygous hemochromatosis will remain asymptomatic and have a normal life span (5,6)[A].

COMMONLY ASSOCIATED CONDITIONS

See "Complications."

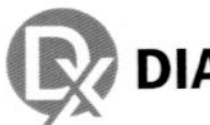

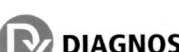

DIAGNOSIS

HISTORY

- Weakness (83%)
- Abdominal pain (58%)
- Arthralgia (43%)
- Loss of libido or potency (38%)
- Amenorrhea (22%)
- Dyspnea on exertion (15%)
- Neurologic symptoms (6%)
- Symptoms of diabetes

PHYSICAL EXAM

- Hepatomegaly (83%)
- Increased skin pigmentation (75%)
- Loss of body hair (20%)
- Splenomegaly (13%)
- Peripheral edema (12%)
- Jaundice (10%)
- Gynecomastia (8%)
- Ascites (6%)
- Testicular atrophy
- Hepatic tenderness

DIFFERENTIAL DIAGNOSIS

- Repeated transfusions
- Hereditary anemias with ineffective erythropoiesis
- Alcoholic cirrhosis
- Porphyria cutanea tarda
- Atransferrinemia
- Excessive ingestion of iron (rare)

DIAGNOSTIC TESTS & INTERPRETATION

- Transferrin saturation (serum iron concentration ÷ total iron-binding capacity × 100): >70% is virtually diagnostic of iron overload; ≥45% warrants further evaluation. Iron supplements and transfusions may elevate serum iron.
- Serum ferritin: >300 μg/L for men and postmenopausal women and 200 μg/L for premenopausal women (7); may be elevated by inflammatory reactions, other forms of liver disease, certain tumors (e.g., acute granulocytic leukemia), and rheumatoid arthritis
- After the diagnosis is established
  - Obtain an oral glucose tolerance test to rule out diabetes and undergo an echocardiogram to rule out cardiomyopathy
  - Urinary iron
  - Increased urine hemosiderin
  - Hyperglycemia
  - Decreased FSH
  - Decreased LH
  - Decreased testosterone
  - Increased serum glutamic-oxaloacetic transaminase
  - Hypoalbuminemia
- If the diagnosis is uncertain after laboratory testing, MRI may be helpful (1).

Diagnostic Procedures/Other

- Liver biopsy for stainable iron is the standard for diagnosis. Presence or absence of cirrhosis also can be ascertained. However, with the availability of genetic testing, liver biopsy is not frequently necessary to confirm the diagnosis (7)[C].
- DNA PCR testing for *HFE* gene mutations C282Y and H63D: present in 85–90% of patients
- Homozygosity for the C282Y mutation or compound heterozygosity for C282Y and H63D with biochemical evidence for iron overload can confirm the diagnosis (8).

Test Interpretation

- Increased hepatic parenchymal iron stores
- Hepatic fibrosis and cirrhosis with hepatomegaly
- Pancreatic enlargement
- Excess hemosiderin in liver, pancreas, myocardium, thyroid, parathyroid, joints, skin
- Cardiomegaly
- Joint deposition of iron

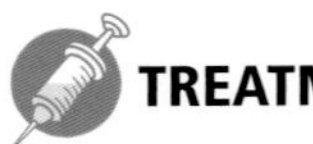

TREATMENT

MEDICATION

- None. Only when phlebotomy is not feasible or in the presence of severe heart disease should the iron-chelating agent deferoxamine (Desferal) be considered.
- Hepatitis A and hepatitis B immunizations should be done if there is no evidence of previous exposure (9).

GENERAL MEASURES

- Remove excess iron by repeated phlebotomy once or twice weekly to establish and maintain a mild anemia (hematocrit of 35–39%) (7)[C].
- When the patient finally becomes iron deficient, a lifelong maintenance program of 2–6 phlebotomies a year to keep storage iron normal; maintain serum ferritin 50–100 μg/L.

INPATIENT CONSIDERATIONS

Admission Criteria/Initial Stabilization

Outpatient treatment

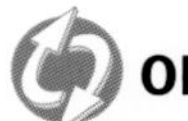

ONGOING CARE

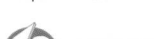

FOLLOW-UP RECOMMENDATIONS

Full activity unless there is significant heart disease

Patient Monitoring

- Measure hematocrit before each phlebotomy; skip phlebotomy if hematocrit <36%.
- Schedule an additional phlebotomy when hematocrit >40%.
- When anemia becomes refractory, repeat transferrin saturation and serum ferritin to confirm depletion of iron stores.
- When iron stores are depleted, 2–6 phlebotomies a year should keep iron stores normal; maintain serum ferritin 50–100 μg/L.
- During maintenance therapy, measure transferrin saturation and serum ferritin yearly.

DIET

- An iron-poor diet is not of significant benefit.
- Avoid alcohol, iron-fortified foods, iron-containing supplements, and uncooked shellfish (increased susceptibility to *Vibrio* sp.).
- Restrict vitamin C to small doses between meals.
- Tea chelates iron and may be drank with meals.

PATIENT EDUCATION

- Iron Disorders Institute, PO Box 675, Taylors, SC 29687
- Iron Overload Diseases Association, Inc., 525 Mayflower Rd, West Palm Beach, FL 33405
- American Hemochromatosis Society, Inc., 4044 W. Lake Mary Blvd., Unit 104, Lake Mary, FL 32746-2012

PROGNOSIS

- Patients diagnosed before cirrhosis develops and treated with phlebotomy have a normal life expectancy.
- Life expectancy is reduced in patients with cirrhosis and DM and in those who require >18 months of phlebotomy therapy to return iron stores to normal.
- Patients with ferritin levels <1,000 μg/L are unlikely to have cirrhosis (3,10).

COMPLICATIONS

- Cirrhosis
- Hepatoma (only in patients with cirrhosis)
- DM
- Cardiomyopathy
- Arthritis
- Hypogonadism

REFERENCES

1. van Bokhoven MA, van Deursen CT, Swinkels DW. Diagnosis and management of hereditary haemochromatosis. *BMJ*. 2011;342:c7251.
2. Sood R, Bakashi R, Hegade VS, et al. Diagnosis and management of hereditary haemochromatosis. *Br J Gen Pract*. 2013;63(611):331–332.
3. Allen KJ, Gurrin LC, Constantine CC, et al. Iron-overload-related disease in HFE hereditary hemochromatosis. *N Engl J Med*. 2008;358(3):221–230.
4. Brandhagen DJ, Fairbanks VF, Baldus W. Recognition and management of hereditary hemochromatosis. *Am Fam Physician*. 2002;65(5):853–860.
5. Bacon BR, Adams PC, Kowdley KV, et al. Diagnosis and management of hemochromatosis: 2011 practice guideline by the American Association for the Study of Liver Diseases. *Hepatology*. 2011;54(1):328–343.
6. Crownover BK, Covey CJ. Hereditary hemochromatosis. *Am Fam Physician*. 2013;87(3):183–190.
7. Qaseem A, Aronson M, Fitterman N, et al. Screening for hereditary hemochromatosis: a clinical practice guideline from the American College of Physicians. *Ann Intern Med*. 2005;143(7):517–521.
8. Cherfane CE, Hollenbeck RD, Go J, et al. Hereditary hemochromatosis: missed diagnosis or misdiagnosis? *Am J Med*. 2013;126(11):1010–1015.
9. Alexander J, Kowdley KV. Hereditary hemochromatosis: genetics, pathogenesis, and clinical management. *Ann Hepatol*. 2005;4(4):240–247.
10. Janssen MC, Swinkels DW. Hereditary haemochromatosis. *Best Pract Res Clin Gastroenterol*. 2009;23(2):171–183.

ADDITIONAL READING

- Fleming RE, Ponka P. Iron overload in human disease. *N Engl J Med*. 2012;366(4):348–359.
- U.S. Preventive Services Task Force. Screening for hemochromatosis: recommendation statement. *Ann Intern Med*. 2006;145(3):204–208.

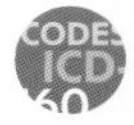

CODES

ICD10

- E83.110 Hereditary hemochromatosis
- E83.118 Other hemochromatosis
- E83.111 Hemochromatosis due to repeated red blood cell transfusions

CLINICAL PEARLS

- The best laboratory tests available to screen a patient initially for hemochromatosis are serum ferritin and transferrin saturation. An elevated transferrin saturation is the earliest abnormality in hemochromatosis. Ferritin is a sensitive measure of iron overload but can be elevated in a variety of infectious and inflammatory conditions without iron overload being present.
- Liver biopsy need not be done to confirm the diagnosis or to check for cirrhosis if the patient is homozygous for C282Y or is heterozygous for C282Y/H63D. If the patient's serum ferritin is <1,000 μg/L, LFTs are normal, and hepatomegaly is not present, cirrhosis is very unlikely, so liver biopsy is not needed.
- Initially, a patient with hemochromatosis should have a phlebotomy weekly until the serum ferritin is 50–100 μg/L and the transferrin saturation falls to <30%. Then, lifelong maintenance therapy of 2–6 phlebotomies a year is mandatory to keep the ferritin 50–100 μg/L and the transferrin saturation <50%.
- Most patients with hemochromatosis go undiagnosed. Because treatment with phlebotomy will prevent all complications when begun early, physicians should consider the diagnosis of hemochromatosis much more frequently. However, the U.S. Preventive Services Task Force recommends against routine screening of asymptomatic average-risk populations.

HEMOPHILIA

Frank J. Domino, MD

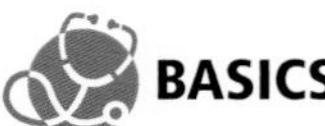

BASICS

DESCRIPTION

- Deficiency of factor VIII (hemophilia A) or factor IX (hemophilia B) coagulation proteins leading to bleeding tendencies in affected individuals. The majority of cases are due to inherited genetic mutations in factor VIII or factor IX coagulation proteins. However, an estimated 30% of all hemophilia cases result from spontaneous mutations.
- Hemophilia A and B are clinically indistinguishable but can be differentiated by assays that detect levels of factors VIII and IX, respectively.
- Disease severity correlates with the relative levels of coagulation factors present in serum analysis:
  - Severe: frequent spontaneous bleeding (factor activity <1%)
  - Moderate: bleeding with mild to moderate trauma (factor activity 1–5%)
  - Mild: bleeding with major trauma, tooth extraction, or surgery (factor activity 5–40%)
- Frequency of bleeding is similar when levels of severity are comparable in hemophilia A and B.
- Synonym(s): Christmas disease (hemophilia B)

EPIDEMIOLOGY

- Worldwide, an estimated 400,000 people are affected with hemophilia.
- Hemophilia A represents 80–85% of the total hemophilia population; hemophilia B comprises the remaining 15–20%.

ETIOLOGY AND PATHOPHYSIOLOGY

- Damage to vascular endothelium leads to exposure of subendothelial tissue factors, which interact with platelets, plasma proteins, and coagulation factors to produce a localized platelet plug contributing to hemostasis. Complexes involving factors VIII and IX participate in the intrinsic coagulation pathway to activate factor X, FXa. Downstream interactions involving FXa culminate in the conversion of prothrombin to thrombin, mediating platelet activation and fibrin deposition necessary for stabilization of the platelet plug.
- Deficiencies of factor VIII or factor IX result in decreased production of FXa, leading to an unstable platelet plug and impaired hemostasis.

Genetics

- Exhibits an X-chromosome linked inheritance pattern. Therefore, males are almost exclusively affected with hemophilia and females are asymptomatic carriers, unless their factor activity is <40% of normal.
- Carriers with symptomatically low clotting factor levels are treated similarly to patients with the trait:
  - Occasional female carrier will bleed at time of surgery.
- Males within the same family share similar deficiencies and level of severity owing to the same genetic defect.

GENERAL PREVENTION

- Hemophilia patients should carry medical ID tags listing their bleeding disorder or factor deficiency, inhibitor status, type of treatment products used, and initial treatment doses for mild, moderate, or severe bleeding.
- Immediate family members of affected patients should have factor VIII and IX levels checked prior to invasive procedures, childbirth, and if bleeding tendencies occur.
- Genetic testing should be offered to at-risk female family members of persons with hemophilia to facilitate genetic counseling or prenatal testing.

DIAGNOSIS

- History and initial presentation
  - 2/3 of presenting hemophilic patients have a positive family history. All male infants born to known carriers should have factor level testing.
  - Prolonged bleeding with circumcision, dental work, surgery, or injury
  - Excessive or easy bruising in early childhood, hematomas, hemarthroses
  - Spontaneous bleeding, especially in joints, muscle, or soft tissue
- Life-threatening bleeds
  - Intracranial hemorrhage: generally resulting from trauma; incidence of 1:10; fatal in 30% of cases
  - Hematomas of bowel wall can cause obstruction or intussusception as well as pain mimicking appendicitis.
  - Neck or throat bleeds: can lead to airway obstruction
- Serious bleeds
  - Hemarthrosis, most commonly of ankles, elbows, and knees
    - Infants may present with irritability or decreased use of limb.
    - Adults may have prodromal stiffness, acute pain, and swelling of joint.
    - Arthropathy results from repeated bleeding into joints, damaging cartilage and subchondral bone:
      - Can result in fixed joints, muscle wasting, and significantly impaired mobility
  - Muscular hematomas most commonly occur in quadriceps, iliopsoas, and forearm:
    - May result in compartment syndrome and ischemic nerve damage, such as femoral nerve neuropathy due to undetected retroperitoneal hemorrhage.
  - Mucous membrane bleeding, such as in the genitourinary tract, leading to hematuria
  - Pseudotumor syndrome: untreated hemorrhage causing a hematoma, which calcifies (named because it can be mistaken for cancer)

DIFFERENTIAL DIAGNOSIS

- Von Willebrand disease
- Vitamin K deficiency, warfarin (Coumadin) therapy (factor IX is vitamin K–dependent)
- Other factor deficiencies, afibrinogenemia, dysfibrinogenemia, fibrinolytic defects, platelet disorders
- Child abuse

DIAGNOSTIC TESTS & INTERPRETATION

Initial Tests (lab, imaging)

- CBC with platelet count, PT, aPTT, platelet function (preferred) or bleed time, vWF, factor VIII:C assay, factor IX assay. Prolonged aPTT: corrected when mixed with pooled normal plasma in absence of inhibitors
- PT, platelet count, and platelet function are normal.
- Diagnosis based on factor VIII:C or IX activity
  - Normal factor levels: 50–150 IU/dL
  - Mild 5–40 IU/dL
  - Moderate 1–5 IU/dL
  - Severe <1 IU/dL

Follow-Up Tests & Special Considerations

Inhibitors to factor VIII and IX (see "Complications"):

- Should be periodically measured using the Nijmegen or Bethesda assay, which quantifies the alloantibody titer.
- Screen before invasive procedures and at regular intervals.

Diagnostic Procedures/Other

Prenatal diagnosis: genetic testing of a sample of chorionic villus or fluid obtained at amniocentesis

Test Interpretation

In affected joints: synovial hemosiderosis, articular cartilage degeneration, thickening of periarticular tissues, bony hypertrophy

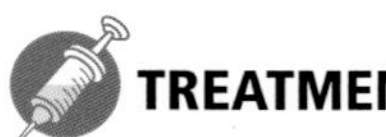

TREATMENT

GENERAL MEASURES

- Avoid aspirin or other NSAIDs
- Treat early; symptoms may occur before bleeding is clinically apparent.
- For surgical prophylaxis
  - If major surgery is undertaken, factor levels should be maintained at >50% for at least 2–3 weeks after the procedure:
    - Fibrin glue products may be beneficial for oozing at extensive incision sites.
  - Dental extractions: Antifibrinolytics (Amicar, tranexamic acid) may be used.
  - Minor procedures: may use desmopressin (DDAVP)
- Hepatitis A and B vaccinations are recommended.
- Encourage physical activity: Patients should avoid high-impact contact sports; restrict activities in proportion to degree of factor deficiency.

MEDICATION

First Line

- Principles of therapy
  - Primary prophylaxis: administration of specific factor replacement therapy in the absence of bleeding to maintain adequate baseline plasma levels sufficient for hemostasis in all categories of severity (1)[A]
    - Lower frequency of acute bleeds and episodes of life-threatening hemorrhage compared to on-demand therapy
    - Standard of care for children with severe hemophilia A to prevent joint bleeds and joint degeneration

- Dosing, frequency, duration of therapeutic regimens tailored to individual patient needs in clinical practice
- Opinions differ about optimal age to initiate prophylaxis, optimal dosing and frequency, and if or when to transition from prophylaxis to on-demand therapy.

  - On-demand therapy: treatment administered in response to occurrence of bleeding
    - Amount and duration of factor replacement depends on location and severity of bleeding:
      - A target factor level of >30% is generally sufficient for mild bleeding episodes.
      - Major hemorrhages and large muscle bleeds require correction to levels between 50% and 100%.
      - Life-threatening bleeds require levels between 80% and 100%, which should be sustained with bolus dosing or continuous infusion.
- Specific agents: Consensus guidelines express no preference for recombinant versus plasma-derived factor concentrates:
  - Hemophilia A: Replacement with factor VIII concentrates is treatment of choice:
    - 2 sources for the factor available:
      - Purified plasma-derived factor VIII: Donor pool is screened and the plasma-derived factor is treated to inactivate viruses (HIV, hepatitis B, and hepatitis C). Theoretical risks still exist.
      - Recombinant factor VIII
        - Dosing: 1 IU of factor VIII (the amount in 1 mL of plasma)/kg body weight administered will raise the plasma level of the recipient by 2%.
  - Hemophilia B: Replacement with factor IX concentrates is treatment of choice:
    - Plasma-derived factor IX and recombinant factor IX (preferred) are commercially available.
      - Dosing: 1 IU/kg body weight administered will raise plasma factor IX levels 1%.
- Hemophilia patients with inhibitors (neutralizing alloantibodies to factors VIII or IX)
  - Inhibitor formation should be suspected when replacement with the deficient factor fails to correct coagulopathy.
  - Low-titer (<5 BU/mL) patients: Replace with high doses of the deficient factor to overcome the circulating inhibitor concentration.
  - High-titer patients: Treat using products that *bypass* the factor neutralized by the alloantibody, or emergently with high doses of the specific deficient factor:
    - 2 bypassing agents available; both are efficacious at providing 80% of bleeding episodes:
      - Anti-inhibitor coagulation complex (AICC)
      - Recombinant activated factor VII (rFVIIa)
  - Immune tolerance induction (ITI): protocols to promote immune tolerance through repeated exposure to high-dose factor VIII therapy over 12–18 months, with or without immunosuppressive therapy (corticosteroids, cyclophosphamide, rituximab). Success rates are 60–80%.

Second Line

- Cryoprecipitate and fresh frozen plasma (FFP): can be used in instances where the specific factor concentrate is unavailable for *emergent hemostasis*
  - FFP: contains all coagulation factors but generally difficult to attain high levels of factors VIII or IX
    - Acceptable starting dose: 15–20 mL/kg
  - Cryoprecipitate: derived from precipitates of cooled FFP; contains significant levels of factor VIII (up to 100 IU/bag) but *not* factor IX:
    - Dosing: 1 mL cryoprecipitate has ~3–5 IU factor VIII.
- Desmopressin (DDAVP): synthetic vasopressin; stimulates endogenous release of factor VIII (*and vWF*) from endothelial stores; used in mild to moderate hemophilia
  - IV or SC: 0.3 μg/kg infused 30 minutes prior to procedure; may repeat if needed
  - Intranasal (150 μg/spray): adult dose, 1 spray to each nostril (300 μg total). Alternate dose if <50 kg: 150 μg once.
  - Adverse effect: hyponatremic seizures, especially in children; restrict fluids and watch sodium levels and urine output.
- Antifibrinolytic agents: inhibit plasminogen activation, thereby stabilizing the clot
  - Effective in controlling mucosal bleeding, such as bleeding in oral cavity, epistaxis, and menorrhagia; can also be used prophylactically (e.g., prior to tooth extractions)
    - Tranexamic acid (25 mg/kg PO q6–8h or 10 mg/kg IV q6–8h)
    - Aminocaproic acid (Amicar) is less frequently used.

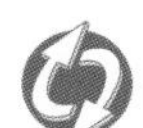

ONGOING CARE

FOLLOW-UP RECOMMENDATIONS

Patient Monitoring

Regular evaluations every 6–12 months, including a musculoskeletal evaluation, an inhibitor screen, liver tests, and tests for antibodies to hepatitis viruses and HIV

PATIENT EDUCATION

- National Hemophilia Foundation: www.hemophilia.org
- World Federation of Hemophilia: www.wfh.org

PROGNOSIS

- Survival is normal for those with mild disease; mortality is increased 2–6-fold in those with moderate to severe disease.
- Intracranial hemorrhage is a leading cause of death in hemophilia.
- Hemophilic arthropathy is the main cause of morbidity in patients with severe hemophilia.

COMPLICATIONS

- Hemophilic arthropathy: Symptoms include pain, limitation of motion, and contractures.
- Theoretical transmission of bloodborne infections, such as hepatitis A, B, C, and D and HIV; this risk has been greatly reduced with current testing of blood products.
- Development of inhibitor autoantibodies
  - More common in hemophilia A (20–30% of patients compared to 5% in hemophilia B) and in patients with severe disease requiring multiple transfusions
  - Risk factors for inhibitor development:
    - Specific genetic defect (family history); null mutations have higher inhibitor incidence.
    - Very low or no circulating factor, therefore requiring multiple transfusions
    - Age of 1st exogenous factor exposure; previous studies report a higher incidence of developing antibodies in those exposed to exogenous factor at <6 months of age, but new studies show this may be due to severity of disease.
    - Concurrent inflammation/infection when administering factor (e.g., surgical prophylaxis)
    - Duration of factor exposure
  - No increased risk of bleeding, but when bleeding occurs, it is more difficult to achieve hemostasis due to decreased response to factor replacement.

REFERENCES

1. Srivastava A, Brewer AK, Mauser-Bunschoten EP, et al. Guidelines for the management of hemophilia. *Haemophilia*. 2013;19(1):e1–e47.

ADDITIONAL READING

- Benson G, Auerswald G, Elezovi I, et al. Immune tolerance induction in patients with severe hemophilia with inhibitors: expert panel views and recommendations for clinical practice. *Eur J Haematol*. 2012;88(5):371–379.
- Berntorp E, Shapiro AD. Modern haemophilia care. *Lancet*. 2012;379(9824):1447–1456.
- Fischer K. Prophylaxis for adults with haemophilia: one size does not fit all. *Blood Transfus*. 2012;10(2): 169–173.
- Franchini M, Mannucci PM. Past, present and future of hemophilia: a narrative review. *Orphanet J Rare Dis*. 2012;7:24.
- Gater A, Thomson TA, Strandberg-Larsen M. Haemophilia B: impact on patients and economic burden of disease. *Thromb Haemost*. 2011;106(3):398–404.
- Leissinger C, Gringeri A, Antmen B, et al. Anti-inhibitor coagulant complex prophylaxis in hemophilia with inhibitors. *N Engl J Med*. 2011; 365(18):1684–1692.
- Ragni MV, Fogarty PJ, Josephson NC, et al. Survey of current prophylaxis practices and bleeding characteristics of children with severe haemophilia A in US haemophilia treatment centres. *Haemophilia*. 2012;18(1):63–68.

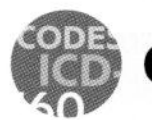

CODES

ICD10

- D66 Hereditary factor VIII deficiency
- D67 Hereditary factor IX deficiency
- D68.1 Hereditary factor XI deficiency

H

HEMORRHOIDS

Juan Qiu, MD, PhD

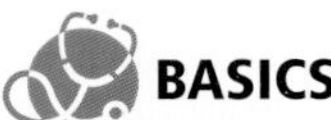

BASICS

DESCRIPTION

- Varicosities of the hemorrhoidal venous plexus
- External hemorrhoids
  - Located below the dentate line (painful)
  - Covered by squamous epithelium
- Internal hemorrhoids
  - Located above the dentate line (painless)
- Both types of hemorrhoids often coexist.
- Classification of internal hemorrhoids (1,2,3)
  - 1st-degree: Hemorrhoids do not prolapse.
  - 2nd-degree: prolapse through the anus on straining but reduce spontaneously
  - 3rd-degree: protrude and require digital reduction
  - 4th-degree: cannot be reduced
- Hemorrhoids often progress from itching, bleeding stage to protrusion with easy reduction, then difficult reduction, and finally rectal prolapse. Thrombosis may occur at any protrusion stage. External hemorrhoids cause pain; internal hemorrhoids generally do not (2,3).

Geriatric Considerations

Hemorrhoids more common in elderly, as is rectal prolapse.

Pediatric Considerations

- Uncommon in infants and children; when discovered, look for underlying cause (e.g., vena caval or mesenteric obstruction, cirrhosis, portal hypertension [HTN]).
- Occasionally, as in adults, hemorrhoids may result from chronic constipation, fecal impaction, and straining at stool. Surgery is rarely required in children.

Pregnancy Considerations

- Common in pregnancy
- Usually resolves after pregnancy
- No treatment required, unless extremely painful.

EPIDEMIOLOGY

- Predominant age: adults; peak between 45 and 65 years
- Predominant sex: male = female

Incidence

Common

Prevalence

~4–5% in general population in the United States

ETIOLOGY AND PATHOPHYSIOLOGY

- There are 3 primary hemorrhoidal cushions located typically in left lateral, right anterior, and right posterior positions. Hemorrhoidal cushions augment anal closure pressure and protect the anal sphincter during stool passage. During Valsalva, intra-abdominal pressure increases raising pressure within the hemorrhoidal cushions helping to preserve anal closure. Mechanisms implicated in symptomatic hemorrhoidal disease include the following:
  - Dilated veins of hemorrhoidal plexus
  - Tight internal anal sphincter
  - Abnormal distention of the arteriovenous anastomosis
  - Prolapse of the cushions and the surrounding connective tissues

Genetics

No known genetic pattern

RISK FACTORS

- Pregnancy
- Pelvic space-occupying lesions
- Liver disease
- Portal HTN
- Constipation
- Occupations that require prolonged sitting
- Loss of perianal muscle tone due to old age, rectal surgery, episiotomy, anal intercourse
- Obesity
- Chronic diarrhea

GENERAL PREVENTION

- Avoid constipation with high-fiber diet and hydration.
- Maintain appropriate weight.
- Avoid prolonged sitting or straining on the toilet.

COMMONLY ASSOCIATED-CONDITIONS

- Liver disease
- Pregnancy
- Portal HTN
- Constipation

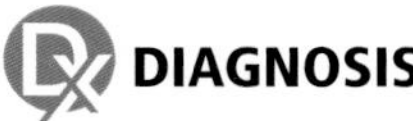

DIAGNOSIS

Diagnosis is typically straightforward through history and inspection of the perineum, rectal exam, and anoscopy.

HISTORY

- Internal/external hemorrhoids
  - Classically, bright red blood per rectum
    - May be scant blood on toilet paper *or*
    - Copious in the toilet bowl
  - Constipation or diarrhea
  - Straining with defecation
- Small or minimal external hemorrhoids
  - Episodic bleeding on stool or toilet paper, pruritus
- More extensive internal hemorrhoids
  - Feeling of incomplete evacuation
- Thrombosed hemorrhoids present as an acute painful mass (2,3).

PHYSICAL EXAM

- Anorectal exam including anoscopy (2,3)
- Inspection following straining at stool
- For protruding hemorrhoids: mass, more prominent bleeding. If not reducible, increased risk of strangulation and/or thrombosis with acute pain
- Abdominal exam to exclude mass
- Peripheral stigmata of cirrhosis and portal hypertension (caput, telangiectasias, palmar erythema)

DIFFERENTIAL DIAGNOSIS

- Rectal or anal neoplasia
- Condyloma
- Skin tag
- Inflammatory bowel disease
- Anal fistula, fissure, or abscess

DIAGNOSTIC TESTS & INTERPRETATION

Diagnostic Procedures/Other

Sigmoidoscopy or colonoscopy depending on risk factors for malignancy in patients with rectal bleeding (3)[A].

TREATMENT

- Prevention
  - Fiber supplements
  - Stool softeners

GENERAL MEASURES

- Hemorrhoids are a recurrent disease, even after surgical excision; preventive measures should be continued indefinitely.
- For mild symptoms or prevention (3)[A]
  - Avoid prolonged sitting during bowel movements.
  - Avoid straining.
  - Avoid constipation by eating a high-fiber diet or by taking fiber supplements; if necessary, take regular stool softeners.
  - Regular exercise
- For pain, Sitz baths warm water or hypertonic Epsom salts (1 cup per 2 quarts of water)
- Pruritus or mild discomfort after stooling responds well to topical hydrocortisone ointment, anesthetic ointments or sprays, and warm Sitz baths.
- Constipation relief, anal hygiene, local ointments, and Sitz baths are effective through the stage of easy reduction (stage 2). More severe stages often require ligation or surgery (3)[A].

MEDICATION

First Line

- Dietary modification with adequate fluid and fiber is the primary 1st-line, nonoperative therapy for symptomatic hemorrhoids (3)[A].
- Pain
  - Hydrocortisone ointment (0.5–1%)
  - Analgesic sprays or ointments: benzocaine, dibucaine (Nupercainal). Use sprays with caution, as they may contain alcohol that can cause burning sensation when applied.
- Pruritus: hydrocortisone (Anusol-HC, Cortifoam) ointment
- Bleeding
  - Astringent suppositories (Preparation H)
  - Hydrocortisone (Anusol; Cortifoam) ointment

Second Line

Treatment for special cases

- Thrombosed external hemorrhoids: Common complication of hemorrhoidal disease. With conservative treatment, the thrombus will be absorbed over the course of weeks and pain improves within 2–3 days (1–3)[A].
- With severe acute pain, prompt excision should be performed under local anesthetic and the wound left open without packing. Use Sitz baths, topical anesthetics, and mild pain relievers for first 7–10 days after excision (1–3)[A].
- Strangulated hemorrhoid: From irreducible 3rd- or 4th-degree hemorrhoid. If untreated, it can progress to ulceration and thrombosis. Treatment requires urgent or emergent hemorrhoidectomy.
- Acute hemorrhoidal bleeding associated with portal HTN can be life-threatening. Treatment should be suture of the bleeding site with incorporation of the mucosa, submucosa, and internal sphincter. Coagulopathy should be corrected.

SURGERY/OTHER PROCEDURES

- Indications: failure of medical and nonoperative therapy, symptomatic stage 3 or stage 4 symptoms in presence of a concomitant anorectal condition requiring surgery, or patient preference (1–3)[A]
- Incision of thrombosed hemorrhoid: for severe pain
- Severe protruding hemorrhoids
  - Rubber band ligation (internal hemorrhoids only) (1–3)[A]
  - Sclerotherapy: for symptomatic prolapsed stage I or II hemorrhoids; care must be taken not to inject near periprostatic parasympathetic nerves. Not for advanced disease or if evidence of infection, inflammation, ulceration is present
    - Cryotherapy is no longer recommended due to high rate of complications.
  - Prolapsed rectum
    - Requires surgical correction
  - Surgical resection
    - Gold standard: Conventional hemorrhoidectomy should be considered for grade III hemorrhoids not responding to banding, mixed internal and external, grade IV hemorrhoids, or when complicated by fissures, fistula, or extensive skin tags (1–3)[A].
- Newer techniques reduce surgical time, early postop pain, urinary retention, and time to return to normal activity.
  - Transanal hemorrhoidal dearterialization (THD): fewer complications and can be used in cases of recurrent diseases (2,3)[A],(4)[B]
  - Stapled hemorrhoidopexy: less painful than traditional surgery but higher incidence of skin tags and recurrent prolapse (2)[A],(4)[B]
  - LigaSure hemorrhoidectomy: reduces operating time, is superior in patient tolerance, and is equally effective as conventional hemorrhoidectomy in long-term symptom control (5,6)[B],(7)[A]

COMPLEMENTARY & ALTERNATIVE MEDICINE

Aloe vera cream on the surgical site after hemorrhoidectomy reduces postoperative pain and decreases healing time and analgesic requirements.

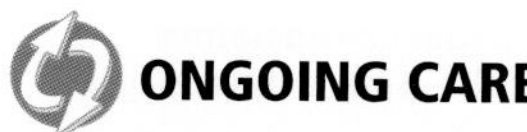

ONGOING CARE

FOLLOW-UP RECOMMENDATIONS

- Encourage physical fitness and appropriate weight management.
- Avoid prolonged sitting and straining on the toilet.

Patient Monitoring

As needed, depending on treatment

DIET

High-fiber with 25–30 g of insoluble fiber/day through sources such as wheat bran cereals, oatmeal, peanuts, artichokes, beans, corn, peas, spinach, potatoes, apples, apricots, blackberries, raspberries, prunes, pears, bananas; adequate fluids (6–8 glasses of water/day); avoid excessive caffeine.

PATIENT EDUCATION

High-fiber diet: Today's Dietitian Top Fiber-Rich Foods List. http://www.todaysdietitian.com/newarchives/063008p28.shtml

PROGNOSIS

- Spontaneous resolution
- Recurrence

COMPLICATIONS

- Thrombosis
- Ulceration
- Anemia (rare)
- Incontinence
- Pelvic sepsis following hemorrhoidectomy

REFERENCES

1. Klein, JW. Common anal problems. *Med Clin N Am*. 2014;98(3):609–623.
2. Hall, JF. Modern management of hemorrhoidal disease. *Gastroenterol Clin N Am*. 2013;42:759–772.
3. Ganz, RA. The evaluation and treatment of hemorrhoids: a guide for the gastroenterologist. *Clin Gastroenterol Hepatol*. 2013:11(6):593–603.
4. Ratto, C. THD Doppler procedure for hemorrhoids: the surgical technique. *Tech Coloproctol*. 2014:18(3):291–298.
5. Michalik M, Pawlak M, Bobowicz M, et al. Long-term outcomes of stapled hemorrhoidopexy. *Wideochir Inne Tech Malo Inwazyjne*. 2014;9(1):18–23.
6. Chen CW, Lai CW, Chang YJ, et al. Results of 666 consecutive patients treated with LigaSure hemorrhoidectomy for symptomatic prolapsed hemorrhoids with a minimum follow-up of 2 years. *Surgery*. 2013;153(2):211–218.
7. Nienhuijs S, de Hingh I. Conventional versus LigaSure hemorrhoidectomy for patients with symptomatic hemorrhoids. *Cochrane Database Syst Rev*. 2009;(1):CD006761.

ADDITIONAL READING

- Castellví J, Sueira A, Espinosa J, et al. Ligasure versus diathermy hemorrhoidectomy under spinal anesthesia or pudendal block with ropivacaine: a randomized prospective clinical study with 1-year follow-up. *Int J Colorectal Dis*. 2009;24(9):1011–1018.
- Giordano P, Gravante G, Sorge R, et al. Long-term outcomes of stapled hemorrhoidopexy vs conventional hemorrhoidectomy: a meta-analysis of randomized controlled trials *Arch Surg*. 2009;144(3):266–272.
- Reese GE, von Roon AC, Tekkis PP. *Haemorrhoids. Clin Evid (Online)*. 2009;2009:pii.0415.
- Rivadeneira DE, Steele SR, Ternent C, et al. Practice parameters for the management of hemorrhoids (revised 2010). *Dis Colon Rectum*. 2011;54(9):1059–1064.

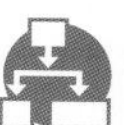

SEE ALSO

Colorectal Cancer; Portal Hypertension

CODES

ICD10

- K64.9 Unspecified hemorrhoids
- K64.0 First degree hemorrhoids
- K64.1 Second degree hemorrhoids

CLINICAL PEARLS

- Hemorrhoids are a very common clinical condition. Internal hemorrhoids are painless. External hemorrhoids are typically painful.
- Anal hygiene and symptomatic pain relief are the treatments of choice for stage 1 and 2 hemorrhoids. Sitz baths with warm water or hypertonic Epsom salts (1 cup per 2 quarts of water) are effective for pain relief.
- More advanced hemorrhoidal disease requires intervention with ligation or surgery.

HENOCH-SCHÖNLEIN PURPURA

Shani Muhammad, MD

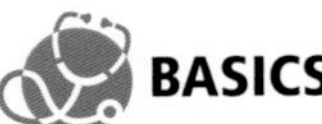

BASICS

DESCRIPTION

- Henoch-Schönlein purpura (HSP) is a nonthrombocytopenic, predominantly IgA-mediated, small vessel vasculitis that affects multiple organ systems and occurs in both children and adults.
- HSP is often self-limited, with the greatest morbidity and mortality attributable to long-term renal damage.
- Characterized by a tetrad of purpuric skin lesions, arthralgia, abdominal pain, and nephropathies

EPIDEMIOLOGY

Incidence

- Annual incidence: 135/1 million children and 3.4–14.3/1 million adults
- Mean age of patients affected is 6 years; 90% <10 years of age but has been reported in patients age 6 months–75 years old
- Gender: Male-to-female ratio is 1.2:1.
- Race/ethnicity: most common in Caucasians and Asians, less common among African Americans

Prevalence

- Annual prevalence: 10–22/100,000 persons
- Year-round occurrence; more common in late fall to early spring

ETIOLOGY AND PATHOPHYSIOLOGY

- Autoimmune disorder in which IgA production is increased in response to trigger(s), IgA1 immune complexes then activate the complement pathway, leading to production of inflammatory cytokines and chemokines.
- Immune complex deposition results in small vessel inflammation; fibrosis; and necrosis within skin, intestinal mucosa, joints, and kidneys.
- No single etiologic agent has been identified.
- Known triggers include infection, drugs, vaccinations, and insect bites.
- Infectious antigens include (but are not limited to) group A Streptococcus (may be present in up to 30% of HSP-associated nephritis), parvovirus B19, *Bartonella henselae*, *Helicobacter pylori*, *Haemophilus parainfluenzae*, coxsackievirus, adenovirus, hepatitis A and B viruses, Mycoplasma, Epstein-Barr virus, varicella, *Campylobacter*, methicillin-resistant *Staphylococcus aureus*.
- Drugs: acetaminophen, quinolones, etanercept, codeine, clarithromycin
- Vaccinations: MMR (measles, mumps, rubella), pneumococcal, meningococcal, influenza, hepatitis B

Genetics

Associated with α_1-antitrypsin deficiency, familial Mediterranean fever, *HLA-DRB1*01*, *HLA-B35*

COMMONLY ASSOCIATED CONDITIONS

- Malignancy (rare): Greatest association is with solid tumors, including lymphoma, prostate cancer, and non–small cell lung cancer, but also associated with multiple myeloma.
- Studies suggest a possible relationship with *H. pylori* infection. (1)

DIAGNOSIS

Palpable purpura and *at least 1* of the following:

- Diffuse abdominal pain
- Biopsy with predominant IgA deposition
- Arthralgia or arthritis
- Renal involvement (hematuria or proteinuria)

HISTORY

- History of exposure to known trigger, including recent infection (particularly upper respiratory infection), vaccination, or offending drug
- Rash (most common presenting symptom): purpuric, palpable; distribution often symmetric on lower extremities and buttocks; may present on upper extremities, trunk, and face; typical duration 3–10 days; no definitive temporal association with other symptoms
- Fatigue
- Low-grade fever
- Nausea/vomiting
- Abdominal pain (diffuse, colicky, may be transient or constant)
- Hematochezia/melena
- Polyarthritis (often symmetric involvement of knees and ankles)
- Gross hematuria
- Rare symptoms: periorbital or scrotal swelling, headache, neuropathy, hemoptysis

PHYSICAL EXAM

- Rash (96% of cases, 74% primary presenting symptom):
  - May start as urticaria, develops into nonblanching purpura, with or without petechiae and ecchymoses, may also be bullous
  - Distribution usually symmetric, most commonly involving the lower extremities but may involve the face and trunk
- Abdominal tenderness (66% of cases, 12% primary presenting symptom):
  - Evidence of GI hemorrhage (28% of cases)
- Joint tenderness (64% of cases, 15% primary presenting symptom):
  - Mainly affects knees or ankles; may have associated warmth and limited range of motion, less commonly effusion; erythema is absent.
  - Mostly nonmigratory, transient, and nondeforming
- Orchitis (5%):
  - Presents as scrotal swelling and tenderness, may have associated torsion
- Renal disease (<1% primary presenting symptom):
  - Hypertension may be present.
- Rarely, patients present with CNS or pulmonary involvement, which may manifest as signs of cerebral hemorrhage or diffuse interstitial pneumonia, respectively.

DIFFERENTIAL DIAGNOSIS

- Infection:
  - Meningococcemia
  - Rocky Mountain spotted fever
  - Bacterial endocarditis
  - Rheumatic fever
- Immune mediated:
  - Polyarteritis nodosa
  - Wegener granulomatosis
  - Systemic lupus erythematosus
  - Kawasaki disease
- Other:
  - Inflammatory bowel disease
  - Idiopathic thrombocytopenic purpura
  - Juvenile rheumatoid arthritis
  - Leukemia
  - Acute surgical abdomen
  - Child abuse

DIAGNOSTIC TESTS & INTERPRETATION

- No single lab test confirms the diagnosis of HSP.
- Labs directed toward excluding other illnesses and assessing degree of renal involvement

Initial Tests (lab, imaging)

The following are generally accepted as initial labs for HSP:

- CBC:
  - Leukocytosis and thrombocytosis may occur. Thrombocytopenia indicates an alternative cause of purpura.
  - Hemoglobin is variable, depending on whether GI hemorrhage occurs.
- Basic serum chemistry panel (electrolytes, BUN, creatinine:
  - Electrolyte imbalances or elevated creatinine indicate renal dysfunction.
- Urinalysis:
  - Gross or microscopic hematuria, proteinuria, and red cell casts indicate renal dysfunction.
- PT and PTT:
  - Normal in HSP
- Imaging is not part of the routine workup for HSP but may be performed to rule out alternative etiologies or for evaluation of suspected complications, particularly in cases of GI and renal involvement. Initial imaging modalities to consider include the following:
  - Abdominal radiographs, with or without barium enema: evaluate for free abdominal air suggestive of bowel perforation
  - Abdominal ultrasound: sensitive for the detection of intramural bleeding in HSP and may also show thickened bowel wall, reduced peristalsis, intussusception
- Renal ultrasound: evaluates for hydronephrosis in cases of renal failure

Follow-Up Tests & Special Considerations

The following labs are also useful in diagnosing HSP:

- Blood culture:
  - To rule out sepsis/bacteremia when diagnosis is unclear
- Acute phase reactants:
  - Expect mild elevation.
- IgA level:
  - Often elevated, although nonspecific, nonsensitive
- Visfatin levels: (2)
- Degree of elevation correlates with disease severity and likelihood of renal involvement (2).
- Complement levels:
  - Normal; sometimes decreased
- Antinuclear antibody/antineutrophil cytoplasmic antibody:
  - Negative
- Antistreptolysin-O titer:
  - Evaluates for preceding streptococcal infection
- Stool guaiac if suspected GI hemorrhage
- CT arteriography may be necessary to identify the location of bleeding in patients with GI hemorrhage.

Diagnostic Procedures/Other
- Renal biopsy: obtain if diagnosis uncertain or if nephrotic range proteinuria. Shows mesangial IgA deposition, mesangial proliferation, or, in severe cases, crescentic glomerulonephritis.
- Skin biopsy of purpura: IgA deposition in the dermis on immunofluorescence
- Endoscopy may be considered in cases of GI hemorrhage given symptomatic overlap of HSP with inflammatory bowel disease.
- Barium enema may be therapeutic in some instances of intussusception, although surgical correction is commonly needed.

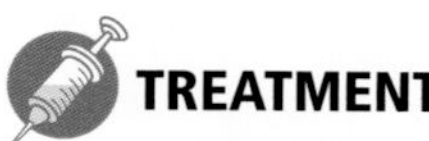

TREATMENT

GENERAL MEASURES
Rest and elevation of affected areas may limit purpura.

MEDICATION
- In the absence of renal dysfunction or complication, HSP is usually self-limited and best managed with supportive care.
- NSAIDs are effective for symptomatic treatment of joint pain. Caution is advised in cases of GI hemorrhage; avoid use in cases of renal involvement and consider acetaminophen as an alternative.
- Steroids given early in disease course using oral prednisone 1–2 mg/kg/day for 1–2 weeks decrease both duration of abdominal pain and severity of joint pain and may have benefit in preventing GI bleeding and causes of surgical abdomen, including intussusception.
- Steroids have benefit in treatment of severe and/or bullous purpura.
- Steroids given early in disease are effective for the acute treatment of crescentic nephritis and may prevent chronic renal disease in such patients.
- Early intervention with steroids has no effect on the prevention or development of renal involvement after 1 year.
- High-dose IV pulse steroids (500 mg–1 g) may be considered in cases of mesenteric vasculitis and severe renal impairment. Evidence is very limited to support use of cyclophosphamide, plasmapheresis, and intravenous immunoglobulin (IVIG) for severe renal and GI involvement, as well as colchicine for severe skin lesions.
- Mycophenolate mofetil (MMF) could be valuable in the treatment of complicated HSP (2,3)[A].

ISSUES FOR REFERRAL
- Consider nephrology referral for renal biopsy if nephrotic range proteinuria at any time or proteinuria >100 mg/mmol for 3 months after diagnosis.
- Dermatology referral for skin biopsy

INPATIENT CONSIDERATIONS
Admission Criteria/Initial Stabilization
- Insufficient oral intake
- Renal insufficiency
- Severe abdominal pain
- Severe GI bleeding
- Altered mental status
- Mobility restriction due to arthritis
- Hypertension (HTN)
- Nephrotic syndrome

IV-Fluids
Hydration should be maintained.

ONGOING CARE

FOLLOW-UP RECOMMENDATIONS
Patient Monitoring
- Patients should be seen weekly during the acute illness. Visits should include history and physical exam to include BP measurement and urinalysis.
- Because ~100% of patients who develop renal involvement will do so within 6 months of HSP diagnosis, all patients should be followed at least monthly with BP and urinalysis for a duration of no less than 6 months.
- Women with a history of HSP should be monitored for proteinuria and HTN during pregnancy.
- Consider workup for occult malignancy in patients with adult-onset HSP.

PATIENT EDUCATION
- American Family Physician handout on HSP available at: www.aafp.org/afp/980800ap/980800b.html
- National Kidney and Urologic Diseases Information Clearinghouse (NKUDIC): http://kidney.niddk.nih.gov/kudiseases/pubs/hsp/

PROGNOSIS
- Long-term prognosis heavily dependent on presence and severity of nephritis
- HSP is self-limited in 94% of children and 89% of adults.
- Most cases of HSP resolve within 4 weeks of diagnosis. Recurrence rate within 6 months of diagnosis is 33%.
- Factors associated with poorer prognosis include age >8 years, fever at presentation, purpura above the waist, elevated ESR or IgA concentration, and increasing severity of renal histology grade.
- Chronic renal disease occurs in up to 20% of children with nephritic and nephrotic syndrome compared with 50% of adults who had any renal involvement. Risk of long-term renal failure is ≤5%.
- Risk factors that may result in renal failure include old age, HTN, elevated serum creatinine, and nephrotic and mixed nephritic–nephrotic syndrome at the onset of disease (2).

COMPLICATIONS
- Nephrotic/nephritic syndrome and renal failure
- HTN
- Hemorrhagic cystitis
- Ureteral obstruction
- Intestinal infarction, perforation, obstruction, stricture
- GI hemorrhage
- Intussusception
- Alveolar hemorrhage
- CNS complications, including cerebral hemorrhage and seizure
- Anterior uveitis
- Myocarditis
- Orchitis
- Testicular torsion

REFERENCES

1. Kutlubay Z, Zara T, Engin B, et al. *Helicobacter pylori* infection and skin disorders. *Hong Kong Med J.* 2014;20(4):317–324.
2. Nikibakhsh AA, Mahmoodzadeh H, Karamyyar M, et al. Treatment of severe henoch-schonlein purpura nephritis with mycophenolate mofetil. *Saudi J Kidney Dis Transpl.* 2014;25(4):858–863.
3. Antoon JW, Keane MW. Migratory polyarthritis in a child. *Clin Pediatr (Phila).* 2012;51(4):401–403.

ADDITIONAL READING

- Batu ED, Ozen S. Pediatric vasculitis. *Curr Rheumatol Rep.* 2012;14(2):121–129.
- Boulis E, Majithia V, McMurray R. Adult onset Henoch-Schonlein purpura with positive c-ANCA (anti-protinease 3): case report and review of literature. *Rheumatology International.* 2013;33(2):493–496.
- Cao N, Chen T, Guo ZP, et al. Elevated serum levels of visfatin in patients with henoch-schönlein purpura. *Ann Dermatol.* 2014;26(3):303–307.
- Dillon MJ, Ozen S. A new international classification of childhood vasculitis. *Pediatr Nephrol.* 2006;21(9):1219–1222.
- González LM, Janniger CK, Schwartz RA. Pediatric Henoch-Schönlein purpura. *Int J Dermatol.* 2009;48(11):1157–1165.
- Hoyer PF. Prevention of renal disease in Henoch-Schonlein purpura: clear evidence against steroids. *Arch Dis Child.* 2013;98(10):750–751.
- Jithpratuck W, Elshenawy Y, Saleh H, et al. The clinical implications of adult-onset Henoch-Schonelin purpura. *Clin Mol Allergy.* 2011;9(1):9.
- Kawasaki Y. The pathogenesis and treatment of pediatric Henoch-Schonlein purpura nephritis. *Clin Exp Nephrol.* 2011;15(5):648–657.
- McCarthy HJ, Tizard EJ. Diagnosis and management of Henoch-Schönlein purpura. *Eur J Pediatr.* 2010;169(6):643–650.
- Ozen S, Pistorio A, Iusan SM, et al. EULAR/PRINTO/PRES criteria for Henoch-Schönlein purpura, childhood polyarteritis nodosa, childhood Wegener granulomatosis and childhood Takayasu arteritis: Ankara 2008. Part II: final classification criteria. *Ann Rheum Dis.* 2010;69(5):798–806.
- Reamy BV, Williams PM, Lindsay TJ. Henoch-Schönlein purpura. *Am Fam Physician.* 2009;80(7):697–704.
- Saulsbury FT. Henoch-Schönlein purpura. *Curr Opin Rheumatol.* 2001;13(1):35–40.
- Sohagia AB, Gunturu SG, Tong TR, et al. Henoch-Schonlein purpura—a case report and review of the literature. *Gastroenterol Res Pract.* 2010;2010:597648.
- Weiss PF, Klink AJ, Localio R, et al. Corticosteroids may improve clinical outcomes during hospitalization for Henoch-Schönlein purpura. *Pediatrics.* 2010;126:674–681.

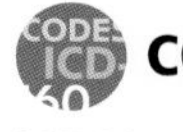

CODES

ICD10
D69.0 Allergic purpura

CLINICAL PEARLS
- HSP is a systemic small vessel vasculitis characterized by clinical tetrad of palpable purpura, abdominal pain, arthralgia, and renal dysfunction.
- The main form of treatment is supportive care, but oral corticosteroids are beneficial in certain circumstances.
- In all patients with HSP, regardless of renal involvement at presentation, it is reasonable to check BP and urinalysis at weekly to monthly intervals for no less than 6 months after diagnosis to monitor for developing renal dysfunction.

HEPARIN-INDUCED THROMBOCYTOPENIA

Rami Farhat, DO • Tipsuda Junsanto-Bahri, MD • Maria A. Pino, PhD, MS, RpH

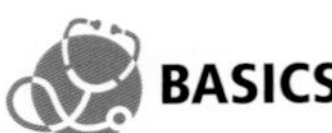

BASICS

DESCRIPTION

- Unexplained decrease in platelet count in a patient treated with heparin
  - Minimum platelet count falls between 30% and 50% from baseline.
- Antibody-mediated prothrombotic disorder initiated by heparin administration
- Unlike other thrombocytopenias, heparin-induced thrombocytopenia (HIT) produces thrombosis rather than bleeding.
- Idiosyncratic reaction
- Two types: nonimmune heparin-associated thrombocytopenia (previously called HIT type I) and HIT (immune induced; previously called HIT type II)
  - Nonimmune heparin-associated thrombocytopenia: more common, onset 1–4 days after starting heparin, mild thrombocytopenia (>100,000), few complications
  - HIT: less common, onset 5–14 days after primary exposure to heparin, thrombocytopenia often <100,000 but usually >20,000; high risk of thrombosis
    - Presentation of thrombocytopenia can be immediate with recent heparin exposure (within past 100 days).

EPIDEMIOLOGY

Incidence

- 10–15% of heparin-treated patients will experience decrease in platelet count.
- 0.3–3% will develop HIT.

ETIOLOGY AND PATHOPHYSIOLOGY

- Nonimmune heparin-associated thrombocytopenia: potentially a result of direct platelet membrane binding with heparin
- HIT: Heparin can cause an increase in the blood concentration of platelet factor 4 (PF4), a chemokine. PF4 will form a complex with heparin.
- This heparin/PF4 complex can, in turn, stimulate the production of specific antiheparin/PF4 complex antibodies. These antibodies cause platelet activation and a prothrombotic state. Ultimately, this hypercoagulable state leads to thromboembolic complications in many patients.

RISK FACTORS

- Postsurgical > medical > obstetric
  - Postcardiopulmonary bypass is the most significant risk factor.
- Bovine unfractionated heparin (UFH) > porcine UFH > low-molecular-weight heparin (LMWH)
- Female > male
- Heparin duration >4 days

GENERAL PREVENTION

- Inquire about recent heparin exposure and any history of HIT.
- Use of LMWH (vs. unfractionated) and for a shorter duration reduce the risk of developing HIT.
- Properly document past HIT reactions in patient's medical record (1)[A].
- No form of heparin should be administered once the diagnosis of HIT is confirmed.

COMMONLY ASSOCIATED CONDITIONS

- Venous thrombosis: deep venous thrombosis (DVT), pulmonary embolism, adrenal vein thrombosis with hemorrhagic infarction
- Arterial thrombosis
- Skin lesions (skin necrosis at site of injection)
- Acute systemic reactions

DIAGNOSIS

- Nonimmune heparin-associated thrombocytopenia: asymptomatic drop in platelet count
- HIT: thrombocytopenia or thrombosis with the presence of heparin-dependent antibodies
  - A clinicopathologic syndrome, meaning the foundation for diagnosis, is based on both clinical and serologic findings.

HISTORY

- Duration of current heparin therapy
- Previous exposure to heparin, including heparin flushes and heparin-coated catheters
- In patients being treated with heparin for thrombosis, in which thrombosis recurs during therapy, consider HIT as a potential cause.
- Pretest probability for HIT can be calculated using the "4 Ts" methodology:
  - **T**hrombocytopenia of new onset
  - **T**iming of thrombocytopenia (5–10 days after exposure)
  - **T**hrombosis of new onset
  - **T**hrombocytopenia by other causes is ruled out.
- The HIT Expert Probability score is an effective pretest probability tool (2,3)[B].

PHYSICAL EXAM

- Signs of venous or arterial thrombosis
- Skin necrosis (begins with erythema, progresses to ecchymosis and necrosis)
- Ischemic changes (signs of limb, renal, splenic, mesenteric ischemia)
- Bleeding (less common)
- Acute systemic reactions after IV bolus of heparin (e.g., signs of anaphylaxis)

DIFFERENTIAL DIAGNOSIS

Other potential causes of thrombocytopenia include (list is not all-inclusive)

- Sepsis and other infections
- Drug reactions
- Autoimmune
- Transfusion reactions
- Physical destruction (e.g., during cardiopulmonary bypass)

DIAGNOSTIC TESTS & INTERPRETATION

- Serial platelet counts in patients receiving heparin who have a possible risk of HIT >1%: Check platelets at baseline and then every 2–3 days from days 4–14 of heparin therapy (4)[B]:
  - Withhold platelet monitoring for patients receiving heparin with risk of HIT <1%.
- Confirmatory lab tests needed for a clinical diagnosis can be divided into two major categories:
  - Antigen assay to detect presence of HIT antibodies:
    - ELISA: up to 99% sensitive, poor specificity; thus, has an excellent negative predictive value for HIT
  - Functional assay to detect evidence of platelet activation in the presence of heparin:
    - Serotonin release assay (SRA), gold standard for diagnosis: high specificity and high sensitivity
    - Heparin-induced platelet activation (HIPA): high specificity and low sensitivity
- Either a functional assay or an antigenic assay alone may not be adequate for clinical diagnosis; their use in combination is usually recommended:
  - Antigenic assay should be the initial test.
- The diagnostic interpretation of these laboratory tests must be made in the context of the clinical estimation of the pretest probability because HIT is a clinicopathologic syndrome. Patients may form heparin-dependent antibodies and still not develop HIT.

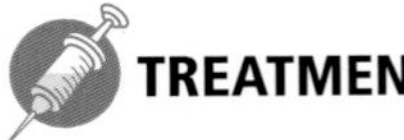

TREATMENT

Treatment is by prompt withdrawal of heparin and replacement with a suitable alternative anticoagulant.

GENERAL MEASURES

- Discontinue all heparin products, including flushes and heparin-coated catheters.
- Nonimmune heparin-associated thrombocytopenia generally resolves when heparin is stopped:
  - Consider a nonheparin alternative such as fondaparinux if pharmacologic DVT prophylaxis is warranted (5)[C].
- Platelet transfusions can increase thrombosis. Give platelet transfusions only if bleeding or during an invasive procedure with a high risk of bleeding.
- Warfarin should not be administered until platelet recovery. If warfarin has been administered, vitamin K should be given.
- Adverse reaction to heparin should be clearly documented in the medical record with instruction to avoid all heparin products.
- For patients with a documented history of HIT, under special circumstances only (such as the need for cardiopulmonary bypass), the use of heparin for a short duration may be acceptable if the absence of heparin/PF4 complex antibodies can be documented (4)[B].
- All patients with a diagnosis of HIT should receive alternative anticoagulation as they are of high thrombotic risk.

MEDICATION

- Most patients require anticoagulation either because of
  - Preexisting thrombosis *or*
  - Risk of thrombosis during 30 days after HIT diagnosis; consider anticoagulation for 30 days.

- Dosing of anticoagulant depends on indication (prophylaxis vs. treatment):
  - In cases with a clinically low suspicion/pretest probability of HIT and laboratory confirmation is pending, it may be appropriate to continue antithrombotic prophylaxis using non-heparin anticoagulants.
  - In cases with high suspicion/pretest probability of HIT and laboratory confirmation is pending, it is appropriate to begin anticoagulation treatment with a non-heparin product (6)[B].
- Direct thrombin inhibitors (DTIs) (argatroban and bivalirudin)
  - Reduce relative risk of thrombosis by 30% and are associated with a 5–10% risk of significant bleeding
  - Can produce misleading elevation in international normalized ratio (INR) (most likely an in vitro reaction)
    - Argatroban > bivalirudin (4)[B]
  - Argatroban
    - Initial dose, 2 μg/kg/min by continuous IV infusion; decrease dose with reduced hepatic function or with critical illness.
    - Dose adjustments based to achieve activated partial thromboplastin time (aPTT) 1.5–3 times the baseline.
  - Bivalirudin
    - Favorable pharmacologic profile; however, evidence for use is insufficient compared to argatroban (limited to case series).
    - Reduced risk of bleeding in patients undergoing percutaneous artery interventions (PCIs) and other cardiac procedures
    - Initial dose of 0.15 mg/kg/hr followed by adjustments to keep aPTT 1.5–2.5 times the baseline. Reduced dose with renal insufficiency (creatinine clearance [CrCl] <30 mL/min)
    - Dose adjustments based on aPTT
- Factor Xa inhibitor (fondaparinux)
  - Reports of its use are theorized to be useful; however, minimal data support its efficacy for HIT, and an ideal dose has yet to be determined.
  - Association with the development of HIT has been reported.
  - Optional agent for thromboembolic prophylaxis when practitioner wants to avoid heparin
  - Contraindicated in patients with renal dysfunction (CrCl <30 mL/min) (6)[C]
- Warfarin
  - Must anticoagulate with an immediate-acting agent before starting warfarin
  - Use of warfarin without other anticoagulants should be avoided because it can cause thrombosis.
  - Begin warfarin after platelet count >150,000.
  - Discontinue other anticoagulant and continue only warfarin after INR is therapeutic (2–3) for at least 5 days. This management differs from the normal heparin-to-warfarin transition in other conditions requiring anticoagulation (5)[C].
- LMWH
  - Although LMWH has a lower risk of initiating a HIT reaction, it should *not* be used when antibodies are already present. These antibodies can cross-react with LMWH and induce thrombosis and thrombocytopenia.

INPATIENT CONSIDERATIONS

Nursing

- Avoid heparin flushes.
- Avoid platelet transfusion.
- Clearly document reaction in all medical records to control the future use of heparin.

ONGOING CARE

FOLLOW-UP RECOMMENDATIONS

- The transition period of anticoagulation with a DTI and warfarin in patients with HIT can be problematic.
- The INR while administering both a DTI and warfarin should be therapeutic (2–3) for at least 5 days before discontinuing the DTI.
- Warfarin therapy should not be commenced until the platelet count has stabilized within a normal range.
- Warfarin therapy should continue for a minimum of 3 months.
- DTIs can prolong INR; therefore, if INR is <4 while on both warfarin and a DTI, temporarily hold the DTI for 4–6 hours and recheck INR; this second INR will represent only the anticoagulant effect of warfarin.
- Monitor use of concurrent drugs with warfarin.

Patient Monitoring

- Serial platelet counts
- Monitor PTT or INR as determined by the anticoagulation agent.

PATIENT EDUCATION

- Patient should inform all health care providers of any previous adverse reaction to heparin.
- HIT information available at: http://medlibrary.org/medwiki/Heparin-induced_thrombocytopenia

PROGNOSIS

- Thrombosis in HIT has 20–30% mortality, with additional morbidity from stroke and limb ischemia.
- Platelet counts normalize within weeks after stopping heparin.
- Risk of delayed thrombosis, especially in the first 30 days

REFERENCES

1. Martel N, Lee J, Wells PS. Risk for heparin-induced thrombocytopenia with unfractionated and low-molecular-weight heparin thromboprophylaxis: a meta-analysis. *Blood*. 2005;106(8):2710–2715.
2. Cuker A, Arepally G, Crowther MA, et al. The HIT Expert Probability (HEP) Score: a novel pre-test probability model for heparin-induced thrombocytopenia based on broad expert opinion. *J Thromb Haemost*. 2010;8(12):2642–2650.
3. Lo GK, Juhl D, Warkentin TE, et al. Evaluation of pretest clinical score (4 T's) for the diagnosis of heparin-induced thrombocytopenia in two clinical settings. *J Thromb Haemost*. 2006;4(4):759–765.
4. Bakchoul T, Greinacher A. Recent advances in the diagnosis and treatment of heparin-induced thrombocytopenia. *Ther Adv Hematol*. 2012;3(4):237–251.
5. Linkins LA, Dans AL, Moores LK, et al. Treatment and prevention of heparin-induced thrombocytopenia: Antithrombotic Therapy and Prevention of Thrombosis, 9th ed: American College of Chest Physicians Evidence-Based Clinical Practice Guidelines. *Chest*. 2012;141(2)(Suppl):e495S–e530S.
6. Shantsila E, Lip GY, Chong BH. Heparin-induced thrombocytopenia: a contemporary clinical approach to diagnosis and management. *Chest*. 2009;135(6):1651–1664.

ADDITIONAL READING

- Dager WE, Dougherty JA, Nguyen PH, et al. Heparin-induced thrombocytopenia: treatment options and special considerations. *Pharmacotherapy*. 2007;27(4):564–587.
- Stone GW, Ware JH, Bertrand ME, et al. Antithrombotic strategies in patients with acute coronary syndromes undergoing early invasive management: one-year results from the ACUITY trial. *JAMA*. 2007;298(21):2497–2506.
- Warkentin TE. Heparin-induced thrombocytopenia: diagnosis and management. *Circulation*. 2004;110(18):e454–e458.
- Warkentin TE, Greinacher A, Craven S, et al. Differences in the clinically effective molar concentrations of four direct thrombin inhibitors explain their variable prothrombin time prolongation. *Thromb Haemost*. 2005;94(5):958–964.
- Warkentin TE, Maurer BT, Aster RH. Heparin-induced thrombocytopenia associated with fondaparinux. *N Engl J Med*. 2007;356(25):2653–2655; discussion 2653–2655.

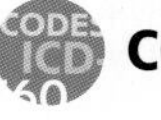

CODES

ICD10

D75.82 Heparin induced thrombocytopenia (HIT)

CLINICAL PEARLS

- Heparin exposure through virtually any preparation (including LMWH), any dose, or any route can cause HIT.
- LMWH is contraindicated in HIT; although LMWH is less likely to cause HIT, once HIT is present, the antibodies will cross-react and continue to cause a HIT reaction.
- If a patient is suspected of HIT (with or without confirmatory testing), immediately discontinue all forms of heparin.
- Patients will require anticoagulation either because of preexisting thrombosis or the risk of thrombosis in first 30 days after HIT.
- A DTI should be used until a patient's INR is therapeutic (2–3) on warfarin for at least 5 days.
- The key to avoiding sequelae from HIT is awareness, vigilance, and a high degree of suspicion.

HEPATIC ENCEPHALOPATHY

Walter M. Kim, MD, PhD • Jyoti Ramakrishna, MD

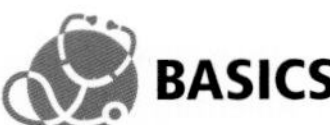

BASICS

DESCRIPTION

- Hepatic encephalopathy (HE) is characterized by reversible altered mental and neuromotor functioning that occurs in association with acute or chronic liver disease and/or portal systemic shunting of blood.
- The prominent features are confusion, impaired arousability, and a "flapping tremor" (asterixis).
- System(s) affected: gastrointestinal; nervous
- Synonym(s): portosystemic encephalopathy; hepatic coma; liver coma

EPIDEMIOLOGY

Predominant sex: male = female (reflecting underlying liver disease)

Prevalence

- Overt HE occurs in 30–45% of cirrhotic patients.
- Occurs in all cases of fulminant hepatic failure
- Present in nearly 1/2 of patients who require liver transplantation
- Parallels the age predominance of fulminant liver disease: peaks in the 40s; cirrhosis peaks in the late 50s; may occur at any age

ETIOLOGY AND PATHOPHYSIOLOGY

- There is no defined pathophysiology for the development of HE. Three classifications have been proposed (1):
  - Type A: resulting from acute liver failure
  - Type B: resulting from portosystemic bypass or shunting
  - Type C: resulting from cirrhosis
- Several metabolic factors have been implicated in the development of HE based on the failure of the liver to detoxify agents noxious to the CNS (e.g., ammonia, mercaptan, fatty acids).
- Increased aromatic and reduced branched chain amino acids in blood may act as false neurotransmitters, possibly interacting with the γ-aminobutyric acid (GABA) receptor and causing clinical symptoms.
- HE presents most commonly in long-standing cirrhosis of the liver with spontaneous shunting of intestinal blood through collateral vessels or surgically constructed portacaval shunts.
- Transjugular intrahepatic portosystemic shunt (TIPS), a widely used radiologically inserted shunt to lower portal pressure, is associated with HE in some cases.

Genetics

- Unknown
- Conditions such as cystic fibrosis, α-1-antitrypsin deficiency, and Wilson disease can contribute to HE.

RISK FACTORS

In patients with underlying liver disease, precipitating factors include the following:

- Infection (overt or occult, including spontaneous bacterial peritonitis)
- GI hemorrhage
- Use of sedative or opiate drugs
- Fluid or electrolyte disturbance (Na^+, K^+, Mg^{2+}, or other electrolyte depletion)
- TIPS
- Constipation

GENERAL PREVENTION

- Recognize early signs and seek prompt treatment.
- Avoid nonessential medications, particularly opiates, benzodiazepines, and sedatives.

COMMONLY ASSOCIATED CONDITIONS

- Occurs rarely with portacaval shunt with normal liver function
- May occur as a complication of acute fatty liver of pregnancy

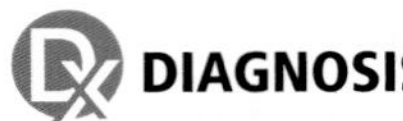

DIAGNOSIS

HISTORY

- Preexisting liver disease
- Confusion
- Impaired arousability

PHYSICAL EXAM

- Age 10–60 years
  - Prominent signs of underlying liver disease (50%); jaundice most common, ascites second most common
  - GI hemorrhage with hematemesis or melena: 20%
  - Systemic infection, urinary tract, or pulmonary: 20%
  - Five grades (West Haven classification) of confusion and degree of obtundation (1):
    - Minimal: psychometric or neuropsychological alterations of testing without mental status changes
    - Grade I: lack of awareness, anxiety, shortened attention span, impairment of arithmetic, altered sleep rhythm
    - Grade II: asterixis lethargy, disorientation to time, personality change, inappropriate behavior
    - Grade III: somnolence, confusion, gross disorientation, bizarre behavior
    - Grade IV: coma
- Age >60 years
  - Signs of underlying liver disease diminish (25%).
  - Confusion more prominent
  - Precipitating GI hemorrhage or infection is less often identified.
  - Progression is slower.
- Age <10 years
  - Signs of underlying liver disease prominent; usually fulminant hepatic failure or extremely advanced cirrhosis
  - Progression through the stages is very rapid, often 6–12 hours.
  - Wilson disease can imitate HE.
- Vital signs:
  - Bradycardia
  - Increased blood pressure suggestive of increased intracranial pressure
- Jaundice, ascites, and other correlates of liver disease
- CNS exam pertaining to stage of HE: Assess short-term memory and presence of asterixis.

DIFFERENTIAL DIAGNOSIS

- Metabolic encephalopathy related to anoxia, hypoglycemia, hypokalemia, hypo- or hypercalcemia, or uremia
- Head trauma, concussion, subdural hematoma
- Transient ischemic attack (TIA), ischemic stroke
- Alcohol withdrawal syndrome
- Alcohol intoxication
- Toxic confusion due to medication or drugs
- Meningitis
- Wilson disease
- Reye syndrome

DIAGNOSTIC TESTS & INTERPRETATION

- The clinical setting and findings are adequate to establish diagnosis in 80% of the cases.
- The treatment response often confirms the diagnosis.
- EEG: shows symmetric slowing of basic (α) rhythm common with other forms of metabolic encephalopathy; useful to a limited extent (2)
- Visual evoked potential: specific in grades II–IV
- Number connection test, line drawing test, clicker flicker frequency (CFF) test, continuous reaction time (CRT) test, inhibitory control test (ICT), and other psychometric tests may be used to assess for minimal HE.

Initial Tests (lab, imaging)

- Liver tests, including aspartate aminotransferase (AST), alanine aminotransferase (ALT), and serum albumin to evaluate severity of underlying liver disease
- Prothrombin time (PT) and international normalized ratio (INR) are elevated in liver failure due to impaired hepatic synthesis of coagulation factors.
- Elevated ammonia often present; levels affected by infusion of amino acid solutions, opiate administration producing severe constipation, uremia, and rapid and severe tissue breakdown, massive burns, trauma, or infection
- CBC to identify anemia and leukocytosis
- Complete metabolic profile to identify hypokalemia, hyperbilirubinemia, altered calcium concentration, hypomagnesemia, and hypoglycemia
- BUN: creatinine >20 suggestive of dehydration or GI bleeding
- Blood, urine, and ascitic fluid cultures to identify infection, if clinically indicated
- Consider arterial blood gas measurement.
- Toxicology screen for illicit drugs
- Useful only to rule out other diagnoses
- CT scan of the head may be the most useful imaging modality to identify frontal cortical atrophy and mild general edema.
- MRI may demonstrate increased T1 signal in globus pallidus.

Diagnostic Procedures/Other

EEG has typical rhythm (see earlier discussion).

Test Interpretation

- Brain edema in 100% of fatal cases
- Glial hypertrophy in chronic encephalopathy

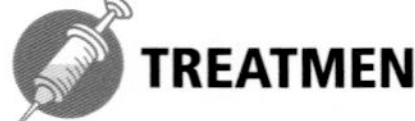

TREATMENT

GENERAL MEASURES

- Identify and vigorously treat precipitating causes: GI bleeding, infection, sedative drugs, and electrolyte imbalance are most common.
- Grade I or higher: Ensure adequate fluid intake and at least 1,000 kcal (4.19 MJ) daily; avoid hypoglycemia.
- Give initial enema to all patients without diarrhea.
- If clumsiness and poor judgment are prominent, be sure the patient has the care needed to avoid falls, cuts on broken glass, smoking burns, and machinery/auto accidents.
- Avoid sedative or opiate medications: benzodiazepine sedatives and opiate derivatives, such as diphenoxylate/atropine.

MEDICATION

First Line

- Lactulose syrup (nonabsorbable disaccharide whose laxative action decreases colonic transit time while bacterial digestion acidifies the colon, thereby promoting excretion of ammonia): 30–45 mL PO up to every hour for goal of 3–6 bowel movements per day. Diminish to 15–30 mL BID when ≥3 bowel movements occur daily (3)[A].
- Lactulose enema (for patients who cannot tolerate oral lactulose or have suspected ileus): 300 mL lactulose plus 700 mL tap water, retained for 1 hour.
- If worsening occurs acutely or no improvement in 2 days, add antibiotics:
  - Rifaximin: 400 mg PO TID (nonabsorbable antibiotic); highly effective in reversing minimal HE as well as prevention of HE recurrence (4)[B]
- Contraindications:
  - Total ileus
  - Hypersensitivity reaction
- Precautions:
  - Hypokalemia
  - Electrolyte imbalance
  - Renal failure

Second Line

- Neomycin: 1–2 g/day PO divided q6–8h, if renal function is within normal limits (5)
- Polyethylene glycol has recently been studied for acute hepatic encephalopathy and appears to be effective.
- Metronidazole is an alternative antibiotic.
- Flumazenil may be of benefit in select patients.

ISSUES FOR REFERRAL

Refer early to a transplant center.

SURGERY/OTHER PROCEDURES

- Artificial liver perfusion devices have proven useful in fulminant hepatic failure to bridge the patient until a donor liver is available for transplantation.
- Grade II–IV patients should be considered for liver transplantation.

COMPLEMENTARY & ALTERNATIVE MEDICINE

Probiotics and prebiotics have been associated with improvement of HE through modulation of gut flora (6)[C] and reduced recurrence of HE in patients with underlying cirrhosis.

INPATIENT CONSIDERATIONS

Admission Criteria/Initial Stabilization

- Monitor closely in grades I and II when diagnosis is clear, and watch for progression.
- Grade II–IV in fulminant hepatic failure is a strong indication for evaluation for liver transplantation; transfer to a transplant center should be considered. These patients require intensive care.

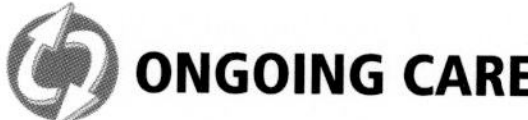

ONGOING CARE

FOLLOW-UP RECOMMENDATIONS

Activity as tolerated once resolved

Patient Monitoring

- To optimize treatment, a trail-making test should be followed (a pencil/paper connect-the-dots according to numbers). Evaluate patients periodically to determine how much maintenance treatment is needed and what diet is appropriate. The test should be run daily at first and then at each visit when changes in drugs and diet are made.
- Patients with changed findings should be seen twice weekly.
- Stable patients should be seen monthly.
- Number connection test or line drawing test at each office visit
- In cirrhosis, evaluate for transplantation and periodically monitor Model for End-stage Liver Disease (MELD) score.

DIET

- Integrate with underlying disease.
- Lower total protein (0.8–1.2 g/kg/day); vegetable protein diets are better tolerated than animal protein diets; special IV/enteral formulations with increased branched chain amino acids are available.
- Grades III–IV patients need parenteral nutrition or jejunal feeds.
- Instruct patient in lower protein diet.

PATIENT EDUCATION

American Association for the Study of Liver Diseases, 1729 King Street, Suite 200, Alexandria, VA 22314; 703-299-9766: www.aasld.org

PROGNOSIS

- With adequate aggressive treatment, disappears without residue or recurrence
- Chronic disease
  - Coma returns.
  - With each recurrence, becomes more and more difficult to treat—the degree of improvement with treatment is increasingly less; the mortality rate is 80%.

COMPLICATIONS

- Recurrence
- With many recurrences, permanent basal ganglion injury (non-Wilsonian hepatolenticular degeneration)
- Hepatorenal syndrome

REFERENCES

1. Vilstrup H, Amodio P, Bajaj J et al. Hepatic encephalopathy in chronic liver disease: 2014 practice guideline by the American Association for the Study of Liver Diseases and the European Association for the Study of the Liver. *Hepatology*. 2014;69(2):715–735.
2. Saxena N, Bhatia M, Joshi YK, et al. Electrophysiological and neuropsychological tests for the diagnosis of subclinical hepatic encephalopathy and prediction of overt encephalopathy. *Liver*. 2002;22(3):190–197.
3. Als-Nielsen B, Gluud LL, Gluud C. Non-absorbable disaccharides for hepatic encephalopathy: systematic review of randomised trials. *Br Med J*. 2004;328(7447):1046–1511.
4. Bass NM, Mullen KD, Sanyal A, et al. Rifaximin treatment in hepatic encephalopathy. *N Engl J Med*. 2010;362(12):1071–1081.
5. Hawkins RA, Jessy J, Mans AM, et al. Neomycin reduces the intestinal production of ammonia from glutamine. *Adv Exp Med Biol* 1994;368:125–134.
6. Liu Q, Duan ZP, Ha DK, et al. Synbiotic modulation of gut flora: effect on minimal hepatic encephalopathy in patients with cirrhosis. *Hepatology*. 2004;39(5):1441–1449.

ADDITIONAL READING

- Agrawal A, Sharma CB, Sharma P, et al. Secondary prophylaxis of hepatic encephalopathy in cirrhosis: an open-label, randomized controlled trial of lactulose, probiotics and no therapy. *Am J Gastroenterol*. 2012:107(7):1043–1050.
- Blei AT, Córdoba J, Practice Parameters Committee of the American College of Gastroenterology. Hepatic encephalopathy. *Am J Gastroenterol*. 2001;96(7):1968–1976.
- Liu Q, Duan ZP, Ha DK, et al. Synbiotic modulation of gut flora: effect on minimal hepatic encephalopathy in patients with cirrhosis. *Hepatology*. 2004;39(5):1441–1449.
- McGee RG, Bakens A, Wiley K, et al. Probiotics for patients with hepatic encephalopathy. *Cochrane Database Syst Rev*. 2011;(11):CD008716.
- Ong JP, Aggarwal A, Krieger D, et al. Correlation between ammonia levels and the severity of hepatic encephalopathy. *Am J Med*. 2003;114(3):188–193.
- Quero Guillén JC, Herrerías Gutiérrez JM. Diagnostic methods in hepatic encephalopathy. *Clin Chim Acta*. 2006;365(1–2):1–8.
- Sidhu SS, Goyal O, Mishra BP, et al. Rifaximin improves psychometric performance and health-related quality of life in patients with minimal hepatic encephalopathy (the RIME Trial). *Am J Gastroenterol*. 2011;106(2):307–316.
- Weissenborn K, Ennen JC, Schomerus H, et al. Neuropsychological characterization of hepatic encephalopathy. *J Hepatol*. 2001;34(5):768–773.

SEE ALSO

Algorithm: Delirium

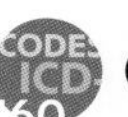

CODES

ICD10

- K72.90 Hepatic failure, unspecified without coma
- K72.91 Hepatic failure, unspecified with coma

CLINICAL PEARLS

- HE is a spectrum of neuropsychiatric findings occurring in patients with significant alterations in normal hepatic function.
- Lactulose remains a cornerstone of therapy for HE.
- Asterixis ("liver flap") is the classic physical finding associated with HE. It is also present in patients with uremia, barbiturate toxicity, and some cases of pulmonary disease. As such, asterixis is not pathognomonic for HE.

HEPATITIS A

Edward Feller, MD, FACP, FACG

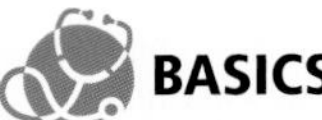

BASICS

DESCRIPTION

Infection with the hepatitis A virus (HAV) primarily involving the liver. One of the world's most common viral diseases

EPIDEMIOLOGY

Pediatric Considerations

- Disease is often milder or asymptomatic in children; severity increases with age (1).
- Infections are asymptomatic in 70% of children age <6 years.
- In 2009, <1/2 of 13–17-year-olds (in the United States) had been vaccinated.
- As many as 1/2 of current HAV infections in the United States are acquired from travel to endemic countries.

Pregnancy Considerations

- Pregnant women with HAV have increased for complications including preterm labor (2).
- Vertical transmission has been reported; fecal-oral transmission during birth is possible.
- Breastfeeding is not contraindicated.

Incidence

- HAV is cause of roughly 50% of reported cases of viral hepatitis in the United States (3).
- 1.4 million cases globally
- Since the hepatitis A vaccine has been in routine use (1995), the incidence of HAV has decreased by >90%.
- 22,000 HAV infections in 2009, lowest ever recorded in the United States (4)
- Incidence in the United States: 0.6/100,000
- Predominant sex: male = female

Prevalence

Serologic evidence of prior HAV infection: 1/3 of United States population. Anti-HAV prevalence related to age, ranging from 9% in children ages 6–11 years to 75% of those >70 years. Related inversely to income

ETIOLOGY AND PATHOPHYSIOLOGY

- Hepatitis A is a single-stranded linear RNA enterovirus of the Picornaviridae family.
- Humans are the only natural host.
- Incubation is 2–6 weeks (mean 4 weeks).
- Greatest infectivity is during 2 weeks before the onset of clinical illness.
- Infection occurs primarily after consuming food or water contaminated with HAV. Also spread via direct contact with HAV-infected person with poor hygiene.
- Food can become contaminated if handled by an infected individual with poor personal hygiene.
- Shellfish (clams and oysters) may be contaminated if harvested from waters contaminated with HAV.
- Blood-borne transmission is rare.
- HAV is not a chronic disease.

Genetics

Autoimmune hepatitis is rarely associated with human leukocyte antigen class II; DR3 and DR4 after active infection with HAV.

RISK FACTORS

- Foreign travel to developing countries accounts for >50% of cases in North America and Europe.
- Employment in health care
- Household exposure
- Intimate exposure, especially men who have sex with men
- Child care centers, schools
- Institutionalized individuals
- Clotting factor disorders, such as hemophilia
- Blood exposure/transfusion (rare)
- No identifiable risk factor in 50%.

GENERAL PREVENTION

- Proper sanitation and personal hygiene, including hand washing, especially for food handlers, health care, and daycare workers
- Active immunization: HAV vaccines: Havrix and Vaqta; Twinrix-combination HAV and HBV
- Vaccine is recommended for travelers, daycare staff/children, custodial facility employees, sewage workers, military, men who have sex with men (MSM), food handlers, and intravenous drug users (IVDUs).
- Vaccine is also recommended for close contacts of children adopted from countries with HAV infection; ideally ≥2 weeks before arrival
- HIV-infected patients who are negative for HAV IgG should receive HAV vaccine series, preferably early in course of HIV infection
  - If CD4 count is <200 cells/mm^3 or the patient has symptomatic HIV disease, defer vaccination until several months after initiation of antiretroviral (ARV) therapy to maximize the antibody response to the vaccine.
- Passive immunization
  - Immunoglobulin is effective for both pre- and postexposure prophylaxis of hepatitis A (5)[A]:
    - 0.02–0.06 mL/kg IM given within 2 weeks after exposure prevents illness in 80–90%.
    - HAV vaccine has similar efficacy to immunoglobulin in postexposure prophylaxis if given within 2 weeks.
    - Use immunoglobulin in cases where travelers need immediate protection, children age <1 year, and pregnant women who will be traveling.
    - Use 0.06 mL/kg q5mo for long-term travelers if they are unable to receive the vaccine.
    - Do not give immunoglobulin with MMR or varicella vaccines.
- HAV is *not* killed by freezing.
- HAV is killed by
  - Heating to 185°F for 60 seconds
  - Chlorine
  - Iodine

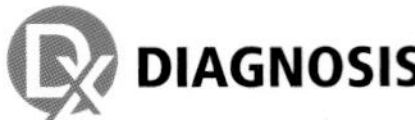

DIAGNOSIS

HISTORY

- Abrupt onset is common.
- Fever, malaise, fatigue, myalgias, anorexia
- Nausea and vomiting, headache
- Dark urine (bilirubinuria)
- Right upper abdominal pain
- Pruritus (suggests cholestasis)
- Symptom severity increases with age.
- Pediatric cases frequently asymptomatic

PHYSICAL EXAM

- Fever
- Jaundice, icterus
- Hepatomegaly (common), splenomegaly (less common)
- Right upper quadrant abdominal tenderness

DIFFERENTIAL DIAGNOSIS

- Hepatitis B, C, D, E
- Not clinically distinguishable from other forms of viral hepatitis; diagnosis may be suspected with typical symptoms during an outbreak.
- Infectious mononucleosis, cytomegalovirus (CMV)
- Primary or secondary hepatic malignancy
- Ischemic hepatitis
- Drug-induced hepatitis; toxin-induced hepatitis
- Alcoholic hepatitis
- Hemochromatosis in adults
- Autoimmune hepatitis; Wilson disease
- Nonhepatobiliary disease (elevated AST/ALT): celiac disease, congestive heart failure, thyroid disease

DIAGNOSTIC TESTS & INTERPRETATION

Initial Tests (lab, imaging)

- AST and ALT elevated: ALT usually > AST (6)[A]
- Alkaline phosphatase: mildly elevated
- Bilirubin: conjugated and unconjugated fractions usually increased. Usually follows rises in ALT/AST.
- Hepatocellular injury pattern
- Anti-HAV IgM: positive at time of onset of symptoms sensitivity and specificity > 95%
- Anti-HAV IgG: appears soon after IgM and generally persists for years
- Prothrombin time and partial thromboplastin time usually remain normal or near normal.
  - Significant rises should raise concern of possible acute hepatic failure or coexistent chronic liver disease.
- CBC: mild leukocytosis; aplasia and pancytopenia are rare.
  - Thrombocytopenia may predict illness severity.
- Albumin, electrolytes, and glucose
- Urinalysis (not clinically necessary): bilirubinuria
- Consider ultrasound (US) to rule out biliary obstruction only if lab pattern is cholestatic.

Follow-Up Tests & Special Considerations
Illness usually resolves within 4 weeks from onset of symptoms. Usually can be managed symptomatically as outpatient

Diagnostic Procedures/Other
Liver biopsy usually not necessary

Test Interpretation
- Positive serum markers in hepatitis A
  - Acute disease: anti-HAV IgM
  - Recent disease: anti-HAV IgM and IgG positive
  - Previous disease: anti-HAV IgM negative and IgG positive
- If liver biopsy obtained, shows portal inflammation; immunofluorescent stains for HAV antigen positive

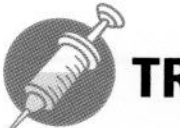

TREATMENT

GENERAL MEASURES
- Maintain appropriate nutrition/hydration.
- Attend to personal hygiene to prevent spread.
- Monitor coagulation defects, fluid and electrolytes, acid–base imbalance, hypoglycemia, and impairment of renal function.
- Report to local public health department.

MEDICATION
Postexposure prophylaxis to persons within 2 weeks of exposure to HAV who have not previously received HAV vaccine (7)[A]

- Administer hepatitis A vaccine to persons between the ages of 1 and 40 years at age-appropriate dose. Separate syringe site from immunoglobulin.
- Administer immunoglobulin (0.02 mL/kg) to persons <1 and >40 years of age.

First Line
- No antiviral medications indicated; spontaneous resolution occurs in almost all patients.
- Steroids are not indicated unless patient has autoimmune hepatitis.

Second Line
- Antiemetics
- IV fluids
- Pruritus: diphenhydramine 50 mg PO/IM q6h and cholestyramine 4 g BID

ISSUES FOR REFERRAL
- Dictated by severity of illness
- Hepatic failure

SURGERY/OTHER PROCEDURES
Liver transplant in fulminant hepatic failure—rare

COMPLEMENTARY & ALTERNATIVE MEDICINE
Avoid botanicals with potential hepatotoxicity, including barberry, comfrey, golden ragwort, groundsel, huang qin, kava kava, pennyroyal, sassafras, senna, valerian, wall germander, and wood sage.

INPATIENT CONSIDERATIONS

Admission Criteria/Initial Stabilization
Treatment is usually outpatient; dictated by severity of illness

IV Fluids
Treat dehydration and any noted electrolyte imbalances.

Nursing
Enteric isolation. Private rooms, gowns, and masks are not necessary. Frequent hand washing. Use gloves when handling material potentially contaminated with feces.

ONGOING CARE

FOLLOW-UP RECOMMENDATIONS
Return to work/school 10–14 days after onset of symptoms with diligence to hygiene.

Patient Monitoring
- Monitor coagulation defects, fluid and electrolytes, acid–base imbalance, hypoglycemia, and impairment of renal function.
- Usually infectious 4 weeks from initial symptoms

DIET
- Adequate balanced nutrition
- Avoid alcohol.
- Avoid hepatotoxic medications.

PATIENT EDUCATION
- Segregate food handlers with HAV.
- HAV immunity persists after infection
- CDC Hepatitis A Fact Sheet Link: http://www.cdc.gov/hepatitis/A/PDFs/HepAGeneralFactSheet_BW.pdf

PROGNOSIS
- Excellent; mortality is 0.2%.
- Risk increased with underlying chronic liver disease and in the elderly

COMPLICATIONS
- Coagulopathy, encephalopathy, and renal failure
- Relapsing HAV: usually milder than the initial case
- Positive anti-HAV IgM. Total duration is usually <9 months.
- Prolonged cholestasis: characterized by protracted periods of jaundice and pruritus (>3 months), resolves without intervention
- Autoimmune hepatitis: good response to steroids
- Hepatic failure: rare (1–2%)
- Postviral encephalitis, Guillain-Barré syndrome, pancreatitis, aplastic or hemolytic anemia, agranulocytosis, thrombocytopenic purpura, pancytopenia, arthritis, vasculitis, and cryoglobulinemia (all rare)

REFERENCES

1. Dorrell CG, Yankey D, Byrd KK, et al. Hepatitis A vaccination coverage among adolescents in the United States. *Pediatrics*. 2012;129(2):213–221.
2. Almashhwari AA, Ahmed KT, Rahman RN, et al. Liver diseases in pregnancy: diseases not unique to pregnancy. *World J Gastroenterol*. 2013;19(43):7630–7638.
3. Matheny SC, Kingery JE. Hepatitis A. *Am Fam Physician*. 2012;86(11):1027–1034.
4. Lu PJ, Euler GL, Hennessey KA, et al. Hepatitis A vaccination coverage among adults aged 18–49 years in the United States. *Vaccine*. 2009;27(9):1301–1305.
5. Liu JP, Nikolova D, Fei Y. Immunoglobulins for preventing hepatitis A. *Cochrane Database Syst Rev*. 2009;(2):CD004181.
6. Woreta TA, Alqahtani SA. Evaluation of abnormal liver tests. *Med Clin North Am*. 2014;98(1):1–16.
7. National Guideline Clearinghouse, Agency for Healthcare Research and Quality. Prevention of secondary disease: preventive medicine. *Viral Hepatitis*. 2011. www.guideline.gov. Accessed 2014.

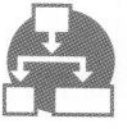

SEE ALSO
- Hepatitis B; Hepatitis C
- Algorithm: Hyperbilirubinemia and Cirrhosis

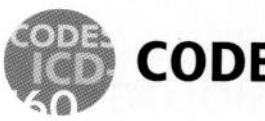

CODES

ICD10
B15.9 Hepatitis A without hepatic coma

CLINICAL PEARLS
- HAV vaccine is indicated for travelers, daycare staff/children, custodial facility employees, sewage workers, military, MSM, food handlers, and IVDUs.
- HAV disease severity directly correlates with age; children are often asymptomatic.
- Check HAV IgG in all HIV-positive patients; immunize all who are negative.

H

HEPATITIS B

Jason Chao, MD, MS

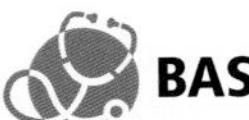

BASICS

DESCRIPTION

Systemic viral infection associated with acute and chronic liver disease and hepatocellular carcinoma (HCC)

EPIDEMIOLOGY

Incidence

- Predominant age: can infect patients of all ages
- Predominant sex: fulminant hepatitis B virus (HBV): male > female (2:1)
- In the United States, estimated 38,000 new infections in 2009, 70% due to IV drug use
- African Americans have the highest rate of acute HBV infection in the United States.
- Overall rate of new infections is down 82% since 1991 (due to national immunization strategy).
- U.S. vaccine coverage for the birth dose of HBV increased from 68.6% in 2011 to 71.6% in 2012.

Prevalence

- In the United States, 800,000–1.4 million people have chronic HBV.
- Asia and the Pacific Islands have the largest populations at risk for HBV.
- Chronic HBV worldwide: 350–400 million persons
  - Per year: 1 million deaths
    - 2nd most important carcinogen behind tobacco
    - Of chronic carriers with active disease, 25% die due to complications of cirrhosis or HCC.
    - Of chronic carriers, 75% are Asian.

ETIOLOGY AND PATHOPHYSIOLOGY

HBV is a DNA virus of the Hepadnaviridae family. Highly infective via blood and secretions for at least a week following exposure.

Genetics

Family history of HBV and/or HCC

RISK FACTORS

- The following high-risk groups should be screened for HBV with HBsAg/sAb and subsequently vaccinated if seronegative (1)[A]:
  - Persons born in endemic areas (45% of world)
  - Hemodialysis patients
  - IV drug users (IVDUs), past or present
  - Men who have sex with men (MSM)
  - HIV- and HCV-positive patients
  - Household members of HBsAg carriers
  - Sexual contacts of HBsAg carriers
  - Inmates of correctional facilities
  - Patients with chronically elevated aspartate aminotransferase/alanine aminotransferase (AST/ALT)
- Additional risk factors:
  - Needle stick/occupational exposure
  - Recipients of blood/products; transplanted organ recipients
  - Intranasal drug users
  - Body piercing/tattoos
  - Survivors of sexual assault

Pediatric Considerations

- Shorter acute course; fewer complications
- 90% of vertical/perinatal infections become chronic.

Pregnancy Considerations

- Universal prenatal screening with HBsAg (1)[A]
- High viral load at 28 weeks should prompt consideration to begin treatment with oral nucleos(t)ide medicines at 32 weeks to reduce perinatal transmission (2)[C].

Marker	Acute infection	Chronic infection	Inactive carrier	Resolved infection	Susceptible to infection	Vaccinated
HBsAg	+	+	+	–	–	–
HBsAb	–	–	–	+	–	+
HBcAb	+IgM	–IgM; +total/IgG	+	+	–	–
HBeAg	+	±	–	–	–	–
HBeAb	–	±	+	±	–	–
HBV DNA	Present	Present	Low–negative	–	–	–
ALT	Marked elevation	Normal to mildly elevated	Normal	Normal		

- Infants born to HBV-infected mothers require HB immune globulin (HBIg) (0.5 mL) and HBV vaccine within 12 hours of birth.
- Breastfeeding is safe if HBIg and HBV vaccine are administered and the areolar complex is without fissures or open sores. Oral nucleos(t)ide medications are not recommended for lactating mothers.
- HIV coinfection significantly increases risk of vertical transmission.
- Continue medications if pregnancy occurs while on an oral antiviral therapy to prevent acute flare.

GENERAL PREVENTION

Most effective: HBV vaccination series (3 doses)

- Vaccinate
  - All infants at birth and during well-child care visits (3-shot series)
  - All at-risk patients (see "Risk Factors")
  - Health care and public safety workers
  - Sexual contacts of HBsAg carriers
  - Household contacts of HBsAg carriers
- Proper hygiene/sanitation by health care workers, IVDU, and tattoo/piercing artists
  - Barrier precautions, needle disposal, sterilization of equipment, cover open cuts
- Do not share personal items exposed to blood (e.g., nail clipper, razor, toothbrush).
- Safe sexual practices (condoms)
- HBsAg carriers cannot donate blood or tissue.
- Postexposure (e.g., needle stick): HBIg 0.06 mL/kg in <24 hours and vaccination

COMMONLY ASSOCIATED CONDITIONS

HIV coinfection, hepatitis C coinfection

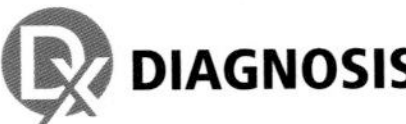

DIAGNOSIS

HISTORY

- Exposure: detailed family and social history
- Acute HBV
  - Fever, malaise, fatigue, arthralgias, myalgias
  - Anorexia, nausea, vomiting
  - Jaundice, scleral icterus
  - Dark urine, pale stools
  - Right upper quadrant (RUQ) abdominal pain
- Chronic HBV: typically asymptomatic

PHYSICAL EXAM

Acute: Ill; jaundice/scleral icterus; RUQ tenderness, hepatomegaly

DIFFERENTIAL DIAGNOSIS

- Epstein-Barr virus (EBV); cytomegalovirus (CMV); hepatitis A, C, or E
- Drug-induced, alcoholic, or autoimmune hepatitis
- Wilson disease or rheumatologic/immunologic disorders

DIAGNOSTIC TESTS & INTERPRETATION

Initial Tests (lab, imaging)

- AST/ALT: marked elevation in acute HBV, (particularly ALT) with levels in the hundreds to several thousand IU/mL. Transaminases may be normal or mildly elevated in chronic HBV:
  - Transaminases elevate before bilirubin
- Bilirubin (conjugated/unconjugated): normal to markedly elevated in acute HBV:
  - Last test to normalize as acute infection resolves
- Alkaline phosphatase: mild elevation
- HBcAb IgM may be the only early finding ("window period," when HBsAg/sAb–).
- For acute hepatitis:
  - Monitor PT, albumin, electrolytes, glucose, CBC
  - If severe acute HBV, check for superinfection with hepatitis D (HDV Ag and HBDV Ab)
  - Hepatitis B serologic markers
- Hepatitis Be antigen (HBeAg+) indicates high replication/infectivity; confirmed with high HBV DNA ($\geq 10^5$ copies/mL); these patients benefit from medical therapy.
- HBV precore mutants have undetectable HBeAg despite active viral replication (confirm with HBV DNA level) as well as antibody to e antigen (HBeAb+).
- Screen for HDV, HIV, HCV, and immunity to hepatitis A virus (HAV Ab total/IgG).
- Ultrasound to document ascites, organomegaly, signs of portal hypertension, hepatic or portal obstruction and to screen for HCC
- Contrast CT or MRI if ultrasound is abnormal or if α-fetoprotein (AFP) is elevated.

Follow-Up Tests & Special Considerations

HBsAg+ persistence >6 months defines chronic HBV:

- Measure HBV DNA level and ALT every 3–6 months.
- If age >40 years and ALT borderline or mildly elevated, consider liver biopsy.
- Measure baseline AFP.
- Follow HBeAg for loss (every 6–12 months).
- Lifetime monitoring for progression, need for treatment, and screening for HCC

Diagnostic Procedures/Other

- Liver biopsy
- Experimental noninvasive tests (Hepascore, Fibro test) or measurement of elastography (Fibroscan) to assess for hepatic fibrosis

Test Interpretation
Liver biopsy in chronic HBV may show interface hepatitis and inflammation, necrosis, cholestasis, fibrosis, cirrhosis, or chronic active hepatitis.

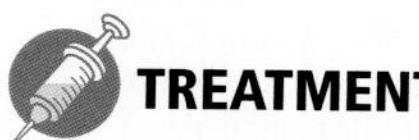

TREATMENT

GENERAL MEASURES
- Vaccinate for HAV if seronegative.
- Monitor CBC, coagulation, electrolytes, glucose, renal function, phosphate.
- Monitor ALT and HBV DNA; increased ALT and reduced DNA implies response to therapy.
- Screen for HCC if HBsAg+.

MEDICATION
First Line
- Acute HBV
  - Supportive care; spontaneously resolves in 95% of immunocompetent adults
  - Antiviral therapy not indicated except for fulminant liver failure or immunosuppressed.
- Precautions:
  - Oral drugs: Renal insufficiency
  - Peg-IFN: coagulopathy, myelosuppression, depression/suicidal ideation

Second Line
Emtricitabine suppresses viral load; not FDA approved.

ISSUES FOR REFERRAL
- Refer all persistent HBsAg+ patients for consideration of antiviral therapy.
- Refer immediately to liver transplant program if fulminant acute hepatitis, end-stage liver disease, or HCC

SURGERY/OTHER PROCEDURES
Liver transplantation, operative resection, radiofrequency ablation for HCC

INPATIENT CONSIDERATIONS
Admission Criteria/Initial Stabilization
- Worsening course (marked increase in bilirubin, transaminases, or symptoms)
- Hepatic failure (high PT, encephalopathy)

Chronic hepatitis B therapy

HBeAg	HBV DNA viral load	ALT*	Recommend
(+)	≥20,000 IU/mL	Elevated	
(−)	≥2,000 IU/mL	Elevated	Consider biopsy or serum fibrosis marker and treatment
(+)	≤20,000 IU/mL	Any	Monitor q6–12mo
(−)	≥2,000 IU/mL	Normal	Biopsy; treat if disease
(+)	≥20,000 IU/mL	Normal	Observe, consider treatment if ALT elevated. Biopsy if age >40 years or ALT is high normal to mild elevation
(−)	≤2,000 IU/mL	Any	Monitor q6–12mo
Cirrhosis	Any	Any	Treat with mono or combination treatment
Liver failure	Any	Any	Treat + refer for transplant

*ALT elevated if >2 × ULN; ULN for male = 30 IU/mL and for female = 19 IU/mL.

- Chronic HBV: Treatment is based on HBeAg status:
  - FDA-approved drugs: lamivudine 100 mg, adefovir 10 mg, entecavir 0.5–1 mg, telbivudine 600 mg, or tenofovir 300 mg, all given PO every day (dose based on renal function); pegylated interferon (peg-IFN) α2a, α2b SC weekly (3)[A]
- Entecavir, tenofovir, and peg-IFN are preferred 1st-line agents (3)[A].
- Oral agents given for extended period (3)[A]:
  - If HBeAg+, treat 6–12 months postloss of HBeAg and gain of HBeAb, and monitor after cessation.
  - If HBeAg−, treat indefinitely or until HBsAg clearance and HBsAb development.
- Change/add drug based on development of resistance:
  - Confirm patient compliance with medications before assuming resistance.
  - Adherence to therapy lowers rate of resistance.
- Dose adjustment made for elevated creatinine
- Standard interferon (Intron A) no longer used in favor of peg-IFN:
  - Peg-IFN (Pegasys) injections given weekly for 48 weeks
  - Best efficacy in genotype A
  - Contraindicated if decompensated cirrhosis
- Goals of therapy: undetectable HBV DNA, normal ALT, loss of HBeAg, gain of HBeAb; loss of HBsAg and gain of HBsAb

ONGOING CARE

FOLLOW-UP RECOMMENDATIONS
Patient Monitoring
- Monitor serial ALT and HBV DNA:
  - High ALT + low HBV DNA associated with favorable response to therapy
- Serologic markers: See chart
- CBC to monitor WBC and platelets for patients on interferon therapy
- Monitor HBV DNA q3–6mo during therapy:
  - Undetectable DNA at week 24 of oral drug therapy associated with low resistance at year 2
- Monitor for complications (ascites, encephalopathy, variceal bleed) in cirrhosis.
- Recommend vaccination for all household members and sexual partners.
- Ultrasound every q6–12mo for HCC screening starting at age 40 years in men and age 50 in women (3)[B]

DIET
Avoid alcohol.

PATIENT EDUCATION
- Acute HBV
  - Review transmission precautions.
- Chronic HBV
  - Alcohol and tobacco use accelerate progression of liver disease.
  - Strict medication compliance to prevent flare
- Patient education materials in English and Spanish available at http://www.cdc.gov/hepatitis/Resources/PatientEdMaterials.htm

PROGNOSIS
- Acute infection: 95% of adults recover
- Severity of encephalopathy predicts survival in fulminant hepatic failure.
- Acute HBV: mortality 1%
- Acute HBV + HDV: mortality 2–20%
- Chronic HBV
  - Spontaneous resolution: 0.5% per year
  - Premature death from cirrhosis or HCC: 25%
  - Risk of HCC rises with rate of viral replication, even if no cirrhosis

COMPLICATIONS
- Acute or subacute hepatic necrosis; cirrhosis; hepatic failure
- HCC (all chronic HBV patients are at risk)
- Severe flare of chronic HBV with corticosteroids and other immunosuppressants: Avoid if possible.
- Reactivation of resolved infection if immunosuppressed (e.g., chemotherapy): prophylactic premedication recommended if HBsAg+ (2,4) or if HBcAb+ and received systemic chemotherapy

REFERENCES

1. Weinbaum CM, Williams I, Mast EE, et al; Centers for Disease Control and Prevention. Recommendations for identification and public health management of persons with chronic hepatitis B infection. *MMWR Recomm Rep*. 2008;57(RR-8):1–20.
2. Borgia G, Carleo MA, Gaeta GB, et al. Hepatitis B in pregnancy. *World J Gastroenterol*. 2012;18(34):4677–4683.
3. McMahon BJ. Chronic hepatitis B virus infection. *Med Clin North Am*. 2014;98(1):39–54.

ADDITIONAL READING

Woo G, Tomlinson G, Nishikawa Y, et al. Tenofovir and entecavir are the most effective antiviral agents for chronic hepatitis B: a systematic review and Bayesian meta-analyses. *Gastroenterology*. 2010;139(4):1218–1229.

SEE ALSO

- Cirrhosis of the Liver; Hepatitis A; Hepatitis C
- Algorithm: Hyperbilirubinemia

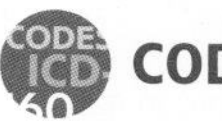

CODES

ICD10
- B19.10 Unspecified viral hepatitis B without hepatic coma
- B16.9 Acute hepatitis B w/o delta-agent and without hepatic coma
- B18.1 Chronic viral hepatitis B without delta-agent

CLINICAL PEARLS
- All patients born in endemic countries should be screened for HBV infection with HBsAg.
- Patients with chronic HBV need lifetime monitoring for disease progression and HCC.

H

HEPATITIS C

David T. O'Gurek, MD

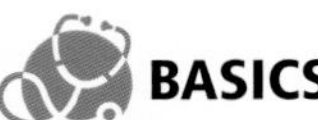

BASICS

DESCRIPTION

Systemic viral infection (acute and chronic) primarily involving liver

EPIDEMIOLOGY

- Highest incidence in ages 20–39 years; highest prevalence ages 30–49 years
- Male = female

Geriatric Considerations

Age >60 years less likely to respond to therapy; treat earlier if able.

Pediatric Considerations

- Prevalence: 0.3%
- Test children born to HCV-positive mothers after 18 months
- Fewer symptoms; fewer abnormal liver tests; more likely to clear spontaneously; slower rate of progression

Pregnancy Considerations

- Vertical transmission occurs in 4 of every 100 births in HCV-positive mothers; risk increases 2–3× if HIV coinfection.
- Breastfeeding safe if no fissures

Incidence

- In 2011, CDC estimated there were 16,500 new cases, of which 1,229 were new cases of *acute* hepatitis C (incidence of 0.4 cases per 100,000 population), the first increase in incidence in 7 years.
- In 2011, 34 states reported 185,979 cases of hepatitis C (past or present; cannot differentiate those who spontaneously cleared). 45–85% are unaware they are infected (1).

Prevalence

- ~3.2 million in United States (1–1.5%) HCV Ab+
- Prevalence is 3.5% in persons born between 1945 and 1965 ("baby boomers").
- ~3 million have chronic HCV (HCV RNA+).
- ~15,000 deaths HCV-related in 2007, overtaking HIV-related deaths
- Most common cause of chronic liver disease and liver transplantation in the United States
- Genotype 1 is predominant form (75% of cases)

ETIOLOGY AND PATHOPHYSIOLOGY

Single-stranded RNA virus of Flaviviridae family

RISK FACTORS

- Exposure risks were as follows:
  - Hemodialysis
  - Tattoo in unregulated setting
  - Blood/blood product transfusion or organ transplantation before 1992
  - Hemophilia treatment before 1987
  - Household or health care–related exposure to infected body fluids
  - History of incarceration
  - Children born to HCV-positive mothers
  - Current sexual partners of HCV-positive persons
- Risk behaviors and/or medical conditions were as follows:
  - Any prior history of injection drug use
  - Intranasal illicit drug use
  - HIV and hepatitis B infection
  - Unexplained chronic liver disease or chronic hepatitis including elevated alanine aminotransferase levels (ALT)

GENERAL PREVENTION

- *Primary prevention*
  - Do not share razors/toothbrushes/nail clippers.
  - Use and dispose of needles properly.
  - Needle/syringe exchange programs
  - Sexual transmission rare in monogamous long-term partners
- *Secondary prevention*
  - CDC/USPSTF/AASLD/IDSA: Screen all adults born between 1945 and 1965 once for hepatitis C.
  - Annual testing for those who inject drugs and for HIV-seropositive men who have sex with men (MSM).
  - No vaccine or postexposure prophylaxis currently available
  - Substance abuse treatment
  - Reinforce use of barrier contraception for HIV-seropositive coinfected with HCV.

COMMONLY ASSOCIATED CONDITIONS

Diabetes, metabolic syndrome, iron overload, depression, substance abuse/recovery, autoimmune and hematologic disease, HIV, and hepatitis B coinfection

DIAGNOSIS

HISTORY

- Determine exposure risk: *detailed* social history
- Chronic HCV: most mildly symptomatic (nonspecific fatigue) or asymptomatic elevated ALT/aspartate aminotransferase (AST)
- Acute HCV: *If* symptoms develop (rare):
  - Onset 2–26 weeks postexposure (mean: 7–8 weeks) and persist 2–12 weeks
  - Jaundice, dark urine, steatorrhea, nausea, abdominal pain (right upper quadrant), fatigue, low-grade fevers, myalgias, arthralgias

PHYSICAL EXAM

- Typically normal unless advanced fibrosis/cirrhosis
- May have right upper quadrant (RUQ) tenderness/hepatomegaly

DIFFERENTIAL DIAGNOSIS

Hepatitis A or B; Epstein-Barr virus (EBV), cytomegalovirus (CMV); alcoholic hepatitis; nonalcoholic steatohepatitis (NASH); hemochromatosis, Wilson disease, α1–antitrypsin deficiency; ischemic, drug-induced, or autoimmune hepatitis

DIAGNOSTIC TESTS & INTERPRETATION

Initial Tests (lab, imaging)

- AST/ALT: Often normal. May be persistently elevated in chronic HCV; ALT usually 1–2 × upper limit of normal (ULN); AST may be normal/elevated, but typically less so than ALT.
  - Acute hepatitis C can cause marked elevation of transminases and bilirubin (direct and indirect).
- AST/ALT ratio ≥1 associated with cirrhosis
  - If AST/ALT ratio >2, rule out alcohol abuse
  - Other liver function tests (alkaline phosphatase, γ-glutamyltransferase, bilirubin, albumin, and prothrombin time) usually elevated with cirrhosis
- HCV antibody (anti-HCV) negative until 8–9 weeks postexposure
  - Positive test indicates current (active) infection, past resolved infection, or false-positive test (autoimmune/rheumatologic disease)
  - HCV nucleic acid test (NAT) or HCV RNA is necessary to confirm (2)[A].
- HCV RNA positive 1–3 weeks postexposure
  - Use to confirm active infection, diagnose acute infection (exposure <6 months ago) (2)[A], and in persons with negative anti-HCV who are immunocompromised (i.e., chronic hemodialysis) (2)[C]
  - Persistent HCV RNA >6 months = chronic HCV

Follow-Up Tests & Special Considerations

- Evaluate for other coinfection with HBV and HIV (2)[B].
- Vaccinate if seronegative for hepatitis A/B (2)[C]
- Pneumococcal polysaccharide vaccine (PPSV23)

Diagnostic Procedures/Other

- Quantitative HCV RNA testing to document baseline viremia prior to treatment (2)[A]
- Test for HCV genotype to guide treatment (2)[A].
- Evaluate for advanced hepatic fibrosis (2)[B]:
  - Liver imaging (ultrasound, CT scan, MRI)
  - Liver elastography
  - Serum fibrosis markers (e.g., FibroTest; AST to platelet ratio index [APRI])
  - Liver biopsy

Test Interpretation

- Biopsy shows periportal lymphocytic inflammation
- Inflammation: grades 0–4; fibrosis: stages 0–4 (Metavir scoring system)

Scoring system for inflammatory activity and fibrosis in HCV

0	Portal/periportal activity (PPA) – none; lobular activity (LA) – none; fibrosis (F) – none
1	PPA – portal inflammation; LA – inflammation no necrosis; F – enlarged fibrotic tracts
2	PPA – mild necrosis; LA – focal necrosis; F – normal architecture but septae present
3	PPA – moderate necrosis; LA – severe focal cell damage; F – architectural distortion, no cirrhosis
4	PPA – severe necrosis; LA – bridging necrosis; F – probable or definite cirrhosis

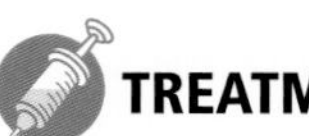

TREATMENT

GENERAL MEASURES

- Report acute cases of HCV to the health department.
- All patients with virologic evidence HCV should be considered for treatment.
- Pretreatment patient counseling is critical and should include thorough behavioral health and substance abuse history.
- Optimize medical therapy for comorbid conditions prior to treatment.
- Pretreatment laboratory evaluation including the following:
  - CBC, BMP, uric acid, serum ferritin, iron saturation, antinuclear antibody (ANA), pregnancy test, ECG (if preexisting cardiac disease)
  - Consider: IL28B genotype (can be used to predict treatment response)

- Discuss individual treatment plan and likelihood of success based on individual factors such as BMI, genotype, race, stage of fibrosis, and viral load.
- Evaluate for Peg-IFN eligibility; IFN-ineligible patients include the following:
  - Autoimmune hepatitis or other autoimmune disorders, hypersensitivity to Peg, decompensated hepatic disease, uncontrolled depression, baseline neutrophil count $<1500/\mu L$, baseline platelet count $<90,000/\mu L$, baseline hemoglobin <10 g/dL, preexisting cardiac disease

MEDICATION

First Line

- Acute HCV: treatment may be delayed until 12 weeks after suspected inoculation to allow chance for spontaneous clearance.
  - Pegylated interferon (Peg-IFN) alone or with low-dose ribavirin (if HIV coinfected) for 12 weeks (genotypes 2–4) and 24 weeks (genotype 1)
- Chronic HCV: Antiviral therapies and length of therapy depend on genotype:
  - Peg-IFN/ribavirin (RBV)
    - Peg-IFN α2b 1.5 μg/kg SC weekly *OR*
    - Peg-IFN α2a 180 μg SC weekly *WITH*
    - Ribavirin 800–1,400 mg PO, divided BID (weight-based)
    - *Side effects*: fatigue, weight loss, insomnia, headache, depression, cognitive changes, nausea, rash, cough, thyroiditis, alopecia
    - Pregnancy Category X
    - Premedicate with acetaminophen or NSAIDs.
  - HCV RNA polymerase inhibitor
    - Sofosbuvir 400 mg daily
  - Protease inhibitors
    - Simeprevir 150 mg daily
    - Telaprevir (TVR) 1,125 mg BID with 20 g of fat (3)[A]
    - Boceprevir (BOC) 800 mg every 7–9 hours with food (4)[A]
    - *Side effects*: skin rash (mild to moderate 50%, DRESS and Stevens-Johnson seen in $<1\%$), anemia, anorectal pain, dysgeusia
  - Duration of therapy: 12–48 weeks based on genotype, cirrhosis, and response-guided therapy with assessment of HCV viral load (VL) (2)[B]
  - TVR and BOC are not FDA approved for acute HCV infection, HIV and HCV coinfection, and non–genotype 1 HCV infection.
  - Sofosbuvir plus simeprevir shows promise as a non–IFN-based regimen and each drug is individually approved; however, the combination treatment is not FDA approved (5)[A].
  - Pretreatment with SSRIs lowers the incidence and severity of IFN-associated depression in chronic hepatitis C infection (6)[A].

ISSUES FOR REFERRAL

- A physician experienced with HCV therapy should be involved in all cases.
- Refer to liver transplant program if fulminant acute hepatitis, at first complication of end-stage disease, or at diagnosis of HCC.

ADDITIONAL THERAPIES

Interferon-alfacon-1 (consensus IFN, Infergen); up to 37% cure rate in nonresponders/relapsers.

COMPLEMENTARY & ALTERNATIVE MEDICINE

- No evidence for effective complementary therapy in HCV/cirrhosis/HCC.
- Milk thistle (silymarin) safe; may reduce ALT but does not eradicate virus or improve outcomes; avoid while on IFN.

ONGOING CARE

FOLLOW-UP RECOMMENDATIONS

- If treatment is deferred, patients should be screened with annual LFTs; monitored for disease progression; and maintain sobriety (if alcohol dependence involved).
- Monitor serial viral load only if on antiviral therapy.
- Consider abdominal ultrasound every 6 months with AFP levels to monitor for hepatocellular carcinoma (expert opinion).

Patient Monitoring

- Serial ALT/AST; fasting glucose and CBCs
- Follow electrolytes, thyroid-stimulating hormone (TSH), renal function, PT
- HCV qualitative RNA negativity at week 4 indicates rapid viral response (RVR) and confers ~90% chance of sustained virologic response (SVR) in all genotypes.
- HCV quantitative RNA negativity (or drop of ≥ 2 log) at week 12 is early virologic response (EVR) and also confers good chance SVR.
- SVR also more likely in following patients: age ≤ 40 years; female gender; white; absence of bridging fibrosis/cirrhosis; HCV RNA $<400,000$ IU/mL; genotypes 2 and 3; BMI <30 kg/m^2; absence of insulin resistance and steatosis; absence of HIV; recent infection (e.g., needle stick).
- HCV RNA $>1,000$ IU/mL at week 4 or week 12 for patients on IFN/RBV and TVR requires discontinuation of therapy (3)[A].
- HCV RNA >100 IU/mL at week 12 for patients on IFN/RBV and BOC requires discontinuation of therapy (4)[A].
- Monitor for decompensation (low albumin, ascites, encephalopathy, GI bleed) in patients with cirrhosis.
- Goal of therapy is SVR: eradication of HCV by negative qualitative RNA (transcription mediated amplification test) 6 months posttreatment (relapse extremely rare after 6 months)

DIET

- Low-fat, high-fiber diet and exercise to treat obesity/fatty liver
- Extra protein and fluids while on IFN therapy

PATIENT EDUCATION

- Avoid alcohol, tobacco, and illicit drugs (including marijuana); refer to rehab/12-step program and monitor for relapse as appropriate.
- Warn against claims of false cures
- Caution with nutritional supplements and hepatotoxic medications (may contain hepatotoxins and contaminants)
- www.cdc.gov/knowmorehepatitis/

PROGNOSIS

- For every 100 persons infected with HCV:
  - 75–85 will develop chronic infection.
  - 60–70 will develop chronic liver disease.
  - 5–20 will develop cirrhosis over 20–30 years (more rapid if older age at infection, male gender, alcohol/substance abuse, HIV/HBV coinfection, or diabetes/insulin resistance).
  - 1–5 will die from consequences (liver cancer or cirrhosis).
- Chronic HCV is *curable* in ~70% of cases; in noncirrhotic genotype 2 or 3, cure rate ~90%.

COMPLICATIONS

Acute/subacute hepatic necrosis, liver failure, hepatocellular carcinoma, transplant and complications, death

REFERENCES

1. Smith BD, Morgan RL, Beckett GA, et al. Recommendations for the identification of chronic hepatitis C virus infection among persons born during 1945-1965. *MMWR Recomm Rep*. 2012;61(RR-4):1–32.
2. American Association for the Study of Liver Disease, Infectious Diseases Society of America. Recommendations for testing, managing, and treating hepatitis C. http://www.hcvguidelines.org. Accessed June 4, 2014.
3. McHutchison JG, Everson GT, Gordon SC, et al. Telaprevir with peginterferon and ribavirin for chronic HCV genotype 1 infection. *N Engl J Med*. 2009;360(18):1827.
4. Bacon BR, Gordon SC, Lawitz E, et al. Boceprevir for previously treated chronic HCV genotype 1 infection. *N Engl J Med*. 2011;364(13):1207.
5. Jacobson IM, Ghalib R, Rodriguez-Tirres M, et al. SVR results of a once-daily regimen of simeprevir plus sofosbuvir with or without ribavirin in cirrhotic and non-cirrhotic HCV genotype 1 treatment-naive and prior null responder patients: the COSMOS study. Paper presented at: 64th annual meeting of the American Association for the Study of Liver Diseases; November 1–5, 2013; Washington, DC.
6. Sarkar S, Schaefer M. Antidepressant pretreatment for the prevention of interferon alfa-associated depression: a systematic review and meta-analysis psychosomatics. *Psychosomatics*. 2014;55(3):221–234.

ADDITIONAL READING

- European Association for the Study of the Liver. EASL clinical practice guidelines: management of hepatitis C virus infection. *J Hepatol*. 2014;60(2):392–420.
- WHO. *Guidelines for the Screening, Care, and Treatment of Persons with Hepatitis C Infection*. Geneva, Switzerland: World Health Organization; 2014.
- Yee HS, Chang MF, Pocha C. Update on the management and treatment of hepatitis C virus infection: recommendations from the Department of Veterans Affairs Hepatitis C Resource Center Program and the National Hepatitis C Program Office. *Am J Gastroenterol*. 2012;107(5):669–689.

SEE ALSO

- Hepatitis A; Hepatitis B; Cirrhosis of the Liver; HIV/AIDS
- Algorithm: Hyperbilirubinemia and Cirrhosis

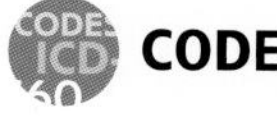

CODES

ICD10

- B19.20 Unspecified viral hepatitis C without hepatic coma
- B17.10 Acute hepatitis C without hepatic coma
- B18.2 Chronic viral hepatitis C

CLINICAL PEARLS

- 1 of 10 patients with hepatitis C has no identifiable risk factors.
- 15–25% of HCV-infected persons spontaneously resolve infection without specific treatment.
- Look for coinfections (HBV/HIV) and comorbid substance abuse in patients infected with HCV.

HEPATOMA

Edward James Kruse, DO • David M. Hardy, MD • Ray S. King, MD, PhD

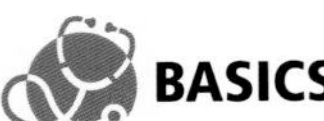

BASICS

DESCRIPTION

Hepatoma, also known as hepatocellular carcinoma (HCC), is the most common primary malignant tumor of the liver, arising from hepatic parenchymal cells (hepatocytes); 80% are associated with underlying chronic liver disease, most commonly cirrhosis related to hepatitis B and C (exception: rare fibrolamellar type).

EPIDEMIOLOGY

Incidence

- Second leading cause of cancer-related death worldwide
- 5th most common malignancy worldwide, >700,000 new cases/year worldwide (1)[A]
- 4–5 new cases/100,000/year of the United States population; 120 new cases/100,000/year in Asia and sub-Saharan Africa
- Among known cirrhotics, 2–5 cases/100 cirrhotics/year
- Incidence increasing since 1980s in the United States (due to increase in hepatitis C infection)
- In the United States, estimate is 28,720 new cases of primary liver cancer will be diagnosed in 2012 and 20,550 deaths.
- Male > female (mean 3.7:1 for incidence and 2:1 for deaths)

Prevalence

- Asians/Pacific Islanders > African Americans > Native American > Hispanics > Caucasians
- Predominant age: median age 65 years in the West, 4th–5th decades in Asia and Africa
- Predominant sex: male > female (3–4:1)

ETIOLOGY AND PATHOPHYSIOLOGY

- Cirrhosis accounts for 80–90% of HCC. Alcoholic cirrhosis is most common in the Western world. Reported risk in patients with alcoholic cirrhosis is 3–10% with micronodular pattern.
- HBV and HCV are independent and synergistic risk factors for HCC.
  - Associated with >70% of cases worldwide
  - Most important factor in Africa and Asia
- Chronic alcohol use
- Chronic tobacco abuse
- Betel nut chewing (common in Asia)
- Mycotoxins (aflatoxins): metabolite of the fungus *Aspergillus flavus* that contaminates foods
- Vinyl polymers associated with angiosarcoma and, less commonly, HCC

Genetics

No known genetic pattern

RISK FACTORS

For HCC

- 80–90% of HCC associated with cirrhosis (2)[B]:
  - Cirrhosis can be from any etiology: hepatitis B and C, alcoholism, hemochromatosis, nonalcoholic steatohepatitis (NASH), α_1–antitrypsin deficiency, biliary cirrhosis, autoimmune hepatitis, Wilson disease, glycogen storage disease
- Fungal aflatoxins (contaminants of grain in Africa and Asia): synergistic effect with other causes of liver disease
- Vinyl chloride
- Thorium dioxide
- Anabolic steroids
- Arsenic
- Nonalcoholic fatty liver disease/nonalcoholic steatohepatitis (3)[C]
- For fibrolamellar type: no identified risk factors
- For angiosarcoma: vinyl chloride

GENERAL PREVENTION

- The major risk factor for HCC is cirrhosis. Prevention of cirrhosis and tumor surveillance in patients with or at risk for cirrhosis are key.
- Prevent hepatitis B virus (HBV) and hepatitis C virus (HCV) infection through safe sexual practices, avoidance of shared IV drug paraphernalia, and HBV vaccination.
- Treat chronic HBV and HCV with lamivudine, adefovir, entecavir, tenofovir, or ribavirin/pegylated interferon, according to guidelines.
- Avoid excessive alcohol use.
- Drink >3 cups of coffee per day (4)[A].
- Statin use is associated with decreased risk of HCC.
- High-risk individuals:
  - Chronic hepatitis with HBV or HCV
  - Alcoholic cirrhosis
  - Genetic hemochromatosis
  - Exposure to vinyl chloride >10 years (screen every 6 months)
  - Primary biliary cirrhosis
  - Morbid obesity
- Screen high-risk patients by US and α-fetoprotein every 6–12 months (5)[B].
- HCC progresses from dysplastic nodules to vascular invasion (after tumor is >2 cm in diameter).

DIAGNOSIS

- In children:
  - Feminization, precocious puberty
  - Palpable liver mass, pain, asymmetrical hepatomegaly
- In adults:
  - Known cirrhosis or clinical signs of cirrhosis: 80%
  - Abdominal pain: 80%; right upper quadrant, dull to severe ache
  - Hepatomegaly: 80–90%; irregular, nodular, firm/hard, tender
  - Weight loss: 30%
  - Hepatic arterial bruit: 20%
  - Paraneoplastic syndromes: hypertrophic osteoarthropathy, carcinoid syndrome, feminization, polycythemia
  - Unexplained deterioration of stable cirrhosis
  - Budd-Chiari syndrome (hepatic vein obstruction)
  - Portal vein thrombosis

DIFFERENTIAL DIAGNOSIS

- Small, asymptomatic tumors or underlying liver conditions,
  - Cirrhosis with regenerative nodules
  - Benign liver nodules
  - Hamartoma
  - Hemangioma
  - Metastatic adenocarcinoma
  - Cholangiocarcinoma
  - Adenomas
- Larger, symptomatic tumor with hepatomegaly:
  - Cirrhosis
  - Hepatic cyst
  - Adenoma
  - Hemangioma
  - Abscess
  - Metastatic malignancy of liver
  - Thrombosis of hepatic veins, portal vein, or inferior vena cava
  - Active viral hepatitis or alcoholic hepatitis
- Ruptured tumor: all causes of acute abdomen
- Traumatic hemoperitoneum

DIAGNOSTIC TESTS & INTERPRETATION

Initial Tests (lab, imaging)

LFTs, alkaline phosphatase, BUN and creatinine, CBC, calcium, α-fetoprotein (AFP)

- Ultrasound (US) (1,5)[B]:
  - Detects tumors >1 cm; performance dependent on examiner, technology, and degree of cirrhosis (decreases sensitivity)
  - Sonographic characteristics include masses with poorly defined margins and irregular internal echoes
  - If <1 cm, repeat US in 3–6 months.
  - More sensitive when combined with AFP level
  - May be useful to follow patients with cirrhosis to help identify hepatocellular cancer at an early tumor stage
  - If >1cm, CT or MRI is performed to confirm (5)[B].
  - May be used as image guidance during percutaneous liver biopsy or other therapy (injection or ablation)
- Helical 3-phase CT scan:
  - Detects <1-cm tumors
  - Valuable in determining extrahepatic spread (most commonly to lung, periportal lymph nodes, bone, brain)
  - Delineates vascular anatomy to guide treatment
- Positron emission tomography (PET)/PET-CT improves CT detection rates.
- MRI:
  - More sensitive than helical CT scan for early detection of HCC
  - Helps differentiate benign from malignant tumors
  - Helpful in delineating the tumor and invasion of vessels
- Arteriography: used rarely because of the accuracy of MRI and CT
- 1–2-cm nodules with typical imaging features have specificities and positive predictive values nearing 100% and sensitivities up to 70%; can be used to identify HCC without tissue diagnosis (1,5)[B].

Follow-Up Tests & Special Considerations

- LFT abnormalities (aspartate aminotransferase, alanine aminotransferase, alkaline phosphatase)
- AFP:
  - Most important lab test for diagnosis of HCC but *not* recommended as a sole screening test (60% sensitivity, 80% specificity) (2)[B]
  - Level of >400 ng/mL (>400 μg/L) is diagnostic. Level of >200 ng/mL is highly suggestive of HCC; level does not correlate with prognosis but is useful in monitoring for recurrence.
  - Fibrolamellar carcinoma usually does not produce AFP.

- Some conditions, such as acute or chronic hepatitis, germ cell tumors, and pregnancy, may cause a slight elevation in AFP.
- Specific treatments will be determined by the degree of liver impairment, commonly using the Child-Pugh classification and/or Model for End-Stage Liver Disease score.
- Rare paraneoplastic syndrome: polycythemia, elevated calcium, low glucose

Diagnostic Procedures/Other

- Percutaneous tissue biopsies should be limited to confirmation of equivocal imaging findings. Tissue confirmation is also useful to rule out liver metastases (5)[B].
- *It is unnecessary to biopsy* a liver mass with typical radiographic features and elevated AFP in the setting of cirrhosis. These findings are diagnostic.
- Liver biopsy: performed using image guidance (US or CT) when nodules are not palpable. This is *not indicated* when a lesion has typical CT/MRI characteristics and an elevated AFP.
- Laparoscopy: to evaluate extent of cirrhosis and perform resection or ablation in skilled centers
- Preoperative workup: evaluation of extrahepatic metastases

Test Interpretation

- Nodular: 75%; usually in cirrhotic liver
- Massive: common in children and noncirrhotic livers; prone to rupture
- Diffuse: rare; usually a large portion of liver is involved
- Hepatocellular: most commonly multicentric and well differentiated; usually superimposed on underlying cirrhosis

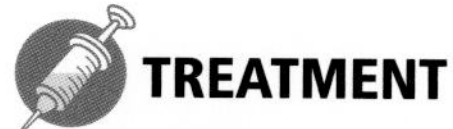

TREATMENT

MEDICATION

- Targeted therapy with sorafenib offers a small survival benefit in patients with disease not amenable to surgical intervention (6)[B].
- Treatment of hepatoma in patients with active HCV with pegylated interferon-α and ribavirin prolongs survival and improves quality of life.

SURGERY/OTHER PROCEDURES

- Surgical resection and liver transplantation offer highest cure rate in HCC (2)[B].
  - Resection should be considered in children and may include up to 1 lobe of the liver.
  - The resected specimen should contain a negative margin of normal liver tissue.
  - Intraoperative US should be performed to survey for additional lesions.
  - Resection is the preferred treatment in noncirrhotic patients with HCC if liver function is preserved and there is no evidence of portal hypertension (2)[B].
    - Varies from segmental to trisegmental resection (up to 80% of the liver)
  - Transplantation is the preferred treatment for cirrhotic patients or unresectable tumors that meet transplantation criteria (2)[B].This modality is limited due to lack of donors relative to number of patients currently awaiting transplant.
  - Advanced liver disease, medical comorbidities, and extrahepatic metastases are common; therefore, only 15–30% of HCC patients are eligible for resection (2)[B].
- The cure rate is high for both surgical options with the presence of ≤3 nodules, each <5 cm.
  - Tumor ablation
  - Tumor ablation in patients not deemed candidates for resection or transplantation is often a safe alternative.
  - Ablation may be chemical with alcohol; cryotherapy with liquid nitrogen probes; or hyperthermic with radiofrequency, microwave, or laser.
  - Ablation may be performed surgically or percutaneously, depending on the location.
  - Radiofrequency ablation (RFA) is considered superior to alcohol injection for localized therapy (7)[B].
  - Recent trials show similar survival rates for RFA versus surgical resection in small HCCs. Insufficient evidence exists to change recommendations favoring surgery at this time.
  - Irreversible electroporation is a newer ablation technique that is undergoing clinical trials.
- Percutaneous treatments are best for unresectable disease as a bridge to surgical resection or transplantation and for early-stage tumors that are not amenable to surgery.
  - Regional transarterial therapy (chemoembolization, which delivers chemotherapy directly to the tumor via its immediate blood supply or selective internal radiation therapy) is used for intermediate-stage tumors or when primary surgery is not planned; these modalities may provide palliation or downstage the tumor, making surgery possible. These 2 approaches can be used together and may yield a better outcome than either treatment alone (8)[B].
- Fibrolamellar variant should be treated by surgical resection; this has shown excellent survival rates.

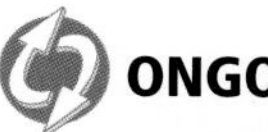

ONGOING CARE

FOLLOW-UP RECOMMENDATIONS

Patient Monitoring

Even after successful resection, there is a high risk of recurrence.

- AFP level every 3 months
- US every 4–6 months or contrast-enhanced CT/MRI scan, depending on local expertise

DIET

Attention to nutrition: high-calorie diet

PATIENT EDUCATION

Emphasize preventive measures and HBV vaccine.

PROGNOSIS

- Depends on amount of tumor replacing normal liver tissue and degree of hepatic impairment
- Unresectable, symptomatic tumors: poor, patients seldom live >6 months
- Resectable, asymptomatic tumors
  - Surgery curative in >70% of children, 40% of adults
  - Surgery curative in >80% of cirrhotic adults with tumors <3 cm
- Transplantation: similar to tumor-free patients with tumors <2 cm; 5-year survival rate of >70% with 1 tumor <5 cm or maximum of 3 lesions <3 cm (United Network of Organ Sharing criteria) (5)[B]

COMPLICATIONS

- Rupture
- Hemoperitoneum
- Liver failure
- Cachexia
- Metastases
- Thrombosis of portal, hepatic, renal veins: variceal bleeding

REFERENCES

1. Forner A, Llovet JM, Bruix J. Hepatocellular carcinoma. *Lancet*. 2012;379(9822):1245–1255.
2. Cha CH, Saif MW, Yamane BH, et al. Hepatocellular carcinoma: current management. *Curr Probl Surg*. 2010;47(1):10–67.
3. Siegel AB, Zhu AX. Metabolic syndrome and hepatocellular carcinoma: two growing epidemics with a potential link. *Cancer*. 2009;115(24): 5651–5661.
4. Bravi F, Bosetti C, Tavani A, et al. Coffee reduces risk for hepatocellular carcinoma: an updated meta-analysis. *Clin Gastroenterol Hepatol*. 2013;11(11):1413–1421.
5. El-Serag HB, Marrero JA, Rudolph L, et al. Diagnosis and treatment of hepatocellular carcinoma. *Gastroenterology*. 2008;134(6):1752–1763.
6. NCCN Clinical Practice Guidelines Version 2.2011. Hepatocellular cancers. www.nccn.org. Accessed 2014.
7. Cho YK, Kim JK, Kim MY, et al. Systematic review of randomized trials for hepatocellular carcinoma treated with percutaneous ablation therapies. *Hepatology*. 2009;49(2):453–459.
8. Garrean S, Hering J, Helton WS, et al. A primer on transarterial, chemical, and thermal ablative therapies for hepatic tumors. *Am J Surg*. 2007;194(1): 79–88.

ADDITIONAL READING

- Cancer Facts and Figures 2012: www.cancer.org
- European Association for the Study of the Liver; European Organisation for Research and Treatment of Cancer. EASL-EORTC clinical practice guidelines: management of hepatocellular carcinoma. *J Hepatol*. 2012;56(4):908–943.

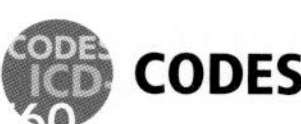

CODES

ICD10

C22.0 Liver cell carcinoma

CLINICAL PEARLS

- With benign liver tumors, most patients will have normal LFTs; 97% with HCC will have >1 abnormal test.
- Hepatitis C is the greatest risk factor, especially if combined with alcohol abuse.
- Aggressive use of hepatitis B vaccination
- Most common cause of cancer death worldwide; in the West, secondary to chronic alcoholism; in rest of world, secondary to hepatitis B and C
- Limit alcohol, treat alcoholism and NASH and drink coffee.

HEPATORENAL SYNDROME

Jerin Mathew, MD • Mony Fraer, MD, FACP, FASN

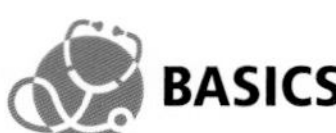

BASICS

DESCRIPTION

- Hepatorenal syndrome (HRS) is kidney failure in decompensated liver disease. It is characterized by decreased effective arterial blood volume (EABV) caused by severe splanchnic vasodilatation (1).
- HRS has a poor prognosis with median survival of weeks (rapidly progressive disease, type 1) to months (slowly progressive disease, type 2) if untreated (1)[B].
- Liver transplant is the preferred treatment for type 1 HRS.
- Vasoconstrictors and albumin have been tried for both type 1 and type 2 with variable results.

EPIDEMIOLOGY

Incidence

- Up to 40% of cirrhotic patients with ascites after 5 years of follow-up
- Higher incidence with progression of end-stage liver disease (ESLD)

ETIOLOGY AND PATHOPHYSIOLOGY

- Portal hypertension leads to splanchnic vasodilatation by increasing nitric oxide production, which reduces EABV.
- Inflammatory response involving mesenteric lymph nodes triggered by bacterial translocation is suspected as an important factor for vasodilatation.
- Reduced EABV, if mild, could be compensated by increase in cardiac output, activation of renin-angiotensin-aldosterone system, or secretion of vasopressin.
- Compensatory mechanisms cannot overcome marked reduction in EABV and resultant renal vasoconstriction further diminishes renal blood flow.

Genetics

- No genetic link to HRS by itself has been found.
- Any primary liver problem culminating in end-stage liver disease can cause hepatorenal syndrome.

RISK FACTORS

- Infections
  - Spontaneous bacterial peritonitis (SBP); ~30% of patients with SBP develop HRS.
  - Systemic infection
- Reduction of EABV in cirrhosis
  - Low mean arterial pressure
  - Excessive diuretics
  - Large-volume paracentesis
  - Diarrhea (e.g., lactulose-induced)
  - Vomiting
  - GI bleeding
  - Low serum albumin level
  - Increased intra-abdominal pressure from ascites

GENERAL PREVENTION

- Early diagnosis and aggressive treatment of infections in cirrhotic patients
- Long-term oral norfloxacin (400 mg/day) reduces HRS in cirrhotic patients with ascites and elevated creatinine.
- Albumin replacement with large-volume paracentesis (8 g/L of ascites removed) is controversial; American Association for the Study of Liver Diseases (AASLD) guidelines consider and European Association for the Study of the Liver (EASL) guidelines recommend.
- Pentoxifylline 400 mg PO TID reduced the incidence of HRS from 32% in the placebo group to 7% in the pentoxifylline group.

DIAGNOSIS

- Major criteria
  - Low GFR: serum creatinine >1.5 mg/dL (>133 mmol/L)
  - No improvement in serum creatinine level (decrease to <1.5 mg/dL [<133 mmol/L]) after >2 days with diuretic withdrawal and volume expansion with albumin (a single infusion of 1 g/kg of body weight, maximum of 100 g)
  - Not in shock
  - Absence of parenchymal kidney disease (proteinuria >500 mg/day, microhematuria [>50 RBC/hpf], and/or abnormal renal US). The presence of underlying renal disease does not rule out evolving hepatorenal syndrome.
- Supportive criteria
  - Urine volume <500mL/day
  - Urine sodium <10 mEq/L
  - Urine osmolality > plasma osmolality
  - Urine RBC <50 per high-power field
  - Serum sodium <130 mEq/L
- Concurrent spontaneous bacterial peritonitis does not exclude hepatorenal syndrome. Therapy for both may be necessary.

HISTORY

- Symptoms of decompensated cirrhosis: fatigue, malaise
- Symptoms of renal failure

PHYSICAL EXAM

- Signs of renal failure:
  - Oliguria
  - Edema
  - Altered mental status
- Signs of reduced EABV:
  - Hypotension
  - Tachycardia
- Signs of decompensated cirrhosis:
  - Ascites
  - Splenomegaly
  - Jaundice
- Palmar erythema
- Asterixis
- Spider nevi; fetor hepaticus
- Edema; clubbing
- Signs of infection:
  - Fever, hypotension, tachycardia
  - Altered mental status
  - Abdominal tenderness

DIFFERENTIAL DIAGNOSIS

Other causes of acute kidney injury (AKI):

- Drug-induced nephrotoxicity (NSAIDs, gentamicin)
- Prerenal failure (intravascular volume depletion)
- Glomerulonephritis
- Postrenal (obstruction)

DIAGNOSTIC TESTS & INTERPRETATION

Other causes of AKI need to be ruled out.

Initial Tests (lab, imaging)

- Serum creatinine, BUN, electrolytes (Na, K, Cl, HCO_3)
- Urinalysis with microscopy
- Urine Na, creatinine, protein
- LFTs, prothrombin time
- Renal US to rule out chronic kidney disease, hydronephrosis, or obstruction
- Abdominal US to confirm ascites

Test Interpretation

- Elevated BUN and creatinine
- Hyponatremia
- Bland urine sediment
- No proteinuria
- Low urine Na (<20 mEq/L)
- Normal renal US
- Paracentesis to exclude spontaneous bacterial peritonitis (SBP) if necessary

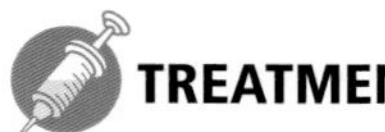

TREATMENT

GENERAL MEASURES

- Discontinue diuretics.
- Avoid NSAIDs, aminoglycosides, or other nephrotoxins.
- Relieve urinary obstruction when present.

MEDICATION

First Line

- Albumin starts with priming dose of 1 g/kg body weight followed by 20–40 g/day.
- Vasoconstrictors:
  - Ornipressin (not available in United States) Synthetic vasopressin with short half-life. Delivered by continuous IV infusion; used in conjunction with albumin (and dopamine)
  - Terlipressin (1 mg q4–6h IV; titrated up to 2 mg q4–6h after 3 days) (2)[C]:
    - Cardiovascular or ischemic complications in ~12% of patients
    - Not available in the United States
  - Midodrine (7.5–15 mg PO TID) and octreotide (100–200 mg SC TID) norepinephrine (0.5–3 mg/hr continuous IV; titrated to increase mean arterial pressure by >10 mm Hg)
  - Some anecdotal evidence that rapid titration of midodrine is more beneficial than stepwise increase
  - N-acetylcysteine (Mucomyst): used to treat acetaminophen overdose. Replenishes hepatic glutathione; unclear mechanism/role in HRS
  - Dopamine (2–5 μg/kg/min): often prescribed to improve renal perfusion; has not been shown to improve outcomes in HRS; may be useful if used in conjunction with ornipressin

ADDITIONAL THERAPIES

Dialysis is indicated only as a supportive measure for patients awaiting liver transplant or in patients with acute, potentially reversible liver failure.

- Not enough data available to determine the best dialysis modality.
- Liver dialysis (e.g., molecular absorbent recirculating systems) has been investigated.
- Antibiotics should be used if infection present. IV cefotaxime for concomitant SBP.

SURGERY/OTHER PROCEDURES

- Liver transplant has a survival rate of 65% in type 1 HRS:
  - High mortality rate while on the waiting list
  - Simultaneous liver and kidney transplant is considered for patients with advanced CKD or on dialysis for >6–8 weeks.
- Transjugular intrahepatic portosystemic shunt (TIPS) has been proposed but very limited data are available.

INPATIENT CONSIDERATIONS

Early nephrology and hepatology consultation should be considered; surgical consultation if transplantation considered

Admission Criteria/Initial Stabilization

- Type 1 HRS requires hospitalization.
- Type 2 HRS may be managed in outpatient setting.

Discharge-Criteria

- Stable renal function
- Following liver transplant

FOLLOW-UP RECOMMENDATIONS

Patient Monitoring

- Monitor renal and hepatic function and serum electrolytes.
- Follow up with a hepatologist and nephrologist.

DIET

Low-sodium (2 g) diet. No need to restrict protein in absence of encephalopathy.

PATIENT EDUCATION

- Avoid NSAIDs and IV contrast exposure.
- Notify clinician about weight gain, lightheadedness, vomiting, diarrhea, GI bleed, or confusion.
- Alcohol abstinence in order to qualify for listing for liver transplantation

PROGNOSIS

- Median survival if untreated is 2 weeks for type 1 HRS and 6 months for type 2 HRS.
- The time and degree of renal recovery after liver transplantation is variable, but a substantial number of patients do show significant renal improvement.

COMPLICATIONS

- Death
- Dialysis dependency/end-stage renal disease
- Fluid overload with congestive heart failure or pulmonary edema
- Hepatic coma
- Secondary infections

REFERENCES

1. Fagundes C, Ginès P. Hepatorenal syndrome: a severe, but treatable, cause of kidney failure in cirrhosis. *Am J Kidney Dis*. 2012;59(6):874–885.
2. Gluud LL, Christensen K, Christensen E, et al. Terlipressin for hepatorenal syndrome. *Cochrane Database Syst Rev*. 2012;9:CD005162.

ADDITIONAL READING

- European Association for the Study of the Liver. EASL clinical practice guidelines on the management of ascites, spontaneous bacterial peritonitis, and hepatorenal syndrome in cirrhosis. *J Hepatol*. 2010;53(3):397–417.
- Fernández J, Navasa M, Planas R, et al. Primary prophylaxis of spontaneous bacterial peritonitis delays hepatorenal syndrome and improves survival in cirrhosis. *Gastroenterology*. 2007;133(3):818–824.
- Skagen C, Einstein M, Lucey MR, et al. Combination treatment with octreotide, midodrine, and albumin improves survival in patients with type 1 and type 2 hepatorenal syndrome. *J Clin Gastroenterol*. 2009;43(7):680–685.
- Runyon BA, AASLD Practice Guidelines Committee. Management of adult patients with ascites due to cirrhosis: an update. *Hepatology*. 2009;49(6):2087–2107.
- Salerno F, Gerbes A, Ginès P, et al. Diagnosis, prevention and treatment of hepatorenal syndrome in cirrhosis. *Gut*. 2007;56(9):1310–1318.
- Singh V, Ghosh S, Singh B, et al. Noradrenaline vs. terlipressin in the treatment of hepatorenal syndrome: a randomized study. *J Hepatol*. 2012;56(6):1293–1298.
- Tyagi P, Sharma P, Sharma BC, et al. Prevention of hepatorenal syndrome in patients with cirrhosis and ascites: a pilot randomized control trial between pentoxifylline and placebo. *Eur J Gastroenterol Hepatol*. 2011;23(3):210–217.

SEE ALSO

- Acetaminophen Poisoning, Treatment; Cirrhosis of the Liver; Hepatitis A; Hepatitis B; Hepatitis C
- Algorithm: Acute Kidney Injury (Acute Renal Failure)

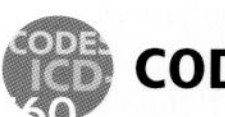

CODES

ICD10

K76.7 Hepatorenal syndrome

CLINICAL PEARLS

- HRS is a diagnosis of exclusion. Other causes of acute renal failure must be ruled out.
- Liver transplantation is the treatment of choice.

H

HERNIA

Margaret Fairhurst, DO • Brian Garrity, DO

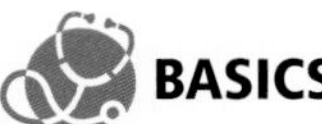

BASICS

DESCRIPTION

Hernias are areas of weakness or frank disruption of the fibromuscular tissues of the body wall through which intracavity structures pass.

- Types
  - Inguinal
    - Direct inguinal: acquired; herniation through defect in transversalis fascia of abdominal wall medial to inferior epigastric vessels; increased frequency with age as fascia weakens
    - Indirect inguinal: congenital; herniation lateral to the inferior epigastric vessels through internal inguinal ring into inguinal canal. A "complete hernia" is one that descends into the scrotum, whereas an "incomplete hernia" remains within the inguinal canal.
  - Pantaloon: combination of direct and indirect inguinal hernia with protrusion of abdominal wall on both sides of the epigastric vessels
  - Femoral: herniation that descends through the femoral canal deep to the inguinal ligament. Because of the narrow neck of a femoral hernia, this type of hernia is especially prone to incarceration and strangulation.
  - Incisional or ventral: herniation through a defect in the anterior abdominal wall at the site of a prior surgical incision
  - Congenital: herniation through fascial defect in abdominal wall, secondary to collagen deficiency disease
  - Umbilical: defect occurs at umbilical ring tissue.
  - Epigastric: protrusion through the linea alba above the level of the umbilicus. These may develop at exit points of small paramidline nerves and vessels or through an area of congenital weakness in the linea alba.
  - Interparietal (e.g., Spigelian hernia): Hernia sac insinuates itself between layers of the abdominal wall; strangulation common, often mistaken for tumor or abscess.
  - Other: obturator, sciatic, perineal
- Definitions
  - Reducible: Extruded sac and its contents can be returned to original intra-abdominal position, either spontaneously or with gentle manual manipulation.
  - Irreducible/incarcerated: Extruded sac and its contents cannot be returned to original intra-abdominal position.
  - Strangulated: Blood supply to hernia sac contents is compromised.
  - Richter: Partial circumference of the bowel is incarcerated or strangulated. Partial wall damage may occur, increasing potential for bowel rupture and peritonitis.
  - Sliding: Wall of a viscus forms part of the wall of the inguinal hernia sac (i.e., R-cecum, L-sigmoid colon).

Geriatric Considerations

Abdominal wall hernias increase with advancing age, with significant increase in risk during surgical repair.

Pregnancy Considerations

- Increased intra-abdominal pressure and hormone imbalances with pregnancy may contribute to increased risk of abdominal wall hernias.
- Umbilical hernias are associated with multiple, prolonged deliveries.

EPIDEMIOLOGY

Incidence

- 75–80% groin hernias: inguinal and femoral
- 2–20% incisional/ventral, depending on whether a prior surgery was associated with infection or contamination
- 3–10% umbilical, considered congenital
- 1–3% other
- Groin
  - 6–27% lifetime risk in adult men
  - 2-peak theory: most inguinal hernias present before 1 year of age or after 55 years of age
  - ~50% of children younger than 2 years of age will have a patent processus vaginalis, decreasing to 40% after age 2 years. Only between 25% and 50% will become clinically significant.
  - Inguinal hernia found in <5% of newborns but male-to-female ratio is 10:1.
  - Increased incidence in premature infants
  - Increased incidence in patients with abdominal aortic aneurysms
  - Femoral <10% of all groin hernias, 40% present as a surgical emergency
- Incisional/ventral: ~10–23% of abdominal surgeries complicated by an incisional hernia, most common in upper midline incisions.
- Incidence ratio: male = female
- Umbilical: 10–20% of newborns; most close by 5 years of age.

Prevalence

- Groin and inguinal hernias are more prevalent in men.
- Femoral and umbilical hernias are more prevalent in women.
- Most inguinal hernias are indirect in both genders.
- Incisional/ventral hernias are more prevalent in obese persons as well as in smokers. The opposite may be true for inguinal hernias.

ETIOLOGY AND PATHOPHYSIOLOGY

Loss of tissue strength and elasticity, especially with aging or congenital defect in abdominal fascia resulting in a defect in the fascia of the abdominal wall. Most pediatric hernias are congenital defects (e.g., patent processus vaginalis), whereas most adult hernias are a result of acquired weakness in the tissues of the anterior abdominal wall.

Genetics

No known genetic pattern

RISK FACTORS

- Increased abdominal pressure, coughing, heavy lifting, constipation, pregnancy, ascites, prostatism, obesity, advancing age (loss of tissue turgor), smoking, steroid use, low birth weight, prematurity
- Age: Femoral and scrotal hernias, along with recurrent groin hernias, are associated with increased risk for acute hernia surgery (1).

COMMONLY ASSOCIATED CONDITIONS

Obesity, chronic obstructive pulmonary disease, multiple abdominal surgeries, pregnancy, advanced age, Ehlers-Danlos syndrome, Marfan syndrome, polycystic kidney disease (PKD), osteogenesis imperfecta, Down syndrome, abdominal aortic aneurysm

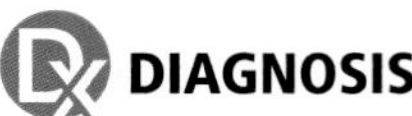

DIAGNOSIS

HISTORY

- Pain, nausea, vomiting, bloating; relieved with reclining; many are asymptomatic.
- May observe protrusion through abdominal wall during increased intra-abdominal pressure (Valsalva maneuver or cough)

PHYSICAL EXAM

- Exam should initially occur with patient standing. During palpation, the patient should be instructed to cough, strain, or perform Valsalva maneuver so the extent of intracavitary content movement can be appreciated. Exam should also be performed with patient in supine position.
- Inguinal (superior to inguinal ligament)
  - Direct inguinal hernia: Finger in inguinal canal finds defect of the transversalis fascia as a deep (posterior to anterior) bulge palpated by pad of finger with increased intra-abdominal pressure.
  - Indirect inguinal hernia: Finger in inguinal canal finds a persistent process vaginalis as a bulge (lateral to medial) palpated by fingertip; it may extend down into scrotum.
- Femoral (inferior to inguinal ligament): bulge in upper middle thigh; neck of the sac will protrude lateral to and below a finger placed on the pubic tubercle.
- Umbilical: palpable protrusion at umbilicus
- Incisional/ventral: palpable protrusion at site of prior abdominal incision or midline superior to the umbilicus
- Epigastric: palpable protrusion that occurs off midline above umbilicus

DIFFERENTIAL DIAGNOSIS

Lymphadenopathy, hydrocele, lipoma, varices, cryptorchidism, abscess, tumor, sports hernia (athletic pubalgia), pelvic fractures, adductor tears, omphalomesenteric duct, urachal cyst

DIAGNOSTIC TESTS & INTERPRETATION

Hernia evaluation rarely requires imaging; reserve for suspected abdominal hernia or unclear diagnosis. Plain radiographs to rule out obstruction

- Ultrasound (US) can be used to assess inguinal hernias.
- CT or tangential radiography for incisional and abdominal wall hernias and postsurgical patients with complaints of abdominal pain
- Herniography is no longer recommended.

Pediatric Considerations

There is insufficient evidence for contralateral exploration in pediatric patients, except using US.

Follow-Up Tests & Special Considerations

For occult hernias not well appreciated on exam or with imaging, diagnostic laparoscopy may be beneficial.

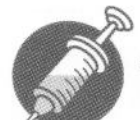

TREATMENT

- Elective setting
  - Elective surgical repair is associated with significantly lower morbidity and mortality.
- Acute setting
  - Pain management is recommended for symptomatic hernias.
  - Strangulated hernias should be surgically repaired as early as possible to prevent complications such as necrosis and viscus perforation.
  - Manual reduction of incarcerated hernia improves outcomes by allowing for elective repair after reduction of acute swelling and inflammation.
  - Complication rate is nearly 20× greater in emergent repair of pediatric inguinal hernias than elective procedures (2)[B].
  - Acute hernia repair carries a higher morbidity and lower survival rate.
  - Laparoscopic repair of incisional/ventral hernia (IVH) is safe, with fewer complications and shorter hospital stays and possibly a shorter surgical time. However, postoperative pain and recurrence rates are similar for both techniques (3)[B].

MEDICATION

- Antibiotics: Antibiotic prophylaxis did not reduce wound infections after groin hernia repairs.
- Pain: Local anesthetic during surgical repair results in significant reduction of postoperative pain. Tension-free procedures, such as Lichtenstein, may be performed under local anesthesia.

ADDITIONAL THERAPIES

Geriatric Considerations

Use of a truss (external supportive device) for direct inguinal hernias is common; no data exist regarding efficacy.

ISSUES FOR REFERRAL

Warn patients of symptoms or signs of incarceration or strangulation (acute abdominal pain, fever, bloody bowel movements), which mandate immediate self-referral to emergency room.

SURGERY/OTHER PROCEDURES

All inguinal hernias should be surgically repaired, but watchful waiting in the asymptomatic patient is a safe option if significant comorbidities may compromise emergent repair.

- Incarceration and strangulation are absolute indications for hernia repair.
- Contraindications: patients who are not surgical candidates based on cardiovascular risk factors
  - Elective repair should be avoided in pregnant patients or those with active infections.
- Special considerations
  - Umbilical hernias <0.5 cm usually obliterate and can be managed by observation.
  - Umbilical hernias in children age 2–4 years may be observed, as there is a high rate of spontaneous closure.
  - Laparoscopic repair of IVHs is associated with fewer complications and shorter hospital stays when compared with open repair. However, postoperative pain and recurrence rates are similar.
  - "Watchful waiting" is recommended in pregnancy. Elective postpartum hernia repair provided similar results to the nonpregnant population without increased risk of incarceration or strangulation before or during delivery.
  - Women had lower recurrence rates with laparoscopic methods than with Lichtenstein open method.
  - Ascites is not a strict contraindication for surgical repair. There is a greater risk of strangulation and complication without repair than the increased risks associated with repair in the presence of ascites.
  - The more emergent hernia operations can be performed using the same methods for nonacute situations. However, incarceration with strangulation may require laparotomy with partial bowel resection.
- Gold standard
  - Inguinal hernia
    - Open: Lichtenstein with mesh (37%) or mesh plug (34%): decreased recurrence rates
    - Laparoscopic (14%) with mesh: decreased hospital stay and postoperative pain
      - Requires general anesthesia
      - Transabdominal preperitoneal (TAPP) versus total extraperitoneal (TEP)
    - Pediatric: recovery and outcome similar after open and laparoscopic repair. Laparoscopic hernia repair associated with increased operation/anesthesia time and postoperative pain (2).
  - Incisional/ventral
    - Laparoscopic repair is effective for most patients with primary or recurrent ventral hernias; it is associated with a <10% recurrence rate.
  - Umbilical
    - Pediatric: open excision and closure with suture
    - Adult: Open repair with mesh or plug may reduce hernia recurrence.
- Newer techniques
  - Prolene hernia system
  - Biologic wound closure system: reduced recurrence in contaminated procedures
- Complications
  - Recurrence
  - Seromas
  - Postoperative pain, temporary or chronic: improved in laparoscopic approach versus open
  - Wound infection
  - Injury to cord structures in inguinal herniorrhaphy; with nerve injury, most symptoms will resolve.

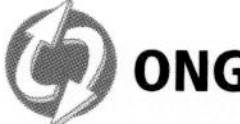

ONGOING CARE

PATIENT EDUCATION

Umbilical hernias: Boston Children's Hospital: www.childrenshospital.org/az/Site1018/mainpageS1018P0.html

PROGNOSIS

- Groin (pediatric): low recurrence rates (<3%) with surgical treatment; may spontaneously resolve in infants
- Groin (adult): ≥1% per year risk of bowel strangulation without surgical treatment; 0–10% postoperative recurrence rates, depending on surgeon's experience level and method
- Incisional/ventral: 3–5% postoperative occurrence: 2–17% postrepair recurrence, increased to 20–46% in larger hernias
- Umbilical (pediatric)
  - High rate of spontaneous resolution
  - Hernia less likely to close further in older children and in children with larger defects
- Umbilical (adult): up to 11% postoperative recurrence rate
- Epigastric: most will ultimately become incarcerated and/or strangulated without surgical treatment. Recurrence is high due to frequency of missed defects during repair.

REFERENCES

1. Abi-Haidar Y, Sanchez V, Itani KM. Risk factors and outcomes of acute versus elective groin hernia surgery. *J Am Coll Surg*. 2011;213(3):363–369.
2. Brandt ML. Pediatric hernias. *Surg Clin North Am*. 2008;88(1):27–43, vii–viii.
3. Sajid MS, Bokhari SA, Mallick AS, et al. Laparoscopic versus open repair of incisional/ventral hernia: a meta-analysis. *Am J Surg*. 2009;197(1):64–72.

ADDITIONAL READING

- Buch KE, Tabrizian P, Divino CM. Management of hernias in pregnancy. *J Am Coll Surg*. 2008;207(4):539–542.
- Matthews RD, Neumayer L. Inguinal hernia in the 21st century: an evidence-based review. *Curr Probl Surg*. 2008;45(4):261–312.
- Ng TT, Hamlin JA, Kahn AM. Herniography: analysis of its role and limitations. *Hernia*. 2009;13(1):7–11.
- Rosemar A, Angerås U, Rosengren A. Body mass index and groin hernia: a 34-year follow-up study in Swedish men. *Ann Surg*. 2008;247(6):1064–1068.
- Snyder CL. Current management of umbilical abnormalities and related anomalies. *Semin Pediatr Surg*. 2007;16(1):41–49.

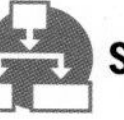

SEE ALSO

Algorithms: Abdominal Pain, Lower; Intestinal Obstruction; Pelvic Pain

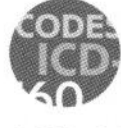

CODES

ICD10

- K46.9 Unspecified abdominal hernia without obstruction or gangrene
- K40.90 Unil inguinal hernia, w/o obst or gangr, not spcf as recur
- K41.90 Unil femoral hernia, w/o obst or gangrene, not spcf as recur

CLINICAL PEARLS

- Inguinal
  - Direct inguinal: acquired; herniation through defect in transversalis fascia of abdominal wall medial to inferior epigastric vessels
  - Indirect inguinal: congenital; herniation lateral to the inferior epigastric vessels; a "complete hernia" descends into the scrotum; an "incomplete hernia" remains within the inguinal canal.
- Pantaloon: combination of direct and indirect inguinal hernia
- Femoral: descends through the femoral canal deep to the inguinal ligament
- Incisional or ventral: iatrogenic, herniation through a defect at site of a prior surgical incision
- Umbilical: Defect occurs at umbilical ring tissue.

H

HERPES EYE INFECTIONS

Rachel Marinch, MD • William Fosmire, MD

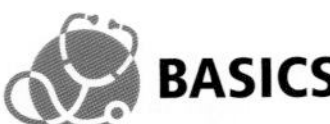

BASICS

DESCRIPTION

- Eye infection (blepharitis, conjunctivitis, keratitis, stromal keratitis, uveitis, retinitis, glaucoma, or optic neuritis) caused by herpes simplex virus (HSV) types 1 or 2 or varicella-zoster virus (VZV, also known as human herpes virus type 3 [HHV3])
- Categories
  - HSV: can affect many parts of the eye but most often affects the cornea (herpes keratoconjunctivitis); HSV1 > HSV2. Can be further divided into primary and recurrent
  - VZV: when VZV is reactivated and affects the ophthalmic division of the 5th cranial nerve, this is known as herpes zoster ophthalmicus (HZO), a type of shingles
- System(s) affected: eye, skin, central nervous system (CNS) (neonatal)

EPIDEMIOLOGY

- Predominant age: HSV-mean age of onset 37.4 years but can occur at any age, including primary infection in newborns; VZV usually advancing age (>50 years)
- Predominant sex: HSV—male = female; HZO—female > male

Incidence

- HSV keratitis: In the United States, approximated at 18.2 per 100,000 person-years. Incidence is 1.5 million per year worldwide (1).
- VZV: 1 million new cases of shingles per year in the United States; 25–40% develop ophthalmic complications. Temporary keratitis is most common.

Prevalence

- Ocular HSV prevalence estimated at 500,000 in the United States (1)
- VZV: prevalence of herpes zoster infection is 20–30%. Ocular involvement in 50% if not treated with antivirals (2). Overall lifetime prevalence of HZO: 1%

ETIOLOGY AND PATHOPHYSIOLOGY

- HSV and VZV are *Herpes viridae* dsDNA viruses
- HSV: primary infection from direct contact with infected person via saliva, genital contact, or birth canal exposure (neonates)
  - Primary infection may lead to severe disease in neonates, including eye, skin, CNS, and disseminated disease.
  - Recurrent infection is more common overall cause of herpetic eye infections.
- VZV: Primary infection from direct contact with infected person may cause varicella ("chickenpox") and/or lead to a latent state within trigeminal ganglia.
  - Reactivation of the virus may affect any dermatome (resulting in herpes zoster or "shingles"), including the ophthalmic branch (HZO).

RISK FACTORS

- HSV: personal history of HSV or close contact with HSV-infected person
  - General risk factors for reactivation: stress, trauma, fever, UV light exposure, other viral infections
  - Risk factors for HSV keratitis: UV laser eye treatment, some topical ocular medications such as prostaglandin analogues and primary/secondary immunosuppression
- HZO
  - History of varicella infection, advancing age (>50 years), sex (female > male), acute/painful prodrome, trauma, stress, immunosuppression (1,3)

ALERT
Consider primary/secondary immunodeficiency disorders in all zoster patients <40 years of age (e.g., AIDS, malignancy).

GENERAL PREVENTION

- Contact precautions with active lesions (HSV and VZV)
- VZV can be spread to those who have not had chickenpox and are not immunized.
- Varicella vaccination (Zostavax) (VZV only): single 0.65 mL SC dose; no booster. Recommended by the CDC for all persons age 60 years and older. Reduces incidence of herpes zoster by 51% and HZO for 49%; also significantly decreases rates of post-herpetic neuralgia (PHN) (4)
- Acyclovir can be used prophylactically to prevent recurrence of ocular HSV.
- HSV immunization currently being researched (1)

ALERT
Zoster vaccination is contraindicated if HIV-positive or other immunocompromised state, pregnancy, or in active untreated tuberculosis (TB).

Pregnancy Considerations

- Pregnant women without history of chickenpox should avoid contact with persons with active zoster.
- Pregnancy increases risk of recurrence of HSV/VZV.
- Live vaccine (Zostavax) is contraindicated during pregnancy.

COMMONLY ASSOCIATED CONDITIONS

Primary and secondary immunocompromised states

DIAGNOSIS

HISTORY

- Varies according to the virus and the ocular structures involved
- History of varicella or herpes simplex infection
- Acute onset, eye pain, headache, photophobia, tearing, ocular redness, decreased or blurry vision (3)[A]
- May present with a prodromal period of fever, malaise, headache, and eye pain before skin eruptions and eye lesions (HZO) (3)[A]

PHYSICAL EXAM

- Varies according to the virus and ocular structures involved
  - HSV most commonly affects the corneal epithelium (1)[A].
  - VZV most commonly affects corneal stroma and uvea (3)[A].
- Typically unilateral in presentation
  - HZO presents as early as 1–2 days after unilateral vesicular eruption in a dermatomal pattern (3)[A].
- Decreased visual acuity
- Conjunctival injection near the limbus
- Decreased corneal sensation
- Slit-lamp exam
  - Fluorescein and rose bengal stain: dendritic corneal lesions most often seen in HSV, followed by stromal keratitis, corneal edema, or infiltrate (2)[C]
  - Stromal keratitis often seen in HZO, although dendritic lesions may form (2)[A]

ALERT
Unilateral dermatomal vesicular rash most commonly in ophthalmic branch (V_1) of trigeminal nerve (VZV):

- Hutchinson sign: vesicular lesion on nose from VZV indicates an increased risk of HZO due to involvement of nasociliary branch of trigeminal nerve, which also innervates the eye (3)[A].

DIFFERENTIAL DIAGNOSIS

- Any other cause of red, painful eye
  - Bacterial, fungal, allergic, or other viral conjunctivitis
  - Acute angle closure glaucoma
- Corneal abrasion, recurrent corneal erosion, toxic conjunctivitis
- Temporal arteritis
- Trigeminal neuralgia

DIAGNOSTIC TESTS & INTERPRETATION

Initial Tests (lab, imaging)

- Typically none needed, as diagnosis is primarily based on history and physical exam (3)[A]
- Other
  - Corneal swab for HSV DNA by polymerase chain reaction (PCR) (PPV = 96%)
  - If vesicle present, can perform a Tzanck smear for VZV or HSV (multinucleated giant cells)
  - Antibody titers to assess exposure only; DFA (direct fluorescent antibody); tissue culture

ALERT
Urgent ophthalmology referral necessary for slit-lamp exam, dilated fundus exam, and intraocular pressure measurement

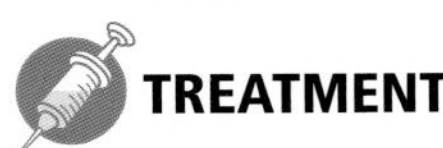

TREATMENT

GENERAL MEASURES

- Avoid contact with nonimmune people.
- No contact lenses should be worn during treatment period.
- Cool compresses
- Artificial tears
- Oral pain medications

MEDICATION

First Line

- HSV corneal epithelial disease
  - Trifluridine 1%: apply 1 drop q2h while awake to a max of 9 drops daily until reepithelialization occurs, then 1 drop q4h for another 7 days
  - Acyclovir: 400 mg PO 5 times per day for 10 days
  - Ganciclovir 0.15% gel: apply 1 drop in eye q3h while awake, ~5× daily, until reepithelialization occurs, then 1 drop q8h for 7 days
  - Vidarabine 3% ointment (Vira-A): apply 0.5 inch into lower conjunctival sac 5× daily q3h, until reepithelialization occurs.

- Trifluridine and acyclovir appear to be more effective than vidarabine (5)[A].
- No significant differences in healing between acyclovir or trifluridine. Evidence lacking to compare to ganciclovir (5)[A]
- Epithelial débridement by an ophthalmologist: may accelerate healing in combination with treatment as above (5)[A]
- Avoid topical steroids.

- HSV stromal keratitis or uveitis (without epithelial disease): combination of antiviral and steroid treatment; requires ophthalmology evaluation
  - Prednisolone acetate: 1% drops QID with slow taper (6)[A]
  - Consider systemic steroids in severe uveitis (6)[A].
  - Trifluorothymidine: 1% drops QID for prophylaxis while on topical steroids
- HZO
  - Valacyclovir (Valtrex) 1 g PO TID for 7–10 days *or* famciclovir (Famvir) 500 mg PO TID for 7–10 days *or* acyclovir 800 mg PO 5× a day for 7–10 days
  - Valacyclovir and famciclovir result in significant reduction in PHN compared to acyclovir (number needed to treat [NNT] = 3) with equivalent efficacy (7)[A]
  - Topical antibiotic ophthalmic ointment to protect ocular surfaces (e.g., Bacitracin, Polymyxin): 0.5-inch ribbon BID–TID for 7–10 days (8)[C]
  - If immunocompromised: acyclovir 10–15 mg/kg IV q8h for 10 days
  - Prednisolone acetate: 1% drops QID with slow taper with an ophthalmologist (8)[C]
- Cycloplegic agent if anterior uveitis present; intraocular pressure-lowering agent if necessary

Second Line

- HSV: acyclovir 2 g/day PO in divided doses over 10 days in patients intolerant of topical antivirals
- Topical idoxuridine, acyclovir, brivudine, although approved internationally, are not approved for use in the United States.
- Concomitant treatment with interferon may also improve outcomes but is not currently available.

ALERT

- HZO: Antiviral therapy is most effective within the first 72 hours of rash onset but should still be initiated >72 hours after onset because of the possible complications of HZO (2)[C].
- Topical antiviral agents
  - Toxic to corneal epithelium, especially after 10–14 days of continuous use
- Acyclovir: reduce dosage in renal insufficiency
- Topical steroids
  - Should only be prescribed by an ophthalmologist
  - Contraindicated with active corneal epithelial disease, which is best monitored with a slit lamp
  - Can increase intraocular pressure, cause corneal thinning, and, with long-term use, cause cataracts
- Prednisone: caution in immunocompromised patients

ISSUES FOR REFERRAL

Emergent or urgent ophthalmology referral, depending on severity of disease

ADDITIONAL THERAPIES

- Recurrent HSV requires suppressive therapy:
  - Acyclovir 400 mg PO every day or BID *or* valacyclovir 500 mg PO daily (9)[C]
- HZO leading to PHN is very common and can be treated with gabapentin or pregabalin, TCAs, opioids, and/or lidocaine gel.

SURGERY/OTHER PROCEDURES

Corneal transplantation for severe scarring or perforation

INPATIENT CONSIDERATIONS

Admission Criteria/Initial Stabilization

- Severe systemic VZV disease
- Systemic HSV in neonates —see topic: HSV, Pediatric

DISCHARGE CRITERIA

Resolution of systemic disease

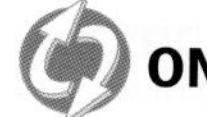

ONGOING CARE

FOLLOW-UP RECOMMENDATIONS

Patient Monitoring

- Monitor with slit-lamp exam q1–2d until improvement, then q3–4d until epithelial defect resolves.
- Weekly after epithelial disease resolves until off topical antivirals

PATIENT EDUCATION

Educate patients about importance of early recognition of recurrent symptoms and need for prompt evaluation and treatment.

PROGNOSIS

- Many cases are self-limited but, depending on the ocular structure involved, can lead to permanent blindness, especially in the setting of recurrent disease.
- Ocular HSV is the number 1 cause of infectious blindness worldwide (1)
- Recurrent ocular HSV
  - HSV epithelial disease without treatment
    - Without sequelae, 40% resolve.
    - With treatment, 90–95% resolve without complication.

Pediatric Considerations

- Neonatal primary HSV often disseminated, with high mortality rate; 37% develop vision worse than 20/200
- Pediatric cases more likely to be bilateral (26%); recurrent (48% in 15 months); and may cause amblyopia

COMPLICATIONS

- Recurrence
- Corneal neovascularization and scarring resulting in poor vision
- Neurotrophic ulcer with perforation
- Secondary bacterial or fungal infection
- Secondary glaucoma in 10%
- Post-herpetic neuralgia in 20–40% with VZV, typically longer lasting in older patients
- Vision loss from optic neuritis or chorioretinitis

REFERENCES

1. Faroog AV, Shukla D. Herpes simplex epithelial and stromal keratitis: an epidemiologic update. *Surv Opththalmol*. 2012;57(5):448–462.
2. Carter WP III, Germann CA, Baumann MR. Ophthalmic diagnoses in the ED: herpes zoster ophthalmicus. *Am J Emerg Med*. 2008;26(5):612–617.
3. Liesegang TJ. Herpes zoster ophthalmicus natural history, risk factors, clinical presentation, and morbidity. *Ophthalmology*. 2008;115(2):S3–S12.
4. Gelb LD. Preventing herpes zoster through vaccination. *Opthalmology*. 2008;115(2)(Suppl):S35–S38.
5. Wilhelmus KR. Antiviral treatment and other therapeutic interventions for herpes simplex virus epithelial keratitis. *Cochrane Database Syst Rev*. 2010;8(12):CD002898.
6. Knickelbein JE, Hendricks RL, Charukamnoetkanok P. Management of herpes simplex virus stromal keratitis: an evidence-based review. *Surv Ophthalmol*. 2009;54(2):226–234.
7. McDonald EM, de Kock J, Ram FS. Antivirals for management of herpes zoster including ophthalmicus: a systematic review of high-quality randomized controlled trials. *Antivir Ther*. 2012;17(2):255–264.
8. Dworkin RH, Johnson RW, Breuer J, et al. Recommendations for the management of herpes zoster. *Clin Infect Dis*. 2007;44(Suppl 1):S1–S26.
9. de Rojas Silva MV, Díez-Feijóo E, Javaloy J, et al. Prophylactic perioperative antiviral therapy for LASIK in patients with inactive herpetic keratitis. *J Refract Surg*. 2006;22(4):404–406.

ADDITIONAL READING

Rowe AM, St Leger AJ, Jeon S, et al. Herpes keratitis. *Prog Retin Eye Res*. 2013;32:88–101.

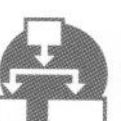

SEE ALSO

- Algorithm: Eye Pain
- Topic: Herpes Simplex
- Topic: Herpes Simplex Virus, Pediatric
- Topic: Herpes Zoster

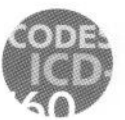

CODES

ICD10

- B00.50 Herpesviral ocular disease, unspecified
- B02.30 Zoster ocular disease, unspecified
- B00.52 Herpesviral keratitis

CLINICAL PEARLS

- HSV and VZV can lead to a wide array of ocular manifestations, ranging from self-limited disease to potentially vision-threatening disease and complications.
- A slit-lamp exam with fluorescein stain should be performed on all patients with possible HSV keratitis or HZO.
- Topical antiviral treatment is appropriate for HSV, but systemic PO antiviral treatment is necessary for HZO.
- An ophthalmologist should be consulted before prescribing topical steroids. All HZO patients should be referred to an ophthalmologist.
- Hutchinson sign (vesicular lesion on nose from VZV) is a strong indicator of HZO.
- Zostavax is effective at preventing zoster and HZO as well as decreasing the duration of PHN.

HERPES SIMPLEX

Sonia Rivera-Martinez, DO, FACOFP

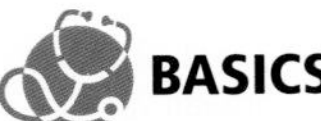

BASICS

DESCRIPTION

- Characteristic vesicular rash primarily located in oral and genital regions as the result of infection with
  - Herpes simplex virus (HSV)-1 primarily associated with blisters on lips, in mouth, face, eyes
  - HSV-2 is primary source of genital herpes, although cross-reactivity is common (with HSV-1 being a cause of genital sores as well, due to oral–genital contact).
- Associated with a wide range of sequelae. Complexity and variation of presentation depends on the age and immune status of host, whether the rash outbreak is primary or recurrent and the degree of dissemination.
- Viral shedding varies but is typically greatest in the first (primary) infection and lessens with recurrences.
- Meningitis/encephalitis and pneumonia are among the serious systemic manifestations associated with HSV infection.

EPIDEMIOLOGY

- Predominant age: affects all ages; however, most HSV-1 is acquired in childhood, and most HSV-2 is acquired in young–middle adulthood.
- Predominant sex: male = female

Incidence

- 29/100,000 office visits per year are for herpes simplex–related codes.
- HSV stays dormant and can reactivate, causing recurrent disease within the same patient.

Prevalence

- Widespread; 0.65–25% of adults may shed HSV-1 or HSV-2 at any given time. Many are potentially unaware of their infection status.
- Prevalence of antibodies to HSV-1 is 90% by adulthood in the general population. 30% of adults have antibodies to HSV-2.

ETIOLOGY AND PATHOPHYSIOLOGY

HSV-1 and 2 are double stranded DNA viruses from the family *Herpesviridae*. HSV-1 and 2 are transmitted by contact with infected skin during periods of viral (re)activation. Transmission can also occur vertically during childbirth. Most often, HSV-1 is associated with oral lesions and HSV-2 with genital lesions, but reverse also occurs.

RISK FACTORS

- Immunocompromised state
  - Chemotherapy, malignancy/chronic disease states such as diabetes or AIDS, older age
- Atopic eczema, especially in children
- Prior HSV infection
- Sexual intercourse with infected person (condoms help minimize HSV transmission, but lesions outside condom-protected areas can spread virus)
- Occupational exposure
  - Dental professionals at higher risk for HSV-1 and resulting herpetic whitlow
- Neonatal herpes simplex: Primary infection is life-threatening and usually acquired by vaginal birth to an infected mother; fetal and neonatal risk are greatest in mothers with primary genital herpes infection ; incubation is usually from 5 to 7 days (rarely 4 weeks); cutaneous, mucous membrane, or ocular signs seen in only 70%.

GENERAL PREVENTION

- Avoid direct contact with immunocompromised people, the elderly, and newborns if lesions present.
- Hand hygiene
- Kissing, sharing beverages, and sharing utensils/toothbrushes can transmit HSV.
- Genital herpes: Avoid sexual contact while disease is active (herpes simplex is also transmitted when disease appears to be inactive), discuss condom benefits and limits, consider antiviral therapy to reduce viral shedding, and encourage safe sex.
- Topical microbicides (not yet commercially available) may prevent transmission of HSV-2.

COMMONLY ASSOCIATED CONDITIONS

- Erythema multiforme: 50% of associated cases are caused by HSV-1 or -2.
- All severe, unusual locations, or treatment-resistant HSV cases should be screened for HIV.

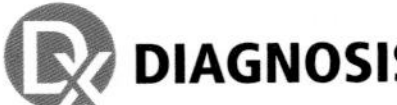

DIAGNOSIS

HISTORY

- Most patients endorse no known exposure, as transmission is often distant or acquired through asymptomatic contacts.
- Prodrome of fatigue, low-grade fever, itching, tingling, or hot skin area for a few days immediately prior to outbreak of characteristic vesicular rash
- In herpes labialis: precipitating events may be sunlight, fever, trauma, menses, and stress; prodrome of pain, burning, and itching may last 6–48 hours before vesicles appear.

PHYSICAL EXAM

- Vesicles: usually cluster and open as painful ulcerated lesions, often with erythematous base
- Primary genital herpes: see "Herpes, Genital."
- Primary herpetic gingivostomatitis and pharyngitis: usually in early childhood; incubation from 2 to 12 days, followed by fever, sore throat, pharyngeal edema, and erythema
  - Small vesicles develop on pharyngeal and oral mucosa, rapidly ulcerate, and increase in number to involve soft palate, buccal mucosa, tongue, floor of mouth, lips, and cheeks; tender, bleeding gums; cervical adenopathy; fever, general toxicity, poor oral intake, and excess salivation contribute to dehydration; autoinoculation of other sites may occur; resolves in 10–14 days.
- Primary herpes keratoconjunctivitis: unilateral conjunctivitis with regional adenopathy, as blepharitis with vesicles on lid margin, as keratitis with dendritic lesions, or with punctate opacities; lasts 2–3 weeks; systemic involvement prolongs process.
- Eczema herpeticum: diffuse poxlike eruption complicating atopic dermatitis; sudden appearance of lesions in typical atopic areas (upper trunk, neck, head); high fever, local edema, adenopathy
- Herpetic whitlow: localized primary infection of affected finger with intense itching and pain, followed by vesicles that may coalesce with swelling and erythema and may mimic pyogenic paronychia; neuralgia and axillary adenopathy sometime occur; heals over 2–3 weeks
- Congenital infection through transplacental transfer may present with jaundice, hepatosplenomegaly, disseminated intravascular coagulation (DIC), encephalitis, seizures, temperature instability, chorioretinitis, and conjunctivitis with or without vesicles.
- Recurrent diseases from endogenous reactivation
  - Herpes labialis: recurrent lesions on lips with HSV-1; usually <1 recurrence/6 months, but 5–25% may have >1 attack/month; vesicles often at vermilion border, then ulcerate and crust within 48 hours; heal within 8–10 days; may have local adenopathy
  - Ocular herpes: may recur as keratitis, blepharitis, or keratoconjunctivitis; dendritic ulcers, decreased corneal sensation, less visual acuity; uveitis may cause permanent visual loss.

DIFFERENTIAL DIAGNOSIS

- Impetigo: straw-colored crusted vesicles
- Aphthous stomatitis: grayish, shallow erosions with ring of hyperemia, of anterior in mouth and lips
- Herpes zoster: unilateral dermatome distribution
- Syphilitic chancre: usually painless ulcer
- Folliculitis: may mimic "shave bumps" in genital area.
- Herpangina: vesicles predominate on anterior tonsillar pillars, soft palate, uvula, and oropharynx but not more anteriorly on lips/gums (usually caused by group A coxsackievirus).
- Stevens-Johnson syndrome

DIAGNOSTIC TESTS & INTERPRETATION

- Screen for other sexually transmitted infections (STIs) in patients with primary genital herpes.
- Viral: HIV, hepatitis B and C, and human papillomavirus (HPV) have crossover.
- Bacterial: screen for concurrent gonorrhea, chlamydia in new primary genital outbreaks.

Initial Tests (lab, imaging)

- Tzanck smear shows multinucleated giant cells with 12–15 nuclei, often with eosinophilic intranuclear inclusions (scrape material from lesion to slide, fix with ethanol/methanol, stain with Giemsa or Wright preparation); varicella (herpes zoster) has identical findings.
- HSV culture: on viral-specific media, swab and sample may need to be refrigerated; can take up to 6 days to be positive. Highly specific, hence, reliable if positive but has 20% false–negative rate.
- HSV type-specific antibody tests distinguish between HSV-1 and HSV-2
  - PCR (polymerase chain reaction), DFA (direct fluorescent antibody), ELISA, and Western blot
  - 3 weeks after infection, 50% of those infected test positive; 6 weeks after infection: 70%; >16 weeks: nearly all infected test positive.

Diagnostic Procedures/Other

Occasionally, a biopsy is needed to confirm diagnosis.

Test Interpretation

- Intraepithelial edema (ballooning degeneration) and intracellular edema
- Brain biopsy (in encephalitis) has hemorrhagic necrosis of gray and white matter with acute and chronic inflammation, thrombosis, and fibrinoid necrosis of parenchymal vessels; intranuclear inclusions in astrocytes, oligodendroglia, and neurons.

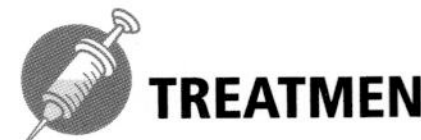

TREATMENT

GENERAL MEASURES

- Intermittent, cool, moist dressings with aluminum acetate solution
- Painful urination and inability to void due to painful genital lesions is helped by pouring a cup of warm water over genitals while urinating or by sitting in a warm bath while urinating (sitz baths).

- Children with gingivostomatitis who resist oral intake due to pain or extensive skin disease (eczema herpeticum) may require IV hydration.

MEDICATION

First Line

- Treatment should begin promptly, preferably in prodromal phase.
- Acyclovir (generic)
  - Mucocutaneous (or genital) HSV
    - Primary/1st infection: 400 mg TID or 200 mg 5 times/day × 7–10 days
    - If severe, start with IV q8h dosing for 1st few days, then complete 10-day course PO route.
    - Recurrence: 400 mg PO TID × 5 days *or* 800 mg BID × 5 days *or* 800 mg TID × 2 days
    - Suppression: 400 mg BID daily (1)[B]
  - Keratitis HSV: 400 mg PO 5 ×/day; however, topical treatment is preferred 1st line.
  - Pediatric dosing: neonatal herpes simplex or encephalitis: 60 mg/kg/day IV divided q8h × 14–21 days (2)[B]
    - Older (>3 months of age) immunocompetent is weight-based dosing (40–80 mg/kg/day [max 1,000 mg/day] divided q8h for 5–7 days).
  - Safe in pregnancy and lactation—Category B
  - Recurrent herpes labialis: 800–1,600 mg/day for prevention (3–5)[B]
- Penciclovir (Denavir): 1% cream. Apply to oral lesions q2h during waking hours × 4 days (6)[B].
- Valacyclovir (Valtrex)
  - Primary genital herpes: 1 g PO BID for 7–10 days. Recurrent genital herpes: 500 mg PO BID for 3 days; suppression: 500–1,000 mg PO daily (depending on frequency of outbreaks); labialis HSV (cold sores/oral lesions): 2,000 mg PO q12h × 1 day (3–5)[B]
  - 500 mg daily dose if suppression is needed/desired
  - Recurrent herpes labialis: 500 mg/day for 4 months for prevention (3,4)[B]
- Famciclovir (Famvir)
  - Primary genital herpes: 250 mg PO TID for 7–10 days
  - Recurrence: 125 mg PO BID for 5 days or 1,000 mg PO BID for 1 day
  - Suppression: 250 mg PO BID
- Precautions
  - Renal dosing required in all oral antivirals
  - Significant possible interactions: Probenecid with IV acyclovir and possibly probenecid with valacyclovir may reduce renal clearance and elevate antiviral drug levels.

Second Line

- Foscarnet
  - Drug of choice for acyclovir resistance in immunocompromised persons with systemic HSV
  - 40 mg/kg IV q8h (assume valacyclovir and famciclovir resistance also if acyclovir resistance occurs)
- Other topicals
  - Ophthalmic preparations for herpes keratoconjunctivitis; acyclovir, vidarabine (Vira-A), ganciclovir, trifluridine
  - Topical acyclovir and penciclovir improve recurrent herpes labialis healing times by ~10% (3)[B].
  - Topical analgesics: Lidocaine 2% or 5% helps reduce pain associated with vulvar and penile outbreaks.
- Over-the-counter topical antivirals: docosanol

ISSUES FOR REFERRAL

Recurrent cases of herpes keratoconjunctivitis should be referred to an ophthalmologist.

INPATIENT CONSIDERATIONS

Admission Criteria/Initial Stabilization

- Pregnancy considerations
  - Caesarean section and/or acyclovir indicated if any active genital lesions (or prodrome) present at time of delivery; consider cesarean delivery if primary genital herpes suspected within previous 4 weeks (6)[B].
  - Daily oral antivirals from 36 weeks onward in women with history of recurrent genital herpes to prevent outbreak near to/at time of delivery
  - Avoid fetal scalp electrodes, forceps, vacuum extractor, and artificial rupture of membranes if mother has history of genital HSV.
  - Risk of viral shedding at delivery from asymptomatic recurrent genital HSV is low (~1.6%); not predicted by monitoring cultures.
- Pediatric considerations
  - Neonates with likely exposure (high index of suspicion) to HSV at birth or with signs of infection should have all bodily fluid sources cultured and immediately begin treatment with IV acyclovir.

ONGOING CARE

FOLLOW-UP RECOMMENDATIONS

- For most typical cases, follow-up is not necessary. Lesions and symptoms resolve rapidly within 10 days. Extensive cases should be rechecked in 1 week; monitor for secondary bacterial infections.
- Consider long-term suppression.

DIET

If oral lesions present, avoid salty, acidic, or sharp foods (e.g., chips and orange juice).

PATIENT EDUCATION

- Explain the natural history, that timing of exposure is difficult to determine, and that the virus will remain in the body indefinitely. Try to minimize psychological impact of this diagnosis (reduce any stigma).
- Emphasize personal hygiene to avoid self-spreading to other body areas (autoinoculation) or exposing others. Frequent hand washing; avoid scratching; cover active, moist lesions.

PROGNOSIS

- Usual duration of primary disease is 5 days–2 weeks.
- Antiviral treatment limits length of disease, reduces complications, and nearly eliminates recurrences (if used daily).
- Viral shedding during recurrence is briefer than with primary disease; frequency of recurrence is variable and depends on individual host factors.
- Newborns/immunocompromised individuals are at highest risk for major morbidity/mortality.
- HSV is never eliminated from the body but stays dormant and can reactivate, causing symptoms.

COMPLICATIONS

- Herpes encephalitis: A brain biopsy may be needed for diagnosis.
- Herpes pneumonia

REFERENCES

1. Gupta R, Warren T, Wald A. Genital herpes. *Lancet*. 2007;370(9605):2127–2137.
2. Pinninti SG, Kimberlin DW. Neonatal herpes simplex virus infections. *Pediatr Clin North Am*. 2013;60(2):351–365. doi:10.1016/j.pcl.2012.12.005.
3. Rahimi H, Mara T, Costella J, et al. Effectiveness of antiviral agents for the prevention of recurrent herpes labialis: a systematic review and meta-analysis. *Oral Surg Oral Med Oral Pathol Oral Radiol*. 2012;113(5):618–627.
4. Harmenberg J, Oberg B, Spruance S. Prevention of ulcerative lesions by episodic treatment of recurrent herpes labialis: a literature review. *Acta Derm Venereol*. 2010;90(2):122–130.
5. Cernik C, Gallina K, Brodell RT. The treatment of herpes simplex infections: an evidence-based review. *Arch Intern Med*. 2008;168(11):1137–1144.
6. Obiero J, Mwethera PG, Wiysonge CS. Topical microbicides for prevention of sexually transmitted infections. *Cochrane Database Syst Rev*. 2012;6:CD007961.

ADDITIONAL READING

Wang X, Zhou F, Zhao J, et al. Elevated risk of opportunistic viral infection in patients with Crohn's disease during biological therapies: a meta analysis of randomized controlled trials. *Eur J Clin Pharmacol*. 2013;69(11):1891–1899.

SEE ALSO

- Herpes, Genital
- Algorithm: Genital Ulcers

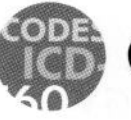

CODES

ICD10

- B00.9 Herpesviral infection, unspecified
- A60.00 Herpesviral infection of urogenital system, unspecified
- B00.1 Herpesviral vesicular dermatitis

CLINICAL PEARLS

- 25–30% of the U.S. population has evidence of genital herpes (HSV-2), and >80% of the U.S. population is seropositive for HSV-1 infection.
- Most individuals are unaware that they have been infected and asymptomatically pass on the virus.
- Chronic viral suppression for patients with frequent recurrences reduces transmission and decreases outbreak frequency. Recurrences also naturally become less frequent over time.

HERPES ZOSTER (SHINGLES)

Robert J. Hyde, MD, MA

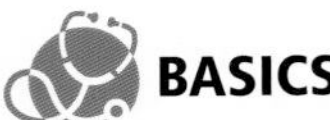

BASICS

DESCRIPTION

- Results from reactivation of latent varicella-zoster virus (human herpesvirus type 3) infection
- Postherpetic neuralgia (PHN) is defined as pain persisting at least 1 month after rash has healed. Because of variable definitions of PHN used in research, the term *zoster-associated pain* is more clinically useful.
- Usually presents as a painful unilateral vesicular eruption within a dermatome
- System(s) affected: nervous; integumentary; exocrine
- Synonym(s): shingles

EPIDEMIOLOGY

Predominant sex: male = female

Incidence

- Incidence increases with age: 2/3 of cases occur in adults age ≥50 years. Incidence is increasing overall as the U.S. population ages.
- Herpes zoster: 4/1,000 person-years (1)
- PHN: 18% in adult patients with herpes zoster; 33% in patients ≥79 years of age

Prevalence

Nearly 1 million new herpes zoster cases yearly

Pregnancy Considerations

May occur during pregnancy

Geriatric Considerations

- Increased incidence of zoster outbreaks
- Increased incidence of PHN

Pediatric Considerations

- Occurs less frequently in children
- Has been reported in newborns primarily infected in utero

ETIOLOGY AND PATHOPHYSIOLOGY

Reactivation of varicella-zoster virus from dorsal root/cranial nerve ganglia. Upon reactivation, the virus replicates within neuronal cell bodies, and virions are carried along axons to dermatomal skin zones, causing local inflammation and vesicle formation.

RISK FACTORS

- Increasing age
- Immunosuppression (malignancy or chemotherapy)
- HIV infection
- Use of immunosuppressant drugs after organ transplant surgery
- Spinal surgery

GENERAL PREVENTION

- Herpes zoster vaccination (Zostavax) is recommended by Advisory Committee on Immunization Practices (ACIP) for patients ≥60 years of age (FDA-approved for patients >50 years) (2–4):
  - Vaccine reduces cases of zoster and the incidence of PHN (5,6).
- Patients with active zoster may transmit virus-causing varicella (chickenpox) to susceptible persons.

COMMONLY ASSOCIATED CONDITIONS

Immunocompromised individuals, HIV infection, posttransplantation, immunosuppressive drugs, and malignancy

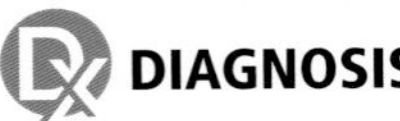

DIAGNOSIS

HISTORY

- Prodromal phase (sensations over involved dermatome prior to rash)
  - Tingling
  - Itching
  - Boring knifelike pain
- Acute phase
  - Constitutional symptoms (e.g., fatigue, malaise, headache, low-grade fever) are variable.
  - Dermatomal rash

PHYSICAL EXAM

- Acute phase
  - Weakness (1% may have weakness in distribution of rash)
  - Rash: initially erythematous and maculopapular; evolves rapidly to grouped vesicles
  - Vesicles become pustular and/or hemorrhagic in 3–4 days.
  - Resolution of rash, with crusts separating by 14–21 days
- Possible sine herpete (zoster without rash) and other chronic disorders associated with varicella-zoster virus without the typical rash
- Herpes zoster ophthalmicus (HZO). Vesicles on tip of nose (Hutchinson sign), indicating involvement of the external branch of cranial nerve V; associated with increased incidence of ocular zoster
- Chronic phase
  - PHN (15% overall; increases with age)
  - A small percentage (1–5%) may affect the motor nerves, causing weakness (called *zoster motorius*); facial nerve (e.g., Ramsay Hunt syndrome); spinal motor radiculopathies.

DIFFERENTIAL DIAGNOSIS

- Rash
  - Herpes simplex virus
  - Coxsackievirus
  - Contact dermatitis
  - Superficial pyoderma
- Pain
  - Cholecystitis
  - Appendicitis
  - Nephrolithiasis
  - Pleuritis
  - Myocardial infarction
  - Diabetic neuropathy

DIAGNOSTIC TESTS & INTERPRETATION

Initial Tests (lab, imaging)

Rarely necessary because clinical appearance is sufficiently distinctive

Follow-Up Tests & Special Considerations

- Viral culture
- Tzanck smear (does not distinguish from herpes simplex, and false-negative results occur)
- Polymerase chain reaction
- Immunofluorescent antigen staining
- Varicella-zoster–specific IgM

Test Interpretation

- Multinucleated giant cells with intralesional inclusion
- Lymphatic infiltration of sensory ganglia with focal hemorrhage and nerve cell destruction

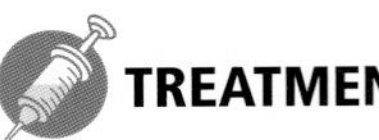

TREATMENT

GENERAL MEASURES

- Treatment is directed to control symptoms and prevent complications.
- Antiviral therapy decreases viral replication, lessens nerve damage and inflammation, and reduces the severity and duration of long-term pain syndromes (7)[A].
- Prompt analgesic control may shorten the duration of zoster-associated pain.
- Lotions, such as calamine and colloidal oatmeal, may help reduce itching and burning sensation.

MEDICATION

First Line

- Acute treatment
  - Antiviral agents initiated within 72 hours of skin lesions may relieve symptoms, speed resolution, and prevent/ameliorate PHN (7,8)[A].
  - Valacyclovir: 1,000 mg PO TID × 7 days
  - Famciclovir: 500 mg PO TID × 7 days
  - Acyclovir: 800 mg q4h (5 doses daily) × 7 days
- Analgesics (acetaminophen, NSAIDs)
- Corticosteroids given acutely during zoster infection are ineffective in preventing PHN (9).
  - PHN and zoster-associated pain (7)
  - Tricyclic antidepressants (TCAs; amitriptyline 25 mg at bedtime and other low-dose TCAs) relieve pain acutely and may reduce pain duration; dose may be titrated up to 75–150 mg/day as tolerated.
  - Lidocaine patch 5% (Lidoderm) applied after skin rash closure over painful areas (limit 3 patches simultaneously or trim a single patch) for up to 12 hours has been reported to be effective in 1 limited trial.

  - Gabapentin: 100–600 mg TID for pain and other quality-of-life indicators; limited by adverse effects
  - Capsaicin cream, and other analgesics may be useful adjuncts. Use opioids sparingly.
  - Pregabalin: 50–100 mg TID reduces pain, but usefulness is limited by side effects.
- Prevention of PHN and zoster-associated pain: No treatment has been shown to prevent PHN completely, but treatment may shorten duration and/or reduce severity of symptoms (10)[A]:
  - Antiviral therapy with valacyclovir, famciclovir, or acyclovir given during acute skin eruption may decrease the duration of pain.
  - Low-dose amitriptyline in the same dosage as for treatment of PHN but started within 72 hours of rash onset and continued for 90 days may reduce PHN incidence/duration.
  - Insufficient evidence to suggest that corticosteroids reduce incidence, severity, or duration of PHN (9).
- Precautions
  - Assess renal function prior to using valacyclovir, famciclovir, or acyclovir.
  - Valacyclovir, famciclovir, and acyclovir are pregnancy Category B.
  - Refer to the manufacturer's profile of each drug.

Second Line

Numerous therapies have been advocated, but good supporting evidence is lacking to routinely recommend.

COMPLEMENTARY & ALTERNATIVE MEDICINE

Studies on cupping therapy (traditional Chinese medicine) show potential benefit, but clear evidence is conflicting (11)[A].

INPATIENT CONSIDERATIONS

Admission Criteria/Initial Stabilization

Outpatient treatment, unless disseminated or occurring as complication of serious underlying disease requiring hospitalization

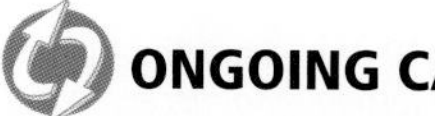

ONGOING CARE

FOLLOW-UP RECOMMENDATIONS

Referral to ophthalmology if concern for involvement of ophthalmic branch of the trigeminal nerve

Patient Monitoring

Follow duration of symptoms—particularly PHN. Consider hospitalization if symptoms are severe; patients are immunocompromised; more than 2 dermatomes are involved; serious bacterial superinfection, disseminated zoster, or meningoencephalitis develops.

DIET

No special diet

PATIENT EDUCATION

- The duration of rash is typically 2–3 weeks.
- Encourage good hygiene and proper skin care.
- Warn of potential for dissemination (dissemination must be suspected with constitutional illness signs and/or spreading rash).
- Warn of potential PHN.
- Warn of potential risk of transmitting illness (chickenpox) to susceptible persons.
- Seek medical attention if any eye involvement.

PROGNOSIS

- Immunocompetent individuals should experience spontaneous and complete recovery within a few weeks.
- Resolution of acute rash within 14–21 days
- PHN may occur in patients age ≥50 years despite treatment with antiviral medications.

COMPLICATIONS

- PHN
- HZO: 10–20%
- Superinfection of skin lesions
- Meningoencephalitis
- Disseminated zoster
- Hepatitis
- Pneumonitis
- Myelitis
- Cranial and peripheral nerve palsies
- Acute retinal necrosis

REFERENCES

1. Yawn BP, Saddier P, Wollan PC, et al. A population-based study of the incidence and complication rates of herpes zoster before zoster vaccine introduction. *Mayo Clin Proc*. 2007;82(11):1341–1349.
2. Centers for Disease Control and Prevention. Adult vaccination coverage—United States, 2010. *MMWR Morb Mortal Wkly Rep*. 2012;61(4):66–72.
3. Schmader KE, Levin MJ, Gnann JW Jr, et al. Efficacy, safety, and tolerability of herpes zoster vaccine in persons aged 50–59 years. *Clin Infect Dis*. 2012;54(7):922–928.
4. Harpaz R, Ortega-Sanchez IR, Seward JF, et al. Prevention of herpes zoster: recommendations of the Advisory Committee on Immunization Practices (ACIP). *MMWR Recomm Rep*. 2008;57(RR-5):1–30.
5. Chen N, Li Q, Zhang Y, et al. Vaccination for preventing postherpetic neuralgia. *Cochrane Database Syst Rev*. 2011;(3):CD007795.
6. Langan SM, Smeeth L, Margolis DJ, et al. Herpes zoster vaccine effectiveness against incident herpes zoster and post-herpetic neuralgia in an older US population: a cohort study. *PLoS Med*. 2013;10(4):e1001420.
7. Mounsey AL, Matthew LG, Slawson DC. Herpes zoster and postherpetic neuralgia: prevention and management. *Am Fam Physician*. 2005;72(6):1075–1080.
8. McDonald EM, de Kock J, Ram FS. Antivirals for management of herpes zoster including ophthalmicus: a systematic review of high-quality randomized controlled trials. *Antivir Ther (Lond)*. 2012;17(2):255–264.
9. Chen N, Yang M, He L, et al. Corticosteroids for preventing postherpetic neuralgia. *Cochrane Database Syst Rev*. 2010;(12):CD005582.
10. Li Q, Chen N, Yang J, et al. Antiviral treatment for preventing postherpetic neuralgia. *Cochrane Database Syst Rev*. 2009;(2):CD006866.
11. Cao H, Li X, Liu J. An updated review of the efficacy of cupping therapy. *PLoS One*. 2012;7(2):e31793.

SEE ALSO

- Bell Palsy; Chickenpox (Varicella Zoster); Herpes Eye Infections; Herpes Simplex
- Algorithm: Genital Ulcers

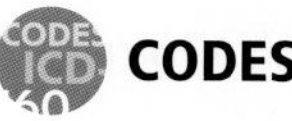

CODES

ICD10

- B02.9 Zoster without complications
- B02.29 Other postherpetic nervous system involvement

CLINICAL PEARLS

- Zoster vaccine is ACIP-recommended for patients ≥60 years of age (and since 2011, FDA-approved for patients >50 years).
- Patients with herpes should begin antiviral therapy within 72 hours of the onset of rash to be most effective.

H

HERPES, GENITAL

Cecilia M. Kipnis, MD

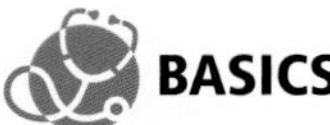

BASICS

DESCRIPTION
- Chronic, recurrent genital infection of any area innervated by the sacral ganglia
- Due to herpes simplex virus (HSV) type 1 or 2
- HSV-1 causes anogenital and orolabial lesions.
- HSV-2 causes anogenital lesions.
- Primary episode: occurs in the absence of preexisting antibodies to HSV-1 or HSV-2
- 1st episode nonprimary: first genital lesion eruption (likely due to HSV-2); preexisting antibodies to HSV-1 are present.
- Reactivation: recurrent episodes
- Synonym(s): herpes genitalis

EPIDEMIOLOGY
- Predominant age: 15–65 years; cases increase with age due to cumulative effect.
- Predominant sex: female > male
- Predominant race: non-Hispanic blacks

Incidence
>700,000 new cases per year

Prevalence
- 50–70% in developed countries and approaching 100% in developing countries (1)
- Overall prevalence of HSV-2 is 10–40% in the general population and up to 60–95% in the HIV-positive population (1).
- Up to 90% of seropositive persons have not been formally diagnosed.
- >50 million are infected with HSV-2 in the United States.

ETIOLOGY AND PATHOPHYSIOLOGY
- HSV is a double-stranded DNA virus of the Herpetoviridae family (1).
- Spread via genital-to-genital contact, oral-to-genital contact, and via maternal–fetal transmission. Viral shedding continues in the absence of lesions (2).
- Incubation is 2–12 days after exposure.

RISK FACTORS
- Risk increases with age, number of lifetime partners and history of sexually transmitted infections (STIs), sexual encounters before the age of 17 years, and partner with HSV-1 or HSV-2.
- Infection with HSV-1 increases the risk of being infected with HSV-2 by 3-fold.
- Immunosuppression, fever, stress, and trauma increase risk of reactivation once already infected.

COMMONLY ASSOCIATED CONDITIONS
Syphilis, HIV, chlamydia, gonorrhea, and other STI

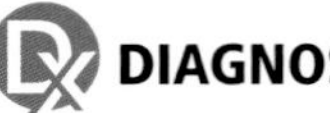

DIAGNOSIS

HISTORY
- Most patients are asymptomatic (74% of HSV-1 and 63% of HSV-2) or do not recognize clinical manifestations of disease (2).
- Symptoms can be more severe, associated with constitutional symptoms and last longer with primary episode.
- Common presenting symptoms (primary episode): multiple bilateral genital ulcers, dysuria, pruritus, fever, tender inguinal lymphadenopathy, headache, malaise, myalgias, cervicitis/dyspareunia, urethritis with watery discharge
- 1st episode, nonprimary: less severe symptoms than a primary episode due to preexisting antibodies to HSV-1 which have some activity against HSV-2
- Common presenting symptoms for recurrent episodes: prodrome of tingling, burning, or shooting pain (2–24 hours before lesion appears); single ulcer; dysuria; pruritus (last 4–6 days on average)
- Less common presentations: constipation (from anal involvement causing tenesmus), proctitis, stomatitis, pharyngitis, sacral paresthesias

PHYSICAL EXAM
- Impossible to differentiate among primary, 1st episode nonprimary, recurrent disease or type of virus (HSV-1 or HSV-2) on basis of symptoms and exam
- Lesions occur in "boxer short" distribution and within anus, vagina, and on cervix.
- Lesion may appear as papular, vesicular, pustular, ulcerated, or crusted; can be in various stages.
- Inguinal lymphadenopathy
- Extragenital manifestations include meningitis, recurrent meningitis (Mollaret syndrome), sacral radiculitis/paresthesias, encephalitis, transverse myelitis, and hepatitis.

Pediatric Considerations
Neonatal infection occurs in 20–50/100,000 live births. 80% of infections result from asymptomatic maternal viral shedding during an undiagnosed primary infection in the 3rd trimester. Transmission ranges from 30–50% if the primary episode is near time of delivery (3). High morbidity and mortality.

Pediatric Considerations
Suspect abuse if genital lesions in children are discovered.

DIFFERENTIAL DIAGNOSIS
- Primary syphilis
- Chancroid
- Herpes zoster
- Ulcerative balanitis
- Granuloma inguinale
- Lymphogranuloma venereum
- HIV
- Cytomegalovirus; Epstein-Barr virus
- Drug eruption
- Trauma
- Behçet syndrome
- Neoplasia

DIAGNOSTIC TESTS & INTERPRETATION

Initial Tests (lab, imaging)
- Viral isolation from lesion (swab or scraping)
  - Culture and PCR are preferred (4)[A].
  - Use Dacron or polyester-tipped swabs with plastic shafts because cotton tips/wood shafts inhibit viral growth and/or replication (1).
  - Culture by unroofing vesicle to obtain fluid sample. Specificity >99%, sensitivity depends on sample: 52–93% for vesicle, 41–72% for ulcer, 19–30% for crusted lesion (1,3,4).
  - Culture requires timely transport of live virus to the laboratory at 4°C (3).
  - PCR has the greatest sensitivity (98%) and specificity (>99%) but is also expensive and not readily available. It can increase detection rates by up to 70% (4). Used primarily for CSF samples (1).
- Type-specific serologic assays
  - Western blot (gold standard) and type-specific IgG antibody (glycoprotein G) enzyme-linked immunosorbent assay (ELISA) are used to discriminate between HSV-1 and HSV-2 (4)[B].
  - Western blot is >97–99% sensitive and specific but labor intensive and not readily available (1,4).
  - ELISA is 81–100% sensitive and 93–100% specific (1,3).
  - Seroconversion occurs 10 days–4 months after infection (4). *Antibody testing is not necessary if a positive culture or PCR has been obtained.*
  - IgM antibody testing is not useful because HSV IgM is often present with recurrent disease and does not distinguish new from old infection.
  - Screening with type-specific antibody in the general population is not recommended (4) but may be considered in
    - Asymptomatic patients with HIV infection
    - Discordant couples (1 partner with known HSV, the other without)

Test Interpretation
Cytopathology is not recommended for diagnosis (1).

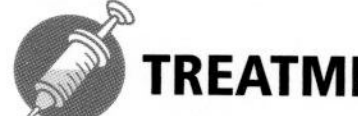

TREATMENT

GENERAL MEASURES

- Cool compresses with aluminum acetate (Domeboro)
- Ice packs to perineum, sitz baths, and topical anesthetics
- Analgesics, NSAIDs

MEDICATION

Antiviral medications should be started within 72 hours of onset of symptoms (including prodrome).

If presentation is >72 hours, antivirals may be helpful if new lesions continue to form or patient is experiencing significant pain.

First Line

- Acyclovir (5)[A]: the most studied antiviral in genital herpes. Decreases pain, duration of viral shedding, and time to full resolution.
  - Primary episode
    - 400 mg PO TID for 7–10 days
    - 200 mg PO 5× a day for 7–10 days
    - longer if needed for incomplete healing
  - Episodic therapy
    - 200 mg 5× per day for 5 days
    - 400 mg TID for 5 days
    - 800 mg BID for 5 days
    - 800 mg TID for 2 days
  - Daily suppression
    - 400 mg BID
  - Severe, complicated infections that require IV therapy
    - 5–10 mg/kg/dose q8h until clinical improvement; switch to PO therapy to complete a 10-day course.
  - HIV infection: 400 mg PO 3–5×/day until clinical resolution is attained
  - Precautions
    - Modify dose in patients with renal insufficiency.
- Valacyclovir (Valtrex) (5)[A]: prodrug of acyclovir, improved bioavailability, less frequent dosing
  - Primary episode
    - 1 g PO BID for 7–10 days
  - Episodic therapy
    - 500 mg PO BID for 3–5 days
    - 1 g PO daily for 5 days
  - Daily suppression
    - 500 mg PO daily or
    - 1 g PO daily
- Famciclovir (Famvir) (5)[A]
  - Primary episode
    - 250 mg PO TID for 7–10 days
  - Episodic therapy
    - 125 mg PO BID for 5 days
    - 1 g PO BID for 1 day
  - Daily suppression: 250 mg PO BID

Second Line

- Used for acyclovir-resistant HSV
- Foscarnet: 40 mg/kg/dose IV q8h in severe disease
  - Associated with significant toxicity
- Cidofovir topical: 0.1–0.3% gel for 5 days

Pregnancy Considerations

ACOG Clinical Management Guidelines (5)[A],(6)[C]:

- SCREENING: Pregnant women who test antibody negative for HSV-1 and HSV-2 should avoid sexual contact in the 3rd trimester if their partner is antibody positive.
- SUPRESSIVE THERAPY: Pregnant women with a history of genital herpes should be offered suppression treatment starting at 36 gestational weeks until delivery to decrease reactivation rate. Goal is to reduce the risk of neonatal infection and C-section. Recommended regimens to continue until delivery:
  - Acyclovir 400 mg PO TID
  - Valacyclovir 500 mg PO BID
- Monitor for outbreaks during pregnancy and examine for any lesions at the onset of labor. C-section is recommended if prodomal symptoms or lesions are present at onset of labor to reduce neonatal transmission.

Pediatric Considerations

- High-risk infants include those with active symptoms or lesions, those delivered vaginally with maternal lesions present, and those born during a primary maternal episode. Monitor closely, obtain specimen for diagnosis, and treat with acyclovir 20 mg/kg IV q8h for 10–14 days (5)[A].
- Low-risk infants who are asymptomatic can be observed while obtaining serum HSV PCR and ocular, nasal, anal, and oral cultures.
- Infants with possible HSV infection should be isolated from other neonates; maternal separation is not necessary and breastfeeding is not contraindicated.

ONGOING CARE

GENERAL PREVENTION

- Use barrier contraception, daily suppressive antiviral therapy, and avoid sexual contact when symptoms are present to decrease transmission.
- Abstinence is the only option to provide complete protection.

FOLLOW-UP RECOMMENDATIONS

- Avoid sexual contact when symptoms or lesions are present.
- Alert sex partners of herpes status prior to sexual activity.
- Concordant couples (i.e., both partners with the same type of herpes [HSV-1 or HSV-2]) may have sex without worry of triggering outbreaks.

Patient Monitoring

Test for other STIs if initial HSV infection.

DIET

PATIENT EDUCATION

- Herpes Resource Center: http://www.ashastd.org/herpes/herpes_overview.cfm
- Warren T. *The Good News About the Bad News: Herpes: Everything You Need to Know*. Oakland, CA: New Harbinger Publications; 2009.
- Centers for Disease Control and Prevention: http://www.cdc.gov/

PROGNOSIS

- Resolution of signs/symptoms: 3–21 days
- Average recurrence rate is 1–4 episodes per year (2).
- Antivirals do not eliminate virus from body but can reduce transmission, shedding, and outbreaks.

Pediatric Considerations

Neonatal infection survival rates: localized >95%; CNS 85%; systemic 30%

COMPLICATIONS

Behavioral issues include lowered self-esteem, guilt, anger, depression, fear of rejection, and fear of transmission to partner.

REFERENCES

1. LeGoff J, Péré H, Bélec L. Diagnosis of genital herpes simplex virus infection in the clinical laboratory. *Virol J*. 2014;11:83.
2. Hofstetter AM, Rosenthal SL, Stanberry LR. Current thinking on genital herpes. *Curr Opin Infect Dis*. 2014;27(1):75–83.
3. Scoular A. Using the evidence base on genital herpes: optimizing the use of diagnostic tests and information provision. *Sex Transm Infect*. 2002;78(3):160–165.
4. Geretti AM. Genital herpes. *Sex Transm Infect*. 2006;82(Suppl 4):iv31–iv34.
5. Centers for Disease Control and Prevention. 2010 STD treatment guidelines. http://www.cdc.gov/std/treatment/2010/. Accessed 2014.
6. American College of Obstetricians and Gynecologist. ACOG practice bulletin no. 82: management of herpes in pregnancy. *Obstet Gynecol*. 2007;109(6):1489–1498.

ADDITIONAL READING

- Centers for Disease Control and Prevention. 2010 STD treatment guidelines. http://www.cdc.gov/std/treatment/2010/. Accessed 2014.
- Money D, Steben M, Society of Obstetricians and Gynaecologists of Canada. SOGC clinical practice guidelines: guidelines for the management of herpes simplex virus in pregnancy. Number 208, June 2008. *Int J Gynaecol Obstet*. 2009;104(2):167–171.
- Sheffield JS, Hollier LM, Hill JB, et al. Acyclovir prophylaxis to prevent herpes simplex virus recurrence at delivery: a systematic review. *Obstet Gynecol*. 2003;102(6):1396–1403.
- Tavares F, Cheuvart B, Heineman T, et al. Meta-analysis of pregnancy outcomes in pooled randomized trials on a prophylactic adjuvanted glycoprotein D subunit herpes simplex virus vaccine. *Vaccine*. 2013;31(13):1759–1764.
- Tobian AA, Grabowski MK, Serwadda D, et al. Reactivation of herpes simplex virus type 2 after initiation of antiretroviral therapy. *J Infect Dis*. 2013;208(5):839–846.

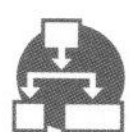

SEE ALSO

Algorithm: Genital Ulcers

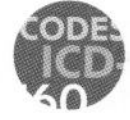

CODES

ICD10

- A60.00 Herpesviral infection of urogenital system, unspecified
- A60.04 Herpesviral vulvovaginitis
- A60.09 Herpesviral infection of other urogenital tract

CLINICAL PEARLS

- Genital herpes infections can be caused by HSV-1 and HSV-2.
- Most seropositive individuals are unaware that they are infected.
- Most primary episodes are asymptomatic.
- Viral shedding occurs in the absence of lesions.

HICCUPS

James H. Lewis, MD, FACP, FACG, AGAF

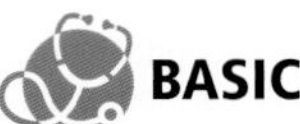

BASICS

DESCRIPTION

- Hiccups are caused by a repetitive sudden involuntary contraction of the inspiratory muscles (predominantly the diaphragm) terminated by abrupt closure of the glottis, stopping the inflow of air and producing a characteristic sound.
- System(s) affected: nervous, pulmonary
- Synonym(s): hiccoughs; singultus

Geriatric Considerations

Can be a serious problem among the elderly

Pregnancy Considerations

- Fetal hiccups are noted as rhythmic fetal movements (confirmed sonographically) that can be confused with contractions.
- Fetal hiccups often recur in subsequent pregnancies.

EPIDEMIOLOGY

- Predominant age: all ages (including fetus)
- Predominant sex: male > female (4:1)

Prevalence

Self-limited hiccups are extremely common, as are intra- and postoperative hiccups.

ETIOLOGY AND PATHOPHYSIOLOGY

- Pathophysiologic significance is unknown; only found in mammalian species; may be a vestigial reflex; hiccups have been associated with >100 underlying disorders (1–3). One theory suggests hiccups function to remove swallowed gas from the stomach as a burping reflex (4).
- Results from stimulation of ≥1 limbs of the hiccup reflux arc (vagus and phrenic nerves) with a "hiccup center" located in the upper spinal cord
- In men, >90% have an organic basis, whereas in women, a psychogenic cause may be more likely.
- Specific underlying causes include the following:
  - Alcohol abuse
  - CNS lesions (brain stem tumors, vascular lesions, Parkinson disease)
  - Diaphragmatic irritation (tumors, pericarditis, eventration, splenomegaly, hepatomegaly, peritonitis)
  - Irritation of the tympanic membrane
  - Pharyngitis, laryngitis
  - Mediastinal and other thoracic lesions (pneumonia, aortic aneurysm, tuberculosis [TB], myocardial infarction [MI], lung cancer, rib exostoses)
  - Esophageal lesions (reflux esophagitis, achalasia, *Candida* esophagitis, carcinoma, obstruction)
  - Gastric lesions (ulcer, distention, cancer)
  - Hepatic lesions (hepatitis, hepatoma)
  - Pancreatic lesions (pancreatitis, pseudocysts, cancer)
  - Inflammatory bowel disease
  - Cholelithiasis, cholecystitis
  - Prostatic disorders
  - Appendicitis
  - Postoperative, abdominal procedures
  - Toxic metabolic causes (uremia, hyponatremia, gout, diabetes)
  - Drug-induced (dexamethasone, methylprednisolone, anabolic steroids, benzodiazepines, α-methyldopa, propofol)
  - Psychogenic causes (hysterical neurosis, grief, malingering)
  - Idiopathic

RISK FACTORS

- General anesthesia; conscious sedation
- Postoperative state
- Genitourinary disorders
- Irritation of the vagus nerve branches
- Structural, vascular, infectious, neoplastic, or traumatic CNS lesions

GENERAL PREVENTION

- Identify and correct the underlying cause if possible.
- Avoid gastric distention.
- Acupuncture is equal or superior to chronic drug therapy to control hiccups.

COMMONLY ASSOCIATED CONDITIONS

See "Etiology."

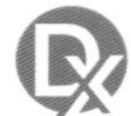

DIAGNOSIS

- Hiccup attacks usually occur at brief intervals and last only a few seconds or minutes. Persistent bouts lasting >48 hours often imply an underlying physical or metabolic disorder.
- Intractable hiccups may occur continuously for months or years (1).
- Hiccups usually occur with a frequency of 4–60 per minute (1).

HISTORY

- Recent surgery (especially genitourinary)
- General anesthesia
- Behavioral health history
- Medications
- Alcoholism
- GI, cardiac, or pulmonary disorders (see "Etiology")
- Malignancy

PHYSICAL EXAM

- Correlate exam with potential etiologies (e.g., rales with pneumonia).
- Examine the ear canal for foreign bodies.

DIFFERENTIAL DIAGNOSIS

Hiccups may rarely be confused with burping (eructation).

DIAGNOSTIC TESTS & INTERPRETATION

- If history suggests an underlying etiology, consider condition-specific testing as appropriate (e.g., CBC, metabolic panel, chest x-ray).
- Fluoroscopy is useful to determine whether 1 hemidiaphragm is dominant.

Diagnostic Procedures/Other

- Upper endoscopy; colonoscopy; CT scan (or other imaging) of brain, thorax, abdomen, and pelvis looking for underlying causes
- The extent of the workup is often in proportion to the duration and severity of the hiccups (1,2).

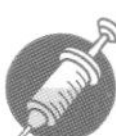

TREATMENT

- Outpatient (usually)
- Inpatient (if elderly, debilitated, or intractable hiccups)
- Most hiccup treatments are purely anecdotal; those with recorded success are described.

GENERAL MEASURES

- Seek medical attention for frequent bouts or persistent hiccups.
- Treat any specific underlying cause when identified (1–3)[C]
  - Dilate esophageal stricture or obstruction.
  - Treat ulcers or reflux disease.
  - Remove hair or foreign body from ear canal
  - Angostura bitters for alcohol-induced hiccups
  - Catheter stimulation of pharynx for operative and postoperative hiccups
  - Antifungal treatment for *Candida* esophagitis
  - Correct electrolyte imbalance.
- Medical measures
  - Relief of gastric distention (gastric lavage, nasogastric aspiration, induced vomiting)
  - Counterirritation of the vagus nerve (supraorbital pressure, carotid sinus massage, digital rectal massage)—use with caution
  - Respiratory center stimulants (breathing 5% CO_2)
  - Behavioral health modification (hypnosis, meditation)
  - Phrenic nerve block or electrical stimulation (or pacing) of the dominant hemidiaphragm
  - Acupuncture
  - Miscellaneous (cardioversion)

MEDICATION

First Line

Possible drug remedies (1,2)

- Baclofen, a GABA analog: 5–10 mg PO TID (2,4–6)[B]
- Chlorpromazine: 25–50 mg PO/IV TID
- Haloperidol: 2–5 mg PO/IM followed by 1–2 mg PO TID
- Phenytoin: 200–300 mg PO HS
- Metoclopramide: 5–10 mg PO QID
- Nifedipine: 10–20 mg PO daily to TID
- Amitriptyline: 10 mg PO TID
- Viscous lidocaine 2% : 5 ml PO daily to TID
- Gabapentin (Neurontin): 300 mg PO HS; may increase up to 1,800 mg/day PO in divided doses (7)[B]
- Contraindications: Refer to manufacturer's literature.
  - Baclofen is not recommended in patients with stroke or other cerebral lesions or in severe renal impairment.
- Precautions: Refer to manufacturer's literature.
  - Abrupt withdrawal of baclofen should be avoided.

Second Line

Possible drug therapies (1,2)[C]

- Amantadine, carbidopa-levodopa in Parkinson disease
- Steroid replacement in Addison disease
- Antifungal agent in *Candida* esophagitis
- Ondansetron in carcinomatosis with vomiting
- Nefopam (a nonopioid analgesic with antishivering properties related to antihistamines and antiparkinsonian drugs) is available outside the United States in both IV and oral formulations.

ISSUES FOR REFERRAL

For acupuncture or phrenic nerve crush, block, or electrostimulation; cardioversion

SURGERY/OTHER PROCEDURES

- Phrenic nerve crush or transaction or electrostimulation of the dominant diaphragmatic leaflet
- Resection of rib exostoses

COMPLEMENTARY & ALTERNATIVE MEDICINE

- Acupuncture is increasingly being used to manage persistent or intractable hiccups, especially in patients with cancer (6,8)[A].
- Simple home remedies (1,2)[C]
  - Swallowing a spoonful of sugar
  - Sucking on hard candy or swallowing peanut butter
  - Holding breath and increasing pressure on diaphragm (Valsalva maneuver)
  - Tongue traction
  - Lifting the uvula with a cold spoon
  - Inducing fright
  - Smelling salts
  - Rebreathing into a paper (not plastic) bag
  - Sipping ice water
  - Rubbing a wet cotton-tipped applicator between hard and soft palate for 1 minute

INPATIENT CONSIDERATIONS

Admission Criteria/Initial Stabilization

Most patients can be managed as outpatients; those with severe intractable hiccups may require rehydration, pain control, IV medications, or surgery.

ONGOING CARE

FOLLOW-UP RECOMMENDATIONS

Patient Monitoring

Until hiccups cease

DIET

Avoid gastric distension from overeating, carbonated beverages, and aerophagia.

PATIENT EDUCATION

See "General Measures."

PROGNOSIS

- Hiccups often cease during sleep.
- Most acute benign hiccups resolve spontaneously or with home remedies.
- Intractable hiccups may last for years or decades.
- Hiccups have persisted despite bilateral phrenic nerve transection.

COMPLICATIONS

- Inability to eat
- Weight loss
- Exhaustion, debility
- Insomnia
- Cardiac arrhythmias
- Wound dehiscence
- Death (rare)

REFERENCES

1. Lewis JH. Hiccups: causes and cures. *J Clin Gastroenterol*. 1985;7(6):539–552.
2. Lewis JH. Hiccups and their cures. *Clin Perspect Gastroenterol*. 2000;3(5):277–283.
3. Chang FY, Lu CL. Hiccup: mystery, nature and treatment. *J Neurogastroenterol Motil*. 2012;18(2):123–130.
4. Ramírez FC, Graham DY. Treatment of intractable hiccup with baclofen: results of a double-blind randomized, controlled, cross-over study. *Am J Gastroenterol*. 1992;87(12):1789–1791.
5. Mirijello A, Addolorato G, D'Angelo C, et al. Baclofen in the treatment of persistent hiccup: a case series. *Int J Clin Pract*. 2013;67(9):918–921.
6. Moretto EN, Wee B, Wiffen PJ, et al. Interventions for treating persistent and intractable hiccups in adults. *Cochrane Database Syst Rev*. 2013;1:CD008768.
7. Thompson DF, Brooks KG. Gabapentin therapy of hiccups. *Ann Pharmacother*. 2013;47(6):897–903.
8. Choi TY, Lee MS, Ernst E. Acupuncture for cancer patients suffering from hiccups: a systematic review and meta-analysis. *Complement Ther Med*. 2012;20(6):447–455.

ADDITIONAL READING

- Bilotta F, Rosa G. Nefopam for severe hiccups. *N Engl J Med*. 2000;343(26):1973–1974.
- Brostoff JM, Birns J, Benjamin E. The "cotton bud technique" as a cure for hiccups. *Eur Arch Otorhinolaryngol*. 2009;266(5):775–776.
- Chen KS, Bullard MJ, Chien YY, et al. Baclofen toxicity in patients with severely impaired renal function. *Ann Pharmacother*. 1997;31(11):1315–1320.
- Chou CL, Chen CA, Lin SH, et al. Baclofen-induced neurotoxicity in chronic renal failure patients with intractable hiccups. *South Med J*. 2006;99(11):1308–1309.
- Howes D. Hiccups: a new explanation for the mysterious reflex. *Bioessays*. 2012;34(6):451–453.
- Kranke P, Eberhart LH, Morin AM, et al. Treatment of hiccups during general anaesthesia or sedation: a qualitative systematic review. *Eur J Anaesthesiol*. 2003;20(3):239–244.
- Landers C, Turner D, Makin C, et al. Propofol associated hiccups and treatment with lidocaine. *Anesth Analg*. 2008;107(5):1757–1758.
- Marinella MA. Diagnosis and management of hiccups in the patient with advanced cancer. *J Support Oncol*. 2009;7(4):122–127,130.
- Miwa H, Kondo T. Hiccups in Parkinson's disease: an overlooked non-motor symptom? *Parkinsonism Relat Disord*. 2010;16(4):249–251.
- Okuda Y, Kitajima T, Asai T. Use of a nerve stimulator for phrenic nerve block in treatment of hiccups. *Anesthesiology*. 1998;88(2):525–527.
- Schiff E, River Y, Oliven A, et al. Acupuncture therapy for persistent hiccups. *Am J Med Sci*. 2002;323(3):166–168.
- Schuchmann JA, Browne BA. Persistent hiccups during rehabilitation hospitalization: three case reports and review of the literature. *Am J Phys Med Rehabil*. 2007;86(12):1013–1018.

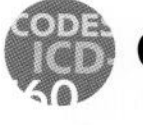

CODES

ICD10

- R06.6 Hiccough
- F45.8 Other somatoform disorders

CLINICAL PEARLS

- Most hiccups resolve spontaneously.
- An organic cause for persistent hiccups is more likely to be found in men.
- Rule out a foreign body in the ear canal as hiccup trigger.
- Baclofen is the only pharmacologic agent proven effective in a clinical trial.
- Acupuncture is effective for persistent hiccups.

HIDRADENITIS SUPPURATIVA

Travis C. Geraci, MD • Siva Vithananthan, MD, FACS

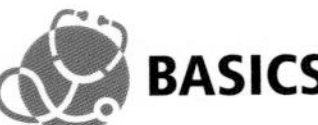

BASICS

DESCRIPTION

- Chronic follicular occlusive disease manifested as recurrent inflammatory nodules, abscesses, sinus tracts, and complex scar formation
- Lesions are tender, malodorous, often with exudative drainage.
- Common in intertriginous skin regions: axillae, groin, perianal, perineal, inframammary skin
- Most common in women, ages 20–30 years
- System affected: skin.
- Synonym(s): acne inversa; Verneuil disease; apocrinitis; hidradenitis axillaris

Geriatric Considerations

Rare after menopause

Pediatric Considerations

Rarely occurs before puberty; occurrence in children associated with premature adrenarche

Pregnancy Considerations

No Accutane (isotretinoin) or tetracycline treatment during pregnancy. Disease may ease during pregnancy and rebound after parturition.

EPIDEMIOLOGY

Predominant sex: female > male (3:1).

Incidence

Peak onset during 2nd and 3rd decades of life

Prevalence

0.3–4%

ETIOLOGY AND PATHOPHYSIOLOGY

- Not fully understood; previously considered a disorder of apocrine glands
- Inflammatory disorder of the hair follicle triggered by follicular plugging within apocrine gland–bearing skin.
- Hormonally induced ductal keratinocyte proliferation leads to a failure of follicular epithelial shedding, causing follicular occlusion.
- Mechanical stress on skin (intertriginous regions) precipitates follicular rupture and immune response.
- Bacterial involvement is a secondary event.
- Rupture and reepithelialization cause sinus tracts to form.
- Obesity and smoking are major risk factors in disease onset and severity.

Genetics

- Familiar occurrences suggest single gene transmission (autosomal dominant), but the condition may also be polygenic.
- Estimated 40% of patients have an affected family member.

RISK FACTORS

- Obesity
- Smoking
- Hyperandrogenism, oral contraceptive pills (OCPs)
- Lithium may trigger onset of or exacerbate this condition.

GENERAL PREVENTION

- Lose weight if overweight or obese.
- Smoking cessation
- Avoid constrictive clothing/synthetic fabrics, frictional trauma, heat exposure, excessive sweating, shaving, depilation, and deodorants.
- Use of antiseptic soaps

COMMONLY ASSOCIATED CONDITIONS

- Acne vulgaris, acne conglobate
- Perifolliculitis capitis abscedens et suffodiens (dissecting cellulitis of scalp)
- Pilonidal disease
- Arthritis and spondyloarthritis (seronegative)
- Obesity (with diabetes, atopy, acanthosis)
- Irritable bowel disease (Crohn disease)
- Squamous cell carcinoma
- PAPASH syndrome (pyogenic arthritis, pyoderma gangrenosum, acne, suppurative hydradenitis)

DIAGNOSIS

HISTORY

- Diagnostic criteria adopted by the 2nd International Conference on Hidradenitis Suppurativa, March 2009, San Francisco, CA
- All 3 criteria must be present for diagnosis:
  - Typical lesions: painful nodules, abscesses, draining sinus, bridged scars, and "tombstone" double-ended pseudocomedones in secondary lesions
  - Typical topography: axillae, groins, perineal and perianal region, buttocks, infra- and intermammary folds
  - Chronicity and recurrences, commonly refractory to initial treatments.

PHYSICAL EXAM

- Tender nodules (dome-shaped) 0.5–3 cm in size are present:
  - Location corresponds with the distribution of apocrine-related mammary tissue and terminal hair follicles dependent on low androgen concentrations.
  - Sites ordered by frequency of occurrence: axillary, inguinal, perianal and perineal, mammary and inframammary, buttock, pubic region, chest, scalp, retroauricular, eyelid
  - Large lesions are often fluctuant; comedones may be present.
  - Possible malodorous discharge
- Hurley clinical staging system
  - Stage I: abscess formation (singular or multiple) without sinus tracts or scarring
  - Stage II: widely separated, recurrent abscesses with tract formation and scarring
  - Stage III: diffuse, multiple interconnected tracts and abscesses
- Sartorius clinical staging system (points attributed)
  - Anatomic region
  - Quantity and quality of lesions
  - Distance between lesions
  - Presence or absence of normal skin between lesions

DIFFERENTIAL DIAGNOSIS

- Acne vulgaris, conglobate
- Furunculosis/carbuncles
- Infected Bartholin or sebaceous cysts
- Lymphadenopathy/lymphadenitis
- Cutaneous Langerhans cell histiocytosis
- Actinomycosis
- Granuloma inguinale
- Lymphogranuloma venereum
- Apocrine nevus
- Crohn disease with anogenital fistula(s) (may coexist with hidradenitis suppurativa)
- Cutaneous tuberculosis
- Fox-Fordyce disease

DIAGNOSTIC TESTS & INTERPRETATION

Initial Tests (lab, imaging)

- Cultures of skin or aspirates of boils are most commonly negative. When positive, cultures are often polymicrobial and commonly grow *Staphylococcus aureus* and *Staphylococcus epidermidis*.
- Lesion biopsy usually unnecessary. Useful to rule out other disorders such as squamous cell carcinoma
- May note increased erythrocyte sedimentation rate (ESR), leukocytosis, decreased serum iron, normocytic anemia, or changes in serum electrophoresis pattern

Follow-Up Tests & Special Considerations

- Consider biopsy of concerning lesions due to increased risk of squamous cell carcinoma.
- If the patient is female, overweight, and/or hirsute, check the following:
  - Dehydroepiandrosterone sulfate
  - Testosterone: total and free
  - Sex hormone-binding globulin
  - Progesterone

Diagnostic Procedures/Other

- Incision and drainage, culture and biopsy
- US may be useful in planning an excision to identify the full extent of sinus tracts.

Test Interpretation

- Dermis shows granulomatous inflammation and inflammatory cells, giant cells, sinus tracts, subcutaneous abscesses, extensive fibrosis.
- Hair follicular dilatation and occlusion by keratinized stratified squamous epithelium

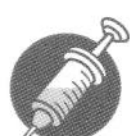

TREATMENT

Treatment goals: Reduce extent of disease, prevent new lesions, remove chronic disease, limit scar formation.

- Conservative treatment includes all items under general prevention, plus use of warm compresses, sitz baths, topical antiseptics for inflamed lesions, and nonopioid analgesics.
- Weight loss and smoking cessation result in marked improvement.
- For stage I–II, attempt medical treatment.
- Short medical trial may be appropriate in stage III prior to moving on to surgical therapies.
- No medications are curative; relapse is almost inevitable, but the disease may be controlled.

GENERAL MEASURES

- Education and psychosocial support
- Appropriate hygiene including avoidance of shearing stress to skin (light clothing), daily cleansing with antibacterial soap
- Diet: Avoid dairy and high glycemic loads.
- Symptomatic treatment for acute lesions.
- Improve environmental factors that cause follicular blockage (see "General Prevention").
- Smoking cessation and weight loss

MEDICATION

First Line

- Stage I disease: Consider either systemic or topical antibiotics:
  - Topical antibiotics (clindamycin has the most evidence) (1)[B]
    - Clindamycin 1% solution BID × 12 weeks with or without Benzoyl peroxide 5–10% solution
    - Chlorhexidine 4% solution

- Systemic antibiotics (initial 7–10 day course)
  - Tetracycline 500 mg BID
  - Doxycycline 100 mg q12h
  - Augmentin 875 mg q8–12h
  - Clindamycin 300 mg BID (2)[B]
- Stage II–III disease
  - Address overlying bacterial infection with broad-spectrum coverage. Base antibiotic selection on disease location, characteristics; longer durations (3–6 months) may be required.
  - Tetracycline 500 mg BID
  - Minocycline 100 mg BID
  - Doxycycline 100 mg BID
  - Minor surgical procedures (punch débridement, local unroofing) to treat individual lesions or sinus tracts
- Other modalities (rarely used):
  - Hormonal therapy: antiandrogenic therapy such as cyproterone acetate (may not be available in the United States), estrogen/norgestrel oral contraceptive, finasteride (5 mg daily) (3)[B]
- Intralesional corticosteroids: accelerates healing, although efficacy not formally evaluated (triamcinolone acetonide 5–10 mg/mL)

Second Line

- Combination antibiotic regimens
  - Clindamycin and rifampin
  - Rifampin, moxifloxacin, and metronidazole
- Dapsone 50–150 mg daily (4)[C]
- Metformin: significant reduction in Sartorius score (5)[B]
- Oral retinoids (Isotretinoin): poor efficacy, limited therapeutic effect (6)[B].
- TNF-alpha inhibitors: clinical efficacy for infliximab, adalimumab, etanercept (7)[A]

ISSUES FOR REFERRAL

- Lack of response to treatment, stage II–III disease, or concern for malignancy (squamous cell carcinoma) is a reason to refer for surgical excision or radiation/laser treatment (stage II).
- If significant psychosocial stress exists secondary to disease, refer for stress management or psychiatric evaluation.
- Suspicion of hyperandrogenic states (e.g., polycystic ovary syndrome [PCOS]) should prompt investigation or referral.
- Severe perianal/perivulvar disease or otherwise very extensive disease may prompt referral to plastic surgeon or reconstructive urologist.

SURGERY/OTHER PROCEDURES

- Important mode of treatment
- Could be used in conjunction with antibiotics or if 1st-line therapy fails
- Various surgical approaches have been used for stage II–III disease (8,9)[B]:
  - Incision and drainage: may be necessary to treat as a temporizing method for acute flare-ups
  - Deroofing and marsupialization of the sinus tracts is often beneficial primarily for Hurley stage I–II disease, as healing time is reduced. Recurrences remain common but usually are smaller than original lesions.
  - Wide full-thickness excision with healing by granulation or flap placement is the most definitive treatment and rarely has local recurrence if all sinus tracts are excised. Rates of local recurrence (within 3–72 months): axillary (3%), perianal (0%), inguinoperineal (37%), submammary (50%)
- Laser therapy for Hurley stage I–II disease (rarely used)
  - Consider monthly treatments with neodymium-doped yttrium aluminum garnet (Nd:YAG) laser for 3–4 months.
  - CO_2 laser ablation with healing by secondary intention

ONGOING CARE

FOLLOW-UP RECOMMENDATIONS

Follow up monthly or sooner to evaluate progress and to assist with symptom management.

DIET

- Avoid dairy, high glycemic loads.
- Healthy diet that promotes weight loss
- May benefit from zinc supplementation

PATIENT EDUCATION

- Severity can range from only 2–3 papules per year to extensive draining sinus tracts.
- Medications are temporizing measures, rarely curative. Attempts at local surgical "cures" do not affect recurrence at other sites.
- Smoking cessation and weight loss can improve symptoms significantly. Hidradenitis Suppurativa Foundation: www.hs-foundation.org

PROGNOSIS

- Individual lesions heal slowly in 10–30 days.
- Recurrences may last for several years.
- Relentlessly progressive scarring and sinus tracts are likely with severe disease.
- Radical wide-area excision, with removal of all hair-bearing skin in the affected area, shows the greatest chance for cure.

COMPLICATIONS

- Contracture and stricturing of the skin after extensive abscess rupture, scarring, and healing; or at sites of surgical excisions
- Lymphatic obstruction, lymphedema
- Psychosocial: anxiety, malaise, depression/self-injury (SI)
- Anemia, amyloidosis, and hypoproteinemia (due to chronic suppuration)
- Lumbosacral epidural abscess, sacral bacterial osteomyelitis
- Squamous cell carcinoma may develop in indolent sinus tracts.
- Disseminated infection or septicemia (rare)
- Urethral, rectal, or bladder fistula (rare)

REFERENCES

1. Jemec GB, Wendelboe P. Topical clindamycin versus systemic tetracycline in the treatment of hidradenitis suppurativa. *J Am Acad Dermatol*. 1998;39(6):971–974.
2. van der Zee HH, Boer J, Prens EP, et al. The effect of combined treatment with oral clindamycin and oral rifampicin in patients with hidradenitis suppurativa. *Dermatology*. 2009;219(2):143–147.
3. Searles GE. Daily oral finasteride 5 mg for hidradenitis suppurativa. Paper presented at: the Annual meeting of the Canadian Dermatology Association. Vancouver, British Columbia, Canada, July 2009.
4. Kaur MR, Lewis HM. Hidradenitis suppurativa treated with dapsone: a case series of five patients. *J Dermatolog Treat*. 2006;17(4):211–213.
5. Verdolini R, Clayton N, Smith A, et al. Metformin for the treatment of hidradenitis suppurativa: a little help along the way. *J Eur Acad Dermatol Venereol*. 2013;27(9):1101–1108.
6. Soria A, Canoui-Pontrine F, Wolkenstein P, et al. Absence of efficacy of oral isotretinoin in hidradenitis suppurativa: a retrospective study based on patient's outcome assessment. *Dermatology*. 2009;218(2):134–135.
7. Blok JL, van Hattem S, Jonkman MF, et al. Systemic therapy with immunosuppressive agents and retinoids in hidradenitis suppurativa: a systematic review. *Br J Dermatol*. 2013;168(2):243–252.
8. Kagan RJ, Yakuboff KP, Warner P, et al. Surgical treatment of hidradenitis suppurativa: a 10-year experience. *Surgery*. 2005;138(4):734–740; discussion 740–741.
9. Mandal A, Watson J. Experience with different treatment modules in hidradenitis suppuritiva: a study of 106 cases. *Surgeon*. 2005;3:23–26.

ADDITIONAL READING

- Alikhan A, Lynch PJ, Eisen DB. Hidradenitis suppurativa: a comprehensive review. *J Am Acad Dermatol*. 2009;60(4):539–561.
- Jemec GB. Clinical practice. Hidradenitis suppurativa. *N Engl J Med*. 2012;366(12):158–164.
- Rambhatla PV, Lim HW, Hamzavi I. A systematic review of treatments for hidradenitis suppurativa. *Arch Dermatol*. 2012;148(4):439–446.
- Slade DE, Powell BW, Mortimer PS. Hidradenitis suppurativa: pathogenesis and management. *Br J Plast Surg*. 2003;56(5):451–461.

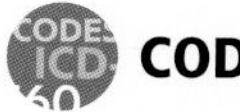

CODES

ICD10

L73.2 Hidradenitis suppurativa

CLINICAL PEARLS

- Chronic inflammatory disease of the skin, often difficult to control with behavior changes and medication alone
- For patients with refractory or severe disease, wide local excision provides the only chance at a cure. Success rates depend on the location and extent of excision.

H

HIRSUTISM

Laura Novak, MD • Imola K. Osapay, MD

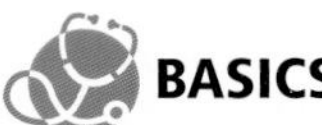

BASICS

DESCRIPTION

- Presence of excessive terminal (coarse, pigmented) hair of body and face, in a male pattern, in women of reproductive age
- May be present in normal adults as an ethnic characteristic or may develop as a result of androgen excess
- Different from hypertrichosis which is vellus (fine, nonpigmented) hair in generalized, nonsexual distribution, independent of androgens
- Most common in polycystic ovarian syndrome (PCOS); may be accompanied by menstrual irregularities, insulin resistance, obesity, or acne
- System(s) affected: dermatologic, endocrine/metabolic, reproductive

Pregnancy Considerations

- May have related infertility. Offer intervention, if desired.
- As hormone balance improves, fertility may increase; provide contraception, as needed.
- Several medications used for treatment are contraindicated in pregnancy.

EPIDEMIOLOGY

Prevalence

5–10% of adult women

ETIOLOGY AND PATHOPHYSIOLOGY

- Hirsutism is due to increased androgenic (male) hormones, either from increased peripheral binding (idiopathic) or increased production from the ovaries, adrenals, or fat. Exogenous medications can also cause hirsutism.
- Androgens determine the type and distribution of hair over the body.
- The effects of androgens are mediated through 5-α reductase (1).

Genetics

Multifactorial

RISK FACTORS

- Family history, race, ethnicity
- Anovulation

GENERAL PREVENTION

- Women with late-onset congenital adrenal hyperplasia (CAH) should be counseled that they may be carriers for the severe early-onset childhood disease.
- Avoid quackery and unlicensed electrolysis.

COMMONLY ASSOCIATED CONDITIONS

- PCOS: most common cause of hirsutism. Variable presentation but commonly presents with some combination of excess androgen, abnormal menses, and insulin resistance. It is estimated that 75% of hirsute women have PCOS.
- Insulin resistance syndromes/metabolic syndrome
  - Presence of associated insulin resistance or PCOS can increase the risk of heart disease.
- Prolonged amenorrhea and anovulation
  - Prolonged amenorrhea may, over time, put the patient at risk for endometrial hyperplasia or carcinoma.
- Hypothyroidism or hyperprolactinemia
- Late-onset CAH (21-hydroxylase deficiency): a genetic enzyme deficiency associated with more severe and earlier onset hirsutism; present in <2% of hirsute, amenorrheic patients
- Tumor: rare (<0.2%); ovarian or adrenal; especially if associated with virilization (rapid onset, clitoromegaly, balding, deepening voice) (2)
- Cushing syndrome: rare; characterized by central obesity, moon facies, striae, hypertension

DIAGNOSIS

HISTORY

- Age of onset (usually gradual), duration of symptoms, and psychosocial impact on patient
- Menstrual and fertility history
- Medication history: Look for use of valproic acid, testosterone, danazol, glucocorticoids, and athletic performance drugs.
- If galactorrhea is present, workup for hyperprolactinemia.
- Family history of PCOS, CAH, DM type 2, male pattern balding before age 30 years

PHYSICAL EXAM

- The Ferriman-Gallwey scale (an instrument that rates hair growth in 9 areas on a scale of 0–4, with >8 being positive) may be used for diagnosis but underrates patient's perception of hirsutism and altered by previous cosmetic treatment (1).
- Increased hair growth on face, chest, and groin
- Check skin for acne, striae, acanthosis nigricans (velvety black skin in the axilla, neck, in insulin resistance)
- An abdominal exam and bimanual exam should be performed to check for palpable masses.
- Virilization: Deep voice, balding, and clitoromegaly can indicate risk of tumor.

DIFFERENTIAL DIAGNOSIS

- PCOS—irregular menses, elevated androgens, polycystic ovaries on US, infertility, insulin resistance
- Idiopathic hyperandrogenemia—elevated androgen levels, with normal menses and ovaries
- Idiopathic hirsutism—hirsutism with normal androgen levels
- Late-onset CAH presents in adolescence with severe hirsutism and irregular menses.
- Androgen-secreting tumor—rapid onset, virilization, resistance to treatment
- Thyroid dysfunction
- Rare endocrine disorders—Cushing (central obesity, stria, and hypertension), acromegaly (enlarging extremities and facial deformity), prolactinoma (amenorrhea and galactorrhea) (2)

DIAGNOSTIC TESTS & INTERPRETATION

- Diagnosis is clinical.
- PCOS is diagnosed by having two out of three signs: menstrual dysfunction, clinical or biochemical hyperandrogenemia, polycystic ovaries on US (2)[C].
- Empiric treatment without lab workup is an acceptable option in mild–moderate hirsutism.
- Lab testing is performed to rule out underlying tumor and pituitary diseases, which are rare.

Initial Tests (lab, imaging)

Basic workup recommended by American Congress of Obstetrician and Gynecologist (ACOG) (3)[C]; total testosterone, thyroid-stimulating hormone (TSH), and, if clinically suspicious, an insulin resistance workup

- Testosterone: random testosterone level is usually sufficient. A morning free testosterone is slightly more sensitive, but the difference is not clinically relevant (1,4): Level >150 (some use 200) ng/dL may indicate tumor (2,3).
- If testosterone is >150 (some use 200) ng/dL, consider ovarian or adrenal tumor. Testosterone is made by both the ovaries and adrenals, so both areas should be scanned. US is best for the ovaries, and CT is best for the adrenals.
- If testosterone is <150 ng/dL, the need for further testing is determined by the clinical findings (see below).
- TSH-elevation indicates hypothyroidism.
- Insulin resistance testing: Results vary with age and ethnicity.
  - Fasting insulin level >20 or fasting glucose-to-insulin ratio <4.5 may indicate resistance.
  - ACOG recommends fasting and 2-hour glucose after 75-g glucose load in PCOS.
- Ovarian US to diagnose PCOS
- If the patient is amenorrheic, check prolactin, FSH, LH, and a pregnancy test in addition.

Follow-Up Tests & Special Considerations

- 17-hydroxyprogesterone (17-OHP)
  - Elevations of 17-OHP (>300) can indicate nonclassic CAH; rare (<2%)
  - Consider in patients with onset in early adolescence or high-risk group (Ashkenazi Jews)
  - If elevated levels, do corticotropin stimulation test.
- If prolactin level is high, image pituitary
- If PCOS is diagnosed, ACOG recommends screening for dyslipidemia and DM type 2 (1)[C].
- Dehydroepiandrosterone sulfate (DHEA-S) is no longer recommended routinely but should be checked in virilization (4)[C].
  - Levels >700 may indicate adrenal tumor.

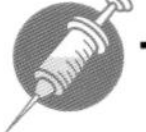

TREATMENT

GENERAL MEASURES

- Treatment in mild hirsutism depends on patient preference and psychosocial effect.
- Cosmetic treatment includes many methods of hair removal; temporary: shaving, chemical depilation, plucking, waxing. Permanent: laser epilation and photoepilation are preferred to electrolysis (3)[C].
- If patient desires pregnancy, induction of ovulation may be necessary.
- Provide contraception, as needed.
- Encourage patient to maintain ideal weight with lifestyle modification.
- Treat accompanying acne.

MEDICATION

First Line

- Treatment goal is to decrease new hair growth and improve metabolic disorders.
- Oral contraceptives are first line (5)[B]; they will decrease androgens, improve metabolic syndrome, and slow but not reverse hair growth. Take 6 months to show effect and are continued for years; any preparation is effective; however, those containing the progestins, norgestimate, desogestrel, or drospirenone may have more androgen-blocking effects (2)[C].
- Progesterone (depot or intermittent oral) can be used if estrogens are contraindicated (3)[C].
- Eflornithine (Vaniqa) HCl cream: apply BID at least 8 hours apart; reduces facial hair in 40% of women (must be used indefinitely to prevent regrowth). Only FDA-approved hirsutism treatment.

Second Line

- Insulin sensitizers (metformin, thioglitazones) are mildly effective but less so than oral contraceptives. May be used in diabetes or if oral contraceptives are contraindicated. Metformin is more effective than thioglitazones (2)[A].
- Antiandrogenic drugs must be used in combination with oral contraceptives to prevent menorrhagia and potential fetal toxicity; will further reduce hirsutism 15–25%. Usually begun after 6 months of 1st-line therapy if results are suboptimal. All should be avoided in pregnancy (4,5)[C].
  - Spironolactone, 50–200 mg/day: onset of action is slow; use with oral contraceptives to prevent menorrhagia. Watch for hyperkalemia, especially with drospirenone-containing OCP (Yasmin); avoid use in pregnancy.
  - Finasteride: 5 mg/day decreases androgen binding; not approved by FDA. Use with contraception (pregnancy category X).
  - Cyproterone, not available in the United States: 12.5–100 mg/day for days 5–15 of cycle combined with ethinyl estradiol 20–50 mcg days 5–25 of cycle
  - Flutamide: nonsteroidal androgen receptor antagonist. Has not been used in the past due to hepatotoxicity and side effects; lower doses (62.5 mg) are not associated with hepatotoxicity, however, diminished efficacy for hirsutism
- Steroids: used in nonclassic congenital adrenal hyperplasia (NCCAH)
  - Dexamethasone: 2 mg/day

COMPLEMENTARY & ALTERNATIVE MEDICINE

- Saw palmetto (*Serenoa repens*): in small studies, decreases hair growth via blocking 5-α reductase activity in the skin. Has similar peripheral action to finasteride (decreasing 5-α reductase), therefore use with contraception (6)[C].
- Spearmint tea: 1 cup BID: In a study of 21 patients, 1 cup BID for 6 months led to decreased hirsutism.
- Licorice: In a small study, 9 women using 3.5 g/day for 2 cycles had benefited. Excess licorice can lead to hypokalemic hypertension (6)[C].

ONGOING CARE

FOLLOW-UP RECOMMENDATIONS

No special activity.

Patient Monitoring

Monitor for known side effects of medications.

DIET

No special diet.

PATIENT EDUCATION

- Hormonal treatment stops further hair growth and will improve but not reverse present hair.
  - Treatment takes 6 months for effect and may need to be lifelong.
- Cosmetic measures may be needed for already present hair (see above).

PROGNOSIS

- Good (with long-term therapy) for halting further hair growth
- Moderate to poor for reversing current hair growth

COMPLICATIONS

- If PCOS is present, dysfunctional uterine bleeding may lead to anemia.
- If PCOS is present, anovulation may increase uterine cancer risk.
- Androgenic excess may adversely affect lipid status, cardiac risk, and bone density.
- Poor self-image

REFERENCES

1. Somani N, Harrison S, Bergfeld WF. The clinical evaluation of hirsutism. *Dermatol Ther*. 2008;21(5):376–391.
2. Bode D, Seehusen DA, Baird D. Hirsutism in women. *Am Fam Physician*. 2012;85(4):373–380.
3. ACOG Clinical Practice Guideline No. 44. *On the Diagnosis and Management of Polycystic Ovarian Syndrome*. Washington, DC: American College of Obstetrics and Gynecology; 2002.
4. Rosenfeld RL. Clinical practice. Hirsutism. *N Eng J Med*. 2005;353(24):2578–2588.
5. Martin KA, Chang RJ, Ehrmann DA, et al. Evaluation and treatment of hirsutism in premenopausal women: an endocrine society clinical practice guideline. *J Clin Endocrinol Metab*. 2008;93(4):1105–1120.
6. Meletis C, Zabriskie N. Natural approaches for treating polycystic ovarian syndrome. *Altern Complement Ther*. 2006;12(4):157–164.

ADDITIONAL READING

- Akdoğan M, Tamer MN, Cüre E, et al. Effect of spearmint (Mentha spicata Labiatae) teas on androgen levels in women with hirsutism. *Phytother Res*. 2007;21(5):444–447.
- Azziz R. The evaluation and management of hirsutism. *Obstet Gynecol*. 2003;101(5, Pt 1):995–1007.
- Brown J, Farquhar C, Lee O, et al. Spironolactone versus placebo or in combination with steroids for hirsutism and/or acne. *Cochrane Database Syst Rev*. 2009;(2):CD000194.
- Harborne L, Fleming R, Lyall H, et al. Metformin or antiandrogen in the treatment of hirsutism in polycystic ovary syndrome. *J Clin Endocrinol Metab*. 2003;88(9):4116–4123.
- National Institute of Health. Evidence-based methodology workshop on PCOS. http://prevention.nih.gov/workshops/2012/pcos/docs/PCOS_Final_Statement.pdf. Accessed 2014.
- Swiglo BA, Cosma M, Flynn DN, et al. Clinical review: antiandrogens for the treatment of hirsutism: a systematic review and metaanalyses of randomized controlled trials. *J Clin Endocrinol Metab*. 2008;93(4):1153–1160.

SEE ALSO

Acne Vulgaris; Infertility; Polycystic Ovarian Syndrome (PCOS)

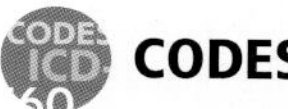

CODES

ICD10

- L68.0 Hirsutism
- E28.2 Polycystic ovarian syndrome

CLINICAL PEARLS

- PCOS is the most common cause of hirsutism.
- Treatment is long term and often lifelong.

HIV/AIDS

Jeremy D. DeFoe, DO • Karen Sue Phelps, MD

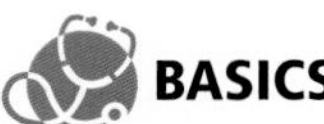

BASICS

DESCRIPTION

HIV is a retrovirus (subgroup lentivirus) that integrates into CD4 T lymphocytes, altering cell-mediated immunity and causing cell death, severe immunodeficiency, opportunistic infections, and malignancies if untreated.

- Because of treatment advances, HIV is now classified as a chronic disease.
- The natural history of untreated HIV infection includes viral transmission, acute retroviral syndrome, recovery and seroconversion, asymptomatic chronic HIV infection, and symptomatic HIV infection or AIDS.
- Without treatment, the average patient develops AIDS ~10 years after transmission.
- All HIV-infected persons with CD4 <200 cells/mm^3 or with AIDS-defining illnesses are categorized as living with AIDS.

EPIDEMIOLOGY

Incidence

- At the end of 2008, an estimated 33.4 million people were living with HIV/AIDS worldwide. 2.7 million new HIV infections and 2 million deaths are attributable to AIDS globally on an annual basis.
- In the United States, HIV incidence has remained relatively stable at about 50,000 infections per year since the mid-1990s.

Prevalence

- Estimated 1.14 million persons in the United States are living with HIV/AIDS as of 2010 (1,2); 16% unaware of their status (2)
- HIV/AIDS cases are disproportionately high among racial/ethnic minority populations (2).
- Transmission of a drug-resistant virus rising
- Younger females particularly vulnerable

ETIOLOGY AND PATHOPHYSIOLOGY

- HIV primarily infects CD4+ cells. HIV is a single-stranded, positive-sense, enveloped RNA virus. It enters target cells, and through the process of reverse transcription, viral RNA is transcribed to DNA and imported to the host cell nucleus and encoded into the cellular DNA. The virus can then become latent or produce new viral RNA and viral proteins that are released to infect other CD4∞ cells. Host CD8+ cells are activated and produce the seroconversion response.
- There are 2 types of HIV. HIV-1 is the virus that was first described and is more virulent. It causes the majority of HIV infections worldwide. HIV-2 is less infective and seen primarily in West Africa.

Genetics

People who lack CCR5, a cell-surface chemokine coreceptor, are highly resistant to HIV infection.

RISK FACTORS

- Sexual activity (70% of transmission): Ulcerative urogenital lesions promote transmission (3).
- Male-to-male sexual contact accounted for 63% of newly diagnosed HIV/AIDS cases in 2010 (2)
- Injection drug abuse (IDA)
- Children of HIV-infected women
  - Maternal HIV-1 RNA level predicts transmission.
  - HIV testing and treatment in pregnancy and infancy has reduced perinatal HIV transmission by >70% (4)[B].
  - Pregnant women should be treated until viral load is undetectable.
  - HIV can also be transmitted by breastfeeding.
- Recipients of blood products from 1975 to 1985
- Occupational exposure

GENERAL PREVENTION

- Avoid unprotected sexual intercourse and IDA.
- Preexposure prophylaxis is recommended for individuals at high risk for transmission (5)[A].

COMMONLY ASSOCIATED CONDITIONS

- Syphilis may be more aggressive if HIV-infected.
- Tuberculosis (TB) is coepidemic with HIV; test all persons with HIV for TB. Dually infected patients have 100× greater risk of developing active TB.
- Patients coinfected with hepatitis C have a more rapid progression to cirrhosis.

DIAGNOSIS

- Acute retroviral syndrome: CD4 lymphocyte count declines with increase in viral load ~1–4 weeks after transmission; confirmed by demonstrating a high HIV RNA in the absence of HIV antibody
- Acute retroviral syndrome presents as a mononucleosis-like syndrome including the following:
  - Fever (97%)
  - Adenopathy
  - Pharyngitis (73%)
  - Rash (77%)
  - Myalgias/arthralgia (58%)
  - Less common: headache, diarrhea, nausea, vomiting, hepatosplenomegaly, weight loss, thrush, and neurologic symptoms (12%)
  - Seroconversion: Positive HIV antibody test occurs 4 weeks to 6 months after exposure.
- Clinical latency (asymptomatic): variable duration (average is 8–10 years) accompanied by a gradual decline in CD4 cell counts and a relatively stable HIV RNA levels (the viral "set point"). Patients often develop persistent generalized lymphadenopathy (>1 cm in ≥2 extrainguinal sites) and may develop fever, weight loss, myalgias, and gastrointestinal problems if they progress (untreated) to symptoms associated with AIDS.
- Symptomatic conditions:
  - Fever or diarrhea >1 month, bacillary angiomatosis, thrush, persistent candidal vulvovaginitis, cervical dysplasia or carcinoma in situ, oral hairy leukoplakia, herpes zoster, idiopathic thrombocytopenic purpura, pelvic inflammatory disease, peripheral neuropathy or myelopathy
- AIDS: defined by a CD4 cell count <200, a CD4 cell percentage of total lymphocytes <14%, or 1 of several AIDS-related opportunistic infections: *Pneumocystis jiroveci* (*carinii*) pneumonia, cryptococcal meningitis, recurrent bacterial pneumonia, candida esophagitis, CNS toxoplasmosis, TB and non-Hodgkin lymphoma (NHL), progressive multifocal encephalopathy, HIV nephropathy, Kaposi sarcoma, NHL, Hodgkin lymphoma, invasive cervical cancer
- Advanced HIV disease: CD4 cell count <50. Most AIDS-related deaths occur at this time. Common late opportunistic infections: cytomegalovirus (CMV) disease (retinitis, colitis) or disseminated *Mycobacterium avium* complex as well as HIV wasting syndrome (>10% weight loss) and HIV encephalopathy/dementia/cognitive–motor disorder.

HISTORY

- Complete medical history, including risk exposures and social/occupational history
- Review of systems: fever, chills, night sweats, diarrhea, weight loss, fatigue, adenopathy, oral sores, odynophagia (esophageal candidiasis), cough, shortness of breath and dyspnea on exertion (early *P. jiroveci* pneumonia), visual changes (CMV retinitis), skin rash, neurologic symptoms (CNS infection, malignancy, or dementia), sinusitis
- Review immunization record.

PHYSICAL EXAM

Focus on weight, skin, retinal exam, oropharynx; lymph nodes; liver, spleen, mental status, sensation, genital, and rectal examinations

DIFFERENTIAL DIAGNOSIS

Burkitt lymphoma; candidiasis; coccidioidomycosis; cryptococcus; CMV; herpes simplex; lymphoma; toxoplasmosis

DIAGNOSTIC TESTS & INTERPRETATION

Initial Tests (lab, imaging)

- 4 generation HIV testing combines antibody/antigen immunoassay for HIV-1, HIV-2 (6)
  - Can be positive within 2–3 weeks of exposure
- Screening: ELISA sensitivity and specificity >98%. Obtain HIV RNA if acute HIV infection is suspected:
  - New rapid oral test available and FDA approved
- Confirmatory: Western blot
  - Positive test is reaction with 2 of these 3 bands: P24, gp 41, and gp 120/160. If indeterminate, repeat test in 3–6 months.
- CD4 cell count and percentage (6)[A]
- HIV RNA viral load (6)[A]
- CBC with differential
- Serum chemistry
- Serologies: hepatitis A, B, and C; syphilis
- Urine screen for STIs (*Neisseria gonorrhoeae, Chlamydia trachomatis*)
- Cervical cytology
- Purified protein derivative (PPD) to screen for latent TB infection
- Glucose-6-phosphate levels
- Lipids at baseline and during highly active antiretroviral therapy (HAART)
- Genotypic tests for resistance to antiretrovirals for patients with pretreatment HIV RNA >1,000 copies/mL (6)[A]
- Chest x-ray if pulmonary symptoms or positive PPD
- Other potential tests/serologies: throat cultures for bacterial/viral respiratory pathogens, Epstein-Barr virus viral capsid antigen IgM/Igg, CMV IgM/IgG, human herpesvirus 6 IgM/IgG

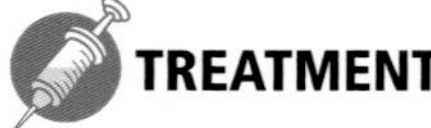

TREATMENT

- Antiretroviral therapy should be initiated in all patients with an AIDS-defining illness or with a CD4 count <350 (6)[A].
- Genotypic testing recommended to guide therapy in patients naïve to antiretroviral therapy

- Antiretroviral therapy should be initiated regardless of CD4 count in pregnancy, HIV-associated nephropathy and HBV coinfections when treatment of hepatitis B virus is indicated (6)[A], rapidly declining CD4 counts (e.g., >100 cells/mm³ decrease per year), and higher viral load (>100,000 copies/mL) (6)[B].
- Antiretroviral therapy is recommended for all patients with CD4 count between 350 and 500 (6)[A].
- Emtricitabine/tenofovir disoproxil fumarate (Truvada) FDA approved for preexposure prophylaxis in adults at high risk (5)

GENERAL MEASURES

- Main goal of HAART: Reduce viral load (ideally to <50 HIV-1 RNA copies/mL) and delay immune suppression. Viral load is the most important indicator of response to HAART.
- Check for transmitted drug resistance before starting HAART (6)[A].
- An adequate CD4 response to therapy is typically defined as an increase in CD4 count from 50 to 150 cells/mm³ per year. An accelerated response is often noted in the first 3 months of therapy (6).
- Prevent HIV-associated complications, short- and long-term adverse drug reactions, HIV transmission, HIV drug resistance, and preservation of HIV treatment options.
- Assess substance abuse, economic factors (unstable housing), social support, mental illness, comorbidities, high-risk behaviors, and factors known to impair adherence and promote transmission.
- Prophylactic antimicrobial agents and vaccines
  - *P. jiroveci*: trimethoprim/sulfamethoxazole (TMP-SMX) 1 DS daily or 1 SS daily indicated if CD4 <200/mm³, prior *P. jiroveci*, thrush, or unexplained fever for >2 weeks
  - *Mycobacterium tuberculosis*: Treat if PPD >5 mm induration without prior prophylaxis or treatment, recent TB contact, or history of inadequately treated TB that healed. Confirmed by culture. Treatment is based on susceptibility.
  - *Toxoplasma gondii*: 33% per year risk of infection in untreated patients with CD4 <100/mm³; prophylaxis: TMP-SMX DS daily
  - *M. avium* complex: 20–40% risk with CD4 <50 and no HAART. Preferred prophylaxis is clarithromycin 500 mg PO BID or azithromycin 1,200 mg PO weekly.
  - Varicella: Seronegative and unexposed are at risk if exposed to chickenpox or shingles. Preferred regimen is VZIG 5 vials within 96 hours but preferably within 48 hours.
  - *Streptococcus pneumoniae*: 50–100 times increased risk of invasive infection compared with general population; pneumovax every 5 years
  - Influenza vaccine annually
  - Hepatitis A and B vaccines for at-risk patients
  - Tetanus: dT vaccine in adults

MEDICATION

- Nucleoside reverse transcriptase inhibitors (NRTIs)
  - Abacavir (ABC, Ziagen), didanosine (DDL, Videx), emtricitabine (FTC, Emtriva), lamivudine (3TC, Epivir), stavudine (d4T, Zerit), tenofovir (Viread), zalcitabine (ddC, Hivid), zidovudine (AZT, Retrovir), zidovudine + lamivudine (Combivir), zidovudine ± lamivudine ± abacavir (Trizivir), tenofovir ± emtricitabine (Truvada), abacavir ± lamivudine (Epzicom)
- Nonnucleoside reverse transcriptase inhibitors (NNRTIs): delavirdine (Rescriptor); efavirenz (Sustiva); nevirapine (Viramune); rilpivirine (Edurant); efavirenz ± Truvada (Atripla); rilpivirine ± Truvada (Complera)
- Protease inhibitors (PIs): amprenavir (Agenerase), atazanavir (Reyataz), darunavir (Prezista), fosamprenavir (Lexiva), indinavir (Crixivan), lopinavir-ritonavir (Kaletra), nelfinavir (Viracept), ritonavir (Norvir), saquinavir (Fortovase, Invirase), tipranavir (Aptivus)
- Fusion inhibitors: enfuvirtide (Fuzeon)
- Entry inhibitors: maraviroc (Selzentry)
- Integrase inhibitors: raltegravir (Isentress) stribild (elvitegravir ± cobicistat ± tenofovir ± emtricitabine)
- Drug failure: Before selecting regimen, review clinical symptoms, history of HAART, and adherence. Perform resistance testing.
- PIs can cause metabolic syndrome.
- HAART, especially the protease inhibitors, have potentially life-threatening interactions.

First Line

- Avoid monotherapy.
- NNRTIs + 2 NRTI (avoid AZT/d4T combination) (7)[A]
- Efavirenz is a preferred NNRTI in 1st-line treatment of HIV, particularly in resource-limited settings (8)[A]; avoid in pregnancy
- PIs (preferably boosted with ritonavir) + 2 NRTI (6)[A]
- Integrase inhibitor + 2 NRTI (6)[A]

ONGOING CARE

FOLLOW-UP RECOMMENDATIONS

Patient Monitoring

- If HIV RNA is detectable at 2–8 weeks, repeat every 4–8 weeks until suppressed to less than level of detection, then every 3–6 months (6).
- Monitor HIV RNA, CD4, CBC every 3–4 months (6).
- Test fasting lipids and fasting glucose annually if normal; basic chemistry, aspartate aminotransferase, alanine aminotransferase, T/D bilirubin every 6–12 months (6)
- HLA-B 5701 if considering abacavir (6)
- Pregnancy test if starting efavirenz (6)

DIET

- Encourage good nutrition and multivitamin use.
- Avoid raw eggs and unpasteurized milk. Severely immunocompromised patients should boil tap water to prevent *Cryptosporidium*.

PATIENT EDUCATION

- Provide nonjudgmental prevention counseling, reviewing high-risk behaviors and viral transmission.
- Emphasize importance of adherence to HAART to prevent resistance.
- National AIDS Hotline: 800-342-2437 [Spanish 800-342-7432]
- National Institute of Health AIDS Clinical Trials Group: 800-874-2572
- American Foundation for AIDS Research: 212-719-0033 (new treatments and research)
- www.aidsinfo.nih.gov

PROGNOSIS

- Untreated HIV infection leading to the diagnosis of AIDS has an associated life expectancy of 3.7 years.
- AIDS-defining opportunistic infections usually do not develop until CD4 <200.
- In untreated HIV infection, CD4 counts decline at a rate of 50–80 per year, with more rapid decline as counts drop <200.
- Adherence failure—not drug resistance—is the most common cause of treatment failure (2)[B].

COMPLICATIONS

- Immunodeficiency
- Opportunistic infections
- Malignancy, including cervical or anal cancer

REFERENCES

1. Centers for Disease Control and Prevention: Diagnoses of HIV infection and AIDS in the United States and Dependent Areas, 2011 HIV Surveillance Report. www.cdc.gov/hiv/surveillance/resources/reports/2008report/. Accessed 2014.
2. Centers for Disease Control and Prevention. HIV in the United States: at a glance. http://www.cdc.gov/hiv/pdf/statistics_basics_factsheet.pdf. Accessed 2014.
3. Quinn TC, Wawer MJ, Sewankambo N, et al. Viral load and heterosexual transmission of human immunodeficiency virus type 1. Rakai Project Study Group. *N Engl J Med*. 2000;342(13):921–929.
4. Mofenson LM. U.S. Public Health Service Task Force recommendations for use of antiretroviral drugs in pregnant HIV-1-infected women for maternal health interventions to reduce perinatal HIV-1 transmission in the United States. *MMWR Recomm Rep*. 2002;51(RR-18):1–38.
5. Centers for Diease Control and Prevention. Preexposure prophylaxis for the prevention of HIV infection in the United States - 2014. A clinical practice guideline. http://www.cdc.gov/hiv/guidelines/index.html. Accessed 2014.
6. U.S. Department of Health and Human Services. Guidelines for the use of antiretroviral agents in HIV-1-infected adults and adolescents. http://aidsinfo.nih.gov/contentfiles/lvguidelines/adultandadolescentgl.pdf. Accessed 2014.
7. Schafer JJ, Short WR. Rilpivirine, a novel non-nucleoside reverse transcriptase inhibitor for the management of HIV-1 infection: a systematic review. *Antivir Ther*. 2012;17(8):1495–1502.
8. Pillay P, Ford N, Shubber Z, et al. Outcomes for efavirenz versus nevirapine-containing regimens for treatment of HIV-1 infection: a systematic review and meta-analysis. *PLoS One*. 2013;8(7):e68995.

ADDITIONAL READING

Simon V, Ho DD, Abdool Karim Q. HIV/AIDS epidemiology, pathogenesis, prevention, and treatment. *Lancet*. 2006;368(9534):489–504.

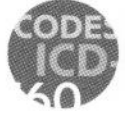

CODES

ICD10

- Z21 Asymptomatic human immunodeficiency virus infection status
- B20 Human immunodeficiency virus [HIV] disease
- R75 Inconclusive laboratory evidence of human immunodef virus

CLINICAL PEARLS

- Acute HIV seroconversion illness mimics mononucleosis and is characterized by fever, sore throat, adenopathy, myalgias, and rash.
- Transmitted drug resistance is increasing. Evaluate patients for resistance before initiating HAART.
- Appropriate vaccination and prophylactic antibiotics should be administered to HIV+ patients based on clinical history and CD4 count.

H

HODGKIN LYMPHOMA

Jennifer J. Gao, MD • Fred J. Schiffman, MD

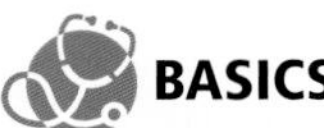

BASICS

DESCRIPTION

Historical background:

- Described in 1832 by Thomas Hodgkin in "On some morbid appearance of the absorbent glands and spleen"
- First neoplasm to be (i) defined by cytologic grounds based on presence of Reed-Sternberg (RS) cells, (ii) clinically staged neoplastic disease, and (iii) treated with chemotherapy and/or radiotherapy
- Neoplastic RS cells of monoclonal lymphoid B-cell origin within inflammatory background of lymphocytes (T-helper type 2 and regulatory T cells), eosinophils, histiocytes, and plasma cells (1,2)
- Two subtypes: classic Hodgkin lymphoma (CHL, 95% of cases) and nodular lymphocyte predominant Hodgkin lymphoma (NLPHL, 3–8% of cases) (1)
  - NLPHL: B cells, neoplastic luteinizing hormone (LH) cells with multilobulated nuclei, small nucleoli, and popcorn-like appearance
  - CHL histologic subdivisions: nodular sclerosing (60%), mixed cellularity (30%), lymphocyte depleted (<10%), lymphocyte rich (<10%)
  - Frequency of lymph node involvement: cervical > mediastinal > axillary > paraaortic

EPIDEMIOLOGY

- Incidence: 2.8/100,000/year
- Predominance: 8% of lymphoid malignancies (1)

Geriatric Considerations

Poorer prognosis if present at ≥60 years:

- Less likely to tolerate intensive chemotherapy
- Less likely to be included in clinical trial

Pediatric Considerations

Young females (<30 years of age) treated with thoracic radiation are at high risk for breast cancer, and early breast cancer screening is recommended.

Pregnancy Considerations

- Abdominal ultrasonography to detect subdiaphragmatic disease
- Treatment:
  - Delay until after delivery if asymptomatic and early-stage.
  - ABVD safely used in 2nd and 3rd trimesters
  - Vinblastine monotherapy to control symptoms
  - 1st trimester: ABVD may or may not cause fetal malformations.

Incidence

- ~9,000 new cases in the United States annually
- Mean age at diagnosis: 38 years

Prevalence

~175,000 living with Hodgkin lymphoma in the United States in 2009

ETIOLOGY AND PATHOPHYSIOLOGY

- RS cells likely derived from germinal center B cells with mutations in immunoglobulin variable chain
- Seasonal features and higher frequencies with Epstein-Barr virus (EBV) suggest environmental factors.
- T-lymphocyte defects persist even after successful treatment.
- Human leukocyte antigen (HLA) strongly associated with increased risk (2)
- EBV positivity associated with increased risk (2)
- Genome-wide association studies identified 19p13.3 at intron 2 of *TCF3*.

Genetics

- First-degree relative: 3–9× risk
- Siblings of younger patients: 7× risk
- Weak correlation between familial HL and HLA class I regions containing HLA A1, B5, B8, B18 alleles

RISK FACTORS

- Immunodeficiency (inherited or acquired)
- Autoimmune disorders
- EBV (2)
- Seasonal factors

COMMONLY ASSOCIATED CONDITIONS

In HIV:

- AIDS-defining illness
- Predominantly mixed-cellularity or lymphocyte-depleted histologic subtypes
- At diagnosis: widespread disease, extranodal involvement, systemic symptoms

DIAGNOSIS

HISTORY

- Asymptomatic lymphadenopathy (cervical/supraclavicular)
- Pel-Ebstein fever
- Constitutional symptoms: night sweats, weight loss, fatigue, anorexia
- Alcohol-induced pain
- Pruritus

PHYSICAL EXAM

Focus on lymph nodes, spleen, and liver

DIFFERENTIAL DIAGNOSIS

Non-Hodgkin lymphoma, infectious lymphadenopathy, solid tumor metastases, sarcoidosis, autoimmune disease, AIDS/HIV, drug reaction

DIAGNOSTIC TESTS & INTERPRETATION

Initial Tests (lab, imaging)

- CBC and electrolytes
- LFT, including hepatitis serologies
- HIV
- Pregnancy test
- Pulmonary function tests (diffusion capacity of the lung for carbon monoxide for ABVD or BEACOPP)
- Chest x-ray
- CT of chest, abdomen, and pelvis
- PET: for initial staging, midtreatment decision making, and end-of-treatment evaluation
- Bone scan, gallium scan, abdominal ultrasound
- EBV (2)

Follow-Up Tests & Special Considerations

- Fertility considerations:
  - Semen cryopreservation if chemotherapy or pelvic radiation therapy
  - In vitro fertilization or ovarian tissue/oocyte cryopreservation
- Radiation therapy (RT) considerations:
  - Splenic RT: pneumococcal, *Haemophilus influenzae*, meningococcal vaccine

Diagnostic Procedures/Other

- Excisional lymph node biopsy
- Immunohistochemistry
- Bone marrow biopsy
- Liver biopsy (in selected cases)

Test Interpretation

RS cell characteristics include the following:

- Diameter: 20–50 μm
- Abundant acidophilic cytoplasm
- Bi- or polylobulated nucleus
- Acidophilic nucleoli
- CD30+, CD15+, CD45−, CD3−, CD20+ in 40% of cases
- RS cells necessary but not sufficient for diagnosis (needs inflammatory background)

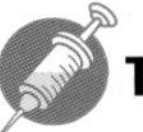

TREATMENT

- Ann Arbor staging with Cotswold modification:
  - Stage I: single lymph node or of a single extralymphatic organ or site
  - Stage II: ≥2 lymph node regions on the same side of diaphragm alone or with involvement of extralymphatic organ or tissue
  - Stage III: node groups on both sides of the diaphragm
  - Stage IV: dissemination involving extranodal organs (except the spleen, which is considered lymphoid tissue)
  - Subclasses: A = no systemic symptoms; B = systemic symptoms (fever, night sweats, weight loss >10% body weight); X = bulky disease (widened mediastinum, > intrathoracic diameter, or >10-cm nodal mass)
  - Pathologic stage at given site denoted by: M = bone marrow, H = liver, L = lung, O = bone, P = pleura, D = skin:
    - Splenectomy, liver biopsy, lymph node biopsy, bone marrow biopsy mandatory for pathologic staging
- Goal: Aim for cure.
- All subsequent treatment and follow-up care recommendations based on National Comprehensive Cancer Network (NCCN) consensus. Please refer to NCCN Practice Guidelines in Oncology for Hodgkin lymphoma.

MEDICATION

First Line

- ABVD: doxorubicin, bleomycin, vinblastine, dacarbazine:
  - Highly emetic, severe phlebitis
  - Monitor cardiac function on doxorubicin
- BEACOPP: bleomycin, etoposide, doxorubicin, cyclophosphamide, vincristine, procarbazine, prednisone:
  - Bleomycin: risk of pulmonary toxicity, death; test dose may be administered prior to first cycle
- Stage I/II with no risk factors: 2 cycles ABVD followed by 20 Gy involved-field radiotherapy (IFRT)
- Stage I/II with risk factors (large mediastinal mass, unfavorable histology, age, extranodal disease, erythrocyte sedimentation rate (ESR), B symptoms, number of nodal areas): 4 cycles chemotherapy (BEACOPP and/or ABVD) followed by 30 Gy IFRT
- Stage III/IV: 4–6 cycles chemotherapy (BEACOPP and/or ABVD) and consider autologous stem cell transplant (SCT) or radiotherapy

- Relapsed and refractory: high-dose conditioning therapy (HDCT) followed by autologous SCT:
  - Maintenance therapy: trials with brentuximab vedotin (anti-CD30) and lenalidomide under way.
  - Brentuximab vedotin: anti-CD30, use in relapsed HL after 2 prior lines of treatment have been tried, side effects include peripheral neuropathy, nausea, fatigue, neutropenia, diarrhea (3)
  - Allogeneic SCT to be considered if failed autologous SCT (used in trials only)

Second Line

- Median survival <3 years if fail 2nd-line therapy, including SCT
- SCT in progressive disease or relapse:
  - High-dose chemotherapy and autologous stem cell transplant (HDCT/autoSCT): improved event-free and progression-free survival compared with conventional chemotherapy but not overall survival; can achieve disease-free survival in 30–40% of patients after alloSCT (4,5)
  - Reduced intensity conditioning (RIC) with bis-chloroethylnitrosourea (BCNU), etoposide, cytarabine, melphalan (BEAM) followed by allogeneic transplant (alloSCT) to induce graft-versus-tumor (GVT) effect in patients who have relapsed after autoSCT, complete response seen in 81%, nonrelapse mortality of 13% at 1 year, 1-year relapse rate of 36% (4,6)
- Rituximab: excellent activity against lymphocyte-predominant variant due to CD20+ lymphocytes
- Brentuximab vedotin: anti-CD30 chimeric antibody conjugated to synthetic antimicrotubule agent monomethyl auristatin E:
  - Approved by U.S. Food and Drug Administration (FDA) in 2011 for patients who failed/not candidate for SCT or failure of two prior multiagent chemotherapy regimens
- Novel agents undergoing studies: NF-κB inhibitors (bortezomib), mammalian target of rapamycin (mTOR) inhibitors (everolimus), immunomodulators (lenalidomide), cell signaling targets histone deacetylase (HDAC) inhibitors (vorinostat, panobinostat, mocetinostat)

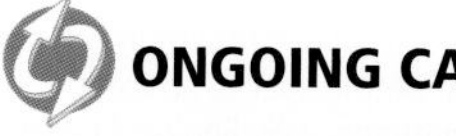

ONGOING CARE

FOLLOW-UP RECOMMENDATIONS

Patient Monitoring

- During therapy: CBC, nutrition, and hydration
- Restage with PET after 2–4 cycles of chemotherapy: sensitive prognostic indicator
- Posttreatment monitoring:
  - History and physical (H&P): q2–4 months for first 2 years, then q3–6 months for next 3–5 years
  - Laboratory studies:
    - CBC, platelets, ESR, chemistry profile q2–4 months for 1–2 years, then q3–6 months for next 3–5 years
    - Thyroid-stimulating hormone (TSH) annually if radiation to neck
  - Imaging:
    - Chest: chest x-ray or CT q6–12 months during first 2–5 years
    - Abdominal/pelvic: CT q6–12 months during first 2–3 years
    - Annual breast mammogram or MRI beginning 8–10 years after therapy or at age 40 years if chest or axillary irradiation
    - Surveillance PET should not be done routinely due to risk of false-positive findings.
- Splenic irradiation or splenectomy as part of Hodgkin treatment increases risk of secondary cancers (leukemia, myelodysplastic syndrome, non-Hodgkin lymphoma, solid cancers) (7).

PATIENT EDUCATION

- Reproductive impact
- Risks of secondary malignancy
- Oral and dental care during therapy
- Leukemia Society of America (www.lls.org)

PROGNOSIS

- Cure rate for classic Hodgkin lymphoma: 80%
- Relapse or progression of disease rate: 5–20%
- Overall survival rates:
  - 1-year survival: 92%
  - 5-year survival: 85%
  - 10-year survival: 81%
- International prognostic score for advanced disease:
  - Age ≥45 years
  - Male gender
  - Albumin <4 g/dL
  - Hemoglobin <10.5 g/dL
  - Lymphocytopenia: <600 lymphocyte cells/dL or lymphocytes <8% of WBC
  - WBC ≥15,000 cells/dL
  - Stage IV disease
- Main cause of death:
  - Initial 5 years: Hodgkin lymphoma
  - After 5–10 years: leukemia, myelodysplastic syndrome
  - After 20 years: second primary malignancy, cardiovascular disease

REFERENCES

1. Goel A, Fan W, Patel AA, et al. Nodular lymphocyte predominant Hodgkin lymphoma: biology, diagnosis and treatment. *Clin Lymphoma Myeloma Leuk*. 2014;14(4):261–270.
2. Cozen W, Timofeeva MN, Li D, et al. A meta-analysis of Hodgkin lymphoma reveals 19p13.3 tcf3 as a novel susceptibility locus. *Nat Commun*. 2014;5:3856.
3. Siddiqi T, Thomas SH, Chen R. Role of brentuximab vedotin in the treatment of relapsed or refractory Hodgkin lymphoma. *Pharmgenomics Pers Med*. 2014;7:79–85.
4. Lim AB, Ritchie DS. Hodgkin lymphoma, allogeneic transplant, and the graft-versus-tumor effect: size does matter. *Leuk Lymphoma*. 2014;55(6): 1223–1224.
5. Rancea M, von Tresckow B, Monsef I, et al. High-dose chemotherapy followed by autologous stem cell transplantation for patients with relapsed or refractory hodgkin lymphoma: a systematic review with meta-analysis. *Crit Rev Oncol Hematol*. 2014; 92(1):1–10.
6. Sobol U, Rodriguez T, Smith S, et al. Seven-year follow-up of allogeneic transplant using BCNU, etoposide, cytarabine and melphalan chemotherapy in patients with Hodgkin lymphoma after autograft failure: importance of minimal residual disease. *Leuk Lymphoma*. 2014;55(6):1281–1287.
7. Mosalpuria K, Loberiza F Jr. Splenectomy and second malignancies in Hodgkin lymphoma patients: is there causal relationship? *Leuk Lymphoma*. 2014;25:1–2.

ADDITIONAL READING

- Armitage JO. Early-stage Hodgkin's lymphoma. *N Engl J Med*. 2010;363(7):653–662.
- Borchmann P, Eichenauer DA, Engert A. State of the art in the treatment of Hodgkin lymphoma. *Nat Rev Clin Oncol*. 2012;9(8):450–459.
- Czuczman M, Straus D, Gribben J, et al. Management options, survivorship, and emerging treatment strategies for follicular and Hodgkin lymphomas. *Leuk Lymphoma*. 2010;51(Suppl 1):41–49.
- Dinner S, Advani R. Targeted therapy in relapsed classical Hodgkin lymphoma. *J Natl Compr Canc Netw*. 2013;11(8):968–976.
- NCCN clinical practice guidelines in oncology. Hodgkin lymphoma. Version 2. 2013. www.nccn.org. Accessed 2014.
- SEER stat fact sheet. Hodgkin lymphoma. http://seer.cancer.gov/statfacts/html/hodg.html. Accessed 2014.
- von Tresckow B, Engert A. Refractory Hodgkin lymphoma. *Curr Opin Oncol*. 2013;25(5):463–469.

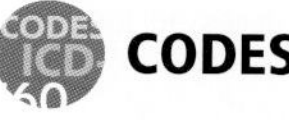

CODES

ICD10

- C81.90 Hodgkin lymphoma, unspecified, unspecified site
- C81.91 Hodgkin lymphoma, unsp, lymph nodes of head, face, and neck
- C81.92 Hodgkin lymphoma, unspecified, intrathoracic lymph nodes

CLINICAL PEARLS

- Neoplastic disease of lymphatics
- RS cells of monoclonal lymphoid B-cell origin within inflammatory background of lymphocytes
- Two subtypes: CHL, 95% of cases and NLPHL, 5% of cases
- Cure rate for CHL: 80%
- Relapse or progression of disease rate: 5–20%

HOMELESSNESS

Dana Sprute, MD, MPH, FAAFP • Jessica Heselschwerdt, MD

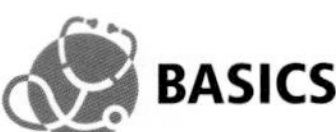

BASICS

DESCRIPTION

"Homeless" or "homeless individual or homeless person" includes the following: (i) an individual who lacks a fixed, regular, and adequate nighttime residence; and (ii) an individual who has a primary nighttime residence that is (a) a supervised publicly or privately operated shelter designed to provide temporary living accommodations (including welfare hotels, congregate shelters, and transitional housing for the mentally ill); (b) an institution that provides a temporary residence for individuals intended to be institutionalized; and (c) a public or private place not designed for, or ordinarily used as, a regular sleeping accommodation for human beings.

EPIDEMIOLOGY

Prevalence

As of January 2013, on any given night, there are 610,042 homeless individuals in the United States: 37% are homeless families, 48% are not chronically homeless individuals; 15% are chronically homeless individuals; and 23% are children (1).

- From 2012 to 2013, overall homelessness decreased by 3.7%, and targeted federal assistance has increased. Risk for becoming homeless remains high (2).
- Although many homeless individuals reside in temporary housing or shelters, 35% live on the streets (2).

RISK FACTORS

- Economic factors
  - Poverty
    - 2014 federal poverty definition: $23,850 annual income for 4-person household (3).
    - In 2012, 15% of the U.S. population fell below federal poverty definition.
  - Unemployment: U.S. rate: 6.3% in May 2014 (U.S. Bureau of Labor Statistics, accessed June 11, 2014)
  - Lack of affordable health care: in 2012, 48 million people in United States are without health insurance:
    - Young adults (ages 19–34 years) are disproportionately uninsured (27%) compared with the average for all ages (15%); the uninsured rate for ages 19–25 years has decreased by 4.2% since 2009, following Affordable Care Act provision allowing individuals in this age group to stay on their parents' insurance plans.
  - Lack of affordable housing: housing is considered affordable if ≤30% of household income
    - Over 6.5 million households are defined by HUD as "severely housing cost burdened" (≥50% of income is spent on housing) (2).
  - Increase in home foreclosures
    - In 2010, there were 2.9 million homes in foreclosure, an increase of 239% since 2005.
- At-risk populations: domestic violence and victims of violence; youth (particularly those aging out of foster care); veterans; rural; addiction; psychiatric illness; disabled due to chronic medical disease, psychiatric illness, or substance use disorder; reentry after incarceration/prison
  - Domestic violence: 63% of homeless women experience domestic violence, and in many cases, domestic violence leads directly to homelessness (4).
  - Youth: each year, 550,000 unaccompanied youths (up to age 24 years) experience an episode of homelessness lasting longer than a week (4).
  - Veterans: 8% of the homeless population; homelessness rate decreased between 2009 and 2013 (1).
  - Addiction disorders: 46% of homeless individuals report alcohol and/or drug use as a major factor contributing to homelessness (4).
  - Psychiatric illness: 45% of homeless report indicators of a mental health issue in the past year; 25% of homeless adults suffer from chronic mental illness (4).
  - Reentry after incarceration: 30–50% of parolees homeless at any given time (4).
- Fundamental issues in homelessness and health care that require ongoing consideration (5)[C]:
  - Unstable housing, limited access to nutritious food and water, lack of transportation
  - Higher risk for abuse and violence
  - Physical/cognitive impairments, behavioral health problems
  - Developmental discrepancies for children: speech delay, chronic ear infection, insufficient opportunity to practice gross and fine motor skills
  - Higher risk for communicable disease
  - Lack of health insurance/resources, discontinuous/inaccessible health care, lack of a medical home, barriers to disability assistance
  - Cultural/linguistic barriers: racial and ethnic groups overrepresented in homeless population
  - Limited education/literacy
  - Lack of social supports: Alienation from family and friends precipitates homelessness.
  - Criminalization of homelessness: frequent arrests for loitering, sleeping in public places

GENERAL PREVENTION

- Policy and funding for community programs that provide emergency/rapid housing, housing stabilization, and case management services to address risk factors
- Affordable Care Act (ACA): in 2010 increased Medicaid eligibility for homeless and expanded home and community-based services and case management to the homeless population (6)
- Department of Housing and Urban Development (HUD): increasing permanent supportive housing units, increasing services for veterans and those with disabilities (6)
- Social Justice Policy Recommendations: permanent affordable housing, foreclosure and homelessness prevention, increased funds for HUD McKinney-Vento programs (emergency, transitional, and permanent housing), rural homeless assistance, universal health care, universal livable income, employment/workforce services, prevention of hate crimes against the homeless, decriminalization of homelessness

COMMONLY ASSOCIATED CONDITIONS

- Hunger
- Medical conditions
  - Worsening of chronic conditions: lack of healthy food, places to store medications, or medical equipment; inability to get restful sleep; decreased health literacy (7)
  - Infectious diseases
    - Tuberculosis (TB), HIV/AIDS, STI (7)
    - Skin/nail infections and infestation (lice and scabies)
    - Liver disease (e.g., hepatitis B or C, or alcohol-related)
- Cognitive impairment: traumatic brain injury (TBI), cerebrovascular accident (CVA), substance use
- Dental problems
- Exposure-related conditions (frostbite, heatstroke)
- Psychiatric illness (5)
- Trauma: increased risk of assault, victims of hate crimes

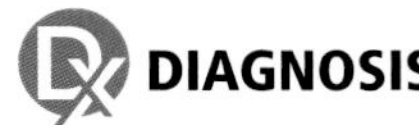

DIAGNOSIS

HISTORY

- Living conditions: location, access to food, restrooms, place to store medicines, safety
- Prior homelessness: what precipitated it, first time, chronic
- Individual/family history of reactive airway disease (RAD), chronic otitis media, anemia, diabetes, cardiovascular disease (CVD), TB, HIV/STIs, hospitalizations
- Family members, especially dependent children
- Medications: include OTC medication, dietary supplements, medication "borrowed" from others
- Prior providers: oral health, primary care, current medical home
- Mental health: stress, anxiety, appetite, sleep, concentration, mood, speech, memory, thought process and content, suicidal/homicidal ideation, insight, judgment, impulse control, social interactions; symptoms of brain injury (headaches, seizures, memory loss, lability, irritability, dizziness, insomnia, poor organizational/decision-making skills)
- Alcohol/nicotine/drug use: amount, frequency, duration
- Gender identity/orientation, behaviors, rape, pregnancies, hepatitis, HIV, other STIs
- History or current abuse: emotional, physical, sexual; patient safety
- Legal problems/violence: history of incarceration
- Regular/strenuous activities: routines (treatment feasibility); level of strenuous activity
- Work: previous types of jobs, length held, veteran status, occupational injuries/toxic exposures; vocational skills, interest
- Education: highest level; ever in special education; assess ability to read/language skills/English fluency.
- Nutrition/hydration: diet, food resources, preparation skills, liquid intake
- Cultural heritage/affiliations: family, friends, faith community, other sources of support
- Strengths: coping skills, resourcefulness, abilities, interests

PHYSICAL EXAM

- Comprehensive exam: height/weight, BMI, especially: liver, dermatologic, oral, feet, neurologic, mental status
- Focused exams: for patients uncomfortable with full-body, unclothed exam at 1st visit
- Dental assessment: age-appropriate teeth, obvious caries, dental/referred pain, diabetes, CVD

DIAGNOSTIC TESTS & INTERPRETATION

- Mental health: Patient Health Questionnaire (PHQ-9, PHQ-2), MHS-III, MDQ
- Cognitive assessment: Mini-Mental Status Exam (MMSE), Traumatic Brain Injury Questionnaire (TBIQ), Repeatable Battery for the Assessment of Neuro-Psychological Status (RBANS)

- Developmental assessment: Ages & Stages Questionnaires, Parents' Evaluation of Developmental Status (PEDS), Denver II or other standard screening tool
- Interpersonal violence: domestic violence, rape, and so forth
- Forensic evaluation: if strong evidence of abuse
- Baseline labs: as needed, to address suspected medical concerns
- Tuberculosis screening: PPD
- STI screening: HIV; chlamydia; gonorrhea; syphilis; hepatitis B antigen; hepatitis C, A, B; trichomonas; bacterial vaginosis; monilia
- Substance abuse: SSI-AOD (Simple Screening Instrument for Alcohol and Other Drugs), urine drug screen

Follow-Up Tests & Special Considerations

- **Reproductive health care and STIs:** obtain detailed sexual history (sexual identity, orientation, behaviors/sexual practices, number of partners). Consider possible exploitation of patient, especially if mental illness/developmental disability suspected. Communicate willingness to initiate contraception first visit without exam. Genital exam recommended, but be sensitive to patient needs if possible sexual abuse history. If pelvic exam is refused, consider empiric treatment for STI (and possibility of multiple orifice infection). Dispense medications on site; ask if partner needs treatment.
- **Pediatric care:** complete exam every visit, use each visit to identify/address problems and provide vaccinations as homeless families may not see a medical provider unless child is sick. Vision and hearing screening at every visit and refer for abnormalities.

TREATMENT

- Establish rapport: sensitivity to prior negative health care experiences
- Enlist resources: mental health and substance abuse programs, free clinics, case management
- Health care maintenance: vaccinations (hepatitis A and B, Pneumovax, Tdap, influenza) cancer and chronic disease screening for adults; Early Periodic Screening, Diagnosis, and Treatment Program (EPSDT) screening and vaccinations for children
- Care plan
  - Basic needs: Food, clothing and housing may be higher priorities than health care.
  - Patient goals and priorities: immediate/long-term health needs. Address patient wants first.
  - Action plan: simple language, portable pocket card
  - After hours: extended clinic hours
  - Safety plan: for violence and abuse suspected; mandatory reporting requirements
  - Emergency plan: location of nearest emergency department (ED), preparation for evacuation
  - Adherence plan: use of interpreter, identification of potential barriers

MEDICATION

- Simple regimen: low pill count, once-daily dosing
- Dispensing: small amounts on-site to promote follow-up, decrease loss/theft/misuse risk. Determine resources for written prescriptions.
- Storage of medications: If no access to refrigeration, avoid medications requiring it.
- Patient assistance: free/low-cost drugs if readily available for continuous use; seek local options for assistance
- Aids to adherence: harm reduction, outreach/case management, directly observed therapy
- Side effects: primary reason for nonadherence (diarrhea, polyuria, nausea, disorientation)
- Analgesia/symptomatic treatment: consider pain contract, single provider for pain medication refills
- Dietary supplements: multivitamins with minerals, nutritional supplements
- Managed care: generics, if possible; assistance getting prescription filled
- Lab monitoring: Monitor patients on antipsychotic medications for metabolic disorders.

ADDITIONAL THERAPIES

- Associated problems/complications
  - Fragmented care: multiple providers. Use electronic medical record (EMR); list prescribed medication on wallet-sized card.
  - Masked symptoms/misdiagnosis: for example, weight loss, dementia, edema, lactic acidosis
  - Focus on immediate concerns, not possible future consequences.
  - Integrated treatment for concurrent mental illness/substance use disorders
  - Support for parent of child abused by others and for abused parent
- Follow-up
  - Reliable phone/e-mail contact for patient/friend/family/case manager
  - Frequent follow-up, incentives, nonjudgmental care regardless of adherence
  - Anticipate/accommodate unscheduled clinic visits.
  - Provide car fare, tokens, and help with transportation services.
  - Monitor school attendance and address health/developmental problems with family/school.

INPATIENT CONSIDERATIONS

Admission Criteria/Initial Stabilization

Homeless likely to benefit from admission if living conditions are suboptimal to treat medical, psychiatric, and substance use disorders.

Discharge Criteria

- Bed rest, extended periods of elevation, rest, or icing are not feasible in most instances.
- Plans requiring multiple return visits likely to fail if no transportation.
- Admission to inpatient rehabilitation if appropriate and possible

ONGOING CARE

FOLLOW-UP RECOMMENDATIONS

- Patients with a history of nonadherence need additional support (e.g., case manager, outreach) to succeed in ongoing care after hospital discharge.
- Limited access to telephones to schedule appointments; may be unable to receive telephone messages with test results or rescheduled appointment times.
- Arrange appointments prior to discharge.
- Document the best way to contact the individual.
- Refer to health care agency designed to address needs of people who are homeless with integrated physical/mental health services and substance use treatment.

PROGNOSIS

Mortality rates for chronically homeless adults are 4 times higher and average life expectancy is 42–52 years compared with 78 years for the general population (7).

REFERENCES

1. U.S. Department of Housing and Urban Development, Office of Community Planning and Development. The 2013 annual homeless assessment report (AHAR) to congress: part 1, point-in-time estimates of homelessness. https://www.hudexchange.info/resources/documents/ahar-2013-part1.pdf. Accessed 2014.
2. National Alliance to End Homelessness. The state of homelessness in America 2014. http://www.endhomelessness.org/library/entry/the-state-of-homelessness-2014. Accessed 2014.
3. U.S. Department of Health and Human Services. 2014 poverty guidelines. http://aspe.hhs.gov/poverty/14poverty.cfm. Accessed June 11, 2014.
4. National Alliance to End Homelessness. www.endhomelessness.org. Accessed July 3, 2013.
5. Bonin E, Brehove T, Carlson T, et al. *Adapting your Practice: General Recommendations for the Care of Homeless Patients*. Nashville, TN: Health Care for the Homeless Clinicians' Network, National Health Care for the Homeless Council, Inc.; 2010.
6. United States Interagency Council on Homelessness. Opening doors: federal strategic plan to prevent and end homelessness, update 2013. http://usich.gov/opening_doors/. Accessed 2014.
7. O'Connell JJ. *Premature Mortality in Homeless Populations: A Review of the Literature*. Nashville, TN: National Health Care for the Homeless Council, Inc.; 2005.

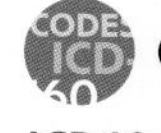

CODES

ICD10

- Z59.0 Homelessness
- Z59.1 Inadequate housing
- Z59.8 Other problems related to housing and economic circumstances

CLINICAL PEARLS

- Ending homelessness requires permanent housing, supportive services, and implementing policies to prevent chronic homelessness.
- Assistance in gaining access to benefits or meeting basic needs may decrease stress, improve therapeutic relationship, and allow individuals to direct attention to physical health.

HORDEOLUM (STYE)

Konstantinos E. Deligiannidis, MD, MPH

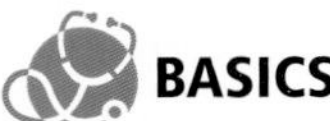

BASICS

DESCRIPTION

- An acute inflammation or infection of the eyelid margin involving the sebaceous gland of an eyelash (external hordeolum) or a meibomian gland (internal hordeolum)
- System(s) affected: skin/exocrine
- Synonym(s): internal hordeolum; external hordeolum; Zeisian stye; meibomian stye; stye

EPIDEMIOLOGY

- Predominant age: none
- Predominant sex: male = female

Incidence

Unknown: Although external hordeolum is common, internal hordeolum is rare.

ETIOLOGY AND PATHOPHYSIOLOGY

- Bacterial infection of sebaceous or meibomian glands, causing an acute inflammatory reaction
- In an internal hordeolum, the meibomian gland may become obstructed, leading to a pustule on the conjunctival surface as opposed to the margin of the eyelid.
- Most commonly caused by *Staphylococcus aureus* (~90–95% of all cases) or by *Staphylococcus epidermidis*.
- Seborrhea can predispose to infections of the eyelid.

Genetics

No known genetic pattern

RISK FACTORS

- Poor eyelid hygiene
- Previous hordeolum
- Contact lens wearers
- Application of makeup
- Predisposing blepharitis (low-grade infections of the eyelid margin)
- Ocular rosacea

GENERAL PREVENTION

Eyelid hygiene

COMMONLY ASSOCIATED CONDITIONS

- Acne
- Seborrhea
- An association may exist between hordeolum during childhood and developing rosacea in adulthood.

DIAGNOSIS

HISTORY

- Localized inflammation (vs. involvement of the entire eyelid or surrounding skin)
- Foreign body sensation in the eye
- Prior episodes are common.

PHYSICAL EXAM

- Localized inflammation of the eyelashes or a small pustule at the margin of the eyelid
- Localized swelling and tenderness on the internal or external aspect of the eyelid with an opening to either side
- To determine if an internal hordeolum is obstructed, the eyelid should be gently everted to examine for a pustule on the tarsal conjunctiva.
- Itching or scaling of the eyelids; collection of discharge, redness, and irritation leading to localized tenderness and pain

DIFFERENTIAL DIAGNOSIS

- Chalazion
- Blepharitis
- Eyelid neoplasms
- Periorbital cellulitis
- Dacryocystitis

DIAGNOSTIC TESTS & INTERPRETATION

Culture of the eyelid margins usually is not necessary.

Diagnostic Procedures/Other

History and eye exam

Test Interpretation

Bacterial contamination and white cells in eyelid discharge

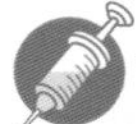

TREATMENT

GENERAL MEASURES

- The hordeolum should not be expressed.
- Warm compresses to the area of inflammation can help increase blood supply and encourage spontaneous drainage.
- Good personal hygiene with attention to cleansing the eyelids on a daily basis helps to prevent recurrent infections.

MEDICATION

First Line

- A Cochrane review found no evidence for or against nonsurgical treatment of internal hordeolum. External hordeola were not considered (1)[A].
- Usually, a hordeolum spontaneously drains, aided by warm compresses to the area.
- Application of an antibiotic ointment (e.g., erythromycin) to the margin of the eyelid after proper cleansing (except in children age <12 years, in whom there is a risk of blurred vision and amblyopia) helps reduce bacterial proliferation. There is little evidence that any topical therapy is effective. Erythromycin ophthalmic ointment may be applied up to 6×/day for 7–10 days or an antibiotic ointment containing bacitracin (2)[C].
- Treat underlying dry eye with artificial tears.

Second Line

- Occasionally, the use of an aminoglycoside ophthalmic ointment, such as gentamicin or tobramycin, may be necessary if condition is refractory to simpler treatment (case reports).
- Oral dicloxacillin or cephalexin for 2 weeks if refractory to topical antibiotics

ISSUES FOR REFERRAL

Consider referral if unresponsive to oral antibiotics.

SURGERY/OTHER PROCEDURES

- If the infection becomes localized to a single gland, incision, drainage, or curettage sometimes is necessary. This is an in-office procedure with a local anesthetic: Exercise caution because ocular perforation has been reported with the injection of an anesthetic to an infected lid.
- Use of combined antibiotic ointment (neomycin sulfate, polymyxin B sulfate, and gramicidin) after surgery was not shown to have any statistically significant benefit compared with artificial tears.

COMPLEMENTARY & ALTERNATIVE MEDICINE

Broncasma berna is a polyvalent antigen vaccine that may be useful in the treatment of recurrent hordeolum.

INPATIENT CONSIDERATIONS

Admission Criteria/Initial Stabilization

Outpatient

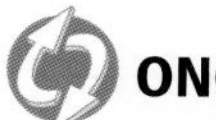

ONGOING CARE

FOLLOW-UP RECOMMENDATIONS

No restrictions

Patient Monitoring

The patient should be seen within several weeks to assess the effectiveness of therapy or should at least call the physician's office with a progress report.

DIET

No special diet

PATIENT EDUCATION

- The patient should be instructed in proper cleansing of the eyelids using a solution of tap water and baby shampoo or a commercially prepared hypoallergenic cleanser.
- The stye should not be squeezed or incised.

PROGNOSIS

- Usually responds well to good hygiene and warm compresses
- Inflammation usually improves within a week.
- Hordeolum tends to recur in some patients.

COMPLICATIONS

An internal hordeolum, if untreated, may lead to chalazion, infections of adjacent glands, or generalized cellulitis of the lid.

REFERENCES

1. Lindsley K, Nichols JJ, Dickersin K. Interventions for acute internal hordeolum. *Cochrane Database Syst Rev.* 2013;(4):CD007742.
2. Wald ER. Periorbital and orbital infections. *Pediatr Rev.* 2004;25(9):312–320.

ADDITIONAL READING

- Bamford JT, Gessert CE, Renier CM, et al. Childhood stye and adult rosacea. *J Am Acad Dermatol.* 2006;55(6):951–955.
- Hirunwiwatkul P, Wachirasereechai K. Effectiveness of combined antibiotic ophthalmic solution in the treatment of hordeolum after incision and curettage: a randomized, placebo-controlled trial: a pilot study. *J Med Assoc Thai.* 2005;88(5):647–650.
- Kim JH, Yang SM, Kim HM, et al. Inadvertent ocular perforation during lid anesthesia for hordeolum removal. *Korean J Ophthalmol.* 2006;20(3):199–200.
- Nakatani M. Treatment of recurrent hordeolum with Broncasma Berna. *Eye.* 1999;13(Pt 5):692.
- Wald ER. Periorbital and orbital infections. *Infect Dis Clin North Am.* 2007;21(2):393–408, vi.

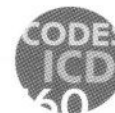

CODES

ICD10

- H00.019 Hordeolum externum unspecified eye, unspecified eyelid
- H00.029 Hordeolum internum unspecified eye, unspecified eyelid
- H00.039 Abscess of eyelid unspecified eye, unspecified eyelid

CLINICAL PEARLS

- A hordeolum should not be expressed.
- Warm compresses to the area of inflammation can encourage spontaneous drainage.
- Application of an antibiotic ointment (e.g., erythromycin) to the margin of the eyelid after proper cleansing helps reduce bacterial proliferation but may have no effect on healing of the stye.
- Good personal hygiene with attention to cleansing the eyelids on a daily basis can prevent recurrent infections.

H

HORNER SYNDROME

Jonathan Giordano, DO, MSc • Deborah A. Lardner, DO, DTM&H • Michael Passafaro, DO, DTM&H, FACEP, FACOEP

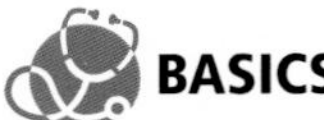

BASICS

DESCRIPTION

- Horner syndrome presents as a classic triad of ipsilateral miosis, eyelid ptosis, and/or anhidrosis of the face and neck (with iris heterochromia in children).
- It is caused by the interruption of sympathetic nerve supply to the head, neck, and eye.
  - Central or preganglionic lesion (complete syndrome): 1st- or 2nd-order neuron
  - Peripheral postganglionic lesion (incomplete syndrome, no anhidrosis): 3rd-order neuron
- System(s) affected: nervous, skin/exocrine
- Synonym(s): Bernard-Horner syndrome; Bernard syndrome; Horner's syndrome; cervical sympathetic syndrome; oculosympathetic syndrome; oculosympathetic paralysis; oculosympathetic deficiency; oculosympathetic paresis

EPIDEMIOLOGY

- Predominant age: none
- Predominant sex: male = female

Incidence

Unknown

Prevalence

Unknown

ETIOLOGY AND PATHOPHYSIOLOGY

- Constellation of signs produced when sympathetic innervation to the head, neck, and eye is interrupted somewhere along the 3-neuron arc
  - Absence of innervation of iris dilator and Müller muscles leads to miosis and slight ptosis, respectively.
  - Sympathetic innervation also controls sweat glands; interruption causes anhidrosis.
- Oculosympathetic pathway
  - 1st-order neuron: Sympathetic nerve fibers originate in the hypothalamus, descend through the brainstem, and synapse at the ciliospinal center (of Budge) located at approximately the C8–T2 levels of the spinal cord.
  - 2nd-order neuron: exits the spinal column at the T1 level primarily, arches over the apex of the lung and under the subclavian artery, ascending to the superior cervical ganglion at the level of the carotid bifurcation and angle of the jaw
  - 3rd-order neuron: ascends along the adventitia of the internal carotid artery, through the cavernous sinus in proximity to cranial nerve [CN] VI, and joins CN V_1 to innervate the iris dilator muscle and Müller muscle in the eye
- Sympathetic fibers innervating sweat glands and vasodilatory muscles branch off before the cervical sympathetic ganglion traveling along the external carotid artery, so distal lesions will not result in anhidrosis.
- Lesions anywhere along this pathway will lead to ipsilateral Horner syndrome.
- Idiopathic (40%), congenital, or acquired
- Best classified by which order neuron is affected and by age (pediatric vs. adult)
- 1st-order neuron (13%)
  - Arnold-Chiari malformation
  - Basal meningitis (e.g., syphilis)
  - Basal skull tumors
  - Cerebral vascular accident: lateral medullary (Wallenberg) syndrome
  - Cervical cord trauma
  - Demyelinating disease (multiple sclerosis)
  - Intrapontine hemorrhage
  - Neck trauma
  - Pituitary tumor
  - Syringomyelia
  - Unintended subdural placement of lumbar epidural catheter
- 2nd-order neuron (44%)
  - Aneurysm/dissection of aorta
  - Central venous catheterization
  - Chest tubes
  - First rib fracture
  - Lymphadenopathy (Hodgkin, leukemia, tuberculosis, mediastinal tumors, sarcoid)
  - Mandibular tooth abscess
  - Neurofibromatosis type I and II
  - Pancoast tumor or infection of lung apex
  - Proximal common carotid artery dissection
  - Trauma/surgical injury
- 3rd-order neuron lesions (43%)
  - Carotid cavernous fistula or other pathology
  - Carotid endarterectomy or carotid artery stenting
  - Cluster headaches
  - Internal carotid artery dissection
  - Herpes zoster
  - Lesions of the middle ear (acute otitis media)
  - Lyme disease
  - Nasopharyngeal cancer
  - Tonsillectomy
  - Raeder paratrigeminal syndrome
- Drugs: acetophenazine, alseroxylon, bupivacaine, butaperazine, carphenazine, chloroprocaine, deserpidine, diacetylmorphine, diethazine, ethopropazine, etidocaine, guanethidine, influenza virus vaccine, levodopa, lidocaine, mepivacaine, mesoridazine, methdilazine, methotrimeprazine, oral contraceptives, perazine, prilocaine, procaine, prochlorperazine, promazine, propoxycaine, reserpine, thioproperazine, thioridazine, trifluoperazine

Genetics

Rare autosomal dominant inheritance

RISK FACTORS

- Most common: apical bronchogenic carcinoma (Pancoast tumor) in smokers
- Aneurysm of the carotid or subclavian artery
- Injuries to the carotid artery high in the neck
- Dissection of the carotid arteries
- Carotid artery occlusion
  - 15% of patients with carotid artery occlusion develop ipsilateral Horner syndrome.
  - May occur without evidence of cerebral ischemia, neck injuries, or operative procedures
- Cluster headaches
  - 20% have an ipsilateral Horner syndrome

Pediatric Considerations

2nd-order neuron lesion is most common etiology: birth trauma to neck and shoulder, chest surgery, neuroblastoma (paraspinal), and vascular anomalies of the carotid arteries

COMMONLY ASSOCIATED CONDITIONS

- Wallenberg syndrome
- Pancoast tumor
- C8 radiculopathy

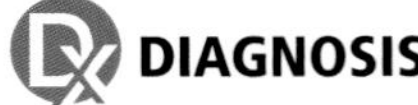

DIAGNOSIS

HISTORY

- Ptosis (typically mild; 1–2 mm)
- Miosis (with an associated dilation lag)
- Anhidrosis or hypohidrosis (often not appreciated by patients or clinicians):
  - Ipsilateral side of the body: central (1st-order neuron)
  - Ipsilateral face: preganglionic (2nd-order neuron)
  - Medial portion of forehead and side of nose: postganglionic (3rd-order neuron after vasomotor and sudomotor fiber have branched off)

Pediatric Considerations

In infants and children, loss of facial flushing is appreciated more than anhidrosis (harlequin sign).

ALERT

Horner syndrome in the presence of pain merits special consideration:

- Axial, shoulder, scapula, arm, or hand pain may be related to Pancoast tumor.
- Acute-onset, ipsilateral facial or neck pain: Consider carotid artery dissection until proven otherwise.
- Paratrigeminal syndromes:
  - Raeder paratrigeminal syndrome type I: orbital pain, miosis, ptosis, with associated ipsilateral lesions of CN III–VI; suspect middle cranial fossa mass lesion.
  - Raeder paratrigeminal syndrome type II: episodic retrobulbar or orbital pain, miosis, ptosis with no CN lesions; suspect migraine variant, syphilis, herpes zoster, hypertension.

PHYSICAL EXAM

- Measure pupillary diameter in dim and bright light and reactivity to light and accommodative response:
  - Anisocoria is greatest in dark, with affected pupil failing to dilate.
  - Redilation (after light is removed) may lag 15–20 seconds on the affected side.
- Examine the upper lids for ptosis (<2 mm).
- Examination of the lower lids for "upside-down ptosis": elevation of lower lid due to Müller muscle weakness
  - Illusion of enophthalmos secondary to narrowing of palpebral fissure
- Ipsilateral impaired flushing may be found.
- Loss of ciliospinal reflex. Pinching the skin on back of the neck normally produces ipsilateral pupil dilation (unreliable).
- Biomicroscopic exam of the papillary margin and iris structure and color
  - In congenital Horner syndrome, long-standing Horner syndrome, or Horner syndrome that occurs in children <2 years: Iris shows reduced pigmentation, blue-gray, and mottling of the affected eye (heterochromia iridis) because formation of iris pigment early in life is under sympathetic control.
- Observe for the presence of nystagmus, facial swelling, lymphadenopathy, or vesicular eruptions.
- Ophthalmoparesis, specifically CN VI palsy with Horner syndrome, is suggestive of cavernous sinus lesion.
- Neurologic and chest exams for associated physical findings

DIFFERENTIAL DIAGNOSIS

- Neurologic diseases
- 3rd nerve palsy
- Unilateral use of miotics
- Unilateral use of mydriatics
- Adie tonic pupil
- Iris sphincter muscle damage

DIAGNOSTIC TESTS & INTERPRETATION

Initial Tests (lab, imaging)

CBC, fluorescent treponemal antibody absorption test, venereal disease research laboratory, purified protein derivative; vanillylmandelic acid, homovanillic acid to rule out neuroblastoma in pediatric patients

- Chest x-ray if patient is a smoker (apical bronchogenic carcinoma)
- CT/MRI/MRA of the brain, chest, and spinal cord
  - If painful, order MRI/MRA to evaluate for carotid artery dissection emergently.
- Ultrasound may be considered for evaluation of internal carotid artery

Pediatric Considerations

In a child of any age without contributory history, MRI brain, neck, and chest to exclude a mass lesion (1)[B]

Diagnostic Procedures/Other

- Confirmation of Horner syndrome
  - Topical 0.5% apraclonidine (2)[A],(3,4)[B]
  - 4–10% topical cocaine
    - Used to confirm diagnosis of Horner syndrome but will not identify location of lesion
    - If the diagnosis is clear clinically, this test is not required.
    - A normal pupil will dilate. The miotic pupil in Horner syndrome (regardless of location of lesion) will not dilate or will dilate poorly after 45 minutes because of the absence of norepinephrine at the nerve endings of the 3rd-order neuron (2)[A].
    - Positive test is anisocoria of ≥1 mm.
    - Cocaine blocks the reuptake of norepinephrine by the neuron.
- Distinguishing a 3rd-order neuron disorder from a 1st- or 2nd-order neuron disorder:
  - Topical 1% hydroxyamphetamine (2)[A]
    - If there is a 1st- or 2nd-order neuron lesion, dilation will take place.
    - Failure of the pupil to dilate, or poor dilation, indicates a 3rd-order neuron lesion (positive when anisocoria increases by ≥1 mm).
    - No pharmacologic test exists to differentiate between a 1st- and 2nd-order neuron lesion.
    - Hydroxyamphetamine causes release of endogenous norepinephrine stored in the postganglionic neuron.
    - Alternative test: 1% topical pholedrine
- Must wait >24 hours between the cocaine and hydroxyamphetamine tests

Pediatric Considerations

Due to transsynaptic degeneration in children, the hydroxyamphetamine test is not reliable.

Test Interpretation

- Brainstem lesion
- Massive hemisphere lesion
- Cervical cord lesion
- Root lesion
- Sympathetic chain lesion

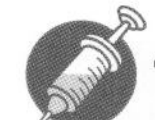

TREATMENT

GENERAL MEASURES

- Horner syndrome in itself does not produce any disability or necessarily require treatment.
- Treat the underlying etiology.
- Search for a tumor or other compressive lesion.

MEDICATION

Carotid artery dissection: Pharmacologic treatment options include thrombolysis, antithrombotic therapy with anticoagulation, or antiplatelet therapy. No randomized control trials have compared these treatment options (5)[C].

ISSUES FOR REFERRAL

- Neurologic, neuro-ophthalmic, oculoplastic
- Neurologic or vascular surgery: interventional in cases of suspected carotid artery dissection or aneurysm
- Neurosurgery, surgical oncology, oncology, or radiotherapy consultation depends on the particular etiology.

SURGERY/OTHER PROCEDURES

- Surgical care depends on etiology.
- Consider ptosis repair surgery (oculoplastics).

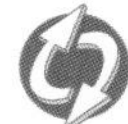

ONGOING CARE

PROGNOSIS

- Postganglionic: usually benign
- Central and preganglionic: poorer prognosis

COMPLICATIONS

- Chronic pupillary constriction
- Cosmesis

REFERENCES

1. Al-Moosa A, Eggenberger E. Neuroimaging yield in isolated Horner syndrome. *Curr Opin Ophthalmol*. 2011;22(6):468–471.
2. Antonio-Santos AA, Santo RN, Eggenberger ER. Pharmacological testing of anisocoria. *Expert Opin Pharmacother*. 2005;6(12):2007–2013.
3. Koc F, Kavuncu S, Kansu T, et al. The sensitivity and specificity of 0.5% apraclonidine in the diagnosis of oculosympathetic paresis. *Br J Ophthalmol*. 2005;89(11):1442–1444.
4. Chen PL, Chen JT, Lu DW, et al. Comparing efficacies of 0.5% apraclonidine with 4% cocaine in the diagnosis of Horner syndrome in pediatric patients. *J Ocul Pharmacol Ther*. 2006;22(3):182–187.
5. Patel RR, Adam R, Maldjian C, et al. Cervical carotid artery dissection: current review of diagnosis and treatment. *Cardiol Rev*. 2012;20(3):145–152.

ADDITIONAL READING

- Ahmadi O, Saxena P, Wilson BK, et al. First rib fracture and Horner's syndrome: a rare clinical entity. *Ann Thoracic Surg*. 2013;95(1):355.
- Almog Y, Gepstein R, Kesler A. Diagnostic value of imaging in Horner syndrome in adults. *J Neuroophthalmol*. 2010;30(1):7–11.
- Bazari F, Hind M, Ong YE. Horner's syndrome–not to be sneezed at. *Lancet*. 2010;375(9716):776.
- Davagnanam I, Fraser CL, Miszkiel K, et al. Adult Horner's syndrome: a combined clinical, pharmacological, and imaging algorithm. *Eye (Lond)*. 2013;27(3):291–298.
- Kong YX, Wright G, Pesudovs K, et al. Horner syndrome. *Clin Exp Optom*. 2007;90(5):336–344.
- Lee JH, Lee HK, Lee DH, et al. Neuroimaging strategies for three types of Horner syndrome with emphasis on anatomic location. *AJR Am J Roentgenol*. 2007;188(1):W74–W81.
- Lyrer PA, Brandt T, Metso TM et al. Clinical import of Horner syndrome in internal carotid and vertebral artery dissection. *Neurology*. 2014;82(18):1653–1659.
- Mahoney NR, Liu GT, Menacker SJ, et al. Pediatric horner syndrome: etiologies and roles of imaging and urine studies to detect neuroblastoma and other responsible mass lesions. *Am J Ophthalmol*. 2006;142(4):651–659.
- Martin TJ. Horner's syndrome, pseudo-Horner's syndrome, and simple anisocoria. *Curr Neurol Neurosci Rep*. 2007;7(5):397–406.
- Reede DL, Garcon E, Smoker WR, et al. Horner's syndrome: clinical and radiographic evaluation. *Neuroimaging Clin N Am*. 2008;18(2):369–385,xi.

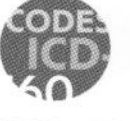

CODES

ICD10

- G90.2 Horner's syndrome
- S14.5XXA Injury of cervical sympathetic nerves, initial encounter

CLINICAL PEARLS

- Horner syndrome triad: ipsilateral miosis, eyelid ptosis, and anhidrosis caused by a lesion of the oculosympathetic pathway
- Ptosis is mild, usually <2 mm.
- Red flags: If associated with pain, suspect central or preganglionic lesion.
- Confirm the diagnosis clinically with topical cocaine to the affected eye.
- Use hydroxyamphetamine to differentiate which order neuron is affected.
- Order imaging studies based on history and physical and hydroxyamphetamine testing.
- Horner syndrome in the presence of acute-onset, ipsilateral facial or neck pain: Consider carotid artery dissection until proven otherwise.

HYDROCELE

Varun Kumar Bhalla, MD • Mohamad Masoumy, MD, MS • Edward James Kruse, DO

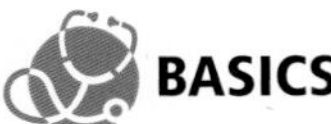

BASICS

DESCRIPTION

A collection of fluid within the scrotum

- Communicating hydrocele
  - Associated with a patent processus vaginalis
  - Has an associated indirect inguinal hernia
- Noncommunicating hydrocele (the processus vaginalis is not patent)
  - Infantile type: often spontaneous resolution
  - Adult type: infrequent resolution
- Hydrocele of the cord: distal portion of the processus vaginalis has closed; midportion patent and fluid filled; proximal portion open or closed
- Acute hydrocele: fluid collection resulting from an acute process within the tunica vaginalis
- System(s) affected: reproductive

Pediatric Considerations

In a communicating hydrocele, consider contralateral inguinal exploration.

EPIDEMIOLOGY

Predominant age: childhood (1)

Incidence

Estimated at 0.7–4.7% of male infants

Prevalence

- 1,000/100,000
- Estimated at 1% of adult men

ETIOLOGY AND PATHOPHYSIOLOGY

- Closure of the processus vaginalis, resulting in trapped peritoneal fluid (noncommunicating)
- Closure of the distal processus, trapping fluid in midportion of the processus vaginalis (hydrocele of the cord)
- Failure of closure of the processus vaginalis (communicating hydrocele)
- Infection
- Tumors
- Trauma
- Ipsilateral renal transplantation

RISK FACTORS

- Ventriculoperitoneal shunt
- Exstrophy of the bladder
- Cloacal exstrophy
- Ehlers-Danlos syndrome
- Peritoneal dialysis

COMMONLY ASSOCIATED CONDITIONS

- Testicular tumors
- Trauma
- Ventriculoperitoneal shunt
- Nephrotic syndrome
- Renal failure with peritoneal dialysis

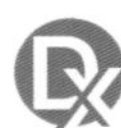

DIAGNOSIS

HISTORY

- Acute or subacute onset of scrotal swelling
- Frequent changes in size of the hydrocele (indicative of a communication)
- Swelling in the scrotum or inguinal canal
- Usually painless
- Sensation of heaviness in the scrotum
- Pain radiating to the flank/back (occasionally)

PHYSICAL EXAM

- Swelling in the scrotum or inguinal canal
- Scrotal mass, usually fluctuant
- Fluctuation in size (communicating hydrocele)
- Scrotal fluid collection that transilluminates

DIFFERENTIAL DIAGNOSIS

- Indirect inguinal hernia
- Orchitis
- Epididymitis
- Traumatic testicular injury
- Testicular torsion or torsion of appendix testes

DIAGNOSTIC TESTS & INTERPRETATION

Lab studies are rarely helpful.

- Inguinoscrotal ultrasound (US): can demonstrate the presence of bowel (e.g., distinguish incarcerated hernia from a hydrocele of the cord) as well as the presence of testicular torsion (2)
- Testicular nuclear scan or Doppler US: can distinguish testicular torsion
- Abdominal radiograph: may be useful to distinguish incarcerated hernias from hydroceles (rarely needed)

Diagnostic Procedures/Other

ALERT

Aspiration of a hydrocele for diagnosis should be discouraged.

Test Interpretation

Patent processus vaginalis in communicating hydroceles

TREATMENT

ISSUES FOR REFERRAL

Recovery should be rapid and complete.

SURGERY/OTHER PROCEDURES

- In children, surgical treatment is generally deferred until 2 years of age because many hydroceles will spontaneously resolve (1)[C].
  - Surgical: an inguinal approach with ligation of the processus vaginalis and excision, distal splitting, or drainage of hydrocele sac in children (in a hydrocele of cord, the sac can be completely removed) (3)[B]
  - Patients age <12 years should undergo an inguinal approach, whereas a scrotal approach can be considered in children age >12 years (4)[C].
- In adults, no therapy is needed unless the hydrocele causes discomfort or unless there is a significant underlying cause such as a tumor (5).
  - Surgical: A scrotal approach with internal drainage of the hydrocele in adults carries the highest recurrence rate (6)[C].

– Surgical: A scrotal approach with resection of hydrocele sac has the highest complication rate but lowest recurrence rate (6)[C].

- Jaboulay-Winkelmann procedure (for a thick hydrocele sac): The hydrocele sac is wrapped posteriorly around cord structures (6)[C],(7)[A].
- Lord procedure (for a thin hydrocele sac): Radial sutures are used to gather the hydrocele sac posterior to testis and epididymis (6)[C],(7)[A].
- Aspiration of the hydrocele with instillation of a sclerosing agent has been successfully used in adults (8)[B].
  – Aspiration with instillation of sodium tetradecyl sulphate was compared prospectively with the Jaboulay procedure (30 patients each group) (9)[B].
    ○ The aspiration instillation group had fewer complications with a lower hospital cost but higher recurrence rates (34%) and more patient dissatisfaction.
  – Aspiration with instillation of 200–400 mg of doxycycline diluted in 10 mL of 0.5% bupivacaine has demonstrated an 84% success rate with a single treatment for nonseptated hydroceles (10)[B].
- Hydrocelectomy may be performed endoscopically via a transscrotal approach; it involves cauterization of the entire parietal surface of the tunical vaginalis (11)[A].

INPATIENT CONSIDERATIONS

Admission Criteria/Initial Stabilization

- Outpatient surgery
- Observation in early infancy until a definite communication is demonstrated or until 2 years of age

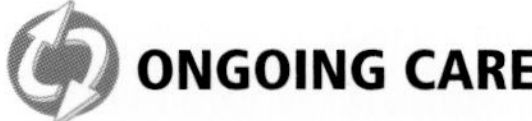

ONGOING CARE

FOLLOW-UP RECOMMENDATIONS

Full activity after surgery

Patient Monitoring

- Follow at 3–6-month intervals until a decision is made for/against surgery
- Postoperative follow-up at 2–4 weeks and subsequent 2–3 month intervals until resolution of any postoperative (traumatic) hydrocele

COMPLICATIONS

- Complication rate for a scrotal approach may reach 30% (12)[C].
- Postoperative traumatic hydrocele is common and usually resolves spontaneously.
- Injury to vas deferens or spermatic vessels
- Suture granuloma
- Hematoma
- Wound infection: Preoperative antibiotics may be beneficial in reducing postoperative infections (12)[C].
- Recurrence
- Tense infantile abdominoscrotal hydrocele may have high complication rate (13)[C].
  – May have significant rate of testicular dysmorphism (including hypoplasia)

REFERENCES

1. Hall NJ, Ron O, Eaton S, et al. Surgery for hydrocele in children—an avoidable excess? *J Pedtr Surg.* 2011;46(12):2401–2405.
2. Clarke S. Pediatric inguinal hernia and hydrocele: an evidence-based review in the era of minimal access surgery. *J Laparoendosc Adv Surg Tech A.* 2010;20(3):305–309.
3. Gahukamble DB, Khamage AS. Prospective randomized controlled study of excision versus distal splitting of hernial sac and processus vaginalis in the repair of inguinal hernias and communicating hydroceles. *J Pedtr Surg.* 1995;30(4):624–625.
4. Wilson JM, Aaronson DS, Schrader R, et al. Hydrocele in the pediatric patient: inguinal or scrotal approach? *J Urol.* 2008;180(4)(Suppl):1724–1727; discussion 1727–1728.
5. de Castilla-Ramírez B, López-Flores SY, del Roció Rábago-Rodríguez M, et al. A clinical guideline for diagnosis and treatment of hydrocele in childhood [in Spanish]. *Rev Med Inst Mex Seguro Soc.* 2011;49(1):101–108.
6. Ku JH, Kim ME, Lee NK, et al. The excisional plication and internal drainage techniques: a comparison of the results for idiopathic hydrocele. *BJU Int.* 2001;87(1):82–84.
7. Miroglu C, Tokuc R, Saporta L. Comparison of an extrusion procedure and eversion procedures in the treatment of hydrocele. *Int Urol Nephrol.* 1994;26(6):673–679.
8. Yilmaz U, Ekmekçioğlu O, Tatlişen A, et al. Does pleurodesis for pleural effusions give bright ideas about the agents for hydrocele sclerotherapy? *Int Urol Nephrology.* 2000;32(1):89–92.
9. Khaniya S, Agrawal CS, Koirala R, et al. Comparison of aspiration-sclerotherapy with hydrocelectomy in the management of hydrocele: a prospective randomized study. *Int J Surg (London).* 2009;7(4):392–395.
10. Francis JJ, Levine LA. Aspiration and sclerotherapy: a nonsurgical treatment option for hydroceles. *J Urol.* 2013;189(5):1725–1729.
11. Emir L, Sunay M, Dadali M, et al. Endoscopic versus open hydrocelectomy for the treatment of adult hydroceles: a randomized controlled clinical trial. *Int Urol Nephrol.* 2011;43(1):55–59.
12. Swartz MA, Morgan TM, Krieger JN. Complications of scrotal surgery for benign conditions. *Urology.* 2007;69(4):616–619.
13. Cozzi DA, Mele E, Ceccanti S, et al. Infantile abdominoscrotal hydrocele: a not so benign condition. *J Urol.* 2008;180(6):2611–2615; discussion 2615.

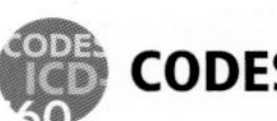

CODES

ICD10

- N43.3 Hydrocele, unspecified
- N43.2 Other hydrocele
- P83.5 Congenital hydrocele

CLINICAL PEARLS

- A hydrocele can usually be diagnosed by physical exam and will transilluminate. Occasionally, US is needed, especially with any concern for an underlying process.
- Aspirating a hydrocele is not recommended as the primary treatment. If a presumed hydrocele is actually an incarcerated inguinal hernia, aspiration may result in significant complications. In addition, hydroceles tend to recur following aspiration unless a sclerosing agent is used.

H

HYDROCEPHALUS, NORMAL PRESSURE

Dennis E. Hughes, DO, FAAFP, FACEP

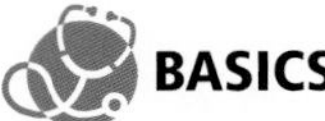

BASICS

DESCRIPTION

- Normal pressure hydrocephalus (NPH) is a clinical triad of gait instability, incontinence, and dementia (mnemonic: *wet, wobbly, wacky*). Originally described by Hakim in 1957, it occurs rarely, but is potentially treatable.
- 2 forms of the disorder: Idiopathic and secondary
- Absence of papilledema on clinical exam and normal CSF pressures at lumbar puncture

Geriatric Considerations

Idiopathic NPH primarily affects persons >60 years; extremely rare before 40 years

EPIDEMIOLOGY

Incidence

- No formal epidemiologic data exist regarding NPH because of the lack of consensus-derived diagnostic criteria. The natural history of untreated NPH has not been studied.
- Idiopathic (iNPH) form primarily affects elderly, at least >40 years of age.
- Secondary form can occur at any age.
- Male = female

Prevalence

- 3.3/100,000 age 50–59 years to 11.7/100,000 age 70–79 years for iNPH and increases to upwards of 5.9% in those 80 years and older
- Estimated to be a contributing factor in 6% of all cases of dementia

ETIOLOGY AND PATHOPHYSIOLOGY

- Idiopathic form is a communicating hydrocephalus, a disorder of decreased CSF absorption (not overproduction). In iNPH, the leading theory suggests that poor venous compliance impairs the subarachnoid granulations' ability to maintain baseline removal of CSF. In secondary NPH, scarring is likely.
- The result is a pressure gradient between the subarachnoid space and ventricular system.
- CSF production decreases in the face of an increased pressure set-point (but still in excess of the amount of CSF absorbed).
- Elevated pressure distends ventricles and compresses the brain parenchyma.
- As a result of compression, ischemic changes occur in the parenchymal vasculature with subsequent tissue damage and loss.
- Some believe that the idiopathic form is a result of persistently insufficient removal of CSF by immature subarachnoid granulations from childhood.
- Secondary NPH may result from the following:
  - Head trauma (most common)
  - Subarachnoid hemorrhage
  - Resolved acute meningitis
  - Chronic meningitis (tuberculosis, syphilis)
  - Paget disease of the skull

RISK FACTORS

- Idiopathic risk is unknown (case reports suggest a possible genetic link but unsubstantiated).
- Secondary form is due to head trauma, subarachnoid hemorrhage, meningitis, or encephalitis.

DIAGNOSIS

Detailed history and careful examination is the key to early diagnosis.

HISTORY

- Insidious and usually progressive; gait instability usually manifests initially, followed by changes in mentation, and eventually, urinary incontinence.
- Behavioral changes noted in many cases: Depression, mania, and psychotic features in many cases precede the physical findings and respond poorly to usual treatment (1)[B].
- Difficulty with initiation of movement: Feet appear "glued to the floor." Gait is wide-based, shuffling, and turning appears "en bloc."
- Inattention, forgetfulness, and lack of spontaneity often are seen with the subcortical dementia of NPH.
- Urinary urgency initially, followed by lack of inhibition and then frank incontinence.
- A minimum duration of at least 3–6 months of symptoms and progression over time
- A remote trauma or infection suggests secondary versus the idiopathic form.
- A lack of psychiatric, neurologic, or other medical conditions to explain the symptoms (including structural reasons for CSF flow restriction) (2)
- Because memory impairment may be present, it is important to include a knowledgeable informant who is familiar with the patient's premorbid state.
- Frontal lobe function is affected disproportionately to the memory impairment (objective testing may lead to an early diagnosis).

PHYSICAL EXAM

- Decreased step height and length
- Reduced speed of walking (cadence)
- Widened standing base
- Swaying of trunk during walking
- Decreased fine motor speed and accuracy
- Recall impaired for recent events
- Impaired ability to do multistep tasks or interpret abstractions

DIFFERENTIAL DIAGNOSIS

- Alzheimer disease (may be a comorbid condition in as many as 75%)
- Parkinson disease
- Chronic alcoholism
- Intracranial infection
- Multi-infarct dementia
- Subdural hematoma
- Carcinomatous meningitis
- Collagen vascular disorders
- Depression
- Syphilis
- B_{12} deficiency
- Urologic disorders
- Other hydrocephalus disorders

DIAGNOSTIC TESTS & INTERPRETATION

Initial Tests (lab, imaging)

- Thyroid-stimulating hormone (TSH)
- Syphilis serology
- CBC
- Serum B_{12}, folate
- Metabolic profile
- Blood alcohol, analysis for drugs of abuse
- Urinalysis
- CSF analysis, including an opening pressure <245 mm H_2O (a value greater than this rules out iNPH by definition)
- Imaging is essential.
  - Either CT or MRI shows the ventriculomegaly (particularly lateral and 3rd ventricles) with preservation of the cerebral parenchyma (as opposed to ventricular enlargement seen in other forms of dementia where brain atrophy is present). A narrow subarachnoid space ("tight convexity") was recently shown to correlate to probable or definite iNPH (3)[A].
  - MRI can allow detection of other features, such as signs of altered brain water content and callosal angles. However, these supportive findings are not independently diagnostic of NPH.

Diagnostic Procedures/Other

CSF removal aids in the definitive diagnosis as well as predicting response to surgical treatment.

- High-volume (30–70 mL) CSF removal via spinal tap on 3 successive days or continuous spinal drainage (150–200 mL/day) for 3 days
- Comparison of gait analysis before and after CSF removal (a ≥20% improvement indicates a positive test) especially when combined with coexisting executive function improvement (4)[B]

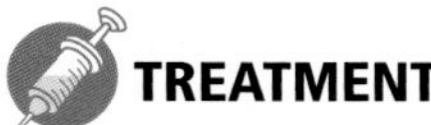

TREATMENT

MEDICATION

- No medication is significantly helpful.
- Use of carbonic anhydrase inhibitors (acetazolamide) with repeat lumbar punctures has provided mild and transient relief but is only supported by anecdotal evidence.
- Use of levodopa to rule out Parkinson disease may be helpful (NPH will display little, if any, significant improvement to dopamine agonist).

ISSUES FOR REFERRAL

- Neurology or neurosurgical consultation is helpful in suspected cases when other reversible medical conditions are ruled out.
- Recent cohort studies have demonstrated clinical improvement after surgical shunts. Perimeters of urinary continence, gait stability, and cognitive scores all improved at 1 year post shunt.

ADDITIONAL THERAPIES

Gait training and use of ambulation assist devices, as indicated, but limited efficacy

SURGERY/OTHER PROCEDURES

- Current therapy is limited to placement of ventriculoperitoneal or ventriculoatrial shunt from a lateral ventricle tunneled SC and drained into the peritoneal cavity (or right atrium). There is no compelling evidence (no randomized controlled trial [RCT]) that this therapy is effective.
- Patients whose symptoms have been present for a shorter period (<2 years) have a greater chance of improvement with shunting. Also, patients with a known cause of NPH tend to respond more favorably. However, improvement has been seen in patients with symptoms present for a long time (5)[B].

INPATIENT CONSIDERATIONS

Admission Criteria/Initial Stabilization

Usually only for planned surgical treatment

ONGOING CARE

FOLLOW-UP RECOMMENDATIONS

- Assessment and modification of environment for fall risks
- Evaluation for ability to operate a motor vehicle safely (if driving)

Patient Monitoring

- Repeat neuropsychological testing to evaluate the status of the dementia after treatment.
- Improvement in the incontinence and walking speed can also be objectively measured.

PATIENT EDUCATION

Information at: http://www.ninds.nih.gov/disorders/normal_pressure_hydrocephalus/normal_pressure_hydrocephalus.htm

PROGNOSIS

Natural history is progressive deterioration. Patient's axial skeletal stability worsens with inability to walk, stand, sit, or turn over in bed.

COMPLICATIONS

- In patients treated surgically, cerebral infarcts, hemorrhage, infection, and seizures (in addition to the usual surgical risks): all usual age-related illnesses (as NPH is a condition affecting those age >65 years)
- Shunt malfunction (especially when symptoms recur after successful shunt placement)
- Falls due to gait instability
- UTIs
- Skin breakdown, pressure ulcers, infections as movement dysfunction progresses

REFERENCES

1. Oliveira MF, Oliveira JR, Rotta JM, et al. Psychiatric symptoms are present in most of the patients with idiopathid normal pressure hydrocephalus. *Arq Neuropsiquiatr*. 2014;72(6):435–438.
2. Williams MA, Relkin NR. Diagnosis and management of idiopathic normal-pressure hydrocephalus. *NeuroClinPract*. 2013;3(5):375–385.
3. Hashimoto M, Ishikawa M, Mori E, et al. Diagnosis of idiopathic normal pressure hydrocephalus is supported by MRI-based scheme: a prospective cohort study. *Cerebrospinal Fluid Res*. 2010;7:18.
4. Allali G, Ladiet M, Beauchet O, et al. Dual-task related gait changes after CSF tapping: a new way to identify idiopathic noral pressure hydrocephals. *J Neuroeng Rehabil*. 2013;10:117.
5. Razay G, Vreughenhil A, Liddell J. A prospective study of ventriculo-peritoneal shunting for idiopathic normal pressure hydrocephalus. *J Clin Neurosci*. 2009;16(9):1180–1183.

ADDITIONAL READING

- Andren K, Wikkelso C, Tisell M, et al. Natural course of idiopathic normal pressure hydrocephalus. *J Neurol Neurosurg Psychiatry*. 2014;85(7):806–810.
- Ghosh S, Lippa C. Diagnosis and prognosis in idiopathic normal pressure hydrocephalus. *Am J Alzheimers Dis Other Demen*. 2014;29(7):583–589.

SEE ALSO

Algorithm: Ataxia

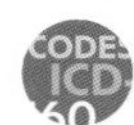

CODES

ICD10

- G91.2 (Idiopathic) normal pressure hydrocephalus
- G91.0 Communicating hydrocephalus

CLINICAL PEARLS

- Consider in unexplained dementia or behavioral change
- Poor prognosis without therapy

H

HYDRONEPHROSIS

Rama Challapalli Sri, MD • Pang-Yen Fan, MD

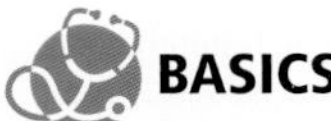

BASICS

DESCRIPTION

- Hydronephrosis refers to a structural finding—dilatation of the renal calyces and pelvis.
  - May occur with urinary tract infection (UTI), vesicoureteric reflux (VUR), high urine output, or physiologic changes in pregnancy
  - Sometimes accompanied with hydroureter
  - Presentation varies from incidental finding to discovery during workup for UTI or for flank or abdominal pain.
- Hydronephrosis should not be used interchangeably with obstructive uropathy, which refers to the damage to renal parenchyma resulting from urinary tract obstruction (UTO).

EPIDEMIOLOGY

- UTO is more common in men than women and in children than adults (congenital anomalies).
- Acute unilateral obstruction is more common than bilateral.

ETIOLOGY AND PATHOPHYSIOLOGY

- Hydronephrosis develops with increased pressure in the urinary collecting system.
- Increased pressure within the renal collecting system can cause calyceal fornix rupture and urinary extravasation.
- Over time, pressures return to normal, but kidney function declines from intense renal vasoconstriction.
- With concomitant urinary infection, bacteria can enter the renal vasculature, resulting in sepsis.
- UTO: may be acute/chronic, partial/complete, uni-/bilateral
  - Intraluminal obstruction: calculi, sloughed renal papillae, blood clot, fungal ball
  - Intrinsic abnormality of the urinary collecting system: transitional cell carcinomas, benign prostatic hypertrophy, prostate cancer, congenital ureteropelvic junction (UPJ) obstruction, ureterocele, neurogenic bladder (functional obstruction), urethral stricture or tuberculosis (TB) (can cause ureteral narrowing)
  - Extrinsic compression of the urinary collecting system: extraurinary malignancy (lymphoma, colon, cervix), aortic/iliac aneurysm, retroperitoneal fibrosis, uterine prolapse (15% affected), endometriosis, ovarian vein syndrome, IgG4-related disease
  - Transplant hydronephrosis: Consider BK virus.
- UTO in transplanted kidneys is commonly due to ureteral strictures, lymphoceles (ureteral compression and bladder dysfunction).
- VUR resulting in varying degrees of hydroureteronephrosis
- Physiologic hydronephrosis of pregnancy
- Hydronephrosis due to high urine output (e.g., diabetes insipidus, psychogenic polydipsia)
- Hydronephrosis of infection: due to bacterial toxins inhibiting smooth muscle contraction of the renal pelvis and ureter

Pediatric Considerations

- Antenatal hydronephrosis is diagnosed in 1–5% of pregnancies, usually by US, as early as the 12th–14th week of gestation.
- Children with antenatal hydronephrosis are at greater risk of postnatal pathology.
- Postnatal evaluation begins with US exam; further studies, such as voiding cystourethrogram (VCUG), based on the severity of postnatal hydronephrosis
- In neonates, it is the most common cause of abdominal mass.
- Common etiologies in children are VUR, congenital UPJ obstruction, neurogenic bladder, and posterior urethral valves.
- Pediatric diagnostic algorithm differs from adult due to different differential diagnosis necessitating age-appropriate testing.

Pregnancy Considerations

- Physiologic hydronephrosis in pregnancy is more prominent on the right than left and can be seen in up to 80% of pregnant women.
- Dilatation is caused by hormonal effects, external compression from expanding uterus, and intrinsic changes in the ureteral wall.
- Despite high incidence, most cases are asymptomatic.
- If symptomatic and refractory to medical management, ureteric calculus should be considered and urinary infection must be excluded.

DIAGNOSIS

Symptoms vary according to cause, chronicity, location, and degree of obstruction.

HISTORY

- Although often asymptomatic, hydronephrosis can be associated with pain ranging from vague, intermittent discomfort to severe renal colic.
- Nausea, vomiting may be associated with severe pain or infection.
- Fever, chills with coexisting infection
- Polyuria may occur due to impaired urinary concentration in partial obstruction, postobstructive diuresis.
- Anuria, if complete bilateral obstruction or complete obstruction of a solitary kidney
- Symptoms of chronic kidney disease: anorexia, malaise, weight gain, edema, shortness of breath, mental state changes, tremors from long-standing bilateral obstruction
- Dietl crisis: sudden attack of flank pain due to distension of renal pelvis caused by rapid ingestion of large amount of liquid or kinking of a ureter, producing temporary occlusion of urine flow
- Symptoms of bladder outlet obstruction: weak urine stream, nocturia, straining to void, overflow incontinence, urgency, and frequency
- General medical and surgical history: malignancy (extrinsic compression), radiotherapy (ureteric stricture/fibrosis), surgery (iatrogenic obstruction), trauma (hematoma or fibrosis), gynecologic disease (endometriosis, ovarian masses, uterine prolapse), smoking (urothelial cancer), drugs (methysergide-induced retroperitoneal fibrosis)

PHYSICAL EXAM

- General signs
  - Volume overload (edema, rales, hypertension [HTN]) from renal failure
  - Diaphoresis, tachycardia, tachypnea with pain
  - High-grade fever, if infection
- Abdominal exam: CVA tenderness, palpable bladder, rarely palpable abdominal mass (may be visible, particularly in thin children)
- Pelvic exam: pelvic mass, uterine prolapse, palpable enlarged prostate (cancer or benign), urethral meatal stenosis, phimosis

DIAGNOSTIC TESTS & INTERPRETATION

- Urinalysis with microscopy: hematuria, proteinuria, crystalluria, pyuria
- Midstream urine culture and sensitivity: Exclude UTI.
- Basic metabolic panel: Elevated urea and creatinine may indicate obstructive uropathy. Hyperkalemic nonanion gap metabolic acidosis may indicate type 4 distal RTA due to obstruction (1).
- CBC: anemia of chronic kidney disease (CKD), leukocytosis, if infection; check platelet count prior to considering ureteral instrumentation.
- Prostate-specific antigen (PSA): adult males age >50 years or with abnormal digital rectal exam or bladder outlet obstruction signs or symptoms
- Urine cytology: for malignant cells in urothelial malignancies
- US and noncontrast CT scanning are effective in diagnosing presence and cause of obstruction in most cases.
- US: screening test of choice for hydronephrosis
  - Sensitivity 90%, specificity 84.5% compared with IVU. Does not assess function and rarely detects cause and level of obstruction. Degree of hydronephrosis does not correlate with duration or severity of the obstruction.
  - Advantages: detects renal parenchymal disease (decreased renal size, increased cortical echogenicity, cortical thinning, cysts). No exposure to radiation or contrast. Safe in pregnancy, contrast allergy, and renal dysfunction.
  - False-positive findings 15.5% (for UTO): normal extrarenal pelvis, parapelvic cysts, VUR, excessive diuresis
  - False-negative findings 10%: dehydration, acute obstruction, calyceal dilatation misinterpreted as renal cortical cysts, and retroperitoneal fibrosis
- Noncontrast helical CT (NHCT): test of choice for suspected nephrolithiasis
  - Reported sensitivity 94–96%, specificity 94–100%. Stone is most commonly found at levels of ureteric luminal narrowing: UPJ, pelvic brim, and the vesicoureteric junction.
  - Typical findings in acute obstruction are hydronephrosis with hydroureter proximal to the level of obstruction, perinephric stranding, and renal swelling. If chronic, renal atrophy may be noted.
  - Advantages: no contrast exposure, time-saving, cost-effective, identifies extraurinary pathology
  - Disadvantages: does not assess function or degree of obstruction; higher radiation exposure, although low radiation dose protocols have shown comparable accuracy.

- DTPA or MAG-3 radionuclide renal scan (diuretic renal scintigraphy)
  - Indicated only for evaluation of hydronephrosis without apparent obstruction
  - Determines presence of true obstruction as well as total and split (right vs. left) renal function
  - Furosemide is given 20 minutes after the tracer and the T1/2 for the tracer's washout is measured. T1/2; <10 minutes is unobstructed, >20 minutes is obstructed, and 10–20 minutes is equivocal; some experts consider <15 minutes normal.
  - Advantages: no contrast exposure, safe in contrast allergy and renal dysfunction
  - False-positive findings: delayed excretion due to renal failure, massive dilatation causing a water-reservoir effect of delayed excretion without obstruction
  - False-negative findings: dehydration or inadequate diuretic challenge
- Multiphase contrast-enhanced CT
  - Nonenhanced phase detects stones and swelling.
  - Parenchymal phase demonstrates decreased enhancement of renal parenchyma with acute obstruction; can identify extraurinary causes of obstruction and determine the relative glomerular filtration rate (GFR) of each kidney with accuracy equal to radionuclide renal scan
  - Delayed phase allows visualization of the collecting system and soft tissue filling defects (e.g., urothelial cancer).
- Magnetic resonance urography (MRU): indicated when US and NHCT are nondiagnostic
  - Provides anatomic, functional, and prognostic information. Sensitivity not superior to US or NHCT for nephrolithiasis (70%) but superior for soft tissue causes including strictures.
  - Advantages: no radiation exposure, safe in young children and pregnant women
  - Disadvantages: more expensive and time-consuming (35 vs. 5 minutes) and less available compared with CT. Gadolinium contraindicated in renal failure due to risk of nephrogenic systemic fibrosis.

Diagnostic Procedures/Other

Cystoscopy, retrograde pyelogram ± ureteroscopy and biopsy are occasionally used to determine the cause of obstruction (e.g., small urothelial cancer missed on imaging) or to confirm a normal distal ureter prior to pyeloplasty. In addition, such procedures are often needed to establish a definitive pathologic diagnosis for mass lesions.

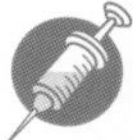

TREATMENT

GENERAL MEASURES

- Medical treatment: correction of fluid and electrolyte abnormalities, pain control, antibiotics as an adjunct to drainage if infection present
- Relief of obstruction: prompt drainage indicated in the presence of UTI, compromised renal function, or uncontrollable/persistent pain
  - Bladder outlet obstruction: urethral or suprapubic catheter
  - Ureteric obstruction: retrograde (cystoscopic) or antegrade (percutaneous) stenting
- VUR is often managed conservatively with antibiotics; surgical management required in severe cases in children or women of childbearing age
- Medical expulsive therapy (MET) with α-blockers or calcium channel blockers indicated for urethral stones <10 mm in patients with controlled pain, no signs of sepsis, with good renal function

SURGERY/OTHER PROCEDURES

- Hydronephrosis due to obstruction
  - Congenital UPJ obstruction: Pyeloplasty (open or laparoscopic) and minimally invasive stricture incision (endopyelotomy) are used with comparable results.
  - Nephrolithiasis: Extracorporeal shock wave lithotripsy (ESWL) is the initial treatment of choice for management of impacted upper urethral stones ≤2 cm. Ureteroscopy with or without intracorporeal lithotripsy has lower retreatment but higher complication rates and longer hospital stay. Ureteral stenting pre ESWL or post ureteroscopy associated with no additional benefit and more discomfort and morbidity (2)[A]
  - Transitional cell cancer: nephroureterectomy
  - Idiopathic retroperitoneal fibrosis: ureterolysis (frees ureters from inflammatory mass)
  - Prostate disorders: various treatment modalities, including transurethral resection of the prostate (TURP) and radical prostatectomy
- Nonobstructed hydronephrosis
  - VUR: ureteric reimplantation, endoscopic suburethral injection

INPATIENT CONSIDERATIONS

Admission Criteria/Initial Stabilization

Obstruction coexisting with infection (pyonephrosis) is a true urologic emergency requiring urgent drainage. Typically, this requires placement of percutaneous nephrostomy tube(s), as retrograde (cystoscopic) stenting is often difficult, but both are equally effective.

ONGOING CARE

FOLLOW-UP RECOMMENDATIONS

- Serial monitoring of kidney function (electrolytes, BUN, and creatinine) and BP until renal function stabilizes. Frequency of monitoring depends on severity of renal dysfunction.
- Follow-up US after stabilization of renal function to assess for resolution of hydronephrosis. If hydronephrosis persists, consider diuretic radionuclide study to rule out persistent obstruction.

PROGNOSIS

- Recovery of renal function depends on etiology, presence or absence of UTI, and degree and duration of obstruction.
- Significant recovery can occur despite days of complete obstruction, although some irreversible injury may develop within 24 hours. Delays in therapy can lead to irreversible renal damage (3).
- Diagnostic testing is of poor predictive value. Course of incomplete obstruction is highly unpredictable.

COMPLICATIONS

- Urine stasis: increased risk of infection and stones formation
- Obstruction causes progressive atrophy of kidney with irreversible loss of function.
- Spontaneous rupture of a calyx may occur with urine extravasation in the perinephric space.
- Postobstructive diuresis: marked polyuria after relief of obstruction
  - Caused mostly by fluid and solute overload but may be exacerbated by impaired renal tubular concentrating ability. Urine output may be >500 mL/hour.
  - Replace urine losses with hypotonic fluid (usually with 0.45% NaCl) and only enough to avoid volume depletion. Replacement of urine output with equal amounts of saline will perpetuate the diuresis.

REFERENCES

1. Batlle DC, Arruda JA, Kurtzman NA. Hyperkalemic distal renal tubular acidosis associated with obstructive uropathy. *N Engl J Med*. 1981;304(7):373.
2. Aboumarzouk OM, Kata SG, Keeley FX, et al. Extracorporeal shock wave lithotripsy (ESWL) versus ureteroscopic management for ureteric calculi. *Cochrane Database Syst Rev*. 2011;(12):CD006029.
3. Cohen EP, Sobrero M, Roxe DM, et al. Reversibility of long-standing urinary tract obstruction requiring long-term dialysis. *Arch Intern Med*. 1992;152(1):177.

ADDITIONAL READING

- Ramsey S, Robertson A, Ablett MJ, et al. Evidence-based drainage of infected hydronephrosis secondary to ureteric calculi. *J Endourol*. 2010;24(2):185–189.
- Seitz C, Liatsikos E, Porpiglia F, et al. Medical therapy to facilitate the passage of stones: what is the evidence? *Eur Urol*. 2009;56(3):455–471.
- Shen P, Jiang M, Yang J, et al. Use of ureteral stent in extracorporeal shock wave lithotripsy for upper urinary calculi: a systematic review and meta-analysis. *J Urol*. 2011;186(4):1328–1335.
- Worster A, Preyra I, Weaver B, et al. The accuracy of noncontrast helical computed tomography versus intravenous pyelography in the diagnosis of suspected acute urolithiasis: a meta-analysis. *Ann Emerg Med*. 2002;40(3):280–286.

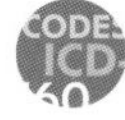

CODES

ICD10

- N13.30 Unspecified hydronephrosis
- N13.39 Other hydronephrosis
- Q62.0 Congenital hydronephrosis

CLINICAL PEARLS

- US and noncontrast CT identify most causes of hydronephrosis.
- Relief of obstruction, when present, is the primary treatment.

HYPERCHOLESTEROLEMIA

Sebastian T. C. Tong, MD, MPH • Wendy Brooks Barr, MD, MPH, MSCE

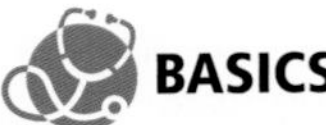

BASICS

DESCRIPTION

- Serum cholesterol >200 mg/dL (5.18 mmol/L)
  - A function of lifestyle and genetic (familial) influences
- Lipoprotein subtypes:
  - Low-density lipoproteins (LDL): primary target of therapy, atherogenic
  - High-density lipoproteins (HDL): atheroprotective
  - Triglycerides (TG)
- High cholesterol is a significant risk factor for atherosclerotic cardiovascular disease (ASCVD).
- System(s) affected: cardiovascular (CV)

EPIDEMIOLOGY

Age: increases with age (female onset delayed by 10–15 years compared with male)

Prevalence

54.9% of men and 46.5% of women in the United States with cholesterol >200 mg/dL

ETIOLOGY AND PATHOPHYSIOLOGY

- Pathophysiology
  - Deposition of cholesterol in vascular walls creating fatty streaks that become fibrous plaques
  - Inflammation causes plaque instability, leading to plaque rupture.
- Etiology
  - Primary: diet, lack of physical activity, obesity
  - Secondary: excessive alcohol intake, hypothyroidism, diabetes, nephrotic syndrome, liver disease, chronic renal failure, medications (thiazide diuretics, carbamazepine, cyclosporine, progestins, anabolic steroids, corticosteroids, protease inhibitors)

Genetics

- Type 2 familial hypercholesterolemia (FH)
  - Most severe familial form: autosomal dominant
  - Prevalence = 1/500 in the United States
  - High cholesterol levels from birth; atherosclerotic disease in early adulthood and high coronary heart disease (CHD) risk in 40s–50s
  - Tendon xanthomas on Achilles and extensor tendons of hands common
  - Early lipid-lowering drug therapy shown to reduce ASCVD risk.
- Other types: mutation in apolipoprotein B-100 gene (*APO-B*) or proprotein convertase subtilisin/kexin type 9 gene (*PCSK9*)
- Early cholesterol testing of family members beneficial

RISK FACTORS

Diet rich in saturated fat and cholesterol, obesity (BMI >30 kg/m^2), physical inactivity, heredity

GENERAL PREVENTION

- Reduced intakes of saturated fat and cholesterol
- Regular physical activity
- Weight control (see "Ongoing Care" section)

COMMONLY ASSOCIATED CONDITIONS

Hypertension, diabetes mellitus (DM), obesity

DIAGNOSIS

Screening recommendations:

- US Preventive Services Task Force (USPSTF): total cholesterol and HDL cholesterol (HDL-C) every 5 years
  - All men age ≥35 years
  - Women age ≥45 years if at increased risk for ASCVD
  - Men aged 20–35 years and women aged 20–45 years if at increased risk for ASCVD (1)[A]
- American Diabetic Association: yearly dyslipidemia screening for diabetics

Pediatric Considerations

National Heart, Lung, and Blood Institute (NHLBI): recommends lipid screening on all children between 9 and 11 years. However, these recommendations are highly controversial and not supported by most other organizations (2)[C].

HISTORY

- Review possible secondary etiologies.
- Review medications that may change lipid levels.
- Assess other ASCVD risk factors.

PHYSICAL EXAM

Nonspecific findings and not important in diagnosis

DIAGNOSTIC TESTS & INTERPRETATION

Initial Tests (lab, imaging)

- Fasting lipid panel: total cholesterol, LDL cholesterol (LDL-C), HDL-C, TG: LDL-C is usually a calculated value and is accurate if TG <350 mg/dL.
- If elevated LDL-C or other form of hyperlipidemia, clinical/laboratory assessment before initiating lipid-lowering therapy: ALT, diabetes screening
- Consider genetic etiology in very high LDL (>190 mg/dL).

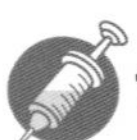

TREATMENT

ALERT

- New 2013 American College of Cardiology/American Heart Association (ACC/AHA) cholesterol guidelines no longer recommend treatment to an LDL goal. Review of evidence suggests there was never strong evidence to support specific LDL targets.
- **United States: ACC/AHA cholesterol guidelines (3)[C]**
  - Four groups benefit from statin therapy:
    - Clinical ASCVD
      - <75 years old: high-intensity statin
      - >75 years old or not candidate for high-intensity statin: moderate-intensity statin
    - Primary elevation of LDL-C >190 mg/dL: high-intensity statin
    - Diabetes (type 1 or 2) ages 40–75 years with LDL-C 70–189:
      - 10-year ASCVD risk <7.5%: moderate-intensity statin
      - 10-year ASCVD risk >7.5%: high-intensity statin
    - Without above but estimated 10-year ASCVD risk >7.5% based on Pooled Cohort Equations (http://my.americanheart.org/cvriskcalculator): moderate- to high-intensity statin
  - Definition of clinical ASCVD:
    - Acute coronary syndrome or history of MI
    - Stable or unstable angina
    - Coronary or other arterial revascularization
    - Stroke or TIA
    - Peripheral arterial disease
  - Significant controversy over recommendation to treat patients with >7.5% 10-year ASCVD risk:
    - Concern that Pooled Cohort Equations significantly overestimate ASCVD risk
    - Concern for significant overtreatment: one study showing 96% of men and 66% of women >55 years of age on statins based on recommendations
  - Many more patients treated and medications used in the United States than elsewhere in the world without substantial evidence for improved outcomes
- **United Kingdom: National Institute for Health and Care Excellence (NICE) cholesterol guidelines (4)[C]**
  - No history of CV disease
    - Current guideline: if 10-year risk of CVD >20%, start simvastatin 40 mg
    - 2014 draft new guideline: if 10-year risk of CVD >10%, start atorvastatin 20 mg
  - History of CV disease or type 2 diabetes
    - Current guideline: start simvastatin 40 mg
    - 2014 draft new guideline: start atorvastatin 80 mg
  - 10-year risk to be calculated using QRISK2: http://www.qrisk.org/
- **European: European Society of Cardiology/European Atherosclerosis Society (ESC/EAS) cholesterol guidelines (5)[C]**
  - Risk stratification to low, moderate, high, and very high risk based on SCORE charts
  - High- and very high-risk patients should be offered drug therapy.

ALERT

Elevated serum TG

- If >500, TG lowering becomes primary target until TG <500 to prevent acute pancreatitis.
  - First line: fibrate + therapeutic life changes; second line, nicotinic acid

MEDICATION

- Therapeutic lifestyle changes are cornerstone therapies to be attempted before drug therapy (diet and regular exercise; see "Ongoing Care").
- Check fasting lipoprotein profile 4–12 weeks after starting medication to evaluate response/compliance.
  - High-intensity statin: should lower LDL-C >50%
  - Moderate-intensity statin: should lower LDL-C 30–50%

First Line

HMG-CoA reductase inhibitors (statins)

- Categorized based on intensity
  - High intensity
    - Atorvastatin 40–80 mg/day
    - Rosuvastatin 20–40 mg/day
  - Moderate intensity
    - Atorvastatin 10–20 mg/day
    - Rosuvastatin 5–10 mg/day
    - Simvastatin 20–40 mg/day
    - Pravastatin 40–80 mg/day
    - Lovastatin 40 mg/day
    - Fluvastatin XL 80 mg/day
    - Fluvastatin 40 mg BID
    - Pitavastatin 2–4 mg/day

- Low intensity
  - Simvastatin 10 mg/day
  - Pravastatin 10–20 mg/day
  - Lovastatin 20 mg/day
  - Fluvastatin 20–40 mg/day
  - Pitavastatin 1 mg/day
- To be taken in the evening or at bedtime for best effect (exception: atorvastatin, rosuvastatin)
- Effect is greatest in lowering LDL-C; shown to decrease CHD incidence and all-cause mortality (secondary prevention; primary prevention less certain, larger numbers needed to treat).
- Contraindications: pregnancy, lactation, or active liver disease
- Drug interactions: cyclosporine, macrolide antibiotics, various antifungal agents, HIV protease inhibitors, fibrates/nicotinic acid (to be used with caution)
- Adverse reactions:
  - Liver transaminase elevations: ALT before therapy to establish baseline; if ALT >3 times upper limit of normal, do not start statin; routine monitoring not recommended; reasonable to measure hepatic function if symptoms suggesting hepatotoxicity occur.
  - Association with increased cases of diabetes: 0.1 excess cases of diabetes per 100 persons on moderate-intensity statin and 0.3 excess cases per 100 persons on high-intensity statin
  - Myopathies (considered rare but not well studied):
    - Creatine kinase (CK) baseline reasonable for those at increased risk for adverse muscle events; routine monitoring not needed unless muscle symptoms occur
    - Instruct patients to report immediately any muscle pain, muscle weakness, or brown urine.
    - If myopathy or rhabdomyolysis suspected, discontinue statin use and draw serum CK, creatinine, urine analysis.
    - Can rechallenge statin at lower dose or different type after resolution of symptoms
    - Mild myalgia relatively common

ALERT

FDA alert: Simvastatin should no longer be prescribed at 80 mg/day doses due to increased risk of myopathy. Patients who have been at this drug dosage for >1 year can continue if no signs of myopathy. Dose restrictions to reduce myopathy risk include:

- Do not exceed simvastatin 10 mg/day with amiodarone, verapamil, and diltiazem.
- Do not exceed simvastatin 20 mg/day with amlodipine and ranolazine.

ALERT

Avoid grapefruit juice.

Pregnancy Considerations

- Statins contraindicated during pregnancy: class X
- Lactation: possibly unsafe

Second Line

- Second-line drugs should rarely be used because none of these medications have been shown to have CV benefit or reduced mortality/morbidity.
- Ezetimibe
  - Can be taken by itself or in combination with a statin: monotherapy (Zetia 10 mg/day) or ezetimibe/simvastatin (Vytorin 10/10, 10/20, 10/40)
  - Effect: lowers LDL-C; no studies to date have shown CV benefit or decreased mortality/morbidity rates. Current indication for use of medication is not clear.
  - Adverse reactions: generally well tolerated
- Fibrates
  - Types: Gemfibrozil (Lopid) 600 mg BID, fenofibrate (Antara, Lofibra, Tricor, Triglide).
  - Effect: most effective in lowering TG with moderate effect in lowering LDL and raising HDL. More recent studies with statins fail to show benefit in most patients.
  - Contraindications: severe hepatic or renal insufficiency
  - Possible interactions: potentiates effects of warfarin and oral hypoglycemic agents. Technically, should be avoided with statins due to increased risk of rhabdomyolysis.
  - Adverse reactions: GI complaints; increased likelihood of gallstones
- Nicotinic acid: effect: most effective lipid-lowering agent for raising HDL levels but no evidence for improved outcomes in statin era, and significant potential harms. Should no longer be used in routine practice (6,7).
- Bile acid sequestrant
  - Types: cholestyramine (Questran) 4–16 g/day; colestipol (Colestid) 5–30 g/day; colesevelam (Welchol) 2.6–3.6 g/day
  - Contraindications: familial dysbetalipoproteinemia; TG >200 mg/dL (relative); TG >400 mg/dL (absolute); complete biliary obstruction; bowel obstruction
  - Possible interactions: can decrease absorption of other drugs (separate from warfarin, digoxin, and amiodarone administration by at least 2 hours)
  - Adverse reactions: constipation, nausea, bloating; rarely used now because poorly tolerated by patients

COMPLEMENTARY & ALTERNATIVE MEDICINE

- Omega-3 fatty acids and fish oil intake: Sources are fish oil (salmon), plant sources (flaxseed, canola oil, soybean oil, nuts); mainly lower TG level but has some benefit in lowering LDL and raising HDL although overall CV benefit and mortality reduction uncertain. Supplements do not reduce overall or cardiovascular mortality. Patients should be advised to eat a variety of oily fish twice a week.
- β-Sitosterols and red yeast rice (contains natural lovastatin-analogue) can reduce total cholesterol and LDL.
- Garlic: appears to have some lipid-lowering effect but more studies needed; effective dose not established but generally 1–2 cloves of raw garlic/day, 300 mg dried garlic powder tablet BID or TID, or 7.2 g of aged garlic extract/day

ONGOING CARE

FOLLOW-UP RECOMMENDATIONS

Exercise: sustained exercise for 30 minutes, 3–4 times per week: increases HDL, lowers total cholesterol, and helps control weight.

Patient Monitoring

- Initially, lipid panel in 4–12 weeks after starting therapy, routine monitoring of LDL levels in patients on statin not necessary
- Routine monitoring of LFTs is no longer recommended if initial ALT is within normal range.

REFERENCES

1. U.S. Preventive Services Task Force. Screening for lipid disorders in adults. Recommendation statement. June 2008. http://uspreventiveservicestaskforce.org/uspstf/uspschol.htm. Accessed 2014.
2. National Heart, Lung, and Blood Institute. Integrated guidelines for cardiovascular health and risk reduction in children and adolescents. December 2011. http://www.nhlbi.nih.gov/guidelines/cvd_ped/index.htm. Accessed 2014.
3. Stone NJ, Robinson JG, Lichtenstein AH, et al. 2013 ACC/AHA guideline on the treatment of blood cholesterol to reduce atherosclerotic cardiovascular risk in adults. *Circulation*. 2014;129(25)(Suppl):S1–S45. doi:10.1016/j.jacc.2013.11.002.
4. National Institute for Health and Care Excellence. Lipid modification: cardiovascular risk assessment and the modification of blood lipids for the primary and secondary prevention of cardiovascular disease. Clinical guideline draft. 2014. http://www.nice.org.uk/guidance/cg181. Accessed 2014.
5. European Association for Cardiovascular Prevention & Rehabilitation, Reiner Z, Catapano AL, et al. ESC/EAS guidelines for the management of dyslipidaemias: the Task Force for the management of dyslipidaemias of the European Society of Cardiology (ESC) and the European Atherosclerosis Society (EAS). *Eur Heart J*. 2011;32(14):1769–1818.
6. Anderson TJ, Boden WE, Desvigne-Nickens P, et al. Safety profile of extended-release niacin in the AIM-HIGH trial. *N Engl J Med*. 2014;371(3):288–290.
7. HPS2-THRIVE Collaborative Group, Landray MJ, Haynes R, et al. Effects of extended-release niacin with laropiprant in high-risk patients. *N Engl J Med*. 2014;371(3):203–212.

ADDITIONAL READING

Taylor F, Huffman MD, Macedo AF, et al. Statins for the primary prevention of cardiovascular disease. *Cochrane Database Syst Rev*. 2013;1:CD004816.

SEE ALSO

- Atherosclerosis; Hypothyroidism, Adult
- Algorithm: Hyperlipidemia

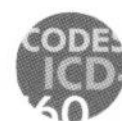

CODES

ICD10

E78.0 Pure hypercholesterolemia

CLINICAL PEARLS

- Hypercholesterolemia is a significant risk factor for ASCVD, but ASCVD is a complex disorder likely dependent on inflammation more than on cholesterol per se.
- Diet and exercise should be tried before pharmaceutical interventions.
- Statins are considered 1st-line medications for hypercholesterolemia. Other medications show little evidence of benefit in modern era.

H

HYPEREMESIS GRAVIDARUM

Emma Brooks, MD • Scott A. Fields, MD, MHA

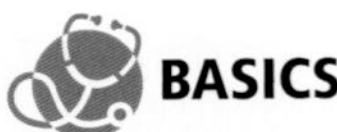

BASICS

DESCRIPTION

- Hyperemesis gravidarum is persistent vomiting in a pregnant woman that interferes with fluid and electrolyte balance as well as nutrition:
  - Usually associated with the 1st 8–20 weeks of pregnancy
  - Believed to have biomedical and behavioral aspects
  - Associated with high estrogen and human chorionic gonadotropin (hCG) levels
  - Symptoms usually begin ~2 weeks after 1st missed period.
- System(s) affected: endocrine/metabolic; gastrointestinal; reproductive
- Synonym(s): morning sickness

Pregnancy Considerations

Common condition during pregnancy, typically in the 1st and 2nd trimesters but may persist into the 3rd trimester

EPIDEMIOLOGY

Incidence

Hyperemesis gravidarum occurs in 1–2% of pregnancies.

Prevalence

Hyperemesis gravidarum is the most common cause of hospitalization in the 1st half of pregnancy and the 2nd most common cause of hospitalization of pregnant women.

ETIOLOGY AND PATHOPHYSIOLOGY

- Unknown
- Possible psychologic factors
- Hyperthyroidism
- Hyperparathyroidism
- Gestational hormones
- Liver dysfunction
- Autonomic nervous system dysfunction
- CNS neoplasm
- Addison disease

RISK FACTORS

- Obesity
- Nulliparity
- Multiple gestations
- Gestational trophoblastic disease
- Gonadotropin production stimulated
- Altered GI function
- Hyperthyroidism
- Hyperparathyroidism
- Liver dysfunction
- Female fetus
- *Helicobacter pylori* infection

GENERAL PREVENTION

Anticipatory guidance in 1st and 2nd trimesters regarding dietary habits in hopes of avoiding dehydration and nutritional depletion

Pregnancy Considerations

- 2% of pregnancies have electrolyte disturbances.
- 50% of pregnancies have at least some GI disturbance.

COMMONLY ASSOCIATED CONDITIONS

Hyperthyroidism

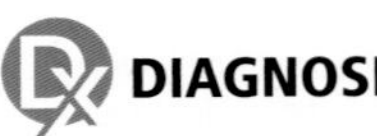

DIAGNOSIS

HISTORY

- Hypersensitivity to smell
- Alteration in taste
- Excessive salivation
- Poor appetite
- Nausea
- Vomiting with retching
- Decreased urine output
- Fatigue
- Dizziness with standing

DIAGNOSTIC TESTS & INTERPRETATION

Initial Tests (lab, imaging)

- Urinalysis: may see glucosuria, albuminuria, granular casts, and hematuria (rare); ketosis more common
- Thyroid-stimulating hormone (TSH), T4
- Electrolytes, BUN, creatinine:
  - Electrolyte abnormalities due to nausea and vomiting and subsequent dehydration
  - Acidosis
- Calcium
- Uric acid
- Hypoalbuminemia
- No imaging is indicated for the diagnosis of hyperemesis gravidarum unless there is concern for hydatidiform mole or multiple gestation, in which case ultrasound may be obtained.

Follow-Up Tests & Special Considerations

- If hypercalcemia, consider checking parathyroid hormone (PTH) for hyperparathyroidism.
- Drugs are unlikely to alter lab results.

Diagnostic Procedures/Other

Indicated only if it is necessary to rule out other diagnoses, as listed in the following section

DIFFERENTIAL DIAGNOSIS

Other common causes of vomiting must be considered:

- Gastroenteritis
- Gastritis
- Reflux esophagitis
- Peptic ulcer disease
- Cholelithiasis
- Cholecystitis
- Pyelonephritis
- Anxiety
- Hyperparathyroidism
- *H. pylori* infection

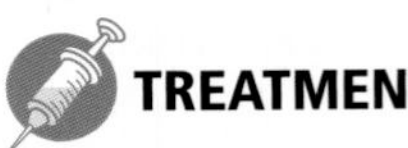

TREATMENT

Pyridoxine and doxylamine (pregnancy Category A) are first-line treatments for hyperemesis gravidarum (1)[C]. This is followed by metoclopramide or ondansetron (pregnancy Category B), then prochlorperazine (pregnancy Category C), methylprednisolone (pregnancy Category C), or promethazine (pregnancy Category C).

GENERAL MEASURES

- Patient reassurance
- Bed rest
- If dehydrated, IV fluids, either normal saline or 5% dextrose normal saline (with consideration for potential thiamine deficiency). Repeat if there is a recurrence of symptoms following initial improvement.
- For severe cases, consider PO thiamine 25–50 mg TID or IV 100 mg in 100 mL of normal saline over 30 minutes once weekly and potential parental nutrition if needed.

- Ondansetron carries an FDA warning regarding concerns for QT prolongation, but this is in the setting of high-dose IV administration and in patients with heart disease. It has unclear risk in the setting of pregnancy. The majority of the current studies appear to show no increased risk of fetal malformation with the use of ondansetron, but this is still an area of controversy (2)[C],(3)[B].

MEDICATION

- Pyridoxine (vitamin B_6) 25 mg PO or IV every 8 hours
- Antihistamines (e.g., diphenhydramine [25–50 mg q4–6h] or doxylamine [12.5 mg PO BID]) (4)[C]
- Combination product Diclegis (sustained-release pyridoxine 10 mg and doxylamine 10 mg) dosed 2 tabs daily-2 BID approved in 2013

- Phenothiazines (e.g., promethazine or prochlorperazine):
  - Precautions: Phenothiazines are associated with prolonged jaundice, extrapyramidal effects, and hyper- or hyporeflexia in newborns.
- Meclizine 25 mg PO q6h
- Metoclopramide 10 mg PO q6–8h
- Methylprednisolone 16 mg PO/IV q8h for 2–3 days, then taper over 2 weeks if initial 3-day treatment effective
- Ondansetron 4–8 mg PO q8h

Pregnancy Considerations

All medications taken during pregnancy should balance the risks and benefits both to the mother and the fetus.

COMPLEMENTARY & ALTERNATIVE MEDICINE

- Ginger 350 mg PO TID may help (5)[A].
- Motion sickness wristbands are another nonpharmacologic intervention that may improve symptoms. Evidence is mixed regarding the impact of acupressure and acupuncture in treating hyperemesis gravidarum (6)[C].
- Medical hypnosis may be a helpful adjunct to the typical medical treatment regimen, but further study is needed (7)[C].

INPATIENT CONSIDERATIONS

Admission Criteria/Initial Stabilization

- Typically outpatient therapy
- In some severe cases, parenteral therapy in the hospital or at home may be required.
- Enteral volume and nutrition repletion may be indicated.

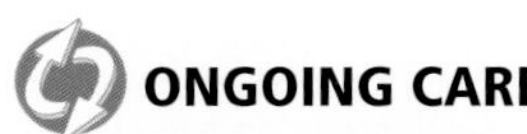

ONGOING CARE

FOLLOW-UP RECOMMENDATIONS

Activity as tolerated after improvement

Patient Monitoring

- In severe cases, follow-up on a daily basis for weight monitoring.
- Special attention should be given to monitor for ketosis, hypokalemia, or acid–base disturbances due to hyperemesis.

DIET

- NPO for first 24 hours if patient is ill enough to require hospitalization
- For outpatient: a diet rich in carbohydrates and protein, such as fruit, cheese, cottage cheese, eggs, beef, poultry, vegetables, toast, crackers, rice. Limit intake of butter. Patients should avoid spicy meals and high-fat foods. Consider cold foods. Encourage small amounts at a time every 1–2 hours.

PATIENT EDUCATION

- Attention should be given to psychosocial issues, such as possible ambivalence about the pregnancy.
- Patients should be instructed to take small amounts of fluid frequently to avoid volume depletion.
- Avoid individual foods known to be irritating to the patient.
- Wet-to-dry nutrients (sherbet, broth, gelatin to dry crackers, toast)

PROGNOSIS

- Self-limited illness with good prognosis if patient's weight is maintained at >95% of prepregnancy weight
- With complication of hemorrhagic retinitis, mortality rate of pregnant patient is 50%.

COMPLICATIONS

- Patients with >5% weight loss are associated with intrauterine growth retardation and fetal anomalies.
- Poor weight gain is associated with slightly increased risk for small for gestational age infant <2,500 g and premature birth <37 weeks (8)[A].
- Hemorrhagic retinitis
- Liver damage
- CNS deterioration, Wernicke encephalopathy secondary to thiamine deficiency, coma

REFERENCES

1. Maltepe C, Koren G. The management of nausea and vomiting of pregnancy and hyperemesis gravidarum—a 2013 update. *J Popul Ther Clin Pharmacol*. 2013;20(2):e184–e192.
2. Doggrell SA, Hancox JC. Cardiac safety concerns for ondansetron, an antiemetic commonly used for nausea linked to cancer treatment and following anesthesia. *Expert Opin Drug Saf*. 2013;12(3):421–431.
3. Pasternak B, Svanstrom H, Hviid A. Ondansetron in pregnancy and risk of adverse fetal outcomes. *N Engl J Med*. 2013;368(9):814–823.
4. Boelig RC, Berghella V, Kelly AJ, et al. Interventions for treating hyperemeisis gravidarum. *Cochrane Database of Systematic Reviews*. 2013;6:CD010607.
5. Viljoen E, Visser J, Koen N, et al. A systematic review and meta-analysis of the effect and safety of ginger in the treatment of pregnancy-associated nausea and vomiting. *Nutr J*. 2014;13:20.
6. Xu J, MacKenzie IZ. The current use of acupuncture during pregnancy and childbirth. *Curr Opin Obstet Gynecol*. 2012;24(2):65–71.
7. McCormack D. Hypnosis for hyperemesis gravidarum. *J Obstet Gynecol*. 2010.2010;30(7):647–653.
8. Veenendaal MV, van Abeelen AF, Painter RC, et al. Consequences of hyperemesis gravidarum for offspring: a systematic review and meta-analysis. *BJOG*. 2011;118(11):1302–1313.

ADDITIONAL READING

- Anderka M, Mitchell AA, Louik C, et al. Medications used to treat nausea and vomiting of pregnancy and the risk of selected birth defects. *Birth Defects Res A Clin Mol Teratol*. 2012;94(1):22–30.
- Jarvis S, Nelson-Piercy C. Management of nausea and vomiting in pregnancy. *BMJ*. 2011;342:d3606.
- Matthews A, Haas DM, O'Mathuna DP, et al. Interventions for nausea and vomiting in early pregnancy. *Cochrane Database Syst Rev*. 2014;3:CD007575.
- McCarthy FP, Lutomski JE, Greene RA. Hyperemesis gravidarum: current perspectives. *Int J Womens Health*. 2014;6:719–725.
- Tan PC, Omar SZ. Contemporary approaches to hyperemesis during pregnancy. *Curr Opin Obstet Gynecol*. 2011;23(2):87–93.

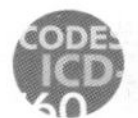

CODES

ICD10

- O21.9 Vomiting of pregnancy, unspecified
- O21.0 Mild hyperemesis gravidarum
- O21.1 Hyperemesis gravidarum with metabolic disturbance

CLINICAL PEARLS

- Do not allow patients to become volume depleted. Once this occurs, it is more difficult to interrupt the process.
- Do not be hesitant to use medications to assist the patient, as this may help avoid volume depletion.
- Consider secondary causes of hyperemesis if it develops after 12 weeks of gestation.

HYPEREOSINOPHILIC SYNDROME

Kristen M. Wyrick, MD

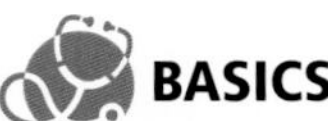

BASICS

DESCRIPTION

- Hypereosinophilic syndrome (HES): a group of disorders characterized by an overproduction of eosinophils that subsequently infiltrate and damage multiple organs
- Hypereosinophilia (HE): with eosinophilia-mediated organ damage
  - Hypereosinophilia
    - A persistent blood eosinophilia >1.5 × 109 cells/L on two examinations separated by at least 1 month and/or tissue HE
    - Exclusion of all other causes of organ damage and eosinophilia ("MAAACP": **m**alignancy, **a**sthma, **a**llergy, **A**ddison disease [AD], **c**onnective tissue disease, **p**arasitic infection).
    - Tissue HE defined by the following:
      - Eosinophils >20% of all nucleated cells on bone marrow section and/or
      - Extensive tissue infiltration on histopathology and/or
      - Marked deposition of eosinophil granular proteins in tissue
- System(s) affected: hematologic, cardiac, cutaneous, pulmonary, neurologic, gastrointestinal (GI); rheumatologic, ocular

EPIDEMIOLOGY

A rare condition, prevalence 0.36–6.3/100,000, typically seen between 20 and 50 years

- Clinically relevant variants:
  - T-cell lymphocytic (L-HES): benign polyclonal hypergammaglobulinemia but may progress to T-cell lymphoma. CD3−/CD4+, interleukin (IL)-5–producing T cells. Prominent skin findings include erythroderma, plaques, and/or urticaria.
  - Myeloproliferative (F/P+HES): almost exclusively in males with *FIP1L1-PDGFRa* fusion (Fip1-like-1 fused with platelet derived growth factor receptor alpha [F/P][2] and increased serum B_{12}, bicytopenia, organomegaly, increased serum tryptase, and positive mast cell abnormalities)
  - Familial HES: AD asymptomatic eosinophilia present at birth
  - Benign HES: hypereosinophilia without end-organ damage
  - Complex HES: multisystem organ involvement
  - Episodic HES: Periodic rise in IL-5 leads to angioedema and eosinophilia; resolves spontaneously; may progress to L-HES
  - Overlap HES: restricted eosinophilia to a single organ (GI, pulmonary, cardiac, vascular)
  - Other clinical situations with hypereosinophilia:
    - Churg-Strauss syndrome (eosinophilic vasculitis that can affect skin, sinuses, heart, lungs, peripheral nerves), Gleich syndrome (episodic HES with pruritus, urticaria, fever, weight gain, increase serum IgM, and leukocytosis)
    - Immunodysregulation (collagen vascular disease, sarcoid, ulcerative colitis, autoimmune lymphoproliferative syndrome, HIV)
    - Hypereosinophilia of undetermined significance (no complications related to tissue eosinophilia)

Incidence

- Peak incidence in 4th decade of life
- Uncommon in children
- Incidence decreases in elderly
- Predominant sex: male > female (9:1)

ETIOLOGY AND PATHOPHYSIOLOGY

- Primary molecular defect resulting in clonal eosinophilic proliferation and/or overproduction or functional abnormalities of eosinophilopoietic cytokines and/or defects in normal suppressive regulation of eosinophilopoiesis
- Three hematopoietic cytokines: IL-3, IL-5, and granulocyte-macrophage colony-stimulating factor (GM-CSF) stimulate bone marrow myeloid progenitors to overproduce eosinophils; IL-5 is most specific for eosinophil differentiation.
- Pathogenesis:
  - HES: Eosinophils infiltrate organs and release toxic granules containing major basic protein, eosinophil peroxidase, eosinophil cationic protein (ECP), eosinophil-derived neurotoxin (EDN), Charcot-Leyden crystals, VIP, and substance P; neurotoxic, cytotoxic, and prothrombotic; creates oxidative burst, reactive oxygen species
  - EDN and ECP activate fibroblasts: fibrosis and organ dysfunction

Genetics

- F/P+HES: Microdeletion at 4q12 causing gene fusion creates constitutively active tyrosine kinase.
- Other *PDGFRA* fusion partners besides *FIP1L1*; *PDGFRb* → translocation at 5q31-33 and *FGFR1* → translocation at 8p11-13
- L-HES: clonal T-cell expansion; mutations such as 16q breakage, partial 6q or 10p deletions, trisomy 7
- Familial eosinophilia: autosomal dominant, at 5q31-q33; eosinophilia at birth, often asymptomatic
- Cardiac disease more in males, carriers of HLA-Bw44

RISK FACTORS

Male gender (F/P+HES)

GENERAL PREVENTION

No known preventive measures

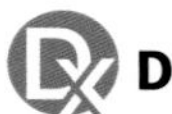

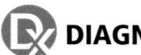

DIAGNOSIS

- A persistently elevated eosinophil count >1.5 × 10^9 cells/L on 2 examinations at least 1 month apart and/or tissue hypereosinophilia (1)[C]
- Eosinophil-mediated organ damage in which other potential causes for the damage have been excluded

HISTORY AND PHYSICAL EXAM

- Dermatologic manifestations (37%) may cause pruritic lichenified eczematous rash with papules and nodules, plus dermatographism, and/or recurrent urticaria and angioedema; may also cause erythroderma. Mucosal ulcerations are more common in patients with *FIP1L1-PDGFRa* fusion.
- Pulmonary manifestations (25%) may cause dyspnea, wheezing, and nonproductive cough.
- GI manifestations (14%): gastritis/enteritis; diarrhea, vomiting, abdominal pain (embolic bowel infarction); hepatic manifestations of hepatitis, Budd-Chiari syndrome
- Cardiac manifestations (5%) may cause endocarditis, myocarditis, shortness of breath, chest pain, ventricular failure, cardiomegaly, and/or restrictive cardiomyopathy; eosinophilic myocarditis more common in patients with *FIP1L1-PDGFRα* fusion
- Asymptomatic hypereosinophilia (6%)
- Neurologic manifestations may result from thromboembolic disease, behavioral changes, memory loss, confusion, and neuropathy.
- Ocular manifestations: blurry vision/blindness from microemboli
- Other: myalgias, arthralgias

DIFFERENTIAL DIAGNOSIS

- Leukemias, lymphomas, paraneoplastic syndromes, *KIT* mutation–associated systemic mastocytosis with eosinophilia, drug hypersensitivity reactions, and helminth infections
- Chronic eosinophilic leukemia: clonality like F/P+HES but differs by having 2–20% blasts peripherally or 5–20% blasts in the marrow
- Acute eosinophilic leukemia: a form of acute myelogenous leukemia (AML) with 50–80% immature eosinophils, >10% blast in marrow; may cause cardiac and neurologic complications

DIAGNOSTIC TESTS & INTERPRETATION

- Hypereosinophilia >1.5 × 10^9 cells/L on 2 occasions; may be discovered incidentally on routine lab testing
- CBC with differential and peripheral smear
  - Leukocytosis of 10,000–30,000 (>90,000 carries poor prognosis)
  - Mature eosinophils ≥1,500 cells/μL (nuclear hypersegmentation, hypo- and hypergranularity): hypogranularity and vacuolization more common with cardiac disease
  - Often normal platelets but may have thrombocytosis or thrombocytopenia in cases with features of myeloproliferative disorder (plus tear drop cells)
  - Normocytic anemia (anemia of chronic disease)
- Genetics
  - Fluorescent in situ hybridization (FISH) analysis or reverse transcription-polymerase chain reaction (RT-PCR): assess *FIP1L1/PDGFRA* translocation/other TK mutations such as *PDGFRA* variants, *PDGFR*B, *FGFR1*
  - Rule out *c-KIT* mutation (mastocytosis)
  - RT-PCR or Southern blot: assess IL-5-producing CD3−/CD4+ T lymphocytes
- Chemistries
  - Increased IgE
  - Increased serum tryptase and B_{12} levels (F/P+myeloproliferative HES)
  - L-HES: increased IL-5, IgG, IgM, thymus and activation-regulated chemokine (TARC) levels
- ECG: T-wave inversion, restrictive cardiomyopathy

Initial Tests (lab, imaging)

- Elevated serum tryptase
  - Peripheral blood screening for *FIP1L1-PDGFRA*
  - If negative, then bone marrow biopsy and cytogenetics for *FIP1L1/PDGFRA, BCR/ABL, c-KIT* translocations; T-lymphocyte phenotyping with flow cytometry and T-cell receptor (TCR) analysis (1)[B]
- If all negative, consider idiopathic HES.
- Echocardiogram
- Abdominal/chest CT: assess end-organ involvement

Diagnostic Procedures/Other

- Tissue biopsy (organ-restricted disease); bone marrow aspirate and biopsy
- Histopathology
  - Organ infiltration with eosinophils and lymphocytes, tissue necrosis, eosinophil degranulation, and microabscesses

TREATMENT

- Consider *FIP1L1/PDGFRA* (F/P) transcript status.
- Initial treatment involves a trial of glucocorticoids alone in all patients *EXCEPT* those with F/P+ (1)[B].

MEDICATION

- F/P+ HES
  - Tyrosine kinase inhibitors (TKIs) in all patients with or without symptoms
  - Danger of heart failure (rapid release of killed eosinophil contents) at start of therapy: Obtain troponin, monitor carefully, treat with corticosteroids 1–2 mg/kg/day concurrently or prior to initiation of therapy if complications arise, cardiac enzymes elevated, abnormal echocardiogram.
  - TKIs induce complete molecular response (no F/P transcript); not yet known to be curative
- F/P− HES
  - Corticosteroids are the mainstay of treatment.
  - A corticosteroid-sparing agent (interferon-alfa, anti-CD52 agents in L-HES, IL-5 inhibitors, chemotherapeutic agents) may be used if steroids are not tolerated or fail to manage disease.
  - May respond to TKI, suggesting non-F/P tyrosine kinase activity

First Line

- F/P+, PDGFRA/B, FGFR1 HES: imatinib mesylate (Gleevec) at 100–400 mg/day
  - 100 mg/day in *PDGFRA*
  - 400 mg/day in *PDGFRB* and *FGFR1*
  - Generally, lower doses needed to induce/maintain remission than with chronic myelogenous (or myeloid) leukemia (CML). Therapy is continued indefinitely.
  - Side effects: thrombocytopenia, anemia, nausea, diarrhea, increased liver function tests (LFTs); avoid pregnancy
  - Resistance: T674I point mutation, similar to CML
- F/P− HES: prednisone: initial challenge of 60 mg once to determine responsiveness, followed by 1 mg/kg/day × 1–2 weeks. A taper should be initiated based on disease severity, persistent eosinophilia:
  - Intolerance should prompt decreasing dose and adding 2nd agent.
  - Once stable, may add corticosteroid-sparing agent

Second Line

- F/P+ HES Patients rarely have shown resistance to imatinib; initiate trial of other TKI such as nilotinib, sorafenib, or dasatinib.
- F/P− HES
  - Imatinib
    - Trial of 400 mg/day once stabilized on steroids or fail to respond/intolerant to steroids
  - Interferon-alfa
    - Effective dose 1–8 million U 3–7 times a week; start low; increase as tolerated.
    - Side effects: flulike symptoms, cytopenia, depression, elevated LFTs, GI disturbances
  - Hydroxyurea
    - Start at 500–1,000 mg/day, increase to 2,000 mg/day
    - Side effects: cytopenia, nausea, rash, alopecia, diffuse pulmonary infiltrates, elevated LFTs, teratogen
  - Mepolizumab (in clinical trials)
    - Anti-IL5 antibody; administered 750 mg IV every 4 weeks; decreases steroid use
    - FDA approved Orphan Drug Designation
    - Side effects: fatigue, headaches, arthralgia, pruritus
  - Alemtuzumab
    - Anti-CD52 antibody, IV administration
    - Effective for relapsed refractory idiopathic HES and chronic eosinophilic leukemia NOS
    - Side effects: infusion reactions and hematologic toxicity with immunosuppression, leading to increased risk of opportunistic infections, especially CMV reactivation

ISSUES FOR REFERRAL

Refer to a hematologist and appropriate specialist depending on target organ involvement.

ADDITIONAL THERAPIES

Investigational:

- *PDGFR* fusion oncogenes proliferate autonomously and differentiate toward eosinophil lineage via nuclear factor (NF)-κB, suggesting treatment potential.
- JAK 1/2 inhibitor, ruxolitinib, may have a role in treatment.

SURGERY/OTHER PROCEDURES

- Allogeneic stem cell transplant
  - Patients failing other treatment modalities and/or those with aggressive disease
  - Patients with L-HES progressing to T-cell lymphoma
  - Role has not been well established
- Cardiac surgery for complications of HES is helpful. If valve replacement is necessary, use porcine valve because of underlying hypercoagulable state.

INPATIENT CONSIDERATIONS

Admission Criteria/Initial Stabilization

- Emergency treatment for eosinophilia >100,000 includes high-dose corticosteroids (prednisone 1 mg/kg).
- If levels fail to decrease in 24 hours: vincristine 1–2 mg/m^2, imatinib 400 mg, or plasmapheresis
- Heart failure, splenic rupture, organ failure; very high eosinophilia

ONGOING CARE

FOLLOW-UP RECOMMENDATIONS

Depends on etiology of disease, response to treatment, and severity of end-organ damage

Patient Monitoring

- Weekly CBC on treatment; longer when stable
- L-HES: increased risk of T-cell lymphoma; CBC every 3 months; flow cytometry biannually to monitor abnormal lymphocytosis
- Patients on imatinib: LFTs and CBC monthly; RT-PCR for the F/P transcript; echocardiogram every 3 months
- Screen for organ involvement every 6 months: cardiac enzymes, pulmonary function tests, LFTs, renal function tests, ECG, echocardiogram
- Anticoagulation unnecessary unless thrombi present

PROGNOSIS

- Better prognosis:
  - Absence of heart disease
  - Presentation with angioedema
  - Corticosteroid responsive
  - No associated indicators of myeloproliferative disease (elevated B_{12} or tryptase, splenomegaly, abnormal lymphocytes, cytogenetic abnormalities)
- Worse prognosis:
  - Concurrent myeloproliferative disorder
  - Male sex
  - Peripheral blood blasts
  - WBC count >100,000

REFERENCES

1. Gotlib J. World Health Organization-defined eosinophilic disorders: 2014 update on diagnosis, risk stratification, and management. *Am J Hematol*. 2014;89(3):325–337.

ADDITIONAL READING

- Chusid MJ, Dale DC, West BC, et al. The hypereosinophilic syndrome: analysis of fourteen cases with review of the literature. *Medicine (Baltimore)*. 1975;54:1–27.
- Montano-Almendras CP, Essaghir A, Schoemans H, et al. ETV6-PDGFRB and FIP1L1-PDGFRA stimulate human hematopoietic progenitor cell proliferation and differentiation into eosinophils: the role of nuclear factor-κB. *Haematologica*. 2012;97(7):1064–1072.
- Ogbogu PU, Bochner BS, Butterfield JH, et al. Hypereosinophilic syndrome: a multicenter, retrospective analysis of clinical characteristics, and response to therapy. *J Allergy Clin Immunol*. 2009;124(6):1319–1325.
- Simon HU, Rothenberg ME, Bochner BS, et al. Refining the definition of hypereosinophilic syndrome. *J Allergy Clin Immunol*. 2010;126(1):45–49.
- Tefferi A, Gotlib J, Pardanani A. Hypereosinophilic syndrome and clonal eosinophilia: point-of-care diagnostic algorithm and treatment update. *Mayo Clin Proc*. 2010;85(2):158–164.
- Valent P, Klion AD, Horny HP, et al. Contemporary consensus proposal on criteria and classification of eosinophilic disorders and related syndromes. *J Allergy Clin Immunol*. 2012;130(3):607–312.
- Verstovsek S, Tefferi A, Kantarjian H, et al. Alemtuzumab therapy for hypereosinophilic syndrome and chronic eosinophilic leukemia. *Clin Cancer Res*. 2009;15(1):368–373.

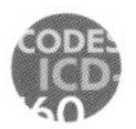

CODES

ICD10

D72.1 Eosinophilia

CLINICAL PEARLS

- HES encompasses a group of diseases with eosinophils >1,500/μL and end-organ damage without an identifiable secondary cause.
- F/P+ transcript status should be determined to help guide the course of treatment.
- Prognosis and treatment depend on subtype.
- Cardiac disease is a dangerous complication of HES and may not be reversible.

HYPERKALEMIA

Ruben Peralta, MD, FACS

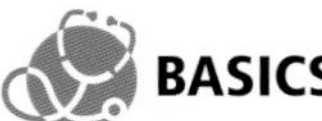

BASICS

DESCRIPTION

- Hyperkalemia is a common electrolyte disorder that may be defined as a plasma potassium (K) concentration >5.5 mEq/L (>5 mmol/L).
- Hyperkalemia depresses cardiac conduction and can lead to fatal arrhythmias.
- Normal K regulation
  - Ingested K enters portal circulation; pancreas releases insulin in response. Insulin facilitates K entry into cells.
  - K in renal circulation causes renin release from juxtaglomerular cells, leading to activation of angiotensin I, which is converted to angiotensin II in lungs. Angiotensin II acts in adrenal zona glomerulosa to stimulate aldosterone secretion. Aldosterone, at the renal collecting ducts, causes K to be excreted and sodium to be retained.
- 4 major causes
  - Increased load: either endogenous from tissue release or exogenous from a high intake, usually in association with impaired excretion
  - Decreased excretion: due to decreased glomerular filtration rate
  - Cellular redistribution: shifts from intracellular space (majority of K is intracellular) to extracellular space
  - Pseudohyperkalemia: related to red cell lysis during collection or transport of blood sample, thrombocytosis, or leukocytosis

Geriatric Considerations

Increased risk for hyperkalemia because of decreases in renin and aldosterone as well as comorbid conditions

EPIDEMIOLOGY

Prevalence

- 1–10% of hospitalized patients
- Predominant sex: male = female
- No age-related predilection

ETIOLOGY AND PATHOPHYSIOLOGY

- Pseudohyperkalemia
  - Hemolysis of red cells in phlebotomy tube (spurious result is most common)
  - Thrombolysis
  - Leukocytosis
  - Thrombocytosis
  - Hereditary spherocytosis
  - Infectious mononucleosis
  - Traumatic venipuncture or fist clenching during phlebotomy (spurious result)
- Transcellular shift (redistribution)
  - Metabolic acidosis
  - Insulin deficiency
  - Hyperglycemia
  - Tissue damage (rhabdomyolysis, burns, trauma)
  - Tumor lysis syndrome
  - Cocaine abuse
  - Exercise with heavy sweating
  - Mannitol
- Impaired K excretion
  - Renal insufficiency/failure
  - Addison disease
  - Mineralocorticoid deficiency
  - Primary hyporeninemia, primary hypoaldosteronism
  - Type IV renal tubular acidosis (hyporeninemic hypoaldosteronism)
- Medication-induced
  - Excess K supplementation
  - Statins
  - ACE inhibitors
  - Angiotensin receptor blockers
  - β-Blockers
  - Cyclosporine
  - Digoxin toxicity
  - Ethinyl estradiol/drospirenone
  - Heparin
  - NSAIDs
  - Penicillin G potassium
  - Pentamidine
  - Spironolactone
  - Succinylcholine
  - Tacrolimus
  - Trimethoprim, particularly with other medications associated with hyperkalemia (3,4)

Genetics

Associated with some inherited diseases and conditions

- Familial hyperkalemic periodic paralysis
- Congenital adrenal hyperplasia

RISK FACTORS

- Impaired renal excretion of K
- Acidemia
- Massive cell breakdown (rhabdomyolysis, burns, trauma)
- Use of K-sparing diuretics
- Excess K supplementation

GENERAL PREVENTION

Diet and oral supplement compliance in those at risk

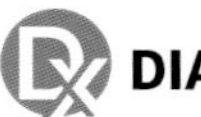

DIAGNOSIS

HISTORY

- Neuromuscular cramps
- Diarrhea
- Abdominal pain
- Myalgias
- Numbness
- Weakness

PHYSICAL EXAM

- Decreased deep tendon reflexes
- Flaccid paralysis of extremities

DIAGNOSTIC TESTS & INTERPRETATION

- Serum electrolytes
- Renal function: BUN, creatinine
- Urinalysis: K, creatinine, osmoles (to calculate fractional excretion of K and transtubular K gradient; both assess renal handling of K)
- Disorders that may alter lab results
  - Acidemia: K shifts from the intracellular to extracellular space.
  - Insulin deficiency
  - Hemolysis of sample
- Cortisol and aldosterone levels to check for mineralocorticoid deficiency when other causes are ruled out

Diagnostic Procedures/Other

EKG

- Peaked T wave in precordial leads (most common, usually earliest EKG change) (5)
- Loss of P wave
- Widened QRS
- Sine wave at very high K

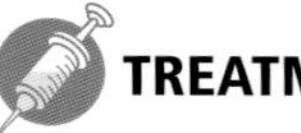

TREATMENT

MEDICATION

- After initial treatment with calcium gluconate IV to stabilize myocardial membranes (if life-threatening hyperkalemia is present), institute measures to decrease total body K:
  - Sodium polystyrene sulfonate (Kayexalate): 15 g PO or 30 g rectally
  - This requires 1–4 hours to lower K and is a definitive treatment. This may be repeated q6h, if necessary.
  - Best used in conjunction with rapidly acting transient therapies listed in the following text
  - Enema form more quickly effective
- Little clinical evidence for the use of diuretics (loop and thiazides) (1)[B]
- Dextrose 50%, 1 amp (if plasma glucose <250 mg/dL) and insulin 10 U IV may drive K intracellularly but does not decrease total body K and may result in hypokalemia (close monitoring advised).
- Nebulized albuterol and other β-agonists also drive K inside cells but does not lower total body K.
- Consider the use of recombinant urate oxidase (rasburicase) in patients with tumor lysis syndrome.
- Hemodialysis is the definitive therapy when other measures are not effective. This may be required particularly when conditions such as digitalis toxicity, rhabdomyolysis, end-stage renal disease, severe chronic kidney disease, or acute kidney injury, are present.

ALERT

- Kayexalate provides a sodium load that may exacerbate fluid overload in patients with cardiac or renal failure.
- Rapid administration of calcium in patients with suspected digitalis toxicity may result in a fatal dysrhythmia. Calcium should be administered slowly over 20–30 minutes in 5% dextrose with extreme caution.
- Calcium and dextrose/insulin are only temporizing measures and do not actually lower total body K levels.
- Sodium bicarbonate is no longer recommended to lower K, although it may be appropriate in patients with severe metabolic acidosis.

INPATIENT CONSIDERATIONS

Admission Criteria/Initial Stabilization

- If hyperkalemia is severe, treat first, and then do diagnostic investigations.
- IV calcium to stabilize myocardium (caution in setting of digoxin toxicity, when calcium may worsen effects of toxicity)
- Insulin (usually 10 U IV, given with 50 mL of 50% glucose to avoid hypoglycemia); consider repeating if elevation persists.
- Inhaled β_2-agonist (nebulized albuterol)
- Discontinue any medications that may increase K (e.g., K-sparing diuretics, exogenous K).
- Admit for cardiac monitoring if EKG changes are present or if K is >6 mEq/L (6 mmol/L).

ONGOING CARE

FOLLOW-UP RECOMMENDATIONS

Patient Monitoring

- Reduction of plasma K should begin within the 1st hour of treatment initiation.
- Serum K levels should be rechecked every 2–4 hours until the patient has stabilized and recurrent hyperkalemia is no longer a threat.
- Identification and elimination of possible causes and risk factors for hyperkalemia are essential.

DIET

≤80 mEq (≤80 mmol) of K/24 hours. Many foods contain K. Those that are particularly high in K (>6.4 mEq/serving) include bananas, orange juice, other citrus fruits and their juices, tomatoes, tomato juice, cantaloupe, honeydew melon, peaches, potatoes, salt substitutes, and many herbal medications.

PATIENT EDUCATION

Consult with a dietitian about a low-K diet.

PROGNOSIS

- Associated with poor prognosis in patients with heart failure
- Associated with poor prognosis in disaster medicine, with trauma, tissue necrosis, K^+ supplementation, metabolic acidosis, if calcium gluconate administered for treatment of hyperkalemia, if AKI, or if prolonged duration of hyperkalemia (1,6)

COMPLICATIONS

- Life-threatening cardiac arrhythmias
- Hypokalemia
- Potential complications of the use of ion-exchange resins for the treatment of hyperkalemia include volume overload and intestinal necrosis (7)[C].

REFERENCES

1. Zimmerman JL, Shen MC. Rhabdomyolysis. *Chest*. 2013;144(3):1058–1065.
2. Howard SC, Jones DP, Pui CH. The tumor lysis syndrome. *N Engl J Med*. 2011;364(19):1844–1854.
3. Antoniou T, Gomes T, Juurlink DN, et al. Trimethoprim-sulfamethoxazole–induced hyperkalemia in patients receiving inhibitors of the renin-angiotensin system: a population-based study. *Arch Intern Med*. 2010;170(12):1045–1049.
4. Weir MA, Juurlink DN, Gomes T, et al. Beta-blockers, trimethoprim-sulfamethoxazole, and the risk of hyperkalemia requiring hospitalization in the elderly: a nested case-control study. *Clin J Am Soc Nephrol*. 2010;5(9):1544–1551.
5. Wong R, Banker R, Aronowitz P, et al. Electrocardiographic changes of severe hyperkalemia. *J Hosp Med*. 2011;6(4):240.
6. Khanagavi J, Gupta T, Aronow WS, et al. Hyperkalemia among hospitalized patients and association between duration of hyperkalemia and outcomes. *Arch Med Sci*. 2014;10(2):251–257.
7. Sterns RH, Rojas M, Bernstein P, et al. Ion-exchange resins for the treatment of hyperkalemia: are they safe and effective? *J Am Soc Nephrol*. 2010;21(5): 733–735.

ADDITIONAL READING

- Bosch X, Poch E, Grau JM. Rhabdomyolysis and acute kidney injury. *N Engl J Med*. 2009;361(1): 62–72.
- Cross NB, Webster AC, Masson P, et al. Antihypertensives for kidney transplant recipients: systematic review and meta-analysis of randomized controlled trials. *Transplantation*. 2009;88(1):7–18.
- Hall AB, Salazar M, Larison DJ. The sequencing of medication administration in the management of hyperkalemia. *J Emerg Nurs*. 2009;35(4):339–342.
- Hollander-Rodriguez JC, Calvert JF Jr. Hyperkalemia. *Am Fam Physician*. 2006;73(2):283–290.
- Jain N, Kotla S, Little BB, et al. Predictors of hyperkalemia and death in patients with cardiac and renal disease. *Am J Cardiol*. 2012;109(10):1510–1513.
- Kim HJ, Han SW. Therapeutic approach to hyperkalemia. *Nephron*. 2002;92(Suppl 1):33–40.
- Noori N, Kalantar-Zadeh K, Kovesdy CP, et al. Dietary potassium intake and mortality in long-term hemodialysis patients. *Am J Kidney Dis*. 2010;56(2): 338–347.
- Pepin J, Shields C. Advances in diagnosis and management of hypokalemic and hyperkalemic emergencies. *Emerg Med Pract*. 2012;14(2):1–17; quiz 17–18.
- Putcha N, Allon M. Management of hyperkalemia in dialysis patients. *Semin Dial*. 20(5):431–439.
- Riccardi A, Tasso F, Corti L, et al. The emergency physician and the prompt management of severe hyperkalemia. *Intern Emerg Med*. 2012;7(Suppl 2): S131–S133.
- Shapiro MI, Badea A, Luchette FA. Rhabdomyolysis in the intensive care unit. *J Intensive Care Med*. 2012;27(6):335–342.
- Stevens MS, Dunlay RW. Hyperkalemia in hospitalized patients. *Int Urol Nephrol*. 2000;32(2): 177–180.

SEE ALSO

- Addison Disease; Hypokalemia
- Algorithm: Hyperkalemia

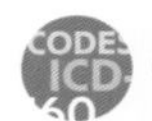

CODES

ICD10

E87.5 Hyperkalemia

CLINICAL PEARLS

- Emergency and urgent management of hyperkalemia takes precedent to a thorough diagnostic workup. Urgent treatment includes stabilization of the myocardium with calcium gluconate to protect against arrhythmias and pharmacologic strategies to move K from the extracellular (vascular) space into cells.
- Multiple herbal medications can also increase K levels, including alfalfa, dandelion, horsetail nettle, milkweed, hawthorn berries, toad skin, oleander, foxglove, and ginseng.
- To lower a patient's risk of developing hyperkalemia, have the patient follow a low-K diet, use selective β_1-blockers, such as metoprolol or atenolol, instead of nonselective β-blockers such as carvedilol. Avoid NSAIDs. Concomitant use of kaliuretic loop diuretics may be useful.

HYPERNATREMIA

Krishna Manda, MD, MRCP • Pang-Yen Fan, MD

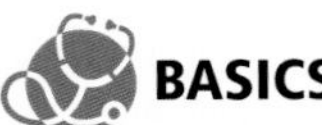

BASICS

DESCRIPTION

- Serum sodium (Na) concentration >145 mEq/L (1)
- Usually represents a state of hyperosmolality (1)
- Na concentration reflects balance between total body water (TBW) and total body Na. Hypernatremia occurs from deficit of water relative to Na.
- Hypernatremia results from net water loss or, more rarely, from primary Na gain (1).
- May exist with hypo-, hyper-, or euvolemia, although hypovolemia is by far most common type
  - Hypovolemic: occurs with a decrease in TBW and a proportionately smaller decrease in total body Na
  - Euvolemic: no change in TBW with a proportionate increase in total body Na
  - Hypervolemic: increase in TBW and a proportionately greater increase in total body Na
- It has been shown to be an indicator for higher mortality in critically ill patients and patients with chronic kidney disease (CKD) (2)[B].

EPIDEMIOLOGY

Incidence

- More common in elderly and young
  - Occurs in 1% of hospitalized elderly patients (3)
  - Seen in about 9% of ICU patients (3)
- Gastroenteritis with diarrhea is the most common cause of hypernatremia in infants.
- Women are at an increased risk due to decreased TBW as compared with men.

ETIOLOGY AND PATHOPHYSIOLOGY

- Pure water loss (total body Na normal) resulting from the following:
  - Adipsia/hypodipsia (e.g., impaired thirst regulation, decreased access to water) (4)
  - Nephrogenic diabetes insipidus (DI) (congenital or due to renal dysfunction, hypercalcemia, hypokalemia, medication-related, particularly lithium)
  - Central DI (due to head trauma, stroke, meningitis) (3)
  - Increased insensible water loss (e.g., fever, hyperventilation, hypermetabolic state, heat exposure, newborns under radiant warmers)
- Hypotonic fluid loss (total body Na decreased) resulting from the following:
  - Loss of fluid containing relatively more water than Na (e.g., excessive sweating, severe burns)
  - Urinary loss
    - Osmotic diuresis: hyperglycemia, mannitol
    - Diuretics, especially loop diuretics
    - Diabetes mellitus, particularly new presentation/decompensated
    - Post acute tubular necrosis (ATN) or post obstructive diuresis
    - Intrinsic renal disease
  - Gastrointestinal loss
    - Diarrhea, especially in children
    - Vomiting, nasogastric (NG) lavage
    - Enterocutaneous fistula
- Excess Na (increase in total body Na) resulting from the following:
  - IV NaCl or $NaHCO_3$ during cardiopulmonary resuscitation, metabolic acidosis, or hyperkalemia (3)
  - Sea water ingestion
  - Excessive use of $NaHCO_3$ antacid
  - Incorrect infant formula preparation
  - Intrauterine NaCl for abortion
  - Excessive Na in dialysate solutions
  - Disorders of the adrenal axis (Cushing syndrome, Conn syndrome, congenital adrenal hyperplasia)
  - Tube feeding

Genetics

Some forms of DI may be hereditary.

RISK FACTORS

- Infants/children
- Old age
- Patients who are intubated/have altered mental status
- Diabetes mellitus
- Prior brain injury
- Surgery
- Diuretic therapy, especially loop diuretics
- Lithium treatment

GENERAL PREVENTION

- Treatment/prevention of underlying cause
- Properly prepare infant formula and never add salt to any commercial infant formula.
- Keep patients well hydrated.

COMMONLY ASSOCIATED CONDITIONS

- Gastroenteritis
- Altered mental status
- Burns
- Hypermetabolic conditions
- Head injury
- Renal dysfunction

DIAGNOSIS

HISTORY

- Excessive thirst, nausea, vomiting, diarrhea, oliguria, polyuria
- Fever, myalgia, muscle weakness
- Neurologic symptoms common: altered mental status, seizure (especially if rapid development of hypernatremia), lethargy, irritability, coma, anophthalmos
- Symptoms tend to develop when Na >160 mEq in adults.
- Obtain list of current and recent medications.
- Review recent illnesses and activities.

PHYSICAL EXAM

- Sinus tachycardia, hypotension, orthostatic hypotension, poor O_2 saturation
- Dry mucous membranes, cool/gray skin
- Neurologic abnormalities: lethargy, weakness, focal deficits (in cases of intracerebral bleeding/lesion), confusion, coma, seizures

DIFFERENTIAL DIAGNOSIS

- DI
- Hyperosmotic coma
- Salt ingestion
- Hypertonic dehydration
- Hypothyroidism
- Cushing syndrome

DIAGNOSTIC TESTS & INTERPRETATION

Initial Tests (lab, imaging)

- Serum Na, potassium, BUN, creatinine, calcium, and osmolality (serum lithium if appropriate)
- Urine Na and osmolality
  - DI: urine osmolality < serum osmolality, and urine Na usually low normal/slightly low (due to dilution) (4)
  - Osmotic diuresis: urine osmolality intermediate, urine Na low/low-normal, total daily osmole excretion high
  - Salt ingestion: increased urine osmolality and high urine Na
  - Hypertonic dehydration: increased urine osmolality and decreased urine Na
- Serum glucose
- Special tests for DI
  - Water deprivation test: In DI, urine osmolality does not increase as it normally should when hypernatremic.
  - Antidiuretic hormone (ADH) stimulation: distinguishes central versus nephrogenic DI
    - Urine osmolality does not increase after ADH or desmopressin (DDAVP) in nephrogenic DI.
- Head CT/MRI in DI to rule out craniopharyngioma, other brain tumor or masses, or median cleft syndrome

Diagnostic Procedures/Other

History, physical, laboratory studies, family history for central DI

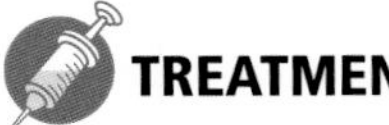

TREATMENT

GENERAL MEASURES

- Goal for corrected Na is 145 mEq/L. Treat underlying cause (1).
- Speed of correction depends on symptom severity/rate of development of hypernatremia. Avoid rapid correction to prevent development of cerebral edema if chronic hypernatremia (>24 hours):
  - Maximum of 0.5 mEq/L/hr or 10 mEq/L/day (5)[C]
  - May correct at up to 1 mEq/L/hr if acute hypernatremia (<24 hours) (1)
- Treat volume depletion first, then hypernatremia:
  - Restore intravascular volume with IV fluids to normalize serum Na levels.
- Replace water orally if patient is conscious.
- Important formulas in determining rate of fluid administration
  - TBW = coefficient × wt (kg), where coefficient = 0.6 for children, 0.5 for nonelderly women and elderly men, 0.45 for elderly women.
  - Calculated free water deficit (liters) = TBW × [1− (Na_t/Na_m)], where Na_t = target Na+, and Na_m = measured Na+. Note: wt = weight in kilograms.
  - Change in serum Na per 1 L infusate = [(infusate Na + infusate K) − serum Na]/(TBW + 1)
- Account for ongoing fluid losses during calculation of rate of fluid administration.
- Dialysis can be considered if acute kidney injury is present concomitantly and if conventional treatment has failed (6)[B].

MEDICATION

First Line

- See "General Measures" below for overall approach.

- Dehydration: Use isotonic fluids initially if signs of hemodynamic compromise, then change to hypotonic fluids when stable:
  - Hypotonic fluids (0.45% NaCl or dextrose 5% in water)
    - Important not to decrease serum Na by >0.5 mEq/L/hr or 10 mEq/L/day to prevent cerebral edema (4)[C]
- Hypervolemia: Give furosemide along with hypotonic fluids. Dose varies depending on desired urine output. Loop diuretics with fluid restriction worsen hypernatremia (4)[C].
- Central DI
  - DDAVP acetate: Use parenteral form for acute symptomatic patients, and use intranasal or oral form for chronic therapy (4).
  - Free water replacement: may use 2.5% dextrose in water if giving large volumes of water in DI to avoid glycosuria
  - May consider sulfonylureas/thiazide diuretics for chronic, but not acute, treatment
- Nephrogenic DI
- Treat with diuretics and NSAIDs
- Lithium-induced nephrogenic DI: hydrochlorothiazide 25 mg PO BID or indomethacin 50 mg PO TID, or amiloride hydrochloride 5–10 mg PO BID (7)
- Precautions
  - Rapid correction of hypernatremia can cause cerebral edema, central pontine myelinosis, seizures, or death (8).
  - Hypocalcemia and more rarely acidosis can occur during correction.
  - DI: High rates of dextrose 5% in water can cause hyperglycemia and glucose-induced diuresis.

Second Line

- Consider NSAIDs in nephrogenic DI.
- Modalities requiring further investigations
  - Continuous renal replacement therapy (CRRT): Multiple case reports and case series have shown success and safety in using CRRT to treat hypernatremia in critically ill patients with CHF and severe burns (6,9).

ISSUES FOR REFERRAL

Underlying renal involvement associated with hypernatremia would benefit from a nephrology referral.

INPATIENT CONSIDERATIONS

Admission Criteria/Initial Stabilization

Symptomatic patient with serum Na >155 mEq/L requires IV fluid therapy.

IV Fluids

Refer to "Medication" section.

Nursing

Bed rest until stable or underlying condition resolved/controlled

Discharge Criteria

Stabilization of serum Na level and symptoms are minimal.

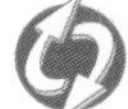

ONGOING CARE

FOLLOW-UP RECOMMENDATIONS

Patient Monitoring

- Frequent reexams in an acute setting
- Frequent electrolytes: initially q6–8h
- Urine osmolality and urine output in DI
- Ensure adequate ingestion of calories because patients may ingest so much water that they feel full and do not eat.
- Daily weights

DIET

- Ensure proper nutrition during acute phase.
- After resolution of acute phase, may want to consider Na-restricted diet for patient
- Low-salt, low-protein diet in nephrogenic DI

PATIENT EDUCATION

Patients with nephrogenic DI must avoid salt and drink large amounts of water.

PROGNOSIS

Most recover, but neurologic impairment can occur.

COMPLICATIONS

- CNS thrombosis/hemorrhage
- Seizures
- Mental retardation
- Hyperactivity
- Chronic hypernatremia: >2 days duration has higher mortality.
- Serum Na >180 mEq/L (>180 mmol/L): often results in residual CNS damage
- More common if rapid development of hypernatremia

REFERENCES

1. Adrogué HJ, Madias NE. Hypernatremia. *N Engl J Med*. 2000;342(20):1493–1499.
2. Kovesdy CP, Lott EH, Lu JL, et al. Hyponatremia, hypernatremia, and mortality in patients with chronic kidney disease with or without congestive heart failure. *Circulation*. 2012;125(5):677–684.
3. Bagshaw SM, Townsend DR, McDermid RC. Disorders of sodium and water balance in hospitalized patients. *Can J Anaesth*. 2009;56(2):151–167.
4. Hannon MJ, Finucane FM, Sherlock M, et al. Clinical review: disorders of water homeostasis in neurosurgical patients. *J Clin Endocrinol Metab*. 2012;97(5):1423–1433.
5. Al-Absi A, Gosmanova EO, Wall BM. A clinical approach to the treatment of chronic hypernatremia. *Am J Kidney Disease*. 2012;60(6):1032–1038.
6. Huang C, Zhang P, Du R, et al. Treatment of acute hypernatremia in severely burned patients using continuous veno-venous hemofiltration with gradient sodium replacement fluid: a report of nine cases. *Intensive Care Med*. 2013;39(8): 1495–1496.
7. Libber S, Harrison H, Spector D. Treatment of nephrogenic diabetes insipidus with prostaglandin synthesis inhibitors. *J Pediatr*. 1986;108(2):305–311.
8. Mastrangelo S, Arlotta A, Cefalo MG, et al. Central pontine and extrapontine myelinosis in a pediatric patient following a rapid correction of hypernatremia. *Neuropediatrics*. 2009;40(3):144–147.
9. Park HS, Hong YA, Kim HG, et al. Usefulness of continuous renal replacement therapy for correcting hypernatremia in a patient with severe congestive heart failure. *Hemodial Int*. 2012;16(4):559–563.

ADDITIONAL READING

Waite MD, Fuhrman SA, Badawi O, et al. Intensive care unit–acquired hypernatremia is an independent predictor of increased mortality and length of stay. *J Crit Care*. 2012;28(4):405–412.

SEE ALSO

- Diabetes Insipidus
- Algorithm: Hypernatremia

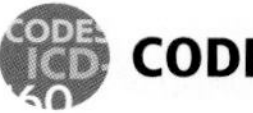

CODES

ICD10

E87.0 Hyperosmolality and hypernatremia

CLINICAL PEARLS

- Occurs from water deficit in comparison to total body Na stores
- Common causes include dehydration, DI, impaired access to fluids.
- Determine if the patient has hypervolemic, euvolemic, or hypovolemic hypernatremia in the differential diagnosis of etiology; most commonly hypovolemic; other entities rare
- Avoid rapid correction of hypernatremia to prevent development of cerebral edema when hypernatremia is chronic (>24 hours).
- Use hypotonic fluids unless patient has hemodynamic compromise, which necessitates use of isotonic fluids.
- Use oral replacement in conscious patients if possible.

H

HYPERPARATHYROIDISM

Robert A. Baldor, MD, FAAFP

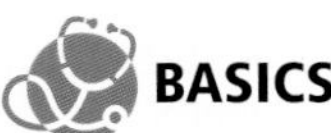

BASICS

DESCRIPTION

A dysfunction of the body's normal regulatory feedback mechanisms resulting in excess production of parathyroid hormone (PTH)

- Primary hyperparathyroidism (HPT): intrinsic parathyroid gland dysfunction resulting in excessive secretions of PTH with a lack of response to feedback inhibition by elevated calcium
- Secondary HPT: excessive secretion of PTH in response to hypocalcemia, which can be caused by vitamin D deficiency or renal failure
- Tertiary HPT: autonomous hyperfunction of the parathyroid gland in the setting of long-standing secondary HPT

EPIDEMIOLOGY

Incidence

Predominant sex: female > male (2:1)

Prevalence

Primary HPT: 1/1000 in the United States

ETIOLOGY AND PATHOPHYSIOLOGY

- PTH is synthesized by the parathyroid glands, which are located behind the 4 poles of the thyroid gland (locations can vary).
- PTH releases calcium from bone by osteoclastic stimulation (bone resorption).
- PTH increases reabsorption of calcium in the distal tubules of the kidneys.
- PTH stimulates conversion of 25-hydroxycholecalciferol (25[OH]D) to 1,25-dihydroxycholecalciferol (1,25$[OH]_2$D or active vitamin D) in the kidneys.
  - 1,25$(OH)_2$D increases calcium absorption from the GI tract, increases calcium and phosphate reabsorption in the kidneys, and stimulates osteoclastic activity and bone resorption.
- Primary HPT: unregulated PTH production and release, causing increase in serum calcium
  - Solitary adenoma (89%)
  - Double adenomas (5%)
  - Diffuse hyperplasia (6%) caused by multiple adenomas, multiple endocrine neoplasia (MEN) types 1 and 2a, and familial hypocalciuric hypercalcemia
  - Parathyroid carcinoma (<2%)
- Secondary HPT: adaptive parathyroid gland hyperplasia and hyperfunction
  - Dietary: vitamin D or calcium deficiency
  - Chronic renal disease resulting in the following:
    - Renal parenchymal loss causing hyperphosphatemia
    - Impaired calcitriol production causing hypocalcemia
    - General skeletal and renal resistance to PTH
- Tertiary HPT: autonomous oversecretion of PTH following prolonged parathyroid stimulation

Genetics

- MEN types 1 and 2a: Patients with multiple gland hyperplasia in the absence of renal disease should be screened for MEN-1 gene mutation.
- Neonatal severe primary HPT
- HPT—jaw tumor syndrome
- Familial hypocalciuric hypercalcemia (FHH): autosomal dominant
- Familial isolated HPT

RISK FACTORS

Chronic kidney disease, increasing age, poor nutrition, radiation, and/or family history

GENERAL PREVENTION

Adequate intake of calcium and vitamin D may help prevent secondary HPT.

COMMONLY ASSOCIATED CONDITIONS

- MEN syndromes type 1 and 2a
- Chronic renal failure

DIAGNOSIS

HISTORY

- History of present illness:
  - 50% of patients are asymptomatic.
  - Bone, abdominal, and flank pain as well as psychosis, which are all classic complaints of hypercalcemia
- Past medical history:
  - The following conditions may be associated with HPT:
    - MEN syndrome (MEN-associated conditions include pancreatic cancer, pituitary adenomas, medullary thyroid cancer, and pheochromocytoma), nephrolithiasis (in 20–30%), nephrocalcinosis, pancreatitis, gastroduodenal ulcer, hypertension, short QT interval, left ventricular hypertrophy, osteitis fibrosa cystica, cystic bone lesions, spontaneous fracture, vertebral collapse, osteoporosis, gout, pseudogout, anxiety, depression, psychosis, coma, conjunctivitis, band keratopathy, conjunctival calcium deposits, radiation to the neck
- Medications: thiazides or lithium
- Review of systems:
  - Possible symptoms include polydipsia, polyuria, flank pain, abdominal pain, constipation, vomiting, anorexia, weight loss, muscle fatigue, pain, weakness, hypotonia, arthralgia, bone pain, fatigue, apathy, and somnolence.

PHYSICAL EXAM

- Limited usefulness; 70–80% of patients have no obvious symptoms or signs of disease.
  - Physical findings may found related to underlying cause of HPT.

DIFFERENTIAL DIAGNOSIS

- Increased PTH: ectopic PTH production
- Nonparathyroid causes:
  - Malignancy: lung (squamous cell) carcinoma, breast carcinoma, multiple myeloma, lymphoma, leukemia, prostate cancer, Paget disease
  - Granulomatous disease: sarcoidosis, tuberculosis, berylliosis, histoplasmosis, coccidioidomycosis
  - Drugs: thiazide diuretics, vitamin D intoxication, vitamin A excess, lithium, milk-alkali syndrome, exogenous calcium intake
  - Endocrine: hyperthyroidism, acute adrenal insufficiency
  - Familial: hypocalciuric hypercalcemia

DIAGNOSTIC TESTS & INTERPRETATION

Initial Tests (lab, imaging)

- Disease is often detected by an incidental finding of hypercalcemia.
- Order serum calcium level and albumin:
  - Calculate plasma albumin–adjusted calcium >2.65 mmol/L on 2 occasions.
- If hypercalcemia is confirmed, follow with intact PTH level (1)[B].
  - High PTH (>3.0 pmol/L) suggests primary HPT.
  - Low PTH (<3.0 pmol/L) suggests non–PTH-mediated hypercalcemia.
- If elevated calcium is inconsistent, elevated ionized serum calcium in the setting of high PTH confirms diagnosis. Other findings may include low serum phosphate, elevated serum chloride, decreased serum CO_2, and abnormal 24-hour urine calcium excretion.
- In secondary HPT, an elevated phosphorus suggests chronic renal failure; a low phosphorus suggests another cause, most commonly vitamin D deficiency.

Follow-Up Tests & Special Considerations

- A 24-hour urine calcium concentration to creatinine clearance ratio >0.02 suggests primary HPT; a ratio <0.01 may be normal or indicate FHH; important because FHH does not require surgery (1)[C]
- Routine measurement of 25(OH)D levels is recommended in all patients with primary HPT. In case of vitamin D deficiency (<20 ng/mL or <50 nmol/L), defer management decisions until levels are maintained >20 ng/mL (50 nmol/L) (2)[C].
- Intraoperative measurement of intact PTH and/or γ-probe localization of abnormal glands with technetium-99m sestamibi scan has aided focused resections for patients with single-gland etiology (3)[C].
- Screening for kidney stones is not recommended in patients without a history of nephrolithiasis (3)[B].

Diagnostic Procedures/Other

- Consider EKG to assess for short QT interval.
- Imaging is not required for diagnosis. It is required for surgical planning, especially for minimally invasive parathyroidectomy (MIP) (4)[C].
  - Imaging is also indicated to localize hyperplasia or an ectopic parathyroid gland in repeat surgery.
- Imaging options for presurgical localization:
  - Technetium-99m sestamibi with single-photon emission computed tomography (SPECT)
    - Has had the greatest reported success in localizing single parathyroid adenomas (5)[B]
  - US
    - Painless, noninvasive, inexpensive, and does not expose the patient to radiation; however, its accuracy is very operator-dependent (6)[C].
  - Positron emission tomography (PET) using C-methionine (MET-PET) is comparable to US and technetium-99m sestamibi with SPECT in terms of diagnostic use (4)[B].
  - Four-dimensional CT (4D-CT) may be more effective for primary localization than both US and sestamibi-SPECT (7)[B].
  - CT and MRI are mostly used to localize ectopic mediastinal glands.
  - Comprehensive cervical US (CCU) used for further localization following a negative sestamibi scan often reveals a single adenoma (8)[C].
    - A negative sestamibi scan likely indicates parathyroid hyperplasia/multiglandular disease and thus requires open neck exploratory surgery.
    - CCU after negative sestamibi result allows more patients who were previously excluded to be candidates for MIP.

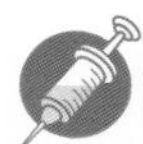

TREATMENT

MEDICATION

- Primary HPT: Operative management is curative. For those awaiting or unable to have surgery
  - Bisphosphonates (alendronate): reduces bone turnover and helps to maintain bone density; avoid in kidney disease.
  - Calcimimetics (cinacalcet): Further studies needed to establish long-term benefit in primary HPT.
  - Selective estrogen receptor modulator therapy (raloxifene)
  - Hormone replacement therapy with estrogens is not recommended as 1st-line treatment; must weigh benefit with risks of known systemic effects
    - Can be used in postmenopausal women who do not undergo or refuse surgery
- Secondary HPT
  - Calcium replacement
  - Vitamin D analogues (paricalcitol and calcitriol)
  - Phosphorus-binding agents (sevelamer)
  - Calcimimetic (cinacalcet) (1)[A]: activates calcium-sensing receptor in parathyroid gland, thereby inhibiting PTH secretion
- Tertiary HPT
  - Medical treatment is not curative and generally not indicated.

SURGERY/OTHER PROCEDURES

- Operative management is curative for patients with primary HPT in 95–98% of patients.
- Indications for parathyroidectomy:
  - Symptomatic primary HPT
    - Nephrolithiasis
    - Nephrocalcinosis
    - Osteitis fibrosa cystica
  - Asymptomatic primary HPT
    - Serum Ca^+ level >1 mg/dL above normal
    - Age <50 years
    - GFR <60 mL/min/1.73 m^2 or creatinine clearance reduced to <60 mL/min
    - Bone density loss with a T-score ≤ -2.5 at the lumbar spine, femoral neck, total hip, or 33% radius
- Tertiary HPT
- Surgical removal of diseased gland or tissue is only proven curative therapy for HPT.
- Surgical options include the following:
  - Bilateral open neck exploratory surgery
  - MIP using preoperative sestamibi scan with SPECT and intraoperative PTH levels result in decreased pain, smaller incisions, improved cosmetic results, lower morbidity, and decreased length of hospital stay when compared with open neck exploratory surgery.
- Follow postoperative serum calcium level (hypocalcemia in "hungry bone" syndrome); patients also at risk for bleeding and airway compromise; keep injectable calcium and seizure medications at bedside.
- Monitor renal function closely.

INPATIENT CONSIDERATIONS

Admission Criteria/Initial Stabilization

Critical hypercalcemia requires IV fluid rehydration, IV bisphosphonate therapy, and SC calcitonin (4 U/kg q12h) for severe symptoms.

ONGOING CARE

FOLLOW-UP RECOMMENDATIONS

Asymptomatic patients with primary HPT require serial monitoring of calcium and PTH.

Patient Monitoring

In patients with primary HPT who are asymptomatic, measurements of serum calcium and creatinine annually and bone density scan every 1–2 years is sufficient.

DIET

- In the presence of hypercalciuria or elevated $1,25(OH)_2D$ levels, dietary calcium restriction is recommended. Otherwise, daily calcium intake should be maintained at up to 1,000 mg.
- Restrict dietary phosphate in secondary HPT.

PATIENT EDUCATION

- Importance of periodic lab testing
- Signs of severe hypercalcemia

PROGNOSIS

Prognosis after surgery is excellent in primary HPT, with resolution of many of the preoperative symptoms.

COMPLICATIONS

Related to high levels of PTH and/or elevated calcium

REFERENCES

1. Fraser WD. Hyperparathyroidism. *Lancet*. 2009;374(9684):145–158.
2. Eastell R, Arnold A, Brandi ML, et al. Diagnosis of asymptomatic primary hyperparathyroidism: proceedings of the third international workshop. *J Clin Endocrinol Metab*. 2009;94(2):340–350.
3. Bilezikian JP, Khan AA, Potts JT Jr, et al. Guidelines for the management of asymptomatic primary hyperparathyroidism: summary statement from the third international workshop. *J Clin Endocrinol Metab*. 2009;94(2):335–339.
4. Caldarella C, Treglia G, Isgrò MA, et al. Diagnostic performance of positron emission tomography using ^{11}C-methionine in patients with suspected parathyroid adenoma: a meta-analysis. *Endocrine*. 2013;43(1):78–83.
5. Caldarella C, Treglia G, Pontecorvi A, et al. Diagnostic performance of planar scintigraphy using ^{99}mTc-MIBI in patients with secondary hyperparathyroidism: a meta-analysis. *Ann Nucl Med*. 2012;26(10):794–803.
6. Udelsman R, Pasieka JL, Sturgeon C, et al. Surgery for asymptomatic primary hyperparathyroidism: proceedings of the third international workshop. *J Clin Endocrinol Metab*. 2009;94(2):366–372.
7. Cheung K, Wang TS, Farrokhyar F, et al. A meta-analysis of preoperative localization techniques for patients with primary hyperparathyroidism. *Ann Surg Oncol*. 2012;19(2):577–583.
8. Kandil E, Malazai AJ, Alrasheedi S, et al. Minimally invasive/focused parathyroidectomy in patients with negative sestamibi scan results. *Arch Otolaryngol Head Neck Surg*. 2012;138(3):223–225.

ADDITIONAL READING

Li D, Shao L, Zhou H, et al. The efficacy of cinacalcet combined with conventional therapy on bone and mineral metabolism in dialysis patients with secondary hyperparathyroidism: a meta-analysis. *Endocrine*. 2012;43(1):68–77.

CODES

ICD10

- E21.3 Hyperparathyroidism, unspecified
- E21.0 Primary hyperparathyroidism
- E21.1 Secondary hyperparathyroidism, not elsewhere classified

CLINICAL PEARLS

- 50% of patients with primary HPT are asymptomatic.
- HPT is often detected by an incidental finding of hypercalcemia on a routine serum chemistry analysis.
- Classic symptoms of hypercalcemia include painful bones, renal stones, abdominal pains, and behavioral changes ("stones, bones, moans, and groans").
- Repeat calcium (elevated), correct for serum albumin, and obtain intact PTH levels to make an initial diagnosis.
- The 2 most commonly used imaging modalities in HPT are technetium-99m sestamibi scan and US.
- Surgery is curative for most cases of primary HPT.

HYPERPROLACTINEMIA

D'Ann Somerall, DNP, MAEd, FNP-BC • William E. Somerall, Jr., MD, MEd

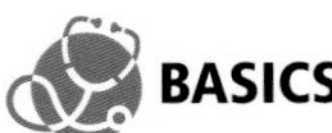

BASICS

DESCRIPTION

Hyperprolactinemia is an abnormal elevation in the serum prolactin level with multiple possible etiologies.

EPIDEMIOLOGY

Prevalence

- Predominant age: reproductive age
- Predominant sex: female > male
- More readily detected in females because a slight elevation in prolactin causes changes in menstruation and galactorrhea

ETIOLOGY AND PATHOPHYSIOLOGY

- Prolactin, which is produced by lactotrophs in the anterior pituitary, is regulated by:
  - Inhibitory factors, primarily dopamine, produced in the hypothalamus and delivered via the hypothalamic-pituitary vessels in the pituitary stalk
  - Stimulatory factors, primarily thyrotropin-releasing hormone (TRH)
- Causes of hyperprolactinemia include the following:
  - Physiologic:
    - Pregnancy
    - Breastfeeding
    - Nipple stimulation
    - Stress, including postoperative state
  - Medications:
    - Dopamine (D_2) blockers: prochlorperazine, metoclopramide
    - Dopamine depleters: α-methyldopa, reserpine
    - Antidepressants: selective serotonin reuptake inhibitors, tricyclic antidepressants
    - Verapamil (but no other calcium channel blockers; thought to decrease hypothalamic synthesis of dopamine)
    - Antipsycotics: haloperidol, fluphenazine, risperidone
  - Hypothyroidism (due to elevated TRH)
  - Chest wall conditions:
    - Herpes zoster
    - After thoracotomy
    - Trauma
  - Prolactin-secreting adenoma, categorized:
    - Microadenoma: ≤1 cm
    - Macroadenoma: >1 cm
  - Pituitary stalk compression/disruption:
    - Craniopharyngioma
    - Rathke cleft cyst
    - Meningioma
    - Astrocytoma
    - Metastases
    - Head trauma
    - Infiltrative/inflammatory disorders
  - Diminished prolactin clearance:
    - Renal failure
    - Cirrhosis
- Cocaine

DIAGNOSIS

HISTORY

- Galactorrhea
- Amenorrhea
- Oligomenorrhea
- Infertility
- Osteoporosis/osteopenia
- Decreased libido, impotence
- Weight gain
- Also may have signs and symptoms of pituitary enlargement:
  - Headache
  - Visual field impairment (bitemporal hemianopsia)
  - Hypopituitarism (secondary to tumor pressure on surrounding structures)
- Also may have signs and symptoms of associated conditions:
  - Hypothyroidism
  - Cushing disease
  - Acromegaly
  - Multiple endocrine neoplasia (MEN)-1 syndrome

PHYSICAL EXAM

- Visual field testing
- Cranial nerve exam

DIFFERENTIAL DIAGNOSIS

Macroprolactinemia: Macroprolactin, a polymer of several units of prolactin, is detected by immunologically based lab tests but is not biologically active. If patient is asymptomatic but found to have elevated prolactin (PRL), consider this diagnosis and notify the lab. No treatment is required.

DIAGNOSTIC TESTS & INTERPRETATION

- Serum prolactin (most accurate results if checked fasting, in morning) <25 μg/L normal; >25 μg/L abnormal; >250 μg/L often indicates a prolactinoma (1)[A].
- Pregnancy test
- Thyroid-stimulating hormone (TSH)
- Luteinizing hormone (LH)/follicle-stimulating hormone (FSH) if amenorrheic
- Chemistry, renal function
- LFTs

Initial Tests (lab, imaging)

A single measurement of serum prolactin; a level above the upper limit of normal confirms the diagnosis.

- Pituitary MRI
- CT scan if MRI is contraindicated
- Levels should be drawn prior to breast exam

Follow-Up Tests & Special Considerations

Formal visual field testing if pituitary adenoma suspected

TREATMENT

GENERAL MEASURES

- Discontinue offending medications, if any (1)[A].
- Treat underlying causes (1)[A].
- For asymptomatic patients with mild PRL elevations, observation alone may be considered (1,2)[A]
- Medications indicated for (1)[A]:
  - Symptoms of hypogonadism, such as decreased libido
  - Galactorrhea (if bothersome to patient)
  - Restoration of fertility
  - Pituitary adenoma
  - Prevention of osteoporosis

MEDICATION

Dopamine agonists:

- Bromocriptine (Parlodel): often 1st-line treatment given. This has longest clinical history: dosed BID; preferred by some clinicians when infertility is an indication for treatment (2,3)[A].
- Cabergoline (Dostinex): dosed twice weekly. Some consider 1st line due to efficacy and better side effect profile. Cabergoline was more effective than bromocriptine in reducing persistent hyperprolactinemia, amenorrhea/oligomenorrhea, and galactorrhea (2)[A]. Has recently been reported to be associated with significant improvements in the body mass index, total HDL and LDL cholesterol levels and insulin sensitivity; decrease in proinflammatory markers; and carotid intima media thickness; indicated with bromocriptine failure or resistance
  - Both are effective for reducing tumor size and improving symptoms (2)[A].
  - SE less with cabergoline than bromocriptine (2)[A]
- Cabergoline has been shown to reduce erectile dysfunction in hyperprolactinemic men (1)[A].
  - Adverse effects (better tolerated if start with low dose, slow titration, given at night with food):
    - Nausea/vomiting
    - Headache
    - Dizziness
    - Fatigue
    - Lightheadedness
    - Postural hypotension (2)[A]
- Pergolide (Permax) is no longer used in the United States. If patient is still on med, do not withdraw abruptly.

ADDITIONAL THERAPIES

Patients with medically and surgically refractory prolactinomas; radiotherapy produced a reduction in prolactin levels in nearly all patients and normalization in over a quarter of patients with low complication rates (2)[A].

SURGERY/OTHER PROCEDURES

- For adenomas, medical treatment will be successful in 80–90% of patients. In some cases, surgery is indicated. (1)
- Indications:
  - Intolerance or resistance to medical treatment
  - Headache
  - Visual field loss
  - CSF leak due to tumor apoplexy or shrinkage
  - Cranial nerve deficit
- Risks:
  - High recurrence rate (up to 40%)
  - CSF leakage
  - Meningitis
  - Transient diabetes insipidus (4)[A]
- Pituitary insufficiency

ONGOING CARE

FOLLOW-UP RECOMMENDATIONS

Patient Monitoring

- Depends on etiology
- After at least 2 years of treatment, no tumor and prolactin levels normal may consider decreasing and stopping medication. Must be followed closely, as tumor may grow back (1).
- Consider:
  - Formal visual field testing yearly (3)[A]
  - Serial MRIs if clinically indicated (3)[A]

Pregnancy Considerations

- If pregnancy is desired in a woman with hyperprolactinemia, dopamine agonists are not approved during pregnancy and should be discontinued once pregnancy is confirmed, but their use is recommended if neurologic findings are present (1)[A].
- With microprolactinoma: Treat with bromocriptine if symptomatic; monthly pregnancy tests; discontinue bromocriptine when pregnancy is confirmed.
- With macroprolactinomas: a definitive, individualized plan is made. Options include discontinuation of bromocriptine at conception and careful monitoring of PRL levels and VS, with or without MRI scan evidence of tumor enlargement; prepregnancy transsphenoidal surgery with debulking of tumor; continuation of bromocriptine throughout gestation, with a risk to the fetus.
- Careful monitoring of visual fields in each trimester. No need to monitor prolactin levels, as they are normally high due to pregnancy (1)[A].

PATIENT EDUCATION

- Discuss risks of untreated hyperprolactinemia:
  - Headache
  - Visual field loss
  - Decreased bone density
  - Infertility
- Patient guide to hyperprolactinemia diagnosis and treatment

PROGNOSIS

- Tends to recur after discontinuation of medical therapy (1)[A]
- Over 10 years, 7% chance of progression of prolactin-secreting microadenoma (3)[A]

COMPLICATIONS

- Depends on underlying cause
- If pituitary adenoma, risk of permanent visual field loss

REFERENCES

1. Hoffman AR, Melmed S, Schlechte J. Patient guide to hyperprolactinemia diagnosis and treatment. *J Clin Endocrinol Metab*. 2011;96(2):35A–36A.
2. Wang AT, Mullan RJ, Lane MA, et al. Treatment of hyperprolactinemia: a systematic review and meta-analysis. *Syst Rev*. 2012;1:33.
3. Casanueva FF, Molitch ME, Schlechte JA, et al. Guidelines of the Pituitary Society for the diagnosis and management of prolactinomas. *Clin Endocrinol (Oxf)*. 2006;65(2):265–273.
4. Bloomgarden E, Molitch ME. Surgical treatment of prolactinomas: cons. *Endocrine*. 2014;47(3):730–733.
5. Sun GE, Pantalone KM, Gupta M, et al. Is chronic nipple associated with hyperprolactinemia? *Pituitary*. 2013,16(3):351–353.

ADDITIONAL READING

- Inancli SS, Usluogullari A, Ustu Y, et al. Effect of cabergoline on insulin sensitivity, inflammation, and carotid intima media thickness in patients with prolactinoma. *Endocrine*. 2013;44(1):193–199.
- Inder WJ, Castle D. Antipsychotic-induced hyperprolactinaemia. *Aust N Z J Psychiatry*. 2011;45(10):830–837.
- Jackson J, Safranek S. What is the recommended evaluation and treatment for elevated serum prolactin? *JFP*. 2006;54(10):897–899.
- Klibanski A. Clinical practice. Prolactinomas. *N Engl J Med*. 2010;362(13):1219–1226.
- Melmed S, Casanueva FF, Hoffman AR, et al. Diagnosis and treatment of hyperprolactinemia: an Endocrine Society clinical practice guideline. *J Clin Endocrinol Metab*. 2011;96(2):273–288.
- Molitch ME. Pituitary gland: can prolactinomas be cured medically? *Nat Rev Endocrinol*. 2010;6(4):186–188.
- Wang AT, Mullan RJ, Lane MA, et al. Treatment of hyperprolactinemia: a systematic review and meta-analysis. *Syst Rev*. 2012;1:33.

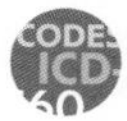

CODES

ICD10

E22.1 Hyperprolactinemia

CLINICAL PEARLS

- If a cause for hyperprolactinemia cannot be found by history, examination, and routine laboratory testing, an intracranial lesion might be the cause and brain MRI with specific pituitary cuts and intravenous contrast media should be performed.
- Treatment of hyperprolactinemia should be targeted at correcting the cause (hypothyroidism, discontinuation of offending medications, etc.).
- There is a difference among antipsychotics in influencing prolactin levels. In general, those with the highest potency D_2 antagonism are most likely to elevate prolactin levels. Among the newer atypical antipsychotics, risperidone has been identified as more likely to elevate prolactin.
- Chronic nipple piercing has not been shown to cause hyperprolactinemia (5)[A].
- High prolactin levels decrease testosterone by inhibiting gonadotropin-releasing hormone (GnRH), LH, and FSH secretion and by decreasing central dopamine activity, both of which are important in mediating sexual arousal.

HYPERSENSITIVITY PNEUMONITIS

Kenia Mansilla-Rivera, MD

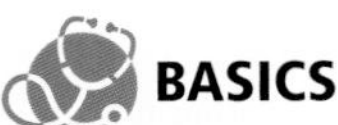

BASICS

DESCRIPTION

- Hypersensitivity pneumonitis (HP) is also called extrinsic allergic alveolitis (EAA), a diffuse inflammatory disease of the lung caused by an immunologic reaction to aerosolized antigenic particles found in a variety of environments, occurring within the pulmonary parenchyma. Classification depends on time frame involved:
  - Acute: fever, chills, diaphoresis, myalgias, nausea; cough and dyspnea common but not necessarily present. Occurs 4–12 hours after heavy exposure to an inciting agent. Symptoms subside within 12 hours to several days after removal from exposure. Complete resolution occurs within weeks.
  - Subacute: mainly caused by continual low-level antigen exposure, could have a low-grade fever in first week, cough, dyspnea, fatigue, anorexia, weight loss—develops over days to weeks
  - Chronic: from recurrent exposure either acute or subacute cases, prolonged and progressive cough, dyspnea, fatigue, weight loss, could lead to fibrosis and respiratory failure
- Farmer's lung is an old term of this disease, a type of HP, particular to the farmer population, where the causative agent is a bacterium found in moldy hay or straw. Farmer's lung now has new and different etiologies due to modernization of farming practices (1,2).

EPIDEMIOLOGY

Not well defined. Tends to occur in adults as a result of occupation-related exposure, but some home environmental exposures are also seen.

Incidence

0.9 per 100,000

Prevalence

- Farmers: 1–19% exposed farmers
- Bird fanciers: 6–20% exposed individuals
- Others: 1–8% exposed

ETIOLOGY AND PATHOPHYSIOLOGY

- Hypersensitivity reaction involving immune complexes: Inhaled antigens bind to IgG, triggering complement cascade (types III and IV immunologic reactions) (3).
- Cellular-mediated reaction: T cell–mediated immune inflammatory response
- Farming, vegetable, or dairy cattle workers (1,2)
  - Moldy hay, grain, silage: thermophilic actinomycetes, such as *Faenia rectivirgula*
  - Mold on pressed sugar cane: *Thermoactinomyces sacchari*, *Thymus vulgaris*
  - Tobacco plants: *Aspergillus* sp., *Scopulariopsis brevicaulis*
  - Mushroom worker's lung: *Saccharopolyspora rectivirgula*, *T. vulgaris*, *Aspergillus* spp.
  - Potato riddler's lung: Thermophilic actinomycetes, *T. vulgaris*, *Faenia rectivirgula*, *Aspergillus* sp.
  - Wine maker's lung: *Mucor stolonifer*
  - Cheese washer's lung: *Penicillium casei*, *Aspergillus clavatus*
  - Coffee worker's lung: coffee bean dust
  - Tea grower's lung: tea plants
- Ventilation and water-related contamination (1,2)
  - Contaminated humidifiers and air conditioners: amoebae, nematodes, yeasts, bacteria
  - Unventilated shower: *Epicoccum nigrum*
  - Hot-tub lung: *Cladosporium* sp., *Mycobacterium avium complex*
  - Sauna taker's lung: *Aureobasidium* sp.
  - Summer-type pneumonitis: *Trichosporon cutaneum*
  - Swimming pool lung (lifeguard) lung: aerosolized endotoxin and *M. avium complex*
  - Contaminated basement pneumonitis: *Cephalosporium* and *Penicillium* spp.
- Bird and poultry handling (1)
  - Bird fancier's lung: droppings, feathers, serum proteins
  - Poultry worker's lung: serum proteins
  - Turkey-handling disease: serum proteins
  - Canary fancier's lung: serum proteins
  - Duck fever: feathers, serum proteins
- Veterinary work and animal handling (1,2)
  - Laboratory worker's lung: urine, serum, pelts, proteins
  - Pituitary snuff taker's disease: dried, powdered neurohypophysis
  - Furrier's lung: animal pelts
  - Bat lung: bat serum protein
  - Fish meal worker's lung: fish meal
  - Coptic lung: cloth wrapping of mummies
  - Mollusc shell HP: sea-snail shell
  - Pearl oyster shell pneumonitis: oyster shells
- Grain and flour (1,2)
  - Grain measurer's lung: cereal grain, grain dust
  - Miller's lung: *Sitophilus granarius*
  - Malt worker's disease: *A. fumigatus*, *A. clavatus*
- Lumber milling, construction, wood stripping, paper, wallboard manufacture (1,2)
  - Wood dust pneumonitis: *Alternaria* sp., *Bacillus subtilis*
  - Sequoiosis: *Graphium*, *Pullularia*, *Trichoderma* sp., *Aureobasidium pullulans*
  - Maple bark disease: *Cryptostroma corticale*
  - Wood trimmer's disease: *Rhizopus* sp., *Mucor* sp.
  - Wood pulp worker's disease: *Penicillium* sp.
  - Suberosis: *T. viridis*, *P. glabrum*
- Plastic manufacturing, painting, electronics, chemicals (1)
  - Chemical HP: diphenyl diisocyanate, toluene diisocyanate
  - Detergent worker's lung: *B. subtilis* enzymes
  - Pauli reagent alveolitis: sodium diazobenzene sulfate
  - Vineyard sprayer's lung: copper sulfate
  - Pyrethrum: *Pyrethrum*
  - Epoxy resin lung: phthalic anhydride
  - Bible printer's lung: moldy typesetting water
  - Machine operator's lung: *Pseudomona fluorescens*, aerosolized metal working fluid
- Textile workers
  - Byssinosis: cotton mill dust
  - Velvet worker's lung: nylon, tannic acid, potato starch
  - Upholstery fabric: aflatoxin-producing fungus, *Fusarium* sp.
  - Lycoperdonosis: puffball spores

Genetics

No evidence of clear genetic susceptibility. Possible genetic predisposition involving tumor necrosis factor alpha (TNF-α) and major histocompatibility complex (MHC) class II genes (1,3)[B]

RISK FACTORS

- Contact with organic antigens increases the risk of developing HP. Viral infection at time of exposure could also increase risk (4).
- Nonsmokers have an increased incidence of HP compared with smokers (nicotine could have a protective effect) (4).
  - Smokers have a diminished antibody response to inhaled antigens.
  - However, smokers that develop disease tend to have the chronic form, and mortality is higher.

GENERAL PREVENTION

Avoidance of offending antigen and/or use of protective equipment

COMMONLY ASSOCIATED CONDITIONS

Constrictive bronchiolitis

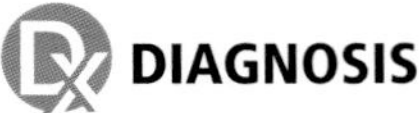

DIAGNOSIS

HISTORY

- Diagnosis criteria most widely used but not validated: (i) history and physical and pulmonary function tests (PFTs) indicating restriction or diffusion disease, (ii) radiologic imaging consent with interstitial lung disease, (iii) exposure to a recognized cause, (iv) proof of sensitization in BAL fluids (serum precipitins and/or lymphocytosis) (2)
- Six significant predictors: exposure to a known antigen, positive precipitating antibodies, recurrent episodes of symptoms, inspiratory crackles, symptoms 4–8 hours after exposure, weight loss (5)
- Acute form: develops 4–12 hours following exposure. Cough, dyspnea without wheezing, fever, chills, diaphoresis, headache, nausea, malaise, chest tightness. Symptoms last hours to days.
- Sequela (prior subacute, chronic): gradual or progressive productive cough, dyspnea, fatigue, anorexia, weight loss can lead to respiratory failure; develops over days, weeks to months.
- Symptomatic improvement when away from work or home

PHYSICAL EXAM

- Acute: fever, tachypnea, diffuse fine rales
- Sequela or chronic: inspiratory crackles, progressive hypoxia, weight loss, diffuse rales, clubbing, rarely wheezing

DIAGNOSTIC TESTS & INTERPRETATION

- Testing for antibodies (Ab): not as helpful or identifiable. Positive serum Ab is a significant predictor of HP. Antigens that cover most cases: pigeon and parakeet sera, dove feather, *Aspergillus sp.*, *Penicillium*, *S. rectivirgula*, and *T. viridans*
- PFTs: Typical profile is a restrictive pattern with low diffusing capacity, could also have an obstructive pattern (5).
- Bronchoalveolar lavage (BAL) with serum precipitins and lymphocytosis: usually with low CD4-to-CD8 ratio. Findings not unique to HP (1,5).
- Positive antigen–specific inhalation challenge testing: reexposure to the environment, inhalation challenge to the suspected antigen in a hospital setting but it lacks standardization (6)
- Chest x-ray (CXR): used to rule out other diseases
  - Acute: ground-glass infiltrates, nodular or striated patchy opacities interstitial pattern in a variety of distributions in lung field. Up to 20% could be normal.
  - Sequela/chronic: upper lobe fibrosis, nodular or ground-glass opacities, volume loss, emphysematous changes
- CT scan of chest: Patterns not specific to HP:
  - Acute: ground-glass opacities, poorly defined centrilobular nodules and ground-glass opacities and air trapping on expiratory images (6,7)
  - Chronic: fibrosis, ground-glass attenuation, irregular opacities, bronchiectasis, loss of lung volume, honeycombing, emphysematous changes (6,7)
- High-resolution CT (HRCT) appearance is a mid-to-upper zone predominance of centrilobular ground glass or nodular opacities with signs of air trapping (6).
- Usually start with CXR; may progress to HRCT based on findings (1,6)

Diagnostic Procedures/Other

Lung biopsy:

- Transbronchial: reveals small, poorly formed noncaseating granulomas near respiratory or terminal bronchioles, large foam cells, peribronchial fibrosis
- Open lung biopsy: highest yield in advanced disease. Reveals varying patterns of organizing pneumonia, centrilobular and perilobular fibrosis, multinucleated giant cells with clefts

DIFFERENTIAL DIAGNOSIS

- Acute: acute infectious pneumonia: influenza (or other viral pneumonia), mycoplasma, *Pneumocystis jiroveci* pneumonia, asthma, aspiration (3)
- Chronic: sarcoidosis, chronic bronchitis, chronic obstructive pulmonary disease, tuberculosis, collagen vascular disease, idiopathic pulmonary fibrosis, lymphoma, fungal infections, *P. jiroveci* pneumonia (3)

ALERT

HP in farmers must be distinguished from febrile, toxic reactions to inhaled dusts (organic dust toxic syndrome [ODTS]). Nonimmunologic reactions occur 30–50% more commonly than HP in farmers. ODTS is associated with intense exposure occurring on a single day.

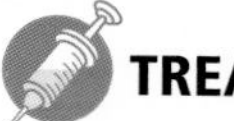

TREATMENT

GENERAL MEASURES

Outpatient, except for acute pneumonitis cases and admission for workup (BAL, lung biopsy)

MEDICATION

First Line

- Avoidance of offending antigen is primary therapy and results in disease regression (1,2).
- Corticosteroids: help control the symptoms of exacerbations but do not improve long-term outcomes
  - Prednisone: 20–50 mg daily (5)
  - For severe symptomatic patients, initial course of 1–2 weeks with taper (5)

Second Line

- Bronchodilators and inhaled corticosteroids may symptomatically improve patients with wheeze and chest tightness (4,5)[B].
- Oxygen may be needed in advanced cases.
- Lung transplantation may be the last resort in severe cases unresponsive to therapy.

ISSUES FOR REFERRAL

Referral to pulmonologist/immunologist

INPATIENT CONSIDERATIONS

Admission Criteria/Initial Stabilization

Supportive management, as needed, to maintain oxygenation and ventilation:

- Unstable ventilation, oxygen requirement, mental status changes
- Need for invasive evaluation (lung biopsy)

ONGOING CARE

FOLLOW-UP RECOMMENDATIONS

Patient Monitoring

- Initial follow-up should be weekly to monthly, depending on severity and course.
- Follow treatments with serial CXR, PFTs, circulating antibody levels.

DIET

No dietary restrictions

PATIENT EDUCATION

Note that chronic exposure may lead to a loss of acute symptoms with exposure (i.e., the patient may lose awareness of exposure–symptom relationship).

PROGNOSIS

- Presence of fibrosis is a poor prognosis factor (1,2).
- Acute: good prognosis with reversal of pathologic findings if elimination of offending antigen early in disease (2,4)
- Sequela/chronic: Corticosteroids have been found to improve lung function acutely but offer no significant difference in long-term outcome (4,5)[C].

COMPLICATIONS

- Progressive interstitial fibrosis with eventual respiratory failure
- Cor pulmonale and right-sided heart failure

REFERENCES

1. Girard M, Cormier Y. Hypersensitivity pneumonitis. *Curr Opin Allergy Clin Immunol*. 2010;10(2):99–103.
2. Costabel U, Bonella F, Guzman J. Chronic hypersensitivity pneumonitis. *Clin Chest Med*. 2012;33(1):151–163.
3. Grunes D, Beasley MB. Hypersensitivity pneumonitis: a review and update of histologic findings. *J Clin Pathol*. 2013;66(10):888–895.
4. Selman M, Buendía-Roldán I. Immunopathology, diagnosis and management of hypersensitivity pneumonitis. *Semin Respir Crit Care Med*. 2012;33(5):543–554.
5. Lacasse Y, Girard M, Cormier Y. Recent advances in hypersensitivity pneumonitis. *Chest*. 2012;142(1):208–217.
6. Ohshimo S, Bonella F, Guzman J, et al. Hypersensitivity pneumonitis. *Immunol Allergy Clin North Am*. 2012;32(4):537–556.
7. Hirschmann JV, Pipavath SN, Godwin JD. Hypersensitivity pneumonitis: a historical, clinical, and radiologic review. *Radiographics*. 2009;29(7):1921–1938.

ADDITIONAL READING

Girard M, Lacasse Y, Cormier Y. Hypersensitivity pneumonitis. *Allergy*. 2009;64(3):322–334.

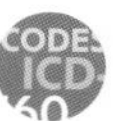

CODES

ICD10

- J67.9 Hypersensitivity pneumonitis due to unspecified organic dust
- J67.0 Farmer's lung
- J67.2 Bird fancier's lung

CLINICAL PEARLS

- Skin testing is not useful for the diagnosis of HP.
- Diagnosis should be suspected in every patient with unexplained cough and dyspnea on exertion, functional impairment (restriction or diffusion defect), and unclear fever, especially if exposure to potential antigens is known (workplace, domestic bird keeping, moldy walls in the home) (2).
- Once the disease is established, smoking does not appear to attenuate its severity, and it may predispose to more chronic and severe course.
- Use of protective gear on individual with high-risk exposure occupations can prevent HP.

HYPERSPLENISM

Frank J. Domino, MD

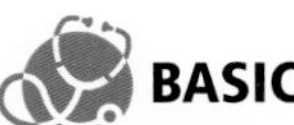

BASICS

DESCRIPTION

- Hypersplenism is defined as overactivity of the spleen and presents as the following:
  - Splenomegaly (commonly but not always)
  - Cytopenias with respective bone marrow hyperplasia of precursors
  - Resolution of cytopenias with splenectomy
- Hypersplenism can usually be diagnosed without splenectomy.
- Splenomegaly is not synonymous with hypersplenism. Overactivity of the spleen can occur without enlargement, as is seen in immune thrombocytopenic purpura (ITP) and autoimmune hemolytic anemia.

EPIDEMIOLOGY

May be as common as 30–70% in patients with cirrhosis and portal hypertension (HTN)

ETIOLOGY AND PATHOPHYSIOLOGY

Enlargement of the spleen results in sequestration of formed blood elements, leading to peripheral cytopenias and concomitant bone marrow precursor hyperplasia.

Many of the common etiologies are listed below. Almost any process involving the spleen or the hematologic system can result in hypersplenism:

- Infectious
  - Tuberculosis
  - Malaria
  - Leishmaniasis
  - Candidiasis
  - Viral
  - Syphilis
  - Schistosomiasis
- Hematologic
  - Myeloproliferative disorders
  - Polycythemia vera
  - Primary hypersplenism
  - ITP
  - Autoimmune hemolytic anemia
- Neoplastic
  - Hematologic malignancies
  - Melanoma
  - Various carcinomas
- Storage diseases
  - Gaucher disease
  - Niemann-Pick disease
  - Amyloidosis
  - Glycogen storage disease
- Inflammatory
  - Sarcoidosis
  - Systemic lupus erythematosus
  - Felty syndrome
- Congestive

DIAGNOSIS

HISTORY

- Patients may complain of abdominal fullness or protrusion of the spleen through the abdominal wall; may complain of early satiety if the spleen is compressing stomach
- Patients may complain of tenderness in the left upper quadrant, especially with viral infections. In lymphoproliferative disorders, spleen may be enlarged but asymptomatic unless there is splenic infarction. Given location of the spleen next to the diaphragm, a sense of fullness may be referred through the phrenic nerve to the C3–C5 dermatomes in the left shoulder.

PHYSICAL EXAM

- Jaundice: if hemolytic anemia is present
- Splenomegaly
  - The normal spleen is usually not palpable. A palpable spleen may indicate pathology such as splenomegaly—and, in turn, hypersplenism in the appropriate clinical context—or may indicate a wandering spleen.
  - Begin by percussing Traube semilunar space, demarcated laterally by left anterior axillary line, inferiorly by the left costal margin, and superiorly by the left 6th rib. This space is usually hollow. Splenic enlargement may cause dullness to percussion in this area. Other processes that may cause dullness include pleural or pericardial effusions. Additionally, if the patient recently ate a large meal, this area may be dull to percussion.
  - With patient supine, rest hand gently on the abdomen to prevent sudden tensing of the abdominal musculature, which may obscure palpation. As the spleen enlarges, it moves caudally and medially. Start by palpating in the right lower quadrant and moving toward the umbilicus, toward the left upper quadrant. If there is doubt about whether the spleen has moved beyond the costal margin, ask patient to take a large breath, which will push the diaphragm, and, in turn, the spleen toward the examiner's hands.

DIAGNOSTIC TESTS & INTERPRETATION

On CBC, any and all cell lines may be decreased, resulting in the following:

- Anemia
- Leukopenia
- Thrombocytopenia

Initial Tests (lab, imaging)

- CBC
- Reticulocyte count if anemia
- If there is hemolysis, there should be an elevated reticulocyte count along with evidence of hyperbilirubinemia.
- US
- CT
- Tc-99m sulfur colloid scintigraphy
- PET
- MRI

Follow-Up Tests & Special Considerations

Based on other historical and exam findings, testing for specific infectious etiologies may be warranted:

- Blood parasite smear for malaria
- EBV serologies
- HIV ELISA with Western blot
- JAK2 mutation in polycythemia vera
- PPD for tuberculosis

Diagnostic Procedures/Other

Bone marrow biopsy

Test Interpretation

Hyperplasia of bone marrow precursors, especially those correlating with the patient's individual cytopenias

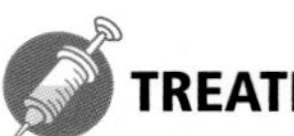

TREATMENT

MEDICATION

- No specific medication can be recommended for patients with hypersplenism. The most important intervention is to treat the underlying disorder.
- If ITP is the cause, the patient may benefit from the following:
  - Prednisone or methylprednisolone
  - IVIG
  - Rituximab
- If an infectious cause is discovered, treatment with appropriate antibiotic therapy may help to improve the cytopenias.

SURGERY/OTHER PROCEDURES

Many patients undergo splenectomy to alleviate severe cytopenias resulting from hypersplenism.

ALERT

- Splenectomized patients should receive immunization to pneumococcus, meningococcus, *Haemophilus influenzae*, and influenza at least 14 days prior to splenectomy (1)[A].
- If this cannot be done (i.e., in cases of emergent splenectomy), wait at least 14 days post splenectomy to immunize.
  - Pneumococcal vaccine
    - Pneumococcal polyvalent-23 vaccine (PPSV23) for use in adults and fully immunized children ≥2 years of age
    - Pneumococcal polyvalent-13 vaccine (PCV13) for infants and young children ≥2 months of age as part of routine immunization schedule (2)[A]
    - PCV13 for adolescents and adults in addition to PPSV23; refer to CDC for timing of administration.
    - Current guidelines recommend single revaccination of PPSV23 5 years after the initial dose.
  - *H. influenzae* vaccine
  - Meningococcal vaccine (3)[A]
    - Meningococcal conjugate vaccine (MCV4) for use in patients between 2 and 55 years
    - Meningococcal polysaccharide vaccine (MPSV4) for use in patients >55 years of age
    - Revaccination is recommended every 5 years.
  - Influenza vaccine should be administered yearly based on prevalent circulating strains. Although patients are not at higher risk from influenza itself, infection with influenza may place patients at higher risk for secondary bacterial infections.
- Radiofrequency ablation (RFA) is becoming more available and can be successful at preventing recurrence of hypersplenism. It is not currently known whether there are differences between RFA and splenectomy in terms of postprocedure infectious risks. Other alternatives to splenectomy include total and partial splenic embolization and shunting, although these techniques are evolving and additional studies are needed to evaluate efficacy and morbidity as compared to splenectomy.

INPATIENT CONSIDERATIONS

Admission Criteria/Initial Stabilization

- Hypersplenism alone generally does not warrant admission. However, all patients should be monitored closely for complications of the resulting cytopenias, including bleeding and infection, as well as complications of splenomegaly, including increased risk of splenic rupture. In some patients, the large spleen compresses the stomach and prevents adequate oral intake.
- Splenectomized patients are at increased risk of infection and postsplenectomy sepsis, especially with *Streptococcus pneumoniae*. Fevers, chills, or pain concerning for underlying infection warrant immediate attention, as clinical decompensation can occur within hours. Empiric broad-spectrum antibiotics should not be delayed while evaluation is ongoing. Common empiric regimens include the following:
  - Ceftriaxone/: 2g IV q24h and vancomycin 1 g IV q12h
  - Levofloxacin: 750 mg IV q24h and vancomycin 1 g IV q12h in β-lactam–allergic patients

ONGOING CARE

- Adult patients who are splenectomized should be advised to monitor closely for fever or rigors at home, which may be an early sign of bacteremia. They should be instructed to begin antibiotics immediately prior to proceeding to a medical facility for evaluation. Early antibiotics have been shown to reduce the mortality from overwhelming postsplenectomy sepsis.
- Controlled trials have not been performed, but some regimens include the following:
  - Amoxicillin-clavulanate: 875 mg PO twice daily
  - Cefuroxime axetil: 500 mg PO twice daily
- Patients allergic to β-lactam antibiotics can be given an extended-spectrum fluoroquinolone such as levofloxacin 750 mg PO *or* moxifloxacin 400 mg PO daily.
- In children with splenectomy, daily antibiotic prophylaxis for overwhelming postsplenectomy sepsis with penicillin VK or amoxicillin is recommended until age 5 or at least 3 years after splenectomy:
  - Age 2 months–5 years: 125 mg PO BID
  - >5 years old: 250 mg PO BID

PATIENT EDUCATION

Patients who are splenectomized should be counseled extensively about the risk of overwhelming postsplenectomy sepsis and the need to obtain prompt medical evaluation in the event of fevers, chills, or any other concerning symptoms.

REFERENCES

1. Advisory Committee on Immunization Practices. Recommended adult immunization schedule: United States, 2012. *Ann Intern Med*. 2012;156(3):211–217.
2. American Academy of Pediatrics. Children with asplenia or functional asplenia. In: Pickering LK, Baker CI, Kimberlin DW, et al, eds. *Red Book: 2009 Report of the Committee on Infectious Diseases*. 28th ed. Elk Grove Village, IL: American Academy of Pediatrics; 2009:72.
3. Centers for Disease Control and Prevention. Updated recommendations for use of meningococcal conjugate vaccines—Advisory Committee on Immunization Practices (ACIP), 2010. *MMWR Morb Mortal Wkly Rep*. 2011;60(3):72–76.

ADDITIONAL READING

- Abdella HM, Abd-El-Moez AT, Abu El-Maaty ME, et al. Role of partial splenic arterial embolization for hypersplenism in patients with liver cirrhosis and thrombocytopenia. *Indian J Gastroenterol*. 2010;29(2):59–61.
- Di Sabatino A, Carsetti R, Corazza GR. Post-splenectomy and hyposplenic states. *Lancet*. 2011;378(9785):86–97.
- Feng K, Ma K, Liu Q, et al. Randomized clinical trial of splenic radiofrequency ablation versus splenectomy for severe hypersplenism. *Br J Surg*. 2011;98(3):354–361.
- Iriyama N, Horikoshi A, Hatta Y, et al. Localized, splenic, diffuse large B-cell lymphoma presenting with hypersplenism: risk and benefit of splenectomy. *Intern Med*. 2010;49(11):1027–1030.
- Jandl JH, Aster RH, Forkner CE, et al. Splenic pooling and the pathophysiology of hypersplenism. *Trans Am Clin Climatol Assoc*. 1967;78:9–27.
- Kapoor P, Singh E, Radhakrishnan P, et al. Splenectomy in plasma cell dyscrasias: a review of the clinical practice. *Am J Hematol*. 2006;81(12):946–954.
- Mourtzoukou EG, Pappas G, Peppas G, et al. Vaccination of asplenic or hyposplenic adults. *Br J Surg*. 2008;95(3):273–280.
- Shatz DV, Schinsky MF, Pais LB, et al. Immune responses of splenectomized trauma patients to the 23-valent pneumococcal polysaccharide vaccine at 1 versus 7 versus 14 days after splenectomy. *J Trauma*. 1998;44(5):760–765; discussion 765–766.

SEE ALSO

Anemia, Autoimmune Hemolytic; Malaria; Polycythemia Vera; Tuberculosis

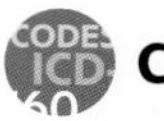

CODES

ICD10

D73.1 Hypersplenism

CLINICAL PEARLS

- Splenectomy is not necessary to make the diagnosis.
- Avoid splenectomy in patients unless absolutely necessary. Splenectomized patients are at lifelong risk for overwhelming postsplenectomy infection and sepsis.
- If splenectomy is to be performed, give immunization for pneumococcus, meningococcus, *Haemophilus*, and influenza at least 14 days prior to surgery. Otherwise, wait until the 14th postop day to immunize.

HYPERTENSION, ESSENTIAL

Lisa M. Schroeder, MD • Rishin Patel, MD

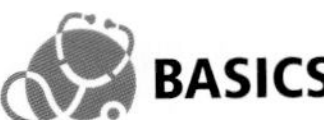

BASICS

DESCRIPTION

- Hypertension (HTN) is defined (JNC VIII) as ≥2 elevated BPs
  - Age 60 years or older: systolic BP (SBP) ≥150 mm Hg and/or diastolic BP (DBP) ≥90 mm Hg at ≥2 visits 1[A]
  - Age <60 years with chronic kidney disease (CKD) or diabetes: SBP ≥140 mm Hg and/or DBP ≥90 mm Hg at ≥2 visits (1)[A]
  - Operationally, any BP at which drug treatment results in a net benefit to a population
- HTN is a strong risk factor for cardiovascular disease.
- Synonym(s): benign, chronic, idiopathic, familial, or genetic HTN; high BP

Geriatric Considerations

- Isolated systolic HTN is common.
- Therapy has been shown to be effective and beneficial at preventing stroke, although target SBP is higher than in younger patients (150 mm Hg systolic), and adverse reactions to medications are more frequent. The benefit of therapy has been conclusively demonstrated in older patients for SBP ≥160 mm Hg.

Pediatric Considerations

- Measure BP during routine exams for >3 years of age.
- Defined as SBP or DBP ≥95th percentile on repeated measurements (2)
- Pre-HTN: SBP or DBP between 90th and 95th percentile (2)[A]

Pregnancy Considerations

- Elevated BP during pregnancy may be either chronic HTN or pregnancy-induced preeclampsia. ACE inhibitors and angiotensin II receptor blockers (ARBs) are contraindicated.
- Maternal and fetal mortality benefit from treatment of severe HTN. Evidence not clear for mild HTN (see topic "Preeclampsia")

EPIDEMIOLOGY

Incidence

- Lifetime risk for men and women aged 55–65 years by age 80–85 years is >90%.
- Predominant age: essential (primary, benign, idiopathic) onset usually in the 20s–30s
- Predominant sex: male > female; males tend to run higher than females and have a significantly higher risk of cardiovascular disease at any given pressure.

Prevalence

In 2009–2010, prevalence in adults was 28.6% (2009–2010 National Health and Nutrition Examination Survey [NHANES])

ETIOLOGY AND PATHOPHYSIOLOGY

- >90% of HTN has no identified cause.
- Secondary causes of HTN (see "Hypertension, Secondary and Resistant"): renal parenchymal: glomerulonephritis, pyelonephritis, polycystic kidneys; endocrine: primary hyperaldosteronism, pheochromocytoma, hyperthyroidism, Cushing syndrome; vascular: coarctation of aorta, renal artery stenosis; chemical: commonly, oral contraceptives, NSAIDs, decongestants, corticosteroids; sleep apnea

Genetics

BP levels are strongly familial, but no clear genetic pattern exists. Familial risk for cardiovascular diseases should be considered.

RISK FACTORS

Family history, obesity, alcohol use, excess dietary sodium, stress, physical inactivity, tobacco abuse, insulin resistance

DIAGNOSIS

HISTORY

- HTN is asymptomatic except in extreme cases or after related cardiovascular complications develop.
- Headache can be seen with higher BP, often present on awakening and occipital in nature.

PHYSICAL EXAM

- Retinopathy: narrowed arteries, arteriovenous (AV) nicking, copper or silver wiring of retinal arterioles
- Increased/louder S_2 (aortic component heart sound)
- Synchronous radial and femoral pulse can help to rule out coarctation of the aorta.

DIFFERENTIAL DIAGNOSIS

Secondary HTN: Because of the low incidence of reversible secondary HTN, special tests should be considered only if the history, physical exam, or basic laboratory evaluation indicate the possibility. (See "Hypertension, Secondary and Resistant.")

DIAGNOSTIC TESTS & INTERPRETATION

ECG to evaluate possible presence of left ventricular hypertrophy (LVH) or rhythm abnormalities affecting therapy

Initial Tests (lab, imaging)

- Hemoglobin and hematocrit or CBC
- Complete urinalysis (may reveal proteinuria)
- Potassium, calcium, creatinine, and uric acid
- Lipid panel (total, HDL, LDL, triglyceride [TG])
- Fasting blood glucose, hemoglobin A1c

Follow-Up Tests & Special Considerations

- Special tests (only if history, physical, or labs indicates) (See "Hypertension, Secondary and Resistant.")
- Ambulatory (24-hour) BP monitoring if "white coat" HTN is suspected.
- Home BP monitoring is effective, especially if white coat HTN is a consideration; elevated home BPs correlate with adverse outcomes, possibly more so than office BPs, and normal readings are reassuring.

Diagnostic Procedures/Other

- Age 60 years or older: SBP (SBP) ≥150 mm Hg and/or DBP ≥90 mm Hg) at ≥2 visits
- Age <60 years with CKD or diabetes: SBP ≥140 mm Hg and/or DBP ≥90 mm Hg at ≥2 visits
- Operationally, any BP at which drug treatment results in a net benefit to a population.
- Assuming proper resting conditions, cuff size, and application are maintained.
- The Joint National Committee VIII (JNC) recommends emphasis on
  - Family or personal history of HTN; cardiovascular, cerebrovascular, renal disease, and diabetes
  - Previous elevated BPs
  - Previous treatment for HTN
  - History of weight gain, exercise activities, sodium and fat intake, and alcohol use
  - Symptoms suggesting secondary HTN
  - Psychosocial and environmental factors affecting BP and risk for cardiovascular disease
  - Other cardiovascular risk factors, such as obesity, smoking, hyperlipidemia, and diabetes
  - Funduscopic exam for arteriolar narrowing, AV compression, hemorrhages, exudates, and papilledema
  - Body mass index (BMI)
  - Waist circumference
  - BP in both arms
  - Complete cardiac and peripheral pulse exam: compare radial and femoral pulse for differences in volume and timing, auscultation for carotid and femoral bruits.
  - Abdominal exam for masses and bruits: listen high in the flanks over the kidneys.
  - Neurologic assessment

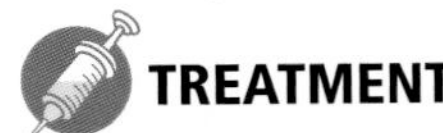

TREATMENT

GENERAL MEASURES

- Treating patients age <60 years or with CKD or diabetes to lower-than-standard BP targets, ≥140/90 mm Hg, does not further reduce mortality or morbidity. Individualize goal pressures based on risk factors.
- Target SBP at or just below 150 mm Hg in patients >60 years of age is acceptable in the general population (1).
- Although primary focus is SBP goal; treatment should accommodate patient preferences (1). Majority of treatment benefit is attained with initial 2–3 medications. Striving for small additional drops in BP to achieve a "target" is less clinically beneficial and more likely to cause side effects.
- Lower DBP targets were not associated with decreased morbidity/mortality (3).
- Aerobic exercise (30 minutes of aerobics 4–5 days per week), weight reduction for obese patients
- Smoking cessation
- Risk stratification from JNC VII no longer addressed in JNC VIII (1)[A]
  - Age 60 years or older: SBP ≥150 mm Hg and/or DBP ≥90 mm Hg at ≥2 visits
  - Age <60 years with CKD or diabetes: SBP ≥140 mm Hg and/or DBP ≥90 mm Hg at ≥2 visits
  - Assess overall risk and individualize decision to treat.
  - Choose from one of 4 classes of medications: (1)[A] ACE inhibitors, ARBs, calcium channel blockers (CCBs), or diuretics.

MEDICATION

- Multiple drugs at submaximal dose may achieve target BP with fewer side effects. In patients on more than one medication, divide between morning and nighttime for better 24-hour antihypertensive effect.
- Sequential monotherapy attempts might be tried with different classes because individual responses vary.
- Many patients will require multiple medications.
- First-line agents for uncomplicated essential HTN include thiazide diuretics, ACE inhibitors, ARBs, and long-acting CCBs (amlodipine, felodipine) (1,4)[A].

- If concomitant conditions, choose 1st-line agent based on comorbidity.
- Combination 1st-line agents: Benazepril combined with amlodipine may be superior to combination with HCTZ in high-risk patients. Some suggest that ACE/ARB + dihydropyridine CCB is first choice after monotherapy.
- β-Blockers had been strongly recommended until recent meta-analyses. Atenolol may be particularly *ineffective* in reducing adverse outcomes of HTN (except in patients with left ventricle hypertrophy undergoing dialysis).
- ACE inhibitors should be used in patients with diabetes, proteinuria, atrial fibrillation, or heart failure with reduced ejection fraction (HFrEF) but *not in pregnancy*.
- α-Adrenergic blockers are not the 1st choice for monotherapy but remain as 2nd line after combination therapy of 1st-line agents; might benefit males with benign prostatic hypertrophy (BPH)
- β-Blockers might benefit patients with ischemic heart disease, CHF, or migraine post ST-segment elevation myocardial infarction (STEMI).
- CCB could be considered in patients with isolated systolic HTN, atherosclerosis, angina, migraine, or asthma; well documented to reduce risk of stroke
- Thiazide diuretics or CCB preferred as 1st line in the general black population.

First Line

- Thiazide diuretics (3)[A]
  - Chlorthalidone: 12.5–25 mg/day (more potent than hydrochlorothiazide but causes more hyponatremia and hypokalemia)
  - Hydrochlorothiazide:12.5–50 mg/day
  - Indapamide: 1.25–2.5 mg/day
- ACE inhibitors
  - Lisinopril: 10–40 mg/day
  - Enalapril: 5–40 mg/day
  - Ramipril: 2.5–20 mg/day
  - Benazepril: 10–40 mg/day
- CCB
  - Diltiazem CD: 180–360 mg/day
  - Nifedipine (sustained release): 30–90 mg/day
  - Verapamil (sustained release): 120–480 mg/day
  - Amlodipine: 2.5–10 mg/day
- ARBs
  - Losartan: 25–100 mg in 1 or 2 doses; has unique but modest uricosuric effect
  - Valsartan: 80–320 mg daily
  - Irbesartan: 75–300 mg daily
  - Candesartan: 4–32 mg daily
  - Renin inhibitor: aliskiren 150–300 mg daily
- Contraindications
  - Diuretics may worsen gout.
  - β-Blockers (relative) in reactive airway disease, heart block, diabetes, and peripheral vascular disease; probably should be avoided in patients with metabolic syndrome or insulin-requiring diabetes
  - Diltiazem or verapamil: do not use with systolic dysfunction or heart block
  - ACE inhibitors can worsen bilateral renovascular disease and are pregnancy Category D.

Second Line

- Many may be combined. Choose additional medications with complementary effects (i.e., ACE inhibitors/ARBs with diuretic or a vasodilator with a diuretic or β-blocker).
- Centrally acting α-2 agonists: clonidine: 0.1–1.2 mg BID or weekly patch 0.1–0.3 mg/day; guanfacine: 1–3 mg daily; or methyldopa: 250–2,000 mg BID
- α-Adrenergic antagonists: prazosin: 1–10 mg BID; terazosin: 1–20 mg/day; or doxazosin: 1–16 mg/day
- Peripherally acting adrenergic inhibitors: rarely used: reserpine: 0.1–0.25 mg/day
- Vasodilators
  - Hydralazine: 10–25 mg QID; risk of tachycardia, so generally combined with β-blocker; also drug-induced systemic lupus erythematosus (SLE)
  - Minoxidil: rarely used due to adverse effects. May be more effective than other medications in renal failure and refractory HTN.
- Loop diuretics (for volume overload): furosemide: 20–320 mg/day *or* bumetanide: 0.5–2 mg/day
- K^+-sparing diuretics in patients with hypokalemia while taking thiazides: amiloride: 5–10 mg/day or triamterene: 50–150 mg/day
- Medication-refractory HTN or suspected aldosteronism: spironolactone: 25–100 mg/day

COMPLEMENTARY & ALTERNATIVE MEDICINE

Biofeedback and relaxation exercise

ONGOING CARE

FOLLOW-UP RECOMMENDATIONS

Patient Monitoring

- Reevaluate patients q3–6mo until stable, then q6–12mo. Consider use of home self-BP monitoring; quality-of-life issues including sexual function should be considered.
- Poor medication adherence is a leading cause of apparent medication failure.
- Annual urinalysis, creatinine, and potassium

DIET

- ~20% of patients will respond to reduced-salt diet (<100 mmol/day; <6 g NaCl or <2.4 g Na).
- Consider Dietary Approaches to Stop Hypertension (DASH) diet: www.nhlbi.nih.gov/health/public/heart/hbp/dash/new_dash.pdf.
- Limit alcohol consumption to <1 oz/day.

PATIENT EDUCATION

- Emphasize the asymptomatic nature of HTN and importance of lifetime treatment.
- Printed aids for high BP education available: www.nhlbi.nih.gov/health/public/heart/index.htm&hbp

COMPLICATIONS

Heart failure, renal failure, LVH, myocardial infarction, retinal hemorrhage, stroke, hypertensive heart disease, drug side effects

REFERENCES

1. James PA, Oparil S, Carter BL, et al. 2014 evidence-based guideline for the management of high blood pressure in adults: report from the panel members appointed to the Eighth Joint National Committee (JNC 8). *JAMA*. 2014;311(5):507–520.
2. Riley M, Bluhm B. High blood pressure in children and adolescents. *Am Fam Physician*. 2012;85(7):693–700.
3. Arguedas JA, Perez MI, Wright JM. Treatment blood pressure targets for hypertension. *Cochrane Database Syst Rev*. 2009;(3):CD004349.
4. Chobanian AV, Bakris GL, Black HR, et al. The seventh report of the Joint National Committee on prevention, detection, evaluation, and treatment of high blood pressure: the JNC 7 report. *JAMA*. 2003;289(19):2560–2572.

ADDITIONAL READING

- The ACCORD Study Group. Effects of intensive blood-pressure control in type 2 diabetes mellitus. *N Engl J Med*. 2010;362(17):1575–1585.
- ALLHAT Officers and Coordinators for the ALLHAT Collaborative Research Group. Major outcomes in high-risk hypertensive patients randomized to angiotensin-converting enzyme inhibitor or calcium channel blocker vs diuretic: the Antihypertensive and Lipid-Lowering Treatment to Prevent Heart Attack Trial (ALLHAT). *JAMA*. 2002;288(23):2981–2997.
- Dorsch MP, Gillespie BW, Erickson SR, et al. Chlorthalidone reduces cardiovascular events compared with hydrochlorothiazide: a retrospective cohort analysis. *Hypertension*. 2011;57(4):689–694.
- Mancia G, Fagard R, Narkiewicz K, et al. 2013 ESH/ESC guidelines for the management of arterial hypertension: the Task Force for the Management of Arterial Hypertension of the European Society of Hypertension (ESH) and of the European Society of Cardiology (ESC). *Eur Heart J*. 2013;34(28):2159–2219.
- National Institute for Health and Care Excellence. Clinical guideline 127. Hypertension: clinical management of primary hypertension in adults. www.nice.org.uk/nicemedia/live/13561/56008/56008.pdf. Accessed 2014.

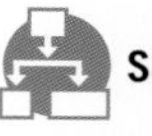

SEE ALSO

Hypertension, Secondary and Resistant; Hypertensive Emergencies; Polycystic Kidney Disease

CODES

ICD10

I10 Essential (primary) hypertension

CLINICAL PEARLS

- Treatment of HTN reduces risk of many serious medical conditions with numbers needed to treat to prevent 1 serious event (e.g., stroke or myocardial infarction) ranging from 20 patients per year for severe HTN to more than several hundred per year for mild HTN.
- Multiple submaximal doses are likely to have fewer side effects and more effectiveness than fewer maximum-dosed drugs.
- In older patients, measure BP standing to avoid overtreatment and syncope.

HYPERTENSION, SECONDARY AND RESISTANT

George H. Maxted, MD

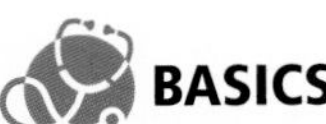

BASICS

DESCRIPTION

Uncontrolled hypertension (HTN) comprises the following entities (see "Alert" below):

- Resistant HTN: defined as blood pressure that remains above goal in spite of the concurrent use of 3 antihypertensive agents of different classes. Ideally, one of the 3 agents should be a diuretic and all agents should be prescribed at optimal dose amounts (1–3)[C].
- Secondary HTN: elevated BP that results from an identifiable underlying mechanism (1–3)
- Both the recent Eight Joint National Committee (JNC8) and AHA/ACC/CDC guidelines recommend a goal BP of <140/90 mm Hg, although JNC8 allows for a goal of <150/90 mm Hg for patients older than age 60 years (4,5)[C].

Geriatric Considerations

- Onset of HTN in adults >60 years of age is a strong indicator of secondary HTN.
- In patients >80 years of age, consider a higher target systolic blood pressure (SBP) of $\geq$150 mm Hg. Be cautious to avoid excessive diastolic lowering.
- Elderly may be particularly responsive to diuretics and dihydropyridine calcium channel blockers.
- Systolic HTN is particularly problematic in the elderly.
- Secondary causes more common in the elderly; include sleep apnea, renal disease, renal artery stenosis, and primary aldosteronism.

ALERT

Pseudoresistance

- Inaccurate measurement of BP
  - Cuff too small
  - Patient not at rest; sitting quietly for 5 minutes
- Poor adherence: In primary care settings, this has been estimated to occur in 40–60% of patients with HTN.
- White coat effect: prevalence 20–40%. Do not make clinical decisions about HTN based solely on measurement in the clinic setting. Home BP monitoring and/or ambulatory BP monitoring is more reliable.
- Inadequate treatment

EPIDEMIOLOGY

- Predominant age: In general, HTN has its onset between ages 30 and 50 years. Patients with resistant HTN are more likely to experience the combined outcomes of death, myocardial infarction, congestive heart failure (CHF), stroke, or chronic kidney disease.
- Depending on etiology, age of onset can vary. Age of onset <20 or >50 years increases likelihood of a secondary cause for HTN.
- The strongest predictors for resistant HTN are age (>75 years), presence of left ventricular hypertrophy (LVH), obesity (body mass index [BMI] >30), and high baseline systolic BP. Other predictors include chronic kidney disease, diabetes, living in the southeastern United States, African American race (especially women), and excessive salt intake.

Prevalence

- Prevalence of resistant HTN is unknown. NHANES analysis indicates only 53% of adults are controlled to a BP of <140/90 mm Hg.
- Secondary HTN occurs in about 5–10% of adults with chronic HTN.

ETIOLOGY AND PATHOPHYSIOLOGY

- Obstructive sleep apnea (OSA): 1 study diagnosed OSA in 83% of treatment-resistant hypertensives.
- Primary hyperaldosteronism (17–22% of resistant HTN cases)
- Chronic renal disease (2–5% of hypertensives)
- Renovascular disease (0.2–0.7%, up to 35% of elderly, 20% of patients undergoing cardiac catheterization)
- Cushing syndrome (0.1–0.6%)
- Pheochromocytoma (0.04–0.1% of hypertensives)
- Other rare causes: hyperthyroidism, hyperparathyroidism, aortic coarctation, intracranial tumor
- Drug-related causes
  - Medications, especially NSAIDs (may also blunt effectiveness of ACE inhibitors), decongestants, stimulants (e.g., amphetamines, attention-deficient hyperactivity disorder [ADHD] medications), anorectic agents (e.g., modafinil, ephedra, guarana, ma huang, bitter orange), erythropoietin, natural licorice (in some chewing tobacco), yohimbine, glucocorticoids
  - Oral contraceptives: unclear association; mainly epidemiologic and with higher estrogen pills
  - Cocaine, amphetamines, other illicit drugs; drug and alcohol withdrawal syndromes
- Lifestyle factors: Obesity and dietary salt may negate the beneficial effect of diuretics. Excessive alcohol may cause or exacerbate HTN. Physical inactivity also contributes.

RISK FACTORS

A recent large cohort study revealed that those with resistant HTN (16.2%) were more likely to be male, Caucasian, older, and diabetic. They were also more likely to be taking β-blockers, calcium channel blockers, and α-adrenergic blockers compared with other drug classes. Factors predictive of resistant or secondary HTN: female sex, African American race, obesity, diabetes, worsening of control in previously stable hypertensive patient, onset in patients age <20 years or >50 years, lack of family history of HTN, significant target end-organ damage, stage 2 HTN (systolic BP >160 mm Hg or diastolic BP >100 mm Hg), renal disease, and alcohol or drug use (3)[A]

GENERAL PREVENTION

The prevention of resistant and secondary HTN is thought to be the same as for primary or essential HTN: Adopting a DASH (Dietary Approaches to Stop Hypertension) diet, a low-sodium diet, weight loss in obese patients, exercise, limitation of alcohol intake, and smoking cessation may all be of benefit. Relaxation techniques may be of help, but data are limited.

DIAGNOSIS

HISTORY

- Ask or review at every visit: "The Big Four" SANS mnemonic: 1. Salt intake, 2. Alcohol intake, 3. NSAID use, 4. Sleep (author's suggestion, based on reference listed).
- Review home BP readings; consider ambulatory BP monitoring.
- History will vary with etiology of HTN.
  - Pheochromocytoma: episodes of headache, palpitations, sweating
  - Cushing syndrome: weight gain, fatigue, weakness, easy bruising, amenorrhea
  - OSA: loud snoring while asleep, daytime somnolence
  - Increased intravascular volume: swelling

PHYSICAL EXAM

- Ensure that the BP is measured correctly. The patient should be sitting quietly with back supported for 5 minutes before measurement. Proper cuff size: bladder encircling at least 80% of the arm. Support arm at heart level. Minimum of 2 readings at least 1 minute apart. Check BP in both arms. Also check standing BP for orthostasis.
- Attention to findings related to possible etiologies: renovascular HTN: systolic/diastolic abdominal bruit. Pheochromocytoma: diaphoresis, tachycardia. Cushing syndrome: hirsutism, moon facies, dorsal hump, purple striae, truncal obesity. Thyroid disease: enlarged thyroid, tremor, exophthalmos, tachycardia. Coarctation of the aorta: upper limb HTN with decreased or delayed femoral pulses.
- Funduscopic exam

DIAGNOSTIC TESTS & INTERPRETATION

- ECG performed as part of the initial workup; LVH is an important marker of resistant HTN.
- Sleep study if history and physical indicate. The Epworth Sleepiness Scale is recommended.
- Home-based polysomnography has been shown to be accurate in screening for OSA. Overnight oximetry is not helpful.

Initial Tests (lab, imaging)

Initial limited diagnostic testing should include urinalysis, CBC, potassium, sodium, glucose, creatinine, lipids, thyroid-stimulating hormone (TSH), and calcium. 50% of patients with hyperaldosteronism may have normal potassium levels.

- Imaging tests listed are necessary only if history, physical, or lab data indicate.
- Abdominal US: if renal disease is suspected
- MR angiography (MRA) of renal vasculature: Preferred test for renovascular HTN. Sensitive but low specificity. Conventional angiography or CT angiography second-line after MRA to look at distal renal artery. Renal arteriography remains gold standard for renovascular disease.
- Adrenal "incidentaloma" frequently arises in this era of multiple CT studies. If present in the setting of resistant HTN, consider hyperaldosterone or hyperadrenalcorticoid states.

Follow-Up Tests & Special Considerations

Further testing for primary aldosteronism (PA) may be considered.

- Empiric treatment with an aldosterone inhibitor may be preferable and more clinically relevant: Spironolactone or eplerenone. Amiloride may be more effective in African Americans.
- Plasma aldosterone-to-renin ratio (ARR) is the preferred lab test, *but* the test is difficult to perform and interpret properly. Consult your reference lab and interpret results with caution.
  - Further testing for pheochromocytoma: plasma
  - Other tests to consider for resistant or secondary HTN: 24-hour urine for free cortisol, calcium, parathyroid hormone (PTH), overnight 1-mg dexamethasone suppression test, urine toxicology screen

Diagnostic Procedures/Other

Consider 24-hour ambulatory BP monitoring, especially if white coat effect is suspected. Home BP monitor results predict mortality, stroke, and other target organ damage better than office BP. Optimal protocol involves 2 paired measurements: morning and evening (4 measurements) over 4–7 days.

- Oscillometric, electronic, upper arm, fully automatic device with memory. Average multiple readings over several days.
- See www.dableducational.org for validated monitors.

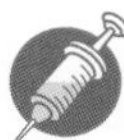

TREATMENT

- Treatment modality depends on etiology of HTN. Please see each etiology listed for information on proper treatment.
- Emphasize Adherence to JNC8 and/or AHA/ACC guidelines, with emphasis on lifestyle modification (4,5)[C].
  - Obese patients, African Americans, and elderly may be particularly responsive to diuretics.
  - Tolerance to diuretics may occur: long-term adaptation to thiazides or the "braking effect." Consider increasing the dose of thiazide or adding an aldosterone inhibitor.
- Treatment specific to certain secondary etiologies
  - Primary aldosteronism: aldosterone receptor antagonist: spironolactone or eplerenone
  - Cushing syndrome: aldosterone receptor antagonist
  - OSA: continuous positive airway pressure (CPAP) ± oxygen, surgery, weight loss
  - Nocturnal hypoxia: oxygen supplementation
  - Earlier studies had suggested benefit from renal sympathetic denervation, but a recent sham study, SYMPLICITY HTN-3, was not supportive (6)[B].

MEDICATION

- Follow treatment guidelines and algorithms by JNC8 and AHA/ACC/CDC, understanding the differences between them (4,5)[C].
- Aldosterone antagonists may offer significant benefit (7,8)[B].
- Central-acting agents (e.g., clonidine) are effective at reducing BP, but outcome data are lacking.

ALERT

- Agents specific for treatment of HTN emergencies should be initiated under a situation in which immediate BP reduction will prevent or limit end-organ damage (see topic "Hypertensive Emergencies").
- Renovascular HTN: Angioplasty is the treatment of choice for fibromuscular dysplasia of a renal artery.
- The recent CORAL study concluded that in patients with atherosclerotic renovascular disease and HTN, renal artery stenting did not improve outcomes over medical therapy alone (9).
- Referral to an HTN specialist or clinic: Retrospective studies indicate improved control rates for patients with resistant HTN referred to special HTN clinics.

First Line

See topic "Hypertension."

INPATIENT CONSIDERATIONS

Admission Criteria/Initial Stabilization

Hospitalization may be necessary for hypertensive urgency or emergency general measures.

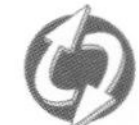

ONGOING CARE

FOLLOW-UP RECOMMENDATIONS

Encourage aerobic activity of 30 min/day, depending on patient condition.

DIET

- Reduced salt may lower BP.
- Recommend the Mediterranean diet or DASH.

PATIENT EDUCATION

Home BP monitoring is recommended.

REFERENCES

1. Calhoun DA, Jones D, Textor S, et al. Resistant hypertension: diagnosis, evaluation, and treatment. A scientific statement from the American Heart Association Professional Education Committee of the Council for High Blood Pressure Research. *Hypertension*. 2008;51(6):1403–1419.
2. Sarafidis PA, Bakris GL. Resistant hypertension: an overview of evaluation and treatment. *J Am Coll Cardiol*. 2008;52(22):1749–1757.
3. Daugherty SL, Powers JD, Magid DJ, et al. Incidence and prognosis of resistant hypertension in hypertensive patients. *Circulation*. 2012;125(13):1635–1642.
4. James PA, Oparil S, Carter BL, et al. 2014 Evidence-based guideline for the management of high blood pressure in adults: report from the panel members appointed to the Eighth Joint National Committee (JNC 8). *JAMA*. 2014;311(5):507–520.
5. Go AS, Bauman MA, Coleman King SM, et al. An effective approach to high blood pressure control: a science advisory from the American Heart Association, the American College of Cardiology, and the Centers for Disease Control and Prevention. *Hypertension*. 2014;63(4):878–885.
6. Bhatt DL, Kandzari DE, O'Neill WW, et al. A controlled trial of renal denervation for resistant hypertension. *N Engl J Med*. 2014;370(15):1393–1401.
7. Calhoun DA. Low-dose aldosterone blockade as a new treatment paradigm for controlling resistant hypertension. *J Clin Hypertens*. 2007;91(Suppl 1):19–24.
8. Gaddam KK, Nishizaka MK, Pratt-Ubunama MN, et al. Characterization of resistant hypertension: association between resistant hypertension, aldosterone, and persistent intravascular volume expansion. *Arch Intern Med*. 2008;168(11):1159–1164.
9. Cooper CJ, Murphy TP, Cutlip DE, et al. Stenting and medical therapy for atherosclerotic renal-artery stenosis. *N Engl J Med*. 2014;370(1):13–22.

ADDITIONAL READING

- Agarwal R, Bills JE, Hecht TJ, et al. Role of home blood pressure monitoring in overcoming therapeutic inertia and improving hypertension control: a systematic review and meta-analysis. *Hypertension*. 2011;57(1):29–38.
- Aronow WS, Fleg JL, Pepine CJ, et al. ACCF/AHA 2011 expert consensus document on hypertension in the elderly: a report of the American College of Cardiology Foundation Task Force on Clinical Expert Consensus documents developed in collaboration with the American Academy of Neurology, American Geriatrics Society, American Society for Preventive Cardiology, American Society of Hypertension, American Society of Nephrology, Association of Black Cardiologists, and European Society of Hypertension. *J Am Coll Cardiol*. 2011;57(20):2037–2114.
- Basner RC. Cardiovascular morbidity and obstructive sleep apnea. *N Engl J Med*. 2014;370(24):2339–2341.
- Ernst ME, Moser M. Use of diuretics in patients with hypertension. *N Engl J Med*. 2009;361(22):2153–2164.
- Johansson JK, Niiranen TJ, Puukka PJ, et al. Optimal schedule for home blood pressure monitoring based on a clinical approach. *J Hypertens*. 2010;28(2):259–264.
- Powers BJ, Olsen MK, Smith VA, et al. Measuring blood pressure for decision making and quality reporting: where and how many measures? *Ann Intern Med*. 2011;154(12):781–788.
- Rimoldi SF, Scherrer U, Messerli FH. Secondary arterial hypertension: when, who and how to screen? *Eur Heart J*. 2014;35(19):1245–1254.

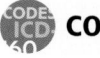

SEE ALSO

Aldosteronism, Primary; Coarctation of the Aorta; Cushing Disease and Cushing Syndrome; Hyperparathyroidism; Hypertension, Essential; Hyperthyroidism; Pheochromocytoma

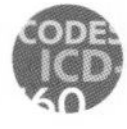

CODES

ICD10

- I15.9 Secondary hypertension, unspecified
- I15.8 Other secondary hypertension
- I15.0 Renovascular hypertension

CLINICAL PEARLS

- Onset of HTN in adults >60 years of age is a strong indicator of secondary HTN.
- Common causes of resistant HTN: obstructive sleep apnea, excessive salt intake, medication nonadherence
- Common secondary causes include sleep apnea, renal disease, renal artery stenosis, and primary aldosteronism.
- Home BP monitoring predicts outcomes better than office monitoring of BP.

HYPERTHYROIDISM

Anup K. Sabharwal, MD, MBA, FACE, CCD • Atil Y. Kargi, MD

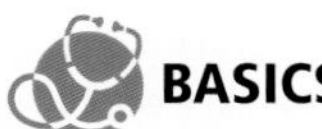

BASICS

Hyperthyroidism or thyrotoxicosis is composed of a spectrum of clinical findings consistent with thyroid hormone excess. The former describes excess from the thyroid gland, whereas the latter can be produced from another source.

DESCRIPTION

- Graves disease (GD): the most common form; diffuse goiter and thyrotoxicosis are common characteristics. Infiltrative orbitopathy is seen in 50% of patients. Infiltrative dermopathy is rare. Autoantibodies are directed at the thyrotropin-stimulating hormone (TSH) receptors.
- Toxic multinodular goiter (TMNG): 2nd most common; a TSH receptor mutation has been found in 60% of patients; patients $>$40 years, insidious onset, frequent in iodine-deficient areas
- Toxic adenoma: younger patients, autonomously functioning nodules
- Iodine-induced hyperthyroidism
- Thyroiditis: transient autoimmune process:
  - Subacute thyroiditis/De Quervain: granulomatous giant cell thyroiditis, benign course; viral infections have been involved.
  - Postpartum thyroiditis
  - Drug-induced thyroiditis: amiodarone, interferon-α, interleukin-2, lithium
  - Miscellaneous: thyrotoxicosis factitia, TSH-secreting pituitary tumors, and functioning trophoblastic tumors (1)[B]
- Subclinical hyperthyroidism: suppressed TSH with normal thyroxine (T_4); may be associated with osteoporosis and atrial fibrillation
- Thyroid storm: rare hyperthyroidism; fever, tachycardia, systolic hypertension, CNS dysfunction (e.g., coma); up to 50% mortality

Geriatric Considerations

- Characteristic symptoms and signs may be absent.
- Atrial fibrillation is common when TSH $<$0.1 mIU/L (2)[A].

Pediatric Considerations

- Neonates and children are treated with antithyroids for 12–24 months.
- Radioactive iodine is controversial in patients $<$15–18 years.

Pregnancy Considerations

Propylthiouracil (PTU) is currently the drug of choice during pregnancy. Treat with lowest effective dose. Avoid treatment-induced hypothyroidism. Radioiodine therapy is contraindicated.

EPIDEMIOLOGY

- 1.3% of population
- Predominant sex: female $>$ male (7–10:1)
- Predominant age: autoimmune thyroid disease in 2nd and 3rd decades. TMNG presents in patients $>$40 years. GD is seen between 40 and 60 years of age.

Incidence

- Female 1/1,000
- Male: 1/3,000

ETIOLOGY AND PATHOPHYSIOLOGY

- GD: autoimmune disease
- TMNG: 60% TSH receptor gene abnormality; 40% unknown
- Toxic adenoma: point mutation in TSH receptor gene with increased hormone production
- Thyroiditis:
  - Hashitoxicosis: autoimmune destruction of the thyroid; antimicrosomal antibodies present
  - Subacute/de Quervain thyroiditis: granulomatous reaction; genetic predisposition in specific human leukocyte antigens; viruses, such as coxsackievirus, adenovirus, echovirus, and influenza virus, have been implicated; self-limited course, 6–12 months
  - Suppurative: infectious
  - Drug-induced thyroiditis: Amiodarone produces an autoimmune reaction and a destructive process. Lithium, interferon-α, and interleukin-2 cause an autoimmune thyroiditis.
  - Postpartum thyroiditis: autoimmune thyroiditis that lasts up to 8 weeks and, in 60% of patients, hypothyroidism manifests in the future

Genetics

Concordance rate for GD among monozygotic twins is 35%.

RISK FACTORS

- Positive family history, especially in maternal relatives
- Female
- Other autoimmune disorders
- Iodide repletion after iodide deprivation, especially in TMNG

COMMONLY ASSOCIATED CONDITIONS

- Autoimmune diseases
- Down syndrome
- Iodine deficiency

DIAGNOSIS

HISTORY

- Thyrotoxicosis is a hypermetabolic state in which energy production exceeds needs, causing increased heat production, diaphoresis, and even fever.
- Thyrotoxicosis affects several different systems:
  - Constitutional: fatigue, weakness, increased appetite, weight loss
  - Neuropsychiatric: agitation, anxiety, emotional lability, psychosis, coma and poor concentration and memory
  - GI: increased appetite, hyperdefecation
  - Gynecologic: oligomenorrhea, amenorrhea
  - Cardiovascular: tachycardia (most common) and chest discomfort that mimics angina

Geriatric Considerations

Apathetic hyperthyroidism in the elderly

PHYSICAL EXAM

- Adults:
  - Skin: warm, moist, pretibial myxedema (GD only)
  - Head, eye, ear, nose, throat (HEENT): exophthalmos, lid lag
  - Endocrine: hyperhidrosis, heat intolerance, goiter, gynecomastia, low libido, and spider angiomata (males)
  - Cardiovascular: tachycardia, atrial fibrillation, cardiomegaly
  - Musculoskeletal: skeletal demineralization, osteopenia, osteoporosis, fractures
  - Neurologic: tremor, proximal muscle weakness, anxiety and lability, brisk deep tendon reflexes
  - Rarely: thyroid acropathy (clubbing), localized dermopathy
- Children:
  - Linear growth acceleration
  - Ophthalmic abnormalities more common

DIFFERENTIAL DIAGNOSIS

- Anxiety
- Malignancy
- Diabetes mellitus
- Pregnancy
- Menopause
- Pheochromocytoma
- Depression
- Carcinoid syndrome

DIAGNOSTIC TESTS & INTERPRETATION

- 95% have suppressed TSH and elevated free T_4. Total T_4 and triiodothyronine (T_3) represent the bound hormone and can be affected by pregnancy and hepatitis (1)[A].
- T_3: elevated, especially in T_3 toxicosis or amiodarone-induced thyrotoxicosis
- T_4: elevated; TSH autoantibodies rarely needed
- Free thyroxine index (FTI): calculated from T_4 and thyroid hormone–binding ratio; corrects for misleading results caused by pregnancy and estrogens
- Inappropriately normal or elevated TSH with high T_4 suspicious for pituitary tumor or thyroid hormone resistance
- Drugs may alter lab results: estrogens, heparin, iodine-containing compounds (including amiodarone and contrast agents), phenytoin, salicylates, steroids (e.g., androgens, corticosteroids)
- Drug precautions: Amiodarone and lithium may induce hyperthyroidism; MMI may cause warfarin resistance.
- Other findings that can occur: anemia, granulocytosis, lymphocytosis, hypercalcemia, transaminase, and alkaline phosphate elevations

Initial Tests (lab, imaging)

- TSH, free T_4, T_4, T_3, thyroid-stimulating immunoglobulin
- TSH receptor antibodies (TSH-R Abs): The routine assay is the TSH-binding inhibitor immunoglobulin assay (TBII). TSH-R Abs are useful in the prediction of postpartum Graves thyrotoxicosis and neonatal thyrotoxicosis.

- Thyroxine/triiodothyronine ratio: The T_4-to-T_3 ratio may be a useful tool when the iodine uptake testing is not available/contraindicated. ~2% of thyrotoxic patients have "T_3 toxicosis."
- Nuclear medicine scanning (^{123}I or ^{131}I): The reference range values for 24-hour radioiodine uptake is between 5% and 25%.
- Increased thyroid iodine uptake is seen with TMNG, toxic solitary nodule, and GD.
- GD shows a diffuse uptake and can have a paradoxical finding of high uptake at 4–6 hours but normal uptake at 24 hours because of the rapid clearance.
- TMNG will show a heterogeneous uptake, whereas solitary toxic nodule will show a warm or "hot" nodule.
- In iodine-deficient areas, an increased uptake is associated with low urine iodine levels.
- Hashimoto thyroiditis can have an increased uptake at an early stage but no increased thyroid hormone production.
- Causes of thyrotoxicosis with low iodine uptake:
  - Acute thyroiditis, thyrotoxicosis factitia, and iodine intoxication with amiodarone or contrast material can cause low-uptake transient thyrotoxicosis. After thyroiditis resolves, the patient can become euthyroid or hypothyroid.
  - Iodine loading can cause iodine trapping and decreased iodine uptake (Wolff-Chaikoff effect).
  - Thyrotoxicosis factitia: Thyroglobulin levels are low in exogenous intake and high in endogenous production.
  - Other extrathyroidal causes include struma ovarii and metastatic thyroid carcinoma.
  - Technetium-99m scintigraphy: controversial because it has a 33% discordance rate with radioactive iodine scanning

Follow-Up Tests & Special Considerations

In severe cases, such as thyroid storm, hospitalize until stable, especially if >60 years of age, because of the risk of atrial fibrillation.

Diagnostic Procedures/Other

Neck US will show increased diffuse vascularity in GD.

Test Interpretation

- GD: hyperplasia
- Toxic nodule: nodule formation

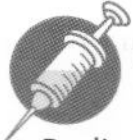

TREATMENT

- Radioactive iodine therapy (RAIT): most common definitive treatment used in the US for GD and TMNG
- Pretreatment with antithyroid drugs is preferred to avoid worsening thyrotoxicosis. MMI is preferred over PTU as pretreatment because of decreased relapse, but it is held 3–5 days before therapy (3)[A].
- There is concern for a slightly higher risk of lymphoma and leukemia in patients treated with RAIT.
- Usually, patients become hypothyroid 2–3 months after therapy; therefore, antithyroid medications are continued after ablation.
- Glucocorticoids: reduce the conversion of active T_4 to the more active T_3. In Graves ophthalmopathy, the use of prednisone before and after RAIT improves outcome (3)[B].
- After RAIT, the release of antigens can worsen the inflammatory reaction and the ophthalmopathy.
- Smoking in GD patients is a risk factor for ophthalmopathy when treated with RAIT.
- For TMNG, the treatment of choice is RAIT. Medical therapy with antithyroid medications has shown a high recurrence rate. Surgery is considered only in special cases (3)[B].
- Treatment for subacute thyroiditis is supportive with NSAIDs and β-blockers. Steroids can be used for 2–3 weeks (3).
- For amiodarone-induced thyrotoxicosis (AIT) type I, the treatment is antithyroid drugs and β-blockers. Thyroidectomy is the last option. AIT type II is self-limited but may use glucocorticoids.
- Graves dermopathy: difficult to treat in the chronic phase. Topical steroids with occlusive dressing may help in acute phase.

MEDICATION

First Line

- Antithyroid drugs: MMI and PTU are thionamides that inhibit iodine oxidation, organification, and iodotyrosine coupling. PTU can block peripheral conversion of T_4 to active T_3. Both can be used as primary treatment for GD and prior to RAIT or surgery (1)[A].
- Duration of treatment: 12–18 months; 50–60% relapse after stopping; treatment beyond 18 months did not show any further benefit. The most serious side effects are hepatitis (0.1–0.2%), vasculitis, and agranulocytosis; baseline CBC recommended:
  - MMI (preferred): adults: 10–15 mg q12h; children aged 6–10 years: 0.4 mg/kg/day PO once daily
  - PTU: adults (preferred in thyroid storm and first trimester of pregnancy): 100–150 mg PO q8h, not to exceed 200 mg/day during pregnancy
- β-Adrenergic blocker: Propranolol in high doses (>160 mg/day) inhibits T_3 activation by up to 30%. Atenolol, metoprolol, and nadolol can be used.
- Glucocorticoids: reduce the conversion of active T_4 to the more active T_3
- Cholestyramine: anion exchange resin that decreases thyroid hormone reabsorption in the enterohepatic circulation; dose: 4 g QID (1)[B]
- Other agents:
  - Lithium: inhibits thyroid hormone secretion and iodotyrosine coupling; use is limited by toxicity.
  - Lugol solution or saturated solution of potassium iodide (SSKI); blocks release of hormone from the gland but should be administered at least 1 hour after thionamide was given; acts as a substrate for hormone production (Jod-Basedow effect)
  - RAIT: See "Treatment" section.

ISSUES FOR REFERRAL

Patients with Graves ophthalmopathy should be referred to an experienced ophthalmologist.

SURGERY/OTHER PROCEDURES

Thyroidectomy for compressive symptoms, masses, and thyroid malignancy may be performed in the 2nd trimester of pregnancy only.

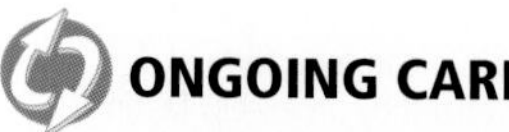

ONGOING CARE

FOLLOW-UP RECOMMENDATIONS

Patient Monitoring

- Repeat thyroid tests once a year, CBC, and LFTs on thionamide therapy; continue therapy with thionamides for 12–18 months.
- After RAIT, thyroid function tests at 6 weeks, 12 weeks, 6 months, and annually thereafter if euthyroid; TSH may remain undetectable for months if patient is euthyroid; follow T_3 and T_4.

DIET

Sufficient calories to prevent weight loss

PROGNOSIS

Good (with early diagnosis and treatment)

COMPLICATIONS

- Surgery: hypoparathyroidism, recurrent laryngeal nerve damage, and hypothyroidism
- RAIT: postablation hypothyroidism
- GD: high relapse rate with antithyroid drug as primary therapy
- Graves ophthalmopathy, worsening heart failure if cardiac condition, atrial fibrillation, muscle wasting, proximal muscle weakness, increased risk of cerebrovascular accident (CVA) and cardiovascular mortality

REFERENCES

1. Nayak B, Hodak SP. Hyperthyroidism. *Endocrinol Metab Clin North Am*. 2007;36(3):617–656.
2. Cappola AR, Fried LP, Arnold AM, et al. Thyroid status, cardiovascular risk, and mortality in older adults. *JAMA*. 2006;295(9):1033–1041.
3. Abraham P, Avenell A, Park CM, et al. A systematic review of drug therapy for Graves' hyperthyroidism. *Cochrane Database Sys Rev*. 2005;153(4):489–498.

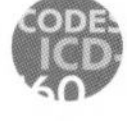

CODES

ICD10

- E05.90 Thyrotoxicosis, unspecified without thyrotoxic crisis or storm
- E05.20 Thyrotxcosis w toxic multinod goiter w/o thyrotoxic crisis
- E06.1 Subacute thyroiditis

CLINICAL PEARLS

- Not all thyrotoxicoses are secondary to hyperthyroidism.
- GD presents with hyperthyroidism, ophthalmopathy, and goiter.
- Medical treatment for GD has a high relapse rate after stopping medications.
- Thyroid storm is a medical emergency that needs hospitalization and aggressive treatment.

H

HYPERTRIGLYCERIDEMIA

S. Lindsey Clarke, MD, FAAFP

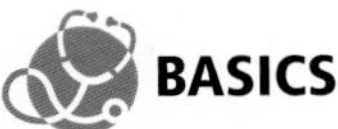

BASICS

DESCRIPTION

- Hypertriglyceridemia is a common form of dyslipidemia characterized by an excess fasting plasma concentration of triglycerides (TGs).
  - TGs are fatty molecules made of glycerols that are esterified by fatty acids at all 3 hydroxyl groups.
  - They occur naturally in vegetable oils and animal fats.
  - In humans, TGs are major sources of dietary energy; they are packaged into chylomicrons and very-low-density lipoproteins.
  - Hypertriglyceridemia is independently associated with cardiovascular disease risk, but the degree to which excess TGs cause atherosclerosis is uncertain and debatable.
- Hypertriglyceridemia is a biomarker of risk for premature coronary artery disease in both men and women at levels ≥200 mg/dL and for pancreatitis at levels ≥1,000 mg/dL.
- Classification of TG levels in adults after a 12-hour fast
  - Normal: <150 mg/dL (1.7 mmol/L)
  - Borderline to high: 150–199 mg/dL
  - High: 200–499 mg/dL
  - Very high: ≥500 mg/dL
  - Divide by 88.5 to convert to millimoles per liter.
- TGs are considered high in children who exceed the 95th percentiles for age and sex.
  - 143 mg/dL for adolescent boys, 126 mg/dL for adolescent girls
  - 111 mg/dL for preadolescent boys, 120 mg/dL for preadolescent girls

EPIDEMIOLOGY

- Predominant gender: male > female
- Predominant race: Hispanic, white > black

Prevalence

- 33% of U.S. population has TG levels ≥150 mg/dL.
- 1.7% has TG levels ≥500 mg/dL.
- Highest prevalence at age 50–70 years
- The most common genetic syndromes with hypertriglyceridemia are familial combined hyperlipidemia and familial hypertriglyceridemia (≤1% of general population each).

ETIOLOGY AND PATHOPHYSIOLOGY

- Primary
  - Familial
  - Acquired (sporadic)
- Secondary
  - Obesity and overweight
  - Physical inactivity
  - Cigarette smoking
  - Excess alcohol intake
  - Very high carbohydrate diets (>60% of total caloric intake)
  - Certain medications
    - Interferon-α
    - Atypical antipsychotics
    - β-Blockers other than carvedilol
    - Bile acid sequestrants
    - Corticosteroids
    - Oral estrogens
    - Protease inhibitors
    - Raloxifene
    - Retinoic acid
    - Tamoxifen
    - Thiazides
  - Medical conditions
    - Type 2 diabetes mellitus
    - Hypothyroidism
    - Chronic renal failure, nephrotic syndrome
    - Autoimmune disorders (e.g., systemic lupus erythematosus)
    - Paraproteinemias (e.g., macroglobulinemia, myeloma, lymphoma, lymphocytic leukemia)
    - Pregnancy (usually physiologic and transient)

Genetics

- Familial hypertriglyceridemia: autosomal dominant
- Familial dysbetalipoproteinemia: autosomal recessive
- Familial combined hyperlipidemia: unknown

RISK FACTORS

- Genetic susceptibility
- Obesity, overweight
- Diabetes
- Alcoholism
- Certain medications (see "Etiology")
- Medical conditions (see "Etiology")

GENERAL PREVENTION

- Weight reduction
- Moderation of dietary fat and carbohydrates
- Regular aerobic exercise

COMMONLY ASSOCIATED CONDITIONS

- Coronary artery disease
- Dyslipidemias
  - Decreased high-density lipoprotein (HDL) cholesterol
  - Increased low-density lipoprotein (LDL), non-HDL, and total cholesterol
  - Small, dense LDL particles
- Nonalcoholic steatohepatitis (NASH)
- Insulin resistance and type 2 diabetes mellitus
- Metabolic syndrome (3 of following):
  - Abdominal obesity (waist circumference >40 inches in men, >35 inches in women)
  - TGs ≥150 mg/dL
  - Low HDL cholesterol (<40 mg/dL in men, <50 mg/dL in women)
  - BP ≥130-/85 mm Hg
  - Fasting glucose ≥100 mg/dL
- Pancreatitis
- Polycystic ovary syndrome

DIAGNOSIS

HISTORY

- Usually asymptomatic
- Patients with chylomicronemia syndrome can have memory loss, headache, vertigo, dyspnea, and paresthesias.
- Pancreatitis: epigastric pain, nausea, and vomiting
- Assess for other cardiac risk factors.
- Family history of coronary artery disease

PHYSICAL EXAM

- Obesity, overweight (body mass index ≥25 kg/m^2)
- Eruptive cutaneous, tuberous, and striate palmar xanthomas
- Lipemia retinalis
- Epigastric tenderness in pancreatitis
- Hepatomegaly in NASH and chylomicronemia

DIFFERENTIAL DIAGNOSIS

Primary and secondary hypertriglyceridemia

DIAGNOSTIC TESTS & INTERPRETATION

Initial Tests (lab, imaging)

- Serum: turbid with milky supernatant
- Fasting lipid profile (12-hour fast)
  - Routine screening every 5 years beginning at age 35 years for men and age 45 years for women
  - Begin screening earlier in those at higher risk for coronary heart disease.
  - For interpretation, see "Description."
- Secondary causes
  - Glycosylated hemoglobin, fasting or postprandial glucose for type 2 diabetes mellitus
  - Creatinine, urinary protein measurement for nephrotic syndrome, renal failure
  - Thyroid-stimulating hormone for hypothyroidism
  - Human chorionic gonadotropin for pregnancy
- Atherosclerosis: cardiac stress imaging, coronary angiography, CT arteriography
- Pancreatitis: CT scan, US of pancreas

Follow-Up Tests & Special Considerations

- Repeat lipid panel after 2 months of therapy.
- High levels of apolipoprotein (APO) B (≥90 mg/dL) are a strong predictor of coronary death in patients whose LDL cannot be calculated because of very high TGs. However, evidence for routine clinical use is lacking.

Test Interpretation

- Chylomicronemia syndrome: lipid-laden macrophage (foam cell) infiltration of visceral organs, bone marrow, and skin
- Atherosclerosis
- Pancreatitis

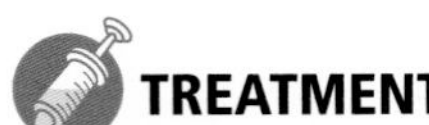

TREATMENT

GENERAL MEASURES

- Therapeutic lifestyle changes, 1st-line interventions for all patients, can reduce TGs by as much as 50% (1)[C]:
  - Dietary modifications can reduce TGs by 20–50% (see "Diet").
  - Moderate-intensity physical activity can reduce TGs by 20–30%.
  - Weight loss of 5–10% can reduce TGs by 20%.
  - Persons with very high TGs should abstain from alcohol.
- Search for correctable secondary causes; treat underlying illness, or remove offending drug.
- Improve glycemic control if diabetic.
- Control other cardiac risk factors such as hypertension, diabetes mellitus, and smoking.
- Primary hypertriglyceridemia: Screen other family members.

- According to current guidelines (2)[C], getting LDL cholesterol to goal takes priority over correction of TGs unless TGs ≥500 mg/dL (1)[C] for lowering TGs. Assessment of LDL "goal" may not be needed in patients treated with moderate- or high-dose statin.
- Usually outpatient; see "Admission Criteria."

MEDICATION

First Line

- Statins if TGs <500 mg/dL and LDL is not at goal (1)[A], although more recent guidelines emphasize decision treatment based on 10-year cardiac risk (ACC/AHA 2013 chooses 7.5% 10-year risk and other clinical factors for initiation of therapy). Although statins are not the most effective at reducing TG, they are the most effective agents in reducing cardiovascular risk; dosing will depend on intensity of statin desired in accordance with guidelines:
  - Atorvastatin (Lipitor): 10–80 mg/day
  - Pravastatin (Pravachol): 10–80 mg/day
  - Rosuvastatin (Crestor): 5–40 mg/day
  - Simvastatin (Zocor): 5–40 mg nightly
  - Adverse reactions: myalgias, myopathy, rhabdomyolysis (especially if combined with fibrates); contraindicated in pregnancy and lactation
- Fibrates if TGs ≥500 mg/dL (1)[C]: Fibrates have been shown to decrease nonfatal myocardial infarction, but not all cause mortality (3)[A]:
  - Fenofibrate (Tricor, others): 35–200 mg daily
  - Gemfibrozil (Lopid): 600 mg BID
  - Adverse reactions: GI upset, hepatotoxicity, cholelithiasis, myalgias, rhabdomyolysis (when combined with a statin), gemfibrozil–warfarin interaction (enhanced anticoagulation)
  - Gemfibrozil should be avoided in combination with statins due to high risk of muscle injury. If combination therapy is needed, use fenofibrate.

Second Line

- Niacin (20–50% reduction in TGs with immediate-release [IR] niacin, 10–30% with extended-release [ER] forms) (4)[B]. Clinical use of niacin should be very limited, as it fails to show outcome benefit in statin users:
  - 1,000–3,000 mg IR daily divided BID–TID; 500–2,000 mg ER nightly
  - Pretreatment with aspirin reduces flushing.
  - Adverse reactions: flushing, pruritus, peptic ulcer disease, hepatotoxicity, fulminant hepatic necrosis (with ER forms), hyperuricemia and gout, hyperglycemia, and toxic amblyopia
- Omega-3 fatty acids (20–50% reduction in TGs)
  - Lovaza: 4 g daily or 2 g BID
  - Epanova: 2–4 g daily (5)[C]
  - Vascepa: 2 g BID with food (6)[C]
  - Safe, well-tolerated but limited outcomes data

ISSUES FOR REFERRAL

- Hypertriglyceridemia refractory to treatment
- Familial hypertriglyceridemia syndromes

INPATIENT CONSIDERATIONS

Admission Criteria/Initial Stabilization

- Acute pancreatitis
- Acute coronary syndrome
- In medical emergencies such as acute hypertriglyceridemic pancreatitis with TG levels >1,000 mg/dL, TGs can be lowered rapidly and safely by apheresis or insulin infusion.

Discharge Criteria

Stabilization of acute complicating illness

ONGOING CARE

FOLLOW-UP RECOMMENDATIONS

2 months after initiation or modification of therapy (repeat fasting lipid profile)

Patient Monitoring

- Fasting lipid profile q6–12mo
- Maintain TGs <1,000 mg/dL to reduce risk of acute pancreatitis (possibly effective, unproven).
- Hepatic transaminases
- Creatine phosphokinase if patient has myalgias

DIET

- Restrict dietary fat to 30% of total caloric intake; restrict further to 15% of caloric intake if TGs ≥1,000 mg/dL (1)[C].
- Limit carbohydrates (especially simple carbohydrates and sugars) to 60% of total caloric intake.
- Mediterranean-style diet reduces TGs 10–15% more than a low-fat diet.
- Increase marine-derived omega-3 polyunsaturated fatty acids (4 g/day reduces TGs by 25–30%, dose-response relationship).
- Eliminate trans fatty acids.
- Increase dietary fiber.
- Avoid concentrated sugars such as fructose.
- Moderate alcohol intake (<1 oz/day or complete abstinence if TGs are very high)

PATIENT EDUCATION

Smoking cessation

PROGNOSIS

- Good with correction of TG levels
- Patients with primary hypertriglyceridemia usually require lifelong treatment.

COMPLICATIONS

- Atherosclerosis
- Chylomicronemia syndrome
- Pancreatitis

REFERENCES

1. Miller M, Stone NJ, Ballantyne C, et al. Triglycerides and cardiovascular disease: a scientific statement from the American Heart Association. *Circulation*. 2011;123(20):2292–2333.
2. Stone NJ, Robinson JG, Lichtenstein AH, et al. 2013 ACC/AHA guideline on the treatment of blood cholesterol to reduce atherosclerotic cardiovascular risk in adults: a report of the American College of Cardiology/American Heart Association Task Force on Practice Guidelines. *Circulation*. 2014;129(25)(Suppl 2):S1–S45.
3. Abourbih S, Filion KB, Joseph L, et al. Effect of fibrates on lipid profiles and cardiovascular outcomes: a systematic review. *Am J Med*. 2009;122(10):962.e1–962.e8.
4. Wi J, Kim JY, Park S, et al. Optimal pharmacologic approach to patients with hypertriglyceridemia and low high-density lipoprotein-cholesterol: randomized comparison of fenofibrate 160 mg and niacin 1500 mg. *Atherosclerosis*. 2010;213(1):235–240.
5. Kastelein JJ, Maki KC, Susekov A, et al. Omega-3 free fatty acids for the treatment of severe hypertriglyceridemia: the EpanoVa fOr Lowering Very high triglyceridEs (EVOLVE) trial. *J Clin Lipidol*. 2014;8(1):94–106.
6. Maki KC, Orloff DG, Nicholls SJ, et al. A highly bioavailable omega-3 free fatty acid formulation improves the cardiovascular risk profile in high-risk, statin-treated patients with residual hypertriglyceridemia (the ESPRIT trial). *Clin Ther*. 2013;35(9):1400–1411.e1–e3.

ADDITIONAL READING

- Berglund L, Brunzell JD, Goldberg AC, et al. Evaluation and treatment of hypertriglyceridemia: an Endocrine Society clinical practice guideline. *J Clin Endocrinol Metab*. 2012;97(9):2969–2989.
- PL Detail-Document. Strategies for lowering triglycerides. *Pharmacist's Letter/Prescriber's Letter*. June 2011.

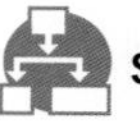

SEE ALSO

- Hypercholesterolemia; Pancreatitis, Acute
- Algorithm: Hypertriglyceridemia

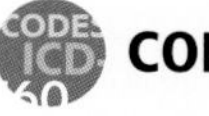

CODES

ICD10

E78.1 Pure hyperglyceridemia

CLINICAL PEARLS

- Hypertriglyceridemia is a risk factor for coronary artery disease at levels ≥200 mg/dL and for pancreatitis at levels ≥1,000 mg/dL.
- Diet and exercise are 1st-line interventions for all patients who have hypertriglyceridemia.
- In patients with TG levels <500 mg/dL, the primary treatment for cardiovascular risk management is statins.
- For patients with TG levels ≥500 mg/dL, the greatest amount of TG lowering is achieved with fibrates, although magnitude of clinical benefit is uncertain.

HYPERTROPHIC CARDIOMYOPATHY

Arka Chatterjee, MD • Nirmanmoh Bhatia, MD • Ihab Hamzeh, MD, FACC

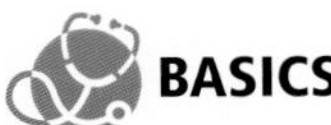

BASICS

DESCRIPTION

- Hypertrophic cardiomyopathy (HCM) is a form of primary myocardial hypertrophy, with or without presence of left ventricular outflow tract (LVOT) obstruction; it is characterized by 4 cardinal features:
  - Idiopathic LV hypertrophy (LVH) in absence of other cardiac or systemic disease causing hypertrophy of such magnitude
  - Cardiac myocyte and myofibrillar disarray
  - Familial occurrence
  - Associated sudden cardiac death
- System(s) affected: cardiovascular
- Synonym(s): hypertrophic obstructive cardiomyopathy (HOCM); muscular subaortic stenosis (MSS), idiopathic hypertrophic subaortic stenosis (IHSS)

EPIDEMIOLOGY

- The disorder may present at any age.
- It is seen in equal frequency in both sexes, although it is often underrecognized in females and African Americans.
- Apical HCM is a variant seen more often in China and Japan (Yamaguchi apical variant).

Incidence

~1% of patients with HCM die annually, but this is no different from the overall population.

Prevalence

- Prevalence of phenotypically expressed HCM in the adult general population is 1:500 (0.2%).
- ~600,000 people are affected with HCM in the United States.

ETIOLOGY AND PATHOPHYSIOLOGY

- LVH
  - ≥1 region of LV wall are thickened: classically at the basal anterior septum but may involve posterior septum or LV free wall and apex
  - Hypertrophy develops usually in adolescence, with an average 100% increase in LV mass.
- Systolic anterior motion (SAM) of the mitral valve
  - Mitral valve abnormalities are primary manifestations of HCM: 1 or both leaflets may be elongated.
  - SAM is the abrupt motion of the MV leaflet toward the septum, which creates dynamic LVOT obstruction on contact with the septum.
  - Caused by drag effect of the high-velocity jet caused by ejection through a narrowed LVOT and/or a Venturi phenomenon
- Disorganized myocardial architecture
  - Myocytes and myofilaments are laid down in disorganized pattern, with increased matrix components causing myocyte disarray.
  - Microvascular disease leads to ischemia and replacement fibrosis.
- Diastolic dysfunction
  - Result of reduced ventricular compliance; contributes predominantly to the symptoms of heart failure, such as dyspnea

Genetics

- Inherited as a mendelian autosomal dominant trait with >50% penetrance and variable expressivity
- 11 sarcomeric gene mutations are known, including, among others, β-myosin heavy chain, myosin-binding protein C, and troponin I and T.

RISK FACTORS

Risk factors for sudden cardiac death (SCD) in patients with IHSS include the following (1):

- A prior history of cardiac arrest or spontaneous sustained ventricular tachycardia (VT)
- Family history of premature SCD (especially in close relative or multiple)
- Unexplained syncope
- Extreme LVH measuring >30 mm hypotensive response to exercise: inability to increase by at least 20 mm Hg or a drop of at least 20 mm Hg
- Nonsustained VT during Holter monitoring
- Other factors that may indicate increased risk are LVOT obstruction (resting gradient >30 mm Hg), LV apical aneurysm, high-risk mutation, delayed enhancement on cardiac MRI

GENERAL PREVENTION

- Avoid strenuous exercise (particularly involving burst exertion) and heavy lifting (induces Valsalva maneuver).
- Maintain hydration to avoid volume depletion.
- Avoid alcohol.
- Certain drugs, such as nitrates, digoxin, β-agonists, vasodilators, and diuretics, are best avoided, particularly in presence of increased LVOT gradient.
- Implantable cardioverter defibrillator (ICD) is recommended for patients at high risk for sudden cardiac death (1,2)[C].

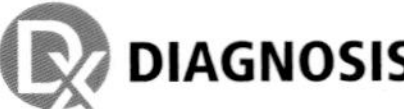

DIAGNOSIS

HISTORY

- Symptoms of heart failure: dyspnea, paroxysmal nocturnal dyspnea, fatigue
- Angina pectoris
- Palpitations
- Exertional syncope or presyncope
- Symptoms may be worsened by anemia, hot and humid weather, a large meal, alcohol, or fever.
- Clinical symptoms correlate poorly with the severity of LVOT obstruction.
- 50% of these patients have positive family history for HCM (and 50% are sporadic).

PHYSICAL EXAM

- A systolic crescendo/decrescendo murmur from LVOT obstruction is best heard at left lower sternal border.
- Intensity of murmur is dynamic and changes with maneuvers that affect the degree of obstruction.
- Maneuvers that decrease venous return (e.g., Valsalva, standing position, amyl nitrite) increase intensity of the murmur.
- Maneuvers that increase LV afterload (e.g., handgrip) will soften the murmur.
- Bisferiens pulse
- Double or triple apical impulse
- Prominent S_4
- Holosystolic murmur of mitral regurgitation may be heard at the apex.

DIFFERENTIAL DIAGNOSIS

- Valvular aortic stenosis
- Hypertensive heart disease, especially in elderly
- Athlete's heart: differentiated by normal/enlarged LV cavity, regression of LVH on deconditioning
- Cardiac amyloidosis
- Noonan syndrome, mitochondrial myopathy, and metabolic storage disorders (e.g., Anderson Fabry disease and Friedrich ataxia)

DIAGNOSTIC TESTS & INTERPRETATION

- ECG: common findings (50–90%):
  - Nonspecific ST-T wave abnormalities
  - LVH: Pediatric-specific criterion of RaVL+SV2 >23 mm may have superiority for screening (3).
- ECG: less common findings (<50%):
  - Prominent and abnormal Q waves in anterior precordial and lateral limbs lead
  - Left atrial enlargement
  - Diffuse, marked, symmetric giant negative T waves in lateral precordial leads seen in patients with apical HCM
- Holter monitoring is recommended (2) and findings may include supraventricular tachycardia (SVT), premature ventricular contractions (PVCs), nonsustained ventricular tachycardia (VT), and atrial fibrillation
- Chest x-ray may show cardiomegaly and left atrial enlargement.
- Echocardiogram helps establish the diagnosis most easily and reliably. Typical echo findings:
  - Asymmetric septal hypertrophy with septal-to-free-wall ratio >1.3:1 classically
  - LVH (especially LV wall thickness in diastole >15 mm)
  - Small LV chamber
  - In patients with apical IHSS, LV cavity looks like a spade.
  - Abnormal systolic anterior motion of mitral valve leaflet
  - Continuous-wave Doppler best measures significant dynamic outflow obstruction.
  - Evidence of diastolic dysfunction
  - Provocative measures, such as inhalation of amyl nitrate/Valsalva/dobutamine/exercise, may be necessary to elicit significant LVOT gradients during echocardiography.
- Stress testing may be used to assess BP response with exercise (2).
- Cardiac MRI is useful if echo images are suboptimal or LV segmental hypertrophy is seen in an unusual location; delayed gadolinium enhancement is increasingly being considered an independent risk factor for mortality (2,4); mitral valve morphology can be better defined and may have a novel role in assessment.

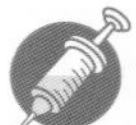

TREATMENT

- These patients must be counseled against competitive athletics, irrespective of LVOT obstruction, presence of ICD, previous septal reduction therapy, and associated symptoms (2).
- Adequate hydration should be maintained.
- Not a high-risk condition for endocarditis prophylaxis
- Genetic counseling may be appropriate.
- Only symptomatic patients will benefit from drug therapy.

MEDICATION

First Line

- β-Blockers
  - First-line drugs for patients with provocable gradient
  - Indicated for treatment of symptoms (angina/dyspnea) in adults with HCM (obstructive or nonobstructive) (2)
  - 1/3–2/3 of patients experience symptomatic improvement.
- Disopyramide
  - Used as an adjunct with β-blockers or calcium channel blockers only, as it may accelerate atrioventricular (AV) conduction (2,5)[B]
- Verapamil
  - Treatment of those who do not tolerate/respond to β-blockers
  - Caution in patients with high gradients/advanced heart failure, given the systemic vasodilatory effects (2).
- Dihydropyridine calcium channel blockers are potentially harmful in HCM patients with resting or provocable obstruction (2)[C].

Second Line

- Atrial fibrillation is common and should be controlled.
- Maintenance of sinus rhythm should be aggressively pursued because of association of atrial fibrillation with heart failure symptoms and embolic phenomena (6)[C].
- Amiodarone is most effective for sinus rhythm maintenance in IHSS-associated atrial fibrillation; disopyramide with concomitant β-blockers or verapamil is an alternative option.

ADDITIONAL THERAPIES

Pregnant patients with HCM:

- Patients who wish to become pregnant should be counseled prenatally regarding its autosomal dominant inheritance.
- In women with HCM who are asymptomatic or whose symptoms are controlled on β-blockers (2)[C]:
  - Pregnancy is reasonable.
  - β-Blockers should be continued, but increased fetal surveillance is warranted for bradycardia or related complications.
  - Expert maternal/fetal medical specialist care, including cardiovascular and prenatal monitoring, is recommended.
- Women with gradient >50 mm Hg or with uncontrolled symptoms have increased risk with pregnancy and referral to high-risk obstetrician is indicated.
- Pregnancy with HCM and advanced heart failure is associated with excess morbidity/mortality.
- Should be monitored closely in a tertiary care center during labor, as peripheral vasodilatation, fluid shift, and epidural analgesia pose a theoretical risk in presence of LVOT obstruction
- Spinal analgesia is contraindicated. Careful administration of epidural analgesia is controversial.

SURGERY/OTHER PROCEDURES

- Ventricular septal myotomy-myectomy (Morrow procedure)
  - The gold standard for drug-refractory symptomatic patients with obstructive IHSS (2)[B] and for relief of obstruction with outflow gradient >50 mm Hg at rest/with provocation
  - 5–10 g of tissue is removed from the proximal septum.
  - Most (about 70%) patients achieve subjective improvement in symptoms lasting ≥5 years following their surgery.
  - Postoperative complications may include left bundle branch block (LBBB), ventricular septal defect (VSD), and aortic regurgitation.
- Percutaneous alcohol septal ablation
  - Controlled alcohol-induced septal myocardial infarction resulting in an akinetic septal segment with instantaneous obliteration of the outflow obstruction and gradient
  - Preferred in patients at high risk from septal myectomy, those who refuse surgical therapy, and those who have failed surgical myectomy
  - Better outcomes reported in patients >65 years, septal diameter <18 mm, and gradient <100 mm Hg (7)
- Implantable cardiac defibrillators for prevention of SCD in patient at high risk (2)[C]
- Ablation of refractory ventricular arrhythmia can be considered; combined endocardial and epicardial approach may be required (8).
- Heart transplant is advocated for HCM patients not amenable to other treatment modalities (2)[B] and children with refractory symptoms due to restrictive physiology not responding to conventional treatment (2)[C].

ONGOING CARE

FOLLOW-UP RECOMMENDATIONS

- Annual follow-up is recommended for stable patients.
- Among the 1st-degree relatives, screening with ECG and echo is recommended q12–18mo between ages 12 and 21 years and every 5 years in adults, particularly if adverse HCM-related events have occurred in the family.
- Genetic testing can be used for index patient and to help screen 1st-degree relatives (2)[B].

PATIENT EDUCATION

Patients with characteristic phenotype of HCM (LVH) are excluded from all competitive sports except those with low static and dynamic intensity (e.g., golf) (2)[C].

PROGNOSIS

Annual mortality of 1% is no different from the general U.S. population. Although HCM may be associated with important symptoms and premature SCD, most of these patients have no or relatively mild disability and normal life expectancy.

COMPLICATIONS

- Sudden death (1% per year), usually due to ventricular arrhythmia
- Atrial fibrillation
- Infective mitral endocarditis
- Progressive heart failure

REFERENCES

1. Maron BJ. Contemporary insights and strategies for risk stratification and prevention of sudden death in hypertrophic cardiomyopathy. *Circulation*. 2010;121(3):445–456.
2. Gersh BJ, Maron BJ, Bonow RO, et al. 2011 ACCF/AHA guideline for the diagnosis and treatment of hypertrophic cardiomyopathy: executive summary: a report of the American College of Cardiology Foundation/American Heart Association Task Force on Practice Guidelines. *Circulation*. 2011;124(24):2761–2796.
3. Brothers MB, Oster ME, Ehrlich A, et al. Novel electrocardiographic screening criterion for hypertrophic cardiomyopathy in children. *Am J Cardiol*. 2014;113(7):1246–1249.
4. Green JJ, Berger JS, Kramer CM, et al. Prognostic value of late gadolinium enhancement in clinical outcomes for hypertrophic cardiomyopathy. *JACC Cardiovasc Imaging*. 2012;5(4):370–377.
5. Sherrid MV, Barac I, McKenna WJ, et al. Multicenter study of the efficacy and safety of disopyramide in obstructive hypertrophic cardiomyopathy. *J Am Coll Cardiol*. 2005;45(8):1251–1258.
6. Maron BJ, Olivotto I, Bellone P, et al. Clinical profile of stroke in 900 patients with hypertrophic cardiomyopathy. *J Am Coll Cardiol*. 2002;39(2):301–307.
7. Sorajja P, Binder J, Nishimura RA, et al. Predictors of an optimal clinical outcome with alcohol septal ablation for obstructive hypertrophic cardiomyopathy. *Catheter Cardiovasc Interv*. 2013;81(1):E58–E67.
8. Dukkipati SR, d'Avila A, Soejima K, et al. Long-term outcomes of combined epicardial and endocardial ablation of monomorphic ventricular tachycardia related to hypertrophic cardiomyopathy. *Circ Arrhythm Electrophysiol*. 2011;4(2):185–194.

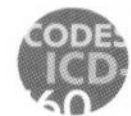

CODES

ICD10

- I42.2 Other hypertrophic cardiomyopathy
- I42.1 Obstructive hypertrophic cardiomyopathy

CLINICAL PEARLS

- HCM should be considered in all patients with a history of unexplained SCD. It is the most common cause of SCD in young athletes in the United States.
- Delayed de novo onset of LVH may occur in midlife.
- Intense competitive sports, strenuous exercise, and heavy lifting should be restricted because of high risk of SCD.

HYPOGLYCEMIA, DIABETIC

Joseph A. Florence, MD • Emily K. Flores, PharmD, BCPS

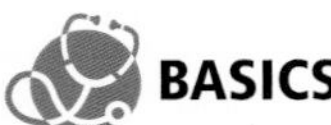

BASICS

DESCRIPTION

- Abnormally low concentration of glucose in circulating blood of a patient with diabetes mellitus (DM); often referred to as an *insulin reaction*
- Classification includes the following (1)[A]:
  - Severe hypoglycemia: an event requiring assistance of another person to actively administer treatment
  - Documented symptomatic hypoglycemia: an event during which typical symptoms are accompanied by a measured plasma glucose of <70 mg/dL (3.9 mmol/L)
  - Asymptomatic hypoglycemia: an event not accompanied by symptoms but a measured glucose of <70 mg/dL (3.9 mmol/L)
  - Probable symptomatic hypoglycemia: event with symptoms but glucose not tested
  - Pseudohypoglycemia: an event with typical symptoms but glucose ≥70 mg/dL (3.9 mmol/L)
- Hypoglycemia is the leading limiting factor in the glycemic management of type 1 diabetes mellitus (T1DM) and type 2 diabetes mellitus (T2DM). Severe or frequent hypoglycemia requires modification of treatment regimens, including higher treatment goals.

ALERT

Hypoglycemia unawareness

- Major risk factor for severe hypoglycemic reactions
- Most commonly found in patients with long-standing T1DM and children age <7 years

EPIDEMIOLOGY

Incidence

- From the Accord Study, the annual incidence of hypoglycemia was the following (2)[A]:
  - 3.14% in the intensive treatment group
  - 1.03% in the standard group
  - Increased risk among women, African Americans, those with less than high school education, aged participants, and those who used insulin at trial entry
- From the RECAP-DM study (3)[A]: Hypoglycemia was reported in 38% of patients with T2DM who added a sulfonylurea or thiazolidinedione to metformin therapy during the past year.

ETIOLOGY AND PATHOPHYSIOLOGY

- Loss of hormonal counterregulatory mechanism in glucose metabolism
- Diet: too little food (skipping or delaying meals), decreased carbohydrate (CHO) intake
- Medication: too much insulin or oral hypoglycemic agent (improper dose, timing, or erratic absorption)
- Exercise/physical activity: unplanned or excessive
- Alcohol consumption
- Vomiting or diarrhea

RISK FACTORS

- Nearly 3/4 of severe hypoglycemic episodes occur during sleep.
- Autonomic neuropathy
- Illness, stress, and unplanned life events
- Duration of DM >5 years, advanced age, renal/liver disease, congestive heart failure (CHF), hypothyroidism, hypoadrenalism, gastroenteritis, gastroparesis (unpredictable CHO delivery)
- Starvation or prolonged fasting
- Alcoholism: Evening consumption of alcohol is associated with an increased risk of nocturnal and fasting hypoglycemia, especially in patients with T1DM.
- Current smokers with T1DM
- Insulin secretagogues: Sulfonylureas (glyburide, glimepiride, glipizide, etc.) and glinide derivatives (repaglinide, nateglinide) stimulate insulin secretion and can cause hypoglycemia.
- Severe hypoglycemia is associated with comorbid conditions in patients age ≥65 years and in users of a long-acting sulfonylurea.
- Hypoglycemia is rare in diabetics not treated with insulin or insulin secretagogues.
- Intensive insulin therapy (further lowering A1C from 7% to 6%) is associated with higher rate of hypoglycemia.

Geriatric Considerations

Oral hypoglycemics with long duration and high potency have greater hypoglycemic risks. American Geriatric Society Beers criteria recommend avoiding glyburide and chlorpropamide due to their prolonged half-life in older adults and risk for prolonged hypoglycemic episodes. Medications should be dosed for age and renal function.

Pediatric Considerations

Children may not realize when they have hypoglycemia, needing increased supervision during times of higher activity. Children may have higher glycemic goals for this reason. Caregivers should be instructed in use of glucagon (1)[A].

Pregnancy Considerations

Hypoglycemia management and avoidance education should be reemphasized and blood glucose monitoring increased due to more stringent glycemic goals and increased risk in early pregnancy.

GENERAL PREVENTION

- Maintain routine schedule of diet (consistent CHO intake), medication, and exercise.
- Regular self-monitoring of blood glucose (SMBG), if taking insulin or secretagogue
  - ≥3× daily testing if multiple injections of insulin, insulin pump therapy, or pregnant diabetic; frequency and timing dictated by needs and treatment goals
  - Particularly helpful for asymptomatic hypoglycemia
- Diabetes treatment and teaching programs (DTTPs) especially for high-risk type 1 patients, which teach flexible insulin therapy to enable dietary freedom
- Hypoglycemia may be prevented with use of insulin analogs, continuous SC insulin infusion (CSII) pumps, and continuous glucose monitoring (CGM) systems.
- If preexercise glucose is <100 mg/dL and taking insulin or secretagogue, then CHO consumption or reduction in medication may prevent hypoglycemia.

COMMONLY ASSOCIATED CONDITIONS

- Autonomic dysfunction
- Neuropathies
- Cardiomyopathies
- Older type 2 diabetics with severe hypoglycemia have a higher risk of dementia.

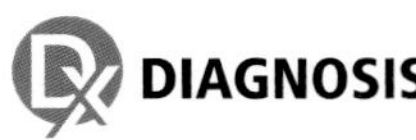

DIAGNOSIS

HISTORY

- Discuss frequency and cause of any severe hypoglycemia episode(s) (4)[A].
- Symptoms vary considerably between individuals.
- Adrenergic symptoms
  - Hunger, trembling, pallor, sweating, shaking, pounding heart, anxiety
- Neurologic symptoms
  - Dizziness, poor concentration, drowsiness, weakness, confusion, lightheadedness, slurred speech, blurred vision, double vision, unsteadiness, poor coordination
- Behavioral symptoms
  - Tearfulness, confusion, fatigue, irritability, aggressiveness
- If altered cognition, consider hypoglycemia

PHYSICAL EXAM

- General: confusion, lethargy
- HEENT: diplopia
- Coronary: tachycardia
- Neurologic: tremulousness, weakness, paresthesias, stupor, seizure, or coma
- Mental status: irritability, inability to concentrate, or short-term memory loss
- Skin: pale, diaphoresis
- End-organ damage: microvascular, macrovascular, ophthalmologic, neurologic, renal

DIFFERENTIAL DIAGNOSIS

- Hypoglycemia may be seen in chronic alcoholics and binge drinkers.
- GI dysfunction causing postprandial hypoglycemia or alimentary reactive hypoglycemia
- Hormonal deficiency states (hormonal reactive hypoglycemia)
- Hypoglycemia of sepsis
- Islet cell tumors
- Factitious hypoglycemia from surreptitious injection of insulin

DIAGNOSTIC TESTS & INTERPRETATION

- Plasma, serum, or whole-blood glucose <70 mg/dL
- SMBG and CGM are especially useful for asymptomatic hypoglycemia (1)[A].
- A hypoglycemic reading from a CGM sensor should be verified by SMBG fingerstick glucose testing prior to treatment (4)[A].
- Suspect hypoglycemic unawareness in T1DM with low/normal HgbA1c (1)[A].
- Chronic hypoglycemia is indicated by low HgbA1c level.
- Disorders that may alter lab results
  - Conditions that affect erythrocyte turnover, such as hemolysis or blood loss, and hemoglobin variants may alter HbgA1c (4)[A].

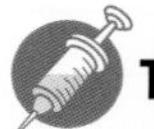

TREATMENT

GENERAL MEASURES

- Glucose: preferred; any form of CHO that contains glucose should be effective (4)[A].
  - Any sugar-containing food or beverage that can be rapidly absorbed: juice or nondiet soda (4–5 oz), candy (5–6 pieces of hard candy), or OTC glucose tablets (4 tablets = 16 g CHO)
- Glucagon should be prescribed to patients at significant risk of severe hypoglycemia. People in close contact with these individuals should be instructed in using an emergency glucagon kit (4)[A].
- α-Glucosidase inhibitors (acarbose, precise) prevent digestion of complex CHOs; therefore, hypoglycemia must be treated with monosaccharides, such as glucose tablets.
- Patients with severe hypoglycemia combined with hypoglycemic unawareness should have glycemic targets raised to avoid hypoglycemia (4)[A].
- Most people with T1DM should use insulin analogs to reduce hypoglycemia risk (4)[A].
- CGM can supplement SMBG in those with hypoglycemia unawareness and/or frequent hypoglycemic episodes (4)[A].
- CGM augmented CSII with automated insulin suspension reduces the combined rate of severe and moderate hypoglycemia in T1DM (4,5)[A].

MEDICATION

- Conscious patients (4)[A]:
  - Glucose (15–20 g) is preferred, although any form of CHO may be used.
    - Takes ~15 minutes for CHOs to be digested and enter bloodstream as glucose
    - Blood glucose value may correct prior to symptoms resolving.
    - "Rul T4-to-T3 e of 15": 15–20 g CHO (~60–80 calories simple CHO) repeated q15min until blood sugar is ≥70 mg/dL
  - Once sugar has normalized, a meal or snack should be consumed to prevent recurrence of hypoglycemia
- Loss of consciousness at home (6)[A]:
  - Administer glucagon.
  - IM or SC in the deltoid or anterior thigh
    - Age <6 years and/or weight <20–25 kg: 0.50 mg
    - Age ≥6 years and/or weight >20–25 kg: 1 mg
    - May repeat dose in 15 minutes if needed
- In unconscious, if emergency medical personnel are present or patient hospitalized (6)[A]:
  - Give 25 grams IV 50% dextrose every 5–10 minutes until patient awakens.
  - Then, feed orally and/or administer 5% dextrose IV at level that will maintain blood glucose >100 mg/dL.
  - Patients with hypoglycemia secondary to oral hypoglycemics should be monitored for 24–48 hours because hypoglycemia may recur after apparent clinical recovery.
- Significant possible interactions:
  - Overtreatment may cause hyperglycemia.
  - Clearance of certain oral hypoglycemics may be prolonged in persons with renal or liver disease.

ISSUES FOR REFERRAL

- Frequent or recurring episodes that do not readily respond to treatment
- Consultant pharmacists in long-term care facilities

INPATIENT CONSIDERATIONS

Admission Criteria/Initial Stabilization

- Any doubt of cause
- Expectation of prolonged hypoglycemia (e.g., caused by sulfonylurea drug)
- Inability to drink
- Treatment has not resulted in prompt sensory recovery.
- Seizures, coma, or altered behavior (e.g., ataxia, disorientation, unstable motor coordination, dysphasia) secondary to documented or suspected hypoglycemia

Discharge Criteria

Normoglycemia and risk of severe hypoglycemia is negligible.

ONGOING CARE

FOLLOW-UP RECOMMENDATIONS

Rest until glucose is normal.

Patient Monitoring

Self-monitoring of blood glucose (SMBG)

DIET

- If alcohol consumed, combine with food to reduce risk of hypoglycemia.
- Protein does not slow absorption of CHOs.
- Fats may slow absorption of CHOs and may retard and then prolong the acute glycemic response (6)[A].

PATIENT EDUCATION

- Always have access to quick-acting CHO.
- For planned exercise, consider a reduced insulin dose; additional CHOs are needed for unplanned exercise.
- Educate patients and their relatives, close friends, teachers, and supervisors to be aware of DM diagnosis and signs/symptoms of hypoglycemia and treatment.
- Teach SMBG and self-adjustment for insulin therapy, diet control, and exercise regimen.
- Wear medical alert identification bracelet or necklace.
- The annual Diabetes Forecast Consumer Guide has a description and list of commercially available products for treating lows: http://www.diabetesforecast.org/2014/Jan/glucose-products-2014.html

PROGNOSIS

Full recovery usually depends on rapidity of diagnosis and treatment.

COMPLICATIONS

- Coma, seizure, myocardial infarction, stroke (especially in elderly)
- Prolonged or severe hypoglycemia may cause permanent neurologic damage and/or cognitive impairment.
- Children with T1DM have a greater vulnerability to neurologic manifestations of hypoglycemia.

ALERT

The ACCORD trial (adults withT2DM) demonstrated that intensively lowering blood glucose below current recommendations increased the risk of death versus standard treatment strategy (2)[A].

REFERENCES

1. Seaquist ER, Anderson J, Childs B, et al. Hypoglycemia and diabetes: a report of a workgroup of the American Diabetes Association and The Endocrine Society. *J Clin Endocrinol Metab*. 2013;98(5):1845–1859.
2. Action to Control Cardiovascular Risk in Diabetes Study Group, Gerstein HC, Miller ME, et al. Effects of intensive glucose lowering in type 2 diabetes. *N Engl J Med*. 2008;358(24):2545–2559.
3. Alvarez Guisasola F, Tofé Povedano S, Krishnarajah G, et al. Hypoglycaemic symptoms, treatment satisfaction, adherence and their associations with glycaemic goal in patients with type 2 diabetes mellitus: findings from the Real-Life Effectiveness and Care Patterns of Diabetes Management (RECAP-DM) Study. *Diabetes Obes Metab*. 2008;10(Suppl 1):25–32.
4. American Diabetes Association. Standards of medical care in diabetes–2014. *Diabetes Care*. 2014;37(Suppl 1):S14–S79.
5. Bergenstal RM, Klonoff DC, Garg SK, et al. Threshold-based insulin-pump interruption for reduction of hypoglycemia. *N Engl J Med*. 2013;369(3):224–232.
6. Cryer PE, Axelrod L, Grossmann AB, et al. Evaluation and management of adult hypoglycemic disorders: an Endocrine Society Clinical Practice Guideline. *J Clini Endocrinol Metab*. 2009;94(3):709–728.

ADDITIONAL READING

- Franz MJ, Powers MA, Leontos C, et al. The evidence for medical nutrition therapy for type 1 and type 2 diabetes in adults. *J Am Diet Assoc*. 2010;110(12):1852–1889.
- Whitmer RA, Karter AJ, Yaffe K, et al. Hypoglycemic episodes and risk of dementia in older patients with type 2 diabetes mellitus. *JAMA*. 2009;301(15):1565–1572.

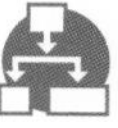

SEE ALSO

- Diabetes Mellitus, Type 1
- Algorithm: Hypoglycemia

CODES

ICD10

- E11.649 Type 2 diabetes mellitus with hypoglycemia without coma
- E10.649 Type 1 diabetes mellitus with hypoglycemia without coma
- E13.649 Oth diabetes mellitus with hypoglycemia without coma

CLINICAL PEARLS

- Hypoglycemia unawareness, which is most common with tightly controlled, long-standing T1DM and children age <7 years, should be recognized and addressed by less aggressive glycemic goals for a period of time and hypoglycemia management.
- Any form of CHO that contains glucose should be effective, such as sugar-containing food or beverage that can be rapidly absorbed:
  - 4–5 oz juice or nondiet soda; 5–6 pieces of hard candy; OTC glucose tablets, liquids, gels, or bits
  - Using the "rule of 15" is an easy way to teach patients to manage hypoglycemia at home.
- Patients with diabetes that use insulin, secretagogues, and/or alcohol are at higher risk for hypoglycemia and should be educated on how to recognize and manage hypoglycemia.
- Newly approved CSII systems with CGM-augmented insulin suspension reduce hypoglycemic events.

HYPOGLYCEMIA, NONDIABETIC

Matthew A. Silva, PharmD, RPh, BCPS • Pablo I. Hernandez Itriago, MD, MS, FAAFP

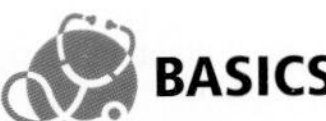

BASICS

DESCRIPTION

- Hypoglycemia defined by the Whipple triad
  - Low plasma glucose level (≤60 mg/dL) with hypoglycemic symptoms that are relieved when glucose is corrected
  - Occurs commonly in patients with diabetes receiving sulfonylurea or insulins; less commonly in patients without diabetes
- Reactive hypoglycemia occurs in response to a meal, drugs, herbal substances, or nutrients and may occur 2–3 hours postprandially or later (1).
  - Symptoms are generally observed with serum glucose ≤60 mg/dL, lower in patients with hypoglycemic unawareness.
  - Also seen after GI surgery (in association with dumping syndrome in some patients)
- Spontaneous (fasting) hypoglycemia may be associated with primary conditions including hypopituitarism, Addison disease, myxedema, or disorders related to hepatic dysfunction or renal failure (1,2).
  - If hypoglycemia presents as a primary disorder, consider hyperinsulinism and extrapancreatic tumors.

EPIDEMIOLOGY

Incidence

- True incidence is unknown.
- 0.5–8.6% of hospitalized patients ≥65 years (3,4,5)
  - Asymptomatic in 25% of cases

Prevalence

True prevalence is unknown:

- Predominant age: older adult
- Predominant sex: female > male

ETIOLOGY AND PATHOPHYSIOLOGY

- Reactive, postprandial
  - Alimentary hyperinsulinism
  - Meals high in refined carbohydrate
  - Certain nutrients, including fructose, galactose, leucine
  - Glucose intolerance (prediabetes)
  - GI surgery
  - Idiopathic (unknown cause)
- Spontaneous
  - Fasting
  - Alcohol or prescription medication–associated (6) (insulin, sulfonylureas, thiazolidinediones, incretin-mimetics, DPP-IV inhibitors, β-blockers, salicylates, quinine, hydroxychloroquine, fluoroquinones, doxycycline, sertraline, disopyramide, pentamidine)
  - Nonprescription over-the-counter (OTC) agents, including performance-enhancing agents. Adulterated versions of phosphodiesterase inhibitors and performance-enhancing agents are routinely imported and may contain sulfonylureas and other hypoglycemic agents.
  - Consider medication errors as a source of unexplained hypoglycemia even in patients without diabetes.
  - Surreptitious drug use (self-injection of insulin or ingestion of oral hypoglycemic medications in patients with diabetes)
  - Natural medicines or herbs (bitter melon, caffeine, cassia cinnamon, chromium, fenugreek, ginseng, guarana, mate, Stevia, vanadium)
  - Postsurgical (e.g., gastrectomy, Roux-en-Y) hypoglycemia/dumping syndrome
  - Islet cell hyperplasia or tumor (insulinoma)
  - Extrapancreatic insulin–secreting tumor
  - Hepatic disease
  - Glucagon deficiency
  - Adrenal insufficiency
  - Catecholamine deficiency
  - Hypopituitarism
  - Hypothyroidism
  - Eating disorders
  - Exercise
  - Fever
  - Pregnancy
  - Renal glycosuria
  - Large tumors
  - Ketotic hypoglycemia of childhood
  - Enzyme deficiencies or defects
  - Severe malnutrition
  - Sepsis
  - Total parenteral nutrition therapy
  - Hemodialysis

Genetics

Some aspects may involve genetics (e.g., hereditary fructose intolerance).

RISK FACTORS

Refer to "Etiology and Pathophysiology."

GENERAL PREVENTION

- Follow dietary and exercise guidelines.
- Patient recognition of early symptoms and knowledge of corrective action

Pediatric Considerations

- Usually divided into 2 syndromes
  - Transient neonatal hypoglycemia
  - Hypoglycemia of infancy and childhood
- Screening infants for hypoglycemia is appropriate when pregnancy was complicated by maternal diabetes.
- Cases of hypoglycemia observed in children taking propranolol for infantile hemangioma
- Associated with indomethacin when treating patent ductus arteriosus

Geriatric Considerations

- More likely to have underlying disorders or be caused by medications
- Iatrogenic hypoglycemia is common in the hospitalized elderly with renal insufficiency.

COMMONLY ASSOCIATED CONDITIONS

- Severe liver disease; alcoholism
- Addison disease; adrenocortical insufficiency
- Myxedema
- Malnutrition (patients with renal failure)
- GI surgery
- Panhypopituitarism
- Insulinoma

DIAGNOSIS

HISTORY

- CNS (neuroglycopenic) symptoms predominate with gradual glucose reduction:
  - Headache
  - Confusion
  - Light-headedness
  - Fatigue and weakness
  - Visual disturbances
  - Changes in personality
- Adrenergic symptoms: more prominent in acute drop in glucose
  - Anxiety
  - Tremulousness
  - Dizziness
  - Diaphoresis
  - Warmth/flushing
  - Heart palpitations
- GI symptoms
  - Hunger
  - Nausea
  - Belching

PHYSICAL EXAM

- CNS (neuroglycopenic) symptoms predominate with gradual glucose reduction:
  - Convulsions
  - Coma
  - Hypotension
- Adrenergic symptoms: more prominent in acute drop in glucose
  - Tremulousness
  - Diaphoresis
  - Warmth/flushing
  - Heart palpitations

DIFFERENTIAL DIAGNOSIS

CNS disorders

- Psychogenic
- Pseudohypoglycemia: Symptoms of hypoglycemia or self-diagnosis in patients in whom low blood glucose may not be detectable and who may be impossible to convince that they do not suffer from hypoglycemia after all tests are found to be normal.

DIAGNOSTIC TESTS & INTERPRETATION

Initial Tests (lab, imaging)

- Blood glucose ≤45 mg/dL (≤2.5 mmol/L) when symptomatic followed by symptom resolution with feeding (2)[C]
- Plasma glucose overnight fasting: ≤60 mg/dL (≤3.33 mmol/L); confirm on ≥2 occasions (2)[C].
- Plasma glucose 72-hour fasting: ≤45 mg/dL (≤2.5 mmol/L) for females; ≤55 mg/dL (≤3.05 mmol/L) for males; fast may be ended when Whipple triad is achieved or hypoglycemia is demonstrated (2)[C].
- Abdominal CT to rule out abdominal tumor

Follow-Up Tests & Special Considerations

- Misinterpretation of glucose tolerance tests may lead to misdiagnosis of hypoglycemia; ≥1/3 of normal patients have hypoglycemia, with or without symptoms, during the 4-hour glucose tolerance test. These patients may be at future risk for type 2 diabetes.
- C-peptide measurement (2)[C]
- Check liver studies, serum insulin, adrenocorticotrophic hormone (ACTH), and cortisol. Serum insulin should be suppressed when glucose is <60 mg/dL.
- Serum β-hydroxybutyrate (2)[C]
- Insulin radioimmunoassay: Elevated insulin levels suggest islet cell hyperplasia or tumor.
- Drugs that may alter lab results: Many drugs can affect glucose levels; refer to drug or laboratory reference.

Diagnostic Procedures/Other

- For definitive diagnosis, patient should have
  - Documented low glucose levels
  - Symptoms when glucose levels are low
  - Evidence that symptoms are relieved specifically by ingestion of sugar or other food
  - Identification of the specific type of hypoglycemia
- Serum β-hydroxybutyrate <2.7 mg/dL in the presence of high serum insulin, C-peptide, and low serum glucose suggests excessive insulin production (2)[C].

TREATMENT

GENERAL MEASURES

- Outpatient except for severe cases; may also be inpatient for testing
- Oral carbohydrate for alert patient without drug overdose (2–3 tbsp of sugar in glass of water or fruit juice, 1–2 cups of milk, piece of fruit, or several soda crackers)
- If unable to swallow: Use glucagon IM or SC.
- If caused by medication or nutrients: Avoid or control causative agents.
- If triggered by meals: Try high-protein diet with carbohydrate restriction.
- Nonhypoglycemic hypoglycemia or pseudohypoglycemia
  - Many patients (often women aged 20–45 years) present with diagnosis of reactive hypoglycemia (self-diagnosed or misinterpretation of tests).
  - Symptoms may pertain to chronic fatigue and somatic complaints (stress often plays a role in these symptoms).
  - Management difficult; listening is important. Try 120-g carbohydrate diet.
  - Counseling may be useful for stress and other problems.

MEDICATION

- Once diagnosis is established, begin therapy appropriate for underlying disorder.
- If unable to swallow: glucagon 1 mg (1 unit) IM or SC. If no response, give IV bolus of 25–50 g of 50% glucose solution followed by continuous infusion until patient able to take by mouth.
- Postsurgical gastrectomy patients unresponsive to dietary changes may benefit from propantheline, psyllium, fiber, or oat bran, which delays gastric emptying.
- Insulinoma

SURGERY/OTHER PROCEDURES

If islet cell tumor (insulinoma) or other insulin-secreting tumor, surgery is treatment of choice; if inoperable, diazoxide may relieve symptoms (1)[C].

INPATIENT CONSIDERATIONS

Admission Criteria/Initial Stabilization

Hypoglycemia unresponsive to oral intake

ONGOING CARE

FOLLOW-UP RECOMMENDATIONS

- Exercise routine or daily activity may need to be reevaluated.
- Patients with recurrent hypoglycemia should have glucose source at hand for immediate ingestion during symptoms.

Patient Monitoring

- Depends on type and severity of symptoms and treatment of underlying cause
- Hypoglycemia from sulfonylureas can last for hours to days depending on half-life and renal function.

DIET

- High protein, high fiber, complex carbohydrates from multigrain and whole foods in moderation
- Frequent small feedings (6 daily)
- Avoid fasting.

PATIENT EDUCATION

- Dietary instruction
- Counseling for stress, if appropriate
- Recognition of early symptoms of hypoglycemia and how to take corrective action

PROGNOSIS

Favorable, with appropriate treatment

COMPLICATIONS

- Insulinoma: If tumor identified and removed, some surgical risk is involved.
- Organic brain syndrome: may occur with extensive, prolonged hypoglycemia

REFERENCES

1. Guettier JM, Gorden P. Hypoglycemia. *Endocrinol Metab Clin North Am*. 2006;35(4):753–766.
2. Service FJ. Hypoglycemic disorders. *N Engl J Med*. 1995;332(17):1144–1152.
3. Kagansky N, Levy S, Rimon E, et al. Hypoglycemia as a predictor of mortality in hospitalized elderly patients. *Arch Intern Med*. 2003;163(15):1825–1829.
4. Mannucci E, Monami M, Mannucci M, et al. Incidence and prognostic significance of hypoglycemia in hospitalized non-diabetic elderly patients. *Aging Clin Exp Res*. 2006;18(5):446–451.
5. Nirantharakumar K, Marshall T, Hodson J, et al. Hypoglycemia in non-diabetic in-patients: clinical or criminal? *PLoS One*. 2012;7(7):e40384.
6. Ben Salem C, Fathallah N, Hmouda H, et al. Drug-induced hypoglycaemia: an update. *Drug Saf*. 2011;34(1):21–45.

ADDITIONAL READING

- Bharmal SV, Moyes V, Ahmed S, et al. Hypoglycaemia: possible mediation by chromium salt medication. *Hormones (Athens)*. 2010;9(2):181–183.
- Cansu DU, Korkmaz C. Hypoglycaemia induced by hydroxychloroquine in a non-diabetic patient treated for RA. *Rheumatology (Oxford)*. 2008;47(3):378–379.
- Carroll MF, Burge MR, Schade DS. Severe hypoglycemia in adults. *Rev Endocr Metab Disord*. 2003;4(2):149–157.
- Chan TY. Outbreaks of severe hypoglycaemia due to illegal sexual enhancement products containing undeclared glibenclamide. *Pharmacoepidemiol Drug Saf*. 2009;18(12):1250–1251.
- Chaubey SK, Sangla KS, Suthaharan EN, et al. Severe hypoglycaemia associated with ingesting counterfeit medication. *Med J Aust*. 2010;192(12):716–717.
- Lawrence KR, Adra M, Keir C. Hypoglycemia-induced anoxic brain injury possibly associated with levofloxacin. *J Infect*. 2006;52(6):e177–e180.
- Murad MH, Coto-Yglesias F, Wang AT, et al. Clinical review: drug-induced hypoglycemia: a systematic review. *J Clin Endocrinol Metab*. 2009;94(3):741–745.
- Pollak PT, Mukherjee SD, Fraser AD. Sertraline-induced hypoglycemia. *Ann Pharmacother*. 2001;35(11):1371–1374.
- Singh M, Jacob JJ, Kapoor R, et al. Fatal hypoglycemia with levofloxacin use in an elderly patient in the post-operative period. *Langenbecks Arch Surg*. 2008;393(2):235–238.
- Yamada C, Nagashima K, Takahashi A, et al. Gatifloxacin acutely stimulates insulin secretion and chronically suppresses insulin biosynthesis. *Eur J Pharmacol*. 2006;553(1–3):67–72.

SEE ALSO

- Hypoglycemia, Diabetic; Insulinoma
- Algorithm: Hypoglycemia

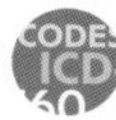

CODES

ICD10

- E16.2 Hypoglycemia, unspecified
- E16.1 Other hypoglycemia
- P70.4 Other neonatal hypoglycemia

CLINICAL PEARLS

- Symptoms coincide with low blood glucose levels and resolve with PO/IV glucose or glucagon.
- Avoid known agents/nutrients that trigger hypoglycemia.
- Treat underlying cause.

HYPOKALEMIA

Ruben Peralta, MD, FACS

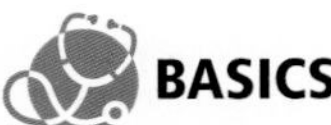

BASICS

DESCRIPTION

Hypokalemia is defined as a serum potassium concentration <3.5 mEq/L (normal range, 3.5–5 mEq/L).

- Mild hypokalemia (serum potassium 3–3.5 mEq/L)
- Moderate hypokalemia (serum potassium 2.5–3 mEq/L)
- Severe hypokalemia (serum potassium <2.5 mEq/L)

EPIDEMIOLOGY

Predominant sex: male = female

Incidence

- Electrolyte abnormality is commonly encountered in clinical practice and in the elderly (1).
- Found in >20% of hospitalized patients (when defined as potassium <3.6 mEq/L)
- Higher incidence (5–20%) in individuals with eating disorders
- >10% of inpatients with alcoholism
- Higher incidence in patients with AIDS
- Higher incidence in patients receiving diuretics
- Associated risk after bariatric surgery

ETIOLOGY AND PATHOPHYSIOLOGY

Most common causes:

- Decreased intake: deficient diet in alcoholics and elderly; anorexia nervosa
- GI loss: vomiting, diarrhea, nasogastric tubes, laxative abuse, fistulas, villous adenoma, ureterosigmoidostomy, malabsorption, chemotherapy, radiation enteropathy, bulimia
- Intracellular shift of potassium: metabolic alkalosis, insulin excess, β-adrenergic catecholamine excess (acute stress, B_2 agonists), hypokalemic periodic paralysis, intoxications (theophylline, caffeine, barium, toluene)
- Renal potassium loss:
  - Drugs: diuretics (especially loop and thiazides), amphotericin B, aminoglycosides
  - Mineralocorticoid excess states: primary hyperaldosteronism; secondary hyperaldosteronism (congestive heart failure [CHF], cirrhosis, nephrotic syndrome, malignant hypertension, renin-producing tumors); renovascular hypertension; Bartter syndrome; Gitelman syndrome; congenital adrenogenital syndromes; exogenous mineralocorticoids (glycyrrhizic acid in licorice, carbenoxolone, steroids in nasal sprays); Liddle syndrome; vasculitis
- Glucocorticoid excess states: Cushing syndrome, exogenous steroids, ectopic adrenocorticotrophic hormone (ACTH) production, II B hydroxysteroid dehydrogenase deficiency
- Renal tubular acidosis (type I and II):
  - Leukemia
  - Magnesium depletion
  - Thyrotoxic hypokalemic paralysis
- Osmotic diuresis (e.g., poorly controlled diabetes)
- Refeeding syndrome

Genetics

Some rare, familial disorders cause hypokalemia:

- Familial hypokalemic periodic paralysis: hypokalemia after a high-carbohydrate or high-sodium meal or after exercise
- Congenital adrenogenital syndromes
- Liddle syndrome: increases K+ secretion
- Familial interstitial nephritis

GENERAL PREVENTION

When initiating a diuretic, especially loop and thiazide diuretics, advice patients to increase their dietary potassium intake (see "Diet").

COMMONLY ASSOCIATED CONDITIONS

- Acute GI illnesses with severe vomiting or diarrhea
- Increased risk of cardiac arrhythmias; atrial fibrillation (2,3)
- Hypokalemia is a predictor of development of severe alcohol withdrawal syndrome (SWAS) (4).

DIAGNOSIS

- Patients with hypokalemia often have no symptoms, especially if the hypokalemia is mild (serum potassium 3–3.5 mEq/L).
- Neuromuscular (most prominent manifestations):
  - Skeletal muscle weakness (proximal > distal muscles, lower limbs > upper limbs) may range from mild weakness to total paralysis, including respiratory muscles; it may lead to rhabdomyolysis and/or respiratory arrest in severe cases.
  - Smooth muscle involvement may lead to GI hypomotility, producing ileus and constipation.
- Cardiovascular:
  - Ventricular arrhythmias; higher risk if underlying CHF, left ventricular failure (LVF), cardiac ischemia
  - Increased risk of atrial fibrillation
  - Hypotension
  - Cardiac arrest
- Renal: polyuria, polydipsia, nocturia owing to impaired ability to concentrate, myoglobinuria
- Metabolic: hyperglycemia

HISTORY

Muscle weakness, hypotension, vomiting, diarrhea, polyuria, polydypsia

PHYSICAL EXAM

Decreased skin turgor in dehydration, hypotension, orthostasis, pulmonary congestion/rales, peripheral edema in heart failure

DIFFERENTIAL DIAGNOSIS

- Spurious hypokalemia: occurs when blood with high WBC count (>100,000/mm^3) is allowed to stand at room temperature (WBCs extract potassium from plasma)
- Thyrotoxicosis

DIAGNOSTIC TESTS & INTERPRETATION

- Serum potassium <3.5 mEq/L (<3.5 mmol/L)
- Disorders that may alter lab results: leukemia and other conditions with high WBCs

Initial Tests (lab, imaging)

- If source of potassium loss not likely to be medications or GI tract: serum electrolytes, urinary potassium, ECG
- Calculate plasma anion gap normal (anion gap = Na – [Cl + HCO_3]); normal values, 12 ± 4 mEq/L. Must correct calculated anion gap for hypoalbuminemia. Increase calculated anion gap by 2.5 mEq/L for each 1 g/dL decrease in albumin <4 g/dL.
- CT scan of adrenal glands if there is evidence of mineralocorticoid excess

Follow-Up Tests & Special Considerations

- Excessive renal potassium loss: In patients with excessive renal potassium loss and hypertension, plasma renin and aldosterone levels should be determined to differentiate adrenal from nonadrenal causes of hyperaldosteronism. In these cases, urinary potassium is >20 mEq/day despite the presence of hypokalemia.
- If hypertension is absent and the patient is acidotic, renal tubular acidosis should be considered.
- If hypertension is absent and serum pH is normal to alkalotic, high urine chloride (>10 mEq/day [>10 mmol/day]) suggests hypokalemia secondary to diuretics or Bartter syndrome; low urine chloride (<10 mEq/day [<10 mmol/day]) suggests vomiting as a probable cause.
- ECG:
  - Hypokalemia increases the myocyte resting potential, which increases the refractory period; this can lead to arrhythmias.
  - Flattening or inversion of T waves
  - Increased prominence of U waves (small, positive deflection after T wave, best seen in V_2 and V_3)
  - Depression of ST segment
  - Ventricular ectopia

Test Interpretation

In severe hypokalemia, necrosis of cardiac and skeletal muscle

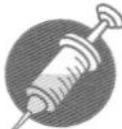

TREATMENT

GENERAL MEASURES

- Underlying cause of hypokalemia should be identified.
- For asymptomatic patients treated with oral replacement, outpatient follow-up is sufficient.
- Patients with cardiac manifestations require IV replacement with cardiac monitoring in an intensive care setting.

MEDICATION

- Nonemergent conditions (serum potassium >2.5 mEq/L [>2.5 mmol/L], no cardiac manifestations):
  - Oral therapy preferred: 40–120 mEq/day (40–120 mmol/day) in divided doses usually is adequate.
  - IV potassium should be given only when oral administration is not feasible (e.g., vomiting, postoperative state). Rate should not exceed 10 mEq/h, and concentration should not exceed 40 mEq/L. Up to 40 mEq in 100 mL over 1 hour can be given safely through a central venous line. The patient's cardiac rhythm should be closely monitored.
  - >Potassium chloride is suitable for all forms of hypokalemia.
  - Other potassium salts may be indicated if a coexisting disorder is present: potassium bicarbonate or bicarbonate precursor (gluconate, acetate, or citrate) in metabolic acidosis or phosphate in phosphate deficiency
- Emergent situations (serum potassium <2.5 mEq/L [<2.5 mmol/L], arrhythmias), IV replacement: Rate of administration should not exceed 20 mEq/hr (20 mmol/hr); maximum recommended concentration, 60 mEq/L (60 mmol/L) of saline for peripheral administration. Administration through central venous lines preferred for rates above 20 mEq/hr.
- Check serum magnesium and replace, if needed; cannot adequately replace potassium in a setting of low magnesium.
- Precautions:
  - Any form of potassium replacement carries the risk of hyperkalemia.
  - Serum potassium should be checked more frequently in groups at higher risk: the elderly, diabetic patients, and patients with renal insufficiency.
  - Patients receiving digitalis and patients with diabetic ketoacidosis in whom intracellular shift in potassium is expected after insulin therapy is initiated must have more aggressive replacement.
- Significant possible interactions: Concomitant administration of potassium-sparing diuretics (spironolactone, triamterene, amiloride, ACE inhibitors) magnifies risk of hyperkalemia.

Geriatric Considerations

May need to correct magnesium depletion

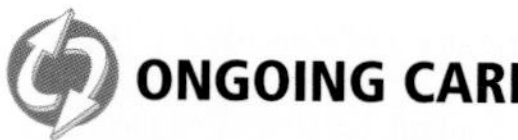

ONGOING CARE

FOLLOW-UP RECOMMENDATIONS

Patient Monitoring

- Patients receiving IV therapy should have cardiac monitoring and serum potassium level checked frequently (q4–6h).
- Patients requiring potassium supplements should have serum potassium studied at intervals and magnesium level dictated by clinical judgment and patient compliance (5)[C].

DIET

In patients with mild hypokalemia (potassium, 3–3.5 mEq/L [3–3.5 mmol/L]) not caused by GI losses, dietary supplementation may be sufficient; potassium-rich foods include oranges, bananas, cantaloupes, prunes, raisins, dried beans, dried apricots, and squash.

PATIENT EDUCATION

- Instructions for appropriate diet
- If potassium supplementation is necessary, stress the need for compliance.

PROGNOSIS

- Associated with higher morbidity and mortality because of cardiac arrhythmias
- Ease of correction of hypokalemia and need for prolonged treatment rest on the primary cause; if it can be eliminated (e.g., resolution of diarrhea, discontinuation of diuretics, removal of adrenal tumor), hypokalemia can be expected to resolve and no further treatment is indicated.

COMPLICATIONS

- Hyperkalemia can occur during the course of treatment.
- Increased risk of digoxin toxicity
- Increased risk of atrial fibrillation (2,3)[B]

REFERENCES

1. Hanlon JT, Semla TP, Schmader KE. Medication misadventures in older adults: literature from 2013. *J Am Geriatr Soc*. 2014;62(10):1950–1953.
2. Kritjthe BP, Heeringa J, Kors JA, et al. Serum potassium levels and the risk of atrial fibrillation: the Rotterdam Study. *Int J Cardiol*. 2013;168(6): 5411–5415.
3. Tran CT, Bundgaard H, Ladefoged SD, et al. Potassium dynamics are attenuated in hyperkalemia and a determinant of QT adaptation in exercising hemodialysis patients. *J Appl Physiol*. 2013;115(4):498–504.
4. Goodson CM, Clark BJ, Douglas IS. Predictors of severe alcohol withdrawal syndrome: a systematic review and meta-analysis. *Alcohol Clin Exp Res*. 2014;38(10):2664–2677.
5. Unwin RJ, Luft FC, Shirley DG, et al. Pathophysiology and management of hypokalemia: a clinical perspective. *Nat Rev Nephrol*. 2011;7(2):75–84.

ADDITIONAL READING

- Arsenault KA, Yusuf AM, Crystal E, et al. Interventions for preventing post-operative atrial fibrillation in patients undergoing heart surgery. *Cochrane Database Syst Rev*. 2013;1:CO003611.
- Asmar A, Mohandas R, Wingo CS. A physiologic-based approach to the treatment of a patient with hypokalemia. *Am J Kidney Dis*. 2012;60(3): 492–497.
- Ben Salem C, Hmouda H, Bouraoui K. Drug-induced hypokalaemia. *Curr Drug Saf*. 2009;4(1):55–61.
- Chan KE, Lazarus JM, Hakim RM. Digoxin associates with mortality in ESRD. *J Am Soc Nephrol*. 2010;21(9):1550–1559.
- Ernst ME, Moser M. Use of diuretics in patients with hypertension. *N Engl J Med*. 2009;361(22): 2153–2164.
- Facchini M, Sala L, Malfatto G, et al. Low-K+ dependent QT prolongation and risk for ventricular arrhythmia in anorexia nervosa. *Int J Cardiol*. 2006;106(2):170–176.
- Jones E. Hypokalemia. *N Engl J Med*. 2004;350(11):1156.
- Osadchii OE. Mechanisms of hypokalemia-induced ventricular arrhythmogenicity. *Fundam Clin Pharmacol*. 2010;24(5):547–559.
- Palmer BF. A physiologic-based approach to the evaluation of a patient with hypokalemia. *Am J Kidney Dis*. 2010;56(6):1184–1190.
- Zietse R, Zoutendijk R, Hoorn EJ. Fluid, electrolyte and acid-base disorders associated with antibiotic therapy. *Nat Rev Nephrol*. 2009;5(4):193–202.

SEE ALSO

- Hyperkalemia
- Algorithm: hypokalemia

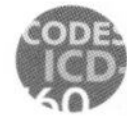

CODES

ICD10

E87.6 Hypokalemia

CLINICAL PEARLS

- In patients without heart disease, a low potassium level will rarely cause cardiac disturbances. In an otherwise healthy patient, gentle repletion using oral potassium or an increase in potassium-rich foods should be adequate.
- In patients with cardiac ischemia, heart failure, or left ventricular hypertrophy, even mild to moderate hypokalemia can cause arrhythmias. These patients should receive potassium repletion as well as cardiac monitoring.
- To safely prevent hypokalemia in diabetic and renal insufficiency patients, ensure adequate dietary potassium intake with foods rich in potassium, including spinach, tomatoes, broccoli, squash, potatoes, bananas, cantaloupe, and oranges. Avoid potassium-sparing diuretics, if possible.
- Uncorrected hypomagnesemia can hinder the correction of hypokalemia. Check magnesium levels and replete as necessary.

HYPONATREMIA

Ruben Peralta, MD, FACS

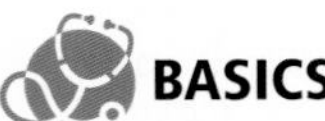

BASICS

DESCRIPTION

- Hyponatremia is a plasma sodium concentration of <135 mEq/L. Hyponatremia itself does not provide information about the "total body water" state of the patient. Patients with hyponatremia may be fluid overloaded, hypovolemic, or euvolemic.
- System(s) affected: endocrine/metabolic

EPIDEMIOLOGY

Incidence

- Most common electrolyte disorder seen in the general hospital population
- Predominant age: all ages
- Predominant sex: male = female

Prevalence

2.5% of hospitalized patients

Geriatric Considerations

The elderly have lower total body water, a decreased thirst mechanism, and decreased urinary concentrating ability; their kidneys are less responsive to antidiuretic hormone (ADH), and they show decreased renal mass, renal blood flow, and glomerular filtration rate, making them at higher risk for hyponatremia.

ETIOLOGY AND PATHOPHYSIOLOGY

- Hypovolemic hyponatremia: decrease in total body water and greater decrease in total body sodium; decreased extracellular fluid volume; orthostatic hypotension and other changes consistent with hypovolemia are present.
- Euvolemic hyponatremia: increase in total body water with normal total body sodium; extracellular fluid volume is minimally to moderately increased but with no edema.
- Hypervolemic hyponatremia: increase in total body sodium and greater increase in total body water; extracellular fluid increased markedly; edema is present.
- Redistributive hyponatremia: shift of water from intracellular compartment to extracellular compartment with resulting dilution of sodium; total body water and total body sodium unchanged; occurs with hyperglycemia
- Pseudohyponatremia: dilution of aqueous phase by excessive proteins, glucose, or lipids; total body water and total body sodium unchanged; occurs in hypertriglyceridemia or multiple myeloma
- Low sodium creates an osmotic gradient between plasma and cells and fluid shifts into cells, causing edema and increased intracranial pressure.
- Hypovolemic hyponatremia: extrarenal loss of sodium (Na <30 mmol/L in urine)
  - GI loss: vomiting, diarrhea
  - 3rd spacing: peritonitis, pancreatitis, burns, rhabdomyolysis
  - Skin loss: burns, sweating, cystic fibrosis
  - Heat-related illnesses
- Hypovolemic hyponatremia: renal loss of sodium (Na >30 mmol/L in urine)
  - Cerebral salt wasting syndrome
  - Adrenal pathology (e.g., Addison disease, hemorrhage, tuberculosis)
  - Diuretics
  - Osmotic diuresis
- Euvolemic hyponatremia (Na >30 mmol/L in urine)
  - Hypothyroidism
  - Hypopituitarism or other cause of glucocorticoid deficiency
  - Medications (e.g., carbamazepine, clofibrate, cyclosporine, levetiracetam, opiates, oxcarbazepine, phenothiazines, SSRIs, tricyclic antidepressants, vincristine) (1)
  - Primary polydipsia
  - Syndrome of inappropriate antidiuretic hormone secretion (SIADH)
  - Iatrogenic (e.g., excess hypotonic IV fluids)
- Hypervolemic hyponatremia (Na <30 mmol/L in urine, except chronic renal failure)
  - Nephrotic syndrome
  - Cirrhosis
  - Congestive heart failure (CHF)
  - Chronic renal failure
- Redistributive hyponatremia
  - Hyperglycemia
  - Mannitol infusion
  - Hypertriglyceridemia
- Multiple myeloma

Genetics

- Polymorphisms have been demonstrated.
- Mutations have been associated with nephrogenic syndrome of inappropriate antidiuresis (NSIAD; SIADH).

GENERAL PREVENTION

Depends on underlying condition

COMMONLY ASSOCIATED CONDITIONS

- Hypothyroidism
- Hypopituitarism
- Adrenocortical hormone deficiency
- HIV patients
- SIADH is associated with cancers, pneumonia, tuberculosis, encephalitis, meningitis, head trauma, cerebrovascular accident, HIV infection.
- Acute neurologic patients, brain injury
- Marathon runners in hot environments

DIAGNOSIS

- Symptoms related to the rate of fall in serum sodium and the degree of hyponatremia
- Mild (130–135 mEq/L): usually asymptomatic
- Moderate (120–130 mEq/L): nausea, vomiting, malaise
- Severe: (115–120 mEq/L): headache, lethargy, restlessness, disorientation
- Severe/rapid decreases can cause seizure, coma, and respiratory arrest and may be fatal.
- Other signs and symptoms: weakness, muscle cramps, anorexia, hiccups, depressed deep tendon reflexes, hypothermia, positive Babinski responses, cranial nerve palsies, orthostatic hypotension

PHYSICAL EXAM

- Volume status: skin turgor, jugular venous pressure, heart rate, orthostatic BP
- Exam for underlying illness: signs of CHF, cirrhosis, hypothyroidism

DIFFERENTIAL DIAGNOSIS

See "Etiology and Pathophysiology."

DIAGNOSTIC TESTS & INTERPRETATION

Initial Tests (lab, imaging)

- Comprehensive metabolic profile (BUN, creatinine, glucose, electrolytes, liver function studies, etc.)
- Thyroid-stimulating hormone (TSH)
- Lipid panel
- Serum osmolality
- Urine sodium and osmolality
- Chest x-ray to rule out pulmonary pathology if SIADH diagnosed

Follow-Up Tests & Special Considerations

- CT scan of head if pituitary problem suspected or if SIADH from CNS problem suspected
- Interpretation of labs: suspect hypovolemic hyponatremia
  - Plasma osmolality low
  - BUN-to-Cr ratio > 20:1
  - If urine sodium >20 mEq/L (>20 mmol/L): renal loss
  - If urine sodium <10 mEq/L (<10 mmol/L): extrarenal loss
  - Serum potassium >5 mEq/L (>5 mmol/L): consider mineralocorticoid deficiency
- Interpretation of labs: suspect euvolemic hyponatremia
  - Plasma osmolality low
  - BUN-to-Cr ratio < 20:1
  - Urine sodium >20 mEq/L (>20 mmol/L)
  - TSH to rule out hypothyroidism
  - Consider 1-hour cosyntropin-stimulation test to rule out adrenal insufficiency
- Interpretation of labs: hypervolemic hyponatremia
  - Plasma osmolality low
  - Urine sodium <10 mEq/L (<10 mmol/L) in nephrotic syndrome, CHF, cirrhosis
  - Urine sodium >20 mEq/L (>20 mmol/L) in acute and chronic renal failure
- Redistributive hyponatremia
  - Plasma osmolality normal or high
  - Glucose or mannitol levels elevated
- Pseudohyponatremia
  - Plasma osmolality normal
  - Triglyceride, glucose, or protein levels elevated

TREATMENT

GENERAL MEASURES

- Assess all medications patient is taking.
- Institute seizure precautions.

MEDICATION

ALERT

Rapid correction of severe symptomatic hyponatremia has been associated with central pontine myelinolysis, a neurologic disorder in which loss of myelin and supportive structures in pons and occasionally in other areas of the brain occurs (2)[C]. This results in irreversible injury. Symptoms are apparent 2–6 days after injury and include seizure, coma, spastic paraparesis, dysarthria, and dysphagia.

- Treatment tailored to clinical situation: The degree of hyponatremia, how rapidly the hyponatremia developed, and whether the patient is symptomatic influence the urgency of correction. Some general principles apply:
  - Expected change in serum Na with selected infusates: ΔNa = [(infusate Na+infusate K-Serum Na)/(TBW+1)] where TBW = a coeff × weight (wt) as in the following text:

Table 1 Total Body Water

Children	0.6 × weight
Women	0.5 × weight
Men	0.6 × weight
Elderly Women	0.45 × weight
Elderly Men	0.5 × weight

  - Formula to determine correction available at http://www.medcalc.com/sodium.html
- Asymptomatic, euvolemic patients can be treated with fluid restriction; the underlying cause also must be addressed.
- For severely hyponatremic/symptomatic patients, it is generally considered safe to increase the serum sodium by 0.6–2 mEq/L each hour, not to exceed 8 mEq/24 hours.
- For mild to moderate hyponatremia, use isotonic saline solution (0.9%). For moderate to severe hyponatremia, consider specialist consultation for use of hypertonic saline (3%) via central line access at a rate of 1–2 mL/kg body weight/hr; increasing serum sodium levels by 0.5 mmol/L/hr and monitoring frequently the plasma sodium level (~q2h).
- In patients with severe hyponatremia (euvolemic and hypervolemic state) who do not respond to the above-mentioned approach, consider the use of vasopressin V2-receptor antagonists, such as tolvaptan, or conivaptan (3)[A].
- Treat underlying condition: heart failure, cirrhosis, etc.
- Chronic hyponatremia resulting from SIADH: demeclocycline (inhibits ADH action at the collecting duct) if fluid restriction alone is not effective
  - Contraindication: can cause nephrotoxicity in patients with liver disease
  - In doses of 600–1,200 mg/day, the drug produces a nephrogenic diabetes insipidus.
  - Significant possible interactions: oral anticoagulants, oral contraceptives, penicillin

ALERT

Caution: If severe, consider hypertonic saline (3% sodium chloride) with central line access; exercise extreme caution and monitor serum sodium as frequently as q1–2h.

INPATIENT CONSIDERATIONS

Admission Criteria/Initial Stabilization

- Admission is mandatory if the patient has acute hyponatremia or is symptomatic; acute hyponatremia (developing over <48 hours) carries the risk of cerebral edema.
- Admission is advised if patient is asymptomatic and has a serum sodium <125 mEq/dL.

ONGOING CARE

DIET

- Euvolemic hyponatremia: Restrict water to 1 L/day.
- Hypervolemic hyponatremia: water and sodium restriction

PROGNOSIS

- In hospitalized patients, hyponatremia is associated with an elevated risk of adverse clinical outcomes and higher mortality (4,5)[B].
- Recently, in community-dwelling, middle-aged, and elderly adults, mild hyponatremia has been shown to be an independent predictor of death.
- Associated with poor prognosis in patients with acute pulmonary embolism
- Associated with poor prognosis in patients with liver cirrhosis and those waiting for liver transplant; it is associated with significant postop risk and short-term graft loss.

COMPLICATIONS

- Occult tumor may present if SIADH is identified
- Hypervolemia if saline used
- Osmotic demyelination (central pontine and extrapontine irreversible myelinolysis) (2,6)[C]
- Hyponatremia is the cause in 30% new onset seizures in intensive care settings.
- Chronic hyponatremia is associated with increased odds of osteoporosis.

REFERENCES

1. Meulendijks D, Mannesse CK, Jansen PA, et al. Antipsychotic-induced hyponatraemia: a systematic review of the published evidence. *Drug Saf.* 2010;33(2):101–114.
2. Singh TD, Fugate JE, Rabinstein AA. Central pontine and extrapontine myelinolysis: a systematic review. *Eur J Neurol.* 2014;21(12):1443–1450.
3. Rozen-Zvi B, Yahav D, Gheorghiade M, et al. Vasopressin receptor antagonists for the treatment of hyponatremia: systematic review and meta-analysis. *Am J Kidney Dis.* 2010;56(2):325–337.
4. Bavishi C, Ather S, Bambhroliya A, et al. Prognostic significance of hyponatremia among ambulatory patients with heart failure and preserved and reduced ejection fractions. *Am J Cardiol.* 2014;113(11):1834–1838.
5. Basu A, Ryder RE. The syndrome of inappropriate antidiuresis is associated with excess long-term mortality: a retrospective cohort analyses. *J Clin Pathol.* 2014;67(9):802–806.
6. Esposito P, Piotti G, Bianzina S, et al. The syndrome of inappropriate antidiuresis: pathophysiology, clinical management and new therapeutic options. *Nephron Clin Pract.* 2011;119(1):c62–c73.

ADDITIONAL READING

- Abraham WT, Hensen J, Gross PA, et al. Lixivaptan safely and effectively corrects serum sodium concentrations in hospitalized patients with euvolemic hyponatremia. *Kidney Int.* 2012;82(11):1223–1230.
- Cowtan T. Thiazide diuretics. *N Engl J Med.* 2010;362(7):659–660.
- De Picker L, Van Den Eede F, Dumont G, et al. Antidepressants and the risk of hyponatremia: a class-by-class review of literature. *Psychosomatics.* 2014;55(6):536–547.
- Ernst ME, Moser M. Use of diuretics in patients with hypertension. *N Engl J Med.* 2009;361(22):2153–2164.
- Friedman B, Cirulli J. Hyponatremia in critical care patients: frequency, outcome, characteristics, and treatment with the vasopressin V2-receptor antagonist tolvaptan. *J Crit Care.* 2013;28(2):219.e1–219.e12.
- Lim YJ, Park EK, Koh HC, et al. Syndrome of inappropriate secretion of antidiuretic hormone as a leading cause of hyponatremia in children who underwent chemotherapy or stem cell transplantation. *Pediatr Blood Cancer.* 2010;54(5):734–737.
- Sood L, Sterns RH, Hix JK, et al. Hypertonic saline and desmopressin: a simple strategy for safe correction of severe hyponatremia. *Am J Kidney Dis.* 2013;61(4):571–578.
- Spasovski G, Vanholder R, Allolio B, et al. Clinical practice guideline on diagnosis and treatment of hyponatraemia. *Eur J Endocrinol.* 2014;170(3):G1–G47.
- Sterns RH, Hix JK, Silver SM. Management of hyponatremia in the ICU. *Chest.* 2013;144(2):672–679.

SEE ALSO

Algorithm: Hyponatremia

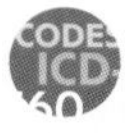

CODES

ICD10

E87.1 Hypo-osmolality and hyponatremia

CLINICAL PEARLS

- Alcohol-dependent individuals with vitamin deficiencies, elderly women taking thiazide diuretics, and people with hypokalemia or burns are at increased risk of central pontine myelinolysis. A longer duration of hyponatremia is also a risk factor.
- Bronchogenic carcinoma, pancreas, duodenal, prostate, thymoma, lymphoma, and mesothelioma are neoplastic diseases associated with SIADH.
- Formulas have been developed (Adrogue and Madias) for safe correction of hyponatremia and are available online (see http://www.medcalc.com/sodium.html).

H

HYPOPARATHYROIDISM

Diana P. Vaca, MD • Felix B. Chang, MD, DABMA, ABIHM

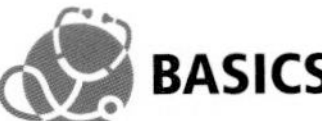

BASICS

DESCRIPTION

- Deficient secretion of parathyroid hormone (PTH)
- Usually asymptomatic
- Acute hypoparathyroidism: tetany, muscle cramps, carpopedal spasm, irritability, altered mental status, convulsion, stridor, and tingling of the circumoral area, hands, and feet
- Chronic: lethargy, personality changes, anxiety, blurry vision, parkinsonism, mental retardation
- System(s) affected: endocrine/metabolic; musculoskeletal; nervous; bones; kidneys; parathyroid

Pediatric Considerations

- May occur in premature infants
- Neonates born to hypercalcemic mothers may experience suppression of developing parathyroid glands.
- Congenital absence of parathyroids
- May appear later in childhood as autoimmune or APS-1

Geriatric Considerations

Hypocalcemia is fairly common in elderly; however, rarely secondary to hypoparathyroidism

Pregnancy Considerations

Use of magnesium as a tocolytic may induce functional hypoparathyroidism.

EPIDEMIOLOGY

More common in women. Affects all ages.

Incidence

Most common after surgical procedure of the anterior neck. Transient hyperparathyroidism is seen after 20% of thyroidectomies, whereas permanent hypoparathyroidism, 0.8–3.0%.

Prevalence

Wide variation. Autosomal dominant hypocalcemia with hypercalciuria (ADHH): 1/70,000 typically in infancy with hypocalcemic seizures

ETIOLOGY AND PATHOPHYSIOLOGY

- PTH is involved in the control of serum ionized calcium levels:
  - Mobilizes calcium and phosphorus from bone stores
  - Stimulates formation of 1,25-dihydroxy-vitamin D
  - Stimulates reabsorption of calcium in the distal convoluted tubule and phosphate excretion in proximal tubule
- Loss of PTH action results in hypocalcemia, hyperphosphatemia, and hypercalciuria.
- Magnesium is crucial for PTH secretion and activation of the PTH receptor; hypo- or hypermagnesemia may result in functional hypoparathyroidism.
- Acquired hypoparathyroidism
  - Surgical: removal or damage to parathyroid glands or their blood supply; thyroid, parathyroid, or radical neck surgery for head and neck cancers (1)
  - Autoimmune: isolated or combined with other endocrine deficiencies in polyglandular autoimmune (PGA) syndrome
  - Deposition of heavy metals in gland: copper (Wilson disease) or iron (hemochromatosis, thalassemias), radiation-induced destruction, and metastatic infiltration
  - Functional hypoparathyroidism: associated with hypomagnesemia; hypermagnesemia
  - Congenital
    - Calcium-sensing receptor (CaSR) abnormalities: hypocalcemia with hypercalciuria
    - HDR or Barakat syndrome: deafness, renal dysplasia
    - Familial: mutations of the *TBCE* gene; abnormal PTH secretions
    - 22q11.2 deletion syndrome
- Autoimmune: genetic gain-of-function mutation in CaSR
- Infiltrative: metastatic carcinoma, hemochromatosis, Wilson disease, granulomas
- Hypo- (alcoholics) or hypermagnesemia: chronic iron overloads

Genetics

- Genetic defects may result in X-linked or in autosomal recessive hypoparathyroidism due to abnormal parathyroid gland development; associated with mutations in the transcription factor glial cell missing B (BCMB)
- Mutations in transcription factors or regulators of parathyroid gland development
  - Component of a larger genetic syndrome (APS-1 or DiGeorge syndrome) or in isolation (X-linked hypoparathyroidism) (2)
  - May be autosomal dominant (DiGeorge), autosomal recessive (APS-1), or X-linked recessive (X-linked hypoparathyroidism) (2)
  - Congenital syndromes
    - 22q11.2 deletion syndrome, familial hypomagnesemia, hypoparathyroidism with lymphedema (2)
    - Hypoparathyroidism with sensorineural deafness
    - ADHH: mutations gain-of-function of the CaSR gene suppressing the parathyroid gland, without elevation of PTH
  - PGA syndrome type 1: mucocutaneous candidiasis, hypoparathyroidism, and Addison disease

RISK FACTORS

Neck surgery and neck trauma, neck malignancies, family history of hypocalcemia, PGA syndrome

GENERAL PREVENTION

Intraoperative identification and preservation of parathyroid tissue

COMMONLY ASSOCIATED CONDITIONS

- DiGeorge syndrome
- PGA syndrome type 1
- Multiple endocrine deficiency autoimmune candidiasis (MEDAC) syndrome
- Juvenile familial endocrinopathy
- Addison disease
- Moniliasis (HAM) syndrome: a polyglandular deficiency syndrome, possibly genetic, characterized by hypoparathyroidism

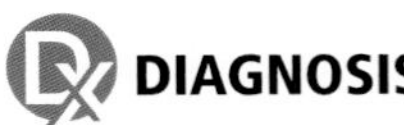

DIAGNOSIS

HISTORY

Often asymptomatic; ask about previous neck trauma or surgery, head or neck irradiation, family history of hypocalcemia, or presence of other autoimmune endocrinopathies.

- Fatigue, circumoral or distal extremity paresthesias
- Muscle cramps, seizures, neuropsychiatric symptoms

PHYSICAL EXAM

- Surgical scar on neck
- Chvostek sign: ipsilateral twitching of the upper lip on tapping the facial nerve on the cheek. 10% normal people have positive Chvostek sign.
- Trousseau sign: painful carpal spasm after 3-minute occlusion of brachial artery with BP cuff. BP cuff inflated to > systolic BP for 3 minutes leads to carpal spasm (flexion of metacarpophalangeal [MCP] joints, extension of interphalangeal [IP] joints, adduction of fingers and thumb).
- Tetany, laryngo- or bronchospasm, cataracts, cardiac arrhythmias, or failure; dry hair, brittle nails
- Loss of deep tendon reflexes
- Dysrhythmias (secondary hypocalcemia)
- Cataracts
- Tooth enamel defects

DIFFERENTIAL DIAGNOSIS

- Vitamin D deficiency/resistance
- Pseudohypoparathyroidism, which presents in childhood, kidney and bone unresponsiveness to PTH; characterized by hypocalcemia, hyperphosphatemia, and, in contrast to hypoparathyroidism, elevated rather than reduced PTH concentrations
- Hypoalbuminemia, renal failure, malabsorption, familial hypocalcemia, hypomagnesemia

DIAGNOSTIC TESTS & INTERPRETATION

Initial Tests (lab, imaging)

- Calcium: total and ionized (low) (correct serum calcium level for albumin)
  - Corrected serum calcium = total serum calcium + 0.8 (4 – serum albumin)
- Phosphorus (high)
- PTH (low or inappropriately normal)
- Magnesium (low or high may cause hypoparathyroidism; may also be normal)
- BUN, creatinine, 25-OH vitamin D level (especially in elderly)

- Urinary calcium (normal or high)
- Calcium should be monitored after thyroid or parathyroid surgery.
- Radiographs may show absent tooth roots, calcification of cerebellum, choroid plexus, or cerebral basal ganglia.

Follow-Up Tests & Special Considerations

- ECG: prolongation of ST and QTc intervals nonspecific repolarization changes, dysrhythmias
- Urine calcium: Creatinine ratio (normal 0.1–0.2) may be low before treatment but should be monitored to prevent stones due to hypercalciuria.
- Gene sequencing: Evaluation of other hormone levels may be required to diagnose APS-1.
- Hungry bone syndrome (transient hypoparathyroidism after parathyroid surgery)
  - Hypocalcemia due to hungry bone syndrome may persist despite recovery of PTH secretion from the remaining normal glands. Thus, serum PTH concentrations may be low, normal, or even elevated.
- Infiltrative: osteoblastic metastasis of prostate, breast, or lung cancer
- Metabolic/nutritional: renal failure, neonatal hypocalcemia, hypoalbuminemia, malabsorption, calcium (Ca^{++}) chelators, hypomagnesemia
- Familial hypocalcemia, acute hyperphosphatemia (rare), vitamin D deficiency
- Autoantibodies against NACHT leucine-rich-repeat protein 5(NALPS) found in 49% of 73 patients with APS-1 and hypoparathyroidisms

Test Interpretation

Parathyroid gland parenchymal tissue completely or almost completely replaced by fat

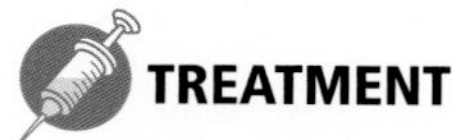

TREATMENT

GENERAL MEASURES

- Monitor ECG during calcium repletion.
- Maintenance therapy: may require lifelong treatment with calcium and calcitriol (2)
  - Maintain serum calcium in low normal range: 8–8.5 mg/dL (2–2.12 mmol/L).
- If hypercalcemia occurs, hold therapy until calcium returns to normal. Treat magnesium deficiency if present.
- Phosphate binders required if high calcium-phosphate product.
- Thiazide diuretics combined with a low-salt diet may be used to prevent hypercalciuria, nephrocalcinosis, and nephrolithiasis.
- Oral calcium administration and vitamin D supplementation after thyroidectomy may reduce the risk for symptomatic hypocalcemia after surgery.

MEDICATION

First Line

- Hypoparathyroid tetany, severe symptoms (tetany, seizures, cardiac failure, laryngospasm, bronchospasm)
  - IV calcium gluconate: 1 or 2 g, each infused over a period of 10 minutes. Central venous catheter preferred because calcium-containing solutions can irritate surrounding tissues. Follow with infusion of 10 g calcium gluconate in 1 L 5% dextrose water at a rate of 1–3 mg calcium gluconate/kg of body weight/hr.
- Maintenance
  - Oral calcium: calcium salts: 1–3 g/day PO
  - Calcitriol: (vitamin D 1,25-dihydroxycholecalciferol): 0.25 μg/day. Doses 0.5–2.0 μg/day are usually required.
- Hypomagnesemia: acutely: 1–2 g IV q6h long-term magnesium oxide tablets (600 mg) once or twice per day

Second Line

Cholecalciferol 10,000–50,000 U duration of action 4–8 weeks

ISSUES FOR REFERRAL

Endocrinologist, nephrologist, ophthalmologist

ADDITIONAL THERAPIES

Parathyroid hormone 1–34 (SC) (3,4)[A]

- May be as effective as calcitriol for maintaining growth and serum calcium levels in children with chronic hypoparathyroidism.

SURGERY/OTHER PROCEDURES

Autotransplantation of cryopreserved parathyroid tissue: restores normocalcemia in 23% of cases

INPATIENT CONSIDERATIONS

Admission Criteria/Initial Stabilization

Laryngospasm, seizures, tetany, QT prolongation

Discharge Criteria

Resolution of hypocalcemic symptoms, patient educated on hypoparathyroidism and treatment

ONGOING CARE

FOLLOW-UP RECOMMENDATIONS

Patient Monitoring

- Goal is a total corrected serum calcium level in low normal range (8–8.5 mg/dL or 2–2.12 mmol/L), 24-hour urine calcium <300 mg, and calcium-phosphate product <55.
- Outpatient measurement of serum calcium, phosphorus, and creatinine weekly to monthly during initial management; measure calcium, phosphate, and creatinine twice yearly when stable.
- Measure urine calcium and creatinine twice yearly.
- Annual slit-lamp and ophthalmologic evaluations are recommended.
- DEXA scan

DIET

Low-phosphate diet in patients with hyperphosphatemia

PATIENT EDUCATION

www.hypopara.org

PROGNOSIS

Hypoparathyroidism following neck surgery is often transient. Length of required treatment may vary depending on origin.

COMPLICATIONS

- Reversible: due to low calcium levels, most likely to improve with adequate treatment
  - Neuromuscular symptoms: paresthesias (circumoral, fingers, toes), tetany, seizures, parkinsonian symptoms; pseudotumor cerebri has been described.
  - Renal: hypercalciuria, nephrocalcinosis, nephrolithiasis
  - Cardiovascular: heart failure; arrhythmias
- Irreversible: when condition starts early in childhood and will not improve with calcium and vitamin D treatment
  - Stunting of growth
  - Enamel defects and hypoplasia of teeth
  - Atrophy, brittleness, and ridging of nails
  - Cataracts and basal ganglia calcifications

REFERENCES

1. Al-Azem, Khan A. Hypoparathyroidism. *Best Pract Res Clin Endocrinol Metab*. 2012;26(4):517–522.
2. Cusano NE, Rubin MR, McMahon DJ, et al. The effect of PTH(1-84) on quality of life in hypoparathyroidism. *J Clin Endocrinol Metab*. 2013;98(6):2356–2361.
3. de la Morena MT, Eitson JL, Dozmorov IM, et al. Signature MicroRNA expression patterns identified in humans with 22q11.2 deletion/DiGeorge syndrome. *Clin Immunol*. 2013;147(1):11–22.
4. Winer KK, Zhang B, Shrader JA, et al. Synthetic human parathyroid hormone 1–34 replacement therapy: a randomized crossover trial comparing pump versus injections in the treatment of chronic hypoparathyroidism. *J Clin Endocrinol Metab*. 2012;97(2):391–399.

ADDITIONAL READING

Cusano NE, Rubin MR, McMahon DJ, et al. The effect pf PTH(1-84) on quality of life in hypoparathyroidism. *J Clin Endocrinol Metab*. 2013;98(6):2356–2361.

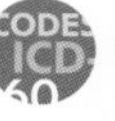

CODES

ICD10

- E20.9 Hypoparathyroidism, unspecified
- P71.4 Transitory neonatal hypoparathyroidism
- E89.2 Postprocedural hypoparathyroidism

CLINICAL PEARLS

Often asymptomatic; consider if hypocalcemic with fatigue and circumoral or distal extremity paresthesias.

- Correct the serum calcium level for albumin level.
- Monitor calcium after thyroid or parathyroid surgery.
- Serum levels of magnesium and 25(OH) should be measured to rule out deficiency that could contribute to reduced serum calcium levels.

HYPOTENSION, ORTHOSTATIC

Zeeshan Hussain, MD • Nirmanmoh Bhatia, MD • Marcus F. Stoddard, MD

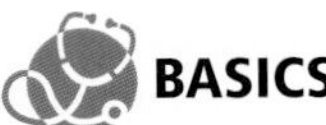

BASICS

Postural or orthostatic hypotension (OH) represents the failure of cardiovascular reflexes to maintain adequate BP on standing from a supine or sitting position.

DESCRIPTION

- OH is defined as a sustained and persistent drop in systolic BP (SBP) ≥20 mm Hg or diastolic BP (DBP) ≥10 mm Hg within 3 minutes of achieving a standing position or head-up tilt to at least 60 degrees on tilt table (1). Delayed OH can infrequently occur with a slow decline in SBP beyond 5 minutes of standing and may be revealed by extending the period of orthostatic stress.
- Symptoms differ greatly in severity and can be precipitated by postural changes, postprandially, or by exertion. Characteristic symptoms of OH are recurrent dizziness, light-headedness, presyncope, or syncope with assumption of an upright posture, typically relieved by achieving a recumbent position and can be incapacitating. In the elderly, OH may be asymptomatic or present with nonspecific complaints of weakness.

EPIDEMIOLOGY

Asymptomatic OH is far more common than symptomatic OH but importantly is an independent risk factor for mortality and cardiovascular disease. OH is also a manifestation of many underlying diseases and may be the initial sign of autonomic failure in many neurodegenerative disorders. The prevalence increases with age, hypertension (HTN), diabetes, and use of medications, particularly antihypertensive and antidepressant medications.

Incidence

80,095 orthostatic-related hospitalizations occurred in the United States in 2004; OH was the primary diagnosis in 35%.

Prevalence

~6% of middle-aged persons and 18% of individuals ≥65 years of age; more common in those living in long-term care facilities (45% vs. 6% living in the community). In those with HTN, prevalence is 13.4–32.1%

ETIOLOGY AND PATHOPHYSIOLOGY

- During standing, 500–1,000 mL of blood pools in the lower extremities and the splanchnic vasculature. This reduces cardiac preload but is opposed by an increase in sympathetic tone and vasopressin release that maintains cerebral perfusion pressure by increasing peripheral vascular resistance. Impairment of these compensatory mechanisms by autonomic dysfunction, or nonneurogenic causes such as medications, hypovolemia, or cardiac pump failure, leads to an inability to maintain effective cerebral perfusion pressure. Autonomic dysfunction also impairs proximal tubule renal sodium reabsorption, which contributes to OH through urinary sodium wasting and a consequent reduction in circulating plasma volume. In older people, vascular stiffening and decreased baroreceptor sensitivity predispose to OH.
- Supine hypertension (SH), due to baroreflex dysfunction and fluid redistribution upon assuming a horizontal position, is common in patients with OH. Increased renal perfusion pressure in the recumbent position also leads to nocturnal natriuresis, which decreases circulating volume, worsening orthostatic tolerance in the morning.
- Medications (iatrogenic causes)
  - Antidepressants (most commonly implicated): TCA, MAOIs
  - Anticholinergics: benztropine, oxybutynin
  - Antihypertensives: of classes including diuretics, alpha-blockers, beta-blockers
  - Dopamine agonists: levodopa, bromocriptine, ropinirole, pramipexole
  - Ethanol
  - Insulin (may exacerbate OH in the setting of diabetic neuropathy)
  - Vasodilators: hydralazine, nitroglycerin
  - Phosphodiesterase inhibitors: sildenafil, tadalfil
  - Opioids/sedatives: morphine, benzodiazepines, barbiturates, promethazine
  - Antipsychotics: thioridazine, iloperidone
  - Neurotoxic drugs: vincristine, cisplatin
- Neurogenic causes
  - Idiopathic OH (1/3 of cases of OH)
  - Central autonomic nervous system diseases: familial dysautonomia (rare, childhood), synucleinopathies such as Lewy body dementia, multisystem atrophy (Shy-Drager syndrome), Parkinson disease (PD): (40% of patients with PD have OH) and pure autonomic failure (rare)
  - Peripheral autonomic nervous system diseases: acute autonomic neuropathy and Guillain-Barré syndrome (acute onset, frequently preceded by viral syndrome); alcoholic polyneuropathy; amyloidosis; autoimmune autonomic ganglionopathy (rare); chronic renal failure: uremic or β-2 microglobulin neuropathy (dialysis). Diabetes: diabetic autonomic neuropathy (very common). Exposure to neurotoxins. Hereditary sensory and autonomic neuropathies: dopamine-β-hydroxylase deficiency (rare). HIV neuropathy. Paraneoplastic autonomic neuropathy: small cell lung cancer (SCLC), nonsmall cell lung cancer (NSCLC), GI neoplasias, prostate, breast, bladder, kidney, testicle, and ovary. Spinal cord pathologies: trauma, myelitis, tumors, tabes dorsalis, multiple sclerosis, syringomyelia, infarction, vitamin B_{12} deficiency
- Nonneurogenic causes
  - Cardiac disorders: heart failure, arrhythmias, pericardial disease, severe aortic stenosis, idiopathic hypertrophic subaortic stenosis (IHSS), hypertrophic obstructive cardiomyopathy (HOCM), acute aortic regurgitation, acute myocardial infarction
  - Deconditioning
  - Intravascular volume depletion: bleeding, diarrhea, diabetes insipidus, diuretics, poor oral intake, vomiting
  - Metabolic: adrenal insufficiency, hypoaldosteronism, pheochromocytoma, carcinoid syndrome, hypokalemia (severe), hypothyroidism, porphyria
  - Sepsis
  - Systemic mastocytosis
  - Venous pooling: heat or vigorous exercise, postprandial splanchnic dilation, prolonged recumbency or standing

RISK FACTORS

- Elderly, particularly in long-term care facilities
- Multiple comorbidities, including HTN, diabetes, neurodegenerative disorders, and neuropathy
- Polypharmacy (See "Epidemiology" section)

GENERAL PREVENTION

Avoid polypharmacy and monitor drug interactions, maintain adequate fluid balance.

COMMONLY ASSOCIATED CONDITIONS

Diabetes mellitus with neuropathy, uncontrolled HTN and antihypertensive treatment, PD, dehydration

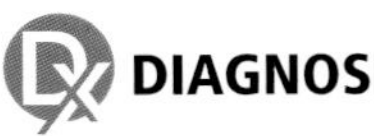

DIAGNOSIS

Initial approach: detailed history and physical examination with a focus on neurodegenerative disorders and neuropathy; thorough medication review; screening for reversible causes: 12-lead ECG, CBC, and BMP

HISTORY

- Postural symptoms: dizziness, light-headedness, palpitations, visual blurring, syncope, or presyncope. Elderly patients may have vague complaints even before frank syncope: generalized weakness, fatigue, nausea, difficulty with concentration or cognition, leg buckling, pure vertigo, visual blurring, headache or "coat-hanger" pattern neck-shoulder pain, orthostatic dyspnea, or angina
- Aggravating factors: warm environments, exertion, prolonged standing, ingestions of large/carbohydrate-rich meals, alcohol intake (vasodilation)
- Volume depletion: vomiting, diarrhea, poor oral intake, polyuria
- Cardiac pump failure: orthopnea, edema, paroxysmal nocturnal dyspnea, angina
- Peripheral neuropathy: numbness, pain, paresthesia, imbalance, or falls
- Associated diseases: diabetes, PD, dementia
- Autonomic symptoms: altered sweating (hyper- or hypohidrosis), GI dysfunction (bloating, nausea, vomiting, constipation), impotence, bladder dysfunction, sicca symptoms
- May be asymptomatic

PHYSICAL EXAM

- Measure BP while supine and standing: Patient should be supine for 5 minutes, then after standing, check the BP at 3 minutes. Use sitting measurements only if the patient is too dizzy or weak to stand. Use fall precautions: Do not check for OH in patients with supine SBP <90 mm Hg (shock) as it adds no useful information. Tachycardic response to standing may be a sign of hypovolemia or cardiac pump failure, whereas minimal or no change in heart rate may suggest a neurogenic cause. Orthostatic tachycardia without a significant drop in BP does not meet criteria for OH and may suggest postural orthostatic tachycardia syndrome (POTS).
- Cardiac exam: jugular venous distention, pulse irregularity, edema, murmurs, S_3
- Neurologic exam: hypomimia, gait, tremor, cogwheel rigidity, motor strength, fine touch, pain sensation, proprioception, Romberg maneuver, cerebellar signs, and myoclonus

DIFFERENTIAL DIAGNOSIS

Neurally mediated (reflex) syncope: vasovagal syncope, situational syncope (cough, micturition, defecation, swallowing), carotid sinus hypersensitivity. Falls related to a neurologic disorder. Postprandial hypotension. POTS. Shock (must have a normal lying BP before testing)

DIAGNOSTIC TESTS & INTERPRETATION

Initial Tests (lab, imaging)

- CBC, BMP (hypokalemia, alkalosis, and renal insufficiency suggesting volume depletion), thyroid-stimulating hormone (TSH) (2)[C]
- ECG and/or Holter monitor/event monitor: to rule out arrhythmias and detect structural heart disease. Echocardiogram: for abnormal ECG, new murmurs, or suspected heart failure (2)[C]. MRI: for suspected neurodegenerative disorders or spinal disease

Follow-Up Tests & Special Considerations

- If neuropathy is found on exam, consider vitamin B_{12} levels and serum and urine protein electrophoresis (amyloidosis) (3)[C]. Nerve conduction studies and electromyography and serologic testing for syphilis may also be considered.
- Adrenal insufficiency and pheochromocytoma evaluation is warranted in OH of uncertain cause: 8 AM cortisol level: if <18 μg/dL, consider cosyntropin testing. 24-hour urinary or plasma fractionated metanephrines: Consider further testing, depending on results.
- Antibodies to the neuronal nicotinic receptor (nAChR) in cases of suspected autoimmune autonomic ganglionopathy

Diagnostic Procedures/Other

- Tilt table testing: indicated if orthostatic symptoms are persistent, significant, and characteristic despite a nondiagnostic clinical examination. Provocation with nitroglycerin or IV isoproterenol is not recommended, as it may cause false-positive results (1,3)[C].
- Autonomic testing: useful in cases where neurally mediated syncope versus orthostatic syncope is unclear and to diagnose subclinical cases. Includes heart rate (HR) and BP variability with deep inspiration and Valsalva maneuver, sudomotor evaluation, orthostatic vascular resistance, plasma norepinephrine response to orthostasis, and pharmacologic challenges (4)[C].

TREATMENT

- Abdominal binder or compression stockings (not thrombo-embolism deterrent [TED] hose), preferably waist high with 20 mm Hg of pressure (worn before rising) (1,3,5)[B]
- Moving gradually when switching to standing from a sitting position (3–5)[C]. Also, physical counter maneuvers (to increase vascular resistance and preload): isometric contraction of leg muscles for 30 seconds at a time, repeated feet dorsiflexion, leg crossing and contraction, squatting, bending at the waist, leg elevation, and respiratory maneuvers, such as inspiration through pursed lips and inspiratory sniffing (1,4,5)[B].
- Moderate exercise (supine or sitting isotonic exercise if symptoms are severe): improves orthostatic tolerance and reduces venous pooling (1,5)[B]
- Increase water and sodium intake: 1.25–2.5 L of fluid a day and up to 6–9 g/day of sodium (if needed, salt tablets starting at 500 mg PO TID may be used). Encourage drinking water with meals and before exercise. Rapid ingestion of two 8-oz glasses of water (500 mL) over 3–4 minutes elicits a marked pressor response lasting for up to 2 hours (1,3,4)[B].
- Elevate the head of the bed 20 degrees (6–9 inches) to reduce supine HTN and nocturnal natriuresis (4,5)[B],(6)[C].
- Avoid: prolonged recumbency; increased intrathoracic pressure (straining, coughing); large meals, especially if high in carbohydrates; and alcohol (4,5)[C]

MEDICATION

First, identify and discontinue all potentially aggravating medications. Medication is indicated only when nonpharmacologic measures are insufficient to control symptoms. Goal of therapy is to improve functional capacity and quality of life without causing excessive supine HTN rather than to eliminate orthostatic drops in BP.

First Line

- Fludrocortisone: synthetic mineralocorticoid that increases sodium and fluid retention and increases peripheral vascular resistance. Starting at 0.1 mg/day, titrate for symptoms every week up to 0.5 mg/day. Contraindicated in patients with heart failure (HF) and chronic renal insufficiency due to volume expansion (1,5,7)[B].
- Midodrine: selective peripheral α-agonist that increases vascular resistance. Only drug currently FDA approved to treat OH. Start at 2.5 mg PO TID and titrate for symptoms up to 10 mg TID. Avoid within 4 hours of bedtime to prevent worsening supine HTN, and use with caution in patients with coronary artery disease (1)[B],(5,7)[A].

Second Line

- Pyridostigmine: acetylcholinesterase inhibitor, increases sympathetic ganglionic neurotransmission, 30–60 mg PO TID (1,5,7)[B]
- Caffeine: methylxanthine with pressor effect due to blockade of adenosine receptors, 100–250 mg PO TID, as tablets or caffeinated beverages, particularly for postprandial hypotension (3)[B]
- Octreotide: likely mechanism splanchnic vasoconstriction and shunting of blood from central circulation (12.5–25 μg SQ BID) (3)[B],(6)[C],(7)[B]
- Erythropoietin: increases RBC mass. Consider only when significant anemia coexists, 25–75 U/kg SQ 3×/wk (maintenance dose may be lower). Iron studies and supplementation usually are required (4,7)[B].
- Ephedrine: mixed α- and β-agonist, 25–50 mg PO TID (avoid within 4 hours before bedtime to prevent worsening supine HTN)
- Pseudoephedrine: mixed α- and β-agonist, 30–60 mg PO TID (avoid within 4 hours before bedtime) (3)[B],(4,6)[C]
- Desmopressin: vasopressin analogue, 5–40 μg/day nasal spray, or 100–800 μg/day PO (4)[C]
- L-dihydroxyphenylserine (Droxidopa): prodrug that is converted to noradrenaline by dopa decarboxylase enzyme, 200–400 mg/day PO divided 3 times/day (6,7)[C]
- Nonsteroidal anti-inflammatory drugs: may supplement treatment with fludrocortisone or a sympathomimetic agent. They are believed to act by limiting the vasodilating effects of circulating prostaglandins.

ADDITIONAL THERAPIES

Consider bedtime nitrates or nifedipine to treat severe, sustained supine HTN; may increase the risk of syncope and falls (4)[C]. Caffeine and octreotide are recommended for postprandial hypotension (3)[B].

ISSUES FOR REFERRAL

Consider cardiology referral if there is significant heart disease or tilt table testing will be required. Consider neurology referral for confirmed or suspected primary neurologic pathologies.

ONGOING CARE

FOLLOW-UP RECOMMENDATIONS

Monitor for significant supine HTN, fluid overload, electrolyte abnormalities, and HF in patients under medical treatment. In patients without an apparent cause of OH, follow-up is essential because OH alone may be the initial presentation of neurologic disorders.

PATIENT EDUCATION

Recognize symptoms and avoid aggravating factors. Educate on nonpharmacologic measures.

COMPLICATIONS

Syncope, falls (hip fracture, head trauma)

REFERENCES

1. Lanier JB, Mote MB, Clay EC. Evaluation and management of orthostatic hypotension. *Am Fam Physician*. 2011;84(5):527–536.
2. Lahrmann H, Cortelli P, Hilz M, et al. EFNS guidelines on the diagnosis and management of orthostatic hypotension. *Eur J Neurol*. 2006;13(9):930–936.
3. Arnold AC, Shibao C. Current concepts in orthostatic hypotension management. *Curr Hypertens Rep*. 2013;15(4):304–312. doi:10.1007/s11906-013-0362-3.
4. Freeman R. Clinical practice. Neurogenic orthostatic hypotension. *N Engl J Med*. 2008;358(6):615–624.
5. Figueroa JJ, Basford JR, Low PA. Preventing and treating orthostatic hypotension: as easy as A, B, C. *Cleve Clin J Med*. 2010;77(5):298–306.
6. Raj SR, Coffin ST. Medical therapy and physical maneuvers in the treatment of the vasovagal syncope and orthostatic hypotension. *Prog Cardiovasc Dis*. 2013;55(4):425–433.
7. Ong AC, Myint PK, Shepstone L, et al. A systematic review of the pharmacological management of orthostatic hypotension. *Int J Clin Pract*. 2013;67(7):633–646. doi:10.1111/ijcp.12122.

ADDITIONAL READING

- Benvenuto LJ, Krakoff LR. Morbidity and mortality of orthostatic hypotension: implications for management of cardiovascular disease. *Am J Hypertens*. 2011;24(2):135–144.
- Goldstein DS, Sharabi Y. Neurogenic orthostatic hypotension: a pathophysiological approach. *Circulation*. 2009;119(1):139–146.

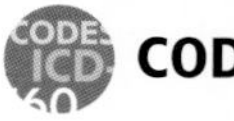

CODES

ICD10

I95.1 Orthostatic hypotension

CLINICAL PEARLS

- OH is a clinical finding, not a disease. Treatment should be guided by symptoms rather than by absolute BP drop.
- Always check the medication list and volume status. Drug-related OH may be a sign of underlying autonomic dysfunction.
- Pharmacologic treatment is indicated only when nonpharmacologic measures are insufficient to control symptoms.

HYPOTHYROIDISM, ADULT

Gisela M. Lopez Payares, MD • Fozia Akhtar Ali, MD

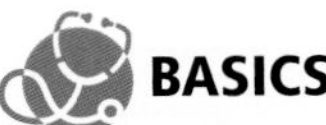

BASICS

DESCRIPTION

- Clinical and metabolic state resulting from decreased circulating levels of free thyroid hormone or from resistance to hormone action
- Can be primary (intrinsic thyroid disease) >95% of cases or secondary (hypothalamic-pituitary disease)
- Subclinical hypothyroidism: elevated thyroid-stimulating hormone upper reference limit, with normal free T_4 (1)[A]
- System(s) affected: endocrine/metabolic
- Synonym(s): myxedema (severe hypothyroidism)

EPIDEMIOLOGY

Incidence

- Women: 3.5 per 1,000 survivors per year
- Men: 0.6 per 1,000 survivors per year
- Risk of developing hypothyroidism in women with positive antibodies and elevated thyroid stimulating hormone (TSH) was 4% per year and 2–3% per year in those with either alone. In men, rate remained well below those in women (1)[A].

Prevalence

- The National Health and Nutrition Examination Survey III (NHANES III), between 1988 and 1994 unselected U.S. population >12 years of age with upper limit TSH 4.5, subclinical was 9.3% and hypothyroidism prevalence of 0.3%
- Framingham study, 5.9% in women and 2.3% in men above 60 years of age, TSH >10 mIU/L.
- Colorado survey, self-selected individuals attending a health fair were tested upper limit TSH 5.0, prevalence of 8.5% and 2.4% subclinical, not taking medications.
- British Whickham survey, 9.3% in women and 1.2% in men, serum TSH >10 (1)[A].

ETIOLOGY AND PATHOPHYSIOLOGY

- Primary: >95% of cases: the most common cause is autoimmune thyroid disease in United States: Hashimoto thyroiditis or chronic autoimmune thyroiditis (AITDs), characterized pathologically by infiltration of the thyroid with sensitized T lymphocytes and serologically by circulating thyroid antibodies. Autoimmunity to the thyroid gland appears to be an inherited defect in immune surveillance, leading to abnormal regulation of immune responsiveness or alteration of presenting antigen in the thyroid (1)[A].
  - Hashimoto thyroiditis (goitrous hypothyroidism)
  - Ord disease (atrophic hypothyroidism)
  - The most common cause worldwide: environmental iodine deficiency (1)[A]
- Secondary
  - Postablative: follows radioactive iodine therapy or thyroid surgery; delayed hypothyroidism may develop in patients treated with thioamide drugs (e.g., propylthiouracil or methimazole) 4–25 years later.
  - Surgical thyroidectomy
  - Radiotherapy for neck malignancies
  - Transient hypothyroidism during the course of subacute or painless thyroiditis (silent thyroditis, most common during postpartum period) and subacute granulomatous thyroiditis
  - Infiltrative disease (fibrous thyroiditis, hemochromatosis, sarcoidosis)
  - Genetics or deficiency of thyrotropin-releasing hormone (TRH) from hypothalamus or TSH from pituitary
- Other causes: heritable biosynthetic defects, iodine deficiency (rare in the United States), or drugs (iodides, lithium, phenylbutazone, acetylsalicylic acid [ASA], amiodarone, aminoglutethimide, and IFN-α)
- No known genetic pattern for idiopathic primary hypothyroidism
- May be associated with type 2 autoimmune polyglandular syndrome, which is associated with HLA-DR3 and -DR4
- Secondary hypothyroidism frequently results from treatment for Graves disease, which may be familial.

RISK FACTORS

- Personal or family history of autoimmune diseases, including type 1 diabetes mellitus, Addison disease, Hashimoto thyroiditis
- Previous postpartum thyroiditis
- Previous head or neck irradiation
- History of Graves disease
- Treatment with lithium, immune modulators, such as IFN-α, or the iodine-containing amiodarone
- More common in persons of Japanese descent

COMMONLY ASSOCIATED CONDITIONS

- Hyponatremia
- Macrocytic anemia
- Idiopathic adrenocorticoid deficiency
- Diabetes mellitus/metabolic syndrome
- Hypoparathyroidism
- Myasthenia gravis
- Vitiligo
- Hypercholesterolemia
- Mitral valve prolapse
- Depression
- Rapid-cycling bipolar disorder
- Ischemic heart disease
- Down syndrome
- Celiac disease
- Elevated creatine kinase

DIAGNOSIS

HISTORY

- Onset may be insidious, subtle
- Weakness, fatigue, lethargy
- Cold intolerance
- Decreased memory, concentration
- Hearing impairment
- Constipation
- Muscle cramps, arthralgias, paresthesias
- Modest weight gain (10 lb [4.5 kg])
- Decreased sweating
- Menorrhagia
- Depression
- Hoarseness
- Carpal tunnel syndrome

PHYSICAL EXAM

- Dry, coarse skin; reduced body and scalp hair
- Dull facial expression
- Coarsening or huskiness of voice
- Periorbital puffiness
- Swelling of hands and feet (nonpitting)
- Bradycardia
- Hypothermia
- Reduced systolic BP; increased diastolic BP
- Delayed relaxation of deep tendon reflexes
- Macroglossia
- Weight gain
- Goiter (particularly in patient with Hashimoto thyroiditis)
- Impalpable thyroid gland (often in Ord disease or atrophic hypothyroidism)

Geriatric Considerations

- Characteristic signs and symptoms frequently changed or absent or sometimes unspecific symptoms
- Diagnosis based on laboratory criteria

DIFFERENTIAL DIAGNOSIS

- Nephrotic syndrome/chronic nephritis
- Neurasthenia
- Depression
- Euthyroid sick syndrome
- Congestive heart failure
- Primary amyloidosis
- Dementia from other causes
- Primary adrenal insufficiency
- Recovery from nonthyroidal illness
- Thyrotropin-secreting pituitary adenoma

DIAGNOSTIC TESTS & INTERPRETATION

Initial Tests (lab, imaging)

Screening test: TSH levels

- Primary hypothyroidism
  - TSH elevated
  - Serum free T_4 decreased
- Central hypothyroidism
  - Assessment only free T_4 or free T_4 index, not TSH (1)[A]
  - Serum free T_4 decreased
  - Impaired TSH response to TRH
  - MRI of brain should be performed.
- Severe hypothyroidism
  - Macrocitic anemia
  - Elevated cholesterol
  - Elevated creatine phosphokinase, lactate dehydrogenase, aspartate aminotransferase
  - Hyponatremia
- Subclinical hypothyroidism
  - TSH elevated (>4.5 mIU/L)
  - Serum free T_4 normal (2)[A]
  - Note: Serum free triiodothyronine (T_3) or total T_3 should not be done to diagnose hypothyroidism (1)[A].

Follow-Up Tests & Special Considerations

- Antithyroid antibodies may define the cause of primary hypothyroidism but are not necessary in all settings.
- Drugs that may alter lab results:
  - Drugs that decrease TSH
    - Thyroid supplement, cortisone, dopamine, octreotide
  - Drugs that increase TSH:
    - Phenytoin, amiodarone, dopamine antagonist (metoclopramide/domperidone, salicylates, oral colecystographic dyes [sodium ipodate]), or estrogen or androgen in excess of replacement
- Disorders that may alter lab results:
  - Any severe illness, pregnancy, chronic protein malnutrition, hepatic failure, or nephrotic syndrome

Test Interpretation

- SCREENING
  - Patient with risks factors
    - H/o autoimmune disease, DM type 1
    - H/o previous radioactive iodine therapy
    - H/o neck or head radiation
    - Family history of thyroid disease
    - Use of medications that may impair thyroid function
    - Clinical evidence of goiter

- Patient with laboratory or imaging abnormalities
  - Substantial hyperlipidemia or change in lipid pattern
  - Hyponatremia, often resulting from inappropriate production of antidiuretic hormone
  - High serum muscle enzyme concentrations
  - Macrocytic anemia
  - Pericardial or pleural effusion
  - Pituitary or hypothalamic disorder
- Pregnant women
  - Personal or family history of thyroid disease
  - DM type 1
  - Personal history of thyroid peroxidase antibodies
  - H/o recurrent miscarriage, morbid obesity, or infertility, thyroid peroxidase antibody (TPOAb) should be considered (1)[A].

• Recommendations by expert groups
  - U.S. Preventive Services Task Force does not recommend routine screening for children or adults (1)[A].
  - ATA recommend screening in all adults at age 35 years and every 5 years thereafter.
  - AACE recommend screening older patients, especially women.

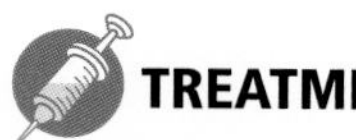

TREATMENT

MEDICATION

First Line

• Levothyroxine (Synthroid, Levothroid)
  - 1.6 μg/kg/day; increase by 12–25 μg/day every 4–6 weeks until TSH in normal range
  - Dosage requirements may vary with age, gender, residual secretory capacity of thyroid gland, other drugs being taken by patient, and intestinal function (1)[A].
  - Elderly patients may require 2/3 of dose used in young adults because clearance is decreased.
  - Levothyroxine should be taken on an empty stomach, ideally an hour before breakfast. Administering at bedtime may result in higher levels than administering in the morning (3)[A].
  - Medications that interfere with its absorption should be taken 4 hours after the T_4 dose: ferrous sulfate, proton pump inhibitors, calcium carbonate, bile acid resins.

• Contraindications
  - Thyrotoxic heart disease
  - Uncorrected adrenocorticoid insufficiency
  - MI, acute
  - TSH suppression, preexisting

• Precautions
  - Start with lower doses, such as 25 μg, in elderly and in patients with heart disease.
  - Diabetic patients may need readjustment of hypoglycemic agents with institution of thyroxine (T_4).
  - Dosage of oral anticoagulants may need adjustment; monitor prothrombin time while initiating treatment.

• Significant possible interactions
  - Oral anticoagulants, insulin, oral hypoglycemic, estrogen, oral contraceptives, cholestyramine, proton pump inhibitors,
  - Ferrous sulfate, calcium carbonate, antacids, laxatives, colestipol, sucralfate, ciprofloxacin, and cholestyramine may decrease absorption.
  - Malabsorption of levothyroxine in celiac disease

• Controversy exists whether subclinical hypothyroidism should be treated. Cochrane Review found no improvement in survival, cardiovascular morbidity, or health-related quality of life. Some evidence indicates improvement in lipid profiles and left ventricular function. Subclinical hypothyroidism should be treated in patients with iron deficiency anemia and in patients with TSH >10 (2,4,5)[B].

Pregnancy Considerations

• Replacement therapy may need adjustment; average dose increase from 25 to 50% (6)[A].
• TSH levels should be monitored monthly during 1st trimester; goal TSH of 2–2.5 mIU/L for 1st trimester, <3.0 mIU/L for 2nd trimester, and <3.5 mIU/L for 3rd trimester (6)[A]
• Postpartum: Check TSH levels at 6 weeks (6)[A].
• Painless subacute thyroiditis may occur in postpartum period, leading to transient hypothyroidism lasting 3 months. Treatment with replacement therapy may be warranted. Up to 30% of these individuals develop permanent hypothyroidism.

Second Line

• No benefit to adding T_3 to T_4 (6)[A]
• Desiccated thyroid hormone is not recommended for the treatment of hypothyroidism (1).

ISSUES FOR REFERRAL

• Children and infants
• Pregnancy
• Patient in whom it is difficult to render and maintain a euthyroid state
• Cardiac disease
• Presence of goiter, nodule, or other structural changes in the thyroid gland
• Presence of adrenal or pituitary disorders (1)[C]

INPATIENT CONSIDERATIONS

Admission Criteria/Initial Stabilization

Myxedema coma, hypothermia

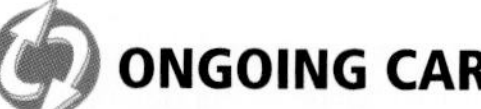

ONGOING CARE

FOLLOW-UP RECOMMENDATIONS

Patient Monitoring

• Monitor TSH and free T_4 every 4–8 weeks after initiating treatment or after change in dose. Once stabilized, periodic TSH level should be done after 6 months and then at 12-month intervals or more frequently if the clinical situation dictates otherwise (1)[B].
• Follow cardiac status closely in older patients.
• Check TSH more frequently in pregnancy, initiation of estrogen supplementation, or after large changes in body weight.
• In central hypothyroidism, TSH unreliable; must monitor free T_4 and T_3
• Thyroid hormones should not be used to treat obesity in euthyroid patients (1)[A].

PATIENT EDUCATION

• Stress importance of compliance with thyroid replacement therapy.
• Explain need for lifelong treatment.
• Instruct to report to physician any signs of infection or heart problems.
• Describe signs of thyrotoxicity.
• High-bulk diet may help avoid constipation.

PROGNOSIS

• Return to normal state is the rule.
• Relapses will occur if treatment is interrupted.
• If untreated, may progress to myxedema coma.

COMPLICATIONS

• Hypothyroid patients (mild to moderate) tolerate surgery, with mortality and complications similar to euthyroid patients.
• If surgery is elective, render patient euthyroid prior to procedure.
• If surgery is urgent, proceed with procedure with individualized replacement therapy preoperatively and postoperatively.
• Treatment-induced congestive heart failure in people with coronary artery disease
• Myxedema coma: mortality 30–60%
• Increased susceptibility to infection
• Megacolon
• Sexual dysfunction
• Organic psychosis with paranoia
• Adrenal crisis with vigorous treatment of hypothyroidism, especially in patients with undiagnosed polyendocrine syndromes
• Infertility
• Hypersensitivity to opiates
• Treatment over long periods can lead to bone demineralization.
• Subclinical hypothyroidism is associated with increased ischemic heart disease and increased all-cause mortality in men but not in women.

REFERENCES

1. Garber JR, Cobin RH, Gharib H, et al. Clinical practice guidelines for hypothyroidism in adult: cosponsored by the American Association of Clinical Endocrinologist and American Thyroid Association. *Thyroid*. 2012;22(12):1200–1235.
2. Cooper DS, Biondi B. Subclinical thyroid disease. *Lancet*. 2012;379(9821):1142–1154.
3. Bolk N, Visser TJ, Nijman J, et al. Effects of evening vs morning levothyroxine intake: a randomized, double blind crossover trial. *Arch Int Med*. 2010; 170(22):1996–2003.
4. Khandelwal D, Tandon N. Overt and subclinical hypothyroidism: who to treat and how. *Drugs*. 2012;72(1):17–33.
5. Villar HC, Saconato H, Valente O, et al. Thyroid hormone replacement for subclinical hypothyroidism. *Cochrane Database Syst Rev*. 2007;(3):CD003419.
6. Alexander EK, Marqusee E, Lawrence J, et al. Timing and magnitude of increases in levothyroxine requirements during pregnancy in women with hypothyroidism. *N Engl J Med*. 2004;351(3):241–249.

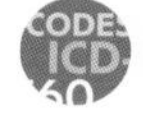

CODES

ICD10

• E03.9 Hypothyroidism, unspecified
• E06.3 Autoimmune thyroiditis
• E89.0 Postprocedural hypothyroidism

CLINICAL PEARLS

Monitor TSH and free T_4 every 4–8 weeks after initiating treatment or after change in dose. Once stabilized, periodic TSH level should be done after 6 months and then at 12 month-intervals or more frequently if the clinical situation dictates otherwise (1)[B].

• Screening test: TSH levels (1)[A]
• Serum free T_3 or total T_3 should not be done to diagnose hypothyroidism (1)[A]

H

ID REACTION

Jeremy Golding, MD, FAAFP

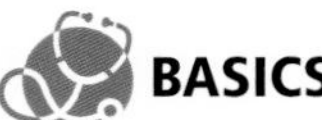

BASICS

DESCRIPTION

A generalized skin reaction associated with various infectious (fungal, bacterial, viral, or parasitic) or inflammatory cutaneous conditions distant from the primary disease site (1)

- "Id" is often combined with a root to reflect the causative factor (i.e., bacterid, syphilid, and tuberculid). Dermatophytid is the most frequently referenced id reaction. A dermatophytid is an autosensitization reaction in which a secondary cutaneous reaction occurs at a site distant to a primary fungal infection. The eruption typically begins within 1–2 weeks of the onset of the main lesion or following exacerbation of the main lesion.
- Most commonly localized vesicular lesions, erythema nodosum, and erythema multiforme
- System(s) affected: skin/exocrine
- Synonym(s): dermatophytid, trichophytid, autoeczematization

EPIDEMIOLOGY

- Predominant age: all ages
- Predominant sex: male = female
- Predominant race: all races

Incidence

Unknown

Prevalence

Common

ETIOLOGY AND PATHOPHYSIOLOGY

Precise pathophysiology is uncertain. Circulating antigens may react with antibodies at sensitized areas of the skin. An abnormal immune recognition of autologous skin antigens may also occur. Inflammation may alter the irritation threshold of the skin and the hematogenous spread of cytokines may also play a role.

- Etiology
  - Infectious
    - Fungal infections: *Trichophyton mentagrophytes*, *Trichophyton rubrum*, *Epidermophyton floccosum*, and *Candida* spp.
    - Bacterial infections: *Streptococcus pyogenes*, *Staphylococcus aureus*, and *Mycobacterium tuberculosis*
    - Viral infections: HSV, *Molluscum contagiosum*, orf, and milker's nodules
    - Parasitic infections: *Sarcoptes scabiei* and *Leishmania* spp.
  - Allergic
    - Id reactions occur in patients with nickel and aluminum allergy.
  - Miscellaneous
    - Id reaction rarely develop due to retained postoperative sutures.
    - Rarely, id reaction has been documented in patients receiving intravesical BCG live therapy for transitional cell carcinoma.

RISK FACTORS

- Fungal infection of the skin, especially tinea pedis
- Stasis dermatitis

GENERAL PREVENTION

- Good skin hygiene (particularly in intertriginous areas) to minimize risk of developing fungal infections
- Promptly treat any developing fungal infection.

COMMONLY ASSOCIATED CONDITIONS

- Primary fungal infection
- Stasis dermatitis

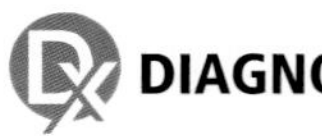

DIAGNOSIS

HISTORY

Itchy rash: Inquire about presence of lesions (typically fungal or bacterial) that could have incited the id reaction in the preceding days to weeks.

PHYSICAL EXAM

- Common
  - Symmetric, pruritic vesicles on the palms and, most commonly, on lateral aspects of fingers
  - Tinea infection on the feet; contact or other eczematous dermatosis; bacterial, fungal, or viral infection of the skin
- Less common
  - Papules
  - Lichenoid eruption
- Eczematoid eruption

DIFFERENTIAL DIAGNOSIS

- Pompholyx (dyshidrotic eczema)
- Contact dermatitis
- Drug eruptions
- Pustular psoriasis
- Folliculitis
- Scabies

DIAGNOSTIC TESTS & INTERPRETATION

- Potassium hydroxide (KOH) or fungal culture of primary lesion
- No fungal elements are present at the site of the id reaction.
- Special tests: Skin shows a positive trichophyton reaction. A wheal >10 mm at 20 minutes and induration >5 mm at 72 hours is a positive response.

Follow-Up Tests & Special Considerations

- The id reaction resolves with successful eradication of the primary skin condition.
- It is important to distinguish dermatophytids from drug-induced allergic reactions, as continued treatment is essential to clear the underlying infection.

Test Interpretation

- Histology
  - Vesicles in the upper dermis
  - Superficial perivascular lymphohistiocytic infiltrate with small numbers of eosinophils and increased granular cell layer
  - No infectious agents present in biopsy specimen

TREATMENT

GENERAL MEASURES

- Outpatient treatment of the underlying infection or eczematous dermatitis
- Symptomatic treatment of pruritus with antihistamines and/or topical steroids if needed (may require class 1 or 2 steroid)
- Treatment for secondary bacterial infection

MEDICATION

First Line

- PO antihistamines for pruritus (2)
  - Chlorpheniramine: 4 mg PO q4–6h PRN; max 24 mg/24 hr; (pediatric: 6–11 years 2 mg PO q4–6h PRN; max 12 mg/24 hr; ≥12 years, refer to adult dosing)
  - Diphenhydramine: 25–50 mg PO q4–6h PRN; max 400 mg/24 hr; (pediatric: 5 mg/kg/24 hr divided q6h PRN; 2–5 years max 37.5 mg/24 hr; 6–11 years max 150 mg/24 hr; ≥12 years, refer to adult dosing)
  - Hydroxyzine: 25–100 mg PO q6–8h PRN; max 600 mg/24 hr; (pediatric: 2 mg/kg/24 hr divided q6h PRN)
- Topical treatments for pruritus
  - Triamcinolone 0.1% ointment TID
  - Hydrocortisone 0.5%, 1%, 2.5%: up to QID
  - Capsaicin 0.025%, 0.075% cream: Apply TID–QID; EMLA (2.5% lidocaine + 2.5% prilocaine) applied 30–60 minutes prior to capsaicin may minimize burning.
  - Doxepin 5% cream: Apply QID for up to 8 days (to max of 10% of the body).
  - Permethrin 5% cream (for scabies)
    - Apply from neck down after bath.
    - Wash off thoroughly with water in 8–12 hours.
    - May repeat in 7 days
  - Permethrin 1% cream rinse (for lice)
    - Shampoo, rinse, towel dry, saturate hair and scalp (or other affected area), leave on 10 minutes, then rinse.
    - May repeat in 7 days
  - White petroleum emollients: Apply after short bath/shower in warm (not hot) water.
- Systemic steroids only if reaction is severe or generalized (e.g., prednisone 20 mg)

Second Line

- Topical and/or systemic antifungals for identified associated fungal infection (common)
  - Tinea cruris/corporis
    - Topical azole antifungal compounds econazole (Spectazole) and ketoconazole (Nizoral): usually applied BID × 2–4 weeks
    - Terbinafine (Lamisil): over-the-counter (OTC) compound; can be applied daily or BID × 1–2 weeks
    - Butenafine (Mentax): applied once daily × 2 weeks; also very effective
  - Tinea capitis
    - PO griseofulvin for *Trichophyton* and *Microsporum* sp.; microsized preparation available; dosage 20–25 mg/kg/day divided BID or as a single dose daily × 6–12 weeks
    - PO terbinafine can be used for *Trichophyton* sp. at 62.5 mg/day in patients weighing 10–20 kg, 125 mg/day if weight 20–40 kg, 250 mg/day if weight >40 kg, and use for 4–6 weeks.
- Topical or systemic antibiotics for any secondary bacterial infection
- Treatment with antiviral agents for erythema multiforme associated with HSV is required.

ONGOING CARE

PATIENT EDUCATION

Avoid hot, humid conditions that promote fungal growth. Aerate susceptible body areas (e.g., wear sandals or open footwear). If possible, wear loose-fitting clothing and undergarments, dry wet skin after bathing, and use powders and antiperspirants to discourage fungal growth. Treat primary dermatitis promptly.

PROGNOSIS

After appropriate treatment, complete resolution in days to weeks

COMPLICATIONS

- Secondary bacterial infection (cellulitis)
- After resolution of dermatophytid, postinflammatory hyperpigmentation is common and disappears without treatment in 1 month.

REFERENCES

1. Ilkit M, Durdu M, Karakaş M. Cutaneous id reactions: a comprehensive review of clinical manifestations, epidemiology, etiology, and management. *Crit Rev Microbiol*. 2012;38(3):191–202.
2. Cotes MES, Swerlick RA. Practical guidelines for the use of steroid-sparing agents in the treatment of chronic pruritus. *Dermatol Ther*. 2013;26(2):120–134.

ADDITIONAL READING

- Elmariah SB, Lerner EA. Topical therapies for pruritus. *Semin Cutan Med Surg*. 2011;30(2):118–126.
- Greaves MW. Recent advances in pathophysiology and current management of itch. *Ann Acad Med Singapore*. 2007;36(9):788–792.
- Paulsen LL, Geller DD, Guggenbiller M. Symmetrical vesicular eruption on the palms. *Am Fam Physician*. 2012;85(8):811–812.
- Stachler RJ, Al-khudari S. Differential diagnosis in allergy. *Otolaryngol Clin North Am*. 2011;44(3):561–590, vii–viii.
- Veien NK. Acute and recurrent vesicular hand dermatitis. *Dermatol Clin*. 2009;27(3):337–353, vii.
- Yosipovitch G, Bernhard JD. Chronic pruritus. *N Engl J Med*. 2013;368(17):1625–1634.

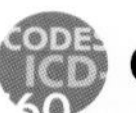

CODES

ICD10

- L30.2 Cutaneous autosensitization
- B35.9 Dermatophytosis, unspecified

CLINICAL PEARLS

- When one skin eruption follows another closely in time, consider an id reaction.
- When assessing an itchy rash, inquire about potential fungal or bacterial lesions in the preceding days to weeks as a potential prelude to the id reaction.

I

IDIOPATHIC THROMBOCYTOPENIC PURPURA

Kyu K. Jana, MD

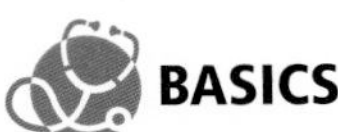

BASICS

DESCRIPTION

- Idiopathic thrombocytopenic purpura (ITP) is an acquired, isolated thrombocytopenia with platelet counts of $<100 \times 10^9$/L caused by accelerated destruction and/or impaired thrombopoiesis by antiplatelet antibodies.
- ITP is classified by the following:
  - Age: adult or pediatric
  - Phases: newly diagnosed (<3 months), persistent, and chronic (>12 months); or acute (<6 months) and chronic ITP (>6 months).
  - Etiology: primary (idiopathic) or secondary when occurring in association with another disorder
- ITP is a relatively common disease of childhood that often follows viral infection or vaccination. Onset is within 1 week, and spontaneous resolution occurs within 2 months in 83% of patients.
- In adults, ITP is usually a chronic disease and spontaneous remission is rare (9% in 1 series).
- System(s) affected: heme, lymphatic, immunologic
- Synonym(s): immune thrombocytopenia; immune thrombocytopenic purpura; and Werlhof disease

EPIDEMIOLOGY

- Peak age
  - Pediatric ITP: 2–4 years
  - Chronic ITP: >50 years with incidence 2 times higher in persons 60 years than those <60 years of age
- Predominant gender
  - Pediatric ITP: male = female
  - Chronic ITP: female > male (1.2–1.7:1)

Incidence

- Pediatric acute ITP, 1.9–6.4/100,000 children/year (1)
- Adult ITP, 3.3/100,000 per year

Prevalence

Limited data. In one population (in Oklahoma) (2):

- Overall prevalence of 11.2/100,000 persons
- In children (<16 years), 8.1/100,000 with average age of 6 years
- In adults (>16 years), 12.1/100,000 persons with average age of 55 years

ETIOLOGY AND PATHOPHYSIOLOGY

- Accelerated platelet uptake and destruction by reticuloendothelial phagocytes results from action of IgG autoantibodies against platelet membrane glycoproteins IIb/IIIa. There is also cell-mediated platelet destruction by $CD8^+$ T cells.
- Autoantibodies interfere with megakaryocyte maturation, resulting in decreased production.

RISK FACTORS

- Autoimmune thrombocytopenia (e.g., Evan syndrome)
- Common variable immune deficiency
- Drug side effect (e.g., quinidine, gold, penicillin, procainamide, methyldopa, sulfamethoxazole)
- Infections: *Helicobacter pylori*, hepatitis C, HIV, varicella zoster
- Vaccination side effect
- Bone marrow transplantation side effect
- Connective tissue disease, such as systemic lupus erythematosus, antiphospholipid antibody syndrome
- Lymphoproliferative disorders

COMMONLY ASSOCIATED CONDITIONS

- Viral infections, such as measles, rubella, varicella, influenza, and EBV
- Live virus vaccinations carry a lower risk than natural viral infection: 2.6/100,000 cases MMR vaccine doses versus 6–1,200/100,000 cases of natural rubella or measles infections.

DIAGNOSIS

A careful history, physical exam, and review of CBC and peripheral blood smear remain the key components of the diagnosis of ITP.

HISTORY

- Often asymptomatic; found incidentally on routine CBC
- Posttraumatic bleeding occurs at counts of 40–60 $\times 10^9$/L.
- With counts $<30 \times 10^9$/L, bruising tendency, epistaxis, menorrhagia, and gingival bleeding are common.
- GI bleeding, hematuria, and hemoptysis are less common.
- Spontaneous bleeding may occur with platelet count $<20 \times 10^9$/L.
- Intracerebral bleeding is rare and may occur with counts $<20 \times 10^9$/L and associated trauma or vascular lesions, resulting in neurologic symptoms.
- Constitutional symptoms are absent except for malaise. Symptoms are varied and most are asymptomatic at time of diagnosis.

PHYSICAL EXAM

- Ecchymoses, petechiae, epistaxis, and bleeding from the gums are common.
- Abnormal uterine bleeding may be present.
- Hemorrhagic bullae on buccal mucosa reflect acute, severe thrombocytopenia.
- Absence of splenomegaly is an essential diagnostic criterion. Also absent: hepatomegaly, lymphadenopathy, stigmata of congenital disease

DIFFERENTIAL DIAGNOSIS

- Acute leukemia
- Thrombotic thrombocytopenic purpura
- Hemolytic uremic syndrome
- Factitious: platelet clumping on peripheral smear
- Thrombocytopenia secondary to sepsis
- Myelodysplastic syndrome, particularly in older patients
- Decreased marrow production: malignancy, drugs, viruses, megaloblastic anemia
- Posttransfusion
- Gestational thrombocytopenia
- Isoimmune neonatal purpura
- Congenital thrombocytopenias
- Disseminated intravascular coagulation
- Alcohol-induced thrombocytopenic purpura

DIAGNOSTIC TESTS & INTERPRETATION

Initial Tests (lab, imaging)

- CBC with differential and peripheral smear:
  - Isolated decreased platelet count $<100 \times 10^9$/L
  - Giant platelets are usually present.
- For patients with history, exam, CBC, and peripheral smear typical of ITP, only the following tests may be needed:
  - PT/PTT is normal.
  - In adults, serologies for hepatitis B, hepatitis C, and HIV infections are recommended (3)[B].
  - In pediatric ITP, immunoglobulin levels to exclude common variable immunodeficiency are commonly obtained (3)[B].
  - Other tests are not necessary for patients with typical ITP presentation (3): antiplatelet, antinuclear, antiphospholipid antibodies; *H. pylori* testing; thrombopoietin; platelet parameters; direct antiglobulin test; reticulocyte count; urinalysis; and thyroid function tests.

Diagnostic Procedures/Other

- Imaging is not necessary.
- Bone marrow aspiration/biopsy
  - Not part of routine workup and not necessary for diagnosis irrespective of age of patients presenting with typical ITP or for children failing first-line therapy (pediatric (3)[B]; adult (3)[C])
  - Can be considered for a patient with atypical symptoms, such as fever and weight loss and multiple abnormalities in blood count

Test Interpretation

- Peripheral smear: normal red and white cells with large or giant platelets but diminished in number
- Marrow reveals abundant megakaryocytes with normal erythroid and myeloid precursors.

TREATMENT

GENERAL MEASURES

- Management with observation alone in children with no or mild bleeding (not more than bruising and petechiae) regardless of platelet count (3)
- Outpatient management unless patient has platelet count $<20 \times 10^9$/L and is at risk for bleeding (3)
- Admit patients with active bleeding.

MEDICATION

First Line

- Pediatric
  - First-line treatment:
    - For children with no or mild bleeding (bruising and petechiae only and no mucosal bleeding), observation alone regardless of platelet count (3)[B]
    - For children with significant bleeding
      - Single-dose intravenous immunoglobulin (IVIG) 0.8–1 g/kg, especially when a more rapid increase in platelet count is desired (3)[B]. Do not administer in patients with IgA deficiencies because of anaphylaxis risk.
      - A short course of corticosteroids (e.g., PO prednisone 2 mg/kg/day for 2 weeks with 3 weeks taper) (3)[B]
      - For nonsplenectomized children who are Rh-positive, single dose of anti-Rho(D) immunoglobulin (anti-D), 50–75 g/kg. Do not use in children with low hemoglobin or evidence of hemolysis (3)[B].
  - Second and other treatments for pediatric and adolescent persons with ITP (3)
    - Splenectomy for chronic or persistent ITP (3)[B]
    - Rituximab (Rituxan) 375 mg/m^2 weekly for 4 weeks (3)[C]
    - High-dose dexamethasone 0.6 mg/kg/day for 4 days every 4 weeks (3)[C]
    - Others without adequate data: azathioprine, cyclosporin A, danazol, mycophenolate mofetil, anti-CD52 monoclonal antibody, and interferon

- Adult
  - First line, adult ITP
    - Treatment is recommended for newly diagnosed patients with platelet count <30 × 10^9/L (3)[C].
    - Longer course of corticosteroids preferred (e.g., PO prednisone 1 mg/kg/day for 21 days then tapered with addition of IVIG to corticosteroids when a more rapid increase in platelet count is required) (3)[B]
    - If corticosteroids are contraindicated
      - IVIG, 1–2 g/kg once, repeating as necessary (3)[C]
      - *OR* anti-D, 50–75 μg/kg once, repeating as necessary for Rh+, nonsplenectomized patients. Do not use anti-D in patients with low hemoglobin or evidence of hemolysis (3)[C].
  - Second line, adult ITP
    - Splenectomy for patients who failed corticosteroid therapy (3)[B]
    - For patients for whom splenectomy is contraindicated, thrombopoietin receptor agonists (3)[B]: eltrombopag (Promacta), 50 mg/day PO *OR* romiplostim (Nplate), 1 μg/kg SC weekly; may be used for patients at high risk of bleeding.
    - Rituximab, 375 mg/m^2 IV weekly for 4 weeks, for patients at high risk of bleeding who have failed one line of therapy or post splenectomy (3)[C]
    - Consider combination therapy with dexamethasone and rituximab (4)[C].
    - Thrombopoietin receptor agonists can be considered for patients at risk of bleeding who failed first line of therapy (3)[C].
    - Others to consider: azathioprine, cyclosporine A, cyclophosphamide, danazol, dapsone, mycophenolate mofetil, and vincristine
    - ITP in pregnancy
  - Preeclampsia or gestational thrombocytopenia may cause thrombocytopenia unrelated to ITP.
  - Corticosteroids or IVIG are considered safe and are considered first line (4)[C].
  - ITP management at time of delivery is based on maternal bleeding risks, and mode of delivery should be based on obstetric indications (4)[C]. Platelet autoantibodies can cross the placenta and cause neonatal thrombocytopenia.
  - Caesarean section can be considered if platelet count >50 × 109/L.
  - Prednisone and/or IVIG may be considered 2–3 weeks prior to delivery.
- ITP secondary to HIV
  - Antivirals should be considered before other treatment (3)[C].
  - If treatment is required, corticosteroids, IVIG, or anti-D are 1st-line options; and splenectomy is a 2nd-line option (3)[C].
- ITP secondary to HCV
  - Antivirals should be considered before other treatment (3)[C].
  - If treatment required, IVIG is initial treatment (3)[C].
- EMERGENCY TREATMENT
  - Patients with intracranial or GI bleeding, massive hematuria, internal hematoma, or who need emergent surgery.
  - IV corticosteroids (e.g., IV methylprednisolone, 1 g/day for 3 days) (3)[B] with caution in patients with GI bleeding and/or IVIG 1 g/kg, repeat following day for count <50 × 109/L (3)[B].
  - Platelet transfusions with IVIG may also be considered for significant bleeding (3)[C].
  - Other agents that may be considered: Recombinant factor VIIa (3)[C] not only promotes hemostasis but also increases risk of thrombosis. Efficacy of antifibrinolytic agents, aminocaproic acids, and tranexamic acid, is unproved; they may be used as adjunctive treatments only. Emergent splenectomy has been reported.

ISSUES FOR REFERRAL

Hematology consultation is recommended for acute bleeding or for those who fail to respond to first-line therapies.

ADDITIONAL THERAPIES

Proprietary traditional Chinese medicines: Dihuang Zhixue (blend of Rehmannia root and others herbs) showed benefit for childhood refractory ITP in a single, small, randomized controlled trial (5); limited evidence for Kami-kihi-to, minor decoction of *Bupleurum*, replenishing qi and tonifying kidney, roasted licorice decoction, Sairei-to, Shengxueling, and Zhinu-I and Zhinu-II (6). Unclear evidence for active hexose correlated compound, berberine, dong quai, ginseng, licorice, melatonin, and periwinkle. (7)

SURGERY/OTHER PROCEDURES

Splenectomy

- Mortality rate is very low (<1%) even in patients with severe thrombocytopenia.
- Necessary vaccinations prior to splenectomy: polyvalent pneumococcal vaccine and quadrivalent meningococcal vaccine every 3–5 years and 1-time *Haemophilus influenzae B* (Hib).
- Consider lifelong prophylactic antibiotics with penicillin or erythromycin.
- Should raise the platelet count to at least 20 × 10^9/L prior to surgery
- Reported 5–10-year efficacy is ~65% for all patients.
- Laparoscopic splenectomy has similar long-term outcomes compared to open splenectomy and has better short-term outcomes (8)[C].

ONGOING CARE

FOLLOW-UP RECOMMENDATIONS

Patient Monitoring

Platelet counts weekly for patients on prednisone and monthly for stable patients are reasonable.

DIET

- Evidence demonstrating benefit of an anti-inflammatory diet in ITP is lacking.
- The following foods and supplements can cause significant bleeding: garlic, ginger, *Gingko biloba*, and saw palmetto.
- Some foods and supplements that may inhibit platelets: evening primrose oil, fish oil, feverfew, ginseng, licorice, soy, vitamin C, vitamin E, and wintergreen.
- Partial list of foods and supplements with coumarin or salicylate components: alfalfa, angelica, anise, asafetida, aspen bark, birch, black cohosh, celery, chamomile, cinnamon, dandelion, fenugreek, heartsease, horse chestnut, meadowsweet, poplar, prickly ash, quassia, sarsaparilla, sweet birch, sweet clover, and willow bark.

PATIENT EDUCATION

- Modified activity to prevent injury or bruising; avoid contact sports.
- Avoid anticoagulants, aspirin and other platelet-inhibiting drugs, and NSAIDs.

PROGNOSIS

- Acute ITP
  - ~80–85% of patients completely recover within 2 months.
  - 15% proceed to chronic ITP.
- Chronic ITP
  - ~10–20% of the patients recover spontaneously.
  - Remainder with diminished platelets for months to years
  - May see spontaneous remissions (5%) and relapses
- ~10% are refractory (fail medical therapy and splenectomy).

COMPLICATIONS

- Related to thrombocytopenia: 1% mortality due to intracranial hemorrhage and severe blood loss
- Related to treatment: for example, corticosteroid adverse effects, anaphylaxis and renal failure with IVIG, hepatotoxicity with eltrombopag, reports of progressive multifocal leukoencephalopathy with rituximab, hemolysis with anti-D, and septicemia for splenectomized patients

REFERENCES

1. Terrell DR, Beebe LA, Vesely SK, et al. The incidence of immune thrombocytopenic purpura in children and adults: a critical review of published reports. *Am J Hematol*. 2010;85(3):174–180.
2. Terrell DR, Beebe LA, Neas BR, et al. Prevalence of primary immune thrombocytopenic purpura in Oklahoma. *Am J Hematol*. 2012;87(9):848–852.
3. Neunert C, Lim W, Crowtha M, et al. The American Society of Hematology 2011 evidence-based practice guideline for immune thrombocytopenia. *Blood*. 2011;117(16):4190–4207.
4. Gudbrandsdottir S, Birgens HS, Frederiksen H, et al. Rituximab and dexamethasone vs dexamethasone monotherapy in newly diagnosed patients with primary immune thrombocytopenia. *Blood*. 2013;121(11):1976–1981.
5. Liu QC, Wu WH, Wu DY, et al. Clinical observation on the treatment of childhood refractory idiopathic thrombocytopenic purpura with Dihuang Zhixue Capsule. *Chin J Integr Med*. 2008;14(2):132–136.
6. http://www.pdsa.org/
7. https://naturalmedicines.therapeuticresearch.com/databases.aspx
8. Qu Y, Xu J, Jiao C, et al. Long-term outcomes of laparoscopic splenectomy versus open splenectomy for idiopathic thrombocytopenic purpura. *Int Surg*. 2014;99(3):286–290.

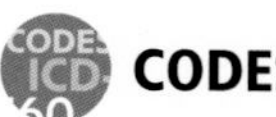

CODES

ICD10

D69.3 Immune thrombocytopenic purpura

CLINICAL PEARLS

- ITP: platelet counts of <100 × 10^9/L caused by accelerated destruction and/or impaired thrombopoiesis by antiplatelet antibodies
- Pediatric ITP: relatively common, with spontaneous remission in 2 months
- Adult ITP: usually persistent; requires treatment, with rare spontaneous remission

I

IGA NEPHROPATHY

Mony Fraer MD, FACP, FASN

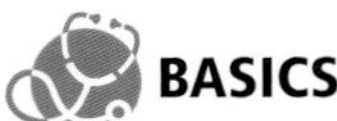

BASICS

DESCRIPTION

- Most common form of glomerulonephritis in the world (particularly high incidence in Asia), resulting from deposition of large amounts of a modified IgA molecule in the glomerular mesangium
- Heterogeneous condition ranging from asymptomatic all the way to end-stage renal disease (ESRD)

EPIDEMIOLOGY

Incidence

30–40% in Asia, 15–20% in Europe, and 5–10% in North America of all renal biopsy performed

Prevalence

- More common in Asians (particularly in Japan and Korea), Caucasians, and American Indians
- Less common in African Americans in the United States and Africa
- Most common in 2nd and 3rd decades of life
- More common in male than female patients

ETIOLOGY AND PATHOPHYSIOLOGY

Autoimmune disease: Underglycated IgA1 deposition within the mesangium leads to an inflammatory reaction (autoantibodies, complement, growth factors) that culminates with glomerular and subsequently renal tubulointerstitial scaring.

Genetics

Rare familial forms of IgA nephropathy exist.

COMMONLY ASSOCIATED CONDITIONS

Diseases associated with glomerular IgA deposition and secondary forms of IgA nephropathy (1)

- Henoch-Schönlein purpura
- Diseases of the liver (alcoholic, primary biliary, or cryptogenic cirrhosis, etc.)
- Diseases of the intestine (celiac disease, inflammatory bowel disease)
- Diseases of the skin (dermatitis herpetiformis, psoriasis)
- Diseases of the lung (sarcoidosis, idiopathic pulmonary hemosiderosis, cystic fibrosis, etc.)
- Malignancy
- Infection (HIV)
- Other systemic or immunologic disorders (systemic lupus erythematosus, rheumatoid arthritis, cryoglobulinemia, etc.)

DIAGNOSIS

HISTORY

- Classically, it presents with a painless recurrent episodes of macroscopic hematuria concurrent to or immediately after viral URIs.
- Wide spectrum from asymptomatic microscopic hematuria to acute renal failure

PHYSICAL EXAM

- Hypertension
- Edema

DIFFERENTIAL DIAGNOSIS

Other conditions associated/presenting with microscopic hematuria:

- Thin basement membrane disease
- Alport syndrome
- Lupus nephritis
- Postinfectious glomerulonephritis
- Nephrolithiasis
- Urinary tract malignancy
- Henoch-Schönlein purpura (also presenting with IgA deposition)

DIAGNOSTIC TESTS & INTERPRETATION

Initial Tests (lab, imaging)

- Serum BUN and creatinine to evaluate for renal insufficiency
- Complement levels should be normal.
- Urinalysis with microscopy to evaluate for proteinuria, hematuria, dysmorphic RBCs and RBC casts
- Spot urine protein to creatinine ratio or 24-hour urine protein
- Imaging may be indicated to rule out other urologic causes of hematuria.

Diagnostic Procedures/Other

Renal biopsy is the gold standard and the only definitive method for the diagnosis IgA nephropathy.

Test Interpretation

- Light microscopy: variable findings ranging from mesangial cell proliferation and expansion to crescentic or chronic sclerosing glomerulonephritis
- Immunofluorescence staining: pathognomonic finding of IgA deposits in a diffuse pattern within the mesangium
- Electron microscopy: electron-dense deposits in the mesangium

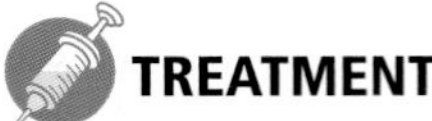

TREATMENT

GENERAL PRINCIPLES

- Therapeutic options are limited to the nonspecific treatment to reduce proteinuria and control blood pressure.
- Monitor low-risk patients with no hypertension, normal GFR, and proteinuria <0.5 g/day.
- Supportive treatment with angiotensin-converting enzyme inhibitor (ACEI) or angiotensin receptor blocker (ARB) is the cornerstone of the treatment.
- Strategies to control intrarenal inflammation include the administration of fish oil and for severe disease, the use of immunosuppressive agents such as cyclophosphamide, glucocorticosteroids, and mycophenolate mofetil.
- Good, randomized clinical trials to determine optimal treatments are still lacking.

MEDICATION

First Line

- Antiproteinuric and antihypertensive ACEI or ARB to achieve BP target of 130/80 mm Hg (125/75 mm Hg if proteinuria is >1 g/day) and decrease proteinuria to <0.5 g/day (2)[A]
- 6-month trial of pulse or oral corticosteroids in addition to RAS blockade in patients with persistent (>3–6 months) proteinuria (>1 g/day) (3,4)[B]
- Cyclophosphamide in combination with steroids has been shown to improve renal survival in patients with crescentic forms of IgA nephropathy if estimated GFR is > 30 mL/min (5)[B].

Second Line

Omega-3 fatty acids in large doses (12 g/day) may be beneficial in preserving renal function for persistent proteinuria despite ACEI/ARB use (6)[B].

ISSUES FOR REFERRAL

Any patients with hematuria, proteinuria, or abnormal renal function should be referred to a nephrologist early.

ADDITIONAL THERAPIES

Prevention of CKD progression and its consequence

- Lipid-lowering therapies with a statin (±ezetimibe)
- Low-salt diet (± diuretics)
- Antihypertensives
- Smoking cessation, etc.

SURGERY/OTHER PROCEDURES

Consider referring for kidney transplant evaluation when the patient is reaching CKD stage 5.

INPATIENT CONSIDERATIONS

Admission Criteria/Initial Stabilization

Acute kidney injury or complications related to CKD

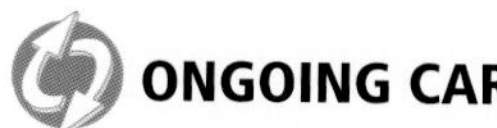

ONGOING CARE

FOLLOW-UP RECOMMENDATIONS

- Patients with mild proteinuria (<500 mg/day), normal renal function, and normal BP may be treated conservatively with regular follow-up at 6-month intervals.
- Patients with more aggressive disease characterized by persistent hematuria, higher grade proteinuria, difficult-to-control hypertension, or decreased GFR will require closer monitoring.

Patient Monitoring

- BP
- Serum electrolytes
- Serum creatinine
- Urine microscopy to evaluate disease activity
- Quantification of urine protein

DIET

Low-sodium diet

PATIENT EDUCATION

- Avoid NSAIDs.
- Avoid IV contrast exposure.
- In patients approaching ESRD, educate the patient regarding options for renal replacement therapy.

PROGNOSIS

- Hypertension, heavy/persistent proteinuria (>1 g/day), decreased GFR, and advanced histologic findings are risk factors for progressing of CKD (7).
- Specific histologic findings also have some prognostic significance.

COMPLICATIONS

- 25–30% of patients will require RRT (e.g., dialysis, transplant) within 20–25 years of presentation (8).
- 1.5% of patients reach ESRD each year (8)
- 5% risk of kidney graft failure secondary to a recurrent IgA nephropathy 5 years after renal transplant (8)

REFERENCES

1. Donavio JV, Grande JP. IgA nephropathy. *N Engl J Med*. 2002;347(10):738–748.
2. Cheng J, Zhang W, Zhang XH, et al. ACEI/ARB therapy for IgA nephropathy: a meta analysis of randomized controlled trials. *Int J Clin Pract*. 2009; 63(6):880–888.
3. Cheng J, Zhang X, Zhang W, et al. Efficacy and safety of glucocorticoids therapy for IgA nephropathy: a meta-analysis of randomized controlled trials. *Am J Nephrol*. 2009;30(4):315–322.
4. Manno C. Randomized controlled clinical trial of corticosteroids plus ACE-inhibitors with long-term follow-up in proteinuric IgA nephropathy. *Nephrol Dial Transplant*. 2009;24(12):3694–3701.
5. Tumlin J. Crescentic, proliferative IgA nephropathy: clinical and histological response to methylprednisolone and intravenous cyclophosphamide. *Nephrol Dial Transplant*. 2003;18(7):1321–1329.
6. Donadio JV Jr, Bergstralh EJ, Offord KP, et al. A controlled trial of fish oil in IgA nephropathy. Mayo Nephrology Collaborative Group. *N Engl J Med*. 1994;331(18):1194–1199.
7. Barbour SJ, Reich HN. Risk stratification of patients with IgA nephropathy. *Am J Kidney Dis*. 2012; 59(6):865–873.
8. Barratt J, Feehally J. IgA nephropathy. *J Am Soc Nephrol*. 2005;16(7):2088–2097.

ADDITIONAL READING

- Floege J, Eitner F. Current therapy for IgA nephropathy. *J Am Soc Nephrol*. 2011;22(10):1785–1794.
- Kidney Disease: Improving Global Outcomes (KDIGO) glomerulonephritis work group. KDIGO Clinical Practice Guideline for Glomerulonephritis. *Kidney Inter*. 2012;(Suppl 2):139–274.

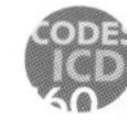

CODES

ICD10

N02.8 Recurrent and persistent hematuria w oth morphologic changes

CLINICAL PEARLS

- IgA nephropathy is the most common cause of glomerulonephritis in the world.
- It has a wide clinical spectrum ranging from asymptomatic microscopic hematuria to ESRD.
- Clinical risk factors for progressive disease are an abnormal GFR, hypertension, and moderate to severe proteinuria.
- Control of proteinuria and hypertension via RAAS blockade with ACE inhibitors or ARBs is the mainstay of therapy.

IMMUNODEFICIENCY DISEASES

Brian P. Peppers, DO, PhD • Robert W. Hostoffer, DO, FACOP, FACOI, FAAP, FCCP

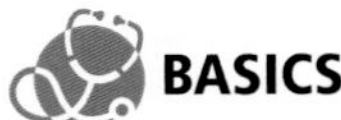

BASICS

DESCRIPTION

- Immunodeficiency can be either primary or secondary (acquired). There are numerous causes; each may lead to increased risk of infections, autoimmune diseases, and cancers.
- Primary immunodeficiency disease (PID): an intrinsic defect in the immune system affecting receptor function, cytoplasmic enzymes, and gene regulatory proteins. These defects affect the maturation and function of B cells, T cells, phagocytes, the complement system, and NK cells. Depending on the defect, effects may be seen directly or indirectly in ≥1 systems.
- B-cells: humoral immunodeficiencies: defects in antibody production that typically present as recurrent sinopulmonary or gastrointestinal infections. Most common form of PID (~2/3). Typically not seen before 6 months of age due to maternal antibodies:
  - IgA deficiency: most common primary immunodeficiency: Clinical symptoms range from asymptomatic/mild to severe. Sporadic more common than inherited. Spanish and Arabian populations more at risk than European (~1:150 to 1:400+). Asians at least risk (~1:2,600–1:18,000). Associated with autoimmune diseases such as rheumatoid arthritis (RA) (at any age) and systemic lupus erythematosus (SLE). Children <5 years presenting with IgA deficiency may outgrow it.
  - Common variable immunodeficiency: a heterogeneous form of severe antibody deficiency. Low immunoglobulins (IgG, IgA, and/or IgM) leave patients susceptible to pyogenic infections. Moderate to severe clinical systems are more common than mild/asymptomatic. Adult onset (mid-20s) more common than childhood. Sporadic (~90%) more common than inherited. Incidence for CVID 1:25,000–1:66,000. Northern European descent higher risk than African, Asian, and Hispanic. Men and women at equal risk. Similar risks and family history as with IgA deficiency. Treatment is important to prevent bronchiectasis, malabsorption, and vitamin deficiencies.
  - X-linked agammaglobulinemia (XLA): Xq22; Bruton tyrosine kinase. Recurrent infections with encapsulated bacteria after birth are common. Growth and development are usually normal. All serum immunoglobulins are extremely low. T and NK cells' function are preserved. Tonsils, adenoids, and peripheral lymph nodes are diminished in size.
  - Hyper-IgM syndrome (HIMG): Similar infections as XLA. *Pneumocystis jiroveci* pneumonia possible as initial. Defect of either B-cell isotype switching from IgM-secreting to IgG, A, or E (HIMG1-4: autosomal recessive [AR], NEMO) or helper T-cell inability to signal/activate B cells (X-linked: Xq26 and formerly a T-cell PID). Serum IgM concentration is polyclonal and normal to elevated.
  - Other examples: defects in Ig heavy chain gene, hypogammaglobulinemia
- T cells (cellular-mediated immunodeficiencies): defects in maturation or function of T-lymphocytes. Predisposed to infections such as *Candida*, parasite, and *P. jiroveci*:
  - 22q11.2 deletion syndrome/DiGeorge syndrome: defect of embryogenesis. Structures involved include thymus, parathyroid, and aortic arch. De novo or autosomal dominant (AD). Prevalence is ~1:4,000. Normally diagnosed in infancy. Characteristics (CATCH 22): cardiac abnormalities, hypognathus, long philtrum, low set ears, hypertelorism, downward slanted eyes, "carp-shaped" mouth, thymic abnormalities (absent thymic shadow), cleft palate, hypoparathyroidism
  - Immune dysregulation polyendocrinopathy enteropathy X- linked (IPEX): classically seen as a syndrome of diarrhea, polyendocrinopathy, and fatal infection in infancy. Involves neonatal-onset diabetes mellitus, hypothyroidism, enteritis (diarrhea/villous atrophy), hemolytic anemia and thrombocytopenia and dermatitis. Death normally occurs by 1–2 years of age. Missense mutations in FOXP3 result in impaired development and function of CD4+CD25 and regulatory T cells and may repress cytokine promoters.
- Combined immunodeficiencies: Defects in the cellular effector and humoral mechanisms directly involving a combination of B and T lymphocytes and NK cells. Typically present as failure to thrive, often associated with diarrhea and severe eczema:
  - Severe combined immunodeficiency (SCID): Depending on genetic mutation, patients may have absent T cells with/without impairment to B cells and/or NK cells. Presents in infancy with failure to thrive, recurrent or persistent thrush, and gastrointestinal illnesses. Prevalence 1/50,000–100,000. If treatment is unsuccessful or delayed, death normally occurs before 1–2 years of age. X-linked, AR, and known mutations in adenosine deaminase deficiency gene, purine nucleoside phosphorylase deficiency gene, interleukin-γ chain, *JAK3*, *CD45*, ZAP70, *RAG1*, and *RAG2*.
  - Others: Wiskott-Aldrich syndrome (X-linked), MHC II deficiency, and ataxia telangiectasia (AR)
- Phagocytic immunodeficiencies: defects in the function and/or quantity of phagocyte cells. Recurrent pyogenic infections such as staphylococcal and *Aspergillus, Klebsiella,* and *Pseudomonas*. Granuloma formation and poor wound healing are common.
  - Chronic granulomatous disease: 90% inherited disorder (X-linked and AR) of phagocytic cells; results from an inability of phagocytes to undergo respiratory burst (key enzyme: NADPH oxidase). Recurrent life-threatening bacterial and fungal infections, often involving lymph nodes, liver, spleen, and skin. Normally occurs early in life. X-linked: mutation of cytochrome gp91 or b558 genes, called CYBB. AR: chromosome 7, NCF1 (p47phox) gene.
  - Leukocyte adhesion deficiency: an AR disorder resulting in a dysfunction of cell surface adhesion. The defect is in CD18, important in stabilizing macrophage interaction with T cells and bacterial opsonization. Delayed separation of the umbilical cord may be seen in the neonatal period. Later in life, recurrent pyogenic infections without pus formation are common.
  - Glucose-6-phosphate dehydrogenase deficiency: X-linked (Xq28) defect preventing generation of NADPH via the hexose monophosphate shunt. Lack of NADPH oxidase produces a clinical picture similar to CGD. Differs by a later age of onset (>10 years); commonly presents as hemolytic anemia
  - Myeloperoxidase deficiency: facilitates the oxidation of chloride and iodide by hydrogen peroxide. Deficiency results in the attenuation of bactericidal PMNs activity. Most individuals are asymptomatic, but some may have recurrent candidal infections. AR: 17q21.3-q23
  - Other examples: Chediak-Higashi syndrome and lazy leukocyte syndrome
- Complement deficiencies: inherited or acquired and complete or partial
  - Classical (C1, C4, C2): immune complex diseases (e.g., discoid or systemic lupus erythematosus, pneumococcal infections)
  - Alternative (properdin, factor B, factor D): severe fulminant pyogenic neisserial infections with a high mortality rate
  - Mannose-binding lectin: recurrent infections, accelerated course of SLE and RA
  - Other examples: C3, factor H, and factor I (pyogenic bacterial infections). Terminal pathway C5–C9 (neisserial and bacterial infections)
- Gene regulatory protein defects
  - (STAT 1) Chronic mucocutaneous candidiasis: a heterogenous group of disorders involving recurrent *Candida* infections. May occur anywhere on the body and at any point in life. Disease can be familial (STAT 1: AD). Although *Candida* is the defining infection, it may expand to incorporate other organisms. Endocrine abnormalities are normally involved.
  - (STAT 3) Hyper-IgE syndrome: Recurrent severe staphylococcal abscesses (skin, lungs, and viscera). Characteristic facial features include prominent forehead, deep-set eyes, broad nasal bridge, wide fleshy nasal tip, mild prognathism, facial asymmetry, and hemihypertrophy. Extremely high serum IgE, elevated serum IgD, and normal concentrations of IgG, IgA, and IgM. STAT3 gene mutation (AD with incomplete penetrance).
- Secondary immunodeficiency disease: either acquired as a result of age, malnutrition, pregnancy, illness (autoimmune, cancers, leukemias, HIV), treatment(s) (chemotherapy, corticosteroids, immunosuppressants, radiation), or injury (burns, trauma). May be transient (newborn) or permanent (HIV). More common than PID and tend to be occur later in life.

GENERAL PREVENTION

- Early identification is key to prevent infection and possible comorbidity. For newborns with known family history, consider genetic counseling and prenatal diagnostic testing
- Proper hygiene and nutrition for all ages regardless of type of immunodeficiency
- For certain secondary immunodeficiencies such as HIV and hepatitis B and C, emphasize safe needle practices and safe sexual practices.

DIAGNOSIS

HISTORY

- Both a complete personal and family history is key to direct diagnosis; limits blood work, radiation exposure, and time invested for both patient and physician. Recurrent respiratory infections are the most common clinical manifestations of PID (1,2).
- 10 signs of possible primary immunodeficiency
  - ≥4 new ear infections in 1 year
  - ≥2 serious sinus infections in 1 year
  - ≥2 months on antibiotics with little effect
  - ≥2 pneumonias within 1 year
  - Failure to thrive
  - Recurrent deep skin or organ abscesses
  - Persistent thrush or fungal infections on skin
  - Need for IV antibiotics to clear an infection
  - ≥2 deep-seated infections (e.g., sepsis)
  - Family history of primary immunodeficiency
- Infection history and possible clues
  - Pneumococcus, *Haemophilus influenzae*, etc.: Think B-cell defect.
  - PCP, *Candida*, parasites: Think T-cell defect.
  - *Aspergillus, Klebsiella, Pseudomonas*: Think PMN defect.
  - Meningococcus: Think complement defect.
- Family history: similar symptoms, known PID, autoimmune diseases, early infant deaths, cancers, or hemolytic diseases
- Newborn screening: SCID testing is currently included in WI, MA, NY, CA, CT, MI, CO, MS, DE, FL, TX, MN, IA, PA, UT, and OH.

PHYSICAL EXAM

Varies with condition. Focus on skin, sinopulmonary, and gastrointestinal exam. Assess for lymphadenopathy.

DIAGNOSTIC TESTS & INTERPRETATION

Initial Tests (lab, imaging)

- Complete blood count with differential
- Serum protein electrophoresis for immunoglobulin levels, including IgG, IgA, IgM, and IgE
- X-rays or CT scans as indicated (if there is concern for SCID or DiGeorge, absent thymic shadow, PNA, abscesses)

Follow-Up Tests & Special Considerations

It is appropriate to consult an immunologist before ordering additional special testing (3,4):

- Flow cytometry to examine lymphocyte subsets (CD4, CD8, CD3, CD19, CD20) (3,5): helps to detect deficiency in T, B, NKT, and NK cells
- B-cell antibody responses to vaccines (e.g., pneumococcus): helps to test the function of the humoral systems response to antigens
- T-cell enumeration, mitogen/antigen stimulation, FISH
- Combined immunodeficiencies: T-cell enumeration, mitogen/antigen stimulation, ADA/PNP activity, ZAP 70, and IL2-γ chain evaluation
- Phagocyte immunodeficiencies: nitroblue tetrazolium test, dihydrorhodamine reductase test, chemiluminescence, biopsy of granules, chemotaxis assay
- Complement deficiencies: CH50, AH 50, individual complement components
- NK cell deficiency: NK-cell function test

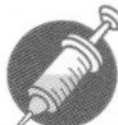

TREATMENT

GENERAL MEASURES

- Live viral vaccines should be avoided in patients with severe cellular or antibody immunodeficiencies. This includes intranasal influenza, varicella, zoster, measles, mumps, rubella, oral polio, smallpox, Bacille Calmette-Guérin, and yellow fever.
- Consult the CDC's Advisory Committee on Immunization Practices (ACIP) regarding vaccine safety for up-to-date recommendations (6).
- Patients receiving (or who have received) immunoglobulin replacement therapy (IgG) in the past 6 months are considered passively immune and do not require vaccination.
- Use irradiated, CMV-negative blood products for transfusion in patients with cellular or combined defects.
- Bone marrow, stem cell, or thymic transplants for certain immunodeficiencies such as SCID, MHC II, etc.

MEDICATION

- Highly variable depending on form and severity of PID or acquired immunodeficiency
- Antibiotics, antivirals, antifungal, antiparasitic agents: Specific to organism if known, broad coverage until known; may need prophylactic or chronic medications
- Immunoglobulin replacement therapy for the humoral deficiencies (e.g., CVID, XLA, HIMG)

ISSUES FOR REFERRAL

All individuals suspected of a primary immunodeficiency should be referred to a clinical immunologist.

ONGOING CARE

FOLLOW-UP RECOMMENDATIONS

Patient Monitoring

- Varies according to deficiency
- Recurrence of infections or failure to fully treat current infection
- Decline in respiratory function
- Patients on IgG should have levels checked regularly (<600 at risk for infections).
- Monitor for comorbid malignancies and/or autoimmune conditions.
- Malnutrition

PATIENT EDUCATION

Immune Deficiency Foundation, 40 West Chesapeake Ave. Suite 308, Towson, MD 21204. Tel: (800) 296-4433. www.primaryimmune.org.

PROGNOSIS

Highly variable; depends on specific deficiency and compliance with preventative and active treatments

COMPLICATIONS

- Immunoglobulin replacement therapy: allergic reactions, increased risk of blood clots
- Transplants: graft-versus-host disease, infection
- Frequent/prophylactic antibiotic use: development of resistant stains

REFERENCES

1. Bonilla FA, Bernstein IL, Khan DA, et al. Practice parameter for diagnosis and management of primary immunodeficiency. *Ann Allergy Asthma Immunol*. 2005;94(5 Suppl 1):S1–S63.
2. Notarangelo LD. Primary immunodeficiencies. *J Allergy Clin Immunol*. 2010;125(2 Suppl 2):S182–S194.
3. Oliveira JB, Fleisher TA. Laboratory evaluation of primary immunodeficiencies. *J Allergy Clin Immunol*. 2010;125(2 Suppl 2):S297–S305.
4. Orange JS, Ballow M, Stiehm ER, et al. Use and interpretation of diagnostic vaccination in primary immunodeficiency: a working group report of the Basic and Clinical Immunology Interest Section of the American Academy of Allergy, Asthma & Immunology. *J Allergy Clin Immunol*. 2012;130(3 Suppl):S1–S24.
5. Meyer-Bahlburg A, Renner ED, Rylaarsdam S, et al. Heterozygous signal transducer and activator of transcription 3 mutations in hyper-IgE syndrome result in altered B-cell maturation *J Allergy Clin Immunol*. 2012;129(2):559–562.
6. Principi N, Esposito S. Vaccine use in primary immunodeficiency disorders. *Vaccine*. 2014;32(30):3725–3731.

ADDITIONAL READING

- Bousfiha AA, Jeddane L, Ailal F, et al. Primary immunodeficiency diseases worldwide: more common than generally thought. *J Clin Immunol*. 2013;33(1):1–7.
- Chinen J, Shearer WT. Secondary immunodeficiencies, including HIV infection. *J Allergy Clin Immunol*. 2010;125(2 Suppl 2):S195–S203.
- DePiero AD, Lourie EM, Berman BW, et al. Recurrent immune cytopenias in two patients with DiGeorge/velocardiofacial syndrome. 1997;131(3):484–486.

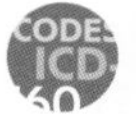

CODES

ICD10

- D84.9 Immunodeficiency, unspecified
- D80.9 Immunodeficiency with predominantly antibody defects, unspecified
- D80.2 Selective deficiency of immunoglobulin A [IgA]

CLINICAL PEARLS

- Patients with immunodeficiencies may appear healthier than they are due to attenuated inflammatory response.
- Patients with humoral deficiencies may have comorbid autoimmune illnesses with normal antibody testing.
- Patients with T-cell deficiencies may not react to purified protein derivative testing for TB.

IMPETIGO

Elisabeth L. Backer, MD

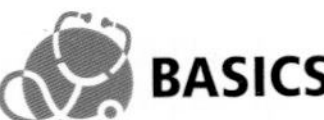

BASICS

DESCRIPTION

- A contagious, superficial, intraepidermal infection occurring prominently on exposed areas of the face and extremities
- Infected patients usually have multiple lesions.
- Cultures are positive in >80% cases for *Staphylococcus aureus* either alone or combined with group A β-hemolytic streptococci; *S. aureus* is the more common pathogen since the 1990s.
- Nonbullous impetigo: most common form of impetigo. Formation of vesiculopustules that rupture, leading to crusting with a characteristic golden appearance; local lymphadenopathy may occur.
- Bullous impetigo: staphylococcal impetigo that progresses rapidly from small to large flaccid bullae (newborns/young children) caused by epidermolytic toxin release; less lymphadenopathy; trunk more often affected; <30% of patients
- Folliculitis: considered by some to be *S. aureus* impetigo of hair follicles
- Ecthyma: a deeper, ulcerated impetigo infection often with lymphadenitis
- System(s) affected: skin/exocrine
- Synonym(s): pyoderma; impetigo contagiosa; impetigo vulgaris; fox impetigo

EPIDEMIOLOGY

Incidence

- Predominant sex: male = female
- Predominant age: children ages 2–5 years

Prevalence

In the United States: not reported but common

Pediatric Considerations

- Poststreptococcal glomerulonephritis may follow impetigo (in young children).
- Impetigo neonatorum may occur due to nursery contamination.

ETIOLOGY AND PATHOPHYSIOLOGY

- Coagulase-positive staphylococci: pure culture ~50–90%; more contagious via contact
- β-hemolytic streptococci: pure culture only ~10% of the time (primarily group A)
- Mixed infections of streptococci and staphylococci common; data suggest increasing importance of staphylococci over past 20 years.
- Direct contact or insect vector
- Can result from contamination at trauma site
- Regional lymphadenopathy

RISK FACTORS

- Warm, humid environment
- Tropical or subtropical climate
- Summer or fall season
- Minor trauma, insect bites, breaches in skin
- Poor hygiene, poverty, crowding, epidemics, wartime
- Familial spread
- Poor health with anemia and malnutrition
- Complication of pediculosis, scabies, chickenpox, eczema/atopic dermatitis
- Contact dermatitis (*Rhus* spp.)
- Burns
- Contact sports
- Children in daycare
- Possibly tobacco exposure
- Carriage of group A *Streptococcus* and *Staphylococcus aureus*

GENERAL PREVENTION

- Close attention to family hygiene, particularly hand washing among children
- Covering of wounds
- Avoidance of crowding and sharing of personal items
- Treatment of atopic dermatitis

COMMONLY ASSOCIATED CONDITIONS

- Malnutrition and anemia
- Crowded living conditions
- Poor hygiene
- Neglected minor trauma
- Any chronic/underlying dermatitis

DIAGNOSIS

HISTORY

- Lesions are often described as painful.
- May be slow and indolent or rapidly spreading
- Most frequent on face around mouth and nose or at site of trauma

PHYSICAL EXAM

- Tender red macules or papules as early lesions (contact dermatitis presents with pruritic lesions)
- Thin-roofed vesicles to bullae: usually nontender
- Pustules
- Weeping, shallow, red ulcers
- Honey-colored crusts
- Satellite lesions
- Often multiple sites
- Bullae on buttocks, trunk, face

DIFFERENTIAL DIAGNOSIS

- Nonbullous
  - Chickenpox
  - Herpes
  - Folliculitis
  - Erysipelas
  - Insect bites
  - Severe eczematous dermatitis
  - Scabies
  - Tinea corporis
- Bullous
  - Burns
  - Pemphigus vulgaris
  - Bullous pemphigoid
- Stevens-Johnson syndrome

DIAGNOSTIC TESTS & INTERPRETATION

Initial Tests (lab, imaging)

- None usually done; cultures of pus/bullae fluid may be helpful if no response to empiric therapy
  - Culture: taken from the base of lesion after removal of crust will grow both staphylococci and group A streptococci
  - Antistreptolysin-O (ASO) titer: can be weak positive for streptococci but overall not useful
  - Antideoxyribonuclease B (anti-Dnase B) and antihyaluronidase (AHT) response more reliable than ASO response
  - Streptozyme: positive for streptococci
- Disorders that may alter lab results: Streptococcal pharyngitis will alter streptococcal enzyme tests.

Follow-Up Tests & Special Considerations

- Monitor for spread of disease and systemic manifestations.
- Serologic testing helpful in context of impetigo with subsequent poststreptococcal glomerulonephritis

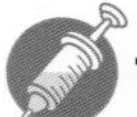

TREATMENT

GENERAL MEASURES

- Treatment speeds healing and avoids spread of disease.
- Prevent with mupirocin or triple antibiotic ointment TID to sites of minor skin trauma.
- Remove crusts; clean with gentle washing 2–3× daily; and clean with antibacterial soap, chlorhexidine, or Betadine.
- Washing of entire body may prevent recurrence at distant sites.

MEDICATION

- In 2005, the Infectious Diseases Society of America (IDSA) recommended topical treatment for limited lesions and oral medication when the disease is more severe/extensive (1)[A].
- Optimal treatment is unclear due to limited quality of evidence. Treatment reduces spread of infection and enhances resolution (2)[C].
- Penicillin and macrolide therapy is no longer recommended. Fluoroquinolones are not indicated due to resistance patterns.
- Consult the local hospital or health department for microbial resistance information.
- Nonbullous (minor spread, treat 7 days; widespread, treat 10 days); bullous (treat 10 days)
  - Retapamulin 1% ointment to be applied BID × 5 days
  - Mupirocin (Bactroban) 2% topical ointment applied TID × 7–10 days (nonbullous only); not as effective on scalp as around mouth
  - Dicloxacillin: adult 250 mg PO QID; pediatric <40 kg: 12–25 mg/kg/day divided q6h; >40 kg: 125–250 q6h
- Dicloxacillin, cephalexin, topical mupirocin, and fusidic acid are effective unless local staphylococcal strains are resistant. (For methicillin-resistant *S. aureus* [MRSA] infections, treatment options include clindamycin, tetracyclines, trimethoprim-sulfamethoxazole, or linezolid.) Oral doses given for 7 days are usually sufficient (3)[C].
- 1st-generation cephalosporins
  - Children
    - Cephalexin 25–50 mg/kg/day divided, q6h–q12h
    - Cefaclor 20–40 mg/kg/day divided q8h
    - Cephradine 25–50 mg/kg/day divided q6h–q12h
    - Cefadroxil 30 mg/kg/day divided BID
  - Adults
    - Cephalexin 250 mg up to QID
    - Cefaclor 250 mg TID
    - Cephradine 500 mg BID
    - Cefadroxil 1 g/day in divided doses
- Clindamycin 300 mg q6h–8h
- Severe bullous disease may require IV therapy such as nafcillin or cefazolin.

ISSUES FOR REFERRAL

If resistant or extensive infections occur, especially in immunocompromised patients

ADDITIONAL THERAPIES

Monitor for microbial resistance patterns.

ONGOING CARE

FOLLOW-UP RECOMMENDATIONS

- Athletes restricted from contact sports
- School and daycare contagious restrictions

Patient Monitoring

If not clear within 7–10 days, culture the lesions.

PATIENT EDUCATION

Avoidance of infection spread is the key; hand washing is vital, especially for reducing spread in children.

PROGNOSIS

- Complete resolution in 7–10 days with treatment
- Antibiotic treatment will not prevent or halt glomerulonephritis, as it will rheumatic fever.
- If not clear within 7–10 days, culture is necessary to find resistant organism.
- Recurrent impetigo: Evaluate for carriage of *S. aureus* in nares (also perineum, axillae, toe web). Apply mupirocin ointment to nares BID × 5 days for clearance/decolonization.

COMPLICATIONS

- Ecthyma
- Erysipelas
- Poststreptococcal acute glomerulonephritis
- Cellulitis
- Bacteremia
- Osteomyelitis
- Septic arthritis
- Pneumonia
- Lymphadenitis

REFERENCES

1. Koning S, van der Sande R, Verhagen AP, et al. Interventions for impetigo. *Cochrane Database Syst Rev*. 2012;1:CD003261.
2. Stevens DL, Bisno AL, Chambers HF, et al. Practice guidelines for the diagnosis and management of skin and soft-tissue infections. *Clin Infect Dis*. 2005;41(10):1373–1406.
3. Del Giudice P, Hubiche P. Community-associated methicillin-resistant *Staphylococcus aureus* and impetigo. *Br J Dermatol*. 2010;162(4):905–906.

ADDITIONAL READING

- George A, Rubin G. A systematic review and meta-analysis of treatments for impetigo. *Br J Gen Pract*. 2003;53(491):480–487.
- Parish LC, Jorizzo JL, Breton JJ, et al. Topical retapamulin ointment (1%, wt/wt) twice daily for 5 days versus oral cephalexin twice daily for 10 days in the treatment of secondarily infected dermatitis: results of a randomized controlled trial. *J Am Acad Dermatol*. 2006;55(6):1003–1013.
- Stanley JR, Amagai M. Pemphigus, bullous impetigo, and the staphylococcal scalded-skin syndrome. *N Engl J Med*. 2006;355(17):1800–1810.

SEE ALSO

Algorithm: Rash, Focal

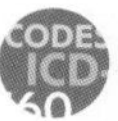

CODES

ICD10

- L01.00 Impetigo, unspecified
- L01.01 Non-bullous impetigo
- L01.03 Bullous impetigo

CLINICAL PEARLS

- Superficial, intraepidermal infection
- Predominantly staphylococcal in origin
- Microbial resistance patterns need to be monitored.
- Topical treatment is recommended for limited lesions and oral medication only when the disease is more severe/extensive.

I

INCONTINENCE, FECAL

Kalyanakrishnan Ramakrishnan, MD

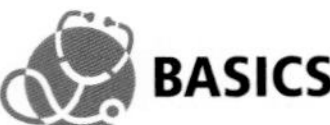

BASICS

Continuous or recurrent involuntary passage of fecal material through the anal canal for >1 month in an individual with a developmental age of at least 4 years

- Involves recurrent, involuntary loss of solid/liquid stool
- Requires careful rectal exam to assess rectal tone, voluntary squeeze, and rule out overflow incontinence from fecal impaction
- Endorectal ultrasound (EUS) is the simplest, most reliable, and least invasive test to detect anatomic defects in the anal sphincters.
- The goal of treatment is to restore continence and/or improve quality of life.

DESCRIPTION

Major incontinence is the involuntary evacuation of feces. Minor incontinence (fecal soilage) includes incontinence to flatus and occasional seepage of liquid stool.

Geriatric Considerations

- The prevalence of fecal incontinence increases with age. It is an important cause of nursing home placement, especially among the elderly.
- Idiopathic fecal incontinence is more common in older women.

EPIDEMIOLOGY

Incidence

Patients underreport fecal incontinence unless specifically queried ("silent affliction"). Studies underestimate the number of patients affected.

Prevalence

- In younger persons: women > men
- 8% of adults overall
- 15% of adults age >70 years
- 56–66% of hospitalized older patients and >50% in nursing home residents
- 50–70% of patients who have urinary incontinence also suffer from fecal incontinence.

Pregnancy Considerations

Obstetric injury to the pelvic floor may result in initial temporary incontinence or incontinence that persists.

Geriatric Considerations

- Fecal impaction and overflow diarrhea leading to fecal incontinence is common in older patients.
- Surgical history
  - Anal surgery, including hemorrhoidectomy, anal fissure repair (sphincterotomy), and anal dilatation, may predispose to fecal incontinence.
  - 3rd- and 4th-degree obstetric lacerations

ETIOLOGY AND PATHOPHYSIOLOGY

- Continence requires complex orchestration of pelvic musculature, nerves, and reflex arcs.
- Stool volume and consistency, colonic transit time, anorectal sensation, rectal compliance, anorectal reflexes, external and internal sphincter muscle tone, puborectalis muscle function, and mental capacity each play a role in maintaining fecal continence.
- Disease processes/structural defects impacting any of these factors may contribute to fecal incontinence.
- Diabetes is the most common metabolic disorder leading to fecal incontinence through pudendal nerve neuropathy.
- Congenital: spina bifida and myelomeningocele with spinal cord damage
- Trauma: anal sphincter damage from vaginal delivery and surgical procedures
- Medical: diabetes, stroke, spinal cord trauma, degenerative disorders of the nervous system, inflammatory conditions, rectal neoplasia

RISK FACTORS

- Physical status
  - Older age, female sex, obesity, limited physical activity
- Neuropsychiatric conditions
  - Multiple sclerosis, spinal cord injury, dementia, depression, stroke, diabetic neuropathy
- Trauma
  - Prostatectomy, radiation
  - Risk factors for perineal trauma at the time of vaginal delivery include occipitoposterior position, prolonged 2nd stage of labor, assisted vaginal delivery (forceps or vacuum-assist), and episiotomy.
- Others
  - Diarrhea, inflammatory bowel disease (IBD), irritable bowel syndrome (IBS), menopause, smoking, constipation
  - Potential association with child abuse and sexual abuse
  - Congenital abnormalities, such as imperforate anus/rectal prolapse
  - Fecal impaction

GENERAL PREVENTION

- Behavioral and lifestyle changes: Obesity, limited physical activity/exercise, poor diet, and smoking are modifiable risk factors.
- Postmeal bowel regimen—scheduling defecation regularly after meals, when gastrocolic reflex assists defecation
- Pelvic floor muscle training during and after pregnancy and pelvic surgery
- Increasing fiber intake

COMMONLY ASSOCIATED CONDITIONS

- Age >70 years
- Urinary incontinence/pelvic organ prolapse
- Chronic medical conditions—diabetes mellitus, dementia, stroke, spinal cord compression, depression, immobility, chronic obstructive pulmonary disease, IBS, and IBD
- Perineal trauma (most commonly obstetric)
- Surgeries in the anorectal area
- History of pelvic/rectal irradiation

DIAGNOSIS

Diagnosis of fecal incontinence is based on clinical history and physical findings.

HISTORY

- Patients seldom volunteer information about fecal incontinence, so direct questioning is important.
- Problem-specific history including the following (1)[C]:
  - Severity of soiling by liquid stool or gross incontinence of solid stool
  - Onset and duration (recent onset vs. chronic)
  - Frequency, presence of constipation/diarrhea
  - Medication review
  - Review diet, medical and obstetric history, lifestyle, and mobility.
- Evaluate for social withdrawal and depression

PHYSICAL EXAM

- Inspect the perineum for chemical dermatitis, hemorrhoids, fistula, surgical scars, skin tags, rectal prolapse, soiling, and ballooning of the perineum (sarcopenia of pelvic musculature).
- A patulous anal orifice may indicate myopathy/neurologic disorder.
- Evaluate the external sphincter response to perineal skin stimulation (anal wink). Absence suggests neuropathy.
- Ask the patient to bear down, preferably in standing position, to assess for rectal prolapse.
- Digital rectal exam to assess anal canal pressure sphincter tone, rectal bleeding, hemorrhoids, neoplasm, fecal consistency, and diarrhea/distal fecal impaction
- General neurologic examination, including perianal sensation (1)[C]
- Evaluation of mental status

DIFFERENTIAL DIAGNOSIS

- Anorectal disorders
  - Inflammatory/infectious disorders
  - Neoplasms, radiation proctitis, ischemic colitis, fistulas
  - Prolapsing internal hemorrhoids/rectal prolapse
  - Trauma: obstetric, surgical, radiation, accidental, sexual
- Neurologic disorders
  - Stroke, dementia, neoplasms, spinal cord injury, and/or diseases causing altered level of consciousness
  - Pudendal neuropathy, neurosyphilis, multiple sclerosis, diabetes mellitus
- Miscellaneous causes
  - Infectious diarrhea, fecal impaction and overflow, IBS, laxative abuse, IBD, short bowel syndrome, myopathies, senescence and frailty, collagen vascular disease, psychological and behavioral problems

DIAGNOSTIC TESTS & INTERPRETATION

History and physical exam are generally sufficient for diagnosis. If uncertainty remains, consider the following:

- EUS: the most reliable and least invasive test for defining anatomic defects in the external and internal anal sphincters, rectal wall, and the puborectalis muscle (1)[B]; can be used to predict therapeutic response to sphincteroplasty.
- Plain abdominal x-ray (impaction, constipation)
- Sigmoidoscopy/anoscopy/colonoscopy (colitis, neoplasm)

Initial Tests (lab, imaging)

- If history of travel, antibiotics, tube feedings, or signs and symptoms of sepsis, the following stool studies may be indicated:
  - Culture
  - Ova and parasites
  - *Clostridium difficile* toxin assay
- Thyroid-stimulating hormone (TSH), electrolytes, and BUN in elderly patients with fecal impaction

- EUS may demonstrate anal sphincters, rectal wall, and the puborectalis muscle structural abnormalities.
- EUS may detect a sphincter injury in over 1/3 of primiparous vaginal deliveries and nearly half of multipara delivering vaginally.
- The approach to fecal incontinence in older patients should be individualized, minimally invasive, and practically feasible.

Follow-Up Tests & Special Considerations
- Defecography can measure the anorectal angle, evaluate pelvic descent, and detect occult/overt rectal prolapse (2)[C].
- MRI defecography (dynamic MRI) can further define pelvic floor anatomy.
- Anorectal manometry: Measure parameters such as maximal resting anal pressure, amplitude and duration of squeeze pressure, the rectoanal inhibitory reflex, threshold of conscious rectal sensation, rectal compliance, and anorectal pressures during straining.
- Pudendal nerve terminal motor latency (PNTML): This technique is operator-dependent and has poor correlation with clinical symptoms and histologic findings.
- Electromyography: sometimes is helpful in evaluating neurogenic/myopathic damage in patients with fecal incontinence

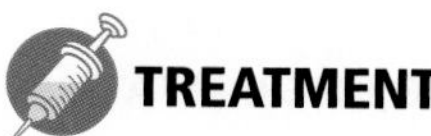

TREATMENT

GENERAL MEASURES
- In ambulatory patients, prompted and scheduled defecation is effective, particularly in patients with overflow incontinence.
- Pelvic floor (Kegel) exercises
- If bed-bound, scheduled osmotic or stimulant laxatives for constipation
- Enemas, laxatives, and suppositories may help promote more complete bowel emptying in impacted patients while minimizing postdefecation leakage.
- Scheduled toileting and use of stool deodorants (Periwash, Derifil, Devrom)

MEDICATION
Limited evidence that antidiarrheals (loperamide, codeine) and drugs enhancing sphincter tone (phenylepinephrine gel, sodium valproate) are of benefit (3)[B]. Cholestyramine, colestipol useful in diarrhea following malabsorption or cholecystectomy; alosetron in diarrhea due to IBS, amitriptyline in idiopathic fecal incontinence

First Line
Specific treatment of underlying disorder (e.g., infectious diarrhea/IBD) may improve fecal continence.

Second Line
- Increasing dietary fiber in milder forms of fecal incontinence reduces symptoms (1)[B]. Stool-bulking agents include high-fiber diet, psyllium products, or methylcellulose.
- Antidiarrheal agents, such as adsorbents or opium derivatives, may reduce fecal incontinence (1)[C].
- Patients with fecal impaction and overflow incontinence should be disimpacted and treated with a bowel regimen to prevent recurrence.

ADDITIONAL THERAPIES
- Biofeedback: initial treatment modality in motivated patients with some voluntary sphincter control (1)[C]; involves teaching patients to recognize rectal distension and contract the external anal sphincter while keeping intra-abdominal pressure low
- Biofeedback plus electrical stimulation is more effective than either alone.
- Patients with systemic neurologic disorders, anal deformities, or frequent episodes of incontinence respond poorly.

SURGERY/OTHER PROCEDURES
- Surgery should be considered only when nonsurgical approaches have failed.
- Sphincter repair should be offered for highly symptomatic patients with well-defined defect of external anal sphincter (1)[A].
- Injectable therapy (tissue-bulking agent injected into the anorectal submucosa or the intersphincteric space) appears safe and effective for patients with internal anal sphincter dysfunction (4)[B].
- Artificial anal sphincter implantation/dynamic graciloplasty (where gracilis muscle transposed into anus as modified sphincter) may be considered in patients with severe fecal incontinence with irreparable sphincter damage (5)[B].
- Stoma (colostomy/ileostomy) creation may be appropriate in patients with disabling fecal incontinence when other available therapeutic options have failed or when preferred by patient (1)[B].
- Anal plugs are another useful alternative, minimizing fecal leakage in patients who do not benefit from other treatment modalities, especially those immobilized, institutionalized, or neurologically disabled; often poorly tolerated (6)[C]
- Sacral nerve stimulation (neuromodulation) via implantation of SC electrodes delivering low-amplitude electrical stimulation to sphincter muscles improves overall rectal tone, especially in patients with a coexistent sphincter defect (7)[B].

INPATIENT CONSIDERATIONS

Admission Criteria/Initial Stabilization
If secondary to fecal impaction, manual evacuation of fecal mass (after lubrication with lidocaine jelly)

Nursing
- Avoid catharsis.
- No hot water, soap, or hydrogen peroxide enemas.

Discharge Criteria
Outpatient care

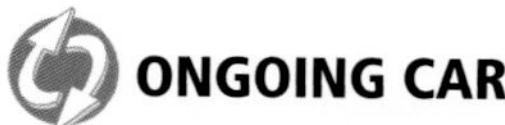

ONGOING CARE

FOLLOW-UP RECOMMENDATIONS
Periodic rectal exam

Patient Monitoring
Fewer than 1 bowel movement every other day with fecal incontinence may suggest impaction.

DIET
- High fiber (25 g/day) and at least 1.5 L fluid daily
- Avoid precipitants (caffeine).

PATIENT EDUCATION
Kegel/sphincter training exercises alone do not work for fecal incontinence but may help.

PROGNOSIS
- Reimpaction likely if bowel regimen discontinued
- 50% failure rate over 5 years following overlapping sphincteroplasty

COMPLICATIONS
- Depression and social isolation
- Skin ulcerations
- Artificial bowel sphincter: infection, erosion, mechanical failure

REFERENCES

1. Tjandra JJ, Dykes SL, Kumar RR, et al. Practice parameters for the treatment of fecal incontinence. *Dis Colon Rectum*. 2007;50(10):1497–1507.
2. Vitton V, Vignally P, Barthet M, et al. Dynamic anal endosonography and MRI defecography in diagnosis of pelvic floor disorders: comparison with conventional defecography. *Dis Colon Rectum*. 2011;54(11):1398–1404.
3. Omar MI, Alexander CE. Drug treatment for faecal incontinence in adults. *Cochrane Database Syst Rev*. 2013;(6):CD002116.
4. Maeda Y, Laurberg S, Norton C. Perianal injectable bulking agents as treatment for faecal incontinence in adults. *Cochrane Database Syst Rev*. 2013;(2):CD007959.
5. Chapman AE, Geerdes B, Hewett P, et al. Systematic review of dynamic graciloplasty in the treatment of faecal incontinence. *Br J Surg*. 2002;89(2):138–153.
6. Deutekom M, Dobben AC. Plugs for containing faecal incontinence. *Cochrane Database Syst Rev*. 2012;(4):CD005086.
7. Ratto C, Litta F, Parello A, et al. Sacral nerve stimulation in faecal incontinence associated with an anal sphincter lesion: a systematic review. *Colorectal Dis*. 2012;14(6):e297–e304.

ADDITIONAL READING

Rao SSC. Fecal incontinence. In: Feldman M, Friedman LS, Brandt LJ, eds. *Sleisenger and Fordtran's Gastrointestinal and Liver Disease*. 9th ed. Philadelphia: Saunders/Elsevier; 2010:247–258.

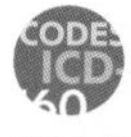

CODES

ICD10
- R15.9 Full incontinence of feces
- R15.2 Fecal urgency
- R15.0 Incomplete defecation

CLINICAL PEARLS
- New onset of fecal incontinence may indicate spinal cord compression when observed with other neurologic symptoms.
- True incontinence must be differentiated from pseudoincontinence (overflow or functional incontinence).
- Scheduled defecation after meals, bulking agents, and scheduled enemas to minimize impaction are helpful in mild/moderate fecal incontinence.

I

INCONTINENCE, URINARY ADULT FEMALE

Cara Marshall, MD

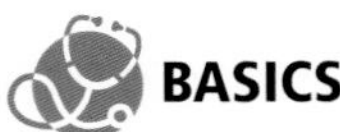

BASICS

DESCRIPTION

- Urinary incontinence: involuntary loss of urine that is objectively demonstrable and is of medical, financial, social, or hygienic concern
- Stress incontinence: associated with increased intra-abdominal pressure such as coughing, laughing, sneezing, or exertion
- Urge incontinence: sudden uncontrollable loss of urine (also known as overactive bladder or detrusor overactivity)
- Mixed incontinence: loss of urine from a combination of stress and urge incontinence
- Overflow incontinence: high residual or chronic urinary retention leading to urinary spillage from an overdistended bladder
- Functional incontinence: loss of urine due to deficits of cognition and/or mobility
- Total incontinence: continuous leakage of urine; leakage without awareness

EPIDEMIOLOGY

- Affects 25% of premenopausal and up to 75% of postmenopausal women (1)
- Women 19–64 years of age have predominantly stress incontinence (12–28%), followed by mixed (7–12%), and urge (5–10%) incontinence.
- In women >65 years of age, mixed is the most common (17%), followed by stress (16%) and urge (12%) incontinence (2).
- Severe or large-volume incontinence is primarily mixed (37%), followed by urge (27%) and stress (15%) (3).

ETIOLOGY AND PATHOPHYSIOLOGY

- Stress incontinence: occurs with increased intra-abdominal pressure. Two types:
  - Anatomic: due to urethral hypermobility from lack of pelvic support
  - Intrinsic sphincter deficiency (ISD): impaired closure of urethra. Urethral mucosal seal and inherent closure from collagen, fibroelastic tissue, smooth and striated muscles, etc., may be lost secondary to surgical scarring, radiation, or hormonal and senile changes.
- Urge incontinence: may be due to detrusor overactivity or may be idiopathic
- Overflow incontinence: urinary retention (usually from neurogenic bladder)
- Total incontinence: constant loss of urine. Ectopic ureters in females usually open in the urethra distal to the sphincter or in the vagina, causing continuous leakage. May also occur with fistulous connections between bladder, ureters, or urethra and vagina or uterus.

RISK FACTORS

Advanced age, impaired functional status, obesity (BMI >30), history of gestational diabetes, pregnancy, vaginal childbirth, pelvic surgery or radiation, urethral diverticula, genital prolapse, smoking, chronic obstructive pulmonary disease (COPD), cognitive impairment, constipation, and pelvic floor dysfunction

GENERAL PREVENTION

Obesity avoidance, smoking cessation, high-fiber diet to reduce constipation

COMMONLY ASSOCIATED CONDITIONS

Pelvic organ prolapse, UTI, COPD, diabetes mellitus, neurologic disease, obesity, chronic constipation, depression, low libido, dyspareunia, and any disease that results in chronic cough

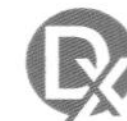

DIAGNOSIS

HISTORY

- Age: Stress incontinence is more common in women aged 19–64 years, whereas mixed incontinence is more common in women >65 years. Onset from childhood indicates congenital causes (e.g., ectopic ureter).
- Amount and frequency of leakage
- Stress incontinence: occurs in small spurts; patients typically remain dry at night in bed.
- Urge incontinence: sudden urge followed by leakage of large amounts, usually associated with frequency and nocturia. Sensory stimuli may trigger (e.g., cold).
- Continuous slow leakage in between regular voiding indicates ectopic ureter, urinary fistula, etc.
- Pain: Suprapubic pain with dysuria implies urinary infection, dyspareunia, interstitial cystitis, etc.
- Medical history
  - Neurologic conditions or suggestive symptomatology: cerebrovascular accident, parkinsonism, multiple sclerosis, myelodysplasia, diabetes, spinal cord injury
  - Radiation to pelvic and vaginal areas: causes ISD, overactive bladder, fibrotic changes of pelvic floor musculature, and low bladder compliance
  - Obstetric history: Weakness of the pelvic floor is more likely in multiparous women.
  - History of smoking and COPD with a chronic cough can aggravate incontinence.
  - Constipation can aggravate incontinence.
- Medications
  - Sympatholytic α-blockers (terazosin, prazosin, doxazosin, tamsulosin, alfuzosin, silodosin) can cause or worsen incontinence.
  - Sympathomimetic agents, tricyclic antidepressants, anticholinergics, and opioids can cause retention with overflow incontinence.
- Surgical history: Pelvic surgery, including gynecologic and bowel surgery, can injure the pelvic floor musculature and affect neurologic function.

PHYSICAL EXAM

- General status
  - Obesity (BMI)
- General neurologic examination
  - Mental status, speech, intellectual performance
  - Motor status: gait, generalized or focal weakness, rigidity, tremor
  - Sensory status: impairment of perineal–sacral area sensation
- Urologic examination
  - Abdomen: masses, incisional scars of previous surgeries
  - Suprapubic tenderness: may indicate cystitis
  - Palpable, distended bladder: chronic urinary retention
- Pelvic examination
  - Examination of the perineum and external genitalia, including tissue quality and sensation
  - Vaginal (half-speculum) examination for prolapse
  - Bimanual pelvic and anorectal examination for pelvic masses, fecal impaction, pelvic floor function, etc.
    - Urethral hypermobility: gauged by palpation of the descent of the proximal urethra on straining
    - Assessment of pelvic floor resting tone and function (ability to isolate and contract pelvic floor musculature) (4)[C]
  - Stress test for urinary incontinence: Patient is asked to cough or strain to reproduce stress incontinence.
  - Cystocele: If evident, stage (grade 0–4).
  - Rectocele: If evident, stage (stage 0–IV).

DIFFERENTIAL DIAGNOSIS

- Nocturnal enuresis: idiopathic, detrusor overactivity, neurogenic, cardiogenic, or sleep apnea
- Continuous leakage: ectopic ureter, urinary fistulas
- Postvoid dribbling: urethral diverticulum, idiopathic, iatrogenic, surgical
- Pelvic pain/dyspareunia: interstitial cystitis
- Pelvic organ prolapse
- Hematuria/recurrent UTI/pelvic mass: malignancy (5)

DIAGNOSTIC TESTS & INTERPRETATION

- Urinalysis and urine culture
- Renal function assessment: recommended if renal impairment is suspected

Initial Tests (lab, imaging)

- Unnecessary in uncomplicated patients
- Bladder scan to evaluate postvoid residual if overflow suspected (<50–100 mL expected) (5)
- Upper tract imaging if upper tract involvement is suspected: scan or renal ultrasound (US)
- International Consultation of Incontinence Modulator Questionnaire (ICIQ) is highly recommended for assessment of patient's perspective of symptoms of incontinence and their impact on quality of life.
- 3IQ Questionnaire helps differentiate between stress and urge incontinence (www.overactivebladder.com/3IQ.aspx) (3).
- Voiding diary to evaluate fluid intake, caffeine intake, timing of leakage, and patient habits

Follow-Up Tests & Special Considerations

Asymptomatic bacteriuria is common. With a positive urine culture, initial treatment is indicated; however, if this is ineffective, repeat treatment is not indicated (4).

Diagnostic Procedures/Other

Urodynamic studies (may consider when initial treatment fails or surgery is planned):

- Cystometric study of detrusor function
- Results on urodynamic testing are not predictive of treatment or surgery success (1).

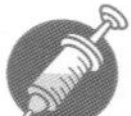

TREATMENT

GENERAL MEASURES

- Treat correctable causes (e.g., UTI).
- Encourage weight loss in obese patients.
- Aggressively correct constipation.
- Treat mixed for primary symptom type.

MEDICATION

First Line

- Stress incontinence
  - Lifestyle changes
    - Weight loss of 8% can reduce frequency of incontinence episodes by 47% (6)[A].
    - Caffeine avoidance (5)[B]
    - Aggressive treatment of constipation: Limit medications that may induce constipation, polyethylene glycol 3350 (PEG 3350), increased fluid intake, etc.
  - Kegel exercises
    - Pelvic floor muscle training
    - At least eight contractions TID (4)[A]
    - Proper technique should be confirmed on exam; training by physical therapists
    - Maintain treatment for at least 3 months (3).
    - 40% improvement (1)[A]
- Urge incontinence
  - Supervised bladder training/scheduled voiding (1)[C]

Second Line

Stress incontinence

- Pelvic floor rehabilitation (4)[A]
- Anticholinergics may be successful in mixed incontinence.
- Duloxetine (Cymbalta) has some limited efficacy (1)[A].
- Estrogen may be beneficial in topical form, but transdermal estrogen may worsen symptoms (1)[B].

Urge incontinence: anticholinergic agents (1)[A]

- Tolterodine (Detrol LA): 2–4 mg/day PO
- Oxybutynin (Ditropan XL): 5–30 mg/day PO
- Solifenacin (Vesicare): 5–10 mg/day PO
- Darifenacin (Enablex): 7.5–15 mg/day PO
- Trospium chloride (Sanctura XR): 60 mg/day PO
- Transdermal oxybutynin gel (Gelnique): 10% applied daily
- Transdermal oxybutynin patch (Oxytrol): twice weekly—available over the counter (OTC)
- Fesoterodine (Toviaz): 4–8 mg/day PO
- Dry mouth, dry eyes, constipation, impaired cognitive function, and other anticholinergic side effects can limit use.
- Avoid with narrow-angle glaucoma, urinary retention (postvoid residual [PVR] >250 mL), impaired gastric emptying, and frail elders (4)[A].
- Number 1 agent has been shown to be superior, with overall 20% continence rates (1)[A].
- Extended-release and transdermal medications cause fewer side effects (6)[B].
- β-3 agonist: mirabegron (Myrbetriq ER): 25–50 mg/day PO (6)[B]; onset of action delayed ~8 weeks; increases BP (avoid use in those with uncontrolled HTN)

Third Line

- Stress incontinence
  - Biofeedback and electrostimulation of pelvic floor muscles
  - Occlusive and supportive devices (e.g., cones, pessaries, and super tampons)
  - Acupuncture (in selected cases)
  - Periurethral injection of bulking agents (provide symptom relief but not permanent cure): collagen, carbon beads, hyaluronic acid, calcium hydroxylapatite, Macroplastique (polydimethylsiloxane) (1)(B)
  - Surgical management for stress incontinence:
    - Midurethral sling (preferral surgical intervention) (5)[A]
      - Retropubic (more perioperative complications)
      - Transobturator (more pain/dyspareunia)
      - Single-incision sling (Mini-arc, Solyx)
    - Abdominal approaches: Marshall-Marchetti-Krantz cystourethropexy, Burch colposuspension, laparoscopic colposuspension (5)[A]
  - Of note: Up to 1/3 of women who have surgery undergo a 2nd procedure during their lifetime. Quality of life improves, but it is rare to have complete resolution of symptoms after surgery.
- Urge incontinence
  - Intradetrusor onabotulinum toxin A (urinary retention common, self-catheterization may be needed) (5)[A]
  - Sacral nerve stimulation: 50% reduction in episodes in 2/3 of patients who have failed other treatments. Invasive with frequent complications (5)[B].
  - Percutaneous tibial nerve stimulation: office-based therapy, requires frequent visits (4)
  - Bladder augmentation (5)[C]

ONGOING CARE

FOLLOW-UP RECOMMENDATIONS

Patient Monitoring

- Postoperative assessment: Rule out UTI, check postvoid residual, check suture lines.
- Periodic long-term follow-up with outcome-based questionnaire surveys

PATIENT EDUCATION

Instructions on self-care and warning signs are available at PubMed Health: Urinary Incontnence at http://www.ncbi.nlm.nih.gov/pubmedhealth/PMH0003629/

PROGNOSIS

Significant improvements are usually obtained with most patients.

COMPLICATIONS

- Prolonged exposure to urine causes skin breakdown and dermatitis, which may lead to ulceration and secondary infection.
- Inability for self-care is the precipitating factor for many nursing home admissions.
- Social isolation/depression
- Weight gain (due to self-limiting exercise from fear of leakage)
- Impaired sexual function
- Impaired quality of life

REFERENCES

1. Seehusen D. Treatments for urinary incontinence in women. *Am Fam Physician*. 2013;87(10):726–728.
2. Shamliyan T, Wyman J, Bliss DZ, et al. Prevention of urinary and fecal incontinence in adults. *Evid Rep Technol Assess (Full Rep)*. 2007;(161):1–379.
3. Myers DL. Female mixed urinary incontinence: a clinical review. *JAMA*. 2014;311(19):2007–2014.
4. Smith A, Bevan D, Douglas HR, et al. Management of urinary incontinence in women: summary of updated NICE guidance. *BMJ*. 2013;347:f5170.
5. Lucas M, Bedretdinova D, Bosch J, et al. Guidelines on urinary incontinence. European Association of Urology 2014. http://www.uroweb.org/gls/pdf/20%20Urinary%20Incontinence_LR.pdf. Accessed 2014.
6. Gormley EA, Lightner DJ, Burgio K, et al. Diagnosis and treatment of overactive bladder (non-neurogenic) in adults: AUA/SUFU guideline. *J Urol*. 2012;188(6)(Suppl):2455–2563.

ADDITIONAL READING

- Abrams P, Andersson KE, Birder L, et al. Fourth International Consultation on Incontinence Recommendations of the International Scientific Committee: evaluation and treatment of urinary incontinence, pelvic organ prolapse, and fecal incontinence. *Neurourol Urodyn*. 2010;29(1):213–240.
- Labrie J, Berghmans BL, Fischer K, et al. Surgery versus physiotherapy for stress urinary incontinence. *N Engl J Med*. 2013;369(12):1124–1133.
- Nygaard I. Clinical practice. Idiopathic urgency urinary incontinence. *N Engl J Med*. 2010;363(12):1156–1162.
- Rogers RG. Clinical practice. Urinary stress incontinence in women. *N Engl J Med*. 2008;358(10):1029–1036.
- Visco AG, Brubaker L, Richter HE, et al. Anticholinergic therapy vs. onabotulinumtoxina for urgency urinary incontinence. *N Engl J Med*. 2012;367(19):1803–1813.

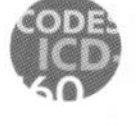

CODES

ICD10

- R32 Unspecified urinary incontinence
- N39.3 Stress incontinence (female) (male)
- N39.41 Urge incontinence

CLINICAL PEARLS

- Urinary incontinence is the involuntary loss of urine that is objectively demonstrable; markedly detrimental to quality of life; and is of medical, financial, social, or hygienic concern.
- Stress incontinence: associated with increased intra-abdominal pressure such as coughing, laughing, sneezing, or exertion
- Urge incontinence: sudden uncontrollable urgency, leading to leakage of urine (also known as overactive bladder or detrusor overactivity)
- Rule out UTI or STI by culture.
- Aggressively treat constipation.
- Assume that a great percentage of women can be significantly helped by treatment.
- For stress incontinence, physical therapy/pelvic floor rehabilitation and midurethral sling surgeries are most commonly used.
- For urge incontinence, if anticholinergic agents fail, intradetrusor onabotulinum toxin A is often beneficial.

INCONTINENCE, URINARY ADULT MALE

Abhijeet Patil, MD, MS

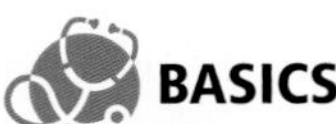

BASICS

DESCRIPTION

- Urinary incontinence (UI) refers to the involuntary loss of urine that presents a medical, financial, social, or hygienic problem; the 2 main types of incontinence: stress incontinence and urge incontinence
- Stress incontinence: involuntary urine leaks secondary to increased intra-abdominal pressure being greater than the sphincter can control; may be precipitated by sneezing, laughing, coughing, exertion
- Urge incontinence: Involuntary leakage of urine associated with urgency is believed to be secondary to uncontrolled contraction of the urinary bladder. It is also called detrusor overactivity.
- Mixed incontinence: involuntary leakage of urine with urgency and with sneezing, laughing, coughing, exertion

EPIDEMIOLOGY

- Stress incontinence in men is rare, unless it is attributable to prostate surgery, neurologic disease, or trauma.
- Reported rates of incontinence range from 1% after transurethral resection to 2–60% after radical prostatectomy, although rates decline with time.

Prevalence

- Systematic reviews have shown prevalence of daily UI in men ranged from 2 to 11%.
- Prevalence of UI in men increases sharply with age: Up to 2.4% of men age <39 years have UI, whereas up to 22% of those age ≥80 years experience symptoms.
- No difference in prevalence between racial/ethnic groups.
- Prevalence of moderate/severe UI is 4.5%.
- Urge UI is most common (40–80%) followed by mixed UI (10–30%) and stress UI (<10%).
- Incontinence in men of all ages is approximately half as prevalent as it is in women.

ETIOLOGY AND PATHOPHYSIOLOGY

- Incontinence secondary to bladder abnormalities
  - Detrusor overactivity results in urge incontinence.
  - Detrusor overactivity commonly is associated with bladder outlet obstruction from benign prostatic hyperplasia (BPH).
- Incontinence secondary to outlet abnormalities
  - Sphincteric damage secondary to pelvic surgery or radiation
  - Sphincteric dysfunction secondary to neurologic disease
- Mixed incontinence is caused by abnormalities of both the bladder and the outlet overflow or by enlarged prostate/bladder neck contracture from prostate surgery.

RISK FACTORS

- Age
- Hypertension
- Neurologic disease
- Prostate surgery
- Pelvic trauma
- History of urinary tract infections
- Major depression
- Diabetes

GENERAL PREVENTION

Proper management of conditions, such as symptomatic bladder outlet obstruction caused by BPH early in the course may prevent continence problems later in life; no evidence for screening in men (1)[B]

COMMONLY ASSOCIATED CONDITIONS

- Neurologic disease (cerebrovascular accident, parkinsonism, multiple sclerosis, myelodysplasia, spinal cord injury)
- Pelvic radiation
- Pelvic trauma
- BPH
- Prostate surgery

DIAGNOSIS

HISTORY

- Voiding symptoms
  - Duration and characteristics of incontinence
  - Stress, urge, total
  - Precipitants and associated symptoms
  - Use of pads, briefs, diapers
  - Fluid intake
  - Alteration in bowel habits
  - Previous treatments and effect on incontinence
  - BPH symptoms
- Diabetes mellitus
- Associated conditions, such as neurologic disease
- Medication use: diuretics, drugs for BPH
- Alcohol and drug use, including caffeine
- Radical pelvic surgery/radiation
  - Abdominoperineal resection
  - Prostatectomy: radical for cancer, open/transurethral for benign disease

PHYSICAL EXAM

- Abdominal examination
  - Suprapubic mass suggests retention.
  - Suprapubic tenderness suggests UTI.
  - Surgical scars suggesting pelvic surgery
  - Skin lesions associated with neurologic disease (e.g., neurofibromatosis and café au lait spots)
- External genitalia
- Prostate
- Spine/back
- Skeletal deformities
- Scars from previous spinal surgery
- Sacral abnormalities may be associated with neurogenic bladder dysfunction:
  - Cutaneous signs of spinal dysraphism
    - SC lipoma
    - Vascular malformation, tuft of hair, or skin dimple on lower back
  - Cutaneous signs of sacral agenesis
    - Low, short gluteal cleft
    - Flattened buttocks
    - Coccyx is not palpable.
- Focal neurologic exam
  - Motor function
    - Inspect muscle bulk for atrophy.
    - Tibialis anterior (L4–S1): dorsiflexion of foot
    - Gastrocnemius (L5–S2): plantarflexion of foot
    - Toe extensors (L5–S2): toe extension
- Sensory function
- Reflexes
  - Anal reflex (S2–S5)
    - Gently stroke mucocutaneous junction of circumanal skin.
    - Absent visible contraction (wink) suggests peripheral nerve/sacral (conus medullaris) abnormality.
  - Bulbocavernosus reflex (BCR) (S2–S4)
    - Elicited by squeezing glans to cause reflex contraction of anal sphincter
    - Absence of BCR suggests sacral nerve damage.

DIFFERENTIAL DIAGNOSIS

- Urge incontinence
- Stress incontinence
- Mixed incontinence
- Overflow incontinence
- Intrinsic sphincter deficiency

DIAGNOSTIC TESTS & INTERPRETATION

- Creatinine if significant retention suspected
- Urinalysis and urine culture to check for glucosuria, infection
- Prostate-specific antigen (PSA)
- Postvoid residual volume
- IV pyelogram, renal ultrasound, or CT of abdomen to confirm normality of upper tracts
- Voiding cystogram in select cases

DIAGNOSTIC PROCEDURES/OTHER

- Urodynamics is useful for confirming bladder outlet obstruction as a possible cause of detrusor overactivity.
- Prostate ultrasound and biopsy if indicated by physical exam or PSA
- Consider referral to a urologist for complicated UI, which includes pelvic pain, prior pelvic surgery/radiation, elevated PSA.

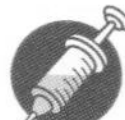

TREATMENT

- Best managed by combining lifestyle modification and medication
- Lifestyle changes: weight loss (especially if overweight), limit fluids (especially at night), toilet on a scheduled basis, eliminate certain foods that may make symptoms worse (e.g., caffeine, acidic foods, alcohol)
- Bladder relaxation techniques (when trained by expert); unclear if pelvic floor exercises (Kegel) are effective for men; biofeedback
- Following radical prostatectomy, it is best to try conservative management and watchful waiting for 6–12 months to allow for spontaneous resolution.

GENERAL MEASURES

- Bladder diaries are invaluable in helping patients understand patterns of incontinence.
- Time voiding to avoid significant bladder distention.

MEDICATION

First Line

- Urge incontinence (all equally efficacious; selection based on side effect tolerance)
- Antimuscarinic agents are the primary treatments for urge incontinence; in men with urgency associated with BPH, consider use of alpha-blockers (i.e., tamsulosin, alfuzosin, silodosin) as monotherapy or in combination with antimuscarinic.
  - Oxybutynin (Ditropan XL) 5–15 mg PO every day
  - Tolterodine (Detrol LA) 2–4 mg PO every day
  - Darifenacin (Enablex) 7.5–15 mg PO every day
  - Solifenacin (Vesicare) 5–10 mg PO every day
  - Trospium chloride (Sanctura XR) 60 mg PO every day
  - Transdermal oxybutynin (Gelnique) 10% apply daily
  - Fesoterodine (Toviaz) 4–8 mg PO every day
- Stress incontinence
  - No generally accepted drug therapy
  - Tricyclics sometimes used: imipramine 10–25 mg PO BID/TID
  - Duloxetine 40 mg PO BID is approved in the European Union.

Second Line

- Urge incontinence
- Tricyclic antidepressants
  - Imipramine 10–25 mg PO BID/TID
- Desmopressin (DDAVP) for nocturnal symptoms
  - 0.1–0.5 mg PO or intranasal at bedtime
- Intradetrusor botulinum toxin injections (not FDA approved)
- Mirabegron (Myrbetriq): new β-3 agonist (FDA approved) 25–50 mg PO daily. *Caution*: HTN

Geriatric Considerations

- Anticholinergics and tricyclics may result in significant cognitive impairment in elderly patients.
- DDAVP should be avoided in patients with known/potential cardiac disease.

ADDITIONAL THERAPIES

- Pelvic floor rehabilitation (Kegel exercises) may significantly reduce both stress and urge incontinence in male patients and should be considered a part of initial management for stress UI.
- Timed voiding is a useful therapy for patients with urge incontinence.
- Overflow incontinence is usually caused by poor bladder contractility with urinary retention:
  - Indwelling catheter
  - Intermittent catheterization
  - Evaluate for outlet obstruction.

SURGERY/OTHER PROCEDURES

- Urge incontinence
  - Sacral neuromodulation
  - Augmentation cystoplasty
  - Botulinum toxin injection via cystoscopy
- Stress incontinence (2)[B]
  - Urethral bulking agents: modest success rates with low cure rates
  - Male sling procedures: promising short-term and intermediate results but no long-term studies
  - Artificial urinary sphincter implant has excellent long-term continence rates and is considered gold standard.

COMPLEMENTARY & ALTERNATIVE MEDICINE

- Acupuncture in selected cases
- Physical therapy in selected cases

ONGOING CARE

FOLLOW-UP RECOMMENDATIONS

Patient Monitoring

Must monitor residual volume after voiding in patients taking anticholinergic medications

PROGNOSIS

Continence can be improved in almost all patients.

COMPLICATIONS

- Dermatitis
- Candidiasis
- Skin breakdown
- Social isolation
- Avoidance of sex
- Weight gain

REFERENCES

1. Landefeld CS, Bowers BJ, Feld AD, et al. National Institutes of Health state-of-the-science conference statement: prevention of fecal and urinary incontinence in adults. *Ann Intern Med*. 2008;148(6):449–458.
2. Herschorn S, Bruschini H, Comiter C, et al. Surgical treatment of stress incontinence in men. *Neurourol Urodyn*. 2010;29(1):179–190.

ADDITIONAL READING

- Bauer RM, Bastian PJ, Gozzi C, et al. Postprostatectomy incontinence: all about diagnosis and management. *Eur Urol*. 2009;55(2):322–333.
- Buckley BS, Lapitan MC; Epidemiology Committee of the Fourth International Consultation on Incontinence, Paris, 2008. Prevalence of urinary incontinence in men, women, and children—current evidence: findings of the Fourth International Consultation on Incontinence. *Urology*. 2010;76(2):265–270.
- Khullar V, Amarenco G, Angulo JC, et al. Efficacy and tolerability of mirabegron, a β(3)-adrenoceptor agonist, in patients with overactive bladder: results from a randomised European-Australian phase 3 trial. *Eur Urol*. 2013;63(2):283–295.
- Markland AD, Goode PS, Redden DT, et al. Prevalence of urinary incontinence in men: results from the national health and nutrition examination survey. *J Urol*. 2010;184(3):1022–1027.
- Stewart WF, Van Rooyen JB, Cundiff GW, et al. Prevalence and burden of overactive bladder in the United States. *World J Urol*. 2003;20(6):327–336.

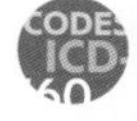

CODES

ICD10

- R32 Unspecified urinary incontinence
- N39.3 Stress incontinence (female) (male)
- N39.41 Urge incontinence

CLINICAL PEARLS

- Think "outside" the lower urinary tract: Comorbid medical illness and impairments are independently associated with UI; treat contributing comorbidities and medicines.
- Always check postvoid residual to rule out overflow incontinence.
- Have patient complete the International Prostate Symptom Score and do uroflow.
- Check PSA.
- Urodynamics can be very helpful.
- Pelvic floor rehabilitation may have a significant effect for male patients.

INFECTIOUS MONONUCLEOSIS, EPSTEIN-BARR VIRUS INFECTIONS

Dennis E. Hughes, DO, FAAFP, FACEP

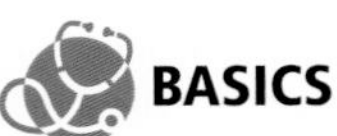

BASICS

DESCRIPTION

- Epstein-Barr virus (EBV) is a member of the herpes virus family.
  - 2 subtypes: ST1 predominates in Western Hemisphere, Southeast Asia; ST1 and ST2 equally prevalent in Africa.
- Primary infection typically occurs in childhood; responsible for infectious mononucleosis (most common disease association) and numerous cancers.
- Other names: glandular fever

EPIDEMIOLOGY

Incidence

Worldwide, infects >90% of people (antibody-positive)

Prevalence

Primary EBV infection

- Military, college students, and others living in cloistered and crowded populations have highest infection rate.
- Predominant age of primary infection is 10–19 years.
  - Primary clinical manifestation is infectious mononucleosis.
  - Early childhood infections are usually asymptomatic.
- By ~20 years of age, 60–90% of persons have a persistent (lifelong) anti-EBV antibody.
- Seroconversion occurs later in childhood in developed countries; there is suggestion of race/ethnicity disparity in the United States with higher seroprevalence in non-Hispanic black, Asian, and Hispanic populations (1).

ETIOLOGY AND PATHOPHYSIOLOGY

- After inoculation, the virus replicates in the nasopharyngeal epithelium with resulting cell lysis, virion spread and viremia. The reticuloendothelial system is affected, resulting in a host response and the appearance of atypical lymphocytes in the peripheral blood.
- A polyclonal B-cell proliferative response follows. Relatively few circulating lymphocytes are infected by EBV (<0.1% of circulating mononuclear cells in the acute illness).
- A persistent (asymptomatic) state ensues with the EBV genome maintained invisible to the immune system.
- A subsequent coinfection is felt to increase risk for developing an EBV-associated condition (e.g., malignancy).
- Either by B-cell stimulation or diminished EBV-specific immune modulation, the previously latent EBV-infected B cells replicate, allowing clinical manifestation of the EBV genome. The proteins produced may either modify host response to or contribute directly to the subsequent malignancy (2).
- Immunosuppression (organ transplant/acquired immune deficiency) can result in transformation and lymphoproliferative disorders.

RISK FACTORS

- Age
- Sociohygienic level
- Geographic location
- Close, intimate contact
- Immunosuppression

GENERAL PREVENTION

- Avoid close physical contact with persons known to be currently symptomatic with EBV/infectious mononucleosis
- Good hand washing and hygiene
- General precautions with potential blood exposure (EBV can be transmitted via blood contamination, as well as transplanted hematopoietic cell and solid organs)
- EBV vaccines are currently undergoing study, but thus far only limited efficacy seen in small studies.

COMMONLY ASSOCIATED CONDITIONS

- Infectious mononucleosis: Symptomatic primary EBV infection common in otherwise healthy older children, adolescents, and young adults.
  - Clinical features vary in severity and duration: In children age <10 years, generally mild; in adolescents and adults, symptoms can be more severe and protracted
  - Incubation period is 30–50 days.
- X-linked lymphoproliferative syndrome (XLP-rare inherited extreme vulnerability to EBV infection)
- Lymphoproliferative syndromes due to EBV infections in transplant recipients
- Lymphomas (B-cell lymphoblastic, T-cell)
- Lymphocytic interstitial pneumonitis
- Hairy leukoplakia of the tongue, leiomyosarcoma, and CNS lymphomas in patients with AIDS
- Burkitt lymphoma (most common childhood tumor in Africa and Papua New Guinea where malaria is also endemic and may be a cofactor)
- Nasopharyngeal carcinoma (particularly in southeast China)
- Parotid carcinoma
- Hodgkin lymphoma (most common EBV-associated malignancy in United States, European Union)
- Postulated to be associated with multiple sclerosis (2–3× incidence in EBV-positive individuals)
- Chronic active Epstein-Barr Virus (CAEBV) due to loss of host control of viral replication

DIAGNOSIS

HISTORY

- May begin abruptly or insidiously
- Syndrome of fatigue, malaise, and sore throat
- In adults, temperature may rise to 103°F (39.4°C) and gradually fall over a variable period of 7–10 days; in severe cases, temperature elevations of 104–105°F (40.0–40.6°C) may persist for 2 weeks.
- Children typically with low-grade fever or afebrile
- Diffuse hyperemia and hyperplasia of oropharyngeal lymphoid tissue
- Gelatinous, grayish-white exudative tonsillitis persists for 7–10 days in 50%.
- Petechiae develop at border of hard and soft palates in 60%.
- Axillary, epitrochlear, popliteal, inguinal, mediastinal, and mesenteric lymphadenopathy (95% of patients)
- Lymph node enlargement subsides over days/weeks.
- Chest pain (myocarditis and pericarditis)

PHYSICAL EXAM

- Fever, lymphadenopathy, pharyngitis in >50%, with palatal petechiae and hepatosplenomegaly in ~10%
- Tender lymphadenopathy (cervical nodes are most commonly enlarged)
- Splenomegaly in 50%
- Skin manifestations in 3–16%
  - Erythematous macular/maculopapular rash
  - Petechial and purpuric exanthems have been reported.
  - Rash location: trunk and upper arms; occasionally the face and forearms are involved

DIFFERENTIAL DIAGNOSIS

- Streptococcal pharyngitis and tonsillitis
- Diphtheria
- Blood dyscrasias
- Rubella
- Measles
- Viral hepatitis
- Cytomegalovirus
- Toxoplasmosis

DIAGNOSTIC TESTS & INTERPRETATION

Initial Tests (lab, imaging)

- CBC with differential
- Lymphocytes and atypical lymphocytes
  - Increased numbers of lymphocytes (especially atypical lymphocytes; may be up to 70% of leukocytes) in peripheral blood
  - In 1st week after onset, WBC count is normal/moderately decreased.
    - By the 2nd week, lymphocytosis develops with >10% atypical lymphocytes.
  - During early illness, atypical lymphocytes are B cells transformed by the EBV; later, atypical cells are primarily T cells.
- Antibodies
  - Heterophile antibodies in 80–90% of adults
  - Heterophile antibody is an IgM response, which appears during the 1st/2nd week of illness and disappears in 4–6 weeks.
  - In general, agglutinin titer is higher in infectious mononucleosis than in other disorders; an unabsorbed heterophile titer >1:128 and ≥1:40 after absorption is significant.
- Specific antibodies to EBV-associated antigens
  - Develop regularly in infectious mononucleosis
  - Viral capsid-specific IgM and IgG are present early in illness.
  - Viral capsid-IgM disappears after several weeks, viral capsid-IgG persists for life.

- Liver tests: hypertransaminasemia, hyperbilirubinemia are common; jaundice is rare.
- Atypical lymphocytes are not specific for EBV infections and may be present in other clinical conditions, including rubella, infectious hepatitis, allergic rhinitis, asthma, and primary atypical pneumonia.
- Abdominal ultrasound to monitor for splenic enlargement is not supported routinely.
- Consider ultrasound for those wishing to return to strenuous activity/contact sports at day 21 of illness to ensure resolution of splenomegaly.

Follow-Up Tests & Special Considerations

- Abnormal hepatic enzymes persist in 80% of patients for several weeks; hepatomegaly in 15–20%
- In transplant recipients, quantitative polymerase chain reaction (PCR) used to monitor EBV loads

Diagnostic Procedures/Other

Chest x-ray

- Hilar adenopathy may be observed in infectious mononucleosis with extensive lymphoid hyperplasia.

Test Interpretation

- Mononuclear infiltrations involve lymph nodes, tonsils, spleen, lungs, liver, heart, kidneys, adrenal glands, skin, and CNS.
- Bone marrow hyperplasia with small granulomas formation may be present; these findings are nonspecific and have no prognostic significance.

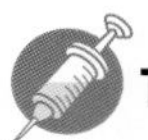

TREATMENT

GENERAL MEASURES

- Treatment is mostly supportive.
- NSAIDs or acetaminophen
- During acute stage, limit activity for 4 weeks to reduce potential complications (e.g., splenic rupture).
- Transplant recipients who develop EBV infection may require reduction in immunosuppression as well as administration of monoclonal anti-CD20 (rituximab).

MEDICATION

- In primary infections:
  - Antimicrobial agents (usually penicillin) only if throat culture is positive for group A β-hemolytic streptococci. Previously, ampicillin rash in presumed group B *Streptococcus* (GBS) was thought to be highly suggestive of infectious mononucleosis. Incidence of rash much lower than historically thought (3)[B].
  - Warm saline gargles for oropharyngeal pain
  - Corticosteroids
    - May provide some symptomatic relief but no improvement in resolution of illness
    - Consider in severe pharyngotonsillitis with oropharyngeal edema and airway encroachment. Dexamethasone 0.3 mg/kg/day may be used for 1–3 days.
    - Also for patients with marked toxicity/major complications (e.g., hemolytic anemia, thrombocytopenic purpura, neurologic sequelae, myocarditis, pericarditis) (4)[B]
- Antiviral medications (acyclovir) have been evaluated in small randomized controlled trials (RCTs) and found to shorten recovery time and improve subjective symptoms in acute EBV infection.

ISSUES FOR REFERRAL

Most cases can be managed as an outpatient without the need for specialty referral. Consider referral for complications such as oropharyngeal edema with airway compromise needing intubation or ventilator support.

SURGERY/OTHER PROCEDURES

- With profound thrombocytopenia, refractory to corticosteroid therapy, splenectomy may be necessary.
- Only current effective treatment for XLP is hematopoietic stem cell transplantation.

INPATIENT CONSIDERATIONS

Admission Criteria/Initial Stabilization

- Inability to eat food or drink fluids
- Immune suppressed
- Splenic rupture

ONGOING CARE

FOLLOW-UP RECOMMENDATIONS

ALERT

Rupture of the spleen may be fatal if not recognized; it requires blood transfusions, treatment for shock, and splenectomy. Occurrence is estimated at 0.1%.

Patient Monitoring

- Avoid contact sports, heavy lifting, and excess exertion until spleen and liver have returned to normal size (ultrasound can verify).
- Eliminate alcohol/exposure to other hepatotoxic drugs until LFTs return to normal.
- Monitor patients closely during the first 2–3 weeks after the onset of symptoms as rates of complications are highest during this period.
- Alert patients that symptoms (malaise, fatigue, intermittent sore throat, lymphadenopathy) may persist for months.

DIET

No restrictions. Hydration during acute phase is very important.

PROGNOSIS

- Most recover in ~4 weeks.
- Fatigue may persist for months.

COMPLICATIONS

- Neurologic (rare)
  - Aseptic meningitis
  - Bell palsy
  - Meningoencephalitis
  - Guillain-Barré syndrome
  - Transverse myelitis
  - Cerebellar ataxia
  - Acute psychosis
- Hematologic (rare)
  - Thrombocytopenia, slight to moderate, early in illness
  - Hemolytic anemia with marked neutropenia during early weeks
  - Aplastic anemia
  - Agammaglobulinemia
- Pneumonitis
- Splenic rupture
  - Rare, but most often occurs in first 21 days of illness

REFERENCES

1. Dowd JB, Palermo T, Brite J, et al. Seroprevalence of Epstein Barr virus infections in the US children ages 6-19, 2003-2010. *PLoS One*. 2013;8(5):e64921.
2. Thorley-Lawson DA, Hawkins JB, Tracy SI, et al. The pathogenesis of Eptein-Barr virus persistent infection. *Curr Opin Virol*. 2013;3(3):227–232.
3. Chovel-Sella A, Ben Tov A, Lahav E, et al. Incidence of rash after amoxicillin treatment in children with infectious mononucleosis. *Pediatrics*. 2013;131(5):e1424–e1427.
4. Odumade O, Hogquist K, Balfour H. Progress and problems in understanding and managing primary Epstein-Barr virus infections. *Clin Microbiol Rev*. 2011;24(1):193–209.

ADDITIONAL READING

- Almohmeed YH, Avenell A, Aucott L, et al. Systematic review and meta-analysis of the sero-epidemiological association between Epstein Barr virus and multiple sclerosis. *PLoS One*. 2013;8(4):e61110.
- Klein G, Klein E, Kashuba E. Interaction of Epstein-Barr virus (EBV) with human B-lymphocytes. *Biochem Biophys Res Comm*. 2010;396(1):67–73.
- Münz C, Moormann A. Immune escape by Epstein-Barr virus associated maligancies. *Semin Cancer Biol*. 2008;18(6):381–387.

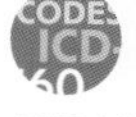

CODES

ICD10

- B27.00 Gammaherpesviral mononucleosis without complication
- B27.09 Gammaherpesviral mononucleosis with other complications
- B27.01 Gammaherpesviral mononucleosis with polyneuropathy

CLINICAL PEARLS

- In cases of acute symptomatic infectious mononucleosis, 98% manifest with fever, sore throat, cervical node enlargement, and tonsillar hypertrophy.
- False-negative monospot (heterophile antibody) common in the first 10–14 days of illness. 90% will have heterophile antibodies by week 3 of illness.
- Lymphocytosis (not monocytosis) common in infectious mononucleosis.

INFERTILITY

Sharon L. Koehler, DO, FACS • Sara Soshnick, DO, MS • David Tegay, DO, FACMG, FACOI

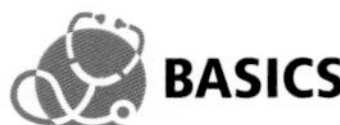

BASICS

DESCRIPTION

- Definition: failure to conceive after ≥12 months of regular unprotected intercourse or after ≥6 months if the woman is ≥35 years. Primary: Couple has never been pregnant. Secondary: Couple has been pregnant.
- Evaluation: warranted if couple fails to conceive after 12 months of unprotected intercourse if patient is ≤35 years and after 6 months if patient is ≥35 years. Evaluation may commence earlier in women ≥40 years. Evaluation of both partners should be simultaneous when applicable.

EPIDEMIOLOGY

Incidence

Incidence is the probability of achieving a pregnancy within 1 year. ~85% of couples will conceive within 12 months of unprotected intercourse.

Prevalence

- In the United States, 5–15% of women currently trying to conceive are infertile.
- ~11.5% of married couples between ages 15 and 34 years and 42% between ages 35 and 44 years meet the criteria for being infertile.
- May increase as more women delay childbearing; 20% of women in the United States have their 1st child >35 years.

ETIOLOGY AND PATHOPHYSIOLOGY

- Most cases multifactorial: Approximately 50% of cases due to female factors (of which 20% are due to ovulatory dysfunction and 30% due to tubal and pelvic pathology), 30% due to male factors, and 20% are of unknown etiology.
- Acquired: Most common cause of infertility in the United States is pelvic inflammatory disease (PID) secondary to chlamydia (causes tubal scarring and Fitz-Hugh-Curtis syndrome), endometriosis, polycystic ovary syndrome (PCOS), premature ovarian failure, and increased maternal age.
- Diminished ovarian reserve (DOR): low fertility due to low quantity or functional quality of oocytes
- Congenital: anatomic and genetic abnormalities

Genetics

- Higher incidence of genetic abnormalities among infertile population, including Klinefelter syndrome (47XXY), Turner syndrome (45X or mosaic), and fragile X syndrome
- Y chromosomal microdeletions are associated with isolated defects of spermatogenesis → found in 16% of men with azo/severe oligospermia.
- Cystic fibrosis transmembrane conductance regulator (CFTR) gene mutation causing congenital bilateral absence of vas deferens (CBAVD)

RISK FACTORS

- Female
- Gynecologic history: irregular/abnormal menses, sexually transmitted infections (STIs), dysmenorrhea, fibroids, prior pregnancy
- Medical history: endocrinopathy, autoimmune disease, undiagnosed celiac disease (1), collagen vascular diseases (2), thrombophilia, obesity, and cancer
- Surgical history: appendicitis, pelvic surgery, intrauterine surgery, tubal ligation
- Social history: smoking, alcohol/substance abuse, eating disorders, exercise, advanced maternal age
- Male
- Medical history: STI, prostatitis, medication use (i.e., β-blockers, calcium channel blocker, antiulcer medication), endocrinopathy, cancer
- Surgical history: orchiopexy, hernia repair, vasectomy with/without reversal
- Social: smoking, alcohol/substance abuse, anabolic steroids, environmental exposures, occupations leading to increased scrotal temperature

GENERAL PREVENTION

Normal diet and exercise, avoid smoking and other substance abuse, decrease risk of STIs

COMMONLY ASSOCIATED CONDITIONS

- Sexual behavior increasing risk for STIs
- Pelvic pathology: endometriosis, ovarian cysts, endometrial polyps, and uterine fibroids
- Endocrine dysfunction (thyroid, glucose metabolism, menstrual cycle abnormalities, prolactin)
- Anovulation is commonly associated with hyperandrogenism and PCOS.

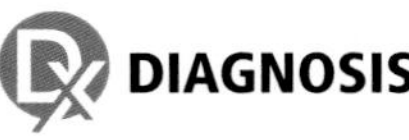

DIAGNOSIS

HISTORY

- Complete reproductive history
  - Age at menarche, regularity of cycles, physical development, previous methods of contraception, history of abnormal Pap smears and treatment
  - History of abortion, D&Cs, bilateral tubal ligation, vasectomy, or other pelvic/abdominal surgery
- Frequency of intercourse and sexual dysfunction
- Abdominal pain or other abdominal symptoms
- STI
- History of endocrine abnormalities
- History of malignancy or chronic illness
- Family history: close relatives with congenital abnormalities or mental retardation; infertility or early menopause in close relatives of female partner
- Medications: drug abuse, allergies, occupation and exposure to environmental hazards

PHYSICAL EXAM

- BMI and distribution of body fat
- Female
  - Pubertal development with Tanner staging
  - Signs of PCOS: androgen excess, obesity, signs of insulin resistance
  - Breast exam: galactorrhea
  - Vaginal exam: describe rugation, discharge, anatomic variation
  - Uterine size/shape, mobility, tenderness
  - Adnexal tenderness infection or mass
- Male
  - Abnormalities of the penis or urethral meatus.
  - Testes: volume, symmetry, masses (varicocele, hydrocele), presence/absence of vas deferens

DIAGNOSTIC TESTS & INTERPRETATION

Initial Tests (lab, imaging)

Evaluation is directed by history:

- Assessment of ovulation
  - Irregular or infrequent menses, not accompanied by consistent premenstrual or moliminal characteristics, which are inconsistent in flow and duration, are indicative of ovulatory dysfunction.
  - Additional tests should focus on determining the underlying cause of ovulatory disturbance.
  - Luteal-phase progesterone ≥3 ng/mL confirms ovulation has recently occurred but does not indicate when it occurred.
  - Luteinizing hormone (LH) testing kit: identifies mid-cycle LH surge, which occurs approximately 14–26 hours prior to ovulation. Greatest fertility on day of LH surge and 2 days after. Only test that predicts time of ovulation in advance so couples can time intercourse.
  - Basal body temperature (BBT): ~1 degree increase in BBT taken upon wakening indicates ovulation has occurred: Greatest fertility spans 7 days PRIOR to rise in BBT. Not preferred.
- Assessment of ovarian reserve
  - Follicle-stimulating hormone (FSH)/estradiol (E_2): FSH and E_2 levels on cycle days (CD) 2–5 are used to predict response to ovulation induction and pregnancy. High FSH levels >10 mIU/mL and high estradiol (>80 pg/mL) indicate a low chance of pregnancy with in vitro fertilization (IVF).
  - Anti-müllerian hormone (AMH) and antral follicle counts (AFCs): The number of antral follicles measured by transvaginal ultrasound (US) at any one time in the ovary is termed the "antral follicle count." AMH is secreted by the granulosa cells of the antral follicles and decreases as a woman approaches menopause. AMH <0.7 μg/dL and total AFC <10 between both ovaries during the follicular phase indicate DOR. Clomiphene challenge test: Measure FSH on CD 3, administer 100 mg clomiphene CDs 5–9, recheck FSH on CD 10. FSH ≥10 mIU/mL on CDs 3 or 10 indicates DOR; may increase the sensitivity of the standard day 3 FSH test
- Semen analysis
  - Warranted in all infertile couples. Semen analysis alone is not used to predict male fertility potential: normal results in 6–27% of infertile males, abnormal results in fertile males
  - Semen collection: collected after 2–5 days of abstinence. Repeat test 2–3× due to inherent variability within the same individual.
  - Parameters for male subfertility: sperm concentration <13.5 mill/mL, sperm motility <32%, sperm morphology <9% normal
- Additional labs
  - Prolactin, thyroid-stimulating hormone, 17-hydroxyprogesterone, androgen levels
  - HIV, HSV 1 and 2, chlamydia gonorrhea antibody, RPR, hepatitis B and C, CMV
  - Genetic testing based on family history
- Transvaginal US for anatomic abnormality
- Hysterosalpingogram (HSG) to evaluate patency of tubes and contour of the cavity; may be both diagnostic and therapeutic.
- Sonohysterography (SHG) may provide a more detailed evaluation of the uterine cavity, if indicated.

Follow-Up Tests & Special Considerations

- Abnormal lab values warrant reevaluation/referral.
- Abnormal imaging may require surgical evaluation.

Diagnostic Procedures/Other

- Hysteroscopy: gold standard, used to directly visualize the endometrial cavity; may be indicated to evaluate filling defects on HSG or SHG
- Laparoscopy: used to directly visualize the peritoneal cavity and may be indicated to evaluate abnormal findings on HSG. It is the only way to definitively diagnose endometriosis.

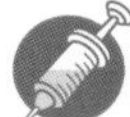

TREATMENT

GENERAL MEASURES

- Be aware of insurance coverage for each patient.
- Infertility and its treatment involve emotional issues. Many patients may benefit from counseling and support measures.
- All female fertility patients should be taking folate supplementation of at least 400 μg/day.
- New evidence is suggesting beneficial effects of antioxidants in decreasing time to pregnancy. Additionally, dietary carotenoids in males may improve sperm quality (3,4).
- IVF is the most effective infertility treatment available:
  - Eggs are removed from the female and fertilized outside the body. The embryo is monitored for 3–5 days and then implanted into the uterus on day 3 or day 5.
  - Is an option for all causes of infertility
  - Anatomic causes should be referred immediately for IVF, although surgical consult may be required.
  - Fewer complications have been reported for individuals undergoing IVF for anatomic causes rather than ovulatory dysfunction (low APGAR scores, DM) (5)[A].
- Male factor
  - Consider lifestyle changes.
  - Intrauterine insemination (IUI): Sperms are placed via a catheter directly in the uterus. IUI effectively increases the sperm count.
  - Intracytoplasmic sperm injection (ICSI) is performed in conjunction with IVF for males with severe abnormalities (i.e., <5 million sperm) or those who have failed to conceive with IUI. A single sperm is injected directly into the cytoplasm of the egg. Fertilization occurs ~70% of the time.
  - Frozen donor sperm can be obtained from banks for severe male factor.

MEDICATION

First Line

- Treatment of infertility depends on the etiology.
- Anovulation: must determine if HYPOgonadotrophic or NORMOgonadotrophic
  - Hypogonadotrophic patients: Standard treatment to induce ovulation consists of daily injections of both FSH and LH, which need to be carefully monitored to avoid overstimulation, resulting in ovarian hyperstimulation syndrome (OHSS).
  - Normogonadotrophic patients: most commonly due to PCOS. Ovulation induction with clomiphene citrate (Clomid). Regimen: 50 mg/day for 5 days beginning typically on CD 5 after spontaneous or progestin-induced withdrawal bleed. If no ovulation, increase dose to 100 mg/day in subsequent cycles; maximum, 150 mg/day. Some will increase dose with ovulation but no pregnancy. Most effective with ~10% body weight loss if obese.
- Unexplained infertility: IVF most effective; IUI, clomiphene, or LH/FSH yield minor improvements; better outcomes in combination
- Coital or cervical problems: IUI
- Endometriosis: either IVF or surgery; medical therapy does not increase pregnancy rates.

Second Line

- If clomiphene fails to induce ovulation:
  - Aromatase inhibitors (i.e., letrozole) may produce a better response.
  - Metformin beneficial in anovulatory women with PCOS; initiate with 500 mg daily and increase to ~1,500 mg/day; monitor renal function. Metformin may take up to 3 months to be effective. Consider also oral contraceptive pills (OCPs) for ≥2 cycles, and then retry the clomiphene immediately after stopping the OCPs.
- Generally in subspecialty care: Gonadotropin therapies (injectable FSH or FSH + LH) are effective, but riskier, treatments for infertility. They are effective for hypothalamic dysfunction for which clomiphene generally is not.

ISSUES FOR REFERRAL

Reproductive endocrinology and/or urology: Specialized lab prep is needed for IUI. FSH + LH therapies and IVF warrant referral in most cases

ADDITIONAL THERAPIES

- Increased age or with poor ovarian reserve, consideration of donor-egg IVF is warranted.
- Consider using surrogate pregnancy if couple is amenable and female cannot conceive.

SURGERY/OTHER PROCEDURES

Reproductive surgery may be necessary in those with anatomic causes of infertility. Polypectomy could be beneficial for large polyps obstructing the lumen of the uterus. Myomectomy may increase pregnancy success rates for intramural fibroids that obstruct or distort the uterine cavity. Salpingectomy is recommended and increases fertility in those with hydrosalpinx.

COMPLEMENTARY & ALTERNATIVE MEDICINE

Acupuncture may increase live birth rates with IVF.

INPATIENT CONSIDERATIONS

Admission Criteria/Initial Stabilization

Rarely needed; however, may be needed occasionally for problems in early pregnancy and OHSS

ONGOING CARE

FOLLOW-UP RECOMMENDATIONS

Patients should be referred to a specialist and consider more aggressive options if not successful after 3–6 cycles of oral ovulation induction.

Patient Monitoring

Cycle monitoring may decrease risks. US can show the number of developing follicles per cycle, which may help to predict OHSS and risk of multiple gestations.

DIET

A diet with sufficient calories to maintain a BMI permissive for ovulation is important. If obese, weight loss is recommended.

PATIENT EDUCATION

- Knowledge of women of reproductive age is lacking regarding the adverse effects of STI, irregular menses, and obesity on reproduction. Infertility treatment should focus on patient education (6)[A].
- American Society for Reproductive Medicine (http://www.asrm.org)
- Resolve: Patient advocacy group (http://www.resolve.org)

PROGNOSIS

Excellent; most couples will achieve a pregnancy. Without therapy, ~50% of couples not yet pregnant will conceive during the 2nd and 3rd years of trying.

COMPLICATIONS

Anxiety (stress levels are high during treatment), multiple pregnancy (rates increase with all medical ovulation induction therapies), OHSS (very rare with oral medications but more common with FSH treatments). Couples with infertility may have a slightly increased risk of congenital abnormalities in offspring.

REFERENCES

1. Tersigni C, Castellani R, de Waure C, et al. Celiac disease and reproductive disorders: meta-analysis of epidemiologic associations and potential pathogenic mechanisms. *Hum Reprod Update*. 2014;20(4):582–593.
2. Hurst BS, Lange SS, Kullstam SM, et al. Obstetric and gynecologic challenges in women with Ehlers-Danlos syndrome. *Obstet Gynecol*. 2014;123(3):506–513.
3. Ruder EH, Hartman TJ, Reindollar RH, et al. Female dietary antioxidant intake and time to pregnancy among couples treated for unexplained infertility. *Fertil Steril*. 2014;101(3):759–766.
4. Zareba P, Colaci DS, Afeiche M, et al. Semen quality in relation to antioxidant intake in a healthy male population. *Fertil Steril*. 2013;100(6):1572–1579.
5. Grigorescu V, Zhang Y, Kissin DM, et al. Maternal characteristics and pregnancy outcomes after assisted reproductive technology by infertility diagnosis: ovulatory dysfunction versus tubal obstruction. *Fertil Steril*. 2014;101(4):1019–1025.
6. Lundsberg LS, Pal L, Gariepy AM, et al. Knowledge, attitudes, and practices regarding conception and fertility: a population-based survey among reproductive-age United States women. *Fertil Steril*. 2014;101(3):767–774.

ADDITIONAL READING

- Fritz MA. The modern infertility evaluation. *Clin Obst Gynecol*. 2012;55(3):692–705.
- Pavone ME, Hirshfeld-Cytron JE, Kazer RR. The progressive simplification of the infertility evaluation. *Obstet Gynecol Surv*. 2011;66(1):31–41.
- The Practice Committee of American Society for Reproductive Medicine. Diagnostic evaluation of the infertile female: a committee opinion. *Fertil Steril*. 2012;98(2):302–307.
- The Practice Committee of American Society for Reproductive Medicine. Diagnostic evaluation of the infertile male: a committee opinion. *Fertil Steril*. 2012;98(2):294–301.

SEE ALSO

- Endometriosis; Amenorrhea; Infertility; Metabolic Syndrome; Polycystic Ovarian Syndrome
- Algorithm: Infertility

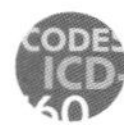

CODES

ICD10

- N97.9 Female infertility, unspecified
- N46.9 Male infertility, unspecified
- N97.1 Female infertility of tubal origin

CLINICAL PEARLS

- Women <35 years of age should be evaluated for infertility after failing to conceive after 1 year of unprotected intercourse; those ≥35 years should receive evaluation after 6 months, and those ≥40 years should receive assistance immediately.
- Medical therapy for endometriosis does not increase pregnancy rates, but surgical treatment does.

I

INFLUENZA

Katherine M. Tromp, PharmD • Hershey S. Bell, MD, MS, FAAFP

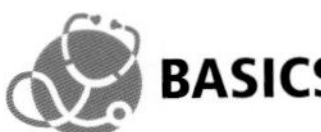

BASICS

DESCRIPTION

- Acute, typically self-limited, febrile infection caused by orthomyxovirus influenza types A and B
- Marked by inflammation of nasal mucosa, pharynx, conjunctiva, and respiratory tract
- Outbreaks have varying degrees of severity and generally peak in winter.
- Influenza virus can undergo antigenic shift (abrupt change) leading to strains of virus to which little immunologic resistance exists in a population, potentially resulting in pandemic outbreak. Minor seasonal variations are called *antigenic drift*.
- System(s) affected: typical cases: head/eyes/ears/nose/throat; pulmonary; complicated cases: cardiac and CNS involvement
- Synonym(s): flu; grippe; acute catarrhal fever

EPIDEMIOLOGY

- Predominant age: children (3 months–16 years) and young adults
  - Morbidity: seasonal morbidity and rates of hospitalization highest in very young (preschool), elderly (>75 years of age), and individuals with comorbid illness (lung disease, malignancy)
- Predominant sex: male = female

Incidence

- Seasonal influenza in preuniversal vaccination: 95 million cases per year, typically fall/winter
- Attack rates in healthy children: 10–40% each year, prior to routine influenza vaccination

ETIOLOGY AND PATHOPHYSIOLOGY

Orthomyxovirus (influenza types A [majority] and B). Influenza A virus subtypes HxNx based on hemagglutinin and neuraminidase.

- Incubation is 1–4 days; infected persons are most contagious during peak symptoms.
- Spread by aerosolized droplets or contact with respiratory secretions
- Hemagglutinin binds to columnar respiratory epithelium where replication occurs, and neuraminidase protein facilitates spread along respiratory epithelium.

RISK FACTORS

- For contracting disease
  - Crowded environments such as nursing homes, schools, and correctional facilities
- For complications
  - Neonates, infants, elderly
  - Pregnancy, especially in 3rd trimester
  - Chronic pulmonary diseases
  - Cardiovascular diseases, including valvular problems and congestive heart failure (CHF)
  - Metabolic disease, morbid obesity
  - Hemoglobinopathies
  - Malignancy
  - Immunosuppression
  - Neuromuscular diseases that limit respiratory function and secretion handling
  - Patients younger than age 19 years of age who are on long-term aspirin therapy

GENERAL PREVENTION

- Vaccination: All persons older than the age of 6 months should be vaccinated annually, with very few exceptions:
  - Inactivated influenza vaccine (IIV) is available with either 3 (IIV3) or 4 (IIV4) strains of influenza. IIV also is available as high-dose, intradermal, cell culture-based (ccIV3), and recombinant hemagglutinin influenza vaccine (RIV3).
  - Live attenuated influenza vaccine (LAIV) is an intranasal quadrivalent vaccine.
- IIV recommended annually for the following:
  - All persons aged ≥6 months
  - Vaccine should be administered annually as soon as the vaccine is available.
  - Protection occurs 1–2 weeks after immunization.
  - Typically mild side effects include low-grade fever and local reaction at vaccination site.
  - Inactivated IM dose: ≥3 years of age: 0.5 mL; children 6–35 months of age: 0.25 mL
  - Intradermal formulation for 18–64-year-olds uses a short 30-gauge needle in a single-use prefilled syringe with 0.1 mL vaccine; somewhat higher local reactions given intradermal
  - Single dose every year except for children <9 years of age, who should receive 2 doses (4 weeks apart) the 1st year they receive influenza vaccine.
  - Vaccine contraindication: Severe allergy such as anaphylaxis to eggs or other IIV components; hives from eggs are not considered a contraindication to IIV due to very low ovalbumin dose in current IIV and good safety information; observe egg-allergic patients for 30 minutes after vaccination; no skin testing with influenza vaccine needed in egg-allergic patients. Egg allergy is a contraindication to LAIV. RIV is safe in patients with an egg allergy.
  - Precaution: Guillain-Barré syndrome within 6 weeks after a previous dose of influenza vaccine
- LAIV recommended annually for the following:
  - Healthy persons 2–49 years old
  - Vaccine contraindications: anaphylaxis to eggs or other vaccine components, immunocompromising conditions, pregnancy, high-risk conditions including asthma or other chronic cardiopulmonary conditions, history of Guillain-Barré syndrome, chronic aspirin therapy in children
  - Single dose every year except for children <9 years of age, who should receive 2 doses (4 weeks apart) the 1st year they receive influenza vaccine
- IIV-HD: high-dose trivalent IIV
  - Contains 4× the antigen concentration of IIV
  - Licensed for persons ≥65 years of age
  - Results in higher antibody levels but somewhat higher rates of local reactions
  - Effectiveness being studied
  - Advisory Committee on Immunization Practices does not express a preference for or against IIV-HD.
- Antiviral prophylaxis depends on current resistance patterns each year; see www.cdc.gov/flu for the current patterns or check with local health department:
  - In high-risk groups that have not been vaccinated or need additional control measures during epidemics. *Not* a substitute for vaccination unless vaccine is contraindicated (1)[B]
  - During influenza season, for those with contraindications to vaccine
  - For staff and residents in nursing home outbreaks
  - For immune-deficient persons who are expected not to respond to vaccination

Pediatric Considerations

- Vaccinate children 6–23 months old with IIV.
- Either IIV or LAIV in healthy children 2–18 years of age; LAIV is the preferred choice in children 2–8 years of age when it is available.
- For prophylaxis, oseltamivir dosage varies by weight and is approved for prophylaxis for children 1 year of age and older; see package insert; zanamivir is approved for prophylaxis for children ≥5 years of age at a dosage of 2 inhalations per day. For prophylaxis, the dosage of amantadine and of rimantadine is 5 mg/kg/day up to 150 mg in 2 divided doses. Currently, amantadine is not recommended due to emerging resistance.

Pregnancy Considerations

- The CDC recommends vaccinating all women who will be pregnant during influenza season.
- If unvaccinated at the time of flu season, pregnant women should receive IIV.
- Oseltamivir, zanamivir, rimantadine, and amantadine are pregnancy category C.

COMMONLY ASSOCIATED CONDITIONS

Bacterial pneumonia

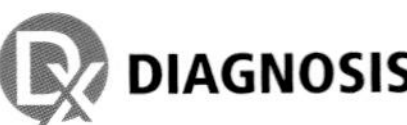

DIAGNOSIS

Rule out influenza by the ABSENCE of the following:

- Systemic symptoms
- Cough
- Not being able to cope with daily activities
- Being confined to bed

HISTORY

Sudden onset of the following:

- Fever (37.7°–40.0°C), especially if combined with presenting within 3 days of illness onset
- Anorexia
- Chills, sweats, malaise, myalgia, arthralgia
- Headache
- Sore throat/pharyngitis
- Nonproductive cough
- Rhinorrhea, nasal congestion

PHYSICAL EXAM

- Physical exam is not specific for influenza.
- Physical examination should exclude complications such as otitis media, pneumonia, sinusitis, and tracheobronchitis.

DIFFERENTIAL DIAGNOSIS

- Respiratory viral infections including respiratory syncytial virus, parainfluenza, adenovirus, enterovirus ("influenza-like-illness")
- Infectious mononucleosis
- Coxsackievirus infections
- Viral or streptococcal tonsillitis
- Atypical mycoplasmal pneumonia
- *Chlamydia pneumoniae*
- Q fever
- Less likely possibilities include severe acute respiratory syndrome, primary HIV infection, acute myeloid leukemia, tuberculosis, anthrax, and malaria.

DIAGNOSTIC TESTS & INTERPRETATION

Initial Tests (lab, imaging)

- During influenza season, diagnosis can solely base on clinical findings. If additional testing is needed
  - Reverse transcription polymerase reaction (RT-PCR) from nasopharyngeal swab or aspirate is the gold standard when diagnostic confirmation needed.
  - CBC: typically shows normal WBC count or mild leukopenia. Leukocytosis may indicate bacterial complications.

- Direct fluorescent antibody or indirect fluorescent antibody staining for influenza antigen; results available within hours but heavily dependent on lab expertise.
- Commercial rapid enzyme-linked immunosorbent assay antigen tests are available. Some rapid tests diagnose influenza A, whereas others diagnose A and B. Sensitivity and specificity vary by manufacturer, strain of influenza, and age of patient. False negatives are fairly common particularly during periods of peak influenza activity in the population being tested.
- Viral isolation not particularly useful except in periods of low influenza activity where making the correct diagnosis is critical.

- Imaging
  - Chest x-ray if pneumonia is suspected

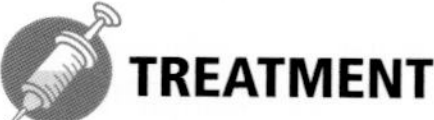

TREATMENT

GENERAL MEASURES

- Symptomatic treatment is typically all that is required (saline nasal spray, analgesic gargle, antipyretics, analgesics).
- Cool-mist or ultrasonic humidifier to increase moisture of inspired air
- Droplet precautions: See www.cdc.gov/flu/professionals/infectioncontrol/index.html.
- 5 days is the average period of viral shedding in immunocompetent hosts.
- Hospitalized patients may require oxygen or ventilatory support.
- Tobacco cessation

MEDICATION

First Line

- Antiviral treatment depends on current resistance patterns each year; check www.cdc.gov/flu or local health department for current patterns. Antivirals are most effective if administered within 1st 48 hours in those with laboratory-confirmed (or highly suspected based on clinical findings) influenza illness.
- Antivirals within 48 hours of symptom onset recommended if at risk of complications (i.e., diabetes, CHD, COPD, asthma, etc.) (2)[B].
- Antivirals recommended if hospitalized (1)[B].
- Antivirals include amantadine, rimantadine, oseltamivir, zanamivir, and (investigational) peramivir.
- Antivirals may be considered for persons not at increased risk of complications from influenza whose onset of symptoms is within the past 48 hours and who wish to shorten the duration of illness and further reduce their relatively low risk of complications.
- Symptomatic treatment is preferred for those patients *without risk factors* and *without* signs of lower respiratory tract infection (3)[A].
- Effect is reduction of symptoms by 24 hours and a reduction in complication rates.
  - Zanamivir dose: 2 inhalations BID for 5 days (age ≥7 years)
  - Rimantadine dose: 100 mg BID for ages 13–64 years; 100 mg/day for >65 years of age
  - Amantadine dose: 100 mg BID for ages 13–64 years; 100 mg/day for >65 years of age
  - Oseltamivir dose: 75 mg PO BID for 5 days (age ≤13 years)
  - If severe renal impairment, 75 mg/day PO
  - Oseltamivir for children ≥1 year of age
    - <15 kg, 30 mg BID
    - >15–23 kg, 45 mg BID
    - >23–40 kg, 60 mg BID
    - >40 kg, 75 mg BID
  - Oseltamivir for children <1 year of age: 3 mg/kg/dose BID
- Antipyretics
  - Acetaminophen: in children
- Precautions
  - Zanamivir may cause bronchospasm if the patient has COPD or asthma; the patient should have a bronchodilator available.
  - Amantadine: has anticholinergic properties and should be used with caution in those with psychiatric, addiction, or neurologic disorders, as it may increase risk for suicide attempts or increase neurologic symptoms
  - Rimantadine may increase the risk of seizures in those with an underlying seizure disorder.
  - Oseltamivir may cause nausea and vomiting; may be less severe if taken with food
- Decrease dose of certain antivirals if creatinine clearance <30 mL/min.

Second Line

- Ibuprofen or other NSAIDs for symptomatic relief
- Aspirin: should not be used in children <16 years due to risk of Reye syndrome

INPATIENT CONSIDERATIONS

Admission Criteria/Initial Stabilization

Outpatient treatment is sufficient except for cases with severe complications or in high-risk groups.

ONGOING CARE

FOLLOW-UP RECOMMENDATIONS

Patient Monitoring

- Mild cases: Usually no follow-up required.
- Moderate or severe cases: Follow until symptoms and any secondary sequelae resolve.

DIET

Increase fluid intake

PATIENT EDUCATION

CDC: www.cdc.gov/flu

PROGNOSIS

Good

COMPLICATIONS

- Otitis media
- Acute sinusitis
- Croup
- Bronchitis
- Pneumonia (primary viral or secondary bacterial)
- Apnea in neonates
- Reye syndrome
- Rhabdomyolysis/myositis
- Postinfluenza asthenia
- COPD or CHF exacerbation
- Encephalopathy, death

Geriatric Considerations

Complications are more likely in elderly who are also more likely to require hospitalization.

REFERENCES

1. Harper SA, Bradley JS, Englund JA, et al. Seasonal influenza in adults and children—diagnosis, treatment, chemoprophylaxis, and institutional outbreak management: clinical practice guidelines of the Infectious Diseases Society of America. *Clin Infect Dis*. 2009;48(8):1003–1032.
2. Lalezari J, Campion K, Keene O, et al. Zanamivir for the treatment of influenza A and B infection in high-risk patients: a pooled analysis of randomized controlled trials. *Arch Int Med*. 2001;161(2):212–217.
3. Center for Disease Control and Prevention. Seasonal influenza. http://cdc.gov/H1N1flu/flu. Accessed 2014.

ADDITIONAL READING

- Centers for Disease Control and Prevention. Advisory Committee on Immunizing Practices (ACIP) recommends a preference for using the nasal spray flu vaccine. http://www.cdc.gov/media/releases/2014/s0625-acip.html. Accessed 2014.
- Ebell MH, White LL, Casault T. A systematic review of the history and physical examination to diagnose influenza. *J Am Board Fam Pract*. 2004;17(1):1–5.
- Grayson ML, Melvani S, Druce J, et al. Efficacy of soap and water and alcohol-based hand-rub preparations against live H1N1 influenza virus on the hands of human volunteers. *Clin Infect Dis*. 2009;48(3):285–291.
- Osterholm MT, Kelley NS, Sommer A, et al. Efficacy and effectiveness of influenza vaccines: a systematic review and meta-analysis. *Lancet Infect Dis*. 2012;12(1):36–44.

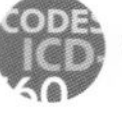

CODES

ICD10

- J11.1 Influenza due to unidentified influenza virus with other respiratory manifestations
- J10.1 Flu due to oth ident influenza virus w oth resp manifest
- J11.00 Flu due to unidentified flu virus w unsp type of pneumonia

CLINICAL PEARLS

- Influenza is an acute, (typically) self-limited, febrile infection caused by influenza virus types A and B.
- With rare exceptions, all persons older than age 6 months should be vaccinated against influenza on an annual basis.
- Complications from influenza are most common in the very young, very old, and those with preexisting comorbidities.
- Hand hygiene either with soap and water (slightly superior) or with alcohol-based hand rubs and covering coughs are simple ways to reduce the spread of influenza.

INGROWN TOENAIL

Steven E. Roskos, MD

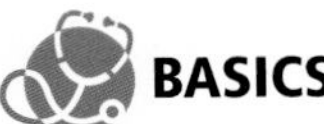

BASICS

DESCRIPTION

- In ingrown toenail, the distal margin of the nail plate grows into the lateral nail fold, causing irritation, inflammation, and sometimes bacterial or fungal infection:
  - Stage 1 (inflammation): erythema, slight edema, tenderness of lateral nail fold
  - Stage 2 (abscess): increased pain, erythema, and edema as well as drainage (purulent or serous)
  - Stage 3 (granulation): further increased erythema, edema and pain, with granulation tissue growing over the nail plate
- Can be recurrent
- Synonym(s): onychocryptosis

EPIDEMIOLOGY

- Great toenail is almost exclusively affected.
- Lateral edge of nail is more commonly affected than the medial edge.
- Most common in males aged 16–25 years
- More common in elderly females than in elderly males
- More common in those with lower incomes

Prevalence

- 24.5/1,000 overall
- 50/1,000 ≥65 years

ETIOLOGY AND PATHOPHYSIOLOGY

- Nail plate penetrates the nail fold.
- This causes a foreign body reaction (inflammation).
- Bacteria or fungi may enter through the opening in the nail fold, causing infection and abscess formation.
- The inflamed and infected tissue hypertrophies, further covering the nail plate.

RISK FACTORS

- Genetic factors:
  - Increased nail fold width
  - Decreased nail thickness
  - Medial rotation of the toe
- Many others proposed; none proven, including the following:
  - Distorted, thickened nail (onychogryphosis)
  - Fungal infection (onychomycosis)
  - Hyperhidrosis
  - Improper trimming of the lateral nail plate
  - Poorly fitting shoes
  - Trauma to nail or nail fold

GENERAL PREVENTION

- Properly fitting shoes
- Proper nail trimming

DIAGNOSIS

HISTORY

- Pain
- Redness
- Swelling
- Drainage

PHYSICAL EXAM

- Tenderness of lateral nail fold
- Erythema
- Edema
- Drainage (serous or purulent)
- Granulation tissue
- Hypertrophy of lateral nail fold

DIFFERENTIAL DIAGNOSIS

- Cellulitis
- Felon (deep abscess on plantar aspect of toe)
- Onychogryphosis (gross thickening and hardening of the nail)
- Onycholysis (separation of nail from nail bed)
- Onychomycosis (fungal infection of the nail)
- Osteomyelitis
- Paronychia
- Subungual exostosis (osteochondroma beneath the nail)

DIAGNOSTIC TESTS & INTERPRETATION

Initial Tests (lab, imaging)

None needed unless patient appears septic. Then consider CBC and blood cultures.

- Consider MRI, x-ray, or bone scan if osteomyelitis is suspected.
- Consider x-ray if subungual exostosis is suspected.

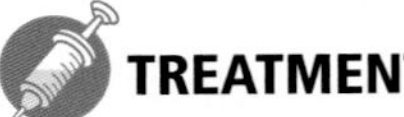

TREATMENT

- Surgical interventions are more effective than nonsurgical interventions in preventing recurrence (1,2)[A].
- The use of phenol for nail bed ablation is probably more effective than nail avulsion alone in preventing recurrence (1,2)[A].
- Nail avulsion techniques (described in the following section) are more effective than nail fold debulking techniques (not described in this topic) (2)[A]. Nonsurgical interventions, such as a flexible gutter splint, are another option for treatment of stage 2 or 3 ingrown nails (3,4)[B].

GENERAL MEASURES

For stage 1:

- Warm water soaks twice a day
- Proper nail trimming
- Properly fitted shoes

MEDICATION

- Neither oral nor topical antibiotics are useful as an adjunct to surgical treatment.
- NSAIDs are usually adequate for analgesia.

ADDITIONAL THERAPIES

- For stage 1 ingrown nails, several treatments are available:
  - Cotton wool
    - Bluntly insert a wisp of cotton under the ingrown portion of the nail.
    - Instruct the patient to reinsert new cotton if the other comes out until the nail grows beyond the nail fold.
    - Consider adding silver nitrate cautery to the nail fold, which the patient then repeats at home.
  - Dental floss
    - Bluntly insert some dental floss to lift the nail away from the lateral nail fold.
    - Instruct the patient to replace the floss as necessary if it comes out or gets dirty.
    - Keep floss in place until the nail grows beyond the nail fold.
  - Taping
    - Apply surgical tape to both sides of toe.
    - Use another piece of tape from 1 side to the other to pull the lateral nail fold away from the nail plate.
    - Instruct the patient to keep taping until the nail grows beyond the fold.
  - Cryotherapy of the lateral nail fold
- For stage 2 ingrown nails, consider attempting conservative treatment, as above, especially cotton, wool, or cryotherapy.

SURGERY/OTHER PROCEDURES

- For stage 2 ingrown nails where conservative treatment has failed, stage 3 ingrown nails, or recurrent ingrown nails, consider either
  - Partial avulsion of the nail with phenol nail matrix ablation
    - Achieve local anesthesia as described in the following text.
    - Place a tourniquet around the base of the toe.
    - Incise the nail longitudinally with scissors or a nail splitter a few millimeters from the ingrown border, starting at the distal edge and proceeding to the matrix.

  - Elevate the ingrown part of the nail from the nail bed with a periosteal (Freer) elevator or hemostat.
  - Pull this portion gently out with a hemostat.
  - Dip a urethral swab in 80–88% phenol solution.
  - Apply the phenol for 1 minute to the nail matrix under the proximal nail fold. Use multiple swabs if necessary.
  - Wash the area with isopropyl (rubbing) alcohol to neutralize phenol.
- Flexible gutter splint
  - Cut a 1–2-cm long piece of sterilized plastic tube, such as IV tubing, 2–3 mm in diameter (alternatively, you may use a cap from a 29-gauge needle).
  - Make a slit in the tubing lengthwise, and cut the end off at an angle.
  - Apply local anesthesia.
  - Release the ingrown edge of the nail from the nail fold with a hemostat.
  - Slide the tube, angled end first, along the ingrown edge of the nail.
  - Consider fixing the tube in place with self-curing formable acrylic resin (used for dentures and sculptured nails), tape, or a single suture through the nail plate.
  - Leave the tube in place until nail has grown beyond the nail fold.

- Other options for nail matrix ablation include the following:
  - Sodium hydroxide (NaOH)
  - Cryotherapy
  - Electrocautery with a special flattened tip coated with Teflon on 1 side to protect the proximal nail fold
  - Curettage
  - Surgical excision
- Local anesthesia can be achieved with either
  - Distal wing block: Infuse 1% lidocaine without epinephrine near the junction of the proximal and lateral nail folds. Continue infusing until the nail folds and the tip of the digit under the distal nail are white from the pressure of the anesthetic.
  - Digital ring block: Infuse 1% lidocaine without epinephrine on the medial and lateral surfaces of the involved digit to anesthetize the plantar and dorsal digital nerves. Lidocaine with epinephrine may be used in selected patients (no peripheral vascular disease, diabetes, cardiac problems, or any evidence of digital infection, gangrene, or bone fracture) (5).

ONGOING CARE

FOLLOW-UP RECOMMENDATIONS

- Dress with antibiotic ointment or sterile petroleum jelly; cover with sterile gauze and tube gauze.
- Postop instructions should include the following:
  - Rest and elevate the foot for 12–24 hours.
  - Take NSAIDs for discomfort.
  - Change dressing and wash with soap and water daily.
  - Expect a sterile exudate for 2–6 weeks.
  - Avulsed nails may take 6–12 months to grow completely out (if no matrix ablation).
  - Call for increasing pain, redness, or swelling.
  - Average time to return to normal activities is 2 weeks.
- Patients treated conservatively should be followed up in the office every 7–10 days until marked improvement is noted.

PATIENT EDUCATION

- Trim nails straight across perpendicular to long axis of the nail (do not round corners) and not too short.
- Wear properly fitting, comfortable shoes.

COMPLICATIONS

- Cellulitis after surgical procedure (uncommon)
- Damage to fascia or periosteum from overly aggressive matrix ablation
- Damage to nail bed
- Distal toe ischemia due to prolonged use of a tourniquet during surgery (rare)
- Nail plate deformity (due to damage to nail matrix)
- Osteomyelitis (rare)
- Permanent narrowing of nail (if matrix ablation is performed)
- Postop wound drainage
- Recurrence (40–80% with avulsion alone, 0.6–14% with matrix ablation, 6–13% with gutter splint)

REFERENCES

1. Eekhof JA, Van Wijk B, Knuistingh Neven A, et al. Interventions for ingrowing toenails. *Cochrane Database Syst Rev*. 2012;(4):CD001541.
2. Park DH, Singh D. The management of ingrowing toenails. *BMJ*. 2012;344:e2089.
3. Arai H, Arai T, Nakajima H, et al. Formable acrylic treatment for ingrowing nail with gutter splint and sculptured nail. *Int J Dermatol*. 2004;43(10):759–765.
4. Nazari S. A simple and practical method in treatment of ingrown nails: splinting by flexible tube. *J Eur Acad Dermatol Venereol*. 2006;20(10):1302–1306.
5. Altinyazar HC, Demirel CB, Koca R, et al. Digital block with and without epinephrine during chemical matricectomy with phenol. *Dermatol Surg*. 2010;36(10):1568–1571.

ADDITIONAL READING

- Bos AM, van Tilburg MW, van Sorge AA, et al. Randomized clinical trial of surgical technique and local antibiotics for ingrowing toenail. *Br J Surg*. 2007;94(3):292–296.
- Chapeskie H. Ingrown toenail or overgrown toe skin?: alternative treatment for onychocryptosis. *Can Fam Physician*. 2008;54(11):1561–1562.
- Reyzelman AM, Trombello KA, Vayser DJ, et al. Are antibiotics necessary in the treatment of locally infected ingrown toenails? *Arch Fam Med*. 2000;9(9):930–932.
- Richert B. Basic nail surgery. *Dermatol Clin*. 2006;24(3):313–322.
- Woo SH, Kim IH. Surgical pearl: nail edge separation with dental floss for ingrown toenails. *J Am Acad Dermatol*. 2004;50(6):939–940.

SEE ALSO

For a video of this Nail Avulsion and Matrixectomy procedure, go to: http://5minuteconsult.com/procedure/1508006

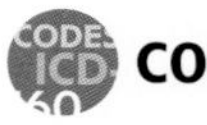

CODES

ICD10

L60.0 Ingrowing nail

CLINICAL PEARLS

- The best treatment for a stage 1 ingrown toenail is to insert a wisp of cotton or dental floss between the nail plate and lateral nail fold.
- The best treatment for a stage 3 ingrown toenail is partial nail avulsion with phenol matrix ablation.
- A patient can prevent ingrown toenails by trimming nails properly and wearing properly fitting shoes.
- Antibiotics are not useful in the treatment of ingrown nails in conjunction with surgical treatment.

INJURY AND VIOLENCE

Jonathan R. Ballard, MD, MPH, MPhil

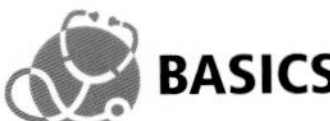

BASICS

DESCRIPTION

- Injury, intentional or not, is considered predictable and preventable (1).
- Unintentional injuries are no longer considered "accidents" given that injuries are preventable (1).
- Unintentional injury is the 5th leading cause of death, and intentional self-harm is the 10th leading cause of death in 2010 in the United States (2).
- Injury is the leading cause of death of people aged 1–44 years and a leading cause of disability for people of all ages, regardless of sex, race/ethnicity, or socioeconomic status (1).
- Violence-related deaths account for 54,103 deaths in the United States in 2009 (3) with 61% suicide, 25% homicide, and 14% deaths of undetermined intent (4).

EPIDEMIOLOGY

Incidence

Leading Cause of Death by Age Group, United States, 2011 (5)

Age	Most Common	Number of Deaths
<1	Congenital anomalies	5,013
1–44	**Unintentional injury**	46,050
45–64	Malignant neoplasm	161,469
65+	Heart disease	475,097

- Children mostly die of unintentional injuries: (in order) motor vehicle accidents (MVAs), fire/burn, drowning, and suffocation (6)
- MVAs are the most common type of unintentional injury in adolescents, followed by firearm-associated injuries (7).
- Suicide is the second leading cause of death for adolescents and young adults age 15–34 years (5).
- Poisoning is particularly deadly for young adults ages 15–59 years, for whom it is the leading cause of unintentional home injury deaths (6).
- Unintentional death by firearm is fourth common cause of death in children ages 5–14 years and third common cause for adolescents and adults ages 15–29 years (6).
- Homicide is the third leading cause of death in 2011 for persons between ages 1 and 4 years, and 15 and 34 years in the United States (5).
- Watch for homicide *as cause of unexplained death in young children*.

ETIOLOGY AND PATHOPHYSIOLOGY

Multifactorial

RISK FACTORS

- MVAs:
  - MVAs account for 35,303 deaths in 2010 in the United States, with an age-adjusted rate of 11 deaths per 100,000 persons (3).
  - More than 2.3 million adult drivers and passengers were treated in emergency departments from MVAs in 2009 (8).
  - Young adults (18–24) have the highest crash-related injury rates of all adults (8).
  - Motorcyclists are found to be 37 times more likely to die in a motor vehicle crash than passenger car occupants and 9 times more likely to be injured (9).
  - Risk factors for involvement in an MVA include high speed; teenage drivers; alcohol consumption; distracted driving, including hand-held mobile phones; and inadequate visibility (10).
  - Risk of death by an MVA increases with male driver, inexperience, nighttime driving, speeding, tailgating, driving with other teenagers, cell phones, unrestrained occupants, use of older cars, nonuse of crash helmets, alcohol and drug use. In elderly, poor vision, medical conditions, and comorbidities increases risk of death by an MVA (8,10).
- Pedestrians:
  - 4,280 pedestrians were killed by motor vehicles in 2010, and about 70,000 were injured in 2010 (8).
  - Pedestrians are 1.5 more times likely than passenger vehicle occupants to be killed in a car crash on each trip (8).
- Bicycles:
  - Risk of death increased from crash with motor vehicle if speed $>$30 km/h ($\sim$18 mph) and cyclist impact with front of vehicle (10).
  - Risk factors for cyclist injury include alcohol consumption, shared use motorways, poor visibility, lack of understanding of road safety, and design/type of impacting vehicle (10).
- Suffocation: increased risk for children $<$1 year, unsafe sleeping environments (11)
- Drowning: increased risk for African American children, unattended children in bathtubs, access to swimming pools and recreational water activities (11)
- Homicide:
  - Third leading cause of death for children 1–4 years and adolescents and young adults ages 15–34 years (5).
  - Lack of access to social capital, community organization, and economic resources; familial instability; community and family violence; access to firearms (4)
  - Homicide and suicide: access to firearms, mental health, alcohol and drug use, exposure to suicidal behavior, history of aggressive behavior, cognitive deficits, poor supervision, exposure to violence, parental drug and alcohol use, poor peer-to-peer interaction, academic failure, poverty, lower socioeconomic class (4)
- Adolescent violence:
  - 33% of students are involved in fights annually; 13% of students participated in $\geq$1 fights at school in the last year (11).
  - 17% of students have carried a weapon in the last 30 days; 6.1% of students have carried a weapon to school. 9% of students have been injured by a weapon at school (11).
- Injury (sports related):
  - High school athletes are at increased risk (12).
  - High school students sustained 1.2 million injuries during the 2008–2009 school year (12).
- Bullying:
  - Prevalence is 30% for children either bullying and/or being bullied in 6th–10th graders (13).
  - Bullying associated with low self-esteem, social isolation, and depression (13)
  - 1:9 middle school students report being cyberbullied (via the Internet or cell phones). $\sim$50% of victims don't know perpetrator's identity (13).
- Interpersonal violence (IPV):
  - 40–70% of female homicides killed by boyfriends or husbands (14)
  - Nearly 31% of women and 26% of men report having some form of IPV in their lifetime (14).
  - Dating violence: Prevalence has been reported to range from 9 to 46% (14).
  - Female, young (33% of rapes occur prior to 12 years of age; 50% by 18 years), history of IPV or sexual assault or child abuse, drugs, marital difficulties, unemployment, depression, minority status, income or educational disparity, poverty, weak legal sanctions (14)
- Falls: poor vision, psychotropic medications and diuretics, arthritis, impaired mobility, inappropriate footwear and walking aids, cognitive impairment, gait imbalance, environmental risk factors (9)
- Poisonings:
  - Poisonings are the second leading cause of unintentional home injury deaths for ages 15–59 years (6).
  - Prescription drug overdose is a leading cause of accidental death in adults (6).
  - A signficant increase in opioid-associated deaths has occurred from 2000 to 2008 (6).
  - Combined use of other sedating drugs (6)
  - Watch for opiod-induced poisonings in unexplained altered mental status.

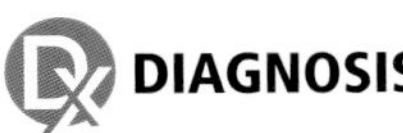

DIAGNOSIS

HISTORY

- Mechanism, timing, and location of injury:
  - Blunt versus penetrating; intentional versus unintentional; others injured versus isolated injury; circumstances (weather, substance use, restrained vs. unrestrained)
  - Does history correlate with level of injury (i.e., level of suspicion for abuse [elderly, child, or partner])?
  - Is further evaluation required (blood and/or urine testing, response to opioid receptor antagonists, imaging)?
- IPV: neurologic deficits, seizures, chronic pain, GI, STI, pregnancy, psychiatric presentations.
  - In January 2013, USPSTF recommends that clinicians screen women of childbearing age for intimate partner violence, such as domestic violence, and provide or refer women who screen positive to intervention services (15)[B].
  - There is insufficient evidence to screen elderly or vulnerable adults for abuse or neglect (15)[C].

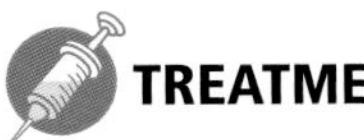

TREATMENT

- Prevention: The primary focus for reducing injury and violence is specific individually tailored preventive measures based on risk factors and population-level prevention (1). Prevention efforts have been framed as "the 5 E's": enhanced education, engineering strategies, economic incentives, and enforcement/enactment of laws (1,9)[C].
- Prevention by level of intervention: primary (i.e., prevent crash), secondary (i.e., prevent injury upon crash), and tertiary (i.e., prevent poor outcomes upon injury) (1,9)[C]

- Acute setting: Follow Basic Life Support (BLS), Advanced Trauma Life Support (ATLS), Advanced Cardiovascular Life Support (ACLS), and Pediatric Advanced Life Support (PALS) guidelines (1,16)[A].
- Motor vehicle injuries:
  - Infants, toddlers, and children: age-appropriate child safety seats and passenger restraints with distribution programs, education programs for parents and caregivers, safety seat checkpoints, harsh penalties for drivers transporting children under the influence of drugs and/or alcohol, legislation regarding restraint of motor vehicle occupants (9)[A]
  - Adolescents and adults: graduated driver licensing programs, blood alcohol concentration laws, minimum drinking age laws, sobriety checkpoints, programs for alcohol servers, zero–alcohol tolerance laws for young drivers, school-based education programs on drinking and driving. Emergency medical services (EMS) response times, engineering cars for rapid extraction, organized trauma systems; collapsible automobile steering columns have been shown to decrease injury mortality and morbidity (9)[B]
  - Older adults: alternative transportation programs, screening for high-risk drivers, gradual curtailment of driving privileges, more frequent license renewal process (9)[B]
  - Bicycle helmets can reduce risk of head injury by 63–88%. Canadian helmet legislation decreased mortality by 52% (9)[B].
  - Pedestrian injury: pedestrian safety education, reflective clothing, use of crosswalks, limit mobile phone use while crossing roads (9)[B]. Street lighting for pedestrians (9)[A]. Fluorescent clothing for pedestrians and cyclists (9)[A]
  - Cyclists injury: flashing lights and reflectors at night (9)[B]. Helmet use (9)[A]. Cyclists separation for motor vehicles (9)[B]
- Falls:
  - Home safety assessments, installation of handrails and grab bars, removal of tripping hazards, nonslip mats, exercise programs such as Tai Chi to improve strength and balance, night lights, cataract surgery, gradual withdrawal of psychotropic medication (9)[B]
  - In May 2012, USPSTF recommended exercise or physical therapy and vitamin D supplementation to prevent falls in community-dwelling adults aged 65 years or older who are at increased risk for falls (15)[B].
  - The USPSTF does not recommend automatically performing an in-depth multifactorial risk assessment in conjunction with comprehensive management of identified risks to prevent falls in community-dwelling adults aged 65 years or older because the likelihood of benefit is small (15)[C].
- Drowning:
  - Improved supervision of young children, especially for those with epilepsy. Swimming lessons in those >4 years, trained lifeguard supervision, fencing, locked gates and pool alarms, no use of alcohol in recreation aquatic activities, personal flotation devices and boating safety awareness; parental and caregiver certification in CPR (9)[B]
- Violence (homicide, suicide, assaults):
  - Primary prevention: Most effective strategies focus on younger age groups to change individual attitudes and risk-taking behaviors (9)[C].
  - Secondary prevention: Detect and identify violence in early stages (9)[B]. The USPSTF recommends that clinicians screen women of childbearing age for intimate partner violence, such as domestic violence, and provide or refer women who screen positive to intervention services (15)[B].
  - Tertiary prevention: IPV reduced by alcoholism treatment for partner, intense advocacy interventions of >12 hours (9)[A]
  - Suicide: access to mental health services, improved family and community support, development of healthy coping and problem-solving skills. USPSTF recommends screening adults for depression when depression care supports are in place to assure accurate diagnosis, effective treatment, and follow-up (15)[B].
  - Dating violence: self-reported dating violence reduced by school and community-based programs for prevention of dating violence (9)[A]
- Sports-related injuries:
  - Proper equipment. Helmets can prevent bicyclist head injuries and mortality (9)[A].
  - Plan of action for dealing with concussion and head injury in young athletes, with guidelines regarding if or when it is safe to return to play (17)[B]
- Poisonings:
  - Follow acute care guidelines. Contact Poison Control Center hotline immediately after discovered ingestion of toxin for recommendations (18)[A].

ONGOING CARE

COMPLICATIONS

Social burden of injury: loss of productivity, emotional loss, nonmedical expenditures, reduced quality of life, litigation, rehabilitation, mental health costs, altered family and peer relationships, chronic pain, substance use and abuse, changes in lifestyle (1,9)

REFERENCES

1. Sleet DA, Dahlberg LL, Basavaraju SV, et al. Injury prevention, violence prevention, and trauma care: building the scientific base. *MMWR Surveill Summ*. 2011;60(Suppl 4):78–85.
2. Murphy SL, Xu J, Kochanek KD. Deaths: final data for 2010. *Nat Vital Stat Rep*. 2013;61(4):1–118.
3. Centers for Disease Control and Prevention, National Center for Injury Prevention and Control. Web-based Injury Statistics Query and Reporting System (WISQARS). www.cdc.gov/ncipc/wisqars. Accessed 2014.
4. Centers for Disease Control and Prevention. Division of Violence Prevention Annual Report 2011. http://www.cdc.gov/violenceprevention/pdf/dvp_annualreport_2011.pdf. Accessed 2014.

Centers for Disease Control and Prevention, National Center for Injury Prevention and Control. Leading Causes of Death 2011. http://www.cdc.gov/injury/wisqars/pdf/leading_causes_of_death_by_age_group_2011-a.pdf. Accessed 2014.

5. Mack KA, Rudd RA, Mickalide AD, et al. Fatal unintentional injuries in the home in the U.S., 2000–2008. *Am J Prev Med*. 2013;44(3):239–246.
6. Centers for Disease Control and Prevention. National Suicide Statistics at a Glance. http://www.cdc.gov/ViolencePrevention/suicide/statistics/index.html. Accessed 2014.
7. Centers for Disease Control and Prevention. Injury Prevention and Control: Motor Vehicle Safety. http://www.cdc.gov/Motorvehiclesafety/. Accessed 2014.
8. Curry P, Ramaiah R, Vavilala MS. Current trends and update on injury prevention. *Int J Crit Illn Inj Sci*. 2011;1(1):57–65.
9. World Health Organization. World report on road traffic injury and prevention. 2004. http://whqlibdoc.who.int/publications/2004/9241562609.pdf?ua=1. Accessed 2014.
10. Committee on Injury, Violence, and Poison Prevention. Policy statement–role of the pediatrician in youth violence prevention. *Pediatrics*. 2009;124(1):393–402.
11. Centers for Disease Control and Prevention. National Action Plan for Child Injury Prevention. 2012. http://www.cdc.gov/safechild/pdf/National_Action_Plan_for_Child_Injury_Prevention.pdf. Accessed 2014.
12. Donnerstein E. Internet bullying. *Pediatr Clin North Am*. 2012;59(3):623–633.
13. Moyer VA. Screening for intimate partner violence and abuse of elderly and vulnerable adults. *Ann Intern Med*. 2013;158(6):478–486.
14. US Preventive Services Task Force. Recommendations. http://www.uspreventiveservicestaskforce.org/recommendations.htm. Accessed 2014.
15. Field JM, Hazinski MF, Sayre MR, et al. Executive summary: 2010 American Heart Association guidelines for cardiopulmonary resuscitation and emergency cardiovascular care. *Circulation*. 2010;122(18)(Suppl 3):S640–S656.
16. Armstrong C. Evaluation and management of concussion in athletes: recommendations from the ANN. *Am Fam Physician*. 2014;89(7).585–7.
17. Mowry JB, Spyker DA, Cantilena LR, et al. 2012 annual report of the American Association of Poison Control Centers' National Poison Data System (NPDS). *Clin Toxicol*. 2013;51(10):949–1229.

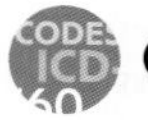

CODES

ICD10

- T14.90 Injury, unspecified
- T14.8 Other injury of unspecified body region
- R29.6 Repeated falls

CLINICAL PEARLS

- Injury and violence are predictable and preventable.
- Unintentional injury is the fifth leading cause of death.
- Injury is the primary source of lost years of productive life for individuals younger than age 44 years.
- MVAs cause most deaths in children and adolescents.
- Children die of unintentional injuries (in order): MVA, drowning, fire/burn, and suffocation
- Nearly 31% of women and 26% of men report having some form of IPV in their lifetime.

INSOMNIA

Susanne Wild, MD

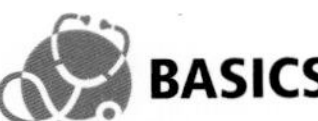

BASICS

DESCRIPTION

- Difficulty initiating or maintaining sleep or non-restorative sleep despite adequate opportunity and circumstances for sleep
- Causes at least one of the following forms of daytime impairment related to nighttime sleep difficulty:
  - Fatigue or malaise
  - Attention, concentration, or memory impairment
  - Social or vocational dysfunction or poor school performance
  - Mood disturbance or irritability
  - Daytime sleepiness
  - Motivation, energy, or initiative reduction
  - Proneness for errors or accidents at work or while driving
  - Tension, headaches, or GI symptoms in response to sleep loss
  - Concerns or worries about sleep

EPIDEMIOLOGY

- Predominant age: increases with age
- Predominant sex: female > male (5:1)

Prevalence

- Insomnia (transient and chronic): 5–35% of the population; 10–15% associated with daytime impairment
- Chronic insomnia: 10% middle-aged adults; 1/3 of people >65 years

ETIOLOGY AND PATHOPHYSIOLOGY

- Transient/intermittent (<30 days)
  - Stress/excitement/bereavement
  - Shift work
  - Medical illness
  - High altitude
- Chronic (>30 days)
  - Medical: gastroesophageal reflux disease, sleep apnea, chronic pain, congestive heart failure, Alzheimer disease, Parkinson disease, chronic fatigue syndrome, irritable bowel syndrome
  - Psychiatric: mood, anxiety, psychotic disorders
  - Primary sleep disorder: idiopathic, psychophysiologic (heightened arousal and learned sleep-preventing associations), paradoxical (sleep state misperception)
  - Circadian rhythm disorder: irregular pattern, jet lag, delayed/advanced sleep phase, shift work
  - Environmental: light (liquid crystal display [LCD] clocks), noise (snoring, household, traffic), movements (partner/young children/pets)
  - Behavioral: poor sleep hygiene, adjustment sleep disorder
  - Substance induced
  - Medications: antihypertensives, antidepressants, corticosteroids, levodopa-carbidopa, phenytoin, quinidine, theophylline, thyroid hormones

Pregnancy Considerations

Transient insomnia occurs secondary to change of sleep position, nocturia, gastritis, back pain, anxiety.

RISK FACTORS

- Age
- Female gender
- Medical comorbidities
- Unemployment
- Psychiatric illness
- Impaired social relationships
- Lower socioeconomic status
- Shift work
- Separation from spouse or partner
- Drug and substance abuse

GENERAL PREVENTION

- Practice consistent sleep hygiene:
  - Fixed wake-up times and bedtimes regardless of amount of sleep obtained (weekdays and weekends)
  - Go to bed only when sleepy.
  - Avoid naps.
  - Sleep in cool, dark, quiet environment.
  - No activities or stimuli in bedroom associated with anything but sleep or sex.
  - 30-minute wind-down time before sleep
  - If unable to sleep within 20 minutes, move to another environment and engage in quiet activity until sleepy.
- Limit caffeine intake to mornings.
- No alcohol after 4 PM
- Fixed eating times
- Avoid medications that interfere with sleep.
- Regular moderate exercise

COMMONLY ASSOCIATED CONDITIONS

- Psychiatric disorders
- Painful musculoskeletal conditions
- Obstructive sleep apnea
- Restless leg syndrome
- Drug or alcohol addiction/dependence

DIAGNOSIS

HISTORY

- Daytime sleepiness and napping
- Unintended sleep episodes (driving, working)
- Insomnia history
  - Duration, time of problem
  - Sleep latency, difficulty in maintaining sleep (repeated awakening), early morning awakening, nonrestorative sleep, or patterns (weekday vs. weekend, with or without bed partner, home vs. away)
- Sleep hygiene
  - Bedtime/wakening time
  - Physical environment of sleep area: LED clocks, TV, room lighting, ambient noise
  - Activity: nighttime eating, exercise, sexual activity
  - Intake: caffeine, alcohol, herbal supplements, diet pills, illicit drugs, prescriptions, over-the-counter (OTC) sleep aids
- Symptoms or history of depression, anxiety, obsessive-compulsive disorder, or other major psychological symptomatology
- Symptoms of restless leg syndrome and periodic limb movement disorder
- Symptoms of heightened arousal
- Snoring and other symptoms of sleep apnea
- Symptoms or history of drug or alcohol abuse
- Current medication use
- Chronic medical conditions
- Acute change or stressors such as travel or shift work
- Sleep diary: sleep log for 7 consecutive days

DIFFERENTIAL DIAGNOSIS

- Sleep-disordered breathing such as obstructive sleep apnea
- CNS hypersomnias (e.g., narcolepsy)
- Circadian rhythm sleep disturbances
- Sleep-related movement disorders (e.g., restless leg syndrome)
- Substance abuse
- Insomnia due to medical or neurologic disorder
- Mood and anxiety disorders such as depression or anxiety

DIAGNOSTIC TESTS & INTERPRETATION

- Diagnostic testing usually not required; consider polysomnography if sleep apnea or periodic limb movement disorder is suspected (1)[C].
- Primary insomnia
  - Symptoms for at least 1 month: difficulty in initiating/maintaining sleep or nonrestorative sleep
  - Impairment in social, occupational, or other important areas of functioning
  - Does not occur exclusively during narcolepsy, breathing-related sleep disorder, circadian rhythm sleep disorder, or parasomnia
  - Does not occur exclusively during major depressive disorder, generalized anxiety disorder, delirium
  - Is not secondary to physiologic effects of substance or general medical condition
  - Sleep disturbance (or resultant daytime fatigue) causes clinically significant distress.
- Secondary insomnia
  - Due to substance abuse, medication induced (diuretics, stimulants, etc.), primary depressive disorder, generalized anxiety disorder or phobias, acute situational stress, posttraumatic stress disorder, pain

Initial Tests (lab, imaging)

Testing to consider based on history and physical exam:

- Thyroid-stimulating hormone
- Urine toxicology

Diagnostic Procedures/Other

Polysomnography or multiple sleep latency test not routinely indicated but may be considered if

- Initial diagnosis is uncertain.
- Treatment interventions have proven unsuccessful.

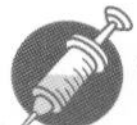

TREATMENT

- Transient insomnia
  - May use medications for short-term use only; benzodiazepines favored
  - Self-medicating with alcohol can increase awakenings and sleep-stage changes.
- Chronic insomnia
  - Treatment of underlying condition (major depressive disorder, generalized anxiety disorder, medications, pain, substance abuse)
  - Advise good sleep hygiene.
  - Cognitive-behavioral therapy is 1st-line treatment for chronic insomnia, especially in >60 years population, especially when sedatives are not advantageous (2)[A].
  - Behavioral therapy effective treatment for insomnia and a potentially more effective long-term treatment than pharmacotherapy (3)[B].
  - Ramelteon is the only agent without abuse potential (4)[B].

MEDICATION

- Reserved for transient insomnia such as with jet lag, stress reactions, transient medical condition
- Nonbenzodiazepine hypnotics
  - Act on benzodiazepine receptor so have abuse potential
    - Zaleplon (Sonata) 5–20 mg; half-life 1 hour
    - Zolpidem (Ambien) 5–10 mg (males); 5 mg (females); half-life 2.5–3 hours
    - Zolpidem (Ambien CR) 6.25–12.5 mg (males); 6.25 mg (females); half-life 2.5–3 hours
    - Eszopiclone (Lunesta) 1–3 mg; half-life 6 hours
- Benzodiazepine hypnotics
  - Intermediate acting
    - Temazepam 7.5–30 mg; half-life 8.8 hours long-acting
      - Lorazepam 1–4 mg; half-life 14 hours
      - Diazepam 5–10 mg; half-life 30–60 hours
- Contraindications/precautions:
  - Not indicated for long-term treatment due to risks of tolerance, dependency, daytime attention and concentration compromise, incoordination, rebound insomnia
  - Long-acting benzodiazepines associated with higher incidence of daytime sedation and motor impairment
  - Avoid in elderly, pregnant, breastfeeding, substance abusers, and patients with suicidal or parasuicidal behaviors.
  - Avoid in patients with untreated obstructive apnea and chronic pulmonary disease.
  - No good evidence for benzodiazepines for patients undergoing palliative care (5)[A].
  - Nonbenzodiazepine benzodiazepine receptor agonists may occasionally induce parasomnias (sleepwalking, sleep eating, sleep driving).
- Melatonin receptor agonist
  - Ramelteon 8 mg; half-life 1–2.6 hours
    - Effective to reduce sleep time onset for short- and long-term use in adults, without abuse potential; no comparative studies with older agents have been completed. Onset of effect may take up to 3 weeks (4)[B].
- Serotonergic antidepressants
  - Trazodone 25–200 mg; half-life 3–9 hours
  - Doxepin 10–50 mg; half-life 15 hours
    - New formulation of medication available at dosage 3–6 mg QHS.
  - Amitriptyline 25–50 mg; half-life 10–26 hours
  - Mirtazapine 7.5–15 mg; half-life 20–40 hours
- Sedating antihistamines are not recommended and should be used conservatively for insomnia due to insufficient evidence of efficacy and significant concerns about risks of these medications.

Geriatric Considerations

Caution (risk of falls and confusion) when prescribing benzodiazepines or other sedative hypnotics; if absolutely necessary, use short-acting nonbenzodiazepine benzodiazepine agonists at half the dosage or melatonin agonists for short-term treatment.

ADDITIONAL THERAPIES

Associated with hypertension, congestive heart failure, anxiety and depression, and obesity; management of these chronic conditions will help with incidence and symptoms of insomnia.

COMPLEMENTARY & ALTERNATIVE MEDICINE

- Melatonin: decreases sleep latency when taken 30–120 minutes prior to bedtime, but there is no good evidence for efficacy in insomnia, and long-term effects are unknown (6)[B].
- Valerian: inconsistent evidence supporting efficacy, and its slow onset of action (2–3 weeks) makes it unsuitable for the acute treatment of insomnia.
- Acupuncture: insufficient evidence on effect of needle acupuncture and its variants (7)
- Cognitive behavioral therapy (including relaxation therapy): effective and considered more useful than medications; recommended initial treatment for patients with chronic insomnia

ONGOING CARE

FOLLOW-UP RECOMMENDATIONS

- Daily exercise improves quality of sleep and may be more effective than medication.
- Avoid exercise within 4 hours of bedtime.

Patient Monitoring

- Reassess need for medications periodically; avoid standing prescriptions.
- Caution patients that nonbenzodiazepine benzodiazepine agonists (zolpidem, zaleplon, eszopiclone), as well as benzodiazepines, can be habit forming.
- Studies suggest an association between receiving a hypnotic prescription and a >3-fold increase in hazards of death, even when prescribed <18 pills per year (8)[B].

DIET

- Avoid caffeine or reserve for morning only.
- Avoid heavy late-night snacks (light snack at bedtime may help)
- Avoid alcohol within 6 hours of bedtime.

PROGNOSIS

- Situational insomnia should resolve with time.
- Treatment of underlying etiology and consistent sleep hygiene are the mainstays of treatment.

COMPLICATIONS

- Transient insomnia can become chronic.
- Daytime sleepiness, cognitive dysfunction
- Pulmonary hypertension if chronic sleep apnea left untreated
- Sleep apnea may lead to hypertension, stroke, or cardiac ischemia.

REFERENCES

1. Kushida CA, Littner MR, Morgenthaler T, et al. Practice parameters for the indications for polysomnography and related procedures: an update for 2005. *Sleep*. 2005;28(4):499–521.
2. Montgomery P, Dennis J. Cognitive behavioural interventions for sleep problems in adults aged 60+. *Cochrane Database Syst Rev*. 2003;(1):CD003161.
3. Ebben MR, Spielman AJ. Non-pharmacological treatments for insomnia. *J Behav Med*. 2009;32(3):244–245.
4. Reynoldson JN, Elliott ES, Nelson LA. Ramelteon: a novel approach in the treatment of insomnia. *Ann Pharmacother*. 2008;42(9):1262–1271.
5. Hirst A, Sloan R. Benzodiazepines and related drugs for insomnia in palliative care. *Cochrane Database Syst Rev*. 2002;(4):CD003346.
6. Verster GC. Melatonin and its agonists, circadian rhythms, and psychiatry. *Afr J Psychiatry (Johannesbg)*. 2009;12(1):42–46.
7. Cheuk DK, Yeung WF, Chung KF, et al. Acupuncture for insomnia. *Cochrane Database Syst Rev*. 2012;9:CD005472.
8. Kripke DF, Langer RD, Kline LE. Hypnotics' association with mortality or cancer: a matched cohort study. *BMJ Open*. 2012;2(1):e000850.

ADDITIONAL READING

Glass J, Lanctôt KL, Herrmann N, et al. Sedative hypnotics in older people with insomnia: meta-analysis of risks and benefits. *BMJ*. 2005;331(7526):1169.

SEE ALSO

- Anxiety; Depression; Fibromyalgia; Sleep Apnea, Obstructive
- Algorithms: Anxiety; Insomnia, Chronic; Restless Leg Syndrome (RLS)

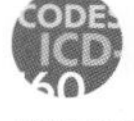

CODES

ICD10

- G47.00 Insomnia, unspecified
- F51.02 Adjustment insomnia
- F51.01 Primary insomnia

CLINICAL PEARLS

- Treatment of underlying etiology of the insomnia and consistent sleep hygiene are keys.
- Most medications are indicated for short-term use only.
- Sedative hypnotics are not recommended in the elderly because risks may outweigh benefits.
- Patients with chronic insomnia benefit from cognitive-behavioral therapy.

INTELLECTUAL DISABILITY (INTELLECTUAL DEVELOPMENTAL DISORDER)

Jennifer L. Ayres, PhD

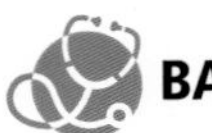

BASICS

- Intellectual disability (ID) is a global deficit in cognitive functioning evidenced by a significant difference between one's mental and chronological ages (also known as *intelligence quotient* [IQ]) and significantly impaired adaptive functioning (1).
- Although these cognitive issues typically have a pervasive impact, patients with ID will display highly variable levels of functioning and subsequent service needs.
- Patients must be evaluated individually. Treatment plans must be tailored to specific needs.
- The term *mental retardation* was deleted from the *DSM-5* and replaced with "intellectual disability" or "intellectual developmental disorder." The rationale was that the term mental retardation is considered pejorative and culturally insensitive.

DESCRIPTION

- ID is defined as an IQ $\leq$70 + 5 and a significant impairment in intellectual functioning, including verbal and nonverbal reasoning, planning, academic learning, problem solving, and experiential learning. The intellectual functioning is confirmed by both IQ testing and clinical assessment (1).
- A diagnosis of ID also requires deficits in adaptive functioning, such as communication, socialization, and independent living (1).
- By definition, ID is a neurodevelopmental disorder that is typically present from birth or determined during early childhood (1).
- Currently, ID is subgrouped according to the patient's level of adaptive functioning and level of support needed. Severity levels: *mild* (typical development in some domains, mild impairment in others), *moderate* (skills are markedly behind same-age peers), *severe* (skills are quite limited, compared to peers), profound (very limited awareness of concepts, language, dependent on others for all aspects of adaptive functioning) (1).
- The 3 most common causes of ID are Down syndrome, fragile X syndrome, and fetal alcohol syndrome (FAS).
- If the ID reflects a loss of previously acquired intellectual skills, comorbid diagnoses of ID and neurocognitive disorder may be appropriate.

ALERT

For some causes of ID, prenatal testing is available.

EPIDEMIOLOGY

Incidence

- 1 of 6 children (2)
- Predominant sex: male > female: 1.6:1 for mild ID, 1.2:1 for severe ID (1)

Prevalence

In the US, 1% of the general population. The prevalence for severe ID is 6/1,000 (1).

ETIOLOGY AND PATHOPHYSIOLOGY

- Causes:
  - Maternal substance abuse (e.g., alcohol); FAS is a leading environmental cause of ID.
  - Maternal infections: TORCH viruses (toxoplasma, other infections, rubella, cytomegalovirus, and herpes simplex)
  - Down syndrome
  - Sex chromosome abnormalities: fragile X, Turner syndrome, Klinefelter syndrome
  - Autosomal dominant conditions: neurocutaneous syndromes (e.g., neurofibromatosis, tuberous sclerosis)
  - Autosomal recessive conditions:
    - Amino acid metabolism (e.g., phenylketonuria, maple syrup urine disease)
    - Carbohydrate metabolism (e.g., galactosemia, fructosuria)
    - Lipid metabolism
    - Tay-Sachs disease
    - Gaucher disease
    - Niemann-Pick disease (e.g., mucopolysaccharidosis)
    - Purine metabolism (e.g., Lesch-Nyhan disease)
    - Other (e.g., Wilson disease)
- Maternal use of prescription medications (e.g., Accutane, dilantin)
- Perinatal factors:
  - Prematurity
  - Birth injuries
  - Perinatal anoxia
- Postnatal factors:
  - Childhood diseases (e.g., meningitis, encephalitis, hypothyroidism, seizure disorders)
  - Trauma (e.g., accidents, physical abuse, hypoxia)
  - Severe deprivation
  - Poisoning (e.g., lead, carbon monoxide, household products)

Genetics

A number of genetic and epigenetic causes are known, and more are under investigation (3).

RISK FACTORS

- Maternal substance abuse during pregnancy
- Maternal infection during pregnancy
- For some causes, family history

GENERAL PREVENTION

- Public health efforts to reduce alcohol and drug use by pregnant women
- Prenatal folic acid supplementation

COMMONLY ASSOCIATED CONDITIONS

- Seizures
- Mood disorders
- Behavioral disorders
- Constipation

DIAGNOSIS

A diagnosis of ID should be made only through a psychodiagnostic assessment conducted by a mental health provider who is trained and licensed to conduct formal psychological testing.

HISTORY

- Children with profound/severe ID are typically diagnosed at birth or during the newborn period and may have dysmorphic features.
- Children with ID often are identified because they fail to meet motor/language milestones.

PHYSICAL EXAM

Careful examination by a physician trained in the assessment of morphologic features suggestive of a specific etiology for ID (e.g., microcephaly) (4)

DIFFERENTIAL DIAGNOSIS

- Brain tumors
- Auditory, visual, and/or speech/language impairment
- Autistic disorder (language and social skills are more affected than other cognitive abilities); however, 75% of individuals with an autistic disorder may meet criteria for a comorbid diagnosis of ID.
- Expressive/receptive language disorders
- Cerebral palsy
- Emotional/behavioral disturbance
- Learning disorders (reading, math, written expression)
- Auditory/sensory processing difficulties
- Lack of environmental opportunities for appropriate development

DIAGNOSTIC TESTS & INTERPRETATION

- Visual and hearing tests to rule out these etiologies as a cause of impairment and provide an assessment of visual and auditory functioning, which are often impaired in children and adults with ID
- Formal testing of intellectual and adaptive functioning:
  - A child's communication skills must be considered in test selection. For example, a patient with auditory processing issues/limited expressive/receptive language skills may need to be assessed using a nonverbal IQ test, such as the Leiter-R, Test of Nonverbal Intelligence, or other nonverbal measures.
  - Commonly used intelligence tests (e.g., Bayley Scales of Infant Development, Stanford-Binet Intelligence Scale, Wechsler Intelligence Scales) are determined by age/developmental level of the child.
  - Common tests of adaptive functioning include the Vineland Adaptive Behavior Scales, 2nd ed., and Adaptive Behavior Assessment System, 2nd ed. These tests assess areas of functioning such as age-appropriate communication, social skills, activities of daily living, and motor skills.
- Metabolic screening is not routine unless history and physical suggest or no newborn screening done (5).
- Lab:
  - Lead (5)[B]
- Thyroid-stimulating hormone if systemic features present/no newborn screening (5)[B]
- Routine cytogenetic testing (karyotype) (5)[B]:
  - Fragile X screening (*FMR1* gene), particularly with a family history of intellectual disability
  - Rett syndrome (*MECP2* gene) in women with unexplained moderate to severe intellectual disability (5)
- Molecular screening, such as array comparative genomic hybridization, is used increasingly and may yield a diagnosis in 10% of undiagnosed cases (4)[B].
- Neuroimaging (MRI more sensitive than CT) is routinely recommended. The presence of physical findings (microcephaly, focal motor deficit) will increase the yield of a specific diagnosis (5)[B].
- MRI may show mild cerebral abnormalities but is unlikely to establish etiology of ID (4).

Follow-Up Tests & Special Considerations

- Electroencephalogram is not routine unless epilepsy or a specific epileptiform syndrome is present (5)[C].
- Assessment of quality of life provides salient information about a patient's general sense of well-being and life satisfaction; however, quality of life may be difficult to assess when significant behavioral issues confound an individual's self-report and socialization.

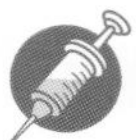

TREATMENT

- Early intervention services tailored to the individual's specific needs
- Caregiver support, including:
  - Training caregiver(s) to address behavioral issues and support socialization development
  - Encouraging caregivers to create a structured home environment that is based on the child's developmental level and specific needs rather than age-appropriate expectations
  - Providing caregiver(s) with an opportunity to address their reactions to the diagnosis and their child's special needs
  - Informing caregivers about advocacy groups and available community, state, and national resources (6,7,8)
  - Encouraging caregiver(s) to seek social support to increase overall sense of well-being
- Individualized education plans and, depending on the level of impairment, social skills and behavioral plans/training
- Refer to job training programs and independent living opportunities, if appropriate.
- Notice all changes in behavior, which may be indicative of pain/illness, particularly in individuals with limited communication skills.
- Assess for abuse and neglect

MEDICATION

Medication may be appropriate for comorbid conditions (e.g., anxiety, ADHD, depression).

ONGOING CARE

The physician should match his or her communication of exam procedures, test results, and treatment recommendations to the patient's level of cognitive functioning and receptive language skills:

- Most patients with ID will fall within the mild range and are fully capable of understanding information if it is provided at the appropriate level.
- Provide oral and written explanations directly to the patient instead of solely to his or her caregivers. The dignity of the patient must be respected at all times. This includes providing honest information, responding to patient's questions with respect, and not infantilizing the patient due to his or her intellectual disability.

FOLLOW-UP RECOMMENDATIONS

- Many adults and children with ID exhibit poor physical fitness. Preliminary studies suggest structured exercise programs are effective to engage this population in healthy activities (9)[A].
- Linkage to community-based resources for job training, independent living, caregiver support, school-based services

Patient Monitoring

- Primary care with attention to associated medical conditions
- Vision testing at least once before age 40 years (age 30 years in Down syndrome) and every 2 years thereafter (10)[B]
- Hearing evaluations every 5 years after age 45 years (every 3 years throughout life in Down syndrome) (10)[B]
- Screen for sexual activity and offer contraception and testing for STIs (10)[B].
- Abuse and neglect of people with ID are common. Screen at least annually and if behavior change is noted. Report abuse/neglect to appropriate protective agencies (10)[B].
- Dysphagia and aspiration are common; consider speech pathology evaluation and swallowing study (11)[B].
- Monitor for and treat constipation (11)[B].
- Osteoporosis: common; low threshold to order imaging studies after traumatic injury (11)[B]

DIET

No restrictions, except in cases of metabolic and storage disorders (e.g., phenylketonuria)

PATIENT EDUCATION

- Association for Retarded Citizens: www.thearc.org
- American Association of Intellectual and Developmental Disabilities: www.aaidd.org
- Family support groups (Parent to Parent, local Down Syndrome or Autism Association)
- Special Olympics: www.specialolympics.org

PROGNOSIS

Although ID is a lifelong diagnosis, individuals with ID are capable of living a fulfilling, purposeful life that includes having a career, living independently, marrying/participating in a committed relationship, and becoming a parent. Also, the level of severity and support needed may vary over the course of the individual's life.

COMPLICATIONS

- Constipation is a commonly overlooked problem and can lead to significant morbidity.
- Polypharmacy, often associated with psychotropic medication use to control behaviors, should be addressed to minimize adverse side effects.

REFERENCES

1. American Psychiatric Association. *Diagnostic and Statistical Manual of Mental Disorders*. 5th ed. Arlington, VA: American Psychiatric Association; 2013.
2. Centers for Disease Control and Prevention. Developmental disabilities. http://www.cdc.gov/ncbddd/dd/. Accessed 2014.
3. Grant ME. The epigenetic origins of mental retardation. *Clin Genet*. 2008;73(6):528–530.
4. van Karnebeek CDM, Jansweijer MCE, Leenders AG, et al. Diagnostic investigations in individuals with mental retardation: a systematic literature review of their usefulness. *Eur J Hum Genet*. 2005;13(1):6–25.
5. Shevell M, Ashwal S, Donley D, et al. Practice parameter: evaluation of the child with global developmental delay: report of the Quality Standards Subcommittee of the American Academy of Neurology and the Practice Committee of the Child Neurology Society. *Neurology*. 2003;60:367–380.
6. Shogren KA, Bradley VJ, Gomez SC, et al. Public policy and the enhancement of desired outcomes for persons with intellectual disability. *Intellect Dev Disabil*. 2009;47(4):307–319.
7. Rizzolo MC, Hemp R, Braddock D, et al. Family support services for persons with intellectual and developmental disabilities: recent national trends. *Intellect Dev Disabil*. 2009;47(2):152–155.
8. Samuel PS, Hobden KL, LeRoy BW, et al. Analysing family service needs of typically underserved families in the USA. *J Intellect Disabil Res*. 2012;56(1):111–128.
9. Heller T, Hsieh K, Rimmer JH. Attitudinal and psychosocial outcomes of a fitness and health education program on adults with down syndrome. *Am J Ment Retard*. 2004;109(2):175–185.
10. Sullivan WF, Heng J, Cameron D, et al. Consensus guidelines for primary health care of adults with developmental disabilities. *Can Fam Physician*. 2006;52(11):1410–1418.
11. Prater CD, Zylstra RG. Medical care of adults with mental retardation. *Am Fam Physician*. 2006;73(12):2175–2183.

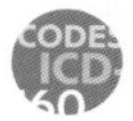

CODES

ICD10

- F79 Unspecified intellectual disabilities
- F70 Mild intellectual disabilities
- F71 Moderate intellectual disabilities

CLINICAL PEARLS

- The term mental retardation may be interpreted as culturally insensitive and disrespectful to patients and their caregivers. Intellectual disability or intellectual developmental disorder is the correct diagnosis.
- Overall functioning with ID is highly variable and influenced by multiple factors, including appropriateness of school placement/special education services, exposure to early intervention, behavioral therapy, parent training, self-esteem, and social skills.
- Previous stereotypes of people with ID (e.g., always happy, poor prognosis, unable to function independently) have been refuted. People with ID are showing a level of functioning variability that parallels what is found in the non-ID population.
- Be aware of the unique parenting needs that caregivers may face. Link families to community and national resources that can provide practical and emotional support when appropriate.
- Because children with developmental disabilities are at higher risk of being abused than their peers without developmental disabilities, discuss with caregivers how to educate children about safety precautions in a developmentally appropriate manner.

INTERSTITIAL CYSTITIS

Montiel Teresa Rosenthal, MD

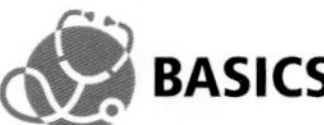

BASICS

DESCRIPTION

- A disease of unknown cause, probably representing a final common pathway from several etiologies
- Likely, pathogenesis is disruption of urothelium, impaired lower urinary tract defenses, and loss of bladder muscular wall elasticity. The symptoms in many patients are insidious, and the disease progresses for years before diagnosis is established.
- Newer research implicates urine and serum inflammatory proteins antiproliferative factor, epidermal growth factor, heparin-binding epidermal growth factor, glycosaminoglycans, and bladder nitric oxide as contributing factors.
- Mild: normal bladder capacity under anesthesia. Ulceration, cracking, or glomerulation of mucosa (or not) with bladder distention under anesthesia. No incontinence. Symptoms wax and wane and may not progress. Interstitial cystitis is a bladder sensory problem.
- Severe: progressive bladder fibrosis. Small true bladder capacity under anesthesia. Poor bladder wall compliance. In 5–10% of cases, Hunner ulcers present at cystoscopy. May have overflow incontinence and/or chronic bacteriuria unresponsive to antibiotics
- System(s) affected: renal/urologic
- Synonym(s): urgency frequency syndrome; IC/bladder pain syndrome (BPS)

Pregnancy Considerations

Unpredictable symptom improvement or exacerbation during pregnancy. No known fetal effects from interstitial cystitis. Usual problems of unknown effect on fetus with medications taken during pregnancy

EPIDEMIOLOGY

- Occurs predominantly among whites
- Predominant sex: female > male (10:1)
- Patients <30 years have predominant symptoms: dysuria, frequency, urinary urgency, pain in external genitals, and dyspareunia; and those >60 years more commonly have nocturia, urinary incontinence, or Hunner ulcer disease.
- Predominant age
  - Mild: 20–40 years
  - Severe: 20–70 years
- Pediatric considerations
  - <10 years old and again at 13–17 years
  - Daytime enuresis, dysuria without infection

Prevalence

In the United States

- Up to 1 million affected, but many cases likely are unreported
- 0.052% but may be higher, up to 10%

ETIOLOGY AND PATHOPHYSIOLOGY

- Unknown but is not primarily psychosomatic
- Possible causes
  - Subclinical urinary infection
  - Damage to glycosaminoglycan mucus layer increasing bladder wall permeability to irritants such as urea
  - Autoimmune
  - Mast cell histamine release
- Neurologic upregulation/stimulation

RISK FACTORS

Unknown

COMMONLY ASSOCIATED CONDITIONS

- Fibromyalgia
- Allergies
- Chronic fatigue syndrome
- Depression
- Vulvodynia
- Sleep disturbance
- Migraines
- Syncope
- Dyspepsia
- Chronic prostatitis
- Chronic pelvic pain
- Irritable bowel syndrome
- Anal/rectal disease

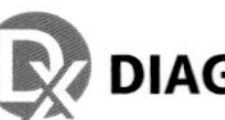

DIAGNOSIS

- Frequent, urgent, relentless urination day and night; >8 voids in 24 hours
- Pain with full bladder that resolves with bladder emptying (except if bacteriuria is present)
- Urge urinary incontinence if bladder capacity is small
- Sleep disturbance
- Dyspareunia, especially with full bladder
- Secondary symptoms from chronic pain and sleeplessness, especially depression

HISTORY

- Pelvic Pain and Urgency/Frequency Patient Symptom Scale: self-reporting questionnaire for screening potential interstitial cystitis patients (1)[B] (http://www.wgcaobgyn.com/files/urgency_frequency_pt_symptom_scale.pdf)
- Frequent UTIs, vaginitis, or symptoms during the week before menses
- O'Leary/Sant Voiding and Pain Indices (http://www.ichelp.org.document.doc?id=306)

PHYSICAL EXAM

- Perineal/prostatic pain in men
- Anterior vaginal wall pain in women

DIFFERENTIAL DIAGNOSIS

- Uninhibited bladder (urgency, frequency, urge incontinence, less pain, symptoms usually decrease when asleep)
- Urinary infection: cystitis, prostatitis
- Bladder neoplasm
- Bladder stone
- Neurologic bladder disease
- Nonurinary pelvic disease (STIs, endometriosis, pelvic relaxation)

DIAGNOSTIC TESTS & INTERPRETATION

Initial Tests (lab, imaging)

- Urinalysis: normal except with chronic bacteriuria (rare)
- Urine culture from catheterized specimen: normal except with chronic bacteriuria (rare) or partial antibiotic treatment
- Urine cytology
  - Normal: reserve for men >40 years old and women with hematuria

Diagnostic Procedures/Other

- Cystoscopy (especially in men >40 years old or women with hematuria)
  - Bladder wall visualization
  - Hydraulic distention: no improved diagnostic certainty over history and physical alone
- No role for urodynamic testing
- K^+ sensitivity test
  - Insert catheter, empty bladder, instill 40 mL H_2O over 2–3 minutes, rank urgency on scale of 0–5 in intensity, rank pain on scale of 0–5 in intensity, drain bladder, instill 40 mL potassium chloride (KCl) 0.4 mol/L solution:
    - If immediate pain, flush bladder with 60 mL H_2O and treat with bladder instillations.
    - If no immediate pain, wait 5 minutes and rate urgency and pain.
- If urgency or pain >2, treat as above.
- Pain or urgency >2 is considered a positive test and strongly correlates with interstitial cystitis if no radiation cystitis or acute bacterial cystitis is present.

Test Interpretation

- Nonspecific chronic inflammation on bladder biopsies
- Urine cytology negative for dysplasia and neoplasia
- Possible mast cell proliferation in mucosa

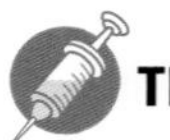

TREATMENT

GENERAL MEASURES

- Appropriate health care: outpatient
- Self-care (eliminate foods and liquids that exacerbate symptoms on individual basis, fluid management)
- Biofeedback bladder retraining

MEDICATION

- Randomized controlled trials of most medications for interstitial cystitis demonstrate limited benefit over placebo; there are no clear predictors of what will benefit an individual. Prepare the patient that treatment may involve trial and error.
- Behavioral therapy combined with oral agents found improved outcomes compared to medications alone.
- Intravesical injections of botulinum toxin are not effective in the treatment of ulcer-type interstitial cystitis.

First Line

- Pentosan polysulfate (Elmiron) 100 mg TID on empty stomach; may take several months (3–6) to become effective; rated as modestly beneficial in systematic drug review (only FDA-approved treatment for interstitial cystitis)
- Amitriptyline: most effective at higher doses (≥50 mg/day); however, initiate with lower doses to minimize side effects (3)[B].
- Hydroxyzine 25–50 mg HS
- Sildenafil 25 mg/day (2)[B]
- Triple drug therapy: 6 months of pentosan, hydroxyzine, doxepin
- Antibacterials for bacteriuria
- Oxybutynin, hyoscyamine, tolterodine, and other anticholinergic medications decrease frequency.
- Prednisone (only for ulcerative lesions)
- Montelukast has shown some benefit.
- NSAIDs for pain and any inflammatory component
- Bladder instillations
  - Lidocaine, sodium bicarbonate, and heparin or pentosan polysulfate sodium
  - Dimethyl sulfoxide (DMSO) every 1–2 weeks for 3–6 weeks, then PRN
  - Heparin sometimes added to DMSO
  - Intravesical liposomes
  - Other agents: steroids, silver nitrate, oxychlorosene (Clorpactin)
- Contraindication
  - No anticholinergics for patients with closed-angle glaucoma
- Significant possible interaction
  - Refer to manufacturer's profile of each drug.

Second Line

- Phenazopyridine, a local bladder mucosal anesthetic, usually is not very effective.
- Intravesicular injection of botulinum type A for nonulcer interstitial cystitis

ISSUES FOR REFERRAL

- Need for clarity with respect to diagnosis
- Surgical intervention

ADDITIONAL THERAPIES

Myofascial physical therapy (targeted pelvic, hip girdle, abdominal trigger point massage) (4)[B]

SURGERY/OTHER PROCEDURES

- Hydraulic distention of bladder under anesthesia: symptomatic but transient relief
- Cauterization of bladder ulcer
- Augmentation cystoplasty to increase bladder capacity and decrease pressure with or without partial cystectomy. Expected results in severe cases: much improved, 75%; with residual discomfort, 20%; unchanged, 5%
- Urinary diversion with total cystectomy only if disease is completely refractory to medical therapy
- Sacral neuromodulation

COMPLEMENTARY & ALTERNATIVE MEDICINE

Guided imagery

ONGOING CARE

FOLLOW-UP RECOMMENDATIONS

Patient Monitoring

Not specifically needed unless symptoms are unresponsive to treatment

DIET

- Variable effects from person to person
- Common irritants include caffeine, chocolate, citrus, tomatoes, carbonated beverages, K^+-rich foods, spicy foods, acidic foods, and alcohol.

PATIENT EDUCATION

Interstitial Cystitis Association, 110 Washington St. Suite 340, Rockville, MD 20850; 1-800-HELPICA: http://www.ichelp.org

PROGNOSIS

- Mild: exacerbations and remissions of symptoms; may not be progressive; does not predispose to other diseases
- Severe: progressive problems that usually require surgery to control symptoms

COMPLICATIONS

Severe, with long-term, continuous high bladder pressure could be associated with renal damage.

REFERENCES

1. Parsons CL, Dell J, Stanford EJ, et al. Increased prevalence of interstitial cystitis: previously unrecognized urologic and gynecological cases identified using a new symptom questionnaire and intravesical potassium sensitivity. *Urology*. 2002;60(4):573–578.
2. Chen H, Wang F, Chen W, et al. Efficacy of daily low-dose sildenafil for treating interstitial cystitis: results of a randomized, double-blind, placebo-controlled trial—treatment of interstitial cystitis/painful bladder syndrome with low-dose sildenafil. *Urology*. 2014;84(1):51–56.
3. Foster HE Jr, Hanno PM, Nickel JC, et al. Effect of amitriptyline on symptoms in treatment naïve patients with interstitial cystitis/painful bladder syndrome. *J Urol*. 2010;183(5):1853–1858.
4. FitzGerald MP, Payne CK, Lukacz ES, et al. Randomized multicenter clinical trial of myofascial physical therapy in women with interstitial cystitis/painful bladder syndrome and pelvic floor tenderness. *J Urol*. 2012;187(6):2113–2118.

ADDITIONAL READING

Rais-Bahrami S, Friedlander JI, Herati AS, et al. Symptom profile variability of interstitial cystitis/painful bladder syndrome by age. *BJU Int*. 2012;109(9):1356–1359.

SEE ALSO

- Urinary Tract Infection (UTI) in Females
- Algorithm: Pelvic Girdle Pain (Pregnancy or Postpartum Anterior Pelvic Pain)

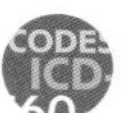

CODES

ICD10

- N30.10 Interstitial cystitis (chronic) without hematuria
- N30.11 Interstitial cystitis (chronic) with hematuria

CLINICAL PEARLS

- The potassium sensitivity test has been the most useful in confirming an initial diagnosis of interstitial cystitis.
- K^+ sensitivity test
  - Insert catheter, empty bladder, instill 40 mL H_2O over 2–3 minutes; rank urgency on scale of 0–5 in intensity; rank pain on scale of 0–5 in intensity; drain bladder; and instill 40 mL KCl 0.4 mol/L solution.
- Submucosal petechial hemorrhages and/or ulceration at the time of bladder distention and cystoscopy further support the diagnosis.
- At present, there is no definitive treatment for IC.
- Most patients with severe disease receive multiple treatment approaches. Regular multidisciplinary follow-up, pharmacologic therapy, avoidance of symptom triggers, and psychological and supportive therapy are all important because this disease tends to wax and wane. Monitor patients for comorbid depression.
- Empowering patients to manage their symptoms, communicate regularly with their physicians, and learn as much as they can about this disease which may help them to optimize their outcome

I

INTERSTITIAL NEPHRITIS

Roger P. Holland, MD, PhD

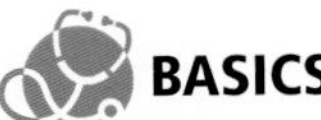

BASICS

DESCRIPTION

- Acute and chronic tubulointerstitial diseases result from the interplay of renal cells and inflammatory cells and their products. Lethal or sublethal injury to renal cells leads to expression of new local antigens, inflammatory cell infiltration, and activation of proinflammatory and chemoattractant cytokines. These cytokines are produced by macrophages and lymphocytes and also by the renal cells (i.e., proximal tubule, vascular endothelial cells, interstitial cells, fibroblasts). The outcome can be acute interstitial nephritis (AIN) or chronic interstitial nephritis (CIN).
- AIN presents as acute kidney injury (AKI) after the use of offending drugs or agents (OFA) and is associated with typical findings of proteinuria, hematuria, and white cell casts. Less frequently, AIN is secondary to infection or systemic diseases (e.g., sarcoidosis, mixed connective tissue disease [MCTD], SLE, Sjögren syndrome).
- System(s) affected: renal/urologic, endocrine/metabolic, immunologic
- Synonym(s): acute interstitial allergic nephritis

EPIDEMIOLOGY

Pediatric Considerations

- Children with history of lead poisoning are more likely to develop CIN as young adults.
- Tubulointerstitial nephritis with uveitis (TINU) presents in adolescent females.

Incidence

- AIN and CIN accounts for 10–15% of kidney disease.
- Peak incidence in women 60–70 years of age

Geriatric Considerations

The elderly have more severe disease and increased risk of permanent damage due to their increased use of OFA.

ETIOLOGY AND PATHOPHYSIOLOGY

- AIN
  - Delayed drug hypersensitivity reactions
  - Causes AKI
  - Renal dysfunction generally is usually partially or completely reversible, possibly reflecting the regenerative capacity of tubules with a preserved basement membrane.
  - Hypersensitivity to drugs (75%): not dose dependent
    - Antibiotics (e.g., penicillins, cephalosporins, sulfonamides, tetracycline, vancomycin, fluoroquinolones, macrolides, TB meds)
    - Antivirals (Indinavir)
    - NSAIDs (all, including Cox-2 inhibitors)
    - Diuretics (thiazide, loop, and triamterene)
    - Proton pump inhibitors
    - Miscellaneous (allopurinol, H_2 blockers, diphenylhydantoin, and 5-aminosaliclates such as azulfidine and mesalamine)
  - Infections: *Legionella*, *Leptospira*, streptococci, CMV, *Mycobacterium tuberculosis* (5–10%)
  - Autoimmune disorders (e.g., SLE, Sjögren syndrome, sarcoidosis, Wegener granulomatosis, cryoglobulinemia) (10–15%)
  - Toxins (e.g., snake bite venom)
- CIN
  - Follows long-term exposure to OFA (e.g., heavy metals, especially lead)
  - Often found on routine labs or evaluation for hypertension (HTN)
  - Characterized by interstitial scarring, fibrosis, and tubular atrophy, resulting in progressive chronic kidney disease (CKD)

GENERAL PREVENTION

- Early recognition and prompt discontinuation of OFA
- Avoid further nephrotoxic substances.

COMMONLY ASSOCIATED CONDITIONS

CIN

- Chronic pyelonephritis
- Abuse of analgesics
- Lithium use
- Gout and gout therapy
- Immune disorders
- Malignancy (lymphoma, multiple myeloma)
- Amyloidosis
- Exposure to heavy metals (e.g., lead, cadmium)
- Renal papillary necrosis

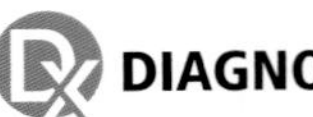

DIAGNOSIS

- AIN: suspected in a patient who presents with nonspecific signs and symptoms of AKI (e.g., malaise, fever, nausea, vomiting) with an elevated serum creatinine and an abnormal urinalysis
  - AKI
    - Elevated creatinine, BUN and electrolyte abnormalities (e.g., hyperkalemia, low serum bicarbonate)
    - Decreased urine output (oliguria in 51%)
    - Signs of fluid overload or depletion
  - Signs of systemic allergy (e.g., fever [27%], maculopapular rash [15%], peripheral eosinophilia [23%], arthralgias [45%], but less commonly found when NSAIDs are the OFA)
  - White cells, red cells, and white cell casts
- CIN
  - HTN
  - Decreased urine output or polyuria
  - Inability to concentrate urine
  - Polydipsia
  - Metabolic acidosis
  - Anemia
  - Fanconi syndrome

HISTORY

- Medications: Onset of AIN following drug exposure ranges from 3 to 5 days (as occurs with a second exposure to an OFA) to as long as several weeks to many months (the latter with NSAIDs, especially) (1).
- Infections: may have symptoms related to an associated infection or systemic condition
- TINU patients present with interstitial nephritis and uveitis and occasionally systemic findings.
- Exposure to heavy metals
- Post organ transplant

PHYSICAL EXAM

- Increased BP
- Fluid retention/extremity swelling/weight gain
- Rash accompanying renal findings in acute AIN
- Lung crackles if fluid overloaded
- Pericardial rub if uremic pericarditis

DIFFERENTIAL DIAGNOSIS

- AKI secondary to other causes:
  - Prerenal (e.g., hypovolemia, shock, sepsis, renal artery emboli)
  - Intrarenal (e.g., acute tubular necrosis, hypertensive nephropathy, DM nephropathy)
  - Postrenal (e.g., obstructive uropathy)
  - Some OFA that cause AIN can produce other forms of AKI as well:
    - NSAIDs can exacerbate prerenal disease.
    - Aminoglycosides can cause acute tubular necrosis.
- CKD secondary to long-standing HTN, diabetes, and chronic pyelonephritis

DIAGNOSTIC TESTS & INTERPRETATION

- Chemistry
  - Elevated plasma creatinine: seen in all patients, with 40% requiring dialysis
  - Hyperkalemia and acidosis
- CBC
  - Eosinophilia (80%): NSAID-induced AIN is only associated with eosinophilia in $\sim$15% of cases.
  - Anemia
- Urinalysis with urine electrolytes
  - Hematuria (95%)
  - Mild and variable proteinuria: usually $<$1 g/24 hr, except in AIN-associated with NSAIDs where it is significantly higher (1)[B]
  - Urine sediment: white cells, red cells, white cell casts. Red blood cell casts are rare.
  - Eosinophiluria but has no clinical utility specific for AIN (2)[C]
  - Fractional excretion of sodium (FENa $>$1%) indicative of tubular damage
  - Normal urinalysis does not rule out AIN.
- CXR to evaluate for pulmonary tuberculosis, sarcoidosis, and other infections
- Serologic testing for immunologic disease (e.g., sarcoidosis, Sjögren syndrome, Wegener granulomatosis, Behçet syndrome) or infectious causes (e.g., histoplasmosis, coccidiomycosis, toxoplasmosis, EBV)
  - Serum levels of angiotensin-converting enzyme and serum Ca^{++} for sarcoidosis
  - Antinuclear antibody (ANA) and dsDNA to exclude SLE
  - Urinary antigen to exclude *Legionella* infection
  - Anti-Ro/SSA, anti-La/SSb antibodies, CRP, and rheumatoid factor to exclude Sjögren syndrome
- Liver function tests: elevated serum transaminase levels in patients with associated drug-induced liver injury
- Renal US may demonstrate kidneys that are normal to enlarged in size with increased cortical echogenicity, but no US findings will reliably confirm or exclude AIN versus other causes of AKI.
- IV pyelography (IVP) and CT scans with contrast are relatively contraindicated because of the associated nephrotoxicity and limited diagnostic yield.

Follow-Up Tests & Special Considerations

Patients who do not recover renal function and those with CIN should receive long-term follow-up care to protect kidneys from further potentially nephrotoxic therapies.

Diagnostic Procedures/Other

- Renal biopsy is the definitive method of establishing the diagnosis of AIN. Ideally, it should be performed to:
  - Patients treated with an OFA known to cause AIN but have normal urinalysis

- Patients who are being considered for steroid therapy
- Patients who are not on glucocorticosteroid therapy initially and do not have spontaneous recovery following cessation of the OFA
- Patients with advanced renal failure of recent onset (<3 months)
- Patients with any features (such as high-grade proteinuria) that makes the diagnosis of AIN uncertain
- Contraindications: Renal biopsy is contraindicated in bleeding diathesis, solitary kidney, end-stage renal disease (ESRD) with small kidneys, uncontrolled HTN and sepsis, or renal parenchymal infection.

Test Interpretation
- Acute
  - Marked interstitial infiltrate consisting of T lymphocytes and monocytes. Eosinophils, plasma cells, and neutrophils also may be found.
  - In general, the urinary findings will distinguish AIN from other causes (e.g., acute tubular necrosis, glomerulonephritis)
- Chronic: CIN is characterized by tubular atrophy, fibrosis, and cellular infiltration with mononuclear cells.

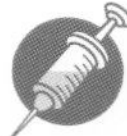

TREATMENT

For AIN, data on corticosteroids' efficacy have been limited (3)[B].

GENERAL MEASURES
- Discontinue offending agent. If topical NSAIDs are in use, discontinue these as well.
- Reduce exposure to other nephrotoxic agents (e.g.,furosemide, aminoglycosides).
- Supportive measures:
  - Maintain adequate hydration.
  - Symptomatic relief for fever, rash, etc.
  - Control of BP and anemia
  - Correct acidosis and electrolyte imbalances.
  - Possible short-term dialysis until recovery of renal function (3)[B]

MEDICATION
- Mainstay of treatment is supportive therapy.
- If patient is taking multiple offending agents, a reasonable clinical approach should include substitution of the suspected drug with another medication.
- If AKI persists after removing the offending agent, attempt medication therapy.

First Line
- Optimal therapy of AIN is unknown because there are no randomized controlled trials (RCTs) or large observational studies.
- Immunosuppressive therapy employed if no subsequent improvement within 3–7 days after discontinuation of OFA
- A renal biopsy is preferred to confirm AIN and to exclude other possible diseases or CIN, where immunosuppressive Rx not indicated.
- Prednisone 1 mg/kg/day PO or equivalent IV dose to a max of 40–60 mg/day × 1–2 weeks, beginning a gradual taper after serum creatinine has returned to near baseline for a duration of 2–3 months, followed by a gradual taper over 3–4 weeks (4)[B].
  - Patients who started steroids within 7 days of withdrawal of offending agent more likely to recover function than those who started later (odds ratio [OR] 6.6)

Second Line
- There is limited experience with treating AIN in patients who are steroid dependent (i.e., relapse during prednisone taper), steroid resistant (as with NSAID-induced disease), or cannot tolerate steroids.
- Mycophenolate mofetil may be considered in these patients who have biopsy-proven AIN (5)[C]. Rx may need to be continued for 1–3 years.
- Lead toxicity: Chelation may improve function.
  - Succimer 10 mg/kg (max 500 mg) PO q8h × 5 days, then q12h × 14 days, or
  - EDTA 2 g IV/IM; if IM, use with 2% lidocaine
- SLE nephritis: steroids + cyclophosphamide or azathioprine
- Urate nephropathy: urate-lowering agents
  - Allopurinol starting at 100 mg/day, increasing to 300 mg/day to achieve serum urate level <6 mg/dL
  - Dose may need to be adjusted down depending on level of renal impairment.
  - Allopurinol itself can be a cause of AIN.
  - Discontinue thiazide.
- Lithium-induced nephritis: Use amiloride as adjunct.
- Indinavir-induced nephritis: Use probenecid as adjunct.

ISSUES FOR REFERRAL
Most patients presenting with AKI, proteinuria, and acid–base and/or electrolyte disorders require consultation with a nephrologist.

INPATIENT CONSIDERATIONS
Patients with AKI and/or with serious electrolyte or acid–base disorders may require inpatient care until stabilization or resolution.

Admission Criteria/Initial Stabilization
- Persistent oliguria or anuria
- Severe acidosis and/or electrolyte abnormalities
- ECG changes

Discharge Criteria
- Stable vitals; correction of all electrolyte imbalances, including magnesium; and resolution of acute ECG changes
- Normal urine production

ONGOING CARE

FOLLOW-UP RECOMMENDATIONS

Patient Monitoring
If patients must remain on nephrotoxic agents, measure renal function, electrolytes, and phosphorus frequently.

DIET
- Low potassium (<2 g/day)
- Low sodium
- Low protein

PATIENT EDUCATION
Printed materials for patients are available at the National Kidney Disease Education Program, (866) 4-KIDNEY, www.nkdep.nih.gov.

PROGNOSIS
- If the associated AIN is detected early (within 1 week of the rise in serum creatinine) and the offending agent is discontinued promptly, the long-term outcome is favorable for a return to baseline or near baseline serum creatinine levels, except in the instance of NSAID-induced AIN.
- Renal biopsy reveals extent of damage.
- AIN
  - Recovery within weeks to months (6)[C]
  - Acute dialysis is needed for 1/3 of patients before resolution.
  - Rarely progresses to ESRD
- CIN: can progress to ESRD
  - Renal disease may remit in 1 year if untreated.
  - TINU has relapsing course, requiring systemic corticosteroids.
- Untreated severe AKI has 45–70% mortality.

COMPLICATIONS
- Chronic tubulointerstitial disease may progress to ESRD, requiring dialysis or transplantation.
- Analgesics increase the risk of transitional cell cancers of the uroepithelium.

REFERENCES

1. Clive DM, Stoff JS. Renal syndromes associated with nonsteroidal antiinflammatory drugs. *N Engl J Med*. 1984;310(9):563.
2. Muriithi AK, Nasr SH, Leung N. Utility of urine eosinophils in the diagnosis of acute interstitial nephritis. *Clin J Am Soc Nephrol*. 2013;8(11):1857.
3. Koselj M, Kveder R, Bren AF, et al. Acute renal failure in patients with drug-induced acute interstitial nephritis. *Ren Fail*. 1993;15(1):69.
4. Clarkson MR. Acute interstitial nephritis: clinical features and response to corticosteroid therapy. *Nephrol Dial Transplant*. 2004;19(11):2778–2783.
5. Preddie DC, Markowitz GS, Radhakrishnan J, et al. Mycophenolate mofetil for the treatment of interstitial nephritis. *Clin J Am Soc Nephrol*. 2006;1(4):718.
6. Rossert J. Drug-induced acute interstitial nephritis. *Kidney Int*. 2001;60(2):804.

ADDITIONAL READING

- Braden GL, O'Shea MH, Mulhern JG. Tubulointerstitial diseases. *Am J Kidney Dis*. 2005;46(3):560–572.
- Fougue D, Laville M. Low-protein diets for chronic kidney disease in nondiabetic adults. *Cochrane Database Syst Rev*. 2009;(3):CD001892.
- Li C, Su T, Chu R, et al. Tubulonephritis with uveitis in Chinese adults. *Clin J Am Soc Nephrol*. 2014;9(1):21.
- Markowitz GS, Perazella MA. Drug-induced renal failure: a focus on tubulointerstitial disease. *Clin Chim Acta*. 2005;351(1–2):31–47.

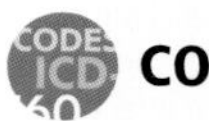

CODES

ICD10
- N12 Tubulo-interstitial nephritis, not spcf as acute or chronic
- N10 Acute tubulo-interstitial nephritis
- N11.9 Chronic tubulo-interstitial nephritis, unspecified

CLINICAL PEARLS
- First step in treatment is to remove OFA.
- A renal biopsy is preferred to confirm AIN.
- Immunosuppressive therapy is employed if no subsequent improvement within 3–7 days after discontinuation of OFA.

INTESTINAL PARASITES

Douglas W. MacPherson, MD, MSc(CTM), FRCPC

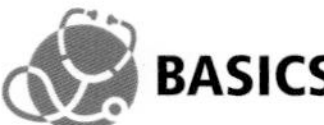

BASICS

DESCRIPTION

- Parasites are divided into 2 groups:
  - Intestinal protozoa: single-cell organisms; typically multiply within the host transmission by direct fecal–oral route; do not cause eosinophilia
  - Helminths (worms): multicellular organisms; rarely multiply within the host (exceptions: *Strongyloides stercoralis*, *Hymenolepis nana*); infection may cause eosinophilia. Level of eosinophilia is associated with the degree of tissue invasiveness. Worms have a limited life span and, without reinfection, most eventually die on their own.
- Most worms require incubation outside the host before being infectious or need a vector for transmission. *Enterobius vermicularis* (pinworm) eggs are infectious shortly after being passed; autoinfection occurs readily.
- Person-to-person transmission of worms is uncommon (except for pinworm).
- System(s) affected: gastrointestinal (GI)

Pediatric Considerations

Most common age group affected

Pregnancy Considerations

Many treatments are contraindicated during pregnancy.

EPIDEMIOLOGY

Acquired through lapse in personal, food, and/or water sanitation and/or migration from high-prevalence area

Incidence

- Predominant sex: male = female
- Predominant age: pediatric

Prevalence

- United States: 5–30% of general population have at least one fecal parasite. Random laboratory testing finds at least 1 GI parasite in 5–10% of all people.
- From daycare surveys: asymptomatic 20–30%; symptomatic 50–80%
- Intestinal protozoa account for most parasitic infections in North America. Helminths account for <10% of GI parasites.
- *Blastocystis hominis* is a commensal enteric fungus of no clinical significance found in 20–30% of stools.

ETIOLOGY AND PATHOPHYSIOLOGY

- The pathophysiology is host–parasite-specific.
- Most intestinal parasitic infections are self-limiting. Most worms have a defined life expectancy in the host. Autoreinfection occurs in few worm infections (e.g., strongyloidiasis, pinworm).
- Protozoan pathogens:
  - *Giardia lamblia*: common
  - *Entamoeba histolytica*, *Cryptosporidium* sp., *Isospora belli*, *Balantidium coli*, *Cyclospora cayetanensis*, *Microsporida*
- Possible protozoan pathogens: *Dientamoeba fragilis*
- Probable nonpathogenic protozoa:
  - Amoebas: all other *Entamoeba* sp., *Endolimax nana*; all other intestinal flagellates
- Helminthic pathogens
  - Nematodes (roundworms): *Enterobius vermicularis*, *Trichuris trichiura*, hookworm (*Necator americanus*, *Ancylostoma duodenale*), *Strongyloides stercoralis*, *Capillaria philippinensis*, *Trichostrongylus* sp.
  - Trematodes (flukes): *Fasciolopsis buski*, *Clonorchis sinensis*, *Opisthorchis viverrini*, *Heterophyes*, *Fasciola hepatica*, *Paragonimus westermani*, *Schistosoma mansoni*, *Schistosoma japonicum*, *Schistosoma haematobium*, *Schistosoma mekongi*
  - Cestodes (tapeworms): *Taenia saginata*, *Taenia solium*, *Diphyllobothrium latum*, *H. nana*, *Hymenolepsis diminuta*, *Dipylidium caninum*

RISK FACTORS

- Age (children most commonly infected)
- Low socioeconomic status and poor sanitation—personal, food, water; crowding: daycare centers, institutional care
- International travel or immigration
- Pregnancy; medical comorbidities: gastric hypoacidity, immunosuppression (AIDS, hypogammaglobulinemias)

GENERAL PREVENTION

- Intestinal parasites are usually acquired through the fecal–oral route via ingestion of contaminated food or water. Rarely, infected arthropod vectors are involved in transmission. Person-to-person transmission may occur through fecal–oral means.
- Safe food and water precautions ("Wash it, cook it, boil it, peel it, or forget it"); enteric and hand hygiene is the gold standard for preventing infections. Public health infrastructure systems for safe food and water processing contribute to the low prevalence of intestinal parasites in developed countries.

COMMONLY ASSOCIATED CONDITIONS

- HIV infection or AIDS, steroid use, immune deficiencies
- Intestinal parasite infection may protect against allergic sensitization (1)[A].

DIAGNOSIS

HISTORY

Historical or physical features alone cannot separate intestinal parasites from other GI infections:

- Acute bacterial or viral GI syndromes tend to be sudden onset and short duration.
- Fever is uncommon with GI parasites unless there is tissue invasion (e.g., amoebiasis, strongyloidiasis).
- Chronic bloating, excessive gas, and intermittent/unpredictable diarrhea without blood is typical of giardiasis.
- Extraintestinal symptoms and signs are uncommon with GI parasites, except invasive strongyloidiasis.
- A water, food, or fecal contamination exposure history (e.g., international travel, migration, high-risk environments [daycare centers, camping]) may suggest a particular parasitic agent.
- Passing a roundworm or tapeworm or a worm segment in the stool
- A family or personal history of inflammatory or irritable bowel syndromes does not exclude GI parasites.

PHYSICAL EXAM

- Will generally appear well even if distressed with GI complaints; usually afebrile
- Diffuse, migratory rash (cutaneous larva currens) with invasive strongyloidiasis; is a medical emergency.
- Weight loss and anorexia may be present (e.g., chronic giardiasis, invasive amoebiasis, chronic helminths).
- Excessive gas: bloating, eructation, flatulence, borborygmi
- Nausea or vomiting: intermittent, recurrent
- Abdominal pain/tenderness
- May have bowel tenderness, but liver and spleen are usually normal
- Diarrhea: persistent and recurrent, chronic but dysentery (i.e., frank GI bleeding) is rare, except with *E. histolytica*, *B. coli*
- Pruritus ani: *E. vermicularis*, *T. trichiura*, *S. stercoralis*, tapeworms; perirectal or vulvar rash

DIFFERENTIAL DIAGNOSIS

- Other nonparasitic intestinal infections
- Food poisoning
- Malabsorption: commonly lactose, gluten enteropathy; rarely celiac disease, tropical or nontropical sprue
- Inflammatory and irritable bowel diseases
- Hemorrhoid or rectal fissure

DIAGNOSTIC TESTS & INTERPRETATION

- Stool specimens (ova and parasites) that are properly collected, preserved, and transported for examination in a qualified and proficient laboratory by a dedicated parasitology technologist team have the highest diagnostic yield.
- Anemia may be present with heavy hookworm infections.
- *Giardia* antigen—fluorescent antibody (FA) and ELISA tests: A single FA or ELISA may be at least as sensitive as 3 stools for ova and parasites.
- Special diagnostics for *Cryptosporidium*, *I. belli*, *Cyclospora*, *Microsporidia*, and *Strongyloides*: Give specific laboratory notice.
- Pinworm paddles provide a greater diagnostic yield for *E. vermicularis*. Multiple tests (2) may be needed to exclude pinworms.
- Parasite culture is possible for *G. lamblia*, *E. histolytica*, and *S. stercoralis* but is rarely indicated; only done in reference laboratories
- Rarely, a biopsy and histology will demonstrate the presence of an invasive helminth on tissue section.
- Tissue biopsies of intestine, liver, or bladder may show granulomatous reactions of schistosome eggs.
- A single stool specimen collected into a preservative (i.e., sodium acetate formalin [SAF]), well mixed to fix and preserve all elements, yields an accurate diagnosis of 90%. Additional specimens improve diagnostic accuracy (3)[A].
- Serology: useful if parasite is not found in stool samples normally or if low numbers of parasites; available only through reference centers; only indicated for *Strongyloides*, amebiasis, schistosomiasis
- Drugs that may alter lab results: Use of antibiotics; oil-based laxatives, and barium in the stool interfere with microscopy.

Initial Tests (lab, imaging)

- Screening blood eosinophilia is not recommended.
- Diagnostic radiology is rarely needed. Exception: invasive disease due to amebiasis for colitis, amebomas, and liver abscesses

Follow-Up Tests & Special Considerations

- A single negative stool examination does not rule out intestinal parasitic infection but when performed under best conditions is highly accurate. Repeat testing may be indicated for primary diagnosis.
- Population-based intestinal parasite screening in North America (e.g., daycare attendees, personal care providers, food handlers, immigrants) has low diagnostic use and is not recommended.

Diagnostic Procedures/Other

- Invasive diagnostic procedures are rarely needed or indicated.
- Egg granulomata of schistosomiasis may be demonstrated in affected tissues.
- With hemorrhagic colitis due to invasive amebiasis, sigmoidoscopy may be diagnostic.
- Upper intestinal endoscopy can yield fluid to be examined for *G. lamblia* trophozoites and *S. stercoralis* larvae.

Test Interpretation

- Most intestinal parasites are not invasive and produce nonspecific or no changes in bowel histology.
- Invasive amebiasis produces a classic endoscopic and histologic picture of ulceration and inflammation in the colon.
- Protozoa or helminths may be seen in bowel biopsy histology.

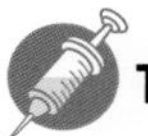

TREATMENT

Specific antiparasitic treatment should be selected based on patient history, parasite biology, and epidemiology.

GENERAL MEASURES

- Not all patients need drug therapy.
- Symptomatic treatment is indicated for patient comfort once specific therapy has been initiated.
- Drugs inhibiting intestinal motility are relatively contraindicated in patients with diarrhea caused by invasive organisms.

MEDICATION

- Protozoa (4)[A]
  - *E. histolytica*: Asymptomatic infection needs individual assessment and may not require drug therapy.
  - Symptomatic intestinal *E. histolytica*: iodoquinol or diloxanide furoate
  - Invasive *E. histolytica*: iodoquinol or diloxanide furoate plus metronidazole alone or metronidazole alone or emetine + chloroquine phosphate
  - *G. lamblia*: metronidazole or tinidazole or furazolidone or quinacrine. *Note*: Albendazole, available in the United States only from manufacturer, may have activity against *G. lamblia*.
- *Cryptosporidium*: none proven effective
- *I. belli* protozoa: trimethoprim-sulfamethoxazole
- *B. coli*: tetracycline or iodoquinol or metronidazole
- *Cyclospora*: sulfamethoxazole-trimethoprim
- *Microsporidia*: albendazole (some species)
- Helminths
  - Nematodes (except *Strongyloides* and *Trichostrongylus*): mebendazole or pyrantel pamoate or piperazine citrate or albendazole (available in the United States only from manufacturer)
  - *Strongyloides* and *Trichostrongylus*: thiabendazole or albendazole (available in the United States only from manufacturer)
  - Cestodes: praziquantel or niclosamide
  - Trematodes: niclosamide or praziquantel

Pediatric Considerations

Giardia: Nitazoxanide 7.5 mg/kg PO BID × 3 days or single-dose tinidazole 50 mg/kg (not available in the United States) may be used.

ISSUES FOR REFERRAL

Treatment failures, complex patients (including drug intolerances or allergies), multiple parasitic infections, and complicated medical (e.g., HIV/AIDS, diabetes, chronic steroid use) or surgical conditions: specialist in tropical medicine or infectious diseases

COMPLEMENTARY AND ALTERNATIVE MEDICINE

Many complementary and alternative therapies exist, but none are effective for primary treatment.

SURGERY/OTHER PROCEDURES

- Surgical procedures play little role, except for amebic liver abscesses, which may need to be drained,
- Surgery possible for bowel or organ obstruction, *Ascaris lumbricoides* migration, or complicated amebic colitis

INPATIENT CONSIDERATIONS

Nosocomial intestinal parasitic infections are rare, as are hospital-based parasitic GI outbreaks.

Admission Criteria/Initial Stabilization

Admission is rarely required except for intestinal obstruction, dysentery, or systemic invasion.

ONGOING CARE

FOLLOW-UP RECOMMENDATIONS

Patient Monitoring

- For most intestinal parasitic infections, testing for clearance is not indicated. Repeat stool examination for clearance should be timed, taking into account the life cycle of the parasite and the risk of reinfection.
- Consequences of intestinal parasitic infections include lactose intolerance, irritable bowel syndrome, or nutritional calorie–protein deficiencies, dehydration, and vitamin B_{12} deficiency.

DIET

Many patients experience symptoms of irritable bowel syndrome and/or lactose intolerance during and following bowel infections, especially with *G. lamblia*.

PATIENT EDUCATION

Personal hygiene and proper food/water sanitation is important to reduce the risk of reinfection or transmission.

COMPLICATIONS

Complications are rare; they include chronic persistent diarrhea, irritable bowel syndrome, and chronic malabsorption.

REFERENCES

1. Feary J, Britton J, Leonardi-Bee J. Atopy and current intestinal parasite infection: a systematic review and meta-analysis. *Allergy*. 2011;66(4):569–578.
2. Strand EA, Robertson LJ, Hanevik K, et al. Sensitivity of a *Giardia* antigen test in persistent giardiasis following an extensive outbreak. *Clin Microbiol Infect*. 2008;14(11):1069–1071.
3. Senay H, MacPherson D. Parasitology: diagnostic yield of stool examination. *CMAJ*. 1989;140(11):1329–1331.
4. Drugs for parasitic infections. In: *The Medical Letter*. On Drugs and Therapeutics. 3rd ed. New York, NY: The Medical Letter; 2013. http://secure.medicalletter.org/para. Accessed 2014.

ADDITIONAL READING

- Centers for Disease Control and Prevention. Parasites. http://www.cdc.gov/parasites/az/index.html. Accessed 2014.
- Escobedo AA, Alvarez G, González ME, et al. The treatment of giardiasis in children: single-dose tinidazole compared with 3 days of nitazoxanide. *Ann Trop Med Parasitol*. 2008;102(3):199–207.
- Leonardi-Bee J, Pritchard D, Britton J. Asthma and current intestinal parasite infection: systematic review and meta-analysis. *Am J Respir Crit Care Med*. 2006;174(5):514–523.
- van Lieshout L, Verweij JJ. Newer diagnostic approaches to intestinal protozoa. *Curr Opin Infect Dis*. 2010;23(5):488–493.

SEE ALSO

Algorithm: Hematemesis (Bleeding, Upper GI)

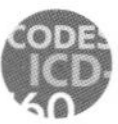

CODES

ICD10

- B82.9 Intestinal parasitism, unspecified
- A07.9 Protozoal intestinal disease, unspecified
- B82.0 Intestinal helminthiasis, unspecified

CLINICAL PEARLS

- GI parasites are relatively common when dealing with relevant GI symptom and a history of travel, recent immigration, children, or other vulnerable populations; chronic or persistent diarrhea; or seeing worms in the stool.
- Properly collected stool specimens detect most intestinal parasites. Exceptions: *S. stercoralis*, *E. vermicularis*, *Cryptosporidium*, *Cyclospora*, and *Microspora* sp.
- Eosinophilia is not a reliable screening method.

I

IRRITABLE BOWEL SYNDROME

Patricia May Lacsina, MD • Fozia Akhtar Ali, MD

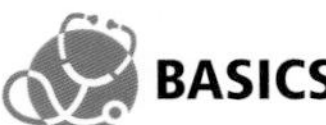

BASICS

DESCRIPTION

- A functional gastrointestinal disorder characterized by
  - Chronic abdominal pain associated with
    - Alteration in bowel habits
    - Absence of organic pathology
- May be characterized as diarrhea predominant or constipation predominant or may alternate between diarrhea and constipation
- Synonym(s): spastic colon; irritable colon

EPIDEMIOLOGY

Irritable bowel syndrome (IBS) accounts for up to 50% of visits to gastroenterologists:

- Second only to upper respiratory infection as cause of lost workdays

Prevalence

Pooled estimate of 11% IBS prevalence internationally; ranges from South Asia (7.0%) to South America (21.0%) (1)

- Predominant age: 20–39 years
- If age >50 years, consider other diagnoses.
- Predominant sex: in the United States, female > male (2:1)
- More common in low socioeconomic communities

ETIOLOGY AND PATHOPHYSIOLOGY

- The etiology is unknown, but patients demonstrate intestinal motility abnormalities with enhanced sensitivity to visceral stimuli.
- The trigger may be luminal or environmental.
- Evidence for the role of small intestine bacterial overgrowth (SIBO) in IBS and subsequent antibiotic therapy is conflicting; older age and female gender are predictors of SIBO in IBS patients.

Genetics

Unknown, but more common in families of IBS patients

RISK FACTORS

- Other family members with similar GI disorder
- History of childhood sexual abuse
- Sexual/domestic abuse (primarily in women)
- Depression
- Gastrointestinal infection

Pregnancy Considerations

No risk to mother or fetus

GENERAL PREVENTION

See "Diet."

COMMONLY ASSOCIATED CONDITIONS

- Chronic migraine
- Urinary frequency and urgency
- Fibromyalgia
- Chronic fatigue syndrome
- Sleep disorders
- Dyspareunia
- Depression
- Posttraumatic stress disorder

DIAGNOSIS

HISTORY

- Abdominal pain/discomfort described as cramping worsened by emotional stress and eating (Rome III criteria)
- Recurrent abdominal pain or discomfort at least 3 days/month in the last 3 months associated with 2 or more
- Improvement with defecation
- Onset associated with a change in frequency of stool
- Onset associated with a change in form (appearance) of stool
- Symptoms can also include the following:
  - Mucus in stools
  - Constipation
  - Bloating
  - Diarrhea
  - Abdominal distention
  - Upper abdominal discomfort after eating
  - Straining for normal consistency stools
  - Urgency of defecation
  - Feelings of incomplete evacuation
  - Abnormal stool form
  - Nausea, vomiting (rarely)
- May have history of abuse or depression
- Patient may note worsening of symptoms with stress or around menses.
- IBS is unlikely in patients with a history of the following:
  - Weight loss
  - Bleeding
  - Nocturnal diarrhea
  - Fever
  - Anemia

PHYSICAL EXAM

- Generally normal
- Performed to exclude other causes
- Vital signs typically normal
- Absence of jaundice, organomegaly, but may have abdominal tenderness to palpation

DIFFERENTIAL DIAGNOSIS

- Inflammatory bowel disease
- Lactose intolerance; fructose malabsorption
- Infections (*Giardia lamblia, Entamoeba histolytica, Salmonella, Campylobacter, Yersinia, Clostridium difficile*)
- Celiac sprue
- Microscopic colitis
- Laxative abuse
- Magnesium-containing antacids
- Hypo-/hyperthyroidism
- Pancreatic insufficiency
- Depression
- Small bowel bacterial overgrowth
- Somatization
- Villous adenoma
- Endocrine tumors
- Diabetes mellitus
- Radiation damage to colon or small bowel

DIAGNOSTIC TESTS & INTERPRETATION

- In the setting of a typical history and in the absence of danger signs, such as anemia or weight loss, obtain baseline labs to rule out other causes and begin treatment.
- In those who do not respond to treatment, further evaluation with imaging studies and endoscopy is warranted to exclude organic pathology.

Initial Tests (lab, imaging)

As needed to rule out other pathology specific to the patient's symptoms:

- Diarrhea-predominant: ESR, CBC, tissue transglutaminase, thyroid-stimulating hormone (TSH), and stool for ova and parasites (2)
- Constipation-predominant: CBC, TSH, electrolytes, calcium (2)
- Abdominal pain: LFTs and amylase
- Abdominal CT scan or abdominal ultrasound to evaluate pain is generally normal.
- Small bowel series or video capsule endoscopy to rule out Crohn disease may be considered and will also be normal.
- Sitz Marker study may be used to evaluate colon transit in patients with constipation.

Follow-Up Tests & Special Considerations

Consider lactulose breath test to assess for small bowel bacterial overgrowth associated with IBS (2)[C].

Diagnostic Procedures/Other

Sigmoidoscopy/colonoscopy may be used to rule out inflammatory bowel disease or microscopic colitis.

ALERT

Colonoscopy should be performed in all persons >50 years of age for colorectal cancer screening.

Test Interpretation

None

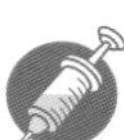

TREATMENT

- Goals: symptomatic relief and improvement of quality of life (3)
  - Determine if diarrhea predominant, constipation predominant, or mixed type
- Lifestyle modification
  - Exercise 3–5 times/week decreases severity (3).
  - Food diary to determine triggers that worsen symptoms (3)
- Medications
  - Fiber supplementation (psyllium) to increase stool bulk; does not relieve abdominal pain; may be used for all types (3,4)[B]
- Medications that improve abdominal pain, global symptoms, and symptom severity in all types are as follows:
  - Antispasmodics such as hyoscyamine (Levsin) and dicyclomine can be used for all types but have adverse effects such as dry mouth, dizziness, and blurred vision (3).
  - Probiotics such as *Lactobacillus*, *Bifidobacterium*, and *Streptococcus* (5)[C]
  - Serotonin antagonists 5-HT3 and 5-4T agonists (alosetron, cilansetron) have been shown to improve IBS symptoms (vs. placebo) (6).

- Diarrhea predominant
  - Antidiarrheal such as loperamide 4–8 mg/day orally divided into once a day to three times a day as needed decreases stool frequency and increases stool consistency but does not help with abdominal pain; may also use Lomotil (diphenoxylate/atropine) (3)
  - Antibiotics such as 2-week course of rifaximin improve bloating, pain, and stool consistency (7).
  - Alosetron (Lotronex 0.5 mg orally twice a day), used for women with severe symptoms but associated with ischemic colitis, constipation, and death in a small number of patients (8)
- Constipation predominant
  - Laxatives such as MiraLAX (polyethylene glycol) may improve stool frequency but not pain.
  - Antibiotics such as neomycin and selective chloride channel activators such as lubiprostone (Amitiza) 8 mg twice a day can improve global symptoms and severity (3,9)[B].
  - Linaclotide (guanylate cyclase-C agonist) has been shown to improve bowel function and reduces abdominal pain and overall severity in adults only (10).
- Mixed
  - May use medications as above for either picture (3)
- Treat underlying behavioral issues:
  - Use of SSRIs such as Prozac, sertraline, Paxil, and tricyclic antidepressants such as imipramine can improve abdominal pain and symptom score (4).
  - Tricyclic antidepressants can help control IBS symptoms in moderate to severe cases (11)[B].
  - Behavioral therapy helps reduce symptoms (7).

ISSUES FOR REFERRAL

- Behavioral health referral for affective or personality disorders
- Gastroenterology referral for difficult to control cases

ADDITIONAL THERAPIES

Probiotics use may result in reducing IBS symptoms and decreasing pain and flatulence. There is no difference among *Lactobacillus*, *Streptococcus*, *Bifidobacterium*, and combinations of probiotics.

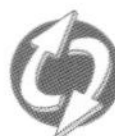

ONGOING CARE

FOLLOW-UP RECOMMENDATIONS

Patient Monitoring

The IBS Severity Scoring (12) is a validated measure to assess the severity of IBS symptoms and can help monitor response to treatment.

IBS Severity Score include following five questions score from 0 to 10:

- How severe has your abdominal pain been over the last 10 days?
- On how many of the last 10 days did you get pain?
- How severe has your abdominal distension (bloating, swollen, or tight) been over the last 10 days?
- How satisfied have you been with your bowel habit (frequency, ease, etc.) over the last 10 days?
- How much has your IBS been affecting/interfering with your life in general over the last 10 days?

DIET

Low FODMAPs diet: This diet contains fermentable oligo-, di-, and monosaccharides and polyols that are carbohydrates (sugars) found in foods. FODMAPs are osmotic, so they may not be digested or absorbed well and could be fermented upon by bacteria in the intestinal tract when *eaten in excess*.

A low FODMAP diet may help reduce symptoms, which will limit foods high in fructose, lactose, fructans, galactans, and polyols.

- Increase fiber slowly to avoid excess intestinal gas production.
- During initial evaluation, may wish to try 2 weeks of lactose-free diet to rule out lactose intolerance.
- Avoid large meals, fatty foods, and caffeine, which can exacerbate symptoms.
- A gluten-free diet resolves symptoms for some patients (especially diarrhea predominant IBS) despite negative testing for celiac disease.

PATIENT EDUCATION

IBS is not a psychiatric illness.

PROGNOSIS

- IBS is a functional disorder that significantly reduces the patient's quality of life. Many patients have behavioral health implications (depression, anxiety) and also more invasive procedures and surgeries to help control symptoms. IBS does not increase mortality (1).
- Expect recurrences, especially when under stress.
- Evidence suggests that "symptom shifting" occurs in some patients, whereby resolution of functional bowel symptoms is followed by the development of functional symptoms in another system (1).

REFERENCES

1. Canavan C, West J, Card T. The epidemiology of irritable bowel syndrome. *Clin Epidemiol*. 2014;6:71–80.
2. Reddymasu SC, Sostarich S, McCallum RW. Small intestinal bacterial overgrowth in irritable bowel syndrome: are there any predictors? *BMC Gastroenterol*. 2010;10:23.
3. Wilkins T, Pepitone C, Alex B, et al. Diagnosis and management of IBS in adults. *Am Fam Physician*. 2012;86(5):419–426.
4. Ruepert L, Quartero AO, de Wit NJ, et al. Bulking agents, antispasmodics and antidepressants for the treatment of irritable bowel syndrome. *Cochrane Database Syst Rev*. 2011;8:CD003460.
5. Ciorba MA. A gastroenterologist's guide to probiotics. *Clin Gastroenterol Hepatol*. 2012;10(9):960–968.
6. Ford AC, Brandt LJ, Young C, et al. Efficacy of 5-HT3 antagonists and 5-HT4 agonists in irritable bowel syndrome: systematic review and meta-analysis. *Am J Gastroenterol*. 2009;104(7):1831–1844.
7. Schey R, Rao SS. The role of rifaximin therapy in patients with irritable bowel syndrome without constipation. *Expert Rev Gastroenterol Hepatol*. 2011;5(4):461–464.
8. Rahimi R, Nikfar S, Abdollahi M. Efficacy and tolerability of alosetron for the treatment of irritable bowel syndrome in women and men: a meta-analysis of eight randomized, placebo-controlled, 12-week trials. *Clin Ther*. 2008;30(5):884–901.
9. Drossman DA, Chey WD, Johanson JF, et al. Clinical trial: lubiprostone in patients with constipation-associated irritable bowel syndrome—results of two randomized, placebo-controlled studies. *Aliment Pharmacol Ther*. 2009;29(3):329–341.
10. Videlock EJ, Cheng V, Cremonini F. Effects of linaclotide in patients with irritable bowel syndrome with constipation or chronic constipation: a meta-analysis. *Clin Gastroenterol Hepatol*. 2013;11(9):1084–1092.e3.
11. Rahimi R, Nikfar S, Rezaie A, et al. Efficacy of tricyclic antidepressants in irritable bowel syndrome: a meta-analysis. *World J Gastroenterol*. 2009;15(13):1548–1553.
12. Francis CY, Morris J, Whorwell PJ. The irritable bowel severity scoring system: a simple method of monitoring irritable bowel syndrome and its progress. *Aliment Pharmacol Ther*. 1997;11(2):395–402.

SEE ALSO

Algorithm: Diarrhea, Chronic

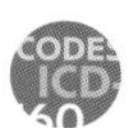

CODES

ICD10

- K58.9 Irritable bowel syndrome without diarrhea
- K58.0 Irritable bowel syndrome with diarrhea

CLINICAL PEARLS

- Use Rome III criteria for diagnosis.
- Goals of treatment are symptomatic relief and improvement of quality of life.
- If patient does not respond to initial treatment, consider further evaluation to exclude organic pathology.

KAWASAKI SYNDROME

Scott P. Grogan, DO, MBA, FAAFP • Matthew V. Fargo, MD, MPH

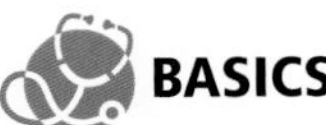

BASICS

DESCRIPTION

- Kawasaki syndrome (KS) is an acute, febrile, systemic vasculitis of small- and medium-sized arteries that predominantly affects patients under age 5 years and is the most prominent cause of acquired coronary artery disease in pediatric populations.
  - Vasculitis of coronary arteries resulting in aneurysms/ectasia, further leading to myocardial infarction (MI)/ischemia or sudden death
- System(s) affected: cardiovascular; gastrointestinal; hematologic/lymphatic/immunologic; musculoskeletal; nervous; pulmonary; renal/urologic; skin/exocrine
- Synonym(s): mucocutaneous lymph node syndrome (MCLS); infantile polyarteritis, Kawasaki disease

ALERT

KS should be considered in any child with extended high fever unresponsive to antibiotics or antipyretics, rash, and nonexudative conjunctivitis.

EPIDEMIOLOGY

Incidence

- Worldwide: affects all races but most prevalent in Asia; Japan annual incidence rate 216/100,000 in children <5 years of age
- In the United States, the annual incidence in children <5 years is 19/100,000. In comparison to Caucasians, African Americans have a 1.5× risk, and Asian Americans have a 2.5× -increased risk. Highest state incidence is in Hawaii.
- Leading cause of acquired heart disease in children in developed countries
  - Predominant age: 1–5 years
  - 85% of cases are children <5 years of age and 50% <2 years of age.
  - Male-to-female ratio = 1.5:1

Prevalence

- Highest to lowest prevalence: Asians > African Americans > Hispanics > Caucasians
- Seasonal variation: increased in winter and early spring in temperate places, summer in Asia, and outbreaks at 2–3-year intervals

ETIOLOGY AND PATHOPHYSIOLOGY

- Acute KS causes inflammation in the smooth muscle layer of medium extraparenchymal arteries, especially the coronary arteries.
- Inflammatory cells in the media secrete cytokines (TNF-α), interleukins, and matrix metalloproteases that cause fragmentation of the internal elastic lamina.
- A prominence of IgA plasma cells and IgA deposits are characteristic features and may be found in the lungs.
- As the process resolves, active inflammatory cells are replaced by fibroblasts and monocytes; tissue repair/remodeling may cause vascular fibrosis and stenosis.
- Unknown; believed to be an exaggerated immune response to infectious agent due to the acute, self-limited nature; community-wide outbreaks; age distribution; seasonality; and laboratory features indicating respiratory route of entry

Genetics

- Siblings of patients in Japan have a 10–30-fold increased risk, and >50% develop KS within 10 days of first case. Increased occurrence of KS in children whose parents also had illness in childhood
- Populations at higher risk and family link suggest a genetic predisposition.

GENERAL PREVENTION

No preventive measures available

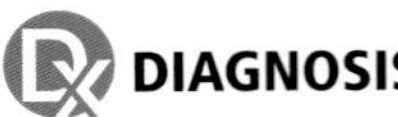

DIAGNOSIS

≥5 days of fever and ≥4 of the following 5 principal clinical features; or <4 features and presence of coronary artery disease on 2D echocardiography:

- Bilateral conjunctival injection with limbic sparing
- Erythematous mouth and pharynx, tongue, and lips
- A polymorphous, generalized, erythematous rash
- Changes in the skin of the peripheral extremities
- Cervical lymphadenopathy

Pediatric Considerations

- Prolonged fever without rash and treated with antibiotics may cause clinicians to believe that later rash development is due to a drug reaction.
- Can be diagnosed on day 4 of illness if ≥4 principal features present
- Incomplete Kawasaki syndrome
  - ≥5 days of fever, ≥2 principal clinical features, labs indicating systemic inflammation, and exclusion of other diseases
  - Incomplete cases that exhibit <4 clinical criteria often occur in infants ≤6 months of age or older children/adolescents. The frequency of coronary artery aneurysms (CAAs) is often higher in patients with missed diagnosis/delayed treatment. Therefore, in infants with prolonged fever and few or no clinical features, consider echocardiography and inflammatory labs.

HISTORY

- Fever is the first sign during the acute phase.
- Symptoms may not occur all at once but usually occur in close proximity.

PHYSICAL EXAM

- High-spiking and remittent fever for ≥5 days
  - Fever is high (102°–105°F [39.4°–40.5°C]) and unresponsive to antibiotics.
  - May be prolonged, up to 3–4 weeks
  - Extreme irritability is a very common feature.
- Bilateral painless nonpurulent conjunctival injection without corneal ulceration, or edema. Limbic sparing is usually seen.
- Changes in lips and oral cavity
  - Redness and swelling of lips in the acute stage; cracking, fissuring, bleeding in subacute phase
  - Strawberry/erythematous tongue
- Extensive erythematous polymorphous rash: within 5 days of fever
  - Morbilliform is most common. May be maculopapular, scarlatiniform; can resemble erythema multiforme, erythroderma, urticarial exanthem; rarely micropustular
  - Perineal desquamation, especially in skin folds
- Extremity changes
  - Reddened palms and soles on days 3–5
  - Edema of hands and feet on days 4–7; painful induration
  - Desquamation of fingers and toes that begins in periungual area at 2–3 weeks
- Acute, unilateral cervical lymphadenopathy (least common symptom)
  - ≥1 lymph nodes >1.5 cm, firm, nonfluctuant, and usually with no to slight tenderness
- Cardiac exam: tachycardia, gallop rhythms, hyperdynamic precordium, innocent flow murmurs, depressed contractility
- Other organ system involvement:
  - Cardiovascular: myocarditis; pericarditis (often subclinical),CAAs, and other medium-sized arterial aneurysms
  - Gastrointestinal: anorexia, abdominal pain, vomiting/diarrhea, acute gallbladder hydrops, hepatic enlargement, jaundice
  - Renal: proteinuria, sterile pyuria
  - Joints: polyarthritis of small joints in acute phase; weight-bearing joints affected after 10th day from onset of fever
  - Neurologic: irritability, aseptic meningitis, peripheral neuropathy (unilateral facial palsy), transient high-frequency hearing loss

DIFFERENTIAL DIAGNOSIS

- Bacterial: staphylococcal scalded-skin syndrome, toxic shock syndrome, scarlet fever, bacterial cervical lymphadenitis, *Mycoplasma* infection, leptospirosis, Lyme disease, Rocky Mountain spotted fever
- Viral: measles, adenovirus, Epstein-Barr virus
- Toxoplasmosis
- Reiter syndrome
- Hypersensitivity drug reactions (erythema multiforme minor, Stevens-Johnson syndrome)
- Juvenile rheumatoid arthritis
- Acrodynia (mercury poisoning)

DIAGNOSTIC TESTS & INTERPRETATION

- Initial workup: CBC with differential, urinalysis (UA)/culture, blood culture; lumbar puncture if signs of meningitis or if <90 days old
  - Leukocytosis (12K–40K cells/mm^3) with immature and mature granulocytes
  - Anemia: normochromic, normocytic
  - Thrombocytosis (500,000–>1,000,000/mm^3) in 2nd and 3rd weeks. Thrombocytopenia during acute phase is associated with CAA and MI.
- Elevated C-reactive protein (CRP) (>35 mg/L in 80% cases), erythrocyte sedimentation rate (ESR) (>60 mm/hr in 60% cases), and α_1-antitrypsin

ALERT

ESR can be artificially high after intravenous immunoglobulin (IVIG) therapy.

- Hyponatremia
- Moderately elevated AST, ALT, GGT, and bilirubin
- Decreased albumin and protein
- CSF pleocytosis may be seen (lymphocytic with normal protein and glucose).
- *N*-terminal brain natriuretic peptide might be elevated in acute phase.
- Sterile pyuria but not seen in suprapubic collection
- Nasal swab to rule out adenovirus

Initial Tests (lab, imaging)

- If KS is suspected, obtain ECG and echocardiogram.
  - ECG may show arrhythmias, prolonged PR interval, and ST/T wave changes.
  - Echocardiography has a high sensitivity and specificity for detection of abnormalities of proximal left main coronary artery, and right coronary artery may show perivascular brightening, ectasia, decreased left ventricular contractility, pericardial effusion, or aneurysms.
  - Cardiac stress test if CAA seen on echocardiogram

- Baseline chest x-ray (CXR): may show pleural effusion, atelectasis, and congestive heart failure (CHF)
- Hydrops of the gallbladder may be associated with abdominal pain or may be asymptomatic.

Diagnostic Procedures/Other

- No laboratory study is diagnostic; diagnosis rests on constellation of clinical features and exclusion of other illnesses.
- Magnetic resonance coronary angiography is noninvasive modality to visualize coronary arteries for stenosis, thrombi, and intimal thickening (1).
- Patients with complex coronary artery lesions may benefit from coronary angiography after the acute inflammatory process has resolved; generally recommended in 6–12 months

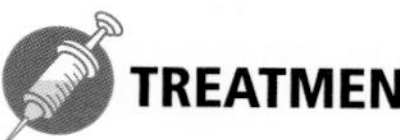

TREATMENT

GENERAL MEASURES

Use antibiotics until bacterial etiologies are excluded (e.g., sepsis or meningitis).

MEDICATION

- Optimal therapy is IVIG 2 g/kg IV over 10 hours with high-dose aspirin preferably within 7–10 days of fever, followed by low-dose aspirin until follow-up echocardiograms indicate a lack of coronary abnormalities.
  - IVIG lowers the risk of CAA and may shorten fever duration.
  - The extreme irritability often resolves very quickly after IVIG is given.
- Retreatment with IVIG if clinical response is incomplete or fever persists/returns >36 hours after start of IVIG treatment
  - ≥10% of patients do not respond to initial IVIG treatment. 2/3 of nonresponders respond to the 2nd dose of IVIG.
  - Nonresponders tend to have ↑ bands, ↓ albumin, and an abnormal echo.
- Aspirin, 80–100 mg/kg/day in 4 doses beginning with IVIG administration. Switch to low-dose aspirin (3–5 mg/kg/day) when afebrile for 48–72 hours, or continue until day 14 of illness. Maintain low dose for 6–8 weeks until follow-up echocardiogram is normal. Continue salicylate regimen in children with coronary abnormalities long term or until documented regression of aneurysm (2)[C].
- Aspirin does not appear to reduce CAA (3)[B].
- Contraindications
  - IVIG: documented hypersensitivity, IgA deficiency, anti-IgE/IgG antibodies, severe thrombocytopenia, coagulation disorders
  - Aspirin: vitamin K deficiency, bleeding disorders, liver damage, documented hypersensitivity, hypoprothrombinemia
- Precautions
  - No statistically significant difference noted between different preparations of IVIG
  - High-dose aspirin therapy can result in tinnitus, decrease of renal function, and increased transaminases.
  - Do not use ibuprofen in children with coronary artery aneurysms who are taking aspirin for antiplatelet effects.
  - Significant possible interactions: Aspirin therapy has been associated with Reye syndrome in children who develop viral infections, especially influenza B and varicella. Yearly influenza vaccination thus is recommended for children requiring long-term treatment with aspirin. Delay any live vaccines for 11 months after IVIG treatment.

Second Line

- Corticosteroids should be used only if ≥2 IVIG treatments have failed. The addition of corticosteroids to IVIG and aspirin during initial treatment might improve CAA outcomes but lacks consistent evidence (4)[C].
- In patients refractory to IVIG and steroids, consider infliximab (5)[B].
- Plasma exchange may decrease likelihood of CAA in IVIG nonresponders (6)[B].

ISSUES FOR REFERRAL

Pediatric cardiologist if abnormalities on echo or if extensive stenosis

ADDITIONAL THERAPIES

- Treatment and prevention of thrombosis are crucial.
- Antiplatelet agents (clopidogrel, dipyridamole), heparin, low-molecular-weight heparin, or warfarin are sometimes added to the low-dose aspirin regimen, depending on severity of coronary involvement.

SURGERY/OTHER PROCEDURES

- Rarely needed; coronary artery bypass grafting for severe obstruction/recurrent MI. Younger patients have a higher mortality rate.
- Coronary revascularization via percutaneous coronary intervention for patients with evidence of ischemia on stress testing

INPATIENT CONSIDERATIONS

IV Fluids

Normal saline (NS) for rehydration and 1/2 NS for maintenance

Discharge Criteria

Discharge if afebrile after IVIG treatment × 24 hours.

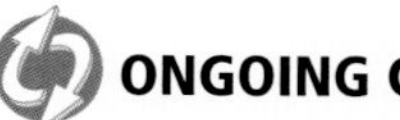

ONGOING CARE

FOLLOW-UP RECOMMENDATIONS

With aneurysms, contact and high-risk sports should be avoided.

Patient Monitoring

- Repeat ECG and echocardiogram at 6–8 weeks. If abnormal, repeat at 6–12 months.
- Patients with complex coronary artery lesions may benefit from coronary angiography at 6–12 months.

PROGNOSIS

- Usually self-limited
- Moderate-sized aneurysms usually regress in 1–2 years, resolving in 50–66% of cases.
- Recurrence (3% in Japan, <1% in the United States)
- Sudden death in early adulthood (rare)

COMPLICATIONS

- 15–25% of untreated patients develop CAAs in convalescent phase.
- 2–7% of treated patients develop aneurysms. 1% develop giant aneurysms.
- Risk factors for aneurysm
  - Male, <1 year of age, ↑ ESR >4 weeks, fever >2 weeks, fever >48 hours after IVIG treatment
- Mortality of 0.08–0.17% is due to cardiac disease.

REFERENCES

1. JCS Joint Working Group. Guidelines for diagnosis and management of cardiovascular sequelae in Kawasaki disease (JCS 2008)—digest version. *Circ J*. 2010;74(9):1989–2020.
2. Baumer JH, Love SJ, Gupta A, et al. Salicylate for the treatment of Kawasaki disease in children. *Cochrane Database Syst Rev*. 2006;(4):CD004175.
3. Lee G, Lee SE, Hong YM, et al. Is high-dose aspirin necessary in the acute phase of Kawasaki disease? *Korean Circ J*. Mar;43(3):182–186.
4. Chen S, Dong Y, Yin Y, et al. Intravenous immunoglobulin plus corticosteroid to prevent coronary artery abnormalities in Kawasaki disease: a meta-analysis. *Heart*. 2013;99(2):76–82.
5. Tremoulet AH, Jain S, Jaggi P, et al. Infliximab for intensification of primary therapy for Kawasaki disease: a phase 3 randomised, double-blind, placebo-controlled trial. *Lancet*. 2014;383(9930):1731–1738.
6. Hokosaki T, Mori M, Nishizawa T, et al. Long-term efficacy of plasma exchange treatment for refractory Kawasaki disease. *Pediatr Int*. 2012;54(1):99–103.

ADDITIONAL READING

- Huang SK, Lin MT, Chen HC, et al. Epidemiology of Kawasaki disease: prevalence from national database and future trends projection by system dynamics modeling. *J Pediatr*. 2013;163(1):126–131. e121.
- Kobayashi T, Saji T, Otani T, et al. Efficacy of immunoglobulin plus prednisolone for prevention of coronary artery abnormalities in severe Kawasaki disease (RAISE study): a randomised, open-label, blinded-endpoints trial. *Lancet*. 2012;379(9826):1613–1620.
- Newburger JW, Takahashi M, Gerber MA, et al. Diagnosis, treatment, and long-term management of Kawasaki disease: a statement for health professionals from the Committee on Rheumatic Fever, Endocarditis and Kawasaki Disease, Council on Cardiovascular Disease in the Young, American Heart Association. *Circulation*. 2004;110(17):2747–2771.
- Oates-Whitehead RM, Baumer JH, Haines L, et al. Intravenous immunoglobulin for the treatment of Kawasaki disease in children. *Cochrane Database Syst Rev*. 2003;(4):CD004000.
- Rowley AH, Shulman ST. Pathogenesis and management of Kawasaki disease. *Expert Rev Anti Infect Ther*. 2010;8(2):197–203.
- Takahashi K, Oharaseki T, Yokouchi Y. Update on etio and immunopathogenesis of Kawasaki disease. *Current Opin Rheumatol*. 2014;26(1):31–36.
- Uehara R, Belay ED. Epidemiology of Kawasaki Disease in Asia, Europe, and the United States. *J Epidemiol*. 2012;22(2):79–85.

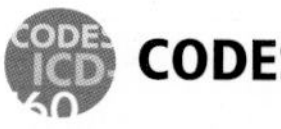

CODES

ICD10

M30.3 Mucocutaneous lymph node syndrome [Kawasaki]

CLINICAL PEARLS

- The diagnosis of KS rests on a constellation of clinical features.
- Once KS is suspected, all patients need an inpatient cardiac evaluation, including ECG and echocardiogram.
- Expert recommendations for optimal therapy is IVIG 2 g/kg IV over 10 hours, with high-dose aspirin 80–100 mg/kg/day in 4 doses.

KELOIDS

Felix Geissler, MD, PhD • Jennifer Pisani, PharmD

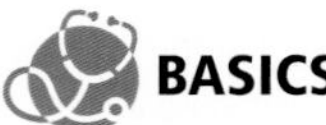

BASICS

DESCRIPTION

- Keloids are benign hyperproliferative growths of dermal fibroblasts characterized by the excessive deposition of extracellular matrix components, especially collagen, fibronectin, elastin, proteoglycans, and growth factors such as transforming growth factor-β (TGF-β).
- Keloids present as abnormal scar tissue proliferations at a site of injury.
- System(s) affected: skin/exocrine

EPIDEMIOLOGY

Incidence

- Predominant age: 10–30 years
- Higher incidence during puberty, early adulthood, and pregnancy

Prevalence

- 5–15% of wounds develop keloid scars.
- 4–16% of the black and Hispanic populations
- Higher incidence in the Asian population
- Data from United Kingdom demonstrated that $<$1% of Caucasians had keloids.

ETIOLOGY AND PATHOPHYSIOLOGY

- The mechanisms of keloid formation include alterations in growth factors, collagen turnover, and skin tension alignment, as well as genetic and immunologic contributions.
- Trauma, foreign-body reactions, infections, and endocrine dysfunctions have all been proposed as risk factors for the development of keloids after surgery in genetically susceptible people.
- Rarely occur in places on body lacking sebaceous glands; thus, sebaceous glands and the body's reaction to this sebum are hypothesized to be an etiologic factor in keloid development. Moreover, humans are the only mammals with sebaceous glands and the only mammals affected by keloids.
- Common sites that develop keloids: shoulders, clavicle and sternum, neck, jaw, and ears
- Wounds: traumatic, surgical, body piercing (foreign body reaction)
- Wound infection
- Burn injury (thermal or chemical)
- Other injuries:
  - Insect bite
  - Pseudofolliculitis barbae and folliculitis keloidalis nuchae
  - Acne
  - Chickenpox
- Vaccination (especially bacille Calmette-Guérin [BCG])
- Increased ratio of type I to type III collagen
- Increased density and proliferation rate of fibroblasts

Genetics

- More common in blacks and Asians (5–16×) than in Caucasians; in all races, more darkly pigmented individuals are at higher risk.
- Both autosomal dominant and autosomal recessive familial inheritance have been reported.
- Several genes have been implicated in the etiology of keloid disease, but no single gene mutation has thus far been found to be responsible.
- High frequency of identical twins both developing keloids strongly supports a role for genetics in keloid etiology.

RISK FACTORS

- Previous keloid
- Family history of keloids
- Race
- Darker skin pigmentation
- Location on the body (e.g., deltoids, chest, neck, earlobes)
- Pregnancy
- Adolescence
- Repeated abnormal wound healing (e.g., earring sites)

GENERAL PREVENTION

- Primary prevention: Avoid elective surgery, body piercing, and tattooing in high-risk patients.
- When feasible, laparoscopic approaches are preferred in keloid formers.
- Compressive pressure dressings may be useful in high-risk (e.g., burn) patients. Local steroid injection postoperatively in high-risk patients is also effective.
- Physicians should be alert to delays in wound healing if erythema or pruritus persists as impending symptoms of possible keloid formation.
- Attempts to reduce inflammation and tension on the skin with appropriate methods are vital for prevention.

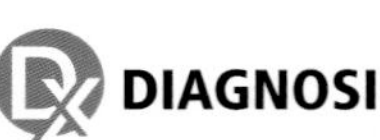

DIAGNOSIS

HISTORY

- Pain
- Tenderness
- Hyperesthesia
- Pruritus and burning (occasional)
- Abnormal growth beyond the border of the original wound
- May be asymptomatic

PHYSICAL EXAM

- Firm, smooth, elevated scar with sharply demarcated borders
- Initially, may be pale or mildly erythematous
- Older lesion hypo- or hyperpigmented
- Scar extends beyond margins of the initial wound.
- Over period of years, keloids may continue to grow and may develop claw-like projections.
- Keloids occur more frequently on the chest, shoulders, upper back, back of the neck, and earlobes.

DIFFERENTIAL DIAGNOSIS

- Hypertrophic scar (usually regresses spontaneously, does not cross wound margins, follows scars linearly, and often appears 4–6 weeks after a traumatic wound) (1)[C]
- Dermatofibroma
- Infiltrating basal cell carcinoma
- Sclerosing metastatic malignancies
- Desmoplastic melanoma
- Sarcoidosis
- Leprosy (nodular LL type)
- Other fibronodular skin diseases (e.g., neurofibromatosis, post–kala-azar dermal leishmaniasis)

DIAGNOSTIC TESTS & INTERPRETATION

Biopsy only if unable to differentiate from carcinoma or infectious disease, as biopsy may increase the keloid's size. Use a 2-mm punch biopsy to minimize trauma (2).

Test Interpretation

Histology shows whorl-like arrangements of hyalinized collagen bundles, with pressure thinning of papillary dermis and minimal elastic tissue. Cellular fibrous bands are also noted (2).

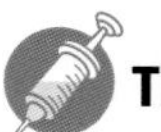

TREATMENT

- Given the high recurrence rates and significant expense associated with treatment, prevention of keloids should take priority (1)[C]. Avoidance of known risk factors such as piercings, tattoos, and elective surgery is highly recommended in people with either a family or personal history of keloids (3)[B].
- There are no uniform treatment protocols (1).
- Combination regimens are the most successful for treatment and prevention of keloid recurrence (1)[C].
- Treatment options should be based on the type of keloid. Characteristics to take into consideration: (i) presence or absence of scar contractures, (ii) size, and (iii) number of keloids (2)[A]
  - Small, single keloids can be treated more aggressively.
  - Large or multiple keloids are typically more complicated to treat and should be evaluated on an individual basis.
  - Earlobe keloids: Use surgery and pressure for treatment (1)[C].
  - Neck, lower limbs: Surgery with immediate radiation has a ≥65% response rate (1)[C].
- Antimitotic drugs described in the literature, such as steroid injection, 5-FU, mitomycin C, and bleomycin, mainly target the fibroblasts in scar tissue (1)[A].

GENERAL MEASURES

- Intralesional corticosteroid injections are most commonly used for treatment (1).
- For refractory keloids, consider combination treatment, which may include radiation, occlusive dressings, surgical excision, or corticosteroid injections (1)[C].
- Pressure bandages must maintain 25–40 mm Hg and should be worn for 6–12 months. Bandages should be worn for 23–24 hr/day (1)[C].
- Pressure clips (Zimmer splints) are useful for earlobes. Designer splints look like fashion earrings (1)[C].
- Cryotherapy may be useful for small keloids (e.g., acne scars) (4).
  - Use 10–20-second freeze–thaw cycles every month; may cause pain and blistering (4)[A]
- Topical agents: No evidence to support efficacy of retinoic acid, vitamin E, allantoin, or onion extract; some evidence for imiquimod (2,5)[A]. Generally, retinoids are tolerated in patients with pigmented skin; however, the treating physician must be cognizant of the development of retinoid dermatitis, which can induce hyperpigmentation (6).

MEDICATION

First Line

- 5-FU (5-fluorouracil) (1)[A]
  - 5-FU tattooing was more effective than intralesional triamcinolone for the treatment of keloids.
  - In 1 study with keloids treated with intralesional 5-FU weekly with a total of 16 injections, ~1/2 of the patients showed >50% flattening. The older keloids (>5 years) were more difficult to treat.
  - Side effects are local erythema, swelling, pain, molting, pigmentation, and occasional ulcers.
  - Effectiveness rate of 5-FU injection alone is 62.5%, whereas the efficacy of 5-FU in combination with glucocorticoids is significantly better at 92%.
- Triamcinolone (Kenalog) suspension 10 mg/mL
  - Other steroids may be used, but triamcinolone is the most commonly used treatment option (3)[A].
  - Cure rate is 80% with use of corticosteroids after keloid excision (1)[C].
  - Likely more effective if combined with cryotherapy, pulsed dye laser, or 5-FU. No difference when combined with excision versus monotherapy (1)[A]
  - Intralesional injections as an outpatient are commonly administered.
  - Use 27–30-gauge needle.
  - General dosing: 0.1–0.2 mL/cm^2 of keloid tissue
  - Reinject every 4–8 weeks until clinical improvement. Several months of treatment are often needed (1)[C].
  - If no response with 10 mg/mL triamcinolone suspension, may increase to 40 mg/mL suspension (3)[A]
  - May mix triamcinolone with local anesthetic for difficult keloids. Contraindications: active skin infection at injection site
  - Precautions: systemic absorption with reversible adrenal suppression, hyperglycemia
    - Local effects: skin atrophy, ulceration, depigmentation, telangiectasias
    - Both types of side effects are more common with 40 mg/mL triamcinolone suspension.
- Silica gel sheeting: 1st-line prophylaxis after surgical procedure or keloid excision
  - Patient compliance limits effectiveness.
  - Sheets are cut to fit and must be worn 12–24 hr/day for 18 months (1)[C].
  - Unclear whether benefit is from silicone or occlusive effect
  - Adverse effects are generally from irritation: pruritus, rash, and breakdown of the skin (1)[C].

Second Line

- Cryotherapy is likely to be more useful in early, smaller lesions (4)[A]. It is not recommended for larger areas or darker skin because of pain and decreased skin pigmentation.
- Verapamil locally may be helpful as an adjuvant following excision and topical silicone (5,6)[A].
- Interferon-α2b may be helpful after excision (5,6)[A].
- Topical imiquimod (Aldara) may be helpful after excision (4)[A].
- Intralesional bleomycin, retinoic acid, mitomycin C, colchicine (1)[A]
- Radiation therapy has greater success rates when used in combination with surgical excision (5)[A]. There are some concerns about precipitating malignant lesions with radiation; however, a direct correlation has not been made (7)[C].

Pregnancy Considerations

Radiation therapy, 5-FU, and bleomycin are unsafe in pregnancy. Triamcinolone should be used with caution.

ISSUES FOR REFERRAL

When intralesional steroids fail, referral to dermatologist or plastic surgeon may be indicated.

ADDITIONAL THERAPIES

- Local radiotherapy may be effective after excision but carries a small risk of carcinogenesis (2)[A].
- Clinical studies are currently investigating the inhibition of the mTOR pathway as possible therapy (8).

SURGERY/OTHER PROCEDURES

- Surgery: High recurrence rate (45–100%) if used alone; therefore, it is used only for the debulking of large keloids or if a lesion is unresponsive to steroid injections or other therapy. Combine with preoperative steroid injection and possibly other modalities. Debulking just enough for symptomatic improvement is recommended (2)[A].
- Pulsed-dye laser surgery: No definitive evidence of efficacy or advantage over other methods. Therefore, use only if other methods fail, and then use in conjunction with them. Some promise is seen in combination with triamcinolone and 5-FU (1)[A].

ONGOING CARE

FOLLOW-UP RECOMMENDATIONS

Patient Monitoring

Monthly visits for up to 1 year for evaluation and possible steroid reinjections

PATIENT EDUCATION

- Stress the possibility of recurrence despite appropriate treatment.
- May require many months of treatment with combined modalities
- Prevention: In those with risk factors or previous keloids, caution against activities or procedures that may entail dermal disruption, and suggest early treatment of any such events.

PROGNOSIS

When treatment is successful, lesions gradually diminish over 6–18 months with therapy, leaving a flat, shiny scar. Although keloids can improve with treatment, cure is unlikely.

COMPLICATIONS

Skin atrophy, ulceration, depigmentation, and telangiectasias can occur as a result of local steroid injections.

REFERENCES

1. Wang XQ, Liu YK, Qing C, et al. A review of the effectiveness of antimitotic drug injections for hypertrophic scars and keloids. *Ann Plast Surg*. 2009;63(6):688–692.
2. Ogawa R. The most current algorithms for the treatment and prevention of hypertrophic scars and keloids. *Plast Reconstr Surg*. 2010;125(2):557–568.
3. Sadeghinia A, Sadeghinia S. Comparison of the efficacy of intralesional triamcinolone acetonide and 5-fluorouracil tattooing for the treatment of keloids. *Dermatol Surg*. 2012;38(1):104–109.
4. Gauglitz GG, Korting HC, Pavicic T, et al. Hypertrophic scarring and keloids: pathomechanisms and current and emerging treatment strategies. *Mol Med*. 2011;17(1–2):113-125.
5. Viera MH, Caperton CV, Berman B. Advances in the treatment of keloids. *J Drugs Dermatol*. 2011;10(5): 468–480.
6. Geria AN, Lawson CN, Halder RM. Topical retinoids for pigmented skin. *J Drugs Dermatol*. 2011;10(5): 483–489.
7. Schneider M, Meites E, Daane SP. Keloids: which treatment is best for your patient? *J Fam Pract*. 2013;62(5):227–233.
8. Syed F, Sherris D, Paus R, et. al. Keloid disease can be inhibited by antagonizing excessive mTOR signalling with a novel dual TORC1/2 inhibitor. *Am J Pathol*. 2012;181(151):1642–1658.

ADDITIONAL READING

- Davison SP, Dayan JH, Clemens MW, et al. Efficacy of intralesional 5-fluorouracil and triamcinolone in the treatment of keloids. *Aesthet Surg J*. 2009;29(1): 40–46.
- Halim AS, Emami A, Salahshourifar I, et al. Keloid scarring: understanding the genetic basis, advances, and prospects. *Arch Plast Surg*. 2012;39(3):184–189.

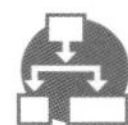

SEE ALSO

Bites, Animal and Human; Burns; Leprosy; Warts

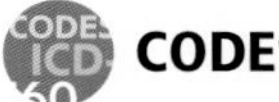

CODES

ICD10

- L91.0 Hypertrophic scar
- L73.0 Acne keloid

CLINICAL PEARLS

- The most successful treatment of hypertrophic scar or keloid is achieved while the scar is still immature, but the overlying epithelium is intact, although this is not as yet confirmed in the literature.
- Differentiation of keloids from hypertrophic scars is vital. Keloids extend beyond the margins of the original wound and do not regress with time, but hypertrophic scars do. Treatment is similar, but keloids are much more likely to recur.
- Closing wounds with a minimum of suture tension, avoiding midsternal incisions and crossing joint lines, and injecting steroids into the incision postoperatively reduce the chance of keloids forming following unavoidable surgery.

KERATOACANTHOMA

Carl Bryce, MD • Matthew Snyder, DO

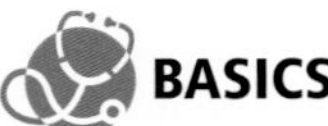

BASICS

DESCRIPTION

- Rapidly proliferating, solitary, dome-shaped, erythematous or flesh-colored papule or nodule with a central keratinous plug, typically reaching 1–2 cm in diameter
- Classified as a variant of a well-differentiated squamous cell carcinoma (SCC); histologic differentiation of a keratoacanthoma (KA) from an SCC may be difficult and unreliable.
- It is highly debated as to whether KA is a benign or malignant variant of SCC.
- Majority are benign and resolve spontaneously, but lesions do have the potential for invasion and metastasis; therefore require treatment
- Three clinical stages of KAs (1)
  - Proliferative: rapid growth of the lesion over weeks to several months
  - Maturation/stabilization: Lesion stabilizes and growth subsides.
  - Involution: spontaneous resolution of the lesion, leaving a hypopigmented, depressed scar; most but not all lesions will enter this stage.
- System(s) affected: integumentary

EPIDEMIOLOGY

- Greatest incidence over the age of 50 years but may occur at any age
- Presentation increased during summer and early fall seasons
- Most frequently on sun-exposed, hair-bearing skin but may occur anywhere
- Predominant sex: male > female (2:1)
- Most commonly in fair-skinned individuals; highest rates in Fitzpatrick I–III
- 104 cases per 100,000 individuals

ETIOLOGY AND PATHOPHYSIOLOGY

- Derived from an abnormality, causing hyperkeratosis within the follicular infundibulum
- Squamous epithelial cells proliferate to extend upward around the keratin plug and proceed downward into the dermis; followed by invasion of elastic and collagen fibers
- Cellular mechanism responsible for the hyperkeratosis is currently unknown.
- Regression may be due to immune cytotoxicity or terminal differentiation of keratinocytes.
- Multiple etiologies have been suggested:
  - UV radiation
  - Trauma: accidental or iatrogenic, including surgery, cryotherapy, laser therapy
  - Viral infections: human papillomavirus (HPV) or Merkel cell polyomavirus
  - Genetic predisposition: Muir-Torre syndrome, xeroderma pigmentosum, Ferguson-Smith syndrome
  - Immunosuppression
  - Chemical carcinogen exposure

Genetics

- Mutation of *p53* or H-*ras*
- Ferguson-Smith (AD)
- Witten-Zak (AD)
- Muir-Torre (AD)
- Xeroderma pigmentosum (AR)
- Gzybowski (sporadic)
- Incontinentia pigmenti (XLD)

RISK FACTORS

- UV exposure/damage: outdoor and/or indoor tanning
- Fitzpatrick skin type I–III
- Trauma (typically appears within 1 month of injury): accidental, surgery, cryotherapy, tattoos
- Chemical carcinogens: tar, pitch, and smoking
- Immunocompromised state
- Discoid lupus erythematosus

GENERAL PREVENTION

Sun protection

COMMONLY ASSOCIATED CONDITIONS

- Frequently, the patient has concurrent sun-damaged skin: solar elastosis, solar lentigines, actinic keratosis, nonmelanoma skin cancers (basal cell carcinoma, SCC)
- In Muir-Torre syndrome, KAs are found with coexisting sebaceous neoplasms and malignancy of the GI and GU tracts.

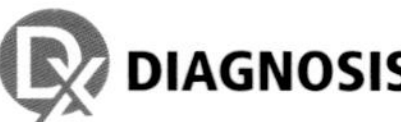

DIAGNOSIS

HISTORY

- Lesion begins as a small, solitary, pink macule that undergoes a rapid growth phase; classically reaching a diameter of 1–2 cm; size may vary.
- Once the proliferative stage has subsided, lesion size remains stable (1)[B].
- May decrease in size, indicating regression
- Asymptomatic, occasionally tender
- If multiple lesions present, important to elicit a family history
- If sebaceous neoplasms present, must review history for signs/symptoms of GI or GU malignancies

PHYSICAL EXAM

- Firm, solitary, erythematous or flesh-colored, dome-shaped papule or nodule with a central keratin plug, giving a crateriform appearance
- Surrounding skin and borders of lesion may show telangiectasia, atrophy, or dyspigmentation.
- Solitary; although multiple lesions can occur.
- Most commonly seen on sun-exposed areas: face, neck, scalp, dorsum of upper extremities, and posterior legs
- May also be seen on areas without sun exposure: buttocks, anus, subungual, mucosal surfaces
- Subungual KAs are very painful and seen on the first 3 digits of the hands.
- Lesion may enlarge up to 30 cm as a KA centrifugum marginatum—extremely rare (2).
- Examine for regional lymphadenopathy due to chance of lesion invasion and metastasis.
- Dermoscopy (3)[B]
  - Central keratin
  - White circles, blood spots
  - Cannot reliably distinguish between AK and SCC

DIFFERENTIAL DIAGNOSIS

- SCC
- Nodular or ulcerative basal cell carcinoma
- Cutaneous horn
- Hypertrophic actinic keratosis
- Merkel cell carcinoma
- Metastasis to the skin
- Molluscum contagiosum
- Prurigo nodularis
- Verruca vulgaris
- Verrucous carcinoma
- Sebaceous adenoma
- Hypertrophic lichen planus
- Hypertrophic lupus erythematosus
- Deep fungal infection
- Atypical mycobacterial infection
- Nodular Kaposi sarcoma

DIAGNOSTIC TESTS & INTERPRETATION

- Excisional biopsy is the diagnostic test of choice (3,4)[C].
  - Important to include the center of the lesion as well as the margin
- A shave biopsy may be insufficiently deep to distinguish KA from an SCC.
  - Questionable as to whether a KA can be reliably differentiated from an SCC
- If unable to perform an excisional biopsy, a deep shave (saucerization) of the entire lesion, extending into the subcutaneous fat, can be done.
- Punch biopsies should be avoided because they give an insufficient amount of tissue to represent the entire lesion.

Initial Tests (lab, imaging)

- Subungual KA: radiograph of the digit to monitor for osteolysis (cup-shaped radiolucent defect)
- Aggressive tumors may need CT with contrast for evaluation of lymph nodes and MRI if there is concern of perineural invasion.
- Most lesions do not need any form of imaging.

Test Interpretation

- Pathology of biopsy: a well-demarcated central core of keratin surrounded by well-differentiated, mildly pleomorphic, atypical squamous epithelial cells with a characteristic glassy eosinophilic cytoplasm
- May see elastic and collagen fibers invading into the squamous epithelium
- KAs have a greater tendency than SCC to display fibrosis and intraepidermal abscesses of neutrophils and eosinophils.
- Regressing KA shows flattening and fibrosis at base of lesion.

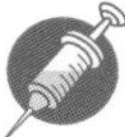

TREATMENT

- Treatment of choice is surgical excision with 3–5-mm surgical margins (4)[C].
- Aggressive tumors (>2 cm) or lesions in cosmetically sensitive areas (face, digits, genitalia) that require tissue sparing, consider Mohs micrographic surgery
  - Mohs is the treatment of choice in cases with perineural or perivascular invasion.
- Small lesions (<2 cm) of the extremities may undergo electrodessication and curettage.
- Immunocompromised patients should receive immediate surgical treatment.

MEDICATION

- Nonsurgical management is a viable and relatively cost-effective option in these select cases not amenable to surgery due to lesion number, size, or location; also for patients with multiple comorbidities who are unwilling or unable to withstand surgery
- Evidence for the following treatments based upon case reports and retrospective reviews:
  - Intralesional methotrexate 12.5–25 mg in 0.5 mL normal saline every 2–3 weeks for one to four treatment sessions (4)[B]
    - Monitor for pancytopenia with complete blood count (5)[C].
  - 5% Imiquimod cream 3×/week for 11–13 weeks (5)[B]
  - Topical 5% 5-fluorouracil cream daily, 61–92% cure rate (4)[B]
  - Intralesional 5-fluorouracil of 50 mg/mL on a weekly basis for three to eight treatment sessions—98% cure rate (4)[B]
  - Intralesional IFN a-2a or a-2b (83%, 100% cure rate, respectively) (4)[B]
  - Intralesional bleomycin—100% cure rate (4)[B]
  - Isotretinoin oral 0.5–1 mg/kg/day

ISSUES FOR REFERRAL

Dermatology referral if lesions are >2 cm, numerous, mucosal, or subungual

ADDITIONAL THERAPIES

- Photodynamic therapy with methyl aminolevulinic acid and red light, successful case reports (6)[B] but also reported aggravation following treatment
- Cryotherapy
- Argon or YAG lasers
- Radiotherapy, primary or adjuvant: KAs may regress with low doses of radiation but may require doses up to 40–50 Gy in 10–20 fractions for possible SCC.
- Erlotinib (EGFR inhibitor) 150 mg daily for 21 days, single case report (7)[B]

SURGERY/OTHER PROCEDURES

Despite spontaneous regression in many cases, KA requires treatment as an SCC (3,4)[C].

ONGOING CARE

FOLLOW-UP RECOMMENDATIONS

After the surgical site has healed or lesion has resolved, patient should be seen every 6 months due to increased risk of developing new lesions or skin cancers, annually at minimum (2)[C].

Patient Monitoring

- Skin self-exams should be routinely performed with detailed instructions (see "Additional Reading").
- If multiple KAs are present in patient or family members, evaluate for Muir-Torre syndrome and obtain a colonoscopy beginning at age 25 years, as well as testing for genitourinary cancer (2)[C].

PATIENT EDUCATION

- Sun protection measures: sun block with SPF >30, wide-brimmed hats, long sleeves, dark clothing, avoiding indoor tanning
- Tar, pitch, and smoking should be avoided.

PROGNOSIS

- Atrophic scarring and hypopigmentation will occur with self-resolution but may be significantly reduced by intervention.
- Very few cases of invasion and metastasis
- 4–8% recurrence
- Mucosal and subungual lesions do not regress, must undergo treatment

REFERENCES

1. Zalaudek I, Bonifazi E, Ferrara G, et al. Keratoacanthomas and spitz tumors: are they both "self-limiting" variants of malignant cutaneous neoplasms? *Dermatology*. 2009;219(1):3–6.
2. Sarabi K, Selim A, Khachemoune A. Sporadic and syndromic keratoacanthomas: diagnosis and management. *Dermatol Nurs*. 2007;19(2):166–170.
3. Rosendahl C, Cameron A, Argenziano G, et al. Dermoscopy of squamous cell carcinoma and keratoacanthoma. *Arch Dermatol*. 2012;148(12): 1386–1392.
4. Chitwood KL, Etzkorn J, Cohen G. Topical and intralesional treatment of nonmelanoma skin cancer: efficacy and cost comparisons. *Dermatol Surg*. 2013;39(9):1306–1316.
5. Jeon HC, Choi M, Paik SH, et al. Treatment of keratoacanthoma with 5% imiquimod cream and review of the previous report. *Ann Dermatol*. 2011;23(3):357–361.
6. Farias M, Hasson A, Navarrete C, et al. Efficacy of topical photodynamic therapy for keratoacanthomas: a case-series of four patients. *Indian J Dermatol Venereol Leprol*. 2012;78(2):172–174.
7. Reid DC, Guitart J, Agulnik M. Treatment of multiple keratoacanthomas with erlotinib. *Int J Clin Oncol*. 2010;15(4):413–415.

ADDITIONAL READING

- The American Academy of Dermatology: http://www.aad.org/spot-skin-cancer/understanding-skin-cancer/how-do-i-check-my-skin/how-to-perform-a-self-exam
- The Skin Cancer Foundation: www.skincancer.org/

SEE ALSO

Squamous Cell Carcinoma, Cutaneous

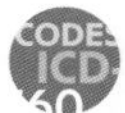

CODES

ICD10

L85.8 Other specified epidermal thickening

CLINICAL PEARLS

- Suspect KA with a solitary, dome-shaped, erythematous or flesh-colored papule or nodule with a central keratinous plug.
- If KA is in the differential diagnosis, elicit time frame of onset during patient encounter; rapid onset supports diagnosis.
- Due to the unreliable histologic differentiation of a KA and an SCC, as well as the ability of KAs to metastasize, a KA should be treated as an SCC with surgical excision as 1st-line therapy.
- Excisional biopsy is the test of choice to diagnose KA.
- Consider KA in subungual lesions if it is painful and does not regress.
- Medical therapy is available for patients who are not surgical candidates or for lesions that are undesirable for surgery.

KERATOSIS, ACTINIC

Zoltan Trizna, MD, PhD

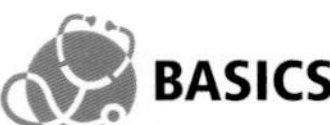

BASICS

DESCRIPTION

- Common, usually multiple, premalignant lesions of sun-exposed areas of the skin. Many resolve spontaneously, and a small proportion progress to squamous cell carcinoma
- Common consequence of excessive cumulative ultraviolet (UV) light exposure
- Synonym(s): solar keratosis

Geriatric Considerations

Frequent problem

Pediatric Considerations

Rare (if child, look for freckling and other stigmata of xeroderma pigmentosum)

EPIDEMIOLOGY

Incidence

- Rates vary with age group and exposure to sun.
- Predominant age: ≥40 years; progressively increases with age
- Predominant sex: male > female
- Common in those with blonde and red hair; rare in darker skin types

Prevalence

- Age-adjusted prevalence rate for actinic keratoses (AKs) in U.S. Caucasians is 6.5%.
- For 65–74-year-old males with high sun exposure: ~55%; low sun exposure, ~18%

ETIOLOGY AND PATHOPHYSIOLOGY

- The epidermal lesions are characterized by atypical keratinocytes at the basal layer with occasional extension upward. Mitoses are present. The histopathologic features resemble those of squamous cell carcinoma (SCC) in situ or SCC, and the distinction depends on the extent of epidermal involvement.
- Cumulative UV exposure

Genetics

The *p53* chromosomal mutation has been shown consistently in both AKs and SCCs. Many new genes have been shown recently to have similar expression profiles in AKs and SCCs.

RISK FACTORS

- Exposure to UV light (especially long-term and/or repeated exposure due to outdoor occupation or recreational activities, indoor or outdoor tanning)
- Skin type: burns easily, does not tan
- Immunosuppression, especially organ transplantation

GENERAL PREVENTION

Sun avoidance and protective techniques are helpful.

COMMONLY ASSOCIATED CONDITIONS

- SCC
- Other features of chronic solar damage: lentigines, elastosis, and telangiectasias

DIAGNOSIS

HISTORY

- The lesions are frequently asymptomatic; symptoms may include pruritus, burning, and mild hyperesthesia.
- Lesions may enlarge, thicken, or become more scaly. They also may regress or remain unchanged.
- Most lesions occur on the sun-exposed areas (head and neck, hands, forearms).

PHYSICAL EXAM

- Usually small (<1 cm), often multiple red, pink, or brown macules, papules, or plaques that are rough to palpation.
- Yellow or brown adherent scale is often present on top of the lesion.
- Several clinical variants exist.
  - Atrophic: dry, scaly macules with indistinct borders and an erythematous base
  - Hypertrophic: Overlying hyperkeratosis (in an extreme form, cutaneous horn) may be impossible to differentiate from SCC clinically.
  - Pigmented: smooth tan/brown plaque, spreading centrifugally
  - Bowenoid: red scaly plaques with distinct borders
  - Actinic cheilitis: inflammatory lesion involving usually the lower lip

DIFFERENTIAL DIAGNOSIS

- SCC (hypertrophic type)
- Keratoacanthoma
- Bowen disease
- Basal cell carcinoma
- Verruca vulgaris
- Less likely: verrucous nevi, warty dyskeratoma, lichenoid keratoses, seborrheic keratoses, porokeratoses, seborrheic dermatitis or psoriasis (near hairline), lentigo maligna, solar lentigo, discoid lupus erythematosus

DIAGNOSTIC TESTS & INTERPRETATION

Diagnostic Procedures/Other

- The diagnosis is usually made clinically, except where there is a suspicion of carcinoma.
- Skin biopsy is especially recommended if large, ulcerated, indurated, or bleeding; or if the lesions are nonresponsive to treatment.

Test Interpretation

- Dysplastic keratinocytes in lower levels of epidermis with a dermal lymphocytic infiltrate
- Neoplastic cells, mostly found in the lower epidermal layers, are cytologically identical to those of SCCs.
- If neoplastic cells extend throughout entire epidermis or into the dermis, the lesions will qualify as an SCC in situ or invasive SCC, respectively.
- Malignant cells are sparse except of the bowenoid variety.
- Hypertrophic, atrophic, bowenoid, acantholytic, and pigmented varieties show the corresponding epidermal findings.

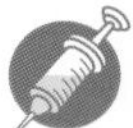

TREATMENT

1st-line treatment is cryotherapy (technically, this is considered surgery, especially by insurance companies) (1,2)[A]. Medical therapy is usually reserved for extensive AKs ("field therapy").

GENERAL MEASURES

- Sun-protective techniques
- Sunscreens and physical sun protection recommended.

MEDICATION

First Line

- Topical treatments target both visible and subclinical lesions.
- With the exception of generic 5-fluorouracil, medication cost is high ($600–$1,200 per course).
- Topical fluorouracil (Efudex, Carac, Fluoroplex cream, Fluoroplex solution)
  - Every day—BID for 3–6 weeks, depending on the brand, concentration, and formulation
  - Can be very irritating
- Topical imiquimod (Aldara) 5% cream
  - Apply 2 days per week at HS for up to 16 weeks to an area not larger than the forehead or 1 cheek.
  - Can be irritating
- Topical imiquimod (Zyclara) 3.75% cream
  - Apply once a day for 2 weeks, followed by no treatment for the next 2 weeks; then apply once a day for another 2 weeks.
  - Can be irritating
- Topical ingenol mebutate (Picato) 0.015% and 0.05% gel
  - Apply to the face and scalp once a day for 3 consecutive days.
  - Apply to the trunk and extremities once a day for 2 consecutive days.
- Diclofenac (Solaraze) 3% gel
  - Apply BID for 60–90 days.

Second Line

- Topical tretinoin (Retin-A) or tazarotene (Tazorac): may be used to enhance the efficacy of topical fluorouracil
- Systemic retinoids: used infrequently

ADDITIONAL THERAPIES

Close monitoring with no treatment is an appropriate option for mild lesions.

SURGERY/OTHER PROCEDURES

- Cryosurgery ("freezing," liquid nitrogen)
  - Most common method
  - Cure rate: 75–98.8%
  - May leave scars
  - May be superior to photodynamic therapy for thicker lesions
- Photodynamic therapy with a photosensitizer (e.g., aminolevulinic acid) and "blue light"
  - May clear >90% of AKs
  - Less scarring than cryotherapy
  - May be superior to cryotherapy, especially in the case of more extensive skin involvement
- Curettage and electrocautery (electrodesiccation and curettage [ED&C]; "scraping and burning")
- Medium-depth peels, especially for the treatment of extensive areas
- CO_2 laser therapy
- Dermabrasion
- Surgical excision (excisional biopsy)

ONGOING CARE

FOLLOW-UP RECOMMENDATIONS

Patient Monitoring

Depends on associated malignancy and frequency with which new AKs appear

PATIENT EDUCATION

- Teach sun-protective techniques.
  - Limit outdoor activities between 10 AM and 4 PM.
  - Wear protective clothing and wide-brimmed hat.
  - Proper use (including reapplication) of sunscreens with SPF >30, preferably a preparation with broad-spectrum (UV-A and UV-B) protection
- Teach self-examination of skin (melanoma, squamous cell, basal cell).
- Patient education materials
  - http://dermnetnz.org/lesions/solar-keratoses.html
  - www.skincarephysicians.com/ actinickeratosesnet /index.html
  - www.skincancer.org/Actinic-Keratosis-and-Other -Precancers.htm

PROGNOSIS

Very good. A significant proportion of the lesions may resolve spontaneously (3), with regression rates of 20–30% per lesion per year.

COMPLICATIONS

- AKs are premalignant lesions that may progress to SCCs. The rate of malignant transformation is unclear; the reported percentages vary (3) but range from 0.1% to a few percent per year per lesion.
- Patients with AKs are at increased risk for other cutaneous malignancies.
- Approximately 60% of SCCs arise from an AK precursor.

REFERENCES

1. Helfand M, Gorman AK, Mahon S, et al. Actinic Keratoses. Rockville, MD: Agency for Healthcare Research and Quality; 2001.
2. de Berker D, McGregor JM, Hughes BR. Guidelines for the management of actinic keratoses. *Br J Dermatol*. 2007;156(2):222–230.
3. Criscione VD, Weinstock MA, Naylor MF, et al. Actinic keratoses: natural history and risk of malignant transformation in the Veterans Affairs Topical Tretinoin Chemoprevention Trial. *Cancer*. 2009;115(11):2523–2530.

ADDITIONAL READING

- Kanellou P, Zaravinos A, Zioga M, et al. Genomic instability, mutations and expression analysis of the tumour suppressor genes p14(ARF), p15(INK4b), p16(INK4a) and p53 in actinic keratosis. *Cancer Lett*. 2008;264(1):145–161.
- Rossi R, Mori M, Lotti T. Actinic keratosis. *Int J Dermatol*. 2007;46(9):895–904.

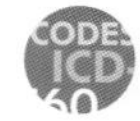

CODES

ICD10

L57.0 Actinic keratosis

CLINICAL PEARLS

- AKs are premalignant lesions.
- Often more easily felt than seen
- Therapy-resistant lesions should be biopsied, especially on the face.

K

KERATOSIS, SEBORRHEIC

Jelaun K. Newsome, DO • Heather O'Mara, DO

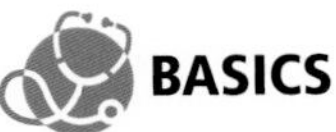

BASICS

DESCRIPTION

- One of the most common benign tumors of the epidermis
- Formed from keratinocytes
- Frequently appears in multiples on the head, neck, and trunk of older individuals but may occur on any hair-bearing area of the body. Lesions spare the palms and soles.
- Typically are light brown to black, sharply demarcated, round, or elongated lesions with a velvety, verrucous-like, "stuck-on" appearance; lesions may also appear waxy yellow or pink.
- Clinical variants include the following:
  - Common seborrheic keratosis
  - Dermatosis papulosa nigra
  - Stucco keratosis
  - Flat seborrheic keratosis
  - Pedunculated seborrheic keratosis
- System(s) affected: integumentary
- Synonym(s): verruca seborrhoica; seborrheic wart; senile wart; basal cell papilloma; verruca senilis; basal cell acanthoma; benign acanthokeratoma

EPIDEMIOLOGY

Incidence

- Predominant age
  - Usually appear after the 3rd decade
  - Most commonly seen during middle and older age
  - Can occasionally arise as early as adolescence
- Predominant sex: male = female
- Most common among Caucasians, except for the dermatosis papulosa nigra variant, which usually presents in darker skinned individuals

Prevalence

- 69–100% in patients >50 years of age
- The prevalence rate increases with advancing age.

ETIOLOGY AND PATHOPHYSIOLOGY

- Seborrheic keratoses are monoclonal tumors.
- Etiology still is largely unclear.
- Ultraviolet (UV) light and genetics are thought to be involved.
- The role of human papillomavirus is uncertain.

Genetics

An autosomal dominant inheritance pattern is suggested.

RISK FACTORS

- Advanced age
- Exposure to UV light and genetic predisposition are possible factors (1).

GENERAL PREVENTION

Sun protection methods may help prevent seborrheic keratoses from developing.

COMMONLY ASSOCIATED CONDITIONS

- Sign of Leser-Trélat: A paraneoplastic syndrome characterized by a sudden eruption of multiple seborrheic keratoses in association with an internal malignancy, most commonly stomach or colon adenocarcinoma. Usually represents a poor prognosis. The validity of this syndrome as a marker for internal malignancy is controversial (2)[B].
- Documentation of other cutaneous lesions, such as basal cell carcinoma, malignant melanoma, Bowen disease, or squamous cell carcinoma, growing adjacent to or within a seborrheic keratosis, has been reported. The exact relationship between lesions is unclear.

DIAGNOSIS

HISTORY

- Usually asymptomatic
- Trauma or irritation of the lesion may result in pruritus, erythema, bleeding, pain, and/or crusting.

PHYSICAL EXAM

- Typically begin as oval- or round-shaped, flat, dull, sharply demarcated patches
- As they mature, may develop into thicker, elevated, uneven, verrucous-like papules, plaques, or peduncles with a waxy or velvety surface, and appear "stuck on" to the skin (3)
- Commonly appear on sun-exposed areas of the body, predominately the head, neck, or trunk but may appear on any hair-bearing skin
- Vary in color from black, brown, tan, gray to white, or skin-colored, and range in size, from 1 mm to 4 cm
- Usually occur as multiples, with patients having >100 lesions is not uncommon.
- May grow along folds on truncal skin, forming a "Christmas tree" pattern
- If irritated, may be bleeding, inflamed, painful, pruritic, or crusted
- Common clinical variants include the following (4):
  - Common seborrheic keratoses: on hair-bearing skin, usually on the face, neck, and trunk; verrucous-like, waxy, or velvety lesions that appear "stuck on" to the skin
  - Dermatosis papulosa nigra: small black papules that usually appear on the face, neck, chest, and upper back; most common in darker skinned individuals, more common in females; most have a positive family history.
  - Stucco keratoses: small gray-white, rough, verrucous papules; usually occur in large numbers on the lower extremities or forearms; more common in men
  - Flat seborrheic keratoses: oval-shaped, brown patches or macules on face, chest, and upper extremities; increases with age
  - Pedunculated seborrheic keratoses: Hyperpigmented peduncles appear on areas of friction (neck, axilla).

DIFFERENTIAL DIAGNOSIS

Consider the following diagnoses if the seborrheic keratosis is:

- Pigmented
  - Malignant melanoma
  - Melanocytic nevus
  - Angiokeratoma
  - Pigmented basal cell carcinoma
- Lightly pigmented
  - Basal cell carcinoma
  - Bowen disease
  - Condyloma acuminatum
  - Fibroma
  - Verruca vulgaris
  - Eccrine poroma
  - Invasive squamous cell carcinoma
  - Acrochordon
  - Acrokeratosis verruciformis of Hopf
  - Follicular infundibulum tumor
- Flat
  - Solar lentigo
  - Verrucae planae juveniles
- Hyperkeratotic
  - Actinic keratosis

DIAGNOSTIC TESTS & INTERPRETATION

Initial Tests (lab, imaging)

Not needed unless internal malignancy is suspected

Diagnostic Procedures/Other

- The diagnosis can usually be made based on clinical appearance.
- Dermoscopy
  - Can aid in diagnosis
  - Common findings are comedo-like openings, fissures, ridges, sharply demarcated borders, milia-like cysts, pseudofollicular openings, hairpin vessels, and horn pseudocysts (5,6).
- Biopsy and histologic exam should be performed if the seborrheic keratosis
  - Is atypical
  - Has inflammation
  - Recently changed in appearance
  - Diagnosis remains unclear.

Test Interpretation

- Histologic findings include the following:
  - Acanthosis and papillomatosis due to basaloid cell proliferation
  - "Squamous eddies" or squamous epithelial cell clusters
  - Hyperpigmentation
  - Hyperkeratosis
  - Horn cysts
  - Pseudocysts
- Several histologic variants exist.

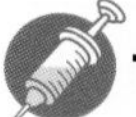

TREATMENT

- Treatment is not usually necessary due to the benign nature of the lesions.
- Removal of seborrheic keratoses may be indicated if
  - Symptomatic
  - Aesthetically displeasing or undesirable (common)
  - There is a question of malignancy.

MEDICATION

Current topical treatments of seborrheic keratoses are less effective than a surgical approach.

ISSUES FOR REFERRAL

- New seborrheic keratoses appear abruptly.
- A seborrheic keratosis becomes inflamed or changes in appearance.

SURGERY/OTHER PROCEDURES

- A surgical approach to treatment is preferred.
- Choice depends on physician preference and availability of the treatment.
- The following procedures are used:
  - Cryotherapy (liquid nitrogen)
    - Spray flat lesions for 5–10 seconds; may require more time or additional treatments if the seborrheic keratosis is thicker
    - Possible complications include scarring, hypopigmentation, recurrence.
  - Curettage
  - Electrodessication
  - Shave excision
  - Excisional biopsy
  - Chemical peel
- Use of following laser treatments have been reported:
  - Ablative CO_2
  - Ablative erbium-YAG
  - Argon
  - 492 nm
  - 510 nm
  - Alexandrite lasers
- No statistically significant differences were found in patient's ratings of cosmetic appearance between cryotherapy and curettage. The majority of patients preferred cryotherapy over curettage due to decreased postoperative wound care, despite the increased discomfort experienced and increased frequency of seborrheic keratosis remaining after cryotherapy when compared to curettage (7)[B].

ONGOING CARE

FOLLOW-UP RECOMMENDATIONS

Patient Monitoring

After initial diagnosis, follow-up is not usually required unless

- Inflammation or irritation develops.
- There is a change in appearance.
- New seborrheic keratoses suddenly appear.

PATIENT EDUCATION

- Sun-protective methods may help reduce seborrheic keratosis development.
- Patient education materials
  - http://www.aad.org/dermatology-a-to-z/diseases-and-treatments/q–t/seborrheic-keratoses
  - www.cdc.gov/cancer/skin/basic_info/prevention.htm

PROGNOSIS

- Seborrheic keratoses generally do not become malignant.
- Sign of Leser-Trélat usually represents a poor prognosis.

COMPLICATIONS

- Irritation and inflammation due to mechanical irritation (i.e., from clothing, jewelry)
- Possible complications of surgical treatment include hypopigmentation, hyperpigmentation, scarring, incomplete removal, and recurrence.
- Misdiagnosis (rare)

REFERENCES

1. Saeed AK, Salmo N. Epidermal growth factor receptor expression in mice skin upon ultraviolet B exposure - seborrheic keratosis as a coincidental and unique finding. *Adv Biomed Res*. 2012;1:59.
2. Ponti G, Luppi G, Losi L, et al. Leser-Trélat syndrome in patients affected by six multiple metachronous primitive cancers. *J Hematol Oncol*. 2010;3:2.
3. Luba MC, Bangs SA, Mohler AM, et al. Common benign skin tumors. *Am Fam Physician*. 2003;67(4):729–738.
4. Noiles K, Vender R. Are all seborrheic keratoses benign? Review of the typical lesion and its variants. *J Cutan Med Surg*. 2008;12(5):203–210.
5. Marghoob AA, Usatine RP, Jaimes N. Dermoscopy for the family physician. *Am Fam Physician*. 2013;88(7):441–450.
6. Takenouchi T. Key points in dermoscopic diagnosis of basal cell carcinoma and seborrheic keratosis in Japanese. *J Dermatol*. 2011;38(1):59–65.
7. Wood LD, Stucki JK, Hollenbeak CS, et al. Effectiveness of cryosurgery vs curettage in the treatment of seborrheic keratoses. *JAMA Dermatol*. 2013;149(1):108–109.

ADDITIONAL READING

- Culbertson GR. 532-nm diode laser treatment of seborrheic keratoses with color enhancement. *Dermatol Surg*. 2008;34(4):525–528; discussion 528.
- Draelos ZD, Rizer RL, Trookman NS. A comparison of postprocedural wound care treatments: do antibiotic-based ointments improve outcomes? *J Am Acad Dermatol*. 2011;64(Suppl 3):S23–S29.
- Garcia MS, Azari R, Eisen DB. Treatment of dermatosis papulosa nigra in 10 patients: a comparison trial of electrodesiccation, pulsed dye laser, and curettage. *Dermatol Surg*. 2010;36(12):1968–1972.
- Georgieva IA, Mauerer A, Groesser L, et al. Low incidence of oncogenic EGFR, HRAS, and KRAS mutations in seborrheic keratosis. *Am J Dermatopathol*. 2014;36(8):635–642.
- Hafner C, Vogt T. Seborrheic keratosis. *J Dtsch Dermatol Ges*. 2008;6(8):664–677.
- Herron MD, Bowen AR, Krueger GG, et al. Seborrheic keratoses: a study comparing the standard cryosurgery with topical calcipotriene, topical tazarotene, and topical imiquimod. *Int J Dermatol*. 2004;43(4):300–302.
- Krupashankar DS, Indian Association of Dermatologists Venereologists and Leprologists Dermatosurgery Task Force. Standard guidelines of care: CO2 laser for removal of benign skin lesions and resurfacing. *Indian J Dermatol Venereol Leprol*. 2008;74(Suppl):S61–S67.
- Rajesh G, Thappa DM, Jaisankar TJ, et al. Spectrum of seborrheic keratoses in South Indians: a clinical and dermoscopic study. *Indian J Dermatol Venereol Leprol*. 2011;77(4):483–488.
- Taylor SC, Averyhart AN, Heath CR. Postprocedural wound-healing efficacy following removal of dermatosis papulosa nigra lesions in an African American population: a comparison of a skin protectant ointment and a topical antibiotic. *J Am Acad Dermatol*. 2011;64(3)(Suppl):S30–S35.

CODES

ICD10

- L82.1 Other seborrheic keratosis
- L82.0 Inflamed seborrheic keratosis

CLINICAL PEARLS

- Seborrheic keratoses are one of the most common benign tumors of the epidermis.
- Prevalence increases with age.
- Underlying internal malignancy should be considered if large numbers of seborrheic keratoses appear suddenly.

KLINEFELTER SYNDROME

Leslie Lemanek, MD • Mary DiGiulio, DO

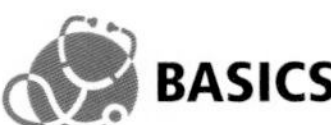

BASICS

DESCRIPTION

- Abnormal body regional proportion, decreased trunk-to-leg ratio, eunuchoid body habitus
- Clinical features of hypergonadotropic hypogonadism: gynecomastia, small firm testicles, decreased facial and pubic hair
- Most common karyotype is 47,XXY.
- Virtually all men are infertile.
- Diagnosis is made during adolescence and adulthood; may remain undiagnosed because symptoms are usually subtle.
- Klinefelter syndrome (KS) has been associated with both increased morbidity and mortality believed to be related to genetic, hormonal, behavioral, and socioeconomic factors (1).

EPIDEMIOLOGY

Prevalence

~1 in 600 males

ETIOLOGY AND PATHOPHYSIOLOGY

- Primary hypergonadotropic hypogonadism
- Unclear whether many aspects of syndrome are caused by hormonal abnormalities or extra X chromosome
- Mutations are spontaneous, and patients have no family history.
- Recurrence risk is that of the general population.

Genetics

- The most common sex chromosome abnormality.
- The classic form of KS (47,XXY) occurs following meiotic nondisjunction of the sex chromosomes during gametogenesis:
  - 40% during spermatogenesis, 60% during oogenesis
- Mosaic forms of KS (46,XY/47,XXY) are thought to result from chromosomal mitotic nondisjunction within the zygote and occur in ~10% of individuals with KS.
- Other chromosome variants of KS (48,XXYY, 48,XXXY) have been identified but are much less common.
- Severity of phenotype is directly correlated with extra number of X-chromosomes, suggesting an effect related to gene dosage:
  - Each extra X is associated with a decrease in IQ of ~15–16 points.

RISK FACTORS

Weakly associated with advanced maternal age; X-chromosome nondisjunction increases with age

Pregnancy Considerations

- Prenatal diagnosis is possible by karyotyping cells obtained from amniocentesis.
- Diagnosis made via amniocentesis is usually incidental.

COMMONLY ASSOCIATED CONDITIONS

- Clinical manifestations of hypogonadism:
  - Infertility (>99%)
  - Azoospermia (>95%)
  - Osteopenia/osteoporosis (50%)
  - Erectile dysfunction
- Neurodevelopmental sequelae:
  - Low IQ
  - Gross motor delay or dysfunction
  - Learning disabilities: speech, language, and reading difficulties
  - Autism spectrum behavior
  - ADHD, attention deficits
  - Emotional and behavior problem
- Cardiovascular and metabolic disorders:
  - Thromboembolic disease
  - Mitral valve prolapse and aortic valve disease
  - Metabolic syndrome (46%) and diabetes (10–39%)
- Autoimmune diseases (uncommon):
  - Rheumatoid arthritis
  - Chronic thyroiditis
- Malignancies (rare):
  - Breast cancer (>50× risk than the general population)
  - Extragonadal germ cell tumors, mainly mediastinal (>65× risk than the general population)

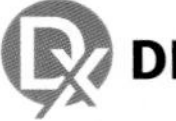

DIAGNOSIS

HISTORY

- Adolescence: delayed or absent puberty or persistent gynecomastia
- Middle age: erectile dysfunction, infertility, decreased libido
- Older age: metabolic syndrome, osteoporosis
- Learning disabilities, psychosocial problems, psychiatric illness

PHYSICAL EXAM

- Small, firm testes (4–6 mL) (95%)
- Eunuchoid body habitus (long legs, short torso, narrow shoulders, broad hips)
- Decreased facial hair (60–80%)
- Gynecomastia (38–75%)
- Decreased muscle strength (70%)
- Decreased pubic hair (30–60%)
- Varicose veins (40%)
- Sparse facial and body hair (88%); female pubic hair distribution (53%)
- Increased fat-to-muscle ratio; abdominal adiposity
- Mitral valve prolapse
- Specific mild dysmorphic features (2)[C]:
  - Clinodactyly (74%)
  - Hypertelorism (69%)
  - Mild elbow dysplasia (36%)
  - High arched palate (37%)

Pediatric Considerations

- <10% diagnosed before puberty
- Cryptorchidism in a prepubescent child with behavioral problems, learning disabilities, and tall stature may indicate the diagnosis (3).

DIFFERENTIAL DIAGNOSIS

- Primary hypogonadism (high follicle-stimulating hormone [FSH]/luteinizing hormone [LH]):
  - Congenital:
    - Pure gonadal dysgenesis
    - Congenital anorchia
    - Hemochromatosis
- Acquired:
  - Mumps orchitis
  - Injury to the testicles
  - Chemotherapy or radiation therapy
- Secondary hypogonadism (low FSH/LH):
  - Kallmann syndrome
  - Pituitary tumor
  - Inflammatory disorders: sarcoidosis, TB, histiocytosis
  - HIV/AIDS
  - Medications: steroids, opiate pain medication
  - Obesity
  - Old age

DIAGNOSTIC TESTS & INTERPRETATION

Initial Tests (lab, imaging)

- Confirm diagnosis of primary hypogonadism:
  - Testosterone levels are low.
  - Elevated gonadotropins: FSH, LH
- Karyotype analysis to confirm genetic abnormality:
  - Cytogenetic analysis (karyotype)
  - Polymerase chain reaction (PCR) looking at the copy number of the androgen receptor (AR) gene (located on Xq11.2–q12) has been described as a screen for KS and other X-chromosome aneuploidies, not commonly used (4)[C].

Follow-Up Tests & Special Considerations

- Fertility:
  - Semen analysis
  - Most men are infertile; although rare, fertility is possible in mosaics.
- Screening for associated conditions:
  - Look for metabolic abnormalities; fasting glucose, lipids, thyroid function.
  - Vitamin D levels
- Adequacy of androgen replacement:
  - Testosterone levels
- Chest x-ray to rule out mediastinal tumor
- Bone density screening
- Echocardiogram to evaluate for valve disease
- Testes and breast ultrasound

Test Interpretation

Testicular biopsy in an adult demonstrates hyalinization of the seminiferous tubules and hyperplasia of Leydig cells.

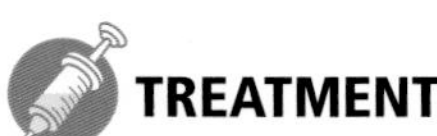

TREATMENT

GENERAL MEASURES

- Preventive dental care
- Calcium and vitamin D supplementation

MEDICATION

First Line

Testosterone therapy:

- Benefits:
  - Develops secondary male sex characteristics:
    - Increases body hair and penis length and improves libido
    - May reduce gynecomastia and abdominal adiposity and increase muscle mass (5)[C] (not replicated in all studies)

- Improves libido/decreases erectile dysfunction
- Metabolic:
  - Improves bone density (5)[C]
  - May lower serum total cholesterol (5) and improve metabolic syndrome (6)[C]
- Other:
  - May improve mood, energy level, cognition, and social functioning and decrease aggression (5)[B]
  - May possibly reduce hypercoagulability (7); improve autoimmune disease (8)[C]
- Risks and side effects:
  - Erythrocytosis
  - Acne
  - Lowering of HDL
  - Worsening of aggression
  - Peliosis hepatitis, hepatic adenomas, and hepatocellular carcinoma
  - Worsening of subclinical prostate cancer
  - May accelerate infertility in adolescents and young men
- Contraindications:
  - Prostate cancer
  - Liver disease
- Dosage:
  - IM injection
  - Transdermal gel
  - Transdermal patch
  - Subcutaneous implant
  - Buccal adhesive

Pediatric Considerations

- Testosterone therapy, beginning at age 11–13 years, is recommended by experts (9)[C].
- Consider postponing testosterone therapy in adolescents wishing to pursue sperm cryopreservation or testicular sperm extraction (TESE), as long-term depot testosterone administration decreases spermatogenesis (3)[C].
- Monitor bone age every 2–3 years (10)[C].
- Perform DXA scan 1–2 times in childhood (10)[C].
- Micropenis in infants and children has been treated with topical or IM testosterone (9)[C].

ISSUES FOR REFERRAL

- Most men have azoospermia at time of diagnosis. Adolescents and young men wishing to preserve fertility should be referred for cryopreservation of existing sperm if sperm are present on semen analysis.
- If viable sperm are noted on semen analysis, fertility treatment may be offered using TESE or micro-TESE followed by intracytoplasmic sperm injection (ICSI).
- Sperm recovery rate = 66% (3)[C]
- Live birth achievement = 45% (3)[C]
- Embryos fertilized using TESE with ICSI are at a modestly increased risk of cytogenetic abnormalities, but most of the resulting pregnancies are healthy.
- Boys born to fathers with KS do not have a higher incidence of KS (3)[C].
- Optimum age at which to attempt TESE is unknown, but success rates decrease with increasing age (3)[C].

ADDITIONAL THERAPIES

Individual or family counseling, if indicated

SURGERY/OTHER PROCEDURES

Mastectomy can be performed to correct gynecomastia and reduce the risk of breast cancer, which can be a cause of psychological strain.

ONGOING CARE

FOLLOW-UP RECOMMENDATIONS

Men who are treated with testosterone will require frequent follow-up.

Patient Monitoring

- Annual lipid and diabetes screening
- Annual clinical breast exam ± breast imaging
- Periodic bone density testing

PATIENT EDUCATION

- Presentation is variable, with most patients appearing physically normal.
- Patients are likely infertile, but there may be options for reproductive therapy.
- There should be careful thought and discussion between the patient and the provider about the risks and benefits of androgen replacement. Patients should know that testosterone can induce puberty and increase libido.
- There is high incidence of learning disabilities and psychiatric illness. Appropriate therapy should be used.
- Risk of diabetes and importance of regular screening and maintaining a healthy weight
- Risk of osteoporosis and importance of calcium, vitamin D, and weight-bearing exercise
- Regular dental care
- American Association for Klinefelter Syndrome Information and Support: www.aaksis.org
- Klinefelter Syndrome Support Group: http://klinefeltersyndrome.org

PROGNOSIS

- Hypogonadism is permanent.
- There is an increased risk for comorbidities associated with KS.
- On average, adults have modestly reduced intelligence, verbal reasoning, language skills, and motor dexterity.
- Increased number of X chromosomes is correlated with increased phenotypic severity.

REFERENCES

1. Bojesen A, Gravholt CH. Morbidity and mortality in Klinefelter syndrome (47,XXY). *Acta Paediatr*. 2011;100(6):807–813.
2. Zeger MP, Zinn AR, Lahlou N, et al. Effect of ascertainment and genetic features on the phenotype of Klinefelter syndrome. *J Pediatr*. 2008;152(5):716–722.
3. Gies I, Unuane D, Velkeniers B, et al. Management of klinefelter syndrome during transition. *Eur J Endocrinol*. 2014;171(2):R67–R77.
4. Ottesen AM, Garn ID, Aksglaede L, et al. A simple screening method for detection of Klinefelter syndrome and other X-chromosome aneuploidies based on copy number of the androgen receptor gene. *Mol Hum Reprod*. 2007;13(10):745–750.
5. Wang C. Long-term testosterone gel (AndroGel) treatment maintains beneficial effects on sexual function and mood, lean and fat mass, and bone mineral density in hypogonadal men. *J Clin Endocrinol Metab*. 2004;89(5):2085–2098.
6. Spark RF. Testosterone, diabetes mellitus, and the metabolic syndrome. *Curr Urol Rep*. 2007;8(6):467–471.
7. Zitzmann M, Junker R, Kamischke A, et al. Contraceptive steroids influence the hemostatic activation state in healthy men. *J Androl*. 2002;23(4):503–511.
8. Koçar IH, Yesilova Z, Ozata M, et al. The effect of testosterone replacement treatment on immunological features of patients with Klinefelter's syndrome. *Clin Exp Immunol*. 2000;121(3):448–452.
9. Bojesen A, Gravholt CH. Klinefelter syndrome in clinical practice. *Nat Clin Pract Urol*. 2007;4(4):192–201.
10. Aksglaede L, Link K, Giwercman A, et al. 47,XXY Klinefelter syndrome: clinical characteristics and age-specific recommendations for medical management. *Am J Med Genet C Semin Med Genet*. 2013;163C(1):55–63.
11. Van Saen D, Gies I, De Schepper J, et al. Can pubertal boys with Klinefelter syndrome benefit from spermatogonial stem cell banking? *Hum Reprod*. 2012;27(2):323–30.

ADDITIONAL READING

- Grouth KA, Skakkebæk A, Høst C, et al. Klinefelter syndrome—a clinical update. *J Clin Endocinol Metab*. 2013;98(1):20–30.
- Radicioni AF, Ferlin A, Balercia G, et al. Consensus statement on diagnosis and clinical management of Klinefelter syndrome. *J Endocrinol Invest*. 2010;33(11):839–850.
- Wattendorf DJ, Muenke M. Klinefelter syndrome. *Am Fam Physician*. 2005;72(11):2259–2262.

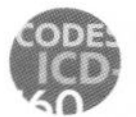

CODES

ICD10

- Q98.4 Klinefelter syndrome, unspecified
- Q98.1 Klinefelter syndrome, male with more than two X chromosomes
- Q98.0 Klinefelter syndrome karyotype 47, XXY

CLINICAL PEARLS

- Klinefelter syndrome males have ≥1 additional X chromosome (XXY karyotype) with associated features of hypergonadotropic hypogonadism.
- Accounts for 3% of male infertility
- Most men do not have "textbook features" and, therefore, frequently remain undiagnosed until adulthood.
- Testosterone therapy, beginning in adolescence, has many benefits.
- Semen cryopreservation or TESE followed by ICSI are current options to achieve fertility.
- Cryopreservation of spermatogonial stem cells (SCCs) banked by prepubescent or pubescent KS patients with in vitro maturation of SCCs followed by ICSI at a later date is a current area of research that may further increase fertility rates (11).

KNEE PAIN

Tara Futrell, MD • J. Herbert Stevenson, MD

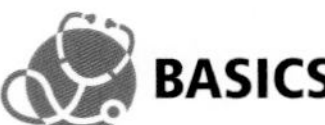

BASICS

DESCRIPTION

Knee pain is a common outpatient complaint with a broad differential diagnosis.

- Knee pain may be acute, chronic, or an acute exacerbation of a chronic condition.
- Trauma, overuse, and degenerative change are frequent causes.
- A detailed history, including patient age, pain onset and location, mechanism of injury, and associated symptoms can help narrow the differential diagnosis.
- A thorough and focused examination of the knee (as well as the back, hips, and ankles) helps to establish the correct diagnosis and determine the appropriate treatment.

EPIDEMIOLOGY

Incidence

- Knee pain accounts for 1.9 million primary care visits annually.
- The incidence of knee osteoarthritis is 240 cases/100,000 person/year.

Prevalence

- The knee is a common site of lower extremity injury.
  - Patellar tendonopathy and patellofemoral syndrome are the most common causes of knee pain in runners (1).
- Osteoarthritis (OA) is one of the leading causes of disability in the United States.

ETIOLOGY AND PATHOPHYSIOLOGY

- Trauma (ligament or meniscal injury, fracture, dislocation)
- Overuse (tendinopathy, patellofemoral syndrome, bursitis, apophysitis)
- Age-related (arthritis, degenerative conditions, apophysitis [young])
- Rheumatologic (rheumatoid arthritis [RA], gout, pseudogout)
- Infectious (bacterial, postviral, Lyme disease)
- Referred pain (hip, back)
- Vascular: popliteal artery aneurysm, deep vein thrombosis
- Others: tumor, cyst, plica

RISK FACTORS

- Obesity
- Malalignment
- Poor flexibility, muscle imbalance or weakness
- Rapid increases in training frequency and intensity
- Improper footwear, training surfaces, technique
- Activities that involve cutting, jumping, pivoting, deceleration, kneeling
- Previous injuries

GENERAL PREVENTION

- Maintain normal body mass index.
- Use appropriate exercise training principles; avoid overtraining.
- Correct postural strength and flexibility imbalances.
- Proper activity-specific techniques and equipment

COMMONLY ASSOCIATED CONDITIONS

- Fracture, contusion
- Effusion, hemarthrosis
- Patellar dislocation/subluxation
- Meniscal or ligamentous injury
- Tendinopathy, bursitis
- Osteochondral injury
- Osteoarthritis, septic arthritis
- Muscle strain

DIAGNOSIS

HISTORY

- Pain:
  - Diffuse pain: OA, patellofemoral pain syndrome (chondromalacia)
  - Pain ascending/descending stairs: meniscal injury, patellofemoral pain syndrome
  - Pain with prolonged sitting, standing from sitting: patellofemoral pain syndrome
  - Mechanical symptoms (locking): meniscal injury
- Mechanism of injury:
  - Hyperextension, deceleration, cutting: anterior cruciate ligament (ACL) injury
  - Hyperflexion, fall on flexed knee, "dashboard injury": posterior cruciate ligament (PCL) injury
  - Lateral force (valgus load): medial collateral injury
  - Twisting on planted foot: meniscal injury
- Effusion:
  - Rapid onset (2 hours): ACL tear, patellar subluxation, tibial plateau fracture. Hemarthrosis is common.
  - Slower onset (24–36 hours), smaller: meniscal injury, ligament sprain
  - Swelling behind the knee: popliteal cyst. Prepatellar: bursitis

PHYSICAL EXAM

- Observe for antalgic gait, patellar tracking abnormalities.
- Inspect for malalignment, atrophy, swelling, ecchymosis, or erythema.
- Palpate for effusion, warmth, and tenderness.
- Evaluate active and passive range of motion (ROM) and flexibility of quadriceps and hamstrings.
- Evaluate strength and muscle tone.
- Note joint instability, locking, and catching.
- Evaluate hip ROM, strength, and stability.
- Special tests:
  - Patellar apprehension test: patellar instability. Patellar grind test: patellofemoral pain or OA (1)
  - Lachman test (more sensitive and specific), pivot shift, anterior drawer: ACL integrity
  - Posterior drawer, posterior sag sign: PCL integrity
  - Valgus/varus stress test: medial/lateral collateral ligament (MCL/LCL) integrity
  - McMurray test, Apley grind, Thessaly test: meniscal injury
  - Ober test: Iliotibial band (ITB) tightness
  - Dial test: positive with posterolateral corner laxity
  - Patellar tilt test and squatting may help suggest patellofemoral pain syndrome, but there is not yet one definitive test.
  - Patella facet tenderness suggests OA or patellofemoral pain syndrome (1)[A].

DIFFERENTIAL DIAGNOSIS

- Acute onset: fracture, contusion, cruciate or collateral ligament tear, meniscal tear, patellar dislocation/subluxation. If systemic symptoms: septic arthritis, gout, pseudogout, Lyme disease, and osteomyelitis.
- Insidious onset: patellofemoral pain syndrome/chondromalacia, iliotibial band syndrome, osteoarthritis, RA, bursitis, tumor, tendinopathy, loose body, bipartite patella, degenerative meniscal tear
- Anterior pain: patellofemoral pain syndrome, patellar injury, patellar tendinopathy, pre- or suprapatellar bursitis, tibial apophysitis, fat pad impingement, quadriceps tendinopathy, OA (1)
- Posterior pain: PCL injury, posterior horn meniscal injury, popliteal cyst or aneurysm, hamstring or gastrocnemius injury, deep venous thrombosis (DVT)
- Medial pain: MCL injury, medial meniscal injury, pes anserine bursitis, medial plica syndrome, OA
- Lateral pain: LCL injury, lateral meniscal injury, ITB syndrome, OA

DIAGNOSTIC TESTS & INTERPRETATION

Initial Tests (lab, imaging)

- Suspected septic joint, gout, pseudogout:
  - Arthrocentesis with cell count, Gram stain, culture, protein/glucose, synovial fluid analysis
- Suspected RA:
  - CBC, erythrocyte sedimentation rate (ESR), rheumatoid factor
- Consider Lyme titer.
- Radiographs to rule out fracture in patients with acute knee trauma (Ottawa rules):
  - Age >55 years *or*
  - Tenderness at the patella or fibular head *or*
  - Inability to bear weight 4 steps *or*
  - Inability to flex knee to 90 degrees
- Radiographs help diagnose OA, osteochondral lesions, patellofemoral pain syndrome:
  - Weightbearing, upright anteroposterior, lateral, merchant/sunrise, notch/tunnel views

Follow-Up Tests & Special Considerations

- MRI is a "gold standard" for imaging soft tissue structures.
- Ultrasound may help diagnose tendonopathy (2)[B].
- CT can further elucidate fracture.

Diagnostic Procedures/Other

Arthroscopy may be beneficial in the diagnosis of certain conditions, including meniscus and ligament injuries.

Geriatric Considerations

OA, degenerative meniscal tears, and gout are more common in middle-aged and elderly populations.

Pediatric Considerations

- 3 million pediatric sports injuries occur annually.
- Look for physeal/apophyseal and joint surface injuries in skeletally immature:
  - Acute: patellar subluxation, avulsion fractures, ACL tear
  - Overuse: patellofemoral pain syndrome, apophysitis, osteochondritis dissecans, patellar tendonitis, stress fracture
  - Others: neoplasm, juvenile RA, infection, referred pain from slipped capital femoral epiphysis

TREATMENT

GENERAL MEASURES

Acute injury: PRICEMM therapy (**p**rotection, **r**elative rest, **i**ce, **c**ompression, **e**levation, **m**edications, **m**odalities)

MEDICATION

First Line

- Oral medications:
  - Acetaminophen: up to 3 g/day. Safe and effective in OA
  - Nonsteroidal anti-inflammatory drugs (NSAIDs):
    - Ibuprofen: 200–800 mg TID
    - Naproxen: 250–500 mg BID:
      - Useful for acute ligament sprains, muscle strains
      - Useful for short-term pain reduction in OA. Long-term use not recommended due to side effects.
      - Not recommended for fracture, stress fracture, chronic muscle injury; lay be associated with delayed healing; low dose and brief course only if necessary
  - Tramadol/opioids: not recommended as 1st-line treatment; can be used with acute injuries
  - Celecoxib: 200 mg QD may be effective in OA with less GI side effects than NSAIDs (3)[A].
- Topical medications:
  - Topical NSAIDs may provide pain relief in OA and are more tolerable than oral medications.
  - Topical capsaicin may be an adjuvant for pain management in OA.
- Injections:
  - Intra-articular corticosteroid injection may provide short-term benefit in knee OA (2)[A].
  - Viscosupplementation may reduce pain and improve function in patients with OA (2)[A], particularly those wishing to delay joint replacement.

ISSUES FOR REFERRAL

- Acute trauma, young athletic patient
- Joint instability
- Lack of improvement with conservative measures
- Salter-Harris physeal fractures (pediatrics)

ADDITIONAL THERAPIES

- Physical therapy is recommended as initial treatment for patellofemoral pain syndrome (4) and tendonopathies (2)[A].
- Muscle strengthening improves outcome in OA.
- Foot orthoses, taping, acupuncture
- May need bracing for stability (4)

SURGERY/OTHER PROCEDURES

- Surgery may be indicated for certain injuries (e.g., ACL tear in competitive athletes).
- Chronic conditions refractory to conservative therapy may require surgical intervention.

COMPLEMENTARY & ALTERNATIVE MEDICINE

May reduce pain and improve function in early OA:

- Glucosamine sulfate (500 mg TID) (5)
- Chondroitin (400 mg TID) (5)
- S-adenosylmethionine (SAMe), ginger extract, methylsulfonylmethane: less reliable improvement and evidence (6)
- Acupuncture

ONGOING CARE

FOLLOW-UP RECOMMENDATIONS

- Activity modification in overuse conditions
- Rehabilitative exercise in OA:
  - Low-impact exercise: walking, swimming, cycling
  - Strength, ROM, and proprioception training

Patient Monitoring

- After initial treatment in acute injury, consider rehabilitation.
- In chronic and overuse conditions, assess functional status, rehabilitation exercise compliance, and pain control at follow-up visit.

DIET

Weight reduction for overweight patient with OA

PATIENT EDUCATION

- Review activity modifications.
- Encourage active role in the rehabilitation process.
- Review medication risks and benefits.

PROGNOSIS

Varies with diagnosis, injury severity, chronicity of condition, patient motivation to participate in rehabilitative exercises, and whether surgical intervention is required

COMPLICATIONS

- Disability
- Arthritis
- Chronic joint instability
- Deconditioning

REFERENCES

1. Hong E, Kraft MC. Evaluating anterior knee pain. *Med Clin North Am*. 2014;98(4):697–717.
2. Ayhan E, Kesmezaca H, Akgun I. Intraarticular injections (corticosteroid, hyaluronic acid, platelet rich plasma) for the knee osteoarthritis. *World J Orthop*. 2014;5(3):351–361.
3. Bijlsma JW, Berenbaum F, Lafeber FP. Osteoarthritis: an update with relevance to clinical practice. *Lancet*. 2011;377(9783):2115–2126.
4. Bolgla LA, Boling MC. An update for the conservative management of patellofemoral pain syndrome: a systematic review. *Int J Sports Phys Ther*. 2011; 6(2):112–125.
5. Henrotin Y, Marty M, Mobashen A. What is the current status of chondroitin sulfate and glucosamine for the treatment of knee osteoarthritis. *Maturitas*. 2014;78(3)184–187.
6. Debbi EM, Agar G, Fichman G, et al. Efficacy of a methylsulfonylmethane supplementation on osteoarthritis of the knee: a randomized control trial. *BMC Complement Altern Med*. 2011;11:50.

ADDITIONAL READING

- Collins NJ, Bissett LM, Crossley KM, et al. Efficacy of nonsurgical interventions for anterior knee pain: systematic review and meta-analysis of randomized trials. *Sports Med*. 2012;42(1):31–49.
- Derry S, Moore RA, Rabbie R. Topical NSAIDs for chronic musculoskeletal pain in adults. *Cochrane Database of Syst Rev*. 2012;9:CD007400.
- Lopes AD, Hespanhol LC, Yeung SS, et al. What are the main running-related musculoskeletal injuries? A systematic review. *Sports Med*. 2012;42(10): 891–905.
- Nunes GS, Stapait EL, Kirsten MH, et al. Clinical test for diagnosis of patellofemoral pain syndrome: systematic review with meta-analysis. *Phys Ther Sport*. 2013;14(1):54–59.
- Ziltener JL, Leal S, Fournier PE. Non-steroidal anti-inflammatory drugs for athletes: an update. *Ann Phys Rehabil Med*. 2010;53(4):278–282.

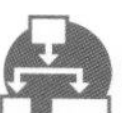

SEE ALSO

Algorithms: Knee Pain; Popliteal Mass

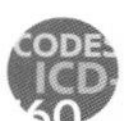

CODES

ICD10

- M25.569 Pain in unspecified knee
- M17.9 Osteoarthritis of knee, unspecified
- M76.50 Patellar tendinitis, unspecified knee

CLINICAL PEARLS

- For patients presenting acutely with knee pain, consider ligamentous injury, meniscal tear, and fracture.
- Consider osteoarthritis, patellofemoral pain, syndrome, tendinopathy, bursitis, and stress fracture in patients presenting with more chronic symptoms.
- Consider physeal, apophyseal or articular cartilage injury in young patients presenting with knee pain.
- The presence of an effusion in a patient <30 years of age indicates a significant injury requiring accurate diagnosis.
- Referred pain from the hip (slipped capital femoral epiphysis, Legg-Calvé-Perthes disease) can present as knee pain.

LABYRINTHITIS

Annie Marian Tubman, MD • Chris Wheelock, MD

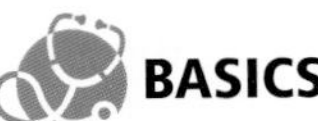

BASICS

DESCRIPTION

- The sudden and persistent onset of vertigo, often accompanied by hearing loss, caused by acute inflammation or infection of the labyrinth
- Labyrinthitis is a clinical diagnosis in absence of neurologic deficits.
- Typically presents with false sense of motion or room-spinning vertigo lasting for hours or days and often sudden unilateral hearing loss
- Often associated with vestibular hypofunction of the involved ear. Peripheral vertigo improves over time with central compensation.
- System(s) affected: nervous; special sensory (auditory and vestibular)
- Synonym(s): acute peripheral vestibulopathy; vestibular neuronitis (vertigo/dizziness only); vestibular neuritis (vertigo/dizziness only)

ALERT

- "Vertigo" and "dizziness" are commonly used terms. Clarify symptoms by giving options of alternative descriptions such as light-headedness, disequilibrium, room-spinning vertigo, or imbalance.
- Hearing loss and duration of symptoms can help narrow the differential diagnosis in patients with vertigo.
- Benign paroxysmal positional vertigo (BPPV) is the most common cause of vertigo. Unlike labyrinthitis, BPPV is episodic, with severe symptoms lasting <1 minute. BPPV is diagnosed using the Dix-Hallpike maneuver. Unlike labyrinthitis, it is not associated with hearing loss.
- Ménière disease presents with the classic triad of episodic vertigo, tinnitus, and sensorineural hearing loss that is often fluctuant (1)[C].

Geriatric Considerations

- Elderly are less likely to compensate fully and may report symptoms of disequilibrium lasting weeks to months after resolution of the acute vertigo.
- Avoid excessive use of scopolamine, meclizine, and other vestibular suppressants following the initial event, as this will delay central compensation.
- Benzodiazepines are preferred vestibular suppressant treatment but do increase the risk of falls in older persons.

Pediatric Consideration

Less common in children, incidence of vestibular vertigo in 10-year olds estimated to be 5.7% (2)[C]

EPIDEMIOLOGY

- 10% of all patients seen for dizziness
- Most common 30–50 years of age (3)
- Predominant sex: female = male

Incidence

- Viral labyrinthitis is the most common etiology.
- Suppurative or serous labyrinthitis secondary to otitis media is increasingly rare.

Prevalence

In the United States, 2nd most common cause of dizziness due to persistent peripheral vestibular hypofunction (9%); benign positional vertigo (40%) is most common. More than one-third of adults see a health care provider for vertigo in their lifetimes (4).

ETIOLOGY AND PATHOPHYSIOLOGY

- Acute inflammation or damage to the inner ear, involving both branches of the vestibulocochlear nerve
- Viruses pass via hematogenous spread into the labyrinth or directly from the middle ear to labyrinth via the round/oval window.
- Bacterial toxins and host inflammatory mediators from a middle ear infection may reach the inner ear.
- Ischemia: ischemic or thromboembolic events involving the labyrinthine artery can cause symptoms that mimic acute labyrinthitis. Often presents with associated neurologic symptoms
- Autoimmune: local or systemic inflammatory processes may affect the inner ear via autoantibodies vasculitis of the labyrinthine artery
  - Wegener granulomatosis, Cogan syndrome, systemic lupus erythematous, polyarteritis nodosa, Behçet disease
- Infections
  - Common viral: cytomegalovirus, mumps, varicella zoster, rubeola, influenza, parainfluenza, herpes simplex, adenovirus, coxsackievirus, respiratory syncytial virus, HIV
  - Common bacterial: *Streptococcus pneumoniae*, *Haemophilus influenzae*, *Moraxella catarrhalis*, *Neisseria meningitidis*, *Streptococcus* spp., *Staphylococcus* spp., *Borrelia burgdorferi*
  - Treponemal: *Treponema pallidum*
- Ototoxic drugs (e.g., aspirin, aminoglycosides, loop diuretics, cisplatin)

Genetics

No known genetic link

RISK FACTORS

- Viral upper respiratory infection
- Otitis media
- Vestibulotoxic/ototoxic medications
- Head trauma
- History of allergies
- Meningitis
- Cerebrovascular disease
- Other risk factors include autoimmune disease, herpes zoster infection, excessive alcohol consumption, and smoking.

GENERAL PREVENTION

- Scheduled immunizations (to prevent common viral pathogens)
- Prevent maternal transmission of pathogens, including syphilis and HIV.

COMMONLY ASSOCIATED CONDITIONS

- Viral upper respiratory infection
- Allergies
- Otitis media
- Cholesteatoma
- Head injury

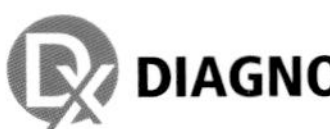

DIAGNOSIS

HISTORY

- Vertigo *AND* (often) hearing loss in 1 ear
- Vertigo is acute in onset and lasts days to weeks.
- Nausea and vomiting are common.
- Fullness of affected ear
- Tinnitus of affected ear (roaring, ringing)
- Upper respiratory tract infection symptoms
- Otorrhea or otalgia (not common with viral causes)
- Severe headache, fever, and nuchal rigidity in the setting of meningitis
- Recurrent symptoms should raise suspicion for autoimmune causes.
- Profound imbalance or associated focal neurologic signs are not typical and should prompt imaging.

PHYSICAL EXAM

- Nystagmus
  - Fast-beating nystagmus toward affected ear (acutely)
  - Fast-beating nystagmus away from affected ear (chronically)
- Symptoms abate in supine position and with eyes closed or with visual fixation.
- Otologic exam may be unremarkable in the setting of viral labyrinthitis.
- Serous/purulent effusion may be present in the middle ear.
- Retraction of the tympanic membrane and keratinaceous debris may be present with cholesteatoma.

DIFFERENTIAL DIAGNOSIS

- Vestibular neuritis/neuronitis (vertigo without hearing loss)
- BPPV: episodic, vertigo lasting seconds/minutes, worse when lying down or looking up
- Ménière disease: episodic vertigo lasting minutes to hours, associated with the triad of episodic vertigo, tinnitus, and hearing loss
- Vestibular migraine
- Autoimmune inner ear disease
- Postconcussive syndrome
- Acute otitis media
- Ototoxicity
- Cardiovascular accident (CVA)/brainstem infarct
- Cerebellopontine-angle tumors (e.g., vestibular schwannoma)
- Less common etiologies: parainfectious encephalomyelitis or cranial polyneuritis, Ramsay Hunt syndrome, HIV infection, syphilis, temporal lobe epilepsy, perilymphatic fistula, superior canal dehiscence, idiopathic sudden single-sided deafness, multiple sclerosis, vasculitis (cerebral or systemic)

DIAGNOSTIC TESTS & INTERPRETATION

- Routine lab studies not helpful in making the diagnosis unless an autoimmune cause is highly suspected.
- Consider culture of otorrhea or middle ear fluid to direct antibiotic choice.
- Consider lumbar puncture only if meningitis is suspected.
- Consider screening for syphilis or HIV when clinically indicated by risk factors or clinical history.
- Imaging is not required for the diagnosis of acute labyrinthitis.
- If associated neurologic symptoms or sensorineural hearing loss are present, an MRI and MR angiography of brain and brainstem is recommended.
- Vertigo usually spontaneously resolves, and there is a low risk of developing Ménière disease or migraines.

Follow-Up Tests & Special Considerations
Labyrinthitis ossificans is fibrosis of the internal auditory canal following bacterial meningitis and is thought to occur due to a suppurative labyrinthitis. This can occur rapidly, especially after *S. pneumoniae* meningitis.

Diagnostic Procedures/Other
- Audiogram should be obtained.
- Vestibular tests are not typically indicated in the acute setting. If vertigo and dizziness persist after expected resolution of symptoms, electronystagmography should be used.

Test Interpretation
- Audiogram may show varying degrees of both hearing loss and discrimination.
- Caloric testing may show relative weakness of the horizontal semicircular canal of the affected side. Sensitivity and specificity of this test are variable within literature.

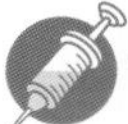

TREATMENT

- Symptom management and reassurance
- Vestibular rehabilitation is the mainstay of treatment and has been shown to be safe and effective management for unilateral peripheral vestibular dysfunction (5)[A].
- Patients should begin exercises as soon as the acute phase resolves and movement is tolerable, generally within 2–3 days of onset.
- Vestibular suppressants as needed (see "Medication") for severe acute attacks of vertigo only. Patients should be advised *NOT* to use these medications as scheduled medications or for prophylaxis without symptoms.
- Sudden single-sided hearing loss (onset within 2 weeks) should be managed with high-dose oral steroids as soon as possible.
- Auricular acupuncture and Ginkgo biloba may be emerging adjunctive therapies to reduce vertiginous symptoms, although research is limited (6)[B],(7)[C].
- For suppurative labyrinthitis, appropriate antibiotics to eradicate infection

GENERAL MEASURES
Vestibular exercises for prolonged symptoms and unilateral vestibular loss have been shown to alleviate postural control.

MEDICATION
Use of the following drugs should be on a PRN basis. Benzodiazepines can also assist with the anxiety associated with vertigo. No patient should take vestibular suppressants as a chronic medication, as they can block central compensation.

- Vestibular suppressants
  - Lorazepam (Ativan): 0.5–2 mg sublingual (SL)/PO BID PRN or diazepam (Valium) 2–5 mg QID PO PRN
  - Meclizine (Antivert, Bonine, Zentrip [dissolvable]) 12.5–25 mg PO BID–TID PRN
  - Dimenhydrinate (Dramamine) 25–50 mg PO q4–6h PRN
- Antiemetics
  - Ondansetron (Zofran) 4–8 mg PO TID PRN or granisetron (Kytril) 1 mg PO TID PRN
  - Meclizine (Antivert, Bonine) 12.5–25 mg PO q4h PRN
  - Promethazine (Phenergan) 12.5–25 mg PO/PR QID PRN or prochlorperazine (Compazine) 25 mg PR BID PRN
  - Metoclopramide (Reglan) 10 mg PO TID PRN
- Antivirals
  - Acyclovir 800 mg PO 5× per day for 7 days can be used in cases associated with herpes.
- Steroids
  - Adults: methylprednisolone initially 100 mg PO daily, then tapered to 10 mg PO daily over 3 weeks
  - Pediatrics: prednisone 1 mg/kg PO daily 3 × 1 week, then taper over 3 weeks
  - Given early in the setting of bacterial meningitis, may decrease the otologic sequelae, specifically labyrinthitis ossificans
  - Used in treatment of labyrinthitis for associated sudden sensorineural hearing loss

Pregnancy Considerations
Dimenhydrinate, diphenhydramine, ondansetron, granisetron, and metoclopramide are pregnancy Category B.

First Line
- Benzodiazepines, which are better vestibular suppressants, are preferred over antihistamine/anticholinergics such as meclizine. Sublingual benzodiazepines are very effective for vertigo and should be considered 1st-line therapy.
- Urgent steroid treatment in acute setting

ISSUES FOR REFERRAL
- Consider neuro-otology referral for other peripheral causes of vertigo or unremitting vertigo.
- Consider neurology referral for suspected central causes of vertigo or dizziness.
- Consider otolaryngology referral for progressive bilateral hearing loss and vertigo after preliminary laboratory workup excluding rheumatologic causes.

INPATIENT CONSIDERATIONS
Admission Criteria/Initial Stabilization
- Patients with systemic infection, young age, or intractable vertigo with nausea and vomiting may need to be hospitalized for intravenous fluids and medications.
- Usually outpatient management

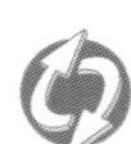

ONGOING CARE

FOLLOW-UP RECOMMENDATIONS
Patient Monitoring
Follow hearing loss weekly with audiograms until hearing stabilizes. Acute vertiginous symptoms may last up to 6 weeks. Residual symptoms have been documented to last months or year (8)[C].

DIET
Avoid alcohol, as this may exacerbate symptoms.

PATIENT EDUCATION
Lie still with eyes closed in a darkened room during acute attacks. Otherwise, encourage activity as tolerated. Minimize rapid head movement until symptoms resolve.

PROGNOSIS
Prognosis depends on cause of labyrinthitis.

COMPLICATIONS
Permanent hearing loss, more common with bacterial causes, and chronic impairment of balance

REFERENCES

1. Post RE, Dickerson LM. Dizziness: a diagnostic approach. *Am Fam Physician*. 2010;82(4):361–368.
2. Jahn K, Langhagen T, Schroeder AS, et al. Vertigo and dizziness in childhood—update on diagnosis and treatment. *Neuropediatrics*. 2011;42(4):129–134.
3. Neuhauser HK, Lempert T. Vertigo: epidemiologic aspects. *Semin Neurol*. 2009;29(5):473–481.
4. Wipperman J. Dizziness and vertigo. *Prim Care*. 2014;41(1):115–131.
5. Hillier SL, McDonnell M. Vestibular rehabilitation for unilateral peripheral vestibular dysfunction. *Cochrane Database Syst Rev*. 2011;(2):CD005397.
6. Sokolova L, Hoerr R, Mischenko T. Treatment of vertigo: a randomized, double blind trial comparing efficacy and safety of Ginkgo biloba extract EGb 761 and betahistine. *Int J Otolaryngol*. 2014;2014:682439.
7. Romoli M, Allais G, Airola G, et al. Ear acupuncture and fMRI: a pilot study for assessing the specificity of auricular points. *Neurol Sci*. 2014;35(Suppl 1):189–193.
8. Lee HK, Ahn SK, Jeon SY, et al. Clinical characteristics and natural course of recurrent vestibulopathy: a long-term follow-up study. *Laryngoscope*. 2012;122(4):883–886.

SEE ALSO

Ménière Disease; Postconcussive Syndrome; Tinnitus

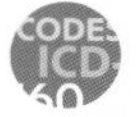

CODES

ICD10
- H83.09 Labyrinthitis, unspecified ear
- H83.01 Labyrinthitis, right ear
- H83.02 Labyrinthitis, left ear

CLINICAL PEARLS

- Ask patients to describe symptoms in their own words, alternative symptoms include light-headedness, vertigo, disequilibrium, or imbalance.
- Benzodiazepines are better vestibular suppressant and are preferred over antihistamine/anticholinergics such as meclizine.
- Episodic vertigo tends to be caused by BPPV or Ménière disease, whereas persistent vertigo is more consistent with labyrinthitis.

LACRIMAL DISORDERS (DRY EYE SYNDROME)

Kinder Fayssoux, MD • Mark Minot, MD

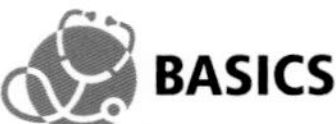

BASICS

DESCRIPTION

- Diseases and abnormalities of tear production and maintenance of tear film
- The most common lacrimal disorder is dry eye syndrome, which is often referred to as dysfunctional tear syndrome.
- Lacrimal duct disorders usually result in overflow tearing.
- System(s) affected: skin/exocrine

EPIDEMIOLOGY

Prevalence

Very common throughout the United States; more often seen in arid climates:

- Predominant gender: female > male
- Predominant age: Dry eye symptoms increase with age and are most often seen in the elderly.

ETIOLOGY AND PATHOPHYSIOLOGY

- Tear film is composed of 3 layers:
  - Mucin layer: allows spread of aqueous tears
  - Thick aqueous layer: produced by lacrimal gland
  - Lipid layer: controls tear evaporation
- Results from poor tear production, rapid tear evaporation, and/or an abnormal concentration of mucin or lipid in tear film
- Most common cause of dry eye symptoms is aqueous tear deficiency.
- Decreased androgens are thought to contribute to a decrease in tear production.

RISK FACTORS

- Exposure to dry environments (e.g., high altitudes)
- Contact lens wear
- Female gender
- Computer use
- Hormonal diseases
- History of collagen vascular disease such as rheumatoid arthritis, Sjögren syndrome, thyroid disease, rosacea, Bell palsy, eyelid abnormalities
- Medications, including oral contraceptives, diuretics, β-blockers, anticholinergics, antihistamines, and antidepressants
- Smoking
- Vitamin A deficiency
- Eye surgery: blepharoplasty, cataract, laser vision correction
- Artificial tears (with preservatives)

GENERAL PREVENTION

- Prevent exposure to eye irritants from pollution, cigarette smoke, and sun exposure.
- Ensure adequate vitamin A intake through diet or as a supplement.
- Patients with prior laser vision correction should wait at least 6 months before undergoing blepharoplasty because of the effects on corneal sensation, tear production, and tear film alteration (1)[C].
- Increasing awareness of this condition among people residing in dry environments
- Decrease or stop contact lens wear.

COMMONLY ASSOCIATED CONDITIONS

- Sjögren syndrome
- Rheumatoid arthritis
- Thyroid disease
- Rosacea
- Pregnancy
- Menopause
- Malnutrition

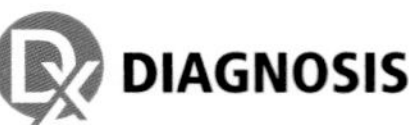

DIAGNOSIS

HISTORY

- Dry sensation in eyes
- Foreign body sensation
- Blurry vision
- Itching
- Ocular pain
- Photophobia
- Burning
- Occasional tearing due to excessive reflex tearing.
  - Patient's symptoms usually worsen in dry, smoky environments, while reading, driving, or using a computer for extended periods.

Pediatric Considerations

Lacrimal duct obstruction should be suspected in an infant presenting with excessive tearing (epiphora).

PHYSICAL EXAM

- Slit-lamp exam reveals decreased tear film and may reveal punctate epithelial defects on cornea.
- Schirmer test can be used to assess tear production.
- Ocular staining may reveal epithelial defects.

DIFFERENTIAL DIAGNOSIS

- Ocular: allergy, conjunctivitis, contact lens complication, exposure keratopathy
- Other: ocular rosacea, thyroid ophthalmopathy, ocular manifestation of HIV, Bell palsy, vitamin A deficiency

DIAGNOSTIC TESTS & INTERPRETATION

Initial Tests (lab, imaging)

Tear production can be measured using a Schirmer filter strip after instillation of topical anesthetic. Wetting of <10 mm of the slip after 5 minutes is indicative of insufficient tear production.

Diagnostic Procedures/Other

- Staining of the ocular surface with fluorescein will show areas of abnormal uptake and patches of drying. It allows the tear break-up time (TBUT) to be calculated. A TBUT of <10 seconds is abnormal.
- Rose bengal will be taken up by dead or dying epithelial cells, and it may be a more sensitive test.

Test Interpretation

In Sjögren syndrome, infiltration of the lacrimal gland with inflammatory cells may be evident.

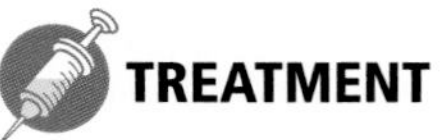

TREATMENT

GENERAL MEASURES

- Those with systemic illnesses predisposed to dry eye should be informed and instructed in the appropriate use of artificial tear supplements. Some artificial tear supplements with preservatives may exacerbate the condition.
- Symptoms of dry eye may decrease with an increase in home humidification and hydration.

MEDICATION

First Line

- Preservative-free artificial tears: 1 drop in each eye several times a day to prevent discomfort (2)[A],(3)[C]
- Ophthalmic lubricating ointment may be used in each eye at bedtime (4)[B].

Second Line

- Dry eye has been identified as having an inflammatory component that responds in refractory cases to topical immunosuppressives such as cyclosporine 0.05% (Restasis), 1 drop to each eye BID (5,6,7)[A].
- Emerging therapies include topical androgens, secretagogues (e.g., oral pilocarpine), cytokine-blocking agents, and a P2Y2 receptor agonist (Diquafosol).

ISSUES FOR REFERRAL
Rheumatology referral if systemic collagen vascular disease is suspected

ADDITIONAL THERAPIES
Lid massage and warm compresses several times a day

Pediatric Considerations
For most babies born with nasolacrimal duct obstructions, the obstructions will clear spontaneously during the 1st year of life. On occasion, surgical probing is necessary.

SURGERY/OTHER PROCEDURES
Punctal occlusion, with either punctal plugs or laser, is used in moderate to severe dry eye if medical therapy fails.

COMPLEMENTARY & ALTERNATIVE MEDICINE
- Fatty acid (omega-3), linoleic acid, and γ-linoleic acid supplements (8)[B]
- Acupuncture has been studied with inconclusice results (9)[A].

ONGOING CARE

FOLLOW-UP RECOMMENDATIONS

Patient Monitoring
- Monitor early to assess efficacy of treatment.
- The viscosity of artificial tears and frequency of use can be increased for symptom relief.

DIET
- Diet rich in omega-3 fatty acids and/or linoleic acids may benefit some patients.
- Adequate vitamin A intake

PATIENT EDUCATION
All individuals with systemic illnesses predisposed to dry eye, postmenopausal women, residing in arid climates, or those >60 years of age should be instructed in the use of artificial tear supplements to combat dry eye symptoms.

PROGNOSIS
- Lacrimal disorders can be adequately managed with artificial tear supplements.
- Blocked tear ducts can be managed with probing and punctal dilation and/or dacryocystorhinostomy procedures in more severe cases.

COMPLICATIONS
Severe dry eye may lead to the following:
- Corneal breakdown
- Secondary invasion by bacteria
- Eye infections

REFERENCES

1. Lee WB, McCord CD, Somia N, et al. Optimizing blepharoplasty outcomes in patients with previous laser vision correction. *Plast Reconstr Surg*. 2008; 122(2):587–594.
2. Ousler GW, Michaelson C, Christensen MT. An evaluation of tear film breakup time extension and ocular protection index scores among three marketed lubricant eye drops. *Cornea*. 2007;26(8):949–952.
3. Karadayi K, Ciftci F, Akin T, et al. Increase in central corneal thickness in dry and normal eyes with application of artificial tears: a new diagnostic and follow-up criterion for dry eye. *Ophthalmic Physiol Opt*. 2005;25(6):485–491.
4. Tauber J. Efficacy, tolerability and comfort of a 0.3% hypromellose gel ophthalmic lubricant in the treatment of patients with moderate to severe dry eye syndrome. *Curr Med Res Opin*. 2007;23(11): 2629–2636.
5. Hardten DR, Brown MJ, Pham-Vang S. Evaluation of an isotonic tear in combination with topical cyclosporine for the treatment of ocular surface disease. *Curr Med Res Opin*. 2007;23(9): 2083–2091.
6. Roberts CW, Carniglia PE, Brazzo BG. Comparison of topical cyclosporine, punctal occlusion, and a combination for the treatment of dry eye. *Cornea*. 2007;26(7):805–809.
7. Sall K, Stevenson OD, Mundorf TK, et al. Two multicenter, randomized studies of the efficacy and safety of cyclosporine ophthalmic emulsion in moderate to severe dry eye disease. CsA Phase 3 Study Group. *Opthalmology*. 2000;107(4):631–639.
8. Barabino S, Rolando M, Camicione P, et al. Systemic linoleic and gamma-linoleic acid therapy in dry eye syndrome with an inflammatory component. *Cornea*. 2003;22(2):97–101.
9. Lee MS, Shin BC, Choi TY, et al. Acupuncture for treating dry eye: a systematic review. *Acta Opthalmol*. 2011;89(2):101–106.

ADDITIONAL READING

- Behrens A, Doyle JJ, Stern L, et al. Dysfunctional tear syndrome: a Delphi approach to treatment recommendations. *Cornea*. 2006;25(8):900–907.
- Dogru M, Nakamura M, Shimazakie J, et al. Changing the trends in the treatment of dry eye disease. *Expert Opin Investig Drugs*. 2013;22(12):1581–1596.
- Galor A, Feuer W, Lee DJ, et al. Prevalence and risk factors of dry eye syndrome in a United States veterans affairs population. *Am J Ophthalmol*. 2011;152(3):377–384.
- Gilbard J. The diagnosis and management of dry eyes. *Otolaryngol Clin N Am*. 2005,38(5): 871–885.
- Moss SE, Klein R, Klein BE, et al. Prevalence and risk factors for dry eye syndrome. *Arch Opthalmol*. 2000; 118(9):1264–1268.
- Tong L, Petznick A, Lee S, et al. Choice of artificial tear formulation for pateints with dry eye; where do we start. *Cornea*. 2012;31(Suppl 1):532–536.

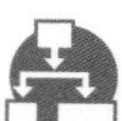

SEE ALSO

Sjögren Syndrome

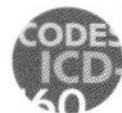

CODES

ICD10
- H04.9 Disorder of lacrimal system, unspecified
- H04.129 Dry eye syndrome of unspecified lacrimal gland
- H04.539 Neonatal obstruction of unspecified nasolacrimal duct

CLINICAL PEARLS
- Dry eye syndrome is common in the United States, affecting postmenopausal women more than any other population.
- Symptoms are usually adequately managed with preservative-free artificial tears and humidified environments.
- Dry eye symptoms that are refractory to medical treatment and/or punctal plugs should raise suspicion of an underlying systemic condition, and a rheumatology consult should be considered.

L

LACTOSE INTOLERANCE

Nihal Patel, MD

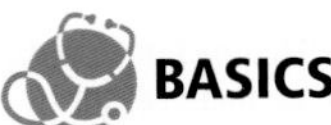

BASICS

DESCRIPTION

- Inability to digest lactose into constituent components (glucose and galactose) due to low levels of lactase in the brush border of the small intestinal mucosa, causing bloating, borborygmi (audible stomach "rumblings"), abdominal pain, and diarrhea
  - Congenital lactose intolerance: very rare
  - Primary lactose intolerance: common in adults who develop a low level of lactase after childhood
  - Secondary lactose intolerance: inability to digest lactose caused by any condition injuring the intestinal mucosa (e.g., infectious enteritis, celiac disease, eosinophilic gastroenteritis, or inflammatory bowel disease) or a reduction of available mucosal surface (e.g., resection)
- Lactase activity peaks at birth then starts to decrease after the first few months of life and continuously during lifetime. 75% of adults' worldwide exhibit decline in lactase activity. *However, only 50% of lactase activity is needed to digest lactose without causing symptoms of lactose intolerance.*
- Lactose malabsorption results from reduction of lactase activity, is asymptomatic, and is as common in healthy patients as in those with functional bowel disorders.
- System(s) affected: endocrine/metabolic, gastrointestinal

Pediatric Considerations

- Primary lactose intolerance usually begins in late childhood.
- No consensus exists on whether young children (<5 years of age) should avoid lactose following diarrheal illness.
- Lactose-free formulas are available.
- Exclude a milk protein allergy.

EPIDEMIOLOGY

Incidence

- ≥50% of infants with acute or chronic diarrheal disease has lactose intolerance, especially with rotavirus infection.
- Lactose intolerance is common with giardiasis and ascariasis, irritable bowel syndrome (IBS), tropical and nontropical sprue, and the AIDS malabsorptive syndrome.

Prevalence

- In South America, Africa, and Asia, rates of lactose intolerance are >50%.
- In the United States, the prevalence is 15% among whites, 53% among Hispanic Americans, and 80% among African Americans.
- In Europe, lactose intolerance varies from 15% in Scandinavian countries to 70% in Italy.
- Predominant age:
  - Primary: teenage and adult
  - Secondary: depends on underlying condition
- Predominant sex: male = female

ETIOLOGY AND PATHOPHYSIOLOGY

- Primary lactose intolerance: Normal decline in the lactase activity in the intestinal mucosa is genetically controlled and permanent after weaning.
- Secondary lactose intolerance: associated with gastroenteritis in children and with nontropical and tropical sprue, regional enteritis, abetalipoproteinemia, cystic fibrosis, inflammatory bowel disease, celiac disease, and immunoglobulin deficiencies in both adults and children

Genetics

- In Caucasians, lactase deficiency has been associated with a single nucleotide polymorphism (SNP) consisting of a nucleotide switch of T for C 13.910. bp on chromosome 2. This results in variants of CC-13910 (lactase nonpersistence) *OR* CT-13910/TT-13910 (lactase persistence) (1).
- SNP (C/T-13910) is associated with lactase persistence in northern Europeans.
- Other SNPs (G/C-14010, T/G-13915, and C/G-13907) have been linked to lactase persistence in Africans.

RISK FACTORS

- Adult-onset lactase deficiency varies widely among countries.
- Age:
  - Signs and symptoms usually do not become apparent until after age 6–7 years; recent studies actually have shown that hypolactasia may begin after age 20 years.
  - Symptoms may not be apparent until adulthood, depending on dietary lactose intake and rate of decline of intestinal lactase activity.
  - Lactase enzyme activity correlates with age, regardless of symptoms.

GENERAL PREVENTION

Lactose avoidance relieves symptoms. Patients can learn what level of lactose is tolerable in their diet.

COMMONLY ASSOCIATED CONDITIONS

- Tropical or nontropical sprue
- Giardiasis
- Inflammatory bowel disease
- Immunoglobulin deficiencies
- Celiac disease
- Cystic fibrosis

DIAGNOSIS

- Evaluation of lactose intolerance includes a careful medical history, review of symptoms, and physical examination. Lactose intolerance is defined as a combination of a positive lactose hydrogen breath test result plus accompanying clinical symptoms.
- Lactose intolerance can mimic symptoms of functional gastrointestinal disorders. Lactose intolerance can also be a coexisting condition.

HISTORY

- Assess patient's daily lactose consumption. A single dose of lactose (12 g, equivalent to 1 cup of milk) consumed alone produces no or minor symptoms in persons with lactose intolerance or maldigestion.
- Lactose doses of 15–18 g are well tolerated with other nutrients. Doses >18 g cause progressively more symptoms, and quantities >50 g elicit symptoms in most individuals.
- Symptoms may arise 30 minutes–2 hours after consumption of lactose-containing products.
- Symptoms include bloating, cramping, abdominal discomfort, vomiting diarrhea or loose stools, and flatulence.
- Symptoms tend to appear 30 minutes–2 hours after eating.
- Abdominal pain may be crampy in nature and often is localized to the periumbilical area or lower quadrant.
- Stools usually are bulky, frothy, and watery.
- Only 1/3–1/5 of individuals with lactose malabsorption develop symptoms.

PHYSICAL EXAM

Borborygmi may be audible on physical examination and to the patient. The exam is otherwise typically nonspecific.

DIFFERENTIAL DIAGNOSIS

- Sucrase deficiency
- Cow's milk protein allergy
- IBS
- Bacterial overgrowth
- Celiac disease
- Inflammatory bowel disease

DIAGNOSTIC TESTS & INTERPRETATION

Initial Tests (lab, imaging)

- The lactose breath hydrogen test (LBT) is the best tool to diagnose lactose intolerance. It is noninvasive, easy to perform, and cost effective. It is limited by suboptimal sensitivity (2)[B]. Intestinal bacteria digest carbohydrates, producing hydrogen and methane that are measured in air exhaled from the lungs:
  - Oral lactose is administered in the fasting state, (2 g/kg; max dose 25 g). Breath hydrogen is sampled at baseline and at 30-minute intervals for 3 hours. The postlactose and baseline values are compared. A breath hydrogen value of 10 ppm is normal. Values between 10 and 20 ppm may be indeterminate unless accompanied by symptoms, values >20 ppm are considered diagnostic of lactose malabsorption.
- The biochemical assay of lactase activity on duodenal sample is as sensitive as LBT in detecting lactase deficiency; it seems to be more accurate than LBT in predicting the clinical response to a lactose-free diet; but cost and invasiveness limit its clinical use as a 1st-line test.
- For patients with symptoms of lactose intolerance undergoing endoscopy for other reasons, a biochemical assay on duodenal biopsies can rule out lactose malabsorption.
- A positive LBT confirms lactose malabsorption but does not define the etiology.

Diagnostic Procedures/Other

Lactose absorption test: alternative to LBT in adults (more invasive and equivalent in sensitivity and specificity to breath test). Following oral administration of a 50-g test dose in adults (2 g/kg in children), blood glucose levels are monitored at 0, 60, and 120 minutes. An increase in blood glucose of $<$20 mg/dL (1.1 mmol/L) with the concurrent development of symptoms is diagnostic. False-negative results may occur in patients with diabetes or bacterial overgrowth.

Test Interpretation

Lactase deficiency in intestinal mucosa may be patchy or focal.

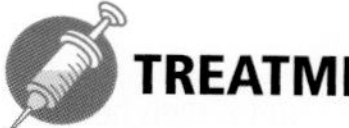

TREATMENT

There is insufficient evidence on treatments including probiotics, colonic adaptation, and other supplements to recommend any as definitive 1st-line.

- Treatment of lactose malabsorption in the absence of a correctable underlying disease includes four general principles (3)[B].
  - Patients should avoid milk and dairy products in order to improve symptoms.
  - Up to 12–15 g of lactose can be tolerated in patients with lactose intolerance without significant symptoms (1 cup of milk).
  - Lactose should be gradually reintroduced along with other nutrients until the patient's threshold for symptoms is reached. Spreading lactose servings throughout the day instead of a single dose has been shown to improve tolerance.
  - If symptoms persist, patients can substitute lactose for fermented and matured milk products.
- Certain strains, concentrations, and preparations of probiotics may alleviate symptoms of lactose intolerance.
- Some studies have looked at treating the symptoms of lactose intolerance with incremental doses of lactose to induce colonic adaptation with limited success.
- To date, insufficient scientific evidence exists to strongly recommend lactose-reduced or hydrolyzed milk, lactase supplements taken with milk, probiotics, or colonic adaptation to treat lactose intolerance, mainly because most studies are small, heterogeneous, and poor in quality. However, use of these supplements should be assessed in a case-by-case fashion.
- It is very important to maintain calcium and vitamin D intake.

MEDICATION

First Line

Lactase (Lactaid, Lactrase):

- Commercially available "lactase" preparations are actually bacterial or yeast β-galactosidases.
- Take 1–2 capsules or tablets prior to ingesting milk products.
- These vary in effectiveness at preventing symptoms.
- Can add tablets or contents of capsules to milk (1–2 caps/tabs per quart of milk) before drinking; also available in milk in some areas
- Not effective for all people with lactose intolerance
- High-quality, large, randomized controlled trials showing efficacy and safety are lacking.

COMPLEMENTARY & ALTERNATIVE MEDICINE

Certain probiotic formulations taken with meals may alleviate some of the symptoms of lactose intolerance (4)[B].

ONGOING CARE

DIET

- Reduce or restrict dietary lactose to control symptoms. This is patient-specific and done as "trial-and-error."
- Yogurt and fermented products such as hard cheese are often better tolerated than milk.
- Supplement calcium in the form of calcium carbonate
- Prehydrolyzed milk (Lactaid) is available.

PATIENT EDUCATION

- Patients must learn to read labels on commercial products because milk sugar is used in many products and may cause symptoms.
- Lactose-intolerant patients may tolerate whole milk or chocolate milk better than skim milk due to slower rate of gastric emptying.
- Lactose consumed with other food products is better tolerated than when consumed alone.
- Primary lactase deficiency is permanent; secondary lactose intolerance usually is temporary, although it may persist for several months after the inciting event.
- 20% of prescription drugs and 6% of over-the-counter (OTC) medicines use lactose as a base.
- Most patients can tolerate 12–15 g of lactose, despite their lactose intolerance or malabsorption.

PROGNOSIS

- Normal life expectancy
- Symptoms can be controlled through diet alone if lactase tablets are ineffective.

COMPLICATIONS

Calcium deficiency: Avoidance of milk and other dairy products can lead to reduced calcium intake, which may increase the risk for osteoporosis and fracture.

REFERENCES

1. Mattar R, de Campos Mazo DF, Carrilho FJ. Lactose intolerance: diagnosis, genetic, and clinical factors. *Clin Exp Gastroenterol*. 2012;5:113–121.
2. Law D, Conklin J, Pimentel M. Lactose intolerance and the role of the lactose breath test. *Am J Gastroenterol*. 2010;105(8):1726–1728.
3. Shaukat A, Levitt MD, Taylor BC, et al. Systematic review: effective management strategies for lactose intolerance. *Ann Intern Med*. 2010;152(12):797–803.
4. Levri KM, Ketvertis K, Deramo M, et al. Do probiotics reduce adult lactose intolerance? A systematic review. *J Fam Pract*. 2005;54(7):613–620.

ADDITIONAL READING

- Almeida CC, Lorena SL, Pavan CR, et al. Beneficial effects of long-term consumption of a probiotic combination of Lactobacillus casei Shirota and Bifidobacterium breve Yakult may persist after suspension of therapy in lactose-intolerant patients. *Nutr Clin Pract*. 2012;27(2):247–251.
- Boettcher E, Crowe SE. Dietary proteins and functional gastrointestinal disorders. *Am J Gastroenterol*. 2013;108(5):728–736.
- Fernández-Bañares F. Reliability of symptom analysis during carbohydrate hydrogen-breath tests. *Curr Opin Clin Nutr Metab Care*. 2012;15(5):494–498.
- Furnari M, Bonfanti D, Parodi A, et al. A comparison between lactose breath test and quick test on duodenal biopsies for diagnosing lactase deficiency in patients with self-reported lactose intolerance. *J Clin Gastroenterol*. 2013;47(2):148–152.
- Tan-Dy CR, Ohlsson A. Lactase treated feeds to promote growth and feeding tolerance in preterm infants. *Cochrane Database Syst Rev*. 2013;3:CD004591.

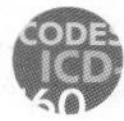

CODES

ICD10

- E73.9 Lactose intolerance, unspecified
- E73.8 Other lactose intolerance
- E73.1 Secondary lactase deficiency

CLINICAL PEARLS

- The diagnosis of lactose intolerance is based on clinical history and most often confirmed by hydrogen breath testing.
- Most patients can tolerate 12–15 g of lactose despite their lactose intolerance or malabsorption.
- Lactose-intolerant patients may tolerate yogurt and fermented products better than milk and cheese.
- A food diary helps identify problematic food sources.
- Patients should read ingredient labels to look for milk, lactose, whey, and curd, which indicate the presence of lactose.
- Lactose-intolerant patients may tolerate whole milk or chocolate milk better than skim milk due to a slower rate of gastric emptying.
- Many patients with lactose intolerance unnecessarily avoid all dairy products, causing inadequate intake of calcium and vitamin D, which may predispose them to osteoporosis.

LARYNGEAL CANCER

Hugh J. Silk, MD, MPH • Sheila O. Stille, DMD

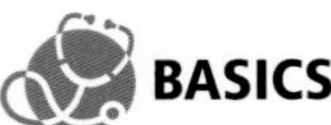

BASICS

DESCRIPTION

- A friable, granular tumor of the larynx that leads to hoarseness, hemoptysis, and cough
- Of all malignant lesions, <1% squamous cell carcinomas constitute 95–98% of all malignant neoplasms of the larynx.
- Laryngeal cancer accounts for <2% of all carcinomas.
- At the time of diagnosis, 62% will have local disease, 26% regional disease, and 8% distant disease in the lungs, liver, and/or bone.
- System(s) affected: pulmonary; ear, nose, throat (ENT)
- Synonym(s): cancer of the larynx; throat cancer; cancer of the voice box

EPIDEMIOLOGY

Incidence

- Per year, 3.4/100,000 (12,630 new cases per year in the United States, 2014; prevalence: 89,000 in 2010); predominately squamous cell carcinomas (1)[A]
- Predominant age
  - Median age of occurrence in 6th and 7th decades
  - <1% of laryngeal cancers arise in patients <30 years.
- Predominant sex: male > female (4–5:1); blacks > whites; increasing incidence in women who smoke; synergistic with alcohol abuse (2)[A]

Prevalence

- About 3,610 deaths from disease in the United States yearly (2)[A]
- 2nd most common site for head and neck cancer (25% of all cases)
- 2–3% of the cancers in whole body
- 11th most common cancer in male

ETIOLOGY AND PATHOPHYSIOLOGY

- Smoking (dose dependent)—most important risk factor
- Heavy alcohol use (3)[C]
- Smoking plus moderate alcohol use—synergistic (3)[C]
- Possibly chronic laryngopharyngeal reflux (small studies)
- Occupational hazards (asbestos, pesticides, polycyclic aromatic hydrocarbons, woodworkers, exposure to radiation) (1,2)[A]
- Bacteria, viruses, for example, HPV (< oropharyngeal; 35% vs. 24%) (4,5)[A]

Genetics

Unknown—possible genetic inheritance

RISK FACTORS

See "Etiology and Pathophysiology."

GENERAL PREVENTION

- Avoid or cease smoking and/or alcohol abuse (85% attributed to smoking or alcohol abuse).
- Wear proper respiratory masks/respirators if chronic exposure to certain chemicals, gases, and wood dust.
- Treat chronic laryngopharyngeal reflux.
- Indirect laryngoscopy for at-risk patients with persistent hoarseness lasting >2–3 weeks

COMMONLY ASSOCIATED CONDITIONS

Up to 10% of patients may have a synchronous squamous cell carcinoma in the lower or upper aerodigestive tract, most notably in the esophagus or lungs.

DIAGNOSIS

- Early laryngeal cancer generally has a good prognosis, with a 5-year disease-specific survival rate of >90% for T1 tumors.
- 57% are diagnosed at this local stage (1)[A].

HISTORY

- Persistent hoarseness or voice change in an elderly or middle-aged cigarette smoker, lasting >3 weeks (6)[C]
- A sore throat, dysphagia, or odynophagia
- Lasting >6 weeks
- Lump in neck
- Dyspnea and/or stridor
- Ipsilateral otalgia
- Chronic cough
- Hemoptysis
- Weight loss due to poor nutrition
- Halitosis due to tumor necrosis factor
- Chronic exposure to known risk factors (see "Etiology and Pathophysiology")

PHYSICAL EXAM

- Visualization of larynx initially by mirror and then a full nasolaryngoscopic exam (7)[A]
- Physical observation of vocal cord mobility, airway patency, and any regional spread
- Cervical lymph node exam and cranial nerve exam
- Mass in the neck from metastatic lymph node
- Laryngeal tenderness secondary to tumor necrosis factor or suppuration
- Broadening of the larynx on palpation with loss of crepitation
- Fullness of the cricothyroid membrane

DIFFERENTIAL DIAGNOSIS

- Acute or chronic laryngitis secondary to allergies, voice overuse, or chemical exposures
- Benign vocal cord lesions such as polyps, nodules, and papillomas
- Tuberculosis or fungal infection (candidiasis) of the larynx (8)[B]

DIAGNOSTIC TESTS & INTERPRETATION

Initial Tests (lab, imaging)

- Endoscopy, CT scan, or MRI to rule out suspected esophagus, chest, liver, or brain metastasis (7)[A]
- Barium swallow
- Chest radiograph
- Bone scan if bone metastasis suspected

Diagnostic Procedures/Other

Indirect and/or direct laryngoscopy and fine needle aspiration biopsy to determine stage of disease, as well as histologic confirmation (6,7)[A]

Test Interpretation

- Laryngoscopy: fungating, friable tumor with heaped-up edges and granular appearance, with multiple areas of central necrosis and exudate surrounding areas of hyperemia
- Squamous cell carcinoma in 95% of cases

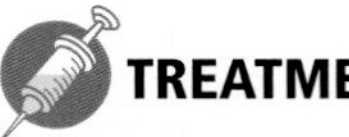

TREATMENT

- Radiotherapy tends to be the treatment of choice in northern Europe, Australasia, and Canada, whereas surgery tends to be the treatment of choice in southern Europe and many centers in the United States.
- Increased use of transoral endoscopic laser microsurgery, improved delivery of radiotherapy, and concomitant chemoradiotherapy have been used over the past 10+ years with promising results (9)[A].
- Radiotherapy and/or surgery, including laser excision surgery, is designed with preserving vocal function (7)[A].

GENERAL MEASURES

- Tracheotomy care, when applicable
- If patient is diagnosed during pregnancy: Natural history of disease and treatment side effects have to be weighed against the possibilities of continuing on to delivery.

MEDICATION

- Opioids may be necessary for pain control during treatment for mucositis (of the mouth) secondary to radiation therapy (RT). Swishing with viscous lidocaine can be helpful as well.
- Nystatin mouth rinses for oral thrush (8)[B]

ISSUES FOR REFERRAL

- ENT for direct visualization of larynx; biopsy and surgery (7)[A]
- Depending on patient's management plan, nutritional and dental consultations are needed.
- Treatment may result in need for voice rehabilitation and be the cause of social isolation, job loss, and depression; therefore, refer to speech therapist, psychology, social work, and/or support groups as indicated (7)[A].

ADDITIONAL THERAPIES

Radiotherapy

- There is increased focus on RT, combined chemotherapy and RT, and function-preserving laryngectomy surgery due to patient fear of voice loss (10)[A].
- Early disease may be treatable by either RT or laser cordectomy on an outpatient basis. No randomized controlled trial has proven superiority of either when last reviewed by Cochrane in 2007. 90% cure rates are the rule (9)[A].
- BCCIP protein (*BRCA2* and *CDKN1A* [p21 (Waf1/Cip1)] interacting protein) can be a prognostic marker for RT, with loss of the protein indicating a worse prognosis (11)[A].

SURGERY/OTHER PROCEDURES

- Tracheotomy may be necessary if a tumor is large enough to cause upper airway obstruction (12)[A].
- More advanced disease needs inpatient care, necessitating partial or total laryngectomy and postoperative RT 4–5 weeks after surgery depending on the stage of disease (7)[A].

INPATIENT CONSIDERATIONS

Admission Criteria/Initial Stabilization

- More advanced disease, surgical intervention, and complication management
- Nutritional or airway issues/complications
- Primarily outpatient care

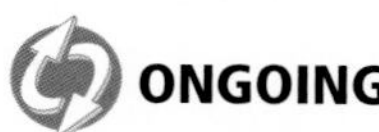

ONGOING CARE

FOLLOW-UP RECOMMENDATIONS

Patient may remain fully active unless debilitated from more advanced disease and/or greater degree of surgery.

Patient Monitoring

- Repeat indirect laryngoscopy and complete head and neck exams periodically for at least 5 years after treatment to detect early recurrence or 2nd primary
- Yearly chest x-rays and liver function test monitoring for metastatic disease
- Patients with dysphagia should undergo barium swallow and/or esophageal endoscopy to rule out 2nd synchronous tumor in the esophagus.
- Patients with unexplained pain should have appropriate radiologic or nuclear medicine bone scans.
- Mental status change warrants CT scan of the brain to rule out brain metastases.

DIET

- Nasogastric or gastrostomy feeding may be necessary if tumor involves esophageal inlet.
- No special diet otherwise

PATIENT EDUCATION

- Material is available from local Cancer Society branch.
- Secondary prevention to address all risk factors especially smoking cessation

PROGNOSIS

- Early disease is expected to have >90% cure rate, with laryngeal and voice preservation.
- If lesion enlarges or metastasizes to regional cervical lymph nodes, the cure rate usually drops by 50%.
- Most recurrences occur within 2 years of initial treatment.

COMPLICATIONS

- Temporary odynophagia or dysphagia secondary to mucositis and/or thrush during RT
- Persistent hoarseness despite adequate treatment, necessitating further adjunctive procedures and/or speech therapy
- Tracheostoma stenosis requiring stenting with laryngectomy tubes or further surgery
- Dysphagia secondary to upper esophageal stricture after total laryngectomy, necessitating dilation
- Aspiration after partial laryngectomy, necessitating complete laryngectomy or tracheotomy
- Inability to decannulate after partial laryngectomy because of laryngeal stenosis and/or aspiration
- Radiation-induced chondronecrosis, which mimics tumor recurrence
- Radiation edema, necessitating emergent tracheotomy
- Hypothyroidism secondary to laryngectomy and RT (13)[C]

REFERENCES

1. Howlader N, Noone AM, Krapcho M, et al, eds. *SEER cancer statistics review, 1975–2010*. Bethesda, MD: National Cancer Institute; 2013. http://seer.cancer.gov/csr/1975_2010/. Accessed 2014.
2. American *Cancer Society. Cancer Facts & Figures 2014*. Atlanta, GA: American Cancer Society; 2014. http://www.cancer.org/acs/groups/content/@research/documents/webcontent/acspc-042151.pdf. Accessed May 21, 2014.
3. La Vecchia C, Zhang ZF, Altieri A. Alcohol and laryngeal cancer: an update. *Eur J Cancer Prev*. 2008;17(2):116–124.
4. Centers for Disease Control and Prevention. Human papillomavirus-associated cancers—United States, 2004–2008. *MMWR Morb Mortal Wkly Rep*. 2012;61:258–261.
5. Bisht M, Bist SS. Human papilloma virus: a new risk factor in a subset of head and neck cancers. *J Cancer Res Ther*. 2011;7(3):251–255.
6. Chu EA, Kim YJ. Laryngeal cancer: diagnosis and preoperative work-up. *Otolaryngol Clin North Am*. 2008;41(4):673–695.
7. National Cancer Institute. Laryngeal cancer treatment (PDQ®). http://www.cancer.gov/cancertopics/pdq/treatment/laryngeal/patient/page1. Accessed 2014.
8. Nunes FP, Bishop T, Prasad ML, et al. Laryngeal candidiasis mimicking alignancy. *Laryngoscope*. 2008;118(11):1957–1959.
9. Samson DJ, Ratko TA, Rothenberg BM, et al. Comparative effectiveness and safety of radiotherapy treatments for head and neck cancer. Rockville, MD: Agency for Healthcare Research and Quality; 2010.
10. Milovanovic J, Jotic A, Djukic V, et al. Oncological and functional outcome after surgical treatment of early glottic carcinoma without anterior commissure involvement. *Biomed Res Int*. 2014;2014:464781.
11. Rewari A, Lu H, Parikh R, et al. BCCIP as a prognostic marker for radiotherapy of laryngeal cancer. *Radiother Oncol*. 2009;90(2):183–188.
12. Sherman EJ, Fisher SG, Kraus DH, et al. TALK score: development and validation of a prognostic model for predicting larynx preservation outcome. *Laryngoscope*. 2012;122(5):1043–1050.
13. Alkan S, Baylancicek S, Ciftçic M, et al. Thyroid dysfunction after combined therapy for laryngeal cancer: a prospective study. *Otolaryngol Head Neck Surg*. 2008;139(6):787–791.

ADDITIONAL READING

- American Society of Clinical Oncology, Pfister DG, Laurie SA, et al. American Society of Clinical Oncology clinical practice guideline for the use of larynx-preservation strategies in the treatment of laryngeal cancer. *J Clin Oncol*. 2006;24(22):3693–3704.
- D'Cruz AK, Sharma S, Pai PS. Current status of near-total laryngectomy: a review. *J Laryngol Otol*. 2012;126(6):556–562.
- Ferlito A, Bradley PJ, Rinaldo A. What is the treatment of choice for TI squamous cell carcinoma of the larynx? *J Laryngol Otol*. 2004;118(10):747–749.
- Huang SH, Lockwood G, Irish J, et al. Truths and myths about radiotherapy for verrucous carcinoma of larynx. *Int J Radiat Oncol Biol Phys*. 2009;73(4):1110–1115.
- Hutcheson KA, Lewin JS. Functional outcomes after chemoradiotherapy of laryngeal and pharyngeal cancers. *Curr Oncol Rep*. 2012;14(2):158–165.

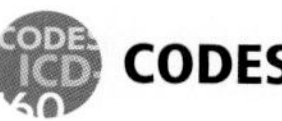

CODES

ICD10

- C32.9 Malignant neoplasm of larynx, unspecified
- C32.8 Malignant neoplasm of overlapping sites of larynx
- C32.3 Malignant neoplasm of laryngeal cartilage

CLINICAL PEARLS

- Persistent hoarseness in an at-risk older person should prompt investigation with indirect and/or direct laryngoscopy.
- RT and multimodal therapies have reduced the need for laryngectomy except in advanced cases. ENT and radiation oncology consultations are recommended.
- Counsel all patients about primary prevention (no smoking, limit alcohol use), and counsel patients with cancer on secondary prevention.

LARYNGITIS

Hugh J. Silk, MD, MPH • Sheila O. Stille, DMD • Alliam Regan, MD

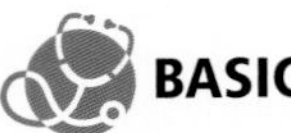

BASICS

DESCRIPTION

- Laryngitis is inflammation, erythema, and edema of the mucosa of the larynx and/or vocal cords characterized by hoarseness, loss of voice, throat pain, or coughing.
- There is a range of severity, but most cases are acute and are associated with viral upper respiratory infection, irritation, or acute vocal strain.
- System(s) affected: pulmonary; ears, eyes, nose, throat (ENT)
- Synonym(s): acute laryngitis; chronic laryngitis; croup or laryngotracheitis (in children)

EPIDEMIOLOGY

- Predominant age: affects all ages
- Children more susceptible than adults due to increased risk of symptomatic inflammation from smaller airways
- Predominant sex: male = female

Incidence

Common

Prevalence

Common

ETIOLOGY AND PATHOPHYSIOLOGY

- Misuse or abuse of voice
- Viral infections: influenza A, B; parainfluenza; adenovirus; coronavirus; rhinovirus; human papillomavirus; cytomegalovirus; varicella-zoster virus; herpes simplex virus; respiratory syncytial virus; coxsackievirus
- Bacterial infections (uncommon): β-hemolytic streptococcus, *Streptococcus pneumoniae*, *Haemophilus influenzae*, tuberculosis (TB), leprosy, *Moraxella catarrhalis*, *Mycoplasma pneumoniae*, *Chlamydophila pneumoniae*
- Fungal infections (rare): histoplasmosis, blastomycosis, *Coccidioides*, *Cryptococcus*, and *Candida*
- Secondary syphilis left untreated
- Leprosy (in 30–55% of those with leprosy, larynx is affected; tropical and warm countries)
- Inhaling irritating substances (e.g., air pollution, cigarette smoke)
- Aspiration of caustic chemicals
- Aging changes: muscle atrophy, loss of moisture in larynx, and bowing of vocal cords
- Gastroesophageal reflux disease (GERD)/ laryngopharyngeal reflux disease (LPRD)
- Excessively dry environment
- Allergy exposures (including pollens)
- Idiopathic
- Iatrogenic: inhaled steroids such as those used to treat asthma; surgical injury; endotracheal intubation nerve
- Vocal cord nodules/polyps ("singer's nodes")
- Local cancer
- Neuromuscular disorder (e.g., myasthenia gravis); stroke
- Rheumatoid arthritis
- Trauma (e.g., blunt or penetrating trauma to neck)

RISK FACTORS

- Acute:
  - Upper respiratory tract infection
  - Voice overuse—excess talking, singing, or shouting
  - Pneumonia
  - Influenza
  - Lack of immunization for pertussis or diphtheria
  - Immunocompromised
  - Recent endotracheal intubation or local surgery
- Chronic:
  - Allergies
  - Chronic rhinitis/sinusitis
  - Voice abuse
  - GERD/LPRD (rare) (1,2)[A]
  - Smoking: primary or secondhand
  - Excessive alcohol use
  - Stroke
  - Constant exposure to dust or other irritants such as chemicals at workplace; environmental pollution
  - Medications: inhaled steroids, anticholinergics, antihistamines, anabolic steroids (3)[B]

Geriatric Considerations

May be more ill, slower to heal

Pediatric Considerations

- Common in this age group
- Consider congenital/anatomic causes.

GENERAL PREVENTION

- Avoid overuse of voice (voice training helpful for vocal musicians/public speakers).
- Influenza virus vaccine is suggested for high-risk individuals.
- Quit smoking, and avoid secondhand smoke.
- Limit or avoid alcohol/caffeine/acidic foods.
- Control GERD/LPRD.
- Maintain proper hydration status.
- Avoid allergens.
- Wear mask around chemical/environmental irritants.
- Good hand washing (infection prevention)

COMMONLY ASSOCIATED CONDITIONS

- Viral pharyngitis
- Diphtheria (rare): Membrane can descend into larynx.
- Pertussis: larynx involved as part of the respiratory system
- Bronchitis
- Pneumonitis
- Croup, epiglottitis, in children

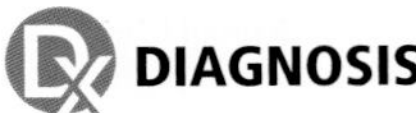

DIAGNOSIS

HISTORY

- Hoarseness, throat tickling, dry cough, and rawness
- Abnormal-sounding voice
- Constant urge to clear the throat
- Possible fever
- Malaise
- Dysphagia/odynophagia
- Regional cervical lymphadenopathy
- Stridor or possible airway obstruction in children (4)[C]
- Cough may be worse at night in children.
- Hemoptysis
- Laryngospasm or sense of choking
- Allergic rhinitis/rhinorrhea/postnasal drip (PND)
- Occupation or other reasons for voice overuse
- Smoking history
- Blunt or penetrating trauma to neck
- GERD/LPRD

PHYSICAL EXAM

- Head and neck exam, including cervical nodes; cranial nerve exam
- ENT referral for persistent symptoms (>2–3 weeks) or concern for foreign body

DIFFERENTIAL DIAGNOSIS

- Diphtheria
- Vocal nodules or polyps
- Laryngeal malignancy
- Thyroid malignancy
- Upper airway malignancy
- Epiglottitis
- Pertussis
- Laryngeal nerve trauma/injury
- Foreign body (in children)

DIAGNOSTIC TESTS & INTERPRETATION

- Rarely needed
- WBCs elevated in bacterial laryngitis
- Viral culture (seldom necessary)

Follow-Up Tests & Special Considerations

- Barium swallow, only if needed for differential diagnosis
- CT scan if foreign body suspected

Diagnostic Procedures/Other

- Fiber-optic or indirect laryngoscopy: looking for red, inflamed, and occasionally hemorrhagic vocal cords; rounded edges and exudate (Reinke edema)
- Consider otolaryngologic evaluation and biopsy: laryngitis lasting >2 weeks in adults with history of smoking or alcohol abuse to rule out malignancy
- pH probe (24-hour): no difference in incidence of pharyngeal reflux as measured by pH probe between patients with chronic reflux laryngitis and healthy adults (5)[C]
- Strobovideo laryngoscopy for diagnosis of subtle lesions (e.g., vocal cord nodules or polyps)

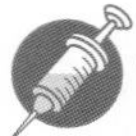

TREATMENT

- Evidence is limited, but good, that treatment beyond supportive care is ineffective.
- Antibiotics appear to have no benefit because it is predominantly viral (6)[A]. The bacterial form is rare.
- Corticosteroids in severe cases of laryngitis to reduce inflammation such as croup
- May need voice training, if voice overuse
- Racemic epinephrine reduces symptoms at 30 minutes, but effect lasts only 2 hours (7)[A].

GENERAL MEASURES

- Acute:
  - Usually a self-limited illness lasting <3 weeks and not severe
  - Antibiotics of no value (6)[A]
  - Avoid excessive voice use, including whispering.
  - Steam inhalations or cool-mist humidifier
  - Increase fluid intake, especially in cases associated with excessive dryness.
  - Avoid smoking (or secondhand exposure).
  - Warm saltwater gargles
- Chronic:
  - Symptomatic treatment as above
  - Voice therapy (for patients with intermittent dysphagia and vocal abuse)
  - Stop smoking.
  - Reduce or stop alcohol intake.
  - Occupational change or modification, if exposure
  - Allergen avoidance
  - Consider discontinuing inhaled corticosteroids.
- Reflux laryngitis: elevate head of bed, diet changes, other antireflux lifestyle change management; proton pump inhibitors

MEDICATION

Usually none

First Line

- Analgesics
- Antipyretics (rare)
- Cough suppressants
- Throat lozenges
- Plenty of fluids

Second Line

- Inhaled corticosteroids (consider if allergy induced)
- Oral corticosteroids: only if urgent need in adults (presenter, singer, actor)
- Oral corticosteroids: Evidence of benefit has been studied with single-dose dexamethasone in children ages 6 months–5 years for moderate-severity croup; reduces symptoms within 6 hours, reduces hospitalizations, hospital length of stay, and revisits to office (8)[A].
- Standard of care is to prescribe proton pump inhibitors for chronic laryngitis if GERD or LPRD is suspected; however, evidence suggests only a modest benefit, if any (9,10)[C].
- Treat nonviral infectious underlying causes.
- Candidal laryngitis:
  - Mild cases: oral antifungal (fluconazole)
  - Amphotericin B or echinocandin can be given in life-threatening cases.

ISSUES FOR REFERRAL

- Consider otolaryngologic evaluation and biopsy for laryngitis lasting >2 weeks in adults, especially in those with history of smoking or alcohol abuse to rule out malignancy.
- Consider GI consult to rule out GERD/LPRD.

SURGERY/OTHER PROCEDURES

- Vocal cord biopsy of hyperplastic mucosa and areas of leukoplakia if cancer or TB is suspected
- Removal of nodules or polyps if voice therapy fails

COMPLEMENTARY & ALTERNATIVE MEDICINE

The following, although not well studied, have been recommended by some experts:

- Barberry, blackcurrant, echinacea, eucalyptus, German chamomile, goldenrod, goldenseal, warmed lemon and honey, licorice, marshmallow, peppermint, saw palmetto, slippery elm, vitamin C, zinc

ONGOING CARE

PATIENT EDUCATION

- Educate on the importance of voice rest, including whispering.
- Provide assistance with smoking cessation.
- Help the patient with modification of other predisposing habits or occupational hazards.

PROGNOSIS

Complete clearing of the inflammation without sequelae

COMPLICATIONS

Chronic hoarseness

REFERENCES

1. Hawkshaw MJ, Pebdani P, Sataloff RT. Reflux laryngitis: an update, 2009–2012. *J Voice*. 2013;27(4):486–494.
2. Hom C, Vaezi MF. Extraesophageal manifestations of gatroesophageal reflux disease. *Gastroenterol Clin North Am*. 2013;42(1):71–91.
3. Ray S, Masood A, Pickles J, et al. Severe laryngitis following chronic anabolic steroid abuse. *J Laryngol Otol*. 2008;122(3):230–232.
4. Gallivan GJ, Gallivan KH, Gallivan HK. Inhaled corticosteroids: hazardous effects on voice—an update. *J Voice*. 2007;21(1):101–111.
5. Johnson DA. Medical therapy of reflux pharyngitis. *J Clin Gastroenterol*. 2008;42(5):589–593.
6. Reveiz L, Cardona AF. Antibiotics for acute laryngitis in adults. *Cochrane Database Syst Rev*. 2013;3:CD004783.
7. Bjornson C, Russell KF, Vandermeer B, et al. Nebulized epinephrine for croup in children. *Cochrane Database Syst Rev*. 2011;(2):CD006619.
8. Russell KF, Liang Y, O'Gorman K, et al. Glucocorticoids for croup. *Cochrane Database Syst Rev*. 2011;(1):CD001955.
9. Tulunay OE. Laryngitis—diagnosis and management. *Otolaryngol Clin North Am*. 2008;41(2):437–452.
10. Kim JH, Sung IK, Hong SN, et al. Is the proton pump inhibitor test helpful in patients with laryngeal symptoms? *Dig Dis Sci*. 2013;58(6):1663–1667.

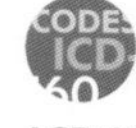

CODES

ICD10

- J04.0 Acute laryngitis
- J37.0 Chronic laryngitis
- J04.2 Acute laryngotracheitis

CLINICAL PEARLS

- Laryngitis is usually self-limited and needs only comfort care. Standard treatment is voice rest.
- Refer to ENT for direct visualization of vocal cords for prolonged laryngitis.
- Corticosteroids have some benefits for children with moderately severe croup.

LAXATIVE ABUSE

Matthew E. Bryant, MD • Shima Syed, MD

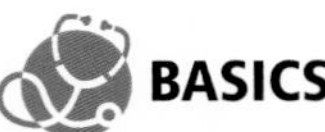

BASICS

DESCRIPTION

- A chronic watery diarrhea caused by intentional or unintentional misuse of laxatives due to self-medication or provider error
- System(s) affected: gastrointestinal, nervous, psychiatric, skin, and renal
- Synonym(s): factitious diarrhea; cathartic colon; as part of Münchausen syndrome (self or by proxy)—most dramatic form

EPIDEMIOLOGY

- Predominant age: 18–40 years associated with bulimia or anorexia nervosa
- Common in the elderly as a result of treatment for constipation, either by health care professional or self-directed (*unintentional*)
- Associated with athletes in sports with weight limits (wrestling)
- Predominant sex (*intentional abuse*): female (90%) > male
- More common in upper socioeconomic classes

Prevalence

Laxative abuse in different groups:

- 0.7–5.5% in the general population
- As many as 15% undergoing evaluation for chronic diarrhea
- Unexplained chronic diarrhea after routine investigations: 4–7%
- Up to 70% of patients with binging/purging anorexia and bulimia nervosa abuse laxatives but rarely as the sole method of purging.
- Chronic use of constipating medications (opioids)

Pediatric Considerations

Children may be given excess laxatives by caregivers (Münchausen syndrome by proxy).

Geriatric Considerations

Elderly in nursing homes are at increased risk for laxative overuse (usually inadvertent).

ETIOLOGY AND PATHOPHYSIOLOGY

- Chronic diarrhea characterized by four types: secretory, osmotic, inflammatory, and fatty. Be certain to rule out other causes of chronic diarrhea because laxative abuse is diagnosis of exclusion (1).
- Chronic ingestion of any laxative agent: four types:
  - Stimulant (most common, rapid onset of action):
    - Diphenylmethane (Bisacodyl)
    - Anthraquinones (Senna, Cascara, Castor oil)
  - Saline and osmotic products (sodium phosphate, magnesium sulfate/citrate and hydroxide, lactulose, polyethelene glycol)
  - Bulking agents (psyllium)
  - Surfactants (docusate)
- Psychologic factors:
  - Bulimia or anorexia nervosa (associated with behavioral pathology)
  - Secondary gain (attention-seeking): disability claims or need for concern, caring from others
  - Inappropriate perceptions of "normal" bowel habits

RISK FACTORS

In patients with eating disorders:

- Longer duration of illness
- Comorbid psychiatric diagnoses (e.g., major depression, obsessive-compulsive disorder, posttraumatic stress disorder, anxiety, borderline personality disorder)
- Early age of appearance of eating disorder symptoms

GENERAL PREVENTION

- Educate patients about proper nutrition, normal bowel function, potential adverse effects of excessive laxative use, and other medications (e.g., magnesium-containing antacids) that can cause diarrhea.
- Ask patients specifically about laxative use; Inadvertent overuse is common.

COMMONLY ASSOCIATED CONDITIONS

- Anorexia nervosa, bulimia nervosa
- Use of constipating medications (opioids, iron supplements)
- Any chronic disorder associated with constipation
- Depression and anxiety
- Borderline personality
- Self-injurious behaviors/suicidal ideation
- Impulsive behavior
- Münchausen syndrome/Münchausen syndrome by proxy (children); may have associated factitious symptoms involving diverse organ systems
- Fictitious disorders
- Patient is dependent on a caregiver.

DIAGNOSIS

HISTORY

- Suspect in patients with undiagnosed, refractory chronic diarrhea.
- Assess over-the-counter medication use, and take thorough dietary history (2).
- Signs and symptoms: increasing frequency of bowel movements; large volume, watery diarrhea; nocturnal bowel movements (typically absent in osmotic diarrhea or in irritable bowel syndrome) (2,3).
- Additional symptoms: abdominal pain, rectal pain, nausea, vomiting, weight loss, malaise, muscle weakness, or chronic constipation.
- Assess "doctor shopping" and potential factitious symptoms.

PHYSICAL EXAM

- No specific findings but may include cachexia, evidence of dehydration, abdominal pain or distension, and edema; fever may be due to self-infected wounds or thermometer manipulation (2)
- Bulimics or anorexics who purge may have Russell sign (excoriation of fingers from repeated self-induced retching) (5); clubbing, cyclic edema, skin pigmentation changes.
- Rarely, severe cases may be associated with renal failure, cardiac arrhythmias, skeletal muscle paralysis, anemia from blood-letting or self-induced skin wounds.

DIFFERENTIAL DIAGNOSIS

Any etiology of chronic diarrhea, especially in high-risk groups

DIAGNOSTIC TESTS & INTERPRETATION

If patient has not had an initial workup for chronic diarrhea, infectious, inflammatory, and malignant causes must be ruled out as appropriate based on patient demographics and risk factors.

Initial Tests (lab, imaging)

- Serum electrolytes hypokalemia, hypernatremia, hyperphosphatemia
  - Acute diarrhea: metabolic acidosis (hypovolemia)
  - Chronic diarrhea: metabolic alkalosis secondary to hypokalemia-induced inhibition of chloride uptake with inhibited bicarbonate secretion
- CBC, stool cultures, *Clostridium difficile* polymerase chain reaction (PCR) to rule out infectious cause if history is suspicious (fecal leukocytes, ova and parasites (O&P)—check for giardia, isospora, and cryptosporidia specifically) (2,3)
- Colonoscopy, small-bowel endoscopy, or imaging studies are not usually necessary for diagnosis of laxative abuse but may be needed to evaluate other causes of chronic diarrhea (2).
- *Melanosis coli* on sigmoidoscopy or colonoscopy indicate overuse of anthracene laxatives.

Follow-Up Tests & Special Considerations

If history and initial lab tests are suspicious, the following algorithm can be used to confirm diagnosis and determine what type of laxative is being used (1,6)[B]:

- Collect 24-hour stool: If stool is solid, workup is over.
- Obtain stool osmolality, stool electrolytes, and calculate osmolal gap ($= 290 - 2(Na^+ + K^+)$, where Na^+ and K^+ are the concentrations from the stool sample.
  - If osmolality >400 mOsm/kg, rule out urine contamination of stool. Measure urea and creatinine of sample.
  - If osmolality <250–400 mOsm/kg, rule out water added to stool (colon cannot dilute stool to osmolality of plasma).
  - If osmolality = 250–400 mOsm/kg, measure osmolal gap.
    - Gap >50: unmeasured solute; check fecal fat and stool magnesium levels.
    - Gap <50: Rule out use of secretory laxative; urinalysis and stool analysis for laxative titers. Do not obtain serum laxative titers, as they peak 1–2 hours after ingestion. Urine titers can be 10× as high as plasma titers.
- Confirm diagnosis with multiple stool analyses before addressing patient with concern for intentional abuse.

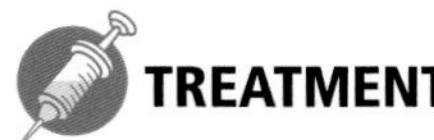

TREATMENT

GENERAL MEASURES

- Psychological support is essential in intentional use.
- Wean patient off laxatives and supplements; substitute high-fiber diet and bulk preparations or short-term saline enemas.
- Treat secondary constipation (3)[C].
- Treat metabolic abnormalities.

MEDICATION

Replace needed fluid, vitamins, electrolytes, and minerals.

First Line

- Patient education on normal bowel habits
- Nonstimulant laxatives if needed to treat constipation (3)[C]:
  - Polyethylene glycol (3)[C]
  - Lactulose (3)[C]
  - High-fiber diet
- Precautions: Patients may be manipulative in attempts to deny problem; may hide laxatives in hospital rooms.
- Significant possible interactions:
  - Increased rate of intestinal motility may affect rate of absorption of medications (e.g., antibiotics, hormones).
  - Docusate sodium may potentiate hepatotoxicity of other drugs.
  - Consider loperamide to improve anal tone and promote rectal inhibitory reflex (7)[C].

ISSUES FOR REFERRAL

In cases of Münchausen syndrome by proxy, legal proceedings must be considered, especially because most victims are children. Behavioral health support for patients with significant psychological comorbidities

SURGERY/OTHER PROCEDURES

Avoid exploratory surgery and repetitive evaluations with invasive procedures.

INPATIENT CONSIDERATIONS

Admission Criteria/Initial Stabilization

- Persistent diarrhea with evidence of hemodynamic instability
- Electrolyte/metabolic complications, including lactic acidosis
- Cardiac arrhythmias

IV Fluids

Resuscitate based on clinical presentation. If patient is hemodynamically stable and without significant abnormalities in serum sodium, give normal saline boluses or oral replacement to correct metabolic alkalosis (chronic) or acidosis (acute) as needed. If patient is hemodynamically unstable, treat volume status as in hypovolemic shock, while monitoring serum electrolytes closely (especially sodium, potassium, and bicarbonate (7,8)[C].

Nursing

If stable, patient does not need continuous telemetry. Depending on psychiatric history, patient may need one-on-one or line-of-sight observation. Special care must be taken to ensure adequate nutrition and control access to laxatives. If surreptitious laxative ingestion is suspected, do not perform unauthorized room searches due to legal constraints.

Discharge Criteria

- Psychological support
- Diet and bowel programs
- Resolution of electrolyte abnormalities/dehydration

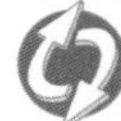

ONGOING CARE

FOLLOW-UP RECOMMENDATIONS

Patient Monitoring

- Ongoing behavioral counseling
- Careful medical support; frequent visits as needed
- Assess serum electrolytes.

DIET

Ensure good nutritional habits:

- Increase fiber intake.
- Avoid constipating substances.
- Adequate calories, especially with bulimia

PROGNOSIS

- Natural history is unclear and varied depending on underlying cause.
- Prognosis is related to psychological response in intentional abuse or underlying etiology when organic disease is present.
- Prognosis is poor with anorexia nervosa; very poor in Münchausen syndrome.
- Cathartic colon is commonly refractory to treatment (8)[C].

COMPLICATIONS

- Risk of multiple tests, procedures, and surgeries (intentional use)
- Malnutrition
- Electrolyte imbalances (hypokalemia, hypermagnesemia, acute phosphate nephropathy) (3)
- Renal failure
- Cardiac arrhythmias/sudden death; fatalities seen, especially in children given laxatives by parents; eating disorders (3)
- Renal calculi
- Cathartic colon with constipation as a consequence of prolonged irritant laxative use; no diarrhea, fever, or blood loss (8)
- Fecal impaction in elderly
- Recurrences are common for factitious abuse, even after confrontation.
- Rebound edema (8)

REFERENCES

1. Thomas PD, Forbes A, Green J, et al. Guidelines for the investigation of chronic diarrhoea, 2nd edition. *Gut*. 2003;52(Suppl 5):v1–v15.
2. Schiller LR. Definitions, pathophysiology, and evaluation of chronic diarrhoea. *Best Pract Res Clin Gastroenterol*. 2012;26(5):551–562.
3. Roerig JL, Steffen KJ, Mitchell JE, et al. Laxative abuse: epidemiology, diagnosis and management. *Drugs*. 2010;70(12):1487–1503.
4. Sweetser S. Evaluating the patient with diarrhea: a case-based approach. *Mayo Clin Proc*. 2012;87(6):596–602.
5. Sim LA, McAlpine DE, Grothe KB, et al. Identification and management of eating disorders in the primary care setting. *Mayo Clin Proc*. 2010;85(8):746–751.
6. Fine KD, Santa Ana CA, Fordtran JS. Diagnosis of magnesium-induced diarrhea. *N Engl J Med*. 1991;324(15):1012–1017.
7. Kent AJ, Banks MR. Pharmacologic management of diarrhea. *Gastroenterol Clin North Am*. 2010;39(3):495–507.
8. Neims DW, McNeill J, Giles TR, et al. Incidence of laxative abuse in community and bulimic populations: a descriptive review. *Int J Eat Disord*. 1995;17(3):211–228.

ADDITIONAL READING

- Abraham BP, Sellin JH. Drug-induced, factitious, and idiopathic diarrhea. *Best Pract Res Clin Gastroenterol*. 2012;26(5):633–648.
- Bytzer P, Stokholm M, Andersen I, et al. Prevalence of surreptitious laxative abuse in patients with diarrhoea of uncertain origin: a cost benefit analysis of a screening procedure. *Gut*. 1989;30(10):1379.
- Shelton JH, Santa Ana CA, Thompson DR, et al. Factitious diarrhea induced by stimulant laxatives: accuracy of diagnosis by a clinical reference laboratory using thin layer chromatography. *Clin Chem*. 2007;53(1):85–90.
- Tozzi F, Thornton LM, Mitchell J, et al. Features associated with laxative abuse in individuals with eating disorders. *Psycosom Med*. 2006;68(3):470–477.

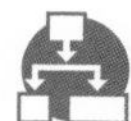

SEE ALSO

Algorithm: Diarrhea, Chronic

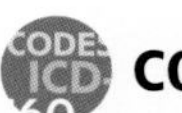

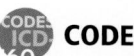

CODES

ICD10

F55.2 Abuse of laxatives

CLINICAL PEARLS

- Laxative abuse may be intentional or unintentional.
- When associated with eating disorders, laxative abuse is associated with more severe disease.
- Consider the diagnosis in patients with watery diarrhea, especially when unexplained or refractory.
- As many as 15% of patients referred to tertiary care centers for unexplained chronic diarrhea abuse laxatives.
- Presentation is diverse and nonspecific, including weight loss, weakness, and hypotension without acknowledgment of diarrhea, when intentional.

L

LEGIONNAIRES' DISEASE

Mark B. Stephens, MD, MS, FAAFP, CAPT, MC, USN

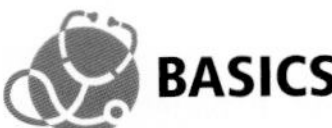

BASICS

DESCRIPTION

- *Legionnaires' disease* was named for an epidemic of lower respiratory tract disease at an American Legion convention in Philadelphia in 1976. The causative bacterium was previously unrecognized. It was isolated, identified, and named *Legionella pneumophila*. The organism primarily causes pneumonia and flulike illness. The bacteria preferentially colonize man-made water systems (e.g., hotels, hospitals, air conditioning cooling towers).
  - Among the 3 most common clinical pneumonias
  - Most common atypical pneumonia
- System(s) affected: gastrointestinal, pulmonary
- Synonym(s): *Legionella* pneumonia; legionellosis

EPIDEMIOLOGY

- Predominant age: 15 months–84 years; increased in patients >50 years
- Predominant gender: male > female

Incidence

- Reported cases increased from 1,310 in 2002 to 2,223 in 2003, with >2,000 cases/year from 2003 to 2005.
- Outbreaks occur most often at the end of the summer and early fall.

ETIOLOGY AND PATHOPHYSIOLOGY

- *L. pneumophila* is a weak gram-negative aerobic saprophytic freshwater bacterium. It is widely distributed in soil and water. Bipolar flagella provide motility; grows optimally at 40–45°C
- Exists as an intracellular protozoan parasite, colonizing surfaces and growing in biofilms, which persist in nematodes.
- Serogroups 1–6 account for clinical disease.
- In the lung, *Legionella* infects alveolar macrophages.
- The organism is transmitted by aspiration, direct transmission (e.g., contaminated respiratory equipment), and (most importantly) by airborne dissemination and aerosolization of contaminated water sources (e.g., contaminated shower water—felt responsible for the inaugural Philadelphia outbreak).
- Recently, community outbreaks have been associated with whirlpools, spas, and fountains.

RISK FACTORS

- Impaired cellular immunity (*Legionella* are intracellular pathogens)
- Smoking
- Alcohol abuse
- Immunosuppression/HIV
- Chronic cardiopulmonary disease
- Advanced age
- Transplant recipients
- Diabetes mellitus
- Use of antimicrobials within the past 3 months

GENERAL PREVENTION

- *Not transmitted person to person* (Isolation is unnecessary.)
- Superheat and flush water systems: Heat water to 70°C, and flush outlets with hot water for 30 minutes (1)[C].
- Ultraviolet light or copper–silver ionization are bactericidal.
- Monochloramine disinfection of municipal water supplies decreases risk for *Legionella* infection.

COMMONLY ASSOCIATED CONDITIONS

Pontiac fever: self-limited flulike illness without pneumonia caused by *Legionella* species

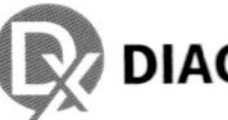

DIAGNOSIS

- Illness ranges from asymptomatic seroconversion and mild febrile illness to severe pneumonia.
- Wound infections with *Legionella* have also been reported.
- Incubation period is 2–14 days.

HISTORY

- Signs and symptoms (with associated percentage):
  - Dry cough: 92%, may become productive
  - Fever/chills: 90%
  - Dyspnea: 62%
  - Pleuritic chest pain: 35%
  - Headache: 48%
  - Myalgia/arthralgia: 40%
  - Watery diarrhea: 50%
  - Nausea and vomiting: 49%
  - Neuropsychiatric symptoms such as encephalopathy, confusion, disorientation, obtundation, depression, hallucinations, insomnia, seizure: 53%
- History of immunosuppression increases risk.

PHYSICAL EXAM

- Fever
- Relative bradycardia (key sign)
  - Defined as a temperature ≥102°F with an inappropriately low pulse pressure <100 beats/minute (normal compensatory reaction to fever is tachycardia >110 beats/minute)
- Rales and signs of consolidation (egophony; tactile fremitus)

DIFFERENTIAL DIAGNOSIS

- Other bacterial pneumonias, especially atypical pneumonias: *Mycoplasma pneumoniae*, Q fever (*Coxiella burnetii*), *Chlamydophila pneumoniae*, *Chlamydophila psittaci*, *Francisella tularensis*
- Viral pneumonias, such as adenovirus, influenza (human, avian, swine), cytomegalovirus (CMV)

DIAGNOSTIC TESTS & INTERPRETATION

Initial Tests (lab, imaging)

- Diagnosis:
  - Gold standard is sputum culture for *Legionella*. Alert lab about diagnostic possibility (sample needs buffered charcoal yeast extract agar). Variable sensitivity (10–80%) and time consuming (up to 7 days for results). Hampered by lack of sputum production in >50% of patients.
  - Urinary antigen test (UAT) detects serogroup 1 (which causes most human disease). Urinary antigen tests are highly specific (99%) but variably sensitive. *Legionella* antigenuria can be detected 1–2 days after onset of disease and persists for days to weeks. Limited by only detecting serogroup 1 (may miss 40% of cases) (2)[C].
    - Indications for UAT: ICU admission, failure of outpatient antibiotic treatment, current alcohol abuse, recent travel (within past 2 weeks), pleural effusion
  - Combination of respiratory cultures and urine *Legionella* antigen is optimal for diagnosis (3)[C].
  - Monoclonal direct fluorescence assay (DFA) on respiratory secretions is diagnostic:
    - Sensitivity 41–94%
    - Limited by lengthy (4–6 weeks) seroconversion
  - Silver/Gimenez stains used for lung specimens.
  - Disorders that may alter lab results: Direct immunofluorescence can cross-react with *Pseudomonas* and *Bacteroides* sp., *Escherichia coli*, and *Haemophilus* sp.
- Other lab abnormalities (often not seen with other forms of pneumonia):
  - Hyponatremia
  - Hypophosphatemia (transient)
  - Lymphopenia
  - Mildly elevated serum transaminases
  - Elevated LDH
  - Elevated creatinine kinase
  - Microscopic hematuria
  - Highly elevated C-reactive protein (CRP) (>30)
  - Highly elevated ferritin (≥2× normal)
- Chest radiograph
  - Not specific for *Legionella*
  - Commonly shows unilateral lower lobe patchy alveolar infiltrate with consolidation
  - Cavitation and abscess formation is more common in immunocompromised patients.
  - Pleural effusion occurs in up to 50%.
  - May take 1–4 months for radiographic findings to resolve. Progression of infiltrate on x-ray can be seen despite antibiotic therapy.

Diagnostic Procedures/Other

Transtracheal aspiration/bronchoscopy occasionally necessary for sputum/lung samples

Test Interpretation

- Multifocal pneumonia with alveolitis and bronchiolitis, and fibrinous pleuritis; may have serous or serosanguineous pleural effusion
- Abscess formation occurs in up to 20% of patients.
- Progression of infiltrates on x-ray (despite appropriate therapy) suggests Legionnaires' disease. Radiographic improvement may not correlate with clinical findings (longer lag times).

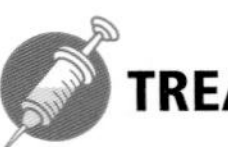

TREATMENT

GENERAL MEASURES

- Severity of illness and available support dictate the appropriate site for care.
- Supportive care:
  - Oxygenation, hydration, and electrolyte balance with antibiotic therapy
- Extrapulmonary complications and higher mortality in patients with AIDS

MEDICATION

First Line

- Antibiotics that achieve high intracellular concentrations (e.g., macrolides, tetracyclines, fluoroquinolones) are most effective; 1st-line treatment is levofloxacin; however, no prospective randomized controlled trials have compared fluoroquinolones to macrolides for the treatment of *Legionella*. In retrospective and observational studies, levofloxacin is associated with more rapid defervescence, fewer complications, and decreased hospital stay compared with macrolide antibiotics. Antibiotics should be initiated parenterally to start route due to the GI symptoms associated with *Legionella*:
  - Levofloxacin is the preferred agent:
    - Levofloxacin 750 mg/day IV (switch to PO when patient is afebrile/tolerating PO) for 5 days or 500 mg/day for 10–14 days
  - Azithromycin may also be used first line. It requires a shorter duration of treatment than levofloxacin due to a longer half-life:
    - Azithromycin 500 mg/day IV (switch to PO when afebrile/tolerating PO) for 7–10 days
- Contraindications: hypersensitivity reactions
- Precautions: liver disease
- Significant possible interactions:
  - Can increase theophylline, carbamazepine, and digoxin levels; can increase activity of oral anticoagulants
  - May decrease the effectiveness of digoxin, quinidine, oral contraceptives, and hypoglycemic agents
- Longer courses of treatment (up to 21 days) may be needed in immunocompromised patients.

Second Line

- Doxycycline 100 mg IV/PO q12h for total 14 days; for severe infections, initial dose is 200 mg IV/PO q12h.
- Doxycycline cannot be used in pregnant patients and is not approved for children <8 years of age.

INPATIENT CONSIDERATIONS

Admission Criteria/Initial Stabilization

- Inability to tolerate oral antibiotics
- Hypoxemia
- Criteria for direct admission to the ICU:
  - Any of the major criteria for severe CAP:
    - Septic shock requiring vasopressor support
    - Acute respiratory failure requiring intubation and/or mechanical ventilation
  - 3 or more of the minor criteria for severe CAP:
    - RR ≥30 breaths/min; PaO_2:FiO_2 ratio ≤250; multilobular infiltrates; confusion/disorientation; uremia (BUN ≥20 mg/dL); leukopenia (WBC <4,000 cells/mm^3); thrombocytopenia (PLT <100 K cells/mm^3); hypothermia (temperature <36°C); hypotension requiring aggressive fluid resuscitation

Discharge Criteria

- Afebrile
- Able to tolerate oral antibiotics
- Normal oxygen saturation

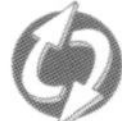

ONGOING CARE

FOLLOW-UP RECOMMENDATIONS

Patient Monitoring

- Monitor respiratory status, hydration, and electrolyte status closely.
- Chest radiography does not help with monitoring clinical response.

PATIENT EDUCATION

- Disease prevention: Eliminate pathogens from water supplies, focusing on low-emission cleaning procedures of cooling towers with control measurements of water and air samples.
- *Legionella* is not spread person-to-person.

PROGNOSIS

- Recovery is variable:
  - Patients may clinically worsen despite treatment early in the course of therapy (first 1–2 days).
  - There is usually rapid improvement with defervescence in 3–5 days and complete recovery in 6–10 days. Some may have a more protracted course despite treatment.
- Mortality approaches 50% with nosocomial infections.

COMPLICATIONS

- Dehydration
- Hyponatremia
- Respiratory insufficiency requiring ventilator support
- Bacteremia/abscess formation in immunocompromised patients
- Extrapulmonary diseases:
  - Encephalitis
  - Cellulitis
  - Sinusitis
  - Pancreatitis
  - Pyelonephritis
  - Endocarditis (most common extrapulmonary site)
  - Pericarditis
  - Perirectal abscess
- Renal failure
- Disseminated intravascular coagulation
- Multiple organ dysfunction syndrome (MODS)
- Coma
- Death occurs in 10% of treated immunocompetent patients and in up to 80% of untreated immunocompromised patients.

REFERENCES

1. Walser SM, Gerstner DG, Brenner B, et al. Assessing the environmental health relevance of cooling towers—a systematic review of legionellosis outbreaks. *Int J Hyg Environ Health*. 2014;217(2–3):145–154.
2. Bartlett JG. Diagnostic tests for agents of community-acquired pneumonia. *Clin Infect Dis*. 2011;52(Suppl 4):S296–S304.
3. Tronel H, Hartemann P. Overview of diagnostic and detection methods for legionellosis and *Legionella* spp. *Lett Appl Microbiol*. 2009;48(6):653–656.

ADDITIONAL READING

- Blázquez Garrido RM, Espinosa Parra FJ, Alemany Francés L, et al. Antimicrobial chemotherapy for Legionnaires disease: levofloxacin versus macrolides. *Clin Infect Dis*. 2005;40:800–806.
- Cunha BA, Klein NC, Strollo S, et al. Legionnaires' disease mimicking swine influenza (H1N1) pneumonia during the "herald wave" of the pandemic. *Heart Lung*. 2010;39(3):242–248.
- Mandell LA, Wunderink RG, Anzueto A, et al. Infectious Diseases Society of America/American Thoracic Society consensus guidelines on the management of community-acquired pneumonia in adults. *Clin Infect Dis* 2007;44:S27–S72.
- Shimada T, Noguchi Y, Jackson JL, et al. Systemic review and metaanalysis: urinary antigen tests for legionellosis. *Chest*. 2009;136(6):1576–1585.
- Yzerman EP, den Boer JW, Lettinga KD, et al. Sensitivity of three urinary antigen tests associated with clinical severity in a large outbreak of Legionnaires' disease in The Netherlands. *J Clin Microbiol*. 2002;40:3232–3236.

SEE ALSO

Pneumonia, Bacterial

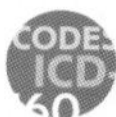

CODES

ICD10

- A48.1 Legionnaires' disease
- A48.2 Nonpneumonic Legionnaires' disease [Pontiac fever]

CLINICAL PEARLS

- *Legionella* is an intracellular organism and must be grown on buffered charcoal yeast extract agar.
- Consider Legionnaires' disease in patients with pneumonia, extrapulmonary findings (atypical CAP) and relative bradycardia, and any 3 of the following: relative lymphopenia, mildly elevated serum transaminases (aspartate aminotransferase/alanine aminotransferase), highly increased ferritin levels, or hypophosphatemia.
- Consider Legionnaires' disease in cases of nosocomial pneumonia.
- Because an increase in *Legionella* antibody titers cannot be detected >3–4 weeks, serology is not useful in early stages of the disease.
- Respiratory specimen cultures combined with urine *Legionella* antigen testing is the preferred strategy for definitive diagnosis.

L

LEUKEMIA, ACUTE LYMPHOBLASTIC IN ADULTS (ALL)

Richard A. Larson, MD

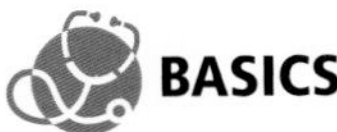

BASICS

DESCRIPTION

- ALL in adults is a malignant proliferation and accumulation of immature lymphocytes.
- ALL is the most common malignancy in children (see "Acute Lymphoblastic Leukemia, Pediatric")
- System(s) affected: hemic/lymphatic/immunologic
- Synonym(s): acute lymphocytic leukemia

Pregnancy Considerations

Many chemotherapy drugs are teratogenic.

EPIDEMIOLOGY

- Predominant age: median age, 35–40 years; incidence increases with age.
- Predominant sex: male > female (slightly)

Incidence

In the United States: 1,000 adult cases per year

ETIOLOGY AND PATHOPHYSIOLOGY

- Unknown
- Epstein-Barr virus is implicated in Burkitt leukemia/lymphoma.

Genetics

- Increased incidence in children with Down syndrome or in rare familial diseases such as ataxia-telangiectasia, Bloom syndrome, Fanconi anemia, Klinefelter syndrome, and neurofibromatosis (1)
- With P53 mutation in Li-Fraumeni syndrome
- Can rarely occur in adult identical twins

RISK FACTORS

- Age >60 years
- Incidence seems to increase after exposure to chemical agents such as benzene, or to radiation, but acute myeloid leukemia (AML) is more common.
- May follow aplastic anemia

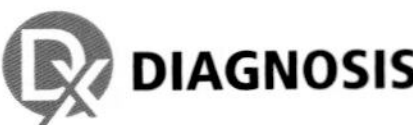

DIAGNOSIS

HISTORY

- Anemia: fatigue, shortness of breath, light-headedness, angina, headache
- Thrombocytopenia: easy bruising
- Neutrocytopenia: fever, infection
- Lymphocytosis: bone pain
- CNS: confusion

PHYSICAL EXAM

- Thrombocytopenia: petechiae, ecchymoses, epistaxis, retinal hemorrhages
- Anemia: pallor
- Neutrocytopenia: fever, infection
- Lymphocytosis: lymphadenopathy, splenomegaly; less often, hepatomegaly
- CNS: cranial nerve palsies, confusion

DIFFERENTIAL DIAGNOSIS

- Malignant disorders: other leukemias, especially AML; chronic myeloid leukemia in lymphoid blast phase; prolymphocytic leukemia; malignant lymphomas; multiple myeloma; bone marrow metastases from solid tumors (breast, prostate, lung, renal); myelodysplastic syndromes
- Nonmalignant disorders: aplastic anemia, myelofibrosis, autoimmune diseases (Felty syndrome, lupus), infectious mononucleosis, pertussis, autoimmune thrombocytopenic purpura, leukemoid reaction to infection

DIAGNOSTIC TESTS & INTERPRETATION

Initial Tests (lab, imaging)

CBC with differential, liver function tests, uric acid, anemia: normochromic, normocytic

- Thrombocytopenia
- Peripheral blood lymphoblasts
- Elevated lactate dehydrogenase
- Elevated uric acid

Follow-Up Tests & Special Considerations

Special tests

- Immunophenotyping of marrow/blood lymphoblasts: B lineage (CD19, CD20, CD22, CD24); T lineage (CD2, cCD3, CD5, CD7); common ALL antigen (CD10); human leukocyte antigen (HLA)-DR; terminal deoxynucleotidyl transferase (TdT); aberrant myeloid antigens (CD13, CD33); stem cell antigen (CD34)
- Cytochemical stains: myeloperoxidase, negative; Sudan black B, usually negative; TdT, positive; periodic acid–Schiff ± is variable, depending on subtype.
- Cytogenetics: Specific recurring chromosomal abnormalities have independent diagnostic and prognostic significance (hyperdiploidy >50 chromosomes or t[14q11q13] are favorable; the Philadelphia chromosome, t[9;22], t[4;11], −7 and +8 are unfavorable). A translocation t(8;14) or t(2;8) or t(8;22) identifies Burkitt-type mature B-cell leukemia that requires specific therapy.
- Reverse transcription polymerase chain reaction for rapid diagnosis of BCR/ABL + ALL
- HLA typing of patient and siblings for hematopoietic cell transplantation
- Chest CT scan and/or chest radiograph to evaluate for mediastinal mass or hilar adenopathy and for pulmonary infiltrates suggestive of infection
- US exam to assess splenomegaly or renal enlargement suggestive of leukemic infiltration

Diagnostic Procedures/Other

- Bone marrow examination with aspiration, biopsy, immunophenotyping, cytochemistry, cytogenetics, and molecular diagnostics
- Lymph node biopsy is rarely necessary but can be diagnostic.
- Lumbar puncture is typically done both for diagnosis of CNS involvement and for intrathecal treatment. It should be done at diagnosis and immediately if neurologic symptoms or signs are present. Repeat lumbar puncture after bone marrow remission is achieved to evaluate occult CNS involvement and continue prophylactic CNS treatment.

Test Interpretation

Diffuse replacement of marrow and lymph node architecture by sheets of malignant lymphoblasts

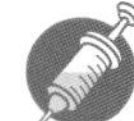

TREATMENT

GENERAL MEASURES

- Appropriate health care
  - Inpatient care during remission induction chemotherapy
  - Postremission therapy is usually outpatient.
- Protective isolation from infection
- Adequate calcium and vitamin D supplementation may reduce bone injury from corticosteroids and avascular necrosis of large joints.

MEDICATION

First Line

Optimal therapy is not yet known (2)[B]. ALL should be treated at a comprehensive oncology center. All treatment regimens are still investigational but clearly effective for some fraction of patients. Younger adults (<40 years old) benefit from pediatric-inspired regimens (3,4)[B]. Cancer and leukemia group B protocol 9111 is an example of therapy (5)[B]:

- Remission induction
  - Cyclophosphamide: 1,200 mg/m^2 IV on day 1 (800 mg/m^2 if ≥60 years old)
  - Daunorubicin: 45 mg/m^2 IV on days 1, 2, and 3 (30 mg/m^2 if ≥60 years old)
  - Vincristine: 2 mg IV on days 1, 8, 15, and 22
  - Asparaginase (L-asparaginase): 6,000 units/m^2 SC or IM on days 5, 8, 11, 15, 18, and 22 (or pegylated asparaginase 2,000 U/m^2 (maximum 3,750 U) given on day 5
  - Prednisone: 60 mg/m^2 on days 1–21 (days 1–7 if ≥60 years old) (or dexamethasone 10 mg/m^2 on days 1–7 and 15–21)
  - Filgrastim, G-CSF: 5 μg/kg/day SC starting on day 4 has been shown to shorten the duration of neutropenia and improve the complete remission rate, especially in older patients.
  - Imatinib mesylate: 600–800 mg/day (or dasatinib 70 mg BID) are effective alone and in combination with chemotherapy for Philadelphia chromosome-positive ALL (6)[B].
- Consolidation (repeat twice in 8 weeks)
  - Cyclophosphamide: 1,000 mg/m^2 IV on day 1
  - Intrathecal (IT) methotrexate: 15 mg with hydrocortisone 50 mg on day 1
  - Mercaptopurine (6-mercaptopurine): 60 mg/m^2/day on days 1–14
  - Cytarabine: 75 mg/m^2/day SC on days 1–4 and 8–11
  - Vincristine: 2 mg IV on days 15 and 22
  - Asparaginase: 6,000 U/m^2 SC or IM on days 15, 18, 22, and 25 (or pegylated asparaginase 2,000 U/m^2 (maximum 3,750 U) on day 15
- CNS prophylaxis and interim maintenance: 24 Gy cranial irradiation
  - IT-methotrexate: 15 mg with hydrocortisone 50 mg on days 1, 8, 15, 22, and 29
  - Mercaptopurine (6-mercaptopurine): 60 mg/m^2/day on days 1–70, taken in the evening
  - Oral methotrexate: 20 mg/m^2 on days 36, 43, 50, 57, and 64
- Late intensification
  - Doxorubicin: 30 mg/m^2 IV on days 1, 8, and 15
  - Vincristine: 2 mg IV on days 1, 8, and 15
  - Dexamethasone: 10 mg/m^2 on days 1–14
  - Cyclophosphamide: 1,000 mg/m^2 IV on day 29
  - Thioguanine (6-thioguanine): 60 mg/m^2 on days 29–42
  - Cytarabine: 75 mg/m^2 SC on days 29–32 and 36–39

- Prolonged maintenance
  - Vincristine: 2 mg/mo IV for 16 months
  - Prednisone: 60 mg/m^2 for 5 days with the vincristine or dexamethasone 10 mg/m^2 on days 1–5
  - Mercaptopurine (6-mercaptopurine): 60 mg/m^2/day for 16 months, taken in the evening
  - Oral methotrexate: 20 mg/m^2/week for 16 months
  - Special: Philadelphia chromosome–positive ALL(6,7)[B]
    - Imatinib mesylate (400–800 mg/day) is effective alone and in combination with chemotherapy.
    - Dasatinib (140 mg/day) is effective in combination with dexamethasone or with chemotherapy.
  - Contraindications: Doses and schedule may need to be altered for older patients and for concurrent infection and organ toxicity (8)[C].
  - Precautions
    - Tumor lysis syndrome (elevated uric acid, potassium, and phosphate with decreased calcium, leading to renal failure, disseminated intravascular coagulation, and cardiac arrhythmias) may be prevented by administering allopurinol 300 mg/day. Begin 2 days before chemotherapy begins. Reduce doses if used with mercaptopurine or azathioprine. Give increased fluids; IV urate oxidase (rasburicase) can be used to treat hyperuricemia rapidly.
    - Oral sulfamethoxazole-trimethoprim or aerosolized pentamidine is given for *Pneumocystis jirovecii* prophylaxis.
    - Profound immunosuppression: Take appropriate precautions when patient is neutropenic.
    - High-dose cyclophosphamide causes severe nausea and vomiting. Use appropriate antiemetic regimen to prevent.
    - Neurotoxicity, ileus with vincristine
    - Asparaginase may cause severe allergic reactions as well as impaired pancreatic and liver function. Monitor serum glucose concentrations frequently and carefully. Pancreatitis or thrombosis may occur. Peg-asparaginase has been approved and can be used IV, SC, or IM in place of native *Escherichia coli* asparaginase.
    - Avascular (osteo)necrosis (AVN) of bone may occur in adolescents and young adults after alkylating agents and corticosteroids.
    - Rituximab (anti-CD20 monoclonal antibody) appears to improve the outcome of patients with ALL if CD20 is expressed on more than 20% of their blast cells.
    - Also note: Burkitt leukemia/lymphoma (mature B-cell ALL-L3)
      - The outcome is clearly better if high-dose methotrexate and alkylating agents are used as part of initial therapy.
      - Only 18 weeks of treatment are required.
      - Rituximab (anti-CD20 monoclonal antibody) improves the outcome of patients with Burkitt leukemia when added to chemotherapy.

Second Line

- Clofarabine has been approved for relapsed childhood ALL. Nelarabine has been approved as a single agent for relapsed T-cell ALL. Pegylated asparaginase (IV or IM) has been used in place of *E. coli*–derived L-asparaginase. Liposomal vincristine has been approved for single-agent use for the treatment of relapsed ALL in adults.
- Other anthracyclines, investigational chemotherapy agents, and monoclonal antibodies (e.g., rituximab; alemtuzumab). Immunoconjugates such as inotuzumab ozogamicin and bifunctional antibodies such as blinatumomab are under investigation.
- Allogeneic hematopoietic stem cell transplantation is recommended for any patient with relapsed ALL or during first remssion if high-risk genetic features are present (9)[B],(10)[A].

ISSUES FOR REFERRAL

ALERT

ALL can become a fatal disorder quickly. As soon as the diagnosis is suspected, patients should be referred immediately to an appropriate oncology center.

SURGERY/OTHER PROCEDURES

Surgical placement of a percutaneous, silastic, double-lumen central venous catheter or a percutaneous intravenous central catheter (PICC)

COMPLEMENTARY & ALTERNATIVE MEDICINE

Unproven; may result in drug interactions with chemotherapy

ONGOING CARE

FOLLOW-UP RECOMMENDATIONS

Ambulatory as tolerated

PATIENT MONITORING

- Daily during induction chemotherapy for metabolic and infectious complications
- Weekly during remission consolidation chemotherapy
- Monthly during maintenance therapy
- Every 3 months thereafter

DIET

- Nutritional support; if needed IV hyperalimentation
- Avoid alcohol.
- Calcium and vitamin D

PATIENT EDUCATION

- Risks of infection, transfusion, chemotherapy
- Stop smoking.

PROGNOSIS

- ~80–95% of adults <60 will achieve a complete remission, and 35–60% will remain free of disease at 5 years.
- Older patients (>60 years) do less well, but 80% may achieve a complete remission.
- Patients with unfavorable cytogenetic subtypes [especially t(9;22) and t(4:11)] should undergo allogeneic stem cell transplantation in 1st remission if an HLA-identical donor is available. Autologous stem cell transplantation should be considered for Ph+ ALL patients who become reverse transcriptase polymerase chain reaction negative for BCR/ABL and lack an allogeneic donor.

COMPLICATIONS

- Infections (*Pneumocystis carinii* pneumonia, bacterial pneumonia or sepsis, fungal pneumonia)
- Bleeding
- Coagulopathy (deep vein thrombosis) from asparaginase therapy
- Need for transfusions
- Sterility from treatment
- Arachnoiditis and CNS effects from intrathecal chemotherapy, high-dose methotrexate and irradiation
- Pancreatitis and liver dysfunction from chemotherapy
- Osteonecrosis of joints (avascular necrosis) related to corticosteroids
- Relapse of ALL in marrow or extramedullary sites (CNS, testis)

REFERENCES

1. Mullighan C. The molecular genetic makeup of acute lymphoblastic leukemia. *Hematology*. 2012;2012:389–396.
2. Bassan R, Hoelzer D. Modern therapy of acute lymphoblastic leukemia. *J Clin Oncol*. 2011;29(5):532–543.
3. Stock W, La M, Sanford B, et al. What determines the outcomes for adolescents and young adults with acute lymphoblastic leukemia treated on cooperative group protocols? A comparison of Children's Cancer Group and Cancer and Leukemia Group B studies. *Blood*. 2008;112:1646–1654.
4. McNeer JL, Raetz EA. Acute lymphoblastic leukemia in young adults: which treatment? *Curr Opin Oncol*. 2012;24(5):487–494.
5. Larson RA, Dodge RK, Linker CA, et al. A randomized controlled trial of filgrastim during remission induction and consolidation chemotherapy for adults with acute lymphoblastic leukemia: CALGB study 9111. *Blood*. 1998;92(5):1556–1564.
6. Stock W. Current treatment options for adult patients with Philadelphia chromosome-positive acute lymphoblastic leukemia. *Leuk Lymphoma*. 2010;51(2):188–198.
7. Foa R, Vitale A, Vignetti M, et al; GIMEMA Acute Leukemia Working Party. Dasatinib as first-line treatment for adult patients with Philadelphia chromosome-positive acute lymphoblastic leukemia. *Blood*. 118(25):6521–6528, 2011.
8. Gokbuget N. How I treat older patients with ALL. *Blood*. 2013;122(8):1366–1375.
9. Mattison RJ, Larson RA. Role of allogeneic hematopoietic cell transplantation in adults with acute lymphoblastic leukemia. *Curr Opin Oncol*. 2009;21(6):601–608.
10. Oliansky DM, Larson RA, Weisdorf D, et al. The role of cytotoxic therapy with hematopoietic stem cell transplantation in the treatment of adult acute lymphoblastic leukemia: update of the 2006 evidence-based review. *Biol Blood Marrow Transplant*. 2012;18:16–17.

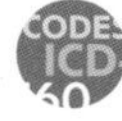

CODES

ICD10

- C91.00 Acute lymphoblastic leukemia not having achieved remission
- C91.01 Acute lymphoblastic leukemia, in remission
- C91.02 Acute lymphoblastic leukemia, in relapse

CLINICAL PEARLS

ALL can become fatal quickly; as soon as diagnosis is suspected, refer the patient to an oncology center. Optimal therapy is not yet known. ALL should be treated at a comprehensive oncology center. All treatment regimens are still investigational but clearly are effective for large fraction of patients.

LEUKEMIA, ACUTE MYELOID

Jan Cerny, MD, PhD, FACP

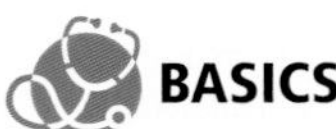

BASICS

DESCRIPTION

- Acute myeloid leukemia (AML) is characterized by proliferation and accumulation of abnormal immature myeloid progenitors (blasts) with reduced capacity to differentiate into more mature cellular elements. This leads to bone marrow failure and results in a variety of systemic symptoms.
- Previously, the French–American–British (FAB) classification system divided AML based on the cell morphology with the addition of cytogenetics (subtypes M0–M7).
- The World Health Organization (WHO) classification attempts to provide more meaningful prognostic information.
  - AML with characteristic genetic abnormalities: translocation t(8;21), t(15;17), and inversion in chromosome 16 inv(16)
  - AML with multilineage dysplasia: presence of a prior myelodysplastic syndrome (MDS) or myeloproliferative neoplasm (MPN) that transformed into AML
  - AML and MDS, therapy related
  - AML not otherwise categorized
  - Acute leukemias of ambiguous lineage (*biphenotypic acute leukemia*)

EPIDEMIOLOGY

- ~13,500 cases diagnosed in 2007; 2nd most common type of leukemia in adults
- Predominant sex: male ≥ female

Incidence

The incidence of AML increases with age, and median age is >70 years.

ETIOLOGY AND PATHOPHYSIOLOGY

Precise causes unknown, but some risk factors have been identified (see "Risk Factors").

Genetics

- Unknown; some are familial.
- Cytogenetics and genetics play an important role in diagnosis and prognosis of AML and have implications for therapy.
- 3 risk groups
  - Good risk: inv(16), t(8;21), t(15;17)
  - Standard risk: normal karyotype
  - Poor risk: monosomy 5 and 7 (typically secondary AML), deletion 5q, abnormalities of 11q23 or complex karyotype
- *FLT3* gene mutations, especially internal transmembrane duplications (FLT3-ITD), have been associated with poor survival in AML. These and growing list of (onco)gene (e.g., *NPM1*, *DNMT3A*, and *P53*) mutations have been studied to further risk-stratify patients (1,2)[A].

RISK FACTORS

- Genetic predisposition (e.g., Down syndrome); other familial disorders are Bloom syndrome (~25% develop AML), Fanconi anemia (52%), neurofibromatosis, Li-Fraumeni syndrome, Wiskott-Aldrich syndrome, Kostmann syndrome, and Diamond-Blackfan anemia.
- Radiation exposure
- Immunodeficiency states
- Chemical and drug exposure (nitrogen mustard and alkylating agents; benzene)
- MDS
- Cigarette smoking

GENERAL PREVENTION

None currently identified, but treatment of high-risk MDS with demethylating agents (Vidaza, 5-azacitidine) has been shown to prolong time to transformation from MDS into AML (3)[A].

COMMONLY ASSOCIATED CONDITIONS

The following are oncologic emergencies:

- Disseminated intravascular coagulopathy (DIC) especially in acute promyelocytic leukemia (APL) but may be seen in any AML
- Leukostasis (high blast number and increased adhesive ability of blasts)
- Tumor lysis syndrome (TLS): spontaneous or in response to chemotherapy

DIAGNOSIS

HISTORY

Fatigue (anemia or tumor burden); bleeding (low platelets or DIC); difficulty clearing infections (neutropenia or immune dysregulation)

PHYSICAL EXAM

- Mostly nonspecific and related to marrow or tissue infiltration
  - Fever
  - Bleeding
  - Pallor
  - Splenomegaly
  - Hepatosplenomegaly
  - Lymphadenopathy (usually reactive)
- If CNS is involved, symptoms of increased intracranial pressure can be present.
- Occasionally, patients will present with prominent extramedullary sites of leukemia (e.g., skin infiltration or ultimately as a myeloid sarcoma).

DIFFERENTIAL DIAGNOSIS

- Virus-induced cytopenia, lymphadenopathy, and organomegaly
- Immune cytopenias (including systemic lupus erythematosus [SLE])
- Drug-induced cytopenias
- Other marrow failure and infiltrative diseases (e.g., aplastic anemia, paroxysmal nocturnal hemoglobinuria, MDSs, Gaucher disease)

DIAGNOSTIC TESTS & INTERPRETATION

- CBC shows subnormal RBCs, neutrophils, and platelets.
- Bone marrow for histology, flow cytometry, and cytogenetics to establish diagnosis and prognosis
- ESR
- Lactate dehydrogenase (LDH) and uric acid can be elevated (e.g., TLS).
- Coagulation profile can be normal or prolonged (e.g., DIC).
- Drugs that may alter lab results: chemotherapy agents, corticosteroids
- Other special tests: Spinal tap may reveal fluid with leukemic cells.
- Ultrasonography or CT scan of the abdomen may discover organomegaly.

Diagnostic Procedures/Other

Bone-marrow studies are usually necessary to make the diagnosis.

- Aspirates: for cell morphology, cytochemistries, immunophenotyping (can confirm differentiation stage of AML); cytogenetics: chromosomal aberration (prognostic value; see "Genetics")
- Biopsies provide valuable information for cellularity, architecture, and so forth.

Test Interpretation

- Marrow is usually hypercellular and the normal architecture effaced; leukemic blast count is 20% or more.
- Liver and spleen may be infiltrated with leukemic cells.

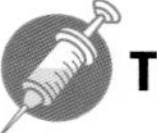

TREATMENT

- Chemotherapy is the backbone of AML therapy; it consists of induction and consolidation phase ± maintenance (APL).
- Bone marrow transplantation (BMT) for high-risk AML
- Only modest improvements have been made in AML induction chemotherapy. Supportive care has improved significantly.

GENERAL MEASURES

- Ongoing assessment of bone marrow, liver, heart, and kidney functions during therapy
- Close monitoring of coagulation parameters (risk for DIC)
- Supportive therapy with
  - Good hydration
  - Transfusions of packed RBCs and platelets based on patient's needs (threshold as for platelets as low as 5,000); use leuko-reduced, irradiated blood products, as all patients can be considered for BMT.
  - Avoid antiplatelet agents (e.g., aspirin products).
  - Follow febrile neutropenic guidelines in neutropenic patient who becomes febrile (even low-grade fever).

Geriatric Considerations

- Older patients (>60–65 years of age) remain a therapeutic challenge. These patients are offered so-called reduced-intensity or nonmyeloablative BMT.
- Adding growth factors (granulocyte-colony stimulating factor [G-CSF]) may reduce toxicity in older patients (but is not broadly accepted).
- Hypomethylating agent, such as 5-azacitidine, significantly prolongs survival in older adults with low marrow blast count (<30%).

Pediatric Considerations

Tolerate intense treatments better

Pregnancy Considerations

Chemotherapy is a viable option in the 2nd and 3rd trimesters.

MEDICATION

First Line

- APL (APL, AML with t[15;17])
  - All-trans retinoic acid (ATRA) and arsenic trioxide both promote maturation to granulocytes.
  - Idarubicin is often added to induction therapy.
- Treatment of AML in younger adults: AML (other than APL)
  - Induction (daunorubicin or idarubicin [anthracycline and cytarabine]): The generally accepted combination is 3 + 7 (anthracycline is given for 3 days and cytarabine for 7 days) or more intensive regimens with high dose of cytarabine (HiDAC) or high dose of anthracycline.
- Remission is typically consolidated in younger patients by the following:
  - In good-risk AML, 3–4 cycles of HiDAC and BMT is reserved for time of recurrence.
  - In poor-risk patients, 1–2 cycles of HiDAC (until donor is identified) are followed by allogeneic BMT.
  - Intermediate-risk AML should be treated based on individual patient's features, donor availability, and access to clinical trials. A meta-analysis showed that even intermediate-risk patients benefit from allogeneic BMT (4)[A].
- Treatment of AML in older adults (>65 years of age) remains a challenge. These patients have poor performance status, more likely secondary AML, higher incidence of unfavorable cytogenetics, comorbidities, shorter remissions, and shorter overall survival.
  - Intensive chemotherapy may be feasible for patients with good performance status; alternative regimens with mitoxantrone, fludarabine, and clofarabine. New drugs (hypomethylating agents as above, FLT3 inhibitors, monoclonal antibodies, etc.) are being studied in clinical trials (5)[A].
- Contraindications: comorbidities; therapy has to be individualized.
- Precautions
  - If organ failure, some drugs may be avoided or dose reduced (e.g., no anthracyclines in patients with preexisting cardiac problems).
  - Patients will be immunosuppressed during treatment. Avoid live vaccines. Administer varicella-zoster or measles immunoglobulin as soon as exposure of patient occurs.
- Significant possible interactions: Allopurinol accentuates the toxicity of 6-mercaptopurine.

Second Line

Healthy, younger patients usually are offered reinduction chemotherapy and allogeneic BMT.

ISSUES FOR REFERRAL

- AML should be managed by specialized team led by a hematologist/oncologist.
- Refer patient to a transplant center early because a search for a donor may be necessary.

SURGERY/OTHER PROCEDURES

- BMT: Decision between myeloablative and nonmyeloablative approach should be based on patient's performance status, comorbidities, and AML risk factors.
  - Allogeneic BMT is acceptable in 1st remission in intermediate- or high-risk AML or in 2nd remission in all other AML patients. Matched related donor used to be preferred over matched unrelated donor (lower risk of graft-versus-host disease); recent data suggest equal outcomes, as allogeneic transplant regimens and posttransplant care have improved significantly.
- Haploidentical transplants and cord blood may be used as alternative sources of hematopoietic stem cells for adults.
- Autologous BMT may be acceptable in specific situations (e.g., no donor is available).

INPATIENT CONSIDERATIONS

Admission Criteria/Initial Stabilization

Induction treatment for AML requires inpatient care, usually on a specialized ward. Episodes of febrile neutropenia typically require admission and IV antibiotics.

IV Fluids

Appropriate hydration to prevent TLS

Nursing

IV may lead to chemical burns in the event of extravasation.

ONGOING CARE

FOLLOW-UP RECOMMENDATIONS

Ambulatory, as tolerated; no intense or contact sports; no aspirin due to risk of bleeding.

Patient Monitoring

- Repeat bone-marrow studies to document remission and also if a relapse is suspected.
- Follow CBC with differential, coagulation studies, uric acid level, and other chemistries related to TLS (creatinine, potassium, phosphate, calcium); monitor urinary function at least daily during induction phase and less frequently later.
- Physical evaluation, including weight and BP, should be done frequently during treatment.

DIET

Ensure adequately balanced calorie/vitamin intake. Total parenteral nutrition (TPN) in case of severe mucositis

PATIENT EDUCATION

- Leukemia Society of America, 600 Third Avenue, New York, NY 10016, 212-573-8484
- National Cancer Institute, Bethesda, MD, has pamphlets and telephone education.
- Baker LS. *You and Leukemia: A Day At a Time*. Philadelphia, PA: Saunders; 1978.

PROGNOSIS

AML remission rate is 60–80%, with only 20–40% long-term survival. The wide variable prognosis is due to prognostic group (age, cytogenetics, and genetics).

COMPLICATIONS

- Acute side effects of chemotherapy, including febrile neutropenia
- TLS
- DIC
- Late-onset cardiomyopathy in patients treated with anthracyclines
- Chronic side effects of chemotherapy (secondary malignancies)
- Graft-versus-host disease in patients who have received allogeneic BMT

REFERENCES

1. Döhner H, Estey EH, Amadori S, et al. Diagnosis and management of acute myeloid leukemia in adults: recommendations from an international expert panel, on behalf of the European LeukemiaNet. *Blood*. 2010;115(3):453–474.
2. Patel JP, Gönen M, Figueroa ME, et al. Prognostic relevance of integrated genetic profiling in acute myeloid leukemia. *N Engl J Med*. 2012;366(12):1079–1089.
3. Fenaux P, Mufti GJ, Hellstrom-Lindberg E, et al. Efficacy of azacitidine compared with that of conventional care regimens in the treatment of higher-risk myelodysplastic syndromes: a randomised, open-label, phase III study. *Lancet Oncol*. 2009;10(3):223–232.
4. Koreth J, Schlenk R, Kopecky KJ, et al. Allogeneic stem cell transplantation for acute myeloid leukemia in first complete remission: systematic review and meta-analysis of prospective clinical trials. *JAMA*. 2009;301(22):2349–2361.
5. Fenaux P, Mufti GJ, Hellström-Lindberg E, et al. Azacitidine prolongs overall survival compared with conventional care regimens in elderly patients with low bone marrow blast count acute myeloid leukemia. *J Clin Oncol*. 2010;28(4):562–569.

ADDITIONAL READING

O'Donnell MR, Appelbaum FR, Coutre SE, et al. Acute myeloid leukemia. *J Natl Compr Canc Netw*. 2008;6(10):962–993.

SEE ALSO

Disseminated Intravascular Coagulation (DIC); Leukemia Acute Lymphoblastic in Adults (ALL); Leukemia, Chronic Myelogenous; Myelodysplastic Syndromes; Myeloproliferative Neoplasms

CODES

ICD10

- C92.00 Acute myeloblastic leukemia, not having achieved remission
- C92.01 Acute myeloblastic leukemia, in remission
- C92.02 Acute myeloblastic leukemia, in relapse

CLINICAL PEARLS

- Prognosis of leukemia depends on the cytogenetic and molecular profile of the disease.
- Allogeneic transplant remains the only therapy with curative potential for patients with intermediate- and high-risk AML.

L

LEUKEMIA, CHRONIC LYMPHOCYTIC

Jan Cerny, MD, PhD, FACP

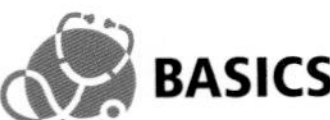

BASICS

DESCRIPTION

- Chronic lymphocytic leukemia (CLL) is a monoclonal disorder characterized by a progressive accumulation of mature but functionally incompetent lymphocytes.
- CLL should be distinguished from prolymphocytic leukemia (PLL); based on percentage of prolymphocytes, the disease may be regarded as CLL (<10% prolymphocytes), PLL (>55% prolymphocytes), or CLL/PLL (>10% and <55% prolymphocytes).
- Small lymphocytic lymphoma is a lymphoma variant of CLL.
- System(s) affected: hematologic; lymphatic; immunologic

EPIDEMIOLOGY

Incidence

- With 15,000–17,000 new cases reported every year, CLL *represents the most common form of leukemia in adults in the United States.*
- In 2013, an estimated 4,580 adults in United States will die from CLL, which makes it the second leading cause of death among adults with leukemia in United States after acute myeloid leukemia (1)[A].
- Predominant age: CLL primarily affects elderly individuals, median age of diagnosis being 70 years. The incidence continues to rise in those age >55 years.
- Predominant sex: male > female (1.7:1)
- The incidence is higher among whites than among African Americans.

ETIOLOGY AND PATHOPHYSIOLOGY

- The cell of origin in CLL is a clonal B cell arrested in the B-cell differentiation pathway, intermediate between pre–B cells and mature B cells. In the peripheral blood, these cells resemble mature lymphocytes and typically show B-cell surface antigens: CD19, CD20, CD21, and CD23. In addition, they express CD5 (usually found on T cells).
- The bcl2 proto-oncogene is overexpressed in B-CLL. Bcl2 is a known suppressor of apoptosis (programmed cell death), resulting in extremely long life of the affected lymphocytes.
  - Unknown, but genetic mutations leading to disrupted function and prolonged survival of affected lymphocytes are suspected.

Genetics

CLL is an acquired disorder, and reports of truly familial cases are exceedingly rare. CLL has been shown; however, to occur at higher frequency among 1st-degree relatives of patients with the disease, and several somatic gene mutations have been identified at significantly higher rates among CLL patients.

RISK FACTORS

- As in the case of most malignancies, the exact cause of CLL is uncertain.
- Possible chronic immune stimulation is suspected but is still being elucidated.
- Monoclonal B-cell lymphocytosis: 1% risk progression to CLL

GENERAL PREVENTION

Unknown

COMMONLY ASSOCIATED CONDITIONS

- Immune system dysregulation is common.
- Autoimmune hemolytic anemia (AIHA) may accompany CLL.
- Immune thrombocytopenic purpura (ITP) may accompany CLL.
- Pure red cell aplasia (PRCA) may accompany CLL.

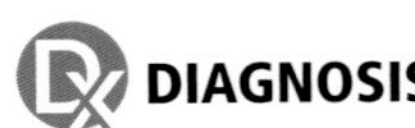

DIAGNOSIS

HISTORY

- Insidious onset; it is not unusual for CLL to be discovered incidentally. Up to 40% of patients are asymptomatic at the time of diagnosis.
- Others may have the following:
  - Repetitive infections (e.g., not only pneumonia but also mucocutaneous herpetic infections)
  - Enlarged lymph nodes
  - Early satiety and/or abdominal discomfort related to an enlarged spleen
  - Mucocutaneous bleeding and/or petechiae due to thrombocytopenia
  - Fatigue-related and/or other symptoms of anemia
  - Fevers, night sweats, >10% weight loss (B symptoms)

PHYSICAL EXAM

- Localized or generalized lymphadenopathy
- Splenomegaly (30–40%)
- Hepatomegaly (20%)
- Mucocutaneous bleeding (thrombocytopenia)
- Skin petechiae (thrombocytopenia)
- Pallor

DIFFERENTIAL DIAGNOSIS

- Infectious causes are the following:
  - Bacterial (tuberculosis)
  - Viral (mononucleosis)
- Malignant causes are the following:
  - Leukemic phase of non-Hodgkin lymphomas
  - Hairy cell leukemia
  - Waldenstrom macroglobulinemia
  - Large granular lymphocytic leukemia

DIAGNOSTIC TESTS & INTERPRETATION

Initial Tests (lab, imaging)

- CBC with differential shows B cell absolute lymphocytosis with >5,000 B lymphocytes/μL. The blood smear also shows ruptured lymphocytes ("smudge" cells) and morphologically mature-appearing small lymphocytes.
- Exam of the blood smear is important in diagnosis of CLL.
- Diagnosis can be confirmed by immunophenotyping: CLL cells are positive for CD19, CD20, and CD24 as well as CD5. They have low levels of surface membrane immunoglobulin (Ig) M or IgD. The monoclonality is proven by the presence of a single immunoglobulin light chain (κ or λ). FMC7 is absent.
- CBC shows anemia and/or thrombocytopenia.
- Plasma β_2-microglobulin may be elevated.
- Serum protein electrophoresis (some patients may have monoclonal gammopathy)
- Lactate dehydrogenase (LDH) may be elevated (due to disease activity or to AIHA).
- Hypogammaglobulinemia
- In cases associated with AIHA, labs consistent with hemolysis may be present (elevated LDH, total bilirubin; reticulocyte count does not have to be elevated due to bone marrow infiltration).
- Liver/spleen ultrasound may demonstrate organomegaly and may also detect enlarged abdominal lymph nodes.
- CT scan of chest/abdomen/pelvis typically is not necessary for staging. However, it may help to identify compression of organs or internal structures from enlarged lymph nodes.
- Positron emission tomography (PET) scan might be helpful to guide biopsy if Richter transformation is suspected (see below).

Follow-Up Tests & Special Considerations

Frequency and type of follow-up depend on severity of symptoms as well as risk factors (see "Prognosis").

Diagnostic Procedures/Other

- Although bone marrow biopsy has its prognostic value (diffuse infiltration is a risk factor), it is not done routinely.
- Consider a lymph node biopsy if lymph node(s) begins to enlarge rapidly in a patient with known CLL to assess the possibility of transformation to a high-grade lymphoma (Richter syndrome), especially when accompanied by fever, weight loss, and pain.

Test Interpretation

- A bone marrow aspirate usually shows >30% lymphocytes.
- Cytogenetic (fluorescence in situ hybridization) may show chromosomal changes, which are prognostic (i.e., del(13q), del(11q), del(17p), trisomy 12, and del(6q)).
- *SF3B1* mutation is associated with rapid disease progression and shorter survival in CLL (2)[A].

TREATMENT

GENERAL MEASURES

Patients with frequent infections associated with hypogammaglobulinemia are likely to benefit from monthly infusions of intravenous immunoglobulin (IVIG).

MEDICATION

First Line

- Most patients are asymptomatic and do not need active treatment unless they have generalized (so-called B) symptoms, progressive marrow failure, AIHA or thrombocytopenia, progressive splenomegaly, massive lymphadenopathy, or progressive lymphocytosis (increase >50% in 2 months or a doubling time of <6 months).
- Low-risk disease, Rai stage 0, and Binet stage A require only periodic follow-up.

- Intermediate-risk group, Rai stages I and II, and Binet stage B could be observed until evidence of disease progression or development of symptoms.
- Treatment should be initiated in high-risk patients, Rai stage III and IV, and Binet stage C.
- Early treatment in low-risk group is not recommended.
- 3 main groups of drugs used are alkylating agents (chlorambucil and, recently, bendamustine), purine analogues (fludarabine and pentostatin), and monoclonal antibodies (rituximab and alemtuzumab).
- Single-agent (fludarabine, bendamustine, or chlorambucil) or combination regimens commonly used
- Fludarabine-based regimens are FC (in combination with cyclophosphamide), FR (fludarabine + rituximab), and FCR (fludarabine + cyclophosphamide + rituximab).
- FCR is the widely used regimen of choice if patient can tolerate it.
- Steroids (prednisone) are useful in patients with autoimmune manifestations of CLL (e.g., AIHA, ITP).

Second Line

- Combinations of chemotherapeutic agents that patient did not fail yet. Occasionally, some patients can be retreated with a drug used previously.
- Alemtuzumab (anti-CD52) has shown activity in relapsed and refractory disease.
- Newer agents, like ofatumumab (novel anti-CD20), lenalidomide, and others, have shown promising activity.
- Ibrutinib, is a Bruton tyrosine kinase (BTK) inhibitor from a novel class of agents, which has a high level of activity in CLL (3)[A].
- Consider splenectomy (surgery/radiation) if massive splenomegaly causes significant anemia and thrombocytopenia.
- Allogenic and autologous stem cell transplant can be considered in high-risk and younger patients (limited data available).

ISSUES FOR REFERRAL

- Surgical consultation for splenectomy in selected patients
- Bone marrow transplant in young patients with refractory disease (however, still considered experimental therapy)
  - Allogeneic hematopoietic stem cell transplant (HSCT) with nonmyeloablative conditioning offers lower treatment-related mortality and may be appropriate for certain patients.

ADDITIONAL THERAPIES

Patients requiring therapy who are high risk for tumor lysis syndrome should be given allopurinol to prevent uric acid nephropathy.

SURGERY/OTHER PROCEDURES

- Splenectomy in selected patients with splenomegaly and refractory cytopenia
- Radiation (if compression symptoms from bulky lymphadenopathy)

INPATIENT CONSIDERATIONS

Admission Criteria/Initial Stabilization

No specific criteria but due to complications of disease (e.g., AIHA) or of therapy (e.g., febrile neutropenia) or significant tumor lysis syndrome after initiation of chemotherapy

ONGOING CARE

FOLLOW-UP RECOMMENDATIONS

Patient Monitoring

Patients with low-risk CLL and/or patients in remission

- CBC with differential (lymphocytosis) every 3–6 months, LDH, β_2-microglobulin, IgG level
- Physical exam (lymphadenopathy, splenomegaly)

DIET

- Ensure adequately balanced calorie/vitamin intake.
- Follow weight.

PATIENT EDUCATION

Leukemia and Lymphoma Society has educational pamphlets: www.webmd.com/cancer/tc/leukemia-topic-overview.

PROGNOSIS

There are 2 staging systems used: the Rai in the United States and the Binet in Europe. Neither is completely satisfactory.

- Rai staging system
  - Stage 0: lymphocytosis only; median survival of 120 months
  - Stage I: lymphocytosis and adenopathy; median survival of 95 months
  - Stage II: lymphocytosis and splenomegaly and/or hepatomegaly; median survival of 72 months
  - Stage III: lymphocytosis and anemia (hemoglobin $<$10 g/dL); median survival of 30 months
  - Stage IV: lymphocytosis and thrombocytopenia (platelets $<100 \times 10^9$/L); median survival of 30 months
- Binet staging system
  - Stage A: hemoglobin $\geq$10 g/dL, platelets 100×10^9, and $<$3 lymph node areas involved (Rai stages 0, I, and II); survival $>$120 months
  - Stage B: hemoglobin and platelet levels as in stage A and 3 or more lymph node areas involved (Rai stages I and II); survival is 61 months.
  - Stage C: hemoglobin $<$100 g/L, platelets $<100 \times 10^9$, or both (Rai stages III and IV); survival is 32 months.
- Adverse risk factors
  - Advanced Rai or Binet stage
  - Peripheral lymphocyte doubling time $<$12 months
  - Diffuse marrow infiltration
  - Increased number of prolymphocytes or cleaved cells
  - Poor response to chemotherapy
  - High β_2-microglobulin and thymidine kinase levels and low micro RNAs (miRNAs)
  - Abnormal karyotyping: deletion 17p (del(17p) *P53* mutation or deletion) and del(11q)
  - New IgVH unmutated status (expression of ZAP-70 $>$20% or CD38 $>$30% evaluated by immunophenotyping are surrogate markers)
  - NOTCH1 mutation (also associated with unmutated IgVH)

COMPLICATIONS

- Acute or long-term effects of chemotherapy
- Richter syndrome (above)
- AIHA (in some cases may be related to the use of fludarabine)
- Slightly increased risk of solid tumors (especially Kaposi sarcoma, malignant melanoma, laryngeal cancers, lung cancers)
- Infection (especially gram negative and encapsulated organisms)
- Membranoproliferative glomerulonephritis (MPGN) or other glomerular pathology

REFERENCES

1. Siegel R, Naishadham D, Jemal A. Cancer statistics, 2013. *CA Cancer J Clin*. 2013;63(1):11–30.
2. Wan Y, Wu CJ. *SF3B1* mutations in chronic lymphocytic leukemia. *Blood*. 2013;121(23):4627–4634.
3. Advani RH, Buggy JJ, Sharman JP, et al. Bruton tyrosine kinase ibrutinib (PCI-32765) has significant activity in patients with relapsed/refractory B-cell malignancies. *J Clin Oncol*. 2013;31(1):88–94.

ADDITIONAL READING

- Chiorazzi N, Rai KR, Ferrarini M. Chronic lymphocytic leukemia. *N Engl J Med*. 2005;352(8):804–815.
- National Comprehensive Cancer Network guidelines: www.nccn.org
- Shanafelt TD, Kay NE. Comprehensive management of the CLL patient: a holistic approach. *Hematology Am Soc Hematol Educ Program*. 2007:324–331.

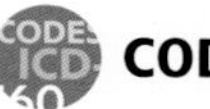

CODES

ICD10

- C91.10 Chronic lymphocytic leuk of B-cell type not achieve remis
- C91.11 Chronic lymphocytic leukemia of B-cell type in remission
- C91.12 Chronic lymphocytic leukemia of B-cell type in relapse

CLINICAL PEARLS

- CLL represents the most common form of leukemia in adults in the United States.
- Predominant age: CLL primarily affects elderly individuals, median age of diagnosis being 70 years. The incidence continues to rise in those age $>$55 years.
- Clinical monitoring of asymptomatic and low-risk patients is a reasonable approach ("watch and wait").
- High-risk patients, bulky disease, or patients who fail fludarabine- and rituximab-based therapies have typically poor prognosis and may require intensive therapies, including allogeneic transplantation.
- Median survival is 3–10 years, depending on stage.

LEUKEMIA, CHRONIC MYELOGENOUS

Jan Cerny, MD, PhD, FACP

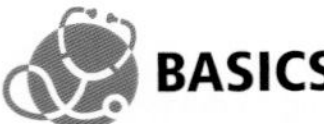

BASICS

DESCRIPTION

- Chronic myelogenous leukemia (CML) is a myeloproliferative neoplasm characterized by clonal proliferation of myeloid precursors in the bone marrow with continuing differentiation into mature granulocytes.
- Hallmark of CML is Philadelphia chromosome [translocation t(9;22)].
- Natural history of the disease evolves in 3 clinical phases: a chronic phase, an accelerated phase, and blast phase or crisis (transformation to acute leukemia).

EPIDEMIOLOGY

Incidence

- Per year, 1.6 cases/100,000 persons
- Predominant age: 50–60 years
- Predominant sex: male > female (1.3:1)

Prevalence

Accounts for 15–20% of adult leukemias

ETIOLOGY AND PATHOPHYSIOLOGY

Philadelphia chromosome is a balanced translocation between *BCR* (on chromosome 22) and *ABL* (on chromosome 9) genes t(9;22)(q34;q11). This fusion gene, *BCR-ABL*, codes for an abnormal constitutively active tyrosine kinase that affects numerous signal transduction pathways, resulting in uncontrolled cell proliferation and reduced apoptosis.

Genetics

Acquired genomic changes

RISK FACTORS

Ionizing radiation exposure (uncommon)

GENERAL PREVENTION

None currently identified

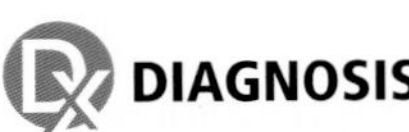

DIAGNOSIS

85–90% of patients present in the chronic phase, and the disease can be found accidentally during routine screening.

HISTORY

- Chronic phase: fatigue, weight loss, night sweats, abdominal fullness owing to enlarged spleen, early satiety, dyspnea, bleeding. Rare: bruising, left upper quadrant abdominal pain, sternal pain (owing to expanding bone marrow), and gouty arthritis; up to 30% of patients are asymptomatic.
- Accelerated phase: progressive splenomegaly and left upper quadrant abdominal pain occasionally referred to the left shoulder (owing to splenic infarction or rupture), progressive weight loss and sweats, unexplained fever or bone pain, chloromas (extramedullary tumors)
- Blast phase: bleeding, bruising, infections, prominent constitutional symptoms

PHYSICAL EXAM

- Splenomegaly (50–90%), hepatomegaly (up to 50%)
- Less common: splenic friction rub, lymphadenopathy

DIFFERENTIAL DIAGNOSIS

- Chronic myelomonocytic leukemia, chronic neutrophilic leukemia, chronic eosinophilic leukemia, juvenile myelomonocytic leukemia, infectious mononucleosis, leukemoid reaction, polycythemia vera, and treatment with granulocyte-stimulating factors
- Acute myelogenous leukemia resembles blast crisis with myeloid blasts, and acute lymphoblastic leukemia resembles blast crisis with lymphoid blasts.
- Atypical CML is a chronic myeloproliferative disorder with a clinical hematologic picture similar to CML, but it lacks Philadelphia chromosome and *BCR-ABL* rearrangement.

DIAGNOSTIC TESTS & INTERPRETATION

- CBC
  - Hematocrit: may be normal, slightly increased, or decreased
  - WBC count: markedly increased (50,000–100,000/μL), with granulocytes in all stages of development, including occasional blasts <10% in chronic phase, basophilia, eosinophilia
  - Platelets: normal, elevated (34%), or occasionally low
  - In accelerated phase: anemia, 10–19% blood or marrow blasts, basophils plus eosinophils >20%, thrombocytopenia
  - Blast phase: blood or marrow blasts >20%
- Genetics
  - Demonstration of the Philadelphia chromosome, t(9;22), by cytogenetic techniques, fluorescence in situ hybridization (FISH), or reverse-transcription-polymerase chain reaction (RT-PCR)
  - Additional cytogenetic abnormalities occur in the accelerated and blast phases [monosomy 7, t(3,21), trisomies 8 and 19, Philadelphia chromosome duplication, abnormalities of chromosome 17 such as monosomy, trisomy, and isochromosome mutations]. These may contribute to resistance to tyrosine kinase inhibitors (TKIs; e.g., imatinib). Further molecular testing (mutations within *BCR-ABL*) is suggested in case of loss of response to therapy.
- Others:
  - Low or absent leukocyte alkaline phosphatase in neutrophils
  - High lactate dehydrogenase (LDH)
  - Elevated uric acid

Initial Tests (lab, imaging)

- CBC, LDH, uric acid, bone marrow biopsy and aspirate, cytogenetics on bone marrow, and FISH for *BCR-ABL*, RT-PCR, LFTs
- Abdominal ultrasound or CT scan shows splenomegaly; not mandatory

Follow-Up Tests & Special Considerations

- Mutation analysis of tyrosine kinase domain of *ABL* kinase, as they may cause resistance to therapy with TKIs
- HLA-A*02 positive is associated with CML, and a protective effect is seen with the HLA-B*35 allele (pooled odds ratio 0.64, 95% confidence interval 0.48–0.86).

Diagnostic Procedures/Other

Bone marrow aspiration and biopsy

Test Interpretation

Myeloid hyperplasia with elevated myeloid: erythroid ratio, normal maturation, marrow basophilia, and increased reticulin fibrosis

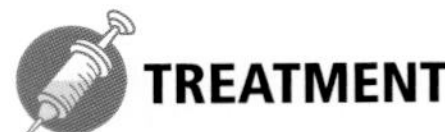

TREATMENT

MEDICATION

- TKIs (e.g., imatinib) provide durable, long-term control of disease.
- The response to TKIs is assessed at specific time points from the beginning of treatment and is categorized as follows:
  - Complete hematologic response (CHR): normalization of peripheral counts, no disease symptoms, no immature cells
  - Minor/partial/complete cytogenetic response (CCR): 1–34%, 35–90%, no Philadelphia-positive metaphases
  - Major molecular response (MMR): decreased level of *BCR-ABL* transcript by PCR 3-log
  - Complete molecular response (CMR): *BCR-ABL* transcript is undetectable by PCR.

First Line

- Imatinib mesylate (Gleevec), an oral TKI, 400 mg/day
- Side effects: thrombocytopenia, anemia, elevated liver enzymes, edema, GI disturbances, rash
- International Randomized Study of Interferon versus STI571 (IRIS) established imatinib as 1st-line therapy (1)[A].

- Imatinib dose can be increased to 600 and 800 mg/day if only suboptimal response is achieved with standard dose.
- 2nd-generation TKIs have shown higher efficacy and fewer side effects and are approved for 1st-line therapy of chronic phase CML: nilotinib (Tasigna) and dasatinib (Sprycel) (2,3)[A].

Second Line

- Dasatinib, 2nd-generation TKI, active against most of *BRC-ABL* mutants, not active in *T315I* mutation
  - 100 mg/day in patients resistant or intolerant to imatinib and 70 mg BID for patients in accelerated or blastic phase
  - Side effects: pleural effusions, cytopenias
- Nilotinib, also 2nd-generation TKI, highly selective and more potent *BCR-ABL* TKI, active against most *BRC-ABL* mutants, not active in *T315I* mutation
  - 400 mg PO BID in patients resistant or intolerant to imatinib in chronic or accelerated phase
  - Side effects: cytopenias, QTc prolongation, pancreatitis
- Bosutinib and omacetaxine are now approved for patient who failed or did not tolerate 2 TKIs previously. Ponatinib has now more restricted approval, but together with omacetaxine they are the only effective agents in patients with *T315I* mutation. Agents targeting leukemic stem cells are being developed for clinical use.

ISSUES FOR REFERRAL

All patients with CML should be referred to a hematologist. Patients with inadequate response to TKIs or with *T315I* mutation should consult with a bone marrow transplant physician.

SURGERY/OTHER PROCEDURES

Allogenic bone marrow transplant (BMT)

- It is the only known cure; however, 71% of patients who achieve CCR with imatinib maintain that response for 7 years, and no patient progressed on the trial between years 5 and 6 of treatment.
- Most effective in patients <50 years of age who are in the chronic phase.
- Initial mortality is higher (related to the use of myeloablative regimens) than medical management but provided higher rates of survival in pre-TKI era.
- Significant improvement in transplant techniques leading to better outcomes, such as alternative sources of stem cells; nonmyeloablative regimens have shown improvements in transplant-related mortality.
- Transplant option should be thoroughly discussed with young patients in chronic phase and considered an alternative to TKIs especially if the patient does not tolerate TKIs or disease is not responding.
- Can be considered in patients who fail to achieve CHR by 3 months, have no cytogenetic response or cytogenetic relapse, or have *T315I* mutation

INPATIENT CONSIDERATIONS

Admission Criteria/Initial Stabilization

Acute abdominal symptoms (infarcted or ruptured spleen); tumor lysis syndrome owing to initial therapy; complications of BMT

- Hydroxyurea might be given, with the goal of reduction of the WBC count, but it has minimal impact on patient response to TKIs.
- Induction chemotherapy (for acute leukemia) in setting of blastic phase
- Allopurinol to prevent tumor lysis syndrome in patients with very high counts; however, probably not necessary when TKIs are used

Discharge Criteria

Abatement of acute symptoms

ONGOING CARE

FOLLOW-UP RECOMMENDATIONS

- Frequency depends on stage at presentation and response to 1st-line therapy.
- Although splenomegaly persists, avoid contact sports or trauma to abdomen.

Patient Monitoring

- CBC with differential: weekly until blood counts stable, then every 2–4 weeks during CHR; once in CCR and stable, patient can be followed less frequently (3-month intervals).
- Bone marrow cytogenetics (evaluation for clonal evolution) every 6 months while in CHR, every 12–18 months while in complete cytogenic response, MMR, CMR
- Quantitative RT-PCR every 3 months (peripheral blood)
- ECGs (concern for QT prolongation), LFTs while on TKIs. Nilotinib, bosutinib, and ponatinib can cause pancreatitis.

PROGNOSIS

- With treatment and good response, the survival is similar to the normal population.
- Without treatment: CML invariably will progress to accelerated phase within 2–5 years and blast phase within several months of the accelerated phase.
- Poor prognosis: patients presenting in accelerated or blastic phase or presenting with very large spleen size, platelets >700,000/μL, and patients resistant to TKIs (*T315I* mutation)

COMPLICATIONS

- Splenic infarct or rupture
- Progression to accelerated or blastic phase
- Thrombotic events owing to elevated platelets
- Bleeding owing to low or dysfunctional platelets
- Sequelae of anemia

REFERENCES

1. O'Brien SG, Guilhot F, Goldman JM, et al. International randomized study of interferon versus STI571 (IRIS) 7-year follow-up: sustained survival, low rate of transformation and increased rate of major molecular response (MMR) in patients (pts) with newly diagnosed chronic myeloid leukemia in chronic phase (CMLCP) treated with imatinib (IM). *ASH Ann Meeting Abstracts*. 2008;112:186.
2. Saglio G, Kim DW, Issaragrisil S, et al. Nilotinib versus imatinib for newly diagnosed chronic myeloid leukemia. *N Engl J Med*. 2010;362(24):2251–2259.
3. Kantarjian H, Shah NP, Hochhaus A, et al. Dasatinib versus imatinib in newly diagnosed chronic-phase chronic myeloid leukemia. *N Engl J Med*. 2010;362(24):2260–2270.

ADDITIONAL READING

- Kantarjian HM, Baccarani M, Jabbour E, et al. Second-generation tyrosine kinase inhibitors: the future of frontline CML therapy. *Clin Cancer Res*. 2011;17(7):1674–1683.
- Kantarjian H, Pasquini R, Hamerschlak N, et al. Dasatinib or high-dose imatinib for chronic-phase chronic myeloid leukemia after failure of first-line imatinib: a randomized phase 2 trial. *Blood*. 2007;109(12):5143–5150.
- Naugler C, Liwski R. Human leukocyte antigen class I alleles and the risk of chronic myelogenous leukemia: a meta-analysis. *Leuk Lymphoma*. 2010;51(7):1288–1292.

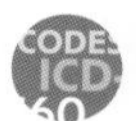

CODES

ICD10

- C92.10 Chronic myeloid leukemia, BCR/ABL-positive, not having achieved remission
- C92.11 Chronic myeloid leukemia, BCR/ABL-positive, in remission
- C92.12 Chronic myeloid leukemia, BCR/ABL-positive, in relapse

CLINICAL PEARLS

- CML belongs to the myeloproliferative disorders group.
- The gold standard for diagnosis of CML is detection of the Philadelphia chromosome or its products, *BCR-ABL* mRNA, and fusion protein.
- TKIs provide durable, long-term control of the disease and have dramatically altered treatment.
- Atypical CML is a form of clinically typical CML but without the presence of the typical *BCR-ABL* translocation.
- Blast crisis is a form of acute leukemia that is a possible complication of CML.

LEUKOPLAKIA, ORAL

Christine K. Jacobs, MD, FAAFP

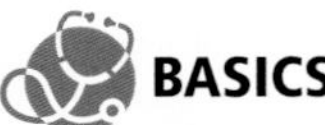

BASICS

DESCRIPTION

- Oral leukoplakia is defined by the World Health Organization as white plaques of questionable risk having excluded (other) known diseases or disorders that carry no increased risk for cancer (1)[C].
- System(s) affected: gastrointestinal

EPIDEMIOLOGY

- Develops in middle age, increases with age
- Most common in India, where more people smoke and chew tobacco and areca nuts

Prevalence

- 1–3% of the adult population is affected.
- Usual age of onset is over 40 years with peak in the 60s.
- Males twice as often as females

Geriatric Considerations

Malignant transformation to carcinoma is more common in older patients.

ETIOLOGY AND PATHOPHYSIOLOGY

Hyperkeratosis or dyskeratosis of the oral squamous epithelium

- Tobacco use in any form
- Alcohol consumption/alcoholism
- Oral infections
- *Candida albicans* infection may induce dysplasia and increase malignant transformation (2)[B].
- Human papillomavirus, types 11 and 15
- Sunlight
- Vitamin deficiency
- Syphilis
- Dental restorations/prosthetic appliances
- Estrogen therapy
- Chronic trauma or irritation
- Epstein-Barr virus (oral hairy leukoplakia)
- Areca nut/betel (Asian populations)
- Mouthwash preparations and toothpaste containing the herbal root extract sanguinaria

Genetics

- Dyskeratosis congenital and epidermolysis bullosa increase the likelihood of oral malignancy (1)[B].
- P53 overexpression correlates with leukoplakia and particularly squamous cell carcinoma (3)[B].

RISK FACTORS

- 70–90% of oral leukoplakia is related to tobacco, particularly smokeless tobacco or areca/betel nut use.
- Repeated or chronic mechanical trauma from dental appliances or cheek biting
- Chemical irritation to oral regions
- Diabetes
- Age
- Socioeconomic status
- Risk factors for malignant transformation of leukoplakia
  - Female
  - Long duration of leukoplakia
  - Nonsmoker (idiopathic leukoplakia)
  - Located on tongue or floor of mouth
  - Size >200 mm^2
  - Nonhomogenous type
  - Presence of *C. albicans*
  - Presence of epithelial dysplasia

GENERAL PREVENTION

- Avoid tobacco of any kind, alcohol, habitual cheek biting, tongue chewing.
- Use well-fitting dental prosthesis.
- Regular dental check-ups to avoid bad restorations
- Diet rich in fresh fruits and vegetables may help to prevent cancer.
- HPV vaccination may be preventive.

COMMONLY ASSOCIATED CONDITIONS

- HIV infection is closely associated with hairy leukoplakia.
- Erythroplakia in association with leukoplakia, "speckled leukoplakia," or erythroleukoplakia is a marker for underlying dysplasia.

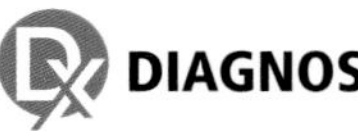

DIAGNOSIS

Leukoplakia is an asymptomatic white patch on the oral mucosa.

HISTORY

- Usually asymptomatic
- History of tobacco or alcohol use or oral exposure to irritants

PHYSICAL EXAM

- Location
  - 50% on tongue, mandibular alveolar ridge, and buccal mucosa
  - Also seen on maxillary alveolar ridge, palate, and lower lip
  - Infrequently seen on floor of the mouth and retromolar areas
  - Floor of mouth, ventrolateral tongue, and soft palate complex are more likely to have dysplastic lesions.
- Appearance
  - Varies from homogeneous, nonpalpable, faintly translucent white areas to thick, fissured, papillomatous, indurated plaques
  - May feel rough or leathery
  - Lesions can become exophytic or verruciform.
  - Color may be white, gray, yellowish white, or brownish gray.
  - Cannot be wiped or scraped off
- World Health Organization classification (1)
  - Homogeneous refers to color.
    - Flat, corrugated, wrinkled or pumice
  - Nonhomogeneous refers to color and texture (more likely to be dysplastic or malignant).
    - Erythroleukoplakia (mixture of red and white)
    - Exophytic: papillary or verrucous texture

DIFFERENTIAL DIAGNOSIS

- White oral lesions that can be wiped away: acute pseudomembranous candidiasis
- White oral lesions that cannot be rubbed off (1)
  - Morsicatio buccarum (habitual cheek-biting), generally benign (4)[C]
  - Chemical injury
  - Acute pseudomembranous candidiasis
  - Traumatic or frictional keratosis (e.g., linea alba)
  - Leukoedema (benign milky opaque lesions that disappear with stretching)
  - Aspirin burn (from holding aspirin in cheek)
  - Lichen planus (bilateral fairly symmetric lesions, reticular pattern of slightly raised gray-white lines)
  - Lichenoid reaction
  - Verrucous carcinoma
  - Discoid lupus erythematosus
  - Skin graft (known history)
  - Squamous cell carcinoma
  - Oral hairy leukoplakia, commonly on the lateral border of the tongue with a bilateral distribution (in HIV patients with Epstein-Barr virus infection)
  - Smoker's palate (leukokeratosis nicotina palati)
  - White sponge nevus (congenital benign spongy lesions)
  - Syphilitic oral lesion
  - Dyskeratosis congenita (a rare inherited multisystem disorder)

DIAGNOSTIC TESTS & INTERPRETATION

Biopsy to rule out carcinoma if lesion is persistent, changing, or unexplained

Initial Tests (lab, imaging)

- Laboratory tests generally are not indicated.
  - Consider saliva culture if *C. albicans* infection is suspected.
- No imaging is indicated.

Follow-Up Tests & Special Considerations

- Biopsy is necessary to rule out carcinoma if lesion is persistent, changing, or unexplained (1).
- Consider CBC, rapid plasma reagin (RPR).

Diagnostic Procedures/Other

- Oral cytology is superior to conventional oral examination (5)[A].
- Computer-assisted cytology or liquid-based cytology is not superior to oral cytology (5)[A].
- Noninvasive brush biopsy and analysis of cells with DNA–image cytometry constitute a sensitive and specific screening method.
- Patients with dysplastic or malignant cells on brush biopsy should undergo more formal excisional biopsy (1).
- Excisional biopsy is definitive procedure.

Test Interpretation

- Biopsy specimens range from hyperkeratosis to invasive carcinoma.
- At initial biopsy, 6% are invasive carcinoma.
- 0.13–6% subsequently undergo malignant transformation.
- Location is important: 60% on floor of mouth or lateral border of tongue are cancerous; buccal mucosal lesions are generally not malignant but require biopsy if not resolving.

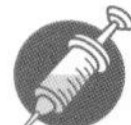

TREATMENT

- All oral leukoplakias should be treated.
- Treatment may include the following:
  - For 2–3 circumscribed lesions, surgical excision
  - For multiple or large lesions where surgery would cause unacceptable deformity, consider cryosurgery, or laser surgery (6)[C].
  - Removal of predisposing habits (alcohol and tobacco)
- Complete excision is standard treatment for dysplasia or malignancy.
- After treatment, up to 30% of leukoplakia recurs, and some leukoplakia still transforms to squamous cell carcinoma (6)[B].

GENERAL MEASURES

- Eliminate habitual lip biting.
- Correct ill-fitting dental appliances, bad restorations, or sharp teeth.
- Stop smoking and using alcohol.
- Some small lesions may respond to cryosurgery.
- Beta-carotene, lycopene, retinoids, and cyclooxygenase 2 (COX-2) inhibitors may cause partial regression.
- For hairy tongue: tongue brushing

MEDICATION

Carotenoids, vitamins A, C, and K, bleomycin, and photodynamic therapy ineffective to prevent malignant transformation and recurrence (7)[A]

ISSUES FOR REFERRAL

Consider otolaryngologist or oral surgery referral for extensive disease.

SURGERY/OTHER PROCEDURES

- Scalpel excision, laser ablation, electrocautery, or cryoablation (8)[C]
- Cryotherapy slightly less effective than photodynamic therapy response (73% vs. 90%) and recurrence (27% vs. 24%) (9)[A]
- CO_2 laser had 20% recurrence and 10% malignant transformation within 5 years (10)[B].

INPATIENT CONSIDERATIONS

Admission Criteria/Initial Stabilization

- Eliminate etiologic factors.
- Reevaluate in 7–14 days.
- Biopsy if lesion is persistent.

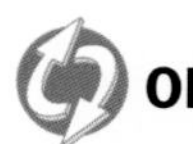

ONGOING CARE

FOLLOW-UP RECOMMENDATIONS

Patient Monitoring

- Regular, close follow-up, even after successful treatment
- Biopsy as needed

DIET

Regular

PATIENT EDUCATION

- If biopsy is negative, stress importance of periodic and careful follow-up.
- Initiate a dental referral to eliminate dental factors.
- Stress importance of stopping tobacco and alcohol use.
- Encourage participation in smoking cessation program.

PROGNOSIS

- Most leukoplakia is benign.
- Leukoplakia may regress, remain stable, or progress.
- 0.13–6% of initially benign lesions subsequently develop into cancer.
- More likely to be cancerous if on floor of mouth or lateral border of tongue

COMPLICATIONS

- New lesions may develop after treatment.
- Risk of malignant transformation to squamous cell carcinoma is approximately 5–17% (11)[B].
- Larger lesions and nonhomogeneous leukoplakia are associated with higher rates of malignant transformation.

REFERENCES

1. Warnakulasuriya S, Johnson N, van der Wall I. Nomenclature and classification of potentially malignant disorders of the oral mucosa. *J Oral Pathol Med*. 2007;36(10):575–580.
2. Cao J, Liu HW, Jin JQ, et al. The effect of oral candida to development of oral leukoplakia into cancer. *Zhonghua Yu Fang Yi Xue Za Zhi*. 2007;41(Suppl):90–93.
3. Duarte EC, Ribeiro DC, Gomez MV, et al. Genetic polymorphisms of carcinogen metabolizing enzymes are associated with oral leukoplakia development and *p53* overexpression. *Anticancer Res*. 2008;28(2A):1101–1106.
4. Cam K, Santoro A, Lee JB, et al. Oral frictional hyperkeratosis (morsicatio buccarum): an entity to be considered in the differential diagnosis of white oral mucosal lesions. *Skinmed*. 2012;10(2):114–115.
5. Fuller C, Camilon R, Nguyen S, et al. Adjunctive diagnostic techniques for oral lesions of unknown malignant potential: systematic review with meta-analysis [published online ahead of print March 5, 2014]. *Head Neck*. doi:10.1002/hed.23667
6. Feller L, Lemmer J. Oral leukoplakia as it relates to HPV infection: a review. *Int J Dent*. 2012;2012:540561.
7. Ribeiro AS, Salles PR, da Silva TA, et al. A review of the nonsurgical treatment of oral leukoplakia. *Int J Dent*. 2010;2010:186018.
8. Kumar A, Cascarini L, McCaul JA, et al. How should we manage oral leukoplakia? *Br J Oral Maxillofac Surg*. 2013;51(5):377–383.
9. Kawczyk-Krupka A, Waśkowska J, Raczkowska-Siostrzonek A, et al. Comparison of cryotherapy and photodynamic therapy in treatment of oral leukoplakia. *Photodiagnosis Photodyn Ther*. 2012;9(2):148–155.
10. Jerjes W, Upile T, Hamdoon Z, et al. CO2 laser of oral dysplasia: clinicopathological features of recurrence and malignant transformation. *Lasers Med Sci*. 2012;27(1):169–179.
11. Rhodus NL, Kerr A, Patel K. Oral cancer leukoplakia, premalignancy, and squamous cell carcinoma. *Dent Clin North Am*. 2014;58(2):315–340.

ADDITIONAL READING

- Lodi G, Sardella A, Bez C, et al. Interventions for treating oral leukoplakia. *Cochrane Database Syst Rev*. 2006;(4):CD001829.
- Nair D, Pruthy R, Pawar U, et al. Oral cancer: premalignant conditions and screening—an update. *J Cancer Res Ther*. 2012;8(Suppl 1):s57–s66.
- Reamy BV, Derby R, Bunt CW. Common tongue conditions in primary care. *Am Fam Physician*. 2010;81(5):627–634.
- Warnakulasuriya S, Dietrich T, Bornstein MM, et al. Oral health risks of tobacco use and effects of cessation. *Int Dent J*. 2010;60(1):7–30.

SEE ALSO

Epstein-Barr Virus Infections; HIV/AIDS

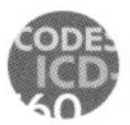

CODES

ICD10

- K13.21 Leukoplakia of oral mucosa, including tongue
- K13.3 Hairy leukoplakia

CLINICAL PEARLS

- Excisional biopsy is indicated for any undiagnosed leukoplakia.
- After treatment, up to 30% of leukoplakia recurs, and some leukoplakia still transforms to squamous cell carcinoma; thus, long-term surveillance is essential.
- To lessen risk of malignant transformation, encourage tobacco and alcohol cessation and consider *C. albicans* eradication.

L

LICHEN PLANUS

Mercedes E. Gonzalez, MD, FAAD • Herbert P. Goodheart, MD

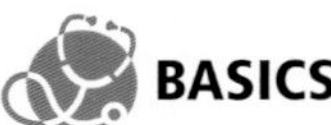

BASICS

Lichen planus (LP) is an idiopathic eruption with characteristic shiny, flat-topped (Latin: *planus*, "flat") purple (violaceous) papules and plaques on the skin, often accompanied by characteristic mucous membrane lesions. Itching may be severe.

DESCRIPTION

- Classic (typical) LP is a relatively uncommon inflammatory disorder of the skin and mucous membranes; hair and nails may also be affected.
  - Skin lesions are small, flat, angular, red-to-violaceous, shiny, pruritic papules and/or plaques with overlying fine, white lines (called Wickham striae) or gray-white puncta; most commonly seen on the flexor surfaces of the upper extremities, extensor surfaces of the lower extremities, the genitalia, and on the mucous membranes
  - On the oral mucosa, lesions typically appear as raised white lines in a lacelike pattern seen most often on the buccal mucosa.
  - Onset is abrupt or gradual. Course is unpredictable; may resolve spontaneously, recur intermittently, or persist for many years.
- Drug-induced LP
  - Clinical and histopathologic findings may mimic those of classic LP. Lesions usually lack Wickham striae (see in the following text), and oral involvement is rare.
  - There is generally a latent period of months from drug introduction until lesions appear.
  - Lesions resolve when the inciting agent is discontinued, often after a prolonged period.
- LP variants
  - Follicular: also called lichen planopilaris; typically seen on the scalp, can lead to scarring alopecia
  - Annular: Papules spread centrifugally as central area resolves; occur on glans penis, axillae, and oral mucosa
  - Linear: may be an isolated finding
  - Hypertrophic: itchy, hyperkeratotic, thick plaques on dorsal legs and feet
  - Atrophic: rare, most often the result of resolved lesions
  - Bullous LP: Intense inflammation in the dermis leads to blistering of epidermis.
  - LP pemphigoides: a combination of LP and bullous pemphigoid (IgG autoantibodies to collagen 17)
  - Nail LP: affects the nail matrix, lateral thinning, longitudinal ridging, and fissuring
- System(s) affected: skin/exocrine
- Synonym(s): lichenoid eruptions

EPIDEMIOLOGY

- Predominant age: 30–60 years old; rare in children and the geriatric population
- Predominant sex: female > male

Prevalence

In the United States, 450/100,000

ETIOLOGY AND PATHOPHYSIOLOGY

LP is considered to be a T-cell–mediated autoimmune response to self-antigens on damaged keratinocytes.

RISK FACTORS

Exposure to certain drugs or chemicals

- Thiazides, furosemide, β-blockers, sulfonylureas, antimalarials, penicillamine, gold salts, and angiotensin-converting enzyme inhibitors
- Rarely: photo-developing chemicals, dental materials, tattoo pigments

COMMONLY ASSOCIATED CONDITIONS

- An association has been noted between LP and hepatitis C virus infection, particularly in certain geographic regions (Asia, South America, the Middle East, Europe) (1)[A]. Hepatitis should be considered in patients with widespread presentations of LP and those with primarily oral disease.
- In addition, chronic active hepatitis, lichen nitidus, and primary biliary cirrhosis have been noted to coexist with LP.
- Association with dyslipidemia has been reported (2)[B].
- LP has also been reported in association with other diseases of altered immunity, more often than would be expected by chance.
  - Bullous pemphigoid
  - Alopecia areata
  - Myasthenia gravis
  - Vitiligo
  - Ulcerative colitis
  - Graft versus host reaction
  - Lupus erythematosus (lupus erythematosus–LP overlap syndrome)
  - Morphea and lichen sclerosis et atrophicus

DIAGNOSIS

LP is most commonly diagnosed by its appearance despite its range of clinical presentations. A skin biopsy should be performed if the diagnosis is in doubt.

HISTORY

A minority of patients have a family history of LP. Affected families have an increased frequency of human leukocyte antigen B7 (HLA-B7). A thorough drug history should be performed.

PHYSICAL EXAM

- Skin (often severe pruritus)
  - Papules: 1–10 mm, shiny, flat-topped (planar) lesions that occur in crops; lesions may have a fine scale.
  - Evidence of scratching (i.e., crusts and excoriations) is usually absent.
  - Color: violaceous, with white lacelike pattern (Wickham striae) on surface of papules. Wickham striae are best seen after topical application of mineral oil and, if present, are virtually pathognomonic for LP.
  - Shape: polygonal or oval. Annular lesions may appear on trunk and mucous membranes. Various shapes and sizes may be noted (polymorphic).
  - Arrangement: may be grouped, linear, or scattered individual lesions
  - Koebner phenomenon (isomorphic response): New lesions may be noted at sites of minor injuries, such as scratches or burns.
  - Distribution: ventral surface of wrists and forearms, dorsa hands, glans penis, dorsa feet, groin, sacrum, shins, and scalp. Hypertrophic (verrucous) lesions may occur on lower legs and may be generalized.
  - Postinflammatory hyperpigmentation: Lesions typically heal, leaving darkly pigmented macules in their wake.
- Mucous membranes (40–60% of patients with skin lesions; 20% have mucous membrane lesions without skin involvement)
  - Most commonly asymptomatic, nonerosive, milky-white lines with an elegant, lacy, netlike streaked pattern
  - Usually seen on buccal mucosa but may appear on tongue, gingiva, palate, or lips
  - Less commonly, LP may be erosive; rarely bullous
  - Painful, especially if ulcers present
  - Lesions may develop into squamous cell carcinoma (1–3%).
  - Glans penis, labia minora, vaginal vault, and perianal areas may be involved.
- Hair/scalp
  - LP of the hair follicle (lichen planopilaris) presents with keratotic plugs at the follicle orifice with a violaceous rim; may result in atrophy and permanent destruction of hair follicles (scarring alopecia)
- Nails (10%)
  - Involvement of nail matrix may cause proximal-to-distal linear grooves and partial or complete destruction of nail bed with pterygium formation.

DIFFERENTIAL DIAGNOSIS

- Skin
  - Lichen simplex chronicus
  - Eczematous dermatitis
  - Psoriasis
  - Discoid lupus erythematosus
  - Other lichenoid eruptions (those that resemble LP)
  - Pityriasis rosea
  - Lichen nitidus
- Oral mucous membranes
  - Leukoplakia
  - Oral hairy leukoplakia
  - Candidiasis
  - Squamous cell carcinoma (particularly in ulcerative lesions)
  - Aphthous ulcers
  - Herpetic stomatitis
  - Secondary syphilis
- Genital mucous membranes
  - Psoriasis (penis and labia)
  - Nonspecific balanitis, Zoon balanitis
  - Fixed drug eruption (penis)
  - Candidiasis (penis and labia)
  - Pemphigus vulgaris, bullous pemphigoid, and Behçet disease (all rare)
- Hair and scalp
  - Scarring alopecia (central centrifugal cicatricial alopecia)

DIAGNOSTIC TESTS & INTERPRETATION

If suggested by history

- Serology for hepatitis
- Liver function tests

Diagnostic Procedures/Other
- Skin biopsy
- Direct immunofluorescence helps to distinguish LP from discoid lupus erythematosus.

Test Interpretation
- Dense, bandlike (lichenoid) lymphocytic infiltrate of the upper dermis
- Vacuolar degeneration of the basal layer
- Hyperkeratosis and irregular acanthosis, increased granular layer
- Basement membrane thinning with "saw-toothing"
- Degenerative keratinocytes, known as colloid or Civatte bodies, are found in the lower epidermis.
- Melanin pigment in macrophages

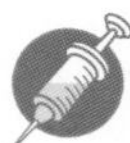

TREATMENT

Although LP can resolve spontaneously, treatment is usually requested by patients who may be severely symptomatic or troubled by its cosmetic appearance.

GENERAL MEASURES
- Goal is to relieve itching and resolve lesions
- Asymptomatic oral lesions require no treatment.

MEDICATION
First Line
- Skin
- Superpotent topical steroids (e.g., 0.05% clobetasol propionate) BID for 2 weeks
  - Potent topical steroids such as triamcinolone acetonide 0.1% or fluocinonide 0.05% under occlusion
  - Intralesional corticosteroids (e.g., triamcinolone [Kenalog] 5–10 mg/mL) for recalcitrant and hypertrophic lesions
  - Antihistamines (e.g., hydroxyzine, 25 mg PO q6h) have limited benefit for itching but may be helpful for sedation at bedtime.
  - "Soak and smear" technique: can lead to a rapid improvement of symptoms in even 1–2 days and may obviate the need for systemic steroids. Soaking allows water to hydrate the stratum corneum and allows the anti-inflammatory steroid in the ointment to penetrate more deeply into the skin. Smearing of the ointment traps the water in the skin because water cannot move out through greasy materials.
    - Soaking is done in a bathtub using lukewarm plain water for 20 minutes, then, without drying the skin, the affected area is immediately smeared with a thin film of the steroid ointment containing clobetasol or another superpotent topical steroid.
    - Soak and smear may be done for 4–5 days or longer, if necessary. The treatments are best done at night because the greasy ointment applied to the skin gets on pajamas (instead of on daytime clothes) and the ointment is on the skin during sleep. A topical steroid cream is applied thereafter during the daytime hours, if necessary.
- Mucous membranes
  - For oral, erosive, painful LP, a Cochrane review found at best weak evidence for the effectiveness of any intervention (3)[A].
    - Topical corticosteroids (0.1% triamcinolone [Kenalog] in Orabase) or 0.05% clobetasol propionate ointment BID
    - Intralesional corticosteroids
    - Topical 0.1% tacrolimus (Protopic ointment) BID or 1% pimecrolimus (Elidel) cream BID. A Cochrane review found no evidence that calcineurin inhibitors are better than placebo (4)[A].
    - Topical retinoids (e.g., 0.05% tretinoin [retinoic acid] in Orabase)

Pediatric Considerations
Children may absorb a proportionally larger amount of topical steroid because of larger skin surface-to-weight ratio.

Second Line
Skin and mucous membranes
- Intralesional corticosteroids
- Topical 0.1% tacrolimus (Protopic ointment) BID or topical 1% pimecrolimus (Elidel) cream BID
- Oral prednisone: used only for a short course (e.g., 30–60 mg/day for 2–4 weeks) or IM triamcinolone (Kenalog) 40–80 mg every 6–8 weeks
  - Precautions with systemic steroids
    - Systemic absorption of steroids may result in hypothalamic-pituitary-adrenal axis suppression, Cushing syndrome, hyperglycemia, or glucosuria.
    - Increased risk with high-potency topical steroids (i.e., use over large surface area, prolonged use, occlusive dressings)
    - In pregnancy: usually safe, but benefits must outweigh the risks
- Oral retinoids: Isotretinoin in doses of 10 mg PO daily for 2 months, acitretin 30 mg, or alitretinoin 30 mg PO daily have resulted in improvement in some refractory cases. Observe carefully for resultant dyslipidemia.
- Oral metronidazole 500 mg BID for 20–60 days can be given as a safer alternative to systemic corticosteroids.
- Cyclosporine may be used in severe cases, but cost and potential toxicity limit its use; topical use for severe oral involvement refractory to other treatments
- Thalidomide
- Psoralen ultraviolet-A (PUVA), broad- or narrow-band ultraviolet-B (UVB) (5)
- Griseofulvin
- Azathioprine
- Mycophenolate mofetil
- Metronidazole

ALERT
Avoid oral and topical retinoids during pregnancy.

INPATIENT CONSIDERATIONS
Admission Criteria/Initial Stabilization
Outpatient care

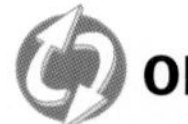

ONGOING CARE

FOLLOW-UP RECOMMENDATIONS
Patient Monitoring
Serial oral examinations for erosive/ulcerative lesions

PATIENT EDUCATION
- Oral, erosive, or ulcerative LP: annual follow-up to screen for malignancy (6)[A]
- Avoid spicy foods, cigarettes, and excessive alcohol.
- Avoid dry crispy foods such as corn chips, pretzels, and toast.

PROGNOSIS
- Spontaneous resolution in weeks is possible, but disease may persist for years, especially oral lesions and hypertrophic lesions on the shins.
- There is a tendency toward relapse.
- Recurrence in 12–20%, especially in those with generalized involvement

COMPLICATIONS
- Alopecia
- Nail destruction
- Squamous cell carcinoma of the mouth or genitals

REFERENCES

1. Shengyuan L, Songpo Y, Wen W, et al. Hepatitis C virus and lichen planus: a reciprocal association determined by a meta-analysis. *Arch Dermatol*. 2009;145(9):1040–1047.
2. Arias-Santiago S, Buendía-Eisman A, Aneiros-Fernández J, et al. Cardiovascular risk factors in patients with lichen planus. *Am J Med*. 2011;124(6):543–548.
3. Cheng S, Kirtschig G, Cooper S, et al. Interventions for erosive lichen planus affecting mucosal sites. *Cochrane Database Syst Rev*. 2012;(2):CD008092.
4. Thongprasom K, Carrozzo M, Furness S, et al. Interventions for treating oral lichen planus. *Cochrane Database Syst Rev*. 2011;(7):CD001168.
5. Pavlotsky F, Nathansohn N, Kriger G, et al. Ultraviolet-B treatment for cutaneous lichen planus: our experience with 50 patients. *Photodermatol Photoimmunol Photomed*. 2008;24(2):83–86.
6. Fitzpatrick SG, Hirsch SA, Gordon SC. The malignant transformation of oral lichen planus and oral lichenoid lesions: a systematic review. *J Am Dent Assoc*. 2014;145(1):45–56.

ADDITIONAL READING

- Fazel N. Cutaneous lichen planus: a systematic review of treatments. *J Dermatolog Treat*. 2014;9:1–4.
- Kolios AG, Marques Maggio E, Gubler C, et al. Oral, esophageal and cutaneous lichen ruber planus controlled with alitretinoin: case report and review of the literature. *Dermatology*. 2013;226(4):302–310.

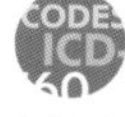

CODES

ICD10
- L43.9 Lichen planus, unspecified
- L43.0 Hypertrophic lichen planus
- L43.1 Bullous lichen planus

CLINICAL PEARLS
- Remember the 7 P's of LP: **p**urple, **p**lanar, **p**olygonal, **p**olymorphic, **p**ruritic (not always), **p**apules that heal with **p**ostinflammatory hyperpigmentation.
- Serial oral or genital exams are indicated for erosive/ulcerative LP lesions to monitor for the development of squamous cell carcinoma.
- An association has been noted between LP and hepatitis C virus infection, chronic active hepatitis, and primary biliary cirrhosis.
- The "soak and smear" technique can lead to a rapid improvement of symptoms in 1–2 days and may obviate the need for systemic steroids.

L

LICHEN SIMPLEX CHRONICUS

Vibin Roy, MD • Manjula Julka, MD, FAAFP

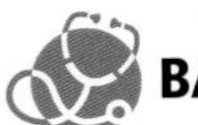

BASICS

DESCRIPTION

- Lichen simplex chronicus (LSC) is a chronic dermatitis resulting from chronic, repeated rubbing or scratching of the skin. Skin becomes thickened with accentuated lines ("lichenification").
- System(s) affected: skin
- Synonym(s): LSC; lichen simplex; localized neurodermatitis; neurodermatitis circumscripta

EPIDEMIOLOGY

Geriatric Considerations

Most common in middle aged and elderly

Pediatric Considerations

Rare in preadolescents

Incidence

- Common
- Peak incidence 35–50 years
- Predominant sex: females > males (2:1)

Prevalence

Common

ETIOLOGY AND PATHOPHYSIOLOGY

- Common triggers are excess dryness of skin, heat, sweat, and psychological stress.
- Scratching may be secondary to habit or a conditioned response to anxiety.
- The formation of an itch–scratch cycle leads to a chronic dermatosis. Repeated scratching or rubbing causes inflammation and pruritus → continued scratching.
- Secondary forms begin as a pruritic skin disease that evolves into neurodermatitis after resolution of the primary dermatitis. Precursor dermatoses include atopic dermatitis, contact dermatitis, lichen planus, stasis dermatitis, psoriasis, fungal infections, and insect bites.
- There is a possible relation between disease development and underlying neuropathy, particularly radiculopathy or nerve root compression.
- Pruritus-specific C neurons are temperature sensitive, which may explain itching that occurs in warm environments.

RISK FACTORS

- Anxiety disorders
- Dry skin
- Insect bites

GENERAL PREVENTION

Avoid common triggers such as psychological distress, environmental factors such as heat and excessive dryness, skin irritation, and the development of pruritic dermatoses.

COMMONLY ASSOCIATED CONDITIONS

- Prurigo nodularis is a nodular variety of the same disease process.
- Atopic dermatitis
- Anxiety, depression, and obsessive-compulsive disorders

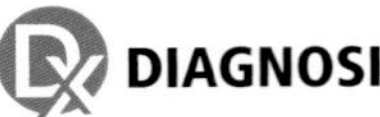

DIAGNOSIS

HISTORY

- Gradual onset
- Begins as a localized area of pruritus
- Most patients acknowledge that they respond with vigorous rubbing, itching, or scratching, which brings temporary satisfaction.
- Pruritus is typically paroxysmal, worse at night, and may lead to scratching during sleep.

PHYSICAL EXAM

- Well-defined plaques of thickened skin with varying amounts of overlying excoriation or scaling
- Accentuation of normal skin lines (lichenification)
- In cases of long-standing duration, hyperpigmentation or hypopigmentation can be seen.
- Scarring may result following ulcer formation or secondary infection.
- Most commonly involves easily accessible areas
  - Lateral portions of lower legs/ankles
  - Nape of neck
  - Vulva/scrotum/anus
  - Extensor surfaces of forearms
  - Scalp

DIFFERENTIAL DIAGNOSIS

- Psoriasis
- Atopic dermatitis
- Contact, irritant, or stasis dermatitis
- Extramammary Paget disease
- Lichen planus
- Mycosis fungoides
- Lichen amyloidosis
- Fungal infection
- Nummular eczema

DIAGNOSTIC TESTS & INTERPRETATION

Initial Tests (lab, imaging)

- None are diagnostic.
- Microscopy (i.e., KOH prep) and culture preparation may be helpful in identifying a superimposed bacterial or fungal infection.

Diagnostic Procedures/Other

- Skin biopsy to identify characteristic changes on pathology can be beneficial if the diagnosis is in question.
- Patch testing may be used to rule out a contact dermatitis.

Test Interpretation

- Hyperkeratosis
- Acanthosis
- Lengthening of rete ridges
- Hyperplasia of all components of epidermis
- Mild to moderate lymphohistiocytic inflammatory infiltrate with prominent lichenification

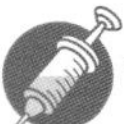

TREATMENT

GENERAL MEASURES

- Patient education
- Treat pruritus to interrupt the scratch–itch cycle (1):
  - Itching may occur at night while the patient is asleep; occlusion may be helpful in these cases.
- Treat underlying pruritic skin conditions.

MEDICATION

First Line

- Reducing inflammation
  - Topical steroids are 1st-line agents (2,3)[C].
  - High-potency steroids alone, such as 0.05% betamethasone dipropionate cream or 0.05% clobetasol propionate cream, can be used initially but not on the face, anogenital region, or intertriginous areas. They should be used on small areas only, for no longer than 2 weeks except under the close supervision of a physician.
  - Switch to intermediate- or low-potency steroids as response allows.
  - An intermediate-potency steroid, such as 0.1% triamcinolone cream, may be used for initial, brief treatment of the face and intertriginous areas, and for maintenance treatment of other areas.
  - A low-potency steroid, such as 1% hydrocortisone cream, should be used for maintenance treatment of the face and intertriginous areas.
  - Steroid tape, flurandrenolide, has optimized penetration and provides a barrier to continued scratching. Change tape once daily.
  - Intralesional steroids, such as triamcinolone acetate, are also safe and effective.
  - Contraindications: High-potency topical steroids should not be used on the face or intertriginous areas.
  - Precautions: Topical steroid therapy can cause epidermal and dermal atrophy, as well as hypopigmentation.
- Preventing the itch–scratch cycle:
  - Antipruritic agents such as 1% menthol preparations and pramoxine
  - 1st-generation oral antihistamines such as diphenhydramine and hydroxyzine for antipruritic and sedative effects
  - Sedating tricyclics, such as doxepin and amitriptyline, for nighttime itching

Second Line

All recommendations

- Topical aspirin has been shown to be helpful in treating neurodermatitis (4).
- Topical 5% doxepin cream has significant antipruritic activity.
- Topical capsaicin cream can be helpful for treatment of early disease manifestations.
- A case report showed that topical 0.1% tacrolimus was effective in treating LSC of the face.

- Topical pimecrolimus may decrease the symptoms of vulvar LSC.
- Gabapentin was found to decrease symptoms in patients who are nonresponsive to steroids.
- Botulinum toxin injected intradermally has been reported to improve symptoms in patients with recalcitrant pruritus (5).
- Transcutaneous electrical nerve stimulation may relieve pruritus in patients for whom topical steroids were not effective (6).
- SSRIs may be effective in controlling compulsive scratching.

ISSUES FOR REFERRAL

- No response to treatment
- Presence of signs and symptoms suggestive of a systemic cause of pruritus
- Consultation with a psychiatrist for patients with severe stress, anxiety, or compulsive scratching
- Consultation with an allergist for patients with multisystemic atopic symptoms

ADDITIONAL THERAPIES

- Cooling of the skin with ice or cold compresses
- Soaks and lubricants to improve barrier layer function
- Provide barrier protection with bandages or Unna boots.
- Nail trimming

COMPLEMENTARY AND ALTERNATIVE MEDICINE

- Cognitive-behavioral therapy may improve awareness and help to identify coping strategies.
- Hypnosis may be beneficial in decreasing pruritus and preventing scratching.
- Homeopathic remedies (i.e., thuja and graphites) have been used.

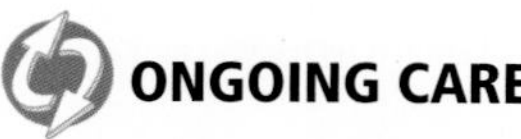

ONGOING CARE

FOLLOW-UP RECOMMENDATIONS

Patient Monitoring

Patients should be followed closely and regularly for response to therapy, complications from therapy, and secondary infections.

DIET

Regular balanced diet

PATIENT EDUCATION

- Patients should understand the cause of this disease and their role in its resolution:
  - Emphasize that scratching and rubbing must stop for lesions to heal.
- Stress reduction techniques can be useful for patients for whom stress plays a role.
- Avoid exposure to known triggers.

PROGNOSIS

- Often chronic and recurrent
- Good prognosis if the itch–scratch cycle can be broken
- After healing, the skin should return to normal appearance but may also retain accentuated skin markings or postinflammatory hyperpigmentation.
- Postinflammatory pigmentary changes may be slow to resolve.

COMPLICATIONS

- Secondary infection
- Scarring is rare.
- Complications related to therapy, as mentioned in medication precautions
- Squamous cell carcinoma within affected regions is rare.

REFERENCES

1. Lotti T, Buggiani G, Prignano F. Prurigo nodularis and lichen simplex chronicus. *Dermatol Ther*. 2008;21(1):42–46.
2. Lynch PJ. Lichen simplex chronicus (atopic/neurodermatitis) of the anogenital region. *Dermatol Ther*. 2004;17(1):8–19.
3. Brunner N, Yawalkar S. A double-blind, multicenter, parallel-group trial with 0.05% halobetasol propionate ointment versus 0.1% diflucortolone valerate ointment in patients with severe, chronic atopic dermatitis or lichen simplex chronicus. *J Am Acad Dermatol*. 1991;25(6, Pt 2):1160–1163.
4. Yosipovitch G, Sugeng MW, Chan YH, et al. The effect of topically applied aspirin on localized circumscribed neurodermatitis. *J Am Acad Dermatol*. 2001;45(6):910–913.
5. Heckmann M, Heyer G, Brunner B, et al. Botulinum toxin type A injection in the treatment of lichen simplex: an open pilot study. *J Am Acad Dermatol*. 2002;46(4):617–619.
6. Yüksek J, Sezer E, Aksu M, et al. Transcutaneous electrical nerve stimulation for reduction of pruritus in macular amyloidosis and lichen simplex. *J Dermatol*. 2011;38(6):546–552.

ADDITIONAL READING

- Aschoff R, Wozel G. Topical tacrolimus for the treatment of lichen simplex chronicus. *J Dermatolog Treat*. 2007;18(2):115–117.
- Engin B, Tufekci O, Yazici A, et al. The effect of transcutaneous electrical nerve stimulation in the treatment of lichen simplex: a prospective study. *Clin Exp Dermatol*. 2009;34(3):324–328.
- Gencoglan G, Inanir I, Gunduz K. Therapeutic hotline: treatment of prurigo nodularis and lichen simplex chronicus with gabapentin. *Dermatol Ther*. 2010;23(2):194–198.
- Goldstein AT, Parneix-Spake A, McCormick CL, et al. Pimecrolimus cream 1% for treatment of vulvar lichen simplex chronicus: an open-label, preliminary trial. *Gynecol Obstet Invest*. 2007;64(4):180–186.
- Hercogová J. Topical anti-itch therapy. *Dermatol Ther*. 2005;18(4):341–343.
- Kirtak N, Inaloz HS, Akçali C, et al. Association of serotonin transporter gene-linked polymorphic region and variable number of tandem repeat polymorphism of the serotonin transporter gene in lichen simplex chronicus patients with psychiatric status. *Int J Dermatol*. 2008;47(10):1069–1072.
- Konuk N, Koca R, Atik L, et al. Psychopathology, depression and dissociative experiences in patients with lichen simplex chronicus. *Gen Hosp Psychiatry*. 2007;29(3):232–235.
- Shenefelt PD. Biofeedback, cognitive-behavioral methods, and hypnosis in dermatology: is it all in your mind? *Dermatol Ther*. 2003;16(2):114–122.
- Solak O, Kulac M, Yaman M, et al. Lichen simplex chronicus as a symptom of neuropathy. *Clin Exp Dermatol*. 2009;34(4):476–480.
- Wu M, Wang Y, Bu W, et al. Squamous cell carcinoma arising in lichen simplex chronicus. *Eur J Dermatol*. 2010;20(6):858–859.

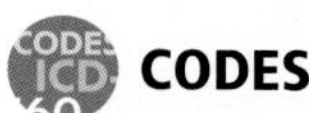

CODES

ICD10

L28.0 Lichen simplex chronicus

CLINICAL PEARLS

- Primary lichen simplex chronicus originates de novo, whereas secondary lichen simplex chronicus occurs in the setting of a pruritic dermatologic condition.
- This is a chronic inflammatory condition that results from repeated scratching and rubbing.
- The diagnosis is made clinically, based on history and skin examination.
- If the diagnosis is unclear, consider empiric treatment with close monitoring or skin biopsy.
- Stopping the itch–scratch cycle through patient education, skin lubrication, and topical antipruritic medications is key.

LIPOMA

Bradley M. Turner, MD, MPH, MHA

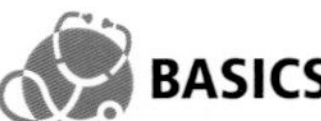

BASICS

DESCRIPTION

- Lipomas are the most common soft tissue tumor (benign or malignant).
- One of several distinct benign lipomatous tumors. In its most conventional (simple) form, lipomas are composed of mature adipose tissue, typically enveloped by a well-defined thin fibrous capsule.
- Not distinguishable histologically from normal adipose tissue
- Several nonconventional forms of lipomas (less commonly encountered) have been described, which may present in multiple locations, contain varying amounts of both adipose and nonadipose tissue, and/or have more atypical cytologic features.
- These nonconventional variants include chondroid lipoma, myolipoma, lipoblastoma, angiolipoma, spindle cell lipoma/pleomorphic lipoma, intramuscular/intermuscular lipoma, lipoma of tendon sheath and joint, lipoma arborescens, lipomatosis of nerve, diffuse lipomatosis, multiple symmetric lipomatosis, adiposis dolorosa, and hibernoma. Typically slow growing, superficial (subcutaneous), and asymptomatic; less commonly presents as a painful (angiolipoma) or deep-seated lesion
- May present as an infiltrative lesion (cellular angiolipoma, diffuse lipomatosis, multiple symmetric lipomatosis (Madelung disease), and adiposis dolorosa (Dercum disease)
- Often found in the upper trunk, especially the shoulders, back, neck, and head, but can be found anywhere in the body
- Lipomas have been reported in anatomic locations as varied as cardiac, intrathoracic, endobronchial, retroperitoneal, breast, calf, thigh, scapular, intraosseous, fingers, palmar, toe, epidural, spinal, intra-articular (knee), parapharyngeal, nasopharyngeal, adrenal, inguinal, bladder, scrotal, ovarian, intracranial, intraneural, and GI tract (most often in the ileum).
- Lipomas can cause respiratory distress due to bronchial obstruction of major airways, GI obstruction or bleeding, neuropathic symptoms from compression in locations such as the forearm or ankle, or cord compression if in dural/medullary components of the spinal cord.
- Must be differentiated from other tumors, particularly liposarcomas, as treatment protocols differ

EPIDEMIOLOGY

- Lipomas can occur at any age but most commonly occur in middle-aged adults, typically in the 40–60-year-old age group.
- Hibernomas typically present in the 3rd decade.
- Conventional lipomas and most variants are rare in children; however, lipoblastoma and diffuse lipomatosis typically present in children younger than 3 years of age.
- No clear gender predilection in conventional lipomas and most variants.
- Females reportedly more commonly diagnosed with: chondroid lipoma, myolipoma, and adiposis dolorosa.
- Males reportedly more commonly diagnosed with spindle cell/pleomorphic lipoma, intramuscular/intermuscular lipoma, lipoblastoma, and multiple symmetric lipomatosis.
- Approximately 5% of patients have multiple lipomas.

Incidence

Has been reported as 2.1 per 1,000 individuals per year; however, incidence is difficult to accurately estimate.

Prevalence

Has been reported as present in ≈1% the population; however, as with incidence, prevalence is difficult to accurately estimate, and is most likely underestimated.

ETIOLOGY AND PATHOPHYSIOLOGY

- The etiology and pathogenesis of lipomas is unclear.
- A pathogenetic link between soft tissue trauma and the formation of lipomas has been suggested.
- Two potential explanations to correlate soft tissue trauma and adipose tissue tumor growth have been proposed:
  - Formation of so-called posttraumatic pseudolipomas by prolapsing adipose tissue through fascia resulting from direct impact
  - Lipoma formation as a result of preadipocyte differentiation and proliferation mediated by cytokine release following soft tissue trauma and hematoma formation

Genetics

- Approximately 2/3 of lipomas are characterized by chromosomal aberrations.
- The most common chromosomal aberrations are rearrangements of the chromatin remodeling gene *HMGA2* on chromosome 12q15 (67%).
- Less common chromosomal aberrations include anomalies of the 13q12–22 region (15%) and rearrangements of the 6p21 region (5%).
- Frequent association of chromosomal aberrations in the long arm of chromosomes 13 and 16 with spindle cell/pleomorphic lipomas
- Consistent chromosomal aberrations identified in the long arm of chromosome 11 with hibernomas
- Various case reports of other chromosomal aberrations exist.

RISK FACTORS

- Because the pathogenesis of lipomas is unclear, risk factors are difficult to qualify.
- Possible risk factors include obesity, alcohol abuse, liver disease, glucose intolerance, and soft tissue trauma (see "Etiology and Pathophysiology").

COMMONLY ASSOCIATED CONDITIONS

May appear as part of a hereditary syndrome: Dercum disease, Madelung syndrome (also known as Launois-Bensaude syndrome), Gardner syndrome, Cowden syndrome, and Bannayan-Riley-Ruvalcaba syndrome (children)

DIAGNOSIS

HISTORY

- Useful questions on history are duration, associated symptoms, tenderness, recurrence, progression, similar lesions, and weight loss.
- Lipomas are generally slow growing—if the presenting lesion is fast growing, suspect another diagnosis.

PHYSICAL EXAM

- Lipomas are usually soft, homogeneous, oval, and nontender, with a rubbery or doughy consistency; if hard, suspect another diagnosis.
- The overlying skin is typically mobile and normal in appearance; if erythematous, suspect another diagnosis such as infection.
- Lipomas are commonly ≤5 cm in diameter. If larger, this raises suspicion for liposarcoma (1), although lipomas can be >10 cm (2,3).

DIFFERENTIAL DIAGNOSIS

- Differential diagnosis includes a variety of benign and malignant tumors (1,4).
- The most common considerations include epidermal inclusion cyst, trichilemmal cysts, hematoma, vasculitis, panniculitis, rheumatic nodules, abscess/infection, and malignant disease.
- Trichilemmal cysts can often be differentiated from lipomas by their characteristic central punctum and surrounding induration.
- An abscess typically has pain, along with overlying induration and erythema.
- Diagnosis may be more challenging with other lesions, particularly deeper-seated lesions.
- Imaging, core needle biopsy, or excision can be useful in further clarifying the diagnosis (1,2,3,4).

DIAGNOSTIC TESTS & INTERPRETATION

Patients presenting with smaller (≤5 cm) subcutaneous lesions that are clinically considered lipomas typically will not receive preoperative imaging. Larger lesions with irregular shape and/or suggestion of myofascial involvement should receive preoperative imaging (1)[A].

Initial Tests (lab, imaging)

- Because of differences in treatment, prognosis, and long-term follow-up, it is important to preoperatively distinguish lipomas from liposarcomas and other malignant lesions (2–6).
- Ultrasonography (US), magnetic resonance imaging (MRI), or computed tomography (CT) can be used in the suspected diagnosis of lipoma (1,2).
- US may be limited with larger lesions or lesions which have atypical patterns (2).
- MRI is the most sensitive imaging modality for lipomatous masses, has a high negative predictive value (1)[A], and can be useful when US is equivocal (2)[A].
- MRI can be extremely helpful in distinguishing a lipoma from a liposarcoma (1,2)[B], although lipoma variants may show characteristics of a liposarcoma due to the presence of decreased adipose tissue, nonadipose tissue, and/or irregular margins.
- MRI findings suggestive of liposarcoma include nonadipose areas, a partially ill-defined margin, neurovascular involvement, enhancing thick/nodular septum, a bright signal intensity on T1 weighted images that are not completely suppressed on T1 fat suppression images, and a high T2 signal within the lesion (1–3).

Diagnostic Procedures/Other

- If diagnosis is in doubt, an open surgical incisional biopsy has traditionally been considered the "gold standard" to obtain a histologic diagnosis (4).
- A core-needle biopsy has been proposed as a preferred biopsy method that can provide accurate diagnosis and assessment of malignant potential if examined by an experienced pathologist (4)[C].
- Fine needle aspiration cytology is not considered appropriate for the initial diagnostic evaluation of mesenchymal tumors (4).

Test Interpretation

- Pathologic interpretation is still generally considered the "gold standard" of diagnosis (1,4).
- Lipomas are typically composed of benign adipose tissue, with inconspicuous nuclei and varying amounts of connective tissue.
- Lipomas are typically surrounded by a fibrous, well-defined thin capsule that is separate from the surrounding tissue; however, this may not be present on the microscopic tissue due to sampling bias.
- Atypical features such as prominent or atypical nuclei, inflammation, fibrosis, and necrosis may be present and may be mistaken for atypical features seen in atypical lipomatous tumor/well differentiated liposarcoma (ALT/WDL) (5).
- Pathologists may overcall a diagnosis of ALT/WDL in lipomas with atypical features (1,5,6).
- Complementary molecular testing may augment histologic diagnosis in challenging cases, as MDM2 gene amplification is not present in benign lipomas but has been reported to be a highly sensitive marker in ALT/WDL (3,5,6)[B].

TREATMENT

- If diagnostically certain that the lesion is a benign lipoma, observation is a consideration.
- Treatment of lipoma typically consists of surgical excision; however, advances in medical treatment can shrink lipomas (1)[A].
- Treatments like steroid injection or liposuction can be cosmetically useful in superficial lesions, particularly in locations where scars should be avoided (1)[A], although liposuction has not always been associated with the best aesthetic outcomes (1)[C].
- A successful trial of lipomas treated with subcutaneous deoxycholate injections has been reported, suggesting that low-concentration deoxycholate may be a relatively safe and effective treatment for small collections of adipose tissue (1)[C].
- Indications for removal of a suspected lipoma include diagnostic uncertainty, cosmetic concerns, nerve impingement, pain, increase in size, irregular characteristics, size >5 cm, samples of a core needle biopsy consistent with atypical features, or features consistent with a sarcoma (1)[A].

SURGERY/OTHER PROCEDURES

- Surgical removal techniques include enucleation/excisional biopsy and open incisional biopsy (1,4).
- In uncomplicated cases, the excision can be performed in the office or in the minor procedure room under local anesthetic.
- Plan the incision to follow skin lines, if possible, to minimize scarring. Use a surgical marker to draw out the palpable margins of the lipoma and the planned incision. The incision should be ≈50–75% of the length of the lipoma along Langer lines (defined as parallel skin creases correlating with the direction of least elasticity) (1)[C].
- After anesthetizing the skin with a local anesthetic, a linear incision is carried out down to the level of the capsule using a number 11 or 15 blade.
- Blunt dissection (curved hemostat) and sharp dissection (iris scissor) are used to separate the fibrous capsule from the surrounding soft tissue. Care must be taken not to invade the capsule to maintain proper aesthetics (1).
- As the lobule is lifted, the dissection is continued to free up the entire tumor.
- Apply pressure to the outside of the lipoma to express it through the skin opening. In many cases, the lipoma will simply pop out. If not, more dissection may be needed, or the incision may need to be lengthened.
- After the lipoma is out, pressure with gauze is usually all that is needed to obtain good hemostasis. If bleeding persists, use electrocoagulation before closing the incision (1).
- If necessary, dead space may be closed with deep absorbable sutures. The skin may be closed with nonabsorbable simple interrupted sutures or skin adhesive.
- A minimal scar technique to facilitate removal from a small incision using segmental dissection of the lipoma has been described (1)[B].
- It is advisable to send all biopsied tissue to pathology (1)[C].

ONGOING CARE

FOLLOW-UP RECOMMENDATIONS

Usual surgical follow-up is needed to monitor for any complications.

PATIENT EDUCATION

Handout: "What are lipomas?" *Am Fam Physician*. 2002;65:905. Available at: http://www.aafp.org/afp/20020301/905ph.html

PROGNOSIS

Most lipomas grow very slowly, are asymptomatic, and remain stable. Recurrence after excision is rare (1–2%), unless the excision was incomplete.

COMPLICATIONS

- Hematoma and seroma formation are the most common complications.
- Infection is rare but possible.
- The risk of recurrence is greatest with intramuscular lipomas and lipomas with infiltrating tendencies (cellular angiolipoma, diffuse lipomatosis, multiple symmetric lipomatosis, and adiposis dolorosa).
- Occasionally a bilobar lipoma may be missed, resulting in "recurrence."

REFERENCES

1. Pandya KA, Radke F. Benign skin lesions: lipomas, epidermal inclusion cysts, muscle and nerve biopsies. *Surg Clin North Am*. 2009;89(3):677–687.
2. Strauss DC, Qureshi YA, Hayes AJ, et al. The role of core needle biopsy in the diagnosis of suspected soft tissue tumours. *J Surg Oncol*. 2010;102(5):523–529.
3. Jaovisidha S, Suvikapakornkul Y, Woratanarat P, et al. MR imaging of fat-containing tumours: the distinction between lipoma and liposarcoma. *Singapore Med J*. 2010;51(5):418–423.
4. Brisson M, Kashima T, Delaney D, et al. MRI characteristics of lipoma and atypical lipomatous tumor/well-differentiated liposarcoma: retrospective comparison with histology and MDM2 gene amplification. *Skeletal Radiol*. 2013;42(5):635–647.
5. Zhang H, Erickson-Johnson M, Wang X, et al. Molecular testing for lipomatous tumors: critical analysis and test recommendations based on the analysis of 405 extremity-based tumors. *Am J Surg Pathol*. 2010;34(9):1304–1311.
6. Weaver J, Downs-Kelly E, Goldblum J, et al. Fluorescence in situ hybridization for MDM2 gene amplification as a diagnostic tool in lipomatous neoplasms. *Mod Pathol*. 2008;21(8):943–949.

ADDITIONAL READING

- Aust MC, Spies M, Kall S, et al. Posttraumatic lipoma: fact or fiction? *Skinmed*. 2007;6(6):266–270.
- Bancroft LW, Kransdorf MJ, Peterson JJ, et al. Benign fatty tumors: classification, clinical course, imaging appearance, and treatment. *Skeletal Radiol*. 2006;35(10):719–733.
- Gaskin CM, Helms CA. Lipomas, lipoma variants, and well-differentiated liposarcomas (atypical lipomas): results of MRI evaluations of 126 consecutive fatty masses. *AJR Am J Roentgenol*. 2004;182(3):733–739.
- Liang CW, Mariño-Enríquez A, Johannessen C, et al. Translocation (Y;12) in lipoma. *Cancer Genetics*. 2011;204(1):53–56.
- Rotunda AM, Ablon G, Kolodney MS. Lipomas treated with subcutaneous deoxycholate injections. *J Am Acad Dermatol*. 2005;53(6):973–978.
- Salam GA. Lipoma excision. *Am Fam Physician*. 2002;65(5):901–904.

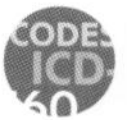

CODES

ICD10

- D17.9 Benign lipomatous neoplasm, unspecified
- D17.79 Benign lipomatous neoplasm of other sites
- D17.0 Ben lipomatous neoplm of skin, subcu of head, face and neck

CLINICAL PEARLS

- Lipomas are slow growing, often asymptomatic, and typically diagnosed without imaging or biopsy.
- Asymptomatic subcutaneous lipomas can be followed clinically unless there is diagnostic uncertainty, they are causing cosmetic or pain problems, are large (>5 cm) or growing rapidly, or causing compression of vital organs/nerves.
- Most symptomatic lipomas are removed surgically. With the appropriate indications, nonsurgical options are available.
- In uncomplicated cases, excision can be performed in the office setting.
- Consider referral to a subspecialist if a lipoma is in a delicate anatomic location, or if there is a concern that the lesion might be malignant.

LONG QT INTERVAL

Carl Bryce, MD • Matthew Snyder, DO

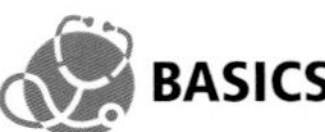

BASICS

DESCRIPTION

- QT interval: electrocardiogram (ECG) measurement that measures the duration of repolarization of myocardial cells. Measured from the onset of the QRS complex to the end of the T wave
- Corrected QT interval (QTc): QT interval corrected for heart rate (interval shortens with increased rate). See formulas.
- Prolonged QTc is generally defined as >440 msec (1):
  - 440–460 msec considered borderline in men
  - 440–470 msec considered borderline in women
  - 440–460 msec considered borderline in children aged 1–15 years old (2)
- Most cases of prolonged QT are acquired, but genetic mutations can also cause hereditary long QT syndromes (LQTS).
- Prolonged QTc from any cause can precipitate polymorphic ventricular tachycardia (VT) called torsade de pointes (TdP), leading to dizziness, syncope, and sudden cardiac death from ventricular fibrillation (VF).

EPIDEMIOLOGY

Incidence

Incidence of medication-induced QTc prolongation and TdP varies with medication and a host of other factors. Exact incidences are difficult to estimate (1).

Prevalence

- Hereditary LQTS is estimated to occur in 1/2,500–1/7,000 births.
- Five thousand people across the United States may die yearly due to LQTS-related cardiac arrhythmia (2).

ETIOLOGY AND PATHOPHYSIOLOGY

- Acquired
  - Electrolyte abnormalities such as hypokalemia, hypomagnesemia
  - Hypothyroidism
  - Underlying heart disease
  - Medications (3)[A]
    - Antiarrhythmic medications (quinidine, procainamide, dofetilide, sotalol, disopyramide, and amiodarone)
    - Antipsychotic medications, especially if given IV (haloperidol*, chlorpromazine*, thioridazine*, pimozide*)
    - Many antidepressants (SSRI's, SNRI's, trazodone, TCA's)
    - Antibiotics/antivirals/antifungals (clarithromycin*, erythromycin* which are also CYP3A4 inhibitors)
    - Antiemetics (metoclopramide, ondansetron, promethazine)
    - Opioids (methadone*, buprenorphine)
    - Antihistamines (cetirizine, hydroxyzine, diphenhydramine)
    - Decongestants (pseudoephedrine, phenylephrine
    - Stimulants (albuterol, phentermine)
    - Misc: chloroquine*, pentamidine*
    - *Denote "high-risk" medication for TdP.
- Congenital
  - Defective membrane proteins that work as channels for sodium and potassium in myocytes
- Pathophysiology
  - Depolarization of the myocardium results from the rapid influx of sodium through sodium channels and causes myocyte contraction, with resulting cardiac muscle contraction and systole (seen on ECG as the QRS complex).
  - During repolarization, there is an efflux of potassium from the cell through both rapid (I_{Kr}) and slow (I_{Ks}) potassium channels. The T wave on an ECG represents myocyte repolarization.
  - Drug-induced QT prolongation is primarily due to blockade of I_{Kr} leading to delayed repolarization (1).
  - Medications, medical conditions, electrolyte disturbances, and genetic mutations that affect functioning of these membrane channels can cause delayed repolarization.
  - Delayed repolarization can lead to a propensity for reentry and initiate TdP.
  - TdP type rhythm may be self-limited but symptomatic (syncope or near syncope). It can also degrade into VF.

Genetics

- 12 different genes have been linked to LQTS (2).
- Incomplete penetrance makes both diagnosis and management of asymptomatic disease challenging.
- LQTS 1 (42–54%) is the most common. Mutation causes a defect in the I_{Ks} transport protein. Arrhythmias can be triggered by tachycardia due to exercise (swimming seems to be especially problematic) and other high catecholamine states.
- LQTS 2 (35–45%) is a defect in the I_{Kr} transport protein that is sensitive to catecholamine surges. Sudden loud noises or emotional arousal can provoke arrhythmias.
- LQTS 3 (8%) is a defect in the sodium channel that allows an excess of sodium into the cell, increasing repolarization time. Arrhythmias tend to manifest more during rest or sleep.
- Jervell and Lange-Nielsen syndrome: Autosomal recessive form of LQTS that features homozygous mutations affect the I_{Ks} channel and presents with severe form of LQTS 1. Features also include deafness.
- Romano-Ward syndrome: autosomal dominant form of LQTS with variable penetrance. Hearing is normal.

RISK FACTORS

For TdP, the feared complication (4) are as follows:

- Female (~2× increased risk)
- QTc >500 msec (2–3× increased risk)
- QTc >60 msec over previous baseline
- History of syncope or presyncope
- History of TdP
- Bradycardia
- Liver or kidney disease (by increasing blood levels of QT prolonging medications)
- Medications that cause QTc prolongation
  - High doses
  - Fast infusions
  - Combination of medications
- Electrolyte abnormalities
  - Hypokalemia
  - Hypomagnesemia
  - Hypocalcemia
- For hereditary LQTS
  - Catecholamine surges from exercise (especially swimming), emotional stress, loud noises

GENERAL PREVENTION

- Avoid (or use with caution) causative medications, including combinations with potentially additive effects. Replete electrolytes (goal Mg >2, K 4.5–5.0) (4)[C].
- Treat underlying medical disease (hypothyroidism, cardiac disease).
- Avoid strenuous sports in LQTS.
- Avoid sudden loud noises in LQTS (alarm clocks, doorbells, telephones).

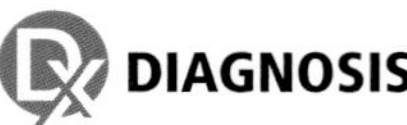

DIAGNOSIS

HISTORY

- Evaluate for syncope, near syncope, and associated precipitating events (such as emotional triggers, swimming, diving).
- Evaluate for history of seizures in patient or in family (Tonic–clonic movement may due to cerebral hypoperfusion during episodes of ventricular arrhythmia or due to seizure-like activity during a syncopal episode.).
- Detailed medication history
- Evaluate for family history of sudden death and syncope.
- Congenital deafness

PHYSICAL EXAM

- Usually normal physical exam
- If underlying cardiac disease present, may have findings specific to cardiac condition
- Evaluate for signs of hypothyroidism.
- Congenital deafness may be present in some forms of LQTS.

DIAGNOSTIC TESTS & INTERPRETATION

Initial Tests (lab, imaging)

- ECG
- Metabolic panel
- Calcium level
- Magnesium level
- TSH

Follow-Up Tests & Special Considerations

- Echocardiogram to evaluate for cardiomyopathy
- Outpatient cardiac rhythm monitoring
- Consider provocative testing (epinephrine infusion, exercise stress testing) to evaluate for QTc interval changes and/or to evaluate for coronary artery disease (2)[C].
  - Genetic testing for LQTS mutations

Test Interpretation

- QTc calculation using ECG is best done by measuring the QT interval in lead II and measuring the RR interval immediately preceding this QT interval. The easiest and most commonly used formula to calculate QTc is the Bazett formula, although it overcorrects for tachycardia and undercorrects for bradycardia (1).
- Bazett formula: $QTc = QT/\sqrt{(RR)}$ (all measurements in seconds, and RR obtained by direct measurement or 60/heart rate)
- Fridericia's formula is similar to Bazett's but uses a cube root instead of a square root of the RR interval. $QTc = QT/(RR)^{1/3}$
- U wave is not included in the calculation unless it is merged in with the T wave and is 50% of the T-wave amplitude.

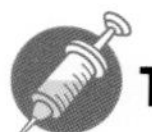

TREATMENT

GENERAL MEASURES

- VT, TdP, and VF should be treated emergently as per ACLS guidelines.
- Cardiac pacing may be needed emergently for drug-induced TdP to prevent bradycardia.
- Withdraw offending agents, correct electrolytes (1)[C].

MEDICATION

First Line

- For torsade de pointes: magnesium sulfate 2 g infused over 2–15 minutes, followed by continuous infusion of 2–4 mg/min if needed. Monitor for magnesium toxicity in those with renal insufficiency (1)[C].
- For hereditary LQTS, to prevent life-threatening arrhythmias: Propranolol initiated at 1.8 mg/kg/day divided twice daily (max 640 mg/day) has been shown to be more efficacious than other β-blockers for management of LQTS 1 and 2. β-Blockers are effective in decreasing but not eliminating the risk of fatal arrhythmias. Minimal effect of β-blockers is seen in those with LQTS 3 (5)[B].
- For high-risk patients or those who remain symptomatic on a β-blocker, implantable cardiac defibrillators (ICDs) with or without pacemaker is an important consideration (2)[B].

Second Line

Nadolol 0.9 mg/kg PO once daily (max 320 mg/day) may also be used (5)[B].

ISSUES FOR REFERRAL

- Refer to cardiologist for establishing diagnosis, especially for hereditary LQTS.
- Symptomatic prolonged QT

SURGERY/OTHER PROCEDURES

- ICD for those with a history of major cardiac events
- Left cervical-thoracic sympathetic denervation was used for symptomatic LQTS prior to the advent of β-blockers. It is still an option for those patients with LQTS who are refractory to β-blocker therapy (2)[B].

INPATIENT CONSIDERATIONS

Admission Criteria/Initial Stabilization

- Patients with TdP, VT, and VF should be promptly treated as per ACLS guidelines. Correct electrolytes on an emergent basis. Evaluate for acquired QT prolongation. If no cause is found, consider hereditary LQTS.
- Patients with prolonged QTc and syncope, near syncope should be monitored on telemetry during evaluation.
- Monitor ECG if initiating medications or combining medications that may prolong QT, suggest at baseline, within 30 days, and then annually (3)[C].
- Monitor electrolytes and urgently treat hypokalemia, hypomagnesemia, and hypokalemia in those with significantly prolonged QT.

Nursing

For those who have LQTS 2, avoid sudden loud noises.

ONGOING CARE

FOLLOW-UP RECOMMENDATIONS

On routine visits, ask about syncope, presyncope and palpitations in those who have QTc prolongation.

- Patient monitoring: Consider ECG and/or outpatient cardiac rhythm monitoring with any medication additions or dosage changes that may cause further prolongation of the QTc.
- For those who may have symptomatic QTc prolongation of any cause, prompt evaluation is warranted.
- Check labs for electrolyte imbalances, correct as needed.

PATIENT EDUCATION

- Educate patients with QTc prolongation about medications side effects and possibility of medication interactions.
- Patients with congenital forms of LQTS should be aware of, and avoid situations that may trigger, torsade (depending on their specific gene mutation)
- Large emotional and psychological impact of diagnosis. Additional reading by Fortescue shares personal impact of LQTS.
- Information and support from groups listed may be helpful.

PROGNOSIS

Untreated, quite poor. Perhaps 20% of untreated patients presenting with syncope die within 1 year, 50% within 10 years (4).

REFERENCES

1. Kallergis EM, Goudis CA, Simatirakis EN, et al. Mechanisms, risk factors, and management of acquired long QT syndrome: a comprehensive review. *ScientificWorldJournal*. 2012;2012:212178.
2. Clarke CJ, McDaniel GM. The risk of long QT syndrome in the pediatric population. *Curr Opin Pediatr*. 2009;21(5):573–578.
3. Isbister GK, Page CB. Drug induced QT prolongation: the measurement and assessment of the QT interval in clinical practice. *Br J Clin Pharmacol*. 2013;76(1):48–57.
4. QT prolongation, torsades de pointes, and medication safety. *Pharmacist's Letter/Prescriber's Letter*. 2010;26(4):260421.
5. Chockalingam P, Crotti L, Girardengo G, et al. Not all beta-blockers are equal in the management of long QT syndrome types 1 and 2: higher recurrence of events under metoprolol. *J Am Coll Cardiol*. 2012;60(20):2092–2099.

ADDITIONAL READING

- Fortescue EB. A piece of my mind. Keeping the pace. *JAMA*. 2014;311(23):2383–2384.
- Levine E, Rosero SZ, Budzikowski AS, et al. Congenital long QT syndrome: considerations for primary care physicians. *Cleve Clin J Med*. 2008;75(8):591–600.
- Morita H, Wu J, Zipes DP. The QT syndromes: long and short. *Lancet*. 2008;372(9640):750–763.
- van Noord C, Eijgelsheim M, Stricker BH. Drug- and non-drug-associated QT interval prolongation. *Br J Clin Pharmacol*. 2010;70(1):16–23.
- Webster G, Berul CI. Congenital long-QT syndromes: a clinical and genetic update from infancy through adulthood. *Trends Cardiovasc Med*. 2008;18(6):216–224.
- Yap YG, Camm AJ. Drug induced QT prolongation and torsades de pointes. *Heart*. 2003;89(11):1363–1372.

SEE ALSO

- http://www.crediblemeds.org (Medication lists and additional resources related to long QT and torsade de pointes)
- Cardiac Arrhythmias Research and Education Foundation (http://www.longqt.org)
- Sudden Arrhythmia Death Syndromes Foundation (http://www.sads.org)

CODES

ICD10

I45.81 Long QT syndrome

CLINICAL PEARLS

- Evaluate for acquired causes before making a diagnosis of hereditary LQTS.
- For accurate diagnosis, calculate QTc manually.
- The ideal management of TdP is prevention; avoid multiple "stacking" risk factors and seek alternates to risky medications, correct electrolytes, and monitor treatment with serial ECGs if no alternatives exist.
- Magnesium sulfate is the treatment of choice during ACLS for TdP.
- β-blockers are initial treatment of choice for hereditary LQTS.

LUMBAR (INTERVERTEBRAL) DISC DISORDERS

Rebecca L. Peebles, DO

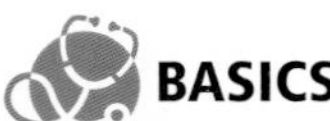

BASICS

DESCRIPTION

- A common age-related degenerative process that can lead to chronic debilitating pain with significant negative effects on quality of life
- Degeneration may be histologically evident as early as 15 years of age with symptoms becoming prevalent during the 3rd–4th decades. Once initiated, the degeneration is a progressive and irreversible process modified by a variety of intrinsic and extrinsic factors.
- Radiologically evident degeneration, herniation, collapse, nerve impingement, intervertebral narrowing, and osteophyte formation are common end states.
- Low back pain may be categorized into four groups: mechanical (80–90%), neurologic involvement (5–15%), specific spinal pathology (1–2%), nonspinal origin (1–3%).
- Chronic low back pain is defined by low back pain that persists of over a 3-month period.
- Predictors of persistent disabling low back pain include maladaptive pain coping skills, nonorganic signs, functional impairment, general health status, and psychiatric comorbidities.
- Primary system(s) affected: musculoskeletal, nervous, psychiatric
- Synonym(s): degenerative disc disease; intervertebral disc dislocation; herniated disc; herniated nucleus pulposus

EPIDEMIOLOGY

Incidence

- 25.9 millions Americans are affected by low back pain each year
- Direct and indirect costs from low back pain are estimated at \$80–\$100 billion per year.
- Accounts for about 2% of all physician visits
- Among patients with acute back pain, only 4% have nerve root symptoms due to a herniated disc.

Prevalence

- An estimated 33% of individuals younger than age 40 years and nearly all individuals 60–80 years have identifiable disc degeneration on MRI. *Most are asymptomatic.*
- Lifetime prevalence of low back pain is 70–80%, with disc degeneration as a common cause.

Pediatric Considerations

May emerge rapidly after adolescence, leading to significant and chronic low back pain

Pregnancy Considerations

Increased incidence of low back pain, sacroiliac dysfunction, and/or sciatica during pregnancy

Geriatric Considerations

Usually multifactorial, disc degeneration, lesions of spine, spondylolisthesis, spinal stenosis, and osteoporotic fractures

ETIOLOGY AND PATHOPHYSIOLOGY

- With age, the nucleus pulposus loses ability to support compressive force, shifting weight onto the annulus fibrosis, which fatigues.
- Over time, fibers of the annulus fibrosus lengthen, weaken, and fray with subsequent protrusion, extrusion, or sequestration of disc fragments.
- Symptomatic degenerative disc disease results from inflammatory irritation of adjacent tissues (ligament, nerve root, and vertebrae) or compression of structures (bulging disc, herniated nucleus pulposus, degenerative changes of the spine). There is no definitive correlation of radiographic findings and symptomatology.

RISK FACTORS

- Smoking
- Genetics
- Elevated BMI
- Osteoporosis
- Occupational risks: prolonged standing, heavy lifting, use of vibrating tools (jackhammer)
- Affective or somatization disorder
- Trauma
- Cancer
- Socioeconomic factors do not contribute to risk of initial injury/degeneration but contribute significantly to subsequent degree of disability

GENERAL PREVENTION

- Most episodes of low back pain are not preventable.
- Modification of occupational risk factors
- Management of bone mineral density, diabetes mellitus, and BMI
- Smoking cessation
- Aerobic and core strengthening exercises

COMMONLY ASSOCIATED CONDITIONS

- Obesity
- Diabetes mellitus
- Osteoarthritis
- Osteoporosis
- Depression/anxiety
- Low job satisfaction

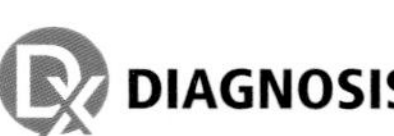

DIAGNOSIS

HISTORY

- Assess location, onset, aggravating/relieving factors, and associated symptoms. Establish baseline pain level and functional deficits.
- Degenerative disc disease usually described as recurrent episodes of pain with periods of complete or near-complete resolution
- Inciting event for pain flare is usually not traumatic; often occurs after exertion (lifting, bending, twisting)
- Radicular pain often greater than back pain with disc herniation
- Pain often exaggerated by Valsalva maneuver
- Red flags
  - Cauda equina syndrome: saddle anesthesia, bladder dysfunction, neurologic deficits in lower extremities
  - Expanding lesion (swelling or tumor growth): progressively worsening symptoms
  - Fracture: major/minor trauma, strenuous lifting, steroid use, osteoporosis
  - Cancer: age $>$50 years or $<$20 years, weight loss, severe nighttime pain
  - Infection: IV drug use, skin infection, UTI, immunosuppression
- Yellow flags: indicate risk for development of prolonged pain
  - Depression, impaired global function, job dissatisfaction, disputed compensation claims

PHYSICAL EXAM

- Assess gait, posture, range of motion, reflexes, sensation (particularly femoral, peroneal, tibial, lateral femoral cutaneous nerves and L2–L5, S1 dermatomes), and strength (assess muscles of hip girdle, knee, ankle, and foot).
- Palpate bony landmarks.
- Paraspinal muscle spasm usually present
- For radiculopathy
  - Straight-leg raise (SLR) test: (sensitivity = 0.91; specificity = 0.26)
  - Crossed SLR test: (sensitivity = 0.29; specificity = 0.88) — if positive, considered pathognomonic for disc herniation
  - Loss of Achilles reflex S1 impingement
  - Combined femoral stretch test, patellar reflex, medial ankle sensation, and crossed femoral stretch test support L4 impingement.

DIFFERENTIAL DIAGNOSIS

- Acute or chronic lumbosacral strain
- Facet joint disease
- Piriformis syndrome
- Spondylosis/spondylolisthesis
- Spinal arthritis
- Sciatica
- Fibromyalgia
- Compression fracture
- Metastatic and primary tumors
- Vertebral infection
- Vertebral vascular insufficiency
- Pain referred from hip, retroperitoneum (i.e., hematoma), aneurysms, intra-abdominal or pelvis (i.e., UTI or urolithiasis); neurogenic claudication
- Cauda equina syndrome

DIAGNOSTIC TESTS & INTERPRETATION

Labs

- Workup indicated if red flags are present or organic causes are suspected: CBC, ESR, or C-reactive protein (infection, autoimmune arthropathy, cancer).
- Serum protein electophoresis (SPEP) and urine protein electophoresis (UPEP) if malignancy suspected
- Urinalysis if suspected urinary system etiology

Imaging

- Lumbosacral plain films often not routinely necessary; obtain if pt $>$50 years of age, history of trauma, presence of neuromuscular deficits, unexplained weight loss, history of drug/EtOH abuse, history of cancer, fever, corticosteroid use, recurrent visits for same complaint, patient seeking compensation
- MRI is imaging of choice for evaluation of disc and nerve root pathology, spinal stenosis, masses, and discitis; consider if red flags present and with severe/progressive neurologic deficits; may also consider if failed conservative treatment after 6 weeks if patient adherent to therapy and clinical suspicion warrants
- Degenerative findings in asymptomatic patients on MRI are not reliably predictive of development or duration of future symptomatology.
- Non-contrast CT: useful if bony abnormality suspected; limited evaluation of neural pathology without use of thecal contrast
- CT myelogram: considered definitive for diagnosis of herniation, stenosis, or osteophytes; invasive and rarely used

- Nerve conduction studies/EMG: helps localize spinal level; only positive after radiculopathy present for 4 or more weeks; doesn't exclude radiculopathy if negative
- Discogram: identifies specific disc pathology but invasive and rarely used

Test Interpretation

Difficult to distinguish the imaging findings of normal aging process of disc degeneration from specific lesions causing low back pain and sciatica; must correlate history, physical exam, and radiologic findings

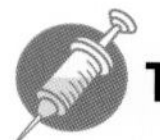

TREATMENT

GENERAL MEASURES

- Conservative therapy is recommended for 6 weeks in absence of red flags: relative rest for 1–3 days, isometric core strengthening (back/abdomen/legs), postural retraining, walking, analgesics, muscle relaxants, massage, avoiding prolonged sitting, lying in semi-Fowler position (1)[B].
- Failed conservative management past 6 weeks, consider reevaluation and imaging studies.
- Patients with significant pain that fails to resolve after 6 weeks of conservative care may be candidates for epidural steroid injections (will not resolve neurologic symptoms).
- Surgery may be an option for patients with chronic low back pain that has failed prolonged conservative care.
- Discussion is recommended at each stage of patient care to address expectations, risks, and short- and long-term benefits.

MEDICATION

First Line

- Analgesia with acetaminophen or NSAIDs (with consideration of side effect profile); muscle relaxants for acute paraspinal muscle spasm only
- If depression is present, it should be treated with 1st-line interventions for improved outcomes and decreased need for narcotic medications.

Second Line

- May consider short- or long-term use of opiates or tramadol
- Epidural steroid injection indicated only for patients with persistent radicular pain
- Gabapentin or pregabalin effective when combined with NSAID or opiate

SURGERY/OTHER PROCEDURES

- Absolute indications: cauda equina syndrome, multiple episodes of radiculopathy, progressive severe neurologic deficit, and persistent dysfunctional pain
- Careful patient selection for surgery improves outcomes.
- Decompressive surgery (open discectomy, microdiscectomy, hemilaminectomy): for patients with neurologic impingement such as spinal stenosis or disc herniation. Most evidence supports minimally invasive approach.
- Disc arthroplasty (disc prosthesis): appropriate for patients with degenerative changes confined to one localized lesion. Contraindications include vertebral abnormalities, nerve root compression, and spinal stenosis.
- Spinal fusion: indicated for unstable vertebral segment caused by severe degenerative changes
- Chemonucleolysis: limited evidence; enzymatic injection to decrease bulge/herniation
- Spinal cord stimulation: limited evidence; indicated for pain refractory to operative management

COMPLEMENTARY & ALTERNATIVE MEDICINE

- Pain should be considered in a biopsychosocial context, incorporating the patient's beliefs, coping strategies, and social interactions.
- Manipulation, physical therapy, exercise, acupuncture, and yoga are beneficial.
- Psychosocial support is important for long-term improvement. Consider referral to a psychiatrist/psychologist.

INPATIENT CONSIDERATIONS

Admission Criteria/Initial Stabilization

Inpatient admission uncommon; for protracted cases, consider pain management consult.

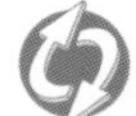

ONGOING CARE

FOLLOW-UP RECOMMENDATIONS

- Follow up immediately if pain or neurologic deficit is increasing.
- Return visit 10 days to 2 weeks following initial visit
- Monitor every 2–4 weeks until fully functional.
- Follow-up visits should focus on pain level, neurologic status, psychosocial factors, and preventive care.

PATIENT EDUCATION

Encourage exercise, proper posture and body mechanics, and avoidance of risk factors.

PROGNOSIS

- Acute low back pain (90%) or radiculopathy (75–90%) can be expected to recover spontaneously within 6 weeks using conservative care.
- 25% of patients treated nonsurgically who had at least 1 month of herniation-induced radicular symptoms report recurrence within 1 year.
- Most patients with chronic radicular and nonradicular discogenic low back pain respond to conservative management. Improved postop outcomes (90%) are associated with careful patient selection, male gender, younger age, active individuals, and exercise program initiated within 4–6 weeks.
- Risk factors for recurrence include return to work before full postop recovery, occupation requiring manual labor, and low education level.
- 4–20% of patients require reoperation.
- Most helpful predictors of persistent disabling low back pain are maladaptive pain coping skills, nonorganic signs, functional impairment, general health status, and psychiatric comorbidities.

COMPLICATIONS

- Foot drop with weakness of anterior tibial, posterior tibial, and peroneal muscles
- Bladder and rectal sphincter weakness, with retention or incontinence
- Limitation of movement, restricted activity, long-term disability, decreased quality of life

REFERENCES

1. Morlion B. Chronic low back pain: pharmacological interventional and surgical strategies. *Nat Rev Neurol*. 2013;9(8):462–473.

ADDITIONAL READING

- Chou R, Loeser JD, Owens DK, et al. Interventional therapies, surgery, and interdisciplinary rehabilitation for low back pain: an evidence-based clinical practice guideline from the American Pain Society. *Spine*. 2009;34(10):1066–1077.
- Chou R, Qaseem A, Snow V, et al. Diagnosis and treatment of low back pain: a joint clinical practice guideline from the American College of Physicians and the American Pain Society. *Ann Intern Med*. 2007;147(7):478–491.
- Schoenfeld AJ, Weiner BK. Treatment of lumbar disc herniation: evidence-based practice. *Int J Gen Med*. 2010;3:209–214.
- Siepe CJ, Heider F, Haas E, et al. Influence of lumbar intervertebral disc degeneration on the outcome of total lumbar disc replacement: a prospective clinical, histological, x-ray and MRI investigation. *Eur Spine J*. 2012;21(11):2287–2299.
- Suri P, Rainville J, Hunter DJ, et al. Recurrence of radicular pain or back pain after nonsurgical treatment of symptomatic lumbar disk herniation. *Arch Phys Med Rehabil*. 2012;93(4):690–695.
- Suri P, Rainville J, Katz JN, et al. The accuracy of the physical examination for the diagnosis of midlumbar and low lumbar nerve root impingement. *Spine*. 2011;36(1):63–73.

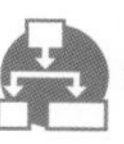

SEE ALSO

- Back Pain, Low
- Algorithm: Low Back Pain, Acute

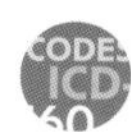

CODES

ICD10

- M51.36 Other intervertebral disc degeneration, lumbar region
- M51.26 Other intervertebral disc displacement, lumbar region
- M51.06 Intervertebral disc disorders with myelopathy, lumbar region

CLINICAL PEARLS

- In the absence of red flags, patients can be managed conservatively with pain management and self-care for 6 weeks. Most will recover spontaneously.
- Routine imaging is rarely indicated. Indications for imaging include red flag symptoms, progressive neurologic deficits, or failure of conservative management at 6 weeks.
- Consider a surgical referral for patients with persistent and disabling pain that fails to resolve after appropriate conservative management.

LUNG, PRIMARY MALIGNANCIES

Maryann R. Cooper, PharmD, BCOP • Gerald Gehr, MD

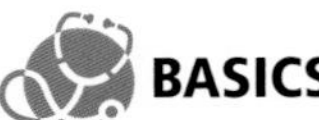

BASICS

DESCRIPTION

- Lung cancers (primary) are the leading cause of cancer-related death in the United States (estimated 159,260 deaths in 2014, 27% of all cancer-related deaths).
- Divided into 2 broad categories
  - Non–small cell lung cancer (NSCLC) (>85% of all lung cancers)
    - Adenocarcinoma (~40% of NSCLC): most common type in the United States, most common type in nonsmokers, metastasizes earlier than squamous cell, poor prognosis; bronchoalveolar, a subtype of adenocarcinoma has better prognosis.
    - Squamous cell carcinoma (<25% of NSCLC): dose-related effect with smoking; slower growing than adenocarcinoma
    - Large cell (~10% of NSCLC): prognosis similar to adenocarcinoma
  - Small cell lung cancer (SCLC) (16% of all lung cancers): centrally located, early metastases, aggressive
- Other: mesothelioma, carcinoid tumor, and sarcoma
- Staging
  - NSCLC: staged from 0 to IV based on: primary tumor (T), lymph node status (N), and presence of metastasis (M)
  - SCLC: staged based on disease location: limited to ipsilateral hemithorax (stages I–IIIB); extensive if metastatic beyond hemithorax (stages IIIB and IV)
- Tumor locations: upper: 60%; lower: 30%; middle: 5%; overlapping and main stem: 5%
- May spread by local extension to involve chest wall, diaphragm, pulmonary vessels, vena cava, phrenic nerve, esophagus, or pericardium
- Most commonly metastasize to lymph nodes (pulmonary, mediastinal), then liver, adrenal, bone (osteolytic), kidney, brain

EPIDEMIOLOGY

Incidence

- Estimated 224,210 new cases in the United States in 2014
- Predominant age: >40 years; peak at 70 years
- Predominant sex: male > female

Prevalence

- Most common cancer worldwide
- Lifetime probability: men: 1 in 13; women: 1 in 16

ETIOLOGY AND PATHOPHYSIOLOGY

Multifactorial; see "Risk Factors."

Genetics

NSCLC

- Oncogenes: Ras family (H-ras, K-ras, N-ras)
- Tumor suppressor genes: retinoblastoma, *p53*

RISK FACTORS

- Smoking (relative risk [RR] 10–30)
- Secondhand smoke exposure
- Radon
- Environmental and occupational exposures
  - Asbestos exposure (synergistic increase in risk for smokers)
  - Air pollution
  - Ionizing radiation
  - Mutagenic gases (halogen ethers, mustard gas, aromatic hydrocarbons)
  - Metals (inorganic arsenic, chromium, nickel)
- Lung scarring from tuberculosis
- Radiation therapy to the breast or chest

GENERAL PREVENTION

- Smoking cessation and prevention programs
- Screening recommended by USPSTF but remains controversial; the risks of screening (e.g., radiation, biopsy) may offset the benefit (1)[A].
- Annual screening with low-dose computed tomography in adults ages 55–80 years who have a 30 pack-year smoking history and currently smoke or have quit within the past 15 years
- Screening should be discontinued once a person has not smoked for 15 years or develops a health problem that substantially limits life expectancy or the ability or willingness to have curative lung surgery.
- Prevention via aggressive smoking cessation counseling and therapy; a 20–30% risk reduction occurs within 5 years of cessation.
- Avoid supplemental β-carotene and vitamin E in smokers.
- Avoid hormone replacement therapy in postmenopausal smokers or former smokers (increased risk of death from NSCLC).

COMMONLY ASSOCIATED CONDITIONS

- Paraneoplastic syndromes: Hypertrophic pulmonary osteoarthropathy, Lambert-Eaton syndrome, Cushing syndrome, hypercalcemia from ectopic parathyroid-releasing hormone, syndrome of inappropriate antidiuretic hormone (SIADH)
- Hypercoagulable state
- Pancoast syndrome
- Superior vena cava syndrome
- Pleural effusion
- Chronic obstructive pulmonary disease (COPD), other sequelae of cigarette smoking

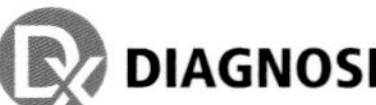

DIAGNOSIS

HISTORY

- May be asymptomatic for most of course
- Pulmonary
  - Cough (new or change in chronic cough)
  - Wheezing and stridor
  - Dyspnea
  - Hemoptysis
  - Pneumonitis (fever and productive cough)
- Constitutional
  - Malaise
  - Bone pain (metastatic disease)
  - Fatigue
  - Weight loss, anorexia
  - Fever
  - Anemia
  - Clubbing of digits
- Other presentations:
  - Chest pain (dull, pleuritic)
  - Shoulder/arm pain (Pancoast tumors)
  - Dysphagia
  - Plethora (redness of face or neck)
  - Hoarseness (involvement of recurrent laryngeal nerve)
  - Horner syndrome
  - Neurologic abnormalities (e.g., headaches, syncope, weakness, cognitive impairment)
  - Pericardial tamponade (pericardial invasion)

PHYSICAL EXAM

- General: pain, performance status, weight loss
- Head, eye, ear, nose, throat (HEENT): Horner syndrome, dysphonia, stridor, scleral icterus
- Neck: supraclavicular/cervical lymph nodes, mass
- Lungs: effusion, wheezing, airway obstruction, pleural effusion
- Abdomen/groin: hepatomegaly or lymphadenopathy
- Extremities: signs of hypertrophic pulmonary osteoarthropathy, deep venous thrombosis (DVT)
- Neurologic: Rule out cognitive and focal motor defects.

DIFFERENTIAL DIAGNOSIS

- COPD (may coexist)
- Granulomatous (tuberculosis, sarcoidosis)
- Cardiomyopathy
- Congestive heart failure (CHF)

DIAGNOSTIC TESTS & INTERPRETATION

Initial Tests (lab, imaging)

- CBC
- BUN, serum creatinine
- Liver function tests (LFTs), lactate dehydrogenase (LDH)
- Electrolytes
  - Hypercalcemia (Paraneoplastic syndrome)
  - Hyponatremia (SIADH)
- Sputum cytology
- Chest x-ray (CXR) (compare with old films)
  - Nodule or mass, especially if calcified
  - Persistent infiltrate
  - Atelectasis
  - Mediastinal widening
  - Hilar enlargement
  - Pleural effusion
- CT scan of chest (with IV contrast material)
  - Nodule or mass (central or peripheral)
  - Lymphadenopathy
- Evaluation for metastatic disease
  - Brain MRI: Lesions may be necrotic, bleeding.
  - CT abdomen: hepatic, adrenal, renal masses
- Positron emission tomography (PET) scan: to evaluate metastasis
- Bone scan: advanced disease or bone pain

Follow-Up Tests & Special Considerations

CBC, BUN, serum creatinine, LFTs prior to each cycle of chemotherapy

Diagnostic Procedures/Other

- Biopsy with pathology review to determine NSCLC versus SCLC
- In patients with advanced NSCLC, determination of epidermal growth factor receptor (EGFR)-activating mutations, *KRAS* mutations, and *ALK* gene rearrangements in patients with nonsquamous or mixed squamous histology
- Pulmonary function tests
- Enlarged mediastinal lymph nodes necessitate staging by mediastinoscopy, video-assisted thoracoscopy, or fine-needle aspiration.
- Transbronchial biopsy (Wang needle)
- Bronchoscopy for surgical planning
- Bone marrow aspirate (small cell)
- Cervical mediastinoscopy (the upper, middle peritracheal, and subcarinal lymph nodes)
- Anterior mediastinotomy (the posterior mediastinum and peritracheal, subazygous, hilar, and aortopulmonary window nodal regions)
- Video-assisted thoracoscopy (associated pleural disease and suspected mediastinal nodal spread)

Test Interpretation

Pathologic changes from smoking are progressive: basal cell proliferation, development of atypical nuclei, stratification, metaplasia of squamous cells, carcinoma in situ, and then invasive disease.

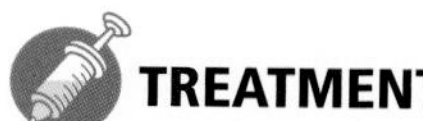

TREATMENT

GENERAL MEASURES

- NSCLC
  - Stage I, stage II, and selected stage III tumors are surgically resectable. Neoadjuvant or adjuvant therapy is recommended for many patients with stages II and III NSCLC. Patients with resectable disease who are not surgical candidates may receive curative radiation therapy.
  - Patients with unresectable or N2, N3 disease are treated with combination chemotherapy and radiation. Selected patients with T3 or N2 disease can be treated effectively with surgical resection and either pre- or postoperative chemotherapy or chemoradiation therapy.
  - Patients with distant metastases (M1) can be treated with radiation therapy or chemotherapy for palliation or best supportive care alone.
- SCLC
  - Limited stage: concurrent chemoradiation
  - Extensive stage: combination chemotherapy
  - Consider prophylactic cranial irradiation (PCI) in patients achieving a complete or partial response (2)[A].
- Quality-of-life assessments: Karnofsky performance scale (KPS), Eastern Cooperative Oncology Group (ECOG)
- Discussions with patient and family about end-of-life care

MEDICATION

- Chemotherapy is the mainstay of treatment.
- Adjuvant chemotherapy following surgery improves survival in patients with fully resected stage II–III NSCLC.
- Palliative measures: analgesics
- Dyspnea: oxygen, morphine

First Line

- NSCLC
  - Stages II–III: neoadjuvant or adjuvant chemotherapy (3,4)[A]
    - Cisplatin-based doublets (combination with paclitaxel, etoposide, vinorelbine, docetaxel, gemcitabine)
    - Carboplatin alternative for patients unlikely to tolerate cisplatin
    - Cisplatin plus pemetrexed (nonsquamous cell)
  - Unresectable stage IIA, IIIB
    - Concurrent chemoradiation
      - Cisplatin plus etoposide, vinblastine, or pemetrexed (nonsquamous cell) plus concurrent radiation
      - Carboplatin plus pemetrexed (nonsquamous cell) plus concurrent radiation
- Stage IV
  - No chemotherapy can be recommended for routine use.
  - Cisplatin-based doublets (5)[A]
  - Carboplatin plus paclitaxel +/− bevacizumab (nonsquamous cell)
  - Cisplatin plus vinorelbine +/− cetuximab
  - Erlotinib or afatinib for patients EGFR mutations
  - Crizotinib for patients with EML4-ALK translocations
    - Ceritinib for patients that fail or are intolerant to crizotinib
  - Maintenance therapy after 4–6 cycles of original regimen in patients achieving a complete response, partial response, or stable disease
    - Continue original regimen, single agent from original regimen, bevacizumab, cetuximab, pemetrexed, erlotinib, or observation.
- SCLC
  - Cisplatin or carboplatin + etoposide

Second Line

- NSCLC
  - Cisplatin-based doublets with or without bevacizumab (nonsquamous cell) or cetuximab
  - Docetaxel or pemetrexed (nonsquamous cell) or erlotinib (EGFR-positive tumors)
- SCLC
  - Topotecan or CAV (cyclophosphamide, doxorubicin, vincristine), gemcitabine, docetaxel, paclitaxel

ADDITIONAL THERAPIES

- Smoking cessation counseling
- Consider IV bisphosphonates or denosumab in patients with bone metastases to reduce skeletal related events.

SURGERY/OTHER PROCEDURES

- Resection for NSCLC, for stages I, II, and IIIa, if medically fit to undergo surgery
- Resection of isolated, distant metastases has been achieved and may improve survival.
- Resection involves lobectomy in 71%, wedge in 16%, and complete pneumonectomy in 18%.
- Resection should be accompanied by lymph node dissection for pathologic staging.

ONGOING CARE

FOLLOW-UP RECOMMENDATIONS

Patient Monitoring

- Depends on clinical history; in general, postoperative visits every 3–6 months in the year after surgery with physical exam and CXR
- Follow-up CT scans, as indicated

PATIENT EDUCATION

- www.cancer.gov/cancertopics
- www.smokefree.gov/

PROGNOSIS

- For combined, all types and stages, 5-year survival rate is 16% (NSCLC: 17%; SCLC 6%).
- NSCLC
  - Localized disease (stages I and II): 49%
  - Regional disease: 16%
  - Distant metastatic disease: 2%
- SCLC
  - Without treatment: median survival from diagnosis of only 2–4 months
  - Limited-stage disease: median survival of 16–24 months; 5-year survival rate: 14%
  - Extensive-stage disease: median survival of 6–12 months; long-term disease-free survival is rare.

COMPLICATIONS

- Development of metastatic disease, especially to brain, bones, adrenals, and liver
- Local recurrence of disease
- Postoperative complications
- Side effects of chemotherapy or radiation

REFERENCES

1. National Lung Screening Trial Research Team, Aberle DR, Adams AM, et al. Reduced lung-cancer mortality with low-dose computed tomographic screening. *N Engl J Med*. 2011;365(5):395–409.
2. Slotman B, Faivre-Finn C, Kramer G, et al. Prophylactic cranial irradiation in extensive small cell lung cancer. *N Engl J Med*. 2007;357(7):664–672.
3. Pignon JP, Tribodet H, Scagliotti GV, et al. Lung adjuvant cisplatin evaluation: a pooled analysis by the LACE Collaborative Group. *J Clin Oncol*. 2008;26(21):3552–3559.
4. Gilligan D, Nicolson M, Smith I, et al. Preoperative chemotherapy in patients with resectable non-small cell lung cancer: results of the MRC LU22/NVALT 2/EORTC 08012 multicentre randomised trial and update of systematic review. *Lancet*. 2007;369(9577):1929–1937.
5. Delbaldo C, Michiels S, Rolland E, et al. Second or third additional chemotherapy drug for non-small cell lung cancer in patients with advanced disease. *Cochrane Database Syst Rev*. 2007;(4):CD004569.

ADDITIONAL READING

- American College of Chest Physicians. Diagnosis and management of lung cancer. *Chest*. 2013;143(Suppl 5):S7–S50.
- Collins LG, Haines C, Perkel R, et al. Lung cancer: diagnosis and management. *Am Fam Physician*. 2007;75(1):56–63.
- National Cancer Institute. General information about non-small cell lung cancer. www.cancer.gov/cancertopics/pdq/treatment/non-small-cell-lung/healthprofessional. Accessed 2014.
- National Cancer Institute. General information about small cell lung cancer. www.cancer.gov/cancertopics/pdq/treatment/small-cell-lung/healthprofessional. Accessed 2014.

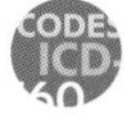

CODES

ICD10

- C34.90 Malignant neoplasm of unsp part of unsp bronchus or lung
- C34.10 Malignant neoplasm of upper lobe, unsp bronchus or lung
- C34.30 Malignant neoplasm of lower lobe, unsp bronchus or lung

CLINICAL PEARLS

- Prognosis and treatment of lung cancer differs greatly between small cell- and non–small cell histologies.
- Adjuvant cisplatin-based chemotherapy improves survival in patients with completely resected stage II-III NSCLC.
- Chemotherapy, with or without radiation, can be offered to patients with advanced NSCLC or SCLC.
- There is little role for surgery in the treatment of SCLC

LUPUS ERYTHEMATOSUS, SYSTEMIC (SLE)

Katherine M. Tromp, PharmD • Hershey S. Bell, MD, MS, FAAFP

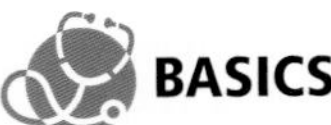

BASICS

DESCRIPTION

- Systemic lupus erythematosus (SLE) is a multisystem autoimmune inflammatory disease characterized by a chronic relapsing/remitting course; can be mild to severe and may be life threatening (CNS and renal forms)
- System(s) affected: mucocutaneous; musculoskeletal; renal; nervous; pulmonary; cardiac; hematologic; vascular; gastrointestinal (GI)
- Synonym(s): SLE; lupus

ALERT

Women with SLE have a 7–50-fold increased risk of coronary artery disease and may present with atypical/nonspecific symptoms.

EPIDEMIOLOGY

Predominant age: 15–45 years

Incidence

- Per year, 1.6–7.6/100,000 and increasing due to better diagnosis
- Most common: African American women (8.1–11.4/100,000/year)
- Least common: Caucasian men (0.3–0.9/100,000/year)

Prevalence

Occurs in 30–50/100,000 and increasing due to increased survival

ETIOLOGY AND PATHOPHYSIOLOGY

- Skin: photosensitivity; scaly erythematous, plaques with follicular plugging, dermal atrophy, and scarring; nonscarring erythematous psoriasiform/annular rash; alopecia; mucosal ulcers
- Musculoskeletal: nonerosive arthritis; ligament and tendon laxity, ulnar deviation, and swan neck deformities; avascular necrosis
- Renal: glomerulonephritis
- Pulmonary: pleuritis, pleural effusion, alveolar hemorrhage, pneumonitis, interstitial fibrosis, pulmonary hypertension, pulmonary embolism (PE)
- Cardiac: nonbacterial verrucous endocarditis, pericarditis, myocarditis, atherosclerosis
- CNS: thrombosis of small intracranial vessels ± perivascular inflammation resulting in micro- or macroinfarcts ± hemorrhage
- Peripheral nervous system: mononeuritis multiplex, peripheral neuropathy
- GI: pancreatitis, peritonitis, colitis
- Hematologic: hemolytic anemia, thrombocytopenia, leukopenia, lymphopenia
- Vascular: vasculitis, thromboembolism
- Most cases are idiopathic with possible environmental factors.
- Drug-induced lupus: hydralazine, D penicillamine, quinidine, procainamide, minocycline, isoniazid, etc.

Genetics

- Identical twins: 24–58% concordance
- Fraternal twins and siblings: 2–5% concordance
- 8-fold risk if 1st-degree relative with SLE
- Major histocompatability complex associations: HLA-DR2, HLA-DR3
- Deficiency of early complement components, especially C1q, C2, and C4
- Immunoglobulin receptor polymorphisms: *FCγR2A* and *FCγR3A*
- Polymorphism in genes associated with regulation of programmed cell death, protein tyrosine kinases, and interferon production

RISK FACTORS

- Race: African Americans, Hispanics, Asians, and Native Americans
- Predominant sex: females > males (8:1)
- Environmental: UV light, infectious agents, stress, diet, drugs, hormones, vitamin D deficiency, and tobacco

COMMONLY ASSOCIATED CONDITIONS

- Overlap syndromes: rheumatoid arthritis (RA), Sjögren syndrome, scleroderma
- Antiphospholipid syndrome; coronary artery disease; nephritis; depression

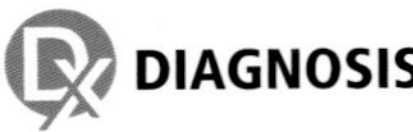

DIAGNOSIS

Consider SLE in multisystem disease including fever, fatigue, and signs of inflammation.

HISTORY

- Fever, fatigue, malaise, weight loss, headache
- Rash (butterfly/*hyperpigmented ears* or *scalp*), photosensitivity, alopecia
- Oral/nasal ulcers (usually painless)
- Arthritis, arthralgia, myalgia, weakness
- Pleuritic chest pain, cough, dyspnea, hemoptysis
- Early stroke (age <50 years), seizure, psychosis, cognitive deficits
- Proteinuria, cellular casts
- Hemolytic anemia, leukopenia, lymphopenia, thrombocytopenia
- Abdominal pain, anorexia, nausea, vomiting
- Raynaud phenomenon

PHYSICAL EXAM

- Vital signs: fever, hypertension
- Malar, discoid, psoriasiform, or annular rash, alopecia
- Oral/nasal ulcers (*often minimally symptomatic*)
- Lymphadenopathy, splenomegaly
- Acrocyanosis
- Inflammatory arthritis, tenosynovitis
- Pleural/pericardial rub, heart murmur
- Bibasilar rales
- Cranial/peripheral neuropathies

DIFFERENTIAL DIAGNOSIS

Undifferentiated connective tissue disease, Sjögren syndrome, fibromyalgia, RA, vasculitis, idiopathic thrombocytopenia purpura, antiphospholipid antibody syndrome, drug-induced lupus

DIAGNOSTIC TESTS & INTERPRETATION

Initial Tests (lab, imaging)

- Antinuclear antibody (ANA)
  - High sensitivity (98%), low specificity
  - False-positive rate of 5–30%: elderly, autoimmune thyroid/liver disease, chronic infection, etc.
  - Low titers <1:160 of limited clinical use
- Anti–double-stranded DNA (dsDNA) and anti-Smith antibodies: high specificity for SLE: predictor of nephritis and hemolytic anemia
  - Correlates with disease activity
- RNA protein antibodies (anti-RNP, anti-Ro, anti-La): less specific for SLE
- False-positive Venereal Disease Research Laboratory (VDRL) test: high sensitivity, low specificity. Surrogate marker of cardiolipin antibody presence
- Low serum complement levels: C3, C4
- Erythrocyte sediment rate (ESR): nonspecific, often high in active disease
- CBC: hemolytic anemia, thrombocytopenia, leukopenia, or lymphopenia
- Serum creatinine: elevated in lupus nephritis
- Urinalysis (UA): proteinuria, hematuria, cellular cast
- Phospholipid antibodies: cardiolipin immunoglobulin (Ig) G/IgM, lupus anticoagulant, β_2-glycoprotein IgG/IgM
- Anti-P (ribosomal autoantibodies) is associated with SLE arthritis and disease activity.
- Initial imaging is dependent on presenting symptoms.
- Radiograph of involved joints
- Chest x-ray: infiltrates, pleural effusion, low lung volumes
- Chest CT scan, ventilation-perfusion (V-Q) scan, duplex ultrasound for PE or deep vein thrombosis
- Head CT scan: ischemia, infarct, hemorrhage
- Brain MRI: focal areas of increased signal intensity
- Echocardiogram: pericardial effusion, valvular vegetations, pulmonary hypertension
- Contrast angiography for medium-size artery vasculitis: mesenteric/limb ischemia, CNS symptom

Follow-Up Tests & Special Considerations

- Hemolytic anemia: elevated reticulocyte count and indirect bilirubin, low haptoglobin, positive direct Coombs test
- Confirm positive phospholipid antibodies results in 12 weeks.
- If phospholipid antibodies are initially negative, but symptoms arise, repeat, as they may become positive over time.
- 24-hour urine collection/spot protein/creatinine to quantify proteinuria
- Histone antibodies present in >95% of drug-induced lupus (vs. 80% of idiopathic SLE)
- Fasting lipid panel and glucose
- Follow vitamin D[25(O)H] levels and replenish PRN.

Diagnostic Procedures/Other

- Renal biopsy to diagnose lupus nephritis (if UA abnormal)
- Skin biopsy with immunofluorescence on involved and uninvolved non–sun-exposed skin (*lupus band test*) may help differentiate SLE rash from others.
- Lumbar puncture in patients with fever and CNS/meningeal symptoms
- EEG for seizures/global CNS dysfunction
- Neuropsychiatric testing for cognitive impairment
- EMG/nerve conduction study (NCS) for peripheral neuropathy and myositis
- Nerve and/or muscle biopsy
- ECG, cardiac enzymes, stress tests
- American College of Rheumatology classification (not diagnostic) criteria: any 4 of the 11 listed (95% specificity and 85% sensitivity):
  - Malar (butterfly) rash
  - Discoid rash
  - Photosensitivity: by patient history/physician observation
  - Oral/nasopharyngeal ulcers

- Nonerosive arthritis: involving ≥2 peripheral joints
- Pleuritis *OR* pericarditis
- Renal disorder: proteinuria (>0.5 g/day or >3+) *OR* cellular casts (red cell, hemoglobin, granular, tubular, or mixed)
- Neurologic disorder: psychosis/seizures
- Hematologic disorder: hemolytic anemia, leukopenia (<4,000/mm^3 on ≥2 tests), lymphopenia (<1,500/mm^3 on ≥2 tests), thrombocytopenia (<100,000/mm^3)
- Immunologic disorder: anti-DNA, anti-Sm, anticardiolipin IgG/IgM, lupus anticoagulant, or false–positive VDRL findings
- Positive ANA in absence of drugs known to cause positive ANA

Test Interpretation

- Skin: vascular/perivascular inflammation, immune-complex deposition at dermal–epidermal junction, mucinosis, basal layer vacuolar changes
  - Similar findings seen in other connective tissue disorders such as dermatomyositis
- Renal: mesangial hypercellularity/matrix expansion, subendothelial/subepithelial immune deposits, glomerular sclerosis, fibrous crescents
  - Vary depending on degree of involvement
- Vascular: immune-complex deposition in vessel walls with fibrinoid necrosis and perivascular mononuclear cell infiltrates, intraluminal fibrin thrombi

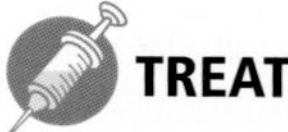

TREATMENT

GENERAL MEASURES

- Education, counseling, and support
- Influenza/pneumococcal vaccines are safe; avoid live vaccines in immunocompromised patients.
- Low-estrogen oral contraceptives safe in mild SLE

MEDICATION

First Line

- *Antimalarial agents and NSAIDs are 1st-line therapy for patients with mild SLE* (1)[A].
  - Hydroxychloroquine for constitutional and musculoskeletal symptoms, rash, mild serositis; may reduce flares and increase long-term survival (2,3)[A]. NSAIDs for musculoskeletal manifestations, mild serositis, headache, and fever (2)[C]
- Systemic glucocorticoids (prednisone or equivalent)
  - Low dose (<0.5 mg/kg) for minor disease activity not responsive to NSAIDs or when NSAIDs are contraindicated (2)[A]
  - High-dose (1–2 mg/kg/day) (2)[A] or IV pulse methylprednisolone for organ-threatening disease, particularly CNS and renal; often combined with immunosuppressive agent (2)[A]
- Topical glucocorticosteroids for skin manifestations

Second Line

- Belimumab as adjunct for preventing flares in patients with active lupus despite 1st-line therapy (4)[A]
  - 10 mg/kg IV every 2 weeks × 3 doses, then monthly
- Methotrexate (2)[A], azathioprine (2)[B], mycophenolate mofetil (2)[C], or leflunomide as steroid-sparing agent for persistent active disease or to maintain remission
  - Requires laboratory monitoring for toxicity
- Treatments under investigation: rituximab, epratuzumab, abatacept, interferon-α inhibitors
- Immunosuppressive agents for severe disease
  - Cyclophosphamide (2)[A]: adequate hydration to reduce risk of hemorrhagic cystitis
  - Mycophenolate mofetil (2)[A]: more efficacious for lupus nephritis (1)[A]

SURGERY/OTHER PROCEDURES

Renal transplant for end-stage renal disease

COMPLEMENTARY & ALTERNATIVE MEDICINE

Biofeedback, visual imagery, cognitive therapy

INPATIENT CONSIDERATIONS

Admission Criteria/Initial Stabilization

- Difficult to differentiate SLE flare from infection; may need to treat both pending full evaluation
- IV pulse Solu-Medrol 1 g/day × 3–5 days for life- or organ-threatening disease (2)[A]

ONGOING CARE

FOLLOW-UP RECOMMENDATIONS

Patient Monitoring

- Clinical evaluation for signs and symptoms
  - Weekly to monthly for active disease
  - Every 3–6 months for mild/inactive disease
- Measures of disease activity and damage: Systemic Lupus Erythematosus Disease Activity Index, British Isles Lupus Assessment Group Index, European Consensus Lupus Activity Measure
- Laboratory studies
  - CBC with differential
  - Serum creatinine, UA
  - Vitamin D
  - Declining C3/C4 and rising DS-DNA and ESR may correlate with disease activity.
- Monitor for adverse effects of treatment
  - NSAIDs: GI bleeding and/or ulceration
  - Glucocorticoids: glucose, lipids, bone density
  - Hydroxychloroquine: ophthalmologic exam every 6–12 months
  - Methotrexate: CBC, creatinine, albumin, aspartate aminotransferase (AST), alanine aminotransferase (ALT) every 2 months
  - Azathioprine and mycophenolate mofetil: CBC every 1–3 months
  - Cyclophosphamide
    - CBC, creatinine, UA every 2 weeks, and liver function tests monthly during treatment
    - UA every 6–12 months for life

DIET

- No special diet unless for complications such as renal failure, diabetes, hyperlipidemia (2)[C]
- Adequate calcium/vitamin D intake in patients on corticosteroids (2)[A]
- Low glycemic index or calorie-restricted diet in patients on corticosteroids

PATIENT EDUCATION

- Avoid UV light exposure: sunscreens (SPF ≥30), protective clothing (2)[B]
- Weight control, smoking cessation, exercise (2)[C]
- Stress avoidance/management

PROGNOSIS

- Permanent treatment-free remission is uncommon.
- 5-year survival after diagnosis is 95%.
- Poor prognostic factor: major organ involvement
- Drug-induced lupus resolves within weeks to months after discontinuation of the offending drug.

COMPLICATIONS

Infections, neoplasms, cardiac disease, nephritis, neuropsychiatric lupus; depression

Pregnancy Considerations

- Exacerbations during pregnancy are less common when in remission for 6 months prior to conception.
- Fetal loss is increased, especially in those with active lupus/antiphospholipid antibodies.
- A 2% risk of congenital heart block if anti-SS-A (Ro) or anti-SS-B (La) antibodies are present.
- See "Antiphospholipid Antibody Syndrome" for recommendations regarding use of aspirin and heparin to prevent pregnancy complications.

REFERENCES

1. Yildirim-Toruner C, Diamond B. Current and novel therapeutics in the treatment of systemic lupus erythematosus. *J Allergy Clin Immunol*. 2011;127(2):303–312.
2. Bertsias G, Ioannidis JP, Boletis J, et al. EULAR recommendations for the management of systemic lupus erythematosus. Report of a task force of the EULAR Standing Committee for International Clinical Studies Including Therapeutics. *Ann Rheum Dis*. 2008;67(2):195–205.
3. Ruiz-Irastorza G, Ramos-Casals M, Brito-Zeron P, et al. Clinical efficacy and side effects of antimalarials in systemic lupus erythematosus: a systematic review. *Ann Rheum Dis*. 2010;69(1):20–28.
4. Navarra SV, Guzman RM, Gallacher AE, et al. Efficacy and safety of belimumab in patients with active systemic lupus erythematosus: a randomised, placebo-controlled, phase 3 trial. *Lancet*. 2011;377(9767):721–731.

ADDITIONAL READING

Lisnevskaia L, Murphy G, Isenberg D. Systemic lupus erythematosus. *Lancet*. 2014;384(9957):1878–1888. doi:10.1016/S0140-6736(14)60128-8.

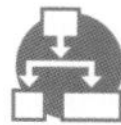

SEE ALSO

Antiphospholipid Antibody Syndrome

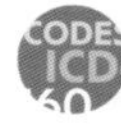

CODES

ICD10

- M32.9 Systemic lupus erythematosus, unspecified
- M32.10 Systemic lupus erythematosus, organ or system involv unsp
- M32.14 Glomerular disease in systemic lupus erythematosus

CLINICAL PEARLS

- *Aggressiveness of therapy should reflect intensity of disease.*
- Most important diagnostic test is the UA: if abnormal, order kidney biopsy; *serum and urine lab values often do not reveal extent of kidney disease.*
- Atherosclerotic and atheroembolic complications are the major cause of death; address modifiable cardiovascular risk factors.

LUPUS NEPHRITIS

Weizhen Tan, MD • Neena R. Gupta, MD

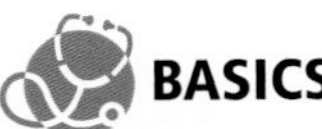

BASICS

DESCRIPTION

- Lupus nephritis (LN) is the renal manifestation of systemic lupus erythematosus (SLE).
- American College of Rheumatology (ACR) criteria: persistent proteinuria >500 mg/day or ≥3 on dipstick and/or presence of cellular casts. Alternatively, spot urine protein-to-creatinine ratio >0.5 and "active urinary sediment" (>5 RBC/hpf, >5 WBC/hpf in absence of infection, or cellular casts—RBC or WBC casts) (1)
- Clinical manifestations primarily due to immune complex–mediated glomerular disease. Tubulointerstitial and vascular involvement often seen. Diagnosed based on clinical findings, urine abnormalities, autoantibodies, and renal biopsy
- Treatment and prognosis depend on International Society of Nephrology/Renal Pathology Society (ISN/RPS) histologic class—risk of end-stage renal disease (ESRD) highest in class IV.
- Delay in diagnosis/treatment increases risk of ESRD.

EPIDEMIOLOGY

- Peak incidence of SLE is 15–45 years of age.
- Predominant sex: female > male (10:1)
- Once SLE develops, LN affects both genders equally; it is more severe in children and men and less severe in older adults.

Incidence

- SLE: 1.4–21.9/100,000 (2)
- Up to 60% of SLE patients develop LN over time, and 25–50% of SLE patients have nephritis as the initial presentation.

Pediatric Considerations

LN is more common and more severe in children: 60–80% have LN at or soon after SLE onset.

Prevalence

SLE: 7.4–159.4/100,000 (2)

ETIOLOGY AND PATHOPHYSIOLOGY

- Immune complex–mediated inflammation injures glomeruli, tubules, interstitium, and vasculature.
- Glomeruli: varying degrees of mesangial proliferation, crescent formation (see "Pathologic Findings"), and fibrinoid necrosis causing reduced glomerular filtration rate (GFR)
- Persistence of inflammation (chronicity) leads to sclerosis and glomerular loss.
- Tubulointerstitial injury (edema, inflammatory cell infiltrate acutely; tubular atrophy in chronic phase) with or without tubular basement membrane immune complex deposition leads to reduced renal function.
- Vascular lesions: immune complex deposition and noninflammatory necrosis in arterioles
- SLE is a multifactorial disease, with a multigenic inheritance; exact etiology is elusive.
- Defective T-cell autoregulation and polyclonal B-cell hyperactivity
- Dysregulated apoptosis and impaired clearance of apoptotic cells inhibits self-tolerance to nuclear antigens.
- Anti-DNA, anti-C1q, anti-α-actin, and other nuclear component autoantibodies develop.
- Deposition of circulating immune complexes or autoantibodies attaching to local nuclear antigens leads to complement activation, inflammation, and tissue injury.
- Interaction of genetic, hormonal, and environmental factors leads to great variability in LN severity.

Genetics

No clear pattern but multigenic inheritance supported by ethnic differences, clustering in families, ~25% concordance in identical twins.

RISK FACTORS

Risk factors for LN include younger age, African American or Hispanic race, more ACR criteria met for diagnosis of SLE, longer disease duration, hypertension, lower socioeconomic status, family history of SLE, anti-dsDNA antibodies.

COMMONLY ASSOCIATED CONDITIONS

Other organ systems, such as skin, hematologic, cerebral, pulmonary, GI, and cardiac, are often involved in SLE.

DIAGNOSIS

HISTORY

Assess for risk factors and other signs/symptoms of SLE: rash, photosensitivity, arthritis, neurologic complaints; fever; weight loss; alopecia.

PHYSICAL EXAM

- Hypertension, fever
- Pleural/pericardial rub
- Skin rash
- Edema
- Arthritis

DIFFERENTIAL DIAGNOSIS

- Primary glomerular disease
- Secondary renal involvement in other systemic disorders such as antineutrophil cystoplasmic autoantibody (ANCA) associated vasculitis, Henoch-Schönlein purpura (HSP), antiglomerular basement membrane disease, and viral infections
- Mixed connective tissue disorder may have glomerulonephritis indistinguishable from LN.

DIAGNOSTIC TESTS & INTERPRETATION

- Clinical data have to be combined with serologic and renal biopsy patterns to differentiate LN from other processes. Renal biopsy is the gold standard for diagnosing and classifying LN
- Active urine sediment suggests nephritis.
- Autoantibodies, low C3, C4, CH50 complement levels
- Renal biopsy is gold standard for diagnosis, treatment, and prognosis.

Initial Tests (lab, imaging)

- Urinalysis may show hematuria, proteinuria, and active urine sediment (3)[C].
- Serum electrolytes, BUN, creatinine, albumin, routine serologic markers of SLE such as antinuclear antibody (ANA), anti-dsDNA, anti-Ro, anti-La, anti-RNP, anti-Sm, antiphospholipid antibody, C3, C4, CH50, CBC with differential, and C-reactive protein (CRP) (3)[C]
- CBC may show anemia, thrombocytopenia, and leukopenia.
- Renal ultrasound (3)[C]

Follow-Up Tests & Special Considerations

- Monitor every 3 months for disease activity (3)[C]: urinalysis for hematuria, proteinuria; blood for C3, C4, anti-dsDNA, serum albumin, and creatinine
- Patients with estimated glomerular filtration rate (eGFR) <60 mL should be managed according to the National Kidney Foundation guidelines for chronic kidney disease.
- Drug level monitoring if on immunosuppressants

Pregnancy Considerations

- Pregnancy leads to worsening of renal function in LN. Risk factors include renal impairment at baseline, active disease, hypertension, and proteinuria.
- Risk factors for fetal loss include elevated serum creatinine, heavy proteinuria, hypertension, and anticardiolipin antibodies.

Test Interpretation

- Adequate renal biopsy (at least 10 glomeruli for light microscopy or total 20–25 glomeruli) is essential. Light, immunofluorescence, and electron microscopy needed for accurate classification.
- On immunofluorescence microscopy: immune complex deposits consisting of IGG, IGA, IGM, C1q, and C3 ("full house") highly suggestive of LN
- Revised ISN/RPS histologic classification guides therapeutic decisions.
- LN is classified as purely mesangial (class I, II), focal proliferative: <50% glomeruli (class III), diffuse proliferative: ≥50% (class IV), membranous (class V), and advanced sclerosis (class VI). Subdivisions for activity (A) and chronicity (C) in class III/IV and for segmental (S) or global (G) glomerular involvement in class IV (Class III A, C, A/C and class IV S[A], G[A], S[A/C], S[C], G[C].
- LN may change to another class over time or with therapy.
- Focal and diffuse proliferative LN (classes III and IV) are common and most likely to progress to ESRD.

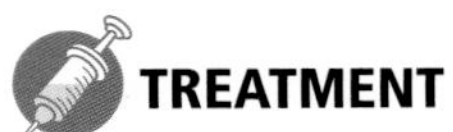

TREATMENT

GENERAL MEASURES

- Monitor bone density, optimize vitamin D and calcium intake in patients on glucocorticoids.
- Low-salt diet for hypertension, edema. For eGFR <60 mL: Follow National Kidney Foundation guidelines for chronic kidney disease.
- Avoid sun or ultraviolet light exposure.

MEDICATION

First Line

- **Class I + II LN**: No specific therapy needed, as long-term renal prognosis is good. Renin-angiotensin system blockade (ACE inhibitors or angiotensin receptor blockers) to manage BP and proteinuria
- **Proliferative LN (Class III, IV, V + III/IV)**: Induce remission by steroids + IV cyclophosphamide or mycophenolate mofetil (MMF) and maintenance of remission by low-dose steroids and azathioprine (AZA) or MMF (1).
- Principles of treatment:
  - Avoid delay in treatment.
  - Inducing remission quickly (3–6 months)
  - Maintaining response and avoiding iatrogenic morbidity (5–10 years)

- **INDUCTION**: steroids + immunosuppressive agent (for mild class III, high-dose steroids may be sufficient):
  - Glucocorticoids: methylprednisolone pulse 0.5–1 g/day for 3 days followed by oral prednisone 0.5–1 mg/kg/day PO (max 60 mg/day, taper after 4–8 weeks) (4,5)[A] *AND*
  - Cyclophosphamide **(CYC)**: IV CYC (high dose = 0.5–1 g/m^2 monthly × 6 doses—NIH regimen; low dose = 0.5 g q2wk × 6 doses—EuroLupus regimen) *OR*
  - Mycophenolate mofetil (MMF): 1–3 g/day PO divided BID (target 3 g/day as tolerated) for 6 months. MMF is as effective as CYC in achieving remission with fewer side effects (6)[A].
- **MAINTENANCE:**
  - Glucocorticoids: oral prednisone tapered to low doses (generally <10 mg/day by 6 months) AND
  - MMF 1–2 g/day divided BID PO OR AZA (azathioprine): 1–2.5 mg/kg/day PO (4,5)[A]
  - In the ALMS (Aspreva Lupus Management Study) MMF shown to be superior than AZA for maintenance therapy in a varied population (7)[A].
  - In the MAINTAIN nephritis trial, MMF shown to be equal to AZA for maintenance therapy in a mostly Caucasian population (8)[A].
  - Cyclophosphamide IV quarterly for 1–2 year after renal remission; not used now due to availability of less toxic regimen
- **Class V LN**: good prognosis in general, treatment not standardized
  - For subnephrotic patients, no specific treatment except renin-angiotensin system blockade.
  - Options for nephrotic patients include steroids with either calcineurin inhibitors, IV CYC, AZA, or MMF (5)[B].
  - Class V LN with presence of class III or class IV biopsy findings needs aggressive combination regimen as for class III/IV.

Second Line
Other treatments in selected patients: rituximab, plasma exchange, IVIG, calcineurin inhibitors. Belimumab was approved by FDA in 2011, but trials excluded patients with severe active LN (9)[C].

ISSUES FOR REFERRAL
Nephrology consults for initial management and relapses

ADDITIONAL THERAPIES
- KDIGO 2012 guidelines for LN state that all patients with LN of any class be treated with hydroxychloroquine (maximum daily dose of 6–6.5 mg/kg ideal body weight), unless they have a specific contraindication to this drug.
- BP control; treat dyslipidemia and other modifiable cardiovascular risk factors
- Anticoagulation for symptomatic antiphospholipid antibody syndrome

SURGERY/OTHER PROCEDURES
- Renal transplant for ESRD when indicated
- Patient and graft survival rates are similar to non-SLE patients (2)[C].
- Risk of recurrent LN in renal transplant recipients ranges between 0 and 30%; graft loss due to recurrence is rare.

INPATIENT CONSIDERATIONS
Admission Criteria/Initial Stabilization
- Uncontrolled hypertension, acute kidney injury
- Severe extrarenal manifestation
- Control hypertension and proteinuria, if present.
- Labs to help confirm SLE/LN, renal ultrasound
- Nephrology for manage input and renal biopsy

IV Fluids
Patients who have nephrotic syndrome or acute kidney injury should be fluid restricted.

Discharge Criteria
Once the patient is stabilized and renal biopsy is performed, management safely as an outpatient.

ONGOING CARE

FOLLOW-UP RECOMMENDATIONS
Patient Monitoring
- Monitor urine protein-to-creatinine ratio, urine microscopy, serum albumin and creatinine, antibody titers (especially anti-dsDNA), C3, C4, BP at least every 3 months for first 2–3 years (3)[C].
- Once stable on maintenance therapy with no active disease, follow-up every 6–12 months (3)[C].
- Cyclophosphamide: CBC, ensure adequate hydration
- MMF: CBC, LFT, SrCr
- Azathioprine: CBC

DIET
Low-salt diet. For eGFR <60 mL: Follow National Kidney Foundation guidelines for chronic kidney disease.

PATIENT EDUCATION
Medication adherence and self-monitoring for symptom relapse

PROGNOSIS
- 10-year survival 88 and 94% in SLE patients with and without renal involvement (1)
- Relapse rate 35%. 10–20% of patients progress to ESRD within 10 years (10).
- 5-year renal survival of class IV LN <30% before 1970; has improved to >80% in last 2 decades (2)
- Early and complete remission with treatment is the best prognostic factor. Predictors of remission include low baseline proteinuria, normal creatinine, Caucasian race, and treatment initiation within 3 months of clinical diagnosis.
- Indicators of poor prognosis: diffuse proliferative LN (especially crescentic), higher activity/chronicity index, African American race, lower socioeconomic status, poor response to treatment, high creatinine at baseline, uncontrolled hypertension, and relapse

COMPLICATIONS
- Risks from immunosuppression: infections, malignancy
- Treatment side effects: Cyclophosphamide causes primary amenorrhea.
- MMF may cause GI upset and nausea and is a teratogen. (Azathioprine recommended for women who desire pregnancy).
- Risk of vascular thromboses (hypercoagulable state from antiphospholipid antibodies)
- About 10–20% of patients develop ESRD from progressive disease refractory to treatment requiring dialysis/kidney transplantation.

REFERENCES

1. Hahn BH, McMahon MA, Wilkinson A, et al. American College of Rheumatology guidelines for screening, treatment, and management of lupus nephritis. *Arthritis Care Res (Hoboken)*. 2012;64(6):797–808.
2. Ortega LM, Schultz DR, Lenz O, et al. Review: lupus nephritis: pathologic features, epidemiology and a guide to therapeutic decisions. *Lupus*. 2010;19(5):557–574.
3. Mosca M, Tani C, Aringer M, et al. European League Against Rheumatism recommendations for monitoring patients with systemic lupus erythematosus in clinical practice and in observational studies. *Ann Rheum Dis*. 2010;69(7):1269–1274.
4. Ponticelli C, Glassock RJ, Moroni G, et al. Induction and maintenance therapy in proliferative lupus nephritis. *J Nephrol*. 2010;23(1):9–16.
5. Bomback AS, Appel GB. Updates on the treatment of lupus nephritis. *J Am Soc Nephrol*. 2010;21(12):2028–2035.
6. Henderson LK, Masson, PM, Craig JC, et al. Induction and maintenance treatment of proliferative lupus nephritis: a meta-analysis of RCTs. *Am J Kidney Dis*. 2013;61(1):74–87.
7. Dooley MA, Jayne D, Ginzler EM, et al. Mycophenolate versus azathioprine as maintenance therapy for lupus nephritis. *N Engl J Med*. 2011;365(20):1886–1895.
8. Morris HK, Canetta PA, Appel GB. Impact of ALMS and MAINTAIN trials on the management of lupus nephritis. *Nephrol Dial Transplant*. 2013;28(6):1371–1376.
9. Lo MS, Tsokos GC. Treatment of systemic lupus erythematosus: new advances in targeted therapy. *Ann N Y Acad Sci*. 2012;1247:138–152.
10. Houssiau FA, Ginzler EM. Current treatment of lupus nephritis. *Lupus*. 2008;17(5):426–430.

ADDITIONAL READING

- Kidney Disease: Improving Global Outcomes (KDIGO) Glomerulonephritis Work Group. KDIGO clinical practice guideline for glomerulonephritis. *Kidney Inter*. 2012;2(Suppl):139–274.
- Weening JJ, D'Agati VD, Schwartz MM, et al. The classification of glomerulonephritis in systemic lupus erythematosus revisited. *J Am Soc Nephrol*. 2004;15(2):241–250.

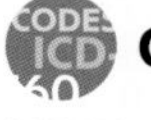

CODES

ICD10
M32.14 Glomerular disease in systemic lupus erythematosus

CLINICAL PEARLS
- Early diagnosis, correct classification by renal biopsy, and rapid treatment improve renal survival in patients with LN.
- Treatment of proliferative/progressive LN consists of a short induction course followed by longer maintenance course using glucocorticoids and immunosuppressants.

LYME DISEASE

Felix B. Chang, MD, DABMA, ABIHM

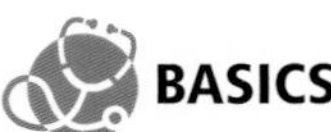

BASICS

DESCRIPTION

- A multisystem infection caused by *Borrelia* spirochetes, transmitted primarily by ixodid ticks
  - *Ixodes scapularis* (deer ticks) in the New England and Great Lakes areas
  - *Ixodes pacificus* in the West, also known as black-legged ticks and Western black-legged ticks
  - *Ixodes ricinus* in Europe
  - *Ixodes persuladas* in Asia and Russia
- Early localized Lyme disease includes a characteristic expanding skin rash (erythema migrans [EM]) (70%) and constitutional flulike symptoms.
- Disseminated Lyme disease presents with involvement of ≥1 organ systems. Neurologic, cardiac, and pauciarticular arthritis are most common.
- Post–Lyme disease syndrome includes arthritis (50%) and chronic neurologic syndromes.
- System(s) affected: hemic/lymphatic/immunologic; musculoskeletal; skin/exocrine; cardiac; neurologic
- Synonym(s): Lyme arthritis; Lyme borreliosis

EPIDEMIOLOGY

Incidence

- 96% of U.S. cases in 2011 were reported from 13 states: New England, New York, New Jersey, Delaware, Pennsylvania, Maryland, Minnesota, and Wisconsin (1).
- In states where Lyme disease is endemic, the incidence is 0.5 per 1,000 but can be substantially higher in local areas.
- Cases have been reported from all 50 states.

Prevalence

- The most reported vector-borne illness in the United States
- Predominant age: most common in children ages 5–14 years and in adults aged 55–70 years of age
- Predominant sex: male > female in the United States

ETIOLOGY AND PATHOPHYSIOLOGY

- Infection with spirochete *Borrelia burgdorferi* in the United States, or *Borrelia afzelii* or *Borrelia garinii* in Europe, transmitted by the bite of ixodid ticks (2)[A]
- Approximately 90% of cases are transmitted during the nymph stage of the tick life cycle.
- If a tick is infected, the chance of transmission increases with time attached: 12% at 48 hours, 79% at 72 hours, and 94% at 96 hours of attachment.
- Primary animal reservoir is the white-footed mouse.
- Spirochetes multiply and spread within dermis. Host response results in characteristic (EM) rash. Hematogenous dissemination results in disease within CNS, cardiovascular, or other organ systems.
- Start ticks (*Amblyomma americanum*), the American dog tick (*Dermacentor variabilis*), the Rocky Mountain wood tick (*Dermacentor andersoni*), and the brown dog tick (*Rhipicephalus sanguineous*) are not known to transmit Lyme Disease.

Genetics

Human leukocyte antigen: Haplotype DR4 or DR2 may be more susceptible to prolonged arthritis.

RISK FACTORS

- Exposure in tick-infested area; most common from April to November
- Those who reside or are employed in endemic areas where ixodid ticks are found are at increased risk.
- Ixodid ticks are commonly found on deer. Hunters may be at an increased risk.

GENERAL PREVENTION

- "Tick checks": Examine skin for ticks after outdoor activities.
- Removing ticks within 36 hours helps limit transmission.
- Wear clothing that covers the ankles in endemic areas.
- Use insect repellants containing DEET.
- Permethrin may be applied to clothes, shoes, tents.
- Antibiotic prophylaxis is recommended for the prevention of Lyme disease in endemic areas following an *Ixodes* tick bite.
- Prophylactic treatment with 1 dose of 200 mg of doxycycline within 72 hours of a tick bite in highly endemic areas is 87% effective. (Contraindicated in pregnancy and in children; no prophylactic agent is approved for these groups.) (2)[A]

COMMONLY ASSOCIATED CONDITIONS

Southern tick–associated rash illness may be mistaken for Lyme disease. It is seen in the southeastern and south central United States and is associated with the bite of the Lone Star tick, *Amblyomma americanum*.

- Coinfection with babesiosis has been reported. Suggested by high fever

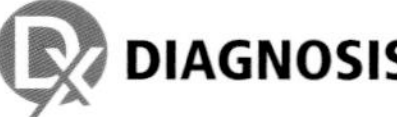

DIAGNOSIS

HISTORY

- History of a tick bite followed by illness with erythema migrans (3)
- Early Lyme disease: incubation period 3–30 days
  - Some patients may be asymptomatic (4).
  - Fever
  - Headache
  - Myalgias
  - Arthralgias
- Disseminated Lyme disease
  - Carditis (pleuritic chest pain; palpitations)
  - Facial palsies or other cranial neuropathies
  - Joint pain (polyarthritis/algias; late disease: monoarthritis-like knee)
  - Iritis, conjunctivitis
  - Migratory musculoskeletal pain
- Late untreated Lyme disease
  - Recurrent synovitis
  - Recurrent tendonitis and bursitis
  - Encephalopathic symptoms
    - Headaches
    - *Cognitive slowing*
    - Confusion
    - Profound fatigue
  - Symptoms mimicking other CNS diseases
    - Multiple sclerosis–like symptoms
    - Stroke-like symptoms
    - Transverse myelitis
  - Peripheral neuropathic symptoms; motor, sensory, or autonomic neuropathies
  - Meningitis

PHYSICAL EXAM

- Early Lyme disease
  - Erythema migrans (4)[A]
- Disseminated Lyme disease
  - Multiple erythema migrans
  - Facial palsies or other cranial neuropathies
  - Heart block—irregular pulse
  - Pericarditis—friction rub
  - Arthritis
  - Other focal neurologic findings

DIFFERENTIAL DIAGNOSIS

- Other rickettsial disease (Rocky Mountain spotted fever [RMSF])
- Juvenile rheumatoid arthritis; systemic lupus erythematosus (SLE); rheumatoid arthritis (RA)
- Viral syndromes
- Contact dermatitis; cellulitis; granuloma annulare (mimic EM)
- Syphilis
- AV block

DIAGNOSTIC TESTS & INTERPRETATION

Initial Tests (lab, imaging)

- Testing and treatment not indicated if tick attached for <48 hours (3)
- Diagnosis is based mainly on clinical findings in endemic areas (4).
- Serology: enzyme-linked immunosorbent assay (ELISA) for immunoglobulin (Ig) M and IgG *B. burgdorferi* antibodies, followed by a Western blot test if positive or equivocal, or an indirect immunofluorescence assay
- Culture of CSF for *B. burgdorferi*
- Plasma polymerase chain reaction (PCR) testing is of little value (only exception is synovial fluid analysis).
- No imaging routinely indicated.

Follow-Up Tests & Special Considerations

Disorders that may alter lab results: False-positive response has been seen with RMSF, syphilis, SLE, and RA.

- Arthritis: Serology + PCR of synovial fluid is both sensitive and specific.
- Neuroborreliosis: serology + CSF pleocytosis (PCR of CSF has a very low sensitivity)
- Late-stage disease with negative serology may be seen in patients who received early antibiotic treatment.
- After an infection, antibodies may persist for months to years. *Serologic tests do not distinguish active from past infection.*
- Antibodies are not protective.

Diagnostic Procedures/Other

Lumbar puncture when neurologic findings are present, with ELISA of CSF for *B. burgdorferi* antibodies. Xenodiagnosis in humans (5)

Test Interpretation

Culture of *B. burgdorferi* from blood or skin biopsy has a very low yield.

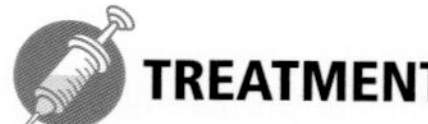

TREATMENT

GENERAL MEASURES

Early and disseminated Lyme disease can usually be treated as an outpatient except in the case of complications, such as carditis or meningitis, requiring parenteral antibiotics.

MEDICATION

First Line

- Erythema migrans
  - Doxycycline (Vibramycin) 100 mg PO BID for 10–21 days (do not use in children <8 or in pregnant women) (6,2)[A]; *or*
  - Amoxicillin 500 mg PO TID for 14–21 days (pediatric dose 50 mg/kg/day); *or*
  - Cefuroxime axetil 500 mg PO BID for 14–21 days
    - Doxycycline has the advantage of covering other tick-borne infections such as ehrlichiosis, anaplasmosis, RMSF.
    - Alternative: azithromycin 500 mg qd for 7–10 days or clarithromycin 500 mg BID for 14–21 days
- Neurologic disease
  - Normal CSF, treat for 14–21 days (2)[A].
  - Doxycycline 100 mg PO BID or amoxicillin 500 mg PO TID
  - Abnormal CSF, treat for 4 weeks: ceftriaxone 2 g qd IV, cefotaxime 2 g q8h, *or* penicillin G 5 mIU q6h
  - Cardiac disease
    - Mild (1st-degree AV block, PR <300 millisecond): doxycycline 100 mg PO BID or amoxicillin 500 mg PO TID for 14–21 days
    - More serious: ceftriaxone 2 g qd IV for 30 days
- Arthritis without neurologic disease (2)[A]
  - Oral treatment for 28 days with doxycycline 100 mg BID or amoxicillin 500 mg TID
  - If oral treatment fails, repeat oral regimen for 28 days or begin IV treatment with ceftriaxone 2 g qd for 2–4 weeks.
- Contraindications
  - Allergy to specific medication
  - Doxycycline is contraindicated in children and in women who are pregnant or breastfeeding.
- Precautions
  - In ~15% of patients treated with IV therapy, a Jarisch-Herxheimer–type reaction develops within 24 hours of initiation of therapy.
- Significant possible interactions
  - Oral anticoagulants may require dose adjustments.
  - Oral contraceptives may be less effective.

Pediatric Considerations

- Amoxicillin is the drug of choice in children.
- Tetracyclines are contraindicated.

Pregnancy Considerations

- Because *B. burgdorferi* can cross the placenta; pregnant patients with active disease should be treated with parenteral antibiotics.
- Doxycycline should not be used in pregnancy.

Second Line

- Azithromycin, 500 mg PO daily for 7 days, can be used for those allergic to β-lactams and unable to take tetracyclines but is less effective (2).
- There is no evidence for meaningful clinical benefit from prolonged treatment or retreatment of patients with persistent unexplained symptoms despite previous antibiotic treatment of Lyme disease.

IN-PATIENT CONSIDERATIONS

Admission Criteria/Initial Stabilization

- Admission is recommended for patients with Lyme carditis and symptoms of chest pain, syncope, or dyspnea, and for those with 2nd- or 3rd-degree heart block or 1st-degree heart block of ≥300 millisecond.
- Admission is also recommended for patients with symptoms of meningitis.

ONGOING CARE

FOLLOW-UP RECOMMENDATIONS

Patient Monitoring

Based on the severity of symptoms, patients with Lyme carditis, neurologic syndromes, or arthritis may require prolonged follow-up.

DIET

No restrictions

PATIENT EDUCATION

- In endemic areas, patients should be advised to protect themselves against tick exposure.
- https://www.rheumatology.org/Practice/Clinical/Patients/Diseases_And_Conditions/Lyme_Disease/

PROGNOSIS

- Early treatment with antibiotics can shorten the duration of symptoms and prevent later disease.
- Response of late-stage disease to treatment is variable. Symptoms may take weeks to resolve after beginning treatment.

COMPLICATIONS

- Recurrent synovitis, tendonitis, bursitis (7)[A]
- Chronic neurologic symptoms
- Peripheral neuropathies
- Posttreatment Lyme disease syndrome: 10–20% lingering symptoms of fatigue, pain, or joint and muscle aches. Can last for 6 months (8)[A]

REFERENCES

1. Centers for Disease Control and Prevention. Statistics on Lyme disease. www.cdc.gov/lyme/stats/index.html. Accessed 2014.
2. Lyme disease. http://www.cdc.gov/lyme. Accessed 2014.
3. Wright WF, Riedel DJ, Talwani R, et al. Diagnosis and management of Lyme Disease. *Am Fam Physician*. 2012;85(11):1086–1093.
4. Duncan CJ, Carle G, Seaton RA. Tick bite and early Lyme borreliosis. *BMJ*. 2012;334:e3124.
5. Marques A, Telford SR III, Turk SP, et al. Xenodiagnosis to detect *Borrelia burgdorferi* infection: a first-in-human study. *Clin Infect Dis*. 2014;58(7):937–945. doi:10.1093/cid/cit939
6. Klempner MS, Baker PJ, Shapiro ED, et al. Source treatment trials for post-Lyme disease symptoms revisited. *Am J Med*. 2013;126(8):665–669.
7. Nadelman R, Hanincová K, Mukherjee P, et al. Differentiation of reinfection from relapse in recurrent Lyme disease. *N Engl J Med*. 2012;367(20):1883–1890.
8. Marques A. Chronic Lyme disease: a review. *Infect Dis Clin North Am*. 2008;22(2):341–360.

ADDITIONAL READING

- Delong A, Blossom B, Maloney EL, et al. Antibiotic retreatment of Lyme disease in patients with persistent symptoms: a biostatistical review of randomized, placebo-controlled, clinical trials. *Contemp Clin Trials*. 2012;33(6):1132–1142.
- Overstreet M. Tick bites and Lyme disease: the need for timely treatment. *Crit Care Nurs Clin North Am*. 2013;25(2):165–172.
- Stanek G, Wormser G, Gray J, et al. Lyme borreliosis. *Lancet*. 2012;379(9814):461–473.

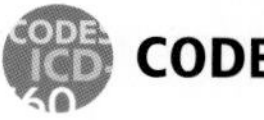

CODES

ICD10

- A69.20 Lyme disease, unspecified
- A69.23 Arthritis due to Lyme disease
- A69.21 Meningitis due to Lyme disease

CLINICAL PEARLS

- The presence of erythema migrans following a tick bite in an area endemic for Lyme disease warrants empiric treatment.
- Repeat episodes of erythema migrans in appropriately treated patients are due to reinfection and not relapse.
- There is no evidence that Lyme disease is transmitted from person to person.
- Lyme disease acquired during pregnancy may lead to infection of the placenta and possible stillbirth. No negative effect on the fetus have been found when mother receives appropriate antibiotic therapy.
- Ticks must be attached for 36–48 hours or more for disease transmission.

LYMPHANGITIS

Amar Kapur, DO, CPT, MC, USA

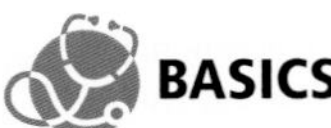

BASICS

DESCRIPTION

Acute or chronic inflammation of lymphatic channels due to a skin breach or local trauma; presents as red, tender streaks extending to regional lymph nodes

- May result from compromised lymphatic drainage due to surgical procedures
- May be infectious or noninfectious

ETIOLOGY AND PATHOPHYSIOLOGY

- Acute infection
  - Usually caused by group A β-hemolytic *Streptococcus*
  - Less commonly caused by the following:
    - *Staphylococcus aureus*
    - *Pasteurella multocida*
    - *Erysipelothrix*
    - *Spirillum minus* (rat bite disease)
    - *Pseudomonas*
    - Other *Streptococcus* sp.
    - Immunocompromised patients can be infected with gram-negative rods, gram-negative bacilli, or fungi.
    - In fresh water exposures, *Aeromonas hydrophila*
- Nodular lymphangitis
  - Also known as sporotrichoid lymphangitis
  - Presents as painful or painless nodular subcutaneous swellings along lymphatic vessels
  - Lesions may ulcerate with accompanying regional lymphadenopathy.
  - Typical of infections from the following: *Sporothrix schenckii*, *Nocardia brasiliensis*, *Mycobacterium marinum*, leishmanisis, tularemia, and systemic mycoses
  - Pathology may show granulomas.
- Noninfectious granulomatous lymphangitis
  - Rare acquired lymphedema of the genitalia in children
  - May be due to atypical Crohn disease or sarcoidosis (1)[C]
- Filarial lymphangitis
  - Parasites in the lymphatic vessels cause inflammation and dilatation; can predispose to secondary bacterial infection
  - Usually caused by *Wuchereria bancrofti*. Other causes are *Brugia malayi* and *Brugia timori*.
- Lymphangitis due to surgery
  - May occur after surgical procedures and lymph node dissection
- Sclerosing lymphangitis of the penis
  - Asymptomatic cord such as swelling around coronal sulcus of penis usually resulting from vigorous sexual activity or masturbation

RISK FACTORS

- Impaired lymphatic drainage due to surgery, nodal dissection, or irradiation
- Diabetes mellitus
- Chronic steroid use
- Peripheral venous catheter
- Varicella infection
- Immunocompromising condition
- Human, animal, or insect bites
- Fungal, bacterial, or mycobacterial skin infections
- Any trauma to the skin
- IV drug abuse
- Residence in endemic areas of filariasis

GENERAL PREVENTION

- Reduce chronic lymphedema with compression devices or by treating underlying process
- Insect repellant
- Proper wound and skin care

COMMONLY ASSOCIATED CONDITIONS

- Lymphedema
- Prior lymph node dissection
- Tinea pedis (athlete's foot)
- Sporotrichosis
- Cellulitis, erysipelas
- Filarial infection (*W. bancrofti*)

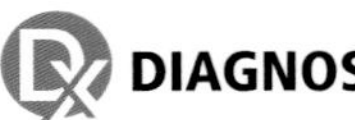

DIAGNOSIS

HISTORY

- History of trauma to skin, cut, abrasion, or fungal infection
- Systemic symptoms:
  - Malaise
  - Fever and chills
  - Loss of appetite
  - Headache
  - Muscle aches
- Travel to a tropical region or region with known filariasis

PHYSICAL EXAM

Local signs:

- Erythematous, macular linear streaks from site of infection toward the regional lymph nodes
- Tenderness and warmth over affected skin or lymph nodes
- May have blistering of affected skin
- Fluctuance, swelling, or purulent drainage
- Nodular lymphangitis can present with subcutaneous swellings along the lymphatic channels.
- Sporotrichosis may present with papulonodular lesions that may ulcerate.
- Sites may be nonpainful.

DIFFERENTIAL DIAGNOSIS

- Superficial thrombophlebitis
  - Thrombus or infection within the thrombosis (septic thrombophlebitis)
- Contact dermatitis
- Allergic reaction: less likely to be allergic if >24 hours after exposure (e.g., insect bite)
- Lymphangitis carcinomatosa
- Malignancy-related inflammation

DIAGNOSTIC TESTS & INTERPRETATION

- CBC may show leukocytosis or blood smear may show filarial infection.
- Blood or wound cultures
- Biopsy cultures

Initial Tests (lab, imaging)

Plain radiology unnecessary; may consider lymphangiography for lymphedema (2)[C]

Diagnostic Procedures/Other

- Swab, aspirate, and/or biopsy primary site, purulent discharge, nodule or distal ulcer for culture, acid fast staining, histology, and microscopy.
- Blood cultures
- Serology (e.g., *Francisella tularensis*, histoplasma)
- Blood film/smear (e.g., filaria)
- Lymphangiography to determine lymphedema or lymphatic obstruction

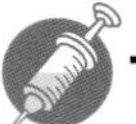

TREATMENT

GENERAL MEASURES

- Hot, moist compresses to affected area
- If lymphedema is involved, compression garments and weight loss may help.
- Abstinence from sexual activity (for sclerosing lymphangitis)

MEDICATION

- Empirically treat common organisms. Use culture and susceptibility to guide subsequent antibiotic treatment (3)[B].

- If mild systemic signs and limited local signs, treat as an outpatient with oral antibiotics
- If no improvement after 48 hours of oral antibiotics, reassess and consider IV antibiotics and/or hospitalization.
- If systemic involvement, start IV antibiotics.
- If necrotizing fasciitis due to group A β-hemolytic *Streptococcus* is suspected, treat aggressively with antibiotics and surgical intervention.

First Line

- Antibiotics for group A streptococcal infection
  - Amoxicillin (if patient known to have only group A *Streptococcus*)
    - Dosing
      - Adults
        - Mild to moderate: 500 mg PO q12h
        - Severe: 875 mg PO q12h or 500 mg PO q8h
      - Children <3 months: 30 mg/kg/day PO divided q12h
      - Children ≥3 months, ≤40 kg
        - Mild to moderate: 25 mg/kg/day PO divided q12h or 20 mg/kg/day divided q8h
        - Severe: 45 mg/kg/day PO divided q12h or 40 mg/kg/day divided q8h
      - Children ≥40 kg same as adult dosing
    - Common adverse effects
      - Diarrhea
    - Serious adverse effects
      - Anaphylaxis, Stevens-Johnson syndrome (SJS), toxic epidermal necrolysis (TEN)
    - Drug interactions
      - Methotrexate, venlafaxine, warfarin, hormonal contraceptives
    - Contraindications
      - Hypersensitivity to penicillin
- Ampicillin/sulbactam
  - Dosing
    - Adults and children ≥40 kg: 1.5–3 g (ampicillin + sulbactam component) IV/IM q6h
    - Children <40 kg: 200 mg/kg/day IV infusion, in divided doses q6h; maximum 8 g ampicillin per day

- Common adverse effects
    - Diarrhea, injection site reactions
- Serious adverse effects
    - *Clostridium difficile* diarrhea, pseudomembranous enterocolitis, dysuria
- Drug interactions
    - Hormonal contraceptives
- Contraindications
    - Hypersensitivity reactions

- Ceftriaxone
  - Dosing
    - Adults: 1–2 g IV/IM q24h
    - Children: 50–75 mg/kg/day IV/IM once daily or in divided doses q12h; maximum 2 g/day
  - Common adverse effects
    - Injection site reactions, diarrhea
  - Serious adverse effects: same as amoxicillin or ampicillin
  - Drug interactions
    - Do not administer calcium-containing IV solutions in the same IV line.
  - Contraindications
    - Hypersensitivity to cephalosporins
    - Concurrent calcium-containing IV fluids
    - Increased risk of kernicterus, salt precipitation in lungs and kidneys in neonates <28 days (use cefotaxime instead)
- Cephalexin
  - Dosing
    - Adults: 500 mg PO q12h
    - Children: 25–50 mg/kg/day divided q12h
  - Common adverse effects
    - Diarrhea
  - Serious adverse effects
    - SJS, TEN, interstitial nephritis, renal failure, pseudomembranous enterocolitis, anaphylaxis
  - Contraindications
    - Hypersensitivity to cephalosporins
- Azithromycin (if penicillin or cephalosporin allergy)
  - Dosing
    - Adults: 500 mg PO on day 1 followed by 250 mg/day PO on days 2–5
    - Children ≥2 years: 12 mg/kg/day PO (maximum dose: 500 mg/day) once daily for 5 days (FDA off-label use for skin infections in children)
  - Common adverse effects
    - Abdominal pain, nausea, vomiting, diarrhea, headache
  - Serious adverse effects
    - Prolonged QT interval, torsades de pointes, liver failure, Lambert-Eaton syndrome, myasthenia gravis, corneal erosion, anaphylaxis
  - Drug interactions
    - Nelfinavir, warfarin, other medications with potential to prolong QT interval
  - Contraindications
    - Hepatic dysfunction or cholestatic jaundice with prior treatment
    - Hypersensitivity to macrolide (azithromycin, erythromycin, clarithromycin)
- Diethylcarbamazine, ivermectin, albendazole, and doxycycline are used to treat filarial infection.
- Acetaminophen or ibuprofen (NSAIDs) for pain and fever

SURGERY/OTHER PROCEDURES

- Incision and drainage of abscess if present
- Necrotizing fasciitis needs surgical evaluation and likely débridement
- Nodular lymphangitis may benefit from I&D
- With severe lymphedema, consider surgical drainage.

INPATIENT CONSIDERATIONS

Admission Criteria/Initial Stabilization

- Admit for signs of serious illness: fluids if in hypotensive shock
- Fever, chills, systemic toxicity
- IV antibiotics
- ICU or surgery as indicated

Discharge Criteria

Patient can be discharged on oral antibiotics after systemic symptoms resolve. Home IV antibiotics are an option depending on clinical setting.

ONGOING CARE

FOLLOW-UP RECOMMENDATIONS

- Elevate affected area.
- 48-hour follow-up to ensure improvement
- Recurrent lymphangitis should prompt workup to ascertain underlying cause (other infectious organism, anatomic abnormality, etc.).

Patient Monitoring

Close follow-up to ensure decreasing inflammation

PATIENT EDUCATION

Instruct patients on proper wound and skin care.

PROGNOSIS

- Good prognosis for uncomplicated cases
- Antimicrobial therapy is effective in 90% of patients.
- Untreated, can spread rapidly, especially group A *Streptococcus*

COMPLICATIONS

- Sepsis, cellulitis, necrotizing fasciitis, myositis

REFERENCES

1. Taylor MJ, Hoerauf A, Bockarie M. Lymphatic filariasis and onchocerciasis. *Lancet*. 2010;376(9747):1175–1185.
2. Falagas ME, Bliziotis IA, Kapaskelis AM. Red streaks on the leg. *Am Fam Physician*. 2006;73(6):1061–1062.
3. Badger C, Seers K, Preston N, et al. Antibiotics/anti-inflammatories for reducing acute inflammatory episodes in lymphoedema of the limbs. *Cochrane Database Syst Rev*. 2004;(2):CD003143.

ADDITIONAL READING

- Babu AK, Krishnan P, Andezuth DD. Sclerosing lymphangitis of the penis—literature review and report of 2 cases. *Dermatol Online J*. 2014;20(7):9.
- Bonnetblanc JM, Bédane C. Erysipelas: recognition and management. *Am J Clin Dermatol*. 2003;4(3):157–163.
- Edlich RF, Winters KL, Britt LD, et al. Bacterial diseases of the skin. *J Long Term Eff Med Implants*. 2005;15(5):499–510.
- Haddad FG, Waked CH, Zein EF. Peripheral venous catheter-related inflammation. A randomized prospective trial. *J Med Liban*. 2006;54(3):139–145.
- Raja A, Seshadri RA, Sundersingh S. Lymphangitis carcinomatosa: report of a case and review of literature. *Indian J Surg Oncol*. 2010;1(3):274–276.
- Schubach A, Barros MB, Wanke B. Epidemic sporotrichosis. *Curr Opin Infect Dis*. 2008;21(2):129–133.

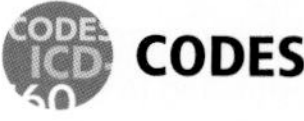

CODES

ICD10

- I89.1 Lymphangitis
- L03.91 Acute lymphangitis, unspecified

CLINICAL PEARLS

- Lymphangitis classically presents with erythematous linear streaks along the skin from inciting site (e.g., bite, cut, abrasion) to regional lymph nodes.
- Patients with prior surgical lymph node dissection are predisposed to lymphangitis.
- Patients with severe systemic symptoms should be admitted and treated with IV antibiotics.
- Parasitic or fungal infections can cause chronic lymphangitis.
- Treatment of underlying skin infection such as tinea pedis may prevent recurrence.

LYMPHEDEMA

Jon S. Parham, DO, MPH • Sandra N. New, DrNP

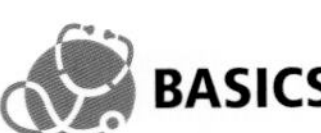

BASICS

DESCRIPTION

- Accumulation of lymphatic fluid in the interstitial tissue causing swelling
- Lymphedema can develop when lymphatic vessels are missing or impaired (primary) or when lymph vessels are damaged or lymph nodes removed (secondary).
- Most common in the lower limb (80%) but also can occur in the arms, face, trunk, and external genitalia

EPIDEMIOLOGY

Incidence

- Predominant sex: female > male
- Predominant age: any age
- 13% of patients with breast cancer treated with surgery; 42% of those treated with surgery and radiation therapy; 25% after GYN cancer surgery
- Milroy disease presents at birth; estimated to be between 1/6,000 and 1/300 live births
- Meige disease develops during puberty.

Prevalence

- 120 million people worldwide are affected with lymphatic filariasis in 73 countries but no primary infections in United States.
- 10 million people are affected by nonfilarial secondary lymphedema in the United States.

ETIOLOGY AND PATHOPHYSIOLOGY

Secondary lymphedema:

- Postoperative: gradual failure of distal lymphatics, which have to "pump" lymph at a greater pressure through damaged proximal ducts
- Risk is higher with postoperative radiation because radiation reduces regrowth of ducts due to fibrous scarring.
- Trauma; recurrent infection; malignancy, including metastatic disease
- Developing countries: Most common cause is filariasis (*Wucheria bancrofti*).

Genetics

- Milroy disease: autosomal dominant; diagnosed either at birth or the 1st year of life
- Lymphedema praecox has onset between the ages of 1 and 35 years.
- Lymphedema tarda occurs in those >35 years of age.

RISK FACTORS

- Filariasis: most common cause worldwide
- Mastectomy
- Prior trauma, infection of affected limb
- History of prior surgical (particularly if lymph nodes were removed) or radiation therapy for malignancy (radiation can damage lymph nodes and cause skin dermatitis)
- Long history of venous insufficiency
- Obesity, DVT

GENERAL PREVENTION

Healthy body weight maintenance; treatment of congestive heart failure (CHF) and venous insufficiency

COMMONLY ASSOCIATED CONDITIONS

Venous disease

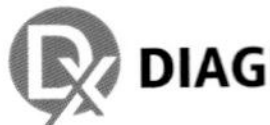

DIAGNOSIS

HISTORY

Recent surgery: Vein stripping can significantly exacerbate mild lymphedema (1)[B]:

- 1st symptom: painless swelling
- Feeling of heaviness in the limb, especially at the end of the day and in hot weather

PHYSICAL EXAM

- Initial: pitting edema, can spread proximally
- Later: nonpitting; after 1st year, does not spread proximally/distally but spreads radially
- Hyperkeratosis (thicker skin)
- Papillomatosis (rough skin)
- Increase in skin turgor
- Positive Stemmer sign (inability to pinch the skin of the dorsum of the 2nd toe between the thumb and forefinger): Exclude heart failure.

DIFFERENTIAL DIAGNOSIS

- CHF, renal failure, lipidemia
- Hypoalbuminemia, protein-losing nephropathy
- DVT, chronic venous disease
- Postoperative complications following ipsilateral surgery
- Cellulitis, Baker cyst, idiopathic edema

DIAGNOSTIC TESTS & INTERPRETATION

- Lack of response to elevation or diuretic therapy may indicate a lymphatic insufficiency (2)[B].
- Diuretics increase excretion of salt and water, thereby decreasing plasma volume, venous capillary pressure, and filtration. Diuretics improve filtration edema but do not improve lymph drainage over the long term.
- Some relevant protein biomarkers for lymphedema have been identified and show promise for early- and latent-stage diagnosis (3)[B].

Initial Tests (lab, imaging)

- Comprehensive chemistry panel: evaluates for hepatic or renal impairment.
- Urinalysis: protein-losing nephropathy
- Ultrasound: evaluates for acute/chronic DVT; gives information about soft tissue changes but does not tell about truncal anatomy of the lymphatics (1)[B]
- Duplex ultrasound: Lymphedema causes gradual impedance of venous return that aggravates the edema; 82% of patients with unexplained limb edema were diagnosed using a combination of duplex ultrasound and lymphoscintigram (4)[A].

Follow-Up Tests & Considerations

- Lymphangiogram: direct cannulation of lymphatics through the skin; risk for infection, local inflammation; not used commonly (4)[C]
- Lymphoscintigram: radiolabeled protein technetium-99m–labeled colloid
  - Measures lymphatic function, lymph movement, lymph drainage, and response to treatment
  - Sensitivity, 73–97%; specificity, 100%
  - Best to use 1 hour and delayed images together (4)[A]
- Indocyanine green lymphography: reported accurately screens post surgically for subclinical lymphedema (5)[B]
- CT scan: calf skin thickening, thickening of the SC compartment, increased fat density, thickened perimuscular aponeurosis; typical honeycomb appearance (4)[B]
- MRI: circumferential edema, increased volume of SC tissue, honeycomb pattern above the fascia between the muscle and subcutis; cannot differentiate primary from secondary lymphedema (4)[B]

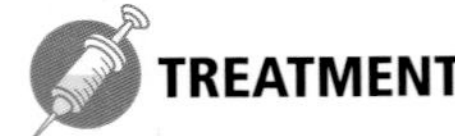

TREATMENT

GENERAL MEASURES

- Seek optimal weight, early treatment of cellulitis, avoid trauma to affected area (direct injury, venipunctures, inept nail care, extreme heat/cold).
- Achieve mechanical reduction and maintenance of limb size: compression garments via professionals.
- Elevate affected limb/area, but avoid stasis.
- Avoid BP cuffs in affected limbs.
- Prevent skin infection with daily cleansing, inspection, and skin care (with emollients).
- Treatment of varicose veins may benefit some.

MEDICATION

- Diuretics of limited benefit and may lead to volume depletion
- Benzopyrenes (flavonoids and coumarin) (not available for prescription use in the United States)
  - Micronized purified flavonoid fraction (Daflon 500 mg) is effective in decreasing venous stasis and idiopathic cyclic edema, chronic venous insufficiency, and postmastectomy lymphedema. It also reduces capillary permeability and the inflammatory component (6)[C].
- Coumarin reduces edema fluid by increasing the number of macrophages and enhancing proteolysis, resulting in the removal of protein, increasing softness in the limbs, and decreasing elevated skin temperature with subsequent symptom improvement and decreased secondary infection. Some reports of hepatotoxicity (6)[C].

ISSUES FOR REFERRAL

- Refer to physical therapist with lymphedema training for manual decongestive therapy.
  - In patients with recurrent or metastatic disease, discuss with oncologist prior to initiation of complete decongestive therapy in order not to promote the spread of cancer.
- Provide education for patient/family for self-administration of therapy in future.
- Education for family about bandaging
- Fitting for compression garments

ADDITIONAL THERAPIES

- Exercise: Lymph flow occurs as a result of inspiratory reduction in the intrathoracic pressure associated with inspiration. Best results are achieved with combination of flexibility, strength, and aerobic training (4)[B]. Compression with custom-made elastic stocking (minimum pressure is 40 mm Hg).
  - Protection against external incidental trauma
  - Decreases the intrinsic trauma on the skin due to chronically increased interstitial pressures, which cause stretch of the skin and SC tissues
  - No data on preference of custom-made versus prefabricated
  - Replace every 3–6 months or when starting to lose elasticity (1)[B].
- Multilayer bandaging: inner layer of tubular stockinette followed by foam and padding to protect the joint flexures and to even out the contours of the limb so that pressure is distributed evenly; outer layer of at least 2 short-stretch extensible bandages; more effective than hosiery alone (1)[B]
- Pneumatic pumps: development of high pressure up to 150 mm Hg; can reduce limb girth by 37–68.6%; wear a compression stocking when not using pump; high risk of genital edema; no metastasis in limb due to risk of spread (1)[B]

SURGERY/OTHER PROCEDURES

- Bypass procedures: creation of lymphatic–venous anastomosis or lymph node transplantation (most effective) via microsurgery showed a reduction in use of conservative compression therapy (7)[B]: reserved for refractory cases only. In a pilot study, low-level laser therapy was shown not to be inferior to manual lymphatic drainage or the combination of the two in arm volume reduction in breast cancer–related lymphedema and required less than or equal to one-half the treatment time (8)[C].
- Debulking procedures (Charles procedure): radical excision of SC tissue with primary or staged skin grafting
  - Men had less improvement than women.
  - Main risk is infection and necrosis of the skin graft.
  - Liposuction is cosmetically preferred to debulking.

COMPLEMENTARY & ALTERNATIVE MEDICINE

Heat therapy: Hot water immersion, microwave, and electromagnetic irradiation may be helpful (1)[C].

INPATIENT CONSIDERATIONS

Admission Criteria/Initial Stabilization

Systemic signs of infection

- May admit to specialized rehabilitation unit for combination treatment in patients with heart failure or severe pulmonary disease
- IV antibiotics for infection

Nursing

- Leg elevation
- Encourage patient mobilization/exercise.
- Patient education for bandaging/wound care

Discharge Criteria

- Resolution of signs/symptoms of infection (e.g., elevated WBC count, fever, abnormal vital signs)
- Clinical improvement in wound appearance

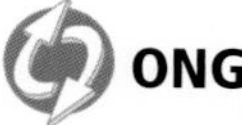

ONGOING CARE

FOLLOW-UP RECOMMENDATIONS

Lymphedema will return in several days if patient stops wearing compression garments during the day and bandaging at night.

Patient Monitoring

- Daily visit to therapist for acute treatment
- Monthly visits for maintenance care

DIET

Low sodium; weight loss oriented if needed

PATIENT EDUCATION

- Use compression garments, especially when exercising.
- Avoid affected limb(s) being dependant for long period of time: Patient should perform daily skin examination.
- http://www.nlm.nih.gov/medlineplus/lymphedema.html

PROGNOSIS

No cure, but treatment can produce good results with daily care

COMPLICATIONS

- Infection (local vs. systemic): common
- Risk of wound formation (venous wounds/abrasions) that are difficult to heal: common
- Lymphangiosarcoma: Found in lymphedematous arms of patients following radical mastectomy; also in patients with Milroy disease. Treatment is radiotherapy with surgery, reserved for patients with discrete nonmetastatic disease.

REFERENCES

1. Warren A, Brorson H, Borud LJ, et al. Lymphedema: a comprehensive review. *Ann Plastic Surg*. 2007;59(4):464–472.
2. Mortimer P. Implications of the lymphatic sytem in CVI-associated edema. *Angiology*. 2000;51(1):3–7.
3. Lin S, Kim J, Lee M-J, et al. Prospective transcriptomic pathway analysis of human lymphatic vascular insufficiency: identification and validation of a circulating biomarker panel. *PLoS One*. 2012;7(12):e52021.
4. Brennan MJ, Miller LT. Overview of treatment options and review of the current role and use of compression garments, intermittent pumps, and exercise in the management of lymphedema. *Cancer*. 1998;83(Suppl 12):2821–2827.
5. Akita S, Mitsukawa N, Rikihisa N, et al. Early diagnosis and risk factors for lymphedema following lymph node dissection for gynecologic cancer. *Plast Reconstr Surg*. 2013;131(2):283–290.
6. Tiwari A, Cheng KS, Button M, et al. Differential diagnosis, investigation, and current treatment of lower limb lymphedema. *Arch Surg*. 2003;138(2):152–161.
7. Basta MN, Gao LL, & Wu LC. Operative treatment of peripheral lymphedema: a systematic meta-analysis of the efficacy and safety of lymphovenous microsurgery and tissue transplantation. *Plast Reconstr Surg*. 2014;133(4):905–913.
8. Ridner SH, Poage-Hooper E, Kanar C, et al. A pilot randomized trial evaluating low-level laser therapy as an alternative treatment to manual lymphatic drainage for breast cancer-related lymphedema. *Oncol Nurs Forum*. 2013;40(4):383–393.

ADDITIONAL READING

Rockson SG. Causes and consequences of lymphatic disease. *Ann NY Acad Sci*. 2010;1207(Suppl 1):e2–e6.

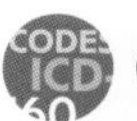

CODES

ICD10

- I89.0 Lymphedema, not elsewhere classified
- Q82.0 Hereditary lymphedema
- I97.89 Oth postproc comp and disorders of the circ sys, NEC

CLINICAL PEARLS

- Use short-stretch bandages for wrapping (not ACE wraps).
- Avoid heat/whirlpool: typically worsens condition.
- Much higher risk for cutaneous-sourced infections than patients with only venous insufficiency

LYMPHOMA, BURKITT

Jennifer Greene Welch, MD

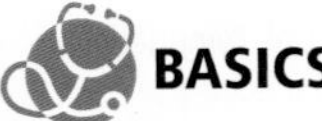

BASICS

DESCRIPTION

- Burkitt lymphoma is a mature B-cell neoplasm arising in lymph node germinal centers.
- Highly aggressive, rapidly growing malignancy
- Can present as lymphoma or leukemia
- 3 distinct forms, differing in epidemiology, clinical presentation, and genetics
  - Endemic or African
  - Sporadic
  - Immunodeficiency-related
    - HIV/AIDS-related
    - Postsolid organ transplant
    - Congenital immunodeficiency
- Associated with Epstein-Barr virus (EBV)
  - Almost 100% of endemic cases
  - Up to 30% of sporadic cases
- Characteristic chromosome translocation (t[8;14])
- Similar disease characteristics to diffuse large B-cell lymphoma (DLBCL)
- System(s) affected: hematologic, lymphatic
- Synonym(s): mature B-cell high-grade lymphoma; mature B-cell acute lymphoblastic leukemia; L3 type (French-American-British [FAB] classification); Burkitt cell leukemia

Pediatric Considerations

Common age group (30% of cases in the United States)

Geriatric Considerations

Unusual in this age group. Toxicity with chemotherapy may be increased in the elderly.

Pregnancy Considerations

With aggressive treatment, good maternal, and fetal outcome

EPIDEMIOLOGY

- Varies by disease form
- Endemic
  - One of most common tumors of childhood in Africa, most frequently occurring in children age 4–7 years
  - Rare in adults
- Sporadic
  - In the United States, trimodal peaks of age incidence around ages 10, 40, and 75 years
  - More common in Caucasians
  - Predominant sex: male > female (3:1 or 4:1)

Incidence

Rare in the United States, incidence 0.27 per 100,000 person-years; 50 times more common in endemic regions of Africa

Prevalence

Composes <1% of adult non-Hodgkin lymphoma (NHL); accounts for 30–40% of NHL in children in the United States and Western Europe

ETIOLOGY AND PATHOPHYSIOLOGY

- Activation and overexpression of *c-myc* oncogene (1)
- Monoclonal proliferation of B lymphocytes resulting from dysregulation of *c-myc*
  - Translocation of *c-myc* to immunoglobulin coding regions results in constitutive expression of gene product.
  - EBV-infected cells in germinal center reactions may increase the risk of translocation.
- Poorly regulated proliferation of genetically unstable B cells increases chance of translocations:
  - Immunodeficient patients with persistent generalized lymphadenopathy and polyclonal B-cell activation

RISK FACTORS

Pediatric Considerations

Endemic: Children with early acquisition of EBV infection are at increased risk. Coinfection with malaria and EBV increases incidence 100-fold.

GENERAL PREVENTION

No known methods to prevent Burkitt lymphoma

COMMONLY ASSOCIATED CONDITIONS

- EBV infection
- Immunodeficiency, especially AIDS

DIAGNOSIS

HISTORY

- Rapidly progressive bulky adenopathy or extranodal mass
- Symptoms of bone marrow involvement
  - Fatigue, exercise intolerance, bruising, epistaxis, other bleeding, fever
- Abdominal presentation
  - Abdominal pain, nausea, vomiting, bowel obstruction, GI bleeding, symptoms mimicking acute appendicitis or intussusception
- Endemic (African): jaw or facial bone tumor, with mouth pain, loose teeth, or jaw mass
- Nonendemic: extranodal disease, abdominal presentation typical
- Can present as acute leukemia (L3-ALL) with predominant bone marrow involvement and no mass lesions
- Renal function impairment and significant metabolic derangement may quickly manifest due to the rapid progression and spread of the tumor.

PHYSICAL EXAM

- Endemic: mass on jaw or facial bone, pallor, petechiae, hepatosplenomegaly
- Sporadic: lymphadenopathy, any mass lesion, abdominal tenderness, pallor, petechiae, hepatosplenomegaly

DIFFERENTIAL DIAGNOSIS

- Other NHLs
  - Burkitt-like lymphoma: intermediate immunophenotype and molecular characteristics between classic Burkitt lymphoma and DLBCL
  - DLBCL: large, irregular cells, often with B-cell lymphoma (BCL) rearrangement
  - Precursor B-lymphoblastic lymphoma
  - Precursor T-lymphoblastic lymphoma
  - Mantle cell lymphoma, blastoid variant
- Hodgkin lymphoma
- Acute lymphoblastic leukemia
- Other causes of lymphadenopathy
  - Infection (e.g., bacterial lymphadenitis, mononucleosis, tuberculosis, atypical mycobacterium, cat-scratch disease)
  - Reactive lymphoid hyperplasia
  - Histiocytosis
- Other primary malignancies of childhood (e.g., Wilms tumor, neuroblastoma, peripheral neuroectodermal tumor)
- Other metastatic malignancies

DIAGNOSTIC TESTS & INTERPRETATION

Initial Tests (lab, imaging)

- Biopsy of mass lesion: diagnosis by cellular morphology on histologic examination
- CBC with differential: anemia, neutropenia, or thrombocytopenia
- Tumor lysis syndrome: hyperkalemia, hyperphosphatemia, hyperuricemia, renal failure. Order electrolytes, BUN, creatinine, calcium, magnesium, phosphorus, serum lactate dehydrogenase (LDH), uric acid
- Consider hepatitis B virus serologies prior to rituximab
- Chest x-ray
- CT scan of chest, abdomen, pelvis
- Consider whole body PET to identify active disease.
- Dedicated imaging of any site suspected to be involved by tumor

Follow-Up Tests & Special Considerations

- Diagnosis requires immunophenotypic and cytogenetic data.
- Immunophenotype studies
  - Cells express surface immunoglobulin (Ig) M- and B-associated antigens (CD19, CD20, CD22, CD79a), as well as CD10, HLA-DR, and CD43
  - Cells also show nuclear staining for BCL-6 protein.
- Cytogenic studies to visualize chromosomal translocation
  - Reciprocal chromosome translocation involving *c-myc* and immunoglobulin heavy chain (IgH) gene (t[8;14]) (80% of cases) or immunoglobulin light chain (IgL) genes (t[2;8] or t[8;22])
  - Fluorescence in situ hybridization (FISH) or long-segment polymerase chain reaction (PCR) may be necessary to identify translocation.
- EBV testing in lesional cells
- Gene expression profiling can help distinguish Burkitt lymphoma from DLBCL.

Diagnostic Procedures/Other

- Bone marrow aspiration and biopsy for morphology and flow cytometry
- Lumbar puncture for CSF cell count, differential, and cytology
- Lymph node biopsy: most lymph nodes suggestive of disease should be selected for excisional biopsy.
  - Frozen sections and needle biopsies discouraged as lymph node architecture helpful for diagnosis.
- Diagnostic laparotomy with resection of localized disease

Test Interpretation

- Monotonous diffuse infiltrate of medium-sized round cells, with round or oval nuclei, several nucleoli, and coarse chromatin. Cytoplasm is intensely basophilic and moderately abundant.
- Mitotic rate is high; close to 100% of viable cells will be actively engaged in cell cycle.
- Classic starry-sky histologic appearance
  - Results from the presence of scattered macrophages with phagocytic cell debris
  - Characteristic of, although not pathognomonic for, Burkitt lymphoma

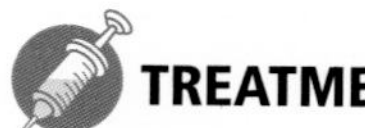

TREATMENT

If available, all patients should be offered participation in an appropriate clinical trial.

MEDICATION

First Line

- Intensive, short-term, multiagent chemotherapy administered in cycles (2)[A]
  - Chemotherapeutic agents include cyclophosphamide, methotrexate, vincristine, prednisone, high-dose methotrexate, high-dose cytarabine, etoposide, isophosphamide, and doxorubicin.
  - Type and extent of therapy depend on stage of disease.
- Rituximab in combination with chemotherapy may improve outcome (3)[B].
- Nonintensive chemotherapy protocols used in developing countries can be effective (4)[B].
  - Cyclophosphamide, methotrexate
  - Areas with limited financial and medical resources
- CNS prophylaxis for most patients
  - Not necessary for limited disease far from CNS
  - Intrathecal methotrexate, with or without IV methotrexate and cytarabine, may be used for CNS prophylaxis.
  - Prophylactic irradiation does not improve outcome.
- Chemotherapy cycles should be initiated as soon as hematologic recovery permits.
  - Delay of chemotherapy may result in regrowth of resistant tumor between cycles.
- Management of tumor lysis syndrome with initial cycle of chemotherapy

Second Line

- Rituximab may be effective if not used previously.
- Hematopoietic stem cell transplantation in combination with high-dose chemotherapy (5,6)[B]

ISSUES FOR REFERRAL

All patients should be treated by a pediatric or adult oncologist.

SURGERY/OTHER PROCEDURES

- Biopsy and staging
  - All patients require a biopsy to establish the diagnosis pathologically.
- Surgical resection
  - Treatment for small, completely resectable abdominal tumors (in addition to chemotherapy)
  - For patients with intestinal obstruction who cannot begin chemotherapy immediately
  - Aggressive upfront resection of disease is not indicated.
- Patients require placement of a central venous line for administration of chemotherapy.

COMPLEMENTARY & ALTERNATIVE MEDICINE

Many complementary therapies exist to assist in management of side effects of chemotherapy.

INPATIENT CONSIDERATIONS

Admission Criteria/Initial Stabilization

- Almost all patients should be admitted to the hospital for initial care.
- Burkitt lymphoma has high-growth fraction and short doubling time
  - Rapid initiation of definitive chemotherapy is essential.
- Management of tumor lysis syndrome with initial cycle of chemotherapy
  - Aggressive hydration without potassium
  - Close monitoring of electrolytes, renal function, and uric acid initially q6–8h
  - Rasburicase (0.2 mg/kg IV once daily for up to 5 days, depending on response to therapy) to break down uric acid
  - Allopurinol (10 mg/kg PO divided 2–3/day) if rasburicase not available
    - Consider alkalization of urine with bicarbonate-containing IV fluids (goal urine pH 7–8) when using allopurinol.
  - Phosphate binder if serum phosphorus becomes elevated
  - Avoid supplemental calcium unless symptomatic hypocalcium develops.
  - Medical management of hyperkalemia

IV Fluids

Aggressive IV hydration with first cycle of chemotherapy

- Typically D5/0.5 NS at 125 mL/m^2/hour (twice the maintenance rate)
- No potassium in IV fluids

ONGOING CARE

FOLLOW-UP RECOMMENDATIONS

Patient Monitoring

- Close monitoring of serum chemistries is critical due to high risk of tumor lysis syndrome and uric acid nephropathy.
- CBC, liver function, and renal function should also be closely monitored throughout chemotherapy.
- Surveillance history and physical exam for detection of recurrence
- Consideration of routine imaging for detection of recurrence (7)[B]
- All patients, particularly children, should be followed indefinitely for long-term effects of chemotherapy.

PATIENT EDUCATION

Educational materials are available online from

- Leukemia and Lymphoma Society (www.leukemia-lymphoma.org)
- CureSearch (www.curesearch.org)

PROGNOSIS

- Low-stage localized disease, 5-year event-free survival >95%
- Aggressive treatment of advanced disease yields >80% 5-year event-free survival (8)
- Recurrent disease more resistant to therapy
- Mortality for endemic form remains high where access to health care is limited.

COMPLICATIONS

- Complications of extensive abdominal disease include obstructive jaundice and pancreatitis, bowel obstruction, and intestinal perforation.
- Tumor lysis syndrome with renal failure (uric acid nephropathy) may occur prior to, and especially following, the start of chemotherapy.
- Rituximab has been associated with reactivation of hepatitis B virus resulting in fulminant liver failure.
- Other effects of chemotherapy include alopecia, myelosuppression, life-threatening infection, nausea, mucositis, infusion reactions, peripheral neuropathy, seizures, infertility, congestive heart failure, and secondary malignancy.

REFERENCES

1. Said J, Lones M, Yea S. Burkitt lymphoma and MYC: what else is new? *Adv Anat Pathol*. 2014;21(3): 160–165.
2. Okebe JU, Skoetz N, Meremikwu MM, et al. Therapeutic interventions for Burkitt lymphoma in children. *Cochrane Database Syst Rev*. 2011;(7): CD005198.
3. Rizzieri DA, Johnson JL, Byrd JC, et al. Improved efficacy using rituximab and brief duration, high intensity chemotherapy with filgrastim support for Burkitt or aggressive lymphomas: cancer and leukemia Group B study 10 002. *Br J Haematol*. 2014;165(1):102–111.
4. Beogo R, Nacro B, Ouedraogo D, et al. Endemic Burkitt lymphoma of maxillofacial region: results of induction treatment with cyclophosphamide plus methotrexate in West Africa. *Pediatr Blood Cancer*. 2011;56(7):1068–1070.
5. Gross TG, Hale GA, He W, et al. Hematopoietic stem cell transplantation for refractory or recurrent non-Hodgkin lymphoma in children and adolescents. *Biol Blood Marrow Transplant*. 2010;16(2):223–230.
6. Maramattom LV, Hari PN, Burns LJ, et al. Autologous and allogeneic transplantation for burkitt lymphoma outcomes and changes in utilization: a report from the center for international blood and marrow transplant research. *Biol Blood Marrow Transplant*. 2013;19(2):173–179.
7. Eissa HM, Allen CE, Kamdar K, et al. Pediatric Burkitt's lymphoma and diffuse B-cell lymphoma: are surveillance scans required? *Pediatr Hematol Oncol*. 2014;31(3):253–257.
8. Costa LJ, Xavier AC, Wahlquist AE, et al. Trends in survival of patients with Burkitt lymphoma/leukemia in the USA: an analysis of 3691 cases. *Blood*. 2013;121(24):4861–4866.

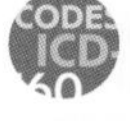

CODES

ICD10

- C83.70 Burkitt lymphoma, unspecified site
- C83.71 Burkitt lymphoma, lymph nodes of head, face, and neck
- C83.73 Burkitt lymphoma, intra-abdominal lymph nodes

CLINICAL PEARLS

- Burkitt lymphoma is an aggressive, mature B-cell malignancy most commonly diagnosed in childhood.
- Burkitt lymphoma is strongly associated with t(8;14) and with EBV and malaria infections.
- Burkitt lymphoma is highly treatable with intense multiagent systemic and intrathecal chemotherapy.

MACULAR DEGENERATION, AGE-RELATED

Richard W. Allinson, MD

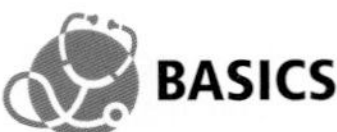

BASICS

DESCRIPTION

- Age-related macular degeneration (ARMD) results in pigmentary changes in the macula or typical drusen associated with visual loss to the 20/30 level or worse, not caused by cataract or other eye disease, in individuals >50 years of age, although some definitions exclude age or visual acuity criteria.
- Leading cause of irreversible, severe visual loss in persons age >65 years
- Stages
  - Atrophic/nonexudative
  - Neovascular/exudative
- System(s) affected: nervous
- Synonym(s): senile macular degeneration; subretinal neovascularization

EPIDEMIOLOGY

- Neovascular/exudative form is rare in blacks and more common in whites.
- Predominant sex: female

Incidence

- In the Framingham Eye Study (FES), drusen were noted in 25% of all participants who were ≥52 years of age. ARMD-associated visual loss was noted in 5.7%.
- Atrophic/nonexudative stage accounts for 20% of cases of severe visual loss
- Neovascular/exudative stage accounts for 80% of cases of severe visual loss

Prevalence

Per FES study:

- People 65–74 years old: 11%
- People ≥75 years old: 27.9%

ETIOLOGY AND PATHOPHYSIOLOGY

- Breaks in the Bruch membrane allow choroidal neovascular membranes (CNVMs) to invade the retinal pigment epithelium (RPE) and grow into the subretinal space.
- Atrophic/nonexudative: drusen and/or pigmentary changes in the macula
- Neovascular/exudative: growth of blood vessels underneath the retina
- Visible light can result in the formation and accumulation of metabolic by-products in the RPE, a pigment layer underneath the retina that normally helps remove metabolic byproducts from the retina. Excess accumulation of these metabolic by-products interferes with the normal metabolic activity of the RPE and can lead to the formation of drusen.
- Neovascular stage generally arises from the atrophic stage.
- Most do not progress beyond the atrophic/nonexudative stage; however, those who do are at a greater risk of severe visual loss.

Genetics

- Genetic susceptibility may be a factor in ARMD: ~25% genetically determined.
- Complement factor H is an important susceptibility gene for ARMD.
- Although the development of ARMD may be predicted by specific alleles, the clinical response to anti–vascular growth factor is not (1)[A].

RISK FACTORS

- Obesity
- Ethnicity: non-Hispanic whites
- Cigarette smoking
- *Chlamydia pneumoniae* infection
- Family history
- Excess sunlight exposure
- Blue or light iris color
- Hyperopia
- History of cardiovascular disease
- Short stature
- Aspirin use

GENERAL PREVENTION

- Ultraviolet (UV) protection for eyes
- Routine ophthalmologic visits
  - Every 2–4 years for patients age 40–64 years
  - Every 1–2 years after age 65 years
- Patients who take statins, which modify lipid profiles, may have a reduced risk.

COMMONLY ASSOCIATED CONDITIONS

- Presumed ocular histoplasmosis syndrome
- Exudative retinal detachment
- Vitreous hemorrhage
- Other causes of CNVMs

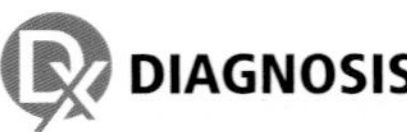

DIAGNOSIS

HISTORY

- Patients frequently notice distortion of central vision.
- Patients may notice straight lines appear crooked (e.g., telephone poles).

PHYSICAL EXAM

- Atrophic/nonexudative stage retinal exam
  - Drusen (small yellowish white lesions)
    - Subtypes: hard drusen and soft drusen
  - Atrophy of the RPE
- Neovascular/exudative stage retinal exam
  - Blood vessels growing underneath the retina from the choroid are called CNVMs or subretinal neovascularization (SRN). The choroid is the vascular layer underneath the RPE.
  - Subretinal fluid or hemorrhage
  - Exudates
  - On Amsler grid testing, the horizontal or vertical lines may become broken, distorted, or missing.
- Disciform scar: an advanced stage resulting in a fibrovascular scar

DIFFERENTIAL DIAGNOSIS

- Idiopathic SRN
- Presumed ocular histoplasmosis syndrome
- Diabetic retinopathy
- Hypertensive retinopathy

DIAGNOSTIC TESTS & INTERPRETATION

Diagnostic Procedures/Other

- Amsler grid testing
- Fluorescein angiography
  - Detection of CNVMs
  - Differentiate between atrophic and neovascular ARMD.
- Indocyanine green video angiography: may identify occult or hidden CNVMs
- Optical coherence tomography (OCT) may be useful in identifying CNVMs, subretinal fluid, and retinal thickening:
  - Fluorescein angiography is better than time-domain OCT in detecting new-onset CNVMs (2)[C]

Test Interpretation

Drusen: deposits of hyaline material between the RPE and Bruch membrane (the limiting membrane between the RPE and the choroid)

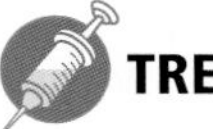

TREATMENT

MEDICATION

First Line

- Ranibizumab (Lucentis)
  - Antibody fragment that inhibits all active forms of vascular endothelial growth factor (VEGF)
  - Approved for neovascular (wet) ARMD
  - Injected intravitreally, at a dose of 0.5 mg, every 4 weeks
  - 1 year after treatment, up to 40% of patients treated with ranibizumab gained at least 3 lines of vision, and ~95% maintained vision.
  - Ranibizumab is superior to verteporfin in the treatment of predominately classic CNVMs.
  - The PrONTO study demonstrated OCT-guided, variable-dosing regimen with ranibizumab resulted in similar results to the MARINA and ANCHOR studies with monthly injections.
  - When comparing ranibizumab and bevacizumab in a multicenter study, both treatments were effective in stabilizing visual loss, and no difference was found in the visual outcome between the 2 treatment groups. A slightly higher rate of serious systemic adverse events was noted in the bevacizumab group (3)[A].
- VEGF Trap-Eye/Aflibercept (Eylea)
  - A decoy VEGF receptor that inhibits all isoforms of VEGF-A and placental growth factor (PlGF), the members of the VEGF family in mammals primarily involved in ocular neovascularization
  - Approved for neovascular (wet) ARMD
  - Injected intravitreally, at a dose of 2 mg, every 4 weeks for 12 weeks then every 8 weeks
  - Dosed as need after the 12-week fixed dosing schedule resulted in a 5.3-letter gain in best corrected visual acuity at 52 weeks (4)[B].
  - Routine use of prophylactic antibiotics after intravitreal injections may be unnecessary (5)[B].
  - Maybe beneficial in patients who are not responding to ranibizumab or bevacizumab (6)[C]

Second Line

- Pegaptanib sodium (Macugen) is a compound that binds to and neutralizes VEGF. Pegaptanib preserves vision rather than improving it. 70% of treated patients lost fewer than 15 letters of visual acuity at 1 year.
- Bevacizumab (Avastin) is a full-length antibody to VEGF, administered intravitreally at a dose of 1.25 mg; it is being evaluated in the treatment of neovascular ARMD. Widely used off-label because of its lower cost.
- Agents that block platelet-derived growth factor (PDGF) are being investigated.

GENERAL MEASURES
Low-vision aids may be helpful.

SURGERY/OTHER PROCEDURES
- Neovascular/exudative macular degeneration
  - The Macular Photocoagulation Study (MPS) demonstrated a treatment benefit for laser treatment of CNVMs that were ≥200 microns (200 microns = 0.2 mm) from the center of the macula.
- Treatment of CNVMs 1–199 microns from the center of the macula has been studied by the Age-Related Macular Degeneration Study-Krypton Laser (ARMDS-K). The benefit of laser treatment was greatest among patients without evidence of hypertension (HTN). No benefit was observed among patients who had highly elevated BP or used antihypertensive medication.
- Vitrectomy has been used to remove CNVMs, but this is generally not recommended.
- CNVMs can bleed spontaneously, leaving blood underneath the retina. Vitrectomy to remove subretinal blood may be of benefit and should be performed within 7 days of the bleed. Tissue plasminogen activator (tPA) instilled into the eye may help remove a subretinal hemorrhage. In some cases, intravitreal gas with or without tPA may displace submacular blood:
  - Intravitreal anti-VEGF monotherapy may be helpful in the treatment of neovascular ARMD associated with a submacular hemorrhage (7)[C].
- Photodynamic therapy (PDT) with verteporfin reduces vision loss in patients with >50% "classic" subfoveal CNVMs. Verteporfin is administered IV, and a diode laser at 689 nm is applied to the CNVM
  - Patients should be informed of a <4% risk of acute, severe vision loss after PDT.
  - Ranibizumab has greater clinical efficacy than PDT.
  - Intravitreal triamcinolone combined with PDT may result in improved visual acuity for patients with CNVMs.
- Combination therapy combining intravitreal ranibizumab with PDT and/or intravitreal triamcinolone is being evaluated.
  - Combination treatment with intravitreal ranibizumab and PDT appears to offer similar gain in visual acuity when compared with ranibizumab monotherapy (8)[B].
  - Combination treatment with ranibizumab and PDT may reduce the number of ranibizumab retreatments.
- Stereotactic radiotherapy is being investigated in the treatment of neovascular ARMD.
- Laser photocoagulation to treat drusen is not recommended.

COMPLEMENTARY & ALTERNATIVE MEDICINE
Free radical formation in the retina, induced by visible light, may play a role in cellular damage that results in atrophic/nonexudative macular degeneration. The Age-Related Eye Disease Study (AREDS) found that a high-dose regimen of antioxidant vitamins and mineral supplements reduced progression of ARMD in some cases.
- Recommended daily doses: vitamin C 500 mg, vitamin E 400 IU, β-carotene 15 mg, zinc oxide 80 mg, and cupric oxide 2 mg
- Exercise caution with β-carotene use in smokers due to potential link to lung cancer.
- The Age-Related Eye Disease Study 2 (AREDS2) found the addition of lutein with zeaxanthin alone or in combination with omega-3 fatty acids had no overall effect in further reducing the risk of progression to advanced ARMD (9)[A].

ONGOING CARE

FOLLOW-UP RECOMMENDATIONS

Patient Monitoring
- Amsler grid can aid in discovering visual disturbances.
- Patients with soft drusen or pigmentary changes in the macula are at an increased risk of visual loss. They should monitor their vision, such as by daily Amsler grid testing, and subjective measures of visual acuity, such as reading ability. If no new symptoms, follow-up examination in 6–12 months.

DIET
- Eating dark green, leafy vegetables (spinach/collard greens), which are rich in carotenoids, may decrease the risk of developing the neovascular/exudative stage.
- Fish consumption with omega-3 fatty acid intake reduces the risk of ARMD.

PATIENT EDUCATION
Instruct visually impaired patients to check with the local low-vision center for aids.

PROGNOSIS
- Patients with bilateral soft drusen and pigmentary changes in the macula, but no evidence of exudation, have an increased likelihood of developing CNVMs and subsequent visual loss.
- Patients with bilateral drusen carry a cumulative risk of 14.7% over 5 years of suffering significant visual loss in 1 eye from the neovascular stage of ARMD.
- Patients with neovascular stage in 1 eye and drusen in the opposite eye are at an annual risk of 5–14% of developing the neovascular stage in the opposite eye with drusen.
- High incidence of recurrence after thermal laser treatment for CNVMs
- After 2 years of monthly ranibizumab injections, visual loss is commonly associated with impaired function of the photoreceptors and RPE and not from active leakage from CNVMs (10)[A].
- The 7-year outcomes after ranibizumab treatment demonstrate 1/3 of patients with good visual outcomes and another third with poor visual outcomes (11)[B].

COMPLICATIONS
- Blindness
- Geographic atrophy developed in approximately 1/5 of patients in the Comparison of Age-Related Macular Degeneration Treatments Trial (CATT) (12)[A].
- The intraocular pressure should be monitored in eyes receiving intravitreal anti-VEGF injections.

REFERENCES

1. Hagstrom SA, Ying GS, Pauer GJ, et al. Parmacogenetics for genes associated with age-related macular degeneration in the Comparison of AMD Treatment Trials (CATT). *Ophthalmology*. 2013;120(3):593–599.
2. Do DV, Gower EW, Cassard SD, et al. Detection of new-onset choroidal neovascularization using optical coherence tomography: the AMD DOC Study. *Ophthalmology*. 2012;119(4):771–778.
3. Comparison of Age-related Macular Degeneration Treatments Trials (CATT) Research Group, Martin DF, Maguire MG, et al. Ranibizumab and bevacizumab for treatment of neovascular age-related macular degeneration: two-year results. *Ophthalmology*. 2012;119(7):1388–1398.
4. Heier JS, Boyer D, Nguyen QD, et al. The 1-year results of CLEAR-IT 2, a phase 2 study of vascular endothelial growth factor trap-eye dosed as-needed after 12-week fixed dosing. *Ophthalmology*. 2011;118(6):1098–1106.
5. Yin VT, Weisbrod DJ, Eng KT, et al. Antibiotic resistance of ocular surface flora with repeated use of a topical antibiotic after intravitreal injection. *JAMA Ophthalmol*. 2013;131(4):456–461.
6. Chang AA, Li H, Broadhead GK, et al. Intravitreal aflibercept for treatment-resistant neovascular age-related macular degeneration. *Ophthalmology*. 2014;121(1):188–192.
7. Shienbaum G, Garcia Filho CA, Flynn HW Jr, et al. Management of submacular hemorrhage secondary to neovascular age-related macular degeneration with anti-vascular endothelial growth factor monotherapy. *Am J Ophthalmol*. 2013;155(6):1009–1013.
8. Larsen M, Schmidt-Erfurth U, Lanzetta P, et al. Verteporfin plus ranibizumab for choroidal neovascularization in age-related macular degeneration: twelve-month MONT BLANC study results. *Ophthalmology*. 2012;119(5):992–1000.
9. The Age-Related Eye Disease Study 2 (AREDS2) Research Group. Lutein + zeaxanthin and omega-3 fatty acids for age-related macular degeneration: the Age-Related Eye Disease Study 2 (AREDS2) randomized clinical trial. *JAMA*. 2013;309(19):2005–2015.
10. Rosenfeld PJ, Shapiro H, Tuomi L, et al. Characteristics of patients losing vision after 2 years of monthly dosing in the phase III ranibizumab clinical trials. *Ophthalmology*. 2011;118(3):523–530.
11. Rofagha S, Bhisitkul RB, Boyer DS, et al. Seven-year outcomes in ranibizumab-treated patients in ANCHOR, MARINA, and HORIZON: a multicenter cohort study (SEVEN-UP). *Ophthalmology*. 2013;120(11):2292–2299.
12. Grunwald JE, Daniel E, Huang J, et al. Risk of geographic atrophy in the comparison of age-related macular degeneration treatments trials. *Ophthalmology*. 2014;121(1):150–161.

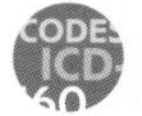

CODES

ICD10
- H35.30 Unspecified macular degeneration
- H35.31 Nonexudative age-related macular degeneration
- H35.32 Exudative age-related macular degeneration

CLINICAL PEARLS
- Patients frequently notice distortion of central vision.
- Patients may notice straight lines appear crooked (e.g., telephone poles).
- Hyperopia is a risk factor for ARMD.
- The AREDS study found that a high-dose regimen of antioxidant vitamins and mineral supplements reduces progression of ARMD in some cases.
- Tobacco cessation should be strongly encouraged.

MALARIA

Paul M. Arguin, MD

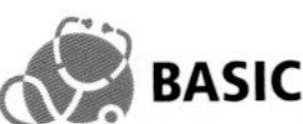

BASICS

DESCRIPTION

- Acute or chronic infection transmitted to humans by *Anopheles* spp. mosquitoes
- Most morbidity and mortality is caused by *Plasmodium falciparum*; responsible for 207 million cases annually, including 627,000 deaths, most of which occur in children <5 years of age in sub-Saharan Africa (1).
- Nonimmune individuals are most susceptible to rapid progression to severe disease.
- System(s) affected: cardiovascular, hematologic, renal, respiratory, cerebral, lymphatic, immunologic

EPIDEMIOLOGY

- Cases imported to the United States: 58% *P. falciparum*; 17% *Plasmodium vivax*; 3% *Plasmodium malariae*; 3% *Plasmodium ovale*; 1% mixed; 17% unknown
- *P. falciparum*, *P. malariae*, *P. vivax*, *P. ovale*, and *P. knowlesi* in parts of Southeast Asia

Incidence

- Most U.S. cases (>99%) are imported.
- ~1,500 cases and 5 deaths per year in the United States (2)

Prevalence

- Predominant age: all ages
- Predominant sex: male = female

ETIOLOGY AND PATHOPHYSIOLOGY

- Malarial parasites digest red blood cell (RBC) proteins and alter the RBC membrane, thereby causing hemolysis, increased splenic clearance, and anemia.
- RBC lysis stimulates release of cytokines and tumor necrosis factor-α (TNF-α).
- *P. falciparum* alters RBC viscosity, causing obstruction and end-organ ischemia.

Genetics

Unknown genetic predilection but inherited conditions may affect disease severity and susceptibility (glucose-6-phosphate deficiency, sickle cell disease or trait, and hereditary elliptocytosis)

RISK FACTORS

- Travel/migration from endemic areas (primarily sub-Saharan Africa)
- Rarely, blood transfusion, mother-to-fetus transmission, and autochthonous transmission

GENERAL PREVENTION

- Mosquito avoidance measures: use of insect repellent, wear clothing that covers exposed skin, use mosquito nets treated with permethrin, and avoid outdoor activity from dusk to dawn.
- *Malarial chemoprophylaxis when in endemic area*
  - Mefloquine: begin at least 2 weeks before arrival and continue for 4 weeks after leaving area. Adults, 250 mg (1 tablet) weekly; children ≤9 kg, 5 mg/kg; children >9–19 kg, 1/4 tablet weekly; children >19–30 kg, 1/2 tablet weekly; children >30–45 kg, 3/4 tablet weekly; children >45 kg as adult
    - Caution: mefloquine-resistant areas
  - Atovaquone/proguanil: begin 1–2 days before arrival and continue for 1 week after leaving area. Adults, 1 adult tablet daily; children 5–8 kg, 1/2 pediatric tablet daily; children 9–10 kg, 3/4 pediatric tablet daily; children 11–20 kg, 1 pediatric tablet daily; children 21–30 kg, 2 pediatric tablets daily; children 31–40 kg, 3 pediatric tablets daily; children >40 kg, 1 adult tablet daily
  - Doxycycline: begin 1–2 days before arrival and continue for 4 weeks after leaving area. Adults, 100 mg daily; children, 2 mg/kg up to 100 mg daily (not for children younger than 8 years old)
  - Chloroquine: begin 1–2 weeks before arrival and continue for 4 weeks after leaving area. Adults, 500 mg (300-mg base) weekly; children, 8.3 mg/kg (5-mg base/kg) weekly up to 300 mg
    - Caution: chloroquine-resistant areas
  - Primaquine: begin 1–2 days before arrival and continue for 1 week after leaving area; adults, 30 mg/day; children, 0.5 mg/kg/day up to adult dose
    - For use only in areas predominantly endemic for *P. vivax*
    - Caution: Glucose-6-phosphate dehydrogenase deficiency must be excluded prior to first use.

COMMONLY ASSOCIATED CONDITIONS

Bacterial coinfections sometimes occur.

DIAGNOSIS

HISTORY

- Initial symptoms of malaria are nonspecific; suspect malaria in anyone ill returning from endemic area who presents with
  - Fever, malaise, myalgias, chills, headache, nausea, splenomegaly (with chronic infection), hypotension, anemia (with chronic or severe disease), thrombocytopenia, jaundice, vomiting, and diarrhea resembling gastroenteritis
- *P. falciparum*
  - Incubation usually 12–14 days, symptoms within 1 month of infection in most individuals (partially immune individuals such as immigrants may become ill up to 1 year after last exposure)
  - Severe disease and complications: vascular collapse, CNS impairment, renal failure, and acute respiratory distress syndrome
- *P. vivax* and *P. ovale*
  - Incubation period 12–18 days for primary infection and up to 12 months (and longer) for relapses; generally presents with fevers
  - Dormant parasites may remain in liver and reactivate years after initial infection.
  - Can be severe
- *P. malariae*
  - Incubation period ~35 days
  - May become chronic; untreated can persist asymptomatically in human host for years
- *P. knowlesi*
  - Incubation period ~12 days
  - Possibly severe

PHYSICAL EXAM

- Often not specific
- General: elevated temperature, fatigue, tachycardia, tachypnea, jaundice
- Neurologic: mental status and motor–sensory exam (cerebral malaria)
- Cardiopulmonary exam: hemodynamic stability and signs of vascular leak (effusion)
- Skin exam: pallor, rash
- Abdominal exam: organomegaly

DIFFERENTIAL DIAGNOSIS

- Infections (disseminated or localized): abscess, viral, gastroenteritis, typhoid/paratyphoid, other bacteremias, rickettsial disease, mycobacteria
- Collagen vascular disease (systemic lupus erythematosus [SLE], vasculitides)
- Neoplasms (lymphoma, leukemia, other blood dyscrasias, other tropical causes of splenomegaly)
- Severe malaria infection may mimic hepatitis, pneumonia, stroke, or sepsis.

DIAGNOSTIC TESTS & INTERPRETATION

- Malarial smear thick and thin preparations
  - Microscopy to evaluate for presence of parasite forms, determine species, and quantify the percentage of RBCs that are infected
  - Test should be performed on site, immediately, with results quickly available.
  - Rapid antigen capture enzyme: can detect the presence of malaria parasites within minutes. Cannot determine species or quantify parasitemia. Positive and negative results must always be confirmed by microscopy.
  - Other tests: species-specific PCR; species confirmation by PCR is encouraged.
- General laboratory findings (nonspecific)
  - In uncomplicated infection
    - Elevated liver function tests and lactate dehydrogenase
    - Thrombocytopenia, anemia, and leukopenia
- Note: a low to low-normal platelet count or a slightly high bilirubin is typical and should alert the clinician to the diagnosis after exposure in an endemic setting.
- Note: Antimalarial prophylactic agents may reduce parasitemia.

Initial Tests (lab, imaging)

- CBC with differential and platelets
- Basic chemistry panel including bilirubin
- Malaria thick and thin blood films (if negative, repeat q12–24h for at least 3 sets)
- Imaging necessary only for respiratory disease (chest x-ray) or cerebral malaria (CT scan prior to lumbar puncture)

Follow-Up Tests & Special Considerations

- Nonimmune individuals with suspected or confirmed *P. falciparum* should be hospitalized.
- Leftover clinical specimens from malaria cases in the United States can be submitted to the Centers for Disease Control and Prevention (CDC) for drug resistance surveillance.

Test Interpretation

Interpretation of microscopy. Blood is obtained from the patient and spread on a microscope slide as a thick/thin prep and stained with Giemsa (most commonly). The slide is viewed under 100X oil immersion to examine for ring, gametocyte, trophozoite, and schizont forms associated with *P. falciparum* infection.

TREATMENT

MEDICATION

First Line

- For uncomplicated chloroquine-resistant *P. falciparum* (most *P. falciparum*), chloroquine-resistant *P. vivax*, or when species is unknown, the following regimens are recommended:
  - Atovaquone-proguanil (Malarone): adult tablet: 250 mg atovaquone and 100 mg proguanil. Pediatric tablet: 62.5 mg atovaquone and 25 mg proguanil. Adults: 4 adult tablets once per day for 3 days. Children 5–8 kg: 2 pediatric tablets once per day for 3 days; children 9–10 kg: 3 pediatric tablets once per day for 3 days; children 11–20 kg: 1 adult tablet once per day for 3 days; children 21–30 kg: 2 adult tablets once per day for 3 days; children 31–40 kg: 3 adult tablets once per day for 3 days; children >40 kg: 4 adult tablets once per day for 3 days
  - Artemether-lumefantrine (Coartem): tablet contains 20 mg artemether and 120 mg lumefantrine. Persons 5–<15 kg: 1 tablet BID for 3 days; persons 15–<25 kg: 2 tablets BID for 3 days; persons 25–<35 kg: 3 tablets BID for 3 days; persons ≥35 kg: 4 tablets BID for 3 days
  - Quinine sulfate plus doxycycline or clindamycin: adults: quinine sulfate 650 mg (salt) TID for 3 days (should be extended to 7 days for infections acquired in southeast Asia). Doxycycline 100 mg BID for 7 days. Clindamycin 20 mg (base)/kg/day divided TID for 7 days. Children: quinine sulfate 10 mg (salt)/kg TID for 3 days (should be extended to 7 days for infections acquires in Southeast Asia) plus clindamycin dosed as above.
  - Mefloquine: adults: 750 mg followed by 500 mg 8 hours later. Children: 15 mg/kg followed by 10 mg/kg 8 hours later (maximum total dose: 1,250 mg)
- PO therapy for *P. ovale, P. malariae*, chloroquine-sensitive *P. falciparum* (rare), and chloroquine-sensitive *P. vivax* (New Guinea has highest rates of chloroquine-resistant *P. vivax*); in addition to the treatment regimens listed above, other options are as follows:
  - Chloroquine: adults: 1 g (600-mg base) followed by 500 mg (300-mg base) at 6, 24, and 48 hours after 1st dose. Children: 16.6 mg/kg (10-mg base/kg) on day 1 (max 1,000 mg [600-mg base]), then 8.3 mg/kg (5-mg/kg base) at 6, 24, and 48 hours after 1st dose
  - Primaquine (should be added to the acute treatment regimen for cure of dormant forms of *P. vivax* and *P. ovale*): adults: 30-mg base (52.6 mg) daily for 2 weeks. Children: 0.6-mg base/kg/day for 2 weeks
- Therapy for severe *P. falciparum*
  - Clinical features defining severe malaria:
    - Impaired level of consciousness (LOC)
    - Respiratory distress, jaundice
    - Repeated convulsions, shock
    - Renal failure
  - Laboratory features:
    - Parasitemia >5%
    - Hypoglycemia
    - Acidosis (usually lactic acidosis)
- Parenteral therapy
  - Quinidine gluconate 10 mg/kg in normal saline over 1–2 hours followed by 0.02 mg/kg/min continuous infusion
  - Intensive care monitoring is necessary, especially when initiating quinidine therapy.
- In severe malaria, CDC should be contacted for assistance; CDC Malaria Branch: 770-488-7100; http://www.cdc.gov/Malaria/
- In 2007, CDC made artesunate available in the United States for severe malaria and in special circumstances under an investigational protocol. Contact the CDC for assistance, as noted above.

ISSUES FOR REFERRAL

Infectious disease or tropical medicine consultation advised. Malaria is a reportable disease (http://www.cdc.gov/malaria/features/new_report_form.html).

ADDITIONAL THERAPIES

None

Pediatric Considerations

- Children are particularly susceptible to severe disease.
- All children, even infants, should receive chemoprophylaxis if traveling to an endemic area.
- Malaria commonly resembles acute gastroenteritis in children.
- Children with severe disease are particularly prone to hypoglycemia. IV fluids with glucose should be used for maintenance and frequent blood glucose measurements taken.

Pregnancy Considerations

- Chloroquine is safe in the doses recommended for prevention and treatment of malaria; FDA pregnancy Category C.
- Mefloquine is safe in the doses recommended for prevention and treatment of malaria; FDA pregnancy Category B
- Atovaquone-proguanil (Malarone) has not been studied in pregnant women; it has not been shown to cause birth defects or other problems in animal studies; FDA pregnancy Category C
- No primaquine (FDA class undetermined) or tetracyclines (FDA pregnancy Category D) in pregnancy
- Quinine/Quinidine (FDA pregnancy Category C, respectively) should be used during pregnancy because benefit outweighs risk.

COMPLEMENTARY & ALTERNATIVE MEDICINE

None. Many deaths have resulted from using unapproved alternatives to medications.

SURGERY/OTHER PROCEDURES

Rarely, splenectomy must be performed in patients with splenic rupture.

INPATIENT CONSIDERATIONS

Initial Stabilization

- Inpatient care for all cases of *P. falciparum* malaria in nonimmune patients or any patient, despite the species, with signs of severe illness; outpatient care for others
- Nonimmune with *P. falciparum* may progress from mild symptoms to death within 12 hours. All patients treated on outpatient basis should have follow-up within 24 hours.

Admission Criteria/Initial Stabilization

- All nonimmune patients with confirmed or suspected *P. falciparum*
- All patients with signs of severe disease (see "Treatment")

IV Fluids

Maintenance IV fluids with glucose because of risk of hypoglycemia are recommended if unable to tolerate fluids by mouth. Excess fluids may result in iatrogenically induced pulmonary edema.

Nursing

Observe for fluid excess, renal insufficiency (urine output), and hypoglycemia.

Discharge Criteria

Clinical improvement and ability to tolerate oral medications and fluids, with documented decreasing parasitemia levels

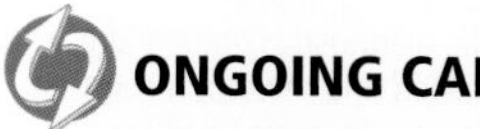

ONGOING CARE

PATIENT EDUCATION

- Malarial chemoprophylaxis prior to travel
- Travel information may be obtained at the CDC travel Web site: http://www.cdc.gov/travel

PROGNOSIS

Malaria infection (particularly *P. falciparum*) can carry a high mortality if untreated. If diagnosed early and treated appropriately, the prognosis is excellent.

COMPLICATIONS

- If not treated early: cerebral malaria, acute renal failure, acute gastroenteritis, respiratory distress syndrome, and massive hemolysis
- Other complications: seizures, anuria, delirium, coma, dysentery, algid malaria, blackwater fever, hyperpyrexia
- *P. malariae*: Nephrotic syndrome may develop in patients with chronic infection.

REFERENCES

1. World Health Organization. *World Malaria Report 2013*. Geneva, Switzerland: WHO Press; 2013.
2. Cullen KA, Arguin PM. Malaria surveillance—United States, 2011. *MMWR Surveil Summ*. 2013;62(5):1–17.

ADDITIONAL READING

- Centers for Disease Control and Prevention. Guidelines for treatment of malaria in the United States. http://www.cdc.gov/malaria/resources/pdf/treatmenttable.pdf. Updated July 1, 2013. Accessed 2014.
- Griffith KS, Lewis LS, Mali S, et al. Treatment of malaria in the United States: a systematic review. *JAMA*. 2007;297(20):2264–2277.
- Steinhardt LC, Magill AJ, Arguin PM. Review: malaria chemoprophylaxis for travelers to Latin America. *Am J Trop Med Hyg*. 2011;85(6):1015–1024.

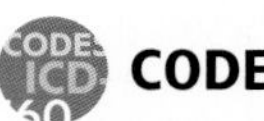

CODES

ICD10

- B54 Unspecified malaria
- B50.9 Plasmodium falciparum malaria, unspecified
- B51.9 Plasmodium vivax malaria without complication

CLINICAL PEARLS

- Persons with malaria despite chemoprophylaxis use (usually incomplete) should be treated with a different regimen than their chemoprophylaxis drug.
- Think malaria in travelers returning from endemic areas who present with fever or nonspecific flulike illness.
- Early identification and aggressive treatment, particularly of nonimmune persons with suspected or confirmed *P. falciparum* malaria, is the key to good clinical outcomes.

MARFAN SYNDROME

Michele Roberts, MD, PhD • Helio Pedro, MD

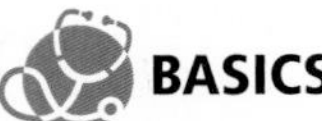

BASICS

DESCRIPTION

- Marfan syndrome (MFS) is an inherited disorder of connective tissue.
- Because many features of MFS appear in the general population, specific diagnostic criteria (Ghent nosology) were established and revised, recognizing a constellation of features with major and minor criteria for establishing the diagnosis (1,2).
- System(s) affected: musculoskeletal, cardiovascular, ocular, pulmonary, skin/integument, connective tissue (dura)

Pediatric Considerations

Careful monitoring, as described. Early surgical intervention may reduce the degree of scoliosis.

Pregnancy Considerations

- Manage pregnancy in MFS as high risk, with a cardiologist; prepregnancy evaluation: screening transthoracic echocardiogram for aortic root dilation
- Consider β-blockers in all pregnancies to minimize risk of aortic dilation throughout the pregnancy.
- 1% complication rate if aortic root diameter <40 mm; 10% if >40 mm. Consider elective surgery before pregnancy if >47 mm.
- Avoid spinal anesthesia due to risk of dural ectasia.

EPIDEMIOLOGY

- Congenital; although clinical manifestations may be apparent in infancy, affected individuals may not present until adolescence or young adulthood.
- No gender, ethnic, or racial predilection; with advanced paternal age, a slightly increased risk of de novo mutation resulting in MFS in offspring.

Prevalence

1/3,000–1/5,000

ETIOLOGY AND PATHOPHYSIOLOGY

Genetic abnormality; mutations of the *FBN1* (fibrillin) gene. Fibrillin is an extracellular matrix protein widely distributed in elastic and nonelastic connective tissue.

Genetics

- Mutations of the fibrillin-1 (*FBN1*) gene on chromosome 15q21.1 OMIM 154700.
- MFS is an autosomal dominant condition with complete penetrance and variable expressivity. Apparent nonpenetrance may be due to lack of recognition of MFS in a mildly affected individual.
- Each child of an affected parent has a 50% chance of inheriting MFS and may be more or less severely affected. 25% of cases result from de novo mutation.

GENERAL PREVENTION

- Prenatal diagnosis is possible in families with a known mutation.

COMMONLY ASSOCIATED CONDITIONS

- High prevalence of obstructive sleep apnea in MFS; may be a risk factor for aortic root dilatation
- Increased prevalence of migraine in MFS

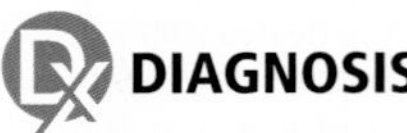

DIAGNOSIS

- In the revised Ghent nosology:
  - Cardiovascular manifestations (aortic root aneurysm/dissection) and ectopia lentis have more weight.
  - Molecular genetic testing for *FBN1* plays a more prominent diagnostic role but is not required.
  - Less specific manifestations were removed or made less influential, thus avoiding obligate thresholds that were not evidence based. Careful follow-up diminishes risk of missed diagnosis.
  - New criteria explicitly allow for alternative diagnoses, when additional features warrant: Shprintzen-Goldberg syndrome (SGS), Loeys-Dietz syndrome (LDS), or vascular-type Ehlers-Danlos syndrome (vEDS).
  - *Z*-score calculator for aortic root enlargement: www.marfan.org
- In the absence of a family history of MFS:
  - Aortic root dilatation or dissection ($Z \geq 2$) (Ao) *and* ectopia lentis (EL): unequivocal diagnosis of MFS, irrespective of systemic features, except when they are diagnostic of SGS, LDS, or vEDS
  - Ao *and* a bona fide *FBN1* mutation: diagnostic of MFS, even in the absence of EL
  - Where Ao is present but EL is absent and the *FBN1* status is negative (or unknown), diagnosis of MFS requires systemic findings score of ≥7 points using new scoring system (see below) and exclusion of SGS, LDS, and vEDS.
  - With EL but without Ao, *FBN1* mutation previously associated with Ao is required for diagnosis of MFS.
- Systemic features, scoring system (see "Physical Exam"):
  - Wrist *and* thumb sign +3 (thumb protrudes from clenched fist); wrist *or* thumb sign +1 (encircles wrist with little finger and thumb of opposite hand)
  - Pectus carinatum deformity +2; pectus excavatum or chest asymmetry +1
  - Hindfoot deformity +2; pes planus +1
  - Pneumothorax +2
  - Dural ectasia +2
  - Protrusio acetabuli +2 by x-ray, CT, or MRI
  - Reduced upper-to-lower segment ratio (US/LS) *and* increased arm/height *and* no severe scoliosis +1
  - Scoliosis or thoracolumbar kyphosis +1
  - Reduced elbow extension +1
  - Facial features (3/5) +1
  - Skin striae +1
  - Myopia >3 diopters +1
  - Mitral valve prolapse (all types) +1
- Maximum: 20 points; score ≥7 indicates systemic involvement
- Positive family history requires a family member independently diagnosed using above criteria.
- With a positive family history, MFS can be diagnosed with ectopia lentis, *or* systemic score ≥7, *or* aortic root dilatation with $Z \geq 2$ in persons >20 years old *or* $Z \geq 3$ in persons <20 years old.
- In persons <20 years old who have negative family history and suggestive findings but who do not meet Ghent criteria, "nonspecific connective tissue disorder" is diagnosed;close follow-up is recommended.
- In the presence of a relevant *FBN1* mutation, "potential MFS" is diagnosed and close follow-up is recommended.
- In adults who have suggestive findings but who do not meet Ghent criteria, consider alternative diagnoses: ectopia lentis syndrome, mitral valve prolapse syndrome, MASS (**M**itral valve prolapse, **A**ortic dilation, **S**kin, and **S**keletal) phenotype.

PHYSICAL EXAM

- Facial features: dolichocephaly (head length longer than expected compared with width), enophthalmos, down-slanting palpebral fissures, malar hypoplasia, micrognathia
- High-arched, narrow palate
- Thumb sign: distal phalanx of thumb protrudes from clenched fist; wrist sign: thumb and 5th digit overlap when circling wrist.
- Pectus carinatum deformity: pectus excavatum or chest asymmetry beyond normal variation
- Hindfoot valgus with forefoot abduction and lowering of the midfoot; distinguish from pes planus
- Reduced upper segment-to-lower segment (US/LS) ratio: 0.93 in unaffected individuals versus ≤0.85 in affected white adults, ≤0.78 in affected black adults. US is measured from the top of the head to the top of the mid-pubic bone; LS is measured from the top of the pubic bone to the sole of the foot. In children, abnormal US/LS: US/LS <1, age 0–5 years; US/LS <0.95, 6–7 years; US/LS <0.9, 8–9 years; <0.85, age ≥10 years.
- Increased arm span to height ratio >1.05
- Scoliosis or thoracolumbar kyphosis is diagnosed if, on bending forward, there is a vertical difference ≥1.5 cm between the ribs of the left and right hemithorax.
- Reduced elbow extension if angle between upper and lower arm measures ≤170 degrees on full extension
- Skin: Striae atrophicae are significant if not associated with significant weight changes (or pregnancy) and if located on midback, lumbar region, upper arm, axilla, or thigh.
- Because of lack of specificity, joint hypermobility, high-arched palate, and recurrent or incisional herniae were removed from diagnostic criteria (1).

DIFFERENTIAL DIAGNOSIS

Clinical manifestations overlapping with MFS in cardiovascular, ocular, and skeletal systems:

- Ectopia lentis syndrome: no aortic root dilatation
- Mitral valve prolapse syndrome: mitral valve prolapse; limited systemic features may include pectus excavatum, scoliosis, mild arachnodactyly; aortic enlargement and ectopia lentis preclude this diagnosis.
- MASS phenotype: mitral valve prolapse; myopia; borderline, nonprogressive *a*ortic enlargement ($Z < 2$); and nonspecific *s*keletal and *s*kin involvement. Aortic involvement in MASS is usually nonprogressive; some risk for more severe vascular involvement
- Shprintzen-Goldberg, Loeys-Dietz, Ehlers-Danlos, Stickler syndromes; congenital contractural arachnodactyly; Weill-Marchesani syndrome, multiple endocrine neoplasia type 2B, fragile X
- Homocystinuria: marfanoid habitus, thrombosis, mental retardation; urine amino acid analysis is diagnostic; lens dislocates downward.
- Familial thoracic aortic aneurysm

DIAGNOSTIC TESTS & INTERPRETATION

- Sequencing of *FBN1* is the preferred method for molecular diagnosis. Mutations can be found in 95% of patients meeting diagnostic criteria for MFS.
- Specific criteria have been established (1) for *FBN1* mutations causative of MFS. *FBN1* mutation is a valuable marker for risk or aortic dissection (3).
- Echocardiography: Measure aortic root at the level of sinuses of Valsalva; check for mitral valve prolapse. The Marfan Foundation has nomograms to calculate aortic root *Z*-score in children (www.marfan.org).
- In patients whose physical exam is suggestive of MFS, measure urinary homocystine to rule out homocystinuria, an inborn error of metabolism.
- Anteroposterior (AP) radiograph: protrusio acetabuli
- Scoliosis: Cobb angle ≥20 degrees on radiographs; imaging for MFS diagnosis or as per clinical exam

- Hindfoot valgus with forefoot abduction and lowering of the midfoot: anterior and posterior views
- MRI or CT to evaluate for dural ectasia and if symptomatic, symptoms highly variable, nonspecific, and include lower back pain

Diagnostic Procedures/Other

- Ectopia lentis is diagnosed on slit-lamp examination after maximal dilatation of the pupil (60%); lens dislocation is most often upward and temporal.
- Myopia: common in the general population; myopia >3 diopters contributes to MFS systemic score.
- Elongated globe, keratoconus, increased risk of vitrious or retinal detachment, glaucoma, and early cataract formation

Test Interpretation

- Cystic medial necrosis of the aorta descriptive, not pathognomonic
- Myxomatous degeneration of cardiac valves

TREATMENT

MEDICATION

- Prevention of aortic complications: β-adrenergic blockers. Dosage adjusted to target heart rate (resting rate 60 bpm, increase to ≤110 bpm after moderate exertion or <100 bpm after submaximal exercise) (1)[C]
- If β-blockers contraindicated: Calcium channel blockers, angiotensin-converting enzyme inhibitors, and angiotensin receptor blockers may retard aortic dilation in children and adolescents (4)[B].
- Recent studies support the use of losartan in addition to β-blockers to prevent progressive aortic root dilation in patients with MFS (5).

ISSUES FOR REFERRAL

Genetics, cardiology, orthopedics, ophthalmology

SURGERY/OTHER PROCEDURES

- When cardiac symptoms develop or aortic root diameter is ≥5 cm, consider surgical intervention (6). Many MFS patients will ultimately require reconstructive cardiovascular surgery:
  - Dissection of ascending aorta (type A) is a surgical emergency. Consider prophylactic surgery when diameter of sinus of Valsalva approaches 5 cm, rate of change approaches 1 cm/year, and with progressive aortic regurgitation (3); other risk factors: family history, other cardiac pathology, pregnancy
  - Dissection of descending thoracic aorta (type B): Surgical indications include intractable pain, limb or organ ischemia, aortic diameter >5.5 cm (or rapidly increasing) (1)
- Mitral valve repair: for severe mitral valve regurgitation or progressive LV dilatation or dysfunction or in patients undergoing valve-sparing root replacement (1)
- Lens subluxation: Incidence of glaucoma is high, so surgery is performed only if the condition cannot be treated with corrective lenses; surgical removal of lens in lens opacity, impending complete luxation, lens-induced glaucoma or uveitis, or anisometropia or refractive error not amenable to optical correction (1)
- Severe pectus excavatum may interfere with pulmonary or cardiac function and require surgery.
- Scoliosis: bracing for curves 20–40 degrees until growth is complete or surgery if >40 degrees
- Surgery for only most severe cases of dural ectasia
- Hip replacement in middle age or later if protrusio acetabuli has led to severe arthritic change

ONGOING CARE

FOLLOW-UP RECOMMENDATIONS

- Avoid sports that can increase aortic root enlargement or pneumothorax; in general, avoid contact sports, Valsalva, breathing against resistance, and exhaustion (7,8)[C].
- Exercise restrictions: Follow recommendation from the National Marfan Foundation (www.marfan.org) and guidelines from the American Heart Association/American College of Cardiology Task Force.

Patient Monitoring

Exams at least twice/year while patient is growing, with attention to the cardiovascular system and to scoliosis.

- Cognitive ability usually normal, but visual and medical difficulties may interfere with learning (7)[C].
- Cardiac
  - Aortic root dilatation in MFS is usually progressive, warrants vigilance even when not seen on initial examination; age <20 years, yearly echocardiogram; adults with repeatedly normal aortic root measurements, echo every 2–3 years (1)[C].
  - Yearly echocardiograms (initially), more frequent if aortic diameter is increasing rapidly (≥5 cm/year) or is approaching surgical threshold (≥4.5 cm in adults)
  - Regular imaging after surgical repair of aorta
- Musculoskeletal
  - Excessive linear growth of long bones, extremities disproportionately long, paucity of muscle mass, peak growth velocity 2 years early. Growth curves for MFS are available (7)[C].
  - Clinical evaluation for scoliosis earlier than in general population; plain radiographs of spine during growth years
  - Evaluate for scoliosis, joint laxity, and pectus deformity every visit to age 1 year, annually age 1–5 years, semiannually age 6–18 years, and yearly thereafter.
  - Bone age in preadolescence: Consider hormonal therapy if with large discrepancy (7)[C].
  - Scoliosis or pectus deformity may progress more rapidly than in those without MFS.
  - Excellent prognosis for scoliosis curves <30 degrees; bracing may be effectifve for curves <35 degrees; rapid progression likely if curve >50 degrees (7)[C]
- Annual ophthalmologic evaluation: ectopia lentis, myopia, cataract, glaucoma, and retinal detachment; myopia is very common in MFS and may have early onset, rapid progression, and high degree of severity; early monitoring, aggressive refraction to prevent amblyopia (1)[C]
- Respiratory: pulmonary function tests (PFTs) for pulmonary complaints; screen for obstructive sleep apnea.
- Review the diagnosis, examine family members, and offer support group information at diagnosis and PRN.
- Provide genetic counseling at diagnosis, discuss pregnancy risks in adolescence, discuss activity restrictions starting age 6 years, and transition planning in early adolescence. Review symptoms of potential catastrophic events: aortic dissection, vision changes, and pneumothorax starting age 6 years.

PATIENT EDUCATION

- National Marfan Foundation, www.marfan.org
- NLM Genetics Home Reference: marfan syndrome http://ghr.nlm.nih.gov/condition/marfan-syndrome

PROGNOSIS

Life-threatening complications involve cardiovascular dysfunction. In 1972, lifespan was 32 years. Currently, lifespan is nearly normal.

COMPLICATIONS

Bacterial endocarditis, aortic dissection, aortic or mitral valve insufficiency, dilated cardiomyopathy, retinal detachment, glaucoma, pneumothorax

REFERENCES

1. Loeys BL, Dietz HC, Braverman AC, et al. The revised Ghent nosology for the Marfan syndrome. *J Med Genet*. 2010;47(7):476–485.
2. Faivre L, Collod-Beroud G, Callewaert B, et al. Pathogenic FBN1 mutations in 146 adults not meeting clinical diagnostic criteria for Marfan syndrome: further delineation of type 1 fibrillinopathies and focus on patients with an isolated major criterion. *Am J Med Genet A*. 2009;149A(5):854–860.
3. Faivre L, Collod-Beroud G, Child A, et al. Contribution of molecular analyses in diagnosing Marfan syndrome and type I fibrillinopathies: an international study of 1009 probands. *J Med Genet*. 2008;45(6):384–390.
4. Williams A, Davies S, Stuart AG, et al. Medical treatment of Marfan syndrome: a time for change. *Heart*. 2008;94(4):414–421.
5. Groenink M, den Hartog AW, Franken R, et al. Losartan reduces aortic dilatation rate in adults with Marfan syndrome: a randomized controlled trial. *Eur Heart J*. 2013;34(45):3491–3500.
6. Benedetto U, Melina G, Takkenberg JJ, et al. Surgical management of aortic root disease in Marfan syndrome: a systematic review and meta-analysis. *Heart*. 2011;97(12):955–958.
7. Tinkle B, Saul HM; Committee on Genetics. Health supervision for children with Marfan syndrome. *Pediatrics*. 2013;132(4):e1059–e1072.
8. Maron BJ, Chaitman BR, Ackerman MJ, et al. Recommendations for physical activity and recreational sports participation for young patients with genetic cardiovascular diseases. *Circulation*. 2004;109(22):2807–2816.

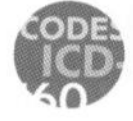

CODES

ICD10

- Q87.40 Marfan's syndrome, unspecified
- Q87.43 Marfan's syndrome with skeletal manifestation
- Q87.418 Marfan's syndrome with other cardiovascular manifestations

CLINICAL PEARLS

- Because many features of MFS appear in the general population, diagnostic criteria have been established. Molecular diagnostic testing for *FBN1* mutations will play an increasing role.
- Screen very tall athletes for aortic root dilatation.
- Early diagnosis of homocystinuria is important because clinical complications can be minimized with appropriate diet and medication.
- Ectopia lentis and aortic root dilatation are best discrimination features, but height ≥3.3 *SD* above the mean is a simple discriminant in primary care.

MARIJUANA (CANNABIS) USE DISORDER

Adriana C. Linares, MD, MPH, DrPH

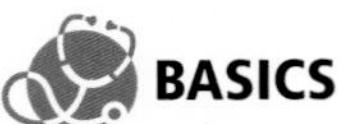

BASICS

DESCRIPTION

Marijuana or cannabis use disorder is classified in *DSM-5* in different categories (mild, moderate, or severe) depending on the presence of criteria for abuse and dependence (1). The criteria are the following:

- Failure to fulfill major obligations
- Use of substances in hazardous situations
- Use of substances even though person is having recurrent social or interpersonal problems
- Tolerance, defined by using increased amounts of cannabis to achieve the desired effect or intoxication or diminished effect with continued use of the same amount of cannabis
- Withdrawal
- Use of substances in greater amounts
- Desire to cut down substances
- Time spent in activities necessary to obtain the substance
- Important activities are given up due to use of substance.
- Continued use of substance even though having problems associated with the use of it
- Presence of craving for the substance

EPIDEMIOLOGY

- The United States is ranked 1st among 17 European and North American countries by the World Health Organization for prevalence of marijuana use.
- Cannabis is the most widely used illicit psychoactive substance in the United States (2).
- ~42% of teens will have tried marijuana by the time they graduate from high school.
- Approximately 30% of students report having used marijuana at college entry (3).
- In the United States, 10% of those who ever used marijuana become daily users, and 20–30% became weekly users.
- In the United States, some states have approved medical marijuana use, and 2 states (Washington and Colorado) have approved recreational use of marijuana.
- Other states in the United States are currently trying to pass legislation to legalize the use of recreational marijuana.

ETIOLOGY AND PATHOPHYSIOLOGY

- Main active ingredient in marijuana: delta-9-tetrahydrocannabinol (THC)
- When marijuana is smoked, THC rapidly passes from the lungs into the blood and to the brain, where it binds to cannabinoid receptors (CBRs).
- CBRs are responsible for memory, thinking, concentration, sensory and time perception, pleasure, movement, and coordination.
- THC artificially stimulates the CBRs, disrupting the function of endogenous cannabinoids. A marijuana "high" results from overstimulation of these receptors.
- Over time, overstimulation alters the function of CBRs, which can lead to addiction and to withdrawal symptoms when drug use stops.
- Effects of smoked marijuana can last 1–3 hours.
- Effects from marijuana consumed in foods or beverages appear later, usually in 30 minutes–1 hour, but can last up to 4 hours.
- Smoking marijuana delivers significantly more THC into the bloodstream than eating or drinking the drug.

RISK FACTORS

- Age (highest use among those 18–25 years)
- Male sex
- Comorbid psychiatric disorders (i.e., bipolar disorder, posttraumatic stress disorder [PTSD])
- Other substance use (i.e., alcohol, cocaine)
- Lower educational achievement (rates of dependence lowest among college graduates)

DIAGNOSIS

- Screen for marijuana use along with other lifestyle questions such as tobacco and alcohol use.
- Ask for frequency and amount used (e.g., "How long does a nickel bag last you?").
- Unexplained deterioration in school or work performance may be a red flag for abuse.
- Problems with, or changes in, social relationships (e.g., spending more time alone or with persons suspected of using drugs) and recreational activities (e.g., giving up activities that were once pleasurable) may indicate abuse.
- If available, information from concerned parents or spouses should be obtained.
- *DSM-5* criteria for cannabis use dependence has been changed from *DSM-IV*. The legal issues associated with use of cannabis were dropped, and the presence of cravings was added.

HISTORY

- Clinical presentation of acute intoxication:
  - Euphoria, elation, laughter, heightened sensory perception, altered perception of time, increased appetite
  - Poor short-term memory, concentration
  - Fatigue, depression
  - Occasionally, distrust, fear, anxiety, panic
  - With large doses, acute psychosis: delusions, hallucinations, loss of sense of personal identity (4)
- Withdrawal symptoms include the following:
  - Nausea
  - Weight loss
  - Decreased appetite
  - Insomnia
  - Depressed mood

PHYSICAL EXAM

- Evaluate for:
  - Conjunctival injection
  - Xerostomia
  - Nystagmus
  - Increased heart rate
  - Altered pulmonary status
  - Altered body temperature
  - Reduced muscle strength
  - Decreased coordination
- Withdrawal findings include the following:
  - Restlessness/agitation
  - Irritability
  - Tremor
  - Diaphoresis
  - Increased body temperature

DIAGNOSTIC TESTS & INTERPRETATION

Positive urine drug screen. Cannabinoids can be detected in urine weeks to months after marijuana use.

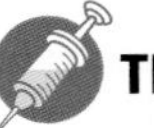

TREATMENT

- 4 methods of behavioral-based interventions:
  - Cognitive-behavioral therapy
  - Motivational interviewing
  - Motivational enhancement therapy
  - Contingency management
- No intervention to date has proved consistently effective for marijuana abuse.
- Despite this, trials on cognitive-behavioral therapy and contingency management have shown better outcomes in reduction in marijuana use and maintaining abstinence.
- For younger persons, family-based interventions may be more effective.
- With marijuana abuse, most prevalent among patients suffering from other psychiatric disorders, studies indicate that treating the mental health disorder may help reduce marijuana use, particularly among heavy users and those with more chronic mental disorders.

- Advice to give to patients for management of withdrawal:
  - Gradually reduce amount of marijuana used before cessation.
  - Delay 1st use of marijuana until later in the day.
  - Consider use of nicotine replacement therapy if planning to stop, separate tobacco use at the same time.
  - Relaxation, distraction
  - Avoid cues and triggers associated with cannabis use.
- Prescribe short-term analgesia and sedation for withdrawal symptoms, if required.
- If irritability and restlessness are marked, consider prescribing very low-dose diazepam for 3–4 days.
- Provide user and family members with information regarding marijuana abuse and withdrawal to increase understanding of the abuse and reduce likelihood of relapse.
- Withdrawal symptoms peak on day 2 or 3, and most are over by day 7. Sleep and vivid dreams can continue for 2–3 weeks.

MEDICATION

- No effective medication for the treatment of marijuana abuse
- One study suggested oral THC could be used to abate marijuana withdrawal in individuals who are trying to quit.
- Another study concluded medications used to treat other drug use disorders, such as buspirone, lithium, and fluoxetine, may have therapeutic benefit.

ONGOING CARE

FOLLOW-UP RECOMMENDATIONS

- Monitor cessation of marijuana use with urine tests over several weeks for the inactive metabolite of cannabis (carboxy-tetrahydrocannabinol).
- Heavy smokers may continue to be positive for marijuana for up to 6 weeks.

PATIENT EDUCATION

To learn more about marijuana abuse, visit the National Institute on Drug Abuse (NIDA) Web site at www.drugabuse.gov. Other NIDA Web sites include the following:

- http://backtoschool.drugabuse.gov
- http://marijuana-info.org
- http://teens.drugabuse.gov

COMPLICATIONS

- Acute adverse effects:
  - Anxiety and panic, especially in naive users
  - Psychotic symptoms at high doses
  - Motor vehicle accidents if a person drives while intoxicated
- Chronic adverse effects:
  - Subtle cognitive impairment
  - Poor educational outcomes, lower income, greater welfare dependence, and unemployment
  - Chronic bronchitis and impaired respiratory function in regular smokers
  - Psychotic symptoms and disorders in heavy users, especially those with a history of psychotic symptoms or a family history of these disorders

REFERENCES

1. American Psychiatric Association. *Diagnostic and Statistical Manual of Mental Disorders*. 5th ed. Arlington, VA: American Psychiatric Association; 2013.
2. National Institute on Drug Abuse. NIDA Website. http://www.drugabuse.gov/. Accesed June 2014.
3. Suerken CK, Reboussin BA, Sutfin EL, et al. Prevalence of marijuana use at college entry and risk factors for initiation during freshman year. *Addict Behav*. 2014;39(1):302–307.
4. Hall W, Degenhardt L. Adverse health effects of non-medical cannabis use. *Lancet*. 2009;374(9698):1383–1391.

ADDITIONAL READING

- Budney A, Vandrey R, Hughes J, et al. Oral delta-9-tetrahydrocannabinol suppresses cannabis withdrawal symptoms. *Drug Alcohol Depend*. 2007;86(1):22–29.
- Denis C, Lavie E, Fatseas M, et al. Psychotherapeutic interventions for cannabis abuse and/or dependence in outpatient settings. *Cochrane Database Syst Rev*. 2006;(3):CD005336.
- Fergusson D, Boden J. Cannabis use and later life outcomes. *Addiction*. 2008;103(6):969–976.
- Hubbard J, Franco S, Onaivi E. Marijuana: medical implications. *Am Fam Physician*. 1999;60(9): 2583–2593.
- National Institute on Drug Abuse. *Research Report Series: Marijuana Abuse*. Bethesda, MD: U.S. Department of Health and Human Services and National Institute of Health; 2010. http://www.drugabuse.gov/publications/research-reports/marijuana/letter-director. Accessed 2015.
- Vandrey R, Haney M. Pharmacotherapy for cannabis dependence: how close are we? *CNS Drugs*. 2009; 23(7):543–553.
- Winstock A, Ford C, Witton J. Assessment and management of cannabis use disorders in primary care. *BMJ*. 2010;340:c1571.

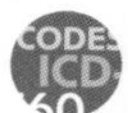

CODES

ICD10

- F12.10 Cannabis abuse, uncomplicated
- F12.20 Cannabis dependence, uncomplicated
- F12.288 Cannabis dependence with other cannabis-induced disorder

CLINICAL PEARLS

- Marijuana abuse may result in poor performance in school or work, legal problems, and arguments with family.
- Patients with schizophrenia are frequently found to be using marijuana and their use hindering the treatment for schizophrenia. Management of these dual diagnoses is important for the successful treatment of schizophrenia.
- Patients should be screened for marijuana use and asked about frequency and amount used.
- Effects of smoked marijuana can last 1–3 hours. Effects from foods or beverages containing marijuana appear later, usually in 30 minutes–1 hour, but can last up to 4 hours.
- Smoking marijuana delivers significantly more THC into the bloodstream than eating or drinking the drug.
- Acute marijuana intoxication is manifested by conjunctival injection, increased heart rate, euphoria, heightened sensory perception, altered perception of time, increased appetite, poor short-term memory and concentration, and fatigue. Large doses may result in acute psychosis, delusions, or hallucinations.
- Inquire of all patients about their use of marijuana. Changes in values and attitudes have made marijuana use more mainstream, and patients do not consider marijuana a substance of abuse.
- Withdrawal symptoms include nausea, weight loss, decreased appetite, insomnia, and depressed mood. Peaks on day 2 or 3 and most are over by day 7.
- Cognitive-behavioral therapy, motivational interviewing, motivational enhancement therapy, and contingency management are 4 methods of behavioral-based interventions used in the treatment of marijuana abuse.

MASTALGIA

Eduardo Lara-Torre, MD • Amanda B. Murchison, MD • Patrice M. Weiss, MD, FACOG

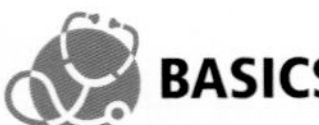

BASICS

DESCRIPTION

- Painful breast tissue, often bilateral, which can be cyclic or noncyclic
  - 2/3 of breast pain is cyclic and usually associated with hormonal changes related to menses, external hormones, pregnancy, or menopause.
  - 1/3 is noncyclic and often is related to a breast or chest wall lesion.
- Synonym(s): mastodynia; breast pain

EPIDEMIOLOGY

Incidence

- Predominant sex: most common in women but occurs occasionally in men
- Predominant age: generally seen from adolescence to menopause
- Frequency of breast cancer with those reporting breast pain ranges from 1.2 to 6.7% (1)[C].
- Up to 70% of women report some degree of breast pain at some point in their lives (2)[B].
- Most describe mild pain, but 11% describe pain as moderate to severe.

ETIOLOGY AND PATHOPHYSIOLOGY

- Causative pathophysiology remains unclear but is thought to be related to hormonal or nutritional factors.
- When fibrocystic disease is the source, growth and distension of the cyst with hormonal fluctuation can cause pain.
- Hormonal factors (e.g., hormone-replacement therapy, oral contraceptives, pregnancy, menses, puberty, and menopause) may influence the diverse conditions that cause mastalgia or may themselves cause breast tenderness and pain.
- Benign breast disorders (e.g., fibrocystic changes)
- Trauma (including sexual abuse/assault)
- Diet and lifestyle (e.g., poor-fitting exercise breast support)
- Lactation problems (e.g., engorgement, mastitis, breast abscess)
- Breast masses, including breast cancer
- Hidradenitis suppurativa
- Costochondritis (Tietze syndrome)
- Postthoracotomy syndrome
- Spinal and paraspinal disorders
- Potential side effects of medications
- Postradiation effects
- Referred pain (e.g., pulmonary, cardiac, or gallbladder disease)
- Ductal ectasia

Genetics

Familial tendency

RISK FACTORS

- Diet high in saturated fats
- Cigarette smoking
- Recent weight gain
- Pregnancy
- Large, pendulous breasts (caused by stretching of Cooper ligaments)
- Exogenous hormones
- Caffeine has been shown not to be a risk factor (3)[A].

GENERAL PREVENTION

- Avoid exposure to risk factors.
- Properly fitted bra support

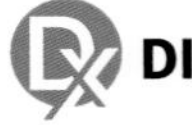

DIAGNOSIS

HISTORY

- Location, duration, frequency, severity, associated symptoms, related activities (e.g., trauma), and aggravating and ameliorating factors
- Complete medical history with focus on gynecologic/obstetric history
- Complete systematic review of systems
- Diet/smoking history
- Detailed family history for risk assessment for breast cancer
- There may be an association with other pain syndromes such as fibromyalgia (4)[B].

PHYSICAL EXAM

- Examine breasts systematically in both standing and sitting positions.
- Assess for skin changes, breast symmetry and contour, dimpling, localized tenderness, bruising, masses, nipple discharge, and lymphadenopathy. Look for signs that are suggestive of breast malignancy.

DIFFERENTIAL DIAGNOSIS

- The most important disease to rule out is breast cancer (although uncommon), particularly if pain is localized.
- Manipulation or trauma also can worsen symptoms.
- Chest wall pain or referred pain resulting from splenomegaly also must be differentiated from mastalgia.
- Sometimes cyclic pain is concurrent with premenstrual syndrome.
- Ductal ectasia of the breast

DIAGNOSTIC TESTS & INTERPRETATION

Initial Tests (lab, imaging)

- If galactorrhea is found, check a fasting prolactin level
- Consider thyroid-stimulating hormone (TSH)
- Consider an ultrasound in women with focal, persistent breast pain
- Mammogram ± ultrasound in women aged ≥30–35 years

Pediatric Considerations

Ultrasound is the imaging test of choice for children and adolescents. A mammogram is not useful.

Diagnostic Procedures/Other

- Cysts may need to be aspirated to relieve symptoms or verify diagnosis.
- Biopsies may be indicated based on the results of examination, ultrasound, or mammography.

Pediatric Considerations

In children and adolescents, do not perform biopsies unless there is suspicion for cancer. Refer to a specialist in pediatric breast disease.

Test Interpretation

- Normal breast tissue
- Benign: fibrocystic changes, duct ectasia, solitary papillomas, simple fibroadenomas
- Small increased risk of breast cancer: ductal hyperplasia without atypia, sclerosing adenosis, diffuse papillomatosis, complex fibroadenomas
- Moderate increased risk: atypical ductal hyperplasia, atypical lobular hyperplasia
- Breast cancer

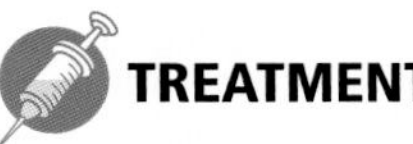

TREATMENT

GENERAL MEASURES

- Stop or modify the current hormonal therapy.
- A repeat examination may help to establish any cyclic nodularity pattern.
- Wear a properly fitted support bra (may be fitted by a professional).
- Reassurance (sufficient for most patients)
- Weight loss for obese patients
- Smoking cessation
- Relaxation training

MEDICATION

First Line

Acetaminophen or NSAIDs, either oral or topical (e.g., diclofenac sodium or piroxicam) (5)[B]

Second Line

- Oral contraceptives may help some patients prevent fibrocystic disease but may worsen pain in some sensitive patients.
- If the patient is on an oral contraceptive, switch to one that has a lower estrogen component.
- In some patients with mastalgia only during their menses, menstrual suppression with continuous oral contraceptives may be of benefit.
- Oral progesterone: 10 mg PO daily
- Other possibilities for patients with refractory symptoms, used infrequently because of potential side effects, include the following:
  - Danazol: 100 mg BID (possibly lower doses) may be the most effective; major adverse effects include menstrual irregularities, weight gain, acne, hirsutism, and voice change; *may be used during luteal phase only;* approved by the FDA for this indication
  - Toremifene: 30 mg PO daily (6)[B]
  - Bromocriptine: 5 mg PO daily and cabergoline 0.5 mg PO weekly, both during the 2nd half of the menstrual cycle are equally effective, but cabergoline has fewer side effects (7)[B].

ADDITIONAL THERAPIES

If the patient is breastfeeding, correct any breastfeeding difficulties; treat underlying mastitis or breast abscess.

Pediatric Considerations

Children and adolescents may require referrals to a specialist.

SURGERY/OTHER PROCEDURES

Some patients may need surgical breast reduction.

COMPLEMENTARY & ALTERNATIVE MEDICINE

- Vitamin E and evening primrose oil have not been found to be of benefit for chronic mastalgia (3)[A].
- Flaxseed oil is not effective for the treatment of mastalgia (3)[C].

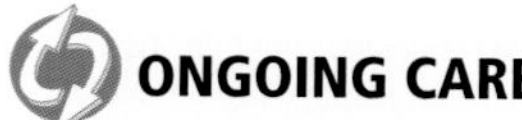

ONGOING CARE

FOLLOW-UP RECOMMENDATIONS

As needed

Patient Monitoring

- As needed for patients not receiving pharmacotherapy
- Time of follow-up will vary by type of pharmacotherapy and patient's particular problems.

DIET

- Decrease fat intake to 20% of total calories.
- No evidence suggests that reduction in caffeine intake may help to decrease the severity or incidence of the disease (3)[A].

PATIENT EDUCATION

Avoid or adjust risk factors.

PROGNOSIS

- Premenstrual mastalgia increases with age and then generally stops at menopause unless the patient is receiving hormone therapy (HT).
- Most patients can control symptoms without receiving HT.
- Several months of HT may provide several more months of relief, but mastalgia may recur.
- Cyclic mastalgia responds better than noncyclic mastalgia to treatment.
- Effects of long-term HT are unknown.

REFERENCES

1. Smith RL, Pruthi S, Fitzpatrick LA. Evaluation and management of breast pain. *Mayo Clinic Proc.* 2004;79(3):353.
2. Ader DN, Shriver CD. Cyclical mastalgia: prevalence and impact in an outpatient breast clinic sample. *J Am Coll Surg.* 1997;185(5):466–470.
3. Chase C, Wells J, Eley S. Caffeine and breast pain: revisiting the connection. *Nurs Womens Health.* 2011;15(4):286–294.
4. Genc V, Genc A, Ustuner E, et al. Is there an association between mastalgia and fibromyalgia? Comparing prevalence and symptom severity. *Breast.* 2011;20(4):314–318.
5. Ahmadinejad M, Delfan B, Haghdani S, et al. Comparing the effect of diclofenac gel and piroxicam gel on mastalgia. *Breast J.* 2010;16(2):213–214.
6. Gong C, Song E, Jia W, et al. A double-blind randomized controlled trial of toremifene therapy for mastalgia. *Arch Surg.* 2006;141(1):43–47.
7. Aydin Y, Atis A, Kaleli S, et al. Cabergoline versus bromocriptine for symptomatic treatment of premenstrual mastalgia: a randomised, open-label study. *Eur J Obstet Gynecol Reprod Biol.* 2010;150(2):203–206.

ADDITIONAL READING

- Blommers J, de Lange-De Klerk ES, Kuik DJ. Evening primrose oil and fish oil for severe chronic mastalgia: a randomized, double-blind, controlled trial. *Am J Obstet Gynecol.* 2002;187(5):1389–1394.
- Brennan M, Houssami N, French J. Management of benign breast conditions. Part 1–painful breasts. *Aust Fam Physician.* 2005;34(3):143–144.
- Colak T, Ipek T, Kanik A. Efficacy of topical nonsteroidal antiinflammatory drugs in mastalgia treatment. *J Am Coll Surg.* 2003;196(4):525–530.
- Miltenburg DM, Speights VO. Benign breast disease. *Obstet Gynecol Clin North Am.* 2008;35(2):285–300, ix.
- Olawaiye A, Withiam-Leitch M, Danakas G, et al. Mastalgia: a review of management. *J Reprod Med.* 2005;50(12):933–939.
- Rosolowich V, Saettler E, Szuck B. *SOGC Clinical Practice Guideline: Mastalgia.* Ottawa, Canada: Society of Obstetricians and Gynaecologists of Canada; 2006. www.sogc.org/guidelines/public/170E-CPG-January2006.pdf. Accessed 2014.

SEE ALSO

- Premenstrual Syndrome (PMS) and Premenstrual Dysphoric Disorder
- Algorithms: Breast Discharge; Breast Pain

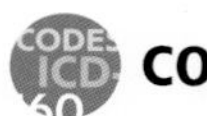

CODES

ICD10

N64.4 Mastodynia

CLINICAL PEARLS

- When evaluating a patient with breast pain, always rule out cancer first.
- In the adolescent population, do not biopsy; instead, refer to a pediatric specialist.
- Premenstrual mastalgia increases with age and then generally stops at menopause unless the patient is receiving HT.

M

MASTITIS

Montiel Teresa Rosenthal, MD

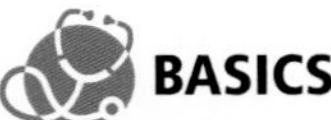

BASICS

DESCRIPTION

- Mastitis is an inflammation of the breast parenchyma and possibly associated tissues (areola, nipple, subcutaneous [SC] fat).
- Usually associated with bacterial infection (and milk stasis in the postpartum mother)
- Usually an acute condition but can become chronic cystic mastitis

EPIDEMIOLOGY

- Predominantly affects females
- Mostly in the puerperium; epidemic form rare in the age of reduced hospital stays for mothers and newborns
- Neonatal form
- Posttraumatic: ornamental nipple piercing increases risk of transmission of bacteria to deeper breast structures: *Staphylococcus aureus* is the predominant organism.

Incidence

- 2.5% of breastfeeding mothers develop non-epidemic mastitis.
- Greatest incidence among breastfeeding mothers 2–3 weeks postpartum
- Neonatal form occurs at 1–5 weeks of age, with equal gender risk and unilateral presentation.
- Pediatric form
- Around or after puberty
- 82% of cases in girls

ETIOLOGY AND PATHOPHYSIOLOGY

- Microabscesses along milk ducts and surrounding tissues
- Inflammatory cell infiltration of breast parenchyma and surrounding tissues
- Nonpuerperal (infectious)
  - *S. aureus*, *Bacteroides* sp., *Peptostreptococcus*, *Staphylococcus* (coagulase neg.), *Enterococcus faecalis*
  - *Histoplasma capsulatum*
  - *Salmonella enterica*
  - Rare case of *Actinomyces europaeus*
- Puerperal (infectious)
  - *Staphylococcus aureus*, *Streptococcus pyogenes* (group A or B), *Corynebacterium* sp., *Bacteroides* sp., *Staphylococcus* (coagulase neg.), *Escherichia coli*, *Salmonella* sp.
  - Methicillin-resistant *S. aureus* (MRSA) (1)
- Rare secondary site for tuberculosis in endemic areas (1% of mastitis cases in these areas): single breast nodule with mastalgia
- *Corynebacterium* sp. associated with greater risk for development of chronic cystic mastitis
- Granulomatous mastitis
  - Idiopathic
    - Predilection for Asian and Hispanic women
    - Association with α-1-antitrypsin deficiency, hyperprolactinemia with galactorrhea, oral contraceptive use, *Corynebacterium* sp. infection, and breast trauma
    - Most women have a history of lactation in previous 5 years.
  - Lupus; autoimmune
- Puerperal
  - Retrograde migration of surface bacteria up milk ducts
  - Bacterial migration from nipple fissures to breast lymphatics
  - Secondary monilial infection in the face of recurrent mastitis or diabetes
  - Seeding from mother to neonate in cyclical fashion
- Nonpuerperal
  - Ductal ectasia
  - Breast carcinoma
  - Inflammatory cysts
  - Chronic recurring SC or subareolar infections
  - Parasitic infections: *Echinococcus*; filariasis; Guinea worm in endemic areas
  - Herpes simplex
  - Cat-scratch disease
- Lupus

RISK FACTORS

- Breastfeeding
- Milk stasis
  - Inadequate emptying of breast
    - Scarring of breast due to prior mastitis
    - Scarring due to previous breast surgery (breast reduction, biopsy, or partial mastectomy)
  - Breast engorgement: interruption of breastfeeding
- Ornamental nipple piercing increases risk of transmission of bacteria to deeper breast structures: *S. aureus* predominant organism
- Neonatal colonization with epidemic *Staphylococcus*
- Neonatal
  - Bottle-fed babies
  - Manual expression of "witch's milk"
  - Can predispose to lethal necrotizing fasciitis
- Maternal diabetes
- Maternal HIV
- Maternal vitamin A deficiency (in animal models)

GENERAL PREVENTION

Regular emptying of both breasts and nipple care to prevent fissures when breastfeeding (2)[A]

COMMONLY ASSOCIATED CONDITIONS

Breast abscess

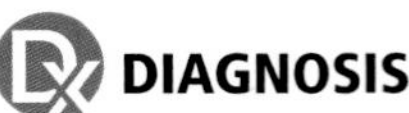

DIAGNOSIS

- Fever and malaise
- Nausea ± vomiting
- Localized breast tenderness, heat, and redness
- Possible breast mass

HISTORY

- Breast pain
- "Hot cords burning in chest wall"

PHYSICAL EXAM

- Breast tenderness
- Localized breast induration, redness, and warmth
- Peau d'orange appearance to overlying skin

DIFFERENTIAL DIAGNOSIS

- Abscess (bacterial, idiopathic granulomatous mastitis, fungal, tuberculosis)
- Tumor
  - Idiopathic granulomatous mastitis
  - Inflammatory breast cancer
  - Wegener granulomatosis
  - Sarcoidosis
  - Foreign body granuloma
- Ductal cyst (ductal ectasia)
- Consider monilial infection in lactating mother, especially if mastitis is recurrent.

DIAGNOSTIC TESTS & INTERPRETATION

Initial Tests (lab, imaging)

Mastitis is typically a clinical diagnosis. Labs rarely needed. In those ill enough to need hospitalization, consider

- CBC
- Blood culture
- In epidemic puerperal mastitis
  - Milk leukocyte count
  - Milk culture
  - Neonatal nasal culture
- No imaging required for postpartum mastitis in a breastfeeding mother that responds to antibiotic therapy.
- Mammography for women with nonpuerperal mastitis
- Breast ultrasound to rule out abscess formation in women
  - Special consideration for this in women with breast implants who have mastitis

Follow-Up Tests & Special Considerations

Lactating mothers produce salty milk from affected side (higher Na and Cl concentrations) as compared with unaffected side.

Diagnostic Procedures/Other

Options if further progression to abscess formation

- Needle aspiration
- Incision and drainage
- Excisional biopsy

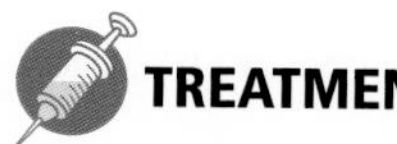

TREATMENT

A recent Cochrane review found that insufficient evidence exists to confirm or refute the effectiveness of antibiotic therapy for the treatment of lactational mastitis (3)[A].

MEDICATION

- Prioritized on the basis of likelihood of MRSA as etiologic factor and clinical severity of condition.
- Treat for 10–14 days.
- For idiopathic granulomatous mastitis and localized infection, usually resolves with antibiotics and drainage

First Line

- Outpatient
  - Dicloxacillin 500 mg QID
  - Cephalexin 500 mg QID
  - Trimethoprim/sulfamethoxazole (TMP/SMX); DS BID (MRSA possible)
  - *Lactobacillus fermentum* or *Lactobacillus salivarius* 9 log 10 CFU/day (4)[B]
- Inpatient
  - Nafcillin 2 g q4h
  - Oxacillin 2 g q4h
  - Vancomycin 1 g q12h (MRSA possible)
- Breastfeeding beyond 1 month
  - Penicillin, ampicillin, or erythromycin

Pediatric Considerations

TMP/SMX given to breastfeeding mothers with mastitis can potentiate jaundice for neonates.

Second Line

- If mastitis is odoriferous and localized under areola, add metronidazole 500 mg TID IV or PO.
- If yeast is suspected in recurrent mastitis, add topical and oral nystatin.

ISSUES FOR REFERRAL

- Abscess formation
- Need for breast biopsy

ADDITIONAL THERAPIES

- Warm packs (or ice packs) to affected breast for comfort
- The use of a breast pump may aid in breast emptying, especially if the infant is unable to assist in doing this.
- Wear supporting bra that is not too tight.

SURGERY/OTHER PROCEDURES

In cases of biopsy-proven idiopathic granulomatous mastitis, surgical removal can result in a 5–50% chance of recurrence, fistula formation, and poor wound healing.

INPATIENT CONSIDERATIONS

If a new mother is admitted to the hospital for treatment of her mastitis, rooming-in of the infant with the mother is mandatory so that breastfeeding can continue (5)[C]. In some hospitals, rooming-in may require hospital admission of the infant.

Admission Criteria/Initial Stabilization

- Failure of outpatient/oral therapy
  - Patient unable to tolerate oral therapy
  - Patient noncompliant with oral therapy
  - Severe illness without adequate supportive care at home
- Neonatal mastitis
- Antibiotics
- Frequent emptying of breasts, if breastfeeding
- Analgesics for pain
  - Acetaminophen
  - Ibuprofen

Nursing

- Breastfeeding/pumping of breasts encouraged
- Start infant with feedings on affected side.
- Abscess drainage is not a contraindication for breastfeeding.

Discharge Criteria

- Afebrile
- Tolerating oral antibiotics well

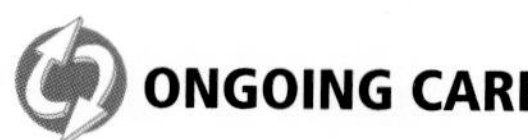

ONGOING CARE

FOLLOW-UP RECOMMENDATIONS

Rest for lactating mothers, up to bathroom

DIET

- Encourage oral fluids
- Multivitamin, including vitamin A

PATIENT EDUCATION

- Encourage oral fluids.
- Rest essential
- Regular emptying of both breasts with breastfeeding
- Nipple care to prevent fissures

PROGNOSIS

- Puerperal
  - Good with prompt (within 24 hours of symptom onset) antibiotic treatment and breast emptying; 96% success rate
  - 11% risk of abscess if left untreated with antibiotics
  - Antibodies develop in breast glands within first few days of infection, which may provide protection against infection or reinfection.
- Rare risk of abscess formation beyond 6 weeks postpartum if no recurrent mastitis

COMPLICATIONS

- Breast abscess
- Recurrent mastitis with resumption of breastfeeding or with breastfeeding after next pregnancy
- Bacteremia
- Sepsis

REFERENCES

1. Gastelum DT, Dassey D, Mascola L, et al. Transmission of community-associated methicillin-resistant *Staphylococcus aureus* from breast milk in the neonatal intensive care unit. *Pediatr Infect Dis J*. 2005;24(12):1122–1124.
2. Crepinsek MA, Crowe L, Michener K, et al. Interventions for preventing mastitis after childbirth. *Cochrane Database Syst Rev*. 2012;10:CD007239.
3. Jahanfar S, Ng CJ, Teng CL, et al. Antibiotics for mastitis in breastfeeding women. *Cochrane Database Syst Rev*. 2013;2:CD005458.
4. Arroyo R, Martín V, Maldonado A, et al. Treatment of infectious mastitis during lactation: antibiotics versus oral administration of lactobacilli isolated from breast milk. *Clin Infect Dis*. 2010;50(12):1551–1558.
5. Academy of Breastfeeding Medicine Protocol Committee. ABM clinical protocol #4: mastitis. Revision, May 2008. *Breastfeed Med*. 2008;3(3):177–180.

ADDITIONAL READING

Spencer JP. Management of mastitis in breastfeeding women. *Am Fam Physician*. 2008;78(6):727–731.

SEE ALSO

Algorithms: Breast Discharge; Breast Pain

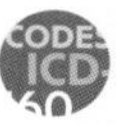

CODES

ICD10

- N61 Inflammatory disorders of breast
- O91.22 Nonpurulent mastitis associated with the puerperium
- O91.23 Nonpurulent mastitis associated with lactation

CLINICAL PEARLS

- Complete emptying of the breasts on a regular schedule, avoiding constrictive clothing or bras that might obstruct breast ducts, meticulous attention to nipple care, "adequate rest," and a liberal intake of oral fluids for the mother can all reduce the risk of a breastfeeding mother's developing mastitis.
- First-line treatment for puerperal mastitis is dicloxacillin 500 mg PO QID × 10–14 days. Most mastitis can be treated with oral therapy.
- Among breastfeeding mothers, if the symptoms of mastitis fail to resolve within several days of appropriate management, including antibiotics, further investigations may be required to confirm resistant bacteria, abscess formation, an underlying mass, or inflammatory or ductal carcinoma.
- More than 2 recurrences of mastitis in the same location or with associated axillary lymphadenopathy warrant evaluation with ultrasound or mammography to rule out an underlying mass.

MASTOIDITIS

Roger Y. Wu, MD, MBA • Jane C. Preotle, MD

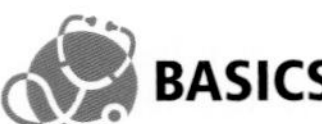

BASICS

Mastoiditis is a suppurative complication of acute otitis media (AOM) affecting the mastoid air cells or posterior process of the temporal bone.

DESCRIPTION

- Inflammatory process of the mastoid bone
- Acute mastoiditis is a suppurative infection that typically presents following AOM. Symptoms are present for <1 month.
- Subdivided into 2 stages
  - Acute mastoiditis with periosteitis: involves the mastoid periosteum and purulence within the mastoid air cells
  - Acute mastoid osteitis (coalescent mastoiditis): destruction of bony septae separating air cells; leading to empyema and more serious head/neck complications
- Subacute mastoiditis (masked mastoiditis): indolent process, may occur with insufficiently treated AOM
- Chronic mastoiditis: due to failed treatment of chronic suppurative otitis media. Usually associated with cholesteatoma; symptoms last months to years.

EPIDEMIOLOGY

- Children > adults
- Most common in children <2 years of age
- In children: males > females
- Incidence reduced after introduction of antibiotics; incidence may be increasing with rise of antibiotic-resistant *Streptococcus pneumoniae*.

Incidence

1–4 cases/100,000/year (1)

ETIOLOGY AND PATHOPHYSIOLOGY

- Subclinical stage begins with AOM causing inflammation of mastoid air cells (likely present in all cases of AOM).
- Obstruction of the aditus ad antrum (connecting the tympanic cavity and mastoid) occurs during severe cases of AOM:
  - Blocks outflow tract of mastoid air cells
  - Edema and accumulation of purulent material with penetration of periosteum (acute mastoiditis with periosteitis)
- Increased pressure from fluid within the air cells leads to destruction of bony septae (acute mastoid osteitis/acute coalescent mastoiditis).
- Acute mastoid osteitis can spread to adjacent areas in head and neck with subsequent abscess formation:
  - Subperiosteal abscess (most common complication), Bezold abscess, suppurative labyrinthitis, suppurative CNS complications
- AOM: *Haemophilus influenzae*, *S. pneumoniae*
- Acute mastoiditis: *Streptococcus pneumoniae* (most common), *Streptococcus pyogenes*, *H. influenzae*, *Staphylococcus aureus* (including methicillin-resistant *Staphylococcus aureus* [MRSA])
  - Introduction of the 7-valent pneumococcal conjugate vaccine in 2,000 associated with increase in multidrug-resistant *S. pneumoniae* serotype 19A
- Chronic mastoiditis: *Pseudomonas aeruginosa*, *S. aureus*, Enterobacteriaceae, anaerobic bacteria, polymicrobials (2)

Genetics

No known genetic pattern

RISK FACTORS

- Cholesteatoma
- Recurrent AOM or chronic suppurative otitis media
- Immunocompromised state

GENERAL PREVENTION

- Pneumococcal conjugate vaccine
- Early referral to ENT for chronic otitis media
- Appropriate diagnosis and treatment of AOM
- Prevention of recurrent AOM
- Treatment of chronic eustachian tube dysfunction (pressure equalization tubes)
- Early identification of cholesteatoma

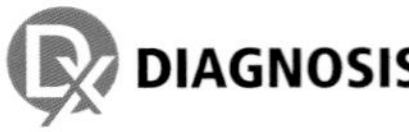

DIAGNOSIS

HISTORY

- Most common symptoms in infancy (1)[A]
  - Lethargy/malaise/irritability
  - Fever
  - Poor feeding/decreased appetite
- Otalgia/possible otorrhea
- Hearing loss
- Headache
- Pain/redness/swelling noted over mastoid.
- At time of admission (1)[A]
  - 42% of children have history of otologic disease.
  - 54% on antibiotic therapy
  - Average duration of symptoms 10 days
- Suspicion for mastoiditis increases when symptoms of AOM persist >2 weeks.

PHYSICAL EXAM

- Postauricular changes: erythema, tenderness, edema, and/or fluctuance (81–85%) (1)[A]
- Bulging, erythematous, or dull tympanic membrane (60–71%)
- Protrusion of auricle (79%)
- Fever (76%)
- Otorrhea if tympanic membrane is perforated
- Edema of external auditory canal
- Tympanic membrane (TM) can be normal in 10% of patients.

DIFFERENTIAL DIAGNOSIS

- Postauricular inflammatory adenopathy
- Severe otitis externa
- Postauricular cellulitis
- Benign neoplasm: aneurysmal bone cyst, fibrous dysplasia
- Malignant neoplasm: rhabdomyosarcoma, neuroblastoma
- Deep neck space infections
- Parotitis

DIAGNOSTIC TESTS & INTERPRETATION

Initial Tests (lab, imaging)

- CBC with differential: increased leukocyte count (3)[C]
- Elevated erythrocyte sedimentation rate (ESR) and C-reactive protein (CRP) (2,3)
- Blood cultures
- Myringotomy/tympanocentesis: Send for cultures, Gram stain, acid-fast stain (1)[B].
- Mastoiditis is often a clinical diagnosis. CT confirms diagnosis and identifies regional complications.
- If obvious physical exam and/or historical findings are absent, temporal bone imaging is recommended for patients with cervical or postauricular findings (4).
- Plain radiographs of mastoid have low diagnostic yield but may show distortion of mastoid outline or clouding of mastoid air cells. This is not diagnostic, as it can also be seen in AOM.
- CT findings (97% sensitivity; 94% positive predictive value) (5)
  - Clouding/opacification of air cells (a finding also present in AOM)
  - Mastoid air cell coalescence
  - Cortical bone erosion
  - Rim-enhancing fluid collections
- CT of temporal bone with contrast is useful for identifying suppurative extension (4)[C].
- Technetium-99m bone scan is more sensitive to osteolytic changes than CT.
- Indications for CT scan in children (5)[C]
  - Neurologic signs
  - Vomiting/lethargy
  - Suspected cholesteatoma
  - Fever after 48–72 hours of therapy
  - Concern for local disease progression
- MRI use increasing; may see increased fluid signal of mastoid air cells on T2-weighted MRI—an incidental finding in the absence of clinical signs

Follow-Up Tests & Special Considerations

Interpret normal WBC with caution in immunocompromised patient with symptoms.

Diagnostic Procedures/Other

- Tympanocentesis to obtain middle ear fluid for culture and sensitivity (1)[B]
- Myringotomy with culture (also therapeutic)
- Audiography if suspected hearing loss
- Obtain CSF if intracranial extension suspected.
- Biopsy tissue protruding through TM or tympanostomy tube

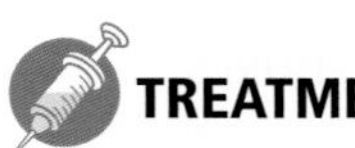

TREATMENT

- IV antibiotics and myringotomy (± tympanostomy tubes) is currently the preferred treatment for uncomplicated acute mastoiditis (reflects a shift away from more invasive surgical treatment).
- Simple mastoidectomy is recommended for nonresponders after 3–5 days to avoid intracranial complications (6)[C].

GENERAL MEASURES

- Inpatient care during acute phase for IV antibiotics
- Keep affected ear dry.

MEDICATION

First Line

- Empiric antibiotics against most common organisms: *S. pneumoniae* (including multiply resistant strains), *S. pyogenes*, *S. aureus* (including MRSA), *P. aeruginosa*
- Use 3rd-generation cephalosporin with additional coverage for resistant strains (4)[C].
- Ceftriaxone 1–2 g IV q24h
  - Pediatric dosing: 50–75 mg/kg/day IV divided q12–24h
  - Precaution: Adjust dose with renal impairment.
- Add clindamycin for coverage of ceftriaxone-resistant *S. pneumoniae* in pediatric patients (4)[C]:
  - Clindamycin pediatric dosing: 20–40 mg/kg/day IV divided q6–8h
- Cefotaxime 1–2 g IV q4–8h, depending on severity
  - Pediatric dosing: 100–200 mg/kg/day divided q6–8h
- Add vancomycin 30–60 mg/kg/day divided q8–12h if concerned for MRSA:
  - Pediatric dosing: 15 mg/kg/dose q6–8h
  - Precaution: Adjust dose with renal impairment.
- For patients with a history of recurrent AOM or recent antibiotic administration, treat with piperacillin–tazobactam 3.375 g IV q6h:
  - Pediatric dosing: 300 mg/kg/day based on piperacillin component divided q6–8h
- For other significant contraindications, precautions, or interactions, please refer to the manufacturer's literature.

Second Line

- Oral antibiotics are given after 7–10 days of IV antibiotics and once myringotomy/blood cultures identify pathogen and sensitivities. Common oral antibiotics include the following:
  - Amoxicillin–clavulanate (Augmentin) or clindamycin + 3rd-generation cephalosporin for 3 weeks or total treatment duration of 4 weeks
- For chronic mastoiditis: Use topical drops, ofloxacin otic solution (0.3%) or neomycin, polymyxin B, hydrocortisone 3 drops, 3–4×/day.

ISSUES FOR REFERRAL

All cases of mastoiditis, both adult and pediatric patients, should be referred to ENT specialists.

SURGERY/OTHER PROCEDURES

- Tympanocentesis should be performed to obtain cultures and guide antibiotic choice (1)[B].
- Myringotomy followed by tympanostomy tubes allow drainage of middle ear (6)[C].
- Mastoidectomy is definitive treatment for patients whose condition fails to improve or progress within 24–48 hours despite IV antibiotics and myringotomy and for those with meningeal or intracranial complications (5,6)[C].
- For management of subperiosteal abscesses, if a trial of conservative therapy with drainage, myringotomy, and IV antibiotics fails, simple mastoidectomy is most effective (7)[C].
- Clean ear canal under microscope to ensure pressure-equalization tube patency and adequate drainage of middle ear.
- Topical antibiotic drops usually used after insertion of pressure-equalization tubes.

INPATIENT CONSIDERATIONS

Admission Criteria/Initial Stabilization

- Clinical or imaging evidence of acute mastoiditis
- Hospitalize any patient with acute mastoiditis; start IV antibiotics immediately.

Nursing

Avoid getting affected ear wet.

Discharge Criteria

- Afebrile for 48 hours before IV antibiotics are discontinued
- Clinical improvement
- Able to take oral antibiotics

ONGOING CARE

FOLLOW-UP RECOMMENDATIONS

- Oral antibiotics for 3 weeks following course of IV antibiotics (total duration of antibiotics is 4 weeks)
- For chronic mastoiditis, consider antimicrobial prophylaxis with amoxicillin for several months.

Patient Monitoring

- Postoperative: audiogram after acute condition has subsided to assess for hearing loss
- Follow-up with ENT, particularly patients with intracranial complications or hearing loss

PATIENT EDUCATION

Precaution about getting affected ear wet

PROGNOSIS

- Depends on severity and stage of disease
- Conductive hearing loss may require reconstructive surgery.
- Most cases of mastoiditis recover fully identified and treated early.

COMPLICATIONS

Total estimated complication rate is 18% (3).

Extracranial

- Subperiosteal abscess (most common complication)
- Bezold abscess (abscess of sternocleidomastoid muscle, insidious, risk of mediastinitis)
- Citelli abscess (osteomyelitis of the calvaria)
- Osteomyelitis of the temporal bone
- Suppurative labyrinthitis (resulting in deafness)
- Facial nerve paralysis

Intracranial

- Intracranial abscess: epidural/subdural/cerebral
- Meningitis/cerebritis/periosteitis
- Gradenigo syndrome (palsy of the 6th cranial nerve, draining ear, and retro-orbital pain)
- Sigmoid sinus thrombosis
- Central venous sinus thrombosis

REFERENCES

1. van den Aardweg MT, Rovers MM, de Ru JA, et al. A systematic review of diagnostic criteria for acute mastoiditis in children. *Otol Neurotol*. 2008;29(6):751–757.
2. Chien JH, Chen YS, Hung IF, et al. Mastoiditis diagnosed by clinical symptoms and imaging studies in children: disease spectrum and evolving diagnostic challenges. *J Microbiol Immunol Infect*. 2012;45(5):377–381.
3. Bilavsky E, Yarden-Bilavsky H, Samra Z, et al. Clinical, laboratory, and microbiological differences between children with simple or complicated mastoiditis. *Int J Pediatr Otorhinolaryngol*. 2009;73(9):1270–1273.
4. Lin HW, Shargorodsky J, Gopen Q, et al. Clinical strategies for the management of acute mastoiditis in the pediatric population. *Clin Pediatr (Phila)*. 2010;49(2):110–115.
5. Bakhos D, Trijolet JP, Morinière S, et al. Conservative management of acute mastoiditis in children. *Arch Otolaryngol Head Neck Surg*. 2011;137(4):346–350.
6. Psarommatis IM, Voudouris C, Douros K, et al. Algorithmic management of pediatric acute mastoiditis. *Int J Pediatr Otorhinolaryngol*. 2012;76(6):791–796.
7. Psarommatis I, Giannakopoulos P, Theodorou E, et al. Mastoid subperiosteal abscess in children: drainage or mastoidectomy? *J Laryngol Otol*. 2012:126(12):1204–1208.

ADDITIONAL READING

- Minks DP, Porte M, Jenkins N. Acute mastoiditis—the role of radiology. *Clin Radiol*. 2013;68(4):397–405.
- Pritchett CV, Thorne MC. Incidence of pediatric acute mastoiditis: 1997–2006. *Arch Otolaryngol Head Neck Surg*. 2012;138(5):451–455.
- Tamir S, Shwartz Y, Peleg U, et al. Shifting trends: mastoiditis from a surgical to a medical disease. *Am J Otolaryngol*. 2009;31(6):467–471.

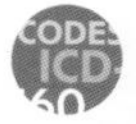

CODES

ICD10

- H70.90 Unspecified mastoiditis, unspecified ear
- H70.009 Acute mastoiditis without complications, unspecified ear
- H70.099 Acute mastoiditis with other complications, unspecified ear

CLINICAL PEARLS

- Suspect mastoiditis when symptoms of AOM persist >2 weeks with a normal TM (TM can be normal in 10% of patients with mastoiditis).
- Hospitalize all patients with acute mastoiditis for IV antibiotics. Consult ENT for drainage procedure.
- Treat with broad-spectrum IV antibiotics; collect middle ear fluid cultures to guide specific therapy.
- If conservative treatment fails after 3–5 days, simple mastoidectomy should be performed to avoid intracranial complications.

MEASLES (RUBEOLA)

Herbert L. Muncie, Jr., MD

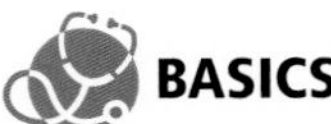

BASICS

DESCRIPTION

- A highly communicable, acute viral illness characterized by an exanthematous maculopapular rash that begins at the head and spreads inferiorly to the trunk and extremities
- Rash is preceded by fever and the classic triad of cough, coryza, and conjunctivitis (3 C's). Koplik spots are pathognomonic lesions of the oral mucosa.
- Public health problem in the developing world, with significant morbidity and mortality
- System(s) affected: hematologic; lymphatic; immunologic; pulmonary; skin
- Synonym(s): rubeola

EPIDEMIOLOGY

- Transmission: direct contact with infectious droplets; highly contagious; 90% of nonimmune close contacts likely to become infected on exposure.
  - Droplets can remain in the air for hours.
- Infectivity is greatest during the prodromal phase.
  - Patients are considered contagious from 4 days before symptoms until 4 days after rash appears.
  - Immunocompromised patients are considered contagious for entire duration of disease.
- Incubation period: averages 12.5 days from exposure to onset of prodromal symptoms (1)
- Predominant age: varies based on local vaccine practices and disease incidence. In developing countries, most cases occur in children <2 years of age.

Incidence

- United States: no longer considered an endemic disease by the CDC; isolated outbreaks still occur.
- In the first half of 2014, the CDC reported 288 confirmed cases of measles.
  - Of these, 97% (280) were imported.
  - Many cases were in vaccine-eligible patients who declined due to philosophic or religious beliefs.
  - Children aged 6–23 months traveling abroad are at increased risk if unvaccinated.
- Worldwide: An estimated 20 million measles cases occur each year, with 164,000 measles deaths in 2008. Large recent outbreaks in southern and eastern Africa. In 2009, 36,000 cases were reported from 46 African countries. In 2010, the number had increased to 172,824. Over 95% of measles deaths occur in poor countries with limited health infrastructure (2).

ETIOLOGY AND PATHOPHYSIOLOGY

Measles virus enters through the respiratory mucosa and replicates locally. It then spreads to regional lymphatic tissues and other reticuloendothelial sites via the bloodstream.

- Measles virus is a spherical, enveloped, nonsegmented, single-stranded, negative-sense RNA virus of genus *Morbillivirus*, family *Paramyxoviridae*.
- Humans are the only natural host.

RISK FACTORS

- For developing measles:
  - Lack of adequate vaccination (2-dose)
  - Travel to countries where measles is endemic
  - Contact with exposed individuals, travelers, or immigrants
- For severe measles or measles complications:
  - Immunodeficiency
  - Malnutrition
  - Pregnancy
  - Vitamin A deficiency
  - Age <5 years or >20 years

GENERAL PREVENTION

- 100% preventable with proper vaccination (3)
- Measles vaccine (active immunization)
  - Vaccine is usually given in combination with mumps and rubella (MMR) or with added varicella (MMR-V; ProQuad)
  - Primary vaccination requires 2 doses (0.05 mL SC)
    - 1st dose given at 12–15 months; 95% develop immunity.
    - 2nd dose given at time of school entry (4–6 years of age) or any time >4 weeks after 1st measles vaccine; the 5% of initial nonresponders almost always develop immunity after second dose.
    - Health care workers should have immunity verified and if not immune receive the vaccine if not contraindicated.
  - Common adverse reactions
    - Fever
    - Febrile seizures are rare (<5%) and occur 6–12 days after vaccination. Risk of febrile seizures increases if immunization is delayed (4)[B].
    - Transient, mild, measles-like rash 7–10 days after vaccination (2%, with decreasing incidence during 2nd vaccination)
    - If hypersensitivity reaction occurs, test for immunity; if immune, 2nd dose not needed
    - There is no substantiated link between MMR vaccine and autism (5)[A].
  - Contraindications
    - Live viral vaccines contraindicated in immunosuppressed patients. For MMR, however, HIV-infected children should be vaccinated if asymptomatic and with adequate CD4 count.
    - Pregnancy: Live vaccine is contraindicated (theoretical risk of fetal infection).
    - Anaphylactic reaction to gelatin or neomycin; consult allergist before vaccination
    - Egg anaphylaxis is not considered a contraindication.

COMMONLY ASSOCIATED CONDITIONS

- Immunosuppression
- Malnutrition

DIAGNOSIS

HISTORY

- Prodromal period: usually 2–3 days before rash (may be up to 8 days)
  - Fever
    - Begins 8–12 days after exposure; persists until 2–3 days after onset of rash
    - Temperature often >102°F (39–40.5°C); can precipitate febrile seizures
    - Fever onset >3 days after rash suggests complicated course.
  - "3-C" triad: cough, coryza, and conjunctivitis
  - Cough may persist for 2 weeks.
  - Prodromal symptoms typically intensify over 2–4 days, peaking on 1st day of rash before subsiding.
- Loose stools, malaise, irritability, photophobia (from iridocyclitis), sore throat, headache, and abdominal pain

PHYSICAL EXAM

- Koplik spots
  - Pathognomonic of prodromal measles
  - 2–3-mm, gray–white, raised lesions on erythematous base that appear on buccal mucosa
  - Occur ~48 hours before measles exanthem
- Exanthematous rash (characteristic but not pathognomonic)
  - Maculopapular, blanches
  - Begins at ears and hairline and spreads head to toe, reaching hips by day 2
  - Discrete erythematous patches become confluent over time, with greater confluence on upper body than lower body.
  - Clinical improvement usually occurs within 48 hours after appearance of rash.
  - 3–4 days after rash appears, it fades and changes to brown color, followed by fine desquamation.
- Lymphadenopathy and pharyngitis may be seen during exanthematous period.

DIFFERENTIAL DIAGNOSIS

- Drug eruptions
- Rubella
- *Mycoplasma pneumoniae* infection
- Infectious mononucleosis
- Parvovirus B19 infection
- Roseola
- Enteroviruses
- Rocky Mountain spotted fever
- Dengue
- Toxic shock syndrome
- Meningococcemia
- Kawasaki disease

DIAGNOSTIC TESTS & INTERPRETATION

Initial Tests (lab, imaging)

- Obtain serum sample and throat (or nasopharyngeal) swab. Molecular testing of serum and respiratory specimens is most accurate means for confirming measles infection. IgM assay and measles RNA by real-time polymerase chain reaction (RT-PCR)
- Measles virus–specific IgM assay from serum and saliva may be undetectable on 1st day of exanthema but usually detectable by day 3.
  - Sensitivity: 77% within 72 hours of rash onset; 100% 4–11 days after rash onset. If negative but rash lasts >72 hours, repeat.
  - IgM falls to undetectable levels 4–8 weeks after rash onset.
- Measles virus–specific IgG may be undetectable up to 7 days after exanthem; peaks 14 days after exanthem.
  - An IgG level by standard serologic assay from at least 7 days after rash onset versus a level 14 days later with a 4-fold increase is confirmatory.
- Measles viral cultures are not commonly performed.
- Mild neutropenia is common.
- Liver transaminases and pancreatic amylase may be elevated, particularly in adults.

ALERT

- Suspected measles cases in the United States must be reported to the local or state health department.
- Chest x-ray (CXR) if suspicious for secondary pneumonia.

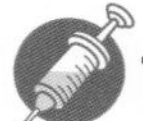

TREATMENT

GENERAL MEASURES

- All patients with measles should be placed in respiratory isolation until 4 days after onset of rash; immunocompromised patients should be isolated for duration of illness.
- Supportive therapy (i.e., antipyretics, antitussives, humidification, increased consumption of oral fluids)

MEDICATION

- No approved antiviral therapy is available. Immunosuppressed children with severe measles have been treated with IV or aerosolized ribavirin, but no controlled trial data exist, and this use is not FDA approved.
- Vitamin A: WHO recommends these daily dosages for 2 consecutive days:
  - Children <6 months of age 50,000 IU
  - Children 6–12 months of age 100,000 IU
  - Children >12 months of age 200,000 IU
- Antibiotics
  - Reserved for patients with clinical signs of bacterial superinfection (pneumonia; purulent otitis; pharyngitis/tonsillitis) (6)
  - A small randomized, double-blinded trial resulted in an 80% (number needed to treat [NNT] = 7) decrease in measles-associated pneumonia with prophylactic antibiotics; consider antibiotic use prophylactically in patients with a high risk of complications (7)[B].
- Outbreak control
  - *The CDC defines an outbreak of measles as a single case.*
  - Immunize contacts (individuals exposed or at risk of having been exposed) within 72 hours.
    - Monovalent vaccine may be given to infants 6 months–1 year of age, but 2 further doses of vaccine after 12 months must be given for appropriate immunization.
    - Monovalent or combination vaccine may be given to all measles-exposed susceptible individuals where not contraindicated.
    - Individuals who have not been immunized within 72 hours of exposure should be excluded from school, child care, and health care settings (social quarantine) until 2 weeks after onset of rash in last case of measles.
  - Immunoglobulin therapy (passive immunity) may be necessary for the following high-risk individuals exposed to measles for whom vaccine is inappropriate:
    - Children age <1 year (Infants 6–12 months of age may receive MMR vaccine in place of IG if given within 72 hours of exposure)
    - Pregnant women
    - Individuals with severe immunosuppression
    - IM immunoglobulin should be given within 6 days of exposure to measles; CDC recommends 0.25 mL/kg to maximum of 15 mL; immunocompromised individuals receive 0.5 mL/kg to a maximum of 15 mL.

INPATIENT CONSIDERATIONS

Outpatient care is appropriate, except where complications develop (e.g., encephalitis, pneumonia).

ONGOING CARE

FOLLOW-UP RECOMMENDATIONS

Signs of complications needing close follow-up include the following:

- Difficulty breathing or noisy breathing
- Changes in vision
- Changes in behavior, confusion
- Chest or abdominal pain

PATIENT EDUCATION

- Emphasize adherence to recommended immunization schedules.
- Avoid exposure to other individuals, particularly unimmunized children and adults, pregnant women, and immunocompromised persons, until 4 days after rash onset.
- Avoid contact with potential sources of secondary bacterial pathogens until respiratory symptoms resolve.
- Centers for Disease Control and Prevention. Measles. www.cdc.gov/measles/about/index.html

PROGNOSIS

- Typically self-limited; prognosis good
- High fatality rates may be seen among malnourished or immunocompromised children, particularly in developing countries.

COMPLICATIONS

- Otitis media (5–15%)
- The immune response to measles infection paradoxically depresses response to non-measles-virus antigens, which renders individuals more susceptible to pneumonia and diarrhea.
- Respiratory complications:
  - Bronchopneumonia (5–10%)
    - Accounts for most measles-related deaths
    - May be viral or bacterial
  - Interstitial pneumonitis: in immunocompromised patients
  - Laryngotracheobronchitis ("measles croup"): occurs in younger age group (<2 years)
- GI complications: diarrhea (may lead to dehydration)
- Neurologic complications
  - Febrile seizures
  - Acute disseminated encephalomyelitis with seizures and variety of neurologic abnormalities (occurs in 1/1,000 cases): presents within 2 weeks of rash, probably an autoimmune response
  - Inclusion body encephalitis is a rare but fatal complication in persons with defective cellular immunity.
  - Subacute sclerosing panencephalitis
    - Rare degenerative CNS disease resulting from persistent measles infection following natural disease, usually fatal
    - Presents 5–15 years after infection
    - Most often in persons infected before age 2 years
- Ocular complications
  - Keratitis
    - Can lead to permanent scarring, blindness
    - Vitamin A deficiency predisposes to more severe keratitis and its complications
- Other secondary bacterial infections
- Death: Results from complications, mainly pneumonia, rather than the virus itself. CDC statistics show that for every 1,000 children who get measles, 1 or 2 will die.

REFERENCES

1. Lessler J, Reich NG, Brookmeyer R, et al. Incubation periods of acute respiratory viral infections: a systematic review. *Lancet Infect Dis*. 2009;9(5):291–300.
2. Moss W, Griffin D. Measles. *Lancet*. 2012;379(9811):153–164.
3. Althouse BM, Bergstrom TC, Bergstrom CT, et al. Evolution in health and medicine Sackler colloquium: a public choice framework for controlling transmissible and evolving diseases. *Proc Natl Acad Sci U S A*. 2010;107(Suppl 1):1696–1701.
4. Rowhani-Rahbar A, Fireman B, Lewis E, et al. Effect of age on the risk of fever and seizures following immunization with measles-containing vaccines in children. *JAMA Pediatr*. 2013;167(12):1111–1117.
5. Demicheli V, Jefferson T, Rivetti A, et al. Vaccines for measles, mumps and rubella in children. *Cochrane Database Syst Rev*. 2005;(4):CD004407.
6. Kabra SK, Lodha R. Antibiotics for preventing complications in children with measles. *Cochrane Database Syst Rev*. 2013;8:CD001477.
7. Garly ML, Balé C, Martins CL, et al. Prophylactic antibiotics to prevent pneumonia and other complications after measles: community based randomised double blind placebo controlled trial in Guinea-Bissau. *BMJ*. 2006;333(7581):1245.

ADDITIONAL READING

- Mulholland EK, Griffiths UK, Biellik R. Measles in the 21st Century. *N Engl J Med*. 2012;366(19):1755–1756.
- Papania MJ, Wallace GS, Rota PA, et al. Elimination of endemic measles, rubella, and congenital rubella syndrome from the western hemisphere: the US experience. *JAMA Pediatr*. 2014;168(2):148–155.

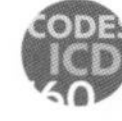

CODES

ICD10

- B05.9 Measles without complication
- B05.2 Measles complicated by pneumonia
- B05.89 Other measles complications

CLINICAL PEARLS

- Measles is a highly communicable viral disease whose natural transmission has been halted in the United States by mass immunization.
- Immunization requires 2 doses: 1 at 12–15 months of age and 1 at school age (4–6 years of age).
- Presentation includes a prodrome of fever, cough, coryza, and conjunctivitis, followed by a descending maculopapular rash beginning on the face and progressing to the chest and lower body (centrifugal).
- Consider measles in the differential diagnosis of a febrile rash illness (especially in unvaccinated individuals with recent international travel).
- Suspected measles cases must be reported to state or local health departments and measures taken to contain outbreak.
- Measles-associated pneumonia is the most common cause of mortality.

MEASLES, GERMAN (RUBELLA)

Ekaterina Brodski-Quigley, MD, EdM

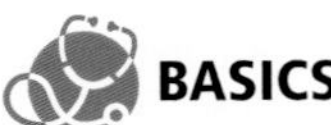

BASICS

DESCRIPTION

- Rubella is a mild, generally self-limited exanthematous viral infection of children and adults, with rare complications. Nonimmune women who become infected with rubella while pregnant may have devastating fetal effects. Up to 50% of rubella infections may be asymptomatic (1,2)[A].
- System(s) affected: hematologic; nervous; pulmonary; exocrine; ophthalmologic; skeletal
- Synonym(s): German measles; 3-day measles

Pregnancy Considerations

- Pregnancy-associated rubella infection may lead to congenital rubella syndrome (CRS) with potentially devastating fetal outcomes.
- CRS is present in up to 90% of fetuses exposed during the 1st trimester (2)[A].
- Screening pregnant women for rubella immunity and vaccinating nonimmune women is the most effective means to prevent CRS (2)[A].
- Although no case of vaccine-associated CRS has been reported, women should not become pregnant for 28 days after vaccination because the vaccine-type virus can cross the placenta (2)[A].
- Polymerase chain reaction (PCR) detection of viral RNA in amniotic fluid and fetal blood sampling allow for rapid diagnosis of fetal infection after 15 weeks' gestation (3)[B].

EPIDEMIOLOGY

- 50–70-nm RNA togavirus of genus *Rubivirus* (1)[A]
- 13 genotypes have been identified (4)[A].
- Live attenuated vaccine (LAV) available in United States since 1969
- Since 2004, all cases of rubella in United States have been imported, typically in travelers with inadequate immunity (1)[A].
- Average incubation: 14 days; range 12–23 days
- Infectious period between 7 days before and 5–7 days after rash onset
- Transmitted by respiratory droplets
- Most common in late winter and early spring
- Humans are only natural hosts (1)[A].

Incidence

- U.S. incidence: <10/100,000 since 2001
- 5 cases were reported in the United States in 2010.
- Still occurs worldwide in developing countries: 100,000 cases of CRS annually worldwide

ETIOLOGY AND PATHOPHYSIOLOGY

- Virus invades the respiratory epithelium, replicates in nasopharynx and regional lymph nodes and spreads hematogenously. Infected patients shed virus from the nasopharynx 3–8 days after inoculation. Shedding lasts 7 or more days after onset of rash.
- Disease progresses from a prodromal stage (1–5 days) to lymphadenopathy (5–10 days) and finally to an exanthematous, pruritic, and maculopapular rash. Rash starts on the face and spreads to the trunk and extremities, sparing the palms and soles (14–17 days after onset of initial symptoms).
- Rubella first described by German scientists in the mid-18th century as a variant form of measles or scarlet fever
- Given the name rubella in 1866
- 1962–1965: global pandemic resulting in an estimated 12.5 million cases in the United States, with 2,000 cases of encephalitis, 11,250 cases of therapeutic or spontaneous abortions, 2,100 neonatal deaths, and 20,000 infants born with CRS (1)[A]
- LAV licensed in the United States in 1969 primarily to prevent CRS

Genetics

Children with CRS and children with type 1 diabetes mellitus (DM) share a high frequency of HLA-DR3 histocompatibility Ag and a high prevalence of islet cell Ab.

RISK FACTORS

Inadequate immunization, inadequate immunity after prior vaccination, immunodeficiency states, immunosuppressive therapy, crowded living/working conditions, international travel (1)[A]

GENERAL PREVENTION

- Vaccination is the most effective preventive strategy.
- Available combined with measles and mumps (MMR) or with varicella (MMR-V). Single rubella vaccine is not available in the United States.
  - A 2-dose schedule combined MMR vaccine recommended for those born after 1957. The 1st dose recommended at ages 12–15 months; 2nd dose recommended either at 4–6 years or at 11–12 years of age. Children with HIV should receive MMR vaccine at 12 months of age if no contraindications exist. In the event of an outbreak, immediate vaccination for infants 6–11 months old is recommended (2)[A].
  - Vaccine is recommended for nonimmune people in the following groups: prepubertal boys and girls, all women of reproductive age, college students, daycare personnel, health care workers, and military personnel.
- Contraindicated: pregnancy, immunodeficiency (except HIV infection), within 3 months of IVIG or blood administration, severe febrile illness, or hypersensitivity to vaccine components. Patients who receive rubella vaccine do not transmit rubella to others, although the virus can be isolated from the pharynx. Breastfeeding is not a contraindication to vaccination (1)[A].
- During outbreaks, serologic screening before vaccination is *NOT* recommended because rapid mass vaccination is necessary to stop disease spread (2)[A].
- The MMR vaccine *is not associated with autism* (5)[A],(6)[B].
- Children who receive the MMR-V vaccine have a 2-fold increase in risk of febrile seizures compared with those who receive MMR and varicella vaccines separately (6)[B].
- Routine rubella antibody screening is recommended during pregnancy by the CDC and ACOG (5)[A].

DIAGNOSIS

Counsel of State and Territorial Epidemiologists (CSTE) Case Definition Classifications of Rubella (1)[A]

- Clinical case definition
  - Acute onset of pink, coalescent macules on the face that spreads to the trunk and extremities, becoming discrete macules; fading in previously affected areas
  - Temperature >99°F (37.2°C), if measured
  - Arthralgia or arthritis, lymphadenopathy, or conjunctivitis
- Laboratory criteria for diagnosis
  - Isolation of virus from throat or nasopharynx, serum, CSF, urine, or cataracts (postmortem)
  - 4-fold rise in acute- and convalescent-phase titers of serum IgG Ab
  - Positive serologic test for IgM Ab
  - PCR positive for virus

HISTORY

- Most cases of postnatal rubella are due to inadequately immunized travelers returning from endemic areas.
- Rubella can spread quickly among persons residing in close quarters.
- Postnatal rubella: low-grade fever, sore throat, nausea, anorexia, arthritis, arthralgia, malaise. 50% may be asymptomatic.
- CRS: parental concerns about hearing or vision impairment, jaundice, or developmental delay
- Deafness could be the only manifestation and not be noticed until 2nd year of life (2)[A].

PHYSICAL EXAM

- Postnatal rubella: low-grade fever, lymphadenopathy (posterior auricular, occipital, posterior cervical), exanthem (mild, pink, discrete 1–4-mm maculopapular rash), soft palate petechiae (Forchheimer sign) (20%) (1)[A]
- CRS: microcephaly, large anterior fontanelle, sensorineural hearing loss (58%), cataracts, glaucoma, microphthalmia, pigmentary retinopathy, purpuric ("blueberry muffin") skin lesions, murmur (50%) consistent with patent ductus arteriosus (PDA), hepatosplenomegaly, jaundice, cryptorchidism, inguinal hernia, radiolucent bone disease (2)[A]

DIFFERENTIAL DIAGNOSIS

- Postnatal rubella
  - Measles virus (rubeola)
  - Scarlet fever (strep A)
  - Infectious mononucleosis
  - Erythema infectiosum (parvovirus B19)
  - Roseola infantum (i.e., exanthem subitum)
  - Toxoplasmosis
  - Drug eruptions
  - Other exanthematous enteroviral infections
- Congenital rubella
  - Measles
  - Parvovirus B19
  - Human herpesvirus 6
  - Other exanthematous entero- or arboviruses

DIAGNOSTIC TESTS & INTERPRETATION

- Because 50% of cases are subclinical, laboratory testing is the best way to confirm the diagnosis (1,2)[A].
- Detection of wild-type virus is the gold standard (1)[A].
- Enzyme immunoassay (EIA): preferred testing for IgM antibodies, which may not be detectable before 5 days after the onset of rash (1)[A]
- Hemagglutination inhibition (HAI) test: A 4-fold increase of IgG Ab levels from acute to convalescent phase is diagnostic for recent infection (1)[A].
- Latex agglutination (LA) test: sensitive and specific but dependent on experience of lab personnel (1)[A]

- Immunofluorescent antibody (IFA) assay: used for detection of viral IgG and IgM Ab (1)[A]
- Avidity test: not routine and should only be performed in reference labs. Used to distinguish between recent and past infections (1)[A]
- Serum collection should be performed within 7–10 days after the onset of the illness. When testing for IgM, repeat collection may be necessary if the sample was taken before day 5. When testing for seroconversion, a 2nd sample for IgG testing should be collected 2–3 weeks after the 1st specimen (acute to convalescent phase). In most cases, IgG is detectable 8 days after rash onset (1)[A].
- Virus may be isolated from 1 week prior to 2 weeks after the onset of rash. Maximal viral shedding occurs up to day 4 after rash onset. Best results are from throat swabs (1)[A].
- Epidemiologically, viral genotyping by reverse transcription (RT)-PCR helps determine the country of origin. Throat swabs should be collected 4 days after the rash onset and sent directly to the CDC (1)[A].
- Viral cultures of CSF are reserved for suspected cases of CRS or rubella encephalitis (1)[A].
- If a pregnant female is exposed, amniotic fluid PCR or fetal blood sampling may be done at 15 weeks' gestation for viral detection. Placental biopsy (less common) may be done at 12 weeks' gestation. If positive, parents should be offered genetic counseling (1)[A].
- As the incidence of rubella decreases, the positive predictive value (PPV) of IgM results decreases. False-positive findings occur in patients with parvovirus B19, mononucleosis, and positive rheumatoid factor (1)[A].
- After reexposure, a person with a low level of Ab from past infection or prior vaccination may experience an acute, small rise in Ab levels. This is not associated with a high incidence of contagion to others or of fetal risk (1)[A].

Follow-Up Tests & Special Considerations

- Reporting: state-dependent. Samples should be sent to the CDC for genotyping. Cases of CRS are reported to the National Congenital Rubella Syndrome Registry (1,2)[A].
- Infants with CRS may shed virus up to 1 year. Observe contact isolation during all hospitalizations until child turns 1 year old (unless child has 2 negative throat cultures and urine specimens a month apart after 3 months of age) (2)[A].

TREATMENT

- Supportive for mild cases
- Isolate patients for 5–7 days after rash onset.
- Postnatal rubella: mild and self-limited; treat symptomatically. Hospitalize for complications: idiopathic thrombocytopenic purpura (ITP) or encephalitis (1)[A].
- CRS: supportive care unless neurologic or hemorrhagic complications develop; phototherapy may be indicated for jaundice; multidisciplinary management of long-term complications (2)[A]

MEDICATION

No specific therapy available for mild cases.

First Line

- Age- and dose-appropriate antipyretics
- NSAIDs can be used for arthritis and arthralgias in adults and infants age >6 months.
- IVIG can be given for severe thrombocytopenia—most cases, however, are self-limited.

ONGOING CARE

FOLLOW-UP RECOMMENDATIONS

Patient Monitoring

- Individuals immune to rubella through natural infection or vaccine may be reinfected when reexposed; such infection is usually asymptomatic and detectable only by serology. Those who have received the vaccine have lower measurable IgG levels than those who had the natural disease.
- In CRS, it is important to detect auditory and visual impairment early (2)[A].
- 2/3 of internationally adopted children have no written record of immunizations (4)[A].

PATIENT EDUCATION

- www.cdc.gov/rubella/
- www.nlm.nih.gov/medlineplus/ency/article/001574.htm
- http://www.who.int/mediacentre/factsheets/fs367/en/

PROGNOSIS

- Postnatal rubella: Complete and full recovery without sequelae is typical.
- CRS
  - Varied and unpredictable spectrum, ranging from stillbirth to normal infancy/childhood (1,2)[A]
  - Detectable levels of IgG persist for years and then may decline (does not drop at the expected 2-fold dilution/month). By age 5 years, 20% have no detectable antibody (2)[A].
  - IgM may not be detectable until 1 month after birth and may persist for 6–12 months (2)[A].
  - Overall mortality (up to 10%) is greatest during first 6 months.
  - 70% of encephalitis cases develop residual neurologic defects, including autistic syndrome.
  - Prognosis is excellent if only minor congenital defects are present.

COMPLICATIONS

- Postinfectious encephalitis (1/5,000 cases)
- Thrombocytopenic purpura (1/3,000 cases)
- CRS: incidence dependent on trimester exposed
- Rubella vaccine may rarely cause encephalitis or ITP.
  - ITP is self-limited and is not a contraindication to vaccination.

REFERENCES

1. Centers for Disease Control and Prevention. Chapter 14—rubella. In: McLean H, Redd S, Abernathy E, et al, eds. *Manual for the Surveillance of Vaccine-Preventable Diseases*. 5th ed. Atlanta, GA: Center for Disease Control and Prevention; 2014. www.cdc.gov/vaccines/pubs/surv-manual/chpt14-rubella.html. Accessed 2014.
2. Centers for Disease Control and Prevention. Chapter 15—congenital rubella syndrome. In: McLean H, Redd S, Abernathy E, et al, eds. *Manual for Surveillance of Vaccine-Preventable Diseases*. 5th ed. Atlanta, GA: Center for Disease Control and Prevention; 2014. www.cdc.gov/vaccines/pubs/surv-manual/chpt15-crs.html. Accessed 2014.
3. Tang J, Aarons E, Hesketh L, et al. Prenatal diagnosis of congenital rubella infection in the second trimester of pregnancy. *Prenat Diagn*. 2003;23(6):509–512.
4. Abernathy E, Hubschen J, Muller C, et al. Status of global virologic surveillance for rubella viruses. *J Infect Dis*. 2011;204(Suppl 1):S524–S532.
5. McLean HQ, Fiebelkorn AP, Temte JL, et al; Centers for Disease Control and Prevention. Prevention of measles, rubella, congenital rubella syndrome, and mumps, 2013: summary recommendations of the Advisory Committee on Immunization Practices (ACIP). *MMWR Recomm Rep*. 2013;62(RR-04):1–34.
6. Lai J, Fay K, Bocchini J. Update on childhood and adolescent immunizations: selected review of US recommendations and literature: part 2. *Curr Opin Pediatr*. 2011;23(4):470–481.

ADDITIONAL READING

- Centers for Disease Control and Prevention. Rubella. In: Atkinson W, Wolfe C, Hamborsky J, eds. *Epidemiology and Prevention of Vaccine-Preventable Diseases*. 12th ed. Atlanta, GA: Centers for Disease Control and Prevention; 2012. www.cdc.gov/vaccines/pubs/pinkbook/rubella.html. Accessed 2014.
- Mongua-Rodriguez N, Díaz-Ortega JL, García-García L, et al. A systematic review of rubella vaccination strategies implemented in the Americas: impact on the incidence and seroprevalence rates of rubella and congenital rubella syndrome. *Vaccine*. 2013;31(17):2145–2151.
- Walling A. Measles, mumps, and rubella in pregnant women. *Am Fam Physician*. 2006;73(5):907–908.

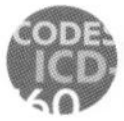

CODES

ICD10

- B06.9 Rubella without complication
- B06.00 Rubella with neurological complication, unspecified
- P35.0 Congenital rubella syndrome

CLINICAL PEARLS

- Rubella is typically a self-limited viral exanthematous infection of children and adults.
- Nonimmune women who are infected with rubella while pregnant may have devastating fetal effects.

M

MEDIAL TIBIAL STRESS SYNDROME (MTSS)/SHIN SPLINTS

Michael Y. Yang, MD • Marc W. McKenna, MD

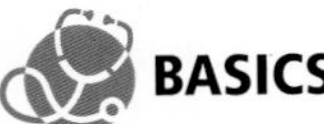

BASICS

DESCRIPTION

- Medial tibial stress syndrome (MTSS) is more commonly known as "shin splints." Aching pain along the inner edge of the tibial shaft, which develops when the muscle attachments to the periosteum in the (lower) leg become irritated by repetitive activity. The condition is part of a continuum of stress-related injuries to the lower leg. MTSS does not encompass pain from ischemia (compartment syndrome) or stress fractures.
- Tendonitis/periostitis of the medial soleus muscles, anterior tibialis, and posterior tibialis muscles
- Synonyms: tibial stress reaction; anterior muscle syndrome; periostitis; perimyositis

EPIDEMIOLOGY

Incidence

Common, can account for between 5 and 32% of running injuries. Frequently occurs bilaterally.

Pediatric Considerations

Shin splints may account for up to 31% of all overuse injuries in high school athletes (1).

ETIOLOGY AND PATHOPHYSIOLOGY

- Multifactorial involving anatomic and biomechanical factors
  - Overuse injuries causing or limited by
    - Microtrauma from repetitive motion leading to periosteal inflammation
    - Overpronation of the subtalar joint and tight gastrocnemius/soleus complex with increased eccentric loading of musculature inserting along medial shin
    - Interosseous membrane pain
    - Periostitis
    - Tears of collagen fibers
    - Enthesopathy
  - Anatomic structures affected include the following:
    - Flexor hallucis longus
    - Tibialis anterior
    - Tibialis posterior
    - Soleus
    - Crural fascia
- Pathogenesis: theorized to be due to persistent repetitive loading, which leads to inadequate bone remodeling and possible microfissures causing pain without evidence of fracture or ischemia

RISK FACTORS:

- Intrinsic or personal risk factors
  - Greater internal and external ranges (>65 degrees) of hip motion
  - Significant over pronation at the ankle
  - Female gender
  - Leaner calf girth
  - Femoral neck anteversion
  - Genu varus
- External or environmental factors:
  - Lack of physical fitness
  - Inexperienced runners—particularly those with rapid increases in mileage and inadequate prior conditioning
  - Excessive overuse or distance running, particularly on hard or inclined surface
  - Prior injury
  - Equipment (shoe) failure
- Other risk factors:
  - Elevated BMI
  - Lower bone mineral density
  - Tobacco use
- Population affected typically include the following:
  - Runners
  - Military personnel—common in recruit/boot camp
  - Gymnasts, soccer, and basketball players
  - Ballet dancers

GENERAL PREVENTION

- Proper technique for guided calf stretching and lower extremity strength training
- Rehabilitation for prior injuries
- Other suggested but unproven recommendations include the following:
  - Foot mechanical analysis and gait training for over pronation
  - Orthotic footwear use.

COMMONLY ASSOCIATED CONDITIONS

- Stress fractures and compartment syndrome are important to exclude.
- Pes planus (flat feet)

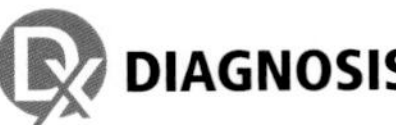

DIAGNOSIS

HISTORY

- Patients typically describe dull, sharp, or deep along the lower leg that is resolved with rest.
- Patients are often able to run through the pain in early stages.
- Pain is commonly associated with exercise (also true with compartment syndrome), but in severe cases, pain may persist with rest.

PHYSICAL EXAM

- Tenderness to palpation is typically elicited along the posteromedial border of the middle-to-distal third of the tibia.
- Pain with plantar flexion.
- Ensure neurovascular integrity of the lower extremity, examining distal pulses, sensation, reflexes, and muscular strength.

DIFFERENTIAL DIAGNOSIS

- Bone
  - Tibial stress fractures
    - Typically, pain persists at rest or with weight bearing activities.
    - Focal tenderness on exam over the anterior tibial surface
- Muscle/soft tissue injury
  - Strain
  - Tear
  - Tendinopathy
  - Muscle hernia
- Fascial
  - Chronic exertional compartment syndrome (2)[C]
    - Complaints of pain without direct tenderness elicited on exam
    - History of increasing pain with exertion but resolution at rest
    - Pain is described as cramping or squeezing pain with possible weakness or paresthesias on exam.
  - Interosseous membrane tear
- Nerve
  - Spinal stenosis
  - Lumbar radiculopathy
  - Common peroneal nerve entrapment with tight fitting clothes
- Vascular
  - DVT
  - Popliteal arterial entrapment (3)[B]
    - Rare but limb-threatening disease
    - History of intermittent unilateral claudication in lower limb
    - Diagnosis with MRI reveals compression of the artery by the medial head of the gastrocnemius muscle.
- Infection
  - Osteomyelitis
- Malignancy
  - Bone tumors

DIAGNOSTIC TESTS & INTERPRETATION

- Plain radiographs help rule out stress fractures if >2 weeks of symptoms (4).
- Bone scintigraphy
  - Diffuse linear vertical uptake in the posterior tibial cortex on the lateral view.
  - Stress fractures demonstrate a focal ovoid uptake.
- High-resolution MRI reveal abnormal periosteal and bone marrow signals, which are useful for early discrimination of tibial stress fractures.
- Increased pain and localized tenderness warrants further imaging with MRI due to concern for tibial stress fracture.
- Concern for compartment syndrome should be excluded using intracompartmental pressure testing.

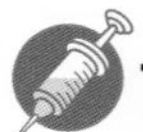

TREATMENT

GENERAL MEASURES

- Activity modification with a gradual return to training based on improvement of symptoms
- Patients should maintain fitness with low-impact activities such as swimming and cycling.
- Continue activity modification until patients are pain-free on ambulation.
- Good supportive footwear is recommended.

MEDICATION

- Analgesia with acetaminophen or other oral nonsteroidal anti-inflammatory agent
- Cryotherapy (ice massage) is also advised to relieve acute-phase symptoms (5)[C].

ADDITIONAL THERAPIES

- Stretching of the gastrocnemius, soleus, and peroneal muscles are treatment mainstays (5)[C].
- Calf stretch, peroneal stretch, TheraBand exercises, and eccentric calf raises may improve endurance and strength.
- Structured running programs with warm up exercises have not been demonstrated to reduce pain in young athletes (6)[B].

SURGERY/OTHER PROCEDURES

- Surgical intervention includes a posterior medial fascial release in individuals with both
  - Severe limitation of physical activity
  - Failure of 6 months of conservative treatment
    - Patient should be counseled that complete return of activity to sport may not be always achieved postoperatively with risks including infection, hematoma, and stress fractures.
- Extracorporeal shock wave therapy (ESWT) may decrease recovery time when added to a running program (7)[B].

COMPLEMENTARY & ALTERNATIVE THERAPIES

- Individualized polyurethane orthoses may be an effective conservative therapy for chronic running injuries (8)[A].
- Special insoles, shock absorbing running shoes, and knee braces have not been shown to decrease the incidence of shin splints (5)[C].
- Ultrasound, acupuncture, aquatic therapy, electrical stimulation, whirlpool baths, cast immobilization, taping, and steroid injection may help improve pain.

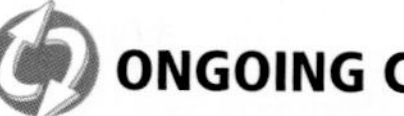

ONGOING CARE

FOLLOW-UP RECOMMENDATIONS

Patient Monitoring

- Patient should be advised against prematurely resuming preinjury pace.
- Stretching and strengthening exercises should be added.
- Preinjury training errors should be identified and a gradual return to activity should be recommended.

PROGNOSIS

The condition is usually self-limiting and most patient respond well with rest and nonsurgical intervention.

COMPLICATIONS

- Stress fractures and compartment syndrome
- Undiagnosed MTSS or chronic exertional compartment syndrome can lead to a complete fracture or tissue necrosis, respectively.

REFERENCES

1. Cuff S, Loud K, O'Riodan MA. Overuse injuries in high school athletes. *Clin Pediatr*. 2010;49(8):731–736.
2. Hutchinson M. Chronic exertional compartment syndrome. *Br J Sports Med*. 2011;45(12):952–953.
3. Politano AD, Bhamidipati CM, Tracci MC, et al. Anatomic popliteal entrapment syndrome is often a difficult diagnosis. *Vasc Endovascular Surg*. 2012;46(7):542–545.
4. Chang GH, Paz DA, Dwek JR, et al. Lower extremity overuse injuries in pediatric athletes: clinical presentation, imaging findings, and treatment. *Clin Imaging*. 2013;37(5):836–846.
5. Fields KB, Sykes JC, Walker KM, et al. Prevention of running injuries. *Curr Sports Med Rep*. 2010;9(3):176–182.
6. Moen MH, Holtslag L, Bakker E, et al. The treatment of medial tibial stress syndrome in athletes; a randomized clinical trial. *Sports Med Arthrosc Rehabil Ther Technol*. 2012;4:12.
7. Moen MH, Rayer S, Schipper M, et al. Shockwave treatment for medial tibial stress syndrome in athletes; a prospective controlled study. *Br J Sports Med*. 2012;46(4):253–257.
8. Hirschmüller A, Baur H, Müller S, et al. Clinical effectiveness of customised sport shoe orthoses for overuse injuries in runners: a randomised controlled study. *Br J Sports Med*. 2011;45(12):959–965.

ADDITIONAL READING

- Cosca DD, Navazio F. Common problems in endurance athletes. *Am Fam Physician*. 2007;76(2):237–244.
- Newman P, Witchalls J, Waddington G, et al. Risk factors associated with medial tibial stress syndrome in runners: a systematic review and meta-analysis. *Open Access J Sports Med*. 2013;4:229–241.
- The Tibalis Anterior Stretch—Kinetic Health: http://youtube/6Z6XM63x2TM. June 19, 2014.

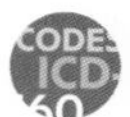

CODES

ICD10

- S86.899A Other injury of other muscle(s) and tendon(s) at lower leg level, unspecified leg, initial encounter
- S86.891A Other injury of other muscle(s) and tendon(s) at lower leg level, right leg, initial encounter
- S86.892A Other injury of other muscle(s) and tendon(s) at lower leg level, left leg, initial encounter

CLINICAL PEARLS

- Medial tibial stress syndrome is the preferred term for "shin splints."
- Diagnosis is based on the history of repetitive overuse.
- Pain that is worsened with activity and relieved with rest is commonly described along the middle and distal third of the posteromedial tibial surface.
- Treatment includes ice, activity modification, analgesics, eccentric stretching, and a gradual return to activity.

MELANOMA

Carl Bryce, MD • Matthew Snyder, DO

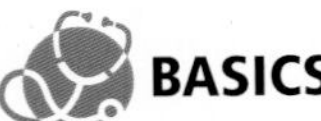 BASICS

DESCRIPTION

- Melanoma is a tumor arising from malignant transformation of cells from the melanocytic system.
  - Most arise in the skin but may also present as a primary lesion in any tissue: ocular, GI, GU, lymph node, and leptomeninges.
  - Metastatic spread to any site in body
- Main types of cutaneous melanoma include the following (1):
  - Superficial spreading melanoma: 50–80% cases; occurs in sun-exposed areas (trunk, back, and extremities); most ~6 mm diameter at diagnosis; when seen in younger patients, presents as a flat, slow growing, irregularly bordered lesion
  - Nodular: 20–30%, present in older patients, often ulcerate and hemorrhage, most commonly thick and pigmented
  - Lentigo maligna (subtype of melanoma in situ) slowest growing; older population; occurs in sun-exposed areas (head, neck, forearms). Lentigo maligna melanoma (LMM) is its invasive counterpart.
  - Amelanotic melanoma (<5%): can be missed and diagnosed at a later stage, as it can mimic benign skin conditions
  - Acral-lentiginous: 2–8% of all melanomas; however, most common melanoma in black or Asian patients, found in palmar, plantar, and subungual areas.
  - Subungual melanoma (0.7–3.5%): dark longitudinal band in nail bed; Hutchinson sign when proximal nail fold involved
  - Desmoplastic melanoma (~1%): sarcoma-like tendencies with increased hematogenous spread
- System(s) affected: skin/exocrine

Geriatric Considerations

Lentigo maligna, slowly enlarging pigmented lesion, is most common in elderly patients. This type is usually found on face, beginning as a circumscribed macular patch of mottled pigmentation showing shades of dark brown, tan, or black.

Pediatric Considerations

Large congenital nevi (>5 cm) are risk factors and have a >2% lifetime risk of malignant conversion. Blistering sunburns in childhood significantly increase risk.

Pregnancy Considerations

No increased risk of melanoma in pregnancy. However, it is suggested waiting 1–2 years if further pregnancy desired in case of recent melanoma. Melanomas can spread to the placenta.

EPIDEMIOLOGY

Incidence

- In 2014, an estimated 76,100 Americans were diagnosed with melanoma, with 9,710 expected deaths (2).
- Predominant age: median age: 62 and 54 years for men and women respectively, >50% of all individuals with melanoma are between 20 and 40 years of age.
- Predominant sex: male > female (1.5×)
- Incidence among whites greater than that among minority groups; ~20× higher than blacks (1)
- Minority groups demonstrate increased rates of metastasis, advanced stages at diagnosis, thicker initial lesions, earlier age at diagnosis, and overall poorer outcomes.
- Low socioeconomic status associated with higher incidence of melanoma

Prevalence

- Lifetime risk: men: 1/37; female: 1/56
- 2% of all cancer deaths
- The most common cancer affecting women age 25–29 years of age and second only to breast cancer in women 30–34 years of age (1).

ETIOLOGY AND PATHOPHYSIOLOGY

- DNA damage by UV-A/UV-B exposure
- Tumor progression: initially may be confined to epidermis with lateral growth, may then grow into dermis with vertical growth

Genetics

- Dysplastic nevus syndrome is a risk factor for development of melanoma. Close surveillance warranted.
- 8–12% of patients with melanoma have a family history of disease.
- Mutation in *CDKN2A (p16)* is found in 1/3 of patients with family incidence of melanoma.
- Mutations in *BRAF (V600E)* implicated in 50–60% of cutaneous melanomas
- Additional susceptibility genes include *NRAS, CKIT, GNAQ/GNA11, BRCA2, MCR1, and OCA1.*

RISK FACTORS

- Genetic predisposition
- UV-A and UV-B exposure
- History of >5 sunburns during lifetime
- History of intense intermittent sun exposure
- Previous pigmented lesions (especially dysplastic melanocytic nevi)
- Fair complexion, freckling, blue eyes, and blond/red hair
- Highest predictor of risk is increased number of nevi (>100).
- Family/personal history of melanoma
- Tanning bed use: 75% increased risk if 1st exposure before age 35 years
- Changing nevus
- Large (>5 cm) congenital nevi
- Other skin cancers
- Chronic immunosuppression (chronic lymphocytic leukemia, non-Hodgkin lymphoma, AIDS, or post-transplant)
- Blistering sunburns in childhood
- Living at high altitude (>700 m or 2,300 ft above sea level)
- Occupational exposure to ionizing radiation
- The HARMM acronym identifies the five most important independent factors for increased likelihood of melanoma. A score of 5 represents high-risk patients versus 0–1 confer a low risk of melanoma.
  - **H**istory of prior melanoma
  - **A**ge older than 50 years
  - Absence of a **R**egular dermatologist
  - A changing **M**ole
  - **M**ale gender

GENERAL PREVENTION

- Avoidance of sunburns, especially in childhood
- Use of sunscreen with at least SPF 30 to all skin exposed to sunlight, reapplying regularly and after toweling or swimming
- Avoid tanning beds; class 1 carcinogen by World Health Organization (WHO)
- Screening of high-risk individuals, especially males older than the age of 50 years
- Education for proper diagnosis plays a large factor in prevention.
- Any suspicious lesions should be biopsied with a narrow excision encompassing the entire breadth plus sufficient depth of the lesion. Options include elliptical excisions, punch, or shave biopsies.

COMMONLY ASSOCIATED CONDITIONS

- Dysplastic nevus syndrome
- >50 nevi. These individuals have higher lifetime risk of melanoma than the general population as 50% of all melanoma arise in preexisting nevi.
- Giant congenital nevus: 6% lifetime incidence of melanoma
- Xeroderma pigmentosum is a rare condition associated with an extremely high risk of skin cancers, including melanoma.
- Psoriasis after psoralen-UV-A (PUVA) therapy

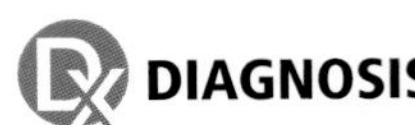 DIAGNOSIS

HISTORY

- Change in a pigmented lesion: either hypo- or hyperpigmentation, bleeding, scaling, ulceration, or changes in size or texture
- Obtain family and personal history of melanoma or nonmelanoma skin cancer.
- Obtain social history on sunbathing, tanning, and other sun exposure.

PHYSICAL EXAM

- ABCDE: **A**symmetry, **B**order irregularity, **C**olor variegation (especially red, white, black, blue), **D**iameter >6 mm, **E**levation above skin surface
- Any new and/or changing nevus, bleeding/ulcerated
- Location on Caucasians is primarily back and lower leg, on African Americans is the hands, feet, and nails
- Individuals at high risk for melanoma should have careful ocular exam to assess for presence of melanoma in the iris and retina.

DIFFERENTIAL DIAGNOSIS

- Dysplastic and blue nevi
- Vascular skin tumor
- Pigmented actinic keratosis
- Traumatic hematoma
- Pigmented squamous cell and basal cell carcinomas, seborrheic keratoses, other changing nevi

DIAGNOSTIC TESTS & INTERPRETATION

- Lactate dehydrogenase (LDH), chest/abdomen/pelvic CT, brain MRI, and/or PET CT at baseline and in monitoring progression in metastatic disease (stage IV) (3)
- Imaging studies only helpful in detecting and evaluating for progression of metastatic disease

Diagnostic Procedures/Other

- Dermoscopy allows for magnification of lesions, allowing for a decreased number of biopsies of benign skin lesions in addition to providing increased sensitivity in detecting melanoma and basal cell carcinoma (4)[B].
- Surgical biopsy remains the standard of care. Any suspicious nevus should be excised, either by elliptical excision; a scoop shave (saucerization) technique may be appropriate, as long as a full-thickness can be achieved (1)[C].
- Sentinel lymph node biopsy discussed in the following texts (3)[A].
- MelaFind is a handheld computerized, point-of-care vision system designed to aid dermatologists in detecting melanoma.

Test Interpretation

- Nodular melanoma is primarily vertical growth, whereas the other 3 types are horizontal.
- Estimated that 1/10,000 dysplastic nevi become melanoma annually.
- Immunohistochemical testing increases sensitivity of lymph node biopsies.
- Staging is based on the tumor-node-metastasis (TNM) criteria by 2010 American Joint Committee on Cancer (AJCC) criteria (3).

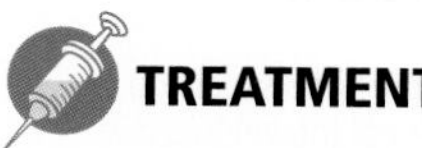

TREATMENT

GENERAL MEASURES

Full surgical excision of melanoma is the standard of care. See below for recommended surgical margins.

MEDICATION

- For stages I–III, surgical excision is curative in most cases; in patients with stage IV disease, systemic treatment with chemotherapy is recommended.
- Preferred regimens (5)[A] include the following:
  - Ipilimumab (Yervoy), monoclonal antibody against CTLA-4, is FDA approved for treatment of advanced melanoma, increased patient survival by 10 months in stage III and IV trials
  - Vemurafenib (Zelboraf), a BRAF inhibitor approved for metastatic, unresectable melanoma expressing BRAFV600E
  - High-dose interleukin-2 (significant toxicity)
  - Referral for enrollment in clinical trials
- Additional active regimens (e.g., dacarbazine [DTIC], temozolomide, paclitaxel, carmustine [BCNU], cisplatin, carboplatin, vinblastine); often limited to those who are not candidates to preferred regimens.
- Imatinib (Gleevec) in tumors with C-KIT mutation
- Interferon-α as adjuvant therapy received FDA approval in 1995 (high dose) and 2011 (pegylated) to treat stage IIB-III melanoma; shown to improve 4-year relapse rate but no overall effect on survival; 1/3 of patients will discontinue due to toxicity (granulocytopenia, hepatotoxicity). Biochemotherapy is advocated by some (i.e., chemo- + immunotherapy combination), although optimal regimen remains uncertain given disease heterogeneity (5)[B].

ISSUES FOR REFERRAL

- Consultation with oncologist for consideration of chemotherapeutic options.
- Plastic surgery sometimes needed after final excision

ADDITIONAL THERAPIES

Immunotherapy using dendritic cell–based vaccinations targeting gp100, tyrosinase, and other antigens have shown promising results in few limited studies (6)[B].

SURGERY/OTHER PROCEDURES

- Standard of care for melanoma includes early surgical excision with the following recommended margins (3)[A]:
  - In situ tumors: 0.5 cm margin has been standard of care but may by insufficient in lentigo maligna (7)[B].
  - Thickness of 1.01–2.00 mm: 1–2 cm margins
  - Thickness of >2.00 mm: 2 cm margins
- Sentinel lymph node biopsy is indicated in patients with T2, T3, and T4 staged melanomas.
  - Selected patients with stage T1b melanoma should also be considered for sentinel lymph node biopsy.
  - Not recommended in melanoma in situ or T1a
- Mohs surgery is often used for lesions with ill-defined borders or lesions of head and neck.
- Radiotherapy can be used to treat lentigo maligna in addition to certain head and neck lesions.
- Palliative radiation therapy can be used with metastatic melanoma.

COMPLEMENTARY & ALTERNATIVE MEDICINE

Molecular and mouse tumor model studies support role of topical silymarin (milk thistle derivative) in decreasing UV radiation–induced inflammation, oxidative stress, and carcinogenesis (7)[B].

INPATIENT CONSIDERATIONS

Admission Criteria/Initial Stabilization

Most surgeries are done as outpatients with no stabilization needed.

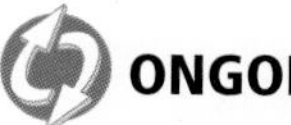

ONGOING CARE

FOLLOW-UP RECOMMENDATIONS

After diagnosis and treatment, close follow-up and skin protection (i.e., sunblock, UV protective clothing) are highly advised.

Patient Monitoring

- Routine screening clinical skin examination annually for all persons older than the age of 40 years is controversial and without proven benefit.
- Total body photography and dermoscopy should be used for surveillance of skin lesions, most commonly used for patients with >5 atypical nevi
- For patients with a history of cutaneous melanoma, specialty guidelines suggest every 3–12 months depending on recurrence risk (3)[C], although a systematic review notes wide variability in this practice (8)[A].
- Lab and imaging tests after diagnosis and treatment of stage I–II melanoma are low yield, have high false-positive rates, and are not recommended (3)[B].

DIET

No data to support specific dietary manipulations; general recommendations from American Cancer Society for cancer prevention

PATIENT EDUCATION

- Teach patients who are at risk, or have had melanoma, the principles of ABCDE examinations.
- High-risk patients should perform monthly skin self-examinations and be taught to examine inaccessible areas.
- Patients with a history of melanoma or dysplastic nevus syndrome should have regular total body examinations.

PROGNOSIS

- Breslow depth (thickness) in millimeters remains among strongest predictors of prognosis.
- Median age at death 68 years
- Highest survival seen in women <45 years of age at diagnosis
- Metastatic melanoma has an average survival of 6–9 months
- Stage I and II, appropriately treated, have 20-year survival rates of 90% and 80%, respectively.

COMPLICATIONS

- Metastatic spread
- Unsatisfactory cosmetic results following the primary surgery

REFERENCES

1. Shenenberger D. Cutaneous malignant melanoma: a primary care perspective. *Am Fam Physician*. 2012; 85(2):161–168.
2. American Cancer Society. What are the key cancer statistics about melanoma skin cancer? http://www.cancer.org/cancer/skincancer-melanoma/detailedguide/melanoma-skin-cancer-key-statistics. Accessed on June 24, 2014.
3. Bichakjian CK, Halpern AC, Johnson TM, et al. Guidelines of care for the management of primary cutaneous melanoma. *J Am Acad Dermatol*. 2011; 65(5):1032–1047.
4. Marghoob AA, Usatine RP, Jaimes N. Dermoscopy for the family physician. *Am Fam Physician*. 2013; 88(7):441–450.
5. Coit DG, Andtbacka R, Anker CJ, et al. Melanoma, version 2.2013: featured updates to the NCCN guidelines. *J Natl Compr Canc Netw*. 2013;11(4): 395–407.
6. Oshita C, Takikawa M, Kume A, et al. Dendritic cell-based vaccination in metastatic melanoma patients: phase II clinical trial. *Oncol Rep*. 2012; 28(4):1131–1138.
7. Erickson C, Miller SJ. Treatment options in melanoma in situ: topical and radiation therapy, excision and Mohs surgery. *Int J Dermatol*. 2010;49(5):482–491.
8. Cromwell K, Ross MI, Xing Y, et al. Variability in melanoma post-treatment surveillance practices by country and physician specialty: a systematic review. *Melanoma Res*. 2012;22(5):1–21.

ADDITIONAL READING

- Markovic SN, Erickson LA, Rao RD, et al. Malignant melanoma in the 21st century, part 1: epidemiology, risk factors, screening, prevention, and diagnosis. *Mayo Clin Proc*. 2007;82(3):364–380.
- Markovic SN, Erickson LA, Rao RD, et al. Malignant melanoma in the 21st century, part 2: staging, prognosis and treatment. *Mayo Clin Proc*. 2007;82(4):490–513.
- MelaFind: www.melasciences.com
- Tuong W, Cheng LS, Armstrong AW, et al. Melanoma: epidemiology, diagnosis, treatment, and outcomes. *Dermatol Clin*. 2012;30(1):113–124, ix.

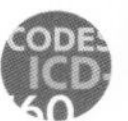

CODES

ICD10

- C43.9 Malignant melanoma of skin, unspecified
- C43.30 Malignant melanoma of unspecified part of face
- C43.4 Malignant melanoma of scalp and neck

CLINICAL PEARLS

- Remember that amelanotic melanomas exist; pigmentation is not required.
- 80% of cutaneous melanomas arise in existing nevi. Any changing nevi should be considered for full-thickness biopsy.
- Excellent prognosis in early detection and treatment, as well as being a common cancer affecting young adult women, require a high clinical suspicion and low threshold for thorough evaluation.

MÉNIÈRE DISEASE

Robert A. Baldor, MD, FAAFP

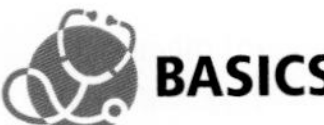

BASICS

DESCRIPTION

- An inner ear (labyrinthine) disorder characterized by recurrent attacks of hearing loss, tinnitus, vertigo, and sensations of aural fullness due to an increase in the volume and pressure of the inner ear endolymph fluid (endolymphatic hydrops)
- Often unilateral initially, nearly half become bilateral over time.
- Severity and frequency of vertigo may diminish with time, but hearing loss is often progressive and/or fluctuating.
- Usually idiopathic (Ménière disease) but may be secondary to another condition causing endolymphatic hydrops (Ménière syndrome)
- System(s) affected: nervous
- Synonym(s): Ménière syndrome; endolymphatic hydrops

EPIDEMIOLOGY

- Predominant age of onset: 40–60 years
- Predominant gender: female > male (1.3:1)
- Race/ethnicity: white, Northern European > blacks

Incidence

Estimates 1–150/100,000 per year

Prevalence

Varies from 7.5 to >200/100,000

ETIOLOGY AND PATHOPHYSIOLOGY

- Not fully understood; theories include increased pressure of the endolymph fluid due to increased fluid production or decreased resorption. This may be caused by endolymphatic sac pathology, abnormal development of the vestibular aqueduct, or inflammation caused by circulating immune complexes. Increased endolymph pressure may cause rupture of membranes and changes in endolymphatic ionic gradient.
- Ménière *syndrome* may be secondary to injury or other disorders (e.g., reduced middle ear pressure, allergy, endocrine disease, lipid disorders, vascular, viral, syphilis, autoimmune). Any disorder that could cause endolymph hydrops could be implicated in Ménière *syndrome*.

Genetics

Some families show increased incidence, but genetic and environmental influences are incompletely understood.

RISK FACTORS

May include

- Stress
- Allergy
- Increased salt intake
- Caffeine, alcohol, or nicotine
- Chronic exposure to loud noise
- Family history of Ménière
- Certain vascular abnormalities (including migraines)
- Certain viral exposures (especially herpes simplex virus [HSV])

GENERAL PREVENTION

Reduce known risk factors: stress; salt, alcohol, and caffeine intake; smoking; noise exposure; ototoxic drugs (e.g., aspirin, quinine, aminoglycosides).

COMMONLY ASSOCIATED CONDITIONS

- Anxiety (secondary to the disabling symptoms)
- Migraines
- Hyperprolactinemia

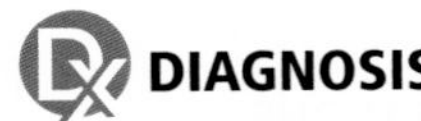

DIAGNOSIS

Diagnosis is clinical (1)[C].

HISTORY

Symptomatic episodes are typically spontaneous but may be preceded by an aura of increasing fullness in the ear and tinnitus. These may occur in clusters, with long periods of symptom-free remissions.

- Formal criteria for diagnosis from American Academy of Otolaryngology–Head and Neck Surgery:
  - At least 2 episodes of rotational-horizontal vertigo >20 minutes in duration
  - Tinnitus or aural fullness
  - Hearing loss: Low frequency (sensorineural) confirmed by audiometric testing.
  - Other causes (e.g., acoustic neuroma) excluded.
  - During severe attacks: pallor, sweating, nausea, vomiting, falling, prostration
  - Symptoms are exacerbated by motion.
- Between attacks, affected patients may experience motion-related imbalance without vertigo.
- *Caution*: Many conditions produce auditory and vestibular findings identical to those of Ménière disease.

PHYSICAL EXAM

- Physical exam rules out other conditions; no finding is unique to Ménière disease.
- Horizontal nystagmus may be seen during attacks.
- Otoscopy is typically normal.
- Triggering of attacks in the office with Dix-Hallpike maneuver suggests diagnosis of benign paroxysmal positional vertigo, not Ménière disease.

DIFFERENTIAL DIAGNOSIS

- Acoustic neuroma or other CNS tumor
- Syphilis
- Perilymphatic fistula
- Viral labyrinthitis
- Transient ischemic attack (TIA), migraine
- Vertebrobasilar disease
- Other labyrinthine disorders (e.g., Cogan syndrome, benign positional vertigo, temporal bone trauma)
- Diabetes or thyroid dysfunction
- Vestibular neuronitis
- Medication side effects
- Otitis media

DIAGNOSTIC TESTS & INTERPRETATION

Testing is done to rule out other conditions but does not necessarily confirm or exclude Ménière disease.

Initial Tests (lab, imaging)

- Consider serologic tests specific for *Treponema pallidum* in at-risk populations (1)[C].
- Thyroid, fasting blood sugar, and lipid studies
- Consider MRI to rule out acoustic neuroma or other CNS pathology, including tumor, aneurysm, and multiple sclerosis (MS).

Diagnostic Procedures/Other

- Auditory
  - Audiometry using pure tone and speech to show low-frequency sensorineural (nerve) loss and impaired speech discrimination. Usually shows low-frequency sensorineural hearing loss
  - Tuning fork tests (i.e., Weber and Rinne) complement audiometry.
  - ABR or MRI to rule out acoustic neuroma
  - Electrocochleography may be useful to confirm etiology (1)[C].
- Vestibular
  - Caloric testing: Electronystagmography may show reduced caloric response. Can obtain reasonably comparable information with use of 0.8 mL of ice water caloric testing. Reduced activity on either side is consistent with Ménière diagnosis but is not itself diagnostic.
  - Drugs that may alter lab results: Any sedating medication may affect and invalidate vestibular testing.

Test Interpretation

Histologic temporal bone analysis (at autopsy). Dilation of inner ear fluid system may be seen.

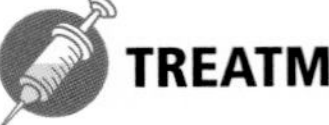

TREATMENT

- Usually managed in outpatient setting
- A paucity of evidence-based guidelines exist; therefore, there is no gold standard treatment.
- Medications are primarily for symptomatic relief of vertigo and nausea.
- During attacks, bed rest with eyes closed prevents falls. Attacks rarely last >4 hours.

MEDICATION

First Line

- Acute attack: Initial goal is stabilization and symptom relief. For severe episodes (2)[C]
  - Benzodiazepines (such as diazepam): decrease vertigo and anxiety
  - Antihistamines (meclizine/dimenhydrinate): decrease vertigo and nausea
  - Anticholinergics (transdermal scopolamine): reduces nausea and emesis associated with motion sickness
  - Antidopaminergic agents (metoclopramide, (promethazine): decrease nausea, anxiety
  - Rehydration therapy and electrolyte replacement
  - Steroid taper for acute hearing loss
- Maintenance (goal is to prevent/reduce attacks)
  - Lifestyle changes (e.g., low-salt diet) are needed.
  - Diuretics may help reduce attacks by decreasing endolymphatic pressure and volume; there is insufficient evidence to recommend routine use (3)[A]:
    - Hydrochlorothiazide; hydrochlorothiazide/triamterene (Dyazide, Maxzide)
    - Acetazolamide (Diamox)

- Contraindications/warnings:
  - Atropine: cardiac disease, especially supraventricular tachycardia and other arrhythmias, prostatic enlargement
  - Scopolamine: children and elderly, prostatic enlargement
  - Diuretics: electrolyte abnormalities, renal disease
- Precautions:
  - Sedating drugs should be used with caution, particularly in the elderly. Patients cautioned not to operate motor vehicles or machinery. Atropine and scopolamine should be used with particular caution.
  - Diuretics: Monitor electrolytes.
- Significant possible interactions: transdermal scopolamine: anticholinergics, antihistamines, tricyclic antidepressants, other

Second Line

- Steroids, both intratympanic and systemic (PO or IV) have been used for longer treatment of hearing loss:
  - Intratympanic administration results in higher steroid levels in the inner ear and may be more effective and safer than systemic (2)[C].
  - Addition of prednisone 30 mg/day to diuretic treatment reduced severity and frequency of tinnitus and vertigo in 1 pilot study.
- In Europe, betahistine, a histamine agonist is routinely used (unavailable in the United States). Other vasodilators, such as isosorbide dinitrate, niacin, and histamine, have also been used; evidence of their effectiveness is incomplete (2)[C].
- Evidence is lacking for routine use of Famvir, may improve hearing more than balance.
- Inner ear perfusion with gentamicin and steroids has been used to control and stabilize vertigo and hearing loss (4)[B].

ISSUES FOR REFERRAL

- Consider ear, nose, throat/neurology referral.
- Patients should have formal audiometry to confirm hearing loss.

ADDITIONAL THERAPIES

- Application of intermittent pressures via a myringotomy using a Meniett device has been shown to relieve dizziness:
  - Safe; requires a long-term tympanostomy tube
- Vestibular rehabilitation may be beneficial for patients with persistent vestibular symptoms (5)[A]:
  - Safe and effective for unilateral vestibular dysfunction

SURGERY/OTHER PROCEDURES

- Interventions that preserve hearing (6)[B]:
  - Endolymphatic sac surgery, either decompression or drainage of endolymph into mastoid or subarachnoid space
    - Less invasive; may decrease vertigo, may influence hearing/tinnitus
    - Insufficient evidence of the beneficial effect of endolymphatic sac surgery in Ménière disease (7)[A]
  - Vestibular nerve section (intracranial procedure)
    - More invasive
    - Decreases vertigo and preserves hearing
  - Tympanostomy tube: may decrease symptoms by decreasing the middle ear pressure
- Interventions for patients with no serviceable hearing (6)[B]:
  - Labyrinthectomy: very effective at controlling vertigo but causes deafness
  - Vestibular neurectomy
  - Many patients may be candidates for cochlear implantation if they have lost serviceable hearing.

COMPLEMENTARY & ALTERNATIVE MEDICINE

Insufficient evidence to support effectiveness, but many integrative techniques have been tried, including the following (2)[C]:

- Acupuncture (8)[A], acupressure, tai chi
- Niacin, bioflavonoids, lipoflavonoids, ginger, ginkgo biloba, and other herbal supplements

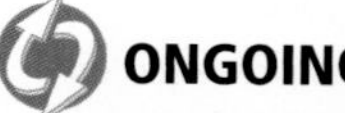

ONGOING CARE

FOLLOW-UP RECOMMENDATIONS

Patient Monitoring

Due to the possibility of progressive hearing loss despite decrease in vertiginous attacks, it is important to monitor changes in hearing and to monitor for more serious underlying causes (e.g., acoustic neuroma).

DIET

- Diet is usually not a factor, unless attacks are brought on by certain foods.
- A low salt is often recommended but not proven effective in randomized controlled trials.

PATIENT EDUCATION

- Limit activity during attacks.
- Between attacks, patient may be fully active but is often limited due to fear or lingering symptoms. This can be severely disabling.
- Vestibular Disorders Association: (www.vestibular.org)
- American Academy of Otolaryngology–Head and Neck Surgery: (www.entnet.org/HealthInformation/menieresDisease.cfm)

PROGNOSIS

- Alert patients about the nature of alternating attacks and remission.
- 50% resolve spontaneously within 2–3 years.
- Some cases last >20 years.
- Severity and frequency of attacks diminish, but hearing loss is often progressive.
- 90% can be treated successfully with medication; 5–10% of patients require surgery for incapacitating vertigo.

COMPLICATIONS

Loss of hearing; injury during attack; inability to work

REFERENCES

1. Sajjadi H, Paparella MM. Meniere's disease. *Lancet*. 2008;372(9636):406–414.
2. Coelho DH, Lalwani AK. Medical management of Ménière's disease. *Laryngoscope*. 2008;118(6):1099–1108.
3. Thirlwall AS, Kundu S. Diuretics for Ménière's disease or syndrome. *Cochrane Database Syst Rev*. 2006;(3):CD003599.
4. Hamid M. Medical management of common peripheral vestibular diseases. *Curr Opin Otolaryngol Head Neck Surg*. 2010;18(5):407–412.
5. Hillier SL, Hollohan V. Vestibular rehabilitation for unilateral peripheral vestibular dysfunction. *Cochrane Database Syst Rev*. 2007;(4):CD005397.
6. van Benthem PP, Giard JL, Verschuur HP. Surgery for Ménière's disease (Protocol). *Cochrane Database Syst Rev*. 2005;3:CD005395.
7. Pullens B, Giard JL, Verschuur HP, et al. Surgery for Ménière's disease. *Cochrane Database Syst Rev*. 2010;(1):CD005395.
8. Long AF, Xing M, Morgan K. Exploring the evidence base for acupuncture in the treatment of Ménière's syndrome—a systematic review. *Evid Based Complement Alternat Med*. 2011;2011:429102.

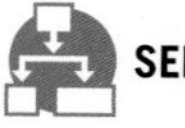

SEE ALSO

- Hearing Loss; Labyrinthitis; Tinnitus
- Algorithm: Vertigo

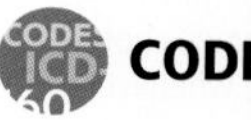

CODES

ICD10

- H81.09 Meniere's disease, unspecified ear
- H81.01 Meniere's disease, right ear
- H81.02 Meniere's disease, left ear

CLINICAL PEARLS

- Ménière disease is a clinical diagnosis based on repeated episodes of vertigo, hearing loss, and tinnitus/aural fullness.
- Multiple medical, surgical, and rehabilitative treatments are available to decrease the severity and frequency of attacks.
- Patients often have progressive hearing loss and fewer vertigo attacks.
- Must exclude acoustic tumor, which produces an identical clinical picture

MENINGITIS, BACTERIAL

Felix B. Chang, MD, DABMA, ABIHM • Kristen M. Wyrick, MD

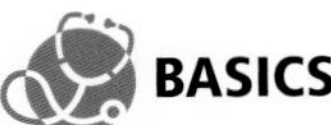

BASICS

DESCRIPTION

- Bacterial meningitis is a potential life-threatening emergency due to bacterial infection and inflammation of the meninges.
- System affected: nervous

EPIDEMIOLOGY

- Predominant age: neonates, infants, and elderly
- Predominant sex: male = female

Incidence

Varies with age (1)[C]

- <2 months: 80/100,000
- 2–23 months: 7/100,000
- 2–10 years: 0.5/100,000
- 11–17 years: 0.4/100,000
- 18–34 years: 0.66/100,000
- 35–49 years: 0.95/100,000
- ≥65 years: 1.92/100,000

Varies with pathogen

- *Streptococcus pneumoniae*: 0.81/100,000
- Group B *Streptococcus*: 0.25/100,000
- *Neisseria meningitidis:* 0.19/100,000
- *Haemophilus influenzae:* 0.08/100,000
- *Listeria monocytogenes:* 0.05/100,000

ETIOLOGY AND PATHOPHYSIOLOGY

Bacterial infection causes inflammation of the pia mater, arachnoid, and the fluid of the ventricles. Age groups with likely pathogens guide empiric choice of antibiotics. Guide therapy by culture whenever possible (1):

- Newborns (<2 months)
  - Group B *Streptoccus*
  - *Escherichia coli*
  - *L. monocytogenes*
- Infants and children
  - *S. pneumoniae*
  - *N. meningitidis*
  - *H. influenzae*
- Adolescents and young adults
  - *N. meningitidis*
  - *S. pneumoniae*
- Immunocompromised adults
  - *S. pneumoniae, L. monocytogenes*, gram-negative bacilli such as *Pseudomonas aeruginosa*
- Older adults
  - *S. pneumoniae* 50%
  - *N. meningitidis* 30%
  - *L. monocytogenes* 5%
  - 10% gram-negatives bacilli*: Escherichia coli, Klebsiella, Enterobacter, P. aeruginosa*

Genetics

Navajo Indians and American Eskimos appear to have genetic or acquired susceptibility to invasive disease.

RISK FACTORS

- Immune compromise
- Alcoholism, diabetes, chronic disease
- Neurosurgical procedure/head injury
- Abdominal surgery
- Neonates: prematurity, low birth weight, premature rupture of membranes, maternal peripartum infection, and urinary tract abnormalities
- Abnormal communication between nasopharynx and subaracnoid space (congenital, trauma)
- Parameningeal source of infection: otitis, sinusitis, mastoiditis.

GENERAL PREVENTION

- Treat infections appropriately.
- Strict aseptic techniques for patients with head wounds or skull fractures.
- Consider CSF fistula in patients with recurrent meningitis.
- Meningitis caused by *H. influenzae* type B has decreased 55% due to routine vaccination.
- Conjugate vaccines against *S. pneumoniae* may reduce the burden of disease in childhood and produce herd immunity among adults.
- Close contacts of patients having meningococcal meningitis should receive chemoprophylaxis (2)[A].

COMMONLY ASSOCIATED CONDITIONS

Conditions associated with a worse prognosis:

- Alcoholism, old age, infancy
- Diabetes mellitus, multiple myeloma
- Head trauma, seizures
- Coma, bacteremia, sepsis

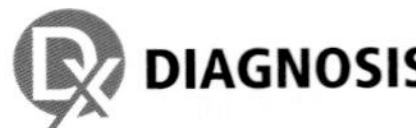

DIAGNOSIS

HISTORY

- Antecedent upper respiratory infection
- Fever, headache, vomiting, photophobia
- Seizures, confusion, nausea, rigors
- Profuse sweats, weakness
- Elderly: subtle findings including confusion
- Infants: irritability, lethargy, poor feeding
- Altered mental status

PHYSICAL EXAM

The triad of fever, neck stiffness, and altered mental status has low sensitivity (44%) (3)[C]. However, 95% of patients present with at least 2 of the following 4 symptoms: headache, fever, neck stiffness, and altered mental status.

- Meningismus
- Focal neurologic deficits
- Meningococcal rash: macular and erythematous at first, then petechial or purpuric
- Papillema
- Brudzinski sign: Passive flexion of neck elicits involuntary flexing of knees in supine patients.
- Kernig sign: resistance or pain to knee extension following 90-degree hip flexion by clinician in supine patients

DIFFERENTIAL DIAGNOSIS

- Bacteremia, sepsis, brain abscess
- Seizures, other nonbacterial meningitides
- Aseptic meningitis
- Drug-induced: NSAIDs, co-trimoxazole, amoxicillin, cephalosporin, isoniazid
- Inflammatory noninfectious: Behcet disease, systemic lupus erythematosus (SLE), sarcoidosis
- Stroke

DIAGNOSTIC TESTS & INTERPRETATION

Initial Tests (lab, imaging)

- Prompt lumbar puncture (1)[A]
  - Head CT first if focal neuro findings, papilledema, or altered mentation
- Typical CSF analysis: turbid
  - Adults
    - >500 cells/mL WBCs
    - Glucose <40 mg/dL
    - <2/3 blood-to-glucose ratio
    - CSF protein >200 mg/dL
    - CSF opening pressure >30 cm
    - Suspect ruptured brain abscess when WBC count is unusually high (>100,000).
- CSF Gram stain and cultures
- Polymerase chain reaction (PCR) of CSF (particularly if culture—in suspected viral meningitis)
- Bacterial antigen tests should be reserved for cases in which the initial CSF Gram stain is negative and CSF culture is negative at 48 hours of incubation.
- Serum blood cultures, serum electrolytes
- Evaluate clotting function if petechiae or purpura are present.
- Chest radiograph may reveal pneumonitis or abscess.
- Later in course: head CT if hydrocephalus, brain abscess, subdural effusions, and subdural empyema are suspected or if no clinical response after 48 hours of appropriate antibiotics
- C-reactive protein: Normal CRP has high negative predictive value for bacterial meningitis (3)[B].

Diagnostic Procedures/Other

Lumbar puncture

- Head CT first if concern for increased intracranial pressure or warning signs of space-occupying lesion (new-onset seizure, papilledema, or brain herniation)
- IDSA CT recommendations: immunocompromised, history of central nervous system disease (stroke, mass lesion, focal infection), papilledema, focal neurologic defect including fixed dilated pupil, gaze palsy, weakness of extremity, visual field cut, new-onset seizure <12 week prior to presentation, abnormal level of consciousness (3)[C]
- Contraindications to LP: signs of increased intracranial preassure (decerebrate posturing, papilledema), skin infection at site of lumbar puncture, CT or MRI evidence of obstructive hydrocephalus, cerebral edema, herniation

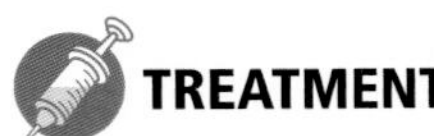

TREATMENT

GENERAL MEASURES

- Initiate empiric antibiotic therapy immediately after lumbar puncture (LP > Abx) or, if head CT scan is needed, then immediately after blood cultures (Abx > CT > LP).
- Vigorous supportive care with constant nursing to ensure prompt recognition of seizures and prevention of aspiration

MEDICATION

Empiric IV therapy, (with dexamethasone when indicated) until culture results available

- Consider local patterns of bacterial sensitivity.

First Line
- Neonates
  - Ampicillin: 150mg/kg/day divided q8h *AND*
  - Cefotaxime 150mg/kg/day divided q8h
- Infants >4 weeks of age (3,4)[A]
  - Ceftriaxone: 100 mg/kg/day divided q12–24h or cefotaxime 225–300 mg/kg/day divided q6–8h *AND*
  - Vancomycin: 60mg/kg/day divided q6h
- Adults (3,4)[A]
  - Vancomycin: loading dose 25–30 mg/kg IV then 15–20 mg/kg q8–12h with goal trough of 15–20 *AND*
  - Ceftriaxone: 2 g IV q12 *OR*
  - Cefotaxime: 2 g IV q4–6h
  - Older than age 50 years, add ampicillin: 2 g IV q4h for *Listeria*
  - Immunocompromised use vancomycin, ampicillin, ceftazidime, *AND* acyclovir.
- Precaution: ototoxicity from aminoglycoside
- Penicillin-allergic patients (3,4)[A]
  - Chloramphenicol: 1 g IV q6h *AND*
  - Vancomycin: loading dose 25–30 mg/kg IV then 15–20 mg/kg q8–12h with goal trough of 15–20
- Treatment duration
  - *S. pneumoniae*: 10–14 days
  - *N. meningitidis*, *H. influenzae*: 7–10 days
  - Group B *Streptococcus* organisms, *E. coli*, *L. monocytogenes*: 14–21 days
  - Neonates: 12–21 days or at least 14 days after a repeated culture is sterile
- Corticosteroids (5)[A]
  - Pediatrics
    - Early treatment with dexamethasone (0.15 mg/kg IV q6h × 2–4 days) decreases mortality and morbidity for patients >1 month of age with acute bacterial meningitis with no increased risk of GI bleeding.
    - Corticosteroids are associated with lower rates of severe hearing loss, any hearing loss, and neurologic sequelae.
  - Adults
    - Initiate in adults, then only continue if CSF Gram stain is gram-positive diplococcus or if blood or CSF positive for *S. pneumoniae*
  - Dexamethasone: 10 mg IV q6h started 15–20 minutes before or with antibiotic for 4 days

Second Line
Antipseudomonal penicillins
- Aztreonam
- Quinolones (e.g., ciprofloxacin)
- Meropenem

ISSUES FOR REFERRAL
Consultation from infectious disease and/or critical care specialist

INPATIENT CONSIDERATIONS
Admission Criteria/Initial Stabilization
Bacterial meningitis requires hospitalization.

Nursing
- ICU monitoring may be needed to recognize changes in consciousness or other neurologic signs and to treat severe agitation effectively.
- Patients with suspected meningococcal infection require respiratory isolation for 24 hours.

Discharge Criteria
Consider home therapy for completion of IV antibiotics once clinically stable and culture/sensitivity results are known.

ONGOING CARE

FOLLOW-UP RECOMMENDATIONS
Patient Monitoring
- Brainstem auditory-evoked response testing for infants before hospital discharge
- Vaccinations
  - Hib conjugate vaccine is recommended during infancy for 4 doses.
  - Meningococcal conjugate vaccine quadrivalent (MCV4) is given to children aged 11–12 years with a booster at 16 years.
  - Immunizing infants <3 months old with MCV4 does not reduce morbidity or mortality, and vaccinating pregnant women does not reduce infant infections.
  - Administer 2 doses MCV4 at least 2 months apart to adults with the following:
    - HIV, functional asplenia
    - Persistent complement deficiencies
  - Administer 1 dose of meningococcal vaccine to the following:
    - Military recruits
    - Microbiologists routinely exposed to isolates of *N. meningitidis*
    - Those who travel to or live in countries where meningitis is hyperendemic or epidemic.
    - First-year college students up through age 21 years who live in residence halls if they have not received a dose on or after their 16th birthday
  - MCV4 is preferred for adults with any of the preceding indications who are ≤55 years of age; meningococcal polysaccharide vaccine (MPSV4) is preferred for adults aged ≥56 years.
  - Revaccination with MCV4 every 5 years is recommended for adults previously vaccinated with MCV4 or MPSV4 who are at increased risk.
- Prophylaxis (2)[A]
  - Only for close contacts of patients
  - Rifampin is effective in eradicating *N. meningitidis* up to 4 weeks after treatment but may lead to resistance.
  - Rifampin: 600 mg PO BID × 2 days
    - Ciprofloxacin and ceftriaxone are effective up to 2 weeks after treatment without leading to resistance.
    - Ciprofloxacin: 500 mg PO × 1 dose
    - Ceftriaxone: 250 mg IM × 1 dose

DIET
Regular, as tolerated, except with syndrome of inappropriate secretion of antidiuretic hormone.

PROGNOSIS
Overall case fatality: 21%
- Fatality rate increases linearly with age.

COMPLICATIONS
- Seizures: 20–30%; focal neurologic deficit
- Cranial nerve palsies (III, VI, VII, VIII)
  - Comprises 10–20% of the cases
  - Usually disappear within a few weeks
- Sensorineural hearing loss: 10% in children
- Neurodevelopmental sequelae: 30% subtle learning deficits
- Obstructive hydrocephalus, subdural effusion
- Syndrome of inappropriate secretion of antidiuretic hormone
- Elevated intracranial pressure: herniation, brain swelling

REFERENCES

1. Centers for Disease Control and Prevention. Meningitis. www.cdc.gov/meningitis/bacterial.html. Accessed 2014.
2. Zalmanovici Trestioreanu A, Fraser A, Gafter-Gvili A, et al. Antibiotics for preventing meningococcal infections. *Cochrane Database Syst Rev*. 2013;10:CD004785. doi:10.1002/14651858.CD004785.pub5
3. Smith L. Management of bacterial meningitis: new guidelines from the IDSA. *Am Fam Physician*. 2005;71(10):2003–2008.
4. Liu C, Bayer A, Cosgrove SE, et al. Clinical practice guidelines by the Infectious Diseases Society of America for the treatment of methicillin-resistant *Staphylococcus aureus* infections in adults and children. *Clin Infect Dis*. 2011;52(3):e18–e55. Correction *Clin Infect Dis*. 2011;53(3):319.
5. Brouwer MC, McIntyre O, Prasad K, et al. Corticosteroids for acute bacterial meningitis. *Cochrane Database Syst Rev*. 2013;6:CD004405.

ADDITIONAL READING

- Kulik DM, Uleryk EM, Maguire JL. Does this child have bacterial meningitis? A systematic review of clinical prediction rules for children with suspected bacterial meningitis. *J Emerg Med*. 2013;45(4):508–519.
- Maconochie IK, Bhaumik S. Fluid therapy for acute bacterial meningitis. *Cochrane Database Syst Rev*. 2014;5:CD004786. doi:10.1002/14651858.CD004786.pub4.
- van de Beek D, Brouwer MC, Thwaites GE, et al. Advance in treatment of bacterial meningitis. *Lancet*. 2012:380(9854):1693–1702.
- Wall E, Ajdukiewicz K, Heyderman RS, et al. Osmotic therapies added to antibiotics for acute bacterial meningitis. *Cochrane Database Syst Rev*. 2013;3:CD008806.

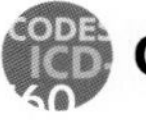

CODES

ICD10
- G00.9 Bacterial meningitis, unspecified
- G00.2 Streptococcal meningitis
- G00.8 Other bacterial meningitis

CLINICAL PEARLS
- Initiate antibiotic therapy immediately (following diagnostic lumbar puncture) if meningitis is suspected.
- Corticosteroids reduce hearing loss and neurologic sequelae but not overall mortality.
- Repeat lumbar puncture if patients don't respond to antimicrobial therapy after 48 hours.
- Classic triad of fever, neck stiffness, and altered mental status has low sensitivity for bacterial meningitis. Meningeal signs are unreliable for diagnosis or ruling out meningitis
- Rapidly evolving petechial rash (purpura fulminans) is more common in meningococcal meningitis.

MENINGITIS, VIRAL

Christine M. Broszko, MD • James E. Hougas, III, MD

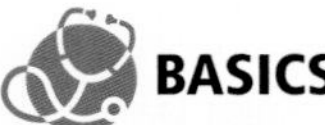

BASICS

DESCRIPTION

- A clinical syndrome characterized by signs/symptoms of acute meningeal inflammation
- Aseptic meningitis has no identifiable bacterial pathogen in CSF. Viral meningitis (VM) is the most common cause of aseptic meningitis.
- System(s) affected: nervous

EPIDEMIOLOGY

Incidence

- Estimated 30,000–75,000 VM cases annually in United States
- Estimated 26,000–42,000 VM hospitalizations annually in United States
- Most common form of infectious meningitis
  - Annual incidence of VM is higher than all other causes of meningitis combined.
- Peaks June 1–October 31
  - Enteroviruses and arthropod-borne viruses predominate in warm months (70% of cases July–October).
  - Mumps usually occurs in the winter and spring, often in epidemics.
- Occurs in both outbreak and sporadic forms

ETIOLOGY AND PATHOPHYSIOLOGY

- First described by Wallgren in 1925
- In immunocompetent hosts, VM is generally caused by a systemic viral infection with neurotropic predilection.
- Less commonly, direct neural transmission occurs from an acute flare of a chonic viral illness (such as HSV) already present in the immunocompetent host.
- 85–95% of cases are caused by enterovirus family; (often transmitted by the fecal–oral route) including coxsackievirus A and B, echovirus, poliovirus, and non–polio E variants: E9 and E30 strains specifically implicated in eastern and western hemispheres, respectively. Most recently, outbreak of E68 in 2014
- Less common: HSV-1, HSV-2, varicella-zoster virus (VZV), adenovirus, lymphocytic choriomeningitis virus (LCMV), cytomegalovirus (CMV), Epstein-Barr virus (EBV), HIV, parvovirus B19, and mumps virus
- Increasing frequency of neonatal morbidity and mortality associated with human parechovirus
- Arthropod-borne viruses: West Nile virus, St. Louis encephalitis virus, and California encephalitis virus
- Recurrent benign lymphocytic (Mollaret) meningitis shows 80% association with HSV-2.

GENETICS

None identified

RISK FACTORS

- Close contact with known cases of VM
- Age (common in children < 5 years)
- Immunocompromised hosts may be more susceptible to CMV, HSV, and adenovirus in particular.
- LCMV is transmitted via exposure to rodent feces, bite, bodily fluids, or nesting materials.

Geriatric Considerations

Cases of VM in the elderly are rare. Consider alternative diagnoses (e.g., carcinomatous meningitis, NSAID- or medication-induced meningitis) in older patients.

GENERAL PREVENTION

Limit exposure to known hosts. Observe hand washing and general hygiene procedures.

COMMONLY ASSOCIATED CONDITIONS

Encephalitis; neurologic deficits; myopericarditis; neonatal enteroviral sepsis

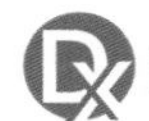

DIAGNOSIS

HISTORY

Predominant symptoms include acute onset (hours to days) of

- Fever (in 76–100% of patients)
- Headache (prominent early symptom)
- Photophobia
- Myalgias
- Nausea
- Vomiting
- Malaise
- Nuchal rigidity (>50%)
- Mental status changes
  - Encephalitis is associated with other neurologic dysfunction, such as behavioral change, focal neurologic deficits, seizure, etc. Therefore, there is a continuum between meningitis and encephalitis that can be labeled as one or the other according to predominant symptom type, or jointly labeled "meningoencephalitis".

Also document the following:

- Travel and exposure history
- Sexual activity (e.g., HSV, HIV)
- Outdoor activities (Lyme disease)
- Exposure to rodent feces and/or urine (LCMV)
- Solid-organ transplant (LCMV, CMV)
- Immunocompromised host (CMV, HSV, adenovirus)
- History of varicella-zoster infection (VZV)
- Immunization status (mumps virus)

PHYSICAL EXAM

- Altered mental status (AMS)
  - AMS generally more common in encephalitis than meningitis
- Fever (>100.4°F/38°C)
- Meningeal signs (should not be used exclusively to diagnose or rule out meningitis):
  - Nuchal rigidity
  - Brudzinski sign: Neck flexion elicits involuntary knee flexion in supine patient.
  - Kernig sign: resistance to knee extension following flexion of hips and knees by physician
  - Jolt accentuation test
- Genital lesions (HSV2: can precede meningeal symptoms by up to a week, however uncommon)
- Parotitis (mumps)
- Asymmetric flaccid paralysis (West Nile virus)
- Mucocutaneous findings
  - Vesicular rash in hand, foot, and mouth disease (coxsackie)
  - Herpangina (coxsackie A)
  - Herpes zoster rash (VZV)
  - Erythema chronicum migrans or cranial neuropathy (Lyme disease [*Borrelia burgdorferi*])
  - Generalized maculopapular rash (Echovirus 9)
  - Oropharyngeal thrush (HIV)
  - Petechial rash (*Neisseria meningitidis*)

DIFFERENTIAL DIAGNOSIS

- Bacterial meningitis (BM)
- Encephalitis
- Other infectious agents:
  - Tuberculosis; syphilis; leptospirosis; Lyme disease; Rocky Mountain spotted fever; ehrlichiosis; *Coccidioides*; *Cryptococcus neoformans*; amebiasis
- Parameningeal infections (e.g., subdural empyema)
- Postinfectious encephalomyelitis
- Viral syndrome (e.g., influenza)
- Leukemia or carcinomatous meningitis
- Migraine/tension headache
- Acute metabolic encephalopathy
- Chemical meningitis
- Drug-induced meningitis (NSAIDs, IVIG, Bactrim)
- Brain/epidural abscess

DIAGNOSTIC TESTS & INTERPRETATION

Initial Tests (lab, imaging)

- Rule out BM:
  - There is debate over whether patients with low suspicion of BM need an lumbar puncture (LP). Some authors contend that if meningeal symptoms have been present >48 hours with a normal neurologic exam in an immunocompetent patient with confirmed normal level of alertness, BM is extremely unlikely and LP is not warranted. Others contend that BM cannot be excluded clinically and to exercise caution discharging meningitic patients without LP.
  - Bacterial Meningitis Score (BMS) to distinguish VM from BM based on Gram stain, CSF neutrophil count, serum neutrophil count, and seizure activity
  - CSF bacterial culture positive in 80–90% of BM patients who have not yet received 2–4 hours of antibiotic treatment (considered "pretreated")
- LP is standard of care in patients with clinical suspicion of BM:
  - If high suspicion of BM, start antibiotic treatment immediately.
  - Contraindications for LP: signs of increased intracranial pressure (e.g., focal neurologic findings, papilledema, altered mental status, vomiting), known ventricular obstruction, new onset seizure, immunocompromised state, local infection over potential LP site or suspected epidural abscess, use of anticoagulation or coagulopathy, and possibility of cardiorespiratory compromise secondary to patient positioning during procedure
  - CSF analysis: glucose, protein, WBC count with differential, RBC count, Gram stain, culture; consider CSF lactate:
    - CSF lactate elevation can differentiate BM from VM (NPV 99%, PPV 82% for BM if >3.8 mmol/L) [1].
- Typical CSF findings in viral meningitis:
  - Elevated WBC count: 10–1,000/mm^3, classically lymphocyte predominance (less consistent in younger patients). May show neutrophil predominance in first 48 hours of disease
  - Decreased or normal glucose (relative to concurrent serum glucose)
  - Protein normal to slightly elevated (<150 mg/dL)
  - Negative Gram stain and bacterial culture
  - Elevated opening pressure
  - RBCs in CSF (Consider HSV meningitis/encephalitis).
  - Pathogen identification
    - Gold standard: CSF viral culture for enteroviruses, HSV, and mumps has low sensitivity (<6%); therefore, viral culture may yield no additional information over nucleic acid amplification alone.

- Polymerase chain reaction (PCR): has a sensitivity of 95–100% for HSV-1 and -2, EBV, and enterovirus
- RT PCR test is approved by the FDA for enteroviral meningitis. Results within 2.5 hour.
- Serology can be performed for many arthropod-borne viruses.

- Other labs: CBC, blood culture, blood glucose; consider serum CRP and procalcitonin (PCT).
  - CBC: normal or mildly elevated WBCs
  - Multiple studies showing PCT correlation with BM. PCT levels of >0.28–0.74 shown to be 94.7–95% sensitive and 100% specific, with NPV 93.9–100% and PPV 97–100% for BM. Also, elevated serum CRP was 96% sensitive and 93% specific, with NPV 99% for BM (1,2).
- Consider EEG if concern for encephalitis.
- Indication for imaging depends on clinical scenario. Perform prior to LP if papilledema, spinal cord trauma, altered mental status, or focal neurologic findings. CT scan may not be clinically necessary in the absence of risk factors.

Follow-Up Tests & Special Considerations

- Disorders that may alter lab results:
  - Diabetes: Consider current blood sugar level to correlate with CSF glucose level.
  - Preexisting neurologic diseases (e.g., intracranial neoplasm, demyelinating disease)

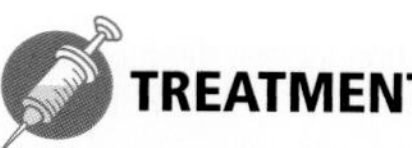

TREATMENT

GENERAL MEASURES

Management is largely supportive care (e.g., pain control, IV fluids).

MEDICATION

First Line

- Analgesics (adult doses)
  - Morphine 2.5–5 mg IV, titrated to pain relief
  - Hydromorphone (Dilaudid: 1–2 mg IV, titrated to pain relief)
  - Hydrocodone (Norco) 5/325 mg 1–2 tablets PO q6h *OR* oxycodone (Percocet) 5/325 mg 1–2 tablets PO q4–6h
- Antiemetics
  - Ondansetron (Zofran) 4–8 mg IV q8h
  - Metoclopramide (Reglan) 10–20 mg IV/IM q4–6h
- Antipyretics: acetaminophen (Tylenol) 650 mg PO or rectal suppository q4h
- Antiviral agents: Initiate empiric acyclovir at 10 mg/kg IV q8h for patients with CSF pleocytosis, negative Gram stain, and suspicion for HSV while awaiting results of definitive (e.g., HSV PCR) testing.
- Antibiotics
  - Not indicated for treatment of VM
  - If unclear etiology, treat symptomatically and follow the patient closely in the hospital setting.
  - If in doubt, initiate an IV or IM broad-spectrum antibiotic with good CSF penetration. Consider especially in elderly, <3 month old, or immunocompromised patient. Empiric treatment in otherwise healthy patient
    - If <1 month, consider ampicillin PLUS cefotaxime (dosing dependent on age and size).
    - If 1 month to 17 years old, consider vancomycin PLUS ceftriaxone OR cefotaxime (dosing dependent on age and size).
    - If 18 years–49 years old, consider vancomycin (15–20 mg/kg/dose q8–12h; also consider loading dose of 25–30 mg/kg) PLUS ceftriaxone (2g q12h) OR cefotaxime (2g q4–6h).
    - In >50 years old, consider vancomycin (15–20 mg/kg/dose q8–12h; also consider loading dose of 25 to 30 mg/kg) PLUS ampicillin (150–250 mg/kg/day divided q3–4h) PLUS ceftriaxone (2g q12h) OR cefotaxime (2g q4–6h).
- Precautions: Avoid aspirin in children and adolescents (potential Reye syndrome).
- If concern for BM, can consider corticosteroids along with antibiotic therapy.

IN-PATIENT CONSIDERATIONS

Admission Criteria/Initial Stabilization

Generally, VM is treated as outpatient. Patients with VM and complications (encephalitis) may be hospitalized. Hospitalize for empiric antibiotic therapy, pain/fluid control, immunocompromised patient, or <1 year old.

- Study of ED visits found that most children diagnosed with VM were hospitalized (91%).

IV Fluids

Crystalloid bolus or continuous infusion, based on hydration status and clinical presentation

Nursing

- Neurologic monitoring for changes in mental status, fever, and other clinical indicators to assess disease progression
- Contact precautions until BM is ruled out
- Private room indicated with sterile precautions
- Encourage hand washing.

Discharge Criteria

Discharge depends on likelihood of BM, CFS WBC count and clinical parameters such as dehydration, functional level, social circumstances, and ability to follow up.

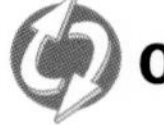

ONGOING CARE

FOLLOW-UP RECOMMENDATIONS

Follow up with primary care physician to ensure resolution.

Patient Monitoring

- Monitor for relapse or exacerbation of symptoms after treatment.
- Monitor for neurologic/neuroendocrine complications:
  - Seizures, cerebral edema, syndrome of inappropriate antidiuretic hormone (SIADH)
  - Assess ability to have companion monitor change in mental/neurologic status if patient discharged.

DIET

Consider NPO if nausea or vomiting, with advancement to clear fluids/regular diet as tolerated.

PATIENT EDUCATION

- Discuss low probability of transmission to contacts.
- Expected duration of illness is 5–10 days. Recurrence of headache, myalgia, weakness possible over 2–3 weeks

PROGNOSIS

- Complete recovery generally within 7–10 days
- Headaches and other symptoms may persist intermittently for 1–2 weeks.
- Only 0.6% of hospitalizations for VM result in death.
- European studies suggest potential residual postmeningeal cognitive impairment.

COMPLICATIONS

- Post-LP headache: 36.5% of patients within 48 hours
- Fatigue
- Irritability
- Muscle weakness
- Seizures (rare)

REFERENCES

1. Viallon A, Desseigne N, Marjollet O, et al. Meningitis in adult patients with a negative direct cerebrospinal fluid examination: value of cytochemical markers for differential diagnosis. *Crit Care*. 2011;15(3):R136.
2. Morales Casado M, Moreno Alonso F, Juarez Belaunde A,, et al. Ability of procalcitonin to predict bacterial meningitis in the emergency department [In Spanish] [published online ahead of print October 3, 2014]. *Neurologia*.

ADDITIONAL READING

- Ciovacco WA, Baraff LJ. Lumbar puncture is not needed for all patients suspected to have viral meningitis. *Ann Emerg Med*. 2012;59(3):228–229.
- Mohseni MM, Wilde JA. Viral meningitis: which patients can be discharged from the emergency department? *J Emerg Med*. 2012;43(6):1181–1187.
- Nigrovic LE, Fine AM, Monuteaux MC, et al. Trends in the viral management of viral meningitis at US children's hospitals. *Pediatrics*. 2013;131(4):670–675.
- Polage CR, Petti CA. Assessment of the utility of viral culture of cerebrospinal fluid. *Clin Infect Dis*. 2006;43(12):1578–1579.
- Studahl M, Lindquist L, Eriksson BM, et al. Acute viral infections of the central nervous system in immunocompetent adults: diagnosis and management. *Drugs*. 2013;73(2):131–158.
- Swadron SP. Pitfalls in the management of headache in the emergency department. *Emerg Med Clin North Am*. 2010;28(1):127–147.
- Talan DA. Bacterial cause of suspected meningitis cannot be safely excluded without cerebrospinal fluid analysis. *Ann Emerg Med*. 2012;59(3):227–228.
- Thomas KE. The diagnostic accuracy of Kernig's sign, Brudzinski's sign, and nuchal rigidity in adults with suspected meningitis. *Clin Infect Dis*. 2002;35(1):46–52.

SEE ALSO

Algorithm: Delirium

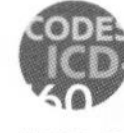

CODES

ICD10

- A87.9 viral meningitis, unspecified
- A87.1 adenoviral meningitis
- A87.0 enteroviral meningitis

CLINICAL PEARLS

- Viral meningitis cannot always be reliably distinguished from BM based on clinical findings. Potential cases of BM should be hospitalized.
- VM is more common than BM in children.
- Antibiotic administration >2–4 hours prior to CSF analysis may result in "partially treated" BM that mimics VM.
- IV acyclovir should be administered when there is high clinical suspicion for HSV.
- If BM is suspected, broad-spectrum antibiotics should be administered until BM has been ruled out.
- Morbidity with VM is low but increases if there is associated encephalitis.

MENINGOCOCCAL DISEASE

Glenn Skow, MD, MPH

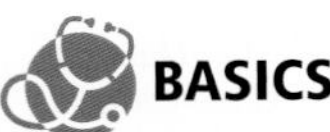

BASICS

DESCRIPTION

- Meningococcemia is a blood-borne infection caused by *Neisseria meningitidis*.
- Bacteremia without meningitis: Patient is acutely ill and may have skin manifestations (rashes, petechiae, and ecchymosis) and hypotension.
- Bacteremia with meningitis: sudden onset of fever, nausea, vomiting, headache, decreased ability to concentrate, and myalgias
- Disease progresses rapidly within a matter of hours.
- Meningococcal bacteremia rarely occurs without frank sepsis.
- Skin manifestations and hypotension may also be present:
  - A petechial rash appears as discrete lesions 1–2 mm in diameter; most frequently on the trunk and lower portions of the body and will be seen in >50% of patients on presentation
  - Purpura fulminans is a severe complication of meningococcal disease and occurs in up to 25% of cases. It is characterized by acute onset of cutaneous hemorrhage and necrosis due to vascular thrombosis and disseminated intravascular coagulopathy.

EPIDEMIOLOGY

Incidence

- The mortality rate is ~13%:
  - 11–19% of survivors suffer serious sequelae, including deafness, neurologic deficit, or limb loss due to peripheral ischemia.
- Disease is seasonal, peaking in December/January.
- Annually, ~1,000 cases of invasive meningococcal disease occur in the United States (1):
  - Most common in adolescents and young adults, followed by infants <1 year

ETIOLOGY AND PATHOPHYSIOLOGY

- *N. meningitidis* is a gram-negative diplococcus with at least 13 serotypes.
- *N. meningitidis* has an outer coat that produces disease—causing endotoxin.
- Major serogroups in the United States: B, C, Y, and W-135
  - Serogroup B is the predominant cause of meningococcemia in children <1 year.
  - Serogroup C is the most common cause of cases in the United States.
  - Serogroup Y is the predominant cause of meningococcemia in the elderly (2).
- Major serogroups worldwide are A, B, C, Y, and W-135:
  - W-135 is the major cause of disease in the "meningitis belt" of sub-Saharan Africa.

Genetics

Late complement component deficiency has an autosomal recessive inheritance.

RISK FACTORS

- Age: 3 months–1 year
- Late complement component deficiency (C5, C6, C7, C8, or C9)
- Asplenia (1)
- Close contacts (e.g., household contacts, nursery/daycare centers, dormitories, military barracks)
- Exposure to active and passive tobacco smoke (1)

GENERAL PREVENTION

- 2 vaccines are currently licensed for use in the United States. Each contains antigens to serogroups A, C, Y, and W-135. Neither provides immunity against serotype B, which is responsible for 1/3 of U.S. cases (2):
  - Meningococcal polysaccharide vaccine (MPSV4): recommended for patients ≥55 years who are at elevated risk (1)
    - Duration of protection is short: 1–3 years for patients <5 years; 3–5 years for adolescents and adults (2)
    - Often used for patients requiring short duration of protection—traveling to endemic areas, college freshmen, community outbreaks (2)
  - Meningococcal conjugate vaccine (MCV4): recommended for patients 2–55 years (1)
- Protective levels of antibody are achieved ~7–10 days after primary immunization (2).
- Vaccine is recommended for all persons 11–18 years and persons 19–55 years at increased risk for the disease:
  - Guillain-Barré syndrome has been associated with the MCV4 vaccine, so a personal history of Guillain-Barré is a relative contraindication for receiving this vaccine.
- CDC International Travel Advisory
  - Vaccine is required by the Government of Saudi Arabia for Hajj pilgrims older than the age of 2 years.
  - The vaccine should be given to travelers to sub-Saharan Africa ("meningitis belt") in dry season.

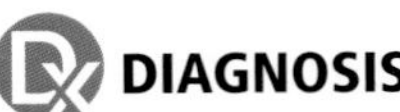

DIAGNOSIS

HISTORY

- Symptoms
  - Sudden onset of fever, nausea, vomiting, headache, myalgias, chills, rigor, and/or sore throat (nonsuppurative)
    - Pharyngitis may be mistaken for streptococcal pharyngitis.
    - Myalgia may be mistaken for severe "flu," with a peak incidence coinciding in winter months.
  - Changes in mental status, decreased ability to concentrate, stiff neck, convulsions
  - Atypical presentations may include acute arthritis or neuritis (3).
- Assess possible exposures.

PHYSICAL EXAM

- Fever, hypotension, tachycardia
- Neurologic: nuchal rigidity, focal neurologic findings, coma, seizure
  - Focal neurologic findings and seizures are more commonly seen with *Haemophilus influenzae* or *Streptococcus pneumoniae*.
- Cardiopulmonary: signs of heart failure with pulmonary edema—gallop; rales
- Dermatologic: maculopapular rash, petechiae, ecchymosis, purpura
- Median time of onset of specific meningitis symptoms (e.g., neck stiffness, photophobia, bulging fontanelle) is as fast as 12–15 hours after onset of illness (4).
- Late signs of meningitis (e.g., unconsciousness, delirium, or seizures) occur ~15 hours in infants <1 year and ~24 hours in older children (4).

DIFFERENTIAL DIAGNOSIS

- Sepsis
- Bacterial meningitis (other organisms)
- Gonococcemia
- Acute bacterial endocarditis
- Rocky Mountain spotted fever
- Hemolytic uremic syndrome
- Gonococcal arthritis dermatitis syndrome
- Influenza

DIAGNOSTIC TESTS & INTERPRETATION

ALERT

- The gold standard for the diagnosis of systemic meningococcal infection is the isolation of *N. meningitidis* from a sterile site (blood or CSF).
- Antibiotic administration may render blood and/or CSF culture negative within 2 hours. Treat, then test.

Initial Tests (lab, imaging)

- CBC with differential
  - Leukocytosis or leukopenia
  - Left shift of leukocytes, toxic granulation
  - Thrombocytopenia
- Lactic acidosis
- Coagulation studies
  - Prolonged prothrombin time/partial thromboplastin time
  - Low fibrinogen
  - Elevated fibrin degradation products
- Blood culture
  - Blood culture positive for *N. meningitidis*
  - Cultures positive in 50–60% of cases
- CSF
  - Grossly cloudy
  - Increased WBCs with polymorphonuclear predominance
  - Gram stain showing gram-negative diplococci
  - Glucose-to-blood glucose ratio <0.4
  - Protein >45 mg/dL
  - Positive for *N. meningitidis* antigen (MAT or PCR)
  - CSF culture for *N. meningitidis*: positive in 80–90% of cases
- CT scan of head if concern for space-occupying lesions

Test Interpretation

- Disseminated intravascular coagulation (DIC)
- Exudates on meninges
- Polymorphonuclear infiltration of meninges
- Hemorrhage of adrenal glands

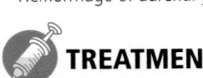

TREATMENT

MEDICATION

First Line

- Antibiotics
  - Treatment for meningococcal meningitis must begin as soon as suspected; coverage for other causes of meningitis must be given until a definitive diagnosis is made.
  - Age influences empiric treatment based on common etiologic organisms:
    - Preterm to <1 month: ampicillin plus cefotaxime or ampicillin plus gentamicin
      - Cefotaxime
        - 0–7 days: 50 mg/kg q12h
        - 8–28 days: 50 mg/kg q8h

- Ampicillin
  - >2,000 g
    - 0–7 days: 50 mg/kg q8h
    - 8–28 days: 50 mg/kg q6h
  - <2,000 g
    - 0–7 days: 50 mg/kg q12h
    - 8–28 days: 50 mg/kg q8h
- 1 month–50 years: cefotaxime or ceftriaxone plus vancomycin
  - If severe penicillin allergy: chloramphenicol plus trimethoprim-sulfamethoxazole (TMP-SMX) plus vancomycin
- >50 years of age or patients with alcoholism, debilitating disease, or impaired immunity: ampicillin plus ceftriaxone plus vancomycin
  - Ampicillin: 2 g IV q4h
  - Ceftriaxone: 2 g IV q12h
  - Vancomycin: 30–45 mg/kg/day IV divided q6h
  - If severe penicillin allergy: TMP-SMX plus vancomycin
- Penicillin G
  - Effective if the isolate is penicillin sensitive
  - Penicillin can be used if the isolate has a penicillin minimum inhibitory concentration (MIC) of <0.1 μg/mL.
  - For isolates with a penicillin MIC of 0.1–1 μg/mL, treatment with high-dose penicillin is effective, but a 3rd-generation cephalosporin is preferred (5).
  - Penicillin G: 4 million units IV q4h (pediatric dose: 0.25 mU/kg/day IV divided q4–6h). *OR* ampicillin: 2 g IV q4h (pediatric dose: 200–300 mg/kg/day IV divided q6h)
- Duration of treatment: 7 days (5)
- Dexamethasone
  - Indications
    - Known or suspected pneumococcal meningitis in selected adults
    - Children with *H. influenzae* type B meningitis
- Dexamethasone is often given initially in adults and children with suspected bacterial meningitis while awaiting microbiologic data.
- Dexamethasone has not been shown to be of benefit in meningococcal meningitis and should be discontinued once this diagnosis is established.
- Dosage
  - Infants and children >6 weeks: IV 0.15 mg/kg/dose q6h for the first 2–4 days of antibiotic treatment
  - Start 10–20 minutes before or with the first dose of antibiotic.
- Chemoprophylaxis
  - Indications
    - Close contacts: those who have had prolonged (>8 hours) contact while in close proximity (<3 feet) to the patient or who have been directly exposed to the patient's oral secretions between 1 week before the onset of the patient's symptoms until 24 hours after initiation of appropriate antibiotic therapy (2)
      - Examples: household members and personnel in nurseries, daycare centers, nursing homes, dormitories, military barracks, correctional facilities and other closed institutional settings
    - No chemoprophylaxis is indicated for casual contacts, including most health care workers, unless there is exposure to respiratory secretion.
  - Timing
    - Ideally <24 hours after case identification
    - Chemoprophylaxis should not be administered if identified more than 14 days after exposure.
  - Prophylactic regimens
    - Rifampin, ciprofloxacin, and ceftriaxone
      - Ceftriaxone
        - Recommended for pregnant women
        - Adults: 250 mg IM as a single dose
      - Rifampin (meningococcal meningitis prophylaxis)
        - Adult: 600 mg IV or PO q12h for 2 days
        - Pediatric
          - <1 month: 10 mg/kg/day in divided doses q12h for 2 days
          - Infants and children: 20 mg/kg/day in divided doses q12h for 2 days (max 600 mg/dose)
      - Ciprofloxacin
        - Adults: 500 mg PO as a single dose (6)[B]
- Vaccination
  - For household contacts (if the case is from a vaccine-preventable serogroup)
- Precautions
  - Adjust the dosage of both medications in patients with severe renal dysfunction.

Second Line

- For meningitis
  - Chloramphenicol: 1 g IV q6h (pediatric dose: 75–100 mg/kg/day divided q6h) or ceftriaxone 2 g IV q12h (pediatric dose: 80–100 mg/kg/day divided q12–24h)
  - In large outbreaks, a single dose of long-acting chloramphenicol has been used. Single-dose ceftriaxone shows equal efficacy in one randomized controlled trial.
- Precautions
  - Ceftriaxone should not be used in patients with a history of anaphylactic reactions to penicillin (e.g., hypotension, laryngeal edema, wheezing, hives).
  - Chloramphenicol may cause aplastic anemia.

ISSUES FOR REFERRAL

Potential complications

- Seizure activity
- DIC
- Acute respiratory distress syndrome
- Renal failure
- Adrenal failure

INPATIENT CONSIDERATIONS

Admission Criteria/Initial Stabilization

- If meningitis is suspected, initiate antibiotics (± corticosteroids), then proceed to an immediate lumbar puncture.
- Droplet isolation for 24 hours from the beginning of antibiotic therapy

IV Fluids

Replace volume as needed; with septic shock, large volumes of crystalloid needed

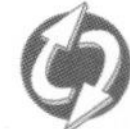

ONGOING CARE

PATIENT EDUCATION

- Educate family and close contacts regarding the risk of contracting meningococcal infections.
- Educate health care personnel who are not at risk of contracting meningococcal infections.

PROGNOSIS

Overall mortality is 13%.

COMPLICATIONS

- DIC
- Acute tubular necrosis
- Neurologic: sensorineural hearing loss, cranial nerve palsy, seizures
- Obstructive hydrocephalus
- Subdural effusions
- Acute adrenal hemorrhage
- Waterhouse-Friderichsen syndrome

REFERENCES

1. Centers for Disease Control and Prevention. Factsheet: meningococcal disease and meningococcal vaccine. http://www.cdc.gov/meningococcal/clinical-info.html. Accessed 2014.
2. Gardner P. Clinical practice. Prevention of meningococcal disease. *N Engl J Med*. 2006;355(14):1466–1473.
3. Rodríguez CL, Octavio JG, Isea C, et al. Acute polyarthritis as sole manifestation of meningococcal disease. *J Clin Rheumatol*. 2012;18(1):42–43.
4. Thompson MJ, Ninis N, Perera R, et al. Clinical recognition of meningococcal disease in children and adolescents. *Lancet*. 2006;367(9508):397–403.
5. Tunkel AR, Hartman BJ, Kaplan SL, et al. Practice guidelines for the management of bacterial meningitis. *Clin Infect Dis*. 2004;39(9):1267–1284.
6. Fraser A, Gafter-Gvili A, Paul M, et al. Antibiotics for preventing meningococcal infections. *Cochrane Database Syst Rev*. 2005;(1):CD004785.

ADDITIONAL READING

- Visintin C, Mugglestone MA, Fields EJ, et al. Management of bacterial meningitis and meningococcal septicaemia in children and young people: summary of NICE guidance. *BMJ*. 2010;340:c3209.
- Wright C, Wordsworth R, Glennie L. Counting the cost of meningococcal disease: scenarios of severe meningitis and septicemia. *Paediatr Drugs*. 2013;15(1):49–58.

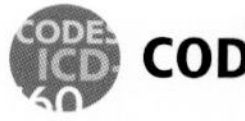

CODES

ICD10

- A39.4 Meningococcemia, unspecified
- A39.0 Meningococcal meningitis
- A39.2 Acute meningococcemia

CLINICAL PEARLS

- Rapid identification of cases with early treatment is essential for good clinical outcomes.
- Chemoprophylaxis should be provided to close contacts.
- Vaccination of at-risk populations is an important preventive measure.

MENISCAL INJURY

Jennifer Schwartz, MD

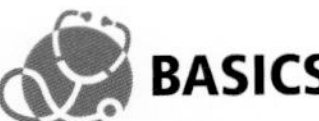

BASICS

DESCRIPTION

- The menisci are fibrocartilaginous structures located intra-articularly between the medial and lateral femoral condyles and tibial plateau.
- Each meniscus has a body, anterior horn, and posterior horn.
- The menisci help stabilize the knee, distribute forces across the joint, and aid in joint lubrication.
- After the age of 10 years, the menisci begin to devascularize.
  - In adults, the outer 1/3 remains vascularized.
  - The inner 2/3 is avascular and heals poorly.
- The medial meniscus is attached to the joint capsule and medial collateral ligament (MCL).

Geriatric Considerations

Meniscal tears in older patients are more likely due to chronic degeneration.

Pediatric Considerations

- Meniscal injuries are rare in children <10 years old (prior to physial fusion)
- Meniscal tears in young children are often due to a *discoid meniscus*:
  - Anatomic variant (thicker and wider) primarily involving the lateral meniscus (incidence of 3.5–5%).
- MRI is less sensitive and specific in diagnosing meniscal tears in children <12 years of age (1)[B].
  - Normal still-vascularized meniscal tissue can be misinterpreted as a tear.

EPIDEMIOLOGY

- More common in the 3rd–5th decades of life
- More common in males.
  - Male > female (2.5:1–4:1)

Incidence

- Medial meniscus more commonly injured because of reduced mobility and increased weight-bearing surface.
- Injuries can be *acute* or *degenerative*.
  - Degenerative tears more likely >40 years of age
  - Acute traumatic tears more likely <40 years of age; 80–90% occur during athletics

Prevalence

One of the most common musculoskeletal injuries; frequency of 24/100,000 per year (2)[B]

ETIOLOGY AND PATHOPHYSIOLOGY

- Acute tears typically occur due to a twisting motion of the knee while the foot is planted. Also can occur with hyperflexion
- Degenerative tears occur with minimal trauma.

Genetics

A congenital abnormality leading to discoid meniscus increases the risk of meniscal tear among children. No specific gene locus has been identified.

RISK FACTORS

- Increased age (>60 years), male
- Obesity
- High degree of physical activity (especially pivot/cutting sports like soccer, football, basketball, and rugby)
- Anterior cruciate ligament (ACL), posterior cruciate ligament (PCL) insufficiency:
  - Waiting >12 months between ACL injury and surgery increases risk of medial meniscal tear (3)[B],(4)[C].

GENERAL PREVENTION

- Treatment and rehabilitation of previous knee injuries, particularly ACL injuries
- Strengthening and increased flexibility of quadriceps and hamstring muscles

COMMONLY ASSOCIATED CONDITIONS

- ACL is concomitantly torn in 1/3 of cases.
- MCL and lateral collateral ligament (LCL) tears
- Tibial plateau or femoral shaft fractures
- Tibiofemoral joint dislocation (rare)

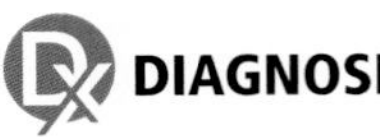

DIAGNOSIS

HISTORY

- Noncontact twisting or hyperflexion mechanism
- Delayed swelling, typically >24 hours after the injury
- Knee pain (on the side of the knee where the meniscal tears is present):
  - Increased with flexion of the knee (i.e., climbing stairs or squatting)
- Locking, catching, popping
- Sensation of buckling or giving out
- Pain typically worse with weight bearing

PHYSICAL EXAM

- Clinical exam by an experienced provider can be valuable and sufficient in diagnosing meniscal injury, especially medial meniscus (5)[B].
- Pertinent findings on physical exam are the following:
  - Effusion (mild–moderate)
  - Joint line tenderness
  - Positive McMurray test:
    - Pain, clicking of meniscus being stressed
  - The Apley grind test for meniscal tear is neither sensitive nor specific.
  - Thessaly test: 98.5% positive predictive value, 86% negative predictive value. Patient stands facing examiner who supports the patient's outstretched hands. Patient rotates knee and body three times with knee flexed 20 degrees. Pain along joint line indicates positive test (1).
  - Decreased range of motion, locking
  - Pain with full flexion (posterior horn tear) or extension (anterior horn tear)

DIFFERENTIAL DIAGNOSIS

- ACL or collateral ligament tear
- Pathologic plica
- Osteochondritis dissecans
- Loose body or fracture
- Osteoarthritis (OA)
- Patellofemoral syndrome
- Gout, pseudogout, rheumatoid arthritis

DIAGNOSTIC TESTS & INTERPRETATION

- Laboratory evaluation generally not indicated unless signs of septic arthritis.
- Plain radiographs can detect fractures, loose bodies, or arthritic changes.

Follow-Up Tests & Special Considerations

- MRI is the primary study for diagnosing meniscal tears.
  - Increased signal within a meniscus corresponds to degenerative changes; signal contacting the articular surface indicates an acute tear.
- Meniscal tears are often found incidentally on MRI and may not be the cause of patient's symptoms.
  - 36–76% of meniscal tears found on MRI were asymptomatic. Asymptomatic tears increase with age and in the setting of OA (2)[B].

Diagnostic Procedures/Other

Arthroscopy may be needed for diagnostic purposes if the MRI is indeterminate.

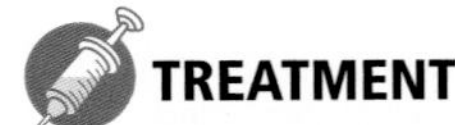

TREATMENT

GENERAL MEASURES

- Treatment depends on the type, location, and extent of the tear, as well as the age and activity level of the patient.
- Conservative treatment (RICE [rest, ice, compression, elevation], activity modification, physical therapy, intra-articular corticosteroid injections) are effective 1st-line options for many patients, especially those with degenerative tears.
  - No increased benefit found to surgery versus physical therapy in treating symptomatic meniscal tears in patients with mild–moderate OA (6,7)[B].
  - Meniscal preservation to decrease future complications of OA is a primary goal of treatment.
  - Small, partial thickness, or peripheral tears may heal on their own or remain asymptomatic.
  - Arthroscopy offers minimal short-term benefit over steroid injections for degenerative tears (8)[C].
- Consider surgical intervention if:
  - Mechanical symptoms, locking
  - Concurrent injuries (i.e., ACL tear)
  - Persistent symptoms following 3–6 months of conservative treatment
  - Young patients (<30 years) or very active patients with an acute tear

MEDICATION

First Line

NSAIDs, opioid analgesics if severe pain

ISSUES FOR REFERRAL

Surgical consult for patients satisfying criteria for operative repair

ADDITIONAL THERAPIES

- Rehabilitation is required for both surgical and nonsurgical patients.
- Electrical stimulation may help improve recovery when coupled with physical therapy (9)[B].
- Weight control: Weight gain is associated with increased cartilage loss and pain in adults with medial meniscal tears.

SURGERY/OTHER PROCEDURES

- Most surgeries can be performed arthroscopically.
- Meniscectomy (partial or total) removes the injured portion of the meniscus.
  - Can lead to articular cartilage degeneration and OA
  - One study found no better outcomes after partial meniscectomy compared to sham procedure.
- Meniscal repairs reapproximate the meniscus with sutures or other fixation techniques.
  - Better functional outcome and decreased risk of OA compared with meniscectomy for isolated, traumatic tears

ONGOING CARE

FOLLOW-UP RECOMMENDATIONS

- Return to play requires that the patient be pain free, have full range of motion, and full strength.
- Following meniscal repair, patients can generally return to all activities in 3–6 months.
- Combined ACL and meniscal repair requires 6 months of postoperative rehabilitation before the patient can return to sports.

PATIENT EDUCATION

Patients should be aware of the risks and benefits of surgery compared with conservative treatment.

PROGNOSIS

- Prognosis better if surgery is done within 8 weeks, patient is <30 years of age, or tear is peripheral/lateral <2.5 cm.
- Young athletes recover faster than older patients.

COMPLICATIONS

- Meniscectomies may eventually lead to OA. Consequently, meniscal repair is preferred to meniscectomy whenever possible.
- Risk of developing OA increases 6-fold 20 years after a meniscectomy.

REFERENCES

1. Harrison BK, Abell BE, Gibson TW. The Thessaly test for detection of meniscal tears: validation of a new physical examin technique for primary care medicine. *Clin J Sport Med*. 2009;19(1):9–12.
2. Carter CW, Kocher MS. Meniscus repair in children. *Clin Sports Med*. 2012;31(1):135–154.
3. Maak TG, Fabricant PD, Wickiewicz TL. Indications for meniscus repair. *Clin Sports Med*. 2012; 31(1):1–14.
4. Snoeker BA, Bakker EW, Kegel CA, et al. Risk factors for meniscal tears: a systematic review including meta-analysis. *J Orthop Sports Phys Ther*. 2013;43(6):352–367.
5. Guenther ZD, Swami V, Dhillon SS, et al. Meniscal injury after adolescent anterior cruciate ligament injury: how long are patients at risk? *Clin Orthop Relat Res*. 2014;472(3):990–997.
6. Siddiqui MA, Ahmad I, bin Sabir A, et al. Clinical examination vs MRI: evaluation of diagnostic accuracy in detecting ACL and meniscal injuries in comparison to arthroscopy. *Polish Orthop Traumatol*. 2013;78:59–63.
7. Rathleff CR, Cavallius C, Jensen HP, et al. Successful conservative treatment of patients with MRI-verified meniscal lesions. *Knee Surg Sports Traumatol Arthrosc*. 2015;23(1):178–183.
8. Katz JN, Brophy RH, Chaisson CE, et al. Surgery versus physical therapy for a meniscal tear and osteoarthritis. *N Engl J Med*. 2013;368(18): 1675–1684.
9. Vermesan D, Prejbeanu R, Laitin S. Arthroscopic debridement compared to intra articular steroids in treating degenerative medial meniscal tears. *Eur Rev Med Pharmacol Sci*. 2013;17(23):3192–3196.

ADDITIONAL READING

- Englund M, Guermazi A, Gale D. Incidental meniscal findings on knee MRI in middle-aged and elderly persons. *N Engl J Med*. 2008;359(11):1108–1115.
- Englund M, Roemer FW, Hayashi D, et al. Meniscus pathology, osteoarthritis and the treatment controversy. *Nat Rev Rheumatol*. 2012;8(7):412–419.
- Ercin E, Kaya I, Sungur I, et al. History, clinical findings, magnetic resonance imaging, and arthroscopic correlation in meniscal lesions. *Knee Surg Sports Traumatol Arthrosc*. 2012;20(5):851–856.
- Herrlin SV, Wange PO, Lapidus G, et al. Is arthroscopic surgery beneficial in treating non-traumatic, degenerative medial meniscal tears? A five year follow-up. *Knee Surg Sports Traumatol Arthrosc*. 2013;21(2): 358–364.
- Imoto AM, Almeida GJ, Saconato H, et al. Effectiveness of electrical stimulation on rehabilitation after ligament and meniscal injuries: a systematic review. *Sao Paulo Med J*. 2011;129(6):414–423.
- Konan S, Rayan F, Haddad FS. Do physical diagnostic tests accurately detect meniscal tears? *Knee Surg Sports Traumatol Arthrosc*. 2009;17(7):806–811.
- LaPrade RF, Wills NJ, Spiridonov SI, et al. A prospective outcomes study of meniscal allograft transplantation. *Am J Sports Med*. 2010;38(9):1804–1812.
- Paxton ES, Stock MV, Brophy RH. Meniscal repair versus partial meniscectomy: a systematic review comparing reoperation rates and clinical outcomes. *Arthroscopy*. 2011;27(9):1275–1288.
- Rosas HG, De Smet AA. Magnetic resonance imaging of the meniscus. *Top Magn Reson Imaging*. 2009;20(3):151–173.
- Sihvonen R, Paavola M, Malmivaara A et al. Arthroscopic partial meniscectomy versus sham surgery for a degenerative meniscal tear. *N Engl J Med*. 2013;369(26):2515–2524.
- Stein T, Mehling AP, Welsch F, et al. Long-term outcome after arthroscopic meniscal repair versus arthroscopic partial meniscectomy for traumatic meniscal tears. *Am J Sports Med*. 2010;38(8): 1542–1548.
- Strouse PJ. MRI of the knee: key points in the pediatric population. *Pediatr Radiol*. 2010;40(4): 447–452.
- Subhas N, Sakamoto FA, Mariscalco MW, et al. Accuracy of MRI in the diagnosis of meniscal tears in older patients. *AJR Am J Roentgenol*. 2012; 198(6):W575–W580.
- Surgery or physiotherapy for meniscal tears? *BMJ*. 2013;346:f1921.
- Teichtahl AJ, Wluka AE, Wang Y, et al. The longitudinal relationship between changes in body weight and changes in medial tibial cartilage, and pain among community-based adults with and without meniscal tears. *Ann Rheum Dis*. 2014;73(9): 1652–1658.

SEE ALSO

Algorithm: Knee Pain

CODES

ICD10

- S83.209A Unsp tear of unsp meniscus, current injury, unsp knee, init
- S83.249A Oth tear of medial meniscus, current injury, unsp knee, init
- S83.289A Oth tear of lat mensc, current injury, unsp knee, init

CLINICAL PEARLS

- MRI is the preferred imaging modality to identify meniscal tears.
- Degenerative meniscal tears are common in patients older than 40 years of age and generally do not require surgical repair.
- Functional outcomes following meniscal injury are improved with a comprehensive plan of rehabilitation involving strengthening and stretching of knee musculature.
- In patients opting for surgery, meniscal preservation should be the goul-meniscal repairs, have a better functional outcome, and decreased risk of OA compared with meniscectomy.
- Improving core strength, proprioception, and quadricep/hamstring flexibility may prevent knee injuries, especially in female athletes.

MENOPAUSE

Anjie Li, MD • Julia V. Johnson, MD

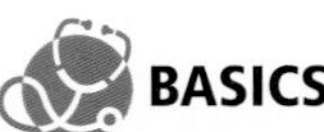

BASICS

DESCRIPTION

- Menopause is defined retrospectively after 12 consecutive months of amenorrhea in a nonpregnant woman ≥40 years of age with no associated pathologic or surgical etiology:
  - Loss of ovarian response to gonadotropins
  - Loss of production of estrogen and progesterone
- Perimenopause/menopausal transition (MT): from the onset of menstrual changes through to the final menstrual cycle. Mean age at start of MT is 47 years, average length of MT is 4 years (1).
- Primary ovarian insufficiency: irregular or cessation of menses before age 40 years

EPIDEMIOLOGY

- Average age of menopause is 51 years.
- 5% of women undergo menopause after age 55 years and 5% between ages 40 and 45 years (2).
- Earlier menopause occurs in Hispanic women and later in Japanese American women as compared with Caucasian women (3).
- Age of menopause for 1st-degree relatives is the best predictor of the age of menopause.

Incidence

Per the CDC, globally, there are about 37.5 million women reaching or currently at menopause.

ETIOLOGY AND PATHOPHYSIOLOGY

- Normal physiologic process: As women age, the number of ovarian follicles decreases: Ovarian production of estrogen has variable decrease, and follicle-stimulating (FSH) hormone production increases:
  - Rise in FSH causes varied production of estradiol and possible perimenopausal menorrhagia
  - Cycles with decreased estradiol production result in absence of the luteinizing hormone (LH) surge and failure to produce progesterone with oligomenorrhea.
  - Eventual decrease in estrogen leads to thinning of endometrial lining and cessation of menses.
- Surgical: Removal of ovaries results in immediate loss of estradiol and progesterone. Hysterectomy results in loss of end organ response to ovarian hormones.

RISK FACTORS

- Age
- Oophorectomy or ovarian surgery
- Sex chromosome abnormalities (e.g., Turner syndrome)
- Age of maternal menopause
- Smoking (earlier age of onset by 2 years)

GENERAL PREVENTION

Goal is not to prevent or treat menopause. Long-term risk of osteoporosis due to loss of estrogen can be prevented:

- Weight-bearing exercise
- Avoid smoking and excessive alcohol intake.
- Calcium intake 1,200 mg/day beginning in adolescence, best from diet and not from supplements
- Adequate vitamin D (800–1,200 IU daily)
- Evaluate risk with FRAX tool and bone mineral density (BMD).

DIAGNOSIS

HISTORY

- Cessation of menses
  - Generally preceded by a period of irregular cycles with heavy or diminished vaginal bleeding
- Vasomotor symptoms: sudden feeling of warmth, most commonly over face, neck, and chest
  - Most commonly reported symptom, prevalence of 50–82% (4). Last approximately 3–4 minutes, occur at unpredictable intervals. Varies across race and ethnicities
  - Frequency and duration varies. 87% of women who report flushes experience them daily, approximately 33% have more than 10 per day. Mean duration of symptoms last 4–10.2 years and may begin during MT and extend well past menopause (5)[A].
  - More common in obese women (6)[B]
- Urogenital atrophy (30–47%)
  - Vaginal/vulvar dryness, discharge, itch, dyspareunia, and possibly sexual dysfunction
  - Alkaline vaginal pH and atrophy increases risk of vaginal infections and UTIs
  - Persists or worsens with aging
  - Urologic symptoms (urgency, frequency, dysuria, incontinence) not clearly correlated with MT
- Anxiety, depression: Some studies show a new diagnosis of depression is 2.5 times more likely to occur during MT as compared to premenopause (7).
- Sleep disturbance: arousal from sleep and chronic insomnia; can be associated with vasomotor symptoms
- Osteopenia and osteoporosis
- Decrease in HDL, possible increased risk of atherosclerotic heart disease
- Change in intensity and severity of migraines
- Skin thinning, hair loss, hirsutism, brittle nails

Geriatric Considerations

Vaginal bleeding in postmenopausal women is abnormal; endometrial cancer must be ruled out.

PHYSICAL EXAM

- Decrease in breast size and change in breast texture
- External, speculum, and bimanual pelvic exams: atrophic vaginal mucosa

DIFFERENTIAL DIAGNOSIS

Pregnancy, hyperthyroidism and other thyroid disease, pituitary adenoma, Sheehan syndrome, hypothalamic dysfunction, anorexia nervosa, Asherman syndrome, obstruction of uterine outflow tract

DIAGNOSTIC TESTS & INTERPRETATION

Initial Tests (lab, imaging)

- Generally none is required; the patient's age and symptoms establish the diagnosis.
- If laboratory confirmation is desired:
  - Elevated serum FSH level indicates decreased ovarian response.
  - Symptoms may precede lab changes.
- Estrogens, androgens, and oral contraceptive pills (OCPs) may alter lab results.
- U.S. Preventive Services Task Force (USPSTF) recommends mammogram every other year from ages 50 to 74 years. United Kingdom (National Health Service [NHS]) guidelines recommend every 3 years.

Follow-Up Tests & Special Considerations

- TSH if thyroid disease suspected
- Brain MRI if pituitary tumor suspected
- Vaginal bleeding in a postmenopausal patient should be evaluated by transvaginal ultrasound (TVUS) and/or endometrial biopsy. If endometrial stripe is <5 mm on TVUS, endometrial carcinoma is unlikely.
- USPSTF recommends BMD screening with dual energy x-ray absorptiometry (DEXA) scan in postmenopausal women >65 years, or <65 years if the risk for fracture is equivalent to that of a 65-year-old woman (using the FRAX tool to assess, http://www.shef.ac.uk/FRAX/). Risk factors include a previous history of fractures, low body weight, cigarette smoking, and family history of osteoporotic fracture.

Test Interpretation

- Abnormal BMD and DEXA scan results in femoral head and spine:
  - T-score on DEXA of −1 to −2.5 = osteopenia
  - T-score < −2.5 = osteoporosis
- *Z*-score measures age-matched mean bone density (not clinically useful).

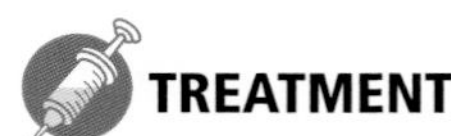

TREATMENT

MEDICATION

First Line

Hormone therapy (HT): Individual risk-benefit profile is considered. Goal of treatment is to minimize menopausal symptoms on quality of life.

- The primary indication for HT is the treatment of moderate to severe vasomotor symptoms.
  - Oral estrogen or combination of estrogen-progestin can have up to 75% reduction in weekly hot flush frequency (8)[A].
- HT also helpful with sleep disorders, urogenital atrophy, and lowers risk of osteoporotic fracture. May help with mood symptoms
- In women with an intact uterus, estrogen should be given with progestin as an unopposed estrogen carries an increased risk of endometrial cancer.
- Treatment regimens include but are not limited to:
  - Standard dose: conjugated equine estrogen (CEE) 0.625 mg/day OR micronized estradiol 17β 1.0 mg/day OR transdermal estradiol 17β 0.05 mg/day
  - Low dose: CEE 0.3–0.45 mg/day OR micronized estradiol 17β 0.5 mg/day OR transdermal estradiol 17β 0.025 mg/day
  - Ultra-low dose: micronized estradiol 17β 0.025 mg/day OR transdermal estradiol 17β 0.014 mg/day
  - ± Medroxyprogesterone acetate (MPA) 2.5 mg/day OR natural micronized progesterone 100 mg/day can be used if progestin is indicated. Can be given cyclically (5 mg or 200 mg respectively) for 12–14 days/month
  - CEE 0.45 mg + bazedoxifene (a new selective estrogen receptor modulator [SERM]) 20 mg (Duavee) approved by FDA for treatment of vasomotor symptoms and osteoporosis. Bazedoxifene opposes action of estrogen in uterus and breast and is not a progestin.

- American Congress of Obstetricians and Gynecologists (ACOG) recommends HT should be individualized with lowest effective dose given for the shortest duration of time needed to relieve vasomotor symptoms. Lower doses have similar symptom reduction profiles for many patients.
- Although generally well tolerated, side effects of HT include breast tenderness, vaginal bleeding, bloating, and headaches. Higher doses can cause hypercoagulability, gallbladder disease, and HTN.
- Discontinuation of HT may result in recurrence of vasomotor symptoms in approximately 50% of women. There is insufficient evidence to recommend 1 method of discontinuation. Per ACOG, the decision to discontinue HT should be individualized.
- Precautions:
  - Women's Health Initiative (WHI) study demonstrated that of every 10,000 women who take CEE with MPA, each year there were 7 more CHD events, 8 more strokes, 8 more PEs, and 8 more invasive breast cancers independent of mammography screening frequency. Absolute risk reductions revealed 6 fewer colorectal cancers and 5 fewer hip fractures.
  - It is recommended that HT should not be used for cardioprotective benefit as studies have shown risk outweighs benefit (9)[A].
  - Association between ovarian cancer and HT use is inconclusive.
- Use caution when using HT in women with estrogen-dependent malignancies, unexplained uterine bleeding, history of thromboembolism or stroke, coronary artery disease (CAD), and active liver disease.
- For osteoporosis: Encourage smoking cessation, vitamin D and weight-bearing exercise. In women with a history of hip or vertebral fracture, or a personal history of osteoporosis, bisphosphonates can be used to inhibit osteoclast action and resorption of bone:
  - Alendronate 70 mg/week or 10 mg/day
  - Risedronate 35 mg/week or 5 mg/day
  - Zoledronic acid 5 mg IV/year
  - Ibandronate 150 mg/month PO or 3 mg IV q3mo
    - The BONE trial demonstrated ibandronate decreased the risk of vertebral fracture but did not show a decrease in the risk of extravertebral fractures.
  - SERMs selectively inhibit or stimulate estrogen-like action in various tissues. The SERMs used for the treatment of osteoporosis include:
  - Raloxifene 60 mg/week: less effective than bisphosphonates or estrogen but can be used in women who cannot tolerate bisphosphonates or estrogen.
- For atrophic vaginitis: Use of vaginal lubricants should be encouraged. Low-dose estrogen therapy with oral CEE (0.3 mg/day) or transdermal estradiol (12.5 μg/day) is effective. Local vaginal estrogen in cream, ring, or tablet formulations are effective. Vaginal estrogen has not been shown to increase risk of endometrial hyperplasia; thus, addition of progestin is not needed. Ospemifene is a SERM approved for dyspareunia associated with vaginal atrophy.

Second Line

- Paroxetine (7.5 mg/day) is the only nonhormonal therapy approved by the FDA for vasomotor symptoms. Venlafaxine, (ER 75 mg/day) and desvenlafaxine (100 mg/day) may result in fewer hot flashes per day (10)[B].
- Gabapentin (600–900 mg/day) has been shown to reduce hot flush frequency by 45%.
- Clonidine (0.1 mg/day) may be used to treat vasomotor symptoms.

COMPLEMENTARY & ALTERNATIVE MEDICINE

- Phytoestrogens including soy show a mixed effect in reducing hot flashes in placebo-controlled trials.
- There is insufficient data to support usage of acupuncture and herbal remedies including black cohost, ginseng, St. John's wort, ginkgo biloba, dang gui bu xue tang, and dong quai to treat vasomotor symptoms.

ONGOING CARE

FOLLOW-UP RECOMMENDATIONS

Patient Monitoring

BMD at age 65 years for all women or for younger women with fracture risk equivalent to age 65 years.

DIET

Encourage calcium-rich diet and vitamin D supplements.

PATIENT EDUCATION

Encourage lifestyle modifications:

- Smoking cessation
- Weight-bearing exercise at least 30 minutes, 3 times a week
- Avoid excess alcohol.
- Address cardiovascular risk factor modification.

PROGNOSIS

If untreated:

- Ultimate disappearance of vasomotor symptoms usually takes several years.
- Vaginal atrophy may continue or worsen over time.
- Osteoporosis: possible fractures of the hip, vertebrae, and wrists

COMPLICATIONS

Osteoporosis: At menopause, women have accelerated bone loss and increased risk of CAD.

REFERENCES

1. Avis NE, McKinlay SM. The Massachusetts Women's Health Study: an epidemiologic investigation of the menopause. *J Am Med Womens Assoc*. 1995;50(2):45–49.
2. McKinlay SM, Brambilla DJ, Posner JG. The normal menopause transition. *Maturitas*. 1992;14(2): 103–115.
3. Henderson KD, Bernstein L, Henderson B, et al. Predictors of the timing of natural menopause in the Multiethnic Cohort Study. *Am J Epidemiol*. 2008;167(11):1287–1294.
4. Feldman BM, Voda A, Gronseth E. The prevalence of hot flash and associated variables among perimenopausal women. *Res Nurs Health*. 1985;8(3):261–268.
5. Politi MC, Schleinitz MD, Col NF. Revisiting the duration of vasomotor symptoms of menopause: a meta-analysis. *J Gen Intern Med*. 2008;23(9):1507–1513.
6. Thurston RC, El Khoudary SR, Sutton-Tyrrell K, et al. Are vasomotor symptoms associated with alterations in hemostatic and inflammatory markers? Findings from the Study of Women's Health Across the Nation. *Menopause*. 2011;18(10):1044–1051.
7. Freeman EW, Sammel MD, Lin H, et al. Associations of hormones and menopausal status with depressed mood in women with no history of depression. *Arch Gen Psychiatry*. 2006;63(4):375–382.
8. MacLennan AH, Broadbent JL, Lester S, et al. Oral oestrogen and combined oestrogen/progestogen therapy versus placebo for hot flushes. *Cochrane Database Syst Rev*. 2004;(4):CD002978.
9. Marjoribanks J, Farquhar C, Roberts H, et al. Long term hormone therapy for perimenopausal and post-menopausal women. *Cochrane Database Syst Rev*. 2012;(7):CD004143.
10. Pinkerton JV, Archer DF, Guico-Pabia CJ, et al. Maintenance of the efficacy of desvenlafaxine in menopausal vasomotor symptoms: a 1-year randomized controlled trial. *Menopause*. 2013;20(1):38–46.

ADDITIONAL READING

- American College of Obstetricians and Gynecologists Practice Bulletin No. 141: management of menopausal symptoms. *Obstet Gynecol*. 2014;123(1):202–216.
- Grady D. Clinical practice. Management of menopausal symptoms. *N Engl J Med*. 2006;355(22):2338–2347.

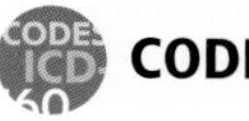

CODES

ICD10

- N95.1 Menopausal and female climacteric states
- Z78.0 Asymptomatic menopausal state
- E28.310 Symptomatic premature menopause

CLINICAL PEARLS

- Menopause is usually diagnosed by history alone.
- HT should be individualized with lowest effective dose given for the shortest duration of time needed to relieve vasomotor symptoms.
- HT can be used short term for relief of moderate to severe vasomotor symptoms and/or vaginal atrophy but should not be used long term for prevention of cardiovascular disease.

M

MENORRHAGIA

Paul Locus, MD • Farhana Rob, DO

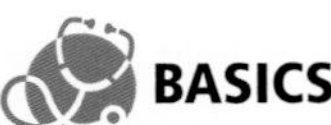

BASICS

DESCRIPTION

- Menorrhagia is an excessive amount or duration of menstrual flow at predictable intervals. Flow ≥80 mL/cycle, compared with normal average of 30–60 mL that lasts for more than 7 days.
- Menorrhagia implies ovulation or regular cyclic menses, not irregular bleeding.
- Distinguishable from, but may overlap with, the following:
  - Metrorrhagia: irregular or frequent flow, noncyclic
  - Menometrorrhagia: frequent, excessive, irregular flow in amount and duration (menorrhagia plus metrorrhagia)
  - Polymenorrhea: frequent flow, cycles of ≤21 days
  - Intermenstrual bleeding: bleeding between regular menses
  - Abnormal uterine bleeding (AUB): abnormal endometrial bleeding of hormonal and other causes related to pregnancy, anovulation (estrogen breakthrough), estrogen or progesterone excess or withdrawal, thyroid disorders, adenomyosis, endometriosis, malignancy, as well as infection and bleeding disorders
- System affected: reproductive

EPIDEMIOLOGY

Prevalence

- The prevalence of menorrhagia is estimated at 30% in the general population during reproductive years and increases with age.
  - Menarche to menopause; ~50% of cases occur in patients age >40 years.
  - Menorrhagia is fairly common in adolescence and in the perimenopausal period.
  - In adolescence, irregular or heavy bleeding due to anovulation and immaturity of the hypothalamic–pituitary–ovarian axis is common.
  - In adolescence, severe menorrhagia may be associated with a bleeding disorder up to 40% of the time, with platelet function defects and von Willebrand disease being the most common.

Pediatric Considerations

Genital bleeding before puberty can result from trauma, foreign bodies, vaginal infection due to abuse, or exogenous hormone administration but is not considered menorrhagia by definition.

Pregnancy Considerations

Bleeding in pregnancy is not menorrhagia. But menorrhagia in a period a couple days late could be a miscarriage.

ETIOLOGY AND PATHOPHYSIOLOGY

- Hypothyroidism if regular menses
- Endometrial proliferation//hyperplasia
  - Anovulation; oligo-ovulation frequently associated with heavy, prolonged, painful periods; called menorrhagia if occurring regularly
  - Ovarian tumor or other estrogen-producing tumor
  - Prolonged use of oral combination pill formulated to allow menses
  - Polycystic ovarian syndrome, (PCOS) (although menses often irregular)
  - Local factors:
    - Abnormal endometrial prostaglandin levels
    - Endometrial polyps
    - Endometrial neoplasia
    - Adenomyosis/endometriosis
    - Uterine myomata (fibroids)
    - Intrauterine device (IUD)
    - Uterine sarcoma
- Coagulation disorders:
  - Thrombocytopenia, platelet disorders
  - von Willebrand disease, factor deficiencies
  - Leukemia
  - Ingestion of aspirin/acetylsalicylic acid or anticoagulants
  - Renal failure/dialysis leading to uremic platelet dysfunction

RISK FACTORS

- Obesity due to estrogen excess
- Infertility/nulliparity
- Anovulation due to chronic unopposed estrogen stimulation (menses usually irregular)
- Family history of endometrial or colon cancer

GENERAL PREVENTION

Combined oral contraceptives help prevent menorrhagia when progesterone is dominant. Lower estrogen doses result in less menstrual bleeding. Ibuprofen inhibits prostaglandin production without permanently affecting platelets and is also noted to decrease blood loss at menses. Progesterone-only contraceptives reduce blood loss but can often convert menorrhagia to unpredictable (although lighter) uterine bleeding.

COMMONLY ASSOCIATED CONDITIONS

Endometriosis, adenomyosis, fibroids, low-grade infection

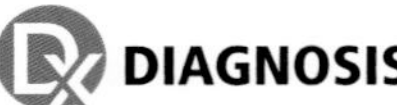

DIAGNOSIS

HISTORY

- Excessive menstrual flow is defined subjectively and varies greatly from woman to woman (1).
- Useful features: Regular bleeding substantially heavier than usual flow (or >80 mL/cycle, if quantified, or changing pads or tampons every 1–2 hours as quantified by patient) lasting >7 days.
  - Significant clotting
  - Symptomatic anemia with no other cause but menses
- Symptoms that suggest cycles are ovulatory:
  - Regular menstrual interval
  - Midcycle pain (mittelschmerz)
  - Premenstrual symptoms: breast soreness, mood changes
- Abdominal pain or cramps at other times of the cycle may be associated with structural causes:
  - Myomas
  - Polyps
  - Ovarian tumors
  - Endometriosis
- Symptoms that may indicate a more general bleeding disorder:
  - Epistaxis, bleeding gums
  - Easy bruising
  - Family history of bleeding disorder
- Review of medications
  - Anticoagulant use in women of childbearing age due to hypercoagulable states

PHYSICAL EXAM

- Hirsutism, acne, or obesity may accompany chronic anovulation such as with PCOS.
- Signs of nongenital or general bleeding, bruising, petechiae
- Pelvic/rectal examination to detect/exclude other causes of bleeding:
  - Cervical or vaginal bleeding
  - Pelvic or adnexal masses
  - Signs of pelvic infection
  - Urethral trauma
  - Gastrointestinal bleeding

DIFFERENTIAL DIAGNOSIS

- Pregnancy complications
  - Early threatened abortion
  - Early incomplete abortion
- Nonendometrial bleeding
  - Cervical neoplasia/polyp
  - Cervical or vaginal trauma/foreign body
- Pelvic inflammatory disease
  - Endometritis
  - Tuberculosis

DIAGNOSTIC TESTS & INTERPRETATION

Initial Tests (lab, imaging)

- Pregnancy test: Always exclude pregnancy first.
- CBC with differential to assess severity of blood loss and to rule out thrombocytopenia and leukemia
- In selected cases:
  - Thyroid-stimulating hormone test, prolactin
  - If suspected anovulation, DHEAS
  - Coagulation panel, with platelet function testing if screen is abnormal
  - Creatinine, BUN to rule out uremia
  - Serum progesterone: 5–20 ng/mL (15.9–63.6 nmol/L) in luteal phase, <1 ng/mL (<3.18 nmol/L) in follicular phase or anovulatory cycle
  - If infectious cause is suspected, aerobic genital culture, wet and KOH preps for microscopic evaluation, or bacterial vaginosis panel and PCR for gonorrhea and chlamydia
- Transvaginal ultrasonography can help distinguish bleeding caused by structural abnormalities versus anovulatory bleeding via assessment of endometrial stripe.
- Abdominopelvic ultrasonography to evaluate suspected adnexal masses or myomas
- Saline infusion sonography for evaluation of small lesions frequently missed on transvaginal ultrasound
- Hysteroscopy to evaluate structural abnormalities more closely (2)[A]
- CT may be used to investigate potentially malignant pelvic masses if needed after ultrasound.

Diagnostic Procedures/Other

- Endometrial biopsy detects hyperplasia, dysplasia, or atrophy. If done before expected menses, it may also help confirm the diagnosis of anovulation or luteal phase defect.
- All women older than age 40 years with unexplained menorrhagia or older than age 35 years with unexplained menometrorrhagia should undergo an endometrial biopsy to rule out cancer.
- Progestins used before endometrial biopsy may cause decidualization but rarely obscure correct diagnosis and often are valuable as an empiric test.

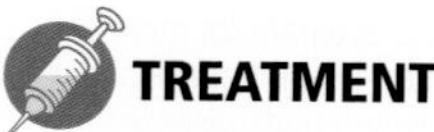

TREATMENT

MEDICATION

First Line

- For acute control of severe bleeding:
  - Estrogen, conjugated (Premarin): 25 mg IV q4h up to 6 doses or 10–20 mg/day PO in four divided doses until bleeding abates; not for use in patients with estrogen contraindications (give with antiemetics).
  - Tranexamic acid 650 mg (3) 3× daily for up to 5 days, expensive but as effective, nonestrogenic but not for those with clotting disorder
- For less severe bleeding (usual case) or after control of acute bleeding has been achieved:
  - Medroxyprogesterone acetate (Provera): 10–30 mg/day for 5–10 days
  - Any combination oral contraceptive (i.e., usually a high-dose oral contraceptive) 1 tablet QID for 5–7 days (usually poorly tolerated, give with antiemetic)
- To prevent heavy bleeding in subsequent cycles:
  - Medroxyprogesterone acetate: 5–10 mg/day for 10 days/month if the problem is due to estrogen excess (2)[A]
  - Cyclic dose of a combination oral contraceptive usually with ≤35 μg of estrogen

Second Line

- Nonsteroidal prostaglandin-synthetase inhibitors (e.g., naproxen, mefenamic acid, ibuprofen) can reduce blood loss ~25% with ovulatory cycles and reduce dysmenorrhea.
- Norethindrone acetate (Aygestin): 2.5–10 mg/day for 10–21 days/month if anovulatory
- Levonorgestrel intrauterine system (Mirena IUD) causes amenorrhea in around 50% and irregular spotting in the other half. A few women experience heavier bleeding.

SURGERY/OTHER PROCEDURES

- Endometrial ablation by laser or electrosurgical, microwave, or thermal means is a conservative alternative to hysterectomy and usually successful, although some patients require additional therapy in the long term (4)[B].
- Uterine artery embolization is a conservative method to treat leiomyomata (5,6)[A].
- Hysterectomy when indicated to treat coexisting conditions (myomas, endometrial dysplasia) or for bleeding unresponsive to other measures

INPATIENT CONSIDERATIONS

Admission Criteria/Initial Stabilization

- Bleeding leading to orthostatic hypotension
- Hematocrit <25% or hemoglobin <8 and symptomatic
- Most cases can be managed as outpatient in an office or emergency department.
- Rule out pregnancy complications and nonuterine bleeding.
- Treat severe or life-threatening bleeding acutely:
  - Circulatory support; transfusion, if necessary
  - IV Premarin (estrogen), tranexamic acid PO
  - Curettage, if necessary
  - Uterine tamponade and hysterectomy in extreme cases

ONGOING CARE

FOLLOW-UP RECOMMENDATIONS

Proceed to identify the underlying cause of bleeding, and treat to prevent recurrence:

- Hormonal therapy
- Dilatation and curettage for cases that fail to respond to hormone therapy
- Consider endometrial ablation, uterine fibroid embolization, or hysterectomy in persistent cases in which fertility is not a concern (4).
- Specific treatment for neoplasia, polyps, systemic disease
- Patients desiring fertility may also need appropriate treatment for anovulation, endometriosis, and myomas (surgical) (1,4,6)[A].

Patient Monitoring

Medical treatment of hyperplastic/dysplastic endometrium should be followed by a repeat biopsy to confirm that histologic structure has returned to normal.

DIET

Iron supplementation may help correct for increased blood loss.

PATIENT EDUCATION

Information about side effects of medications should be provided as well as risks and benefits of procedures.

PROGNOSIS

Most patients with hormonal imbalances will respond to hormonal manipulation.

COMPLICATIONS

- Anemia
- Asherman syndrome from vigorous dilation and curettage
- Estrogen may precipitate acute, intermittent porphyria or cholestatic jaundice in susceptible patients.
- Prolonged treatment with Depo-Provera may lead to bone loss, but clinical significance is uncertain; rapid regain after discontinuation is usual.
- Even with acute bleeding, estrogen should not be used in patients with coronary artery disease, significant carotid narrowing, active liver disease, thrombophilias, estrogen-dependent cancer history, or pregnancy.

REFERENCES

1. Matteson KA, Munro MG, Fraser IS. The structured menstrual history: developing a tool to facilitate diagnosis and aid in symptom management. *Semin Reprod Med*. 2011;29(5):423–435.
2. Sweet MG, Schmidt-Dalton TA, Weiss PM, et al. Evaluation and management of uterine bleeding in premenopausal women. *Am Fam Physician*. 2012;85(1):35–43.
3. Bouchard P. Current and future medical treatments for menometrorrhagia during the premenopause. *Gynecol Endocrinol*. 2011;27(Suppl 1):1120–1125.
4. Karimi-Zarichi M, Dehghani-Firoozabadi R, Tabatabaie A, et al. A comparison of the effect of levonorgestrel IUD with oral medroxyprogesterone acetate on abnormal uterine bleeding with simple endometrial hyperplasia and fertility preservation. *Clin Exp Obstet Gynecol*. 2013;40(3):421–424.
5. Osayande AS, Mehulic S. Diagnosis and initial management of dysmenorrhea. *Am Fam Physician*. 2014;89(5):341–346.
6. van der Kooij SM, Bipat S, Hehenkamp WJ, et al. Uterine artery embolization versus surgery in the treatment of symptomatic fibroids: a systematic review and metaanalysis. *Am J Obstet Gynecol*. 2011;205(4):317.e1–317.e18.

SEE ALSO

- Abnormal Pap and Cervical Dysplasia; Amenorrhea; Cervical Malignancy; Cervical Polyps; Cervicitis, Ectropion, and True Erosion; Abnormal (Dysfunctional) Uterine Bleeding; Dysmenorrhea; Menopause; Polycystic Ovarian Syndrome (PCOS); Uterine Myomas
- Algorithm: Menorrhagia (Excessive Bleeding)

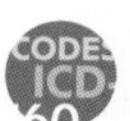

CODES

ICD10

- N92.0 Excessive and frequent menstruation with regular cycle
- N92.1 Excessive and frequent menstruation with irregular cycle
- N93.8 Other specified abnormal uterine and vaginal bleeding

CLINICAL PEARLS

- Menorrhagia is defined as an excessive amount or duration of menstrual flow at regular intervals.
- Pregnancy should be ruled out as part of the initial evaluation.
- Because endometrial carcinoma is a significant cause of bleeding in women age >35 years, an endometrial biopsy to rule out endometrial carcinoma is recommended if the bleeding remains undiagnosed, especially if not confined to regular cyclic menses.
- Remember that estrogen should not be used in patients with coronary artery disease, carotid stenosis, liver disease, thrombophilias, and family history of estrogen-dependent cancer (breast and endometrial).

MERKEL CELL CARCINOMA

Cindy J. Chambers, MD, MAS, MPH • Ronald G. Chambers, Jr., MD, FAAFP • Victoria R. Sharon, MD, DTMH

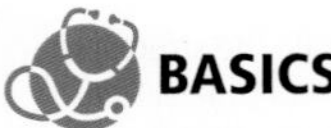

BASICS

- Rare, highly aggressive, cutaneous neuroendocrine carcinoma classically found on the head and neck of elderly individuals
- System(s) affected: skin
- Synonym(s): primary neuroendocrine carcinoma of the skin; trabecular carcinoma; anaplastic carcinoma of the skin; primary small cell carcinoma of the skin; cutaneous apudoma

EPIDEMIOLOGY

Incidence

- Age-adjusted incidence estimated to be 0.24/100,000 person-years in the United States (1).
- Incidence has tripled since 1986, with an average annual increase of 8% (2).
- Highest in the elderly: Median age at diagnosis is 71 years in immunocompetent and 60 years in immunosuppressed (3).
- Increased incidence likely secondary to aging population, increased sun exposure, and number of immunocompromised individuals (2)
- Rarely, <1% of all skin cancers in the United States
- 1,500 cases diagnosed in 2007 (2).

ETIOLOGY AND PATHOPHYSIOLOGY

- Tumor shares several ultrastructural, morphologic, and immunohistologic features with Merkel cells (slowly adapting fine-touch mechanoreceptors in the basal epidermis) as well as with other extracutaneous neuroendocrine tumors. Despite these shared features from which the tumor was originally named, there is little evidence for direct relationship between Merkel cells and MCC. As such the term "primary cutaneous neuroendocrine tumor" has been suggested but not yet widely adopted (4).
- Some suggest derivation from immature pluripotent cells in dermis.
- Merkel cell polyomavirus (MCPyV) likely contributes to development of Merkel cell carcinoma (MCC) and has been detected in 80% of tumors tested (5,6).

RISK FACTORS

- UV exposure (natural or artificial)
- History of prior skin cancer
- Fair skin
- Age >65 years
- Chronic immune suppression (HIV, leukemia, organ transplantation)
- MCPyV

GENERAL PREVENTION

Avoid sun exposure; early biopsy of suspicious rapidly growing lesion; early referral for further management

COMMONLY ASSOCIATED CONDITIONS

Increased risk for developing other malignancies, including lymphomas and other skin cancers

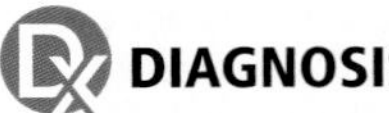

DIAGNOSIS

Complete examination of skin and regional lymph nodes, followed by biopsy. Sentinel lymph node biopsy should be considered for all patients, as even small tumors have been shown to have a ≥15% risk of lymph node disease.

HISTORY

Rapidly growing, painless nodule

PHYSICAL EXAM

- Distribution
  - Favors chronically sun-exposed skin such as head and neck, followed by extremities, buttocks
- Morphology
  - Nonspecific appearance; may be mistaken for more common skin lesions, including BCC, cyst or abscess
  - Classically presents as a rapidly enlarging red pink to violaceous solitary dome-shaped nodule or firm plaque
  - May be shiny and have telangiectasias similar to basal cell carcinoma (BCC)
- Associated signs
  - Grows rapidly, rarely can ulcerate

DIFFERENTIAL DIAGNOSIS

- Clinical DDx:
  - Cyst
  - BCC
  - Abscess
  - Squamous cell carcinoma (SCC)
  - Amelanotic melanoma
  - Lymphoma cutis
  - Kaposi sarcoma
  - Pyogenic granuloma
  - Adnexal tumor
  - Dermatofibrosarcoma protuberans
  - Angiosarcoma
  - Lymphoma
- Histologic DDx:
  - Small cell/oat cell carcinoma of the lung
  - Metastatic neuroblastoma
  - Primary peripheral primitive neuroectodermal tumor
  - Ewing sarcoma
  - Melanoma
  - Poorly differentiated SCC

DIAGNOSTIC TESTS & INTERPRETATION

- Biopsy with histologic stains (see below) (2)[C]
- In cases of confirmed MCC, evaluate for metastatic disease. This includes clinical lymph node examination evaluating for gross lymph node disease and sentinel lymph node biopsy to evaluate for microscopic lymph node disease. Radiologic imaging can be used to evaluate for distant metastases if indicated.
- CT/MRI/PET scans are most valuable in cases of confirmed lymph node disease to evaluate for visceral or bone metastases. Imaging may also be used to evaluate patients with primary lesions >2 cm who are known to have a higher risk of metastasis and/or to monitor for disease progression.

Follow-Up Tests & Special Considerations

MRI may help plan target volume for radiation therapy.

Diagnostic Procedures/Other

Skin biopsy

Test Interpretation

- Morphology
  - Small, uniformly round, blue cells; 2–3× larger than lymphocytes; basophilic nuclei; minimal cytoplasm; finely dispersed chromatin; frequent mitoses; extensive necrosis, high apoptotic index
  - Dermal tumor nodule frequently extending into subcutaneous fat, fascia, and muscle usually sparing papillary dermis and adnexa
  - Similar histologic appearance as small cell lung cancer, small cell melanoma, lymphoma
- Immunohistochemistry
  - Stains positive for epithelial and neuroendocrine markers, negative for lymphoid and melanoma markers including S-100 (differentiates melanoma from MCC) and leukocyte common antigen
  - CK20 staining in perinuclear dot pattern (low-molecular-weight intermediate filament) is highly sensitive for MCC and can help differentiate from BCC.
  - TTF-1 negativity (thyroid transcription factor-1) differentiates MCC from small cell carcinoma of the lung (2)[C].

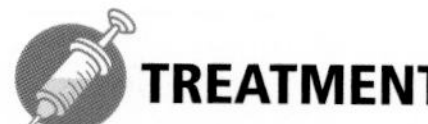

TREATMENT

Primary: wide local excision followed by locoregional radiation, including affected lymph node basin (2)[C]

GENERAL MEASURES

- Wide local excision (>1 cm for lesions <2 cm in size and 2 cm for lesions >2 cm) with pathologically clear margins and sentinel lymph node biopsy (2)[C]
- Adjuvant radiation to primary site ± draining regional nodes decreases locoregional recurrence and improves survival.
- Radiation may be used as monotherapy in inoperable disease and has been used alone to control local disease.

ISSUES FOR REFERRAL

Early referral to dermatologist if MCC is suspected. Recommend multidisciplinary tumor board with surgeon and radiation oncologist.

ADDITIONAL THERAPIES

- Chemotherapy reserved for palliative care for patients with stage IV disease; can shrink advanced metastatic disease but may not increase survival
- The discovery of MCVyV has led to the investigation of antivirals including interferon as well as other potential immunotherapeutic agents in the treatment of MCC.

SURGERY/OTHER PROCEDURES

Mohs surgery may be indicated for MCC on the head, where it may not be possible to obtain a margin of at least 2 cm (2)[C].

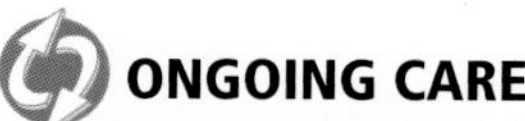

ONGOING CARE

FOLLOW-UP RECOMMENDATIONS

- Regular follow-up appointments with dermatologist every 1–3 months for the 1st year, every 3–6 months in 2nd year, and annually thereafter (2)[C]
- CT scans every 6 months after a high-risk diagnosis

Patient Monitoring

Patients should perform routine skin checking for any new nodules or pigmentary changes at surgical site to suggest local recurrence or distant cutaneous metastasis.

PATIENT EDUCATION

- http://www.merkelcell.org
- http://www.cancer.gov/cancertopics/pdq/treatment/merkelcell/Patient/page1

PROGNOSIS

- 70–80% of patients with MCC present with localized disease (3).
- Locoregional recurrence usually develops within 8 months of diagnosis and is associated with distant metastasis in the future (2).
- 2- and 5-year mortality rate is 30% to 50%, respectively (2).
- Distant metastasis found at mean of 18 months: mean survival <6 months (2)

COMPLICATIONS

Metastasizes via lymphatics, commonly to skin, liver, lung, bone, and brain

REFERENCES

1. Agelli M, Clegg LX. Epidemiology of primary Merkel cell carcinoma in the United States. *J Am Acad Dermatol*. 2003;49(5):832–841.
2. Nicolaidou E, Mikrova A, Antoniou C, et al. Advances in Merkel cell carcinoma pathogenesis and management: a recently discovered virus, a new international consensus staging system and new diagnostic codes. *Br J Dermatol*. 2012;166(1):16–21.
3. Schwartz JL, Bichakjian CK, Lowe L, et al. Clinicopathologic features of primary Merkel cell carcinoma: a detailed descriptive analysis of a large contemporary cohort. *Dermatol Surg*. 2013;39(7):1009–1016.
4. Sibley RK, Dehner LP, Rosai J. Primary neuroendocrine (Merkel cell?) carcinoma of the skin. I. A clinicopathologic and ultrastructural study of 43 cases. *Am J Surg Pathol*. 1985;9(2):95–108.
5. Feng H, Shuda M, Chang Y, et al. Clonal integration of a polyomavirus in human Merkel cell carcinoma. *Science*. 2008;319(5866):1096–1100.
6. Faust H, Andersson K, Ekström J, et al. Prospective study of Merkel cell polyomavirus and risk of Merkel cell carcinoma. *Int J Cancer*. 2014;134(4):844–848.

ADDITIONAL READING

- Albores-Saavedra J, Batich K, Chable-Montero F, et al. Merkel cell carcinoma demographics, morphology, and survival based on 3870 cases: a population based study. *J Cutan Pathol*. 2010;37(1):20–27.
- Coursaget P, Samimi M, Nicol JT, et al. Human Merkel cell polyomavirus: virological background and clinical implications. *APMIS*. 2013;121(8):755–769.
- Miller SJ, Alam M, Andersen J, et al. Merkel cell carcinoma. *J Natl Compr Canc Netw*. 2009;7(3):322–332.
- Schrama D, Ugurel S, Becker JC. Merkel cell carcinoma: recent insights and new treatment options. *Curr Opin Oncol*. 2012;24(2):141–149.
- Schwartz JL, Griffith KA, Lowe L, et al. Features predicting sentinel lymph node positivity in Merkel cell carcinoma. *J Clin Oncol*. 2011;29(8):1036–1041.
- Schwartz JL, Wong SL, McLean SA, et al. NCCN Guidelines implementation in the multidisciplinary Merkel Cell Carcinoma Program at the University of Michigan. *J Natl Compr Canc Netw*. 2014;12(3):434–441.

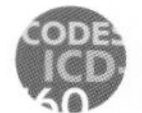

CODES

ICD10

- C4A.9 Merkel cell carcinoma, unspecified
- C4A.30 Merkel cell carcinoma of unspecified part of face
- C4A.4 Merkel cell carcinoma of scalp and neck

CLINICAL PEARLS

- MCC is a rare, cutaneous neuroendocrine carcinoma that classically presents as a rapidly enlarging red pink to violaceous solitary dome-shaped nodule or firm plaque on the head and neck of elderly individuals.
- Clinically, MCC may be mistaken for less aggressive or even benign skin lesions; however, MCC is a highly aggressive tumor with a 5-year disease-specific survival rate of approximately 50% portending a poorer prognosis than melanoma.
- Disease recurrence ranges from 40 (extremities) to 77% (head and neck) typically within 2 years of diagnosis.
- Early detection is critical—Biopsy any rapidly growing suspicious lesion.
- Optimal management often requires involvement of multiple specialists, including pathologists, dermatologists, surgeons, and radiation and medical oncologists.

MESENTERIC ADENITIS

Anne Walsh, MMSc, PA-C, DFAAPA • Kashyap Trivedi, MD

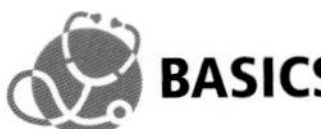

BASICS

Mesenteric adenitis involves inflammation of the mesenteric lymph nodes and is a common cause of self-limited RLQ abdominal pain.

DESCRIPTION

- Characterized by benign inflammation of the mesenteric lymph nodes
- Acute and chronic mesenteric adenitis are both described.
- May be primary or secondary
- May clinically mimic acute appendicitis

EPIDEMIOLOGY

- Commonly misdiagnosed, making definite incidence unknown
- Most common cause of appendicitis-like pain in children (1)
  - ~20% in patients presenting for appendectomy (2)
- More common in children <15 years of age than in adults
  - Primary adenitis is more common in children.
  - Secondary adenitis is more common in adults:
    - Rule out associated diverticulitis, appendicitis, Crohn disease, or systemic infectious/inflammatory disease (e.g. HIV, SLE).

Prevalence

- Affects males and females equally
  - Adenitis secondary to *Yersinia* infection is more prevalent in boys than girls.
    - The prevalence *Yersinia enterocolitica* is most common in North America, Eastern Europe, and Australia.

ETIOLOGY AND PATHOPHYSIOLOGY

- In infectious etiologies, pathogens are ingested, translocate through the intestinal epithelium via Peyer patches, and gain access to mesenteric lymph nodes via intestinal lymphatics. Subsequent inflammatory reaction within mesenteric lymph nodes causes symptoms and clinical disease.

  Infectious agents include the following:
  - *Y. enterocolitica*
  - β-Hemolytic *Streptococcus* spp.
  - *Staphylococcus* spp.
  - *Streptococcus viridans*
  - *Escherichia coli*
  - *Mycobacterium tuberculosis*
  - Giardia lamblia
  - Epstein–Barr virus (EBV)
  - Acute HIV infection
  - Rubeola virus
  - Cat-scratch disease
  - Adenovirus species

Genetics

No known genetic susceptibility

RISK FACTORS

- Typically preceded by upper respiratory infection or pharyngitis
- History of ingesting undercooked pork particularly in areas where *Yersinia* is endemic (parts of Europe)

GENERAL PREVENTION

Minimize risk by eating fully cooked foods, especially meat.

COMMONLY ASSOCIATED CONDITIONS

- Appendicitis
- Diverticulitis
- Crohn disease
- Acute gastroenteritis
- Systemic inflammatory/autoimmune disease

DIAGNOSIS

HISTORY

- The onset of symptoms is variable; nausea or abdominal pain is usually the initial presenting symptom. Generally, symptoms are nonspecific.
- Nausea and vomiting (may precede abdominal pain)
- Abdominal pain, periumbilical; RLQ
- Malaise or fatigue
- Diarrhea
- Fever
- Anorexia
- Recent history of upper respiratory tract infection

PHYSICAL EXAM

- Fever
- Abdominal tenderness; (with or without rebound and often in the RLQ)
- Peripheral/generalized lymphadenopathy
- Toxic appearance
- Rectal tenderness
- Rhinorrhea
- Hyperemic pharynx

DIFFERENTIAL DIAGNOSIS

- Appendicitis, intussusception, intestinal duplication, regional enteritis (Crohn disease), or ulcerative colitis
- Epiploic appendagitis, mesenteric ischemia
- UTI, pyelonephritis
- Salpingitis, pelvic inflammatory disease, ectopic pregnancy

DIAGNOSTIC TESTS & INTERPRETATION

Initial Tests (lab, imaging)

- CBC: leukocytosis
- Basic metabolic panel: may show electrolyte disturbances and azotemia if dehydrated and/or alkalotic from recalcitrant vomiting
- Stool cultures if diarrhea
- Serologic testing if specific infectious agent suspected
- Blood cultures if septic
- CT scan: enlarged mesenteric lymph nodes (larger in size, number, and distribution compared with appendicitis)
  - Specific CT appearance includes ≥3 clustered lymph nodes measuring at least 5 mm in the short axis, most commonly located to the right of the psoas muscle (3)[B].
  - May or may not have evidence of ileal or ileocecal wall thickening
  - Appendix appears normal.
- US: less sensitive; used for exclusion of other potential differential diagnoses
  - Preferred imaging modality in children, younger patients, and women (1)[C]
  - Used to evaluate for signs of appendicitis (96% positive predictive value in children) (2)[B]

Diagnostic Procedures/Other

Lymph node biopsy: applicable only for those patients already subjected to laparotomy, to isolate the causative organism

Test Interpretation

- On gross inspection, lymph nodes are enlarged and soft.
- Adjoining mesentery may be edematous and may or may not present with fluid collections.
- Microscopically
  - Lymph nodes display nonspecific hyperplasia. If a suppurative infection is present, lymph nodes may contain necrotic material with pus formation.
  - Lymphatic sinuses may be enlarged.
  - In cases of *Y. enterocolitica* infection, lymph node capsules may be thickened, with surrounding edema present. There may be lymph node hyperplasia, with plasma cell infiltration.

TREATMENT

MEDICATION

First Line

- Supportive and symptomatic treatment for uncomplicated cases
- IV fluid resuscitation for patients with clinical evidence of hypovolemia
- Correction of any underlying electrolyte aberrations

Second Line

- Broad-spectrum antibiotic therapy for moderately to severely ill patients if diagnosis is unclear pending workup and/or surgical evaluation
- Treatment duration is variable based on cause and severity of illness. For uncomplicated cases, antibiotic treatment is not necessary.

SURGERY/OTHER PROCEDURES

Surgery is usually indicated in cases of suppuration and/or abscess formation, with signs of peritonitis, or if acute appendicitis cannot be excluded with certainty.

INPATIENT CONSIDERATIONS

Admission Criteria/Initial Stabilization

- Indicated for patients with complications and hemodynamic instability
- Volume resuscitation as needed and correction of any underlying electrolyte abnormalities

IV Fluids

- IV fluid hydration may be indicated for patients who cannot tolerate PO intake due to nausea or vomiting.
- Aggressive fluid hydration is indicated for patients who show evidence of sepsis.

Discharge Criteria

Hemodynamic stability, able to tolerate PO diet, able to follow up in the outpatient setting

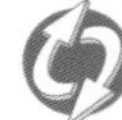

ONGOING CARE

FOLLOW-UP RECOMMENDATIONS

Patient Monitoring

Close outpatient monitoring is needed to ensure total resolution of symptoms.

DIET

There are no specific dietary recommendations. Oral intake can be temporarily held until nausea and vomiting resolve. Advance diet slowly as tolerated.

PATIENT EDUCATION

In cases of *Yersinia* infection, patients should avoid unpasteurized milk, raw pork, and contaminated water.

PROGNOSIS

- Generally self-limiting and benign condition
- Increased morbidity/mortality for patients presenting with sepsis

COMPLICATIONS

- Increased GI losses leading to hypovolemia and electrolyte imbalance
- Abscess formation
- Peritonitis
- Sepsis
- Latent extraintestinal manifestations, including arthralgias, truncal and extremity rashes, and erythema nodosum in instances of *Y. enterocolitica* infection
- Postinfectious chronic complications of *Yersinia* infection including reactive arthritis, conjunctivitis, and urethritis

REFERENCES

1. Millet I, Alili C, Pages E, et al. Infection of the right iliac fossa. *Diagn Interv Imaging*. 2012;93(6): 441–452.
2. Toorenvliet B, Vellekoop A, Bakker R, et al. Clinical differentiation between acute appendicitis and acute mesenteric lymphadenitis in children. *Eur J Pediatr Surg*. 2011;21(2):120–123.
3. Purysko A, Remer E, Filho H, et al. Beyond appendicitis: common and uncommon gastrointestinal causes of right lower quadrant abdominal pain at multidetector CT. *Radiographics*. 2011;31(4): 927–947.

ADDITIONAL READING

- Ikeda Y, Ikeda Y, Nakai T, et al. A case of mesenteric lymphadenitis with long-acting symptom, showing marked response to corticosteroid. *Nihon Shokakibyo Gakkai Zasshi*. 2007;104(9):1371–1376.
- Zganjer M, Roic G, Cizmic A, et al. Infectious ileocecitis—appendicitis mimicking syndrome. *Bratisl Lek Listy*. 2005;106(6–7):201–202.

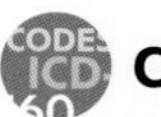

CODES

ICD10

I88.0 Nonspecific mesenteric lymphadenitis

CLINICAL PEARLS

- This is a self-limited inflammatory process involving the mesenteric lymph nodes, and it may mimic appendicitis.
- Mesenteric adenitis is more common in children than adults and may follow an upper respiratory tract infection.
- Treatment is mainly supportive.

METABOLIC SYNDROME

Deepali Nivas Tukaye, MD, PhD

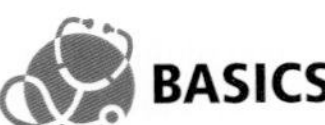

BASICS

DESCRIPTION

- A cluster of metabolic abnormalities that confer an increased risk factor for type 2 diabetes mellitus (T2DM), cardiovascular disease, stroke, fatty liver, and certain cancers
- Involves the following metabolic abnormalities:
  - Intra-abdominal obesity
  - Dyslipidemia
  - Hypertension
  - Insulin resistance with or without impaired glucose tolerance
  - Proinflammatory state
  - Prothrombotic state

EPIDEMIOLOGY

- Predominant age: >60 years old (~50% of cases)
- Predominant sex: male = female
- Ethnicity: Mexican Americans (highest risk)

Prevalence

- Affects 34% of U.S. adults aged >20 years; increasing with the aging population and the prevalence of obesity
- Data vary among populations, depending on the criteria used, but available literature suggests that metabolic syndrome is a rapidly growing epidemic worldwide.

Pediatric Considerations

- Obese children and adolescents are at high risk of metabolic syndrome (prevalence of 6.4% in the United States). Risk factors in children and adolescents include heredity, low birth weight, childhood weight gain and obesity, endocrine abnormalities, hostility, maternal gestational diabetes, and poor health habits.
- International Diabetes Federation consensus report defined criteria in three age groups (6–≤10 years; 10–≤16 years; 16+ years, adult criteria applicable) (1)[C]. Obesity defined by waist circumference ≥90th percentile; rest of the diagnostic criteria (triglycerides [TGs], high-density lipoprotein cholesterol [HDL-C], hypertension [HTN], and fasting blood sugar/T2DM) are largely the same as in adults for children ≥10 years, with some exceptions, and warrant treatment. Clinical significance of metabolic syndrome in pediatric population is not well established. Focus on established risk factors rather than diagnosis.

ETIOLOGY AND PATHOPHYSIOLOGY

- Adipose tissue dysfunction and insulin resistance
- Decreased levels of adiponectin, an adipocytokine, known to protect against T2DM, HTN, atherosclerosis, and inflammation
- Increase in intra-abdominal and visceral adipose tissue
- Abnormal fatty acid metabolism, endothelial dysfunction, systemic inflammation, oxidative stress, elevated renin-angiotensin system activation, and a prothrombotic state (increased tissue plasminogen activator inhibitor-1) are also associated.
- The main etiologic factors are the following:
  - Obesity (particularly abdominal)/excess adipose tissue
  - Insulin resistance
  - Other contributing factors:
    - Advancing age
    - Proinflammatory state
    - Genetics
- Endocrine (e.g., postmenopausal state)

Genetics

Genetic factors contribute significantly to causation. Most identified genes are transcription factors or regulators of transcription and translation. It is a multifactorial disease with evidence of complex interactions between genetics and environment.

RISK FACTORS

- Obesity/intra-abdominal obesity
- Insulin resistance
- Older age
- Ethnicity
- Family history
- Physical inactivity
- High-carbohydrate diet
- Smoking
- Postmenopausal status
- Low socioeconomic status
- Alteration of gut flora

GENERAL PREVENTION

- Effective weight loss and maintenance of normal body weight long term
- Regular and sustained physical activity
- Diet low in saturated fats and simple sugars

COMMONLY ASSOCIATED CONDITIONS

- Polycystic ovary syndrome
- Fatty liver disease (nonalcoholic steatohepatitis)
- Chronic renal disease
- Obstructive sleep apnea
- Gallstones (cholesterol)
- Erectile dysfunction (in men)
- Hyperuricemia and gout

DIAGNOSIS

HISTORY

- Family history of metabolic syndrome, T2DM, and cardiovascular disease
- Symptoms indicating cardiovascular disease or diabetes
- Comprehensive lifestyle history:
  - Diet, including intake of carbohydrates and fats
  - Weight history, including onset of obesity and previous weight loss attempts
  - Exercise regimen
  - Alcohol intake
- Cigarette smoking
- Assess cardiovascular risk with Framingham risk assessment tool.

PHYSICAL EXAM

Various criteria-based definitions have been proposed (2)[A]. According to guidelines from the National Heart, Lung, and Blood Institute (NHLBI) and the American Heart Association (AHA) (3)[A], a diagnosis of metabolic syndrome can be made when ≥3 of the following 5 characteristics are present:

- Abdominal obesity: men >102 cm, women >88 cm (ATP III recommends lowering threshold in population susceptible to insulin resistance, especially Asian Americans)
- BP ≥130/85 mm Hg
- TGs ≥150 mg/dL
- HDL: men >40 mg/dL, women <50 mg/dL
- Fasting glucose ≥100 mg/dL

DIFFERENTIAL DIAGNOSIS

Individual components of the syndrome may be present without fulfilling all the ATP III diagnostic criteria.

DIAGNOSTIC TESTS & INTERPRETATION

Initial Tests (lab, imaging)

- Fasting lipids (particularly TGs and HDL)
- Fasting glucose

Follow-Up Tests & Special Considerations

- Formal 75-mg oral glucose tolerance test for diagnosis of impaired fasting glucose/impaired glucose tolerance (IGT)
- Serum free testosterone, sex hormone–binding globulin
- liver function tests
- Measurement of insulin levels is controversial.
- None necessary to diagnose metabolic syndrome

Diagnostic Procedures/Other

- May require 24-hour BP monitoring (rules out white coat hypertension)
- ECG, stress test, and coronary angiography may be used for diagnosis of cardiovascular disease arising as a complication of the syndrome.

Test Interpretation

- Microalbuminuria
- Increased WBC count
- Increased C-reactive protein
- Increased fibrinogen
- Increased proinflammatory cytokines (e.g., tumor necrosis factor-α)
- Increased uric acid
- Increased homocysteine
- T2DM
- Fatty liver (complicated by end-stage liver disease and hepatocellular carcinoma)
- Hypertensive and/or diabetic eye disease
- Renal impairment/failure
- Peripheral vascular disease
- Coronary artery disease
- Cerebrovascular disease

TREATMENT

Primary therapeutic goal is to prevent or reduce obesity. Aggressive lifestyle modification (diet and exercise) is considered first-line therapy.

GENERAL MEASURES

- Aggressive treatment of individual risk factors
- Avoid or stop smoking.
- Avoid excess alcohol intake.

MEDICATION

- Daily treatment with aspirin is recommended for patients with cardiovascular disease or those at high risk.
- Consult clinical guidelines for treatment of dyslipidemia, hypertension, IGT, and diabetes.
- Multiple medications usually are required to achieve adequate BP control.
- Diagnosis and treatment of insulin resistance is controversial.

First Line

Lifestyle modification alone as initial strategy is applicable to individuals with low 10-year Framingham risk for coronary artery disease (CAD). In individuals with higher 10-year risk, more aggressive risk factor–based approach is recommended in addition to lifestyle modifications:

- Obesity: Lifestyle changes are the cornerstone of treatment. Aim for a gradual ~5–10% weight reduction. Any amount of weight loss is associated with significant benefits.
  - Phentermine–topiramate (delayed release) (Qsymia) (4)[A] and lorcaserin (Belviq) (5)[A] have been approved by the FDA for management of obesity with promising outcomes on weight, BP, dylipidemia, and other metabolic/glycemic parameters. Long-term safety data is awaited.
- Physical activity (6)[A]: 30–60 minutes of moderate-intensity aerobic activities such as brisk walking 5–7 days/week; increase in daily lifestyle activities and resistance training 1–2 days/week. In patients with established CAD, assess detailed history of physical activity and exercise tolerance to guide activity prescription. Advise medically supervised programs for high-risk population (recent acute coronary syndrome [ACS], congestive heart failure, recent revascularization). Cumulative exercise time over the day contributes to health benefit.
- Dyslipidemia: Drug therapy can be commenced after 6 weeks of lifestyle modification. Therapy to be guided by 2013 ACC/AHA lipid guidelines (7)[A], following determination of which treatment group the patient belongs to:
  - Individuals with clinical atherosclerotic cardiovascular disease (ASCVD): high-intensity statin therapy—rosuvastatin 20–40 mg or atorvastatin 40–80 mg—should be used to achieve at least a 50% reduction in LDL cholesterol.
  - Individuals with LDL cholesterol levels ≥190 mg/dL such as those with familial hypercholesterolemia: High-intensity statin should be used with the goal of achieving at least a 50% reduction in LDL cholesterol levels.
  - Individuals with diabetes aged 40–75 years old with LDL cholesterol levels 70–189 mg/dL and without evidence of ASCVD: Moderate-intensity statin, defined as a drug that lowers LDL cholesterol 30–49%, should be used, whereas a high-intensity statin is a reasonable choice if the patient also has a 10-year risk of ASCVD exceeding 7.5% (using the new ACC/AHA global risk assessment tool).
  - Individuals without evidence of cardiovascular disease or diabetes but who have LDL cholesterol levels between 70 and 189 mg/dL and a 10-year risk of ASCVD ≥7.5%: a moderate- or high-intensity statin
  - In individuals who don't fit into any of the four groups, additional factors can be considered if the decision to start statin therapy is unclear: (a) family history of premature (ASCVD) in a first-degree relative, (b) high-sensitivity C-reactive protein (CRP) >2 mg/L, (c) calcification on a coronary artery calcium (CAC) scan, and (d) an ankle-brachial index <0.9.
- HTN: Aim for similar targets to patients with diabetes (<140/80 mm Hg based on ADA guidelines).
  - ACE inhibitor or angiotensin receptor blocker (e.g., losartan 50 mg/day if ACE inhibitor intolerance) is usually prescribed for patients with diabetes.
- Impaired glucose tolerance
  - Current guidelines emphasize that treatment should be with diet and exercise. The role of oral hypoglycemic agents to prevent diabetes in patients with the metabolic syndrome is unclear. Metformin, 500 mg–1 g, 1–2× daily, may be considered.
- Prothrombotic state: Low-dose aspirin for patients with 10-year risk for CAD ≥10% or known atherosclerotic CAD or T2DM or others in high-risk category. Use clopidogrel if aspirin is contraindicated in these groups.
- If CAD or T2DM is already evident, treat as per guidelines. Use ASA 81 mg for primary prevention of CAD if benefits outweigh bleeding risk.

ISSUES FOR REFERRAL
- Nutrition
- Exercise program
- Smoking cessation

SURGERY/OTHER PROCEDURES
- Surgery to treat obesity in severely obese patients who have failed trials of lifestyle modification and pharmacotherapy; surgery recommended if body mass index (BMI) >40 or BMI >35 with obesity-related comorbidities
- Liposuction of abdominal adipose tissue does not reduce insulin resistance or cardiovascular risk factors.

COMPLEMENTARY & ALTERNATIVE MEDICINE
Fish oils and plant sterol esters for cardioprotective effects

INPATIENT CONSIDERATIONS
Management usually does not require admission.

Admission Criteria/Initial Stabilization
Serious complications (e.g., ACS, hypertensive crisis, diabetic coma)

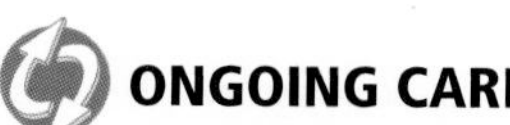

ONGOING CARE

FOLLOW-UP RECOMMENDATIONS
- Regular 30-minute exercise will improve all components of the metabolic syndrome. Cumulative small periods of exercise over the day provide significant health benefits.
- Encourage changing sedentary activity choices (e.g., driving car, taking elevator, and the like) to more active ones (e.g., walking, cycling).
- Regular monitoring of weight, abdominal circumference measurements, BP, fasting lipids, and sugar levels

Patient Monitoring
- Regular monitoring of weight, abdominal circumference measurements, BP, fasting lipids, and sugar levels
- Fasting lipids, fasting sugar, and/or oral glucose tolerance test should be checked annually.

DIET
- Weight reduction to correct abdominal obesity is a primary goal achieved by reduction of energy intake and increased physical activity. Reduction by 500 calories/day will usually achieve a weight loss of 0.5 kg/week.
- Current recommendations include saturated fats <7% total calories, reduction in trans fats, dietary cholesterol <200 mg/day, and total fat 25–35% of total calories. Diet composed of unsaturated fat with limitation of simple sugars. Encourage salt restriction, increased consumption of fresh fruits and vegetables, alcohol moderation, and increased fiber and whole grains.

PROGNOSIS
Increased risk of T2DM (~5-fold), CAD (~1.5–3-fold), acute myocardial infarction (~2.5-fold), and all-cause mortality (~1.5-fold)

COMPLICATIONS
Long-term complications are primarily CAD and T2DM. Recent evidence demonstrates an increased risk of nonalcoholic fatty liver disease, stroke, and an increased risk of developing certain cancers, especially breast cancer in postmenopausal women.

REFERENCES

1. Zimmet P, Alberti KG, Kaufman F, et al. The metabolic syndrome in children and adolescents—an IDF consensus report. *Pediatr Diabetes*. 2007;8(5):299–306.
2. National Cholesterol Education Program Expert Panel on Detection, Evaluation, and Treatment of High Blood Cholesterol in Adults. Third Report of NCEP Expert Panel on Detection, Evaluation, and Treatment of High Blood Cholesterol in Adults (Adult Treatment Panel III) final report. *Circulation*. 2002;106(25):3143–3421.
3. Grundy SM, Cleeman JI, Daniels SR, et al. Diagnosis and management of the metabolic syndrome. *Crit Pathw Cardiol*. 2005;4(4):198–203.
4. Shin JH, Gadde KM. Clinical utility of phentermine/topiramate (Qsymia™) combination for the treatment of obesity. *Diabetes Metab Syndr Obes*. 2013;6:131–139.
5. Chan EW, He Y, Chui CS, et al. Efficacy and safety of lorcaserin in obese adults: a meta-analysis of 1-year randomized controlled trials (RCTs) and narrative review of short-term RCTs. *Obes Rev*. 2013;14(5):383–392.
6. Slentz CA, Duscha BD, Johnson JL, et al. Effects of the amount of exercise on body weight, body composition, and measures of central obesity: STRRIDE—a randomized controlled study. *Arch Intern Med*. 2004;164(1):31–39.
7. Stone NJ, Robinson JG, Lichtenstein AH, et al. 2013 ACC/AHA guideline on the treatment of blood cholesterol to reduce atherosclerotic cardiovascular risk in adults. *Circulation*. 2014;129(25)(Suppl 2):S1–S45.

ADDITIONAL READING

- Kassi E, Pervanidou P, Kaltsas G, et al. Metabolic syndrome: definitions and controversies. *BMC Med*. 2011;9:48.
- National Institutes of Health. Clinical guidelines on the identification, evaluation, and treatment of overweight and obesity in adults: the evidence report. *Obes Res*. 1998;6(Suppl 2):51S–209S.

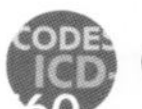

CODES

ICD10
E88.81 Metabolic syndrome

CLINICAL PEARLS
- Abdominal circumference should be measured as part of a cardiovascular risk assessment.
- Prevention or reduction of obesity is the cornerstone of management of metabolic syndrome. Cumulative physical activity over the day significantly adds to the benefit of regular 30–60-minute exercise regimen.
- Aggressive lifestyle modification is 1st-line lifelong treatment for all patients.

METATARSALGIA

Kenneth M. Bielak, MD, FACSM, FAAFP, CAQ-SM • Tanika M. Pinn, MD

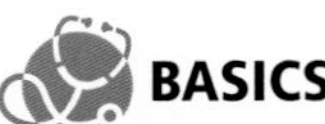

BASICS

DESCRIPTION

- Metatarsalgia generally refers to pain in the forefoot in the region of the metatarsal heads.
- System affected: musculoskeletal

EPIDEMIOLOGY

Incidence

Especially common in athletes engaging in high-impact sports (running, jumping, dancing) and in rock climbers (12.5%)

Prevalence

Common

ETIOLOGY AND PATHOPHYSIOLOGY

- The 1st metatarsal head bears significant weight when walking or running. A normal metatarsal arch also ensures this balance. The 1st metatarsal head has adequate padding to accommodate increased forces.
- Reactive tissue can build up a callus around the metatarsal head, which compounds the pain.
  - Excessive or repetitive stress. Forces are transmitted to the forefoot during several stages (midstance and push-off) during walking and running. These forces are translated across the metatarsal heads reaching nearly 3× body weight (1)[C].
  - A pronated splayfoot disturbs this balance, causing equal weight bearing on all metatarsal heads.
  - Any foot deformity also changes distribution of weight to areas of the foot that do not have sufficient padding.
  - Soft tissue dysfunction: intrinsic muscle weakness, laxity in the Lisfranc ligament
  - Abnormal foot posture: forefoot varus or valgus, cavus or equinus deformities, loss of the metatarsal arch, splayfoot, pronated foot
  - Dermatologic: warts, calluses
- Great toe
  - Hallux valgus (bunion), either varus or rigidus
- Lesser metatarsals
  - Freiberg infraction (i.e., aseptic necrosis of the metatarsal head usually due to trauma in adolescents who jump or sprint)
  - Hammer toe or claw toe
  - Morton syndrome (i.e., long 2nd metatarsal)

RISK FACTORS

- Obesity
- High heels, narrow shoes, or overly tight-fitting shoes (rock climbers typically wear small shoes)
- Competitive athletes in weight-bearing sports (e.g., ballet, basketball, running, soccer, baseball, football)
- Foot deformities (e.g., pes planus, pes cavus, tight Achilles tendon, tarsal tunnel syndrome, hallux valgus, prominent metatarsal heads, excessive pronation, hammer toe deformity, tight toe extensors)

Geriatric Considerations

- Often concomitant arthritis
- Metatarsalgia is common in older athletes.
- Age-related atrophy of the metatarsal fat pad may increase the risk for metatarsalgia.

Pediatric Considerations

- Muscle imbalance disorders (e.g., Duchenne muscular dystrophy) cause foot deformities in children.
- In adolescent girls, consider Freiberg infraction (aseptic necrosis of the metatarsal head usually due to trauma in adolescents who jump or sprint).
- Salter I injuries may affect subsequent growth and healing of the epiphysis.

Pregnancy Considerations

- Forefoot pain during pregnancy usually results from change in gait, center of mass, and joint laxity.
- Wear properly fitted, low-heeled shoes.

GENERAL PREVENTION

- Wear properly fitted shoes with good padding.
- Start weight-bearing exercise programs gradually.

COMMONLY ASSOCIATED CONDITIONS

- Arthritis
- Morton neuroma
- Sesamoiditis
- Plantar keratosis

DIAGNOSIS

HISTORY

- Pain gradually develops and persists over the heads of 1 or more metatarsals, usually on the plantar surface
- Pain is often chronic (rather than acute in onset).
- Predisposition with pes cavus deformity and hyperpronation
- Pain often described as walking with a pebble in the shoe; aggravated during midstance or propulsion phases of walking or running

PHYSICAL EXAM

- Point tenderness over plantar metatarsal heads
- Pain in the interdigital space or a positive metatarsal squeeze test suggests Morton neuroma.
- Plantar keratosis (callus formation) often noted
- Tenderness of the metatarsal head(s) with pressure applied by the examiner's finger and thumb
- Erythema and swelling (occasionally)

DIFFERENTIAL DIAGNOSIS

- Stress fracture (most commonly 2nd metatarsal)
- Morton neuroma (i.e., interdigital neuroma)
- Sesamoiditis or sesamoid fracture
- Salter I fracture in pediatric population
- Arthritis (e.g., gouty, rheumatoid, inflammatory, osteoarthritis, septic, calcium pyrophosphate dihydrate crystal deposit disease [CPPD])
- Lisfranc injury
- Avascular necrosis of the metatarsal head
- Ganglion cyst
- Foreign body
- Vasculitis (diabetes)

DIAGNOSTIC TESTS & INTERPRETATION

Initial Tests (lab, imaging)

- Only if diagnosis is in question:
  - Erythrocyte sedimentation rate or C-reactive protein
  - Rheumatoid factor
  - Uric acid
  - Glucose
  - CBC with differential
- Weight-bearing radiographs: anteroposterior, lateral, and oblique views:
  - Occasionally, metatarsal or sesamoid axial films (to rule out sesamoid fracture) or skyline view of the metatarsal heads to assess the plantar declination of the metatarsal heads: obtained with the metatarsophalangeal joints in dorsiflexion (to evaluate alignment)
- Ultrasound and MRI in recalcitrant cases (2)[C]
- MR arthrography of the metatarsophalangeal (MTP) joint can delineate capsular tears, typically of the distal lateral border of the plantar plate, an often underrecognized cause of metatarsalgia.
- Bone scan if high index of suspicion of stress fracture exists

Diagnostic Procedures/Other

Plantar pressure distribution analysis may help distinguish pressure distribution patterns due to malalignment.

TREATMENT

Treatment for metatarsalgia is typically conservative.

MEDICATION

- NSAIDs (ibuprofen 800 mg TID 7–14 days or naproxen 500 mg BID 7–14 days)
- Contraindications: GI bleeding or ulcer
- Precautions in patients with:
  - Renal disease
  - Hepatic disease
  - Coagulation disorders
- Significant possible interactions:
  - Anticoagulants
  - Digoxin
  - Lithium
  - Methotrexate
  - Cyclosporin

ISSUES FOR REFERRAL

High-level athletes may benefit from early podiatric or orthopedic evaluation.

ADDITIONAL THERAPIES

- Physical therapy to restore normal foot biomechanics
- Low-heeled (<2 cm height) wide-toe-box shoes
- Metatarsal bars, pads, and arch supports. Metatarsal bars may be more effective than pads.
- Orthotics/rocker bar (prescriptive orthotics have been shown to be effective treatment)
- Thick-soled shoes
- Shaving the callus may provide temporary relief but should not be excised.
- Improve flexibility and strength of the muscles of the foot with:
  - Exercises (e.g., towel grasps, pencil curls)
  - Physical therapy to maintain range of motion and restore normal biomechanics

SURGERY/OTHER PROCEDURES

- If no improvement with conservative therapy for 3 months, referral to foot/ankle orthopedic or surgical podiatrist may be necessary.
- Surgery may help correct anatomic abnormality: bunionectomy, partial osteotomy, or surgical fusion. Success rates vary depending on procedure.
- Direct plantar plate repair (grade II tear) combined with Weil osteotomy can restore normal alignment of the MTP joint, leading to diminished pain with improved functional scores.
- The Weil osteotomy (distal metatarsal oblique osteotomy) is safe and effective for metatarsalgia.
- Callus removal is generally not recommended (callus is a response to pressure change—not the cause).
- Interdigital nerve block offers temporary relief for Morton neuroma. Morton neurectomy or ultrasound-guided alcohol ablation of Morton neuroma are other options (3)[C].
- Surgery only as a last resort if no anatomic abnormality is present

COMPLEMENTARY & ALTERNATIVE MEDICINE

Magnetic insoles not effective for chronic nonspecific foot pain

INPATIENT CONSIDERATIONS

Admission Criteria/Initial Stabilization

- Relieve pain
- Ice initially
- Rest: temporary alteration of weight-bearing activity; use of cane or crutch. For more physically active patients, suggest an alternative exercise or cross-training:
  - Moist heat later
  - Taping or gel cast
  - Stiff-soled shoes will act as a splint
- Relieve the pressure beneath the area of maximal pain by redistributing the pressure load of the foot, which can be achieved by weight loss.

ONGOING CARE

FOLLOW-UP RECOMMENDATIONS

Patient Monitoring

If stress fracture has been ruled out and patient's condition has not improved >3 months of conservative treatment, consider surgical evaluation.

PATIENT EDUCATION

- Instruct about wearing proper shoes and gradual return to activity.
- Cross-training until symptoms subside. Goal is to restore normal foot biomechanics, relieve abnormal pressure on the plantar metatarsal heads, and relieve pain (4)[C].

PROGNOSIS

Outcome depends on the severity of the problem and whether surgery is required to correct it.

COMPLICATIONS

- Back, knee, and hip pain due to change in gait
- Transfer metatarsalgia following surgical intervention, which subsequently transfers stress to other areas

REFERENCES

1. Hockenbury RT. Forefoot problems in athletes. *Med Sci Sports Exerc*. 1999;31(7)(Suppl):S448–S458.
2. Iagnocco A, Coari G, Palombi G, et al. Sonography in the study of metatarsalgia. *J Rheumatol*. 2001; 28(6):1338–1340.
3. Musson RE, Sawhney JS, Lamb L, et al. Ultrasound guided alcohol ablation of Morton's neuroma. *Foot Ankle Int*. 2012;33(3):196–201.
4. Espinosa N, Brodsky JW, Maceira E. Metatarsalgia. *J Am Acad Orthop Surg*. 2010;18(8):474–485.

ADDITIONAL READING

- Birbilis T, Theodoropoulou E, Koulalis D. Forefoot complaints–the Morton's metatarsalgia. The role of MR imaging. *Acta Medica (Hradec Kralove)*. 2007;50(3):221–222.
- Buda R, Di Caprio F, Bedetti L, et al. Foot overuse diseases in rock climbing: an epidemiologic study. *J Am Podiatr Med Assoc*. 2013;103(2):113–120.
- Burns J, Landorf KB, Ryan MM, et al. Interventions for the prevention and treatment of pes cavus. *Cochrane Database Syst Rev*. 2007;4:CD006154.
- Clinical Practice Guideline Forefoot Disorders Panel, Thomas JL, Blitch EL IV, et al. Diagnosis and treatment of forefoot disorders. Section 2. Central metatarsalgia. *J Foot Ankle Surg*. 2009;48(2):239–250.
- Deshaies A, Roy P, Symeonidis PD, et al. Metatarsal bars more effective than metatarsal pads in reducing impulse on the second metatarsal head. *Foot (Edinb)*. 2011;21(4):172–175.
- Janisse DJ, Janisse E. Shoe modification and the use of orthoses in the treatment of foot and ankle pathology. *J Am Acad Orthop Surg*. 2008;16(3): 152–158.
- Ko PH, Hsiao TY, Kang JH, et al. Relationship between plantar pressure and soft tissue strain under metatarsal heads with different heel heights. *Foot Ankle Int*. 2009;30(11):1111–1116.
- Nery C, Coughlin MJ, Baumfeld D, et al. Lesser metatarsophalangeal joint instability: prospective evaluation and repair of plantar plate and capsular insufficiency. *Foot Ankle Int*. 2012;33:301–311.
- Pace A, Scammell B, Dhar S, et al. The outcome of Morton's neurectomy in the treatment of metatarsalgia. *Int Orthop*. 2010;34(4):511–515.
- Thomson CE, Gibson JN, Martin D. Interventions for the treatment of Morton's neuroma. *Cochrane Database Syst Rev*. 2004;3:CD003118.

SEE ALSO

Morton Neuroma

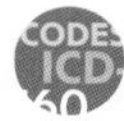

CODES

ICD10

- M77.40 Metatarsalgia, unspecified foot
- G57.60 Lesion of plantar nerve, unspecified lower limb
- M77.42 Metatarsalgia, left foot

CLINICAL PEARLS

- Metatarsalgia refers to pain of the plantar surface of the forefoot in the region of the metatarsal heads.
- Metatarsalgia is common in athletes participating in high-impact sports involving the lower extremities.
- Pain is often described as walking with a pebble in the shoe and aggravated during midstance or propulsion phases of walking or running.
- The most common physical finding is point tenderness over plantar metatarsal heads.
- Pregnant patients should wear properly fitted, low-heeled shoes to reduce incidence of metatarsalgia.

M

METHICILLIN RESISTANT STAPHYLOCOCCUS AUREUS (MRSA) SKIN INFECTIONS

Stephen A. Martin, MD, EdM • Paul P. Belliveau, PharmD, RPh

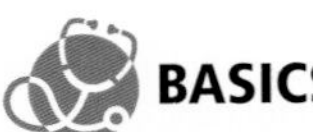

BASICS

DESCRIPTION

- Community-acquired methicillin-resistant *Staphylococcus aureus* (CA-MRSA) has unique properties allowing the organism to cause skin and soft tissue infections (SSTIs) in otherwise healthy hosts:
  - CA-MRSA has a different virulence and disease pattern than hospital-acquired MRSA (HA-MRSA).
- CA-MRSA infections are acquired by persons who have not been recently (<1 year) hospitalized or had a medical procedure (e.g., dialysis, surgery, catheters).
- *The prevalence of CA-MRSA is rapidly increasing in the United States.*
- CA-MRSA typically causes mild to moderate SSTIs, particularly abscesses, furuncles, and carbuncles:
  - Severe or invasive disease from CA-MRSA is less frequent but can include the following:
    - Necrotizing pneumonia with abscesses
    - Necrotizing fasciitis
    - Septic thrombophlebitis
    - Sepsis
    - Osteomyelitis
- Although less frequent, HA-MRSA can still cause SSTIs in the community. One study showed no significant difference in hospitalization rates among CA-MRSA, HA-MRSA, and methicillin-sensitive *S. aureus* (MSSA) infections.
- System(s) affected: skin, soft tissue

EPIDEMIOLOGY

- Predominant age: all ages, generally younger
- Predominant sex: female > male

Incidence

- 316/100,000/year (2004–2005)
- 46/100,000/year pediatric MRSA SSTI hospitalizations (2009)

PREVALENCE

- Significantly affected by local epidemiology
- 25–30% of U.S. population are colonized with *S. aureus*; up to 7% are colonized with MRSA.
- CA-MRSA isolated in ~60% of SSTIs presenting to emergency departments (range 15–74%). In 1993, 1.5 million SSTIs were seen in U.S. emergency rooms. In 2005, this had increased to 3.4 million. Hospital admission data indicate a 29% increase in SSTIs from 2000 to 2004.
- CA-MRSA accounts for up to 75% of all community staphylococcal infections in children.

ETIOLOGY AND PATHOPHYSIOLOGY

- First noted in 1980, current U.S. CA-MRSA epidemic began in 1999. The USA 300 clone is predominant.
- CA-MRSA is distinguished from HA-MRSA by
  - Lack of a multidrug-resistant phenotype
  - Presence of exotoxin virulence factors
  - Type IV *Staphylococcus* cassette cartridge (contains the methicillin-resistance gene *mecA*)

RISK FACTORS

- ~50% of patients with CA-MRSA do not have an obvious risk factor.
- Any antibiotic use in the past month
- Presence of an abscess
- Reported "spider bite"
- History of MRSA infection
- Close contact with a similar infection
- Children, particularly in daycare centers
- Competitive athletes
- Incarceration
- High prevalence in the community
- Hospitalization in the past 12 months (although *S. aureus* can colonize for years)

GENERAL PREVENTION

- Colonization (particularly of the anterior nares) is a risk factor for subsequent *S. aureus* infection. It is not yet clear whether this is also the case for CA-MRSA. Oropharyngeal and inguinal colonization are equally prevalent.
- CA-MRSA may be transmitted much more through environmental and household contact (1)[B].
- Health care workers are a major vector of MRSA for hospitalized patients, reinforcing the need for aggressive cleaning of hands and equipment.
- Research for a vaccine is underway.
- CDC guidance for prevention of MRSA in athletic community: http://www.cdc.gov/mrsa/community/team-hc-providers/advice-for-athletes.html

COMMONLY ASSOCIATED CONDITIONS

Many patients are otherwise healthy.

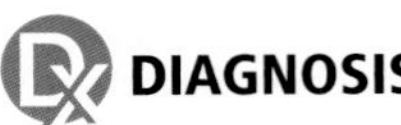

DIAGNOSIS

HISTORY

- Review potential risk factors.
- "Spider bite" is commonly confused with MRSA—patients may report an unclear history of spider bite.
- Prior MRSA skin infection
- Risk factors alone cannot rule in or rule out a CA-MRSA infection.

PHYSICAL EXAM

- Furuncles and/or carbuncles, sometimes with surrounding cellulitis. A nonsuppurative cellulitis is also possible, although it is a less common presentation of CA-MRSA.
- Erythema
- Increased warmth
- Tenderness
- Swelling
- Fluctuance
- Infected wound
- Folliculitis, pustular lesions
- Appearance like an insect or spider bite
- Tissue necrosis

DIFFERENTIAL DIAGNOSIS

SSTIs due to another cause.

DIAGNOSTIC TESTS & INTERPRETATION

Initial Tests (lab, imaging)

- Wound cultures establish definitive diagnosis. Recent guidelines recommend cultures only when a purulent lesion is accompanied by systemic signs of illness or immunocompromise (2)[B].
- Susceptibility testing; many labs use oxacillin instead of methicillin.
- A "D-zone disk-diffusion test" evaluates for inducible clindamycin resistance in CA-MRSA resistant to erythromycin.
- In unclear cases, ultrasound may help identify abscesses (3,4)[A].
- Although CT or MRI may show fascial plane edema in necrotizing fasciitis, do not delay surgical intervention waiting for imaging, particularly in ill patients.

Diagnostic Procedures/Other

Purulent lesions should be incised and drained (I&D); needle aspiration is not recommended (2).

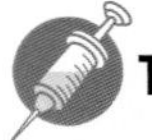

TREATMENT

- A recent guideline recommends antibiotics active against MRSA for patients with carbuncles or abscesses who failed initial antibiotic treatment, have markedly impaired host defenses, or present with systemic inflammatory response (SIRS) and hypotension (2).
- Routine use of agents to eliminate MRSA colonization for patients with active infection or their close contacts is not currently recommended.
- Most CA-MRSA infections are localized SSTIs and not requiring hospitalization or vancomycin.
- Initial empirical antibiotic coverage should be based on local CA-MRSA prevalence and individual patient risk factors.
- http://www.cdc.gov/mrsa/pdf/Flowchart_pstr.pdf

GENERAL MEASURES

- Modify therapy based on culture and susceptibility.
- Determine if household or other close contacts have SSTI or other infections and evaluate accordingly.
- Treat underlying condition (e.g., tinea pedis).
- Restrict contact if wound cannot be covered.
- Elevate affected area.

MEDICATION

ALERT

For purulent infections, basic principles include surgical drainage and debulking, wound culture, and narrow-spectrum antimicrobials:

- *Successful I&D may have more impact than antibiotics in mild cases for both adults and children.*
- Moist heat may work for small furuncles.
- Patients with an abscess are frequently cured by incision and drainage alone.
- Packing does not appear to improve outcomes (3)[A].

First Line

CA-MRSA SSTIs: Treat with a 7–14-day course of one of the following agents (duration of therapy depends on severity and clinical response):

- Trimethoprim/sulfamethoxazole (TMP-SMX): DS (160 mg TMP and 800 mg of SMX) 1–2 tablet(s) PO BID daily (8–12 mg/kg/day of trimethoprim component in 2 divided doses for children)
- Doxycycline or minocycline: 100 mg PO BID (children >8 years and <45 kg; 2–5 mg/kg/day PO in 1–2 divided doses, not to exceed 200 mg/day; children >8 years and >45 kg, use adult dosing), taken with a full glass of water

- Clindamycin: 300–450 mg PO QID (30–40 mg/kg/day PO in 3 divided doses for children), taken with full glass of water. Check D-zone test in erythromycin-resistant, clindamycin-susceptible *S. aureus* isolates (if the test is positive, this shows induced resistance and a new antibiotic should be chosen).
- CA-MRSA is resistant to β-lactams (including oral cephalosporins and antistaphylococcal penicillins) and often macrolides, azalides, and quinolones.
- Although most CA-MRSA isolates are susceptible to rifampin, this drug should *never* be used as a single agent because of concerns of resistance. The role of combination therapy with rifampin in CA-MRSA SSTIs is not clearly defined.
- There has been increasing resistance to clindamycin, both initial (~33%) and induced.
- Although CA-MRSA isolates are susceptible to vancomycin, oral vancomycin cannot be used for CA-MRSA SSTIs due to limited GI absorption.

Second Line

For treatment of severe CA-MRSA SSTIs requiring hospitalization or for HA-MRSA SSTIs, consider 1 of the following:

- Vancomycin: Generally, 1 g IV q12h (30 mg/kg/day IV in 2 divided doses; in children: 40 mg/kg/day IV in 4 divided doses) vancomycin-like antibiotics that require only 1 or 2 doses may soon be more broadly available (5)[A].
- Linezolid: 600 mg IV/PO BID (uncomplicated: children <5 years of age, 30 mg/kg/day in 3 divided doses; 20 mg/kg/day IV/PO in 2 divided doses for children 5–11 years of age; children >11 years, use adult dosing. Complicated: birth to 11 years, 30 mg/kg/day IV/PO in 3 divided doses; older, use adult dosing)
  - Linezolid seems to be more effective than vancomycin for treating people with SSTIs, but current studies have high risk of bias.
- Clindamycin: 600 mg IV TID; in children, 10–13 mg/kg/dose q6–8h up to 40 mg/kg/day
- Daptomycin: 4 mg/kg/day IV (safety/efficacy not established in patients <18 years of age) if no pulmonary involvement
- Ceftaroline 600 mg BID IV (for adults)

Pediatric Considerations

- Tetracyclines not recommended <8 years of age
- TMP-SMX not recommended <2 months

Pregnancy Considerations

- Tetracyclines are contraindicated.
- TMP-SMX not recommended in 1st or 3rd trimester

Geriatric Considerations

A recent review notes no prospective trials in this age group and recommends use of general adult guidelines.

ISSUES FOR REFERRAL

Consider consultation with infectious disease in cases of

- Refractory CA-MRSA infection
- Plan to attempt decolonization

SURGERY/OTHER PROCEDURES

Progression to serious SSTIs, including necrotizing fasciitis, is possible and mandates prompt surgical evaluation.

INPATIENT CONSIDERATIONS

Admission Criteria/Initial Stabilization

Consider admission in patients either

- Systemically ill (e.g., febrile) with stable comorbidities, or
- Systemically well with comorbidities that may delay or complicate resolution of their SSTI
- Depends on severity of SSTI, presence of SSTI complications (sepsis, necrotizing fasciitis), and comorbidities

Nursing

Contact precautions

Discharge Criteria

If admitted for IV therapy, assess the following before discharge:

- Afebrile for 24 hours
- Clinically improved
- Able to take oral medication
- Has adequate social support and is available for outpatient follow-up

ONGOING CARE

FOLLOW-UP RECOMMENDATIONS

Patient Monitoring

For outpatients:

- Return promptly with systemic symptoms, worsening local symptoms, or failure to improve within 48 hours. Consider a follow-up within 48 hours of initial visit to assess response and review culture.

PATIENT EDUCATION

- Keep wounds that are draining covered with clean, dry bandages.
- Clean hands regularly with soap and water or alcohol-based gel. Hot shower daily with soap.
- Do not share items that may be contaminated (including razors or towels).
- Clean clothes, towels, and bed linens.

The CDC has gathered information for health care professionals, including clinical guides, via the National MRSA Education Initiative: www.cdc.gov/mrsa/.

PROGNOSIS

- In outpatients, improvement should occur within 48 hours.

Data are limited as to risk of recurrence.

COMPLICATIONS

- Necrotizing pneumonia or empyema (after an influenza-like illness)
- Necrotizing fasciitis
- Sepsis syndrome
- Pyomyositis and osteomyelitis
- Purpura fulminans
- Disseminated septic emboli
- Endocarditis

REFERENCES

1. Uhlemann AC, Dordel J, Knox JR, et al. Molecular tracing of the emergence, diversification, and transmission of S. aureus sequence type 8 in a New York community. *Proc Natl Acad Sci U S A*. 2014;111(18):6738–6743.
2. Stevens DL, Bisno AL, Chambers HF, et al. Practice guidelines for the diagnosis and management of skin and soft tissue infections: 2014 update by the Infectious Diseases Society of America. *Clin Infect Dis*. D014;59(2):e10–e52.
3. Mistry RD. Skin and soft tissue infections. *Pediatr Clin North Am*. 2013;60(5):1063–1082. doi:10.1016/j.pcl.2013.06.011.
4. Singer AJ, Talan DA. Management of skin abscesses in the era of methicillin-resistant *Staphylococcus aureus*. *N Engl J Med*. 2014;370(11):1039–1047. doi:10.1056/NEJMra1212788.
5. Chambers HF. Pharmacology and the treatment of complicated skin and skin-structure infections. *N Engl J Med*. 2014;370(23):2238–2239.

ADDITIONAL READING

- Breen JO. Skin and soft tissue infections in immunocompetent patients. *Am Fam Physician*. 2010;81(7):893–899.
- Chen LF, Chastain C, Anderson DJ. Community-acquired methicillin-resistant *Staphylococcus aureus* skin and soft tissue infections: management and prevention. *Curr Infect Dis Rep*. 2011;13(5):442–450.
- Chuck EA, Frazee BW, Lambert L, et al. The benefit of empiric treatment for methicillin-resistant *Staphylococcus aureus*. *J Emerg Med*. 2010;38(5):567–571.
- Dryden MS. Complicated skin and soft tissue infection. *J Antimicrob Chemother*. 2010;65(Suppl 3):iii35–iii44.
- Fitch MT, Manthey DE, McGinnis HD, et al. Videos in clinical medicine. Abscess incision and drainage. *N Engl J Med*. 2007;357(19):e20. doi:10.1056/NEJMvcm071319.
- Gurusamy KS, Koti R, Toon CD, et al. Antibiotic therapy for the treatment of methicillin-resistant *Staphylococcus aureus* (MRSA) infections in surgical wounds. *Cochrane Database Syst Rev*. 2013;(8):CD009726.

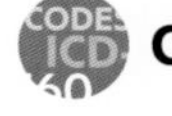

CODES

ICD10

- L08.89 Oth local infections of the skin and subcutaneous tissue
- A49.02 Methicillin resis staph infection, unsp site
- Z22.322 Carrier or suspected carrier of methicillin resis staph

CLINICAL PEARLS

- Incise and drain purulent lesions and send for wound culture if abscess is present.
- Prevalence and susceptibilities of CA-MRSA dictates treatment in different location. The CDC has a helpful algorithm for outpatient treatment of CA-MRSA: http://www.cdc.gov/mrsa/pdf/Flowchart_pstr.pdf.
- A mixture of 1/4-cup household bleach diluted in 1 gallon of water can be used to clean surfaces.

MILD COGNITIVE IMPAIRMENT

Birju B. Patel, MD, FACP, AGSF • N. Wilson Holland, MD, FACP, AGSF

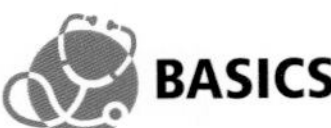

BASICS

DESCRIPTION

- Mild cognitive impairment (MCI) is defined as significant cognitive impairment in the absence of dementia, as measured by standard memory tests:
  - Concern regarding change in cognition
  - Preservation of independence in functional activities (ADLs)
  - Impairment in ≥1 cognitive domains (attention, executive dysfunction, memory, visuospatial, language) (1)
  - Other terms used in the literature relating to MCI: isolated memory impairment; cognitive impairment not dementia (CIND); predementia; mild cognitive disorder; age-associated memory impairment; age-related cognitive decline; benign senescent forgetfulness. Some of these conditions do not progress to dementia (i.e., benign senescent forgetfulness, age-associated memory impairment, age-related cognitive decline). *DSM-5* mentions "mild neurocognitive disorder" (NCD) which may be a precursor to Alzheimer disease and has many of the same features as MCI (2).
- Annual rates of conversion of MCI to dementia are 2–15% in the elderly.

EPIDEMIOLOGY

Incidence

- Predominant sex: male > female (3)
- Predominant age:
  - Higher in older persons and in those with less education
  - 12–15/1,000 person-years in those age ≥65 years
  - 54/1,000 person-years in those age ≥75 years

Prevalence

- MCI is more prevalent than dementia in the United States.
- 3–5% for those age ≥60 years
- 15% for those age ≥75 years

ETIOLOGY AND PATHOPHYSIOLOGY

- Subtypes of MCI:
  - Single-domain amnestic
  - Multiple-domain amnestic
  - Nonamnestic single-domain
  - Nonamnestic multiple-domain
- The amnestic subtype is higher risk for progression to Alzheimer disease (4).
- Vascular, degenerative, traumatic, metabolic, psychiatric, or a combination

Genetics

Apolipoprotein (APO) E4 genotype: Various pathways exist leading to amyloid accumulation and deposition thought to be associated with dementia.

RISK FACTORS

- Age
- Diabetes
- Hypertension
- Hyperlipidemia
- Cerebrovascular disease
- Smoking
- Sleep apnea
- APO E4 genotype

COMMONLY ASSOCIATED CONDITIONS

See "Risk Factors" (5)

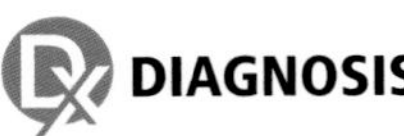

DIAGNOSIS

HISTORY

- Focus on cognitive deficits and impairment.
- Review all medications that may affect cognition; give particular emphasis to anticholinergic medications (patients on these may mistakenly be classified as having MCI).
- Rule out depression.
- Assess function (ADLs, instrumental ADLs) and subtle changes in daily function (e.g., in the workplace).
- Impact on interpersonal relationships and caregiver stress
- Assess vascular risk factors (hypertension, diabetes, hyperlipidemia, and cerebrovascular disease)
- Assess behavioral changes.

PHYSICAL EXAM

- A general exam focusing on clinical clues to identifying vascular disease (e.g., bruits, abnormal BP)
- Neurologic exam to rule out reversible CNS causes cognitive impairment or other causes of cognitive impairment (e.g., Parkinson disease).
- Office measures of cognitive function, depression, and functional status

DIFFERENTIAL DIAGNOSIS

- Delirium
- Dementia
- Depression
- "Reversible" cognitive impairment
  - Medications (anticholinergics and medications with anticholinergic properties)
  - Hypothyroidism
  - Vitamin B_{12} deficiency
- Reversible CNS conditions
- Give consideration to sleep conditions, especially sleep apnea, that can contribute to cognitive deficits.

DIAGNOSTIC TESTS & INTERPRETATION

Initial Tests (lab, imaging)

- CBC
- Comprehensive metabolic profile
- Thyroid-stimulating hormone
- Vitamin B_{12}
- Lipids
- Consider HIV testing in the appropriate risk setting.
- Imaging tests are helpful when there are focal neurologic deficits or rapid or atypical presentations:
  - CT scan can detect structural CNS conditions leading to cognitive impairment:
    - Subdural hematoma
    - Normal pressure hydrocephalus
    - Metastatic disease
  - MRI further evaluates vascular, infectious, neoplastic, and inflammatory conditions.
- Rule out reversible causes of cognitive impairment.
- Cognitive testing is important (e.g., Montreal Cognitive Assessment [MOCA] and Saint Louis University Mental Status [SLUMS]); MOCA may be more sensitive for detecting and following MCI.
- Neuropsychological testing for complex and atypical presentations
- Vascular risk factor reduction and treatment

Follow-Up Tests & Special Considerations

- Document progression of functional impairment, cognitive decline, concurrent depression, and comorbid conditions.
- Advanced planning while patient is competent.
- Early education of caregivers on safety, maintaining structure, managing stress, and future planning

Test Interpretation

- Little is known about MCI pathology due to a lack of longitudinal studies.
- Alzheimer dementia pathophysiology:
  - Neurofibrillary tangles in hippocampus
  - Senile plaques (amyloid deposition)
  - Neuronal degeneration
- Those with MCI have intermediate amounts of pathologic findings of Alzheimer disease with amyloid deposition and neurofibrillary tangles in the mesial temporal lobes compared with those with dementia.
- Amnestic MCI is associated with white matter hyperintensity volume on MRI, whereas nonamnestic MCI is associated with infarcts.

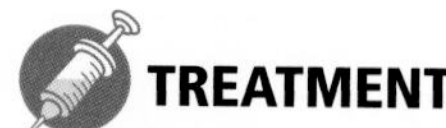

TREATMENT

GENERAL MEASURES

Atherosclerotic risk factors should be treated aggressively.

MEDICATION

The use of cholinesterase inhibitors (ChEIs) in MCI is not associated with any delay in the onset of Alzheimer disease or dementia. Moreover, the safety profile showed that the risks associated with ChEIs are significant. Therefore, ChEIs are not recommended routinely (6)[A],(7)[C].

ISSUES FOR REFERRAL

Consider referral to a memory specialist (i.e., geriatrician, neurologist, geropsychiatrist, neuropsychologist) to evaluate and differentiate subtypes of MCI and specific cognitive deficits.

COMPLEMENTARY & ALTERNATIVE MEDICINE

- No evidence suggests the efficacy of vitamin E in the prevention or treatment of people with MCI. More research is needed to identify the role of vitamin E, if any, in the management of cognitive impairment.
- Long-term use of ginkgo biloba extract has shown to have no benefit in the treatment of MCI and in terms of progression to dementia. In addition, ginkgo biloba can be associated with increase in bleeding risk including CNS bleeds (8)[B].

INPATIENT CONSIDERATIONS

- Delirium is more common in patients hospitalized with all forms of cognitive impairment.
- Avoid medications that may worsen or precipitate cognitive decline (e.g., anticholinergics, antihistamines).
- Patients may be extremely sensitive to the hospital environment:
  - Moderate level of stimulation is best.
  - Avoid sensory deprivation. Make sure that patients have access to hearing aids and eyeglasses.
  - Use frequent cueing and have caregivers or family in the room whenever possible with patient.
  - Frequently orient patients to date and time.

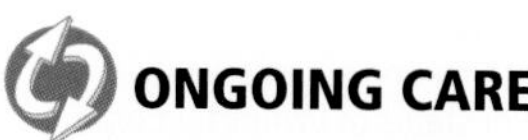

ONGOING CARE

FOLLOW-UP RECOMMENDATIONS

Patients should be reevaluated every 6–12 months to determine if symptoms are progressing.

Patient Monitoring

Appropriate cognitive and functional testing should be used to evaluate progression, along with clinical history and exam. If a medication is started, patients need to be followed more frequently to evaluate for efficacy, side effects, dose titration, and so forth. Declining executive function may be an early marker to progression of MCI to dementia, and clinicians should monitor and advise patients and families proactively to look for this. Impairments in ADL function is a good clue to progression to dementia from MCI.

DIET

Diets that are promoted by the American Heart Association to minimize atherosclerotic risk factors should be emphasized.

PATIENT EDUCATION

- Encourage lifestyle changes:
  - Physical activity, such as walking 30 minutes daily on most days of the week
  - Mental activity that stimulates language skills and psychomotor coordination should be encouraged. Computer activities, reading books, crafts, crossword puzzles, and games may be linked to decreased risk of development of MCI (9)[C],(10)[B].
- Cognitive rehabilitation strategies may be beneficial in helping with daily activities relating to memory tasks in MCI.
- Participation in exercise programs modestly improved some measures of cognition in some studies.
- Treatment of vascular risk factors (hypertension, diabetes, cerebrovascular disease, and hyperlipidemia) is important in lowering risk of progression to dementia.

PROGNOSIS

- Conversion rates from MCI to dementia range from 5 to 15% annually.
- Amnestic subtypes of MCI are most likely to progress to dementia.

REFERENCES

1. Petersen RC. Clinical practice. Mild cognitive impairment. *N Engl J Med*. 2011;364(23):2227–2234.
2. Peterson RC, Caracciolo B, Brayne C, et al. Mild cognitive impairment: a concept in evolution. *J Intern Med*. 2014;275(3):214–228.
3. Petersen RC, Roberts RO, Knopman DS, et al. Prevalence of mild cognitive impairment is higher in men. The Mayo Clinic Study of Aging. *Neurology*. 2010;75(10):889–897.
4. Albert MS, DeKosky ST, Dickson D, et al. The diagnosis of mild cognitive impairment due to Alzheimer's disease: recommendations from the National Institute on Aging-Alzheimer's Association workgroups on diagnostic guidelines for Alzheimer's disease. *Alzheimers Dement*. 2011;7(3):270–279.
5. Li J, Wang YJ, Zhang M, et al. Vascular risk factors promote conversion from mild cognitive impairment to Alzheimer disease. *Neurology*. 2011;76(17):1485–1491.
6. Russ TC, Morling JR. Cholinesterase inhibitors for mild cognitive impairment. *Cochrane Database Syst Rev*. 2012;(9):CD009132.
7. Patel BP, Holland NW. Adverse effects of acetylcholinesterase inhibitors clinical geriatrics. *Clin Geriatr*. 2011;19:27–30.
8. Vellas B, Coley N, Ousset PJ, et al. Long-term use of standardised ginkgo biloba extract for the prevention of Alzheimer's disease (GuidAge): a randomised placebo-controlled trial. *Lancet Neurol*. 2012;11(10):851–859.
9. Marshall GA, Rentz DM, Frey MT, et al. Executive function and instrumental activities of daily living in mild cognitive impairment and Alzheimer's disease. *Alzheimers Dement*. 2011;7(3):300–308.
10. Nagamatsu LS, Handy TC, Hsu CL, et al. Resistance training promotes cognitive and functional brain plasticity in seniors with probable mild cognitive impairment. *Arch Intern Med*. 2012;172(8):666–668.

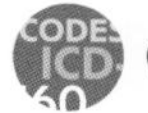

CODES

ICD10

G31.84 Mild cognitive impairment, so stated

CLINICAL PEARLS

- Amnestic MCI affects primarily memory and is more likely to progress to Alzheimer dementia.
- Screen for reversible factors, particularly anticholinergic medications, depression, and sleep disorders.
- Look closely at vascular risk factors and modify them as best as possible.
- ChEIs should not be used routinely unless memory complaints are affecting quality of life in patients. Potential side effects of these medications should be thoroughly discussed with patients and their families. A baseline EKG should be done prior to initiation of ChEIs due to risk of bradycardia and syncope.
- Encourage both physical and mental exercises.

MITRAL REGURGITATION

Yongkasem Vorasettakarnkij, MD, MSc

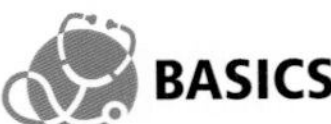

BASICS

DESCRIPTION

- Disorder of mitral valve (MV) closure, either primary or secondary (functional), resulting in a backflow of the left ventricular (LV) stroke volume into the left atrium (LA); uncompensated, this leads to LV and LA enlargement, elevated pulmonary pressures, atrial fibrillation, heart failure, and sudden cardiac death.
- Types of mitral regurgitation (MR)
  - Acute versus chronic
  - Primary versus secondary (functional)
    - Primary: MV structures include not only the mitral annulus, MV leaflets, chordae tendineae, and papillary muscles but also posterior LA wall and LV wall.
    - Secondary: No valvular abnormalities are found. The abnormal and dilated LV causes papillary muscle displacement, resulting in leaflet tethering with annular dilatation that prevents coaptation.
- System(s) affected: cardiac; pulmonary

EPIDEMIOLOGY

Moderate to severe MR affects 2.5 million people in the United States (2000 data). It is the most common valvular disease, and its prevalence is expected to double by 2030 (1).

Prevalence

- By severity on echocardiography
  - Mild MR: 19% (up to 40% if trivial jets included)
  - Moderate MR: 1.9%
  - Severe MR: 0.2%
- By category (1)
  - Degenerative (myxomatous disease, annular calcification): 60–70%
  - Ischemic: 20%
  - Endocarditis: 2–5%
  - Rheumatic: 2–5%

ETIOLOGY AND PATHOPHYSIOLOGY

- Acute MR: Acute damage to MV leads to sudden LA and LV volume overload. Sudden rise in LV volume load without compensatory LV remodeling results in impaired forward cardiac output and possible cardiogenic shock.
- Chronic MR: LV eccentric hypertrophy compensates for increased regurgitant volume to maintain forward cardiac output and alleviate pulmonary congestion. However, ongoing LV remodeling can result in LV dysfunction. Simultaneously, LA compensatory dilatation for the larger regurgitant volume predisposes patients to develop atrial fibrillation (AF).
- Ischemic MR: papillary muscle rupture, ischemia during acute myocardial infarction (MI), and incomplete coaptation of valve leaflets or restricted valve movement resulting from ischemia
- Acute MR
  - Flail leaflet: myxomatous disease, infective endocarditis, or trauma
  - Ruptured chordae tendineae: trauma, spontaneous rupture, infective endocarditis, or rheumatic fever
  - Ruptured or displaced papillary muscle: acute MI, severe myocardial ischemia, or trauma
- Chronic MR
  - Primary
    - Degenerative: mitral annular calcification, mitral valve prolapse (MVP)
    - Infective endocarditis
    - Rheumatic heart disease (RHD)
    - Inflammatory diseases: lupus, eosinophilic endocardial disease
    - Anorectic drugs
    - Congenital (cleft leaflet)
  - Secondary (functional)
    - Ischemic: coronary artery disease (CAD)/MI
    - Nonischemic: cardiomyopathy, LV dysfunction from any cause, hypertrophic cardiomyopathy

RISK FACTORS

Age, hypertension, RHD, endocarditis, anorectic drugs

GENERAL PREVENTION

- Risk factor modification for CAD
- Antibiotic prophylaxis for poststreptococcal RHD
- Endocarditis prophylaxis for MR is no longer recommended.

COMMONLY ASSOCIATED CONDITIONS

MVP with MR common in Marfan syndrome

DIAGNOSIS

HISTORY

- Associated conditions: RHD, prior MI, connective tissue disorder
- Acute MR
  - Sudden onset of dyspnea
  - Orthopnea, paroxysmal nocturnal dyspnea
  - Chronic MR
    - Exertional dyspnea
    - Fatigue
    - Palpitation: paroxysmal/persistent AF

PHYSICAL EXAM

- Acute MR
  - Rapid and thready pulses
  - Sign of poor tissue perfusion with peripheral vasoconstriction
  - Hyperdynamic precordium without apical displacement
  - S_3 and S_4 (if in sinus rhythm)
  - Systolic murmur at left sternal border and base
    - Early, middle, or holosystolic murmur
    - Often soft, low-pitched decrescendo murmur
  - Rales
- Chronic MR
  - Brisk upstroke of arterial pulse
  - Leftward displaced LV apical impulse
  - Systolic thrill at the apex (suggests severe MR)
  - Soft S_1 and widely split S_2, S_3 gallop
  - Loud P_2 (if pulmonary hypertension)
  - Holosystolic murmur at apex that radiates to axilla
  - Ankle edema, jugular venous distension, and ascites, if development of right-sided heart failure

DIFFERENTIAL DIAGNOSIS

- Aortic stenosis (AS): usually midsystolic but can be long; difficult to distinguish from holosystolic, at apical area, and radiating to the carotid arteries (unlike MR)
- Tricuspid regurgitation: holosystolic but at left lower sternal border; does not radiate to axilla or increase in intensity with inspiration (unlike MR)
- Ventricular septal defect (VSD): harsh holosystolic murmur at lower left sternal border but radiates to right sternal border (not axilla)

DIAGNOSTIC TESTS & INTERPRETATION

- Chest x-ray (CXR)
  - Acute MR: pulmonary edema, normal heart size
  - Chronic MR: LA and LV enlargement
- ECG
  - Acute MR
    - Varies depending on etiologies (e.g., acute MI)
  - Chronic MR
    - P mitrale from LA enlargement, AF
    - LV hypertrophy
    - Q waves from prior MI

Initial Tests (lab, imaging)

- Cardiac enzymes and brain natriuretic peptide (BNP), if appropriate
- Transthoracic echocardiogram (TTE)
  - Indications for TTE (2)
    - Baseline evaluation of LV function, right ventricular and LA size, pulmonary artery pressure, and severity of MR
    - Delineation of mechanism of MR
    - Surveillance of asymptomatic moderate to severe LV dysfunction (ejection fraction [EF] and end-systolic dimension [ESD])
    - Evaluate MV apparatus and LV size and function after a change in signs/symptoms in a patient with MR.
    - Evaluate after MV repair or replacement.
  - Findings in acute MR
    - Evidence of etiology: flail leaflet or infective vegetations
    - Normal LA and LV size
  - Findings in chronic MR
    - Evidence of degenerative, rheumatic, ischemic, congenital, and other causes
    - Enlarged LA and LV

Follow-Up Tests & Special Considerations

- Intervals for follow up TTE: See "Follow-Up Recommendations."
- Cardiovascular magnetic resonance (CMR)
  - TTE results are not satisfactory to assess LV and RV volumes, function, or MR severity (2)[C].
- Transesophageal echocardiogram (TEE)
  - Intraoperatively to define severity/cause of MR and/or LV function (2)[C]
  - Nondiagnostic information about severity, mechanism, and/or status of LV function from noninvasive imaging (2)[C]
- Exercise Doppler echo
  - Assess exercise tolerance and the effects of exercise on pulmonary artery pressure in asymptomatic patients with severe MR.
- Noninvasive imaging (stress nuclear/position emission tomography, CMR, stress echocardiography), cardiac CT angiography, or cardiac catheterization, including coronary angiography
  - To establish etiology of chronic secondary MR and/or to assess myocardial viability (2)[C]

Diagnostic Procedures/Other

Cardiac catheterization (2)

- Hemodynamic measurements: Pulmonary pressure is discordant to the severity of MR as assessed by noninvasive testing.

- Left ventriculography and hemodynamic measurement
  - Noninvasive tests are inconclusive regarding severity of MR.
  - Regurgitant severity is discordant between clinical and noninvasive findings.
- Coronary angiography: prior to MV surgery in patients at risk for CAD

Test Interpretation

Quantification of severe MR requires integration of the following:

- Structural parameters
  - LA size: dilated, unless acute
  - LV size: dilated, unless acute
  - Leaflets: abnormal
- Doppler parameters
- Quantitative parameter

TREATMENT

MEDICATION

- Acute, severe MR
  - Medical therapy has a limited role and is aimed primarily to stabilize hemodynamics preoperatively.
  - Vasodilators (nitroprusside, nicardipine): to improve hemodynamic compensation but is often limited by systemic hypotension (2)
- Chronic MR
  - Primary
    - Asymptomatic: no proven long-term medical therapy
    - Symptomatic: diuretics, β-blockers (carvedilol, metoprolol),angiotensin-converting enzyme inhibitors (ACEIs) or angiotensin receptor blockers (ARBs), and possibly aldosterone antagonists as indicated in standard therapy for heart failure (2)[C]
  - Secondary: LV dysfunction or symptomatic (stages B–D)
    - ACEIs or ARBs, β-blockers, diuretics, and possibly aldosterone antagonists as indicated in standard therapy for heart failure (2)[C]

SURGERY/OTHER PROCEDURES

- Isolated MV surgery is not indicated for patients with mild to moderate MR.
- Acute, severe MR secondary to acute MI
  - Acute rupture of papillary muscle: emergency MV repair/replacement
  - Papillary muscle displacement
    - Aggressive medical stabilization and intra-aortic balloon pump
    - Valve surgery usually required in addition to revascularization.
- Chronic severe MR
  - MV repair in an experienced center is recommended over MV replacement in most circumstances (3):
    - Survival rate: Early and overall mortality were lower after MV repair than after MV replacement.
    - 10-year rate of stroke: 10% (repair) versus 12% (bioprosthetic valve replacement) versus 23% (mechanical valve replacement)
    - Risk of endocarditis: 1.5% at 15 years versus 0.3–1.2% per year
    - Overall rates of reoperation are similar.
  - Severe primary MR (2)
  - MV surgery
    - Symptomatic patients (stage D)
      - Absence of severe LV dysfunction (EF ≥30%) (2)[C]
      - Severe LV dysfunction (EF <30%) (2)[C]
    - Asymptomatic patients
      - Mild to moderate LV dysfunction (EF 30–60% and/or ESD ≥40 mm, stage C2) (2)[C]
      - MV repair is reasonable for asymptomatic patients (stage C1) with preserved LV function (EF >60% and ESD <40 mm):
        - The likelihood of successful repair without residual MR is >95% and expected mortality <1% when performed at a heart valve center of excellence (2)[C].
        - Nonrheumatic MR with new onset AF or resting pulmonary hypertension (pulmonary artery systolic pressure [PASP] >50 mm Hg) and the likelihood of a successful and durable repair is high (2)[C].
    - Transcatheter MV repair: may be considered for severely symptomatic patients (NYHA class III/IV) despite optimal GDMT for HF, who have a reasonable life expectancy but a prohibitive surgical risk because of severe comorbidities (2)[C]
  - Severe secondary MR (2)
  - MV surgery
    - Undergoing coronary artery bypass graft (CABG) or aortic valve replacement (AVR) (2)[C]
    - Persistent symptom (NYHA class III-IV) despite optimal GDMT for HF (2)[C]
  - Cardiac resynchronization therapy with biventricular pacing is recommended for symptomatic patients (stage B–D) who meet the indications for device therapy (2)[C].

Geriatric Considerations

- Medical therapy alone for patients >75 years of age with MR is preferred, owing to increased operative mortality and decreased survival (compared with those with AS), especially with preexisting CAD or need for MV replacement.
- MV repair is preferable to MV replacement.

INPATIENT CONSIDERATIONS

Admission Criteria/Initial Stabilization

Acute MR: Stabilize ABCs (airway, breathing, circulation). Initiate IV, O_2, and monitoring. Nitroprusside (+dobutamine and/or aortic balloon counterpulsation if hypotensive). Treat underlying causes (e.g., MI). Treat acute pulmonary edema with furosemide, morphine. Obtain urgent surgical consultation.

ONGOING CARE

FOLLOW-UP RECOMMENDATIONS

Chronic MR: asymptomatic

- Mild MR with normal LV size and function and no pulmonary hypertension: annual clinical evaluation to assess symptom progression and TTE every 3–5 years to assess MR severity, LV size and function
- Moderate MR: annual clinical evaluation and TTE every 1–2 years
- Severe MR: clinical evaluation and TTE every 6–12 months
- Consider serial CXRs and ECGs, and consider stress test if exercise capacity is doubtful.

PATIENT EDUCATION

- Exercise after MV repair: Avoid sports with risk for bodily contact or trauma. Low-intensity competitive sports are allowed.
- Competitive athletes with MR
  - Asymptomatic with normal LV size and function, normal pulmonary artery pressures, and sinus rhythm: no restrictions
  - Mildly symptomatic and those with LV dilatation: Activities with low to moderate dynamic and static cardiac demand allowed
- AF and anticoagulation: no contact sports

PROGNOSIS

- Acute, severe MR: Mortality risk with surgery is 50%; mortality risk with medical therapy alone, 75% in first 24 hours; 95% at 2 weeks
- Chronic MR: asymptomatic severe MR with normal LVEF: 10% yearly rate of progression to symptoms and subnormal resting LVEF. Symptomatic severe MR: 8-year survival rate, 33% without surgery; mortality rate, 5% yearly

Pregnancy Considerations

MR with NYHA functional class III–IV at high risk for maternal and/or fetal risk

COMPLICATIONS

Acute pulmonary edema, CHF, AF, bleeding risk with anticoagulation, endocarditis, sudden cardiac death

REFERENCES

1. Enriquez-Sarano M, Akins CW, Vahanian A. Mitral regurgitation. *Lancet*. 2009;373(9672):1382–1394.
2. Nishimura RA, Otto CM, Bonow RO, et al. 2014 AHA/ACC guideline for the management of patients with valvular heart disease. *Circulation*. 2014;129(23):e521–e643.
3. Foster E. Clinical practice. Mitral regurgitation due to degenerative mitral-valve disease. *N Engl J Med*. 2010;363(2):156–165.

ADDITIONAL READING

- Acker MA, Parides MK, Perrault LP, et al. Mitral-valve repair versus replacement for severe ischemic mitral regurgitation. *N Engl J Med*. 2014;370(1):23–32.
- Feldman T, Young A. Percutaneous approaches to valve repair for mitral regurgitation. *J Am Coll Cardiol*. 2014;63(20):2057–2068.
- Vahanian A, Alfieri O, Andreotti F, et al. Guidelines on the management of valvular heart disease (version 2012). *Eur Heart J*. 2012;33(19):2451–2496.
- Yancy CW, Jessup M, Bozkurt B, et al. 2013 ACCF/AHA guideline for the management of heart failure. *Circulation*. 2013;128(16):e240–e327.

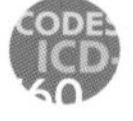

CODES

ICD10

- I34.0 Nonrheumatic mitral (valve) insufficiency
- I05.1 Rheumatic mitral insufficiency
- Q23.3 Congenital mitral insufficiency

CLINICAL PEARLS

- Follow-up for mild to moderate MR: serial exam and/or echo unless LV structural changes
- Severe MR is usually managed with MV repair.
- Endocarditis prophylaxis is not recommended.

MITRAL STENOSIS

Zeeshan Hussain, MD • Nirmanmoh Bhatia, MD • Marcus F. Stoddard, MD

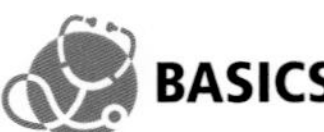

BASICS

DESCRIPTION

- Mitral stenosis (MS) presents as resistance to diastolic filling of the left ventricle (LV) due to narrowing of mitral valve (MV) orifice.
- Normal valve orifice 4–6 cm^2; symptoms typically seen when orifice is $<$2.5 cm^2.
- Hemodynamic consequences are due to passive transmission of left atrial (LA) pressure to the pulmonary circulation. May coexist with mitral regurgitation and aortic valvulopathies
- Stages vary from A (with risk factors), B (hemodynamically obstruction), C (severe but no symptoms) to D (symptomatic) (1).

EPIDEMIOLOGY

- Most common acquired valvular disease secondary to rheumatic heart disease (60% of cases)
- Predominant age: Symptoms primarily occur in 4th–7th decades.
- Predominant sex: female $>$ male (2:1)

Incidence

Decreased incidence of MS is seen in the United States because of decreased incidence of rheumatic fever (primarily shift in prevalence away from rheumatogenic strains of group A streptococci [GAS] and also treatment of GAS infection). However, global burden remains significant (2).

ETIOLOGY AND PATHOPHYSIOLOGY

- Obstruction between LA and LV impairs LV filling during diastole and leads to increased LA pressure.
- Increased LA pressure is transmitted passively ("back pressure") to the pulmonary circulation; over time, pulmonary hypertension (HTN) results.
- Over time, LA pressure overload can dilate the chamber and interrupt the cardiac conduction system, resulting in atrial fibrillation.
- Pulmonary HTN can also cause increased collateralization between pulmonary and bronchial circulation, resulting in intraparenchymal hemorrhage with hemoptysis.
- Rheumatic fever: most common (see "Risk Factors")
- Aging (extension of mitral annular calcification)
- Rare causes
  - Congenital (associated with mucopolysaccharidoses)
  - Autoimmune: systemic lupus erythematosus (SLE), rheumatoid arthritis
  - Malignant carcinoid
  - Other acquired: LA myxoma, LA thrombus. Endomyocardial fibrosis

RISK FACTORS

- Rheumatic fever is the greatest risk factor:
  - 30–40% of rheumatic fever patients eventually develop MS, presenting an average of 20 years after diagnosis of rheumatic fever.
  - Acute rheumatic fever occurs 2–3 weeks after episode of untreated GAS pharyngitis caused by rheumatogenic organism in a genetically susceptible host.
  - Low socioeconomic status (i.e., crowded conditions) favors the spread of streptococcal infection.
- Aging (increasing valvular calcification)
- Chest irradiation (increasing tissue fibrosis)

GENERAL PREVENTION

- Prompt recognition and treatment of GAS infection; recognition of cardinal signs and symptoms of acute rheumatic fever via Jones criteria
- Modified Jones criteria for Acute Rheumatic Fever: Diagnosis requires evidence of streptococcal infection plus 2 major criteria or 1 major plus 2 minor criteria.

Evidence of streptococcal infection	Antistreptolysin O titer or positive throat culture
Major criteria	Carditis, polyarthritis, Sydenham chorea, erythema marginatum, subcutaneous nodules
Minor criteria	Migratory arthralgias, fever, acute phase reactants (elevated erythrocyte sedimentation rate [ESR], leukocytosis), prolonged PR interval on ECG

COMMONLY ASSOCIATED CONDITIONS

- Atrial fibrillation (30–40% of symptomatic patients)
- Associated valve lesions due to chronic inflammation (aortic stenosis, aortic insufficiency)
- Pulmonary congestion and pulmonary HTN
- Right heart failure
- Systemic embolism, pulmonary embolism (10%)
- Infection, including Infectious endocarditis (1–5%)

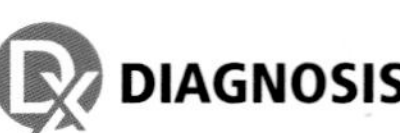

DIAGNOSIS

HISTORY

- History of rheumatic fever
- Severity of presentation depends on valve area; most early cases will be asymptomatic.
- Mean age of presentation is usually 50–60 years (3).
- Presenting features usually due to pulmonary vascular congestion: Palpitations, dyspnea on exertion, fatigue, pulmonary edema, and paroxysmal nocturnal dyspnea may cause chest pain.
- Atrial fibrillation, embolic event
- In advanced disease, symptoms of HTN and right heart failure predominate: jugular venous distention, hepatomegaly, ascites, and peripheral edema.
- Other presentations: hemoptysis, hoarseness (compression of recurrent laryngeal nerve by enlarged pulmonary artery or LA), dysphagia (compression), rarely as infective endocarditis
- Infection, atrial fibrillation with rapid rate, exercise, or pregnancy may exacerbate symptoms.

PHYSICAL EXAM

- Reduced peripheral pulses
- Auscultation
  - Classic murmur: accentuated S_1, opening snap, apical early decrescendo diastolic rumble with presystolic accentuation
  - Murmur variability seen in severe stenosis:
    - With mobile, noncalcified valve, murmur persists throughout diastole and S_1, and the opening snap remains loud.
    - With a heavily calcified valve, murmur often is difficult to hear. S_1 and the opening snap may be soft to absent.
    - In contrast to tricuspid stenosis, the intensity of the murmur from MS increases with inspiration and a prominent *a* wave in jugular venous pulse.
- If HTN is present: Right ventricle (RV) lift, increased P_2, high-pitched decrescendo diastolic murmur of pulmonic insufficiency (Graham Steell murmur) may have signs of right heart failure.
- May also find associated aortic or, less commonly, tricuspid murmurs due to aortic or tricuspid valve involvement from rheumatic heart disease

DIAGNOSTIC TESTS & INTERPRETATION

Initial Tests (lab, imaging)

- ECG (4,5)[C]
  - LA enlargement (manifested by broad, notched P waves in lead II [P mitrale] with a negative terminal deflection of the P wave in lead V_1)
  - Atrial fibrillation common
  - Right ventricular hypertrophy (RVH), right axis deviation, and a large R wave in V_1 possible
- Chest radiograph (4,5)[C]
  - LA enlargement, straightening of the left heart border, a "double density," and elevation of the left main stem bronchus
  - Prominent pulmonary arteries at the hilum with rapid tapering, RVH
  - Pulmonary edema pattern with Kerley B lines (late presentation)
- ECG indications (1)[B],(5)[C]:
  - Class I
    - Diagnosis of MS
    - Assess severity.
    - Reassess after change in symptoms.
    - Exercise Doppler for discrepancies between symptoms and echo findings.
    - During evaluation for commissurotomy
    - TEE when transthoracic echo nondiagnostic, to exclude thrombus in left atrium or to evaluate severity of MR (1)[B]
  - Class II
    - Reassess asymptomatic patients.
    - Very severe ($<$1.0 cm^2) MS: yearly
    - Severe $\leq$1.5 (cm^2) MS: every 1–2 years
    - Mild or moderate MS: every 3–5 years
  - Class III
    - Satisfactory result of transthoracic echo
- ECG findings:
  - MV anterior leaflet doming, immobility of the posterior leaflet
  - Echo can demonstrate alternative causes of MS if not rheumatic.
  - MV area defined (1)
    - Normal: 4–6 cm^2
    - Progressive MS: $>$1.5 cm^2
    - Severe MS: $<$1.5 cm^2
    - Very severe: $<$1.0 cm^2
- Cardiac catheterization indications (1,5)[C]:
  - Class I recommendations:
    - When echo is inconclusive
    - Discrepancy between echo and symptoms
    - Discrepancy between echo and valve area
  - Class II recommendations:
    - To assess response of LA and pulmonary artery pressures to exercise when symptoms and echo findings do not match
    - Assess cause of severe HTN out of proportion to echo results.
  - Class III recommendations: satisfactory result of echo

Follow-Up Tests & Special Considerations

- If valve area $>$1.5 cm^2 and mean pressure gradient $<$5 mm Hg, then no further initial workup is needed.
- If valve area is $<$1.5 cm^2, then do further workup prior to surgical correction.

Diagnostic Procedures/Other

Exercise or dobutamine stress test (1,5)[C]:

- When symptoms are severe but echo findings are mild
- To determine if surgery is needed

Test Interpretation

Rheumatic fever–induced pathologic changes: leaflet thickening, leaflet calcification, commissural fusion, chordal shortening

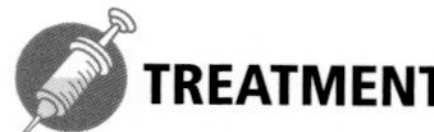

TREATMENT

GENERAL MEASURES

- Exercise
  - Patients with mild MS are usually asymptomatic even with strenuous exercise.
  - Usually recommend low-level aerobic exercise, limited by symptoms of dyspnea (5)[C]
- Counsel patients that MS usually is slowly progressive but can have sudden onset of atrial fibrillation, which could become rapidly fatal. Call 911 for marked worsening of symptoms.
- Atrial fibrillation accompanying MS impairs LV filling, especially with a rapid ventricular response:
  - Rate control with β- or calcium channel blockers (1)[C].
  - Cardioversion for medical failure or if patient is unstable (6)[B].
  - If the atrial fibrillation has been present for >24–48 hours, then anticoagulate for 3 weeks then cardiovert, or alternatively, heparinize, perform TEE, and, if no atrial thrombus, then cardiovert (6)[B].
  - After cardioversion, patient needs long-term anticoagulation.
  - These patients can critically decompensate due to loss of atrial contractility, causing an inability to fill the LV.

MEDICATION

First Line

- Because MS is a mechanical anomaly, medical management is always considered adjunctive to interventional management when the latter is indicated.
- Antibiotic prophylaxis against rheumatic fever and/or carditis is recommended for patients with history of rheumatic fever (1)[C]:
  - Penicillin V PO or penicillin G IM: IM is more effective than PO (7)[A].
  - Sulfadiazine
  - Macrolides: Take antibiotic continuously to prevent recurrence of rheumatic fever or carditis.
  - Duration of rheumatic fever prophylaxis:
    - Rheumatic fever without carditis: Take for 5 years or until age 21 years, whichever is longer.
    - Rheumatic fever with carditis but no residual heart disease: Take for 10 years or well into adulthood, whichever is longer.
    - Rheumatic fever with carditis plus residual heart disease: Take for 10 years or until 40 years old, whichever is longer.
- Antibiotic prophylaxis against infective endocarditis is not routinely recommended (1)[B].
- β-Blockers or calcium channel blockers for tachycardia or exertional symptoms (1)[B]
- Diuretics for congestive symptoms (5)[C]
- Digitalis for atrial fibrillation if LV or RV dysfunction (5)[C]
- Anticoagulation (1)[B]
  - Class I recommendations:
    - MS and atrial fibrillation or history of atrial fibrillation
    - MS and prior embolic event
    - MS and LA thrombus
  - Class IIB recommendations:
    - Asymptomatic MS but with severe MS and LA dimension >54 mm by echo
    - Severe MS, enlarged LA, and spontaneous contrast on echo
- Warfarin (international normalized ratio) range 2–3
- Heparin in the acute atrial fibrillation setting
- The new oral anticoagulants (factor Xa inhibitor and direct thrombin inhibitor) are not approved for use in atrial fibrillation that is secondary to MS.

Second Line

Amiodarone for rate control if β-blockers or calcium channel blockers cannot be used (5)[C]

SURGERY/OTHER PROCEDURES

- Balloon valvotomy: symptomatic patients with NYHA class II, III, or IV symptoms with valves that look favorable and with favorable comorbidities (1)[A]
- MV surgery: when MS is severe and balloon valvotomy is contraindicated due to unfavorable anatomy (1)[B],(8)[C]

Pregnancy Considerations

Volume expansion during pregnancy can exacerbate heart failure symptoms. Hence, MS often presents during the intrapartum period. For patients with known severe MS, intervention should be pursued before pregnancy. Such patients have a high rate of both maternal and fetal complications, including death. Percutaneous balloon valvotomy can be performed in symptomatic pregnant patients.

ONGOING CARE

FOLLOW-UP RECOMMENDATIONS

- Ascertain the valve gradient and pulmonary arterial pressure with ECG.
- Follow-up will depend on the severity of the MS and the patient's symptoms:
  - Asymptomatic patients: annual history and examination; follow-up serial echocardiography based on the severity of MS
  - Symptomatic patients are reviewed according to individual therapy, symptoms, and signs; ECG to evaluate for changes (1)[C]

DIET

Salt restriction for pulmonary congestion

PROGNOSIS

Natural history

- Asymptomatic latent period after rheumatic fever for 10–30 years. 10-year survival for asymptomatic or minimally symptomatic patients is 80%. 10-year survival after onset of symptoms is 50–60%.
- Symptoms typically become debilitating 10 years after onset.
- 10-year survival after onset of debilitating symptoms is only 0–15%.
- Mean survival with significant HTN is <3 years.
- The severity of MS progresses over time in almost all patients. There are no known definitive medical therapies, apart from prevention of recurrent rheumatic fever, that alter its natural history. When symptoms develop, balloon valvotomy, open mitral commissurotomy, or closed mitral commissurotomy provides effective means of reducing stenosis but is not curative. Restenosis sometimes occurs and can be early (<5 years) or late (>20 years).
- Appropriate medical treatment can delay necessity for surgery, and surgical treatment substantially prolongs survival in patients with severe MS.

COMPLICATIONS

Left and right heart failure, atrial fibrillation and systemic embolization, pulmonary HTN, bacterial endocarditis

REFERENCES

1. Nishimura RA, Otto CM, Bonow RO, et al. 2014 AHA/ACC guideline for the management of patients with valvular heart disease: a report of the American College of Cardiology/American Heart Association Task Force on Practice Guidelines. *J Thorac Cardiovasc Surg*. 2014;148(1):e1–e132.
2. Ray S. Changing epidemiology and natural history of valvular heart disease. *Clin Med*. 2010;10(2):168–171.
3. Ramakrishna CD, Khadar SA, George R, et al. The age-specific clinical and anatomical profile of mitral stenosis. *Singapore Med J*. 2009;50(7):680–685.
4. Maganti K, Rigolin VH, Sarano ME, et al. Valvular heart disease: diagnosis and management. *Mayo Clin Proc*. 2010;85(5):483–500.
5. Bruce CJ, Nishimura RA. Newer advances in the diagnosis and treatment of mitral stenosis. *Curr Probl Cardiol*. 1998;23(3):125–192.
6. Anderson JI, Halperin JL, Albert NM, et al. Management of patients with atrial fibrillation (compilation of 2006 ACCF/AHA/ESC and 2011 ACCF/AHA/HRS recommendations): a report of the American College of Cardiology/American Heart Association Task Force on Practice Guidelines. *J Am Coll Cardiol*. 2013;61(18):1935–1944.
7. Manyemba J, Mayosi BM. Penicillin for secondary prevention of rheumatic fever. *Cochrane Database Syst Rev*. 2002;(3):CD002227.
8. Zakkar M, Amirak E, Chan KM, et al. Rheumatic mitral valve disease: current surgical status. *Prog Cardiovasc Dis*. 2009;51(6):478–481.

ADDITIONAL READING

- Chandrashekhar Y, Westaby S, Narula J. Mitral stenosis. *Lancet*. 2009;374(9697):1271–1283.
- Guérios EE, Bueno R, Nercolini D, et al. Mitral stenosis and percutaneous mitral valvuloplasty (part 1). *J Invasive Cardiol*. 2005;17(7):382–386.

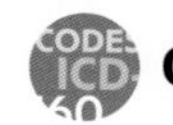

CODES

ICD10

- I05.0 Rheumatic mitral stenosis
- I05.8 Other rheumatic mitral valve diseases
- I34.2 Nonrheumatic mitral (valve) stenosis

CLINICAL PEARLS

- Asymptomatic patients may be followed clinically with yearly exams for development of symptoms, with periodic echo to evaluate valve area.
- Once symptoms of MS develop, initiate appropriate medical therapy, but advise patient that, for most, surgical therapy will be needed to prolong survival. Almost all cases of MV stenosis progress in severity over time.
- MS often presents during the intrapartum period. For patients with known severe MS, intervention should be pursued prior to pregnancy. Pregnancy in a patient with severe MS has a high rate of both maternal and fetal complications, including death.

MITRAL VALVE PROLAPSE

Zeeshan Hussain, MD • Wasiq Faraz Rawasia, MD • Marcus F. Stoddard, MD

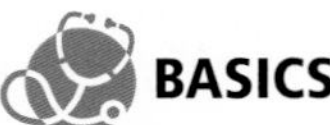

BASICS

DESCRIPTION

- Mitral valve prolapse (MVP) is a systolic billowing of 1 or both mitral leaflets into the left atrium (LA) during systole ± mitral regurgitation (MR).
- More specifically, MVP is a single or bileaflet prolapse of at least 2 mm superior displacement into the LA during systole on the parasternal long-axis annular plane of the valve on echocardiogram ± leaflet thickening:
  - Classic: prolapse with >5 mm of leaflet thickening
  - Nonclassic: prolapse with <5 mm of leaflet thickening (1)
- Synonym(s): systolic click-murmur syndrome; billowing mitral cusp syndrome; myxomatous mitral valve; floppy valve syndrome; redundant cusp syndrome; Barlow syndrome

EPIDEMIOLOGY

Incidence

- Predominant age: MVP has been described in all age groups.
- Initial descriptions based on clinical examinations suggested a 2:1 female predominance. Using modern echocardiogram criteria, men and women are affected equally (2).
- The most serious consequences of hemodynamically significant MR occur in men age >50 years.

Prevalence

MVP is the most common valvular abnormality, affecting 1–2.5% of the general population, depending on the precise definition (2,3).

ETIOLOGY AND PATHOPHYSIOLOGY

- The pathology causing MVP is multifactorial and includes the following:
  - Abnormal valve tissue
    - Myxomatous degeneration: redundant layers of leaflet "hooding" the cords, chordal elongation, and annular dilatation
    - Myxoid leaflets are more elastic and less stiff than normal valves.
    - Chordal rupture is more common.
  - Disparity in size between the mitral valve and the left ventricle (LV)
  - Connective tissue disorders (1)
- MVP is often associated with variable degrees of MR.
- Frequently, there is enlargement of the LA and LV.
- Mitral annulus is often dilated.
- Involvement of other valves may occur (tricuspid valve prolapse 40%, pulmonic prolapse and aortic prolapse 2–10%).
- Possible increased vagal tone
- Possible increased urine epinephrine and norepinephrine
- MVP patients often have orthostatic hypotension and tachycardia.
- Genetics causes proliferation of the spongiosa layer of the leaflets (3).
- Fibrosis on surface of leaflets (3)
- Thinning and elongation of chordae tendineae
- The mitral valve differentiates during days 35–42 of fetal development, the same time as differentiation of the vertebrae and ribs.

Genetics

- Familial MVP is inherited as an autosomal dominant trait but with variable expressivity and incomplete penetrance.
- 2 genetic loci identified
  - *MMVP1* on chromosome 16p11.2–p12.1
  - *MMVP2* on chromosome 11p15.4

RISK FACTORS

- MVP is a primary cardiovascular disorder.
- MVP is more likely to occur in patients with connective tissue disorders (see "Commonly Associated Conditions").
- Physical characteristics associated with MVP
  - Straight thoracic spine
  - Pectus excavatum
  - Asthenic body habitus
  - Low body mass index (BMI)
  - Scoliosis or kyphosis
  - Hypermobility of the joints
  - Arm span > height
  - Narrow anteroposterior (AP) diameter of the chest

COMMONLY ASSOCIATED CONDITIONS

- Marfan syndrome (91% of Marfan syndrome patients have MVP, although large majority of MVP patients do not meet criteria for Marfans.) (1)
- Ehlers-Danlos syndrome
- Hypertrophic cardiomyopathy
- Pseudoxanthoma elasticum
- Osteogenesis imperfecta
- von Willebrand disease
- Primary hypomastia

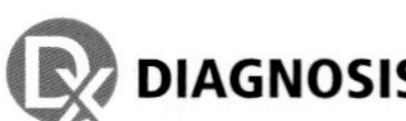

DIAGNOSIS

Physical exam and echocardiography

HISTORY

- Most patients are asymptomatic.
- The most frequent symptom is palpitations.
- Symptoms related to autonomic dysfunction
  - Anxiety and panic attacks
  - Arrhythmias
  - Exercise intolerance
  - Palpitations and chest pains that are atypical for coronary artery disease (CAD)
  - Fatigue
  - Orthostasis, syncope, or presyncope
  - Neuropsychiatric symptoms
- Symptoms related to progression of MR
  - Fatigue
  - Dyspnea
  - Exercise intolerance
  - Orthopnea
  - Paroxysmal nocturnal dyspnea
  - Congestive heart failure (CHF)
- Symptoms occur as a result of an associated complication (stroke, arrhythmia).

PHYSICAL EXAM

- Auscultatory examination
  - Mid- to late systolic click
    - May vary in timing and intensity based on ventricular beat-to-beat volume variations
    - At low ventricular volumes, the valve may prolapse earlier during systole and further into the LA than during volume overload.
    - It may or may not be followed by a high-pitched, mid- to late systolic murmur at the cardiac apex.
  - Murmur: a mid- to late crescendo systolic murmur best heard at apex, middle- to high-pitched, occasionally musical or honking in quality
  - Occasionally, only the ejection click is present.
  - The duration of the murmur corresponds with the severity of MR.
- Dynamic auscultation
  - Maneuvers that move the click and murmur toward S_1
    - Arterial vasodilation
    - Amyl nitrite
    - Valsalva
    - Augmented contractility
    - Decreased venous return (which can be induced by standing up)
  - Maneuvers that move the click and murmur toward S_2
    - Squatting
    - Leg raise
    - Isometric exercise
  - Valsalva maneuver may help differentiate hypertrophic obstructive cardiomyopathy (HOCM) from MVP because it increases the intensity of the murmur in HOCM while it makes it longer but not louder in MVP.

DIFFERENTIAL DIAGNOSIS

- MR
- Tricuspid regurgitation
- Tricuspid valve prolapse
- Papillary muscle dysfunction
- Hypertrophic cardiomyopathy
- Ejection clicks (do not change timing with systole)

DIAGNOSTIC TESTS & INTERPRETATION

Initial Tests (lab, imaging)

- Echocardiogram (test of choice) (4)[B],(5)[C]
  - In asymptomatic individuals with physical signs of MVP, an echocardiogram is indicated for diagnosis (4)[B].
  - Follow-up echocardiograms are not indicated for asymptomatic patients who have MVP with no changes clinically, even if they had mild MR (4,5)[C].
  - Parasternal long-axis view is most specific for diagnosis (4).
  - Findings that may be seen with MVP
    - Anterior leaflet billowing
    - Leaflet thickening of ≥5 mm
    - Leaflet redundancy
    - MR
    - Posterior leaflet displacement
  - Nondiagnostic transthoracic echocardiogram: ≤10%
  - Transesophageal echocardiography particularly with 3D imaging may be considered to further visualize the anatomy if an intervention is being planned (6)[B].
  - Stress echocardiograms may reveal exercise-induced MR or latent LV dysfunction (1,5)[C].
- Angiography
  - Rarely used for diagnostic purposes
  - MVP may be incidentally seen on a catheterization.
- ECG is usually normal:
  - May be nonspecific ST-T wave changes
  - T-wave inversions, prominent Q waves, or prolonged QT may also occur.

- A chest x-ray (CXR) is not necessary for diagnosis:
  - Typically, the CXR is normal.
  - Other findings
    - Possible pulmonary edema: Pulmonary edema may be asymmetric with acute chordal rupture and flail leaflet.
    - Possible calcification of the mitral annulus
- Holter monitoring is optional if patient has palpitations. Order Holter monitoring as usual for syncope or dizziness.
- Tilt table testing may be of value in patients with MVP who presents with syncope of unknown etiology.

Follow-Up Tests & Special Considerations

Patients with a family history of MVP should be screened with echocardiography (4)[B].

Test Interpretation

- Myxomatous proliferation of the middle layer (spongiosa) of the valve, resulting in increased mucopolysaccharide deposition and myxomatous degeneration
- By electron microscopy, the collagen fibers in the valve leaflets are disorganized and fragmented.
- With increased stroma deposition, the valve leaflets enlarge and become redundant.
- The endothelium is usually noncontiguous and a frequent site for thrombus or infective vegetation.

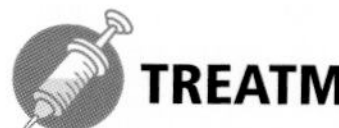

TREATMENT

GENERAL MEASURES

Treat MVP with orthostatic symptoms by liberalizing fluid and salt intake. If severe, mineralocorticoids may rarely be used. Support stockings may also be beneficial.

MEDICATION

- Asymptomatic MVP is treated with reassurance; normal lifestyle and regular exercise is encouraged.
- MVP and transient ischemic attacks are treated with aspirin 75–325 mg daily (Class I recommendation) (4)[C].
- MVP with history of cryptogenic stroke, or atrial fibrillation with $CHADS_2$ (acronym for **C**ongestive heart failure, **H**ypertension, **A**ge >75 years, **D**iabetes mellitus, and prior **S**troke or transient ischemic attack) score <2, is generally treated with aspirin 75–325 mg daily (4)[C].
- MVP with atrial fibrillation with $CHADS_2$ score ≥2 is treated with warfarin (4)[C].
- MVP with high-risk echocardiographic features (thickening >5 mm or valve redundancy) and a history of stroke, warfarin therapy may be considered (4)[C].
- MVP with palpitations is treated with β-blockers and/or recommendation to discontinue alcohol, cigarettes, and caffeine (5)[C].

ADDITIONAL THERAPIES

- Endocarditis prophylaxis is no longer recommended for MVP.
- Patients with prior endocarditis undergoing dental, respiratory tract, infected skin, or musculoskeletal procedures should receive prophylaxis for endocarditis with amoxicillin 30–60 minutes prior to procedure. Ampicillin, cefazolin, or ceftriaxone IM or IV may be used if unable to tolerate oral medications (4)[B].

SURGERY/OTHER PROCEDURES

- Referral for surgery is recommended for patients with severe MR with impaired LV systolic function or flail leaflet owing to ruptured chordae tendineae (4)[C].
- Minimally invasive mitral valve repair patients have shorter postoperative hospital stay compared with conventional median sternotomy open repair for patients with bileaflet prolapse and severe MR (7)[B].
- Surgical repair of MR due to isolated posterior leaflet prolapse is associated with a low reoperation rate (8)[A].
- Asymptomatic patients with atrial fibrillation or pulmonary hypertension should be considered for intervention as well (3)[C].

ONGOING CARE

FOLLOW-UP RECOMMENDATIONS

- Asymptomatic MVP patients with no significant MR can be followed clinically every 3–5 years (4)[C].
- Patients who are symptomatic or have high-risk features on initial echocardiogram, including moderate to severe MR, may need serial echocardiograms and should be followed clinically once per year (4)[C].
- Patients with MVP and severe MR may require coronary angiography and transesophageal echocardiography if cardiac surgical referral is planned (4)[C].

PATIENT EDUCATION

- No contraindication to pregnancy
- Restriction from competitive sports if patient has MVP with one of the following features (9):
  - A history of syncope associated with document arrhythmia
  - A family history of MVP-related sudden cardiac death
  - Sustained or repetitive and nonsustained supraventricular tachycardia or frequent and/or complex ventricular tachyarrhythmias on ambulatory Holter monitoring
  - Severe MR
  - A prior embolic event
  - LV systolic dysfunction
- Explain the hereditary nature of familial MVP.

PROGNOSIS

- Excellent prognosis for asymptomatic patients
- For patients with severe MR or reduced ejection fraction, the prognosis is similar to that for nonischemic MR.

COMPLICATIONS

- Sudden cardiac death: not clearly established. May be secondary to ventricular arrhythmias especially if significant MR is present (1,5).
- Chordae rupture with acute mitral insufficiency (higher risk of cardiac death; up to 2% per year)
- Infectious endocarditis (risk increased if murmur present) (5)
- Cerebrovascular ischemic event (1)
- Fibrin emboli
- Heart failure with progressive MR
- Arrhythmias such as atrial and ventricular premature beats, paroxysmal supraventricular tachycardias may all be seen. Risk increases with coexistent MR (5).
- Pulmonary hypertension

REFERENCES

1. Hayek E, Gring CN, Griffin BP. Mitral valve prolapse. *Lancet*. 2005;365(9458):507–518.
2. Freed LA, Levy D, Levine RA, et al. Prevalence and clinical outcome of mitral-valve prolapse. *N Engl J Med*. 1999;341(1):1–7.
3. Verma S, Mesana TG. Mitral-valve repair for mitral-valve prolapse. *N Engl J Med*. 2009;361(23):2261–2269.
4. Bonow RO, Carabello BA, Chatterjee K, et al. 2008 focused update incorporated into the ACC/AHA 2006 guidelines for the management of patients with valvular heart disease: a report of the American College of Cardiology/American Heart Association Task Force on Practice Guidelines (Writing Committee to revise the 1998 guidelines for the management of patients with valvular heart disease). *J Am Coll Cardiol*. 2008;52(13):e1–e142.
5. Sims JM, Miracle VA. An overview of mitral valve prolapse. *Dimens Crit Care Nurs*. 2007;26(4):145–149.
6. Shah PM. Current concepts in mitral valve prolapse—diagnosis and management. *J Cardiol*. 2010;56(2):125–133.
7. Speziale G, Nasso G, Esposito G, et al. Results of mitral valve repair for Barlow disease (bileaflet prolapse) via right minithoracotomy versus conventional median sternotomy: a randomized trial. *J Thorac Cardiovasc Surg*. 2011;142(1):77–83.
8. Johnston DR, Gillinov AM, Blackstone EH, et al. Surgical repair of posterior mitral valve prolapse: implications for guidelines and percutaneous repair. *Ann Thorac Surg*. 2010;89(5):1385–1394.
9. Maron BJ, Ackerman MJ, Nishimura RA, et al. Task Force 4: HCM and other cardiomyopathies, mitral valve prolapse, myocarditis, and Marfan syndrome. *J Am Coll Cardiol*. 2005;45(8):1340–1345.

ADDITIONAL READING

Zuppiroli A, Mori F, Favilli S, et al. Arrhythmias in mitral valve prolapse: relation to anterior mitral leaflet thickening, clinical variables, and color Doppler echocardiographic parameters. *Am Heart J*. 1994;128(5):919–927.

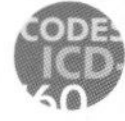

CODES

ICD10

I34.1 Nonrheumatic mitral (valve) prolapse

CLINICAL PEARLS

- MVP patients may have orthostatic hypotension and tachycardia.
- Asymptomatic MVP patients with no significant MR can be followed clinically every 3–5 years. Patients who are symptomatic or have high-risk features on initial echocardiogram, including moderate to severe MR, may need serial echocardiograms and should be followed clinically once per year.
- Endocarditis prophylaxis is no longer recommended for MVP.

MOLLUSCUM CONTAGIOSUM

Erica Pearce, PharmD, BCPS, BCACP • Rupal Trivedi, MD

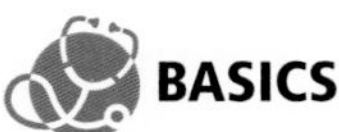

BASICS

DESCRIPTION

Molluscum contagiosum is a common, benign, viral (poxvirus) skin infection, characterized by small (2–5 mm), waxy white or flesh-colored, dome-shaped papules with central umbilication. When lesions are opened, a creamy, white-gray material can be expressed. Molluscum contagiosum is highly contagious and spreads by autoinoculation, skin-to-skin contact, sexual contact, and shared clothing/towels. Molluscum contagiosum is a self-limited infection in immunocompetent patients but difficult to treat and disfiguring in immunocompromised patients.

EPIDEMIOLOGY

Prevalence

- 1% in the United States, occurring mainly in children 2–15 years and sexually active young adults
- 5–18% HIV population

ETIOLOGY AND PATHOPHYSIOLOGY

- DNA virus; Poxviridae family
- 4 genetic virus types, clinically indistinguishable
- Virions invade and replicate in cytoplasm of epithelial cells causing abnormal cell proliferation
- Genome encodes proteins to evade host immune system.
- Incubation period: 2–6 weeks
- Not associated with malignancy
- No cross-hybridization or reactivation by other poxviruses

RISK FACTORS

- Skin-to-skin contact with infected person
- Contact sports
- Sexual activity with infected partner
- Immunocompromised: HIV, chemotherapy, corticosteroid therapy, transplant patients

GENERAL PREVENTION

- Avoid skin-to-skin contact with host (e.g., contact sports, sexual activity).
- Avoid sharing clothing and towels.

COMMONLY ASSOCIATED CONDITIONS

- Atopic dermatitis
- Immunosuppression medications: corticosteroids, chemotherapy
- HIV/AIDS

DIAGNOSIS

HISTORY

- Contact with known infected person
- Participation in contact sports
- Sexual activity

PHYSICAL EXAM

- Perform thorough skin exam including conjunctiva and anogenital area
- Discrete, firm papules with a central umbilication
- Umbilication not obvious in small children
- White curdlike core under umbilicated center
- Lesions are flesh, pearl, or red in color.
- May have surrounding erythema or dermatitis
- Immunocompetent hosts: average of 11–20 lesions, 2–5 mm diameter (range: 1–10 mm)
- Hosts with HIV/AIDS: hundreds of widespread lesions
- Children: trunk, extremities, face, anogenital region
- Sexually active: inner thighs, anogenital area

Pediatric Considerations

- Infants $<$3 months, consider vertical transmission
- Children: fever, $>$50 lesions, limited response to therapy, consider immunodeficiency
- Children: anogenital lesions, consider autoinoculation/possible sexual abuse

DIFFERENTIAL DIAGNOSIS

- AIDS patients: cryptococcus, penicilliosis, histoplasmosis, coccidioidomycosis
- Basal cell carcinoma
- Benign appendageal tumors: syringomas, hydrocystomas, ectopic sebaceous glands
- Condyloma acuminatum
- Dermatofibroma
- Eyelid: abscess, chalazion, foreign-body granuloma
- Folliculitis/furunculosis
- Keratoacanthoma
- Oral squamous cell carcinoma
- Trichoepithelioma
- Verruca vulgaris
- Warty dyskeratoma

DIAGNOSTIC TESTS & INTERPRETATION

Initial Tests (lab, imaging)

- Virus cannot be cultured.
- Culture lesion if concern is secondary infection.
- Sexual transmission: Test for other sexually transmitted infections, including HIV.
- Microscopy: scrape lesion
  - Core material has characteristic Henderson-Paterson intracytoplasmic viral inclusion bodies.
  - Crush prep with 10% potassium hydroxide will show characteristic inclusion bodies as well.
  - Alternatively, hematoxylin-eosin–stained formalin-fixed tissue shows same confirmatory features.

Diagnostic Procedures/Other

Clinical; using magnifying lens

Test Interpretation

Molluscum cytoplasmic inclusion bodies within keratinocytes

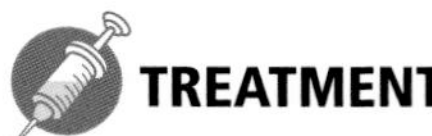

TREATMENT

GENERAL MEASURES

- In healthy patients, molluscum contagiosum is generally self-limited and heals spontaneously; however, some patients many opt for treatment.
- No single intervention is shown to be convincingly more effective than any other in treating molluscum contagiosum (1)[B].
- No treatment is FDA-approved for treatment of molluscum contagiosum
- Three categories of treatment: destructive, immune-enhancing and anti-viral

MEDICATION

First Line

- Cantharidin 0.7–0.9% solution: In office application to lesions, cover with dressing; wash off in 2–6 hours or sooner if blistering. Repeat treatment every 2–4 weeks until lesions resolve (1)[B],(2,3)[C].
  - Not commercially available in the United States but may be obtained from Canada
  - Adverse effects: blistering, erythema, pain, pruritus
  - Precautions: Do not use on face or on genital mucosa

Second Line

- Benzoyl peroxide 10% cream: apply to each lesion twice daily for 4 weeks (1)[B]
  - Adverse effects: mild dermatitis
- For immunocompromised patients with refractory lesions, consider
  - Starting or maximizing HAART therapy in patients with HIV/AIDS (4)[C].
  - Cidofovir
    - 3% cream applied to lesions once daily, 5 days/week for 8 weeks (4)[C]

 - ○ 1% cream applied to lesions once daily, 5 days/week for 2 weeks, repeat in 1 month, if necessary (4)[C]
 - ○ Adverse effects with topical use: erythema, pain, pruritus, erosions
 - ○ 3–5 mg/kg IV weekly for 1–2 weeks, followed by IV infusions every other week, until clinical clearance or up to 9 infusions (5)[C]
 - ○ Adverse effects with IV use: nephrotoxicity, neutropenia
 - ○ Monitoring with IV use: renal function and complete blood counts prior to and 24–48 hours after infusions
 - ○ Precaution: must coadminister oral probenecid and provide IV hydration with each IV infusion; refer to cidofovir manufacturer's recommendations on dosing
- – Ingenol mebutate 0.015% gel applied to lesions once daily for 3 days; may repeat once if needed (6)[C]
  - ○ Adverse effects: erythema, irritation

SURGERY/OTHER PROCEDURES

- Cryotherapy: 5–10 seconds with 1–2-mm margins; repeat every 3–4 weeks as needed until lesions disappear (7)[B]
  - – Adverse effects: erythema, edema, pain, blistering
  - – Contraindications: cryoglobulinemia, Raynaud disease
- Curettage under local or topical anesthesia (1)[A],(8)[B]
  - – Adverse effects: pain, scarring

COMPLEMENTARY & ALTERNATIVE MEDICINE

- Australian lemon myrtle oil: Apply 10% solution once daily for 21 days (9)[B].
- Potassium hydroxide 5–10% solution: apply 1–2 times a day until the lesions disappeared completely (10,11)[B]

Pediatric Considerations

- Surgical interventions: 2nd line in small children due to associated pain
- Pain control: Pretreat with topical lidocaine or EMLA before surgical treatment.
- Note: Adverse effect:
  - – Lidocaine or EMLA over large body surface area: Methemoglobinemia and CNS toxicity. Refer to manufacturer's recommendations on dosing and use in children.

Pregnancy Considerations

Safe in pregnancy: curettage, cryotherapy, incision, and expression

ONGOING CARE

FOLLOW-UP RECOMMENDATIONS

Patient Monitoring

Depends on type of treatment

PATIENT EDUCATION

- Cover lesions to prevent spread.
- Avoid scratching.
- Avoid contact sports.
- Avoid sharing towels and clothing.
- Avoid sexual activity when lesions present.

PROGNOSIS

- Immunocompetent: self-limited, resolves in 3–12 months (range: 2 months–4 years)
- Immunocompromised: lesions difficult to treat; may persist for years

COMPLICATIONS

- Secondary infection
- Scarring, hyper-/hypopigmentation

REFERENCES

1. van der Wouden JC, Menke J, Gajadin S, et al. Interventions for cutaneous molluscum contagiosum. *Cochrane Database Syst Rev.* 2006;(2):CD004767.
2. Moye V, Cathcart S, Burkhart CN, et al. Beetle juice: a guide for the use of cantharidin in the treatment of molluscum contagiosum. *Dermatol Ther.* 2013;26(6):445–451.
3. Silverberg NB, Sidbury R, Mancini AJ. Childhood molluscum contagiosum: experience with cantharidin therapy in 300 patients. *J Am Acad Dermatol.* 2000;43(3):503–507.
4. Chen X, Anstey AV, Bugert JJ. Molluscum contagiosum virus infection. *Lancet Infect Dis.* 2013;13(10):877–888.
5. Erikson C, Driscoll M, Gaspari A. Efficacy of intravenous cidofovir in the treatment of giant molluscum contagiosum in a patient with human immunodeficiency virus. *Arch Dermatol.* 2011;147(6):652–654.
6. Javed S, Tyring SK. Treatment of molluscum contagiosum with ingenol mebutate. *J Am Acad Dermatol.* 2014;70(5):e105.
7. Al-Mutairi N, Al-Doukhi A, Al-Farag S, et al. Comparative study on the efficacy, safety, and acceptability of imiquimod 5% cream versus cryotherapy for molluscum contagiosum in children. *Pediatr Dermatol.* 2010;27(4):388–394.
8. Hanna D, Hatami A, Powell J, et al. A prospective randomized trial comparing the efficacy and adverse effects of four recognized treatments of molluscum contagiosum in children. *Pediatr Dermatol.* 2006;23(6):574–579.
9. Burke BE, Baillie JE, Olson RD. Essential oil of Australian lemon myrtle *(Backhousia citriodora)* in the treatment of molluscum contagiosum in children. *Biomed Pharmacother.* 2004;58(4):245–247.
10. Rajouria EA, Amatya A, Karn D. Comparative study of 5% potassium hydroxide solution versus 0.05% tretinoin cream for molluscum contagiosum in children. *Katmandu Univ Med J.* 2011;9(36):291–294.
11. Handjani F, Behazin E, Sadati MS. Comparison of 10% potassium hydroxide solution versus cryotherapy in the treatment of molluscum contagiosum: an open randomized clinical trial. *J Dermatolog Treat.* 2014;25(3):249–250.

ADDITIONAL READING

- Brown J, Janniger CK, Schwartz RA, et al. Childhood molluscum contagiosum. *Int J Dermatol.* 2006;45(2):93–99.
- Dohil MA, Lin P, Lee J, et al. The epidemiology of molluscum contagiosum in children. *J Am Acad Dermatol.* 2006;54(1):47–54.
- Ting PT, Dytoc MT. Therapy of external anogenital warts and molluscum contagiosum: a literature review. *Dermatol Ther.* 2004;17(1):68–101.

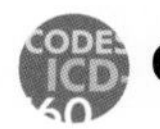

CODES

ICD10

B08.1 Molluscum contagiosum

CLINICAL PEARLS

- Natural resolution is preferred treatment in healthy patients.
- Reassure parents that lesions will heal naturally and generally resolve without scarring.
- No specific treatment has been identified as superior to any other.
- Consider topical corticosteroids for pruritus or associated dermatitis.

M

MORTON NEUROMA (INTERDIGITAL NEUROMA)

Catherine Mygatt, MD • J. Herbert Stevenson, MD

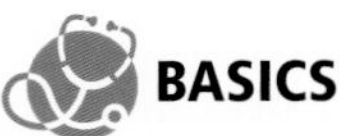

BASICS

DESCRIPTION

- Perineural fibrosis of the common digital nerve as it passes between metatarsals
  - The interspace between the 3rd and 4th metatarsals is most commonly affected.
  - Between the 2nd and 3rd metatarsals is the next most common site.
- System(s) affected: musculoskeletal, nervous
- Synonym(s): plantar digital neuritis; Morton metatarsalgia; intermetatarsal neuroma

EPIDEMIOLOGY

Prevalence

- Unknown
- Mean age: 45–50 years
- Predominant sex: female > male (8:1)

ETIOLOGY AND PATHOPHYSIOLOGY

- Lateral plantar nerve joins a portion of medial plantar nerve, creating a nerve with a larger diameter than those going to other digits.
- Nerve lies in SC tissue, deep to the fat pad of foot, just superficial to the digital artery and vein.
- Overlying the nerve is the strong, deep transverse metatarsal ligament that holds the metatarsal bones together.
- With each step the patient takes, the inflamed nerve becomes compressed between the ground and the deep transverse metatarsal ligament. This can generate perineural fibrotic reaction with subsequent neuroma formation.

RISK FACTORS

- High-heeled shoes
  - Transfer more weight to the forefoot
- Shoes with tight toe boxes
  - Cause lateral compression
- Pes planus (flat feet)
  - Pulls nerve medially, increasing irritation
- Obesity
- Ballet dancing, basketball, aerobics, tennis, running, and similar activities

GENERAL PREVENTION

- Wear properly fitting shoes.
- Avoid high heels and shoes with narrow toe boxes.

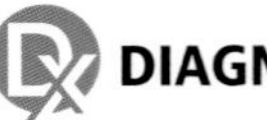

DIAGNOSIS

HISTORY

- Most common complaint is pain localized to interspace between 3rd and 4th toes.
- Pain is less severe when not bearing weight.
- Pain, cramping, or numbness of the forefoot during weight bearing or immediately after strenuous foot exertion
- Radiation of pain to the toes
- Pain is relieved by removing shoes and massaging the foot.
- Patients often complain of "walking on a marble."
- Burning pain in the ball of the foot radiating to the toes
- Tingling or numbness in the toes
- Aggravated by wearing tight or narrow shoes

PHYSICAL EXAM

- Intense pain when pressure applied between metatarsal heads, sometimes with a palpable nodule.
- Assess midfoot motion and digital motion to determine if arthritis or synovitis.
- Palpate along metatarsal shafts to assess for metatarsalgia or stress fractures.

DIFFERENTIAL DIAGNOSIS

- Stress fracture
- Hammer toe
- Metatarsophalangeal synovitis
- Metatarsalgia
- Arthritis
- Bursitis
- Foreign body

DIAGNOSTIC TESTS & INTERPRETATION

Initial Tests (lab, imaging)

- Predominantly a clinical diagnosis; imaging should be reserved for when the diagnosis is unclear or more than one web space is involved (1)[A],(2)[B].
- Radiographs may help to rule out osseous pathology if diagnosis is in question, but films usually are normal in patients with a Morton neuroma (1)[A].
- US has a 79% specificity and a 99% sensitivity for Morton neuromas but is poor at assessing the size of the lesion. Specificity declines to 50% for lesions less than 6 mm (1)[A].
- MRI can rule out an osseous tumor and help determine how much of the nerve to resect surgically; it has a sensitivity of 83% and a specificity of 99% (1)[A].

Diagnostic Procedures/Other

- Five special tests have been described: web space tenderness, foot squeeze test, toe tip sensation deficit, plantar percussion test, and Mulder sign.
- Mulder sign is a "click" and pain produced by squeezing the metatarsal heads together and simultaneously compressing the neuroma between the thumb and index finger of the other hand; 40–84% sensitive (1)[A].
- More than 1 of the above tests being positive increases the diagnostic accuracy (3)[B].

Test Interpretation

Chronic fibrosis and thickening of the digital nerve

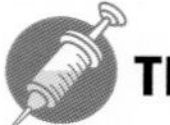

TREATMENT

GENERAL MEASURES

- Wear flat shoes with a roomy toe box.
- Plantar pads may help with alignment of metatarsal heads and provide relief.
- NSAIDs for temporary symptom relief

MEDICATION

First Line

Injectable steroids (e.g., betamethasone phosphate/acetate or methylprednisolone): use if general measures fail; number needed to treat (NNT) for significant benefit over conservative measures = 2.3 (4)[A]

Second Line

- US-guided alcohol ablation therapy to sclerose the nerve is safe, reduces pain, and may offer an alternative to surgery (5,6)[B].
- A pilot study has demonstrated that injection with onabotulinumtoxinA is of possible usefulness to relieve the pain and improve function in Morton neuroma (7)[B].
- There is no evidence for the use of supinatory insoles (8)[A].

ISSUES FOR REFERRAL

Continued pain despite conservative treatments and injections

SURGERY/OTHER PROCEDURES

Surgical removal of the neuroma or shortening of the metatarsals, with or without release of the transverse metatarsal ligament, have a 61–100% success rate defined by satisfaction scores (9)[A].

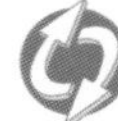

ONGOING CARE

FOLLOW-UP RECOMMENDATIONS

At diagnosis or if no improvement after 3 months of conservative treatment, consider corticosteroid injection.

- Repeat injection if no improvement after 2–4 weeks.

PATIENT EDUCATION

Wear properly fitted comfortable shoes.

PROGNOSIS

- 40–50% improve with 3 months of conservative treatment.
- 45–60% improve with steroid injection (9)[A].
- 96% improve with surgery.

COMPLICATIONS

Hip and knee pain related to gait changes

REFERENCES

1. Sharp RJ, Wade CM, Hennessy MS, et al. The role of MRI and ultrasound imaging in Morton's neuroma and the effect of size of lesion on symptoms. *J Bone Joint Surg Br*. 2003;85(7):999–1005.
2. Pastides P, El-Sallakh S, Charalambides C. Morton's neuroma: a clinical versus radiological diagnosis. *Foot Ankle Surg*. 2012;18(1):22–24.
3. Owens R, Gougoulias N, Guthrie H, et al. Morton's neuroma: clinical testing and imaging in 76 feet, compared to a control group. *Foot Ankle Surg*. 2011;17(3):197–200.
4. Saygi B, Yildirim Y, Saygi EK, et al. Morton's neuroma: comparative results of two conservative methods. *Foot Ankle Int*. 2005;26(7):556–559.
5. Musson RE, Sawhney JS, Lamb L, et al. Ultrasound guided alcohol ablation of Morton's neuroma. *Foot Ankle Int*. 2012;33(3):196–201.
6. Climent JM, Mondéjar-Gómez F, Rodríguez-Ruiz C, et al. Treatment of Morton neuroma with botulinum toxin A: a pilot study. *Clin Drug Investig*. 2013;33(7):497–503.
7. Thomson CE, Gibson JN, Martin D. Interventions for the treatment of Morton's neuroma. *Cochrane Database Syst Rev*. 2004;(3):CD003118.
8. Akermark C, Crone H, Skoog A, et al. A prospective randomized controlled trial of plantar versus dorsal incisions for operative treatment of primary Morton's neuroma. *Foot Ankle Int*. 2013;34(9):1198–1204.
9. Thomson CE, Beggs I, Martin DJ, et al. Methylprednisolone injections for the treatment of Morton neuroma: a patient-blinded randomized trial. *J Bone Joint Surg Am*. 2014;95(9):790–798.

ADDITIONAL READING

- Jain S, Mannan K. The diagnosis and management of Morton's neuroma: a literature review. *Foot Ankle Spec*. 2013;6(4):307–317.
- Schreiber K, Khodaee M, Poddar S, et al. Clinical inquiry. What is the best way to treat Morton's neuroma? *J Fam Pract*. 2011;60(3):157–158, 168.

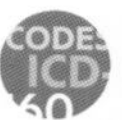

CODES

ICD10

- G57.60 Lesion of plantar nerve, unspecified lower limb
- G57.61 Lesion of plantar nerve, right lower limb
- G57.62 Lesion of plantar nerve, left lower limb

CLINICAL PEARLS

- Morton neuroma is usually a clinical diagnosis.
- Footwear modification is the mainstay of treatment.
- Corticosteroid injection into or US-guided alcohol ablation of the neuroma may be helpful.
- Neurectomy is the definitive treatment. Patients should be aware of the likelihood of postoperative dysesthesias.

M

MOTION SICKNESS

Courtney I. Jarvis, PharmD • Allison Hargreaves, MD

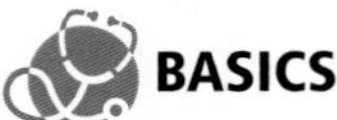

BASICS

DESCRIPTION

- Motions sickness is not a true sickness but a normal response to a situation in which sensory conflict about body motion exists among visual receptors, vestibular receptors, and body proprioceptors.
- Also can be induced when patterns of motion differ from those previously experienced
- System affected: nervous
- Synonym(s): car sickness; sea sickness; air sickness; space sickness; physiologic vertigo

EPIDEMIOLOGY

Incidence

Predominant sex: female > male

Prevalence

Estimation is complex; syndrome occurs in ~25% due to travel by air, ~29% by sea, and ~41% by road. Estimates for vomiting are 0.5% by air, 7% by sea, and 2% by road.

ETIOLOGY AND PATHOPHYSIOLOGY

- Precise etiology unknown; thought to be due to a mismatch of vestibular and visual sensations.
- Nausea and vomiting occur as a result of increased levels of dopamine and acetylcholine, which stimulate chemoreceptor trigger zone and vomiting center in CNS.

Genetics

Heritability estimates range from 55 to 75%.

RISK FACTORS

- Motion (auto, plane, boat, amusement rides)
- Travel
- Visual stimuli (e.g., moving horizon)
- Poor ventilation (fumes, smoke, carbon monoxide)
- Emotions (fear, anxiety)
- Zero gravity
- Pregnancy, menstruation, oral contraceptive use
- History of migraine headaches, especially vestibular migraine
- Other illness or poor health

GENERAL PREVENTION

See "General Measures."

Pediatric Considerations

- Rare in children <2 years of age
- Incidence peaks between 3 and 12 years of age.
- Antihistamines may cause excitation in children.

Geriatric Considerations

- Age confers some resistance to motion sickness.
- Elderly are at increased risk of anticholinergic side effects from treatment.

Pregnancy Considerations

- Pregnant patients are more likely to experience motion sickness.
- Treat with medications thought to be safe during morning sickness (e.g., meclizine, dimenhydrinate) (1)[C].

COMMONLY ASSOCIATED CONDITIONS

Migraine headache

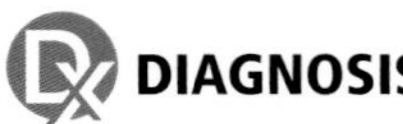

DIAGNOSIS

HISTORY

Presence of the following signs and symptoms in the context of a typical stimulus (2)[C]:

- Nausea
- Vomiting
- Diaphoresis
- Pallor
- Hypersalivation
- Yawning
- Hyperventilation
- Anxiety
- Panic
- Malaise
- Fatigue
- Weakness
- Confusion
- Dizziness

PHYSICAL EXAM

No specific findings

DIFFERENTIAL DIAGNOSIS

- Mountain sickness
- Vestibular disease, central and peripheral
- Gastroenteritis
- Metabolic disorders
- Toxin exposure

DIAGNOSTIC TESTS & INTERPRETATION

None indicated

TREATMENT

- Follow guidelines under "General Measures" section to prevent motion sickness (2)[C].
- Premedicate before travel with antidopaminergic, anticholinergic, or antihistamine agents (2)[A]:
  - For extended travel, consider treatment with scopolamine transdermal patch (3)[A].
  - Second-generation (nonsedating) antihistamines are not effective at preventing motion sickness (4)[B].
  - Serotonin (5-HT3) antagonists (e.g., ondansetron) do not appear effective in preventing motion sickness (5)[B].
- Conflicting data exist on the efficacy of acupressure for nausea and vomiting associated with motion sickness (6)[B].
- Benzodiazepines suppress vestibular nuclei but would not be considered first line due to sedation and addiction potential (7)[C].

GENERAL MEASURES

- Minimize exposure (sit in middle of plane or boat, front of car).
- Improve ventilation; avoid noxious stimuli.
- Use semirecumbent seating or lying supine.
- Fix vision on horizon; avoid fixation on moving objects; keep eyes fixed on still, distant objects.
- Avoid reading while actively traveling.
- Frequent and graded exposure to stimulus that triggers nausea (habituation)
- Minimize food intake before travel; avoid alcohol.
- Increase airflow around face.
- Acupressure on point PC6 has been shown to reduce feelings of nausea but not the incidence of vomiting during pregnancy, after surgery, and in cancer chemotherapy. However, conflicting evidence of efficacy has been found for motion sickness. Point PC6 (*Neiguan* on pericardium meridian): 2 cm proximal of transverse crease of palmar side of wrist between tendons of the palmaris longus and the flexor carpi radialis (6)[B]

MEDICATION

First Line

- Scopolamine transdermal patch: Apply 2.5-cm^2 (4 mg) patch behind ear at least 4 hours (preferably 6–12 hours) before travel, and replace every 3 days (3)[A]:
  - Scopolamine may also be given in tablets, capsules, or oral solution; all are more effective than placebo (3)[A].

- Dimenhydrinate (Dramamine): take 30–60 minutes before travel
  - Adults and adolescents: 50–100 mg q4–6h, maximum 400 mg/day
  - Children 6–12 years of age: 25–50 mg q6–8h, maximum 150 mg/day
  - Children 2–6 years of age: 12.5–25 mg q6–8h, maximum 75 mg/day
- Meclizine (Antivert): take 30–60 minutes before travel. Adults and adolescents >12 years of age: 12.5–25 mg q12–24h
- Cyclizine (Marezine): take 30–60 minutes before travel
  - Adults and adolescents: 50 mg q4–6h, maximum 200 mg/day
  - Children 6–12 years of age: 25 mg up to TID
- Promethazine (Phenergan): take 30–60 minutes before travel
  - Adults and adolescents: 25 mg q12h; 25–50 mg IM if already developed severe motion sickness
  - Children 2–12 years of age: 0.5 mg/kg q12h, maximum 25 mg BID. *Caution:* increased risk of dystonic reaction in this age group
- Contraindications: patients at risk for acute-angle closure glaucoma
- Precautions:
  - Young children
  - Elderly
  - Pregnancy
  - Urinary obstruction
  - Pyloric-duodenal obstruction
- Adverse reactions:
  - Drowsiness
  - Dry mouth
  - Blurred vision
  - Confusion
  - Headache
  - Urinary retention
- Significant possible interactions:
  - Sedatives (antihistamines, alcohol, antidepressants)
  - Anticholinergics (belladonna alkaloids)

Second Line

- Benzodiazepines: take 1–2 hours before travel
  - Diazepam 2–10 mg PO q6–12h
  - Lorazepam 1–2 mg PO q8h
- Contraindications:
  - Severe respiratory dysfunction
  - Severe liver dysfunction
- Precautions:
  - Alcohol/drug abuse
  - Elderly
  - Sedation
  - Addiction is possible.

COMPLEMENTARY & ALTERNATIVE MEDICINE

Ginger: 940 mg or 1 g; take 4 hours before travel (evidence controversial) (8)[B]

ONGOING CARE

FOLLOW-UP RECOMMENDATIONS

- Semirecumbent seating
- Avoid reading while actively traveling.

DIET

- Decrease oral intake or take frequent small feedings.
- Avoid alcohol.

PROGNOSIS

- Symptoms should resolve when motion exposure ends.
- Resistance to motion sickness seems to increase with age.

COMPLICATIONS

- Hypotension
- Dehydration
- Depression
- Panic
- Syncope

REFERENCES

1. Carroll ID, Williams DC. Pre-travel vaccination and medical prophylaxis in the pregnant traveler. *Travel Med Infect Dis*. 2008;6(5):259–275.
2. Committee to Advise on Tropical Medicine and Travel. Statement on motion sickness. *Can Commun Dis Rep*. 2003;29:1–12.
3. Spinks A, Wasiak J, Bernath V. Scopolamine (hyoscine) for preventing and treating motion sickness. *Cochrane Database Syst Rev*. 2011;(6):CD002851.
4. Cheung BS, Heskin R, Hofer KD. Failure of cetirizine and fexofenadine to prevent motion sickness. *Ann Pharmacother*. 2003;37(2):173–177.
5. Hershkovitz D, Asna N, Shupak A, et al. Ondansetron for the prevention of seasickness in susceptible sailors: an evaluation at sea. *Aviat Space Environ Med*. 2009;80(7):643–646.
6. Streitberger K, Ezzo J, Schneider A. Acupuncture for nausea and vomiting: an update of clinical and experimental studies. *Auton Neurosci*. 2006;129(1–2):107–117.
7. Zajonc TP, Roland PS. Vertigo and motion sickness. Part II: pharmacologic treatment. *Ear Nose Throat J*. 2006;85(1):25–35.
8. White B. Ginger: an overview. *Am Fam Physician*. 2007;75(11):1689–1691.

ADDITIONAL READING

Murdin L, Golding J, Bronstein A. Managing motion sickness. *BMJ*. 2011;343:d7430.

SEE ALSO

Algorithm: Vertigo

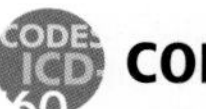

CODES

ICD10

T75.3XXA Motion sickness, initial encounter

CLINICAL PEARLS

- The scopolamine patch should be applied at least 4 hours before travel, although it may be more effective if placed 6–12 hours before departure.
- Oral medications should be administered 30–60 minutes before departure.
- Although acupressure wristbands have been found to be effective by systematic reviews in postoperative and chemotherapy-induced nausea and vomiting, conflicting data exist for motion sickness.

MULTIPLE MYELOMA

Jasmine S. Beria, DO, MPH • Maria M. Plummer, MD

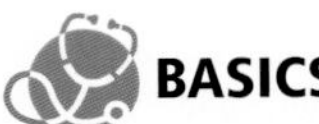

BASICS

DESCRIPTION

- Multiple myeloma (MM) is a clonal proliferation of malignant plasma cells.
- This clonal proliferation in the bone marrow can cause extensive skeletal destruction with osteolytic lesions and pathologic fractures.
- The malignant plasma cells produce monoclonal protein in the blood and urine.
- MM is also characterized by hypercalcemia, increased susceptibility to infections, renal impairment, and end-organ damage (1).
- Monoclonal gammopathy of undetermined significance (MGUS) is a common disorder with limited monoclonal plasma cell proliferation that progresses to MM at rate of ~1% per year.
- MGUS progresses to smouldering or asymptomatic MM and eventually to symptomatic MM.
- Synonym(s): plasma cell myeloma, plasma cell leukemia

EPIDEMIOLOGY

- Accounts for ~1.9% of all cancers and slightly >10% of hematologic malignancies in the United States
- Median age of diagnosis is 69 years; 62.2% diagnosed at age ≥65 years.
- Slight male predominance. Blacks about 2–3× more commonly affected than whites. Less common in Asians.

Incidence

6.1 new cases/100,000 annually

Prevalence

In 2011, there were 83,367 cases in the United States (2).

ETIOLOGY AND PATHOPHYSIOLOGY

- Clonal proliferation of plasma cells derived from postgerminal center B cells (3)
- Plasma cells undergo multiple chromosomal mutations to progress to MM.
- Genetic damage in developing B lymphocytes at time of isotype switching, transforming normal plasma cells into malignant cells, arising from single clone
- Earliest chromosomal translocations involve immunoglobulin heavy chains on chromosome 14q32, with the translocation at t(4;14) having a poor prognosis.
- Malignant cells multiply in bone marrow, suppressing normal bone marrow cells and producing large quantities of monoclonal immunoglobulin (M) protein.
- There is suppression of humoral and cell-mediated immunity and increased cell-mediated immunity with increased interleukin 6 (IL-6) (1).
- Malignant cells stimulate osteoclasts that cause bone resorption and inhibit osteoblasts that form new bone, causing lytic bone lesions.

Genetics

Rare family clusters

RISK FACTORS

- Most cases have no known risks associated.
- Older age; immunosuppression; and chemicals like dioxin, herbicides, insecticides, petroleum, heavy metals, plastics, and ionizing radiation increase the risk of MM.
- MGUS stage consistently precedes MM.

COMMONLY ASSOCIATED CONDITIONS

Secondary amyloidosis commonly due to MM

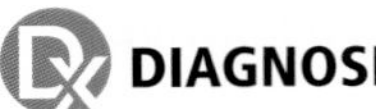

DIAGNOSIS

HISTORY

- 34% of patients are asymptomatic at the time of presentation.
- Hypercalcemia (28%): anorexia, nausea, somnolence, and polydipsia
- Renal failure (20–50%)
- Anemia (73%)
- Bony lesions (80%): lytic lesions causing bone pain (58%) (3), osteoporosis or pathologic fracture (26–34%)
- Other symptoms: fatigue (32%), peripheral neuropathy, weight loss (24%), recurrent infections, hyperviscosity syndrome, and cord compression

PHYSICAL EXAM

- Dehydration
- Skin findings of amyloidosis: waxy papules, nodules, or plaques that may be evident in the eyelids, retroauricular region, neck, or inguinal and anogenital regions; petechiae and ecchymosis; "pinch purpura"
- Extramedullary plasmacytomas can present as large, purplish, subcutaneous masses.
- Hyperviscosity syndrome in 7%: retinal hemorrhages, prolonged bleeding, neurologic changes
- Tender bones and masses

DIFFERENTIAL DIAGNOSIS

- MGUS
- Smouldering MM
- Metastatic carcinoma (kidney, breast, non-small cell lung cancer)
- Waldenström macroglobulinemia
- AL amyloidosis
- Solitary plasmacytoma
- Polyneuropathy, organomegaly, endocrinopathy, M protein, skin changes (POEMS) syndrome

DIAGNOSTIC TESTS & INTERPRETATION

Criteria for diagnosis: The diagnosis of MM requires all of the following (3)[A]:

- Bone marrow (BM) involvement with ≥10% of plasma cells (PC) or the presence of a plasmacytoma
- Monoclonal protein (M-spike) in the blood and/or urine
- Presence of one or more of the following: calcium elevation (>11.5 g/dL), renal insufficiency (creatinine >2 mg/dL), anemia (hemoglobin <10 g/dL or 2 g/dL < normal), bone disease (lytic or osteopenic)

Initial Tests (lab, imaging)

- CBC with differential to evaluate anemia and other cytopenias with evaluation of peripheral blood smear
- BUN, creatinine (elevated creatinine due to myeloma cast nephropathy)
- Serum electrolytes, serum albumin, serum calcium
- Serum lactate dehydrogenase (LDH), β_2-microglobulin
- Serum protein electrophoresis (SPEP), serum immunofixation electrophoresis (SIFE): M protein level elevated
- Quantitative serum immunoglobulin levels: immunoglobulin (Ig) G, IgA, and IgM
- Quantitative serum free light chain (FLC) levels: κ and λ chains
- Elevated ESR, C-reactive protein
- Urine analysis: 24-hour urine for protein, urine protein electrophoresis (UPEP), urine immunofixation electrophoresis (UIFE); 20% positive urine protein (3)[A]:
  - Urinalysis dip is often negative for protein, as this test identifies albumin, and the protein in MM is Bence-Jones (BJ) monoclonal protein.
- Bone marrow aspirate and biopsy for histology, immunohistochemistry, flow cytometry, cytogenetics, and fluorescence in situ hybridization (FISH)
- Skeletal survey: for lytic bone lesions, osteopenia, osteoporosis, or compression fractures
- MRI for any back pain or earliest signs/symptoms of spinal cord compression

Follow-Up Tests & Special Considerations

- CT scan: if high suspicion for bone lesions despite normal skeletal survey; can differentiate malignant from benign vertebral compression fractures in patients who are not MRI candidates
- PET scans: used if bone involvement is suspected despite a normal skeletal survey, MRI, and CT
- Baseline bone densitometry may be indicated (3)[A].
- Bone marrow aspirate and biopsy to monitor response to treatment
- SPEP with SIFE: M protein helps to track progression of myeloma and response to treatment.
- Serum immunoglobulins and free light chains can be used to monitor response or relapse.
- Plasma cell labeling index may be helpful to identify the fraction of the myeloma cell population that is proliferating (3)[A].

Diagnostic Procedures/Other

Staging:

- Durie Salmon stage
  - Stage I: low cell mass: $<0.6 \times 10^{12}$ cells/m^2 plus all of the following: hemoglobin >10 g/dL, serum IgG <5 g/dL, serum IgA <3 g/dL, normal serum calcium, urine BJ protein >12 g/24 hr, no generalized lytic bone lesions
  - Stage II: neither stage I nor stage III
  - Stage III: high cell mass: $>1.2 \times 10^{12}$ cells/m^2 plus one or more of the following: hemoglobin <8.5 g/L, serum calcium >12 mg/dL, bone lesions, IgG >7 g/dL, IgA >5 g/dL, urine BJ protein >12 g/24 hr, advanced lytic bone lesions
- International staging system (ISS)
  - Stage I: albumin ≥3.5 g/dL and β_2-microglobulin <3.5 μg/mL
  - Stage II: neither stage I nor stage III
  - Stage III: β_2-microglobulin ≥5.5 μg/mL
- Mayo Clinic risk stratification (mSMART)
  - Standard risk: t(11:14), t(6:14), and hyperdiploidy
  - Intermediate risk: t(4:14), del 13q by cytogenetics, hypodiploidy
  - High risk: t(14:16), t(14,20), del 17 p, and plasma cell labeling index >3%

Test Interpretation

Bone marrow involvement with plasma cells ≥10%; Russell bodies

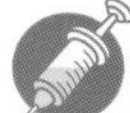

TREATMENT

- Treatment varies depending on level of disease activity and stage of MM.
- Treatment for smoldering MM is close monitoring at 3-month intervals. Early treatment with lenalidomide and dexamethasone delays progression and increases overall survival (4)[B].
- Key determinant factor in choosing chemotherapy regimen is to establish if the patient is an autologous stem cell transplant (ASCT) candidate or not.
- Treatment protocols vary by institution and patient.
- ASCT following induction chemotherapy is standard of care for patients with symptomatic disease.

GENERAL MEASURES

Maintain adequate hydration to prevent renal insufficiency. All patients receiving primary melanoma therapy should be given bisphosphonates initially (3)[A].

MEDICATION

- Induction chemotherapy for ASCT eligible patients (5)[C]:
  - Standard risk: (lenalidomide/low-dose dexamethasone)
  - Intermediate risk: (bortezomib/cyclophosphamide/dexamethasone)
  - High risk: (bortezomib/lenalidomide/dexamethasone)
  - After ASCT, maintenance can include a bortezomib compound for the high- or intermediate-risk group; lenalidomide can be considered for the standard group. Maintenance lenalidomide after ASCT has shown to improve progression-free survival (PFS) of 41 versus 23 months with placebo (6)[A].
- Induction chemotherapy for ASCT-ineligible patients:
  - Same regimens as ASCT eligible patients; however, the number of treatment cycles are increased (5)[C].

First Line

- Bortezomib
  - A proteasome inhibitor, it blocks the ubiquitin-proteasome catalytic pathway in cells by binding to the 20S proteasome complex.
  - Toxicity: peripheral neuropathy, cytopenia, nausea
  - Consider herpes simplex virus (HSV) prophylaxis.
- Cyclophosphamide
  - Nitrogen mustard–derivative alkylating agent
  - Often used in combination with prednisone or thalidomide in cases of relapsed disease
  - Toxicity: cytopenia, anaphylaxis, interstitial pulmonary fibrosis, secondary malignancy, impaired fertility
- Immunomodulators
  - Thalidomide and lenalidomide
    - Works by antiangiogenesis inhibition, immunomodulation, and inhibition of tumor necrosis factor
    - Toxicity: birth defects, deep vein thrombosis (DVT), neuropathy, rash, nausea, bradycardia
    - DVT prophylaxis, usually with aspirin
- Dexamethasone
  - Low doses (40 mg/week) superior to higher doses
  - Increases risk of DVT
- Bisphosphonates (7)[A]
  - No effect on mortality but decrease pain, pathologic vertebral fractures, and fractures of other bones
  - IV pamidronate or zoledronic acid can be used; evidence that zoledronic acid may be superior in preventing skeletal-related events.
  - Dose-adjust/monitor renal function.
  - Monitor for osteonecrosis of jaw.
- Alternative options:
  - As 1st-line treatment for transplant-ineligible patients with newly diagnosed MM, bortezomib/melphalan/prednisone was associated with significantly increased PFS compared with melphalan/prednisone (8)[A].

Second Line

- May be treated with any of the agents not already used
- The following agents can be used as salvage therapy to treat relapsed or refractory MM:
  - Bortezomib/lenalidomide
  - Liposomal doxorubicin
  - Carfilzomib: 2nd-generation selective proteasome inhibitor
- Emerging options: pomalidomide, thalidomide analog
- Interferon-α may be appropriate in selected patients, but because of its toxicity and availability of better alternatives, it has a limited role in treating MM.

ISSUES FOR REFERRAL

For spinal or other bone pathology, refer to orthopedics for support.

ADDITIONAL THERAPIES

- Local radiation therapy for bone pain
- ASCT (investigational)
- Effective pain management: Avoid NSAIDs due to nephrotoxicity.
- Kyphoplasty/vertebroplasty: consider for symptomatic vertebral compressions
- Plasmapheresis: for hyperviscosity syndrome (a rare complication)
- Erythropoietin: for selected patients with anemia
- Patients should receive vaccines for pneumococcus and influenza.
- Do not administer zoster vaccine and other live-virus vaccines.

INPATIENT CONSIDERATIONS

Admission Criteria/Initial Stabilization

Indications: pain, infections, cytopenia, renal failure, bone complications, spinal cord compression

- Avoid IV radiographic contrast materials due to risk for contrast-induced nephropathy.
- Adequate hydration
- Manage hypercalcemia and control hyperuricemia.

ONGOING CARE

PATIENT EDUCATION

- www.myeloma.org
- www.nccn.org/patients/patient_guidelines/myeloma/index.html

PROGNOSIS

- Median survival overall is 3 years. The 5-year survival rate is around 35%.
- Median survival by ISS stage:
  - Stage I: 62 months
  - Stage II: 44 months
  - Stage III: 29 months
- Median survival in patients with high-risk multiple myeloma (see staging for definition) is <2–3 years, even after ASCT; standard risk have median overall survival of 6–7 years.

COMPLICATIONS

Many, including infection, pain, lytic bone lesions, hypercalcemia, hyperuricemia, spinal cord compression, anemia, hyperviscosity syndrome, amyloidosis, renal insufficiency

REFERENCES

1. Attal M, Lauwers-Cances V, Marit G, et al. Lenalidomide maintenance after stem-cell transplantation for multiple myeloma. *N Engl J Med*. 2012;366(19):1782–1791.
2. Howlader N, Noone AM, Krapcho M, et al. *SEER Cancer Statistics Review, 1975-2011*. Bethesda, MD: National Cancer Institute. http://seer.cancer.gov/csr/1975_2011/. Accessed 2014.
3. Mhaskar R, Redzepovic J, Wheatley K, et al. Bisphosphonates in multiple myeloma: a network meta-analysis. *Cochrane Database Syst Rev*. 2012;5:CD003188.
4. Mateos MV, Hernández MT, Giraldo P, et al. Lenalidomide plus dexamethasone for high-risk smoldering multiple myeloma. *N Engl J Med*. 2013;369(5):438–447.
5. Palumbo A, Anderson K. Multiple myeloma. *N Engl J Med*. 2011;364(11):1046–1060.
6. Palumbo A, Hajek R, Delforge M, et al. Continuous lenalidomide treatment for newly diagnosed multiple myeloma. *N Engl J Med*. 2012;366(19):1759–1769.
7. Rajkumar SV. Multiple myeloma: 2013 update on diagnosis, risk-stratification, and management. *Am J Hematol*. 2013;88(3):226–235.
8. San Miguel JF, Schlag R, Khuageva NK, et al. Persistent overall survival benefit and no increased risk of second malignancies with bortezomib-melphalan-prednisone versus melphalan-prednisone in patients with previously untreated multiple myeloma. *J Clin Oncol*. 2013;31(4):448–455.

ADDITIONAL READING

National Comprehensive Cancer Network. NCCN multiple myeloma clinical practice guidelines in oncology (Version 2.2014). National Comprehensive Cancer Network Web site. Published 2014. www.nccn.org. Accessed 2014.

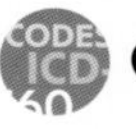

CODES

ICD10

- C90.00 Multiple myeloma not having achieved remission
- C90.01 Multiple myeloma in remission
- C90.02 Multiple myeloma in relapse

CLINICAL PEARLS

- MM is a plasma cell malignancy that causes end-organ damage.
- Look for presence of "CRAB" (hypercalcemia, renal insufficiency, anemia, and bone lesions).
- Suspect MM if high total protein-to-albumin ratio is present.
- Maintain high index of suspicion for spinal cord compression.
- Avoid nephrotoxins (radiographic contrast material, NSAIDs, dehydration).
- Patients with MM are immunocompromised.

MULTIPLE SCLEROSIS

Hayden Tran, DO, MS • Carmen Tran, MD • Matthew J. Goldman, MD

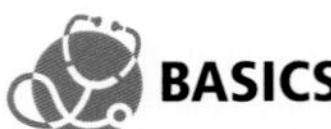

BASICS

DESCRIPTION

- An autoinflammatory disease causing demyelination, neuronal loss, and scarring within the white matter of the brain and spinal cord
- 4 recognized forms of multiple sclerosis (MS) (1):
  - Relapsing-remitting multiple sclerosis (RRMS) (85%): episodic flare-ups occurring over days to weeks between periods of neurologic stability. During attacks, new symptoms may present, whereas previous symptoms may worsen. Complete recovery or residual deficits may ensue following each bout.
  - Secondary progressive multiple sclerosis (SPMS): beginning as RRMS, progressive deterioration in neurologic function, unassociated with attacks, eventually ensues (progression may continue or halt). $\sim$2% risk per year of RRMS becoming SPMS
  - Primary progressive multiple sclerosis (PPMS) ($\sim$15%): steady decline of neurologic function from onset of disease without episodic flares
  - Progressive relapsing multiple sclerosis (PRMS) ($\sim$5%): steady decline of neurologic function from onset of disease with episodic flare-ups

Pregnancy Considerations

- Most patients experience lower exacerbation rates during pregnancy. Following delivery however, the immune system reverts and MS flares become more likely.
- Breastfeeding does not affect the risk of MS relapse.
- Relapse during postpartum can be safely treated by IVIG and corticosteroids (2)[C].

EPIDEMIOLOGY

- Age: Peak incidence occurs between 20 and 40 years (slightly earlier in women than men).
- Gender: Women are $\sim 3\times$ more likely to develop MS than men.
- Latitude: Prevalence tends to rise with increasing distance from the equator, although newer data reveals this latitude gradient may be declining (3,4).

Incidence

- Women (worldwide): 3.6 cases/100,000 person-years
- Men (worldwide): 2.0 cases/100,000 person-years

Prevalence

- United States: $\sim$350,000 MS patients.
- Worldwide: $\sim$2,500,000 MS patients

ETIOLOGY AND PATHOPHYSIOLOGY

- MS lesions: Inflammatory cells, mainly T lymphocytes and macrophages, surround vasculature within the CNS, creating sites of inflammation. These cells then disrupt the blood–brain barrier and infiltrate the surrounding white matter, meanwhile preserving the vessel wall. B lymphocytes, as well as myelin-specific autoantibodies also infiltrate the CNS and cause degeneration of the myelin sheaths.
- Following demyelination, faster salutatory nerve conduction velocities (impulses jumping between nodes of Ranvier) are replaced with considerably slower continuous nerve velocities.
- Astrocytes begin to proliferate and cause gliosis.
- Oligodendrocytes, which have survived, or ones formed from precursor cells, are able to partially remyelinate stripped axons, producing irreversible scars.
- In each MS lesion, axonal damage may occur, but it is the cumulative axonal loss over time that is responsible for the progressive and irreversible neurologic disability seen in MS patients.
- Most axons are typically lost from the lateral corticospinal (motor) tracts of the spinal cord.

Genetics

- Strong predisposition: HLA DRB1 (5)
- Proposed predisposition: IL2RA and IL7RA
- Race: Caucasian > Africans or Asians

RISK FACTORS

- Genetic: DRB1 locus on chromosome 6 has strongest MS risk association; DRB1*15 and *16 produce major histocompatibility complexes (MHC) with high binding affinity to myelin basic proteins (MPBs) (3,5).
- Geographic: Sun exposure to the skin provides the ultraviolet B (UVB) radiation necessary for endogenous vitamin D production. Insufficient UVB radiation exposure, especially in higher latitudes during winter months, is more common in temperate zones (3).
- Infectious: Epstein-Barr virus, human herpes virus (3,5)
- Race: Caucasian > African or Asian (5)
- Others: tobacco smoking (6)

GENERAL PREVENTION

Further research is required to determine prevention from environmental risk factors. A goal of therapy is to prevent new attacks and disability.

COMMONLY ASSOCIATED CONDITIONS

- Internuclear ophthalmoplegia (INO): Injury to the medial longitudinal fasciculus (MLF) causes impaired adduction to the affected eye.
- Optic neuritis: inflammation of optic nerve resulting in loss of vision
- Uhthoff phenomenon: Symptoms worsen with exposure to higher than usual temperature.
- Lhermitte sign: electric-like shocks extending down spine caused by neck movement, especially flexion

DIAGNOSIS

- A person with MS can present with a number of neurologic signs and symptoms depending on the locations of the lesions within the CNS (5)[C].
- Clinical diagnosis: $\geq$2 attacks; objective clinical evidence of $\geq$2 lesions or objective clinical evidence of 1 lesion with history of a previous episode. Flare-up duration must be at least >24 hours. Relapses must be separated by $\geq$1 month. $\geq$1 out of 2 neurologic signs must be present. The second clinical sign may be obtained through an abnormal paraclinical exam such as MRI or evoked potentials or may be supported by an abnormal paraclinical exam (5,7)[C].
- For patients with steady decline of neurologic function for $\geq$6 months without flares, intrathecal IgG may be used to support the diagnosis (5)[C].

HISTORY

Symptoms may include fatigue, depression, emotional instability, epilepsy, memory loss, diplopia, sudden vision loss, facial palsy, dysarthria, dysphagia, muscle weakness or spasms, ataxia, vertigo, falls, hyperesthesia or paresthesia, pain, bowel or bladder incontinence, urinary frequency or retention, or impotence (5)[C].

PHYSICAL EXAM

- Optic disc swelling or pallor
- Internuclear ophthalmoplegia
- Nystagmus in abducting eye
- Ataxia
- Intention tremor
- Hypesthesia or paresthesia
- Cerebellar dysarthria (scanning speech)
- Spasticity (especially in lower extremities)

DIFFERENTIAL DIAGNOSIS

- Lyme disease
- Systemic lupus erythematosus (SLE)
- Antiphospholipid antibody syndrome
- Epilepsy
- Progressive multifocal leukoencephalopathy (PML)
- CNS neoplasms
- Guillain-Barré syndrome
- Metachromatic leukodystrophy
- Sarcoidosis
- Stroke
- Vascular malformation
- HIV, neurosyphilis
- Cobalamin (B_{12}) deficiency
- Acute disseminated encephalomyelitis (ADEM)
- Behçet disease

DIAGNOSTIC TESTS & INTERPRETATION

- CSF: Increased monocyte cell count and intrathecally formed IgG levels. Total protein within CSF may be normal or increased. The presence of oligoclonal bands (OCB) is used to determine amount of IgG intrathecally synthesized. $\geq$2 OCBs is diagnostic (5)[B].
- Tests used for exclusion of alternative diagnoses: antinuclear antibodies (ANAs), serum cobalamin level, erythrocyte sedimentation rate (ESR), and testing for syphilis
- MRI of head/spine (more sensitive than CT):
  - T2 (spin-echo) image: hyperintense lesions
  - T2 image: hypointense lesions
  - Gadolinium (Gd): Given IV, leakage of Gd into the parenchyma represents an increase in BBB permeability due to vascular breakdown.
- McDonald criteria (5):
  - Dissemination in space: $\geq$1 T2 lesion on MRI in at least 2 out of 4 CNS regions typically affected by MS: periventricular, juxtacortical, infratentorial, or spinal cord or by waiting for another clinical attack implying a different CNS location
  - Dissemination in time: simultaneous presentation of asymptomatic Gd-enhanced and nonenhancing lesions at any moment or a new T2 and/or Gd-enhanced lesion on an MRI when compared baseline scans

Diagnostic Procedures/Other

Evoked potentials (EPs): assess function in visual, auditory, and somatosensory or motor CNS pathways by measuring CNS electric potentials evoked by stimulation of either the brain or selected peripheral nerves; a marked delay in a provoked CNS EP, without a clinical manifestation, is suggestive of a demyelinating disorder (5).

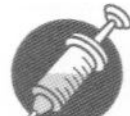

TREATMENT

Currently, there is no treatment for promoting remyelination or neuronal repair.

GENERAL MEASURES

- 3 main categories currently exist for MS treatment: treatment for acute relapses, treatment for reducing MS-related activity using disease-modifying agents and symptomatic therapy (2,5)[B].
- For apparent acute relapse, rule out infectious etiology prior to treatment.

MEDICATION

- Acute relapses (2)[B]
  - Methylprednisolone 1 g/day IV for 3–5 days; without subsequent oral tapering; a second course may be given.
    - Adverse effects: fluid retention, potassium loss, weight gain, GI disturbances, acne, and emotional lability
- Reduction of MS biologic activity (1,5,8)
  - Interferon-β (IFN-β):
    - Avonex (IFN-β_{1a}) 30 μg IM weekly
    - Rebif (IFN-β_{1a}) 22 or 44 μg SC 3×/week
      - Betaseron (IFN-β_{1b}) 0.25 mg SC every other day, Extavia (IFN-β_{1b}) 0.25 mg SC every other day
        - CBC w/ diff., Plt, LFTs at 1, 3, and 6 months after starting Tx
        - TFTs every 6 months if Hx of thyroid dysfunction
  - Glatiramer acetate
    - Copaxone 20 mg SC daily or 40 mg 3 times per week
      - Common adverse reactions: injection site reaction, nausea, chest pain, hypertonia, diaphoresis
      - No routine monitoring tests recommended
  - Natalizumab (Tysabri): 300 mg IV every 4 weeks
    - Restricted distribution in the United States; call 1-800-456-2255 for more info.
    - MRI at baseline
  - Fingolimod (Gilenya): 0.5 mg PO daily
    - EKG at baseline
    - Serious adverse reactions: QT prolongation, AV block; 6-hour observation following first dose
  - Teriflunomide (Aubagio): 7–14 mg PO daily
    - Avoid pregnancy, teratogenic; pregnancy test at baseline
    - Use reliable contraception during Tx.
- Symptomatic therapies (5)[B]:
  - Ataxia: clonazepam, propranolol, ondansetron
  - Spasticity: baclofen, diazepam, tizanidine, dantrolene, cyclobenzaprine hydrochloride
  - Pain: NSAIDs, carbamazepine, gabapentin, phenytoin, amitriptyline, mexiletine
  - Bladder dysfunction: (urgency) propantheline bromide, oxybutynin, tolterodine tartrate; (retention) phenoxybenzamine, terazosin hydrochloride, bethanechol
  - Constipation: high-fiber diets, fluids, natural or other laxatives, stool softeners, bulk-producing agents, suppositories
  - Sexual dysfunction: tadalafil, sildenafil, vardenafil
  - Weakness/fatigue: dalfampridine, amantadine, methylphenidate
  - Tremors: clonazepam, β-blockers, primidone
  - Depression: fluoxetine other SSRIs, tricyclic antidepressants, nontricyclic antidepressants

ADDITIONAL THERAPIES

- Cognitive-behavioral therapy
- Physical and occupational therapy
- Water therapy: Swimming, in cool water, is typically well-tolerated.

COMPLEMENTARY & ALTERNATIVE MEDICINE

- Omega-3: immunomodulary properties
- Vitamin D supplementation, sunlight exposure

ONGOING CARE

FOLLOW-UP RECOMMENDATIONS

Treat relapses with corticosteroids to minimize disease progression and duration of relapse. Maintain regular activity, but avoid overwork and fatigue. Rest during periods of acute relapse (2)[B].

Patient Monitoring

Assessing the severity of neurologic impairment from MS can be done using the Kurtzke Expanded Disability Status Score (EDSS): 0 indicates a normal neurologic exam and 10 indicates death due to MS. The EDDS uses a functional status (FS) score, covering the following: pyramidal symptoms, cerebellar, brainstem, sensory, bowel and bladder, visual/optic and cerebral/mental functions. EDDS scoring system (9)[C]:

- 0.0 – Normal neurologic examination
- 1.0 – No disability, minimal signs in 1 FS
- 1.5 – No disability, minimal signs in >1 FS
- 2.0 – Minimal disability in 1 FS
- 2.5 – Minimal disability in 2 FS
- 3.0 – Moderate disability in 1 FS or mild disability in 3–4 FS, but fully ambulatory
- 3.5 – Moderate disability in 1 FS and 1–2 FS grade 2 or 2 FS grade 3 or 5 FS grade 2, but fully ambulatory
- 4.0 – Ambulatory without aid or rest for ~500 m
- 4.5 – Ambulatory without aid or rest for ~300 m
- 5.0 – Ambulatory without aid or rest for ~200 m
- 5.5 – Ambulatory without aid or rest for ~100 m
- 6.0 – Intermittent or constant unilateral assistance (cane, crutch or brace) required to walk 100 m with or without rest
- 6.5 – Constant bilateral (cane, crutch or brace) required to walk 20 m with or without rest
- 7.0 – Unable to walk beyond 5 m with even aid, essentially restricted to wheelchair, wheels self and transfers alone; active in wheelchair for 12 hours/day
- 7.5 – Unable to take more than several steps, restricted to wheelchair and may require aid to transfer
- 8.0 – Essentially restricted to bed, chair, or wheelchair, but may be out of bed most of the day; retains self-care functions, generally effective use of arms
- 8.5 – Essentially restricted to bed most of the day, some effective use of arms and retains some self-care functions
- 9.0 – Helpless, bed-bound, patient but can communicate, eat
- 9.5 – Unable to effectively communicate, eat/swallow
- 10.0 – Death due to MS

DIET

High-fiber diet with bulk laxatives and plenty of fluids to prevent constipation

PATIENT EDUCATION

National Multiple Sclerosis Society: 1-800-344-4867 or www.nationalmssociety.org/

PROGNOSIS

- Differs in each individual; depends on the form of MS, the individual's sex and age, the initial presentation of the disease, and the amount of disability
- Average life expectancy is 5–10 years less than unaffected people.
- Specific clinical features suggest a more favorable course: early onset, RRMS form, female sex, <2 relapses within first year of diagnosis, and minimal functional decline after 5 years (5).
- Mortality secondary to an MS relapse is unusual; death is more commonly associated with a complication of MS such as an infection in a person who is more disabled.

COMPLICATIONS

Depression or emotional instability, paraplegia, chronic pain, sexual dysfunction, delirium, impaired vision (9)

REFERENCES

1. Compston A, Coles A. Multiple sclerosis. *Lancet*. 2008;372(9648):1502–1517.
2. Thrower BW. Relapse management in multiple sclerosis. *Neurologist*. 2009;15(1):1–5.
3. Ascherio A, Munger KL. Environmental risk factors for multiple sclerosis. Part I: the role of infection. *Ann Neurol*. 2007;61(4):288–299.
4. Alonso A, Hernán MA. Temporal trends in the incidence of multiple sclerosis: a systematic review. *Neurology*. 2008;71(2):129–135.
5. Rejdak K, Jackson S, Giovannoni G. Multiple sclerosis: a practical overview for clinicians. *Br Med Bull*. 2010;95(1):79–104.
6. Ascherio A, Munger KL. Environmental risk factors for multiple sclerosis. Part II: noninfectious factors. *Ann Neurol*. 2007;61(6):504–513.
7. Polman CH, Reingold SC, Banwell B, et al. Diagnostic criteria for multiple sclerosis: 2010 revisions to the McDonald criteria. *Ann Neurol*. 2011;69(2):292–302.
8. Zintzaras E, Doxani C, Mprotsis T, et al. Network analysis of randomized controlled trials in multiple sclerosis. *Clin Ther*. 2012;34(4):857–869.e9.
9. Kurtzke JF. Rating neurologic impairment in multiple sclerosis: an expanded disability status scale (EDSS). *Neurology*. 1983;33(11):1444–1452.

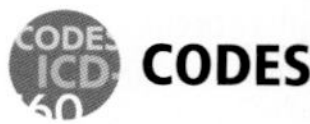

CODES

ICD-10

G35 Multiple sclerosis

CLINICAL PEARLS

- Immune-mediated inflammatory disease causing demyelination, neuronal loss, and scarring within the white matter of the CNS
- Charcot classical MS triad: nystagmus, intention tremor, and dysarthria
- Acute relapses are treated with steroids; disease-modifying medications are used for chronic treatment; currently, there is no treatment for promoting remyelination or neuronal repair.

MUMPS

Frances Y. Wu, MD

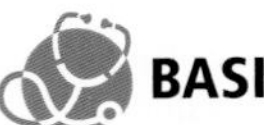

BASICS

Mumps is an acute, generalized paramyxovirus infection typically presenting with unilateral or bilateral parotitis.

DESCRIPTION

- Up to1/3 of individuals with mumps are asymptomatic.
- Painful parotitis occurs in 95% of symptomatic mumps cases. Epidemics in late winter and spring. Transmission by respiratory secretions
- Incubation period is 14–24 days.
- System(s) affected: hematologic/lymphatic/immunologic, reproductive, skin, exocrine
- Synonym(s): epidemic parotitis; infectious parotitis

EPIDEMIOLOGY

- Predominant age: 85% of mumps case occur before age 15 years:
  - Adult cases are typically more severe.
- Predominant sex: male = female
- Geriatric population: Most adults are immune.
- Acute epidemic mumps
  - Most cases occur in unvaccinated children aged 5–15 years.
  - Recent (2006) U.S. epidemic in vaccinated college students aged 18–24 years: 5,700 U.S. cases:
    - Another U.S. epidemic in 2009–2010 in New York/New Jersey: >1,500 cases
  - Mumps is unusual in children <2 years of age and most infants <1 year are immune.
  - Period of maximal communicability is 24 hours before to 72 hours after onset of parotitis

Incidence

- 796 cases in the United States in January 2014 to June 2014
- 438 cases in the United States in 2013 (1)
- Occasional epidemic outbreaks in a given region

Prevalence

- 0.0064/100,000 persons
- 90% of adults are seropositive even without history.

ETIOLOGY AND PATHOPHYSIOLOGY

Mumps virus replicates in glandular epithelium of parotids, pancreas, and testes, leading to interstitial edema and inflammation.

- Interstitial glandular hemorrhage may occur.
- Pressure caused by edema of the testes against the tunica albuginea can lead to necrosis and loss of function.

RISK FACTORS

- Foreign travel: 38% of other nations do *not* vaccinate for mumps, including most of Africa and South Asia.
- Crowded environments such as dormitories, barracks, or detention facilities
- Immunity wanes after single-dose vaccination:
  - After 2 doses, immunity drops from 95 to 86% in 9 years.
  - Genotypic variation from original vaccine strain may have a role in decreased vaccine efficacy (2).

GENERAL PREVENTION

- Vaccination
  - 2 doses of live mumps vaccine or measles-mumps-rubella (MMR) vaccine recommended, 1st at 12–15 months and 2nd at 4–6 years of age.
  - 95% effective in clinical studies, but field trials show 68–95% efficacy, which may be below level needed for herd immunity to prevent epidemic spread.
  - Scandinavian data suggest that successful prevention may require 95% 1st-dose and >80% 2nd-dose adherence.
  - Adverse effects: Most common proven effect is idiopathic thrombocytopenic purpura (ITP), with incidence of 3.3/100,000 doses.
  - *No relationship between MMR vaccine and autism*
- Immunoglobulin (Ig) is not effective in preventing mumps.
- Postexposure vaccination does not protect from recent exposure (3)[B]
- Isolate hospitalized patients for 5 days after onset.
- Isolate nonimmune individuals for 26 days after last case onset (social quarantine).

Pregnancy Considerations

- Live viral vaccines typically contraindicated in pregnancy; however, vaccination of children should not be delayed due to a pregnant family member.
- Immunization of contacts protects against future (but not current) exposures.

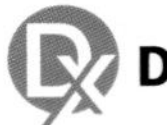

DIAGNOSIS

HISTORY

Parotid swelling peaks in 1–3 days and lasts 3–7 days.

- Up to 1/3 of individuals with mumps are asymptomatic.
- Rare prodrome of fever, neck muscle ache, and malaise
- Sour foods cause pain in parotid gland region.
- Moderate fever, usually not >104°F (40°C):
  - High fever frequently is associated with complications.

PHYSICAL EXAM

- Painful parotid swelling (unilateral or bilateral) obscures angle of mandible and elevates earlobe.
- Meningeal signs in 15%, encephalitis in 0.5%
- Rarely arthritis, orchitis, thyroiditis, mastitis, pancreatitis, oophoritis, myocarditis
- Rare maculopapular, erythematous rash
- Up to 50% of cases may be very mild
- Redness at opening of Stensen duct but no pus
- Swelling in sternal area; rare, but pathognomonic of mumps

DIFFERENTIAL DIAGNOSIS

- If not epidemic, other viruses are more common: parainfluenza parotitis, Epstein-Barr virus, coxsackievirus, adenovirus, parvovirus B19
- Suppurative parotitis: often associated with *Staphylococcus aureus* (presence of Wharton duct pus on massaging parotid gland nearly excludes diagnosis of mumps)
- Recurrent allergic parotitis
- Salivary calculus with intermittent swelling
- Lymphadenitis from any cause, even HIV infection
- Cytomegalovirus parotitis in immunocompromised patients
- Mikulicz syndrome: chronic, painless parotid and lacrimal gland swelling of unknown cause that occurs in tuberculosis, sarcoidosis, lupus, leukemia, lymphosarcoma, and malignant or benign salivary gland tumors
- Sjögren syndrome, diabetes mellitus, uremia, malnutrition
- Drug-related parotid enlargement (iodides, guanethidine, phenothiazine)
- Other causes of the complications of mumps (meningoencephalitis, orchitis, oophoritis, pancreatitis, polyarthritis, nephritis, myocarditis, prostatitis)
- Mumps orchitis must be differentiated from testicular torsion and from chlamydial or bacterial orchitis. (Testicular sonogram can be useful.)

DIAGNOSTIC TESTS & INTERPRETATION

- 3 special tests used to confirm an outbreak—if positive must be reported to health department (1)[A]
  - IgM titer (positive by day 5 in 100% of nonimmunized patients)
  - Swab of parotid duct or other affected salivary ducts for viral culture
  - Rise in IgG titer samples; test should be ordered if patient previously immunized: 1st sample within 5 days of onset, and 2nd, 2 weeks later.
- Other potential findings: Serum amylase may be elevated; CSF leukocytosis and leukopenia may be present.
- Testicular ultrasound may be useful to differentiate mumps orchitis from testicular torsion.
- Clinical diagnosis (swelling of one or both parotid glands):
  - Lasting ≥2 days
  - No other apparent cause
  - Rare presentation of meningitis without parotitis (1–10%)

Diagnostic Procedures/Other

If meningitis is present, lumbar puncture to exclude bacterial process. CSF pleocytosis, usually lymphocytes, is found in 65% of patients with parotitis.

Test Interpretation

Periductal edema and lymphocytic infiltration in affected glands on biopsy

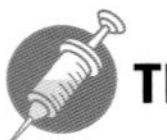

TREATMENT

- No specific antiviral therapy, only supportive care (1) [A],(4)[C]

- Analgesics to relieve pain
- Avoid corticosteroids for mumps orchitis because they can reduce testosterone concentrations and increase testicular atrophy.
- IVIG only successful for certain autoimmune-based sequelae:
  - Postinfectious encephalitis
  - Guillain-Barré syndrome
  - ITP
- Interferon-α2b improved severe bilateral orchitis but did not decrease testicular atrophy in small studies (5)[B].

GENERAL MEASURES

- Rarely need to hospitalize patients with high fever, pancreatitis, or CNS symptoms for supportive care, steroids, or interferon using appropriate isolation precautions
- Orchitis
  - Ice packs to scrotum can help to relieve pain.
  - Scrotal support with adhesive bridge while recumbent and/or athletic supporter while ambulatory

MEDICATION

First Line

- Analgesics and anti-inflammatory medications (acetaminophen; non-steroidal anti-inflammatory drugs [NSAIDs]) may diminish pain and swelling in acute orchitis and arthritis mumps.
- May use acetaminophen for fever and/or pain
- Precautions: Avoid aspirin for pain in children as previouslyassociated with Reye syndrome.

Second Line

- Interferon-α2b
- Chinese medicinal herbs and acupuncture have not shown proven benefit in randomized controlled trials (6,7).

INPATIENT CONSIDERATIONS

Admission Criteria/Initial Stabilization

- Hospitalize only if CNS symptoms occur.
- Outpatient supportive care if no complications

IV Fluids

If severe nausea or vomiting accompanies pancreatitis

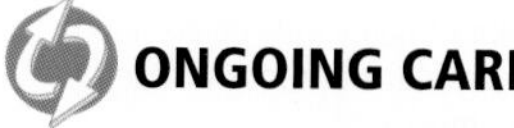

ONGOING CARE

FOLLOW-UP RECOMMENDATIONS

Mumps orchitis:

- Bed rest and local supportive clothing (e.g., 2 pairs of briefs) or adhesive-tape bridge
- Must be out of school until no longer contagious: about 9 days after onset of pain

Patient Monitoring

Most cases will be mild. Monitor hydration status.

DIET

Liquid diet if cannot chew

PATIENT EDUCATION

Orchitis is common in older children but rarely results in sterility, even after bilateral orchitis.

PROGNOSIS

- Complete recovery is usual; immunity is lifelong.
- Transient sensorineural hearing loss occurs in 4% of adults.
- Rare recurrence after 2 weeks may be recurrent nonepidemic parotitis.

COMPLICATIONS

- May precede, accompany, or follow salivary gland involvement and may occur (rarely) without primary involvement of the parotid gland
- Orchitis is common (30%) in postpubertal boys:
  - It starts within 8 days after parotitis.
  - Impaired fertility in 13%, but absolute sterility is rare.
- Meningitis (1–10%) or encephalitis (0.1%) may present 5–10 days after 1st symptoms of illness. Aseptic meningitis typically is mild, but meningoencephalitis may lead to seizures, paralysis, hydrocephalus, or, in 2% of encephalitis patients, death.
- Acute cerebellar ataxia has been reported after mumps infections; self-resolving in 2–3 weeks.
- Oophoritis in 7% of postpubertal females; no decreased fertility
- Pancreatitis, usually mild
- Nephritis, thyroiditis, and arthralgias are rare.
- Myocarditis: usually mild, but may depress ST segment; may be linked to endocardial fibroelastosis
- Deafness: 1/15,000 unilateral nerve deafness; may not be permanent
- Inflammation about the eye (keratouveitis) is rare.
- Dacryoadenitis, optic neuritis

Pediatric Considerations

- Orchitis is more common in adolescents.
- Young children are less likely to develop complications.
- Most complications occur in postpubertal group.
- Avoid aspirin use in children with viral symptoms.

Pregnancy Considerations

Disease may increase the rate of spontaneous pregnancy loss in 1st trimester. Perinatal mumps may also have a benign course.

REFERENCES

1. Centers for Disease Control and Prevention. Overview of mumps. http://www.cdc.gov/mumps/about/disease-overview.html. Accessed 2014.
2. Gouma S, Sane J,Gijselaar D, et al. Two major mumps genotype G variants dominated recent mumps outbreaks in the Netherlands (2009–2012). *J Gen Virol*. 2014;95(Pt 5):1074–1082.
3. Fiebelkorn AP, Lawler J, Curns A, et al. Mumps postexposure prophylaxis with a third dose of measles-mumps-rubella vaccine, Orange County, New York, USA. *Emerg Infect Dis*. 2013;19(9):1411–1417.
4. Davis NF, McGuire BB, Mahon JA.The increasing incidence of mumps orchitis: a comprehensive review. *BJU Int*. 2010;105(8):1060–1065.
5. Yapanoglu T, Kocaturk H, Aksoy Y, et al. Long-term efficacy and safety of interferon alpha-2B in patients with mumps orchitis. *Int Urol Nephrol*. 2010;42(4):867–871.
6. Shu M, Zhang YQ, Li Z, et al. Chinese medicinal herbs for mumps. *Cochrane Database Syst Rev*. 2012;(9):CD008578.
7. He J, Zheng M, Zhang M, et al. Acupuncture for mumps in children. *Cochrane Database Syst Rev*. 2012;(9):CD008400.

ADDITIONAL READING

- Centers for Disease Control and Prevention. Update: mumps outbreak—New York and New Jersey, June 2008–Jan 2010. *MMWR Morb Mortal Wkly Rep*. 2010;59(5):125–129.
- Flaherty DK. The vaccine-autism connection: a public health crisis caused by unethical medical practices and fraudulent science. *Ann Pharmacother*. 2011;45(10):1302–1304.
- MacDonald N, Hatchette T, Elkout L, et al. Mumps is back: why is mumps eradication not working? *Adv Exp Med Biol*. 2011;697:197–220.
- Shirts BH, Welch RJ, Couturier MR. Seropositivity rates for measles, mumps, and rubella IgG and costs associated with testing and revaccination. *Clin Vaccine Immunol*. 2013;20(3):443–445.

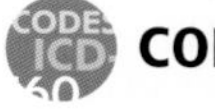

CODES

ICD10

- B26.9 Mumps without complication
- B26.1 Mumps meningitis
- B26.2 Mumps encephalitis

CLINICAL PEARLS

- Mumps is diagnosed clinically, based on swelling of ≥1 parotid glands for ≥2 days without other obvious cause. Confirmatory testing must be done in epidemic setting.
- Ultrasound is useful to distinguish testicular torsion from testicular pain related to mumps orchitis.
- A history of vaccination with MMR does not exclude mumps as field trials suggest the MMR vaccine is 68–95% effective.

MUSCULAR DYSTROPHY

Nimmy Thakolkaran, MD • George G.A. Pujalte, MD, FACSM

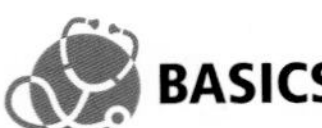

BASICS

- Primary inherited myopathies caused by dysfunctional proteins of muscle fibers and extracellular matrix
- Distribution of weakness, other associated symptoms, and disease prognosis depend on the specific gene affected and severity of the mutation.

DESCRIPTION

- Duchenne muscular dystrophy (DMD)
  - Highest incidence muscular dystrophy, X-linked inheritance, early onset, progressive
  - Patients are wheelchair-dependent prior to age 13 years
- Becker muscular dystrophy (BMD)
  - Less severe phenotype than Duchenne, also caused by mutation in *DMD* gene; later onset and milder clinical course
  - Distinction from DMD is clinical: Patients are wheelchair-dependent after age 16 years.
  - Collectively referred to as dystrophinopathies
- Myotonic muscular dystrophy (MMD)
  - Myotonia (slow relaxation after muscle contraction), distal and facial weakness
  - 2nd most common inherited muscle disease
- Facioscapulohumeral muscular dystrophy (FSHMD)
  - Facial and shoulder muscles most affected
  - 3rd most common inherited muscle disease
- Limb-girdle muscular dystrophy (LGMD)
  - Proximal weakness and atrophy, variable prognosis with many different identified mutations
- Oculopharyngeal muscular dystrophy (OPMD)
  - Usually adult onset, affects extraocular and pharyngeal muscles. Presents with ptosis and dysphagia
- Emery-Dreifuss muscular dystrophy (EDMD)
  - Triad of early development of joint contractures, slowly progressive muscle wasting, and cardiomyopathy. Serious cardiac manifestion can present as sudden death in apparently healthy young adults (1).
- Congenital muscular dystrophies (CMD)
  - Heterogeneous group of autosomal recessive myopathic diseases presenting in infancy with generally poor prognosis
  - Includes Fukuyama CMD, Ullrich CMD, Walker-Warburg syndrome, muscle-eye-brain disease

EPIDEMIOLOGY

Incidence

- Duchenne: 1/4,000 male births (2)
- Myotonic dystrophy: 1/10,000 births
- Other muscular dystrophies vary widely by population but are generally rare.

ETIOLOGY AND PATHOPHYSIOLOGY

Mutations affect proteins connecting cytoskeleton to cell membrane and extracellular matrix, causing muscle fibers to become fragile and easily damaged; muscle weakness and atrophy result.

- DMD/BMD
  - Defective protein is dystrophin, product of the largest human gene, *DMD*; Duchenne phenotype results from mutations that cause profound loss of dystrophin, the protein involved in calcium transport in muscle cells.
  - Becker phenotype results from less severe mutations in *DMD* gene; patients have low but detectable levels of functional dystrophin.
- MMD: Trinucleotide repeat expansion in the untranslated region of the gene *DMPK* on chromosome 19; encodes myotonin–protein kinase
- LGMD: mutations in genes encoding proteins associated with dystrophin: calpain-, dysferlin-, and fukutin-related proteins are affected most commonly.
- EDMD: Dysfunctional proteins are associated with the nuclear membrane in muscle fibers; emerin in X-linked form, lamin A/C in autosomal forms
- OPMD: Trinucleotide repeat expansion in *PABPN1* results in nuclear inclusions in muscle cells by hampering normal transport of mRNA from the nucleus.
- FSHMD: Deletion in untranslated region of chromosome 4; function of deleted genes is unclear, although the most accepted concept is that they likely affect the expression of multiple genes by epigenetic effects.

Genetics

- X-linked
  - Duchenne and Becker muscular dystrophies
  - Gene located at Xp21
    - 30% of affected males have a de novo mutation (mother is not a carrier).
    - 20% of female carriers have some manifestation of the mutation (usually mild muscle weakness or cardiomyopathy).
- Autosomal dominant
  - Generally later onset and less severe than diseases with recessive or X-linked inheritance
  - FSHMD, OPMD, some forms of LGMD and EDMD
  - Myotonic dystrophy
    - Trinucleotide repeat expansion with more severe phenotype in subsequent generations due to accumulation of repeats
- Autosomal recessive
  - Most types of CMD

GENERAL PREVENTION

Genetic counseling for carriers and prenatal diagnosis

COMMONLY ASSOCIATED CONDITIONS

- Decreased IQ: on average, 1 *SD* below the mean in DMD; speech and language delay
- Dilated cardiomyopathy and conduction abnormalities
  - Can be severe in EDMD
  - Can affect otherwise asymptomatic female carriers of DMD
  - Progressive scoliosis

DIAGNOSIS

HISTORY

- DMD: normal attainment of early motor milestones with subsequent abnormal gait and slowing gross motor development; clumsiness, waddling gait, frequent falls, difficulty running or climbing stairs
- BMD: progressive difficulty with ambulation and frequent falls in later childhood
- MMD: slurred speech, muscle wasting, difficulty with ambulation; often with family history
- LGMD: back pain, lordosis/inability to rise from a chair, climb stairs, and use arms overhead
- FSHMD: facial weakness, inability to close eyes completely
- EDMD: contractures of elbows and ankles, difficulty with ambulation in teenage years
- OPMD: ptosis and dysphagia; often with family history

PHYSICAL EXAM

- DMD/BMD
  - Proximal muscle weakness; Gower sign: use of arms to push upper body into standing posture from lying prone
  - Trendelenburg gait (hip waddling)
  - Hyporeflexia/areflexia
  - Winged scapulae and lordosis
  - Pseudohypertrophy of the calf (caused by proliferation of fat and connective tissue)
  - Contractures of lower extremity joints and elbows
- MMD
  - Characteristic facial appearance: narrow face, open triangular mouth, high-arched palate, concave temples, drooping eyelids, frontal balding in males
  - Myotonia: inability to relax muscles after contraction
  - Distal muscle weakness and wasting
- CMD
  - Arthrogryposis (multiple joint contractures); diffuse hypotonia and muscle wasting in an infant

DIFFERENTIAL DIAGNOSIS

- Glycogen storage diseases and other metabolic myopathies
- Mitochondrial myopathies: MELAS (**M**itochondrial **E**ncephalopathy, **L**actic **A**cidosis, and **S**troke-like episodes), MERRF (**M**yoclonus with **E**pilepsy and **R**agged-**R**ed **F**ibers)
- Inflammatory myopathies: polymyositis, dermatomyositis, inclusion-body myositis
- Neuromuscular junction diseases: myasthenia gravis, Lambert-Eaton syndrome
- Motor neuron diseases: amyotrophic lateral sclerosis, spinal muscular atrophy
- Charcot-Marie-Tooth disease
- Friedreich ataxia

DIAGNOSTIC TESTS & INTERPRETATION

Initial Tests (lab, imaging)

- Creatine kinase (CK): initial screening test if MD is suspected (3)[A]
- Elevated in DMD (10–100×); elevated at birth, peaks at time of presentation and falls during illness
- Initial detected lab abnormality may be elevated aspartate transaminase/alanine transaminase (AST/ALT) originating from muscle
- Genetic testing
  - For definitive diagnosis in patient with characteristic presentation and elevated CK
  - Deletion and duplication analysis will identify most patients; can sequence *DMD* gene for point mutations (4)[A]
  - Genetic testing is available clinically for most other muscular dystrophies.

Diagnostic Procedures/Other

- Muscle biopsy: rarely performed in DMD (dystrophin protein absent), may be helpful in other cases (4)[A]
- Electromyography and nerve conduction studies are not necessary unless considering alternative diagnoses.
- ECG: abnormalities found in >90% of males and up to 10% of female carriers of DMD; Q waves in anterolateral leads, tall R waves in V_1, shortened PR interval, arrhythmias, resting sinus tachycardia

Test Interpretation

- Heterogenic muscle fibers: atrophy and hypertrophy of fibers with proliferation of connective tissue in muscle
- Immunohistochemical staining for dystrophin protein
  - DMD: no detectable dystrophin in most fibers; occasional revertant fibers with normal dystrophin
  - BMD: highly variable staining for dystrophin throughout muscle

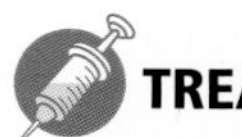

TREATMENT

Trials of agents that affect gene expression, such as antisense oligonucleotides, and small molecules that cause skipping of premature stop codons (ataluren) are ongoing; however, steroid treatment is the only clinically available therapy that affects disease progression.

GENERAL MEASURES

- Ambulation prolonged by knee-ankle-foot orthoses
- Serial casting to treat contractures
- Diagnose sleep apnea with polysomnography; treat with noninvasive ventilation
- Adaptive devices to improve function
- Avoid overexertion and strenuous exercise

MEDICATION

- Prednisone 0.75 mg/kg/day (4)[A]
  - Slows the decline in muscle function, progression to scoliosis and degradation of pulmonary function; prolongs functional ambulation; prolongs lifespan; improved cardiac outcomes
  - Initiate therapy when there is no longer progress in motor skills but prior to decline (3).
  - Monitor adverse effects
    - Consider bisphosphonates for preventing loss of bone density; annual exam for cataracts; monitor hypertension; avoid NSAIDs due to risk of peptic ulcer disese (PUD); stress-dose steroids during surgeries and illnesses due to adrenal suppression
    - Patients should be aware of immune suppression and notify emergency providers.
- Deflazacort (0.9 mg/kg) is an alternative oral steroid that is also considered 1st-line therapy in DMD; not available in the United States
- ACE inhibitors
  - Treatment of cardiomyopathy; may be used in conjunction with β-blockers

ISSUES FOR REFERRAL

- Refer to neuromuscular diseases center for definitive diagnosis and coordinated multidisciplinary care (4).
- Cardiology for management of cardiomyopathy
- Pulmonology for monitoring of pulmonary function and clearance regimen
- Physical medicine and rehabilitation for management of adaptive devices
- Nutrition/swallowing: for normal weight gain, attention for dysphagia
- Psychosocial: learning/behavior and coping assessment, social development (3)

SURGERY/OTHER PROCEDURES

- Spinal surgery for scoliosis—diminishes rate of deformity progression (2)[A],(5)
- Scapular fixation for scapular winging may be beneficial; also lacking clinical trials
- Consider surgical treatment of ankle/knee contractures
- Surgical procedures should be performed at a center experienced in DMD; total IV anesthesia should be used.

ONGOING CARE

- Individualized education plan and developmental evaluation for school accommodations
- Maintenance of current influenza and pneumococcal vaccination status

FOLLOW-UP RECOMMENDATIONS

Patient Monitoring

- Electrocardiogram (ECG), echocardiogram, and consultation with a cardiologist at diagnosis and annually after age 10 years
  - Female carriers of DMD mutation should be monitored every 5 years.
- Annual spinal radiography for scoliosis
- Dual-energy x-ray absorptiometry (DEXA) scanning and serum marker testing for osteoporosis
- Pulmonary function testing twice yearly if no longer ambulatory
- Psychosocial: coping, emotional adjustment, depression

DIET

- Obesity is common due to steroid treatment and wheelchair confinement: weight control can improve quality of life
- Diet may be limited by dysphagia; swallow evaluation can determine appropriate foods; may require gastrostomy
- Calcium and vitamin D supplementation for patients on steroids; monitor vitamin D levels

PATIENT EDUCATION

- Muscular Dystrophy Association: http://www.mda.org
- Parent Project Muscular Dystrophy: http://www.parentprojectmd.org

PROGNOSIS

- DMD/BMD
  - Progressive weakness, contractures, inability to walk
  - Kyphoscoliosis and progressive decline in respiratory vital capacity with recurrent pulmonary infections
  - Significantly shortened lifespan (DMD: 16 ± 4 years; BMD: 42 ± 16 years). Respiratory failure cause of death in 90%; remaining due to myocardial disease (heart failure and dysrhythmia) (5)
- Other types: slow progression and near-normal lifespan with functional limitations

COMPLICATIONS

- Cardiac arrhythmia, cardiomyopathy
- Dysphagia, gastroesophageal reflux disease (GERD), constipation
- Scoliosis, joint contractures
- Obstructive sleep apnea
- Malignant hyperthermia–like reaction to anesthesia
- Respiratory failure and early death

REFERENCES

1. Emery AE. The muscular dystrophies. *Lancet*. 2002;359(9307):687–695.
2. Van Ruiten HJ, Straub V, Bushby K, et al. Improving recognition of Duchenne muscular dystrophy: a retrospective case note review. *Arch Dis Child* 2014;99(12):1074–1077.
3. Bushby K, Finkel R, Birnkrant DJ, et al. Diagnosis and management of Duchenne muscular dystrophy, part 1: diagnosis, and pharmacological and psychosocial management. *Lancet Neurol*. 2009;9(1):77–93.
4. Bushby K, Finkel R, Birnkrant DJ, et al. Diagnosis and management of Duchenne muscular dystrophy, part 2: implementation of multidisciplinary care. *Lancet Neurol*. 2010;9(2):177–189.
5. Roberto R, Fritz A, Hagar Y, et al. The natural history of cardiac and pulmonary function decline in patients with Duchenne muscular dystrophy. *Spine*. 2011;36(15):E1009–E1017.

ADDITIONAL READING

- American Academy of Pediatrics Section on Cardiology and Cardiac Surgery. Cardiovascular health supervision for individuals affected by Duchenne or Becker muscular dystrophy. *Pediatrics*. 2005;116(6):1569–1573.
- Cheuk DKL, Wong V, Wraige E, et al. Surgery for scoliosis in Duchenne muscular dystrophy. *Cochrane Database Syst Rev*. 2013;2:CD005375.
- Cossu G, Sampaolesi M. New therapies for Duchenne muscular dystrophy: challenges, prospects and clinical trials. *Trends Mol Med*. 2007;13(12):520–526.
- Fairclough RJ, Bareja A, Davies KE. Progress in therapy for Duchenne muscular dystrophy. *Exp Physiol*. 2011;96(11):1101–1113.
- Ishikawa Y, Bach JR, Minami R. Cardioprotection for Duchenne's muscular dystrophy. *Am Heart J*. 1999;137(5):895–902.
- Manzur AY, Kuntzer T, Pike M, et al. Glucocorticoid corticosteroids for Duchenne muscular dystrophy. *Cochrane Database Syst Rev*. 2008;(1):CD003725.
- Orrell RW, Copeland S, Rose MR. Scapular fixation in muscular dystrophy. *Cochrane Database Syst Rev*. 2010;(1):CD003278.
- Schram G, Fournier A, Leduc H, et al. All-cause mortality and cardiovascular outcomes with prophylactic steroid therapy in Duchenne muscular dystrophy. *J Am Coll Cardiol*. 2013;61(9):948–954.
- Takami Y, Takeshima Y, Awano H, et al. High incidence of electrocardiogram abnormalities in young patients with Duchenne muscular dystrophy. *Pediatr Neurol*. 2008;39(6):399–403.
- van der Kooi EL, Lindeman E, Riphagen I. Strength training and aerobic exercise training for muscle disease. *Cochrane Database Syst Rev*. 2005;(1):CD003907.

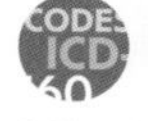

CODES

ICD10

- G71.0 Muscular dystrophy
- G71.11 Myotonic muscular dystrophy
- G71.2 Congenital myopathies

CLINICAL PEARLS

- Primary care providers should have a low threshold to obtain serum CK as a screening test in the face of gross motor delay/muscular weakness, especially in boys.
- Steroids should be initiated in patients with DMD when gross motor function ceases to progress.
- High-quality care of patients requires a medical home; a multidisciplinary team of physicians, therapists, and other providers; and extensive patient and family support.

MYASTHENIA GRAVIS

Melody A. Jordahl-Iafrato, MD

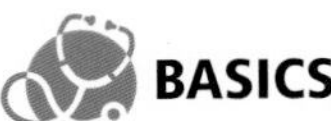

BASICS

DESCRIPTION

Primary disorder of neuromuscular transmission characterized by fluctuating muscle weakness:

- Ocular myasthenia gravis (MG) (15%): weakness limited to eyelids and extraocular muscles
- Generalized MG (85%): commonly affects ocular as well as a variable combination of bulbar, proximal limb, and respiratory muscles
- 50% of patients who present with ocular symptoms develop generalized MG within 2 years.
- Onset may be sudden and severe, but it is typically mild and intermittent over many years, maximum severity reached within 3 years for 85%.
- System(s) affected: neurologic; hematologic; lymphatic; immunologic; musculoskeletal

EPIDEMIOLOGY

Occurs at any age but a bimodal distribution to the age of onset:

- Female predominance: 20–40 years
- Male predominance: 60–80 years

Incidence

Estimated annual incidence 2–21/1 million

Prevalence

In the United States, 200/1 million; increasing over the past 5 decades

Pediatric Considerations

A transient form of neonatal MG seen in 10–20% of infants born to mothers with MG. It occurs as a result of the transplacental passage of maternal antibodies that interfere with function of the neuromuscular junction. Resolves in weeks to months

ETIOLOGY AND PATHOPHYSIOLOGY

- Reduction in the function of acetylcholine receptors (AChR) at muscle endplates, resulting in insufficient neuromuscular transmission
- Antibody-mediated autoimmune disorder
- Antibodies present in most cases of MG.
  - Seropositive/antiacetylcholine receptor (anti-AChR): a humoral, antibody-mediated, T-cell–dependent attack of the AChRs or receptor-associated proteins at the postsynaptic membrane of the neuromuscular junction. Found in 85% of generalized MG and 50% of ocular MG. Thymic abnormalities common (1)
  - Muscle-specific kinase (MuSK). 5% of generalized MG patients. Typically females. Is a severe form, respiratory and bulbar muscles involved. Thymic abnormalities rare (1)
  - In remainder of seronegative, 12–50% with anti-LRP4, a molecule that forms a complex with MuSK, clinical phenotype not well defined (1)
  - Seronegative MG (SNMG): 5%. May have anti-AChR detectable by cell-based assay. Clinically similar to anti-AChR, thypic hyperplasia may be present (1)
- Also documented immediately after viral infections (measles, Epstein-Barr virus [EBV], HIV, and human T-lymphotropic virus [HTLV])

Genetics

- Congenital MG syndrome describes a collection of rare hereditary disorders. This condition is not immune-mediated but instead, results from the mutation of a component of the neuromuscular junction (autosomal recessive).
- Familial predisposition seen in 5% of cases.

RISK FACTORS

- Familial MG
- D-penicillamine (drug-induced MG)
- Other autoimmune diseases

COMMONLY ASSOCIATED CONDITIONS

- Thymic hyperplasia (60–70%)
- Thymoma (10–15%)
- Autoimmune thyroid disease (3–8%)

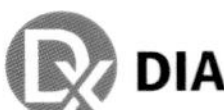

DIAGNOSIS

Myasthenia Gravis Foundation of America Clinical Classification (2)[C]:

- Class I: any eye muscle weakness, possible ptosis, no other evidence of muscle weakness elsewhere
- Class II: eye muscle weakness of any severity; mild weakness of other muscles:
  - Class IIa: predominantly limb or axial muscles
  - Class IIb: predominantly bulbar and/or respiratory muscles
- Class III: eye muscle weakness of any severity; moderate weakness of other muscles:
  - Class IIIa: predominantly limb or axial muscles
  - Class IIIb: predominantly bulbar and/or respiratory muscles
- Class IV: eye muscle weakness of any severity; severe weakness of other muscles:
  - Class IVa: predominantly limb/axial muscles
  - Class IVb: predominantly bulbar and/or respiratory muscles (can also include feeding tube without intubation)
- Class V: intubation needed to maintain airway

HISTORY

The hallmark of MG is fatigability.

- Fluctuating weakness, often subtle, that worsens during the day and after prolonged use of affected muscles, may improve with rest
- Early symptoms are transient with asymptomatic periods lasting days or weeks.
- With progression, asymptomatic periods shorten, and symptoms fluctuate from mild to severe.
- >50% of patients present with ocular symptoms (ptosis and/or diplopia). Eventually, 90% of patients with MG develop ocular symptoms.
- Ptosis might be unilateral, bilateral, or shifting from eye to eye.
- 15% present with bulbar symptoms.
- <5% present with proximal limb weakness alone.

ALERT

Myasthenic crisis: respiratory muscle weakness producing respiratory insufficiency and pending respiratory failure

PHYSICAL EXAM

- Ptosis may worsen with propping of opposite eyelid (curtain sign) or sustained upward gaze.
- "Myasthenic sneer," in which the midlip rises but corners of mouth do not move.
- Muscle weakness is usually proximal and symmetric.
- Test for muscle fatigability by repetitive or prolonged use of individual muscles.
- Important to test and monitor respiratory function.

DIFFERENTIAL DIAGNOSIS

- Thyroid ophthalmopathy
- Oculopharyngeal muscular dystrophy
- Myotonic dystrophy
- Kearns-Sayre syndrome
- Chronic progressive external ophthalmoplegia
- Brainstem and motor cranial nerve lesions
- Botulism
- Motor neuron disease (e.g., amyotrophic lateral sclerosis [ALS])
- Lambert-Eaton myasthenic syndrome
- Drug-induced myasthenia
- Congenital myasthenic syndrome
- Dermatomyositis/polymyositis
- Neurosarcoidosis
- Tolosa-Hunt syndrome

DIAGNOSTIC TESTS & INTERPRETATION

Initial Tests (lab, imaging)

- Anti-AChR antibody (74–85% are seropositive):
  - Generalized myasthenia: 75–85%
  - Ocular myasthenia: 50%
  - MG and thymoma: 98–100%
  - Poor correlation between antibody titer and disease severity (1)
  - False–positive results in thymoma without MG, Lambert-Eaton myasthenic syndrome, small cell lung cancer, and rheumatoid arthritis treated with penicillamine
- Anti-MuSK antibody:
  - Used if MG suspected, patient seronegative
  - Strong correlation between titer and disease severity (1)
- LRP4 and clustered anti-AChR:
  - Used if MG suspected, patient seronegative
- Thyroid and other autoimmune testing antistriated muscle (anti-SM) antibody:
  - Present in 84% of patients with thymoma who are <40 years of age
  - Can be present without thymoma in patients >40 years of age
- Chest radiographs or CT scans may identify a thymoma.
- MRI of brain and orbits to rule out other causes of cranial nerve deficit

Diagnostic Procedures/Other

- Tensilon (Edrophonium) test:
  - Initial 2-mg IV dose, followed by another 2 mg every 60 seconds up to a maximum dose of 10 mg
  - A positive test shows improvement of strength within 30 seconds of administration.
  - Sensitivity 80–90% (3)[C]

- Cardiac disease and bronchial asthma are relative contraindications, especially in elderly.
- Atropine: 0.4–0.6 mg IV may rarely be required as antidote; must be available.
- Can also do trial of other cholinesterase inhibitors (neostigmine or oral) and monitor response
- Ice pack test:
  - Ice pack applied to closed eyelid for 60 seconds, then removed; extent of ptosis immediately assessed
  - Ice will decrease the ptosis induced by MG.
  - Sensitivity 80% in patients with prominent ptosis
- Electrophysiology testing:
  - Repetitive nerve stimulation (RNS):
    - Widely available, most frequently used
    - Moderately sensitive for both generalized MG (75%) and ocular MG (50%) (3)[C]
  - Single-fiber electromyogram (SFEMG):
    - Assesses temporal variability between 2 muscle fibers within same motor unit (jitter)
    - Sensitive (90–95%) but less specific
    - Technically difficult to perform; limited availability, use if suspected and negative RNS (3)[C]

Test Interpretation

- Lymphofollicular hyperplasia of thymic medulla occurs in 65% of patients with MG, thymoma in 15%.
- Immunofluorescence: IgG antibodies and complement on receptor membranes in seropositive patients

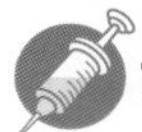

TREATMENT

GENERAL MEASURES

- Treatment based on age, gender, and disease severity and progression
- 3 basic approaches: symptomatic, immunosuppressive, and supportive. Few should receive a single therapeutic modality.

MEDICATION

First Line

Symptomatic treatments (anticholinesterase agents):

- Pyridostigmine bromide (Mestinon):
  - *Most commonly prescribed because available in oral tablet*
  - Starting dose of 30 mg PO TID with food
  - Maximum dose: 120 mg q3–4h
  - Long-acting available, but effect not consistent
- Neostigmine methylsulfate (Prostigmin):
  - Starting dose of 0.5 mg SC or IM q3h
  - Titrate dosage to clinical need.
- Patients with anti-MuSK may not respond well to these meds.

Second Line

- Immunosuppressants: Oral corticosteroids are 1st choice of drugs when immunosuppression is necessary.
  - Prednisone: Start as inpatient with a 60 mg/day PO; taper the dosage every 3 days; switch to alternate-day regimen within 2 weeks. Taper very slowly to establish the minimum dosage necessary to maintain remission (4)[B].
  - Cyclophosphamide: adults: 1–5 mg/kg/day PO; children: 2–8 mg/kg/day PO (5)[B]
  - Cyclosporine: adults: 5 mg/kg/day PO (nephrotoxicity and drug interactions) (5)[B]
  - Mycophenolate: 1 g PO or IV BID
  - Azathioprine: 100–200 mg/day PO (5)[B]
    - *Most frequently used for long-term immunomodulation*, similar efficacy to steroids and IVIG
    - Benefit may not be apparent for up to 18 months after initiation of therapy.
    - Prednisolone + azathioprine may be effective when used as a corticosteroid-sparing agent.
- Acute immunomodulating treatments:
  - Plasmapheresis: bulk removal of 2–3 L of plasma 3× per week, repeated until rate of improvement plateaus (6)[B]
    - Improves weakness in nearly all and can last up to 3 months
  - Immunoglobulin: 2 g/kg IV over 2–5 days (5)[B]
  - *Plasmapheresis and immunoglobulin have comparable efficacy in treating moderate to severe MG* (6)[C].
  - Rapid onset of effect but short duration of action
  - Used for acute worsening of MG to improve strength prior to surgery, prevent acute exacerbations induced by corticosteroids, and as a chronic intermittent treatment to provide relief in refractory MG.
- Other immunosuppressant therapies:
  - Tacrolimus
  - Rituximab:
    - Seronegative MuSK-antibody positive MG patients may have better response to rituximab than conventional therapies.

ALERT

Use caution with drugs that can precipitate weakness: aminoglycosides, fluoroquinolones, β-blockers, calcium channel blockers, neuromuscular blockers, statins, diuretics, oral contraceptives, gabapentin, phenytoin, lithium, among others.

SURGERY/OTHER PROCEDURES

- Thymectomy recommended for patients with thymic abnormalities
- No clear clinical benefit if onset at ≥60 years of age unless thymoma present.

Pediatric Considerations

- Infants with severe weakness from transient neonatal myasthenia may be treated with oral pyridostigmine; general support is necessary until the condition clears.
- Corticosteroids limited only to severe disease

INPATIENT CONSIDERATIONS

Admission Criteria/Initial Stabilization

- Management of pulmonary infections
- Myasthenic/cholinergic crises
- Plasmapheresis
- IV γ-globulin

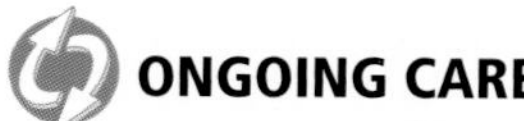

ONGOING CARE

PATIENT EDUCATION

MG Foundation of America (MGFA): www.myasthenia.org

PROGNOSIS

- Overall good but highly variable
- Myasthenic crisis associated with substantial morbidity and 4% mortality
- Seronegative patients are more likely to have purely ocular disease, and those with generalized SNMG have a better outcome after treatment.

COMPLICATIONS

Acute respiratory arrest; chronic respiratory insufficiency

REFERENCES

1. Berrih-Aknin S, Frenkian-Cuvelier M, Eymard B. Diagnostic and clinical classification of autoimmune myasthenia gravis. *J Autoimmun*. 2014;48–49:143–148.
2. Jaretzki A III, Barohn RJ, Ernstoff RM, et al. Myasthenia gravis: recommendations for clinical research standards. Task Force of the Medical Scientific Advisory Board of the Myasthenia Gravis Foundation of America. *Neurology*. 2000;55(1):16–23.
3. Meriggioli MN, Sanders DB. Myasthenia gravis: diagnosis. *Semin Neurol*. 2004;24(1):31–39.
4. Schneider-Gold C, Gajdos P, Toyka KV, et al. Corticosteroids for myasthenia gravis. *Cochrane Database Syst Rev*. 2005;(2):CD002828.
5. Hart IK, Sathasivam S, Sharshar T. Immunosuppressive agents for myasthenia gravis. *Cochrane Database Syst Rev*. 2007;(4):CD005224.
6. Barth D, Nabavi Nouri M, Ng E, et al. Comparison of IVIg and PLEX in patients with myasthenia gravis. *Neurology*. 2011;76(23):2017–2023.

ADDITIONAL READING

- Angelini C. Diagnosis and management of autoimmune myasthenia gravis. *Clin Drug Investig*. 2011;31(1):1–14.
- Chan KH, Lachance DH, Harper CM, et al. Frequency of seronegativity in adult-acquired generalized myasthenia gravis. *Muscle Nerve*. 2007;36(5):651–658.
- Deymeer F, Gungor-Tuncer O, Yilmaz V, et al. Clinical comparison of anti-MuSK- vs anti-AChR-positive and seronegative myasthenia gravis. *Neurology*. 2007;68(8):609–611.
- McConville J, Farrugia ME, Beeson D, et al. Detection and characterization of MuSK antibodies in seronegative myasthenia gravis. *Ann Neurol*. 2004;55(4):580–584.
- Merrigioli MN. Myasthenia gravis: immunopathogenesis, diagnosis, and management. *Continuum Lifelong Learning Neurology*. 2009;15(1):35–62.

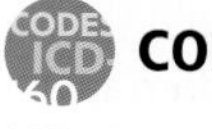

CODES

ICD10

- G70.00 Myasthenia gravis without (acute) exacerbation
- G70.01 Myasthenia gravis with (acute) exacerbation
- P94.0 Transient neonatal myasthenia gravis

CLINICAL PEARLS

- An autoimmune disease, marked by abnormal fatigability and weakness of selected muscles, which is relieved by rest
- Anticholinesterase medication and a thymectomy lessen symptom severity.
- Steroid therapy, plasma exchange, or immunoglobulin can be used in severely affected patients.

MYELODYSPLASTIC SYNDROMES

Richard A. Larson, MD

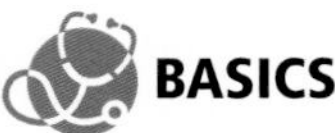

BASICS

DESCRIPTION

Myelodysplastic syndromes (MDSs) constitute a heterogeneous group of acquired hematopoietic stem cell disorders characterized by cytologic dysplasia in the bone marrow and blood and by various combinations of anemia, neutropenia, and thrombocytopenia:

- The natural progression of disease evolves as cellular maturation becomes more arrested and blast cells accumulate. There is an overlap between arbitrary diagnostic subgroups (1)[C],(2)[A],(3)[C].

- World Health Organization (WHO) classification
  - Refractory cytopenia with unilineage dysplasia
    - Refractory anemia (RA); refractory neutropenia; refractory thrombocytopenia
    - <5% blasts and <15% ring sideroblasts in marrow; <1% blasts in blood
  - Refractory anemia with ring sideroblasts (RARS)
    - <5% blasts in marrow; ≥15% of erythroid precursors are ring sideroblasts; no blasts in blood
    - Also known as acquired idiopathic sideroblastic anemia
  - RA with ring sideroblasts and marked thrombocytosis
  - Refractory cytopenia with multilineage dysplasia:
    - Marked trilineage dysplasia, but without excess blasts in marrow; no Auer rods; <1% blasts in blood
  - Refractory cytopenia with multilineage dysplasia and ring sideroblasts
  - RA with excess blasts-1 (RAEB-1):
    - 5–9% blasts in marrow; no Auer rods; <5% blasts in blood; <1,000 monocytes/mm^3
  - RAEB-2
    - 10–19% blasts in marrow; 5–19% blasts in blood; ±Auer rods; <1,000 monocytes/mm^3
  - MDS associated with isolated del(5q)
    - RA with erythroid hyperplasia, increased megakaryocytes with hypolobated nuclei, and normal or increased platelets; <5% blasts in marrow; <1% blasts in blood
  - Acute MDS with sclerosis:
    - RAEB with marked myelosclerosis
  - Chronic myelomonocytic leukemia (CMMoL) is now grouped with myelodysplastic/myeloproliferative disorders:
    - <20% blasts and promonocytes in marrow and blood with >1,000 monocytes/mm^3
  - RAEB in transformation is now considered acute myeloid leukemia (AML):
    - 20–30% blasts in marrow; >20% blasts in blood
    - Incidence: 2:1 (female > male)
  - Therapy-related MDS (t-MDS):
    - Seen 3–7 years after treatment with alkylating agents and/or radiotherapy
    - Evolves to AML over ~6 months
    - Classified by the WHO as therapy-related myeloid neoplasm
- System(s) affected: hematologic; lymphatic; immunologic
- Synonym(s): dysmyelopoietic syndrome; hemopoietic dysplasia; preleukemia; smoldering or subacute myeloid leukemia

Pediatric Considerations

Pediatric presentations of MDS

- Monosomy 7 syndrome
- Juvenile chronic myelogenous leukemia

EPIDEMIOLOGY

- Predominant age: median age, >65 years; uncommon in children and young adults
- Predominant sex: male = female

Incidence

Apparent increased incidence (1–2/100,000 per year) in recent years may be due to improved diagnosis; incidence increases markedly with older age.

Genetics

- Most are clonal neoplasms by cytogenetics, G6PD isoenzyme analysis, or restriction fragment length polymorphism analysis.
- Mutations in *RAS* oncogene
- Mutations in *RPS14* gene on chromosome 5q
- Mutations in *TET2, SF3B1, SRSF2, U2AF1, DNMT3A, ASXL1*

RISK FACTORS

- Primary MDS is associated with older age, occupational exposure to petroleum solvents (benzene, gasoline), and smoking.
- Secondary (therapy-related) MDS is associated with prior treatment with alkylating agents or radiotherapy.

COMMONLY ASSOCIATED CONDITIONS

- Anemia
- Neutropenia
- Thrombocytopenia
- Pancytopenia
- Opportunistic infections
- Bleeding, bruising
- Sweet syndrome (neutrophilic dermatosis)

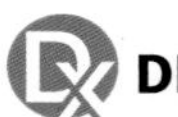

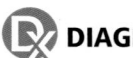

DIAGNOSIS

HISTORY

- Fatigue
- Fever
- Easy bruising

PHYSICAL EXAM

- Anemia
  - Fatigue
  - Shortness of breath
  - Light-headedness
  - Angina
- Leukopenia
  - Fever
  - Infection
- Thrombocytopenia
  - Ecchymoses
  - Petechiae
  - Epistaxis
  - Purpura
- Splenomegaly (uncommon)
  - Mild to moderate enlargement may be encountered, particularly in CMMoL.
- Skin infiltrates
  - Sweet syndrome

DIFFERENTIAL DIAGNOSIS

- Other malignant disorders
  - Evolving AML or erythroleukemia
  - Chronic myeloproliferative disorders
  - Polycythemia vera
  - Myeloid metaplasia with myelofibrosis
  - Malignant lymphoma
  - Metastatic carcinoma
- Nonmalignant disorders
  - Aplastic anemia
  - Autoimmune disorders (Felty syndrome, lupus, hemolytic anemia)
  - Nutritional deficiencies (vitamin B_{12}, pyridoxine, copper, protein malnutrition)
  - Heavy metal intoxication
  - Alcoholism
  - Chronic liver disease
  - Hypersplenism
  - Chronic inflammation
  - Recent cytotoxic therapy or irradiation
  - HIV infection
  - Paroxysmal nocturnal hemoglobinuria

DIAGNOSTIC TESTS & INTERPRETATION

Initial Tests (lab, imaging)

- CBC with differential and peripheral smear
- Reticulocyte count and serum erythropoietin level if anemia were present
- Review of the peripheral blood smear for the presence of dysplasia
- Liver/spleen scan or CT, although rarely necessary, may disclose occult splenomegaly or lymphadenopathy
- Cytogenetics
  - At least 50% of patients with primary MDS and nearly all with t-MDS have clonal chromosomal abnormalities: +8, −7, del(5q), del(7q), del(20q), iso(17), various others, and complex karyotypes.
  - Detection of clonal abnormality establishes a diagnosis of neoplasm and rules out a nutritional, toxic, or autoimmune disorder.
  - Cytogenetic analysis of metaphase cells from a bone marrow aspirate provides more information than fluorescence in situ hybridization analysis on blood cells.
- Granulocyte function tests: abnormal in 50% (decreased myeloperoxidase activity, phagocytosis, chemotaxis, and adhesion)
- Platelet function tests: impaired aggregation
- Marrow colony assays in vitro
  - Results are variable and correlate poorly with clinical course.
  - Poor clonal growth may suggest more rapid evolution to AML.
- Immunophenotyping
  - Nonspecific myeloid markers are present.
  - Occasionally, evidence can be found for concomitant lymphoproliferative disorder.
  - Loss of CD59 expression suggests paroxysmal nocturnal hemoglobinuria (PNH).

Follow-Up Tests & Special Considerations

- Anemia: often macrocytic; occasional poikilocytosis, anisocytosis; variable reticulocytosis
- Granulocytopenia: hypogranular or agranular neutrophils with poorly condensed chromatin; Pelger-Huet anomaly with hyposegmented nuclei
- Thrombocytopenia: occasionally giant platelets or hypogranular platelets
- Fetal hemoglobin may be elevated.
- Flow cytometry to detect loss of CD59 on RBCs, CD16 on granulocytes, and CD14 on monocytes; typical of PNH
- Direct antiglobulin (Coombs) test
- Paraprotein: present in some
- Erythropoietin: usually normally elevated given the degree of anemia unless renal failure is present
- Increased serum and tissue iron (ferritin), especially if anemia has been long-standing
- Serum copper level

Diagnostic Procedures/Other
- Review peripheral blood smear.
- Bone marrow aspiration, biopsy, and cytogenetics
- Myeloid gene mutation array

Test Interpretation
- Ineffective hematopoiesis with dysplasia in 1 or more cell lineages dominates the bone marrow picture in MDS.
- Marrow cellularity usually is normal or increased for the patient's age but may be hypoplastic in ~10%.
- Reticulin fibrosis usually is minimal except in t-MDS and acute MDS with sclerosis.
- Myeloblasts may be clustered in the intertrabecular spaces with abnormal localization of immature precursors.

TREATMENT

GENERAL MEASURES
- Immunize for pneumococcal pneumonia, pertussis, influenza, and hepatitis B (4)[C].
- RBC transfusions to alleviate symptoms
- Platelet transfusions only for bleeding or before surgery to avoid alloimmunization
- Early use of antibiotics for fever, even while culture results are pending, due to quantitative and qualitative granulocyte disorder
- Iron chelation therapy to avoid iron overload from chronic transfusions

MEDICATION
First Line
- Epoetin alfa or darbepoetin can increase hemoglobin levels in MDS patients who have low serum erythropoietin levels at baseline (5)[C].
- Only azacitidine, decitabine, and lenalidomide have been approved by the FDA for MDS.
- Azacitidine and decitabine have been proven in randomized controlled trials to be more effective for these heterogeneous disorders than only supportive care, with antibiotics, and transfusions.
- Vitamins, iron, corticosteroids, androgens, or thyroid hormone are rarely helpful, unless evidence of a specific deficiency exists.
- Clinical trials show azacitidine, 75 mg/m^2/d SC for 7 days and repeated every 28 days, decreases RBC transfusion requirements, yields longer times to AML or death, and improves quality of life.
- Decitabine was approved with a continuous IV schedule that usually requires hospitalization. More commonly, it is given at 20 mg/m^2 IV over 1 hour daily for 5 days as an outpatient, repeated every 4 weeks.
- Lenalidomide, 10 mg PO daily for 21 days every 4 weeks has yielded complete remission in patients with MDS and del(5q). It is less effective in patients with MDS without del(5q) (6)[B].
- Intensive chemotherapy
  - Younger patients with MDS may benefit from AML chemotherapy, especially if Auer rods are present, but toxicity may be severe for older patients.
  - Remission durations are variable (median, ~1 year).
- Allogeneic hematopoietic stem cell transplantation:
  - Recommended for younger patients with HLA antigen–matched donors to eradicate the malignant clone and resupply normal hematopoietic stem cells (7)[A].
- Aminocaproic acid (epsilon-aminocaproic acid) or tranexamic acid may benefit patients with chronic, severe thrombocytopenia and bleeding.
- Contraindications: Cytotoxicity of chemotherapy may increase the risk of bleeding and infection and the need for transfusion support.
- Precautions: Aspirin, salicylates, and NSAIDs should be avoided.

Second Line
- Danazol or prednisone may be of benefit for concomitant autoimmune thrombocytopenia.
- Investigational agents
  - Low doses of cytarabine, tretinoin (all-trans retinoic acid), 13-cis retinoic acid, arsenic trioxide, histone/protein deacetylase inhibitors, interferon, cyclosporine, antithymocyte globulin, filgrastim, and interleukin-3
  - Agents, such as thalidomide, that inhibit the production of tumor necrosis factor in the marrow
- Amifostine may stimulate the proliferation of normal hematopoiesis.

ISSUES FOR REFERRAL
- Refer younger adults for allogeneic hematopoietic cell transplantation.
- Refer patients with symptoms or transfusion requirements for clinical trials.

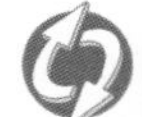

ONGOING CARE

FOLLOW-UP RECOMMENDATIONS
Usually outpatient, except when necessary to hospitalize for the treatment of infection, blood transfusions, or intensive chemotherapy

Patient Monitoring
- At least monthly during supportive care
- More frequently if receiving treatment

DIET
Reduce alcohol use and iron intake (unless patient is iron-deficient).

PATIENT EDUCATION
- Stop smoking.
- Seek early medical attention for fever, bleeding, or symptoms of anemia.
- Advise about the risks of chronic transfusion therapy.

PROGNOSIS
- Median survival for RA and RARS is 5 years, but it may extend much longer (8)[B].
- RA with del(5q) syndrome is favorable.
- Median survival for RAEB, RCMD, and CMMoL is ~1 year; 50% of patients evolve to AML and the other 50% die of infection or bleeding.

COMPLICATIONS
- Infection
- Bleeding
- Complications of anemia and transfusions

REFERENCES

1. Malcovati L, Hellström-Lindberg E, Bowen D, et al. Diagnosis and treatment of primary myelodysplastic syndromes in adults: recommendations from the European Leukemia Net. *Blood*. 2013;122(17):2943–2964.
2. Swerdlow SH, Campo E, Harris NL, et al., eds. *WHO Classification of Tumours of Haematopoietic and Lymphoid Tissues*. Lyon, France: IARC Press; 2008.
3. Greenberg PL. The multifaceted nature of myelodysplastic syndromes: clinical, molecular, and biological prognostic features. *J Natl Compr Canc Netw*. 2013;11(7):877–885.
4. Larson RA. Myelodysplasia: when to treat and how. *Best Pract Res Clin Haematol*. 2006;19(2):293–300.
5. Fenaux P, Adès L. How we treat lower-risk myelodysplastic syndromes. *Blood*. 2013;121(21):4280–4286.
6. List A, Dewald G, Bennett J, et al. Lenalidomide in the myelodysplastic syndrome with chromosome 5q deletion. *N Engl J Med*. 2006;355(14):1456–1465.
7. Koreth J, Pidala J, Perez WS, et al. Role of reduced-intensity conditioning allogeneic hematopoietic stem-cell transplantation in older patients with de novo myelodysplastic syndromes: an international collaborative decision analysis. *J Clin Oncol*. 2013;31(21):2662–2670.
8. Voso MT, Fenu S, Latagliata R, et al. Revised International Prognostic Scoring System (IPSS) predicts survival and leukemic evolution of myelodysplastic syndromes significantly better than IPSS and WHO Prognostic Scoring System: validation by the Gruppo Romano Mielodisplasie Italian Regional Database. *J Clin Oncol*. 2013;31(21):2671–2677.

ADDITIONAL READING

- Cheson BD, Greenberg PL, Bennett JM, et al. Clinical application and proposal for modification of the International Working Group (IWG) response criteria in myelodysplasia. *Blood*. 2006;108(2):419–425.
- Nybakken GE, Bagg A. The genetic basis and expanding role of molecular analysis in the diagnosis, prognosis, and therapeutic design for myelodysplastic syndromes. *J Mol Diagn*. 2014;16(2):145–158.
- Larson RA, Le Beau MM. Therapy-related myeloid leukaemia: a model for leukemogenesis in humans. *Chem Biol Interact*. 2005;153–154:187–195.
- Singh ZN, Huo D, Anastasi J, et al. Therapy-related myelodysplastic syndrome: morphologic subclassification may not be clinically relevant. *Am J Clin Pathol*. 2007;127(2):197–205.

CODES

ICD10
- D46.9 Myelodysplastic syndrome, unspecified
- D46.4 Refractory anemia, unspecified
- D46.B Refract cytopenia w multilin dysplasia and ring sideroblasts

CLINICAL PEARLS
- MDS constitutes a heterogeneous group of acquired, hematopoietic stem cell disorders characterized by cytologic dysplasia in the bone marrow and blood and by various combinations of anemia, neutropenia, and thrombocytopenia.
- The natural progression of disease evolves as cellular maturation becomes more arrested and blast cells accumulate.

MYELOPROLIFERATIVE NEOPLASMS

Frank J. Domino, MD

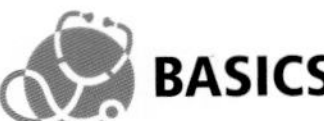

BASICS

DESCRIPTION

- Myeloproliferative neoplasms (MPNs) are defined as disorders of the pluripotent hematopoietic stem cells of bone marrow.
- MPNs are characterized by proliferation of a specific stem cell lineage such as myeloid, erythroid, or megakaryocyte; resulting in granulocytosis, erythrocytosis, or thrombocytosis, respectively.
- The "classic" MPNs include chronic myelogenous leukemia (CML), polycythemia vera (PV), essential thrombocythemia (ET), and primary myelofibrosis (PMF). The classification now includes the "nonclassic" conditions of chronic neutrophilic leukemia, chronic eosinophilic leukemia not otherwise specified (CEL-NOS), systemic mastocytosis, and myeloproliferative neoplasm unclassifiable. This topic focuses on the classic MPNs.
- CML is classified as a Philadelphia-positive MPN, whereas ET, PMF, and PV are classified as Philadelphia-negative MPNs.
- CML: characterized by uninhibited growth and production of granulocytes at varying stages, primarily neutrophils, leading to granulocytosis
- PMF: progressive fibrosis of the bone marrow due to clonal stem cell proliferation that has become hypersensitive to the effects of cytokines, leading to extramedullary hematopoiesis
- ET: characterized by a clonal proliferation of megakaryocytes, leading to thrombocytosis
- PV: trilineage growth of hematopoietic stem cells with erythroid precursors predominating, leading to erythrocytosis

EPIDEMIOLOGY

Incidence

- CML: 0.6–2.0/100,000/year; median age at diagnosis 66 years; male > female (1.6:1)
- PMF: 0.5–1.5/100,000/year; median age at diagnosis 65 years; male = female
- ET: 0.6–2.5/100,000/year; median age at diagnosis 60 years, 2nd peak in younger patients at ~30 years; female > male (2:1)
- PV: 1–2/100,000/year; male > female (1.3:1)

ETIOLOGY AND PATHOPHYSIOLOGY

- CML: *BCR-ABL1* gene leads to increased and unrestrained activity of tyrosine kinase resulting in activity of downstream signaling pathways, unchecked proliferation, incomplete differentiation, inhibition of apoptosis and extended survival of hematopoietic cells, as well as mobilization of progenitor cells, leading to the neutrophilic changes seen in CML.
- PMF: Hematopoietic stem cells become hyperreactive to the effects of circulating cytokines, causing clonal proliferation of the stem cells leading to bone marrow fibrosis and resultant extramedullary hematopoiesis, accounting for most of the signs/symptoms of PMF.
- ET: Thrombopoietin binds to a pluripotent stem cell receptor to induce proliferation of a megakaryocyte and eventually a platelet; this process is normally regulated by a negative feedback loop, which is nonfunctioning in ET, leading to unrestrained growth and development of platelets.
- PV: Gain-of-function mutation (*JAK2*) leads to increased erythrocyte production regardless of an intact negative feedback mechanism (normal expression of cell surface receptors and decreased renal production of erythropoietin).
- Unknown; familial component described in PV, ET, and PMF

Genetics

- Philadelphia chromosome (*BCR-ABL1* gene): translocation and fusion of the *BCR* gene on chromosome 22 and the *ABL* gene on chromosome 9; seen in all patients with CML
- *JAK2* mutations: point mutations in the tyrosine kinase domain of *JAK2*, causing a substitution of valine for phenylalanine at position 617 (*JAK2V617F*); leading to unrestrained *JAK2* activation with a deactivation of typical feedback mechanism:
  - Seen in >95% of PV cases; 50% of ET and PMF cases
- Myeloproliferative leukemia virus (*MPL*) gene: Mutations found in 5–10% of patients with PMF and in 3–5% of those with ET.

RISK FACTORS

- Rare familial cases have been reported.
- CML: exposure to ionizing radiation

COMMONLY ASSOCIATED CONDITIONS

- Progression to acute myeloid leukemia; most common with CML
- Thrombosis/hemorrhage

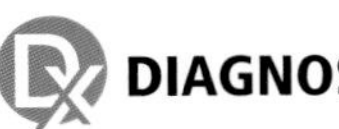

DIAGNOSIS

HISTORY

- Many MPN cases are found incidentally on routine blood work.
- CML: Most patients are asymptomatic at time of diagnosis:
  - Fatigue, malaise, weight loss, excessive perspiration, abdominal fullness, early satiety, bleeding episodes
- PMF: Symptoms depend on the degree of anemia and splenomegaly:
  - Fatigue, shortness of breath, early satiety, constitutional symptoms, cachexia, Budd-Chiari syndrome, splenic infarcts, osteosclerosis
- ET: characterized by thrombotic and hemorrhagic events
  - Thrombotic events (deep vein thrombosis, pulmonary embolism, Budd-Chiari syndrome), microvascular occlusive events (digital ischemia, erythromelalgia), major/minor hemorrhagic events; headaches, dizziness, syncope, tingling, visual changes, transient ischemic attacks
- PV: Symptoms are due to level of erythrocytosis and the resultant increased blood viscosity.
  - Erythromelalgia, pruritus after hot baths, headaches, tinnitus, paresthesias, gout attacks

PHYSICAL EXAM

- CML: splenomegaly, hepatomegaly
- PMF: splenomegaly seen in nearly all patients, hepatomegaly, paleness
- ET: possible petechiae, purpura, ecchymosis
- PV: cyanotic blush (lips, nose, ears, distal extremities), increased blood pressure, splenomegaly, epistaxis, ecchymosis

DIFFERENTIAL DIAGNOSIS

- CML: leukemoid reaction (elevated LAP), juvenile myelomonocytic leukemia, chronic myelomonocytic leukemia (CMML), chronic eosinophilic leukemia, chronic neutrophilic leukemia
- PMF: other MPNs, lymphoma, hairy cell leukemia, multiple myeloma, metastatic cancer, connective tissue disease, rickets, renal osteodystrophy
- ET: reactive thrombocytosis, CML, PV, PMF, and myelodysplastic syndromes
- PV: hypoxic states (e.g., chronic obstructive pulmonary disease [COPD], anemia), renal cell carcinoma, Wilms tumor, hepatoma, polycystic kidney disease, exogenous androgens

DIAGNOSTIC TESTS & INTERPRETATION

- CML: White blood cell count $>100,000 \times 10^9$/L with differential showing increased neutrophils at varying stages of development and an increased percentage of myelocytes; neutrophils have decreased leukocyte alkaline phosphatase; platelet count $>600,000 \times 10^9$/L and a normochromic, normocytic anemia.
- PMF (1)[A] (World Health Organization [WHO] criteria): Diagnosis requires meeting all 3 major criteria and >2 minor criteria:
  - *Major criteria*: (i) Megakaryocyte proliferation and atypia accompanied by either reticulin or collagen fibrosis. (ii) Not meeting WHO criteria for CML, PV, MDS, or other myeloid neoplasm. (iii) Demonstration of *JAK2V617F* or other clonal marker or absence of marker with no evidence of secondary marrow fibrosis
  - *Minor criteria*: (i) Leukoerythroblastosis. (ii) Increased serum lactate dehydrogenase level. (iii) Anemia. (iv) Palpable splenomegaly
- ET (1)[A] (WHO criteria): Diagnosis requires meeting all 4 major criteria:
  - *Major criteria*: (i) Thrombocytosis with persistent platelet level $\geq 450 \times 10^9$/L. (ii) Megakaryocyte proliferation with large and mature morphology. (iii) Not meeting WHO criteria for CML, PV, PMF, MDS, or other myeloid neoplasm. (iv) Demonstration of *JAK2V617F* or other clonal marker or absence of clonal marker with no evidence of reactive thrombocytosis
- PV (1)[A] (WHO criteria): Diagnosis requires either both major criteria and 1 minor criterion or the first major criterion and 2 of the minor criteria:
  - *Major criteria*: (i) Hemoglobin >18.5 g/dL in men, >16.5 g/dL in women or other evidence of increased red cell volume. (ii) Presence of *JAK2V617F* or other functionally similar mutation (e.g., *JAK2* exon 12 mutation) (1)[B]
  - *Minor criteria*: (i) Bone marrow biopsy showing hypercellularity for age with trilineage myeloproliferation. (ii) Low serum erythropoietin level. (iii) Endogenous erythroid colony formation in vitro

Initial Tests (lab, imaging)

If clinical suspicion of MPN, obtain a CBC and peripheral blood smear; if positive, obtain bone marrow biopsy.

- PMF: radiographic osteosclerosis in 25–66%
- ET: ultrasonic imaging if venous thrombosis suspected

Diagnostic Procedures/Other

- CML: diagnosis with identification of Philadelphia chromosome: Karyotyping of metaphase chromosomes is the gold standard for diagnosis; fluorescence in situ hybridization used when karyotypic analysis is negative/inconclusive; polymerase chain reaction for monitoring response to tyrosine kinase inhibitors
  - Bone marrow biopsy: granulocytic hyperplasia with dwarf megakaryocytes
- PMF, ET, and PV: genotypic analysis and bone marrow biopsy as described in above WHO criteria; "dry tap" for bone marrow aspiration in PMF
- Risk stratification
  - CML: 3 phases of CML
    - (i) Chronic phase (85% patients at diagnosis; <5% blast counts). (ii) Accelerated phase (poorly controlled regardless of treatment, 10–19% blast counts). (iii) Blast crisis (resembles acute leukemia, >20% blast counts)
  - PMF: International Prognostic Scoring System (IPSS) at diagnosis and Dynamic IPSS (DIPSS-plus) throughout disease
    - IPSS: age >65 years, constitutional symptoms, hemoglobin <10 g/dL, leukocyte count $>25 \times 10^9$, circulating blasts >1%
      - Low risk = 0 of above; intermediate-1 risk = 1 of above; intermediate-2 risk = 2 of above; high risk = ≥3 of above
    - DIPSS-plus: same 5 risk factors in the IPSS + the need for red cell transfusion, platelets $<100 \times 10^9$/L and unfavorable karyotype
      - Low risk = 0 of above; intermediate-1 risk = 1 of above; intermediate-2 risk = 2–3 of above; high risk = ≥4 of above
  - ET: low risk = age <40 years, no prior thromboembolic events, no cardiovascular risk factors, platelet count $<1{,}500 \times 10^9$/L; intermediate risk = age 40–59 years, presence of cardiovascular risk factors, platelet count $<1{,}500 \times 10^9$/L; high risk = age ≥60 years and/or prior thromboembolic or hemorrhagic episode and/or platelet count $>1{,}500 \times 10^9$/L
  - PV: low risk = age <60 years, no history of thrombosis/cardiovascular risk factors; intermediate risk = platelets $>1{,}000 \times 10^9$/L and cardiovascular risk factors; high risk = age >60 years or a history of thrombosis

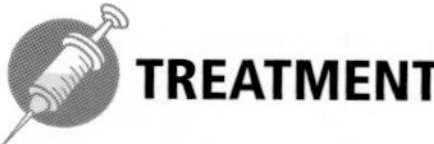

TREATMENT

GENERAL MEASURES

Splenectomy has no impact on mortality but is occasionally carried out for symptomatic relief (2)[B].

MEDICATION

First Line

- CML
  - Chronic phase: Imatinib mesylate (Gleevec): 400 mg/day, a potent tyrosine kinase inhibitor (TKI)
  - Accelerated or blast phase: Increase imatinib to 800 mg/day and consider allogeneic stem cell transplant (aSCT).
  - While awaiting confirmation of diagnosis, hydroxyurea can be used to lower the WBC count.
- PMF: Main goal is symptomatic relief:
  - Low and intermediate-1 risk: no drug therapy indicated, palliative measures if necessary
  - Intermediate-2 and high risk: hydroxyurea or consider aSCT
  - Palliative treatment
    - Anemia (keep hemoglobin >10 g/dL): transfusions, low-dose prednisone; erythropoiesis-stimulating agents, androgens, danazol, or thalidomide 50 mg/day
    - Splenomegaly: hydroxyurea, splenectomy or IV cladribine monthly for refractory cases
    - Thrombosis: hydroxyurea and low-dose aspirin
- ET low and intermediate risk: "Watch and wait" + low-dose aspirin if microvascular disturbances present and no contraindications; high risk: hydroxyurea 15 mg/kg/day in divided doses to reduce platelet count to $<450 \times 10^9$/L
- PV
  - Low and intermediate risk: phlebotomy and low-dose aspirin
  - High risk (or those who do not tolerate phlebotomy): hydroxyurea 500–1,000 mg/day

Second Line

- CML: Only curable treatment is aSCT; reserved for accelerated/blast phase due to high rates of morbidity and mortality with aSCT
  - 2nd-generation TKIs: dasatinib, nilotinib, and bosutinib; increasing evidence for improved, deeper responses with these medications; ongoing studies assessing role of 2nd-generation TKIs for 1st-line therapy
- ET: If resistant/intolerant to hydroxyurea, use anagrelide:
  - If resistant/intolerant to hydroxyurea or anagrelide, pregnant or age <40 years: Use interferon-α.
- PMF: Only curable treatment is aSCT; reserved for intermediate-2 or high-risk patients age <50 years
  - If unresponsive to hydroxyurea, use pegylated interferon-α; tolerance may be an issue.
- Ongoing investigations for *JAK2* inhibitors in the treatment of PV, PMF, and ET
  - Ruxolitinib, a JAK2 Inhibitor, has completed phase III trials for the treatment of PMF.

ISSUES FOR REFERRAL

Patients with MPNs are usually referred to hematology/oncology. May consult palliative care or surgical/radiation oncology if necessary.

SURGERY/OTHER PROCEDURES

May require splenectomy/palliative radiation for foci of extramedullary hematopoiesis

INPATIENT CONSIDERATIONS

Admission Criteria/Initial Stabilization

- Severe cachexia; renal failure and hepatomegaly secondary to extramedullary hematopoiesis; massive splenomegaly requiring treatment; severe thrombotic/hemorrhagic episodes; anemia; tumor lysis syndrome
  - Treatment aimed at symptom relief and pain control

IV Fluids

Optimal hydration to prevent tumor lysis syndrome

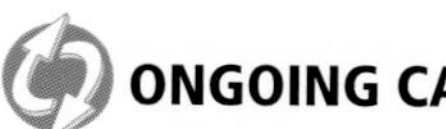

ONGOING CARE

PROGNOSIS

- CML: 10-year survival rate ~80% from time of diagnosis; 85% will die in blast crisis; 12- to 18-month median survival for accelerated phase; 3- to 6-month median survival for blast phase
- PMF: worst prognosis of the MPNs; drug therapy does not modify disease course but treats the symptoms; median survival for low risk = 135 months, intermediate-1 risk = 95 months; intermediate-2 risk = 48 months; high risk = 27 months
- ET and PV: near-normal life expectancy

COMPLICATIONS

- CML: blast crisis, transformation to acute leukemia, gout, or nephropathy due to hyperuricemia
- PMF: 10% develop acute myeloid leukemia; anemia, massive hepatosplenomegaly, thrombohemorrhagic events, osteosclerosis, secondary gout, splenic infarcts, paraspinal/epidural extramedullary hematopoiesis
- ET: <10% develop post-ET myelofibrosis, 2% develop acute myeloid leukemia; thrombohemorrhagic events
- PV: erythromelalgia, pruritus, secondary gout, headaches, vascular occlusive events

REFERENCES

1. Sonbol MB, Firwana B, Zarzour A, et al. Comprehensive review of JAK inhibitors in myeloproliferative neoplasms. *Ther Adv Hematol*. 2013;4(1):15–35.
2. Koopmans SM, van Marion AM, Schouten HC. Myeloproliferative neoplasia: A review of clinical criteria and treatment. *Neth J Med*. 2012;70(4):159–167.

ADDITIONAL READING

- Bittencourt RI, Vassallo J, Chauffaille Mde L, et al. Philadelphia-negative chronic myeloproliferative neoplasms. *Rev Bras Hematol Hemoter*. 2012;34(2):140–149.
- Cervantes F. Management of essential thrombocythemia. *Hematology Am Soc Hematol Educ Program*. 2011;2011:215–221.
- Ferdinand R, Mitchell SA, Batson S, et al. Treatments for chronic myeloid leukemia: a qualitative systematic review. *J Blood Med*. 2012;3:51–76.
- Tohami T, Nagler A, Amariglio N. Laboratory tools for diagnosis and monitoring response in patients with chronic myeloid leukemia. *Isr Med Assoc J*. 2012;14(8):501–507.
- Vannucchi AM. Management of myelofibrosis. *Hematology Am Soc Hematol Educ Program*. 2011;2011:222–230.

SEE ALSO

Leukemia, Chronic Myelogenous; Polycythemia Vera

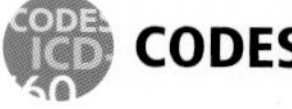

CODES

ICD10

- D47.1 Chronic myeloproliferative disease
- C92.10 Chronic myeloid leukemia, BCR/ABL-positive, not having achieved remission
- D45 Polycythemia vera

CLINICAL PEARLS

MPNs are defined as disorders of the pluripotent hematopoietic stem cells of bone marrow.

NARCOLEPSY

Jeffrey F. Minteer, MD

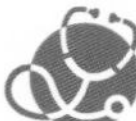

BASICS

DESCRIPTION

- Disorder of unknown etiology characterized by excessive daytime sleepiness typically associated with cataplexy (sudden bilateral weakness of skeletal muscles) and other rapid eye movement (REM) sleep phenomena, such as sleep paralysis and hypnagogic hallucinations (e.g., vivid auditory or visual perceptions without an external stimulus that occur as one is falling asleep)
- Frequently overlooked disorder, with an average of 15 years of symptoms prior to diagnosis
- System affected: nervous

EPIDEMIOLOGY

Incidence

- Onset usually in teenage years
- Bimodal distribution peak at 15 and 36 years of age
- Predominant sex: male > female (1.6:1)
- Occurrence: 1 in 3,000 persons

Pediatric Considerations

Uncommon in childhood

Prevalence

25–50 cases/100,000 people

ETIOLOGY AND PATHOPHYSIOLOGY

- Unknown
- Neurodegenerative disorder resulting from selective loss of neurons containing hypocretin (orexin) in the hypothalamus; may be autoimmune (associated with influenza A, H1N1 vaccine, and *Streptococcus pyogenes*)
- Orexin neurons also regulate metabolism, feeding, reward and autonomic tone; weight gain especially in children from reduction of metabolism
- 85% of patients with narcolepsy and cataplexy have low hypocretin in CSF.
- Possible involvement of immune system and environmental influences

Genetics

- Increased incidence in families with positive history: 1–2% in 1st-degree relative of index case (10–40× the general population)
- Twin concordance is 25–31% (suggests environmental contribution).
- Most are sporadic.
- 85–95% of patients with narcolepsy and cataplexy have biologic human leukocyte antigen (HLA) DQB1*0602; 40% of patients with narcolepsy without cataplexy express this antigen. HLA DQB1*0602 is present in 24% of the general population.
- Autosomal-recessive inheritance pattern
- 12% of Asians, 25% of whites, and 38% of African Americans are gene carriers.

RISK FACTORS

- Head trauma
- CNS infectious disease
- Anesthesia
- Psychological stress
- Pregnancy
- Family history
- High BMI

COMMONLY ASSOCIATED CONDITIONS

Obstructive sleep apnea (up to 25%), obesity, anxiety

DIAGNOSIS

HISTORY

- Classic tetrad of excessive daytime sleepiness, cataplexy, sleep paralysis, and hypnagogic hallucinations (4 most common symptoms): Only 10–20% of patients have all 4 symptoms.
- 3 general forms
  - Narcolepsy without cataplexy: 40%
  - Narcolepsy with cataplexy: 60%
  - Narcolepsy due to a medical condition: unknown (e.g., Parkinson disease with sleep disturbance)
- Excessive daytime sleepiness and sleep attacks (cardinal symptom)
  - Primary symptom and required for diagnosis
  - Instantaneous, irresistible REM sleep
  - First and most disabling symptom
  - Tendency to take naps lasting 5–10 minutes
  - Episodes last minutes to hours
  - 1–8 naps/day but normal 24-hour sleep duration
  - Associated with dreaming
  - Nap restores wakefulness for several hours
  - More likely in a monotonous, warm environment, after a large meal, or with strong emotions
- Cataplexy: auxiliary symptom (60%; cardinal symptom)
  - Pathognomonic if present
  - Sudden bilateral weakness of skeletal muscles
  - Provocation by sudden strong wave of emotion
  - Consciousness and memory are not impaired.
  - Short duration (less than a few minutes)
  - Can be limited to a particular muscle group (e.g., jaw droop with inability to speak; arm, neck, or leg weakness, eye muscles not affected)
  - Status cataplecticus: in children or on withdrawal of drugs
- Sleep paralysis: auxiliary symptom (25–50%)
  - When falling asleep or on awakening, the patient wants to but cannot move; this can end abruptly when the patient is touched or spoken to.
  - Brain wakes from sleep while body remains paralyzed in REM sleep.
  - Lasts seconds to minutes
  - Patients are aware of events around them but cannot open eyes or move.
  - Can be preceded by hallucinatory phenomena
  - 50% of the normal population have ≥1 episodes (thus, this symptom is nonspecific).
- Hypnagogic hallucinations: auxiliary symptom (30–60%)
  - Vivid, frightening visual or auditory illusions or hallucinations at onset of sleep
  - Dreamlike experiences that occur during wakefulness or suddenly at sleep onset
  - Characteristic hallucinations include seeing human or animal faces or feeling that someone else is in the room.
  - Hallucinations also can be auditory.
- Disturbed nocturnal sleep (66%)
  - Normal total sleep with decreased sleep efficiency
  - More frequent transitions from wakefulness to sleep
  - Retrograde amnesic and automatic behavior lasting minutes to hours
  - Increased periodic leg movements (50%)
  - Depression (18–37%)
  - Automatic behavior: activity without memory of the event

PHYSICAL EXAM

- A complete exam is useful to rule out other causes of hypersomnia.
- If cataplexy is witnessed, examiner will be unable to elicit deep tendon reflexes.

DIFFERENTIAL DIAGNOSIS

Excessive daytime sleepiness is present in 4% of the general population, although most individuals are not narcoleptic. Possible etiologies include the following:

- Sleep apnea syndromes (40–50% of those with excessive somnolence); increased incidence in narcolepsy, up to 26% prevalence
- Epileptic seizures and syncope
- Idiopathic CNS hypersomnolence (5–10% of those with excessive somnolence)
- Nocturnal myoclonus
- Psychomotor seizures
- Niemann-Pick type C
- Recurrent hypersomnia that lasts days to weeks and recurs months later
- Hypersomnia related to a medical condition, such as Parkinson disease

DIAGNOSTIC TESTS & INTERPRETATION

Initial Tests (lab, imaging)

- Nighttime polysomnography (PSG): Monitoring of patients in a sleep laboratory will usually document fragmented sleep with a normal amount of REM sleep but a pattern of sleep-onset REM. The PSG is useful to rule out other causes of excessive daytime sleepiness, including sleep apnea syndromes and nocturnal myoclonus.
- Multiple sleep latency test (MSLT): begins ≥90 minutes after nighttime test
  - The patient is monitored during 4–5 naps taken at 2-hour intervals; rapidity of sleep onset and type of sleep pattern are documented. The supportive test includes mean sleep latency (time to fall asleep) of ≤8 minutes and ≥1 sleep-onset REM periods.
  - Sensitivity 77%; specificity 97%; positive predictive value 73%

Follow-Up Tests & Special Considerations

- HLA typing for DQB1 in ambiguous cases
- Low CSF hypocretin-1 level: 99% specificity, 87% sensitivity in patients with cataplexy; useful in children unable to do an MSLT (described below)

Diagnostic Procedures/Other

- Diagnostic criteria according to the International Classification of Sleep Disorders 2nd edition (1)[C]
  - Narcolepsy with cataplexy
    - Excessive daytime sleepiness daily for 3 months
    - Cataplexy
    - MSLT latency <8 min with 2 or more sleep-onset REM periods or CSF hypocretin-1 level <110
    - Hypersomnia not better explained by another sleep disorder
  - Narcolepsy without cataplexy—all above without the cataplexy and low hypocretin-1
  - Low CSF hypocretin-1 level <110 pg/mL; use if unable to do MSLT, especially in children

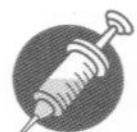

TREATMENT

GENERAL MEASURES

- None of the currently available medications enables people with narcolepsy to consistently maintain a fully normal state of alertness.
- Drug therapy should be supplemented by various behavioral strategies.
- Well-timed 20-minute naps may be helpful.
- Avoid sedative drugs.
- Use safety precautions, particularly when driving. People with untreated narcoleptic symptoms are involved in automobile accidents roughly 10× more frequently than the general population. However, accident rates are at normal levels among patients who have received appropriate medication therapy.

MEDICATION

First Line

- Excessive daytime sleepiness
  - Modafinil (Provigil):
    - Structurally distinct from amphetamines
    - 200–400 mg/d in the morning; start with 100 mg/d and increase over 3–4 days (2)[A].
    - 1st-line treatment: 60% effective and 20% partially effective
    - Half-life of 14 hours, can dose daily
    - No decrease in cataplexy
  - Armodafinil (Nuvigil):
    - Enantiomeric form of modafinil with slightly longer half-life of 15 hours
    - 150–250 mg every morning
  - Sodium oxybate (Xyrem):
    - 2.5–9 mg; may take 3 months to achieve full response
    - Preferred treatment for narcolepsy with cataplexy and disturbed nocturnal sleep
    - Give 1/2 dose at bedtime and 1/2 dose 4 hours later.
    - One of the date rape drugs; abuse potential (2)[A]
    - Can use with modafinil in severe cases
    - May worsen sleep-disordered breathing in patients with obstructive sleep apnea
    - Expensive with short half-life
- Cataplexy:
  - Sodium oxybate: See above
  - Serotonin-norepinephrine reuptake inhibitors
    - Venlafaxine: 75–375 mg/d
  - Tricyclic antidepressants
    - High side-effect profile
    - Abrupt withdrawal causes rebound cataplexy.
    - Protriptyline: 2.5–10 mg/d
  - Amphetamines
    - Methylphenidate (Ritalin): initial dose 30 mg/day divided BID or TID; maximum dose 100 mg/day (2)[B], short-acting
    - Dextroamphetamine: initial dose 15 mg/day divided BID or TID; maximum dose 100 mg/day (2)[B]
- Auxiliary symptoms (e.g., cataplexy, hypnagogic hallucination, sleep paralysis (3)[C]):
  - Antidepressants suppress REM sleep
    - Imipramine: 75–150 mg/d
    - Protriptyline: 10–40 mg/d
    - Clomipramine: 150–250 mg/d
    - Fluoxetine: 20–60 mg/d
    - Venlafaxine: 75–150 mg BID
  - Although often used, quality evidence is lacking to demonstrate improvement in cataplexy symptoms from antidepressants (3)[A].
- Contraindications: stimulants in hypertensive patients
- Precautions
  - Amphetamines
    - If the patient develops a tolerance to stimulants, switch drugs rather than increase dose; there is little cross-tolerance.
    - Headaches, irritability, hypertension (HTN), psychosis, anorexia, habituation, rebound hypersomnia
    - Pemoline: fewer cardiovascular side effects, longer acting, liver toxicity, little abuse potential
  - Other
    - Imipramine: dry mouth, sedation, urinary retention, impotence
    - Modafinil: less rebound hypersomnia; may become drug of choice; does not affect BP; tolerance limited; best if initial treatment; does not treat cataplexy; main side effect is headache; increased metabolism of oral contraceptives (use 50-μg pill)
    - The patient may develop a tolerance to the anticataplectic effect of tricyclic antidepressants (TCAs) and can have rebound cataplexy when a drug is withdrawn.
- Significant possible interactions: Combination of TCAs and stimulants can lead to significant HTN.

Second Line

- Excessive daytime sleepiness
  - Amphetamines
    - Methylphenidate (Ritalin): initial dose 20–30 mg/day divided BID or TID; maximum dose 60 mg/day (2)[B], short-acting, most potent amphetamine available
    - Dextroamphetamine: initial dose 15 mg/day divided BID or TID; maximum dose 60 mg/d (2)[B]
  - Selegiline: selective MAO-B inhibitor; anticataplectic effective for excessive daytime sleepiness; 20–40 mg/d divided morning and noon (2)[B]
- Contraindications: stimulants in hypertensive patients
- Precautions
  - Amphetamines
    - If the patient develops a tolerance to stimulants, switch drugs rather than increase dose; there is little cross-tolerance.
    - Headaches, irritability, HTN, psychosis, anorexia, habituation, rebound hypersomnia
  - Other: selegiline: Doses >20 mg require a low-tyramine diet because the drug begins to lose selectivity.
  - The patient may develop a tolerance to the anticataplectic effect of antidepressants and can have rebound cataplexy when a drug is withdrawn.

ISSUES FOR REFERRAL

- Unresponsive to primary medications
- Patient support groups can be very beneficial.

ONGOING CARE

FOLLOW-UP RECOMMENDATIONS

Patient Monitoring

Frequent BP checks and regular follow-ups (approximately every 6 months) are recommended.

DIET

Selegiline: Doses >20 mg require a low-tyramine diet because the drug begins to lose selectivity.

PATIENT EDUCATION

- Narcolepsy information from the National Institute of Neurological Disorders and Stroke at www.ninds.nih.gov/disorders/narcolepsy/narcolepsy.htm
- Narcolepsy Network, Inc., North Kingstown, RI 02852; www.narcolepsynetwork.org

PROGNOSIS

Narcolepsy is a lifelong disease. Symptoms can worsen with aging. In women, symptoms can improve after menopause.

REFERENCES

1. American Academy of Sleep Medicine. *International classification of sleep disorders: Diagnostic and coding manual*. 2nd ed. Westchester, IL: American Academy of Sleep Medicine; 2005.
2. Mohsenin V. Narcolepsy–master of disguise: evidence-based recommendations for management. *Postgrad Med*. 2009;121(3):99–104.
3. Vignatelli L, D'Alessandro R, Candelise L. Antidepressant drugs for narcolepsy. *Cochrane Database Syst Rev*. 2010;(1):CD003724.

ADDITIONAL READING

- Dauvilliers Y, Arnulf I, Mignot E. Narcolepsy with cataplexy. *Lancet*. 2007;369(9560):499–511.
- Leschziner G. Narcolepsy: a clinical review. *Pract Neurol*. 2014;14(5):323–331.
- Vignatelli L, D'Alessandro R, Candelise L. Antidepressant drugs for narcolepsy. *Cochrane Database Syst Rev*. 2008;(1):CD003724.
- Zaharna M, Dimitriu A, Guilleminault C. Expert opinion on pharmacotherapy of narcolepsy. *Expert Opin Pharmacother*. 2010;11(10):1633–1645.

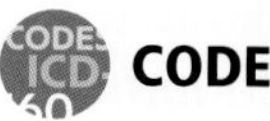

CODES

ICD10

- G47.419 Narcolepsy without cataplexy
- G47.411 Narcolepsy with cataplexy
- G47.429 Narcolepsy in conditions classified elsewhere w/o cataplexy

CLINICAL PEARLS

- Narcolepsy is a frequently missed disorder, with an average of 15 years of symptoms before a definitive diagnosis is made.
- The classic tetrad of symptoms includes excessive daytime sleepiness, cataplexy, sleep paralysis, and hypnagogic hallucinations.
- The International Classification of Sleep Disorders has specific diagnostic criteria for narcolepsy.
- Medications are helpful but not curative.

NASAL POLYPS

Julissa Mendoza, MD • Stephen J. Conner, MD

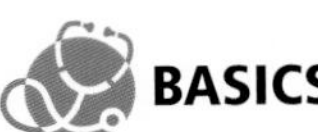

BASICS

DESCRIPTION

- Chronic inflammatory lesion of nasal mucosa
- Appearance of edematous pedunculated mass in the nasal cavity or within the paranasal sinus
- Often causes symptoms of blockage, discharge, or loss of smell
- Most commonly bilateral; suspect tumor, such as inverted papilloma, if unilateral

EPIDEMIOLOGY

Incidence

- Estimated to be ~1–4% in adults
- Much rarer in children: ~0.1%
- Increases with age

Prevalence

- Estimated to be 1–4% in general population
- Predominant sex: female > male (2:1)

ETIOLOGY AND PATHOPHYSIOLOGY

- No clearly delineated pathway; research has demonstrated separate TH1- and TH2-driven pathways (1,2)[B].
- Remains unclear; multiple inflammatory and infectious pathways resulting from chronic rhinosinusitis is most common (1,3)[B].

RISK FACTORS

- Chronic sinusitis
- Asthma
- Allergic fungal sinusitis
- Aspirin sensitivity
- Cystic fibrosis
- Primary ciliary dyskinesia (Kartagener syndrome)
- Laryngopharyngeal reflux (4)[B]

GENERAL PREVENTION

Use of intranasal corticosteroids after polyp removal surgery has shown effectiveness against recurrence.

COMMONLY ASSOCIATED CONDITIONS

- Bronchial asthma
- Aspirin hypersensitivity
- Allergic rhinitis (4)[B]

DIAGNOSIS

HISTORY

- Two or more symptoms, one of which is either nasal blockage/obstruction/congestion OR nasal discharge (5)[A].
- Nasal obstruction/restricted nasal airflow: persistent mouth breathing (5)[A]
- Nasal discharge:
  - Anterior discharge–rhinorrhea
  - Postnasal drip
- Reduction/loss of smell
- Dull headaches
- Facial pain/pressure
- Symptoms of acute, recurrent, or chronic rhinosinusitis (5)[A]

PHYSICAL EXAM

- Anterior rhinoscopy looking for a pale translucent mass of tissue
  - Most commonly from lateral wall of middle meatus
  - Otoscope with nasal speculum or even otologic speculum is typically used (5)[A].
- Flexible/rigid endoscopy is required to assess the nasal cavity fully (5)[A].
  - Endoscopy is the gold standard for diagnosis.
  - Topical anesthesia nasal spray should be used prior to the endoscopy if patient is awake.
- Tympanic membrane examination for eustachian tube dysfunction secondary to large posterior nasal polyps (5)[A].
- Examine the posterior pharynx via oral cavity for large posterior polyps (5)[A].

DIFFERENTIAL DIAGNOSIS

- Antrochoanal polyp
- Benign or malignant tumor:
  - Papilloma
  - Intranasal glioma
  - Encephalocele
  - Rhabdomyosarcoma
  - Mycetoma

DIAGNOSTIC TESTS & INTERPRETATION

Initial Tests (lab, imaging)

- Allergy testing (3)[B]:
  - Skin prick test
  - Immunocap testing
  - Radioallergosorbent test (RAST)
- Testing for cystic fibrosis in children with multiple benign polyps: sweat test: often requires repeat tests (3)[B]
- CT scanning (3)[B]:
  - May be helpful to corroborate history and endoscopic findings
  - Unable to differentiate polyp from other soft tissue masses
- MRI (3)[B]:
  - May aid in unilateral polyposis if concern for neoplasia, mycetoma, or encephalocele

Follow-Up Tests & Special Considerations

Histologic exam to exclude malignancy if unilateral polyp

Diagnostic Procedures/Other

- Diagnosis is made by the combination of rhinoscopy, endoscopy, and CT scanning.
- CT reveals extent of disease and is necessary to formulate a plan for surgical intervention (3)[B].

Test Interpretation

- Ciliated pseudostratified columnar epithelium: with areas of transitional or squamous epithelium
- Chronic infiltration of inflammatory cells
- Eosinophils are the predominant cells in most patients (4)[B].

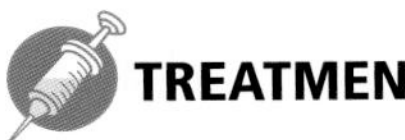

TREATMENT

MEDICATION

First Line

- Intranasal corticosteroid use has been demonstrated to reduce polyp size and recurrence, as well as improvement in nasal congestion based on controlled studies (2,5)[A],(6)[B].
- Treat for a minimum of 12 weeks; minimal systemic absorption, side effects rare—minor nose bleeding is most common (2,5)[A].
  - Budesonide 256 μg/day
  - Beclomethasone dipropionate 320 μg/day
  - Fluticasone dipropionate 400 μg/day
  - Mometasone furoate 200 μg BID

Second Line

- Oral systemic corticosteroids: less definitive benefit; more systemic adverse effects; use with caution in patients with diabetes mellitus, hypertension, or peptic ulcer disease (2,5)[A]
- Prednisolone
  - Weight-based dosing burst with taper
- Perioperative use oral prednisone 30 mg daily 5–7 days prior to surgery (2)[A]
  - Decrease nasal mucosa inflammation
  - Improves surgical field
  - Shorter surgical time
  - Improves post-op results
  - Weight-based dosing burst with taper

ISSUES FOR REFERRAL

Patients with severe obstruction symptoms should be referred for surgery (5)[A].

ADDITIONAL THERAPIES

Antileukotrienes: clinical improvement without aspirin hypersensitivity (2,5)[A],(3)[B]:

- Aspirin desensitization may have a role in reducing recurrence of nasal polyposis.
- Anti-interleukin-5 immunomodulators: may benefit those with T_H2 eosinophilic disease process

SURGERY/OTHER PROCEDURES

- Indicated for patients with 4 or more episodes in 1 year of acute rhinosinusitis refractory to medical therapy (5)[A]
  - Disease must be documented endoscopically or on CT during symptomatic period prior to surgical intervention.
- Most surgeries are approached endonasally.
  - Endoscopic sinus surgery has become the mainstay of treatment.
  - The external (Caldwell-Luc) approach is used for more difficult cases but carries higher risk of complications.
- Functional endonasal sinus surgery has slightly lower revision rate than intranasal polypectomy. Both modalities provide effective symptom relief.
- Postoperative use of nasal corticosteroids delay the recurrence of nasal polyps and hence the timing of revision surgery (2)[A],(6)[B].
- Postoperative use of steroid releasing stents to prevent polyp recurrence by decreasing mucosal inflammation (2)[A],(6)[B].
- Intrapolyp steroid injection may be considered in cases refractory to other interventions but has risk of visual loss.

ONGOING CARE

COMPLICATIONS

- Acute/chronic sinus infection
- Heterotropic bone formation within the sinus cavity
- Recurrence:
  - Of patients, 5–10% with severe disease
  - Twice as likely in those with asthma (4)[B]

REFERENCES

1. Tomassen P, Van Zele T, Zhang N, et al. Pathophysiology of chronic rhinosinusitis. *Proc Am Thorac Soc.* 2011;8(1):115–120.
2. Poetker DM, Jakubowski LA, Lal D, et al. Oral corticosteroids in the management of adult chronic rhinosinusitis with and without nasal polyps: an evidence-based review with recommendations. *Int Forum Allergy Rhinol.* 2013;3(2):104–120.
3. DeMarcantonio MA, Han JK. Nasal polyps: pathogenesis and treatment implications. *Otolaryngol Clin North Am.* 2011;44(3):685–695,ix.
4. Kariyawasam H, Rotiroti G. Allergic rhinitis, chronic rhinosinusitis and asthma: unravelling a complex relationship. *Curr Opin Otolaryngol Head Neck Surg.* 2013;21(1):79–86.
5. Fokkens WJ, Lund VJ, Mullol J, et al. EPOS 2012: European position paper on rhinosinusitis and nasal polyps 2012. A summary for otorhinolaryngologists. *Rhinology.* 2012;50(1):1–12.
6. Rudmik L, Schlosser RJ, Smith TL, et al. Impact of topical nasal steroid therapy on symptoms of nasal polyposis: a meta-analysis. *Laryngoscope.* 2012;122(7):1431–1437.

ADDITIONAL READING

- Aouad RK, Chiu AG. State of the art treatment of nasal polyposis. *Am J Rhinol Allergy.* 2011;25(5):291–298.
- Bachert C. Evidence-based management of nasal polyposis by intranasal corticosteroids: from the cause to the clinic. *Int Arch Allergy Immunol.* 2011;155(4):309–321.
- Hopkins C, Slack R, Lund V, et al. Long-term outcomes from the English national comparative audit of surgery for nasal polyposis and chronic rhinosinusitis. *Laryngoscope.* 2009;119(12):2459–2465.
- Small CB, Stryszak P, Danzig M, et al. Onset of symptomatic effect of mometasone furoate nasal spray in the treatment of nasal polyposis. *J Allergy Clin Immunol.* 2008;121(4):928–932.
- Stjärne P, Olsson P, Alenius M. Use of mometasone furoate to prevent polyp relapse after endoscopic sinus surgery. *Arch Otolaryngol Head Neck Surg.* 2009;135(3):296–302.

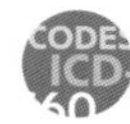

CODES

ICD10

- J33.9 Nasal polyp, unspecified
- J33.0 Polyp of nasal cavity
- J33.8 Other polyp of sinus

CLINICAL PEARLS

- Intranasal corticosteroid use has been demonstrated to reduce polyp size and recurrence, as well as improvement in nasal congestion.
- Treat for a minimum of 12 weeks.
- Allergy testing can be helpful.
- Nasal polyposis associated with asthma and aspirin hypersensitivity known as Samter triad or aspirin exacerbated respiratory disease (AERD) (1,3)[B]
- Patients with severe obstruction should be referred for surgery.
- Unilateral nasal polyp needs malignancy workup (MRI).

N

NEPHROTIC SYNDROME

Jeremy D. DeFoe, DO • Karen Sue Phelps, MD

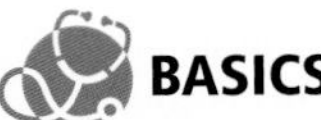

BASICS

DESCRIPTION

- A clinical syndrome of heavy proteinuria (>3.5 g/1.73 m^2/24 hours), hypoalbuminemia, hyperlipidemia, and edema
- Includes both primary and secondary forms
- Associated with many types of kidney disease

EPIDEMIOLOGY

Based on definitive diagnosis

- Diabetic nephropathy: most common cause of secondary nephrotic syndrome (1)
- Minimal change disease (MCD)
  - Most common nephrotic syndrome in children, peaks at 2–8 years
  - Associated with drugs or lymphoma in adults
- Amyloidosis: rare
- Lupus nephropathy (LN): Adult women are affected about 10× more often than men.
- Focal segmental glomerulosclerosis (FSGS)
  - 25% of nephrotic syndrome in adults
  - Most common primary nephrotic syndrome in African Americans
  - Has both primary and secondary forms
- Membranous nephropathy
  - Most common primary nephrotic syndrome in Caucasians
  - Associated with malignancy and infection
- Membranoproliferative glomerulonephritis (MGN)
  - May be primary or secondary
  - May present in the setting of a systemic viral or rheumatic illness

ETIOLOGY AND PATHOPHYSIOLOGY

- Increased glomerular permeability to protein molecules, especially albumin
- Edema results primarily from renal salt retention, with arterial underfilling from decreased plasma oncotic pressure playing an additional role.
- Hyperlipidemia is thought to be a consequence of increased hepatic synthesis resulting from low oncotic pressure and urinary loss of regulatory proteins.
- The hypercoagulable state that can occur in some nephrotic states is likely due to loss of antithrombin III in urine.
- Primary renal disease:
  - MCD
  - FSGS
  - MGN
  - IgA nephropathy
- Secondary renal disease (associated primary renal disease shown in parentheses):
  - Diabetic nephropathy
  - Amyloidosis
  - LN
  - FSGS
  - Infections (MGN)
  - Cancer (MCD or MGN)
  - Drugs (MCD or MGN)

Genetics

Genetic factors are likely to play a role in susceptibility to the various nephrotic syndromes, although these have not been sufficiently defined to be useful clinically.

RISK FACTORS

- Drug addiction (e.g., heroin [FSGS])
- Hepatitis B and C, HIV, other infections
- Immunosuppression
- Nephrotoxic drugs
- Vesicoureteral reflux (FSGS)
- Cancer (usually MGN, may be MCD)
- Chronic analgesic use/abuse
- Preeclampsia
- Diabetes mellitus

GENERAL PREVENTION

In general, there are few preventive measures, except avoidance of known causative medications.

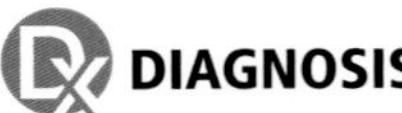

DIAGNOSIS

HISTORY

- Inquire about signs or symptoms of systemic disease: joint complaint, rash, edema, infectious complaint, fevers, anorexia, oliguria, foamy urine, acute flank pain, hematuria
- Obtain a recent drug history for medications that may be causative, especially NSAIDs.
- Assess for risk factors.

PHYSICAL EXAM

A complete physical exam may discover clues to systemic disease as a potential cause and/or may suggest the severity of disease.

- Fluid retention: abdominal distention, abdominal fluid shift, extremity edema, puffy eyelids, scrotal swelling, weight gain, shortness of breath. Pericardial rub and decreased breath sounds with pleural effusions may develop.
- Hypertension
- Orthostatic hypotension

ALERT
The potential for thromboembolic disease leading to pulmonary embolism is one of the most life-threatening aspects of a patient who is actively nephrotic.

DIFFERENTIAL DIAGNOSIS

- Edema and proteinuria: see "Etiology and Pathophysiology."
- Edema alone: Other diseases to rule out in patients who have edema without proteinuria include congestive heart failure, cirrhosis, hypothyroidism, nutritional hypoalbuminemia, protein-losing enteropathy.

DIAGNOSTIC TESTS & INTERPRETATION

Initial Tests (lab, imaging)

- Confirm proteinuria is present: by urine dipstick initially, and then quantitate by 24-hour urine or spot urine protein-to-creatinine ratio
- Rule out urine infection with urine culture.
- Full blood count and coagulation screen
- Renal function tests: BUN, creatinine with estimated glomerular filtration rate (GFR)
- Glucose to rule out overt diabetes
- Consider blood cultures to rule out a postinfectious process.
- Lipid panel
- Liver function tests to exclude liver disease or infection
- Look for autoimmune disease.
  - Antinuclear antibody and/or antidouble-stranded DNA positivity suggest lupus.
  - Complement levels: A low C3 may suggest a postinfectious or membranoproliferative process, whereas both low C3 and C4 point to lupus.
- Serum protein electrophoresis/urine immune electrophoresis to rule in a paraproteinemia
- Hepatitis B and C screen
- HIV and syphilis testing
- Urinalysis to evaluate for the presence of cellular casts
- Renal US to verify the presence of 2 kidneys of normal shape and size
- Chest x-ray to detect presence of pleural effusion or infection
- If thrombosis suspected:
  - Doppler US of the legs
  - MRI or venography for renal vein thrombosis
  - Ventilation/perfusion nuclear medicine lung scan and/or CT may be required to rule out pulmonary embolism.

Diagnostic Procedures/Other

Renal biopsy

- Rarely done in children with 1st episode of nephrotic syndrome, as MCD is common and empiric steroid therapy is the standard of care.
- Required to confirm the clinical diagnosis in adults and assist with making a treatment plan (1)

Test Interpretation

- Light microscopy
  - May see nothing (e.g., MCD)
  - Sclerosis (e.g., FSGS or diabetic nodules in diabetes)
  - Diffuse hypercellularity suggests a proliferative disease such as IgA nephropathy, LN, or postinfectious glomerulonephritis (GN).
- Immunofluorescence: Mesangial IgA suggests IgA nephropathy, Henoch-Schönlein; other staining patterns are specific for other disease processes.
- Electron microscopy: The location of immunoglobulin deposits is useful in pointing to a particular diagnosis.

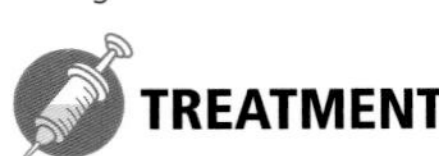

TREATMENT

MEDICATION

First Line

- Edema: salt restriction and salt-wasting diuretics (loop and thiazide diuretics):
  - Salt restriction to <2 g sodium per day
  - Restrict fluid intake to <1.5 L/day if hyponatremic.
  - Target weight loss of 0.5–1 kg/day (1–2 lb/day)
- Statins have been shown to improve endothelial function (2)[A] and may decrease proteinuria (3)[A], but effect on GFR and preservation of renal function is small. The major role for statin use is in cardiovascular risk reduction.
- ACE inhibitors or angiotensin II receptor blockers thought to reduce proteinuria, hyperlipidemia, thrombotic tendencies, progression of renal failure, and to control hypertension, if present (2,4)[A].
- For steroid-responsive disease (MCD and FSGS), steroids dosed in consultation with nephrologist.

Second Line

- Many of the nephrotic diseases will require escalation in therapy above steroids. These include rapidly relapsing forms, as well as MGN, LN, and IgA nephropathy. Bolus steroids and other immunosuppressives are required in this circumstance (cyclophosphamide, mycophenolate mofetil, chlorambucil, cyclosporine) (5)[A].
- Rituximab, combined with steroids or other immunosuppressive agents, has demonstrated early promise in the treatment of refractory nephrotic syndrome (6)[B].
- Randomized controlled data have been insufficient to determine which patients require prophylactic anticoagulation (7)[A]. Common practice is to anticoagulate with heparin and then warfarin in patients who have persistent nephrotic-range proteinuria. This decision is made based on the patient's history of edema, hypoalbuminemia, thromboembolism, or immobility.
- Hypocalcemia from vitamin D loss should be treated with oral vitamin D.

ISSUES FOR REFERRAL

Consultation with a nephrologist is often required to assist with renal biopsy to confirm diagnosis and to assist with management of edema. Cytotoxic medications may be called for, depending on the disease process, and this may best be handled by a nephrologist.

ADDITIONAL THERAPIES

Ambulation or range-of-motion exercises to lower risk of deep vein thrombosis (DVT)

INPATIENT CONSIDERATIONS

Admission Criteria/Initial Stabilization

Respiratory distress, sepsis/severe infection, thromboses, renal failure, hypertension, or other complications

Discharge Criteria

Hemodynamically, stable patients without complications may be managed as outpatients.

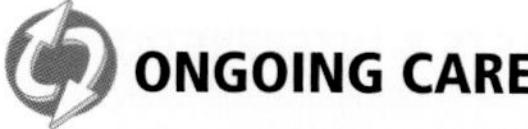

ONGOING CARE

FOLLOW-UP RECOMMENDATIONS

Patient Monitoring

- Frequent monitoring is required for relapse, disease progression, and for detecting signs of toxicity of medical management.
- Reevaluate for azotemia, urine protein, hypertension, edema, loss of renal function, cholesterol, and weight.

DIET

- Normal protein (1 g/kg/day)
- Low fat (cholesterol)
- Reduced sodium
- Supplemental multivitamins and minerals, especially vitamin D and iron
- Fluid restriction if hyponatremic

PATIENT EDUCATION

- Printed material for patients: National Kidney Foundation, 30 E. 33rd Street, Suite 1100, New York, NY 10016; 800-622-9010
  - Childhood nephrotic syndrome
  - Diabetes and kidney disease
  - Focal glomerulosclerosis
- Web site: National Institutes of Health: nephrotic syndrome

PROGNOSIS

Nephrotic syndrome in children (MCD) is typically self-limited and carries a good prognosis. In the adult, the prognosis is variable. Complete remission is expected if the basic disease is treatable (infection, malignancy, drug-induced); otherwise, a relapsing and remitting course is possible, with progression to dialysis seen in more aggressive forms (diabetic glomerulosclerosis).

COMPLICATIONS

- Thromboembolism:
  - Deep vein, renal vein, or central venous thrombosis may occur.
  - The risk appears to be greater the lower the serum albumin.
  - Pulmonary embolism is a known complication.
- Pleural effusion
- Ascites
- Hyperlipidemia, cardiovascular disease
- Acute renal failure, progressive renal failure
- Protein malnutrition/muscle wasting
- Infection secondary to low serum IgG concentrations, reduced complement activity, and depressed T-cell function: peritonitis, pneumonia, or cellulitis
- Loss of vitamin D (vitamin D–binding protein loss in urine) leading to bone disease

REFERENCES

1. Kodner C. Nephrotic syndrome in adults: diagnosis and management. *Am Fam Physician*. 2009;80(10):1129–1134.
2. Randomised placebo-controlled trial of effect of ramipril on decline in glomerular filtration rate and risk of terminal renal failure in proteinuric, non-diabetic nephropathy. The GISEN Group (Gruppo Italiano di Studi Epidemiologici in Nefrologia). *Lancet*. 1997;349(9069):1857–1863.
3. Fried LF, Orchard TJ, Kasiske BL. Effect of lipid reduction on the progression of renal disease: a meta-analysis. *Kidney Int*. 2001;59(1):260–269.
4. Kunz R, Friedrich C, Wolbers M, et al. Meta-analysis: effect of monotherapy and combination therapy with inhibitors of the renin angiotensin system on proteinuria in renal disease. *Ann Intern Med*. 2008;148(1):30–48.
5. Hodson EM, Willis NS, Craig JC. Interventions for idiopathic steroid-resistant nephrotic syndrome in children. *Cochrane Database Syst Rev*. 2010;(11):CD003594.
6. Kamei K, Okada M, Sato M, et al. Rituximab treatment combined with methylprednisolone therapy and immunosuppressants for childhood steroid resistant nephrotic syndrome. *Pediatr Nephrol*. 2014;29(7):1181–1187.
7. Kulshrestha S, Grieff M, Navaneethan SD. Interventions for preventing thrombosis in adults and children with nephrotic syndrome (protocol). *Cochrane Database Syst Rev*. 2006;(2):CD006024.

ADDITIONAL READING

- Cadnapaphornchai MA, Tkachenko O, Shchekochikhin D, et al. The nephrotic syndrome: pathogenesis and treatment of edema formation and secondary complications. *Pediatr Nephrol*. 2014;29(7):1159–1167.
- Madaio MP, Harrington JT. The diagnosis of glomerular diseases: acute glomerulonephritis and the nephrotic syndrome. *Arch Intern Med*. 2001;161(1):25–34.
- Meyrier A. An update on the treatment options for focal segmental glomerulosclerosis. *Expert Opin Pharmacother*. 2009;10(4):615–628.

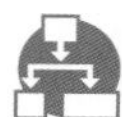

SEE ALSO

- Amyloidosis; Diabetes Mellitus, Type 1; Diabetes Mellitus, Type 2; Glomerulonephritis, Acute; HIV/AIDS; Lupus Erythematosus, Discoid; Multiple Myeloma
- Algorithm: Acute Kidney Injury (Acute Renal Failure)

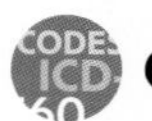

CODES

ICD10

- N04.9 Nephrotic syndrome with unspecified morphologic changes
- N04.1 Nephrotic syndrome w focal and segmental glomerular lesions
- N04.2 Nephrotic syndrome w diffuse membranous glomerulonephritis

CLINICAL PEARLS

- Nephrotic syndrome is a clinical syndrome of >3.5 g/day proteinuria, hypoalbuminemia, hyperlipidemia, and edema often associated with diabetes and NSAIDs use.
- Pediatric nephrotic syndrome typically carries a good prognosis and is more easily treated with steroids, although recurrences are common.
- Nondiabetic adults with nephrotic syndrome will require a renal biopsy to determine cause.
- Have a high index of suspicion for symptoms that may represent an embolic event in patients with nephrotic syndrome.

NEUROFIBROMATOSIS TYPE 1

Rayna Goldstein, MD • Michele Roberts, MD, PhD

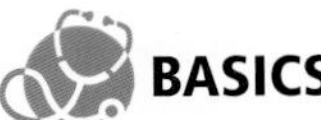

BASICS

DESCRIPTION

- Neurofibromatosis types 1 (NF1) and 2 (NF2) are neurocutaneous syndromes (phakomatoses). Although they share a name, they are distinct and unrelated conditions with genes on different chromosomes.
  - NF2 is a rare condition that causes bilateral vestibular schwannomas.
  - NF1 is a multisystem disorder that may affect any organ. It is the most common of the phakomatoses.
- System(s) affected: musculoskeletal; nervous; skin/exocrine; cardiovascular; neuroophthalmologic
- Synonym(s): von Recklinghausen disease, formerly peripheral NF

EPIDEMIOLOGY

Incidence

- Predominant sex for NF1: male = female
- Birth incidence NF1: 1:2,500–3,000

Prevalence

1:3,000–1:4,000

ETIOLOGY AND PATHOPHYSIOLOGY

- Neurofibromin is a guanosine triphosphatase–activating protein that acts as a tumor suppressor by downregulating a cellular protooncogene, *p21-ras*, which enhances cell growth and proliferation.
- Neurofibromata are benign tumors composed of Schwann cells, fibroblasts, mast cells, and vascular components that develop along nerves.
- The 2-hit hypothesis has been invoked to explain malignant transformation in *NF1*.

Genetics

- Online Mendelian Inheritance in Man 162200
- Caused by a mutation in the *NF1* gene on chromosome 17q11.2; autosomal dominant inheritance; protein product is called *neurofibromin*.
- 50% of cases are due to new mutations. Prenatal diagnosis possible if family history is positive.
- Penetrance is nearly 100%; expressivity is highly variable.
- Gene is large, with a variety of mutations causing NF1. Molecular technology can detect 95% of clinically important *NF1* mutations, but it is usually not indicated because clinical diagnosis frequently can be made in childhood.
- ~5% of individuals with NF1 have a large deletion of the entire *NF1* gene (or nearly so); they usually have a more severe phenotype.
- *Segmental NF* (an NF1 variant) is limited to a single body region and is caused by mosaicism for the *NF1* mutation.

RISK FACTORS

- Having an affected 1st-degree relative is a diagnostic criterion for NF1, although relatives may be unaware of their condition.
- Affected individuals with a positive family history, as well as those with a new mutation, have a 50% risk of transmitting NF1 to each of their offspring; 1 in 12 will be severely affected.
- Individuals with segmental NF1 may have gonadal mosaicism and may be at risk for transmission of the mutated gene.

COMMONLY ASSOCIATED CONDITIONS

Congenital heart disease, pulmonary stenosis, hypertension, renal artery stenosis

DIAGNOSIS

- NF1 can be diagnosed by routine exam by age 4 years, with attention to skin stigmata; diagnostic criteria include ≥2 of the following (1):
  - ≥6 café au lait (light brown) macules, ≥5 mm in prepubertal individuals or ≥15 mm in adults
  - ≥2 neurofibromata of any type or 1 plexiform (noncircumscribed) neurofibroma
  - Axillary or inguinal freckling
  - ≥2 Lisch nodules (benign iris hamartomas, asymptomatic)
  - Optic glioma by MRI
  - Characteristic osseous lesions: sphenoid dysplasia, long-bone cortical thinning, ribbon ribs, angular scoliosis
  - 1st-degree relative with NF1 by above criteria
- Prenatal diagnosis is possible with known mutation or by linkage testing (with positive family history), although not predictive of clinical course.

HISTORY

- Family history of a 1st-degree relative with NF1
- Manifestations generally are not visible at birth, although plexiform neurofibromata usually are congenital and tibial bowing is congenital.
- In addition to cutaneous lesions, NF1 may present with painful neurofibromata, pathologic fractures, or headaches secondary to hypertension caused by pheochromocytomas.
- Optic gliomata may present as involuntary eye movement, squinting, loss of vision, or as diencephalic syndrome.

PHYSICAL EXAM

- Skin
  - Café au lait macules develop during the first 3 years of childhood and are usually the presenting feature of NF1. Evenly pigmented, irregularly shaped (coast-of-California), light brown macules present in 97% of patients with NF1; many unaffected individuals have 1–3 such macules.
  - Neurofibromata: can be cutaneous, SC, or plexiform and may be soft or firm; buttonhole invagination is pathognomonic. Cutaneous neurofibromata usually begin to appear during late childhood or adolescence.
  - Plexiform neurofibromata are present in up to 50% of individuals with NF1:
    - Usually congenital; may be subtle in infancy
    - Freckling or hypertrichosis may be present over plexiform neurofibromata; may affect underlying structures or cause focal hyperplasia
    - Many are internal, not obvious on exam.
    - Most grow slowly over many years but can have rapid growth, especially in early childhood
  - Evaluate for new lesions and progression of preexisting ones. Rapidly growing cutaneous lesions should be evaluated thoroughly.
  - Axillary freckling (Crowe sign) or inguinal freckling (91%)
- Ophthalmologic
  - Lisch nodules (benign iris hamartomas) in 30%: well-defined, dome-shaped, gelatinous hamartomatous lesions projecting from the iris, varying from clear yellow to brown
  - Essentially unique to NF, Lisch nodules are asymptomatic and are significant only for diagnosis.
  - Pallor or atrophy of optic disc, bulging of orbit, loss of vision may be signs of optic glioma.
- Skeletal
  - Scoliosis and vertebral angulation
  - Localized bone hypertrophy, especially of the face
  - Limb abnormalities:
    - Pseudoarthrosis of the tibia
    - Tibial dysplasia (anterolateral bowing of the tibia) is congenital, if present.
    - Nonossifying fibromas of the long bones in adolescents and adults are uncommon but can increase risk of fracture.
- Pay particular attention to neurologic examination or new focal pain.
- Measure BP yearly. Hypertension is more common in patients with NF1 and could be secondary to renal artery stenosis, aortic stenosis, or pheochromocytoma.
- Evaluate neurodevelopmental progress in children. Learning disabilities occur in 50–75%.

DIFFERENTIAL DIAGNOSIS

Familial café au lait spots (autosomal dominant, no other NF1 features), Watson syndrome, LEOPARD syndrome, McCune-Albright syndrome, neurocutaneous melanosis, proteus syndrome, lipomatosis

Geriatric Considerations

In NF1, cutaneous lesions and tumors increase in size and number with age.

Pediatric Considerations

- Children who have inherited the *NF1* gene of an affected parent usually are identified by age 1 year, but external stigmata may be subtle. If there are no stigmata by age 2 years, NF is unlikely, but the child should be reexamined within the next few years. Definite diagnosis can be made by age 4 years using National Institute of Health (NIH) criteria (1).
- Young children with multiple café au lait spots, but no other stigmata after careful physical and ophthalmologic evaluation, should be followed clinically as if they have NF1 (2).
- Molecular confirmation may be appropriate, especially with atypical presentation (3).

DIAGNOSTIC TESTS & INTERPRETATION

- DNA sequence and deletion/duplication analysis of the *NF1* gene can identify mutations in ~96% of those with a clinical diagnosis.
- Molecular genetic testing is available, although often not necessary for diagnosis. Diagnostic laboratory information: www.genetests.org
- Confirmatory genetic testing is appropriate in those who are suspected of having NF1 but do not fulfill diagnostic criteria or for prenatal diagnosis or preimplantation genetic diagnosis (PGD) (4).

Initial Tests (lab, imaging)

- Characteristic radiographic findings: Sphenoid dysplasia, long bone cortical thinning, ribbon ribs, and angular scoliosis. Screening radiographs of the knees in adolescents is controversial. CT can demonstrate bony changes.
- MRI findings of the orbits, brain, or spine (86%). Routine head MRI scanning in asymptomatic individuals with NF1 is controversial. Optic gliomata (seen on MRI, 11–15%) may lead to blindness. Although areas of increased T2 signal intensity (unidentified bright objects) are common on brain MRI, they are not diagnostic of NF1 and are of no clinical significance.

- The NIH Consensus Development Conference does not recommend routine neuroimaging as a means of establishing a diagnosis, although modification of diagnostic criteria is discussed (1)[C].

Diagnostic Procedures/Other

- Ophthalmologic evaluation, including slit-lamp exam of the irides; visual field testing to evaluate optic gliomata
- Neuropsychological testing: Intelligence usually normal but may have significant deficits in language, visuospatial skills, and neuromotor skills.

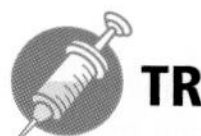

TREATMENT

MEDICATION

First Line

There are no specific therapeutic agents approved; individual aspects are treated as they arise (i.e., - anticonvulsants for seizures, medications for ADHD, management of blood pressure).

Second Line

Multiple clinical trials for NF1 are recruiting patients (see www.clinicaltrials.gov).

ISSUES FOR REFERRAL

- Patients with more than minimal manifestations of NF1: Refer to a multidisciplinary NF clinic.
- Referral for psychosocial issues of family and affected individuals
- Educational intervention for children with learning disabilities or ADHD (40%)
- Early referral to orthopedics for congenital tibial bowing

ADDITIONAL THERAPIES

- Occupational therapy for children with NF1 who present with fine motor difficulties
- There is no evidence supporting laser therapy for café au lait spots.
- The Children's Tumor Foundation (CTF) has established the NF Clinical Trials Consortium and the CTF NF Clinic Network to facilitate future clinical trials and help identify best practices (5).

SURGERY/OTHER PROCEDURES

Surgical treatment for severe scoliosis, plexiform neurofibromata, or malignancy

ONGOING CARE

FOLLOW-UP RECOMMENDATIONS

NF1 health supervision 2008 guidelines:

- Infancy to 1 year (6)[C]
  - Growth and development: mild short stature, macrocephaly (increased brain volume); aqueductal stenosis/obstructive hydrocephalus, hydrocephalus
  - Check for focal neurologic signs or asymmetric neurologic exam.
  - Skeletal abnormalities, especially spine and legs
  - Neurodevelopmental progress
- 1–5 years (6)[C]
  - Café au lait spots and axillary freckling have no clinical significance.
  - Annual ophthalmologic exam
  - Brain MRI for visual changes, persistent headaches, seizures, marked increase in head size, plexiform neurofibroma of the head
  - Assess speech and language: hypernasal speech due to velopharyngeal insufficiency and delayed expressive language development
  - Developmental evaluation of learning and motor abilities; may benefit from speech/language and/or motor therapy, and special education
  - Monitor BP annually.
- 5–13 years (6)[C]
  - Evaluate for skin tumors causing disfigurement and obtain consultation if surgery is desired to improve appearance or function.
  - Evaluate for premature or delayed puberty. If sexual precocity is noted, evaluate for an optic glioma or hypothalamic lesion. Review the effects of puberty on NF.
  - Evaluate for learning disabilities and ADHD.
  - Evaluate social adjustment, development, and school placement.
  - Monitor ophthalmologic status yearly until age 8 years; complete eye exam every 2 years
  - Monitor BP annually.
  - Refer patient to a clinical psychologist or child psychiatrist for problems with self-esteem.
  - Discuss growth of neurofibromata during adolescence and pregnancy.
  - Counsel parents about discussing diagnosis with child.
- 13–21 years (6)[C]
  - Examine the adolescent for abnormal pubertal development.
  - Perform a thorough skin examination for plexiform neurofibromata and a complete neurologic exam for findings suggestive of deep plexiform neurofibromata; seek surgical consultation for signs of pressure on deep structures.
  - Continue to monitor BP yearly.
  - Continue ophthalmologic examination every 2 years until age 18 years.
  - Discuss genetics of NF1 or refer for genetic counseling.
  - Discuss sexuality, contraception, and reproductive options.
  - Discuss effects of pregnancy on NF1, if appropriate. Neurofibromata may enlarge and new tumors may develop during pregnancy.
  - Review prenatal diagnosis or refer the patient to a geneticist.

PATIENT EDUCATION

- Genetic counseling and patient education regarding future complications about family planning
- The CTF: www.CTF.org. Support groups are important.

PROGNOSIS

Variable; most patients have a mild expression of NF1 and lead normal lives.

COMPLICATIONS

- Disfigurement: Skin neurofibromata develop primarily on exposed areas. The number tends to increase with puberty or pregnancy.
- Scoliosis: 10–30% (most cases mild); bowing of long bones, 2%; osteopenia and osteoporosis
- A large head is common but rarely associated with hydrocephalus.
- Increased risk of malignancy: malignant peripheral nerve sheath tumor (MPNST) (5–10%) usually in adults (1), especially within the field of previous radiotherapy for plexiform neurofibroma
- CNS tumors (5–15%), especially optic pathway glioma (most common CNS tumor), most often asymptomatic, but if symptomatic, usually presents before age 6 years. Symptomatic lesions are usually stable or only slowly progressive.
- High relative risk (RR) for some uncommon malignancies
- Increased risk for pheochromocytoma, rhabdomyosarcoma, leukemia, Wilms tumor
- RR for cancer of the esophagus (3.3), stomach (2.8), colon (2.0), liver (3.8), lung (3.0), bone (19.6), thyroid (4.9), malignant melanoma (3.6), non-Hodgkin lymphoma (3.3), chronic myeloid leukemia (6.7), female breast (2.3), and ovary (3.7)
- Learning disability: ~50%; may be associated with ADHD; mental retardation in 4–8%
- GI neurofibromata may cause GI disturbances.
- Seizures: 6–7%
- Hypertension is a frequent finding in adults and may occur during childhood.
- Disorders of puberty

Pregnancy Considerations

Increased risk of perinatal complications, stillbirth, intrauterine growth constriction; risk of cord compression, and outlet obstruction by pelvic neurofibromata

REFERENCES

1. DeBella K, Szudek J, Friedman JM. Use of the National Institutes of Health Criteria for diagnosis of neurofibromatosis 1 in children. *Pediatrics*. 2000;105(3, Pt 1):608–614.
2. Nunley KS, Gao F, Albers AC, et al. Predictive value of café au lait macules at initial consultation in the diagnosis of neurofibromatosis type 1. *Arch Dermatol*. 2009;145(8):883–887.
3. Burkitt Wright EM, Sach E, Sharif S, et al. Can the diagnosis of NF1 be excluded clinically? A lack of pigmentary findings in families with spinal neurofibromatosis demonstrates a limitation of clinical diagnosis. *J Med Genet*. 2013;50(9):606–613.
4. National Institutes of Health Consensus Development Conference statement: neurofibromatosis. Bethesda, Md., USA, July 13–15, 1987. *Neurofibromatosis*. 1988;1:172–178.
5. Williams VC, Lucas J, Babcock MA, et al. Neurofibromatosis type 1 revisited. *Pediatrics*. 2009;123(1):124–133.
6. Hersh JH; American Academy of Pediatrics Committee on Genetics. Health supervision for children with neurofibromatosis. *Pediatrics*. 2008;121(3):633–642.

SEE ALSO

Tuberous Sclerosis Complex; Von Hippel-Lindau Syndrome

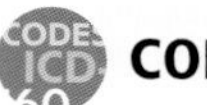

CODES

ICD10

Q85.01 Neurofibromatosis, type 1

CLINICAL PEARLS

- Marked clinical variability. External stigmata may be subtle or absent in young children. Minimally affected children may become severely affected adults.
- A single café au lait spot is of no concern in a child, but having ≥6 is a diagnostic criterion for NF1.

NEUROLEPTIC MALIGNANT SYNDROME

Robert A. Baldor, MD, FAAFP

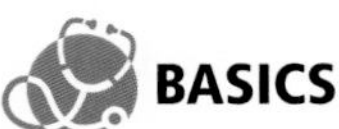

BASICS

DESCRIPTION

- Neuroleptic malignant syndrome (NMS) is a life-threatening condition that may develop during treatment with neuroleptic medications; most cases develop within the first 2 weeks of initiating therapy.
- Nonneuroleptic medications that have antidopaminergic activity have also been implicated.
- Characterized by muscular rigidity due to dopamine antagonism in the nigrostriatal pathway
- Hyperthermia from the blockage of hypothalamic thermoregulation (more likely in the setting of benzodiazepine withdrawal); autonomic stability; cognitive changes and elevations of serum creatine phosphokinase are other hallmarks.
- May be indistinguishable from other causes of drug-induced hyperthermia (e.g., malignant hyperthermia, serotonin syndrome, lethal catatonia, anticholinergic toxins, or sympathomimetic poisoning); detailed history can help differentiate between these causes.

EPIDEMIOLOGY

Incidence

- Variably reported as 0.01–3%
- 2,000 new cases annually in the United States
- Predominant sex: male > female
- Predominant age: <40 years

Prevalence

0.15% ± 0.05% among patients receiving neuroleptics

ETIOLOGY AND PATHOPHYSIOLOGY

- Exact mechanism unknown
- Most likely due to central dopaminergic blockade of nigrostriatal, hypothalamic, mesocortical/limbic pathways
- Sympathoadrenal hyperactivity and defects in neuronal calcium regulatory proteins may also contribute.
- Most commonly seen in treatment with typical antipsychotics: phenothiazines (e.g., fluphenazine), butyrophenones (e.g., haloperidol), and thiothixene
- May also be seen with atypical antipsychotics (e.g., clozapine, risperidone, olanzapine)
- Nonneuroleptic agents with antidopaminergic activity (e.g., metoclopramide, promethazine, and droperidol) have also been implicated.
- Rare cases have occurred with usage of medications not known to have any central antidopaminergic activity (e.g., lithium, phenelzine, and desipramine).
- Also associated with withdrawal from dopamine agonists in Parkinson disease, CNS shunt failure, and functional hemispherectomy

Genetics

- Some studies show a genetic predisposition to NMS.
- Polymorphisms: loss of del allele in 141C Ins/Del of the dopamine D_2 receptor gene and *Ser9Gly* in the dopamine D_3 receptor gene

RISK FACTORS

- High-potency neuroleptic medications; newly administered medication or a rapid increase in the dose of an existing agent
- Intramuscular or depot administration of medications
- Concurrent use of multiple neuroleptic agents
- Administration of neuroleptics with other drugs known to cause NMS, such as lithium
- Previous episodes of NMS
- Exposure to heat
- Dehydration/malnutrition
- Presence of an underlying structural/functional brain disorder (tumor, encephalitis, delirium/dementia)
- Postpartum women may be at an increased risk of developing NMS.

DIAGNOSIS

HISTORY

- Neuroleptic use or an increase in dose
- Discontinuation of antiparkinsonian drug
- Mental status changes are common.

PHYSICAL EXAM

- Extrapyramidal symptoms: dysphagia, short shuffling gait, resting tremor, and significant skeletal muscle rigidity—lead-pipe rigidity (these symptoms are less likely with clozapine-induced NMS) (1)[C]
- Hyperthermia (temperature may be as high as 106–107°F [41°C])
- Altered level of consciousness (ranging from mild drowsiness, agitation, or confusion to a severe delirium/coma)
- Autonomic instability (e.g., diaphoresis, flushing, skin pallor, tachycardia, tachypnea, labile BP, urinary incontinence)

DIFFERENTIAL DIAGNOSIS

- Infectious: meningitis, encephalitis, brain abscess, pneumonia/sepsis
- Metabolic: acute renal failure, thyrotoxicosis, pheochromocytoma
- Malignant hyperthermia, severe dystonic reaction
- Serotonin syndrome
- Anticholinergic poisoning, salicylate poisoning
- Sympathomimetic poisoning
- Acute hydrocephalus or spinal cord injury
- Tetanus; rabies
- Heat stroke
- Strychnine poisoning
- Cerebrovascular accident
- Acute intermittent porphyria
- Nonconvulsive status epilepticus
- Drug withdrawal: from alcohol, benzodiazepines, baclofen, sedatives, and hypnotics

DIAGNOSTIC TESTS & INTERPRETATION

- CBC (evaluate for leukocytosis)
- Elevated creatine phosphokinase (CPK)
- Serum electrolyte abnormalities (hypocalcemia, hypomagnesemia, hypo-/hypernatremia, hyperkalemia, metabolic acidosis)
- Consider: lactate dehydrogenase levels, liver function tests, urine myoglobin, BUN and creatinine, uric acid, serum iron, and coagulation studies

Initial Tests (lab, imaging)

- Chest x-ray (if aspiration pneumonia is suspected)
- Head CT scan (before lumbar puncture and to rule out underlying brain etiology)
- MRI to detect restricted diffusion in cerebellar hemispheres, basal ganglia, and cerebellum (2)[C]

Diagnostic Procedures/Other

- Lumbar puncture (rule out other causes of fever/altered mental status)
- Urinalysis (rule out UTI)
- Blood culture (as part of sepsis workup)
- Urinary drug screen
- Electroencephalography (rule out nonconvulsive status epilepticus)

TREATMENT

- NMS is a medical emergency. Discontinue offending agent immediately.
- Treat hyperthermia aggressively with cooling baths or ice packs.
- Provide supportive care (3)[C]:
  - Hydration
  - Maintain renal function.

GENERAL MEASURES

- Patients often require ICU admission to control volume status, correct electrolyte abnormalities, protect renal function, and ameliorate muscle rigidity.
- Recognize complications (e.g., rhabdomyolysis, respiratory failure, acute renal failure); mortality can be as high as 50%.

MEDICATION

- Dopamine agonists can be used, but their role in NMS is still uncertain:
  - Bromocriptine: 2.5 mg PO every 8–12 hours up to max of 40 mg/day; recommended to continue for 10 days and then slowly tapered
  - Amantadine: 100 mg PO BID; increase, as needed, to a max of 400 mg/day.
- Skeletal muscle relaxant: dantrolene—1–2.5 mg/kg IV; may be repeated up to max of 10 mg/kg/day
- Benzodiazepines
  - Diazepam: 5 mg IV q5min
  - Lorazepam: 1 mg IV q5min
- Electroconvulsive therapy may be used for refractory symptoms not responding to medical treatment.
- Neither bromocriptine nor dantrolene has a rapid onset, and neither has been demonstrated to alter outcome.
- If symptoms are due to CNS insult and do not subside on alleviation of insult, consider use of intrathecal baclofen (4,5)[C].

ISSUES FOR REFERRAL

- Involve psychiatry for withdrawal or change of neuroleptic medications.
- All patients should be transferred to an acute care facility where intensive monitoring is available.
- Nephrology should be consulted in the setting of renal failure.

INPATIENT CONSIDERATIONS

Admission Criteria/Initial Stabilization

- All patients with the diagnosis of NMS should be admitted, often for intensive care.
- Airway intervention and circulatory support, as needed; ventilation may be difficult because of chest wall rigidity.
- IV fluids, supplemental O_2, cardiac monitor
- Immediate IV benzodiazepines (e.g., diazepam, lorazepam); may require repeated large doses to control agitation
- If symptoms are not controlled within a few minutes, rapid-sequence intubation and neuromuscular blockade are necessary; nondepolarizing neuromuscular blockers (e.g., vecuronium, rocuronium, pancuronium) are preferable to succinylcholine.
- Cool the patient (ice packs, cooling blankets, ice baths) as quickly as possible.
- Treat symptoms, such as seizures and high blood pressure, appropriately.
- Aggressive IV fluid therapy with lactated Ringer solution or NS, and alkalinization of urine to prevent renal failure from rhabdomyolysis (high CPK levels)
- Monitor for hyperosmolar hyperglycemic state (HHS).
- Administer heparin/low-molecular-weight heparin to prevent deep venous thrombosis.

IV Fluids

Hydration with IV NS

ONGOING CARE

FOLLOW-UP RECOMMENDATIONS

- Allow 2 weeks after recovery to consider rechallenge neuroleptic; rechallenge should not be with the medication implicated in the original NMS episode; consider lower potency neuroleptic agent. Involve psychiatry for appropriate medication selection and titration.
- For pregnant women, untreated psychosis by discontinuing neuroleptics in the setting of NMS can lead to adverse effect such as miscarriage, stillbirth, prematurity, and small size for gestational age; consider risk and benefit before restarting neuroleptic therapy.
- Start at low dose and titrate gradually.
- Carefully monitor for signs and symptoms of recurrent NMS.

PATIENT EDUCATION

- Discuss risk-to-benefit ratio of restarting therapy versus a recurrence of NMS.
- NMS information service: www.nmsis.org

PROGNOSIS

- Mortality rate is estimated at 5–11.6% (25% in 1984).
- Poor prognostic include temperature >104°F, renal failure, HHS, and cardiopulmonary complications.
- In the absence of complications, the prognosis for recovery is good; most patients recover in 15 days.
- Prognosis is better when NMS is detected early.

COMPLICATIONS

- Rhabdomyolysis (causing acute renal failure and, possibly, disseminated intravascular coagulation)
- Cardiac arrest (cardiac arrhythmia, myocardial infraction)
- Respiratory failure (aspiration pneumonia, pulmonary embolism, chest wall rigidity)
- Dehydration and electrolyte disturbances
- Deep venous thrombophlebitis/thrombosis (due to immobilization)
- Seizure
- Hepatic failure
- Sepsis
- Uncontrolled psychosis; persistent neuropsychiatric complications
- Death

REFERENCES

1. Trollor JN, Chen X, Sachdev PS. Neuroleptic malignant syndrome associated with atypical antipsychotic drugs. *CNS Drugs*. 2009;23(6):477–492.
2. Lyons JL, Cohen AB. Selective cerebellar and basal ganglia injury in neuroleptic malignant syndrome. *J Neuroimaging*. 2013;23(2):240–241.
3. Seitz DP, Gill SS. Neuroleptic malignant syndrome complicating antipsychotic treatment of delirium or agitation in medical and surgical patients: case reports and a review of the literature. *Psychosomatics*. 2009;50(1):8–15.
4. Wait SD, Ponce FA, Killory BD. Neuroleptic malignant syndrome from central nervous system insult: 4 cases and a novel treatment strategy. Clinical article. *J Neurosurg Pediatr*. 2009;4(3):217–221.
5. Strawn JR, Keck PE, Caroff SN. Neuroleptic malignant syndrome. *Am J Psychiatry*. 2007;164(6): 870–876.

ADDITIONAL READING

- Berman BD. Neuroleptic malignant syndrome: a review for neurohospitalists. *Neurohospitalist*. 2011;1(1):41–47.
- Halloran LL, Bernard DW. Management of drug-induced hyperthermia. *Curr Opin Pediatr*. 2004;16(2):211–215.
- Neuhut R, Lindenmayer JP, Silva R, et al. Neuroleptic malignant syndrome in children and adolescents on atypical antipsychotic medication: a review. *J Child Adolesc Psychopharmacol*. 2009;19(4):415–422.
- Perry PJ, Wilborn CA. Serotonin syndrome vs neuroleptic malignant syndrome: a contrast of causes, diagnoses, and management. *Ann Clin Psychiatry*. 2012;24(2):155–162.
- Rock W, Elias M, Lev A, et al. Haloperidol-induced neuroleptic malignant syndrome complicated by hyperosmolar hyperglycemic state. *Am J Emerg Med*. 2009;27(8):1018.e1–e1018.e3.

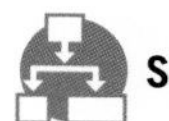

SEE ALSO

Algorithms: Coma; Delirium

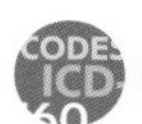

CODES

ICD10

G21.0 Malignant neuroleptic syndrome

CLINICAL PEARLS

- NMS is a medical emergency.
- 2/3 of NMS cases occur within the 1st week of starting a neuroleptic therapy.
- Elevated serum creatinine kinase is the most consistent lab abnormality in patients with NMS.

N

NEUROPATHIC PAIN

Pamela L. Grimaldi, DO, FAAFP

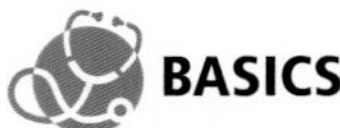

BASICS

DESCRIPTION

- Neuropathic pain is a complex pain state that arises as a direct consequence of injured, damaged, or dysfunctional nerve fibers of the somatosensory system.
- Can arise from damage to the nerve pathways at any point from the terminals of the peripheral nociceptors to the cortical neurons in the brain
- Distinct from nociceptive pain in the way that the latter is induced by activation of peripheral nociceptor nerve fibers
- May be triggered by direct nerve injury, infection, metabolic dysfunction, autoimmune disease, neoplasm, drugs, radiation, and neurovascular disorders
- May reflect the pathologic operation of a dysfunctional nervous system rather than a manifestation of any underlying pathology itself (i.e., phantom limb pain, complex regional pain syndrome [CRPS])
- Patients may paradoxically experience pain and hypersensitivity in an area of denervation (1)[A].

EPIDEMIOLOGY

Incidence

Epidemiologic data are limited. Depending on the inclusion criteria: Radiculopathies, peripheral neuropathy, >3 million Americans suffer from painful diabetic neuropathy.

- 1 million Americans suffer from postherpetic neuralgia (1)[A].

Prevalence

Estimated at 1.5% of the population

ETIOLOGY AND PATHOPHYSIOLOGY

- Positive symptoms due to changes in peripheral nerves, loss of inhibitory mechanisms in CNS, and central sensitization
- Negative symptoms likely due to axonal or neuronal loss
- Associated with a predisposing factor
- Risk factors:
  - Demyelinating disorders (multiple sclerosis [MS], Guillain-Barré)
  - Neoplasm (primary/metastatic)
  - Neurovascular (central poststroke syndrome, diabetes, trigeminal neuralgia)
  - Autoimmune disease (Sjögren syndrome, polyarteritis nodosa)
- Structural disease (herniated disc disease) (1)[A]

RISK FACTORS

- Radiculopathy
- Polyneuropathy (diabetes mellitus, alcohol-induced, postchemotherapy, heritable neuropathies)
- Trauma (nerve entrapment, postsurgical, nerve injury)
- Infection (HIV, herpes zoster, Lyme disease)
- Central mechanisms (stroke, MS, spinal cord injury, limb amputation)
- Nutritional deficiencies (B_{12}, folate)
- Medications (AIDS medications DDC and DDI, antibiotics metronidazole and isoniazid, some chemotherapeutics, amiodarone, hydralazine, phenytoin, nitrofurantoin) (1)[A]

COMMONLY ASSOCIATED CONDITIONS

- Depression/anxiety
- Sleep disturbance
- Fibromyalgia (1)[A]

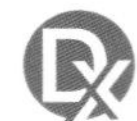

DIAGNOSIS

HISTORY

- May have history of nerve trauma; however, absence does not exclude the diagnosis of neuropathic pain.
- Clinical manifestation can include both negative and positive sensory symptoms and signs. Motor dysfunction is rare.
- Pain is often described as burning, shocklike, tingling, numbing, or intensely hot or cold; decreased proprioception (1)[A]

PHYSICAL EXAM

- Positive signs/symptoms:
  - Hyperalgesia: an exaggerated pain response to a noxious stimulus
  - Allodynia: perception of pain due to a nonnoxious stimuli; for instance, gentle mechanical pressure, light pinprick, hot or cold stimuli, and vibration cause pain.
- Negative signs/symptoms: reduced sensation to touch, pinprick, temperature, or vibration; decreased proprioception
- Motor signs and symptoms: Signs may include hypotonia, tremor, dystonia, ataxia, hypo-/hyperreflexia, or motor neglect. Motor symptoms include weakness, fatigability, decreased range of motion, joint stiffness, and spontaneous muscle spasm (1)[A].

DIAGNOSTIC TESTS & INTERPRETATION

Initial Tests (lab, imaging)

None specifically for neuropathic pain but can rule in or out a cause of symptoms

- Serum B_{12}
- 25-hydroxyvitamin D
- Thyroid-stimulating hormone (TSH)
- Rapid plasma reagin (RPR) or Venereal Disease Research Laboratory (VDRL) test
- Fasting glucose, creatinine
- Lyme serology
- EMG
- Used to rule in or out causes for neuropathic pain
- Consider imaging based on affected area: MRI shows greatest anatomic detail for spine.
- PET and SPECT scans and standard and functional MRI all have been used to map synaptic activity in the thalamus and somatosensory cortex. Initial studies using these imaging techniques have suggested maladaptive reorganization of the thalamus and somatosensory cortex; used more for clinical research, not diagnostically

Follow-Up Tests & Special Considerations

Studies may include nerve conduction, electromyography, evoked potentials, quantitative sensory testing, thermography, and radiologic imaging.

Diagnostic Procedures/Other

If these procedures help with pain, it helps with the diagnosis.

- Sympathetic nerve blocks
- Epidural steroids
- Peripheral nerve blocks
- Dorsal column stimulator and peripheral nerve stimulator

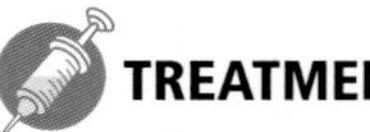

TREATMENT

GENERAL MEASURES

- Use heat or cold packs on painful area.
- Stay active.
- Learn ways to relax body and mind.

MEDICATION

First Line

Effective at least 25% of the time

- Calcium channel alpha-2-delta ligands
  - Gabapentin
    - Efficacy for postherpetic neuralgia (PHN) and painful diabetic neuropathy (PDN)
    - Dosing: start 300 mg PO daily ×1 day, then 300 mg PO BID ×1 day, then 300 mg PO TID; max: 3,600 mg/day
    - Taper over >7 days to discontinue.
    - An adequate trial can require ≥2 months before considering failure.
    - Adverse effects: dizziness, somnolence, ataxia, fatigue, tremor, blurred vision, asthenia, GI symptoms, peripheral edema, headache, weight gain, xerostomia (2)[A]
  - Pregabalin
    - Used for the treatment of PDN, spinal cord injury, PHN, fibromyalgia (3)[A]
    - Dosing: diagnosis dependent; max 300 mg/day
    - Precaution: in elderly patients, renal impairment, NYHA class III or IV HF, angioedema history or risk, depression or history, CNS depressant use or EtoH use
    - Adverse effects: dizziness, somnolence, GI symptoms, peripheral edema
- Tricyclic antidepressants
  - Nortriptyline, amitriptyline
    - Secondary amines (nortriptyline) tolerated better than amitriptyline
    - Dosing: start at 10–25 mg at bedtime, then titrate up to ~75 mg/day as tolerated
    - Adequate trial: 6–8 weeks, including 2 weeks at the highest dose tolerated; onset of analgesia may be after 1 week.
    - Adverse effects: QT interval abnormalities, arrhythmias, sedation, dry mouth, constipation, sexual dysfunction, weight gain, postural hypotension, urinary retention
    - Obtain a pretreatment ECG for documentation/monitoring any arrhythmias if concern for conduction abnormalities (4)[A].
- Serotonin norepinephrine reuptake inhibitors (SNRIs)
  - Duloxetine
    - Effective in the treatment of PDN, fibromyalgia, and more recently chronic low back pain
    - Dosing: 60 mg PO daily
    - Increased risk for serotonin syndrome
    - Adverse effects: GI symptoms, dizziness, somnolence, insomnia, fatigue, anorexia, blurred vision, headache, erectile dysfunction, tremor, weight changes, elevated BP, postural hypotension (5)[A]

- Venlafaxine (Effexor XR)
  - Efficacy in PDN and painful polyneuropathies of different origins but not in PHN
  - Dosages evaluated varied considerably based on etiology of chronic pain conditions in the range of 75–225 mg/day; onset of relief may occur in 1–2 weeks or take up to 6 weeks for full benefit.
  - Adverse effects: anxiety, insomnia, bleeding risk, HTN, hypercholesteremia, sexual dysfunction (6)[A]
- Anticonvulsants
  - Oxcarbazepine: shown to be helpful in diabetic neuropathy and radiculopathy and is better tolerated and more efficacious than carbamazepine (7)[A]
  - Local anesthetic: IV lidocaine, or PO analogs: mexiletine and tocainide (8)[A]

Second Line

Effective but needs further research

- Topical treatments
  - Lidocaine patches: may be more efficacious if used in conjunction with gabapentin (9)[A].
  - Capsaicin cream: low dose questionable effectiveness; high dose (8%) applied under local anesthesia has been effective for up to 3 months (10)[A].
- Opioids
  - Limited effectiveness compared to risk of side effects and addiction and dependency
  - If used, should be in conjunction with gabapentin
  - Controlled-release opioids recommended (oxycodone, morphine, transdermal fentanyl) (11)[A]
- Tramadol
  - Norepinephrine and serotonin inhibitor with a major metabolite that acts as an opioid (μ-receptor) agonist
  - Dosage: 50–100 mg every 4–6 hours, max 400 mg/day
  - Precautions: avoid in those with seizure history
  - Adverse effects: dizziness, nausea, constipation, somnolence, orthostatic hypotension (12)[A]

Third Line

Insufficient evidence for effectiveness

- Low-dose capsaicin, valproic acid, levetiracetam, imipramine, desipramine
- Drugs proven not effective
  - Topiramate, Lamictal, Klonopin, phenytoin

ISSUES FOR REFERRAL

Referral to pain clinic if refractory to initial treatment or neurosurgery is appropriate.

ADDITIONAL THERAPIES

- Transcutaneous electrical nerve stimulation (TENS) may be helpful; but more research is needed (13,14)[C].
- Noninvasive brain stimulation, showing some efficacy but needs more study (15)[C]
- Osteopathic manipulative treatment (OMT) has been shown to help with trigeminal and peripheral neuropathy (16)[C].
- Cognitive-behavioral therapy has been shown to help with fibromyalgia (17)[A].
- Acupuncture: needs more research; Cochrane review pending
- Herbal supplements need more research; Cochrane review pending

SURGERY/OTHER PROCEDURES

Nerve destructive procedures haven't shown effectiveness and have serious side effects.

- Caution, as more studies needed
  - Sympathetectomy dorsal root entry zone lesion (dorsal rhizotomy)
  - Lateral cordotomy
  - Trigeminal nerve ganglion ablation (18)[A]

ONGOING CARE

FOLLOW-UP RECOMMENDATIONS

- Multidisciplinary team
- Opioid contracts to prevent abuses if used

Patient Monitoring

- Random urinalysis for specific prescribed drug and all drugs of abuse for patients receiving opioid therapy
- ECG monitoring if on a tricyclic

PROGNOSIS

Chronic course of pain symptoms often requires management with numerous medications and adjunctive therapies.

COMPLICATIONS

Long-term disability and drug addiction are possible.

REFERENCES

1. Finnerup NB, Sindrup SH, Jensen TS. The evidence for pharmacological treatment of neuropathic pain. *Pain*. 2010;150(3):573–581.
2. Moore RA, Wiffen PJ, Derry S, et al. Gabapentin for chronic neuropathic pain and fibromyalgia in adults. *Cochrane Database Syst Rev*. 2011;(3):CD007938.
3. Moore RA, Straube S, Wiffen PJ, et al. Pregabalin for acute and chronic pain in adults. *Cochrane Database Syst Rev*. 2009;(3):CD007076.
4. Moore RA, Derry S, Aldington D, et al. Amitriptyline for neuropathic pain and fibromyalgia in adults. *Cochrane Database Syst Rev*. 2012;12:CD008242.
5. Lunn MPT, Hughes RAC, Wiffen PJ. Duloxetine for treating painful neuropathy or chronic pain. *Cochrane Database Syst Rev*. 2010;(4):CD007115.
6. Saarto T, Wiffen PJ. Antidepressants for neuropathic pain: a Cochrane review. *J Neurol Neurosurg Psychiatry*. 2010;81(12):1372–1373.
7. Zhou M, Chen N, He L, et al. Oxcarbazepine for neuropathic pain. *Cochrane Database Syst Rev*. 2013;2:CD007963.
8. Challapalli V, Tremont-Lukats IW, McNicol ED, et al. Systemic administration of local anesthetic agents to relieve neuropathic pain. *Cochrane Database Syst Rev*. 2009;(4):CD003345.
9. Derry S, Wiffen PJ, Moore RA, et al. Topical lidocaine for neuropathic pain. *Cochrane Database Syst Rev*. 2014;7:CD010958.
10. Derry S, Sven-Rice A, Cole P, et al. Topical capsaicin (high concentration) for chronic neuropathic pain in adults. *Cochrane Database Syst Rev*. 2013;2:CD007393.
11. The Cochrane pain and palliative and support care group. Oxycodone for neuropathic pain. *Cochrane Database Syst Rev*. 2014;7.
12. Hollingshead J, Dühmke RM, Cornblath DR. Tramadol for neuropathic pain. *Cochrane Database Syst Rev*. 2006;(3):CD003726.
13. Nnoaham KE, Kumbang J. Transcutaneous electrical nerve stimulation (TENS) for chronic pain. *Cochrane Database Syst Rev*. 2008;(3):CD003222.
14. Mulvery MR, Bagnall AM, Johnson MI, et al. Transcutaneous electrical nerve stimulation (TENS) for phantom pain and stump pain following amputation. *Cochrane Database Syst Rev*. 2010;5:CD007264.
15. O'Connell NE, Ward BM, Marston L, et al. Non-invasive brain stimulation for the treatment of chronic pain. *Cochran Database Syst Rev*. 2014;4:CD008208.
16. Galluzzi KE. Managing neuropathic pain. *J Am Osteopath Assoc*. 2007;107(10)(Suppl 6):ES39–ES48.
17. Bernardy K, Klose P, Busch AJ, et al. Cognitive behavioral therapy for fibromyalgia. *Cochrane Database Syst Rev*. 2013;9:CD009796.
18. Straube S, Derry S, Moore RA, et al. Cervico-thorasic or lumbar sympathectomy for neuropathic pain and complex regional syndrome. *Cochrane Database Syst Rev*. 2013;9:CD002918.

ADDITIONAL READING

Wiffen PJ, Derry S, Moore RA. Lamotrigine for acute and chronic pain. *Cochrane Database Syst Rev*. 2011;(2):CD006044.

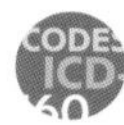

CODES

ICD10

- M79.2 Neuralgia and neuritis, unspecified
- E10.40 Type 1 diabetes mellitus with diabetic neuropathy, unsp
- E11.40 Type 2 diabetes mellitus with diabetic neuropathy, unsp

CLINICAL PEARLS

- Opioids should be reserved for selected patients with moderate to severe pain that adversely impacts function or quality of life.
- Lamotrigine, topiramate, Klonopin, and phenytoin do not have a significant place in therapy based on available evidence.

N

NEUROPATHY, PERIPHERAL

Amy Chen, MD, PhD • David N. Herrmann, MBBCh

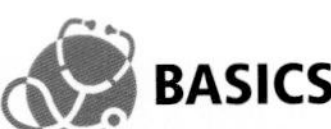

BASICS

DESCRIPTION

- Peripheral neuropathy (PN) is a functional or structural disorder of the peripheral nervous system (PNS).
- PN affects any combination of motor, sensory, or autonomic nerves.
- The motor PNS comprises spinal cord motor neurons, their nerve roots that combine to form plexus, and branches that form individual nerves innervating skeletal muscles. Peripheral motor involvement causes muscle atrophy, weakness, cramps, and fasciculations.
- The sensory PNS consists of sensory organs, which transmit touch, vibration, and position sensation in larger diameter myelinated fibers and pain and temperature in small-diameter, lightly myelinated and unmyelinated C fibers to the dorsal root ganglia. Sensory signals are relayed to the central nervous system (CNS) for integration. Disorders of sensory nerves produce negative phenomena (loss of sensibility, lack of balance) or heightened phenomena (tingling or pain). Large sensory fiber dysfunction impairs touch and vibration sensation, whereas small fiber sensory neuropathy (SFN) affects pin and thermal sensation and causes neuropathic pain.
- The autonomic nervous system (ANS) includes the sympathetic and parasympathetic systems. ANS dysfunction causes cardiovascular, gastrointestinal, and sudomotor symptoms.
- The PNS can be affected from the cell body (sensory ganglionopathy or motor neuronopathy), root (radiculopathy), or plexus (plexopathy) to the nerve (demyelinating or axonal neuropathy).

EPIDEMIOLOGY

Prevalence

Approximately 2.4% of general population, or 8% of people older than age 55 years, are affected by distal symmetric PN, the most common form of PN.

ETIOLOGY AND PATHOPHYSIOLOGY

- PN can be acquired or hereditary.
- The most common cause of acquired PN is diabetes.
- Other categories of acquired PN with illustrative examples are the following:
  - Vascular: ischemia, vasculitis
  - Infectious: HIV, hepatitis C, cryoglobulinemia, Lyme disease
  - Traumatic
  - Autoimmune: rheumatoid arthritis, Sjögren, postinfectious Guillain-Barré syndrome (GBS), chronic inflammatory demyelinating polyneuropathy (CIDP)
  - Metabolic: diabetes, renal failure, hypothyroidism, vitamin B_{12} deficiency, celiac disease
  - Iatrogenic/toxic: chemotherapy, platinum, taxanes, metronidazole, colchicine, infliximab, alcoholism
  - Idiopathic: 30% of PN
  - Neoplastic/paraneoplastic: paraproteinemia, Waldenstrom macroglobulinemia, multiple myeloma, amyloidosis, neurofibromatosis
- PN occurs due to demyelination or axonal degeneration.
- Demyelination results from Schwann cell dysfunction, mutations in myelin protein genes, or direct damage to myelin sheaths.
- Axonal degeneration occurs when injury/dysfunction occurs at the cell body or axon.

Genetics

- Approximately 50% of undiagnosed PN is hereditary.
- Currently, there are over 70 known genetic causes of hereditary PN.
- Charcot-Marie-Tooth (CMT) neuropathies: the most common hereditary PN
  - *CMT1A* (duplication of the *PMP22* gene) is the most common CMT.
  - A *PMP22* deletion causes PN with liability to pressure palsy (HNPP)

RISK FACTORS

Systemic disorders predispose to PN.

GENERAL PREVENTION

- Healthy nutrition and avoidance of alcoholism and of pressure at nerve entrapment sites
- Surveillance for glucose dysmetabolism and tight glycemic control may prevent diabetic PN.

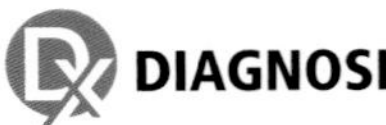

DIAGNOSIS

HISTORY

- A detailed inquiry for symptoms of sensory, motor, or autonomic dysfunction:
  - Numbness, tingling, prickling, burning pain, a "tightly wrapped" sensation, and an "unsteady gait"
  - Distal weakness manifests as foot drop (tripping, foot slapping) or difficulty with grip; proximal weakness (e.g., difficulty arising from a chair) is less common.
  - Orthostatic dizziness, abnormal sweating, constipation, or voiding difficulties
- Symptom onset:
  - Acute: Consider infection (e.g., Lyme disease), postinfectious dysimmune process (e.g., GBS), ischemia (e.g., vasculitis), toxin, or trauma.
  - Subacute: Consider metabolic, neoplastic, paraneoplastic, or dysimmune processes.
  - Chronic: Consider dysimmune process (CIDP), idiopathic, or hereditary.
- Progression: stable or indolent; slowly or rapidly progressive; monophasic or relapsing or remitting
- Anatomic pattern: focal, multifocal, diffuse

ALERT

Hemibody symptoms suggest CNS rather than PNS pathology.

PHYSICAL EXAM

- Based on exam, a functional (*sensory*: small-fiber vs. large-fiber vs. mixed, *sensorimotor*, *motor*, *autonomic*) and anatomic pattern of PN (*distal symmetric*, *multifocal*, or *focal*) should be established.
- Cognition preserved in isolated PN.
- Cranial nerves may be involved with focal or multifocal PN (e.g., bifacial weakness may occur with GBS, Lyme disease, sarcoidosis, among other causes).
- Stocking/glove sensory loss is typical of distal symmetric sensory PN (e.g., diabetes).
- Isolated reduced pin or thermal sensation or allodynia suggests a pure small-fiber neuropathy (SFN).
- Reduced vibration and joint position sense suggests large-fiber sensory neuropathy; when severe, a Romberg sign is present, and gait is wide-based or ataxic.
- Distal muscle atrophy and weaknesses of toe extension and finger abduction are often present with distal symmetric axonal PN.
- In acquired demyelinating PN (e.g., GBS or CIDP), weakness is commonly both proximal and distal.
- Deep tendon reflexes may be reduced or absent, distally at the ankles in large-fiber axonal PN, or diffusely in demyelinating PN.
- High arched or flat feet or hammer toes suggest hereditary PN.

ALERT

Hemibody deficits or sensory loss below a spinal cord level suggest a CNS process.

ALERT

Hyperreflexia and spasticity are upper motor neuron signs not seen with isolated PN.

DIFFERENTIAL DIAGNOSIS

The following categories of PN can be identified (differential diagnosis [DDx] listed when applicable):

- Pure sensory neuropathy
  - DDx: SFN, sensory ganglionopathy, polyradiculopathy
- Distal symmetric sensorimotor axonal PN
  - Most common type of PN
  - DDx: distal acquired demyelinating symmetric PN (DADS)
- Motor predominant PN
  - DDx: motor neuron disease, polyradiculopathy, immune-mediated multifocal motor neuropathy (MMN)
- Mononeuropathy
  - Most likely due to compression, entrapment, or trauma
  - DDx: monoradiculopathy
- Mononeuropathy multiplex
  - DDx: plexopathy, polyradiculopathy

DIAGNOSTIC TESTS & INTERPRETATION

Initial Tests (lab, imaging)

- Nerve conduction studies and electromyography (NCS/EMG)
  - Best performed by physicians with specialty training in electrodiagnostic medicine
  - Delineate axonal versus demyelinating, anatomic pattern, chronicity, and severity of PN.
- Blood tests
  - CBC, BUN, creatinine, fasting glucose, HgA1C, vitamin B_{12}, serum protein electrophoresis, and immunofixation
- Specialized skin biopsy
  - In clinically suspected SFN if NCS/EMG normal
  - Analysis of lower limb epidermal nerve fiber density (ENFD) (1)[A]
- Autonomic tests
  - Not routinely done but useful to characterize autonomic PN
- Neuroimaging
  - Generally not indicated in evaluation of PN but useful in evaluation of brachial plexopathies, radiculopathies, or where findings are attributable to the CNS

Follow-Up Tests & Special Considerations

- Additional blood tests are tailored to the medical history, the PN type, and NCS/EMG findings.
- Genetic testing for diagnosis of hereditary PN should be ordered by neurologists with expertise in PN.
- Screen patients with distal symmetric PN for unhealthy alcohol use with CAGE-AID or AUDIT-C.

ALERT
Ordering of laboratory batteries (e.g., peripheral nerve antibody panels) without careful consideration of the clinical and NCS/EMG features should be avoided.

Diagnostic Procedures/Other

- Nerve biopsy (sural or superficial peroneal nerve): useful if vasculitis, amyloidosis, granulomatous disorders, or neoplastic infiltration is suspected; rarely helpful in late-onset chronic, slowly progressive distal symmetric PN
- Lumbar puncture
  - Cytoalbuminemic dissociation in GBS or CIDP
  - Infection, inflammation, or neoplasia in polyradiculopathies

Test Interpretation

- Demyelinating PN: disproportionate slowing of conduction velocities on NCS
- Axonal PN: reduced amplitude in sensory or motor responses, with relatively preserved conduction velocities on NCS
- Reduced ENFD on distal leg skin biopsies is supportive of SFN.

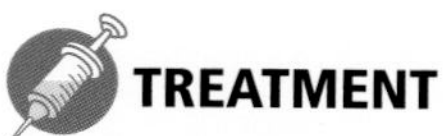

TREATMENT

GENERAL MEASURES

Manage associated medical conditions; disease-modifying therapy for specific forms of PN (e.g., CIDP); symptomatic relief of pain and dysautonomia; rehabilitation to optimize function.

MEDICATION

First Line

- Treatment of neuropathic pain: evidence of efficacy derived from clinical trials in diabetic painful neuropathy (DPN) and postherpetic neuralgia (PHN):
- Pregabalin: for DPN and PHN
- Duloxetine: for DPN
- Lidocaine patch: for PHN
- Gabapentin: (off-label) for DPN
- Tricyclic antidepressants: (off-label) for DPN
- Venlafaxine: (off-label) for DPN
- Tramadol: (off-label) for DPN
- Targeted treatment for underlying systemic conditions:
  - Glycemic control, thyroid hormone supplementation, vitamin supplementation, antimicrobial therapy (e.g., Lyme disease, HIV), glucocorticoids for sarcoidosis, and cytotoxic therapy for vasculitis
- Immunotherapy for dysimmune PN
  - Intravenous immunoglobulin (IVIG): within the first 2 weeks of GBS to hasten recovery (2)[A]; as a 1st-line alternative for CIDP (3)[A]; and for prevention of secondary axonal loss in multifocal motor neuropathy (MMN) (4)[A]
    - Loading dose 2 g/kg body weight divided into 2–5 days; maintenance regimen variable for CIDP and MMN
    - Adverse effects (AE): headache, fever, hypertension, and rarely pulmonary embolism
  - Plasma exchange: 1st agent shown to improve functional outcome for patients with GBS (5)[A]; short-term benefit in CIDP (6)[A]
    - AE: catheter complication, hypotension, and others
  - Corticosteroids: 1st agent used in treatment of CIDP (7)[C]
- Treatment of autonomic symptoms
  - Compression stockings, hydration, midodrine, and fludrocortisone for orthostatic hypotension
  - Pyridostigmine for immune-mediated dysautonomia (off-label)

ISSUES FOR REFERRAL

- Rapidly progressive symptoms, suspected demyelinating PN, or hereditary PN should be referred to a neurologist with expertise in neuromuscular disorders.
- Patients with vasculitic PN should be referred to rheumatology.
- Patients with paraproteinemia should have a skeletal bone survey and be referred to hematology.
- Patients with imbalance, ataxia, or falls should be referred to physical therapy for gait and balance training.

ADDITIONAL THERAPIES

- Combination therapy (e.g., gabapentin with TCA or venlafaxine or tramadol) can be more effective than monotherapy for neuropathic pain.
- Long-acting opiates can be considered for refractory neuropathic pain.
- Additional immunosuppressant agents (e.g., cyclophosphamide) may be used in refractory chronic dysimmune PN.

ALERT
Opiates have significant side effects and may cause rebound headaches, tolerance, and dependence.

SURGERY/OTHER PROCEDURES

- Decompressive surgery for entrapment neuropathy (e.g., carpal tunnel syndrome)
- Foot and ankle surgery to improve symptoms or function in hereditary PN
- Radiation, surgery, or bone marrow transplantation for plasmacytoma or osteosclerotic myeloma or POEMS syndrome
- Liver transplantation for amyloidotic PN

COMPLEMENTARY & ALTERNATIVE MEDICINE

Low-intensity transcutaneous electrical nerve stimulation (TENS), acupuncture, mediation

ALERT
Vitamin B_6 supplementation may cause peripheral neurotoxicity and should be avoided except for a deficiency state

INPATIENT CONSIDERATIONS

Admission Criteria/Initial Stabilization

- Patients with suspected GBS should be admitted for diagnosis, monitoring (30–60% may develop cardiovascular or respiratory failure), and for acute treatment.
- Elective intubation may be required in GBS when forced vital capacity is <15 mL/kg body weight.
- Other rapidly progressive undiagnosed PNs that impair independent ambulation may require admission.

ONGOING CARE

FOLLOW-UP RECOMMENDATIONS

- Physical therapy and gait assistive devices as needed
- Flu vaccination should be avoided in the 1st year following GBS.

PROGNOSIS

- Late onset idiopathic distal symmetric axonal PN are indolent.
- 80% of GBS have a near complete or good recovery. 80% of CIDP have moderate or good response with treatment but can be relapsing.

REFERENCES

1. Lauria G, Hwieh ST, Johansson O, et al. European Federation of Neurological Societies/ Peripheral Nerve Society Guideline on the use of skin biopsy in the diagnosis of small fiber neuropathy. Report of a joint task force of the European Federation of Neurological Societies and the Peripheral Nerve Society. *Eur J Neurol*. 2010;17(7):903–912.
2. Hughes RA, Swan AV, van Doorn PA. Intravenous immunoglobulin for Guillain-Barré syndrome. *Cochrane Database Syst Rev*. 2012;7:CD002063.
3. Hughes RA, Donofrio P, Bril V, et al; ICE Study Group. Intravenous immune globulin (10% caprylate–chromatography purified) for the treatment of chronic inflammatory demyelinating polyradiculoneuropathy (ICE study): a randomised placebo-controlled trial. *Lancet Neurol*. 2008;7(2):136–144.
4. Cats EA, van der Pol WL, Piepers S, et al. Correlates of outcome and response to IVIg in 88 patients with multifocal motor neuropathy. *Neurology*. 2010;75(9):818–825.
5. Plasmapheresis and acute Guillain-Barré syndrome. The Guillain-Barré syndrome Study Group. *Neurology*. 1985;35(8):1096–1104.
6. Dyck PJ, Daube J, O'Brien P, et al. Plasma exchange in chronic inflammatory demyelinating polyradiculoneuropathy. *N Engl J Med*. 1986;314(8):461–465.
7. Dyck PJ, O'Brien PC, Oviatt KF, et al. Prednisone improves chronic inflammatory polyradiculoneuropathy more than no treatment. *Ann Neurol*. 1982;11(2):136–141.

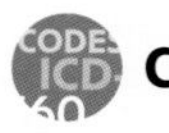

CODES

ICD10

- G62.9 Polyneuropathy, unspecified
- G60.9 Hereditary and idiopathic neuropathy, unspecified
- G60.8 Other hereditary and idiopathic neuropathies

CLINICAL PEARLS

- There are many causes of PN. Diagnosis is made by history and physical exam, targeted laboratory testing, NCS/EMG, skin biopsy, or ANS testing.
- Consider hereditary neuropathy if patient has an early age of PN symptom onset, family history of PN, or foot deformity.
- GBS is monophasic and progresses for up to 4 weeks; CIDP progresses beyond 8 weeks, and untreated usually has a progressive course.

NICOTINE ADDICTION

Benjamin N. Schneider, MD • Brett White, MD

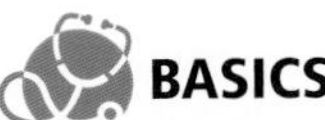

BASICS

DESCRIPTION

Nicotine addiction is characterized by signs of dependence and compulsive use despite knowledge of its adverse effects.

EPIDEMIOLOGY

Incidence

20–25% of the U.S. population use nicotine.

Prevalence

70 million in the United States ≥12 years of age reported current use of tobacco (58.7 million smoked cigarettes, 13.3 million cigars, 2.1 million pipes, and 8.6 million used smokeless tobacco) (1).

Pediatric Considerations

Nicotine use is common and underrecognized in this population. Use of cigarettes or smokeless tobacco in the past month: 8th graders: 4.9% and 2.8%, 10th graders: 10.8% and 6.4%, 12th graders: 17.1% and 7.9% (2)

ETIOLOGY AND PATHOPHYSIOLOGY

- Nicotine causes changes in brain nicotinic acetylcholine receptors (nAChRs) during smoking that initiate addiction, including nicotine-induced upregulation in nAChR binding sites.
- Nicotine has both stimulating and depressing effects within the CNS; relaxing and euphoric effects may contribute to psychological dependence. It is likely that endogenous opioid peptides and their receptors play an important role in the psychoactive properties of nicotine.
- Polymorphisms in neuronal nAChR genes could be associated with increased susceptibility to tobacco dependence.

Genetics

- Mutation in the α_4 subunit of nAChRs expressed by neurons was found to lower the threshold for the induction of nicotine dependence.
- SNP mutations in the nAChR have been associated with smoking heaviness as well as reduced abstinence despite pharmacotherapy.
- Specific genes have been isolated that are associated with nicotine dependence, including *CHRNB3*, the β_3 nicotine receptor subunit gene.
- T-variant gene associated with decreased activity of CYP2B6 (enzyme that breaks down nicotine in the brain); may lead to increased craving during smoking cessation. These patients are also 1.5 times more likely to resume smoking during treatment.

RISK FACTORS

- Mental illness (depression, posttraumatic stress disorder, bipolar disorder, and schizophrenia)
- Low socioeconomic status
- Low educational status
- Early 1st-hand nicotine experience increases risk for chronic abuse.
- Environmental factors are critical for smoking initiation; genetic factors contribute to smoking persistence and difficulty quitting.

GENERAL PREVENTION

- The U.S. Preventive Services Task Force (USPSTF) strongly recommends clinicians screen all:
  - Adults for tobacco use and provide tobacco cessation interventions for those who use tobacco products.
  - Pregnant women for tobacco use and provide augmented pregnancy-tailored counseling to those who smoke.
- The USPSTF gives an I recommendation for or against routine screening for tobacco use or interventions to prevent and treat tobacco use among children or adolescents.

Pregnancy Considerations

- Carbon monoxide and nicotine may interfere with fetal oxygen supply, resulting in growth restriction and decreased birth weight.
- Maternal smoking adversely affects offspring lung development, with lifelong decreases in pulmonary function and increased asthma risk.
- Smoking may increase the incidence of spontaneous abortion and sudden infant death syndrome (SIDS) as well as learning on behavioral problems and an increased risk of obesity in children.

COMMONLY ASSOCIATED CONDITIONS

- Chronic obstructive pulmonary disease (COPD) (emphysema and chronic bronchitis)
- Cancers (lung, oral/pharyngeal, kidney, bladder, cervical, anal)
- Coronary artery disease
- Periodontal disease

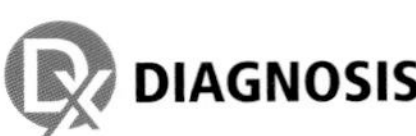

DIAGNOSIS

HISTORY

- Amount and duration of smoking
- Previous attempts to quit

PHYSICAL EXAM

Cardiovascular exam

DIFFERENTIAL DIAGNOSIS

- Depression
- COPD
- α_1-Antitrypsin deficiency
- Asthma
- Congestive heart failure (CHF)
- Respiratory infections
- Lung cancer
- Cystic fibrosis

DIAGNOSTIC TESTS & INTERPRETATION

Spirometry: decreased FEV_1 only if COPD suspected—not screening

Diagnostic Procedures/Other

- American College of Chest Physicians Lung Cancer Screening Recommendations 2013
  - Low-dose CT screening for individuals aged 55–75 years with a history of 30 or more pack-years who are still smoking or have quit within the past 15 years in settings that can deliver the comprehensive care provided to National Lung Screening Trial participants.
  - Screening is not recommended for individuals with a smoking history of fewer than 30 pack-years, those who fall outside the age guidelines, or those with comorbidities that might limit their life expectancy.

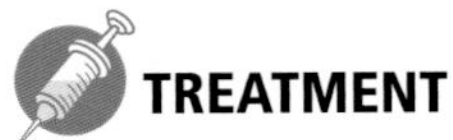

TREATMENT

Counseling (3)[A]

- Advice from medical providers helps improve quit rates (number needed to treat [NNT] 75).
- Providing brief, simple advice about cessation increases the likelihood of quitting and remaining a nonsmoker at 12 months. More intensive advice (i.e., motivational interviewing) may result in higher rates of quitting. Providing follow-up support may increase quit rates slightly.
- The USPSTF strongly recommends screening all adults for tobacco use and providing cessation interventions for those using tobacco products (Level A recommendation).

GENERAL MEASURES

- Brief strategies to help the patient willing to quit tobacco use—the "5 As" (4)[A]
  - Ask the patient if he or she uses tobacco.
  - Advise him or her to quit.
  - Assess willingness to make a quit attempt.
  - Assist those willing to make a quit attempt.
  - Arrange for follow-up contact to prevent relapse.
- Enhancing motivation to quit—the "5 Rs" (4)[A]
  - Relevance: Encourage patient to indicate why quitting is personally relevant.
  - Risks: Ask patient to identify potential negative consequences of use.
  - Rewards: Ask patient to identify potential benefits of cessation.
  - Roadblocks: Ask patient to identify barriers or impediments to quitting and provide treatment (e.g., problem-solving counseling or medication) that could address barriers.
  - Repetition: The motivational intervention should be repeated each visit.

MEDICATION

- There are 7 FDA-approved medications for tobacco use and all are efficacious: bupropion SR, nicotine gum, inhaler, lozenge, nasal spray, patch, and varenicline.
- Varenicline and combination nicotine replacement therapy (NRT; long-acting patch + PRN short-acting agent) should be considered first line as they have been shown to be more effective than nicotine patch alone.
- All medications for cessation have side effects and some have FDA warnings; providers should be familiar with these.

First Line

- Varenicline (Chantix) is a nicotinic acetylcholine partial agonist for the treatment of nicotine addiction. Trials have suggested this agent may be more efficacious than bupropion (5)[A]. Longer term therapy (up to 24 weeks) may delay or prevent relapse:
  - Starter pack: 0.5 mg/day for 3 days, 0.5 mg BID for 4 days, 1 mg/day starting on day 7
  - Maintenance pack 1 mg BID continue for 12 weeks total; if successful in quitting, may continue for another 12 weeks
- Combination NRT: All forms of NRT increase the rate of quitting (6)[A] by 50–70%. No overall difference in effectiveness of different forms of NRT and combining long- with short-acting NRTs has been shown to be more effective than using the patch alone (e.g., patch + inhaler, patch + gum). Heavier smokers may need higher doses. Starting NRT before planned quit date may increase the chances of success.
  - Nicotine gum (Nicorette): for >25 cigarettes/day habit, 4-mg gum q1–2h for 6 weeks; for <25 cigarettes/day habit, 2-mg gum q1–2h for 6 weeks; decrease dosing by q1–2h for 3 weeks; chew then tuck between cheek and gingiva.

- Nicotine transdermal (NicoDerm CQ): for >10 cigarettes/day habit, 21-mg patch/day for 6 weeks, then 14-mg patch/day for 2 weeks, then 7-mg patch/day for 2 weeks; for <10 cigarettes/day habit, 14-mg patch/day for 6 weeks, then 7-mg patch/day for 2 weeks
- Nicotine lozenge (Commit): for patients who have 1st cigarette within 30 minutes of waking, 4-mg lozenge PO q1–2h for 6 weeks; 1st cigarette >30 minutes after waking, 2-mg lozenge PO q1–2h for 6 weeks; decrease dosing by q1–2h for 3 weeks.
- Nicotine nasal (Nicotrol NS): 1–2 sprays (0.5 mg/spray) each nostril q1hr for 8 weeks, then taper; max 10 sprays/hr and 80 sprays/day
- Nicotine inhaler (Nicotrol inhaler): 6–16 cartridges inhaled (4 mg/cartridge) per day for 6–12 weeks, then taper

ALERT

- Varenicline (Chantix) carries a boxed warning for risks of serious neuropsychiatric events, including changes in behavior, hostility, agitation, depressed mood, and suicidal thoughts or actions. It should be used with extreme caution in patients with serious psychiatric disorders (bipolar disorder, depression, or schizophrenia); use may exacerbate these conditions. Varenicline may also increase the risk of certain cardiovascular adverse events in patients with cardiovascular disease.
- Varenicline + bupropion has not been shown to be more effective than either agent alone but with increased side effects.

Second Line

- Single-agent NRT: See earlier section for Rx information.
- Bupropion SR (Zyban): An antidepressant; start 150 mg/day PO for 3 days, then 150 mg PO BID; stop smoking 5–7 days after starting treatment; continue 7–12 weeks.
  - 1:1,000 risk of seizure
- Nortriptyline: tricyclic antidepressant; start 25 mg/day, gradually increase to target dose of 75–100 mg/day; stop smoking 2–4 weeks after starting treatment; continue for 12 weeks:
  - Contraindications: narrow-angle glaucoma or heart disease (acute myocardial infarction, atrioventricular or bundle-branch block, QT prolongation)
  - Caution: pregnancy Category D

ADDITIONAL THERAPIES

Some Internet-based interventions can assist smoking cessation, especially if the information is appropriately tailored to the users and frequent automated contacts with the users are ensured.

- Other interventions
  - Smokers who get support from partners and other people are more likely to quit.
  - Group programs double cessation rates more than self-help materials without face-to-face instruction and group support. It is unclear whether groups are better than individual counseling or other advice, but they are more effective than no treatment. Not all smokers making a quit attempt want to attend meetings, but for those who do, they are likely to be helpful.
- Smokers should be given a choice of quitting methods, either reducing smoking before quitting or abruptly quitting, as neither has demonstrated superior quit rates.
- E-cigarettes: Currently, there are questions from the FDA and others around safety, consistency of nicotine dose, and possible benefits from these devices. Thus far, results looking at efficacy and safety have been mixed. Given the limited available evidence on the risks and benefits of e-cigarette use, large, randomized controlled trials are urgently needed to definitively establish their potential for smoking cessation.

Pregnancy Considerations

- Interventions are effective in helping women to stop smoking during pregnancy (overall by ~6%). The most effective intervention appears to be providing incentives, which helped ~24% of women to quit smoking during pregnancy. The smoking cessation interventions reduced the number of babies with low birth weight and preterm births.
- NRT is metabolized faster in pregnant women, so higher doses may be required. A 2012 Cochrane review found insufficient evidence for efficacy or change in adverse birth outcomes.

COMPLEMENTARY & ALTERNATIVE MEDICINE

- Acupuncture: no consistent evidence of efficacy
- Hypnotherapy: no consistent evidence of efficacy

INPATIENT CONSIDERATIONS

- Programs to stop smoking that begin during a hospital stay and include follow-up support for at least 1 month after discharge are effective. Programs are effective when administered to all hospitalized smokers, regardless of admitting diagnosis (7)[A].
- Consider NRT to all inpatients who smoke to decrease withdrawal symptoms (7)[A].

 ONGOING CARE

FOLLOW-UP RECOMMENDATIONS

- Patients motivated to quit smoking and who have initiated therapy should follow up routinely with the physician to monitor response and observe for any medication side effects.
- Encourage routine exercise as a component of smoking-cessation treatment.

DIET

Weight gain (4–5 kg over 10 years) possible after smoking cessation

PATIENT EDUCATION

- http://www.smokefree.gov
- http://women.smokefree.gov/
- http://teen.smokefree.gov
- http://www.nicotine-anonymous.org
- http://quitnet.com
- 1-877-44U-QUIT (1-877-448-7848)

PROGNOSIS

>85% of those who try to quit on their own relapse, most within a week.

REFERENCES

1. National Institute on Drug Abuse. *Tobacco Addiction*. NIH Publication Number 09-4342. Bethesda, MD: National Institute of Health; 2009.
2. Johnston LD, O'Malley PM, Bachman JG, et al. *Monitoring the Future National Results on Adolescent Drug Use: Overview of Key Findings, 2011*. Ann Arbor, MI: Institute for Social Research, University of Michigan; 2012.
3. Stead LF, Bergson G, Lancaster T. Physician advice for smoking cessation. *Cochrane Database Syst Rev*. 2008;(2):CD000165.
4. National Guideline Clearinghouse (NGC). Guideline synthesis: Tobacco use cessation. In: *National Guideline Clearinghouse (NGC)*. Rockville, MD: Agency for Healthcare Research and Quality (AHRQ); 2001. http://www.guideline.gov.
5. Cahill K, Stead LF, Lancaster T. Nicotine receptor partial agonists for smoking cessation. *Cochrane Database Syst Rev*. 2008;(3):CD006103.
6. Stead LF, Perera R, Bullen C, et al. Nicotine replacement therapy for smoking cessation. *Cochrane Database Syst Rev*. 2008;(1):CD000146.
7. Rigotti NA, Clair C, Munafò MR, et al. Interventions for smoking cessation in hospitalised patients. *Cochrane Database Syst Rev*. 2012;(5):CD001837.

ADDITIONAL READING

- Benowitz NL. Nicotine addiction. *N Engl J Med*. 2010;362(24):2295–2303.
- Centers for Disease Control and Prevention. Smoking and tobacco use. http://www.cdc.gov/tobacco/index.htm.
- Clinical Practice Guideline Treating Tobacco Use and Dependence 2008 Update Panel, Liaisons, and Staff. A clinical practice guideline for treating tobacco use and dependence: 2008 update. A U.S. Public Health Service Report. *Am J Prev Med*. 2008;35(2):158–176.
- Civljak M, Sheikh A, Stead LF, et al. Internet-based interventions for smoking cessation. *Cochrane Database Syst Rev*. 2010;(9):CD007078.
- Wilson JF. In the clinic. Smoking cessation. *Ann Intern Med*. 2007;146(3):ITC2-1–ICT2-16.

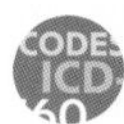 CODES

ICD10

- F17.200 Nicotine dependence, unspecified, uncomplicated
- F17.201 Nicotine dependence, unspecified, in remission
- F17.203 Nicotine dependence unspecified, with withdrawal

CLINICAL PEARLS

- Smoking cessation should be encouraged for all patients who smoke.
- No single type of NRT is best; they are equally effective. Choice, therefore, should be based on patient preference and risk factors for side effects.
- Consider NRT for all hospitalized patients who smoke to decrease withdrawal symptoms.

NONALCOHOLIC FATTY LIVER DISEASE (NAFLD)

Jill T. Wei, MD • Daniel T. Lee, MD, MA

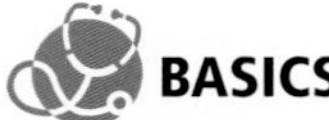

BASICS

- Nonalcoholic fatty liver disease (NAFLD) represents a spectrum of fatty liver diseases not due to excess alcohol consumption ranging from nonalcoholic fatty liver (NAFL) to steatohepatitis and cirrhosis with hepatocyte injury with/without fibrosis.
- Leading cause of chronic liver disease; may be implicated in up to 90% of patients with asymptomatic, mild aminotransferase elevation not caused by alcohol, viral hepatitis, or medications

DESCRIPTION

- NAFL (1):
  - Reversible condition in which large vacuoles of triglyceride fat accumulate in hepatocytes
  - Liver biopsy: fatty deposits in >30% of liver cells, no ballooning of hepatocytes, no necrosis, no fibrosis
  - Alanine aminotransferase/aspartate aminotransferase (ALT/AST) enzymes usually normal but may be elevated, rarely >3–4× upper limit of normal.
  - Minimal risk of progression to cirrhosis and liver failure
  - Synonym: steatosis
- Nonalcoholic steatohepatitis (NASH): progressive form of NAFL (1)
  - Liver biopsy: fatty deposits in >50% of liver cells with ballooning, acute and chronic inflammation, ± fibrosis
  - ALT and AST elevated, generally <3–4× upper limit of normal
  - May progress to cirrhosis, liver failure, and rarely hepatocellular cancer; incomplete data to assess natural history; some data suggest that 30% with NASH have progression of fibrosis over 5 years.
  - Synonym: steatohepatitis
- NASH cirrhosis (1):
  - Presence of cirrhosis with current or previous histologic evidence of steatosis or steatohepatitis

EPIDEMIOLOGY

- NAFLD: most common chronic liver disease globally; usually benign, asymptomatic
- NASH may be symptomatic with progressive inflammation and fibrosis.
  - Predominant age: 40s–50s; does occur in children
  - Predominant sex: male > female (slight)

Incidence

Limited studies with high variability: estimates from 31–86 cases of NAFLD per 10,000 person-years to 29 cases of NAFLD per 100,000 person-years (1)

Prevalence

- United States estimate: 6–24% (1)
- Worldwide: 6–33%, median 20% (1)
- Present in 58–74% of obese persons (BMI >30) and 90% of morbidly obese persons (BMI >39) (1)
- Among individuals with T2DM, rate of 69–87%; in patients with dyslipidemia, rate of 50% (1)

ETIOLOGY AND PATHOPHYSIOLOGY

Primary mechanism is *insulin resistance,* which leads to increased lipolysis, triglyceride synthesis, and increased hepatic uptake of fatty acids.

- NAFLD: excessive triglyceride accumulation in the liver and an impaired ability to remove fatty acids
- NASH: "2-hit" hypothesis involving (1) macrovesicular steatosis due to increased hepatic lipid synthesis, reduced transfer of lipids, and increased insulin resistance with hepatic oxidative stress and (2) mitochondrial damage leading to impaired restoration of ADT stores, lipid peroxidation, and increased iron stores (1)

Genetics

Largely unknown: Data suggest familial clustering and slight increased heritability. NAFL: more 1st-degree relatives with cirrhosis than matched controls; NASH: 18% with affected 1st-degree relative. Carriers of hemochromatosis gene are more likely to be affected. Genetic variants in apolipoprotein *C3* gene may play a role in NAFLD, hypertriglyceridemia, and insulin resistance (1).

RISK FACTORS

- Obesity (BMI >30), visceral obesity (waist circumference >102 cm for men or >88 cm for women), T2DM, hypertension, dyslipidemia, high serum triglycerides and low serum high-density lipoprotein (HDL) levels, metabolic syndrome
- Possible associations with hypothyroidism, hypopituitarism, hypogonadism, obstructive sleep apnea, pancreatoduodenal resection, and polycystic ovary syndrome
- Increasing age associated with increased prevalence, severity, advanced fibrosis, and mortality
- Protein–calorie malnutrition; total parenteral nutrition (TPN) >6 weeks
- Severe acute weight loss (starvation, bariatric surgery)
- Organic solvent exposure (e.g., chlorinated hydrocarbons, toluene); vinyl chloride; hypoglycin A
- Gene for hemochromatosis/other conditions with increased iron stores
- Drugs: tetracycline, glucocorticoids, tamoxifen, methotrexate, valproic acid, fialuridine, many chemotherapy regimens, and nucleoside analogues

Pregnancy Considerations

Acute fatty liver of pregnancy: Rare but serious complication in 3rd trimester. 50% of cases are associated with preeclampsia (2).

- Symptoms: nausea, vomiting, headache, fatigue, right upper quadrant or epigastric gain, jaundice
- Elevated ALT and AST >300 IU/L but usually <1,000 IU/L; elevated bilirubin
- Liver biopsy confirms diagnosis but should not delay treatment.
- Early recognition and prompt delivery is key for successful management.
- Recurrence is rare but can occur in subsequent pregnancies (2).

Pediatric Considerations

- Increasing prevalence of NAFLD among children parallels rise in pediatric obesity.
- Reports of NAFLD as early as age 2 years and NASH-related cirrhosis as early as age 8 years
- Treat with intensive lifestyle modification, possible benefit of Vitamin E.
- Reye syndrome: fatty liver syndrome with encephalopathy usually following viral illness, for example, varicella or influenza
  - Vomiting with dehydration
  - Confusion, progressive CNS damage
  - Hepatomegaly with extensive fatty vacuolization
  - Hypoglycemia (3)
- Etiology unknown; viral URIs and drugs (especially salicylates) have been implicated.
- Mortality rate: 50%
- Treat with mannitol, IV glucose, and FFP.

GENERAL PREVENTION

- Avoid excess alcohol: ≤3 standard drinks/day (men); ≤2 standard drinks/day (women).
- Maintain appropriate BMI.
- Prevention and optimally manage diabetes
- Avoid hepatotoxic medications.
- HAV and HBV vaccination if not immune
- Pneumococcal and (annual) influenza vaccinations

COMMONLY ASSOCIATED CONDITIONS

Central obesity; HTN; T2DM; insulin resistance; hyperlipidemia; preeclampsia in pregnancy; possible associations with hypothyroidism, hypogonadism, and obstructive sleep apnea

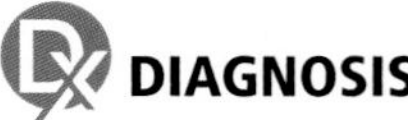

DIAGNOSIS

- Routine screening not currently recommended
- Consider NAFLD in patients with asymptomatic aminotransferase elevations (1)[A].
- Can also occur with normal/fluctuating AST/ALT levels (1)[A]
- NAFLD has no distinguishing historical/laboratory features to distinguish from other chronic liver disorders.
- Index of suspicion is higher with risk factors such as metabolic syndrome, insulin resistance, or obesity.
- May present as cryptogenic cirrhosis
- Noninvasive biomarkers of steatosis/fibrosis are not sufficiently reliable. Liver biopsy is the definitive diagnostic test but should only be considered when results are likely to change management.

HISTORY

- Typically asymptomatic
- Possible fatigue and/or abdominal fullness
- Vague right upper quadrant pain
- History of medication and alcohol use, family history

PHYSICAL EXAM

Most common signs (all are infrequent):

- Liver tenderness
- Mild to marked hepatomegaly
- Splenomegaly
- In advanced cases: cutaneous stigmata of chronic liver disease or portal hypertension, for example, palmar erythema, spider angiomata, ascites

DIFFERENTIAL DIAGNOSIS

- Viral hepatitis
- Alcoholic fatty liver
- Drug- or toxin-induced hepatitis
- Metabolic liver disease
- Autoimmune hepatitis
- Celiac disease
- Muscle disease, if nonhepatic cause of elevated enzymes are possible

DIAGNOSTIC TESTS & INTERPRETATION

Initial Tests (lab, imaging)

- Both ALT and AST may be elevated:
  - Nonalcoholic, usually ALT:AST >1
  - If alcohol-induced, usually AST:ALT ≥2
  - If advanced cirrhosis is present, nonspecific enzyme abnormalities may exist or may be normal (1).
- Level of enzyme elevation does NOT correlate with degree of fibrosis (1).
- Serum ferritin (1.5× normal), alkaline phosphatase (2–3× normal), and total and direct bilirubin may be elevated (1).

- Severity and chronicity in acute liver disease are characterized by defects in ability to produce plasma proteins (serum albumin, PT) and thrombocytopenia (1).
- Lipids abnormalities are common and include elevated cholesterol, low-density lipoprotein (LDL), and triglyceride and decreased HDL (1).
- Biomarkers of inflammation, increased oxidative stress, or hepatocyte apoptosis such as leptin, adiponectin, CRP, serum caspase, and cytokeratin 18 may help differentiate NASH from NAFLD (1)[B].
- Serologic studies to exclude other etiologies of liver disease, for example, celiac, alpha-1-antitrypsin, iron, copper, HepA IgG, HepB Sag, HepC SAb, anti–smooth muscle antibody, ANA, serum gammaglobulin (1)[B]
- Ultrasound (US) is the 1st-line imaging modality for assessment of liver chemistry abnormalities: fatty liver is hyperechoic on US. MRI/CT may also be used (1)[B].

Follow-Up Tests & Special Considerations

- Imaging modalities such as FibroScan (which detects tissue elasticity in cases of suspected hepatic fibrosis) and MR spectroscopy (to assess changes in hepatic fat) are currently being evaluated to help better characterize NAFLD (4)[B].
- No imaging modality can distinguish simple steatosis from steatohepatitis.

Diagnostic Procedures/Other

- Liver biopsy is the gold standard for diagnosis. Biopsy must have reasonable likelihood of changing management as a precondition to the procedure (1)[B].
- NAFLD fibrosis score age (>50 years), BMI (>30), platelet count, albumin, and AST/ALT ratio identifies patients at risk of developing fibrosis and/or cirrhosis (5)[B].

Test Interpretation

- Liver biopsy is the gold standard to differentiate fatty liver with good prognosis from NASH (1).
- In NASH, steatosis, ballooning, and lobular inflammation are minimal criteria for diagnosis. Other common findings include mild to moderate portal inflammation, acidophil bodies, perisinusoidal zone 3 fibrosis, megamitochondria, and Mallory-Denk bodies (hyaline) in hepatocytes (1).
- Staging is based largely on the extent of fibrosis. (1)

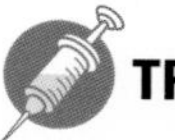

TREATMENT

- Sustained weight loss through lifestyle modification of at least 3–5% of body weight is most successful treatment (1,5)[A].
- Currently no effective medication treatment (1,5)[A].
- Foregut bariatric surgery not yet proven to specifically treat NASH (1)[B]

GENERAL MEASURES

- Aerobic exercise 3× weekly for 20–45 minutes with reduced calorie intake/diet modifications (1)[B]
- Tight control of diabetes (1,5)[B]
- Treatment of metabolic syndrome—hypertension, dyslipidemia, and obesity (1,5)[B]
- Limit alcohol consumption (<21 drinks/week for men and <14 drinks/week for women) (5)[A].
- Avoid hepatotoxic medications (1)[B].

MEDICATION

No specific therapy. Several promising agents include the following:

- Drugs that improve insulin resistance may decrease aminotransferase levels and histologic damage: thiazolidinediones (specifically pioglitazone) (1)[B].
- Vitamin E (800 IU/day) has shown improvement in treating hepatic steatosis and inflammation in nondiabetic NASH (1)[B].
- Other drugs studied in small studies (1,5)[B]:
  - Statins, but study excluded cases with AST and AST >1.5× normal limit
  - Gemfibrozil
  - Omega-3 fatty acids
  - Netaine
  - Angiotensin receptor blockers
  - Ursodeoxycholic acid, high dose in association with glitazones or vitamin E

ISSUES FOR REFERRAL

Persistent AST/ALT elevations 2–3× above upper limit of normal without diagnosis or those with fibrosis on biopsy benefit from hepatology evaluation (1)[A].

COMPLEMENTARY & ALTERNATIVE MEDICINE

Be wary of potential hepatotoxicity of complementary medications and dietary supplements.

SURGERY/OTHER PROCEDURES

Bariatric procedures: NAFLD is not a contraindication in otherwise eligible obese patients. There is a lack of data to definitively assess benefits and harms of surgery in treating patients with NASH (1)[B].

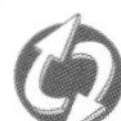

ONGOING CARE

FOLLOW-UP RECOMMENDATIONS

Patient Monitoring

- Annual monitoring of LFTs (1,5)[B]
- Consider surveillance monitoring with US or CT scan to evaluate disease progression/improvement (5)[B]. When seen, these improvements can provide major motivation to continue lifestyle changes.
- Routine liver biopsy is not recommended but may be repeated 5 years after baseline biopsy if fibrosis progression is suspected (1,5)[B].

DIET

Low in saturated and trans fat; low in simple carbohydrates; avoid alcohol (protective effect of light/moderate consumption still inconclusive).

PATIENT EDUCATION

Extensive counseling on sustained lifestyle changes in nutrition, exercise, and alcohol use.

PROGNOSIS

Within the spectrum of NALFD, only NASH has been shown to be progressive, potentially leading to cirrhosis, hepatocellular carcinoma, cholangiocarcinoma, and/or liver failure (6):

- Cirrhosis develops in up to 2–13% of patients with NASH within 5 years of diagnosis (6).
- Transplantation is effective, but NASH may recur after transplantation.

COMPLICATIONS

Progressive disease may lead to decompensated cirrhosis and portal hypertension with complications such as ascites, encephalopathy, bleeding varices, and hepatorenal or hepatopulmonary syndromes.

REFERENCES

1. Chalasani N, Younossi Z, Lavine JE, et al. The Diagnosis and management of non-alcoholic fatty liver disease: practice guideline by the American Gastroenterological Association, American Association for the Study of Liver Diseases, and American College of Gastroenterology. *Gastroenterology*. 2012;142(7):1592–1609.
2. Ahmed KT, Almashhrawi AA, Rahman RN, et al. Liver diseases in pregnancy: diseases unique to pregnancy. *World J Gastroenterol* 2013;19(43): 7638–7646.
3. Hurwitz ES, Nelson DB, Davis C, et al. National surveillance for Reye syndrome: a five-year review. *Pediatrics*. 1992;70(6):895–900.
4. Browning JD. New imaging techniques for nonalcoholic steatohepatitis. *Clin Liver Dis*. 2009;13(4): 607–619.
5. Nascimbeni F, Pais R, Bellentani S, et al. From NAFLD in clinical practice to answers from guidelines. *J Hepatol*. 2013;59(4):859–871.
6. White DL, Kanwal F, El-Serag HB. Association between nonalcoholic fatty liver disease and risk for hepatocellular cancer, based on systematic review. *Clin Gastroenterol Hepatol*. 2012;10(12): 1342–1359.

ADDITIONAL READING

- Edmison J, McCullough AJ. Pathogenesis of nonalcoholic steatohepatitis: human data. *Clin Liver Dis*. 2007;11(1):75–104, ix.
- Kleiner DE, Brunt EM. NAFLD: pathologic patterns and biopsy evaluation in clinical research. *Semin Liver Dis*. 2012;32(1):3–13.
- Schwimmer JB, Pardee PE, Lavine JE, et al. Cardiovascular risk factors and the metabolic syndrome in pediatric nonalcoholic fatty liver disease. *Circulation*. 2008;118(3):277–283.
- Thoma C, Day CP, Trenell MI. Lifestyle interventions for the treatment of non-alcoholic fatty liver disease in adults: a systematic review. *J Hepatol*. 2012;56(1):255–256.

SEE ALSO

Alcohol Abuse and Dependence; Cirrhosis of the Liver; Diabetes Mellitus, Type 2; Metabolic Syndrome

CODES

ICD10

- K76.0 Fatty (change of) liver, not elsewhere classified
- K75.81 Nonalcoholic steatohepatitis (NASH)

CLINICAL PEARLS

- NAFLD: major cause of liver disease. Spectrum ranges from NAFL to NASH, advanced fibrosis, and (rarely) progression to cirrhosis.
- NAFLD: most common chronic liver disease in children; parallel rise in childhood obesity and NAFLD
- Lifestyle changes with targeted weight loss are the cornerstones of therapy for NAFLD.
- NAFLD is a common cause of asymptomatic mild serum aminotransferase elevation.

NOSOCOMIAL INFECTIONS

Cheryl Durand, PharmD • Edward L. Yourtee, MD, FACP

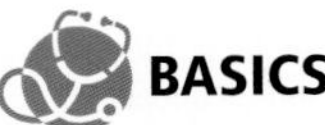

BASICS

DESCRIPTION

- Also known as health care–associated infections (HAIs)
- Infection must not have been present or incubating on admission to a health care facility.
- CDC categories:
  - Catheter-associated urinary tract infection (CAUTI)
  - Surgical site infection (SSI)
  - Ventilator-associated pneumonia (VAP)
  - Central line–associated bloodstream infection (CLABSI)
  - *Clostridium difficile* infection (C. diff, *C. difficile*, CDAD, CDI)
- The National Healthcare Safety Network (NHSN) at www.cdc.gov/nhsn monitors emerging HAI pathogens and their mechanisms of resistance to promote current prevention strategies.
- *Medicare and Medicaid will not pay for the treatment of certain HAI including CAUTIs, CLABSIs, and SSIs.*

EPIDEMIOLOGY

- General
  - 13/1,000 patient-days in the ICU (1)
  - 6.9/1,000 patient-days in high-risk nurseries
  - 2.6/1,000 patient-days in nurseries (1)
  - Estimated cost of HAIs is $20 billion per year (2).
- Infection specific
  - CAUTI
    - Hospital stay increased by 1–3 days.
    - Cost up to $600/infection
  - VAP
    - Hospital stay increased by 6 days.
    - Cost up to $5,000/infection
  - CLABSI
    - Hospital stay increased by 7–20 days.
    - Cost up to $56,000/infection
  - SSI
    - Hospital stay increased by 7.3 days.
    - Cost >$3,000/infection
    - May not be apparent until 1 month after surgery
  - *C. difficile* infection (see topic "*Clostridium difficile* Infection")

Incidence

- 1 out of 25 inpatients in the United States has at least one HAI (3).
  - 722,000 HAIs in U.S. acute care hospitals in 2011 (3)
  - UTI: 13% of HAIs (3)
  - Pneumonia: 22% of HAIs (3)
  - Bloodstream infection: 10% of HAIs (3)
  - SSI: 22% of HAIs (3)
  - Gastrointestinal infection: 17% HAIs (3)
- Infections caused by gram-negative rods resistant to almost all antibiotics are increasing. Up to 70% of nosocomial infections are resistant to at least one previously active antimicrobial.

ETIOLOGY AND PATHOPHYSIOLOGY

- Endogenous spread: Patient host flora causes invasive disease (most common).
- Exogenous spread: flora acquired from within health care facility
- Causative organisms:
- UTI: *Escherichia coli*, *Klebsiella* spp., *Serratia* spp., *Enterobacter*, *Pseudomonas aeruginosa*, *Enterococcus* spp., *Candida albicans* (3)
- Pneumonia: aerobic gram-negative bacilli, *Staphylococcus aureus*, *P. aeruginosa*, *Streptococcus* spp. (3)
  - Bloodstream infection: *Staphylococcus* spp., *Candida spp.*, *Enterococcus spp.*, gram-negative bacilli (3)
  - SSI: *Staphylococcus aureus*, gram-negative bacilli, *Enterococcus* spp., *Streptococcus* spp., *Enterobacter* spp., *Bacteroides* spp. (3)

RISK FACTORS

- Extremes of age
- Invasive surgical procedures (abdominal surgeries; orthopedic surgeries, urogynecologic surgeries; neurosurgery)
- Use of indwelling medical devices
- Chronic disease (including diabetes, renal failure, and malignancy)
- Immunodeficiency
- Malnutrition
- Medications (recent antibiotics, proton pump inhibitors, and sedatives)
- Colonization with pathogenic strains of flora
- Breakdown of mucosal/cutaneous barriers, including trauma and battle wounds
- Anesthesia

GENERAL PREVENTION

- Prevention should target both patient-specific and facility-related risk factors.
- Hand hygiene—thoroughly wash hands (4)[C]:
  - Upon entering and leaving any patient room (4)
  - After contact with blood, excretions, body fluids, wound dressings, nonintact skin, mucous membranes (4)
  - Before using and after removing gloves (gloves are permeable to bacteria)
  - When moving hands from contaminated to clean body site (4)
  - Alcohol-based products are satisfactory per se when hands are not visibly soiled (4).
  - Soap and water should be used when surfaces are visibly soiled or when contact with spores is anticipated.
- Antibiotic stewardship—appropriate selection of antimicrobial therapy includes the following:
  - Judicious use of antibiotics to reduce the emergence of multidrug-resistant organisms and the occurrence of *C. difficile* infection (2)
  - Use of narrow-spectrum early-generation antibiotics when possible
  - Taking an antibiotic "time out" at 72 hours to review the patient's clinical status and culture results and eliminate ("streamline") any redundant or unnecessary antibiotics
  - Use of shorter courses of antibiotics where appropriate
- Hospital-based surveillance programs and antibiograms
- Infection control programs with specially trained employees (4)[C]
- Employee education on HAIs (4)[C]
- Disinfection of hospital rooms with hydrogen peroxide vapor or UV irradiation in addition to standard cleaning reduces environmental contamination and the risk of infection with multidrug-resistant organisms.
- Minimize invasive procedures.
- Caregiver stethoscope cleaning:
  - Stethoscope bacterial contamination is common. Regular cleaning with alcohol-based preparations reduces bacterial load. Evidence is lacking to confirm whether stethoscope contamination causes nosocomial infections.
- Isolation of known pathogen carriers (4)[A]:
  - Contact precautions:
    - Institute for known pathogens spread by direct contact including methicillin-resistant *Staphylococcus aureus* (MRSA), vancomycin-resistant *Enterococcus* (VRE), *C. difficile*, extended-spectrum β-lactamase–producing gram-negative rods, and carbapenemase-producing gram-negative rods.
    - Glove when entering room (4)[B].
    - Gown if clothing will touch patient or environment (4)[B].
  - Droplet precautions:
    - Infectious particles measure >5 μm.
    - Institute for pathogens shed via talking, coughing, sneezing, mucosal shedding, airway suctioning, bronchoscopy. These include *Neisseria meningitidis*, influenza virus infection, *Haemophilus influenzae*, *Corynebacterium diphtheriae*, and *Bordetella pertussis*.
    - Mask when entering room (4)[B].
  - Airborne precautions:
    - Infectious particles measure <5 μm.
    - Institute for pathogens shed via coughing including tuberculosis, varicella-zoster virus, measles.
    - Fit-tested National Institute of Occupational Safety and Health (NIOSH)–approved ≥N-95 respirator on entering room (4)[B]
- Infection-specific measures:
  - CAUTI
    - Employee education on urinary catheters (indications, placement, maintenance)
    - Sterile catheter placement technique (5)[C]
    - Closed urine collection system (5)[C]
    - Use of catheter only for necessary duration, removing catheter as early as possible (5)[B]
    - Use of nurse-driven protocols for guideline-driven catheter removal
    - Do not confuse catheter-associated asymptomatic bacteriuria with CAUTI.
    - Do not screen for bacteriuria by routinely performing a urine culture when the catheter is withdrawn.
  - VAP
    - Intubation only when clinically necessary (6)[C]
    - Perform oral decontamination with oral chlorhexidine (7)[A].
    - Avoid nasotracheal intubation (6)[B].
    - Inline suctioning (6)[C]
    - Elevate patient's head to 30–45 degrees (6)[C].
  - CLABSI
    - Educate staff about appropriate use of IV catheters (indications, placement, maintenance) (8)[A]
    - Place catheters using sterile technique (including chlorhexidine prep and maximal barrier precautions) (8)[A].
    - Use order "bundles" to improve adherence to catheter insertion guidelines.
    - Promptly remove catheter when no longer clinically needed (8)[A].
    - Hand hygiene in addition to glove use (8)[A]
    - Regularly monitor catheter site (8)[A].

- SSI
  - Proper surgical hand hygiene (2)[B]
  - Prophylactic antibiotic therapy when indicated (2)[A]; eliminate underlying infections before surgery if possible (2)[A].
  - Remove hair with electric clippers/depilatory agent prior to incision (2)[B].
  - Poor postoperative blood sugar control increases risk of infection.
- *C. difficile* infection
  - Hand hygiene with soap and water (spores are resistant to alcohol-based products) (2)
  - Restrict use of fluoroquinolones, cephalosporins, and clindamycin when possible (2).
  - *C. difficile* is associated with the use of proton pump inhibitors: H_2 blockers preferred for acid suppression (9)[A].
  - Probiotics may reduce nonspecific antibiotic-associated diarrhea; the effectiveness of probiotics for prevention of *C. difficile* is unclear (9).
- Bloodstream infections
  - Use of chlorhexidine-impregnated washcloths to bathe ICU patients reduces bloodstream infections by 28% (10)[B].
  - Routine surveillance for systemic inflammatory response syndrome (SIRS) using established criteria

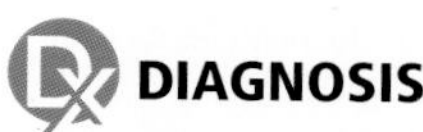

DIAGNOSIS

Consistent with nature of infection

HISTORY

- Exposure to health care facility
- Recent surgery/open wounds
- History of invasive procedure
  - Urinary catheter placement
  - Indwelling vascular catheter
- Recent intubation/mechanical ventilation
- History of past infections (MRSA, VRE, etc.)

PHYSICAL EXAM

Consistent with nature of infection; site-specific exam for infections of skin, catheter sites, wounds, signs of sepsis, or pneumonia

DIFFERENTIAL DIAGNOSIS

- Community-acquired infection
- Sepsis/SIRS
- Other causes of infectious diarrhea

DIAGNOSTIC TESTS & INTERPRETATION

Specific to condition:

- CBC, blood culture
- Wound culture
- Urine culture
- Chest x-ray

Test Interpretation

Consistent with underlying infection

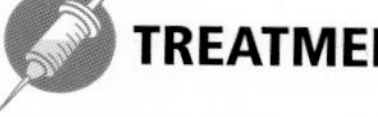

TREATMENT

GENERAL MEASURES

- Treat the underlying infection with appropriate antimicrobial selection.
- Protocol order bundles improves adherence to sepsis guidelines and improves survival.
- UTI: Remove urinary catheters.
- CLABSI: Remove IV catheter.
- *C. difficile*: Stop all antibiotics not being used to treat *C. difficile* infection.

MEDICATION

First Line

- Targeted antimicrobial therapy
- Several new agents recently approved for the treatment of antibiotic-resistant gram-positive infections:
  - Linezolid, daptomycin, telavancin, tigecycline, dalbavancin, ceftaroline

ISSUES FOR REFERRAL

- Failure to respond clinically to initial therapy
- Some emerging resistant gram-negative infections are resistant to nearly all antibiotics and require expert consultation for management.

SURGERY/OTHER PROCEDURES

- Screening for nasal carriage and isolation reduce the nosocomial spread of MRSA.
- Treating proven nasal carriers of *Staphylococcus* or MRSA with mupirocin prevents *S. aureus* nosocomial infections after surgery, as long as the prevalence of mupirocin resistance is low (11)[B].

INPATIENT CONSIDERATIONS

IV Fluids

As needed for hemodynamic support

Nursing

- Hand washing should be performed on entering and exiting the patient room even with no direct contact with the patient.
- Isolation precautions as indicated

Discharge Criteria

When infection has resolved or patient is stable and not an infectious risk

ONGOING CARE

FOLLOW-UP RECOMMENDATIONS

Patient Monitoring

Risk for recurrence is generally low in immunocompetent patients. Manage underlying comorbidities (risk factors).

PROGNOSIS

- 99,000 deaths in 2002 in the United States (1)
- Bloodstream infection mortality: 27%
- Pneumonia mortality: 33–50%
- SSI mortality: 11%

COMPLICATIONS

Related to specific nature of infection

REFERENCES

1. Klevens RM, Edwards JR, Richards CL Jr, et al. Estimating health care-associated infections and deaths in U.S. hospitals, 2002. *Public Health Rep*. 2007;122(2):160–166.
2. Yokoe DS, Mermel LA, Anderson DJ, et al. A compendium of strategies to prevent healthcare-associated infections in acute care hospitals. *Infect Control Hosp Epidemiol*. 2008;29(Suppl 1):S12–S21.
3. Magill SS, Edwards JR, Bamberg W, et al. Multistate point-prevalence survey of health-care associated infections. *N Engl J Med*. 2014;370(13):1198–1208.
4. Siegel JD, Rhinehart E, Jackson M, et al. 2007 guideline for isolation precautions: preventing transmission of infectious agents in health care settings. *Am J Infect Control*. 2007;35(10)(Suppl 2):S65–S164.
5. Hooton TM, Bradley SF, Cardenas DD, et al. Diagnosis, prevention, and treatment of catheter-associated urinary tract infection in adults: 2009 international clinical practice guidelines from the Infectious Disease Society of America. *Clin Infect Dis*. 2010;50(5):625–663.
6. Tablan OC, Anderson LJ, Besser R, et al. Guidelines for preventing health-care associated pneumonia, 2003: recommendations of CDC and the Healthcare Infection Control Practices Advisory Committee. *MMWR Recomm Rep*. 2004;53(RR-3):1–40.
7. Chan EY, Ruest A, Meade MO, et al. Oral decontamination for prevention of pneumonia in mechanically ventilated adults: systematic review and meta-analysis. *BMJ*. 2007;334(7599):889.
8. O' Grady NP, Alexander M, Burns LA, et al. Guidelines for the prevention of intravascular catheter-related Infections, 2011. www.cdc.gov/hicpac/BSI/01-BSI-guidelines-2011.html. Accessed June 28, 2011.
9. Surawicz CM, Brandt LJ, Binion DG, et al. Guidelines for diagnosis, treatment, and prevention of *Clostridium difficile* Infections. *Am J Gastroenterol*. 2013;108(4):478–498.
10. Climo MW, Yokoe DS, Warren DK, et al. Effect of daily chlorhexidine bathing on hospital-acquired infection. *N Engl J Med*. 2013;368(6):533–542.
11. van Rijen M, Bonten M, Wenzel R, et al. Mupirocin ointment for preventing *Staphylococcus aureus* infections in nasal carriers. *Cochrane Database Syst Rev*. 2009;(4):CD006216.

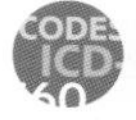

CODES

ICD10

- T83.51XA Infect/inflm reaction due to indwell urinary catheter, init
- T81.4XXA Infection following a procedure, initial encounter
- J95.851 Ventilator associated pneumonia

CLINICAL PEARLS

- Nosocomial infections increase mortality, length of hospital stay, and cost of hospitalization.
- Preventive efforts must address patient-specific and facility-related risk factors.
- Proper use of an alcohol-based hand product should be carried out before and after each patient encounter, even when gloves are used. Alcohol-based hand rubs are not effective for killing spores formed by *C. difficile*. Hand washing with soap and water after exposure to spores is the appropriate alternative.
- Contact, droplet, or airborne precautions should be used when appropriate to reduce the spread of infection.
- The risk of developing a resistant nosocomial infection can be reduced by antibiotic streamlining, use of narrow-spectrum antibiotics, and frequent patient reevaluation to ensure the necessity of continuing antibiotics.

NOVEL INFLUENZA A (H1N1; H7N9; H5N1)

Sumanth Gandra, MD, MPH

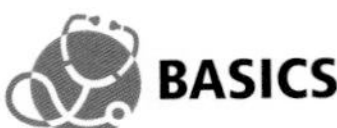

BASICS

DESCRIPTION

Novel influenza

- 2009 H1N1 virus, a novel influenza A virus originated from a reassortment of influenza viruses that circulated in North American and Eurasian pig herds.
- The 2009 H1N1 pandemic started in March 2009 in Mexico and then spread to many countries, including the United States.
- The pandemic was declared over in August 2010 by the World Health Organization (WHO) (1).
- Although the pandemic is over, 2009 H1N1 virus still exists and continues to cause disease.
- According to CDC, 2009 H1N1 accounted for 98% of 784 laboratory-confirmed seasonal influenza cases between December 2, 2013 and January 23, 2014 (2).
- Typically presents with influenza-like symptoms, but patients may be symptomatic with diarrhea and vomiting.
- Susceptible to neuraminidase inhibitors but resistant to adamantine antiviral agents
- Since 2009, several other novel influenza A strains have been reported (H7N9 and H5N1).
- 2009 H1N1 was the predominant influenza A strain during the 2013–2014 United States flu season.

EPIDEMIOLOGY

- The CDC estimates that between 43 million and 89 million cases of 2009 H1N1 occurred between April 2009 and April 2010 in the United States, including ~274,000 hospitalizations and 12,470 deaths.
- 90% of the reported cases were accounted for by patients younger than the age of 64 years.
- Predominant sex: male = female
- Affected mostly young people
- Older people protected by preexisting antibodies that cross-react with 2009 H1N1

ETIOLOGY AND PATHOPHYSIOLOGY

- 2009 H1N1 influenza was a quadruple reassortant strain with individual gene segments of the virus originating from humans, birds, North American pigs, and Eurasian pigs.
- Reservoirs included infected human and pig populations.

RISK FACTORS

- Similar to regular influenza transmission with respiratory secretions accounting for the primary mechanism of spread
- Close contact (<6 feet) with confirmed case increases the risk for spread of respiratory droplets.
- Risk factors for complications of or severe illness with 2009 H1N1 virus infection:
  - Age <5 or >65 years
  - Pregnancy
  - Morbid obesity
  - Chronic medical conditions (diabetes, chronic cardiovascular conditions, cirrhosis, end-stage renal disease [ESRD] on hemodialysis [HD])
  - Chronic lung disorders (chronic obstructive pulmonary disease [COPD], asthma, cystic fibrosis)
  - Immunosuppression (associated with HIV infection, organ transplantation, receipt of chemotherapy or corticosteroids, or malnutrition)
  - Immunoglobulin (Ig) G2 subclass deficiency
  - Sickle cell disease
  - Native Americans/Alaska Natives
  - Persons aged <19 years on long-term aspirin therapy
  - Residents of nursing homes and other chronic care facilities

GENERAL PREVENTION

- 2009 H1N1 vaccination, monovalent or trivalent: The 2011–2012, 2012–2013, and 2013-2014 seasonal influenza vaccines included 2009 H1N1 virus.
- CDC recommends 2009 H1N1 vaccine for all person ≥6 months.
- No safety concerns were identified with 2009 H1N1 vaccine among pregnant women, infants, and children.
- Observe hand hygiene and appropriate cough etiquette.
- Health care personnel must observe droplet precautions (surgical mask or N95 mask and protective goggles) in addition to contact precautions for patients presenting with symptoms of an influenza-like illness (fever with cough or sore throat).
- When leaving exam or hospital rooms, symptomatic patients should be outfitted with a surgical mask to contain their respiratory secretions.

DIAGNOSIS

HISTORY

- Incubation period: 1.5–3 days; may be up to 7 days
- Close contact with a suspected or confirmed case
- Clinical spectrum ranges from afebrile upper respiratory illness to fulminant viral pneumonia.
- Symptoms similar to regular seasonal influenza; most patients present with the following (3):
  - Fever
  - Sore throat
  - Cough
  - Myalgias
  - Nasal congestion
  - Rhinorrhea
- GI symptoms (more common than with seasonal influenza):
  - Nausea
  - Vomiting
  - Diarrhea
- Extrapulmonary complications include the following:
  - Hepatitis
  - Myocarditis
  - Rhabdomyolysis
  - Renal failure
  - Systemic or pulmonary vascular thrombosis
  - Reactive hemophagocytosis
  - In children, acute necrotizing encephalopathy or encephalopathy

DIFFERENTIAL DIAGNOSIS

- Seasonal influenza
- Respiratory viral infections from agents such as coronavirus, rhinovirus, and adenovirus
- Croup
- Pneumonia (typical and atypical)
- Infectious mononucleosis
- Pharyngitis (viral or streptococcal)
- HIV syndrome

DIAGNOSTIC TESTS & INTERPRETATION

- Rapid flu tests:
  - The rapid antigen test and direct fluorescent antibody (DFA) have low sensitivities to detect 2009 H1N1 (17.8% and 46.7%, respectively).
- Viral culture and polymerase chain reaction (PCR) test are highly sensitive (88.9% vs. 97.8%).
- Reverse transcription-polymerase chain reaction (RT-PCR; respiratory viral panel) is the test of choice (4,5)[A].

Initial Tests (lab, imaging)

- Routine testing often not necessary depending on patient's clinical presentation. If laboratory testing is ordered, consider CBC with differential, complete metabolic panel, and blood cultures.
- Chest x-ray (CXR): Among those hospitalized for 2009 H1N1 infection, 50% had infiltrates on CXR.

Test Interpretation

Most consistent histopathologic findings are varying degrees of diffuse alveolar damage with hyaline membranes and septal edema, tracheitis, and necrotizing bronchiolitis.

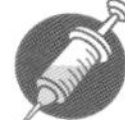

TREATMENT

- Most infections are self-limited and uncomplicated.
- Treatment for seasonal influenza with neuraminidase inhibitors is most effective when administered within 48 hours of symptom onset.
- Neuraminidase inhibitor treatment has been shown to reduce mortality in patients admitted to hospital with pandemic influenza (2009 H1N1) virus infection (6)[A]. Antiviral treatment is therefore recommended as soon as possible (even if patient presents >48 hours after illness onset) for all requiring hospitalization or to those who have progressive, complicated illness; and persons with suspected or confirmed 2009 H1N1 infection regardless of previous health or vaccination status.
- Hospitalized patients of all ages, organ transplant recipients, and pregnant women with 2009 H1N1 who were treated with oseltamivir had faster resolution of symptoms and a more rapid clearance of viral shedding.
- Delayed oseltamivir therapy in severe cases of 2009 H1N1 has been associated with worse outcomes.
- High-risk patients with confirmed or suspected 2009 H1N1 should also be treated with antiviral agents, preferably within 48 hours of symptom onset.

- Consider antiviral treatment for high-risk patients with persistent symptoms who have a positive 2009 H1N1 test result even if specimen was obtained >48 hours after symptom onset.

MEDICATION

- 2009 H1N1 is susceptible to the neuraminidase inhibitors oseltamivir (Tamiflu) and zanamivir (Relenza).
- Oseltamivir resistance is reported in <2% of strains tested globally, due to *H275Y* mutation. These strains remained susceptible to zanamivir.
- Genetic sequencing indicates increasing patterns of resistance to adamantine.

First Line

- Oseltamivir (5)[A]:
  - Adult dosage: 75 mg PO BID × 5 days
  - Pediatric dosage (safety and efficacy not established for children <1 year):
    - ≤15 kg: 30 mg PO BID × 5 days; 16–23 kg: 45 mg PO BID × 5 days; 24–40 kg: 60 mg PO BID × 5 days; >40 kg: 75 mg PO BID × 5 days
  - Infant dosage (<1 year old): 3 mg/kg PO BID × 5 days
  - Longer treatment courses can be considered for patients who are hospitalized and remain severely ill after 5 days of treatment.
  - Adverse effects:
    - Most common symptoms include nausea and vomiting, occurring in 9–10% of patients.
    - Neuropsychiatric events (e.g., hallucinations, delirium, and abnormal behavior) are rare symptoms.
    - Other rare symptoms include anaphylaxis and severe skin reactions such as Stevens-Johnson syndrome and toxic epidermal necrolysis.
  - Other considerations: metabolized by liver
  - Pregnancy class C medication
- Zanamivir (not recommended for patients with respiratory conditions such as COPD or asthma) (5)[A]:
  - Adult dosage: 10 mg (two 5-mg inhalations) BID × 5 days
  - Pediatric dosage: >7 years old: 10 mg (two 5-mg inhalations) BID × 5 days
  - Limited quantities of IV zanamivir were made available.
  - Adverse effects:
    - Most notably may cause bronchospasm, especially in patients with preexisting respiratory illnesses
    - Common adverse symptoms include headache, nausea, dizziness, and cough.
    - Rare symptoms are similar to those of oseltamivir, including neuropsychiatric symptoms, anaphylaxis, and severe skin reactions.
  - Other considerations: metabolized by liver
  - Pregnancy class C medication
- Peramivir:
  - FDA issued emergency use authorization (EUA) for peramivir, an investigational neuraminidase inhibitor for treatment of severely ill cases of confirmed or suspected cases of 2009 H1N1.
  - Administered IV
  - EUA for peramivir expired in June 2010

ADDITIONAL THERAPIES

- Broad-spectrum antibiotics as needed for treatment of bacterial coinfections
- In patients with 2009 H1N1 with acute respiratory distress syndrome (ARDS), extracorporeal membrane oxygenation may be necessary.

COMPLICATIONS

- ARDS
- Rapidly progressive pneumonia
- Respiratory failure
- Bacterial superinfection
- Encephalitis/encephalopathy
- Seizures

REFERENCES

1. World Health Organization. In focus: H1N1 now in the post-pandemic period. www.who.int/csr/disease/swineflu/en/index.html. Accessed August 10, 2010.
2. Flannery B, Thaker SN, Clippard J, et al; Centers for Disease Control and Prevention (CDC). Interim estimates of 2013-14 seasonal influenza vaccine effectiveness—United States, February 2014. *MMWR Morb Mortal Wkly Rep*. 2014;63(7):137–142.
3. Cheng VC, To KK, Tse H, et al. Two years after pandemic influenza A/2009/H1N1: what have we learned? *Clin Microbiol Rev*. 2012;25(2):223–263.
4. Ginocchio CC, Zhang F, Manji R, et al. Evaluation of multiple test methods for the detection of the novel 2009 influenza A (H1N1) during the New York City outbreak. *J Clin Virol*. 2009;45(3):191–195.
5. Fiore AE, Fry A, Shay D, et al. Antiviral agents for the treatment and chemoprophylaxis of influenza—recommendations of the Advisory Committee on Immunization Practices (ACIP). *MMWR Recomm Rep*. 2011;60(1):1–24.
6. Muthuri SG, Venkatesan S, Myles PR, et al; PRIDE Consortium Investigators. Effectiveness of neuraminidase inhibitors in reducing mortality in patients admitted to hospital with influenza A H1N1pdm09 virus infection: a meta-analysis of individual participant data. *Lancet Respir Med*. 2014;2(5):395–404.

ADDITIONAL READING

- Marshall HS, Collins J, Sullivan T, et al. Parental and societal support for adolescent immunization through school based immunization programs. *Vaccine*. 2013;31(30):3059–3064.
- Novel Swine-Origin Influenza A (H1N1) Virus Investigation Team, Dawood FS, Jain S, et al. Emergence of a novel swine-origin influenza A (H1N1) virus in humans. *N Engl J Med*. 2009;360(25):2605–2615.
- Tooher R, Collins JE, Street JM, et al. Community knowledge, behaviours and attitudes about the 2009 H1N1 influenza pandemic: a systematic review. *Influenza Other Respi Viruses*. 2013;7(6):1316–1327.

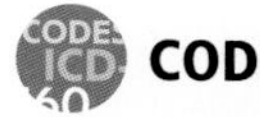

CODES

ICD10

- J09.X2 Flu due to ident novel influenza A virus w oth resp manifest
- J10.1 Flu due to oth ident influenza virus w oth resp manifest

CLINICAL PEARLS

- 2009 H1N1 pandemic started in March 2009 and was declared over in August 2010.
- Although the 2009–2010 pandemic is over, 2009 H1N1 virus still exists and is responsible for a majority of seasonal influenza cases during 2013–2014 in the United States. Most cases are self-limited and uncomplicated.
- Up to 25% of patients with 2009 H1N1 report vomiting and diarrhea in addition to fever, headache, sore throat, and cough.
- RT-PCR (respiratory viral panel) is the viral test of choice.
- 2009 H1N1 is susceptible to neuraminidase inhibitors (oseltamivir and zanamivir) but resistant to adamantine.

OBESITY

Maya Leventer-Roberts, MD, MPH

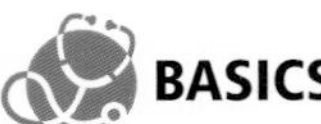

BASICS

DESCRIPTION

- Obesity is the state of excess adipose tissue. Weight status can be defined using the body mass index (BMI = body weight [kg]/[body height (m)]^2) and classified as underweight, normal weight, overweight, or obese:
  - For adults, a BMI ≥30 kg/m^2 is consistent with obesity.
- Obesity is associated with negative health outcomes (1), and the highest risk for increased morbidity and mortality is found in the context of abdominal obesity.
- System(s) affected: endocrine/metabolic, cardiac, respiratory, gastrointestinal, musculoskeletal, dermatologic, mental health
- Synonym(s): overweight; adiposity

Geriatric Considerations

BMI associated with the lowest risk of mortality increases as age increases.

EPIDEMIOLOGY

- Predominant age: Incidence rises in the early 20s.
- Predominant sex: female > male

Prevalence

- Mean prevalence of obesity among adults is 35% in the United States (2).
- Overweight: 40% of men and 25% of women
- Obese: 20% of men and 25% of women

Pediatric Considerations

- Pediatric obesity is categorized as ≥95th percentile, as established by CDC growth curves, by age and sex.
- Obesity during adolescence and young adulthood is strongly associated with obesity in adulthood.
- Risk factors include insufficient physical activity, consumption of sweetened beverages, and excess screen time.

ETIOLOGY AND PATHOPHYSIOLOGY

- Obesity is caused by an imbalance among food intake, absorption, and energy expenditure.
- Underlying organic causes may be psychiatric disturbances, hypothyroidism, hypothalamic disorders, insulinoma, and Cushing syndrome.
- Medications can contribute to obesity, including corticosteroids, neuroleptics (particularly atypical antipsychotics), and antidepressants

Genetics

- Genetic syndromes such as Prader-Willi and Bardet-Biedl are responsible for a minor percentage of people with obesity.
- Studies are insufficiently powered to isolate genes as predictors of obesity.

RISK FACTORS

- Parental obesity
- Sedentary lifestyle
- Consumption of calorie-dense food
- Low socioeconomic status
- >2 hours per day of television viewing

GENERAL PREVENTION

- Encourage at least 1 hour of daily exercise, limited television viewing, and moderation in portion size.
- Avoid calorie-dense and nutrient-poor foods such as sweetened beverages and processed foods.

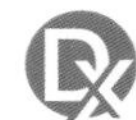

DIAGNOSIS

HISTORY

- Prior attempts at weight loss
- Reported readiness to change lifestyle
- Social support and resources
- Diet and exercise habits
- Associated risk factors: diabetes mellitus type 2, hypertension, hyperlipidemia, sleep apnea
- Psychiatric history
- Symptoms suggesting hypothyroidism, Cushing syndrome, genetic syndromes

PHYSICAL EXAM

Elevated BMI and excess adipose tissue

- BMI = body weight (kg)/body height (m^2):
  - Overweight: BMI = 25–29.9 kg/m^2
  - Obese: BMI ≥30 kg/m^2
- BMI obesity threshold by height

Height	BMI = 25 Weight (lb/kg)	BMI = 27 Weight (lb/kg)	BMI = 30 Weight (lb/kg)
5′0	128/58	138/63	153/70
5′2	136/61	147/67	164/74
5′4	145/66	157/71	174/79
5′6	155/70	167/76	186/84
5′8	164/74	177/81	197/89
5′10	174/79	188/85	209/95
6′0	184/83	199/90	221/100
6′2	194/88	210/95	233/106
6′4	205/92	221/101	246/112

- Fat distribution pattern
  - Abdominal obesity is assessed by measuring around the abdomen at the level of the umbilicus and defined as >40 inches (102 cm) for men and >35 inches (88 cm) for women.

DIAGNOSTIC TESTS & INTERPRETATION

- Yearly screening and laboratory assessment (3)[C]
- Screen for underlying physiologic causes as well as associated comorbid conditions.
- Labs should be done while fasting, although nonfasting labs within normal limits do not need to be repeated.
- Preserved glucose, total insulin, hemoglobin A1C
- Serum lipid panel
- Thyroid function tests
- LFTs
- Imaging interpretation
  - Hypertrophy and/or hyperplasia of adipocytes
  - Cardiomegaly
  - Hepatomegaly

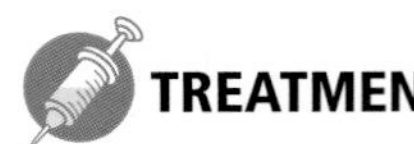

TREATMENT

GENERAL MEASURES

- Begin with the following assessment:
  - Degree of health risk from BMI and waist circumference (see "Diagnosis")
- Motivation to lose weight (4)[A]
  - Patient-specific goals of therapy
  - Referral for intensive counseling for diet, exercise, and behavior modification
  - Long-term follow-up
- Goal for therapy is to achieve and sustain long-term weight loss up of at least 10% of body weight.
- Tracking of caloric intake and exercise
- Goal is to limit total calories.
- Behavior therapy and cognitive-behavioral methods can result in modest weight loss but are most effective when combined with dietary and exercise treatments.
- Use of commercial weight loss programs (e.g., Weight Watchers) can be more effective than "standard of care" counseling (5)[B].

MEDICATION

- National Institute of Health guidelines suggest nonpharmacologic treatment for at least 6 months (4)[C].
- Medication treatment may be initiated for unsatisfactory weight loss in those with a BMI ≥30 or with a BMI ≥27 combined with associated risk factors (e.g., coronary artery disease, diabetes, sleep apnea, hypertension, hyperlipidemia).
- Diet, exercise, and behavior therapy *must* be included with pharmacologic treatment for those without comorbid conditions.
- Relapse may occur after discontinuation of drug.

First Line

- Medications may produce modest weight loss (6)[B].
- The lipase inhibitor orlistat (Xenical) decreases the absorption of dietary fat. Dose: 120 mg PO TID with meals containing fat; omit dose if meal is skipped or does not contain fat. Patients must avoid taking fat-soluble vitamin supplements within 2 hours of taking orlistat. The FDA has approved orlistat (Alli) 60 mg PO TID to be sold over the counter as a weight loss aid (7)[B]; adverse effects mainly GI (cramps, flatus, fecal incontinence)
- Contraindications
  - Orlistat: chronic malabsorption syndromes, cholestasis, pregnancy

Second Line

- Appetite suppressants recommended for short-term treatment (≤6 months) (8)[A]
- Only beneficial in patients who exercise and eat reduced calorie diet
  - Naltrexone/bupropion (Contrave): 8 mg naltrexone/90 mg bupropion per tablet; slow titration up to 2 tablets PO BID by week 4; contraindicated if uncontrolled HTN, seizure disorder, chronic opioid use, pregnancy
  - Liraglutide (Saxenda): 1.203 mg SQ once daily; GLP-1 agonist recently approved for obesity; discontinue if weight loss is <4% after 16 weeks

– Topiramate: initiate with 25 mg BID and increase by 50 mg/week up to 100 mg PO BID; not FDA approved for the treatment of obesity, but effective; tolerance is a concern (paresthesias, somnolence, difficulty concentrating)

- Schedule IV drugs
  – Lorcaserin (Belviq) 10 mg PO BID (D/C if weight loss is <5% after 12 weeks); works as serotonin agonist; avoid in those with CrCl <30 mL/min; contraindicated in pregnancy; avoid use with other serotonergic drugs
  – Phentermine: 15, 30, 37.5 mg PO every morning; discontinue if tolerance or no response after 4 weeks; contraindicated if history of CV disease, hyperthyroidism, history of substance abuse, pregnancy
  – Phentermine/topiramate (3.75–23 mg, 7.5–46 mg, 11.25–69 mg, 15–92 mg); initiate 3.75–23 mg PO once daily; requires enrollment into Risk Evaluation and Mitigation Strategy (REMS); women of child-bearing age require negative pregnancy test prior to initiation and monthly thereafter
  – Diethylpropion: 25 mg PO before meals TID; discontinue if no response after 4 weeks. Contraindicated if severe HTN, hyperthyroidism, history of substance abuse

Pregnancy Considerations

During pregnancy, obese women should gain fewer pounds than recommended for nonobese women.

SURGERY/OTHER PROCEDURES

Patients meeting criteria should be evaluated for gastric bypass or lap band procedures (9)[C].

- Requires complex presurgical evaluation, surgery, and follow-up in a skilled treatment center
- Surgical treatment is the most effective long-term weight-loss treatment available for morbidly obese patients, but there is insufficient evidence on long-term outcomes (10)[A].

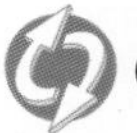

ONGOING CARE

FOLLOW-UP RECOMMENDATIONS

- Exercise is an integral part of any weight loss program, yet exercise alone rarely results in significant weight loss.
- Combination of weight training and aerobic activity is preferred over aerobic activity alone.

Patient Monitoring

Long-term routine follow-up may prevent relapse after weight loss or further weight gain.

DIET

- Long-term studies suggest net calorie reduction of 500–1,000 kcal/day and ease of use are more important than the diet composition for long-term results (11)[A]:
  – A reduction of 500 kcal/day intake can result in ~1 lb (0.45 kg) weight loss per week.
  – Portion-controlled servings are recommended.
- Very low-calorie diet (400–800 kcal/day consumption)
  – Can result in more rapid weight loss than higher calorie diets but are less effective in the long term
  – Complications can include dehydration, orthostatic hypotension, fatigue, muscle cramps, constipation, headache, cold intolerance, and relapse after discontinuation.
  – Contraindications: recent myocardial infarction or cerebrovascular accident, renal disease, cancer, pregnancy, insulin-dependent diabetes mellitus, and some psychiatric disturbances

PATIENT EDUCATION

- Emphasize the value of a healthy BMI.
- Recommended Web site:
  – www.nal.usda.gov/fnic/foodcomp/search for the FDA nutritional content in common foods

PROGNOSIS

- Lowest mortality associated with a BMI of 22
- Long-term maintenance of weight loss is extremely difficult.
- A motivated patient is most likely to achieve successful weight loss.

COMPLICATIONS

- Cardiovascular disease
- Stroke (in men)
- Thromboembolism
- Heart failure
- Hypertension
- Hypoventilation and sleep apnea syndromes
- Higher death rates from cancer: colon, breast, prostate, endometrial, gallbladder, liver, kidney
- Diabetes mellitus
- Skin changes
- Hyperlipidemia
- Gallbladder disease
- Osteoarthritis
- Gout
- Poor self-esteem
- Discrimination
- Increased sick leave

REFERENCES

1. Flegal K, Graubard B, Williamson D, et al. Excess deaths associated with underweight, overweight, and obesity. *JAMA*. 2005;293(15):1861–1867.
2. Ogden CL, Carroll MD, Flegal KM. Prevalence of obesity in the United States. *JAMA*. 2014;312(2): 189–190. doi:10.1001/jama.2014.6228.
3. National Heart, Lung and Blood Institute, National Institutes of Health, U.S. Department of Health and Human Services. *Clinical Guidelines on the Identification, Evaluation, and Treatment of Overweight and Obesity in Adults: The Evidence Report*. Bethesda, MD: National Institutes of Health; 1998. NIH publication 98-4083.
4. Shaw K, O'Rourke P, Del Mar C, et al. Psychological interventions for overweight or obesity. *Cochrane Database Syst Rev*. 2005;(2):CD003818.
5. Jebb SA, Ahern AL, Olson AD, et al. Primary care referral to a commercial provider for weight loss treatment versus standard care: a randomised controlled trial. *Lancet*. 2011;378(9801): 1485–1492.
6. Padwal R, Li SK, Lau DCW. Long-term pharmacotherapy for obesity and overweight (Cochrane Review). *Cochrane Library*. Issue 4. Chichester, UK: Wiley & Sons; 2005.
7. Kramer CK, Leitão CB, Pinto LC, et al. Efficacy and safety of topiramate on weight loss: a meta-analysis of randomized controlled trials. *Obes Rev*. 2011;12(8):e338–e347.
8. Dombrowski SU, Knittle K, Avenell A, et al. Long term maintenance of weight loss with non-surgical interventions in obese adults: systematic review and meta-analyses of randomised controlled trials. *BMJ*. 2014;348:g2646. doi:10.1136/bmj.g2646.
9. Colquitt J, Clegg A, Loveman E, et al. Surgery for morbid obesity. *Cochrane Database Syst Rev*. 2005;(4):CD003641.
10. Puzziferri N, Roshek TB III, Mayo HG, et al. Long-term follow-up after bariatric surgery: a systematic review. *JAMA*. 2014;312(9):934–942. doi:10.1001/jama.2014.10706.
11. Thomas DE, Elliott EJ, Baur L. Low glycaemic index or low glycaemic load diets for overweight and obesity. *Cochrane Database Syst Rev*. 2007;(3):CD005105.

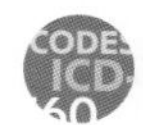

CODES

ICD10

- E66.9 Obesity, unspecified
- E66.3 Overweight
- R63.5 Abnormal weight gain

CLINICAL PEARLS

- Drug treatment with a 1st-line medication may be indicated when nonpharmacologic treatment for 6 months has been ineffective and the patient has a BMI >30 or a BMI >27 with associated risk factors. Medications produce (at most) a modest long-term weight loss.
- Surgical treatment may be indicated in patients with a BMI >40 who have failed more conservative treatment, particularly when there are associated risk factors, such as diabetes mellitus.
- No convincing evidence indicates that any specific diet is more effective than any other diet of equivalent caloric content.

OBSESSIVE-COMPULSIVE DISORDER (OCD)

Anila Khaliq, MD • Mahpara Khaliq, MD • Komel Khaliq, MBBS

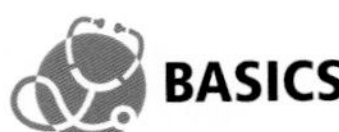

BASICS

DESCRIPTION

- A psychiatric condition classified as an anxiety disorder characterized by obsessions (recurrent intrusive thoughts, ideas, or images) and compulsions (repetitive, ritualistic behaviors or mental acts) causing significant patient distress
- Not to be confused with obsessive-compulsive personality disorder

EPIDEMIOLOGY

Incidence

- Predominant age: mean age of onset 22–36 years
  - Male = female (males present at younger age)
  - Child/adolescent onset in 33% of cases
  - 1/3 of cases present by age 15 years
  - 85% of cases present at <35 years of age
  - Diagnosis rarely made at >50 years of age
- Predominant gender: male > female (3:1)

Pediatric Considerations

Insidious onset; consider brain insult in acute presentation of childhood obsessive-compulsive disorder (OCD).

Geriatric Considerations

Consider neurologic disorders in new-onset OCD in the elderly.

Prevalence

- 2.3% lifetime in adults
- 1–2.3% prevalence in children/adolescents

ETIOLOGY AND PATHOPHYSIOLOGY

- Exact pathophysiology unknown
- Dysregulation of serotonergic pathways
- Dysregulation of corticostriatal-thalamic-cortico (CSTC) pathway
- Exact etiology unknown
- Genetic and environmental factors
- Pediatric autoimmune disorder associated with streptococcal infections

Genetics

- Greater concordance in monozygotic twins
- Positive family history: prevalence rates of 7–15% in 1st-degree relatives of children/adolescents with OCD

RISK FACTORS

- Exact cause of OCD is not fully elucidated.
- Combination of biologic and environmental factors likely involved the following:
  - Link between low serotonin levels and development of OCD
  - Link between brain insult and development of OCD (i.e., encephalitis, pediatric streptococcal infection, or head injury)

GENERAL PREVENTION

- OCD cannot be prevented.
- Early diagnosis and treatment can decrease patient's distress and impairment.

COMMONLY ASSOCIATED CONDITIONS

- Major depressive disorder
- Panic disorder
- Phobia/social phobia
- Tourette syndrome
- Substance abuse
- Eating disorder/body dysmorphic disorder

DIAGNOSIS

HISTORY

- Patient presents with either obsessions or compulsions, which cause marked distress, are time-consuming (>1 hr/day), and cause significant occupational/social impairment.
- 4 criteria support diagnosis of obsessions:
  - Patients are aware that they are thinking the obsessive thoughts; thoughts are not imposed from outside (as in thought insertion).
  - Thoughts are not just excessive worrying about real-life problems.
  - Recurrent thoughts are persistent, intrusive, and inappropriate, causing significant anxiety and distress.
  - Attempts to suppress intrusive thoughts are made with some other thought/activity.
- 2 criteria support a diagnosis of compulsions:
  - The response to an obsession is to perform repetitive behaviors (e.g., hand washing) or mental acts (e.g., counting silently) rigidly.
  - Although done to reduce stress, the responses are either not realistically connected with the obsession or they are excessive.
  - In children, check for precedent streptococcal infection.

PHYSICAL EXAM

- Dermatologic problems caused by excessive hand washing may be observed.
- Hair loss caused by compulsive pulling/twisting of the hair (trichotillomania) may be observed.

DIFFERENTIAL DIAGNOSIS

- Obsessive-compulsive personality disorder
  - In personality disorder, traits are ego-syntonic and include perfectionism and preoccupation with detail, trivia, or procedure and regulation. Patients tend to be rigid, moralistic, and stingy. These traits are often rewarded in the patient's job as desirable.
- Impulse-control disorders: compulsive gambling, sex, or substance abuse: The compulsive behavior is not in response to obsessive thoughts, and the patient derives pleasure from the activity.
- Major depressive disorder
- Eating disorder
- Tics (in tic disorder) and stereotyped movements
- Schizophrenia: Patient perceives thought to be true and coming from an external source.
- Generalized anxiety disorder, phobic disorders, separation anxiety: similar response on heightened anxiety, but presence of obsessions and rituals signifies OCD diagnosis
- Anxiety disorder due to a general medical condition: Obsessions/compulsions are assessed to be a direct physiologic consequence of a general medical condition.

DIAGNOSTIC TESTS & INTERPRETATION

According to *DSM-5*, diagnostic criteria for OCD are (1)[C]:

- Presence of obsessions, compulsions, or both
  - Recurrent or persistent thoughts, urges, or images that are experienced at sometime during the disturbance, as intrusive and unwanted, and that in most individuals cause marked anxiety or distress
  - The individual attempts to ignore or suppress such thoughts, urges, or images or to neutralize them with some other thought or actions (i.e., by performing compulsion).

Compulsions are defined by the following:

- Repetitive behavior (e.g., hand washing, ordering, checking) or mental acts (e.g., praying, counting, repeating words silently) that the individual feels driven to perform in response to an obsession or according to rules that must be applied rigidly.
- The behavior or mental acts are aimed at preventing or reducing anxiety or distress or preventing some dreaded event or situation. However, these behavior or mental acts are not connected in a realistic way with what they are designed to neutralize or prevent or are clearly excessive.
- The obsessions or compulsions are time-consuming (e.g., take more than 1 hour per day) or cause clinically significant distress or impairment in social, occupational, or other important areas of functioning.
- The obsessive-compulsive symptoms are not attributable to the physiologic effects of a substance (e.g., a drug of abuse, a medication, or other medical condition).
- The disturbance is not better explained by the symptoms of another mental disorder (e.g., excessive worries, as in generalized anxiety disorder, preoccupation with appearance, as in body dysmorphic disorder, etc.)
- Specify if:
  - With good or fair insight: The individual recognizes the OCD beliefs are definitely or probably not true or that they may or may not be true.
  - With poor insight: The individual thinks that OCD beliefs are probably true.
  - With absent insight/delusional beliefs: The individual is completely convinced that OCD beliefs are true.
- Specify if:
  - Tic related: The individual has a current or past history of tic disorder.

Diagnostic Procedures/Other

- Yale-Brown Obsessive-Compulsive Scale (Y-BOCS) or CY-BOCS for children (2)[C]
- Maudsley Obsessive-Compulsive Inventory (MOCI) (3)[C]

Test Interpretation

- Compulsions are designed to relieve the anxiety of obsessions; they are not inherently enjoyable (egodynastic) and do not result in completion of a task.
- Common obsessive themes
  - Harm (i.e., being responsible for an accident)
  - Doubt (i.e., whether doors/windows are locked or the iron is turned off)
  - Blasphemous thoughts (i.e., in a devoutly religious person)
  - Contamination, dirt, or disease
  - Symmetry/orderliness
- Common rituals or compulsions
  - Hand washing, cleaning
  - Checking
  - Counting
  - Hoarding
  - Ordering, arranging
  - Repeating
- Neither obsessions nor compulsions are related to another mental disorder (i.e., thoughts of food and presence of eating disorder).
- 80–90% of patients with OCD have obsessions and compulsions.
- 10–19% of patients with OCD are pure obsessional.

TREATMENT

GENERAL MEASURES

- Combined medications and cognitive-behavioral therapy (CBT) is most effective (1,2)[A].
- Family psychoeducation
- Parent behavior management training if patient is a child/adolescent

MEDICATION

First Line

- Adequate trial at least 10–12 weeks
- Doses may exceed typical doses for depression.
- SSRIs recommended 1st-line agents (4,5)[A]
  - Fluoxetine (Prozac)
    - Adults: 20 mg/day; increase by 10–20 mg every 4–6 weeks until response; range: 20–80 mg/day
    - Children (7–17 years of age): 10 mg/day; increase 4–6 weeks until response; range: 20–60 mg/day
- Sertraline (Zoloft)
  - Adults: 50 mg/day; increase by 50 mg every 4–7 days until response; range: 50–200 mg/day; may divide if above 100 mg/day
  - Children (6–17 years of age): 25 mg/day; increase by 25 mg every 7 days until response; range: 50–200 mg/day
- Paroxetine (Paxil)
  - Adults: 20 mg/day; increase by 10 mg every 4–7 days until response; range: 40–60 mg/day
  - Children: Safety and effectiveness in patients <18 years have not been established.
- Fluvoxamine (Luvox)
  - Adult: 100 mg/day; increase by 50 mg every 4–7 days until response; range: 200–300 mg/day
  - Children (8–17 years of age): 25 mg/day; increase by 25 mg every 4–7 days until response; range: 50–200 mg/day
- Absolute SSRI contraindications
  - Hypersensitivity to SSRIs
  - Concomitant use within 14 days of monoamine oxidase inhibitor (MAOI)
- Relative SSRI contraindications
  - Severe liver impairment
  - Seizure disorders (lower seizure threshold)
- Precautions
  - Watch for suicidal behavior/worsening depression during 1st few months of therapy/after dosage changes with antidepressants, particularly in children, adolescents, and young adults.
  - Long half-life of fluoxetine (>7 days) may be troublesome if patient has an adverse reaction.
  - May cause drowsiness and dizziness when therapy initiated; warn patients about driving and heavy-equipment hazards.

Pregnancy Considerations

All SSRIs are pregnancy Category C, except paroxetine, which is Category D.

Second Line

- Try switching to another SSRI.
- Tricyclic acid (TCA), clomipramine (Anafranil)
  - Adults: 25 mg/day; increase gradually over 2 weeks to 100 mg/day, then to 250 mg/day (max dose) over next several weeks, as tolerated.
  - Children (10–17 years of age): 25 mg/day; titrate as needed and tolerated up to 3 mg/kg/day or 200 mg/day (whichever is less).
  - Absolute clomipramine contraindications
    - Within 6 months of a myocardial infarction (MI)
    - Hypersensitivity to clomipramine or other TCA
    - Concomitant use within 14 days of an MAOI
    - 3rd-degree atrioventricular (AV) block
  - Relative clomipramine contraindications
    - Narrow-angle glaucoma (increased intraocular pressure)
    - Prostatic hypertrophy (urinary retention)
    - 1st- or 2nd-degree AV block, bundle-branch block, and congestive heart failure (proarrhythmic effect)
    - Pregnancy Category C
  - Precautions
    - Dangerous in overdose
    - Pretreatment ECG for patients >40 years of age
    - Watch for suicidal behavior/worsening depression during 1st few months of therapy or after dosage changes with antidepressants, particularly in children, adolescents, and young adults.
    - May cause drowsiness and dizziness when therapy is initiated; warn patients about driving and heavy equipment hazards.

ISSUES FOR REFERRAL

- Psychiatric referral for CBT (in vivo exposure and prevention of compulsions)
- Psychiatric evaluation if obsessions and compulsions significantly interfere with patient's functioning in social, occupational, or educational situations

ADDITIONAL THERAPIES

Dopamine receptor antagonists (antipsychotic agents) alone are not effective in treatment of OCD. They can be used as augmentation to SSRI therapy for treatment-resistant OCD; they also can worsen OCD symptoms (5)[C]. Some evidence show that addition of quetiapine or risperidone to antidepressants will increase efficacy; data with olanzapine too limited to draw conclusions (6)[A].

- Haloperidol (Haldol): initial dose: 0.5 mg/day; target dose: 0.5–6 mg/day
- Risperidone (Risperdal): initial dose: 0.5 mg/day; target dose: 0.5–2 mg/day
- Olanzapine (Zyprexa): initial dose: 1.25 mg/day; target dose: 1.25–30 mg/day
- Quetiapine (Seroquel): initial dose: 25 mg/day; target dose: 600 mg/day

ONGOING CARE

FOLLOW-UP RECOMMENDATIONS

Y-BCOS or MOCI surveys to track progress

Patient Monitoring

Monitor for decrease in obsessions and time spent performing compulsions.

DIET

No dietary modifications/restrictions recommended

PATIENT EDUCATION

- Importance of medication adherence
- Importance of psychotherapy (CBT)
- International OCD Foundation, Boston, MA 617-973-5801; http://www.ocfoundation.org
- Obsessive Compulsive Anonymous, New Hyde Park, NY http://obsessivecompulsiveanonymous.org

PROGNOSIS

- Chronic waxing and waning course in most patients:
  - 24–33% fluctuating course
  - 11–14% phasic periods of remission
  - 54–61% chronic progressive course
- Early onset a poor predictor

COMPLICATIONS

- Depression in 1/3 patients with OCD
- Avoidant behavior (phobic avoidance)
  - Children may drop out of education.
  - Adults may become homebound.
- Anxiety and panic-like episodes associated with obsessions

REFERENCES

1. American Psychiatric Association. *Diagnostic and Statistical Manual of Mental Disorders*. 5th ed. Washington, DC: American Psychiatric Association.
2. http://www.cnsforum.com
3. S ánchez-Meca J, Lopez-Pina JA, Lopez-Lopez JA, et al. The Maudsley Obsessive-Compulsive Inventory. *Int J Clin Health Psychol*. 2011;11(3):473–493.
4. Gava I, Barbui C, Aguglia E, et al. Psychological treatments versus treatment as usual for obsessive compulsive disorder (OCD). *Cochrane Database Sys Rev*. 2007;(2):CD005333.
5. Stein DJ, Denys D, Gloster AT, et al. Obsessive-compulsive disorder: diagnostic and treatment issues. *Psychiatr Clin North Am*. 2009;32(3):665–685.
6. Komossa K, Depping AM, Meyer M, et al. Second-generation antipsychotics for obsessive compulsive disorder. *Cochrane Database Sys Rev*. 2010;(12):CD008141.

ADDITIONAL READING

- Koran LM, Hanna GL, Hollander E, et al. Practice guideline for the treatment of patients with obsessive-compulsive disorder. *Am J Psychiatry*. 2007; 164(7 Suppl):5–53.
- Kurlan R, Kaplan EL. The pediatric autoimmune neuropsychiatric disorders associated with streptococcal infection (PANDAS) etiology for tics and obsessive-compulsive symptoms: hypothesis or entity? Practical considerations for the clinician. *Pediatrics*. 2004;113(4):883–886.
- Nestadt G, Grados M, Samuels JF. Genetics of obsessive-compulsive disorder. *Psychiatr Clin North Am*. 2010;33(1):141–158.

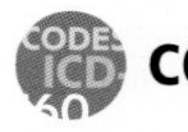

CODES

ICD10

- F42 Obsessive-compulsive disorder
- F63.9 Impulse disorder, unspecified
- F63.3 Trichotillomania

CLINICAL PEARLS

- CBT is the initial treatment of choice for mild OCD.
- CBT plus an SSRI or an SSRI alone is the treatment choice for more severe OCD.
- >65–70% of patients with OCD respond to 1st SSRI treatment.
- Improvement in symptoms is often incomplete, ranging from 25 to 60%.

OCULAR CHEMICAL BURNS

Robert J. Hyde, MD, MA

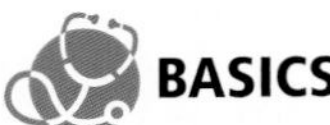

BASICS

DESCRIPTION

- Chemical exposure to the eye can result in rapid, devastating, and permanent damage and is one of the true emergencies in ophthalmology.
- Separate alkaline from acid chemical exposure
  - Alkali burns: more severe. Alkaline compounds are lipophilic, penetrating rapidly into eye tissue; saponification of cells leads to necrosis and may produce injury to lids, conjunctiva, cornea, sclera, iris, and lens (cataracts).
  - Acid burns: Acid usually does not damage internal structures because its associated anion causes protein denaturation, creating a barrier to further acid penetration. (Hydrofluoric acid is an exception to this rule; see below.) Injury is often limited to lids, conjunctiva, and cornea.
- System(s) affected: nervous; skin/exocrine
- Synonym(s): chemical ocular injuries

EPIDEMIOLOGY

- Predominant age: can occur at any age, peak from 16 to 25 years of age
- Predominant sex: male > female

Incidence

- Estimated 300/100,000 per year
- Alkali burns twice as common as acid burns

ETIOLOGY AND PATHOPHYSIOLOGY

- Acidic compounds
  - Anion leads to protein denaturing and protective barrier formation by coagulation necrosis forming an eschar. This more superficial mechanism of injury tends to have prominent scarring that may lead to vision loss:
    - Hydrofluoric acid is an exception. In its nonionized form, it behaves like an alkaline substance, capable of penetrating the corneal stroma and leading to extensive anterior segment lesions. When ionized, it may combine with intracellular calcium and magnesium to form insoluble complexes, leading to potassium ion movements and cell death. Once systemically absorbed, severe hypocalcemia can occur.
- Alkaline compounds
  - Lipophilic compounds that penetrate into deep structures on disassociation into cations and OH^-
  - OH^- causes saponification of fatty acids in cell membranes, leading to cell death.
  - Cation causes hydration of glycosaminoglycans, leading to corneal opacification and hydration of collagen, resulting in rapid shortening and thickening of collagen fibrils that leads to elevated intraocular pressure secondary to distortion of trabecular meshwork.
  - Penetration into deep structures may also affect perfusing vessels, leading to ischemia of affected area.

Sources of alkaline and acidic compounds

Alkaline compounds	**Typical sources**
Calcium hydroxide (lime)	Cement, whitewash
Sodium hydroxide (lye)	Drain cleaner, airbags
Potassium hydroxide (lye)	Drain cleaner
Ammonia	Cleaning agents
Ammonium hydroxide	Fertilizers
Acidic compounds	**Typical sources**
Sulfuric acid	Car batteries
Sulfurous acid	Bleach
Hydrochloric acid	Chem labs, swimming pools
Acetic acid	Vinegar
Hydrofluoric acid	Glass polish

RISK FACTORS

- Construction work (plaster, cement, whitewash)
- Use of cleaning agents (drain cleaners, ammonia)
- Automobile battery explosions (sulfuric acid)
- Industrial work (many possible agents)
- Alcoholism
- Any risk factor for assault (~10% of injuries due to deliberate assault)

GENERAL PREVENTION

Safety glasses to safeguard eyes

COMMONLY ASSOCIATED CONDITIONS

Facial (including eyelids) cutaneous chemical or thermal burns

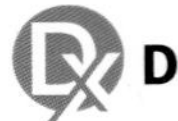

DIAGNOSIS

HISTORY

- Most often complaints of pain, photophobia, blurred vision, and a foreign body sensation
- In alkali burns, can have initial pain that later diminishes
- Mild burns: pain and blurred vision
- Moderate to severe burns: severe pain and markedly reduced vision

PHYSICAL EXAM

- Acidic compound may present with a ground-glass appearance secondary to superficial scar formation.
- Alkaline compounds may present with corneal opacification secondary to glycosaminoglycan hydration; however, severe acid burns may also present with this finding.
- Mild burns
  - Blurry vision
  - Eyelid skin erythema and edema
  - Corneal epithelial defects or superficial punctate keratitis
  - Conjunctival chemosis, hyperemia, and hemorrhages without perilimbal ischemia
  - Mild anterior chamber reaction
- Moderate to severe burns
  - Reduced vision
  - 2nd- and 3rd-degree burns of eyelid skin
  - Corneal edema and opacification
  - Corneal epithelial defects
  - Marked conjunctival chemosis and perilimbal blanching
  - Moderate anterior chamber reaction
  - Increased intraocular pressure
  - Local necrotic retinopathy

DIFFERENTIAL DIAGNOSIS

- Thermal burns
- Ocular cicatricial pemphigoid
- Other causes of corneal opacification
- Ultraviolet radiation keratitis

DIAGNOSTIC TESTS & INTERPRETATION

Not necessary unless suspicion of intraocular or orbital foreign body is present. In this case, CT should be used and MRI is contraindicated.

Diagnostic Procedures/Other

- Measure pH of tear film with litmus paper or electronic probe:
  - Irrigating fluid with nonneutral pH (e.g., normal saline has pH of 4.5) may alter results.
- Careful slit-lamp exam, fundus ophthalmoscopy, tonometry, and measurement of visual acuity
- Full extent of damage from alkali burns may not be apparent until 48–72 hours after exposure.

Test Interpretation

- Corneal epithelial defects or superficial punctate keratitis, edema, opacification
- Conjunctival chemosis, hyperemia, and hemorrhages
- Perilimbal ischemia
- Anterior chamber reaction
- Increased intraocular pressure

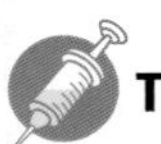

TREATMENT

Copious irrigation and removal of corneal or conjunctival foreign bodies are always the initial treatment (1,2,3)[A]:

- Passively open patient's eyelid and have patient look in all directions while irrigating.
- Be sure to remove all reservoirs of chemical from the eyes.
- Continue irrigation until the tear film and superior/inferior cul-de-sac is of neutral pH (7 ± 0.1) and pH is stable (2)[C]:
  - Severe burns should be irrigated for at least 15 minutes to as much as 2–4 hours; this irrigation should not be interrupted during transportation to hospital (2)[C].
  - Irrigation via Morgan lens (polymethylmethacrylate scleral lens) is a good way to achieve continuous irrigation over a prolonged period of time.
  - It is impossible to overirrigate.
- Initial pH testing should be done on both eyes even if the patient claims to only have unilateral ocular pain/irritation so that a contralateral injury is not neglected.

- Use whatever nontoxic fluid is available for irrigation on scene. In hospital, sterile water, normal saline, normal saline with bicarbonate, balanced salt solution (BSS), or lactated Ringer solution may be used:
  - No therapeutic difference in effectiveness has been noted between types of solutions (1)[C].
- A topical anesthetic can be used to provide patient comfort (e.g., proparacaine, tetracaine).
- Sweep the conjunctival fornices every 12–24 hours to prevent adhesions (2)[C].
- Eye patching may relieve pain but has not been shown to improve outcomes (4)[C].

MEDICATION

First Line

- Further treatment (depending on severity and associated conditions)
  - Topical prophylactic antibiotics: any broad-spectrum agent (e.g., bacitracin–polymyxin B [Polysporin] ointment q2–4h, ciprofloxacin [Ciloxan] drops q2–4h, chloramphenicol [Chloroptic] ointment q2–4h) (1)[C]:
    - Some experts suggest that systemic tetracycline 250 mg PO q6h and especially derivatives such as doxycycline 100 mg PO BID may be beneficial to encourage healing of persistent corneal epithelial defects by inhibiting metalloproteinases (5)[C].
  - Tear substitutes: hydroxypropyl methylcellulose (HypoTears PF, Refresh Plus) drops q4h, carboxymethylcellulose (Refresh PM) ointment at bedtime (1)[C]:
    - Most beneficial in those with impaired tear production (elderly patients)
  - Cycloplegics for photophobia and/or uveitis: cyclopentolate 1% TID or scopolamine 1/4% BID (1)[C]
  - Antiglaucoma for elevated intraocular pressure: latanoprost (Xalatan) 0.005% q24h, timolol (Timoptic) 0.5% BID, *or* levobunolol (Betagan) 0.5% BID, *and/or* acetazolamide (Diamox) 125–250 mg PO q6h, *or* methazolamide (Neptazane) 25–50 mg PO BID, *and/or* IV mannitol 20% 1–2 g/kg as needed (1)[C]
  - Corticosteroids for intraocular inflammation: prednisolone (Pred-Forte) 1% or equivalent q1–4h for 7–10 days; if severe, prednisone 20–60 mg PO daily for 5–7 days. Taper rapidly if epithelium is intact by this time (1)[C]:
    - Use of corticosteroids >10 days may do harm by inhibiting repair and cause corneoscleral melt (1,6)[C].
  - Consider vitamin C (ascorbic acid) 500 mg PO QID *and/or* acetylcysteine (Mucomyst) 10–20% topically q4h if corneal melting occurs (1)[C].
- Precautions
  - Timolol and levobunolol: history of heart failure (HF) or chronic obstructive pulmonary disease (COPD)
  - Acetazolamide and methazolamide: history of nephrolithiasis or metabolic acidosis
  - Mannitol: history of HF or renal failure
  - Scopolamine: history of urinary retention
  - Topical corticosteroids must be used with caution in the presence of damaged corneal epithelium because iatrogenic infection can occur. Daily follow-up or consultation with an ophthalmologist is recommended.

SURGERY/OTHER PROCEDURES

- Goal of subacute treatment is restoration of the normal ocular surface anatomy, control of glaucoma, and restoration of corneal clarity.
- Surgical options include the following:
  - Débridement of necrotic tissue (1)[C]
  - Conjunctival/tenon advancement (tenoplasty) to restore vascularity in severe burns (1)[C]
  - Tissue adhesive (e.g., isobutyl cyanoacrylate) for impending or actual corneal perforation of
    - Tectonic keratoplasty for acute perforation >1 mm (1)[C]
  - Limbal autograft transplantation for epithelial stem cell restoration (1)[C]
  - Amniotic membrane transplantation to promote epithelial regeneration (6)[C]
  - Conjunctival or mucosal membrane transplant to restore ocular surface in severe injury (1)[C]
  - Lamellar or penetrating keratoplasty for tectonic stabilization or visual rehabilitation (1)[C]

INPATIENT CONSIDERATIONS

Admission Criteria/Initial Stabilization

Based on ophthalmologic consultation and concomitant burn injuries

ONGOING CARE

FOLLOW-UP RECOMMENDATIONS

Patient Monitoring

- Depending on severity of ocular injury
  - From daily to weekly visits initially
- May be inpatient
- If on mannitol or prednisone, consider frequent serum electrolytes.

PATIENT EDUCATION

- Safety glasses
- Need for immediate ocular irrigation with any available water following chemical exposure to the eyes

PROGNOSIS

- Depends on severity of initial injury: Increased limbal involvement in clock hours and greater percentage of conjunctival involvement correlate with poorer prognosis (Dua classification system).
- For mildly injured eyes, complete recovery is the norm.
- For severely injured eyes, permanent loss of vision is not uncommon.

COMPLICATIONS

- Orbital compartment syndrome
- Persistent epitheliopathy
- Fibrovascular pannus
- Corneal ulcer/perforation
- Corneal scarring
- Progressive symblepharon and entropion
- Neurotrophic keratitis
- Lid malposition secondary to cicatricial changes
- Glaucoma
- Cataract
- Hypotony
- Phthisis bulbi
- Blindness

REFERENCES

1. Wagoner MD. Chemical injuries of the eye: current concepts in pathophysiology and therapy. *Surv Ophthalmol*. 1997;41(4):275–313.
2. Kuckelkorn R, Schrage N, Keller G, et al. Emergency treatment of chemical and thermal eye burns. *Acta Ophthalmol Scand*. 2002;80(1):4–10.
3. Chau JP, Lee DT, Lo SH. A systematic review of methods of eye irrigation for adults and children with ocular chemical burns. *Worldviews Evid Based Nurs*. 2012;9(3):129–138.
4. Spector J, Fernandez WG. Chemical, thermal, and biological ocular exposures. *Emerg Med Clin North Am*. 2008;26(1):125–136, vii.
5. Ralph RA. Tetracyclines and the treatment of corneal stromal ulceration: a review. *Cornea*. 2000;19(3):274–277.
6. Fish R, Davidson RS. Management of ocular thermal and chemical injuries, including amniotic membrane therapy. *Curr Opin Ophthalmol*. 2010;21(4):317–321.

ADDITIONAL READING

- Gicquel JJ. Management of ocular surface chemical burns. *Br J Ophthalmol*. 2011;95(2):159–161.
- Lin A, Patel N, Yoo D, et al. Management of ocular conditions in the burn unit: thermal and chemical burns and Stevens-Johnson syndrome/toxic epidermal necrolysis. *J Burn Care Res*. 2011;32(5):547–560.
- Roblin I, Urban M, Flicoteau D, et al. Topical treatment of experimental hydrofluoric acid skin burns by 2.5% calcium gluconate. *J Burn Care Res*. 2006;2(6):889–894.

SEE ALSO

Burns

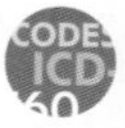

CODES

ICD10

- T26.50XA Corrosion of unsp eyelid and periocular area, init encntr
- T26.60XA Corrosion of cornea and conjunctival sac, unsp eye, init
- S05.00XA Inj conjunctiva and corneal abrasion w/o fb, unsp eye, init

CLINICAL PEARLS

- Prompt irrigation of all chemical burns, even prior to arrival to the emergency department, is essential to ensure best outcomes. It is impossible to overirrigate.
- All patients with chemical injuries to their eyes should have urgent ophthalmology consultation and/or referral.

ONYCHOMYCOSIS

Lauren M. Simon, MD, MPH, FAAFP, FACSM

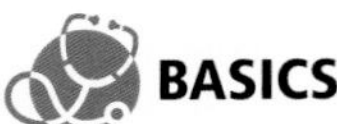

BASICS

DESCRIPTION
- Fungal infection of fingernails/toenails
- Caused mostly by dermatophytes but also yeasts and nondermatophyte molds
- Toenails more commonly affected than fingernails
- System(s) affected: skin; exocrine
- Synonym(s): tinea unguium; ringworm of the nail

EPIDEMIOLOGY

Prevalence
- Occurs in 2–10 in general population
- Predominant age: 20% in adults >60 years of age
- Rare before puberty
- Prevalence 15–40% in persons with human immunodeficiency infection (1)

ETIOLOGY AND PATHOPHYSIOLOGY
- Dermatophytes: *Trichophyton* (*Trichophyton rubrum* most common), *Epidermophyton*, *Microsporum*
- Yeasts: *Candida albicans* (most common), *Candida parapsilosis*, *Candida tropicalis*, *Candida krusei*
- Molds: *Scopulariopsis brevicaulis*, *Hendersonula toruloidea*, *Aspergillus sp.*, *Alternaria tenuis*, *Cephalosporium*, *Scytalidium hyalinum*
- Dermatophytes cause 90% of toenail and most of fingernail onychomycoses.
- Fingernail onychomycosis is more often caused by yeasts, especially *Candida*.
- Dermatophytes can invade normal keratin, whereas nondermatophyte molds invade altered keratin (dystrophic/injured nails).

RISK FACTORS
- Older age
- Tinea pedis
- Concurrent fungal infections
- Cancer/diabetes/psoriasis
- Peripheral vascular disease
- Cohabitation with others with onychomycosis
- Immunodeficiency
- Communal swimming pools
- Smoking
- Peripheral vascular disease
- History of nail trauma
- Autosomal dominant genetic predisposition

COMMONLY ASSOCIATED CONDITIONS
- Immunodeficiency/chronic metabolic disease (e.g., diabetes)
- Tinea pedis/manuum

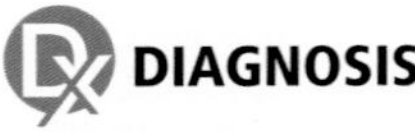

DIAGNOSIS

PHYSICAL EXAM
- Dermatophytes: commonly preceded by dermatophyte infection at another site; 80% involve toenails, especially hallux; simultaneous infection of fingernails and toenails is rare. Five clinical forms occur.
  - Distal/lateral subungual onychomycosis (most common): mainly due to *T. rubrum*. Spreads from distal/lateral margins to nail bed to nail plate; subungual hyperkeratosis; onycholysis; nail dystrophy; discoloration—yellow-white or brown-black, yellow streaking laterally; can progress proximally, *bois vermoulu* ("worm-eaten wood"); onychomadesis
  - Proximal subungual onychomycosis (rare <1% of cases): hands/feet; leukonychia—begins at proximal part of nail plate, appearing to occur from the proximal underside of the nail (or direct invasion of the nail plate from above); spreads to nail plate and lunula; seen with immunosuppressive conditions
  - Superficial (formerly known as superficial white onychomycosis) about 10% of cases: hallux preferentially affected; infection of outer surface of nail plate; opaque white spots on nail plate eventually merge to involve entire surface of the nail. Most commonly due to *Trichophyton mentagrophytes*
  - Endonyx onychomycosis involves interior of nail plate, sparing nail bed. Nail develops milky white appearance with indentations. Subungual hyperkeratosis is absent.
  - Totally dystrophic onychomycosis causes complete destruction of nail plate by fungus, resulting in thickened and ridged nail bed covered with keratotic debris.
- Candidal
  - Hands, 70%, especially for the dominant hand
  - Middle finger most common
  - Pain mild, unless secondarily infected
  - Increases on prolonged contact with water
  - Primarily affects tissue surrounding nail
  - Begins with cuticle detachment
  - White or white-yellow nail discoloration
  - Secondary ungual changes: convex, irregular, striated nail plate with dull, rough surface
  - Onycholysis, especially on hands
  - Distal subungual onychomycosis may occur.
  - Primary involvement of the nail plate is uncommon (thin, crumbly, opaque, brownish nail plate deformed by transverse grooves).
  - Periungual edema/erythema may occur (club-shaped, bulbous fingertips).
- Molds
  - More common in those >60 years of age
  - More common in nails of hallux
  - Resembles distal and lateral onychomycosis

Pediatric Considerations
- Candidal infection presents more commonly as superficial onychomycosis.
- The U.S. Food and Drug Administration (FDA) has not approved any systemic antifungal agents for treatment of onychomycosis in children. Efficacy and safety profiles in children for some systemic antifungals are similar to those previously reported in adults (2).

DIFFERENTIAL DIAGNOSIS
- Psoriasis (most common alternate diagnosis)
- Traumatic dystrophy
- Lichen planus
- Onychogryphosis ("ram's horn nails")
- Eczematous conditions
- Hypothyroidism
- Drugs and chemicals
- Yellow nail syndrome
- Neoplasms (0.7–3.5%) of all melanoma cases are subungual. In a brownish yellow nail, if dark pigment extends into periungual skin fold, consider subungual melanoma.

DIAGNOSTIC TESTS & INTERPRETATION
- Accurate diagnosis requires both laboratory and clinical evidence.
- About 50% of nail dystrophy seen on visual inspection is not fungal in origin, so laboratory assessment improves diagnostic accuracy.
- If onychomycosis is suspected clinically and initial diagnostic laboratory tests are negative, the tests should be repeated.
- A nail plate biopsy or partial/full removal of nail with culture is needed to diagnose proximal subungual onychomycosis.

Initial Tests (lab, imaging)
- Direct microscopy with potassium hydroxide (KOH) preparation (1)[C]
  - Clean nail with 70% isopropyl alcohol.
  - Using sterile clippers, remove diseased, discolored nail plate.
  - Collect debris from stratum corneum of most proximal area (beneath nail or crumbling nail itself) with 1-mm curette/scalpel
  - Larger sample improves sensitivity.
  - Place sample on microscope slide with drop of 5–10% KOH. View after 5 minutes.
  - Gentle heat applied to slide can enhance keratin breakdown.
  - High sensitivity if >2 preparations examined
  - Look for hyphae, pseudohyphae, or spores.
- Cultures: false-negative finding in 30% (secondary to loss of dermatophyte viability; improved by immediate culture on Sabouraud cell culture medium); results may take 3–6 weeks
- In office dermatophyte test, medium culture indicates dermatophyte growth with yellow-to-red color change of the medium; results in 3–7 days; limited studies.
- Histologic examination of nail clippings/nail plate punch biopsy: proximal lesions; stain both with periodic acid–Schiff (PAS) stain (1)[C]
- KOH-treated nail clipping stained with PAS: significantly higher rates of detection of onychomycosis as compared with standard methods of KOH preparation and fungal culture (3)[C]
- Polymerase chain reaction (PCR) increases sensitivity of detection of dermatophytes in nail specimen, results available within 3 days can be used as complementary to direct microscope exam and fungal culture. Not widely available.
- Fluorescence microscopy can be used as a rapid screening tool for identification of fungi in nail specimens.
- Commercial laboratories may use KOH with calcofluor white stain to improve view of fungal elements in fluorescent microscopy.
- Discontinue all topical medication for at least 1 week before obtaining a sample.

Test Interpretation
Pathogens within the nail keratin

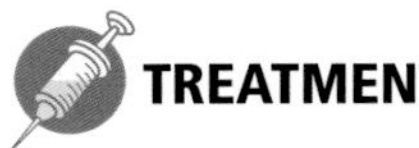

TREATMENT

GENERAL MEASURES
- Avoid factors that promote fungal growth (i.e., heat, moisture, occlusion, tight-fitting shoes).
- Treat underlying disease risk factors.
- Treat secondary infections.

MEDICATION

Pregnancy Considerations
Oral antifungals and ciclopirox are pregnancy category B (terbinafine, ciclopirox) or C (itraconazole, fluconazole, and griseofulvin). Griseofulvin is not advised in pregnancy due to risks of teratogenicity and conjoined twins). Ideally postpone treatment of onychomycosis until after pregnancy.

First Line

- Oral antifungals are preferred due to higher rates of cure but have systemic adverse effects and many drug–drug interactions.
- Terbinafine: 250 mg/day PO × 6 weeks for fingernails and 12 weeks for toenails; most effective in cure and prevention of relapse compared with other antifungals and with itraconazole pulse in meta-analysis for toenail onychomycosis I (4)[C]
- Itraconazole pulse: 200 mg PO BID × 1 week, then 3 weeks off, repeat for 2 cycles for fingernails and 3–4 cycles for toenails more effective than terbinafine for *Candida* and molds; does not need to monitor liver function tests (LFTs) with pulse dosing.
- Itraconazole continuous: 200 mg/day PO × 6 weeks for fingernails and 12 weeks for toenails (less effective than itraconazole pulse for dermatophytes, more effective than terbinafine for *Candida* and molds)

Second Line

- Fluconazole pulse: 150–300 mg PO weekly × 6 months (lower cure rate). Not FDA-approved for onychomycosis
- Griseofulvin: 500–1,000 mg/day PO for up to 18 months (lower cure rate, continue until the diseased nail is replaced)
- Posaconazole: 100, 200, or 400 mg once daily for 24 weeks; 400 mg once daily for 12 weeks; higher cost limit
- Topical agents
- Ciclopirox: 8% nail lacquer: Apply once daily to affected nails (if without lunula involvement) for up to 48 weeks; remove lacquer with alcohol every 7 days, then file away loose nail material and trim nails (low-cure rate, avoids systemic adverse effects, less cost-effective). Application after PO treatment may reduce recurrences. Systematic review >60% failure rate after 48 weeks of use (5)[C],(6)
- Amorolfine: 8% nail lacquer once a week until cure is achieved. Not available in United States.
- Efinaconazole solution 10% approved for use for toenail onychomycosis by FDA in June 2014.
- Contraindications for oral antifungals
  - Hepatic disease
  - Pregnancy (see "Pregnancy Considerations")
  - Current/ history of congestive heart failure (CHF) (itraconazole)
  - Ventricular dysfunction (itraconazole)
  - Porphyria (griseofulvin)
- Other treatments
  - Vicks VapoRub application to nails daily for 48 weeks has been found safe and cost-effective alternative for toenail onychomycosis.
  - Not available in United States: albaconazole: 100–400 mg once a week for 24 or 36 weeks
- Precautions/adverse effects
  - Oral antifungals
    - Hepatotoxicity/neutropenia
    - Hypersensitivity
    - Photosensitivity, lupus-like symptoms, proteinuria (griseofulvin)
    - Chronic kidney disease (avoid terbinafine for patients with creatine clearance (CrCl) <50 mL/min, decrease fluconazole dose)
    - CHF, peripheral edema, pulmonary edema (itraconazole)
    - Rhinitis (itraconazole)
- Ciclopirox: rash, nail disorders; avoid contact with skin except along nail edge; caution with broken skin or vascular compromise
- Numerous significant drug–drug interactions. Need to check each medication:
  - Terbinafine (inhibits cytochrome P450 2D6 isozyme [CYP2D6]): e.g., β-blockers, monoamine oxidase inhibitors (MAOIs), SSRIs, tricyclic antidepressants (TCAs), warfarin, oxycodone,
  - Itraconazole, fluconazole (inhibit CYP3A4): e.g., antiarrhythmics, benzodiazepines, ergot alkaloids, 3-hydroxy-3-methylglutaryl coenzyme A (HMG-CoA) reductase inhibitors, calcium channel blockers, corticosteroids, hydrochlorothiazide, hypoglycemics, oral contraceptives (OCPs), warfarin, zolpidem
  - Griseofulvin: e.g., OCPs, salicylates, warfarin

SURGERY/OTHER PROCEDURES

- Nail débridement to remove infected keratin (efficacy not well studied): Use for few nails involved or if not, for candidate of systemic therapy.
  - Mechanical: Soften with occlusive dressing with 40% urea gel; detach from nail bed with tweezers, file with abrasive stone or curette.
  - Chemical: Protect peripheral tissue with adhesive strips; apply ointment of 30% salicylic acid, 40% urea, or 50% potassium iodide under occlusive dressing.
  - Débridement may be combined with topical antifungal therapy.
  - Surgical avulsion if few nails involved. For pain control
- Laser treatment has shown some positive results but limited efficacy data.
- Photodynamic therapy using topical photosensitizing agents and irradiation with appropriate light source some success for treatment of superficial nail infections. Limited data

COMPLEMENTARY AND ALTERNATIVE MEDICINE

Melaleuca alternifolia (tea tree oil) Cochrane review found no evidence of benefit (5)

ONGOING CARE

FOLLOW-UP RECOMMENDATIONS

- Formation of a new fingernail takes 4–6 months, and a new toenail takes 12–18 months.
- Cure defined as:
  - Clinical cure, 100% absence of clinical signs, and/or
  - Mycotic cure, negative mycology with ≥1 of the following clinical signs:
    - Distal subungual hyperkeratosis/onycholysis leaving <10% of the nail plate affected
    - Nail plate thickening that does not improve with treatment because of comorbid condition

Patient Monitoring

- Topical agents: slow response expected; visits every 6–12 weeks
- Terbinafine, griseofulvin: baseline, and as needed, LFTs and CBC
- Itraconazole continuous: baseline, and as needed, LFTs.

PATIENT EDUCATION

- Advise patient to:
  - Keep affected area clean and dry.
  - Avoid rubber/other occlusive, tight-fitting footwear.
  - Wear absorbent cotton socks.
  - Launder clothing and towels frequently in hot water.
  - Avoid sharing nail implements or use on both normal and abnormal nails.
- Cure of all toenails may not be attainable.
- Nails may not appear normal after cure.

PROGNOSIS

- Complete clinical cure in 25–50% (higher mycologic cure rates)
- Recurrence is 10–50% (relapse/reinfection).
- Poor prognostic factors
  - Areas of nail involvement >50%
  - Significant proximal/lateral disease
  - Subungual hyperkeratosis >2 mm
  - White/yellow or orange/brown streaks in the nail (includes dermatophytoma)
  - Total dystrophic onychomycosis (with matrix involvement)
  - Nonresponsive organisms (e.g., *Scytalidium* mold)
  - Patients with immunosuppression
  - Diminished peripheral circulation

COMPLICATIONS

- Secondary infections with progression to soft tissue infection/osteomyelitis
- Toenail discomfort/pain that can limit physical mobility or activity
- Anxiety, negative self-image

REFERENCES

1. Westerberg DP, Voyack MJ. Onychomycosis: current trends in diagnosis and treatment. *Am Fam Physician*. 2013;88(11):762–770.
2. Gupta AK, Paquet M. Systemic antifungals to treat onychomycosis in children: a systematic review. *Pediatr Dermatol*. 2013;30(3):294–302.
3. Eisman S, Sinclair R. Fungal nail infection: diagnosis and management. *BMJ*. 2014;348:g1800.
4. Gupta AK, Ryder JE, Johnson AM. Cumulative meta-analysis of systemic antifungal agents for the treatment of onychomycosis. *Br J Dermatol*. 2004;150(3):537–544.
5. Crawford F, Hollis S. Topical treatments for fungal infections of the skin and nails of the foot. *Cochrane Database Syst Rev*. 2007;(3):CD001434.
6. Gupta AK, Paquet M, Simpson FC. Therapies for the treatment of onychomycosis. *Clin Dermatol* 2013;31(5):544–554.

ADDITIONAL READING

- Crawford F, Young P, Godfrey C, et al. Oral treatments for toenail onychomycosis: a systematic review. *Arch Dermatol*. 2002;138(6):811–816.
- Haghani I, Shokohi T, Hajheidari Z, et al. Comparison of diagnostic methods in the evaluation of onychomycosis. *Mycopathologia*. 2013;175(3–4):315–321.

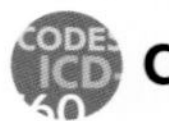

CODES

ICD10

- B35.1 Tinea unguium
- B37.2 Candidiasis of skin and nail

CLINICAL PEARLS

- Psoriasis and chronic nail trauma are commonly mistaken for fungal infection.
- Diagnosis should be based on both clinical and mycologic laboratory evidence.
- Oral antifungals more effective than topical antifungals; important to check for drug–drug interactions
- LFT monitoring is necessary for most oral antifungal regimens.

OPTIC NEURITIS

Olga M. Ceron, MD • Pablo I. Hernandez Itriago, MD, MS, FAAFP

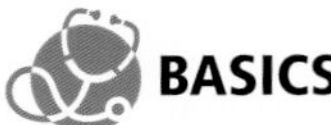

BASICS

DESCRIPTION

- Inflammation of the optic nerve (cranial nerve II)
- Most common form is acute demyelinating optic neuritis (ON), but other causes include infectious disease and systemic autoimmune disorders.
- Optic disc may be normal in appearance at onset (retrobulbar ON, 67%) or swollen (papillitis, 33%).
- Key features:
  - Abrupt visual loss (typically monocular)
  - Periorbital pain with eye movement (90%)
  - Pain in the distribution of the first division of the trigeminal nerve
  - Dyschromatopsia: color vision deficits
  - Relative afferent pupillary defect (RAPD)
- Usually unilateral in adults; bilateral disease more common in children
- Presenting complaint in 25% of patients with multiple sclerosis (MS)
- In children, headaches are common.
- System(s) affected: nervous
- Synonym(s): papillitis; demyelinating optic neuropathy; retrobulbar optic neuritis

EPIDEMIOLOGY

Incidence

- 1–5/100,000 cases per year
- More common in Northern latitudes
- More common in whites than in other races
- Predominant age: 18–45 years; mean age 30 years
- Predominant sex: female > male (3:1)

ETIOLOGY AND PATHOPHYSIOLOGY

- In both MS-associated and isolated monosymptomatic ON, the cause is presumed to be a demyelinating autoimmune reaction.
- Possible mechanisms of inflammation in immune-mediated ON are the cross-reaction of viral epitopes and host epitopes and the persistence of a virus in CNS glial cells.
- Neuromyelitis optica (NMO) IgG autoantibody, which targets the water channel aquaporin-4
- Primarily idiopathic
- MS
- Viral infections: measles, mumps, varicella-zoster, coxsackievirus, adenovirus, hepatitis A and B, HIV, herpes simplex virus, cytomegalovirus
- Nonviral infections: syphilis, tuberculosis, meningococcus, cryptococcosis, cysticercosis, bacterial sinusitis, streptococcus B, *Bartonella*, typhoid fever, Lyme disease, fungus
- Systemic inflammatory disease: sarcoidosis, systemic lupus erythematosus, vasculitis
- Local inflammatory disease: intraocular or contiguous with the orbit, sinus, or meninges
- Toxic: lead, methanol, arsenic, radiation
- Vascular lesions affecting the optic nerve
- Posterior uveitis (i.e., birdshot retinochoroidopathy, toxoplasmosis, toxocariasis)
- Tumors
- Medications: ethambutol, chloroquine, isoniazid, chronic high-dose chloramphenicol, tumor necrosis factor α-antagonist, infliximab (Remicade), adalimumab (Humira), etanercept (Enbrel)

COMMONLY ASSOCIATED CONDITIONS

- MS (common): ON is associated with an increased risk of MS.
- Other demyelinating diseases: Guillain-Barré syndrome, Devic neuromyelitis optica, multifocal demyelinating neuropathy, acute disseminated encephalomyelitis

DIAGNOSIS

HISTORY

- Decreased visual acuity, deteriorating in hours to days, usually reaching lowest level after 1 week
- Usually unilateral but can also be bilateral
- Brow ache, globe tenderness, deep orbital pain exacerbated by eye movement (92%)
- Retro-orbital pain may precede visual loss.
- Desaturation of color vision (dull or faded colors), especially red tones
- Apparent dimness of light intensities
- Impairment of depth perception (80%); worse with moving objects (Pulfrich phenomenon)
- Transient increase in visual symptoms with increased body temperature and exercise (Uhthoff phenomenon)
- May present with a recent flulike viral syndrome
- Detailed history and review of systems, looking for a history of demyelinating, infectious, or systemic inflammatory disease

PHYSICAL EXAM

Complete general exam, full neurologic exam, and ophthalmologic exam looking for the following:

- Decreased visual acuity and color perception
- Central, cecocentral, arcuate, or altitudinal visual field deficits
- Papillitis: swollen disc ± peripapillary flame-shape hemorrhage or often normal disc exam
- Temporal disc pallor seen later at 4–6 weeks (1)[A]
- Relative afferent pupillary defect (Marcus-Gunn pupil): The pupil of the affected eye dilates with a swinging light test unless disease is bilateral.

DIFFERENTIAL DIAGNOSIS

- Demyelinating disease, especially MS
- Infectious/systemic inflammatory disease
- Neuroretinitis: virus, toxoplasmosis, *Bartonella*
- Toxic or nutritional optic neuropathy
- Acute papilledema (bilateral disc edema)
- Compression:
  - Orbital tumor/abscess compressing the optic nerve
  - Intracranial tumor/abscess compressing the afferent visual pathway
  - Orbital pseudotumor
  - Carotid–ophthalmic artery aneurysm
- Temporal arteritis or other vasculitides
- Trauma or radiation
- Neuromyelitis optica (Devic disease)
- Anterior ischemic optic neuropathy
- Leber hereditary optic neuropathy
- Kjer-type autosomal dominant optic atrophy
- Severe systemic hypertension
- Diabetic papillopathy

DIAGNOSTIC TESTS & INTERPRETATION

Initial Tests (lab, imaging)

- In typical presentations, ESR is standard, but other labs are unnecessary. Antinuclear antibodies (ANAs), angiotensin-converting enzyme level, fluorescent treponemal antibody absorption (FTA-ABS), and chest radiograph have been shown to have no value in typical cases. (1)[A].
- In atypical presentations, including absence of pain, a very swollen optic nerve, >30 days without recovery, or retinal exudates, labs may be indicated to rule out underlying disorders:
  - CBC
  - ANA test
  - Rapid plasma reagin test
  - FTA-ABS test
- MRI of brain and orbits: thin cuts (2–3 mm) gadolinium-enhanced and fat-suppression images to look for Dawson fingers of MS (periventricular white matter lesions oriented perpendicular to the ventricles) and also to look for enhancement of the optic nerve
- CT scan of chest to rule out sarcoidosis if clinical suspicion is high
- OCT (ocular coherence tomography) of the retinal nerve fiber layer (RNFL); a noninvasive imaging technique of the optic nerve. May serve as a diagnostic tool to quantify thickness of the nerve fiber layer objectively and, thus, monitor structural change (axonal loss) of the optic nerve in the course of the disease

Follow-Up Tests & Special Considerations

- Visual field test (Humphrey 30–2) to evaluate for visual field loss: diffuse and central visual loss more predominant in the affected eye at baseline (2)[A]
- Low-contrast visual acuity (as a measure of disease progression)
- A novel blood test called *NMO-IgG* checks for antibodies for neuromyelitis optica.

Diagnostic Procedures/Other

- In atypical cases, including bilateral deficits, young age, or suspicion of infectious etiology, lumbar puncture (LP) with neurology consultation is indicated.
- LP for suspected MS is a physician-dependent decision. Some studies indicate that it may not add value to MRI for MS detection (1)[A] but no consensus on the subject exists.

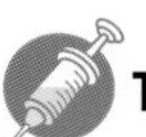

TREATMENT

Most persons with optic neuritis recover spontaneously.

MEDICATION

First Line

- IV methylprednisolone has been shown to speed up the rate of visual recovery but without significant long-term benefit; consider for patients who require fast recovery (i.e., monocular patients or those whose occupation requires high-level visual acuity). For significant vision loss, parenteral corticosteroids may be considered on an individualized basis: ONTT (Optic Neuritis Treatment Trial):
  - Observation and corticosteroid treatment are both acceptable courses of action.
  - High-dose IV methylprednisolone (250 mg q6h × 3 days) followed by oral corticosteroids (1 mg/kg/day PO × 11 days, taper over 1–2 weeks) (3)[A]
- Others use IV Solu-Medrol infusion (1 g in 250 mL D_5 1/2 normal saline infused over 1 hour daily for 3–5 days):
  - No evidence of long-term benefit (1)[A],(4)[B]
  - May decrease recovery time (3)[A],(4)[B]
  - May decrease risk of MS at 2 years but not 5 years (3)[A]
- Give antiulcer medications with steroids.

Second Line

- Disease-modifying agents, such as *interferon-β1a* (IFN-β1a; Avonex, Rebif) and IFN-β1b (Betaseron), are used to prevent or delay the development of MS in people with ON who have ≥2 brain lesions evident on MRI.
  - These medications have been proposed for use in patients with 1 episode of ON (clinically isolated syndrome) at high risk of developing MS (1+ lesion on brain MRI).
- The Controlled High Risk Avonex Multiple Sclerosis (CHAMPS) trial study has shown that IFN-β1a reduces the conversion to clinically definite MS in high-risk patients by ~50% (5)[A].
- Decisions should be made individually with neurology consultation.

ALERT

Never use oral prednisone alone as the primary treatment because this may increase the risk for recurrent ON (3)[A].

Pediatric Considerations

- No systematic study defining high-dose corticosteroids in children with ON have been conducted.
  - Consensus recommends: 3–5 days of IV methylprednisolone (4–30 mg/kg per day), followed by a 2–4 week taper of oral steroids (6)[C]
- Optic disc swelling and bilateral disease are more common in children as is severe loss of visual acuity (20/200 or worse).
- Consider infectious and postinfectious causes of optic nerve impairment.

ISSUES FOR REFERRAL

Referral to a neurologist and/or ophthalmologist

ONGOING CARE

FOLLOW-UP RECOMMENDATIONS

Patient Monitoring

Monthly follow-up to monitor visual changes and steroid side effects

PATIENT EDUCATION

- Provide reassurance about recovery of vision.
- If the disease is believed to be secondary to demyelinating disease, patient should be informed of the risk of developing MS.
- For patient education materials favorably reviewed on this topic, contact:
  - National Eye Institute, Information Officer, Department of Health and Human Services, 9000 Rockville Pike, Bethesda, MD 20892, 301-496-5248
  - North American Neuro-Ophthalmology Society (NANOS), 5841 Cedar Lake Road, Suite 204, Minneapolis, MN 55416, 952-646-2037, fax: 952-545-6073, www.nanosweb.org

PROGNOSIS

- Orbital pain usually resolves within 1 week.
- Visual acuity
  - Rapid spontaneous improvement at 2–3 weeks and continues for several months (may be faster with IV corticosteroids)
  - Often returns to normal or near-normal levels (20/40 or better) within 1 year (90–95%), even after near blindness
- Other visual disturbances (e.g., contrast sensitivity, stereopsis) often persist after acuity returns to normal.
- Recurrence risk of 35% within 10 years: 14% affected eye, 12% contralateral, 9% bilateral; recurrence is higher in MS patients (48%)
- ON is associated with an increased risk of developing MS; 35% risk at 7 years, 58% at 15 years (7)[A]:
  - Brain MRI helps to predict risk:
    - 0 lesions: 16%
    - 1–2 lesions: 37%
    - 3+ lesions: 51%
- Poor prognostic factors:
  - Absence of pain
  - Low initial visual acuity
  - Involvement of intracanalicular optic nerve
- Children with bilateral visual loss have a better prognosis than adults.

COMPLICATIONS

Permanent loss of vision

REFERENCES

1. Vedula SS, Brodney-Folse S, Gal RL, et al. Corticosteroids for treating optic neuritis. *Cochrane Database Syst Rev*. 2007;(1):CD001430.
2. Keltner JL, Johnson CA, Cello KE, et al. Visual field profile of optic neuritis: a final follow-up report from the optic neuritis treatment trial from baseline through 15 years. *Arch Ophthalmol*. 2010;128(3):330–337.
3. Simsek I, Erdem H, Pay S, et al. Optic neuritis occurring with anti-tumour necrosis factor alpha therapy. *Ann Rheum Dis*. 2007;66(9):1255–1258.
4. Gleicher N. *Principles and Practice of Medical Therapy in Pregnancy*. 3rd ed. Norwalk, CT: Appleton & Lange; 1998:1396–1399.
5. Galetta SL. The controlled high risk Avonex multiple sclerosis trial (CHAMPS Study). *J Neuroophthalmol*. 2001;21(4):292–295.
6. Bonhomme GR, Mitchell EB. Treatment of pediatric optic neuritis. *Curr Treat Options Neurol*. 2012;14(1):93–102.
7. Optic Neuritis Study Group. Visual function 15 years after optic neuritis: a final follow-up report from the Optic Neuritis Treatment Trial. *Ophthalmology*. 2008;115(6):1079–1082.e5.
8. Kaufman DI, Trobe JD, Eggenberger ER, et al. Practice parameter: the role of corticosteroids in the management of acute monosymptomatic optic neuritis. Report of the Quality Standards Subcommittee of the American Academy of Neurology. *Neurology*. 2000;54(11):2039–2044.
9. Arnold AC. Evolving management of optic neuritis and multiple sclerosis. *Am J Ophthalmol*. 2005;139(6):1101–1108.
10. Balcer LJ. Clinical practice. Optic neuritis. *N Engl J Med*. 2006;354(12):1273–1280.

SEE ALSO

Multiple Sclerosis

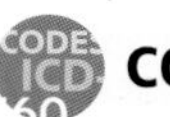

CODES

ICD10

- H46.9 Unspecified optic neuritis
- H46.00 Optic papillitis, unspecified eye
- H46.10 Retrobulbar neuritis, unspecified eye

CLINICAL PEARLS

- MRI is the procedure of choice for determining relative risk and possible therapy for MS prevention.
- The ONTT showed that high-dose IV methylprednisolone followed by oral prednisone accelerated visual recovery but did not improve the 6-month or 1-year visual outcome compared with placebo, whereas treatment with oral prednisone alone did not improve the outcome and was associated with an increased rate of recurrence of ON (1,2,8)[A],(9)[B],(10)[C].

ORAL REHYDRATION

Garrett W. Huck, MD, Capt, USAF • J. David Honeycutt, MD

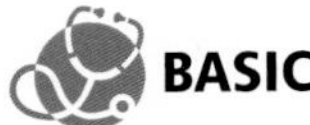

BASICS

DESCRIPTION

- Oral rehydration therapy (ORT) is a clinically useful, cost-effective, and safe technique to treat mild and moderate dehydration from diarrheal illness.
- ORT is as effective as IV hydration and the treatment of choice for children with mild to moderate dehydration caused by diarrhea.
- ORT should be divided into rehydration and maintenance phases.
- ORT should have an osmolality of ~245 mOsm/kg, a sodium (Na) content of ~75 mEq/L, and a glucose concentration of ~75 mmol/L (13.5 g/L) (1)[A].
- Fruit juices, soda, popsicles, sports drinks, and broth have inappropriate Na and/or electrolyte concentrations for ORT.
- Although ORT can be prepared at home, commercially prepared solutions eliminate the potential major errors that can occur from homemade solutions.
- System(s) affected: endocrine/metabolic; gastrointestinal

EPIDEMIOLOGY

Incidence

- Diarrheal disease is a leading cause of childhood morbidity and mortality in the world, causing ~2 million deaths per year (2).
- Diarrhea and the resulting dehydration is the source of >200,000 hospitalizations annually in the United States and >1.5 million outpatient visits (2).
- Predominant age: Primarily infants and children, but ORT is effective for all ages.

ETIOLOGY AND PATHOPHYSIOLOGY

This therapy takes advantage of the preserved coupled transport of Na and glucose in the small intestine during infectious gastroenteritis. Water follows osmotically after Na entry. Potassium is passively absorbed via solvent drag. An equimolar concentration of glucose and Na is most effective for ORT.

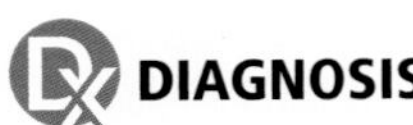

DIAGNOSIS

HISTORY

- Vomiting: duration and amount
- Diarrhea: duration and amount
- Fever
- Weight loss: amount
- Frequency and volume of urination
- Exposure to others with gastroenteritis
- Travel
- Recent antibiotic use
- ast medical history of short gut, or carbohydrate labsorption

CAL EXAM

ent of the degree of dehydration (Table 1)

st useful of these signs to predict tion may be prolonged capillary normal skin turgor (LR 2.5), and ry pattern (LR 2.0).

cale is shown to be better at han physician gestalt (3)[B].

Table 1 Clinical dehydration scale

Characteristic	0	1	2
General appearance	Normal	Thirsty, restless, lethargic, although irritable when touched	Drowsy, lethargic, cold, sweaty and/or comatose
Eyes	Normal	Slightly sunken	Very sunken
Mucous membranes	Moist	"Sticky"	Dry
Tears	Tears	Decreased tears	Absent tears

Scoring: 0: no dehydration: 3%, 1–4: some dehydration: 3–6%, 5–8: moderate dehydration: >6%.

DIAGNOSTIC TESTS & INTERPRETATION

Initial Tests (lab, imaging)

- Most with mild dehydration from diarrheal illness do not need lab tests (2).
- For some with moderate dehydration and all with severe dehydration, obtain Na (hypernatremia), potassium (hyperkalemia), bicarbonate (decreased), chloride, glucose (increased), BUN (increased), and creatinine (increased) (2)[C].

TREATMENT

GENERAL MEASURES

- The composition of oral rehydration solution (ORS) according to the WHO and UNICEF recommendations from 2002 include the following:
  - Total osmolality: 245 mmol/L
  - Equimolar concentrations of glucose and Na
  - Glucose: 1.35%
  - Na concentration: 75 mEq/L
  - Potassium concentration: 20 mEq/L
  - Citrate concentration: 10 mmol/L
  - Chloride concentration: 65 mEq/L (1)[A]
- See Table 2 for composition of common solutions (1)
- ORS is not to be diluted.
- Begin feeding as soon as rehydration is achieved. After rehydration is complete, ORT should not continue as the only fluid intake because the high Na content may lead to hypernatremia (4)[C].
- Effective at all ages
  - If child refuses because of taste, flavor with a commercial flavoring such as sugar-free grape-flavored drink mix and use ~1/4 tsp to 4 oz ORS, although it does not lead to increased intake (5)[B].

MEDICATION

First Line

- ORT can be used for both rehydration and maintenance hydration.
- The overall approach is to perform initial rehydration over 3–4 hours, followed by maintenance hydration.
- Initial rehydration requirements (5)[C]
  - Mild dehydration (3–5% weight loss): 50 mL/kg
  - Moderate dehydration: (6–9%): 100 mL/kg
  - Severe: (>10% estimated): IV hydration, then 100 mL/kg ORS once tolerating
- In the rehydration phase, ORT should be given as frequent, small amounts by spoon or syringe (4)[C].
- 5 mL every 1–2 minutes is often well tolerated and supplies 150–300 mL/hr.
- During the maintenance hydration stage, the fluid goals are as follows (4)[C]:
  - First 0–10-kg body weight: 4 mL/kg/hr
  - Next 10–20-kg: additional 2 mL/kg/hr
  - Additional body weight >20 kg: additional 1 mL/kg/hr
- In addition to the standard volumes of hydration provided, in both rehydration and maintenance phases, ongoing losses should be additionally replaced with 10 mL/kg body weight of ORT for each watery/loose stool or each episode of emesis (4)[C].
- Example: An 18-kg child who has moderate dehydration would require the following:
  - Rehydration phase: 100 mL/kg = 1,800 mL over 3–4 hours = 450–600 mL/hr = ~15–20 mL every 2 minutes
  - Maintenance phase: 56 mL/hr [(10 kg × 4 mL/hr) + (8 kg × 2 mL/hr)] = ~15 mL every 15 minutes
  - The child should receive additional ORT for any ongoing losses.
- Contraindications
  - Conditions predisposing to risk of aspiration
    - Significantly depressed level of consciousness, seizure activity
    - Severe dehydration, for which IV fluids should be started
    - Underlying disorders of intestinal absorption
- Precautions
  - The ingredients should be provided in premixed packets to avoid iatrogenic errors in mixing. In the United States, Pedialyte premixed powder packets are to be diluted in 8 oz (240 mL) of water. Many comparable generic formulations are available.
  - If water contamination is a concern, it should be boiled/treated for purification.
  - Discard the solution after 12 hours if held at room temperature or 24 hours if refrigerated.
- Risks
  - Symptomatic hyponatremia: rare, <1%
  - Hyperglycemia in diabetics

Table 2 Comparison of effective oral dehydration products

Solution	Osmolality (mOsm/kg H_2O)	Na^+ (mEq/L)	K^+ (mEq/L)	HCO_3 (mEq/L)	Carbohydrate (g/L)
WHO	245	75	20	10	13.5
Pedialyte	250	45	20	25	25
Enfalyte	200	50	25	34	30
Rehydralyte	310	75	20	30	25

– Fluid overload if overcorrect in at-risk patients
– Failure (requiring IVF): 4% (5)[B]

Second Line

- For inability to drink adequate amounts of ORS
  – Nasogastric (NG) administration of ORS has similar efficacy as IVF for moderate dehydration. Failure rates (requiring IVF) is around 2% (6)[A].
  – IV fluids if ORS and NG have failed (6)[A]
- WHO recommends supplementation zinc for 10–14 days in developing countries, which shortens the course of diarrhea and lessens costs; 20 mg PO daily for >6 months old, 10 mg for <6 months (5)[A]
- For children with vomiting, ondansetron (0.1–0.15 mg/kg) decreases vomiting, allows easier administration of ORT, and decreases the need for IV fluids. Ondansetron ODT can be particularly effective based on its ease of administration and tolerance in the vomiting child (2)[A].
- Probiotics have been shown to shorten diarrhea by about 1 day, decreasing amount of ORS needed (4)[A].

INPATIENT CONSIDERATIONS

Admission Criteria/Initial Stabilization

Caregivers who are unable to adequately administer ORS at home may encounter intractable vomiting, poor ORS intake by mouth or NG in ER, profuse diarrhea, unusual irritability or drowsiness, or failure to improve with 24 hours of ORS at home (4).

IV Fluids

To be used for initial resuscitation in severe cases or for ORS failure

Nursing

If vomiting occurs, small amounts of ORS given frequently are usually effective.

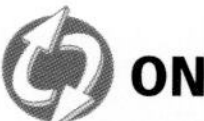

ONGOING CARE

FOLLOW-UP RECOMMENDATIONS

- Primarily outpatient
- Designed to be administered by family members

DIET

- For breastfeeding infants, the mother should continue nursing.
- For bottle-fed babies, there should be an early institution of formulas. Lactose-free formulas rarely are required.
- Age appropriate
  – Complex carbohydrate-rich (e.g., rice, bread, potato, cereal), low-fat foods should be offered as soon as the dehydration deficit is replaced.
- Cow's milk can be added to diet after several days.

PATIENT EDUCATION

- Awareness and availability of ORT markedly diminishes morbidity from gastroenteritis.
- Early use of ORT at home for children with diarrhea reduces outpatient visits, hospitalizations, and costs.
- Travelers concerned with severe diarrhea should carry ORT packets on trips.

PROGNOSIS

- Rapid clinical improvement despite continuing diarrhea is the usual course.
- The overall complication rate for oral rehydration is similar to that for parenteral rehydration in cases of mild and moderate dehydration.

COMPLICATIONS

Change to IV hydration if the patient has increasing weight loss (fluid deficit), clinical deterioration, or intractable vomiting.

REFERENCES

1. Suh JS, Hahn WH, Cho BS. Recent advances of oral rehydration therapy (ORT). *Electrolyte Blood Press*. 2010;8(2):82–86.
2. Niescierenko M, Bachur R. Advances in pediatric dehydration therapy. *Curr Opin Pediatr*. 2013;25(3):304–309.
3. Jauregui J, Nelson D, Choo E, et al. External validation and comparison of three pediatric clinical dehydration scales. *PLoS ONE*. 2014;9(5):e95739.
4. Churgay CA, Aftab Z. Gastroenteritis in children: part II. Prevention and management. *Am Fam Physician*. 2012;85(11):1066–1070.
5. Atia AN, Buchman AL. Oral rehydration solutions in non-cholera diarrhea: a review. *Am J Gastroenterol*. 2009;104(10):2596–2604.
6. Rhouhani S, Meloney L, Ahn R, et al. Alternative rehydration methods: a systematic review and lessons for resource-limited care. *Pediatrics*. 2011;127(3):e748.

ADDITIONAL READING

- Alhashimi D, Al-Hashimi H, Fedorowicz Z. Antiemetics for reducing vomiting related to acute gastroenteritis in children and adolescents. *Cochrane Database Syst Rev*. 2009;(2):CD005506.
- American Academy of Pediatrics, Provisional Committee on Quality Improvement, Subcommittee on Acute Gastroenteritis. Practice parameter: the management of acute gastroenteritis in young children. *Pediatrics*. 1996;97(3):424–435.
- Bryce J, Boschi-Pinto C, Shibuya K, et al; WHO Child Health Epidemiology Reference Group. WHO estimates of the causes of death in children. *Lancet*. 2005;365(9465):1147–1152.
- Canani RB, Cirillo P, Terrin G, et al. Probiotics for treatment of acute diarrhoea in children: randomised clinical trial of five different preparations. *BMJ*. 2007;335(7615):340.
- Duggan C, Fontaine O, Pierce NF. Scientific rationale for a change in the composition of oral rehydration solution. *JAMA*. 2004;291(21):2628–2631.
- Fonseca BK, Holdgate A, Craig JC. Enteral vs intravenous rehydration therapy for children with gastroenteritis: a meta-analysis of randomized controlled trials. *Arch Pediatr Adolesc Med*. 2004;158(5):483–490.
- Hahn S, Kim S, Garner P. Reduced osmolarity oral rehydration solution for treating dehydration caused by acute diarrhoea in children. *Cochrane Database Syst Rev*. 2002;(1):CD002847.
- Hartling L, Bellemare S, Wiebe N, et al. Oral versus intravenous rehydration for treating dehydration due to gastroenteritis in children. *Cochrane Database Syst Rev*. 2006;(3):CD004390.
- Lazzerini M, Ronfani L. Oral zinc for treating diarrhoea in children. *Cochrane Database Syst Rev*. 2008;(3):CD005436.
- Murphy CK, Hahn S, Volmink J. Reduced osmolarity oral rehydration solution for treating cholera. *Cochrane Database Syst Rev*. 2004;(4):CD003754.
- Santosham M, Keenan EM, Tulloch J, et al. Oral rehydration therapy for diarrhea: an example of reverse transfer of technology. *Pediatrics*. 1997;100(5):E10.
- Spandorfer PR, Alessandrini EA, Joffe MD, et al. Oral versus intravenous rehydration of moderately dehydrated children: a randomized, controlled trial. *Pediatrics*. 2005;115(2):295–301.
- Steiner MJ, DeWalt DA, Byerley JS. Is this child dehydrated? *JAMA*. 2004;291(22):2746–2754.
- Victora CG, Bryce J, Fontaine O, et al. Reducing deaths from diarrhoea through oral rehydration therapy. *Bull World Health Organ*. 2000;78(10):1246–1255.
- World Health Organization. Reduced osmolarity oral rehydration salts (ORS) formulation. New York, NY: UNICEF House; 2001. http://www.who.int/child-adolescent-health/New_Publications/NEWS/Expert_consultation.thm. Accessed 2014.

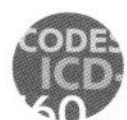

CODES

ICD10

- E86.0 Dehydration
- A09 Infectious gastroenteritis and colitis, unspecified
- K52.9 Noninfective gastroenteritis and colitis, unspecified

CLINICAL PEARLS

- ORT is as effective as and less costly than IV hydration for mild and moderate dehydration, yet it is underused in the developed world.
- ORT should not be diluted.
- The addition of ondansetron can augment the effectiveness of ORT.

OSGOOD-SCHLATTER DISEASE

David Sealy, MD

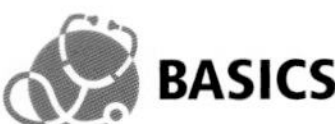

BASICS

DESCRIPTION

- A syndrome associated with traction apophysitis and patellar tendinosis
  - Most common in adolescent boys and girls
  - Pain and swelling of the tibial tubercle
- System(s) affected: musculoskeletal

EPIDEMIOLOGY

Incidence

Incidence in girls increasing with increased participation in organized youth sports

Prevalence

- The most common apophysitis in childhood and adolescence
- Common in adolescent athletes (21%) and in nonathletes (4.5%) (1,2)[B]

ETIOLOGY AND PATHOPHYSIOLOGY

Traction apophysitis of the tibial tubercle due to repetitive strain on the secondary ossification center of the tibial tuberosity, concurrent patellar tendinosis, and proximal tibial apophysis disruption

- Basic etiology unknown, exacerbated by exercise
  - Jumping and pivoting sports place highest strain on the tibial tubercle—repetitive trauma is the most likely inciting factor.
- Possible association with tight hip flexors and tight quadriceps; increased quadriceps strength in adolescence relative to hamstring strength
- Early sports specialization likely increases the risk for Osgood-Schlatter disease (OSD) (1)[B].

RISK FACTORS

- Ages 8–18 years
  - Girls 8–12 years
  - Boys 10–18 years
- Slightly more common in males
- Rapid skeletal growth
- Involvement in repetitive-jumping sports and sports with heavy quadriceps activity such as
  - Football, volleyball, basketball, hockey, soccer, skating, gymnastics
  - Ballet (2-fold risk compared with nonathletes)
- 1 study showed increased risk of OSD in adolescents with ADD/ADHD (3)[C].

GENERAL PREVENTION

- Avoid sports with heavy quadriceps loading (especially deceleration activities—eccentric loading).
- Patients may compete if pain is minimal.
- Increase hamstring and quadriceps flexibility.

COMMONLY ASSOCIATED CONDITIONS

- Shortened (tight) rectus femoris found in 75% with OSD
- Possible association with ADD/ADHD; known increased injury risk in adolescents with diagnosis

DIAGNOSIS

HISTORY

- Unilateral or bilateral (30%) tibial tuberosity pain
- Pain exacerbated by exercise, especially jumping and landing after jumping
- Pain upon kneeling on the affected side(s)
- Antalgic or straight-legged gait

PHYSICAL EXAM

- Knee pain with squatting or crouching
- Absence of effusion or condyle tenderness
- Tibial tuberosity swelling and tenderness
- Pain increased with knee extension against resistance or kneeling
- Erythema over tibial tuberosity
- Functional testing: Single-leg squat (SLS) and standing broad jump reproduce pain (3)[C].

DIFFERENTIAL DIAGNOSIS

- Stress fracture of the proximal tibia
- Pes anserinus bursitis
- Quadriceps tendon avulsion
- Patellofemoral stress syndrome
- Chondromalacia patellae (retropatellar pain)
- Proximal tibial neoplasm
- Osteomyelitis of the proximal tibia
- Tibial plateau fracture
- Sinding-Larsen-Johansson syndrome (patellar apophysitis)—pain over inferior patellar tendon
- Patellar fracture
- Infrapatellar bursitis
- Patellar tendinitis—pain over inferior patellar tendon and inferior pole of patella

DIAGNOSTIC TESTS & INTERPRETATION

Initial Tests (lab, imaging)

- Generally a clinical diagnosis. No blood tests are indicated unless other diagnostic considerations are entertained.
- Radiographic imaging of the proximal tibia and knee may show heterotopic calcification in the patellar tendon:
  - X-rays are rarely diagnostic, but appearance of a separate fragment at the tibial tuberosity increases potential for surgical intervention.
  - Calcified thickening of the tibial tuberosity with irregular ossification at insertion of tendon to tibial tubercle (4)[B]

Diagnostic Procedures/Other

- Bone scan may show increased uptake in the area of the tibial tuberosity:
  - Increased uptake in apophysis exists in any child, but with OSD *may be more than the opposite side*.
- Ultrasound is becoming an excellent alternative, with characteristic findings and marked thickening of the distal patellar tendon.
- MRI has characteristic findings of fragmentation of the tibial tubercle and bone edema.

Test Interpretation

Biopsy is not necessary but would show osteolysis and fragmentation of the tibial tubercle.

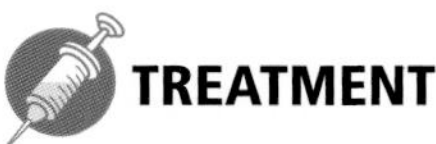

TREATMENT

GENERAL MEASURES

- Frequent ice applications 2–3×/day for 15–20 minutes
- Rest and activity modification—avoid activities that increase pain and/or swelling.
- Knee immobilization in extension (severe cases)
- Physical therapy can help with programs for strengthening and stretching exercises for the hamstrings and quadriceps.
- Open- and closed-chain eccentric quadriceps strengthening
- Avoid aggressive stretching if pain is significant to avoid risk of tibial tubercle avulsion (1)[B].

- If tibial tuberosity fracture or complete avulsion is present, entertain orthopedic evaluation for surgery.
- Electrical stimulation and iontophoresis are not proven but may be beneficial (1)[B].
- Patients with marked pronation may benefit from orthotics.
- 1 older study showed benefit from an infrapatellar strap and many experts recommend the use of a knee brace with an H- or U-shaped buttress (1)[C].

MEDICATION

First Line

- None in particular, but all analgesics may be considered.
- NSAIDs are of minimal benefit but may help control pain.
- Opioids are generally not recommended.

Second Line

- More potent analgesics, such as opioids, may be considered for short-term use or in extreme situations.
- Injectable corticosteroids not recommended
- Hypertonic glucose and/or xylocaine injections have recently been shown of benefit (5)[C].

ISSUES FOR REFERRAL

When conservative therapy is unsuccessful, consideration of surgery warrants referral.

SURGERY/OTHER PROCEDURES

- Débridement of a thickened, cosmetically unsatisfactory tibial tubercle (rare) or removal of mobile heterotopic bone
- Surgical excision of a painful tibial tubercle is rarely needed (<5%).
- 75% return to normal sport activity and 89% are not restricted from competition due to recurrent pain.

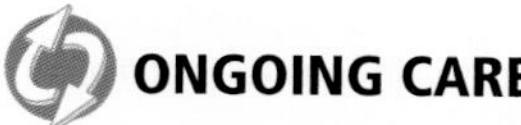

ONGOING CARE

FOLLOW-UP RECOMMENDATIONS

- Athletes may return to play if able to tolerate pain.
- Presence of pain does not preclude competition.

Patient Monitoring

With worsening of symptoms only

PATIENT EDUCATION

- Consider avoidance of jumping sports or reduction of any activities that increase pain and swelling.
- Assure family that symptoms and findings will diminish with time and rest.
- Can play sports with mild pain
- Quadriceps stretching and strengthening important

PROGNOSIS

- Except in rare complicated cases, this is a self-limiting illness that resolves within 2 years of full skeletal maturation.
- Up to 60% of adults with prior OSD will report occasional symptoms and pain with kneeling.
- Most persons with OSD will have residual "knots" of tibial tubercles that never completely resolve.

COMPLICATIONS

Rarely, the heavily fragmented and inflamed tibial ossicle will avulse and require surgery.

REFERENCES

1. Kabiri L, Tapley H, Tapley S. Evaluation and conservative treatment for Osgood-Schlatter disease: a critical review of the literature. *Intl J Ther Rehab*. 2014;21(2):91–96.
2. de Lucena GL, dos Santos GC, Guerra RO. Prevalence and associated factors of Osgood-Schlatter syndrome in a population based sample of Brazilian adolescents. *Am J Sports Med*. 2011;39(2):415–420.
3. Guler F, Kose O, Koparan C, et al. Is there a relationship between attention deficit/hyperactivity disorder and Osgood-Schlatter disease? *Arch Orthop Trauma Surg*. 2013;133(9):1303–1307.
4. Sailly M, Whiteley R, Johnson A. Doppler ultrasound and tibial tuberosity maturation status predicts pain in adolescent male athletes with OSD: a case series with comparison group and clinical interpretation. *Br J Sports Med*. 2013;47(2):93–97.
5. Topol GA, Podesta LA, Reeves KD, et al. Hyperosmolar dextrose injection for recalcitrant Osgood-Schlatter disease. *Pediatrics*. 2011;128(5):e1121–e1128.

ADDITIONAL READING

- Hall R, Barber Foss K, Hewett TE, et al. Sports specialization's association with an increased risk of developing anterior knee pain in adolescent female athletes. *J Sport Rehabil*. 2015;24(1):31–35.
- Kaya DO, Toprak U, Baltaci G, et al. Long-term functional and sonographic outcomes in OSD. *Knee Surg Sports Traumatol Arthrosc*. 2013;21(5):1131–1139.
- Nierenberg G, Falah M, Keren Y, et al. Surgical treatment of residual Osgood-Schlatter disease in young adults: role of the mobile osseous fragment. *Orthopedics*. 2011;34(3):176.
- Pihlajamäki HK, Visuri TI. Long-term outcome after surgical treatment of unresolved Osgood Schlatter disease in young men: surgical technique. *J Bone Joint Surg Am*. 2010;92(Suppl 1, Pt 2):258–264.
- Weiler R, Ingram M, Wolman R. 10 minute consultation: Osgood-Schlatter disease. *BMJ*. 2011;343:d4534.

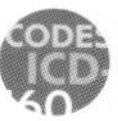

CODES

ICD10

- M92.50 Juvenile osteochondrosis of tibia and fibula, unsp leg
- M92.51 Juvenile osteochondrosis of tibia and fibula, right leg
- M92.52 Juvenile osteochondrosis of tibia and fibula, left leg

CLINICAL PEARLS

- Infrapatellar pain in an athlete during rapid growth spurt is OSD, patellar tendinosis, or Sinding-Larsen-Johansson syndrome.
- Always consider lumbar disc disease, osteogenic sarcoma, or hip etiologies in the differential diagnosis of OSD.
- OSD is generally self-limited. Athletes should modify activity based on pain.
- Treatment focuses on strengthening and stretching of the hamstrings and quadriceps.

OSTEOARTHRITIS

Patrick Wakefield Joyner, MD, MS, LCDR

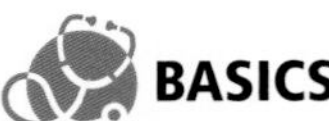

BASICS

DESCRIPTION

- Progressive loss of articular cartilage and reactive changes at joint margins and in subchondral bone
- Primary
  - Idiopathic: categorized by clinical features (localized, generalized, erosive)
- Secondary
  - Posttraumatic
  - Childhood anatomic abnormalities (e.g., congenital hip dysplasia, slipped capital femoral epiphysis [SCFE], Legg-Calvé-Perthes disease)
  - Inheritable metabolic disorders (e.g., Wilson disease, alkaptonuria, hemochromatosis)
  - Neuropathic arthropathy (Charcot joints)
  - Hemophilic arthropathy
  - Endocrinopathies: acromegalic arthropathy, hyperparathyroidism, hypothyroidism
  - Paget disease
  - Noninfectious inflammatory arthritis (e.g., rheumatoid arthritis [RA], spondyloarthropathies)
  - Gout, calcium pyrophosphate deposition disease (pseudogout)
  - Septic or tuberculous arthritis
- System(s) affected: musculoskeletal
- Synonym(s): osteoarthrosis; degenerative joint disease (DJD)

EPIDEMIOLOGY

- Symptomatic disease most common in patients >40 years of age
- Leading cause of disability in patients >65 years of age
- Radiographic evidence (estimates): 33%–~90% in patients >65 years of age
- Predominant sex: male = female
- 90% of hip osteoarthritis (OA) is primary and is more common in whites.

Prevalence

- ~60 million patients
- Increases with age, radiographic evidence of OA is nearly universally present in patients >65 years of age.
- Moderate to severe hip OA in 3–6% of whites; <1% in East Indians, blacks, Chinese, and Native Americans

ETIOLOGY AND PATHOPHYSIOLOGY

- Failure of chondrocytes to maintain the balance between degradation and synthesis of extracellular collagen matrix. Collagen loss results in alteration of proteoglycan matrix and increased susceptibility to degenerative change.
- Biomechanical, biochemical, inflammatory, and immunologic factors contribute to cartilage loss and attempts at repair that most commonly manifest as osteophyte formation.

Genetics

- Up to 65% of OA may have a genetic link.
- The heritability of end-stage hip OA has been estimated to be as high 27%.
- Twin studies in women show 50 (hip; knee)–65% (hip) heritability rates of OA.

RISK FACTORS

- Increasing age: >50 years
- The effect of age as a risk factor is greatest for hip and knee OA, especially after 70 years of age.
- Hand OA has greatest prevalence in postmenopausal women.
- Obesity (weight-bearing joints)
- Prolonged occupational or sports stress
- Injury to a joint from trauma, infection, or preexisting inflammatory arthritis
- Female gender (knee and hand)

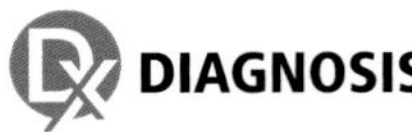

DIAGNOSIS

HISTORY

- Distinguish OA from other types of arthritis by the following:
  - Absence of systemic findings
  - Minimal articular inflammation
  - Distribution of involved joints (e.g., distal and proximal interphalangeal joints, not wrist and metacarpophalangeal joints)
- Slowly developing joint pain that typically follows use of a joint. Pain often described as aching or burning in nature. Anecdotally, many patients describe pain changes with alterations in weather conditions.
- Transient stiffness (especially after awakening in morning and after sitting) that tends to lessen 10–15 minutes after some movement and mobility of the joint
- OA more commonly affects hands, spine, and large weight-bearing joints (hip, knee).

PHYSICAL EXAM

- Joint bony enlargement (Heberden nodules of distal interphalangeal joints; Bouchard nodes of proximal interphalangeal joints)
- Decreased range of motion of affected joints
- Tenderness usually absent; may occur along joint margin if synovitis is persistent
- Crepitation present as a late sign.
- Weakness and wasting of muscles around the joint
- Local pain and stiffness with OA of spine, with radicular pain (if compression of nerve roots)
- Changes in joint alignment (genu varus [bow-legged] and genu valgum [knock-kneed])

DIFFERENTIAL DIAGNOSIS

- Crystalline arthropathies (gout; pseudogout): inflammatory arthritides (rheumatoid arthritis); spondyloarthropathies (reactive arthritis; psoriatic arthritis); septic arthritis.
- Fibromyalgia; avascular necrosis; Lyme disease

DIAGNOSTIC TESTS & INTERPRETATION

Initial Tests (lab, imaging)

- Routine chemistries are not helpful in diagnosis.
- X-ray films usually normal early in disease process
- As OA progresses, plain films show the following:
  - Narrowed, asymmetric joint space
  - Osteophyte formation
  - Subchondral bony sclerosis
  - Subchondral cyst formation
- Erosions may occur on surface of distal and proximal interphalangeal joints (erosive OA).

Follow-up Tests & Special Considerations

- May be useful in monitoring treatment with NSAIDs (renal insufficiency and GI bleeding)
- In secondary OA, underlying disorder may have abnormal lab results (e.g., hemochromatosis [abnormal iron studies]).

Diagnostic Procedures/Other

- Joint aspiration
  - May help to distinguish OA from chronic inflammatory arthritis
  - OA: cell count usually <500 cells/mm^3, predominantly mononuclear
  - Inflammatory: cell count usually >2,000 cells/mm^3, predominantly neutrophils
  - Birefringent crystals in gout (−) and pseudogout (+)

Test Interpretation

- Macroscopic patchy cartilage damage and bony hypertrophy
- Histologic phases:
  - Extracellular matrix edema and cartilage microfissures
  - Subchondral fissuring and pitting
  - Erosion and formation of osteocartilaginous loose bodies
- Subchondral bone trabecular microfractures and sclerosis with osteophyte formation
- Degradation secondary to release of proteolytic and, collagenolytic enzymes, prostaglandins, and associated immune response

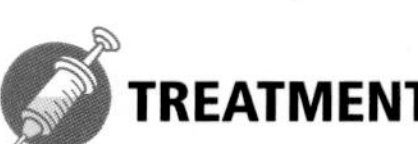

TREATMENT

GENERAL MEASURES

- Weight reduction if overweight
- Heat or cold applications for symptomatic relief
- Physical therapy to maintain or regain joint motion and muscle strength
  - Quadriceps-strengthening exercises relieve knee pain and disability.
- Muscle strengthening exercises improve pain.
- Aerobic exercise improves long-term functional outcomes.
- Exercise must be maintained; benefits are lost 6 months after exercise cessation.
- Protect joints from overuse; ambulatory aides are beneficial (e.g., cane, crutches, walker) as is proper fitting footwear.
- Assess for bracing, joint supports, or insoles in patients with biomechanical joint pain or instability:
  - Bracing is more beneficial in patients with unicompartmental disease of the knee.
  - Knee OA
- For knee OA in particular, *nonpharmacologic modalities are strongly recommended*: aerobic, aquatic, and/or resistance exercise and weight loss.
- Nonpharmacologic modalities that are conditionally recommended for knee OA include medial wedge insoles for valgus knee OA, subtalar strapped lateral insoles for varus knee OA, medially directed patellar taping, manual therapy, walking aids, thermal agents, tai chi, self-management programs, and psychosocial intervention.

MEDICATION

First Line

- Manage pain and inflammation:
  - Acetaminophen up to 1,000 mg TID–QID: effective for pain relief in OA of knee and hip
  - Topical NSAID gels, creams have short-term (<4 weeks) benefits. Topical NSAIDs should be a core treatment for knee and hand OA.
  - If acetaminophen or topical NSAIDs are insufficient, the addition or substitution of an oral NSAID/COX-2 inhibitor should be considered. Use at the lowest effective dose for the shortest time possible. Use is associated with renal insufficiency, hypertension, edema, and GI bleeding.
  - May use nonacetylated salicylates (e.g., salsalate, choline-magnesium salicylate) or low-dose ibuprofen ≤1,600 mg/day
  - Topical NSAIDs and capsaicin effective as adjunctives and alternatives to PO analgesic/anti-inflammatory agents in knee OA.
- NSAID contraindications:
  - All PO NSAIDs/COX-2 inhibitors have analgesic effects of a similar magnitude but vary in their potential GI and cardiorenal toxicity.
  - NSAIDs should be avoided in patients with renal disease, CHF, HTN, active peptic ulcer disease, and previous hypersensitivity to an NSAID or aspirin (asthma, nasal polyps, hypotension, urticaria/angioedema).
  - Combination of NSAIDs and aspirin is contraindicated due to risk of adverse reactions.
  - In patients at high cardiovascular risk: Combination of a nonselective NSAID and low-dose aspirin is recommended.
  - Oral or parenteral corticosteroids are contraindicated.
- Precautions:
  - If PO NSAID/COX-2 inhibitor use is necessary for a patient aged >65 years or a patient <65 years with increased GI-bleeding risk factors, proton-pump inhibitors are recommended.
  - Significant possible interactions:
    - NSAIDs reduce effectiveness of ACE inhibitors and diuretics.
    - Aspirin and NSAIDs (except COX-2 inhibitors) may increase effects of anticoagulants.
    - Salicylates reduce effectiveness of spironolactone (Aldactone) and uricosurics.
    - Corticosteroids and some antacids increase salicylate excretion, whereas ascorbic acid and ammonium chloride reduce salicylate excretion and may cause toxicity.

Pregnancy Considerations

- ASA and NSAIDs have reported fetal risk during 1st and 3rd trimesters of pregnancy.
- Compatible with breastfeeding

Second Line

- Topical capsaicin can be considered as an adjunct therapy for knee and hand OA; may cause local burning
- Topical NSAIDs (e.g., diclofenac gel) can lower gastric and renal risks associated with oral NSAIDs.
- Rubefacients (e.g. Oil of Wintergreen) are not recommended.
- Physical therapy: Core strengthening for hip OA and knee muscle strengthening for knee OA decrease joint reactive forces on the affected joint.
- Bracing: Medial and lateral unloader braces are effective, long leg alignment x-rays can help with determining which brace is appropriate (1).

Third Line

- Intra-articular corticosteroid injections can be used for acute flares and for patients failing 1st- and 2nd-line treatments. Minimize injections (<2/joint/year).
- Intra-articular viscosupplementation with hyaluronic acid (HA) may provide pain relief and improve function at earlier stages of knee. OA HA injections are permitted every 6 months.
- CS and HA injections have similar clinical benefits.
- Both single and staged HA injections are effective (2)[A].
- Platelet-rich plasma (PRP) is more effective than HA injections for early stage knee OA (3).
- No difference in patient outcome scores between PRP and HA injections in hip OA (4)
- TENS is effective for pain relief in large joint OA.
- Ultrasound improves injection accuracy.
- Opioids may be considered in recalcitrant cases.

ADDITIONAL THERAPIES

Address psychosocial factors (i.e., self-efficacy, coping skills). Screen for and appropriately treat anxiety and depression. Improve social support.

SURGERY/OTHER PROCEDURES

Surgery (e.g., osteotomy, débridement, removal of loose bodies, joint replacement, fusion) may be indicated in advanced disease.

COMPLEMENTARY & ALTERNATIVE MEDICINE

- Nutritional supplements (glucosamine and chondroitin sulfate) may benefit some patients and have low toxicity. There is lack of standardized outcome assessments. If no response is apparent within 6 months, treatment should be discontinued.
- A 2010 meta-analysis showed glucosamine +/− chondroitin do not reduce joint pain or joint space narrowing compared with placebo.
- TENS units and acupuncture have shown benefit.

ONGOING CARE

FOLLOW-UP RECOMMENDATIONS

Patient Monitoring

- Follow range of motion and functional status at regular intervals.
- Monitor for GI blood loss, cardiac, renal, and mental status in older patients on NSAIDs or aspirin.
- Periodic CBC, renal function tests, stool for occult blood in patients on chronic NSAID therapy

PATIENT EDUCATION

- American College of Rheumatology: http://www.rheumatology.org/public/factsheets/index.asp?aud = pat
- Arthritis Foundation: http://www.arthritis.org

PROGNOSIS

- Progressive disease: early in course, pain relieved by rest; later, pain may persist at rest and at night.
- Joint effusions and enlargement may occur, (especially in knees) as disease progresses.
- Osteophyte (spur) formation, especially at joint margins
- Advanced stage with full-thickness loss of cartilage down to bone at which point joint replacement is a consideration

COMPLICATIONS

- Leading cause of musculoskeletal pain and disability
- Decompensated CHF, GI bleeding, decreased renal function on chronic NSAID or aspirin therapy

REFERENCES

1. Dessery Y, Belzile EL, Turmel S, et al. Comparison of three knee braces in the treatment of medial knee osteoarthritis. *Knee*. 2014;21(6):1107 -1114.
2. Zoboli AA, de Rezende MU, de Campos GC, et al. Propspective randomized clinical trial: single and weekly viscosupplementation. *Acta Ortop Bras*. 2013;21(5):271–275.
3. Guler O, Mutlu S, Isyar M, et al. Comparison of short-term results of intraarticular platelet-rich plasma (PRP) and hyaluronic acid treatments in early-stage gonarthosis patients [published online ahead of print August 2, 2014]. *Eur J Orthop Surg Traumatol*.
4. Battaglia M, Guaraldi F, Vannini F, et al. Efficacy of ultrasound-guided intra-articular injections of platelet-rich plasma versus hyaluronic acid for hip osteoarthritis. *Orthopaedics*. 2013;36(12): e1501–e1508.

ADDITIONAL READING

- Chen WL, Hsu WC, Lin YJ, et al. Comparison of intra-articular hyaluronic acid injections with transcutaneous electric nerve stimulation for the management of knee osteoarthritis: a randomized controlled trial. *Arch Phys Med Rehabil*. 2013;94(8):1482–1489.
- Jiang L, Tian W, Wang Y, et al. Body mass index and susceptibility to knee osteoarthritis: a systematic review and meta-analysis. *Joint Bone Spine*. 2012; 79(3):291–297.
- Shimizu M, Higuchi H, Takagishi K, et al. Clinical and biochemical characteristics after intra-articular injection for the treatment of osteoarthritis of the knee: prospective randomized study of sodium hyaluronate and corticosteroid. *J Orthop Sci*. 2010; 15(1):51–56.

CODES

ICD10

- M19.90 Unspecified osteoarthritis, unspecified site
- M19.91 Primary osteoarthritis, unspecified site
- M19.93 Secondary osteoarthritis, unspecified site

CLINICAL PEARLS

- Patients with OA typically have morning stiffness lasting for less than 15 minutes.
- OA has distal predominance in the hands.
- Limit intra-articular steroid injections.
- Consider PRP for early stage knee OA.
- Long-term therapy should be based on individual patient goals and expectations, particularly regarding pain management and activity level.

OSTEOCHONDRITIS DISSECANS

Matthew Kendall Hawks, MD • J. David Honeycutt, MD

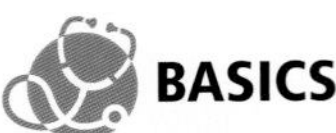

BASICS

DESCRIPTION

- Osteochondritis dissecans (OCD) is a lesion of the subchondral bone that may cause separation and instability of the overlying articular cartilage.
- The loose piece of bone and cartilage may migrate into the joint causing instability, pain, or a locking sensation.
- OCD is the most common cause of an intra-articular loose body in adolescents.
- Knee is the most commonly affected joint.
- OCD can also occur in any other diarthrodial joint, including the following in decreasing order of frequency:
  - Elbow (capitulum)
  - Ankle (talar dome or tibial plafond)
  - Tarsal navicular
  - Hip (femoral capital epiphysis)
  - Shoulder (humeral head or glenoid)
  - Wrist (scaphoid)
- System(s) affected: musculoskeletal

EPIDEMIOLOGY

Incidence

- Unknown: estimated 2–5:10,000 persons
- Predominant age: 10–40 years
- Juvenile type (JOCD) in children and adolescents prior to physeal closure
- Predominant sex: male > female (2:1) with female incidence increasing (1)

ETIOLOGY AND PATHOPHYSIOLOGY

- Loss of subchondral bone support leads to degenerative cartilage changes: softening and fibromatous fissuring
- A fragment may detach and become a loose body within the affected joint.
- Cartilage is avascular and heals by vascular supply to underlying bone, which stimulates inflammation, repair, and remodeling. Primary in OCD is to the underlying bone with secondary cartilage damage due to focal bony necrosis.
- Difficult to predict which lesions will go on to heal and remodel
- Precice etiology is unclear, but theories include the following:
  - Trauma or repetitive microtrauma
  - Ischemia
  - Familial predisposition
  - Fragile blood supply of the physeal line
  - Epiphyseal abnormalities
  - Endocrine imbalance
- Currently, the most credited theory is repetitive microtrauma with resultant vascular insufficiency.
- Most commonly affected joints are the following:
  - Knee: overuse, and with patellar dislocation and injury to the anterior cruciate ligament; bilateral involvement noted in up to 30% of patients
  - Elbow: overuse injury in overhead throwers and racket sports, as well as gymnasts
  - Ankle: frequently associated with history of previous ankle sprain
- Relationship between adult (physeal closure) and juvenile (physeal open) forms of OCD remains unclear.
- Juvenile OCD is more likely to heal spontaneously than adult OCD (2).

Genetics

No genetic patterns have been identified, but bilateral lesions have been noted in up to 25% of patients (3). Case reports of bilateral involvement in twins exist, but this is rare.

RISK FACTORS

- Trauma
- High physical activity level (children and adults)
- Participating in multiple sports, especially gymnastics and overhead sports
- Abnormal mechanical axis of the leg
  - Varus axis and medial condyle OCD
  - Valgus axis and lateral condyle OCD

Pediatric Considerations

Although still idiopathic, the mean age in JOCD is decreasing, and the prevalence in girls is increasing with changes in athletic participation by children (1).

GENERAL PREVENTION

There is no clear way to avoid the development of OCD.

DIAGNOSIS

HISTORY

- Insidious (most common) or posttraumatic onset of pain, which improves with rest
- Pain usually is described as a deep and vague ache.
- Pain may be associated with clicking, swelling, locking (usually with a loose body), and stiffness.

PHYSICAL EXAM

- May be associated with secondary muscle atrophy, mild effusion, decreased range of motion (ROM), joint-line tenderness, or tenderness over the lesion
- Wilson test is poorly sensitive—only 16% of positive exams in patients with radiographically proven OCD lesions (4)[A].

DIFFERENTIAL DIAGNOSIS

- Pathology specific to the knee
  - Meniscal tear
  - Patellofemoral pain syndrome
  - Gout
- Osteoarthritis
- Stress fracture
- Tendinopathy
- Avascular necrosis
- Acute fracture
- Neoplasm

DIAGNOSTIC TESTS & INTERPRETATION

Initial Tests (lab, imaging)

No specific laboratory tests are helpful in the diagnosis of OCD.

- The diagnosis is usually made radiographically (4)[C].
- Typical findings include small articular surface radiolucency/irregularity with bony fragmentation and partial or complete separation of the articular cartilage.
  - Knee: anteroposterior (AP), lateral, sunrise, and tunnel views (most likely location for abnormality in the posterolateral portion of the medial femoral condyle [4])
  - Elbow: routine AP and lateral elbow series (common involvement of the humeral capitellum)
  - Ankle: AP, lateral, and mortise views (lesions most commonly involve the posteromedial or anterolateral talar dome)
- MRI can delineate the bony lesion, involvement of cartilage, and any fluid behind the fragment and is useful to detect the stability or instability (fractured cartilage or separation from underlying suchondral bone) of the lesion (4)[C].
- MRI also allows for staging of adult lesions (2)[C].
- Current MRI classification systems lack validity in evaluating juvenile OCD (3)[C],(4)[B].
- CT scan provides architectural description of the bony lesion but is clinically less helpful than MRI.
- Bone scan may help evaluate healing potential (controversial).

TREATMENT

GENERAL MEASURES

- Goals of treatment
  - Maintain a smooth, congruous joint surface.
  - Alleviate pain.
  - Prevent degenerative joint disease.
  - Promote revascularization of necrotic fragment and regeneration of affected cartilage.
- There are no randomized, controlled trials comparing treatment modalities and outcomes, but in JOCD, initial nonsurgical treatment is the standard of care (4)[C].
- Treatment options include periods of immobilization (potential casting), activity modification, and non–weight bearing. Type and duration of immobilization remain controversial (4)[C].
- Follow closely for at least 12 weeks to ensure healing (4,5)[C].

MEDICATION

First Line

- No specific medications for OCD other than symptomatic treatment.
- Acetaminophen 650 mg q4–6 hours PRN; peds: (15 mg/kg/dose q4–6hrs PRN)
- NSAIDs (e.g., ibuprofen 600–800 mg q6–8 hours PRN; peds: 10 mg/kg/dose q6-8 hours PRN)

ISSUES FOR REFERRAL

- Physeal closure (2)[C]
- Unstable lesions with mechanical symptoms (4)[C]
- Failure of conservative treatment after 3–6 months (4)[C]

SURGERY/OTHER PROCEDURES

- Surgical treatment is used when:
  - Conservative measures have failed (4)[C].
  - Physeal closure (adult form) present (2)[C]
  - Unstable lesions with mechanical symptoms (4)[C]
- Arthroscopic surgery is preferred. Arthroscopy can evaluate lesion stability and visualize articular cartilage (4,5)[C].
- Surgical treatments include fragment excision, microfracture technique (drilling) to increase blood supply, screw fixation of the loose fragment, allograft insertion, and autologous chondrocyte implantation. No single technique is superior (4)[C].

ONGOING CARE

FOLLOW-UP RECOMMENDATIONS

- Outpatient care is the usual course.
- Inpatient treatment for surgical intervention

Patient Monitoring

- If followed radiographically, 6 weeks intervals are appropriate to assess for fragment displacement (4)[C].
- Healing is often seen within 6 months (4)[C].
- If postoperative patient remains symptomatic, may be followed with MRI or SPECT/CT to evaluate healing

DIET

Vitamin D supplementation may be considered.

PATIENT EDUCATION

Patients should be encouraged to comply with rehabilitative treatment recommendations in both nonoperative and operative cases.

PROGNOSIS

- Factors associated with good prognosis
  - Younger age
  - Open growth plate
  - Stable lesions
  - Non–weight-bearing location of the lesion
- An incongruous joint surface may lead to degenerative changes in the future.
- Clinical improvement may proceed radiographic healing.

COMPLICATIONS

- Failure to revascularize and heal
- Displacement of a fragment becoming a loose body within a joint
- Predisposition for early osteoarthritis in the affected joint

REFERENCES

1. Abouassaly M, Peterson D, Salci L, et al. Surgical management of osteochondritis dissecans of the knee in the paediatric population: a systematic review addressing surgical techniques. *Knee Surg Sports Traumatol Arthrosc*. 2014;22(6):1216–1224.
2. Pape D, Filardo G, Kon E, et al. Disease-specific clinical problems associated with the subchondral bone. *Knee Surg Sports Traumatol Arthrosc*. 2010;18(4):448–462.
3. McKay S, Chen C, Rosenfeld S. Orthopedic perspective on selected pediatric and adolescent knee conditions. *Pediatr Radiol*. 2013;43(Suppl 1):S99–S106.
4. Edmonds EW, Polousky J. A review of knowledge in osteochondritis dissecans: 123 years of minimal evolution from König to the ROCK study group. *Clin Orthop Relat Res*. 2013;471(4):1118–1126.
5. Kocher MS, Tucker R, Ganley TJ, et al. Management of osteochondritis dissecans of the knee: current concepts review. *Am J Sports Med*. 2006;34(7):1181–1191.

ADDITIONAL READING

- Chambers HG, Shea KG, Anderson AF, et al; American Academy of Orthopaedic Surgeons. American Academy of Orthopaedic Surgeons clinical practice guideline on: the diagnosis and treatment of osteochondritis dissecans. *J Bone Joint Surg Am*. 2012;94(14):1322–1324.
- Hirschmann MT, Davda K, Rasch H, et al. Clinical value of combined single photon emission computerized tomography and conventional computer tomography (SPECT/CT) in sports medicine. *Sports Med Arthrosc Rev*. 2011;19(2):174–181.
- Jacobi M, Wahl P, Bouaicha S, et al. Association between mechanical axis of the leg and osteochondritis dissecans of the knee: radiographic study on 103 knees. *Am J Sports Med*. 2010;38(7):1425–1428.
- Parikh SN, Allen M, Wall EJ, et al. The reliability to determine "healing" in osteochondritis dissecans from radiographic assessment. *J Pediatr Orthop*. 2012;32(6):e35–e39.
- Quatman CE, Quatman-Yates CC, Schmitt LC, et al. The clinical utility and diagnostic performance of MRI for identification and classification of knee osteochondritis dissecans. *J Bone Joint Surg Am*. 2012;94(11):1036–1044.
- Ramirez A, Abril JC, Chaparro M. Juvenile osteochondritis dissecans of the knee: perifocal sclerotic rim as a prognostic factor of healing. *J Pediatr Orthop*. 2010;30(2):180–185.
- Shea KG, Jacobs JC Jr, Carey JL, et al. Osteochondritis dissecans knee histology studies have variable findings and theories of etiology. *Clin Orthop Relat Res*. 2013;471(4):1127–1136.
- Vasiliadis HS, Danielson B, Ljungberg M, et al. Autologous chondrocyte implantation in cartilage lesions of the knee: long-term evaluation with magnetic resonance imaging and delayed gadolinium-enhanced magnetic resonance imaging technique. *Am J Sports Med*. 2010;38(5):943–949.

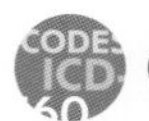

CODES

ICD10

- M93.20 Osteochondritis dissecans of unspecified site
- M93.269 Osteochondritis dissecans, unspecified knee
- M93.229 Osteochondritis dissecans, unspecified elbow

CLINICAL PEARLS

- OCD is an acquired lesion of the subchondral bone, causing separation of the overlying articular cartilage; it may become unstable and require surgical intervention; the knee is the most commonly affected joint.
- Stable juvenile OCD lesions often heal without surgical intervention if patients adhere to appropriate conservative rehabiliitaion program.
- Compliance with conservative therapy and avoidance of further trauma are important elements to ensure proper healing, especially with younger athletes.
- 6-week follow-up intervals are appropriate to assess treatment progress.
- In adult patients with unstable lesions, surgery may be considered as an early treatment option.

OSTEOMYELITIS

Tricia Elaine VanWagner, MD

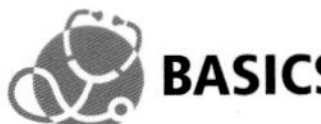

BASICS

DESCRIPTION

- An acute or chronic infection and inflammation of the bone; can occur as a result of hematogenous seeding, contiguous spread of infection, or direct inoculation into intact bone (trauma or surgery)
- 2 major classification systems:
  - Lew and Waldvogel classification
    - Classified according to the duration of the disease (acute or chronic) and the mechanism of infection (hematogenous contiguous)
  - Cierny-Mader classification
    - Based on the portion of bone affected, the physiologic status of the host, and other risk factors
    - Stage 1: medullary bone (typically monomicrobial)
    - Stage 2: bony surface (deep soft tissue infection or ulcer)
    - Stage 3: advance local infection (polymicrobial); often associated with open fracture or infected orthopedic hardware
    - Stage 4: Extensive disease (multiple tissue layers) requires combination medical and surgical therapy.
    - Class A host: otherwise normal
    - Class B host: immunocompromised
    - Class C host: Treatment risk outweighs benefit.
- Special situations
  - Vertebral osteomyelitis
    - Acute, subacute, or chronic
    - May result from hematogenous seeding, direct inoculation, or contiguous spread
    - Back pain is most common initial symptom.
    - Lumbar spine is most commonly involved, followed by thoracic spine.
  - Infections of prosthetic joints
    - Obtaining specific diagnosis and targeted therapy quicker (easy access)
    - X-ray of joint initially done, then 3-phase bone scan, because MRI/CT scans are of limited use in this circumstance
    - Treat with combination of antibiotics, including rifampin, especially in prosthetic joint infections.
  - Posttraumatic infections
    - Depends on type of fracture, level of contamination, and severity of tissue injury
    - Tibia most commonly involved
- System(s) affected: musculoskeletal

EPIDEMIOLOGY

- Predominant age: more common in older adults
- Predominant sex: male > female
- Hematogenous osteomyelitis
  - Adults (most >50 years of age): vertebral
  - Children: long bones
- Contiguous osteomyelitis: related to trauma and surgery in younger adults and decubitus ulcers and infected total joint arthroplasties in older adults

Incidence

Generally low; normal bone is resistant to infection.

Prevalence

Up to 66% of diabetics with foot ulcers

ETIOLOGY AND PATHOPHYSIOLOGY

- Infection is caused by biofilm bacteria, which protects bacteria from antimicrobial agents and host immune responses.
- Acute: suppurative infection of bone with edema and vascular compromise leading to sequestra
- Chronic: presence of necrotic bone or sequestra or recurrence of previous infection
- Hematogenous osteomyelitis (typically monomicrobial)
  - *Staphylococcus aureus* (most common)
  - Coagulase-negative staphylococci and aerobic gram-negative bacteria
  - *Salmonella* sp. (sickle cell disease)
  - *Mycobacterium tuberculosis* and fungi (rare) in endemic areas or in immunocompromised hosts
- Contiguous focus osteomyelitis (commonly polymicrobial)
  - Diabetes or vascular insufficiency
    - Coagulase-positive and coagulase-negative staphylococci
    - Streptococci, gram-negative bacilli, anaerobes (*Peptostreptococcus* sp.)
  - Prosthetic device
    - Coagulase-negative staphylococci and *S. aureus*

RISK FACTORS

- Diabetes mellitus
- Recent trauma/surgery
- Foreign body (e.g., prosthetic implant)
- Neuropathy and vascular insufficiency
- Immunosuppression
- Sickle cell disease
- Injection drug use
- Previous osteomyelitis

GENERAL PREVENTION

- Antibiotic prophylaxis
  - Clean bone surgery
    - Antibiotics should be administered IV within 1 hour prior to skin incision and continued no longer than 24 hours after the operation.
  - Closed fractures
    - Cephazolin, cefuroxime, clindamycin (β-lactam allergy), or vancomycin (β-lactam allergy or MRSA infection)
  - Open fractures
    - In patients who can receive antibiotics within 3 hours of injury with prompt operative treatment, 1st-generation cephalosporins are preferred (clindamycin or vancomycin if allergy exists). Add aminoglycoside if type III fracture and penicillin for anaerobic coverage if farm injury or possible bowel contamination.
- All diabetic patients should have an annual foot examination.

COMMONLY ASSOCIATED CONDITIONS

See "Risk Factors."

DIAGNOSIS

HISTORY

- Fever, chills, lethargy (particularly in children)
- Pain, swelling, erythema in affected area
- Hematogenous osteomyelitis
  - Elicit a history of conditions predisposing to bacteremia (diabetes, renal insufficiency, invasive procedures, IV drug use)
- Contiguous osteomyelitis and vascular insufficiency
  - Recent trauma/surgery within 1–2 months
  - Presence of prosthetic device
  - History of diabetes
- Chronic osteomyelitis
  - History of acute osteomyelitis

PHYSICAL EXAM

- Fever
- Restriction of movement of the involved extremity or refusal to bear weight
- Pain or tenderness in the infected area
- Signs of localized inflammation
- Motor and sensory deficits (vertebral infection)
- Visible defect: probe bone ("positive probe-to-bone test")
- Ulcer >2 cm wide and >3 mm deep increases likelihood in diabetic foot ulcers.
- In patients with diabetes, classic signs and symptoms of infection may be masked due to vascular disease and neuropathy.

DIFFERENTIAL DIAGNOSIS

- Systemic infection from other source
- Aseptic bone infarction
- Localized inflammation or infection of overlying skin and soft tissues (e.g., gout)
- Brodie abscess (subacute osteomyelitis)
- Neuropathic joint disease (Charcot foot)
- Fractures/trauma
- Tumor

DIAGNOSTIC TESTS & INTERPRETATION

Initial Tests (lab, imaging)

Labs

- WBC is not reliable indicator (can be normal even when infection is present).
- CRP is usually elevated but nonspecific.
- ESR is high in most cases:
  - ESR >70 mm/hr increases likelihood of diabetic lower extremity ulcer.
- Drugs that may alter lab results: antimicrobial agents given prior to culture
- Disorders that may alter lab results: immunosuppression (including diabetes), chronic inflammatory disease, other/adjacent sites of infection (1)[C]
- Routine radiography is standard 1st-line imaging: Classic triad for osteomyelitis is demineralization, periosteal reaction, and bone destruction:
  - Bone destruction is not apparent on plain films until after 10–21 days of infection.
  - Bone must undergo 30–50% destruction before damage is evident on films.
- MRI
  - For visualization of septic arthritis, spinal infection, and diabetic foot infections (1)[C]
  - T1-weighted image: low signal intensity
  - T2-weighted image: high signal intensity
  - MRI with gadolinium: sensitivity and specificity range from 60–100% to 50–90%, respectively
- CT
  - Better than standard radiography in fragments and sequestration, but inferior to MRI in soft tissue and bone marrow assessment
  - Useful to define surrounding soft tissues and identify sequestra
  - Bone scan is typically first test after plain x-ray in setting of joint prosthesis.

Follow-Up Tests & Special Considerations

- A persistently elevated CRP (4–6 weeks) can be associated with persistent osteomyelitis.

- Patients receiving prolonged antimicrobial therapy should have the following tests to monitor for adverse reactions:
  - Weekly CBC
  - Liver and kidney function tests
- Radionuclide scanning (e.g., technetium, indium, or gallium) is useful when diagnosis is ambiguous or extent of disease is in question but is limited by low sensitivity and specificity.
- MRI is not helpful in assessing the response to therapy due to persistence of bony edema.

Diagnostic Procedures/Other

- Cultures
  - Definitive diagnosis is made by blood culture (hematogenous) or by needle aspiration/bone biopsy, with subsequent demonstration of the microorganism by culture and sensitivity or histology.
  - Patients with positive blood culture combined with radiographic evidence may not need bone culture.
  - Wound swabs and sinus tract cultures correlate well with the presence of *S. aureus* in deep cultures.
- Image-guided bone biopsy for vertebral osteomyelitis (unless positive blood culture and positive radiographic evidence)

Test Interpretation

Inflammatory process of bone with pyogenic bacteria, necrosis

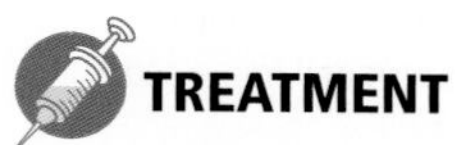

TREATMENT

GENERAL MEASURES

- Adequate nutrition
- Smoking cessation
- Control diabetes

MEDICATION

- Empiric therapy should be directed toward most probable organism and tailored once culture results are available.
- Optimal antimicrobial concentration at infection site is essential (consider vascular perfusion to site).
- Antibiotic dosing altered for renal function
- Duration of therapy 4–6 weeks for acute osteomyelitis and generally >8 weeks for chronic osteomyelitis or MRSA infection
- In children, evidence suggests that early transition from IV to oral therapy, after 3–4 days in patients responding well, followed by oral therapy to a total of 3 weeks may be as effective as longer courses for uncomplicated acute osteomyelitis (2)[B].
- Resistance to fluoroquinolones develops quickly; considered as oral options for chronic suppression

First Line

- *S. aureus* or coagulase-negative staphylococci
  - MSSA: β-lactam at high dose (nafcillin or oxacillin 2 g IV q4h) *or* cefazolin 2 g IV q8h
  - MRSA: vancomycin 15 mg/kg IV q8–12h (use q8h interval if CrCl >70 mL/min) with target trough of 15–20 μg/mL
- *Streptococcus* sp.
  - Ceftriaxone 2 g IV q24h or cefazolin 2 g IV q8h
- *Enterobacter* sp.
  - Fluoroquinolone (levofloxacin 750 mg IV/PO q24h) *or* ceftriaxone 2 g IV q24h
- *Pseudomonas aeruginosa*
  - Cipro 750 mg PO BID or levofloxacin 750 mg PO q24h
- Anaerobes
  - Clindamycin 600 mg IV q8h (300–450 mg PO q6–8h)

Second Line

- *S. aureus*
  - MSSA: fluoroquinolone plus rifampin (levofloxacin 750 mg IV/PO q24h plus rifampin 300 mg PO q12h *or* 600 mg PO q24h)
  - MRSA: linezolid 600 mg PO/IV q12h *or* daptomycin 6 mg/kg IV q24h
- *Streptococcus* sp.
  - Penicillin G 4 million U q4–6h
- *Enterobacter* sp. (quinolone-resistant, including extended-spectrum β-lactamase–producing *Escherichia coli*)
  - Carbapenem (imipenem/cilastatin) 500 mg IV q6h
- *P. aeruginosa*
  - Cefepime or ceftazidime 2 g IV q8h (consider adding aminoglycoside)
- Anaerobes
  - Metronidazole 500 mg IV/PO q6–8h

ADDITIONAL THERAPIES

- Hyperbaric oxygen therapy may be a useful adjunct.
- Negative pressure wound therapy is also a possible adjunctive treatment.

SURGERY/OTHER PROCEDURES

Surgical drainage, dead space management, adequate soft tissue coverage, restoration of blood supply, and removal of necrotic tissues improve cure rates in surgical cases.

Pediatric Considerations

Medullary osteomyelitis (stage 1) in children may be treated without surgical intervention (2)[B].

INPATIENT CONSIDERATIONS

Admission Criteria/Initial Stabilization

Correct electrolyte imbalances, hyperglycemia, azotemia, and acidosis; control pain.

Nursing

Bed rest and immobilization of the involved bone and/or joint

Discharge Criteria

Clinical and laboratory evidence of resolving infection and appropriate outpatient therapy

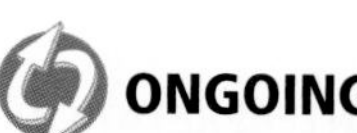

ONGOING CARE

FOLLOW-UP RECOMMENDATIONS

Patient Monitoring

Blood levels of antimicrobial agents, ESR, CRP, and repeat plain radiography as clinical course dictates

PATIENT EDUCATION

Diabetic glycemic control and foot care

PROGNOSIS

- Superficial and medullary osteomyelitis treated with antimicrobial and surgical therapy have a response rate of 90–100%.
- Up to 36% recurrence rate in diabetics
- Increased mortality after amputation

COMPLICATIONS

- Abscess formation
- Bacteremia
- Fracture/nonunion
- Loosening of prosthetic implant
- Postoperative infection
- Sinus tract formation can be associated with neoplasms, especially in presence of long-standing infection.

REFERENCES

1. Malhotra R, Chan CS, Nather A. Osteomyelitis in the diabetic foot. *Diabet Foot Ankle*. 2014;5. doi:10.3402/dfa.v5.24445.
2. Howard-Jones AR, Isaacs D. Systematic review of duration and choice of systemic antibiotic therapy for acute haematogenous bacterial osteomyelitis in children. *J Paediatr Child Health*. 2013;49(9):768–768.

ADDITIONAL READING

- Bhavan KP, Marschall J, Olsen MA, et al. The epidemiology of hematogenous vertebral osteomyelitis: a cohort study in a tertiary care hospital. *BMC Infect Dis*. 2010;10:158.
- Dinh MT, Abad CL, Safdar N. Diagnostic accuracy of the physical examination and imaging tests for osteomyelitis underlying diabetic foot ulcers: meta-analysis. *Clin Infect Dis*. 2008;47(4):519–527.
- Fraimow HS. Systemic antimicrobial therapy in osteomyelitis. *Semin Plast Surg*. 2009;23(2):90–99.
- Sia IG, Berbari EF. Infection and musculoskeletal conditions: osteomyelitis. *Best Pract Res Clin Rheumatol*. 2006;20(6):1065–1081.
- Stumpe KD, Strobel K. Osteomyelitis and arthritis. *Semin Nucl Med*. 2009;39(1):27–35.
- Vardakas KZ, Kontopidis I, Gkegkes ID, et al. Incidence, characteristics, and outcomes of patients with bone and joint infections due to community-associated methicillin-resistant *Staphylococcus aureus*: a systematic review. *Eur J Clin Microbiol Infect Dis*. 2013;32(6):711–721.
- Zimmerli W. Clinical practice. Vertebral osteomyelitis. *N Engl J Med*. 2010;362(11):1022–1029.

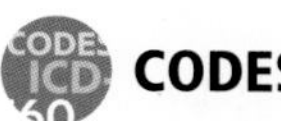

CODES

ICD10

- M86.9 Osteomyelitis, unspecified
- M86.00 Acute hematogenous osteomyelitis, unspecified site
- M86.10 Other acute osteomyelitis, unspecified site

CLINICAL PEARLS

- Hematogenous osteomyelitis is usually monomicrobial, whereas osteomyelitis due to contiguous spread or direct inoculation is usually polymicrobial.
- Acute osteomyelitis typically presents with gradual onset of pain.
- Treatment of osteomyelitis often requires both surgical débridement and at least 6 weeks of antimicrobial therapy.

OSTEOPOROSIS

Nora Gimpel, MD

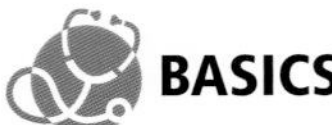

BASICS

DESCRIPTION

A skeletal disease characterized by compromised bone strength that predisposes an individual to an increased risk of fracture

EPIDEMIOLOGY

- Predominant age: elderly >60 years of age
- Predominant sex: female > male (80%/20%)

Incidence

Of persons age >50 years, 9% had osteoporosis at either the femoral neck or lumbar spine.

Prevalence

- 12 million Americans older than 50 years have osteoporosis.
- Women >50 years of age: 24%
- Men >50 years of age: 7.5%
- 50% of postmenopausal women will have an osteoporotic fracture during their lifetime and 15% will experience a hip fracture.

ETIOLOGY AND PATHOPHYSIOLOGY

- Imbalance between bone resorption and bone formation
- Trabecular bone (vertebral) more active than cortical (hip) bone
- Aging
- Hypoestrogenemia

Genetics

- Familial predisposition
- More common in Caucasians and Asians than in African Americans and Hispanics

RISK FACTORS

- Nonmodifiable
  - Advanced age (>65 years)
  - Female gender
  - Caucasian or Asian
  - Family history of osteoporosis
  - History of atraumatic fracture
- Modifiable
  - Low body weight (58 kg or body mass index [BMI] <21)
  - Calcium/vitamin D deficiency
  - Inadequate physical activity
  - Cigarette smoking
  - Excessive alcohol intake (>3 drinks/day)
  - Medications: chronic corticosteroids, excessive thyroid hormone replacement, medroxyprogesterone acetate, heparin, proton pump inhibitors

GENERAL PREVENTION

The aim in the prevention and treatment of osteoporosis is to prevent fracture:

- Depending on the severity of the osteoporosis, between 9 and 60 patients need to be treated for 3 years to prevent 1 vertebral fracture.
- Regularly perform weight-bearing exercise.
- Evidence is insufficient to assess the balance of the benefits and harms of combined vitamin D and calcium supplementation for the primary prevention of fractures in premenopausal women or in men [I statement].
- Evidence is insufficient to assess the balance of the benefits and harms of daily supplementation with greater than 400 IU of vitamin D_3 and greater than 1,000 mg of calcium for the primary prevention of fractures in noninstitutionalized postmenopausal women (1)[B].
- USPSTF recommends against daily supplementation with 400 IU or less of vitamin D_3 and 1,000 mg or less of calcium for the primary prevention of fractures in noninstitutionalized postmenopausal women (1).
- Avoid smoking.
- Limit alcohol consumption (<3 drinks/day).
- Take measures to avoid falls.
- Screen:
  - All women ≥65 years of age (1)[B]
  - Screen women <60 years of age with ≥10-year fracture risk (using the WHO's Fracture Risk Assessment Tool [FRAX]) >9.3%
  - The National Osteoporosis Foundation recommends screening men age >70 years.

COMMONLY ASSOCIATED CONDITIONS

- Malabsorption syndromes: gastrectomy, inflammatory bowel disease, celiac disease
- Hypoestrogenism: menopause, hypogonadism, eating disorders, elite athletes
- Chronic liver disease, hemochromatosis
- Endocrinopathies: hyperparathyroidism, hyperthyroidism, hypercortisolism
- Multiple myeloma, multiple sclerosis, osteomalacia, rheumatoid arthritis, chronic obstructive pulmonary disease (COPD), HIV/AIDS
- Medications: antiepileptics, aromatase inhibitors (raloxifene), SSRI, warfarin, thyroid hormone (in supraphysiologic doses)

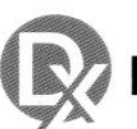

DIAGNOSIS

HISTORY

- Review risk factors.
- Online risk factor assessment tools are available:
  - FRAX (www.sheffield.ac.uk/FRAX)
  - Garvan (http://garvan.org.au/promotions/bone-fracture-risk/calculator/)
- Often no clinical findings until fracture occurs

PHYSICAL EXAM

- Thoracic kyphosis
- Height loss >1.5 cm

DIFFERENTIAL DIAGNOSIS

- Multiple myeloma/other neoplasms
- Osteomalacia
- Type I collagen mutations
- Osteogenesis imperfecta

DIAGNOSTIC TESTS & INTERPRETATION

Dual-energy x-ray absorptiometry (DEXA) of the lumbar spine/hip is considered the gold standard for osteoporosis diagnosis.

Initial Tests (lab, imaging)

Consider in screening for secondary osteoporosis:

- Serum 25-hydroxyvitamin D
- CBC
- Serum chemistry, including serum calcium, phosphorus, total protein, albumin, liver enzymes, creatinine, alkaline phosphatase, electrolytes
- Urinalysis (24-hour collection) for calcium, sodium, and creatinine (to identify calcium malabsorption of hypercalciuria)
- DEXA of the lumbar spine/hip is the gold standard for measuring bone mineral density (BMD) and making a diagnosis of osteoporosis.
- A minimum of 2 years may be needed to reliably measure a change in BMD.
- BMD is expressed in terms of T-scores and *Z*-scores:
  - T-score is the number of standard deviations (*SDs*) a patient's BMD deviates from the mean for young, normal (age 25–40 years) control individuals of the same sex.
  - WHO defines normal BMD as a T-score ≥−1, osteopenia as a T-score between −1 and −2.5, and osteoporosis as a T-score ≤−2.5.
  - WHO thresholds can be used for postmenopausal women and men >50 years of age.
  - The *Z*-score is a comparison of the patient's BMD with an age-matched population.
  - A *Z*-score <−2 should prompt evaluation for causes of secondary osteoporosis.
- Ultrasound densitometry is not as accurate as DEXA, and no studies support its use in determining therapy.
- Plain radiographs lack sensitivity to diagnose osteoporosis, but an abnormality (e.g., widened intervertebral spaces, rib fractures, vertebral compression fractures) should prompt evaluation.

Follow-Up Tests & Special Considerations

Further labs depending on initial evaluation, *Z*-score −2.5 or lower or young age:

- Parathyroid hormone (PTH) and ionized calcium
- Thyroid-stimulating hormone (TSH)
- Testosterone levels (hypogonadism in men)
- Serum protein electrophoresis and free κ and λ light chains (multiple myeloma)
- Urinary-free cortisol (Cushing disease)
- Tissue transglutaminase antibodies (celiac disease)
- Markers of bone resorption (urine *N*-telopeptides of type 1 collagen, serum C-telopeptides of type 1 collagen, serum *N*-terminal propeptide of type 1 procollagen): no prospective studies supporting use in osteoporosis diagnosis and management; potential role for identifying patients at high risk for fracture and monitoring response to therapy

Diagnostic Procedures/Other

Bone biopsy recommended for patients with bone disease and renal failure to establish the correct diagnosis.

Test Interpretation

- Reduced skeletal mass; trabecular bone thinned or lost more than cortical bone
- Osteoclast and osteoblast number variable
- No evidence of other metabolic bone diseases and no increase in unmineralized osteoid
- Bone marrow normal/atrophic

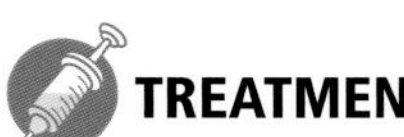

TREATMENT

- Patients with a T-score ≤−2.5 with no risk factors
- All postmenopausal women who have had an osteoporotic vertebral/hip fracture
- All postmenopausal women who have BMD values consistent with osteoporosis (T-score ≤2.5) at the lumbar spine, femoral neck, or total hip region.
- Postmenopausal women with T-scores from −1.0 to −2.5 and a 10-year risk, based on the FRAX calculator, of a major osteoporotic fracture (spine, hip, shoulder, and wrist) of at least 20% or hip of at least 3%
- Treat men >50 years of age who present with a hip or vertebral fracture or a T-score <−2.5 after appropriate evaluation; however, evidence for the effectiveness of treatment of osteoporosis in men is limited.

MEDICATION
Vitamin D 800 IU/day

First Line
- Bisphosphonates
  - Alendronate 10 mg PO daily or 70 mg PO weekly
  - Risedronate 5 mg PO daily, 35 mg PO weekly, 75 mg PO twice monthly, or 150 mg PO monthly
  - Ibandronate 150 mg PO once monthly or 3 mg IV every 3 months
  - Zoledronic acid 5 mg IV yearly
- These drugs become incorporated into skeletal tissue, where they inhibit the resorption of bone by osteoclasts (2,3).
- The evidence on the risk for atrial fibrillation with bisphosphonates is conflicting.
- Osteonecrosis of the jaw has been associated with bisphosphonates, particularly in patients with cancer who receive high doses (4).
- Possible risk of midfemur fractures in patients receiving bisphosphonates for more than 5 years (5)
- Avoid oral bisphosphonates in patients with
  - Delayed esophageal emptying owing to esophageal abnormalities such as achalasia/stricture
  - Inability to stand/sit upright for at least 30–60 minutes after taking the bisphosphonates
  - Hypocalcemia (correct prior to initiating therapy)
  - Severe renal impairment (creatine clearance [CrCl] ≤30 mL/min for risedronate and ibandronate and ≤35 mL/min for alendronate and zoledronic acid)
  - Ibandronate increases bone density but does not appear to decrease fractures.

Second Line
- Raloxifene 60 mg PO daily
  - Selective estrogen receptor modulator with positive effects on BMD and fracture risk but no stimulatory action on breasts/uterus
  - Nonvertebral or hip fracture efficacy has not been demonstrated; increases risk of thromboembolism
  - Additional side effects include menopausal symptoms (hot flashes and night sweats).
- Teriparatide 20 mg SC daily
  - Recombinant formulation of PTH
  - Works anabolically to stimulate the growth of bone through osteoblastic activation
  - Primarily indicated for those with severe osteoporosis that necessitates aggressive therapy
  - Studies have shown a reduction in the incidence of vertebral fractures by 65% and nonvertebral fractures by 54%.
  - No data exist on its safety and efficacy after >2 years of use (6).
- Denosumab: 60 mg SQ every 6 months
  - Human monoclonal antibody receptor activator of nuclear factor kappa-B ligand (RANKL) receptor
  - Inhibits osteoclast formation
- Estrogen 0.625 mg PO daily (with progesterone if patient has a uterus): effective in prevention and treatment of osteoporosis (35% reduction in hip and vertebral fractures after 5 years of use), but the risks (e.g., increased rates of myocardial infarction, stroke, breast cancer, pulmonary embolus, and deep vein thrombosis) must be weighed against the benefits and have decreased interest in this regimen
- Strontium 2 g PO daily
  - Appears to inhibit bone resorption and increase bone formation
  - Available for use in Europe
- Calcitonin
  - PTH antagonist that reduces osteoclastic activity, therefore decreasing bone turnover
  - Has been shown to increase BMD, but no studies have shown conclusively a reduction in the occurrence of fractures
  - Recent FDA panel recommended calcitonin should no longer be used due to minimal evidence of efficacy and association with increased risk of cancer.
  - May decrease acute vertebral compression fracture pain (analgesic)

ISSUES FOR REFERRAL
Endocrinology for recurrent bone loss/fracture

ADDITIONAL THERAPIES
- Weight-bearing exercise 30 minutes 3×/week
- Smoking cessation
- Physical therapy to help with muscle strengthening

SURGERY/OTHER PROCEDURES
Options for patients with painful vertebral compression fractures failing medical treatment:
- Vertebroplasty: Orthopedic cement is injected into the compressed vertebral body.
- Kyphoplasty: A balloon is expanded within the compressed vertebral body to reconstruct volume of vertebrae. Cement is injected into the space.

COMPLEMENTARY & ALTERNATIVE MEDICINE
- Isoflavones not better than placebo for fracture risk
- Beneficial effect of Chinese herbal medicines in improving BMD is still uncertain.

INPATIENT CONSIDERATIONS

Admission Criteria/Initial Stabilization
Inpatient care for pain control of acute back pain secondary to new vertebral fractures and for acute treatment of femoral and pelvic fractures

Discharge Criteria
Rehabilitation, nursing home, or home care may be needed following peripheral fractures.

ONGOING CARE

FOLLOW-UP RECOMMENDATIONS

Patient Monitoring
- Weight-bearing exercises, such as walking, jogging, stair climbing, and tai chi, have been shown to decrease falls.
- All successful studies on the treatment of osteoporosis involve weight-bearing exercise.
- BMD should be tested no earlier than 2 years after starting bisphosphonate. It is uncertain whether repeat DEXA scanning is of value.
- For many women, 5 years of treatment with a bisphosphonate is as good as 10 years of treatment. Those at high risk for vertebral fracture or with very low BMD may benefit by continuing treatment beyond 5 years.
- Physicians prescribing bisphosphonates should advise patients of the small risk of osteonecrosis and encourage dental examinations (7).
- Limited data to guide decision making about "drug holiday." Drug holiday may not be justified for patients at high risk but could be done for patients at low risk.

DIET
- Diet to maintain normal body weight
- Vitamin D (see "General Prevention")

PATIENT EDUCATION
National Osteoporosis Foundation: www.nof.org

PROGNOSIS
- With treatment, 80% of patients stabilize skeletal manifestations, increase bone mass and mobility, and have reduced pain.
- 15% of vertebral and 20–40% of hip fractures may lead to chronic care and/or premature death.

COMPLICATIONS
Severe, disabling pain

REFERENCES

1. http://www.uspreventiveservicestaskforce.org/uspstf/uspsvitd.htm. Accessed 2014.
2. Christenson ES, Jiang X, Kagan R, et al. Osteoporosis management in postmenopausal women. *Minerva Ginecol*. 2012;64(3):181–194.
3. Poole KE, Compston JE. Bisphosphonates in the treatment of osteoporosis. *BMJ*. 2012;344:e3211.
4. Heng C, Badner VM, Johson R, et al. Bisphosphonates-related osteonecrosis of the jaw in patients with osteoporosis. *Am Fam Physician*. 2012;85(12):1134–1141.
5. McClung M, Harris S, Miller P, et al. Bisphosphonates therapy for osteoporosis: benefits, risk, and drug holiday. *Am J Med*. 2013;126(1):13–20.
6. Rao SS, Budhwar N, Ashfaque A, et al. Osteoporosis in men. *Am Fam Physician*. 2010;82(5):503–508.
7. Gómez-de Diego R, Mang-de la Rosa M, Romero-Pérez MJ, et al. Indications and contraindications of dental implants in medically compromised patients: update. *Med Oral Patol Oral Cir Bucal*. 2014;19(5):e483–e489.

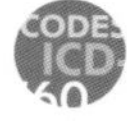

CODES

ICD10
- M81.0 Age-related osteoporosis w/o current pathological fracture
- M80.00XA Age-rel osteopor w current path fracture, unsp site, init
- M80.08XA Age-rel osteopor w current path fracture, vertebra(e), init

CLINICAL PEARLS
- Screen all women ≥65 years of age with DEXA scans.
- Screen both men and women ≥60 years of age at increased risk for osteoporosis with DEXA scans.
- Premenopausal women with osteoporosis should be screened for secondary causes, such as malabsorption syndromes, hyperparathyroidism, hyperthyroidism, and medication sensitivity.
- Evaluate and treat all patients presenting with fractures from minimal trauma.
- If the patient is not responding to treatment, consider screening for a secondary, treatable cause of osteoporosis.

OTITIS EXTERNA

Douglas S. Parks, MD

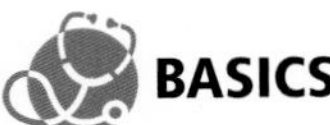

BASICS

DESCRIPTION

Inflammation of the external auditory canal:

- Acute diffuse otitis externa: the most common form; an infectious process, usually bacterial, occasionally fungal (10%)
- Acute circumscribed otitis externa: synonymous with furuncle; associated with infection of the hair follicle, a superficial cellulitic form of otitis externa
- Chronic otitis externa: same as acute diffuse but of longer duration (>6 weeks)
- Eczematous otitis externa: may accompany typical atopic eczema or other primary skin conditions
- Necrotizing malignant otitis externa: an infection that extends into the deeper tissues adjacent to the canal; may include osteomyelitis and cellulitis; rare in children
- System(s) affected: skin/exocrine
- Synonym(s): swimmer's ear

EPIDEMIOLOGY

Incidence

- Unknown; higher in the summer months and in warm, wet climates
- Predominant age: all ages
- Predominant sex: male = female

Prevalence

- Acute, chronic, and eczematous: common
- Necrotizing: uncommon

ETIOLOGY AND PATHOPHYSIOLOGY

- Acute diffuse otitis externa
  - Traumatized external canal (e.g., from use of cotton swab)
  - Bacterial infection (90%): *Pseudomonas* (67%), *Staphylococcus, Streptococcus*, gram-negative rods
  - Fungal infection (10%): *Aspergillus* (90%), *Candida, Phycomycetes, Rhizopus, Actinomyces, Penicillium*
- Chronic otitis externa: bacterial infection: *Pseudomonas*
- Eczematous otitis externa (associated with primary skin disorder)
  - Eczema
  - Seborrhea
  - Psoriasis
  - Neurodermatitis
  - Contact dermatitis
  - Purulent otitis media
  - Sensitivity to topical medications
- Necrotizing otitis externa
  - Invasive bacterial infection: *Pseudomonas*, increasing incidence of methicillin-resistant *Staphylococcus aureus* (MRSA)
  - Associated with immunosuppression

RISK FACTORS

- Acute and chronic otitis externa
  - Traumatization of external canal
  - Swimming
  - Hot, humid weather
  - Hearing aid use
- Eczematous: primary skin disorder
- Necrotizing otitis externa in adults
  - Advanced age
  - Diabetes mellitus (DM)
  - Debilitating disease
  - AIDS
  - Immunosuppression
- Necrotizing otitis externa in children (rare)
  - Leukopenia
  - Malnutrition
  - DM
  - Diabetes insipidus

GENERAL PREVENTION

- Avoid prolonged exposure to moisture.
- Use preventive antiseptics (acidifying solutions with 2% acetic acid [white vinegar] diluted 50/50 with water or isopropyl alcohol, or 2% acetic acid with aluminum acetate [less irritating]) after swimming and bathing.
- Treat predisposing skin conditions.
- Eliminate self-inflicted trauma to canal with cotton swabs and other foreign objects.
- Diagnose and treat underlying systemic conditions.
- Use ear plugs when swimming.

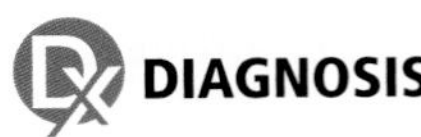

DIAGNOSIS

HISTORY

Variable-length history of itching, plugging of ear, ear pain, and discharge from ear

PHYSICAL EXAM

- Ear canal red, containing purulent discharge and debris
- Pain on manipulation of the pinnae
- Possible periauricular adenitis
- Possible eczema of pinna
- Cranial nerve (VII, IX–XII) involvement (extremely rare)

DIFFERENTIAL DIAGNOSIS

- Idiopathic ear pain
- Otitis media with perforation
- Hearing loss
- Cranial nerve (VII, IX–XII) palsy with necrotizing otitis externa
- Wisdom tooth eruption
- Basal cell or squamous cell carcinoma

DIAGNOSTIC TESTS & INTERPRETATION

- Gram stain and culture of canal discharge (occasionally helpful)
- Antibiotic pretreatment may affect results.
- Radiologic evaluation of deep tissues in necrotizing otitis externa with high-resolution CT scan, MRI, gallium scan, and bone scan

Test Interpretation

- Acute and chronic otitis externa: desquamation of superficial epithelium of external canal with infection
- Eczematous otitis externa: pathologic findings consistent with primary skin disorder; secondary infection on occasion
- Necrotizing otitis externa: vasculitis, thrombosis, and necrosis of involved tissues; osteomyelitis

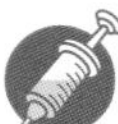

TREATMENT

Outpatient treatment, except for resistant cases and necrotizing otitis externa

GENERAL MEASURES

- Cleaning the external canal may facilitate recovery.
- Analgesics as appropriate for pain
- Antipruritic and antihistamines (eczematous form)
- Ear wick (Pope) for nearly occluded ear canal

MEDICATION

- Resistance is an increasing problem. *Pseudomonas* is the most common bacteria, and it is more susceptible to fluoroquinolones such as ciprofloxacin or ofloxacin, whereas *Staphylococcus* is equally susceptible to both fluoroquinolones and polymyxin B combinations (1)[B]. If a patient has recurring episodes or is not improved in 2 weeks, change the class of antibacterial and consider cultures and sensitivities.
- Oral antibiotics are indicated only if there is associated otitis media. Oral antibiotics alone are not effective and markedly increase the risk of progressing to chronic otitis externa.
- Analgesics as needed; narcotics may be necessary. Recurrent otitis externa may be prevented by applying equal parts white vinegar and isopropyl alcohol (over-the-counter [OTC] rubbing alcohol) to external auditory canals after bathing and swimming.

First Line

- Acute bacterial and chronic otitis externa
  - Ciprofloxacin 0.3% and dexamethasone 0.1% suspension: 4 drops BID × 7 days or ofloxacin: 0.3% solution 10 drops once a day × 7 days (2)[A]. Less ototoxicity and reported antibiotic resistance (3)[A], but branded drugs are far more expensive.
  - Neomycin/polymyxin B/hydrocortisone (Cortisporin): 5 drops QID If the tympanic membrane is ruptured, use the suspension; otherwise, the solution may be used; may be ototoxic and resistance-developing in *Staphylococcus* and *Streptococcus* sp. (4)[B]; least expensive.
  - Acetic acid 2% with hydrocortisone 1%: 3–5 drops q4–6 hours × 7 days; may cause minor local stinging. This is as effective as neomycin–polymyxin B (5)[B] but is expensive. It may take up to 2 days longer to achieve resolution of symptoms (2)[A]. A wick may be helpful in severe cases by keeping the canal open and keeping antibiotic solution in contact with infected skin (6)[C].
- Fungal otitis externa
  - Topical therapy, antiyeast for *Candida* or yeast: 2% acetic acid 3–4 drops QID; clotrimazole 1% solution; itraconazole oral
  - Parenteral antifungal therapy: amphotericin B
  - Patients with Ramsay-Hunt syndrome: acyclovir IV
- Eczematous otitis externa: topical therapy
  - Acetic acid 2% in aluminum acetate
  - Aluminum acetate (5%; Burow solution)
  - Steroid cream, lotion, ointment (e.g., triamcinolone 0.1% solution)
  - Antibacterial, if superinfected

- Necrotizing otitis externa
  - Parenteral antibiotics: antistaphylococcal and antipseudomonal
  - 4–6 weeks of therapy
  - Flouroquinolones PO × 2–4 weeks

Second Line

- Acute bacterial and chronic otitis externa
  - Betamethasone 0.05% solution may be as effective as a polymyxin B combination without the risk of ototoxicity or antibiotic resistance. However, the data are not very robust, and more study is needed (2)[A].
- Azole antifungals for fungal otitis externa

ISSUES FOR REFERRAL

Resistant cases or those requiring surgical intervention

SURGERY/OTHER PROCEDURES

For necrotizing otitis externa or furuncle

COMPLEMENTARY AND ALTERNATIVE MEDICINE

- OTC white vinegar; 3 drops in affected ear for minor case
- Tea tree oil in various concentrations has been used as an antiseptic (7)[B]. Ototoxicity has been reported in animal studies at very high doses.
- Grapefruit seed extract in various concentrations has been described as useful in the lay literature.

INPATIENT CONSIDERATIONS

Admission Criteria/Initial Stabilization

Necrotizing otitis media requiring parenteral antipseudomonal antibiotics

Discharge Criteria

Resolution of infection

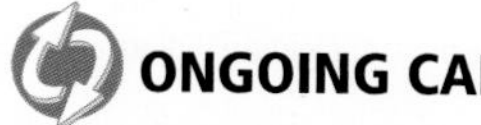

ONGOING CARE

FOLLOW-UP RECOMMENDATIONS

No restrictions

Patient Monitoring

- Acute otitis externa
  - 48 hours after therapy instituted to assess improvement
  - At the end of treatment
- Chronic otitis externa
  - Every 2–3 weeks for repeated cleansing of canal
  - May require alterations in topical medication, including antibiotics and steroids
- Necrotizing otitis externa
  - Daily monitoring in hospital for extension of infection
  - Baseline auditory and vestibular testing at beginning and end of therapy

DIET

No restrictions

PROGNOSIS

- Acute otitis externa: rapid response to therapy with total resolution
- Chronic otitis externa: With repeated cleansing and antibiotic therapy, most cases will resolve. Occasionally, surgical intervention is required for resistant cases.
- Eczematous otitis externa: Resolution will occur with control of the primary skin condition.
- Necrotizing otitis externa: usually can be managed with débridement and antipseudomonal antibiotics; recurrence rate is 100% when treatment is inadequate. Surgical intervention may be necessary in resistant cases or if there is cranial nerve involvement. Mortality rate is significant, probably secondary to the underlying disease.

COMPLICATIONS

- Mainly a problem with necrotizing otitis externa; may spread to infect contiguous bone and CNS structures
- Acute otitis externa may spread to pinna, causing chondritis.

REFERENCES

1. Dohar JE, Roland P, Wall GM, et al. Differences in bacteriologic treatment failures in acute otitis externa between ciprofloxacin/dexamethasone and neomycin/polymyxin B/hydrocortisone: results of a combined analysis. *Curr Med Res Opin.* 2009;25(2):287–291.
2. Kaushik V, Malik T, Saeed SR. Interventions for acute otitis externa. *Cochrane Database Syst Rev.* 2010;(1):CD004740.
3. Mösges R, Nematian-Samani M, Hellmich M, et al. A meta-analysis of the efficacy of quinolone containing otics in comparison to antibiotic-steroid combination drugs in the local treatment of otitis externa. *Curr Med Res Opin.* 2011;27(10):2053–2060.
4. Cantrell HF, Lombardy EE, Duncanson FP, et al. Declining susceptibility to neomycin and polymyxin B of pathogens recovered in otitis externa clinical trials. *South Med J.* 2004;97(5):465–471.
5. van Balen FA, Smit WM, Zuithoff NP. Clinical efficacy of three common treatments in acute otitis externa in primary care: randomised controlled trial. *BMJ.* 2003;327(7425):1201–1205.
6. Block SL. Otitis externa: providing relief while avoiding complications. *J Fam Pract.* 2005;54(8):669–676.
7. Farnan TB, McCallum J, Awa A, et al. Tea tree oil: in vitro efficacy in otitis externa. *J Laryngol Otol.* 2005;119(3):198–201.

ADDITIONAL READING

Rosenfeld RM, Schwartz SP, Cannon CR, et al. Clinical practice guideline: acute otitis externa. *Otolaryngol Head Neck Surg.* 2014;150(1)(Suppl);S1–S24.

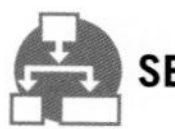

SEE ALSO

Algorithm: Ear Pain

CODES

ICD10

- H60.90 Unspecified otitis externa, unspecified ear
- H60.339 Swimmer's ear, unspecified ear
- H60.509 Unsp acute noninfective otitis externa, unspecified ear

CLINICAL PEARLS

- Acute diffuse otitis externa is the most common form: bacterial (90%), occasionally fungal (10%).
- Acute circumscribed otitis externa is associated with infection of a hair follicle.
- Chronic otitis externa is the same as acute diffuse but of longer duration (>6 weeks).
- Eczematous otitis externa may accompany typical atopic eczema or other primary skin conditions.
- Necrotizing malignant otitis externa is an infection that extends into the deeper tissues adjacent to the canal. It may include osteomyelitis and cellulitis; it is rare in children.

OTITIS MEDIA

Robert A. Baldor, MD, FAAFP

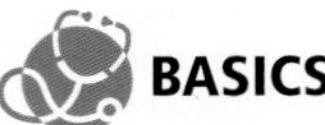

BASICS

DESCRIPTION

- Inflammation of the middle ear; usually accompanied by fluid collection
- Acute otitis media (AOM): inflammation of the middle ear. Rapid onset; cause may be infectious, either viral (AOM-v) or bacterial (AOM-b), but there is also a sterile etiology (AOM-s).
- Recurrent AOM: ≥3 episodes in 6 months or ≥4 episodes in 1 year
- Otitis media with effusion (OME): persistent middle ear fluid that is associated with AOM but can arise without prior AOM
- Chronic otitis media with or without cholesteatoma
- System(s) affected: nervous; ENT
- Synonym(s): secretory or serous otitis media

EPIDEMIOLOGY

Incidence

- AOM
  - Predominant age: 6–24 months; declines >7 years; rare in adults
  - Predominant sex: male > female
  - By age 7 years, 93% of children have had ≥1 episodes of AOM; 39% have had ≥6.
  - Placement of tympanostomy tubes is 2nd only to circumcision as the most frequent surgical procedure in infants.
  - Increased incidence in the fall and winter
- OME
  - By age 4 years, 90% of children have had at least 1 episode

Prevalence

- Most common infection for which antibacterial agents are prescribed in the United States
- Diagnosed 5 million times per year in the United States

ETIOLOGY AND PATHOPHYSIOLOGY

- AOM-b (bacterial): usually, a preceding viral upper respiratory infection (URI) produces eustachian tube dysfunction
  - *Streptococcus pneumoniae*: 20–35%, *Haemophilus influenzae*: 20–30%, *Moraxella* (*B.*) *catarrhalis*: 15%, group A streptococci: 3%, *Staphylococcus aureus*: 12% produce β-lactamases that hydrolyze amoxicillin and some cephalosporins.
- AOM-v (viral): 15–44% of AOM infections are caused primarily by viruses (e.g., respiratory syncytial virus, parainfluenza, influenza, enteroviruses, adenovirus, human metapneumovirus, and parechovirus).
- AOM-s (sterile/nonpathogens): 25–30%
- OME: Eustachian tube dysfunction; allergic causes are rarely substantiated.

Genetics

- Strong genetic component in twin studies for recurrent and prolonged AOM
- May be influenced by skull configuration or immunologic defects

RISK FACTORS

- Premature birth
- Bottlefeeding while supine
- Routine daycare attendance
- Frequent pacifier use after 6 months of age
- Smoking in household; environmental smoke exposure
- Male gender
- Native American/Inuit ethnicity
- Low socioeconomic status
- Family history of recurrent otitis
- AOM before age 1 year is a risk for recurrent AOM
- Presence of siblings in the household
- Underlying ENT disease (e.g., cleft palate, Down syndrome, allergic rhinitis)

GENERAL PREVENTION

- Pneumococcal vaccine (PCV)-7 immunization reduces the number of cases of AOM by about 6–28% (however, evidence shows that this is offset by an increase in AOM caused by other bacteria). The effect of the introduction of the PCV-13 vaccine on the incidence of AOM has yet to be studied (1)[B].
- Influenza vaccine reduces AOM.
- Breastfeeding for ≥6 months is protective.
- Avoiding supine bottlefeeding, passive smoke, and pacifiers >6 months may be helpful.
- Secondary prevention: Adenoidectomy and adenotonsillectomy for recurrent AOM has limited short-term efficacy and is associated with its own adverse risks.
- Vitamin D supplementation (1,000 U/day to maintain vitamin D levels >30) may be helpful in reducing recurrent AOM (2)[B].

COMMONLY ASSOCIATED CONDITIONS

URI

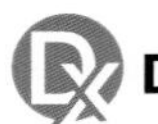

DIAGNOSIS

HISTORY

- AOM: acute history, signs, and symptoms of middle ear inflammation and effusion
  - Earache
  - Preceding or accompanying URI symptoms
  - Decreased hearing
- In adults, earache without fever or hearing loss may be the only presenting feature.

ALERT

- AOM in infants and toddlers:
  - May cause few symptoms in the 1st few months of life
  - Irritability may be the only symptom.
- OME: usually asymptomatic
  - Decreased hearing

PHYSICAL EXAM

- Infectious AOM:
  - Fever (although it is debatable whether OM itself causes fever or fever is due to accompanying viral illness)
  - Decreased eardrum mobility (with pneumatic otoscopy)
  - Eardrum bulging, cloudy, distinctly red; presence of air-fluid level behind the tympanic membrane
  - Redness alone is not a reliable sign.
  - Otorrhea if eardrum is perforated
- OME:
  - Eardrum often dull but not bulging
  - Decreased eardrum mobility (pneumatic otoscopy)
  - Presence of air-fluid level
  - Weber test is positive to affected ear for an ear with effusion.

DIFFERENTIAL DIAGNOSIS

- Tympanosclerosis
- Trauma
- Referred pain from the jaw, teeth, or throat
- TMJ in adults
- Otitis externa
- Otitis-conjunctivitis syndrome
- Temporal arteritis in adults

DIAGNOSTIC TESTS & INTERPRETATION

Initial Tests (lab, imaging)

WBC count may be higher in bacterial AOM than in sterile AOM, but this is almost never useful.

Diagnostic Procedures/Other

- To document the presence of middle ear fluid, pneumatic otoscopy can be supplemented with tympanometry and acoustic reflex measurement.
- Hearing testing is recommended when hearing loss persists for ≥3 months or at any time suspecting language delay, significant hearing loss, or learning problems.
- Language testing should be performed for children with hearing loss.
- Tympanocentesis for microbiologic diagnosis is recommended for treatment failures; may be followed by myringotomy

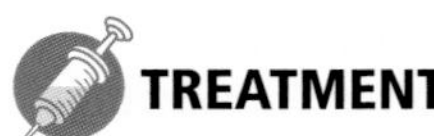

TREATMENT

- Significant disagreement exists about the usefulness of antibiotic treatment for this often self-resolving condition. Studies suggest that ~15 children need to be treated with antibiotics to prevent 1 case of persisting AOM pain at 1–2 weeks; the number needed to treat to cause harm (primarily diarrhea) is 8–10.
- If antibiotics are not used, 81% of patients >2 years of age are better in 1 week versus 94% if antibiotics are used.
- Delay of antibiotics found a modest increase in mastoiditis from 2/100,000 to 4/100,000.
- American Academy of Pediatrics/American Academy of Family Physicians (AAP/AAFP) guidelines recommend the following for observation versus antibacterial therapy, although these guidelines are not rigorously evidence based:
  - <6 months of age: Antibacterial therapy should be administered to any child, regardless of the degree of diagnostic certainty.
  - >6 months: Antibacterial therapy is recommended when the diagnosis of AOM is certain and the illness is severe (i.e., moderate to severe otalgia or fever ≥39°C in the previous 24 hours).
  - Observation is an option when the diagnosis is certain, but illness is not severe, and in patients with an uncertain diagnosis.
- OME: Watchful waiting for 3 months per AAP/AFPP guidelines for those not at risk (see "Complications"). Of these cases, 25–90% will recover spontaneously over this period. No benefit of antihistamines or decongestants or antibiotics or systemic steroids. Autoinflation may be beneficial (3)[A],(4)[B].

GENERAL MEASURES

- Assess pain.
- Although unusual in adults, the treatment is the same.
- Acetaminophen, ibuprofen, benzocaine drops (additional but brief benefit over acetaminophen)

MEDICATION

First Line

- AOM: AAP/AAFP consensus guideline recommends amoxicillin, 80–90 mg/kg/day in 2 divided doses; (5)[A] *OR*

- Amoxicillin-clavulanate 90 mg/kg/day of amoxicillin, with 6.4 mg/kg/day of clavulanate in 2 divided doses; recommended in children who have taken amoxicillin in the previous 30 days and those with concurrent conjunctivitis or history of AOM unresponsive to amoxicillin
- Treatment duration: 10-day course for children <2 years; 7-day course for children 2–5 years; 5–7-day course for children 6 years and older
- If penicillin allergic:
  - Non–type 1 hypersensitivity reaction: cefdinir, 14 mg/kg/day in 1–2 doses; cefpodoxmine, 10 mg/kg/day BID; or cefuroxime 30 mg/kg/day BID
  - Type 1 hypersensitivity to penicillin: azithromycin (10 mg/kg/day [max dose 500 mg/day] as a single dose on day 1 and 5 mg/kg/day [max dose 250 mg/day] for days 2–5)
- A single dose of parenteral ceftriaxone (50 mg/kg) is as effective as a full course of antibiotics in uncomplicated AOM.
- A single dose of azithromycin has been approved by the FDA, but studies did not include otitis-prone children or have criteria for AOM diagnosis.

- Consider treatment of children between ages 6 months and 2 years with antibiotics to reduce duration of symptoms (6)[A].

- OME: See "General Measures"; no benefit to treatment. Medications promote transitory resolution in 10–15%, but the effect is short-lived.

Second Line

- Alternative antibiotics are indicated for the following AOM patients:
  - Persistent symptoms after 48–72 hours of amoxicillin
  - AOM within 1 month of amoxicillin therapy
  - Severe earache
  - Age <6 months with high fever
  - Immunocompromised
    - Amoxicillin-clavulanate, 90 mg/kg–6.4 mg/kg/day, divided BID
    - Ceftriaxone, 50 mg/kg IM or IV q24h for 3 consecutive days can be reserved for those who are too sick to take oral medications or who unsuccessfully took amoxicillin-clavulanate. Neither erythromycin-sulfisoxazole nor trimethoprim-sulfamethoxazole should be used as a second-line agent in treatment failures.
- Recurrent AOM: Antibiotic prophylaxis for recurrent AOM (>3 distinct, well-documented episodes in 6 months) is not recommended.

SURGERY/OTHER PROCEDURES

- Recurrent AOM: Consider referral for surgery if ≥3 episodes of well-documented AOM within 6 months, ≥4 episodes within 12 months, or AOM episodes occur while on chemoprophylaxis.

- Tympanostomy tubes may be effective in selective patients, particularly children age <2 years with recurrent AOM (7)[A].

- Adenoidectomy has limited or no effect.
- Adenotonsillectomy reduced the rate of AOM by 0.7 episode per child only in the 1st year after surgery and had a 15% complications rate.
- OME: Referral for surgery for tympanostomy should be individualized. It can be considered if >4–6 months of bilateral OME and/or >6 months of unilateral OME and/or hearing loss >25 dB or for high-risk individuals at any time.

- Tympanostomy tubes may reduce recurrence of AOM minimally, but it does not lower the risk of hearing loss (8)[A].

- Adenoidectomy is indicated in specific cases; tonsillectomy or myringotomy is never indicated.

COMPLEMENTARY & ALTERNATIVE MEDICINE

- It is unclear whether alternative and homeopathic therapies are effective for AOM, including mixed evidence about the effectiveness of zinc supplementation of reducing AOM.
- Xylitol, probiotics, herbal ear drops, and homeopathic interventions may be beneficial in reducing pain duration, antibiotic use, and bacterial resistance.

INPATIENT CONSIDERATIONS

Admission Criteria/Initial Stabilization

Outpatient, except if surgery is indicated, or for AOM in febrile infants age <2 months or children requiring ceftriaxone who also require monitoring for 24 hr

ONGOING CARE

FOLLOW-UP RECOMMENDATIONS

Patients with otitis media who do not respond within 48–72 hours should be reevaluated:

- If therapy was delayed and diagnosis is confirmed, start therapy with high-dose amoxicillin.
- If therapy was initiated, consider changing the antibiotic; options are limited because macrolides have limited benefit against *Haemophilus influenzae* over amoxicillin, and most oral cephalosporins have no improved outcomes.

Patient Monitoring

- AOM: Up to 40% may have persistent middle ear effusion at 1 month, with 10–25% at 3 months.
- OME: Repeat otoscopic or tympanometric exams at 3 months, as indicated, as long as OME persists or sooner if there are red flags (see earlier discussion).

PROGNOSIS

- See "General Measures."
- Recurrent AOM and OME: usually subsides in school-aged children; few have complications.

COMPLICATIONS

- AOM: Serious complications are rare: tympanic membrane perforation/otorrhea, acute mastoiditis, facial nerve paralysis, otitic hydrocephalus, meningitis, hearing impairment.
- OME: Speech and language disabilities may occur. Hearing loss is not caused by OME, but in children who are at risk for speech, language, or learning problems (e.g., autism spectrum, syndromes, craniofacial disorders, developmental delay, and children already with speech/language delay), it could lead to further problems because they are less tolerant of a hearing impairment.
- Recurrent AOM and OME: atrophy and scarring of eardrum, chronic perforation and otorrhea, cholesteatoma, permanent hearing loss, chronic mastoiditis, other intracranial suppurative complications

REFERENCES

1. Eskola J, Kilpi T, Palmu A. Efficacy of a pneumococcal conjugate vaccine against acute otitis media. *N Engl J Med*. 2001;344(6):403–409.
2. Marchioso P, Consonni D, Baggi E. Vitamin D supplementation reduces the risk of acute otitis media in otitis-prone children. *Pediatr Infect Dis J*. 2013;32(10):1055–1060.
3. Coleman C, Moore M. Decongestants and antihistamines for acute otitis media in children. *Cochrane Database Syst Rev*. 2008;(3):CD001727.
4. Perera R, Glasziou PP, Heneghan CJ, et al. Autoinflation for hearing loss associated with otitis media with effusion. *Cochrane Database Syst Rev*. 2013;5:CD006285.
5. Thanaviratananich S, Laopaiboon M, Vatanasapt P. Once or twice daily versus three times daily amoxicillin with or without clavulanate for the treatment of acute otitis media. *Cochrane Database Syst Rev*. 2008;(4):CD004975.
6. Hoberman A, Paradise JL, Rockette HE, et al. Treatment of acute otitis media in children under 2 years of age. *N Engl J Med*. 2011;364(2):105–115.
7. Kujala T, Alho OP, Luotonen J, et al. Tympanostomy with and without adenoidectomy for the prevention of recurrences of acute otitis media: a randomized controlled trial. *Pediatr Infect Dis J*. 2012;31(6):565–569.
8. Lous J, Burton MJ, Felding JU. Grommets (ventilation tubes) for hearing loss associated with otitis media with effusion in children. *Cochrane Database Syst Rev*. 2005;(1):CD001801.

ADDITIONAL READING

Gould JM, Matz PS. Otitis media. *Pediatr Rev*. 2010;31(3):102–116.

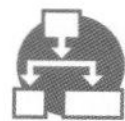

SEE ALSO

Algorithm: Ear Pain

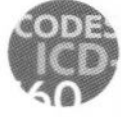

CODES

ICD10

- H66.90 Otitis media, unspecified, unspecified ear
- H66.40 Suppurative otitis media, unspecified, unspecified ear
- H65.199 Other acute nonsuppurative otitis media, unspecified ear

CLINICAL PEARLS

- Pneumatic otoscopy is the single most specific and clinically useful test for diagnosis.
- Consider a delay of antibiotics for 24–48 hours in uncomplicated presentations (>2 years of age) who do not have severe illness.
- First-line treatment is amoxicillin, 80–90 mg/kg/day for 10 days for children age <2 years; consider a 5–7-day course in >2 years of age.
- Erythema and effusion can persist for weeks.
- Antibiotics, antihistamines, and steroids are not indicated for OME.
- OME rarely develops in adults. Persistent unilateral effusion should be investigated to rule out neoplasm, particularly if there is a cranial nerve palsy.

OTITIS MEDIA WITH EFFUSION

Robyn Heidenreich, MD • Hobart Lee, MD

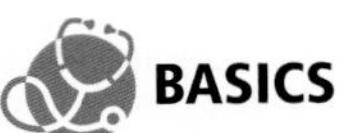

BASICS

DESCRIPTION

- Also called serous otitis media, mucoid otitis media, or "glue ear"
- Otitis media with effusion (OME) is defined as the presence of fluid in the middle ear in the absence of acute signs or symptoms of infection.
- More commonly, a pediatric disease
- May occur spontaneously from poor eustacian tube function or as an inflammatory response after acute otitis media

EPIDEMIOLOGY

Incidence

Approximately 90% of children have OME before school age, mostly between the ages of 6 months and 4 years.

Prevalence

- Approximately 2.2 million new cases annually in the United States
- Less prevalent in adults and is usually associated with an underlying disorder

ETIOLOGY AND PATHOPHYSIOLOGY

- Chronic inflammatory condition where an underlying stimulus causes an inflammatory reaction with increased mucin production creating a functional blockage of the eustachian tube and thick accumulation of mucin-rich middle ear effusion
- Young children are more prone to OME due to shorter and more horizontal eustachian tubes, which become more vertical around 7 years of age.
- Biofilms, anatomic variations, and acute otitis media (AOM) caused by viruses or bacteria have been implicated as stimuli causing OME. The common pathogens causing AOM include nontypeable *Haemophilus influenzae*, *Streptococcus pneumoniae*, and *Moraxella catarrhalis*.
- In adults, OME is often associated with paranasal sinus disease (66%), smoking-induced nasopharyngeal lymphoid hyperplasia and adult onset adenoidal hypertrophy (19%), or head and neck tumors (4.8%).

RISK FACTORS

- Risk factors include a family history of OME, early daycare, exposure to cigarette smoke, bottle-feeding, and low socioeconomic status (1).
- Eustachian tube dysfunction may be a predisposing factor, though the evidence is unclear (2).
- Gastroesophageal reflux is associated with OME (2).

GENERAL PREVENTION

OME is generally not preventable, although lowering smoke exposure, breastfeeding, and avoiding daycare centers at an early age may decrease the risk (3).

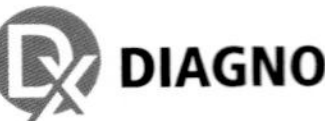

DIAGNOSIS

HISTORY

- OME is transient and asymptomatic in many pediatric patients.
- Most common reported symptom is hearing loss (2). There may be mild discomfort present in the ear, fullness, or "popping" (1).
- Infants may have ear rubbing, excessive irritability, sleep problems, or failure to respond appropriately to voices or sounds (1).
- Clinical features may include "a history of hearing difficulties, poor attention, behavioral problems, delayed speech and language development, clumsiness, and poor balance" (2).
- There may be a history of recent or recurrent episodes of acute otitis media or a recent upper respiratory tract infection (2).

PHYSICAL EXAM

- Cloudy tympanic membrane (TM) with distinctly impaired mobility. Air-fluid level or bubble may be visible in the middle ear (1,2).
- Color may be abnormal (yellow, amber, or blue), and the TM may be retracted or concave (2).
- Distinct redness of the tympanic membrane may be present in approximately 5% of OME cases (1).
- Clinical signs and symptoms of acute illness should be absent in patients with OME (1).

DIFFERENTIAL DIAGNOSIS

- Acute otitis media
- Bullous myringitis
- Tympanosclerosis (may cause decreased/absent motion of the TM)
- Sensorineural hearing loss

DIAGNOSTIC TESTS & INTERPRETATION

Diagnostic Procedures/Other

- The primary standard to make the diagnosis is pneumatic otoscopy, which demonstrates reduced/absent mobility of the TM secondary to fluid in the middle ear. Pneumatic otoscopy has 94% sensitivity and 80% specificity for diagnosing OME. Accuracy of diagnosis with an experienced examiner is between 70% and 79% (1)[C].
- Myringotomy is the gold standard but is not practical for clinical use (2)[C].
- Tympanometry may also be used to support or exclude the diagnosis in infants older than 4 months old, especially when the presence of middle ear effusion is difficult to determine (1)[C].
- Acoustic reflectometry (64% specificity and 80% sensitivity) may be considered instead of tympanometry (4)[B].
- Audiogram may show mild conductive hearing loss (2)[C].
- Hearing tests are recommended for OME lasting more than 3 months (1)[C].
- Language testing is recommended for children with abnormal hearing tests (1)[C].

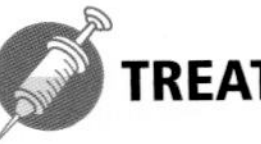

TREATMENT

- OME improves or resolves without medical intervention in most patients within 3 months, especially if secondary to AOM (1)[C].
- Current guidelines support a 3-month period of observation with optional serial exams, tympanometry, and language assessment during that wait time (1,2)[C].
- Adults found to have OME should be screened for an underlying disorder and treated accordingly (2)[C].

MEDICATION

- The 2004 AAFP/AAOHNS/AAP guideline and a 2012 Cochrane review recommend against routine use of antibiotics in treatment of OME. No long-term benefits of antibiotics have been proven, and often prescribed antibiotics have adverse side effects such as diarrhea, vomiting, rashes, and allergic reactions (1)[C],(6)[A].
- The 2004 AAFP/AAOHNS/AAP and a 2006 Cochrane review found that antihistamines and decongestants have no benefit over placebo in the treatment of OME with possible adverse side effects such as insomnia, hyperactivity, and drowsiness (1)[C],(6)[A].
- The 2004 AAFP/AAOHNS/AAP guideline recommends against administering oral or intranasal corticosteroids. No long-term benefit was shown and adverse side effects such as weight gain and behavioral changes are possible (1)[C].
- In adults, eustachian tube dysfunction secondary to allergic rhinitis or recent upper respiratory infection can be the cause of OME. It is unknown whether decongestants, antihistamines, or nasal steroids improve outcomes in adults.

ISSUES FOR REFERRAL

The following are indications for referral to a surgeon for evaluation of tympanostomy tube placement (8)[C]:

- Chronic bilateral OME (≥3 months) with hearing difficulty
- Chronic OME with symptoms (e.g. vestibular problems, poor school performance, behavioral issues, ear discomfort, or reduced quality of life)
- At-risk children (speech, language, or learning problems due to baseline sensory, physical, cognitive, or behavioral factors) with chornic OME or type B (flat) tympanogram

ADDITIONAL THERAPIES

- Hearing aids may be an acceptable alternative to surgery (2)[C].
- Autoinflation, which refers to the process of opening the eustachian tube by raising intranasal pressure (e.g., by forced exhalation with closed mouth and nose) may be beneficial in improving patients' tympanogram or audiometry results beyond 1 month (8)[A].

SURGERY/OTHER PROCEDURES

- Tympanostomy tubes are recommended as initial surgery. Risks include purulent otorrhea, myringosclerosis, retraction pockets, and persistent tympanic membrane perforations (1,2)[C].
- Adenoidectomy with myringotomy has similar efficacy to tympanostomy tubes in children older than 4 years of age but with added surgical and anesthesic risks (1)[C].
- Adenoidectomy should not be performed in children with persistent OME alone unless there is a distinct indication for the procedure for another problem (e.g., adenoiditis/chronic sinusitis/nasal obstruction) (1)[C].
- Adenoidectomy (and concurrent tube placement) may be considered when repeat surgery for OME is necessary (e.g., when effusion recurs after tubes have fallen out or are removed). In these cases, adenoidectomy has been shown to decrease the need for future procedures for OME (1,2)[C].
- Tonsillectomy or myringotomy alone is not recommended for treatment (1)[C].

ONGOING CARE

FOLLOW-UP RECOMMENDATIONS

Patient Monitoring

- Children who are at risk for speech, language, or learning problems and whose OME persists for ≥3 months should undergo hearing evaluation (1)[C].
- Reevaluation and repeat hearing tests should be performed every 3–6 months until the effusion has resolved or until the child develops an indication for surgical referral (1)[C].

PROGNOSIS

Approximately 50% of children older than 3 years of age have OME resolution within 3 months.

COMPLICATIONS

- The most significant complication of OME is permanent hearing loss, leading to possible language, speech, and developmental delays.
- Underventilation of the middle ear can cause a cholesteatoma (1)[C].

REFERENCES

1. American Academy of Family Physicians, American Academy of Otolaryngology-Head and Neck Surgery, American Academy of Pediatrics Subcommittee on Otitis Media With Effusion. Otitis media with effusion. *Pediatrics*. 2004;113(5):1412–1429.
2. Qureishi A, Lee Y, Belfield K, et al. Update on otitis media - prevention and treatment. *Infect Drug Resist*. 2014;10:15–24.
3. Owen MJ, Baldwin CD, Swank PR, et al. Relation of infant feeding practices, cigarette smoke exposure, and group child care to the onset and duration of otitis media with effusion in the first two years of life. *J Pediatr*. 1993;123(5):702–711.
4. Shekelle P, Takata G, Chan, LS, et al. Diagnosis, natural history, and late effects of otitis media with effusion. *Evid Rep Technol Assess (Summ)*. 2002;(55):1–5.
5. van Zon A, Van der Heijden GJ, van Dongen TM, et al. Antibiotics for otitis media with effusion in children. *Cochrane Database Syst Rev*. 2012;9:CD009163.
6. Griffin G, Flynn CA. Antihistamines and/or decongestants for otitis media with effusion (OME) in children. *Cochrane Database Syst Rev*. 2011;(9):CD003423.
7. Rosenfeld RM, Schwartz SR, Pynnonen MA, et al. Clinical practice guideline: tympanostomy tubes in children. *Otolaryngol Head Neck Surg*. 2013;149(Suppl 1):8–16.
8. Perera R, Haynes J, Glasziou P, et al. Autoinflation for hearing loss associated with otitis media with effusion. *Cochrane Database Syst Rev*. 2006;(4):CD006285.

ADDITIONAL READING

- Browning GG, Rovers MM, Williamson I, et al. Grommets (ventilation tubes) for hearing loss associated with otitis media with effusion in children. *Cochrane Database Syst Rev*. 2010;(10):CD001801.
- Casselbrant ML, Mandel EM, Rockette HE, et al. Adenoidectomy for otitis media with effusion in 2-3-year-old children. *Int J Pediatr Otorhinolaryngol*. 2009;73(12):1718–1724.
- Simpson SA, Lewis R, van der Voort J, et al. Oral or topical nasal steroids for hearing loss associated with otitis media with effusion in children. *Cochrane Database Syst Rev*. 2011;(5):CD001935.

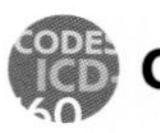

CODES

ICD10

- H65.90 Unspecified nonsuppurative otitis media, unspecified ear
- H65.00 Acute serous otitis media, unspecified ear
- H65.20 Chronic serous otitis media, unspecified ear

CLINICAL PEARLS

- Otitis media with effusion (OME) is defined as the presence of a middle ear effusion in the absence of acute signs of infection.
- In children, OME most often arises following an acute otitis media. In adults, it often occurs in association with eustachian tube dysfunction.
- The primary standard for diagnosis is pneumatic otoscopy.
- There is no benefit to the the routine use of antibiotics, antihistamines, decongestants, or corticosteroids for the treatment of OME in children.
- Management includes watchful waiting and surgery (when indicated); which strategy is chosen depends on many factors, including the risk/presence of any associated speech, language, or learning delays and on the severity of any associated hearing loss.

OVARIAN CANCER

Susan Zweizig, MD • Celeste Straight, MD

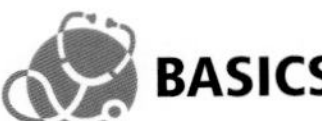

BASICS

There are >22,000 new cases of ovarian cancer annually, and >15,000 women will die of their disease, making this the most lethal of gynecologic cancers.

DESCRIPTION

Malignancy that arises from the epithelium (90%), stroma, or germ cells of the ovary; also, tumors metastatic to the ovary; histologic types include the following:

- Epithelial
  - Serous (tubal epithelium)
  - Mucinous (cervical and GI mucinous epithelium)
  - Endometrioid (endometrial epithelium)
  - Clear cell (mesonephroid)
  - Brenner (transitional cell epithelium)
  - Carcinosarcoma
- Stromal
  - Granulosa cell tumor
  - Theca cell tumor
  - Sertoli–Leydig cell tumors
  - Gynandroblastoma
  - Lipid cell tumor
- Germ cell
  - Teratoma (immature)
  - Dysgerminoma
  - Embryonal carcinoma
  - Gonadoblastoma
  - Endodermal sinus tumor
  - Embryonal carcinoma
  - Choriocarcinoma
- Metastatic disease from the following:
  - Breast
  - Endometrium
  - Lymphoma
  - GI tract (Krukenberg tumor)
  - Primary peritoneal
- System(s) affected: GI; reproductive; endocrine; metabolic

EPIDEMIOLOGY

Incidence

- 21,990 new cases/year in the United States; 15,460 deaths/year
- Leading cause of gynecologic cancer death in women; mortality from ovarian cancer has decreased only slightly during the past 4 decades (1)[A]
- 75% diagnosed at advanced stage
- Predominant age
  - Epithelial: mid 50s
  - Germ cell malignancies: usually observed in patients <20 years of age

Prevalence

Lifetime risk for general population: 1 in 70 women develop ovarian cancer.

ETIOLOGY AND PATHOPHYSIOLOGY

- Malignant transformation of the ovarian epithelium from repeated trauma during ovulation may lead to this change. Many of these cancers originate in the distal fallopian tube.
- Most ovarian cancer (75%) presents as advanced disease. Metastatic disease may develop at the same time as the primary tumor (1).

Genetics

- Hereditary breast/ovarian cancer syndrome: early-onset breast or ovarian cancer, autosomal dominant transmission, usually associated with *BRCA-1* or *BRCA-2* mutation
- Lynch II syndrome: autosomal dominant inheritance; increased risk for colorectal, endometrial, stomach, small bowel, breast, pancreas, and ovarian cancers; defect in mismatch repair genes

RISK FACTORS

- 90% of ovarian cancer is sporadic and not inherited, but family history is the most significant risk factor. Multiple relatives with breast or ovarian cancer increases risk: Refer these patients for genetic counseling. Individuals in families with familial cancer syndromes have 20–60% risk of developing ovarian cancer.
- Nulligravidity (or infertility), early menarche, late menopause, endometriosis
- Environmental (talc, smoking, obesity)

GENERAL PREVENTION

For epithelial cancer, frequency of ovulation appears to be important. The following factors are *protective* (1)[A]:

- Use of oral contraceptives: 5 years of use decreases risk by 20%; 15 years by 50%.
  - The progestin component of oral contraceptive preparations (OCPs) may protect against ovarian cancer by regulating apoptosis of the ovarian epithelium (2)[A].
- Multiparity
- Breastfeeding
- Tubal ligation or hysterectomy
- Recent studies have shown no clear association exists between ovarian cancer and use of ovulation-induction agents such as clomiphene, but more long-term studies are necessary.
- NSAIDs and acetaminophen use have been shown to reduce risk of ovarian cancer.
- Recommendations for high-risk (family history of a hereditary ovarian cancer syndrome) population
  - Women should undergo pelvic examinations, CA-125 level measurement, and transvaginal US every 6–12 months beginning at age 25–35 years.
  - Women with family histories of ovarian cancer or premenopausal breast cancer should be referred for genetic counseling.
  - Prophylactic oophorectomy is advised for mutation carriers after childbearing is completed or by age 35 years.
    - Risk of primary peritoneal carcinoma is 1% after prophylactic oophorectomy.
- Screening: No effective screening exists for ovarian cancer (1)[A].
  - Routine use of CA-125 and transvaginal US for screening in women of average risk is discouraged. Annual pelvic examinations are recommended, particularly in postmenopausal women. An adnexal mass in a premenarchal female or a palpable adnexa in a postmenopausal female warrants further evaluation.

COMMONLY ASSOCIATED CONDITIONS

- Ascites
- Pleural effusion
- Decrease of serum albumin
- Breast carcinoma
- Bowel obstruction
- Carcinomatosis

DIAGNOSIS

HISTORY

- Bloating
- Early satiety, anorexia, dyspepsia
- Sense of abdominal fullness, increased abdominal size
- Abdominopelvic pain or cramping
- Urinary frequency or urgency in absence of infection
- Fatigue
- Dyspareunia
- Weight loss
- Severe pain secondary to ovarian rupture or torsion; most frequent in germ cell tumors
- Precocious puberty (choriocarcinoma, embryonal carcinoma) (3)[B]

PHYSICAL EXAM

- Ascites
- Cul-de-sac and/or pelvic nodularity
- Pelvic mass
- Pleural effusion
- Omental mass
- Cachexia
- Adenopathy
- Hirsutism in androgen-secreting germ cell tumors

DIFFERENTIAL DIAGNOSIS

- GI, fallopian, or endometrial malignancies
- Irritable bowel syndrome
- Colitis
- Hepatic failure with ascites
- Diverticulitis
- Pelvic kidney
- Tubo-ovarian abscess or hydrosalpinx
- Uterine fibroids
- Endometriomas
- Physiologic cysts
- Benign or borderline neoplasms

DIAGNOSTIC TESTS & INTERPRETATION

Initial Tests (lab, imaging)

- Obtain with confirmed or suspected disease.
- CA-125 (not specific for ovarian cancer)
- Liver function tests (LFTs) to rule out hepatic disease
- CBC
- Urinalysis
- Serum albumin
- Carcinoembryonic antigen (CEA) if GI primary suspected
- If nonepithelial tumor suspected: chorionic gonadotropin (β-hCG [dysgerminoma, choriocarcinoma, embryonal carcinoma]), α-fetoprotein (endodermal sinus tumor, embryonal carcinoma), lactate dehydrogenase (LDH [dysgerminoma]), or inhibin (granulosa cell tumor)
- Pelvic US
- CXR
- Abdominopelvic CT scan with contrast material

Follow-Up Tests & Special Considerations

Disorders that may alter lab results: CA-125 may be elevated from gynecologic causes (e.g., menses, pregnancy, endometriosis, peritonitis, myomas, pelvic inflammatory disease) and with ascites, pleural effusion, congestive heart failure (CHF), pancreatitis, systemic lupus erythematosus (SLE), or liver disease.

- Patients with ovarian cancer need current mammography.
- Barium enema or colonoscopy if a colon primary is suspected

Diagnostic Procedures/Other

- Endometrial biopsy if abnormal bleeding present
- Surgery is necessary for definitive diagnosis.
- Paracentesis if patient with symptomatic ascites and not an operative candidate

Test Interpretation

Epithelial ovarian cancer commonly involves the peritoneal surfaces of the abdomen and pelvis, especially the cul-de-sac, paracolic gutters, and diaphragmatic surfaces.

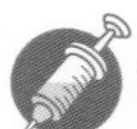

TREATMENT

MEDICATION

First Line

- After surgery, most patients will require chemotherapy. Stage 1a, grade 1 and most stage 1b, grade 1 tumors do not require adjuvant therapy. Patients with clear cell carcinomas, grade 3 tumors, or tumors staged 1c or worse require adjuvant therapy. Patients should be encouraged to participate in clinical trials whenever possible.
- Paclitaxel (Taxol) or docetaxel are recommended in combination with platinum-based therapy (carboplatin or cisplatin) as the 1st-line treatment of epithelial ovarian cancer.
- Intraperitoneal (IP) chemotherapy in combination with IV chemotherapy improves survival in advanced ovarian cancer. IP chemotherapy is associated with more toxicity (4)[A].
- Germ cell cancers: bleomycin, etoposide, platinum agent
- Contraindications: poor functional status, excessive toxicity, hypersensitivity
- Precautions: All regimens cause bone marrow suppression. Cisplatin is associated with ototoxicity, renal toxicity, and peripheral neuropathy. Taxol can cause neutropenia and neuropathy.
- Antiemetic: ondansetron (Zofran), dronabinol (Marinol), metoclopramide (Reglan), prochlorperazine (Compazine), promethazine (Phenergan)

Second Line

- Liposomal doxorubicin
- Carboplatin/gemcitabine
- Topotecan
- Etoposide
- Bevacizumab
- Cyclophosphamide
- Tamoxifen may be used in recurrent disease when chemotherapy is not appropriate (5)[A].

ADDITIONAL THERAPIES

Some patients with advanced disease and poor functional status and/or extreme tumor burden are managed with preoperative chemotherapy (neoadjuvant treatment) followed by interval cytoreductive surgery. These patients receive more chemotherapy after tumor debulking.

SURGERY/OTHER PROCEDURES

- Surgical exploration with staging and debulking is critical. Maximal cytoreduction of tumor burden enhances effectiveness of adjuvant therapy and is associated with longer survival.
- For epithelial malignancies, careful staging, tumor excision/debulking includes the following:
  - Cytologic evaluation of peritoneal fluid (or washings from peritoneal lavage)
  - Bilateral salpingo-oophorectomy with hysterectomy and tumor reductive surgery
  - Excision of omentum
  - Inspection and palpation of peritoneal surfaces
  - Cytologic smear of right hemidiaphragmatic surface
  - Biopsy of adhesions or any suspicious areas
  - Biopsy of paracolic recesses, pelvic sidewalls, posterior cul-de-sac, and bladder peritoneum
  - Pelvic and para-aortic lymph node biopsies
- Germ cell cancers (less likely to be bilateral): salpingo-oophorectomy (unilateral if only 1 ovary involved) in young patient

ONGOING CARE

FOLLOW-UP RECOMMENDATIONS

Patient Monitoring

- Physical exam every 3 months for the first 2 years after diagnosis; every 6 months until 5 years and then annually thereafter
- If CA-125 elevated at diagnosis, follow levels after treatment to detect recurrence (is often elevated 2–5 months before clinical detection of relapse).
- Germ cell/sex-cord stromal cancer: physical exam and tumor markers every 3 months for the first 2 years after diagnosis
  - Tumor markers for sex-cord stromal cancers should be checked every 6 months for 10 years, as recurrences can occur remote from initial diagnosis.
- CT scan of chest, abdomen, and pelvis and/or PET scan when recurrence suspected
- Screening with CXR, MRI, CT, or PET not recommended; insufficient data to support (6)[B]

PROGNOSIS

- Recurrence rates
  - Early-stage disease: 25%
  - Advanced disease: >80%
- 5-year survival rates for ovarian cancer based on International Federation of Gynecology and Obstetrics (FIGO) data
- For most recent FIGO staging criteria, see "References" (7)[A].

Stage I	a 90%	b 86%	c 83%
Stage II	a 71%	b 66%	c 71%
Stage III	a 47%	b 42%	c 33%
Stage IV	19%		

COMPLICATIONS

- Pleural effusion
- Pseudomyxoma peritonei
- Ascites
- Toxicity of chemotherapy
- Bowel obstruction
- Malnutrition
- Electrolyte disturbances
- Fistula formation

REFERENCES

1. Schorge JO, Modesitt SC, Coleman RL, et al. SGO white paper on ovarian cancer: etiology, screening and surveillance. *Gynecol Oncol*. 2010;119(1):7–17.
2. Collaborative Group on Epidemiological Studies of Ovarian Cancer, Beral V, Doll R, et al. Ovarian cancer and oral contraceptives: collaborative reanalysis of data from 45 epidemiological studies including 23,257 women with ovarian cancer and 87,303 controls. *Lancet*. 2008;371(9609):303–314.
3. Goff BA, Mandel LS, Drescher CW, et al. Development of an ovarian cancer symptom index. *Cancer*. 2007;109(2):221–227.
4. Armstrong DK, Bundy B, Wenzel L, et al. Intraperitoneal cisplatin and paclitaxel in ovarian cancer. *N Engl J Med*. 2006;354(1):34–43.
5. Orlando M, Costanzo MV, Chacon RD, et al. Randomized trial of combination chemotherapy (combo) versus monotherapy (mono) in relapsed ovarian carcinoma (ROC): a meta-analysis of published data. *J Clin Oncol*. 2007;25:5524.
6. Gadducci A, Cosio S, Zola P, et al. Surveillance procedures for patients treated for epithelial ovarian cancer: a review of the literature. *Int J Gynecol Cancer*. 2007;17(1):21–31.
7. Prat J; FIGO Committee on Gynecologic Oncology. Staging classification for the cancer of the ovary, fallopian tube, and peritoneum. *Int J Gynecol Obstetr*. 2014;124(1):1–5.

ADDITIONAL READING

- Salani R, Backes F, Fung M, et al. Posttreatment surveillance and diagnosis of recurrence in women with gynecologic malignancies: Society of Gynecologic Oncologists recommendations. *Am J Obstet Gynecol*. 2011;204(6):466–478.
- Schumer ST, Cannistra SA. Granulosa cell tumor of the ovary. *J Clin Oncol*. 2003;21(6):1180–1189.

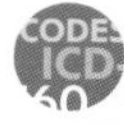

CODES

ICD10

- C56.9 Malignant neoplasm of unspecified ovary
- C56.1 Malignant neoplasm of right ovary
- C56.2 Malignant neoplasm of left ovary

CLINICAL PEARLS

- Family history of ovarian cancer or early-onset breast cancer is the most significant risk factor for the development of ovarian cancer, yet the vast majority of cases remain sporadic.
- The diagnosis of ovarian cancer should be suspected in women with persistent bloating, upper abdominal discomfort, or GI symptoms of unknown etiology.
- Surgery is the mainstay of diagnosis and treatment for ovarian cancer. Many patients benefit from adjuvant chemotherapy.
- The prognosis of advanced ovarian cancer is poor and requires close follow-up by physical exam, tumor markers, and imaging when indicated.

OVARIAN CYST, RUPTURED

Jeremy Golding, MD, FAAFP

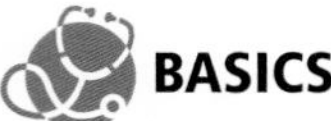

BASICS

- Ovarian cysts are very common. Women of reproductive age develop ovarian cysts with each ovulatory cycle.
- Ovarian cyst rupture and hemorrhage (of follicle or corpus luteum) occur on a physiologic continuum.
- A ruptured ovarian cyst is usually asymptomatic but sometimes causes pain ranging from mild to severe due to peritoneal irritation (blood and sebaceous material most irritating).
- Symptomatic ruptured ovarian cysts can usually be managed conservatively but occasionally require surgical intervention.

DESCRIPTION

Types of ovarian cysts that may rupture fall into 2 groups:

Physiologic:

- Physiologic (functional) cysts result from hormonal stimulation of the ovary. Most are asymptomatic and spontaneously resolve in 60–90 days:
  - Follicular cysts form when a growing follicle fails to rupture and release an egg:
    - Most common type of functional cyst
    - Unilateral and filled with serous fluid
  - Corpus luteum cysts occur when an egg is released and pregnancy does not occur. The residual structure does not regress and may hemorrhage internally (hemorrhagic cysts).
  - Theca lutein cysts result from excessive stimulation of β-human chorionic gonadotropin (infertility patients, molar pregnancies, or choriocarcinoma). These cysts are also susceptible to internal hemorrhage.

Pathologic

- Pathologic cysts are caused by a process other than normal hormonal stimulation. These cysts remain stable in size or may grow:
  - Endometriomas are cysts or collections of blood clots resulting from cycling endometrial tissue on the ovary. Also called "chocolate cysts" due to their appearance.
  - Mature cystic teratoma (dermoid) develop from totipotent germ cells:
    - Most commonly, they contain mucinous material and hair.
    - Up to 14% are bilateral; can grow very large.
    - <1% rupture spontaneously potentially leading to hemorrhage, shock, and acute peritonitis.
  - Cystadenomas may have solid or mucinous areas. They are typically benign and rarely rupture.
  - Other cystic-appearing adnexal structures include paratubal cysts, tubo-ovarian abscess, hydrosalpinx, and ectopic pregnancy.

EPIDEMIOLOGY

- The exact incidence is difficult to determine due to the asymptomatic nature of most cysts.
- Annual incidence of acute pelvic pain attributed to ovarian cysts in the United States estimated at 65,000
- 4% of women have been admitted to a hospital with an ovarian cyst by age 65 years.

RISK FACTORS

Increased risk of developing physiologic cysts associated with:

- Smoking
- Levonorgestrel IUD
- Tamoxifen

GENERAL PREVENTION

For patients with painful, recurrent ovarian cysts, oral contraceptive pills help suppress ovulation: This may prevent the formation of new cysts but will not impact cysts that have already formed.

DIAGNOSIS

- A ruptured ovarian cyst may be asymptomatic or present as acute abdominal pain (mild to severe).
- The broad range of presentations can prove to be a diagnostic dilemma for many physicians.

HISTORY

- A general past medical and surgical history should be reviewed.
- Specific reproductive history:
  - Possibility of pregnancy
  - Menstrual history, with attention to symptoms suggestive of endometriosis or history of cysts
  - STD history
  - Levonorgestrel-containing intrauterine device (up to 12% of users experience ovarian cysts)
  - Infertility treatment
- Features of pain due to rupture include
  - Pain often begins during strenuous activity (exercise or intercourse).
  - Sudden-onset, unilateral pelvic pain that becomes more dull and generalized over time
  - Pain is worse with movement.
- Other causes of acute abdominal pain should also be considered, including GI and urologic etiologies.

ALERT

Patients with bleeding diathesis or undergoing anticoagulation therapy may experience significant bleeding from hemorrhagic cysts.

PHYSICAL EXAM

- Vital signs are typically normal unless significant blood loss has occurred. Then signs of hypovolemic shock such as hypotension and tachycardia are present (uncommon).
- Low-grade fever may be present.
- Tenderness in unilateral lower quadrant (right side more common)
- Peritoneal signs may be present depending on degree of peritoneal irritation.
- On bimanual exam, unilateral adnexal mass may be palpable.
- May have cervical motion tenderness

DIFFERENTIAL DIAGNOSIS

Should include all causes of acute abdominal pain, both gynecologic and nongynecologic

ALERT

The first objective should be to exclude ectopic pregnancy. It has a similar presentation and can be life threatening.

Other considerations include the following:

- Ovarian torsion
- Pelvic inflammatory disease tubo-ovarian abscess
- Ovarian hyperstimulation syndrome (OHSS)
- Ovarian cancer with ascites
- Appendicitis
- Diverticulitis
- Nephrolithiasis
- Bowel obstruction or perforation

DIAGNOSTIC TESTS & INTERPRETATION

- Pregnancy test to rule out ectopic pregnancy.
- CBC to assess hematocrit (compare to baseline if possible) and WBC count (L shift may indicate infection)
- Testing for gonorrhea and chlamydia if pelvic inflammatory disease is suspected
- Urinalysis (infection or stones)
- Blood type and cross-matching if the patient is hemodynamically unstable and surgery is planned
- Tumor markers (i.e., CA-125): not recommended for initial evaluation; not likely to help in diagnosis or management
- Transvaginal US is first-line imaging modality to identify adnexal mass (cyst/tumor) and free fluid within the pelvis
- CT scan is second-line; most useful for excluding nongynecologic pathology
- MRI can distinguish a ruptured ovarian cyst from other gynecologic etiologies, such as tubo-ovarian abscess but is expensive and rarely necessary.

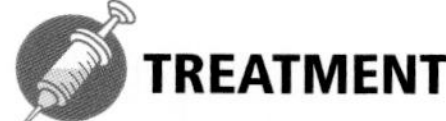

TREATMENT

MEDICATION

- Uncomplicated cyst ruptures (absence of hemodynamic instability, acute abdomen, enlarging hemoperitoneum, or US evidence of malignancy) can generally be managed conservatively.
- Pain due to an uncomplicated cyst rupture is usually self-limiting and can be managed on an outpatient basis with pain medication and rest.

First Line

NSAIDs are the most effective at relieving pain due to peritoneal irritation.

Second Line

Opioid pain medications may also be necessary acutely.

ISSUES FOR REFERRAL

- Most ruptured ovarian cysts in reproductive-age women are the result of functional cysts, and the risk of malignancy is very low.
- Referral to a gynecologic oncologist should be made in any postmenopausal woman with an adnexal mass that has concerning US findings; an elevated CA-125; ascites; a nodular, fixed pelvic mass; and a family history of breast or ovarian cancer.

SURGERY/OTHER PROCEDURES

Decision for surgery should be based on clinical presentation. For complicated ovarian cyst rupture (hemodynamic instability, significant hemoperitoneum, concern for ovarian torsion) or if patient is deteriorating, surgical evaluation is recommended:

- Laparoscopy is typically preferred but approach should be based on surgeon's comfort and expertise and patient factors (clinical condition, body habitus, previous abdominal surgeries, etc.) (1,2).
- Surgical intervention includes suction evacuation of any fluid or blood found in the pelvis, as well as achieving hemostasis, if needed, at the site of the cyst: If a cyst wall is present, it should be removed.
- In most cases, oophorectomy is not necessary.
- Laparoscopic excision of the cyst and capsule of endometriomas substantially decreases risk of recurrence.

INPATIENT CONSIDERATIONS

Inpatient management may include IV hydration, monitoring of vital signs, serial hematocrits, and pain control.

ONGOING CARE

FOLLOW-UP RECOMMENDATIONS

- Patients should have follow-up US in 6 weeks.
- Most functional cysts resolve spontaneously without treatment, and watchful waiting with serial transvaginal US for 2–3 cycles is appropriate.
- If cysts fail to resolve or develop concerning US findings (increasing size or complexity, nodules, septations, excrescences), surgical evaluation is recommended.
- With an uncomplicated cyst rupture, fluid typically resorbs in 24 hours and symptoms resolve within 2–3 days.
- Hormonal contraceptives do not hasten resolution of established cysts (3)[A].

Pregnancy Considerations

Ovarian cysts in pregnancy:

- With the widespread use of US during pregnancy, up to 4% of pregnant women are found to have adnexal masses, most of which are follicular cysts that spontaneously resolve by 16 weeks' gestation.
- <2% will spontaneously rupture or torse during pregnancy; however, this can lead to preterm labor and delivery, which may cause poor obstetric outcomes.
- If cysts are painful, large (>8 cm), or have US characteristics that are concerning for malignancy, consider surgical evaluation.

PATIENT EDUCATION

Educate patient on physiologic nature of process and risk factors associated with recurrence.

REFERENCES

1. Legendre G, Catala L, Morinière C, et al. Relationship between ovarian cysts and infertility: what surgery and when? *Fertil Steril*. 2014;101(3):608–614.
2. Falcone T. Risk of complications from gynecological surgery is lower with laparoscopy than with laparotomy. *Evidence Based Obstet Gynecol*. 2004;4:185–186A.
3. Grimes DA, Jones LB, Lopez LM, et al. Oral contraceptives for functional ovarian cysts. *Cochrane Database Syst Rev*. 2009;2:CD006134.

ADDITIONAL READING

- American College of Obstetricians and Gynecologists. ACOG practice bulletin. Management of adnexal masses. *Obstet Gynecol*. 2007;110(1):201–214.
- Bottomley C, Bourne T. Diagnosis and management of ovarian cyst accidents. *Best Pract Res Clin Obstet Gynaecol*. 2009;23(5):711–724.
- Falcone T. Risk of complications from gynecological surgery is lower with laparoscopy than with laparotomy. *Evidence Based Obstet Gynecol*. 2004;4:185–186A.
- Hart RJ, Hickey M, Maouris P, et al. Excisional surgery versus ablative surgery for ovarian endometriomata. *Cochrane Database Syst Rev*. 2008;2:CD004992.
- Hoo WL, Yazbek J, Holland T, et al. Expectant management of ultrasonically diagnosed ovarian dermoid cysts: is it possible to predict outcome? *Ultrasound Obstet Gynecol*. 2010;36(2):235–240.
- Huchon C, Staraci S, Fauconnier A, et al. Adnexal torsion: a predictive score for pre-operative diagnosis. *Hum Reprod*. 2010;25(9):2276–2280.
- Kruszka PS, Kruszka SJ. Evaluation of acute pelvic pain in women. *Am Fam Physician*. 2010;82(2):141–147.
- Mirena [package insert]. Wayne, NJ: Bayer HealthCare Pharmaceuticals Inc; 2009.
- Møller LM. Complications of gynaecological operations. A one-year analysis of a hospital database [in Danish]. *Ugeskr Laeg*. 2005;167:4654–4659.
- Raziel A, Ron-El R, Pansky M, et al. Current management of ruptured corpus luteum. *Eur J Obstet Gynecol Reprod Biol*. 1993;50(1):77–81.
- Roch O, Chavan N, Aquilina J, et al. Radiologic appearances of gynaecologic emergencies. *Insights Imaging*. 2012;3(3):265–275.
- Saunders BA, Podzielinski I, Ware RA, et al. Risk of malignancy in sonographically confirmed septated cystic ovarian tumors. *Gynecol Oncol*. 2010;118(3):278–282.
- Stany MP, Hamilton CA. Benign disorders of the ovary. *Obstet Gynecol Clin North Am*. 2008;35(2):271–284, ix.
- Suzuki S, Yasumoto M, Matsumoto R, et al. MR findings of ruptured endometrial cyst: comparison with tubo-ovarian abscess. *Eur J Radiol*. 2012;81:3631–3637.

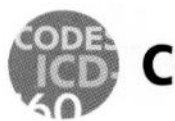

CODES

ICD10

- N83.20 Unspecified ovarian cysts
- N83.0 Follicular cyst of ovary
- N83.1 Corpus luteum cyst

CLINICAL PEARLS

- Functional ovarian cysts are very common in reproductive-age women and usually resolve spontaneously in 60–90 days.
- Always exclude ectopic pregnancy.
- If a cyst does rupture, the pain is usually self-limited and can be treated with oral pain medications on an outpatient basis.
- Surgery may be necessary if pain is extreme or if the patient is hemodynamically unstable. Surgery involves evacuating irritating fluid and blood from the abdominal cavity, achieving hemostasis, and removing the cyst wall if possible.

OVARIAN TUMOR, BENIGN

Kristin D'Orsi, DO • Mark J. Manning, DO, MsMEL

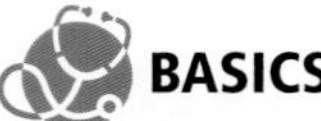

BASICS

DESCRIPTION

- The ovaries are a source of many tumor types (benign and malignant) because of the histologic variety of their constituent cells.
- Benign ovarian tumors create difficulties in differential diagnosis because of the need to identify malignancy and discriminate tumor from cysts, infectious lesions, ectopic pregnancy, and endometriomas.
- Tumors are often clinically silent until well developed; may be solid, cystic, or mixed; and they may be functional (producing sex steroids as with arrhenoblastomas and gynandroblastomas) or nonfunctional.
- System(s) affected: endocrine/metabolic; reproductive

Geriatric Considerations

Because incidence of malignancy increases with age, postmenopausal patients warrant comprehensive evaluation and follow-up.

Pediatric Considerations

Malignancy must be ruled out in premenarchal patients. Early neonatal cysts are rare.

EPIDEMIOLOGY

Incidence

- 30% of regularly cycling females
- 50% of women without regular cycles
- Predominant age: Premenarchal girls have a 6–11% risk of cancer in an ovarian tumor, and postmenopausal women have a 29–35% risk. A high percentage of ovarian tumors are malignant in girls <15 years of age.

ETIOLOGY AND PATHOPHYSIOLOGY

- Endometriosis with localized, repeated ovarian hemorrhage
- Physiologic cysts
- Tumorigenesis, with genetics as yet poorly defined

RISK FACTORS

- Cigarette smoking doubles the relative risk for developing functional ovarian cysts.
- Possible contributory factors are early menarche, obesity, infertility, and hypothyroidism.
- Tamoxifen increases risk of ovarian cyst formation (15–30%) (1).
- Risks for ovarian cancer include age >60 years; early menarche; late menopause; nulligravidity infertility; endometriosis; polycystic ovarian syndrome; family history of ovarian, breast, or colon cancer; a personal history of breast/colon cancer; or *BRCA* mutation.
- Risk for ovarian cancer is decreased in women who have used oral contraceptive pills (OCPs), are multiparous, have a history of a tubal ligation, or who have breastfed.

GENERAL PREVENTION

- OCPs do not appear to increase rates of cyst resolution, they do decrease the risk for forming new ovarian cysts (1).
- Resection of benign cysts has no impact on future risk for ovarian cancer.
- A case-control study of 299 women found no evidence that ovulation-induction treatment predisposes women to the development of borderline ovarian growths (2).

DIAGNOSIS

- A careful history is important.
- Usually asymptomatic
- Pain is related to torsion, endometriosis, or rupture.

HISTORY

- Early satiety
- Dyspepsia/bloating
- Increased abdominal girth
- Bowel pressure or bladder pressure sensations
- Menstrual irregularities
- Dyspareunia
- Deepening of the voice
- Hormonal status (OCPs, hormone replacement therapy [HRT] or fertility drugs)

PHYSICAL EXAM

- Severe acne
- Examine lymph nodes for enlargement.
- Chest auscultation can reveal a pleural effusion.
- Abdominal exam may identify ascites, masses, or increased abdominal girth.
- Hirsutism/sexual precocity
- Pelvic exam
- Rectovaginal exam
- Virilization

DIFFERENTIAL DIAGNOSIS

- Ovarian malignancies
- Endometrioma
- Uterine leiomyoma
- Appendicular cysts
- Diverticulitis/bowel abscess
- Pelvic inflammatory disease (PID) with tubo-ovarian abscess
- Distended urinary bladder
- Ectopic pregnancy
- Hydrosalpinx
- Paraovarian cyst
- Peritoneal inclusion cysts
- Functional cysts (follicular and corpus luteum cysts)
- Polycystic ovaries
- Ovarian lipoma

DIAGNOSTIC TESTS & INTERPRETATION

Initial Tests (lab, imaging)

- CBC for WBCs helpful if PID or ovarian torsion suspected
- Serum β-human chorionic gonadotropin (β-hCG)
- Urinalysis
- Serum estrogens and androgens if signs of androgen excess (although only as part of polycystic ovarian [PCO] workup)
- Serum tumor markers may be considered but often confuse rather than help to resolve diagnosis; choose carefully (3)[B].
  - CA-125 should not be ordered in a premenopausal patient for screening purposes. If an ovarian tumor in a premenopausal patient is highly suspicious for cancer by ultrasound, a CA-125 level >200 U is concerning. In a postmenopausal patient, cancer must be ruled out and a CA-125 >35 U is concerning (value is lab dependent) (4)[B].
  - α-Fetoprotein and hCG can be ordered for suspected germ cell tumor.
- Human epididymis protein 4 (HE4) may offer superior specificity compared to CA-125 for the differentiation of benign and malignant adnexal masses in premenopausal women (2)[B].
- Disorders that may alter lab results are the following:
  - CA-125: endometriosis, peritonitis, PID, Meigs syndrome, uterine fibroids, hepatitis, pancreatitis, systemic lupus erythematosus (SLE), diverticulitis
  - β-hCG: pregnancy, hydatidiform mole
  - α-Fetoprotein: hepatocellular carcinoma, hepatic cirrhosis, acute/chronic hepatitis
- Transvaginal ultrasound is the best means to determine the architecture of an ovarian cyst or mass (5)[B].
- Transvaginal ultrasonography may differentiate tumors from other pelvic lesions and identify features that place the patient at greater risk for malignancy (e.g., solid component; palpillations; multiple septations; ascites, bilaterality, fixed and irregular, rapidly enlarging, accompanied by cul-de-sac nodules).
- Transabdominal ultrasonography can help identify ascites.
- Color-flow Doppler evaluation also may be helpful. Color flow to the solid component of the tumor is concerning for cancer. Gray scale may be an important method of differential diagnosis of ovarian growths.
- MRI with apparent diffusion coefficient mapping may be useful in the differential diagnosis of cystic masses. MRI can be helpful in better defining masses in women with low risk of ovarian cancer, but who have an "indeterminant" mass on ultrasound. Usually not necessary, as decision for surgery can proceed without MRI if indicated. Can add greatly to cost of care

- Cystoscopy if hematuria is present in the absence of infection or if IV pyelogram reveals intravesical surface irregularity
- Abdominopelvic CT scan with contrast material, if MRI unavailable, although ultrasound still far superior (6)

Diagnostic Procedures/Other

Exploratory laparoscopy/laparotomy

Test Interpretation

- Follicular (fluid distension of atretic follicle) and corpus luteum cysts (corpus luteum hematoma). Follicular cysts are the most common ovarian cysts in the premenopausal nonpregnant female.
- Endometrioma (extrauterine endometrial tissue)
- Pregnancy luteoma (composed of hyperplastic stromal theca–lutein cells)
- Serous and mucinous cystadenomas and mixed serous/mucinous cystadenomas
- Granulosa cell tumors
- Benign connective tissue tumors (thecomas, fibromas, Brenner tumors)
- Cystic teratoma (dermoid cyst); teratomas are the most common benign neoplasms
- Germinal inclusion cyst (regarded by some as the precursor for epithelial ovarian cancer)

Pregnancy Considerations

- Most cysts discovered during pregnancy are corpus luteum/follicular cysts.
- The 2 most commonly encountered tumors during pregnancy are cystadenomas (serous/mucinous) and dermoid cysts.

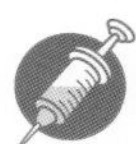

TREATMENT

GENERAL MEASURES

- In premenopausal patients cystic lesions <10 cm in diameter, simple observation for 4–6 weeks is acceptable.
- Premenopausal women should have a repeat ultrasound ideally during their follicular phase (day 3–10 of cycle) (7)[C].
- In premenopausal patients, simple and hemorrhagic cysts <3 cm are not suspicious and do not likely need follow-up (7)[C].
- If a large cyst remains unchanged after 4–6 weeks of observation, then surgical exploration is indicated.
- In postmenopausal patients cysts <1 cm are likely benign (7)[C].

MEDICATION

Oral contraceptives decrease the risk for forming new ovarian cysts. They do not aid in resorption of current ovarian cysts (8)[B].

First Line

NSAIDs or opioids may be helpful for discomfort.

SURGERY/OTHER PROCEDURES

- Cystectomy/wedge resection for cyst with benign features
- Surgical removal of tumor to establish diagnosis when:
  - Premenopausal cysts >5 cm that persist >12 weeks
  - Mass is solid.
  - Mass is >10 cm.
  - Mass in a premenarchal/postmenopausal female
  - Suspicion of torsion/rupture
  - Postmenopausal cysts
  - Cysts with worrisome features on ultrasound (e.g., papillations)
  - For masses that are worrisome for cancer, consider referral to a gynecologist/oncologist for initial surgery.

ONGOING CARE

FOLLOW-UP RECOMMENDATIONS

Patient Monitoring

- Most require only yearly exams.
- Varies by diagnosis

PATIENT EDUCATION

A variety of excellent patient education materials (e.g., "Ovarian Cyst") can be downloaded from the American Association of Family Physicians and American College of Obstetricians and Gynecologists Internet sites: www.aafp.org/afp and www.acog.com.

PROGNOSIS

Complete cure

COMPLICATIONS

Complications of untreated dermoid and mucinous cysts may include rupture and pseudomyxoma peritonei.

REFERENCES

1. Cusidó M, Fábregas R, Pere BS, et al. Ovulation induction treatment and risk of borderline ovarian tumors. *Gynecol Endocrinol*. 2007;23(7):373–376.
2. Holcomb K, Vucetic Z, Miller MC, et al. Human epididymis protein 4 offers superior specificity in the differentiation of benign and malignant adnexal masses in premenopausal women. *Am J Obstet Gynecol*. 2011;205(4):358.e1–e6.
3. Maggino T, Gadducci A, D'Addario V, et al. Prospective multicenter study on CA 125 in postmenopausal pelvic masses. *Gynecol Oncol*. 1994;54(2):117.
4. National Institutes of Health Consensus Development Conference Statement. Ovarian cancer: screening, treatment, and follow-up. *Gynecol Oncol*. 1994;55(2, Pt 3):S4.
5. Myers ER, Bastian LA, Havrilesky LJ, et al. Management of Adnexal Mass. Evidence Report/Technology Assessment No.130. Rockville, MD: Agency for Healthcare Research and Quality; 2006. (Prepared by the Duke Evidence-based Practice Center under Contract No. 290-02-0025) AHRQ Publication No. 06-E004.
6. Iyer VR, Lee SI. MRI, CT, and PET/CT for ovarian cancer detection and adnexal lesion characterization. *AJR Am J Roentgenol*. 2010;194(2):311–321.
7. Levine D, Brown D, Andreotti RF, et al. Management of asymptomatic ovarian and other adnexal cysts imaged at US: Society of Radiologists in Ultrasound Consensus Conference Statement. *Radiology*. 2010;256(3):943–954.
8. Holt VL, Cushing-Haugen KL, Daling JR. Oral contraceptives, tubal sterilization, and functional ovarian cyst risk. *Obstet Gynecol*. 2003;102(2):252–258.

ADDITIONAL READING

- American College of Obstetricians and Gynecologists. ACOG Practice Bulletin. Management of adnexal masses. *Obstet Gynecol*. 2007;110(1):201.
- Crayford TJ, Campbell S, Bourne TH, et al. Benign ovarian cysts and ovarian cancer: a cohort study with implications for screening. *Lancet*. 2000;355(9209):1060–1063.
- Givens V, Mitchell G, Harraway-Smith C, et al. Diagnosis and management of adnexal masses. *Am Fam Physician*. 2009;80(8):815–822.
- Kirilovas D, Schedvins K, Naessén T, et al. Conversion of circulating estrone sulfate to 17beta-estradiol by ovarian tumor tissue: a possible mechanism behind elevated circulating concentrations of 17beta-estradiol in postmenopausal women with ovarian tumors. *Gynecol Endocrinol*. 2007;23(1):25–28.
- Labarge PY. Short-term morbidity and long-term recurrence rate of ovarian dermoid cysts treated by laparoscopy vs. laparotomy. *J Obstet Gynecol Can*. 2006;28(9):789–793.
- Marchesini AC, Magrio FA, Berezowski AT, et al. A critical analysis of Doppler velocimetry in the differential diagnosis of malignant and benign ovarian masses. *J Womens Health (Larchmt)*. 2008;17(1):97–102.

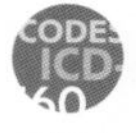

CODES

ICD10

- D27.9 Benign neoplasm of unspecified ovary
- D27.0 Benign neoplasm of right ovary
- D27.1 Benign neoplasm of left ovary

CLINICAL PEARLS

- In perimenopausal patients, follicles and simple cysts <3 cm are normal physiologic findings.
- Transvaginal pelvic ultrasound is the imaging test of choice to initially determine the architecture of an ovarian cyst or mass.
- Malignancy must be ruled out in both premenarchal and postmenopausal patients.
- Do not order CA-125 on premenopausal patients with an ovarian mass unless it is highly suspicious for cancer.

PAGET DISEASE OF THE BREAST

Jordan W. Neighbors, DO • Tracy O. Middleton, DO

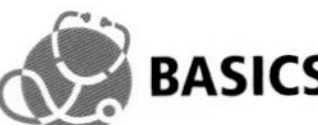

BASICS

DESCRIPTION

- Rare disease of the nipple-areolar complex typically associated with underlying in situ or invasive carcinoma
- Characterized by eczematous changes of the nipple, erythema, ulceration, crusting, bleeding, and/or itching
- Divided into 3 categories (1)
  - Paget disease of the nipple without ductal carcinoma in situ (DCIS)
  - Paget disease of the nipple with associated DCIS in the underlying lactiferous ducts of the nipple-areolar complex
  - Paget disease of the nipple with associated DCIS in the underlying lactiferous ducts of the nipple-areolar complex and associated DCIS or invasive breast cancer elsewhere in the breast at least 2 cm from the nipple-areolar complex
- System(s) affected: skin/exocrine

EPIDEMIOLOGY

Incidence

- 1–3% of breast cancers in females (2)
- Incidence of Paget disease of the breast has been decreasing since 1988, despite an increased incidence of breast cancer (3).
- Median age at diagnosis = 64 years (3)
- Extremely uncommon in males but prognosis is worse in men (4)

Prevalence

<1% of population

ETIOLOGY AND PATHOPHYSIOLOGY

Cause is unknown, but risk factors for Paget disease are similar to those for developing breast cancer in general (see below).

- Epidermotropic theory
  - Ductal carcinoma cells migrate from underlying mammary ducts to epidermis of the nipple to become Paget cells (4,5).
- Transformation theory (not favored)
  - Epidermal cells of nipple/areola transform into Paget cells that can invade the basement membrane into the dermis (4,5).

Genetics

No known genetic pattern, although studies suggest up to 88% display *Her2/Neu* overexpression (2)[B]

RISK FACTORS

Same risk factors apply as for noninherited breast cancers.

- Female gender
- Age >40 years
- Previous breast cancer
- Benign breast disease (atypical ductal/lobular hyperplasia, fibroadenoma, sclerosing adenosis, intraductal papilloma)
- 1st-degree relative with history of breast cancer
- Jewish/Caucasian
- Menarche <12 years of age
- Menopause >50 years of age
- Nulliparity or 1st child after age 34 years
- History of ionizing radiation exposure
- History of alcohol abuse

COMMONLY ASSOCIATED CONDITIONS

- Largest study, using surveillance, epidemiology, and end result (SEER) data representing 1,763 women with confirmed Paget disease, reports an underlying in situ or invasive breast cancer in 87% of patients, although there is often no associated breast mass or mammographic abnormality (3).
- The underlying carcinomas are multifocal/multicentric in 32–41% of patients (2)[B].

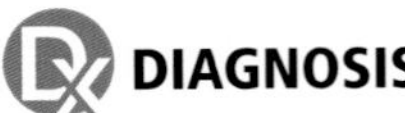

DIAGNOSIS

HISTORY

- Scaly, raw, vesicular, or ulcerated lesion that begins on the nipple and then spreads to the areola
- Pain, burning, and pruritus may be present even before clinically evident disease.
- Nipple/areolar skin changes that have not responded to conservative topical treatment
- Median duration of symptoms is 9 months prior to histologic diagnosis.

PHYSICAL EXAM

- Eczematous nipple changes
- Nipple erythema and scaling
- Nipple erosion or ulceration
- Bloody or serous nipple discharge
- Nipple retraction
- Nipple fissures with crusting
- Palpable breast mass is noted in approximately 50% of patients; when present, mass is often >2 cm from nipple-areolar complex (4)[C].
- Thickening in breast tissue without nipple change

DIFFERENTIAL DIAGNOSIS

- Eczema/atopic dermatitis
- Contact dermatitis
- Duct ectasia
- Psoriasis
- Bowen disease
- Squamous cell carcinoma
- Basal cell carcinoma
- Superficially spreading malignant melanoma
- Lichen simplex chronicus
- Erosive adenomatosis of the nipple

DIAGNOSTIC TESTS & INTERPRETATION

- Bilateral breast imaging should be performed in all cases to evaluate for synchronous invasive cancer or DCIS (1)[C].
- Mammographic appearance can be normal in 22–50% of cases (1)[C].
- If mammography and US negative or inconclusive, further evaluation with MRI is recommended (1,4,5)[C],(6)[B].
- Sensitivity for detecting invasive cancer and DCIS are 79% and 39%, respectively, for mammogram; 74% and 19%, respectively, for US; and 100% and 44%, respectively, for MRI (6)[B].
- Due to increased sensitivity in detecting multifocal or multicentric breast cancer, MRI is becoming a diagnostic standard. Despite higher false-positive rate, some recommend MRI for all new Paget disease patients (4)[C],(6)[B].
- MRI is also suggested in those patients with abnormalities limited to the central breast tissue on mammogram or US (1)[C],(6)[B].
- If considering breast-conserving surgery, MRI greatly aids preoperative planning (1,4,5)[C],(6)[B].
- In one study, 57% of cancers diagnosed with MRI were missed on mammography during initial workup (4)[C].

Diagnostic Procedures/Other

Full-thickness biopsy of breast lesions is the diagnostic standard; provides definitive diagnosis and should be performed in all patients presenting with a skin lesion suspicious for Paget disease (4)[C].

Test Interpretation

- Histologic evidence of Paget cells with abundant pale cytoplasm and hyperchromatic nuclei
- Immunohistochemistry positive for cytokeratin 7, carcinoembryonic antigen (CEA), and epithelial membrane antigen (EMA) and about 50% positive for hormone receptor expression (5)[C]

TREATMENT

MEDICATION

Systemic adjuvant chemotherapy and/or endocrine therapy is based on the stage and hormone receptor status of the associated cancer.

- In Paget disease without an associated cancer, or in estrogen-receptor positive DCIS, consider tamoxifen (7)[C].
- In Paget disease with associated invasive breast cancer, treat per oncology study protocols. See "http://www.nccn.org" for the most recent guidelines (7)[C].
- Possible agents include the following:
  - Tamoxifen
  - Anastrozole, letrozole, or exemestane
  - Doxorubicin
  - Cyclophosphamide
  - Paclitaxel
  - Docetaxel
  - Carboplatin
  - Trastuzumab

ISSUES FOR REFERRAL

- Surgery
- Medical oncology
- Radiation oncology

ADDITIONAL THERAPIES

Possible breast reconstructive surgery with plastic surgery, physical therapy, counseling services, support groups

SURGERY/OTHER PROCEDURES

- Mastectomy with axillary dissection or breast conservation therapy followed by adjuvant radiation therapy, depending on extent and location of malignancy (1)[C],(2)[B],(4)[C],(5)[C]
- Patients with isolated Paget disease of the nipple should undergo excision of the nipple-areolar complex followed by adjuvant radiation (2)[B].
- Multicentric lesions or diffuse calcifications require mastectomy.
- Sentinel node biopsy (SNB)
  - Can avoid side effects seen with full axillary dissection, such as lymphedema, pain, and infection

- Recommended in patients with biopsy-proven or MRI evidence of invasive cancer (4)[C],(6)[B]
- Recommended in patients without clinical or MRI evidence of nodal involvement who are undergoing mastectomy (4)[C],(6)[B]
- Considered for patients with underlying DCIS; use still not clear (4)[C]
- Consider SNB in all confirmed cases of Paget disease due to high likelihood of underlying malignancy, even with negative radiographic studies (8)[B].
- Patients with axillary node metastases diagnosed preoperatively should undergo axillary clearance instead of SNB (6)[B].
- Studies show no difference in long-term survival or disease-free interval with mastectomy versus breast-conserving surgery on carefully selected surgical candidates (3)[B],(4,5)[C].

INPATIENT CONSIDERATIONS

Admission Criteria/Initial Stabilization

Dependent on cancer histology, size, and stage (see topic on "Breast Cancer")

- Surgery
- Radiotherapy
- Chemotherapy
- Hormone therapy

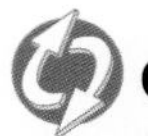

ONGOING CARE

FOLLOW-UP RECOMMENDATIONS

Oncology consultation

Patient Monitoring

- After successful treatment for Paget disease of the breast, patients should start an individualized cancer surveillance program to include regular history, physical examination, and mammograms.
- Routine screening for average-risk women who have never been diagnosed with breast cancer or Paget disease is per USPSTF guidelines.
  - Biennial screening mammography for women ages 50–74 years.

PATIENT EDUCATION

- National Cancer Institute, Department of Health and Human Services, Public Inquiries Section, Office of Cancer Communications, Building 31, Room 101-18, 9000 Rockville Pike, Bethesda, MD 20892; 301-496-5583
- http://www.cancer.gov/cancertopics/factsheet/Sites-Types/paget-breast

PROGNOSIS

- Factors of unfavorable prognosis (2)
  - Palpable breast mass
  - Multifocal disease
  - Lymph node enlargement
  - Vascular invasion/invasive disease
  - Higher stage of disease
  - *Her2/Neu* overexpression
  - Age <60 years
- Prognosis by presence/absence of palpable mass
  - 22% 10-year survival if palpable mass present prior to excision
  - 82% 10-year survival if no palpable mass prior to excision
- Prognosis by lymph node status
  - 47% 10-year survival if positive nodes
  - 93% 10-year survival if negative nodes
- Prognosis by stage of underlying breast carcinoma
  - (See www.cancer.org for breast cancer staging descriptions) (7)

Stage	5-yr relative survival
I	96%
II	78%
III	46%
IV	14%

COMPLICATIONS

Risk factors for recurrence

- Axillary lymph node metastases
- Underlying invasive cancer
- Palpable mass on presentation
- Negative hormone receptor expression
- Her2/Neu overexpression

REFERENCES

1. Lim HS, Jeong SJ, Lee JS, et al. Paget disease of the breast: mammographic, US, and MR imaging findings with pathologic correlation. *Radiographics*. 2011;31(7):1973–1987.
2. Caliskan M, Gatti G, Sosnovskikh I, et al. Paget's disease of the breast: the experience of the European Institute of Oncology and review of the literature. *Breast Cancer Res Treat*. 2008;112(3):513–521.
3. Chen CY, Sun LM, Anderson BO. Paget disease of the breast: changing patterns of incidence, clinical presentation, and treatment in the U.S. *Cancer*. 2006;107(7):1448–1458.
4. Trebska-McGowan K, Terracina KP, Takabe K. Update on the surgical management of Paget's disease. *Gland Surg*. 2013;2(3):137–142.
5. Karakas C. Paget's disease of the breast. *J Carcinog*. 2011;10:31.
6. Siponen E, Hukkinen K, Heikkilä P, et al. Surgical treatment in Paget's disease of the breast. *Am J Surg*. 2010;200(2):241–246.
7. National Comprehensive Cancer Network. NCCN clinical practice guidelines in oncology and breast cancer (version 3.2013). www.nccn.org.
8. Sukumvanich P, Bentrem DJ, Cody HS III, et al. The role of sentinel lymph node biopsy in Paget's disease of the breast. *Ann Surg Oncol*. 2007;14(3):1020–1023.

ADDITIONAL READING

- American Cancer Society. How is breast cancer staged? http://www.cancer.org/Cancer/BreastCancer/DetailedGuide/breast-cancer-staging. Accessed 2014.
- Ceccherini AF, Evans AJ, Pinder SE, et al. Is ipsilateral mammography worthwhile in Paget's disease of the breast? *Clin Radiol*. 1996;51(1):35–38.
- Dalberg K, Hellborg H, Wärnberg F. Paget's disease of the nipple in a population based cohort. *Breast Cancer Res Treat*. 2008;111(2):313–319.
- Kanitakis J. Mammary and extramammary Paget's disease. *J Eur Acad Dermatol Venereol*. 2007;21(5):581–590.
- Kawase K, Dimaio DJ, Tucker SL, et al. Paget's disease of the breast: there is a role for breast-conservative therapy. *Ann Surg Oncol*. 2005;12(5):391–397.
- Kim HS, Seok JH, Cha ES, et al. Significance of nipple enhancement of Paget's disease in contrast enhanced breast MRI. *Arch Gynecol Obstet*. 2010;282(2):157–162.
- Kothari AS, Beechey-Newman N, Hamed H, et al. Paget's disease of the nipple: a multifocal manifestation of a higher-risk disease. *Cancer*. 2002;95(1):1–7.
- Laronga C, Hasson D, Hoover S, et al. Paget's disease in the era of sentinel lymph node biopsy. *Am J Surg*. 2006;192(4):481–483.
- Lohsiriwat V, Martella S, Rietjens M, et al. Paget's disease as a local recurrence after nipple-sparing mastectomy: clinical presentation, treatment, outcome, and risk factor analysis. *Ann Surg Oncol*. 2012;19(6):1850–1855.
- Marshall JK, Griffith KA, Haffty BG, et al. Conservative management of Paget disease of the breast with radiotherapy: 10- and 15-year results. *Cancer*. 2003;97(9):2142–2149.
- Morrogh M, Morris EA, Liberman L, et al. MRI identifies otherwise occult disease in select patients with Paget disease of the nipple. *J Am Coll Surg*. 2008;206(2):316–321.
- National Cancer Institute. Paget disease of the breast. http://www.cancer.gov/cancertopics/factsheet/Sites-Types/paget-breast. Accessed 2014.
- Sanders MA, Dominici L, Denison C, et al. Paget disease of the breast with invasion from nipple skin into the dermis: an unusual type of skin invasion not associated with an adverse outcome. *Arch Pathol Lab Med*. 2013;137(1):72–76.
- Sandoval-Leon AC, Drews-Elger K, Gomez-Fernandez CR, et al. Paget's disease of the nipple. *Breast Cancer Res Treat*. 2013;141(1):1–12.
- Sek P, Zawrocki A, Biernat W, et al. HER2 molecular subtype is a dominant subtype of mammary Paget's cells. An immunohistochemical study. *Histopathology*. 2010;57(4):564–571.
- Zakhireh J, Gomez R, Esserman L. Converting evidence to practice: a guide for the clinical application of MRI for the screening and management of breast cancer. *Eur J Cancer*. 2008;44(18):2742–2752.

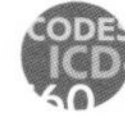

CODES

ICD10

- C50.019 Malignant neoplasm of nipple and areola, unsp female breast
- C50.011 Malignant neoplasm of nipple and areola, right female breast
- C50.012 Malignant neoplasm of nipple and areola, left female breast

CLINICAL PEARLS

- Any chronic or nonhealing nipple or breast lesions should be biopsied to rule out malignancy.
- Further imaging is indicated to rule out additional underlying breast malignancy.
- Breast mammography and ultrasound are not as sensitive as MRI in detecting potential occult breast lesions.
- Treatment is evaluated on a case-by-case basis and is guided by extent of disease, staging, and tumor location.

PALLIATIVE CARE

Suzana K. Everett Makowski, MD, MMM, FACP, FAAHPM

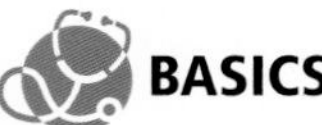

BASICS

Palliative care is a specialty that focuses on preventing and alleviating suffering of patients and their families living with life-limiting illness at any stage of that illness.

DESCRIPTION

- Palliative care's principal aim is to prevent and alleviate suffering—whether physical (pain, breathlessness, nausea, etc.), emotional, social, or spiritual regardless of underlying diagnosis.
- The goal of palliative care is to improve or maintain quality of life of both patient and family despite serious illness.
- Palliative care is available for patients with serious, life-limiting illness, at any stage of their disease, with or without concurrent curative care.
- Location of care: Patients and their families may access palliative care services in hospital; rehabilitative, skilled nursing facility; or ambulatory settings (1).
- Hospice: For patients living in the United States whose average life expectancy is 6 months or less and whose principal goal is to stay home, avoiding hospitalizations and disease-directed care with curative intent, hospice is available. Unlike regular nursing home care services, hospice does not require a patient to be homebound and offers backup support for patients 24 hours a day and 7 days per week.

COMMONLY ASSOCIATED CONDITIONS

Symptoms/syndromes commonly treated in palliative care:

- Pain
  - Chronic pain
  - Headache
  - Neuropathic pain
  - Pain from bone metastases
  - Pruritus
- GI symptoms (~60% incidence)
  - Ascites
  - Anorexia/cachexia (2)
  - Nausea (and vomiting) (3)[A]
    - Think of the underlying etiology and treat accordingly.
      - GI causes: constipation, bowel (full or partial) obstruction, ileus, heart burn, reflux, inflammation
      - Intrathoracic causes: cardiac, effusions (cardiac, pulmonary), mediastinal causes, esophageal
      - Autonomic dysfunction
      - Centrally mediated: change intracranial pressure, inflammation, cerebellar, vestibular, medication or metabolic stimulating vomiting center and/or chemoreceptor trigger zone
  - Bowel obstruction
  - Constipation and impaction of stool (4)[A]
  - Diarrhea
  - Dysphagia
  - Mucositis/stomatitis
  - Sialorrhea
- General medical
  - Delirium (40–85%)
- Pulmonary symptoms
  - Cough, chronic
  - Breathlessness or dyspnea (60%): often due to heart failure, COPD, lung cancer, etc.
    - In addition to treating the underlying cause of breathlessness, as disease advances, there is evidence that low-dose opioids may be beneficial to patients (5,6)[A].
    - Pleural effusion
- Psychological symptoms
  - Anxiety (7)[A]
  - Depression
  - Insomnia
- Skin
  - Decubitus ulcer
  - Pruritus (8)
  - Complex wounds (fungating tumors, etc.)

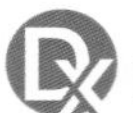

DIAGNOSIS

The PEACE tool evaluates the following:

- Physical symptoms
- Emotive and cognitive symptoms
- Autonomy and related issues
- Communication: contribution to others and closure of life affairs–related issues
- Economic burden and other practical issues, also transcendent and existential issues

HISTORY

- A comprehensive palliative care assessment includes addressing the following (9):
  - Underlying medical conditions and their associated physical symptoms
  - Comprehensive pain and symptom assessment and review of systems. Consider use of Edminton Symptom Assessment Tool.
  - Psychological symptom assessment
  - Cultural, social, and practical concerns
  - Spiritual and existential issues
    - FICA assessment (Faith, Importance and Influence, Community, Address—how does the patient wish to be addressed?) (10)
    - HOPE (sources of **H**ope/strength/comfort, **O**rganized religion's role, **P**ersonal spirituality and practices, **E**ffects on medical care and end-of-life care) (11)
  - Patient's identified presence and sources of suffering: personhood concerns
  - Goals of care: including posthospital care, practical needs, hopes, and fears
  - Prognosis: including functional status and patient's interest in knowing prognosis (12,13)

PHYSICAL EXAM

Comprehensive physician examination is warranted, especially as directed by underlying diagnosis, symptoms, and functional decline.

DIAGNOSTIC TESTS & INTERPRETATION

Initial Tests (lab, imaging)

Per diagnosis and symptoms

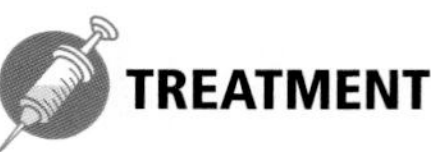

TREATMENT

GENERAL MEASURES

- Targetted interventions to maximize quality of life and minimize symptom burden while taking into consideration the patient's values, goals, fears, and social setting.
- Treatment should involve an interdisciplinary team—addressing potential and realized suffering, whether physical, emotional, social, or spiritual.

MEDICATION

- Attempt to minimize polypharmacy when possible.
- Continue to use appropriate disease-modifying medications especially if they lessen symptom burden and enhance immediate quality of life.
- Medication should focus on symptom management.
- Consider trimming medications that offer little improvement in the quality of life.
- Assure compliance by addressing patient/caregiver understanding and written consensus.
- *Pain*
  - Use immediate-release opioids PO/IV/SC and titrate to control.
  - Once pain is controlled, convert to long-acting **opioids** with short-acting agents made available as tolerance develops and/or patient develops breakthrough pain.
- Bone pain: NSAIDs added to narcotics are more effective than narcotics alone.

- *Vomiting* associated with a particular opioid may be relieved by substitution with an equianalgesic dose of another opioid or a sustained-release formulation. Dopamine receptor antagonists (metoclopramide, prochlorperazine, promethazine) are commonly used.
- Droperidol: insufficient evidence to advise on the use for the management of nausea and vomiting
- *Constipation*: prophylactic stool softeners (docusate) and stimulants (Bisacodyl or senna).

ALERT

Polyethylene glycol should be started when opioid treatment is begun to avoid constipation.

- SC methylnaltrexone is effective in inducing bowel movements without inducing withdrawal with opioid-induced constipation.
- *Dyspnea*: oxygen, narcotics, and, if congestive heart failure (CHF), diuretics and/or long-acting nitrates, **benzodiazepines**
  - Immediate-release **opioids** PO/IV treat dyspnea effectively and typically at doses lower than necessary for the relief of moderate pain.
- *Delirium*: lowest doses necessary of **benzodiazepines** or **antipsychotics** (Haldol, etc.)
- Patient safety and nonpharmacologic strategies to assist orientation (clocks, calendars, environment, and redirection)
- When cause of delirium cannot be identified/corrected rapidly, consider neuroleptics (haloperidol or risperidone).
- Pruritus: no optimal therapy; may try diphenhydramine
- Anxiety: insufficient data for recommendations of specific medication, but anxiolytics and/or other agents may be tried
- Megestrol acetate improves appetite and slight weight gain (7).

ALERT

Avoid morphine in patients with renal failure, as this can lead to delirium, hyperalgesia, agitation, and seizures.

ISSUES FOR REFERRAL

- Referral to palliative care
  - Any patient with a serious, life-limiting illness who could benefit from help with burdensome symptoms or suffering and/or complex goals of care discussion (14)
  - Early referral to palliative care may improve quality of life and longevity for patients with advanced cancer (15,16)[B].
- Referral to hospice care
- Any patient with an average life expectancy of 6 months or less. Consider the question, "Would you be surprised if the patient died within the next 6 months?" If the answer is no, they likely meet prognostic criteria for hospice.
  - Consider patients who (a) spend greater than 50% of daytime hours resting and (b) have multiple hospitalizations and/or emergency department visits in the prior 6 months.
  - Refer to local hospice guidelines for additional disease-specific criteria.

REFERENCES

1. Gomes B, Calanzani N, Curiale V, et al. Effectiveness and cost effectiveness of home palliative care services for adults with advanced illness and their caregivers. *Cochrane Database Syst Rev*. 2013;6:CD007760.
2. Ruiz Garcia V, Lòpez-Briz E, Carbonell Sanchis R, et al. Megestrol acetate for treatment of anorexia-cachexia syndrome. *Cochrane Database Syst Rev*. 2013;3:CD004310.
3. Smith HS, Smith JM, Smith AR. An overview of nausea/vomiting in palliative medicine. *Ann Palliat Med* 2012;1(2):103–114.
4. Candy B, Jones L, Goodman ML, et al. Laxatives or methylnaltrexone for the management of constipation in palliative care patients. *Cochrane Database Syst Rev*. 2011;(1):CD003448.
5. Lorenz KA, Lynn J, Dy SM, et al. Evidence for improving palliative care at the end of life: a systematic review. *Ann Intern Med*. 2008;148(2):147–159.
6. Ben-Aharon I, Gaffer-Gvili A, Paul M, et al. Interventions for alleviating cancer-related dyspnea: a systematic review. *J Clin Oncol*. 2008;26(14):2396–2404.
7. Candy B, Jackson KC, Jones L, et al. Drug therapy for symptoms associated with anxiety in adult palliative care patients. *Cochrane Database Syst Rev*. 2012;10:CD004596.
8. Xander C, Meerpohl JJ, Galandi D, et al. Pharmacological intervention for pruritus in adult palliative care patients. *Cochrane Database Syst Rev*. 2013;6:CD008320.
9. Emanuel LL, et al. Study module 1: comprehensive assessment. EPEC-O (Education in Palliative and End-of-life Care for Oncology). http://www.cancer.gov/cancertopics/cancerlibrary/epeco/selfstudy/module-1/module-1-pdf. Accessed October 24, 2014.
10. Puchalski C, Romber AL. Taking a spiritual history allows clinicians to understand patients more fully. *J Palliat Med*. 2000;31:129–137
11. Anandarajah G, Hight E. Spirituality and medical practice: using the HOPE questions as a practical tool for spiritual assessment. *Am J Fam Phys*. 2001;63(1):81–89.
12. Chan EY, Wu HY, Chan YH. Revisiting the Palliative Performance Scale: change in scores during disease trajectory predicts survival. *Palliat Med*. 2013;27(4):367–374.
13. Moss AH, Ganjoo J, Sharma S, et al. Utility of the "surprise" question to identify dialysis patients with high mortality. *Clin J Am Soc Nephrol*. 2008;3(5):1379–1384.
14. Weissman DE, Meier DE. Identifying patients in need of a palliative care assessment in the hospital setting: a consensus report from the Center to Advance Palliative Care. *J Palliat Med*. 2011;14(1):17–23.
15. Haun MW, Estel S, Rücker G, et al. Early palliative care for improving quality of life and survival time in adults with advanced cancer. *Cochrane Database of Syst Rev*. 2014;5:CD011129.
16. Temel JS, Greer JA, Muzikansky A, et al. Early palliative care for patients with metastatic non-small-cell lung cancer. *NEJM*. 2010;363(8):733–741.

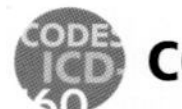

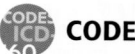

CODES

ICD10

Z51.5 Encounter for palliative care

CLINICAL PEARLS

- Early referral to palliative care may help enhance the quality of life and potential longevity of patients living with serious illness.
- Bone pain: NSAIDs added to narcotics are more effective than narcotics alone.

ALERT

Polyethylene glycol should be started when opioid treatment is begun to avoid constipation.

PANCREATIC CANCER

Edward Feller, MD, FACP, FACG

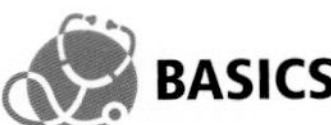

BASICS

DESCRIPTION

- Carcinoma of the exocrine pancreas is the 4th most common cause of cancer death in the United States (1).
- Rarely curable: overall 1-year and 5-year relative survival rates of 25% and 5%, respectively.
- 60–70% occur in the head, 15% in the body, 5% in the tail, 20% diffusely involve the gland.
- <20% are localized at diagnosis. For localized, small cancers (<2 cm) with no lymph node metastases and no extension beyond the capsule, surgical resection has 5-year survival of 18–24%.
- Majority of tumors have metastasized at diagnosis and are thus, largely incurable.
- In apparently resectable disease, 20–40% have unresectable lesions at surgery.
- Ampullary, duodenal, or distal bile duct tumors may mimic pancreatic carcinoma and are more likely to be resectable and curable.
- For advanced or unresectable cancers, survival is <1% at 5 years; most patients die within 1 year.

EPIDEMIOLOGY

During 2003–2007, median age at diagnosis = 72 years; rare younger than age 45 years; after 45 years of age, occurrence rises (2).

Incidence

- An estimated 42,470 people diagnosed in 2009 (21,040 men and 21,420 women); 35,240 deaths
- More common in black and white races, 16.7 and 10.3 in 100,000 men and 14.4 and 10.3 in 100,000 women, respectively. Among Hispanic and Asian/Pacific Islanders, there is an incidence of 10.9 and 8.3 in 100,000 men and 10.1 and 8.3 in 100,000 women, respectively.

Prevalence

In 2008, in the United States, ~34,600 men and women (16,811 men and 17,846 women) were alive who had a history of pancreatic cancer.

RISK FACTORS

- Smoking: relative risk (RR) = 1.5; correlates with amount smoked
- Diabetes: RR = 2.1 (95% confidence interval, 1.6–2.8); as many as 1 in 6 become diabetic within 6 months before diagnosis
- Prior partial gastrectomy or cholecystectomy: 2–5-fold increased risk 15–20 years after gastrectomy
- Familial aggregation/genetic factors: 5–10% of patients have a 1st-degree relative with the disease, which confers a 9-fold increase in risk versus the general population; subgroup may carry germline mutations of DNA repair genes (*BRCA2*) (3).
- Hereditary chronic pancreatitis (autosomal dominant, highly penetrant): cumulative risk by ages 50 and 75 years is 10% and 54%, respectively.
- Peutz-Jeghers syndrome
- Chronic pancreatitis: tropical and nontropical
- Non-O blood type
- High intake of dietary fat and obesity
- Alcohol: Recent data indicate a modest increase in risk confined to heavy alcohol consumers.
- Coffee intake and NSAID use *NOT* regarded as risk factors.

GENERAL PREVENTION

Routine screening is not recommended. Even with a strong family history or predisposition syndromes, use and cost-effectiveness of screening are unclear.

COMMONLY ASSOCIATED CONDITIONS

- Chronic pancreatitis; diabetes mellitus; cystic fibrosis (4)
- Subsets of familial pancreatic cancer involve germline cationic trypsinogen or *PRSS1* mutations (hereditary pancreatitis), *BRCA2* mutations (usually with hereditary breast–ovarian cancer syndrome), *CDKN2* mutations (familial atypical mole, multiple melanoma), or DNA repair gene mutations (e.g., *ATM* and *PALB2*, apart from *BRCA2*).
- However, the vast majority of familial pancreatic cancers do not have their genetic underpinnings identified (3).

DIAGNOSIS

HISTORY

- Dependent on tumor location; majority become symptomatic late in disease. Majority develop in the pancreatic head and may block the periampullary bile duct, causing obstructive jaundice.
- Weight loss 90%; pain 75% (progressive midepigastric dull ache that often radiates to the back); malnutrition 75%; jaundice 70%; anorexia 60%; pruritus 40%; diabetes mellitus 15%; weakness, fatigue, malaise 30–40%; alcoholic stools, dark urine, steatorrhea; depression is common.
- Pancreatic cancer is a consideration in acute pancreatitis in the elderly and with new-onset diabetes, but most new-onset diabetes is not associated with cancer; thus, evaluation for cancer is warranted only in selected cases.
- Uncommon: unexplained thrombophlebitis; acute pancreatitis from tumor obstruction of the pancreatic duct; duodenal obstruction or GI bleeding

PHYSICAL EXAM

- Muscle wasting and malnutrition are common; skin lesions are indicative of pruritus. Exam can be normal.
- Palpable abdominal mass or ascites in 20%
- Jaundice: 70% if tumor obstructs bile duct; 10% with body or tail carcinoma
- Courvoisier sign (painless jaundice with a palpable gallbladder): uncommon; usually associated with pancreatic head tumors, periampullary or primary bile duct tumors; hepatomegaly in advanced disease
- Virchow node (left supraclavicular) and Sister Mary Joseph node (umbilical) in metastatic disease; palpable rectal shelf (nonspecific sign of carcinomatosis)
- Migratory thrombophlebitis (uncommon); due to hypercoagulability in mucin-producing pancreatic cancer
- GI bleeding from tumor erosion into adjacent viscera (colon); portal hypertension-related bleeding (uncommon)
- Pancreatic panniculitis: subcutaneous areas of nodular fat necrosis

DIFFERENTIAL DIAGNOSIS

- Duodenal cancer, cholangiocarcinoma, lymphoma, islet cell tumor, sarcoma, cystic neoplasms, tumor metastatic to pancreas (rare)
- Nonmalignant conditions: choledocholithiasis, acute or chronic pancreatitis, biliary tract stricture, adenoma; chronic mesenteric ischemia
- Tuberculosis or fungal abscess in AIDS
- Patients may present with back pain mimicking musculoskeletal disease.

DIAGNOSTIC TESTS & INTERPRETATION

- Cross-sectional imaging: (usually CT scan as 1st-line choice) to evaluate symptoms or abnormal lab results
- Endoscopic ultrasound-guided biopsy: best modality for tissue diagnosis; sensitivity 75–90%; specificity ~100% for diagnosis of a mass
- Routine laboratory tests may reveal elevated serum bilirubin and alkaline phosphatase (cholestasis), anemia, or decreased serum albumin (malnutrition).

Initial Tests (lab, imaging)

- Most patients do not require measurement of serum tumor markers (CA19-9) for diagnosis or management. Some evidence suggests use in predicting outcome and response to adjuvant chemotherapy (5)[A].
- Elevated CA19.9 antigen: 80% sensitivity; 90% specificity; individuals with Lewis-negative blood group antigen phenotype (5–10%) are unable to synthesize CA19-9. Elevations can occur in benign pancreatic or biliary diseases and in nonpancreatic malignancy. Not recommended as a screening test.

Follow-Up Tests & Special Considerations

- During therapy, increase in CA19-9 may identify progressive tumor growth. Normal CA19-9 does not exclude recurrence.
- CT scan (pancreatic protocol) using thin section, multiphase multidetector helical CT with a pancreatic protocol is the choice for diagnosis and staging: 85–90% sensitivity; 90–95% specificity; useful for evaluation of distant metastasis and prediction of resectability (6)[A].
- Abdominal ultrasound: common initial test to assess jaundice and duct dilatation; less sensitive than CT for pancreatic masses
- Endoscopic ultrasound (EUS) is accurate for tissue biopsy, local tumor and node staging, predicting vascular invasion (90% specificity; 73% sensitivity), and when no mass is identified on CT.
- Endoscopic retrograde cholangiopancreatography (ERCP): invasive procedure with 90% sensitivity; 95% specificity for ductal cancer; useful if endoscopic stent is indicated for biliary obstruction; generally confined to high probability for therapeutic intervention on biliary or pancreatic ductal systems
- MRI: no advantage over contrast-enhanced CT

P

- MR cholangiopancreatography: noninvasive: 90% sensitivity; 95% specificity. Preferred in specific settings: gastric outlet or duodenal stenosis or after surgical rearrangement (Billroth II) or ductal disruption; to detect bile duct obstruction, after attempted ERCP is unsuccessful or provides incomplete information
- Cystic pancreatic lesions may be benign or malignant; must be differentiated from pancreatic pseudocysts. Cystadenocarcinomas have different prognoses than typical pancreatic cancers (7).

Diagnostic Procedures/Other

- Percutaneous fine-needle biopsy with US or CT guidance: 80–90% sensitivity; 98–100% specificity
- EUS-guided biopsy: 85–90% sensitivity; virtually 100% specificity for pancreatic mass
- Staging laparoscopy and US: 92% sensitivity; 88% specificity; 89% accuracy
- Positive peritoneal cytology has a positive predictive value of 94%; specificity of 98%; sensitivity of 25% for determining unresectability.
- PET scan: 90% sensitivity but 70% specificity; limited anatomic information
- Tumor staging
  - Stage I: tumors limited to the pancreas
  - Stage II: regionally invasive; may involve lymph nodes but without celiac or mesenteric artery involvement
  - Stage III: direct involvement of celiac or superior mesenteric artery involvement
  - Stage IV: distant metastases

Test Interpretation

- Duct cell carcinoma: 90%
- Others: acinar, papillary mucinous, signet ring, adenosquamous, mucinous, giant or small cell, cystadenocarcinoma, undifferentiated, unclassified carcinoma

ALERT
Chronic pancreatitis can present with similar pain, weight loss, jaundice, and an inflammatory mass on imaging.

TREATMENT

- Surgical resection: only chance of cure; no role for resection in metastatic disease. As few as 15–20% are candidates for resection (8)[A].
- Criteria for unresectability: extrapancreatic spread, encasement or occlusion of major vessels, distant metastases
- New combination chemotherapy regimens may offer advantages over gemcitabine-based therapies.
- Standard therapies remain unsatisfactory; thus, patients should be considered for clinical trials (9).

MEDICATION

- Analgesics
- Stages I and II
  - Radical pancreatic resection + chemotherapy
  - ESPAC-3 trial after resection: compared with 5-fluorouracil (5-FU) and folinic acid, gemcitabine did not improve overall survival.
  - Currently, postoperative gemcitabine alone or in combination with 5-FU–based chemoradiation is the current standard of care; preoperative neoadjuvant treatment trials are in progress.
- Stage III
  - Standard: Chemotherapy with gemcitabine-based regimens; added chemoradiation is controversial; recent data suggest efficacy in advanced disease
  - Palliation of biliary obstruction by endoscopic, surgical, or radiologic methods
  - Intraoperative radiation therapy and/or implantation of radioactive substances
- Stage IV
  - Chemotherapy: gemcitabine with erlotinib, a platinum agent, or a fluoropyrimidine may modestly prolong survival compared with gemcitabine alone.
  - Pain-relieving procedures (celiac or intrapleural block); supportive care; palliative decompression

ADDITIONAL THERAPIES

- For resected tumors: postoperative radiation therapy with other chemotherapeutic agents
- Intraoperative radiation therapy and/or implantation of radioactive substances (ongoing trials)
- Biliary decompression with endoprosthesis or transhepatic drainage
- Celiac axis and intrapleural nerve blocks can provide effective pain relief for some patients.
- Opiates may be needed for pain control.

SURGERY/OTHER PROCEDURES

- Standard treatment options
  - Pancreaticoduodenectomy, Whipple procedure, en bloc resection of the head of the pancreas, distal common bile duct, duodenum, jejunum, and gastric antrum
  - Total pancreatectomy
  - Distal pancreatectomy for body and tail tumors
- Nonstandard surgeries
  - Pylorus-preserving pancreaticoduodenectomy, regional pancreatectomy
  - Palliative bypass
    - Biliary decompression; gastrojejunostomy for gastric outlet obstruction; duodenal endoprosthesis for obstruction

ONGOING CARE

DIET

- Anorexia, asthenia, pain, and depression may contribute to cachexia.
- Fat malabsorption due to exocrine pancreatic insufficiency may contribute to malnutrition; pancreatic enzyme replacement may help to alleviate symptoms.
- Fat-soluble vitamin deficiency may require replacement therapy.

PROGNOSIS

- Median survival: 10–20 months
- 5-year survival: ~30% if node-negative; 10% if node-positive
- Metastatic cancer: 1–2% 5-year survival
- For localized disease and small cancers (<2 cm) with no lymph node involvement and no extension beyond the capsule, complete surgical resection can yield a 5-year survival of 18–24%.
- Detection of curable precursor lesions is a focus of current efforts to improve diagnosis and prognosis.

COMPLICATIONS

- Diabetes mellitus, malabsorption, thrombophlebitis
- Duodenal or distal bile duct obstruction
- Surgical complications: intra-abdominal abscess, postgastrectomy syndromes, pancreaticojejunostomy, gastric and biliary anastomotic leaks; operative mortality varies

REFERENCES

1. Lennon AM, Wolfgang CL, Canto MI, et al. The early detection of pancreatic cancer: what will it take to diagnose and treat curable neoplasia? *Cancer Res*. 2014;74(13):3381–3389.
2. Yadav D, Lowenfels AB. The epidemiology of pancreatitis and pancreatic cancer. *Gastroenterology*. 2013;144(6):1252–1261.
3. Rustgi A. Familial pancreatic cancer. *Genes Dev*. 2014; 28(1): 1–7.
4. De La Cruz M, Young AP, Ruffin MT. Diagnosis and management of pancreatic cancer. *Am Fam Physician*. 2014;89(8):626–632.
5. Winter JM, Yeo CJ, Brody JR. Diagnostic, prognostic, and predictive biomarkers in pancreatic cancer. *J Surg Oncol*. 2013;107(1):15–22.
6. Kinney T. Evidence-based imaging of pancreatic malignancies. *Surg Clin North Am*. 2010;90(2): 235–249.
7. Verbesey JE, Munson JL. Pancreatic cystic neoplasms. *Surg Clin North Am*. 2010;90(2):411–425.
8. Oberstein PE, Olive KP. Pancreatic cancer: why is it so hard to treat? *Ther Adv Gastroenterol*. 2013; 6(4):321–337.
9. Saif MW. Advancements in management of pancreatic cancer: 2013. *JOP*. 2013;14(2):112–118.

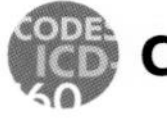

CODES

ICD10

- C25.9 Malignant neoplasm of pancreas, unspecified
- C25.0 Malignant neoplasm of head of pancreas
- C25.1 Malignant neoplasm of body of pancreas

CLINICAL PEARLS

- Sudden onset of diabetes mellitus in nonobese adults aged >40 years may warrant consideration of pancreatic cancer in selected cases.
- Cancer of the exocrine pancreas is rarely curable; overall 5-year survival rate of <4%. Fewer than 20% of cases are localized at diagnosis.
- Be wary of chronic pancreatitis, which can present with similar pain pattern, weight loss, jaundice, and an inflammatory mass on imaging.

PANCREATITIS, ACUTE

Robert L. Frachtman, MD, FACG • Marni Martinez, APRN

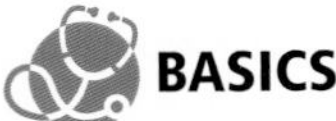

BASICS

DESCRIPTION

Acute inflammatory process of the pancreas with variable involvement of regional tissue or remote organ systems

- Inflammatory episode with symptoms related to intrapancreatic activation of enzymes with pain, nausea, and vomiting and associated intestinal ileus
- Varies widely in severity, complications, and prognosis, accounting for 280,000 hospital admissions per year in the United States
- Complete structural and functional recovery, provided no necrosis or pancreatic ductal disruption

EPIDEMIOLOGY

Incidence

- 1–5/10,000
- Predominant age: none
- Predominant sex: male = female

PREVALENCE

Acute: 19/10,000

ETIOLOGY AND PATHOPHYSIOLOGY

- Alcohol
- Gallstones (including microlithiasis)
- Trauma/surgery
- Acute discontinuation of medications for diabetes or hyperlipidemia
- Following endoscopic retrograde cholangiopancreatography (ERCP)
- Medications (most common, not an exhaustive list)
  - ACE inhibitors
  - Angiotensin receptor blockers (ARBs)
  - Thiazide diuretics and furosemide
  - Antimetabolites (mercaptopurine and azathioprine) (1)
  - Corticosteroids
  - Glyburide
  - Exenatide (Byetta) (2)
  - Mesalamine
  - Pentamidine
  - Sulfamethoxazole/trimethoprim
  - Valproic acid
  - HMG CoA reductase inhibitors, especially simvastatin (1)
  - When a patient presents with pancreatitis, review all medications and continue only if the benefit outweighs risk, especially medication causally implicated.
- Metabolic causes:
  - Hypertriglyceridemia (>1,000 mg/dL)
  - Hypercalcemia
  - Acute renal failure
  - Diet with high glycemic load (3)[B]
  - Systemic lupus erythematosus/polyarteritis
  - Autoimmune pancreatitis, associated with elevated IgG4
  - Infections (list not exhaustive)
    - Mumps, coxsackie, cryptosporidiosis
- Penetrating peptic ulcer (rare)
- Cystic fibrosis and *CFTR* gene mutations
- Tumors (e.g., ampullary)
- Pancreas divisum
- Sphincter of Oddi dysfunction
- Scorpion venom
- Vascular disease
- Acute fatty liver of pregnancy
- Idiopathic/autoimmune
- Pathophysiology—enzymatic "autodigestion" of the pancreas, interstitial edema with severe interstitial acute fluid accumulation ("3rd spacing"), hemorrhage, necrosis, release of vasoactive peptides (within 6 weeks), pseudocyst or acute necrotic collection (>6 weeks), pancreatic ductal disruption, injury to surrounding vascular structures—splenic vein (thrombosis) and splenic artery (pseudoaneurysm)

Genetics

Hereditary pancreatitis is rare. Autosomal dominant

GENERAL PREVENTION

- Avoid excess alcohol consumption.
- Tobacco cessation
- Correct underlying metabolic processes (hypertriglyceridemia or hypercalcemia).
- Discontinue offending medications.
- Cholecystectomy (symptomatic cholelithiasis)
- Diet with low glycemic load (3)[B]

COMMONLY ASSOCIATED CONDITIONS

- Alcohol withdrawal, alcoholic hepatitis, diabetic ketoacidosis, and ascending cholangitis
- Obesity increases severity, local complications, and mortality (4).

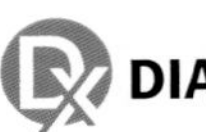

DIAGNOSIS

Symptoms do not always correlate linearly with objective findings (imaging, amylase/lipase).

HISTORY

- Acute onset of "boring" epigastric pain, which may radiate posteriorly toward the back
- Nausea/vomiting
- Alcohol use
- History or family history of gallstones
- Medication use
- Abdominal trauma
- Recent significant rapid weight loss

PHYSICAL EXAM

- Vital signs—assess hemodynamic stability; fever
- Abdominal findings: epigastric tenderness, loss of bowel sounds
- Other findings, jaundice, rales/percussive dullness
- Rare (with hemorrhagic pancreatitis)
  - Flank discoloration (Grey-Turner sign) or umbilical discoloration (Cullen sign)

DIAGNOSTIC TESTS & INTERPRETATION

- Laboratory and radiographic findings should be interpreted within the context of the clinical history, as there are often false-positive and false-negative findings.
- APACHE II scoring is most accurate but difficult to apply (5). BISAP, SIRS (temp, pulse, resp, and WBC), and HAPS are newer, more rapidly applicable calculations.
- *Ranson criteria* historically used to predict mortality
- On admission: age >55 years, WBCs >16,000/mm, blood glucose >200 mg/dL (11.1 mmol/L), serum lactate dehydrogenase (LDH) >350 IU/L, aspartate aminotransferase (AST) >250 IU/L
- Within 48 hours: hematocrit decreases >10%, serum calcium <8 mg/dL, BUN increase >8 mg/dL, arterial PO_2 <60 mm Hg, base deficit >4 mEq/L, fluid retention >6 L.
- Elevated serum amylase >3× upper limit of normal (ULN) (severity is not related to degree of elevation)
- Elevated serum lipase >3× ULN (may stay elevated longer than amylase in mild cases)
- Elevated total bilirubin. If greater than 3 mg/dL consider common bile duct obstruction.
- Transaminases rise quickly with acute bile duct obstruction. They also fall rapidly as alkaline phosphatase rises; a 3-fold elevation in the alanine aminotransferase (ALT) in the setting of acute pancreatitis has a 95% positive predictive value for gallstone pancreatitis. Triglyceride levels >1,000 mg/dL suggest hypertriglyceridemia as the cause.
- Glucose is increased in severe disease.
- Calcium is decreased in severe disease.
- WBC elevation to 10,000–25,000/μL possible and not indicative of active infection
- Rising hemoglobin is a poor prognostic sign (severe 3rd spacing-hemoconcentration). Rising blood urea nitrogen (BUN) and creatinine imply volume depletion or acute renal failure.

DIFFERENTIAL DIAGNOSIS

- Penetrating peptic ulcer
- Acute cholecystitis or cholangitis
- Macroamylasemia, macrolipasemia
- Mesenteric vascular occlusion and/or infarction
- Perforation of a viscus
- Intestinal obstruction
- Aortic aneurysm (dissecting or rupturing)
- Inferior wall myocardial infarction
- Lymphoma

Initial Tests (lab, imaging)

- Use follow-up labs to assess renal function, hydration, sepsis, biliary obstruction, and tissue oxygenation status.
- Plain film of abdomen helps rule out mechanical small bowel obstruction. Ileus is common.
- Chest x-ray (CXR) to evaluate for early acute respiratory distress syndrome (ARDS) and pleural effusion. Can also rule out free subdiaphragmatic air.
- Ultrasound to rule out cholelithiasis; choledocholithiasis can occasionally be seen.
- CT scan
  - Confirms the diagnosis, assesses severity, establishes a baseline, and rules out other possibilities. CT does not rule out noncalcified cholelithiasis.
  - IV contrast is not essential on the initial CT scan and should be avoided in volume-depleted patients.
  - If not contraindicated, a CT scan with IV contrast at day 3 can assess the degree of necrosis when necrotizing pancreatitis is suspected because of O_2 saturation <90%, systolic BP <90 mm Hg, etc.
- MRCP helps assess for choledocholithiasis, pancreas divisum, a dilated pancreatic duct, and chronic ductal changes.
- Esophagogastroduodenoscopy (EGD) may be necessary to rule out a penetrating duodenal ulcer or an obstructing ampullary neoplasm if suggested by laboratory or imaging studies.

- ERCP may be necessary to decompress common bile duct due to an impacted stone.
- Endoscopic ultrasonography (EUS) is useful when a patient with "idiopathic pancreatitis" has 2nd episode.
- FNA may be added to EUS if autoimmune pancreatitis is suspected (6)[C].

Follow-Up Tests & Special Considerations

If renal function is stable, a contrast-enhanced CT scan at day 3 to assess for necrosis. Later in the course, if there is a spike in the temperature, CT aspiration can be done to assess for secondary infection.

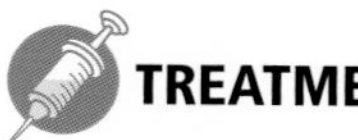

TREATMENT

MEDICATION

First Line

- Analgesia: no consensus; guidelines vary widely on types and dosing for analgesia (7).
  - Hydromorphone (Dilaudid) 0.5–1 mg IV q1–2h PRN
  - AVOID Demerol due to the potential of accumulation of a toxic metabolite.
- Antibiotics
  - The use of prophylactic antibiotics is no longer recommended, even with necrotizing pancreatitis, without evidence of infection.
  - In patients with ascending cholangitis or necrotizing pancreatitis, β-lactam/β-lactamase inhibitor (e.g., piperacillin/tazobactam 4.5 g IV q8h) can be considered for initial treatment, before cultures (especially of aspirated collections) return, if there is a strong suspicion of active infection.
  - Or levofloxacin 500 mg QD IV if cholangitis and there is an allergy to penicillin
  - Be vigilant for monilial superinfections when giving prophylactic antibiotics.

GENERAL MEASURES

Most cases of acute pancreatitis require hospitalization; ICU if multiorgan dysfunction or hypotension/respiratory failure. Acute pancreatitis often progresses from mild to severe (including persistent organ failure) in 15–20% of cases.

- Fluid resuscitation
  - Significant volume deficit due to 3rd spacing
  - Infuse bolus of 1,000–2,000 mL (lactated Ringer may be better than normal saline, unless hypercalcemic), followed by 250–300 mL/hr, adjusted on the basis of age, weight, hemodynamic response, and comorbid conditions.
  - Target urine output should be 0.5–1 mL/kg/hr. Lower infusion rate when this goal is achieved or once BUN decreases, 4 L should be the maximum fluid on day 1.
- Eliminate unnecessary medications, especially those potentially causing pancreatitis.
- Nasogastric (NG) tube for intractable emesis
- Follow renal function, volume status, calcium, and oxygenation. Organ failure is more important prognostic indicator than pancreatic necrosis.
- Intermittent pneumatic compression device
- Begin oral alimentation after pain, tenderness, and ileus have resolved; small amounts of high-carbohydrate, low-fat, and low-protein foods; advance as tolerated; NPO or NG tube if vomiting persists
- Enteral nutrition at level of ligament of Treitz if oral feeding not be possible within 5–7 days (preferable to total parenteral nutrition [TPN] due to decreased infection rate and decreased mortality). Discontinue with increases in pain, amylase/lipase levels, or fluid retention.
- TPN (without lipids if triglycerides are elevated) if oral or nasoenteric feedings are not tolerated (8).

ISSUES FOR REFERRAL

Refer to a tertiary center if pancreatitis is severe or actively evolving and when advanced imaging or endoscopic therapy is being considered.

SURGERY/OTHER PROCEDURES

- Consider cholecystectomy before discharge in patients with cholelithiasis and nonnecrotizing pancreatitis to reduce risk of recurrent acute gallstone pancreatitis.
- Necrosectomy should be performed nonsurgically for either infected or noninfected necrosis. Walled off necrosis should be observed for 4 weeks (treated with antibiotics if infected), followed by percutaneous or dual-modality drainage if available (9)[B].
- ERCP early if evidence of acute cholangitis or at 72 hours if evidence of ongoing biliary obstruction. ERCP with pancreatic ductal stent placement, if ductal disruption persists longer than 1–2 weeks
- Resection or embolization for bleeding pseudoaneurysms
- Plasma exchange with insulin if necrotizing pancreatitis secondary to hypertriglyceridemia

INPATIENT CONSIDERATIONS

Discharge Criteria

- Pain controlled
- Tolerating oral diet
- Alcohol rehabilitation and tobacco cessation
- Low-grade fever and mild leukocytosis do not necessarily indicate infection and may take weeks to resolve. Infections may occur even after 10 days (33% of patients with necrotizing pancreatitis) due to secondary infection of necrotic material, requiring surgical débridement.

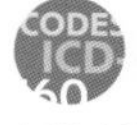

ONGOING CARE

FOLLOW-UP RECOMMENDATIONS

- Follow-up imaging studies in several weeks, if the original CT scan showed a fluid collection or necrosis or if the amylase/lipase continues to be elevated. Follow-up finding may include:
  - Pseudocyst (occurs in 10%) or abscess (sudden onset of fever): Conservative management is an option for asymptomatic pseudocysts up 6 cm in diameter.
  - Splenic vein thrombosis (gastric variceal hemorrhage rarely occurs)
  - Pseudoaneurysm (splenic, gastroduodenal, intrapancreatic) hemorrhage can be life-threatening.
- Mild exocrine and endocrine dysfunction is usually subclinical. Patients with necrotizing pancreatitis, steatorrhea, or ductal obstruction, however, should receive enzyme supplementation.

DIET

Continue to advance diet as tolerated. Dietary modification to reduce dietary fats, alcohol and added sugars

PROGNOSIS

- 85–90% of cases of acute pancreatitis resolve spontaneously; 3–5% mortality (17% in necrotizing pancreatitis)
- BISAP criteria: BUN > 25mg/dL; impaired mental status, ≥2 SIRS criteria; age >60 years; pleural effusion (1 point for each. Patients with score of 5 have 22% mortality.)

REFERENCES

1. Nitsche CJ, Jamieson N, Lerch MM, et al. Drug induced pancreatitis. *Best Pract Res Clin Gastroenterol*. 2010;24(2):143–155.
2. Wang SQ, Li SJ, Feng QX, et al. Overweight is an additional prognostic factor in acute pancreatitis: a meta-analysis. *Pancreatology*. 2011;11(2):92–98.
3. Oskarsson V, Sadr-Azodi O, Orsini N, et al. High dietary glycemic load increases the risk of non-gallstone-related acute pancreatitis: a prospective cohort study. *Clin Gastroenterol Hepatol*. 2014;12(4):676–682.
4. Wu BU, Conwell DL. Acute pancreatitis part I: approach to early management. *Clin Gastroenterol Hepatol*. 2010;8(5):410–416.
5. Lu X, Aoun E. Complications of acute pancreatitis. *Pract Gastroenterol*. 2012;36:11–26.
6. Iwashita T, Yasuda I, Doi S, et al. Use of samples from endoscopic ultrasound-guided 19-gauge fine-needle aspiration in diagnosis of autoimmune pancreatitis. *Clin Gastroenterol Hepatol*. 2012;10(3):316–322.
7. Oláh A, Romics L Jr. Evidence-based use of enteral nutrition in acute pancreatitis. *Langenbecks Arch Surg*. 2010;395(4):309–316.
8. Gravante G, Garcea G, Ong SL, et al. Prediction of mortality in acute pancreatitis: a systematic review of the published evidence. *Pancreatology*. 2009;9(5):601–614.
9. Ross AS, Irani S, Gan SI, et al. Dual-modality drainage of infected and symptomatic walled-off pancreatic necrosis: long-term clinical outcomes. *Gastrointest Endosc*. 2014;79(6):929–935.

ADDITIONAL READING

- Fisher JM, Gardner TB. The "golden hours" of management in acute pancreatitis. *Am J Gastroenterol*. 2012;107(8):1146–1150.
- Wu BU, Banks PA. Clinical management of patients with acute pancreatitis. *Gastroenterology*. 2013;144(6):1272–1281.

CODES

ICD10

- K85.9 Acute pancreatitis, unspecified
- K85.8 Other acute pancreatitis
- K85.2 Alcohol induced acute pancreatitis

CLINICAL PEARLS

- BISAP score is easier to apply than Ranson criteria and just as accurate in predicting mortality.
- Review all medications upon admission and discontinue implicated as causing pancreatitis.
- Patients with mild pancreatitis can progress to severe pancreatitis over the initial 48 hours, often due to inadequate fluid replacement.
- Referral to tertiary center is needed if acute pancreatitis is severe or evolving/worsening.

PANCREATITIS, CHRONIC

Robert L. Frachtman, MD, FACG • Marni Martinez, APRN

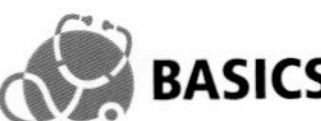

BASICS

DESCRIPTION

- Long-standing and progressive destruction of the pancreas due to persistent inflammation
- Results in exocrine and/or endocrine insufficiency
- Major features
  - Pain
  - Malabsorption
  - Diabetes mellitus (type 3)
  - Increased risk of pancreatic cancer

EPIDEMIOLOGY

Incidence

Predominant age

- 35–45 years (usually related to alcohol)
- Predominant sex: male > female
- Hospitalization more common for blacks than whites

Prevalence

8/10,000

Genetics

Hereditary pancreatitis is a rare condition with an autosomal dominant inheritance pattern. Mutations in *PRSSI* gene and *SPINKI* gene

GENERAL PREVENTION

- Avoid tobacco.
- Avoid excess alcohol.

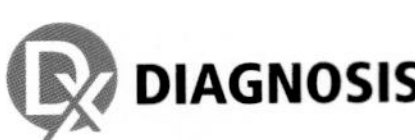

DIAGNOSIS

As with acute pancreatitis, symptoms and objective findings (imaging, amylase/lipase) do not always directly correlate.

HISTORY

- Epigastric pain, often radiating to the back
- Flare-ups may mimic acute pancreatitis.
- Persistent nausea and vomiting
- Chronic vague abdominal pain; may worsen postprandially or with alcohol consumption
- Alcohol use
- Cigarette smoking
- Steatorrhea and/or diarrhea
- Weight loss
- Children
  - Recurrent postprandial epigastric pain
  - Family history of chronic pancreatitis
  - Growth failure
  - Diabetes

PHYSICAL EXAM

- Acute superimposed on chronic pancreatitis
  - See "Pancreatitis, Acute"
  - Epigastric tenderness
  - Loss of bowel sounds
  - Fever
  - Tachycardia
  - Hypotension/shock
  - Jaundice
  - Rales/percussive dullness
- Chronic pancreatitis
  - Mild, diffuse tenderness
  - Ascites

DIAGNOSTIC TESTS & INTERPRETATION

The laboratory and radiographic findings in chronic pancreatitis must be interpreted within the context of each patient presentation due to common false-positive and false-negative fingings.

Initial Tests (lab, imaging)

Features and considerations:

- Amylase and lipase usually normal or near normal
- Hyperglycemia
- Steatorrhea (fecal fat >7 g/day on 100 g of fat per day diet), with other malabsorptive consequences such as low B_{12} level
- Elevated alkaline phosphatase and bilirubin imply obstruction of the intrapancreatic common bile duct Autoimmune pancreatitis: elevated serum IgG4 (type I, not type II), autoantibodies to lactoferrin and carbonic anhydrase (1)
- Pancreatic insufficiency: fecal elastase-1 <200 μg/g in moderate to severe pancreatic insufficiency
- Plain film of abdomen: might show pancreatic calcification if severe
- Ultrasound (US): helps assess common bile duct diameter, less useful for visualizing pancreas
- CT scan of abdomen: pseudocysts, pancreatic duct dilation, and calcifications, which are most commonly associated with alcohol, cigarette smoking, and hereditary pancreatitis and may take 5–10 years to develop (1)
- Magnetic resonance cholangiopancreatography (MRCP): pancreatic ductal deformities/strictures (with or without pancreatic ductal stones), retained common bile duct stones
- Endoscopic US (EUS): might help identify pancreatic cancer

Follow-Up Tests & Special Considerations

Disorders that alter results for amylase or lipase:

- Biliary tract disease
- Penetrating peptic ulcer
- Intestinal obstruction
- Intestinal ischemia/infarction
- Ruptured ectopic pregnancy
- Renal insufficiency
- Burns
- Macroamylasemia
- Macrolipasemia

DIFFERENTIAL DIAGNOSIS

- Pancreatic cancer
- Lymphoma
- Other malabsorptive processes, such as bacterial overgrowth or celiac disease

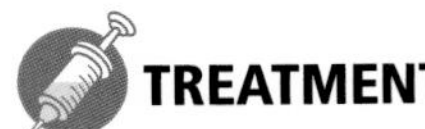

TREATMENT

MEDICATION

First Line

- Analgesics (no consensus on specific medications or doses)
  - Tramadol 50 mg q6h PO is commonly used as a first-line.
  - Chronic opioid (morphine, fentanyl) therapy may be required in some patients.
  - Gabapentin, pregabalin, SNRIs, or TCAs may be used as adjunctive therapy.
- Traditional pancreatic enzyme supplements are microencapsulated and do not require acid inhibition for protection. Dosage is 25–40,000 IU at the beginning of the meal.
- Some experts believe that uncoated enzymes (Viokase) are more efficacious for pain control (when given with proton pump inhibitors [PPIs] to protect their integrity) compared with coated enzymes (2,3). There is a theoretical benefit to using PPIs, even with coated enzymes, in patients with vitamin deficiency to allow faster release of enzymes into the proximal duodenum where fat soluble vitamin absorption occurs (1).
- Octreotide 25–50 mcg/H IV infusion can be supplemental therapy for pancreatic ductal fistulae, which can later be changed to long-acting depo version SQ administration.
- Individualized doses of corticosteroids for autoimmune pancreatitis

GENERAL MEASURES

- Discontinue cigarette smoking, which can exacerbate chronic pancreatitis (4).
- Analgesia: Consider pain management consultation for chronic opioid management.
- Exocrine and endocrine replacement therapy (enzymes and insulin, respectively)

- Consider more advanced therapy for pain: celiac ganglion block via EUS and endoscopic or surgical decompression of partially obstructed pancreatic duct.

SURGERY/OTHER PROCEDURES

- Pseudocyst drainage
  - Conservative approach if asymptomatic
  - Endoscopic (via EUS) or surgical approach if mature wall
  - Percutaneous approach if rapidly enlarging or if thin wall
  - Endoscopic drainage and percutaneous drainage have similar clinical success rates, but percutaneous drainage requires more reintervention and longer hospital stay (5)[C].
- Pancreatic ascites with disruption of the main pancreatic duct
  - Endoscopic placement of pancreatic ductal stent is preferred, if possible.
  - Lateral pancreaticojejunostomy if endoscopic therapy is not possible
- Biliary obstruction (secondary to chronic pancreatitis, not choledocholithiasis)
  - Placement of retrievable metal stent or multiple plastic stents, if possible
  - Choledochojejunostomy if endoscopic therapy is not possible
- Pancreatic ductal obstruction by stone
  - Endoscopic pancreatic sphincterotomy with stone extraction
- Total pancreatectomy and islet autotransplantation
  - Favorable outcomes with pain reduction
  - Indication for timing of procedure uncertain

INPATIENT CONSIDERATIONS

Discharge Criteria

- Pain control
- Resolution of problems secondary to ductal disruption, if present
- Alcohol rehab and smoking cessation, if needed

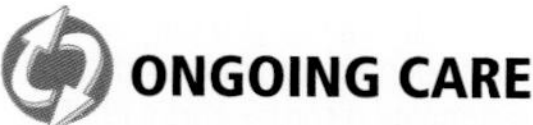

ONGOING CARE

FOLLOW-UP RECOMMENDATIONS

Depends on the source of the pain and whether a ductal disruption exists

DIET

- Small meals high in protein, ~20 g/day of fat; adjust if diabetes mellitus is present. Patients with decreased endocrine function from chronic pancreatitis can be prone to hyper- or hypoglycemia (6)[C].
- Pancreatic enzyme replacement therapy (coated/microencapsulated if treating pancreatic insufficiency, but noncoated with PPI if treating pancreatic pain)
- Vitamin A and vitamin E deficiency are not very common—levels should be checked and supplements provided only if deficiencies are noted (6)[C].

PROGNOSIS

- Patients with recurrent episodes of acute pancreatitis are more likely to develop chronic pancreatitis.
- May "burn out" with resolution of symptoms
- Narcotic addiction occurs frequently.
- Pancreatic exocrine and/or endocrine insufficiency may occur years later.
- Patients with chronic pancreatitis have an increased mortality, particularly from pancreatic cancer (7).
- 25% of patients with chronic pancreatitis have osteoporosis, and almost 2/3 have either osteoporosis or osteopenia. Bone health assessment should be performed routinely (8)[A].

REFERENCES

1. Forsmark CE. Management of chronic pancreatitis. *Gastroenterology*. 2013;144(6):1282–1291.
2. Slaff J. Protease-specific suppression of pancreatic exocrine secretion. *Gastroenterology*. 1984;87(1):44–52.
3. Puylaert M, Kapural L, Van Zundert J, et al. Pain in chronic pancreatitis. *Pain Pract*. 2011;11(5):492–505.
4. Yadav D, Hawes RH, Brand RE, et al; North American Pancreatic Study Group. Alcohol consumption, cigarette smoking, and the risk of recurrent acute and chronic pancreatitis. *Arch Intern Med*. 2009;169(11):1035–1045.
5. Akshintala VS, Saxena P, Zaheer A, et al. A comparative evaluation of outcomes of endoscopic versus percutaneous drainage for symptomatic pancreatic pseudocysts. *Gastrointest Endosc*. 2014;79(6):921–928.
6. Duggan S, Conlon K. A practical guide to the nutritional management of chronic pancreatitis. *Practical Gastroenterol*. 2013;37:24–32.
7. Bang UC, Benfield T, Hyldstrup L, et al. Mortality, cancer, and comorbidities associated with chronic pancreatitis: a Danish nationwide matched-cohort study. *Gastroenterology*. 2014;146(4):989–994.
8. Duggan SN, Smyth ND, Murphy A, et al. High prevalence of osteoporosis in patients with chronic pancreatitis: a systematic review and meta-analysis. *Clin Gastroenterol Hepatol*. 2014;12(2):219–228.

ADDITIONAL READING

- Bornman PC, Botha JF, Ramos JM, et al. Guideline for the diagnosis and treatment of chronic pancreatitis. *S Afr Med J*. 2010;100(12, Pt 2):845–860.
- Bramis K, Gordon-Weeks AN, Friend PJ, et al. Systematic review of total pancreatectomy and islet autotransplantation for chronic pancreatitis. *Br J Surg*. 2012;99(6):761–766.
- Giuliano CA, Dehoorne-Smith ML, Kale-Pradhan PB. Pancreatic enzyme products: digesting the changes. *Ann Pharmacother*. 2011;45(5):658–666.
- Kozarek R, Ball TJ, Patterson DJ, et al. Endoscopic transpapillary therapy for disrupted pancreatic duct and peripancreatic fluid collections. *Gastroenterology*. 1991;100(5, Pt 1):1362–1370.
- Niemann T, Madsen LG, Larsen S, et al. Opioid treatment of painful chronic pancreatitis. *Int J Pancreatol*. 2000;27(3):235–240.
- Yadav D, O'Connell M, Papachristou GI. Natural history following the first attack of acute pancreatitis. *Am J Gastroenterol*. 2012;107(7):1096–1103.

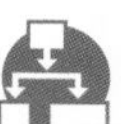

SEE ALSO

Choledocholithiasis; Peptic Ulcer Disease; Substance Use Disorders; Lupus Erythematosus, Systematic (SLE)

CODES

ICD10

- K86.1 Other chronic pancreatitis
- K86.0 Alcohol-induced chronic pancreatitis

CLINICAL PEARLS

- EUS can help differentiate chronic pancreatitis from pancreatic cancer.
- Pancreatic enzyme replacement therapy and the avoidance of cigarettes and alcohol are the cornerstone of therapy for chronic pancreatitis.

PANIC DISORDER

Anub G. John, MD • Hugh Peterson, MD, FACP

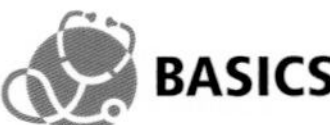

BASICS

DESCRIPTION

- A classic panic attack is characterized by rapid onset of a brief period of sympathetic nervous system hyperarousal accompanied by intense fear.
- In panic disorder, multiple panic attacks occur (including at least 1 without a recognizable trigger). Worried anticipation of additional attacks, which can be disabling, is present for at least 1 month, and, often, maladaptive (e.g., avoidance) behaviors develop.

EPIDEMIOLOGY

Incidence

- Predominant age: all ages; in school-aged children, panic disorder can be confused with conduct disorder and school avoidance
- Peak age of onset is early to mid-20s.
- Predominant sex: female > male (2:1)

Prevalence

- Lifetime prevalence: 4.7% (1)
- 4–8% of patients in a primary care practice population have panic disorder.
- Of patients presenting with chest pain in the emergency room, 25% have panic disorder.
- Chest pain is more likely due to panic if atypical, younger age, female, and known problems with anxiety.

ETIOLOGY AND PATHOPHYSIOLOGY

Unknown

- Biologic theories focus on limbic system malfunction in dealing with anxiety-evoking stimuli.
- Psychological theories posit deficits in managing strong emotions such as fear and anger.
- Noradrenergic neurotransmission from the locus coeruleus causes increased sympathetic stimulation throughout the body.
- Current neurobiologic research focuses on abnormal responses to anxiety-producing stimuli in the hippocampus, amygdala, and prefrontal cortex; for example, there appears to be limbic kindling in which an original frightening experience dominates future responses even when subsequent exposures are not objectively threatening.
- Brain pH disturbances (e.g., excess lactic acid) from normal mentation in genetically vulnerable patients may activate the amygdala and generate unexpected fear responses.

Genetics

Twin and family studies support a genetic predisposition.

RISK FACTORS

- Life stressors of any kind can precipitate attacks.
- History of sexual abuse and physical abuse, anxious and overprotective parents
- Substance abuse, bipolar disorder, major depression, obsessive-compulsive disorder (OCD), and simple phobia

COMMONLY ASSOCIATED CONDITIONS

- Of patients with panic disorder, >70% also have ≥1 other psychiatric diagnoses: PTSD (recalled trauma precedes panic attack), social phobia (fear of scrutiny precedes panic attack), simple phobia (fear of something specific precedes panic), major depression, bipolar disorder, substance abuse, OCD, separation anxiety disorder.
- Panic disorder is more common in patients with asthma, migraine headaches, hypertension, mitral valve prolapse, reflux esophagitis, interstitial cystitis, irritable bowel syndrome, fibromyalgia, nicotine dependence, and suicidality.

DIAGNOSIS

- Panic attack: an abrupt surge of intense fear, reaching a peak within minutes in which ≥4 of the following symptoms develop abruptly: (a) palpitations, pounding heart, or accelerated heart rate; (b) sweating; (c) trembling or shaking; (d) sensations of shortness of breath or feeling smothered; (e) a choking sensation; (f) chest pain or discomfort; (g) nausea or abdominal distress; (h) feeling dizzy, unsteady, lightheaded, or faint; (i) derealization (feelings of unreality) or depersonalization (feeling detached from oneself); (j) fear of losing control or going crazy; (k) fear of dying; (l) paresthesias; (m) chills or hot flushes (2)[C]
- Panic disorder: recurrent unexpected panic attacks not better accounted for by another psychiatric condition (e.g., PTSD, OCD, separation anxiety disorder, social anxiety disorder, or specific phobia) *and* not induced by drugs of abuse, medical conditions, or prescribed drugs *and* with >1 month of at least 1 of the following: (a) worry about additional attacks; (b) worry about the implications of the attack (e.g., losing control, having a heart attack, "going crazy"); and/or (c) a significant maladaptive change in behavior related to the attacks (2)[C]
- Unlike *DSM-IV*, *DSM-5*, defines agoraphobia as separate from panic disorder (2)[C].

HISTORY

- The best way to get a good history is through tactful, nonjudgmental questioning after the worst of the attack is over. Use open-ended questions and be unhurried. Interviewing family members may also be helpful.
- A thorough medication and substance abuse history is important.
- Patients must have a month of fear of out-of-the-blue panic attacks to diagnose panic disorder.

PHYSICAL EXAM

- During an attack, there will be tachycardia, hyperventilation, and sweating.
- Check the thyroid for fullness or nodules.
- Cardiac exam to check for a murmur or arrhythmias
- Lung exam to rule out asthma (limited airflow, wheezing)

DIFFERENTIAL DIAGNOSIS

- Medication use may mimic panic disorder and create anxiety: Antidepressants to treat panic may paradoxically initially cause panic; antidepressants in bipolar patients can cause anxiety/mania/panic; short-acting benzodiazepines (alprazolam), β-blockers (propranolol), and short-acting opioids can cause interdose rebound anxiety; benzodiazepine treatment causes panic when patients take too much and run out of these medicines early; bupropion, levodopa, amphetamines, steroids, albuterol, sympathomimetics, fluoroquinolones, and interferon can cause panic.
- Substances of abuse: alcohol withdrawal, benzodiazepine withdrawal, opioid withdrawal, caffeine, marijuana (panic with paranoia), amphetamine abuse, MDMA, hallucinogens (PCP, LSD), dextromethorphan abuse, synthetic cathinones (bath salts) abuse
- Medical conditions: hypo-/hyperthyroidism, asthma/chronic obstructive pulmonary disease (COPD), reflux esophagitis with hyperventilation, tachyarrhythmias, premenstrual dysphoric disorder, menopause, pregnancy, hypoglycemia (in diabetes), hypoxia, inner ear disturbances (labyrinthitis), myocardial infarction, pulmonary embolus, transient ischemic attacks (TIAs), carcinoid syndrome, pre- and postictal states (e.g., in TLE), autoimmune disease, pheochromocytoma, Cushing syndrome, hyperaldosteronism, Wilson disease
- Psychiatric conditions that have overlapping symptomatology include mood, anxiety, and personality disorders such as major depression, bipolar disorder, PTSD, borderline personality disorder, social phobia, OCD, and generalized anxiety disorder. In PTSD, there is always a recollection or visual image that precedes the panic attack. In social phobia, fear of scrutiny precedes the panic attack. In bipolar disorder, major depression, borderline personality disorder, and particularly substance abuse, the patient often complains first of panic symptoms and anxiety and minimizes other potentially relevant symptoms and behaviors.
- Somatic symptom disorder is also an illness of multiple unexplained medical symptoms, but the presenting picture is usually one of chronic symptoms rather than the acute, dramatic onset of a panic attack. Somatic symptom disorder and panic disorder can be (and often are) diagnosed together.

P

DIAGNOSTIC TESTS & INTERPRETATION

Consider ECG and pulse oximetry to rule out certain serious causes of panic; consider Holter monitoring. No specific lab tests are indicated except to rule out conditions in the differential diagnosis.

- Finger-stick blood sugar in acute setting in a diabetic patient
- Thyroid-stimulating hormone (TSH), electrolytes, CBC
- Consider ordering echocardiogram if you suspect mitral valve prolapse.

Diagnostic Procedures/Other

If a medical cause of anxiety is strongly suspected, do the workup appropriate for that condition.

TREATMENT

Combined antidepressant therapy and psychotherapy is superior to either alone during initial treatment (3)[A]. Cognitive-behavioral therapy (CBT) provides long-lasting treatment, often without subsequent need for medications.

GENERAL MEASURES

CBT, tailored for panic disorder, consists of several steps: education, changing cognitions about the attack and the illness, relaxation and controlled breathing techniques, and, if appropriate, exposure to anxiety-provoking conditions coupled with in vivo relaxation exercises.

MEDICATION

- Medication management is indicated if psychotherapy is not successful (or not available) and may be combined with psychotherapy.
- Patient preference plays a big part in this decision.
- Because patients typically are anxious about their treatment, the therapeutic alliance is critical for the chronic care of this disorder.
- If medications are started, they should be maintained for at least 6 months after symptom control.

First Line

- FDA-approved choices for the treatment of panic disorder include sertraline, paroxetine, fluoxetine, alprazolam, and clonazepam, but avoid giving benzodiazepines to those with a history of substance abuse or who are currently abusing alcohol or benzodiazepines, unless following a detoxification protocol.
- All antidepressants except bupropion can treat panic disorder, but fluoxetine and selegiline patch can cause more initial nervousness than other antidepressants.
- In nonbipolar patients, start a low-dose SSRI (e.g., 5 mg escitalopram, 25 mg sertraline, 10 mg paroxetine) and consider doubling the dose after 2 or 3 weeks; while waiting for the antidepressant to work, schedule frequent visits, give the patient reassurance, teach a relaxation technique, encourage the patient to do vigorous aerobic exercise as soon as a panic attack begins (if medically appropriate and in an appropriate situation); refer the patient to a competent therapist for CBT (4)[A].
- In bipolar patients, panic symptoms often resolve when treated with a mood stabilizer rather than an antidepressant (which may cause mania).

Second Line

- Tricyclic antidepressants, particularly imipramine (start 25 mg/day in the evening and increase up to 25 mg every 3 days to a maximum of 200 mg/day); slower titration and lower doses are often as effective. Imipramine is as efficacious as SSRIs in the treatment of panic. Tricyclic antidepressants are considered second line because of difficulty in dosing, more side effects, and greater risk associated with overdose compared with SSRIs (5)[A].
- Alprazolam (0.5–1 mg) and lorazepam (0.5–1 mg) can be given as a single dose to help with panic symptoms. If antidepressants are only partially effective, consider adding a longer-acting benzodiazepine like clonazepam (0.5–1.5 mg BID).
- Benzodiazepines, particularly longer-acting benzodiazepines like clonazepam, can be considered as single agents to treat panic in patients with bipolar disorder and those with no mood symptoms or anxiety symptoms other than panic.

ISSUES FOR REFERRAL

Consider referral to a psychiatrist for panic disorder that is comorbid with bipolar disorder, borderline personality disorder, schizophrenia, suicidality, alcohol, or substance abuse.

ADDITIONAL THERAPIES

Aerobic exercise reduces symptoms better than placebo (6)[B].

INPATIENT CONSIDERATIONS

Admission Criteria/Initial Stabilization

- If certain life-threatening mimics of panic disorder have not been ruled out, such as a myocardial infarction (MI) or pulmonary embolus (PE), hospitalize patient to complete the evaluation.
- If a panic disorder patient has concrete suicidal ideation, a psychiatric admission is indicated.

ONGOING CARE

PATIENT EDUCATION

- www.nlm.nih.gov/medlineplus/panicdisorder.html
- Patient information handouts in *American Family Physician*. 2005;71:740 and 2006;74:1393.
- http://www.nimh.nih.gov/health/publications/panic-disorder-when-fear-overwhelms/index.shtml

PROGNOSIS

- Most patients recover with treatment.
- It can recur, but treatment of recurrence is usually successful.

COMPLICATIONS

- Iatrogenic benzodiazepine dependence
- Iatrogenic mania in bipolar patients treated for panic with unopposed antidepressants
- Misdiagnosis of more difficult-to-treat psychiatric conditions as panic and vice versa

REFERENCES

1. Kessler RC, Chiu WT, Demler O, et al. Prevalence, severity, and comorbidity of 12-month *DSM-IV* disorders in the National Comorbidity Survey Replication. *Arch Gen Psychiatry*. 2005;62(6):617–627.
2. American Psychiatric Association. *Diagnostic and Statistical Manual of Mental Disorders*, 5th ed. Arlington, VA: American Psychiatric Association; 2013.
3. Furukawa TA, Watanabe N, Churchill R. Combined psychotherapy plus antidepressants for panic disorder with or without agoraphobia. *Cochrane Database Syst Rev*. 2007;(1):CD004364.
4. Otto MW, Tuby KS, Gould RA et al. An effect-size analysis of the relative efficacy and tolerability of serotonin selective reuptake inhibitors for panic disorder. *Am J Psychiatry*. 2001;158(12):1989–1992.
5. Bakker A, van Balkom AJ, Spinhoven P. SSRIs vs. TCAs in the treatment of panic disorder: a meta-analysis. *Acta Psychiatr Scand*. 2002;106(3):163–167.
6. Broocks A, Bandelow B, Pekrun G, et al. Comparison of aerobic exercise, clomipramine, and placebo in the treatment of panic disorder. *Am J Psychiatry*. 1998;155(5):603–609.

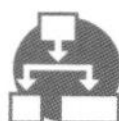

SEE ALSO

Algorithm: Anxiety

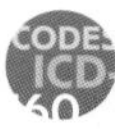

CODES

ICD10

- F41.0 Panic disorder without agoraphobia
- F40.01 Agoraphobia with panic disorder
- F43.0 Acute stress reaction

CLINICAL PEARLS

Encouraging patients (who are medically able) to do 10 minutes of vigorous aerobic exercise the moment a panic attack seems to be starting is often a very effective way to help patients feel safe during panic attacks. Always evaluate a patient with panic for suicidality. Patients with panic disorder are at increased risk for suicide, particularly if depressed.

PARKINSON DISEASE

Robert A. Baldor, MD, FAAFP

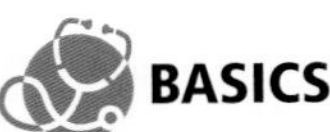

BASICS

DESCRIPTION

- Parkinson disease (PD) is a progressive neurodegenerative disorder caused by degeneration of dopaminergic neurons in the substantia nigra pars compacta.
- Cardinal symptoms include resting tremor, rigidity, bradykinesia, and postural instability.
- Diagnosis is based primarily on history and examination.

EPIDEMIOLOGY

Incidence

- Average age of onset: ~60 years
- Slightly more common in men than women

Prevalence

- Second most common neurodegenerative disease after Alzheimer disease
- 0.3% of general population and 1–2% of those ≥60 years of age and up to 4% of those ≥80 years of age
- Affects approximately 1 million people in the United States and 5 million worldwide

ETIOLOGY AND PATHOPHYSIOLOGY

Dopamine depletion in the substantia nigra and the nigrostriatal pathways results in the major motor complications of PD.

- Pathologic hallmark: selective loss of dopamine-containing neurons in the pars compacta of the substantia nigra
- Loss of neurons accompanied by presence of Lewy bodies, pale bodies (predecessor of the Lewy body), and Lewy neuritis

Genetics

Mutations in multiple autosomal dominant and autosomal recessive genes have been linked to PD/parkinsonian syndrome particularly when the age at symptom onset is younger than 50 years. Genes investigated in PD include *MAPT*, *SNCA*, *HLA-DRB5*, *BST1*, *GAK*, and *LRRK2*.

RISK FACTORS

- Age and family history of PD or tremor are the greatest risk factors.
- History of smoking as well as coffee and caffeine intake may reduce risk.
- Weak association with exposure to toxins (herbicides and insecticides); however, relationship is not clear

COMMONLY ASSOCIATED CONDITIONS

Non–motor-associated symptoms include cognitive abnormalities, autonomic dysfunction (e.g., constipation, urinary urgency), sleep disturbances, mental status changes (depression, psychosis, hallucinations, dementia), orthostatic hypotension, and pain.

DIAGNOSIS

- Diagnosis is based on clinical impression.
- Gold standard for diagnosis is neuropathologic exam.
- Generally, bradykinesia plus either tremor or rigidity must be present in order to make the diagnosis of idiopathic PD.
- Clinical features supportive of the diagnosis include unilateral onset, resting tremor, persistent asymmetry with the side of onset most affected, and significant response to dopaminergic therapy.

HISTORY

Symptoms often subtle or attributed to aging:

- Decreased emotion displayed in facial features
- General motor slowing and stiffness (1 or both arms do not swing with walk)
- Resting tremor (often initially 1 hand)
- Speech soft/mumbling
- Falls/difficulty with balance (tends to occur with disease progression)

PHYSICAL EXAM

- Tremor
  - Resting tremor (4–6 Hz) that is often asymmetric
  - Disappears with voluntary movement
  - Frequently emerges in a hand while walking and may present as pill rolling
  - May also present in jaw, chin, lips, tongue
- Bradykinesia
- Rigidity: cogwheel (catching and releasing) or lead pipe (continuously rigid)
- Postural instability

DIFFERENTIAL DIAGNOSIS

- Essential tremor: Bradykinesia is not present; often symmetric and occurs mostly during action or when holding hands outstretched
- SWEDD: scans without evidence of dopaminergic deficit; isolated upper extremity resting and postural tremor resembling PD but failing to progress to generalized PD
- Dementia with Lewy bodies: characterized clinically by visual hallucinations, fluctuating cognition, and parkinsonism
- Multiple system atrophy: presets with parkinsonism but with varying degrees of dysautonomia, cerebellar involvement, and pyramidal signs
- Progressive supranuclear palsy: impairment in vertical eye movements (particularly down gaze), hyperextension of neck, and early falling
- Idiopathic basal ganglia calcification
- Associated neurodegenerative disorders: late stages of Alzheimer disease, Huntington disease, frontotemporal dementia, spinocerebellar ataxias
- Secondary parkinsonism
  - Drug-induced: reversible; may take weeks/months after offending medication is stopped
    - Neuroleptics (most common cause)
    - Antiemetics (e.g., prochlorperazine and promethazine), metoclopramide
    - SSRIs
    - Calcium channel blockers (e.g., flunarizine and cinnarizine)
    - Amiodarone
    - Lithium
    - Cholinergics
    - Chemotherapeutics
    - Amphotericin B
    - Estrogens
    - Valproic acid

DIAGNOSTIC TESTS & INTERPRETATION

Initial Tests (lab, imaging)

- Diagnosis is mainly clinical and there are no physiologic or blood tests to confirm the diagnosis.
- Excellent response to an acute dopaminergic challenge test supports the diagnosis
- MRI of brain is nondiagnostic but can be used to rule out structural abnormalities.
- DaTscan: Striatal dopamine transporter imaging can distinguish PD and other parkinsonian syndromes but cannot differentiate between them.
- PET and single-photon emission CT may be helpful with diagnosis but are not required.

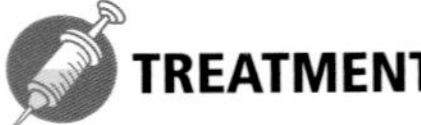

TREATMENT

GENERAL MEASURES

- Multidisciplinary rehabilitation with standard physical and occupational therapy components to improve functional outcomes
- Physiotherapy to help with gait reeducation, enhancement of aerobic capacity, improvement in movement initiation, improvement in functional independence, and help with home safety

MEDICATION

- PD goal: Improve motor and nonmotor deficits.
- Agents are chosen based on patient age and symptoms present.

First Line

- 1st-line agents in early PD: levodopa, dopamine agonists, monoamine oxidase B (MAO-B) inhibitors (1)[A]
  - Levodopa combined with carbidopa is still the most effective treatment for symptoms of Parkinson disease (2)[A].
  - Levodopa versus dopamine agonist is controversial (3)[B]:
    - Most patients eventually will develop motor fluctuations with levodopa. Younger patients are more likely to develop motor fluctuations. Some recommend delaying initiation of levodopa to decrease drug-induced motor fluctuations early in the disease.
    - Older patients often are unable to tolerate the adverse events of dopamine agonists.
    - All patients eventually will require levodopa.
  - MAO-B inhibitors (rasagiline) should be considered as initial monotherapy; investigated for potential neuroprotective effects (3)[B]
- Carbidopa + levodopa (carbidopa inhibits peripheral conversion of levodopa)
  - Immediate release (Sinemet)
    - Tablets (mg): 10/100, 25/100, 25/250
    - Usual initial maintenance dose: 25/100 mg PO TID. Most patients require 25 mg of carbidopa to inhibit peripheral conversion of levodopa.
    - Watch for nausea/vomiting, orthostatic hypotension, sedation, vivid dreams

- Orally disintegrating (Parcopa)
  - Tablets (mg): 10/100, 25/100, 25/25
- Sustained release (Sinemet CR):
  - Tablets (mg): 25/100, 50/200
  - Dose agents initially BID
- Carbidopa + levodopa + entacapone (Stalevo)
  - Tablets (mg): 12.5/50/200, 18.75/75/200, 25/100/200, 31.25/125/200, 37.5/150/200, 50/200/200
  - Addition of entacapone as a single agent should be initiated prior to use of this combination:
    - Once-daily dose of carbidopa/levodopa has been identified; may convert to Stalevo
    - Dose of levodopa may need to be decreased with the addition of entacapone.
  - Side effects are the same, plus diarrhea and brownish orange urine.
- Dopamine agonists (nonergot): side effects: nausea, vomiting, hypotension, sedation, edema, vivid dreaming, compulsive behavior, confusion, light-headedness, and hallucinations:
  - Pramipexole (Mirapex): tablets (mg): 0.125, 0.25, 0.5, 1, 1.5
    - Start with 0.125 mg TID, gradually increase every 5–7 days; usual maintenance of 0.5–1.5 mg TID
    - CrCl 30–59 mL/min 0.125 mg PO BID
    - CrCl 15–29 mL/min 0.125 mg PO daily
  - Pramipexole ER (Mirapex ER): tablets (mg): 0.375, 0.75, 1.5, 3, 4.5; start with 0.375 PO daily
  - Ropinirole (Requip): tablets (mg): 0.25, 0.5, 1, 2, 3, 4, 5; start with 0.25 mg TID, increase gradually to 3–8 mg TID
  - Requip XL: tablets (mg): 2, 4, 6, 8, 12; start at a 2-mg dose once daily, increase in 1–2 weeks
- Selective MAO-B inhibitors: side effects insomnia, jitteriness, hallucinations; mostly found with selegiline; rasagiline similar adverse events as placebo in clinical trials. Rasagiline is metabolized via *CYP1A2;* caution with other medications using this enzyme system (e.g., ciprofloxacin):
  - Both agents contraindicated with meperidine and numerous other agents metabolized via *CYP1A2*
  - At therapeutic doses, unlikely to induce a "cheese reaction" (tyramine storm)
- Selegiline (Eldepryl)
  - Tablets: 5 mg; initiate 5 mg PO BID
  - Orally disintegrating tablet (Zelapar): 1.25 mg; 1.25 mg PO daily for 6 weeks; increase as needed to max of 2.5 mg daily
- Rasagiline (Azilect): tablets: 0.5 mg, 1.0 mg; initiate 0.5–1 mg daily

Second Line

- Second-line agents in early PD: β-adrenergic antagonists (postural tremor), amantadine, anticholinergics (young patients with tremor); there is lack of good evidence for symptom control (1)[A].
- Dopamine agonists (ergot): increased adverse event profile makes these agents nonpreferred to nonergot dopamine agonists; bromocriptine (Parlodel)
- Treatment of levodopa-induced motor complications
  - End of dose wearing off
    - Entacapone (with each levodopa dose) or rasagiline preferred (4)[B]
    - May also consider dopamine agonist, apomorphine, selegiline (5)[B]
  - Dyskinesias
    - Typically occur at peak dopamine level
    - Amantadine may be considered; however, its efficacy is questionable (1)[B].
- Anticholinergic agents: usually avoided due to lack of efficacy (only useful for tremor) and increased adverse event profile, including blurred vision, confusion, constipation, dry mouth, memory difficulty, sedation, and urinary retention
  - Trihexyphenidyl
    - Tablets: 2 mg, 5 mg
    - Start with 1–2 mg daily, increase by 2 mg every 3–5 days until usual dose is 6–10 mg in 3–4 divided doses
  - Benztropine (Cogentin)
    - Tablets: 0.5 mg, 1 mg, 2 mg
    - Start with 0.5–1 mg in 1–2 divided doses; increase by 0.5 mg every 5–6 days; usual dose is 1–2 mg/d divided
- *N*-methyl-D-aspartic acid antagonist: Exact mechanism is unknown and efficacy is questionable; however, it may be useful for dyskinesias. Side effects include confusion, dizziness, dry mouth, livedo reticularis, and hallucinations:
  - Amantadine (Symmetrel)
    - Tablets: 100 mg
    - Start with 100 mg BID; may increase to 300 mg daily in divided doses; renally adjusted
- Catechol-O-methyl transferase (COMT) inhibitors: entacapone preferred due to hepatotoxicity associated with tolcapone. Adverse events include nausea and orthostatic hypotension:
  - Entacapone (Comtan)
    - Tablets: 200 mg
    - 200 mg with each dose of carbidopa/levodopa; max dose, 1,600 mg/day
  - Tolcapone (Tasmar)
    - Tablets: 100 mg, 200 mg
    - Start 100 mg TID; max dose 600 mg/day; must be taken with carbidopa/levodopa
    - Requires LFT monitoring
- Apomorphine (Apokyn): nonergot-derived dopamine agonist given SC for off episodes in advanced disease; adverse events: nausea, vomiting, dizziness, hallucinations, orthostatic hypotension, somnolence
  - Only for "off" episodes with levodopa therapy
  - Requires initial "test" dose (2 mg); monitor for orthostatic hypotension after initial dose; this is a potent emetic, so initiate an antiemetic (e.g., trimethobenzamide) 3 days prior to start and continue for 2 months. Avoid ondansetron (combination contraindicated due to profound hypotension) and dopamine antagonists, such as prochlorperazine and metoclopramide.
  - Effective dose ranges from 2 to 6 mg/injection.

ISSUES FOR REFERRAL

Early specialty referral for patients with suspected PD for an accurate diagnosis and management

ADDITIONAL THERAPIES

- Emotional and psychological support of patient family.
- Physical therapy and manual medicine has been shown to improve balance, muscle strength, and walking speed.
- Speech therapy: may be helpful in improving speech volume and maintaining voice quality

SURGERY/OTHER PROCEDURES

Deep brain stimulation (bilateral subthalamic nucleus/globus pallidus interna) is an effective therapeutic option for patients with motor complications refractory to best medical treatment who are healthy, have no significant comorbidities, are responsive to levodopa, and do not have depression or dementia.

ONGOING CARE

DIET

- Increase dietary fluids and fiber and increase activity for constipation.
- For dysphagia, consider soft food, swallowing evaluation, and increased time for meals.
- Avoid large, high-fat meals that slow digestion and interfere with medication absorption.

PATIENT EDUCATION

- www.apdaparkinson.org
- www.parkinson.org
- www.michaeljfox.org

PROGNOSIS

PD is a chronic progressive disease; prognosis varies based on patient-specific symptoms.

COMPLICATIONS

Most commonly the result of adverse effects of medications used to treat

REFERENCES

1. Gazewood JD, Richards DR, Clebak K. Parkinson disease: an update. *Am Fam Physician.* 2013;87(4):267–273.
2. Drugs for Parkinson's disease. Treatment Guidelines from The Medical Letter. 2013;11(135). http://secure.medicalletter.org/cannotaccess?ac=1&a=135a&t=article&n=11927&p=tg&title=Drugs%20for%20Parkinson%27s%20Disease&i=135. Accessed 2014.
3. International Parkinson Disease Genomics Consortium, Nalls MA, Plagnol V, et al. Imputation of sequence variants for identification of genetic risks for Parkinson's disease: a meta-analysis of genome-wide association studies. *Lancet.* 2011;377(9766):641–649.
4. Pahwa R, Factor SA, Lyons KE, et al. Practice parameter: treatment of Parkinson disease with motor fluctuations and dyskinesia (an evidence-based review): report of the Quality Standards Subcommittee of the American Academy of Neurology. *Neurology.* 2006;66(7):983–995.
5. Diaz NL, Waters CH. Current strategies in the treatment of Parkinson's disease and a personalized approach to management. *Expert Rev Neurother.* 2009;9(12):1781–1789.

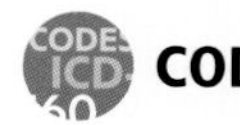

CODES

ICD10

- G20 Parkinson's disease
- G21.9 Secondary parkinsonism, unspecified
- G31.83 Dementia with Lewy bodies

CLINICAL PEARLS

- Emphasize the importance of exercise and movement to help preserve function.
- Pharmacotherapeutic regimens need to be individualized based on patient-specific symptoms and age.

PARONYCHIA

Arvind R. Ankireddypalli, MD • Sherly Abraham, MD, FAAFP

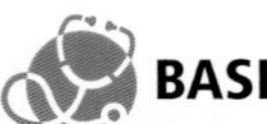

BASICS

DESCRIPTION

- Superficial inflammation of the lateral and posterior folds of skin surrounding the fingernail or toenail
  - Acute: characterized by pain, erythema, and swelling; usually a bacterial infection, appears after trauma. It can progress to abscess formation.
  - Chronic: characterized by swelling, tenderness, cuticle elevation, and nail dystrophy and separation.
  - May be considered work-related among bartenders, waitresses, nurses, and others who often wash their hands
- System(s) affected: skin and nail bed
- Synonym(s): eponychia; perionychia

Pediatric Considerations

Less common in pediatric age groups. Thumb/finger-sucking is a risk factor (anaerobes and *Escherichia coli* may be present).

EPIDEMIOLOGY

Incidence

- Common in the United States
- Predominant age: all ages
- Predominant sex: female > male

ETIOLOGY AND PATHOPHYSIOLOGY

- Acute: *Staphylococcus aureus* (1) most common and *Streptococcus pyogenes* (1); less frequently, *Pseudomonas pyocyanea* and *Proteus vulgaris*. In digits exposed to oral flora especially in pediatric age group, consider *Eikenella corrodens*, *Fusobacterium*, and *Peptostreptococcus*.
- Chronic: eczematous reaction with secondary *Candida albicans* (~95%) (2)
- A paronychial infection commonly starts in the lateral nail fold.
- If the infection includes the complete margin of skin around the nail plate, it results in mechanical separation of the nail plate from the perionychium (3).
- Early in the course, cellulitis alone may be present. An abscess can form if the infection does not resolve quickly.
- Chronic infections most likely represent eczematous skin reaction with superimposed secondary infection and multifocal etiology.

RISK FACTORS

- Acute: trauma to skin surrounding nail-like ingrown nails, manicure/sculptured nails, nail biting, and thumb sucking and predisposing conditions such as diabetes mellitus (DM)
- Chronic: frequent immersion of hands in water with excoriation of the lateral nail fold (e.g., cooks, chefs, bartenders, housekeepers, swimmers), DM, immunosuppression (reported association with antiretroviral therapy for HIV and with use of epidermal growth factor inhibitors) (4)

GENERAL PREVENTION

- Acute: Avoid trauma such as nail biting; prevent thumb sucking.
- Chronic: Avoid allergens; keep fingers/hands dry; wear rubber gloves with a cotton liner. Prevent excoriation of the skin.
- Good diabetic control

COMMONLY ASSOCIATED CONDITIONS

- DM
- Eczema or atopic dermatitis
- Certain medications: antiretroviral therapy (4) (especially protease inhibitors and lamivudine, in which toes more commonly involved) (4)
- Immunosuppression (3)

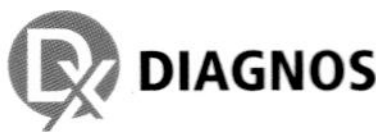

DIAGNOSIS

HISTORY

- Localized pain or tenderness, swelling, and erythema
  - Acute: fairly rapid onset
  - Chronic: 4–6 weeks' duration
- Previous trauma (bitten nails, ingrown nails, manicured nails)
- Contact with herpes infections
- Contact with allergens or irritants (frequent water immersion, latex) (3)

PHYSICAL EXAM

- Acute: red, warm, tender, tense nail fold ± abscess
- Chronic: swollen, tender, boggy nail fold ± abscess
- Occasional elevation of nail bed
- Separation of nail fold from nail plate
- Red, painful swelling of skin around nail plate
- Fluctuance, purulence at the nail margin, or purulent drainage
- Secondary changes of nail plate–like discoloration
- Suspect *Pseudomonas* if with green changes in nail (5).
- Positive fluctuation when mild pressure over the area causes blanching and demarcation of the abscess
- Chronic: retraction of nail fold and absence of adjacent healthy cuticle, thickening of nail plate with prominent transverse ridges known as Beau lines and discoloration

DIFFERENTIAL DIAGNOSIS

- Contact dermatitis
- Herpetic whitlow (similar in appearance, very painful, often associated with vesicles)
- Felon (abscess of fingertip pulp; urgent diagnosis required)
- Acute osteomyelitis of the distal phalanx
- Psoriasis especially acute flare
- Allergic contact dermatitis (latex, acrylic)
- Reiter disease
- Pustular psoriasis
- Proximal/lateral onychomycosis
- Malignancy: squamous cell carcinoma, malignant melanoma, metastatic disease

DIAGNOSTIC TESTS & INTERPRETATION

None required unless condition is severe; resistant to treatment or if recurrence or methicillin-resistant *S. aureus* (MRSA) is suspected, then

- Gram stain
- Culture and sensitivity
- Potassium hydroxide wet mount plus fungal culture especially in chronic
- Drugs that may alter lab results: use of over-the-counter antimicrobials or antifungals

Diagnostic Procedures/Other

- Incision and drainage recommended for suppurative cases or cases not responding to conservative management or empiric antibiotics.
- Tzanck testing or viral culture in suspected viral cases
- Biopsy in cases not responding to conservative management or when malignancy suspected

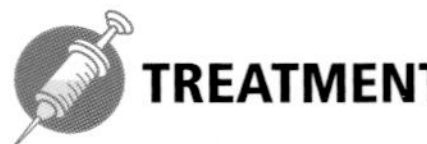

TREATMENT

GENERAL MEASURES

- Acute: warm compresses, elevation, splint protection if pain severe
- Chronic: Keep fingers dry; apply moisturizing lotion after hand washing; avoid exposure to irritants; improved diabetic control

MEDICATION

First Line

- Tetanus booster when indicated
- Acute (mild cases)
  - Antibiotic cream alone or in combination with a topical steroid (6)[B]
  - Antibiotic cream applied TID–QID after warm soak (e.g., mupirocin or gentamicin/neomycin/polymyxin B) for 5–10 days
  - If eczematous: low potent topical steroid applied BID (e.g., betamethasone 0.05% cream) for 7–14 days (7)[B]
- Acute (exposure to oral flora)
  - Amoxicillin clavulanate potassium: 875 mg/125 mg BID or 500 mg/125 mg TID for 7 days; pediatric, 45 mg/kg q12h (for <40 kg)
  - Clindamycin 300–450 mg TID–QID for 7 days; pediatric, 10 mg/kg q8h; *plus* either doxycycline or trimethoprim/sulfamethoxazole
- Acute (no exposure to oral flora)
  - Dicloxacillin 250 mg TID for 7 days
  - Cephalexin 500 mg TID–QID for 7 days
- Acute (suspected MRSA)
  - Trimethoprim/sulfamethoxazole 160 mg/800 mg BID for 7 days
  - Doxycycline 100 mg BID for 7 days
- Chronic
  - Topical steroids: betamethasone 0.05%; applied BID for 7–14 days (8)[B]
  - Topical antifungal: clotrimazole or nystatin; applied topically TID for up to 30 days
  - Other topical: Tacrolimus 0.1% ointment BID for up to 21 days has been shown to be effective but is more expensive.

P

Second Line

- Systemic antifungals (rarely needed)
  - Itraconazole 200 mg/day for 90 days (may have longer action because it is incorporated into nail plate); pulse therapy may be useful (i.e., 200 mg BID for 7 days, repeated monthly for 2 months) (1)[C],(8)
  - Terbinafine 250 mg/day for 6 weeks (fingernails) or 12 weeks (toenails)
  - Fluconazole 150 mg/week for 4–6 months
- Antipseudomonal drugs (e.g., ceftazidime, aminoglycosides) when pseudomonas is suspected

ISSUES FOR REFERRAL

Chronic; in treatment failure, consider biopsy and/or, in cases of chronic paronychia, referral for possible partial excision of the nail fold or eponychial marsupialization with or without complete nail removal.

SURGERY/OTHER PROCEDURES

- Incision and drainage of abscess, if present
- A subungual abscess or ingrown nail requires partial or complete removal of nail with phenolization of germinal matrix.

ONGOING CARE

FOLLOW-UP RECOMMENDATIONS

Chronic: Avoid frequent immersion, triggers, allergens, or nail biting and finger sucking.

DIET

If patient is diabetic, appropriate dietary and medication changes for better control

PATIENT EDUCATION

- Avoid trimming cuticles; avoid nail trauma; and stress importance of good diabetic control and diabetic education.
- Avoid contact irritants; use rubber gloves with cotton liners to avoid exposure to excess moisture.
- Use moisturizing lotion after washing hands; do not bite nails/suck on fingers.

PROGNOSIS

- With adequate treatment and prevention, healing can be expected in 1–2 weeks.
- If no response in chronic lesions, rarely benign or malignant neoplasm may be present and referral should be considered.

COMPLICATIONS

- Acute: subungual abscess
- Chronic: nail thickening, discoloration of nail, and nail loss

REFERENCES

1. Rigopoulos D, Larios G, Gregoriou S, et al. Acute and chronic paronychia. *Am Fam Physician*. 2008;77(3):339–346.
2. Shroff PS, Parikh DA, Fernandez RJ, et al. Clinical and mycological spectrum of cutaneous candidiasis in Bombay. *J Postgrad Med*. 1990;36(2):83–86.
3. Barlow AJ, Chattaway FW, Holgate MC, et al. Chronic paronychia. *Br J Dermatol*. 1970;82(5):448–453.
4. Tosti A, Piraccini BM, D'Antuono A, et al. Paronychia associated with antiretroviral therapy. *Br J Dermatol*. 1999;140(6):1165–1168.
5. Hengge UR, Bardeli V. Images in clinical medicine. Green nails. *N Engl J Med*. 2009;360(11):1125.
6. Wollina U. Acute paronychia: comparative treatment with topical antibiotic alone or in combination with corticosteroid. *J Eur Acad Dermatol Venereol*. 2001;15(1):82–84.
7. Rigopoulos D, Gregoriou S, Belyayeva E, et al. Efficacy and safety of tacrolimus ointment 0.1% vs. betamethasone 17-valerate 0.1% in the treatment of chronic paronychia: an unblinded randomized study. *Br J Dermatol*. 2009;160(4):858–860.
8. Tosti A, Piraccini BM, Ghetti E, et al. Topical steroids versus systemic antifungals in the treatment of chronic paronychia: an open, randomized double-blind and double dummy study. *J Am Acad Dermatol*. 2002;47(1):73–76.

ADDITIONAL READING

- Shaw J, Body R. Best evidence topic report. Incision and drainage preferable to oral antibiotics in acute paronychial nail infection? *Emerg Med J*. 2005;22(11):813–814.
- Rockwell PG. Acute and chronic paronychia. *Am Fam Physician*. 2001;63(6):1113–1116.

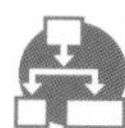

SEE ALSO

Onychomycosis

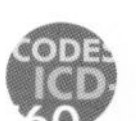

CODES

ICD10

- L03.019 Cellulitis of unspecified finger
- L03.039 Cellulitis of unspecified toe

CLINICAL PEARLS

- Consider tetanus booster when indicated.
- Consider incision and drainage when appropriate.
- For chronic paronychia, topical steroid is 1st-line treatment. Consider other differentials in nonresponders.
- For chronic nonhealing lesion, consider dermatology referral.

PAROTITIS, ACUTE AND CHRONIC

Binny Chokshi, MD • Kathleen Ferrer, MD, FAAP, AAHIVS

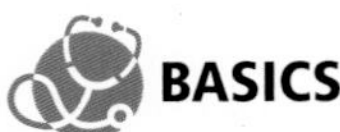

BASICS

DESCRIPTION

- Parotitis is inflammation of the parotid gland caused by infection (viral or bacterial), noninfectious systemic illnesses, mechanical obstruction, or medications.
- Parotitis can be unilateral or bilateral, acute or chronic. Unilateral parotitis is usually associated with duct obstruction, whereas bilateral parotitis more commonly indicates a systemic cause.
- The parotid gland is the largest of the salivary glands, located lateral to the masseter muscle anteriorly and extending posteriorly over the sternocleidomastoid muscle behind the angle of the mandible. It produces exclusively serous secretions, which lack the bacteriostatic properties of mucinous secretions, making the parotid gland more susceptible to infection than other salivary glands.
- The parotid duct, also called Stensen duct, pierces the buccinator muscle to enter the buccal mucosa just opposite the 2nd maxillary molar.
- The branches of the 7th cranial nerve or "facial nerve" divide the gland into lobes.
- The parotid gland contains lymph nodes.

EPIDEMIOLOGY

- Prior to widespread vaccination, parotitis was primarily caused by mumps virus, with 150,000 cases of parotitis per year; in 2011, 370 cases occurred.
- Acute bacterial parotitis occurs more frequently in elderly patients, neonates (especially preterm infants), and postoperative patients.
- Neonatal parotitis and juvenile recurrent parotitis are more common in males than females.
- Juvenile recurrent parotitis is the 2nd most common inflammatory cause of parotitis in the United States after viral parotitis; 1st episode usually occurs between the ages of 3 and 6 years.
- Chronic parotitis mainly affects adults, more often females. The average age of presentation is between 40 and 60 years.
- Chronic bilateral parotid enlargement is a common manifestation of HIV infection; for perinatally HIV-infected children, the average age of onset for parotid enlargement is 5 years.

RISK FACTORS

- Acute viral parotitis: lack of mumps, measles, rubella (MMR) vaccination
- Acute bacterial parotitis
  - Conditions that predispose to salivary stasis such as dehydration, debilitation, poor oral hygiene, Sjögren syndrome, cystic fibrosis, bulimia/anorexia, sialolithiasis (stones), ductal stenosis, trauma
  - Immunosuppression, HIV, chemotherapy, radiation, malnutrition, alcoholism
- Neonatal parotitis: prematurity, low birth weight, ductal obstruction, oral trauma, structural abnormalities, immunosuppression
- Juvenile recurrent parotitis: dental malocclusion, congenital duct malformation, genetic factors, immunologic anomalies
- Drug-induced parotitis: medications such as anticholinergics, antihistamines, diuretics, tricyclic antidepressants, antipsychotics, antineoplastic agents, and iodine
- Chronic parotitis: ductal stenosis, HIV, tuberculosis, Sjögren syndrome, and sarcoidosis

GENERAL PREVENTION

- MMR vaccination with the 1st dose between 12 and 15 months and 2nd dose between 4 and 6 years of age; of note, mumps vaccination does not guarantee prevention, possibly due to waning immunity in adolescence
- Maintain adequate hydration and good dental hygiene.
- Suck on hard or sour candy and use hot compresses with parotid massages to stimulate salivary flow and prevent salivary stasis.
- Smoking cessation, abstinence from alcohol, and avoidance of chronic purging

ETIOLOGY AND PATHOPHYSIOLOGY

- Acute viral parotitis begins as a systemic infection that localizes to the parotid gland, resulting in inflammation and swelling of the gland.
  - Mumps, or paramyxovirus, has a predilection for the parotid gland and classically has been linked to parotitis.
- Acute bacterial parotitis results from stasis of salivary flow that allows retrograde introduction of bacterial pathogens into the parotid gland, resulting in localized infection.
- Acute parotitis pathogens
  - Viral
    - Paramyxovirus (mumps), parainfluenza virus types 1 and 3, influenza A, coxsackie viruses, Epstein-Barr virus (EBV)
    - Cytomegalovirus (CMV) and adenovirus have been seen in patients with HIV.
  - Bacterial
    - *Staphylococcus aureus* and anaerobes (oral flora) are most commonly seen.
    - *Streptococcus pneumoniae*, viridans streptococci, *Escherichia coli*, and *Haemophilus influenza* (less common)
    - Gram-negative rods such as *E. coli*, *Klebsiella*, *Enterobacter*, and *Pseudomonas* can be seen in chronically ill or hospitalized patients.
  - Fungal
    - *Candida* has been isolated in chronically ill or hospitalized patients.
    - *Actinomyces* can be found in patients with a history of trauma or dental caries.
- Acute, recurrent parotitis
  - Juvenile recurrent parotitis may be secondary to chronic inflammation; etiology is unknown, but a genetic predisposition may exist.
  - Mechanical: sialolithiasis, ductal stenosis; repeated sialolith formation can lead to ductal wall damage, fibrosis, and stricture formation, which further decreases salivary flow and perpetuates obstruction
  - Pneumoparotitis may occur when air is trapped in the ducts of the parotid gland; may be seen in wind instrument players, glass blowers, scuba divers, and with dental cleaning.
  - Medications: anticholinergics, antihistamines, tricyclic antidepressants, antipsychotics (especially phenylbutazone, thioridazine, clozapine), iodine (especially contrast media), and l-asparaginase (1)[C]
  - Other: diabetes, alcoholism, bulimia, "anesthesia mumps" (possible mechanisms include transient mechanical compression of Stensen duct by airway devices, loss of muscle tone around the Stensen orifice after neuromuscular relaxants, increased salivary secretion, and increased flexion or rotation of the head during general anesthesia)
- Chronic parotitis may occur due to chronic ductal stenosis but is often due to a chronic infectious or inflammatory condition
  - HIV
  - Tuberculosis, syphilis (rare)
  - Autoimmune: Sjögren syndrome (parotid enlargement, xerostomia, and keratoconjunctivitis)
  - Inflammatory: sarcoidosis
    - Heerfordt syndrome (parotid enlargement, facial palsy, and uveitis) is a rare manifestation of sarcoidosis.
- Chronic parotitis in HIV-infected patients can be due to the presence of benign lymphoepithelial cysts, follicular hyperplasia of parotid lymph nodes, or diffuse infiltrative lymphocytosis syndrome (DILS), causing infiltration of the parotid gland by CD8 cells.
  - Parotitis may also be secondary to immune reconstitution after initiation of combination antiretroviral therapy in HIV-infected patients.

COMMONLY ASSOCIATED CONDITIONS

HIV, Sjögren syndrome, sarcoidosis, sialolithiasis

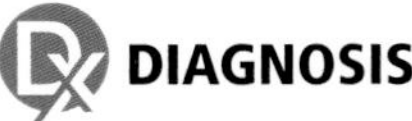

DIAGNOSIS

HISTORY

- Acute parotitis presents with sudden-onset pain and swelling of the cheek usually extending to and obscuring the angle of the mandible.
  - Viral parotitis is usually bilateral and accompanied by a prodrome of malaise, anorexia, headaches, myalgias, arthralgias, and fever; typically, overlying skin is not warm or erythematous, and no pus is reported at the opening of Stensen duct.
  - Bacterial parotitis is typically unilateral with induration, warmth, and erythema over the affected cheek; fever is often present.
  - Juvenile recurrent parotitis is usually unilateral; pain and swelling usually resolve within 2 weeks, and exacerbations occur until puberty; purulent exudate is not typical, but superinfection may occur.
  - Sialolithiasis is characterized by recurrent acute swelling and pain, exacerbated by eating; sialolithiasis affects the submandibular gland more frequently.
  - Other frequently reported symptoms include trismus (inability to open mouth), pain exacerbated by chewing or worsened by foods that stimulate production of saliva (i.e., sour candies), dry mouth with abnormal taste, difficulty with drinking/eating, anorexia, or dehydration.
- Chronic parotitis presents with recurrent or chronic nontender swelling of one or both parotid glands; can have periods of remission lasting weeks to years.
  - Sjögren syndrome, sarcoidosis, HIV, tuberculosis
  - Chronic parotitis may predispose to superinfection, which would present similarly to an acute parotitis.

PHYSICAL EXAM

- Parotitis is characterized by swelling or enlargement of the parotid gland(s) overlying the masseter muscle; it may obscure the angle of the mandible or cause the ear to protrude upward and outward.
- Palpation of the parotid gland is best done by using 1 hand to start at the attachment of the earlobe and palpating anteriorly and inferiorly along the mandibular ramus while the other hand simultaneously palpates the Stensen duct orifice.
  - Tender and bilateral suggests viral etiology, whereas tender, erythematous, warm, and unilateral suggests bacterial etiology.
  - Nontender in HIV, tuberculosis, Sjögren sydrome, sarcoidosis

- Trismus may be noted.
- Pus from Stensen duct is suggestive of bacterial parotitis or superinfection; opening of duct may appear edematous and erythematous in both bacterial and viral parotitis.
- In juvenile recurrent parotitis, Stensen duct is often enlarged, dilated, erythematous, and swollen.
- Halitosis and dental decay are often associated with acute exacerbations.
- Facial nerve palsy can be seen in severe cases.

DIFFERENTIAL DIAGNOSIS

- Lymphoma, neoplasm, lymphangitis, cervical adenitis, otitis externa, dental abscess, odontogenic infections, Ludwig angina, and cellulitis should be considered in the differential.
- Parotid swelling or enlargement typically obscures the angle of the mandible (unlike cervical adenitis).
- Involvement of Stensen duct is unique to parotitis.

DIAGNOSTIC TESTS & INTERPRETATION

- History and physical exam are usually sufficient for diagnosis of parotitis.
- Performing aerobic culture and Gram stain of purulent drainage from Stensen duct or aerobic and anaerobic culture from needle aspiration of gland or abscess can be helpful to identify causative organism.
  - Anaerobic culture from Stensen duct will likely contain oropharyngeal contamination; hence, it is recommended to perform anaerobic cultures only from needle aspirate fluid.
- Acute bacterial parotitis often demonstrates an elevated white blood cell count and amylase.
- For suspected mumps, obtain mumps IgM antibody or mumps reverse transcription-polymerase chain reaction (RT-PCR). A 4-fold increase of mumps IgG antibody indicates infection.
- Consider sending EBV titers and respiratory virus PCR panel if viral parotitis suspected; CMV titers should be sent in immunocompromised patients.
- For chronic, recurrent, or nontender parotitis, obtain HIV test, PPD, SS-A SS-B antibodies, rheumatoid factor, and antinuclear antibodies to evaluate for underlying etiology.
- Consider obtaining ultrasound or CT scan of parotid area to assess for abscess, cystic masses, parotid tumors, ductal stenosis, or sialolithiasis if no response to initial treatment.
- Consider sialography with chronic parotitis to assess the anatomy and functional integrity of the gland; can be diagnostic and therapeutic.

Diagnostic Procedures/Other

Consider performing a biopsy or fine-needle aspiration of gland if there is suspicion for tuberculosis, Sjögren syndrome, or sarcoidosis.

Test Interpretation

- Findings characteristic of HIV are described in the "Etiology and Pathophysiology" section.
- Noncaseating granulomas may be seen in sarcoidosis, and caseating granulomas may be found in tuberculosis.

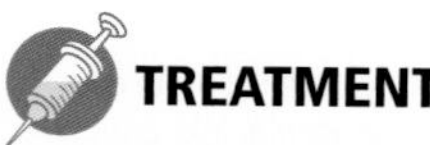

TREATMENT

GENERAL MEASURES

- Usually a self-limiting course that requires primarily supportive treatment with rest, adequate hydration, analgesia, and antipyretics
  - Can stimulate glands to produce saliva by sucking on hard candies or glycerin swabs
  - Local heat and gentle massage of gland can provide symptomatic relief.
  - For chronic presentations, encourage good dental hygiene and treat underlying etiology of parotitis (HIV, Sjögren syndrome, etc.).
- Patients diagnosed with mumps should be isolated with standard and droplet precautions for 5 days after onset of parotid swelling.

MEDICATION

- Viral parotitis: with an uncertain diagnosis or toxic presentation, can empirically initiate antibiotics to cover *Staphylococcus aureus*, anaerobes (oral flora), and *Streptococcus pneumoniae*
- Acute bacterial parotitis
  - Outpatient management: amoxicillin/clavulanate, 1st-generation cephalosporin, clindamycin
  - Chronically ill or hospitalized: ampicillin/sulbactam or clindamycin and nafcillin; if methicillin resistance is probable, consider vancomycin or linezolid
- Pilocarpine and cevimeline can stimulate saliva production and inhibit ascending infection as well as provide symptomatic relief for patients with underlying Sjögren syndrome.

SURGERY/OTHER PROCEDURES

- Consider needle aspiration for bacterial parotitis with abscess formation or clinical deterioration with increasing pain, erythema, and swelling not responding to medication.
- May perform serial drainage for symptomatic cysts
- Consider superficial parotidectomy for severe recurrent parotid infections in patients with underlying predisposing etiology (such as Sjögren syndrome).
- Sialendoscopy has been shown to be both a diagnostic and therapeutic tool for recurrent parotitis and can allow for cortisone irrigation for anti-inflammatory effects (2)[C].
- For sialolithiasis, ductal stenosis, or for patients with >1 recurrence per year, consult otolaryngology for possible duct ligation, ductoplasty, or parotidectomy.
- Sclerotherapy with methyl violet or tetracycline has been shown to be effective in the treatment of cysts in HIV parotitis and is also considered definitive treatment for chronic parotitis (3)[C].

INPATIENT CONSIDERATIONS

Admission is recommended for patients with comorbidities, systemic involvement, and inability to tolerate PO, as well as neonates and patients for whom close outpatient follow-up is not feasible.

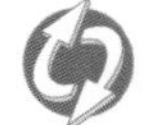

ONGOING CARE

FOLLOW-UP RECOMMENDATIONS

Antibiotic therapy initiated at diagnosis combined with adequate hydration should result in improvement within 48 hours. If not, patient should be reevaluated.

DIET

- Ensure adequate fluid intake.
- Hard or sour candies to promote salivary flow

PROGNOSIS

- Viral infection in immunocompetent individuals often resolves with excellent prognosis.
- Parotid cysts found in HIV-infected patients are usually benign lymphoepithelial lesions with infrequent malignant transformation.
- Increased incidence of malignant lymphoma or lymphoepithelial carcinoma may be seen in patients with Sjögren syndrome.

COMPLICATIONS

- For mumps, potential complications include orchitis, oophoritis, mastitis, meningitis, pancreatitis, sensorineural hearing loss, and nephritis.
- Untreated bacterial parotitis can lead to local extension, abscess formation, and facial paralysis.

REFERENCES

1. Brooks KG, Thompson DF. A review and assessment of drug-induced parotitis. *Ann Pharmacother*. 2012;46(12):1688–1699.
2. Schneider H, Koch M, Künzel J, et al. Juvenile recurrent parotitis: a retrospective comparison of sialdenoscopy versus conservative therapy. *Laryngoscope*. 2014;124(2):451–455.
3. Berg EE, Moore CE. Office-based sclerotherapy for benign parotid lymphoepithelial cysts in the HIV-positive patient. *Laryngoscope*. 2009;119(5): 868–870.

ADDITIONAL READING

- Armstrong MA, Turturro MA. Salivary gland emergencies. *Emerg Med Clin North Am*. 2013;31(2):481–499.
- Brook I. The bacteriology of salivary gland infections. *Oral Maxillofac Surg Clin North Am*. 2009;21(3):269–274.
- Capaccio P, Sigismund PE, Luca N, et al. Modern management of juvenile recurrent parotitis. *J Laryngol Otol*. 2012;126(12):1254–1260.
- Hackett A, Baranano C, Reed M, et al. Sialoendoscopy for the treatment of pediatric salivary gland disorders. *Arch Otolaryngol Head Neck Surg*. 2012;138(10):912–915.
- Harbison JM, Liess BD, Templer JW, et al. Chronic parotitis: a challenging disease entity. *Ear Nose Throat J*. 2011;90(3):E13–E16.
- Ortega KL, Ceballos-Salobreña A, Gaitán-Cepeda LA, et al. Oral manifestations after immune reconstitution in HIV patients on HAART. *Int J STD AIDS*. 2008;19(5):305–308.
- Patel A, Karlis V. Diagnosis and management of pediatric salivary gland infections. *Oral Maxillofac Surg Clin North Am*. 2009;21(3):345–352.

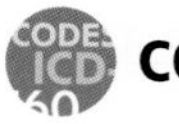

CODES

ICD10

- K11.20 Sialoadenitis, unspecified
- K11.21 Acute sialoadenitis
- K11.23 Chronic sialoadenitis

CLINICAL PEARLS

- History and physical exam are usually sufficient for diagnosis (parotid swelling and tenderness with or without purulent drainage from Stensen duct).
- In recurrent or chronic cases, consider other underlying etiologies such as HIV.
- *S. aureus* and anaerobes (oral flora) are the most common organisms isolated in acute bacterial parotitis.
- Encouraging good oral hygiene and adequate hydration in chronically ill, debilitated, and hospitalized patients can reduce parotitis occurrence.

PARVOVIRUS B19 INFECTION

David C. Krulak, MD, MPH, MBA, FAAFP

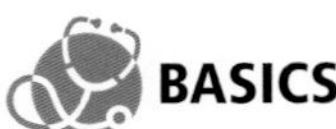

BASICS

DESCRIPTION

- Human parvovirus B19 is the primary cause of acute erythema infectiosum (EI, or fifth disease).
- Complications in susceptible individuals with increased RBC turnover (e.g., sickle cell anemia) include transient aplastic crisis (TAC). In immunocompromised individuals, pure red cell aplasia (PRAC) and chronic anemia are significant complications. In normal hosts, arthritis and arthralgias are common.
- System(s) affected by parvovirus B19 infection: hemic/lymphatic/immunologic, musculoskeletal, skin/exocrine, possibly central nervous system, cardiac, renal

PREGNANCY CONSIDERATIONS

Acute infection during pregnancy should prompt referral to a maternal–fetal medicine specialist. Maternal B19 infection between 9 and 20 weeks' gestation may carry a significant risk for developing fetal anemia and other complications.

EPIDEMIOLOGY

- Infection is common in childhood.
- EI has an extremely low mortality rate
- Peak age for EI is 4–12 years.
- Males and females are equally affected.
- Adult females are more likely to develop postinfectious arthritis.
- No known racial predilection
- In temperate climates, infections often occur from late winter to early summer.
- Local outbreaks may occur every 2–4 years.

Prevalence

Extremely common in the United States. Based on IgG serology

- 1–5 years of age: 2–15% seropositive
- 6–15 years of age: 20–40% seropositive
- 16–40 years of age: 50–60% seropositive
- >40 years of age: 70–85% seropositive

ETIOLOGY AND PATHOPHYSIOLOGY

- Small (20–25 mm), nonenveloped, single-stranded DNA virus in Parvoviridae family
  - Only known parvovirus to infect humans; does not cross-infect dogs or cats.
- Natural host of B19 is human erythroid progenitor.
- Respiratory, hematogenous, and vertical transmission are sources of human spread.
- 4–14-day incubation. Rash and joint symptoms occur 2–3 weeks after initial infection.
- Most contagious 5–10 days after exposure
- EI rash is felt to be autoimmune due to IgM complexes concurrent with viral clearance.
- Cytotoxic infection of proerythroblasts reduces RBC production.

Genetics

Erythrocyte P antigen–negative individuals are resistant to infection.

RISK FACTORS

- School-related epidemic and nonimmune household contacts have a secondary attack rate of 20–50%.
- Highest secondary attack rates are for daycare providers and school personnel in contact with affected children.
- Those with increased cell turnover (e.g., hemoglobinopathy, sickle cell [SS] anemia, thalassemia) are at risk for TAC.
- Immunodeficiency (e.g., HIV, congenital) increases risk of PRAC and chronic anemia.
- As many as 40% of pregnant women are not immune. 1.5% seroconversion rate per year.

GENERAL PREVENTION

- Parvovirus B19 is transmitted via the respiratory route. Standard measures including hand washing and barrier protection help prevent spread.
- Difficult to avoid exposure completely because the period of maximal contagion is prior to clinical symptoms (rash).
- Pregnant health care workers should avoid caring for patients with TAC.
- No significant risk of infection based on occupational exposure. Exclusion from the workplace is neither necessary nor is it recommended.
- No vaccine is available to prevent the disease.
- Droplet precautions recommended around patients with TAC, chronic infection, or anemia.

COMMONLY ASSOCIATED CONDITIONS

- Nondegenerative arthritis
  - In adults, 80% of patients may manifest polyarthritis and/or arthralgia (female > male).
  - In children, joint symptoms are less common.
  - Knees, hands, wrists, and ankles (frequently symmetric) are most commonly involved.
  - Joint symptoms usually subside within 3 weeks but may persist for months. Routine radiography is not necessary. No joint erosion are seen on x-ray if obtained.
- TAC
  - Involves patients with increased RBC turnover, such as sickle cell anemia, spherocytosis, thalassemia, or decreased RBC production (iron deficiency anemia).
  - Patients present with fatigue, weakness, lethargy, and pallor (anemia).
  - Aplastic event may be life threatening but is typically self-limited. Reticulocytes typically reappear in 7–10 days and full recovery in 2–3 weeks.
  - In children with sickle cell hemoglobinopathies and heredity spherocytosis, fever is the most common symptom (73%). Rash is uncommon in these patients.
- Chronic anemia
  - Seen in immunocompromised individuals (HIV, cancer, transplant) with poor IgM response
  - Usually no clinical manifestations such as fever, rash, or joint symptoms.
- Fetal/neonatal infection (1)
  - Risk of transplacental spread of virus is around 33% in infected mothers.
  - A pregnant woman with a rash or arthralgias consistent with parvovirus B19 should be tested.
  - Clinical manifestations vary. Many patients seroconvert without symptoms and have a normal pregnancy. Other patients develop variable degrees of fetal hydrops. Second- and 3rd-trimester pregnancy loss can occur without hydrops.
  - B19 infection should be suspected in cases of nonimmune fetal hydrops.
  - Fetal bone marrow is primarily impacted. RBC survival is shortened, resulting in anemia and (potentially) high-output cardiac failure.
  - >95% of fetal complications (fetal hydrops and death) occur within 12 weeks of acute maternal parvovirus B19 infection.
  - Risk of fetal loss in pregnancy is highest (2–5%) with B19 infections in the 1st trimester.
  - Infants requiring intrauterine transfusions due to parvovirus B19 infection are at risk for long-term neurodevelopmental impairment.
- Papular purpuric gloves and socks syndrome (PPGSS) is an uncommon dermatosis associated with parvovirus B19 infection. It results in a petechial and ecchymotic rash of the hands and feet associated with febrile tonsillopharyngitis and oral ulcerations (2).

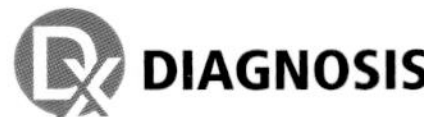

DIAGNOSIS

HISTORY

- Rash
- Headache
- Pharyngitis
- Coryza and rhinorrhea
- Arthralgias and arthritis
- Nausea and GI disturbances are more frequent and severe in adults (nonspecific flulike illness).
- Pruritus (especially soles of feet)
- Fever, myalgia, and malaise

PHYSICAL EXAM

- "Slapped-cheek" appearance is well-known facial rash that spares the nasolabial folds.
- A lacy, reticular rash on the trunk, buttocks, and limbs often follows 1–4 days later lasting 1–6 weeks.
- The rash may be pruritic and recurrent, exacerbated by bathing, exercise, sun exposure, heat, or emotional stress.
- B19 may manifest as painful pruritic papules and purpura on the hands and feet.

DIFFERENTIAL DIAGNOSIS

- Rubella
- Enteroviral disease
- Systemic lupus erythematosus
- Drug reaction
- Lyme disease
- Rheumatoid arthritis

DIAGNOSTIC TESTS & INTERPRETATION

Initial Tests (lab, imaging)

- No need for routine lab studies in typical cases. Diagnosis is clinical; illness is mild and self-limiting.
- IgG and IgM serology preferred in immunocompetent patients.
- B19-specific DNA polymerase chain reaction (PCR) testing for fetal infection (via cord blood or amniotic fluid) as well as for patients with chronic infection or immunocompromised status
- PCR increases diagnostic sensitivity and specificity to confirm infections in patients who are IgM negative.
- For patients with TAC, CBC with reticulocyte count shows anemia and reticulocytopenia. IgM antibodies are present by day 3, and IgG antibodies are detectable at time of clinical recovery. PCR shows high levels of viremia.
- Pregnant women exposed to B19 require serial IgG and IgM serology to assess fetal risk.

Follow-Up Tests & Special Considerations
Fetal/neonatal infection (3)[C]

- To exclude congenital B19 in infants with negative B19 IgM, IgG serology should be followed over the 1st year of life.
- Maternal serum α-fetoprotein may be increased in fetuses with hydrops fetalis.
- Documented acute maternal infection in the 1st trimester warrants serial fetal ultrasound to assess for hydrops: ascites, pericardial effusion, oligohydramnios, cardiomegaly, and placental thickening.
- Weekly peak systolic velocity measurements of the middle cerebral artery by Doppler US is recommended to evaluate for heart failure fetal anemia and the potential need for intrauterine transfusion (>1.5 MoM).
- Cerebral MRI to explore CNS damage in infected neonates with prolonged hydrops fetalis or hematocrit <15%.

Diagnostic Procedures/Other

- Skin biopsy usually normal but may show mild inflammation consisting of perivascular infiltrations of mononuclear cells.
- In stillbirths related to maternal B19 infection, virus can be detected in all tissues.
- In hydrops fetalis, nucleated RBCs may have intranuclear inclusion bodies.

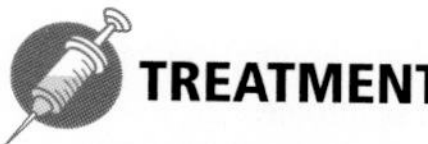

TREATMENT

GENERAL MEASURES

- No therapy is usually needed (4)[C].
- Cessation of immunosuppressive therapy has allowed some patients to clear chronic infections.
- B19-associated anemia in HIV-positive patients may resolve with highly active antiretroviral therapy.

MEDICATION

First Line

- Anti-inflammatory agents to alleviate arthritic symptoms
- Antipyretics for fever. Avoid aspirin in children.

Second Line

- RBC transfusions for aplastic crisis
- Intravenous immunoglobulin (IVIG) for B19-related refractory anemia or PRAC, especially in immunodeficient states (5)[C]
- Intrauterine RBC transfusions reduce mortality in cases of fetal hydrops.

ISSUES FOR REFERRAL

- Acute infection during pregnancy should prompt referral to a maternal–fetal medicine specialist.
- TAC patients require treatment by a hematologist.
- Patients with chronic or abnormal B19 infections may benefit from consultation with immunology or infectious disease specialists.

INPATIENT CONSIDERATIONS

Admission Criteria/Initial Stabilization

- Outpatient management is typical for EI.
- Inpatient management for aplastic crisis, which may require RBC transfusions

ONGOING CARE

FOLLOW-UP RECOMMENDATIONS

Patient Monitoring

Periodic blood counts for anemic patients

PATIENT EDUCATION

- Parvovirus B19 (fifth disease): www.cdc.gov/parvovirusB19/fifth-disease.html
- Parvovirus B19: What You Should Know: www.aafp.org/afp/2007/0201/p377.html
- Parvovirus B19 infection and pregnancy: www.cdc.gov/parvovirusB19/pregnancy.html
- March of Dimes Fifth Disease and Pregnancy: www.marchofdimes.com/pregnancy/complications_fifthdisease.html
- Counsel pregnant women regarding prevention of maternal B19 infection.
- Pregnant women should avoid exposure to patients with active/chronic infections. Exclusion of pregnant women from the workplace where EI is occurring is not recommended as they have likely been exposed.
- Children with typical rash are no longer infectious and may attend childcare or school.

PROGNOSIS

- Usually self-limited
- Joint symptoms subside in weeks (often by 2 weeks but may last months).
- ~20% of infections result in delayed virus elimination and viremia persisting for several months to years.
- Full recovery from aplastic crisis in 2–3 weeks

COMPLICATIONS

Conditions associated with B19 but where causality is unconfirmed.

- Chronic fatigue syndrome
- Glomerulonephritis, nephrotic syndrome, and other renal diseases
- Hepatitis
- Neurologic manifestations/stroke/meningoencephalitis
- Henoch-Schönlein purpura, idiopathic thrombocytopenic purpura, and vasculitis
- Myocarditis and pericarditis
- Hemophagocytic syndrome

REFERENCES

1. De Jong EP, de Haan TR, Kroes AC, et al. Parvovirus B19 infection in pregnancy. *J Clin Virol*. 2006;36(1):1–7.
2. Santonja C, Nieto-González G, Santos-Briz A, et al. Immunohistochemical detection of parvovirus B19 in "gloves and socks" papular purpuric syndrome: direct evidence for viral endothelial involvement. *Am J Dermatopathol*. 2011;33(8):790–795.
3. De Jong EP, Walther FJ, Kroes AC, et al. Parvovirus B19 infection in pregnancy: new insights and management. *Prenat Diagn*. 2011;31(5):419–425.
4. Servey JT, Reamy BV, Hodge J. Clinical presentations of parvovirus B19 infection. *Am Fam Physician*. 2007;75(3):373–376.
5. Orange JS, Hossny EM, Weiler CR, et al. Use of intravenous immunoglobulin in human disease: a review of evidence by members of the Primary Immunodeficiency Committee of the American Academy of Allergy, Asthma and Immunology. *J Allergy Clin Immunol*. 2006;117(4)(Suppl):S525–S553.

ADDITIONAL READING

- Azevedo KM, Setúbal S, Camacho LA, et al. Parvovirus B19 seroconversion in a cohort of human immunodeficiency virus-infected patients. *Mem Inst Oswaldo Cruz*. 2012;107(3):356–361.
- Beigi RH, Wiesenfeld HC, Landers DV, et al. High rate of severe fetal outcomes associated with maternal parvovirus b19 infection in pregnancy. *Infect Dis Obstet Gynecol*. 2008;2008:524601.
- Centers for Disease Control and Prevention. Risk associated with human parvovirus B19 infection. *MMWR Morb Mortal Wkly Rep*. 1989;38(6):81–88, 93–97.
- De Jong EP, Lindenburg IT, van Klink JM, et al. Intrauterine transfusion for parvovirus B19 infection: long-term neurodevelopmental outcome. *Am J Obstet Gynecol*. 2012;206(3):204.e1–204.e5.
- Heegaard ED, Brown KE. Human parvovirus B19. *Clin Microbiol Rev*. 2002;15(3):485–505.
- Lamont RF, Sobel JD, Vaisbuch E, et al. Parvovirus B19 infection in human pregnancy. *BJOG*. 2011;118(2):175–186.
- Snyder M, Wallace R. Clinical inquiry: what should you tell pregnant women about exposure to parvovirus? *J Fam Pract*. 2011;60(12):765–766.
- Young NS, Brown KE. Parvovirus B19. *N Engl J Med*. 2004;350(6):586–597.

CODES

ICD10

- B34.3 Parvovirus infection, unspecified
- B08.3 Erythema infectiosum [fifth disease]

CLINICAL PEARLS

- Parvovirus B19 infection is usually a benign, self-limited illness with no long-term effects.
- The rash of EI, initially presenting with a "slapped cheeks appearance," signifies that the patient is no longer infectious.
- Patients with increased RBC turnover (SS, thalassemia) are at risk for TAC.
- Immunocompromised patients may be at risk for chronic anemia.
- Documentation of acute infection <20 weeks' gestation warrants maternal–fetal consultation for serial monitoring of fetal well-being for 3 months via ultrasound.

PATELLOFEMORAL PAIN SYNDROME

Rathna Nuti, MD • Robert J. Dimeff, MD

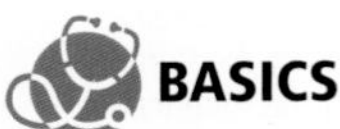

BASICS

DESCRIPTION

- Pain in or around the patella that increases after prolonged sitting, squatting, kneeling, and stair climbing (1)
- Synonyms: retropatellar pain syndrome
- System(s) affected: musculoskeletal

EPIDEMIOLOGY

Prevalence

- Most frequent presenting condition in patients <50 years old with knee complaints (1)
- Women have higher incidence than men (1,2).
- More predominant among female adolescents and physically active young adults (3)
- Higher incidence in physically active populations (3)
- Incidence between 15 and 25% in the general population (3)
- Accounts for 25% of all knee injuries (4)

ETIOLOGY AND PATHOPHYSIOLOGY

- Multifactorial etiology (1)
- Direct relationship with hip weakness and poor functional control of the femur during weight-bearing tasks (5)
- Structural anomalies and lower extremity malalignment contribute (1).
- Increased contact forces between the retropatellar cartilage and the trochlear groove due to musculoskeletal imbalances resulting in abnormal patellar tracking (4)

Genetics

Unknown

RISK FACTORS

- Decreased quadriceps strength (1)
- Female gender (1)
- Q angle >20 degrees (1)
- Limited quadriceps and gastrocnemius flexibility (6)
- Excessive knee valgus during landing phase of gait with subtalar hyperpronation (6)
- Shortened iliotibial (IT) band and lateral retinaculum (6)
- Decreased strength or timing of the medial quadriceps and the gluteus medius (6)
- Decreased hamstring flexibility (5)
- Decreased explosive strength (5)
- Inadequate equipment (5)
- Decreased trochlear groove depth (5)
- Increased medial patellar mobility (5)
- Patella alta (5)
- Tight IT band (5) with weak vastus medialis
- Increased medial tibial intercondylar distance (5)

GENERAL PREVENTION

- 1st step is to identify possible risk factors (1)
- Strengthening exercises particularly terminal extension of the quadriceps (1)
- Reduction in training volume (7)

COMMONLY ASSOCIATED CONDITIONS

- Overuse
- Knee ligament injury/surgery
- Patellar tendinopathy
- Prolonged synovitis
- IT band friction syndrome

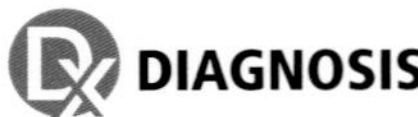

DIAGNOSIS

HISTORY

- An accurate history to differentiate between pain and instability (pain quality and location, swelling, giving way, mechanical symptoms locking and grinding, inciting events, overuse, and history of trauma)
- Most common symptom: anteromedial knee pain exacerbated by physical activity or an increase in physical activity
- Pain often exacerbated when squatting or with prolonged sitting ("theater sign") (3)[A]
- Anterior knee pain when descending/ascending stairs, ambulating over uneven surfaces, or running
- Pain during or after activity

PHYSICAL EXAM

- Observe gait and symmetry of musculature around both knees (atrophy, antalgia).
- Measure Q angle (particularly in females)
- Patellar tilt test: While keeping patient supine, grasp patella between thumb and forefinger and try to lift up the outside edge of the patella using the thumb (3)[A].
- Squatting (3)[A]
- Vastus medialis coordination test: Although patient is laying down supine, place fist under patient's knee and ask the patient to extend the knee slowly without pressing down or lifting away from you (3)[A].
- Apprehension sign: Compress the patella against the femur and ask the patient to contract quadriceps muscles; pain upon contraction is consistent with patellofemoral pain syndrome, although pain may be present in normal individuals as well (3)[A].
- Compression test: reproduction of pain with compression of patella against the trochlea (3)[A]

DIFFERENTIAL DIAGNOSIS

- Prepatellar bursitis
- Patellar and quadriceps tendinitis/tendinopathy
- Patellofemoral arthrosis
- Patellar subluxation and dislocation
- Knee ligamentous and meniscal pathology
- IT band syndrome
- Plica syndrome
- Patellofemoral osteoarthritis
- Chondromalacia patella/osteochondral defect
- Sinding-Larsen-Johansson syndrome
- Osgood-Schlatter disease
- Referred pain from hip or spine

DIAGNOSTIC TESTS & INTERPRETATION

- None indicated. *In general, imaging is unnecessary and not helpful in diagnosis of patellofemoral pain syndrome*. If imaging is indicated because of severity, atypical symptoms, or persistence of symptoms despite treatment, plain films with 4 views of the knee are recommended to view patellar tilt and to rule out other etiologies of anterior knee pain:
  - Lateral
  - Merchant (also called sunrise)
  - Standing anteroposterior
  - Posteroanterior tunnel views
- CT can be used to grade patellar malalignment.
- Radiographic findings may not correlate with symptoms.

Follow-Up Tests & Special Considerations
Radiographic images may be normal until late stages, when the posterior patellar surface becomes irregular and cartilage erosion is radiographically detectable.

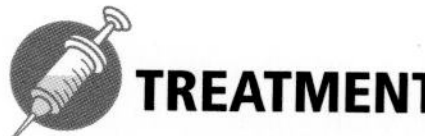

TREATMENT

Conservative therapy is preferred (5)[A].

GENERAL MEASURES

- Stretching and strengthening exercises (especially hip, core, and vastus medialis strengthening) (5)[A]
- Taping and bracing (5)[A]
- Activity modification (5)[A]
- Supervised exercise therapy and neuromuscular training program including hip and quadriceps training (1)[A]
- Patellar taping and foot orthoses may offer some relief (8)[A].
- Electrotherapy and biofeedback (8)[A]

MEDICATION

- NSAIDs for pain management (5)[A]
- The evidence for glycosaminoglycan polysulfate is conflicting and is not routinely recommended for treatment of patellofemoral pain.
- Nandrolone may be effective but is not routinely recommended for treatment.

ISSUES FOR REFERRAL

Referral for surgery is a last resort after all conservative measures fail. Surgery is rarely needed.

ADDITIONAL THERAPIES

Ice packs after activity have been found to improve clinical symptoms.

SURGERY/OTHER PROCEDURES

- No additional benefits of surgery compared to conservative treatment (8)[A]
- Attempts to correct maltracking of the patellofemoral joint with a lateral retinacular release or tibial tubercle transposition have shown variable results (5)[A].
- Rarely indicated

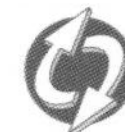

ONGOING CARE

PATIENT EDUCATION

Patient education and exercises: http://familydoctor.org/online/famdocen/home/healthy/physical/injuries/479.html

PROGNOSIS

Often improves with rest and physical therapy

REFERENCES

1. Lankhorst NE, Bierma-Zeinstra SM, van Middelkoop M. Risk factors for patellofemoral pain syndrome: a systematic review. *J Orthop Sports Phys Ther*. 2012;42(2):81–94.
2. Lankhorst NE, Bierma-Zeinstra SM, van Middelkoop M. Factors associated with patellofemoral pain syndrome: a systematic review. *Br J Sports Med*. 2013;47(4):193–206.
3. Nunes GS, Stapait EL, Kirsten MH, et al. Clinical test for diagnosis of patellofemoral pain syndrome: systematic review with meta-analysis. *Phys Ther Sport*. 2013;14(1):54–59.
4. Barton CJ, Lack S, Malliaras P, et al. Gluteal muscle activity and patellofemoral pain syndrome: a systematic review. *Br J Sports Med*. 2013;47(4):207–214.
5. Carry PM, Kanai S, Miller NH, et al. Adolescent patellofemoral pain: a review of evidence for the role of lower extremity biomechanics and core instability. *Orthopedics*. 2010;33(7):498–507.
6. Pappas E, Wong-Rom WM. Prospective predictors of patellofemoral pain syndrome: a systemic review with meta-analysis. *Sports Health*. 2012;4(2):115–120.
7. Tenforde AS, Sayres LC, McCurdy ML, et al. Overuse injuries in high school runners: lifetime prevalence and prevention strategies. *PM R*. 2011;3(2):125–131.
8. Peters JS, Tyson NL. Proximal exercises are effective in treating patellofemoral pain syndrome: a systematic review. *Int J Sports Phys Ther*. 2013;8(5):689–700.

ADDITIONAL READING

- Callaghan MJ, Selfe J. Patellar taping for patellofemoral pain syndrome in adults. *Cochrane Database Syst Rev*. 2012;(4):CD006717.
- Collado H, Fredericson M. Patellofemoral pain syndrome. *Clin Sports Med*. 2010;29(3):379–398.
- Dixit S, DiFiori JP, Burton M, et al. Management of patellofemoral pain syndrome. *Am Fam Physician*. 2007;75(2):194–202.
- Fredericson M, Yoon K. Physical examination and patellofemoral pain syndrome. *Am J Phys Med Rehabil*. 2006;85(3):234–243.
- Frye JL, Ramey LN, Hart JM. The effects of exercise on decreasing pain and increasing function in patients with patellofemoral pain syndrome: a systematic review. *Sports Health*. 2012;4(3):205–210.
- Heintjes E, Berger MY, Bierma-Zeinstra SM, et al. Pharmacotherapy for patellofemoral pain syndrome. *Cochrane Database Syst Rev*. 2004;(3):CD003470.
- Waryasz GR, McDermott AY. Patellofemoral pain syndrome (PFPS): a systematic review of anatomy and potential risk factors. *Dyn Med*. 2008;7:9.

SEE ALSO

Algorithm: Knee Pain

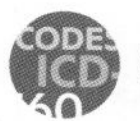

CODES

ICD10

- M25.569 Pain in unspecified knee
- M25.561 Pain in right knee
- M25.562 Pain in left knee

CLINICAL PEARLS

- Patellofemoral pain syndrome is the most common cause of anterior knee pain in active adults.
- The clinical diagnosis is made by history and physical exam.
- Well-designed exercises geared at quadriceps strengthening, hamstring, and IT band flexibility and hip stabilizers are the most effective evidence-based treatment.

PEDICULOSIS (LICE)

Kaelen C. Dunican, PharmD • Cynthia Jeremiah, MD

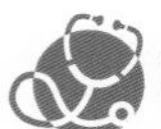

BASICS

DESCRIPTION

- A contagious parasitic infection caused by ectoparasitic blood-feeding insects (lice)
- 2 species of lice infest humans:
  - *Pediculus humanus* has 2 subspecies: the head louse (var. *capitis*) and the body louse (var. *corporis*). Both species are 1–3 mm long, flat, and wingless and have 3 pairs of legs that attach closely behind the head.
  - *Phthirus pubis* (pubic or crab louse): resembles a sea crab and has widespread claws on the 2nd and 3rd legs
- System(s) affected: skin/exocrine
- Synonym(s): lice; crabs

EPIDEMIOLOGY

Incidence

- In the United States: 6–12 million new cases per year
- Predominant age
  - Head lice: most common in children 3–12 years of age; more common in girls than boys
  - Pubic lice: most common in adults

Prevalence

Head lice: 1–3% in industrialized countries

ETIOLOGY AND PATHOPHYSIOLOGY

- Infestation by lice: *P. humanus* (var. *capitis*), *P. humanus* (var. *corporis*), or *P. pubis*
- Characteristics of lice:
  - Adult louse is dark grayish and moves quickly but does not jump or fly.
  - Eggs (nits) camouflage with the individuals' hair color and are cemented to the base of the hair shaft (within 4 mm of the scalp).
  - Nits (empty egg casings) appear white (opalescent) and remain cemented to the hair shaft.
  - Lice feed solely on human blood by piercing the skin, injecting saliva (anticoagulant properties to allow for blood meal), and then sucking blood.
  - Itching is a hypersensitivity reaction to the saliva of the feeding louse.
- Transmission: direct human-to-human contact
  - Head lice: direct head-to-head contact or contact with infested fomite (less common)
  - Body lice: contact with contaminated clothing or bedding
  - Pubic lice: typically transmitted sexually (fomite transmission much less likely)

RISK FACTORS

- General: overcrowding and close personal contact
- Head lice
  - School-aged children, gender (girls; longer hair)
  - Sharing combs, hats (including helmets), clothing, and bed linens
  - African Americans rarely have head lice; theories include twisted hair shaft and increased use of pomades
- Body lice: poor hygiene, homelessness
- Pubic lice: promiscuity (very high transmission rate)

GENERAL PREVENTION

- Environmental measures: Wash, dry-clean, or vacuum all items that may have come in contact with infected individuals.
- Screen and treat affected household contacts.
- Head lice: Follow-up by school nurses may help to prevent recurrence and spread.
- Pubic lice: Limit the number of sexual partners (Condoms do not prevent transmission nor does shaving pubic hair.).
- Body lice: proper hygiene

COMMONLY ASSOCIATED CONDITIONS

Up to 1/3 of patients with pubic lice have at least 1 concomitant STI.

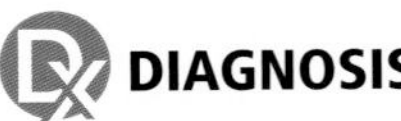

DIAGNOSIS

HISTORY

- Pruritus is common, mostly at night.
- Often associated with "outbreak" in school settings
- Investigate contacts of infected individuals.

PHYSICAL EXAM

- Diagnosis is confirmed clinically by visualization of live lice.
- *P. capitis* (head lice)
  - Found most often on the back of the head and neck and behind the ears (warmer areas)
  - Eyelashes may be involved.
  - Eggs, found cemented on the base of a hair shaft, are difficult to remove.
  - Pruritus may be accompanied by local erythema and small papules.
  - May see excoriations around hairline
  - Scratching can cause inflammation and secondary bacterial infection.
  - Pyoderma and lymphadenopathy may occur in severe infestation.
- *P. corporis* (body lice)
  - Poor general hygiene
  - Adult lice and nits in the seams of clothing
  - Intense pruritus involving area covered by clothing (trunk, axillae, and groin)
  - Uninfected bites present as erythematous macules, papules, and wheals.
  - Pyoderma and excoriation may be seen.
- *P. pubis* (pubic louse)
  - Pubic hair is the most common site, but lice may spread to hair around anus, abdomen, axillae, chest, beard, eyebrows, and eyelashes.
  - Eggs are present at the base of hair shafts.
  - Anogenital pruritus
  - Blue macules may be seen in surrounding skin.
  - Delay in treatment may lead to development of groin infection and regional adenopathy.

DIFFERENTIAL DIAGNOSIS

- Scabies and other mite species that can cause cutaneous reactions in humans
- Dandruff and other hair debris sometimes look like head lice eggs and nits but is less adherent to hair shafts than eggs and nits.

DIAGNOSTIC TESTS & INTERPRETATION

- Diagnosis is based on visualization of live louse.
- Head lice: Comb hair thoroughly with a fine-toothed louse comb (0.2–0.3 mm between teeth) to identify live lice (1)[C]. Simple visual inspection is of similar sensitivity to wet combing but ~25% as effective as dry combing with a metal comb (2).
- Body lice: Examine the seams of clothing to locate lice and their eggs (3).
- Carefully examine hair shafts under the microscope; lice and eggs can be seen easily under a microscope.
- In contrast to dandruff, eggs and nits cannot be removed easily from a hair shaft.

Follow-Up Tests & Special Considerations

- Empty nits will remain on hair shafts for months after eradication of the live infestation. On Wood lamp exam, live nits fluoresce white and empty nits fluoresce gray.
- Pubic lice: Patients should be evaluated for concurrent STIs.

TREATMENT

MEDICATION

Permethrin (over the counter [OTC]), synergized pyrethrin (OTC), spinosad (Rx), benzyl alcohol (Rx), malathion (Rx), and topical ivermectin (Rx) are effective for head lice (1)[A],(2)[C]. Permethrin, synergized pyrethrin, and malathion are effective for pubic lice (2)[C]:

- Permethrin may be preferred because it has residual activity for up to 3 weeks. However, newer shampoos and conditioners may reduce the residual effect (1)[C].
- Malathion and spinosad are considered second line for head lice but may not require a second application due to ovicidal activity (1)[B],(2)[C].
- Ivermectin 0.5% lotion is also effective for head lice (2)[C].

First Line

- Head and pubic lice
- Pyrethrum insecticides: permethrin 1% cream rinse (Nix) or pyrethrins 0.33% with piperonyl butoxide 4% (synergized pyrethrin, Rid, Pronto): Apply for 10 minutes, then wash:
  - Reapplication in 7–10 days (day 9 is optimal) is always required with use of synergized pyrethrin and may be necessary with use of permethrin, if live lice are observed.
  - Side effects: application-site erythema, ocular erythema, and application-site irritation
- Body lice: best treated with synergized pyrethrin lotion applied once and left on for several hours
- Eyelash infestation: Apply petroleum jelly BID × 10 days.
- Precautions
  - Pyrethrin: Avoid in patients with ragweed allergy (may cause respiratory symptoms).
  - Pediculicides should never be used to treat eyelash infections.

Second Line

Head lice and pubic lice

- Malathion 0.5% lotion (Ovide)
  - Apply for 8–12 hours, then wash off.
  - Excipients isopropyl alcohol (78%) and terpineol (12%) may contribute to its efficacy:
    - Flammable and has a bad odor
    - Despite ovicidal activity, a 2nd application may be necessary after 7–10 days (day 9 is optimal) if live lice are observed.
  - Lindane 1% shampoo: Apply for 4 minutes, then wash (should *not* be repeated):
    - Side effects: neurotoxicity (seizures, muscle spasms), aplastic anemia

- Contraindications: uncontrolled seizure disorder, premature infants
- Precautions: Do not use on excoriated skin, in immunocompromised patients, conditions that increase seizure risk, or with medications that decrease seizure threshold.
- Possible interactions: concomitant use with medications that lower the seizure threshold

- Head lice
  - Spinosad 0.9% lotion (Natroba)
    - Apply to dry hair and scalp for 10 minutes, then rinse with warm water. Repeat in 7 days if live lice are observed.
    - Side effects: application-site erythema, ocular erythema, and application-site irritation
  - Benzyl alcohol 5% lotion (Ulesfia)
    - Apply to dry hair using a sufficient amount to saturate scalp and hair (amount depends on hair length), rinse after 10 minutes, and repeat in 7 days.
    - Side effects: pruritus, erythema, pyoderma, ocular irritation, application-site irritation
  - Ivermectin 0.5% lotion (Sklice)
    - Apply to dry hair by using a sufficient amount to saturate the scalp and hair (max. 4 oz) then rinse after 10 minutes.
    - Side effects: burning sensation at application site, dandruff, dry skin, eye irritation
  - Mechanical removal of lice and nits by wetting hair and then systematically combing with a fine-toothed comb every 3–4 days × 2 weeks to remove all lice as they hatch

ALERT

Lindane: FDA black box warning of severe neurologic toxicity (use only when 1st-line agents have failed). The National Pediculosis Association strongly advises against using lindane at all.

GENERAL MEASURES

- Head lice: Wash all bedding, towels, clothes, headgear, combs, brushes, and hair accessories in hot water (60°C).
- Vacuum furniture and carpets
- Any personal articles that cannot be washed in hot water, dry cleaned, or vacuumed should be sealed in a plastic bag and stored for at least 2 weeks.
- All household members and close contacts should be examined and treated concurrently if infested.
- Insecticide sprays are not necessary.
- Pubic lice: Avoid sexual activity until both partners are successfully treated.
- Nit and egg removal
  - It is important to remove eggs that are within 1 cm of the scalp to prevent reinfestation.
  - After treatment with shampoo or lotion, eggs and nits remain in the scalp or pubic hair until mechanically removed.
  - Eggs and nits are best removed with a very fine nit comb.

Pediatric Considerations

- Avoid synergized pyrethrin and permethrin in infants <2 months of age; benzyl alcohol, topical ivermectin, and spinosad in children <6 months of age; and malathion in children <2 years of age
- Lindane: not recommended in patients who weigh <50 kg, including infants

Pregnancy Considerations

Permethrin, synergized pyrethrin, malathion, spinosad, and benzyl alcohol are pregnancy Category B. Lindane and topical ivermectin are Category C.

ADDITIONAL THERAPIES

- For "difficult to treat" cases of head lice, oral ivermectin 400 μg/kg (not approved by the FDA for lice), given twice at a 7-day interval, superior to topical 0.5% malathion lotion (4)[B]
- Ivermectin: 200 μg/kg PO repeated in 7–10 days
  - Should not be used in children weighing <15 kg; pregnancy Category C
  - Not approved by the FDA for lice
- Dual therapy with 1% permethrin and oral trimethoprim/sulfamethoxazole (TMP/SMX) only for cases of multiple treatment failures or suspected cases of lice-related resistance to therapy (TMP/SMX is not approved by the FDA for lice.)

COMPLEMENTARY & ALTERNATIVE MEDICINE

Head lice

- Dry-on, suffocation-based pediculicide: Nuvo or Cetaphil lotion
  - Apply thoroughly to hair, comb, dry with hair dryer, shampoo after 8 hours.
  - Repeat once a week until cured, up to a maximum of 3 applications.
  - Not approved by the FDA for lice
- Dimethicone 4% lotion: Apply to hair for 8 hours; repeat in 1 week (not approved by the FDA for lice).
- No home remedies (e.g., vinegar, isopropyl alcohol, olive oil, mayonnaise, melted butter, and petroleum jelly) have been proven effective to treat head lice infestations.
- Herbal shampoos and pomades have not been evaluated in clinical trials and are not approved by the FDA for lice.
- Lavender oil and tea tree oil have been implicated in triggering prepubertal gynecomastia in boys and should not be used to treat lice.

ONGOING CARE

FOLLOW-UP RECOMMENDATIONS

Children may return to school after completing topical treatment, even if nits remain in place. No-nit policies are not necessary.

Patient Monitoring

Drug resistance should be suspected if no dead lice are observed in 8–12 hours after treatment.

PATIENT EDUCATION

- National Pediculosis Association: www.headlice.org
- CDC: www.cdc.gov/parasites/lice/
- http://www.guideline.gov/content.aspx?id=46429&search=lice

PROGNOSIS

- With appropriate treatment, >90% cure rate
- Recurrence common, mainly from reinfection or treatment nonadherence, although resistance to synthetic pyrethroids is increasing

COMPLICATIONS

- Poor sleep due to pruritus
- Persistent itching may be caused by too frequent use of the pediculicide.
- Missed school; social stigma
- Secondary bacterial infections
- Body lice can transmit typhus and trench fever.

REFERENCES

1. Frankowski BL, Bocchini JA Jr; Council on School Health and Committee on Infectious Disease. Head lice. *Pediatrics*. 2010;126(2):392–403.
2. Burgess IF. Current treatments for pediculosis capitis. *Curr Opin Infect Dis*. 2009;22(2):131–136.
3. Gunning K, Pippitt K, Kiraly B, et al. Pediculosis and scabies: a treatment update. *Am Fam Physician*. 2012;86(6):535–541.
4. Chosidow O, Giraudeau B, Cottrell J, et al. Oral ivermectin versus malathion lotion for difficult-to-treat head lice. *N Engl J Med*. 2010;362(10):896–905.

ADDITIONAL READING

- Cole SW, Lundquist LM. Spinosad for treatment of head lice infestation. *Ann Pharmacother*. 2011;45(7–8):954–959.
- Durand R, Bouvresse S, Berdjane Z, et al. Insecticide resistance in head lice: clinical, parasitological and genetic aspects. *Clin Microbiol Infect*. 2012;18(4):338–344.
- Pariser DM, Meinking TL, Bell M, et al. Topical 0.5% ivermectin lotion for treatment of head lice. *N Engl J Med*. 2012;367(18):1687–1693.

SEE ALSO

Arthropod Bites and Stings; Scabies

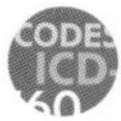

CODES

ICD10

- B85.0 Pediculosis due to Pediculus humanus capitis
- B85.1 Pediculosis due to Pediculus humanus corporis
- B85.3 Phthiriasis

CLINICAL PEARLS

- No-nit policies are not necessary because empty nits may remain on hair shafts for months after eradication.
- Proper product application is essential; improper product application should be considered when assessing treatment failure.
- Prevalence of resistant infestations is increasing, so if no dead lice are observed in 8–12 hours after treatment, suspect resistance and use an alternative agent.
- Routine retreatment on day 9 is recommended for nonovicidal products (permethrin and synergized pyrethrin).
- With all treatment options, patients' hair should be reinspected after 7–9 days and, if live lice are detected, treatment should be repeated on day 9.

PELVIC INFLAMMATORY DISEASE

Fozia Akhtar Ali, MD • Paula A. Shelton, MD

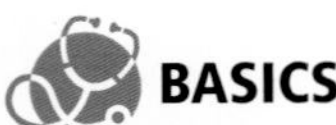

BASICS

DESCRIPTION

- Pelvic inflammatory disease (PID) is an infectious and inflammatory disorder of the upper female genital tract, including the uterus, fallopian tubes, ovaries, and adjacent pelvic structures. It is community acquired from sexually transmitted organisms (1).
- Salpingitis is the most important component due to its impact on future fertility.
- Diagnosis may be challenging and incorrect in up to 1/3 of cases. No set of criteria is both sensitive and specific for the disease.
- System(s) affected: reproductive

EPIDEMIOLOGY

- Predominant age: 15–25 years; this number has remained constant since early 1900s.
- Predominant sex: female only (1)

Incidence

Over 770,000 cases of acute PID are diagnosed annually in the United States. Incidence decreased from 1885 to 2001. The CDC has estimated that more than 1 million women experience an episode of PID every year. The disease leads to approximately 2.5 million office visits, 200,000 hospitalizations, and 100,000 surgical procedures yearly. The cost of PID is approximately $2 billion annually; however, costs have decreased over the past decade (2).

ETIOLOGY AND PATHOPHYSIOLOGY

Multiple organisms may be etiologic agents in PID. Most cases are polymicrobial:

- *Chlamydia trachomatis*, *Neisseria gonorrhoeae*, genital tract mycoplasmas (particularly *Mycoplasma genitalium*), aerobic and anaerobic (*Bacteroides fragilis*), and vaginal flora (e.g., *Prevotella*, *Peptostreptococci*, *Gardnerella vaginalis*, *Escherichia coli*, *Haemophilus influenzae*) are recognized as etiologic agents (1,3,4).
- Many nongonococcal, nonchlamydial microorganisms recovered from upper genital tract in acute PID are associated with bacterial vaginosis (especially *Prevotella bivius*, *Prevotella disiens*, and *Prevotella capillosus*) (2).
- The precise mechanism by which microorganisms ascend from the lower genital tract is unclear. Possible mechanisms include the following: (i) travel from cervix to endometrium to salpinx to peritoneal cavity; (ii) lymphatic spread via infection of the parametrium (from an IUD); and (iii) hematogenous route, although this is rare.
- Of cases, 75% occur within 7 days of menses, when cervical mucus favors ascent of organisms.

RISK FACTORS

- Sexually active and age <25 years (5)
- First sexual activity at young age (<15 years)
- New/multiple sexual partners
- Nonbarrier contraceptive methods (i.e., oral contraceptive pills)
- Previous history of PID; 20–25% will have a recurrence.
- Cervical ectopy
- History of *C. trachomatis*; 10–40% will develop PID.
- History of gonococcal cervicitis; 10–20% will develop PID.
- Gynecologic procedures such as endometrial biopsy, curettage, and hysteroscopy break the cervical barrier, predisposing women to ascending infections.

GENERAL PREVENTION

- Educational programs about safer sex practices such as barrier contraceptives, especially condoms and spermicidal creams or sponges, provide some protection (5).
- The U.S. Preventive Services Task Force recommends screening for chlamydia in all sexually active women younger than 25 years and in those 25 years and older at increased risk (new sex partner/multiple sex partners).
- Routine STI screening in pregnancy
- Early medical care with occurrence of genital lesions or abnormal discharge

COMMONLY ASSOCIATED CONDITIONS

- If PID is suspected in a patient with an IUD and a pelvic abscess is present, an *Actinomyces* infection requiring penicillin treatment may be present.
- Rupture of an adnexal abscess is rare but life threatening. Early surgical exploration is mandatory (3).
- Chlamydial or gonococcal perihepatitis may occur with PID. This combination is called Fitz-Hugh-Curtis (FHC) syndrome and is characterized by severe pleuritic right upper quadrant pain. FHC syndrome complicates 10% of PID cases.
- Plasma cell endometritis has also been seen in the majority of females with PID; the density of plasma cell infiltration has been related to severity of symptoms (3).

DIAGNOSIS

- The diagnosis of PID is based primarily on clinical evaluation. Clinical diagnosis alone is 87% sensitive and 50% specific.
- Physicians must consider PID in the differential diagnosis in women 15–44 years of age who present with lower abdominal or pelvic pain and cervical motion or pelvic tenderness, even if these symptoms are mild.
- The CDC recommends empiric treatment for PID if ≥1 of the following minimum criteria are present on pelvic exam in an at-risk patient: cervical motion tenderness, uterine tenderness, and adnexal tenderness in the presence of lower abdominal or pelvic pain.
- Additional criteria used to enhance specificity: fever >101°F, new/abnormal vaginal discharge, presence of abundant numbers of WBCs on wet prep, elevated ESR, and laboratory documentation of cervical infection with *N. gonorrhoeae* or *C. trachomatis* (1,6)
- Most specific criteria for diagnosing PID: Endometrial biopsy reveals endometritis/plasma cells; transvaginal ultrasound showing thickened, fluid-filled salpinges; and laparoscopic abnormalities consistent with PID (1).

HISTORY

- Lower abdominal or pelvic pain: typically described as dull, aching or crampy, bilateral, and constant; accentuated by motion, exercise, or coitus
- New/abnormal vaginal discharge (~75% of cases)
- Fever, chills, cramping, dyspareunia
- Low back pain
- Urinary discomfort
- Unanticipated vaginal bleeding, often postcoital, is reported in about 40% of cases.
- Recent hysterosalpingogram (HSG)
- IUD insertion within the past 21 days (1,3)

PHYSICAL EXAM

- Fever
- Lower abdominal pain and particularly cervical motion tenderness
- Findings of cervicitis with/without vaginal discharge (1)

DIFFERENTIAL DIAGNOSIS

- Appendicitis
- Constipation
- Gastroenteritis
- Ectopic pregnancy
- Ovarian tumor/torsion
- Hemorrhagic/ruptured ovarian cyst
- Endometriosis/dysmenorrhea
- Functional pelvic pain
- Inflammatory bowel disease
- Diverticulitis
- UTI/pyelonephritis
- Nephrolithiasis (1)

DIAGNOSTIC TESTS & INTERPRETATION

Initial Tests (lab, imaging)

- Pregnancy test: must be performed to rule out ectopic pregnancy and complications of an intrauterine pregnancy
- Specific testing for chlamydia and gonorrhea (usually nucleic acid amplification test [NAAT] and/or ligase chain reaction)
- Urinalysis (3,4)
- Saline microscopy of vaginal fluid (for WBC)
- Consider CBC: WBC count ≥10,500/mm^3, although ≤50% of PID cases present with leukocytosis
- Consider transvaginal ultrasound: not necessary for diagnosis; may show thickened, fluid-filled tubes (hydrosalpinges) ± free fluid, or tubo-ovarian abscess (TOA)

Follow-Up Tests & Special Considerations

- ESR >15 mm/hr or elevated C-reactive protein used in some diagnostic criteria
- Consider HIV testing in patients with PID.
- Follow-up ultrasound as outpatient for resolution of adnexal abscess.

Diagnostic Procedures/Other

- Culdocentesis with culture is rarely necessary.
- Laparoscopy is best used for confirming, as opposed to making, the diagnosis of PID and should be reserved for the following situations:
  - Ill patient with competing diagnosis (e.g., appendicitis)
  - Ill patient who has failed outpatient treatment
  - Any patient not improving after 72 hours of inpatient treatment
- Endometrial biopsy (rarely indicated): reveals endometritis/plasma cells (3)

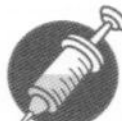

TREATMENT

- Outpatient treatment, if appropriate
- Criteria for hospitalization and parenteral treatment are described below.

GENERAL MEASURES

Avoid intercourse until treatment is completed. IUD removal is NOT required for mild PID.

MEDICATION

First Line

- Several antibiotic regimens are highly effective, with no single regimen of choice (3)[A].
- Outpatient treatment regimen
  - Ceftriaxone 250 mg IM single dose *plus*
  - Doxycycline 100 mg PO BID × 14 days ±
  - Metronidazole 500 mg PO BID × 14 days
- On the basis of the recent emergence of fluoroquinolone-resistant gonococci, the CDC no longer recommends the use of fluoroquinolones for the treatment of gonococcal infections and associated conditions such as PID.
- Metronidazole should be considered in cases where risk of infection with anaerobic organisms is considered high.

Second Line

- Because of emerging resistance in gonococcus, resistance testing and confirmation of treatment success is advisable (3).
- Outpatient treatment regimen
  - Cefoxitin 2 g IM single dose and probenecid 1 g PO administered concurrently in single dose *plus*
  - Doxycycline 100 mg PO BID × 14 days +/−
  - Metronidazole 500 mg PO BID × 14 days
- In persons with documented severe allergic reactions to penicillin or cephalosporins, azithromycin or spectinomycin might be an option for therapy of uncomplicated gonococcal infections.
- Special consideration:
  - Refer sex partners for appropriate evaluation and treatment if they had sexual contact with patient during preceding 60 days or most recent sexual contact. Partners should be treated, irrespective of evaluation, with regimens effective against chlamydia and gonorrhea (3).

SURGERY/OTHER PROCEDURES

Reserved for failures of medical treatment and for suspected ruptured adnexal abscess with resulting acute surgical abdomen

INPATIENT CONSIDERATIONS

Admission Criteria/Initial Stabilization

- Hospitalization recommended in the following (3)[C]:
  - Surgical emergencies (e.g., appendicitis)
  - Suspected pelvic abscess
  - Pregnancy
  - Severe illness, nausea, vomiting, or high fever
  - Intolerance/inability to adhere to outpatient regimen
  - Failure to respond to outpatient therapy
- For inpatient treatment of PID, the CDC also lists 2 currently accepted treatment regimens (6):
  - Parenteral regimen A
    - Cefotetan 2 g IV q12h or cefoxitin 2 g IV q6h + doxycycline 100 mg PO or IV q12h
    - Parenteral therapy × 24 hours after clinical improvement. Continue doxycycline for a total of 14 days.
  - Parenteral regimen B
    - Clindamycin 900 mg IV q8h + gentamicin loading dose IV or IM (2 mg/kg of body weight) followed by a maintenance dose (1.5 mg/kg) q8h
    - Parenteral therapy for 24 hours after clinical improvement; continue doxycycline as aforementioned or clindamycin 450 mg PO QID for a total of 14 days.
- During pregnancy: PID is rare in pregnant patients; however, may appear prior to 12 weeks' gestation before mucous plug appears. Change doxycycline to azithromycin + second-generation cephalosporin (6).

ONGOING CARE

FOLLOW-UP RECOMMENDATIONS

Patient Monitoring

- Review at 72 hours is recommended particularly for patients with moderate or severe clinical presentation.
- Close observation of clinical status, particularly for fever, symptoms, degree of peritonitis, serum WBC.
- Retest for gonorrhea and chlamydia in 3–6 months. The likelihood of reinfection is high.
- Follow adnexal abscess size and position with serial ultrasound (6).

PATIENT EDUCATION

- Abstinence from any type of sexual contact until treatment of patient/partner (if necessary) is complete
- Consistent and correct condom use should be enforced.
- Hepatitis B and human papilloma virus (HPV) vaccines should be given to patients who meet criteria.
- Advise comprehensive STI screening (6).

PROGNOSIS

- Wide variation with good prognosis if early, effective therapy is instituted and further infection is avoided
- Poor prognosis related to late therapy and continued high-risk sexual behavior
- Nongonococcal nonchlamydial PID is more often associated with severe PID and with worse prognosis for future fertility (2).

COMPLICATIONS

- Tubo-ovarian abscess will develop in ~7–16% of patients with PID.
- Recurrent infection occurs in 20–25% of patients.
- Risk of ectopic pregnancy is increased 7–10-fold among women with a history of PID.
- Tubal infertility occurs in 8%, 19.5%, and 40% of women after 1, 2, and 3 episodes of PID, respectively.
- Chronic pelvic pain occurs in 20% of cases and is related to adhesion formation, chronic salpingitis, or recurrent infection (1,2).

REFERENCES

1. Gradison M. Pelvic inflammatory disease. *Am Fam Physician*. 2012;85(8):791–796.
2. Lareau SM, Beigi RH. Pelvic inflammatory disease and tubo-ovarian abscess. *Infect Dis Clin North Am*. 2008;22(4):693–708, vii.
3. Judlin P. Current concepts in managing pelvic inflammatory disease. *Curr Opin Infect Dis*. 2010;23(1):83–87.
4. Weinstein SA, Stiles BG. A review of the epidemiology, diagnosis and evidence-based management of *Mycoplasma genitalium*. *Sex Health*. 2011;8(2):143–158.
5. Sweet RL. Treatment of acute pelvic inflammatory disease. *Infect Dis Obstet Gynecol*. 2011;2011:561909.
6. Workowski KA, Berman S; Centers for Disease Control and Prevention. Sexually transmitted diseases treatment guidelines, 2010. *MMWR Recomm Rep*. 2010;59(RR-12):1–110.

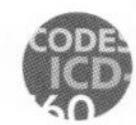

CODES

ICD10

- N73.9 Female pelvic inflammatory disease, unspecified
- N73.0 Acute parametritis and pelvic cellulitis
- N70.93 Salpingitis and oophoritis, unspecified

CLINICAL PEARLS

- Most often, PID starts with gonorrhea or chlamydia, but it can be polymicrobial.
- Physicians should treat on the basis of clinical judgment without waiting for confirmation from laboratory or imaging tests. PID is a common cause of infertility.
- Complications include hydrosalpinx, adhesions, pelvic pain, and 10-fold increased risk of ectopic pregnancy.
- 3 major predictors of preserved post-PID fertility: (i) short duration of symptoms (<72 hours) prior to initiation of treatment, (ii) first episode of PID, and (iii) nongonococcal PID

PEMPHIGOID, BULLOUS

Jeffrey D. Mailhot, MD

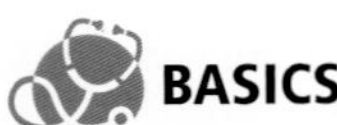

BASICS

DESCRIPTION

- Bullous pemphigoid (BP) is a chronic acquired autoimmune subepidermal blistering skin disorder caused by linear deposition of autoantibodies against the epithelial basal membrane zone.
- Pruritic, tense, symmetric, localized, widespread bullae or urticarial plaques
- Flexural surface (80%), axillary, inguinal folds, and abdomen (20%)
- Oral lesions develop in 10–20% of cases, rarely affecting mucosae of eyes, nose, pharynx, and anogenital zones.

EPIDEMIOLOGY

- Most common autoimmune blistering disease
- Typical between 60 and 80 years old, but juvenile bullous pemphigoid can occur
- Affects both females and males, possibly with higher incidence in females
- No association with race or geographic location

Incidence

- BP is probably the only autoimmune disease that increases in likelihood with age (1).
- 6–13 new cases/million per year

ETIOLOGY AND PATHOPHYSIOLOGY

- Autoantibodies react against hemidesmosomal proteins: the 230-kDa BP antigen (BPAg1) within basal keratinocytes and 180-kDa (BPAg2 or type XVII collagen) in the basement membrane zone (BMZ).
- IgG is usually the predominant autoantibody leading to C3 complement activation, recruitment of inflammatory cells, and liberation of proteolytic enzymes that break down the dermoepidermal junction.
- The noncollagenous 16A domain (NC16A) located at the membrane proximal region of BP180 is considered the major target epitope and is recognized in 80–90% of BP patients.
- It has recently been shown that IgE antibodies correlate with a severe form of BP, and those who test positive for IgE anti-BP180 antibodies required longer duration for remission and therapy.

Genetics

- Certain class II antigens of the major histocompatibility complex (MHC) alleles DQB1*0301 predominate.
- Expression of this allele on antigen-presenting cells is thought to be involved in the presentation to autoreactive T cells in patients with BP.
- Molecular mimicry has been proposed as a mechanism by which exogenous agents may trigger the immune response.

RISK FACTORS

- Advanced age
- No clear precipitating factors but can be related to infections such as hepatitis B, hepatitis C, *Helicobacter pylori*, *Toxoplasma gondii*, cytomegalovirus (CMV).
- Associated with autoimmune disorders and inflammatory dermatoses like lichen planus, psoriasis, and other forms of bullous disease
- Increased risk in patients with neurologic disorders such as multiple sclerosis, dementia, stroke, Parkinson disease, and psychiatric disorders
- Although drug-induced BP is rare, chronic intake of neuroleptics, aldosterone antagonists, furosemide, dopaminergic drugs, opioids, salicylates, NSAIDs, and phenacetin have been associated.
- Less frequent: trauma, burns, surgical scars, UV radiation, and x-ray therapy

COMMONLY ASSOCIATED CONDITIONS

- Underlying malignancy can be found in patients with BP, but it may be age related, and the correlation is marginal.
- Several autoimmune disorders such as rheumatoid arthritis, Hashimoto thyroiditis, dermatomyositis, lupus erythematosus, inflammatory dermatoses–like psoriasis, and lichen planus have been reported but are rare.

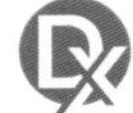

DIAGNOSIS

HISTORY

- BP occurs sporadically without any obvious trigger factor.
- Prodromal nonbullous phase: mild to severe pruritus, associated with excoriated, eczematous, and often urticarial plaques
- Mucosal lesions can be mild, transient, and are often seen with extensive cutaneous disease.
- Bullous stage: single or numerous tense bullae on erythematous, noninflammatory, urticarial skin
- Unusual clinical presentations
  - Localized form: 30% of cases (e.g., disease limited to lower leg, anogenital region, site of trauma)
  - Vegetative form: uncommon, vegetating plaques in intertriginous areas
  - Lichen planus pemphigoides: rare variant, bullae on site of previously normal skin or mucosa, after the onset of lichen planus

PHYSICAL EXAM

- Lesions usually are 1–3 cm round or oval, tense blisters localized on either normal or inflamed skin.
- 80–90% appear in the lower trunk, axilla, and groin, and 10–20% in oral and intertriginous spaces.
- Blister rupture leads to painful erosions that may become crusted and occasionally invaded by organisms.
- Fluid is clear but sometimes presents with hemorrhagic exudates.
- Negative active acantholysis (Nikolsky sign) and no extension of bullae into the surrounding, unblistered skin when vertical pressure is applied to the top of the bulla (Asboe-Hansen sign) support the diagnosis.

DIFFERENTIAL DIAGNOSIS

- Blistering diseases with antibodies: pemphigus, cicatricial pemphigoid, pemphigoid gestationis, epidermolysis bullosa acquisita, linear IgA dermatosis, dermatitis herpetiformis, bullous erythema multiforme
- Blistering diseases without antibodies: erythema multiforme, toxic epidermal necrolysis, porphyria, epidermolysis bullosa, allergic contact dermatitis, bullous impetigo, staphylococcal scaled-skin syndrome, friction blisters

DIAGNOSTIC TESTS & INTERPRETATION

Initial Tests (lab, imaging)

- Diagnosis of BP is based on a combination of clinical features, and the key is immunopathologic findings on skin biopsy.
- Half of patients will have elevated total serum IgE.
- ~50% of patients have peripheral blood eosinophilia that does not correlate with serum IgE levels.
- Diagnosis of atypical and nonbullous variants relies on findings of direct and indirect immunofluorescence from specific circulating antibodies.
- Considerations
  - BP has a waxing and waning course with spontaneous remission in the absence of treatment.
  - ELISA for the NC16A domain of BP180 is available at some centers, reported sensitivity 82–94%; specificity 93–99.9%
  - Old age and poor general health along with presence of anti-BP180 have been related with poor prognosis.

Diagnostic Procedures/Other

- Diagnosis is made by skin biopsy with direct immunofluorescence exam.
- Histopathology: 4-mm punch biopsy from the edge of an intact bulla (perilesional skin). Staining shows subepidermal blister and multiple eosinophils.
- Immunohistochemistry: Studies have suggested that the detection of C3d deposits at the dermoepidermal junction in formalin-fixed tissue is helpful for the diagnosis and is the most consistent finding.
- Direct immunofluorescence (DIF): Second 4-mm perilesional punch biopsy will show linear deposition of IgG and/or C3 along BMZ.
- Serologic studies: Indirect immunofluorescence (IIF) and ELISA are done when DIF is negative, there is a strong suspicion of BP, and when the skin biopsy cannot be performed. Both detect circulating IgG antibodies against 230BP (specificity 96%) and 180BP (specificity 90%).

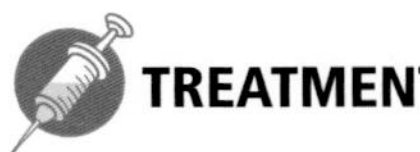

TREATMENT

GENERAL MEASURES

- Discontinue trigger factors.
- In oral lesions: Avoid hard consistency, spicy, and hot food. Soft and liquid meals should be given instead.
- Strict control of wounds to avoid complications

MEDICATION

First Line

- Treatment of BP depends on the extent of the disease.
- Potent topical corticosteroids should be considered in the management of localized and moderate disease.
  - Topical clobetasol propionate 0.05% cream: 40 g/day used twice daily, noted to be as effective as 0.5 mg/kg prednisone (2)[B]
  - Side effects: skin atrophy, striae, hypertrichosis, acne, and ecchymosis
- Systemic therapy
  - Oral prednisolone: 0.5 mg/kg/day for disease control. Goal is to achieve the lowest maintenance dosage that will prevent new lesion formation and reduce adverse reactions.
  - Clinical response is usually obtained within 1–2 weeks and is indicated by healing of existing lesions and cessation of new blister formation.
  - Evidence shows that higher doses >0.75 mg/kg/day do not improve healing rate but do increase mortality.
  - Taper the dose gradually within 1–2 years to avoid relapse; consider transition to steroid-sparing agent.
  - Side effects: cutaneous atrophy, osteoporosis, GI ulcers, Cushing syndrome, diabetes mellitus, hypertension
  - Tetracycline and nicotinamide may be beneficial in disease control and longer remission period (3)[C].

Second Line

- Immunosuppressive agents like azathioprine, mycophenolate mofetil, and methotrexate are used in severe cases; they may be beneficial especially in patients taking systemic corticosteroids.
  - Addition of azathioprine to prednisone regimen reduces the total maintenance dose of prednisone by 45% without increasing serious side effects or mortality.
  - Azathioprine: 0.5–2.5 mg/kg/day, most common side effect: myelosuppression; caution for lethal hypersensitivity syndrome
  - Mycophenolate mofetil: 1.5–2 g/day, most common side effect: GI disturbance
- Methotrexate: 5–20 mg/week, low dose usually initiated (5 mg/week) plus folic acid replacement. Adverse effects: myelosuppression, hepatotoxicity. Higher rate of remission with the use of prednisone
- Dapsone: 25–50 mg daily, most common side effect: hemolytic anemia, watch for agranulocytosis (4)[C].

Third Line

- Cyclosporine: caution with renal disease
- Plasmapheresis: Reduce the amount of prednisolone required to achieve disease control.
- Omalizumab: used in patients who have high levels of IgE antibodies
- IVIG: for patients who did not respond to 1st-line therapy or at risk of potentially fatal side effects from conventional therapy. The recommended dose is 1–2 g/kg divided over a 3- or 5-day cycle every 3–4 weeks.
- Rituximab has limited data (5)[C].

ISSUES FOR REFERRAL

- Dermatology for systemic management and/or scarring, which may suggest mucous membrane pemphigoid
- Gastroenterology, otorhinolaryngology referral in patients who have esophageal, pharyngeal, laryngeal involvement
- Ophthalmologic consult when patient complains of burning sensation, itching, visual changes, and in those patients who require high doses of steroids

INPATIENT CONSIDERATIONS

Admission Criteria/Initial Stabilization

Extensive denuding of skin, dehydration, and electrolyte imbalance requiring IV fluid reposition

ONGOING CARE

FOLLOW-UP RECOMMENDATIONS

Patient Monitoring

- Taper medication when disease is stable and control side effects.
- Perform periodic skin examination for new lesions.
- Frequent bacterial cultures of cutaneous erosions are essential to identify early infections.

DIET

- Liquid or soft diet with active oral lesions
- After lesions are resolved, advance diet. Avoid hard or crunchy foods, as they may cause flare ups.
- Supplement with calcium and vitamin D for patients on systemic corticosteroids

PATIENT EDUCATION

- Symptoms of infection, worsening lesions
- Education in good skin hygiene and wound care
- Wash clothing and linens if they come in contact with oozing, crusting, or infected skin.
- Protect from sun exposure and physical trauma to the skin.

PROGNOSIS

- Disease length can persist from weeks to years even under treatment.
- Around 47% of patients experience relapse within 1 year of therapy, and ~50% of patients can achieve remission within 2.5–6 years.
- Yearly mortality varies from 6 to 40%.
- Poor prognosis and high mortality: old age, poor general condition, and the presence of antibodies in serum
- Other factors that may be included are age >80 years, prednisolone dose >37 mg/day after hospitalization, serum albumin levels of <3.6 g/dL, ESR >100 mm/hr.

COMPLICATIONS

- Most often secondary to medication: osteoporosis, cataracts, adrenal insufficiency, bone marrow suppression
- Skin infections
- Dehydration and electrolytes imbalance

REFERENCES

1. Marazza G, Pham HC, Schärer L, et al. Incidence of bullous pemphigoid and pemphigus in Switzerland: a 2-year prospective study. *Br J Dermatol*. 2009;161(4):861–868.
2. Joly P, Roujeau JC, Benichou J, et al. A comparison of oral and topical corticosteroids in patients with bullous pemphigoid. *N Engl J Med*. 2002;346(5):321–327.
3. Fivenson DP, Breneman DL, Rosen GB, et al. Nicotinamide and tetracycline therapy of bullous pemphigoid. *Arch Dermatol*. 1994;130(6):753–758.
4. Venning VA, Millard PR, Wojnarowska F. Dapsone as first line therapy for bullous pemphigoid. *Br J Dermatol*. 1989;120(1):83–92.
5. Saouli Z, Papadopoulos A, Kiafa G, et al. A new approach on bullous pemphigoid therapy. *Ann Oncol*. 2008;19(4):825–826.

ADDITIONAL READING

- Garcia-Romero MT, Werth VP. Randomized controlled trials needed for bullous pemphigoid intervention. *Arch Dermatol*. 2012;148(2):244–246.
- Gürcan HM, Ahmed AR. Analysis of current data on the use of methotrexate in the treatment of pemphigus and pemphigoid. *Br J Dermatol*. 2009;161(4):723–731.
- Kirtschig G, Middleton P, Bennett C, et al. Interventions for bullous pemphigoid. *Cochrane Database Syst Rev*. 2010;(10):CD002292.
- Marzano AV, Tedeschi A, Berti E, et al. Activation of coagulation in bullous pemphigoid and other eosinophil-related inflammatory skin diseases. *Clin Exp Immunol*. 2011;165(1):45–50.
- Mutasim DF. Autoimmune bullous dermatoses in the elderly: an update on pathophysiology, diagnosis and management. *Drugs Aging*. 2010;27(1):1–19.
- Schmidt E, della Torre R, Borradori L. Clinical features and practical diagnosis of bullous pemphigoid. *Dermatol Clin*. 2011;29(3):427–438.
- Ujiie H, Nishie W, Shimizu H. Pathogenesis of bullous pemphigoid. *Dermatol Clin*. 2011;29(3):439–446.
- Venning VA, Taghipour K, Mohd Mustapa MF, et al. British Association of Dermatologists' guidelines for the management of bullous pemphigoid 2012. *Br J Dermatol*. 2012;167(6):1200–1214.

CODES

ICD10

L12.0 Bullous pemphigoid

CLINICAL PEARLS

- Tense bullae differentiates the lesions of bullous pemphigoid from the flaccid bullae of pemphigus vulgaris.
- Low doses of potent topical steroid have been shown to be just as effective as larger amounts in the initial therapy of BP.

PEMPHIGUS VULGARIS

Laura S. Ball DO • Samantha L. Pyle, MD, MAJ, MC

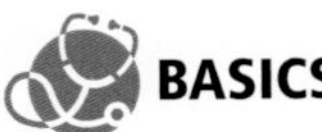

BASICS

Pemphigus is derived from the Greek word *pemphix* meaning "bubble" or "blister."

DESCRIPTION

- Rare, potentially fatal autoimmune mucocutaneous blistering disease that involves the skin and the mucous membranes
- Flaccid, painful, nonhealing bullae or ulcerations that appear spontaneously on the skin and mucosal surfaces, typically begin in the oropharynx, and then may spread to the skin, having a predilection for the scalp, face, chest, axillae, groin, and pressure points.
- Patient often presents with erosions and no intact bullae.
- System(s) affected: skin; GI; genitourinary

EPIDEMIOLOGY

Incidence

- Disease of the middle-aged population, typically occurring after the age of 50 years, although some cases have been reported in younger adults and children.
- Affects both sexes equally
- 0.1–3.2 cases per 100,000 individuals annually worldwide

Prevalence

- Uncommon, affects <200,000 people in the United States
- Seen more frequently in people of Mediterranean decent and Ashkenazi Jew

ETIOLOGY AND PATHOPHYSIOLOGY

- Autoantibodies (IgG) are directed against desmoglein (Dsg) 1 and 3 adhesion molecules. Dsgs interact with desmosomes, which hold epidermal cells together. The antibodies against Dsg molecules cause intraepidermal blister formation and acantholysis.
- Dsg 3 is predominantly expressed in oral epithelium, whereas both Dsg 1 and Dsg 3 are expressed in the skin.
- Dsg 1 is expressed more intensely in the superficial layer, whereas Dsg 3 is found more abundantly in basal and suprabasal layers.
- Additionally, autoantibodies against Dsg 4, the acetylcholine receptor, and pemphaxin have been identified in patients with pemphigus vulgaris (PV). The exact pathogenesis of pemphigus has yet to be fully explained and is likely a "multiple hit" process. Autoimmune; stimulus is unknown.
- Inducing factors include physical trauma, such as thermal burns, UV light, and ionizing radiation; neoplasm, emotional stress, drugs, and infections. Most patients lack a recognized inducing factor.

Genetics

Strong association with certain human leukocyte antigens (HLA), especially HLA DR4, DR14, DQ1, and DQ3, although the susceptibility gene differs depending on ethnic origin.

COMMONLY ASSOCIATED CONDITIONS

- Thymoma
- Myasthenia gravis
- Paraneoplastic pemphigus is a type of pemphigus defined by the fact that the patient has a malignancy at the time the pemphigus is diagnosed.
- Gastric adenocarcinoma

DIAGNOSIS

HISTORY

- Multiple, painful, nonhealing ulcers in the mouth—commonly the buccal and labial mucosa, palate, and tongue (1)[C]
- Progression (weeks to months) to small, clear fluid–filled blisters on the skin—commonly the scalp, face and upper torso. Blisters rupture easily, forming ulcerations (1)[C].
- Consider laryngeal and nasal involvement in patients with hoarseness, odynophagia, or nasal congestion (1)[C].
- Drug-induced: penicillamine, ACE inhibitors, thiol-containing compounds, rifampin

PHYSICAL EXAM

- Mucosal lesions: intact bullae rare; commonly are ill-defined, irregularly shaped gingival, buccal, or palatine erosions that are painful and slow-healing; most often affected area is the oral cavity; may involve conjunctiva, oropharynx esophagus, labia, vagina, cervix, penis, urethra, and anus (1)[C]
- Cutaneous lesions: Painful, flaccid blisters with clear fluid found on normal skin or on erythematous base; fragile bullae rupture easily, forming painful, superficial, coin-sized, sharply demarcated erosions (1)[C]. Nails: Acute or chronic paronychia, onychomadesis, subungual hematomas, and nail dystrophies may be present.
- Nikolsky sign: Involves application of pressure to skin causing intraepidermal cleavage that allows the superficial skin to slip free from the deeper layers, producing an erosion; can be elicited on normal skin or at the margin of a blister (1)[C]
- Asboe-Hansen sign: Lateral pressure on the edge of a blister may spread the blister into clinically unaffected skin.

DIFFERENTIAL DIAGNOSIS

- Predominance of oral mucous lesions: herpes simplex virus (HSV), aphthous ulcers, lichen planus, erythema multiforme
- Predominance of widespread cutaneous lesions: bullous pemphigoid, cicatricial pemphigoid, bullous drug eruptions, pemphigus erythematosus, pemphigus foliaceus, paraneoplastic pemphigus, impetigo, contact dermatitis, dermatitis herpetiformis, erythema multiforme, Stevens-Johnson syndrome, toxic epidermal necrolysis, pemphigoid gestationis, and linear IgA dermatosis

DIAGNOSTIC TESTS & INTERPRETATION

Diagnosis is achieved via three different parameters: perilesional tissue biopsy, histologic, and immunologic examinations.

Initial Tests (lab, imaging)

- Shave or 4-mm punch biopsy of edge of fresh bullous lesion
- A second 4-mm punch biopsy of the perilesional skin is sent for direct immunofluorescence (DIF).
- Serum for indirect immunofluorescence (IDIF) is positive for circulating autoantibodies against Dsgs in 80–90% if DIF is positive.
- ELISA testing can be used to distinguish pemphigus from the other blistering disorders. In order to distinguish PV from BP, immunoblot assay is needed. These tests are not widely available so may not be accessible by all institutions.

Follow-Up Tests & Special Considerations

IDIF corresponds loosely to disease activity and may be useful to gauge disease activity.

Test Interpretation

- Light microscopy: intradermal blister; loss of cohesion between epidermal cells (acantholysis) with an intact basement membrane; "row of tombstones appearance"
- DIF looking for deposits of IgG between epidermal cells

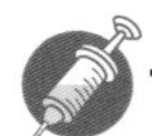

TREATMENT

Reduce inflammatory response and autoantibody production by suppression of the immune system to decrease blister formation and promote healing of blisters and erosions.

GENERAL MEASURES

- Minimize activities that may cause trauma to skin and precipitate blisters.
- Avoid use of dental plates, dental bridges, dental floss or contact lenses that may precipitate or exacerbate mucosal disease.
- Wound care: Daily gentle cleaning, topical agents to promote wound healing, and use of nonadhesive dressings. Clobetasol propionate 0.05% ointment 2× daily in conjunction with systemic steroids for hard to treat lesions
- Oral analgesics: Use before eating for painful oral lesions (viscous lidocaine, Benadryl).

MEDICATION

First Line

- High-dose systemic glucocorticoids (e.g., prednisone 1–2 mg/kg/day) are the mainstay of treatment (2)[B],(3)[C],(4)[A].
- Glucocorticoids can be used alone; however, combination with other steroid-sparing immunosuppressive drugs is most effective (azathioprine—most commonly used [starting at 1 mg/kg/day and increasing by 0.5 mg/kg/day every 2–3 weeks to reach a maintenance dose of 2.5 mg/kg/day]; other nonsteroidal adjunctive therapies include dapsone [50–200 mg/day] or mycophenolate mofetil [MMF] [2–3 g/day]) (4)[A].
- Rituximab is becoming a 1st-line treatment and may be a safer alternative to steroids. Dosing: 4 weekly infusions 375 mg/m^2 or 1,000 mg ×2 separated by 2 weeks (3)[C].
- For mild to moderate disease: Combination therapy of nonsteroidal adjunctive treatment and prednisone is an effective treatment regimen to achieve rapid and complete control of PV. For those patients who fail treatment, rituximab is an efficacious alternative therapy (5)[C].
- Rapidly progressive lesions necessitate high prednisone dose (1.5–2.5 mg/kg/day) for early and adequate control of the disease. Patients with impaired physical status, especially those with relatively stable lesions at baseline, might safely and effectively be treated with low-dose oral prednisone on alternate days plus azathioprine every day (Lever's minitreatment [LMT]) for oral pemphigus (2)[B].

- For oropharyngeal disease: Perilesional/intralesional triamcinolone acetonide injections combined with conventional immunosuppressive therapy shortened the time of complete clinical remission and reduced the total amount of corticosteroids used.

Second Line

For refractory disease

- Rituximab alone or in combination with intravenous immunoglobulin (IVIG) is an effective therapy for patients with refractory PV (6)[A].
- Other options: methotrexate (10–20 mg/week), hydroxychloroquine, gold, plasmapheresis (3)[C]
- Cyclosporine (2.5–5 mg/kg/day) may be ineffective as a steroid-sparing agent (4)[A].
- Tumor necrosis factor (TNF)-α antagonist, etanercept, may be an effective therapeutic agent and may reduce healing time of skin lesions in PV and for patients presenting with recalcitrant disease (4)[A].
- IVIG is a recommended and effective treatment for patients who are not able to tolerate the standard treatment (7)[A].
- For persistent lesions: intralesional triamcinolone acetonide (20 mg/mL)

ISSUES FOR REFERRAL

- Ophthalmologist referral in suspected ocular involvement and prolonged use of high-dose steroids
- Referral to a dentist and/or otolaryngologist for patients with extensive oral disease

INPATIENT CONSIDERATIONS

Admission Criteria/Initial Stabilization

- Secondary infections requiring IV antibiotics
- Severe oral lesions leading to dehydration requiring fluid resuscitation

ONGOING CARE

A minority of (10%) achieve complete remission after initial treatment and do not need continued drug therapy; most require maintenance therapy to stay in remission.

FOLLOW-UP RECOMMENDATIONS

- Patients taking steroids long-term should be screened for osteopenia/osteoporosis, avascular necrosis, HPA-axis suppression, cataract, cushingoid features, hyperlipoproteinemia, myopathy, mood changes, and immunosuppression. Patients on systemic steroids should maintain adequate vitamin D and calcium intake through diet and supplements.
- Patients taking azathioprine should have CBC, Cr, LFT checked at baseline and every 2 weeks the first 3 months then every 3 months after.
- PV can be exacerbated by sun exposure, dental work, trauma, stress, and radiographs. Patients undergoing dental work should be treated prophylactically with 20 mg of prednisone per day for 5–7 days in addition to their regular treatment regimen.
- Avoidance of sun exposure, use of broad-spectrum sunscreen, and wearing protective clothing should be recommended.

Patient Monitoring

Seek medical care for any unexplained blisters and if treated for PV and develop any of the following symptoms:

- Fever, chills
- General ill feeling
- Myalgias, joint pain
- New blisters or ulcers

DIET

- Patients with active oral lesions may benefit from liquid or soft diet and then advance as tolerated.
- Avoid spicy and acidic food when oral ulcers are present.
- Hard food that may cause mechanical trauma to epithelium, such as nuts, chips, and hard vegetables and fruits, may be best avoided in cases of active oral disease.

PATIENT EDUCATION

- Minimize activities that may cause trauma to skin and precipitate blisters, such as contact sports. Nontraumatic exercises, such as swimming, may be helpful.
- Explain wound care of erosions: daily gentle cleaning, covering open areas with clean petrolatum and nonadhesive dressings.
- Educate patients about the chronicity of the disease and the need for long-term follow up:
  - For oral pemphigus:
    - Soft diets and soft toothbrushes help to minimize local trauma.
    - Explain the need for meticulous oral hygiene to prevent dental decay. Encourage gentle tooth brushing, dental flossing, and visits to the dentist/dental hygienist at least every 6 months.
    - Discuss how dental plates, dental bridges, or contact lenses may precipitate or exacerbate mucosal disease.
    - Topical analgesics or anesthetics (e.g., benzydamine hydrochloride 0.15% or viscous lidocaine) may be useful in alleviating oral pain, particularly prior to eating or tooth brushing.

PROGNOSIS

- Mortality rate with combination therapy is ~5%, with most deaths due to drug-induced complications, including sepsis.
- 10% of patients achieve complete remission after initial treatment; most require maintenance therapy to stay in remission.
- Morbidity and mortality are related to the extent of disease, the maximum dose of oral steroids required to induce remission, and the presence of other diseases. Prognosis is worse in older persons and patients with extensive disease.
- Most deaths occur during the 1st few years of the disease; if a patient survives 5 years, prognosis is good.

COMPLICATIONS

- Secondary infection, localized to skin or systemic, may occur because of impaired immune response due to use of immunosuppressive drugs. Most frequent cause of death is *Staphylococcus aureus* septicemia.
- Within the first year, patients are at the highest risk for the development of secondary infections. Older patients and potentially diabetic patient carry an increased risk.
- Consider secondary infections to include bacterial, fungal and viral; particularly herpes simplex in nonhealing ulcers when the patient is receiving adequate treatment.
- Osteoporosis in patients requiring long-term systemic steroids
- Adrenal insufficiency has been reported following prolonged use of glucocorticoids.
- Bone marrow suppression and malignancies have been reported in patients receiving immunosuppressants, with an increased incidence of leukemia and lymphoma.
- Growth retardation has been reported in children taking systemic corticosteroids and immunosuppressants.

REFERENCES

1. Bystryn JC, Rudolph JL. Pemphigus. *Lancet*. 2005;366(9479):61–73.
2. Chaidemenos G, Apalla Z, Koussidou T, et al. High dose oral prednisone vs. prednisone plus azathioprine for the treatment of oral pemphigus: a retrospective, bi-centre, comparative study. *J Eur Acad Dermatol Venereol*. 2011;25(2):206–210.
3. Santoro F, Stoopler E, Werth VP. Pemphigus. *Dent Clin North Am*. 2013;57(4):597–610.
4. Singh S. Evidence-based treatments for pemphigus vulgaris, pemphigus foliaceus, and bullous pemphigoid: a systematic review. *Indian J Dermatol Venereol Leprol*. 2011;77(4):456–469.
5. Strowd LC, Taylor SL, Jorizzo JL, et al. Therapeutic ladder for pemphigus vulgaris: emphasis on achieving complete remission. *J Am Acad Dermatol*. 2011;64(3):490–494.
6. Zakka LR, Shetty SS, Ahmed AR. Rituximab in the treatment of pemphigus vulgaris. *Dermatol Ther*. 2012;2(1):17.
7. Ishii N, Hashimoto T, Zillikens D, et al. High-dose intravenous immunoglobulin (IVIG) therapy in autoimmune skin blistering diseases. *Clin Rev Allergy Immunol*. 2010;38(2–3):186–195.

ADDITIONAL READING

- Khandpur S, Sharma VK, Sharma A, et al. Comparison of enzyme-linked immunosorbent assay test with immunoblot assay in the diagnosis of pemphigus in Indian patients. *Indian J Dermatol Venereol Leprol*. 2010;76(1):27–32.
- Kljuic A, Bazzi H, Sundberg JP, et al. Desmoglein 4 in hair follicle differentiation and epidermal adhesion: evidence from inherited hypotrichosis and acquired pemphigus vulgaris. *Cell*. 2003;113(2):249–260.
- Leshem YA, Gdalevich M, Ziv M, et al. Opportunistic infections in patients with pemphigus. *J Am Acad Dermatol*. 2014;71(2):284–292.

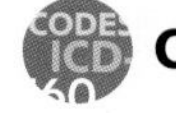

CODES

ICD10

L10.0 Pemphigus vulgaris

CLINICAL PEARLS

Pemphigus vulgaris is a rare, chronic, potentially fatal autoimmune vesiculobullous disease of the mucous membranes and skin. Biopsy immediately with rush processing. When clinical suspicion is high, initiate therapy without delay using systemic corticosteroids. Minimize activities that may cause trauma to skin and precipitate blisters, such as contact sports.

PEPTIC ULCER DISEASE

Fozia Akhtar Ali, MD • Paula A. Shelton, MD

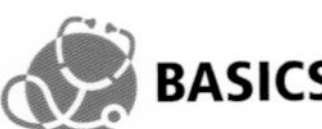

BASICS

DESCRIPTION

- Duodenal ulcer
  - Most common form of peptic ulcer
  - Usually located in the proximal duodenum
  - Multiple ulcers or ulcers distal to the second portion of duodenum raise possibility of gastrinoma (Zollinger-Ellison syndrome).
- Gastric ulcer
  - Less common than duodenal ulcer in absence of NSAID use
  - Commonly located along lesser curvature of the antrum
- Esophageal ulcers
  - Located in the distal esophagus; usually secondary to gastroesophageal reflux disease (GERD); also seen with gastrinoma
- Ectopic gastric mucosal ulceration
  - May develop in patients with Meckel diverticulum (1)

GENERAL PREVENTION

- NSAID ulcers: Avoid salicylates and NSAIDs (1).
  - Alternatives include acetaminophen and tramadol. COX-2 inhibitor use is controversial due to potential cardiac safety risks.
  - If NSAIDs are needed, adjust to decrease risk of ulcerogenesis, and add a proton pump inhibitor (PPI) or misoprostol.
  - To reduce ulcer risk, consider testing for and eradicating *Helicobacter pylori* before starting therapy with NSAIDs.
- Maintenance therapy with PPIs or H_2 blockers is indicated for patients with a history of ulcer complications, recurrences, refractory ulcers, or persistent *H. pylori* infection.
- Should also consider maintenance PPI treatment in patients with *H. pylori*-negative, non–NSAID-induced ulcer
- Imbalance between aggressive factors (e.g., gastric acid, pepsin, bile salts, pancreatic enzymes) and defensive factors maintaining mucosal integrity (e.g., mucus, bicarbonate, blood flow, prostaglandins, growth factors, cell turnover)
- May be multifactorial
- *H. pylori* infection: 90% of duodenal ulcers and 70–90% of gastric ulcers
  - Lifetime risk for peptic ulcer disease (PUD) in *H. pylori*-infected people: 10–20%
  - Annual risk of developing duodenal ulcer in *H. pylori*-infected people: ≤1%
- Ulcerogenic drugs (e.g., NSAIDs)
- Hypersecretory syndromes (e.g., gastrinoma)
- Retained gastric antrum
- Less common: Crohn disease, vascular insufficiency, radiation therapy, cancer chemotherapy, smoking

EPIDEMIOLOGY

Incidence

- Predominant sex: male = female
- Predominant age
  - 70% of ulcers occur in patients ages 25–64 years.
  - Ulcer incidence increases with age.
- Peptic ulcer: 500,000 new cases/year
- Recurrence: 4 million/year
- Global incidence rate: 0.1–0.19%

Prevalence

- Peptic ulcer: 1.8% in the United States
- Lifetime prevalence is 5–10% for patients not infected with *H. pylori*; 10–20% if infected

Genetics

Increased incidence of PUD in families is likely due to familial clustering of *H. pylori* infection and inherited genetic factors reflecting response to the organism (1).

RISK FACTORS

- *H. pylori* infection (1)
- NSAID use (5–20%)
- Smoking cigarettes
- Family history of ulcers
- Stress (after acute illness, ventilator support, extensive burns, head injury)
- Gastrinoma
- Alcohol
- Medications: corticosteroids (high-dose and/or prolonged therapy), bisphosphonates, potassium chloride, chemotherapeutic agents (e.g., IV fluorouracil)

COMMONLY ASSOCIATED CONDITIONS

- Gastrinoma (Zollinger-Ellison syndrome)
- Multiple endocrine neoplasia type 1
- Carcinoid syndrome
- Chronic illness: Crohn disease, chronic obstructive pulmonary disease (COPD), chronic renal failure, hepatic cirrhosis, cystic fibrosis
- Hematopoietic disorders (rare): systemic mastocytosis, myeloproliferative disease, hyperparathyroidism, polycythemia rubra vera

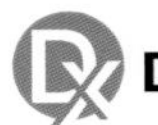

DIAGNOSIS

HISTORY

- Signs and symptoms:
  - Episodic gnawing or burning epigastric pain
  - Pain occurring after meals or on an empty stomach
  - Nocturnal pain
  - Pain relieved by food intake (duodenal), antacids, or antisecretory agents
  - Nonspecific dyspeptic complaints: indigestion, nausea, vomiting, loss of appetite, and heartburn, epigastric fullness
- Alarm symptoms:
  - Anemia, hematemesis, melena, or heme-positive stool suggest bleeding
  - Vomiting and early satiety suggest obstruction
  - Anorexia/weight loss
  - Persisting upper abdominal pain radiating to the back suggests penetration
  - Severe, spreading upper abdominal pain suggests perforation
  - Jaundice, dysphagia
  - Previous gastric surgery
- NSAID-induced ulcers are often silent; perforation/bleeding may be the initial presentation (1).

PHYSICAL EXAM

Physical exam for uncomplicated peptic ulcer may be unreliable and nonspecific: vital signs for hemodynamic stability, conjunctival pallor (anemia); epigastric tenderness (absent in at least 30% of older patients); guaiac-positive stool from occult blood loss (1)

DIFFERENTIAL DIAGNOSIS

Functional dyspepsia, gastritis, GERD, biliary colic, pancreatitis, cholecystitis, Crohn disease, intestinal ischemia, cardiac ischemia, GI malignancy

DIAGNOSTIC TESTS & INTERPRETATION

Initial Tests (lab, imaging)

- Routine lab tests to consider when evaluating PUD:
  - CBC: Rule out anemia.
  - Fecal occult blood test
  - If multiple/refractory ulcers: Consider fasting serum gastrin to rule out gastrinoma (1).
- Indications for *H. pylori* testing: new-onset PUD, history of PUD, persistent symptoms after empirical antisecretory therapy, gastric mucosa–associated lymphoid tissue (MALT) lymphoma, noninvestigated dyspepsia in patients <50 years of age without alarm symptoms (2)
- *H. pylori* diagnostic tests: False-negative results may occur if patient was recently treated with antibiotics, bismuth, or PPIs; or in patients with active bleeding. Diagnostic yield improved by checking 2 different tests in a patient with an ulcer to be sure *H. pylori* is not present:
  - Noninvasive tests (2)[A]:
    - Serology antibody: commonly used in primary care, slow to normalize after treatment, cannot be used to document successful eradication (sensitivity, 85%; specificity, 79%)
    - Urea breath test: identifies active *H. pylori* infection; also used for posttreatment testing (sensitivity, >95%; specificity, >90%)
    - Stool antigen: can be used for screening and posttreatment testing (sensitivity, 91%; specificity, 94%)
  - Invasive tests:
    - Upper endoscopy with gastric biopsy, which can be evaluated with Steiner stain for direct visualization of organism (sensitivity, >95%; specificity, >95%)
    - Rapid urease test: conducted on gastric biopsies (sensitivity, 93–97%; specificity, 95%)
- Barium or Gastrografin contrast radiography (double-contrast hypotonic duodenography): indicated when endoscopy is unsuitable or not feasible

Diagnostic Procedures/Other

Indications for upper endoscopy: patients with suspected peptic ulcers who are >55 years of age, those who have alarm symptoms, and those with ulcers that do not respond to treatment (3)[B]

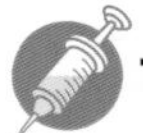

TREATMENT

MEDICATION

First Line

- Acid suppression: PPIs
  - Omeprazole 20 mg/day PO; lansoprazole 30 mg/day PO; rabeprazole 20 mg/day PO; esomeprazole 40 mg/day PO; *or* pantoprazole 40 mg/day PO
  - Administer PPIs before breakfast.
- H_2 blockers: ranitidine or nizatidine 150 mg PO BID or 300 mg PO at bedtime; cimetidine 400 mg PO BID or 800 mg PO at bedtime; famotidine 20 mg PO BID or 40 mg PO at bedtime (4)
- Treat ulcers for 8–12 weeks or until healing is confirmed in patients with complicated ulcers (4).
- PPIs heal peptic ulcers more rapidly (4).
- Precautions:
  - Renal insufficiency: Decrease H_2 blocker dosage by 50% if CrCl <50 mL/min (2).
  - Cimetidine: Use caution with theophylline, warfarin, phenytoin, and lidocaine.

- PPIs may decrease bone density. Obtain interval bone densitometry with long-term PPI use (5).
- PPIs may cause hypomagnesemia. Consider baseline and interval levels in patients, especially for long-term use and in patients taking diuretics.
- PPIs may be associated with increased risk of *Clostridium difficile* infection (5). Short-term use associated with development of community-acquired pneumonia; long-term use does not appear to have an increased risk.
- Despite earlier concerns, PPIs do not appear to decrease the efficacy of clopidogrel (5).

- NSAID-induced ulcers
  - Discontinue NSAID use.
  - Treat acutely with PPIs for 8–12 weeks; may use longer as maintenance for patients with recurrent, complicated, or idiopathic ulcers; or in patients who require long-term aspirin or NSAID use.
- *H. pylori*–induced ulcers
  - *H. pylori* eradication regimens: Preferred duration of therapy is 14 days.
  - Triple therapy: Standard dose PPI given BID + clarithromycin 500 mg PO BID + amoxicillin 1 g PO BID or metronidazole 500 mg PO BID in patients with allergy to amoxicillin (2).
- Bacterial resistance: clarithromycin 10%; amoxicillin 1.4%; metronidazole 37%: Culture-guided choice of triple therapy is more clinically and cost-effective (6).

Second Line

- For *H. pylori* eradication: Use 2nd-line therapy if 1st-line fails (6):
  - Bismuth quadruple therapy × 14 days
    - Bismuth subsalicylate 525 mg PO QID +
    - Metronidazole 250 mg PO QID +
    - Tetracycline 500 mg PO QID +
    - Standard dose PPI PO twice daily
- Sequential therapy
  - Standard dose PPI PO twice daily + amoxicillin 1,000 mg PO QID × 5 days followed by
  - Standard dose PPI PO twice daily + clarithromycin 500 mg PO BID + tinidazole (or metronidazole) 500 mg PO BID × 5 days
    - Levofloxacin 250 mg PO BID may be substituted in those with PCN allergy or in areas of high clarithromycin resistance rates.
  - Another alternative salvage therapy:
    - Rifabutin 300 mg PO daily +
    - Amoxicillin 1,000 mg PO BID +
    - PPI orally BID
  - Alternative ulcer-healing drugs:
    - Sucralfate and antacids are additional options; however, antisecretory options are preferred.
- Significant possible interactions:
  - Cimetidine inhibits cytochrome P450 isozymes (avoid with theophylline, warfarin, phenytoin, and lidocaine).
  - Omeprazole may prolong elimination of diazepam, warfarin, and phenytoin.
  - Sucralfate reduces absorption of tetracycline, norfloxacin, ciprofloxacin, and theophylline; it leads to subtherapeutic levels.

Pregnancy Considerations

PPIs are *not* associated with an increased risk for major congenital birth defects, spontaneous abortions, or preterm delivery.

Breastfeeding

Both ranitidine and esomeprazole are secreted in breastmilk; however, at considerably lower doses than those used for treatment in infants with reflux disease. Use in breastfeeding women is generally regarded as safe (7).

SURGERY/OTHER PROCEDURES

- Endoscopy indicated for patients age >50 years with new onset of dyspeptic symptoms, those who do not respond to treatment, and those of any age with alarm symptoms, such as bleeding and weight loss (8)[B].
- At endoscopy:
  - Biopsy of stomach for *H. pylori* testing (Clo test)
  - Biopsy of margin of gastric ulcer to confirm benign etiology
  - Interventions to stop active bleeding or prevent rebleeding in those with certain stigmata, include injection with epinephrine, heater probe treatment, or placement of endoscopic clips (3).
- Indications for surgery: Ulcers that are refractory to treatment and patients at high risk for complications (e.g., transplant recipients, patients dependent on steroids/NSAIDs); surgery also may be needed acutely for treatment of perforation and bleeding that is refractory to endoscopic therapy (8).
- Surgical options:
  - Duodenal ulcers: truncal vagotomy and drainage (pyloroplasty/gastrojejunostomy), selective vagotomy (preserving the hepatic and/or celiac branches of the vagus) and drainage, or highly selective vagotomy (3)
  - Gastric ulcers: partial gastrectomy, Billroth I or II
  - Perforated ulcers: laparoscopy/open patching (3)

INPATIENT CONSIDERATIONS

Admission Criteria/Initial Stabilization

- Discontinue ulcerogenic agents (e.g., NSAIDs) (1).
- Bleeding peptic ulcers
  - Stable: Give PPI to reduce transfusion requirements, need for surgery, and duration of hospitalization (9).
  - Unstable: fluid/packed RBC resuscitation followed by emergent esophagogastroduodenoscopy (EGD); use IV PPI.
  - Insufficient evidence for concluding superiority, inferiority, or equivalence of high-dose PPI treatment over lower doses in peptic ulcer bleeding (5)[A]
- After endoscopic therapy, oral PPIs are as effective as IV (9).
- Perforated peptic ulcers: Free peritoneal perforation with bacterial peritonitis is a surgical emergency (3).

ONGOING CARE

FOLLOW-UP RECOMMENDATIONS

Patient Monitoring

- *H. pylori* eradication: expected in >90% (with double antibiotic regimen): Confirm eradication by urea breath test.
- Acute duodenal ulcer: Monitor clinically.
- Acute gastric ulcer: Confirm healing via endoscopy after 12 weeks if biopsy is not done initially to confirm that the lesion is benign.

PROGNOSIS

After *H. pylori* eradication (10):

- Low ulcer relapse rate; if relapse, consider surreptitious use of NSAIDs.
- Reinfection rates <1% per year
- Low risk of rebleeding
- Decreased NSAID ulcer recurrence (10)

COMPLICATIONS

- Hemorrhage: up to 25% of patients (initial presentation in 10%)
- Perforation: <5% of patients
- Gastric outlet obstruction: up to 5% of duodenal or pyloric channel ulcers; male predilection found
- Risk of gastric adenocarcinoma increased in *H. pylori*–infected patients (2).

REFERENCES

1. Ramakrishnan K, Salinas RC. Peptic ulcer disease. *Am Fam Physician*. 2007;76(7):1005–1012.
2. Saad R, Chey WD. A clinician's guide to managing Helicobacter pylori infection. *Cleve Clin J Med*. 2005;72(2):109–110,112–113,117–118.
3. Bertleff MJ, Lange JF. Perforated peptic ulcer disease: A review of history and treatment. *Dig Surg*. 2010;27(3):161–169.
4. Gill SK, O'Brien L, Einarson TR. The safety of proton pump inhibitors (PPIs) in pregnancy: a meta-analysis. *Am J Gastroenterol*. 2009;104(6):1541–1545.
5. Neumann I, Letelier LM, Rada G, et al. Comparison of different regimens of proton pump inhibitors for acute peptic ulcer bleeding. *Cochrane Database Syst Rev*. 2013;6:CD007999.
6. Luther J, Higgins PD, Schoenfeld PS, et al. Empiric quadruple vs. triple therapy for primary treatment of Helicobacter pylori infection: systematic review and meta-analysis of efficacy and tolerability. *Am J Gastroenterol*. 2010;105(1):65–73.
7. Marshall JK, Thompson AB, Armstrong D. Omeprazole for refractory gastroesophageal reflux disease during pregnancy and lactation. *Can J Gastroenterol*. 1998; 12(3):225–227.
8. Laine L, Jensen DM. Management of patients with ulcer bleeding. *Am J Gastroenterol*. 2012;107(3):345–360; quiz 361.
9. Yen HH, Yang CW, Su WW, et al. Oral versus intravenous proton pump inhibitors in preventing re-bleeding for patients with peptic ulcer bleeding after successful endoscopic therapy. *BMC Gastroenterology*. 2012;12:66.
10. Gisbert JP, Calvet X, Cosme A, et al. Long-term follow-up of 1,000 patients cured of *Helicobacter pylori* infection following an episode of peptic ulcer bleeding. *Am J Gastroenterol*. 2012;107(8):1197–1204.

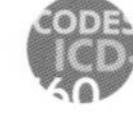

CODES

ICD10

- K27.9 Peptic ulc, site unsp, unsp as ac or chr, w/o hemor or perf
- K26.9 Duodenal ulcer, unspecified as acute or chronic, without hemorrhage or perforation
- K25.9 Gastric ulcer, unspecified as acute or chronic, without hemorrhage or perforation

CLINICAL PEARLS

- In patients with PUD, *H. pylori* should be eradicated to assist in healing and to reduce the risk of gastric and duodenal ulcer recurrence.
- Upper endoscopy is indicated in patients with suspected peptic ulcers who are >55 years of age, those who have alarm symptoms, and those who do not respond to treatment.

PERFORATED TYMPANIC MEMBRANE

Sarah E. Mowry, MD • Brian Ho, MD

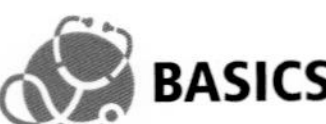

BASICS

DESCRIPTION

- The ear drum or "tympanic membrane" (TM) is a thin barrier that separates the external auditory canal (EAC) from the middle ear and vibrates in response to sound waves, creating amplification as well as providing protection to the middle ear space.
- Rupture of the TM can disrupt hearing while also allowing pathogens to access the middle ear space from the EAC.
- Perforations are classified by location:
  - *Central:* not involving the annulus (the tendon-like structure that attaches the TM to the ear canal), can occur after a case of acute otitis media that leads to perforation (welding injuries)
  - *Marginal:* involves the annulus and may be associated with cholesteatoma and are unlikely to heal spontaneously
  - *Subtotal*: a large defect surrounded with an intact annulus; requires surgery to close
- Classification of perforations by etiology:
  - Infectious: acute/chronic suppurative otitis media
  - Traumatic: barotrauma, (e.g., diving), acoustic trauma, (e.g., explosion), self-inflicted/penetrating (cotton tips)
  - Middle ear mass: cholesteatoma or neoplasm
  - Iatrogenic: persistent perforation after myringotomy tube placement or secondary acquired cholesteatoma
- The TM possesses the ability for spontaneous closure resulting in formation of a dimeric membrane (outer squamous and inner mucosal). However, if this does not occur, a persistent perforation will result.

EPIDEMIOLOGY

Incidence in the general population is unknown because many perforations heal spontaneously.

Genetics

Genetic susceptibility has been reported for recurrent acute otitis media (AOM) and chronic otitis media with effusion (COME), 2 of the etiologies of perforations (1).

GENERAL PREVENTION

- Avoid ear trauma or self-inserted foreign objects in the EAC.
- Treat otitis media in a timely fashion prior to resultant TM perforation.

ETIOLOGY AND PATHOPHYSIOLOGY

- Chronic eustachian tube dysfunction or chronic negative middle ear pressure can lead to OM.
- Insertion of foreign objects into ear (cotton swabs)
- Otitis media: A purulent, serous, or mucoid fluid builds up behind the tympanic membrane leading to therapeutic perforation.
- A ruptured TM that chronically drains painlessly may be due to cholesteatoma.
- Iatrogenic: For the treatment of chronic eustachian tube dysfunction, a myringotomy is performed and tympanostomy tubes are placed; after tubes are extruded, a chronic perforation may result.

COMMONLY ASSOCIATED CONDITIONS

- Chronic eustachian tube dysfunction (e.g., cleft palate)
- OME
- Cholesteatoma
- Tympanosclerosis
- Ossicular chain damage (if traumatic perforation)

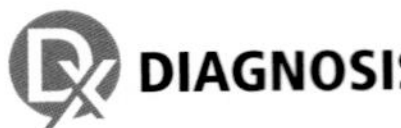

DIAGNOSIS

HISTORY

- Otorrhea or drainage from the ear (pus, blood, or clear fluid)
- Otalgia or earache consistent with AOM, followed by sudden relief of symptoms (because of TM rupture)
- Tinnitus or buzzing
- Self-audible whistling from the ear with Valsalva maneuver or nose blowing
- Hearing loss (can be due to loss of amplification from large TM perforation or from concomitant ossicular chain discontinuity due to trauma)
- Vertigo
- Nausea and vomiting
- History of ear infections as a child or difficulty equalizing pressure during flights (chronic eustachian tube dysfunction)
- Ear surgery (prior placement of PE tubes)
- Recurrent ear infections

PHYSICAL EXAM

- Otoscopic exam: Pay attention to location, purulent drainage, and involvement of annulus or of the malleus. Also, inspect ear canal to look for concomitant otitis externa.
- Pneumatic otoscopy will reveal no motion because air passes freely into the middle ear space, possible to induce vertigo indicating a positive "fistula" sign.
- Note foreign bodies (cotton swabs, PE tubes). Batteries are an emergency and ENT should be consulted for immediate removal.
- Retraction pocket (chronic eustachian tube dysfunction and resultant cholesteatoma) typically in the superior quadrant
- Thinned tympanic membrane (prior perforations or severe chronic retraction)
- Keratin debris consistent with cholesteatoma (pearl white mass or chronically draining ear)
- Mass in the middle ear space behind the TM (cholesteatoma, paragangliomas, CN7 schwannomas, etc.)
- Ulcerations in the EAC, which carry on to the annular surface causing perforations should lead to suspicion of squamous cell carcinoma (ENT consult).
- If history of hearing loss on that side: Weber (512-khz tuning fork to center of forehead; if conductive hearing loss, sound should lateralize to the perforated side) and Rinne tests (place tuning fork to mastoid; when vibration no longer heard, transfer tuning fork next to outside ear canal; air conduction should be greater than bone conduction)
- Facial nerve palsy is uncommon to have with an isolated TM perforation. This is likely due to more occult pathology, and ENT consult should be placed.
- Inspection of oropharynx noting tonsillar asymmetry or neoplasms that can cause eustachian tube obstruction leading to unilateral AOM and TM perforation
- Hemotympanum will resolve spontaneously.

DIAGNOSTIC TESTS & INTERPRETATION

- Audiogram can reveal normal hearing or a mild conductive hearing loss:
  - A simple perforation will typically result in a low-frequency conductive hearing loss.
  - An audiogram that demonstrates a worse-than-expected conductive hearing loss or sensorineural hearing loss is more suspicious for ossicular chain damage or middle ear pathology.
- Tympanometry demonstrates an increased volume in the ear and decreased pressure (can demonstrate perforation even if not present on otoscopic exam); acoustic immittance demonstrates a volume >2 mL.
- MRI and CT imaging are not indicated for routine TM perforations.
- If there is suspicion for cholesteatoma or CN VII palsy, then obtain noncontrasted CT of the temporal bone as initial imaging study.
- Follow-up should be established with an otolaryngologist for proper management, possible débridement, identification of cholesteatoma, and possible surgery for chronic perforations.

DIFFERENTIAL DIAGNOSIS

- Tympanosclerosis
- Dimeric membrane from prior perforation (thin membrane may be hard to discern)
- Otitis externa can obscure a perforation.
- Cholesteatoma causing chronic drainage
- Iatrogenic: previous ear surgery
- Trauma (baro or foreign body)
- Infectious: AOM/OME (rare pathogens such as TB)

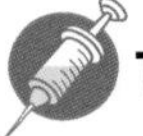

TREATMENT

- Most TM perforations are nonurgent and do not require immediate evaluation by an otolaryngologist. Often, these can be managed as an outpatient with drops and pain control to decrease inflammation; ENT follow-up in few days to a week
- A significant portion of TM perforations heal spontaneously without intervention because of the TM's regenerative abilities.
- Most are uncomplicated with minimal hearing loss (<40 dB) and lack vestibular complaints.
- Observation of >3 months is a feasible option in select patients with uncomplicated, small perforations.
- Debate exists over dry-ear precautions. But conservatively, patients should avoid getting water into the external auditory canal and into middle ear space. Typical showering is less of an issue, but swimming in rivers/swimming pools should be avoided until the perforation has healed.
- Treatment of purulence with topical antibiotic drops will reduce otorrhea.
- If significant bleeding, topical Afrin can also be instilled in the ear canal.

- Perforations with hearing loss >40 dB, any degree of ipsilateral facial weakness, those associated with vestibular symptoms, or those associated with cholesteatoma require referral to ENT; for traumatic perforation, obtain evaluation within 48 hours.

MEDICATION

- Some topical antibiotics (gentamicin, neomycin sulfate, or tobramycin) may rarely cause ototoxicity with TM perforations because they absorb through the round window into the inner ear.
- Topical drops are the mainstay of treatment for acute otitis media with perforation. These can be used for 5–7 days. Topical antibiotic drops should be continued if persistent otorrhea; may need evaluation by an otolaryngologist if drainage does not resolve with ototopical medication
- Nonototoxic drops are preferred, but cost and availability may be relevant considerations given the rarity of oto- and vestibulotoxicity (2)[C].
- Oral antibiotics are not recommended for AOM with perforations because antibiotic drops are more effective. Oral antibiotics should be used in AOM prior to perforation.
- Oral antibiotics are not indicated for the isolated TM perforation.

First Line

- Ciprofloxacin ear drops ± dexamethasone
- Ofloxacin ear drops

ADDITIONAL THERAPIES

- Some authors advocate dry ear precautions (cotton ball with petroleum jelly while showering and use of hairdryer to dry out ear if water enters the EAC).
- Most authors agree that dry ear precautions should be used if patients will be swimming in lakes/rivers.

GENERAL MEASURES

- For some patients with chronic eustachian tube dysfunction, having a perforated tympanic membrane is a favorable situation because it allows for the equalization of pressure in the middle ear that would otherwise be more difficult because of the decreased eustachian tube function, thus obviating the need for tympanostomy tube placement later. For these patients, dry ear precautions are recommended.
- For patients who participate in water sports as a part of daily life, such as swimmers and divers, repair is recommended to provide the patient a "safe ear."
- Because there is a connection from the outer ear to the middle ear, dry ear precautions are needed to prevent a nidus of infection such as using a cotton ball in the ear during showers and gentle hairdryer use over ear if water enters the ear canal.
- A case-by-case risk–benefit analysis must be performed in cases of conductive hearing loss because surgery entails the risk of hearing loss.
- Prevent infection primarily with eardrops or oral antibiotics as a secondary measure.

SURGERY/OTHER PROCEDURES

- Myringoplasty can be performed if the perforation is small and appears to be favorable. This is often performed with gel or paper patch, which provides a scaffold across which the TM can heal.
- Tympanoplasty is performed for larger perforations, persistent perforations, or anteriorly based perforations. Perichondrium, fat, cartilage, pericranium, and temporalis fascia are often used in reconstructing the tympanic membrane.
- A combined tympanoplasty/mastoidectomy surgery might be required for large perforations, chronic draining ears, presence of cholesteatoma, damage to the ossicular chain, or with evidence of mastoid disease.
- Surgery is often outpatient procedure and may be done under sedation and local anesthesia. General anesthesia can also be used.
- Patients can receive mastoid compressive dressings and instructions for postoperative antibiotics.
- Potential major complications of surgery include worsening of hearing, facial nerve damage, CSF leak, bleeding, and repair failure.
- Ossiculoplasty might also be performed if pathology involves the ossicular chain; full repair of the ossicular chain can be performed at primary procedure or as a second look.
  - If ossicular chain discontinuity is repaired, patients will require postoperative audiogram to evaluate airbone gap.

INPATIENT CONSIDERATIONS

Inpatient care is generally not required for tympanic membrane perforation. The presence of comorbid disease like mastoiditis or meningitis would require inpatient stabilization with IV antibiotics/imaging and appropriate care for those disorders.

ONGOING CARE

FOLLOW-UP RECOMMENDATIONS

Patient Monitoring

- Follow-up should be established with an otolaryngologist to confirm tympanic membrane healing and to obtain an audiogram.
- It is vital to reexamine the ear, especially after an episode of infection associated with a perforation, to rule out underlying cholesteatoma or chronic eustachian tube dysfunction, which may be contributing to the perforation.
- Follow-up after surgery is necessary.

DIET

No dietary restrictions

PATIENT EDUCATION

- Dry ear precautions
- Avoid cotton swabs in the ear.
- Call physician for worsening hearing loss, vertigo, **facial nerve palsy**, fever, or persistent drainage.

PROGNOSIS

- Most perforations will heal spontaneously; however, large perforations and those associated with a chronic draining ear often require surgery.
- Mortality associated with this condition is low, but there is a potential for infection to spread to the mastoid, leading to meningitis, if proper aural care is not maintained.

COMPLICATIONS

- Nonhealing perforation
- Infection (otitis media, mastoiditis, meningitis)
- Conductive hearing loss
- Facial paralysis (rare and likely due to additional pathology)
- Ossicular chain disruption (traumatic induced)

REFERENCES

1. Rye MS, Blackwell JM, Jamieson SE. Genetic susceptibility to otitis media in childhood. *Laryngoscope*. 2012;122(3):665–675.
2. Haynes DS, Rutka J, Hawke M, et al. Ototoxicity of ototopical drops—an update. *Otolaryngol Clin North Am*. 2007;40(3):669–683, xi.

ADDITIONAL READING

- Jensen RG, Koch A, Homøe P. Long-term tympanic membrane pathology dynamics and spontaneous healing in chronic suppurative otitis media. *Pediatr Infect Dis J*. 2011;31(2):139–144.
- Lou ZC, Lou ZH, Zhang QP. Traumatic tympanic membrane perforations: a study of etiology and factors affecting outcome. *Am J Otolaryngol*. 2012;33(5):549–555.
- Morris PS, Leach AJ. Acute and chronic otitis media. *Pediatr Clin North Am*. 2009;56(6):1383–1399.

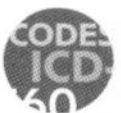

CODES

ICD10

- H72.90 Unsp perforation of tympanic membrane, unspecified ear
- H72.00 Central perforation of tympanic membrane, unspecified ear
- H72.2×9 Other marginal perforations of tympanic membrane, unsp ear

CLINICAL PEARLS

- To evaluate a patient with a suspected tympanic membrane perforation, history and physical exam will usually suffice and does not require imaging.
- Nonhealing perforations associated with malodorous or recurrent infections are often associated with cholesteatoma and an otolaryngology consultation is recommended.
- Retraction pockets and history of AOM are suspicious for chronic eustachian tube dysfunction.
- Tympanoplasty surgery might be required for a perforation that does not spontaneously heal.
- If the presentation is a sudden sensorineural hearing loss, this should warrant referral and initiation of steroid therapy the same day.
- If presentation is also with sudden facial paralysis, this should warrant urgent referral and initiation of steroid therapy ± antiviral treatment.

PERICARDITIS

Veronica J. Ruston, DO • Angela M. Riegel, DO

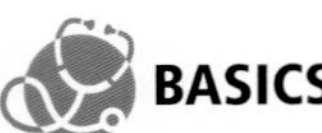

BASICS

DESCRIPTION

Inflammation of the pericardium, with or without associated pericardial effusion. Myopericarditis or perimyocarditis refers to cases that have myocardial involvement in addition to the pericardial sac.

EPIDEMIOLOGY

Incidence

Epidemiologic studies are lacking. Exact incidence unknown but occurs in up to 5% of patients evaluated in the ER for chest pain without myocardial infarction (MI); appears to be a slightly increased prevalence in men

ETIOLOGY AND PATHOPHYSIOLOGY

- Inflammation of the pericardial sac can be *acute* or *chronic* (recurrent). Chronic/recurrent inflammation may result in constrictive pericarditis.
- Can produce serous/purulent fluid/dense fibrinous material (depending on etiology), which may or may not lead to hemodynamic compromise.

Genetics

No known genetic factors:

- Idiopathic: 85–90% of cases. Likely related to viral infection, which may trigger immune-related process.
- Infectious
  - Viral: coxsackievirus, echovirus, adenovirus, Epstein-Barr virus, cytomegalovirus, hepatitis viruses, influenza virus, HIV, measles, mumps, varicella
  - Bacterial: gram-positive and gram-negative organisms
  - Fungal (more common in immunocompromised populations): *Blastomyces dermatitidis, Candida* sp., *Histoplasma capsulatum*
  - Mycobacterial: *Mycobacterium tuberculosis*
  - Parasites: *Echinococcus*
- Noninfectious causes
  - Acute MI (2–4 days after MI), Dressler syndrome (weeks to months after MI)
  - Aortic dissection
  - Renal failure, uremia, dialysis-associated
  - Malignancy (e.g., breast cancer, lung cancer, Hodgkin disease, leukemia, lymphoma)
  - Radiation therapy
  - Trauma
  - Postpericardiotomy
  - After cardiac procedures (e.g., catheterization, pacemaker placement, ablation)
  - Autoimmune disorders: connective tissue disorders, systemic lupus erythematosus (SLE), rheumatoid arthritis, scleroderma, hypothyroidism, inflammatory bowel disease, spondyloarthropathies, Wegener granulomatosis
  - Sarcoidosis
- Medication induced: dantrolene, doxorubicin, hydralazine, isoniazid, mesalamine, methysergide, penicillin, phenytoin, procainamide, rifampin

COMMONLY ASSOCIATED CONDITIONS

Depends on etiology

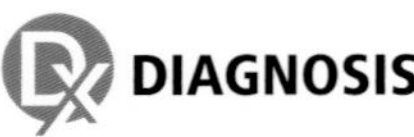

DIAGNOSIS

HISTORY

- Prodrome of fever, malaise, myalgias
- Acute, sharp, stabbing chest pain
- Duration typically hours to days
- Pleuritic pain
- Pain reduced by leaning forward, worsened by lying supine
- Shortness of breath

PHYSICAL EXAM

- Heart rate is usually rapid and regular.
- Pericardial friction rub: coarse, high-pitched sound best heard during end expiration at left lower sternal border with patient leaning forward. Highly specific for diagnosis (but not sensitive); may be transient and mono-, bi-, or triphasic
- New S_3 may suggest myopericarditis.
- Cardiac tamponade
- Diagnostic clinical criteria
  - Acute pericarditis (at least 2 of 4 criteria)
    - Typical (pleuritic) chest pain
    - Pericardial friction rub
    - ECG changes with widespread ST elevation
    - New/increasing pericardial effusion
  - Myopericarditis
    - Definite pericarditis *plus*
    - Symptoms (dyspnea, chest pain, or palpitations) *and* ECG changes not previously documented (ST/T-wave abnormalities, supraventricular/ventricular tachycardia) *or* focal/diffuse depressed left ventricular (LV) function documented on imaging study
    - Absence of evidence of other cause
    - 1 of the following: elevated cardiac enzymes (creatine kinase [CK]-MB, troponin I or T) *or* new focal/diffuse depressed LV function *or* abnormal imaging consistent with myocarditis (MRI with gadolinium, gallium-67 scanning, antimyosin antibody scanning)
  - Case definitions
    - *Suspected myopericarditis*: criteria 1, 2, and 3
    - *Probable myopericarditis*: criteria 1, 2, 3, and 4
    - *Confirmed myopericarditis*: histopathologic evidence of myocarditis by endomyocardial biopsy (EMB) or autopsy (Note: In the clinical setting, for self-limited cases with predominantly pericarditis, EMB is rarely indicated.)

DIAGNOSTIC TESTS & INTERPRETATION

Initial Tests (lab, imaging)

- It is not necessary to order tests for uncomplicated cases or when the diagnosis is clear. Following labs may be helpful (1)[C]:
  - CBC: typically shows leukocytosis
  - Inflammatory markers: elevated erythrocyte sedimentation rate (ESR), C-reactive protein (CRP), and lactodehydrogenase (LDH)
  - Cardiac biomarkers: typically elevated creatine kinase, troponins
    - Elevated troponins associated with younger age, male sex, pericardial effusion at presentation, and ST-segment elevation on ECG
    - Adverse outcomes not predicted by elevated troponin
- ECG: Findings include widespread upward concave ST-segment elevation and PR-segment depression that may evolve through 4 stages. ECG may be normal/show nonspecific abnormalities:
  - Stage 1: diffuse ST-segment elevation and PR-segment depression
  - Stage 2: Normalization of the ST and PR segments and T waves begin to flatten and invert.
  - Stage 3: widespread T-wave inversions
  - Stage 4: normalization of T waves; may have persistent inversions if chronic pericarditis
- ECG may demonstrate low voltage and electrical alternans with tamponade.
- Transthoracic echocardiogram recommended to evaluate for the presence of pericardial effusion, tamponade, or myocardial disease (presence of effusion helps to confirm diagnosis of pericarditis) (1)[C]
- Chest x-ray (CXR) is performed to rule out pulmonary/mediastinal pathology. Enlarged cardiac silhouette suggests large pericardial effusion (at least 200 mL).
- CT and MRI allow visualization of pericardium to assess for complications or if initial workup is inconclusive (1)[C].
- Additional testing (if clinically appropriate based on history or atypical presentation or course) may include tuberculin skin test, sputum cultures, rheumatoid factor, antinuclear antibody, and HIV serology (1)[C].
- Viral cultures and antibody titers rarely clinically useful (1)[C]

Diagnostic Procedures/Other

- Pericardiocentesis indicated for cardiac tamponade; for suspected purulent, tuberculous, or neoplastic pericarditis; and for effusions >20 mm on echocardiography (2)[C]
- Surgical drainage with pericardial biopsy recommended if recurrent tamponade, ineffective pericardiocentesis, or hemodynamic instability (2)[C]

Test Interpretation

- Microscopic examination may reveal hyperemia, leukocyte accumulation, or fibrin deposition.
- Purulent fluid with neutrophilic predominance if bacterial etiology
- Lymphocytic predominance in viral, tuberculous, and neoplastic pericarditis

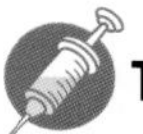

TREATMENT

- Goal of treatment is to relieve pain and reduce complications (e.g., recurrence, tamponade, chronic restrictive pericarditis).
- Outpatient therapy is reported to be successful in 85% patients with low-risk features.

GENERAL MEASURES

Specific therapy directed toward underlying disorder for patients with identified cause other than viral/idiopathic disease.

MEDICATION

First Line

- NSAIDs are considered the mainstay of therapy for acute pericarditis:
  - Ibuprofen 400–800 mg TID × 1–2 weeks (2–4 weeks for recurrence) then taper (3)[C]
  - Aspirin 650–975 mg TID–QID × 1–2 weeks (2–4 weeks for recurrence) then taper; preferable for patients with recent MI because other NSAIDs impair scar formation in animal studies (4)[C]
  - Indomethacin 50 mg TID × 1–2 weeks (2–4 weeks for recurrence) then taper; should avoid in elderly due to flow restrictions to coronaries (3)[C]
  - Ketorolac 15–30 mg IV/IM every 6 hours while inpatient; maximum duration of 5 days (3)[C]
  - GI protection should be provided (3)[C].
  - Tapering should be done only if the patient is asymptomatic and CRP/ESR are normal and are done every 1–2 weeks (3)[C].

P

- Treatment duration using NSAIDs for initial attacks is 1–2 weeks, but for recurrences, consider 2–4 weeks of therapy (3)[C].
- Monitoring: NSAIDs: CBC and CRP at baseline and weekly until CRP normalizes
- Contraindications: hypersensitivity to aspirin or NSAIDs, active peptic ulcer/GI bleeding
- Precautions: Use with caution in patients with asthma, 3rd-trimester pregnancy, coagulopathy, and renal/hepatic dysfunction.

- Colchicine: common practice to use in combination with NSAIDs; 0.6 mg BID for up to 3 months (up to 6 months for recurrence); taper not required. Efficacious as therapy for initial occurrence and if multiple recurrences. This is the only agent proven to prevent recurrences in RCTs. Adjunctive therapy can reduce rate of recurrence by 50% (2)[A]. Monitoring: Consider CBC, CRP, transaminases, creatine kinase, and creatinine at baseline and at least after 1 month.
- Pregnant: <20 weeks' gestation: Aspirin is 1st choice, but NSAIDs and prednisone are also allowed; >20 weeks' gestation: Prednisone is allowed with avoidance of NSAIDs, aspirin, and colchicine (1)[C].

Second Line

- Corticosteroid treatment is indicated in connective tissue disease, tuberculous pericarditis, or severe recurrent symptoms unresponsive to NSAIDs or colchicine; should be avoided in uncomplicated acute pericarditis. *Corticosteroid use alone has been found to be an independent risk factor for recurrence* (4)[C].
- If steroids are used, consider low dose (0.25–0.5 mg/kg/day × 2 weeks for 1st attack, 0.25–0.5 mg/kg/day × 2–4 weeks for recurrence) with slow taper (>50 mg: 10 mg/day every 1–2 weeks; 50–25 mg: 5–10 mg/day every 1–2 weeks; 25–15 mg: 2.5 mg/day every 2–4 weeks; <15 mg/day: 1–2.5 mg/day every 2–6 weeks) following remission. Remember adequate prophylaxis treatment for osteoporosis prevention (4)[C].
- If unable to taper from steroids, resume lowest steroid dose and begin slow taper of 1–2 mg every 2–4 weeks (3)[C].
- Intrapericardial administration of steroids may be effective and limits systemic side effects.

ISSUES FOR REFERRAL

- Refractory cases include those on unacceptably high long-term steroid doses (>25 mg/day).
- Consider trial of aspirin and/or NSAIDs + steroid and colchicine.
- Uremic or dialysis-related cases require more frequent or urgent dialysis without significant benefit from pharmacologics (1)[C].

SURGERY/OTHER PROCEDURES

- Pericardiocentesis is indicated in cases of cardiac tamponade, high likelihood of tuberculous/purulent/neoplastic pericarditis, and large symptomatic effusions refractory to medical therapy.
- Pericardial biopsy may be considered for diagnosis in those with persistent worsening pericarditis without a definite diagnosis.
- Pericardioscopy for targeted diagnostic imaging may be performed at experienced tertiary referral centers in refractory and difficult cases.
- Pericardial window may be performed in cases of recurrent cardiac tamponade with large pericardial effusion despite medical therapy and severe symptoms.
- Pericardiectomy can be considered. The 2004 European Society of Cardiology guidelines recommend pericardiectomy (Class IIa) for frequent and highly symptomatic recurrences of pericarditis refractory to medical therapy. However, this is rarely performed in the United States and has high morbidity and mortality (1)[C].

INPATIENT CONSIDERATIONS

Admission Criteria/Initial Stabilization

Inpatient therapy recommended for pericarditis associated with clinical predictors of poor prognosis:

- Major predictors: fever >38°C, subacute onset, large pericardial effusion, cardiac tamponade, lack of response to NSAID/aspirin therapy after at least 1 week (5)[C]
- Minor predictors: immunosuppressed state, trauma, oral anticoagulation therapy, myopericarditis (5)[C]

IV-Fluids

IV fluids considered for hypotension or in the setting of pericardial tamponade

Discharge Criteria

- Response to therapy with symptom improvement
- Hemodynamic stability

ONGOING CARE

FOLLOW-UP RECOMMENDATIONS

- 7–10 days to assess response to treatment
- 1 month to check CBC and CRP and thereafter if symptoms continue to be present
- Those with clinical predictors of poor prognosis may require closer follow-up based on lab data and echocardiographic findings.

Patient Monitoring

Myopericarditis

- Use lower doses of anti-inflammatory drugs to control symptoms for 1–2 weeks while minimizing deleterious effects on myocarditic process.
- Exercise restrictions for 4–6 weeks or until symptoms resolved and biomarkers normalized (2)[C].
- Echocardiographic monitoring at 1, 6, and 12 months (especially in those with left ventricular dysfunction)

DIET

No restrictions

PROGNOSIS

Overall good prognosis; disease usually benign and self-limiting. Purulent and tuberculosis pericarditis with high mortality.

COMPLICATIONS

- Recurrent pericarditis: occurs in ~30% of patients, with most instances resulting from idiopathic, viral, or autoimmune pericarditis; inadequate treatment of the initial attack; and, less commonly, neoplastic etiologies. Recurrence usually within 1st weeks following initial episode but may occur months to years later; rarely associated with tamponade/constriction
- Cardiac tamponade: rare complication with increased incidence in neoplastic, purulent, and tuberculous pericarditis
- Effusive-constrictive pericarditis: Reported in 24% of patients undergoing surgery for constrictive pericarditis and in 8% of patients undergoing pericardiocentesis and cardiac catheterization for cardiac tamponade. Failure of right atrial pressure to fall by 50% or to a level below 10 mm Hg after pericardiocentesis is diagnostic.
- Constrictive pericarditis: rare complication in which rigid pericardium produces abnormal diastolic filling with elevated filling pressures. Pericardiectomy remains definitive therapy.

REFERENCES

1. Maisch B, Seferović PM, Ristić AD, et al. Guidelines on the diagnosis and management of pericardial diseases executive summary: the task force on the diagnosis and management of pericardial diseases of the European Society of Cardiology. *Eur Heart J*. 2004;25(7):587–610.
2. Imazio M, Brucato A, Belli R, et al. Colchicine for the prevention of pericarditis: what we know and what we do not know in 2014—systemic review and meta-analysis. *J Cardiovas Med*. 2014:15(12):840–846.
3. Lilly L. Treatment of acute and recurrent pericarditis. *Circulation*. 2013;127(16):1723–1726.
4. Imazio M, Brucato A, Trinchero R, et al. Diagnosis and management of pericardial diseases. *Nat Rev Cardiol*. 2009;6(12):743–751.
5. Snyder M, Bepko J, White M. Acute pericarditis: diagnosis and management. *Am Fam Physician*. 2014:89(7):553–560.

ADDITIONAL READING

- Imazio M, Brucato A, Cemin R, et al. A randomized trial of colchicine for acute pericarditis. *N Engl J Med*. 2013;369(16):1522–1528.
- Imazio M, Spodick DH, Brucato A, et al. Controversial issues in the management of pericardial diseases. *Circulation*. 2010;121(7):916–928.
- Khandaker MH, Espinosa RE, Nishimura RA, et al. Pericardial disease: diagnosis and management. *Mayo Clin Proc*. 2010;85(6):572–593.

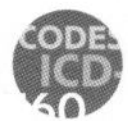

CODES

ICD10

- I31.9 Disease of pericardium, unspecified
- I30.9 Acute pericarditis, unspecified
- I30.1 Infective pericarditis

CLINICAL PEARLS

- Consider *major* predictors and *minor* predictors in deciding which patients should be admitted.
- Therapy aimed at symptomatic relief and NSAIDs are first-line treatment. Colchicine is recommended as an adjunct to NSAIDs.
- Pericardiocentesis is recommended in the setting of cardiac tamponade or possible purulent pericarditis.

PERIODIC LIMB MOVEMENT DISORDER

Donald E. Watenpaugh, PhD • John R. Burk, MD

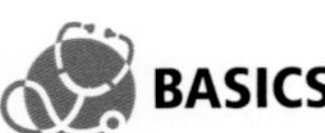

BASICS

DESCRIPTION

- Sleep-related movement disorder with these features:
  - Episodes of periodic limb movements (PLMs) during sleep
  - Movements consist of bilateral ankle dorsiflexion, sometimes with knee and hip flexion.
  - Arm or more generalized movements occur less commonly.
  - Movements may cause brief microarousals from sleep unbeknownst to the patient.
  - Complaints include insomnia, unrestorative sleep, daytime fatigue, and/or somnolence.
  - Bed partner may complain of movements.
  - Another sleep disorder (e.g., obstructive sleep apnea) does not cause the PLMs.
- System(s) affected: musculoskeletal, nervous
- Synonym(s): nocturnal myoclonus; sleep myoclonus; periodic leg movements of sleep

EPIDEMIOLOGY

Incidence

- Increases with age: 1/3 of patients >60 years exhibit PLMs but not necessarily periodic limb movement disorder (PLMD).
- Predominant sex: male = female
- PLMs in 15% of insomnia patients

Prevalence

- PLMs in sleep: common and often of no clinical consequence
- PLMs constituting PLMD (causing sleep complaints and/or daytime consequences) much less common: <5% of adults (but underdiagnosed)

ETIOLOGY AND PATHOPHYSIOLOGY

- Unstudied
- Primary: probable CNS dopaminergic impairment
- Secondary:
  - Iron deficiency
  - Peripheral neuropathy
  - Arthritis
  - Renal failure
  - Synucleinopathies (multiple-system atrophy)
  - Spinal cord injury
  - Pregnancy
  - Medications:
    - Most antidepressants (not bupropion or desipramine)
    - Some antipsychotic and antidementia medications
    - Antiemetics (metoclopramide)
    - Antihistamines

Genetics

Unstudied, but see "Restless Legs Syndrome" (RLS)

RISK FACTORS

- Family history of RLS
- Iron deficiency and associated conditions (e.g., pregnancy, gastric surgery, renal disease)
- Attention-deficit hyperactivity disorder (ADHD)
- Aging
- Peripheral neuropathy
- Arthritis, orthopedic problems
- Chronic limb pain or discomfort

GENERAL PREVENTION

- Regular physical activity
- Adequate nightly sleep
- Avoid causes of secondary PLMD.
- Avoid causes of RLS.

COMMONLY ASSOCIATED CONDITIONS

- RLS
- Rapid eye movement (REM) sleep behavior disorder
- Narcolepsy
- Iron deficiency
- Renal failure
- Cardiovascular disease; stroke
- Gastric surgery
- Pregnancy
- Arthritis
- Synucleinopathies (multiple-system atrophy)
- Lumbar spine disease; spinal cord injury
- Peripheral neuropathy
- Insomnia, insufficient sleep
- ADHD
- Depression

Pediatric Considerations

- PLMD may precede overt RLS by years.
- Association with RLS is more common than in adults.
- Symptoms may be more consequential than in adults.
- Associated with ADHD

Pregnancy Considerations

- May be secondary to iron or folate deficiency
- Most severe in 3rd trimester
- Usually subsides after delivery

Geriatric Considerations

- May become a significant source of sleep disturbance
- May cause or exacerbate circadian disruption and "sundowning"
- Many medications given to the elderly cause or exacerbate PLMs, which can lead to PLMD or RLS.

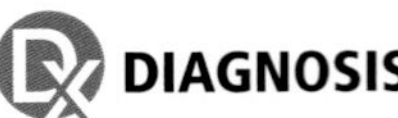

DIAGNOSIS

HISTORY

- Episodes of PLMs during sleep (often reported by bed partner) (1)[A]
- Insomnia: difficulty maintaining sleep
- Unrestorative sleep
- Daytime fatigue, tiredness, and/or somnolence
- Oppositional behaviors
- Memory impairment
- Depression
- ADHD, particularly in children

PHYSICAL EXAM

No specific findings

DIFFERENTIAL DIAGNOSIS

- When PLMs occur along with RLS, REM sleep behavior disorder, or narcolepsy, those disorders are diagnosed as "with PLMs," and PLMD is not diagnosed separately.
- Obstructive sleep apnea: Limb movements (LMs) occur during microarousals from apneas; treatment of sleep apnea eliminates these LMs.
- Sleep starts: nonperiodic, generalized, occur only at wake–sleep transition, <0.2 seconds duration
- Sleep-related leg cramps: isolated and painful
- Fragmentary myoclonus: 75–150 ms of EMG activity, minimal movement, no periodicity
- Nocturnal seizures: epileptiform EEG, motor pattern incongruent with PLMs
- Fasciculations, tremor: no sleep association
- Sleep-related rhythmic movement disorder: voluntary movement during wake–sleep transition; higher frequency than PLMs

DIAGNOSTIC TESTS & INTERPRETATION

- Polysomnography with finding of repetitive, stereotyped LMs (1)[A]:
  - Tibialis anterior electromyographic (EMG) activity lasting 0.5–10 seconds
  - EMG amplitude increases >8 μV from baseline.
  - Movements occur in a sequence of ≥4 at intervals of 5–90 seconds.
  - Children: ≥5 movements/hr; adults, 15
  - Movement may also involve arms.
  - Associated with heart rate variability from autonomic-level arousals
  - Most PLM episodes occur in the first hours of non-REM sleep.
  - Significant night-to-night PLM variability
- Serum ferritin to assess for iron deficiency

P

Diagnostic Procedures/Other
- Ankle actigraphy for in-home use
- EMG or nerve conduction studies for peripheral neuropathy/radiculopathy

Test Interpretation
Serum ferritin <75 ng/mL

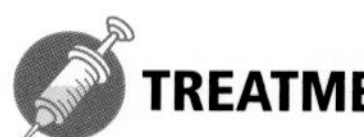

TREATMENT

- Daily exercise
- Adequate nightly sleep
- Treatment paradigm similar to that for RLS, except that all medications are off-label for PLMD

GENERAL MEASURES
- Daily exercise
- Adequate nightly sleep
- Warm the legs (long socks, leg warmers, electric blanket, etc.).
- Hot bath before bedtime
- Avoid nicotine and evening caffeine and alcohol.

MEDICATION
- Use minimum effective dose.
- Consider risks, side effects, and interactions individually (e.g., benzodiazepines in elderly).
- Daytime sleepiness is unusual with the doses and timing employed for PLMD

First Line
- Dopamine agonists: Take 1 hour before bed; titrate weekly to optimal dose (1–3)[B]:
  - Pramipexole (Mirapex): 0.125–0.5 mg; titrate by 0.125 mg
  - Ropinirole (Requip): 0.25–4 mg; titrate by 0.25 mg
  - Transdermal rotigotine (Neupro): 1–3 mg/24 hr patch; initiate with 1 mg/24 hr; titrate by 1 mg weekly to effectiveness.
- Avoid dopamine agonists in psychotic patients, especially if taking dopamine antagonists.

Second Line
- Anticonvulsants: useful for associated neuropathy (1,2)[B]:
  - Gabapentin enacarbil (Horizant): 600 mg/day
  - Pregabalin (Lyrica): 50–300 mg/day
- Opioids: low risk for tolerance with bedtime dose
  - Hydrocodone: 5–20 mg/day
  - Oxycodone: 2.5–20 mg/day
- Benzodiazepines and agonists (1–3)[B]:
  - Clonazepam (Klonopin): 0.5–3 mg/day
  - Zaleplon, zolpidem, temazepam, triazolam, alprazolam, diazepam

Pediatric Considerations
- First-line treatment is nonpharmacologic.
- Consider low-dose clonidine or clonazepam.

Pregnancy Considerations
- Initial approach: Fe supplementation, nonpharmacologic therapies
- Most medications are class C or D.
- In 3rd trimester, low-dose opioids may be considered.

Geriatric Considerations
In weak or frail patients, avoid medications that may cause dizziness or unsteadiness.

ADDITIONAL THERAPIES
- If iron-deficient, iron supplementation:
  - 325 mg ferrous sulfate with 200 mg vitamin C between meals TID
  - Repletion may require months.
  - Symptoms continue without other treatment.
- Vitamin/mineral supplements, including calcium, magnesium, B_{12}, folate
- Clonidine: 0.05–0.1 mg/day
- Relaxis leg vibration device

SURGERY/OTHER PROCEDURES
Correction of orthopedic, neuropathic, or peripheral vascular problems

INPATIENT CONSIDERATIONS
- Control during recovery from orthopedic procedures
- Addition or withdrawal of medications that affect PLMD
- Changes in medical status may require medication changes (e.g., Mirapex contraindicated in renal failure and Requip contraindicated in liver disease).

IV Fluids
- Consider iron infusion when oral supplementation is ineffective, not tolerated, or contraindicated.
- When NPO, consider IV opiates.

Nursing
- Evening walks, hot baths, leg warming
- Sleep interruption risks prolonged wakefulness.

ONGOING CARE

FOLLOW-UP RECOMMENDATIONS
Patient Monitoring
- At monthly intervals until stable
- Annual and PRN follow-up thereafter
- If Fe-deficient, remeasure ferritin to assess repletion.

DIET
Avoid caffeine and alcohol late in the day.

PATIENT EDUCATION
National Sleep Foundation: sleepfoundation.org

PROGNOSIS
- Primary PLMD: lifelong condition with no current cure
- Secondary PLMD: may subside with resolution of cause(s)
- Current therapies usually control symptoms.
- PLMD often precedes emergence of RLS.

COMPLICATIONS
- Tolerance to medications requiring increased dose or alternatives
- Augmentation (increased PLMs and sleep disturbance, emergence of RLS) from prolonged use of dopamine agonists:
  - Higher doses increase risk.
  - Fe deficiency increases risk.
  - Add alternative medication, then detitrate dopaminergic agent.
- Iatrogenic PLMD (from antidepressants, etc.)

REFERENCES

1. Garcia-Borreguero D, Stillman P, Benes H, et al. Algorithms for the diagnosis and treatment of restless legs syndrome in primary care. *BMC Neurol*. 2011;11:28.
2. Aurora RN, Kristo DA, Bista SR, et al. The treatment of restless legs syndrome and periodic limb movement disorder in adults—an update for 2012: practice parameters with an evidence-based systematic review and meta-analyses: an American Academy of Sleep Medicine Clinical Practice Guideline. *Sleep*. 2012;35(8):1039–1062.

ADDITIONAL READING

Picchietti DL, Rajendran RR, Wilson MP, et al. Pediatric restless legs syndrome and periodic limb movement disorder: parent-child pairs. *Sleep Med*. 2009;10(8):925–931.

SEE ALSO

Restless Legs Syndrome

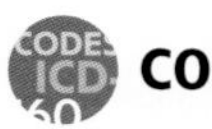

CODES

ICD10
G47.61 Periodic limb movement disorder

CLINICAL PEARLS

- Many patients with PLMs may not require treatment; however, when sleep disturbance from PLMs causes insomnia and/or daytime consequences, PLMD exists and should be treated.
- Many antidepressants and some antihistamines cause or exacerbate PLMs.
- Accumulating data indicate that sleep disturbance, including that from PLMs, may cause or exacerbate ADHD.

PERIORAL DERMATITIS

Heather Summe, MD • Nikki A. Levin, MD, PhD

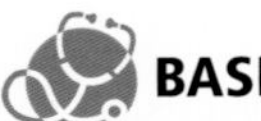

BASICS

DESCRIPTION

- A common facial eruption of women and children
- Presents as tiny, flesh-colored, or erythematous monomorphic papules or pustules around the mouth with characteristic sparing of the area immediately adjacent to the vermilion border
- May also involve the periocular, perinasal, and glabellar regions of the face
- Etiology is unknown, but a relation to topical steroid use has been suggested.
- Without treatment, the course is usually fluctuating and chronic.
- Variants in children include granulomatous periorificial dermatitis (GPD) and facial Afro-Caribbean childhood eruption.
- Synonym(s): periorificial dermatitis (POD); chronic papulopustular facial dermatitis; granulomatous perioral dermatitis; light-sensitive seborrhea; lupus-like perioral dermatitis; papulopustular facial dermatitis; rosacea-like dermatitis; stewardess disease

EPIDEMIOLOGY

- Occurs worldwide, especially in fair-skinned populations
- Predominantly affects children between 6 months and 16 years and women aged 17–45 years
- ~90% of adult cases are in women (1).
- Childhood cases may be more common in boys.
- All races are affected, but the granulomatous form is more common in African American and dark-skinned children.
- Some believe the number of cases peaked in the 1960s–1970s and decreased in the 1980s–1990s when the side effects of topical steroids were recognized. Others believe that cases are still increasing.

Incidence

- Peak incidence is in the 2nd and 3rd decades of life.
- In children, peak incidence is in the prepubertal period.

Prevalence

- Represents ~2% of patients presenting to dermatology clinics (2)
- ~3% of children using inhalational steroids develop some form of POD (3).

ETIOLOGY AND PATHOPHYSIOLOGY

- Exposure to an irritant results in breakdown of the epidermal barrier and subsequent water loss and sensation of dryness; this encourages use of facial products and corticosteroids, which may worsen the condition.
- This inflammatory cycle eventually leads to clinical features of the disease.
- The exact cause is unknown, and there may be more than 1 contributing factor.
- The most widely cited factor implicated in POD is use of potent topical corticosteroids on the face.
- Inhaled corticosteroids, especially when used with a spacer and nebulizer or mask, have also been reported to cause POD.
- Intranasal steroids have been associated with POD beginning in the nasolabial folds.
- Two cases associated with systemic steroid use have been reported in children (4).
- Use of foundation, moisturizer, and night cream was associated with a 13-fold increased risk of POD in 1 study (5).
- Other factors implicated but not proven:
  - Drugs: oral contraceptives
  - Toothpastes: fluoridated, tartar control, whitening
  - Physical factors: UV light, heat, wind, salivary leakage
  - Infectious factors: fusiform bacteria, *Candida* species, *Demodex folliculorum*
  - Miscellaneous factors: atopy, GI disturbances, stress, contact allergy, lip-licking, immunosuppression, bubble gum, formaldehyde, varicella vaccination

Genetics

55% of pediatric patients with POD have a family history of atopy (5).

RISK FACTORS

See "Etiology and Pathophysiology."

GENERAL PREVENTION

- Avoid using potent topical corticosteroids on the face.
- Avoid using excessive foundation, moisturizer, and night cream.
- Avoidance of tartar-control and whitening toothpastes may also be helpful.

COMMONLY ASSOCIATED CONDITIONS

Atopic dermatitis

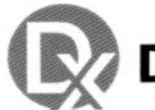

DIAGNOSIS

HISTORY

- Patient reports a history of facial rash, which may improve with use of topical corticosteroids and flare with discontinuation.
- Affected skin may be pruritic or have a burning sensation.
- Course may be chronic and fluctuating.
- Recent topical, inhaled, or systemic steroid use in 72% of patients (6)
- May worsen with sun exposure

PHYSICAL EXAM

- Monomorphic, minute, flesh-colored to erythematous papules or pustules, sometimes surmounted with scale, in a perioral distribution, often asymmetrical, with sparing of the vermilion border 3–5 mm around the lips
- Granulomatous form can usually be distinguished clinically by the absence of pustules and the presence of yellow-brown papules.
- Common locations are alar creases, nasolabial folds, chin, periocular skin, eyelids, and glabella.
- Diameter of lesions is usually 1–2 mm.
- Distribution (2)
  - Perioral area (39%)
  - Perinasal (13%)
  - Periocular (1%)
  - Perioral and perinasal (14%)
  - Perioral and periocular (6%)
  - Perinasal and periocular (6%)
  - Perioral, perinasal, and periocular (10%)
- Lupus-like variant diagnosed by yellowish discoloration of lesions on diascopy

DIFFERENTIAL DIAGNOSIS

- Acne vulgaris
- Contact dermatitis
- Rosacea
- Seborrheic dermatitis
- Lip-licker's dermatitis
- Papular sarcoidosis
- *Demodex* infestation
- Acrodermatitis enteropathica
- Biotin deficiency
- Glucagonoma syndrome
- Xanthomas
- Eruptive syringomas
- Polymorphous light eruption
- Acne agminata
- Lupus miliaris disseminatus faciei
- Haber syndrome (familial rosacea-like dermatosis)

DIAGNOSTIC TESTS & INTERPRETATION

Diagnosis is usually clinical.

- No laboratory abnormalities expected.
- Prick tests and IgE testing may show evidence of atopy but are not routinely done.
- Patch testing may be used to rule out contact dermatitis.
- Scrapings for *Demodex* mites

Diagnostic Procedures/Other

Skin biopsy is not routinely performed but can be helpful in atypical cases.

Test Interpretation

Histopathology of skin biopsy

- Mild, nonspecific inflammation with variable perifollicular or perivascular lymphohistiocytic infiltrate
- Eczematous changes, acanthosis, parakeratosis, and spongiosis
- Occasionally, follicular abscesses are seen.
- Older lesions may contain diffuse hypertrophy of connective tissue and hyperplasia of sebaceous follicles with occasional noncaseating granulomas in the dermis (1).
- Caseating granulomas are seen with granulomatous variant.

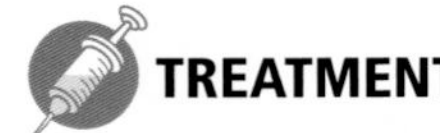

TREATMENT

GENERAL MEASURES

"Zero therapy" can be an effective treatment in adherent patients (2)[B]:

- Reduce use of facial soaps, makeup, and moisturizers, and wash with only water.
- Discontinue use of potent topical corticosteroids on the face.
  - This may result in a flare.
  - Flares may be decreased with use of less-potent topical steroids, calcineurin inhibitors, or IM steroid injection.
- Discontinue use of fluoridated, whitening, and tartar-control toothpaste.

MEDICATION

Based on disease severity and patient's tolerance for adverse effects

First Line

- Severe disease
  - Oral antibiotics
    - Tetracycline has been proven as an effective treatment (2)[A].
    - 250–500 mg BID for 8–10 weeks
    - Dose may be halved after 3–4 weeks if improvement noted.
    - Contraindicated in children <8 years of age and pregnant women.
    - Common side effects: photosensitivity, GI upset, rash, candidiasis, headache, dizziness, and tinnitus
  - Doxycycline or minocycline (5)[C]
    - 50–100 mg BID for 6–8 weeks
    - Dose may be halved after 3–4 weeks if improvement noted.
    - Contraindicated in children <8 years of age and pregnant women.
    - Common side effects of doxycycline: GI upset, esophagitis, joint pain, upper respiratory infection (URI) symptoms, rash, dysmenorrhea, candidiasis, headache, dizziness, photosensitivity, and elevated BUN
    - Common side effects of minocycline: GI upset, lightheadedness, vertigo, ataxia, headache, fatigue, tinnitus, rash, urticaria, candidiasis, and hyperpigmentation
- Alternatively, doxycycline 40 mg/day modified-release capsule may achieve the anti-inflammatory effect without the microbial activity that promotes emergence of resistant bacterial strains (7)[C].
- Erythromycin (5)[C] may be used when tetracycline are contraindicated or not tolerated.
  - 250 mg BID–TID for 6–8 weeks
  - Dose may be halved after 3–4 weeks if improvement noted.
  - May be used in children or pregnant women
  - Common side effects: GI upset, diarrhea, rash, and urticaria
  - Rarer serious side effects: erythema multiforme, pancreatitis, convulsions, QT prolongation, and ventricular arrhythmias
- Moderate disease
  - Topical antibiotics
    - May be slower than systemic antibiotics in clearing lesions
    - Metronidazole cream 0.75% BID (2)[B]
    - Erythromycin 2% gel, solution, or ointment BID (2)[B]
    - Clindamycin 1% gel, lotion, or cream BID
- Mild disease
  - Zero therapy (see "General Measures") (2)[B]

Second Line

- Severe disease
  - Clarithromycin (250 mg/day) may be used when tetracycline and erythromycin are contraindicated or not tolerated (2)[C].
    - Common side effects: GI upset, headache, rash, abnormal taste sensation, and urticaria
  - Oral isotretinoin may be useful in granulomatous cases that are not responsive to a full dose of tetracycline (1)[C].
    - 0.2 mg/kg initially, followed by 0.1 mg/kg after notable improvement
    - Isotretinoin is a pregnancy Category X drug and may cause severe birth defects. Use with caution with in women of reproductive age. Physician and patient must register with iPLEDGE program.
    - Common side effects: dry skin, cheilitis, arthralgias/myalgias, hypertriglyceridemia, elevated liver function tests (LFTs), hair loss, visual disturbances, depression, and tinnitus
  - Pimecrolimus 1% cream may accelerate healing (2)[A], and tacrolimus 0.1% ointment use has been reported with success (2).
    - Rare cases of lymphoma and skin malignancies have been reported. Avoid long-term use.
- Moderate disease
  - Topical therapies
    - Antiacne drugs, such as azelaic acid and adapalene, may be helpful (2).
    - Ichthyol (ammonium bituminosulfonate) (2)

ADDITIONAL THERAPIES

A number of other therapies have been reported in the literature, including photodynamic therapy with 5-aminolevulinic acid (2), radiotherapy, and liquid nitrogen. There has also been a case reported of oral metronidazole (250 mg BID) resulting in complete clearance of GPD without scarring after 1 month of use (8). Most recently, a randomized controlled trial showed significant improvement after 4 weeks of treatment with praziquantel 3% ointment BID (9).

COMPLEMENTARY & ALTERNATIVE MEDICINE

Compress with chamomile tea or physiologic solution may be used if the patient struggles with zero therapy (1).

ONGOING CARE

DIET

No restrictions

PATIENT EDUCATION

- Lesions may take many weeks to resolve.
- Symptoms may temporarily worsen, especially with discontinuance of steroids.
- Recurrence is rare.
- Topical corticosteroid use on the face should be avoided in the future.

PROGNOSIS

- Most cases resolve without recurrence.
- Oral or topical antibiotics usually lead to remission within 6–10 weeks.
- Untreated disease may persist for months to years and be characterized by unpredictable flares.
- Disease is not associated with significant morbidity.

COMPLICATIONS

- Most cases resolve without complications.
- Emotional stress can result from bothersome appearance of lesions and chronic course of disease.
- Scarring may be problematic with lupus-like variant.

REFERENCES

1. Lipozencic J, Ljubojevic S. Perioral dermatitis. *Clin Dermatol*. 2011;29(2):157–161.
2. Wollenberg A, Bieber T, Dirschka T, et al. Perioral dermatitis. *J Dtsch Dermatol Ges*. 2011;9(5):422–427.
3. Henningsen E, Bygum A. Budesonide-induced periorificial dermatitis presenting as chalazion and blepharitis. *Pediatr Dermatol*. 2011;28(5):596–597.
4. Clementson B, Smidt AC. Periorificial dermatitis due to systemic corticosteroids in children: report of two cases. *Pediatr Dermatol*. 2012:29(3):331–332.
5. Vanderweil SG, Levin NA. Perioral dermatitis: it's not every rash that occurs around the mouth. *Dermatol Nurs*. 2009;21(6):317–320, 353; quiz 321.
6. Nguyen V, Eichenfield LF. Periorificial dermatitis in children and adolescents. *J Am Acad Dermatol*. 2006;55(5):781–785.
7. Rosso JQ. Management of papulopustular rosacea and perioral dermatitis with emphasis on Iatrogenic causation or exacerbation of inflammatory facial dermatoses: use of doxycycline-modified release 40 mg capsule once daily in combination with properly selected skin care as an effective therapeutic approach. *J Clin Aesthet Dermatol*. 2011;4(8):20–30.
8. Rodriguez-Caruncho C, Bielsa I, Fernandez-Figueras MT, et al. Childhood granulomatous periorificial dermatitis with a good response to oral metronidazole. *Pediatr Dermatol*. 2013;30(5):e98–e99.
9. Bribeche MR, Fedotov VP, Jillella A, et al. Topical praziquantel as a new treatment for perioral dermatitis: results of a randomized vehicle-controlled pilot study. *Clin Exp Dermatol*. 2014;39(4): 448–453.

ADDITIONAL READING

- Hafeez ZH. Perioral dermatitis: an update. *Int J Dermatol*. 2003;42(7):514–517.
- Kim YJ, Shin JW, Lee JS, et al. Childhood granulomatous periorificial dermatitis. *Ann Dermatol*. 2011;23(3):386–388.
- Peralta L, Morais P. Perioral dermatitis—the role of nasal steroids. *Cutan Ocul Toxicol*. 2012;31(2): 160–163.
- Weber K, Thurmayr R. Critical appraisal of reports on the treatment of perioral dermatitis. *Dermatology (Basel)*. 2005;210(4):300–307.

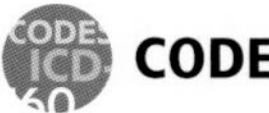

CODES

ICD10

L71.0 Perioral dermatitis

CLINICAL PEARLS

- Suspect POD when an acneiform eruption involves the perioral, perinasal, or periocular areas with characteristic sparing of the skin immediately adjacent to the vermilion border.
- Ask patients about a history of recent corticosteroid use, facial product use, and use of fluoridated, whitening, or tartar-control toothpastes.
- Substitution of low-potency steroids may allow patients to discontinue higher potency steroids while avoiding a rebound flare.

PERIPHERAL ARTERIAL DISEASE

Zhen Lu, MD

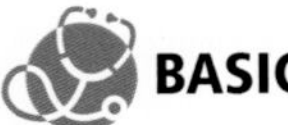

BASICS

DESCRIPTION

Peripheral arterial disease (PAD) is a manifestation of systemic atherosclerosis in which there is partial or total blockage in the arteries, exclusive of the coronary and cerebral vessels. Objectively, PAD is defined as a resting ankle-brachial index (ABI) of <0.90.

EPIDEMIOLOGY

- Predominant age: >40 years
- Predominant sex: male > female (2:1), based on the Framingham study
- Patients with symptomatic PAD have a 5-year mortality rate of 30%.
- Highly prevalent syndrome that affects 8–12 million individuals in the United States

Incidence

Incidence overall: 1–2.7/1,000/year

Prevalence

- U.S. prevalence: 2.7–4.1%
- Age-adjusted prevalence of PAD is close to 12%.
- Up to 29% among patients in primary care practices

ETIOLOGY AND PATHOPHYSIOLOGY

- In patients with PAD, arterial stenoses cause inadequate blood flow in distal limbs, which fails to meet the metabolic demand during exertion:
  - The degree of ischemia is proportional to the size and proximity of the occlusion to the end organ.
  - Acidic products of anaerobic metabolism build up within the muscle and result in claudication clinically.
  - Arterial occlusion also causes significantly diminished distal pressure in patients with PAD due to atherosclerotic lesions.
- Most common cause of arterial stenoses is atherosclerosis.

Genetics

Current NIH-funded research focuses on single-nucleotide polymorphisms in candidate genes that are regulated in the vasculature in an attempt to explore genetic factors responsible for PAD.

RISK FACTORS

- Age >40 years
- Cigarette smoking
- Diabetes mellitus
- Obesity
- Hypertension
- Hyperlipidemia
- Hyperhomocysteinemia

GENERAL PREVENTION

Control risk factors.

COMMONLY ASSOCIATED CONDITIONS

- See "Risk Factors."
- Associated with other common complications of atherosclerosis, including myocardial infarction (MI), transient ischemic attack, stroke, and limb amputation
- Occurs in ~40% of patients with cardiovascular disease

DIAGNOSIS

HISTORY

- Intermittent claudication, with symptoms typically resolving within 2–5 minutes of rest (although it is regarded as the classic symptom for PAD, intermittent claudication is present in only 10% of patients with PAD)
- Rest leg pain (especially in a supine position)
- Skin ulceration (in advanced PAD)
- Gangrene (in advanced PAD)
- Impotence

PHYSICAL EXAM

- Skin pallor when leg is elevated above the level of the heart (in mild PAD)
- Dependent rubor
- Dry and scaly skin
- Poor nail growth
- Hair loss
- Reduced/absent extremity pulses (in advanced PAD)

DIFFERENTIAL DIAGNOSIS

- Arterial embolism
- Deep venous thrombosis
- Thromboangiitis obliterans (Buerger disease)
- Osteoarthritis
- Restless legs syndrome
- Peripheral neuropathy
- Spinal stenoses (pseudoclaudication)
- Intervertebral disc prolapse

DIAGNOSTIC TESTS & INTERPRETATION

Serum glucose is recommended screening for diabetes mellitus in suspected or confirmed PAD.

Initial Tests (lab, imaging)

- Fasting lipid profile is indicated for risk assessment of hyperlipidemia.
- Duplex ultrasonography and Doppler color-flow imaging, which are useful in detecting stenosed segments and assessing lesion severity, are initial imaging tests of choice.
- Magnetic resonance angiography, coupled with 3D reconstruction, is highly sensitive and specific for the localization of occluded lesions.
- CT scanning has a limited role in the evaluation of PAD.
- Angiography remains the gold standard in the diagnosis of PAD.

Diagnostic Procedures/Other

- Doppler ABI measures the ratio of the higher systolic BPs between the dorsalis pedis and the posterior tibial artery versus the higher of the systolic BPs in the 2 brachial arteries: Values for the ABI should be reported as "incompressible" if >1.40, "normal" if 1.00–1.40, "borderline" if 0.91–0.99, and "abnormal" if ≤0.90. ABI <0.4: severe ischemia
- Segmental limb pressures: usually obtained if abnormal ABI measurement is identified; a ≤20-mm Hg reduction in pressure is considered significant for PAD.
- Treadmill exercise test assesses the severity of claudication and the response to treatment.
- Segmental volume plethysmography: often used in conjunction with segmental limb pressures to measure the volume changes in an organ or limb; the study is indicated for calcified vessel when the ABI cannot be applied diagnostically.

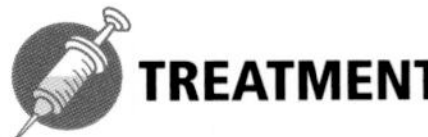

TREATMENT

GENERAL MEASURES

- Claudication exercise rehabilitation program: patient to walk until symptoms develop, then rest and start again, for a total of 30 minutes initially; walking then is increased by 5 minutes until 50 minutes of intermittent walking is achieved.
- Modification of risk factors, including smoking cessation, diabetes mellitus, hypertension, and hyperlipidemia:
  - Weight loss is associated with a decrease in the risk of cardiovascular disease but has not been shown to improve PAD.
  - Antiplatelet therapy (aspirin) is recommended for patients with PAD when there is no other contraindication; however, neither the addition of an anticoagulant nor anticoagulant therapy alone has demonstrated superior outcome in PAD patients.
  - Lipid-lowering therapy with moderate-intensity statin; simvastatin (20–40 mg/day) has been shown to reduce the incidence of new intermittent claudication from 3.6% to 2.3% in patients with coronary artery disease (CAD).
  - No statistical significance for overall improvement of exercise performance or reduction in claudication symptoms for patients on niacin ER–lovastatin combined therapy.
  - β-Adrenergic antagonists should be used with caution in individuals with severe PAD.
  - Smoking cessation is likely to reduce the severity of claudication.

MEDICATION

First Line

Antiplatelet therapy has been the mainstay treatment to prevent ischemic events in patients with PAD. However:

- The effect of aspirin on the risk reduction of overall ischemic events is inconclusive. Some suggest that aspirin delays disease progression and reduces the need for surgical intervention. AHA/ACCF guidelines (1)[A] note that the use of antiplatelet therapy to reduce cardiovascular risks in asymptomatic patients with borderline ABIs is characterized as "not well-established." Aspirin is recommended to reduce the risk of MI, stroke, and vascular death in symptomatic patients with PAD.
- Low-dose aspirin (75–150 mg/day) is as effective as higher doses of aspirin.

Second Line

- Clopidogrel (75 mg/day) is approved by the FDA for the secondary prevention of thrombotic events in patients with symptomatic lower extremity PAD and is recommended as an alternative to aspirin.

- Vorapaxar (Zontivity) 2.08 mg PO daily is a platelet aggregation inhibitor different in mechanism from existing antiplatelet drugs (TRAP inhibitor). It is contraindicated if history of CVA, TIA, or intracranial hemorrhage; concern for bleeding risk; and is expensive
- Other medications that may improve symptoms of claudication include pentoxifylline (1.2 g/day), cilostazol (100 mg BID), and naftidrofuryl (600 mg/day).
- Neither vasodilators nor anticoagulant therapy (e.g., heparin, low-molecular-weight heparin, or oral anticoagulant) has shown any clinically proven efficacy for the treatment of claudication and may be harmful.
- Cilostazol (100 mg BID) improves walking distance in people with intermittent claudication secondary to PAD. There is currently insufficient data on whether taking cilostazol results in a reduction of all-cause mortality and cardiovascular events or an improvement in quality of life (2)[A].
- Other medications that may reduce claudication include pentoxifylline (1.2 g/day), naftidrofuryl (600 mg/day), and prostaglandins (120 μg/day). Ticlopidine (250 mg BID) reduces the risk of MI, stroke, and death in patients with PAD, but it has a complication of thrombocytopenia in 2–3% of patients.

ADDITIONAL THERAPIES

- Weight reduction, smoking cessation, and BP control are essential in treating claudication.
- Exercise programs are of significant benefit compared with placebo or usual care in improving walking time and distance in people with leg pain from intermittent claudication who were considered to be fit for exercise intervention (3)[A]. A walking program should include walking at least 3× per week for 30–60 minutes each time and has been shown to improve quality of life as much as or more so than medication.
- A healthy diet high in complex carbohydrates (e.g., whole grains and pastas), fruits and vegetables, and low in salt and animal fats

SURGERY/OTHER PROCEDURES

Surgical interventions, such as revascularization, are warranted for individuals who have debilitating intermittent claudication, ischemic rest pain, or tissue loss:

- Transluminal balloon angioplasty is a percutaneous method of dilating arterial stenoses or recanalizing occluded vessels with or without stents (reserved for short, isolated, and hemodynamically significant lesions of the iliac or proximal superficial femoral artery).
- Bypass surgery is the standard operative treatment for lower extremity peripheral occlusive disease.

COMPLEMENTARY & ALTERNATIVE MEDICINE

- Acupuncture, biofeedback, chelation therapy, and supplements such as Ginkgo biloba, omega-3 fatty acids, and vitamin E have been studied.
- Ginkgo biloba modestly reduces the symptoms of intermittent claudication (120 mg/day for up to 6 months) and can be considered as an adjunct to exercise therapy. Inconclusive evidence exists for the use of vitamin E.

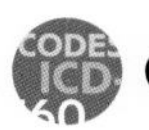

ONGOING CARE

FOLLOW-UP RECOMMENDATIONS

- An exercise training program composed of walking/bicycle riding improves maximal treadmill walking distance and, therefore, enhances functional capacity.
- However, little added benefit exists from Ginkgo biloba treatment when added to supervised exercise training in patients with PAD as compared with patients in exercise training program alone.

DIET

A low-fat cardiac diet is recommended.

PROGNOSIS

- Among patients with intermittent claudication, 15–20% will experience worsening claudication; 5–10% will undergo lower extremity bypass surgery; and 2–5% will need primary amputation (rates for smokers and diabetics are much higher).
- 30,000–50,000 people in the United States undergo amputations annually because of PAD.

REFERENCES

1. Rooke TW, Hirsch AT, Misra S, et al. 2011 ACCF/AHA focused update of the guideline for the management of patients with peripheral artery disease (updating the 2005 guideline): a report of the American College of Cardiology Foundation/American Heart Association Task Force on Practical Guidelines. *J Am Coll Cardiol*. 2011;58(19):2020–2045.
2. Bedenis R, Stewart M, Cleanthis M, et al. Cilostazol for intermittent claudication. *Cochrane Database Syst Rev*. 2014;10:CD003748.
3. Lane R, Ellis B, Watson L, et al. Exercise for intermittent claudication. *Cochrane Database Syst Rev*. 2014;7:CD000990.

ADDITIONAL READING

- Duprez DA. Pharmacological interventions for peripheral artery disease. *Expert Opin Pharmacother*. 2007;8(10):1465–1477.
- Gey DC, Lesho EP, Manngold J. Management of peripheral arterial disease. *Am Fam Physician*. 2004;69(3):525–532.
- Hankey GJ, Norman PE, Eikelboom JW. Medical treatment of peripheral arterial disease. *JAMA*. 2006;295(5):547–553.
- Hiatt WR, Hirsch AT, Creager MA, et al. Effect of niacin ER/lovastatin on claudication symptoms in patients with peripheral artery disease. *Vasc Med*. 2010;15(3):171–179.
- Wang J, Zhou S, Bronks R, et al. Supervised exercise training combined with ginkgo biloba treatment for patients with peripheral arterial disease. *Clin Rehabil*. 2007;21(7):579–586.

CODES

ICD10

- I73.9 Peripheral vascular disease, unspecified
- I70.209 Unsp athscl native arteries of extremities, unsp extremity
- I70.219 Athscl native arteries of extrm w intrmt claud, unsp extrm

CLINICAL PEARLS

- Screening of a general medical population for PAD is not recommended. Studies have indicated that screening for PAD among asymptomatic adults in the general population could lead to false-positive results and unnecessary workups. The prevalence among the general public who are asymptomatic is low.
- A patient already receiving medical treatment should be referred for further surgical evaluation for any of the following scenarios:
  - Unsatisfactory results despite medical therapy
  - No definitive diagnosis can be made.
  - Critical limb ischemia is present, such as rest pain, gangrene, or ulceration.
- The clopidogrel (75 mg/day) versus aspirin (325 mg/day) study in the patients at risk of ischemic events (CAPRIE) trial found a 23.8% relative risk ratio for MI, stroke, or cardiovascular death in PAD patients treated with clopidogrel compared with aspirin but no statistically significant difference in overall mortality reduction. Clopidogrel is much more expensive than aspirin.

PERITONITIS, ACUTE

Jessica Davis, MD • Justin Thomas Ertle, BS, MD • Marie L. Borum, MD, EdD, MPH

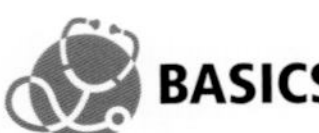

BASICS

DESCRIPTION

- Definition: inflammation of the peritoneum
- Classification
  - Aseptic: due to chemical irritation or systemic inflammation of peritoneum
  - Bacterial: due to infection of peritoneal fluid
- Bacterial peritonitis types
  - Primary/spontaneous bacterial peritonitis (SBP): infection of ascitic fluid without known source; typically monomicrobial
  - Secondary bacterial peritonitis: infection of peritoneal fluid from a detectable intra-abdominal source (i.e., perforation); typically polymicrobial
  - Tertiary bacterial peritonitis: persistent infection despite adequate therapy

EPIDEMIOLOGY

Incidence

- In patients with ascites, the incidence of SBP in a 1-year period is 10–25% (1).
- Secondary bacterial peritonitis: correlates with incidence of the underlying pathology (e.g., colitis, appendicitis, diverticulitis, PUD)
- 57% of patients with secondary bacterial peritonitis progressed to tertiary peritonitis (2).

Prevalence

- SBP: In asymptomatic patients with cirrhosis and ascites, the prevalence is <3.5% in outpatients and 8–36% the nosocomial setting (3).
- In patients with cirrhosis and ascites, 5% of peritonitis is secondary rather than SBP (4).

ETIOLOGY AND PATHOPHYSIOLOGY

- Mechanism
  - SBP
    - Primary mechanism is bacterial translocation via lymphatic spread through mesenteric lymph nodes into ascitic fluid.
    - Cirrhotic patients have multiple secondary mechanisms.
      - Small intestinal bacterial overgrowth (SIBO) and increased intestinal mucosal permeability to bacteria both increase bacterial translocation.
      - Decreased cellular and humoral immunity increases susceptibility to bacterial translocation.
  - Secondary bacterial peritonitis
    - Spillage/translocation of bacteria from inflamed or perforated intraperitoneal organs or introduction of bacteria through instrumentation—e.g., peritoneal dialysis, intraperitoneal chemotherapy
  - Tertiary bacterial peritonitis
    - Occurs in secondary peritonitis with inadequacy of source control or altered host immunity
- Microbiology
  - SBP
    - *Escherichia coli* (46%), *Streptococcus* spp. (30%), Klebsiella (9%), *and Staphylococcus* (6%). Increasing rate of gram-positive and resistant organisms (e.g., extended-spectrum β-lactamase-producing [ESBL] *E. coli*, MRSA, *Enterococcus*) in the nosocomial setting
  - Secondary bacterial peritonitis
    - *E. coli, Klebsiella, Proteus, Streptococcus, Enterococcus, Bacteroides, Clostridium*

RISK FACTORS

- SBP: advanced cirrhosis with ascites, bacterascites, malnutrition, upper GI bleed, PPI usage, prior SBP
  - Acid suppression with PPIs been shown to promote SIBO increasing SBP (3); hospitalized cirrhotics receiving PPIs are 3 times as likely to get SBP.
  - 70% of cases of SBP are seen in patients with Child-Pugh class C cirrhosis (1).
- Secondary bacterial peritonitis: factors associated with perforation or fluid translocation, for example, peritoneal dialysis, *Helicobacter pylori* and NSAIDs causing ulcers, vascular disease causing bowel ischemia, EOH abuse causing pancreatitis

GENERAL PREVENTION

SBP prophylaxis

- Prior SBP: prophylactic norfloxacin or TMP/SMX PO daily (5)[A]
- Cirrhosis and GI bleed: 7-day course of ceftriaxone 2 g IV daily or norfloxacin 400 mg BID, IV while bleeding, PO as tolerated (5)[A]
- Cirrhotic ascites with low ascitic fluid protein (<1.5 g/dL) and either renal impairment (creatinine ≥ 1.2, BUN ≥ 25 or serum Na ≤ 130) or liver failure (Child score ≥ 9, bilirubin ≥ 3): prophylactic norfloxacin PO daily (3,5)[A]

DIAGNOSIS

HISTORY

- SBP: history of cirrhosis or ascites. fever, mental status changes, abdominal pain, chills, nausea/vomiting, GI bleed
- Secondary bacterial peritonitis: history of perforation, abscess or peritoneal dialysis, acute abdominal pain, nausea, vomiting, anorexia, fever, mental status changes
- Tertiary: persistent signs and symptoms despite initial treatment, or history of recurrent peritonitis

ALERT

30% of patients are asymptomatic (1)[C].

Geriatric Considerations

Signs and symptoms are frequently absent, particularly in pediatric and elderly patients (1)[B].

PHYSICAL EXAM

- Tachycardia, fever, tachypnea, altered mental status
- Abdominal distention, ascites, abdominal wall guarding and rigidity, rebound tenderness, hypoactive/absent bowel sounds

DIFFERENTIAL DIAGNOSIS

- Liver disease: acute hepatitis, decompensated cirrhosis
- Luminal disease: abscess formation, ileus, volvulus, intussusception, mesenteric adenitis, pancreatitis, cholecystitis, malignancy, peritoneal carcinomatosis
- Extraluminal disease: ruptured ectopic pregnancy, tubo-ovarian abscess, PID, severe UTI, and/or pyelonephritis
- Systemic disease: tuberculosis, pneumonia, MI, porphyria, SLE

DIAGNOSTIC TESTS & INTERPRETATION

Initial Tests

ALERT

Early diagnosis is essential to reducing mortality. Paracentesis should be performed in any patient with new ascites, including suspected SBP (5)[B].

- Immediate evaluation
  - Perform paracentesis, blood, and urine cultures before administration of antibiotics (5,1)[B].
  - Ascitic fluid studies should minimally include culture (use aerobic and anaerobic blood culture bottles), Gram stain, cell count with differential, and albumin (1)[B]; if assessing for secondary peritonitis, also include LDH, total protein, and glucose.
- Lab interpretation

ALERT

Ascitic fluid culture is negative in up to 50% of patients with SBP (1)[A].

- SBP: bacterascites and ascitic fluid PMN >250 cells/mm^3
- Culture-negative neutrocytic ascites: negative ascites culture, ascitic fluid PMN >250 cells/mm^3
- Nonneutrocytic bacterascites: positive ascites culture, ascitic fluid PMN <250 cells/mm^3
- Secondary peritonitis: PMN >250 cells/mm^3 on ascitic fluid analysis, with any of the following criteria:
  - Polymicrobial culture or 2 of the following: ascitic fluid total protein >1 g/dL, glucose <50 mg/dL, or LDH >225 mU/mL. Sensitivity for perforation 96%, sensitivity for nonperforation secondary peritonitis 50% (5)[B]
  - Secondary peritonitis with perforation is likely with alkaline phosphatase >240 U/l or CEA >5 ng/ml, sensitivity 92% (5)[B]
- Imaging

ALERT

Criteria or clinical suspicion for secondary peritonitis necessitates emergent CT scan. CT diagnostic for secondary peritonitis in 85% (5)[B]

- Ultrasound or CT scan with enteral and IV contrast shows intra-abdominal mass, ascites, abscess, or extravasation of contrast in secondary peritonitis.
- Abdominal or chest x-ray may show free air in peritoneal cavity, large/small bowel dilatation, intestinal wall edema in secondary peritonitis.

Follow-Up Tests & Special Considerations

- If asymptomatic bacterascites, recent antibiotic exposure, nosocomial atypical organism, or no clinical improvement, repeat paracentesis in 48 hours to resolution, defined as decrease in PMNs of 25% or negative cultures (1)[C]
- In hemorrhagic ascites, PMN count can be corrected by subtracting 1 PMN per 250 RBCs (3)[A]
- Leukocyte esterase reagent strips (LERS) are not yet recommended for diagnosis of peritonitis, as ascites-calibrated strips are not yet confirmed in large trials (3)[C].
- Bacterial DNA, procalcitonin, lactoferrin, CRP are not yet recommended diagnostics tests in peritonitis (3)[C].

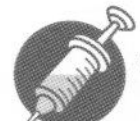

TREATMENT

GENERAL MEASURES

- For SBP, control the effects of cirrhosis/ascites with salt restriction, spironolactone +/− furosemide, albumin infusion after large volume paracentesis, and/or lactulose for encephalopathy (5)[A].
- β-Blockers may reduce long-term risk of SBP (5)[B].
- Limit use of PPIs to data proven indications (5)[B].
- Avoid nephrotoxic medications (e.g. NSAIDs) or other renal insults (5)[C].

MEDICATION

- SBP empiric 1st-line treatment
  - Community-acquired SBP without recent β-lactam antibiotic use: third-generation cephalosporins, preferably, cefotaxime, 2 g IV q8h × 5 days (5)[A]
  - SBP in absence of previous quinolone use/prophylaxis, vomiting, shock, hepatic encephalopathy, or serum creatinine >3 mg/dL: Ofloxacin 400 mg PO can be substituted for cefotaxime (5)[B].
  - Nosocomial SBP or recent β-lactam antibiotic empiric therapy based on local susceptibility of patients with cirrhosis for resistant bacteria (e.g., ESBL enterobacteriaceae, MRSA) (6)[B]
  - Symptomatic bacterascites with PMN count <250 cells/mm^3: cefotaxime 2 g IV q8h while awaiting sensitivities (5)[B]
  - SBP with renal or hepatic impairment (serum creatinine >1 mg/dL, BUN >30 mg/dL or total bilirubin >4 mg/dL): Add albumin 1.5 g/kg within 6 hours and 1 g/kg on day 3 (5)[B].
  - 2nd-line antibiotic regimens include fluoroquinolones (levofloxacin), piperacillin/tazobactam, or vancomycin (5)[C].
- Secondary bacterial peritonitis
  - Empiric broad-spectrum antibiotic coverage for polymicrobial infection
  - In peritoneal dialysis associated infection, intraperitoneal route superior to IV (6)[A].
- Tertiary bacterial peritonitis
  - If no unrepaired perforations or leaks, conservative medical management. This includes antibiotics and early enteral nutrition to prevent atrophy and maintain immunocompetence (2)[B].
  - In recurrent or persistent peritoneal dialysis–associated infection, remove PD catheter (6)[A].

SURGERY/OTHER PROCEDURES

- SBP: medical management
- Secondary bacterial peritonitis: Emergent surgical management including source control with open laparotomy to repair any perforated viscus and eradicate infected material is 1st-line treatment (2)[A],(5)[B].
- Tertiary bacterial peritonitis
  - If no unrepaired perforations or leaks, additional surgery for severe abdominal infection is correlated with deterioration and significant mortality (2).

ALERT

Mortality of SBP approaches 80% if a patient receives unnecessary exploratory laparotomy, whereas mortality of approaches 100% if not treated surgically (1,3).

INPATIENT CONSIDERATIONS

Admission Criteria/ Initial Stabilization

- Acute peritonitis warrants inpatient admission.
- Patients who present with peritonitis can be severely hypovolemic. In these cases, volume resuscitation with crystalloid or colloid fluids is critical to reduce the risk of secondary organ dysfunction; albumin is preferred in SBP (5)[B].
- In patients with cardiogenic or septic shock, invasive monitoring with early goal-directed fluid therapy.
- Nasogastric tube placement can prevent aspiration in patients with vomiting or GI bleeding.

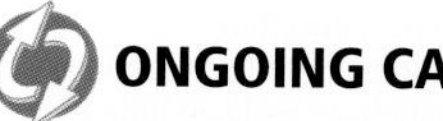

ONGOING CARE

FOLLOW-UP RECOMMENDATIONS

Patient Monitoring

Normalization of vital signs with resolution of leukocytosis indicates improvement.

- SBP: If follow-up paracentesis is performed after 48 hours to evaluate resolution, PMN decrease ≥25% is expected.
- Development of leukopenia indicates immune exhaustion and poor prognosis.

DIET

- NPO, total parental nutrition as necessary
- Resume enteral feeding after return of bowel function.
- Sodium restriction can reduce future ascites (3)[A].

PROGNOSIS

- SBP
  - For inpatients with first episode of SBP, mortality ranges from 10 to 50% (3).
  - Patients with prior SBP have 1-year recurrence rate of 40–70% and 1-year mortality of 31–93% (1,3).
  - Strongest negative prognostic indicator is renal insufficiency.
  - Other poor prognostic factors include nosocomial acquisition, old age, high Child-Pugh-Turcotte or MELD score, malnutrition, malignancy, peripheral leukopenia, and antibiotic resistance (3).
  - Prognosis is improved if antibiotics are started early, prior to onset of shock or renal failure.
- Secondary bacterial peritonitis
  - In-hospital mortality of treated patients is 67% (4).
  - Mortality approaches 100% if not treated surgically, especially if secondary to perforation (2,4).
  - Prognosis is worse in perforated etiologies.

COMPLICATIONS

- Renal failure, liver failure, encephalopathy, coagulopathy
- Secondary infection, iatrogenic infection, abscess, fistula formation, abdominal compartment syndrome
- Sepsis/septic shock, cardiovascular collapse, adrenal insufficiency, respiratory failure, ARDS

REFERENCES

1. Alaniz C, Regal RE. Spontaneous bacterial peritonitis: a review of treatment options. *P T*. 2009;34(4):204–210.
2. Panhofer P, Izay B, Riedl M, et al. Age, microbiology and prognostic scores help to differentiate between secondary and tertiary peritonitis. *Langenbecks Arch Surg*. 2009;394(2):265–271.
3. Wiest R, Krag A, Gerbes A. Spontaneous bacterial peritonitis: recent guidelines and beyond. *Gut*. 2012;61(2):297–310.
4. Soriano G, Castellote J, Alvarez C, et al. Secondary bacterial peritonitis in cirrhosis: a retrospective study of clinical and analytical characteristics, diagnosis and management. *J Hepatol*. 2010;52(1):39–44.
5. Runyon BA. Introduction to the revised American Association for the Study of Liver Diseases Practice Guideline management of adult patients with ascites due to cirrhosis 2012. *Hepatology*. 2013;57(4):1651–1653.
6. Ballinger AE, Palmer SC, Wiggins KJ, et al. Treatment for peritoneal dialysis-associated peritonitis. *Cochrane Database Syst Rev*. 2014;4:CD005284.

ADDITIONAL READING

- Bajaj JS, O'Leary JG, Wong F, et al. Bacterial infections in end-stage liver disease: current challenges and future directions. *Gut*. 2012;61(8):1219–1225.
- Cheong HS, Kang CI, Lee JA, et al. Clinical significance and outcome of nosocomial acquisition of spontaneous bacterial peritonitis in patients with liver cirrhosis. *Clin Infect Dis*. 2009;48(9):1230–1236.
- Deshpande A, Pasupuleti V, Thota P, et al. Acid-suppressive therapy is associated with spontaneous bacterial peritonitis in cirrhotic patients: a meta-analysis. *J Gastroenterol Hepatol*. 2013;28(2):235–242.
- Jain P. Spontaneous bacterial peritonitis: few additional points. *World J Gastroenterol*. 2009;15(45):5754–5755.
- Koulaouzidis A, Bhat S, Karagiannidis. Spontaneous bacterial peritonitis. *Postgrad Med J*. 2007;83(980):379–383.
- Koulaouzidis A, Bhat S, Saeed AA. Spontaneous bacterial peritonitis. *World J Gastroenterol*. 2009;15(9):1042–1049.

SEE ALSO

Appendicitis, Acute; Cirrhosis of the Liver; Diverticular Disease; Peptic Ulcer Disease

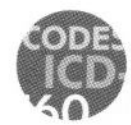

CODES

ICD10

- K65.0 Generalized (acute) peritonitis
- K65.2 Spontaneous bacterial peritonitis
- K65.8 Other peritonitis

CLINICAL PEARLS

- Maintain a high index of suspicion for SBP in cirrhotic patients with ascites. SBP occurs in preexisting ascites and carries a high mortality, especially if presenting with GI bleed.
- Early diagnosis is essential to reducing mortality.
- Paracentesis is necessary to establish the diagnosis of SBP.
- Emergent CT scan should be performed if there is suspicion of secondary bacterial peritonitis.
- Distinguishing SBP from secondary bacterial peritonitis is essential, as SBP treatment consists of antibiotic therapy, whereas secondary bacterial peritonitis necessitates emergent surgical intervention.
- Renal function is the most important prognostic indicator for SBP. Albumin administration decreases the incidence of renal failure and mortality after large-volume paracentesis, and decreases mortality in SBP with renal or hepatic impairment.

PERSONALITY DISORDERS

Moshe S. Torem, MD

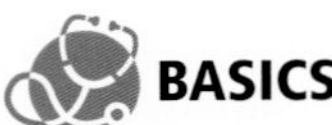

BASICS

DESCRIPTION

- Personality disorders (PDs) are a group of conditions, with onset at or before adolescence, characterized by enduring patterns of maladaptive and dysfunctional behavior that deviates markedly from one's culture and social environment, leading to functional impairment and distress to the individual, coworkers, and family.
  - These behaviors are perceived by patients to be "normal" and "right," and they have little insight as to their ownership, responsibility, and abnormal nature of these behaviors.
  - These conditions are classified based on the predominant symptoms and their severity.
- System(s) affected: nervous/psychiatric
- Synonym(s): character disorder; character pathology

Geriatric Considerations

Coping with the stresses of aging is challenging.

Pediatric Considerations

A history of childhood neglect, abuse, and trauma is not uncommon.

Pregnancy Considerations

Pregnancy adds pressure in coping with the activities of daily living (ADLs).

EPIDEMIOLOGY

Prevalence

- General population: 15% (1)
- Cluster A: 5.7%
- Cluster B: 6.0%
- Cluster C: 9.1%
- Outpatient psychiatric clinic: 3–30% (2)
- In male prisoners, the prevalence of antisocial personality disorder is ~60%.
- Predominant age: starts in adolescence and early 20s and persists throughout patient's life
- Predominant sex: male = female; some personality disorders are more common in females, and others are more common in males.

ETIOLOGY AND PATHOPHYSIOLOGY

- Environmental and genetic factors (3)
- Criteria for a PD includes an enduring pattern of the following:
  - Inner experience and behavior that deviates markedly from the expectations of one's culture in ≥2 of the following areas: cognition, affectivity, interpersonal functioning, or impulse control
  - Inflexibility and pervasiveness across a broad range of personal and social situations
  - Significant distress or impairment in social or occupational functioning
  - The pattern is stable and of long duration
  - The enduring pattern is not better explained as a manifestation of another psychiatric disorder
  - The enduring pattern is not attributable to the effects of a drug or a medical condition
- PDs are classified into 3 major clusters:
  - Cluster A: eccentricism and oddness
    - *Paranoid PD*: unwarranted suspiciousness and distrust of others
    - *Schizoid PD*: emotional, cold, or detached; socially isolated
    - *Schizotypal PD*: eccentric behavior, odd belief system/perceptions, social isolation, and general suspiciousness
  - Cluster B: dramatic, emotional, or erratic behavioral patterns
    - *Antisocial PD*: aggressive, impulsive, irritable, irresponsible, dishonest, deceitful
    - *Borderline PD:* unstable interpersonal relationships, high impulsivity from early adulthood, intense fear of abandonment, mood swings, poor self-esteem, chronic boredom, and feelings of inner emptiness
    - *Histrionic PD:* needs to be the center of attention, with self-dramatizing behaviors and attention seeking in a variety of contexts
    - *Narcissistic PD*: grandiose sense of self-importance and preoccupation with fantasies of success, power, brilliance, beauty, or ideal love; lack of empathy for other people's pain or discomfort
  - Cluster C: anxiety, excessive worry, fear, and unhealthy patterns of coping with emotions
    - *Avoidant PD*: social inhibition, feelings of inadequacy, hypersensitivity to negative evaluation, avoidance of occupational and interpersonal activities that involve the risk of criticism by others, views self as socially inept and personally unappealing or inferior to others
    - *Dependent PD*: excessive need to be taken care of, leading to submissive and clinging behavior with fears of separation, avoids expressing disagreements with others due to fear of losing support and approval, usually seeks out strong and confident people as friends or spouses and feels more secure in such relationships
    - *Obsessive-compulsive PD*: preoccupation with cleanliness, orderliness, perfectionism; preoccupation with excessive details, rules, lists, order, organization, and schedules to the extent that the major point of the activity is lost
  - Personality change due to another medical condition: It is a persistent personality disturbance that is caused by the physiologic effects of a medical condition such as frontal lobe lesion, epilepsy, MS, Parkinson disease, lupus, etc.
  - Other specified *PD and unspecified PD*: A category provided for 2 situations: (i) the individual's personality pattern meets the general criteria for PD and traits of several PDs are present, but the criteria for any specific PD are not met; (ii) the individual's personality pattern meets the general criteria for PD, but the individual is considered to have a PD that is not included in *DSM-5* classification such as passive-aggressive PD, depressive PD, masochistic PD, and dangerous and severe PD.

Genetics

Major character traits are inherited; others result from a combination of genetics and environment.

RISK FACTORS

- Positive family history
- Pregnancy risk factors
  - Nutritional deprivation
  - Use of alcohol or drugs
  - Viral and bacterial infections
- Dysfunctional family with child abuse/neglect

COMMONLY ASSOCIATED CONDITIONS

Depression, other psychiatric disorders in patient and family members

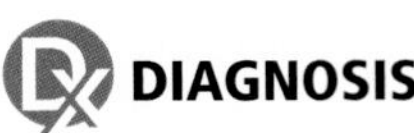

DIAGNOSIS

HISTORY

- Comprehensive interview and mental status examination
- Screen to rule out alcohol and drug abuse
- Interview of relatives and friends helpful in establishing an enduring pattern of behavior.

DIAGNOSTIC TESTS & INTERPRETATION

Psychological testing (e.g., MMPI-II)

Initial Tests (lab, imaging)

- CBC
- Comprehensive metabolic panel
- Thyroid-stimulating hormone
- HIV
- Toxicology screen for substance abuse

Follow-Up Tests & Special Considerations

- EEG to rule out a chronic seizure disorder
- CT and MRI of the brain may be necessary in newly developed symptoms to rule out organic brain disease (e.g., frontal lobe tumor).

DIFFERENTIAL DIAGNOSIS

- Medical disorders with behavioral changes
- Other psychiatric disorders with similar symptoms
  - In obsessive-compulsive disorder (OCD), symptoms are ego-dystonic (i.e., perceived as foreign and unwanted). In addition, OCD has a pattern of relapse and partial remission.
  - In obsessive-compulsive personality disorder (OCPD), symptoms are perceived as desirable behaviors (ego-syntonic) that the patient feels proud of and wants others to emulate. In addition, OCPD has a lifelong pattern (i.e., without significant relapse or remission).

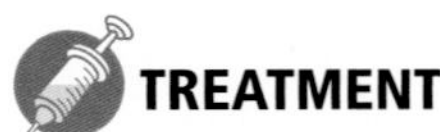

TREATMENT

Psychotherapy with family involvement is the foundation of treatment. No specific drugs are indicated to treat PDs; some medications can reduce the intensity, frequency, and dysfunctional nature of certain behaviors (4)[B].

GENERAL MEASURES

- Long-term psychotherapy and cognitive-behavioral therapy (5)[B]
- Group therapy is helpful in the use of therapeutic confrontation and increasing one's awareness of and insight regarding the damaging effects of dysfunctional behavior patterns (6)[B].

MEDICATION

Medications are effective in the treatment of comorbid conditions such as anxiety and depression.

First Line

- Symptom management (7)[B]
  - Minipsychosis (associated with paranoid, schizoid, borderline, and schizotypal PDs): atypical antipsychotics: risperidone (Risperdal), quetiapine (Seroquel), olanzapine (Zyprexa), ziprasidone (Geodon), aripiprazole (Abilify), asenapine (Saphris), lurasidone (Latuda); start with a low dose, gradually adjusting to the patient's needs
  - Anxiety: anxiolytics (benzodiazepines, buspirone [BuSpar], and serotonin reuptake inhibitors)
  - Depressed mood: antidepressants
- Many patients with borderline PD respond well to small doses of atypical neuroleptics and mood stabilizers (8)[B].
- Precautions: Some atypical neuroleptic drugs may be associated with hyperglycemia and insulin-resistant metabolic syndrome.

Second Line

Mood stabilizers: lithium carbonate, lamotrigine (Lamictal), carbamazepine (Tegretol, Equetro), and valproate (Depacon, Depakene, Depakote) (9)[B]

ISSUES FOR REFERRAL

- When psychiatric comorbidity of Axis I disorders is present (e.g., mood disorders, anxiety disorders, substance abuse, etc.)
- Suicidal ideation or attempts

ADDITIONAL THERAPIES

- Dialectical behavior therapy
- Psychoanalytic therapy
- Interactive psychotherapy
- Group therapy

INPATIENT CONSIDERATIONS

Admission Criteria/Initial Stabilization

Disorders with complications of suicide attempts

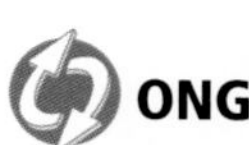

ONGOING CARE

FOLLOW-UP RECOMMENDATIONS

Continue outpatient treatment, potentially long term

Patient Monitoring

- Regular physical exercise (e.g., 30–45 min/day, helps with stress and the ADLs)
- If substance abuse is suspected, check drug screens.
- Infrequent sessions with relatives or friends are helpful in monitoring behavioral progress.

DIET

Emphasize variety of healthy foods; avoid obesity

PATIENT EDUCATION

- Bibliotherapy and writing therapy, specific assignments, and watching certain movies to better understand the nature and origin of one's specific condition are helpful:
  - Kreger R. *The Essential Family Guide to Borderline Personality Disorder*. Center City, MN: Hazelden; 2008.
  - Mason PT, Kreger R. *Stop Walking on Eggshells*. Oakland, CA: New Harbinger Publishers; 2010.
- The movie *As Good as It Gets* illustrates someone with obsessive-compulsive behaviors and their impact on ADLs and relationships with family and friends.
- The movie series *The Godfather* includes several characters with antisocial PD and shows how this affects their interpersonal relationships and their own physical and mental health.
- The movie *What About Bob?* illustrates the challenges involved in treating certain patients with a borderline PD, especially in the management of boundaries in the doctor–patient relationship.
- The movie *A Streetcar Named Desire* illustrates an example of a woman with a histrionic PD.
- The movie *Wall Street* illustrates an example of a person with a narcissistic PD.
- The movie *The Caine Mutiny* illustrates an example of a person with a paranoid PD.
- The movie *Four Weddings and a Funeral* illustrates an example of a person with an avoidant PD.

PROGNOSIS

PDs are enduring patterns of behavior throughout one's lifetime and are not readily responsive to treatment.

COMPLICATIONS

- Disruptive family life with frequent divorces and separations, alcoholism, substance abuse, and drug addiction
- Disruptive behaviors in the workplace may cause absenteeism and loss of productivity.
- Violation of the law and disregard for the concerns and rights of others

REFERENCES

1. American Psychiatric Association. *Diagnostic and Statistical Manual of Mental Disorders*. 5th ed. Arlington, VA: American Psychiatric Association; 2013:645–684.
2. Angstman K, Rasmussen NH. Personality disorders: review and clinical application in daily practice. *Am Fam Physician*. 2011;84(11):1253–1260.
3. Reichborn-Kjennerud T. Genetics of personality disorders. *Clin Lab Med*. 2010;30(4):893–910.
4. Hadjipavlou G, Ogrodniczuk JS. Promising psychotherapies for personality disorders. *Can J Psychiatry*. 2010;55(4):202–210.
5. Clarkin JE. An integrated approach to psychotherapy techniques for patients with personality disorder. *J Pers Disord*. 2012;26(1):43–62.
6. Livesley WJ. Integrated treatment: a conceptual framework for an evidence-based approach to the treatment of personality disorder. *J Pers Disord*. 2012;26(1):17–42.
7. Ripoll LH, Triebwasser J, Siever LJ. Evidence-based pharmacotherapy for personality disorders. *Int J Neuropsychopharmacol*. 2011;14(9):1257–1288.
8. Ripoll LH. Clinical psychopharmacology of borderline personality disorder: an update on the available evidence in light of the *Diagnostic and Statistical Manual of Mental Disorders*—5. *Curr Opin Psychiatry*. 2012;25(1):52–58.
9. Lieb K, Völlm B, Rücker G, et al. Pharmacotherapy for borderline personality disorder: Cochrane systematic review of randomised trials. *Br J Psychiatry*. 2010;196(1):4–12.

ADDITIONAL READING

- Borschmann R, Henderson C, Hogg J, et al. Crisis interventions for people with borderline personality disorder. *Cochrane Database Syst Rev*. 2012;6:CD009353.
- Cosci F. Assessment of personality in psychosomatic medicine: current concepts. *Adv Psychosom Med*. 2012;32:133–159.
- Feurino L III, Silk KR. State of the art in the pharmacologic treatment of borderline personality disorder. *Curr Psychiatry Rep*. 2011;13(1):69–75.
- Kealy D, Ogrodniczuk JS. Narcissistic interpersonal problems in clinical practice. *Harv Rev Psychiatry*. 2011;19(6):290–301.
- Leichsenring F, Leibing E, Kruse J, et al. Borderline personality disorder. *Lancet*. 2011;377(9759):74–84.
- Mauchnik J, Schmahl C. The latest neuroimaging findings in borderline personality disorder. *Curr Psychiatry Rep*. 2010;12(1):46–55.
- Molina JD, López-Muñoz F, Stein DJ, et al. Borderline personality disorder: a review and reformulation from evolutionary theory. *Med Hypotheses*. 2009;73(3):382–386.
- Paris J. Modernity and narcissistic personality disorder. *Personal Disord*. 2014;5(2):220–226.
- Ronningstam E. Narcissistic personality disorder: a current review. *Curr Psychiatry Rep*. 2010;12(1):68–75.
- Stoffers J, Völlm BA, Rücker G, et al. Pharmacological interventions for borderline personality disorder. *Cochrane Database Syst Rev*. 2010;6:CD005653.

SEE ALSO

Obsessive-Compulsive Disorder

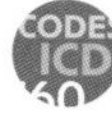

CODES

ICD10

- F60.9 Personality disorder, unspecified
- F60.0 Paranoid personality disorder
- F60.1 Schizoid personality disorder

CLINICAL PEARLS

- PDs are enduring patterns of behavior throughout one's lifetime and are not readily responsive to treatment.
- No specific drugs treat PDs; however, specific medications can reduce the intensity, frequency, and dysfunctional nature of certain behaviors, thoughts, and feelings.
- Most patients with a PD require a well-trained and experienced mental health professional.
- A stable, trustful alliance with the patient is the foundation for any therapeutic progress.

PERTUSSIS

Mary Cataletto, MD, FAAP, FCCP • Margaret J. McCormick, MS, RN

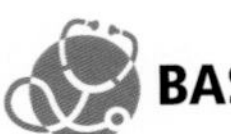

BASICS

Highly contagious disease; aka whooping cough

DESCRIPTION

- Human host: adults most common reservoir
- Can affect all ages
- Worldwide distribution
- May be endemic or epidemic with outbreaks every 3–5 years
- Seasonality: can occur year-round; peaks late summer–autumn
- Transmission: person to person via aerosolized respiratory droplets
- Effective vaccine available but neither vaccine nor infection confer lifelong or 100% immunity
- System(s) affected: respiratory
- Synonym(s): whooping cough

EPIDEMIOLOGY

Incidence

- Worldwide: estimated 48.5 million cases and nearly 295,000 deaths/year (1,2)
- United States: 27,550 cases in 2010; 18,719 in 2011

ETIOLOGY AND PATHOPHYSIOLOGY

- Toxin mediated
- Infectious process with predilection for ciliated respiratory epithelium
- *Bordetella pertussis* (responsible for ~95% of cases)
- *Bordetella parapertussis*

RISK FACTORS

- Exposure to a confirmed case
- Non- or underimmunized infants and children
- Pregnancy
- Premature birth
- Chronic lung disease
- Immunodeficiency (e.g., AIDS)
- Infants <6 months of age account for ~90% pediatric pertussis hospitalizations (1).

GENERAL PREVENTION

- Public health measures
  - Surveillance activities
  - Prevention programs
  - Outbreak management
- Care of exposed persons
  - Household and close contacts
  - Child care workers
  - Health care workers
- Immunization
  - Vaccine products
  - Boosters
- CDC and the Advisory Committee on Immunization Practices recommends 1 Tdap (tetanus toxoid, reduced diphtheria toxoid, and acellular pertussis) vaccination to all adolescents 11–12 years of age and one dose of Tdap for all adults age 18 years and older to provide increased herd immunity.

Pediatric Considerations

- Primary immunization series against pertussis followed by boosters
- Adult immunization and cocooning are alternative strategies to protect unimmunized infants.

ALERT

Tdap vaccine recommended with each pregnancy, preferably after 20 weeks' gestation regardless of Tdap/Td history

Geriatric Considerations

The incidence of pertussis in individuals age 50 years and older has increased between 2006 and 2010.

COMMONLY ASSOCIATED CONDITIONS

- Apnea
- Secondary bacterial pneumonia
- Sinusitis
- Seizures
- Encephalopathy
- Urinary incontinence

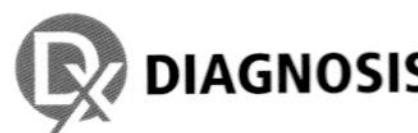

DIAGNOSIS

HISTORY

- Exposure to pertussis
- Incubation period 7–10 days (range 5–21 days)
- Classic symptoms are more common in adults and adolescents and include paroxysmal cough, posttussive whoop, and/or vomiting.
- Infants with pertussis may present with apnea or sudden death.

PHYSICAL EXAM

- Classic pertussis has 3 phases, which occur over 6–10 weeks:
  - Catarrhal phase: rhinorrhea, mild cough, low-grade fever
  - Paroxysmal phase: Cough occurs in bursts, with increased intensity and frequency, often followed by an inspiratory whoop and/or posttussive vomiting.
  - Convalescent phase: Coughing paroxysms decrease in frequency and intensity.
- In the absence of paroxysms or complications, the physical exam may be normal.

ALERT

Infants <6 months of age may have atypical presentations.

DIFFERENTIAL DIAGNOSIS

- *B. parapertussis*
- *Mycoplasma pneumoniae*
- *Chlamydia trachomatis*
- *Chlamydophila pneumoniae*
- *Bordetella bronchiseptica*
- Respiratory syncytial virus
- Adenovirus

DIAGNOSTIC TESTS & INTERPRETATION

Initial Tests (lab, imaging)

- Nasopharyngeal culture (gold standard): 100% specific and permits strain identification and antimicrobial resistance testing. Collect secretions from the back of the throat through the nose, using a Dacron or calcium alginate swab or syringe filled with saline. For best results, collect specimen during the first 2 weeks of cough—sensitivity decreases after 2 weeks.
- Polymerase chain reaction (PCR) assays: Frequently used because they are quick and sensitive. Specificity may vary between assays and must be interpreted within clinical context and local pertussis epidemiology. CDC "Best Practice" guidelines exist for PCR assays, although they have not yet received FDA approval. 6 accurate results can be obtained during the first 3 weeks from onset of cough. Dacron swabs should be used as calcium alginate swabs are inhibitory to PCR (2,3).
- Serology: available commercially; however, there is no FDA-approved test or standardization
  - The CDC uses single point serology obtained between 2 and 8 weeks following cough onset when titers are expected to be at their peak (3).

Follow-Up Tests & Special Considerations

- Evaluation and follow-up for associated conditions and complications
- Chest radiograph (2 views) to evaluate for the presence of pneumonia
- EEG/neuroimaging may be considered in infant with seizures or acute life-threatening events (ALTEs).
- Infants <1 month of age who are treated with macrolides should be monitored for the possible development of hypertrophic pyloric stenosis.

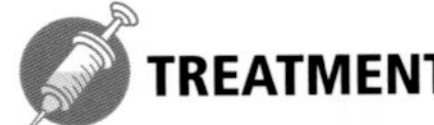

TREATMENT

GENERAL MEASURES

Waiting rooms, during transport and procedures: Patients with suspected pertussis should wear masks.

MEDICATION

Pertussis illness may be less severe only if antibiotics are started early, that is, before the onset of paroxysms or during the catarrhal phase (1,2). Antibiotics can also help to prevent the spread of pertussis to close contacts and is necessary for stopping the spread of pertussis.

First Line

- Empiric antibiotic therapy should be initiated at the time diagnostic testing is performed if sufficient clinical suspicion for pertussis is present.
- One of the following (dosing is age dependent):
  - Azithromycin
  - Erythromycin
  - Clarithromycin

P

- Postexposure prophylaxis treatments are identical to treatment and recommended for those with close contact to patient.
- If administered during catarrhal stage, these antibiotics may ameliorate disease.
- If administered after cough is established, antibiotics will have no individual benefit but may help to limit spread (3)[C].

ALERT
Risk of infantile hypertrophic pyloric stenosis has been associated with the use of macrolides in infants <1 month of age. Consultation and monitoring are recommended.

ALERT
Due to reports of *fatal cardiac dysrhythmias* with azithromycin, consider alternate drugs in the elderly and in those with cardiovascular disease.

Second Line

TRIMETHOPRIM SULFAMETHOXAZOLE (TMP-SMX) (for persons >2 months of age) if

- They cannot tolerate macrolides OR
- They are infected with a macrolide-resistant strain

ALERT
- TMP-SMX is *contraindicated* in infants <2 months of age (3).
- Clarithromycin is not recommended in infants <1 month of age (3).

ISSUES FOR REFERRAL

Evaluation and treatment of infants <6 months of age, especially those born prematurely, who are unimmunized and those who require hospitalization

ADDITIONAL THERAPIES

Symptomatic treatment of the cough in pertussis (e.g., corticosteroids, B2 adrenergic agonists, pertussis-specific immunoglobulin, antihistamine, and leukotriene receptor antagonist) have not shown consistent benefit (4)[B].

INPATIENT CONSIDERATIONS

Admission Criteria/Initial Stabilization

- Small, frequent meals may be necessary to ensure adequate nutrition.
- Correct fluid and electrolyte abnormalities.
- Infants may require IV fluids.

IV Fluids

Indicated for dehydration and when oral fluids are either contraindicated or poorly tolerated

Nursing

- In addition to standard precautions, hospitalized patients should be isolated with respiratory precautions for 5 days after the initiation of effective antibiotic treatment and for 3 weeks after onset of paroxysms in older patients if antibiotics are not used.
- Gentle suctioning of nasal secretions
- Avoid stimuli that trigger paroxysms.
- Respiratory monitoring including pulse oximetry
- Educate each family about the importance of immunizations.
- Discuss chemoprophylaxis with each family.

Discharge Criteria

- Clinically stable
- Able to tolerate oral feedings

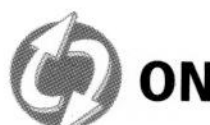

ONGOING CARE

Supportive

FOLLOW-UP RECOMMENDATIONS

- Monitor infants who received EES or azithromycin for pyloric stenosis.
- Neurologic and/or pulmonary follow-up as necessary

Patient Monitoring

ICU care may be necessary for severely ill or compromised patients.

DIET

IV fluids/nutrition may be required to treat dehydration or supplement poor oral intake.

PATIENT EDUCATION

- American Academy of Pediatrics http://www.aap.org
- Centers for Disease Control and Prevention: http://www.cdc.gov

PROGNOSIS

- Complete recovery in most cases
- Most severe morbidity and highest mortality in infants <6 months of age

COMPLICATIONS

- Highest and most severe in infants; may include apnea, cyanosis, and sudden death
- In children: may include conjunctival hemorrhage, inguinal hernia, pneumonia, and seizures
- More frequent in adults than adolescents: may include sinusitis, otitis media, pneumonia, weight loss, fainting, rib fracture, urinary incontinence, seizures, encephalopathy, and death

REFERENCES

1. Lopez MA, Crug AT, Kowalkowski MA, et al. Trends in hospitalizations and resource utilization for pediatric pertussis. *Hosp Pediatr*. 2014;4(5):269–275.
2. Centers for Disease Control and Prevention. *Best Practices for Healthcare Professionals on the use of Polymerase Chain Reaction (PCR) for diagnosing pertussis*. Atlanta, GA: Centers for Disease Control and Prevention; 2011.
3. Pickering LK, Baker CJ, Kimberlin DW, et al, eds. *Red Book: 2012 Report of the Committee* on Infectious Diseases. 29th ed. Elk Grove Village, IL: American Academy of Pediatrics; 2012.
4. Bettiol S, Wang K, Thompson MJ, et al. Symptomatic treatment of the cough in whooping cough. *Cochrane Database Syst Rev*. 2012;5:CD003257.

ADDITIONAL READING

- American College of Obstetrics and Gynecology. ACOG Committee Opinion No. 521: update on immunization and pregnancy: tetanus, diphtheria, and pertussis vaccination. *Obstet Gynecol*. 2012;19(3):690–691.
- Balderston-McGuiness C, Hill J, Fonseca E, et al. The disease burden of pertussis in adults 50 years old and older in the United States: a retrospective study. *BMC Infect Dis*. 2013;13:32.
- Centers for Disease Control and Prevention. Pertussis (whooping cough). http://www.cdc.gov/pertussis. Accessed 2014.
- Snyder J, Fisher D. Pertussis in childhood. *Pediatr Rev*. 2012;33(9):412–421.
- Wallace AS, Ryman TK, Dietz V. Overview of global, regional, and national routine vaccination coverage trends and growth patterns from 1980 to 2009: implications for vaccine-preventable disease eradication and elimination initiatives. *J Infect Dis*. 2014;210(Suppl 1):S514–S522.
- Wiley KE, Zuo Y, Macartney KK, et al. Sources of pertussis infection in young infants: a review of key evidence informing targeting of the cocoon strategy. *Vaccine*. 2013;31(4):618–625.

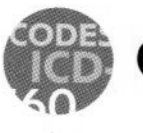

CODES

ICD10

- A37.90 Whooping cough, unspecified species without pneumonia
- A37.80 Whooping cough due to other Bordetella species w/o pneumonia
- A37.10 Whooping cough due to Bordetella parapertussis w/o pneumonia

CLINICAL PEARLS

- Pertussis is a highly contagious infection.
- A high index of suspicion is needed. During the primary or catarrhal phase, the presentation may be nonspecific.
- Immunization (primary series and boosters), isolation, and early treatment of affected cases as well as chemoprophylaxis are key components to controlling the spread of pertussis.

PHARYNGITIS

Jimmy J. Brown, DDS, MD, FACS • Brian Ho, MD

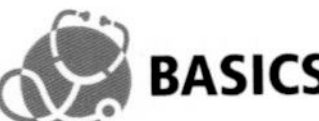

BASICS

DESCRIPTION

- Acute or chronic Inflammation of the pharynx
- Most commonly caused by acute viral infection
- Group A *Streptococcus* pharyngitis is a common clinical focus due to its potential for preventable rheumatic autoimmune sequelae (e.g., cardiac/renal).
- Synonym(s): sore throat; tonsillitis; "strep throat"
- Generally infection mediated but can be due to caustic injury, allergies, gastroesophageal reflux disease (GERD), smoking, endotracheal intubation, or trauma-related

EPIDEMIOLOGY

- Estimated 30 million cases diagnosed yearly
- 12–25% of all sore throats are thought to prompt visits to physicians or other care provider.
- All age groups, but some etiologies may predilect specific age groups
- No gender predilection

Incidence

- Respiratory infections account for 38% of the 129 million physician visits per year in the United States. This accounts for ~200 visits to a physician per 1,000 population in the United States annually (1).
- Most commonly viral (40–60%)
- Group A *Streptococcus* is the most common bacterial cause of acute pharyngitis, accounting for ~15–30% of pediatric cases and 5–10% of adults.
- Rheumatic fever is rare in the United States; 112 cases reported to the CDC in 1994 (the last year this was a reportable disease) due to the preponderance of early antibiotic intervention

Pediatric Considerations

Rheumatic fever has its greatest incidence in children aged 5–18 years, but is currently a rare sequela of streptococcal pharyngitis in modern medicine.

ETIOLOGY AND PATHOPHYSIOLOGY

- Acute, viral (lower grade fever)
  - Rhinovirus
  - Adenovirus (associated with conjunctivitis)
  - Parainfluenza virus
  - Coxsackievirus (hand-foot-mouth disease)
  - Coronavirus
  - Echovirus
  - Herpes simplex virus (vesicular lesions)
  - Epstein-Barr virus (EBV/mononucleosis)
  - Cytomegalovirus
  - HIV
- Acute, bacterial (higher fevers)
  - Group A β-hemolytic streptococci <10% of adult pharyngitis
  - *Neisseria gonorrhoeae*
  - *Corynebacterium diphtheriae* (diphtheria)
  - *Haemophilus influenzae*
  - *Moraxella (Branhamella) catarrhalis*
  - Groups C and G *Streptococcus*, rarely
- Chronic
  - More likely noninfectious
  - Chemical irritation (GERD)
  - Smoking
  - Neoplasms
  - Vasculitis
  - Radiation changes

Genetics

Patients with a positive family history of rheumatic fever have a higher risk of rheumatic sequelae following an untreated group A β-hemolytic streptococcal infection.

RISK FACTORS

- Epidemics of group A β-hemolytic streptococcal disease occurrence
- Age (i.e., younger patients are more susceptible)
- Family history
- Living at close quarters, such as in military recruits
- Immunosuppression
- Fatigue
- Smoking
- Oral sex
- Diabetes mellitus
- Recent illness (secondary postviral bacterial infection)
- Chronic colonization of bacteria in tonsils/adenoids

GENERAL PREVENTION

Avoid contact with infectious patients (viral and bacterial).

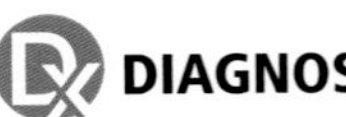

DIAGNOSIS

- Group A (β-hemolytic) *Streptococcus* is almost always not associated with cough.
- Modified Centor clinical prediction rule for group A streptococcal infection (2)[A]:
  - +1 point: tonsillar exudates
  - +1 point: tender anterior chain cervical adenopathy
  - +1 point: fever by history
  - +1 point: age <15 years
  - 0 point: age 15–45 years
  - −1 point: age >45 years
  - −1 point: cough
- Scoring:
  - If 3–4 points, positive predictive value of ~80%; treat empirically.
  - If 2 points, positive predictive value of ~50%, rapid strep antigen + culture; treat if either positive.
  - If 1 point, positive predictive value <50%, positive rapid strep. antigen or culture likely false-positive finding
  - If 0 or −1 point, positive predictive value <20%; do not test; close follow-up as needed
- Coryza (nasal congestion), hoarseness, cough, diarrhea, conjunctivitis, or rash highly suggestive of viral cause

HISTORY

- Sore throat (odynophagia)
- Cough
- Hoarseness
- Fever
- Anorexia
- Chills
- Malaise
- Contacts with similar symptoms or diagnosed infection

PHYSICAL EXAM

- Enlarged tonsils (tonsillar exudate or possible peritonsillar abscess/deep neck space infection)
- Pharyngeal erythema
- Tonsillar/soft palate petechiae (suggest EBV)
- Cervical adenopathy
- Fever (higher in bacterial infections)
- Pharyngeal ulcers (CMV, HIV, Crohn, other autoimmune vasculitides)
- Scarlet fever rash: punctate erythematous macules with reddened flexor creases and circumoral pallor (suggestive of streptococcal pharyngitis)
- Gray oral pseudomembrane found in diphtheria and, occasionally, infectious mononucleosis
- Characteristic erythematous-based clear vesicles are found in herpes simplex virus infection.
- Conjunctivitis is found more commonly with adenovirus infections.

DIFFERENTIAL DIAGNOSIS

- Viral syndrome
- Streptococcal infection
- Allergic rhinitis
- GERD
- Malignancy (lymphoma or squamous cell carcinoma)
- Irritants/chemicals (detergent/caustic ingestion)
- Atypical bacterial (e.g., gonococcal, syphilis, pertussis, diphtheria)
- Oral candidiasis (patients typically complain mostly of dysphagia)

DIAGNOSTIC TESTS & INTERPRETATION

- Testing, if performed, is usually for the presence of group A β-hemolytic streptococci (GAS). Options include the following:
  - Rapid screening for streptococci can be done from throat swab with antigen agglutination kits; 5–10% false-negative results
  - Blood agar throat culture from swab. Bacitracin disk sensitivity of hemolytic colonies suggests group A streptococci.
  - Antistreptolysin-O (carrier state suspected if positive culture, and unchanged ASO titers)
- Special tests usually are done only if history is suggestive of a different diagnosis.
- Screening for gonococcal infection requires warm Thayer-Martin plate or antigen testing.
- Viruses can be cultured in special media (e.g., herpes simplex) but rarely indicated as well as expensive.
- Mono spot test for EBV
- Recent American Heart Association (AHA) scientific statement is "some form of microbiological confirmation, with either a throat culture or a rapid antigen detection test, is required for the diagnosis of GAS pharyngitis" (3).

Test Interpretation

Culture of pathogens may help to identify which is causative, but are not cost-effective or influence outcome. Cultures should be considered when patients fail primary treatment.

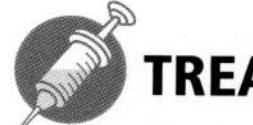

TREATMENT

- Clinicians should remember that acute pharyngitis is caused considerably more often by viruses rather than by bacteria. 1st-line therapy is conservative management (hydration/NSAIDs, etc.).
- Empirical therapy leads to overuse of antibiotics (4).
- Streptococcal infections should be treated to prevent rheumatic fever. Each episode should be documented to support need for patient to undergo tonsillectomy/adenoidectomy.
- Ulcers related to autoimmune diseases usually require steroids systemically or steroid injections into ulcers.
- HIV-related ulcers are due to decreasing counts of CD4 and respond when patients' CD4 titers increase.
- Guidelines in 2000, updated by American Academy of Otolaryngology, states tonsillectomy is indicated for 3 or more strep-positive infections/year or if a patient misses >2 weeks of school/work per year.

CONSERVATIVE MEASURES

- Salt water gargles
- Viscous lidocaine 2% 5–10 mL PO q4h swish/spit
- Acetaminophen 10–15 mg/kg/dose (pediatric) q4h for analgesia. In adults, they should not exceed >3 g of acetaminophen/24 hr
- Anesthetic lozenges
- Cool-mist humidifier
- PO or IV fluid resuscitation
- Opioids are not recommended in the pediatric population due to black box warnings.

MEDICATION

First Line

For streptococcal pharyngitis, penicillin is the standard therapy. Only penicillin has been proven to prevent rheumatic fever. Other antibiotics use streptococcal eradication as a proxy of effectiveness due to the low incidence of rheumatic fever and the ethics of further controlled studies. Treatment duration recommended to be 10 days (5)[A]:

- Penicillin V children: 250 mg PO twice daily or three times daily; adolescents and adults: 500 mg PO twice daily *or*
- Amoxicillin children: 50 mg/kg PO once daily (max 1,000 mg); alternative: 25 mg/kg (max 500 mg) twice daily; adults: 1,000 mg PO once daily or 500 mg PO twice daily. Use with caution if diagnosis is unclear because amoxicillin and *EBV infection may induce rash*.
- For patients allergic to penicillin
  - Cephalexin children: 20 mg/kg/dose PO twice daily (max 500 mg/dose); adults: 500 mg PO twice daily
  - Clindamycin children: 7 mg/kg/dose three times daily (max 300 mg/dose); adults: 300 mg PO three times daily

Second Line

- Penicillin is the most documented treatment to prevent rheumatic sequelae, but cephalosporins have a lower rate of antimicrobial failure.
- Other cephalosporins are generally effective for streptococcal pharyngitis but more expensive than cephalexin.
- Newer macrolides, azithromycin and clarithromycin; although effective against streptococcal pharyngitis, they are more expensive and unproven at preventing rheumatic complications.
- Macrolide-resistant strains of GAS are currently <10% in the United States but more prevalent worldwide.
- If tonsillar hypertrophy, may consider short steroid burst in addition to antibiotic therapy.

ONGOING CARE

FOLLOW-UP RECOMMENDATIONS

- Patient must complete antibiotic course for strep, regardless of symptom response.
- Patients may consider themselves noninfectious after 24 hours of antibiotic therapy.
- Follow-up culture is not recommended.

DIET

As tolerated. Encourage the consumption of fluids.

PROGNOSIS

- Streptococcal pharyngeal infection runs a 5–7-day course with peak fever at 2–3 days.
- Symptoms will resolve spontaneously without treatment, but rheumatic complications are still possible.

COMPLICATIONS

- Rheumatic fever (e.g., carditis, valve disease, arthritis)
- Poststreptococcal glomerulonephritis
- Peritonsillar abscess: also called as quinsy tonsillitis; considered a clinical diagnosis and does not warrant ultrasound/computed tomography. Will generally require percutaneous, commonly transoral, drainage. Surgery may also involve a so-called, quinsy tonsillectomy, which is merely a tonsillectomy in the setting of acute infection. This is generally not advocated unless for special circumstances, as most otolaryngologists recommend infectious resolution followed then by surgery.
- Acute airway compromise (rare) can typically be bypassed with nasal trumpets (requires consult to anesthesiology/otolaryngology).
- Strep "carriage" recurrently positive strep testing without strep symptoms; consider clindamycin or amoxicillin-clavulanate for 10 days.

REFERENCES

1. Armstrong GL, Pinner RW. Outpatient visits for infectious diseases in the United States, 1980 through 1996. *Arch Intern Med*. 1999;159(21):2531–2536.
2. McIsaac WJ, Kellner JD, Aufricht P, et al. Empirical validation of guidelines for the management of pharyngitis in children and adults. *JAMA*. 2004;291(13):1587–1595.
3. Gerber MA, Baltimore RS, Eaton CB, et al. Prevention of rheumatic fever and diagnosis and treatment of acute streptococcal pharyngitis. A scientific statement from the American Heart Association Rheumatic Fever, Endocarditis, and Kawasaki Disease Committee of the Council on Cardiovascular Disease in the Young, the Interdisciplinary Council on Functional Genomics and Translational Biology, and the Interdisciplinary Council on Quality of Care and Outcomes Research: endorsed by the American Academy of Pediatrics. *Circulation*. 2009;119(11):1541–1551.
4. Humair JP, Revaz SA, Bovier P, et al. Management of acute pharyngitis in adults: reliability of rapid streptococcal tests and clinical findings. *Arch Intern Med*. 2006;166(6):640–644.
5. Spinks A, Glasziou PP, Del Mar CB. Antibiotics for sore throat. *Cochrane Database Syst Rev*. 2013;11:CD000023.

ADDITIONAL READING

Pichichero ME, Cohen R. Shortened course of antibiotic therapy for acute otitis media, sinusitis and tonsillopharyngitis. *Pediatr Infect Dis*. 1997;16(7):680–695.

SEE ALSO

- Herpes Simplex; Infectious Mononucleosis, Epstein-Barr Virus (EBV) Infections; Rheumatic Fever
- Algorithm: Pharyngitis

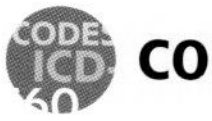

CODES

ICD10

- J02.9 Acute pharyngitis, unspecified
- J02.0 Streptococcal pharyngitis
- J31.2 Chronic pharyngitis

CLINICAL PEARLS

- Most cases of pharyngitis are viral.
- Risk of missed case of GAS is rheumatic fever, a very rare complication (112 cases reported to CDC in 1994; last year it was reported).
- Use Modified Centor Score to guide testing and treatment.
- Presence of coryza (nasal congestion), hoarseness, cough, diarrhea, conjunctivitis, or viral rash highly suggests viral cause.

PHEOCHROMOCYTOMA

Maya Campara, PharmD, BCPS • Anna C. Porter, MD

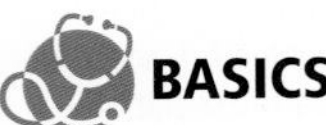

BASICS

DESCRIPTION

- A pheochromocytoma is a rare neuroendocrine tumor arising from the adrenal or extra-adrenal chromaffin tissue and, less commonly, the sympathetic ganglia.
- These tumors are catecholamine-producing: norepinephrine (NE) $>$ epinephrine (EPI) $>>>$ dopamine
- System(s) affected: endocrine; nervous; cardiovascular
- Synonym(s): chromaffin tumors; paragangliomas

EPIDEMIOLOGY

Incidence

- 500–1,000 cases per year diagnosed in the United States.
- $<$0.2% of people with severe hypertension (HTN)

Prevalence

- 1:6,500–1:2,500 in Western countries
- Affects all genders and ages; usually diagnosed in 4th–5th decades of life, familial cases diagnosed 1 decade earlier

ETIOLOGY AND PATHOPHYSIOLOGY

Pheochromocytoma is a tumor that releases catecholamines into the circulation. Catecholamines bind to adrenergic receptors to produce various effects that could induce severe or lethal cardiovascular and cerebrovascular complications.

- Stimulation of α_1 receptors (NE $>$ EPI) causes smooth muscle constriction resulting in high BP (arteriolar vasoconstriction).
- Stimulation of α_2 receptors (EPI $>$ NE) causes smooth muscle contraction, cardiac muscle relaxation, and inhibition of hormones, such as insulin, resulting in elevated blood glucose levels.
- Stimulation of β_1 receptors (EPI = NE) causes heart muscle contraction resulting in increased heart rate.
- Stimulation of β_2 receptors (EPI $>>$ NE) causes smooth muscle relaxation.
- In 80% of cases, it is a sporadic disease of unknown etiology.
- In 20% of cases, it has familial origin and is a component of 1 of the following 4 autosomal dominant diseases.
  - Multiple endocrine neoplasia type 2 (MEN-2)
  - von Hippel-Lindau syndrome (VHL)
  - Hereditary paraganglioma syndrome (PGL)
  - Neurofibromatosis type 1 (NF-1)
- Tumor location
  - 80% are solitary and unilateral.
  - 20% are divided between bilateral lesions and extra-adrenal masses (organ of Zuckerkandl, neck, mediastinum, abdomen, pelvis).

Genetics

Genetic testing is recommended; genes identified in the pathogenesis.

- Rearranged during transfection (*RET*) protooncogene
- von Hippel-Lindau disease tumor suppressor gene (*VHL*)
- Neurofibromatosis type 1 tumor suppressor gene (*NF-1*)
- Genes encoding 4 succinate dehydrogenase complex (*SDH*) subunits
- Gene encoding the enzyme responsible for flavination of the SDHA subunit
- Tumor suppressor *TMEM127* gene

RISK FACTORS

- Familial pheochromocytoma
- Familial paraganglioma
- MEN-2
- VHL disease
- von Recklinghausen NF-1

COMMONLY ASSOCIATED CONDITIONS

- MEN-2A (medullary thyroid carcinoma and primary hyperparathyroidism)
- MEN-2B (medullary thyroid carcinoma and mucosal neuromas)
- VHL disease (retinal angiomas, cerebellar hemangioblastomas, renal cysts, carcinomas, pancreatic cysts, epididymal cystadenomas)
- NF-1
- Sturge-Weber syndrome
- Tuberous sclerosis
- Carney syndrome (gastric epithelioid leiomyosarcoma, pulmonary chondroma, extra-adrenal paraganglioma)
- Familial paraganglioma
- Ataxia-telangiectasia
- Renal artery stenosis

DIAGNOSIS

HISTORY

- Classic "triad" of symptoms includes headache, palpitations, and diaphoresis.
- 5 P's mnemonic
  - Paroxysmal spells
  - Pressure: sudden increase in BP
  - Pain: headache, chest, abdominal pain
  - Perspiration (profuse sweating common in children)
  - Palpitations and pallor
- Additional symptoms: constipation, tremor, weight loss, anxiety, paresthesias, flushing, shortness of breath, nausea/vomiting
- Sudden death may occur in patients with an undiagnosed tumor who undergo surgery or biopsy due to lethal hypertensive crises and multiorgan failure.
- Dopamine-secreting pheochromocytomas lack the classic presentation of catecholamine excess.

PHYSICAL EXAM

- HTN: paroxysmal in 50% of affected patients; most common clinical sign
- Tachyarrhythmias
- Orthostatic hypotension
- Café au lait spots and Lisch nodules of the eye (*in neurofibromatosis*)
- Grades II–IV retinopathy
- Transient ischemic attacks/stroke
- Cardiomyopathy
- GI crisis
- Diabetes mellitus/insipidus
- Fever
- Hypercalcemia
- Erythrocytosis

DIFFERENTIAL DIAGNOSIS

- Labile essential HTN
- Anxiety and panic attacks
- Paroxysmal cardiac arrhythmia
- Thyrotoxicosis
- Menopausal syndrome
- Hypoglycemia
- Withdrawal of adrenergic-inhibiting medications
- Angina
- Hyperventilation
- Migraine headache
- Amphetamine or cocaine use
- Sympathomimetic ingestion/overdose

DIAGNOSTIC TESTS & INTERPRETATION

Initial Tests (lab, imaging)

Diagnosis is typically confirmed by measurements of urine catecholamines and their metabolites (NE/EPI $\rightarrow$ [nor]metanephrine, NE/EPI $\rightarrow$ vanillylmandelic acid [VMA], dopamine $\rightarrow$ homovanillic acid). Their amount in the urine correlates with tumor size.

- Elevated metanephrine and catecholamines in 24-hour urine collection (sensitivity, 90%; specificity, 98%)
  - A positive test is considered to be a 2-fold elevation above the upper limit of normal in urine.
- Elevated plasma fractionated metanephrine (sensitivity, 97%; specificity, 85%)
  - Measured while patient is at rest
  - Pheochromocytoma cannot be excluded if normal catecholamine values are obtained when the patient is normotensive and asymptomatic (record BP at time of blood draw).
- Elevated VMA in 24-hour urine collection (sensitivity, 64%; specificity, 95%)
- Dopamine-secreting pheochromocytomas are often missed if urine or plasma dopamine is not included as part of the catecholamine screening. Urine and plasma dopamine are the most widely used methods in the diagnosis of dopamine-secreting tumors.
- Proceed with imaging after positive laboratory evaluation.
  - Abdominal imaging with MRI/CT has similar specificity and sensitivity.
  - If CT/MRI is negative, but clinical suspicion is high, imaging can be done with 123-I-metaiodobenzylguanidine (MIBG) scan/pentetreotide scan.

Follow-Up Tests & Special Considerations

- Drugs that may increase measured levels of catecholamines and metabolites should be discontinued at least 2 weeks before assessment (1)[C].
  - Tricyclic antidepressants
  - Monoamine oxidase inhibitors (MAOIs)
  - Levodopa, methyldopa
  - Drugs containing adrenergic receptor agonists (e.g., decongestants)

- Amphetamines
- Cocaine
- Buspirone and most psychoactive agents (but not SSRIs)
- Prochlorperazine
- Reserpine
- Withdrawal from clonidine and other drugs
- Ethanol
- Acetaminophen (may increase measured levels of fractionated plasma metanephrine in some assays)
- Drugs that may decrease measured levels of catecholamines and metabolites
  - Reserpine
  - Centrally acting α_2 -receptor agonists (dexmedetomidine, clonidine, tizanidine, guanfacine)
- Conditions that may alter lab results include major physical stress due to surgery, stroke, myocardial infarction, congestive heart failure, and so forth.

Diagnostic Procedures/Other

Clonidine-suppression test distinguishes between pheochromocytoma and essential HTN when urine and plasma tests are equivocal. In essential HTN, plasma and urine catecholamines decrease 3 hours after oral clonidine; in pheochromocytoma, they do not.

Test Interpretation

Pathology shows a tumor that demonstrates staining for chromogranin-A (catecholamine secretory granules).

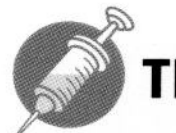

TREATMENT

MEDICATION

First Line

Surgical resection of the tumor is the treatment of choice. Medical management of BP is essential prior to surgery.

- Preoperative control of BP (target <120/80 mm Hg) achieved first with α-adrenergic blockade followed by β-adrenergic blockade starting 1 week before surgical removal of pheochromocytoma (longer for patients with recent history of cardiovascular complication) (2)[B]. Never initiate β-adrenergic blockade before α-adrenergic blockade, as unopposed α-stimulation will result in worsened HTN.
  - α-Adrenergic blockade is achieved with the nonselective α-blocker phenoxybenzamine starting at a dose of 10 mg PO BID and increasing by 10–20 mg every 2 days as needed and tolerated for BP control (normal dose 100 mg/day, but up to 240 mg/day has been reported). Warn patient of postural hypotension.
  - After adequate α-adrenergic blockade, β-blockade is initiated at low doses using short-acting agent propranolol 10 mg PO q6h that can be titrated up until resting heart rate of 60–80 beats/min is achieved (max dose 120 mg/day). Avoid β-blockers in acute decompensated heart failure, bradycardia, and patients with uncontrolled asthma.

Second Line

- Treat hypertensive crisis with nitroprusside, nicardipine, or phentolamine.
- For inoperable tumors requiring long-term medical management, specific α_1 -blocking agents can be used due to a more favorable side effect profile: prazosin, terazosin, doxazosin
- Selective β_1 blockers (no β_2 activity): atenolol, metoprolol, nadolol
- Combined β- and α-blockers: labetalol and carvedilol
- Catecholamine synthesis inhibitor: metyrosine only if intolerant to 1st-line treatment (Mayo Clinic protocol). Avoid long-term use due to adverse reactions (sedation, depression, diarrhea, crystalluria or urolithiasis, and extrapyramidal signs).

SURGERY/OTHER PROCEDURES

- Removal of pheochromocytoma is treatment of choice.
- It is a high-risk surgical procedure requiring experienced surgical and anesthesia teams.
- Laparoscopic approach for tumors in the adrenal gland may result in shorter hospitalization.
- Cortical-sparing subtotal adrenalectomy may preserve adrenocortical function in those with bilateral disease.

INPATIENT CONSIDERATIONS

Admission Criteria/Initial Stabilization

- Severe/refractory HTN
- Control of HTN and replacement of volume with IV normal saline

Nursing

Monitor BP closely.

Discharge Criteria

When hemodynamically stable

ONGOING CARE

FOLLOW-UP RECOMMENDATIONS

Patient Monitoring

- Monitor BP daily before surgery.
- Invasive hemodynamic monitoring intraoperatively
- Monitor urine metanephrine and catecholamine 2 weeks postoperatively and, if normal, recheck annually.
- Ensure resolution of HTN and normalization of blood glucose.

DIET

- Preoperatively, after initiation of α-blocker, encourage high-sodium diet (>5,000 mg/day) to increase blood volume and prevent orthostasis. May be contraindicated in setting of renal or heart failure.
- Postoperatively, resume general diet.

PATIENT EDUCATION

National Adrenal Disease Foundation (NADF), 505 Northern Blvd., Great Neck, NY 11021; 516-487-4992; e-mail: nadfmail@aol.com

PROGNOSIS

- Survival after surgical removal of a benign tumor is similar to age-matched controls.
- Recurrence rate is 8–15%.
- 5-year survival for malignant disease is <50% (3)[A].

COMPLICATIONS

- The most common lethal complications are myocardial infarction and cerebrovascular accident.
- Postural hypotension due to α-blockade can be ameliorated with saline volume expansion/high-sodium diet.
- Intraoperative hypertensive crisis can be managed with IV nitroprusside, nicardipine, and phentolamine.

REFERENCES

1. Karagiannis A, Mikhailidis DP, Athyros VG, et al. Pheochromocytoma: an update on genetics and management. *Endocr Relat Cancer*. 2007;14(4):935–956.
2. Bruynzeel H, Feelders RA, Groenland TH, et al. Risk factors for hemodynamic instability during surgery for pheochromocytoma. *J Clin Endocrinol Metab*. 2010;95(2):678–685.
3. Scholz T, Eisenhofer G, Pacak K, et al. Clinical review: current treatment of malignant pheochromocytoma. *J Clin Endocrinol Metab*. 2007;92(4):1217–1225.

SEE ALSO

Hypertension, Essential; Multiple Endocrine Neoplasia

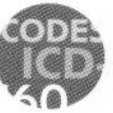

CODES

ICD10

- D35.00 Benign neoplasm of unspecified adrenal gland
- D35.02 Benign neoplasm of left adrenal gland
- D35.01 Benign neoplasm of right adrenal gland

CLINICAL PEARLS

- Rare catecholamine-secreting tumor with serious and potentially lethal cardiovascular complications.
- Clinical presentation is variable, but classic triad consists of episodic headaches, diaphoresis, and tachycardia/palpitations in association with HTN.
- Diagnosis by urine screen for catecholamines and their metabolites followed by imaging studies (CT, MRI)
- Surgical removal of tumor is standard therapy that must be preceded by a period of BP stabilization with nonselective α-adrenergic blockade, followed by β-adrenergic blockade several days later.
- High-salt diet is initiated after α-blockade to minimize orthostasis and ensure volume expansion.
- Never initiate a β-blocker before adequate α-blockade is achieved.

PHOTODERMATITIS

Aamir Siddiqi, MD

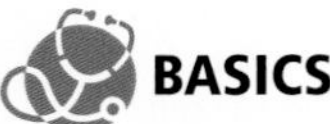

BASICS

DESCRIPTION

- Light-induced eruptions seen in a pattern of photodistribution
  - Phototoxic reactions: result of an acute toxic effect on skin of ultraviolet (UV) light alone (sunburn) or together with a photosensitizing substance (nonallergic) (1)
  - Photoallergic eruptions: a form of allergic dermatitis resulting from combined effects of a photosensitizing substance (drugs or chemical) plus UV light (immunologic/delayed hypersensitivity)
  - Polymorphous light eruption (PLE): chronic, intermittent, light-induced eruption with erythematous papules, urticaria, or vesicles on areas exposed to sunlight
- System(s) affected: skin/exocrine
- Synonym(s): sun poisoning; sun allergy

EPIDEMIOLOGY

Incidence

- PLE usually occurs after the first intense exposure to the sun in the spring or summer.
- Predominant age: all ages
- Predominant sex: male = female

Prevalence

May be as high as 20% in some areas

ETIOLOGY AND PATHOPHYSIOLOGY

- Sunlight
- Phenothiazines
- Diuretics
- Tetracyclines, sulfonamides
- Oral contraceptives
- Topicals: psoralens, coal tars, photoactive dyes (eosin, acridine orange)
- 5-Fluorouracil
- Quinine
- Sunscreens containing *para*-aminobenzoic acid (PABA)
- In the United States, ~115 chemical agents used topically are known to cause photodermatitis.

Genetics

Predisposition occurs in inbred populations (e.g., Pima Indians).

RISK FACTORS

- Job-related exposure to sunlight
- Light and fair-colored skin

GENERAL PREVENTION

- Sunlight avoidance/protective clothing
- Identification and avoidance of causative drugs (see "Etiology and Pathophysiology")
- Sunscreens: Apply before exposure:
  - Zinc oxide: opaque, cosmetically less acceptable
  - Chemical: Use sun-protective factor (SPF) >30 for maximum protection; substantively resistant to sweat and swimming; cosmetically more acceptable (2)
- Avoid direct sun exposure.
- Wear appropriate gear to avoid sunlight exposure.

COMMONLY ASSOCIATED CONDITIONS

- Sunlight aggravation of systemic lupus erythematosus (SLE)
- Persistent light reactivity
- Actinic reticuloid

DIAGNOSIS

HISTORY

Pruritic and often painful rash developing in sun-exposed areas

PHYSICAL EXAM

- Phototoxic (3)
  - Erythema
  - With increasing severity: vesicles and bullae
  - Classic example: sunburn
  - Nails may exhibit onycholysis.
  - Chronic: epidermal thickening, elastosis, telangiectasia, and pigmentary changes
  - Sharp lines of demarcation between involved and uninvolved skin (sunlight exposure)
  - Phototoxic eruption due to topicals: area of application
  - Usually develops shortly after sun exposure
  - Hyperpigmentation may follow resolution.
  - Pain
- Photoallergic (3)
  - Papules with erythema and occasionally vesicles
  - Area exposed to light with less distinct borders
  - Usually delayed ≥24 hours after exposure
  - May spread to unexposed areas
  - Pruritus
- PLE
  - Erythematous papules
  - Occasionally urticaria or vesicles
  - Scattered over sun-exposed areas with normal skin in between
  - Can spread to nonexposed areas
  - Often flares in spring or early summer
  - Desensitization effect (lessens over the course of the summer)
  - Burning or pruritus may precede lesions.

DIFFERENTIAL DIAGNOSIS

SLE

DIAGNOSTIC TESTS & INTERPRETATION

Follow-Up Tests & Special Considerations

Antinuclear antibody to rule out SLE if suspected

Diagnostic Procedures/Other

- Phototesting: exposing patient to UV light
- Photopatch testing: applying suspected agents and chemicals to patient's skin
- Skin biopsy: to rule out other disorders if necessary

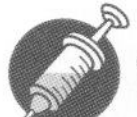

TREATMENT

GENERAL MEASURES

- Appropriate health care: outpatient
- Avoid sunlight/limit exposure.
- Protective clothing/sunscreens
- Ice packs/cold water compresses

MEDICATION

Topical corticosteroids (triamcinolone acetonide 0.25%, 0.1%, 0.5%; betamethasone valerate 0.1% cream, others)

ALERT

Limit use of fluorinated steroids on face; use hydrocortisone ointments.

- NSAIDs (ibuprofen 600 mg QID, indomethacin 25 mg PO TID, aspirin, others)
- Prednisone for severe reactions (0.5–1 mg/kg/day PO) × 3–10 days
- Antihistamines for pruritus (hydroxyzine 25–50 mg PO QID)
- Sunscreens (>30 SPF) for prevention: Use broad-spectrum sunscreen to block both UVA and UVB. PABA may aggravate photodermatitis in sensitized patients (due to the sulfa moiety).
- Aspirin or ibuprofen taken orally or NSAID applied topically (diclofenac) before sun exposure may modestly reduce erythema and pain of sunburn.

Geriatric Considerations

More likely to experience adverse reactions to causative drugs

COMPLEMENTARY & ALTERNATIVE MEDICINE

- PO β-carotene seems to modestly reduce the risk of sunburn in individuals who are sensitive to sun exposure.
- Omega-3 fatty acid intake may decrease the sensitivity of skin to UV exposure (4).
- Compresses made from tea bags steeped in a small amount of water may reduce itching and burning of sunburn (5).

ONGOING CARE

FOLLOW-UP RECOMMENDATIONS

Avoid direct sunlight.

PATIENT EDUCATION

- Avoidance of direct sunlight exposure
- Avoidance of photosensitizing drugs
- Protective clothing (e.g., hats, long sleeves)
- Sunscreens >30 SPF

PROGNOSIS

Good with avoidance/protection measures

COMPLICATIONS

Rare (secondary bacterial infection)

REFERENCES

1. Smith E, Kiss F, Porter RM, et al. A review of UVA-mediated photosensitivity disorders. *Photochem Photobiol Sci*. 2012;11(1):199–206.
2. Kalia S, Laurentiu Haiducu M. Sunscreen and sun protection: shedding light on recent advances. *J Cutan Med Surg*. 2011;15(Suppl 1):S382–S386.
3. Glatz M, Hofbauer GF. Phototoxic and photoallergic cutaneous drug reactions. *Chem Immunol Allergy*. 2012;97:167–179.
4. Pilkington SM, Watson RE, Nicolaou A, et al. Omega-3 polyunsaturated fatty acids: photoprotective macronutrients. *Exp Dermatol*. 2011;20(7):537–543.
5. Saraf S, Gupta A, Kaur CD, et al. Dermatological consequences of photosensitization with an approach to treat them naturally. *Pak J Biol Sci*. 2014;17(2):167–172.

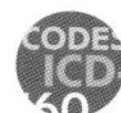

CODES

ICD10

- L56.8 Oth acute skin changes due to ultraviolet radiation
- L57.8 Oth skin changes due to chr expsr to non-ionizing radiation
- L56.4 Polymorphous light eruption

CLINICAL PEARLS

- Choose a sunscreen with an SPF of at least 30 with full-spectrum protection (UVA and UVB) for the best efficacy.
- The most common medications that predispose to photosensitivity include tetracyclines and sulfonamide. However, many other medications may cause photosensitivity.

PILONIDAL DISEASE

Tam Nguyen, MD, FAAFP

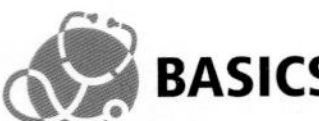

BASICS

DESCRIPTION

- Pilonidal disease results from an abscess, or sinus tract, in the upper part of the natal (gluteal) cleft.
- Synonym(s): jeep disease

EPIDEMIOLOGYS

Incidence

- 16–26/100,000 per year
- Predominant sex: male > female (3–4:1)
- Predominant age: 2nd–3rd decade, rare >45 years
- Ethnic consideration: whites > blacks > Asians

Prevalence

Surgical procedures show male:female ratio of 4:1, yet incidence data are 10:1.

ETIOLOGY AND PATHOPHYSIOLOGY

Pilonidal means "nest of hair"; hair in the natal cleft allows hair to be drawn into the deeper tissues via negative pressure caused by movement of the buttocks (50%); follicular occlusion from stretching, and blocking of pores with debris (50%).

- Inflammation of SC gluteal tissues with secondary infection and sinus tract formation
- Polymicrobial, likely from enteric pathogens given proximity to anorectal contamination

Genetics

- Congenital dimple in the natal cleft/spina bifida occulta
- Follicular-occluding tetrad: acne conglobata, dissecting cellulitis, hidradenitis suppurativa, pilonidal

RISK FACTORS

- Sedentary/prolonged sitting
- Excessive body hair
- Obesity/increased sacrococcygeal fold thickness
- Congenital natal dimple
- Trauma to coccyx

GENERAL PREVENTION

- Weight loss
- Trim hair in/around gluteal cleft weekly
- Hygiene
- Ingrown hair prevention/follicle unblocking

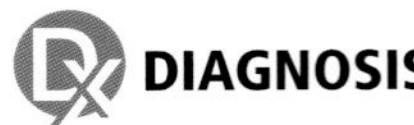

DIAGNOSIS

HISTORY

3 distinct clinical presentations

- Asymptomatic: painless cyst or sinus at the top of the gluteal cleft
- Acute abscess: severe pain, swelling, discharge from the top of the gluteal cleft that may or may not have drained spontaneously
- Chronic abscess: persistent drainage from a sinus tract at the top of the gluteal cleft

PHYSICAL EXAM

- Common: inflamed cystic mass at the top of the gluteal cleft with limited surrounding erythema ± drainage or a sinus tract
- Less common: significant cellulitis of the surrounding tissues near the gluteal cleft

DIFFERENTIAL DIAGNOSIS

- Furunculosis
- Hidradenitis suppurativa
- Anal fistula
- Perirectal abscess
- Crohn disease

DIAGNOSTIC TESTS & INTERPRETATION

Initial Tests (lab, imaging)

- Consider CBC and wound culture but generally not necessary for less-severe infections.
- MRI might be considered to differentiate between perirectal abscess and pilonidal disease.

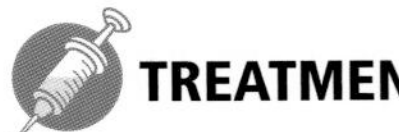

TREATMENT

GENERAL MEASURES

Shave area; remove hair from crypts weekly.

MEDICATION

- Antibiotics not indicated unless there is significant cellulitis (1).
- If antibiotics are needed, a culture to direct therapy might be useful.
- Cefazolin plus metronidazole or amoxicillin-clavulanate are often used empirically if cellulitis is suspected.

ISSUES FOR REFERRAL

- Patients who cannot comply with frequent dressing changes required after incision and drainage (I&D)
- Patients who have recurrence after I&D
- Patients who have complex disease with multiple sinus tracts

ADDITIONAL THERAPIES

- I&D with only enough packing to allow the cyst to drain; overpacking not indicated
- Antibiotics only if significant cellulitis; temporizing, not curative
- Negative pressure wound therapy (2)[A]
- Laser epilation of hair in the gluteal fold (3,4)[B]

SURGERY/OTHER PROCEDURES

6 levels of care based on severity or recurrence of disease; recent innovations in technique are aimed at expediting healing and minimizing recurrence

- I&D, remove hair, curette granulation tissue (5,6)[A].
- Excision of midline "pits" allows drainage of lateral sinus tracts (pit picking) (7,8)[A].
- Pilonidal cystotomy: Insert probe into sinus tract, excise overlying skin, and close wound (7,9)[B].
- Marsupialization: Excise overlying skin and roof of cyst, and suture skin edges to cyst floor (5,10)[B].
- Excision: use of flap closure. No clear benefit for open healing over surgical closure (11)[B]
- Off-midline surgical excision (cleft lift or modified Karydakis procedure): A systematic review showed a clear benefit in favor of off-midline rather than midline wound closure. When closure of pilonidal sinuses is the desired surgical option, off-midline closure should be the standard management (5,7,12)[A].

INPATIENT CONSIDERATIONS

Admission Criteria/Initial Stabilization

- Severe cellulitis
- Large area excision

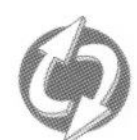

ONGOING CARE

FOLLOW-UP RECOMMENDATIONS

- Frequent dressing changes required after I&D
- Follow-up wound checks to assess for recurrence.

Patient Monitoring

Monitor for fever, more extensive cellulitis.

PATIENT EDUCATION

- Wash area briskly with washcloth daily.
- Shave the area weekly.
- Remove any embedded hair from the crypt.
- Avoid prolonged sitting.

PROGNOSIS

- Simple I&D has a 55% failure rate; median time to healing is 5 weeks.
- More extensive surgical excisions involve hospital stays and longer time to heal.

COMPLICATIONS

Malignant degeneration is a rare complication of untreated chronic pilonidal disease.

REFERENCES

1. Mavros MN, Mitsikostas PK, Alexiou VG, et al. Antimicrobials as an adjunct to pilonidal disease surgery: a systematic review of the literature. *Eur J Clin Microbiol Infect Dis*. 2013;32(7):851–858.
2. Farrell D, Murphy S. Negative pressure wound therapy for recurrent pilonidal disease: a review of the literature. *J Wound Ostomy Continence Nurs*. 2011;38(4):373–378.
3. Loganathan A, Arsalani Zadeh R, Hartley J. Pilonidal disease: time to reevaluate a common pain in the rear! *Dis Colon Rectum*. 2012;55(4):491–493.
4. Oram Y, Kahraman F, Karincao lu Y, et al. Evaluation of 60 patients with pilonidal sinus treated with laser epilation after surgery. *Dermatol Surg*. 2010;36(1):88–91.
5. Humphries AE, Duncan JE. Evaluation and management of pilonidal disease. *Surg Clin North Am*. 2010;90(1):113–124, Table of Contents.
6. Kement M, Oncel M, Kurt N, et al. Sinus excision for the treatment of limited chronic pilonidal disease: results after a medium-term follow-up. *Dis Colon Rectum*. 2006;49(11):1758–1762.
7. Al-Khamis A, McCallum I, King PM, et al. Healing by primary versus secondary intention after surgical treatment for pilonidal sinus. *Cochrane Database Syst Rev*. 2010;(1):CD006213.
8. Iesalnieks I, Deimel S, Kienle K, et al. Pit-picking surgery for pilonidal disease [in German]. *Chirurg*. 2011;82(10):927–931.
9. da Silva JH. Pilonidal cyst: cause and treatment. *Dis Colon Rectum*. 2000;43(8):1146–1156.
10. Aydede H, Erhan Y, Sakarya A, et al. Comparison of three methods in surgical treatment of pilonidal disease. *ANZ J Surg*. 2001;71(6):362–364.
11. Washer JD, Smith DE, Carman ME, et al. Gluteal fascial advancement: an innovative, effective method for treating pilonidal disease. *Am Surg*. 2010;76(2):154–156.
12. Ates M, Dirican A, Sarac M, et al. Short and long-term results of the Karydakis flap versus the Limberg flap for treating pilonidal sinus disease: a prospective randomized study. *Am J Surg*. 2011;202(5):568–573.

ADDITIONAL READING

- Aygen E, Arslan K, Dogru O, et al. Crystallized phenol in nonoperative treatment of previously operated, recurrent pilonidal disease. *Dis Colon Rectum*. 2010;53(6):932–935.
- Bradley L. Pilonidal sinus disease: a review. Part one. *J Wound Care*. 2010;19(11):504–508.
- Harlak A, Mentes O, Kilic S, et al. Sacrococcygeal pilonidal disease: analysis of previously proposed risk factors. *Clinics (Sao Paulo)*. 2010;65(2):125–131.
- Rao MM, Zawislak W, Kennedy R, et al. A prospective randomised study comparing two treatment modalities for chronic pilonidal sinus with a 5-year follow-up. *Int J Colorectal Dis*. 2010;25(3):395–400.
- Theodoropoulos GE, Vlahos K, Lazaris AC, et al. Modified Bascom's asymmetric midgluteal cleft closure technique for recurrent pilonidal disease: early experience in a military hospital. *Dis Colon Rectum*. 2003;49(9):1286–1291.

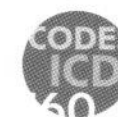

CODES

ICD10

- L05.91 Pilonidal cyst without abscess
- L05.92 Pilonidal sinus without abscess
- L05.01 Pilonidal cyst with abscess

CLINICAL PEARLS

- Avoid prolonged sitting.
- Lose weight.
- Trim hair in gluteal cleft weekly.
- Refer recurring infections for more definitive surgical management.

PINWORMS

Jonathan MacClements, MD, FAAFP

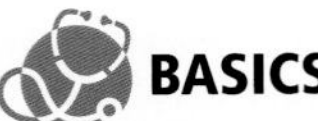

BASICS

DESCRIPTION

- Intestinal infection with *Enterobius vermicularis*
  - Characterized by perineal and perianal itching
  - Usually worse at night
- System(s) affected: gastrointestinal; skin/exocrine
- Synonym(s): enterobiasis

EPIDEMIOLOGY

Predominant age: 5–14 years

Prevalence

- Most common helminthic infection in the United States
  - 20–42 million people harboring the parasite
- ~30% of children are infected throughout the world.

Pediatric Considerations

More common in children, who are more likely to become reinfected

ETIOLOGY AND PATHOPHYSIOLOGY

- Small white worms (2–13 mm) inhabit the cecum, appendix, and adjacent portions of the ascending colon following ingestion.
- Female worms migrate to the perineal areas at night to deposit eggs; this causes local irritation and itching of the perianal area.
- Scratching of the perianal and perineal areas leads to autoingestion of the eggs and continuation of pinworm's life cycle in the host. Eggs incubate 1–2 months in the host small intestine. When mature, female pinworm then migrate to colon where they lay eggs around the anus at night and the lifecycle continues.
- Infestation by the intestinal nematode *E.* (*Oxyuris*) *vermicularis*

RISK FACTORS

- Institutionalization
- Crowded living conditions
- Poor hygiene
- Warm climate
- Handling of infected children's clothing or bedding

GENERAL PREVENTION

- Hand hygiene, especially after bowel movements
- Clip and maintain short fingernails.
- Wash anus and genitals at least once a day, preferably during shower.
- Avoid scratching anus and putting fingers near nose (pinworm eggs can also be inhaled) or mouth.

COMMONLY ASSOCIATED CONDITIONS

Pruritus ani

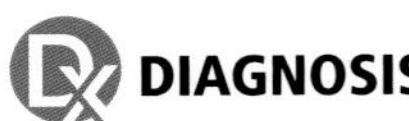

DIAGNOSIS

HISTORY

Many patients are asymptomatic. Common symptoms include the following:

- Perianal or perineal itching
- Vulvovaginitis
- Dysuria
- Abdominal pain (rare)
- Insomnia (typically due to pruritus)

PHYSICAL EXAM

Perineal and perianal exam. Particularly in early morning to look for evidence of migrating worms.

DIFFERENTIAL DIAGNOSIS

- Idiopathic pruritus ani (1)[A]
- Atopic dermatitis
- Contact dermatitis
- Psoriasis
- Lichen planus
- Infection with human papillomavirus
- Herpes simplex
- Fungal infections
- Erythrasma
- Scabies
- Vaginitis
- Hemorrhoids

DIAGNOSTIC TESTS & INTERPRETATION

- Adhesive tape test (2)[A]
  - A piece of transparent cellophane tape is stuck to the perianal skin in the early morning before bathing and then affixed to a microscope slide after removal to look for pinworm eggs.
  - If performed on 3 consecutive mornings, this test has 90% sensitivity.
  - Alternatively, anal swabs or a pinworm paddle coated with adhesive material also can be useful.
  - Scrapings from under fingernails of affected individuals can also reveal pinworm eggs.
- Digital rectal exam with saline slide preparation of stool on gloved finger
- Stool samples are not helpful.
- *Routine stool examination for ova and parasites is positive in only 10–15% of infected patients.*

Test Interpretation

Identification of ova on low-power microscopy or direct visualization of the female worm (10-mm long); ova are asymmetric, flattened on 1 side, and measure $56 \times 27\ \mu m$.

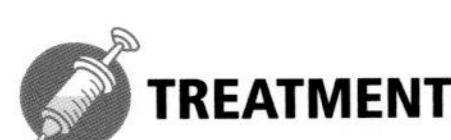

TREATMENT

MEDICATION

First Line

- Treatment options include any of the following:
  - Mebendazole (Vermox): chewable 100-mg tablet as a single dose in adults and children >2 years of age; may repeat in 2–3 weeks; use with caution in children <2 years of age (3,4)[A].
  - Albendazole (Albenza): 400 mg PO as a single dose in adults and children >2 years of age; may repeat in 2–3 weeks; 200 mg PO as a single dose repeated in 7 days in children ≤2 years of age (3,4)[A].

– Pyrantel pamoate (Pin-X, Reese's Pinworm Medicine): oral liquid or tablet 11 mg/kg as a single dose in adults and children >2 years of age; maximum dose 1 g. Use with caution in children <2 years of age (3,4)[A].

- Repeat treatment after 2 weeks is often recommended due to the high frequency of reinfection. Refractory cases may (rarely) require retreatment every 2 weeks for 4–6 cycles.
- All symptomatic family members should be treated.

Pregnancy Considerations

Drug therapy should be avoided in pregnancy. Treatment should be delayed until after delivery (3,4)[A].

ONGOING CARE

FOLLOW-UP RECOMMENDATIONS

Unnecessary unless symptoms do not abate following initial drug therapy

PATIENT EDUCATION

- Take medicine with food.
- Practice good hygiene: hand washing and perineal/perianal hygiene; particularly after bowel movements
- Encourage frequent and careful hand washing
- Clip fingernails.
- Clothing and bedding should be washed after diagnosis to prevent reinfection. Do not shake linen and clothing before laundering because this may spread the eggs.
- Do not share washcloths.
- Do not allow children to co-bathe during treatment and for 2 weeks after the final treatment; showering is preferred.

PROGNOSIS

- Asymptomatic carriers are common.
- Drug therapy is curative in over 90% of symptomatic infections.
- Reinfection is common, especially among children.

COMPLICATIONS

- Perianal scratching may lead to bacterial superinfection.
- Females: vulvovaginitis, urethritis, endometritis, and salpingitis (5)[A]
- UTIs
- Rarely, ectopic disease involving granulomas of the pelvis, urinary tract, female genitourinary tract, and appendix

REFERENCES

1. Stermer E, Sukhotnic I, Shaoul R. Pruritus ani: an approach to an itching condition. *J Pediatr Gastroenterol Nutr*. 2009;48(5):513–516.
2. Kucik CJ. Common intestinal parasites. *Am Fam Physician*. 2004;69(5):1161–1168.
3. Enterobius vermicularis. In: *Drugs for Parasitic Infections. Treatment guidelines from The Medical Letter*, Vol. 8 (Suppl), 2010.
4. CDC Resources for Health Professionals. Parasites—Enterobiasis (also known as Pinworm Infection). www.cdc.gov/parasites/pinworm/health_professionals/index.html. Accessed 2014.
5. Dennie J. Distressing perineal and vaginal pain in prepubescent girsl: an aetiology. *J Paediatr Child Health*. 2013;49(2):138–140.

ADDITIONAL READING

- Cram EB. Studies on oxyuriasis, 28. Summary and conclusions. *Am J Dis Child*. 1943;65:46–59.
- Hamblin J. Pinworms in pregnancy. *J Am Board Fam Pract*. 1995;8(4):321–324.
- Johansson J, Ignatova S. Pinworm infestation mimicking Crohns' disease. *Case Rep Gastrointest Med*. 2013;2013:706197.
- Lamps LW. Infectious causes of appendicitis. *Infect Dis Clin North Am*. 2010;24(4):995–1018.
- Xiao SH, Utzinger J, Tanner M, et al. Advances with the Chinese anthelminthic drug tribendimidine in clinical trials and laboratory investigations. *Acta Trop*. 2013;126(2):115–126.

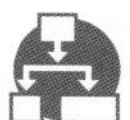

SEE ALSO

Pruritus Ani

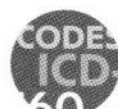

CODES

ICD10

B80 Enterobiasis

CLINICAL PEARLS

- Nocturnal or early morning perianal itch (often manifest as restless sleep or insomnia), particularly in children, is hallmark of symptomatic pinworm infection.
- Treatment for pinworms includes use of mebendazole, albendazole, or pyrantel pamoate.
- Close contacts should be treated as well.
- Retreatment after 2 weeks is typically recommended.

PITUITARY ADENOMA

Anup K. Sabharwal, MD, MBA, FACE, CCD • Lewis S. Blevins, Jr., MD

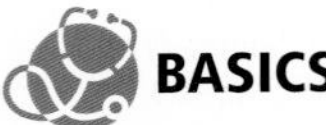

BASICS

DESCRIPTION

Typically benign, slow-growing tumors that arise from cells in the pituitary gland

- Pituitary adenomas have been identified as the 3rd most frequent intracranial tumor; accounts for 10–25%.
- Subtypes (hormonal): prolactinoma (PRL) 50%, nonfunctioning pituitary adenomas 30%, somatotroph adenoma (growth hormone [GH]) 15–20%, corticotroph adenoma (adrenocorticotrophic hormone [ACTH]) 5–10%, thyrotroph adenoma (thyroid-stimulating hormone [TSH]) <1%, gonadotropinoma (luteinizing hormone/follicle-stimulating hormone [LH/FSH]), mixed
- Defined as microadenoma <10 mm and macroadenoma ≥10 mm
- May secrete hormones and/or cause mass effects

EPIDEMIOLOGY

- Predominant age: Age increases incidence.
- Predominant sex: female > male (3:2) for microadenomas (often delayed diagnosis in men)

Incidence

- Autopsy studies have found microadenomas in 3–27% and macroadenomas in <0.5% of people without any pituitary disorders.
- MRI scans illustrate abnormalities consistent with pituitary adenoma in 1/10 persons.
- Clinically apparent pituitary tumors are seen in 18/100,000 persons.

ETIOLOGY AND PATHOPHYSIOLOGY

- Monoclonal adenohypophysial cell growth
- Hormonal effects of functional microadenomas often prompt diagnosis before mass effect.
- Prolactin increased by functional prolactinomas or inhibited dopaminergic suppression by stalk effect

Genetics

- Carney complex
- Familial isolated pituitary adenomas: ~15% have mutations in the aryl hydrocarbon receptor–interacting protein gene (*AIP*); present at a younger age and are larger in size (1)
- McCune-Albright syndrome
- Multiple endocrine neoplasia type 1 (MEN1)–like phenotype (MEN4): germline mutation in the cyclin-dependent kinase inhibitor 1B (CDKN1B) (1)

RISK FACTORS

Multiple endocrine neoplasias

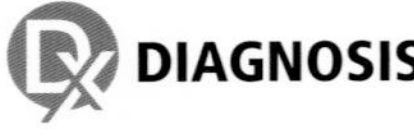

DIAGNOSIS

HISTORY

- Common
  - Hyperprolactinemia: infertility, amenorrhea, galactorrhea, gynecomastia, impotence
  - Headache (sellar expansion)
  - Visual disturbances: bitemporal hemianopsia
- Less common
  - Hypersomatotropinemia: acromegaly (coarse facial features, hand/foot swelling, carpal tunnel syndrome, hyperhidrosis, left ventricular hypertrophy)
  - Hyposomatotropinemia: failure to thrive (FTT) (children), asymptomatic (adults)
  - Intracranial pressure (ICP) elevation: headache, nausea, seizures
  - Hypercorticotropinemia: Cushing disease (supraclavicular/dorsocervical fat pad thickening, moon face, hirsutism, acne, plethora, abdominal striae, centripetal obesity with thin limbs, easy bruising and bleeding, hyperglycemia)
- Rare
  - Apoplexy: headache, sudden collapse
  - Secondary hyperthyroidism: palpitations, diaphoresis, heat intolerance, diarrhea
  - Secondary adrenal insufficiency: weakness, irritability, anorexia, nausea/vomiting
- Hypothalamic compression: temperature, thirst/appetite disorders

PHYSICAL EXAM

- Common
  - Visual disturbances: bitemporal hemianopsia
  - Hyperprolactinemia: hypogonadism, galactorrhea, gynecomastia
  - Hypersomatotropinemia: acromegaly (coarse features, hand/foot swelling, diaphoresis)
  - Hyposomatotropinemia: FTT (children)
- Less common
  - ICP elevation: papilledema, dementia
  - Cushing disease: centripetal obesity, supraclavicular fat pad thickening, moon face, hirsutism, acne
- Rare
  - Apoplexy: hypotension, hypoglycemia, tachycardia, oliguria
  - Secondary hyperthyroidism: tachycardia, tachypnea, diaphoresis, warm/moist skin, tremor
  - Adrenal crisis: orthostatic hypotension
- Hypothalamic compression: temperature dysregulation, obesity, increased urination

DIFFERENTIAL DIAGNOSIS

Pituitary hyperplasia (e.g., pregnancy, primary hypothyroidism, menopause), Rathke cleft cyst, granulomatous disease (e.g., tuberculosis), lymphocytic hypophysitis, metastatic tumor, germinoma, craniopharyngioma

DIAGNOSTIC TESTS & INTERPRETATION

Select based on dysfunction(s) suspected

- Somatotrophic (GH secreting: 40–130/million)
  - Acromegaly/hypersomatotropinemia: serum IGF-1 elevated; oral glucose tolerance test with GH given at 0, 30, and 60 minutes (normally suppresses GH to <1 g/L)
  - Hyposomatotropinemia: low growth hormone–releasing hormone response
- Corticotropic
  - Cushing disease/hypercorticotropinemia
  - 24-hour urinary-free cortisol >50 μg
  - Overnight low-dose dexamethasone suppression test (DMST): normal plasma cortisol (FPC) >1.8 μg/dL at 8 AM (after 1 mg given at 11 PM on night prior)
  - ACTH level assay (if DMST results abnormal): <20 pg/mL = adrenal tumor; ≥20 pg/mL = ectopic/pituitary source
  - Hypocorticotropinemia/secondary glucocorticoid deficiency: high-dose corticotropin stimulation test: FPC <10 g/dL at baseline, with an increase of <25% 1 hour after 250 μg; metyrapone test: 11-deoxycortisol <150 ng/L after 2 g given (prepare to give steroids because test may worsen insufficiency)
- Gonadotrophic/hypogonadotropinism: gonadotropin-releasing hormone stimulation of LH/FSH blunted in pituitary hypergonadism but increased in primary hypogonadism
- Lactotrophic (prolactin secreting): hyperprolactinemia: serum PRL >20 ng/mL
- Thyrotrophic (TSH secreting): hyper-/hypothyroidism: TSH and free T_4 both increased for pituitary hyperthyroidism and both decreased for pituitary hypothyroidism

Initial Tests (lab, imaging)

- A typical panel for asymptomatic tumors: prolactin, GH, IGF-1, ACTH, 24-hour urinary-free cortisol or overnight DMST, βHCG, FSH, LH, TSH, free T_4
- Screening for *AIP* mutations may be offered to families of patients with pituitary adenoma, where available.
- MRI preferred (>90% sensitivity and specificity) after biochemically confirmed
- Octreotide scintigraphy is useful in identifying tumors with somatostatin receptors (2)[B].

Diagnostic Procedures/Other

Inferior petrosal sinus sampling: ACTH sampled from inferior petrosal sinuses to distinguish Cushing disease (pituitary source) from ectopic ACTH

Test Interpretation

- Cell types identified by immunohistochemistry
- Light microscope: eosinophilic (GH, PRL), basophilic (FSH/LH, TSH, ACTH), chromophobic

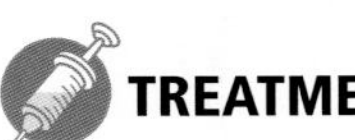

TREATMENT

Medical therapy is primary therapy for prolactinomas and adjunct for other tumors.

MEDICATION

First Line

- Hyperprolactinemia: Dopamine agonists increase dopaminergic suppression of PRL.
  - Cabergoline (Dostinex): D_2 receptor–specific
    - Initial dose: 0.25 mg PO once or twice weekly
    - Maintenance dose: Increase q4wk by 0.25 mg 2 times/week per PRL (max 2 mg/week).
    - Contraindications: hypersensitivity (ergots), uncontrolled hypertension (HTN), pregnancy
    - Precautions: caution with liver impairment
    - Interactions: may be inhibited by tricyclic antidepressants, phenothiazines, opiates
    - Adverse reactions: orthostatic hypotension, vertigo, dyspepsia, hot flashes
  - Bromocriptine (Parlodel): D_2 receptor–specific
    - Initial dose: 1.25–2.5 mg PO daily (give with food)
    - Maintenance dose: increase by 2.5 mg/day q2–7d (max 15 mg/day)
    - Contraindications: hypersensitivity (ergots), uncontrolled HTN, pregnancy; preferred over cabergoline if required
    - Precautions: Caution with liver impairment.
    - Interactions: may be inhibited by tricyclic antidepressants, phenothiazines, opiates
    - Adverse reactions: orthostatic hypotension, seizures, hallucinations, stroke, myocardial infarction
- Somatotropinoma
  - Long-acting analogues of somatostatin (Sandostatin LAR and lanreotide Autogel)
    - Sandostatin LAR: 20 mg q28d (2)[A]; lanreotide Autogel 90 mg q28d; titrate per package insert.
    - Contraindication: hypersensitivity

P

- Precautions: Caution with biliary, thyroid, cardiac, liver, or kidney disease.
- Interactions: pimozide increases risk of QT prolongation; variable effects with β-blockers, diuretics, oral glycemic agents
- Adverse reactions: ascending cholangitis, arrhythmias, congestive heart failure, glycemic instability
- More effective as adjuvant than as primary treatment for somatotropinomas

– Pegvisomant (Somavert): growth hormone receptor antagonist
- Initial dose: 40 mg SC × 1, then 10 mg daily and titrate by 5 mg every 4–6 weeks based on IGF-1 levels (maximum 30 mg/day maintenance dose)
- Contraindication: hypersensitivity
- Precautions: caution if GH-secreting tumors, diabetes mellitus, impaired liver function
- Interactions: NSAIDs, opiates, insulins, oral glycemic agents
- Adverse reactions: hepatitis, tumor growth, GH secretion

- Corticotropinemia: peripheral inhibitors
  - Mitotane (Lysodren)
    - Initial dose: 2–6 g/day divided PO TID (max 19 g/day)
    - Maintenance dose: 2–16 g TID
    - Contraindication: hypersensitivity
    - Precautions: Caution with liver dysfunction and brain damage.
    - Interactions: contraindicated with rotavirus vaccine; caution with other vaccines.
    - Adverse reactions: HTN, orthostatic hypotension, hemorrhagic cystitis, rash
  - Ketoconazole
    - Dosing: 200 mg PO TID (max 1,200 mg/day)
    - Contraindications: hypersensitivity, achlorhydria, fungal meningitis, impaired liver function
    - Precautions: Caution with liver dysfunction.
    - Interactions: contraindicated with dronedarone, methadone, statins, pimozide, sirolimus; caution with other antifungals.
    - Adverse reactions: adrenal insufficiency, thrombocytopenia, hepatic failure, hepatotoxicity, anaphylaxis, leukopenia, hemolytic anemia
  - Signifor (pasireotide)
    - Dosing: initially, 0.6–0.9 mg twice daily, then 0.3–0.9 mg twice daily
    - Contraindication: none
    - Precautions: hypocortisolism, hyperglycemia, bradycardia or QT prolongation, liver test elevations, cholelithiasis, and other pituitary hormone deficiencies
  - Korlym (mifepristone):
    - Dosing: Administer PO once daily with a meal. The recommended starting dose is 300 mg once daily. Not to exceed 600 mg daily in renal impairment.
  - Contraindication: pregnancy, use of simvastatin or lovastatin and CYP3A substrates with narrow therapeutic range, concurrent long-term corticosteroid use, women with history of unexplained vaginal bleeding, women with endometrial hyperplasia with atypia or endometrial carcinoma
  - Precautions: adrenal insufficiency, hypokalemia, vaginal bleeding and endometrial changes, QT interval prolongation, use of strong CYP3A inhibitors
  - Interactions: potential interactions with drugs metabolized by CYP3A, CYP2C8/9, CYP2B6, and hormonal contraceptives. Nursing mothers should discontinue drug or discontinue nursing.
  - Adverse reactions: most common adverse reactions in Cushing syndrome (≥20%): nausea, fatigue, headache, decreased blood potassium, arthralgia, vomiting, peripheral edema, HTN, dizziness, decreased appetite, endometrial hypertrophy
- Gonadotropinemia
  - Bromocriptine: See earlier discussion.
- Thyrotropinemia
  - Somatostatin analogues: See earlier discussion.

Second Line

- Corticotropinemia: peripheral inhibitors
  - Metyrapone
    - Dose: 250 mg PO QID
    - Contraindication: porphyria
    - Precautions: Caution in liver/thyroid disease.
    - Interactions: Dilantin increases metabolism.
    - Adverse reactions: nausea, hypotension
- Gonadotropinemia
  - Octreotide: See earlier discussion.

ISSUES FOR REFERRAL

- Neurosurgery consultation for symptomatic tumors (except for prolactinoma)
- Ophthalmologist evaluation prior to surgery

ADDITIONAL THERAPIES

- Fractionated radiotherapy: often effective as adjunctive when surgery is inadequate (3)[B]
- Stereotactic radiosurgery: alternative to surgery in high-risk patients or as adjunct (3)[B]

SURGERY/OTHER PROCEDURES

- Most are now done endoscopically via translabial/transsphenoidal approach (4)[A].

- Indications: symptoms or treatment-resistant
- Follow-up: serial neurologic/hormonal evaluations to evaluate complications (e.g., diabetes insipidus, CNS damage) and need for more treatment
- Remission rates: 72–87% for microadenoma but only 50–56% for macroadenomas

INPATIENT CONSIDERATIONS

Admission Criteria/Initial Stabilization

Outpatient management unless apoplexy or adrenal crisis

- Treat pituitary apoplexy immediately to prevent death (see "Complications") (4)[A].

- Consider stress-dose steroids in frail or hemodynamically unstable patients.
- Maintain BP with fluids and/or pressor agents.
- Check serum sodium, serum osmolality, and urine specific gravity if polyuric or electrolytes are imbalanced.
- Contact neurosurgery.

IV Fluids

- Diabetes insipidus: hyposmolar IV fluids
- Adrenal crisis: normal saline

Nursing

- Pituitary apoplexy: Monitor inputs/outputs (I/Os), central venous pressure, and ICP and do frequent neurologic checks.
- Adrenal crisis: Monitor BP and I/Os.

Discharge Criteria

Keep as inpatient postoperatively until diabetes insipidus and/or adrenal insufficiency is managed.

ONGOING CARE

FOLLOW-UP RECOMMENDATIONS

Patient Monitoring

- Follow-up MRIs at 6 and 12 months after discharge
- Involved hormone(s) are followed postoperatively, especially after radiation, because hypopituitarism may develop 10–15 years after treatment.

PROGNOSIS

Depends on type, size, symptoms, therapy

COMPLICATIONS

- Postoperative diabetes insipidus and/or hypogonadism (usually transient/common)
- Pituitary apoplexy (acute/uncommon): acute hemorrhagic pituitary infarction; adrenal crisis with severe headache; surgical decompression required to prevent shock, coma, and death
- Nelson syndrome (subacute/uncommon): rapid adenoma growth postadrenalectomy
- Pituitary hormone insufficiency (chronic/uncommon): often years after treatment
- Optic nerve neuropathy and brain necrosis after >60 Gy radiotherapy (chronic/rare)

REFERENCES

1. Georgitsi M, Raitila A, Karhu A. Molecular diagnosis of pituitary adenoma predisposition caused by aryl hydrocarbon receptor-interacting protein gene mutations. *Proc Natl Acad Sci U S A*. 2007;104(10):4101–4105.
2. Tichomirowa MA, Daly AF, Beckers A. Treatment of pituitary tumors: somatostatin. *Endocrine*. 2005;28(1):93–100.
3. Mondok A, Szeifert GT, Mayer A. Treatment of pituitary tumors: radiation. *Endocrine*. 2005;28(1):77–85.
4. Buchfelder M. Treatment of pituitary tumors: surgery. *Endocrine*. 2005;28(1):67–75.

SEE ALSO

Cushing Disease and Cushing Syndrome; Galactorrhea

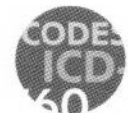

CODES

ICD10

D35.2 Benign neoplasm of pituitary gland

CLINICAL PEARLS

- An incidentaloma is an asymptomatic microadenoma found on imaging. General labs include PRL, GH, IGF-1, ACTH, 24-hour urinary-free cortisol/overnight DMST, β-subunit FSH, LH, TSH, and free T_4. Obtain follow-up MRIs at 6 and 12 months if normal, but consult endocrinology if not.
- Initial treatment selected for symptomatic pituitary adenoma includes a dopamine agonist for prolactinomas and surgical resection for all others.
- Pituitary apoplexy is a rapid hemorrhagic pituitary infarction due to compression of the blood supply. It is fatal within hours unless surgically decompressed.

PLACENTA PREVIA

Jeremy Golding, MD, FAAFP

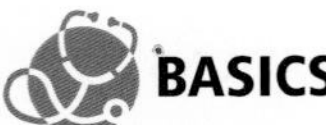

BASICS

DESCRIPTION

- Placental implantation in the lower uterine segment in advance of presenting fetal part and in proximity to/covering the internal os
- Complete/total previa: Placenta covers entire internal cervical os.
- Partial previa: Placenta covers part of internal cervical os.
- Marginal previa: Placental edge is adjacent to cervical os by US, but not overlapping, usually within 2 cm of os.
- Low-lying placenta: placental edge located in the lower uterine segment, but does not encroach on/cover the os; has been defined as within 2–3 cm of cervical os by US
- System(s) affected: cardiovascular; reproductive

EPIDEMIOLOGY

- Average gestational age of 1st bleed, 27–36 weeks
- Most common cause of minimally painful bleeding after 20 weeks' gestational age
- 10% of low-lying placentas at 10–20 weeks persist to term.

Incidence

- 0.4% of primiparous pregnancies, with increasing incidence with cesarean deliveries/other uterine scarring
- Up to 5% incidence in grand multiparous (>5 deliveries) women

Prevalence

- Prevalence decreases from early pregnancy to midpregnancy.
- Placenta previa complicates 0.3–0.5% of deliveries.

ETIOLOGY AND PATHOPHYSIOLOGY

- Not well understood
- Uterine scaring may predispose to placental implantation in the lower uterine segment.
- As lower uterine segment expands and the trophoblastic tissue expands toward the fundus, many marginal or low-lying placentas will resolve to a safe distance from the cervix to allow vaginal delivery.

Genetics

No genetic links have been identified.

RISK FACTORS

- History of placenta previa (relative risk [RR] = 8)
- Advanced maternal age (RR = 9 if >40 years of age)
- Multiparity (5% if >5 deliveries) (RR = 1.1–1.7)
- Assisted reproductive technology (RR = 2)
- Multiple gestation
- Smoking (RR = 1.4–3)
- Cocaine use
- Male fetus (RR = 1.4)
- Asian (RR = 1.9)
- Previous cesarean deliveries:
  - 1 previous C-section: RR = 4.5 (95% CI 3.6–5.5)
  - 4 previous C-sections: RR = 44.9 (95% CI 13.5–15)
- Induced/spontaneous abortion/curettage (Asherman syndrome) (RR = 1.6)
- Leiomyoma/history of lower uterine segment surgery

GENERAL PREVENTION

Once pregnancy is diagnosed, risk factors are not modifiable. If patient has any risk factors for previa and anatomic survey is suggestive of previa, serial US should be performed for monitoring purposes. Patient should be counseled regarding potential bleeding and should be triaged with all bleeding episodes.

COMMONLY ASSOCIATED CONDITIONS

- Abnormal presentations (e.g., oblique and/or transverse fetal lie)
- Antepartum/intrapartum/postpartum hemorrhage (RR = 9.81 for antepartum bleeding)
- Small for gestational age/intrauterine growth restriction (up to 16% in some reports after controlling for confounders)
- Vasa previa/velamentous insertion of the cord (particularly after resolution of early placenta previa)
- Premature rupture of membranes
- Evidence that shortened cervical length in the 3rd trimester is an independent risk factor for bleeding episodes
- Placenta previa is an independent risk factor for placenta accreta (OR = 54; 95% CI = 18–166):
  - Placenta accreta encompasses various types of abnormal placentations in which chorionic villi attach directly to/invade the myometrium.
  - Placenta previa in cases of prior cesarean delivery increases risk of accreta.
  - Elective delivery may be planned earlier (34–36 weeks) if accreta is suspected.

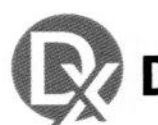

DIAGNOSIS

HISTORY

- Painless, bright-red vaginal bleeding in 2nd/3rd trimester (classic presentation)
- Painful bleeding if contractions are also present
- Decreased fetal movement/nonreassuring fetal heart tracing

PHYSICAL EXAM

ALERT

- Do not perform digital cervical exam in any woman with a complaint of bleeding until placental position has been verified.
- Careful sterile speculum exam can be performed to evaluate for vaginal/cervical source of bleeding.
- Evaluate for rupture of membranes as cause for bleeding.

DIFFERENTIAL DIAGNOSIS

- Abruptio placentae
- Vasa previa
- Labor
- Vaginal and cervical pathology, including polyps, erosion, cancer, trauma, or infections

DIAGNOSTIC TESTS & INTERPRETATION

- Transvaginal/translabial US is gold standard to identify placental position accurately (1).
- Transabdominal US may be performed bedside if skilled sonographer is not available.
- Contraction and fetal heart rate monitoring should be performed during evaluation.

Initial Tests (lab, imaging)

- Maternal blood type and antibody screen
- CBC: Normocytic, normochromic anemia may be present with acute bleeding.
- Prothrombin time (PT)/international normalization ratio (INR), and partial thromboplastin time (PTT): Coagulopathy is rare but may occur with significant blood loss.
- Fibrinogen is optional, and disseminated intravascular coagulation (DIC) panel is often inconclusive.
- Kleihauer-Betke test: Positive test indicates fetal–maternal transfusion may be present and can determine Rho(D) immunoglobulin dosing in Rh-negative patients.
- Cross-match at least 4 units of packed RBCs if clinically significant bleeding:
  - Development of US, especially the transvaginal scan, has helped in the definitive diagnosis and management of placenta previa.
  - External abdominal US with full, then empty bladder: Full bladder can cause compression of lower uterine segment causing a false appearance of previa.
  - Careful assessment may still miss some posterior previas if fetal vertex is low.
  - Vaginal probe sonography using 8.4-MHz transducer to define placental position further. Translabial US may also be used, but may not be able to discern specifically the characteristics of previas.
  - 3D US may help define placenta to cervical os distance for management of delivery.
- Given increased risk of accreta, the placental–uterine interface should be closely examined for evidence of lakes/other abnormal vasculature.
- MRI if concerned for placenta accreta without definitive US diagnosis; important also for surgical planning

Follow-Up Tests & Special Considerations

- Repeat hemoglobin/hematocrit determinations as needed to assess blood loss.
- Previas found on US before 35 weeks should have a repeat US prior to delivery:
  - 10% of previas at 10–20 weeks persist until term.
  - 62% of previas at 28–31 weeks persist until term.
  - 75% of previas at 32–35 weeks persist until term.

Test Interpretation

Placental pathology often shows giant trophoblasts at placental interface, evidence of abruption.

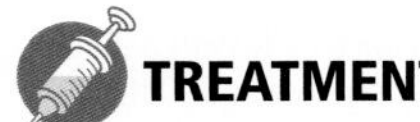

TREATMENT

GENERAL MEASURES

- Many patients with placenta previa will have no antepartum bleeding, and delivery may be electively planned between 36 and 38 weeks (2)[A],(3).
- Avoid vaginal exams, sexual intercourse, douching, or other vaginal manipulation.
- Amniocentesis can determine fetal lung maturity for elective delivery before 38 weeks but not recommended to guide the timing of delivery.
- A trial of labor may be considered in a tertiary care institution with placenta position >2 cm away from the cervix.

- Blood volume is increased in pregnancy; patient can lose >30% maternal blood volume before shock develops.
- Rh-negative women should receive 300 μg Rho(D) immunoglobulin (RhoGAM).

MEDICATION

First Line

- Oxygen supplementation if needed
- Adequate IV access via large-bore catheters
- Aggressive IV fluids/blood products as needed: fresh-frozen plasma, platelets, and packed RBCs
- Antenatal corticosteroids for symptomatic women between 23 and 34 weeks' gestation
- Tocolytics for uterine contractions may be used with caution, especially to allow for steroids for fetal lung maturity if possible. Calcium channel blockers such as nifedipine, loading dose of 10 mg PO q20min × 3, then q4–6h:
  - Watch for placental hypoperfusion (late decelerations on the fetal heart tracing).
  - Contraindications: term fetus/unstable maternal/fetal cardiovascular status

Second Line

Alternative tocolytics:

- Magnesium sulfate: 4–6 g IV load over 20 minutes, then 2g/hr continuous infusion; watch for toxicity: loss of reflexes, pulmonary edema, cardiac arrest.

ISSUES FOR REFERRAL

- Maternal–fetal medicine consult for delivery decisions regarding stable patients
- Neonatal ICU team should be alerted for high-risk delivery and consulted for preterm delivery.
- Appropriate interdisciplinary planning with blood bank, anesthesia, nursing staff in anticipation of placenta previa delivery
- Hospitals with obstetric units should consider massive transfusion protocols and staff training.

ADDITIONAL THERAPIES

Recombinant factor VII is an alternative blood product for DIC when fresh-frozen plasma and cryoprecipitate fail.

SURGERY/OTHER PROCEDURES

- Cesarean delivery is indicated for partial/complete previa.
- Timing of delivery depends on maternal stability and fetal lung maturity.
- Threshold for delivery is lower after 34 completed weeks' gestation and is planned by 38 weeks.

INPATIENT CONSIDERATIONS

Admission Criteria/Initial Stabilization

- Heavy vaginal bleeding warrants inpatient observation at least until 48 hours resolved.
- First bleed usually is self-limited. Patients should be observed and steroids for fetal lung maturity administered at gestational age 24–34 weeks. Once stable, preterm patients may be observed on an outpatient basis without difference in outcome.
- Patients managed outpatient should have reliable, rapid (within 20 minutes) transportation available to a tertiary care OB center.
- Multiple large bleeds may necessitate admission until scheduled delivery between 34 and 36 weeks, depending on institutional guidelines.
- May consider transfer to high-risk perinatology service based on patient condition, local services, and concern for accreta
- Bed rest and NPO until delivery decision made
- 2 large-bore IV sites and IV fluids as needed for resuscitation
- Continuous fetal heart and contraction monitoring

Nursing

- Continuous fetal heart and contraction monitoring
- Frequent vital signs, including fluid intake and output
- Monitor pad count, amount of vaginal bleeding.

Discharge Criteria

- Demonstration of fetal well-being by fetal heart tracing/biophysical profile
- Demonstration of maternal hemodynamic stability: no active bleeding for >48 hours
- Proximity of patient to health care facility and patient reliability
- Final determination made based on number of bleeding episodes, gestational age, and other mitigating factors

ONGOING CARE

FOLLOW-UP RECOMMENDATIONS

- Repeat US of placenta location if last US was done at <37 weeks' gestational age.
- Placentas should be sent for pathologic evaluation.

DIET

No restrictions once stable; NPO if delivery possible

PATIENT EDUCATION

www.nlm.nih.gov/medlineplus/ency/article/000900.htm

PROGNOSIS

- Maternal mortality 0.03% with placenta previa
- Greatest fetal risk is preterm delivery and consequences of hypoxemia if delay in delivery with fetal tracing abnormalities.

COMPLICATIONS

- Peripartum hysterectomy (RR = 33)
  - Increased risk with prior C-section
- Blood transfusion (RR = 10)
- DIC risk is low unless massive bleeding is present.
- Fetal anemia and Rh isoimmunization
- Intra- and postpartum hemorrhage due to placental insertion into noncontractile lower uterine segment

REFERENCES

1. Simon EG, Fouche CJ, Perrotin F. Three-dimensional transvaginal sonography in third-trimester evaluation of placenta previa. *Ultrasound Obstet Gynecol*. 2013;41(4):465.
2. Neilson JP. Interventions for suspected placenta praevia. *Cochrane Database Syst Rev*. 2003;(2):CD001998.
3. American College of Obstetricians and Gynecologists. ACOG committee opinion no. 560: medically indicated late-preterm and early-term deliveries. *Obstet Gynecol*. 2013;121(4):908.

ADDITIONAL READING

- Alfirevic Z, Elbourne D, Pavord S, et al. Use of recombinant activated factor VII in primary postpartum hemorrhage: the Northern European registry 2000–2004. *Obstet Gynecol*. 2007;110(6):1270–1278.
- Belfort MA; Publications Committee, Society for Maternal-Fetal Medicine. Placenta accreta. *Am J Obstet Gynecol*. 2010;203(5):430–439.
- Bhide A, Prefumo F, Moore J, et al. Placental edge to internal os distance in the late third trimester and mode of delivery in placenta praevia. *BJOG*. 2003;110(9):860–864.
- Briggs GG, Wan SR. Drug therapy during labor and delivery, part 2. *Am J of Health Syst Pharm*. 2006;63(12):1131–1139.
- Oyelese Y, Smulian JC. Placenta previa, placenta accreta, and vasa previa. *Obstet Gynecol*. 2006;107(4):927–941.
- Predanci M. A sonographic assessment of different patterns of placenta previa "migration" in the third trimester of pregnancy. *J Ultrasound Med*. 2005;24(6):773.
- Sharma A, Suri V, Gupta I. Tocolytic therapy in conservative management of symptomatic placenta previa. *Int J Gynaecol Obstet*. 2004;84(2):109–113.
- Stafford IA, Dashe JS, Shivvers SA, et al. Ultrasonographic cervical length and risk of hemorrhage in pregnancies with placenta previa. *Obstet Gynecol*. 2010;116(3):595–600.

SEE ALSO

Abruptio Placentae

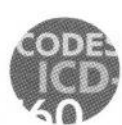

CODES

ICD10

- O44.10 Placenta previa with hemorrhage, unspecified trimester
- O44.11 Placenta previa with hemorrhage, first trimester
- O44.13 Placenta previa with hemorrhage, third trimester

CLINICAL PEARLS

- Placenta previa is a major cause of antepartum bleeding in the 2nd and 3rd trimesters.
- Do *not* perform digital cervical exam, only careful speculum exam.
- US, both transvaginal and transabdominal, is used to verify placenta location and diagnosis.
- Delivery is by cesarean section with rare exceptions.

PLANTAR FASCIITIS

Alan J. Williamson, MD • Katie M. Crowder, Maj, USAF, MC

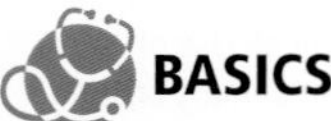

BASICS

DESCRIPTION

- Degenerative change of plantar fascia at origin on medial tuberosity of calcaneus
- Pain on plantar surface, usually at calcaneal insertion of plantar fascia upon weight bearing, especially in morning or on initiation of walking after prolonged rest

EPIDEMIOLOGY

Prevalence

- Lifetime: 10–15% of population
- Data suggest persistence with BMI >30.
- Condition is self-limiting; typically resolves within 10 months

ETIOLOGY AND PATHOPHYSIOLOGY

- Repetitive microtrauma and collagen degeneration of plantar fascia
- Chronic degenerative change (-osis/-opathy rather than -itis) of plantar fascia generally at insertion on medial tuberosity of calcaneus

RISK FACTORS

- Dancers, runners, court sport athletes
- Obesity (BMI >30)
- Pes planus (flat feet), pes cavus (high arch), overpronation, leg length discrepancy
- Occupations with prolonged standing, especially on hard surfaces (nurses, letter carriers, warehouse/factory workers)
- Female, pregnancy
- Age (>40–60 years)
- Tightness of calf and hamstring tendons
- Decreased ankle range of motion in dorsiflexion (tight heel chord; <15 degrees of dorsiflexion)
- Systemic connective tissue disorders

GENERAL PREVENTION

- Maintain normal body weight.
- Avoid prolonged standing on bare feet, sandals, or slippers.
- Avoid training errors (increasing intensity, distance, duration, and frequency of high-impact activities too rapidly).
- Proper footwear (appropriate cushioning and arch support)
- Runners should replace footwear after every 250–500 miles.
- Avoid overtraining.

COMMONLY ASSOCIATED CONDITIONS

- Usually isolated
- Heel spurs common but not marker of severity
- Posterior tibial neuropathy

DIAGNOSIS

HISTORY

- Pain on plantar surface of foot, usually at fascial insertion at calcaneus (medial calcaneal tubercle), but can have pain anywhere along length of plantar fascia
- Pain is typically worse with 1st few steps in the morning or after prolonged rest (poststatic dyskinesia).
- Pain typically improves after 1st few steps only to recur toward the end of the day.
- Pain can be dull and constant in chronic plantar fasciitis.
- Pain with prolonged ambulation or standing
- Limp with excessive toe walking
- Numbness and burning of medial hindfoot when associated with posterior tibial nerve compression

PHYSICAL EXAM

- Point tenderness on medial tuberosity of calcaneus at insertion of plantar fascia
- Pain along plantar fascia with foot dorsiflexion
- Windlass test: pain with passive dorsiflexion of the toes; high specificity, low sensitivity; sensitivity improves (13.5→31.8%) if performed while standing.
- Decreased passive range of motion with dorsiflexion of ankle
- Evaluate for pes planus, pes cavus, overpronation
- Loss of heel fat pad suggests heel fat pad syndrome.
- Point tenderness on posterosuperior aspect of heel suggests Achilles' tendinopathy.

DIFFERENTIAL DIAGNOSIS

- Calcaneal stress fracture
- Heel fat pad syndrome (painful or atrophic heel pad)
- Longitudinal arch strain
- Nerve entrapment (posterior tibial nerve—tarsal tunnel syndrome, medial calcaneal branch of posterior tibial nerve, abductor digiti quinti)
- Achilles' tendinopathy
- Calcaneal contusion
- Plantar calcaneal bursitis
- Tendonitis of posterior tibialis
- Plantar fascia tear
- Calcaneal apophysitis (Sever disease)—adolescents

DIAGNOSTIC TESTS & INTERPRETATION

- None necessary; typically a clinical diagnosis
- Consider further imaging only if diagnosis is in question.
- 2 radiographic views of foot can rule out fracture, tumor, cyst, periostitis, bony erosions; weight-bearing films preferred
- Ultrasound: demonstrates signs of inflammation at insertion (hypoechoic), including thickened plantar fascia (≥4 mm)
- MRI can evaluate for other soft tissue etiologies.
- CT or technetium-99 bone scan can rule out calcaneal stress fracture and evaluate for infection.
- Nerve conduction studies can rule out nerve entrapment.

TREATMENT

- Nonoperative management is mainstay of treatment.
- No treatment has the highest quality level of evidence.

GENERAL MEASURES

- Supportive footwear with stable midfoot; avoid wearing sandals or walking barefoot.
- Relative rest/activity modification
- Stretching: plantar fascial stretches more effective than Achilles' tendon/gastrocnemius-soleus stretches
- Weight reduction if BMI >25
- Orthotics
  - Custom orthotics show no benefit over prefabricated orthotics and are more costly.
  - Improved effectiveness of night splints when used in association with orthotics
- Strengthening of calf and interosseous muscles, using the towel drag/pick-up exercise
- Night splints: can be uncomfortable for the 1st few nights but generally become less bothersome with time; especially effective with calf and Achilles' tightness
- Ice (frozen water bottle roll)
- Massage (golf ball roll)

MEDICATION

First Line

Use only as an adjunct to general measures to control pain and increase compliance

- NSAIDs: naproxen 500 mg PO BID *or* ibuprofen 600–800 mg PO TID PRN for pain
- Acetaminophen 1,000 mg PO TID PRN for pain

Second Line

None

ISSUES FOR REFERRAL

- Podiatry, surgery: Consider referral for more invasive treatments if conservative measures fail after 3–6 months.
- Consider physical therapy referral for patient instruction on proper stretching and strengthening techniques.

ADDITIONAL THERAPIES

- Corticosteroid injections (1)[A]
  - Short-term pain relief
  - Recommend ultrasound guidance, although more painful
  - Risk for plantar fascial rupture and calcaneal fat pad atrophy with resultant permanent heel pain
  - Can cause injection pain and postinjection pain for up to 5–7 days
- Extracorporeal shock wave therapy (ESWT) (2,3)[B]
  - Growing body of evidence showing benefit
  - Multiple meta-analyses and systematic reviews show level I evidence of benefit; moderate and high-intensity treatments may be more beneficial.
  - Uncomfortable to patients but less risk than injection or surgery
  - Consider prior to surgical options; possibly consider prior to steroid injection
  - May be more effective in patients with an obvious spur on x-ray
  - Delivery method not yet standardized
- Some orthopedic surgeons prefer casting in severe cases but avoid this option in overweight patients.
- Low-dye taping
  - Limited evidence
  - Less effective in severe cases
- Promising therapies with inconsisting supporting evidence
  - Platelet-rich plasma injections (4)[B]: Limited, but growing body of evidence shows benefit. Level I evidence (prospective randomized comparative series) comparing PRP to steroid injection showed PRP to be superior at 3, 6, 12, and 24 months.

- Botulinum toxin (BT) A injection (5)[B]
  - RCT comparing steroid injection to BT injection showed similar results in pain reduction and other measures of foot function at 1 month; improvements in these areas persisted at 6 months more so with BT than with steroid injection
  - Randomized, multicenter, double-blind, placebo-controlled study comparing BT injection to placebo showed no statistical difference in pain and global assessment.
- Radiofrequency nerve ablation (6)[B]: Prospective, RCT with sham treatment and crossover demonstrated efficacy; also, retrospective case series demonstrated benefit at 1 and 2 years after treatment.
- Myofascial trigger point manual therapy
- Intralesional autologous blood injection
- Plantar iontophoresis

SURGERY/OTHER PROCEDURES

- Only necessary in a small percentage of patients (<10%)
- Recommended if conservative treatment fails after 6–12 months and pain is unrelenting
- Open/endoscopic plantar fasciotomy (less risk and complications with endoscopic technique but requires specialized equipment and skills and is not widely used)
- Calcaneal spur resection
- More likely beneficial in severely obese
- No RCTs support surgery

COMPLEMENTARY & ALTERNATIVE MEDICINE

- Heel cup with magnet has proven ineffective.
- Acupuncture shows limited benefit in a few studies.

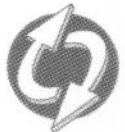

ONGOING CARE

FOLLOW-UP RECOMMENDATIONS

- Ensure patient is adhering to proper stretching exercises.
- Following 3–6 months of unsuccessful conservative treatment, consider additional therapies or referrals

PATIENT EDUCATION

- Weight reduction if BMI >25
- Proper footwear (adequate cushion and arch support)
- Stretch plantar fascia: Pull toes into dorsiflexion prior to walking after prolonged sitting or sleep.
- Ice the foot using a frozen water bottle: Roll foot over bottle for 10 minutes in the morning and after work.
- Massage plantar fascia: Roll foot over a golf ball.
- Strengthen foot muscles: Grab cloth or carpet by plantar flexing the toes.
- Decrease repetitive stress.
- Video overview for patients: www.youtube.com/watch?v=Pnithn4EYQk

PROGNOSIS

- Generally good
- Self-limited condition (resolves within 2 years) in up to 85–90% of patients

COMPLICATIONS

- Rupture of plantar fascia (more common with repeated corticosteroid injections)
- Chronic pain
- Gait abnormality

REFERENCES

1. McMillan AM, Landorf KB, Gilheany MF, et al. Ultrasound guided corticosteroid injection for plantar fasciitis: randomized controlled trial. *BMJ*. 2012;344:e3260:1–12.
2. Chang KV, Chen SY, Chen WS, et al. Comparative effectiveness of focused shock wave therapy of different intensity levels and radial shock wave therapy for treating plantar fasciitis: a systematic review and network meta-analysis. *Arch Phys Med Rahabil*. 2012;93(7):1259–1268.
3. Speed C. A systematic review of shockwave therapies in soft tissue conditions: focusing on the evidence. *Br J Sports Med*. 2014;48(21):1538–1542. doi:10.1136/bjsports-2012-091961.
4. Monto RR. Platelet-rich plasma efficacy versus corticosteroid injection treatment for chronic severe plantar fasciitis. *Foot Ankle Int*. 2014;35(4): 313–318.
5. Jabbari B, Machado D. Treatment of refractory pain with botulinum toxins—an evidence-based review. *Pain Med*. 2011;12(11):1594–1606.
6. Landsman AS, Catanese DJ, Wiener SN, et al. A prospective, randomized, double-blinded study with crossover to determine the efficacy of radio-frequency nerve ablation for the treatment of heel pain. *J Am Podiatr Med Assoc*. 2013;103(1):8–15.

ADDITIONAL READING

- Akşahin E, Doğruyol D, Yüksel HY, et al. The comparison of the effect of corticosteroids and platelet-rich plasma (PRP) for the treatment of plantar fasciitis. *Arch Orthop Trauma Surg*. 2012;132(6):781–785.
- Aqil A, Siddiqui MR, Solan M, et al. Extracorporeal shock wave therapy is effective in treating chronic plantar fasciitis: a meta-analysis of RCTs. *Clin Orthop Relat Res*. 2013;471(11):3645–3652.
- Crawford F, Thomson CE. Interventions for treating plantar heel pain. *Cochrane Database Syst Rev*. 2010;(1):CD000416.
- Digiovanni BF, Nawoczenski DA, Malay DP, et al. Plantar fascia-specific stretching exercise improves outcomes in patients with chronic plantar fasciitis. A prospective clinical trial with two-year follow-up. *J Bone Joint Surg Am*. 2006;88(8):1775–1781.
- Donley BG, Moore T, Sferra J, et al. The efficacy of oral nonsteroidal anti-inflammatory medication (NSAID) in the treatment of plantar fasciitis: a randomized, prospective, placebo-controlled study. *Foot Ankle Int*. 2007;28(1):20–23.
- Goff JD, Crawford R. Diagnosis and treatment of plantar fasciitis. *Am Fam Physician*. 2011;84(6): 676–682.
- Hawke F, Burns J, Radford JA, et al. Custom-made foot orthoses for the treatment of foot pain. *Cochrane Database Sys Rev*. 2008;(3):CD006801.
- Healey K, Chen K. Plantar fasciitis: current diagnostic modalities and treatments. *Clin Podiatr Med Surg*. 2010;27(3):369–380.
- Huang YC, Wei SH, Wang HK, et al. Ultrasonographic guided botulinum toxin type A treatment for plantar fasciitis: an outcome-based investigation for treating pain and gait changes. *J Rehabil Med*. 2010;42(2):136–140.
- Ibrahim MI, Donatelli RA, Schmitz C, et al. Chronic plantar fasciitis treated with two sessions of radial extracorporeal shock wave therapy. *Foot Ankle Int*. 2010;31(5):391–397.
- Peterlein CD, Funk JF, Hölscher A, et al. Is botulinum toxin A effective for the treatment of plantar fasciitis? *Clin J Pain*. 2012;28(6):527–533.
- Ragab EM, Othman AM. Platelets rich plasma for treatment of chronic plantar fasciitis. *Arch Orthop Trauma Surg*. 2012;132(8):1065–1070.
- Renan-Ordine R, Alburquerque-Sendin F, de Souza DP, et al. Effectiveness of myofascial trigger point manual therapy combined with a self-stretching protocol for the management of plantar heel pain: a randomized controlled trial. *J Orthop Sports Phys Ther*. 2011;41(2):43–50.
- Thomas JL, Christensen JC, Kravitz SR, et al. The diagnosis and treatment of heel pain: a clinical practice guideline—revision 2010. *J Foot Ankle Surg*. 2010;49(3)(Suppl):S1–S19.
- Uden H, Boesch E, Kumar S. Plantar fasciitis—to jab or to support? A systematic review of the current best evidence. *J Multidiscip Healthc*. 2011;4:155–164.
- van de Water AT, Speksnijder CM. Efficacy of taping for the treatment of plantar fasciosis: a systematic review of controlled trials. *J Am Podiatr Med Assoc*. 2010;100(1):41–51.
- Young C. In the clinic. Plantar fasciitis. *Ann Intern Med*. 2012;156(1, Pt 1):ITC1-1–ITC1-15; quiz ITC1-16.

SEE ALSO

Algorithm: Heel Pain

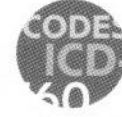

CODES

ICD10

M72.2 Plantar fascial fibromatosis

CLINICAL PEARLS

- Degeneration of plantar fascia at origin (medial calcaneal tuberosity)
- Plantar pain with weight bearing especially 1st few steps in the morning or after prolonged rest is hallmark presentation.
- Conservative treatment is preferred. Wear supportive footwear to avoid excess pronation and provide adequate cushion. Modify activity, stretch plantar fascia, ice (water bottle roll), massage (golf ball roll), and provide arch support.

PLEURAL EFFUSION

Felix B. Chang, MD, DABMA, ABIHM

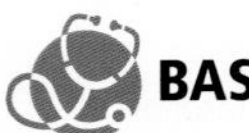

BASICS

Abnormal accumulation of fluid in the pleural space

DESCRIPTION

Types: transudate, exudate

- Congestive heart failure 40%: transudate
- Pneumonia 25%, malignancy 15%, and pulmonary embolism (PE) 10% account for exudative effusions.
- Malignant: lung cancer and metastases of breast, ovary, and lymphoma

EPIDEMIOLOGY

Incidence

Estimated 1.5 million cases/year in the United States; CHF: 500,000; pneumonia: 300,000; malignancy: 150,000; PE: 150,000; cirrhosis: 150,000; TB: 2,500; pancreatitis: 20,000; collagen vascular disease: 6,000

Prevalence

- Estimated 320 cases/100,000 people in industrialized countries; in hospitalized patients with AIDS, prevalence is 7–27%.
- No gender predilection: ~2/3 of malignant pleural effusions occurs in women.

ETIOLOGY AND PATHOPHYSIOLOGY

- Pleural fluid formation exceeds pleural fluid absorption.
- Transudates result from imbalances in hydrostatic and oncotic forces.
  - Increase in hydrostatic and/or low oncotic pressures; increase in pleural capillary permeability; lymphatic obstruction or impaired drainage; movement of fluid from the peritoneal or retroperitoneal space
- Transudates:
  - CHF: 40% of transudative effusions; 80% bilateral. Constrictive pericarditis, atelectasis; superior vena cava syndrome
  - Cirrhosis (hepatic hydrothorax); nephrotic syndrome, hypoalbuminemia; myxedema
  - Urinothorax, central line misplacement; peritoneal dialysis
- Exudates:
  - Lung parenchyma infection, bacterial (parapneumonic, tuberculous pleurisy) fungal, viral, parasitic (amebiasis, *Echinococcus*)
  - Cancer: lung cancer, metastases (breast, lymphoma, ovaries), mesothelioma
  - PE: 25% of PEs are transudate.
  - Collagen vascular disease: rheumatoid arthritis, systemic lupus erythematosus, Wegener granulomatosis, sarcoidosis, Churg-Strauss
  - GI: pancreatitis, esophageal rupture, abdominal abscess, after liver transplant. Chylothorax: thoracic duct tear, malignancy
  - Hemothorax: trauma, PE, malignancy, coagulopathy, aortic aneurysm
  - Others: after coronary artery bypass graft; Dressler syndrome; uremia, asbestos exposure, radiation; drug-induced: nitrofurantoin, bromocriptine, amiodarone, procarbazine, methysergide, hydralazine, procainamide, quinidine, methotrexate, and methysergide
  - Meigs syndrome; yellow nail syndrome; ovarian stimulation syndrome; lymphangiomatosis; acute respiratory distress syndrome (ARDS)
  - Chylothorax: thoracic duct tear, malignancy, associated with lymphoma

RISK FACTORS

- Occupational exposures/drugs
- PE; TB; bacterial pneumonias
- Opportunistic infections (in HIV patients when CD4 count is <150 cells/μL)

COMMONLY ASSOCIATED CONDITIONS

Hypoproteinemia, heart failure, cirrhosis

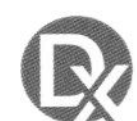

DIAGNOSIS

Presumptive diagnosis in 50% of cases. Small pleural effusions, radiographic area <2 intercostal spaces (<300 mL) are asymptomatic.

HISTORY

Dyspnea, fever, malaise, and weight loss; chest pain, cough, hemoptysis, and dull pain

PHYSICAL EXAM

- Pleural effusion >300 mL: tachypnea, asymmetric expansion of the thoracic cage; decrease/absent tactile fremitus; dullness to percussion; decreased/inaudible breath sounds, egophony, pleural friction rub
- Ascites suggest the following: hepatic hydrothorax, ovarian cancer, and Meigs syndrome.
- Unilateral swelling in lower extremity may suggest PE.

DIFFERENTIAL DIAGNOSIS

Empyema, malignancy, inflammatory, fungal, tubercular, others

DIAGNOSTIC TESTS & INTERPRETATION

Initial Tests (lab, imaging)

Pleural fluid: appearance, pH, WBC differential, total protein, lactate dehydrogenase (LDH), glucose, Gram stain and culture, and acid-fast bacilli staining. Consider polymerase chain reaction (PCR) for *Mycobacterium tuberculosis* and *Streptococcus pneumoniae* (1,2)[A].

- By scenario: amylase, triglycerides, cholesterol, lupus erythematosus (LE) cells, cytology, antinuclear antibodies (ANAs), adenosine deaminase, tumor markers, rheumatoid factor, cytology, creatinine (3)[A]
- Light criteria, transudate versus exudate (98% sensitivity; 80% specificity) fluid is considered an exudate if any of the following (4)[A]:
  - Ratio of pleural fluid-to-serum protein levels >0.5; ratio of pleural fluid-to-serum LDH levels >0.6; pleural fluid LDH level >2/3 the upper limit for serum LDH level (4)[A]
- Other exudate criteria (2)[A]:
  - Serum-effusion albumin gradient ≤1.2 (sensitivity 87%; specificity 92%); cholesterol effusion >45 mg/dL and LDH effusion >200 mg/dL (sensitivity 90%; specificity 98%)

- Empyema: pus, putrid odor; culture; a putrid odor suggests an anaerobic empyema: LDH levels >1,000 IU/L (normal serum = 200 IU/L); glucose, <60 mg/dL; low pH
- Malignancy: cytology, red, bloody; glucose, normal to low, depending on the tumor burden; RBCs, >100,000/mm^3
- Lupus pleuritis: LE cells present; pleural fluid-to-serum ANAs ratio >1; glucose <60 mg/dL; pleural fluid-to-serum glucose ratio <0.5
- Fungal: positive KOH, culture; peritoneal dialysis: protein, <1 g/dL; glucose, 300–400 mg/dL
- Urinothorax: creatinine: pleural/blood >0.5; high LDH pleural fluid, with low protein levels
- Hemothorax: hematocrit: pleural/blood >0.5; benign asbestos effusion: unilateral, exudative; have elevated eosinophil count
- TB pleuritis: lymphocytes >80% predominance effusion; elevated levels of adenosine deaminase >50 U/L and interferon-γ >140 pg/mL; positive acid-fast bacillus (AFB) stain, culture; total protein >4 g/dL
- Chylothorax: milky; triglycerides >110 mg/dL; lipoprotein electrophoresis (chylomicrons)
- Amebic liver abscess: anchovy paste effusion; Waldenström macroglobulinemia and multiple myeloma: protein >7 g/dL
- Esophageal rupture: high salivary amylase; pleural fluid acidosis, pH <6; amylase-rich: acute pancreatitis, chronic pancreatic pleural effusion, malignancy, esophageal rupture; rheumatoid pleurisy: glucose <60 mg/dL; pleural fluid/serum glucose <0.5
- Lymphocytosis: tuberculous pleurisy, lymphoma, sarcoidosis, chronic rheumatoid pleurisy, yellow nail syndrome, or chylothorax (80–95% of the nucleated cells). Carcinomatosis in half of cases (50–70% are lymphocytes)
- Pleural fluid eosinophilia (>10% of total nucleated cells): pneumothorax, hemothorax, malignancy, drugs, pulmonary infarction, fungal (coccidiomycosis, cryptococcosis, histoplasmosis), benign asbestos pleural effusion
- Low glucose (<60 mg/dL): TB, malignancy, rheumatoid pleurisy, parapneumonic, empyema, hemothorax, paragonimiasis, Churg-Strauss syndrome
- RBC count >100,000/mm^3: trauma, malignancy, PE, injury after cardiac surgery, asbestos pleurisy, pancreatitis, TB
- Pleural fluid LDH >1,000 IU/L: suggests empyema, malignant effusion, rheumatoid effusion, or pleural paragonimiasis
- pH >7.3: rheumatoid pleurisy, empyema, malignant effusion, TB, esophageal rupture, or lupus nephritis
- Mesothelial cells in exudates: TB is unlikely if there are >5% of mesothelial cells.
- *Streptococcus pneumoniae* accounts for 50% of cases of parapneumonic effusions in AIDS patients, followed by *Staphylococcus aureus*, *Haemophilus influenzae*, *Mycoplasma pneumoniae*, *Legionella*, *Nocardia*, and *Bordetella bronchiseptica*. Exudate with low count of nucleated cells
- *Pneumocystis jiroveci* is an uncommon cause in HIV. Usually it is a small effusion, unilateral or bilateral, serous to bloody in appearance. Demonstration of the trophozoite or cyst is mandatory.
- Cancer-related HIV pleural effusion: Kaposi sarcoma, Castleman disease, and primary effusion lymphoma. Kaposi sarcoma: mononuclear predominance, exudate, pH >7.4; LDH, 111–330 IU/L; glucose >60 mg/dL.
- Chest x-ray (CXR): posteroanterior–anteroposterior views
  - Upright x-rays show a concave meniscus in the costophrenic angle that suggests >250 mL of pleural fluid; homogeneous opacity, with visibility of pulmonary vessels through diffuse haziness and absence of air bronchogram; 75 mL of fluid will obliterate the posterior costophrenic sulcus.

– Lateral x-rays show blunting of the posterior costophrenic angle and the posterior gutter; decubitus x-rays to exclude a loculated effusion and underlying pulmonary lesion or pulmonary thickening
– Supine x-rays show costophrenic blunting, haziness, obliteration of the diaphragmatic silhouette, decreased visibility of the lower lobe vasculature, and widened minor fissure.
- Ultrasonography (US): detects as 5–50 mL of pleural fluid; identifies loculated effusions; site for thoracocentesis, pleural biopsy, or pleural drainage
- Chest CT scan with contrast for patients with undiagnosed pleural effusion. CT pulmonary angiography if pulmonary embolism is suspected.

Follow-Up Tests & Special Considerations
- 75% of patients with exudative effusions have a non-CHF cause.
  – NT-ProBNP: biomarker of CHF-associated effusion; >1,500 pg/mL; sensitivity and specificity 94% (3)[A]
  – Observation in uncomplicated asymptomatic patients (i.e., CHF, cirrhosis), viral pleurisy, thoracic or abdominal surgery

Diagnostic Procedures/Other
Diagnostic thoracentesis indicated for the following:
- Clinically significant pleural effusion (>10 mm thick on US or lateral decubitus x-ray with no known cause)
- CHF: asymmetric effusion, fever, chest pain, or failure to resolve after diuretics
- Parapneumonic effusions

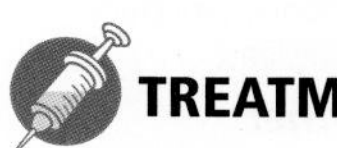

TREATMENT

Oxygen support

GENERAL MEASURES
- Therapeutic thoracentesis, if symptomatic
- Chest tube thoracostomy drainage: >1/2 hemithorax; complicated parapneumonic effusion (positive Gram stain or culture, pH <7.2, or glucose <60 mg/dL); empyema; hemothorax. Recommended limit is 1,000–1,500 mL in a single thoracentesis procedure (5)[B].

MEDICATION
First Line
CHF: diuretics (75% clearing in 48 hours); parapneumonic effusion: antibiotics; rheumatologic conditions/inflammation: steroids and NSAIDs

Second Line
Symptomatic nonmalignant effusions that are refractory to treatment may be managed with repeated therapeutic thoracentesis or pleurodesis.

ISSUES FOR REFERRAL
- Uncertain etiology; malignant effusion; high-risk diagnostic thoracentesis; decortication
- Video-assisted thoracoscopy for sclerosis; peritoneal shunts for symptomatic recurrence

ADDITIONAL THERAPIES
- Pleurodesis for symptomatic patients whose pleural effusion reaccumulates too quickly for repeat therapeutic thoracentesis
- Tunneled pleural catheter is the preferred treatment for patients with malignant pleural effusion and limited survival (6)[A].
- Sclerosing agents for malignant effusions: doxycycline, bleomycin, talc, and minocycline; talc is more efficacious. The relative risk of nonrecurrent effusion was 1.34 (95% confidence interval 1.16–1.55) in favor of talc compared with bleomycin, tetracycline, or mustine.

SURGERY/OTHER PROCEDURES
- Percutaneous pleural biopsy if a cause is not clear after thoracentesis
  – Close pleural biopsy: Pleura is diffusely involved (TB pleuritis, noncaseating granuloma in rheumatoid pleuritis).
  – CT-guided needle biopsy: pleural mass; video-assisted thoracoscopic pleural biopsy: negative percutaneous biopsy, patchy disease, or CT scan does not show obvious mass.
- Parapneumonic effusion should be sampled if free-flowing, but layer is >10 mm on a lateral decubitus film. Loculated, thickened pleura on a contrast-enhanced CT scan, clearly delineated by US Open pleural biopsy by thoracotomy
- Contraindications for thoracocentesis: anticoagulation, bleeding diathesis, thrombocytopenia <20,000/mm^3, mechanical ventilation
- Bronchoscopy: when malignancy is suspected (pulmonary infiltrate or mass on CXR or CT scan, hemoptysis, massive pleural effusion, or shift of the mediastinum toward the side of effusion)
- Thoracoscopy

INPATIENT CONSIDERATIONS
Admission Criteria/Initial Stabilization
Treat any underlying medical disorder.

ONGOING CARE

FOLLOW-UP RECOMMENDATIONS
Patient Monitoring
- Check for the amount and quality of fluid drained, air leak (bubbling), and oscillation.
- Repeat a CXR when drainage decreases to <100 mL/day to evaluate complete clearing.
- For a large effusion, reevaluate catheter position; if positioned appropriately, consider fibrinolytics.

DIET
Cardiac diet in patients with heart failure; correct hypoproteinemia.

PROGNOSIS
- Malignant effusion: poor
- Low-pH malignant effusions have shorter survival and poorer response to chemical pleurodesis than those with pH >7.3 (6)[A].
- Low pleural fluid pH (≤7.15): high likelihood of pleural space drainage

COMPLICATIONS
- Pleural effusion: constrictive fibrosis, pleurocutaneous fistula
- Thoracentesis: pneumothorax (5–10%); hemothorax (~1%); empyema; spleen/liver laceration; reexpansion pulmonary edema (if >1.5 L is removed)

REFERENCES

1. McGrath EE, Anderson PB. Diagnosis of pleural effusion: a systematic approach. *Am J Crit Care*. 2011;20(2):119–127.
2. Wilcox ME, Chong CA, Stanbrook MB, et al. Does this patient have an exudative pleural effusion? The rational clinical examination systematic review. *JAMA*. 2014;311(23):2422–2431.
3. Saquil A, Wyrick K, Hallgren J. Diagnostic approach to pleural effusion. *Am Fam Physician*. 2014;90(2):99–104.
4. Light RW. Pleural effusions. *Med Clin North Am*. 2011;95(6):1055–1070.
5. Mahmood K, Wahidi MM. Straightening out chest tubes: what size, what type, and when. *Clin Chest Med*. 2013;34(1):63–71.
6. Clive A, Bhatnagar R, Preston NJ, et al. Interventions for the management of malignant pleural effusions. *Cochrane Database Syst Rev*. 2013;5:CD010529.

ADDITIONAL READING

- Bielsa S, Porcel JM, Castellote J, et al. Solving the Light's criteria misclassification rate of cardiac and hepatic transudates. *Respirology*. 2012;17(4):721–726.
- Davies HE, Mishra EK, Kahan BC, et al. Effect of an indwelling pleural catheter vs chest tube and talc pleurodesis for relieving dyspnea in patients with malignant pleural effusion: the TIME2 randomized controlled trial. *JAMA*. 2012;307(22):2383–2389.

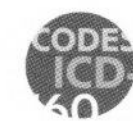

CODES

ICD10
- J90 Pleural effusion, not elsewhere classified
- J91.0 Malignant pleural effusion
- J94.0 Chylous effusion

CLINICAL PEARLS
- All patients with pleural effusion >1 cm of unknown origin should have thoracentesis.
- Thoracocentesis warranted in patients with unknown cause of pleural effusion or patient with known cause and atypical features suggesting second cause
- Bilateral pleural effusion suggest malignancy in absence of cardiomegaly.
- Loculation suggest pleural inflammation and may occur with the following: empyema, hemothorax, and TB.
- Parapneumonic effusion should be tapped ASAP (cannot exclude infection clinically).
- Lateral decubitus views are more sensitive, may detect >25 mL.

PNEUMONIA, BACTERIAL

Rahele Lameh, MD

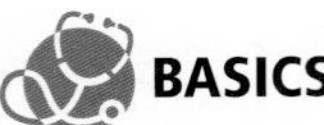

BASICS

Bacterial pneumonia is an infection of the pulmonary parenchyma by a bacterial organism.

DESCRIPTION

Bacterial pneumonia can be classified as the following:

- Community-acquired pneumonia (CAP): lower respiratory tract infection not acquired in a hospital, long-term care facility, or during other recent contact with the health care system
- Medical care–associated pneumonia
  - Hospital-acquired pneumonia (HAP): pneumonia that occurs ≥48 hours after admission and did not appear to be incubating at the time of admission
  - Ventilator-associated pneumonia (VAP): pneumonia that develops >48–72 hours after endotracheal intubation
  - Health care–associated pneumonia (HCAP): pneumonia that occurs in a nonhospitalized patient with extensive health care contact, such as the following:
    - IV therapy/wound care within the past 30 days
    - Residing in a nursing home/long-term care facility
    - Hospitalization in an acute care hospital for ≥2 days within the past 90 days
    - Visited a hospital/hemodialysis clinic within the past 30 days (1,2)

EPIDEMIOLOGY

- Influenza and pneumonia are the 8th leading cause of death in the United States, with about 53,692 deaths in 2010.
- HAP is the leading cause of death among hospital-acquired infections and is the primary cause of death in the ICU.
- Rates of infection are 3 times higher in African Americans than in whites and are 5–10 times higher in Native American adults and 10 times higher in Native American children (2).

Incidence

- CAP: 5–11 cases/1,000 persons with increased incidence occurring in the winter months
- HAP: 5–10 cases/1,000 admissions; incidence increase 6–20-fold in ventilated patients (3)[A].

ETIOLOGY AND PATHOPHYSIOLOGY

- Adults, CAP
  - Typical (85%): *Streptococcus pneumoniae*, *Haemophilus influenzae*, *Staphylococcus aureus*, group A *Streptococcus*, *Moraxella catarrhalis*
  - Atypical (15%): *Legionella* sp., *Mycoplasma pneumoniae*, *Chlamydophila pneumoniae*
- Adults, HCAP/HAP/VAP
  - Aerobic gram-negative bacilli: *Pseudomonas aeruginosa*, *Escherichia coli*, *Klebsiella pneumoniae*, and *Acinetobacter* sp.
  - Gram-positive cocci: *Streptococcus* sp. and *S. aureus* (including MRSA)
- Children
  - Birth to 20 days: *E. coli*, group B streptococci, *Listeria monocytogenes*
  - 3 weeks to 3 months: *Chlamydia trachomatis*, *S. pneumoniae*
  - 4 months to 18 years
    - Typical: *S. pneumoniae*
    - Atypical: *C. pneumoniae*, *M. pneumoniae*

RISK FACTORS

CAP

- Age >65 years
- HIV/immunocompromised
- Recent antibiotic therapy/resistance to antibiotics
- Asthma, CAD, COPD, chronic renal failure, CHF, diabetes, liver disease, neoplasm's VAP, HAP, HCAP
- Hospitalization for ≥2 days during past 90 days
- Severe illness
- Antibiotic therapy in the past 6 months
- Poor functional status as defined by activities of daily living living score
- Immunosuppression (including steroid users)

GENERAL PREVENTION

- All children 2–59 months of age should be routinely vaccinated with PCV-13; given at 2, 4, and 6 months of age; a 4th at 12–15 months of age. PCV-13 is now currently FDA approved for those >50 years of age.
- 23-valent pneumococcal polysaccharide vaccine is recommended for the following: (4)
  - Age ≥65 years: 2nd dose recommended if patient received vaccine 5 years prior and was <65 years at the time of the 1st vaccination
  - Age 19–64 years with chronic cardiovascular disease, chronic pulmonary disease (including asthma), diabetes mellitus, chronic liver disease, CSF leaks, cochlear implants, alcoholism, or who smoke cigarettes/live in chronic care facilities. Revaccination not recommended <65 years of age.
  - Age 19–64 years who are immunocompromised: 2nd dose recommended if ≥5 years have elapsed since 1st dose
- Annual influenza vaccine is recommended according to current guidelines.

DIAGNOSIS

HISTORY

- Fever, chills, rigors, malaise, fatigue
- Dyspnea
- Cough, with/without sputum
- Pleuritic chest pain
- Myalgias
- GI symptoms

ALERT

High fever (>104°F [40°C]), male sex, multilobar involvement, and GI and neurologic abnormalities have been associated with CAP caused by *Legionella* infection.

Geriatric Considerations

Older adults with pneumonia often present with weakness, mental status change, or history of falls.

PHYSICAL EXAM

- Fever >100.4°F (38°C), tachypnea, tachycardia
- Rales, rhonchi, egophony, increased fremitus, bronchial breath sounds, dullness to percussion, asymmetric breath sounds, abdominal tenderness

DIFFERENTIAL DIAGNOSIS

Bronchitis, asthma exacerbation, pulmonary edema, lung cancer, pulmonary tuberculosis, pneumonitis

DIAGNOSTIC TESTS & INTERPRETATION

Initial Tests (lab, imaging)

- Routine laboratory testing to establish an etiology in outpatients with CAP is usually unnecessary.
- For hospitalized patients with CAP, a CBC, sputum Gram stain, and 2 sets of blood cultures
- More extensive diagnostic testing in patients with CAP is recommended if
  - Blood cultures: ICU admission, cavitary infiltrates, leukopenia, alcohol abuse, chronic severe liver disease, asplenia, positive pneumococcal urine antigen test (UAT), pleural effusion
  - Sputum Gram stain and cultures: ICU admission, failure of outpatient treatment, cavitary infiltrates, alcohol abuse, severe COPD/structural lung disease, positive legionella UAT, positive pneumococcal UAT, pleural effusion
  - Legionella UAT: ICU admission, failure of outpatient treatment, alcohol abuse, travel in past 2 weeks, pleural effusion
  - Pneumococcal UAT: ICU admission, failure of outpatient treatment, leukopenia, alcohol abuse, chronic severe liver disease, asplenia, pleural effusion
- A chest x-ray (CXR) is indicated when pneumonia is suspected or with an acute respiratory infection and
  - Vital signs: temperature >100°F (37.8°C); heart rate (HR) >100 beats/min; respiratory rate (RR) >20 breaths/min
  - At least 2 of the following clinical findings: decreased breath sounds, rales, absence of asthma
- Early in the course of the disease, a CXR may be negative.
- Evidence of necrotizing/cavitary pneumonia should raise suspicion for MRSA pneumonia, especially with history of prior MRSA skin lesions.

Diagnostic Procedures/Other

- For VAP/HAP: By bronchoscopic or nonbronchoscopic means, obtain a lower respiratory tract sample for culture prior to initiation/change of therapy. Serial evaluations may be needed (3)[A].
- Safe cessation of antibiotics can be done from a good quality negative sputum culture.

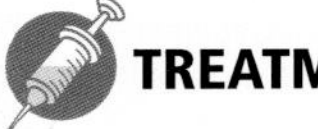

TREATMENT

MEDICATION

First Line

- Adults
  - CAP, outpatient
    - No significant differences in efficacy between antibiotic option in adults (5)[A]
    - Previously healthy, no antibiotics in past 3 months
      - Azithromycin 500 mg PO 1 time, then 250 mg PO daily for 4 days; clarithromycin 500 mg PO BID for 10 days; erythromycin 500 mg PO BID for 10 days, or
      - Doxycycline 100 mg PO BID for 10 days
    - Comorbid conditions, immunosuppressed, antibiotic use in past 3 months
      - Levofloxacin 750 mg PO daily for 5 days; moxifloxacin 400 mg PO daily for 10 days; or
      - Amoxicillin 1 g PO TID; amoxicillin-clavulanate 2 g PO BID + macrolide
      - Treatment may be stopped if
        - Afebrile for >48 hours
        - Supplemental oxygen no longer needed
        - No more than 1 of the following:
          - A. Heart rate >100 beats/min
          - B. Respiratory rate >24 breaths/min
          - C. Systolic BP ≤ 90 mm Hg

- CAP, inpatient (non-ICU)
  - IV antibiotics initially, then switch to oral after clinical improvement
  - Cefotaxime; ceftriaxone; ampicillin-sulbactam + macrolide (clarithromycin; erythromycin) for 14 days or
  - Moxifloxacin; levofloxacin for 14 days
  - If *Pseudomonas* is a consideration:
    - Piperacillin-tazobactam; cefepime; imipenem; meropenem + levofloxacin or
    - Piperacillin-tazobactam; cefepime; imipenem; meropenem + aminoglycoside and azithromycin or
    - Piperacillin-tazobactam; cefepime; imipenem; meropenem + aminoglycoside + levofloxacin
  - If MRSA is a consideration
    - Add vancomycin or linezolid.
- HCAP/HAP/VAP
  - Use IV antibiotics
  - Early onset (<5 days) and no risk factors for multidrug-resistant pathogens
    - Ceftriaxone; ampicillin-sulbactam; ertapenem or
    - Levofloxacin; moxifloxacin
  - Late onset (≥5 days) or risk factors for multidrug-resistant pathogens (antibiotic therapy in preceding 90 days; high frequency of antibiotic resistance in community/hospital; immunosuppressive disease/therapy; risk factors for HCAP)
    - MRSA coverage: linezolid or vancomycin + β-lactam cefepime; ceftazidime; imipenem; meropenem; piperacillin-tazobactam + either fluoroquinolone (levofloxacin) or aminoglycoside (amikacin; gentamicin; tobramycin) (level II)
    - Short-course versus prolonged-course antibiotic therapy for HAP in critically ill adults is only as effective and reduced recurrence of VAP-associated multidrug resistance (6).
    - Drug-resistant *S. pneumoniae* should be treated with high-dose amoxicillin, amoxicillin/clavulanate, cefpodoxime with a macrolide, or a respiratory fluoroquinolone.
- Adult IV antibiotic doses
  - β-Lactams (ampicillin-sulbactam 3 g q6h; aztreonam 2 g q6h; cefepime 1–2 g q8–12h; cefotaxime 1 g q6–8h; ceftazidime 2 g q8h; ceftriaxone 1 g daily; imipenem 500 mg q6h; meropenem 1 g IV q8h)
  - Aminoglycosides (amikacin 20 mg/kg daily; gentamicin 7 mg/kg daily; tobramycin 7 mg/kg daily)
  - Fluoroquinolones (levofloxacin 750 mg daily; moxifloxacin 400 mg daily)
  - Macrolides (azithromycin 500 mg daily; clarithromycin 500 mg daily; erythromycin 500–1,000 mg q6h)
  - Vancomycin 15 mg/kg q12h
  - Linezolid 600 mg q12h

- Pediatric, outpatient (≥3 months)
  - Antibiotic treatment in preschool-aged children is not routinely required because viral pathogens are more common (7)[A].
  - Oral antibiotics are as efficacious as IV antibiotics in CAP (length of stay and oxygen requirement were reduced in those given oral antibiotics).
  - Typical bacterial pneumonia
    - Amoxicillin 90 mg/kg/day PO BID (max 4 g/day) (7)[A]
    - Amoxicillin-clavulanate 90 mg/kg/day PO BID (max 4 g/day) (7)[A]
    - Alternative: levofloxacin 16–20 mg/kg/day PO BID for children 6 months to 5 years, 10 mg/kg/day daily for children ≥5 years (max 750 mg/day) (7)[C]
  - Atypical bacterial pneumonia
    - Azithromycin 10 mg/kg PO on day 1 (max 500 mg), then 5 mg/kg/day (max 250 mg) on days 2–5 (6)[C]
    - Clarithromycin 15 mg/kg/day PO BID (max 1 g/day) (6)[C]
    - Erythromycin 40 mg/kg/day PO daily (6)[C]

INPATIENT CONSIDERATIONS

Admission Criteria/Initial Stabilization

Clinical judgment and use of a validated severity of illness score are recommended to determine if inpatient management is indicated.

- The Pneumonia Severity Index (PSI) is a clinical prediction rule used to calculate the probability of morbidity and mortality among patients with CAP. PSI is risk stratified from I to V. PSI risk class from I to III can be treated as outpatients and IV–V should be hospitalized. PSI can be calculated at http://pda.ahrq.gov/clinic/psi/psicalc.asp.
- The CURB-65 or CRB 65 (confusion, urea nitrogen, respiratory rate, blood pressure, age >65 years) (www.mdcalc.com/curb-65-severity-score-community-acquired-pneumonia/) is a severity of illness score for stratifying adults with CAP into different management groups (5).
- The SMART-COP (systolic BP, multilobar chest radiography, albumin, respiratory rate, tachycardia, confusion, oxygen level, arterial pH) is a new method to predict which patients will require intensive respiratory/vasopressor support. A score of ≥3 has sensitivity of 92% to identify those patients who will receive intensive treatment (5).
- Patients with COPD or CHF are more likely to require ICU admission when suffering from CAP.
- Clinical prediction tools do not replace a physician's clinical judgment.

Pediatric Considerations

Inpatient treatment of children is recommended in the following settings: infants ≤3–6 months; presence of respiratory distress (tachypnea, dyspnea, retractions, grunting, nasal flaring, apnea, altered mental status, O_2 sat <90%); or if known to have CAP as result of a virulent pathogen such as community-associated MRSA should be hospitalized (8).

Discharge Criteria

Clinical stability: temperature ≤100°F (37.8°C); HR ≤100 beats/min; RR ≤24 beats/min; systolic BP ≤90 mm Hg; O_2 sat ≥90% or pO_2 ≥60 mm Hg on room air; ability to maintain oral intake; normal mental status

ONGOING CARE

FOLLOW-UP RECOMMENDATIONS

Patient Monitoring

Consider chest CT if patient is failing to improve on current management.

PATIENT EDUCATION

Smoking cessation, vaccinations

COMPLICATIONS

Necrotizing pneumonia, respiratory failure, empyema, abscesses, cavitation, bronchopleural fistula, sepsis

REFERENCES

1. Marrie TJ, Huang JQ. Epidemiology of community-acquired pneumonia in Edmonton, Alberta: an emergency department-based study. *Can Respir J*. 2005;12(3):139.
2. Davidson M, Parkinson AJ, Bulkow LR, et al. The epidemiology of invasive pneumococcal disease in Alaska, 1986-1990—ethnic differences and opportunities for prevention. *J Infect Dis*. 1994;170(2):368–376.
3. File TM. Recommendations for treatment of hospital-acquired and ventilator-associated pneumonia: review of recent international guidelines. *Clin Infect Dis*. 2010;51(Suppl 1):S42–S47.
4. Vila-Corcoles A, Ochoa-Gondar O, Guzmán JA, et al. Effectiveness of the 23-valent polysaccharide pneumococcal vaccine against invasive pneumococcal disease in people 60 years or older. *BMC Infect Dis*. 2010;10:73.
5. Watkins RR, Lemonovich LT. Diagnosis and management of community-acquired pneumonia in adults. *Am Fam Physician*. 2011;83(11):1299–1306.
6. Pugh R, Grant C, Cooke RP, et al. Short-course versus prolonged-course antibiotic therapy for hospital-acquired pneumonia in critically ill adults. *Cochrane Database Syst Rev*. 2011;(10):CD007577.
7. Bradley JS, Byington CL, Shah SS, et al. The management of community-acquired pneumonia in infants and children older than 3 months of age: clinical practice guidelines by the Pediatric Infectious Diseases Society and the Infectious Diseases Society of America. *Clin Infect Dis*. 2011;53(7):e25–e76.
8. Delvitt M. PIDS and IDSA issue management guidelines for community-acquired pneumonia in infants and young children. *Am Fam Physician*. 2012;86(2):196–202.

ADDITIONAL READING

Schrock-Stuckey K, Hayes LB, George MC. Community-acquired pneumonia in children. *Am Fam Physician*. 2012;86(7):661–667.

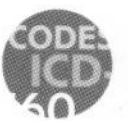

CODES

ICD10

- J15.9 Unspecified bacterial pneumonia
- J15.4 Pneumonia due to other streptococci
- J14 Pneumonia due to Hemophilus influenzae

CLINICAL PEARLS

- Bacterial pneumonia can usually be treated empirically based on its classification as CAP or HCAP/HAP/VAP.
- A severity of illness score is helpful in determining the need for hospitalization of adult patients but does not replace a physician's clinical judgment.

PNEUMONIA, MYCOPLASMA

Rebecca M. Wight, MD • Aaron M. Winnick, MD, FACS

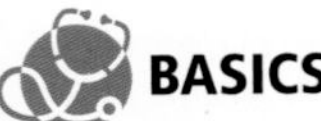

BASICS

DESCRIPTION

- Bronchopulmonary infection caused by the *Mycoplasma* species, *Mycoplasma pneumoniae*
- Smallest free-living organism; fastidious and slow-growing; first isolated in cattle in 1898
- Most frequently affects children/young adults but can also occur in the elderly; often causes epidemics in close communities
- Infection may be asymptomatic, most often confined to the upper respiratory tract; however, may progress to pneumonia (5–10%)
- Course is usually acute with an incubation period of 2–3 weeks.
- Synonym(s): primary atypical pneumonia (PAP); Eaton agent pneumonia; cold agglutinin–positive pneumonia; walking pneumonia

Geriatric Considerations

Uncommonly isolated as a single agent in elderly patients

Pediatric Considerations

- Unusual in infants and children <5 years; (pneumonia <5 years is more commonly viral)
- Increased incidence of asthma exacerbation in older children
- All infants 3–6 months with suspected bacterial pneumonia should be hospitalized.

EPIDEMIOLOGY

Incidence

- Estimated 1 million cases per year in the United States
- Responsible for 20% of community-acquired pneumonia (CAP) requiring hospitalizations annually
- Seasonal variation is low; however, infection is more common in late summer/fall months, accounting for up to 50% of pneumonia cases in summer.

Prevalence

- Predominant sex: male = female
- Predominant age group affected: 5–20 years
  - May occur at any age
  - Rare in children <5 years of age
- Responsible for 15–20% of all cases of CAP yearly
  - Most common cause of pneumonia in school children and young adults who do not have a chronic underlying condition

ETIOLOGY AND PATHOPHYSIOLOGY

- *M. pneumoniae* is a short-rod mucosal pathogen, which lacks a cell wall and thus not visible on Gram stain.
- Can grow under both aerobic and anaerobic conditions
- Highly contagious, *M. pneumoniae* is transmitted by contact and aerosols.
- Pathogenicity linked to its filamentous tips, which adhere selectively to respiratory epithelial cell membrane proteins with production of H_2O_2 and superoxide radicals, damaging cilia
- Toll-like receptor-2 binding involved in activating cytokine pathways causing inflammation
- Decreased ciliary movement produces prolonged paroxysmal, hacking cough.

ALERT

- Macrolide-resistant *M. pneumoniae* has emerged in cases of adult CAP and pediatric pneumonias.
- Infection by *M. pneumoniae* has come to be recognized as a worldwide cause of CAP.

RISK FACTORS

- Immunocompromised state (e.g., HIV, transplant recipients, chemotherapy)
- Smoking
- Close community living (e.g., military bases, prisons, hospitals, fraternity houses, schools, household contacts)

GENERAL PREVENTION

Consider droplet isolation of active cases.

COMMONLY ASSOCIATED CONDITIONS

- Asthma exacerbations as a result of proinflammatory cytokine release
- Chronic obstructive pulmonary disease

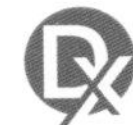

DIAGNOSIS

HISTORY

- Infection may be asymptomatic.
- Gradual onset of headache, malaise, low-grade fevers, chills
- Symptoms of upper respiratory infection then occur, including incessant, nonproductive, worsening cough (which may become mildly productive late in the disease); rhinorrhea, pharyngitis, and sinusitis (1)[A]
- Pneumonia may occur with associated pleural effusion; however, dyspnea is rare.
- The presence of pleuritic chest pain warrants a higher suspicion of *M. pneumoniae* (1)[A].
- Extrapulmonary findings may develop in 5–10% of patients, including arthralgias, skin rashes, cervical adenopathy, hemolysis, congestive heart failure (CHF), and cardiac conduction abnormalities.
- Neurologic symptoms develop more commonly in children and may include encephalitis, aseptic meningitis, cranial nerve palsies, cerebellar ataxia, ascending paralysis, and coma (2)[C].
- Persistent cough is common during convalescence; other sequelae are rare.

PHYSICAL EXAM

- Patients generally appear nontoxic.
- Hacking/pertussis-like cough may be present along with fever and lassitude.
- Normal lung findings with early infection, but rhonchi, rales, and/or wheezes may develop several days later (1)[A].
- Mild pharyngeal injection without exudates
- Minimal/no cervical adenopathy
- Erythematous tympanic membranes or bullous myringitis in patients >2 years of age is an uncommon, but unique, sign.
- Some patients may develop a pleural friction rub.
- Various exanthems, including erythema multiforme and Stevens-Johnson syndrome

DIFFERENTIAL DIAGNOSIS

- Viral/bacterial/fungal pneumonia
- Tuberculosis
- Other atypical pneumonias, including *Chlamydia pneumoniae*, *Chlamydophila psittaci*, *Coxiella burnetii* (Q fever), *Francisella tularensis* (tularemia), *Pneumocystis jiroveci*, *Legionella pneumophila*

DIAGNOSTIC TESTS & INTERPRETATION

- Labs are typically not necessary to make a diagnosis, but they may be indicated depending on the clinical presentation.
- Serology (ELISA) is the mainstay of laboratory diagnosis.

Initial Tests (lab, imaging)

- WBC count may be normal or elevated.
- Hemolytic anemia has been described but is rare.
- Elevated erythrocyte sedimentation rate (ESR) may be present but is nonspecific.
- Positive Coombs test with cold agglutinin titers are elevated in >50% of patients; however, also nonspecific.
- When available, polymerase chain reaction (PCR) for *M. pneumoniae* DNA in respiratory secretions, CSF, and tissue samples may be the most sensitive and specific
- CXR shows reticulonodular pattern with patchy areas of lower lobe consolidation, may be bilateral. Small pleural effusion may be present in 10–15% cases.

Follow-Up Tests & Special Considerations

- Sputum Gram stains are not helpful because *M. pneumoniae* lacks a cell wall and cannot be stained.
- *M. pneumoniae* is difficult to culture and requires 7–21 days to grow; culturing is successful in 40–90% of cases but does not provide information to guide treatment, thus infrequently performed.
- Complement fixation serologic assay shows 4-fold rise in IgM antibody titer at 2–4 weeks after symptom onset; this is an older technique.
- Positive cold agglutinins (titer of ≥1:128 or rising 4-fold) in 50% of infections but can take 1–2 weeks to develop; not sensitive/specific; not routinely recommended
- CT of chest may show a combination of patchy tree-in-bud opacities with segmental ground glass opacities.

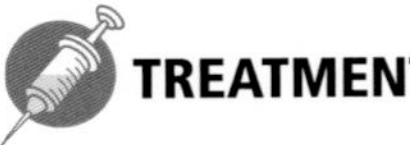

TREATMENT

GENERAL MEASURES

- Avoid sick contacts.
- Treatment is usually empiric and must be comprehensive to cover all likely pathogens in the context of the clinical setting.
- Calculation of pneumonia severity score (CAP score: www.mdcalc.com/psi-port-score-pneumonia-severity-index-adult-cap) may be helpful in determining inpatient versus outpatient treatment.

ALERT

There is insufficient evidence regarding the efficacy of antibiotics in pediatric patients infected with *M. pneumoniae*. However, some studies show benefit to treating with a macrolide and amoxicillin to cover *M. pneumoniae* in addition to other likely agents causing CAP (3,4)[A].

Pregnancy Considerations

- Azithromycin: pregnancy Category B (preferred treatment)
- Clarithromycin and levofloxacin: pregnancy Category C
- Doxycycline: pregnancy Category D

P

MEDICATION

First Line

- Azithromycin
  - <3 months of age: not established
  - >3 months of age: day 1, 10 mg/kg PO × 1 (not to exceed 500 mg); days 2–5: 5 mg/kg PO daily (not to exceed 250 mg/day)
  - Adults: 500 mg PO × 1 followed by 250 mg PO daily × 4 days (5)[A]
- Erythromycin
  - Children: 20–50 mg/kg/day (base) PO divided q6–8h × 10–14 days
  - Adults: 500 mg (base) PO q6h × 10–14 days (5)[A],(6)[B]
- Clarithromycin
  - Children <6 months of age: not established
  - Patients >6 months of age: 15 mg/kg/day PO divided q12h × 10–14 days
  - Adults: 250–500 mg PO BID × 10–14 days
- Doxycycline
  - Children <8 years of age: not recommended
  - Children >8 years of age (≤45 kg): 2–4 mg/kg/day up to 200 mg/day PO divided BID × 10–14 days
  - Children >8 years of age (≥45 kg): Refer to adult dosing.
  - Adults: 100 mg PO BID × 7–14 days (5)[A],(6)[B]

Second Line

- Levofloxacin
  - Children <18 years of age: not recommended
  - Adults: 500 mg PO daily × 7–10 days (5)[A]
- Moxifloxacin
  - Children <18 years of age: not recommended
  - Adults: 400 mg/day PO × 7–10 days
- Levofloxacin and moxifloxacin show good activity against *M. pneumoniae*. Consider use with comorbid conditions and other pneumonia pathogens.

ADDITIONAL THERAPIES

- Albuterol inhaler: 2 puffs q4–6h as needed for wheezing
- Dexamethasone may downregulate cytokine release (7)[B].
- Acetaminophen/ibuprofen as needed for fever
- Up to 10.9% of hospitalized patients may require mechanical ventilation.
- Plasmapheresis in cases of severe hemolytic anemia

INPATIENT CONSIDERATIONS

Admission Criteria/Initial Stabilization

- CAP score risk class IV/V
- Advanced age with comorbidities
- Complicating neoplastic disease
- Significant cerebrovascular, cardiac, renal, liver, or GI symptoms
- Altered mental status
- Inability to maintain oxygen saturation
- Tachycardia/tachypnea
- Hypotension
- Neurologic symptoms
- Signs of Stevens-Johnson syndrome
- Significant hemolysis (autoimmune hemolytic anemia, cold agglutinin disease)

Discharge Criteria

- Change from IV to PO antibiotic may be made when
  - Respiratory distress and hypoxia have resolved.
  - Patients are tolerating oral hydration.
  - No significant complications present.
- Generally, no need for 24-hour observation on PO antibiotics prior to discharge.

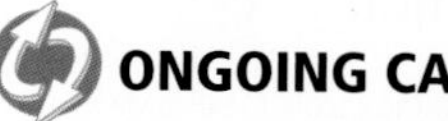

ONGOING CARE

FOLLOW-UP RECOMMENDATIONS

- Clearing of condition on CXR should be documented in patients >50 years of age (4)[A].
- In smokers, document a clear CXR in 6–8 weeks.
- Worsening symptoms/development of rash or meningeal/neurologic signs should prompt immediate presentation to medical attention.
- Antibiotic prophylaxis for exposed contacts is not routinely recommended.
- For household contacts who may be predisposed to severe mycoplasmal infection, macrolide or doxycycline prophylaxis should be used.

DIET

- No special diet considerations
- Ensure adequate hydration.

PATIENT EDUCATION

- Smoking cessation
- Contact and droplet precautions
- Adequate hand washing techniques

PROGNOSIS

- Symptoms usually resolve in 2 weeks.
- Some constitutional symptoms may persist for several weeks.
- With correct therapy, even most severe cases can expect complete recovery.

COMPLICATIONS

- All complications are rare, except reactive airway disease, hemolytic anemia, and erythema multiforme.
- Reactive airway disease may persist indefinitely and can cause acute chest syndrome in patients with sickle cell anemia.
- Meningoencephalitis
- Aseptic meningitis
- Peripheral neuropathy
- Transverse myelitis/acute transverse myelitis
- Cerebellar ataxia
- Acute disseminated encephalomyelitis
- Guillain-Barré syndrome
- Encephalitis (especially in children)
- Polyneuritis/polyarthritis
- Stevens-Johnson syndrome
- Pericarditis/myocarditis
- Respiratory distress syndrome
- Cerebral ataxia
- Thromboembolic phenomena
- Pleural effusion
- Nephritis
- Occasional deaths occur primarily among the elderly and persons with sickle cell disease.

REFERENCES

1. Wang K, Gill P, Perera R, et al. Clinical symptoms and signs for the diagnosis of *Mycoplasma pneumoniae* in children and adolescents with community-acquired pneumonia. *Cochrane Database Syst Rev*. 2012;10:CD009175.
2. Meyer-Sauteur PM, Jacobs BC, Spuesens EMB, et al. Antibody responses to *Mycoplasma pneumoniae*: role in pathogenesis and diagnosis of encephalitis. *PLoS Pathog*. 2014;10(6):e1003983.
3. Mulholland S, Gavranich JB, Gillies MB, et al. Antibiotics for community-acquired lower respiratory tract infections secondary to *Mycoplasma pneumoniae* in children. *Cochrane Database Syst Rev*. 2012;9:CD004875.
4. Bradley JS, Byington CL, Shah SS, et al. The management of community-acquired pneumonia in infants and children older than 3 months of age: clinical practice guidelines by the Pediatric Infectious Diseases Society and the Infectious Diseases Society of America. *Clin Infect Dis*. 2011;53(7):e25–e76.
5. Mandell LA, Wunderink RG, Anzueto A, et al. Infectious Diseases Society of America/American Thoracic Society consensus guidelines on the management of community-acquired pneumonia in adults. *Clin Infect Dis*. 2007;44(Suppl 2):S27–S72.
6. Spindler C, Strålin K, Eriksson L, et al. Swedish guidelines on the management of community-acquired pneumonia in immunocompetent adults—Swedish Society of Infectious Diseases 2012. *Scand J Infect Dis*. 2012;44(12):885–902.
7. Remmelts HHE, Meijvis SCA, Biesma DH, et al. Dexamethasone downregulates the systemic cytokine response in patients with community-acquired pneumonia. *Clin Vaccine Immunol*. 2012;19(9):1532–1538.

ADDITIONAL READING

- Atkinson TP, Balish MF, Waites KB. Epidemiology, clinical manifestations, pathogenesis and laboratory detection of *Mycoplasma pneumoniae* infections. *FEMS Microbiol Rev*. 2008;32(6):956–973.
- Carbonara S, Monno L, Longo B. Community-acquired pneumonia. *Curr Opin Pulm Med*. 2009;15(3):261–273.
- Eliakim-Raz N, Robenshtok E, Shefet D, et al. Empiric antibiotic coverage of atypical pathogens for community-acquired pneumonia in hospitalized adults. *Cochrane Database Syst Rev*. 2012;9:CD004418.
- Kashyap S, Sarkar M. *Mycoplasma pneumonia*: clinical features and management. *Lung India*. 2010;27(2):75–85.
- Torres A, Blasi F, Peetermans WE, et al. The aetiology and antibiotic management of community-acquired pneumonia in adults in Europe: a literature review. *Eur J Clin Microbiol Infect Dis*. 2014;33(7):1065–1079.

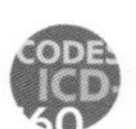

CODES

ICD10

J15.7 Pneumonia due to Mycoplasma pneumoniae

CLINICAL PEARLS

- Most common atypical respiratory pathogens include *M. pneumoniae*, *C. pneumoniae*, and *L. pneumophila*.
- Atypical pneumonia is typically a clinical diagnosis; if labs are indicated, serology is the mainstay of diagnosis.
- Watch closely for complicating symptoms that could indicate worsening disease.

PNEUMONIA, PNEUMOCYSTIS JIROVECI

Thomas J. Hansen, MD

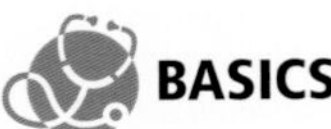

BASICS

DESCRIPTION

- The fungus that causes this pneumonia in humans was previously called *Pneumocystis carinii*.
- The name was formally changed to *Pneumocystis jiroveci* in 2001, following the discovery that the fungus that infects humans is unique and distinctive from the fungus that infects animals (1).
- *P. jiroveci* causes pneumonia primarily in immunocompromised patients.
- *P. jiroveci* is extremely resistant to traditional antifungal agents, including both amphotericin and azole agents (2).
- To prevent confusion, the term PCP, which used to represent *P. carinii* pneumonia, now represents *Pneumocystis* pneumonia (3).

ALERT

No combination of symptoms, signs, blood chemistries, or radiographic findings is diagnostic of *P. jiroveci* pneumonia (4).

EPIDEMIOLOGY

- *P. jiroveci* has a worldwide distribution, and most children have been exposed to the fungus by 2–4 years (5).
- The reservoir and mode of transmission for *P. jiroveci* is still unclear:
  - Human studies favor an airborne transmission model, with person-to-person spread being the most likely mode of infection acquisition (4).

Incidence

- Infants with HIV infection have a peak incidence of PCP between 2 and 6 months (5).
- HIV-infected infants have a high mortality rate, with a median survival of only 1 month.

Prevalence

- The prevalence of *P. jiroveci* colonization among healthy adults is 0–20% (2).
- Recent studies have demonstrated the transient nature of *P. jiroveci* colonization in asymptomatic, immunocompetent patients (4).
- 50% of patients with PCP are coinfected with ≥2 strains of *P. jiroveci* (5).
- Evidence that distinct strains are responsible for each episode in patients who develop multiple episodes of PCP (5).

ETIOLOGY AND PATHOPHYSIOLOGY

Mode of transmission is unknown; respiratory likely important

RISK FACTORS

Individuals at risk (4)

- Patients with HIV/AIDS infection, especially if not receiving prophylactic treatment for PCP
- Patients who are receiving high doses of glucocorticoids
- Patients who have an altered immune system not due to HIV
- Patients who are receiving chronic immunosuppressive medications
- Patients who have hematologic or solid malignancies resulting in malignancy-related immune depression

GENERAL PREVENTION

- Medication
  - Trimethoprim-sulfamethoxazole (TMP-SMX)
    - Adults: one double-strength tablet daily or one double-strength tablet 3× week
    - Children >2 months: 150 mg TMP/m²/day in divided doses q12h for 3 days per week
  - Atovaquone suspension
    - Adults: 1,500 mg PO once daily with food
    - Children: not to exceed 1,500 mg/day
      - 1–3 months: 30 mg/kg/day PO once daily
      - 4–24 months: 45 mg/kg/day PO once daily
      - >24 months: 30 mg/kg/day PO once daily
      - Adolescents ≥13 years: Refer to adult dosing.
  - Dapsone
    - Adults only: 50 mg BID or 100 mg once daily
  - Pentamidine
    - Adults only: 300 mg aerosolized every 4 weeks
- Indications for prophylaxis
  - HIV-infected adults (5)
    - Should start when CD4 count is <200 cells/μL or if the patient develops oropharyngeal candidiasis
  - HIV-infected children (5)
    - Prophylaxis should be provided for children ≥6 years based on adult guidelines.
    - For children aged 1–5 years, start when CD4 count is <500 cells/μL.
    - For infants <12 months, start when the CD4 percentage is <15%.
  - Non–HIV-infected adults receiving immunosuppressive medications or with underlying immune system deficits should receive PCP prophylaxis, but currently there are no specific guidelines on when to start this.
- Discontinuation of prophylaxis
  - When CD4+ cell counts are >200 cells/μL for a period of 3 months in the adult population (2)[C]
  - There are no clear guidelines for discontinuation of prophylaxis in children.

COMMONLY ASSOCIATED CONDITIONS

- HIV/AIDS
- Chronic obstructive pulmonary disease (COPD)
- Interstitial lung disease
- Connective tissue diseases treated with corticosteroids
- Cancer and organ transplant patients on immunosuppressive medication

DIAGNOSIS

HISTORY

- HIV-infected patients
  - Subacute onset over several weeks
    - Progressively worsening dyspnea
    - Tachypnea
    - Cough: nonproductive or productive of clear sputum
    - Low-grade fever, chills
    - Weakness, fatigue, malaise
- Non–HIV-infected immunocompromised patients
  - More acute onset with fulminant respiratory failure
    - Abrupt tachypnea, dyspnea
    - Fever
    - Dry cough

PHYSICAL EXAM

- Fever
- Tachypnea
- Tachycardia
- Lung exam is normal or near normal.

DIFFERENTIAL DIAGNOSIS

- Tuberculosis
- Bacterial pneumonia
- Fungal pneumonia
- Viral pneumonia

DIAGNOSTIC TESTS & INTERPRETATION

P. jiroveci cannot be cultured. Therefore, a diagnosis relies on detection of the organism by colorimetric or immunofluorescent stains or by polymerase chain reaction (PCR) (5)[C].

- ABG: reveals hypoxemia and increased alveolar–arterial gradient that varies with severity of disease
- LDH: Serum lactate dehydrogenase is frequently increased (nonspecific; likely due to underlying lung inflammation and injury).
- CD4 cell count is generally <200 in HIV-infected patients with PCP.

- S-adenosylmethionine levels are significantly lower in a patient with PCP. The levels increase with successful treatment (6)[B].

- Comprehensive metabolic profile
- Chest x-ray (CXR) (4)[C]
  - Bilateral, symmetric, fine, reticular interstitial infiltrates involving perihilar areas. Becomes more homogeneous and diffuse as severity of infection progresses
  - Less common patterns include upper lobe involvement in patients receiving aerosolized pentamidine, solitary or multiple nodular opacities, lobar infiltrates, pneumatoceles, and pneumothoraces.
  - May be normal in up to 30% of patients with PCP (3)[C]
- High-resolution CT is more sensitive than CXR.

Diagnostic Procedures/Other

- Fiber-optic bronchoscopy with bronchoalveolar lavage (BAL) is the preferred diagnostic procedure to obtain samples for direct fluorescent antibody staining:
  - Sensitivities range from 89 to >98%.
- *Pneumocystis* trophic forms or cysts obtained from induced sputum, BAL fluid, or lung tissue, which can be visualized using conventional stains
- PCR can detect *Pneumocystis* from respiratory sources, but the potential remains for false positives (4)[C].

TREATMENT

The recommended duration of therapy differs in patients who are with/without AIDS:

- In patients with PCP who do not have AIDS, the typical duration of therapy is 14 days.
- Treatment of PCP in patients who have AIDS was increased to 21 days due to the risk for relapse after only 14 days of treatment (4)[C].

MEDICATION

- TMP-SMX (2,4)[C]
- Adult dosing
  - TMP: 15–20 mg/kg/day, PO or IV, divided into four doses
- Pediatric dosing (>2 months) (4)[C]
  - TMP: 15–20 mg/kg/day in divided doses q6–8h
- Reduce doses of TMP-SMX in patients with renal failure.
- Treatment response to *Pneumocystis* therapy often requires at least 7–10 days before clinical improvement is documented (2)[C].
- Pregnancy risk factor: Category C (4)[C]
- Precautions
  - History of sulfa allergy
  - There is an emergence of drug-resistant PCP, especially against TMP-SMX.

Second Line

- Pentamidine (for moderate to severe cases)
  - Adults and children: 4 mg/kg IV or IM once daily
- Dapsone + trimethoprim (adults only)
  - Dapsone 100 mg PO once daily, *plus*
  - Trimethoprim 5 mg/kg PO TID
    - Check the glucose-6-phosphate dehydrogenase level before beginning dapsone, as hemolysis may result.
- Clindamycin + primaquine (adults only)
  - Clindamycin 600–900 mg IV q8h or 300–450 mg PO QID, *plus*
  - Primaquine 30 mg PO once daily
- Atovaquone
  - Adults: 750 mg PO BID (>13 years of age)
  - Children: 40 mg/kg/day PO divided BID (max 1,500 mg)
- Note: Pentamidine has greater toxicity than TMP-SMX: hypotension, hypoglycemia, pancreatitis (4)[C]

ADDITIONAL THERAPIES

Adjunctive corticosteroid (prednisone or methylprednisolone) (4)[C],(7)[A]

- Adjunctive corticosteroids are shown to provide benefits in patients who have AIDS and symptoms of moderate to severe PCP.
- Corticosteroids provide the greatest benefit to HIV patients who have hypoxemia manifested as a partial pressure of arterial oxygen <70 mm Hg or an alveolar–arterial gradient >35 mm Hg on room air.
- Adults and children >13 years of age: prednisone, 40 mg PO BID on days 1–5; 40 mg daily on days 6–11; 20 mg daily on days 12–21

INPATIENT CONSIDERATIONS

- No set criteria for hospital admission
- Five predictors of mortality in HIV-associated *Pneumocystis* pneumonia (8)
  - Increased age of the patient
  - Recent IV drug use
  - Total bilirubin >0.6 mg/dL
  - Serum albumin <3 g/dL
  - Alveolar–arterial oxygen gradient ≥50 mm Hg (8)[C]

ONGOING CARE

FOLLOW-UP RECOMMENDATIONS

In patients with HIV/AIDS: Patients with previous episodes of PCP should receive lifelong secondary prophylaxis unless they respond well to highly active antiretroviral therapy (HAART) and have a CD4 count >200 cells/μL for at least 3 months.

Patient Monitoring

Serum lactate dehydrogenase levels, pulmonary function test results, and ABG measurements generally normalize with treatment.

DIET

No special diet needed

PATIENT EDUCATION

- Centers for Disease Control and Prevention: www.cdc.gov/ncidod/dpd/parasites/pneumocystis/default.htm
- FamilyDoctor.org: http://familydoctor.org/online/famdocen/home/common/sexinfections/hiv/475.html

REFERENCES

1. Catherinot E, Lanterneier F, Bougnoux ME. *Pneumocystis jirovecci* pneumonia. *Infect Dis Clin North Am*. 2010;24(1):107–138.
2. Limper AH, Knox KS, Sarosi GA, et al. An official American Thoracic Society statement: treatment of fungal infections in adult pulmonary and critical care patients. *Am J Respir Crit Care Med*. 2011;183(1):96–128.
3. D'Avignon LC, Schofield CM, Hospenthal DR. *Pneumocystis* pneumonia. *Semin Respir Crit Care Med*. 2008;29(2):132–140.
4. Krajicek BJ, Thomas CF, Limper AH. Pneumocystis pneumonia: current concepts in pathogenesis, diagnosis, and treatment. *Clin Chest Med*. 2009;30(2):265–278, vi.
5. Kovacs JA, Masur H. Evolving health effects of *Pneumocystis*: one hundred years of progress in diagnosis and treatment. *JAMA*. 2009;301(24):2578–2585.
6. Skelly MJ, Holzman RS, Merali S. S-adenosylmethionine levels in the diagnosis of *Pneumocystis carinii* pneumonia in patients with HIV infection. *Clin Infect Dis*. 2008;46(3):467–471.
7. Briel M, Bucher H, Boscacci R, et al. Adjunctive corticosteroids for *Pneumocystis jiroveci* pneumonia in patients with HIV-infection. *Cochrane Database Syst Rev*. 2006;(3):CD006150.
8. Fei WM, Kim EJ, Sant CA, et al. Predicting mortality from HIV-associated *Pneumocystis* pneumonia at illness presentation: an observational cohort study. *Thorax*. 2009;64(12):1007–1076.

ADDITIONAL READING

- Centers for Disease Control and Prevention. Guidelines for preventing opportunistic infections among HIV-infected persons—2002 recommendations of the U.S. Public Health Service and the Infectious Disease Society of America. *MMWR*. 2002;51(RR-8):1–46.
- Centers for Disease Control and Prevention. Treating opportunistic infections among HIV-infected adults and adolescents: recommendations from CDC, the National Institutes of Health, and the HIV Medicine Association/Infectious Disease Society of America. *MMWR*. 2004;53(RR-15):1–112.
- Green H, Paul M, Vidal L, et al. Prophylaxis for *Pneumocystis* pneumonia (PCP) in non-HIV immunocompromised patients. *Cochrane Database Syst Rev*. 2007;(3):CD005590.
- Shankar SM, Nania JJ. Management of *Pneumocystis jiroveci* pneumonia in children receiving chemotherapy. *Paediatr Drugs*. 2007;9(5):301–309.
- Stringer JR, Beard CB, Miller RF, et al. A new name (*Pneumocystis jiroveci*) for *Pneumocystis* from humans. *Emerg Infect Dis*. 2002;8(9):891–896.

SEE ALSO

HIV/AIDS

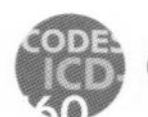

CODES

ICD10

B59 Pneumocystosis

CLINICAL PEARLS

- Colonization with *P. jiroveci* is common in the pediatric population.
- PCP only occurs in immunocompromised patients.
- Patients with HIV are at risk once their CD4 count is <200. At that time, TMP-SMX should be initiated as prophylaxis. Prophylaxis may end after HAART has been initiated and the CD4 count is >200 for 3 months.
- Patients who are immunocompromised are also at risk. Currently, no clear clinical guidelines are available as to when to initiate or end prophylaxis.
- The 1st-line treatment is TMP-SMX. The typical duration of therapy is 14 days in non–AIDS-infected patients and 21 days in AIDS-infected patients.

PNEUMONIA, VIRAL

Aaron Lambert, MD

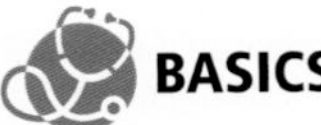

BASICS

DESCRIPTION

- Inflammatory disease of the lungs due to a viral infection
- Most viral pneumonia results from exposure infection in the form of aerosolized secretions.
- Hematogenous and direct spread also possible.

Geriatric Considerations

High rates of morbidity and mortality in the elderly

Pediatric Considerations

- Adenoviral infections in children are serious.
- More serious respiratory viral infections are almost always seen in infants and in immunocompromised patients.

Pregnancy Considerations

- Pregnant patients should avoid contact with anyone who has a viral infection.
- Influenza vaccination is recommended for all pregnant women during the influenza season.

EPIDEMIOLOGY

Incidence

- Predominant age: children <5 years
- Predominant sex: male = female

Prevalence

- Prevalence is variable with seasonal outbreaks, but the disease is more common during winter months.
- ~90% of all cases of childhood pneumonias have a viral cause.
- Between 4 and 39% of pneumonia diagnosed in adults has been attributed to viral causes.

ETIOLOGY AND PATHOPHYSIOLOGY

Overall: Influenza A and respiratory syncytial virus (RSV) are leading causes followed by adenovirus and the parainfluenza viruses:

- Adults
  - Influenza A, B, and C
  - Influenza H1N1
  - Adenovirus
  - Parainfluenza
  - Coronavirus/SARS
- Children
  - Influenza A, B, and C
  - Influenza H1N1
  - Rhinovirus
  - Adenovirus
  - Parainfluenza
  - Rubeola (measles)
  - RSV (particularly for those born prematurely)
- Miscellaneous
  - Cytomegalovirus (CMV) (particularly in immunocompromised patients)
  - Varicella
  - Herpes simplex virus (HSV)
  - Enterovirus
  - Rubeola
  - Epstein-Barr virus
  - Hantavirus
  - Human metapneumovirus

Genetics

No known genetic pattern has been recognized.

RISK FACTORS

- Seasonal: epidemic upper respiratory illness
- Living in close quarters
- Recent upper respiratory infection
- Travel to endemic area
- Nonvaccinated person
- Age >65 years or <5 years
- Altered mental status (due to dysphagia)
- Cardiac disease
- Chronic pulmonary disease (e.g., COPD, emphysema)
- Immunocompromised (HIV, transplant recipient, medication-induced)
- Cystic fibrosis
- Kartagener syndrome

GENERAL PREVENTION

- General hand-hygiene techniques are the 1st-line prevention in transmission of infectious particles.
- Influenza vaccination: Routine vaccination is now recommended for ALL persons aged ≥6 months.
  - Children who are 6 months to 8 years of age and receiving seasonal vaccination for the *first* time should receive 2 doses 4 weeks apart.
  - Children who are 6 months to 8 years of age who received 2 doses of the influenza vaccine should receive 1 dose of the seasonal influenza vaccine the following year.
  - See the CDC guidelines (1)[A] regarding the use of live attenuated vaccine versus inactivated vaccine.
- For those patients who are unable to receive influenza vaccine (e.g., with an egg allergy or other) and are at very high risk because of age, comorbid illness, or another risk factor, oseltamivir or zanamivir may be used for the duration of the season, with special recognition for potential viral resistance.
- For those who did not receive the vaccine and have been exposed to influenza, use of oseltamivir or zanamivir is recommended for up to 10 days following exposure.

COMMONLY ASSOCIATED CONDITIONS

- Rate of mixed viral–bacterial coinfection is ~20% and can lead to more severe illness or hospitalization.
- Fungal infection and *Pneumocystis jiroveci* pneumonia in immunocompromised patients

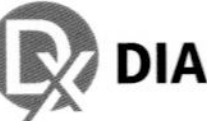

DIAGNOSIS

HISTORY

- Gradual onset
- May have preceding URI symptoms
- Fever/chills
- Headache
- Myalgias
- Malaise
- Anorexia/decreased feeding in adults/infants
- Cough (with or without purulent sputum production)
- Dyspnea
- Rhinorrhea
- Pharyngitis
- Pleurisy
- Upper abdominal pain in children

PHYSICAL EXAM

- Fever
- Tachypnea
- Tachycardia
- Hypoxemia with severe disease
- Altered breath sounds (bronchophony, tactile fremitus, whispered pectoriloquy)
- Pulmonary rales and rhonchi
- Friction rub
- Possible associated rash (i.e., measles, HSV)

DIFFERENTIAL DIAGNOSIS

- Bacterial pneumonia (especially atypical etiologies: *Chlamydophila pneumoniae* and *C. psittaci*, *Mycoplasma pneumoniae*, *Legionella pneumophila*)
- Pulmonary edema
- *Pneumocystis pneumonia/P. jiroveci* pneumonia
- Aspiration pneumonia
- Hypersensitivity pneumonitis
- Bronchiolitis obliterans, with organizing pneumonia
- Pulmonary embolus/infarction
- Cystic fibrosis (in infants)
- Severe acute respiratory syndrome or severe acute respiratory syndrome–associated coronavirus

DIAGNOSTIC TESTS & INTERPRETATION

- No standard labs to diagnose viral pneumonia
- Specific lab investigations should be based on the clinical scenario.

Initial Tests (lab, imaging)

- CBC
  - Normal or near normal granulocyte count, occasionally leukopenic with increased lymphocyte percentage
  - Hemoconcentration (hantavirus)
- Chest x-ray (CXR): interstitial or alveolar infiltrates, peribronchial thickening, pleural effusion
- ESR/CRP may be helpful in children.

Follow-Up Tests & Special Considerations

Clinicians can also consider additional testing, as clinically indicated:

- Appropriate direct fluorescent antibody or enzyme immunoassay from throat nasopharyngeal washings (children) or swab (adults), tracheal aspirate, or bronchoalveolar lavage specimens (HSV, varicella-zoster virus, influenza viruses A and B, RSV, adenovirus)
- Viral culture
  - Limitations: Results take 3–14 days. False-negative results occur with lower viral titers.
  - Rapid antigen detection: nasopharyngeal swab for rapid influenza testing
  - Cytopathology (cytoplasmic inclusion bodies [CMV], HSV, measles virus)

- Serology (4-fold rise in acute compared with convalescent titers): Confirm diagnosis retrospectively but not clinically useful.
- Serologic testing for hantavirus: enzyme immunoassay if available from health departments
- Polymerase chain reaction (PCR) detection if modality available:
  - Highly sensitive and specific, but a positive result does not imply causality
- Sputum Gram stain and culture to identify bacterial copathogens, if present
- Chest CT may show consolidations surrounded by ground glass opacities.

Diagnostic Procedures/Other

Bronchoscopy with bronchoalveolar lavage

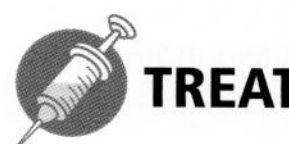

TREATMENT

- Outpatient treatment for most patients
- Inpatient treatment for infants <4 months of age, elderly, or for any patient with diffuse, severe infection (e.g., hypoxemia, hypercarbia, hypotension or shock, acute respiratory distress syndrome [ARDS]) or significant comorbidity (e.g., congestive heart failure [CHF], coronary artery disease, COPD)
- The Pneumonia Severity Index Calculator (2)[A] (http://pda.ahrq.gov/clinic/psi/psicalc.asp) from the Agency for Healthcare Research and Quality may be used to assess the need for hospitalization as well as mortality risk.
- Consider concomitant treatment for bacterial coinfection if severely ill or not responding to treatment.

MEDICATION

First Line

- Influenza viruses A and B
  - Oseltamivir (Tamiflu): Adults and children >40 kg, 75 mg PO q12h for 5 days; dosage adjusted to 75 mg PO q24h in cases where creatinine clearance rate is <30 mL/min. Children <40 kg, weight-based effectiveness is maximal when started within 48 hours of symptom onset.
  - Zanamivir (Relenza): patients >7 years of age, 2 inhalations (10 mg) q12h for 5 days
    - Shown to shorten symptoms by ~12 hours but not risk of complications (3)[B]
- Varicella-zoster virus
  - Acyclovir
    - Adults: for immunocompetent patients, 800 mg PO 5 times per day for 5–7 days
    - Children >2 years: for immunocompetent patients, 80 mg/kg/day PO divided q6h for 5 days. Start within 24 hours of symptom onset; immunocompromised patients 30 mg/kg/day PO divided q6h for 5 days. Start within 24 hours of symptom onset; immunocompromised patients 30 mg/kg/day IV divided q8h for 7–10 days.
- CMV or HSV
  - Acyclovir
    - Immunocompromised adults: 5 mg/kg IV q8h for 7 days
    - Children: Contact an infectious disease specialist or an experienced pharmacist regarding dosing.
  - Ganciclovir: Use should be in conjunction with infectious disease consultation.
- RSV
  - Ribavirin: Indicated in few, select cases (20 mg/mL via continuous aerosol administration for 12–18 h/day for 3–7 days). Ribavirin is teratogenic and should not be administered by pregnant health care personnel: Its cost is high and benefits are marginal.

Second Line

- Influenza: Amantadine and rimantadine are no longer recommended due to high levels of resistance among circulating influenza A viruses (4)[B].
- CMV, HSV, varicella virus infections
  - Foscarnet (Foscavir): 60 mg/kg/dose IV q8h in conjunction with infectious disease consultation

GENERAL MEASURES

- Most healthy individuals will only require symptomatic treatment.
- Encourage coughing and deep breathing exercises to clear secretions.
- Careful disposal of secretions/universal precautions
- Hydration
- Respiratory isolation with negative pressure room for varicella virus, which is highly contagious

ONGOING CARE

FOLLOW-UP RECOMMENDATIONS

Patient Monitoring

- Physical exams
- Repeat a CXR only if warranted by clinical presentation. A CXR may take weeks to resolve after clinical illness has resolved.
- Oxygenation if illness severe enough for hospitalization

PATIENT EDUCATION

- For patient education materials on this topic, contact American Lung Association, 1301 Pennsylvania Avenue, NW, Suite 800, Washington, DC 20004; 800-LUNG-USA
- Centers for Disease Control and Prevention. Seasonal influenza (flu). http://www.cdc.gov/flu.

PROGNOSIS

- Usually favorable prognosis, with illness lasting several days to a week
- Postviral fatigue is common.
- Death can occur, especially in pediatric or bone marrow transplant recipients with adenovirus infections or in older people with influenza.
- The 2009 H1N1 influenza pandemic resulted in higher-than-usual mortality rates among the pediatric, young adult, and pregnant populations.

COMPLICATIONS

- Superimposed bacterial infections, such as *Streptococcus pneumoniae*, *Staphylococcus aureus*, *Haemophilus influenzae*, and others
- Respiratory failure requiring mechanical ventilation
- ARDS
- Reye syndrome after influenza in children (avoid aspirin)

REFERENCES

1. Centers for Disease Control and Prevention. Seasonal influenza (flu). http://www.cdc.gov/flu. Accessed 2014.
2. Agency for Healthcare Research and Quality. *Pneumonia Severity Index Calculator: About. December 2003*. Rockville, MD. http://pda.ahrq.gov/psiabout.htm. Accessed 2014.
3. Heneghan CJ, Onakpoya I, Thompson M, et al. Zanamivir for influenza in adults and children: systematic review of clinical study reports and summary of regulatory comments. *BMJ*. 2014;348:g2547.
4. Centers for Disease Control and Prevention. Prevention and control of influenza with vaccines: recommendations of the Advisory Committee on Immunization Practices (ACIP), 2011. *MMWR Morb Mortal Wkly Rep.* 2011;60(33):1128–1132.

ADDITIONAL READING

- Fiore AE, Uyeki TM, Broder K, et al; Centers for Disease Control and Prevention. Prevention and control of influenza with vaccines: recommendations of the Advisory Committee on Immunization Practices (ACIP) 2010. *MMWR Recomm Rep.* 2010;59(RR-8):1–62.
- Marcos MA, Esperatti M, Torres A. Viral pneumonia. *Curr Opin Infect Dis.* 2009;22(2):143–147.
- Ruuskanen O, Lahti E, Jennings LC, et al. Viral pneumonia. *Lancet.* 2011;377(9773):1264–1275.

SEE ALSO

Bronchiolitis Obliterans and Organizing Pneumonia; Respiratory Distress Syndrome, Acute

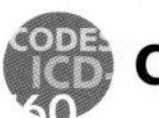

CODES

ICD10

- J12.9 Viral pneumonia, unspecified
- J12.0 Adenoviral pneumonia
- J12.1 Respiratory syncytial virus pneumonia

CLINICAL PEARLS

- Laboratory testing may confirm the diagnosis of viral pneumonia, but this may not change therapy and must not replace clinical judgment.
- Influenza vaccination is recommended for all persons age ≥ 6 months.
- Most patients recover with conservative therapy.
- Monitor for concomitant bacterial infections.
- Amantadine and rimantadine are no longer recommended for use against influenza.

POLYARTERITIS NODOSA

Katherine S. Upchurch, MD • Youmna Lahoud, MD

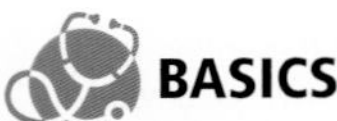

BASICS

DESCRIPTION

- Polyarteritis nodosa (PAN) is an antineutrophil cytoplasmic antibody (ANCA)-negative necrotizing arteritis of medium or small arteries without glomerulonephritis or vasculitis of arterioles, capillaries, or venules (1).
- Most commonly involves GI tract, peripheral nervous system (sensory and motor) and central nervous system (CNS), renal (without glomerulonephritis), skin, testes/epididymis, cardiac (1,2,3)
- Features depend on location of vasculitis: mesenteric ischemia–related symptoms, new onset or worsening hypertension, mononeuritis multiplex, purpuric or nodular skin lesions, or livedo reticularis (3).
- Renal disease in PAN usually manifests as hypertension (HTN) and mild proteinuria with/without azotemia. Renal infarction may occur (3).
- PAN formerly encompassed several distinct entities (classic PAN, microscopic PAN, cutaneous PAN). With the advent of ANCA testing, microscopic PAN appears not to be related to the other 2 pathophysiologically.
  - Patients with classic PAN (commonly referred to as PAN) are *typically ANCA-negative* (1,4).
  - Patients with microscopic PAN have ANCAs directed against myeloperoxidase (MPO) and (generally) involvement of small arterioles (microscopic polyangiitis [MPA]) and is now classified as ANCA-associated vasculitis (1).
  - Cutaneous (or limited) PAN is a chronic disease with cutaneous lesions with characteristic histopathologic features of PAN. There are few systemic manifestations, although myalgias and peripheral motor neuropathy (mononeuritis multiplex) or sensory neuropathy may be present. ANCA positivity is variable (5).
- Synonym(s): periarteritis; panarteritis; necrotizing arteritis

EPIDEMIOLOGY

Incidence

- Predominant age: Peak onset is in the 5th–6th decade, and incidence rises with age.
- 1.5:1 male predominance (6)

Prevalence

Rare: 2–33 cases/1 million adults (6)

ETIOLOGY AND PATHOPHYSIOLOGY

- Segmental, transmural, necrotizing inflammation of medium and small muscular arteries, with intimal proliferation, thrombosis, and ischemia of the organ/tissue supplied by the affected arteries. Aneurysm formation vessel bifurcations vessels (3)
- Hepatitis B–related PAN results in direct injury to the vessel due to viral replication or deposition of immune complexes, with complement activation and subsequent inflammatory response (3).
- Most cases are idiopathic; 20% are related to hepatitis B or C infection (7).
- In patients with PAN and hepatitis B, hepatitis B antigen has been recovered from involved vessel walls (7).

Genetics

Mutations of adenosine deaminase 2 (ADA 2) have been identified in families with multiple members who have PAN with variable clinical expression (8).

RISK FACTORS

Hepatitis B infection >> hepatitis C infection (cutaneous PAN) (7)

COMMONLY ASSOCIATED CONDITIONS

- Hepatitis B (strong association with classic PAN) (7)
- Hepatitis C (less strongly linked to cutaneous PAN)
- Hairy cell leukemia
- 27 existing case reports of systemic PAN following hepatitis B vaccination (9)
- Case reports also associating PAN with amphetamines, minocycline, and interferon (9)

DIAGNOSIS

There are no formal diagnostic criteria for PAN (1,3). Suspect PAN in patients with the following:

- Acute, sometimes fulminant multisystem disease with a relatively short prodrome (i.e., weeks to months)
- Vasculitic skin rash with sensorimotor symptoms/findings
- Recent-onset HTN with systemic symptoms
- Unexplained sensory and/or motor neuropathy with systemic symptoms
- Hepatitis B infection with multisystem disease

HISTORY

General: systemic symptoms with multiorgan involvement (3):

- Constitutional symptoms (fever, weight loss, malaise)
- Organ-specific symptoms:
  - Focal muscular weakness/extremity numbness
  - Myalgia and arthralgia
  - Rash
  - Recurrent postprandial pain, intestinal angina, nausea, vomiting, and bleeding
  - Altered mental status, headaches, mononeuritis multiplex
  - Testicular/epididymal pain, neurogenic bladder (rare)

PHYSICAL EXAM

Related to organ system involved by vasculitic process (may dominate clinical picture and course) (2,3)

- Peripheral nervous system: mononeuritis multiplex, peripheral neuropathy
- Renal: HTN
- Skin: purpura, urticaria, polymorphic rashes, subcutaneous nodules (uncommon, but characteristic), livedo reticularis; deep skin ulcers, especially in lower extremities; Raynaud phenomenon (rare)
- GI: acute abdomen; rebound, guarding, tenderness
- CNS: seizures, altered mental status, papillitis
- Lung: signs of pleural effusion-dullness to percussion; decreased breath sounds
- Cardiac: signs of congestive heart failure and/or myocardial infarction- S3 gallop; pericarditis (friction rub-rare)
- Genitourinary: testicular/epididymal tenderness
- Musculoskeletal: arthritis (usually large joint in lower extremities)

DIFFERENTIAL DIAGNOSIS

- Other forms of vasculitis (ANCA-associated, such as GPA, Churg-Strauss syndrome, and MPA; Henoch-Schönlein purpura, drug-induced vasculitis, cryoglobulinemia, Goodpasture syndrome)
- Buerger disease
- Systemic lupus erythematosus (SLE)
- Embolic disease (atrial myxoma, cholesterol emboli)
- Thrombotic disease (antiphospholipid antibody syndrome)
- Dissecting aneurysm
- Ehlers-Danlos syndrome
- Multiple sclerosis, systemic amyloidosis
- Infection (subacute endocarditis, HIV infection, trichinosis, rickettsial diseases)

DIAGNOSTIC TESTS & INTERPRETATION

- No specific laboratory abnormalities. Confirm diagnosis with biopsy if possible (4)[C].
- Angiography (conventional, CT angiography, or MR angiography) may help reveal microaneurysms and/or beading of bifurcating blood vessels.
- Avoid contrast in renal disease.
- Nonspecific laboratory abnormalities:
  - Elevated ESR and CRP
  - Mild proteinuria, elevated creatinine
  - Hepatitis B surface antigen positive in 10–50%
  - Hepatitis C antibody/hepatitis C virus RNA may be positive.
  - ANCA, antiproteinase 3 (PR3), anti-MPO are negative. Positive ANCA argues against PAN.
  - Rheumatoid factor may be positive.
  - Anemia of chronic disease (3,4)

Initial Tests (lab, imaging)

Lab tests performed to look for evidence of systemic disease and rule out other causes (3,4):

- CBC, ESR, CRP (elevated) (4)[C]
- Chemistries: elevated creatinine/BUN (4)[C]
- Hepatitis B serology: often positive; hepatitis C less commonly positive
- LFTs: abnormal if involving the liver/biliary tract
- Urinalysis: proteinuria/hematuria, generally no cellular casts or active urinary sediment (4)[C]
- ANA, cryoglobulins (4)[C]
- ANCA, anti-MPO, and anti-PR3 (4)[A]
- Complement levels (C3, C4)
- Angiographic demonstration of aneurysmal changes/beading of small and medium-sized arterie

Diagnostic Procedures/Other

- Electromyography and nerve conduction studies in patients with suspected mononeuritis multiplex. If abnormal, consider a sural nerve biopsy.
- Arterial/tissue biopsy
- Skin biopsy from edges of ulcers; include deep dermis and subcutaneous (SC) fat to assess small muscular artery involvement (excisional *not* punch biopsy) (3,4)

Test Interpretation

- Necrotizing inflammation with fibrinoid necrosis of small and medium-sized muscular arteries; segmental, often at bifurcations and branchings. Involvement of venules is not seen in classic PAN.
- Capillaritis/other lung parenchymal involvement by vasculitis *strongly suggests* another process (microscopic PAN, granulomatosis with polyangiitis [GPA; formerly known as Wegener granulomatosis], Churg-Strauss syndrome, or antiglomerular basement membrane disease).
- Acute lesions with infiltration of polymorphonuclear cells through vessel walls into perivascular area; necrosis, thrombosis, infarction of involved tissue
- Aneurysmal dilatations, including aortic dissection

- Peripheral nerves: 50–70% (vasa nervorum with necrotizing vasculitis)
- GI vessels: 50% (at autopsy) with bowel necrosis; gallbladder and appendix vasculature: 10%
- Muscle vessels: 50%
- Testicular vessels involved in symptomatic males
- *The key differences from other necrotizing vasculitides are lack of granuloma formation and sparing of veins and pulmonary arteries* (2,3).

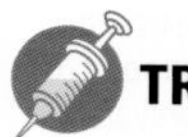

TREATMENT

GENERAL MEASURES

Aggressively treat HTN to prevent associated complications (stroke, myocardial infarction, heart failure)

MEDICATION

First Line

- Severe (life-threatening) disease: corticosteroids (CS) (high-dose prednisone or parenteral Solu-Medrol) (4,10)[A]
  - Only 50% of patients achieve and maintain remission with CS. Other patients require additional immunosuppressive therapy.
  - Cyclophosphamide (CTX) in combination with CS: improves survival and spares use of chronic steroids in moderate/severe PAN (4,10)[A]
    - CTX has associated risk of infertility and malignancy.
  - Plasma exchange for refractory and renal disease (4,7)[A]
  - Rituximab use for refractory disease has been suggested by its efficacy in ANCA + vasculitis (4,11,12)[C].
- Less severe disease: CS alone ± other immunosuppressive agents: azathioprine, (4)[A] methotrexate, mycophenolate mofetil (4,10,13)[B]
- HBV-associated PAN: antiviral agents, short-term CS, plasma exchange (no large evidence-based trials (7,10)[C]

Second Line

- Tumor necrosis factor inhibitors have been anecdotally reported to be of use in PAN (14).
- PAN disease activity correlates with serum IL-6 levels; tocilizumab, an inhibitor of IL-6 approved for use in rheumatoid arthritis; no evidence-based studies yet support this approach in PAN (15).

ADDITIONAL THERAPIES

- For patients receiving IV CTX, concurrent administration of mercaptoethane sulfonate (Mesna) reduces bladder exposure to carcinogenic metabolites (4)[C].
- Prophylactically treat patients on CTX, against *Pneumocystis jiroveci* (*carinii*) pneumonia using trimethoprim sulfamethoxazole (or atovaquone in patients who are intolerant/allergic) (4).

INPATIENT CONSIDERATIONS

Admission Criteria/Initial Stabilization

Depends on extent and involvement of specific organs

ONGOING CARE

FOLLOW-UP RECOMMENDATIONS

Patient Monitoring

- CBC, urinalysis, renal and hepatic function tests
- Acute-phase reactants (e.g., ESR, CRP) may help monitor disease activity.
- Be alert for the following:
  - Treatment specific side effects of CS and immunosuppressant medications
  - Delayed appearance of neoplasms after treatment, especially bladder malignancy in patients treated with CTX. (Check annual U/A, urinary cytology with urologic evaluation if microscopic hematuria.) (4)[C]
  - Steroid-induced osteoporosis

DIET

Low salt (HTN)

PATIENT EDUCATION

- Patient education materials are available from the Arthritis Foundation, 1314 Spring St, N.W., Atlanta, GA 30309; 800-283-7800
- ACR website: www.rheumatology.org

PROGNOSIS

- Expected course of untreated PAN is poor, with an estimated 5-year survival of 13% (16).
- Steroid and cytotoxic treatment increase 5-year survival rate to 75–80% (3,16).
- Survival is greater for hepatitis B–related PAN as a result of the introduction of antiviral treatments (7).
- Patients presenting with proteinuria, renal insufficiency, GI tract involvement, cardiomyopathy, or CNS involvement have a worse prognosis.

COMPLICATIONS

- End-organ damage from ischemia
- Complications of treatment with immunosuppressive agents

REFERENCES

1. Jennette JC, Falk RJ, Bacon PA, et al. 2012 revised International Chapel Hill Consensus Conference Nomenclature of Vasculitides. *Arthritis Rheum*. 2013;65(1):1–11.
2. Ebert EC, Hagspiel KD, Nagar M, et al. Gastrointestinal involvement in polyarteritis nodosa. *Clin Gastroenterol Hepatol*. 2008;6(9):960–966.
3. Pagnoux C, Seror R, Henegar C, et al. Clinical features and outcomes in 348 patients with polyarteritis nodosa: a systematic retrospective study of patients diagnosed between 1963 and 2005 and entered into the French Vasculitis Study Group Database. *Arthritis Rheum*. 2010;62(2):616–626.
4. Mukhtyar C, Guillevin L, Cid M, et al. EULAR recommendations for the management of primary small and medium vessel vasculitis. *Ann Rheum Dis*. 2009;68(3):310–317.
5. Nakamura T, Kanazawa N, Ikeda T, et al. Cutaneous polyarteritis nodosa: revisiting its definition and diagnostic criteria. *Arch Dermatol Res*. 2009;301(1):117–121.
6. Phillip R, Luqmani R. Mortality in systemic vasculitis: a systematic review. *Clin Exp Rheumatol*. 2008;26(5)(Suppl 51):94–104.
7. Guillevin L, Mahr A, Callard P, et al. Hepatitis B virus-associated polyarteritis nodosa: clinical characteristics, outcome, and impact of treatment in 115 patients. *Medicine (Baltimore)*. 2005;84(5):313–322.
8. Navon Elkan P, Pierce SB, Segel R, et al. Mutant adenosine deaminase 2 in a polyarteritis nodosa vasculopathy. *N Engl J Med*. 2014;370(10):921–931.
9. de Carvalho JF, Pereira RM, Shoenfeld Y. Systemic polyarteritis nodosa following hepatitis B vaccination. *Eur J Intern Med*. 2008;19(8):575–578.
10. de Menthon M, Mahr A. Treating polyarteritis nodosa: current state of the art. *Clin Exp Rheumatol*. 2011;29(1)(Suppl 4):S110–S116.
11. Stone JH, Merkel PA, Spiera R, et al. Rituximab versus cyclophosphamide for ANCA-associated vasculitis. *N Engl J Med*. 2010;363(3):221–232.
12. Specks U, Merkel PA, Seo P, et al. Efficacy of remission-induction regimens for ANCA-associated vasculitis. *N Engl J Med*. 2013;369(5):417–427.
13. Ribi C, Cohen P, Pagnoux C, et al. Treatment of polyarteritis nodosa and microscopic polyangiitis without poor-prognosis factors: a prospective randomized study of one hundred twenty-four patients. *Arthritis Rheum*. 2010;62(4):1186–1197.
14. Chan M, Lugmani R. Pharmacotherapy of vasculitis. *Expert Opin Pharmacother*. 2009;10(8):1273–1289.
15. Murakami M, Nishimoto N. The value of blocking IL-6 outside of rheumatoid arthritis: current perspective. *Curr Opin Rheumatol*. 2011;23(3):273–277.
16. Bourgarit A, Le Toumelin P, Pagnoux C, et al. Deaths occurring during the first year after treatment onset for polyarteritis nodosa, microscopic polyangiitis, and Churg-Strauss syndrome: a retrospective analysis of causes and factors predictive of mortality based on 595 patients. *Medicine (Baltimore)*. 2005;84(5):323–330.

SEE ALSO

Hepatitis B; Hepatitis C

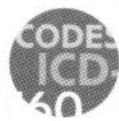

CODES

ICD10

- M30.0 Polyarteritis nodosa
- M30.1 Polyarteritis with lung involvement [Churg-Strauss]
- M30.8 Other conditions related to polyarteritis nodosa

CLINICAL PEARLS

- PAN is a necrotizing vasculitis of small to medium-sized muscular arteries with lack of granuloma formation that spares of veins and the pulmonary arteries.
- Clinical features of PAN depend on affected target organs.
- Perform skin biopsies at ulcer edges to include deep dermis and SC fat and improve diagnostic yield.
- Check hepatitis B and C serologies.
- ANCA is negative in classic PAN.

POLYCYSTIC KIDNEY DISEASE

Maricarmen Malagon-Rogers, MD

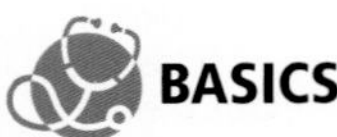

BASICS

DESCRIPTION

- A group of monogenic disorders that results in renal cyst development
- The most frequent are 2 genetically distinct conditions: autosomal dominant polycystic kidney disease (ADPKD) and autosomal recessive polycystic kidney disease (ARPKD).
- ADPKD is one of the most common human genetic disorders.

EPIDEMIOLOGY

- ADPKD is generally late onset:
  - Mean age of end-stage kidney disease (ESKD) 57–69 years
  - More progressive disease in men than in women
  - Up to 90% of adults have cysts in the liver.
- ARPKD usually presents in infants:
  - A minority in older children and young adults may manifest as liver disease.
  - Nonobstructive intrahepatic bile dilatation is sometimes seen.
  - Found on all continents and in all races

Incidence

- Mean age of ESKD: *PKD1 mutation*, 54.3 years versus *PKD2 mutation*, 74 years
- ARPKD affects 1/20,000 live births; carrier level is 1/70.
- ADPKD affects 1/400–1,000 live births.

Prevalence

As ESKD, ADPKD: 8.7/1 million in the United States; 7/1 million in Europe

ETIOLOGY AND PATHOPHYSIOLOGY

- ADPKD
  - PKD1 and PKD2 mutations disrupt the function of polycystins on the primary cilium, forming fluid-filled cysts that progressively increase in size, leading to gross enlargement of the kidney and distortion of the renal architecture.
  - Glomerular hyperfiltration compensates for the progressive loss of healthy glomeruli, and therefore, by the time GFR decline becomes detectable, as much as one-half of the original functional glomeruli are irreversibly lost.
  - The majority of patients with ADPKD ultimately progress to ESKD (1).
- ARPKD
  - *PKHD1* product fibrocystin is also located in cilia.
- ADPKD: Cysts arise from only 5% of nephrons:
  - Autosomal dominant pattern of inheritance but a molecularly recessive disease with the 2-hit hypothesis
  - Requires genetic and environmental factors
- ARPKD: Mutations are scattered throughout the gene with genotype–phenotype correlation.

Genetics

- ADPKD
  - Autosomal dominant inheritance
  - 50% of children of an affected adult are affected.
  - 100% penetrance; genetic imprinting and genetic anticipation are seen as well.
  - 2 genes isolated
    - *PKD1* on chromosome 16p13.3 (85% of patients) encodes polycystin 1
    - *PKD2* on chromosome 4q21 (15% of patients) encodes polycystin 2
    - Presumed *PKD3* not yet identified
- ARPKD
  - Autosomal recessive inheritance
  - Siblings have a 1:4 chance of being affected; gene *PKHD1* on chromosome 6p21.1–p12 encodes fibrocystin.

RISK FACTORS

- Large inter- and intrafamilial variability
- A more rapidly progressive clinical course is predicted by onset of ESKD at <55 years, development of stage 3 CKD at <40 years old, onset of hypertension (HTN) at <18 years, total kidney volume greater than the expected for a given age, or presence of multiple complications (gross hematuria, microalbuminuria) (1).

GENERAL PREVENTION

Genetic counseling

COMMONLY ASSOCIATED CONDITIONS

- ADPKD
  - Cysts in other organs
    - Polycystic liver disease in 58% of young age group to 94% of 45-year-olds
    - Pancreatic cysts: 5%
    - Seminal cysts: 40%
    - Arachnoid cysts: 8%
  - Vascular manifestations
    - Intracerebral aneurysms in 6% of patients without family history and in 16% with family history
    - Aortic dissections
  - Cardiac manifestations: mitral valve prolapse: 25%
  - Diverticular disease
- ARPKD: liver involvement: affected in inverse proportion to renal disease; congenital hepatic fibrosis with portal HTN

DIAGNOSIS

HISTORY

- ADPKD
  - Positive family history
  - Flank pain: 60%
  - Hematuria
  - UTI
  - HTN: 50% aged 20–34 years; 100% with ESKD
  - Renal failure
- ARPKD
  - 30% of affected neonates die:
    - Enlarged echogenic kidneys and oligohydramnios are diagnosed in utero.
    - Later in childhood: HTN
  - Adolescents and adults present with complications of portal HTN: esophageal varices
  - Hypersplenism

PHYSICAL EXAM

- HTN
- Flank masses

DIFFERENTIAL DIAGNOSIS

- ADPKD and ARPKD
- Tuberous sclerosis: prevalence 1/6,000
- Von Hippel–Lindau syndrome: prevalence 1/36,000
- Nephronophthisis: accounts for 10–20% of cases of renal failure in children; medullary cystic kidney disease
- Renal cystic dysplasias: multicystic dysplastic kidneys: grossly deformed kidneys; most common type of bilateral cystic diseases in newborns (prevalence: 1/4,000)
- Simple cysts: most common cystic abnormality
  - Localized or unilateral renal cystic disease
  - Medullary sponge kidney
  - Acquired renal cystic disease
- Renal cystic neoplasms: benign multilocular cyst (cystic nephroma)

DIAGNOSTIC TESTS & INTERPRETATION

Electrolytes, BUN/creatinine, urine analysis plus urinary citrate

Initial Tests (lab, imaging)

- ADPKD
  - Renal dysfunction
    - Impaired renal concentration (2), hypocitraturia aciduria
    - Hyperfiltration
    - Elevated creatinine
  - Urinalysis: hematuria and mild proteinuria
- ARPKD
  - Electrolyte abnormalities and renal insufficiency
  - Anemia, thrombocytopenia, leukopenia
- ADPKD
  - US: diagnostic method of choice
    - Renal enlargement is universal.
    - In at-risk patients: By age 30 years, 2 renal cysts (bilateral or unilateral) are 100% diagnostic. In children, it sometimes appears similar to ARPKD; may be diagnosed in utero
    - Presence of hepatic cysts in young adults is pathognomonic for ADPKD.
    - In the absence of family history, bilateral renal enlargement and cysts make the diagnosis.
  - CT scan/MRI
    - Kidney volume assessed by CT or MRI is a main predictor of progression.
    - Helpful in identifying cysts in other organs
- ARPKD
  - US: Kidneys are enlarged, homogeneously hyperechogenic (cortex and medulla).
  - CT scan is more sensitive if diagnosis is in doubt.
  - Presence of hepatic fibrosis helps the diagnosis.

Follow-Up Tests & Special Considerations

- Diagnosis and prevention of secondary problems because of renal and liver abnormalities
- Follow-up of combined renal volume to assess disease severity
- Beyond age 2 years, renal size decreases in ARPKD but continues to grow in ADPKD at an average rate of 5.27% per year.

P

Diagnostic Procedures/Other
- Genetic testing is available for *PKD1* and *PKD2* in ADPKD when imaging results are equivocal and for potential living related donors (3).
- For *PKHD1* in ARPKD, a prenatal diagnosis is feasible in about 72% of patients.

Test Interpretation
- ADPKD
  - Kidneys are diffusely cystic and, although enlarged, retain their general shape.
  - Cysts range from a few millimeters to several centimeters and are distributed evenly throughout the cortex and medulla.
  - They arise in all segments of the nephron, although they arise initially from the collecting ducts.
  - 1 kidney may be larger than the other.
- ARPKD
  - Disease is a spectrum, ranging from severe renal disease with mild liver damage to mild renal disease with severe liver damage.
  - Renal enlargement is due to fusiform dilatation of the collecting ducts in the cortex and medulla in the newborn period.
  - Liver lesion is diffuse but limited to fibrotic portal areas.

TREATMENT

GENERAL MEASURES
- HTN: moderate sodium restriction, weight control, and regular exercise
- Medications: ACE inhibitors; angiotensin receptor blockers (ARBs)
- Pain: narcotics and other analgesics; bed rest; limit NSAIDs (they worsen renal function).
- Urolithiasis: treated with alkalinization of urine and hydration therapy; surgery as needed
- UTIs/infections of cysts: lipid-soluble antibiotics more effective (e.g., trimethoprim-sulfamethoxazole and chloramphenicol); fluoroquinolones also useful
- Dialysis for ESKD patients
- Hematuria: Reduce physical activity.

MEDICATION
- No specific drug therapy is yet available for PKD, although several studies are being conducted for specific treatments (4).
- HTN: should be very well controlled to prevent complications. ACE inhibitors preferred if no contraindications present.
- The use of antihypertensive medications has been found to decrease mortality (4,5).
- Hyperlipidemia: statins preferred

ISSUES FOR REFERRAL
- Nephrologist primary management
- Urologic consultation for management of symptomatic/infected cysts
- Genetic counseling is critical.

SURGERY/OTHER PROCEDURES
- Indications for surgical intervention
  - Uncontrollable HTN
  - Severe back and loin pain, abdominal fullness
  - Renal deterioration due to enlarging cysts
  - Hematuria/hemorrhage or recurrent UTI
- Open and laparoscopic cyst unroofing: may decrease pain and narcotics requirements; has not been proven to prevent renal failure or to prolong current renal function
- Percutaneous cyst aspiration ± injection of sclerosing agent; not usually performed secondary to recurrent fluid accumulation
- Renal transplant for ESKD

INPATIENT CONSIDERATIONS

Admission Criteria/Initial Stabilization
Severe pain, gross hematuria with clots

ONGOING CARE

FOLLOW-UP RECOMMENDATIONS
None in early stages of the disease; avoid vigorous activity if disease advances. Recurrent gross hematuria is secondary to trauma, associated with faster decline of renal function.

Patient Monitoring
- Monitor BP and renal function. Encourage hydration. Treat UTI and stone disease aggressively.
- Avoid nephrotoxic drugs.
- Creatinine and BP monitoring at least twice a year; more often as needed
- Screening for intracranial aneurysms (6)

DIET
- Low-protein diet may retard renal insufficiency.
- Limit caffeine, because this might increase cyst growth.
- High water intake to decrease ADH >3 liters a day (4)

PROGNOSIS
- Renal failure in 2% by age 40 years; 23% by age 50 years; 48% by age 73 years
- ADPKD accounts for 10–15% of dialysis patients.
- No increased incidence of renal cell cancer

COMPLICATIONS
- Cyst rupture, infection, or hemorrhage
- Progression to renal failure
- Renal calculi

REFERENCES

1. Schrier RW, Brosnahan G, Cadnapaphornchai MA, et al. Predictors of autosomal dominant polycystic disease progression. *J Am Soc Nephrol*. 2014;25(11):2399–2418.
2. Zittema D, Boertien WE, van Beek AP, et al. Vasopressin, copeptin, and renal concentrating capacity in patients with autosomal dominant polycystic kidney disease without renal impairment. *Clin J Am Soc Nephrol*. 2012;7(6):906–913.
3. Harris PC, Rossetti S. Molecular diagnostics for autosomal dominant polycystic kidney disease. *Nat Rev Nephrol*. 2010;6(4):197–206.
4. Mahnensmith RL. Novel treatments of autosomal dominant polycystic kidney disease. *Clin J Am Soc Nephrol*. 2014;9(5):831–836.
5. Patch C, Charlton J, Roderick PJ, et al. Use of anti-hypertensive medications and mortality of patients with autosomal dominant polycystic kidney disease: a population-based study. *Am J Kidney Dis*. 2011;57(6):856–862.
6. Rozenfeld MN, Ansari SA, Shaibani A, et al. Should patients with autosomal dominant polycystic kidney disease be screened for cerebral aneurysms? *AJNR Am J Neuroradiol*. 2014;35(1):3–9.

ADDITIONAL READING

- Chapman AB, Bost JE, Torres VE, et al. Kidney volume and functional outcomes in autosomal dominant polycystic kidney disease. *Clin J Am Soc Nephrol*. 2012;7(3):479–486.
- Harris PC, Torres VE. Polycystic kidney disease. *Annu Rev Med*. 2009;60:321–337.
- Torres VE, Chapman AB, Devuyst O, et al. Tolvaptan in patients with autosomal dominant polycystic kidney disease. *N Engl J Med*. 2012;367(25):2407–2418.
- Torres VE, Harris PC. Polycystic kidney disease in 2011: connecting the dots toward a polycystic kidney disease therapy. *Nat Rev Nephrol*. 2012;8(2):66–68.
- Torres VE, Harris PC, Pirson Y. Autosomal dominant polycystic kidney disease. *Lancet*. 2007;369(9569):1287–1301.
- Wilson PD. Polycystic kidney disease. *N Engl J Med*. 2004;350(2):151–164.

SEE ALSO

Kidney Failure, Chronic; Nephrolithiasis

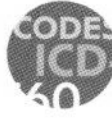

CODES

ICD10
- Q61.3 Polycystic kidney, unspecified
- Q61.19 Other polycystic kidney, infantile type
- Q61.2 Polycystic kidney, adult type

CLINICAL PEARLS
- Most PKD patients eventually develop ESKD. No specific treatment has been proven to prevent ESKD, but hydration and control of BP are reasonable goals and should be started soon.
- Patients may benefit from a nephrology consultation after the initial diagnosis to counsel regarding disease progression prevention. They then can be followed by primary care if the disease was an incidental finding or no significant kidney dysfunction is present.

POLYCYSTIC OVARIAN SYNDROME (PCOS)

Maria De La Luz Nieto, MD

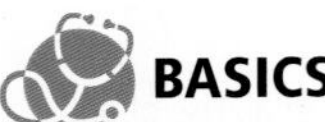

BASICS

DESCRIPTION

- Polycystic ovarian syndrome (PCOS) is a common endocrine disorder with heterogeneous manifestations that affects up to 7% of the U.S. population.
- Hyperandrogenism leading to anovulation, typically presenting as amenorrhea or oligomenorrhea
- Diagnosis is based on clinical assessment and ultrasound findings.
- Diagnostic clinical characteristics include menstrual dysfunction, infertility, hirsutism, acne, obesity, and metabolic syndrome. The ovaries are often polycystic on imaging.
- The etiology of PCOS is unknown but can be modified by lifestyle factors.
- System(s) affected: reproductive, endocrine/metabolic, skin/exocrine
- Synonym(s): Stein-Leventhal syndrome; polycystic ovary disease

ALERT

- Condition may begin at puberty.
- Pregnancy does not resolve the syndrome.
- Predisposes to and is associated with obesity, hypertension, diabetes, metabolic syndrome, hyperlipidemia, infertility, insulin-resistance syndrome

EPIDEMIOLOGY

Prevalence

- Incidence and prevalence are still highly debated due to a wide spectrum of diagnostic features: The National Institutes of Health (NIH) criteria require chronic anovulation in addition to clinical or biochemical signs of hyperandrogenism. The prevalence based on NIH criteria is 6.5–8%.
- Predominant age: reproductive age
- Predominant sex: females only

ETIOLOGY AND PATHOPHYSIOLOGY

- PCOS is a multifactorial functional disorder of unclear etiology.
- Recent evidence points to a primary role for insulin resistance with hyperinsulinemia.
- Androgenism: Ovaries are the main source of excess androgens. Polycystic ovaries have thickened thecal layers, which secrete excess androgens in response to luteinizing hormone (LH). LH receptors are overexpressed in thecal and granulosa cells of polycystic ovaries.
- Ovarian follicles: Abnormal androgen signaling may account for abnormal folliculogenesis causing polycystic ovaries. The mechanism that determines abnormal number of follicles is unknown but may be due to abnormal androgen signaling on the ovarian stroma.
- Insulin resistance: Women with PCOS have insulin resistance similar to that in type 2 diabetes. Elevated levels of insulin decrease sex hormone–binding protein (SHBG), increasing bioavailability of testosterone. Insulin may also act directly on adrenal, ovary, and hypothalamus to regulate androgen and gonadotropin release. Insulin resistance causes elevated insulin levels.
- Insulin resistance may cause the frequently associated metabolic syndrome and frank diabetes mellitus.

Genetics

Ultimate expression is likely a combination of polygenic and environmental factors.

RISK FACTORS

See "Commonly Associated Conditions"; cause and effect are difficult to extricate in this disorder.

GENERAL PREVENTION

None known; focus on early diagnosis and treatment to prevent long-term complications.

COMMONLY ASSOCIATED CONDITIONS

- Infertility
- Obesity
- Obstructive sleep apnea
- Hypertension
- Diabetes mellitus
- Endometrial hyperplasia/carcinoma
- Fatty liver disease
- Mood disturbances and depression

DIAGNOSIS

HISTORY

- A comprehensive history, including a family history of diabetes and premature onset of cardiovascular disease, is important in the differential diagnosis.
- Focus on the onset and duration of the various signs of androgen excess, menstrual history, and concomitant medications, including the use of exogenous androgens (1).

PHYSICAL EXAM

- Vital signs: body mass index (BMI), high BP
- General appearance: central obesity, deepened voice, hirsutism, acne
- Skin: hair pattern and growth, acne, seborrhea, acanthosis nigricans
- Genitalia: clitoromegaly and ovarian enlargement

ALERT

Look specifically for signs of virilization, such as hair pattern, deepened voice, and clitoromegaly.

DIFFERENTIAL DIAGNOSIS

- Cushing syndrome
- HAIR-AN syndrome
- Testosterone-producing ovarian or adrenal tumor
- Prolactin-producing pituitary adenoma
- Hyperthecosis
- Adult-onset adrenal hyperplasia
- Partial congenital adrenal hyperplasia (21-hydroxylase deficiency)
- 11β-hydroxylase deficiency
- 17β-hydroxysteroid dehydrogenase deficiency
- Acromegaly
- Drug-induced hirsutism, oligo-ovulation (e.g., danazol, steroids, valproic acid)
- Thyroid disease

DIAGNOSTIC TESTS & INTERPRETATION

- The value of measurement of circulating androgens to document PCOS is uncertain but should include measuring free testosterone concentration directly by equilibrium dialysis.
- Most common diagnostic criteria used is Rotterdam criteria (need 2 of 3):
  - Oligo- or anovulation
  - Clinical and/or biochemical signs of hyperandrogenism
  - Transvaginal ultrasonographic polycystic ovaries and exclusion of other etiologies; therefore, consider exclusion of Cushing disease, congenital adrenal hyperplasia, and androgen-secreting tumors.
- More recent criteria also focus on similar criteria while acknowledging that there may be forms of PCOS without overt evidence of hyperandrogenism (2,3)[C].

Initial Tests (lab, imaging)

- Screening workup should include human chorionic gonadotropin (hCG), TSH, prolactin, FSH (exclude premature ovarian failure), DHEAS, 17-OH progesterone, and testosterone level.
- LH determination may be ordered but is not usually necessary:
  - Hirsute women should have a testosterone or free testosterone determination and a DHEAS determination.
  - Consider 17-OH progesterone if congenital adrenal hyperplasia is a possibility.
- LH/FSH level $\geq$2.5–3/L in ~50% of women with PCOS, but LH testing is not generally necessary.
- Testosterone increased but <200 ng/dL (6.94 nmol/L)
- Typical findings in PCOS include mild elevation in DHEAS but <800 μg/dL (20.8 μmol/L), mild increase in 17-OH progesterone level, increased estrogen level, and decreased SHBG.
- Drugs that may alter lab results:
  - Oral contraceptives (OCs)
  - Steroids
  - Antidepressants
- Transvaginal ultrasound findings: 1 or both ovaries with $\geq$12 follicles measuring 2–9 mm or increased ovarian volume to 10 cm^3

Follow-Up Tests & Special Considerations

- Consider fasting serum glucose, insulin level, and plasminogen activator inhibitor-1 determinations to establish presence of insulin resistance and glucose intolerance, especially if diagnosis is in doubt.
- Overnight dexamethasone suppression test (Decadron 1 mg PO at 11:00 PM and fasting serum cortisol at 8:00 AM the next morning) to rule out Cushing syndrome in the appropriate setting
- Endometrial biopsy to rule out hyperplasia and/or carcinoma, if indicated
- If the syndrome is diagnosed, determination of fasting glucose and fasting lipid levels should be performed and formal glucose tolerance test considered.

Test Interpretation

- Ovary usually enlarged with a smooth white glistening capsule
- Ovarian cortex lined with follicles in all stages of development, but most atretic
- Thecal cell proliferation with an increase in the stromal compartment

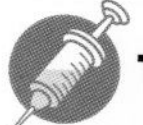

TREATMENT

GENERAL MEASURES

- No ideal treatment exists.
- Therapy must be individualized according to the needs and desires of each patient.

MEDICATION

Drug costs related to this condition are high.

First Line

- The goal of treatment in PCOS depends on symptoms and patient's goals for fertility.
- Treatment can be divided into 5 main categories: Lifestyle changes including appropriate nutrition and exercise to decrease body weight can restore ovulation and increase insulin sensitivity (4)[A],(5)[C].
- Menstrual irregularity when pregnancy not desired:
  - Low-dose OCs (30–35 μg); newer formulations containing progestins with lower androgenicity (e.g., norethindrone, desogestrel, norgestimate, drospirenone) may be particularly beneficial, but all OCs increase SHBG and decrease excess androgen and estrogen. If unable to tolerate OCs, then intermittent medroxyprogesterone (Provera) 10 mg PO × 10 days given every 1–2 months.
  - Metformin may help to correct metabolic abnormalities in women who are shown to be insulin resistant. Initial dose is 500 mg daily × 1 week, increasing by 500 mg/wk to a total of 1,500–2,000 mg/day divided BID; take with food
    - Overall, data support the usefulness of metformin on both cardiometabolic risk and reproduction assistance in PCOS women.
    - Thiazolidinediones may increase likelihood of ovulation and treat insulin resistance.
- If pregnancy desired (6)[B]:
  - Ovulation induction with clomiphene (Clomid, Serophene) and/or exogenous gonadotropins. Birth rate with Clomid is 22.5%, 7.2% with metformin, and 26.8% in women who use both medications.
  - Metformin: 500–2,000 mg PO divided BID has been shown to improve hyperandrogenism and restore ovulation. Many times the drug is continued throughout the 1st trimester or the entire pregnancy if there is a history of spontaneous abortion or glucose intolerance. It does improve clinical pregnancy rates but does not improve live birth rates alone or in combination with clomiphene when used for ovulation induction.
  - Has been demonstrated that metformin reduces the incidence of gestational diabetes

Second Line

- Spironolactone for androgen excess hirsutism not addressed by OC therapy
- Cosmetic issues due to hyperandrogenism: Acne may respond best with OCs with low doses of cyproterone or drospirenone.
- Eflornithine hydrochloride 13.9% cream to inhibit hair growth

ADDITIONAL THERAPIES

Weight loss in overweight women results in biochemical and symptomatic improvement in most.

ISSUES FOR REFERRAL

- To reproductive endocrinologist for all women who cannot achieve pregnancy with Clomid
- High-risk pregnancies
- To endocrinologist if Cushing syndrome, congenital adrenal hyperplasia, or adrenal or ovarian tumors are found during the workup

SURGERY/OTHER PROCEDURES

- Ovarian wedge resection and laparoscopic laser drilling are controversial and rarely used today.
- Mechanical means of hair removal, including electrolysis, waxing, and depilatory, may improve cosmesis.

COMPLEMENTARY & ALTERNATIVE MEDICINE

Acupuncture assists with cycle normalization and weight loss.

ONGOING CARE

FOLLOW-UP RECOMMENDATIONS

Follow-up at 6-month intervals to evaluate response to therapy and to monitor weight as well as medication side effects.

Patient Monitoring

- Counsel patient about the risk of endometrial and breast carcinoma, insulin resistance, and diabetes, as well as obesity and its role in infertility.
- See patient frequently throughout the menstrual cycle, depending on which drug combination is used to induce ovulation.

DIET

In overweight patients, weight loss is the most successful therapy because it improves cardiovascular risk, insulin sensitivity, and menstrual patterns: Counsel on lifestyle dietary changes; consider referral to nutritionist and weight center.

PATIENT EDUCATION

- Provide patient with information about PCOS, such as from www.acog.org.
- Discuss the chronic nature of this condition and the risks and benefits and side effects of potential treatments.
- Review the importance of weight loss, if applicable. Modest weight loss of 5–10% of initial body weight has been demonstrated to improve many of the features of PCOS.

PROGNOSIS

- Fertility prognosis is good but may need assisted reproductive technologies.
- Proper follow-up and screening can prevent endometrial carcinoma.
- Early detection of diabetes may decrease morbidity and mortality associated with cardiovascular risk factor.

COMPLICATIONS

- Reproductive: infertility
- Metabolic: insulin resistance, diabetes mellitus, cardiovascular disease
- Psychosocial: increased anxiety, mood disorder, eating disorder, depression

REFERENCES

1. Azziz R, Carmina E, Dewailly D, et al. The Androgen Excess and PCOS Society criteria for the polycystic ovary syndrome: the complete task force report. *Fertil Steril*. 2009;91(2):456–488.
2. Carmina E, Oberfield SE, Lobo RA, et al. The diagnosis of polycystic ovary syndrome in adolescents. *Am J Obstet Gynecol*. 2010;203(3):201.e1–201.e5.
3. Chang RJ. A practical approach to the diagnosis of polycystic ovary syndrome. *Am J Obstet Gynecol*. 2004;191(3):713–717.
4. Tang T, Lord JM, Norman RJ, et al. Insulin-sensitising drugs (metformin, rosiglitazone, pioglitazone, D-chiro-inositol) for women with polycystic ovary syndrome, oligo amenorrhoea and subfertility. *Cochrane Database Syst Rev*. 2010;1:CD003053.
5. Rotterdam ESHRE/ASRM Sponsored PCOS Consensus Workshop Group. Revised 2003 consensus on diagnostic criteria and long-term health risks related to polycystic ovary syndrome. *Fertil Steril*. 2004;81(1):19–25.
6. Legro RS, Barnhart HX, Schlaff WD, et al. Clomiphene, metformin, or both for infertility in the polycystic ovary syndrome. *N Engl J Med*. 2007;356(6):551–566.

ADDITIONAL READING

- Diamanti-Kandarakis E, Economou F, Palimeri S, et al. Metformin in polycystic ovary syndrome. *Ann N Y Acad Sci*. 2010;1205:192–198.
- Lim CE, Wong WS. Current evidence of acupuncture on polycystic ovarian syndrome. *Gynecol Endocrinol*. 2010;26(6):473–478.
- Moran LJ, Misso ML, Wild RA, et al. Impaired glucose tolerance, type 2 diabetes and metabolic syndrome in polycystic ovary syndrome: a systematic review and meta-analysis. *Hum Reprod Update*. 2010;16(4):347–363.

SEE ALSO

Algorithm: Amenorrhea

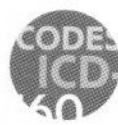

CODES

ICD10

- E28.2 Polycystic ovarian syndrome
- L68.0 Hirsutism

CLINICAL PEARLS

- In the United States, 40% of women with PCOS are not obese.
- Chronic anovulation should be treated because chronic estrogen stimulation in absence of progesterone may lead to endometrial hyperplasia.
- Specific therapies must be individualized according to the needs and desires of each patient.

POLYCYTHEMIA VERA

Richrd D. Detheridge, MD • Roger P. Holland, MD, PhD

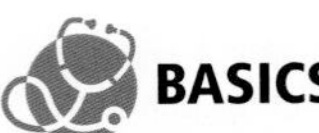

BASICS

DESCRIPTION

- Polycythemia vera (PV) is a chronic myeloproliferative clonal stem cell disorder marked by increased production of red blood cells (erythrocytosis) with excessive erythroid, myeloid, and megakaryocytic elements in the bone marrow.
- Morbidity and mortality are primarily related to complications from blood hyperviscosity or thrombosis development as well as malignant transformation. Myelofibrosis can develop in the bone marrow, leading to progressive hepatosplenomegaly.
- Synonym(s): primary polycythemia; Vaquez disease; Waldenstrom disease; primary PV; PV rubra; polycythemia, splenomegalic; Vaquez-Osler disease

EPIDEMIOLOGY

Incidence

- Predominant age: 50–75 years, 5% are younger than 40 years
- Predominant sex: male > female (slightly)
- Incidence in the United States in 2012: 2.8/100,000 population of men and 1.3/100,000 population of women

Prevalence

In the United States in 2010, estimates ranged from 45–57 cases per 100,000 patients.

ETIOLOGY AND PATHOPHYSIOLOGY

JAK2 V617F mutation associated with clonal proliferative disorder

Genetics

JAK2 V617F (tyrosine kinase) mutation: More than 97% of patients with PV have an activating mutation; this is helpful in differentiating from secondary erythrocytosis. Homozygote carriers will have higher incidence of symptoms such as pruritus but will not have higher incidence of disease than heterozygotes.

RISK FACTORS

- PV is more prevalent among Jews of Eastern European descent than other Europeans or Asians.
- Familial history is rare.

COMMONLY ASSOCIATED CONDITIONS

- Budd-Chiari syndrome
- Mesenteric artery thrombosis
- Myocardial infarction
- Cerebrovascular accident or transient ischemic attack
- Venous thromboembolism and pulmonary embolism

DIAGNOSIS

HISTORY

- Patients may be asymptomatic or present with nonspecific complaints, including fatigue, malaise, and/or subjective weakness.
- Erythromelalgia (burning pain of feet/hands, occasionally with erythema, pallor, cyanosis, or paresthesias)
- Arterial and venous occlusive events
- Headaches
- Blurred vision or blind spots
- Pruritus, especially after the shower
- Spontaneous bruising/bleeding
- Peptic ulcer disease (due to alterations in gastric mucosal blood flow)
- Bone pain (ribs and sternum)
- Tinnitus

PHYSICAL EXAM

- Hypertension
- Facial plethora
- Splenomegaly
- Hepatomegaly
- Bone tenderness (especially ribs and sternum)
- Skin excoriations from significant pruritus
- Gouty tophi or arthritis

DIFFERENTIAL DIAGNOSIS

- Secondary polycythemias
- Hemoglobinopathy
- Ectopic erythropoietin production
- Spurious polycythemia

DIAGNOSTIC TESTS & INTERPRETATION

CBC; if suspicion is high, then obtain erythropoietin level and gene testing for *JAK2 V617F*.

Initial Tests (lab, imaging)

- 2008 World Health Organization diagnostic criteria requires two major criteria and one minor or the first major criterion with two minor criteria (1).
  - Major criteria:
    - Hemoglobin (Hgb) >18.5 g/dL (men); Hgb >16.5 g/dL (women); or Hgb >17 g/dL (men) or Hgb >15 g/dL (women) if associated with a sustained increase of ≥2 g/dL from baseline that cannot be attributed to correction of iron deficiency
    - Presence of *JAK2 V617F* or similar mutation
  - Minor criteria:
    - Bone marrow trilineage myeloproliferation
    - Subnormal serum erythropoietin level
    - Endogenous erythroid colony (EEC) growth
- Diagnosis can be made reliably based on clinical symptoms, presence of *JAK2 V617* mutation, and low EPO (2).
- Other lab findings that are common but not specific
  - Hyperuricemia
  - Hypercholesterolemia
  - Elevated serum vitamin B_{12} levels
- CT or US to assess for splenomegaly, although not necessary for diagnosis
- Causes of secondary erythrocytosis:
  - Sleep apnea
  - Emphysema
  - Cigarette smoking
  - Renal artery stenosis
  - Carbon monoxide poisoning

Diagnostic Procedures/Other

- Bone marrow aspiration shows increased cellularity.
- Cytogenetic testing (*JAK2 V617F*)

Test Interpretation

- If *JAK2 V617F* mutation testing is negative and the erythropoietin level is normal or high, then PV is excluded; investigate causes of secondary erythrocytosis.
- Other causes of erythrocytosis such as ectopic erythropoietin production from a renal tumor, hypoxia from chronic lung or cyanotic heart disease can be excluded with low or undectectable serum erythropoietin level and normal oxygen saturation.

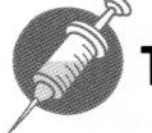

TREATMENT

GENERAL MEASURES

- Risk factors: age, disease duration, disease phenotype, complications, disease activity
- Phlebotomy and low-dose aspirin is 1st-line therapy for low-risk patients.
- Phlebotomy reduces the blood hyperviscosity, improve platelet functions, restore systemic pressures, and decrease risk of thrombosis.
- Phlebotomy:
  - Reduce hematocrit to <45%; will significantly lower rate of cardiovascular death and major thrombosis (3)[A].
  - Performed as often as every 2–3 days until normal hematocrit reached; phlebotomies of 250–500 mL. Reduce to 250–350 mL in elderly patients or patients with cerebrovascular disease.
  - May require concurrent myelosuppressive agent if at high risk for thrombosis
- Complications of phlebotomy: chronic iron deficiency (symptomatology: pica, angular stomatitis, and glossitis), possible muscle weakness, and dysphagia
- Other therapies:
  - Maintain hydration.
  - Pruritus therapy: H_1 and H_2 blockers, ataractics
  - Uric acid reduction therapy

MEDICATION

First Line

- Primary therapies:
  - Low-dose aspirin 81 mg PO has been associated with a statistically nonsignificant reduction in the risk of fatal thrombotic events without increasing bleeding complications when used in conjunction with phlebotomy (4)[A].
  - Hydroxyurea is recommended for patients at high risk for thrombosis (age >60 years or history of thrombotic event) and with splenomegaly and hepatomegaly. Common starting dose 500–1,500 mg PO daily, titrating to control hematocrit and platelet count. Be aware that hydroxyurea can lead to higher risk of leukemic transformation (5)[A].
  - Radioactive phosphorous (^{32}P) may control hemoglobin level and platelet count by destroying overactive marrow cells. May take up to 3 months before affecting cells. Consider for patients intolerant or nonadherent to hydroxyurea or short expected survival due to mutagenic potential.
  - Tyrosine kinase inhibitor imatinib 400–800 mg daily was shown to have moderate cytoreductive effects in PV (6)[B].
  - Pegylated interferon α2a is effective in controlling erythrocytosis, although dosing is generally limited secondary to intolerable side effects (7)[B].
  - Refer to hematologist/oncologist for further dosing and instructions.
- Symptomatic/adjunctive:
  - Allopurinol 300 mg/day PO for uric acid reduction
  - Cyproheptadine 4–16 mg PO daily as needed for pruritus
  - H_2-receptor blockers or antacids for GI hyperacidity; cimetidine is also used for pruritus.
  - SSRIs (paroxetine or fluoxetine) have shown some efficacy in controlling pruritus.
  - Ultraviolet light may help with pruritus.

Second Line

Myelosuppression: chlorambucil or busulfan; busulfan at 2–4 mg daily may be effective option for elderly patients with advanced PV refractory or intolerant to hydroxyurea, but significant rate of transformation was observed.

ISSUES FOR REFERRAL

Referral to a hematologist to assist in diagnosis and management

ONGOING CARE

FOLLOW-UP RECOMMENDATIONS

Patient Monitoring

Monitor hematocrit often and phlebotomize as needed to maintain target goal.

DIET

- Avoid high-sodium diet, can cause fluid retention.
- Avoid iron supplement, a permissive chronic state of iron deficiency can help decrease blood production.

PATIENT EDUCATION

- Perform leg and ankle exercises to prevent clots.
- Continuous education regarding possible complications and seeking treatment early for any change or increase in symptoms

PROGNOSIS

- PV cannot be cured but can be controlled with treatment.
- Survival is >15 years with treatment.
- Patients are at risk for developing postpolycythemic myelofibrosis (PPMF) and an increased risk of malignant transformation.

COMPLICATIONS

- Splenomegaly or hepatomegaly
- Budd-Chiari syndrome
- Vascular thrombosis (major cause of death)
- Transformation to acute leukemia
- Transformation to myelofibrosis
- Hemorrhage
- Peptic ulcer
- Uric acid stones
- Secondary gout
- Increased risk for complications and mortality from surgical procedures. Assess risk/benefits and ensure optimal control of disorder before any elective surgery.

REFERENCES

1. Tefferi A, Thiele J, Vardiman JW. The 2008 World Health Organization classification system for myeloproliferative neoplasms: order out of chaos. *Cancer.* 2009;115:3842–3847.
2. Tefferi A. Polycythemia vera and essential thrombocythemia: 2013 update on diagnosis, risk-stratification, and management. *Am J Hematol.* 2013;88(6):507–516.
3. Marchioli R, Finazzi G, Specchia G, et al. Cardiovascular events and intensity of treatment in polycythemia vera. *N Engl J Med.* 2013;368(1):22–33.
4. Squizzato A, Romualdi E, Passamonti F, et al. Antiplatelet drugs for polycythaemia vera and essential thrombocytaemia. *Cochrane Database Syst Rev.* 2013;4:CD006503.
5. Mascarenhas J, Mughal TI, Verstovsek S. Biology and clinical management of myeloproliferative neoplasms and development of the JAK inhibitor ruxolitinib. *Curr Med Chem.* 2012;19(26):4399–4413.
6. Merx K, Fabarius A, Erben P, et al. Effects of imatinib mesylate in patients with polycythemia vera: results of a phase II study. *Ann Hematol.* 2013;92(7):907–915.
7. Quintás-Cardama A, Kantarjian H, Manshouri T, et al. Pegylated interferon alfa-2a yields high rates of hematologic and molecular response in patients with advanced essential thrombocythemia and polycythemia vera. *J Clin Oncol.* 2009;27(32): 5418–5424.

ADDITIONAL READING

- Passamonti F. How I treat polycythemia vera. *Blood.* 2012;120(2):275–284.
- Tefferi A, Fonseca R. Selective serotonin reuptake inhibitors are effective in the treatment of polycythemia vera-associated pruritus. *Blood.* 2002; 99(7):2627.

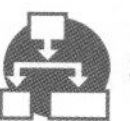

SEE ALSO

Myeloproliferative Neoplasms

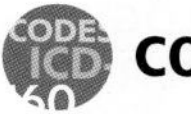

CODES

ICD10

- D45 Polycythemia vera
- D75.1 Secondary polycythemia

CLINICAL PEARLS

- *JAK2* mutations are an important component of myeloproliferative disorders.
- Common complications include thrombosis, malignant transformation, and myelofibrosis.
- Phlebotomy is 1st-line treatment, and consultation with an experienced hematologist is recommended.

POLYMYALGIA RHEUMATICA

Ronald G. Chambers, Jr., MD, FAAFP • Megan Babb, DO

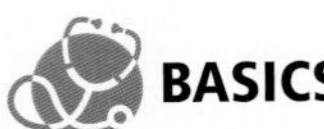

BASICS

DESCRIPTION

- Polymyalgia rheumatica (PMR) is a clinical syndrome characterized by pain and stiffness of the shoulder, hip girdles, and neck.
- Primarily impacts the elderly, associated with morning stiffness and elevated markers of inflammation
- System(s) affected: musculoskeletal; hematologic/lymphatic/immunologic
- Synonym(s): senile rheumatic disease; polymyalgia rheumatica syndrome; pseudo-polyarthrite rhizomélique

Geriatric Considerations

- Incidence increases with age.
- Average age of onset ~70 years

Pediatric Considerations

Almost never occurs in patients <50 years of age. The peak incidence of PMR occurs between ages 70 and 80 years (1).

EPIDEMIOLOGY

Incidence

- Incidence increases after age 50 years. Incidence of PMR and giant cell arteritis (GCA) in the United States population is 50 and 18 per 100,000 people.
- Predominant sex: female > male (2–3:1) (2)
- Most common in Caucasians, especially those of northern European ancestry

Prevalence

Prevalence in population >50 years old: 700/100,000 people

ETIOLOGY AND PATHOPHYSIOLOGY

- Unknown. Symptoms appear to be related to enhanced immune system activity and periarticular inflammatory activity.
- Pathogenesis
  - Polygenic where multiple environmental and genetic factors play a role
  - Significant association found between histologic evidence of GCA and parvovirus B19 DNA in temporal artery specimen

Genetics

Associated with human leukocyte antigen determinants (HLA-DRB1*04 and DRB1*01 alleles) (3)

RISK FACTORS

- Age >50 years
- Presence of GCA

COMMONLY ASSOCIATED CONDITIONS

GCA (temporal arteritis) may occur in 15–30% of patients, more commonly in females than males with PMR.

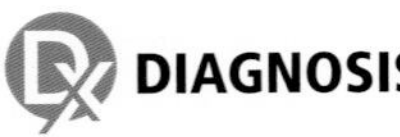

DIAGNOSIS

- Suspect PMR in elderly patients with new onset of proximal limb pain and stiffness (neck, shoulder, hip).
- Difficulty rising from chair or combing hair are signs of proximal muscle involvement.
- Nighttime pain
- Difficulty arising from a chair or raising the arms
- Systemic symptoms in ~25% (fatigue, weight loss, low-grade fever)

PHYSICAL EXAM

- Decreased range of motion (ROM) of shoulders, neck, and hips
- Muscle strength is usually normal, although it may be limited by pain.
- Muscle tenderness
- Disuse atrophy
- Synovitis of the small joints and tenosynovitis
- Coexisting carpal tunnel syndrome

DIFFERENTIAL DIAGNOSIS

- Rheumatoid arthritis
- Palindromic rheumatism
- Late-onset seronegative spondyloarthropathies (e.g., psoriatic arthritis, ankylosing spondylitis)
- Systemic lupus erythematosus; Sjögren syndrome; fibromyalgia
- Polymyositis-dermatomyositis (check creatine phosphokinase, aldolase)
- Thyroid disease
- Hyperparathyroidism, hypoparathyroidism
- Hypovitaminosis D
- Viral myalgia
- Osteoarthritis
- Rotator cuff syndrome; adhesive capsulitis
- RS3PE syndrome (remitting seronegative symmetrical synovitis with pitting edema)
- Occult infection or malignancy (e.g., lymphoma, leukemia, myeloma, solid tumor)
- Myopathy (e.g., steroid, alcohol, electrolyte depletion)
- Depression

DIAGNOSTIC TESTS & INTERPRETATION

- Consider PMR in patients older than 50 years of age with proximal pain and stiffness. Obtain laboratory work recommended in the following text and consider a diagnostic/therapeutic trial of low-dose steroids.
- Temporal artery biopsy if symptoms of GCA are present
- ESR (Westergren) elevation >40 mm/hr
  - ESR is elevated in most patients, sometimes >100 mm/hr.
  - ESR may be normal (<40 mm/hr) in 7–22% of patients.
- Elevated C-reactive protein
- Normochromic/normocytic anemia
- Anticyclic citrullinated peptide (anti-CCP) antibodies usually negative (in contrast to elderly-onset rheumatoid arthritis [RA])
- Rheumatoid factor: negative (5–10% of patients >60 years of age will have positive rheumatoid factor without RA)
- Mild elevations in liver function tests, especially alkaline phosphatase
- Antibodies to ferritin peptide may be a useful marker.
- Drugs that may alter lab results: prednisone
- Disorders that may alter lab results: other disorders causing elevation of the sedimentation rate (e.g., infection, neoplasm, renal failure)
- Normal EMG
- Normal muscle histology

Initial Tests (lab, imaging)

- ESR (usually >40 mm/hr)
- C-reactive protein
- CBC
- MRI is not necessary for diagnosis but may show periarticular inflammation, tenosynovitis, and bursitis.
- US may show bursitis, tendinitis, and synovitis.
- MRI, PET, and temporal artery US may all play a role in diagnosis of PMR.

Diagnostic Procedures/Other

If patients have symptoms suggestive of GCA, a temporal artery biopsy is indicated.

Test Interpretation

A scoring algorithm was devised consisting of the following: morning stiffness >45 minutes (2 points), hip pain/limited ROM (1 point), absence of rheumatoid factor and anti-citrullinated protein antibody (ACPA) (2 points), and absence of peripheral joint pain (1 point). A score of **>4** has been associated with 68% sensitivity and 78% specificity. Sensitivity and specificity increase with a positive temporal artery US.

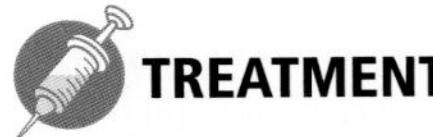

TREATMENT

GENERAL MEASURES

- Document diagnosis because glucocorticoids can mask symptoms of other diseases.
- Address risk of steroid-induced osteoporosis.
  - Obtain dual energy x-ray absorptiometry and check 25-OH vitamin D levels if necessary.
  - Consider antiresorptive therapies (bisphosphonates) based on recommendations for treatment of corticosteroid-induced osteoporosis.
- Encourage adequate calcium (1,500 mg/day) and vitamin D (800–1,000 U/day) supplementation.
- Physical therapy for ROM exercises, if needed

MEDICATION

First Line

- Prednisone: 10–20 mg/day PO initially; typically, expect a dramatic (diagnostic) response within days. 15 mg/day is effective in almost all patients.
  - May increase to 20 mg/day if no immediate response
  - If no response to 10–20 mg/day within a week, reconsider diagnosis.
- Divided-dose steroids (BID or TID) may be useful initially (especially if symptoms recur in the afternoon).
- Consider using delayed-release prednisone taken at bedtime, which may be more efficient in treating morning stiffness compared to conventional immediate-release prednisone.
- Begin slow taper by 2.5 mg decrements every 2–4 weeks to a dose of 7.5–10 mg/day. Below this dose, taper by 1 mg/month to prevent relapse.
- Increase prednisone for recurrence of symptoms (relapse common).
- Corticosteroid treatment often lasts at least 1–2 years.
- May be stopped at 6–12 months if patient is symptom free and there is a normal ESR on maintenance dose

- Contraindications
  - Use steroids with caution in patients with chronic heart failure, diabetes mellitus (or other immunocompromised state), and systemic fungal or bacterial infection.
  - Must treat infections concurrently if steroids are absolutely necessary
- Precautions
  - Long-term steroid use (>2 years) is associated with adverse effects, including sodium and water retention, exacerbation of chronic heart failure, hypokalemia, increased susceptibility to infection, osteoporosis, fractures, hypertension, cataracts, glaucoma, avascular necrosis, depression, and weight gain.
  - Patients may develop temporal arteritis while on low-dose corticosteroid treatment for polymyalgia. This requires an increase in dose to 40–60 mg.
  - Alternate-day steroids are not effective.

Second Line

- NSAIDs usually are not adequate for pain relief.
- Methotrexate has a modest effect in reducing relapse rate and lowering the cumulative dose of steroid therapy.
- There is conflicting evidence for antitumor necrosis factor agents (anti-TNF) (infliximab, etanercept) regarding steroid-sparing effects.
- Corticosteroid injection in the shoulder may help reduce pain and duration of morning stiffness and allow for increased levels of activity.

ONGOING CARE

FOLLOW-UP RECOMMENDATIONS

Patient Monitoring

- Evaluate patients monthly initially and during medication taper; every 3 months otherwise.
- Follow ESR as steroids are tapered; both ESR and CRP should decline as symptoms improve.
- Follow-up with patient for symptoms of GCA. Educate patient to report such symptoms immediately (e.g., headache, visual loss, and diplopia).
- Monitor side effects of corticosteroid therapy such as osteoporosis, hypertension, and hyperglycemia.
- If patient is asymptomatic, do not treat elevated ESR (i.e., do not increase the steroid dose in an attempt to normalize the ESR).

DIET

- Regular diet
- Aim for adequate calcium and vitamin D.

PATIENT EDUCATION

- Review adverse effects of corticosteroids.
- Discuss the symptoms of GCA and instruct the patient to present immediately if any occur.
- Contact physician if symptoms recur during the steroid taper.
- Instruct the patient to never abruptly stop taking steroids.
- Counsel patients on calcium and vitamin D requirements.
- Resources for patients
  - Arthritis Foundation: www.arthritis.org/
  - American College of Rheumatology: http://www.rheumatology.org/Practice/Clinical/Patients/Diseases_And_Conditions/Polymyalgia_Rheumatica/

PROGNOSIS

- Most patients require at least 2 years of corticosteroid treatment.
- Exacerbation is common if steroids are tapered too quickly.
- Prognosis is very good with proper treatment.
- Relapse is common (in 25–50% of patients).
- Higher age at diagnosis, female sex, high baseline ESR, increased plasma viscosity, increased levels of soluble IL-6 receptor, or high initial steroid dose have been associated with a prolonged disease course and greater number of disease flares.

COMPLICATIONS

- Complications related to chronic steroid use
- Exacerbation of disease with taper of steroids; development of GCA (may occur when PMR is being treated adequately)

REFERENCES

1. Salvarani C, Gabriel SE, O'Fallon WM, et al. Epidemiology of polymyalgia rheumatica in Olmsted County, Minnesota, 1970–1991. *Arthritis Rheum*. 1995;38(3):369–373.
2. Liozon E, Ouattara B, Rhaiem K, et al. Familial aggregation in giant cell arteritis and polymyalgia rheumatica: a comprehensive literature review including 4 new families. *Clin Exp Rheumatol*. 2009;27(1 Suppl 52):S89–S94.
3. Weyand CM, Hunder NN, Hicok KC, et al. HLA-DRB1 alleles in polymyalgia rheumatica, giant cell arteritis, and rheumatoid arthritis. *Arthritis Rheum*. 1994;37(4):514–520.

ADDITIONAL READING

- Aikawa NE, Pereira RM, Lage L, et al. Anti-TNF therapy for polymyalgia rheumatica: report of 99 cases and review of the literature. *Clin Rheumatol*. 2012;31(3):575–579.
- Buttgereit F, Gibofsky A. Delayed-release prednisone: a new approach to an old therapy. *Expert Opin Pharmacother*. 2013;14(8):1097–1106.
- Camellino D, Cimmino MA. Imaging of polymyalgia rheumatica: indications on its pathogenesis, diagnosis and prognosis. *Rheumatology (Oxford)*. 2012;51(1):77–86.
- Dasgupta B, Borg FA, Hassan N, et al. BSR and BHPR guidelines for the management of polymyalgia rheumatica. *Rheumatology (Oxford)*. 2010;49(1):186–190.
- Dasgupta B, Cimmino MA, Maradit-Kremers H, et al. 2012 provisional classification criteria for polymyalgia rheumatica: a European League Against Rheumatism/American College of Rheumatology collaborative initiative. *Ann Rheum Dis*. 2012;71(4):484–492.
- Hernández-Rodríguez J, Cid MC, López-Soto A, et al. Treatment of polymyalgia rheumatica: a systematic review. *Arch Intern Med*. 2009;169(20):1839–1850.
- Kreiner F, Galbo H. Effect of etanercept in polymyalgia rheumatica: a randomized controlled trial. *Arthritis Res Ther*. 2010;12(5):R176.
- Kremers HM, Reinalda MS, Crowson CS, et al. Relapse in a population based cohort of patients with polymyalgia rheumatica. *J Rheumatol*. 2005;32(1):65–73.
- Michet CJ, Matteson EL. Polymyalgia rheumatica. *BMJ*. 2008;336(7647):765–769.
- Régent A, Ly KH, Blet A, et al. Contribution of antiferritin antibodies to diagnosis of giant cell arteritis. *Ann Rheum Dis*. 2013;72(7):1269–1270.
- Salvarani C, Cantini F, Olivieri I, et al. Corticosteroid injections in polymyalgia rheumatica: a double-blind, prospective, randomized, placebo controlled study. *J Rheumatol*. 2000;27(6):1470–1476.
- Spies CM, Burmester GR, Buttgereit F. Methotrexate treatment in large vessel vasculitis and polymyalgia rheumatica. *Clin Exp Rheumatol*. 2010;28(5)(Suppl 61):S172–S177.

SEE ALSO

Arteritis, Temporal; Osteoarthritis; Arthritis, Rheumatoid; Depression; Fibromyalgia; Polymyositis-Dermatomyositis

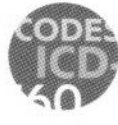

CODES

ICD10

- M35.3 Polymyalgia rheumatica
- M31.5 Giant cell arteritis with polymyalgia rheumatica

CLINICAL PEARLS

- Consider PMR in patients older than 50 years of age who present with proximal limb (hip, neck, shoulder) pain and stiffness.
- A normal ESR does not exclude the diagnosis of PMR.
- If there is not a dramatic and rapid response to steroids, reconsider the diagnosis.
- Adjust steroids according to patient symptoms, not the ESR.

POLYMYOSITIS/DERMATOMYOSITIS

Christopher M. Wise, MD

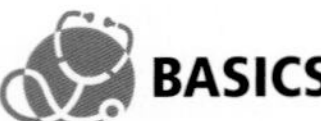

BASICS

DESCRIPTION

- Systemic connective tissue disease characterized by inflammatory and degenerative changes in proximal muscles, sometimes accompanied by characteristic skin rash
  - If skin manifestations (Gottron sign [symmetric, scaly, violaceous, erythematous eruption over the extensor surfaces of the metacarpophalangeal and interphalangeal joints of the fingers]; heliotrope [reddish violaceous eruption on the upper eyelids]) are present, it is designated as dermatomyositis.
  - Different types of myositis include the following:
    - Idiopathic polymyositis
    - Idiopathic dermatomyositis
    - Polymyositis/dermatomyositis as an overlap (usually with lupus or systemic sclerosis or as part of mixed connective-tissue disease)
    - Myositis associated with malignancy
    - HIV-associated myopathy
- Inclusion-body myositis (IBM), a variant with atypical patterns of weakness and biopsy findings
- System(s) affected: cardiovascular, musculoskeletal, pulmonary, skin/exocrine
- Synonym(s): myositis; inflammatory myopathy; antisynthetase syndrome (subset with certain antibodies)

EPIDEMIOLOGY

Incidence

- Estimated at 0.5–0.8/100,000 population/year
- Predominant age: 5–15 years, 40–60 years, peak incidence in mid-40s
- Predominant sex: female > male (2:1)

Prevalence

1–2 patients/100,000 population

Geriatric Considerations

Elderly patients with myositis or dermatomyositis are at increased risk of neoplasm.

Pediatric Considerations

Childhood dermatomyositis is likely a separate entity associated with cutaneous vasculitis and muscle calcifications.

ETIOLOGY AND PATHOPHYSIOLOGY

- Inflammatory process, mediated by T cells and cytokine release, leading to damage to muscle cells (predominantly skeletal muscles)
- In patients with IBM, degenerative mechanisms may be important.
- Unknown; potential viral, genetic factors

Genetics

Mild association with human leukocyte antigen (HLA)–DR3, HLA-DRw52

RISK FACTORS

Family history of autoimmune disease (e.g., systemic lupus, myositis) or vasculitis

COMMONLY ASSOCIATED CONDITIONS

- Malignancy (in 15–25%)
- Progressive systemic sclerosis
- Vasculitis
- Systemic lupus erythematosus (SLE)
- Mixed connective-tissue disease

DIAGNOSIS

HISTORY

- Symmetric proximal muscle weakness (1) causing difficulty when
  - Arising from sitting or lying positions
  - Climbing stairs
  - Raising arms
- Joint pain/swelling
- Dysphagia
- Dyspnea
- Rash on face, eyelids, hands, arms

PHYSICAL EXAM

Proximal muscle weakness

- Shoulder muscles
- Hip girdle muscles (trouble standing from seated or squatting position, weak hip flexors in supine position)
- Muscle swelling, stiffness, induration
- Distal muscle weakness is seen only in patients with IBM.
- Rash over face (eyelids, nasolabial folds), upper chest, dorsal hands (especially knuckle pads), fingers ("mechanic's hands")
- Periorbital edema
- Calcinosis cutis (childhood cases)
- Mesenteric arterial insufficiency/infarction (childhood cases)
- Cardiac impairment; arrhythmia, failure

DIFFERENTIAL DIAGNOSIS

- Vasculitis
- Progressive systemic sclerosis
- SLE
- Rheumatoid arthritis
- Muscular dystrophy
- Eaton-Lambert syndrome
- Sarcoidosis
- Amyotrophic lateral sclerosis
- Endocrine disorders
  - Thyroid disease
  - Cushing syndrome
- Infectious myositis (viral, bacterial, parasitic)
- Drug-induced myopathies
  - Cholesterol-lowering agents (statins)
  - Statin-associated autoimmune myopathy (2)
  - Colchicine
  - Corticosteroids
  - Ethanol
  - Chloroquine
  - Zidovudine
- Electrolyte disorders (magnesium, calcium, potassium)
- Heritable metabolic myopathies
- Sleep-apnea syndrome

DIAGNOSTIC TESTS & INTERPRETATION

- Diagnosis of muscle component (myositis) usually relies on 4 findings:
  - Weakness
  - Creatine kinase (CK) and/or aldolase elevation
  - Abnormal electromyogram (EMG)
  - Findings on muscle biopsy
- Presence of compatible skin rash of dermatomyositis

Initial Tests (lab, imaging)

- Increased CK, aldolase
- Increased serum AST (aspartate aminotransferase)
- Increased LDH (lactate dehydrogenase)
- Myoglobinuria
- Increased ESR
- Positive rheumatoid factor (<50% of patients)
- Positive ANA (antinuclear antibody) (>50% of patients)
- Leukocytosis (<50% of patients)
- Anemia (<50% of patients)
- Hyperglobulinemia (<50% of patients)
- Myositis-specific antibodies (antisynthetase antibodies) described in a minority of patients:
  - Anti-Jo-1 is the most common but has been found in <20% of patients.
  - Associated with an increased incidence of interstitial lung disease
- Chest radiograph as part of initial evaluation to assess for associated pulmonary involvement or malignancy

Follow-Up Tests & Special Considerations

- Changes in muscle enzymes (CK or aldolase) correlate with improvement and worsening.
- MRI to assess muscle edema and inflammation may be used in some patients to determine best biopsy site or response to therapy.

Diagnostic Procedures/Other

- EMG: muscle irritability, low-amplitude potentials, polyphasic action potentials, fibrillations
- Muscle biopsy (deltoid or quadriceps femoris)

Test Interpretation

- Microscopic findings:
  - Muscle fiber degeneration
  - Phagocytosis of muscle debris
  - Perifascicular muscle fiber atrophy
  - Inflammatory cell infiltrates in adult form
  - Via electron microscopy: inclusion bodies (IBM only)
  - Sarcoplasmic basophilia
- Muscle fiber increased in size
- Vasculopathy (childhood polymyositis/dermatomyositis)

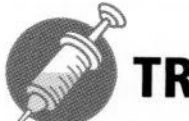

TREATMENT

GENERAL MEASURES

General evaluation for malignancy in all adults, particularly with dermatomyositis, at initial evaluation and during follow-up

MEDICATION

First Line

- Prednisone
  - 40–80 mg/day PO in divided doses (3)[B]
  - Consolidate doses and reduce prednisone slowly when enzyme levels are normal.
  - Probably need to continue 5–10 mg/day for maintenance in most patients
- For steroid-refractory or steroid-dependent patients: azathioprine 1 mg/kg PO (arthritis dose) once daily or BID
  - Methotrexate 10–25 mg PO weekly, useful in most steroid-resistant patients
- Rash of dermatomyositis may require topical steroids or oral hydroxychloroquine.
- Patients with IBM have very poor response to steroids and other 1st- and 2nd-line drugs in general.

Second Line

- Other immunosuppressant drugs (e.g., cyclophosphamide, chlorambucil, cyclosporine, mycophenolate, tacrolimus) can be added to steroids.
- Combination methotrexate and azathioprine also may be useful in refractory cases.
- IVIG (4)[B] and rituximab (5)[B] have been reported to be helpful in a small series of patients with refractory disease.
- Contraindications: Methotrexate is contraindicated with previous liver disease, alcohol use, pregnancy, and underlying renal disease (use with extreme caution in patients with serum creatinine >1.5 mg/dL in general).
- Precautions
  - Prednisone: Adverse effects associated with long-term steroid use include adrenal suppression, sodium and water retention, hypokalemia, osteoporosis, cataracts, and increased susceptibility to infection.
  - Azathioprine: Adverse effects include bone marrow suppression, increased liver function tests, and increased risk of infection.
  - Methotrexate: Adverse effects include stomatitis, bone marrow suppression, pneumonitis, and risk of liver fibrosis and cirrhosis with prolonged use.

ISSUES FOR REFERRAL

- Diagnostic uncertainty, usually related to elevated muscle enzymes without typical symptoms of findings of muscle weakness
- Poor response to initial steroid therapy
- Excessive steroid requirement (unable to taper prednisone to <20 mg/day after 4–6 months)

SURGERY/OTHER PROCEDURES

None indicated, other than initial biopsy

INPATIENT CONSIDERATIONS

Admission Criteria/Initial Stabilization

- Inability to stand, ambulate
- Respiratory difficulty
- Fever or other signs of infection
- Inpatient evaluation seldom needed

ONGOING CARE

FOLLOW-UP RECOMMENDATIONS

Patient Monitoring

- Follow muscle enzymes along with muscle strength and functional capacity.
- Monitor for steroid-induced complications (e.g., hypokalemia, hypertension, and hyperglycemia).
- Bone densitometry and consideration of calcium, vitamin D, and bisphosphonate therapy
- If azathioprine, methotrexate, or other immunosuppressant is used, appropriate laboratory monitoring should be done periodically (e.g., hematology, liver enzymes, and creatinine).
- Attempt to decrease and/or discontinue steroid dose as patient responds to therapy.
- Maintain immunosuppression until patient's muscle strength stabilizes for prolonged period depending on individual patient parameters, risks of medication, risk of relapse; time period undefined (months, years).

DIET

Moderation of caloric and sodium intake to avoid weight gain from corticosteroid therapy.

PATIENT EDUCATION

- Curtail excess physical activity in early phases when muscles enzymes are markedly elevated.
- Emphasize range-of-motion exercises.
- Gradually introduce muscle strengthening when muscle enzymes are normal or improved and stable (6)[B].

PROGNOSIS

- Residual weakness: 30%
- Persistent active disease: 20%
- 5-year survival 65–75%, but mortality is 3-fold higher than general population (7,8).
- Survival is worse for women and African Americans and those with dermatomyositis, IBM, or cancer.
- Most patients improve with therapy.
- Patients with IBM respond poorly to most therapies (9).
- 20–50% have full recovery

COMPLICATIONS

- Pneumonia
- Infection
- Myocardial infarction
- Carcinoma (especially breast, lung)
- Severe dysphagia
- Respiratory impairment due to muscle weakness, interstitial lung disease
- Aspiration pneumonitis
- Steroid myopathy
- Steroid-induced diabetes, hypertension, hypokalemia, osteoporosis

REFERENCES

1. Khan S, Christopher-Stine L. Polymyositis, dermatomyositis, and autoimmune necrotizing myopathy: clinical features. *Rheum Dis Clin North Am*. 2011;37(2):143–158, v.
2. Mohassel P, Mammen AL. The spectrum of statin myopathy. *Curr Opin Rheumatol*. 2013;25(6):747–752.
3. Aggarwal R, Oddis CV. Therapeutic approaches in myositis. *Curr Rheumatol Rep*. 2011;13(3):182–191.
4. Wang DX, Shu XM, Tian XL, et al. Intravenous immunoglobulin therapy in adult patients with polymyositis/dermatomyositis: a systematic literature review. *Clin Rheumatol*. 2012;31(5):801–806.
5. Oddis CV, Reed AM, Aggarwal R, et al. Rituximab in the treatment of refractory adult and juvenile dermatomyositis and adult polymyositis: a randomized, placebo-phase trial. *Arthritis Rheum*. 2013;65(2):314–324.
6. Alemo Munters L, Dastmalchi M, Andgren V, et al. Improvement in health and possible reduction in disease activity using endurance exercise in patients with established polymyositis and dermatomyositis: a multicenter randomized controlled trial with a 1-year open extension followup. *Arthritis Care Res*. 2013;65(12):1959–1968.
7. Marie I. Morbidity and mortality in adult polymyositis and dermatomyositis. *Curr Rheumatol Rep*. 2012;14(3):275–285.
8. Schiopu E, Phillips K, MacDonald PM, et al. Predictors of survival in a cohort of patients with polymyositis and dermatomyositis: effect of corticosteroids, methotrexate and azathioprine. *Arthritis Res Ther*. 2012;14(1):R22.
9. Machado P, Brady S, Hanna MG. Update in inclusion body myositis. *Curr Opin Rheumatol*. 2013;25(6):763–771.

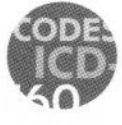

CODES

ICD10

- M33.20 Polymyositis, organ involvement unspecified
- M33.90 Dermatopolymyositis, unspecified, organ involvement unspecified
- M33.92 Dermatopolymyositis, unspecified with myopathy

CLINICAL PEARLS

- Corticosteroids alone may be sufficient in patients who have rapid improvement in weakness and muscle enzymes. However, most patients require azathioprine, methotrexate, or other immunosuppressive medications.
- The risk of associated malignancy is higher in patients >50 years and in those with cutaneous manifestations.
- Elevated muscle enzymes (e.g., CK and aldolase) are seen frequently as transient phenomena in patients with febrile illness and injuries; may return to normal on repeat.
- In patients with persistently elevated muscle enzymes and symptoms and findings of muscle weakness, EMG followed by muscle biopsy should be the initial studies considered.
- Suspect IBM in older patients with very slow onset and progression of symptoms, poor response to steroids and immunosuppressive therapy, and atypical patterns (asymmetric, sometimes distal) of muscle weakness.

P

POPLITEAL (BAKER) CYST

Chris Wheelock, MD

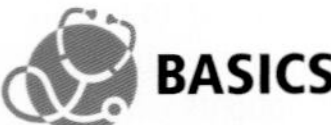

BASICS

DESCRIPTION
- A fluid-filled synovial sac arising in the popliteal fossa as a distention of (typically) the gastrocnemial-semimembranous bursa. Not a true cyst.
- Can be unilateral or bilateral
- Most frequent cystic mass around the knee (1)
- Primary cysts are a distention of the bursa arising independently without an intra-articular disorder.
- Secondary cysts occur if a communication exists between the bursa and knee joint, allowing articular fluid to fill the cyst. Pathologic joint processes can also be transmitted in this manner.
- Associated with synovial inflammation

EPIDEMIOLOGY
Incidence
- Bimodal distribution
  - Children ages 4–7 years
  - Adults increasing with age
- Primary cysts usually seen in children <15 years of age
- Secondary cysts seen in adults

Prevalence
- Studies report variable adult prevalences of 19–47% in symptomatic knees and 2–5% in asymptomatic knees.
- In children: 6.3% in symptomatic knees; 2.4% in asymptomatic knees

ETIOLOGY AND PATHOPHYSIOLOGY
Associated intra-articular pathology includes the following:
- Meniscal tears, mostly of the posterior horn
- Anterior cruciate ligament (ACL) insufficiency
- Degenerative articular cartilage lesions
- Rheumatoid arthritis (20%)
- Osteoarthritis (50%)
- Osteochondritis
- Gout (14%)
- Other potential factors:
  - Infectious arthritis
  - Polyarthritis
  - Villonodular synovitis
  - Lymphoma
  - Sarcoidosis
  - Connective tissue diseases (2)
- Extension or herniation of synovial membrane of the knee joint capsule or connection of normal bursa with the joint capsule
- May result from increased intra-articular pressure
- Commonly seen with knee effusions
- Direct trauma to the bursa is likely the primary cause in children because of no communication between the bursa and the joint.
- A valve-like mechanism allowing 1-way passage of fluid from the joint to the bursal connection has been described.

RISK FACTORS
- Osteoarthritis of knee (most common) (3)[B]
- Rheumatoid arthritis
- Meniscal degeneration or tear
- Advancing age
- Ligamentous insufficiency

COMMONLY ASSOCIATED CONDITIONS
Any condition causing knee joint effusion

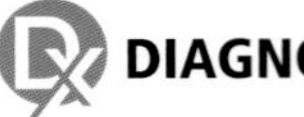

DIAGNOSIS

HISTORY
- Painless mass arising in the popliteal fossa
- Most cysts are asymptomatic.
- Dull ache if cyst is large enough to impede joint motion—typically a restriction of flexion
- Painful if cyst ruptures
- Large cysts may cause entrapment neuropathy of the tibial nerve.
- Vascular compression, most commonly of the popliteal vein, may produce claudication or thrombophlebitis.
- Activity alters the cyst size.

PHYSICAL EXAM
- Examine in full extension and 90 degrees of flexion.
- Foucher sign: Mass increases with extension and disappears with flexion.
- Most commonly found in medial aspect of popliteal fossa lateral to the head of the gastrocnemius and medial to the neurovascular bundle
- Cyst is easiest to palpate when knee is slightly flexed and may occasionally be fluctuant or tender.
- Transillumination can distinguish cyst from solid mass.
- Ruptured cysts are typically painful with associated swelling over calf and medial malleolus, pseudothrombophlebitis, and, rarely, compartment syndrome (4).

DIFFERENTIAL DIAGNOSIS
- Infection/abscess
- Lipoma, liposarcoma
- Fibroma, fibrosarcoma
- Hematoma
- Deep venous thrombosis
- Vascular tumor
- Popliteal vein varices
- Xanthoma
- Aneurysm (rare)
- Ganglion cyst
- Thrombophlebitis
- Muscular herniation (rare, related to trauma)

DIAGNOSTIC TESTS & INTERPRETATION
Initial Tests (lab, imaging)
- CBC, sedimentation rate if suspecting septic arthritis
- If aspiration is done, first ensure not a popliteal aneurysm. Send aspirate for cell count and culture to determine nature of effusion: infectious, inflammatory, or mechanical
- Ultrasound confirms presence and size; with Doppler, can differentiate Baker cysts from popliteal vessel aneurysms or soft tissue tumors
- MRI is useful to assess for causal derangements of internal joint structures and to identify cyst leakage or rupture.

Follow-Up Tests & Special Considerations
- In children, consider observation before invasive testing.
- Radiographs may show soft tissue density posteriorly.
- Arthrography may demonstrate communication with joint capsule or rupture.
- CT–arthrography together is superior in visualizing cystic details and can help separate lipomas, aneurysms, and malignancies from cysts.

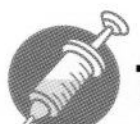

TREATMENT

GENERAL MEASURES

- No treatment if cyst is asymptomatic.
- Treat underlying conditions.
- Compressive wrap or sleeve may be used for comfort.

MEDICATION

Once etiology is identified from cellular fluid examination, treat the underlying condition.

First Line

Analgesics, NSAIDs for symptomatic relief

ADDITIONAL THERAPIES

- Physical therapy improves knee ROM and strength, particularly with coexisting pathology.
- Temporary relief with needle aspiration; recurrence common
- Improvement in joint ROM, knee pain, swelling, accompanied reduction in bursa size has been shown after aspiration and intra-articular or intracystic corticosteroid injection (5)[B]
- The best improvements in terms of pain, functionality, and reduction in cyst size were achieved with combination of physical therapy and corticosteroid injection (6)[A].
- Sclerotherapy injections of ethanol or dextrose/sodium morrhuate shown to have good results in studies with small sample sizes (7)[B].

SURGERY/OTHER PROCEDURES

- Consider excision when symptoms persist despite treatment or no etiology is found.
- Surgery usually not required in children
- Recurrence after standard surgery is common and is highest when chondral lesions are present. Arthroscopic surgery, when the valvular mechanism is identified and intra-articular pathology is treated, is highly successful (8,9)[B].
- A modified surgical technique in children has proved effective without recurrence (10)[B].
- Excision via arthroscopy or open procedure often requires concomitant treatment of underlying pathology (11)[B].

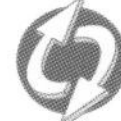

ONGOING CARE

PROGNOSIS

- Variable; many cysts remain asymptomatic.
- Some cysts resolve with treatment of underlying etiology (e.g., gout, rheumatoid arthritis).
- In children, most cysts resolve without treatment because there is rarely internal derangement.

COMPLICATIONS

- Compartment syndrome in ruptured cyst
- Thrombophlebitis from compression of the popliteal vein
- Infection of popliteal cyst
- Hemorrhage into cyst if on anticoagulants

REFERENCES

1. Marra MD, Crema MD, Chung M, et al. MRI features of cystic lesions around the knee. *Knee.* 2008;15(6):423–438.
2. Liao ST, Chiou CS, Chang CC. Pathology associated to the Baker's cysts: a musculoskeletal ultrasound study. *Clin Rheumatol.* 2010;29(9):1043–1047.
3. Chatzopoulos D, Moralidis E, Markou P, et al. Baker's cysts in knees with chronic osteoarthritic pain: a clinical, ultrasonographic, radiographic and scintigraphic evaluation. *Rheumatol Int.* 2008;29(2):141–146.
4. Sanchez JE, Conkling N, Labropoulos N. Compression syndromes of the popliteal neurovascular bundle due to Baker cyst. *J Vasc Surg.* 2011;54(6):1821–1829.
5. Acebes JC, Sánchez-Pernaute O, Diaz-Oca A, et al. Ultrasonographic assessment of Baker's cysts after intra-articular corticosteroid injection in knee osteoarthritis. *J Clin Ultrasound.* 2006;34(3):113–117.
6. Di Sante L, Paoloni M, Dimaggio M, et al. Ultrasound-guided aspiration and corticosteroid injection compared to horizontal therapy for treatment of knee osteoarthritis complicated with Baker's cyst: a randomized, controlled trial. *Eur J Phys Rehabil Med.* 2012;48(4):561–567.
7. Centeno CJ, Schultz J, Freeman M. Sclerotherapy of Baker's cyst with imaging confirmation of resolution. *Pain Physician.* 2008;11(2):257–261.
8. Rupp S, Seil R, Jochum P, et al. Popliteal cysts in adults. Prevalence, associated intraarticular lesions, and results after arthroscopic treatment. *Am J Sports Med.* 2002;30(1):112–115.
9. Lie CW, Ng TP. Arthroscopic treatment of popliteal cyst. *Hong Kong Med J.* 2011;17(3):180–183.
10. Chen JC, Lu CC, Lu YM, et al. A modified surgical method for treating Baker's cyst in children. *Knee.* 2008;15(1):9–14.
11. Handy JR. Popliteal cysts in adults: a review. *Semin Arthritis Rheum.* 2001;31(2):108–118.

ADDITIONAL READING

- Akagi R, Saisu T, Segawa Y, et al. Natural history of popliteal cysts in the pediatric population. *J Pediatr Orthop.* 2013;33(3):262–268.
- Akgul O, Guldeste Z, Ozgocmen S. The reliability of the clinical examination for detecting Baker's cyst in asymptomatic fossa. *Int J Rheum Dis.* 2014;17(2):204–209.

SEE ALSO

Algorithm: Knee Pain

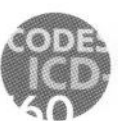

CODES

ICD10

- M71.20 Synovial cyst of popliteal space [Baker], unspecified knee
- M71.21 Synovial cyst of popliteal space [Baker], right knee
- M71.22 Synovial cyst of popliteal space [Baker], left knee

CLINICAL PEARLS

- In children, conservative treatment of Baker cysts is preferred as most will spontaneously resolve.
- Treatment of underlying cause may resolve Baker cysts in adults.
- Pain and swelling over the medial malleolus is classic for cyst rupture, also known as pseudothrombophlebitis.
- Presence of a Baker cyst is not associated with the severity of intra-articular pathology.

PORTAL HYPERTENSION

Walter M. Kim, MD, PhD • Jyoti Ramakrishna, MD

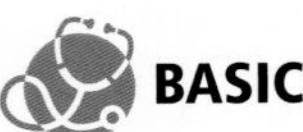

BASICS

DESCRIPTION

- Increased portal venous pressure >5 mm Hg that occurs in association with splanchnic vasodilatation, portosystemic collateral formation, and hyperdynamic circulation
- Most commonly secondary to elevated hepatic venous pressure gradient (HVPG; the gradient between portal and central venous pressures)
- Course is generally progressive, with risk of complications including acute variceal bleeding, ascites, encephalopathy, and hepatorenal syndrome.

EPIDEMIOLOGY

Incidence

- Prevalence: <200,000 persons in the United States
- Predominant age: adult
- Predominant sex: male > female

ETIOLOGY AND PATHOPHYSIOLOGY

- Causes generally classified as follows:
  - Prehepatic (portal vein thrombosis or obstruction)
  - Intrahepatic (most commonly cirrhosis)
  - Posthepatic (hepatic vein thrombosis, Budd-Chiari syndrome, right-sided heart failure)
- Cirrhosis accounts for 90% of intrahepatic cases; may be due to the following:
  - Virus (hepatitis B, hepatitis C, hepatitis D)
  - Alcoholism
  - Schistosomiasis
  - Wilson disease
  - Hemochromatosis
  - Primary biliary cirrhosis (PBC)
  - Sarcoidosis
- Increased HVPG results in venous collateral formation in the distal esophagus, proximal stomach, rectum, and umbilicus.
- Gastroesophageal variceal formation is found in 40% of patients with portal hypertension.
- Progression of portal hypertension results in splanchnic vasodilation and angiogenesis.

Genetics

No known genetic patterns except those associated with specific hepatic diseases that cause portal hypertension

RISK FACTORS

See "Etiology"

Pediatric Considerations

In children, portal vein thrombosis is the most common extrahepatic cause; intrahepatic causes are more likely to be biliary atresia, viral hepatitis, and metabolic liver disease.

DIAGNOSIS

HISTORY

- Weakness/fatigue
- Jaundice
- Symptoms of heart failure including chest pain, shortness of breath, and/or edema
- Hematemesis
- Melena
- Oliguria
- History of chronic liver disease
- Alcoholic hepatitis
- Alcohol abuse

PHYSICAL EXAM

- Exam findings may be general or related to specific complications.
- General
  - Pallor
  - Icterus
  - Digital clubbing
  - Palmar erythema
  - Splenomegaly
  - Caput medusa
  - Spider angiomata
  - Umbilical bruit
  - Hemorrhoids
  - Gynecomastia
  - Testicular atrophy
- Gastroesophageal varices
  - Hypotension
  - Tachycardia
- Ascites
  - Distended abdomen
  - Fluid wave
  - Shifting dullness with percussion
- Hepatic encephalopathy
  - Confusion/coma
  - Asterixis
  - Hyperreflexia

DIFFERENTIAL DIAGNOSIS

Usually related to specific presentations

- Gastroesophageal varices with hemorrhage
  - Portal hypertensive gastropathy
  - Hemorrhagic gastritis
  - Peptic ulcer disease
  - Mallory-Weiss tear
- Ascites
  - Spontaneous bacterial peritonitis (SBP)
  - Pancreatic ascites
  - Peritoneal carcinomatosis
  - Tuberculous peritonitis
  - Nephrotic syndrome
  - Fluid overload from heart failure
  - Hepatic malignancy
- Hepatic encephalopathy
  - Delirium tremens
  - Intracranial hemorrhage
  - Sedative abuse
  - Uremia
- Hepatorenal syndrome
  - Drug nephrotoxicity
  - Renal tubular necrosis

DIAGNOSTIC TESTS & INTERPRETATION

Initial Tests (lab, imaging)

Direct calculation of HVPG (approximation of the gradient in pressure between portal vein and IVC):

- HVPG = wedged hepatic venous pressure (WHVP) − free hepatic venous pressure (FHVP)
- HVPG >10, esophageal varices generally develop.
- WHVP is estimated by occlusion of the hepatic vein by a balloon catheter and measurement of the proximal static column of blood.
- FHVP is estimated by direct measurement of the patent hepatic vein, infra-abdominal inferior vena cava, or right atrium.
- Nonspecific changes associated with underlying disease:
  - Hypersplenism: anemia (also may be due to malnutrition or bleeding), leukopenia, thrombocytopenia
  - Hepatic dysfunction
    - Hypoalbuminemia
    - Hyperbilirubinemia
    - Elevated alkaline phosphatase
    - Elevated liver enzymes (AST, ALT)
    - Abnormal clotting (prothrombin time, international normalized ratio, partial thromboplastin time)
  - GI bleeding
    - Iron deficiency anemia
    - Elevated serum ammonia
    - Fecal occult blood
    - Thrombocytopenia
  - Hepatorenal syndrome
    - Elevated serum creatinine (Cr), blood urea nitrogen (BUN)
    - Urine Na <5 mEq/L (<20 mmol/L)
  - US and CT scan/MRI may detect cirrhosis, splenomegaly, ascites, and varices.
  - US/duplex Doppler
    - Can determine presence and direction of flow in portal and hepatic veins
    - Useful in diagnosing portal vein thrombosis, shunt thrombosis, or the presence of ascites
  - CT scan/MRI: angiographic measurement of hepatic venous wedge pressure via jugular or femoral vein
    - Correlates with portal pressure
    - Risk of variceal bleeding is increased if hepatic venous pressure gradient >12 mm Hg.
  - Upper GI series may outline varices in esophagus and stomach.

Diagnostic Procedures/Other

Endoscopy can diagnose esophageal and gastric varices and portal hypertensive gastropathy.

Test Interpretation

Specific for underlying disease

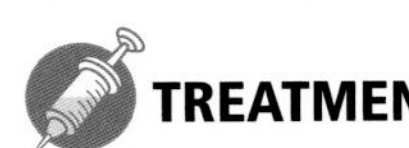

TREATMENT

GENERAL MEASURES

- Avoid sedatives that may precipitate encephalopathy.
- Limit sodium intake because cirrhotic patients avidly retain sodium.
- Restrict protein only if encephalopathic.

MEDICATION

Therapy for encephalopathy: See "Hepatic Encephalopathy."

First Line

- Prophylaxis against variceal bleeding (1,2)[A]:
  - Nonselective β-blockade
    - Propranolol: start with 10–20 mg/day PO BID–TID
    - Nadolol: 40–80 mg/day PO once-daily dosing
  - Doses may be titrated up as tolerated to maximum recommended doses; goal resting HR of 55–60 bpm
- Therapy for acute variceal hemorrhage:
  - Vasopressin: start with 0.2–0.4 U/min IV; increase to maximum dose 0.8 U/min as needed; pediatric dose: 0.002–0.005 U/kg/min; do not exceed 0.01 U/kg/min. After bleeding stops, continue at same dose for 12 hours and then taper off over 24–48 hours.
  - Somatostatin: 250 μg IV bolus, followed by 250 μg/hr continuous infusion; continue for 2–5 days if successful
  - Octreotide: 50μg IV bolus, followed by 25–50 μg/hr continuous infusion; pediatric dose: 1 μg/kg bolus followed by 1 μg/kg/hr is used traditionally; treat for up to 5 days
- For prevention of recurrence and for overall reduction in mortality:
  - Propranolol: 10–60 mg/day PO BID–QID; pediatric dose: 0.5–1 mg/kg/day PO divided q6–8h
  - Nadolol: 40–80 mg/day PO reduces portal venous blood inflow by blocking the adrenergic dilatation of the mesenteric arterioles.
  - Tetrandrine, a calcium channel blocker, also has been found to reduce the rate of rebleeding with fewer side effects.
- Treatment for ascites (along with salt and fluid restriction):
  - Furosemide: 20–40 mg/day PO; pediatric dose: 1–2 mg/kg/dose PO $\pm$ IV albumin infusion
  - Spironolactone: 50–100 mg/day PO; pediatric dose: 1–3 mg/kg/day PO

Second Line

- Terlipressin (2 mg IV q4h; titrate down to 1 mg IV q4h once hemorrhage is controlled; may be used for up to 48 hours) is a more selective splanchnic vasoconstrictor and may be associated with fewer complications. It is currently used when standard therapy with somatostatin or octreotide fails.
- Addition of nitrates, such as nitroglycerin or isosorbide mononitrate, reduces portal pressures and bleeding rates and has been shown to reduce mortality. Because the risk–benefit ratio is not clear, nitrates are not considered 1st-line treatment.
- Studies are ongoing for possible benefits of other agents including simvastatin, clonidine, verapamil, and losartan.

ISSUES FOR REFERRAL

Patients with portal hypertension should be managed longitudinally by both a primary care physician and a gastroenterologist.

SURGERY/OTHER PROCEDURES

- Treatments available for specific complications of portal hypertension (in addition to or if refractory to medications):
  - Gastroesophageal varices with hemorrhage
    - Endoscopic variceal banding or sclerosis (the 1st-line treatment in many cases for acute hemorrhage)
    - Balloon tamponade (not used commonly when endoscopic treatment is available)
    - Transjugular intrahepatic portosystemic shunt (TIPS)
    - Portocaval shunting
  - Ascites refractory to medical management
    - Large-volume paracentesis
    - Peritoneovenous shunt
    - TIPS
- Liver transplantation should be considered for patients with advanced disease.

INPATIENT CONSIDERATIONS

- Acute GI bleeding should be managed in the inpatient setting, either on the regular medical floor if the patient is hemodynamically stable or occasionally in the ICU if the patient is unstable.
- Patients with mental status changes from encephalopathy need to be evaluated in the inpatient setting.

Admission Criteria/Initial Stabilization

- Acute bleeding from the intestinal tract, either vomiting or per rectum
- Acute confusional state/mental status changes
- If acute variceal bleeding:
  - Type and cross patient's blood.
  - Initial resuscitation with isotonic fluid until packed RBCs are available
  - Correct coagulopathy with vitamin K and fresh-frozen plasma (FFP).
  - Endoscopy as soon as the patient is stabilized (for diagnosis and treatment)
- Avoid sedatives that may precipitate encephalopathy.
- Limit sodium administration because cirrhotic patients avidly retain sodium.
- Restrict protein only if encephalopathic.

ALERT
If the patient is an active alcohol drinker, watch for signs and symptoms of withdrawal. Follow inpatient protocols for alcohol withdrawal management.

IV Fluids

Use isotonic fluid for hydration.

Discharge Criteria

- For GI bleeding:
  - No active bleeding in 24 hours
  - Stable hemoglobin and hematocrit
  - Hemodynamically stable (especially heart rate)
- For encephalopathy: improvement in or resolution of mental status changes to baseline

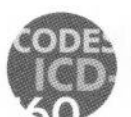

ONGOING CARE

DIET

- In patients with cirrhosis, sodium restriction is important because cirrhotic patients avidly retain sodium.
- Restrict protein only in patients who are encephalopathic.

PATIENT EDUCATION

Refrain from drinking alcohol. Resources for patients who have difficulty with not drinking alcohol can be obtained from Alcoholics Anonymous at www.aa.org.

PROGNOSIS

- Hepatic reserve defined by Child-Pugh classification: rating based on encephalopathy, ascites, bilirubin, albumin, prothrombin
- Variceal bleeding
  - 1/3 of patients with known varices will bleed eventually.
  - 50% rebleed, usually within 2 years, unless portal pressure is reduced by surgical or TIPS procedure.
  - 15–20% mortality rate
- Ascites and encephalopathy often recur.
- Prognosis of patients with ascites is poor: 50% 1-year survival without liver transplant (compared with 90% for patients with cirrhosis and no ascites)

REFERENCES

1. Hayes PC, Davis JM, Lewis JA et al. Meta-analysis of value of propanolol in prevention of variceal hemorrhage. *Lancet*. 1990;336(8708):153–156.
2. Garcia-Tsao G, Sanyal AJ, Grace ND, et al. Prevention and management of gastroesophageal varices and variceal hemorrhage in cirrhosis. *Hepatology*. 2007;46(3):922–938.

ADDITIONAL READING

- Abraldes JG, Angermayr B, Bosch J. The management of portal hypertension. *Clin Liver Dis*. 2005;9(4):685–713.
- Bloom S, Kemp W, Lubel J. Portal hypertension—pathophysiology, diagnosis and management. *Intern Med J*. 2015;45(1):16–26. doi:10.1111/imj.12590.
- Bosch J, Berzigotti A, Garcia-Pagan JC, et al. The management of portal hypertension: rational basis, available treatments and future options. *J Hepatology*. 2008;48(Suppl 1):S68–S92.
- Sanyal AJ, Bosch J, Blei A, et al. Portal hypertension and its complications. *Gastroenterology*. 2008;134(6):1715–1728.

CODES

ICD10
K76.6 Portal hypertension

CLINICAL PEARLS

- Endoscopic treatment is successful for acute variceal hemorrhage 85% of the time.
- Prognosis of patients with ascites is poor: 50% 1-year survival without liver transplant (compared with 90% for patients with cirrhosis and no ascites).
- Advantages and disadvantages of balloon tamponade for acute variceal bleed:
  - Advantages include rapid and often effective control of bleeding and common availability of device.
  - Disadvantages include recurrence of bleeding when balloon is deflated, patient discomfort, and risk of esophageal perforation.

POSTCONCUSSION SYNDROME (MILD TRAUMATIC BRAIN INJURY)

Tyler Wheeler, MD

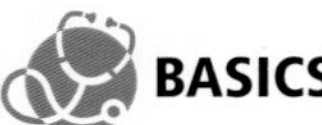

BASICS

DESCRIPTION

- Postconcussion syndrome (PCS) is an evolving clinical diagnosis involving physical, cognitive, and/or behavioral symptoms that develop 2–12 weeks after a concussion and persist for weeks to months.
- Symptoms of PCS (1)[C]
  - Cognitive
    - Poor focus
    - Poor organization
    - Diminished academic/intellectual performance
    - Slowed response time
  - Physical
    - Headache
    - Nausea
    - Visual changes
    - Light and nose sensitivity
    - Tinnitus
    - Dizziness and balance problems
    - Fatigue and sleep disturbance
  - Behavioral
    - Depression
    - Irritability/emotional lability
    - Apathy
    - Increased sensitivity to alcohol
- Diagnosis is a clinical one based on history and clinical symptoms and signs.

EPIDEMIOLOGY

Incidence

The reported range of mild traumatic brain injury (MTBI) in patients who develop PCS varies widely between 5 and 80%.

- The variation is due to difficulty in differentiating normal postconcussion *symptoms* from postconcussion *syndrome*.
- Consensus from the 3rd International Conference on Concussion in Sport (2008) is that 80–90% of concussion victims recover from postconcussion *symptoms* within 7–10 days, or maybe slightly longer in children/adolescents (2)[C].

Prevalence

- MTBI accounts for most head trauma seen in emergency departments.
- Predominant sex: Female > male, although female gender is not universally considered a risk factor.

ETIOLOGY AND PATHOPHYSIOLOGY

- Controversial; exact mechanism(s) unknown
- It is postulated that microscopic axonal injury from shearing forces leads to inflammation that causes the secondary brain injury.
- Conflicting data on structural brain damage and the correlation of imaging findings with physical symptoms (1,3–6)
- Debate regarding correlation between existing psychiatric disease and development of PCS
  - PCS symptoms develop in patients with non–brain trauma at similar rates to those with MTBI. These findings suggest a psychiatric component underlying PCS (5,6)[B].
  - Preexisting psychiatric conditions may masquerade as PCS symptoms, making the diagnosis challenging and leading some to question psychiatric dysfunction as a PCS risk factor (3)[C].
- Because the pathophysiology of PCS is still not well understood and because of significant symptom overlap with other psychiatric conditions, PCS remains a difficult condition to diagnose and to manage.
  - Only some people with MTBI develop PCS; it is unclear what causes PCS symptoms to occur and to persist (5,6).
  - As above, psychiatric factors are commonly associated with, and may play a role in, the development of PCS. It can be a challenge to differentiate pure psychiatric dysfunction from true PCS (3)[C],(5–7)[B].

RISK FACTORS

- Amnesia, migraine, self-reported cognitive decline, noise and light sensitivity, depression/anxiety developing or worsening in the 1st day to weeks after MTBI are thought to be the major risk factors (1,3,4)[A].
- Preexisting psychiatric disease including depression, anxiety, personality disorder, and posttraumatic stress disorder (PTSD)
- Preexisting expectation of poor outcomes in patients following concussion/MTBI (1,3,4)[B]
- Unclear if previous history of concussion(s) is likely a risk factor for PCS (1)[C]
- Poor coping strategies, namely premature return to play following MTBI ("all-or-nothing behavior") (1,4)[B]
- Low socioeconomic status

GENERAL PREVENTION

- Education of players, coaches, parents, and athletic trainers about concussion, PCS, and following game safety rules designed to protect players
- Head injury precautions with activities are advised, but no good evidence that these decrease incidence of MTBI or PCS.
- Early screening and intervention(s) for anxiety and depression

COMMONLY ASSOCIATED CONDITIONS

- PTSD
- Depression
- Anxiety
- Fibromyalgia
- Personality disorders (namely, compulsive, histrionic, and narcissistic)

DIAGNOSIS

HISTORY

- Detailed history of recent impact/closed head injury, including the following:
  - Mechanism
  - Amount and type of force
  - Timing of injury related to symptoms
  - Previous head injuries, including concussion, and timing of those injuries
  - Previous medical, psychiatric, or social history
- Report of neurologic, cognitive, or behavioral symptoms by patient/family

PHYSICAL EXAM

Complete neurologic exam, including the following:

- Glasgow Coma Scale (GCS)
- Depression/anxiety screening
  - Patient Health Questionnaire-9 (PHQ-9)
  - Generalized Anxiety Disorder 7-item (GAD-7) scale
- Sport Concussion Assessment Tool, NFL Sideline Concussion Assessment Tool, or computerized neuropsychological (CNP) testing both pre- and post-MTBI is common practice, although data are limited on validity (2)[C]. More info regarding CNP below

DIFFERENTIAL DIAGNOSIS

- PTSD
- Anxiety/depression
- Personality disorder
- Migraine headaches
- Chronic fatigue syndrome, fibromyalgia
- Evolving intracranial hemorrhage
- Exposure to toxins, including prescription and recreational drugs
- Endocrine/metabolic abnormality

DIAGNOSTIC TESTS & INTERPRETATION

Initial Tests (lab, imaging)

If clinically warranted, consider evaluation for infection, intoxication, and endocrine/metabolic abnormality.

- Brain imaging both on initial evaluation of MTBI and PCS is generally neither fruitful nor indicated.
- Consider the use of cervical imaging when concomitant cervical spine injury is suspected.

Follow-Up Tests & Special Considerations

- Several CNP testing programs can be used to guide decisions regarding return to play. Consensus is that baseline testing should be done and scores used as controls against scores achieved after MTBI. However, data is limited. Formal neuropsychiatric evaluations are likely superior when available. None of these tests should be used alone in decision making, especially if a patient is still having symptoms despite improving or "baseline" scores (2,3)[C].
- Common neuropsychological testing programs for PCS
  - Immediate Post-Concussion Assessment and Cognitive Testing (ImPACT)
  - Axon Sports Computerized Cognitive Assessment Tool (CCAT)
  - Post Concussion Symptom Scale (PCSS)
  - Balance Error Scoring System (BESS)
  - Automated Neuropsychological Assessment Metrics (ANAM)

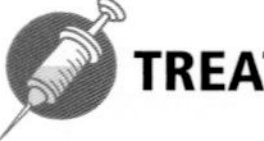

TREATMENT

GENERAL MEASURES

- Return to play guidelines (2,3)[C]
  - Stage 1. No activity: complete physical and relative cognitive rest, until symptom free
    - Consider school/work accommodations to allow earlier return to school/work in an attempt to prevent patients from getting too far behind (3)[C].
    - Some data suggesting that complete rest beyond 3 days is detrimental (7,8)[B]
    - Emerging data that subthreshold exercise may hasten recovery (7,8)[B]
  - Stage 2. Light aerobic exercise: walking, swimming, or stationary cycling keeping intensity $<70\%$ max predicted heart rate. No resistance training
  - Stage 3. Sport-specific exercise: drills (e.g., skating in ice hockey, running in soccer). No head impact activities

- Stage 4. Noncontact training drills: progression to more complex training drills (e.g., passing drills in football and ice hockey). May start progressive resistance training
- Stage 5. Full-contact practice: Following medical clearance, participate in normal training activities.
- Stage 6. Return to play: normal game play
- Each step should take 24 hours. If PCS symptoms occur at any step, the patient should drop back to the previous asymptomatic level and try to progress again after 24 hours of rest (2)[C].
- Persons with concussion or PCS should be restricted from sport activity until they are off all medications that may mask PCS symptoms and the clinical symptoms of PCS have resolved (1,2,3)[C].

MEDICATION

First Line

Headache/neck pain

- Nonopioid pain control (e.g., NSAIDs)
  - Sedation may obscure cognitive evaluation.
  - Possible association with use of opiates and increased risk of depression and anxiety in PCS patients (5)[B]
  - Consider occipital nerve block.

ALERT

Avoid opiates and benzodiazepines (5)[B].

- Depression/sleep disorders
  - Depression/anxiety screening starting in the 1st week post MTBI
    - SSRIs
    - Tricyclic antidepressants, or trazodone if there is concomitant sleep disturbance, may be beneficial.
- Consider referral to mental health specialist(s).
- Cognitive disorders (6)
  - Evaluation by neuropsychiatrist
  - Some evidence suggests CNP testing and rehab programs are beneficial.
  - Methylphenidate may be considered (9).
  - SSRIs may be considered, especially if concomitant depression/anxiety (9).

Second Line

- Dopaminergic agents such as amantadine, levodopa, and bromocriptine (1)[B]
- Dehydroepiandrosterone sulfate (DHEAS) (10)

ISSUES FOR REFERRAL

- Psychiatric treatment, including behavioral therapy for anxiety and depression symptoms. Specifically, neuropsychiatric therapy can be of benefit.
- Occupational therapy for vocational rehabilitation, if needed
- Neurology referral if primary care interventions for seizures, headache, vertigo, or cognition are unsuccessful.
- Comprehensive cognitive evaluation for potential TBI rehabilitation
- Substance abuse counseling, if needed

COMPLEMENTARY & ALTERNATIVE MEDICINE

Massage therapy/osteopathic manipulative treatment for headache and neck pain

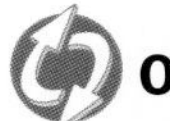

ONGOING CARE

FOLLOW-UP RECOMMENDATIONS

Schedule regular follow-up to evaluate for persistent symptoms, efficacy of/need for neuropsychiatric evaluation, and the efficacy of/need for pharmacologic therapy.

Patient Monitoring

- Consider serial neuropsychological testing.
- Follow return to play guidelines.

PATIENT EDUCATION

- NCAA concussion program: http://www.ncaa.org/wps/wcm/connect/public/NCAA/Health+and+Safety/Concussion+homepage/Concussion+Landing+Page
- Centers for Disease Control and Prevention: http://www.cdc.gov/concussion/sports
- Mayo Clinic Health Information: http://www.mayoclinic.com/health/post-concussion-syndrome/DS01020
- Brain Injury Association of America: www.biausa.org; (800) 444-6443

PROGNOSIS

- Prognosis generally is good.
- Young children may recover more slowly than young adults.

COMPLICATIONS

- Repeat head injury/return to play before resolution of PCS symptoms can worsen/prolong symptoms.
- Case studies of 2nd-impact syndrome, a rare but fatal condition owing to a 2nd head injury soon after the 1st, have been reported.

REFERENCES

1. Jotwani V, Harmon KG. Postconcussion syndrome in athletes. *Curr Sports Med Rep*. 2010;9(1):21–26.
2. McCrory P, Meeuwisse W, Johnston K, et al. Consensus statement on concussion in sport 3rd International Conference on Concussion in Sport held in Zurich, November 2008. *Clin J Sport Med*. 2009;19(3):185–200.
3. Harmon KG, Drezner JA, Gammons M, et al. American Medical Society for Sports Medicine position statement: concussion in sport. *Br J Sports Med*. 2013;47(1):15–26.
4. Hou R, Moss-Morris R, Peveler R, et al. When a minor head injury results in enduring symptoms: a prospective investigation of risk factors for postconcussional syndrome after mild traumatic brain injury. *J Neurol Neurosurg Psychiatry*. 2012;83(2):217–223.
5. Silverberg ND, Iverson GL. Etiology of the post-concussion syndrome: physiogenesis and psychogenesis revisited. *NeuroRehabilitation*. 2011;29(4):317–329.
6. Meares S, Shores EA, Batchelor J, et al. The relationship of psychological and cognitive factors and opioids in the development of the postconcussion syndrome in general trauma patients with mild traumatic brain injury. *J Int Neuropsychol Soc*. 2006;12(6):792–801.
7. Leddy J, Willer B. Use of graded exercise testing in concussion and return-to-activity management. *Curr Sports Med Rep*. 2013;12(6):370–376.
8. Leddy JJ, Cox JL, Baker JG, et. al. Exercise treatment for postconcussion syndrome: a pilot study of changes in functional magnetic resonance imaging activation, physiology, and symptoms. *J Head Trauma Rehabil*. 2013;28(4):241–249.
9. Lee H, Kim S, Kim J, et al. Comparing effects of methylphenidate, sertraline and placebo on neuropsychiatric sequelae in patients with traumatic brain injury. *Hum Psychopharmacol*. 2005;20(2):97–104.
10. Milman A, Zohar O, Maayan R, et al. DHEAS repeated treatment improves cognitive and behavioral deficits after mild traumatic brain injury. *Eur Neuropsychopharmacol*. 2008;18(3):181–187.

ADDITIONAL READING

- Barlow M, Schlabach D, Peiffer J, et al. Differences in change scores and the predictive validity of three commonly used measures following concussion in the middle school and high school aged population. *Int J Sports Phys Ther*. 2011;6(3):150–157.
- Broglio SP, Ferrara MS, Macciocchi SN, et al. Test-retest reliability of computerized concussion assessment programs. *J Athl Train*. 2007;42(4):509–514.
- Leddy JJ, Kozlowski K, Donnelly JP, et al. A preliminary study of subsymptom threshold exercise training for refractory post-concussion syndrome. *Clin J Sport Med*. 2010;20(1):21–27.
- Leddy JJ, Snadhu H, Sodhi V, et al. Rehabilitation of concussion and post-concussion syndrome. *Sports Health*. 2012;4(2):147–154.
- Nampiaparampil DE. Prevalence of chronic pain after traumatic brain injury: a systematic review. *JAMA*. 2008;300(6):711–719.
- Stroth S, Hille K, Spitzer M, et al. Aerobic endurance exercise benefits memory and affect in young adults. *Neuropsychol Rehabil*. 2009;19(2):223–243.
- Stulemeijer M, van der Werf S, Borm GF, et al. Early prediction of favourable recovery 6 months after mild traumatic brain injury. *J Neurol Neurosurg*. 2008;79(8):936–942.

SEE ALSO

Concussion (Mild Traumatic Brain Injury)

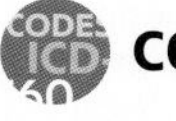

CODES

ICD10

- F07.81 Postconcussional syndrome
- S06.9X0A Unsp intracranial injury w/o loss of consciousness, init
- S06.9X9A Unsp intracranial injury w LOC of unsp duration, init

CLINICAL PEARLS

- Imaging rarely useful for PCS; head CT scan is the test of choice for acute injury to exclude intracranial bleeding.
- Coordinate multidisciplinary treatment plans for patients with persistent symptoms, namely mental health professionals.
- Return to play/activity should not occur until symptom free and off all medications that may mask PCS symptoms. Any return to activity with persistent symptoms should be discussed in detail with the patient and the patient's family.

POSTTRAUMATIC STRESS DISORDER (PTSD)

Rachel Bramson, MD • Michael L. Brown, MD • Suzanne Shurtz, MLIS, AHIP

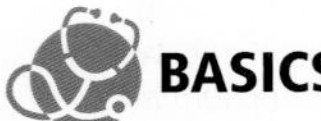

BASICS

DESCRIPTION

- Posttraumatic stress disorder (PTSD) is an anxiety disorder defined as a reaction that can occur after exposure to an extreme traumatic event involving death, threat of death, serious physical injury, or a threat to physical integrity.
- This reaction has 3 cardinal characteristics:
  - Reexperiencing the trauma
  - Avoidance of anything related to the traumatic event and/or numbing of general responsiveness
  - Increased arousal
- Traumatic events that may trigger PTSD include natural/human disasters, serious accidents, war, sexual abuse, rape, torture, terrorism, hostage-taking, or being diagnosed with life-threatening disease.
- PTSD can be the following:
  - Acute: symptoms lasting <3 months
  - Chronic: symptoms lasting ≥3 months
  - Delayed onset: 6 months (from event to symptom onset) in 25% of diagnosed cases

EPIDEMIOLOGY

- ~30% of men and women who have spent time in a war zone experience PTSD.
- Current estimates of PTSD in military personnel who served in Iraq range from 12 to 20%.
- 16% children and adolescents exposed to trauma develop PTSD (high of girls with interpersonal trauma 33%; low of boys with noninterpersonal trauma 8%) (1).

Incidence

~7.7 million American adults aged ≥18 years (3.5% of this age group) are diagnosed with PTSD each year.

Prevalence

Lifetime prevalence for PTSD is 8–9%.

ETIOLOGY AND PATHOPHYSIOLOGY

- During trauma, the locus coeruleus mediates sympathetic outflows to the amygdala (rapid effect) and adrenal medulla (sustained effect). The adrenal medulla then releases catecholamines, which stimulate peripheral afferent vagal β-receptors. Vagal afferents innervate the nucleus tractus solitarius (NTS) in the brainstem medulla. NTS fibers innervate the amygdala with norepinephrine (NE).
- With an increase in NE, the amygdala mediates coupling of emotional valence to declarative memories via long-term potentiation, forming deeply engraved trauma memories and leading to intrusive memories and emotions, potentially leading to PTSD.
- The orbitoprefrontal cortex (which usually exerts an inhibiting effect on this activation) appears less capable of inhibiting this activation due to stress-induced atrophy of specific nuclei in this region.

Genetics

- Monozygotic twins exposed to combat in Vietnam were at increased risk of the cotwin having PTSD compared with twins who were dizygotic.
- Some data suggest an association between dopamine transporter gene (DAT) *SLC6A3 3'* (VNTR) polymorphism and PTSD.

RISK FACTORS

- Pretrauma environment
  - Female sex
  - Younger age
  - Psychiatric history
  - Sexual abuse
- Peritrauma environment
  - Severity of the trauma
  - Peritrauma emotionality
  - Perception of threat to life
  - Perpetration of the trauma
- Posttrauma environment
  - Perceived injury severity
  - Medical complications
  - Perceived social support
  - Persistent dissociation from traumatic event
- Subsequent exposure to trauma-related stimuli

GENERAL PREVENTION

- There is moderate evidence for hydrocortisone (2) and some evidence for propranolol (3) reducing development of full posttraumatic syndrome.
- Compulsory psychological debriefing immediately after a trauma (critical incident stress management) does not prevent PTSD and may be harmful (4).

COMMONLY ASSOCIATED CONDITIONS

- Major depressive disorder
- Alcohol/substance abuse
- Panic disorder
- Obsessive-compulsive disorder
- Agoraphobia and/or social phobia
- Traumatic brain injury
- Smoking (especially with assaultive trauma)
- Major neurocognitive disorders, dementia or amnesia

Pediatric Considerations

Oppositional defiant disorder and separation anxiety are common comorbid conditions.

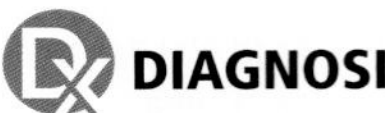

DIAGNOSIS

HISTORY

Diagnosis is based on *DSM-5* criteria:

- Criterion A: exposure to trauma (≥1 of the following)
  - Direct experience of a traumatic event
  - In-person witnessing of a traumatic event
  - Learning of a traumatic event involving a close friend or family member
  - Repeated exposure to details of a traumatic event
- Criterion B: intrusive symptoms associated with the traumatic event (≥1 of the following)
  - Recurrent, involuntary, and intrusive distressing memories of the event
  - Recurrent distressing dreams related to the event
  - Dissociative reactions that simulate a recurrence of the event
  - Intense or prolonged distress to stimuli that resemble an aspect of the event
- Criterion C: avoidance of stimuli associated with the trauma (≥1 of the following)
  - Avoidance of memories, thoughts, or feelings about the event
  - Avoidance of external reminders that trigger memories, thoughts, or feelings about the event
- Criterion D: negative cognitive and mood changes associated with the trauma (≥2 of the following)
  - Inability to remember aspects of event
  - Persistent and exaggerated negative opinion of self, others, or the world
  - Distorted beliefs about the cause or consequences of the event
  - Negative emotional state
  - Diminished interest in significant activities
  - Feeling detached from others
  - Inability to experience positive emotions
- Criterion E: hyperarousal (≥2 of the following)
  - Difficulty sleeping/falling asleep
  - Decreased concentration
  - Hypervigilance
  - Outbursts of anger/irritable mood
  - Exaggerated startle response
  - Self-destructive behavior
- Criterion F: Duration of the relevant criteria symptoms should be >1 month.
- Criterion G: clinically significant distress/impairment in functioning
- Criterion H: relevant criteria not attributed to substance effects or other medical conditions

Pediatric Considerations

- Memories of the traumatic event may not appear distressing and may be seen as play reenactment.
- Frightening dreams of children may not have content attributable to the traumatic event.
- Reactions can include a fear of being separated from a parent, crying, whimpering, screaming, immobility and/or aimless motion, trembling, frightened facial expressions, excessive clinging, and regressive behavior.
- Older children may show extreme withdrawal, disruptive behavior, and/or an inability to pay attention. Regressive behaviors, nightmares, sleep problems, irrational fears, irritability, refusal to attend school, outbursts of anger, fighting, somatic complaints with no medical basis, and decline in schoolwork performance are often seen. Furthermore, depression, anxiety, feelings of guilt, and emotional numbing are often present.
- Parental posttraumatic stress has been shown to be a robust predictor of pediatric PTSD (5)[A].

PHYSICAL EXAM

- Patients may present with physical injuries from the traumatic event.
- Mental status examination
  - Thoughts and perceptions (e.g., hallucinations, delusions, suicidal ideation, phobias)
  - General appearance: disheveled, poor hygiene
  - Behavior: agitation; startle reaction extreme
  - Psychological numbness
  - Orientation may be affected.
  - Memory: forgetfulness, especially concerning the details of the traumatic event
  - Poor concentration
  - Poor impulse control
  - Altered speech rate and flow
  - Mood and affect may be changed: depression, anxiety, guilt, and/or fear

Pediatric Considerations

Elevated heart rate immediately following trauma is associated with development of PTSD (5)[A].

DIFFERENTIAL DIAGNOSIS

- Acute stress disorder (symptoms <4 weeks)
- Generalized anxiety disorder
- Adjustment disorder
- Obsessive-compulsive disorder
- Schizophrenia
- Major depressive disorder
- Mood disorder with psychotic features
- Substance abuse

- Personality disorders
- Dissociative disorders
- Conversion disorder

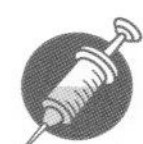

TREATMENT

Better prognosis if treated with a combination of psychotherapy and pharmacotherapy, initiated soon after the trauma

MEDICATION

First Line

- SSRIs: depression, panic attacks, startle response, sleep disruption (6)[A]. All commonly used SSRIs have been shown to be effective in the treatment of PTSD and are the 1st-line treatment:
  - Sertraline: starting dose: 15–50 mg every day; may be increased as tolerated up to 200 mg/day
  - Paroxetine: starting dose: 10 mg every day; may be increased in 10-mg increments at intervals ≥1 week up to 50 mg/day
  - Fluoxetine: starting dose: 20 mg every day; may be increased as tolerated up to 60 mg/day (demonstrates some efficacy for all 3 symptom clusters)
- Sleep disruption: Sleep disruption due to hyperarousal is ubiquitous in PTSD. Medications such as trazodone 50–200 mg at bedtime, mirtazapine 7.5–15 mg QHS, or amitriptyline 25–100 mg QHS may be tried.
- Nightmares/nighttime hyperarousal: prazosin: Initiate with 1 mg HS; may increase as tolerated to 2–15 mg QHS (7)[A], clonidine 0.1–0.2 mg QHS, amitriptyline 25–100 mg QHS.

Second Line

Refractory/residual symptoms: Consider augmentation with the following:

- Depression: mirtazapine 15–45 mg/day; consider switch to a serotonin-norepinephrine reuptake inhibitor (SNRI) such as venlafaxine XR 37.5–300 mg/day, duloxetine 40–60 mg/day or desvenlafaxine 50 mg/day. Nefazodone 300–600 mg/day in divided doses can be very effective but requires quarterly LFTs.
- Reexperiencing/intrusive thoughts: 1st-/2nd-generation antipsychotic medications: aripiprazole 5–15 mg/day, risperidone 0.5–2 mg/day, olanzapine 2.5–10 mg/day, quetiapine 50–400 mg/day (8)[A]. 2nd-generation Rx less prone to extrapyramidal symptoms (EPS), cognitive dulling
- Hyperarousal: clonidine: Start 0.1 mg–0.2 mg/day; guanfacine 1–3 mg/day in divided doses (long-acting forms of both clonidine and guanfacine now available). Also consider 2nd-generation antipsychotics quetiapine, risperidone, and olanzapine as above. Divided doses often more helpful.
- Impulsivity/explosiveness: Anticonvulsants may be tried; supporting data limited: valproic acid 500–2,000 mg/day, carbamazepine 200–600 mg/day, topiramate 50–200 mg/day
- Anxiety: benzodiazepines (see "Alert"), including clonazepam, 1–4 mg/day in divided doses for a limited duration. Consider also hydroxyzine 25–50 mg TID/QID PRN or risperidone 0.25–0.5 mg TID PRN.

ALERT

Given risk of substance abuse and questionable benefit in PTSD, recommended benzodiazepines be avoided (9)[A]. Short-acting benzodiazepines present the greatest risk.

ADDITIONAL THERAPIES

- Psychotherapeutic interventions
  - Exposure therapies have shown the highest effectiveness for treatment of PTSD (10)[A]:
    - Behavioral and cognitive-behavioral therapy (CBT): Early CBT has been shown to speed recovery. CBT is currently considered the standard of care for PTSD by the U.S. Department of Defense.
    - 1-week intensive CBT was as effective as 3-month weekly CBT in one study (11)[A].
    - Internet-based CBT has shown benefit in reduction of PTSD symptoms.
    - Prolonged exposure therapy: Reexperience distressing trauma–related memories and reminders to facilitate habituation and successful emotional processing of memory.
    - EMDR (eye movement desensitization and reprocessing) has been shown to benefit patients with PTSD (12)[A].
  - Stress-reduction techniques
    - Immediate symptom reduction (e.g., rebreathing in a bag for hyperventilation)
    - Early recognition and removal from a stress
    - Relaxation, meditation, and exercise techniques are also helpful in reducing the reaction to stressful events.
- Interpersonal psychotherapy
  - Supportive psychotherapy with an emphasis on the here and now
- Social
  - Establish the social framework of the problem. Clarifying this allows the patient to begin viewing it within the proper context (e.g., change of job/relocation of adult-dependent offspring).

INPATIENT CONSIDERATIONS

Inpatient care is necessary only if the patient becomes suicidal/homicidal or for treatment of comorbid conditions (e.g., depression, substance abuse).

ONGOING CARE

PATIENT EDUCATION

National Center for PTSD: www.ptsd.va.gov

PROGNOSIS

- Varies significantly from patient to patient
- In 50% of cases, the symptoms spontaneously remit after 3 months; however, in other cases, symptoms may persist, often for many years, and cause long-term impairment in life functioning.
- Factors associated with a good prognosis include:
  - Rapid engagement of treatment
  - Early and ongoing social support
  - Avoidance of retraumatization
  - Positive premorbid function
  - Absence of other psychiatric disorders/substance abuse

COMPLICATIONS

- Increased risk for panic disorder, agoraphobia, obsessive-compulsive disorder, social phobia, specific phobia, major depressive disorder, somatization disorder; impulsive behavior, suicide, and homicide. Victims of sexual assault are at especially high risk for developing mental health problems and committing suicide.
- Benzodiazepines lead to abuse and dependence.
- Avoidance of stimuli associated with the trauma can generalize to wide-ranging avoidance. This leads to a far greater negative impact on the patient's life.

REFERENCES

1. Alisic E, Zalta AK, van Wesel F, et al. Rates of post-traumatic stress disorder in trauma-exposed children and adolescents: meta-analysis. *Br J Psychiatry*. 2014;204:335–340.
2. Amos T, Stein DJ, Ipser JC. Pharmacological interventions for preventing post-traumatic stress disorder (PTSD). *Cochrane Database Syst Rev*. 2014;7:CD006239.
3. Searcy CP, Bobadilla L, Gordon WA, et al. Pharmacoloical prevention of combat-related PTSD: a literature review. *Mil Med*. 2012;177(6):649–654.
4. Rose S, Bisson J, Churchill R, et al. Psychological debriefing for preventing post traumatic stress disorder (PTSD). *Cochrane Database Syst Rev*. 2002;(2):CD000560.
5. Brosbe MS, Hoefling K, Faust J. Predicting posttraumatic stress following pediatric injury: a systematic review. *J Pediatr Psychol*. 2011;36(6):718–729.
6. Stein DJ, Ipser JC, Seedat S. Pharmacotherapy for post traumatic stress disorder (PTSD). *Cochrane Database Syst Rev*. 2006;(1):CD002795.
7. Writer BW, Meyer EG, Schillerstrom JE. Prazosin for military combat-related PTSD nightmares: a critical review. *J Neuropsychiatry Clin Neurosci*. 2014;26(1):24–33.
8. Han C, Pae CU, Wang SM, et al. The potential role of atypical antipsychotics for the treatment of posttraumatic stress disorder. *J Psychiatr Res*. 2014;56:72–81.
9. Jeffreys M, Capehart B, Friedman MJ. Pharmacotherapy for posttraumatic stress disorder: review with clinical applications. *J Rehabil Res Dev*. 2012;49(5):703–715.
10. Kornør H, Winje D, Ekeberg Ø, et al. Early trauma-focused cognitive-behavioural therapy to prevent chronic post-traumatic stress disorder and related symptoms: a systematic review and meta-analysis. *BMC Psychiatry*. 2008;8:81.
11. Ehlers A, Hackmann A, Grey N, et al. A randomized controlled trial of 7-day intensive and standard weekly cognitive therapy for PTSD and emotion-focused supportive therapy. *Am J Psychiatry*. 2014;171(3):294–304.
12. Goodson J, Helstrom A, Halpern JM, et al. Treatment of posttraumatic stress disorder in U.S. combat veterans: a meta-analytic review. *Psychol Rep*. 2011;109(2):573–599.

ADDITIONAL READING

American Psychiatric Association. *Diagnostic and Statistical Manual of Mental Disorders*. 5th ed. Washington, DC: American Psychiatric Association; 2013.

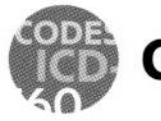

CODES

ICD10

- F43.10 Post-traumatic stress disorder, unspecified
- F43.11 Post-traumatic stress disorder, acute
- F43.12 Post-traumatic stress disorder, chronic

CLINICAL PEARLS

- Treatment is often best accomplished with a combination of psychotherapy and pharmacotherapy.
- The sooner therapy is initiated after the trauma, the better the prognosis.

PREECLAMPSIA AND ECLAMPSIA (TOXEMIA OF PREGNANCY)

Konstantinos E. Deligiannidis, MD, MPH

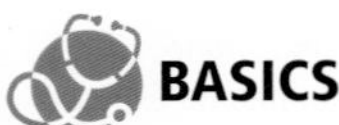

BASICS

DESCRIPTION

- Preeclampsia is a disorder of pregnancy developing at the 20th week (or beyond), with hypertension (HTN) and proteinuria or impaired organ function:
  - May progress from mild to life threatening in hours to days
  - The disorder is reversible by delivery if at term or, if maternal/fetal health are in danger, by preterm delivery.
  - Eclampsia is defined as new-onset grand mal seizure activity in a patient with preeclampsia without underlying neurologic disease.
  - Most postpartum cases occur within 48 hours of delivery but can occur up to 4 weeks postpartum.
- System(s) affected: cardiovascular, renal, reproductive, fetoplacental, CNS, hepatic
- Synonym(s): toxemia of pregnancy

EPIDEMIOLOGY

Incidence

- Predominant age
  - Most cases occur in younger women because of the higher incidence of preeclampsia in younger (nulliparous) women.
  - However, older (>40 years) patients with preeclamsia have 4× the incidence of seizures compared with patients in their 20s.
- Pregnancy-induced HTN: 6% of pregnancies
- Preeclampsia: 5–7%
- Eclampsia develops in 1/2,000 deliveries in developed countries. In developing countries, estimates range from 1/100 to 1/1,700.
- 40% of eclamptic seizures occur before delivery; 16% occur >48 hours after delivery.

ETIOLOGY AND PATHOPHYSIOLOGY

Systemic derangements in eclampsia include the following:

- Cardiovascular: generalized vasospasm
- Hematologic: decreased plasma volume, increased blood viscosity, hemoconcentration, coagulopathy
- Renal: decreased glomerular filtration rate
- Hepatic: periportal necrosis, hepatocellular damage, subcapsular hematoma
- CNS: cerebral vasospasm and ischemia, cerebral edema, cerebral hemorrhage

Genetics

Increased incidence in pregnant women whose mothers/sisters had the disease

RISK FACTORS

- Nulliparity: 3:1 (relative risk [RR])
- Age >40 years: 2:1 (RR)
- High body mass index: 2:1 (RR)
- Chronic HTN, chronic renal disease, or both
- Diabetes: 3.5:1 (RR)
- Multifetal pregnancy: 3:1 (RR)
- Preeclampsia during a previous pregnancy
- Family history of preeclampsia: 3:1 (RR)
- Systemic lupus erythematosus
- In vitro fertilization (1)[C]

GENERAL PREVENTION

- Adequate prenatal care: Women who do not receive prenatal care are 7× more likely to die from complications.
- Good control of preexisting HTN
- Recent systematic reviews, meta-analyses, and task force recommendations show that low-dose aspirin (60–80 mg) started early in pregnancy may lower the risk of developing preeclampsia in moderate- to high-risk patients and the rate of preterm delivery and neonatal death and has no significant effect on the rate of placental abruption/neonatal bleeding complications. The number needed to treat (NNT) to prevent 1 case of preeclampsia ranges from 18 to 118 depending on risk population, but more info is required to see which women would benefit and when to start therapy (2–4)[A]. It may be recommended in those with preeclampsia in >1 prior pregnancy or with a history of preeclampsia and preterm delivery (1)[C].
- Low-dose calcium supplementation has been shown to reduce the risk of preeclampsia (RR = 0.38) (5)[A].
- Although some evidence suggests vitamin C (1,000 mg/day) and vitamin E (400 U/day) may reduce the risk for preeclampsia, recent guidelines recommend against their use (1)[C],(6).

COMMONLY ASSOCIATED CONDITIONS

- Abruptio placenta
- Placental insufficiency
- Fetal growth restriction
- Preterm delivery
- Fetal demise
- Maternal seizures (eclampsia)
- Maternal pulmonary edema
- Maternal liver/kidney failure
- Maternal death

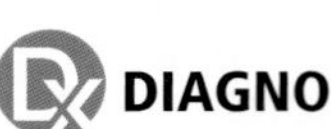

DIAGNOSIS

Diagnosis depends on new-onset elevated BP (SBP ≥140 mm Hg or DBP ≥90 mm Hg on 2 occasions at least 4 hours apart or ≥160/110 mm Hg) after 20 weeks of gestation and proteinuria or new-onset thrombocytopenia, renal insufficiency, impaired liver function, pulmonary edema, or cerebral/visual symptoms (1)[C].

HISTORY

May be asymptomatic. In some cases, rapid excessive weight gain (>5 lb/week; >2.3 kg/week); more severe cases are associated with epigastric pain, headache, altered mental status, and visual disturbance.

PHYSICAL EXAM

- Preeclampsia
  - Mild: elevated BP ≥140/90 mm Hg on 2 occasions at least 4 hours apart or ≥160/110 mm Hg, proteinuria (>300 mg/24 hr or protein-to-creatinine ratio ≥0.3)
  - Severe: elevated BP ≥160 systolic mm Hg or 110 mm Hg diastolic on 2 BP readings 4 hours apart while the patient is on bed rest
    - Platelets <100,000/μL
    - >2 times normal liver transaminase levels, severe persistent right upper quadrant (RUQ)/epigastric pain, or both
    - Creatinine >1.1 mg/dL or doubling of serum creatinine levels
    - Pulmonary edema
    - Cerebral or visual symptoms
- Eclampsia
  - Headache, visual disturbance, and epigastric or RUQ pain often precede seizure.
  - Tonic–clonic seizure activity (focal/generalized)
  - Seizures may occur once/repeatedly.
  - Postictal coma, cyanosis (variable)
  - Temperatures >39°C, consistent with CNS hemorrhage
  - Normal BP, even in response to treatment, does not rule out potential for seizures. Up to 30% may not have edema; 20% may not have proteinuria.

DIFFERENTIAL DIAGNOSIS

- Chronic HTN: HTN before pregnancy; high BP before the 20th week
- Gestational HTN: increased BP first discovered during pregnancy, near term, with no proteinuria; normal BP by 12 weeks postpartum
- Seizures in pregnancy: epilepsy, cerebral tumors, meningitis/encephalitis, ruptured cerebral aneurysm. Until other causes are proven, however, all pregnant women with convulsions should be considered to have eclampsia.

DIAGNOSTIC TESTS & INTERPRETATION

Initial Tests (lab, imaging)

- Routine spot urine testing for protein should be done at each prenatal visit.
- CBC, including platelets
- Creatinine
- Serum transaminase levels
- Uric acid
- Coagulation profiles: Abnormalities suggest severe disease.
- 24-hour urine or protein-to-creatinine ratio
- Daily fetal movement monitoring by mother ("kick counts")
- US imaging is used to monitor growth and cord blood flow; perform, as indicated, based on clinical stability and laboratory findings.
- Nonstress test (NST) at diagnosis and then twice weekly until delivery
- Biophysical profile if NST is nonreactive (1)[C]
- US imaging for growth progress every 3 weeks and amniotic fluid volume at least once weekly (1)[C]
- With seizures, CT scan and MRI should be considered if focal findings persist or uncharacteristic signs/symptoms are present.

Follow-Up Tests & Special Considerations

Disseminated intravascular coagulation, thrombocytopenia, liver dysfunction, and renal failure can complicate preeclampsia associated with HELLP syndrome.

Test Interpretation

CNS: cerebral edema, hyperemia, focal anemia, thrombosis, and hemorrhage: Cerebral lesions account for 40% of eclamptic deaths.

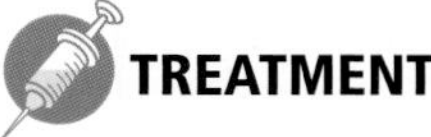

TREATMENT

- Mild ("without severe features")
  - Outpatient care, delivery at 37 weeks' gestation
  - Maternal: daily home BP monitoring; daily weights; weekly labs (24 hour protein, platelet count, creatinine, LFTs)
  - Fetal
    - Patient-measured: daily "kick counts"
    - Medical provider–measured: NST (see imaging section)
- Severe
  - Inpatient care if patient condition deteriorates (BP ≥160/110 mm Hg; severe headache; visual changes [scotoma or "flashing lights"]; impaired mentation; pulmonary edema; epigastric/RUQ

pain; increasing LFTs; oliguria; thrombocytopenia) or if fetal status is deemed "nonreassuring"
- Maternal: daily labs, adding coagulation tests; IV magnesium sulfate as anticonvulsive prophylaxis; IV labetalol or hydralazine and oral sustained-release nifedipine antihypertensive therapy titrated to keep systolic BP <155 mm Hg and diastolic BP <105 mm Hg. Keep diastolic BP >90 mm Hg to avoid hypoperfusing the uterus.
- Fetal: continuous heart monitoring; daily US with BP, amniotic fluid levels, fetal growth assessment as deemed necessary

GENERAL MEASURES

Management by gestational age of severe preeclampsia:
- <23 weeks: Offer to terminate pregnancy.
- At 23–32 weeks: antihypertensives; evaluate maternal–fetal condition; steroids to enhance fetal lung maturity; plan delivery at 34 weeks with magnesium sulfate prophylaxis or for worsening maternal/fetal jeopardy.
- At 33–34 weeks: steroids, magnesium sulfate, and delivery
- At >34 weeks: magnesium sulfate and delivery

ALERT
- Regardless of gestational age, emergent delivery is recommended if there are signs of maternal hypertensive crisis, abruptio placentae, uterine rupture, or fetal distress (7).
- Seizures
  - Control of convulsions, correction of hypoxia and acidosis, lowering of BP, steps to effect delivery as soon as convulsions are controlled
  - See "Medication" section.

MEDICATION

First Line
- For seizure prophylaxis: magnesium sulfate: loading dose 4 g IV in 200 mL normal saline over 20–30 minutes; maintenance dose 1–2 g/hr IV continuous infusion
- For HTN
  - Nifedipine sustained-release (PO): 30–120 mg/day (caution with combination of nifedipine and magnesium sulfate resulting in hypotension and neuromuscular blockade) +
  - Labetalol (IV): 20 mg over 2 minutes followed at 10-minute intervals with doses of 20–80 mg titrated to keep BP <155/105 mm Hg; max of 2,400 mg/day; antihypertensives are inadvisable for mild HTN/preeclampsia.
- For eclampsia/seizures
  - In recent randomized trials, magnesium sulfate was found to be superior to phenytoin in the treatment and prevention of eclampsia and probably more effective and safer than diazepam.
  - Magnesium sulfate for seizures
    - 4–6 g IV over 15–20 minutes followed by 1–3-g/hr infusion
    - Further boluses of magnesium may be given for recurrent convulsions with the amount given based on the neurologic examination and patellar reflexes.
  - Levels of 6–8 mEq/mL are considered therapeutic, but clinical status is most important and must ensure that
    - Patellar reflexes are present.
    - Respirations are not depressed.
    - Urine output is ≥25 mL/hr.
  - May be given safely, even in the presence of renal insufficiency
- Fluid therapy
  - Ringer lactated solution with 5% dextrose at 60–120 mL/hr, with careful attention to fluid–volume status
- HTN, if present and severe (e.g., >160/110 mm Hg), also should be treated:
  - Hydralazine: 5 mg IV then 5–10 mg boluses as needed q20min *or*
  - Labetalol: 10–20 mg IV then double dose at 10-minute intervals up to 80 mg; maximum total cumulative dose of 220–230 mg (e.g., 20–40–80–80 or 10–20–40–80–80)
- Precautions: Do not use diuretics. Carefully monitor neurologic status, urine output, respirations, and fetal status.
- Calcium carbonate (1 g, administered slowly IV) may reverse magnesium-induced respiratory depression.

Second Line
- Diazepam 2 mg/min until resolution or 20 mg given *or*
- Lorazepam 1–2 mg/min up to total of 10 mg *or*
- Phenytoin 15–20 mg/kg at a maximum rate of 50 mg/min *or*
- Phenobarbital 20 mg/kg infused at 50 mg/min; may repeat with additional 5–10 mg/kg after 15 min

ONGOING CARE

FOLLOW-UP RECOMMENDATIONS
- Mild: restricted activity
- Severe: restricted activity, in hospital

DIET
- Salt restriction is inadvisable because the patient often is experiencing intravascular hypovolemia (1)[C].
- Calcium supplementation may be recommended for women who have low calcium intake (<600 mg/day) (6).

PATIENT EDUCATION

American College of Obstetricians and Gynecologists, 409 12th St. SW, Washington, DC 20024-2188; (800) 762-ACOG; www.acog.org

PROGNOSIS
- For nulliparous women with preeclampsia before 30 weeks of gestation, the recurrence rate for the disorder may be as high as 40% in future pregnancies (8).
- Multiparous women have higher rates of recurrence.
- 25% of eclamptic women will have HTN during subsequent pregnancies, but only 5% of these will be severe and only 2% will be eclamptic again.
- Eclamptic, multiparous women may be at higher risk for subsequent essential HTN; they also have higher mortality during subsequent pregnancies than do primiparous women.

COMPLICATIONS
- Most women do not have long-term sequelae from eclampsia, although many may have transient neurologic deficits.
- A history of preeclampsia is equivalent to traditional risk factors for cardiovascular disease. Women with a history of preeclampsia should be strongly advised to avoid obesity and smoking. Other signs of metabolic syndrome should be closely monitored as well (9).
- Maternal and/or fetal death

REFERENCES

1. American College of Obstetricians and Gynecologists, Task Force on Hypertension in Pregnancy. Hypertension in pregnancy. Report of the American College of Obstetricians and Gynecologists' Task Force on Hypertension in Pregnancy. *Obstet Gynecol*. 2013;122(5):1122–1131.
2. Gauer R, Atlas M, Hill J. Clinical inquiries. Does low-dose aspirin reduce preeclampsia and other maternal-fetal complications? *J Fam Pract*. 2008;57(1):54–56.
3. Villa PM, Kajantie E, Räikkönen K, et al. Aspirin in the prevention of pre-eclampsia in high-risk women: a randomised placebo-controlled PREDO Trial and a meta-analysis of randomised trials. *BJOG*. 2013;120(1):64–74.
4. Duley L, Henderson-Smart DJ, Meher S, et al. Antiplatelet agents for preventing pre-eclampsia and its complications. *Cochrane Database of Syst Rev*. 2007;(2):CD004659. doi:10.1002/14651858.CD004659.pub2.
5. Hofmeyr G, Belizán J, von Dadelszen P, et al. Low-dose calcium supplementation for preventing pre-eclampsia: a systematic review and commentary. *BJOG*. 2014;121(8):951–957.
6. Magee LA, Helewa M, Moutquin J-M, et al. Diagnosis, evaluation, and management of the hypertensive disorders of pregnancy. *J Obstet Gynaecol Can*. 2008;30(3)(Suppl):S1–S48.
7. Sibai BM. Diagnosis and management of gestational hypertension and preeclampsia. *Obstet Gynecol*. 2003;102(1):181–192.
8. Report of the National High Blood Pressure Education Program Working Group on high blood pressure in pregnancy. *Am J Obstet Gynecol*. 2000;183(1):S1–S22.
9. Carty DM, Delles C, Dominiczak AF. Preeclampsia and future maternal health. *J Hypertens*. 2010;28(7):1349–1355.

ADDITIONAL READING

- Hofmeyr GJ, Duley L, Atallah A. Dietary calcium supplementation for prevention of pre-eclampsia and related problems: a systematic review and commentary. *BJOG*. 2007;114(8):933–943.
- Rumbold A, Duley L, Crowther CA, et al. Antioxidants for preventing pre-eclampsia. *Cochrane Database Syst Rev*. 2008;(1):CD004227.

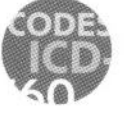

CODES

ICD10
- O14.90 Unspecified pre-eclampsia, unspecified trimester
- O14.10 Severe pre-eclampsia, unspecified trimester
- O15.9 Eclampsia, unspecified as to time period

CLINICAL PEARLS
- Management of preeclampsia depends on both the severity of the condition and the gestational age of the fetus.
- Diagnosis no longer requires presence of proteinuria.

PREMENSTRUAL SYNDROME (PMS) AND PREMENSTRUAL DYSPHORIC DISORDER (PMDD)

Courtney I. Jarvis, PharmD • Allison Hargreaves, MD

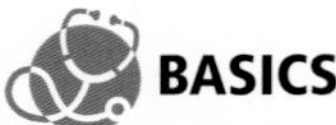

BASICS

DESCRIPTION

- Premenstrual syndrome (PMS), a complex of physical and emotional symptoms sufficiently severe to interfere with everyday life, occurs cyclically during the luteal phase of menses.
- Premenstrual dysphoric disorder (PMDD) is a severe form of PMS characterized by severe recurrent depressive and anxiety symptoms, with premenstrual (luteal phase) onset, that remits a few days after the start of menses.
- PMDD is now included as a full diagnostic category in the 5th edition of the *Diagnostic and Statistical Manual of Mental Disorders* (*DSM-5*).
- System(s) affected: endocrine/metabolic, nervous, reproductive

EPIDEMIOLOGY

Prevalence

- Many women have some physical and psychic symptoms before menses (this is not PMS).
- 30% of menstruating women suffer from PMS; 3–8% of menstruating women have PMDD.

ETIOLOGY AND PATHOPHYSIOLOGY

Not well understood. Leading theories postulate metabolites of progesterone interact with central neurotransmitter receptors (serotonin and γ-aminobutyric acid [GABA]), provoking downstream effects of decreased GABA-mediated inhibition and decreased serotonin levels. Women with PMS/PMDD have similar levels of progesterone but seem to have an increased sensitivity to its metabolites, compared with women without PMS/PMDD.

Genetics

- Role of genetic predisposition is controversial; however, twin studies do suggest a genetic component.
- Involvement of gene coding for the serotonergic *5HT1A* receptor and allelic variants of the estrogen receptor-α gene (*ESR1*) is suggested.

RISK FACTORS

- Age: usually present in late 20s to mid-30s
- History of mood disorder (major depression, bipolar disorder), anxiety disorder, personality disorder, or substance abuse
- Family history
- Low parity
- Tobacco use
- Psychosocial stressors/history of trauma
- High BMI

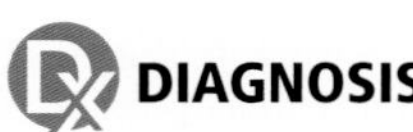

DIAGNOSIS

HISTORY

DSM-5 criteria (1)

- Symptoms occur 1 week before menses, improve in the 1st few days after menses begin, and are minimal/absent in the week following menses (over most menstrual cycles during the past year).
- ≥5 of the following (1 must be among the first 4):
  - Marked depressed mood, feelings of hopelessness, or self-deprecating thoughts
  - Marked anxiety, tension, and/or feelings of being keyed up or on edge
  - Marked affective lability (mood swings)
  - Marked irritability or anger or increased interpersonal conflicts
  - Decreased interest in usual activities and social withdrawal
  - Lethargy, easy fatigability, or lack of energy
  - Appetite change, overeating, food cravings
  - Hypersomnia or insomnia
  - Feeling out of control or overwhelmed
  - Subjective difficulty concentrating
  - Physical symptoms, such as abdominal bloating, breast tenderness, headaches, weight gain, and joint/muscle pain
- For PMDD, emotional symptoms must be sufficiently severe to interfere with work, school, usual social activities, or relationships with others.
- Symptoms may be superimposed on an underlying psychiatric disorder but may not be an exacerbation of another condition, such as panic disorder/major depression.
- Criteria should be confirmed by prospective patient record of symptoms for a minimum of 2 consecutive menstrual cycles (without confirmation, "provisional" should be noted with diagnosis).
- Use the Daily Record of Severity of Problems (available online at http://www.aafp.org/afp/2011/1015/p918-fig1.pdf) or similar inventory (2)[A].
- Symptoms should not be attributable to drug abuse, medications, or other medical conditions.

PHYSICAL EXAM

No specific physical exam required; may consider thyroid and pelvic exams if indicated by additional patient symptoms.

DIFFERENTIAL DIAGNOSIS

- Premenstrual exacerbation of underlying psychiatric disorder
- Psychiatric disorders (especially bipolar disorder, major depression, anxiety)
- Thyroid disorders
- Perimenopause
- Premenstrual migraine
- Chronic fatigue syndrome
- Irritable bowel syndrome (painful symptoms)
- Seizures
- Anemia
- Endometriosis (painful symptoms)
- Drug/alcohol abuse

DIAGNOSTIC TESTS & INTERPRETATION

- The repetitive nature of symptoms precludes need for labs if a classic history is present.
- Consider
  - Hemoglobin to rule out anemia
  - 25-OH vitamin D level to exclude deficiency, although precise relationship of deficiency with the disorder is unclear
  - Serum thyroid-stimulating hormone (TSH) to rule out hypothyroidism
- Imaging with pelvic ultrasound to diagnose causes of pelvic pain and dysmenorrhea may be needed.

TREATMENT

GENERAL MEASURES

Although evidence is lacking for aerobic exercise in treating PMS/PMDD, it is often recommended as part of an integrated care plan.

MEDICATION

First Line

- SSRIs show a small to moderate effect in the treatment of physical, functional, and behavioral symptoms of PMS and PMDD compared to placebo (3)[A]:
  - Both intermittent luteal phase dosing and continuous full-cycle dosing are effective with no clear evidence of difference between modes of administration (3)[A].
  - All SSRIs tested appeared effective (3)[A].
  - SSRIs are effective at low doses. Higher doses have increased effect but are accompanied by increased side effects (3)[A].
- Fluoxetine (Prozac, Sarafem) 20 mg/day every day or 20 mg/day only during luteal phase, or 90 mg once a week × 2 weeks in luteal phase
- Sertraline (Zoloft) 50–150 mg/day every day or 50–150 mg/day only during luteal phase
- Citalopram (Celexa) 10–30 mg/day every day or 10–30 mg/day only during luteal phase
- Adverse effects (number needed to harm [NNH] with moderate-dose SSRI): nausea (NNH = 7), asthenia (NNH = 9), somnolence (NNH = 13), fatigue (NNH = 14), decreased libido (NNH = 14), and sweating (NNH = 14) (3)[A].
- Contraindications: patients taking monoamine oxidase inhibitors (MAOIs)
- Precautions
  - Increased risk of suicidal thinking and behavior in children and adolescents with depressive disorders; uncertain if this risk applies to those taking SSRIs for PMDD
  - Bipolar disorder
  - Seizure disorder
  - Hepatic dysfunction
  - Renal dysfunction
- Possible interactions
  - MAOIs
  - Selegiline
  - Pimozide
  - Thioridazine

Second Line

Alternative therapies should be considered if no response to SSRIs:

- Spironolactone (Aldactone) 50–100 mg/day × 7–10 days during luteal phase; helpful for fluid retention. Adverse reactions: lethargy, headache, irregular menses, hyperkalemia
- Oral contraceptive pills (OCPs)
  - OCPs can cause adverse effects similar to PMDD symptoms (4)[B].
  - Extended-cycle use of OCPs (e.g., 12 weeks on and 1 week off) or a shorter placebo interval (e.g., 24 active pills with 4 placebo days [24/4] compared with 21/7 preparations) may be beneficial (4)[B].

- OCPs containing the progestin drospirenone (structurally similar to spironolactone) may improve physical symptoms and mood changes associated with PMDD (5)[A]. Caution: Risk of venous thromboembolism may be modestly higher than with other OCPs (4)[B].
- Continuous administration of levonorgestrel/ethinyl estradiol may improve patient symptoms in PMDD (4)[B].
  - Suggested OCP formulations:
    - Ethinyl estradiol 0.02–0.03 mg/drospirenone 3 mg (Yasmin/Yaz/Gianvi/Loryna/Ocella/Syeda/Vestura/Zarah): 1 tablet/day
    - Ethinyl estradiol 0.02–0.03 mg/drospirenone 3 mg/levomefolate 0.451 mg (Beyaz/Safyral): 1 tablet/day
    - Levonorgestrel 90 μg/ethinyl estradiol 20 μg (Amethyst/Lybrel): 1 tablet/day

- Anxiolytics
  - Alprazolam (Xanax) 0.25 mg TID–QID only during luteal phase; taper at onset of menses (other benzodiazepines not studied for PMDD). Caution: addictive potential
  - Buspirone (BuSpar) 10–30 mg/day divided BID–TID in the luteal phase
- Ovulation inhibitors
  - Gonadotropin-releasing hormone (GnRH) agonists: leuprolide (Lupron) depot 3.75 mg/month IM
    - Precautions: Menopause-like side effects (e.g., osteoporosis, hot flashes, headaches, muscle aches, vaginal dryness, irritability) limit treatment to 6 months; may be 1st step if considering bilateral oophorectomy for severe, refractory PMDD
  - Danazol (Danocrine) 300–400 mg BID; adverse reactions: androgenic and antiestrogenic effects (e.g., amenorrhea, weight gain, acne, fluid retention, hirsutism, hot flashes, vaginal dryness, emotional lability)
  - Estrogen, transdermal preferred, 100–200 μg:
    - Precautions: increased risk of blood clot, stroke, heart attack, and breast cancer
    - Requires concomitant progesterone add-back therapy to protect against uterine hyperplasia and endometrial cancer
- Progesterone: insufficient evidence to support use (6)[A]

ISSUES FOR REFERRAL

Referral to psychiatrist may be indicated for mood/anxiety disorders if patient has no symptom-free period.

ADDITIONAL THERAPIES

Cognitive-behavioral therapy (CBT) is theoretically helpful for PMS/PMDD given its application for symptom reduction in other mood disorders, but direct evidence is lacking.

SURGERY/OTHER PROCEDURES

Bilateral oophorectomy, usually with concomitant hysterectomy, is an option for rare, refractory cases with severe, disabling symptoms.

COMPLEMENTARY & ALTERNATIVE MEDICINE

- Acupuncture demonstrated superiority to progestins, anxiolytics, and sham acupuncture with no evidence of harm (7)[A].
- Some data support the use of the following (8)[A]:
  - Calcium: 600 mg BID
  - Vitamin B_6: 50–100 mg/day
  - Chasteberry (*Vitex agnus-castus*): 4 mg/day of extract containing 6% of agnuside (or 20–40 mg/day of fruit extract)
  - Omega-3 fatty acids 2 g/day
- Data insufficient regarding the following (8)[A]:
  - Magnesium: 200–400 mg/day
  - Vitamin D: 2,000 IU/day
  - Vitamin E: 400 IU/day
  - Manganese: 1.8 mg/day
  - St. John's wort: 900 mg/day
  - Soy: 68 mg/day isoflavones
  - Ginkgo: 160–320 mg/day
  - Saffron: 30 mg/day
- Evidence supporting efficacy and/or safety of herbal products is lacking; the following products/interventions have *not* been found useful for PMS/PMDD, although not all studies are of high quality and able to eliminate possibility of benefit completely (8)[A]:
  - Evening primrose oil
  - Black currant oil
  - Black cohosh
  - Wild yam root
  - Dong quai
  - Kava kava
  - Light-based therapy

ONGOING CARE

FOLLOW-UP RECOMMENDATIONS

Patient Monitoring

Increased risk of suicidal thinking and behavior in children and adolescents with depressive disorders on initiation of SSRIs; uncertain if this risk applies to those taking SSRIs for PMDD

DIET

- Reduce consumption of salt, sugar, caffeine, dairy products, and alcohol (anecdotal reports).
- Eat small, frequent portions of food high in complex carbohydrates (limited data).

PATIENT EDUCATION

- Counsel patients to eat a balanced diet rich in calcium, vitamin D, and omega-3 fatty acids and low in saturated fat and caffeine.
- Counsel women that they are not "crazy." PMDD is a real disorder with a physiologic basis.
- Although incompletely understood, successful treatment is often possible.

PROGNOSIS

- Many patients can have their symptoms adequately controlled. PMS disappears at menopause.
- PMS can continue after hysterectomy, if ovaries are left in place.

REFERENCES

1. American Psychiatric Association. *Diagnostic and Statistical Manual of Mental Disorders*, 5th ed. Washington, DC: American Psychiatric Association; 2013.
2. Borenstein JE, Dean BB, Yonkers KA, et al. Using the daily record of severity of problems as a screening instrument for premenstrual syndrome. *Obstet Gynecol*. 2007;109(5):1068–1075.
3. Marjoribanks J, Brown J, O'Brien PM, et al. Selective serotonin reuptake inhibitors for premenstrual syndrome. *Cochrane Database Syst Rev*. 2013;(6):CD001396.
4. Freeman EW, Halbreich U, Grubb GS, et al. An overview of four studies of a continuous oral contraceptive (levonorgestrel 90 mcg/ethinyl estradiol 20 mcg) on premenstrual dysphoric disorder and premenstrual syndrome. *Contraception*. 2012;85(5):437–445.
5. Lopez LM, Kaptein A, Helmerhorst FM. Oral contraceptives containing drospirenone for premenstrual syndrome. *Cochrane Database Syst Rev*. 2012;(2):CD006586.
6. Ford O, Lethaby A, Roberts H, et al. Progesterone for premenstrual syndrome. *Cochrane Database Syst Rev*. 2012;(3):CD003415.
7. Kim SY, Park HJ, Lee H, et al. Acupuncture for premenstrual syndrome: a systematic review and meta-analysis of randomised controlled trials. *BJOG*. 2011;118(8):899–915.
8. Whelan AM, Jurgens TM, Naylor H. Herbs, vitamins and minerals in the treatment of premenstrual syndrome: a systematic review. *Can J Clin Pharmacol*. 2009;16(3):e407–e429.

ADDITIONAL READING

- Biggs WS, Demuth RH. Premenstrual syndrome and premenstrual dysphoric disorder. *Am Fam Physician*. 2011;84(8):918–924.
- Nevatte T, O'Brien PM, Bäckström T, et al. ISPMD consensus on the management of premenstrual disorders. *Arch Womens Ment Health*. 2013;16(4):279–291.
- Rapkin AJ, Akopians AL. Pathophysiology of premenstrual syndrome and premenstrual dysphoric disorder. *Menopause Int*. 2012;18(2):52–59.

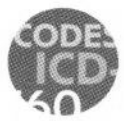

CODES

ICD10

N94.3 Premenstrual tension syndrome

CLINICAL PEARLS

- Have the patient keep a daily log of her symptoms and menses. Symptoms beginning in the week before menses and abating before the end of menses, occurring over at least 2 months, and sufficiently severe to interfere with daily functioning are diagnostic of PMS.
- The difference between PMS and PMDD is that PMDD is a severe form of PMS characterized by recurrent depressive and anxiety symptoms with luteal phase onset, sufficiently severe to disrupt social and occupational functioning. These symptoms remit a few days after the onset of menses.
- PMDD is not the same as more generalized depressive/anxiety disorders. PMDD-associated symptoms of depression and anxiety begin to resolve within the 1st few days of menses.
- Luteal phase treatment only is likely as effective as continuous-cycle treatment with SSRIs but has fewer adverse effects.

PRENATAL CARE AND TESTING

Fozia Akhtar Ali, MD • Teny Anna Philip, MD

BASICS

- The goal of prenatal care is to ensure the birth of a healthy baby with minimal risk for the mother by the following:
  - Identifying the patient who is at risk for complications
  - Estimating the gestational age (GA) as accurately as possible
  - Evaluating the health status of mother and fetus
  - Encouraging and empowering the patient to do her part to care for herself and her baby-to-be
  - Intervening when fetal abnormalities are present to prevent morbidity

GENERAL PREVENTION

- A recommended prenatal care schedule consists of the following:
  - Monthly visits to a health care professional for weeks 4–28 of pregnancy
  - Visits twice monthly from 28 to 36 weeks
  - Weekly after week 36 (delivery at week 38–40)
- Recommendations for use of dietary supplements in pregnancy:
  - Folic acid supplementation (0.4–0.8 mg) prior to conception; 4 mg for secondary prevention
  - Calcium: 1,000–1,300 mg/day; supplement may be beneficial for women with high risk for gestational hypertension or communities with low dietary calcium intake.
  - Iron: Screen for anemia (Hgb/Hct) and treat if necessary. Recommend 30 mg/day of iron in pregnant women.
  - Vitamin A: Pregnant women in industrialized countries should limit to <5,000 IU/day.
  - Vitamin D: Consider supplementation in women with limited exposure to sunlight.
- Routine thyroid screening and vitamin D deficiency during pregnancy is not recommended.

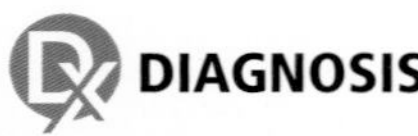

DIAGNOSIS

HISTORY

At the initial visit, a complete medical, obstetrical, family, and psychosocial history should be obtained and updated throughout the pregnancy.

- Assess and counsel as appropriate regarding the following:
  - Lifestyle; nutrition; safety of medications (teratogenicity, category); tobacco, alcohol, and drug use; toxins; relationship issues/domestic violence; stressors/supports; work environment; risk factors
- Domestic violence
  - ACOG guidelines recommend that physicians screen *all* pregnant patients for intimate partner domestic violence:
    - At the 1st prenatal visit
    - At least once per trimester
    - At the postpartum checkup

PHYSICAL EXAM

- A full physical exam should be performed at the 1st prenatal appointment.
- At each subsequent prenatal visit, the following should be recorded:
  - Weight: Total weight gain range (lb) should be 25–35 lb, except in obese women, for whom weight gain should be <15 lb.
  - BP
    - ACOG defines hypertension as BP >140 mm Hg systolic or >90 mm Hg diastolic (1,2).
    - Monitor BP especially closely in patients with chronic hypertension (predating pregnancy), preeclampsia/eclampsia, or gestational hypertension.
  - UA for glucose and protein; 24-hour protein excretion is the gold standard but not practical.
  - Fundal height
  - Fetal heart rate: usually audible by 12 weeks' GA with a Doppler instrument
  - Routine fetal movement counts *not* recommended
  - Fetal position by abdominal palpation at 36 weeks
  - Pelvic/cervical exam if indicated

DIAGNOSTIC TESTS & INTERPRETATION

Cervical cancer screening

- A Pap smear should be obtained when indicated by standard Pap screening guidelines, regardless of gestation (ACOG, USPSTF, ASCCP, ACS, and ASCP guidelines state that women <21 years should not be screened regardless of age of sexual initiation or other risk factors).
- Squamous intraepithelial lesions can progress during pregnancy but often regress postpartum.
- Colposcopy only to exclude the presence of invasive cancer in high-risk women
- Cervical biopsy should be avoided unless a malignancy is suspected. Endocervical sampling is contraindicated.
- 1st prenatal visit:
  - Lab tests:
    - Hematocrit or hemoglobin
    - Blood type: A, B, AB, or O [C]
    - Rhesus type and antibody screen: Rh(+) or Rh(−)
    - Hemoglobin electrophoresis for patients at risk for sickle cell disease or thalassemia
    - Urine testing for glucose and protein
    - Urine culture
    - Rubella titer
    - Syphilis test
    - Gonorrhea/chlamydia screening
    - Hepatitis B surface antigen
    - HIV testing (patient may "opt out" if chooses to decline)
    - Routine screening for bacterial vaginosis, toxoplasmosis, CMV, and parvovirus not recommended
    - Cystic fibrosis screening (information should be made available to all couples)
      - Cystic fibrosis carrier screening should be offered before conception or early in pregnancy when 1 partner is of Caucasian, European, or Ashkenazi Jewish descent (3).
      - It is reasonable to offer cystic fibrosis carrier screening to all couples regardless of race or ethnicity as an alternative to selective testing.
- Screening tests (for birth defects), noninvasive:
  - U/S nuchal translucency (NT): measures thickness at the back of the neck of the fetus
  - Blood screens: human chorionic gonadotropin (hCG), pregnancy-associated plasma protein A (PAPP-A), quad screen: α-fetoprotein (AFP), unconjugated estriol (UE3), hCG, inhibin-A (INH-A)
  - Cell-free DNA testing should be offered as an alternative noninvasive method of screening for fetal aneuploidies to high-risk pregnant women between 10 and 22 weeks' gestation. Women who elect cell-free DNA testing will also need an α-fetoprotein test for neural tube defects. The assay also allows screening for aneuploidy, rhesus typing in Rh(D) -negative women, and single-gene disorders (limited to detection of paternally inherited mutation). Because of a small but real risk for false-positive results, most experts advise using these assays as screening tests and confirming positive result with invasive prenatal diagnostics.
  - 1st-trimester screening between 11 and 14 weeks' GA using both NT and hCG/PAPP-A blood testing is an effective protocol in the general population and is more effective than NT alone, with an 83% detection rate for Down syndrome, with false-positive rate of 5%. Detects trisomy 21 (Down syndrome) and trisomy 18 (Edward syndrome). May be performed either as a single combined stand-alone test (U/S NT + blood [HCG and PAPP-A]) or as part of a sequential "step-by-step" 1st- and 2nd-trimester screening process (see the following discussion)
  - 2nd-trimester screening protocols:
    - Obtain "multiple marker"/quad screen between 15 and 21 weeks' GA, optimally between 16 and 18 weeks; ~84% detection rate for trisomy 21, trisomy 18, and neural tube defects (NTDs), with false-positive rate of 5%, *or*
    - 2-step integrated screening protocol: combines information collected during the 1st and 2nd trimesters of the pregnancy to determine the risk of Down syndrome, trisomy 18, or open NTD:
      - 2 options: stepwise sequential integrated screen (~91% detection rate with false-positive rate 3.3%):
        - 1st trimester: NT measurement, plus blood (hCG, PAPP-A):
          - If calculated risk for Down syndrome is ≥1:30, then additional steps are recommended (genetic counseling, U/S, and chorionic villi sampling [CVS]).
          - If calculated risk for Down syndrome is <1:30 *then*
        - 2nd-trimester quad screen (AFP, UE3, hCG, INH-A) is required, *or*
      - Serum integrated screen: 88% detection rate with false-positive rate of 4.5%; requires a 1st-trimester PAPP-A blood test without NT measurement, *and* a 2nd-trimester (16–18-week quad screen)
- Diagnostic tests (for birth defects), invasive:
  - ACOG guidelines: All pregnant women, not just women ≥35 years, should be offered invasive prenatal diagnostic testing, such as CVS and amniocentesis to detect possible genetic abnormalities in their fetuses (4)[C].
  - Women found to be at increased risk of having a baby with Down syndrome with 1st-trimester screening should be offered genetic counseling and the option of CVS or midtrimester amniocentesis. If screening tests show increased risk of birth defect, there are 2 possible diagnostic tests:
    - CVS: 1st trimester: usually done after 10 weeks (10–12 weeks). Small sample of the placenta; chorionic tissue sample obtained either transcervical (TC) or transabdominal (TA). Complication: pregnancy loss rate of 1.0–1.5%
    - Amniocentesis
      - 1st trimester: usually at 11–13 weeks but higher rate of pregnancy loss and complication

than either CVS or early 2nd-trimester procedures; therefore, not recommended
    - 2nd trimester: usually done after 15 weeks (15–18 weeks). The prenatal diagnostic technique associated with the lowest risk of pregnancy loss. Small sample of amniotic fluid from the amniotic sac surrounding the developing fetus is obtained by an US-guided TA approach. Complication: pregnancy loss rate of ≤0.5%
- 24–28 weeks
  - Obtain diabetes screen (see the following discussion), repeat hematocrit or hemoglobin, and repeat antibody screen in Rh-negative mother prior to receiving prophylactic Rh immunoglobulin:
    - Gestational diabetes mellitus (GDM) screening: universal recommendation for ideal approach for screening and diagnosis of GDM remains elusive. In 2010, the International Association of Diabetes and Pregnancy Study Group proposed a new system in which diabetes in pregnancy is classified as overt versus gestational diabetes. The American Diabetes Association reaffirmed this in 2010 and 2013. Presently, this system is not endorsed by ACOG because there is no evidence that 1-step screening using this criteria leads to clinically significant improvements in maternal and fetal outcomes but would lead to significant increase in health care costs.
    - Overt diabetes (test when women first present for prenatal care): fasting blood sugar ≥126 mg/dL or HbA1c ≥6.5%, or random ≥200 mg/dL that is confirmed with subsequent fasting blood sugar or HbA1c. (These thresholds were chosen due to correlation with adverse vascular events, e.g., retinopathy and CAD.)
    - Gestational diabetes: fasting plasma glucose >92 mg/dL but is <126 mg/dL at any GA. At 24–28 weeks of gestation, a 75 g 2-hour oral glucose tolerance test with at least 1 abnormal result: FBG ≥92 mg/dL but <126 mg/dL, or 1-hour ≥180 mg/dL, or 2-hour ≥153 mg/dL
    - The prevalence of gestational diabetes in the United States can be 2–25%, greater in African Americans, Hispanics, Native Americans, and Asians than in Caucasians. Using the IADPSG criteria for overt versus gestational diabetes, ~18% of women would be diagnosed with diabetes during pregnancy.
    - The following guidelines for GDM are established by ACOG:
      - Specified cutoffs define GDM:
        - A value of >130 mg/dL will identify 90% of women with GDM, but 20–25% of all women screened will need to continue to the 3-hour oral glucose tolerance test (OGTT) (1,2).
        - Raising the value to >140 mg/dL will identify only 80% of women with GDM but decrease to 14–18% the number of women who will need to continue to the 3-hour OGTT (5).
      - Screening test: 1-hour OGTT (nonfasting)
        - 50 g PO glucose load with blood glucose testing 1 hour later
        - Carpenter and Coustan positive screen: >130 mg/dL
        - National Diabetes Data Group (NDDG) positive screen: >140 mg/dL
      - Diagnostic test: 3-hour OGTT (fasting):
        - If abnormal 1-hour OGTT screening test, may be followed by a 3-hour OGTT
        - 100 g PO glucose load with blood drawn: fasting, 1, 2, and 3 hours after ingestion of glucose
        - Either the plasma or serum glucose level designated by Carpenter and Coustan or by the NDDG are appropriate to use:
          - *A positive diagnosis of GDM requires that ≥2 thresholds be exceeded:
            - Carpenter and Coustan standard:
              - *>95 (fasting), >180 (1-hour), >155 (2-hour), >140 (3-hour)
            - National Diabetes Data Group standard:
              - *105 (fasting), >190 (1-hour), >165 (2-hour), >145 (3-hour)
- 35–37 weeks
  - Group B Streptococcus (GBS) culture: Universal screening for GBS colonization at 35–37 weeks of gestation remains the sole strategy for intrapartum antibiotic prophylaxis.
  - High-risk patients: High-risk patients should be screened again for gonorrhea, chlamydia, HIV, and syphilis.
- Postterm pregnancy
  - Rate of stillbirth increases with GA, 1/3,000 per week at 37 weeks, 3/3,000 per week at 42 weeks, 6/3,000 at 43 weeks. In 1 meta-analysis, routine induction of labor at 41 weeks' gestation reduced rates of perinatal death without increased rates of cesarean delivery.
  - For gestational periods beyond 42 weeks, fetal well-being should be assessed with nonstress testing and US assessment of amniotic fluid volume.

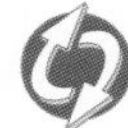

TREATMENT

ISSUES FOR REFERRAL

Abnormal screening labs or imaging may prompt referral to maternal–fetal medicine specialist or other medical specialist, as indicated.

ONGOING CARE

PATIENT EDUCATION

- Immunizations during pregnancy: The following vaccines are considered safe per CDC (6):
  - Women should get (Tdap) during each pregnancy. Ideally, the vaccine should be given between 27 and 36 weeks of pregnancy Hep B, and influenza; possibly include meningococcal, rabies. Contraindicated during pregnancy or safety not established: live vaccines including BCG, MMR, and varicella.
  - Patients should be made aware of the tests that are performed routinely, as well as other tests that might be elected (e.g., CVS or amniocentesis), as well as the choices that would be available if testing were abnormal (pregnancy termination, preparation for the birth of an infant with congenital anomalies, further testing).
- Prevention:
  - Preconception counseling offers the opportunity to discuss individualized risks.
- To decrease the risks of NTDs, preconception folate supplementation is indicated.
- Recommendations:
  - Airline travel: generally safe until up to 4 weeks from EDD. Lengthy trips associated with increased risk of thrombosis
  - Caffeine: Limit to <200 mg/day. Correlation between IUGR and miscarriage with caffeine is undetermined at this time.
  - Exercise: Healthy women with uncomplicated pregnancies should continue to exercise.
  - Seat belts/air bags: ACOG recommends that pregnant women wear lap and shoulder seatbelts and should not turn off air bags.
  - Sexual activity: Intercourse is not associated with adverse outcomes.
- Alcohol, cigarettes, and illicit drugs are injurious to fetal and maternal health.
  - Pregnancy-safe medications (teratogenicity)

REFERENCES

1. American College of Obstetricians and Gynecologists. Screening tools—domestic violence. http://www.acog.org/ACOG_Departments/Violence_Against_Women/Screening_Tools-Domestic-Violence. Accessed August 7, 2012.
2. Committee on Obstetric Practice. Committee Opinion No. 514: emergent therapy for acute-onset, severe hypertension with preeclampsia or eclampsia. *Obstet Gynecol*. 2011;118(6):1465–1468.
3. American College of Obstetricians and Gynecologists Committee on Genetics. ACOG Committee Opinion No. 486: update on carrier screening for cystic fibrosis. *Obstet Gynecol*. 2011;117(4):1028–1031.
4. American College of Obstetricians and Gynecologists. ACOG Practice Bulletin No. 88, December 2007. Invasive prenatal testing for aneuploidy. *Obstet Gynecol*. 2007;110(6):1459–1467.
5. Berger H, Crane J, Farine D, et al. Screening for gestational diabetes mellitus. *J Obstet Gynaecol Can*. 2002;24(11):894–912.
6. http://www.cdc.gov/groupbstrep/guidelines/newdifferences.html.2010guidelines

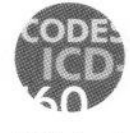

CODES

ICD-10

- Z34.90 Encntr for suprvsn of normal pregnancy, unsp, unsp trimester
- Z36 Encounter for antenatal screening of mother
- Z34.00 Encntr for suprvsn of normal first pregnancy, unsp trimester

CLINICAL PEARLS

Prenatal care and screening are best accomplished using standardized flow sheets and checklists to ensure that the complex sequence of evaluations and education is performed consistently and properly.

PREOPERATIVE EVALUATION OF THE NONCARDIAC SURGICAL PATIENT

Andrew Grimes, MD • Stacy Jones, MD

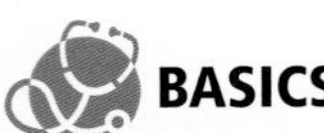

BASICS

DESCRIPTION

- Preoperative medical evaluation should determine the presence of established or unrecognized disease or other factors that may increase the risk of perioperative morbidity and mortality in patients undergoing surgery.
- Specific assessment goals include the following:
  - Conducting a thorough medical history and physical exam to assess the need for further testing and/or consultation
  - Recommending strategies to reduce risk and optimize patient condition prior to surgery
  - Encouraging patients to optimize their health for possible improvement of both perioperative and long-term outcomes
- Synonym(s): preoperative diagnostic workup; preoperative preparation; preoperative general health assessment

EPIDEMIOLOGY

Overall patient morbidity and mortality related to surgery is low. One large study of inpatients looking at 30-day mortality in the United States showed a rate of 1.32%. This rate varies by type of procedure and varies by country. Preoperative patient evaluation and subsequent optimization of perioperative care can reduce both postoperative morbidity and mortality.

RISK FACTORS

- Functional capacity (1): Exercise tolerance is one of the most important determinants of cardiac risk:
  - Self-reported exercise tolerance may be an extremely useful predictive tool when assessing risk. Patients unable to meet a 4 metabolic equivalent (MET) demand (defined in the "Diagnosis" section) during daily activities have increased perioperative cardiac and long-term risks.
  - Patients who report good exercise tolerance require minimal, if any, additional testing.
- Levels of surgical risk
  - High: aortic, major vascular, and peripheral vascular surgery
  - Intermediate: intraperitoneal, intrathoracic, carotid endarterectomy, head/neck, orthopedic, and prostate surgery
  - Low: endoscopic, superficial, cataract, breast, and ambulatory surgery
- Clinical risk factors (1): history of ischemic heart disease, the presence of compensated heart failure or a history of prior congestive heart failure (CHF), cerebrovascular disease, diabetes mellitus (DM), and renal insufficiency; these risk factors plus surgical risk can dictate the need for further cardiac testing.
- Age: Patients >70 years of age are at higher risk for perioperative complications and mortality and have a longer length of stay in the hospital postoperatively. (Likely attributed to increasing medical comorbidities with increasing age.) Age alone should not be a deciding factor in the decision to proceed or not proceed with surgery.

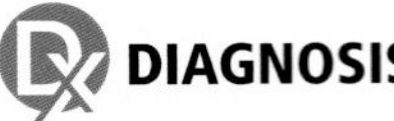

DIAGNOSIS

HISTORY

- Evaluate pertinent medical records and interview the patient. Many institutions provide standard patient questionnaires that screen for preoperative risk factors:
  - History of present illness and treatments
  - Past medical and surgical history
  - Patient and family anesthetic history and associated complications
  - Current medications (including over-the-counter [OTC] medications, vitamins, supplements, and herbals) as well as reasons for use
  - Allergies (including specific reactions)
  - Social history: tobacco, alcohol, drug use, and cessation
  - Family history: prior illnesses and surgeries
- Systems (both history and current status)
  - Cardiovascular: Inquire about exercise capacity.
    - 1 MET: can take care of self, eat, dress, and use toilet; walk around house indoors; walk a block or 2 on level ground at 2–3 mph
    - 4 METs: can climb flight of stairs or walk uphill, walk on level ground at 4 mph, run a short distance, do heavy work around house, participate in moderate recreational activities
    - 10 METs: can participate in strenuous sports such as swimming, singles tennis, football, basketball, or skiing
  - Note presence of CHF, cardiomyopathy, ischemic heart disease (stable vs. unstable), valvular disease, hypertension (HTN), arrhythmias, murmurs, pericarditis, history of pacemaker or implantable cardioverter defibrillator (ICD):
    - Rhythm management devices (pacemakers and automatic ICDs [AICD]) affect the perioperative course. Most importantly, the following information need to be available for proper management: name of cardiologist who manages the device, type of device, manufacturer, last interrogation, and any problems that have occurred recently. Based on this information and the location and type of surgery, a perioperative plan of management will be made (2).
    - Stents: Patients with coronary stents are maintained on antiplatelet therapy with a thienopyridine, such as clopidogrel, frequently in combination with aspirin. Premature discontinuation of antiplatelet therapy markedly increases the risk of acute stent thrombosis, the results of which can be catastrophic. Elective surgery should be delayed and antiplatelet therapy continued for 4–6 weeks after bare metal stent placement and for at least 12 months after placement of drug-eluting stents. Even after this time period, any perioperative disruption in the patient's antiplatelet regimen should be discussed with the patient's cardiologist and surgeon. The risk of perioperative bleeding must be weighed against the risks associated with discontinuation of antiplatelet drugs prior to surgery.
  - Pulmonary: Chronic and active disease processes should be addressed: chronic infections, bronchitis, emphysema, asthma, wheezing, shortness of breath, cough (productive or otherwise):
    - Sleep apnea: Patients with obstructive sleep apnea (OSA) are at increased risk for perioperative adverse events. Because of the high incidence of undiagnosed sleep apnea in perioperative patients, many authors are recommending screening questionnaires such as the Berlin or STOP-BANG (3,4). The American Society of Anesthesiologists (ASA) has practice guidelines based on expert review that take into account the severity of sleep apnea, the invasiveness of surgery, and the projected need for postoperative opioids (5).
    - Patients with OSA frequently are at increased risk for obesity, coronary disease, HTN, atrial fibrillation, CHF, and pulmonary HTN. Optimizing the management of these comorbidities may be the 1st important step in the preoperative management of patients with OSA. Often, patients with an existing diagnosis of OSA who use continuous positive airway pressure (CPAP) at night are asked to bring their CPAP machine to the hospital or surgery center when they are admitted for surgery.
    - Some studies suggest that even short periods (3 weeks) of treatment with CPAP can improve some indicies of ventilation and therefore may reduce postoperative morbidity.
  - GI: hepatic disease, gastric ulcer, inflammatory bowel disease, hernias (especially hiatal), significant weight loss, nausea, vomiting, history of postoperative nausea and vomiting: Any symptoms consistent with gastroesophageal reflux disease (GERD) should be optimally treated.
  - Hematologic: anemia, serious bleeding, clotting problems, blood transfusions, hereditary disorders
  - Renal: kidney failure, dialysis, infections, stones, changes in bladder function
  - Endocrine: nocturia, parathyroid, pituitary, adrenal disease, thyroid disease
    - Diabetes: Evidence that hyperglycemia in the perioperative period is associated with increased perioperative complications. Although recommendations vary, most experts recommend keeping perioperative blood glucose levels <180.
  - Neurologic/psychiatric: seizures, stroke, paralysis, tremor, migraine headaches, nerve injury, multiple sclerosis, extremity numbness, psychiatric disorders (e.g., anxiety, depression)
  - Musculoskeletal: arthritis, lower back pain
  - Reproductive: possibility of pregnancy in women of childbearing potential
- Mouth/upper airway: dentures, crowns, partials, bridges, teeth (loose, chipped, cracked, capped)

PHYSICAL EXAM

- Assess vital signs, including arterial BP bilaterally.
- Check carotid pulses; auscultate for bruits.
- Examine lungs by auscultating all lung fields and listening for rales, rhonchi, wheezes, or other sounds indicating disease.
- Examine cardiovascular system by auscultating heart and noting any irregular rhythms or murmurs; precordial palpation.
- Palpate abdomen.
- Examine airway and mouth for ease of intubation, neck mobility, and size of tongue; note any lesions or dental deformities.
- If a regional anesthesia technique is being contemplated, perform a relevant, focused neurologic exam.

DIAGNOSTIC TESTS & INTERPRETATION

Initial Tests (lab, imaging)

- Laboratory testing should not be obtained routinely prior to surgery unless indicated (6)[C]. Specific tests should be requested if the evaluator suspects findings from the clinical evaluation that may influence perioperative patient management.
- Labs performed within the past 4 months prior to evaluation are reliable unless the patient has had an interim change in clinical presentation or is taking medications that require monitoring of plasma level or effect.
- CBC (6)[C]
  - Hemoglobin: if a patient has symptoms of anemia or is undergoing a procedure with major blood loss; extremes of age; liver or kidney disease
  - WBC count: if symptoms suggest infection or myeloproliferative disorder or the patient is at risk for chemotherapy-induced leukopenia
  - Platelet count: if history of bleeding, myeloproliferative disorder, liver or renal disease, or the patient is at risk for chemotherapy-induced thrombocytopenia
- Serum chemistries (electrolytes, glucose, renal and liver function tests): should be obtained for extremes of age; in known renal insufficiency, CHF, liver dysfunction, or endocrine abnormalities; or the patient is on medications that alter electrolyte levels, such as diuretics
- PT/PTT: if history of a bleeding disorder, chronic liver disease, or malnutrition, or those with recent or chronic antibiotic or anticoagulant use
- Urinalysis: Routine urinalysis is not recommended preoperatively.
- Pregnancy test: controversial; should be *considered* for all female patients of childbearing age
- CXR is not generally indicated. It can be considered in patients with recent upper respiratory tract infection and in those with suspected cardiac or pulmonary disease (because there is a likelihood for unanticipated findings), but these indications are not considered unequivocal.

Diagnostic Procedures/Other

- ECG (6)[C]
  - Evidence indicates that the incidence of ECG abnormalities may be higher in older patients and in patients with multiple cardiac risk factors. In these instances, a preoperative ECG may be warranted. Age alone, however, is not necessarily an indication for a preoperative ECG.
  - ECGs are not indicated for asymptomatic patients undergoing low-risk procedures.
- Further cardiac testing should be considered in patients with poor or unknown functional capacity and 3+ clinical risk factors if the surgery is high risk and testing will change management (e.g., dipyridamole-thallium scan).
- PFTs: Definitive data regarding the efficacy of preoperative testing are lacking. The most important factor is preoperative optimization of patients with chronic obstructive pulmonary disease (COPD) or reactive airways disease with indicated use of antibiotics, bronchodilators, and inhaled corticosteroids. Spirometry can help guide therapy. Upper abdominal and thoracic surgery have a higher risk of postoperative pulmonary complications.

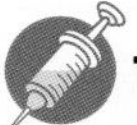

TREATMENT

MEDICATION

- Reducing cardiac risk
  - Elective surgery should be delayed or canceled if the patient has any of the following: unstable coronary syndromes (unstable or severe angina), recent myocardial infarction (MI) (<30 days), decompensated heart failure, significant arrhythmias, or severe valvular disease.
  - Active HF should be treated with diuretics, afterload reduction, and β-adrenergic blockers.
  - Perioperative β-blockade has been shown to reduce mortality and the incidence of perioperative MIs in high-risk patients. Studies conflict, however, in which patients need to be treated, the dosage and timing of treatment, and for what surgeries. *Patients chronically on β-blockers should have the medication continued in the perioperative period.* When β-blockers are discontinued in the perioperative period, 30-day mortality increases. β-Blockers are reasonable for vascular surgery patients with at least 1 clinical risk factor.
  - Perioperative statin use may have a protective effect on reducing cardiac complications. Currently, the American Heart Association (AHA) has a class I indication for perioperative statin therapy for patients already on statins prior to their surgery. There is also evidence that vascular surgery patients benefit from perioperative statins.
  - A recent review looked at prophylactic use of aspirin in the perioperative period and did not find a significant effect on perioperative mortality or risk for MI in patients undergoing noncardiac surgery and may be associated with an increased risk of perioperative bleeding. There were important exclusion criteria including patients with recent stent placement (7).
- Reducing pulmonary risk
  - Recommend cigarette cessation for at least 8 weeks prior to elective surgery.
  - Patients with asthma should not be wheezing and should have a peak flow of at least 80% of their predicted or personal-best value.
  - Treatment of COPD and asthma should focus on maximally reducing airflow obstruction and is identical to treatment of nonsurgical patients.
  - Lower respiratory tract infections (bacterial) should be treated with appropriate antibiotic therapy.

REFERENCES

1. American College of Cardiology Foundation/American Heart Association Task Force on Practice Guidelines, American Society of Echocardiography, American Society of Nuclear Cardiology, et al. 2009 ACCF/AHA focused update on perioperative beta blockade. *J Am Coll Cardiol*. 2009;54(22):2102–2128.
2. Crossley GH, Poole JE, Rozner MA, et al. The Heart Rhythm Society (HRS)/American Society of Anesthesiologists (ASA) Expert Consensus Statement on the perioperative management of patients with implantable defibrillators, pacemakers and arrhythmia monitors: facilities and patient management. *Heart Rhythm*. 2011;8(7):1114–1154.
3. Adesanya AO, Lee W, Greilich NB, et al. Perioperative management of obstructive sleep apnea. *Chest*. 2010;138(6):1489–1498.
4. Chung SA, Yuan H, Chung F. A systematic review of obstructive sleep apnea and its implications for anesthesiologists. *Anesth Analg*. 2008;107(5):1543–1563.
5. American Society of Anesthesiologists Task Force on Perioperative Management of Patients with Obstructive Sleep Apnea. Practice guidelines for the perioperative management of patients with obstructive sleep apnea: an updated report by the American Society of Anesthesiologists Task Force on Perioperative Management of patients with obstructive sleep apnea. *Anesthesiology*. 2014;120(2):268–286.
6. Committee on Standards and Practice Parameters, Apfelbaum JL, Connis RT, et al. Practice advisory for preanesthesia evaluation: an updated report by the American Society of Anesthesiologists Task Force on Preanesthesia Evaluation. *Anesthesiology*. 2012;116(3):522–538.
7. Devereaux PJ, Mrkobrada M, Sessler DI, et al. Aspirin in patients undergoing noncardiac surgery. *N Engl J Med*. 2014;370(16):1494–1503.

ADDITIONAL READING

- Akhtar S, Barash PG, Inzucchi SE, et al. Scientific principles and clinical implications of perioperative glucose regulation and control. *Anesth Analg*. 2010;110(2):478–497.
- Chung F, Subramanyam R, Liao P, et al. High STOP-Bang score indicates a high probability of obstructive sleep apnoea. *Br J Anaesth*. 2012;108(5):768–775.
- Lander JS, Coplan NL. Statin therapy in the perioperative period. *Rev Cardiovasc Med*. 2011;12(1):30–37.
- Pearse RM, Moreno RP, Bauer P, et al. Mortality after surgery in Europe: a 7-day cohort study. *Lancet*. 2012;380(9847):1059–1065.
- Semel ME, Lipsitz SR, Funk LM, et al. Rates and patterns of death after surgery in the United States, 1996 and 2006. *Surgery*. 2012;151(2):171–182.

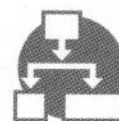

SEE ALSO

Algorithm: Preoperative Evaluation of the Noncardiac Surgical Patient

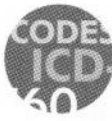

CODES

ICD10

- Z01.818 Encounter for other preprocedural examination
- Z01.811 Encounter for preprocedural respiratory examination
- Z01.812 Encounter for preprocedural laboratory examination

CLINICAL PEARLS

- The preoperative evaluation should include medical record evaluation, patient interview, and physical exam.
- The minimum for the physical exam includes airway, pulmonary, and cardiovascular exams.
- Functional capacity, the level of surgical risk, and clinical risk factors determine if further cardiac testing is needed.
- No preoperative tests are routine.
- Active cardiac conditions should lead to delay or cancellation of nonemergent surgery.

PRESBYCUSIS

Brian Ho, MD • Michael W. Groves, MD, FACS

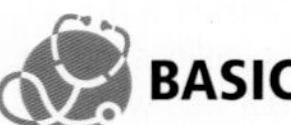

BASICS

DESCRIPTION

- Age-related, bilateral sensorineural hearing loss (SNHL) typically symmetric
- Represents a lifetime of insults to the auditory system from toxic noise exposure and natural decline
- Initially presents as high-frequency SNHL with tinnitus (ringing)
- Impacts the "clarity" of sounds (i.e., ability to detect, identify, and localize sounds)
- Due to mild and progressive nature, presbycusis is often treated with amplification alone.
- Can lead to adverse effects on physical, cognitive, emotional, behavioral, and social function in the elderly (e.g., depression, social isolation)

EPIDEMIOLOGY

Incidence

According to recent community-based epidemiologic study, the 5-year incidence of hearing loss (HL) are as follows (1):

- Age 48–59 years: M (19.1%), F (7%); all (11.6%)
- Age 60–69 years: M (35%), F (18.1%); all (23.1%)
- Age 70–79 years: M (59.1%), F (45.2%); all (4%)
- Age 80–92 years: M (100%), F (94.7%); all (95.5%)

Prevalence

- 10% of the population develops SNHL severe enough to impair communication.
- Increases to 40% in the population >65 years of age
- 80% of HL cases occur in elderly patients.
- Only 10–20% of older adults with HL have ever used hearing aids.
- Predominant sex: male > female
- Hearing levels are poorer in industrialized societies than in isolated or agrarian societies.

ETIOLOGY AND PATHOPHYSIOLOGY

- The external ear transmits sound energy to the tympanic membrane. The middle ear ossicles amplify and conduct the sound waves into the inner ear (cochlea) via the oval window. The organ of Corti, located in the cochlea, contains hair cells that detect these vibrations and depolarize, producing electrical signals that travel through the auditory nerve to the brain. Toxic noise exposure traumatizes the hair cells and leads to cell death and hearing loss. New research also suggests that overexcitation of the neurosynapses causes increased glutamate, which is also neurotoxic.
  - Sensory presbycusis: primary loss of the hair cells in the basal end of the cochlea (high frequency loss)
  - Neural presbycusis: loss of spiral ganglion cells (nerve cells induced by hair cells to produce action potentials to travel to the brainstem)
  - Strial (metabolic) presbycusis: atrophy of the stria vascularis (the cochlear tissue that generates the endocochlear electrical potential)
  - Cochlear conductive (mechanical) presbycusis: no morphologic findings (presumed stiffening of the basilar membrane)
  - Mixed presbycusis: combinations of hair cell, ganglion cell, and stria vascularis loss
  - Indeterminate presbycusis: no morphologic findings (presumed impaired cellular function)
- Presbycusis is caused by the accumulated effects of noise exposure, systemic disease, ototoxic drugs, and genetic susceptibility.

Genetics

Presbycusis has a clear familial aggregation (2):

- Heritability estimates show 35–55% of the variance of sensory presbycusis is from genetic factors; even greater percentage in strial presbycusis
- Heritability is stronger among women than men.

RISK FACTORS

- Noise exposure (military, industrial, etc.)
- Ototoxic substances
  - Organic solvents
  - Heavy metals
  - Carbon monoxide
- Drugs
  - Aminoglycosides
  - Cisplatin
  - Salicylates
  - Diuretics
- Tobacco smoking
- Alcohol
- Lower socioeconomic status
- Family history of presbycusis
- Head trauma (temporal bone fractures)
- Cardiovascular disease (hypertension, atherosclerosis, hyperlipidemia); labyrinthine artery is terminal artery to the cochlea.
- Diabetes mellitus
- Autoimmune disease (auto-cochleitis/labyrinthitis)
- Metabolic bone disease
- Endocrine medical conditions: levels of aldosterone
- Alzheimer disease
- Otologic conditions (e.g., Ménière disease or otosclerosis)

GENERAL PREVENTION

- Avoid hazardous noise exposure.
- Use hearing protection.
- Maintain healthy diet and exercise.
- Screening
  - In the only published RCT on screening for HL, hearing aid use was significantly higher in 3 screened groups (4.1% in those using a questionnaire, 6.3% using handheld audiometry, and 7.4% using both modalities) versus unscreened control participants (3.3%) at 1-year follow-up (3)[B].
  - Based on a 2011 review, according to the USPSTF, there is insufficient evidence to assess the relative benefits and harms of HL screening in adults ≥50 years (4)[A].

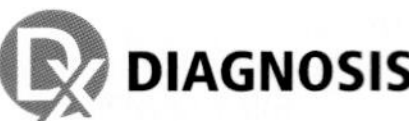

DIAGNOSIS

HISTORY

- Reduced hearing sensitivity and speech understanding in noisy/public environments
- Impaired localization of sound sources
- Increased difficulty understanding conversations, especially with women, due to higher frequency of spoken voice
- Presents bilaterally and symmetrically
- Additional history if HL is suspected or detected (5)
  - Time course of HL
  - Symptoms of tinnitus, otalgia, otorrhea, or vertigo
  - History of noise exposure, ear trauma, or head trauma
  - Presence of any neurologic deficit
- Reports from patient/family/caregiver (5)
  - Confusion in social situations
  - Excessive volume of television/radio/computer
  - Social withdrawal
  - Anxiety in group settings

PHYSICAL EXAM

- Rinne and Weber test are helpful for determining conductive versus sensorineural hearing loss
- Pneumatic otoscopy to evaluate for simple middle ear effusion as cause of conductive hearing loss

DIFFERENTIAL DIAGNOSIS

- Acute noise-induced traumatic loss (explosion)
- Autoimmune HL
- Perilymph fistula (trauma/iatrogenic)
- Ménière disease
- Acoustic neuroma
- Complete canal occlusion (cerumen)
- Otitis externa
- Chronic otitis media or effusion
- Otosclerosis/osteogenesis imperfecta
- Large middle ear tumors (e.g., facial nerve schwannomas, paragangliomas)
- Vascular anomaly
- Cholesteatoma

DIAGNOSTIC TESTS & INTERPRETATION

- Handheld audiometry; insert probe in ear (sealing canal) and have patient indicate if tones can be heard.
  - Positive likelihood ratio (LR) range, 3.1–5.8; negative LR range, 0.03–0.40 (6)
- Screening audiometry
  - Symmetric high-frequency hearing loss in descending slope pattern
  - SNHL frequencies > 2 KHz initially
  - Essential to determine if etiology is conductive hearing loss versus SNHL, pseudohypacusis, and global clinical hearing status

P

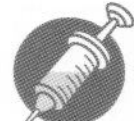

TREATMENT

- Hearing aids (HAs)
  - Types
    - Analog HA: picks up sound waves through a microphone; converts them into electrical signals; amplifies and sends them through the ear canal to the tympanic membrane
    - Digital HA: programmable; may reduce acoustic feedback, reduce background noise, detect and automatically accommodate different listening environments, control multiple microphones
  - HAs have an average decibel gain of 16.3 dB
  - Associated with hypersensitivity to loud sounds ("loudness recruitment")
- Hearing-assistive technologies (HATs) (7)[A]
  - Can be used along or in combination with HAs (for difficult listening conditions)
  - Addresses face-to-face communication, broadcast or other electronic media (radio, TV), telephone conversation, sensitivity to alerting signals and environment stimuli (doorbell, baby's cry, alarm clock, etc.)
  - Includes personal FM systems, infrared systems, induction loop systems, hardwired systems, telephone amplifier, telecoil, TDD (telecommunication device for the deaf), situation-specific devices (e.g., television), alerting devices
- Aural rehabilitation (also known as audiologic orientation or auditory training) (5)[A]
  - Adjunct to HA or HATs
  - Involves education regarding proper use of amplification devices, coaching on how to manage the auditory environment, training in speech perception and communication, and counseling for coping strategies to deal with the difficulties of HAs or HATs

ISSUES FOR REFERRAL

Refer to audiologist for formal evaluation and optimal fitting of HAs and/or HATs.

- Individuals receiving postfitting orientation/education have significantly fewer HA returns.
- Individuals receiving >2 hours of education and counseling report higher levels of satisfaction.

SURGERY/OTHER PROCEDURES

- Cochlear implants (CIs) (8)[B]
  - Indications include hearing no better than identifying ≤50% of key words in test sentences in the best aided condition in the worst ear and 60% in the better ear.
  - Works by bypassing the ear canal, middle ear, and hair cells in the cochlea to provide electric stimulation directly to the auditory nerve
  - Incoming sounds are received through the microphone in the audio processor component (resembles a small HA), which converts them into electrical impulses and sends them to the magnetic coil (located on the skin). The impulses transmit these across intact skin via radio waves to the implanted component (directly subjacent to the coil). The pulses travel to the electrodes in the cochlea and stimulate the cochlea at high rates.
  - Receiving a unilateral CI is most common; some may receive bilateral CIs (either sequentially or in the same surgery). Others may wear a CI in 1 ear and an HA in the contralateral ear (bimodal fit).
- Active middle ear implants (AMEIs) (8)[B]
  - Suitable for elderly adults who cannot wear conventional HAs for medical or personal (cosmetic) reasons and whose HL is not severe enough for a CI
  - Comes in different models and may include components that are implantable under the skin
- Electric acoustic stimulation: use of CI and HA together in 1 ear
  - Addresses the specific needs of patients presenting with good low-frequency hearing (a mild to moderate sensorineural HL in frequencies up to 1,000 Hz) but poorer hearing in the high frequencies (sloping to 60 dB or worse HL above 1,000 Hz) (8)[B]
    - Contraindications: progressive HL, autoimmune disease; HL related to meningitis, otosclerosis, or ossification; malformation of the cochlea; a gap in air conduction and bone conduction thresholds of >15 dB; external ear contraindications, active infection, or unwillingness to use amplification devices (8)

ONGOING CARE

FOLLOW-UP RECOMMENDATIONS

Patient Monitoring

- During follow-up visits, check for compliance of HA use.
  - 25–40% of adults will either stop wearing them or use them only occasionally.
- Assess perceived benefit of HA and, if ineffective, for indications for possible surgical treatments.
- Annual audiograms
- Can follow up with audiologists for HA fittings if HA becomes uncomfortable
- Asymmetric hearing loss should have evaluation via MRI for acoustic neuroma.
- Sudden SNHL is atypical and warrants urgent otolaryngologic evaluation/audiometry. The most recent recommendations by the American Academy of Otolaryngology recommend steroids empirically.

PATIENT EDUCATION

- Educate the patient that conversations should be face-to-face, spoken clearly and unhurriedly, without competing background noise (e.g., radio, TV), and include a confirmation that the message is received.
- Formal speech reading classes may be beneficial; however, availability may be limited.

REFERENCES

1. Nash SD, Cruickshanks KJ, Klein R, et al. The prevalence of hearing impairment and associated risk factors: the Beaver Dam Offspring Study. *Arch Otolaryngol Head Neck Surg*. 2011;137(5):432–439.
2. Huang Q, Tang J. Age-related hearing loss or presbycusis. *Eur Arch Otorhinolaryngol*. 2010;267(8):1179–1191.
3. Yueh B, Collins MP, Souza PE, et al. Long-term effectiveness of screening for hearing loss: the screening for auditory impairment—which hearing assessment (SAI-WHAT) randomized trial. *J Am Geriatr Soc*. 2010;58(3):427–434.
4. Chou R, Dana T, Bougatsos C, et al. Screening adults aged 50 years or older for hearing loss: a review of the evidence for the U.S. Preventive Services Task Force. *Ann Intern Med*. 2011;154(5):347–355.
5. Pacala J, Yueh B. Hearing deficits in the older patient: "I didn't notice anything." *JAMA*. 2012;307(11):1185–1194.
6. Bagai A, Thavendiranathan P, Detsky AS. Does this patient have hearing impairment? *JAMA*. 2006;295(4):416–428.
7. Valente M. Summary guidelines: audiological management of adult hearing impairment. *Audio Today*. 2006;18:32–37.
8. Sprinzl GM, Riechelmann H. Current trends in treating hearing loss in elderly people: a review of the technology and treatment options—a mini-review. *Gerontology*. 2010;56(3):351–358.

CODES

ICD10

- H91.10 Presbycusis, unspecified ear
- H91.13 Presbycusis, bilateral
- H91.11 Presbycusis, right ear

CLINICAL PEARLS

- Presbycusis is age-related HL, showing increased incidence with age. It is often bilateral and initially begins as high-frequency HL. It presents as difficulty communicating in noisy conditions.
- There are more affected males than females.
- Compliance is only from 25 to 40% for those who own HAs. A referral to an audiologist is key for optimal evaluation, fitting for HAs, and consideration for HATs or surgical treatment.
- Indication for CIs include hearing no better than identifying ≤50% key words in test sentences in the best aided condition in the worst ear and 60% in the better ear.

PRESSURE ULCER

Amy M. Zack, MD, FAAFP

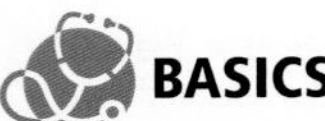

BASICS

DESCRIPTION

- A localized area of soft tissue injury resulting from pressure between an external surface and a bony prominence that causes local tissue breakdown classified in stages according to the National Pressure Ulcer Advisory Panel (NPUAP) classification.
  - Stage I: erythema of localized area, usually non-blanching over bony surface
  - Stage II: partial loss of dermal layer, resulting in pink ulceration
  - Stage III: full dermal loss often exposing subcutaneous tissue and fat
  - Stage IV: full-thickness ulceration exposing bone, tendon, or muscle. Osteomyelitis may be present.
- Synonym(s): decubitus ulcer; bed sores

EPIDEMIOLOGY

Incidence

2.5 million pressure ulcers treated yearly in United States in acute care facilities (1)[A]

Prevalence

- Acute care 0.4–38%; long-term care 2.2–23.9%; home care 0–17%
- Majority occur in patients older than 65 years: 36% with hip fracture, 50% in ICU care (2)[A].

ETIOLOGY AND PATHOPHYSIOLOGY

- Pathophysiology of pressure ulcers is changing, differs depending on stage of ulceration
- Stages I–II result largely from prolonged moisture and friction and may not even be related to pressure and hypoxia, as previously believed (3)[A].
- Stages III–IV likely begin with compressive forces, causing muscle damage and tissue hypoxia and leading to reperfusion injury of the deep tissue. The skin ulcer forms after significant deep tissue damage is already under way (3)[A].
- Shearing and friction forces are also components of some ulcer formation, resulting in localized skin damage and early-stage ulcers (3)[A].

RISK FACTORS

- Immobility: greatest risk factor regardless of patient, temporary or permanent immobility (4)[A]
- Urinary and fecal incontinence present in >80% of immobile patients with pressure ulcers
- Poor nutritional status: Hypoalbuminemia and low BMI are markers for poor ulcer outcome (4)[A].
- Poor skin perfusion, including vascular disease, diabetes, anemia, and tobacco use, increases risk.
- Extended stay in hospital/nursing home, inadequate staffing (5)[C]
- Other risks include history of previous ulcer, age-related skin changes, immunocompromise, impaired skin sensation, and impaired awareness.
- Assessment scales commonly used for risk evaluation include Braden and Norton scales. The use of these does not decrease incidence, but they are more accurate than clinical judgment alone (6)[B].

GENERAL PREVENTION

- Up to 95% are preventable; identification of at-risk patients is essential, with early multidisciplinary care.
- Pressure relief with proper patient positioning and the use of mattresses, cushions, heel protectors, and other devices to minimize pressure and friction. Regular turning of patients, including the use of angles and rotation of extremities, helps to minimize pressure.
- Minimize duration of immobility; adequate physical and occupational therapies when appropriate
- Aggressive moisture prevention with management of incontinence and maintenance of clean resting area
- Nutrition: Assess nutritional status and form plan for improving/maintaining adequate nutrition, particularly protein intake and albumin levels.
- Manage skin health, clean and dry with mild cleansers, skin protection where appropriate

COMMONLY ASSOCIATED CONDITIONS

See "Risk Factors."

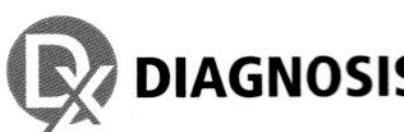

DIAGNOSIS

HISTORY

- Risk factors
- Date of ulcer diagnosis
- Treatment course

PHYSICAL EXAM

- Do full skin examination on admission to hospital or extended-care facility and repeatedly throughout admission, best with bathing/bed changes.
- 83% of hospitalized patients with decubitus ulcers develop them in first 5 days of hospitalization.
- Classify ulcer based on NPUAP stages (see "Description").

DIFFERENTIAL DIAGNOSIS

- Venous stasis ulcers
- Arterial ulcers resulting from poor vascular supply
- Diabetic ulcers
- Pyoderma gangrenosum, cancers, vasculitides, and other dermatologic conditions

DIAGNOSTIC TESTS & INTERPRETATION

Initial Tests (lab, imaging)

- Wound culture: Do not culture surface drainage. Do deep tissue culture/bone biopsy.
- If systemic infection or that of bone, muscle is suspected: Add infectious workup, including inflammatory markers, CBC, blood cultures, x-ray. MRI may be necessary to confirm osteomyelitis.
- Nutritional assessment: BMI, protein and calorie intake, albumin, prealbumin, CBC for anemia. No clear evidence in support of specific nutritional supplements including zinc and vitamin C (7)[A],(8)[B].

Follow-Up Tests & Special Considerations

Additional tests may be indicated when additional medical illness complicates assessment. This may include testing for diabetes, vascular disease, and other dermatologic diagnoses.

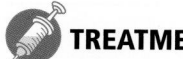

P

TREATMENT

GENERAL MEASURES

- Pressure reduction, minimize immobility, manage incontinence, and improve nutritional status and skin health (as described in "Prevention").
- Wound management by stage of ulcer
  - Stage I: aggressive preventive measures, thin film dressings for protection
  - Stage II: occlusive dressing to maintain healing, transparent films, hydrocolloids
  - Stages III–IV: débridement of necrotic tissue. Exudative ulcers will benefit from absorptive dressings such as calcium alginates, foams, hydrofibers. Dry ulcers require occlusive dressing to maintain moisture, including hydrocolloids and hydrogels.
  - Debridement: Type depends on extent of necrosis or eschar. Incisional with scalpel when extensive, dry. Mechanical with wet-dry dressings; enzymatic debridement is also frequently used.
  - Surgical closure may be necessary in advanced wounds.
- Vacuum-assisted closure
  - Negative pressure reduces wound edema and improves local tissue perfusion.
  - Removes necrotic debris and reduces bacterial load
  - Literature review demonstrates the efficacy of negative-pressure wound therapy (9)[A].

MEDICATION

First Line

- See "General Measures" for first-line treatment.
- Pain control
- Aggressive management of contributing medical conditions
- Infection: If suspected, treat appropriately for cellulitis or osteomyelitis.

Second Line

Nutritional interventions as determined by nutritional assessment

ISSUES FOR REFERRAL

- Vascular surgery is a consideration for improvement of blood flow to wound via vascular bypass.
- Plastic surgery is a consideration for skin graft/flap.

ADDITIONAL THERAPIES

Whirlpool/PulseVac aids in wound débridement.

COMPLEMENTARY AND ALTERNATIVE MEDICINE

- Nutritional support as needed
- Ultrasound and electrical stimulation create new vasculature in affected region (9)[C].

INPATIENT CONSIDERATIONS

Admission Criteria/Initial Stabilization

Refractory cellulitis, osteomyelitis, systemic infection, advanced nutritional decline, suspected patient mistreatment, inability to care for self

Nursing

- Dressing changes 1–3 × daily based on wound assessment and plan of care
- Assess risk factors according to scales.
- Assess for new or changing wounds.

Discharge Criteria

Clinical improvement in wound and systemic illness; when applicable, safe and appropriate location for discharge

ONGOING CARE

FOLLOW-UP RECOMMENDATIONS

Weekly assessment by nurse with wound experience; biweekly assessment by physician

Patient Monitoring

- Home health nursing
- Change in plan of care if no improvement in 2–3 weeks

DIET

- 1–1.5 kg/day of protein
- Good glycemic control
- Include supply of micronutrients in diet or as supplements

PATIENT EDUCATION

- Check skin regularly
- Signs and symptoms of infection
- Report new or increased pain
- Prevention of new wound where old wound healed
- Skin care, moisture prevention

PROGNOSIS

Variable, depending on the following:

- Removal of pressure
- Nutrition
- Wound care

COMPLICATIONS

- Infection
- Amputation

REFERENCES

1. Reddy M, Gill S, Rochon P. Preventing pressure ulcers: a systematic review. *JAMA*. 2006;296(8): 974–984.
2. Baumgarten M, Margolis DJ, Orwig DL, et al. Pressure ulcers in elderly patients with hip fracture across the continuum of care. *J Am Geriatr Soc*. 2009;57(5):863.
3. Sibbald RG, Krasner DL, Woo KY. Pressure ulcer staging revisited: superficial changes and deep pressure framework. *Adv Skin Wound Care*. 2011;24(12):571–580.
4. Cakmak S, Gül U, Ozer S, et al. Risk factors for pressure ulcers. *Adv Skin Wound Care*. 2009:22(9): 412–415.
5. European Pressure Ulcer Advisory Panel and National Pressure Ulcer Advisory Panel. *Treatment of Pressure Ulcers: Quick Reference Guide*. Washington, DC: National Pressure Ulcer Advisory Panel; 2009.
6. Pancorbo-Hidalgo PL, Garcia-Fernandez FP, Lopez-Medina IM, et al. Risk assessment scales for pressure ulcer prevention: a systematic review. *J Adv Nurs*. 2006:54(1):94–110.
7. Langer G, Schloemer G, Knerr A, et al. Nutritional interventions for preventing and treating pressure ulcers. *Cochrane Database Syst Rev*. 2003;(4):CD003216.
8. Jamshed N, Schneider E. Is the use of supplemental vitamin C and zinc for the prevention and treatment of pressure ulcers evidence based? *Ann Long-Term Care Med*. 2010;18(3):28–32.
9. Gregor S, Maegele M, Sauerland S, et al. Negative pressure wound therapy: a vacuum of evidence? *Arch Surg*. 2008;143(2):189–196.

ADDITIONAL READING

Stansby G, Avita L, Jones K, et al. Prevention and management of pressure ulcers in primary and secondary care: summary of NICE guidelines. *BMJ*. 2014;348:g2592.

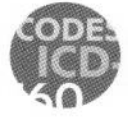

CODES

ICD10

- L89.95 Pressure ulcer of unspecified site, unstageable
- L89.91 Pressure ulcer of unspecified site, stage 1
- L89.92 Pressure ulcer of unspecified site, stage 2

CLINICAL PEARLS

Identify risk, reduce pressure, maximize nutrition, regular skin checks and assess and treat wound appropriately.

PRETERM LABOR

Kara M. Coassolo, MD • John C. Smulian, MD, MPH

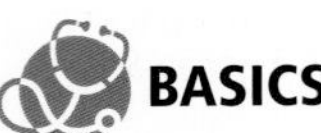

BASICS

DESCRIPTION

Contractions occurring between 20 and 36 weeks' gestation at a rate of 4 in 20 minutes or 8 in 1 hour with at least 1 of the following: cervical change over time or dilation ≥2 cm

EPIDEMIOLOGY

Preterm birth is the leading cause of perinatal morbidity and mortality in the United States.

Incidence

10–15% of pregnancies experience at least 1 episode of preterm labor.

Prevalence

~12% of all births in the United States are preterm (9% spontaneous preterm births and 3% indicated preterm births).

ETIOLOGY AND PATHOPHYSIOLOGY

- Premature formation and activation of myometrial gap junctions
- Inflammatory mediator–stimulated contractions
- Weakened cervix (structural defect or extracellular matrix defect)
- Abnormal placental implantation
- Systemic inflammation/infections (e.g., UTI, pyelonephritis, pneumonia, sepsis)
- Local inflammation/infections (intra-amniotic infections from aerobes, anaerobes, *Mycoplasma*, *Ureaplasma*)
- Uterine abnormalities (e.g., cervical insufficiency, leiomyomata, müllerian anomalies, diethylstilbestrol exposure)
- Overdistension (by multiple gestation or polyhydramnios)
- Preterm premature rupture of membranes
- Trauma
- Placental abruption
- Immunopathology (e.g., antiphospholipid antibodies)
- Placental ischemic disease (preeclampsia and fetal growth restriction)

Genetics

Familial predisposition

RISK FACTORS

- Demographic factors, including single parent, poverty, and black race
- Short interpregnancy interval
- No prenatal care
- Prepregnancy weight <45 kg (100 lb), body mass index <20
- Substance abuse (e.g., cocaine, tobacco)
- Prior preterm delivery (common)
- Previous 2nd-trimester dilation and evacuation (D&E)
- Cervical insufficiency or prior cervical surgery (cone biopsy or loop electrosurgical excision procedure [LEEP])
- Abdominal surgery/trauma during pregnancy
- Uterine structural abnormalities such as large fibroids or müllerian abnormalities
- Serious maternal infections/diseases
- Bacterial vaginosis
- Bacteriuria
- Vaginal bleeding during pregnancy
- Multiple gestation
- Select fetal abnormalities
- Intrauterine growth restriction
- Placenta previa
- Premature placental separation (abruption)
- Polyhydramnios
- Ehlers-Danlos syndrome

GENERAL PREVENTION

- Patient education at each visit in 2nd and 3rd trimesters for those at risk and periodically in the last 2 trimesters for the general population
- If previous preterm birth, evaluate if etiology is likely to recur and target intervention to specific condition.
  - Weekly injections of 17α-hydroxyprogesterone (250 mg IM every week) from 16 to 36 weeks if previous spontaneous preterm birth
  - Consider cerclage placement before 24 weeks' gestation for those at high risk because of cervical insufficiency or significant or progressive cervical shortening (1)[A],(2)[C].
- For women with a short cervix in the 2nd trimester (<20 mm on transvaginal US), progesterone 200 mg/day per vagina × 24–34 weeks may decrease the risk of preterm delivery (3)[A].

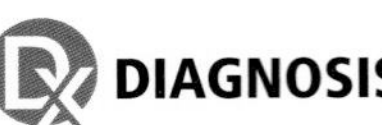

DIAGNOSIS

Diagnosis is generally based on a combination of significant cervical changes (such as dilation, effacement) with regular contractions. However, there is no single test that will reliably diagnose or predict true preterm labor. The diagnosis is based on a combination of physical findings and diagnostic tests that are interpreted in the context of the degree of risk to the patient.

HISTORY

- Address risk factors, especially etiologies of previous preterm birth.
- Regular uterine contractions or cramping
- Dull, low backache or pain
- Intermittent lower abdominal pain
- Increased low pelvic pressure
- Change in vaginal discharge
- Vaginal bleeding
- Fluid leakage

PHYSICAL EXAM

- Sterile speculum exam for membrane rupture evaluation, cultures, and cervical inspection.
- Bimanual cervical exam if intact membranes: dilation of the cervix >1 cm and/or effacement of the cervix >50%

ALERT

Avoid bimanual examination when possible if rupture of the membranes is suspected.

DIFFERENTIAL DIAGNOSIS

- Braxton-Hicks contractions/false labor
- Round ligament pain
- Lumbosacral muscular back pain
- Urinary tract or vaginal infections
- Adnexal torsion
- Degenerating fibroid
- Appendicitis
- Dehydration
- Viral gastroenteritis
- Nephrolithiasis

DIAGNOSTIC TESTS & INTERPRETATION

Initial Tests (lab, imaging)

- In symptomatic women from 22 to 34 weeks' gestation with intact membranes and no intercourse or bleeding in past 24 hours, obtain a fetal fibronectin (FFN) swab from the posterior vaginal fornix. FFN must be obtained prior to digital cervical exam (4)[C].
  - If results are positive (≥50 ng/mL), patient is at a modest increased risk of preterm birth (positive predictive value [PPV] 13–30% for delivery within 2 weeks).
  - If results are negative, more than 97% of patients will not deliver in 14 days, so can consider avoiding complicated or high-risk interventions.
- Urinalysis and urine culture
- Cultures for gonorrhea and chlamydia
- Wet prep for bacterial vaginosis evaluation (although evidence for improved outcomes with treatment is weak)
- Vaginal introitus and rectal culture for group B *Streptococcus*
- pH and Ferning test of vaginal fluid to evaluate for rupture of membranes
- CBC with differential
- Drug screen when appropriate
- US to identify number of fetuses and fetal position, confirm gestational age, estimate fetal weight, quantify amniotic fluid, and look for conditions making tocolysis contraindicated.
- Transvaginal US to evaluate cervical length, funneling, and dynamic changes after obtaining FFN (if clinical assessment of the cervix is uncertain or if the cervix is closed on digital exam).

Follow-Up Tests & Special Considerations

- Repeat FFN as indicated by symptoms.
- After successful treatment, progressive changes of the cervix on repeat examination or US (in 1–2 weeks) may indicate need for hospitalization.

Diagnostic Procedures/Other

- Monitor contractions with external tocodynamometer.
- Consider amniocentesis at any preterm gestational age to evaluate for intra-amniotic infection (cell count with differential, glucose, Gram stain, aerobic, anaerobic, *Mycoplasma*, *Ureaplasma* cultures).
- Consider amniocentesis if ≥32 weeks' gestation for evaluation of fetal lung maturity (e.g., lecithin/sphingomyelin [L:S] ratio and phosphatidylglycerol [PG]). If L:S ratio >2:1 (nondiabetic) and PG is present, hyaline membrane disease is unlikely, so tocolysis may be withheld.

Test Interpretation

- Placental inflammation
  - Acute inflammation usually caused by infection
  - Chronic inflammation caused by immunopathology
- Abruption

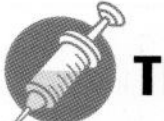

TREATMENT

GENERAL MEASURES

- Treat underlying risk factors (e.g., antibiotics for infections, hydration for dehydration).
- Liquids only or NPO if delivery imminent
- Hospitalization is necessary if the patient is on IV tocolysis.

MEDICATION

Tocolysis may allow time for interventions such as transfer to tertiary care facility and administration of corticosteroids but may not prolong pregnancy significantly (5)[A].

First Line

- Tocolysis
  - Nifedipine: 30 mg PO loading dose; then 10–20 mg q6h × 24 hours; then 10–20 mg PO q8h (do not use sublingual route); check BP often and avoid hypotension. Concurrent use with magnesium sulfate should be avoided to avoid theoretic risk of neuromuscular blockade.
  - Indomethacin: 50–100 mg PO initial dose; then 25–50 mg q6–8h × 24 hours (or, if available, 100-mg suppository per rectum q12h for 2 doses); then 25 mg q6–8h; use for no longer than 72 hours due to risk of premature closure of ductus arteriosus, oligohydramnios, and possibly neonatal necrotizing enterocolitis. Use with caution in patients with platelet dysfunction, liver dysfunction, or allergy to aspirin.
  - Contraindications to tocolysis: severe preeclampsia, hemorrhage, chorioamnionitis, advanced labor, intrauterine growth retardation, fetal distress, or lethal fetal abnormalities
- Antibiotics: antibiotics for group B *Streptococcus* prophylaxis if culture positive or unknown
- Steroids: If mother is at 23–34 weeks' gestation with no evidence of systemic infection, give glucocorticoids to decrease neonatal respiratory distress, intraventricular hemorrhage, necrotizing enterocolitis, and overall perinatal mortality. Betamethasone 12 mg IM × 2 doses 24 hours apart (preferred choice) *or* dexamethasone 6 mg IM q12h for 4 doses (6)[A]

Second Line

- Magnesium sulfate by IV infusion has not been shown to be superior to placebo in prolonging pregnancy beyond 48 hours. The side effects are generally greater compared with calcium channel blockers or NSAIDs. Therefore, this agent should be used cautiously if at all (standard dosages for tocolysis start with a 4–6-g IV bolus over 20 minutes followed by 2–3 g/hr infusion until contractions stop) (7)[C].
  - Magnesium may decrease the risk of cerebral palsy when 12-hour course is given prior to an anticipated preterm birth.
  - Relative contraindications to magnesium sulfate include myasthenia gravis, hypocalcemia, renal failure, or concurrent use of calcium channel blockers.
- Terbutaline 0.25 mg SC q30min for up to 3 doses until contractions stop, then 0.25 mg SC q6h for 4 doses (optional); if contractions persist or pulse >120 bpm, change to another tocolytic agent (may be poorly tolerated by mothers)
- Terbutaline PO or by infusion pump has been used in the past for treatment or prevention of preterm labor. Due to reports of serious cardiovascular events and maternal deaths, PO or long-term SC administration of terbutaline should not be given.
- Significant possible interactions include pulmonary edema from crystalloid fluids and tocolytic agents, especially magnesium sulfate.
- PO maintenance therapy with any agent is controversial, and its use is limited.

ISSUES FOR REFERRAL

- If delivery is inevitable but not immediate, consider transport to a tertiary care center or hospital equipped with a neonatal ICU.
- Consider consultation with maternal–fetal medicine specialist.

ADDITIONAL THERAPIES

- Pelvic rest (e.g., no douching or intercourse) and activity restriction are often recommended; however, data to prove the efficacy are lacking. Some reduction in physical activity may be reasonable; this should be individualized.
- Strict bed rest has not been demonstrated to be effective in most situations.

SURGERY/OTHER PROCEDURES

- For malpresentation or fetal compromise, consider cesarean delivery if labor is progressing.
- Cerclage for cervical insufficiency (until 24 weeks' gestation)

INPATIENT CONSIDERATIONS

Admission Criteria/Initial Stabilization

Suspected/threatened preterm labor

- IV access
- Continuous fetal and contraction monitoring
- Assess cervix for dilatation and effacement.

IV Fluids

Hydrate with 500 mL 5% dextrose normal saline solution or 5% dextrose lactated Ringer solution for 1st half hour; then at 125 mL/hour.

Nursing

Monitor for fluid overload (input/output monitoring, symptoms, lung auscultation, pulse oximetry), especially with tocolysis and multiple gestations.

Discharge Criteria

- Regular contractions and cervical change resolve.
- If cervix is dilated ≥3 cm or FFN is positive, individualize decision to discharge by gestational age and patient circumstances.

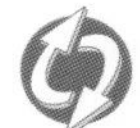

ONGOING CARE

FOLLOW-UP RECOMMENDATIONS

Patient Monitoring

- Weekly office visits with contraction monitoring, cervical checks, or cervical US if at high risk for recurrence
- Routine use of maintenance tocolysis is ineffective in preventing preterm birth.

DIET

Regular

PATIENT EDUCATION

Call physician or proceed to hospital whenever regular contractions last >1 hour, bleeding, increased vaginal discharge or fluid, decreased fetal movement.

PROGNOSIS

- If membranes are ruptured and no infection is confirmed, delivery often occurs within 3–7 days.
- If membranes are intact, 20–50% deliver preterm.

COMPLICATIONS

Labor resistant to tocolysis, pulmonary edema, infection with preterm rupture of membranes

REFERENCES

1. Tita AT, Rouse DJ. Progesterone for preterm birth prevention: an evolving intervention. *Am J Obstet Gynecol*. 2009;200(3):219–224.
2. Simhan HN, Caritis SN. Prevention of preterm delivery. *N Engl J Med*. 2007;357(5):477–487.
3. Berghella V, Rafael TJ, Szychowski JM, et al. Cerclage for short cervix on ultrasonography in women with singleton gestations and previous preterm birth: a meta-analysis. *Obstet Gynecol*. 2011;117(3):663–671.
4. Goldenberg RL, Goepfert AR, Ramsey PS. Biochemical markers for the prediction of preterm birth. *Am J Obstet Gynecol*. 2005;192(5)(Suppl):S36–S46.
5. Haas DM, Caldwell DM, Kirkpatrick P, et al. Tocolytic therapy for preterm delivery: systematic review and network meta-analysis. *Br Med J*. 2012;345:e6226.
6. Roberts D, Dalziel S. Antenatal corticosteroids for accelerating fetal lung maturation for women at risk of preterm birth. *Cochrane Database Syst Rev*. 2006;(3):CD004454.
7. American College of Obstetricians and Gynecologists Committee on Obstetric Practice; Society for Maternal-Fetal Medicine. Committee opinion no. 455: magnesium sulfate before anticipated preterm birth for neuroprotection. *Obstet Gynecol*. 2010;115(3):669–671.

CODES

ICD10

- O60.00 Preterm labor without delivery, unspecified trimester
- O60.02 Preterm labor without delivery, second trimester
- O60.03 Preterm labor without delivery, third trimester

CLINICAL PEARLS

- Treatment of preterm labor may delay delivery to facilitate short-term interventions.
- Steroids improve neonatal outcomes.
- Progesterone therapy can prevent recurrence of preterm birth in next pregnancy.

PRIAPISM

Shenelle Wilson, MD • Kelvin A. Moses, MD, PhD

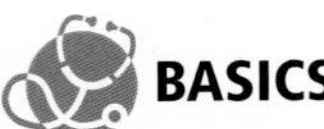

BASICS

DESCRIPTION

- Penile erection that lasts for >4 hours and is unrelated to sexual stimulation or excitement
- Classified into ischemic and nonischemic types
- Ischemic (low-flow) priapism is painful and requires urgent clinical intervention.
- Stuttering priapism is recurrent episodes of short-lived, self-limiting ischemic priapism over an extended period.
- Nonischemic (high-flow) priapism is painless, could be related to prior trauma, and does not require urgent treatment.
- Malignant priapism is a rare condition resulting most commonly from penile metastases from primary bladder, prostatic, rectosigmoid, and renal tumors.
- System(s) affected: reproductive

Pediatric Considerations

In children, nearly all priapism is caused either by sickle cell anemia or trauma (1).

EPIDEMIOLOGY

Incidence

In the United States, 1 study estimates 1,868–2,960 cases of priapism each year. They also noted an increasing incidence from 1998 to 2006, specifically in those from nonhematologic causes (2):

- Mean age: 33.7 years. There has been an age shift in recent years toward men in their 40s.
- Other studies have found the incidence of priapism to double in men aged >40 years (2.9 vs. 1.5/100,000 person-years) (3).
- Race: 61.1% black, 30% white, 6.3% Hispanic
- Associations: sickle cell anemia (41.9%), drug abuse (7.9%), sickle cell trait (2.5%)
- Anatomy and physiology
  - The penis consists of three longitudinally oriented corpora: two dorsolaterally paired corpora cavernosa that are responsible for penile erection and a single ventral corpus spongiosum that surrounds the glans penis and extends distally to form the glans penis
  - In general, the penile artery (which is a branch of the internal pudendal artery that, in turn, is a branch from the internal iliac artery) supplies the penis. It divides into three branches: dorsal artery, bulbar artery (supplies the corpus spongiosum), and cavernosal artery (the main blood supply to the erectile tissue).
  - During an erection, smooth muscle relaxation of the cavernosal arterioles results in high-volume inflow to the sinusoids, resulting in compression of the exiting venules. This leads to significant volume expansion of the corpora cavernosa.
  - During the flaccid resting state, the sympathetic nervous system is predominantly in control. Penile tumescence and erection are driven by the parasympathetic nervous system through the generation of nitric oxide (NO).
  - Smooth muscle relaxation occurs via usage of the phosphodiesterase type 5 (PDE-5A) pathway, which generates cyclic guanosine monophosphate (cGMP).

ETIOLOGY AND PATHOPHYSIOLOGY

- In ischemic priapism, decreased venous outflow results in increased intracavernosal pressure. This leads to erection, decreased arterial inflow, blood stasis, local hypoxia, and acidosis (a compartment syndrome). Eventually, penile tissue necrosis and fibrosis may occur. The exact mechanism is unknown and may involve trapping of erythrocytes in the veins, draining the erectile bodies.
- In nonischemic priapism, there is increased arterial flow without decreased venous outflow. There is increased inflow and outflow, which results in a sustained, nonpainful, partially rigid erection.
- Aberrations in the PDE-5A pathway have been proven in mice to be one mechanism of priapism (4).
- Ischemic priapism
  - Idiopathic, estimated to about 50% (1)
  - Intracavernosal injections of vasoactive drugs for erectile dysfunction
  - Oral agents for erectile dysfunction
  - Pelvic vascular thrombosis
  - Prolonged sexual activity
  - Sickle cell disease and trait
  - Leukemia from infiltration of the corpora
  - Other blood dyscrasias (G6PD deficiency, thrombophilia)
  - Pelvic hematoma or neoplasia (penis, urethra, bladder, prostate, kidney, rectal)
  - Cerebrospinal tumors
  - Asplenism
  - Fabry disease
  - Tertiary syphilis
  - Total parenteral nutrition, especially 20% lipid infusion (results in hyperviscosity)
  - Bladder calculus
  - Trauma to penis
  - UTIs, especially prostatitis, urethritis, cystitis
  - Several drugs suspected as causing priapism (e.g.,chlorpromazine, prazosin, cocaine, trazodone, and some corticosteroids); anticoagulants (heparin and warfarin); phosphodiesterase inhibitors (sildenafil, others); immunosuppressants (tacrolimus); and antihypertensives (hydralazine, propranolol, guanethidine)
  - Intracavernous fat emulsion
  - Hyperosmolar IV contrast
  - Spinal cord injury
  - General or spinal anesthesia
  - Heavy alcohol intake or cocaine use
- Nonischemic priapism
  - The most common cause is penile or perineal trauma resulting in a fistula between the cavernous artery and the corpora.
  - Acute spinal cord injury
  - Rarely, iatrogenic causes for the management of ischemic priapism can result in nonischemic priapism.
  - Certain urologic surgeries have also resulted in nonischemic priapism.

RISK FACTORS

- Sickle cell anemia, lifetime risk of ischemic priapism 29–42% (1)
- Dehydration

GENERAL PREVENTION

- Avoid dehydration.
- Avoid excessive sexual stimulation.
- Avoid causative drugs (see "Etiology and Pathophysiology") when possible.
- Avoid genital and pelvic trauma.

COMMONLY ASSOCIATED CONDITIONS

- Sickle cell anemia or sickle cell trait
- Drug abuse
- G6PD deficiency
- Leukemia
- Neoplasm

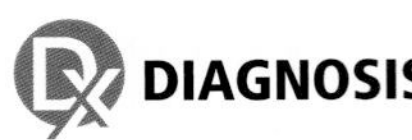

DIAGNOSIS

HISTORY

- Penile erection that is persistent, prolonged, painful, and tender (ischemic)
- Duration of erection, degree of pain
- Perineal or penile trauma
- Prior episodes of priapism
- Urination difficult during erection
- History of any hematologic abnormalities
- Cardiovascular disease
- Medications
- Recreational drugs
- Loss of erectile function if treatment is not prompt and effective

PHYSICAL EXAM

- Ischemic priapism
  - Penis is fully erect, corpora cavernosa are rigid and tender, and corpora spongiosum and glans are flaccid. Usually associated with tenderness and pain
- Nonischemic priapism
  - Penis is partially erect and the corpora cavernosa are semirigid and nontender, with the glans and corpora spongiosum flaccid. Usually not tender or painful
- Perineum, abdomen, and lymph node exam also valuable to rule out underlying condition
- A complete penile and scrotal exam is necessary. Determine if a penile prosthesis is present.

DIAGNOSTIC TESTS & INTERPRETATION

- CBC with reticulocyte count to detect leukemia or platelet abnormalities
- Sickling hemoglobin (Hgb) solubility test and Hgb electrophoresis
- Coagulation profile
- Platelet count
- Urinalysis
- Urine toxicology if illicit drugs suspected
- Corporal blood gas (CBG) should be used to distinguish ischemic from nonischemic priapism.
- A color duplex ultrasound of the penis and perineum may be necessary to differentiate ischemic from nonischemic priapism. In ischemic priapism, there is no blood flow in the cavernosal arteries, whereas in nonischemic patients there is high blood flow (1); may also see fistulas or pseudoaneurysms suggestive of nonischemic priapism
- Penile arteriography can be used to identify the presence and site of fistulas in patients with nonischemic priapism.

Diagnostic Procedures/Other

A physical exam is usually able to distinguish ischemic from nonischemic priapism; however, CBG is the most definitive method.

Test Interpretation

- Pelvic vascular thrombosis
- Partial thrombosis of corpora cavernosa of the penis
- Corpus spongiosum, glans penis: no involvement
- Arterial priapism will show arteriocavernous fistula.

TREATMENT

- Ischemic priapism requires immediate treatment to preserve future erectile function (a longer delay in treatment means a higher chance of future impotence).
  - Cavernosal aspiration with a large bore needle with irrigation (success rate $\sim$30%) (1,5)
  - Cavernosal injection of phenylephrine (α-adrenergic sympathomimetic) with monitoring of patient's BP and pulse (success rate $\sim$65%) (5). Inject q5–10min until detumescence.
  - Continue aspiration, irrigation, and phenylephrine for several hours. If this fails, shunt procedures are considered (1st a distal shunt).
- Nonischemic priapism
  - Initial observation
  - If this fails, arteriography and embolization with absorbable materials (5% rate of impotence vs. 39% with permanent materials) or surgical ligation as a last resort (5)
- Treat the underlying condition (i.e., sickle cell disease). Do not delay intracavernous treatment.

GENERAL MEASURES

- Reassure the patient about the outcome, if warranted.
- Provide continuous caudal or spinal anesthesia if the etiology is neurogenic.
- Treat any underlying cause.
- In sickle cell anemia: IV hydration; supplemental oxygen; partial exchange or repeated transfusions to reduce percentage of sickle cells to $<$50%
- Relieve the patient's pain.
- Initiating proper management depends on whether the priapism is ischemic or nonischemic.

MEDICATION

- Opioids for pain, if needed
- Intracavernous injection of phenylephrine is recommended by the American Urological Association for ischemic priapism (5).
- Phenylephrine minimizes risk of cardiovascular side effects that are more common with other sympathomimetics terbutaline has been studied and may be effective (uncontrolled trials showed a 65% resolution rate) for priapism caused by self-injection of agents to treat erectile dysfunction (5).
- For stuttering priapism, a trial of gonadotropin-releasing hormone (GnRH) agonists or antiandrogens is effective; self-injection of phenylephrine is also effective.
- PDE-5 inhibitors also have a role in the prevention of priapism in patients suffering from stuttering priapism (6).

ISSUES FOR REFERRAL

A urologist should be consulted in all cases of suspected priapism to ensure the highest likelihood of preserved erectile function.

SURGERY/OTHER PROCEDURES

- For ischemic priapism, introduction of 18- or 19-gauge needle into corpora cavernosa (best done by urologist if available) at 9 o'clock and 3 o'clock positions with aspiration of 20–30 mL of blood from corpus cavernosum. May follow with intracavernous injection of 100–500 μg phenylephrine (mix 0.2 mL [200 μg] of 1% phenylephrine in 9.8 mL of normal saline.) 1 mL injections given every 3–5 min for $\sim$1 hour before determining if treatment is successful. If this fails, consider shunts.
- Distal shunts
  - Percutaneous: Ebbehoj, Winter, or T-shunt (7,8,9)
  - Open: Al-Ghorab or corporal snake (10,11)
- Proximal shunts
  - Open: Quackles or Sacher (12,13)
  - Saphenous vein shunt (14)
  - Deep dorsal vein shunt (15)

ONGOING CARE

FOLLOW-UP RECOMMENDATIONS

Bed rest until priapism resolves

Patient Monitoring

Close follow-up with a urologist is required after surgical treatments for priapism.

PATIENT EDUCATION

- Information about long-term outlook, referral for counseling
- Reduction of vasoactive drug therapy if responsible for priapism and elimination of offending drugs if causal

PROGNOSIS

- Even with excellent treatment for a prolonged priapism, detumescence may require several weeks secondary to edema (1).
- Impotence due to irreversible corporal fibrosis is likely in ischemic priapism and is up to 90% if the priapism lasts $>$24 hours.
- Despite early intervention, ischemic priapism is likely to result in impotence in up to 50% of men.

COMPLICATIONS

Erectile dysfunction (i.e., impotence)

REFERENCES

1. Huang YC, Harraz AM, Shindel AW, et al. Evaluation and management of priapism: 2009 update. *Nat Rev Urol*. 2009;6(5):262–271.
2. Chrouser KL, Ajiboye OB, Oyetunji TA, et al. Priapism in the United States: the changing role of sickle cell disease. *Am J Surg*. 2011;201(4): 468–474.
3. Eland IA, van der Lei J, Stricker BH, et al. Incidence of priapism in the general population. *Urology*. 2001;57(5):970–972.
4. Champion HC, Bivalacqua TJ, Takimoto E, et al. Phosphodiesterase-5A dysregulation in penile erectile tissue is a mechanism of priapism. *Proc Natl Acad Sci USA*. 2005;102(5):1661–1666.
5. Montague DK, Jarow J, Broderick GA, et al. American Urological Association guideline on the management of priapism. *J Urol*. 2003;170(1, Pt 4):1318–1324.
6. Muneer A, Minhas S, Arya M, et al. Stuttering priapism—a review of the therapeutic options. *Int J Clin Pract*. 2008;62(8):1265–1270.
7. Ebbehoj J. A new operation for priapism. *Scand J Plast Reconstr Surg*. 1974;8(3):241–242.
8. Winter CC. Cure of idiopathic priapism: new procedure for creating fistula between glans penis and corpora cavernosa. *Urology*. 1976;8(4):389–391.
9. Brant WO, Garcia MM, Bella AJ, et al. T-shaped shunt and intracavernous tunneling for prolonged ischemic priapism. *J Urol*. 2009;181(4): 1699–1705.
10. Borrelli M, Mitre AI, Alfer Júnior W, et al. Surgical treatment of priapism using Al-Ghorab's technic [in Portuguese]. *Rev Paul Med*. 1983;101(1): 27–28.
11. Burnett AL, Pierorazio PM. Corporal "snake" maneuver: corporoglanular shunt surgical modification for ischemic priapism. *J Sex Med*. 2009;6(4):1171–1176.
12. Quackels R. Treatment of a case of priapism by cavernospongious anastomosis [in French]. *Acta Urol Belg*. 1964;32:5–13.
13. Sacher EC, Sayegh E, Frensilli F, et al. Cavernospongiosum shunt in the treatment of priapism. *J Urol*. 1972;108(1):97–100.
14. Grayhack JT, Mccullough W, O'Conor VJ, et al. Venous bypass to control priapism. *Invest Urol*. 1964;1:509–513.
15. Barry JM. Priapism: treatment with corpus cavernosum to dorsal vein of penis shunts. *J Urol*. 1976;116(6):754–756.

ADDITIONAL READING

- Burnett AL. Pathophysiology of priapism: dysregulatory erection physiology thesis. *J Urol*. 2003;170(1):26–34.
- Pryor J, Akkus E, Alter G. Priapism. *J Sex Med*. 2004;1(1):116–120.
- Salonia A, Eardley I, Giuliano F, et al. European association of urology guidelines on priapism. *Eur Urol*. 2014;65(2):480–489.

SEE ALSO

Anemia, Sickle Cell; Erectile Dysfunction

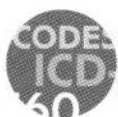

CODES

ICD10

- N48.30 Priapism, unspecified
- N48.39 Other priapism
- N48.31 Priapism due to trauma

CLINICAL PEARLS

- Priapism is a prolonged penile erection that lasts $>$4 hours and is unrelated to sexual stimulation.
- In evaluating priapism, the clinician must distinguish ischemic from nonischemic priapism by history and physical exam, as well as blood gas and possibly ultrasound, if needed.
- Ischemic priapism is an emergent condition that requires immediate urologic evaluation and treatment.
- The most common causes of ischemic priapism are idiopathic, related to treatments for erectile dysfunction, or related to use of substances (medicinal or recreational).
- If an underlying medical condition is identified (sickle cell anemia), proper concomitant treatment is necessary to increase the efficacy of treatment.

PROSTATE CANCER

Frank J. Domino, MD

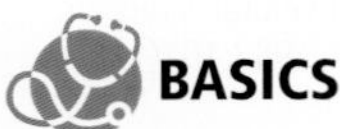

BASICS

DESCRIPTION

- The prostate gland is often likened in size to a walnut, typically averaging 20–25 g in volume in an adult male; tends to become larger with age
- 3 distinct zones delineate the functional anatomy of the prostate: peripheral zone (largest, neighbors rectal wall, palpable on DRE), central zone (contains the ejaculatory ducts), and transition zone (located centrally, adjacent to the urethra).
- Common metastatic locations (most to least common): pelvic lymph nodes, bone, lung, and liver
- Clinical staging is an objective evaluation of disease extent based on pretreatment criteria including imaging, DRE, PSA, and biopsy.
- Pathologic stage is determined only once the prostatic tissue and accompanying lymph nodes have been analyzed histologically.
- Staging: tumor, node, metastasis (TNM) classification: clinical:
  - Tx: Primary tumor cannot be assessed.
  - T0: no evidence of primary tumor
  - T1: clinically inapparent tumor not palpable or visible by imaging. T1a: tumor incidental histologic finding in ≤5% of tissue resected (by transurethral resection of prostate [TURP]). T1b: tumor incidental histologic finding in >5% of tissue resected (by TURP). T1c: tumor identified by needle biopsy (e.g., because of elevated PSA).
  - T2: tumor confined within prostate, found in 1 or both lobes. T2a: Tumor involves ≤1/2 of 1 lobe. T2b: Tumor involves >1/2 of 1 lobe. T2c: both lobes.
  - T3: Tumor extends through the prostatic capsule (invasion into the prostatic apex or into, but not beyond, the prostatic capsule is still T2). T3a: extracapsular extension (unilateral or bilateral). T3b: Tumor invades seminal vesicle(s).
  - T4: Tumor is fixed or invades adjacent structures other than seminal vesicles (e.g., bladder neck, external sphincter, rectum, levator muscles, and/or pelvic wall).
- Pathologic staging based on histologic findings, pT2–pT4 with analogous groupings. Also includes N (nodes) and M (metastasis). Nodes range from Nx (not assessed) to N0 (no nodes) to N1 (metastasis to regional nodes). Metastasis: Mx (not assessed); M0 (no metastasis); and M1 (distant metastasis) including M1a (regional mets), M1b (bones), and M1c (other sites w/o bone disease)
- Gleason grade: Tumors are graded from 1 (well differentiated) to 5 (poorly differentiated) based on the degree of glandular differentiation and structural architecture, although only scores 3–5 are reported as cancers. Primary and secondary scores are reported and combined to form the combined Gleason score.
- Gleason score is now recognized by the American Joint Committee on Cancer (AJCC) as the preferred grading system, and this score is an important variable used to risk stratify patients with localized prostate cancer.

EPIDEMIOLOGY

Incidence

Mortality from carcinoma of the prostate (CaP) is decreasing. Based on 5 years of mortality data (2006–2010), the overall cancer death rate decreased by 3.1% per year.

Prevalence

- According to the National Cancer Institute, an estimated 238,590 men in the US will be newly diagnosed with CaP in 2013.
- ~29,720 men in the US will die of CaP in 2013.
- Mean age at diagnosis is 66 years.
- Prostate cancer is the most commonly diagnosed non–skin cancer in men in the US (~15.3% lifetime risk) and 2nd leading cause of cancer death in men (only ~3% of all CaP results in CaP-related death).
- Autopsy studies find foci of latent CaP in 50% of men in their 8th decade.
- Probability of invasive CaP 12.54% (1 in 8) in men aged ≥70 years

ETIOLOGY AND PATHOPHYSIOLOGY

- Adenocarcinoma: >95%; nonadenocarcinoma: <5% (most common transitional cell carcinoma)
- Cells often stain positive for PSA and prostatic acid phosphatase (PAP).
- Location of CaP: 70% peripheral zone, 20% transitional zone, 5–10% central zone

Genetics

Risk doubled if 1st-degree relative <50 years of age affected

RISK FACTORS

- Age >50 years, African American race
- Incidence is 152.0/100,000 in Caucasians versus 228.5/100,000 in African Americans.
- Age is the most important risk factor.
- Testosterone therapy does not increase CaP recurrence rates postprostatectomy, even in men with high-risk disease.

GENERAL PREVENTION

- Finasteride reduced the risk of prostate cancer by 24.8% *but was associated with an increased risk of high-grade disease* and there were no differences in rates of overall survival with finasteride.
- Dutasteride reduces risk *without* increased risk of high-grade tumors.
- 5-α-Reductase inhibitors are currently not FDA approved for CaP prevention.
- No ↓ risk of CaP with selenium or vitamin E supplements; ↑ CaP risk with vitamin E

ALERT

- U.S. Preventive Services Task Force (USPSTF) recommends against PSA-based screen for prostate cancer; concluded harm of screening outweighs benefit (1)[A]
- For men ages 55–69, the AUA panel recommends shared decision making between physician and patient regarding PSA screening.

DIAGNOSIS

HISTORY

- Inquire about family history of CaP, symptoms of bladder outlet obstruction, and other voiding symptoms.
- Anorexia and weight loss, bone pain (with metastasis), hematuria, hematospermia (rare)

PHYSICAL EXAM

If clinical suspicion (dysuria, hematuria, hematospermia), DRE to assess for prostatic masses/firmness/asymmetry

ALERT

Most patients with CaP are asymptomatic.

DIFFERENTIAL DIAGNOSIS

BPH, benign nodular prostatic growth, subacute prostatitis, prostatic intraepithelial neoplasia (PIN), prostate stones, atypical small acinar proliferation (ASAP)

- The high predictive value of ASAP for subsequent adenocarcinoma warrants repeat biopsy.

DIAGNOSTIC TESTS & INTERPRETATION

Initial Tests (lab, imaging)

- PSA is produced by prostatic epithelial cells.
- Age/race-adjusted "normal" PSA values (ng/mL):

Age	Asians	Blacks	Whites
40–49	0–2.0	0–2.0	0–2.5
50–59	0–3.0	0–4.0	0–3.5
60–69	0–4.0	0–4.5	0–4.5
70–79	0–5.0	0–5.5	0–6.5

- Total PSA ≥4 ng/mL (sensitivity 21%, specificity 91%); 1st-time PSA >4 ng/mL alone not indication for biopsy:
  - Rectal manipulation will not significantly ↑ PSA.
  - Other benign conditions can affect PSA and cause increase (infection, inflammation, normal growth).
- 5-α-Reductase inhibitors decrease PSA ~50%.
- Other PSA metrics used to aid in CaP diagnosis: PSA velocity, PSA doubling time, PSA density, percentage free PSA
  - Total PSA velocity: ≥0.75 ng/mL/year increases CaP suspicion if PSA >4.0 ng/mL.
  - Free PSA and age/race-adjusted PSA helpful in evaluating risk when total PSA is 4–10 ng/mL
  - Consider CaP if PSAD (PSA density) ≥0.15 or if PSA rises even while on 5-α-reductase inhibitors.
- PSA/free PSA and probability of cancer:

PSA (ng/dL)	Cancer rate	% Free PSA	Cancer rate
0–2	1%	0–10%	56%
2–4	15%	10–15%	28%
4–10	25%	15–20%	
>10	>50%	20–25%	16%
		>25%	8%

- Abnormal DRE, PSA, PSA kinetics (i.e., velocity), and all may trigger transrectal ultrasound (TRUS)–guided biopsy of the prostate.
- Patient-specific models to predict pathologic stage based on PSA, TRUS biopsy results, and estimated clinical stage have been validated.

Test Interpretation

Small, closely packed glandular tissue, loss of basement membrane, perineural invasion, and smaller prostate size are associated with higher grade disease.

Follow-Up Tests & Special Considerations

- If life expectancy ≤5 years and patient is asymptomatic, no further workup is needed (if high risk, may consider androgen deprivation therapy [ADT] or radiation therapy [RT] in select patients).
- Bone scan: if T1 and PSA >20, if T2 and PSA >10, if Gleason ≥8, T3 or T4, or symptomatic
- Pelvic CT or MRI: if T3, T4, or T1–T2 with >10% nomogram indicated probability of lymph node involvement
- Biopsy if suspicious nodal findings
- Alkaline phosphatase associated with bony mets
- *PCA3* (prostate cancer gene 3) urine testing used in conjunction with PSA may decrease the unnecessary repeat prostate biopsies. Using a *PCA3* cutoff of 10, the number of false-positive CaP diagnoses may be reduced by >35%.

- Risk categories:
  - D'Amico et al. classify men with localized CaP into categories based on risk of biochemical recurrence (BCR) after definitive treatment: low, intermediate, or high.
  - Must meet all 3 criteria to be low risk; any 1 criterion moves patient to a higher risk group.

Risk category	Clinical stage	Serum PSA	Gleason score
Very low*	T1c		
Low	T1–T2a	<10 ng/mL	≤6
Intermediate	T2b–T2c	>10 and ≤20 ng/mL	7
High	T3a	>20 ng/mL	8–10
Very high	T3b–T4		

*Very low category also includes PSA density <0.15 ng/mL/g and <3 prostate biopsy cores positive (<50% CaP in any core).

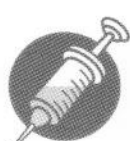

TREATMENT

A treatment decision should be reached after a discussion about options, risks, and benefits. Initial decisions are based on PSA, Gleason score, volume of disease, life expectancy, and patient preference.

- Active surveillance: close monitoring of PSA, DRE, and repeat biopsy at regular intervals (2)[B]
- Prostatectomy: retropubic, robotic-assisted laparoscopic ± pelvic lymph node dissection (PLND); nerve-sparing surgery is possible if there is no extracapsular extension.
- Radiation therapy: external beam and/or brachytherapy—seed implantation
- Brachytherapy: radioactive implants placed in prostate; popular option for early clinical stage localized to the prostate
- Androgen deprivation therapy (see next section)
- Treatment guidelines for clinically localized CaP:
  - Very low risk: active surveillance (if other risk factors, consider moving to low risk)
  - Low risk: active surveillance, external beam RT, brachytherapy, or radical prostatectomy ± PLND
  - Intermediate risk: if life expectancy <10 years: active surveillance, RT ± short-term ADT, brachytherapy. If >10 years, radical prostatectomy ± PLND or RT.
  - High risk: external beam radiotherapy *with* long-term ADT, external beam radiotherapy with brachytherapy ± ADT, or radical prostatectomy with PLND
- Low-volume, high-grade CaP may warrant adjuvant ADT.
- Locally advanced:
  - Very high risk: RT with long-term ADT, RT with brachytherapy ± ADT, radical prostatectomy with PLND, or ADT
- Metastatic: ADT or RT with long-term ADT

MEDICATION

Medications are generally indicated for advanced, high-risk, or metastatic disease.

First Line

- ADT is for patients at high risk of recurrence or those with metastatic disease who are not candidates for local therapy.
- ADT consists of 2 equally effective options:
  - Bilateral orchiectomy (surgical castration)
  - Gonadotropin-releasing hormone (GnRH) agonist or antagonist (medical castration)
- GnRH agonists include leuprolide or goserelin.
- Side effects of ADT: osteoporosis, gynecomastia, erectile dysfunction (ED), decreased libido, obesity, lipid alterations, greater risk of diabetes and cardiovascular disease
- Flare phenomenon (disease flare: hot flashes, fatigue) can occur owing to transient increase in testosterone levels on initiation of GnRH agonist therapy. It can be avoided by giving preceding or concurrent antiandrogen therapy for at least 7 days.
- GnRH antagonist, degarelix: an alternative to GnRH agonists; suppresses testosterone production and avoids flare phenomenon observed with GnRH agonists

Second Line

- Combined androgen blockade with GnRH agonist and antiandrogen (e.g., bicalutamide, nilutamide, or flutamide)
- Castration-recurrent disease: Most patients develop continued disease after androgen deprivation (either castration or GnRH therapy); continued hormonal treatment may be beneficial.
- Chemotherapy with a docetaxel-based regimen has shown survival benefit and is the preferred 1st-line chemotherapy in metastatic castration-resistant prostate cancer (CRPC). Mitoxantrone-based regimen is another option.
- Abiraterone (Zytiga): 1,000 mg/day PO given with prednisone 5 mg BID (NNT 25 for additional 4 months of overall survival) for metastatic CRPC patients who have received prior chemotherapy containing docetaxel
- Cabazitaxel is another FDA-approved medication for men with metastatic CRPC previously treated with a docetaxel regimen.
- Sipuleucel-T is an immunotherapeutic agent that can prolong overall survival.
- Bisphosphonate (zoledronic acid) every 4 weeks is recommended together with ADT or systemic chemotherapy for CRPC. This may prevent disease-related skeletal complications.

ADDITIONAL THERAPIES

- Adjuvant RT should be considered for men with ≥2 adverse features (Gleason 8–10, pT3, positive margins).
- Cryoablation: argon gas–based freezing of tissue

ONGOING CARE

FOLLOW-UP RECOMMENDATIONS

- CT/bone scan if suspected recurrence
- Prostatectomy: PSA/DRE every 6 months for 5 years; yearly thereafter; PSA >0.2 ng/mL after surgery is suggestive of recurrence.
- XRT: PSA/DRE every 3 months for 1 year; every 3–6 months for 4 years; yearly thereafter; PSA ≥2 ng/mL from post-XRT nadir is suggestive of recurrence.

PROGNOSIS

- Localized disease should be curable; advanced disease has a favorable prognosis if lesions are hormone-sensitive.
- 3-year CaP survival by stage: local 100%, regional 99.1%, distant 33.1%, unstaged 79.2%
- Recurrence risk increased if extracapsular extension, seminal vesicle invasion, positive surgical margins

COMPLICATIONS

- Urinary incontinence, mild colitis, ED, radiation cystitis, and hematuria are the most common.
- Treatment options for postop ED: PDE5 inhibitors, intracavernosal injections, penile prosthesis
- Skeletal-related events due to bone metastases

REFERENCES

1. Lin K, Lipsitz R, Miller T, et al. Benefits and harms of prostate-specific antigen screening for prostate cancer: an evidence update for the U.S. Preventive Services Task Force. *Ann Intern Med*. 2008;149(3):192–199.
2. Klotz L. Active surveillance for low-risk prostate cancer. *F1000 Med Rep*. 2012;4:16.

ADDITIONAL READING

- Crawford ED, Rove KO, Trabulsi EJ, et al. Diagnostic performance of PCA3 to detect prostate cancer in men with increased prostate specific antigen: a prospective study of 1,962 cases. *J Urol*. 2012;188(5):1726–1731.
- D'Amico AV, Whittington R, Schultz D, et al. Outcome based staging for clinically localized adenocarcinoma of the prostate. *J Urol*. 1997;158(4):1422–1426.
- Klein EA, Thompson IM Jr, Tangen CM, et al. Vitamin E and the risk of prostate cancer: the Selenium and Vitamin E Cancer Prevention Trial (SELECT). *JAMA*. 2011;306(14):1549–1556.
- Lowrance WT, Scardino PT. Predictive models for newly diagnosed prostate cancer patients. *Rev Urol*. 2009;11(3):117–126.
- National Comprehensive Cancer Network. Clinical practice guidelines: prostate cancer. 2012. www.nccn.org. Accessed 2014.
- Nomiya T, Tsuji H, Toyama S, et al. Management of high-risk prostate cancer: radiation therapy and hormonal therapy. *Cancer Treat Rev*. 2013;39(8):872–878.
- Pastuszak AW, Pearlman AM, Lai WS, et al. Testosterone replacement therapy in patients with prostate cancer after radical prostatectomy. *J Urol*. 2013;190(2):639–644.
- Thompson IM Jr, Goodman PJ, Tangen CM, et al. Long-term survival of participants in the prostate cancer prevention trial. *N Engl J Med*. 2013;369(7):603–610.

CODES

ICD10

C61 Malignant neoplasm of prostate

CLINICAL PEARLS

- Prostate cancer is clinically diverse, ranging from low-risk/indolent disease to high-risk/aggressive disease.
- Most men with CaP are asymptomatic.
- The incidence of CaP is high, yet the mortality is low and a large percentage are thought to be clinically insignificant.
- The use of PSA for CaP screening is controversial and necessitates an open conversation between medical provider and patient regarding benefits/risks.
- Active surveillance is an important treatment option to consider for low-risk patients.
- The Gleason score is the most commonly used classification system for the histologic grading of CaP.
- In patients taking 5-α-reductase inhibitors, must use PSA level times 2 to estimate actual PSA

PROSTATIC HYPERPLASIA, BENIGN (BPH)

David E. Longstroth, MD

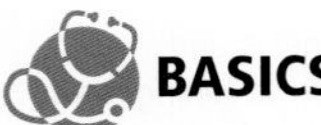

BASICS

- Progressive condition where an increase in number of cells (both stroma and epithelial cell lines) within prostate, ultimately increase its size
- As it grows in volume, the central urethra may become compressed and narrowed, causing symptoms of obstruction, which results in clinical symptoms (difficulty initiating urination, frequency, dysuria). Treatment depends on severity of lower urinary tract symptoms (LUTS) (1)[A].
- Progression may result in upper and lower tract infections and may progress to direct bladder outlet obstruction (BOO), and acute renal failure (ARF).

DESCRIPTION
- Benign prostatic hyperplasia (BPH) is one of the most common diseases of older men (age >45 years).
- Diagnosed histologically, clinically managed by LUTS, which affect quality of life
- Treatment is focused on alleviating symptoms and slowing progression of the disease.

EPIDEMIOLOGY
Near universal development in men; age dependent

Prevalence
From 8% in men aged 31–40 years; to 40–50% in men 51–60 years; and >80% in men >80 years

ETIOLOGY AND PATHOPHYSIOLOGY
- Older age and functional Leydig cells in testes
- BPH is rare in men with hypogonadism onset before age 40 years not treated with androgens.
- Develops in prostatic periurethral or transition zone
- Hyperplastic nodules of stromal and epithelial components increase glandular components.

COMMONLY ASSOCIATED CONDITIONS
- LUTS
  - LUTS can be divided into 2 groups: filling/storage symptoms, and voiding symptoms.
    - Filling/storage symptoms include frequency, nocturia, urgency, and urge incontinence.
    - Voiding: irritative: frequency, urgency, dysuria, nocturia. Obstructive symptoms: poor stream, hesitancy, terminal dribbling, incomplete voiding, overflow incontinence
- BPH symptoms are strong and independent risk factors for sexual dysfunction, including erectile dysfunction and ejaculatory disorders.

Genetics
- 1st-degree relative with BPH increases risk.
- Black men <65 years may need surgical treatment more often than white men.
- Asians have a lower risk for nocturia, whereas risks for African American and Caucasian men are similar.

RISK FACTORS
- Increased risk of BPH with higher free prostate-specific antigen (PSA) levels, heart disease, and use of β-blockers
- Decreased risk with higher physical activity
- Conflicting data that tobacco use may lower risk of surgery for BPH symptoms
- No evidence of increased or decreased risk with smoking, alcohol, or any dietary factors
- Low androgen levels from cirrhosis/chronic alcoholism can reduce the risk of BPH.

GENERAL PREVENTION
The disease appears to be part of the aging process.

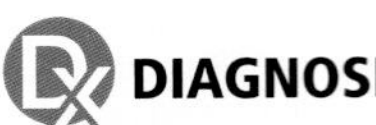

DIAGNOSIS

HISTORY
- International Prostate Symptom Score (IPSS) of LUTS, patient filled survey to follow severity (2)[A]:
  - Questionnaire: Over the past month, how often have you:
    - 1. Had the sensation of not emptying your bladder completely after you finished urinating?
    - 2. Had to urinate again <2 hours after you finished urinating?
    - 3. Found you stopped and started again several times when you urinated?
    - 4. Found it difficult to postpone urination?
    - 5. Had a weak urinary stream?
    - 6. Had to push or strain to begin urination?
    - 7. Been up to urinate from the time you went to bed at night until the time you got up in the morning?
    - 8. How would you feel if you were to spend the rest of your life with your current symptoms?
  - Scoring of the questionnaire:
    - Questions 1–6: no symptoms = 0 points, 1 in 5 times = 1 point, less than half = 2 points, about half = 3 points, more than half = 4 points, most of the time = 5 points
    - Question 7: no occurrence = 0 points, 1 time = 1 point, 2 times = 2 points, 3 times = 3 points, 4 times = 4 points, and 5 times or more = 5 points
    - Question 8: 0 = Delighted, 1 = Pleased, 2 = Mostly satisfied, 3 = Mixed, 4 = Mostly dissatisfied, 5 = Unhappy, 6 = Terrible
    - Symptoms are classified as mild (total score 0–7), moderate (total score 8–19), and severe (total score 20–35).
- Nocturia >2× per night, warrants a frequency/volume chart for 2–3 days to detect urinary patterns.
- Important to include in the history:
  - Gross hematuria
  - History of type 2 diabetes, which can cause nocturia and is a risk factor for BPH; chronically elevated glucose can cause neurogenic bladder
  - Symptoms of neurologic disease
  - Sexual dysfunction
  - History of urethral trauma, urethritis, or urethral instrumentation that could lead to urethral stricture
  - Family history of BPH and prostate cancer
  - Treatment with drugs that can impair bladder function (anticholinergic drugs) or increase outflow resistance (sympathomimetic drugs)

PHYSICAL EXAM
- Digital rectal exam finding of enlarged prostate, but *size does not always correlate with symptoms*
- Abdominal percussion to detect distended bladder
- Signs of renal failure due to obstructive uropathy (edema, pallor, pruritus, ecchymoses, nutritional deficiencies)

DIFFERENTIAL DIAGNOSIS
- Obstructive
  - Prostate cancer
  - Urethral stricture or valves
  - Bladder neck contracture (usually secondary to prostate surgery)
  - Prostatitis
  - Inability of bladder neck or external sphincter to relax appropriately during voiding
- Neurologic
  - Spinal cord injury
  - Stroke
  - Parkinsonism
  - Multiple sclerosis
- Medical
  - Poorly controlled diabetes mellitus
  - Congestive heart failure (CHF)
- Pharmacologic
  - Diuretics
  - Sympathomimetics (e.g., cold medications)
  - Anticholinergics
- Other:
  - Bladder carcinoma
  - Overactive bladder
  - Nocturnal Polyuria
  - Bladder calculi
  - UTI

DIAGNOSTIC TESTS & INTERPRETATION

Initial Tests (lab, imaging)
- Postvoid residual to detect obstruction
- PSA may be elevated but usually <10 ng/mL (10 μg/L) although nonspecific. Acute urinary retention, prostatitis, urinary tract instrumentation, or prostatic infarction may elevate PSA.
- Urinalysis: Pyuria if stones or infection present, pH changes due to chronic residual urine.
- BUN and creatinine (if concerns for uremia)

Follow-Up Tests & Special Considerations
- Uroflow: volume voided per unit time (peak flow <10 mL/s is abnormal)
- Postvoid residual: either with catheterization or bladder ultrasound (>100 mL demonstrates incomplete emptying)
- Transrectal ultrasound: assessment of gland size; not necessary in the routine evaluation
- Abdominal ultrasound: can demonstrate increased postvoid residual or hydronephrosis; not necessary in the routine evaluation

Geriatric Considerations
Drugs to use with caution: anticholinergics, antihistamines, sympathomimetics, tricyclic antidepressants, opioids, and skeletal muscle relaxants

Diagnostic Procedures/Other
- Pressure-flow studies (urine flow vs. voiding pressures) to determine etiology of symptoms
  - Obstructive pattern shows high voiding pressures with low flow rate.
- Cystoscopy
  - Demonstrates presence, configuration, cause (stricture, stone), and site of obstructive tissue
  - May help determine therapeutic option
  - Not recommended in initial evaluation unless other factors, such as hematuria, are present

Test Interpretation
Confirmation obtained by biopsy, resection, or surgery

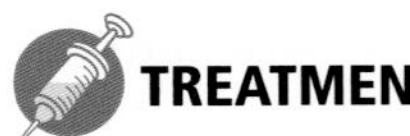

TREATMENT

GENERAL MEASURES
- Focus on modifiable factors, regulation of fluid intake, exercise, diet, and concomitant drug use.
- Watchful waiting is recommended on patient with mild to moderate symptoms without complications.

- Medical treatment requires interval follow-up of 2–4 weeks for α-blockers and 3 months for 5-α-reductase inhibitors until symptoms improved, then annually.
- Patients with complications including obstruction and urinary retention require bladder drainage. If catheterization if difficult, consider coude' catheter or flexible cystoscopy.
- With postobstructive diuresis, monitor electrolytes.

MEDICATION

The American Urological Association (AUA) recommends watchful waiting for patients without bothersome LUTS (AUA-SI score <8) who have not developed a serious complication. Lifestyle modifications are employed.

First Line

- α-Adrenergic antagonists affect contraction of prostatic smooth muscle and are more effective than other methods alone. They reduce prostatic volume, cause dizziness, and may affect blood pressure; requires dose titration, and blood pressure monitoring.
  - Nonselective, reduce prostatic smooth muscle tone, improving urinary flow:
    - Terazosin (Hytrin): 1–10 mg/day PO
    - Doxazosin (Cardura): 1–8 mg/day PO
  - Selective, may produce fewer side effects; generally more expensive:
    - Tamsulosin (Flomax): 0.4–0.8 mg/day PO
    - Alfuzosin (Uroxatral): 10 mg/day PO
    - Silodosin (Rapaflo): 8 mg/day PO
- 5-α-reductase inhibitors reduce prostatic volume (useful if prostatic enlargement):
  - Finasteride (Proscar): 5 mg/day PO
  - Dutasteride (Avodart): 0.5 mg/day PO
  - Also useful in controlling prostatic bleeding
- Anticholinergic agents are appropriate for irritative LUTS without an elevated postvoid residual (PVR).
- Combination therapy of α-blocker plus 5-α-reductase inhibitor is equal to α-blocker therapy, but superior to monotherapy among men with large prostates. Combination therapy is superior to monotherapy to prevent progression but increase risk of drug-related adverse events.
- 5-α-reductase inhibitor's should not be used in men with LUTS without prostatic enlargement.
- Phophodiesterase-5 inhibitor (PDE-5)
- Tadalafil (Cialis): 5 mg/day PO
- Avoid use in combination with α-blockers.
- Avoid in those with CrCl <30 mL/min.
- Contraindications:
  - α-Blockers can cause orthostatic hypotension; less risk with tamsulosin, silodosin, and alfuzosin
  - See specific recommendations for α-blocker use with phosphodiesterase type-5 inhibitors (for erectile dysfunction).
  - α-Blockers should be avoided in men planning cataract surgery until after the surgery (risk for floppy iris syndrome).
  - Avoid anticholinergics in patients with elevated PVR >250mL.

ALERT

5-α-reductase inhibitors reduce PSA by 1/2, so the PSA result should be doubled for purposes of screening for prostate cancer.

ISSUES FOR REFERRAL

- Failure to respond to medical therapy
- Recurrent UTIs or hematuria
- Abnormal PSA or prostate exam
- Any history of urethral trauma or stricture, or neurologic disease of the bladder/urinary system.

SURGERY/OTHER PROCEDURES

- Indications for surgery:
  - Urinary retention due to prostatic obstruction, recurrent, no improvement with medications
  - Intractable symptoms due to prostatic obstruction AUA score >8 and symptoms
  - Obstructive uropathy (renal insufficiency)
  - Recurrent or persistent UTIs due to prostatic obstruction
  - Recurrent gross hematuria due to enlarged prostate
  - Bladder calculi
- Surgical procedures:
  - Minimally invasive: transurethral needle ablation (TUNA) and transurethral microwave thermotherapy (TUMT)—useful on small prostate
  - Transurethral resection of the prostate (TURP) and transurethral vaporization of the prostate (TUVP)
  - Open prostatectomy: treatment of choice for patients with extremely large prostates (>100 g)
  - Transurethral incision of the prostate (TUIP): treatment of choice for men with obstruction and small prostates
  - Transurethral laser ablation: holmium laser ablation of the tissue (HoLAP); useful in patients on anticoagulant therapy
  - Transurethral holmium laser enucleation of the prostate (HoLEP)
  - Photoselective vaporization of prostate (PVP)
- Common complications of TURP:
  - Bleeding can be significant.
  - TUR syndrome: hyponatremia secondary to absorption of hypotonic irrigant
  - Retrograde ejaculation
  - Urinary incontinence

COMPLEMENTARY & ALTERNATIVE MEDICINE

Saw palmetto *(Serenoa repens)* has been thoroughly studied in a subject in Cochrane review, and did not improve LUTS. Similarly, stinging nettle (*Urtica dioica*) shows no improvement. Neither are recommended for use.

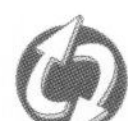

ONGOING CARE

FOLLOW-UP RECOMMENDATIONS

The patient is more likely to void after surgery or illness when able to stand over toilet.

Patient Monitoring

- Symptom index (IPSS) monitored every 3–12 months
- Digital rectal exam yearly
- PSA yearly: should not be checked while patient is in retention, recently catheterized, or within a week of any surgical procedure to the prostate
- Consider monitoring PVR, if elevated.

DIET

Avoid large boluses of oral or IV fluids or alcohol intake.

PATIENT EDUCATION

National Kidney and Urologic Diseases Information Clearinghouse, Box NKUDIC, Bethesda, MD 20893; 301-468-6345

PROGNOSIS

- Symptoms improve or stabilize in 70–80% of patients.
- 25% of men with LUTS will have persistent storage symptoms after prostatectomy.
- Of men with BPH, 11–33% have occult prostate cancer.

COMPLICATIONS

- Urinary retention (acute or chronic)
- Bladder stones
- Prostatitis
- Renal failure
- Hematuria

REFERENCES

1. American Urological Association Guidelines: guideline on the management of benign prostatic hyperplasia (BPH): updated 2010. www.AUAnet.org. Accessed 2014.
2. Rosen R, Altwein J, Boyle P. Lower urinary tract symptoms and male sexual dysfunction: the multinational survey of the aging male (MSAM-7). *Eur Urol*. 2003;44(6):637–649.

ADDITIONAL READING

- Hollingsworth JM, Wei JT. Does the combination of an alpha1-adrenergic antagonist with a 5alpha-reductase inhibitor improve urinary symptoms more than either monotherapy? *Curr Opin Urol*. 2010;20(1):1–6.
- Neal RH, Keister D. What's best for your patient with BPH? *J Fam Pract*. 2009;58(5):241–247.
- Rich KT. FPIN's clinical inquiries. Medical treatment of benign prostatic hyperplasia. *Am Fam Physician*. 2008;77(5):665–666.
- Tacklind J, MacDonald R, Rutks I, et al. *Serenoa repens* for benign prostatic hyperplasia. *Cochrane Database Syst Rev*. 2009;(2):CD001423.
- Wilt TJ. Tamsulosin for benign prostatic hyperplasia. *Cochrane Database Syst Rev*. 2003;(1):CD002081.
- Wilt TJ. Terazosin for benign prostatic hyperplasia. *Cochrane Database Syst Rev*. 2002;(4):CD003851.

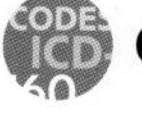

CODES

ICD10

- N40.0 Enlarged prostate without lower urinary tract symptoms
- N40.1 Enlarged prostate with lower urinary tract symptoms

CLINICAL PEARLS

- Although medical therapy has changed the management of BPH, it has only delayed the need for TURP by 10–15 years, not eliminated it.
- Urinary retention, obstructive uropathy, recurrent UTIs, bladder calculi, and recurrent hematuria are indications for surgical management of BPH.
- Indications for referral include recurrent UTIs, elevated PSA, failure of medical therapy, hematuria, retention, and patient desire.

PROSTATITIS

Anne Newbold, DO

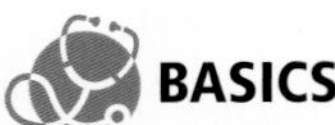

BASICS

DESCRIPTION

- Inflammatory or painful condition affecting the prostate gland; variety of etiologies
- National Institutes of Health's (NIH) prostatitis classification
  - *Class I: Acute bacterial prostatitis*: febrile illness with perineal pain, dysuria, and obstructive symptoms
  - *Class II: Chronic bacterial prostatitis*: chronic or recurrent bacterial infection with pain and voiding disturbances
  - *Class III: Chronic abacterial prostatitis/chronic pelvic pain syndrome*
    - Inflammatory (subtype IIIa): chronic symptoms and significant inflammatory cells in prostatic secretions, urine, or semen; no bacterial infection
    - Noninflammatory (subtype IIIb): chronic symptoms without evidence of inflammation or bacterial infection; insignificant number of inflammatory cells
  - *Class IV: Asymptomatic inflammatory prostatitis*: incidental finding during prostate biopsy for infertility, cancer workup
- System(s) affected: renal/urologic; reproductive

EPIDEMIOLOGY

Incidence

- Two million cases annually in the United States
- Predominant age: 30–50 years, sexually active; chronic more common in those >50 years
- Bacterial prostatitis occurs more frequently in patients with HIV.

Prevalence

2.2–9.7% of the male population (1)

ETIOLOGY AND PATHOPHYSIOLOGY

- Extension of UTI
- May occur following manipulation/biopsy of prostate or urethra
- Ascending infection through urethra
- Infectious: NIH classes I and II
  - Aerobic gram-negative bacteria (e.g., *Escherichia coli*, *Klebsiella*, *Proteus*, *Pseudomonas*, *Neisseria gonorrhoeae*, *Burkholderia pseudomallei*)
  - *E. coli* most common
  - Miscellaneous: *Chlamydia trachomatis*, *Ureaplasma*, trichomoniasis
  - Gram-positive bacteria (*Streptococcus faecalis*, *Staphylococcus aureus*)
  - Organisms suspected but unproven (*Staphylococcus epidermidis*, *S. micrococci*, non–group D *Streptococcus*, diphtheroids)
  - Uncommon: *Mycobacterium tuberculosis*, parasitic, mycoses (blastomycosis, coccidioidomycosis, cryptococcus, histoplasmosis, paracoccidioidomycosis, candidiasis)
- Nonbacterial: cause unknown: Leading theory suggests nonrelaxation (spasm) of the internal urinary sphincter and pelvic floor striated muscles leading to increased prostatic urethral pressure and intraprostatic urinary reflux.

RISK FACTORS

- Age >50 years
- Prostate biopsy (especially in patients with prior exposure to quinolones) (2)
- Prostatic calculi
- UTI
- Trauma (e.g., bicycle, horseback riding)
- Dehydration
- Sexual abstinence
- Chronic indwelling catheter
- Intermittent catheterization
- HIV infection
- Urethral stricture
- Cystoscopy
- Urethral dilatation
- Transurethral resection of prostate

GENERAL PREVENTION

Antibiotic prophylaxis and enema prior to prostatic biopsy

COMMONLY ASSOCIATED CONDITIONS

- Prostatic hypertrophy
- Cystitis
- Urethritis
- Pyelonephritis
- Sexual dysfunction

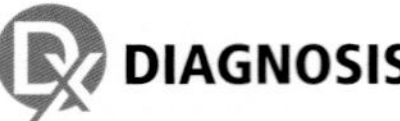

DIAGNOSIS

HISTORY

- Acute prostatitis (NIH class I):
  - Fever, chills, malaise
  - Low back pain, myalgias
  - Prostatodynia, perineal pain
  - Obstructive voiding symptoms
  - Frequency, urgency, dysuria, nocturia
- Chronic prostatitis (NIH classes II and III):
  - Prostatodynia, perineal pain
  - Dysuria, irritative voiding
  - Lower abdominal pain
  - Low back, scrotal, and/or penile pain
  - Pain on ejaculation
  - Hematospermia

PHYSICAL EXAM

- Very tender, boggy prostate on rectal exam
- Prostate may be warm, swollen, firm, or irregular.

ALERT

Avoid massage of the prostate in acute bacterial prostatitis; may induce iatrogenic bacteremia.

DIFFERENTIAL DIAGNOSIS

- Cystitis (bacterial, interstitial)
- Urethritis
- Pyelonephritis
- Malignancy
- Obstructive calculus
- Foreign body
- Acute urinary retention

DIAGNOSTIC TESTS & INTERPRETATION

Initial Tests (lab, imaging)

- Suspected acute prostatitis (NIH class I)
  - Urinalysis, urine and blood cultures, urine Gram stain
  - CBC with differential
- Suspected chronic bacterial prostatitis or abacterial prostatitis (NIH class II or III)
  - Fractional urine exam (4-glass test) (3)[A]
    - Voided bladder 1 (VB1): Initial 10 mL urine from urethra
    - VB2: Next 200 mL discarded; then midstream urine from bladder
    - Expressed prostate secretion (EPS): after prostate massage
    - VB3: Urine *after* prostate massage
  - Post-VB3 semen culture increases sensitivity and specificity (3)[A].
  - Many clinicians employ 2-glass test (VB2 and VB3) only.
  - Specimen handling
    - Culture, sensitivities, Gram stain on all samples
    - pH of EPS
    - Bacterial antigen-specific IgA and IgG levels in EPS
    - Wet mount of EPS
  - Interpretation
    - 10–15 WBCs per high-powered field in VB3 suggest bacterial prostatitis.
    - Macrophages containing fat (oval bodies) suggest bacterial prostatitis.
    - A positive culture in EPS, VB3, or post-VB3 semen sample, but not VB1 or VB2, is diagnostic of bacterial prostatitis.
    - In acute bacterial prostatitis, serum and EPS fluid bacterial antigen-specific IgA and IgG can be detected immediately after the onset of the infection. Level declines over 6–12 months after successful antibiotic therapy.
    - Bacteria count is less in chronic prostatitis.
    - In chronic bacterial prostatitis, no serum IgG elevation is seen, whereas EPS fluid IgA and IgG levels are increased. With antibiotic therapy, IgG levels return to normal in several months, but IgA levels remain elevated for 2 years.
    - Prostatic fluid is alkaline in chronic bacterial prostatitis.
    - Inflammatory cells (WBCs) with a negative culture (although false-negative cultures are not uncommon) suggest abacterial prostatitis.
    - No abnormal findings with chronic prostatitis without inflammation (this misnomer refers to patients with symptoms such as perineal pain, ejaculatory pain, and lower abdominal pain but no inflammatory changes on lab studies)
    - Prostate-specific antigen (PSA) level is increased with acute prostatitis (do not order until at least 1 month after prostatitis is treated).
- Drugs that may alter lab results: antibiotics
- Imaging not required in most cases
- CT or MRI if malignancy or abscess suspected
- Transrectal US if prostatic calculi or abscess suspected

Follow-Up Tests & Special Considerations

- Acute bacterial: urinalysis and culture 30 days after initiating treatment
- Chronic bacterial: urinalysis and culture every 30 days (may take several months of treatment to clear)

Diagnostic Procedures/Other

- Needle biopsy or aspiration for culture
- Urodynamic testing (prostatodynia)
- Cystoscopy (in persistent nonbacterial prostatitis to rule out bladder cancer, interstitial cystitis)

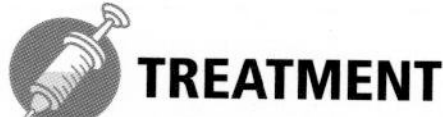

TREATMENT

GENERAL MEASURES

- Analgesics/antipyretics/stool softeners
- Hydration
- Sitz baths to relieve pain and spasm
- Suprapubic catheter for urinary retention
- Anxiolytics, antidepressants

MEDICATION

First Line

- Acute bacterial (outpatient) (4)[A]
  - Fluoroquinolone (ciprofloxacin 500 mg PO q12h or levofloxacin 500 mg PO once daily) × 2–4 weeks *or*
  - Trimethoprim-sulfamethoxazole 1 DS tab PO q12h × 2–4 weeks *or*
  - If gram-positive cocci are seen in initial urine Gram stain, start with amoxicillin 500 mg PO q8h. Adjust antibiotics once culture and sensitivities report is available.
  - Local sensitivity pattern should guide therapy.
  - Ceftriaxone 250 mg IM × 1 dose plus doxycycline 100 mg PO q12h daily for 1 week or azithromycin 1 gram PO single dose if at risk for STD pathogens
- Acute bacterial (inpatient)
  - Ampicillin 2g IV q6h or fluoroquinolone (ciprofloxacin 400 mg IV q12h or levofloxacin 500 mg q24h) begin oral therapy after afebrile for 24–48 hours.
- Chronic bacterial (NIH class II) (5)[B]
  - Fluoroquinolone (e.g., levofloxacin 500 mg PO once daily for 4 weeks (6,7)[A], *or* ciprofloxacin 500 mg PO q12h for 4–12 weeks
  - Combination therapy with azithromycin may help to eradicate unusual pathogens.
  - Anti inflammatory agents for pain symptoms and α-adrenergic receptor antagonists for urinary symptoms
- Chronic abacterial prostatitis (NIH class III)
  - No universally effective treatment
  - Treatment choice is usually by trial and error (8).
    - α-Blockers, antibiotics, and combinations of these therapies achieve greatest improvement in clinical symptom scores (9)[A].
    - α-Blockers better than placebo in some trials
    - Tamsulosin 0.4 mg PO once daily at bedtime for at least 6 months. Continue if there is a response (10)[A].
- Contraindications: drug allergies
- Precautions
  - Renal disease
  - Hepatic disease
  - Glucose-6-phosphate dehydrogenase deficiency may manifest with sulfonamides or NSAIDs.
  - Significant possible interactions: fluoroquinolones, magnesium/aluminum antacids, theophylline, probenecid, NSAIDs, warfarin

Second Line

- Piperacillin or ticarcillin with aminoglycoside, erythromycin, tetracycline, cephalexin, fluoroquinolones, dicloxacillin, nafcillin IV, vancomycin IV
- Finasteride (in patients >45 years, category IIIa inflammatory chronic prostatitis/chronic pelvic pain syndrome, and enlarged prostate glands)
- Nonbacterial: May benefit from erythromycin, doxycycline, trimethoprim-sulfamethoxazole.

ISSUES FOR REFERRAL

Urology referral for surgical drainage if an abscess persists after ≥1 week of therapy, persistent symptoms, hematuria, or elevated PSA

ADDITIONAL THERAPIES

Psychotherapy if sexual dysfunction

COMPLEMENTARY & ALTERNATIVE MEDICINE

- Neuromodulation, acupuncture, heat therapy; limited data to support
- Myofascial release (11)

SURGERY/OTHER PROCEDURES

Surgical resection for intractable chronic disease or to drain an abscess

INPATIENT CONSIDERATIONS

Admission Criteria/Initial Stabilization

- Proven or suspected abscess
- Unstable vital signs (sepsis)
- Immunocompromised

ONGOING CARE

FOLLOW-UP RECOMMENDATIONS

- Most improve in 3–4 weeks.
- Consider prostatic abscess in patients who do not respond well to therapy.

Patient Monitoring

NIH Chronic Prostatitis Symptom Index (www2.niddk.nih.gov): 13 items tabulated into 3 domain scores:

- Pain
- Urinary symptoms
- Quality of life

PROGNOSIS

- Often prolonged and difficult to cure; 55–97% cure rate depending on population and drug used
- 20% have reinfection or persistent infection.

COMPLICATIONS

- Prostatic abscess (common in HIV-infected)
- Gram-negative sepsis, bacteremia
- Urinary retention
- Epididymitis
- Chronic bacterial prostatitis (with acute prostatitis)
- Metastatic infection (spinal, sacroiliac)

REFERENCES

1. Krieger JN, Lee SW, Jeon J, et al. Epidemiology of prostatitis. *Int J Antimicrob Agents*. 2008;31(Suppl 1):S85–S90.
2. Mosharafa AA, Torky MH, Said WM, et al. Rising incidence of acute prostatitis following prostate biopsy: fluoroquinolone resistance and exposure is a significant risk factor. *Urology*. 2011;78(3):511–514.
3. Magri V, Wagenlehner FM, Montanari E, et al. Semen analysis in chronic bacterial prostatitis: diagnostic and therapeutic implications. *Asian J Androl*. 2009;11(4):461–477.
4. Lipsky BA, Byren I, Hoey CT, et al. Treatment of bacterial prostatitis. *Clin Infect Dis*. 2010;50(12):1641–1652.
5. Murphy AB, Macejko A, Taylor A, et al. Chronic prostatitis: management strategies. *Drugs*. 2009;69(1):71–84.
6. Paglia M, Peterson J, Fisher AC, et al. Safety and efficacy of levofloxacin 750 mg for 2 weeks or 3 weeks compared with levofloxacin 500 mg for 4 weeks in treating chronic bacterial prostatitis. *Current Med Res Opin*. 2010;26(6):1433–1441.
7. Naber KG, Roscher K, Botto H, et al. Oral levofloxacin 500 mg once daily in the treatment of chronic bacterial prostatitis. *Int J Antimicrob Agents*. 2008;32(2):145–153.
8. McNaughton CM, Mac Donald R, Wilt T. Interventions for abacterial prostatitis. *Cochrane Database Syst Rev*. 2001;(1):CD002080.
9. Anothaisintawee T, Attia J, Nickel JC, et al. Management of chronic prostatitis/chronic pelvic pain syndrome: a systematic review and network meta-analysis. *JAMA*. 2011;305(1):78–86.
10. Chen Y, Wu X, Liu J, et al. Effects of a 6-month course of tamsulosin for chronic prostatitis/chronic pelvic pain syndrome: a multicenter, randomized trial. *World J Urol*. 2011;29(3):381–385.
11. Anderson RU, Wise D, Sawyer T, et al. 6-day intensive treatment protocol for refractory chronic prostatitis/chronic pelvic pain syndrome using myofascial release and paradoxical relaxation training. *J Urol*. 2011;185(4):1294–1299.

SEE ALSO

- Prostate Cancer; Prostatic Hyperplasia Benign (BPH); Urinary Tract Infection (UTI) in Males
- Algorithm: Hematuria

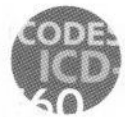

CODES

ICD10

- N41.9 Inflammatory disease of prostate, unspecified
- N41.0 Acute prostatitis
- N41.1 Chronic prostatitis

CLINICAL PEARLS

- Prostatic massage is contraindicated in acute prostatitis.
- Antibiotic therapy is not proven to be effective in chronic abacterial prostatitis (NIH class III).
- At least 30 days of antibiotic therapy is required for acute prostatitis.

PROTEIN C DEFICIENCY

Maissaa Janbain, MD • Rebecca Kruse-Jarres, MD, MPH

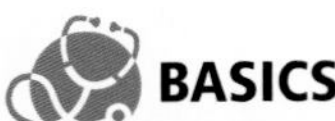

BASICS

DESCRIPTION

- Protein C is a vitamin K–dependent factor made by the liver that becomes activated when thrombin binds to the endothelial receptor thrombomodulin.
- Activated protein C, with protein S as a cofactor, inactivates factors Va and VIIIa.
- Patients with protein C deficiency have a thrombotic disorder that primarily affects the venous system but can also affect the arterial system.
- System(s) affected: cardiovascular, hemic/lymphatic/ immunologic, pulmonary

EPIDEMIOLOGY

Prevalence

- 0.3% of normal individuals
- 4–5% of persons with venous thrombosis (VT)
- Predominant age: Mean age of first thrombosis is 45 years.
- Predominant sex: male = female

ETIOLOGY AND PATHOPHYSIOLOGY

- Polymorphisms in the promoter region of the protein C gene can affect antigen levels. At least 150 mutations have been described in the protein C gene that can lead to functional deficiency.
- New mutations have been described associated with late-onset cerebral thrombosis (1).
- Acquired protein C deficiency can occur with liver disease, ARDS, DIC, chemotherapy with L-asparaginase, 5-FU, methotrexate, and cyclophosphamide, as well as postoperative state and severe infections, especially meningococcemia. Also, rare patients can develop inhibitors to activated protein C. Neonates have lower levels of protein C than adults.

Genetics

Patients heterozygous for protein C deficiency who start warfarin without concomitant heparin can develop warfarin-induced skin necrosis because the half-life of other vitamin K–dependent clotting factors, prothrombin, factor IX, and factor X is much longer than that of protein C (4–8 hours). These patients develop extremely low levels of protein C and subsequently increased thrombin generation, leading to necrosis of the skin over central areas of the body such as the breast, abdomen, buttocks, and genitalia (2)[A].

GENERAL PREVENTION

Because protein C deficiency is a congenital disease, there are no preventive measures.

COMMONLY ASSOCIATED CONDITIONS

- Deep and superficial venous thrombosis, often spontaneous
- Up to 50% of homozygotes will have thrombosis.
- Homozygosity is associated with catastrophic thrombotic complications at birth (e.g., *purpura fulminans*)
- Sites of thrombosis can be unusual, including the mesentery and cerebral veins, especially when combined with other risk factors such as oral contraceptives.
- Arterial thrombosis is rare.
- Skin necrosis can be seen in patients on warfarin.
- Recurrent pregnancy losses

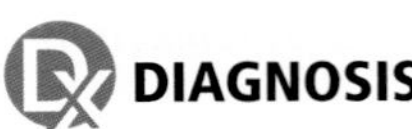

DIAGNOSIS

HISTORY

- VT at <40 years of age without another etiology
- Thrombosis in unusual locations (e.g., mesentery, sagittal sinus, portal vein)
- Family history of thrombosis or spontaneous abortion

PHYSICAL EXAM

Normal

DIFFERENTIAL DIAGNOSIS

- Factor V Leiden (causes resistance to activated protein C, not a deficiency of protein C)
- Protein S deficiency
- Antithrombin deficiency
- Dysfibrinogenemia
- Dysplasminogenemia
- Homocystinemia
- Prothrombin 20210 mutation
- Elevated factor VIII levels

DIAGNOSTIC TESTS & INTERPRETATION

Initial Tests (lab, imaging)

- For evaluation of new clot in patient at risk (see "History"): CBC with peripheral smear, PT/INR, aPTT, thrombin time, lupus anticoagulant, antiphospholipid antibodies, factor VIII, anticardiolipin antibody, anti-β_2-glycoprotein I antibody, activated protein C resistance, protein S antigen and resistance, antithrombin III assay, fibrinogen, factor V Leiden, prothrombin G20210A, homocysteine
- Protein C activity assay using a snake venom protease to activate protein C
- Immunoassay for quantitative assessment of protein C level
- Drugs that may alter lab results
  - Oral contraceptives can raise protein C levels.
  - Warfarin reduces protein C levels.
  - Patients should be off warfarin for 2–3 weeks before reliable testing (3)[C].
- Disorders that may alter lab results
  - Liver disease reduces protein C levels.

ALERT

Acute thrombosis can lower protein C levels. Repeat confirmatory test of low protein C level at a separate time is advisable. If a normal level of protein C is obtained at presentation, then deficiency can be excluded.

TREATMENT

Treat active thrombosis; follow-up.

GENERAL MEASURES

- Routine anticoagulation for asymptomatic patients with protein C deficiency is not recommended (2)[A].
- Anticoagulation for 6–12 months is recommended for patients with protein C deficiency and a first thrombosis.
- Some argue for lifetime anticoagulation; data are limited.
- Anticoagulation for life is indicated for patients with protein C deficiency and recurrent thromboses.
- The role of family screening for protein C deficiency is unclear because most patients with this mutation do not have thrombosis. Screening should be considered for women considering using oral contraceptives or pregnancy and who have a family history of protein C deficiency (4)[B].
- Treatment with LMWH is recommended over unfractionated heparin, unless the patient has severe renal failure (5)[B].
- Treat as outpatient, if possible (5)[B].
- Initiate warfarin together with LMWH on the first treatment day and discontinue LMWH after minimum of 5 days and two consecutive INRs >2 (5)[A].
- For pregnant women with no prior history of venous thromboembolism (VTE), we suggest antepartum and postpartum clinical vigilance. Postpartum prophylaxis for 6 weeks with prophylactic- or intermediate-dose LMWH is reserved only for patients with positive family history of VTE (3)[C],(5).

P

MEDICATION

First Line

- Low-molecular-weight heparin (LMWH) (2)[A]: initially for a minimum of 5 days and 2 consecutive INRs between 2 and 3
  - Enoxaparin (Lovenox) 1 mg/kg SC BID or enoxaparin 1.5 mg/kg/day SC
  - Tinzaparin (Innohep): 175 anti-Xa IU/kg/day SC
  - Dalteparin (Fragmin) 200 units/kg/day
- Factor Xa inhibitors
  - Fondaparinux (Arixtra) <50 kg: 5 mg/day SC; 50–100 kg: 7.5 mg/day SC; >100 kg: 10 mg/day SC; contraindicated if CrCl <30 mL/min
- Oral anticoagulant: warfarin (Coumadin), per the most recent Chest guidelines, 5 mg/day PO then adjusted to an INR of 2–3 for at least 3–6 months (2)[A],(5).
- Contraindications
  - Active bleeding precludes anticoagulation; risk of bleeding is a relative contraindication to long-term anticoagulation.
  - Warfarin is contraindicated in patients with a prior history of warfarin-induced skin necrosis.
- Precautions
  - Observe patient for signs of embolization, further thrombosis, or bleeding.
  - Avoid IM injections.
  - Periodically, check stool and urine for occult blood; monitor CBC, including platelets.
  - Heparin: thrombocytopenia and/or paradoxical thrombosis with thrombocytopenia
  - Warfarin: necrotic skin lesions (typically breasts, thighs, and buttocks)
  - LMWH: Adjust dose in renal insufficiency.
- Significant possible interactions
  - Agents that intensify the response to oral anticoagulants: alcohol, allopurinol, amiodarone, anabolic steroids, androgens, many antimicrobials, cimetidine, chloral hydrate, disulfiram, all NSAIDs, sulfinpyrazone, tamoxifen, thyroid hormone, vitamin E, ranitidine, salicylates, acetaminophen
  - Agents that diminish the response to oral anticoagulants: aminoglutethimide, antacids, barbiturates, carbamazepine, cholestyramine, diuretics, griseofulvin, rifampin, oral contraceptives

Second Line

- Heparin 80 mg/kg IV bolus followed by 18 mg/kg/hr; adjust dose depending on PPT.
- In patients requiring large daily doses of heparin, measure an anti-Xa level for dose guidance.
- Alternatively, and for outpatients, unfractionated heparin can be given at 333 units/kg then 250 units/kg SC, without monitoring (5)[C].

ISSUES FOR REFERRAL

Patients with suspected protein C deficiency should be seen by a hematologist.

However, screening and therefore prophylactic treatment of asymptomatic family members is not justified. (6)

SURGERY/OTHER PROCEDURES

- Anticoagulation must be held for surgical interventions.
- In patients with acute proximal DVT of the leg *and* an absolute contraindication to anticoagulation, inferior vena cava (IVC) filters are recommended; otherwise the use of an IVC filter in addition to anticoagulants is not recommended in most patients with acute DVT of the leg (2)[B],(5).

INPATIENT CONSIDERATIONS

Admission Criteria/Initial Stabilization

- Life-threatening VT
- Significant bleeding while on anticoagulant therapy

Nursing

Look for signs of bleeding while on anticoagulation therapy.

ONGOING CARE

FOLLOW-UP RECOMMENDATIONS

Patient Monitoring

- Warfarin requires periodic (monthly after initial stabilization) monitoring of the INR to maintain a range of 2–3.
- LMWH is the treatment of choice in pregnancy. Periodic monitoring with anti-Xa levels is recommended in these patients.

DIET

Unrestricted

PATIENT EDUCATION

- Patients should be educated about use of oral anticoagulant therapy if taking such.
- Avoid NSAIDs while on warfarin.

PROGNOSIS

- When compared with normal individuals, persons with protein C deficiency have normal life spans.
- By age 45 years, 50% of the people heterozygous for protein C deficiency will have VT; half will be spontaneous.

COMPLICATIONS

Recurrent thrombosis (requires indefinite anticoagulation)

REFERENCES

1. Yang LH, Wang MS, Zheng FX, et al. Different impact of two mutations of a novel compound heterozygous protein C deficiency with late onset thrombosis. *Genet Mol Res*. 2014;13(2): 2969–2977.
2. Bick RL. Prothrombin G20210A mutation, antithrombin, heparin cofactor II, protein C, and protein S defects. *Hematol Oncol Clin North Am*. 2003;17(1):9–36.
3. Moll S. Thrombophilias—practical implications and testing caveats. *J Thromb Thrombolysis*. 2006;21(1):7–15.
4. Langlois NJ, Wells PS. Risk of venous thromboembolism in relatives of symptomatic probands with thrombophilia: a systematic review. *Thromb Haemost*. 2003;90(1):17–26.
5. Guyatt GH, Akl EA, Crowther M, et al. Executive summary: antithrombotic therapy and prevention of thrombosis, 9th ed: American College of Chest Physicians evidence-based clinical practice guidelines. *Chest*. 2012;141(2 Suppl):7S–47S.
6. Hornsby LB, Armstrong EM, Bellone JM, et al. Thrombophilia screening. *J Pharm Pract*. 2014;27(3):253–259.

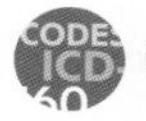

CODES

ICD10

D68.59 Other primary thrombophilia

CLINICAL PEARLS

- Asymptomatic patients with protein C deficiency do not need prophylactic anticoagulation because the risk of thrombosis is low (6).
- Patients with protein C deficiency who have DVT should be anticoagulated for at least 6 months.

PROTEIN S DEFICIENCY

Maissaa Janbain, MD • Rebecca Kruse-Jarres, MD, MPH

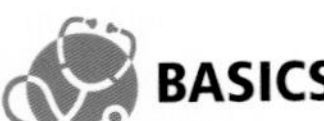

BASICS

DESCRIPTION

- Protein S is a vitamin K–dependent factor made principally by the liver that acts as a cofactor for protein C.
- Protein C becomes activated when thrombin binds to the endothelial receptor, thrombomodulin.
- Activated protein C, with protein S as a cofactor, inactivates clotting factors Va and VIIIa, and it enhances fibrinolysis.
- Protein S is also able to directly inhibit factors Va, VIIa, and Xa independently of activated protein C.
- Patients with protein S deficiency have a thrombotic disorder that primarily affects the venous system.
- System(s) affected: cardiovascular, hematologic/lymphatic/immunologic, pulmonary

EPIDEMIOLOGY

Incidence

- Predominant age: Mean age of 1st thrombosis is the 2nd decade.
- Predominant sex: male = female

Prevalence

- 0.3% of normal individuals
- Found in 3% of persons with VT

ETIOLOGY AND PATHOPHYSIOLOGY

- >131 mutations in the protein S gene leading to an inherited protein S deficiency have been described. Protein S reversibly binds to the C4b-binding protein. Only the free form acts as a cofactor for activated protein C. This leads to conditions in which free protein S is low, but total protein S is normal. These individuals are prone to thrombosis.
- Acquired protein S deficiency from decreased free protein S can occur during pregnancy; in patients taking oral contraceptives or warfarin; and in DIC, liver disease, nephrotic syndrome, inflammation, L-asparaginase chemotherapy, and acute thrombosis.
- Transient autoantibodies can develop to protein S in patients with acute varicella (1)[C].

Genetics

Autosomal dominant. Heterozygotes have an odds ratio (OR) of venous thrombosis (VT) of 1.6–11.5. Arterial thrombosis is more frequent in patients with protein S deficiency who smoke. Homozygotes can have a fulminant thrombotic event in infancy, termed *neonatal purpura fulminans*. Homozygosity or compound heterozygosity, if untreated, is usually incompatible with adult life.

RISK FACTORS

- Oral contraceptives, pregnancy, and the use of HRT increase the risk of VT in patients with protein S deficiency (2)[A].
- Patients with protein S deficiency and another prothrombotic state, such as factor V Leiden, have further increased rates of thrombosis (2)[A].
- Patients heterozygous for protein S deficiency who are initiated on warfarin without concomitant heparin can develop warfarin-induced skin necrosis because the half-life of other vitamin K–dependent clotting factors (e.g., prothrombin, factor IX, and factor X) is much longer than the anticoagulant protein S (4–8 hours), leading to a transient hypercoagulable state when protein S becomes depleted. These patients develop extremely low levels of protein S and develop necrosis of the skin over central areas of the body such as the breast, abdomen, buttocks, and genitalia (2)[A].

Pregnancy Considerations

Increased thrombotic risk in patients with protein C deficiency

GENERAL PREVENTION

Because protein S deficiency is a congenital disease, there are no preventive measures.

COMMONLY ASSOCIATED CONDITIONS

- Deep and superficial VT, often spontaneous
- Up to 50% of homozygotes will have thrombosis.
- Homozygosity is associated with catastrophic thrombotic complications at birth: *neonatal purpura fulminans*.
- Sites of thrombosis can be unusual, including the mesentery, cerebral veins, and axillary veins.
- Arterial thrombosis is rare but reported in several case reports.
- Skin necrosis can be seen in patients on warfarin.
- Recurrent pregnancy losses (3)

DIAGNOSIS

HISTORY

Order testing for patients with VT at age <40 years without another etiology; thrombosis in unusual locations (e.g., mesentery, sagittal sinus, portal vein) with a family history of thrombosis or spontaneous abortion

PHYSICAL EXAM

Normal

DIFFERENTIAL DIAGNOSIS

- Factor V Leiden
- Protein C deficiency
- Antithrombin deficiency
- Dysfibrinogenemia
- Dysplasminogenemia
- Homocystinemia
- Prothrombin 20210 mutation
- Elevated factor VIII levels

DIAGNOSTIC TESTS & INTERPRETATION

Initial Tests (lab, imaging)

- For evaluation of new clot in patient at risk: CBC with peripheral smear, PT/INR, aPTT, thrombin time, lupus anticoagulant, antiphospholipid antibodies, factor VIII, anticardiolipin antibody, anti-β_2-glycoprotein I antibody, activated protein C resistance, protein S antigen and resistance, antithrombin III assay, fibrinogen, factor V Leiden, prothrombin G20210A, homocysteine
- Protein S activity assay (mainly after obtaining APC resistance)
- Immunoassay for quantitative assessment of total and free protein S levels
- Disorders that may alter lab results: Liver disease and pregnancy reduce protein S levels.
- Total protein S levels are markedly decreased in newborns and young infants; use age-adjusted norms.

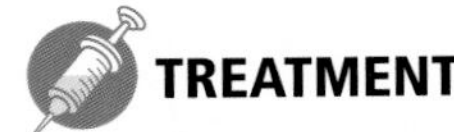

TREATMENT

GENERAL MEASURES

- Routine anticoagulation for asymptomatic patients with protein S deficiency is not recommended (2)[A].
- Anticoagulation for 6–12 months is recommended for patients with protein S deficiency and a 1st thrombosis.
- Some argue for lifetime anticoagulation; data are limited.
- Anticoagulation for life is indicated for patients with protein S deficiency and recurrent thrombosis.
- The role of family screening for protein S deficiency is unclear because most patients with this mutation do not have thrombosis. Screening should be considered for women considering using oral contraceptives or pregnancy, and who have a family history of protein S deficiency (4)[B].
- Treatment of thrombosis with low-molecular-weight heparin (LMWH) is recommended over unfractionated heparin, unless the patient has severe renal failure (5)[B].

- Treat as outpatient, if possible (5)[B].
- Initiate warfarin together with LMWH on the 1st treatment day, and discontinue LMWH after a minimum of 5 days and two consecutive INRs >2 (5)[A].

- For pregnant women with no prior history of VTE, we suggest antepartum and postpartum clinical vigilance. Postpartum prophylaxis is reserved for patients with positive family history only; in that case, we suggest prophylactic- or intermediate-dose LMWH for 6 weeks (1)[C],(5).

MEDICATION

First Line

- LMWH (2)[A] initially for a minimum of 5 days and two consecutive INRs between 2 and 3, at which time it can be stopped
  - Enoxaparin (Lovenox) 1 mg/kg SC BID:
    - Alternatively, 1.5 mg/kg/day SC.
  - Tinzaparin (Innohep) 175 anti-Xa IU/kg/day SC
  - Dalteparin (Fragmin) 200 IU/kg/day
- Factor Xa Inhibitor
  - Fondaparinux (Arixtra) <50 kg: 5 mg/day SC; 50-100 kg: 7.5 mg/day SC; >100 kg: 10 mg/day SC; contraindicated if CrCl <30 mL/min

- Oral anticoagulant: warfarin (Coumadin): 5 mg/day PO then adjusted to an INR of 2–3 for at least 6 months (5)[A]

- Contraindications
  - Active bleeding precludes anticoagulation; risk of bleeding is a relative contraindication to long-term anticoagulation.
  - Warfarin is contraindicated in patients with a prior history of warfarin-induced skin necrosis.
- Precautions
  - Observe patient for signs of embolization, further thrombosis, or bleeding.
  - Avoid IM injections.
  - Periodically, check stool and urine for occult blood; monitor CBC, including platelets.
  - Heparin: thrombocytopenia and/or paradoxical thrombosis with thrombocytopenia
  - Warfarin: necrotic skin lesions (typically breasts, thighs, and buttocks)
  - LMWH: Adjust dose in renal insufficiency.
- Significant possible interactions
  - Agents that intensify the response to oral anticoagulants: alcohol, allopurinol, amiodarone, anabolic steroids, androgens, many antimicrobials, cimetidine, chloral hydrate, disulfiram, all NSAIDs, sulfinpyrazone, tamoxifen, thyroid hormone, vitamin E, ranitidine, salicylates, acetaminophen
  - Agents that diminish the response to oral anticoagulants: aminoglutethimide, antacids, barbiturates, carbamazepine, cholestyramine, diuretics, griseofulvin, rifampin, oral contraceptives

Second Line

Heparin 80 mg/kg IV bolus, followed by 18 mg/kg/hr; adjust dose depending on aPTT:

- In patients requiring large daily doses of heparin, measure an anti-Xa level for dose guidance.
- Alternatively, in outpatients, unfractionated heparin can be given at 333 units/kg then 250 units/kg SC, without monitoring (5)[C].
- It does not alter plasma protein S concentration.

ISSUES FOR REFERRAL

- Patients with suspected protein S deficiency should be seen by a hematologist.
- Screening and prophylactic treatment of asymptomatic family members is not justified (6).

SURGERY/OTHER PROCEDURES

- Anticoagulation must be held for surgical interventions.

- For most patients with DVT, recommendations are against routine use of vena cava filter in addition to anticoagulation; IVC is only recommended in case of contraindication to anticoagulation (5)[A].

INPATIENT CONSIDERATIONS

Admission Criteria/Initial Stabilization

- Life-threatening VT
- Significant bleeding while on anticoagulant therapy

Nursing

Look for signs of bleeding while on anticoagulation therapy.

ONGOING CARE

FOLLOW-UP RECOMMENDATIONS

Patient Monitoring

- Warfarin requires periodic (monthly after initial stabilization) monitoring of the INR.
- Periodic measurement of INR to maintain a range of 2–3
- LMWH is the treatment of choice in pregnancy. Periodic monitoring with anti-Xa levels is recommended in some cases, such as overweight and borderline renal failure.

DIET

Unrestricted

PATIENT EDUCATION

- Patients should be educated about use of oral anticoagulant therapy if taking such.
- Avoid NSAIDs while on warfarin.

PROGNOSIS

- Persons with protein S deficiency have normal life spans.
- By age 45 years, 50% of the people heterozygous for protein S deficiency will have VT; half will be spontaneous.

COMPLICATIONS

Recurrent thrombosis (requires indefinite anticoagulation)

REFERENCES

1. Moll S. Thrombophilias–practical implications and testing caveats. *J Thromb Thrombolysis*. 2006;21(1):7–15.
2. Bick RL. Prothrombin G20210A mutation, antithrombin, heparin cofactor II, protein C, and protein S defects. *Hematol Oncol Clin North Am*. 2003;17(1):9–36.
3. Parand A, Zolghadri J, Nezam M. Inherited thrombophilia and recurrent pregnancy loss. *Iran Red Crescent Med J*. 2013;15(12):e13708.
4. Langlois NJ, Wells PS. Risk of venous thromboembolism in relatives of symptomatic probands with thrombophilia: a systematic review. *Thromb Haemost*. 2003;90:17–26.
5. Guyatt GH, Akl EA, Crowther M, et al. Executive summary: Antithrombotic Therapy and Prevention of Thrombosis, 9th ed: American College of Chest Physicians Evidence-Based Clinical Practice Guidelines. *Chest*. 2012;141(Suppl 2):7S–47S.
6. Hornsby LB, Armstrong EM, Bellone JM, et al. Thrombophilia screening. *J Pharm Pract*. 2014;27(3):253–259.

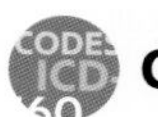

CODES

ICD10

D68.59 Other primary thrombophilia

CLINICAL PEARLS

- Asymptomatic patients with protein S deficiency do not require prophylactic anticoagulation because the risk of thrombosis is low; asymptomatic patients do not require anticoagulation (6).
- Patients with protein S deficiency and DVT should be anticoagulated for at least 6 months, especially if first episode.

PROTEIN-ENERGY MALNUTRITION

Robert A. Baldor, MD, FAAFP

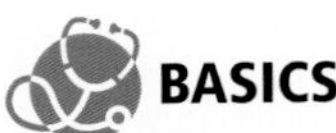

BASICS

DESCRIPTION

- Protein-energy malnutrition (PEM) is present when sufficient energy and/or protein is not available to meet metabolic demands, leading to impairment in normal physiologic processes. It is highly associated with systemic inflammation.
- Malnutrition in children is a major underlying factor in ~5 million preventable deaths annually, with 2 distinct phenotypes.
  - Marasmus: a wasting condition due to deficiency of calories and protein
  - Kwashiorkor: distinguished by generalized edema and ascites, associated with low protein relative to caloric intake
- System(s) affected: immunologic; gastrointestinal; endocrine/metabolic; hematologic; musculoskeletal; integumentary; neurologic

EPIDEMIOLOGY

- Children
  - Most commonly <5 years of age
  - Prevalent sex: males = females
  - Globally, malnutrition increases morbidity and mortality from other common childhood diseases.
- Older patients
  - Highest risk group >age 75 years, affecting 5–10% of nursing home residents and up to 50% of older patients on hospital discharge
  - Increased mortality and morbidity, including pressure ulcers, infection, and cognitive status changes
- Malnutrition may be common, but it is difficult to recognize in hospital populations.

Prevalence

- Worldwide, >70 million children suffer from moderate and severe acute malnutrition.
- Prevalence in older patients is between 29% and 61%.

ETIOLOGY AND PATHOPHYSIOLOGY

- Inadequate dietary intake
- Increased metabolic demands
- Increased nutrient losses

RISK FACTORS

- Starvation-related malnutrition
  - Prolonged and severe reduction of intake
  - Anorexia nervosa
- Mild to moderate inflammatory conditions
  - Chronic inflammatory states (rheumatoid arthritis, chronic cardiac or lung disease, and cancer)
  - Metabolic disorders (diabetes, hyperthyroidism)
  - Malabsorptive and maldigestive states (celiac disease and pancreatic insufficiency)
  - Protein-losing enteropathy, nephrotic syndrome, enteric fistulas
  - Sarcopenic obesity
- Marked inflammatory conditions: acute disease, fever, infection, trauma, burns, closed head injury
- Other states in which caloric requirements are increased: pregnancy and lactation, childhood growth and development

ALERT

- Functional, financial, and social factors may limit access to an adequate diet, particularly in geriatric and pediatric populations.
- Elders with delirium, dementia, or depression or long periods spent NPO or with prolonged hospitalization are at high risk for malnutrition.
- Extreme high or low BMI individuals are also at increased risk.

GENERAL PREVENTION

- Observation and recording of patients' nutritional intake and BMI
- In children, routine record of anthropomorphic measurements and developmental milestones
- Early recognition of increased nutritional requirements during stress, infection, and other medical illness
- Frequent interactions among physician, nurse, and dietitian to assess nutritional needs
- Emphasis on food security and nutritional education

COMMONLY ASSOCIATED CONDITIONS

- Infection: weakened immune system, predisposing to bacterial, viral, and parasitic infections
- Electrolyte disturbances: loss of cellular integrity, diminished transmembrane pump activity, renal dysfunction
- Hypoglycemia: decreased glycogen stores, increased glucose use (as in infection or trauma)
- Micronutrient deficiencies: vitamins, including B complex, folic acid, iron, magnesium
- Wounds: pressure ulcers in older patients (increased incidence if reduced mobility)

DIAGNOSIS

HISTORY

- Diagnostic historical criteria for malnutrition
  - Inadequate nutrient intake, based on estimated energy needs versus measured energy consumed (24-hour recall or calorie count)
  - Weight loss
- Presence of ≥2 diagnostic criteria (historical criteria above or exam criteria below) support the diagnosis of malnutrition (1)[C].
- Other historical features
  - GI tract disorders: early satiety, constipation, vomiting, diarrhea, dysphagia, dental and oral health problems
  - Decreased urine output (assess for dehydration)
  - Chronic medical illness
  - Impaired work capacity, endurance, and muscle strength
  - Falls and/or reduced physical activity
  - Impaired concentration/cognitive function, delirium, or lethargy
  - Delayed wound healing and recovery
  - In children: delayed puberty, diminished cognitive and psychosocial development
  - Medications that cause nausea, dry mouth, loss of appetite, or taste distortion

PHYSICAL EXAM

- Diagnostic exam criteria for malnutrition (1)[C]
  - Localized or generalized fluid accumulation
  - Loss of muscle mass or subcutaneous fat
  - Decreased handgrip strength
- Other possible features: glossitis, cheilosis, loss of vibratory or position sense, sparse hair, nail spooning, night blindness, Bitot spots, loss of taste (2)[C]
- Subnormal heart rate, BP, and core body temperature
- Anthropomorphic measurements
  - Weight (W) and height (H): In children, measure W:H; in adults, BMI <18.5 kg/m^2 in PEM.
  - Mid–upper arm circumference (MUAC): In adults, MUAC <200 mm is suggestive of PEM.
  - Triceps skin-fold thickness
- Bioelectrical impedance analysis to estimate total body water and fat-free body mass
- Marasmic children: thin, little subcutaneous fat; wasting at the shoulders, buttocks, arms, and thighs
- Children with Kwashiorkor are irritable, with anasarca, and sparse and brittle hair:
  - They can develop a "flaky paint" dermatosis characterized by blackish discoloration and excoriation.
  - Hepatomegaly from fatty infiltration may be present.

ALERT

- Commonly used markers of dehydration (dry mucous membranes, lack of tears, skin tenting) are not reliable in PEM.
- Poor immune function may make identification of superimposed infection difficult. Fevers, swelling, and redness are often absent.
- Fluid accumulation may mask weight loss (1)[C].

DIFFERENTIAL DIAGNOSIS

- In children, secondary growth failure due to malabsorption, congenital defects, or deprivation
- Pellagra (niacin deficiency = "4 Ds"): diarrhea, dermatitis, dementia, death
- Nephritis or nephrosis
- Hypo- or hyperthyroidism
- Hyperparathyroidism
- Cardiac failure
- Neoplasm
- Viral or parasitic infection

DIAGNOSTIC TESTS & INTERPRETATION

Initial Tests (lab, imaging)

- Pediatric patients
  - Serum chemistries: hypernatremia, hypokalemia, hypocalcemia, hypophosphatemia, hypomagnesemia
  - Hypoglycemia/hyperglycemia
  - Anemia, decreased lymphocyte count
  - BUN: decreased
  - Plasma transferrin: decreased
  - Plasma cortisol, growth hormone: increased, but insulin is low.
- Adult and elderly patients
  - Serum albumin and prealbumin, inflammatory markers, are affected by acute illness:
    - They do not correlate directly with nutritional status or improve with feeding interventions.
    - Lower albumin levels do, however, correlate with increased mortality.

- Serum prealbumin measures PEM risk level
  - Normal >15 mg/dL
  - Increased risk 5–10 mg/dL:
  - Significant risk <5 mg/dL: poor prognosis, high mortality
- Elevation of serum alkaline phosphatase and C-reactive protein
- Chest x-ray (CXR): evaluate for coexisting pneumonia, neoplasm, or tuberculosis. Cardiomegaly may be present from cardiac failure or marked anemia.

Follow-Up Tests & Special Considerations

In critically ill patients, blood glucose levels >180 mg/dL are associated with increased morbidity and mortality (3)[C].

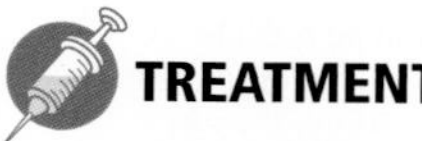

TREATMENT

GENERAL MEASURES

- Slowly restore and maintain fluid and electrolyte balance.
- Initiate oral iron and folate supplements (begin iron therapy ~2 weeks after initiation of dietary treatment to avoid promotion of bacterial infection).
- Administer blood transfusion in the presence of severe anemia (hemoglobin <4–6 g/dL) or symptomatic moderate anemia.
- Ensure that immunizations are up to date (PEM is not a contraindication to vaccination).

MEDICATION

- Diet prescription in conjunction with a dietician or nutritionist
- Appetite stimulants (e.g., megestrol acetate, mirtazapine, dronabinol, others) may be appropriate for short-term treatment of anorexia in adults, but megestrol may increase thromboembolic risk.
- Medications that have weight gain as a side effect (atypical antipsychotics, carbamazepine, gabapentin, corticosteroids, valproic acid, SSRIs, sulfonylureas, injectable medroxyprogesterone) may be used if otherwise indicated in patients with comorbid conditions.

ISSUES FOR REFERRAL

Consider dentistry referral for oral disorders and speech therapy referral for dysphagia.

INPATIENT CONSIDERATIONS

Admission Criteria/Initial Stabilization

- Hemodynamic instability
- Alteration of consciousness (delirium)
- Unsafe living environment (evidence of child/elder mistreatment)
- Profound hypokalemia or hypocalcemia
- Cardiac abnormalities/arrhythmia
- Anemia (hemoglobin <10 g/dL in older patients)
- Reversal of fluid and electrolyte imbalance should occur before IV nutrition, if any, is started.
- Continuous cardiac rhythm monitoring (telemetry) is recommended when electrolyte imbalance or acidosis is present.

IV Fluids

Parenteral (IV) nutrition, which carries a high risk of associated infection, should be reserved for use in patients with severe GI tract dysfunction or anatomic disturbance (3)[C].

Nursing

- Patients should be assessed for risk of pressure ulcer (using a Braden scale or other tool) and a skin care protocol initiated.
- Any patient admitted to the hospital with malnutrition should have a nutritionist consult, if available.
- Physical therapy should be initiated once the patient is stable for assessment.

Geriatric Considerations

Older patients may require assistance with basic activities of daily living (ADLs) and are at high risk of injury due to falls.

Discharge Criteria

- Basic electrolyte abnormalities corrected to tolerance
- Patient demonstrates ability to maintain adequate oral intake of a nutritionally sound diet.
- Social and financial considerations have been identified and addressed.

Geriatric Considerations

Patient may need transfer to alternative level of care (e.g., skilled nursing home, rehabilitation center) temporarily for continued care, depending on level of disability before returning safely home.

ONGOING CARE

FOLLOW-UP RECOMMENDATIONS

Children are discharged from a nutritional rehabilitation program when W:H ratio is >85%, at least 1 week of consistent weight gain has been achieved, and all disease conditions associated with PEM have been addressed.

Patient Monitoring

Frequent assessment until weight stabilized (BMI >18.5 kg/m^2)

DIET

- Slow refeeding of amino acid constituent and calorie-to-BMI-adjusted diet, in consultation with a nutritionist/dietician
- For children, initiate 100 kcal/kg/day with 3 g/kg/day protein. When tolerated, advance to at least 200 kcal/kg/day with 5 g/kg/day protein.
  - Small, frequent feedings are preferred.
  - Consider low-lactose formulas to decrease diarrhea from disaccharidase deficiency.
  - Target growth: 10–15 g/kg/day
  - Supplement with vitamins and micronutrients, especially vitamin A and zinc.

PATIENT EDUCATION

- Emphasis on diet education
- In older patients, caregiver education and supervision may be relevant.

PROGNOSIS

- Excellent when PEM is identified early and managed aggressively.
- Mortality varies between 15% and 40%.
- Compromised immune function returns to normal with recovery.
- Behavioral and mental issues may persist following treatment of severe cases.
- Insufficient evidence indicates that enteral tube feeding in patients with advanced dementia improves survival or lowers the prevalence of pressure ulcers.

COMPLICATIONS

- Fatalities in the early days of treatment usually result from electrolyte imbalance, infection, hypothermia, or circulatory failure. Lethargy, anorexia, stupor, and petechiae are ominous signs.
- Patients who develop PEM have greater risk of hospital-acquired infection.

Pregnancy Considerations

Pregnant women with PEM are at risk of delivering a growth-restricted infant.

REFERENCES

1. White JV, Guenter P, Jensen G, et al. Consensus statement: Academy of Nutrition and Dietetics and American Society for Parenteral and Enteral Nutrition: characteristics recommended for the identification and documentation of adult malnutrition (undernutrition). *JPEN J Parenter Enteral Nutr*. 2012;36(3):275–283.
2. Ziegler TR. Parenteral nutrition in the critically ill patient. *N Engl J Med*. 2009;361(11):1088–1097.
3. Sampson EL, Candy B, Jones L. Enteral tube feeding for older people with advanced dementia. *Cochrane Database Syst Rev*. 2009;(2):CD007209.

ADDITIONAL READING

- Morley JE. Undernutrition in older adults. *Fam Pract*. 2012;29(Suppl 1):i89–i93.
- Soeters PB, Schols AM. Advances in understanding and assessing malnutrition. *Curr Opin Clin Nutr Metab Care*. 2009;12(5):487–494.
- Ziegler TR. Parenteral nutrition in the critically ill patient. *N Engl J Med*. 2009;361(11):1088–1097.

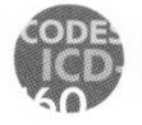

CODES

ICD10

- E46 Unspecified protein-calorie malnutrition
- E41 Nutritional marasmus
- E40 Kwashiorkor

CLINICAL PEARLS

- Older patients may experience elevated BUN levels from excessive protein supplementation; routine monitoring is suggested.
- Decreased muscle mass in patients with malnutrition may lower creatinine level and lead to overestimation of the glomerular filtration rate.
- Malnourished patients have a higher risk of toxicity from fat-soluble or protein-bound drugs due to weight loss and decrease in albumin.

PROTEINURIA

Andrew Allegretti, MD

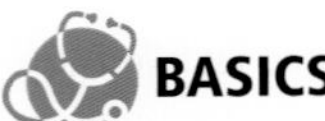

BASICS

DESCRIPTION

Urinary protein excretion of >150 mg/day

- Nephrotic-range proteinuria: urinary protein excretion of >3.5 g/day; also called *heavy proteinuria*
- 3 pathologic types:
  - Glomerular proteinuria: increased permeability of proteins across glomerular capillary membrane
  - Tubular proteinuria: decreased proximal tubular reabsorption of proteins
  - Overflow proteinuria: increased production of low-molecular-weight proteins

Pediatric Considerations

- Proteinuria: Normal is daily excretion of up to 100 mg/m^2 (body surface area).
- Nephrotic-range proteinuria: daily excretion of >1,000 mg/m^2 (body surface area)

Pregnancy Considerations

- Proteinuria in pregnancy beyond 20 weeks' gestation is a hallmark of preeclampsia/eclampsia and demands further workup.
- Proteinuria in pregnancy before 20 weeks' gestation is suggestive of underlying renal disease.

ETIOLOGY AND PATHOPHYSIOLOGY

- Glomerular proteinuria: increased filtration/larger proteins (albumin) due to the following:
  - Increased size of glomerular basement membrane pores and
  - Loss of proteoglycan negative charge barrier
- Tubular proteinuria: Tubulointerstitial disease prevents proximal tubular reabsorption of smaller proteins (β_2-microglobulin, immunoglobulin [Ig] light chains, retinol-binding protein, amino acids).
- Overflow proteinuria: proximal tubular reabsorption overwhelmed by increased production of smaller proteins
- Glomerular proteinuria
  - Primary glomerulonephropathy
    - Minimal-change disease
    - Idiopathic membranous glomerulonephritis
    - Focal segmental glomerulonephritis
    - Membranoproliferative glomerulonephritis
    - IgA nephropathy
  - Secondary glomerulonephropathy
    - Diabetic nephropathy
    - Autoimmune/collagen vascular disorders (e.g., lupus nephritis, Goodpasture syndrome)
    - Amyloidosis
    - Preeclampsia
    - Infection (HIV, hepatitis B and C, poststreptococcal, endocarditis, syphilis, malaria)
    - Malignancy (GI, lung, lymphoma)
    - Renal transplant rejection
    - Structural (reflux nephropathy, polycystic kidney disease)
    - Drug-induced (NSAIDs, penicillamine, lithium, heavy metals, gold, heroin)
- Tubular proteinuria
  - Hypertensive nephrosclerosis
  - Tubulointerstitial disease (uric acid nephropathy, hypersensitivity, interstitial nephritis, Fanconi syndrome, heavy metals, sickle cell disease, NSAIDs, antibiotics)
  - Acute tubular necrosis
- Overflow proteinuria
  - Multiple myeloma (light chains; also tubulotoxic)
  - Hemoglobinuria
  - Myoglobinuria (in rhabdomyolysis)
  - Lysozyme (in acute monocytic leukemia)
- Benign proteinuria
  - Functional (fever, exercise, cold exposure, stress, CHF)
  - Idiopathic transient
  - Orthostasis (postural)

RISK FACTORS

- Hypertension
- Diabetes
- Obesity
- Strenuous exercise
- CHF
- UTI
- Fever

Genetics

No known genetic pattern

GENERAL PREVENTION

Control of weight, BP, and blood glucose reduces the risk of proteinuria.

COMMONLY ASSOCIATED CONDITIONS

- Hypertension (common)
- Diabetes mellitus (common)
- Preeclampsia (common)
- Multiple myeloma (rare)

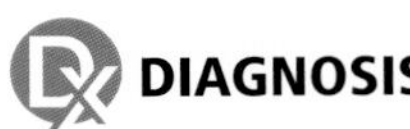

DIAGNOSIS

HISTORY

- Frothy/foamy urine
- Change in urine output
- Blood- or cola-colored urine
- Recent weight change
- Swelling
- Rule out systemic illness: diabetes, heart failure, autoimmune, poststreptococcal infection

PHYSICAL EXAM

- BP
- Weight
- Peripheral edema
- Periorbital/facial edema
- Ascites
- Palpation of kidneys
- Check lungs, heart for signs of CHF

DIFFERENTIAL DIAGNOSIS

Includes all causes listed under "Etiology and Pathophysiology"

DIAGNOSTIC TESTS & INTERPRETATION

Screening for proteinuria is not cost-effective unless directed at groups with hypertension/diabetes, older persons, and so forth.

Initial Tests (lab, imaging)

- Urinalysis (UA) quantitatively estimates proteinuria:
  - Only sensitive to albumin; will not detect smaller proteins of overflow/tubular etiologies
  - False-positive finding if urine pH >7, highly concentrated (specific gravity [SG] >1.015), gross hematuria, mucus, semen, leukocytes, iodinated contrast agents, penicillin analogues, sulfonamide metabolites
  - False-negative finding if urine is dilute (SG 1.005), albumin excretion <20–30 mg/dL, protein is nonalbumin
  - Sensitivity, 32–46%; specificity, 97–100%
  - Also can perform sulfosalicylic acid test to detect nonalbumin protein
- If UA positive, perform urine microscopy. Refer to nephrologist if positive for signs of glomerular disease.
- If UA shows trace to 2+ protein, rule out transient proteinuria with repeat UA at another visit:
  - More common than persistent proteinuria
  - Causes include exercise, fever, CHF, UTI, and cold exposure
  - Reassure patient that transient proteinuria is benign and requires no further workup.
- If initial UA shows 3+ to 4+ protein or repeat UA is positive, measure creatinine clearance and quantify proteinuria with 24-hour urine collection (gold standard) or spot urine protein-to-creatinine (P/C) ratio (acceptable practice) (1)[A]:
  - Numerical P/C ratios correlate with total protein excreted in grams per day (i.e., ratio of 0.2 correlates with 0.2 g during a 24-hour collection).
  - Patients age <30 years with 24-hour urine excretion of <2 g/day and normal creatinine clearance should be tested for orthostatic proteinuria:
    - Benign condition is present in 2–5% of adolescents.
    - Diagnosed with a normal urine P/C ratio in 1st morning void and an elevated urine P/C ratio in a 2nd specimen taken after standing for several hours
- If protein excretion >2 g/day, consider nephrology referral and begin workup for systemic/renal disease.
- Patients with persistent proteinuria not explained by orthostatic changes should undergo renal ultrasound to rule out structural abnormalities (e.g., reflux nephropathy, polycystic kidney).

Follow-Up Tests & Special Considerations

Renal/systemic disease workup can include the following:

- CBC, ferritin, ESR, serum iron
- Electrolytes, LFTs
- Lipid profile (ideally, fasting)
- Prothrombin time/international normalized ratio
- Antinuclear antibodies: elevated in lupus
- Antistreptolysin O titer: elevated after streptococcal glomerulonephritis

- Complement C3/C4: low in most glomerulonephritis
- HIV, syphilis, and hepatitis serologies: all associated with glomerular proteinuria
- Serum and urine protein electrophoresis: abnormal in multiple myeloma
- Blood glucose: elevated in diabetes
- All patients with diabetes should be screened for microalbuminuria.
- Patients with nephrotic-range proteinuria are at increased risk for hypercholesterolemia and thromboembolic events (~25% of adult patients) with highest risk in membranous nephropathy. Optimal duration of prophylactic anticoagulation is unknown but may extend for the duration of the nephrotic state (2).
- Proteinuric pregnant patients beyond 20 weeks' gestation should be examined for other signs/symptoms of preeclampsia (e.g., hypertension, thrombocytopenia, elevated liver transaminases).

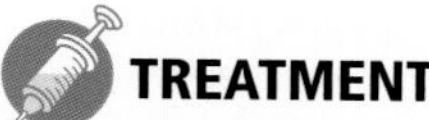

TREATMENT

- BP goals for both diabetic and nondiabetic adults is ≤140/90 mm Hg (3)[C].
- Proteinuria goal is <0.5 g/day (4)[A].

GENERAL MEASURES

- Limit protein intake to 0.8 g/kg/day in adults with DM or without DM and glomerular filtration rate (GFR) <30 mL/min/1.73 m^2. Soy protein may be renoprotective. Monitor protein intake with 24-hour urine urea excretion (4)[A].
- Limit sodium chloride intake to <2 g/day to optimize antiproteinuric medications (3)[B]. Effect on BP is further protective (4)[A].
- Limit fluid intake for urine output goal of <2 L/day. Larger urine volumes are associated with increased proteinuria and later GFR decline (4)[B].
- Smoking cessation: Smoking is associated with increased proteinuria and faster kidney disease progression (4)[B].
- Encourage supine posture (up to 50% reduction vs. upright) (4)[B].
- Discourage severe exertion (4)[B].
- Encourage weight loss (4)[B].

MEDICATION

First Line

- ACE inhibitors: 1st choice; use maximally tolerated doses; use even if normotensive (4)[A]
- Angiotensin receptor blockers (ARBs): proven antiproteinuric and renoprotective; ARBs are 1st choice if ACE inhibitors are not tolerated (4)[A].
- Combination ACE inhibitor and ARB should not be used. Although shown to reduce proteinuria, combination does not reduce poor CV outcomes and does increase risk of adverse drug reactions (5,6)[A].

Second Line

- β-Blockers: antiproteinuric and cardioprotective (4)[A]
- Dihydropyridine calcium channel blockers (DHCCBs): should be avoided unless needed for BP control; not antiproteinuric (4)[A]
- Non-DHCCB: antiproteinuric, may be renoprotective (4)[B]
- Aldosterone antagonists: antiproteinuric independent of BP control (4)[B]
- NSAIDs: antiproteinuric, but also nephrotoxic; generally should be avoided (4)[C]

ISSUES FOR REFERRAL

Consider nephrology referral for possible renal biopsy if

- Impaired creatinine clearance
- Nephrotic-range proteinuria
- Unclear etiology of nonnephrotic-range proteinuria
- Diabetics with microalbuminuria

COMPLEMENTARY & ALTERNATIVE MEDICINE

- Corticosteroids: No proven benefit in mortality or need for renal replacement in adults with nephrotic syndrome, although steroids are recommended in some patients who do not respond to conservative treatment. Classically, children with nephrotic syndrome respond better than adults, especially those with minimal-change disease (7)[A].
- Estrogen/progesterone replacement: may be renoprotective in premenopausal women but should be avoided in postmenopausal women (4)[B]
- Antioxidant therapy: may be antiproteinuric in diabetic nephropathy (4)[C]
- Sodium bicarbonate: not antiproteinuric but may block tubular injury caused by proteinuria; correcting metabolic acidosis may decrease protein catabolism (4)[C].
- Avoid excessive caffeine consumption: antiproteinuric in diabetic rat models 4)[C]
- Avoid iron overload (4)[C].
- Pentoxifylline: prevents progression of renal disease by unclear mechanisms (4)[C]
- Mycophenolate mofetil: antiproteinuric and renoprotective in animal models (4)[C]

ONGOING CARE

FOLLOW-UP RECOMMENDATIONS

Patient Monitoring

All patients with persistent proteinuria should be followed with serial BP checks, UA, and renal function tests in the outpatient setting. Intervals depend on underlying etiology.

PROGNOSIS

- Transient and orthostatic proteinuria are benign conditions that do not convey a poor prognosis.
- Clinical significance of persistent proteinuria varies greatly and depends on underlying etiology.
- Degree of proteinuria is associated with disease progression in chronic kidney disease.
- Independent of GFR, higher levels of proteinuria likely convey an increased risk of mortality, myocardial infarction, and progression to kidney failure (8).

COMPLICATIONS

- Progression to chronic renal failure and the need for dialysis/renal transplant
- Hypercholesterolemia
- Hypercoagulable state

REFERENCES

1. National Kidney Foundation. K/DOQI clinical practice guidelines for chronic kidney disease: evaluation classification, and stratification: guideline 5. Assessment of proteinuria. http://www2.kidney.org/professionals/KDOQI/guidelines_ckd/toc.htm. Accessed 2014.
2. Kerlin BA, Ayoob R, Smoyer WE. Epidemiology and pathophysiology of nephrotic syndrome-associated thromboembolic disease. *Clin J Am Soc Nephrol*. 2012;7(3):513–520.
3. James PA, Oparil S, Carter BL, et al. 2014 evidence-based guideline for the management of high blood pressure in adults: report from the panel members appointed to the Eighth Joint National Committee (JNC 8). *JAMA*. 2014;311(5):507–520.
4. Wilmer WA, Rovin BH, Hebert CJ, et al. Management of glomerular proteinuria: a commentary. *J Am Soc Nephrol*. 2003;14(12):3217–3232.
5. Fried LF, Emanuele N, Zhang JH, et al. Combined angiotensin inhibition for the treatment of diabetic nephropathy. *N Engl J Med*. 2013;369(20):1892–1903.
6. ONTARGET Investigators, Yusuf S, Teo KK, et al. Telmisartan, ramipril, or both in patients at high risk for vascular events. *N Engl J Med*. 2008; 358(15):1547–1559.
7. Kodner C. Nephrotic syndrome in adults: diagnosis and management. *Am Fam Physician*. 2009;80(10):1129–1134.
8. Tonelli M, Muntner P, Lloyd A, et al. Using proteinuria and estimated glomerular filtration rate to classify risk in patients with chronic kidney disease: a cohort study. *Ann Intern Med*. 2011;154(1):12–21.

CODES

ICD10

- R80.9 Proteinuria, unspecified
- R80.2 Orthostatic proteinuria, unspecified
- R80.1 Persistent proteinuria, unspecified

CLINICAL PEARLS

- Transient and orthostatic proteinuria are benign conditions that do not convey a poor prognosis.
- Proteinuria >2 g/day likely represents glomerular malfunction and warrants a nephrology consultation.
- Clinical course varies greatly but, in general, the degree of proteinuria correlates with kidney disease progression.
- First-line therapy for persistent proteinuric patients is a high-dose ACE inhibitor.

PROTHROMBIN 20210 (MUTATION)

Maissaa Janbain, MD • Rebecca Kruse-Jarres, MD, MPH

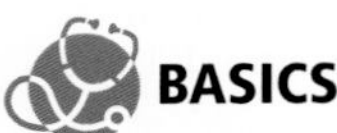

BASICS

DESCRIPTION

- Prothrombin 20210 mutation is the 2nd most common inherited risk factor for venous thromboembolism after factor V Leiden mutation.
- Polymorphism (replacement of G by A) in the 3′ untranslated end of the prothrombin gene causes increased translation, resulting in elevated synthesis and secretion of prothrombin. This leads to a 2.8-fold increased risk for venous thrombosis.
- System(s) affected: cardiovascular; hemic/lymphatic/immunologic; nervous; pulmonary; reproductive
- Synonym(s): prothrombin G20210A mutation; prothrombin G20210 gene polymorphism; prothrombin gene mutation; FII A^{20210} mutation

EPIDEMIOLOGY

- Found largely in Caucasian populations. Found in 2–5% of European and Middle Eastern populations, but rarely in nonwhites. Found in 4–8% of persons with venous thromboembolism and in up to 18% of patients with recurrent thrombosis.
- Predominant age: Mean age of 1st thrombosis is in the 2nd decade.
- Predominant gender: male = female

Prevalence

3–5% of the population

ETIOLOGY AND PATHOPHYSIOLOGY

- Replacement of G for A in the 3′ untranslated region of the prothrombin gene resulting in relatively higher plasma prothrombin activity, leading to increased risk for venous thrombosis
- Gene mutation

Genetics

Autosomal dominant

RISK FACTORS

- Patients with prothrombin 20210 and another prothrombotic state, such as factor V Leiden, have increased rates of thrombosis (1).
- The risk of venous thrombosis in patients with prothrombin 20210 mutation increases when added to the use of oral contraceptives, pregnancy, and the use of hormone replacement therapy as well as any status associated with prolonged immobilization (1).

Pregnancy Considerations

- Increased thrombotic risk in patients with prothrombin 20210.
- A new mutation C20209T has been described recently in women with recurrent pregnancy loss; the clinical and biochemical implications of this mutation are not fully understood yet (2).

GENERAL PREVENTION

Patients with prothrombin 20210 without thrombosis do not require prophylactic anticoagulation (3)[A]; except for pregnant ladies with family history of venous thromboembolism, who require then antepartum and 6-week postpartum prophylaxis with low-molecular-weight heparin (LMWH) (4)[B].

COMMONLY ASSOCIATED CONDITIONS

Venous thromboembolism

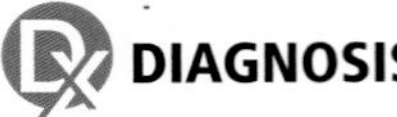

DIAGNOSIS

HISTORY

- Previous thrombosis
- Family history of thrombosis
- Family history of factor prothrombin 20210 mutation

PHYSICAL EXAM

Arterial thrombosis is rare in adults with prothrombin 20210 gene mutation.

DIFFERENTIAL DIAGNOSIS

- Factor V Leiden mutation
- Protein C deficiency
- Protein S deficiency
- Antithrombin deficiency
- Other causes of activated protein C resistance (e.g., antiphospholipid antibodies)
- Dysfibrinogenemia
- Dysplasminogenemia
- Homocystinemia
- Elevated factor VIII levels

DIAGNOSTIC TESTS & INTERPRETATION

Test patients with thrombosis, at age <50 years, history of recurrent idiopathic thrombosis, those with thrombosis in unusual locations, or those with strong family history.

Initial Tests (lab, imaging)

- For evaluation of a new clot in patients at risk: CBC with peripheral smear, PT/INR, aPTT, thrombin time, lupus anticoagulant, antiphospholipid antibodies, factor VIII, anticardiolipin antibody, anti-B2 glycoprotein I antibody, activated protein C resistance, protein S antigen and resistance, antithrombin III assay, fibrinogen, factor V Leiden, prothrombin G20210A, homocysteine
- DNA analysis for mutation
- Testing is reliable during acute thrombosis and on any kind of anticoagulation, as it is a gene analysis (5).
- As appropriate for suspected site of thrombosis: US, CT scan, and V/Q scan

Follow-Up Tests & Special Considerations

Although prothrombin levels are elevated, this is not a sensitive test to make the diagnosis.

Diagnostic Procedures/Other

Magnetic resonance angiography (MRA), venography, or arteriography to detect thrombosis

Test Interpretation

Venous thrombus

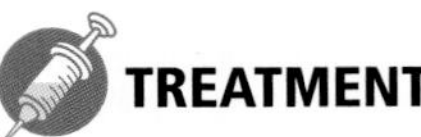

TREATMENT

For acute thrombosis

GENERAL MEASURES

- Patients with prothrombin 20210 mutation and a 1st thrombosis should receive anticoagulation medication initially with heparin or LMWH (1)[A].
- Treatment with LMWH is recommended over unfractionated heparin, unless the patient has severe renal failure (5)[A].
- Treat as outpatient, if possible (5)[B]
- Initiate warfarin on day 1 or 2 of LMWH therapy; discontinue LMWH after minimum of 5 days and 2 consecutive INRs >2 (5)[A].
- Patients should be maintained on warfarin with an INR of 2–3 for at least 3 months (4)[A].
- Recurrent thrombosis requires indefinite anticoagulation (1)[B].

MEDICATION

First Line

- LMWH (3)[A]
  - Enoxaparin (Lovenox): 1 mg/kg SC BID; tinzaparin (Innohep): 175 anti-Xa IU/kg SC daily; dalteparin (Fragmin): 200 IU/kg SC daily
  - Initiate warfarin on day 1 or 2 of LMWH therapy; continue LMWH for a minimum of 5 days and 2 consecutive INRs >2.
  - Fondaparinux (Arixtra): <50 kg: 5 mg SC daily; 50–100 kg: 7.5 mg SC daily; >100 kg: 10 mg SC daily
- Oral anticoagulant
  - Warfarin (Coumadin) 5 mg PO daily; then adjusted to an INR of 2–3 (4)
- Contraindications:
  - Active bleeding precludes anticoagulation (3)[A].
  - Risk of bleeding is a relative contraindication to long-term anticoagulation (3)[A].
  - Warfarin is contraindicated in patients with history of warfarin skin necrosis (3)[A].
  - Fondaparinux: severe renal impairment (CrCl <30 mL/min)

P

- Precautions:
  - Observe patient for signs of embolization, further thrombosis, or bleeding.
  - Avoid IM injections. Periodically check stool and urine for occult blood; monitor CBCs, including platelets.
  - Heparins: thrombocytopenia
  - Warfarin: necrotic skin lesions (typically breasts, thighs, or buttocks)
  - LMWH: Adjust dosage in renal insufficiency.
- Significant possible interactions:
  - Agents that intensify the response to oral anticoagulants: alcohol, allopurinol, amiodarone, anabolic steroids, androgens, many antimicrobials, cimetidine, chloral hydrate, disulfiram, all NSAIDs, sulfinpyrazone, tamoxifen, thyroid hormone, vitamin E, ranitidine, salicylates, acetaminophen
  - Agents that diminish the response to anticoagulants: aminoglutethimide, antacids, barbiturates, carbamazepine, cholestyramine, diuretics, griseofulvin, rifampin, oral contraceptives

Second Line

- Heparin 80 mg/kg IV bolus followed by 18 g/kg/hr continuous infusion
- Adjust dose, depending on aPTT.
- In patients requiring large daily doses of heparin, measure an anti-Xa level for dose guidance.
- Alternatively, unfractionated heparin can be given for outpatients at 333 U/kg then 250 U/kg SC (4)[A].

ISSUES FOR REFERRAL

- Recurrent thrombosis on anticoagulation
- Difficulty anticoagulating
- Genetic counseling

SURGERY/OTHER PROCEDURES

- Anticoagulation must be held for surgical interventions.
- For most patients with deep venous thrombosis (DVT), recommendations are against routine use of vena cava filter in addition to anticoagulation, except in case with contraindication to anticoagulation (4)[A].
- Thrombectomy may be necessary in some cases.

COMPLEMENTARY & ALTERNATIVE MEDICINE

Compression stockings for prevention

INPATIENT CONSIDERATIONS

Admission Criteria/Initial Stabilization

Complicated thrombosis, such as pulmonary embolus; heparin

Discharge Criteria

Stable on anticoagulation

ONGOING CARE

FOLLOW-UP RECOMMENDATIONS

Patient Monitoring

- Warfarin use requires periodic (monthly after initial stabilization) INR measurements, with a goal of 2–3 (3)[A].
- Heterozygous prothrombin 20210 mutations increase the risk for recurrent venous thromboembolism (VTE) only slightly once anticoagulation is stopped and should have the same length of anticoagulation as in someone without the mutation.

DIET

- No restrictions
- Foods rich in vitamin K may interfere with warfarin anticoagulation.

PATIENT EDUCATION

- Patients should be educated about the following:
  - Use of oral anticoagulant therapy
  - Avoidance of NSAIDs while on warfarin
- The role of family screening is unclear, as most patients with this mutation do not have thrombosis. In a patient with a family history of prothrombin 20210, consider screening during pregnancy or if considering oral contraceptive use.

PROGNOSIS

When compared with normal individuals, persons with prothrombin 20210 have normal lifespans.

COMPLICATIONS

- Recurrent thrombosis
- Bleeding on anticoagulation

REFERENCES

1. Girolami A, Simioni P, Scarano L, et al. Prothrombin and the prothrombin 20210 G to A polymorphism: their relationship with hypercoagulability and thrombosis. *Blood Rev*. 1999;(4)13:205–210.
2. Prat M, Morales-Indiano C, Jimenez C, et al. "20209C-T" a variant mutation of prothrombin gene mutation in a patient with recurrent pregnancy loss. *Ann Clin Lab Sci*.2014;44(3):334–336.
3. Guyatt GH, Akl EA, Crowther M, et al. Executive summary: Antithrombotic Therapy and Prevention of Thrombosis, 9th ed: American College of Chest Physicians Evidence-Based Clinical Practice Guidelines. *Chest*. 2012;141(2)(Suppl):7S–47S.
4. Moll S. Thrombophilias–practical implications and testing caveats. *J Thromb Thrombolysis*. 2006;21(1):7–15.

ADDITIONAL READING

Seligsohn U, Lubetsky A. Genetic susceptibility to venous thrombosis. *N Engl J Med*. 2001;344(16): 1222–1231.

SEE ALSO

Antithrombin Deficiency; Deep Vein Thrombophlebitis (DVT); Factor V Leiden; Protein C Deficiency; Protein S Deficiency

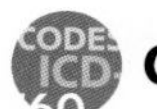

CODES

ICD10

D68.52 Prothrombin gene mutation

CLINICAL PEARLS

- Prothrombin 20210 mutation is the 2nd most common inherited risk factor for VTE after factor V Leiden mutation.
- Asymptomatic patients with prothrombin 20210 mutation do not need anticoagulation.
- Testing for the prothrombin G20210 mutation may be done while the patient is anticoagulated, as it is a genetic assay.
- For pregnant women homozygous for factor V Leiden, or heterozygous for factor V and prothrombin G20210 mutation, but no prior history of VTE, postpartum prophylaxis with prophylactic or intermediate-dose LMWH or vitamin K antagonists with target INR 2–3 for 6 weeks is recommended. Antepartum prophylaxis is added if there is positive family of VTE.

PRURITUS ANI

Pia Prakash, MD • Jessica Davis, MD • Marie L. Borum, MD, EdD, MPH

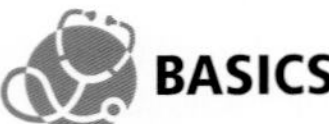

BASICS

DESCRIPTION
- Intense and often unpleasant anal and perianal itching and/or burning
- Usually acute
- Can be classified as idiopathic (primary) pruritus ani (50–90%) or secondary to anorectal pathology (1)

EPIDEMIOLOGY

Incidence
- 1–5% of the general population (1)
- Predominant age: 30–60 years (1)
- Predominant sex: male >female (4:1) (1)

Prevalence
Difficult to estimate, as often unreported or related to hemorrhoidal disease

ETIOLOGY AND PATHOPHYSIOLOGY
- Perianal itching (primary or secondary) incites itch–scratch cycle that may self-perpetuate, as resulting lichenification worsens pruritus.
- Etiologies of primary pruritus ani
  - Poor anal hygiene
  - Loose or leaking stool that makes hygiene difficult—of note, patients with abdominal ostomy bags typically do not complain of pruritus (1)
  - Internal sphincter laxity
  - Idiopathic
- Etiologies of secondary pruritus ani
  - Inflammatory dermatologic disorders
    - Allergic contact dermatitis (soaps, perfumes or dyes in toilet paper, topical anesthetics, oral antibiotics)
    - Psoriasis: Lesions tend to be poorly demarcated, pale, and nonscaling.
    - Atopic dermatitis ± lichen simplex chronicus: Patients likely to have asthma and/or eczema.
    - Eczema from dietary elements (citrus, vitamin C supplements, milk products, coffee, tea, cola, chocolate, beer, wine)
    - Seborrheic dermatitis
    - Lichen planus: may be seen in patients with ulcerative colitis and myasthenia gravis
  - Colorectal and anal pathology: rectal prolapse, hemorrhoids, fissures or fistulas, chronic diarrhea/constipation, papillomas, condyloma, polyps, cancer
  - Malignancies: uncommon, but pruritus ani may be presenting symptom of Bowen or Paget disease
  - Infectious etiologies: dermatophytes (*Tinea*), bacteria (*Staphylococcus aureus*, β-hemolytic *Streptococcus*, *Corynebacterium minutissimum* [Erythrasma], gonorrhea, syphilis), viruses (herpes simplex virus [HSV], human papillomavirus [HPV], molluscum), parasites (pinworms, rarely scabies, or pediculosis)
  - Mechanical factors: vigorous cleaning and scrubbing, tight-fitting clothes, synthetic undergarments
  - Systemic diseases: diabetes mellitus (most common), chronic liver disease, renal failure, leukemia or lymphoma, hyperthyroidism, anemia
  - Chemical irritants: chemotherapy, diarrhea (often from antibiotic use)
  - Psychogenic factors: anxiety–itch–anxiety cycle

RISK FACTORS
- Obesity
- Excess perianal hair growth, excessive perspiration
- Underlying anorectal pathology
- Underlying anxiety disorder
- Caffeine intake has been correlated with symptoms.

GENERAL PREVENTION
- Good perianal hygiene
  - Absorb excess sweat with talcum powder or cornstarch.
- Avoid mechanical irritation of skin (vigorous cleaning or rubbing, harsh soaps or perfumed products, excessive cleansing with dry toilet paper or "baby wipes," scratching with fingernails, or tight/synthetic undergarments).
- Wear cotton gloves at night to control nocturnal scratching (1).
- Minimize moisture in perianal area (absorbent cotton in anal cleft may help keep area dry).
- Avoid laxative use (loose stool is an irritant).

COMMONLY ASSOCIATED CONDITIONS
See earlier listing of conditions causing perianal irritation.

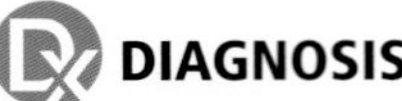

DIAGNOSIS

HISTORY
- Patient presents with complaint of anal and/or perianal itching, burning, or excoriations.
- Inquire about:
  - Melena or hematochezia
  - Frequency of cleansing and products used on affected area
  - Change in bowel habits
  - Recent antibiotic use
  - Medical history (diabetes in particular)
  - Skin disorders (psoriasis, eczema)
  - Rectal or vaginal discharge
  - Caffeine use and dietary history
  - Family history of colorectal cancer
  - Anal receptive intercourse
  - Change in toiletry products
  - Household members with itching (possible pinworms)
  - Clothing preference (tight, synthetic) (1)[C]

PHYSICAL EXAM
- Perianal inspection for erythema, hemorrhoids, anal fissures, maceration, lichenification, rashes, warts, excoriations, neoplasia
- Digital rectal exam to check for masses and to evaluate internal sphincter tone
- Anoscopy to evaluate for hemorrhoids, fissures, other internal lesions
- Classification based on gross appearance
  - Stage 1: erythema, inflamed appearance
  - Stage 2: lichenification
  - Stage 3: lichenification, coarse skin, potential fissures or ulcerations (2,1)[C]

DIFFERENTIAL DIAGNOSIS
- Psoriasis, eczema
- Infections (dermatophytes, bacterial, viral)
- Allergies (topical agents)
- Colorectal pathology: fistulas, fissures, rectal prolapse, sphincter weakness, hemorrhoids, tumor/malignancy
- Skin cancer: squamous cell cancer, extramammary Paget disease, Bowen disease, melanoma
- Systemic illness such as diabetes, uremia, cholestasis

DIAGNOSTIC TESTS & INTERPRETATION

Initial Tests (lab, imaging)
Depending on patient's history and exam, consider the following:
- Blood glucose and hemoglobin A1C to assess for diabetes
- Pinworm tape test; stool for ova and parasites
- CBC, comprehensive metabolic panel, thyroid studies to identify underlying systemic disease
- Wood lamp examination >48 hours after washing will show coral-red fluorescence in erythrasma (1).
- Skin scraping with potassium hydroxide (KOH) prep for dermatophytes or candidiasis (as etiology or as superinfection) and mineral oil prep for scabies
- Perianal skin culture (bacterial superinfection)
- Hemoccult testing of stool

Pediatric Considerations
Pinworms are common in children.

Follow-Up Tests & Special Considerations
Anal DNA polymerase chain reaction (PCR) probe for gonorrhea and anal Pap smear for HPV (*if receptive anal intercourse*)

Diagnostic Procedures/Other
- Biopsy suspicious lesions (e.g., lichenification, ulcerated epithelium, refractory cases) to exclude neoplasia.
- Consider colonoscopy if history, exam, or testing suggests colorectal pathology (family history of colorectal disease, especially if age >40 years, weight loss, rectal bleeding, change in bowel habits).

Geriatric Considerations
- Stool incontinence may be a predisposing factor.
- Consider systemic disease.
- Higher likelihood of colorectal pathology

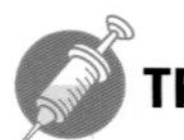

TREATMENT

GENERAL MEASURES
- Educate patients regarding proper anal hygiene and avoidance of chemical and mechanical irritants (1).
- High-fiber diet and/or bowel regimen to maintain regular bowel movements (1)
- Avoid tight-fitting clothing; use cotton undergarments.

MEDICATION

First Line
- Treat underlying infections: fungal or dermatophyte infection with topical imidazoles, bacterial infection with topical antibacterials.

- Break itch–scratch cycle with low-potency steroid cream such as hydrocortisone 1% ointment applied sparingly up to 4× daily (1)[A]. Discontinue when itching subsides. Recommended not to use >12 weeks due to risk of skin atrophy.
- If no response with low-potency steroid, consider high-potency steroid cream.
- Antihistamines may be useful until local measures take effect, particularly sedating antihistamines, which will reduce nighttime itching (3)[C].
- Zinc oxide can be used after completing steroid course for barrier protection (2)[C]; petroleum jelly is another barrier treatment.
- Although trial data are mixed, topical capsaicin cream may be used in combination with steroid cream if refractory itch or hypersensitized skin (1,4)[A].
- A small RCT showed benefit with 0.1% tacrolimus ointment; this may be a good choice in patients with skin thinning at risk for atrophy from prolonged steroid use (5)[C].
- Several small case series have shown symptomatic benefit with methylene blue injection; this may be an additional option for patients with refractory symptoms (6)[C].

Second Line

Radiation may be used to destroy nerve endings (create permanent anesthesia) in intractable cases. This is almost never indicated but is very effective (3)[C].

ISSUES FOR REFERRAL

- Intractable pruritus: Consider referral to gastroenterology (for colonoscopy) or dermatology (for additional treatment, possibly injections). Refractory or persistent symptoms should signal the possibility of underlying neoplasia, as pruritus ani of long duration is associated with a greater likelihood of colorectal pathology.
- If risks or red flags for colon cancer are present, refer for colonoscopy.

SURGERY/OTHER PROCEDURES

None unless malignancy identified

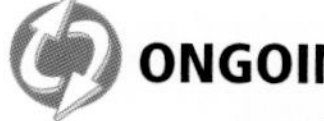

ONGOING CARE

FOLLOW-UP RECOMMENDATIONS

See patient in 2 weeks if not improving. Check for persistent lichenification. With refractory pruritus or lichenification that does not resolve, consider underlying malignancy.

DIET

- Trial elimination of foods and beverages known or suspected to exacerbate symptoms: coffee, tea, chocolate, beer, cola, vitamin C tablets in excessive doses, citrus fruits, tomatoes, or spices
- Eliminate foods or drugs contributing to loose bowel movements. Add fiber supplementation to bulk stools and prevent fecal leakage in patients who have fecal incontinence or partially formed stools.

PATIENT EDUCATION

- Review proper anal hygiene:
  - Resist overuse of soap and rubbing.
  - Avoid toiletry products with irritating perfumes and dyes.
  - Avoid use of ointments to the area, including witch hazel.
  - Wear loose, light cotton clothing.
  - If moisture is a problem, unmedicated talcum powder or cornstarch to keep the area dry.
  - Cleanse perianal area after bowel movements with water-moistened cotton.
  - Dry area after bathing by patting with a soft towel or by using a hair dryer (1).
- Avoid medications that cause diarrhea or constipation.
- Avoid foods implicated in pruritus ani: caffeine, cola, chocolate, citrus, tomatoes, tea, beer/wine (2)[A].
- Use barrier protection if engaging in anal intercourse.
- If unable to completely empty rectum with defecation, use small plain-water enema (infant bulb syringe) after each bowel movement to prevent soiling and irritation.

PROGNOSIS

- Conservative treatment is successful in ~90% of patients.
- Idiopathic pruritus ani often is chronic, waxing and waning. Regardless of etiology, however, pruritus ani may be persistent and recurrent.

COMPLICATIONS

- Bacterial superinfection at site of excoriations and potential abscess formation or penetrating infection via self-inoculation with colonic pathogens
- Lichenification

REFERENCES

1. Markell KW, Billingham RP. Pruritus ani: etiology and management. *Surg Clin North Am*. 2010;90(1):125–135.
2. Nasseri YY, Osborne MC. Pruritus ani: diagnosis and treatment. *Gastroenetrol Clin North Am*. 2013;42(4):801–813.
3. Schubert MC, Sridhar S, Schade R, et al. What every gastroenterologist needs to know about common anorectal disorders. *World J Gastroenterol*. 2009;15(26):3201–3209.
4. Gooding SM, Canter PH, Coelho HF, et al. Systematic review of topical capsaicin in the treatment of pruritus. *Int J Dermatol*. 2010;49(8):858–865.
5. Suys, E. Randomized study of topical tacrolimus ointment as possible treatment for resistant idiopathic pruritus ani. *J Am Acad Dermatol*. 2012;66(2):327–328.
6. Samalavicius NE, Poskus T, Gupta RK et al. Long-term results of single intradermal 1% methylene blue injection for intractable idiopathic pruritus ani: a prospective study. *Tech Coloproctol*. 2012;16(4):295–299.

ADDITIONAL READING

- Al-Ghnaniem R, Short K, Pullen A, et al. 1% Hydrocortisone ointment is an effective treatment of pruritus ani: a pilot randomized controlled crossover trial. *Int J Colorectal Dis*. 2007;22(12):1463–1467.
- Handa Y, Watanabe O, Adachi A, et al. Squamous cell carcinoma of the anal margin with pruritus ani of long duration. *Dermatol Surg*. 2003;29(1): 108–110.
- Lysy J, Sistiery-Ittah M, Israelit Y, et al. Topical capsaicin—a novel and effective treatment for idiopathic intractable pruritus ani: a randomised, placebo controlled, crossover study. *Gut*. 2003;52(9):1323–1326.
- Rucklidge JJ, Saunders D. Hypnosis in a case of long-standing idiopathic itch. *Psychosom Med*. 1999;61(3):355–358.
- Siddiqi S, Vijay V, Ward M, et al. Pruritus ani. *Ann R Coll Surg Engl*. 2008;90(6):457–463.
- Ucak H, Demir B, Cicek D, et al. Efficacy of topical tacrolimus for the treatment of persistent pruritus ani in patients with atopic dermatitis. *J Dermatolog Treat*. 2013;24(6):454–457.
- Weichert GE. An approach to the treatment of anogenital pruritus. *Dermatol Ther*. 2004;17(1): 129–133.
- Zuccati G, Lotti T, Mastrolorenzo A, et al. Pruritus ani. *Dermatol Ther*. 2005;18(4):355–362.

SEE ALSO

Pinworms; Pruritus Vulvae

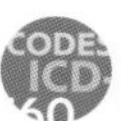

CODES

ICD10

L29.0 Pruritus ani

CLINICAL PEARLS

- Pruritus ani is characterized by intense and often unpleasant anal and perianal itching and/or burning.
- Usually idiopathic or related to skin irritation with subsequent scratch–itch–scratch cyle
- Conservative treatment and reassurance are successful in 90% of patients.
- Consider trial of dietary elimination of citrus, vitamin C supplements, milk products, coffee, tea, cola, chocolate, beer, and wine as adjuvant measure to proper perianal hygiene.
- Consider infection in immunosuppressed patients.
- Consider underlying malignancy with refractory pruritus.

PRURITUS VULVAE

Laura K. Randolph, DO, MS • Michael P. Hopkins, MD, MEd

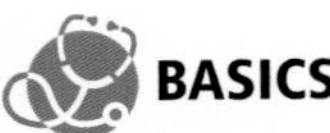

BASICS

DESCRIPTION

- Pruritus vulvae is a symptom, as well as a primary diagnosis:
  - The symptom may indicate an underlying pathologic process.
  - Only when no underlying disease is identified may this be used as a primary diagnosis.
- Pruritus vulvae as a primary diagnosis may also be more appropriately documented as vulvodynia (see "Vulvodynia" topic) and burning vulva syndrome.

EPIDEMIOLOGY

Symptoms may occur at any given age during a woman's lifetime:

- Young girls most commonly have infectious or hygiene etiology.
- The primary diagnosis is more commonly seen in postmenopausal women.

Incidence

The exact incidence is unknown. However, most women complain of vulvar pruritus at some point in their lifetime.

ETIOLOGY AND PATHOPHYSIOLOGY

Vulvar tissue is more permeable than exposed skin due to differences in structure, occlusion, hydration, and susceptibility to friction. It is particularly vulnerable to irritants (1):

- Perfumes
- Soaps
- Laundry detergent
- Douches
- Toilet paper
- Sanitary napkins

RISK FACTORS

- High-risk sexual behavior
- Immunosuppression
- Obesity

GENERAL PREVENTION

- Attention should be paid to personal hygiene and avoidance of possible environmental factors.
- Tight-fitting clothing should be avoided.
- Only cotton underwear should be worn.

COMMONLY ASSOCIATED CONDITIONS

- Infectious etiology
  - Vaginal or vulvar candida
  - *Gardnerella vaginalis*
  - *Trichomonas*
  - Human papillomavirus
  - Herpes simplex virus
- Vulvar vestibulitis
- Lichen sclerosis
- Lichen planus
- Lichen simplex chronicus (squamous cell hyperplasia)
- Malignant or premalignant conditions
- Psoriasis
- Fecal or urinary incontinence
- Excessive heat with sweat
- Dietary: methylxanthines (e.g., coffee, cola), tomatoes, peanuts
- Autoimmune progesterone dermatitis: perimenstrual eruptions
- Irritant or allergic contact dermatitis
- Atopic dermatitis

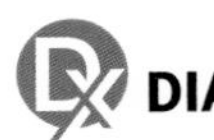

DIAGNOSIS

Pruritus vulvae is a diagnosis of exclusion.

HISTORY

- Persistent itching
- Persistent burning sensation over the vulva or perineum
- Change in vaginal discharge
- Postcoital bleeding
- Dyspareunia

PHYSICAL EXAM

- Visual inspection of the vulva, vagina, perineum, and anus
  - Superior surfaces of the labia majora—extending from mons to the anal orifice are most involved.
  - Vulvar skin is leathery or lichenified in appearance.
  - Papillomatosis may be a sign of chronic inflammation.
- Light touch identification of affected areas
- Cotton swab–applied pressure to vestibular glands

DIAGNOSTIC TESTS & INTERPRETATION

- Sodium chloride: *Gardnerella* or *Trichomonas*
- 10% potassium hydroxide: *Candida*
- Viral culture and polymerase chain reaction (PCR): herpes simplex virus
- Directed biopsy: human papillomavirus, lichen, malignancy
- Colposcopy with acetic acid or Lugol solution of vagina and vulva

Follow-Up Tests & Special Considerations

- A patch test may be performed by a dermatologist to assist in identifying a causative agent if contact dermatitis is suspected.
- Exam-directed biopsies are essential in the postmenopausal population to rule out malignancy.

Diagnostic Procedures/Other

Biopsies should be collected from any ulceration, discoloration, raised areas, macerated areas, and the area of most intense pruritus.

Test Interpretation

- Only in the absence of pathologic findings can the primary diagnosis of pruritus vulvae be made.
- In 1 study, a specific clinicopathologic diagnosis was obtained in 89% of patients by using the most recent 2006 International Society for the Study of Vulvar Diseases (ISSVD) classifications (2).

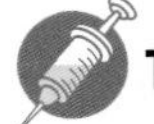

TREATMENT

Identify the underlying cause or disease to target treatment:

- Stop all potential irritants (i.e., excessive body hygiene).
- Eliminate bacterial and fungal infection.
- Cool the affected area: Use cool gel packs (not ice packs, which may cause further injury).
- Sitz baths and bland emollients to soothe fissured or eroded skin

MEDICATION

First Line

- 1st-generation antihistamines (3)[C]
  - Hydroxyzine: Initiate with 10 mg before bedtime (slow increase up to 100 mg).

- Doxepin: Initiate with 10 mg before bedtime (slow increase up to 100 mg).
- 2nd-generation antihistamines are of little benefit.
- SSRIs (3)[C]
  - Citalopram 20–40 mg in the morning may be helpful for daytime symptoms.
- Topical steroids (4)[C]
  - Triamcinolone 0.1% applied daily for 2–4 weeks, then twice weekly
  - Hydrocortisone 1–2.5% cream applied 2–4 times daily (5)
  - Avoid long-term use due to risk of atrophy.
  - One randomized, controlled trial showed no difference between topical triamcinolone and placebo cream (6).

Second Line

Topical pimecrolimus 1% cream applied BID for 3 weeks (7)[B]

- May lead to an 80% reduction of pruritus

ISSUES FOR REFERRAL

- Persistent symptoms should prompt additional investigation and referral to a gynecologist or gynecologist oncologist.
- Gynecology oncology referral for proven or suspected malignancy
- Dermatology referral for patch testing to evaluate for contact dermatitis

ADDITIONAL THERAPIES

- SC triamcinolone injections (8)[B]
- Alcohol nerve block (9)[B]
- Laser therapy (10)[B]
- GnRH analogue (11)[C]

ONGOING CARE

- Frequent evaluation, repeat cultures, and biopsies are necessary for cases resistant to treatment.
- Refractory cases may require referral to gynecologist or gynecology oncology for further management.

DIET

Dietary alterations include avoidance of the following:

- Coffee and other caffeine-containing beverages
- Tomatoes
- Peanuts

PATIENT EDUCATION

- American Congress of Obstetricians and Gynecologists: www.acog.org
- National Vulvodynia Foundation: www.nva.org

PROGNOSIS

Conservative measures and short-term topical steroids control most patients' symptoms.

COMPLICATIONS

Malignancy

REFERENCES

1. Farage M, Maibach HI. The vulvar epithelium differs from the skin: implications for cutaneous testing to address topical vulvar exposures. *Contact Dermatitis*. 2004;51(4):201–209.
2. Kelecki KH, Adamhasan F, Gencdal S, et al. The impact of the latest classification system of benign vulvar diseases on the management of the women with chronic vulvar pruritus. *Indian J Dermatol Venereol Leprol*. 2011;77(3):294–299.
3. Margesson LJ. Overview of treatment of vulvovaginal disease. *Skin Therapy Lett*. 2011;16(3):5–7.
4. Weichert GE. An approach to the treatment of anogenital pruritus. *Dermatol Ther*. 2004;17(1):129–133.
5. Pincus SH. Vulvar dermatoses and pruritus vulvae. *Dermatol Clin*. 1992;10(2):297–308.
6. Lagro-Janssen AL, Sluis S. Effectiveness of treating non-specific pruritus vulvae with topical steroids: a randomized controlled trial. *Eur J Gen Pract*. 2009;15(1):29–33.
7. Sarifakioglu E, Gumus II. Efficacy of topical pimecrolimus in the treatment of chronic vulvar pruritus: a prospective case series—a non-controlled, open-label study. *J Dermatolog Treat*. 2006;17(5):276–278.
8. Kelly RA, Foster DC, Woodruff JD. Subcutaneous injection of triamcinolone acetonide in the treatment of chronic vulvar pruritus. *Am J Obstet Gynecol*. 1993;169(3):568–570.
9. Woodruff JD, Babaknia A. Local alcohol injection of the vulva: discussion of 35 cases. *Obstet Gynecol*. 1979;54(4):512–514.
10. Ovadia J, Levavi H, Edelstein T. Treatment of pruritus vulvae by means of CO_2 laser. *Acta Obstet Gynecol Scand*. 1984;63(3):265–267.
11. Banerjee AK, de Chazal R. Chronic vulvovaginal pruritus treated successfully with GnRH analogue. *Postgrad Med J*. 2006;82(970):e22.

ADDITIONAL READING

- Boardman LA, Botte J, Kennedy CM. Recurrent vulvar itching. *Obstet Gynecol*. 2005;105(6):1451–1455.
- Bohl TG. Overview of vulvar pruritus through the life cycle. *Clin Obstet Gynecol*. 2005;48(4):786–807.
- Farage MA, Miller KW, Ledger WJ. Determining the cause of vulvovaginal symptoms. *Obstet Gynecol Surv*. 2008;63(7):445–464.
- Foster DC. Vulvar disease. *Obstet Gynecol*. 2002;100(1):145–163.
- Petersen CD, Lundvall L, Kristensen E, et al. Vulvodynia. Definition, diagnosis and treatment. *Acta Obstet Gynecol Scand*. 2008;87(9):893–901.
- Sener AB, Kuscu E, Seckin NC, et al. Postmenopausal vulvar pruritus–colposcopic diagnosis and treatment. *J Pak Med Assoc*. 1995;45(12):315–317.

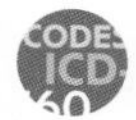

CODES

ICD10

- L29.2 Pruritus vulvae
- N94.819 Vulvodynia, unspecified

CLINICAL PEARLS

- Most women complain of pruritus vulvae at some point in their lifetime.
- Pruritus vulvae is a diagnosis of exclusion once other causes of itching have been ruled out.
- Exam-directed biopsies from any ulceration, discoloration, raised areas, macerated areas, and the area of most intense pruritus are essential to rule out malignancy.
- Initial treatment is conservative.

PSEUDOFOLLICULITIS BARBAE

Maurice Duggins, MD

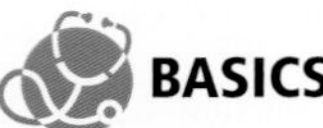

BASICS

DESCRIPTION

- Foreign-body inflammatory reaction from an ingrown hair resulting in the appearance of papules and pustules. This is found mainly in the bearded area (*barbae*) but may occur in other hairy locations such as the scalp, axilla, or pubic areas where shaving is done (1).
- A mechanical problem: extrafollicular and transfollicular hair penetration
- System(s) affected: skin/exocrine
- Synonym(s): chronic sycosis barbae; pili incarnate; folliculitis barbae traumatica; razor bumps; shaving bumps; tinea barbae; pseudofolliculitis barbae (PFB)

EPIDEMIOLOGY

- Predominant age: postpubertal, middle age (14–25) (2)
- Predominant sex: male > female (can be seen in females of all races who wax/shave)

Incidence

- Adult male African Americans: unknown
- Adult male whites: unknown

Prevalence

- Widespread in Fitzpatrick skin types IV–VI (darker complexions) who shave
- 45–83% of African American soldiers who shave (1)

ETIOLOGY AND PATHOPHYSIOLOGY

- Transfollicular escape of the low-cut hair shaft as it tries to exit the skin is accompanied by inflammation and often an intraepidermal abscess.
- As the hair enters the dermis, more severe inflammation occurs, with downgrowth of the epidermis in an attempt to sheath the hair.
- A foreign-body reaction forms at the tip of the invading hair, followed by abscess formation.
- Shaving too close
- Plucking/tweezing or wax depilation of hair may cause abnormal hair growth in injured follicles.

Genetics

- People with curly hair have an asymmetric accumulation of acidic keratin hHa8 on hair shaft.
- Single-nucleotide polymorphism (disruption Ala12Thr substitution) affects keratin of hair follicle.

RISK FACTORS

- Curly hair
- Shaving too close or shaving with multiple razor strokes
- Plucking/tweezing hairs
- South Mediterranean/American, Middle Eastern, Asian, or African descent (skin types IV–VI)

GENERAL PREVENTION

- Prior to shaving, rinse face with warm water to hydrate and soften hairs.
- Use adjustable hair clippers that leave very low hair length above skin.
- Shave with either a manual adjustable razor at coarsest setting (avoids close shaves), a single-edge blade razor (e.g., Bump Fighter), a foil-guarded razor (e.g., PFB razor), or electric triple "O-head" razor.
- Empty razor of hair frequently.
- Shave in the direction of hair growth. Do not overstretch skin when shaving.
- Use a generous amount of the correct shaving cream/gel (e.g., Ef-Kay Shaving Gel, Edge Shaving Gel, Aveeno Therapeutic Shave Gel, Easy Shave Medicated Shaving Cream).
- Daily shaving reduces papules/pruritus.
- Regular use of depilatories

COMMONLY ASSOCIATED CONDITIONS

- Keloidal folliculitis
- Pseudofolliculitis nuchae

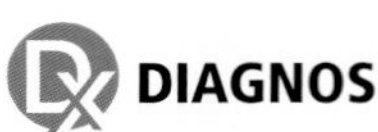

DIAGNOSIS

HISTORY

Pain on shaving; pruritus of shaved areas, irritated "razor bumps"

PHYSICAL EXAM

- Tender, exudative, erythematous follicular papules or pustules in beard area (less commonly in scalp, axilla, and pubic areas); range from 2–4 mm
- Hyperpigmented "razor or shave bumps"
- Alopecia
- Lusterless, brittle hair

DIFFERENTIAL DIAGNOSIS

- Bacterial folliculitis
- Impetigo
- Acne vulgaris
- Tinea barbae
- Sarcoidal papules

DIAGNOSTIC TESTS & INTERPRETATION

Initial Tests (lab, imaging)

- Clinical diagnosis
- Culture of pustules: usually sterile; may show coagulase-negative staphylococcal epidermidis (normal skin flora)
- Additional hormonal testing may be indicated in females with hirsutism and/or polycystic ovary syndrome: dehydroepiandrosterone sulfate, luteinizing hormone (LH)/follicle-stimulating hormone (FSH), and free and total testosterone (3)[C].

Test Interpretation

Follicular papules and pustules

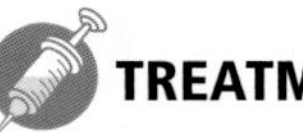

TREATMENT

- Mild cases
  - Stop shaving or avoid close shaving for 30 days while keeping beard groomed and clean (1,2)[C].
  - Consider 5% benzoyl peroxide after shaving and application of 1% hydrocortisone cream at bedtime (or LactiCare HC lotion after shaving) (2)[C].
  - Tretinoin 0.025% cream; apply daily(1)[C]
- Moderate cases
  - Chemical depilatories (barium sulfide; Magic Shave powder); first test on forearm for 48 hours (for irritation) (1,2,3)[B]
  - Consider eflornithine HCl cream (Vaniqa) to reduce hair growth and stiffness in combination with other therapies (1,4)[B].
- Severe cases
  - Laser therapy: Longer wavelength laser (e.g., neodymium [Nd]:YAG) is safer for dark skin (5)[B].
  - Avoid shaving altogether; grow beard (1,2,3)[C].

GENERAL MEASURES

Acute treatment

- Dislodge embedded hair with sterile needle/tweezers.
- Discontinue shaving until red papules have resolved (minimum 3–4 weeks; longer if moderate or severe); can trim to length >0.5 cm during this time.
- Massage beard area with washcloth, coarse sponge, or a soft brush several times daily.
- Hydrocortisone 1–2.5% cream to relieve inflammation
- Selenium sulfide if seborrhea is present and to help reduce pruritus
- Systemic antibiotics if secondary infection is present

Pregnancy Considerations
Do not use tretinoin (Retin-A), tetracycline, or benzoyl peroxide.

MEDICATION
First Line
- Topical or systemic antibiotic for secondary infection
  - Application of clindamycin (Cleocin T) solution BID or topical erythromycin
  - Low-dose erythromycin or tetracycline 250–500 mg PO BID for more severe inflammation
  - Benzoyl peroxide 5%–clindamycin 1% gel BID: Administer until papule/pustule resolves.
- Mild cases: tretinoin 0.025% cream at bedtime; combination of the above therapies
- Moderate disease/chemical depilatories
  - Disrupt cross-linking of disulfide bonds of hair to produce blunt (less sharp) hair tip.
  - Apply no more frequently than every third day: 2% barium sulfide (Magic Shave) or calcium thioglycollate (Surgex); calcium hydroxide (Nair)
- Contraindications
  - Clindamycin: hypersensitivity history; history of regional enteritis or ulcerative colitis; history of antibiotic-associated colitis
  - Erythromycin, tetracycline, tretinoin: hypersensitivity history
- Precautions
  - Clindamycin: colitis, eye burning and irritation, skin dryness; pregnancy category B
  - Erythromycin: Use cautiously in patients with impaired hepatic function; GI side effects, especially abdominal cramping; pregnancy category B (erythromycin base formulation).
  - Chemical depilatories: Use cautiously; frequent use and prolonged application may lead to irritant contact dermatitis and chemical burns.
  - Tetracycline: Avoid in pregnancy.
  - Tretinoin: severe skin irritation; avoid in pregnancy
  - Benzoyl peroxide: skin irritation and dryness, allergic contact dermatitis
  - Hydrocortisone cream: local skin irritation, skin atrophy with prolonged use, lightening of skin color
- Significant possible interactions
  - Erythromycin: increases theophylline and carbamazepine levels; decreases clearance of warfarin
  - Tetracycline: depresses plasma prothrombin activity

Second Line
Chemical peels with either glycolic acid or salicylic acid

ISSUES FOR REFERRAL
- Worsening or poor response to the above therapies after 4–6 weeks should prompt dermatology consultation.
- Occupational demands may also prompt earlier referral to dermatology for more aggressive therapy.

SURGERY/OTHER PROCEDURES
Laser treatment with long-pulsed Nd:YAG is helpful for severe cases.

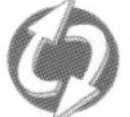

ONGOING CARE

FOLLOW-UP RECOMMENDATIONS
Patient Monitoring
- As needed
- Educate patient on curative and preventive treatment.

DIET
- No restrictions
- No dietary studies available

PATIENT EDUCATION
- Medlineplus.com
- Uptodate.com

PROGNOSIS
- Good, with preventive methods
- Prognosis is poor in the presence of progressive scarring and foreign-body granuloma formation.

COMPLICATIONS
- Scarring (occasionally keloidal)
- Foreign-body granuloma formation
- Disfiguring postinflammatory hyperpigmentation (use sunscreens; can treat with hydroquinone 4% cream, Retin A, clinical peels)
- Impetiginization of inflamed skin
- Epidermal (erythema, crusting, burns with scarring) and pigmentary changes with laser

REFERENCES

1. Bridgeman-Shah S. The medical and surgical treatment of pseudofolliculitis barbae. *Dermatol Ther*. 2004;17(2):158–163.
2. Perry PK. Defining pseudofolliculitis barbae in 2001: a review of the literature and current trends. *J Am Acad Dermatol*. 2002;46(2)(Suppl): S113–S119.
3. Quarles FN, Brody H, Johnson BA, et al. Pseudofolliculitis barbae. *Dermatol Ther*. 2007;20(3): 133–136.
4. Xia Y, Cho S, Howard RS, et al. Topical eflornithine hydrochloride improves the effectiveness of standard laser hair removal for treating pseudofolliculitis barbae: a randomized, double-blinded, placebo-controlled trial. *J Am Acad Dermatol*. 2012;67(4):694–699.
5. Weaver SM, Sagaral EC. Treatment of pseudofolliculitis barbae using the long-pulse Nd:YAG laser on skin types V and VI. *Dermatol Surg*. 2003;29(12):1187–1191.

ADDITIONAL READING

- Cook-Bolden FE. Twice daily application of benzoyl peroxide 5% clindamycin 1% gel versus vehicle in treatment of pseudofolliculitis barbae. *Cutis*. 2004;73(6)(Suppl):13–24.
- Daniel A, Gustafson CJ, Zuprosky PJ, et al. Shave frequency and regimen variation effects on the management of pseudofolliculitis barbae. *J Drugs Dermatol*. 2013;12(4):410–418.
- Kindred C, Oresajo CO, Yatskayer M, et al. Comparative evaluation of men's depilatory composition versus razor in black men. *Cutis*. 2011;88(2):98–103.
- Kundu RV, Patterson S. Dermatologic conditions in skin of color: part II. Disorders occurring predominantly in skin of color. 2013;87(12):859–865.

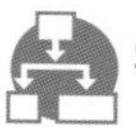

SEE ALSO

Folliculitis; Impetigo

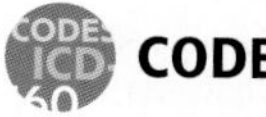

CODES

ICD10
- L73.1 Pseudofolliculitis barbae
- B35.0 Tinea barbae and tinea capitis
- L73.8 Other specified follicular disorders

CLINICAL PEARLS

- Electrolysis is not recommended as a treatment. It is expensive, painful, and often unsuccessful.
- Combination of laser therapy with eflornithine is more effective than laser alone.
- Use Bump Fighter razor from American Safety Razor Company (www.asrco.com).
- Men may prefer the convenience of the Bump Fighter razor over depilatory products.
- The aversive smell of sulfur could be a problem with some depilatory products.
- Have patient test for skin sensitivity with a small (coin-sized) amount of the depilatory on the bearded area or forearm.

PSEUDOGOUT (CALCIUM PYROPHOSPHATE DIHYDRATE)

Mark B. Stephens, MD, MS, FAAFP, CAPT, MC, USN

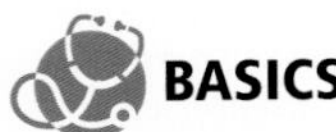

BASICS

DESCRIPTION

- Autoinflammatory disease triggered by calcium pyrophosphate dihydrate (CPPD) crystal deposition in the joints
- 1 of many diseases associated with pathologic mineralization and ossification
  - Although chondrocalcinosis and pseudogout are characterized by CPPD crystal deposition, ankylosing spondylitis, osteoarthritis, and vascular calcification are characterized by hydroxyapatite deposition.
- CPPD crystal deposition may cause a progressive degenerative arthritis in numerous joints:
  - Primarily affects the elderly
  - Usually involves large joints
- Symptom onset is insidious, resulting in symmetric polyarthritis similar to rheumatoid arthritis (RA).
- Definitive diagnosis requires the presence of CPPD crystals in synovial fluid.
- System(s) affected: endocrine/metabolic; musculoskeletal
- Synonyms: pseudogout; CPPD; chondrocalcinosis—when calcification visibly seen within tissues on imaging

EPIDEMIOLOGY

Prevalence

- Predominant age: 80% of patients >60 years
- Predominant sex: male > female 1.4: 1
- Chondrocalcinosis is present in 1:10 adults age 60–75 years and 1:3 by >80 years, however, only a small percentage develop arthropathy (1)[C].

ETIOLOGY AND PATHOPHYSIOLOGY

- Arthropathy results from an acute autoinflammatory reaction to CPPD crystals in the synovial cavity.
- Neutrophils engulf CPPD crystals, inducing the formation of extracellular traps, which cause cellular damage and synovitis (2)[C].
- Physical and chemical changes in aging cartilage favor crystal growth.

Genetics

Uncommonly seen in familial pattern with autosomal dominant inheritance (<1% of patients); most cases are sporadic. Mutation in ANKH gene increased risk for calcium crystal formation.

RISK FACTORS

- Advanced age
- Traumatic injury
- CPPD often may occur as a complication in patients hospitalized for other medical and surgical illnesses.

GENERAL PREVENTION

Colchicine 0.6 mg BID may be used prophylactically to reduce frequency of episodes in recurrent CPPD.

COMMONLY ASSOCIATED CONDITIONS

- Hyperparathyroidism
- Hemochromatosis
- Gout
- Hypophosphatasia
- Hypothyroidism
- Ochronosis
- Wilson disease
- Amyloidosis
- Hypomagnesemia

DIAGNOSIS

HISTORY

- Presentation often similar to gout (thus the term "pseudogout").
- Acute pain and swelling of ≥1 or more joints; knee involved in 50% of all attacks; ankle, wrist, and shoulder are also commonly involved.
- May present as a chronic progressive arthritis with superimposed acute inflammatory attacks
- Progressive degenerative arthritis in numerous joints, including wrists, metacarpophalangeal, hips, shoulders, elbows, and ankles
- Low-grade inflammatory arthritis with multiple symmetric joint involvement (mimicking RA) in <5% of cases
- Can present in proximal joints (mimicking polymyalgia rheumatica), often accompanied by tibiofemoral and ankle arthritis and tendinous calcifications
- May develop after intra-articular injection of hyaluronic acid (Hyalgan, Synvisc)

PHYSICAL EXAM

- Inflammation, joint effusion, decreased range of motion
- 50% associated with fever
- Any synovial joint may be involved, including 1st metatarsophalangeal joint

DIFFERENTIAL DIAGNOSIS

- Illnesses that may cause acute inflammatory arthritis in a single or multiple joint(s):
  - Gout
  - Septic arthritis
  - Trauma
- Other illnesses that may present with an acute inflammatory arthritis:
  - Reiter syndrome
  - Lyme disease
  - Acute RA

DIAGNOSTIC TESTS & INTERPRETATION

Initial Tests (lab, imaging)

Synovial fluid analysis consistent with an inflammatory effusion:

- Cell count 2,000–100,000 WBCs/mL
- Differential predominantly neutrophils (80–90%)
- >50,000 WBC count increases likelihood of septic arthritis, 11% prevalence; number needed to treat (NNT) = 9; >100,000 WBCs/mL, 22% prevalence
- Wet prep with polarized microscopy may demonstrate small numbers of rhomboid-shaped weakly *positively birefringent* crystals in the fluid and within neutrophils; false-negative rate is high. Gout crystals are needle-shaped and negatively birefringent.
- The following metabolic studies should be obtained in patients <50 years of age and considered in the elderly to exclude underlying disease:
  - Serum calcium
  - Serum phosphorus
  - Serum alkaline phosphatase
  - Serum parathormone (i-PTH)
  - Serum iron, total iron-binding capacity, and serum ferritin
  - Serum magnesium
  - Serum thyroid-stimulating hormone (TSH) level
- Plain radiograph
  - Radiographic findings in pseudogout are neither sensitive nor specific.
  - Punctate and linear calcifications may be visualized in articular hyaline or fibrocartilage.
  - Knees, hips, symphysis pubis, and wrists are most commonly affected.
  - Patients with chronic CPPD may demonstrate subchondral cysts and loose bodies (osseous fragmentation with formation of intra-articular radiodense bodies) in joints not typically affected by degenerative joint disease (osteoarthritis).
- Ultrasound
  - US may be more useful than plain radiography for the diagnosis of pseudogout in peripheral joints, with a positive predictive value of 92% and negative predictive value of 93% (3)[C].
  - US imaging characteristics of pseudogout include the following: joint effusion, synovial thickening, and hyperechoic deposits.
- MRI
  - Chondrocalcinosis may be evident as hypointense lesions on MRI, particularly in association with the menisci of the knee.

Diagnostic Procedures/Other

Aspiration of joint fluid with synovial fluid analysis and demonstration of CPPD crystals is required for diagnosis; aspiration may relieve symptoms and speed resolution of the inflammatory process.

Test Interpretation

CPPD crystal deposition in articular cartilage, synovium, ligaments, and tendons

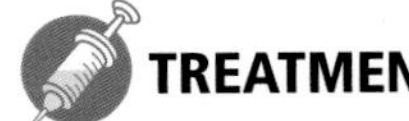

TREATMENT

GENERAL MEASURES

Current regimens target symptom relief (reduce inflammation):

- Rest and elevate affected joint(s).
- Apply ice/cool compresses to affected joints.
- Nonweight bearing on affected joint while painful; Use crutches or a walker.

MEDICATION

First Line

- A combination of pharmacologic and nonpharmacologic measures is recommended.
- Acute attacks should be treated with cool packs, rest, and joint aspiration/steroid injection.
- Chronic inflammatory CPPD arthropathy should be managed prophylactically with oral NSAIDs and/or colchicine (4)[C].
- Oral NSAIDs
  - Ibuprofen (Motrin) 600–800 mg PO TID–QID with food; maximum 3.2 g/day
  - Naproxen (Naprosyn) 500 mg PO BID with food
  - Other NSAIDs at anti-inflammatory doses are effective, although indomethacin has higher complication rates (relative risk [RR] = 2.2) compared with ibuprofen (RR = 1.2).
- Contraindications:
  - History of hypersensitivity to NSAIDs or aspirin
  - Active peptic ulcer disease or history of recurrent upper GI lesions
  - Avoid in renal insufficiency.
  - Serious GI bleeding can occur without warning; patient should be instructed on signs/symptoms. Administer proton pump inhibitor (PPI) or misoprostol 200 μg PO QID in patients at risk for NSAID-induced gastric ulcers.
- Oral colchicine
  - 0.6 mg QID or 0.6 mg hourly until symptoms relieved or vomiting/diarrhea develops; maximum dose per attack 4–6 mg; 0.5–1 mg/day may be used; avoid with significant renal insufficiency.
- Intra-articular steroid injection
  - Prednisolone–sodium phosphate 4–20 mg or triamcinolone diacetate 2–40 mg administered with local anesthetic

ALERT

Significant possible interactions for NSAIDs:

- May elevate BP in treated hypertensives
- May blunt antihypertensive effects of ACE inhibitors
- May prolong prothrombin time (PT) in patients taking oral anticoagulants
- Avoid concomitant aspirin use.
- May blunt diuretic effect of furosemide and hydrochlorothiazide
- May increase plasma lithium level in patients taking lithium carbonate

Second Line

- Oral prednisone: 30–50 mg/day for 7–10 days.
- IM triamcinolone acetonide 40 mg; may repeat in 1–4 days
- Methotrexate may have a role in severe disease resistant to traditional therapy.
- Ethylene diamine tetraacetic acid (EDTA) has been proposed as a therapy to decrease calcium deposition (binds divalent cations including calcium).
- Surgical excision for large space-occupying tophaceous lesions

ISSUES FOR REFERRAL

Consider consultation with orthopedist or rheumatologist if septic joint is a serious consideration or patient is not responding.

ADDITIONAL THERAPIES

Physical therapy

- Isometric exercises to maintain muscle strength during the acute stage (e.g., quadriceps isometric contractions, leg lifts if knee affected)
- Begin joint range-of-motion (ROM) exercises as inflammation and pain subside.
- Resume weight bearing when pain subsides.

SURGERY/OTHER PROCEDURES

Perform arthrocentesis and joint fluid analysis.

INPATIENT CONSIDERATIONS

Admission Criteria/Initial Stabilization

Consider admission for septic arthritis if:

- Synovial fluid WBC count >50,000/mL
- Strongly consider if >100,000/mL.
- Treat with appropriate antibiotics pending culture results.

ONGOING CARE

FOLLOW-UP RECOMMENDATIONS

Patient Monitoring

Reevaluate patient for response to therapy 48–72 hours after treatment instituted; reexamine 1 week later, then as needed.

DIET

No known relationship to diet

PATIENT EDUCATION

- Rest affected joint.
- Symptoms usually resolve in 7–10 days.

PROGNOSIS

- Acute attack usually resolves in 10 days; prognosis for resolution of acute attack is excellent.
- Patients may experience progressive joint damage with functional limitation.

COMPLICATIONS

- Recurrent acute attacks
- Erosive destructive arthritis

Geriatric Considerations

Elderly patients treated with NSAIDs require careful monitoring and are at higher risk for GI bleeding and acute renal insufficiency.

REFERENCES

1. Macmullan P, McCarthy G. Treatment and management of pseudogout: insights for the clinician. *Ther Adv Musculoskelet Dis*. 2012;4(2):121–131.
2. Panq L, Hayes CP, Buac K, et al. Pseudogout-associated inflammatory calcium pyrophosphate dihydrate microcrystals induce formation of neutrophil extracellular traps. *J Immunol*. 2013;190(12):6488–6500.
3. Zhang W, Doherty M, Bardin T, et al. European League Against Rheumatism recommendations for calcium pyrophosphate deposition. Part I: terminology and diagnosis. *Ann Rheum Dis*. 2011;70(4):563–570.
4. Zhang W, Doherty M, Pascual E, et al. EULAR recommendations for calcium pyrophosphate deposition. Part II: management. *Ann Rheum Dis*. 2011;70(4):571–575.

ADDITIONAL READING

- Announ N, Guerne PA. Treating difficult crystal pyrophosphate dihydrate deposition disease. *Curr Rheumatol Rep*. 2008;10(3):228–234.
- Chollet-Janin A, Finckh A, Dudler J, et al. Methotrexate as an alternative therapy for chronic calcium pyrophosphate deposition disease: an exploratory analysis. *Arthritis Rheum*. 2007;56(2):688–692.
- Demertzis JL, Rubin DA. MR imaging assessment of inflammatory, crystalline-induced, and infectious arthritides. *Magn Reson Imaging Clin North Am*. 2011;19(2):339–363.
- Pego-Reigosa JM, Rodriguez-Rodriguez M, Hurtado-Hernandez Z, et al. Calcium pyrophosphate deposition disease mimicking polymyalgia rheumatica: a prospective followup study of predictive factors for this condition in patients presenting with polymyalgia symptoms. *Arthritis Rheum*. 2005;53(6):931–938.
- Richette P, Bardin T, Doherty M. An update on the epidemiology of calcium pyrophosphate dihydrate crystal deposition disease. *Rheumatology (Oxford)*. 2009;48(7):711–715.
- Shah K, Spear J, Nathanson LA, et al. Does the presence of crystal arthritis rule out septic arthritis? *J Emerg Med*. 2007;32(1):23–26.
- Wise CM. Crystal-associated arthritis in the elderly. *Clin Geriatr Med*. 2005;21(3):491–511, v–vi.

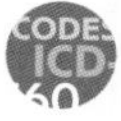

CODES

ICD10

- M11.20 Other chondrocalcinosis, unspecified site
- M11.29 Other chondrocalcinosis, multiple sites
- M11.269 Other chondrocalcinosis, unspecified knee

CLINICAL PEARLS

- Suspect in arthritis cases with a pattern of joint involvement not usually affected by degenerative joint disease (e.g., metacarpophalangeal joints, wrists).
- Perform joint fluid aspiration and analysis to evaluate acute arthritis.
- If septic arthritis is considered, treat presumptively with antibiotics until culture results are available.
- NSAID therapy is preferred treatment.
- Oral steroids are useful if NSAIDs are contraindicated.
- Intra-articular steroids can be used *if* septic arthritis has been excluded.

PSORIASIS

Edwin A. Farnell, IV, MD • Michael O. Needham, MD, CPT, MC, USA

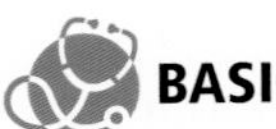

BASICS

DESCRIPTION

- A chronic, multisystem inflammatory disorder most commonly characterized by cutaneous erythematous papules and plaques with silvery scale. A complex genetic and immune-mediated disorder with flares related to systemic, psychological, infectious, and environmental factors. Skin disease with multiple different phenotypic variations and degrees of severity.
- Clinical phenotypes:
  - Plaque (vulgaris): most common variant (>80% of cases); well-demarcated, scaly, pink-to-red plaques of various sizes; symmetrically distributed on scalp, extensor surfaces of extremities, and trunk.
  - Guttate: <2% of psoriasis patients, usually in patients <30 years of age; presents abruptly with 1-mm–10-mm droplet-shaped pink papules and fine scale over trunk and extremities; often preceded by group A β-hemolytic streptococcal infection 2–3 weeks earlier
  - Inverse: affects intertriginous areas and flexural surfaces; pink-to-red plaques with minimal scale; absence of satellite pustules distinguishes it from candidiasis although may coexist.
  - Erythrodermic: ~1–2.25% of psoriasis patients; generalized erythema and scaling, affecting >75% of body surface area; associated with desquamation, hair loss, nail dystrophy, and systemic symptoms such as fever, chills, malaise, or high-output cardiac failure; may require hospital admission for management of dehydration, electrolyte abnormalities, and high risk of infection
  - Pustular: sterile pustules; several forms including generalized pustular psoriasis, annular pustular psoriasis, and impetigo herpetiformis; generalized type can result in life-threatening bacterial superinfections, sepsis, and dehydration if left untreated.
  - Nail disease: pitting, oil spots, and thickening; nails involved in up to 50% of patients with psoriasis with lifetime incidence of 80–90%
  - Psoriatic arthritis: seronegative inflammatory spondyloarthropathy; mono and asymmetric oligoarthritis

EPIDEMIOLOGY

Incidence

Predominant sex: male = female. Predominant age: two peaks in incidence between the ages of 20–30 years and 50–60 years

Prevalence

- 2–4.7%—similar prevalence in all races
- ~80% of patients have mild to moderate disease (1).

ETIOLOGY AND PATHOPHYSIOLOGY

Antigenic triggers activate dendritic cells and T cells; dendritic cells produce type I interferon, and interleukin (IL)-20, which speeds keratinocyte proliferation; myeloid dendritic cells release IL-23 in lymph nodes, recruiting TH1 and TH17 cells to the lesions; T cells produce numerous cytokines, including interferon-γ, IL-17, and IL-22 that stimulate keratinocytes to proliferate and produce proinflammatory antimicrobial peptides and cytokines, which recruit neutrophils to the epidermis and activate dermal fibroblasts.

Genetics

- Genetic predisposition (probably polygenic)
- 40% have psoriasis in a 1st-degree relative.
- Increased incidence of specific human leukocyte antigens (e.g., HLA-Cw6)
- Multiple susceptibility loci contain genes involved in immune system regulation (e.g., psoriasis-susceptibility [*PSORS1*] locus on chromosome 6p21; polymorphisms in the IL-12/IL-13 receptor, the p40 subunit of IL-12 and IL-23, and the p19 subunit of IL-12) (2)

RISK FACTORS

- Family history
- Local trauma; local irritation (exacerbation)
- HIV; streptococcal infection
- Mental stress (exacerbation)
- Medications (lithium, antimalarials, β-blockers, interferon, withdrawal of steroids)
- Smoking

GENERAL PREVENTION

Avoid triggers, including trauma, sunburns, smoking, and exposure to certain medications (as mentioned earlier), alcohol, and stress; weight loss if obese

COMMONLY ASSOCIATED CONDITIONS

- Psoriatic arthritis
- Obesity, metabolic syndrome, diabetes, CKD
- Cardiovascular disease; atherosclerotic disease
- Nonalcoholic fatty liver disease (NAFLD)
- Autoimmune: alopecia areata, celiac disease, Crohn disease, systemic sclerosis
- Psychiatric/psychological: depression, suicide, emotional burden/anxiety, alcohol abuse (3)
- Malignancy: lymphoma, nonmelanoma skin cancer with psoralen–UVA (PUVA) therapy

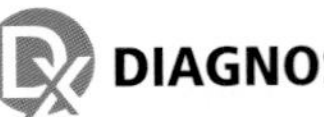

DIAGNOSIS

HISTORY

- May include sudden onset of clearly demarcated, erythematous plaques with overlying silvery scales exacerbation of chronic plaques; especially on extensor surfaces and scalp; typically no or mild pruritus; triggers may include streptococcal/viral infection or trauma.
- Family history of similar condition

PHYSICAL EXAM

- Well-demarcated salmon pink-to-red erythematous papules and plaques; silvery scale
- Distribution favors scalp, auricular conchal bowls and postauricular area; extensor surface of extremities, especially knees and elbows; umbilicus, lower back, intergluteal cleft, and nails
- Nail findings: pitting, oil spots, onycholysis, splinter hemorrhages, subungual hyperkeratosis
- Auspitz sign: underlying pinpoints of bleeding following scraping of plaques
- Koebner phenomenon: new psoriatic lesions arising at sites of skin injury/trauma
- Genitals affected up to 40% of patients (4)
- Sebopsoriasis: Psoriasis can overlap with seborrheic dermatitis as greasy scales on the eyebrows, nasolabial folds, and postauricular and presternal areas

DIFFERENTIAL DIAGNOSIS

- Plaque: seborrheic dermatitis, nummular eczema, atopic dermatitis, contact dermatitis, lichen planus, lichen simplex chronicus, tinea, pityriasis rubra pilaris, subacute/discoid lupus erythematosus, squamous cell carcinoma in situ
- Guttate: pityriasis rosea, pityriasis lichenoides chronica, lichen planus, secondary syphilis, small plaque parapsoriasis
- Pustular: subcorneal pustulosis, acute generalized exanthematous pustulosis, folliculitis, pemphigus foliaceous
- Erythrodermic: cutaneous T-cell lymphoma, drug-induced erythroderma, ichthyosiform erythroderma

DIAGNOSTIC TESTS & INTERPRETATION

Initial Tests (lab, imaging)

Clinical diagnosis based on history and physical exam. May include negative rheumatoid factor, normal erythrocyte sedimentation rate (ESR), and C-reactive protein (elevated in pustular/erythrodermic variants); uric acid level may be elevated in pustular psoriasis; sterile fluid from pustules with neutrophilic infiltrate; fungal studies in hand and foot psoriasis

Diagnostic Procedures/Other

- Psoriasis Area and Severity Index (PASI) evaluates overall severity and body surface area (BSA) involvement.
- Physicians Global Assessment: Target plaque score and the percentage BSA together; 4-mm punch biopsy from affected skin, if necessary
- Dermatology Life Quality Index (DLQI)

Test Interpretation

Biopsy: Thickening of the stratum corneum (hyperkeratosis) with retention of nuclei (parakeratosis); elongation, thickening, and clubbing of rete ridges; dilated tortuous capillary loops in the dermal papillae; perivascular lymphocytic infiltrate, Munro microabscesses: neutrophils in stratum corneum

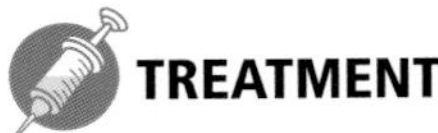

TREATMENT

GENERAL MEASURES

Adequate topical hydration (emollients), sun exposure (avoid sunburns), stress relief

MEDICATION

First Line

- Mild to moderate disease
  - Emollients BID: petrolatum/ointments to maintain skin hydration and minimize pruritus and risk of koebnerization
  - Topical corticosteroids:
    - Anti-inflammatory, antiproliferative, immunosuppressive, and vasoconstrictive effects; tachyphylaxis develops over time, may alternate to prevent.
    - Local side effects: skin atrophy, hypopigmentation, striae, acne, folliculitis, and purpura. Systemic side effects: Risk is higher with higher potency formulations used over a large surface for a prolonged period; pregnancy Category C
    - Applications are typically twice daily until lesions flatten/resolve, then taper to PRN use for maintenance.
    - Scalp: strong potency in solution/foam vehicle; shampoos and sprays also available
    - Face, intertriginous areas, infants: low-potency corticosteroids: 1% hydrocortisone
    - Adult initial therapy: medium-potency corticosteroids daily (e.g., 0.1% mometasone or triamcinolone); strong-potency corticosteroids: 0.05% betamethasone or fluocinonide daily; superpotency corticosteroids: clobetasol, halobetasol; limit use to 2–4 weeks; avoid occlusive dressings; reserved for recalcitrant plaques

P

- Vitamin D analogues: calcipotriene 0.005% ointment daily–BID; limits keratinocyte hyperproliferation; may be highly effective for short-term control in combination with a superpotent corticosteroid; should not be used with products that can alter pH, such as topical lactic acid; local side effects: burning, pruritus, edema, peeling, dryness, and erythema; pregnancy Category C
- Topical retinoids: tazarotene 0.05% or 0.1% (Tazorac) daily; normalizes abnormal keratinocyte differentiation and diminishes hyperproliferation; may be combined with corticosteroids; side effects: local irritation, photosensitivity; pregnancy Category X
- Topical calcineurin inhibitors: tacrolimus 0.1% or pimecrolimus 1% may be used as steroid-sparing agents, especially in facial and intertriginous areas
- Comparison of topical therapies: vitamin D analogues have slower onset of action than topical corticosteroids, but longer disease-free periods for body plaques. For scalp, potent and superpotency steroids more effective (5)[A]
- Combination of superpotent steroids and vitamin D analogs has better efficacy than either as monotherapy or come in combination compounds (6)[A].

• Severe disease: may need combination therapy

- Light therapy: Locally immunosuppressive and antiproliferative. Natural sunlight; UVB (broad/narrow band [BB, NB]) or PUVA: Treatment protocols are skin type–dependent: PUVA most effective, followed by NB-UVB, then BB-UVB (7)[A]; well-tolerated, but increased risk of nonmelanoma skin cancers with >350 treatments
- Systemic therapies:
  ○ Methotrexate: blocks DNA synthesis and inhibits proliferation of lymphoid tissue; start 7.5–15 mg/week IV, PO, IM, or SC, then increase 2.5 mg every 2–3 weeks, up to 25 mg; contraindicated in pregnancy; supplement with folic acid 1–5 mg/day to protect against side effects: hepatotoxicity, pulmonary toxicity, bone marrow suppression; baseline chest x-ray, monitor LFTs, renal function, CBC, testing for latent tuberculosis (TB); consider liver biopsy when cumulative dose reaches 3.5–4 g; avoid alcohol and medications that interfere with folic acid metabolism, including Bactrim, sulfamethoxazole, or hepatotoxic agents (e.g., retinoids).
  ○ Cyclosporine: inhibits T-cell activation; start 2.5 mg/kg/day; if insufficient response after 4 weeks, increase by 0.5 mg/kg/day; additional dosage increases every 2 weeks (max dose: 4 mg/kg/day pregnancy category C; side effects: renal toxicity and hypertension, limit long-term use: monitor renal function, CBC with Mg^{2+} and K^+, and BP.
  ○ Acitretin (Soriatane): systemic retinoid; onset ranges from 3 to 6 months; start 25–50 mg/day given with the main meal; effective for pustular psoriasis and as a maintenance therapy after stabilization with other agents; sometimes combined with UV-B/PUVA; pregnancy Category X: pregnancy test before starting; 2 forms of contraception 1 month before, during, and for at least 3 years after treatment; avoid alcohol (may convert acitretin to etretinate); side effects: alopecia, xerosis, cheilitis, hepatotoxicity, hyperlipidemia, cataracts; monitor LFTs, renal function, lipid profile, CBC; regular eye exams
- Biologics: general guidelines: Screen for latent TB at baseline and yearly, hepatitis panel at baseline, avoid live vaccines; monitor CBC with differential, signs/symptoms of infections, heart failure, malignancy, drug-induced lupus, inflammatory bowel disease, demyelinating disorder. Some concern for "biologic fatigue" phenomenon, or loss of PASI 75 over time. All should be considered effective 1st-line treatments (8)[A],(9). Pregnancy Category B
  ○ TNF-α inhibitors: eternacept (Enbrel): Begin at 50 mg SC twice a week × 3 months then maintenance of 50 mg/week. Adalimumab (Humira): Dosing starts at 80 mg SC × 1 week, then 40 mg SC every other week. Infliximab (Remicade): TNF inhibitor: 5 mg/kg IV at weeks 0, 2, and 6; maintenance doses of 5 mg/kg every 8 weeks thereafter; adjust interval, as needed; anaphylaxis-like infusion reaction occurs in <1% of patients.
  ○ IL-12/IL-23 antagonist: ustekinumab (Stelara): patients <100 kg: 45 mg SC at weeks 0 and 4, then every 12 weeks; >100 kg: 90 mg can be given.

Second Line

Immunosuppressives: azathioprine, hydroxyurea, 6-thioguanine, fumaric acid esters, and topicals: salicylic acid; anthralin

ISSUES FOR REFERRAL

Psoriasis >20% of BSA, severe extremity involvement, particularly hands and feet

SURGERY/OTHER PROCEDURES

Psoriasis and psoriatic medications can affect wound healing postoperatively; methotrexate: Monitor for postoperative infections; hold cyclosporine for 1 week before and after; some surgeons may prefer to hold therapy with biologics for up to 1 month before and after surgery.

INPATIENT CONSIDERATIONS

Admission Criteria/Initial Stabilization

Generalized pustular psoriasis/erythrodermic psoriasis: Rule out sepsis; restoration of barrier function of skin with cleaning and bandaging; intensive topical corticosteroid therapy, phototherapy, systemic therapy, particularly medications with a quick onset such as oral cyclosporine; management of electrolytes

ONGOING CARE

FOLLOW-UP RECOMMENDATIONS

Measure BSA involvement to determine if therapy is working; change therapy or add agent if no improvement is seen.

DIET

Well-balanced diet and exercise to limit cardiovascular risk factors and decrease risk of associated conditions, including obesity, metabolic syndrome, diabetes, and atherosclerosis.

PATIENT EDUCATION

National Psoriasis Foundation: www.psoriasis.org; 800-723-9166

PROGNOSIS

Guttate form may be self-limited and remit after 4 months; chronic plaque type is lifelong, with intermittent spontaneous remissions and exacerbations; erythrodermic and generalized pustular forms may be severe and persistent

COMPLICATIONS

Psoriatic arthritis, generalized pustular psoriasis, erythrodermic psoriasis

REFERENCES

1. Menter A, Korman NJ, Elmets CA, et al. Guidelines of care for the management of psoriasis and psoriatic arthritis: section 6. Guidelines of care for the treatment of psoriasis and psoriatic arthritis: case-based presentations and evidence-based conclusions. *J Am Acad Dermatol*. 2011;65(1):137–174.
2. Villasenor-Park J, Wheeler D, Grandinetti L. Psoriasis: evolving treatment for a complex disease. *Cleve Clin J Med*. 2012;79(6):413–423.
3. Brenaut E, Pouplard C, Barnetche C, et al. Alcohol consumption and psoriasis: a systemic literature review. *J Eur Acad Dermatol Venereol*. 2013;7(Suppl 3):30–35.
4. Meeuwis K, de Hullu J, Massuger L, et al. Genital psoriasis: a systemic literature review on this hidden skin disease. *Acta Derm Venereol*. 2011:91(1):5–11.
5. Mason AR, Mason J, Cork M, et al. Topical treatment for chronic plaque psoriasis. *Cochrane Database Syst Rev*. 2013;3:CD005028.
6. Hendricks A, Keijsers R, Jong E, et al. Efficacy and safety of combinations of first-line topical treatments in chronic plaque psoriasis: a systematic literature review. *J Eur Acad Dermatol Venereol*. 2013;27(8):931–951.
7. Almutawa F, Alnomair N, Wang Y. Systematic review of UV-based therapies for psoriasis. *Am J Clin Derm*. 2013;14(2):87–109.
8. Galván-Banqueri M, Marín Gil R, Santos Ramos B, et al. Biologic treatments for moderate-to-severe psoriasis: indirect comparison. *J Clin Pharm Ther*. 2013;38(2):121–130.
9. Menter A, Gottlieb A, Feldman SR, et al. Guidelines of care for the management of psoriasis and psoriatic arthritis: section 1. Overview of psoriasis and guidelines of care for the treatment of psoriasis with biologics. *J Am Acad Dermatol*. 2008;58(5):826–850.

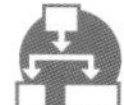

SEE ALSO

Arthritis, Psoriatic

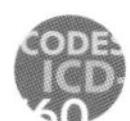

CODES

ICD10

• L40.9 Psoriasis, unspecified
• L40.50 Arthropathic psoriasis, unspecified
• L42 Pityriasis rosea

CLINICAL PEARLS

Chronic lifelong inflammatory skin condition with remissions and exacerbations; set realistic expectations with patient. Disease burden not limited to skin. If 1 medication does not work, use/combine with another agent.

PSYCHOSIS

Michael Golding, MD • Robert A. Baldor, MD, FAAFP

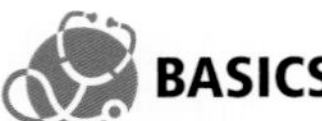

BASICS

DESCRIPTION

Syndrome seen with schizophrenia, schizoaffective disorder, mood disorder, substance use, medical problems, delirium, and dementia; symptoms include the following:

- Positive symptoms: hallucinations and delusions (fixed false and often paranoid beliefs created as the patient loses the ability to correct errors in thinking)
- Negative symptoms: apathy, avolition, withdrawal
- Disorganized speech/behavior
- Cognition: decreased working memory, difficulty with attention, poor and slow information interpretation

EPIDEMIOLOGY

Prevalence

- Schizophrenia: peak onset 18–25 years in men; women peak onset 25–35 years
  - 1% of the U.S. population; thought to be similar worldwide
- Delusional disorder: 0.03% of population
- Bipolar type I: 1% of population
- Prevalence in major depression not known

ETIOLOGY AND PATHOPHYSIOLOGY

- Neurodevelopmental predisposition + 1st/3rd trimester in utero insult (e.g., 1st trimester infection or 3rd trimester birth hypoxia) leads to exaggerated neuronal apoptosis in late adolescence with subsequent thalamic sensory overload. Increased dopaminergic mesolimbic transmission may contribute to delusions and hallucinations in schizophrenia. Dopamine deficiency in mesocortical pathways may contribute to frontal lobe hypoactivity often associated with apathy and withdrawal in schizophrenia. Glutamate, neurosteroids, and neurodevelopmental abnormalities are active areas of research.
- Postulated stress-diathesis model: Individuals biologically at risk develop psychosis when under stress.

Genetics

Schizophrenia: 50% concordance for monozygotic twins, little or no shared environmental effect; multiple candidate genes involving disruption of neurodevelopment

RISK FACTORS

Substance abuse (particularly marijuana), family history of psychosis, lower socioeconomic status

GENERAL PREVENTION

Community interventions for early detection and treatment of prodromal symptoms show promise.

COMMONLY ASSOCIATED CONDITIONS

- Serious mental illness is associated with metabolic syndrome, autonomic dysfunction, and sudden cardiac death.
- Cancer mortality: particularly breast and lung cancer
- Substance abuse disorders, including nicotine dependence

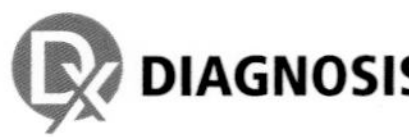

DIAGNOSIS

First, rule out delirium: Psychosis should not have fluctuating consciousness/reduced clarity of awareness.

HISTORY

- Delusions (fixed false beliefs): persecutory (being monitored), bizarre (involving impossible states), somatic (fixed belief in nonexistent serious illness), referential (getting messages from TV, radio, or thoughts inserted/deleted by others), grandiose (belief that one has special powers)
- Hallucinations: auditory, visual, tactile
- Bipolar illness, depression, and dementia are all associated with psychosis, so screen for symptoms of depression, mania, and memory loss
- Screen for toxidromes of drugs of abuse
- Screen for history of epileptiform activity
- Suicidality: higher risk with comorbid depression/mania, previous suicide attempts, drug abuse, agitation/akathisia, poor compliance

PHYSICAL EXAM

- Mental status exam: disorganized idea sequencing and/or error correction, not incorrect thought content, is the *condicio sine qua non* of schizophrenia. Patients often have negative symptoms (e.g., social withdrawal, lack of initiative, poverty of thought) and disorganized behavior.
- Attention to neurologic focalities, antipsychotic-induced parkinsonism, tardive dyskinesia, and akathisia
- May rarely present with catatonia: extreme excitement/lack of movement; posturing, mutism, grimacing, waxy flexibility

DIFFERENTIAL DIAGNOSIS

- Schizophrenia: positive symptoms (psychosis) and negative symptoms (flat affect), prodrome of social withdrawal, cognitive impairment; schizophreniform disorder: psychotic/prodromal symptoms in <6 months; schizoaffective disorder: manic/depressive mood disorder with hallucinations/delusions that persist even when euthymic; schizotypal personality disorder: no true psychosis but distance in relationships and odd beliefs; delusional disorder: nonbizarre delusion (e.g., erotomanic, grandiose, jealous, persecutory, somatic), no negative/mood symptoms
- Mood disorder with psychotic features: can occur in mania/depression. Delusions often mood-congruent; psychosis remits when mood improves.
- Substance-induced psychosis: alcohol and benzodiazepine withdrawal, intoxication with cocaine, bath salts, PCP, cannabis, amphetamines, hallucinogens, and alcohol. May persist beyond acute intoxication.
- Borderline personality disorder: During extreme stress, patients often experience auditory/visual hallucinations (psychosis NOS).
- Posttraumatic stress disorder: psychosis associated with traumatic recollections. Often visual hallucinations (vs. more auditory in schizophrenia).
- Psychosis due to general medical condition: delirium, stroke, infection, collagen vascular disease, head injury, tumor, interictal, porphyria, syphilis, etc.
- Medication-induced psychosis: common causes: steroids, L-dopa, anticholinergic medication, antidepressants in bipolar patients, interferon, digoxin, stimulants

DIAGNOSTIC TESTS & INTERPRETATION

Test for causes of delirium mimicking psychosis, if uncertain.

- Broad screen for medical causes: CBC, metabolic panel, LFTs, thyroid-stimulating hormone (TSH), rapid plasma reagin (RPR), HIV, vitamin B_{12}, U/A, and screens for subclinical infection in elderly
- Screen for drugs of abuse.
- No imaging necessary for diagnosis. Consider MRI/CT to evaluate for medical cause of symptoms, especially if new onset or in elderly. In research studies, schizophrenia is associated with enlarged lateral ventricles and less frontal activity.

Follow-Up Tests & Special Considerations

Because of elevated risk related to schizophrenia and psychotropic medications, screen for metabolic syndrome.

- Consider: Wilson disease, porphyria, metachromatic leukodystrophy, inflammatory conditions
- Consider ECG: Antipsychotics can prolong corrected QT (QTc) interval, particularly ziprasidone, thioridazine, droperidol, IV haloperidol
- Consider lumbar puncture if unable to distinguish from delirium and/or unexplained rapid-onset psychosis.
- Consider electroencephalogram (EEG) for partial complex seizures and psychosis associated with preictal and postictal events.

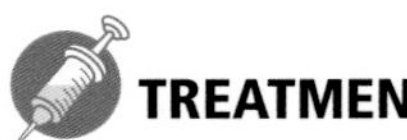

TREATMENT

Before antipsychotic treatment, lipid profile, fasting blood sugar, LFTs, metabolic panel, weight (1)[B]

MEDICATION

- Antipsychotics are the mainstay of treatment (1)[B].
- Classified as typical versus atypical. Dopamine-2 (D_2) antagonists with varied affinity for the receptor. Atypicals also block serotonin 5-HT2A receptors. Help positive symptoms more than negative. Nonspecific effect on agitation begins early; antipsychotic effect takes 1–6 weeks.
- For mania with psychotic features, a mood stabilizer may be used with an antipsychotic.
- For major depression with psychotic features, antidepressant and antipsychotic medications yield better response rate than either medication alone.
- In delirium, must treat underlying cause
- Risks of antipsychotic medications include the following:
  - Acute dystonia: Use 1–3 mg IM/IV benztropine initially, then 0.5–2 mg BID–TID or diphenhydramine 50–100 mg IM/IV BID–TID max 400 mg/day.
  - Parkinsonism: Lower antipsychotic dose; switch to atypical (particularly, quetiapine, olanzapine, or clozapine) or add benztropine 0.5–2 mg PO BID–TID, diphenhydramine 25–50 mg BID–TID.
  - Akathisia: intense restlessness, especially legs. Lower antipsychotic dose; treat with β-blocker, anticholinergic, or benzodiazepine; may switch to antipsychotic with lower risk for akathisia such as quetiapine, olanzapine, iloperidone, or clozapine
  - Tardive dyskinesia: 20% of those treated long-term with typicals. Switch to clozapine or quetiapine. If cannot, minimize dose.
  - Neuroleptic malignant syndrome: potentially fatal; rigidity, tremor, fever, autonomic instability, mental status changes; discontinue neuroleptic; ICU; volume resuscitation; cooling blankets; no anticholinergics/antihistaminics; consider dantrolene, amantadine, bromocriptine electroconvulsive therapy (ECT)
  - Metabolic syndrome, sudden cardiac death (risk higher IM/IV droperidol, IV haloperidol), stroke (elderly), QTc prolonged, pulmonary embolus

First Line

- Benefits of some of the atypical antipsychotics include low risk of extrapyramidal symptoms (quetiapine, olanzapine, iloperidone, or clozapine) and tardive dyskinesia (clozapine, quetiapine); possibly more effective for negative symptoms
- Greater risk of weight gain, new-onset diabetes, and hyperlipidemia with olanzapine and clozapine compared with typicals and some of the other atypicals (ziprasidone, aripiprazole)
- Acute psychotic agitation: olanzapine 5–10 mg IM with up to three 10-mg injections over a 24-hour period, care with subsequent benzodiazepines; ziprasidone 10 mg IM q2h or 20 mg q4h; max 40 mg over a 24-hour period; haloperidol/lorazepam 5 mg/2 mg IM often with 1 mg IM benztropine, max 20 mg haloperidol, and 8 mg lorazepam over a 24-hour period
- Psychosis in schizophrenia
  - Olanzapine: Start 5–10 mg at bedtime, target dose 5–20 mg/day within 2 days and up to 40 mg/day in treatment-refractory schizophrenia. More likely weight gain, hyperlipidemia, and hyperglycemia than other oral atypicals except clozapine; may have lower rates of discontinuation and rehospitalization than several other atypicals but likely not more efficacy than clozapine. Sedation initially.
  - Quetiapine: Start 25 mg BID 25–50 mg BID–TID on days 2 and 3, up to 300–400 mg in divided doses by day 4. Within 2 weeks, up to 400–800 mg/day divided BID–TID; less parkinsonism, useful in Parkinson disease psychosis; more weight gain than aripiprazole, lurasidone, ziprasidone; sedation, restless legs syndrome; more gradual titration tolerated better. Quetiapine XR can start 300 mg/day. Dose increases can be within 1 day and up to 300 mg/day, but slower start and titration may be better; target dose 300–800 mg at bedtime
  - Risperidone: Start 1–2 mg/day; target dose of 2–6 mg/day to be reached over 1–2 weeks; doses >6 mg rarely more effective and higher risk of parkinsonism. Higher risk of prolactinemia/parkinsonism than clozapine, quetiapine, olanzapine.
  - Paliperidone: Start 3–6 mg/day target dose 6–12 mg/day; titrate over 1–2 weeks. Higher risk of prolactinemia/parkinsonism than clozapine, quetiapine, olanzapine.
  - Ziprasidone: Start 20–40 mg PO BID, with target dose of 100–200 mg/day in divided doses over 2 weeks; prolongs QTc; less likely to cause weight gain than other atypicals; higher risk of akathisia/parkinsonism than clozapine, quetiapine, olanzapine. Requires meal. Often sedation.
  - Aripiprazole: Start 10–15 mg/day, may increase up to 30 mg/day over a week or 2; less weight gain but higher rates of akathisia/parkinsonism than clozapine, quetiapine, olanzapine
  - Asenapine: Start 5 mg at bedtime or BID sublingually, increase to 10 mg BID if needed over a week or 2; less weight gain than some, higher rates of akathisia/parkinsonism than clozapine, quetiapine, olanzapine; sedation, orthostatic hypotension, numb tongue, nausea, bad taste
  - Lurasidone: Start 20–40 mg once daily with food (at least 350 calories), increase to 80/120 mg at bedtime if needed over 2–4 weeks. Less weight gain than some but higher rates of akathisia/parkinsonism than clozapine, quetiapine, olanzapine; not antihistaminic but α-blocking sedation and serotonergic nausea.
  - Iloperidone: Start 1 mg BID, may increase by 2 mg BID each day, but slower can be better due to significant orthostasis. Increase to max 12 mg BID. Little akathisia/parkinsonism, less weight gain than olanzapine or clozapine but slower efficacy due to long titration, orthostasis, sedation.

Geriatric Considerations

Increased risk of cerebrovascular accident when antipsychotics are used in the elderly with dementia 3[B]

Second Line

- Clozapine: more effective for reducing symptoms, preventing relapse, decreasing tardive dyskinesia, and decreasing suicidality than other antipsychotics but 2nd line given risk of fatal agranulocytosis. National registry for all patients on clozapine, weekly CBC and absolute neutrophil count (ANC) for 6 months then every 2 weeks for 6 months, then every 4 weeks. More weight gain, hyperlipidemia, hyperglycemia, seizures, myocarditis, pulmonary embolus, and sedation but low rate of parkinsonism, tardive dyskinesia. Useful in treatment-refractory psychosis and in Parkinson disease psychosis.
- Despite association with more weight gain than other antipsychotics, clozapine and olanzapine do not appear to increase risk of cardiac and all-cause mortality (4,5)[B].
- Long-acting preparations: available for 2 typicals (haloperidol and fluphenazine) and 4 atypicals (risperidone, paliperidone, olanzapine, aripiprazole; olanzapine requires registration due to rare delirium syndrome). Test tolerability with oral medication first. Long-acting antipsychotics promote compliance.
- Long-acting haloperidol, paliperidone, olanzapine, aripiprazole administered every 4 weeks; long-acting risperidone and fluphenazine administered every 2 weeks

ISSUES FOR REFERRAL

Encourage contact with advocacy groups for families and patients (National Alliance for the Mentally Ill).

ADDITIONAL THERAPIES

Cognitive-behavioral therapy (CBT) is an effective adjuvant to antipsychotics (1)[B].

INPATIENT CONSIDERATIONS

Admission Criteria/Initial Stabilization

At risk for harm to self or others; extreme functional impairment; unable to care for self; new-onset psychosis

Discharge Criteria

No longer a danger to self or others and adequate outpatient treatment in place

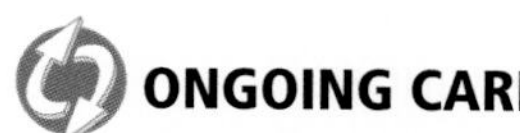

ONGOING CARE

FOLLOW-UP RECOMMENDATIONS

Close follow-up for inpatient discharge (high risk for suicide), use CBT, exercise, teach smoking cessation

PATIENT EDUCATION

National Alliance on Mental Illness: www.nami.org/

PROGNOSIS

Schizophrenia: fluctuating course, 70% first-episode psychosis patients improve in 3–4 months; 7% will die of suicide; 20–40% will attempt suicide.

REFERENCES

1. National Institute for Health and Care Excellence. Psychosis and schizophrenia in adults: treatment and management. http://www.nice.org.uk/guidance/cg178. Accessed 2014.
2. McEvoy JP, Lieberman JA, Stroup TS. Effectiveness of clozapine versus olanzapine, quetiapine, and risperidone in patients with chronic schizophrenia who did not respond to prior atypical antipsychotic treatment. *Am J Psychiatry*. 2006;163(4):600–610.
3. van Iersel MB, Zuidema SU, Koopmans RT. Antipsychotics for behavioural and psychological problems in elderly people with dementia: a systematic review of adverse events. *Drugs Aging*. 2005;22(10):845–858.
4. Tilhonen J, Lönnqvist J, Wahlbeck K, et al. 11-year follow-up mortality in patients with schizophrenia: a population-based cohort study. *Lancet*. 2009;374(9690):620–627.
5. Strom BL, Faich G, Eng SM. Comparative mortality associated with ziprasidone and olanzapine in real-world use: the Ziprasidone Observational Study of Cardiac Outcomes (ZODIAC). *Eur Psychiatry*. 2008;23:158.

SEE ALSO

Delirium; Schizophrenia

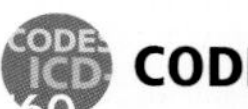

CODES

ICD10

- F29 Unsp psychosis not due to a substance or known physiol cond
- F20.9 Schizophrenia, unspecified
- F39 Unspecified mood [affective] disorder

CLINICAL PEARLS

- Antipsychotics are the mainstay of treatment; evidence corroborates decreased all-cause mortality in patients who are adherent to these medications.
- Clozapine and long-acting preparations are likely underused in schizophrenia in the United States and may increase adherence, whereas newer atypicals (quetiapine, lurasidone, aripiprazole, olanzapine-fluoxetine combination) may help with depressive symptoms in psychosis.

PULMONARY ARTERIAL HYPERTENSION

Urooj Najm, MBBS • Najm Hasan Siddiqui, MD

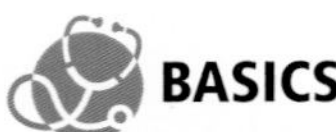

BASICS

DESCRIPTION

- Pulmonary arterial hypertension (PAH) is a category of pulmonary hypertension (PH) characterized by abnormalities in the small pulmonary arteries (precapillary PH) that produce increased pulmonary arterial pressure (PAP) and vascular resistance, eventually resulting in right-sided heart failure. PAH is a progressive disorder associated with increased mortality.
  - Previously, PH was classified as primary PH (without cause: now idiopathic pulmonary arterial hypertension [IPAH]) or secondary PH (with cause or associated condition); now it is clear that some types of secondary PH closely match primary PH (IPAH) in their histology, natural history, and response to treatment. Therefore, WHO classifies PH into five groups based on mechanism, with PAH as group 1 in this classification.
- PAH is diagnosed by right heart catheterization and defined by:
  - Mean PAP ≥25 mm Hg at rest
  - Pulmonary capillary wedge pressure ≤15 mm Hg (to exclude PH owing to left heart disease i.e., group 2 PH)
  - Mild or absent chronic lung disease or other causes of hypoxemia (excludes PH owing to lung disease or hypoxemia; i.e., group 3 PH)
  - Absent venous thromboembolic disease (excludes chronic thromboembolic PH; i.e., group 4 PH)
  - Absent systemic disorder (like sarcoidosis), hematologic disorders (like myeloproliferative disease), and metabolic disorders (like glycogen storage disease). Purpose is to exclude group 5 PH.
- PAH is divided into following main categories:
  - Idiopathic: sporadic, with no family history or risk factors
  - Heritable: IPAH with mutations or familial cases with or without mutations
  - Drug- or toxin induced: mostly associated with anorectics (e.g., fenfluramine), rapeseed oil, L-tryptophan, and illicit drugs such as methamphetamine and cocaine
  - Associated: connective tissue diseases (e.g., systemic lupus erythematosus, rheumatoid arthritis, scleroderma); HIV infection; portal hypertension; congenital heart disease; schistosomiasis; chronic hemolytic anemia (e.g., sickle cell disease)
  - Pulmonary veno-occlusive disease (PVOD) and/or pulmonary capillary hemangiomatosis (PCH) and persistent pulmonary hypertension of the newborn (PPHN) are classified as separate categories due to more differences than similarities with PAH.
    - PVOD and/or PCH: rare cause of PH characterized by extensive diffuse occlusion of the pulmonary veins (unlike PAH which involves the small mascular pulmonary arterioles)
  - PPHN
- System(s) affected: pulmonary; cardiovascular

EPIDEMIOLOGY

- Age: can occur at any age; mean age, 37 years
- Sex (IPAH): female > male (~4:1)

Incidence

- Overall PAH: 5–52 cases/million
- IPAH: low, ~2–6 per million
- Drug-induced PAH: 1/25,000 with >3 months of anorectic use
- HIV associated: 0.5/100
- Portal hypertension associated: 1–6/100
- Scleroderma associated: 6–60%

Prevalence

- PAH: ~15–50 cases per million
- IPAH: ~6 cases per million

ETIOLOGY AND PATHOPHYSIOLOGY

- Pulmonary: Inflammation, vasoconstriction, endothelial dysfunction, and remodeling of pulmonary arteries produced by increased cell proliferation and reduced rates of apoptosis lead to obstruction.
- Cardiovascular: right ventricular hypertrophy (RVH), eventually leading to right-sided heart failure
- IPAH: by definition, unknown. True IPAH is mostly sporadic or sometimes familial in nature.
- Pulmonary arteriolar hyperactivity and vasoconstriction, occult thromboembolism, or autoimmune (high frequency of antinuclear antibodies)

GENETICS

- 75% of heritable pulmonary arterial hypertension (HPAH) cases and 25% of IPAH cases have mutations in *BMPR2* (autosomal dominant).
- Mutations in *ALK1* and endoglin (autosomal dominant) also are associated with PAH.

RISK FACTORS

- Female sex
- Previous anorectic drug use
- Recent acute pulmonary embolism
- Commonly associated conditions
- First-degree relatives of patient with familial PAH

COMMONLY ASSOCIATED CONDITIONS

See associated PAH, earlier discussed.

DIAGNOSIS

Symptoms of PAH are nonspecific, which can lead to missed or delayed diagnosis of this serious disease.

HISTORY

Dyspnea, weakness, syncope, dizziness, chest pain, palpitations, lower extremity edema

PHYSICAL EXAM

- Pulmonary component of S_2 (at apex in >90% of patients)
- Right ventricular (RV) lift
- Early systolic click of pulmonary valve
- Pansystolic murmur of tricuspid regurgitation
- Diastolic murmur of pulmonic insufficiency (Graham-Steell murmur)
- RV S3 or S4
- Edema as jugular vein distention, ascites, hepatomegaly, or peripheral edema

DIFFERENTIAL DIAGNOSIS

Other causes of dyspnea:

- Pulmonary parenchymal disease such as chronic obstructive pulmonary disease
- Pulmonary vascular disease such as pulmonary thromboembolism
- Cardiac disease such as cardiomyopathy
- Other disorders of respiratory function such as sleep apnea

DIAGNOSTIC TESTS & INTERPRETATION

- ECG: RVH and right axis deviation
- Pulmonary function testing and/or arterial blood gas: arterial hypoxemia, reduced diffusion capacity, hypocapnia
- Ventilation–perfusion ratio (V/Q) scan: must rule out proximal pulmonary artery emboli and chronic thromboembolic PH (CTEPH)
- Exercise test: reduced maximal O_2 consumption, high minute ventilation, low anaerobic threshold, increased PO_2 alveolar–arterial gradient; correlation to severity of disease with 6-minute walk test
- Antinuclear antibody positive (up to 40% of patients)
- LFTs to evaluate for portopulmonary HTN, a complication of chronic liver disease
- HIV test, thyroid function tests, sickle cell disease screening
- Elevated brain natriuretic peptide (BNP) and N-terminal-proBNP may be useful for early detection of PAH in young, otherwise healthy patients with mild symptoms. It can also be used to assess disease severity and prognosis.
- Chest radiograph
  - Prominent central pulmonary arteries with peripheral hypovascularity of pulmonary arterial branches
  - RV enlargement is a late finding.
- Echo Doppler
  - Should be performed with suspicion of PAH; recent studies show some inaccuracy compared with right-sided heart catheterization
  - Most commonly used screening tool
    - Estimates mean PAP and assesses cardiac structure and function, excludes congenital anomalies
    - Echo suggests, but does not diagnose, PAH. Invasive hemodynamic evaluation confirms PAH diagnosis.
- Right atrial and ventricular enlargement; tricuspid regurgitation
- Important to rule out underlying cardiac disease such as atrial septal defect with secondary PH or mitral stenosis
- Cardiac magnetic resonance is not commonly used.

Diagnostic Procedures/Other

- Pulmonary angiography
  - Should be done if V/Q scan suggests CTEPH
  - Use caution; can lead to hemodynamic collapse; use low osmolar agents, subselective angiograms.
- Right-sided cardiac catheterization (gold standard for diagnosis of PAH)
  - Essential first step to confirm diagnosis and determine severity and prognosis by measuring pulmonary arterial pressures and hemodynamics
  - Rule out underlying cardiac disease (e.g., left-sided heart disease) and response to vasodilator therapy
- Lung biopsy: not recommended unless primary pulmonary parenchymal disease exists
- 6-minute walk test: classifies severity of PAH and estimates prognosis

Test Interpretation

- Distal arterioles show medial hypertrophy, proliferative/fibrotic intima, complex lesions, and thrombosis.
- Pulmonary veins usually are not affected.

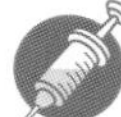

TREATMENT

- Treat underlying diseases/conditions that may cause PAH to relieve symptoms and improve quality of life and survival.
- PAH-specific treatment has been studied mostly in IPAH.

GENERAL MEASURES

Oxygen supplementation to O_2 >90% is indicated for rest, exercise, or nocturnal hypoxemia.

MEDICATION

- Acute vasodilator test (performed during cardiac catheterization) for all IPAH patients who are potential candidates for long-term oral calcium channel blocker (CCB) therapy
  - Screens for pulmonary vasoreactivity/responsiveness using inhaled nitrous oxide; IV epoprostenol, or IV adenosine: Positive response may be a prognostic indicator.
  - Contraindicated in right-sided heart failure or hemodynamic instability
- Chronic vasodilator therapy
  - If IPAH with positive response to acute vasodilator test (a fall in mean PAP of ≥10 mm Hg and to a value <40 mm Hg, with unchanged/increased cardiac output), use CCBs (1)[C]
    - ~13% will initially respond. Long-term clinical response to CCB therapy is small (~7%) (1)[C].
    - CCBs include nifedipine (long-acting), diltiazem, amlodipine.
    - Avoid verapamil due to its significant negative inotropic effect.
    - CCBs are contraindicated in patients with a cardiac index of <2 L/min/m^2 or a right atrial pressure >15 mm Hg.
  - PAH with negative response to acute vasodilator test or worsening on therapy; specific vasodilator choice based on risk stratification (1)[C].
    - Higher risk (NYHA class III–IV): prostacyclins: improve exercise capacity, cardiopulmonary hemodynamics: epoprostenol (IV) (only drug with demonstrated survival benefit and treatment of choice for most ill; i.e., NYHA functional class IV patients) (1)[B]; treprostinil (IV, SC, or inhaled); iloprost (inhaled); inhaled products associated with bronchospasm
    - FDA recently approved treprostinil extended-release tablets for PAH to improve exrcise capacity.
    - Lower risk (NYHA class I–III)
      - Endothelin receptor antagonists: Improve exercise capacity; reducing mortality has been noted (2)[A]: bosentan (PO); ambrisentan (PO). Pregnancy Category X; monitor LFTs monthly
      - Phosphodiesterase-5 inhibitors: suggested improvement in exercise capacity, cardiopulmonary hemodynamics, and symptoms (1)[C]: sildenafil (PO); tadalafil (PO)
      - Guanylate cyclase stimulant: stimulators of the nitric oxide receptor, improves exercise capacity (3)[B]: riociguat (PO)
      - It is unclear whether any of the above separate classes of drugs significantly reduces mortality; however, pooling all the vasodilators in a recent systematic review shows 39% reduction in mortality (4)[A]; another recent meta-analysis shows that only prostanoid class has survival benefit, particularly IV prostacyclins (1)[B].
      - If one agent fails, vasodilator combination therapy (CT) using two vasodilators (e.g., epoprostenol + sildenafil) is currently being studied. A recent meta-analysis found CT did not improve outcomes compared with monotherapy (MT). Only 6-minute walk distance was improved when using CT versus MT (5)[A].
- Anticoagulation
  - Improved survival originally suggested in patients with IPAH only. Newer studies show some evidence for favorable effects of anticoagulation on survival in IPAH, HPAH, or PAH associated with anorexigens (1)[B].
  - Warfarin with international normalized ratio of 1.5–2.5
    - Contraindications: Avoid in patients with syncope or significant hemoptysis; consider drug interactions.
- Diuretics indicated in patients with RV volume overload (e.g., peripheral edema or ascites) (1)[B]
- Digoxin has little long-term data in PAH: used in RV failure and/or atrial dysrhythmias, increases cardiac output and preserves RV contractility

ISSUES FOR REFERRAL

Refer to a pulmonologist and/or a cardiologist for further evaluation/treatment if PAH is suspected.

SURGERY/OTHER PROCEDURES

- Patients with documented large-vessel thromboembolic disease should be considered for pulmonary thrombectomy.
- Balloon atrial septostomy for severe PAH with right-sided heart failure despite optimized medical therapy to relieve symptoms prior to lung transplant or as a treatment on its own
- Heart–lung or lung transplantation

INPATIENT CONSIDERATIONS

Admission Criteria/Initial Stabilization

- Medical therapy is primarily palliative.
- Hospitalization with invasive monitoring is needed to screen vasodilator responsiveness and initiate vasodilator therapy.
- National registry has been established by the National Heart, Lung, and Blood Institute.

ONGOING CARE

FOLLOW-UP RECOMMENDATIONS

- Pneumococcal and influenza vaccines
- Exercise: walking or low-level aerobic activity, as tolerated, once stable; respiratory training

Patient Monitoring

Frequently evaluate disease progression and therapeutic efficacy. Objective tests to measure treatment response include 6-minute walk test and cardiopulmonary exercise test.

DIET

Fluid and salt restrictions, especially with RV failure

PATIENT EDUCATION

Discuss disease, prognosis, lifestyle changes, and all therapeutic options (including transplant).

PROGNOSIS

- Median survival is 2–3 years from diagnosis; 5-year survival rate is 34% for National Institutes of Health registry; newer studies show 5-year survival near 70% with new treatment.
- Mode of death: right-sided heart failure (most common), pneumonia, sudden death, cardiac death
- Poor prognostic factors
  - Rapid symptom progression
  - Clinical evidence of RV failure
  - WHO functional PAH class 4 (or NYHA functional class III or IV)
  - 6-minute walk distance <300 m
  - Peak VO_2 during cardiopulmonary exercise testing <10.4 mL/kg/min
  - Echocardiography with pericardial effusion, significant RV enlargement/dysfunction, right atrial enlargement
  - Mean right atrial pressure >20 mm Hg
  - Cardiac index <2 L/min/m^2
  - Elevated mean PAP
  - Significantly elevated BNP and NT-proBNP; other markers also show promise in predicting survival: RDW, GDF-15, interleukin-6, creatinine
  - Scleroderma spectrum of diseases

COMPLICATIONS

- Thromboembolism, heart failure, pleural effusion, and sudden death
- Pregnancy should be avoided due to high maternal mortality (30–50%) and fetal wastage.

REFERENCES

1. Badesch DB, Abman SH, Simonneau G, et al. Medical therapy for pulmonary arterial hypertension: updated ACCP evidence-based clinical practice guidelines. *Chest*. 2007;131(6):1917–1928.
2. Liu C, Chen J, Gao Y, et al. Endothelin receptor antagonists for pulmonary arterial hypertension. *Cochrane Database Syst Rev*. 2009;(3):CD004434.
3. Ghofrani HA, GalièN, Grimminger F, et al. Riociguat for the treatment of pulmonary arterial hypertension. *N Engl J Med*. 2013;369(4):330–340.
4. Macchia A, Marchioli R, Tognoni G, et al. Systematic review of trials using vasodilators in pulmonary arterial hypertension: why a new approach is needed. *Am Heart J*. 2010;159(2):245–257.
5. Fox BD, Shimony A, Langleben D. Meta-analysis of monotherapy versus combination therapy for pulmonary arterial hypertension. *Am J Cardiol*. 2011;108(8):1177–1182.

SEE ALSO

Cor Pulmonale; Pulmonary Embolism

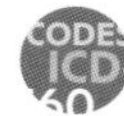

CODES

ICD10

- I27.0 Primary pulmonary hypertension
- I27.2 Other secondary pulmonary hypertension

CLINICAL PEARLS

- PAH involves abnormalities in the small pulmonary arteries (precapillary PH) that produce increased PAP and vascular resistance, eventually resulting in right-sided heart failure.
- In patients with PAH, a V/Q scan should be performed to rule out CTEPH; a normal scan effectively excludes a diagnosis of CTEPH.
- CCBs are 1st-line agents to manage IPAH.

PULMONARY EDEMA

Melissa S. Jefferis, MD, FAAFP

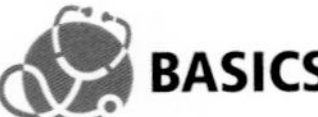

BASICS

DESCRIPTION

- Pulmonary capillaries leak fluid into the lung interstitium and alveoli, leading to hypoxia and respiratory distress.
- Fluid accumulation results from cardiogenic causes (e.g., heart failure), leading to imbalanced hydrostatic and oncotic pressures within pulmonary capillaries or from noncardiogenic causes (e.g., acute lung injury) that increase alveolar membrane permeability.

EPIDEMIOLOGY

Incidence

- Annual heart failure incidence: 650,000 cases
- Heart failure incidence increases with age
  - Age 35–64 years: 2 cases per 1,000
  - Age 65–69 years: 20 cases per 1,000
  - Age >85 years: >80 cases per 1,000
- Disparities in heart failure incidence by race and sex:
  - Blacks (16.3/1,000) versus whites (11.9/1,000)
  - Men (15.8/1,000) versus women (11.7/1,000)
- Acute respiratory distress syndrome (ARDS): 190,000 cases annually in United States

Prevalence

Heart failure syndromes: 5.8 million U.S. adults

ETIOLOGY AND PATHOPHYSIOLOGY

- Cardiogenic causes will increase hydrostatic pressure in the pulmonary capillaries, leading to increased transvascular filtration of a protein-poor fluid into lung interstitium.
- Systolic dysfunction is due to decreased contractility of the left ventricle (LV), leading to decreased cardiac output, which in turn stimulates the renin–angiotensin system and increases fluid retention. Diastolic dysfunction is often due to decreased LV compliance secondary to hypertrophy.
- Cardiogenic (left-sided heart failure)
  - Impaired contractility
    - Ischemic heart disease
    - Dilated cardiomyopathy
    - Myocarditis
    - Volume overload
    - Alcoholic cardiomyopathy
  - Increased LV afterload
    - Systemic hypertension (HTN)
    - Aortic stenosis
    - Cocaine abuse
  - Poor diastolic filling
    - LV hypertrophy
    - Hypertrophic cardiomyopathy
    - Mitral stenosis
    - Atrial fibrillation
  - Valvular dysfunction
    - Mitral regurgitation
    - Acute papillary muscle rupture
  - High cardiac output states
    - Thyrotoxicosis
    - Systemic arteriovenous fistulas
    - Anemia
  - Noncompliance with medications or diet
  - Medications with negative inotropic effects
- Noncardiogenic causes will increase permeability of the lung vasculature, leading to accumulation of protein-rich fluid in the lung interstitium and air spaces. Many causes of this vascular permeability are associated with ARDS.
- Noncardiogenic
  - ARDS
  - Acute lung injury
  - Transfusion-related acute lung injury
  - Preeclampsia
  - Rapid ascent to high altitude (>2,500 m)
  - Drug toxicity (salicylates, opiates)
  - Embolism (thrombus, fat, air, amniotic fluid)
  - Neurogenic (after head trauma/surgery)
  - Reexpansion (after pneumothorax/thoracentesis)

Genetics

Multifactorial

RISK FACTORS

- Cardiogenic: HTN, valvular disease, hyperlipidemia, atherosclerosis, diabetes mellitus, obesity, excessive alcohol intake, physical inactivity, dietary choices, and smoking.
- Noncardiogenic: sepsis, aspiration, pneumonia, trauma, inhaled toxins, DIC

GENERAL PREVENTION

Early detection and treatment of risk factors, including high blood pressure, diabetes, alcohol intake, obesity, and tobacco abuse (1)[A].

COMMONLY ASSOCIATED CONDITIONS

See "Etiology and Pathophysiology."

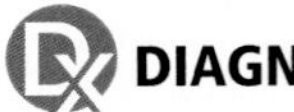

DIAGNOSIS

HISTORY

- Past medical history
  - Underlying comorbidities, including prior heart failure or prior myocardial infarction (MI)
  - Recent trauma
  - Drug or alcohol abuse
  - Dietary or medication noncompliance
  - Recent weight gain or increasing edema
  - Recent use of negative inotropic agents (calcium channel blockers)
  - Recent use of NSAIDs (increase water retention)
- Symptoms
  - Fever or other symptoms of infection
  - Progressive dyspnea
  - Orthopnea and paroxysmal nocturnal dyspnea
  - Cough
  - Fatigue and generalized weakness
  - Pink frothy sputum
  - Chest pain

PHYSICAL EXAM

- Vital signs: tachypnea, tachycardia, and hypoxemia. Patients may be hypotensive or hypertensive.
- General: respiratory distress, diaphoresis
- HEENT (head, eyes, ears, nose, throat): frothy oral secretions, cyanosis
- Cardiac: S_3 or S_4, jugular venous distension, murmurs suggestive of valvular disease
- Pulmonary: crackles or wheezing
- Extremities: edema, cyanosis, mottled skin

DIFFERENTIAL DIAGNOSIS

- COPD
- Pneumonia
- Pulmonary embolism
- Asthma/reactive airway disease
- Pneumothorax
- Cardiac tamponade
- Asphyxiant or toxic gas exposure
- Inhalational burns

DIAGNOSTIC TESTS & INTERPRETATION

Initial Tests (lab, imaging)

- CBC/differential to screen for anemia or infection
- Chemistry panel to screen for acute kidney injury, hyponatremia (associated with severe heart failure), or electrolyte disturbances leading to dysrhythmias
- Troponin may be elevated from recent infarction causing acute heart failure or from myocardial ischemia secondary to elevated ventricular strain. Elevated cardiac enzymes carry a strongly negative prognosis in heart failure.
- In settings of clinical uncertainty, B-type natriuretic peptide (BNP), or N-terminal pro-BNP, can add to clinical judgment in patients with symptoms suggestive of heart failure (1,2)[A]. BNP >500 pg/mL suggests heart failure, and BNP <100 pg/mL suggests alternative causes. BNP may also be elevated due to atrial fibrillation, renal failure, severe valvular disease, or pulmonary HTN.
- Liver function tests (LFTs) to check for elevated transaminases, which can suggest hepatic congestion from heart failure or may indicate heavy alcohol use contributing to cardiomyopathy
- Drug levels (aspirin, opiates, cocaine, alcohol)
- Arterial blood gas to measure pO_2 and A-a gradient
- Serum lipase if suspicious for pancreatitis
- TSH if suspicious for thyrotoxicosis
- Blood/urine cultures and lactic acid if concerned for severe sepsis or septic shock
- Urinalysis to check for nephrotic syndrome or UTI
- Chest x-ray to evaluate for the following:
  - Pneumothorax
  - Cardiomegaly
  - Infiltrate suggestive of pneumonia
  - Increased interstitial markings, perihilar alveolar edema, or pleural effusion
- CT pulmonary angiography if concerned for pulmonary emboli
- ECG to evaluate for ischemia or dysrhythmias
- Echocardiography to assess ventricular function and size, valve function, and for presence of a pericardial effusion or wall motion abnormalities (2)[C].

Follow-Up Tests & Special Considerations

Emergent echocardiography if considering cardiogenic shock, tamponade, or papillary muscle rupture

Diagnostic Procedures

- If cause of pulmonary edema is unknown, a pulmonary artery catheter (or Swan-Ganz) can be inserted to measure the pulmonary artery capillary wedge pressure. A wedge pressure less than 18 mm Hg favors acute lung injury over cardiogenic pulmonary edema.
- Patients with new-onset or worsening heart failure (without determined cause) should have further evaluation for myocardial ischemia. The pretest probability of underlying ischemic cardiomyopathy should guide the decision on which testing modality to use (1)[C].

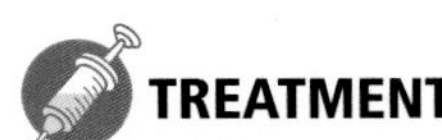

TREATMENT

GENERAL MEASURES

- Guide all treatment based on the suspected cause.
- Start with supplemental oxygen.

MEDICATION

Cardiogenic pulmonary edema

P

First Line

- Diuretics: reduce preload for acute cardiogenic edema; used in low doses daily for chronic heart failure to manage volume overload. If on chronic diuretics, start IV dose at or above home dose and titrate for acute cardiogenic edema. Onset 15–30 minutes for IV loop diuretics. Monitor for electrolyte derangement and renal dysfunction. Use very carefully in patients with aortic stenosis.
  - Acute: furosemide 40–80 mg IV, torsemide 10mg IV, or bumetanide 1mg IV
  - Chronic: furosemide 20–80 mg q6–8h, torsemide 20mg/day, or bumetanide 1 mg q12h
- ACE inhibitors or angiotensin receptor blockers (ARBs): reduce afterload for systolic heart failure. Maintenance therapy may be cautiously continued during exacerbation. Avoid in acutely ill patients with hypotension, acute kidney insult, hyperkalemia, or poor diuresis. Use ARBs in patients who are ACE inhibitor intolerant.
  - Target dose for chronic heart failure: lisinopril 20–40 mg/day, enalapril 10–20 mg q12h, captopril 50 mg q8h, candesartan 32 mg/day, valsartan 160 mg q12h, losartan 100 mg/day
- β-Blockers: reduce afterload for systolic heart failure. Maintenance therapy may be continued for mild decompensation; hold or reduce dose for moderate to severe decompensation. Avoid if patients are hypotensive or recently received inotropic therapy. Do not initiate until recovery from acute exacerbation of heart failure.
  - Target dose for chronic heart failure: carvedilol 25 mg q12h, metoprolol ER 200 mg/day, bisoprolol 10 mg/day
- Inotropes: improve contractility in hypotensive patients with severe systolic heart failure and signs of systemic hypoperfusion (2)[B]. Inotropes increase myocardial oxygen demand and may damage the ischemic myocardium.
  - Dobutamine: 5–10 μg/kg/min IV, titrate
  - Milrinone: loading dose (optional): 50 μg/kg IV over 10 minutes, then infuse 0.375–0.75 μg/kg/min, titrate
  - Dopamine: 5–10 μg/kg/min IV, titrate
  - Norepinephrine: 2–4 μg/min IV for acute cardiogenic shock following acute MI; not for use in acute decompensated heart failure
- Nitrates: Acute cardiogenic pulmonary edema use IV nitrate vasodilators. Rapid onset. Nitroglycerin IV 5–10 μg/min, titrate 5–10 μg/min q3–5min to max 200 μg/min until distress resolved or onset of hypotension. For severe HTN, consider IV nitroprusside 5–10 μg/min, titrate. Max 400 μg/min. Use <48 hours due to risk of cyanide toxicity.
  - For patients who are not tolerant of ACE inhibitors or ARBs, hydralazine and an oral nitrate should be started (1)[C].
- Precaution: Monitor the additive hypotensive effects of diuretics, nitrates, and afterload reducers.

Second Line

- Thiazide diuretics: hydrochlorothiazide (HCTZ) 25–50 mg/day PO, metolazone 2.5–10 mg/day PO
- Spironolactone: 25–50 mg/day PO; recheck renal function and electrolytes in 7–10 days.
- Digoxin: 125 μg/day PO, titrate to serum concentration of 0.5–0.8 ng/mL
- Noncardiogenic pulmonary edema
  - High-altitude pulmonary edema
    - Descent is the single best treatment (3)[A].
    - Adjunctive therapy: supplemental oxygen. Consider nifedipine ER 30 mg PO q12h or sildenafil 50 mg PO q8h or tadalafil 10 mg PO q12h (3)[C].

ISSUES FOR REFERRAL

- Cardiology referral for underlying cardiac disease
- Patients with ARDS should be carefully monitored in an ICU setting.

ADDITIONAL THERAPIES

- Noninvasive positive-pressure ventilation (NPPV) should be considered early for emergency department patients with acute respiratory distress from cardiogenic pulmonary edema/congestive heart failure (CHF). NPPV decreases preload and afterload, thereby alleviating symptoms and potentially avoiding intubation by allowing time for medications to work. Use cautiously if patients are hypotensive (4)[A].
- Early invasive ventilation should be considered for patients with noncardiogenic pulmonary edema secondary to acute respiratory distress syndrome.

SURGERY/OTHER PROCEDURES

- Extracorporeal membrane oxygenation (ECMO) for severe refractory hypoxia/ARDS
- Intra-arterial balloon pump for cardiogenic shock
- Implantable cardioverter defibrillator (ICD) for sudden cardiac death prevention in patients with prior cardiac arrest or ischemic/dilated cardiomyopathy and LVEF <30% (2)[B]
- Cardiac resynchronization therapy (CRT) may be useful for LVEF ≤35%, sinus rhythm, and QRS >0.15 m/s (2)[B].
- LV assist device (LVAD) for severe systolic dysfunction as bridge to a heart transplant (2)[B].

INPATIENT CONSIDERATIONS

Admission Criteria/Initial Stabilization

- Hypotension
- Acute kidney injury
- Altered mental status
- Dyspnea at rest
- O_2 saturation <90%
- Acute coronary syndromes
- Arrhythmias (i.e., new-onset atrial fibrillation)
- Mild distress: oxygen by nonrebreather mask
- Significant hypoxia
- Intubation for patients with apnea, altered mental status, or hypoxia despite NPPV

IV Fluids

Use crystalloid infusions cautiously. Limit free water.

Nursing

- Daily weights, strict input/output
- Assess for functional improvement.

Discharge Criteria

- Underlying condition treated, fluid status optimized
- Started β-blocker and ACE inhibitor in patients with CHF (1)[B].
- Patient and family educated about diet/medications

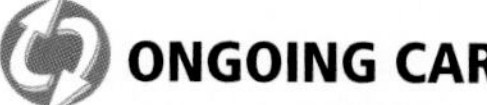

ONGOING CARE

FOLLOW-UP RECOMMENDATIONS

Patient Monitoring

- Strict input/output measurement, daily weights
- Posthospitalization appointment in 7–10 days

DIET

Low-sodium diet (<2 g/day), fluid restriction (<2 L/day) (2)[C].

PATIENT EDUCATION

- Dietary precautions
- Early signs and symptoms of fluid overload
- Adjust diuretic dose based on recent weight gain.

PROGNOSIS

Mortality: 30–60% for noncardiogenic edema/ARDS; up to 80% for cardiogenic causes

COMPLICATIONS

- Acute hypoxic respiratory failure
- CHF increases long-term risk for dysrhythmias and sudden cardiac death.
- ARDS increases short-term risk for pneumonia and pneumothorax. Long-term complications include risks of pulmonary HTN and fibrosis.

REFERENCES

1. Heart Failure Society of America, Lindenfeld J, Albert NM, et al. HFSA 2010 comprehensive heart failure practice guideline. *J Card Fail*. 2010;16(6):e1–e194.
2. Yancy CW, Jessup M, Bozkurt B, et al. 2013 ACCF/AHA guideline for the management of heart failure: a report of the American College of Cardiology Foundation/American Heart Association Task Force on Practice Guidelines. *J Am Coll Cardiol*. 2013;62(16):e147–e239.
3. Luks AM, McIntosh SE, Grissom CK, et al. Wilderness Medical Society consensus guidelines for the prevention and treatment of acute altitude illness. *Wilderness Environ Med*. 2010;21(2):146–155.
4. Vital FM, Saconato H, Ladeira MT, et al. Non-invasive positive pressure ventilation (CPAP or bilevel NPPV) for cardiogenic pulmonary edema. *Cochrane Database Syst Rev*. 2008;(3):CD005351.

ADDITIONAL READING

Putensen C, Theuerkauf N, Zinserling J, et al. Meta-analysis: ventilation strategies and outcome of the acute respiratory distress syndrome and acute lung injury. *Ann Intern Med*. 2009;151(8):566–576.

SEE ALSO

Altitude Illness; Congestive Heart Failure: Differential Diagnosis; Respiratory Distress Syndrome, Acute (ARDS)

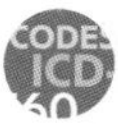

CODES

ICD10

- J81.1 Chronic pulmonary edema
- J81.0 Acute pulmonary edema

CLINICAL PEARLS

- Diagnosis of the underlying etiology is essential.
- Initial treatment of acute cardiogenic edema among hypertensive/normotensive patients includes IV diuretics, IV nitrates, and NPPV.
- Hypotensive patients with pulmonary edema due to CHF will require careful use of inotropes and vasopressor to improve hemodynamic stability.
- Pulmonary edema from ARDS has very high mortality and requires ICU-level care. Home dietary and medication management are critical for long-term treatment of CHF.

PULMONARY EMBOLISM

Alfonso Tafur, MD, MS, RPVI • Ana I. Casanegra, MD, RPVI, FSVM

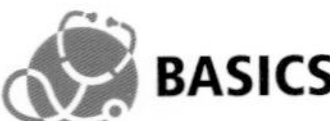

BASICS

DESCRIPTION

- Pulmonary embolism (PE) is the obstruction of the pulmonary arteries, typically due to a thrombus that formed at another site and traveled in the bloodstream until it lodged.
- Venous thromboembolism (VTE) refers to both PE and deep vein thrombosis (DVT).

EPIDEMIOLOGY

The case fatality rate ranges from 1 to 60% depending on the severity of the clinical presentation.

Incidence

- Incidence increases with age.
- ~23–69 new PE cases per 100,000 per year
- 250,000 hospitalizations per year in the United States, 10–60% in hospitalized patients:
  - Highest risk for orthopedic patients
  - 1:1,000 pregnancies (including postpartum)

ETIOLOGY AND PATHOPHYSIOLOGY

- Venous stasis, endothelial damage, and changes in the coagulation properties of the blood trigger the formation of thrombus.
- PE causes increased pulmonary vascular resistance, impaired gas exchange, and decreased pulmonary compliance.
- DVT in the proximal veins is the most common source of PE.
- Upper extremity DVT and pelvic vein thrombi can also cause PE.

Genetics

- Responsible for 20% of all patients with VTE
- Factor V Leiden: the most common thrombophilia. +5.5% in Caucasian, 2.2% in Hispanics, 1.2% in African American, 0.5% in Asian
- Prothrombin G20210A: 3% of Caucasians; rare in African American, Asian, and Native American; 6% in patients with VTE

RISK FACTORS

- Acquired: age, immobilization, surgery, cancer, oral contraceptives, hormonal replacement therapy, pregnancy/puerperium, previous thrombosis, paroxysmal nocturnal hemoglobinuria, antiphospholipid syndrome, prolonged travel
- Inherited: antithrombin deficiency, protein C deficiency, protein S deficiency, factor V Leiden, prothrombin gene mutation *G20210A*, dysfibrinogenemia

GENERAL PREVENTION

- Prevention strategies must be tailored to patient VTE risk and patient bleeding risk.
- Mechanical thromboprophylaxis includes early ambulation after surgery, graduated compression stockings, and intermittent pneumatic compression.
- Intermediate risk: medical patients, general surgery, and gynecologic and urologic surgery. Pharmacologic prophylaxis is recommended with low-molecular-weight heparin (LMWH), unfractionated heparin (UFH), or fondaparinux (1,2)[A].
- High risk: hip or knee arthroplasty, pharmacologic prophylaxis with LMWH, fondaparinux, apixaban, dabigatran, rivaroxaban, or low-dose UFH: hip fracture surgery, LMWH, fondaparinux, UFH, or vitamin K antagonists (VKA); major trauma, spinal cord injury, LMWH, or UFH (3)[A]
- Long-distance travel (>8 hours): hydration, avoidance of constrictive clothing, and calf exercises; if additional risk factors are present, graduated compression stockings below knee
- Patients with factor V Leiden and prothrombin *G20210A* with no previous thrombosis do not need long-term daily prophylaxis.

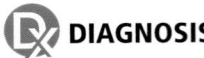

DIAGNOSIS

Establish a pretest probability based on clinical criteria such as Wells score or Geneva score:

- Wells score:
  - Clinical signs and symptoms of DVT +3
  - Alternative diagnosis is less likely than PE +3
  - Heart rate >100 +1.5
  - Immobilization/surgery in previous 4 weeks +1.5
  - Previous DVT/PE +1.5
  - Hemoptysis +1
  - Malignancy +1:
    - 4 or <4 unlikely, >4 likely

HISTORY

- Provoked or idiopathic
- Presence of risk factors and family history
- Bleeding risk (previous anticoagulation, history of bleeding, recent interventions/surgeries, liver disease)
- Dyspnea (82%), chest pain (49%), cough (20%), syncope (14%), hemoptysis (7%)

PHYSICAL EXAM

- Tachycardia, tachypnea, accentuated pulmonary component in S2
- Pleuritic chest pain, pleural friction rub, rales
- Leg swelling, tenderness along a vein, visible collateral veins
- Signs of right ventricular (RV) failure may be present (rare): jugular vein distention, 3rd or 4th sound, systolic murmur at left sternal edge, hepatomegaly.

ALERT

- Massive PE: acute PE with sustained hypotension, pulselessness, or persistent profound bradycardia
- Submassive PE: acute PE without systemic hypotension but with either RV dysfunction or myocardial necrosis:
  - RV dysfunction: RV dilation or RV systolic dysfunction on echocardiography, RV dilation (4-chamber RV diameter divided by left ventricle diameter 0.9) on CT, elevation of BNP or troponins, ECG changes
- Low-risk PE: acute PE without criteria; massive or submassive PE

DIFFERENTIAL DIAGNOSIS

- Pulmonary: pneumonia, bronchitis, pneumonitis, chronic obstructive pulmonary disease (COPD) exacerbation, pulmonary edema, pneumothorax
- Cardiac: myocardial infarction (angina pectoris), pericarditis, congestive heart failure (CHF)
- Vascular: dissection of the aorta
- Musculoskeletal: rib fracture(s), musculoskeletal chest wall pain

DIAGNOSTIC TESTS & INTERPRETATION

- D-dimer: In patients with low pretest probability; D-dimer can rule out PE if result is negative (high negative predictive value [NPV]). It is not diagnostic if positive (low positive predictive value [PPV]), and it is not helpful if pretest probability is likely.
- CBC, creatinine, aPTT and PT, ABG
- In young patients with idiopathic VTE, recurrent VTE, or significant family history of VTE, consider testing for hypercoagulable tests:
  - All patients with intermediate/high pretest probability and low probability with elevated D-dimer need further diagnostic testing.
- Chest x-ray (CXR): suggestive findings: Westermark sign (lack of vessels in an area distal to the embolus), Hampton hump (wedge-shaped opacity with base in pleura), Fleischner sign (enlarged pulmonary arteries), atelectasis, pleural effusion, pulmonary infarct, hemidiaphragm elevation
- ECG: right heart strain, nonspecific rhythm abnormalities, S1Q3T3
- CT pulmonary angiography: sensitivity 96–100%, specificity 86–89%. NPV 99.8%; requires IV iodine contrast (4)[A]
- Ventilation/perfusion scintigraphy (V/Q scan): Use if CT angiography is not available or contraindicated. A high-probability V/Q scan makes the diagnosis of PE; a normal V/Q scan excludes PE (4)[A].
- Pulmonary angiogram: gold standard but invasive and technically difficult: 2% morbidity and <0.01 mortality risk
- Echocardiogram: helpful to assess RV function
- Magnetic resonance angiography: lower sensitivity and specificity than CT angiography
- Compression ultrasound (CUS): noninvasive. 1/3 of the patients with PE will have a DVT.
- CT venography: can be done at the same time as CT angiography; increases diagnostic yield. Requires IV iodinated contrast.

ALERT

If your preclinical probability is intermediate or high and the patient has a low bleeding risk, start the treatment while waiting for the diagnostic results.

ALERT

Do not test for protein C, S, factor VIII, and antithrombin in the acute setting or while on treatment. Results may be falsely abnormal.

Follow-Up Tests & Special Considerations

Elevated troponin I or T and elevated BNP are markers for higher risk patients.

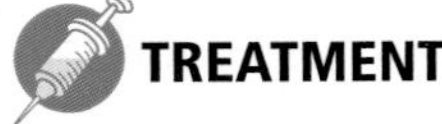

TREATMENT

MEDICATION

- If the clinical suspicion is high and there are no contraindications, start treatment as soon as possible.
- Start LMWH, fondaparinux, and UFH as initial therapy. VKA can be started the 1st day and must overlap with parenteral treatment for a minimum of 5 days and the international normalized ratio (INR) is 2–3 for 24 hours (4)[A].
- Rivaroxaban can be used for initial and long-term treatment (5)[A].
- Patients with massive PE with low bleeding risk: Consider systemic thrombolytics if they have no contraindications (6)[A].
- Patients <75 years with submassive PE and low bleeding risk: Consider thrombolysis (6)[A].

P

First Line

- UFH:
  - IV bolus of 80 U/kg or 5,000 U followed by continuous infusion (initially at 18 U/kg/hr or 1,300 U/hr) with dose adjustments to maintain an aPTT that corresponds to antiactivated factor X (anti-Xa) levels of 0.3–0.7
  - SC injection: 2 options:
    - Monitored: 17,500 U or 250 U/kg BID with dose adjustments to maintain an aPTT that corresponds to anti-Xa levels of 0.3–0.7 measured 6 hours after a dose
    - Fixed dose: 333 U/kg initial dose, followed by 250 U/kg BID
- LMWH:
  - Enoxaparin (Lovenox) 1 mg/kg/dose SC q12h
  - Dalteparin (Fragmin) 200 U/kg SC q24h
  - Fondaparinux (Arixtra): 5 mg (body weight <50 kg), 7.5 mg (body weight 50–100 kg), or 10 mg (body weight >100) SC q24h
- Maintenance therapy: VKA; warfarin: Start on day 1, if possible; 5 mg/day for 3 days for most patients; adjust dose to maintain an INR of 2–3; needs to overlap with UFH, LMWH, or fondaparinux 5–7 days and 2 consecutive therapeutic INR
- Rivaroxaban: 15 mg twice daily for 3 weeks and then 20 mg once daily to complete treatment

ALERT

Contraindications:

- Active bleeding is a contraindication for any anticoagulation.
- Heparin: heparin-induced thrombocytopenia (HIT)
- LMWH: HIT, renal failurer
- Fondaparinux: renal failure (reduced dose)
- Warfarin: pregnancy
- Rivaroxaban: avoid if CrCl <30

Pregnancy Considerations

- Warfarin is teratogenic and should not be used in pregnant patients (especially in 1st trimester); safe while breastfeeding
- Dalteparin, enoxaparin, and fondaparinux are Category B for pregnancy; heparin is Category C.
- Rivaroxaban is Category C. No adequate studies.

Second Line

Massive PE: Evaluate the risks and benefits. Consider thrombolytics if the patient has hemodynamic compromise and a low bleeding risk:

- Tissue plasminogen activator (tPA) 100 mg infused through a peripheral vein over 2 hours
- Absolute contraindications: intracranial hemorrhage, known intracranial cerebrovascular or malignant disease, ischemic stroke within 3 months, suspected aortic dissection, bleeding diathesis, active bleeding, recent neurosurgery, recent major trauma
- Thrombolysis is associated with lower mortality. Number needed to treat (NNT) 59 but higher risk of major bleeding and intracranial hemorrhage: number needed to harm (NNH) 18 and 78, respectively. The risk–benefit balance is more favorable in patients younger than 65 years of age (NNT 51, NNH 176 vs. NNT64, NNH 11 in patients older than 65 years)

SURGERY/OTHER PROCEDURES

- Inferior vena cava (IVC) filter placement in patients with contraindication for anticoagulation
- Emergency surgical embolectomy can be considered if the patient has massive PE with contraindications for thrombolysis and surgical resources are available.
- Consider catheter-based interventions if the patient has massive PE and either contraindications to thrombolytics or if patient remains unstable despite the use of thrombolytics.

INPATIENT CONSIDERATIONS

Admission Criteria/Initial Stabilization

May require ICU-level care if hemodynamically unstable

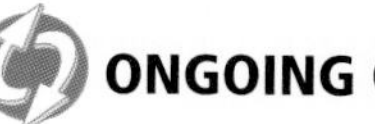

ONGOING CARE

Duration of anticoagulation:

- Provoked PE (and the trigger is no longer present): 3 months
- Unprovoked (idiopathic) PE: a minimum of 3 months, but consider long-term or prolonged secondary prophylaxis if the bleeding risk is low
- Cancer-related PE: LMWH for the 1st 3–6 months, followed by long-term anticoagulation with LMWH or VKA. LMWH dose can be reduced to 75% after the first 6 months.
- Recurrent PE: long-term anticoagulation
- Low-dose aspirin can be used in patients with unprovoked PE and high bleeding risk after completing anticoagulation.

FOLLOW-UP RECOMMENDATIONS

Consider retrieval of retrievable IVC filters in anticoagulated patients.

Patient Monitoring

- INR should be checked at regular intervals. Target INR is 2–3 for therapy.
- aPTT needs to be monitored if the patient is on adjustable SC UFH.
- Anti-Xa can be checked in special circumstances in patients treated with LMWH.

DIET

Patients on warfarin need education for a vitamin K–consistent diet.

PROGNOSIS

- Severity at presentation affects mortality: massive PE 50% versus nonmassive PE 8–14%
- Abbreviated Pulmonary Embolism Severity Index score predicts acute mortality (any one of the following variables defines high risk: age >80 years, history of cancer, chronic cardiopulmonary disease, heart rate ≥110/min, systolic blood pressure <100 mm Hg, O_2 saturation <90%).

COMPLICATIONS

- 1 in 25 PE patients will develop chronic thromboembolic pulmonary hypertension.
- Recurrent DVT or PE
- Complications of the treatment, such as anticoagulation-associated bleeding. Incidence of major hemorrhage associated with thrombolytics is 8%; intracerebral bleed is 2% (fatal in 1/2 of cases).

REFERENCES

1. Kahn SR, Lim W, Dunn AS, et al. Prevention of VTE in nonsurgical patients: antithrombotic therapy and prevention of thrombosis, 9th ed: American College of Chest Physicians Evidence-Based Clinical Practice Guidelines. *Chest*. 2012;141(Suppl 2):e195S–e226S.
2. Gould MK, Garcia DA, Wren SM, et al. Prevention of VTE in nonorthopedic surgical patients: antithrombotic therapy and prevention of thrombosis, 9th ed: American College of Chest Physicians Evidence-Based Clinical Practice Guidelines. *Chest*. 2012;141(Suppl 2):e227S–e277S.
3. Falck-Ytter Y, Francis CW, Johanson NA, et al. Prevention of VTE in orthopedic surgery patients: antithrombotic therapy and prevention of thrombosis, 9th ed: American College of Chest Physicians Evidence-Based Clinical Practice Guidelines. *Chest*. 2012;141(Suppl 2):e278S–e325S.
4. Kearon C, Akl EA, Comerota AJ, et al. Antithrombotic therapy for VTE disease: antithrombotic therapy and prevention of thrombosis, 9th ed: American College of Chest Physicians Evidence-Based Clinical Practice Guidelines. *Chest*. 2012;141(Suppl 2):e419S–e494S.
5. EINSTEIN–PE Investigators, Büller HR, Prins MH, et al. Oral rivaroxaban for the treatment of symptomatic pulmonary embolism. *N Engl J Med*. 2012;366(14):1287–1297.
6. Chatterjee S, Chakraborty A, Weinberg I, et al. Thrombolysis for pulmonary embolism and risk of all-cause mortality, major bleeding, and intracranial hemorrhage: a meta-analysis. *JAMA*. 2014;311(23):2414–2421.

ADDITIONAL READING

- Anderson DR, Kahn SR, Rodger MA, et al. Computed tomographic pulmonary angiography vs ventilation-perfusion lung scanning in patients with suspected pulmonary embolism: a randomized controlled trial. *JAMA*. 2007;298(23):2743–2753.
- Douma RA, Mos IC, Erkens PM, et al. Performance of 4 clinical decision rules in the diagnostic management of acute pulmonary embolism: a prospective cohort study. *Ann Intern Med*. 2011;154(11):709–718.
- Jaff MR, McMurtry MS, Archer SL, et al. Management of massive and submassive pulmonary embolism, iliofemoral deep vein thrombosis, and chronic thromboembolic pulmonary hypertension: a scientific statement from the American Heart Association. *Circulation*. 2011;123(16):1788–1830.
- PIOPED II Investigators; Stein PD, Fowler SE, Goodman LR, et al. Multidetector computed tomography for acute pulmonary embolism. *N Engl J Med*. 2006;354(22):2317–2327.
- Sadigh G, Kelly AM, Cronin P, et al. Challenges, controversies, and hot topics in pulmonary embolism imaging. *AJR Am J Roentgenol*. 2011;196(3):497–515.

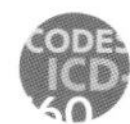

CODES

ICD10

- I26.99 Other pulmonary embolism without acute cor pulmonale
- I27.82 Chronic pulmonary embolism

CLINICAL PEARLS

- PE can be excluded in patients who have a low pretest probability and negative D-dimer testing.
- Unless contraindicated, CT angiogram can reliably be used to diagnose or rule out PE in the majority of cases.
- Perform cancer-oriented review of systems and age- and gender-appropriate cancer screening in patients >40 years of age, recurrent VTE, upper extremity DVT (not related to catheter or lines), bilateral lower extremity DVT, intra-abdominal DVT, and resistance to treatment.
- In patients with a prolonged baseline aPTT, adjust the heparin dose with anti-Xa levels (therapeutic range 0.3–0.7).

PULMONARY FIBROSIS

Anna Rudnicki, MD

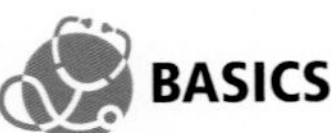

BASICS

DESCRIPTION

- Characterized by fibrosis of the lung parenchyma
- Chest CT shows reticular pattern and honeycombing, with subpleural and lower lobe predominance.
- Lung biopsy shows "usual interstitial pneumonia" pattern.
- Classified based on etiology
  - Idiopathic
  - Nonidiopathic

EPIDEMIOLOGY

Incidence

- Incidence of IPF is 7–16/100,000 person-years.
- Idiopathic pulmonary fibrosis (IPF) is more common in men.
- Most patients with IPF are >60 years.
- Incidence of nonidiopathic pulmonary fibrosis is unknown.

Prevalence

- Prevalence of IPF is 2–39 cases/100,000 people.
- Prevalence of nonidiopathic pulmonary fibrosis is unknown.

ETIOLOGY AND PATHOPHYSIOLOGY

- Postulated that microinjury to alveolar epithelial cells causes release of cytokines that activates fibroblasts, which in turn leads to excess production of extracellular matrix.
- Causes of the nonidiopathic form include the following:
  - Occupational exposure
  - Environmental exposure
  - Drugs
  - Systemic connective tissue diseases
  - Granulomatous diseases

Genetics

- <5% of IPF is familial and may involve mutations in surfactant protein A2 and C and/or abnormal telomere shortening.
- Most likely mode of transmission is autosomal dominant with variable penetrance.

RISK FACTORS

- Family history of pulmonary fibrosis
- Gastroesophageal reflux disease (GERD)
- Smoking
- Exposure to birds, livestock, dust from metals or wood, solvents

GENERAL PREVENTION

Avoid the risk factors mentioned above, such as smoking, certain occupational exposures, or drugs that induce pulmonary fibrosis.

COMMONLY ASSOCIATED CONDITIONS

- Pulmonary hypertension: occurs in 30–80% of patients with IPF, likely as a result of hypoxemic vasoconstriction
- GERD
- Nonidiopathic pulmonary fibrosis may be associated with connective tissue diseases (e.g., rheumatoid arthritis and scleroderma).

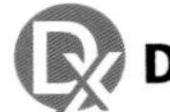

DIAGNOSIS

HISTORY

- Slowly progressive dyspnea
- Dry cough

PHYSICAL EXAM

- Tachypnea
- Fine inspiratory crackles
- Possible clubbing

DIFFERENTIAL DIAGNOSIS

- Asbestosis
- Berylliosis
- Coal worker's pneumoconiosis
- Chronic hypersensitivity pneumonitis
- Sarcoidosis
- Silicosis

DIAGNOSTIC TESTS & INTERPRETATION

Initial Tests (lab, imaging)

- High-resolution chest computed tomography (HRCT) is required to make diagnosis. Characteristic findings include a reticular pattern, traction bronchiectasis, and honeycombing. There is a subpleural and lower lobe predominance. There is minimal to no evidence of active inflammation (1,2).
- If the patient has characteristic findings of pulmonary fibrosis on chest CT, then lung biopsy may not necessarily be required (1).
- HRCT is needed as part of initial workup (as above).

Follow-Up Tests & Special Considerations

- Surgical lung biopsy should be considered if clinical presentation and HRCT are not entirely characteristic of pulmonary fibrosis (1).
- Blood work to rule out associated collagen vascular disease (1)
- Bronchoscopy with bronchoalveolar lavage may help rule out other types of interstitial lung disease and concurrent infection (1).

Diagnostic Procedures/Other

- Pulmonary function testing (PFT): initially, may see only decrease in diffusing capcacity; later in disease, may develop decrease in lung volumes as well
- Echocardiogram to evaluate for concomitant pulmonary hypertension
- Resting and exercise pulse oximetry to determine need for supplemental oxygen

Test Interpretation

Usual interstitial pneumonitis: shows interstitial scarring, honeycombing, and fibroblastic foci. There is temporal heterogeneity, meaning there may be areas of normal lung adjacent to fibrosed or inflamed lung.

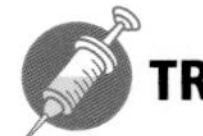

TREATMENT

GENERAL MEASURES

- Pulmonary rehabilitation (1)[C]
- Consider treating for GERD, even if asymptomatic (1)[B].
- Consider lung transplant evaluation.

MEDICATION

First Line

Supplemental oxygen, if needed (1)[C]

ISSUES FOR REFERRAL

- Patients should be evaluated and cared for longitudinally by a pulmonologist.
- If any uncertainty in diagnosis, then consider referral to thoracic surgery for lung biopsy (3,4).
- Depending on patient age, comorbidities, and preference may consider referral for lung transplant

ADDITIONAL THERAPIES

- Recent studies have shown a benefit with the antifibrotic agent pirfenidone and the tyrosine kinase inhibitor nintedanib for slowing the progression of IPF. These drugs are not available for this purpose in the United States (4,5).
- Phosphodiesterase inhibitors (sildenafil) may be of benefit in those developing pulmonary hypertension.
- A recent study showed an increase in mortality in patients treated with a combination of prednisone, azathioprine, and *N*-acetylcysteine when compared with those receiving placebo or *N*-acetylcysteine alone (3).
- Many other clinical trials are currently under way. Some of the targets being studied include TGF-β; connective tissue growth factor; IL-13; CCL2; CXCR4; and CXCL12, ACE, and angiotensin II (6).

P

SURGERY/OTHER PROCEDURES
Lung transplant carries a 5-year survival of 50–56%.

COMPLEMENTARY & ALTERNATIVE MEDICINE
None

INPATIENT CONSIDERATIONS
Admission Criteria/Initial Stabilization
Worsening shortness of breath and/or increased oxygen requirements:
- Provide adequate supplemental oxygen.
- Workup for other possible causes of respiratory decompensation
- If no other cause for respiratory decompensation found, then consider administration of high-dose steroids

Nursing
Supplemental oxygen to keep saturations >90%

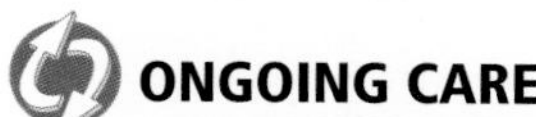

ONGOING CARE

FOLLOW-UP RECOMMENDATIONS
Patient should follow up with a pulmonologist.

Patient Monitoring
Disease progression can be monitored by periodic PFTs and HRCT.

DIET
No specific dietary requirements

PATIENT EDUCATION
- Patients should be counseled extensively regarding the prognosis of this diagnosis and given as much support as possible. Information about support groups in the local community and online may be helpful.
- American Lung Association: http://www.lungusa.org/lung-disease/pulmonary-fibrosis/
- Pulmonary Fibrosis Foundation: http://www.pulmonaryfibrosis.org/, which includes information about active pulmonary fibrosis clinical trials

PROGNOSIS
- Median survival time was thought to be 2–3 years from time of diagnosis. However, recent data from clinical trials suggest that this may be an underestimate.
- Some patients may deteriorate quickly, whereas others can remain stable for an extended period of time. Acute exacerbations carry a high mortality, and ICU treatment (mechanical ventilation) is mostly unsuccessful.
- A higher extent of fibrosis increases the risk of death, whereas a higher percentage-predicted diffusing capacity of lung for carbon monoxide reduced the risk of death.

COMPLICATIONS
- Respiratory failure
- Infection
- Pulmonary hypertension
- Rib fractures secondary to prolonged coughing (especially in elderly patients with decreased bone density)

REFERENCES

1. Raghu G, Collard HR, Egan JJ, et al. An official ATS/ERS/JRS/ALAT statement: idiopathic pulmonary fibrosis: evidence-based guidelines for diagnosis and management. *Am J Respir Crit Care Med*. 2011;183(6):788–824.
2. Lynch DA, Godwin JD, Safrin S, et al. High-resolution computed tomography in idiopathic pulmonary fibrosis: diagnosis and prognosis. *Am J Respir Crit Care Med*. 2005;172(4):488–493.
3. Idiopathic Pulmonary Fibrosis Clinical Research Network. Prednisone, azathioprine, and N-acetylcysteine for pulmonary fibrosis. *N Engl J Med*. 2012;366(21):1968–1977.
4. King TE Jr, Bradford WZ, Castro-Bernardini S, et al. A phase 3 trial of pirfenidone in patients with idiopathic pulmonary fibrosis. *N Engl J Med*. 2014;370(22):2083–2092.
5. Richeldi L, du Bois RM, Raghu G, et al. Efficacy and safety of nintedanib in idiopathic pulmonary fibrosis. *N Engl J Med*. 2014;370(22):2071–2082.
6. Rafii R, Juarez MM, Albertson TE, et al. A review of current and novel therapies for idiopathic pulmonary fibrosis. *J Thorac Dis*. 2013;5(1):48–73.

ADDITIONAL READING

- Castriotta RJ, Eldadah BA, Foster WM, et al. Workshop on idiopathic pulmonary fibrosis in older adults. *Chest*. 2010;138(3):693–703.
- Coward WR, Saini G, Jenkins G. The pathogenesis of idiopathic pulmonary fibrosis. *Ther Adv Respir Dis*. 2010;4(6):367–388.
- Hoo ZH, Whyte MK. Idiopathic pulmonary fibrosis. *Thorax*. 2012;67(8):742–746.
- Lee JS, McLaughlin S, Collard HR. Comprehensive care of the patient with idiopathic pulmonary fibrosis. *Curr Opin Pulm Med*. 2011;17(5):348–354.
- O'Connell OJ, Kennedy MP, Henry MT. Idiopathic pulmonary fibrosis: treatment update. *Adv Ther*. 2011;28(11):986–999.
- Rafii R, Juarez MM, Albertson TE, et al. A review of current and novel therapies for idiopathic pulmonary fibrosis. *J Thorac Dis*. 2013;5(1):48–73.
- Spagnolo P, Del Giovane C, Luppi F, et al. Non-steroid agents for idiopathic pulmonary fibrosis. *Cochrane Database Syst Rev*. 2010;(9):CD003134.

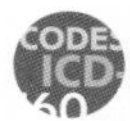

CODES

ICD10
- J84.10 Pulmonary fibrosis, unspecified
- J84.112 Idiopathic pulmonary fibrosis

CLINICAL PEARLS

- Pulmonary fibrosis can usually be diagnosed based on characteristic chest CT findings, which include a reticular pattern, traction bronchiectasis, and honeycombing with a peripheral and basilar predominance.
- There are idiopathic and nonidiopathic forms of pulmonary fibrosis.
- Treatment options for pulmonary fibrosis are very limited and, at best, serve to slow the progression of disease.

PYELONEPHRITIS

Stephen A. Martin, MD, EdM

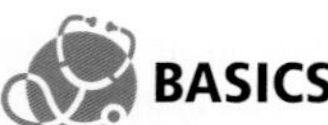

BASICS

DESCRIPTION

- Acute pyelonephritis is a syndrome caused by an infection of the renal parenchyma and renal pelvis, often producing localized flank/back pain combined with systemic symptoms, such as fever, chills, and nausea. It has a wide spectrum of presentation, from mild illness to septic shock.
- Chronic pyelonephritis is the result of progressive inflammation of the renal interstitium and tubules, due to recurrent infection, vesicoureteral reflux, or both.
- Pyelonephritis is considered uncomplicated if the infection is caused by a typical pathogen in an immunocompetent patient who has normal urinary tract anatomy and renal function.
- System(s) affected: renal; urologic
- Synonym: acute upper urinary tract infection (UTI)

Geriatric Considerations

- May present as isolated confusion; absence of fever is common in this age group.
- Elderly patients with diabetes and pyelonephritis are at higher risk of bacteremia, long hospitalization, and mortality.
- The high prevalence of asymptomatic bacteriuria in the elderly makes the use of urine dipstick less reliable in diagnosing UTI (1)[A].

Pregnancy Considerations

- Most common medical complication requiring hospitalization
- Affects 1–2% of all pregnancies. Morbidity does not differ between trimesters.
- Urine culture as test of cure 1–2 weeks after therapy

Pediatric Considerations

- UTI is present in ~5% of patients age 2 months–2 years with fever and no apparent source on history and physical exam.
- Treatment (oral or IV; inpatient or outpatient) should be based on the clinical situation and patient toxicity.

EPIDEMIOLOGY

Incidence

Community-acquired acute pyelonephritis: 28/10,000/year

Prevalence

Adult cases: 250,000/year, with 100,000 hospitalizations

ETIOLOGY AND PATHOPHYSIOLOGY

- *Escherichia coli* (>80%)
- Other gram-negative pathogens: *Proteus*, *Klebsiella*, *Serratia*, *Clostridium*, *Pseudomonas*, and *Enterobacter*
- *Enterococcus*
- *Staphylococcus*: *Staphylococcus epidermis*, *Staphylococcus saprophyticus* (number 2 cause in young women), and *Staphylococcus aureus*
- *Candida*

RISK FACTORS

- Underlying urinary tract abnormalities
- Indwelling catheter/recent urinary tract instrumentation
- Nephrolithiasis
- Immunocompromise, including diabetes
- Elderly, institutionalized patients (particularly women)
- Prostatic enlargement
- Childhood UTI
- Acute pyelonephritis within the prior year
- Frequency of recent sexual intercourse/spermicide use
- Stress incontinence
- Pregnancy
- Hospital-acquired infection
- Symptoms >7 days at time of presentation

COMMONLY ASSOCIATED CONDITIONS

- Indwelling catheters
- Renal calculi
- Benign prostatic hyperplasia

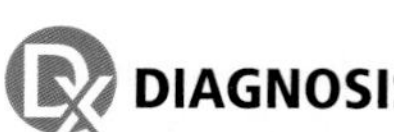

DIAGNOSIS

HISTORY

- In adults
  - Fever
  - Flank pain
  - Nausea ± vomiting
  - Malaise, anorexia
  - Myalgia
  - Dysuria, urinary frequency, urgency
  - Suprapubic discomfort
- In infants and children
  - Irritability
  - GI symptoms

PHYSICAL EXAM

- In adults
  - Fever: ≥37.8°C (100°F)
  - Costovertebral angle tenderness
  - Presentation ranges from no physical findings to septic shock.
  - A pelvic exam may be necessary in female patients to exclude pelvic inflammatory disease.
- In infants and children
  - Sepsis
  - Fever
  - Poor skin perfusion
  - Inadequate weight gain/weight loss
  - Jaundice to gray skin color

DIFFERENTIAL DIAGNOSIS

- Obstructive uropathy
- Acute bacterial pneumonia (lower lobe)
- Cholecystitis
- Acute pancreatitis
- Appendicitis
- Perforated viscus
- Aortic dissection
- Pelvic inflammatory disease
- Kidney stone
- Ectopic pregnancy
- Diverticulitis

DIAGNOSTIC TESTS & INTERPRETATION

Initial Tests (lab, imaging)

- Urinalysis: pyuria ± leukocyte casts, hematuria, nitrites, and mild proteinuria
- Urine leukocyte esterase positive
- Urine Gram stain; urine culture (>10,000 colony-forming units/mL) and sensitivities
- CBC, BUN, creatinine, and glomerular filtration rate
- In one study of hospitalized patients, C-reactive protein levels were found to correlate with prolonged hospitalization and infection recurrence; in another, serum albumin <3.3 g/dL had the strongest association with admission.
- Imaging not necessary in straightforward cases
- Pediatrics: Recent guidelines recommend renal/bladder US, (not voiding cystourethrogram) after 1st UTI.

Follow-Up Tests & Special Considerations

- To obtain reliable pediatric urine cultures, catheterization/suprapubic aspirate should be used to obtain samples from non–toilet-trained children.
- In some geriatric patients, obtaining a clean catch specimen may also be difficult and catheterization may be necessary.
- Blood culture(s): indicated in diagnostic uncertainty, immunosuppression, or a suspected hematogenous source
- Recent antibiotic use may alter lab results.
- If patient's condition does not improve within 72 hours or if obstruction/anatomic abnormality suspected, consider the following:
  - CT scan of abdomen and pelvis ± contrast material
  - US, renal with kidneys, ureter, bladder
  - Cystoscopy with ureteral catheterization

Test Interpretation

- Acute: abscess formation with neutrophil response
- Chronic: fibrosis with reduction in renal tissue

TREATMENT

- 7 days of treatment is equivalent to longer treatment regimens in patients without urogenital abnormalities (2)[A].
- IV antibiotics are indicated for inpatients who are toxic or unable to tolerate oral antibiotics.

GENERAL MEASURES

- Broad-spectrum antibiotics initially, tailoring therapy to culture and sensitivity results
- Analgesics and antipyretics
- Consider urinary analgesics (e.g., phenazopyridine 200 mg TID) for severe dysuria.

MEDICATION

- For empirical oral therapy, a fluoroquinolone is recommended. Should fluoroquinolone resistance exceed 10%, a single initial IV dose of a long-acting antibiotic such as ceftriaxone 1 g is recommended in addition.
- For parenteral therapy, a fluoroquinolone, aminoglycoside ± ampicillin, an extended-spectrum cephalosporin or an extended-spectrum penicillin with or without an aminoglycoside.
- Contraindications:
  - Known drug allergy
  - Fluoroquinolones are contraindicated in children, adolescents, and pregnant women.
  - Nitrofurantoin does not achieve reliable tissue levels for treatment of pyelonephritis.
- Precautions:
  - Most antibiotics require adjustments in dosage in patients with renal insufficiency.
  - Monitor aminoglycoside levels and renal function.
  - If *Enterococcus* is suspected based on Gram stain, ampicillin + gentamicin is a reasonable empirical choice, unless patient is penicillin-allergic; then use vancomycin. If outpatient, add amoxicillin to fluoroquinolone, pending culture results and sensitivity. Do not use a 3rd-generation cephalosporin for suspected/proven enterococcal infection.

First Line

- Adults
  - Severe illness: IV therapy until afebrile 24–48 hours and tolerating oral hydration and medications, then oral agents to complete 2-week course. Adult doses:
  - IV (assuming normal creatine clearance [CrCl])
    - Ciprofloxacin: 400 mg q12h
    - Levofloxacin: 500 mg/day
    - Cefotaxime: 1 g q8–12h up to 2 g q4h
    - Ceftriaxone: 1–2 g/day
    - Cefoxitin: 2 g q4–8h
    - Gentamicin: 5–7 mg/kg of body weight daily (± ampicillin 2 g q6h for *Enterococcus*)
  - Oral (initial outpatient treatment)
    - Ciprofloxacin: 500 mg q12h for 7 days
    - Ciprofloxacin XR: 1,000 mg/day for 7 days
    - Levofloxacin: 750 mg/day for 5 days
    - Trimethoprim/sulfamethoxazole (TMP-SMX) (160/800 mg): 1 tab PO BID for 14 days provided uropathogen known to be susceptible and ceftriaxone 1 g initial IV dose given
- Pediatric
  - IV (general indication for IV therapy is age <2 months/clinical concern in other ages)
    - Ceftriaxone: 50–100 mg/kg/day (also can be used IM in outpatient setting)
    - Ampicillin: 100 mg/kg/day IV divided in 4 doses + gentamicin 7.5 mg/kg/day divided in 3 doses
  - Oral: cefdinir: 14 mg/kg/day PO × 10–14 days; ceftibuten 9 mg/kg/day PO × 10–14 days

Second Line

Adults

- IV
  - Piperacillin–tazobactam: 3.375 g q6–8h
  - Ticarcillin–clavulanate: 3.1 g q4–6h
- Oral
  - Oral β-lactams should be used with caution to treat pyelonephritis due to inferior efficacy and higher relapse rates; if used, provide an initial IV dose of ceftriaxone.
  - Longer courses of therapy (10–4 days) recommended
  - Cefpodoxime (Proxetil): 200 mg q12h
  - Amoxicillin–clavulanate: 875/125 mg q12h or 500/125 mg TID
  - TMP-SMX: 60–800 mg q12h (up to 30% *E. coli* strains are resistant to ampicillin and TMP-SMX in community-acquired infections)

Pediatric Considerations

- Children <2 years of age and children with febrile or recurrent UTI are usually treated for 10 days.
- Initial empiric coverage should include *E. coli*. Ampicillin should be added if *Enterococcus* is suspected.
  - Oral antibiotics (ceftibuten, and amoxicillin/clavulanic acid) may be used alone, *or*
  - IV antibiotics (single daily dosing with aminoglycoside) for 2–4 days, followed by oral antibiotics (3)[A]
- If patient is treated as an outpatient, antibiotic course must be completed in entirety.

ISSUES FOR REFERRAL

- Acute pyelonephritis unresponsive to therapy
- Chronic pyelonephritis
- Abnormal urogenital anatomy

SURGERY/OTHER PROCEDURES

Perinephric abscess may require surgical drainage.

INPATIENT CONSIDERATIONS

Admission Criteria/Initial Stabilization

- Inpatient therapy for severe illness (e.g., high fevers, severe pain, marked debility, intractable vomiting, possible urosepsis), risk factors for complicated pyelonephritis, or extremes of age
- Outpatient therapy if mild to moderate illness (not pregnant, no nausea/vomiting; fever and pain not severe), uncomplicated, and tolerating oral hydration and medications. Most such patients can be selected for outpatient management.

IV Fluids

As indicated for dehydration or renal calculi

Discharge Criteria

Discharge on oral agent (see earlier discussion) after patient is afebrile 24–48 hours to complete 2 weeks.

ONGOING CARE

FOLLOW-UP RECOMMENDATIONS

- Women: Routine follow-up cultures not recommended unless symptoms recur after 2 weeks; then, urologic evaluation is necessary.
- Men, children, adolescents, patients with recurrent infections, patients with risk factors: repeat cultures 1–2 weeks after completing therapy; urologic evaluation after 1st episode of pyelonephritis and with recurrences

Patient Monitoring

- No response within 48 hours (5% of patients): Reevaluate and review cultures, CT scan, or US to review anatomy; adjust therapy as needed; may need urologic consult. The 2 most common causes of failure to respond are a resistant organism and nephrolithiasis.
- Mild to moderate illness: oral therapy for 2 weeks as outpatient
- Maintained with parents to monitor response in children

DIET

Encourage fluid intake.

PROGNOSIS

95% of treated patients respond within 48 hours.

COMPLICATIONS

- Kidney abscess
- Metastatic infection: skeletal system, endocardium, eye, meningitis with subsequent seizures
- Septic shock and death
- Acute/chronic renal failure

REFERENCES

1. Ninan S, Walton C, Barlow G. Investigation of suspected urinary tract infection in older people. *BMJ*. 2014;349:g4070.
2. Eliakim-Raz N, Yahav D, Paul M, et al. Duration of antibiotic treatment for acute pyelonephritis and septic urinary tract infection—7 days or less versus longer treatment: systematic review and meta-analysis of randomized controlled trials. *J Antimicrob Chemother*. 2013;68(10):2183–2191.
3. Strohmeier Y, Hodson EM, Willis NS, et al. Antibiotics for acute pyelonephritis in children. *Cochrane Database Syst Rev*. 2014;7:CD003772.

ADDITIONAL READING

- Beetz R, Westenfelder M. Antimicrobial therapy of urinary tract infections in children. *Int J Antimicrob Agents*. 2011;38(Suppl):42–50.
- Colgan R, Williams M, Johnson JR. Diagnosis and treatment of acute pyelonephritis in women. *Am Fam Physician*. 2011;84(5):519–526.
- Gupta K, Hooton TM, Naber KG, et al. International clinical practice guidelines for the treatment of acute uncomplicated cystitis and pyelonephritis in women: a 2010 update by the Infectious Diseases Society of America and the European Society for Microbiology and Infectious Diseases. *Clin Infect Dis*. 2011;52(5):e103–e120.
- Hooton TM. Clinical practice. Uncomplicated urinary tract infection. *N Engl J Med*. 2012;366(11):1028–1037.
- Roberts KB, Subcommittee on Urinary Tract Infection, Steering Committee on Quality Improvement and Management. Urinary tract infection: clinical practice guideline for the diagnosis and management of the initial UTI in febrile infants and children 2 to 24 months. *Pediatrics*. 2011;128(3):595–610.
- Takhar SS, Moran GJ. Diagnosis and management of urinary tract infection in the emergency department and outpatient settings. *Infect Dis Clin North Am*. 2014;28(1):33–48.
- Wang A, Nizran P, Malone MA, et al. Urinary tract infections. *Prim Care*. 2013;40(3):687–706.

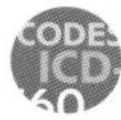

CODES

ICD10

- N12 Tubulo-interstitial nephritis, not spcf as acute or chronic
- N10 Acute tubulo-interstitial nephritis
- N11.9 Chronic tubulo-interstitial nephritis, unspecified

CLINICAL PEARLS

- Pyelonephritis can present with isolated confusion or mental status changes (no fever) in the elderly.
- The most common causes of poor response to treatment include antibiotic resistance and coexisting nephrolithiasis.
- Oral β-lactams are less effective for treating pyelonephritis. Fluroquinolones are the initial drugs of choice.

PYLORIC STENOSIS

Ruben Peralta, MD, FACS

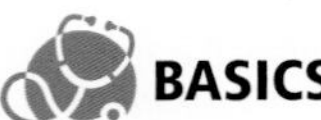

BASICS

DESCRIPTION

- Progressive narrowing of the pyloric canal, occurring in infancy
- Synonym(s): infantile hypertrophic pyloric stenosis

EPIDEMIOLOGY

- Predominant age: infancy
  - Onset usually at 3–6 weeks of age; rarely in the newborn period or as late as 5 months of age
- Considered the most common condition requiring surgical intervention in the 1st year of life.
- A recent decline in its incidence has been reported in a number of countries.
- Predominant sex: male > female (4:1)

Incidence

In Caucasian population, 2–5:1,000 babies; less common in African American and Asian populations

Prevalence

National prevalence level is 1–2:1,000 infants, ranging from 0.5 to 4.21:1,000 live births.

ETIOLOGY AND PATHOPHYSIOLOGY

- Abnormal relaxation of the pyloric muscles leads to hypertrophy.
- Redundant mucosa fills the pyloric canal.
- Gastric outflow is obstructed, leading to gastric distension and vomiting.
- The exact cause remains unknown, but multiple genetic and environmental factors have been implicated (1,2)[B],(3)[C].
- A recent surveillance study of a population-based birth defects registry identified an association between pyloric stenosis and the use of fluoxetine in the 1st trimester of pregnancy, even after adjustment for maternal age and smoking. The adjusted odds ratio was 9.8 (95% CI: 1.5–62) (4)[B].

Genetics

Recent studies have identified linkage to chromosome 11 and multiple loci and chromosome 16 (1,2)[B], (3)[C].

RISK FACTORS

- Incidence higher in firstborn boys
- 5× increased risk with affected 1st-degree relative
- Strong familial aggregation and heritability (2)

COMMONLY ASSOCIATED CONDITIONS

Associated anomalies present in ~4–7% of infants with pyloric stenosis.

- Hiatal and inguinal hernias (most commonly)
- Other anomalies include the following:
  - Congenital heart disease
  - Esophageal atresia
  - Tracheoesophageal fistula
  - Renal abnormalities
  - Turner syndrome and trisomy 18
  - Cornelia de Lange syndrome
  - Smith-Lemli-Opitz syndrome
- A common proposed genetic link between breast cancer, endometriosis, and pyloric stenosis has been observed in families.

DIAGNOSIS

HISTORY

- Nonbilious projectile vomiting after feeding, increasing in frequency and severity
- Emesis may become blood-tinged from vomiting-induced gastric irritation.
- Hunger due to inadequate nutrition
- Decrease in bowel movements
- Weight loss

PHYSICAL EXAM

- Firm, mobile ("olivelike") mass palpable in the right upper quadrant (70–90% of the time)
- Epigastric distention
- Visible gastric peristalsis after feeding
- Late signs: dehydration, weight loss
- Rarely, jaundice when starvation leads to decreased glucuronyl transferase activity resulting in indirect hyperbilirubinemia

DIFFERENTIAL DIAGNOSIS

- Inexperienced or inappropriate feeding
- GERD
- Gastritis
- Congenital adrenal hyperplasia, salt-losing
- Pylorospasm
- Gastric volvulus
- Antral or gastric web

DIAGNOSTIC TESTS & INTERPRETATION

Metabolic disturbances are late findings and are uncommon in present era of early diagnosis and intervention.

- If prolonged vomiting, then check electrolytes for the following:
  - Hypokalemia
  - Hypochloremia
  - Metabolic alkalosis
- Elevated unconjugated bilirubin level (rare)
- Paradoxical aciduria: The kidney tubules excrete hydrogen to preserve potassium in face of hypokalemic alkalosis.
- Abdominal US is the study of choice.
  - US shows thickened and elongated pyloric muscle and redundant mucosa.
- Upper GI series reveals strong gastric contractions; elongated, narrow pyloric canal (string sign); and parallel lines of barium in the narrow channel (double-tract sign or railroad track sign).

Test Interpretation

Concentric hypertrophy of pyloric muscle

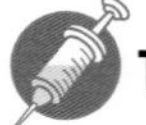

TREATMENT

SURGERY/OTHER PROCEDURES

- Ramstedt pyloromyotomy is curative. The entire length of hypertrophied muscle is divided, with preservation of the underlying mucosa.
- Surgical approaches include open (traditional right upper quadrant transverse) incision, more contemporary circumumbilical incision, and laparoscopic techniques.
- A recent review concluded that the laparoscopic approach results in less postoperative pain and can be performed with no increase in operative time or complications (5,6)[A].
- Conservative approach
  - Conservative management of infantile hypertrophic pyloric stenosis with atropine can be effective in approximately six out of seven cases but has a lower success rate and longer duration of therapy than surgery (7)[B].
  - Atropine therapy may be considered as an alternative to pyloromyotomy for patients unsuitable or at high risk for surgery and in areas of the world where surgery on small infants is unavailable or unsafe (7)[B].

INPATIENT CONSIDERATIONS

Admission Criteria/Initial Stabilization

- Prompt treatment to avoid dehydration and malnutrition
- Correct acid–base and electrolyte disturbances. Surgery should be delayed until alkalosis is corrected.
- Patients need pre- and postop apnea monitoring. They have a tendency toward apnea to compensate with respiratory acidosis for their metabolic alkalosis.

IV Fluids

To correct dehydration and metabolic abnormalities

ONGOING CARE

FOLLOW-UP RECOMMENDATIONS

Patient Monitoring

- Routine pediatric health maintenance
- Postoperative monitoring, including monitoring for pain, emesis, apnea

DIET

- No preoperative feeding
- Initiate feeding 12–24 hours after surgery, with goal of advancing to full oral feedings within 36–48 hours of surgery.

PROGNOSIS

Surgery is curative.

COMPLICATIONS

No long-term morbidity. Duodenal perforation is a known, but uncommon, complication of surgery. In a recent systematic review and meta-analysis addressing major complication rates between open and laparoscopic pyloromyotomy, the author found no major difference in complications, but the laparoscopic group showed faster time to full feed and a shorter hospital stay.

REFERENCES

1. Feenstra B, Geller F, Carstensen L, et al. Plasma lipids, genetic variants near APOA1, and the risk of infantile hypertrophic pyloric stenosis. *JAMA*. 2013;310(7):714–721.
2. Krogh C, Fischer TK, Skotte L, et al. Familial aggregation and heritability of pyloric stenosis. *JAMA*. 2010;303(23):2393–2399.
3. Ranells JD, Carver JD, Kirby RS. Infantile hypertrophic pyloric stenosis: epidemiology, genetics, and clinical update. *Adv Pediatr*. 2011;58(1):195–206.
4. Bakker MK, De Walle HE, Wilffert B, et al. Fluoxetine and infantile hypertrophic pylorus stenosis: a signal from a birth defects-drug exposure surveillance study. *Pharmacoepidemiol Drug Saf*. 2010;19(8):808–813.
5. Sola JE, Neville HL. Laparoscopic vs open pyloromyotomy: a systematic review and meta-analysis. *J Pediatr Surg*. 2009;44(8):1631–1637.
6. Oomen MW, Hoekstra LT, Bakx R, et al. Open versus laparoscopic pyloromyotomy for hypertrophic pyloric stenosis: a systematic review and meta-analysis focusing on major complications. *Surg Endosc*. 2012;26(8):2104–2110.
7. Mercer AE, Phillips R. Question 2: can a conservative approach to the treatment of hypertrophic pyloric stenosis with atropine be considered a real alternative to surgical pylomyotomy? *Arch Dis Child*. 2013;98(6):474–477.

ADDITIONAL READING

- Ein SH, Masiakos PT, Ein A. The ins and outs of pyloromyotomy: what we have learned in 35 years. *Pediatr Surg Int*. 2014;30(5):467–480.
- Everett KV, Capon F, Georgoula C, et al. Linkage of monogenic infantile hypertrophic pyloric stenosis to chromosome 16q24. *Eur J Hum Genet*. 2008;16(9):1151–1154.
- Everett KV, Chioza BA, Georgoula C, et al. Genome-wide high-density SNP-based linkage analysis of infantile hypertrophic pyloric stenosis identifies loci on chromosomes 11q14-q22 and Xq23. *Am J Hum Genet*. 2008;82(3):756–762.
- Georgoula C, Gardiner M. Pyloric stenosis a 100 years after Ramstedt. *Arch Dis Child*. 2012;97(8):741–745.
- National Birth Defects Prevention Network. Selected birth defects data from population-based birth defects surveillance programs in the United States, 2003–2007. *Birth Defects Res A Clin Mol Teratol*. 2010;88(12):1062–1174.
- Owen RP, Almond SL, Humphrey GM. Atropine sulphate: rescue therapy for pyloric stenosis [published online ahead of print August 2, 2012]. *BMJ Case Rep*.
- Sommerfield T, Chalmers J, Youngson G, et al. The changing epidemiology of infantile hypertrophic pyloric stenosis in Scotland. *Arch Dis Child*. 2008;93(12):1007–1011.
- Wyrick DL, Smith SD, Dassinger MS. Surgeon as educator: bedside ultrasound in hyperthrophic pyloric stenosis. *J Surg Educ*. 2014;156(3):650.

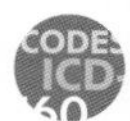

CODES

ICD10

Q40.0 Congenital hypertrophic pyloric stenosis

CLINICAL PEARLS

- Pyloric stenosis is the most common condition requiring surgical intervention in the 1st year of life.
- The condition classically presents between 1 and 5 months of life, with projectile vomiting after feeds and a firm, mobile mass in the right upper quadrant.
- Abdominal US is the study of choice.
- Surgery (laparoscopic Ramstedt pyloromyotomy is the preferred method) is curative.

RABIES

Alan M. Ehrlich, MD

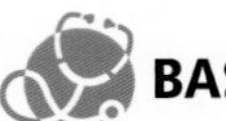

BASICS

DESCRIPTION

- A rapidly progressive CNS infection caused by a ribonucleic acid (RNA) rhabdovirus affecting mammals, including humans
- Generally considered to be 100% fatal once symptoms develop
- System(s) affected: nervous
- Synonym(s): hydrophobia (inability to swallow water)

EPIDEMIOLOGY

Incidence

- Most cases are in developing countries.
- Estimated 55,000 deaths worldwide per year
- Only 1 death in the United States in 2007
- Only 3 cases in the United States in 2006
- Predominant age: any
- Predominant sex: male = female

ETIOLOGY AND PATHOPHYSIOLOGY

Lyssavirus, which is an RNA virus in the family Rhabdoviridae

- Rabies virus is a neurotropic virus present in saliva of infected animals.
- Transmission occurs via bites from infected animals or when saliva from an infected animal comes in contact with an open wound or mucous membranes.
- In the United States, bats are most common reservoir.

RISK FACTORS

- Professions or activities exposing individuals to potentially infected (wild or domestic) animals (e.g., animal handlers, lab workers, veterinarians, cave explorers)
- In the United States, most cases are associated with bat exposure.
- Internationally, rabies remains widespread in both domestic and feral dogs.
- Human-to-human transmission has occurred through cornea, solid organs, and other tissue transplantation.
- Travel to countries where canine rabies is endemic

GENERAL PREVENTION

- Preexposure vaccination for high-risk groups such as veterinarians, animal handlers, and certain laboratory workers
- Consider preexposure vaccination for travelers to areas, such as North Africa, that have increased risk of rabies from domestic animals.
- Immunization of dogs and cats
- Contact animal control and avoid approaching or handling wild (or domestic) animals exhibiting strange behaviors.
- Avoid wild and unknown domestic animals.
- Seek treatment promptly if bitten, scratched, or in contact with saliva from potentially infected animal.
- Infection can be prevented by prompt postexposure treatment.
- Consider postexposure prophylaxis for individuals in direct contact with bats, unless it is known that an exposure did not occur.

DIAGNOSIS

HISTORY

- History of animal exposure
- Most patients in the United States do not recall exposure.
- 5 stages (may overlap)
  - Incubation period: time between bite and 1st symptoms: usually 10 days to 1 year (average of 20–60 days). Incubation is shortest in patients with extensive bites in the head or trunk.
  - Prodrome: lasts 1–14 days; symptoms include pain or paresthesia at bite site and nonspecific flulike symptoms, including fever and headache.
  - Acute neurologic period: lasts 2–10 days. CNS symptoms dominate; generally 1 of 2 forms: (i) furious rabies: brief (~5 minute) episodes of hyperactivity with hydrophobia, aerophobia, hyperventilation, hypersalivation, and autonomic instability; (ii) paralytic rabies: Paralysis dominates; may be ascending (as in Guillain-Barré syndrome) or may affect ≥1 limbs differentially
  - Coma: lasts hours to days; may evolve over several days following acute neurologic period; may be sudden, with respiratory arrest
  - Death: usually occurs within 3 weeks of onset as result of complications

PHYSICAL EXAM

Findings range from normal exam up to severe neurologic findings, including paralysis and coma, depending on the stage of rabies at the time of presentation.

DIFFERENTIAL DIAGNOSIS

- Any rapidly progressive encephalitis; important to exclude treatable causes of encephalitis, especially herpes
- Transverse myelitis

DIAGNOSTIC TESTS & INTERPRETATION

Initial Tests (lab, imaging)

- Lumbar puncture. WBC count is normal or show moderate pleocytosis; protein normal or moderately elevated
- Skin biopsy to detect rabies antigen in hair follicles
  - Available at state and federal reference labs
- Rabies antibody titer on serum and CSF
- Skin biopsy from nape of neck for direct fluorescent antibody examination
- Viral isolation from saliva or CSF
- Corneal smear stains are positive by immunofluorescence in 50% of patients.
- Hyponatremia common
- Head CT scan: normal or nonspecific findings consistent with encephalitis
- MRI can help rule out other forms of encephalitis.

Follow-Up Tests & Special Considerations

Submit brain of the biting animal for testing if possible.

Test Interpretation

Encephalitis may be found on brain biopsy. Other abnormal findings (e.g., brainstem, midbrain, cerebellum) often found only postmortem.

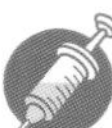

TREATMENT

Thorough wound cleansing with soap and water is first line of treatment. Irrigate wound with virucidal agent, such as povidone-iodine, if available.

GENERAL MEASURES

- Evaluate risk based on possible exposure to rabies and consult local or state public health officials about the need for rabies prophylaxis.
- In the United States, raccoons, skunks, bats, foxes, and coyotes are the animals most likely to be infected, but any carnivore can carry the disease.
- Before initiating specific antirabies treatment, consider the following:
  - Type of exposure (bite or nonbite)
  - Epidemiology of rabies in species involved
  - Circumstances surrounding exposure (provoked vs. unprovoked bite)
  - Vaccination status of offending animal

MEDICATION

ALERT

- Immunosuppression alters immunity after vaccination. Immunosuppressive drugs should be avoided during postexposure prophylaxis if possible. If postexposure prophylaxis is given to an immunosuppressed person, check serum samples for the presence of rabies virus–neutralizing antibody to assess response to vaccination (1)[C].
- Clean wounds thoroughly, regardless of postexposure prophylaxis status.
- Assess need for postexposure prophylaxis based on circumstances of possible exposure.
- Increased risk associated with the following:
  - Bites involving skin puncture are high risk; saliva exposure is a risk only if it comes in contact with an open wound or mucous membranes.
  - Wild or domestic animals unavailable for quarantine
  - Bat exposure
  - Hybrid animals of wild and domestic species (e.g., wolf-dog)
  - Unprovoked attack (Feeding a wild animal is considered a provoked attack.)
- Management based on type of animal as follows:
  - Bites from cats, dogs, and ferrets that can be watched for 10 days do not require prophylaxis unless animal shows signs of illness.
  - Skunks, foxes, bats, raccoons, and most carnivores are high risk, and prophylaxis should begin promptly unless animal can be captured and euthanized for pathologic evaluation.
  - For rodents or livestock, consult local public health authorities before initiating prophylaxis.
- Postexposure prophylaxis (2)[B]
  - Passive vaccination: rabies immunoglobulin (RIG, Hyperab) 20 IU/kg administered once. RIG should be infiltrated around the wound if possible. Administer remaining RIG IM. Do not administer RIG using the same syringe or into the same anatomic site as vaccine.

- Active vaccination: rabies vaccine, human diploid cell vaccine (HDCV) or rabies vaccine adsorbed (RVA) or purified chick embryo cell vaccine IM in the deltoid. Give the first dose, 1 mL, as soon as possible after exposure. The day of the 1st dose is designated day 0. Give additional 1-mL doses on days 3, 7, and 14. If immunocompromised, give 5th dose on day 28. For children, use the anterolateral aspect of the thigh and avoid the gluteal area.
- For previously vaccinated patients, administer an initial 1-mL IM dose of vaccine immediately and an additional 1-mL dose 3 days later. RIG is not necessary in these patients (2)[B].
- Preexposure vaccination: for people in high-risk groups, such as veterinarians, animal handlers, certain laboratory workers, and those spending time in foreign countries where rabies is enzootic (3)[B]:
  - Primary preexposure: three IM 1-mL injections of HDCV or RVA in deltoid area on days 0, 7, and 21, or 28
  - Preexposure boosters: For people at risk of exposure to rabies, serum should be tested every 2 years. Administer preexposure booster of 1.0 mL IM if immunity is waning. If titer cannot be obtained, a booster can be administered instead.
- Contraindications: none for postexposure treatment

Pregnancy Considerations

- Pregnancy is not a contraindication to postexposure prophylaxis.
- Rabies vaccination is not associated with a higher incidence of spontaneous abortion, premature births, or fetal abnormalities.

INPATIENT CONSIDERATIONS

Admission Criteria/Initial Stabilization

Clinical rabies

- Comfort care and sedation for all patients.
- Milwaukee Protocol: experimental treatment using ketamine, midazolam, and amantadine (originally included ribavirin but no longer recommended) (1,4)[C]
- Control cerebral artery vasospasm (with an agent such as nimodipine) (4,5)[C].
- Fludrocortisone and hypertonic saline if needed to maintain normal sodium level (5)[C]

ONGOING CARE

FOLLOW-UP RECOMMENDATIONS

After primary vaccination, serologic testing is necessary only if the patient has a disease or takes immunosuppresive medication.

PATIENT EDUCATION

Homes should be secured from bats by using screens over ventilation areas in the roof. Avoid exposure to wild mammalian species known to carry rabies and report potential exposures immediately.

PROGNOSIS

- No postexposure failures reported in the United States since the 1970s.
- Rabies has the highest case fatality rate of any infectious disease if untreated; generally considered to be 100% fatal once symptoms develop
- There have only been a small number of cases of successful recovery from rabies. Almost all received some form of pre- or postexposure immunization.
- One patient who did not receive pre- or postexposure prophylaxis recovered from clinical rabies in 2004 after being treated with medically induced coma and amantadine in what has become known as the Milwaukee Protocol (1)[C].

COMPLICATIONS

0.6% of people develop mild serum sickness reaction following HDCV boosters. Mild local and systemic reactions are common following vaccination. Mild reactions should not be a cause for interruption of immunization.

REFERENCES

1. Willoughby RE Jr, Tieves KS, Hoffman GM, et al. Survival after treatment of rabies with induction of coma. *N Engl J Med*. 2005;352(24):2508–2514.
2. Rupprecht CE, Briggs D, Brown CM, et al. Use of a reduced (4-dose) vaccine schedule for postexposure prophylaxis to prevent human rabies: recommendations of the Advisory Committee on Immunization Practices. *MMWR Recomm Rep*. 2010;59(RR-2):1–9.
3. Manning SE, Rupprecht CE, Fishbein D, et al. Human rabies prevention—United States, 2008: recommendations of the Advisory Committee on Immunization Practices. *MMWR Recomm Rep*. 2008;57(RR-3):1–28.
4. Aramburo A, Willoughby RE, Bollen AW, et al. Failure of the Milwaukee protocol in a child with rabies. *Clin Infect Dis*. 2011;53(6):572–574.
5. Hu WT, Willoughby RE Jr, Dhonau H, et al. Long-term follow-up after treatment of rabies by induction of coma. *N Engl J Med*. 2007;357(9):945–946.

ADDITIONAL READING

- Centers for Disease Control and Prevention. Recovery of a patient from clinical rabies—California, 2011. *MMWR Morb Mortal Wkly Rep*. 2012;61(4):61–65.
- De Serres G, Skowronski DM, Mimault P, et al. Bats in the bedroom, bats in the belfry: reanalysis of the rationale for rabies postexposure prophylaxis. *Clin Infect Dis*. 2009;48(11):1493–1499.
- Eckerle I, Rosenberger KD, Zwahlen M, et al. Serologic vaccination response after solid organ transplantation: a systematic review. *PLoS One*. 2013;8(2):e56974.
- Hemachudha T, Ugolini G, Wacharapluesadee S, et al. Human rabies: neuropathogenesis, diagnosis, and management. *Lancet Neurol*. 2013;12(5):498–513.
- Vora NM, Basavaraju SV, Feldman KA, et al; Transplant-Associated Rabies Virus Transmission Investigation Team. Raccoon rabies virus variant transmission through solid organ transplantation. *JAMA*. 2013;310(4):398–407.

SEE ALSO

Bites

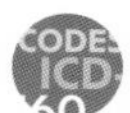

CODES

ICD10

- A82.9 Rabies, unspecified
- Z20.3 Contact with and (suspected) exposure to rabies

CLINICAL PEARLS

- Rabies is rare in the United States but more common in other areas of the world.
- Seek immediate treatment if exposed to scratch, bite, or saliva of potentially infected animal (e.g., feral dog, bat, fox, raccoon, or other wild mammals).
- Postexposure prophylaxis consists of 3 steps: local wound cleansing, passive immunization with rabies immunoglobulin, and active immunization with HDCV.
- Consider postexposure prophylaxis for those reporting direct contact with bats, unless it can be determined that an exposure did not occur.

R

RAPE CRISIS SYNDROME

Jocelyn F. Blackwell, MD, MAJ, MC

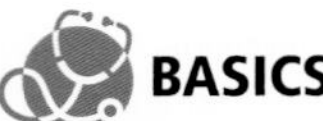

BASICS

DESCRIPTION

- Definitions (legal definitions may vary from state to state)
  - Sexual contact: intentional touching of a person's intimate parts (including thighs) or the clothing covering such areas, if it is construed as being for the purpose of sexual gratification
  - Sexual conduct: vaginal intercourse between a male and female, or anal intercourse, fellatio, or cunnilingus between persons, regardless of sex
  - Rape: any sexual penetration, however slight, using force or coercion against the person's will
  - Sexual imposition: similar to rape but without penetration or the use of force (i.e., nonconsensual sexual contact)
  - Gross sexual imposition: nonconsensual sexual contact with the use of force
  - Corruption of a minor: sexual conduct by an individual age ≥18 years with an individual <16 years of age
- Most states have expanded rape statutes to include marital rape, date rape, and shield laws.
- System(s) affected: nervous; reproductive
- Synonym(s): sexual assault; rape trauma

EPIDEMIOLOGY

- Anyone can be sexually assaulted, but some populations are especially vulnerable.
  - Adolescents and young women
  - People with disabilities
  - Poor and homeless people
  - Sex workers
  - Those living in institutions/areas of conflict
- Predominant age
  - The incidence of sexual assault peaks in those 16–19 years of age, with the mean occurring at 20 years of age.
    - Adolescent sexual assault has a greater frequency of anogenital injuries.
- Predominant sex: female > male
  - For males
    - 69% of male victims were 1st raped before age 18 years.
    - 41% of male victims were raped before age 12 years.

Incidence

- 125,910 rapes and sexual assaults reported in 2009 in the United States, a drop of 38% from 2008 (1).
- Estimated that only a fraction of sexual assaults are reported to law enforcement.
- 18% of American women will be sexually assaulted during their lifetime (2).
  - Between 20 and 25% of females will experience rape/attempted rape during their college years.
- 1.4% of American men will be sexually assaulted during their lifetime.
- Most rape victims either know or have some acquaintance with their attacker.

RISK FACTORS

- In general, adults are assaulted in their own homes, whereas adolescents are assaulted in their assailant's residence.
- Most perpetrators of sexual violence are males, with all acts against females >90%.
- Most acts against males are >65% male perpetrators.

GENERAL PREVENTION

- Scope of rape prevention is very complex and broad.
- The public health approach should include both prevention and avoidance of vulnerability factors and implementation of protective factors.
- Females may benefit from assertiveness training and self-defense training.
- Universal screening by health care providers for interpersonal violence does assist in identifying victims.

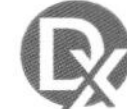

DIAGNOSIS

- In adults
  - History of sexual penetration
  - Sexual contact/conduct without consent and/or with the use of force
- In children
  - Actual observation/suspicion of sexual penetration, sexual contact, or sexual conduct
  - Signs include evidence of the use of force and/or evidence of sexual contact (e.g., presence of semen and/or blood).

HISTORY

- Avoid questioning that implies the patient is at fault.
- Record answers in patient's own words insofar as possible. Include date, approximate time, and general location as best as possible. Document physical abuse other than sexual. Describe all types of sexual contact, whether actual/attempted. Take history of alcohol and/or drug use before or after alleged incident; note that some states require specific forms for documenting history.
- Document time of last activity that could possibly alter specimens (e.g., bath, shower, douche).
- Thorough gynecologic history is mandatory, including last menstrual period, last consenting sexual contact, contraceptive practice, and prior gynecologic surgery (3)[C].

PHYSICAL EXAM

- Use of drawings and/or photographs is encouraged; note that some states require specific forms for documenting physical exam.
- Document all signs of trauma/unusual marks.
- Document mental status/emotional state.
- Use UV light (Wood lamp) to detect seminal stains on clothing/skin.

ALERT

- A forensic kit or "rape kit" contains swabs that are collected from the vagina and rectum, and instructions are given with the kit regarding proper collection.
- Many states and emergency departments across the country are using a Sexual Assault Nurse Examiner (SANE) when available. This has led to more consistent and more accurate collection of evidence in alleged rape cases.
- Complete genital–rectal exam, including evidence of trauma, secretions, or discharge
  - Use of a nonlubricated, water-moistened speculum is mandatory because commonly used lubricants may destroy evidence.
  - Testing and/or specimen collection, as indicated, and in compliance with state requirements (4)

DIFFERENTIAL DIAGNOSIS

Consenting sex among adults

DIAGNOSTIC TESTS & INTERPRETATION

- In females, obtain a serum or urine pregnancy test.
- Record results of wet mount, screening for vaginitis, but also note the presence/absence of sperm and, if present, whether it is motile/immotile.
- Drug/alcohol testing as indicated by history and/or physical findings

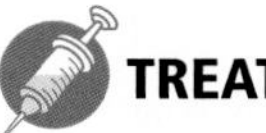

TREATMENT

GENERAL MEASURES

- Providing health care to victims of sexual assault/abuse requires special sensitivity and privacy.
- All such cases *must* be reported immediately to the appropriate law enforcement agency.
- With the victim's permission, enlist the help of personnel from local support agencies (e.g., rape crisis center). When available, use of in-house social services is extremely helpful to victim and family.
- SANE programs have been shown to be beneficial, especially in large cities and metropolitan areas with multiple emergency departments of varying capability and staff training/experience.
- Give sedation and tetanus prophylaxis when indicated.
- Discuss possible pregnancy and pregnancy termination with the victim. If hospital policy precludes such a discussion, then information about this option should be offered to the victim via follow-up mechanisms.
- Discuss suspected HIV and hepatitis B exposure and testing with the victim in accordance with hospital, regional, and state policies/protocols. The initial HIV test should be completed within 7 days of the suspected exposure.

MEDICATION

First Line

- Controversy exists regarding empiric antibiotic prophylaxis for victims of sexual assault. However, the Centers for Disease Control and Prevention (CDC) recommends empiric antibiotic prophylaxis of potential sexually transmitted infections (specifically, gonorrhea, chlamydia, trichomoniasis, and potentially syphilis), as many patients will not return for a follow-up visit and many patients prefer immediate treatment (5)[C].
- Cultures are *not* required before initiating treatment but can be considered as part of routine evidence collection.
- Gonorrhea: ceftriaxone 250 mg IM once. Note: Be aware that drug resistance is on the rise in several major cities. Quinolones are no longer recommended for treatment of gonorrhea.
- Chlamydia: azithromycin 1 g PO single dose, or doxycycline 100 mg PO BID × 7 days, *or* erythromycin base 500 mg PO QID × 7 days, *or* erythromycin ethylsuccinate 800 mg PO QID × 7 days
- Syphilis: benzathine penicillin G 2–4 million units IM once, or doxycycline 100 mg PO BID × 14 days. Some suggest ceftriaxone 1 g/day, either IM/IV, × 8–10 days, but treatment failures have been reported in several geographic areas.
- Trichomoniasis and bacterial vaginosis, if present (if cultures/wet mount were collected): metronidazole 2 g PO once, *or* metronidazole 500 mg PO BID × 7 days (consider single dose to maximize compliance), *or* metronidazole gel 0.75% 1 full applicator (5 g) intravaginally every day × 5 days;

or clindamycin cream 2% 1 full applicator (5 g) intravaginally at bedtime × 7 days (considered less efficacious than PO metronidazole)

- If pregnancy prophylaxis is indicated, use levonorgestrel 1.5 mg once (Plan B, progestin-only), efficacious for up to 5 days after the incident.
  - Levonorgestrel alone has proved more effective than the Yuzpe regimen, a method of emergency contraception.
  - *Alternatively*, ethinyl estradiol/levonorgestrel (Yuzpe) 100 mcg/0.5 mg once and repeated in 12 hours can be used.
  - Alternatively, ulipristal acetate (Ella) 30 μg once can be used.
  - Alternatively, a copper intrauterine device can be inserted up to 5 days after the earliest predicted date of ovulation in that cycle (6)[C].
- HIV: Currently, there is a low likelihood of HIV transmittance, but the CDC still recommends postexposure prophylaxis (PEP) for victims of sexual assault. Regimen is PEP × 3–7 days, with short-term follow-up for further counseling, with a specialist familiar with PEP regimens.
  - Most effective if started within 4 hours and could reduce transmission by as much as 80%; unlikely to be beneficial if started after 72 hours.
- Hepatitis B: if prevalent in area or assailant known to be high risk: hepatitis B immunoglobulin 0.06 mL/kg IM, single dose, and initiate 3-dose hepatitis B virus immunization series. No treatment if the victim has had a complete hepatitis B vaccine series, with documented levels of immunity (7)[C].

Second Line

Pregnancy Considerations

Conduct baseline pregnancy test; discuss pregnancy prevention and termination with patient.

Pediatric Considerations

Assure the child that she or he is a good person and was not the cause of the incident.

INPATIENT CONSIDERATIONS

Admission Criteria/Initial Stabilization

- Contact appropriate social services agency.
- Most adult victims can be treated as outpatients, unless associated trauma (physical/mental) requires admission.
- Most pediatric sexual assault/abuse victims will require admission/outside placement until appropriate social agency can evaluate home environment (8)[C].

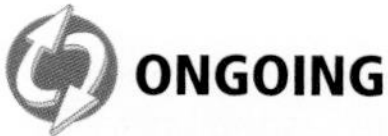

ONGOING CARE

FOLLOW-UP RECOMMENDATIONS

Patient Monitoring

- Patient should be seen in 7–10 days for follow-up care, including pregnancy testing and counseling.
- Close exam for vaginitis and treatment if necessary
- Follow-up test for gonorrhea should occur in 1–2 weeks.
- Follow-up testing for syphilis, HIV, and hepatitis B should occur at 6 weeks, 3 months, and 6 months.
- Provide telephone numbers of counseling agency(ies) that can provide counseling/legal services to the patient.
- Strongly consider SANE, if available (9)[C].

PATIENT EDUCATION

- Local rape crisis support organizations
- National Sexual Violence Resource Center, 123 Enola Drive, Enola, PA 17025; (877) 739-3895; www.nsvrc.org
- National Domestic Violence Hotline at (800) 799-SAFE(7233) or TTY (800) 787-3224 or www.thehotline.org

PROGNOSIS

- Acute phase (usually 1–3 weeks following rape): shaking, pain, wound healing, mood swings, appetite loss, crying. Also feelings of grief, shame, anger, fear, revenge, or guilt
- Late/chronic phase (also called "reorganization"): Female victim may develop fear of intercourse, fear of men, nightmares, sleep disorders, daytime flashbacks, fear of being alone, loss of self-esteem, anxiety, depression, posttraumatic stress syndrome, and somatic complaints (e.g., nonspecific abdominal pain).
- Recovery may be prolonged. Patients who are able to talk about their feelings seem to have a faster recovery. It is unclear if pharmaco- or psychotherapy results in better outcomes.

COMPLICATIONS

Sequelae include the following:

- Trauma (physical and mental)
- STIs, including HIV
- Unwanted pregnancy (with the possibility of abortion)
  - The rape-related pregnancy rate in the United States is 5%/rape among victims of reproductive age, resulting in >32,000 unwanted pregnancies each year.
  - Adolescents are at highest risk of pregnancy.
- Depression
- Posttraumatic stress disorder
- Substance abuse

REFERENCES

1. Rand M, Truman J. Criminal Victimization, 2009. Bureau of Justice Statistics Web site. http://www.bjs.gov/index.cfm?ty=pbdetail&iid=2217. Updated December 7, 2010. Accessed 2014.
2. Tjaden P, Thoennes N. *Extent, Nature, and Consequences of Rape Victimization: Findings from the National Violence Against Women Survey*. Washington, DC: National Institute of Justice and the Centers for Disease Control and Prevention; 2006. https://www.ncjrs.gov/pdffiles1/nij/210346.pdf. Accessed 2014.
3. Linden, JA. Clinical practice. Care of the adult patient after sexual assault. *N Engl J Med*. 2011;365(9):834–841.
4. U.S. Department of Justice, Office on Violence Against Women. *A National Protocol for Sexual Assault Medical Forensic Examinations (Adults/Adolescents)*. 2nd ed. Washington, DC: U.S. Department of Justice; April 2013.
5. Workowski KA, Berman S. Sexually transmitted diseases treatment guidelines, 2010. *MMWR Recomm Rep*. 2010;59(RR-12):1–110.
6. Cheng L, Che Y, Golmezuglu A. Interventions for emergency contraception. *Cochrane Database Syst Rev*. 2012;8:CD001324.
7. Mast EE, Weinbaum CM, Fiore AE, et al. A comprehensive immunization strategy to eliminate transmission of hepatitis B virus infection in the United States: recommendations of the Advisory Committee on Immunization Practices (ACIP) Part II: immunization of adults. *MMWR Recomm Rep*. 2006;55(RR-16):1–33; quiz CE1–CE4.
8. DeVore HK, Sachs CJ. Sexual assault. *Emerg Med Clin North Am*. 2011;29(3):605–620.
9. ACOG Educational Bulletin. Sexual assault. Number 242, November 1997 (replaces no. 172, September 1992). American College of Obstetricians and Gynecologists. *Int J Gynaecol Obstet*. 1998;60(3):297–304.

ADDITIONAL READING

- Centers for Disease Control and Prevention. *Sexual Violence: Facts at a Glance*. Atlanta, GA: Centers for Disease Control and Prevention; 2012.
- Toohey JS. Domestic violence and rape. *Med Clin North Am*. 2008;92(5):1239–1252, xii.
- Welch J, Mason F. Rape and sexual assault. *BMJ*. 2007;334(7604):1154–1158.

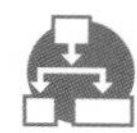

SEE ALSO

Chlamydia Infection (Sexually Transmitted); Gonococcal Infections; Hepatitis B; Hepatitis C; HIV Infection/AIDS; Posttraumatic Stress Disorder (PTSD); Syphilis

CODES

ICD10

- T74.21XA Adult sexual abuse, confirmed, initial encounter
- T74.22XA Child sexual abuse, confirmed, initial encounter
- Z04.41 Encounter for exam and obs following alleged adult rape

CLINICAL PEARLS

- *Rape* is a legal term, and the examining physician is encouraged to use terminology such as *alleged rape* or *alleged sexual conduct*.
- Marital rape is a federal offense in all 50 states and the District of Columbia; in some states, also applies to unmarried cohabiting couples.
- Because "consent defense" is common, documentation of evidence supporting the use of force or the administration of drugs/alcohol is imperative.
- Use of a protocol is encouraged to assure every victim a uniform, comprehensive evaluation, regardless of the expertise of the examiner. The protocol must ensure that all evidence is properly collected and labeled, chain of custody is maintained, and the evidence is sent to the most appropriate forensic laboratory.
- All medical records must be well documented and legible.
- All medical personnel must be willing and able to testify on behalf of the patient.

The views expressed in this chapter are those of the author and do not reflect the official policy or position of the Department of the Army, Department of Defense, or the U.S. government. Opinions, interpretations, conclusions, and recommendations herein are those of the author and are not necessarily endorsed by the U.S. Army.

R

RAYNAUD PHENOMENON

Herbert L. Muncie, Jr., MD

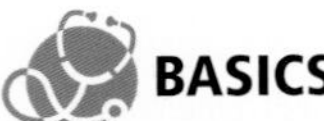

BASICS

DESCRIPTION

- Idiopathic intermittent episodes of vasoconstriction of digital arteries, precapillary arterioles, and cutaneous arteriovenous shunts in response to cold temperatures or emotional stress
  - A triphasic color change of the fingers (occasionally the toes, rarely nipples) is the physical manifestation of the episodes.
    - The initial color is *white* from extreme pallor, then *blue* from cyanosis, and finally with warming and vasodilatation the skin appears *red*.
    - Thumbs are rarely involved.
  - Swelling, throbbing, and paresthesias are associated symptoms.
  - Primary
    - 80% of patients have primary disease.
    - Episodes are bilateral and nonprogressive.
    - Diagnosis confirmed only if after 2 years of symptoms, no underlying connective tissue disease develops.
  - Secondary
    - Progressive and asymmetric
    - Spasm is more frequent and more severe with time. Ulceration is rare; gangrene does not develop; 13% progress to digital fat pad atrophy and ischemic fingertip.
    - Typically associated with an underlying connective tissue disorder
- System(s) affected: hematologic; lymphatic; immunologic; musculoskeletal; dermatologic; exocrine

Pregnancy Considerations

- Raynaud phenomenon can appear as breast pain in lactating women (1).
- Bacterial culture of breast milk distinguishes mastitis from Raynaud phenomenon.

Geriatric Considerations

Initial appearance of Raynaud phenomenon after age 40 years often indicates an underlying connective tissue disease.

Pediatric Considerations

Associated with systemic lupus erythematosus (SLE) and scleroderma

EPIDEMIOLOGY

Incidence

- Primary
  - Predominant age: 14 years; ~1/4 begin >40 years.
  - Predominant sex: female > male (4:1)
- Secondary
  - Predominant age: >40 years
  - Predominant sex: no gender predilection

Prevalence

- Primary: 3–12.5% of men; 6–20% of women (based on clinical history)
- Secondary: ~1% of population

ETIOLOGY AND PATHOPHYSIOLOGY

Unknown. Dysregulation of control mechanisms of vascular motility leads to imbalance between vasodilation and vasoconstriction. 5-HT_2 serotonin receptors may be involved in secondary Raynaud phenomenon. Platelet and blood viscosity abnormalities in secondary contribute to ischemic pathology.

Genetics

Some studies suggest dominant inheritance pattern. ~1/4 of primary patients has a 1st-degree relative with Raynaud phenomenon.

RISK FACTORS

- Existing autoimmune or connective tissue disorder
- Smoking is not associated with increased risk of Raynaud phenomenon.
- End-stage renal disease with hemodialysis may increase risk if a steal phenomenon associated with the arterial-venous shunt develops.
- Primary and secondary disease associated with elevated homocysteine levels

GENERAL PREVENTION

- Avoid exposure to cold.
- Tobacco cessation
- No relationship has been established between Raynaud phenomenon and occupational vibratory tool use.

COMMONLY ASSOCIATED CONDITIONS

Secondary Raynaud

- Scleroderma
- SLE
- Polymyositis
- Sjögren syndrome
- Occlusive vascular disease
- Cryoglobulinemia

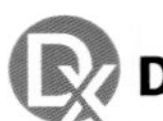

DIAGNOSIS

HISTORY

- Primary
  - Symmetric attacks involving fingers
  - Family history of connective tissue disorder
  - Rule out secondary Raynaud phenomenon.
  - Absence of tissue necrosis, ulceration, or gangrene
  - If after ≥2 years of symptoms, no abnormal clinical or laboratory signs have developed, secondary disease is highly unlikely.
- Secondary
  - Onset typically > age 40 years
  - Asymmetric episodes more intense and painful
  - Arthritis, myalgias, fever, dry eyes and/or mouth, rash, or cardiopulmonary symptoms
  - History of medication and/or recreational drug use
  - Exposure to toxic agents
  - Repetitive trauma

PHYSICAL EXAM

Pallor (whiteness) of fingertips with cold exposure, followed by cyanosis (blue), then redness and pain with warming

- Ischemic attacks evidenced by demarcated or cyanotic skin limited to digits; usually starts on one digit and spreads symmetrically to remaining fingers of both hands. The thumb is typically spared.
- Beau lines: transverse linear depressions in nail plate of most or all fingernails that can occur after exposure to cold temperature or any disease serious enough to disrupt normal nail growth
- Livedo reticularis: mottling of the skin of the arms and legs. Benign and reverses with warming
- Primary
  - Normal physical exam
  - Nail bed capillaries: Place 1 drop of grade B immersion oil on skin at base of fingernail and view capillaries with handheld ophthalmoscope at 10–40 diopters. Normal appearance
- Secondary
  - Clinical features suggestive of connective tissue disease, skin changes, arthritis, abnormal lung findings
  - Ischemic skin lesions: ulceration of finger pads (autoamputation in severe, prolonged cases)
  - Nail bed capillaries distortion

DIFFERENTIAL DIAGNOSIS

- Thromboangiitis obliterans (Buerger disease): primarily affects men; smoking-related
- Rheumatoid arthritis (RA)
- Progressive systemic sclerosis (scleroderma): Raynaud phenomenon precedes other symptoms.
- SLE
- Carpal tunnel syndrome
- Thoracic outlet syndrome
- Hypothyroidism
- CREST syndrome (calcinosis cutis, Raynaud phenomenon, esophageal dysmotility, sclerodactyly, and telangiectasias)
- Cryoglobulinemias
- Waldenström macroglobulinemia
- Acrocyanosis
- Polycythemia
- Occupational (e.g., especially from vibrating tools, masonry work, exposure to polyvinyl chloride)
- Drug-induced (e.g., clonidine, ergotamine, methysergide, amphetamines, bromocriptine, bleomycin, vinblastine, cisplatin, cyclosporine)

DIAGNOSTIC TESTS & INTERPRETATION

Unnecessary to perform provocative test (e.g., ice water immersion)

- Primary
  - Antinuclear antibody: negative
  - ESR: normal
- Secondary
  - Tests for secondary causes (e.g., CBC, ESR)
  - Positive autoantibody has low positive predictive value for an associated connective tissue disease (30%).
  - Antibodies to specific autoantigens more suggestive of secondary disease (e.g., scleroderma with anticentromere or antitopoisomerase antibodies)
  - Videocapillaroscopy is gold standard (200× magnification) (2)[C].

Follow-Up Tests & Special Considerations

Periodic assessments to determine presence of a connective tissue disorder

Diagnostic Procedures/Other

Diagnosis is determined by history and physical exam.

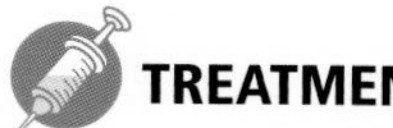

TREATMENT

The effects of treatment can be assessed using a Raynaud Condition Score (3).

GENERAL MEASURES

- Dress warmly, wear gloves, and avoid cold.
- During attacks, rotating the arms in a windmill pattern or placing the hands under warm water or in a warm body fold may help alleviate symptoms.
- Tobacco cessation
- Avoid β-blockers, amphetamines, ergot alkaloids, and sumatriptan.
- Temperature-related biofeedback may help patients increase hand temperature. 1-year follow-up is no better than control.
- Finger guards to protect ulcerated fingertips

MEDICATION

First Line

- Calcium channel blockers (CCBs). Nifedipine is best studied and most frequently used.
- Nifedipine: 30–180 mg/day (sustained-release form); seasonal (winter) use effective with up to 75% of patients experiencing improvement (4)[A].
- Is compatible with breastfeeding
- Contraindications: allergy to drug, pregnancy, CHF
- Precautions: may cause headache, dizziness, lightheadedness, edema, or hypotension
- Significant possible interactions
  - Increases serum level of digoxin; monitor digoxin levels closely after nifedipine is added.

Second Line

- Amlodipine (5–10 mg/day) and nicardipine appear to be effective and may have fewer adverse effects.
- No data exist to support use of another CCB if initial one is ineffective.
- Small studies support benefit from losartan and fluoxetine.
- Phosphodiesterase type-5 inhibitors (sildenafil, vardenafil) may reduce symptoms without increasing blood flow.
- Parenteral iloprost, a prostacyclin, even in low doses (0.5 ng/kg/min over 6 hours), has improved ulcerations with severe Raynaud phenomenon when CCBs failed. Oral prostacyclin has not proved to be useful.
- Nitroglycerin patches may be helpful, but use is limited by the incidence of severe headache. Nitroglycerin gel has shown promise as a topical therapy (5)[B].
- Prazosin (1–2 mg TID) is the only well-studied α_1-adrenergic receptor blocker with modest effect, but adverse effects may outweigh any benefit.
- ACE inhibitors are no longer recommended.

ISSUES FOR REFERRAL

If an underlying disease is suspected, consider rheumatology consultation for evaluation and treatment.

ADDITIONAL THERAPIES

- Botulinum toxin has shown some effect in reducing vasospastic episodes (6)[C].
- Aspirin
- Digital or wrist block with lidocaine or bupivacaine (without epinephrine) to help control pain
- Short-term anticoagulation with heparin if persistent critical ischemia, evidence of large-artery occlusive disease, or both

SURGERY/OTHER PROCEDURES

Surgical intervention is rarely indicated or used for Raynaud phenomenon. Effect of cervical sympathectomy is transient; symptoms return in 1–2 years.

COMPLEMENTARY & ALTERNATIVE MEDICINE

- Well-designed studies have not been done yet.
- *Ginkgo biloba* may reduce the frequency of attacks but did not in one randomized trial (7)[B].
- Fish oil supplements may increase digital systolic pressure and time to onset of symptoms after exposure to cold but was not proven in controlled trials.
- Evening primrose oil reduced severity of attacks in one study (8)[B].
- Oral arginine is no better than placebo.
- Biofeedback is not helpful (9)[A].

ONGOING CARE

FOLLOW-UP RECOMMENDATIONS

Avoid exposure to cold situations; reassess for underlying secondary cause.

Patient Monitoring

Management of fingertip ulcers, including rapid treatment of infection

DIET

No special diet

PATIENT EDUCATION

- Emphasize tobacco cessation.
- Discuss possibility of avoiding aggravating factors (e.g., trauma, vibration, cold).
- Dress warmly; wear gloves.
- Warm hands when experiencing vasospasm.

PROGNOSIS

- Attacks may last from several minutes to a few hours.
- 2/3 of attacks resolve spontaneously.
- ~13% of Raynaud phenomenon patients develop a secondary disorder; most are connective tissue diseases.

COMPLICATIONS

- Primary: very rare
- Secondary: gangrene, autoamputation of fingertips

REFERENCES

1. Barrett ME, Heller MM, Stone HF, et al. Raynaud phenomenon of the nipple in breastfeeding mothers: an underdiagnosed cause of nipple pain. *JAMA Dermatol*. 2013;149(3):300–306.
2. Herrick AL, Cutolo M. Clinical implications from capillaroscopic analysis in patients with Raynaud's phenomenon and systemic sclerosis. *Arthritis Rheum*. 2010;62(9):2595–2604.
3. Khanna PP, Maranian P, Gregory J, et al. The minimally important difference and patient acceptable symptom state for the Raynaud's condition score in patients with Raynaud's phenomenon in a large randomised controlled clinical trial. *Ann Rheum Dis*. 2010;69(3):588–591.
4. Goundry B, Bell L, Langree M, et al. Diagnosis and management of Raynaud's phenomenon. *BMJ*. 2012;344:e289.
5. Chung L, Shapiro L, Fiorentino D, et al. MQX-503, a novel formulation of nitroglycerin, improves the severity of Raynaud's phenomenon: a randomized, controlled trial. *Arthritis Rheum*. 2009;60(3):870–877.
6. Iorio ML, Masden DL, Higgins JP. Botulinum toxin A treatment of Raynaud's phenomenon: a review. *Semin Arthritis Rheum*. 2012;41(4):599–603.
7. Bredie SJ, Jong MC. No significant effect of ginkgo biloba special extract EGb 761 in the treatment of primary Raynaud phenomenon: a randomized controlled trial. *J Cardiovasc Pharmacol*. 2012;59(3):215–221.
8. Belch JJ, Shaw B, O'Dowd A, et al. Evening primrose oil (Efamol) in the treatment of Raynaud's phenomenon: double blind study. *Thromb Haemost*. 1985;54(2):490–494.
9. Malenfant D, Catton M, Pope JE, et al. The efficacy of complementary and alternative medicine in the treatment of Raynaud's phenomenon: a literature review and meta-analysis. *Rheumatology (Oxford)*. 2009;48(7):791–795.

ADDITIONAL READING

- Herrick AL. Contemporary management of Raynaud's phenomenon and digital ischaemic complications. *Curr Opin Rheumatol*. 2011;23(6):555–561.
- Huisstede BM, Hoogvliet P, Paulis WD, et al. Effectiveness of interventions for secondary Raynaud's phenomenon: a systematic review. *Arch Phys Med Rehabil*. 2011;92(7):1166–1180.

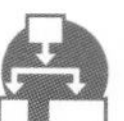

SEE ALSO

Algorithm: Raynaud Phenomenon

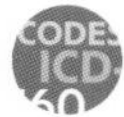

CODES

ICD10

- I73.00 Raynaud's syndrome without gangrene
- I73.01 Raynaud's syndrome with gangrene

CLINICAL PEARLS

- Initial presentation of Raynaud phenomenon after age 40 years suggests underlying (secondary) disease.
- Raynaud phenomenon is a cause of breast pain in lactating women.
- Primary Raynaud phenomenon is symmetric; secondary is asymmetric.
- Digital ulcers are not normal and always merit a workup for secondary disease.

REACTIVE ARTHRITIS (REITER SYNDROME)

Douglas W. MacPherson, MD, MSc(CTM), FRCPC

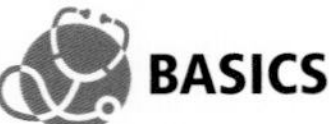

BASICS

Reiter syndrome is a seronegative, multisystem, inflammatory disorder classically involving joints, the eye, and the lower genitourinary (GU) tract. Axial joint (e.g., spine, sacroiliac joints) and dermatologic manifestations are common (1)[C].

DESCRIPTION

The classic triad include arthritis, conjunctivitis/iritis, and either urethritis or cervicitis ("can't see; can't pee; can't bend my knee").

- The epidemiology is similar to other reactive arthritis syndromes, characterized by sterile inflammation of joints associated with infections originating at nonarticular sites. A fourth feature (dermatologic involvement) may include buccal ulceration, balanitis, or a psoriaform skin eruption. (Having only 2 features does not rule out the diagnosis.)
- 2 forms of Reiter syndrome:
  - Sexually transmitted: Symptoms emerge 7–14 days after exposure to *Chlamydia trachomatis* and other urethral/cervical pathogens acquired during sexual contact.
  - Postenteric infection (including traveler's diarrhea)
- In individuals with new or frequent sexual partners, the triggering infection is more likely to be sexually transmitted than enteric.
- In individuals with a history of recent enteric illness, the triggering event is more likely to be a bacterial enteric infection than sexually transmitted.
- System(s) affected: musculoskeletal, renal/urologic, dermatologic/exocrine
- Synonym(s): idiopathic blennorrheal arthritis; arthritis urethritica; urethro-oculosynovial syndrome; Fiessinger-Leroy-Reiter disease; reactive arthritis

Pediatric Considerations

Juvenile rheumatoid arthritis has many of the same clinical features of Reiter syndrome.

Pregnancy Considerations

No special considerations; usual precautions concerning pharmaceutical therapies

EPIDEMIOLOGY

Incidence

- Predominant age: 20–40 years
- Predominant sex: male > female
- 0.24–1.5% incidence after epidemics of bacterial dysentery
- Complicates 1–2% of all cases of nongonococcal urethritis

ETIOLOGY AND PATHOPHYSIOLOGY

- The pathophysiology of all the seronegative reactive arthritis syndromes and the immunologic role of infectious diseases as precipitants for clinical illness are incompletely understood.
- Avoiding precipitant infections and early management of multiorgan inflammation is important. Antibiotic treatment following onset of syndrome does not appear to benefit inflammatory joint, eye, or urinary tract symptoms.
- *C. trachomatis* is the most common sexually transmitted infection associated with Reiter syndrome.
- Dysentery-associated Reiter syndrome follows infection with *Shigella*, *Salmonella*, *Yersinia*, and *Campylobacter* spp. Enteric-associated Reiter syndrome is more common in women, children, and the elderly than the postvenereal form.

Genetics

- HLA-B27 tissue antigen present in 60–80% of patients.
- A family history of seronegative or reactive arthritis syndromes suggests a genetic predisposition.

RISK FACTORS

- New or high-risk sexual contacts 7–14 days before the onset of clinical presentation; the primary infection may be subclinical and undiagnosed.
- Food poisoning or bacterial dysentery

GENERAL PREVENTION

- The immune-response characteristics of this syndrome make specific avoidance of infectious precipitants the most important general precaution and potentially the most difficult to achieve.
- Safe sexual practices and proper food and water hygiene

COMMONLY ASSOCIATED CONDITIONS

- Enteric disease
  - Shigellosis
  - Salmonellosis
  - Camplyobacteriosis
  - Enteric infection with *Yersinia* spp.
- Urogenital infection
  - *Chlamydia* urethritis/cervicitis (2)[C]
  - *Mycoplasma* or *Ureaplasma* spp.
- Infection with HIV

DIAGNOSIS

- Based on the clinical presentation of joint, eye, and GU inflammation ("classic triad") and negative serologic testing for rheumatoid factor
- These three symptoms and signs may not all be evident at the same time.
- HLA-B27 testing is not required for diagnosis.

HISTORY

The presence of the clinical syndrome plus the following:

- Diarrhea, dysentery, urethritis, or genital discharge and risk events for enteric or STIs
- Include a risk history, including travel or migration history and potential exposure to a precipitating infectious agent
- Arthritis associated with urethritis for >1 month (84% sensitive; 98% specific for diagnosis)

PHYSICAL EXAM

- Musculoskeletal
  - Asymmetric arthritis (especially knees, ankles, and metatarsophalangeal joints)
  - Enthesopathy (inflammation at tendinous insertion into bone, such as plantar fasciitis, digital periostitis, and Achilles tendinitis)
  - Spondyloarthropathy (spine and sacroiliac joint involvement)
- Urogenital tract
  - Urethritis
  - Prostatitis
  - Occasionally, cystitis
  - Balanitis
  - Cervicitis: usually asymptomatic
- Eye
  - Conjunctivitis of one or both eyes
  - Occasionally, scleritis, keratitis, and corneal ulceration
  - Rarely, uveitis and iritis
- Skin
  - Mucocutaneous lesions (small, painless, superficial ulcers on oral mucosa, tongue, or glans penis)
  - Keratoderma blennorrhagica (hyperkeratotic skin lesions of palms and soles and around nails—can be mistaken for psoriasis)
- Cardiovascular: occasionally, pericarditis, murmur, conduction defects, and aortic incompetence
- Nervous system: rarely, peripheral neuropathy, cranial neuropathy, meningoencephalitis, and neuropsychiatric changes
- Constitutional
  - Fever, malaise, anorexia, and weight loss
  - Patient can appear seriously ill (e.g., fever, rigors, tachycardia, and exquisitely tender joints).

DIFFERENTIAL DIAGNOSIS

- Rheumatoid arthritis (RA)
- Ankylosing spondylitis
- Arthritis associated with inflammatory bowel disease
- Psoriatic arthritis
- Juvenile RA
- Bacterial arthritis, including gonococcal

DIAGNOSTIC TESTS & INTERPRETATION

- Blood
  - Negative rheumatoid factor
  - Leukocyte count: 10,000–20,000 cells/mm^3
  - Neutrophilic leukocytosis
  - Elevated ESR and/or CRP
  - Moderate normochromic anemia
  - Hypergammaglobulinemia
- Synovial fluid
  - Leukocyte count: 1,000–8,000 cells/mm^3
  - Bacterial culture negative
- Supportive test results
  - Cultures, antigens, or PCR positive for *Chlamydia trachomatis* or stool test positive for *Salmonella*, *Shigella*, *Yersinia*, or *Campylobacter* spp. supports the diagnosis.
  - HIV serology positive (acute retroviral syndrome)
  - HLA-B27-positive status (*not required for diagnosis*)
  - Drugs that may alter lab results: Antibiotics may affect isolation of the bacterial pathogens.
- X-ray
  - Periosteal proliferation, thickening
  - Articular bony spurs
  - Erosions at articular margins
  - Residual joint destruction
  - Syndesmophytes (spine)
  - Sacroiliitis

Diagnostic Procedures/Other

HLA-B27 histocompatibility antigen: positive result in 60–80% of cases in non–HIV-related Reiter syndrome; HLA testing is not required or recommended for diagnosis. Rheumatoid factor is negative.

- Screen for STI if clinically indicated.
- Screening for enteric infections is rarely useful and generally not indicated.

Test Interpretation

- A seronegative spondyloarthropathy (similar to ankylosing spondylitis, enteric arthritis, and psoriatic arthritis)
- Villous formation in joints with hyperemia and inflammation
- Prostatitis and seminal vesiculitis
- Skin biopsy similar to psoriasis
- Nonspecific conjunctivitis

TREATMENT

GENERAL MEASURES

Treatment is determined by symptoms.

- Conjunctivitis does not require specific treatment.
- Iritis requires treatment.
- Mucocutaneous lesions do not require treatment.
- Physical therapy (PT) aids recovery.
- Arthritis may become prominent and disabling during the acute phase.

MEDICATION

First Line

- Symptomatic management: NSAIDs, including indomethacin, naproxen, and others; intra-articular or systemic corticosteroids for refractory arthritis and enteritis
  - Contraindications
    - GI bleeding
    - Patients with peptic ulcer, gastritis, or ulcerative colitis
    - Renal insufficiency
- Specific treatment of pathogenic microorganism may be attempted if isolated.
  - *C. trachomatis*: doxycycline 100 mg PO BID × 7–14 days (*Note*: All STIs should be treated whether associated with Reiter syndrome or not.)
  - *Salmonella, Shigella, Yersinia,* and *Campylobacter* infections: ciprofloxacin 500 mg PO BID × 5–10 days (*Note*: Emerging antimicrobial resistance may limit this agent's effectiveness in treatment and bacterial clearance. Antibiotic treatment does not reduce GI symptoms or duration of infection or prevent carrier state.)
  - Trials of antibiotic treatment for reactive arthritis have produced mixed results, so the efficacy of antibiotics is uncertain.
- GI upset: antacids
- Iritis: intraocular steroids
- Keratitis: topical steroids

Second Line

- Aspirin or other NSAIDs
- Sulfasalazine is promising but not approved for this indication by the FDA.
- Methotrexate or azathioprine in severe cases (such usage is still experimental and not approved or agreed to be effective); immunosuppressive therapy is relatively contraindicated if patient suffers from HIV-related Reiter syndrome.
- Consultation with specialist is recommended, particularly when considering immunomodulatory agents such as sulfasalazine, methotrexate, or azathioprine or for treatment with anti-TNF medications (etanercept and infliximab) which have shown benefit in isolated case reports.
- Role of antibiotics has been under investigation. They are currently unproven in effectiveness in seronegative arthritis syndromes.
- No published evidence supports the beneficial effect of antibiotics on development of this syndrome or the long-term outcome in patients with Reiter syndrome.

ISSUES FOR REFERRAL

Joint and eye complications; complex management

INPATIENT CONSIDERATIONS

Admission Criteria/Initial Stabilization

- Severity, complications, and degree of disability
- Inpatient care may be needed during acute phase.

ONGOING CARE

FOLLOW-UP RECOMMENDATIONS

Activity modification until joint inflammation subsides

Patient Monitoring

Monitor clinical response to anti-inflammation medications. Observe for complications of therapy, particularly sulfasalazine and immunosuppressive drugs.

PATIENT EDUCATION

- Educate on risk factors for exposure, occurrence, and recurrence.
- Home physical therapy regimen
- American Academy of Family Physicians Foundation, P.O. Box 8418, Kansas City, MO 64114, 800-274-2237, ext. 4400.
- Arthritis Foundation, 1314 Spring Street NW, Atlanta, GA 30309, 404-872-7100
- National Institute of Arthritis and Musculoskeletal and Skin Diseases: www.nih.gov/niams/301-496-8188

PROGNOSIS

- Urethritis occurs 1–15 days after sexual exposure to causative agent.
- Reiter syndrome onset within 10–30 days of either enteric infection or STI
- Mean duration of symptoms is 19 weeks.
- Prognosis is poor in cases involving the heel, eye, or heart.

COMPLICATIONS

- Chronic or recurrent disease in 5–50% of patients
- Ankylosing spondylitis develops in 30–50% of patients who test positive for HLA-B27 antigen.
- Urethral strictures
- Cataracts and blindness
- Aortic root necrosis

REFERENCES

1. Selmi C, Gershwin ME. Diagnosis and classification of reactive arthritis. *Autoimmun Rev*. 2014;13(4–5):546–549.
2. Zeidler H, Hudson AP. New insights into *Chlamydia* and arthritis. Promise of a cure? *Ann Rheum Dis*. 2014;73(4):637–644.

ADDITIONAL READING

- Barber CE, Kim J, Inman RD, et al. Antibiotics for treatment of reactive arthritis: a systematic review and metaanalysis. *J Rheumatol*. 2013;40(6):916–928.
- Carter JD, Inman RD. Chlamydia-induced reactive arthritis: hidden in plain sight? *Best Pract Res Clin Rheumatol*. 2011;25(3):359–374.
- Contini C, Grilli A, Badia L, et al. Detection of Chlamydophila pneumoniae in patients with arthritis: Significance and diagnostic value. Rheumatol Int. 2011;31(10):1307–1313
- Curry JA, Riddle MS, Gormley RP, et al. The epidemiology of infectious gastroenteritis related reactive arthritis in U.S. military personnel: a case-control study. *BMC Infect Dis*. 2010;10:266.
- Kim PS, Klausmeier TL, Orr DP. Reactive arthritis: a review. *J Adolesc Health*. 2009;44(4):309–315
- National Guideline Clearinghouse. British Association of Sexual Health and HIV (BASHH) United Kingdom national guideline on management of sexually acquired reactive arthritis. 2009.www.bashh.org/guidelines. Accessed 2014.
- Pope JE, Krizova A, Garg AX, et al. Campylobacter reactive arthritis: a systematic review. *Semin Arthritis Rheum*. 2007;37(1):48–55.
- Porter CK, Thura N, Riddle MS. Quantifying the incidence and burden of postinfectious enteric sequelae. *Mil Med*. 2013;178(4):452–469.
- Siegel DM. Chronic arthritis in adolescence. *Adolesc Med State Art Rev*. 2007;18(1):47–61, viii.
- Wilson G, Folzenlogen DD. Spondyloarthropathies: new directions in etiopathogenesis, diagnosis and treatment. *Mo Med*. 2012;109(1):69–74.

SEE ALSO

Ankylosing Spondylitis; Arthritis, Psoriatic; Behçet Syndrome

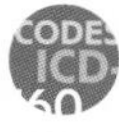

CODES

ICD10

M02.30 Reiter's disease, unspecified site

CLINICAL PEARLS

- Diagnosis of Reiter syndrome is based on the clinical presentation of the classic triad of joint, eye, and GU inflammation and negative serologic testing for rheumatoid factor (signs and symptoms may not all be present at the same time).
- Screen for STI (including HIV) if sexually acquired. Enteric studies are rarely indicated clinically.
- Patients with a chronic or recurrent course or those who have clinical complications benefit from referral to a specialist.

REFRACTIVE ERRORS

Robert M. Kershner, MD, MS, FACS

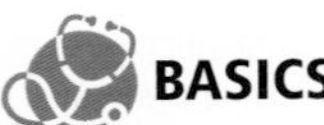

BASICS

DESCRIPTION

- Refraction is the bending of a wave of light as it passes through the optical system of the eye. The degree of bending is dependent on the index of refraction among the air, cornea, and lens and is described quantitatively by Snell law. A refractive error refers to the inability of the eye to produce a focused image on the fovea or central part of the retina.
- Emmetropia: When light rays are in perfect focus, the image being viewed is seen clearly.
- Ametropia: any refractive error of the eye that prevents normal focusing of the image
- Hyperopia: When the cornea of the eye is too flat or the eye is too short, light rays fall in focus behind the retina, and the individual is "farsighted."
- Myopia: When the cornea is too steep or the length of the eyeball is too long, the focal point for light rays lies short of the retina, and the individual is "nearsighted."
- Presbyopia: The natural tendency of the crystalline lens to harden/become sclerotic with age, limiting the focusing of the eye on near objects (accommodation). By the age of 40 years, most people do not have enough room within the eye to allow normal excursion of the lens and accommodation; viewing of near objects is blurred, and reading glasses are required.
- Astigmatism: When the cornea is steeper in 1 meridian more than the other or the globe is not round (i.e., is oval or almond shaped), visual blurriness occurs.
- Anisometropia: an unequal refractive error between the two eyes
- System(s) affected: nervous

Geriatric Considerations

Presbyopia occurs after the age of 40 years.

Pediatric Considerations

Refractive errors can be detected early in life.

EPIDEMIOLOGY

- Predominant age: Refractive errors may be present at birth and can increase in magnitude with age until the eye is fully developed. Often they are not detected until puberty.
- Predominant gender: male = female
- Individuals >40 years of age are more likely to experience presbyopia/the normal loss of accommodation that occurs with age, necessitating the use of reading glasses for close work.

Prevalence

Of the general U.S. population, 70% have some form of ametropia.

ETIOLOGY AND PATHOPHYSIOLOGY

- Developmental (most common)
- Ocular trauma
- Iatrogenic (e.g., postcataract removal)

Genetics

Inherited

GENERAL PREVENTION

No exercises; lenses can prevent/worsen refractive error.

COMMONLY ASSOCIATED CONDITIONS

- Patients with diabetes mellitus have fluctuating myopia as a result of poorly controlled blood glucose and concomitant swelling of the crystalline lens
- Those who have a pathologic steepening of the cornea due to structural weakness (keratoconus) may have increasing myopia and astigmatism throughout life.

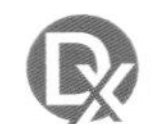

DIAGNOSIS

HISTORY

- Difficulty seeing objects at a distance
- Difficulty focusing on near objects
- Difficulty reading
- Squinting
- Headaches (from squinting)
- In children
  - Rubbing of the eyes
  - Sitting close to TV/computer screen
  - Problems in sports, particularly declining performance
  - Declining grades
  - Preference for front-row seating
  - Covering of an eye while reading

PHYSICAL EXAM

Snellen eye chart (developed by Dr. Hermann Snellen in 1862)

- Test each eye separately.
- The smallest row of letters that the patient can read determines visual acuity in the uncovered eye.
- The standard convention is visual acuity measured at 20 feet with a Snellen chart. A person with "normal" acuity will see letters clearly at 20 feet as recorded 20/20 (6/6 in meters). A person with 20/200 vision would be considered legally blind and able only to see a letter at 20 feet that a person with normal vision could see clearly at 200 feet.

DIAGNOSTIC TESTS & INTERPRETATION

- Pinhole vision test: To distinguish a refractive error from an organic cause of visual blurring, have the patient look through a pinhole in a card without a corrective lens.
- Patients with a pure refractive error have improved vision because the pinhole blocks nonparallel and unfocused rays of light.
- There are no lab tests for measuring visual acuity.
- A number of digital imaging systems exist for measuring refractive error.
  - The use of US can determine the length of the eye (A-Scan Biometry).
  - Autorefractors can measure myopia, hyperopia, and astigmatism using a projected light into the eye and measuring its return.
  - Corneal topography quantitatively and qualitatively measures the amount of curvature on the surface of the cornea that affects the bending and focusing of light on the retina.
  - Wavefront corneal analysis measures the reflected rays of light as they pass into and out of the entire optical system (cornea, lens, and retina).
- Most corneal and refractive imaging techniques are reserved for individuals who are contemplating refractive surgical correction (intraocular lenses or excimer laser surgery "LASIK").

Follow-Up Tests & Special Considerations

Corneal and refractive imaging are used to monitor changing refractive errors postsurgically and to follow pathologic changes such as in keratoconus.

Diagnostic Procedures/Other

- Methods
  - Objective streak retinoscopy may be used to measure the degree of refractive error in spherocylinder correction for the proper spectacle/contact lens.
  - Antimuscarinic agents, such as cyclopentolate (Cyclogyl) or tropicamide (Mydriacyl), applied topically paralyze the ciliary body, preventing accommodation. Cycloplegic refraction can then be performed.
  - α-Adrenergic agents, such as phenylephrine (Neo-Synephrine), can be used concomitantly to stimulate and dilate the pupillary dilator muscle, making measurements easier. They have no effect on cycloplegia.
- Age-related testing
  - Newborns should be examined for general eye health; ophthalmologic evaluation is indicated for any problems discovered.
  - Vision screening should occur at each well-child visit.
  - Visual acuity testing and motility testing should be performed at ~3.5 years of age or at any time that a malposition of the eyes or difficulty following objects is observed.
  - Visual acuity must be performed by age 5 years or prior to the child entering school to screen for and pick up refractive errors early before they lead to amblyopia.
  - Visual acuity should be retested prior to obtaining a driver's license, at age 40 years, and every 2–4 years until age 65 years, after which age evaluations are recommended every 1–2 years.

DIFFERENTIAL DIAGNOSIS

- Corneal disease
- Cataract
- Retinal abnormalities
- Diseases of the optic nerve
- Neuromuscular disorders
- Neurologic impairment

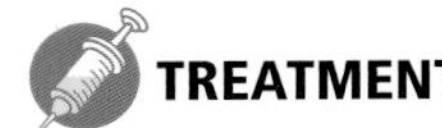

TREATMENT

GENERAL MEASURES

- Spectacle lenses (glasses)
- Soft/hard contact lenses

MEDICATION

Precaution: Antimuscarinic agents may induce acute glaucoma via acute-angle closure in susceptible individuals. The elderly and those with high hyperopia or a history of angle closure should not be tested with these agents.

First Line

No medical treatment for refractive error exists.

Second Line

Cycloplegia is sometimes used to "fog/blur" the better seing eye in cases of amblyopia.

ISSUES FOR REFERRAL

Any individual who fails a basic screening visual acuity test should be promptly referred to an eye care professional for evaluation. Children do not outgrow refractive errors. Left untreated, refractive errors can lead to permanent visual loss.

ADDITIONAL THERAPIES
Eye exercises and visual training may improve hand-to-eye coordination and visual awareness but do not treat refractive error.

SURGERY/OTHER PROCEDURES
- Astigmatic keratotomy with a surgical diamond blade has been performed either as an isolated procedure or as a part of the cataract surgical procedure to effectively flatten the steep corneal meridian (1,2)[C].
- Manual astigmatic keratotomy is being superceeded by the femtosecond laser whereby the surgeon applies the laser to perform the limbal corneal relaxing incisions (LRIs) instead of the surgical diamond blade (3)[C].
- Laser-assisted in-situ keratomileusis (LASIK) was approved by the FDA in 1997. A superficial corneal flap is created with a mechanical keratome/femtosecond laser, under which the excimer laser removes a small amount of tissue corresponding to the correction of refractive error, thus reshaping the cornea. LASIK can be used for all refractive errors but not in all patients. Healing is rapid because reepithelialization is not required. Surgery is reserved for those with a stable refractive error and a cornea that is thick enough to allow safe removal of tissue. The procedure is permanent.
- Implantable contact lens (ICL): A thin plastic lens is permanently implanted either in the anterior chamber and anchored to the iris (FDA-approved in 2005, VERISYES) or in the posterior chamber (Visian ICL, FDA-approved 2006) between the iris and the human crystalline lens. All refractive errors can be corrected. Risks include damage to the natural lens during surgery, cataract formation, and intraocular inflammation/infection.
- Excimer laser photorefractive keratectomy: The laser photoablates corneal tissue from the central visual axis, flattening it. Following the procedure, the cornea must reepithelialize. Healing takes several months, during which there is a mild haze and blurring of vision; FDA-approved October 1995.
- Other modifications:
  - LASIK and epipolis laser in situ keratomileusis (EPI LASIK) involve removing just the superficial epithelium before laser application.
  - IntraLASIK is a femtosecond laser that is used to create the flap as an alternative to a mechanical keratome.
  - Custom ablation: uses the information from a wavefront map of the cornea and eye to tailor the ablation to remove higher orders of refractive errors.
- Older methods now superseded by LASIK:
  - Radial keratotomy: With topical anesthesia, a surgical keratome is used to incise multiple (4–8) radial incisions into the peripheral cornea to a depth of ≥85%. The incisions cause gaping and thus flatten the central, optical zone of the cornea. Radial keratotomy is safe and effective, corrects nearsightedness and astigmatism but has been replaced by excimer laser surgery for its improved accuracy and stability of correction.
  - Photorefractive keratectomy: Surface corneal tissue is removed with the excimer laser to reshape the cornea, correcting nearsightedness, farsightedness, or astigmatism. Risks and disadvantages include pain, keratitis, and potential scarring. Healing requires 3 months with topical antibiotics and steroids, with associated risks of glaucoma, cataract, chronic inflammation, and scarring.
- Several scleral expansion procedures have been under investigation to attempt to increase the space within the ciliary body by surgical means to restore lens movement and accommodation. The results have been unsatisfactory.
- Bifocal intraocular lenses (several types have been approved by the FDA: AcrySof IQ ReSTOR, ReZOOM-AMO, TECNIS-AMO) are implanted in the posterior chamber. They increase the depth of field to allow viewing objects both at near and at distance. Side effects include decreased contrast, glare, ghosting of images, and problems with night vision.
- Accommodative intraocular lenses (Crystalens): first FDA-approved intraocular lens; several others under clinical investigation. The accommodative intraocular lens moves in response to ciliary body movement to allow focusing at different focal lengths. Side effects are minimal. Present lenses have limited range of focus.

ONGOING CARE

FOLLOW-UP RECOMMENDATIONS
Patient Monitoring
- Exams recommended when starting school, entering college, with any change in vision quality, and at the age of onset of presbyopia (the need for reading glasses)
- Individuals with any of the known risks of eye disease or conditions that could affect the eyes (e.g., diabetes) need annual ocular examinations
- Family history of eye diseases/refractive errors necessitates annual reexam.

DIET
Although refractive error is unaffected by diet, diet has been shown to be important for retinal health. Diets high in fats, cholesterol, along with cigarette smoking or diabetes can lead to an increased risk of age-related macular degeneration (AMD), a potentially blinding disease of the retina. Diets high in vegetables, low in meats, and high in the antioxidants (e.g., lutein, β-carotene, vitamins A, C, and E, zinc, and omega-3 fatty acids) have been shown to be protective for retinal degeneration. The age-related eye disease study (AREDS) formulation, which has been proven effective in numerous clinical trials, includes a specific daily amount of 500-mg vitamin C, 400 IU of vitamin E, 15 mg of β-carotene (often labeled as the equivalent of 25,000-IU vitamin A), 80 mg of zinc as zinc oxide, and 2 mg of copper as cupric oxide to prevent copper-deficiency anemia and is taken with meals in two equally divided doses in the morning and evening.

PATIENT EDUCATION
- All patients should have their eyes examined when starting school and periodically thereafter.
- The options of eyeglasses, contact lenses, and permanent surgical correction of refractive errors can be considered.
- Encourage aggressive control of diabetes mellitus and annual exams by an ophthalmologist. These individuals are at increased risk of blindness from their disease and should not undergo refractive corrective surgery.

PROGNOSIS
- Good, if discovered early and corrected appropriately.
- It is not unusual for refractive errors to be temporarily worsened during pregnancy because of hormonal changes in tear function and corneal swelling.
- It is common that refractive errors worsen as a child ages until complete adult growth has been achieved (this is around age 18–20 years for girls and 20–25 years for boys). This is a common source of concern for parents. Reassurance that refractive change is often seen with growth spurts, especially at puberty, is advised.
- Any refractive change that is increasing/worsening each year should prompt further investigation by an ophthalmologist.

COMPLICATIONS
- Amblyopia or permanent loss of vision that is not correctable with glasses or contact lenses
- Poor school performance
- Inability to pass a drivers license examination

R

REFERENCES

1. Kershner RM. Keratolenticuloplasty. In Gills JP, Sanders DR, eds. *Surgical Treatment of Astigmatism*. Thorofare, NJ: Slack; 1994:143–155.
2. Kershner RM. *Refractive Keratotomy for Cataract Surgery and the Correction of Astigmatism*. Thorofare, NJ: Slack; 1994:141.
3. Abbey A, Ide T, Kymionis GD, et al. Femtosecond laser-assisted astigmatic keratotomy in naturally occurring high astigmatism. *Br J Ophthalmol*. 2009;93(12):1566–1569.

ADDITIONAL READING

- American Academy of Opthalmology. Policy statement: frequency of occular exams. San Francisco, CA: American Academy of Opthalmology; 2009.
- American Academy of Opthalmology, Strabismus, American Academy of Pediatrics. Joint policy statement: vision screening for infants and children. San Francisco, CA: American Academy of Ophthalmology; 2007. http://www.one.aao.org/.../vision-screening-for-infants-and-children-2013-pdf. Accessed 2014.
- Fax-on-Demand service of American Academy of Ophthalmology for policy statement and patient education materials: (908) 935–2761.
- National Eye Institute. Age-related eye disease study results—summary. Bethesda, MD: National Eye Institute; 2006. www.nei.nih.gov/amd/summary.asp. Accessed 2014.
- National Eye Institute. Facts about refractive errors. http://www.nei.nih.gov/health/errors/errors.asp. Bethesda, MD: National Eye Institute; 2009. Accessed 2014.

CODES

ICD10
- H52.7 Unspecified disorder of refraction
- H52.00 Hypermetropia, unspecified eye
- H52.10 Myopia, unspecified eye

CLINICAL PEARLS
- Vision screening should occur at each well-child visit.
- Visual acuity testing should be performed at ~3.5 years of age or at any time that the physician or parent is concerned about the child's eye movements, ability to see, or track objects.
- Children *never* grow out of a refractive error. All suspected refractive errors should be referred to the appropriate eye care professional for evaluation to prevent permanent loss of vision from amblyopia.

RENAL CELL CARCINOMA

Jonathon M. Firnhaber, MD

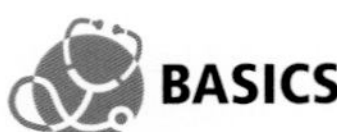

BASICS

DESCRIPTION

- Renal cell carcinoma (RCC; also called hypernephroma or Grawitz tumor) accounts for 3–4% of all adult cancers and 2.3% of all cancer deaths—seventh most common malignant tumor in men and ninth in women.
- Characterized by obscure and varied presentations, including paraneoplastic syndromes, vascular findings, and uncommon metastatic sites
- Early, aggressive surgical management provides the best opportunity for cure.
- System(s) affected: renal/urologic

EPIDEMIOLOGY

Incidence

- Predominant age: patients in 5th–7th decades; median age at diagnosis is 66 years
- Predominant sex: male > female (1.6:1)
- Age-adjusted incidence increasing 3% per year, likely due in part to increased detection as an incidental finding on imaging studies.
- In males, 10.7 new cases of RCC per 100,000 population per year versus 6.5 in females

ETIOLOGY AND PATHOPHYSIOLOGY

Unknown

Genetics

- 2–3% of cases are familial, with several autosomal dominant syndromes described.
- Oncogenes localized to the short arm of chromosome 3 may have etiologic implications. Chromosome 3p12–p26 is specific for clear cell RCC.
- People with HLA types Bw44 and DR8 are prone to develop RCC. These are rare familial RCCs.
- Hereditary papillary RCC is an autosomal dominant form of disease associated with multifocal papillary renal tumors and a 5:1 male predominance.

RISK FACTORS

- Smoking, active and passive (increases relative risk by 2–3)
- Obesity (linear relationship in women)
- Hypertension (antihypertensive medications are not independently associated with RCC)
- End-stage renal failure
- Acquired renal cystic disease
- Tuberous sclerosis
- HIV infection
- Urban environment
- Heavy metal exposure (cadmium, lead)
- Environmental toxin exposure (asbestos, petroleum by-products, chlorinated solvents)

GENERAL PREVENTION

Smoking may contribute to 1/3 of all cases.

COMMONLY ASSOCIATED CONDITIONS

- Von Hippel–Lindau disease: 30–45% of these patients develop clear cell tumors.
- Tuberous sclerosis: associated primarily with angiomyolipoma and clear cell tumors
- Sickle cell trait: With few exceptions, renal medullary tumor is seen in young African American males with sickle cell trait.
- Adult polycystic kidney disease
- Horseshoe kidney
- Acquired renal cystic disease from chronic renal failure

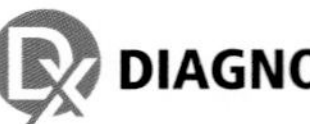

DIAGNOSIS

HISTORY

>70% of RCCs are incidentally discovered in asymptomatic patients due to increased use of ultrasound, CT scanning, and MRI.

PHYSICAL EXAM

- Classic triad of hematuria, abdominal mass, and flank pain in <10%
- Hematuria: 50–60%
- Flank pain: 35–40%
- Palpable mass: 25%
- Hypertension: 22–38%
- Weight loss: 28–36%
- Pyrexia: 7–17%
- Nonmetastatic hepatic dysfunction (Stauffer syndrome): 10–15%
- Neuromyopathy: 3%
- Scrotal varicoceles: 2–11% (most are left sided)
- Patients with vena cava thrombus present with lower extremity edema, new varicocele, dilated superficial abdominal veins, albuminuria, pulmonary emboli, right atrial mass, or nonfunction of the involved kidney.

DIFFERENTIAL DIAGNOSIS

- Benign renal masses (e.g., renal hamartomas)
- Hydronephrosis
- Pyelonephritis
- Renal abscess
- Polycystic kidneys
- Renal tuberculosis
- Renal calculi
- Renal infarction
- Benign renal cyst
- Transitional cell carcinoma of the renal pelvis
- Wilms tumor
- Metastatic disease, especially melanoma

DIAGNOSTIC TESTS & INTERPRETATION

Initial Tests (lab, imaging)

- Increased ESR: 50–60%
- Anemia: 21–41%
- Hypercalcemia: 3–6%
- Erythrocytosis: 3–4%
- Hematuria
- Urinary neoplastic cells
- Alkaline phosphate may be elevated.
- Increased renin
- Increased plasma fibrinogen
- Ultrasonography: Determine if mass is solid or cystic; simple cystic may be observed or subjected to percutaneous aspiration; solid lesions require further imaging.
- Abdominal/pelvic CT, using 3-phase imaging, with and without IV contrast, is the optimal imaging modality to evaluate the kidneys; it is nearly 100% sensitive for detecting a renal mass >15 mm in diameter. A solid renal mass with >15–20 Hounsfield units change on multiphase CT has an 80% likelihood of being an RCC. A predominantly cystic mass with an irregular, nodular, or enhancing wall; calcifications; and/or septa >2-mm thick has a >70% likelihood of being a cystic RCC.

Follow-Up Tests & Special Considerations

- MRI with pre- and postgadolinium phases is superior to ultrasound in evaluating adenopathy, diagnosing intracaval and renal venous thrombus, and demonstrating bony metastases.
- Chest CT scan if initial chest x-ray suggests metastatic disease; brain CT scan if the patient has neurologic symptoms.
- Bone scan is indicated if the alkaline phosphatase level is elevated, or the patient has bone pain.
- CT or MR angiography for staging evaluation; vascular information helpful in planning resection
- PET is of limited use because of RCC's inconsistent uptake of fluorodeoxyglucose, the most commonly used radiotracer, although this variable uptake may be an asset in predicting response to some targeted agents.

Diagnostic Procedures/Other

- No need to aspirate simple cyst unless symptomatic.
- Calcified cysts may contain RCC, requiring open renal biopsy of the cyst wall or partial nephrectomy.
- Hemorrhagic cyst: Aspiration cytology may be helpful, but needle biopsy of solid masses is discouraged, particularly if the patient has a normal contralateral kidney.
- Doppler-flow ultrasound of the renal veins or CT scan that shows the renal vein entering the vena cava can be used to rule out tumor thrombus.

Test Interpretation

- RCC tends to bulge out from the cortex, producing a mass effect.
- 48% of RCCs measure <5 cm, are grossly yellow to yellow-orange due to high lipid content in the clear cell variety. Average size has been decreasing due to incidental discovery and is now ~3.6 cm.
- Small tumors are typically homogeneous.
- Large tumors may have areas of necrosis and hemorrhage.
- About 5–10% of RCCs extend into the venous system as tumor thrombi.
- Five distinct subtypes
  - Clear cell: 70–80%; proximal tubule, typically solitary
  - Papillary renal cell (previously termed chromophilic): 10–15%; proximal tubule; tumors tend to be bilateral and multifocal; type 1 and more aggressive type 2 variant
  - Chromophobic: 3–5%; intercalated cells; tend to have a less aggressive course
  - Medullary: <1%; typically affect younger patients; most are at an advanced stage with metastases at time of diagnosis; occur almost exclusively in patients with sickle cell trait
  - Collecting duct: <1%

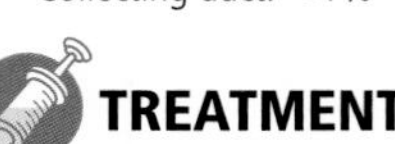

TREATMENT

Among small (<4 cm) renal masses, approximately 20% are benign, 60% represent indolent variants of RCC, and only 20% are potentially aggressive tumors.

MEDICATION

First Line

- Antiangiogenic agents (AAs)—agents that target neoplastic neoangiogenesis by directly blocking the vascular endothelial growth factor (VEGF), or its receptor (e.g., tyrosine kinase inhibitors; TKSs) offer greater efficacy compared to interferon, however radiologic complete response to therapy is rare (1)[A].
- Sunitinib represents front-line standard treatment for the good and intermediate prognosis groups of patients with clear cell RCC (2)[C].
- Sunitinib and sorafenib are both oral inhibitors of the tyrosine kinase portion of the VEGF family of receptors. Sunitinib is considered 1st-line treatment in advanced RCC and in patients refractory or intolerant to cytokine therapy. Sunitinib demonstrated improved response (31% vs. 6%; number needed to treat [NNT] = 4) and longer median progression-free survival (11 vs. 5 months) over interferon-alfa in a randomized study of 750 patients (3)[B].
- Bevacizumab is a monoclonal antibody that binds and neutralizes circulating VEGF protein. Combined with interferon-alfa, bevacizumab offers patients with metastatic RCC a hazard ratio for progression-free survival of 0.63 (95% confidence interval 0.52–0.75; $p = .0001$) compared with interferon alone (4)[B].
- Sunitinib, sorafenib, and bevacizumab have demonstrated superior progression-free survival in patients with metastatic RCC when compared to interferon or placebo (5)[B].
- A 2008 phase III trial of 410 patients comparing everolimus, an mTOR inhibitor, with placebo was stopped early after disease progression was seen in 37% of patients receiving everolimus versus 65% receiving placebo (hazard ratio = 0.30, 95% confidence interval 0.22–0.40; $p < .0001$) (6)[B]. Temsirolimus has also shown benefit.

Second Line

- Response rates with traditional chemotherapeutic agents are typically <15%.
- Despite occasional reports of responses, a review of medroxyprogesterone, the most widely studied progestational agent, concluded that RCCs are neither hormone dependent nor hormone responsive.

ADDITIONAL THERAPIES

RCC is considered radioresistant, but radiation therapy may be useful to treat a single or limited number of metastases, particularly brain or bone metastases or painful recurrences in the renal bed.

SURGERY/OTHER PROCEDURES

- Surgery is curative in most patients with nonmetastatic RCC and is the preferred treatment for all but the most extensive disease.
- There is no current role for adjuvant therapy after nephrectomy for clinically localized disease.
- Assuming a normal contralateral kidney, radical nephrectomy, which can be done laparoscopically and involves node dissection and complete removal of the kidney and Gerota fascia, is the typical preferred approach.
- Partial nephrectomy has shown equal long-term, cancer-specific survival for small to medium (<7 cm) tumors when compared with radical nephrectomy. Partial nephrectomy, however, is a more technically challenging procedure.
- Better cancer-specific quality of life has been reported in patients who underwent radical versus partial nephrectomy and in those who underwent laparoscopic versus open surgery (7)[B].
- Surgical intervention in metastatic disease
  - Metastasectomy in those with limited metastatic disease versus cytoreductive nephrectomy (debulking) prior to systemic therapy
  - Transitional cell carcinoma of the renal pelvis or calyces: nephroureterectomy
  - Wilms tumor in adults: radical nephrectomy for unilateral disease
  - Cortical adenoma <3 cm (7–22% at autopsy): wedge resection

ONGOING CARE

FOLLOW-UP RECOMMENDATIONS

Patient Monitoring

- CT scan of the abdomen/renal fossa 3–6 months after surgery, to monitor recurrences
- For partial nephrectomy: renal ultrasound every 6 months for 3 years, then annually
- CXR or CT scan quarterly for 2 years, then periodically
- Skeletal x-rays and bone scan should be obtained only if patient complains of bone pain or if alkaline phosphatase is elevated.
- Postoperative follow-up with plasma transcobalamin II or serum haptoglobin level to detect or monitor recurrences
- Small (<3 cm), incidentally detected tumors may have an indolent behavior; immediate treatment in poor-risk patients may not be of benefit, and active surveillance may be a viable management strategy.

DIET

Red meat intake may increase the risk of RCC. Higher intakes of heterocyclic amines and polycyclic aromatic hydrocarbons generated in the processing and cooking of red meat have been associated with a 2-fold increase in the risk of papillary RCC and a 20–30% increase in the overall risk of RCC (8)[B].

PROGNOSIS

- 5-year survival in the absence of metastases >50%; in the presence of distant metastases, 5-year survival decreases to 10%
- Median survival for metastatic RCC is in the range of 10–12 months.
- Performance status at diagnosis and histologic grade of tumor also influence prognosis.

COMPLICATIONS

- Paraplegia can result with little warning from spinal vertebral metastasis.
- CNS metastases are not uncommon.
- ~30% of patients with RCC have metastatic disease when the diagnosis is established. Most common sites of metastasis are the lung (50–60%), bone (30–40%), regional nodes (15–30%), brain (10%), and adjacent organs (10%).

REFERENCES

1. Coppin C, Kollmannsberger C, Le L, et al. Targeted therapy for advanced renal cell cancer (RCC): a Cochrane systematic review of published randomised trials. *BJU Int*. 2011;108(10):1556–1563.
2. Di Lorenzo G, Buonerba C, Biglietto M, et al. The therapy of kidney cancer with biomolecular drugs. *Cancer Treat Rev*. 2010;36(Suppl 3):S16–S20.
3. Motzer RJ, Hutson TE, Tomczak P, et al. Sunitinib versus interferon alfa in metastatic renal-cell carcinoma. *N Engl J Med*. 2007;356(2):115–124.
4. Escudier B, Bellmunt J, Négrier S, et al. Phase III trial of bevacizumab plus interferon alfa-2a in patients with metastatic renal cell carcinoma (AVOREN): final analysis of overall survival. *J Clin Oncol*. 2010;28(13):2144–2150.
5. Heng DY, Bukowski RM. Anti-angiogenic targets in the treatment of advanced renal cell carcinoma. *Curr Cancer Drug Targets*. 2008;8(8):676–682.
6. Motzer RJ, Escudier B, Oudard S, et al. Efficacy of everolimus in advanced renal cell carcinoma: a double-blind, randomised, placebo-controlled phase III trial. *Lancet*. 2008;372(9637):449–456.
7. Parker PA, Swartz R, Fellman B, et al. Comprehensive assessment of quality of life and psychosocial adjustment in patients with renal tumors undergoing open, laparoscopic and nephron sparing surgery. *J Urol*. 2012;187(3):822–826.
8. Daniel CR, Cross AJ, Graubard BI, et al. Large prospective investigation of meat intake, related mutagens, and risk of renal cell carcinoma. *Am J Clin Nutr*. 2012;95(1):155–162.

ADDITIONAL READING

- Delahunt B, Srigley JR, Montironi R, et al. Advances in renal neoplasia: recommendations from the 2012 International Society of Urological Pathology Consensus Conference. *Urology*. 2014;83(5):969–974.
- Escudier B. Emerging immunotherapies for renal cell carcinoma. *Ann Oncol*. 2012;23(Suppl 8):viii35–40.
- Iacovelli R, Alesini D, Palazzo A, et al. Targeted therapies and complete responses in first line treatment of metastatic renal cell carcinoma. A meta-analysis of published trials. *Cancer Treat Rev*. 2014;40(2):271–275.

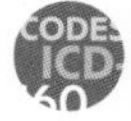

CODES

ICD10

- C64.9 Malignant neoplasm of unsp kidney, except renal pelvis
- C64.1 Malignant neoplasm of right kidney, except renal pelvis
- C64.2 Malignant neoplasm of left kidney, except renal pelvis

CLINICAL PEARLS

- RCC represents 3–4% of all cancers and 2% of all cancer deaths; most patients have clear cell histology and do not respond to standard chemotherapy.
- Diverse and obscure presentations are typical; most RCCs are found incidentally during radiologic studies.
- At presentation, up to 30% of patients with RCC have metastatic disease; recurrence develops in ~40% treated for localized disease.
- Only 20% of renal masses <4 cm represent potentially aggressive tumors.
- Surgery is curative in most patients with nonmetastatic RCC and is the preferred treatment for all but the most extensive disease.
- Multiple pharmacologic options are considered first-line for metastatic RCC; sequential treatments are likely to be pursued for most patients.

RENAL TUBULAR ACIDOSIS

Jason Kurland, MD

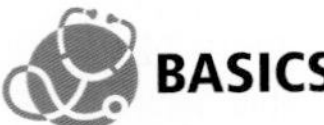

BASICS

DESCRIPTION

- Renal tubular acidosis (RTA) is composed of a group of disorders characterized by an inability of the kidney to resorb bicarbonate/secrete hydrogen ions, resulting in normal anion gap metabolic acidosis. Renal function (glomerular filtration rate [GFR]) must be normal or near normal.
- Several types have been identified:
  - Type I (distal) RTA: inability of the distal tubule to acidify the urine due to impaired hydrogen ion secretion, increased back leak of secreted hydrogen ions, or impaired sodium reabsorption (interfering with the generation of negative luminal charge required for hydrogen/potassium secretion). Urine pH >5.5.
  - Type II (proximal) RTA: defect of the proximal tubule in bicarbonate (HCO_3) reabsorption. Proximal tubular HCO_3 reabsorption absent; plasma HCO_3 concentration stabilizes at 12–18 mEq/L due to compensatory distal HCO_3 reabsorption. Urine pH <5.5 unless plasma HCO_3 brought above reabsorptive threshold.
  - Type III RTA: extremely rare autosomal recessive syndrome with features of both type I and type II (may be due to carbonic anhydrase II deficiency).
  - Type IV RTA (hypoaldosteronism): due to aldosterone resistance/deficiency that results in hyperkalemia. Urine pH usually <5.5.

EPIDEMIOLOGY

Incidence

- Predominant age: all ages
- Predominant sex: male > female (with regard to type II RTA with isolated defect in bicarbonate reabsorption)

ETIOLOGY AND PATHOPHYSIOLOGY

- Type I RTA
  - Genetic: autosomal dominant, autosomal recessive associated with sensorineural deafness
  - Sporadic
  - Other familial disorders: Ehlers-Danlos syndrome, glycogenosis type III, Fabry disease, Wilson disease
  - Autoimmune diseases: Sjögren syndrome, rheumatoid arthritis (RA), systemic lupus erythematosus (SLE), thyroiditis (1)
  - Hematologic diseases: sickle cell disease (hyperkalemic), hereditary elliptocytosis
  - Medications: amphotericin B, lithium, ifosfamide, foscarnet, amiloride, triamterene, trimethoprim, pentamidine
  - Toxins: toluene, glue
  - Hypercalciuria, diseases causing nephrocalcinosis
  - Vitamin D intoxication
  - Medullary cystic disease
  - Obstructive uropathy (hyperkalemic)
  - Hypergammaglobulinemic syndrome
  - Chronic pyelonephritis
  - Chronic renal transplant rejection
  - Leprosy
  - Chronic active hepatitis, primary biliary cirrhosis
  - Malnutrition
- Type II RTA
  - Familial (cystinosis, tyrosinemia, hereditary fructose intolerance, galactosemia, glycogen storage disease type I, Wilson disease, Lowe syndrome, inherited carbonic anhydrase deficiency)
  - Sporadic
  - Multiple myeloma, other dysproteinemic states
  - Amyloidosis
  - Heavy metal poisoning (e.g., cadmium, lead, mercury, copper)
  - Medications: acetazolamide, ifosfamide, tenofovir, sulfanilamide, outdated tetracycline, topiramate (2), aminoglycosides
  - Interstitial renal disease
  - Paroxysmal nocturnal hemoglobinuria
  - Defects in calcium metabolism (hyperparathyroidism)
- Type IV RTA
  - Medications: NSAIDs, ACE inhibitors, ARBs, heparin/low-molecular-weight heparin, ketoconazole, calcineurin inhibitors (tacrolimus, cyclosporine—by decreasing expression of mineralocorticoid receptor [3])
  - Diabetic nephropathy
  - Nephrosclerosis due to hypertension
  - Tubulointerstitial nephropathies
  - Primary adrenal insufficiency
  - Pseudohypoaldosteronism (PHA) (end-organ resistance to aldosterone)
    - PHA type 1
    - PHA type 2 (Gordon syndrome)

Genetics

- Type I RTA: Hereditary forms due to mutations affecting intercalated cells in collecting tubules (4). May occur in association with other genetic diseases (e.g., Ehlers-Danlos syndrome, hereditary elliptocytosis, or sickle cell nephropathy). The autosomal recessive form is associated with sensorineural deafness.
- Type II RTA: Autosomal dominant form is rare. Autosomal recessive form is associated with ophthalmologic abnormalities and mental retardation. Occurs in Fanconi syndrome, which is associated with several genetic diseases (e.g., cystinosis, Wilson disease, tyrosinemia, hereditary fructose intolerance, Lowe syndrome, galactosemia, glycogen storage disease, metachromatic leukodystrophy).
- Type IV RTA: Some cases are familial, such as PHA type I (autosomal dominant).

GENERAL PREVENTION

Careful use/avoidance of causative agents

COMMONLY ASSOCIATED CONDITIONS

- Type I RTA in children: hypercalciuria leading to rickets, nephrocalcinosis
- Type I RTA in adults: autoimmune diseases (Sjögren syndrome, RA, SLE), hypercalciuria
- Type II RTA: Fanconi syndrome (generalized proximal tubular dysfunction resulting in glycosuria, aminoaciduria, hyperuricosuria, phosphaturia, bicarbonaturia)
- Type II RTA in adults: multiple myeloma, carbonic anhydrase inhibitors (acetazolamide) (5)
- Type IV RTA: diabetic nephropathy

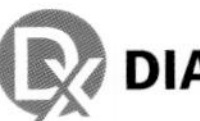

DIAGNOSIS

HISTORY

- Often asymptomatic (particularly type IV)
- In children: failure to thrive, rickets
- Anorexia, nausea/vomiting, constipation
- Weakness or polyuria (due to hypokalemia)
- Polydipsia
- Osteomalacia in adults

DIFFERENTIAL DIAGNOSIS

- Plasma anion gap should be normal. If not, evaluate for causes of anion-gap metabolic acidosis. (MUDPILES: **m**ethanol, **u**remia, **d**iabetic ketoacidosis, **p**ropylene glycol/paraldehyde, **i**ron/isoniazid ingestion, **l**actic acidosis, **e**thylene glycol, **s**alicylates)
- Extrarenal HCO_3 losses
  - Diarrhea
  - Small bowel, pancreatic, or biliary fistulas
  - Urinary diversion (e.g., ureterosigmoidostomy, ileal conduit)
- Acidosis of chronic renal failure (develops when GFR ≤20–30 mL/min)
- Excessive administration of acid load via chloride salts (NaCl, HCl, NH_4Cl, lysine HCl, $CaCl_2$, $MgCl_2$)

DIAGNOSTIC TESTS & INTERPRETATION

- Electrolytes reveal hyperchloremic metabolic acidosis.
- Plasma anion gap normal (anion gap = Na − [Cl + HCO_3]). Normal values (in mEq/L): neonates ≤16; infants/children ≤14–16; adolescents/adults 8 ± 4). Must correct calculated anion gap for hypoalbuminemia. Increase calculated anion gap by 2.5 mEq/L for each 1 g/dL decrease in albumin below 4 g/dL.
- Plasma K^+: Low in type I (if due to impaired distal H^+ secretion/increased H^+ back leak), type II; high in type IV, type I (if due to impaired distal Na^+ reabsorption)
- Plasma HCO_3 (in untreated RTA): type I: <10–20 mEq/L; type II: 12–18 mEq/L (1); type IV: >17 mEq/L
- BUN/Cr normal or near normal (rules out renal failure as cause of acidosis)
- Urinalysis: Urine pH inappropriately alkaline (>5.5) despite metabolic acidosis in type I/II if HCO_3 above reabsorptive threshold (12–18 mEq/L)
- Urine culture: Rule out UTI with urea-splitting organism (may elevate pH) and chronic infection.
- Urine anion gap (urine Na^+, K^+, and Cl^- on random urine): reflects unmeasured urine anions, so inversely related to urine NH_4^+ (or acid) excretion. Positive urine anion gap in an acidemic patient indicates impaired renal acid excretion. Urine Na^+ >25 mEq/L required for accurate interpretation of urine anion gap. Results tend to be
  - Negative in HCO_3 losses due to diarrhea, UTI caused by urea-splitting organisms, and other extrarenal causes of nonanion gap metabolic acidosis
  - Variable in type II RTA
  - Positive in type I RTA (6), type IV RTA
  - Positive in impaired acid excretion due to renal failure

- Urine calcium
  - High in type I
  - Typically normal in type II
- Drugs that may alter lab results
  - Diuretics
  - Sodium bicarbonate (and other alkali)
  - Cholestyramine

Initial Tests (lab, imaging)

Serum electrolytes; consider urinalysis, urine culture

Diagnostic Procedures/Other

- Helpful to measure urine pH on fresh sample with pH meter for increased accuracy instead of dipstick. Pour film of oil over urine to avoid loss of CO_2 if pH cannot be measured quickly.
- Urine NH_4^+ excretion (anion gap only provides a qualitative estimate)
- Urinary acidification (impaired in type I RTA) can be assessed by oral administration of furosemide and fludrocortisone; patients with type I RTA unable to reduce urine pH to <5.3 (7)
- Fractional excretion of HCO_3 >15% during HCO_3 infusion (type II RTA) (1)

Test Interpretation

- Nephrocalcinosis
- Nephrolithiasis
- Rickets
- Osteomalacia, osteopenia (8)
- Findings of an underlying disease causing RTA

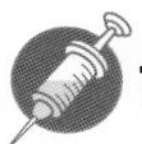

TREATMENT

MEDICATION

First Line

- Provide oral alkali to raise serum HCO_3 to normal. Start at a low dose and increase until HCO_3 is normal. Give as sodium bicarbonate (7.7 mEq $NaHCO_3$/650 mg tab), sodium citrate (oral solution, 1 mEq HCO3 equivalent/mL), sodium/potassium citrate (oral solution), or potassium citrate (tablet, powder, or oral solution: 2 mEq K/mL, 2 mEq HCO_3/mL), depending on need for potassium.
- Type I RTA: Typical doses 1–2 mEq/kg/day (in adults), 3–4 mEq/kg/day (in children) PO alkali divided 3–4 × per day (require much higher doses if HCO_3 wasting is present). May require K^+ supplementation.
- Type II RTA: Typical doses 10–15 mEq/kg/day alkali, divided 4–6 × per day. Very difficult to restore plasma HCO_3 to normal, as renal HCO_3 losses increase once plasma HCO_3 is corrected above resorptive threshold. Exogenous HCO_3 increases K^+ losses, requiring supplemental K^+. Often need supplemental PO_4 and vitamin D due to proximal PO_4 losses. May add thiazide diuretic to induce mild hypovolemia, which increases proximal Na^+/HCO_3^- reabsorption.
- Type IV RTA: Avoid inciting medications; restrict dietary K^+. May augment K^+ excretion with loop diuretic, thiazide diuretic, or Kayexalate. Correcting hyperkalemia increases activity of the urea cycle, augmenting renal ammoniagenesis and adding substrate for renal acid excretion. If necessary, 1–5 mEq/kg/day alkali divided 2–3 × per day. If mineralocorticoid deficiency, fludrocortisone: 0.1–0.3 mg/day.
- Precautions
  - Sodium-containing compounds will increase urinary calcium excretion, potentially increasing the risk of nephrolithiasis.
  - Mineralocorticoids and sodium-based alkali may lead to hypertension and/or edema.
  - Aluminum-containing medications (antacids, sucralfate) should be avoided if solutions containing citric acid are prescribed, as citric acid increases aluminum absorption.
  - Sodium bicarbonate may cause flatulence because CO_2 is formed, whereas citrate is metabolized to HCO_3 in the liver, avoiding gas production.

Second Line

Thiazide diuretics may be used as adjunctive therapy in type II RTA (after maximal alkali replacement) but are likely to further increase urinary K^+ losses.

SURGERY/OTHER PROCEDURES

If distal RTA is due to obstructive uropathy, surgical intervention may be required.

INPATIENT CONSIDERATIONS

Admission Criteria/Initial Stabilization

Generally managed as outpatient; inpatient if acidosis severe, patient unreliable, emesis persistent, or infant with severe failure to thrive

ONGOING CARE

FOLLOW-UP RECOMMENDATIONS

Patient Monitoring

- Electrolytes 1–2 weeks following initiation of therapy, monthly until serum HCO_3 corrected to desired range, then as clinically indicated
- Monitor underlying disease as indicated.
- Poor compliance common due to 3–6 × per day alkali dosing schedule

DIET

Varies based on serum K^+ level and volume status

PATIENT EDUCATION

- National Kidney & Urologic Diseases Information Clearinghouse, Box NKUDIC, Bethesda, MD 20893, 301-468-6345; www.niddk.nih.gov/health/kidney
- National Kidney Foundation: www.kidney.org

PROGNOSIS

- Depends on associated disease; otherwise, good with therapy
- Transient forms of all types of RTA may occur.

COMPLICATIONS

- Nephrocalcinosis, nephrolithiasis (type I)
- Hypercalciuria (type I)
- Hypokalemia (type I, type II if given bicarbonate)
- Hyperkalemia (type IV, some causes of type I)
- Osteomalacia (type II due to phosphate wasting), osteopenia (due to buffering of acid in bone)

REFERENCES

1. Reddy P. Clinical approach to renal tubular acidosis in adult patients. *Int J Clin Pract*. 2011;65(3):350–360.
2. Liamis G, Milionis HJ, Elisaf M. Pharmacologically-induced metabolic acidosis: a review. *Drug Saf*. 2010;33(5):371–391.
3. Heering PJ, Kurschat C, Vo DT, et al. Aldosterone resistance in kidney transplantation is in part induced by a down-regulation of mineralocorticoid receptor expression. *Clin Transplant*. 2004;18(2):186–192.
4. Batlle D, Haque SK. Genetic causes and mechanisms of distal renal tubular acidosis. *Nephrol Dial Transplant*. 2012;27(10):3691–3704.
5. Casaletto JJ. Differential diagnosis of metabolic acidosis. *Emerg Med Clin North Am*. 2005;23(3):771–787.
6. Goswami RP, Mondal S, Karmakar PS, et al. Type 3 renal tubular acidosis. *Indian J Nephrol*. 2012;22(6):466–468.
7. Walsh SB, Shirley DG, Wrong OM, et al. Urinary acidification assessed by simultaneous furosemide and fludrocortisone treatment: an alternative to ammonium chloride. *Kidney Int*. 2007;71(12):1310–1316.
8. Domrongkitchaiporn S, Pongskul C, Sirikulchayanonta V, et al. Bone histology and bone mineral density after correction of acidosis in distal renal tubular acidosis. *Kidney Int*. 2002;62(6):2160–2166.

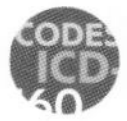

CODES

ICD10

N25.89 Oth disorders resulting from impaired renal tubular function

CLINICAL PEARLS

- Consider RTA in cases of normal anion gap metabolic acidosis with normal/near-normal renal function.
- Type I RTA: urine pH >5.5 in setting of acidemia; positive urine anion gap; acidemia can be severe.
- Type II RTA: urine pH <5.5 unless HCO_3 raised above reabsorptive threshold (12–18 mEq/L)
- Type IV RTA: most common subtype; hyperkalemia; urine pH <5.5; acidemia usually mild
- Treatment includes avoidance of inciting causes, provision of oral alkali (HCO_3 or citrate), and measures to supplement (type II, many type I) or restrict (type IV) potassium.

RESPIRATORY DISTRESS SYNDROME, ACUTE (ARDS)

Muhammad Imran Khan, MD • Najm Hasan Siddiqui, MD

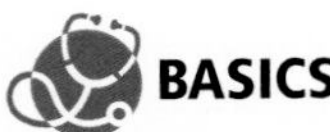

BASICS

DESCRIPTION

- ARDS is an acute, diffuse, inflammatory lung injury that leads to increased pulmonary vascular permeability, increased lung weight, and a loss of aerated tissue (1) with clinical hallmarks of severe hypoxemia and bilateral pulmonary infiltrates.
  - Absence of left atrial hypertension (HTN)
  - By consensus, $PaO_2/FiO_2 < 200$
  - Most severe form of acute lung injury
- System(s) affected: pulmonary; cardiovascular
- Synonym(s): shock lung; wet lung; noncardiac pulmonary edema

EPIDEMIOLOGY

Incidence

ARDS: 13–23 cases/100,000 annually (2).

ETIOLOGY AND PATHOPHYSIOLOGY

3 phases

- Acute exudative phase: characterized by profound hypoxia and associated with inflammation with infiltration of inflammatory and proinflammatory mediators and diffuse alveolar damage
- Fibrosing alveolitis phase: coincides with recovery or after ~1–2 weeks; patients continue to be hypoxic and have increased dead space and decreased compliance
- Resolution may require 6–12 months.
- Several mediators are involved in the initiation and perpetuation of ARDS.
  - Cytokines
  - Complement activation
  - Coagulation activation
  - Platelet-activating factor
  - Oxygen free radicals
  - Lipooxygenase pathways
  - Neutrophil proteases
  - Nitric oxide
  - Endotoxin
  - Cyclooxygenase pathway products
- Systemic inflammatory response with activation of the previous mediators can occur with direct or indirect injury to the lung.
  - Direct
    - Aspiration
    - Pulmonary infections
    - Air, fat, or amniotic fluid emboli
    - Near-drowning
    - Pulmonary contusion
    - Inhalation of toxic gases and dusts
  - Indirect
    - Sepsis
    - Shock
    - Transfusion
    - Trauma
    - Overdose
    - Pancreatitis, severe
    - Eclampsia

RISK FACTORS

- Severe infection (localized or systemic) most common
- Aspiration of gastric contents
- Shock
- Infection
- Trauma with or without lung contusion
- Pneumonia
- Toxic inhalation
- Pancreatitis
- Fat embolism
- Near drowning
- Multiple blood transfusions

GENERAL PREVENTION

No effective measures have been identified.

COMMONLY ASSOCIATED CONDITIONS

- Severe sepsis
- Trauma
- Shock

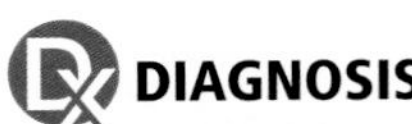

DIAGNOSIS

HISTORY

- No history of heart disease
- Precipitating event (see "Commonly Associated Conditions"): abrupt onset of respiratory distress

PHYSICAL EXAM

- Tachypnea and tachycardia during the first 12–24 hours; respiratory distress
- Lethargy, obtundation
- Flat neck veins
- Hyperdynamic pulses
- Physiologic gallop
- Absence of edema
- Moist, cyanotic skin
- Manifestations of underlying disease

DIFFERENTIAL DIAGNOSIS

- Left ventricular failure
- Interstitial and airway diseases
- Hypersensitivity pneumonitis
- Venoocclusive disease
- Mitral stenosis: intravascular volume overload
- Toxic shock syndrome

DIAGNOSTIC TESTS & INTERPRETATION

Initial Tests (lab, imaging)

- Arterial blood gases (ABGs) show evidence of severe hypoxemia.
- $PaO_2/FiO_2 < 200$
- ECG: sinus tachycardia; nonspecific ST-T–wave changes
- Pulmonary artery wedge pressure (PAWP) <15 mm Hg
- Cardiac index >3.5 L/min/m^2
- Chest x-ray (CXR): normal heart size; fluffy, bilateral infiltrates; air bronchograms common
- Chest CT scan: diffuse interstitial opacities and bullae

Follow-Up Tests & Special Considerations

- Serial blood gases
- Monitor for and treat multisystem organ failure when it occurs.
- Serial CXRs

Diagnostic Procedures/Other

Invasive monitoring of vital signs, cardiac output, and PAWP has been questioned by large clinical trials.

Test Interpretation

- Lungs show exudative, early proliferative, or late proliferative phases.
- Interstitial and alveolar edema is present.
- Inflammatory cells and erythrocytes spill into the interstitium and the alveolus.
- Type 1 cells are destroyed, leaving a denuded basement membrane.
- Protein-rich fluid fills the alveoli.
- Type 2 alveolar cells initially appear unaltered.
- Type 2 cells begin to proliferate within 72 hours of initial insult and cover the denuded basement membrane.
- Aggregates of plasma proteins, cellular debris, fibrin, and surfactant remnants form hyaline membranes.
- Over the next 3–10 days, alveolar septum thickens by proliferating fibroblasts, leukocytes, and plasma cells.
- Capillary injury begins to occur.
- Hyaline membranes begin to reorganize.
- Fibrosis becomes apparent in respiratory ducts and bronchioles.

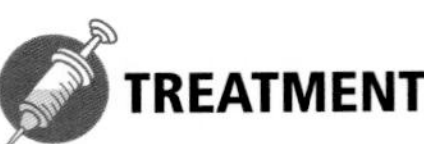

TREATMENT

GENERAL MEASURES

- Ensure adequate oxygenation.
- Ventilatory support generally requires endotracheal intubation and use of positive end-expiratory pressure (PEEP) (3)[A].
- Provide appropriate cardiorespiratory monitoring.
- Fluid management

MEDICATION

- No single drug or combination of drugs prevents or treats full-blown ARDS. Treatment is supportive while addressing the underlying cause.
- Supplemental oxygen
- Ventilatory support
  - Most often requires endotracheal intubation with emphasis on lower tidal volumes per weight and optimization of PEEP
  - High-frequency oscillation ventilation seems not to increase the risk of barotrauma or hypotension and reduces the risk of oxygenation failure, it does not improve survival in adult ARDS patients (4)[A].

ISSUES FOR REFERRAL

- All patients with ARDS should be cared for in an ICU with appropriately trained staff.
- Pregnant patients with ARDS also should be followed by a high-risk perinatologist or obstetrician.

ADDITIONAL THERAPIES

- Inotropic agents: dobutamine to maintain adequate cardiac output after appropriate fluid resuscitation fails to restore perfusion
- Corticosteroids: Short-term use during the acute phase has not been shown to be effective. However, recent data suggest that sustained therapy in patients with full-blown, established ARDS may be beneficial (5)[A].
- Vasodilators: Inhaled nitric oxide (INO) is not recommended for patients with ARDS. INO results in a transient improvement in oxygenation but does not reduce mortality and may be harmful (6)[A].
- Pulmonary surfactant: successful in neonatal respiratory distress syndrome; investigational outside this age group
- Inhaled β_2-agonists may be helpful during the resolution phase.

- There is no current evidence to support or refute the routine use of aerosolized prostacyclin for patients with ARDS (7)[A].
- There is no effect on mortality with granulocyte-macrophage colony–stimulating factor, late low-dose methylprednisolone, neutrophil elastase inhibitors, intravenous salbutamol, surfactant, or N-acetylcysteine (8)[A].
- Early use of neuromuscular-blocking agent treatment of patients with severe sepsis and severe ARDS cannot only improve the severity but also reduce 21-day mortality (9)A].
- Antioxidants (e.g., Procysteine) have produced conflicting results.
- Activated protein-C may be helpful in patients with sepsis.
- Deep vein thrombosis (DVT) prophylaxis
- Ulcer prophylaxis

Pregnancy Considerations

Supportive care while identifying the underlying cause of ARDS continues to be important in the management of pregnant women with ARDS. However, fetal well-being, possible need for delivery, and physiologic changes associated with pregnancy must be considered.

INPATIENT CONSIDERATIONS

Admission Criteria/Initial Stabilization

All patients with ARDS should be managed in an ICU setting.

- Consider prone positioning.
- Identify and treat underlying condition.
- Circulatory support, adequate fluid volume, and nutritional support
- Supplemental oxygen
- Monitoring blood gases, pulse oximetry, bedside pulmonary function test
- Support ventilation using lung-protective strategies and PEEP.
- Monitor for systemic hypotension and hypovolemia without fluid overload.
- BP support, if necessary
- Vasopressor agents
- Fluid management with IV crystalloid solutions while monitoring pulmonary status
- Pulmonary catheter pressure monitoring
- Treat underlying disease process.
- Prevent complications.

IV Fluids

- Maintain the intravascular volume at the lowest level consistent with adequate perfusion (assessed by metabolic acid–base balance and renal function).
- If perfusion is inadequate after restoration of intravascular volume (e.g., septic shock), vasopressor therapy is indicated.
- Increase oxygen content with packed erythrocyte transfusions as necessary.
- Provide appropriate nutritional support with enteral or parenteral nutrition.
- Steroid therapy

Nursing

May include any or all of the following:

- Skin, eye, and mouth care
- DVT prophylaxis
- GI prophylaxis
- Suctioning
- Ensure adequate level of sedation and/or paralysis while on mechanical ventilation.
- Oxygen supplementation
- Nebulizer therapy
- Chest physiotherapy
- Tracheostomy care
- Explain all procedures to patient and family; reduce anxiety.

Discharge Criteria

- Supplemental oxygen
- Nutrition counseling
- Family monitoring of signs and symptoms of respiratory distress

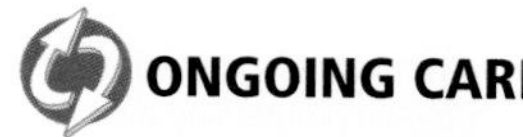

ONGOING CARE

FOLLOW-UP RECOMMENDATIONS

Patient Monitoring

- Vital capacity and static lung compliance are important measures of lung mechanics.
- Daily labs are needed until the patient is no longer critical.
- CXRs to assess endotracheal tube placement, the presence of progressing infiltrates, catheter placement, and complications of mechanical ventilation (e.g., air leaks)
- A Swan-Ganz catheter to assess oxygen delivery, oxygen consumption, and cardiac output may be helpful but has not been shown to improve survival.

DIET

- Nutritional support
- Conservative fluid management shortens ventilator and ICU time but does not affect survival.

PATIENT EDUCATION

ARDS support center and brochure titled "Learn About ARDS." www.ards.org

PROGNOSIS

- Mortality rate is 43% (10).
- Survivors may have pulmonary sequelae with mild abnormalities in oxygenation, diffusion, and lung mechanics, as well as some pulmonary symptoms of cough and dyspnea.
- The prognosis worsens with elevated cardiac troponin-T levels in ARDS patients (11).

COMPLICATIONS

- Permanent lung disease
- Oxygen toxicity
- Barotrauma
- Superinfection
- Multiple organ dysfunction syndrome
- Death

REFERENCES

1. ARDS Definition Task Force, Ranieri VM, Rubenfeld GD, et al. Acute respiratory distress syndrome: the Berlin definition. *JAMA*. 2012;307(23):2526–2533.
2. Lewandowski K, Lewandowski M. Epidemiology of ARDS. *Minerva Anestesiol*. 2006;72(6):473–477.
3. Petrucci N, Iacovelli W. Ventilation with lower tidal volumes versus traditional tidal volumes in adults for acute lung injury and acute respiratory distress syndrome. *Cochrane Database Syst Rev*. 2004;(2):CD003844.
4. Gu XL, Wu GN, Yao YW, et al. Is high-frequency oscillatory ventilation more effective and safer than conventional protective ventilation in adult acute respiratory distress syndrome patients? A meta-analysis of randomized controlled trials. *Crit Care*. 2014;18(3):R111.
5. Ruan SY, Lin HH, Huang CT, et al. Exploring the heterogeneity of effects of corticosteroids on acute respiratory distress syndrome: a systematic review and meta-analysis. *Critical Care*. 2014;18(2):R63.
6. Afshari A, Brok J, Møller AM, et al. Inhaled nitric oxide for acute respiratory distress syndrome (ARDS) and acute lung injury in children and adults. *Cochrane Database Syst Rev*. 2010;(7):CD002787.
7. Afshari A, Brok J, Møller AM, et al. Aerosolized prostacyclin for acute lung injury (ALI) and acute respiratory distress syndrome (ARDS). *Cochrane Database Syst Rev*. 2010;(8):CD007733.
8. Duggal A, Ganapathy A, Mohana Ratnapalan M, et al. Pharmacological treatments for acute respiratory distress syndrome: systematic review [published online ahead of print June 17, 2014]. *Minerva Anestesiol*.
9. Lyu G, Wang X, Jiang W, et al. Clinical study of early use of neuromuscular blocking agents in patients with severe sepsis and acute respiratory distress syndrome [in Chinese]. *Zhonghua Wei Zhong Bing Ji Jiu Yi Xue*. 2014;26(5):325–329.
10. Zambon M, Vincent JL. Mortality rates for patients with acute lung injury/ARDS have decreased over time. *Chest*. 2008;133(5):1120–1127.
11. Rivara MB, Bajwa EK, Januzzi JL, et al. Prognostic significance of elevated cardiac troponin-T levels in acute respiratory distress syndrome patients. *PLoS ONE*. 2012;7(7):e40515.

ADDITIONAL READING

- Cole DE, Taylor TL, McCullough DM, et al. Acute respiratory distress syndrome in pregnancy. *Crit Care Med*. 2005;33(10)(Suppl):S269–S278.
- Wheeler AP, Bernard GR. Acute lung injury and the acute respiratory distress syndrome: a clinical review. *Lancet*. 2007;369(9572):1553–1564.

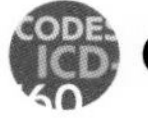

CODES

ICD10

- J80 Acute respiratory distress syndrome
- J98.4 Other disorders of lung
- J95.2 Acute pulmonary insufficiency following nonthoracic surgery

CLINICAL PEARLS

- ARDS is a syndrome characterized by an abrupt onset of diffuse lung injury with severe hypoxemia and bilateral pulmonary infiltrates.
- Treatment of ARDS requires aggressive supportive care in an ICU setting while also addressing the underlying cause.
- The benefit of invasive monitoring of vital signs, cardiac output, and PAWP has been questioned by large clinical trials.

RESPIRATORY DISTRESS SYNDROME, NEONATAL

Mary Cataletto, MD, FAAP, FCCP • Margaret J. McCormick, MS, RN

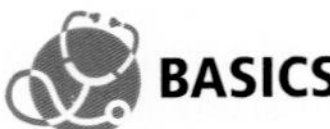

BASICS

DESCRIPTION

- Neonatal respiratory distress syndrome (NRDS) is a serious disorder of prematurity with a clinical manifestation of respiratory distress.
- Pulmonary surfactants that are deficient at birth and an overly compliant chest wall cause diffuse lung atelectasis.
- System(s) affected: pulmonary
- Synonym(s): hyaline membrane disease; surfactant deficiency

ALERT

A disorder of the neonatal period

EPIDEMIOLOGY

Incidence

- In 2007, accounted for ~3% of neonatal deaths
- Predominant age: 93% incidence in infants born at or before 28 weeks' gestational age
- Inversely proportional to gestational age and birth weight
- Predominant sex: slight male predominance

Prevalence

Common disorder in premature infants, especially those born <28 weeks' gestation

ETIOLOGY AND PATHOPHYSIOLOGY

- Structurally immature lungs and surfactant deficiency lead to diffuse atelectasis.
- Exposure to high FiO_2 and barotrauma associated with mechanical ventilation trigger proinflammatory cytokines that further damage alveolar epithelium.
- Decreased lung compliance leads to alveolar hypoventilation and ventilation–perfusion mismatch.
- Impaired surfactant synthesis and secretion

Genetics

No known genetic pattern

RISK FACTORS

- Premature birth
- Infants of diabetic mothers
- Perinatal asphyxia
- History of RDS in a sibling

GENERAL PREVENTION

- Prevention of premature birth with education and regular prenatal care
- Antenatal corticosteroids
- Manage any medical issues appropriately.
- Healthy behaviors including diet and exercise
- Avoid exposure to tobacco smoke, alcohol, and illegal drugs.

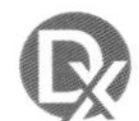

DIAGNOSIS

HISTORY

Preterm neonates with worsening respiratory distress beginning shortly after birth and progressing over 1st few hours of life.

PHYSICAL EXAM

- Tachypnea
- Grunting
- Nasal flaring
- Subcostal and intercostal retractions
- Decreased breath sounds
- Cyanosis

DIFFERENTIAL DIAGNOSIS

- Early-onset group B streptococcal pneumonia and/or sepsis
- Transient tachypnea of newborn
- Meconium aspiration pneumonia

DIAGNOSTIC TESTS & INTERPRETATION

- CBC and blood culture to rule out sepsis and pneumonia
- Electrolytes: Monitor for hypoglycemia and hypocalcemia.
- Arterial blood gases (ABGs)
  - Hypoxemia (which responds to supplemental oxygen)
  - Features of respiratory and metabolic acidosis
- Chest x-ray (CXR):
  - Diffuse reticulogranular pattern (ground-glass appearance)
  - Air bronchograms
  - Low lung volumes

Diagnostic Procedures/Other

Echocardiogram: Consider if murmur is present to evaluate for patent ductus arteriosus (PDA) and contribution to lung disease due to L → R shunting.

Test Interpretation

- Macroscopically: uniformly ruddy, airless appearance of lungs
- Microscopically: diffuse atelectasis and hyaline membranes (eosinophilic and fibrinous membrane lining air spaces)

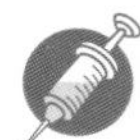

TREATMENT

- Along with antenatal steroids, surfactants improve survival for preterm infants.
- Surfactants are now recommended routinely as early in the course of RDS as possible.

GENERAL MEASURES

- Warm, humidified, oxygen-enriched gases if the neonate is ventilating effectively.
- Continuous positive airway pressure (CPAP) if infant is active and breathing spontaneously (1)[A]
- Positive-pressure ventilation per ETT via conventional mechanical ventilator (CMV) or high-frequency oscillation ventilator (HFOV) if respiratory failure occurs (i.e., respiratory acidosis, apnea, or hypoxia despite nasal CPAP)
- Transcutaneous monitors to measure CO_2 tension as necessary
- Pulse oximetry
- Umbilical artery catheter placement for continuous BP monitoring and sampling ABGs

MEDICATION

- Pulmonary surfactant (2–4)[A]
- Side effects: bradycardia, hypotension, airway obstruction/endotracheal tube blockage with administration; rapid changes in tidal volume due to increased compliance can cause a pneumothorax and small risk of pulmonary hemorrhage.
- Precautions: Transient adverse effects seen with the administration of surfactant may require stopping administration and alleviating situation; may proceed with dosing when stable

- Contraindications: presence of congenital anomalies incompatible with life beyond neonatal period; infant with laboratory evidence of lung maturity
- Perform frequent clinical and laboratory checks so that oxygen and ventilatory support can be modified to respond to respiratory changes.

ISSUES FOR REFERRAL

Comorbid conditions associated with prematurity may require consultation during the course of the infant's NICU admission, including PDA (cardiology consult), necrotizing enterocolitis (NEC) (gastroenterology), retinopathy of prematurity (ROP) (ophthalmology), etc.

ADDITIONAL THERAPIES

Treat associated problems of prematurity.

INPATIENT CONSIDERATIONS

Admission Criteria/Initial Stabilization

All neonates with respiratory distress require evaluation, monitoring, and treatment in a NICU; treatment may be required in the delivery room.

IV Fluids

- To maintain blood pressure and perfusion, when necessary
- To provide optimal fluid balance, provide nutritional support

Nursing

- Supportive care
- Thermoneutral environment
- Respiratory monitoring
- Establish relationship with family to provide education and emotional support.

Discharge Criteria

- Should have stable vital signs and pulse oximetry before discharge
- Medical home and support services should be in place.

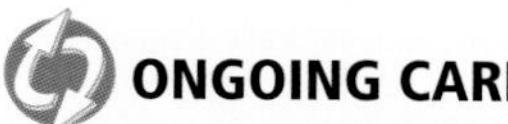

ONGOING CARE

FOLLOW-UP RECOMMENDATIONS

Following discharge, infants should be followed closely by their physicians to monitor growth and respiratory symptomatology.

DIET

As clinically indicated

PATIENT EDUCATION

- Educate parents regarding the risks in subsequent pregnancies.
- Advise parents regarding potential issues with chronic lung disease.
- For patient education materials favorably reviewed on this topic, go to Boston Children's Hospital Web site (www.childrenshospital.org) and search for respiratory distress syndrome in the "My Child Has" window.

PROGNOSIS

Prognosis and outcome highly dependent on gestational age and birth weight.

COMPLICATIONS

- Complications specific to NRDS
  - Pneumothorax
  - Chronic lung disease, bronchopulmonary dysplasia (BPD)
  - Pulmonary interstitial edema (PIE)
- Additional complications may occur related to therapeutic interventions and comorbid conditions.

REFERENCES

1. Support Study Group of the Eunice Kennedy Shriver NICHD Neonatal Research Network, Finer NN, Carlo WA, Walsh MC, et al. Early CPAP versus surfactant in extremely preterm infants. *N Engl J Med*. 2010;362(21):1970.
2. Engle WA, American Academy of Pediatrics Committee on Fetus and Newborn. Surfactant-replacement therapy for respiratory distress in the preterm and term neonate. *Pediatrics*. 2008;121(2):419–432.
3. Moya F. Synthetic surfactants: where are we? Evidence from randomized, controlled clinical trials. *J Perinatol*. 2009;29(Suppl 2):S23–S28.
4. Soll RF. Multiple versus single dose natural surfactant extract for severe neonatal respiratory distress syndrome. *Cochrane Database Syst Rev*. 1999;(2):CD000141.

ADDITIONAL READING

- Hamrick SE, Hansmann G. Patent ductus arteriosus of the preterm infant. *Pediatrics*. 2010;125(5):1020–1030.
- Jain NJ, Kruse LK, Demissie K, et al. Impact of mode of delivery on neonatal complications: trends between 1997 and 2005. *J Matern Fetal Neonatal Med*. 2009;22(6):491–500.
- Ramachandrappa A, Jain L. Health issues of the late preterm infant. *Pediatr Clin North Am*. 2009;56(3): 565–577.
- Sekar KC, Corff KE. To tube or not to tube babies with respiratory distress syndrome. *J Perinatol*. 2009;29(Suppl 2):S68–S72.
- Stoll BJ, Hansen NI, Bell EF, et al. Neonatal outcomes of extremely preterm infants from the NICHD Neonatal Research Network. *Pediatrics*. 2010;126(3):443.
- Sweet DG, Halliday HL. The use of surfactants in 2009. *Arch Dis Child Educ Pract Ed*. 2009;94(3):78–83.

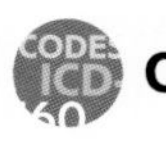

CODES

ICD10

P22.0 Respiratory distress syndrome of newborn

CLINICAL PEARLS

- Surfactants are used routinely as early in the course of RDS as possible.
- If an infant has a murmur, consider an echocardiogram to rule out PDA and shunting.
- Prognosis and outcome are highly dependent on gestational age and birth weight.

RESPIRATORY SYNCYTIAL VIRUS INFECTION

Elizabeth C. McKeen, MD

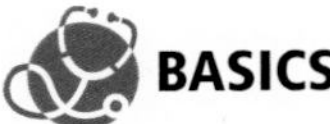

BASICS

Respiratory syncytial virus (RSV) is a medium-sized, membrane-bound ribonucleic acid (RNA) virus that causes acute respiratory tract illness in all ages, with the most clinically significant disease occurring in infants and young children.

DESCRIPTION

A major cause of respiratory illness, either of the upper respiratory tract (URT) or of the lower respiratory tract (LRT/bronchiolitis)

- In adults, RSV causes URT infections (URTIs).
- In infants and children, RSV causes URTIs and LRT infections (bronchiolitis and pneumonia).

Pediatric Considerations

- 90–95% of children are infected at least once by the age of 24 months; reinfection is common.
- Leading cause of pediatric bronchiolitis (50–90%)
- Premature infants are at increased risk for severe acute RSV infection.

EPIDEMIOLOGY

- Seasonality: Highest incidence of RSV in the United States occurs between December and March.
- Morbidity: RSV infection leads to over 100,000 annual hospitalizations.

ETIOLOGY AND PATHOPHYSIOLOGY

- RSV-induced bronchiolitis causes acute inflammation, edema, and necrosis of small airway epithelium, air trapping, bronchospasm, and increased mucus production.
- RSV develops in the cytoplasm of infected cells and matures by budding from the plasma membrane.
- Infection through droplets, either airborne or personal contact, that inoculate the nose of a susceptible individual

Genetics

- A genetic predisposition to severe RSV infections may be associated with polymorphisms in cytokine- and chemokine-related genes, including *CCR5*, *IL4*, and affiliated receptors, *IL8*, *IL10*, and *IL13*.
- Infants with transplacentally acquired antibody against RSV are not protected against infection but may have milder symptoms.

RISK FACTORS

- Risk factors for severe disease
  - Prematurity
  - Age <12 weeks
  - Underlying cardiopulmonary disease
  - Immunodeficiency
- Other risk factors
  - Low socioeconomic status
  - Exposure to environmental air pollutants
  - Child care attendance
  - Severe neuromuscular disease
  - Adult, occupational exposure to young children: hospital staff, teachers, and daycare workers

GENERAL PREVENTION

- Hand hygiene is the most important step to prevent spread of RSV.
  - Alcohol-based rubs are preferred; an alternative is hand washing with soap (1)[B].
- Exposure to passive tobacco smoke should be avoided, especially in infants and children (2)[A].
- Patients with proven or suspected RSV should be isolated.
- Palivizumab (Synagis), a monoclonal antibody directed against the F (fusion) protein of RSV, is indicated as prophylaxis for the following groups:
  - Infants and children <24 months of age with
    - Chronic lung disease of prematurity requiring medical therapy within 6 months of the start of RSV season
    - Hemodynamically significant cyanotic or acyanotic congenital heart disease
    - Congenital abnormalities of the airway or neuromuscular disease that compromises handling airway secretions
  - Infants born at ≤28 weeks' gestation if they are younger than 12 months of age at the start of the RSV season; prophylaxis should be maintained through the end of the RSV season.
  - Infants born at 29–32 weeks' gestation if they are younger than 6 months of age at the start of the RSV season; prophylaxis should be maintained through the end of the RSV season.
  - Infants born at 32–35 weeks' gestation who are younger than 3 months of age at the start of the RSV season or who are born during the RSV season if they have one of the following 2 risk factors:
    - Infant attends child care, or
    - ≥1 more siblings or other children <5 years of age living permanently in the child's household
- Dosage: maximum of 5 monthly doses beginning in November or December at 15 mg/kg per dose administered IM
- For most current palivizumab guidelines, see the most current edition of *Red Book*.

COMMONLY ASSOCIATED CONDITIONS

- Asthma
- Otitis media
- Serious bacterial infection (SBI) in infants and children with concurrent RSV infection is rare.

DIAGNOSIS

ALERT

In most cases, diagnosis should be made by history and physical exam alone. Laboratory and radiologic studies are not routinely necessary (1)[B].

HISTORY

- Rhinorrhea and upper respiratory congestion
- Difficulty feeding in infants (due to respiratory effort)
- Increased respiratory rate or signs of increased work of breathing (grunting, flaring, retracting)
- Wheezing
- Cough
- Fever
- History of prematurity, secondhand tobacco exposure, daycare
- Immunization history
- Family history of respiratory disease

PHYSICAL EXAM

- Vital signs: fever, signs of increased work of breathing (tachypnea, grunting, flaring, retracting), pulse rate; pulse oximetry ("5th vital sign") to assess oxygenation
- Ear, nose, throat: rhinorrhea, dry mucous membranes (dehydration)
- Serous otitis or acute otitis; pulmonary: wheezing, crackles
- Skin turgor
- Repeat examination over time to assess status.

Pediatric Considerations

Young infants with bronchiolitis may develop apnea, which is associated with increased risk of prolonged hospitalization, ICU admission, and mechanical ventilation.

DIFFERENTIAL DIAGNOSIS

- Mild illness/URTI
  - Other respiratory viral infections rhinovirus, human metapneumovirus, influenza virus, human bocavirus
  - Allergic rhinitis
  - Sinusitis
- Severe illness/LRTI
  - Bronchiolitis
  - Asthma
  - Pneumonia
  - Foreign body aspiration

DIAGNOSTIC TESTS & INTERPRETATION

Initial Tests (lab, imaging)

- Routine laboratory testing is not necessary.
  - If obtained, WBC count may be normal or elevated.
  - Virologic tests for RSV, despite high predictive value, rarely change management decisions or outcomes for patients with clinically diagnosed bronchiolitis.
- Given the low risk of SBI, full septic workups are not necessary unless child appears toxic.
- Chest x-ray (CXR) does not predict disease severity or change patient outcomes but may be helpful if a patient does not improve as expected, if the severity of the disease requires further investigation, or if another diagnosis is suspected.
- When obtained, typical CXR findings include the following:
  - Hyperinflation and peribronchiolar thickening
  - Atelectasis
  - Interstitial infiltrates
  - Segmental or lobar consolidation

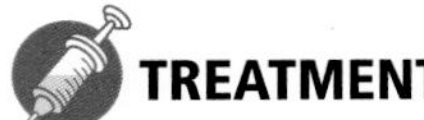

TREATMENT

GENERAL MEASURES

- Clinicians must promptly assess hydration status and ability to take fluids orally. Dehydration must be treated adequately with an oral or IV fluid, with special attention to infants.
- Supplemental oxygen is indicated if pulse oximetry (SpO_2) falls persistently <90% in previously healthy patients.

MEDICATION

First Line

No 1st-line medication for RSV infections; treatment is usually supportive; oxygen as needed

Second Line

- Bronchodilators show small, short-term improvements in clinical scores, but this small benefit should be weighed against the costs and adverse effects of these agents.
  - Bronchodilators do not improve oxygen saturation, reduce hospital admission after outpatient treatment, shorten the duration of hospitalization, or reduce the time to resolution of illness at home.
  - Routine use not recommended
- Nebulized epinephrine is superior compared with placebo for short-term outcomes for outpatients, particularly in the first 24 hours of care.
  - Evidence shows the effectiveness and superiority of adrenaline for outcomes of most clinical relevance among outpatients with acute bronchiolitis, and evidence from a single precise trial for combined adrenaline and dexamethasone (3)[A].
- Current evidence does not support a clinically relevant effect of systemic or inhaled glucocorticoids on admissions or length of hospitalization (4)[A].
  - Some data suggest that the combination of dexamethasone and epinephrine may reduce outpatient admissions (4)[A].
- A recent study found that montelukast (Singulair) has no effect on the clinical course of acute bronchiolitis (5)[C].
- Ribavirin, a nucleoside analogue and antiviral agent, has not been shown to be efficacious in the treatment of RSV, particularly in immunocompromised patients (6)[A].
- There is no current evidence that nebulized rhDNase changes clinical outcomes in children <24 months of age who are hospitalized with acute RSV bronchiolitis (7)[B].
- Use of antibacterial agents should be reserved for patients who have specific findings that suggest a coexisting SBI (8)[B].
- Nebulized 3% saline may reduce the length of stay and improve the clinical severity score in infants hospitalized with acute viral bronchiolitis (9)[A].

ADDITIONAL THERAPIES

Bulb suctioning of the nares may provide some comfort to infants and allow for easier feeding.

Pediatric Considerations

Parents must be reminded that the American Academy of Pediatrics strongly recommends against the use of over-the-counter (OTC) cough and cold medications in children <6 years of age due to lack of efficacy and the risk of life-threatening side effects.

COMPLEMENTARY & ALTERNATIVE MEDICINE

No complementary, alternative, or integrative therapies have been proven to be of benefit in the prevention or treatment of RSV bronchiolitis.

INPATIENT CONSIDERATIONS

Admission Criteria/Initial Stabilization

- Clinical judgment of the patient's degree of respiratory distress is the most important consideration. Ill-appearing infants should be hospitalized.
- Significant respiratory distress and/or oxygen requirement to keep SpO_2 >90% merits admission as does the inability to hydrate orally.
- Mechanical ventilation is required in about 5% of infants hospitalized with RSV and 20% of children with underlying congenital heart disease, chronic lung disease, or immunosuppression and should be instituted in the case of respiratory failure.

IV Fluids

See "Treatment."

Discharge Criteria

No set criteria for discharge exists but the following guidelines may be helpful:

- Stable respiratory status with no oxygen requirement
- Adequate ability to maintain oral intake and sustain hydration
- Home resources adequate to support use of any necessary home therapies, including caretaker ability to clear the infant's airway with bulb suctioning if needed
- Adequate follow-up and patient education ensured.

ONGOING CARE

FOLLOW-UP RECOMMENDATIONS

Follow-up with primary health care provider to ensure resolution.

PATIENT EDUCATION

Bronchiolitis and Your Child, available at http://familydoctor.org/online/famdocen/home/children/parents/common/common/020.html

PROGNOSIS

Most patients with RSV infection recover fully within 7–10 days. Reinfection is common.

COMPLICATIONS

- Infants hospitalized for RSV may be at increased risk for recurrent wheezing and reduced pulmonary function, particularly during the 1st decade of life.
- Overall mortality for infants and children <24 months of age is <1%.
- Although the relationship between RSV and asthma is unclear, RSV bronchiolitis in infancy has been linked to subsequent asthma.

REFERENCES

1. American Academy of Pediatrics Subcommittee on Diagnosis and Management of Bronchiolitis. Diagnosis and management of bronchiolitis. *Pediatrics*. 2006;118(4):1774–1793.
2. DiFranza JR, Masaquel A, Barrett AM, et al. Systematic literature review assessing tobacco smoke exposure as a risk factor for serious respiratory syncytial virus disease among infants and young children. *BMC Pediatrics*. 2012;12(1):81.
3. Hartling L, Fernandes RM, Bialy L, et al. Steroids and bronchodilators for acute bronchiolitis in the first two years of life: systematic review and meta-analysis. *BMJ*. 2011;342:d1714.
4. Fernandes RM, Bialy LM, Vandermeer B, et al. Glucocorticoids for acute viral bronchiolitis in infants and young children. *Cochrane Database Syst Rev*. 2010;(10):CD004878.
5. Amirav I, Luder AS, Kruger N, et al. A double-blind, placebo-controlled, randomized trial of montelukast for acute bronchiolitis. *Pediatrics*. 2008;122(6):e1249–e1255.
6. Hynicka LM, Ensor CR. Prophylaxis and treatment of respiratory syncytial virus in adult immunocompromised patients. *Ann Pharmacother*. 2012;46(4):558–566.
7. Enriquez A, Chu IW, Mellis C, et al. Nebulised deoxyribonuclease for viral bronchiolitis in children younger than 24 months. *Cochrane Database Syst Rev*. 2012;11:CD008395.
8. Spurling GK, Fonseka K, Doust J, et al. Antibiotics for bronchiolitis in children. *Cochrane Database Sys Rev*. 2007;(1):CD005189.
9. Zhang L, Mendoza-Sassi RA, Wainwright C, et al. Nebulized hypertonic saline solution for acute bronchiolitis in infants. *Cochrane Database Syst Rev*. 2008;(4):CD006458.

ADDITIONAL READING

- American Academy of Pediatrics. Section 3: respiratory syncytial virus. In: Pickering LK, Baker CJ, Kimberlin DW, et al., eds. *Red Book: 2012 Report of the Committee on Infectious Diseases*. 29th ed. Elk Grove Village, IL: American Academy of Pediatrics; 2012.
- Gadomski AM, Brower M. Bronchodilators for bronchiolitis. *Cochrane Database Syst Rev*. 2010;(12):CD001266.

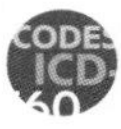

CODES

ICD10

- B97.4 Respiratory syncytial virus causing diseases classd elswhr
- J06.9 Acute upper respiratory infection, unspecified
- J21.0 Acute bronchiolitis due to respiratory syncytial virus

CLINICAL PEARLS

- RSV causes 50–90% of pediatric bronchiolitis.
- Hand sanitation is key for prevention in the general population.
- Palivizumab should be used to prevent RSV in high-risk patients.
- The diagnosis of RSV is clinical in most cases. Routine lab testing is not necessary.
- Treatment of RSV is usually supportive.

RESTLESS LEGS SYNDROME

Donald E. Watenpaugh, PhD • John R. Burk, MD

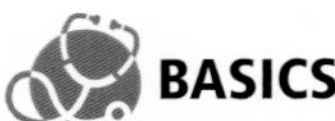

BASICS

DESCRIPTION

- Sensorimotor disorder consisting of a strong urge to move the legs, usually with paresthesia (1)[A]
- Symptoms emerge during inactivity.
- Movement relieves symptoms, but they soon recur with inactivity.
- Symptoms occur preferentially in the evening/night.
- Symptoms may involve the arms or be more generalized.
- Patient may also report involuntary leg jerks (1)[A].
- Associated with insomnia and/or functional impairment(s)
- Not solely accounted for by another disorder
- System(s) affected: musculoskeletal; nervous
- Synonym(s): Willis-Ekbom disease

EPIDEMIOLOGY

Incidence

- Onset at any age; increases with age
- Predominant sex: male = female (nulliparous); female (parous) 2× > male (2)[B]

Prevalence

- 4–15% of Caucasian adults; underdiagnosed
- 1–3% in children and adolescents
- Increases with age
- Lower in non-Caucasians

Pregnancy Considerations

10–30% prevalence; exacerbates existing restless legs syndrome (RLS)

ETIOLOGY AND PATHOPHYSIOLOGY

- Primary (early-onset) RLS: subcortical dopamine deficiency/dysmetabolism
- Late-onset (often secondary) RLS:
  - Iron deficiency and associated conditions
  - Chronic extremity tissue pathology/inflammation
  - Medications
    - Most antidepressants (exceptions: bupropion and desipramine)
    - Dopamine-blocking antiemetics (e.g., metoclopramide, prochlorperazine)
    - Some antiepileptic agents (e.g., phenytoin)
    - Phenothiazine antipsychotics; donepezil
    - Theophylline and other xanthines
    - Antihistamines/over-the-counter (OTC) cold preparations (e.g., pseudoephedrine)
    - Adrenergics, stimulants

Genetics

- Early-onset RLS heritability: ~50%
- Genetically heterogenous
  - Susceptibility loci: 2p14, 2q, 6p21.2, 9p, 12q, 14q, 15q23, and 20p
  - Genes: *MEIS1*, *MAP2K5*/LBXCOR1, and *BTBD9*

RISK FACTORS

- Family history (3,4)
- Aging
- Chronic inactivity
- Inadequate sleep
- Associated conditions (see "Commonly Associated Conditions")
- Certain medications (see "Etiology")

GENERAL PREVENTION

- Regular physical activity/exercise
- Adequate sleep
- Avoid evening caffeine, alcohol, tobacco.
- Avoid late-day use of medications that cause RLS.

COMMONLY ASSOCIATED CONDITIONS

- Periodic limb movements of sleep, insomnia, sleep walking, other parasomnias, delayed sleep phase
- Iron deficiency, renal disease/uremia/dialysis, gastric surgery, liver disease
- Parkinson disease, multiple sclerosis, peripheral neuropathy, migraine
- Orthopedic problems, arthritis, fibromyalgia
- Venous insufficiency/peripheral vascular disease, erectile dysfunction
- Pulmonary hypertension, lung transplantation, chronic obstructive pulmonary disease (COPD)
- ADHD, anxiety/depression, "sundowning"
- Pregnancy (especially if Fe- or folate-deficient)

DIAGNOSIS

- Depends on history, yet often "difficult to describe"
- May go undiagnosed for years by multiple doctors

HISTORY

- Signs/symptoms (see also "Description") (1)[A]
  - Limited to evening, night
  - Example descriptions: burning, achy, itching, antsy, "can't get comfortable"
  - Painful in ~35% of patients
  - Discomfort associated with overwhelming urge to move and relieved by movement
  - Urge to move may be the only "discomfort."
  - Movement frequency every 10–90 seconds (mean ~25 seconds)
  - Some patients must get up and walk.
  - May involve arms or, rarely, whole body
  - Periodic movements in sleep in ~80% of patients.
  - Insomnia, fatigue, anxiety
- Severity range: from rare, minor problem to daily severe impact on quality of life
- Early-onset RLS (before age 45 years) progresses slowly.
- Late-onset RLS (1)[A]
  - Sometimes secondary to other factors
  - Tends to progress more rapidly
  - May resolve to extent that cause(s) resolve

Pediatric Considerations

Consider child's own words in describing symptoms and these additional supportive findings (1)[A]:

- Insomnia or sleep disturbance
- RLS in immediate biologic relative
- Periodic limb movements during sleep

Geriatric Considerations

For diagnosis in the cognitively impaired

- Rubbing or kneading the legs in evening
- Evening hyperactivity (foot tapping, pacing, fidgeting, tossing/turning in bed)

DIFFERENTIAL DIAGNOSIS

- Claudication: Movement does not relieve pain and may worsen it.
- Motor neuron disease fasciculation/tremor: no discomfort or circadian pattern
- Peripheral neuropathy: usually no circadian pattern; unresponsive to dopamine agonists
- Dermatitis/pruritus: movement only to scratch; no circadian pattern
- Sleep-related leg cramps: isolated and very painful muscle contracture
- Periodic limb movement disorder: no wakeful movements
- Sleep starts: isolated involuntary events
- Rhythmic movement sleep disorder: movement periodicity faster than RLS
- Growing pains: no urge to move or relief by movement; circadian pattern opposite RLS
- ADHD: no sleep disorders or complaints in diagnostic criteria

DIAGNOSTIC TESTS & INTERPRETATION

Serum ferritin to assess for iron deficiency

Diagnostic Procedures/Other

- Sleep study helpful but not required
  - Frequent, periodic movements during wake
- Suggested immobilization test
  - Conducted before nocturnal polysomnography
  - Patient attempts to sit still in bed for 1 hour
  - >40 movements per hour suggests RLS.
- Ankle actigraphy for in-home use
- Electromyography, nerve conduction studies for peripheral neuropathy, radiculopathy

Test Interpretation

- Serum ferritin: <75 ng/mL
- Transferrin saturation: <16%

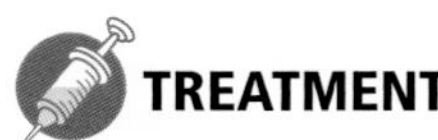

TREATMENT

First-line treatments

- Prescribed daily exercise (3)[B]; adequate sleep
- Correct iron deficiency.
- Dopaminergic medications
- For secondary RLS, treat cause(s).
- Multiple possible causes are *not* mutually exclusive.

GENERAL MEASURES

- If iron deficient, supplement
  - 325 mg $FeSO_4$ TID
  - Repletion requires months.
- Daily exercise
- Unusual activity may exacerbate symptoms.
- Regular and replete sleep
- Hot bath and leg massage
- Warm the legs (long heavy socks, electric blanket).
- Intense mental activity (games, puzzles, etc.)

MEDICATION
- Use minimum effective dose.
- Preferentially use longer acting/extended-release options.
- Daytime sleepiness unusual with doses and timing for RLS
- Severe/refractory RLS may require combination therapy (4,5)[A].

First Line
- Dopamine agonists (4,5)[A]; titrate every 3 days to minimum necessary dose:
  - Pramipexole (Mirapex): 0.125–0.5 mg 1 hour before symptoms; titrate by 0.125 mg
  - Ropinirole (Requip): 0.25–4 mg 1 hour before symptoms; titrate by 0.25 mg
  - Divide dose for evening and bedtime symptoms.
  - Transdermal rotigotine (Neupro): 1–3 mg/24 hr patch; initiate with 1 mg/24 hr; titrate by 1 mg weekly
  - Avoid dopamine agonists in psychotic patients, particularly if taking dopamine antagonists.
  - Add a different class of medication before exceeding dopamine agonist recommended dose.
- Gabapentin enacarbil (Horizant): 600 mg every day ~5:00 PM (4,5)[A]
- All other medications off-label

Second Line
- Anticonvulsants (for comorbid neuropathy)
  - Pregabalin (Lyrica): 50–300 mg/day
  - Carbamazepine: 200–800 mg/day
- Opioids (low risk of tolerance/addiction at bedtime)
  - Hydrocodone: 5–20 mg/day
  - Tramadol: 50 mg/day
  - Oxycodone: 2.5–20 mg/day
- Benzodiazepines and agonists (for associated insomnia or anxiety)
  - Clonazepam (Klonopin): 0.5–3 mg/day
  - Temazepam, triazolam, alprazolam, zaleplon, zolpidem, and diazepam
- Dopamine agonists
  - Carbidopa-levodopa (Sinemet or Sinemet CR): 10/100–25/250; PRN for sporadic symptoms

Pregnancy Considerations
- Initial approach: nonpharmacologic therapies, iron supplements
- Avoid medications class C or D.
- In 3rd trimester, low-dose opioids may be considered.

Pediatric Considerations
- First-line treatment: nonpharmacologic
- Low-dose clonidine or clonazepam may be considered.

Geriatric Considerations
- Avoid medications that cause dizziness or unsteadiness.
- Many medications given to elderly cause/exacerbate RLS.

ISSUES FOR REFERRAL
- Severe, intractable symptoms
- Augmentation response to dopaminergic therapy
- Peripheral neuropathy; orthopedic problems
- Peripheral vascular disease; intransigent iron deficiency

ADDITIONAL THERAPIES
- Vitamin, mineral supplements: Ca, Mg, B_{12}, folate
- Clonidine: 0.05–0.1 mg/day
- Baclofen: 20–80 mg/day
- Methadone: 5–10 mg/day
- Prescription or OTC hypnotics

SURGERY/OTHER PROCEDURES
For orthopedic, neuropathic, or leg vascular disease (laser ablation, sclerotherapy, etc.)

COMPLEMENTARY & ALTERNATIVE MEDICINE
- Relaxis leg vibration device (FDA-approved; see www.sensorymedical.com)
- Sequential pneumatic leg compression
- Enhanced external counterpulsation
- Acupuncture
- MicroVas therapy
- Near-infrared light

INPATIENT CONSIDERATIONS
- Control RLS after orthopedic procedures.
- Addition/withdrawal of medications affecting RLS (e.g., narcotics)
- Changes in medical status may require medication changes.

IV Fluids
- Iron infusion when oral Fe fails or contraindicated.
- When NPO, consider IV opiates.

Nursing
- Evening walks, hot baths, leg massage, and warming
- Sleep interruption risks prolonged wakefulness.

ONGOING CARE

FOLLOW-UP RECOMMENDATIONS
Patient Monitoring
- At 2-week intervals until stable, then annually
- If taking iron, remeasure ferritin.
- If status changes, assess for associated conditions and medications.

DIET
Avoid evening caffeine and alcohol.

PATIENT EDUCATION
- Willis-Ekbom Disease Foundation: www.rls.org
- National Sleep Foundation: sleepfoundation.org

PROGNOSIS
- Early-onset: lifelong condition with no current cure
- Late-onset/secondary: may subside with resolution of precipitating factors
- Current therapies usually control symptoms.

COMPLICATIONS
- Augmentation of symptoms from prolonged dopaminergic therapy
  - Symptoms increase in severity, occur earlier, and/or spread.
  - Higher doses increase risk.
  - Highest risk from daily levodopa or Sinemet
  - Iron deficiency increases risk.
  - Add alternative medication then slowly down-titrate dopamine agonist.
- Obsessive-compulsive or impulse-control disorders from dopamine agonists
- Vicious cycle between sleep loss from RLS and exacerbation of RLS by sleep loss
- Iatrogenic RLS (from antidepressants, etc.)

REFERENCES

1. Allen RP, Picchietti DL, Garcia-Borreguero D, et al. Restless legs syndrome/Willis-Ekbom disease diagnostic criteria: updated International Restless Legs Syndrome Study Group (IRLSSG) consensus criteria—history, rationale, description, and significance. *Sleep Med*. 2014;15(8):860–873.
2. Manconi M, Ulfberg J, Berger K, et al. When gender matters: restless legs syndrome. Report of the "RLS and woman" workshop endorsed by the European RLS Study Group. *Sleep Med Rev*. 2012;16(4):297–307.
3. Aukerman MM, Aukerman D, Bayard M, et al. Exercise and restless legs syndrome: a randomized controlled trial. *J Am Board Fam Med*. 2006;19(5):487–493.
4. Aurora RN, Kristo DA, Bista SR, et al. The treatment of restless legs syndrome and periodic limb movement disorder in adults—an update for 2012: practice parameters with an evidence-based systematic review and meta-analyses: an American Academy of Sleep Medicine Clinical Practice Guideline. *Sleep*. 2012;35(8):1039–1062.
5. Ferini-Strambi L, Marelli S. Pharmacotherapy for restless legs syndrome. *Expert Opin Pharmacother*. 2014;15(8):1127–1138.

ADDITIONAL READING

- Picchietti MA, Picchietti DL. Advances in pediatric restless legs syndrome: iron, genetics, diagnosis and treatment. *Sleep Med*. 2010;11(7):643–651.
- Spiegelhalder K, Hornyak M. Restless legs syndrome in older adults. *Clin Geriatr Med*. 2008;24(1):167–180, ix.
- Yeh P, Walters AS, Tsuang JW. Restless legs syndrome: a comprehensive overview on its epidemiology, risk factors, and treatment. *Sleep Breath*. 2012;16(4):987–1007.

SEE ALSO

- Periodic Limb Movement Disorder
- Algorithm: Restless Leg Syndrome (RLS)

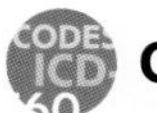

CODES

ICD10
G25.81 Restless legs syndrome

CLINICAL PEARLS
- Insomnia with frequent tossing/turning and difficulty "getting comfortable" is often RLS.
- Many antidepressants, antipsychotics, antiemetics, and antihistamines cause or exacerbate RLS.
- RLS may interfere with use of positive airway pressure to treat obstructive sleep apnea.
- RLS and other sleep disorders may cause ADHD.

RETINAL DETACHMENT

Richard W. Allinson, MD

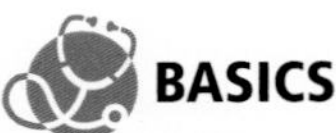

BASICS

DESCRIPTION

- Separation of the sensory retina from the underlying retinal pigment epithelium
- Rhegmatogenous retinal detachment (RRD): most common type; occurs when the fluid vitreous gains access to the subretinal space through a break in the retina (Greek *rhegma*, "rent")
- Exudative or serous detachment: occurs in the absence of a retinal break, usually in association with inflammation or a tumor
- Traction detachment: Vitreoretinal adhesions mechanically pull the retina from the retinal pigment epithelium. The most common cause is proliferative diabetic retinopathy.
- System(s) affected: nervous

EPIDEMIOLOGY

Incidence

- Predominant age: Incidence increases with age.
- Predominant sex: male > female (3:2)
- Per year: 1/10,000 in patients who have not had cataract surgery

Prevalence

After cataract surgery, 1–3% of patients will develop a retinal detachment.

ETIOLOGY AND PATHOPHYSIOLOGY

- Traction from a posterior vitreous detachment (PVD) causes most retinal tears. With aging, vitreous gel liquefies, leading to separation of the vitreous from the retina. The vitreous gel remains attached at the vitreous base, in the retinal periphery, resulting in vitreous traction that produces tears in the retinal periphery. There is an ~15% chance of developing a retinal tear from a PVD.
- PVD associated with vitreous hemorrhage has a high incidence of retinal tears.
- Exudative detachment
  - Tumors
  - Inflammatory diseases (Harada, posterior scleritis)
  - Miscellaneous (central serous retinopathy, uveal effusion syndrome, malignant hypertension)
- Traction detachment
  - Proliferative diabetic retinopathy
  - Cicatricial retinopathy of prematurity
  - Proliferative sickle-cell retinopathy
- Penetrating trauma

Genetics

- Most cases are sporadic.
- There is an increased risk of RRD if a sibling has been affected by this condition. The risk increases with higher levels of myopia in the family history.

RISK FACTORS

- Myopia (>5 diopters)
- Aphakia or pseudophakia: In patients undergoing small-incision coaxial phacoemulsification with high myopia (axial length ≥26 mm), the incidence of retinal detachment is 2.7%.
- PVD and associated conditions (e.g., aphakia, inflammatory disease, and trauma)
- Trauma
- Retinal detachment in fellow eye
- Lattice degeneration: a vitreoretinal abnormality found in 6–10% of the general population
- Glaucoma: 4–7% of patients with retinal detachment have chronic open-angle glaucoma.
- Vitreoretinal tufts: Peripheral retinal tufts are caused by focal areas of vitreous traction.
- Meridional folds: Redundant retina usually is found in the supranasal quadrant.

GENERAL PREVENTION

Patients at risk for retinal detachment should have regular ophthalmologic exams.

Geriatric Considerations

- PVD
- Cataract surgery

Pediatric Considerations

Usually associated with underlying vitreoretinal disorders and/or retinopathy of prematurity

COMMONLY ASSOCIATED CONDITIONS

- Lattice degeneration
- High myopia
- Cataract surgery
- Glaucoma
- History of retinal detachment in the fellow eye
- Trauma

Pregnancy Considerations

Preeclampsia/eclampsia may be associated with exudative retinal detachment. No intervention is indicated, provided hypertension is controlled. Prognosis is usually good.

DIAGNOSIS

HISTORY

- Sudden flashes (photopsia)
- Shower of floaters
- Visual field loss: "curtain coming across vision"
- Central vision will be preserved if the macula is not detached.
- Poor visual acuity (20/200 or worse), with loss of central vision when macula is detached

PHYSICAL EXAM

- Slit-lamp exam
- Dilated fundus exam with binocular indirect ophthalmoscopy

DIFFERENTIAL DIAGNOSIS

Retinoschisis (splitting of the retina)

- Vitreous cells and vitreous hemorrhage are found rarely in the vitreous with retinoschisis, whereas they are seen commonly in RRD.
- Retinoschisis usually has a smooth surface and is dome shaped, whereas RRD often has a corrugated, irregular surface.

DIAGNOSTIC TESTS & INTERPRETATION

Visual field testing: differentiates RRD from retinoschisis. An absolute scotoma is seen in retinoschisis, whereas RRD causes a relative scotoma.

Initial Tests (lab, imaging)

- US can demonstrate a detached retina and may be helpful when the retina cannot be visualized directly (e.g., with cataracts).
- Fluorescein dye leakage can be seen in exudative retinal detachment; caused by central serous retinopathy and other inflammatory conditions

Test Interpretation

- Elevation of the neurosensory retina from the underlying retinal pigment epithelium
- Elevation of retina associated with ≥1 retinal tears in RRD or elevation of the retina without tears in exudative detachment
- In 3–10% of patients with presumed RRD, no definite retinal break is found.
- Tenting of the retina without retinal tears in traction detachment
- Pigmented cells within the vitreous ("tobacco dust")

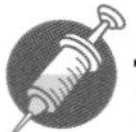

TREATMENT

GENERAL MEASURES

- Not all retinal tears or breaks need to be treated:
  - Flap or horseshoe tears in symptomatic patients (e.g., patients with flashes or floaters) are treated frequently.
  - Operculated holes in symptomatic patients are treated sometimes.
  - Atrophic holes in symptomatic patients are treated rarely.
- Lattice degeneration with or without holes within the lattice in an asymptomatic patient with prior retinal detachment in the fellow eye may be treated prophylactically.
- Flap retinal tears in asymptomatic patients frequently are treated prophylactically.
- Exudative detachments usually are managed by treating underlying disorder.
- Traction detachments usually are managed by observation. If the fovea is involved, a vitrectomy is needed.

MEDICATION

First Line

- Intraocular gases
  - Air
  - Perfluoropropane (C_3F_8)
  - Sulfur hexafluoride (SF_6)
- Perfluorocarbon liquids
- Silicone oil
- Contraindications to intraocular gas: patients with poorly controlled glaucoma
- Precautions with intraocular gas: Expanding intraocular gas bubble increases intraocular pressure; therefore, avoid higher altitudes.
- Significant possible interactions with intraocular gas: Nitrous oxide used in general anesthesia can expand an intraocular gas bubble.

Second Line

Steroids may cause worsening of central serous retinopathy.

SURGERY/OTHER PROCEDURES

- Timing of repairs
  - Macula attached: within 24 hours. If the detachment is peripheral and does not have features suggestive of rapid progression (e.g., large and/or superior tears), repair can be performed within a few days.

- Macula recently detached: within 10 days of development of a macula-off retinal detachment (1)[B]
  - Old macular detachment: elective repair within 2 weeks
- If a retinal break has led to the development of a retinal detachment, surgery is needed. Surgical options (and combinations) include the following:
  - Demarcation laser treatment
  - Pneumatic retinopexy: Head positioning is required postoperatively.
  - Scleral buckle
  - Vitrectomy
  - Perfluorocarbon liquids for giant tears (circumferential tears ≥90°)
  - Silicone oil for complex repairs
- Anesthesia: local or general
- RRD may have >1 break. If any retinal break is not closed at the time of surgery, the surgery will fail.
- Additional surgery may be required if the retina redetaches secondary to a new retinal break or because of proliferative vitreoretinopathy (PVR).
- Adjuvant combination therapy using 5-fluorouracil (5-FU) and low-molecular-weight heparin (LMWH) may reduce the incidence of PVR in patients undergoing vitrectomy for RRD who are at a greater risk of developing PVR, such as patients with uveitis, but does not seem to be of benefit in cases of established PVR.
- If a vitreous hemorrhage is present, presumably from a retinal tear, and the fundus cannot be well visualized, consideration can be given for early vitrectomy (2)[C].
- There is a trend toward primary vitrectomy in the management of RRD. Eyes undergoing pars plana vitrectomy (PPV) for primary RRD repair may not need the addition of a scleral buckle (3)[B].
- There is no statistical difference in the primary reattachment rate between eyes treated with PPV or scleral buckle for RRD in both phakic and pseudophakic/aphakic eyes (4)[A].
- There is a reduced incidence of intraoperative retinal tear formation using a transconjunctival cannulated PPV system compared to the standard 20-gauge system requiring suture closure.

INPATIENT CONSIDERATIONS

Admission Criteria/Initial Stabilization

- Recognition of condition is key (see "Diagnosis").
- Refer to an ophthalmologist for exam and treatment, if indicated.

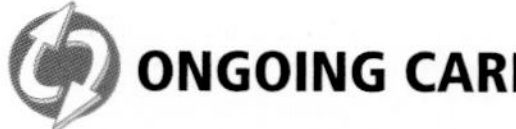

ONGOING CARE

FOLLOW-UP RECOMMENDATIONS

- Bed rest prior to surgery.
- Postoperatively, if intraocular gas has been used, the patient may need specific head positioning and should not travel to high altitudes.

Patient Monitoring

- Alert ophthalmologist if there is new onset of floaters or flashes, increase in floaters or flashes, sudden shower of floaters, curtain or shadow in the peripheral visual field, or reduced vision.
- Patients with acute symptomatic PVD should be reexamined by the ophthalmologist in 3–4 weeks. The development of a retinal detachment is unlikely if no retinal tears are present on reexamination in 3–4 weeks.
- If acute symptomatic PVD is associated with gross vitreous hemorrhage that interferes with complete visualization of the retinal periphery by indirect ophthalmoscopy, the patient should be reexamined at short intervals with indirect ophthalmoscopy until the entire retinal periphery can be observed.
- If the examiner is not certain whether the retina is detached in the presence of opaque medium, US should be performed.

DIET

NPO if surgery is imminent

PATIENT EDUCATION

American Academy of Ophthalmology, 655 E. Beach Street, San Francisco, CA 94109-1336

PROGNOSIS

- RRD
  - 90% of retinal detachments can be reattached successfully after ≥1 surgical procedures. Postoperative visual acuity depends primarily on the status of the macula preoperatively. Also important is the length of time between the detachment and the repair (75% of eyes with macular detachments of <1 week will obtain a final visual acuity of 20/70 or better).
  - 87% of eyes with a retinal detachment not involving the macula attain a visual acuity of 20/50 or better postoperatively. 37% of eyes with a detached macula preoperatively attain 20/50 or better vision postoperatively.
  - In 10–15% of successfully repaired retinal detachments not involving the macula preoperatively, visual acuity does not return to the preoperative level. This decrease is secondary to complications such as macular edema and macular pucker.
- Tractional retinal detachment: When not involving the fovea, the patient usually can be observed because it is uncommon for these to extend into the fovea.
- Exudative retinal detachment
  - Management is usually nonsurgical.
  - The presence of shifting fluid is highly suggestive of an exudative retinal detachment. Fixed retinal folds, which are indicative of PVR, are seen rarely in exudative retinal detachment. If the underlying condition is treated, the prognosis generally is good.

COMPLICATIONS

- PVR is the most common cause of failed retinal detachment repair; 10–15% of retinas that reattach initially after retinal surgery will redetach subsequently, usually within 6 weeks, as a result of cellular proliferation and contraction on the retinal surface.
- Partial or total loss of vision due to macular detachment and/or PVR
- Moderate to severe forms of PVR usually are treated with PPV and fluid–gas exchange. If a segmental scleral buckle was placed at the initial procedure, it may need to be revised.
- Primary retinectomy can be used in cases of PVR without a scleral buckle (5)[C].
- Scleral buckles may erode the overlying conjunctiva and lead to an infection.
- Optic neuropathy after PPV for macula-sparing primary RRD

REFERENCES

1. Hassan TS, Sarrafizadeh R, Ruby AJ, et al. The effect of duration of macular detachment on results after the scleral buckle repair of primary, macula-off retinal detachments. *Ophthalmology*. 2002;109(1):146–152.
2. Tan HS, Mura M, Bijl HM. Early vitrectomy for vitreous hemorrhage associated with retinal tears. *Am J Ophthalmol*. 2010;150(4):529–533.
3. Kinori M, Moisseiev E, Shoshany N, et al. Comparison of pars plana vitrectomy with and without scleral buckle for the repair of primary rhegmatogenous retinal detachment. *Am J Ophthalmol*. 2011;152(2):291–297.
4. Soni C, Hainsworth DP, Almony A. Surgical management of rhegmatogenous retinal detachment: a meta-analysis of randomized controlled trials. *Ophthalmology*. 2013;120(7):1440–1447.
5. Tan HS, Mura M, Oberstein SY. Primary retinectomy in proliferative vitreoretinopathy. *Am J Ophthalmol*. 2010;149(3):447–452.

ADDITIONAL READING

- Alio JL, Ruiz-Moreno JM, Shabayek MH, et al. The risk of retinal detachment in high myopia after small incision coaxial phacoemulsification. *Am J Ophthalmol*. 2007;144(1):93–98.
- Bansal AS, Hsu J, Garg SJ, et al. Optic neuropathy after vitrectomy for retinal detachment: clinical features and analysis of risk factors. *Ophthalmology*. 2012;119(11):2364–2370.
- Covert DJ, Henry CR, Bhatia SK, et al. Intraoperative retinal tear formation and postoperative rhegmatogenous retinal detachment in transconjunctival cannulated vitrectomy systems compared with the standard 20-gauge system. *Arch Ophthalmol*. 2012;130(2):186–189.
- Mitry D, Williams L, Charteris DG, et al. Population-based estimate of the sibling recurrence risk ratio for rhegmatogenous retinal detachment. *Invest Ophthalmol Vis Sci*. 2011;52(5):2551–2555.

SEE ALSO

Retinopathy, Diabetic

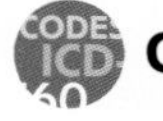

CODES

ICD10

- H33.001 Unspecified retinal detachment with retinal break, right eye
- H33.019 Retinal detachment with single break, unspecified eye
- H33.20 Serous retinal detachment, unspecified eye

CLINICAL PEARLS

- If a patient complains of the new onset of floaters or flashes of light, the patient should undergo a dilated eye exam to rule out a retinal tear or retinal detachment.
- There is an increased risk of retinal detachment after cataract surgery.
- PVR can result in redetachment of the retina after an initially successful repair.

RETINOPATHY, DIABETIC

Richard W. Allinson, MD

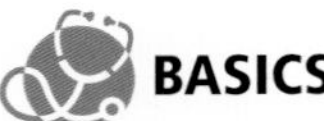

BASICS

DESCRIPTION

- Noninflammatory retinal disorder characterized by retinal capillary closure and microaneurysms. Retinal ischemia leads to release of a vasoproliferative factor, stimulating neovascularization on retina, optic nerve, or iris.
- Most patients with diabetes mellitus (DM) will develop diabetic retinopathy (DR). It is the leading cause of new cases of legal blindness among residents in the United States between the ages of 20 and 64 years.
- DR can be divided into 3 stages.
  - Nonproliferative (background)
  - Severe nonproliferative (preproliferative)
  - Proliferative
- System(s) affected: nervous

Geriatric Considerations

Prevalence will increase, as population generally ages and patients with diabetes live longer.

Pregnancy Considerations

- Pregnancy can exacerbate condition.
- Pregnant diabetic women should be examined in 1st trimester, then every 3 months until delivery.

EPIDEMIOLOGY

Incidence

- Peak incidence of type 1, juvenile-onset DM is between the ages of 12 and 15 years.
- Peak incidence of type 2, adult-onset DM is between the ages of 50 and 70 years.
- Incidence of DR is directly related to the duration of diabetes.
- <10 years of age, it is unusual to see DR, regardless of DM duration.

Prevalence

- 6.6% of the U.S. population between ages of 20 and 74 years has DM.
- ~25% of the diabetic population has some form of DR.
- Predominant age
  - Risk increases after puberty.
  - 2/3 of juvenile-onset diabetics who have had DM for at least 35 years will develop proliferative DR and will develop macular edema. Proportions are reversed for adult-onset diabetes.
- Predominant sex: male = female (type 1, juvenile-onset DM); female > male (type 2)

ETIOLOGY AND PATHOPHYSIOLOGY

- Related to development of diabetic microaneurysms and microvascular abnormalities
- Reduction in perifoveal capillary blood flow velocity, perifoveal capillary occlusion, and increased retinal thickness at the central fovea in diabetic patients are associated with visual impairment in patients with diabetic macular edema.

RISK FACTORS

- Duration of DM (usually >10 years)
- Poor glycemic control
- Pregnancy
- Renal disease
- Systemic hypertension (HTN)
- Smoking
- Elevated lipid levels associated with increased risk of retinal lipid deposits (hard exudates)
- Myopic eyes (eyes with longer axial length) have a lower risk of DR.

GENERAL PREVENTION

- Monitor and control of blood glucose.
- Schedule yearly ophthalmologic eye exams.

COMMONLY ASSOCIATED CONDITIONS

- Glaucoma
- Cataracts
- Retinal detachment
- Vitreous hemorrhage
- Disc edema (diabetic papillopathy); may occur in type 1/type 2 DM

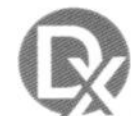

DIAGNOSIS

HISTORY

Diabetic patients should be encouraged to have an annual ophthalmologic exam because early changes are asymptomatic.

PHYSICAL EXAM

- Eye exam: measurement of visual acuity and documentation of the status of the iris, lens, vitreous, and fundus
- Nonproliferative (background) DR
  - Microaneurysms
  - Intraretinal hemorrhage
  - Macular edema causing decrease in central vision
  - Lipid deposits
- Severe nonproliferative (preproliferative) DR
  - Nerve fiber layer infarctions ("cotton wool spots")
  - Venous beading
  - Venous dilatation
  - Intraretinal microvascular abnormalities
  - Extensive retinal hemorrhage
- Proliferative DR
  - New blood vessel proliferation (neovascularization) on the retinal surface, optic nerve, and iris
  - Visual loss caused by vitreous hemorrhage, traction retinal detachment

GENERAL MEASURES

- The Diabetes Control and Complications Trial (DCCT) recommended that for most patients with insulin-dependent DM, blood glucose levels should be as close to the nondiabetic range as is safe to reduce the risk and rate of progression of DR.
  - In the DCCT, insulin-dependent DM patients were randomly assigned into either conventional or intensive insulin treatment. Conventional treatment consisted of 1–2 daily insulin injections, with daily self-monitoring of urine/blood glucose. Intensive treatment consisted of insulin administered ≥3× daily by injection/an external pump, with self-monitored blood glucose levels measured at least 4×/day.
  - The DCCT demonstrated that intensive insulin therapy reduced the risk of macular edema and retinal neovascularization. The benefit of intensive insulin therapy and the reduced risk of DR-associated microvascular complications persist for at least 10 years.
  - In the DCCT, intensive insulin therapy was more effective in reducing the risk of progression of DR in the less advanced stages. However, advanced DR also benefited from the intensive insulin therapy.
- The Early Treatment Diabetic Retinopathy Study demonstrated that aspirin therapy did not prevent the development of proliferative DR or reduce the risk of visual loss associated with DR.
- Microvascular complications, including proliferative DR, are increased when blood sugar levels are ≥200 mg/dL.
- Poor glycemic control is associated with an increased risk both for development and progression of DR, regardless of the type of DM; that hyperglycemia itself is causative is not established, especially for type 2 DM
- Cataracts are more common among those with DM. Try to delay cataract surgery in DM patients with retinopathy until the symptoms are severe. Cataract surgery can cause retinopathy to worsen and increase the risk for development of diabetic macular edema.
- HTN has a detrimental effect on DR and must be controlled.

DIFFERENTIAL DIAGNOSIS

Other causes of retinopathy (e.g., radiation, retinal venous obstruction, HTN)

DIAGNOSTIC TESTS & INTERPRETATION

Diagnostic Procedures/Other

- Fluorescein angiography demonstrates retinal nonperfusion, retinal leakage, and proliferative DR.
- Optical coherence tomography (OCT) can be used to help detect diabetic macular edema by measuring retinal thickness.

Test Interpretation

- Increased capillary permeability
- Microaneurysms
- Hemorrhages in retina
- Exudates in retina
- Capillary nonperfusion

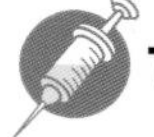

TREATMENT

MEDICATION

- Treatment with the angiotensin-receptor blocker candesartan has been shown to result in regression of DR in some patients (1)[B].
- Under evaluation: Protein kinase C-β is activated by hyperglycemia and is associated with the development of vascular dysfunction. Inhibition of this enzyme could help to reduce the retinal vascular complications from DM.

- Nutritional antioxidant intake of vitamins C and E and of β-carotene has no protective effect on DR.
- Atorvastatin may reduce the severity of lipid deposits with clinically significant diabetic macular edema in type 2 DM and dyslipidemia.

SURGERY/OTHER PROCEDURES

- Laser photocoagulation treatment: recommended for patients with proliferative DR and for those with clinically significant macular edema; destroys leaking blood vessels and areas of neovascularization
- The Diabetic Retinopathy Study demonstrated that panretinal photocoagulation reduced overall rate of severe visual loss from 15.9% in untreated eyes to 6.4% in treated eyes. In certain subgroups, the incidence of severe visual loss in untreated eyes was as high as 36.9% within 2 years.
- The Early Treatment Diabetic Retinopathy Study demonstrated that eyes with significant diabetic macular edema benefited from focal laser treatment. Clinically significant diabetic macular edema (CSDME) is defined as the following:
  - Thickening of the retina within 500 μm of the center of the macula
  - Hard exudates within 500 μm of the center of the macula associated with thickening of the adjacent retina
  - Zone of retinal thickening $\geq$1 disc area within 1 disc diameter of the center of the macula
- Patients with CSDME and high-risk proliferative disease can have simultaneous focal and panretinal photocoagulation without adversely affecting the visual outcome.
- Vitrectomy may benefit some with diffuse macular edema. This may apply especially to eyes with vitreomacular traction found on OCT and with persistent CSDME.
- Intravitreal triamcinolone may be used for DM-related macular edema that fails laser treatment. No long-term benefit of intravitreal triamcinolone relative to focal/grid photocoagulation in patients with CSDME. This is an off-label use (2)[C].
- Ranibizumab, an antibody fragment that binds vascular endothelial growth factor (VEGF), can be used to treat CSDME when injected intravitreally. Ranibizumab 0.3 mg given monthly to treat CSDME resulted in improved vision and reduced central foveal thickness (3)[A].
  - Anti-VEGF therapy is the preferred method of treatment for moderate to severe visual impairment resulting from diabetic macular edema (DME). Anti-VEGF treatment results in superior clinical outcomes compared to laser photocoagulation for DME (4)[A].
  - Intravitreal ranibizumab treatment for diabetic macular edema may also improve DR severity and reduce the risk of DR progression (5)[A].
- Bevacizumab, a full-length antibody that binds VEGF, can be used to treat CSDME when injected intravitreally. This is an off-label use.
  - Intravitreal bevacizumab and ranibizumab have comparable efficacy in treating diabetic macular edema (6)[C].
- Aflibercept, a soluble decoy receptor for VEGF, is being investigated in the treatment of CSDME when injected intravitreally. This is an off-label use (7)[C].
- Preoperative bevacizumab can be used as an adjuvant to vitrectomy for complications of proliferative DR. This is an off-label use:
  - At ~10 days after intravitreal injection of bevacizumab, the vascular component of proliferation is markedly reduced, and the contractile components are not yet very significant. Patients with dense fibrovascular proliferation need to be monitored closely for evidence of traction retinal detachment (8)[C].
- Cryoretinopexy can be used instead of laser treatment in certain patients to decrease the neovascular stimulus and treat proliferative DR.
- Vitrectomy: recommended for patients with severe proliferative DR, traction retinal detachment involving the macula, and nonclearing vitreous hemorrhage
  - A transvitreal fibrinoid response can occur after diabetic vitrectomy and present as a pseudoendophthalmitis (9)[C].

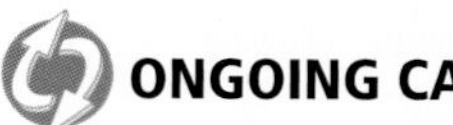

ONGOING CARE

FOLLOW-UP RECOMMENDATIONS

Patient Monitoring

Scheduled ophthalmologic eye exams

- Yearly follow-up if no retinopathy
- Every 6 months with background DR
- At least every 3–4 months with preproliferative DR
- Every 2–3 months with active proliferative DR

DIET

Follow prescribed diet for patients with diabetes.

PATIENT EDUCATION

- Patient education should include regular ophthalmic exams.
- Stress importance of strict blood glucose control through diet, exercise, drugs/insulin, and monitoring of blood glucose.

PROGNOSIS

If the condition is diagnosed and treated early in development, outlook is good. If treatment is delayed, blindness may result.

COMPLICATIONS

Blindness

REFERENCES

1. Sjølie AK, Klein R, Porta M, et al. Effect of candesartan on progression and regression of retinopathy in type 2 diabetes (DIRECT-Protect 2): a randomised placebo-controlled trial. *Lancet*. 2008;372(9647):1385–1393.
2. Diabetic Retinopathy Clinical Research Network, Beck RW, Edwards AR, et al. Three-year follow-up of a randomized trial comparing focal/grid photocoagulation and intravitreal triamcinolone for diabetic macular edema. *Arch Ophthalmol*. 2009;127(3):245–251.
3. Brown DM, Nguyen QD, Marcus DM, et al. Long-term outcomes of ranibizumab therapy for diabetic macular edema: the 36-month results from two phase III trials: RISE and RIDE. *Ophthalmology*. 2013;120(10):2013–2022.
4. Mitchell P, Wong TY; Diabetic Macular Edema Treatment Guideline Working Group. Management paradigms for diabetic macular edema. *Am J Ophthalmol*. 2014;157(3):505–513. e1–e8
5. Ip MS, Domalpally A, Hopkins JJ, et al. Long-term effects of ranibizumab on diabetic retinopathy severity and progression. *Arch Ophthalmol*. 2012;130(9):1145–1152.
6. Nepomuceno AB, Takaki E, Paes de Allmeida FP, et al. A prospective randomized trial of intraviteal bevacizumab versus ranibizumab for the management of diabetic macular edema. *Am J Ophthamol*. 2013;156(3):502–510.
7. Do DV, Nguyen QD, Boyer D, et al. One-year outcomes of the da Vinci Study of VEGF Trap-Eye in eyes with diabetic macular edema. *Ophthalmology*. 2012;119(8):1658–1665.
8. El-Sabagh HA, Abdelghaffar W, Labib AM, et al. Preoperative intravitreal bevacizumab use as an adjuvant to diabetic vitrectomy: histopathologic findings and clinical implications. *Ophthalmology*. 2011;118(4):636–641.
9. Luo C, Ruby A, Neuwelt M, et al. Transvitreal fibrinoid pseudoendophthalmitis after diabetic vitrectomy. *Retina*. 2013;33(10):2069–2074.

ADDITIONAL READING

- Rajendram R, Fraser-Bell S, Kaines A, et al. A 2-year prospective randomized controlled trial of intravitreal bevacizumab or laser therapy (BOLT) in the management of diabetic macular edema: 24-month data: report 3. *Arch Ophthalmol*. 2012;130(8):972–979.
- White NH, Sun W, Cleary PA, et al. Prolonged effect of intensive therapy on the risk of retinopathy complications in patients with type 1 diabetes mellitus: 10 years after the Diabetes Control and Complications Trial. *Arch Ophthalmol*. 2008;126(12):1707–1715.

SEE ALSO

Diabetes Mellitus, Type 1; Diabetes Mellitus, Type 2.

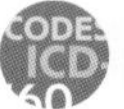

CODES

ICD10

- E11.319 Type 2 diabetes mellitus with unspecified diabetic retinopathy without macular edema
- E10.319 Type 1 diabetes mellitus with unspecified diabetic retinopathy without macular edema
- E10.329 Type 1 diab w mild nonprlf diabetic rtnop w/o macular edema

CLINICAL PEARLS

- Options for the treatment of diffuse macular edema include focal laser treatment, intravitreal triamcinolone, intravitreal ranibizumab, intravitreal bevacizumab, and vitrectomy.
- High BP should be controlled to reduce the risk of diabetic eye complications.
- Blood glucose levels should be well controlled to help reduce the risk and rate of DR progression.
- Schedule yearly ophthalmologic eye exams.

RH INCOMPATIBILITY

Jeremy D. DeFoe, DO • Scott P. Grogan, DO, MBA, FAAFP

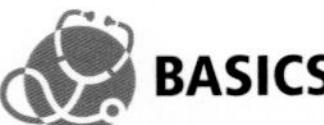

BASICS

DESCRIPTION

- Antibody-mediated destruction of red blood cells (RBCs) that bear Rh surface antigens in individuals who lack the antigens and have become isoimmunized (sensitized) to them
- System(s) affected: hematologic/lymphatic/immunologic
- Synonym(s): Rh isoimmunization; Rh alloimmunization; Rh sensitization

EPIDEMIOLOGY

Incidence

Predominant age and sex: affects fetuses/neonates of isoimmunized, childbearing females

ETIOLOGY AND PATHOPHYSIOLOGY

- Circulating antibodies to Rh antigens (transplacentally transferred antibodies in the case of a fetus/newborn) attach to Rh antigens on RBCs.
- Immune-mediated destruction of RBCs leads to hemolysis, anemia, and increased bilirubin production.
- Transfusion of Rh-positive blood to Rh-negative recipient
- Maternal exposure to fetal Rh antigens, either antepartum or intrapartum
- Most commonly seen in the Rh-positive fetus or infant of an Rh-negative mother

Genetics

- Complex autosomal inheritance of polypeptide Rh antigens; 3 genetic loci with closely related genes carry an assortment of alleles: Dd, Cc, and Ee.
- Individuals who express the D antigen (also called *Rho* or *Rho[D]*) or its weak D (D^u) variant are considered Rh-positive. Individuals lacking the D antigen are Rh-negative.
- Another variant D antigen, DEL, has been identified in some individuals (predominantly Asians) who are classified as Rh-negative by the usual assays. Although testing Rh-negative, these individuals are not likely to be sensitized by exposure to Rh-D antigens through pregnancy or transfusion and should be considered clinically Rh-positive (1).
- Antibodies may be produced to C, c, D, E, or e in individuals lacking the specific antigen; only D is strongly immunogenic (2).
- Isoimmunization to Rh antigens in susceptible individuals is acquired, not inherited.

RISK FACTORS

- ~15% of the white population and smaller fractions of other races are Rh-negative and susceptible to sensitization (3).
- Any Rh-positive pregnancy in an Rh-negative woman can result in sensitization.
- Native risk of isoimmunization after Rh-positive pregnancy had been estimated at ≤15% but seems to be decreasing.
- The risk of isoimmunization antepartum is only 1–2%.
- The risk of isoimmunization is 1–2% after spontaneous abortion and 4–5% after induced abortion (4).
- Use of Rho(D) immunoglobulin prophylaxis has reduced incidence of isoimmunization to <1% of susceptible pregnancies (5)[A].

GENERAL PREVENTION

- Blood typing (ABO and Rh) on all pregnant women and prior to blood transfusions
- Antibody screening early in pregnancy
- Rh immunoglobulin prevents only sensitization to the D antigen.
- For prophylaxis, Rho(D) immunoglobulin (RhIG, RhoGAM, HyperRHO, RHOphylac) given to unsensitized, Rh-negative women after the following:
  - Spontaneous abortion
  - Induced abortion
  - Ectopic pregnancy
  - Antepartum hemorrhage
  - Trauma to abdomen
  - Amniocentesis
  - Chorionic villus sampling
  - Within 72 hours of delivery of an Rh-positive infant
  - Given routinely at 28 weeks' gestation
- Prophylaxis is to prevent sensitization affecting a subsequent pregnancy and has little effect on the current pregnancy.
- Dose for prophylaxis
  - 50-μg dose for events up to 12 weeks' gestation
  - 300-μg dose for events after 12 weeks' gestation
  - Higher doses may be required in the event of a large fetal–maternal hemorrhage (>30 mL of whole blood).

COMMONLY ASSOCIATED CONDITIONS

- Hemolytic disease of newborn
- Hydrops fetalis
- Neonatal jaundice
- Kernicterus
- See "Erythroblastosis Fetalis" topic.

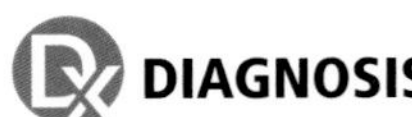

DIAGNOSIS

PHYSICAL EXAM

- Jaundice of newborn
- Kernicterus
- Fetal hydrops or fetal death in utero if severe (see "Erythroblastosis Fetalis" topic)

DIFFERENTIAL DIAGNOSIS

- ABO incompatibility
- Other blood group (non-Rh) isoimmunization
- Nonimmune fetal hydrops
- Hereditary spherocytosis
- RBC enzyme defects

DIAGNOSTIC TESTS & INTERPRETATION

Initial Tests (lab, imaging)

- Positive indirect Coombs test (antibody screen) during pregnancy
- Paternal blood type
- Kleihauer-Betke (fetal hemoglobin acid elution, Hb F slide elution) test to quantify an acute fetal–maternal bleed
- Flow cytometry using antibody to Hemoglobin F is emerging as an alternative to the Kleihauer-Betke test to detect or quantify fetal–maternal bleed (6).
- Congenital or fetal anemia
- Blood type, direct Coombs test in newborn

Follow-Up Tests & Special Considerations

Prior administration of Rho(D) may lead to weakly (false-) positive indirect Coombs test in mother and direct Coombs test in infant.

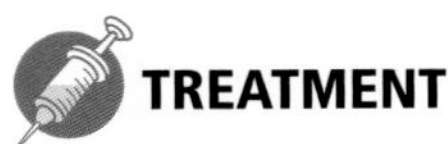

TREATMENT

GENERAL MEASURES

- Depending on severity of involvement, treatment of fetus may include the following:
  - Intrauterine transfusion (7)[C]
  - Early delivery
- Treatment of newborn may include the following:
  - Exchange transfusion
  - Transfusion after delivery
  - Phototherapy
  - Diuretics and digoxin for hydrops
  - Immunoglobulin infusion has reduced the need for exchange transfusion in a few studies (8)[B].

ISSUES FOR REFERRAL

Because of the specialized, somewhat hazardous treatment measures involved, pregnancies in Rh-sensitized women are usually managed at tertiary-care facilities.

INPATIENT CONSIDERATIONS

Admission Criteria/Initial Stabilization

Initial monitoring of the newborn is inpatient or in special care nursery if treatment interventions are needed.

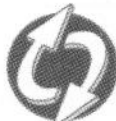

ONGOING CARE

FOLLOW-UP RECOMMENDATIONS

Patient Monitoring

- In most cases, outpatient ambulatory management is appropriate during the antepartum period.
- Antibody titer measured at 20 weeks and every 4 weeks thereafter during pregnancy; a titer of ≥1:16 indicates the need for further testing (9)
- If the patient had a previously affected infant, an Rh-positive fetus in the current pregnancy should be considered at risk regardless of antibody titers (10).
  - Fetal heart rate testing/US to assess fetal status
  - Doppler US measurement of cerebral blood flow is now a suitable alternative to invasive tests (amniocentesis, cordocentesis) for diagnosing fetal anemia (10).
  - Umbilical blood sampling (cordocentesis) for fetal blood type, hematocrit, reticulocyte count, and presence of erythroblasts (9)
  - Amniocentesis for amniotic fluid bilirubin levels (9)
  - Amniocentesis for fetal lung maturity if early delivery is a treatment option (9)

PROGNOSIS

- With appropriate monitoring and treatment, infants born of severely affected pregnancies have a survival rate of >80% (9).
- Even with severe disease, the neurologic outcome of survivors is generally good (7)[C].
- Fetuses with hydrops have a higher mortality rate and higher risk of neurologic impairment (7)[C].
- Disease is likely to be more severe in affected subsequent pregnancies.

COMPLICATIONS

- Pregnancy loss from umbilical blood sampling
- Pregnancy loss from intrauterine transfusion
- Fetal distress requiring emergent delivery (9)

REFERENCES

1. Shao C, Xu H, Xu Q, et al. Antenatal Rh prophylaxis is unnecessary for "Asia type" DEL women. *Transfus Clin Biol*. 2010;17(4):260–264.
2. Agre P, Cartron JP. Molecular biology of the Rh antigens. *Blood*. 1991;78(3):551–563.
3. Bianchi DW, Avent ND, Costa JM, et al. Noninvasive prenatal diagnosis of fetal Rhesus D: ready for prime(r) time. *Obstet Gynecol*. 2005;106(4):841–844.
4. Bowman J. Thirty-five years of Rh prophylaxis. *Transfusion*. 2003;43(12):1661–1666.
5. Crowther CA, Middleton P, McBain RD. Anti-D administration in pregnancy for preventing Rhesus alloimmunisation (review). *Cochrane Database Syst Rev*. 2013;2:CD000020.
6. Kim YA, Makar RS. Detection of fetomaternal hemorrhage. *Am J Hematol*. 2012;87(4):417–423.
7. Lindenberg IT, Smits-Wintjens VE, van Klink JM, et al. Long-term developmental outcome after intrauterine transfusion of the fetus/newborn: the LOTUS study. *Am J Obstet Gynecol*. 2012;206(2):141.e1–e8.
8. Elalfy MS, Elbarbary NS, Abaza HW. Early intravenous immunoglobulin (two-dose regimen) in the management of severe Rh hemolytic disease of newborn—a prospective randomized controlled trial. *Euro J Pediatr*. 2011;170(4):461–467.
9. American College of Obstetricians and Gynecologists. Management of alloimmunization during pregnancy. ACOG Practice Bulletin 75. Washington, DC: American College of Obstetricians and Gynecologists; 2006
10. Moise KJ. Management of rhesus alloimmunization in pregnancy. *Obstet Gynecol*. 2008;112(1):164–176.

ADDITIONAL READING

American College of Obstetricians and Gynecologists. Prevention of Rh D alloimmunization. ACOG Practice Bulletin 4. Washington, DC: American College of Obstetricians and Gynecologists; 1999, reaffirmed 2009.

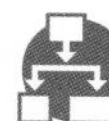

SEE ALSO

Anemia, Autoimmune Hemolytic; Erythroblastosis Fetalis; Jaundice

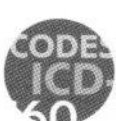

CODES

ICD10

- P55.0 Rh isoimmunization of newborn
- O36.0990 Maternal care for other rhesus isoimmunization, unspecified trimester, not applicable or unspecified
- T80.40XA Rh incompat react due to tranfs of bld/bld prod, unsp, init

CLINICAL PEARLS

- If paternity is certain, determining that the father does not carry the Rh(D) blood group antigen eliminates the need to give RhIG prophylaxis during pregnancy or the need for special fetal surveillance if the mother is already sensitized.
- Attempts have been made to determine the fetal blood type noninvasively by detecting fetal DNA in the maternal blood. Because Rh antigens are polymorphic among racial groups, this technique has both false-positive and false-negative results and should be considered experimental.
- The weak D antigen, formerly called D^u, is a weakly reacting variant of the D antigen. A "weak D–positive" mother or infant should be managed as any other D-positive mother or infant, respectively.
- The dose of RhIG for prophylaxis is affected by gestational age. The fetal blood volume is only a few milliliters at 12 weeks' gestation. Therefore, a 50-μg dose of RhIG may be used for threatened, spontaneous, or induced abortions up to 12 weeks' gestation, instead of the standard 300-μg dose.

RHABDOMYOSARCOMA

Ankur Goel, MD • Olusola Fasusi, MD • Edward James Kruse, DO

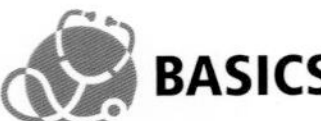

BASICS

DESCRIPTION

- Rhabdomyosarcoma (RMS) is the most common soft tissue sarcoma in children younger than 20 years of age. (It is exceedingly rare in adults, representing 3% of all soft tissue sarcomas.)
  - 50% occur in the 1st decade of life.
- Overall, it is an uncommon malignancy that arises from myoblasts.
- Common anatomic sites
  - Head and neck (most common primary site in children)
  - Genitourinary
  - Musculoskeletal (Extremities are the most common primary sites in adults.)
- Subtypes
  - Alveolar (ARMS): 23% of cases
    - More common in the trunk and extremities. Clinically more aggressive
  - Embryonal (ERMS): early onset. 57% of cases (most common subtype in children)
    - More likely to occur in the head, neck, and genitourinary areas
      - Classic: comprises 50% of cases
      - Botryoid: Sarcoma botryoids is typically seen in girls <4 years of age. 6% of cases
      - Spindle cell: 3% of cases pleomorphic: usually occurs in adults. 1% of cases
- Sarcoma (not otherwise specified): comprises 11% of all cases of RMS (most common subtype in adults, reflects inability for pathologists to characterize tumor)
- Undifferentiated: comprises 8% of all cases of RMS
- Associated term(s): soft tissue sarcoma

EPIDEMIOLOGY

Incidence

- 4.5 cases of RMS per 1 million patients <20 years old per year
  - 50% occur within 1st decade of life.
- In adults, RMS represents 3% of all soft tissue sarcomas in adults.

Prevalence

- RMS comprises 3% of all childhood cancers.
- Predominant sex: male > female (1.37:1)

Genetics

- Alveolar: *PAX3-FOXO1* or *PAX7-FOXO1* fusion genes as a result of t(2;13) and t(1;13), respectively; found in 75% of ARMS
- Embryonal: Loss of alleles on chromosome 11 may be seen.

RISK FACTORS

Smoking, advanced maternal age, in utero x-ray exposure, maternal recreational drug use, and history of stillbirths

COMMONLY ASSOCIATED CONDITIONS

- Neurofibromatosis (NF1) 1: 20-fold increased risk of RMS in patients with NF1
- Li-Fraumeni syndrome: p53 mutations predispose to multiple tumors, including RMS.

DIAGNOSIS

HISTORY

- Presents as a progressive painless mass of the head and neck, genitourinary tissue, trunk, or extremities
- RMS of genitourinary tissue may present as vaginal bleeding in females.
- Other symptoms may be noted due to mass effect of the primary or metastatic lesions.
- Family history of genetic syndromes (i.e., NF1, Li-Fraumeni syndrome)

PHYSICAL EXAM

- Painless, enlarging mass
- Polypoid mass protruding from vagina (botryoid)
- Exophthalmos and chemosis (orbital involvement)
- Abdominal pain
- Compression symptoms (i.e., seizures, visual field defects, nerve palsy, headaches)

DIAGNOSTIC TESTS & INTERPRETATION

Initial Tests (lab, imaging)

- Ultrasound: used for differentiation of cystic versus solid mass
- MRI/CT: used to evaluate tumor
- Staging tests: chest x-ray, CT thorax, fluorodeoxyglucose (FDG)-PET
  - Most common site of metastasis is lung; evaluated by CT
  - FDG-PET scans may be useful to detect lymph node or distant metastases; not readily evident on CT or MRI scans

Diagnostic Procedures/Other

- Core needle biopsy, incisional biopsy, or excisional biopsy (based on size of mass)
  - The presence of rhabdomyoblast indicates the diagnosis.
- Immunohistochemical markers
  - Myogenin: commonly expressed in ARMS
  - Desmin: associated with multiple subtypes of RMS
- Pathology
  - Alveolar: rhabdomyoblasts arranged in what grossly appears to mimic pulmonary alveoli
  - Embryonal
  - Classic: rhabdomyoblasts configured in sheets without alveolar pattern
  - Botryoid: "grape-like" appearance of rhabdomyoblasts with notable clustering in the subepithelium forming the cambium layer
  - Spindle cell: rhabdomyoblasts with a spindle-like appearance
- Undifferentiated: rhabdomyoblast arrangement that cannot be classified as any other subtype
- Staging
  - Based on site, size, regional nodal involvement, and distance spread
  - See table.

Stage	Site	T	Tumor diameter	N	M
1	Orbit; head and neck (excluding parameningeal); genitourinary—nonbladder and nonprostate; biliary tract	T1 or T2	a or b	N0 or N1 or NX	M0
2	Bladder or prostate; extremity; cranial parameningeal; other (includes trunk, retroperitoneum, etc.)	T1 or T2	a	N0 or NX	M0
3	Bladder or prostate; extremity; cranial parameningeal; other (includes trunk, retroperitoneum, etc.)	T1 or T2	a	N1	M0
			0 or N1 or NX	M0	
4	All sites	T1 or T2	a or b	N0 or N1	M1

Note: a, ≤5 cm in diameter; b, >5 cm in diameter; M0, no distant metastasis present; M1, metastasis present; N0, regional nodes not clinically involved; N1, regional nodes clinically involved by neoplasm; Nx, clinical status of regional nodes unknown; T1, confined to site of origin; T2, extension and/or fixation to surrounding tissue.

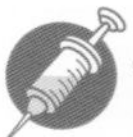

TREATMENT

The 3 tenets of treatment for adults and children consist of surgical resection, radiation therapy, and chemotherapy. Patients should be referred to a multidisciplinary treatment team with expertise in oncology for definitive treatment.

SURGERY/OTHER PROCEDURES

- Wide local resection of tumor. If possible, resect metastasis as well.
- However, wide resection may not be feasible in cases where grossly impaired functionality results.
  - All children receive chemotherapy (1)[B].
  - In North America, the 3-drug combination of vincristine, dactinomycin, and cyclophosphamide (VAC) is the standard regimen:
    - Vincristine
      - Adverse reactions: alopecia, constipation, peripheral neuropathy
    - Actinomycin-D
      - Adverse reactions: pancytopenia, hepatotoxicity
    - Cyclophosphamide
      - Adverse reactions: hemorrhagic cystitis (mesna for prophylaxis), sterility, transitional cell carcinoma
- In addition, ifosfamide, topotecan, doxorubicin, etoposide, and irinotecan may also be used.
- Duration of chemotherapy is dependent on risk stratification and ranges from 6 to 12 months.
- Chemotherapy has been less commonly used in adults, who generally undergo treatment with resection and radiation therapy.
- Radiotherapy is currently used for those whose tumor cannot be completely resected.

ONGOING CARE

FOLLOW-UP RECOMMENDATIONS

Patients should follow up with their multidisciplinary treatment team. Long-term follow-up is necessary for detection of recurrence, metastatic disease, and development of secondary malignancies. Follow-up consists of physical exam, chest x-ray, and imaging of the primary tumor site every 3–6 months for the 1st 3 years.

PROGNOSIS

- RMS (all cases): 62% 5-year survival
- ARMS: 48% 5-year survival
- ERMS: 73% 5-year survival
- Prognosis in adults is worse, it is unclear whether this is related to subtype of tumor or lack of clear guidelines for adults; this is a rare presentation in adults.

COMPLICATIONS

- Recurrence
- Secondary neoplasm
- Growth abnormalities
- Treatment side effects

REFERENCES

1. Ray A, Huh WW. Current state-of-the-art systemic therapy for pediatric soft tissue sarcomas. *Curr Oncol Rep*. 2012;14(4):311–319.

ADDITIONAL READING

- Arndt CA, Rose PS, Folpe AL, et al. Common musculoskeletal tumors of childhood and adolescence. *Mayo Clin Proc*. 2012;87(5):475–487.
- Hawkins DS, Spunt SL, Skapek SX. Children's Oncology Group's 2013 blueprint for research: soft tissue sarcomas. *Pediatr Blood Cancer*. 2013;60(6):1001–1008.
- Kapoor G, Das K. Soft tissue sarcomas in children. *Indian J Pediatr*. 2012;79(7):936–942.
- Klem ML, Grewal RK, Wexler LH, et al. PET for staging in rhabdomyosarcoma: an evaluation of PET as an adjunct to current staging tools. *J Pediatr Hematol Oncol*. 2007;29(1):9–14.
- Malempati S, Hawkins DS. Rhabdomyosarcoma: review of the Children's Oncology Group Soft-Tissue Sarcoma Committee experience and rationale for current COG studies. *Pediatr Blood Cancer*. 2012;59(1):5–10.
- Ognjanovic S, Linabery AM, Charbonneau B, et al. Trends in childhood rhabdomyosarcoma incidence and survival in the United States, 1975–2005. *Cancer*. 2009;115(18):4218–4226.
- Parham DM, Ellison DA. Rhabdomyosarcomas in adults and children. *Arch Pathol Lab Med*. 2006;130(10):1454–1465.
- Sultan I, Qaddoumi I, Yaser S, et al. Comparing adult and pediatric rhabdomyosarcoma in the surveillance, epidemiology and end results program, 1973 to 2005: an analysis of 2,600 patients. *J Clin Oncol*. 2009;27(20):3391–3397.

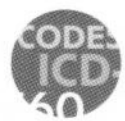

CODES

ICD10

- C49.9 Malignant neoplasm of connective and soft tissue, unsp
- C49.0 Malignant neoplasm of connective and soft tissue of head, face and neck
- C49.5 Malignant neoplasm of connective and soft tissue of pelvis

CLINICAL PEARLS

- RMS is the most common soft tissue sarcoma in children.
- They can arise at any site and in any tissue except bone.
- All persistent soft tissue masses should be evaluated with imaging (ultrasound to rule out cystic vs. solid, then MRI/CT).
- Fine-needle aspiration may be helpful but core needle versus incisional/excisional biopsy for confirmation.

RHEUMATIC FEVER

Jonathan Schimmel, MD • Achyut B. Kamat, MD, FACEP

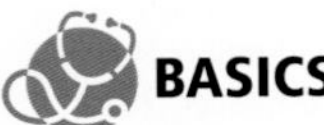

BASICS

DESCRIPTION

- Acute rheumatic fever (ARF) is a delayed inflammatory sequela of group A *Streptococcus* (GAS) tonsillopharyngitis that affects multiple organ systems.
- Can lead to rheumatic heart disease (RHD)
- Recurrence in adults and children is common if antibiotic prophylaxis is withheld.
- Systems affected: cardiovascular, nervous, hematologic/lymphatic/immunologic, skin/exocrine, musculoskeletal

Pediatric Considerations

Can affect any age but most common ages 5–15 years

EPIDEMIOLOGY

- ARF and RHD are now largely restricted to developing countries and some poor populations of wealthy countries.
- Male = female, but females more likely to develop chorea.
- Can occur as an epidemic

Incidence

- Worldwide, incidence (new cases) has been declining for decades due to increasing antibiotic use and improved living conditions.
- In early studies, ARF developed in 3% of children with untreated GAS pharyngitis (1).
- Incidence of ARF in the United States in the 1960s was 13.3/100,000 and is currently <1/100,000 (1).
- 95% of cases currently occur in developing countries (1).

Prevalence

Worldwide, 15.6 million people have RHD, and prevalence has been rising due to improved medical care and longer survival (despite decreasing incidence of ARF) (1).

ETIOLOGY AND PATHOPHYSIOLOGY

- Preceded by tonsillopharyngitis of GAS, also known as *Streptococcus pyogenes*, a gram-positive organism
- Molecular mimicry: Antibodies against M protein on GAS cross-reacts with cardiac and vessel endothelial proteins, leading to an inflammatory cascade (2).

Genetics

- Susceptibility is associated with certain genetic polymorphisms, including toll-like receptors, cytokines, and human leukocyte antigen genes (2).
- Increased susceptibility in certain populations, including Australian aborigines and Pacific Islanders

RISK FACTORS

Genetic susceptibility, possible increased risk with iron deficiency or low serum albumin

GENERAL PREVENTION

- Primary prevention: Antibiotics are effective at reducing incidence of ARF after known or suspected GAS pharyngitis. Number needed to treat is 100 (3).
- Secondary prevention: long-term antibiotic prophylaxis to prevent recurrence

DIAGNOSIS

- Requires evidence of preceding GAS infection (see "Initial Tests")
- Modified Jones criteria for diagnosis
  - 2 major OR 1 major + 2 minor

Major Criteria	Minor Criteria
• Carditis/valvulitis	• Fever
• Polyarthritis	• Arthralgia
• Sydenham chorea	• AV block on ECG
• Erythema marginatum	• ↑ inflammatory markers (ESR, CRP)
• Subcutaneous nodules	

- Can diagnose ARF without Jones criteria if isolated chorea, isolated indolent carditis after GAS infection, recurrent ARF with history of ARF (4)

HISTORY

- ARF presents 1–4 weeks following GAS tonsillopharyngitis.
- Polyarthritis is often first, affecting the knees, ankles, elbows, and wrists. Each resolves in days, thus seems to "migrate."
- Fever
- Erythema marginatum rash
- Pancarditis or valvulitis can be asymptomatic or symptomatic.
- Sydenham chorea (clinical diagnosis) (5)
  - 1–6 months after infection, in 10–30% of patients. More common ages 5–15 years, more common in females
  - Improves or ceases during sleep
  - Psychiatric symptoms may have onset prior to chorea, with emotional lability and obsessive-compulsive symptoms.
  - Usually self-resolves over several months, can relapse

PHYSICAL EXAM

- Neuro: Sydenham chorea: Involuntary movements may be general or unilateral and may involve the face. "Milkmaid grip" is intermittent hypotonia appreciated on test of grip strength.
- Cardiac: pericardial friction rub, blowing holosystolic murmur, rarely diastolic, or new or changing murmur. Rarely evidence of heart failure
- Skin
  - Subcutaneous nodules: firm, painless, up to 2 cm, over bony surfaces or tendons, usually extensor surfaces. More common in severe ARF, remains up to several weeks
  - Erythema marginatum (5–13%): nonpruritic evanescent, pale red macular transitions to central clearing, found on trunk and occasionally limbs, accentuated by warming the skin

DIFFERENTIAL DIAGNOSIS

- Systemic lupus erythematosus
- Poststreptococcal reactive arthritis
- Juvenile rheumatoid arthritis
- Infectious arthritis
- Viral myocarditis
- Innocent cardiac murmur
- Tourette syndrome
- Kawasaki syndrome
- Pediatric autoimmune neuropsychiatric disorders associated with streptococcal infections (PANDAS)

DIAGNOSTIC TESTS & INTERPRETATION

Initial Tests (lab, imaging)

- CBC with differential: leukocytosis, possible normocytic anemia
- ESR and CRP are acute-phase reactants that increase.
- Bacteriologic/serologic evidence of GAS infection
  - Rapid streptococcal antigen test
  - Throat culture (sensitivity 25% by time of ARF)
  - Antistreptolysin O (ASO) titer peaks ~1 month post infection (5).
  - If ASO negative, check anti-DNAse B (peaks ~2.5 months, remains elevated up to 9 months), streptokinase, and antihyaluronidase (5).
- Complement levels normal (do not need to check)
- ECG: AV block of any degree, signs of pericarditis
- Arthrocentesis of affected joints shows sterile inflammatory fluid with 10–100,000 WBC/mm^3.
- Chest x-ray: may have cardiomegaly from myocarditis
- Echocardiogram: Assess chamber size and function, pericardial effusion, and valve disease.
- Antimyosin scintigraphy can detect carditis (nonspecific).

Follow-Up Tests & Special Considerations

- ESR and CRP are useful to monitor rebound inflammation.
- Repeat echocardiograms to monitor evolution of valvular lesions.
- Household contacts should be screened with throat culture even if asymptomatic, and if positive, treated with antibiotics.

Test Interpretation

Prior treatment with aspirin or steroids may alter lab results.

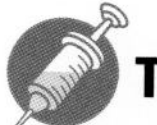

TREATMENT

GENERAL MEASURES

- Antibiotic
- Anti-inflammatory agent (aspirin or naproxen)
- Manage cardiac manifestations as needed in addition to standard ARF treatment (dysrhythmia, pericarditis, myocarditis, valvular disease, heart failure, etc.).

MEDICATION

First Line

- Eradication: Treat initially as if active GAS infection, and then begin prophylaxis.
  - Penicillin V PO × 10 days or benzathine PCN G IM × 1, or amoxicillin PO × 10 days (preferred in children), or 1st-generation cephalosporin PO × 10 days (6)[A]
  - If allergic to penicillins: azithromycin PO × 5 days, clindamycin PO × 10 days, or clarithromycin PO × 10 days (6)[B]
- If there is heart failure, AV block 3rd degree, or other severe manifestations of carditis, appropriate traditional management should be initiated.
- Start aspirin 80–100 mg/kg/day in children and 4–8 g/day in adults × 4–6 weeks until symptoms resolve and ESR, CRP normalize. Aspirin is effective for treatment of arthritis and fever (7)[B]. Efficacy has not been shown to reduce or improve cardiac manifestations (8)[B].
- If severe carditis present, can consider prednisone, although not shown to prevent or reduce cardiac manifestations (8)[B]
- Chorea generally self-resolves and does not require treatment, but if symptoms is severe, can use valproic acid, carbamazepine, or if resistant, an antipsychotic (5)[B]. If still resistant, can use prednisone, which unlike cardiac disease has been shown effective for Sydenham chorea (5)[B]

Second Line

See above

ISSUES FOR REFERRAL

A cardiologist should be involved in management of ARF.

SURGERY/OTHER PROCEDURES

Valve stenosis is a late sequela that can result from fibrosis and calcification; it may require surgical correction (valve repair preferred over replacement).

INPATIENT CONSIDERATIONS

Admission Criteria/Initial Stabilization

- Initial hospitalization may be helpful for diagnosis and to ensure stability.
- Heart failure requires prompt hospitalization.

IV Fluids

Only if signs of dehydration or to augment preload; use caution if heart failure present.

Nursing

Bed rest initially, with gradual return to activity as symptoms subside

ONGOING CARE

FOLLOW-UP RECOMMENDATIONS

- ARF patients should be on a prophylactic antibiotic throughout childhood until age 21 years and possibly indefinitely depending on cardiac damage because recurrence can worsen prognosis (9)[C].
  - 1st-line prophylaxis is long-acting penicillin G monthly IM injections (9)[A].
  - Penicillin V PO 250 mg BID is an alternative but has risk of nonadherence (9)[B].
  - If penicillin allergy, treat with sulfadiazine (9)[B].
  - If penicillin and sulfa drug allergy, treat with azithromycin (9)[C].
- Routine antibiotic prophylaxis for dental procedures is no longer recommended for patients with RHD (10).
- Have low threshold to test and treat episodes of acute tonsillopharyngitis

Patient Monitoring

Initially weekly, then every 6 months

Pediatric Considerations

Use aspirin with caution in children, given risk of Reye syndrome. Naproxen has been found safe and effective in ARF and has fewer side effects than aspirin (7)[B].

Pregnancy Considerations

May exacerbate valve disease, particularly mitral stenosis. Refer pregnant patients to a cardiologist.

DIET

- Regular diet
- Low-sodium if heart failure present

PATIENT EDUCATION

American Heart Association: http://www.heart.org

PROGNOSIS

Sequelae are limited to the heart and depend on the severity of carditis during an acute attack.

COMPLICATIONS

- Recurrence of ARF due to GAS reinfection
- RHD can occur 10–20 years after ARF, with mitral more common than aortic regurgitation, can lead to stenosis. Heart failure is worst complication.
- Jaccoud arthropathy is chronic and involves painless deformities of hands/feet.

REFERENCES

1. Chang C. Cutting edge issues in rheumatic fever. *Clin Rev Allergy Immunol*. 2012;42(2):213–237.
2. Guilherme L, Köhler KF, Postol E, et al. Genes, autoimmunity and pathogenesis of rheumatic heart disease. *Ann Pediatr Cardiol*. 2011;4(1):13–21.
3. Del Mar CB, Glasziou PP, Spinks AB, et al. Antibiotics for sore throat. *Cochrane Database Syst Rev*. 2006;(4):CD000023.
4. Ferrieri P. Proceedings of the jones criteria workshop. *Circulation*. 2002;106(19):2521–2523.
5. Oosterveer DM, Overweg-Plandsoen WC, Roos RA. Sydenham's chorea: a practical overview of the current literature. *Pediatr Neurol*. 2010;43(1):1–6.
6. Shulman ST, Bisno AL, Clegg HW, et al. Clinical practice guideline for the diagnosis and management of group A streptococcal pharyngitis: 2012 update by the Infectious Diseases Society of America. *Clin Infect Dis*. 2012;55(10):e86–e102.
7. Hashkes PJ, Tauber T, Somekh E, et al. Naproxen as an alternative to aspirin for the treatment of arthritis of rheumatic fever: a randomized trial. *J Pediatr*. 2003;143(3):399–401.
8. Cilliers AM, Manyemba J, Saloojee H, et al. Anti-inflammatory treatment for carditis in acute rheumatic fever. *Cochrane Database Syst Rev*. 2003;(2):CD003176.
9. Gerber MA, Baltimore RS, Eaton CB, et al. Prevention of rheumatic fever and diagnosis and treatment of acute streptococcal pharyngitis: a scientific statement from the American Heart Association Rheumatic Fever, Endocarditis, and Kawasaki Disease Committee of the Council on Cardiovascular Disease in the Young, the Interdisciplinary Council on Functional Genomics and Translational Biology, and the Interdisciplinary Council on Quality of Care and Outcomes Research: endorsed by the American Academy of Pediatrics. *Circulation*. 2009;119(11):1541–1551.
10. Wilson W, Taubert KA, Gewitz M, et al. Prevention of infective endocarditis guidelines from the American Heart Association: a guideline from the American Heart Association Rheumatic Fever, Endocarditis, and Kawasaki Disease Committee, Council on Cardiovascular Disease in the Young, and the Council on Clinical Cardiology, Council on Cardiovascular Surgery and Anesthesia, and the Quality of Care and Outcomes Research Interdisciplinary Working Group. *Circulation*. 2007;116(15):1736–1754.

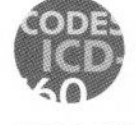

CODES

ICD10

- I00 Rheumatic fever without heart involvement
- I01.9 Acute rheumatic heart disease, unspecified
- I01.0 Acute rheumatic pericarditis

CLINICAL PEARLS

- ARF is an inflammatory disease that affects multiple organ systems including the heart.
- Modified Jones criteria for diagnosis include 2 major or 1 major + 2 minor manifestation in the context of a preceding documented GAS infection.
- Treatment involves aspirin and antibiotic eradication followed immediately by long-term antibiotic prophylaxis.

RHINITIS, ALLERGIC

Naureen Bashir Rafiq, MBBS, MD

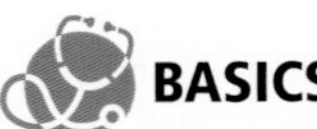

BASICS

Allergic rhinitis is the collection of symptoms, involving mucous membranes of nose, eyes, ears, and throat after an exposure to allergens like pollen, dust, or dander.

DESCRIPTION

- IgE-mediated inflammation of the nasal mucosa following exposure to an extrinsic protein; an immediate symptomatic response is characterized by sneezing, congestion, and rhinorrhea followed by a persistent late phase dominated by congestion and mucosal hyperreactivity.
- Allergic rhinitis can be classified into seasonal or perennial and can be intermittent or persistent.
- Seasonal responses are usually due to outdoor allergens like tree pollen, flowering shrubs in spring, grasses and flowering plants in summer, and ragweed and mold in fall.
- Perennial responses, or year-round symptoms, are usually associated with indoor allergens like dust mites, mold, and animal dander.
- Occupational allergic rhinitis is caused by allergens at the workplace and can be sporadic or year-round.
- Nonallergic rhinitis (e.g., vasomotor, rhinitis of pregnancy, and rhinitis medicamentosa) can occur.

Pediatric Considerations

Chronic nasal obstruction can result in facial deformities, dental malocclusions, and sleep disorders.

Pregnancy Considerations

Physiologic changes during pregnancy may aggravate all types of rhinitis, frequently in the 2nd trimester.

EPIDEMIOLOGY

- Onset usually in first 2 decades, rarely before 6 months of age, with tendency declining with advancing age.
- The mean age of onset is 8–11 years, and about 80% of cases have established allergic rhinitis by age 20 years.

Prevalence

- ~10–25% of the U.S. adult population and 9–42% of the U.S. pediatric population are affected.
- 44–87% of patients with allergic rhinitis have mixed allergic and nonallergic rhinitis, which is more common than either pure form (1).
- Scandinavian studies have demonstrated cumulative prevalence rate of 14% in men and 15% in women.

ETIOLOGY AND PATHOPHYSIOLOGY

- Aeroallergen-driven mucosal inflammation due to resident and infiltrating inflammatory cells, as well as vasoactive and proinflammatory mediators (e.g., cytokines)
- Inhalant allergens:
  - Perennial: house dust mites, indoor molds, animal dander, cockroach/insect detritus
  - Seasonal: tree, grass, and weed pollens; outdoor molds
  - Occupational: latex, plant products (e.g., baking flour), sensitizing chemicals, and certain animals for people working in farms and vet clinics

Genetics

Complex but strong genetic predilection present (80% have family history of allergic disorders)

RISK FACTORS

- Family history of atopy, with a greater risk if both parents have atopy
- Higher socioeconomic status
- Tobacco smoke can exacerbate symptoms and increase risk of developing asthma in patients with allergic rhinitis.
- Having other allergies like asthma
- Unclear evidence regarding risk due to early, repeated exposure to offending allergen and early introduction of solid food.
- Pets in house and houses infested with cockroaches can cause perennial allergic rhinitis.

GENERAL PREVENTION

- Primary prevention of atopic disease has not been proven effective by maternal diet or maternal allergen avoidance (2).
- Exclusive breastfeeding to 6 months of age lowers risk of some atopic disorders
- Symptomatic control by environmental avoidance is the "1st-line treatment."
- No evidence to support use of acaricides with mite-proof mattress and pillow covers, carpet and drape removal, removal of plants in the home, and pet control (2,3)[B].
- Air conditioning and limited outside exposure during allergy season (1)[B].
- HEPA air cleaners and vacuum bags of unclear efficacy.
- Close doors and windows during allergy season.
- Use a dehumidifier to reduce indoor humidity.

COMMONLY ASSOCIATED CONDITIONS

Other IgE-mediated conditions: asthma, atopic dermatitis, allergic conjunctivitis, food allergy

DIAGNOSIS

Diagnosis is made primarily by history and physical exam.

HISTORY

- Evaluation of nature, duration, and time course of symptoms
- History of atopic dermatitis and/or food allergies
- History of nasal congestion; rhinorrhea; pruritus of nose, eyes, ears, and/or palate; sneezing; itching; and watering eyes
- Family history of allergic diseases
- History of environmental and occupational exposure and various nasal stimuli can help differentiate between allergic and vasomotor rhinitis.

PHYSICAL EXAM

Many findings are suggestive of but not specific for allergic rhinitis:

- Dark circles under eyes, "allergic shiners" (infraorbital venous congestion)
- Transverse nasal crease from rubbing nose upward; typically seen in children
- Rhinorrhea, usually with clear discharge
- Pale, boggy, blue-gray nasal mucosa
- Postnasal mucus discharge
- Oropharyngeal lymphoid tissue hypertrophy

DIFFERENTIAL DIAGNOSIS

- Infectious rhinitis: usually viral, commonly with secondary bacterial infection
  - Usually associated with sinusitis and is known as rhinosinusitis
  - Viral rhinitis averages 6 episodes/year from ages 2–6 years.
  - IgA deficiency with recurrent sinusitis
  - Rhinitis medicamentosa:
    - Rebound effect associated with continued use of topical decongestant drops and sprays
    - ACE inhibitors, reserpine, β-blockers, oral contraceptive pills (OCPs), guanethidine, methyldopa
    - Aspirin, NSAIDs
  - Vasomotor (idiopathic) rhinitis caused by numerous nasal stimuli like warm or cold air, scents and odors, light or particulate matter
  - Hormonal: pregnancy, thyroid, OCPs
  - Nonallergic rhinitis with eosinophilia syndrome (NARES)
  - Gustatory: watery rhinorrhea in response to alcohol or food
  - "Skier's nose": watery rhinorrhea in response to cold air
- Conditions associated with rhinitis:
  - Nasal polyps, tumor
  - Septal/anatomic obstruction
    - Adenoidal hypertrophy, particularly in children
    - Septal abnormality or deflected nasal septum (DNS) in adults

DIAGNOSTIC TESTS & INTERPRETATION

- Lab tests rarely needed
- Skin testing is done to identify the allergen for immunotherapy.

Initial Tests (lab, imaging)

- Testing is rarely indicated.
- If diagnosis implies other causes, consider the following:
  - CBC with differential may show elevated eosinophils.
  - Increased total serum IgE level
  - Nasal probe smear may show elevated eosinophils.
- Medications that may alter lab results
  - Corticosteroids may decrease eosinophilia.
  - Antihistamines suppress reactivity to skin tests; stop antihistamines 7 days before testing.
- CT scan of sinuses is not routinely done, but can be used to check for complete opacity, fluid level, and mucosal thickening.

Diagnostic Procedures/Other

- Consider testing in only those cases where allergic symptoms do not respond to treatment and/or considering immunotherapy.
- Specific allergen sensitivity with allergen skin testing or radioallergosorbent testing (RAST); clinical correlation based on history is essential in interpreting results.
- Diagnostic allergen prick tests are used to select agent to determine appropriate environmental control measures, as well as to direct immunotherapy:
  - Prick or puncture: superficial injury to epidermis with application of test antigen
  - Intradermal
- RAST: more expensive and less sensitive than skin testing; typically used in patients in whom skin testing is not practical or a severe reaction is possible
- Rhinoscopy: useful to visualize intranasal anatomy and posterior pharyngeal structures, including adenoids, polyps, and larynx

Test Interpretation

- Nasal washing/scraping: Eosinophils predominate but may see basophils, mast cells.
- Nasal mucosa: submucosal edema but without destruction; eosinophilic infiltration; congested mucous glands and goblet cells

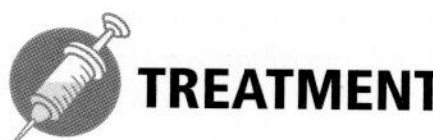

TREATMENT

There are 3 mainstays of treatment of allergic rhinitis:

- Allergen avoidance
- Medication
- Allergy immunotherapy

GENERAL MEASURES

- Establish specific cause(s) by history and appropriate testing.
- Limit exposure to offending allergen.
- Allergen immunotherapy (desensitization)
  - Reserved when symptoms are uncontrollable with medical therapy or have a comorbidity (e.g., asthma)
  - Specific allergen extract is injected SC in increasing doses to induce patient tolerance.

MEDICATION

Oral medication and intranasal sprays are commonly used.

First Line

- Mild symptoms: 2nd-generation nonsedating antihistamines are 1st-line therapy for mild to moderate allergic rhinitis (1,4).
- Adverse effects: mild sedation, mild anticholinergic effects
- Generic (cetirizine, fexofenadine, loratadine; most to least effective)
  - Levocetirizine is a new 2nd-generation nonsedating antihistamine that is effective, but costly.
- Intranasal corticosteroids are 1st-line therapy for moderate to severe allergic rhinitis (1,4)[A]:
  - Most effective drug class for symptoms of allergic rhinitis
  - Use nasal sprays after showering and direct spray away from septum to improve deposition on mucosal surface.
  - May be used as needed; however, less effective than regular use (1)
  - Adverse effects: nosebleed, nasal septal perforation, and systemic corticosteroid effects
- Systemic steroids should be considered only in urgent cases and only for short-term use.

Second Line

1st-generation antihistamines, such as the following:

- Brompheniramine: 12–24 mg PO BID
- Chlorpheniramine: 4 mg PO q4–6h PRN
- Clemastine: 1–2 mg PO BID PRN
- Diphenhydramine: 25–50 mg PO q4–6h PRN:
  - May precipitate urinary retention in men with prostatism and/or hypertrophy
  - Adverse effects: sedation, prolonged QT interval, performance impairment, and anticholinergic effect
- Nasal antihistamines effective but may be systemically absorbed and thus cause sedation: azelastine, olopatadine
- Decongestants
  - Phenylephrine: 10 mg PO q4h PRN
  - Pseudoephedrine: 60 mg PO q4–6h PRN
  - Oxymetazoline nasal spray (Afrin): 2–3 sprays per nostril q10–12h PRN (max 3 days). Intranasal agents should not be used for >3 days due to rebound rhinitis. Discourage use in patients with hypertension (HTN) or cardiac arrhythmia.
- Intranasal anticholinergics such as ipratropium nasal spray 2 sprays per nostril BID–TID
  - Intranasal anticholinergics can increase efficacy in combination with steroid use.
- Leukotriene antagonists such as montelukast 10 mg/day PO
  - Should generally be used as an adjunct, not monotherapy
- Mast cell stabilizers such as cromolyn nasal spray 1 spray per nostril TID–QID
  - May take 2–4 weeks of therapy for optimal efficacy
  - May be ineffective in patients with nonallergic rhinitis and nasal polyps

ISSUES FOR REFERRAL

Refer to allergist for consideration of immunotherapy.

ADDITIONAL THERAPIES

- Immunotherapy, either by injection (5)[A] or sublingually, which may be better tolerated by children (6)[A]
- Nasal saline use has evidence of efficacy as sole agent or as adjunctive treatment (1,7)[A].

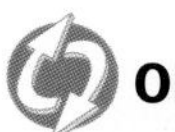

ONGOING CARE

FOLLOW-UP RECOMMENDATIONS

No specific restrictions on activity; emphasize avoiding activity where exposure to the allergen is likely.

Patient Monitoring

Initiation of patient education is critical.

DIET

- No special diet unless concomitant food reactions are suspected and evaluated.
- Some patients with severe sensitivity to seasonal pollens may have oral allergy syndrome, which is associated with itching in the mouth with the ingestion of fresh fruits that may cross-react with the allergens.

PATIENT EDUCATION

- Asthma & Allergy Foundation of America, 1717 Massachusetts Ave., Suite 305, Washington, DC 20036; (800) 7-ASTHMA: www.aafa.org
- Other helpful information available at www.acaai.org and www.aaaai.org

PROGNOSIS

- Acceptable control of symptoms is the goal.
- Treatment is helpful to reduce the risk of comorbidities, such as sinusitis and asthma.

COMPLICATIONS

- Secondary infection such as otitis media or sinusitis
- Epistaxis
- Nasopharyngeal lymphoid hyperplasia
- Airway hyperreactivity with allergen exposure
- Asthma
- Facial changes, especially in children who are mouth breathers
- Sleep disturbance

REFERENCES

1. Wallace DV. The diagnosis and management of rhinitis: an updated practice parameter. *J Allergy Clin Immunol*. 2008;122 (2)(Suppl):S1–S84.
2. Kramer MS, Kakuma R. Maternal dietary antigen avoidance during pregnancy or lactation, or both, for preventing or treating atopic disease in the child. *Cochrane Database Syst Rev*. 2012;9:CD000133.
3. Sheikh A, Hurwitz B, Nurmatov U, et al. House dust mite avoidance measures for perennial allergic rhinitis. *Cochrane Database Syst Rev*. 2010;(7):CD001563.
4. Plaut M, Valentine MD. Clinical practice. Allergic rhinitis. *N Engl J Med*. 2005;353(18):1934–1944.
5. Calderon MA, Alves B, Jacobson M, et al. Allergen injection immunotherapy for seasonal allergic rhinitis. *Cochrane Database Syst Rev*. 2007;(1):CD001936.
6. Wilson DR, Lima MT, Durham SR. Sublingual immunotherapy for allergic rhinitis: systematic review and meta-analysis. *Allergy*. 2005;60(1):4–12.
7. Harvey R, Hannan SA, Badia L, et al. Nasal saline irrigations for the symptoms of chronic rhinosinusitis. *Cochrane Database Syst Rev*. 2007;(3):CD006394.

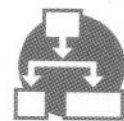

SEE ALSO

Conjunctivitis, Acute

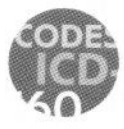

CODES

ICD10

- J30.9 Allergic rhinitis, unspecified
- J30.1 Allergic rhinitis due to pollen
- J30.2 Other seasonal allergic rhinitis

CLINICAL PEARLS

- Nasal saline irrigation (flushing 6–8 oz) may be very helpful in clearing upper airway of secretions and may precede the use of nasal corticosteroids.
- 2nd-generation antihistamines and intranasal corticosteroids are 1st-line therapies for allergic rhinitis.
- Referral to allergist is appropriate for identification of offending allergens and consideration of immunotherapy for inadequate symptom control.

ROCKY MOUNTAIN SPOTTED FEVER

Ginny H. Lee, MD • Alison Southern, MD, MS, FACEP

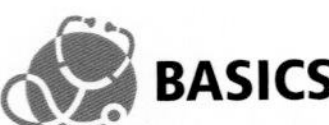

BASICS

DESCRIPTION

- Rocky Mountain spotted fever (RMSF) is a potentially fatal tick-borne systemic small vessel vasculitis caused by the bacterium *Rickettsia rickettsii*.
- RMSF is the most common (and most lethal) rickettsial disease in the United States.
- Typically characterized by fever, headache, and myalgias followed by a centripetal (moving inward from the extremities toward the trunk) rash
- System(s) affected: cardiovascular, musculoskeletal, skin, CNS, renal, hepatic, and pulmonary

EPIDEMIOLOGY

Incidence

- In the United States, the incidence of RMSF increased from <2 cases per million persons in 2000 to >8 per million in 2008 (1).
- Reported in all states except Hawaii, Alaska, and Maine
- North Carolina, Tennessee, Oklahoma, Arkansas, and Missouri account for ~60% of cases. RMSF also found in areas of Canada and in Central and South America (2).
- Predominant age: All ages are susceptible; highest prevalence in children 5–9 years of age (2,3).
- Predominant sex: male > female, likely a product of outdoor exposure (3,4).
- Peak incidence occurs with tick exposure, typically in late spring and summer (3).

Prevalence

In the United States, about 2,000 cases are reported annually (2).

- <0.1% of ticks carry virulent Rickettsial species.

ETIOLOGY AND PATHOPHYSIOLOGY

- Infected ticks are primarily the American dog tick, *Dermacentor variabilis* in the eastern United States; the Rocky Mountain wood tick, *Dermacentor andersoni* in the western United States; and the Brown dog tick, *Rhipicephalus sanuineus* in the southwest (1,2).
- An adult tick releases *Rickettsia rickettsii* from its salivary glands after 6–10 hours of feeding (1).
- Rickettsiae proliferate inside endothelial cells by binary fission and invade contiguous vascular endothelial cells, causing a small-vessel vasculitis and the characteristic rash.
- Subsequent increased vascular permeability can lead to edema, hypovolemia, and hypoalbuminemia, with subsequent end-organ injury.
- Platelets are consumed locally due to vascular injury, but coagulopathy or disseminated intravascular coagulation (DIC) is rare (4).
- Incubation time: 2–14 days, with a median of 4–7 days.
- Transplacental transmission of infection has not been demonstrated.
- RMSF can rarely be caused by direct inoculation of tick blood into open wounds or conjunctivae.

RISK FACTORS

- Known tick bite, engorged tick, or presence of tick for >20 hours; *likelihood of infection increases with duration of tick attachment*
- Crushed tick during its removal
- Accumulated outdoor exposure or residence in a wooded area
- Contact with outdoor pets or wild animals

GENERAL PREVENTION

In known tick-prone areas (2,4,5)

- Limit time spent in tall grasses, open areas of low bushy vegetation, and wooded areas.
- Cover exposed skin; wear a hat, long sleeves, pants and closed-toed shoes.
- Use DEET-containing insect repellents on exposed skin. Permethrin can be used on clothing.
- "Tick checks": Carefully inspect the entire body after possible exposure, especially the scalp, neck, and axillae. Ticks are commonly hidden by hair. Closely inspect legs, groin, external genitalia, and waistlines.
- Remove attached ticks in their entirety with fine-tipped tweezers. Grasp the tick close to the skin and gently pull upward. If mouth-parts separate, try to remove gently. Nail polish, petrolatum jelly, and heating do not aid in tick removal. Wear gloves if possible.
- Wash hands and site of bite thoroughly after tick removal to avoid potential mucosal inoculation.
- Prophylactic antibiotic treatment is not recommended.

DIAGNOSIS

Delay in presentation and initiation of therapy increases risk of long-term sequelae and mortality.

HISTORY

Consider RMSF in acute febrile illness, especially with history of potential tick exposure within previous 14 days, travels to an endemic area, and presentation in the late spring or summer. *The painless tick bite goes unnoticed 30–50% of the time, so many patients will not report a bite* (2,4).

- Early disease (days 1–3) presents like a viral illness with frontal headache, fever, malaise, body aches, nausea, and vomiting. RMSF is easily mistaken for gastroenteritis, pharyngitis, or mononucleosis.
- Signs and symptoms associated with RMSF and their frequency of occurrence
  - Fever, usually >102°F (99–100%)
  - Rash, macular/maculopapular/petechial, blanching (88–90%)
  - Headache (79–91%)
  - "Classic triad" of headache, fever, and rash (50–60%)
  - Myalgias (72–83%)
  - Nausea/vomiting (56–60%)
  - Abdominal pain, particularly in children (35–52%)
  - Cough, nonproductive (33%)
  - CNS dysfunction, stupor/confusion/coma/focal abnormalities (10–30%)
  - Patients may also have malaise, restlessness, arthralgia, conjunctivitis, and peripheral or periorbital edema.

PHYSICAL EXAM

On days 3–4, a centripetal rash usually forms (80% of adults), involving the palms and soles, spreading centrally to arms, legs, and trunk. The rash typically starts as an erythematous, macular, or maculopapular exanthem; 50% become petechial or purpuric, blanchable.

- About 20% never develop the "classic" rash, which may delay diagnosis and result in a more severe outcome. Rash may also be difficult to visualize on dark-skinned patients.
- Rash appearance may be variable. *Do not rely solely on the presence or absence of the typical rash for diagnosis*.
- In severe cases, the rash can involve the entire body and mucosal membranes and may progress to necrotic or gangrenous lesions.
- The rash is not associated with pruritus or urticaria; their presence makes RMSF less likely.
- Hepatosplenomegaly (12–16%)
- Lymphadenopathy (27%)

DIFFERENTIAL DIAGNOSIS

- Viral exanthems (e.g., measles, rubella, roseola)
- Meningoencephalitis (viral meningitis or encephalitis, bacterial meningitis)
- Meningococcemia
- Typhus
- Ehrlichiosis
- Lyme disease
- Leptospirosis
- Toxic shock syndrome
- Adenovirus infection
- Drug reaction or serum sickness
- Mononucleosis
- Kawasaki disease

DIAGNOSTIC TESTS & INTERPRETATION

Diagnosis is often clinical in patients with exposure history in an endemic area. Retrospective confirmation is attained by serology. Treatment should not be delayed awaiting confirmatory serology.

Initial Tests (lab, imaging)

- Specific laboratory diagnosis
  - Serum indirect fluorescent antibody (IFA): Titer of >1:64 is diagnostic. A 4-fold increase of acute and convalescent titers helps confirm an active case of RMSF (1).
  - Antibodies usually develop 7–10 days after onset of symptoms; optimal time for testing, therefore, is 14–21 days after onset of symptom onset. *Do not delay treatment*.
  - Early treatment may limit antibody formation.
  - Seropositivity is related to increasing age in endemic states. Positive spotted fever group *Rickettsia* antibody does not necessarily signify an acute infection.
- Nonspecific laboratory changes (incidence) (4)
  - WBC count: variable and frequently normal
  - Thrombocytopenia (32–52%)
  - Hyponatremia, mild (19–56%)

- Anemia, mild (5–24%)
- Azotemia (12–14%)
- Elevated AST (36–62%)
- Coagulation derangements are uncommon, despite vascular damage.
- CSF is usually normal; some patients may have mononuclear pleocytosis, elevated protein, and normal glucose.
- Other than occasional nonspecific pneumonic infiltrates on chest radiograph, imaging procedures are rarely helpful.

Diagnostic Procedures/Other

Skin biopsy of a rash lesion can offer definitive diagnosis. A 3-mm punch biopsy is sufficient to perform a rapid direct fluorescent antibody (DFA) test (sensitivity 70%, specificity 100%). Electron microscopy (EM) can also identify rickettsiae within endothelial cells. Western immunoblotting is necessary to confirm the specific spotted fever group species (1,2,4).

Test Interpretation

- Rickettsiae can be demonstrated within endothelial cells by DFA or EM.
- Petechiae due to the vasculitis may be seen on various organ surfaces (e.g., liver, brain, or epicardium).
- Secondary thromboses and tissue necrosis may be seen.

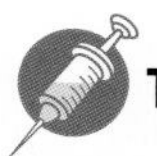

TREATMENT

MEDICATION

First Line

Doxycycline is the treatment of choice in both adults and children (1,2,3,4).

- Untreated rickettsial infections have a high rate of morbidity and mortality. Other antibiotics are considerably less effective.
- The ONLY contraindication to doxycycline is severe allergy.
- For adults: 100 mg PO or IV q12h × 7 days, lengthened to 2 days after the patient has become afebrile.
- For children weighing <45 kg (100 lbs): 2.2 mg/kg/dose (max 200 mg) q12h; those ≥45 kg; refer to adult dosing (4)
- Fever should subside within 24–72 hour with early treatment; may take longer if patient is severely ill.
- If patient has no response to doxycycline, consider an alternate diagnosis. Rickettsial resistance to doxycycline has NOT been documented.
- Side effects of doxycycline
  - Dyspepsia. Take medication with food and water. Avoid dairy products, iron preparations, or antacids, as they may inhibit drug absorption.
  - Photosensitivity may occur. Minimize sun exposure and use sunscreen.
  - Long courses of medication can result in staining teeth in children <9 years old. Risk of dental staining is minimal if short courses are administered.

Second Line

- Chloramphenicol: 50 mg/kg/day IV divided q6h (4 g/day max); same dose in renal failure
  - Associated with aplastic anemia and an increased case mortality
- Fluoroquinolones have not been evaluated clinically in RMSF, but they have shown in vitro activity against *R. rickettsii*.
- Sulfa-containing drugs may worsen tick-borne infections and are contraindicated.

Pregnancy Considerations

- Doxycycline is appropriate for this life-threatening infection in pregnancy if suspicion is high, despite the potential risk to fetal bones/teeth.
- Chloramphenicol may be considered during the first 2 trimesters but should be avoided in the 3rd trimester due to potential for gray baby syndrome.

ISSUES FOR REFERRAL

Consider infectious disease consult.

ADDITIONAL THERAPIES

Patients with neurologic injury or loss of limbs caused by gangrene may require prolonged physical and cognitive therapy.

INPATIENT CONSIDERATIONS

Admission Criteria/Initial Stabilization

- CNS dysfunction
- Nausea/vomiting preventing oral antibiotic therapy
- Immunocompromised patients
- Specific acute organ failure
- Failure of oral pain management
- ICU placement for acutely ill patients with shock

IV Fluids

Aggressive fluid resuscitation and electrolyte management may be required in critically ill patients.

Discharge Criteria

- Resolution of fever
- Ability to take oral therapy and nutrition

ONGOING CARE

FOLLOW-UP RECOMMENDATIONS

- Patients with moderate to severe disease typically should be hospitalized.
- Patients with mild disease may be treated as outpatients. Close follow-up is important to identify complications.
- Infection does not confer lifelong immunity.

Patient Monitoring

- Outpatients should be seen every 2–3 days until symptoms resolve.
- Consider tracking CBC, electrolytes, and LFTs, when clinically indicated.

DIET

Consider nutritional supplementation if intake is poor.

PROGNOSIS

- Prognosis is closely related to timely administration of appropriate antibiotics. Treatment before day 5 of illness can prevent morbidity and mortality (6).
- When treated promptly, prognosis is usually excellent with resolution of symptoms over several days and no sequelae.
- If complications develop (see "Complications"), course may be more severe and long-term sequelae (especially neurologic sequelae) may be present (6).
- Children age 5–9 years and elderly >70 years are at higher risk of morbidity and/or mortality (4,6).
  - Black males with G6PD deficiency are at highest risk for fulminant RMSF, in which death can occur within 5 days (4).

COMPLICATIONS

- Encephalopathy (30–40%); most commonly transient impaired level of consciousness or meningismus
- Seizures, focal neurologic deficit (10%)
- Renal injury (10%)
- Hepatitis (10%)
- Congestive heart failure (CHF) (5%)
- Respiratory failure (5%)
- Also proximal muscle weakness, changes in personality, paresthesias, distal necrosis, and deafness

REFERENCES

1. Lin L, Decker CF. Rocky Mountain spotted fever. *Dis Mon*. 2012;58(6):361–369.
2. Pujalte GG, Chua JV. Tick-borne infections in the United States. *Prim Care*. 2013;40(3): 619–635.
3. Dahlgren FS, Holman RC, Paddock CD, et al. Fatal Rocky Mountain spotted fever in the United States, 1999–2007. *Am J Trop Med Hyg*. 2012;86(4):713–719.
4. Woods CR. Rocky Mountain spotted fever in children. *Pediatr Clin North Am*. 2013;60(2): 455–470. doi:10.1016/j.pcl.2012.12.001.
5. Minniear TD, Buckingham SC. Managing Rocky Mountain spotted fever. *Expert Rev Anti Infect Ther*. 2009;7(9):1131–1137.
6. Botelho-Nevers E, Raoult D. Host, pathogen and treatment-related prognostic factors in rickettsioses. *Eur J Clin Microbiol Infect Dis*. 2011;30(10):1139–1150.

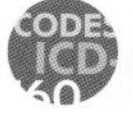

CODES

ICD10

A77.0 Spotted fever due to Rickettsia rickettsii

CLINICAL PEARLS

- Diagnosis of RMSF requires a high index of clinical suspicion. Painless tick bites often go unnoticed, and some patients may never develop a rash.
- Treatment should begin immediately in suspected cases. Doxycycline is indicated for treatment of RMSF in both adults AND children. The only absolute contraindication is severe allergy to the drug.
- Lab testing is nonspecific and frequently normal.
- Although prevalence is highest in central and southeastern United States, cases have been reported in almost all states.

ROSEOLA

Katie L. Westerfield, DO • Hillery Bavani, DO, CPT, USA

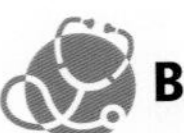

BASICS

DESCRIPTION

- Acute infection of infants or very young children (1)
- Causes a high fever followed by a skin eruption as the fever resolves (1)
- Transmission via contact with salivary secretions or vertical transmission (1% population) (1); incubation period of 9–10 days (2)
- System(s) affected: skin/exocrine; metabolic; gastrointestinal; respiratory; neurologic
- Synonym(s): exanthem subitum; pseudorubella; sixth disease; 3-day fever (3)

Pediatric Considerations

A disease of infants and very young children (4)

EPIDEMIOLOGY

- Predominant age
  - Infants and very young children (<2 years old) (5)
  - Peak age human herpesvirus-6 (HHV-6) infection 9 months, rarely congenital or perinatal infection (1)
- Predominant sex: male = female (1)

Incidence

- Common—accounts for 20% ED visits for febrile illness among children 6–8 months (6)

Prevalence

- Peak prevalence is between 9 and 21 months (5).
- Nearly 100% population carrying human herpesvirus 6 (HHV-6) by 3 years (1)
- >90% population with HHV-7 by 10 years (1)
- Approximately 20% patients with primary HHV-6 have roseola (6).

ETIOLOGY AND PATHOPHYSIOLOGY

- HHV-6 and HHV-7 (4)
- Majority of cases (60–74%) due to HHV-6
  - HHV-6B > HHV-6A (4)
  - HHV-6 binds to CD46 receptors on all nucleated cells (4).
- Latent or persistent asymptomatic infection occurs after primary infection (1).
  - 80–90% population intermittently sheds HHV-6/HHV-7 in salivary glands (4).
  - Patients are viremic from 2 days prior to fever until defervescence and onset of rash.
  - HHV-6 latency also implicated in CSF (6)

Genetics

No known genetic pattern

RISK FACTORS

- Female gender (5)
- Having older siblings (5)
- At-risk adults: immunocompromised (7)
  - Renal, liver, other solid organ, and bone marrow transplant (BMT) (5)
  - HHV-6 reactivation can occur in first week post-transplant (7). HHV-6 viremia occurs in 30–45% of BMT within the first several weeks after transplantation (6).
    - Usually asymptomatic (6)
    - Up to 82% of HHV-6 reactivation/reinfection in solid organ transplant (7)
- Nonrisk factors (5)
  - Child care attendance
  - Method of delivery
  - Breastfeeding
  - Maternal age
  - Season

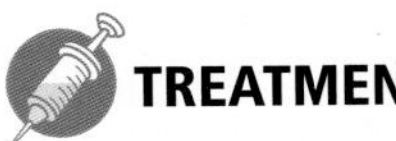

DIAGNOSIS

HISTORY

- Irritability (6)
- ± 3–5 days abrupt fever 102.2°–104°F (39°–40°C) (1)
- Sudden drop of fever (1)
  - After 3–5 days, fever disappears, skin rash appears.
  - ± Rash on trunk then spreads centrifugally mainly to neck, possibly also to peripheral extremities, and face.
- Diarrhea (5)
- Mild upper respiratory symptoms (5)
- Rhinorrhea (5)
- Febrile seizure occurs in 13% of cases (1).

PHYSICAL EXAM

- Rash (exanthem subitum) (1)
  - Rose-pink macules and/or papules
  - First appears on the neck and trunk then peripherally
  - May occur up to 3 days after fever resolves (1)
  - Fades within 2 days
  - Occurs in as few as 13% of patients
- Inflammation of tympanic membrane (6)
- Erythematous papules on soft palate and uvula (Nagayama spots) (1)
- Cervical lymphadenopathy (1)
- Periorbital edema (4)

DIFFERENTIAL DIAGNOSIS

- Enterovirus infection (8)
- Adenovirus infection (1)
- Epstein-Barr virus
- Fifth disease-parvovirus B19 (8)
- Rubella (8)
- Scarlet fever (8)
- Drug eruption (1)
- Measles (1)

DIAGNOSTIC TESTS & INTERPRETATION

- A clinical diagnosis (1)
- Tests often cannot differentiate latent or active disease (9).

Initial Tests (lab, imaging)

- HHV-6 and HHV-7 by PCR (1,7)
  - Serum, whole blood, CSF, or saliva
  - Becoming more widely available
- HHV-6 IgM immunofluorescence (1)
  - Diagnostic for acute infection
  - Check within first week.
- HHV-6 IgG immunofluorescence (1)
  - Check at diagnosis and then 2 weeks later.
  - Use with IgM to show primary infection.
  - Negative initial test and rise on follow-up suggests primary infection.
- Viral culture (7)
  - Rarely done
  - No clinical use (very time consuming)

Diagnostic Procedures/Other

- Urine culture: to rule out UTI as source of fever (2)
- Chest x-ray (CXR): if a child has respiratory symptoms

TREATMENT

No treatment necessary, resolves without sequelae (1)[C].

GENERAL MEASURES

- Symptomatic relief including antipyretics (1)[C]
- Anticonvulsant if there is a seizure

MEDICATION

First Line

- No specific 1st-line treatment in immunocompetent hosts beyond supportive measures (4)[C].
  - Antivirals not suggested in immunocompetent
- No approved antiviral treatment in immunocompromised (4).
- 2nd-line IV ganciclovir, cidofovir, foscarnet tested in vitro studies in stem cell transplant patients.
  - HHV-6B susceptible: ganciclovir and foscarnet (7)[C]
  - HHV-6A and HHV-7: more resistant to ganciclovir (7)
- Antivirals suggested in individual cases of encephalitis (associated with reactivation of HHV-6) (7).

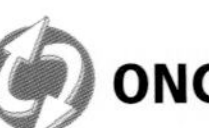

ONGOING CARE

FOLLOW-UP RECOMMENDATIONS

Patient Monitoring

- None after typical rash appears and fever resolves
- Mean duration of illness is 6 days (6).
- If febrile seizures occur, they will cease after fever subsides and will not likely recur (6).
- Symptomatic reactivation in immunocompromised (1)

DIET

Encourage fluids

PATIENT EDUCATION

- Parental reassurance that this is usually a benign, self-limited disease (1)
- There is no specific recommended period of exclusion from out-of-home care for affected children.
- Patient is viremic a few days prior to fever until time of defervescence and rash onset.

PROGNOSIS

- Course: acute, complete recovery without sequelae (1)
- Reactivation in immunocompromised patients is common (6).

COMPLICATIONS

- Febrile seizures
  - 13% patients with roseola (1,6)
  - Accounts for 1/3 of primary seizures in children $<$2 years old (1)
- Medication hypersensitivity syndromes (drug reaction with eosinophilia and systemic symptoms) (4)
- Reactivation can occur in transplant patients, HIV-1 infection (6).
- Meningioencephalitis occurs in immunocompetent and in immunosuppressed patients (6). Poor association with multiple sclerosis (6)
- Pityriasis rosea (1)
- Possible association with progressive multifocal leukoencephalopathy (6)

REFERENCES

1. Stone RC, Micali GA, Schwartz RA. Roseola infantum and its causal human herpesviruses. *Int J Dermatol*. 2014;53(4):397–403.
2. Watkins J. Diagnosing rashes, part 4: generalized rashes with fever. *Practice Nursing*. 2013;24: 335–340.
3. Ely JW, Stone MS. The generalized rash: part I. Differential diagnosis. *Am Fam Physician*. 2010;81(6):726–734.
4. Wolz MM, Sciallis GF, Pittelkow MR. Human herperviruses 6, 7, and 8 from a dermatologic perspective. *Mayo Clin Proc*. 2012; 87(10): 1004–1014.
5. Zerr DM, Meier AS, Selke SS, et al. A population-based study of primary human herpesvirus 6 infection. *N Engl J Med*. 2005;352(8):786–776.
6. Caserta MT, Mock DJ, Dewhurst S. Human herpervirus 6. *Clin Infect Dis*. 2001;33(6):829–833.
7. Le J, Gantt S; AST Infectious Diseases Community of Practice. Human herpesvirus 6, 7, and 8 in solid organ transplantation. *Am J Transplant*. 2012;13(Suppl 4):128–137.
8. Ely JW, Stone MS. The generalized rash: part II. Diagnostic approach. *Am Fam Physician*. 2010;81(6):735–739.
9. Dreyfus DH. Herpesviruses and the microbiome. *J Allergy Clin Immunol*. 2013;132(6):1278–1284.

ADDITIONAL READING

- Ablashi DV, Devin CL, Yoshikawa T, et al. Review part 3: human herpesvirus-6 in multiple non-neurological diseases. *J Med Virol*. 2010;82(11): 1903–1910.
- Caselli E, Di Luca D. Molecular biology and clinical associations of Roseoloviruses human herpesvirus 6 and human herpesvirus 7. *New Microbiol*. 2007;30(3):173–187.
- Dockrell DH, Smith TF, Paya CV. Human herpesvirus 6. *Mayo Clin Proc*. 1999;74(2):163–170.
- Dyer JA. Childhood viral exanthems. *Pediatr Ann*. 2007;36(1):21–29.
- Evans CM, Kudesia G, McKendrick M. Management of herpesvirus infections. *Int J Antimicrob Agents*. 2013;42(2):119–128.
- Folster-Holst R, Kreth HW. Viral exanthems in childhood-infectious (direct) exanthems. Part 1: classic exanthems [in German]. *J Dtsch Dermatol Ges*. 2009;7(4):309–316.
- Huang CT, Lin LH. Differentiating roseola infantum with pyuria from urinary tract infection. *Pediatr Int*. 2013;55(2):214–218.
- Leach CT. Human herpesvirus-6 and -7 infections in children: agents of roseola and other syndromes. *Curr Opin Pediatr*. 2000;12(3):269–274.
- Lowry, M. Roseola infantum. *Pract Nurse*. 2013;43:40–42.
- Stoeckle MY. The spectrum of human herpesvirus 6 infection: from roseola infantum to adult disease. *Ann Rev Med*. 2000;51:423–430.
- Vianna RA, de Oliveira SA, Camacho LA, et al. Role of human herpesvirus 6 infection in young Brazilian children with rash illnesses. *Pediatr Infect Dis J*. 2008;27(6):533–537.

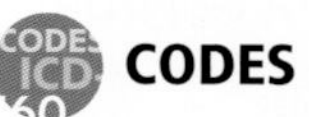

CODES

ICD10

- B08.20 Exanthema subitum [sixth disease], unspecified
- B08.21 Exanthema subitum [sixth disease] due to human herpesvirus 6
- B08.22 Exanthema subitum [sixth disease] due to human herpesvirus 7

CLINICAL PEARLS

- Roseola infection should be suspected if a young child presents with a high temperature.
- As the fever abates, a macular rash will be seen on the neck and trunk, with eventual spread to the face and extremities.
- Roseola is a clinical diagnosis, and laboratory testing is not necessary for most children with classic roseola.
- For atypical presentations, complications, and immunocompromised hosts, several laboratory tools are available, including serologic testing for antibody, viral PCR testing, and viral culture.
- Infection is typically self-limiting and without sequelae.
- Usually only symptomatic treatment is needed.

ROTATOR CUFF IMPINGEMENT SYNDROME

Faren H. Williams, MD, MS • Minjin Fromm, MD

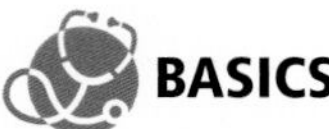

BASICS

DESCRIPTION

- Compression of rotator cuff tendons and subacromial bursa between the humeral head and the structures that make up the coracoacromial arch and humeral tuberosities
- Most common cause of atraumatic shoulder pain in patients age >25 years
- Typical symptom is pain that is most severe with arm abducted between 60 and 120 degrees (the "painful arc").
- Classically divided into three stages
  - Stage I: acute inflammation, edema, or hemorrhage of the underlying tendons due to overuse (typically in those age <25 years)
  - Stage II: progressive tendinosis that leads to partial rotator cuff tear along with underlying thickening or fibrosis of surrounding structures (commonly, ages 25–40 years)
  - Stage III: full-thickness tear (typically in patients age >40 years)

EPIDEMIOLOGY

Incidence

- Shoulder pain accounts for 1% of all primary care visits.
- Peak incidence of 25/1,000 patients/year occurs in patients aged 42–46 years.
- Impingement recorded as causal in 18–74% of patients with shoulder pain.

Prevalence

Prevalence of shoulder pain in general population ranges from ~7 to 30%.

RISK FACTORS

- Repetitive overhead motions, including throwing, swimming
- Glenohumeral joint instability or muscle imbalance
- Acromioclavicular arthritis or, osteophytes
- Thickened coracoacromial ligament
- Shoulder trauma
- Increasing age
- Smoking

GENERAL PREVENTION

- Proper throwing and lifting techniques
- Proper strengthening and balance of rotator cuff and scapula stabilizer muscles

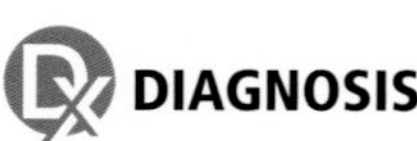

DIAGNOSIS

HISTORY

- Gradual increase in shoulder pain with overhead activities (sudden onset of sharp pain suggests a tear)
- Night pain is common, exacerbated by lying on the affected shoulder or sleeping with the affected arm above the head.
- Anterolateral shoulder pain with overhead activities
- May progress to weakness and decreased range of motion if shoulder is not used through full range of motion

PHYSICAL EXAM

- Neer impingement test: Examiner stabilizes the scapula and moves the affected upper extremity through a flexion arc. Patient reports pain with flexion of the shoulder. Sensitivity: 78%. Specificity: 58% (1)[A]
- Hawkins-Kennedy impingement test: Examiner places the arm in 90 degrees of forward flexion and then gently internally rotates the arm. End point for internal rotation is when the patient feels pain or when the rotation of the scapula is felt or observed by the examiner. Test is positive when patient experiences pain during the maneuver. Sensitivity: 74%. Specificity: 57% (1)[A]
- Empty can test (supraspinatus): Examiner asks the patient to elevate and internally rotate the arm with thumbs pointing downward in the scapular plane. Elbow should be fully extended. Examiner applies downward pressure on upper surface of the arm. Test is positive when patient complains of pain with resistance. Sensitivity: 69%. Specificity: 62% (1)[A]
- Lift-off test (subscapularis): Patient internally rotates the shoulder, placing the hand on ipsilateral buttock, then lifts hand off buttock against resistance. A tear in the subscapularis muscle produces weakness of this action. Sensitivity: 42%. Specificity: 97% (1)[A]
- Drop-arm test: Patient fully elevates arm and then slowly reverses the motion. If the arm is dropped suddenly or the patient has extreme pain, the test is positive for a possible rotator cuff tear. Sensitivity: 21%. Specificity: 92% (1)[A]
- Resisted external rotation: weakness suggestive of infraspinatus and/or teres minor tendon involvement
- Examine cervical spine to rule out cervical pathology as source of shoulder pain.
- Neurovascular exam of the upper extremity

DIFFERENTIAL DIAGNOSIS

- Labral injury
- Acromioclavicular arthritis (more common in older patients; positive cross-arm test)
- Adhesive capsulitis (rotator cuff tendonitis leads to decreased use and atrophy of rotator cuff muscles, followed by contracture of joint; may be related to prior trauma and has been linked to diabetes)
- Anterior shoulder instability (owing to trauma; more common in those age <25 years)
- Multidirectional instability
- Biceps tendonitis or rupture (perform Speed and Yergeson tests and look for visible or palpable defect of biceps)
- Calcific tendonitis
- Cervical radiculopathy (spinal or foraminal stenosis, can test with Spurling maneuver)
- Glenohumeral arthritis (evaluate with plain films)
- Suprascapular nerve entrapment (look for focal muscle atrophy of supra- or infraspinatus)
- Traumatic rotator cuff tear

DIAGNOSTIC TESTS & INTERPRETATION

Initial Tests (lab, imaging)

- Plain-film radiographs of the shoulder (three views): anteroposterior, axillary, scapular Y views
- Plain film may reveal the following:
  - Osteoarthritis of the acromioclavicular and glenohumeral joints
  - Superior migration of the humeral head (indicative of a large rotator cuff tear)
  - Cystic change of the humeral head and sclerosis of the inferior acromion (indicative of chronic rotator cuff disease)
  - Calcific tendonitis
- MRI is used to assess rotator cuff tendinopathy, partial tears, and complete tears.
- MR arthrogram is preferred test for detecting suspected labral pathology.
- Ultrasound is sensitive and specific for rotator cuff tears but is highly operator-dependent.
- CT scan is the preferred imaging study for bony pathology or for those unable to undergo MRI.
- Arthrogram is the modality for people who are suspected of having a rotator cuff tear.

Diagnostic Procedures/Other

- Lidocaine injection test
  - Inject lidocaine into the subacromial space:
    - Repeat impingement tests; if pain is completely relieved and range of motion is improved, likely impingement syndrome.
  - Allows for more accurate strength testing on physical examination:
    - If strength is intact, rules out rotator cuff tear
    - If range of motion does not improve in any plane, more likely adhesive capsulitis
  - Some pain relief and improved range of motion occurs after lidocaine injection with the following:
    - Glenoid labral tear
    - Capsular strain
    - Glenohumeral osteoarthritis
    - Glenohumeral instability
- A lack of any pain relief suggests other sources or inappropriate placement of injection.

Test Interpretation

May have tendinosis, tendonitis, or muscle/tendon tear

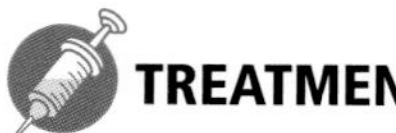

TREATMENT

Anti-inflammatory agents + aggressive rehabilitation can improve and fully resolve rotator cuff tendonitis in most patients.

GENERAL MEASURES
- Rest
- Ice or heat for symptom relief
- Activity modification, with avoidance of aggravating activities, particularly overhead motions
- Range-of-motion exercises
- Rotator-cuff and adjacent muscle strengthening to enhance stability and prevent further injuries

MEDICATION
First Line
NSAIDs or other analgesic, often for 6–12 weeks

ISSUES FOR REFERRAL
Failure of conservative treatment, persistent pain, weakness, or complete tear of rotator cuff

ADDITIONAL THERAPIES
- Supervised- or home-exercise regimens have been shown to provide clinically significant pain reduction and improved function (2)[A].
- Physical therapy has demonstrated evidence of effectiveness for short-term and long-term recovery with respect to function (3)[A]:
  - Initial goal is to restore range of motion.
  - After pain resolves, gradually strengthen rotator cuff muscles in internal rotation, external rotation, and abduction.

COMPLEMENTARY & ALTERNATIVE MEDICINE
Possible benefit of acupuncture when used with physical therapy, reducing pain and improving function, with benefit maintained for up to 1 year (4)[A]

SURGERY/OTHER PROCEDURES
- Steroid injections may have a significant benefit on pain and function in the short term but do not appear to have a significant long-term effect (5)[A]:
  - No apparent significantly increased risk for rotator cuff tears in those receiving subacromial steroid injections (6)[C].
- No evidence that surgical treatment is superior to conservative management, or that one surgical technique is superior to another to treat impingement syndrome (7)[A].
- Platelet-rich therapies for musculoskeletal soft tissue injuries
  - No apparent effect of platelet-rich plasma injection during arthroscopic rotator cuff repair on overall retear rates or shoulder-specific outcomes (8)[A],(9).
- Extracorporeal shock wave therapy is currently under study as an emerging treatment for calcific tendonitis (10).

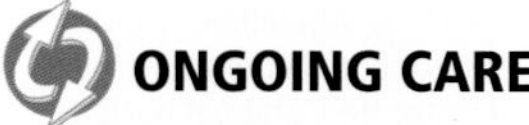

ONGOING CARE

PATIENT EDUCATION
- Patient must understand that physical rehabilitation may be necessary, both in conservative course of treatment (i.e., NSAIDs, physical therapy, home exercises) and with surgical decompression. An aggressive trial of rehabilitation should be encouraged prior to extensive testing or surgical intervention.
- Symptoms often recur if not fully addressed.

PROGNOSIS
- Variable, depends on underlying pathology
- Most patients improve with conservative management, but recovery is often slow.
- Having clinical symptoms for >1 year, and increased severity of symptoms are reported to be prognostic factors for a negative outcome on conservative intervention.

COMPLICATIONS
- Progression of injury
- Tendon retraction in complete rotator cuff tear

REFERENCES

1. Alqunaee M, Galvin R, Fahey T, et al. Diagnostic accuracy of clinical tests for subacromial impingement syndrome: a systematic review and meta-analysis. *Arch Phys Med Rehabil*. 2012;93(2):229–236.
2. Kuhn JE. Exercise in the treatment of rotator cuff impingement: a systematic review and a synthesized evidence-based rehabilitation protocol. *J Shoulder Elbow Surg*. 2009;18(1):138–160.
3. Green S, Buchbinder R, Hetrick S. Physiotherapy interventions for shoulder pain. *Cochrane Database Syst Rev*. 2003;(2):CD004258
4. Vas J, Ortega C, Olmo V, et al. Single-point acupuncture and physiotherapy for the treatment of painful shoulder: a multicentre randomized controlled trial. *Rheumatology (Oxford)*. 2008;47(6):887–893.
5. Gaujoux-Viala C, Dougados M, Gossec L. Efficacy and safety of steroid injections for shoulder and elbow tendonitis: a meta-analysis of randomised controlled trials. *Ann Rheum Dis*. 2009;68(12):1843–1849.
6. Bhatia M, Singh B, Nicolaou N, et al. Correlation between rotator cuff tears and repeated subacromial steroid injections: a case-controlled study. *Ann R Coll Surg Engl*. 2009;91(5):414–416.
7. Gebremariam L, Hay EM, Koes BW, et al. Effectiveness of surgical and postsurgical interventions for the subacromial impingement syndrome: a systematic review. *Arch Phys Med Rehabil*. 2011;92(11):1900–1913.
8. Chahal J, Van Thiel GS, Mall N, et al. The role of platelet-rich plasma in arthroscopic rotator cuff repair: a systematic review with quantitative synthesis. *Arthroscopy*. 2012;28(11):1718–1727.
9. Moraes VY, Lenza M, Tamaoki MJ, et al. Platelet-rich therapies for musculoskeletal soft tissue injuries. *Cochrane Database Syst Rev*. 2013;(12):CD010071. doi:10.1001/14651858.CD010071.pub2.
10. Ioppolo, F, Tattoli M, Di Sante L, et al. Clinical improvement and resorption of calcifications in calcific tendinitis of the shoulder after shock wave therapy at 6 months' follow-up: a systemic review and meta-analysis. *Arch Phys Med Rehabil*. 2013;94(9):1699–1706.

ADDITIONAL READING

- Baumgarten KM, Gerlach D, Galatz LM, et al. Cigarette smoking increases the risk for rotator cuff tears. *Clin Orthop Relat Res*. 2010;468(6):1534–1541.
- Burbank KM, Stevenson JH, Czarnecki GR, et al. Chronic shoulder pain: part I. Evaluation and diagnosis. *Am Fam Physician*. 2008;77(4):453–460.
- Burbank KM, Stevenson JH, Czarnecki GR, et al. Chronic shoulder pain: part II. Treatment. *Am Fam Physician*. 2008;77(4):493–497.
- Cumpston M, Johnston R, Wengier L, et al. Topical glyceryl trinitrate for rotator cuff disease. *Cochrane Database Syst Rev*. 2009;(3):CD006355.
- Hanchard NC, Lenza M, Handoll HH, et al. Physical tests for shoulder impingements and local lesions of bursa, tendon or labrum that may accompany impingement. *Cochrane Database Syst Rev*. 2013;(4):CD007427
- Hegedus EJ, Goode A, Campbell S, et al. Physical examination tests of the shoulder: a systematic review with meta-analysis of individual tests. *Br J Sports Med*. 2008;42(2):80–92; discussion 92.
- Kennedy DJ, Visco CJ, Press J. Current concepts for shoulder training in the overhead athlete. *Curr Sports Med Rep*. 2009;8(3):154–160.

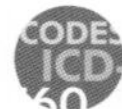

CODES

ICD10
- M75.40 Impingement syndrome of unspecified shoulder
- M75.110 Incmpl rotatr-cuff tear/ruptr of unsp shoulder, not trauma
- M75.120 Complete rotatr-cuff tear/ruptr of unsp shoulder, not trauma

CLINICAL PEARLS
- Consider impingement syndrome in patients with repetitive overhead arm motion (e.g., swimming, throwing).
- Shoulder pain in middle age without trauma may be secondary to rotator cuff tendonitis.
- Supraspinatus tendon most commonly affected
- Use Neer and Hawkins tests to check for shoulder impingement.
- Use empty can test to test for weakness of supraspinatus muscle.
- Drop-arm test is highly specific for rotator cuff tear.
- Physical therapy over 6–12 weeks promotes return to function.
- Most patients respond to conservative management, nonresponders should be referred for surgical treatment.

SALIVARY GLAND CALCULI/SIALADENITIS

Jason Cohn, DO, MS • Mark Weitzel, DO • Mahmoud Ghaderi, DO

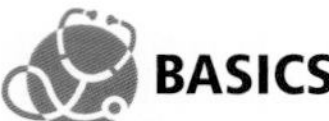

BASICS

DESCRIPTION

- Inflammation and/or calculi (stones) involving ≥1 salivary gland
- Sialolithiasis is the cause of ~90% of all obstructive salivary gland diseases.
- Salivary obstruction is clinically characterized by a food-related painful swelling of the affected gland, known as "mealtime syndrome."
- The submandibular gland is more commonly affected (80–90% of cases) by sialolithiasis and infection compared to the parotid gland. Submandibular stones occur more commonly due to higher mucinous content of saliva, longer course of Wharton duct, slow salivary flow, and saliva flow against gravity.
- Can be acute or chronic
  - Types: infectious, obstructive (sialolithiasis), and autoimmune

EPIDEMIOLOGY

Incidence

- A review of British patients showed an incidence of symptomatic sialolithiasis of 27–59/1 million population per year.
- Predominant sex: male > female
- Predominant age: Peak incidence is 30–60 years.
- Most common in debilitated and dehydrated patients
- 49% men and 51% women, average age 47.5 years; 82% submandibular stones and 18% parotid stones, 44% had a positive smoking history, and 20% of patients were taking diuretics.

Prevalence

- Salivary calculi can be found in 1.2% of the adult population.
- Only 5% of all cases occur in the pediatric population.
- In those with sialographic evidence of benign intraductal obstruction, the obstruction is caused by salivary calculi in 73.2% of cases.

ETIOLOGY AND PATHOPHYSIOLOGY

- Decreased salivary outflow from anticholinergics, dehydration, or radiation is thought to allow bacterial infection of salivary glands.
- Salivary calculi form by deposition of calcium phosphate around an organic matrix consisting of altered salivary mucins, bacteria, and desquamated epithelial cells. Predisposing factors include salivary stasis, retrograde bacterial contamination from the oral cavity, increased alkalinity of saliva, and physical trauma to salivary duct or gland.
- Systemic abnormalities of calcium metabolism do not cause salivary stones. Gout is the only systemic disease known to be associated with salivary stone development. In gout, sialoliths are composed of uric acid.
- Sialadenitis occurs by recurrent inflammatory reactions that result in progressive acinar destruction with fibrous replacement and sialectasis.
- Bacterial sialadenitis: *Staphylococcus aureus, Streptococcus viridans, Streptococcus pyogenes, Haemophilus influenzae, Escherichia coli, Pseudomonas aeruginosa*, and group B streptococci (neonates and prepubescent children)
- Viral sialadenitis: mumps, cytomegalovirus (CMV), Epstein-Barr virus (EBV), HIV, and enteroviruses

Pediatric Considerations

The two most common causes of sialadenitis in children are paramyxovirus infection (most commonly mumps) and juvenile recurrent parotitis (JRP).

Genetics

Polygenic cause, with several loci under investigation

RISK FACTORS

- Dehydration
- Anticholinergic use
- Antihistamine use
- Diuretic use
- Poor oral hygiene
- Malnutrition
- Head/neck radiation
- Tuberculosis (TB)
- HIV
- Failure to immunize (mumps)
- Gout
- Diabetes mellitus
- Hypothyroidism
- Renal failure
- Duct strictures
- Previous intraoral procedures

GENERAL PREVENTION

- Adequate postoperative hydration
- Maintain proper oral care and hygiene.
- Avoid antihistamines, anticholinergics, and other causes of xerostomia, especially if predisposed to risk factors.

COMMONLY ASSOCIATED CONDITIONS

- Postoperative dehydration
- Radiation-induced xerostomia
- Drug-induced xerostomia
- Sjögren syndrome
- Hypercalcemia

DIAGNOSIS

HISTORY

- Acute onset of pain and swelling over the affected salivary gland, especially postprandial
- Dental pain, discharge, foul breath (halitosis), and pain with chewing
- Fever, unintentional weight loss
- Xerostomia
- Recent dental work, surgery
- Immunization history
- Radiation, TB, and HIV exposure
- History of alcoholism, bulimia, and malnutrition (suggest sialadenosis)

PHYSICAL EXAM

- Palpate all salivary glands, floor of mouth, tongue, and neck to assess symmetry, tenderness, induration, edema, presence of stones, and lymphadenopathy.
- Examine duct openings for purulent discharge.
- Palpate gland gently to express purulent material.
- Examine eyes for interstitial keratitis.
- Note lingual papillary atrophy and loss of tooth enamel.

Pediatric Considerations

Stones in children are traditionally smaller in size, within the duct distally, and present with a shorter symptom duration.

DIFFERENTIAL DIAGNOSIS

- Acute bacterial parotitis
- Chronic bacterial parotitis
- Dental abscess
- Mumps
- TB
- HIV (in pediatric populations)
- EBV, CMV, enteroviruses
- Tularemia
- Cystic fibrosis
- Lupus
- Sjögren syndrome
- Alcoholism
- Bulimia
- Hypothyroidism
- Pleomorphic adenoma
- Lymphoma
- Sarcoidosis
- Collagen vascular disease
- Metal poisoning

DIAGNOSTIC TESTS & INTERPRETATION

Initial Tests (lab, imaging)

- CBC, electrolytes
- Culture and sensitivity of any expressed pus
- CT scan with IV contrast is the preferred imaging modality.
- Ultrasound can localize abscesses as well as stones. Ultrasound can differentiate between solid and cystic disease and extraglandular disease. Stones appear hyperechoic with posterior shadowing (1)[B].
- Sonopalpation (concurrent ultrasound with transoral palpation) proved to have a sensitivity and specificity of 96.6% and 90% in finding a calculi compared with physical examination alone (83% and 60%) and ultrasound alone (91% and 80%) (2)[B].

Follow-Up Tests & Special Considerations

- If autoimmune process is suspected, consider ordering appropriate labs, such as autoantibody titers: Sjögren syndrome A (SS-A) and Sjögren syndrome B (SS-B), rheumatoid factor (RF), and antinuclear antibodies (ANAs). Erythrocyte sedimentation rate (ESR) may also be conducted.
- Consider serial CT scans with contrast to evaluate disease resolution.
- Ultrasound can identify indicators of persistent obstruction in patients undergoing sialolithotomy (1)[B].

Diagnostic Procedures/Other
- Sialography to evaluate sialolithiasis and other obstructive lesions
- Sialoendoscopy to find and remove sialoliths. In one study, sialendoscopy confirmed 221 (79%) parotid and 812 (93%) submandibular stones (3)[A].

Test Interpretation
In chronic sialadenitis, loss of acini, fibrosis, and periductal lymphocytosis are evident; degree indicates chronicity.

TREATMENT

GENERAL MEASURES
- Maintain hydration.
- Apply warm compresses with massage.
- Maintain good oral hygiene.
- Antibiotics if indicated by diagnosis

MEDICATION

First Line
- Antistaphylococcal penicillins (nafcillin, dicloxacillin) are indicated in areas where methicillin-resistant *Staphylococcus aureus* (MRSA) is not predominant.
- Penicillin-allergic: Use clindamycin 300 mg PO q8h.
- MRSA: vancomycin
- Gram negative: third-generation cephalosporin or fluoroquinolone
- Anaerobic: metronidazole or clindamycin
- Antibiotic coverage should be narrowed once culture and sensitivity are available.
- Continue antibiotic therapy for 10–14 days.

Second Line
1st-generation cephalosporin (cephalexin or cefazolin) or clindamycin is also indicated for empiric coverage.

ISSUES FOR REFERRAL
In the case of poor dentition and dental abscess, refer patient to a dentist.

ADDITIONAL THERAPIES
In the case of chronic sialadenitis with strictures, consider sialostent placement.

SURGERY/OTHER PROCEDURES
- Submandibular stones found in the anterior floor of the mouth can be excised intraorally, whereas those in the hilum require gland excision. Parotid stones usually require parotidectomy. Superior results in symptom relief and safety have been reported with removal of stones using sialoendoscopy (4)[A].
- Incision and drainage of parotid abscess is indicated after failing 3–5 days of medical management. Sialoliths and stenoses can be successfully treated by radiologically or fluoroscopically controlled or sialendoscopically based methods in ~80% of cases. Extracorporeal shock wave lithotripsy (ESWL) is successful in up to 50% of cases. Transoral duct slitting is an important method for extraparenchymal submandibular stones, with a success rate of 90%.
- Recent evidence shows that larger stones can be successfully and safely treated with holmium:YAG laser lithotripsy (5,6)[B].
- The size of a parotid stone can dictate treatment. In one study, larger parotid stones (52%) required ESWL. Smaller stones could be removed with salivary gland endoscopy alone (22%). The remainder underwent combined endoscopy and shock wave lithotripsy (26%) or parotidectomy (4%). The majority of submandibular stones (92%) only required transoral stone removal. The remainder underwent endoscopy (5%), surgical removal of the gland (4%), and endoscopy combined with shock wave lithotripsy (3%) (3)[A].

Pediatric Considerations
The most effective diagnostic and therapeutic modality for children with sialadenitis is sialendoscopy with stone retrieval (7)[B].

COMPLEMENTARY & ALTERNATIVE MEDICINE
Consider lemon drops or other sialogogues to promote salivation. In one study, postoperative use of sialogogues nearly halved rates of sialadenitis (8)[C].

INPATIENT CONSIDERATIONS

Admission Criteria/Initial Stabilization
- Parotid abscess
- Sepsis
- Inability to tolerate PO intake
- Airway, breathing, circulation
- Check vital signs, with particular attention to blood pressure, as patient may be septic secondary to abscess formation.
- Evaluate airway patency.

Nursing
Responsibilities may include ensuring excellent oral hygiene and avoiding administration of drugs that cause decreased production or flow of saliva.

Discharge Criteria
- Exclude abscess or sepsis
- Ensure ability to tolerate PO intake
- Stable vital signs

ONGOING CARE

FOLLOW-UP RECOMMENDATIONS
- Provide regular follow-up visits for patients with chronic sialadenitis.
- Avoid prescribing medications that cause xerostomia.

Patient Monitoring
Continue to monitor patients with chronic sialadenitis, as decreased salivary gland function due to fibrosis and loss of acini can lead to acute exacerbations.

DIET
- Avoid sialogogues during acute attacks.
- Maintain adequate hydration on an outpatient basis.

PATIENT EDUCATION
- Educate patients on maintaining excellent oral hygiene.
- Educate patients on maintaining good hydration.

PROGNOSIS
- Generally excellent, with acute symptoms resolving in about a week with appropriate treatment
- Patients with autoimmune etiology may have prolonged course due to systemic involvement.

COMPLICATIONS
Abscess, dental caries, recurrent sialadenitis, facial nerve impingement, Ludwig angina

REFERENCES

1. Joshi AS, Lohia S. Ultrasound indicators of persistent obstruction after submandibular sialolithotomy. *Otolaryngol Head Neck Surg*. 2013;149(6):873–877.
2. Patel NJ, Hashemi S, Joshi AS. Sonopalpation: a novel application of ultrasound for detection of submandibular calculi. *Otolaryngol Head Neck Surg*. 2014;151(5):770–775.
3. Zenk J, Koch M, Klintworth N, et al. Sialendoscopy in the diagnosis and treatment of sialolithiasis: a study of more than 1000 patients. *Otolaryngol Head Neck Surg*. 2012;147(5):858–863.
4. Wilson KF, Meier JD, Ward PD. Salivary gland disorders. *Am Fam Physician*. 2014;89(11):882–888.
5. Sionis S, Caria RA, Trucas M, et al. Sialendoscopy with and without holmium:YAG laser-assisted lithotripsy in the management of obstructive sialadenitis of major salivary glands. *Br J Oral Maxillofac Surg*. 2014;52(1):58–62.
6. Phillips J, Withrow K. Outcomes of holmium laser-assisted lithotripsy with sialendoscopy in treatment of sialolithiasis. *Otolaryngol Head Neck Surg*. 2014;150(6):962–967.
7. Francis CL, Larsen CG. Pediatric sialadenitis. *Otolaryngol Clin North Am*. 2014;47(5):763–778.
8. Nakada K, Ishibashi T, Takei T, et al. Does lemon candy decrease salivary gland damage after radioiodine therapy for thyroid cancer? *J Nucl Med*. 2005;46(2):261–266.

ADDITIONAL READING

- Alyas F, Lewis K, Williams M, et al. Diseases of the submandibular gland as demonstrated using high resolution ultrasound. *Br J Radiol*. 2005;78(928):362–369.
- Huoh KC, Eisele DW. Etiologic factors in sialolithiasis. *Otolaryngol Head Neck Surg*. 2011;145(6):935–939.
- Koch M, Zenk J, Iro H. Algorithms for treatment of salivary gland obstructions. *Otolaryngol Clin North Am*. 2009;42(6):1173–1192.

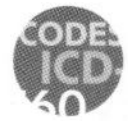

CODES

ICD10
- K11.5 Sialolithiasis
- K11.20 Sialoadenitis, unspecified
- K11.21 Acute sialoadenitis

CLINICAL PEARLS
- Sialadenitis occurs mainly in debilitated patients who lack ability to control hydration.
- Sialadenitis is associated with conditions that predispose patient to xerostomia.
- Mainstay of treatment is hydration, good oral hygiene, sialogogues, and possible surgical excision.
- Many cases are now being successfully and safely treated with sialendoscopy.

SALMONELLA INFECTION

Pia Prakash, MD • Jason P. Glass, MD • Marie L. Borum, MD, EdD, MPH

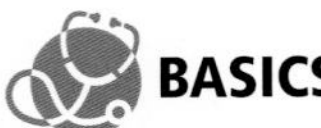

BASICS

DESCRIPTION

- Disease caused by any serotype of the bacterial genus *Salmonella*, a gram-negative bacillus
- *Salmonella enterica*
  - 2,500 different serotypes
  - Most pathogenic species in humans
- Nontyphoidal *Salmonella* has a number of agricultural animal hosts and is an important cause of foodborne infection.
- Clinical syndromes
  - Gastroenteritis (75%)
  - Bacteremia (10%)
  - Enteric fever (10%) (see "Typhoid Fever")
  - Localized infection outside GI tract (5%)
  - Chronic carrier state (<1%)
- Chronic carrier state is defined as a positive stool culture >1 year.

Geriatric Considerations

Patients >65 years of age have increased risk of developing invasive disease. Elderly patients often have comorbid conditions (atherosclerotic endovascular lesions, prostheses, etc.) that increase risk of seeding and bacteremia.

Pediatric Considerations

Neonates (<3 months) are more susceptible to invasive disease and subsequent complications, including CNS infection.

Pregnancy Considerations

Pregnancy does not increase risk or severity of infection.

EPIDEMIOLOGY

Incidence

- Incidence of laboratory-confirmed *Salmonella* infection in the United States (2009)
  - 16 cases per 100,000 in 2012 according to CDC
  - Incidence has been stable over past 6 years.
  - 42,000 cases reported to CDC each year; actual number likely greater (unreported cases)
  - Highest incidence in children <4 years of age
  - Hospitalization rates higher in patients ≥50 years of age
- Peak frequency: July–November
- *Salmonella* is the major cause of bacterial diarrheal disease in the United States.
- *Salmonella* is a common cause of traveler's diarrhea.

ETIOLOGY AND PATHOPHYSIOLOGY

- Ingestion of contaminated food (e.g., poultry, beef, eggs, tomatoes, dairy products, commercially prepared nuts and nut products) or water accounts for 95% of cases.
- Organisms are ingested, invade the gut mucosa, and produce inflammatory and cytotoxic response. Organisms can disseminate into systemic circulation via the lymphatic system.
- Person-to-person and/or fecal–oral spread
- Contact with chronic carrier (daycare center)
- Contact with exotic pets with high fecal carriage rates for *Salmonella*, especially reptiles
- Iatrogenic contamination (e.g., blood transfusion, endoscopy)

RISK FACTORS

- Recent travel outside the United States
- Chicken and egg consumption
- Contact with reptiles or live poultry
- Impaired gastric acidity: H_2 receptor blockers, antacids, proton pump inhibitors (PPIs), gastrectomy, achlorhydria
- Reticuloendothelial blockade: sickle cell disease, malaria, bartonellosis
- Immunosuppression: AIDS, diabetes, corticosteroid use, immunosuppressant use, chemotherapy

GENERAL PREVENTION

- Proper hygiene in production, transport, and storage of food (e.g., refrigerating eggs, thoroughly cooking eggs prior to consumption)
- Control of animal reservoirs: Avoid contact with animal feces and polluted waters.
- Hand hygiene
- Updated reports of *Salmonella* outbreaks are available on CDC Web site (http://www.cdc.gov/salmonella/).

COMMONLY ASSOCIATED CONDITIONS

- Gastroenteritis: typically associated with normal immune function
- Bacteremia: more often seen in immunocompromised patients or those with underlying medical conditions or complications (e.g., cholelithiasis, prostheses)

DIAGNOSIS

HISTORY

- *Salmonella* infections typically result in mild, self-limited gastroenteritis or are completely asymptomatic (1)[C].
- Exposure history: travel; reptiles (4" rule—restriction on sale of turtles with carapaces under 4"); poultry; food preparation
- Symptoms when they occur usually appear 12–72 hours after ingestion of contaminated food and resolve within 4–10 days (2)[A].
- Acute uncomplicated illness
  - Sudden onset of nausea, vomiting, diarrhea (1)[C],(3)[A]
  - Abdominal cramping (1)[C],(3)[A]
  - Headache (1)[C],(3)[A]
  - Myalgias (1)[C],(3)[A]
  - Fever (1)[C],(3)[A]

PHYSICAL EXAM

- Fever (1)[A],(3)[A]
- Evidence of hypovolemia (1)[C],(3)[A]
- Abdominal tenderness (1)[C],(3)[A]
- Heme-positive stool (1)[C],(3)[A]
- Rash in 5–30% of cases (3)[A]

DIFFERENTIAL DIAGNOSIS

- Viral gastroenteritis
- Bacterial enteritis due to other organisms
- Pseudomembranous colitis
- Inflammatory bowel disease

DIAGNOSTIC TESTS & INTERPRETATION

Initial Tests (lab, imaging)

- Gastroenteritis
  - Stool culture should evaluate for *Salmonella*, *Escherichia coli*, *Shigella*, and *Campylobacter* (1)[C].
  - Indications for stool culture include the following:
    - Severe diarrhea (≥6 loose stools daily) (1)[C]
    - Diarrhea >1 week in duration (1)[C]
    - Fever (1)[C]
    - Diarrhea containing blood or mucous (1)[C]
    - Multiple cases of illness suggestive of an outbreak (1)[C]
  - Fecal leukocytes: positive
  - CBC: leukocytosis or normal WBC count
- Bacteremia
  - Blood cultures: positive for *Salmonella* (1)[C],(3)[A]
  - Stool cultures: may also be positive because a percentage of patients with gastroenteritis develop bacteremia (1)[C]
- Local infections
  - CBC: polymorphonuclear leukocytosis
  - Wound culture: may be positive for *Salmonella*
- Chronic carrier state
  - Stool culture positive for >1 year (3)[A]
  - Urine culture may be positive as well.
- Endovascular infection is uncommon but possible in nontyphoidal *Salmonella* bacteremia. Consider angiography in patients >50 years of age with bacteremia if aortic or vascular source is suspected (2)[A].
- Consider CT or MRI for soft tissue or bone infections.

Follow-Up Tests & Special Considerations

- Asymptomatic excretion of *Salmonella* bacilli may occur for weeks after infection.
- Diarrhea lasting >10 days should prompt a search for other causes.
- Serotyping of isolates can be performed at public health laboratories.
- Early, empiric antibiotics may lead to false-negative culture and blunted immunologic response.

Test Interpretation

- Mucosal ulceration, hemorrhage, and necrosis seen on biopsy specimens along with reticuloendothelial hypertrophy/hyperplasia
- Focal organ and soft tissue abscesses

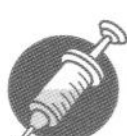

TREATMENT

- Treatment for nonsevere *Salmonella* gastroenteritis is supportive because the illness is typically self-limited in immunocompetent patients (1)[C].
- Antibiotics should be considered in an immunocompetent host with severe diarrhea, high fever, or requiring hospitalization (1)[C].
- Certain populations are at increased risk of bacteremia and benefit from antibiotics.
  - Infants <3 months of age (1)[C]
  - Persons >65 years of age (1)[C]
  - Patients with hemoglobinopathies, underlying atherosclerotic lesions, and prosthetic valves, grafts, or joints or any immunosuppressed state (1)[C],(2)[A]
- Chronic carriage of nontyphoidal *Salmonella*
  - 4–6 weeks of antimicrobial therapy
  - Prophylactic therapy in immunocompromised patients (2)[A]

GENERAL MEASURES

Precautions: Avoid antimotility drugs in patients with fever or dysentery (Lomotil, Imodium). Antimotility drugs may increase contact time of the enteropathogen within the gut mucosa (1)[C].

MEDICATION

First Line

- Gastroenteritis, uncomplicated: No specific medication are necessary (1)[A].
- Gastroenteritis, complicated (risk factors listed earlier)
  - Adults (treat for 14 days if immunocompromised)
    - Levofloxacin (or other fluoroquinolone) 500 mg/day PO × 7–10 days (1)[C]; or
    - Bactrim: 160/800 mg PO BID × 7–10 days *or*
    - Amoxicillin: 500 mg PO TID × 7–10 days *or*
    - Ceftriaxone: 1–2 g/day IV × 7–10 days *or*
    - Azithromycin: 500 mg/day PO × 7 days (1)[C]
  - Children
    - Ceftriaxone: 100 mg/kg/day IV or IM in 2 equally divided doses × 7–10 days (1)[C]; *or*
    - Azithromycin: 20 mg/kg/day PO daily × 7 days (1)[C]
- Bacteremia: Due to resistance trends, life-threatening infections in adults should be treated with a fluoroquinolone *and* a 3rd-generation cephalosporin until susceptibilities are determined (2)[A].
  - Adults
    - Ciprofloxacin (or other fluoroquinolone): 400 mg IV BID × 10–14 days; *or*
    - Ceftriaxone: 1–2 g/day IV × 10–14 days
    - Cefotaxime: 2 g IV q8h × 10–14 days
  - Children
    - Ampicillin: 200 mg/kg/day in 4 divided doses × 10–14 days; *or*
    - Trimethoprim-sulfamethoxazole: 8–12 mg/kg/day of trimethoprim component in 2 divided doses × 10–14 days; *or*
    - Ceftriaxone: 50–75 mg/kg/day (max 1 g) once per day × 10–14 days
- Localized infection (e.g., septic arthritis, osteomyelitis, cholangitis, and pneumonia)
  - Same as for bacteremia
  - In sustained bacteremia, prolonged local infection, or immunocompromised patients, antibiotics can be given PO for 4–6 weeks (2)[A].
- Chronic carrier state (shedding >1 year duration)
  - Amoxicillin: 1 g/day PO TID × 12 weeks; *or*
  - Trimethoprim-sulfamethoxazole 160 mg/800 mg PO BID × 12 weeks; *or*
  - Ciprofloxacin: 500 mg PO BID × 4 weeks, *or* levofloxacin 500 mg/day × 4 weeks *or* norfloxacin 400 mg PO BID × 4 weeks if gallstones are present
- Antimicrobial resistance rates
  - Strains resistant to ampicillin, chloramphenicol, and trimethoprim-sulfamethoxazole have been increasing over the past 15 years. Some strains are rapidly becoming multidrug resistant (4)[B].
  - Fluoroquinolone resistance has been observed in serotypes common to swine and humans (4)[B].
  - Extended-spectrum cephalosporin resistance has been reported in the United States with increasing frequency. 2.5% of invasive serotypes isolated from 1996–2007 in the United States demonstrated resistance to ceftriaxone (4)[B].

Second Line

- Aztreonam is an alternative agent that may be useful in patients with multiple allergies or organisms with unusual resistance patterns (2)[A].
- Fluoroquinolones are now routinely given to children for 5–7 days in areas of the world where multidrug-resistant *Salmonella typhi* is common (2)[A].

SURGERY/OTHER PROCEDURES

- Surgical excision and drainage for infected tissue sites, followed by a minimum of 2 weeks antimicrobial therapy (2)[A]
- If biliary tract disease is present, a preoperative 10–14-day course of parenteral antibiotics followed by cholecystectomy is standard.

ONGOING CARE

FOLLOW-UP RECOMMENDATIONS

Patient Monitoring

- Follow-up fecal cultures are generally not indicated for patients with uncomplicated gastroenteritis. Requirements may differ during a *Salmonella* outbreak (2)[A].
- Criteria may vary by state and local regulations. For example, some public health departments require negative stool cultures for health workers and food handlers prior to returning to work. Shedding may last 4–8 weeks (2)[A].

DIET

Easily digestible foods (1)[C]

PATIENT EDUCATION

- Meticulous hand hygiene; caution handling raw meat, poultry, and eggs (5)[A]
- Fruits and vegetables should be thoroughly washed prior to consumption (5)[A].
- Thoroughly cooking meats eliminates *Salmonella*.
- Caution when handling animals (e.g., reptiles) with high fecal carriage rates (5)[A]
- For more details, visit: www.cdc.gov/salmonella/general/prevention.html.

PROGNOSIS

- Most cases of *Salmonella* gastroenteritis are self-limited and have an excellent prognosis (3)[A].
- Increased mortality is seen in the young (<3 months), the elderly (>65), and immunocompromised patients (1)[C].
- Mortality is increased with multidrug-resistant strains (3)[A].

COMPLICATIONS

Toxic megacolon, hypovolemic shock, metastatic abscess formation, endocarditis, infectious endarteritis, meningitis, septic arthritis, osteomyelitis, pneumonia, appendicitis, cholecystitis (1)[C],(2,3)[A]

REFERENCES

1. DuPont HL. Clinical practice. Bacterial diarrhea. *N Engl J Med*. 2009;361(16):1560–1569.
2. Hohmann EL. Nontyphoidal salmonellosis. *Clin Infec Dis*. 2001;32(2): 263–269.
3. Parry CM, Hien TT, Dougan G, et al. Typhoid fever. *N Engl J Med* 2002; 347(22):1770.
4. Crump JA, Medalla FM, Joyce KW, et al; Emerging Infections Program NARMS Working Group. Antimicrobial resistance among invasive nontyphoidal *Salmonella enterica* isolates in the United States: National Antimicrobial Resistance Monitoring System, 1996 to 2007. *Antimicrob Agents Chemother*. 2011;55(3):1148–1154.
5. Lee MB, Greig JD. A review of nosocomial *Salmonella* outbreaks: infection control interventions found effective. *Public Health*. 2013;127(3):199–206.

S

ADDITIONAL READING

- Centers for Disease Control and Prevention. Preliminary FoodNet data on the incidence of infection with pathogens transmitted commonly through food—10 states, 2009. *MMWR Morb Mortal Wkly Rep*. 2010;84(14):418–422.
- Onwuezobe IA, Oshun PO, Odigwe CC. Antimicrobials for treating symptomatic non-typhoidal *Salmonella* infection. *Cochrane Database Syst Rev*. 2012;(11):CD001167.
- Shah N, DuPont HL, Ramsey DJ. Global etiology of travelers' diarrhea: systematic review from 1973 to the present. *Am J Trop Med Hyg*. 2009;80(4): 609–614.

SEE ALSO

Gastroenteritis; Typhoid Fever

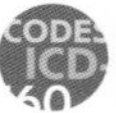

CODES

ICD10

- A02.9 Salmonella infection, unspecified
- A02.0 Salmonella enteritis
- A02.1 Salmonella sepsis

CLINICAL PEARLS

- Nontyphoidal *Salmonella* is a foodborne infection associated with poultry, eggs, and fresh produce.
- Clinical syndromes include gastroenteritis, bacteremia, enteric fever (typhoid fever), localized infection outside the GI tract, or a chronic carrier state.
- Those at greatest risk of complications from *Salmonella* infection include the young, the elderly, and immunocompromised patients.
- Treatment of uncomplicated gastroenteritis in healthy populations is generally supportive.
- Antibiotics should be used in infants, the elderly, and immunocompromised patients.

SARCOIDOSIS

Donnah Mathews, MD, FACP

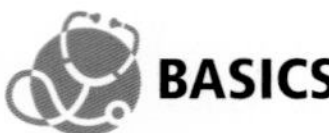

BASICS

DESCRIPTION

- Sarcoidosis is a noninfectious, multisystem granulomatous disease of unknown cause, commonly affecting young and middle-aged adults.
  - Frequently presents with hilar adenopathy, pulmonary infiltrates, ocular and skin lesions
  - In ~50% of cases, it is diagnosed in asymptomatic patients with abnormal chest x-rays (CXRs).
  - Almost any organ may be involved.
- System(s) affected: primarily pulmonary but also cardiovascular; gastrointestinal; hematologic/lymphatic; endocrine; renal; neurologic; dermatologic; ophthalmologic; musculoskeletal
- Synonym(s): Löfgren syndrome (erythema nodosum, hilar adenopathy, fever, arthralgias); Heerfordt syndrome (uveitis, parotid enlargement, facial palsy, fever); Besnier-Boeck disease; Boeck sarcoid; Schaumann disease (1,2)[C]

EPIDEMIOLOGY

Incidence

Estimated 6/100 person-years (3)

Prevalence

- Estimated 10–20/100,000 persons
- <15% of patients with active disease >60 years of age
- Rare in children (3)

ETIOLOGY AND PATHOPHYSIOLOGY

- Despite extensive research, mostly unknown
- Thought to be due to exaggerated cell-mediated immune response to unknown antigen(s)
- In the lungs, the initial lesion is CD4+ T-cell alveolitis, causing noncaseating granulomata, which may resolve/undergo fibrosis.
- "Immune paradox" with affected organs showing an intense immune response and yet anergy exists elsewhere (4)[C].

Genetics

- Reports of familial clustering, with genetic linkage to a section within MHC on the short arm of chromosome 6.
- 3–4× more common in African Americans
- Although worldwide in distribution, increased prevalence in Scandinavians, Japanese, African Americans, and women (3)

RISK FACTORS

Exact etiology and pathogenesis remain unknown.

GENERAL PREVENTION

None

COMMONLY ASSOCIATED CONDITIONS

None

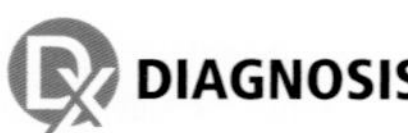

DIAGNOSIS

HISTORY

- Patients may be asymptomatic.
- Patients may have nonspecific complaints, such as the following:
  - Nonproductive cough
  - Shortness of breath
  - Fever
  - Night sweats
  - Weight loss
  - General fatigue
  - Eye pain
  - Chest pain/palpitations
  - Skin lesions
  - Polyarthritis
  - Renal calculi
  - Facial droop due to Bell palsy
  - Encephalopathy, seizures, hydrocephalus (rare)
  - Patients >70 years more likely to have systemic symptoms (4).

PHYSICAL EXAM

- Many patients have a normal physical exam.
- Lungs may reveal wheezing/fine interstitial crackles in advanced disease.
- ~30% of patients have extrapulmonary manifestations (1), which may include the following:
  - Uveitis
  - Other eye findings: conjunctival nodules, lacrimal gland enlargement, cataracts, glaucoma, papilledema
  - Cranial nerve palsies
  - Salivary gland swelling
  - Lymphadenopathy
  - Arrhythmias
  - Hepatosplenomegaly
  - Polyarthritis
  - Rashes (5)[A]
    - Maculopapular of nares, eyelids, forehead, base of neck at hairline, and previous trauma sites
    - Waxy nodular of face, trunk, and extensor surfaces of extremities
    - Plaques (lupus pernio) of nose, cheeks, chin, and ears
    - Erythema nodosum (component of Löfgren syndrome)
    - Atypical lesions

DIFFERENTIAL DIAGNOSIS

- Infectious granulomatous disease such as tuberculosis and fungal infections
- Hypersensitivity pneumonitis
- Lymphoma
- Other malignancies associated with lymphadenopathy
- Berylliosis

DIAGNOSTIC TESTS & INTERPRETATION

No definitive test for diagnosis, but diagnosis is suggested by the following:

- Clinical and radiographic manifestations
- Exclusion of other diagnoses
- Histopathologic detection of noncaseating granulomas

Initial Tests (lab, imaging)

- CBC: Anemia/leukopenia ± eosinophilia can be seen.
- Hypergammaglobulinemia can exist.
- LFTs: Abnormal liver function and increased alkaline phosphatase can be encountered with hepatic involvement.
- Calcium: Hypercalciuria occurs in up to 10% of patients, with hypercalcemia less frequent.
- Serum ACE inhibitors elevated in >75% of patients but is not diagnostic or exclusionary.
  - Drugs may alter lab results: Prednisone will lower serum ACE and normalize gallium scan. ACE inhibitors will lower serum ACE level.
  - Disorders may alter lab results: Hyperthyroidism and diabetes will increase serum ACE level.
- CXR or CT scan may reveal granulomas/hilar adenopathy. Routine CXRs are staged using Scadding classification.
  - Stage 0 = Normal
  - Stage 1 = Bilateral hilar adenopathy alone
  - Stage 2 = Bilateral hilar adenopathy + parenchymal infiltrates
  - Stage 3 = Parenchymal infiltrates alone (primarily upper lobes)
  - Stage 4 = Pulmonary fibrosis (6)
- Chest CT scan may enhance appreciation of lymph nodes.
- High-resolution chest CT scan may reveal peribronchial disease.
- Gallium scan will be positive in areas of acute disease/inflammation but is not specific.
- Positron emission tomography (PET) scan can indicate areas of disease activity in lungs, lymph nodes, and other areas of the body but does not differentiate between malignancy and sarcoidosis.
- Cardiac PET scan may detect cardiac sarcoidosis (7)[B].

Diagnostic Procedures/Other

- Pulmonary function tests (PFTs) may reveal restrictive pattern with decreased carbon monoxide–diffusing capacity (DLCO).
- Characteristically in active disease, bronchioalveolar lavage fluid has an increased CD4-to-CD8 ratio.
- Ophthalmologic examination may reveal uveitis, retinal vasculitis, or conjunctivitis.
- ECG
- Tuberculin skin test
- Biopsy of lesions should reveal noncaseating granulomas.
- If lungs are affected, bronchoscopy with biopsy of central and peripheral airways is helpful. Endobronchial US (EBUS)-guided transbronchial needle aspiration may potentially have a better diagnostic yield.
- Kveim test (ongoing research): Suspension of sterilized splenic cells from a patient with sarcoidosis is injected in an intradermal skin test to evoke a sarcoid granulomatous response over 3 weeks, similar to a tuberculin skin test.

ALERT

If signs indicate Löfgren syndrome, it is not necessary to perform a biopsy because prognosis is good with observation alone, and biopsy would not change management.

Test Interpretation

Noncaseating epithelioid granulomas without evidence of fungal/mycobacterial infection

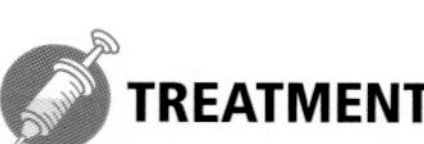

TREATMENT

- Many patients undergo spontaneous remission. It is difficult to assess disease activity and severity, however, making it challenging to develop guidelines.
- No treatment may be necessary in asymptomatic individuals, but treatment may be needed for specific indications, such as cardiac, CNS, renal, or ocular involvement.
- No treatment is indicated for asymptomatic patients with stage I–III radiographic changes with normal/mildly abnormal lung function, although close follow-up is recommended.

- Treatment of pulmonary and skin manifestations is done on the basis of impairment. The symptoms that necessitate systemic therapy remain controversial.
  - Worsening pulmonary symptoms
  - Deteriorating lung function
  - Worsening radiographic findings

MEDICATION

Systemic therapy is clearly indicated for hypercalcemia, cardiac disease, neurologic disease, and eye disease not responding to topical therapy.

First Line

- Systemic corticosteroids in the symptomatic individual (dyspnea, cough, hemoptysis) or in the individual with worsening lung function or radiographic findings
  - The optimal dose of glucocorticoids is not known.
  - Usually prednisone initially, 0.3–0.6 mg/kg ideal body weight (20–40 mg/day) × 4–6 weeks.
  - If stable, taper by 5 mg/week to 10–20 mg/day over the next 6 weeks.
  - If no relapse, 10–20 mg/day × 8–12 months
  - Relapse is common.
  - Higher doses (80–100 mg/day) may be warranted in patients with acute respiratory failure, cardiac, neurologic, or ocular disease.
- In patients with skin disease, topical steroids may be effective.
- Inhaled steroids (budesonide 800–1,600 μg BID) may be of some clinical benefit in early disease with mild pulmonary symptoms.
  - Contraindications: patients with known problems with corticosteroids
  - Precautions: careful monitoring in patients with diabetes mellitus and/or hypertension
  - Significant possible interactions: Refer to the manufacturer's profile of each drug.

Second Line

- All alternative agents to glucocorticoids carry substantial risk for toxicity, including myelosuppression, hepatotoxicity, and opportunistic infection.
- Methotrexate: initially 7.5 mg/week, increasing gradually to 10–15 mg/week
- Azathioprine: 50–100 mg/day
- Leflunomide: 20 mg/day
- Use of immunosuppressants, such as methotrexate or azathioprine, will require regular monitoring of CBC and LFTs.
- Antimalarial agents such as chloroquine or hydroxychloroquine
- Tumor necrosis factor antagonists, such as infliximab, have been useful in refractory cases (8)[C].

ISSUES FOR REFERRAL

May be followed by a pulmonologist, with referrals to other specialists as dictated by involvement of other organ systems

SURGERY/OTHER PROCEDURES

Lung transplantation in severe, refractory cases; long-term outcomes unknown

COMPLEMENTARY & ALTERNATIVE MEDICINE

None known to be effective

ONGOING CARE

FOLLOW-UP RECOMMENDATIONS

There is limited data on indications for the specific tests and optimal frequency of monitoring of disease activity. Suggestions follow.

PATIENT MONITORING

- Patients on prednisone for symptoms should be seen q1–2mo while on therapy.
- Patients not requiring therapy should be seen regularly (q3mo) for at least the first 2 years after diagnosis, obtaining a thorough history and physical exam, laboratory testing tailored to sites of disease activity, PFTs, and ambulatory pulse oximetry.
- If active disease
  - Every 6–12 months, obtain ophthalmologic exam if on hydroxychloroquine.
  - Annually, CBC, creatinine, calcium, LFTs, ECG, 25-hydroxy vitamin D and 1,25 dihydroxy vitamin D, CXR
- Other testing per individual patient's symptoms, including HRCT, echocardiogram, Holter monitoring, urinalysis (UA), thyroid-stimulating hormone (TSH), bone density, MRI of brain
- The serum ACE level is used by some physicians to follow the disease activity. In patients with an initially elevated ACE level, it should fall toward normal while on the therapy or when the disease resolves.
- If inactive disease, follow annually with history and physical exam, PFTs, ambulatory pulse oximetry, CBC, creatinine, calcium, liver enzymes, 1,25 dihydroxy vitamin D, EKG, ophthalmologic exam.

DIET

No special diet

PATIENT EDUCATION

- The American Lung Association at www.lungusa.org/lung-disease/sarcoidosis/?gclid=CPX6zuipm6MCFQxW2godISFepQ
- Sarcoidosis by Medline Plus at www.nlm.nih.gov/medlineplus/sarcoidosis.html

PROGNOSIS

- 50% of patients will have spontaneous resolution within 2 years.
- 25% of patients will have significant fibrosis, but no further worsening of the disease after 2 years.
- 25% of patients (higher in some populations, including African Americans) will have chronic disease.
- Patients on corticosteroids for >6 months have a greater chance of having chronic disease.
- Overall death rate: <5%

COMPLICATIONS

- Patients may develop significant respiratory involvement, including cor pulmonale.
- Pulmonary hemorrhage from infection with aspergillosis in the damaged lung is possible.
- Other organs, especially the heart (congestive heart failure, arrhythmias), eyes (rarely blindness), and CNS can be involved with serious consequences. Cardiac, ocular, and CNS involvement usually manifests early on in patients with these complications of the disease.

REFERENCES

1. Holmes J, Lazarus A. Sarcoidosis: extrathoracic manifestations. *Dis Mon*. 2009;55(11):675–692.
2. King CS, Kelly W. Treatment of sarcoidosis. *Dis Mon*. 2009;55(11):704–718.
3. Rybicki BA, Iannuzzi MC, Frederick MM, et al. Familial aggregation of sarcoidosis. A case-control etiologic study of sarcoidosis (ACCESS). *Am J Respir Crit Care Med*. 2001;164(11):2085–2091.
4. Dempsey OJ, Paterson EW, Kerr KM, et al. Sarcoidosis. *BMJ*. 2009;339:b3206.
5. Lodha S, Sanchez M, Prystowsky S. Sarcoidosis of the skin: a review for the pulmonologist. *Chest*. 2009;136(2):583–596.
6. Statement on sarcoidosis. Joint Statement of the American Thoracic Society (ATS), the European Respiratory Society (ERS) and the World Association of Sarcoidosis and Other Granulomatous Disorders (WASOG) adopted by the ATS Board of Directors and by the ERS Executive Committee, February 1999. *Am J Respir Crit Care Med*. 1999;160(2):736–755.
7. Tremblay A, Stather DR, Maceachern P, et al. A randomized controlled trial of standard vs endobronchial ultrasonography-guided transbronchial needle aspiration in patients with suspected sarcoidosis. *Chest*. 2009;136(2):340–346.
8. Iannuzzi M, Fontana J. Sarcoidosis: clinical presentation, immunopathology, and therapeutics. *JAMA*. 2011;305(4):391–399.

ADDITIONAL READING

- Hoang DQ, Nguyen ET. Sarcoidosis. *Semin Roentgenol*. 2010;45(1):36–42.
- Polychronopoulos VS, Prakash UB. Airway involvement in sarcoidosis. *Chest*. 2009;136(5):1371–1380.

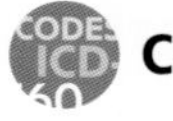

CODES

ICD10

- D86.9 Sarcoidosis, unspecified
- D86.0 Sarcoidosis of lung
- D86.86 Sarcoid arthropathy

CLINICAL PEARLS

- Sarcoidosis is a noninfectious, multisystem granulomatous disease of unknown cause, typically affecting young and middle-aged adults.
- Any organ can be affected.
- Diagnosis is based on clinical findings, exclusion of other disorders, and pathologic detection of noncaseating granulomas.
- Most patients do not need systemic treatment, and the disease resolves spontaneously; a few will have life-threatening progressive organ dysfunction.

SCABIES

Kaelen C. Dunican, PharmD • Brandi Hoag, DO

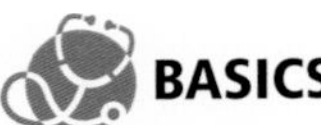

BASICS

DESCRIPTION

- A contagious parasitic infection of the skin caused by the mite *Sarcoptes scabiei*, var. *hominis*
- System(s) affected: skin/exocrine
- Synonym(s): sarcoptic mange

EPIDEMIOLOGY

Incidence

Predominant age: children and young adults

Prevalence

- Global prevalence is estimated at 300 million cases.
- May be more prevalent in urban areas and areas of overcrowding

ETIOLOGY AND PATHOPHYSIOLOGY

Itching is a delayed hypersensitivity reaction to the mite saliva, eggs, or excrement.

S. scabiei, var. *hominis*

- An obligate human parasite
- Female mite lays eggs in burrows in the stratum corneum and epidermis.
- Primarily transmitted by human-to-human direct skin contact
- Infrequently transmitted via fomites (e.g., bedding, clothing, or furnishings)

RISK FACTORS

- Personal skin-to-skin contact (e.g., sexual promiscuity, crowding, nosocomial infection)
- Poor nutritional status, poverty, and homelessness
- Hot, tropical climates
- Seasonal variation: Incidence may be higher in the winter than in the summer (may be due to overcrowding).
- Immunocompromised patients, including those with HIV/AIDS, are at increased risk of developing severe (crusted/Norwegian) scabies.

GENERAL PREVENTION

Prevent outbreaks by prompt treatment and cleansing of fomites (see "Additional Treatment").

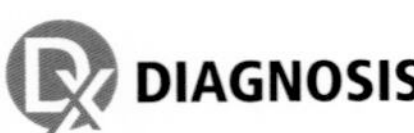

DIAGNOSIS

HISTORY

- Generalized itching is often severe and worse at night.
- Determine any contact with infected individuals.
- Initial infection may be asymptomatic.
- Symptoms may develop after 3–6 weeks.

PHYSICAL EXAM

- Lesions (inflammatory, erythematous, pruritic papules) most commonly located in the finger webs, flexor surfaces of the wrists, elbows, axillae, buttocks, genitalia, feet, and ankles
- Burrows (thin, curvy, elevated lines in the upper epidermis that measure 1–10 mm in length) may be seen in involved areas—a pathognomonic sign of scabies.
- Secondary erosions or excoriations from scratching
- Pustules (if secondarily infected)
- Pruritic nodules in covered areas (buttocks, groin, axillae) resulting from an exaggerated hypersensitivity reaction
- Crusted scabies (Norwegian scabies) is a psoriasiform dermatosis occurring with hyperinfestation with thousands of mites (more common in immunosuppressed patients).

Geriatric Considerations

The elderly often itch more severely despite fewer cutaneous lesions and are at risk for extensive infestations, perhaps related to a decline in cell-mediated immunity. There may be back involvement in those who are bedridden.

Pediatric Considerations

Infants and very young children often present with vesicles, papules, and pustules and have more widespread involvement, including the hands, palms, feet, soles, body folds, and head (rare for adults).

DIFFERENTIAL DIAGNOSIS

- Atopic dermatitis
- Contact dermatitis
- Folliculitis/impetigo
- Tinea corporis
- Dermatitis herpetiformis
- Eczema
- Insect bites
- Papular urticaria
- Pediculosis corporis
- Pityriasis rosea
- Prurigo
- Psoriasis (crusted scabies)
- Pyoderma
- Seborrheic dermatitis
- Syphilis

DIAGNOSTIC TESTS & INTERPRETATION

- The diagnosis should be suspected based on history and physical exam, but definitive diagnosis is based on microscopic identification of mites, eggs, or feces (1,2).
- A failure to find mites does not rule out scabies.

Initial Tests (lab, imaging)

CBC is rarely needed but may show eosinophilia.

Diagnostic Procedures/Other

- Examination of skin with magnifying lens
  - Look for typical burrows in finger webs and on flexor aspect of the wrists and on the penis.
  - Look for a dark point at the end of the burrow (the mite).
  - Presumptive diagnosis is based on clinical presentation, skin lesions, and identification of burrow (1,3).
  - The mite can be extracted with a 25-gauge needle and examined microscopically.
- Mineral oil mounts
  - Place a drop of mineral oil over a suspected lesion. Nonexcoriated papules or vesicles also may be sampled.
  - Scrape the lesion with a surgical blade.
  - Examine under a microscope for mites, eggs, egg casings, or feces (2)[C].
  - Scraping from under fingernails often may be positive.
- Potassium hydroxide (KOH) wet mount not recommended because it can dissolve mite pellets.
- Burrow ink test
  - If burrows are not obvious, apply blue–black ink to an area of rash. Wash off the ink with alcohol. A burrow should remain stained and become more evident.
  - Then apply mineral oil, scrape, and observe microscopically, as noted previously (1)[C].
- Epiluminescence microscopy and high-resolution video dermatoscopy are expensive and have not been proven to be more sensitive than skin scraping (3)[C].

Test Interpretation

Skin biopsy of a nodule (although performed rarely) will reveal portions of the mite in the corneal layer.

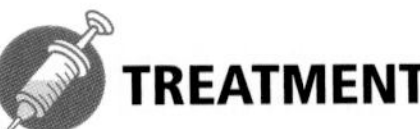

TREATMENT

GENERAL MEASURES

- Treat all intimate contacts and close household and family members.
- Wash all clothing, bed linens, and towels in hot (60°C) water and dry in hot dryer.
- Personal items that cannot be washed should be sealed in a plastic bag for at least 3–5 days.
- Some itching and dermatitis may persist for up to 6 weeks and can be treated with oral antihistamines and/or topical or oral corticosteroids.

MEDICATION

First Line

Permethrin 5% cream (Elimite) is the most effective topical agent for scabies (4)[A].

- After bathing or showering, apply cream from the neck to the soles of the feet paying particular attention to areas that are most involved; then wash off after 8–14 hours. A second application 1 week later is recommended if new lesions develop.
- The adult dose is usually 30 g.
- Side effects include itching and stinging (minimal absorption).

- Crusted scabies may require more frequent application (q2–3d for 1–2 weeks) in combination with repeated doses of PO ivermectin on days 1, 2, 8, 9, and 15 (2,5)[C].

Pediatric Considerations

Permethrin may be used on infants >2 months of age. In children <5 years of age, the cream should be applied to the head and neck as well as to the entire body.

Second Line

- Ivermectin (Stromectol)
  - Not FDA approved for scabies
  - 200–250 μg/kg PO as single dose; repeated in 1 week
  - Take with food to improve bioavailability and enhance penetration into the epidermis.
  - May need higher doses or may need to use in combination with topical scabicide for HIV-positive patients
- Crotamiton (Eurax) 10% cream
  - Apply from the neck down for 24 hours, rinse off, then reapply for an additional 24 hours, and then thoroughly wash off.
  - Nodular scabies: Apply to nodules for 24 hours, rinse off, reapply for an additional 24 hours, then thoroughly wash off.
- Precipitated sulfur 5–10% in petrolatum
  - Not FDA approved for scabies
  - Apply to the entire body from the neck down for 24 hours, rinse by bathing, then repeat for 2 more days (3 days total). It is malodorous and messy but is thought to be safer than lindane, especially in infants <6 months of age, and safer than permethrin in infants <2 months of age.
- Lindane (γ-benzene hexachloride, Kwell) 1% lotion
  - Apply to all skin surfaces from the neck down and wash off 6–8 hours later.
  - 2 applications 1 week apart are recommended but may increase the risk of toxicity.
  - 2 oz is usually adequate for an adult.
    - Side effects: neurotoxicity (seizures, muscle spasms), aplastic anemia
    - Contraindications: uncontrolled seizure disorder, premature infants
    - Precautions: Do not use on excoriated skin, on immunocompromised patients, in conditions that may increase risk of seizures, or with medications that decrease seizure threshold.
    - Possible interactions: concomitant use with medications that lower the seizure threshold

ALERT

Lindane: FDA black box warning of severe neurologic toxicity; use only when 1st-line agents have failed.

Pediatric Considerations

- The FDA recommends caution when using lindane in patients who weigh <50 kg. It is not recommended for infants and is contraindicated in premature infants.
- PO ivermectin should be avoided in children <5 years and in those weighing <15 kg.

Pregnancy Considerations

- Permethrin is pregnancy Category B, and lindane, ivermectin, and crotamiton are Category C.
- Permethrin is considered compatible with lactation, but if permethrin is used while breastfeeding, the infant should be bottlefed until the cream has been thoroughly washed off.

ADDITIONAL THERAPIES

- Crusted scabies may require use of keratolytics to improve penetration of permethrin.
- Benzyl benzoate lotion (not available in the United States but used widely in developing countries)
  - Not FDA approved for scabies.
  - Dose for adults is 25–28%; dilute to 12.5% for children and 6.25% for infants.
  - After bathing, apply lotion from the neck to soles of feet for 24 hours.
- Topical ivermectin 1% lotion (investigational, not available for use in the United States) (6)
  - Not FDA approved for scabies.
  - Apply to affected sites and wash off 8 hours later.

COMPLEMENTARY & ALTERNATIVE MEDICINE

Herbal products such as tea tree oil, eugenol compounds, toto soap, and lippie oil may be effective but require additional evidence to establish efficacy (7).

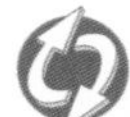

ONGOING CARE

FOLLOW-UP RECOMMENDATIONS

Patient Monitoring

Recheck patient at weekly intervals only if rash or itching persists. Scrape new lesions and retreat if mites or products are found.

PATIENT EDUCATION

- Patients should be instructed on proper application and cautioned not to overuse the medication when applying it to the skin.
- A patient fact sheet is available from the CDC: http://www.cdc.gov/parasites/scabies/

PROGNOSIS

- Lesions begin to regress in 1–2 days, along with the worst itching, but eczema and itching may persist for up to 6 weeks after treatment.
- Nodular lesions may persist for several weeks, perhaps necessitating intralesional or systemic steroids.
- Some instances of lindane-resistant scabies have now been reported. These cases do respond to permethrin.

COMPLICATIONS

- Poor sleep due to pruritus
- Social stigma
- Secondary bacterial infection (group A streptococci and *Staphylococcus aureus*)
- Sepsis
- Glomerulonephritis
- Eczema
- Pyoderma
- Postscabetic pruritus
- Nodules (nodular scabies) may persist for weeks to months after treatment.

REFERENCES

1. Hicks MI, Elston DM. Scabies. *Dermatol Ther*. 2009;22(4):279–292.
2. Gunning K, Pippitt K, Kiraly B, et al. Pediculosis and scabies: a treatment update. *Am Fam Physician*. 2012;86(6):535–541.
3. Leone PA. Scabies and pediculosis pubis: an update of treatment regimens and general review. *Clin Infect Dis*. 2007;44(Suppl 3):S153–S159.
4. Strong M, Johnstone P. Interventions for treating scabies. *Cochrane Database Syst Rev*. 2007;(3):CD000320.
5. Currie BJ, McCarthy JS. Permethrin and ivermectin for scabies. *N Engl J Med*. 2010;362(8):717–725.
6. Chhaiya SB, Patel V, Dave J, et al. Comparative efficacy and safety of topical permethrin, topical ivermectin, and oral ivermectin in patients of uncomplicated scabies. *Indian J Dermatol Venereol Leprol*. 2012;78(5):605–610.
7. Hay RJ, Steer AC, Engelman D, et al. Scabies in the developing world—its prevalence, complications, and management. *Clin Microbiol Infect*. 2012;18(4):313–323.

S

SEE ALSO

Arthropod Bites and Stings; Pediculosis (Lice)

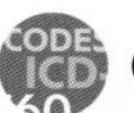

CODES

ICD10

B86 Scabies

CLINICAL PEARLS

- Prior to diagnosis, use of a topical steroid to treat pruritic symptoms may mask symptoms and is termed *scabies incognito*.
- Environmental control is recommended. All linens, towels, and clothing used in the previous 4 days should be washed in hot water or dry-cleaned. Personal items that cannot be washed or dry-cleaned should be sealed in a plastic bag for 3–5 days.
- All members of the affected household may require treatment, especially close contacts (those sharing the same bed or who have intimate contact).
- Eczema and itching may persist for up to 6 weeks after treatment, causing many patients to falsely believe that they have failed treatment or are being reinfected.
- In patients with actual reinfection, either the patient has not applied the medication properly or, more likely, the index patient has not been identified and treated.
- Some experts recommend routine reapplication of permethrin between days 8 and 15.

SCARLET FEVER

John C. Huscher, MD

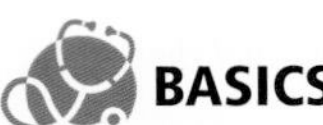

BASICS

DESCRIPTION

- A disease (typically in childhood) characterized by fever, pharyngitis, and rash caused by group A β-hemolytic *Streptococcus pyogenes* (GAS) that produces erythrogenic toxin
- Incubation period: 1–7 days
- Duration of illness: 4–10 days
- Rash usually appears on the second day of illness.
- Rash first appears on the upper chest and flexural creases and then spreads rapidly all over the body.
- Rash clears at the end of the first week and is followed by several weeks of desquamation.
- System(s) affected: head; eyes; ears; nose; throat; skin/exocrine
- Synonym(s): scarlatina

EPIDEMIOLOGY

Incidence

- Rare in infancy because of maternal antitoxin antibodies
- Predominant age: 6–12 years
- Peak age: 4–8 years
- Predominant sex: male = female
- Rare in the United States in persons >12 years because of high rates (>80%) of lifelong protective antibodies to erythrogenic toxins
- Increased rates noted in United Kingdom in 2013.

Prevalence

- 5–30% of cases of pharyngitis in children are due to GAS.
- <10% of children with streptococcal pharyngitis develop scarlet fever.

ETIOLOGY AND PATHOPHYSIOLOGY

- Erythrogenic toxin production is necessary to develop scarlet fever.
- Three toxin types: A, B, C
- Toxins damage capillaries (producing rash) and act as superantigens, stimulating cytokine release.
- Antibodies to toxins prevent development of rash but do not protect against underlying infection.
- Site of streptococcal infection is usually tonsils, but scarlet fever may also occur with infection of skin, surgical wounds, or uterus (puerperal scarlet fever).

RISK FACTORS

- Winter/spring seasonal increase
- More common in school-aged children
- Contact with infected individual(s)
- Crowded living conditions (e.g., lower socioeconomic status, military, child care, schools)

GENERAL PREVENTION

- GAS is spread by contact with airborne respiratory droplets.
- Asymptomatic contacts do not require cultures/prophylaxis.
- Symptomatic contacts may be treated with or without culture.
- Children should not return to school/daycare until they have received 24 hours of antibiotic therapy.

COMMONLY ASSOCIATED CONDITIONS

- Pharyngitis
- Impetigo
- Rheumatic fever
- Glomerulonephritis

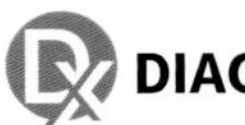

DIAGNOSIS

HISTORY

Prodrome 1–2 days

- Sore throat
- Headache
- Myalgias
- Malaise
- Fever (>38°C [100.4°F])
- Vomiting
- Abdominal pain (may mimic acute abdomen)
- Rash
- Cough, conjunctivitis, hoarseness, and rhinorrhea are more commonly associated with viral infections.

PHYSICAL EXAM

- Oral exam
  - Beefy red tonsils and pharynx with/without exudate
  - Petechiae on palate
  - White coating on tongue: White strawberry tongue appears on days 1–2. This sheds by days 4–5, leaving a red strawberry tongue, which is shiny and erythematous with prominent papillae.
- Exanthem (appears within 1–5 days)
  - Scarlet macules with generalized erythema; blanches when pressed
  - Orange-red punctate skin eruption with sandpaper-like texture, "sunburn with goose pimples"
  - Coarse "sandpaper" rash—helpful in dark-skinned individuals
  - Initially, rash appears on chest and axillae. It then spreads to abdomen and extremities; prominent in skin folds, flexural surfaces (e.g., axillae, groin, buttocks), with sparing of palms and soles.
  - Flushed face with circumoral pallor, red lips
  - Pastia lines: transverse red streaks in skin folds of abdomen, antecubital space, and axillae
  - Desquamation begins on face after 7–10 days and proceeds over trunk to hands and feet; may persist for 6 weeks.
  - In severe cases, small vesicular lesions (miliary sudamina) may appear on abdomen, hands, and feet.

DIFFERENTIAL DIAGNOSIS

- Viral exanthem: measles; rubella; roseola
- Infectious mononucleosis
- *Mycoplasma* pneumonia
- Secondary syphilis
- Toxic shock syndrome
- Staphylococcal scalded-skin syndrome
- Kawasaki disease
- Drug hypersensitivity
- Severe sunburn

DIAGNOSTIC TESTS & INTERPRETATION

- Testing for GAS pharyngitis by rapid antigen detection test (RADT) and/or culture with pharyngeal swab because clinical features alone do not reliably discriminate between GAS and viral pharyngitis.
- Testing for GAS pharyngitis is *not recommended* for patients with symptoms suggesting a viral etiology (e.g., cough, rhinorrhea, hoarseness, oral ulcers).

Initial Tests (lab, imaging)

- RADT: diagnostic if positive, 95% specific; sensitivity approaches that of culture. Negative RADT should be confirmed by throat culture, especially if <16 years. Positive RADTs do not require backup culture (1)[C].
- Throat culture: β-hemolytic colonies that are catalase negative and sensitive to bacitracin; culture is gold standard for confirming streptococcal infection (99% specific, 90–97% sensitive; 5–10% of healthy individuals are carriers) (1).
- Serologic tests (antistreptolysin O titer and streptozyme tests, antihyaluronidase): Confirm recent GAS infection; not helpful or recommended for diagnosis of acute disease.
- Gram stain: Gram-positive cocci in chains
- CBC may show elevated WBC count (12,000–16,000/mm^3); eosinophilia later (second week).
- Follow-up (posttreatment) throat cultures or RADT not routinely recommended
- Diagnostic testing and empiric treatment of asymptomatic household contacts of patients with acute streptococcal pharyngitis is not routinely recommended (2)[B].
- Appropriately symptomatic patients >3 years old with a family member recently diagnosed with laboratory-confirmed GAS pharyngitis may be treated without screening (3)[C].

Follow-Up Tests & Special Considerations

- Recent antibiotic therapy may result in negative throat culture.
- Within 5 days of symptoms, antibiotics can delay/abolish antistreptolysin O response.

Test Interpretation

Skin lesions reveal characteristic inflammatory reaction, specifically hyperemia, edema, and polymorphonuclear cell infiltration.

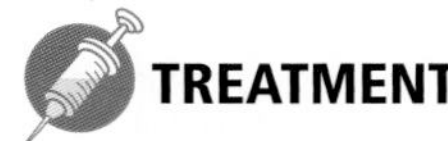

TREATMENT

GENERAL MEASURES

Supportive care. Analgesic/antipyretics such as acetaminophen or an NSAID, for treatment of moderate to severe symptoms or control of fever

MEDICATION

First Line

The main reason for treating GAS is to decrease the risk of acute rheumatic fever. Early treatment decreases symptom duration of symptoms by 1–2 days and decreases the period of contagiousness (3)[B].

- Penicillin (PO; penicillin V and others) for 10 days
  - 250 mg PO BID or TID for ≥27 kg (60 lb); 500 mg BID or TID for >27 kg (60 lb) adolescents and adults(1,4,5)[A]
  - If compliance is questionable, use penicillin G, benzathine: single IM dose 600,000 U for ≥27 kg (60 lb); 1.2 mU for those >27 kg.
- Amoxicillin (PO) 50 mg/kg once daily or 25 mg/kg twice daily for 10 days (use only for definitive GAS because it can induce rash with some viral infections) (6)[A]
  - Contraindications: penicillin allergy
- Acetaminophen for fever and pain
- Precautions: Avoid in patients with penicillin allergy (anaphylaxis).

Second Line

- For patients allergic to penicillin
  - Azithromycin (Zithromax, Z pack): 12 mg/kg/day (max 500 mg) for 5 days (4)[A]
  - Clarithromycin (Biaxin): children >6 months: 7.5 mg/kg BID for 10 days; adults: 250 mg BID for 10 days
- Oral cephalosporins: Many are effective, but first-generation cephalosporins are less expensive:
  - Cephalexin 25–50 mg/kg/day divided every 12 hours × 10 days; max 500 mg every 12 hours (1)[A]
  - Cefadroxil 30 mg/kg/day divided BID; max 500 mg BID × 10 days (1)
- Clindamycin 20 mg/kg/day divided TID × 10 days (4)[B]
- Tetracyclines and sulfonamides should not be used.

ALERT

Avoid aspirin in children due to risk of Reye syndrome.

ISSUES FOR REFERRAL

Development of peritonsillar abscess/shock symptoms: hypotension, disseminated intravascular coagulation (DIC), cardiac, liver, renal dysfunction

SURGERY/OTHER PROCEDURES

- Tonsillectomy may be recommended with recurrent bouts of pharyngitis (≥6 positive strep cultures in 1 year).
- Children still may get strep throat after a tonsillectomy, but for some children with recurring strep throat, tonsillectomy reduces the frequency and severity of strep throat infections.

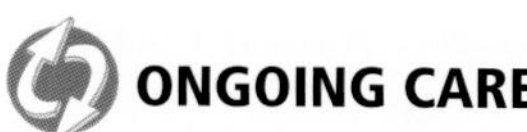

ONGOING CARE

FOLLOW-UP RECOMMENDATIONS

Follow-up throat culture is not needed unless the patient is symptomatic.

Patient Monitoring

Because GAS is uniformly susceptible to penicillin, bacteriologic treatment failures are possible due to the following:

- Poor compliance
- β-Lactamase oral flora hydrolyzing penicillin
- GAS carrier state and concurrent viral rash (requires no treatment)
- Repeat exposure to carriers in family: Streptococci persist on nonrinsed toothbrushes and orthodontic appliances for up to 15 days.
- Penicillin is the drug of choice for treatment.
- Recurrent GAS pharyngitis after a recent oral antibiotic course can be re-treated with the same agent, an alternative oral agent or IM penicillin G.

DIET

No special diet

PATIENT EDUCATION

- Brief delay in initiating treatment while awaiting throat culture results does not increase the risk of rheumatic fever.
- Take antibiotics for recommended course.
- Children should not return to school/daycare until they have received >24 hours of antibiotic therapy.
- Can spread person to person: Attend to personal hygiene (wash hands, don't share utensils).
- "Recurring strep throat: When is tonsillectomy useful?" (www.mayoclinic.com/health/recurring-strep-throat/AN01626)

PROGNOSIS

- Symptoms shortened by 12–24 hours with penicillin.
- Recurrent attacks are possible (different erythrogenic toxins).

COMPLICATIONS

- Suppurative
  - Sinusitis
  - Otitis media/mastoiditis
  - Cervical adenitis
  - Peritonsillar abscess/retropharyngeal abscess
  - Pneumonia
  - Bacteremia with metastatic infectious foci: meningitis, brain abscess, osteomyelitis, septic arthritis, endocarditis, intracranial venous sinus thrombosis, necrotizing fasciitis
- Nonsuppurative
  - Rheumatic fever: Therapy prevents rheumatic fever when started as long as 10 days after onset of acute GAS infection.
  - Glomerulonephritis: due to nephritogenic strain of *Streptococcus*; prevention even after adequate treatment of GAS is less certain.
  - Streptococcal toxic shock syndrome: fever; hypotension; DIC; and cardiac, liver, and/or kidney dysfunction related to other toxin-mediated sequelae
  - Cellulitis
  - Weeks to months later, may develop transverse grooves in nail plates and hair loss (telogen effluvium)

REFERENCES

1. Choby B. Diagnosis and treatment of streptococcal pharyngitis. *Am Fam Physician*. 2009;79(5):383–390.
2. Shulman ST, Bisno AL, Clegg HW, et al. Clinical practice guideline for the diagnosis and management of group A streptococcal pharyngitis: 2012 update by the Infectious Diseases Society of America. *Clin Infect Dis*. 2012;55(10):e86–e102.
3. University of Michigan Health System. *Pharyngitis*. Ann Arbor, MI: University of Michigan Health System; 2013. National Guideline Clearinghouse Guideline Summary NGC-9967.
4. Gerber MA, Baltimore RS, Eaton CB, et al. Prevention of rheumatic fever and diagnosis and treatment of acute streptococcal pharyngitis. *Circulation*. 2009;119(11):1541–1551.
5. van Driel ML, De Sutter AI, Keber N, et al. Different antibiotic treatments for group A streptococcal pharyngitis. *Cochrane Database Syst Rev*. 2013;(4):CD004406.
6. Lennon DR, Farrell E, Martin DR. Once-daily amoxicillin versus twice-daily penicillin V in group A beta-haemolytic streptococcal pharyngitis. *Arch Dis Child*. 2008;93(6):474–478.

SEE ALSO

- Pharyngitis
- Algorithm: Tonsillar Exudates

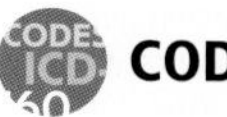

CODES

ICD10

- A38.9 Scarlet fever, uncomplicated
- J02.0 Streptococcal pharyngitis
- A38.0 Scarlet fever with otitis media

CLINICAL PEARLS

- Consider scarlet fever in the differential diagnosis of children with fever and an exanthematous rash.
- Key clinical findings include strawberry tongue, circumoral pallor, and a coarse sandpaper rash.
- Desquamation may last for several weeks following acute illness in scarlet fever.
- Throat culture remains the diagnostic test of choice to document streptococcal illness.

SCHIZOPHRENIA

Maja Skikic, MD • Jeffrey G. Stovall, MD

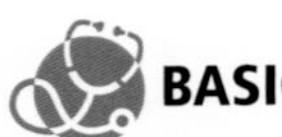

BASICS

Schizophrenia is a chronic, severe, and disabling psychiatric condition characterized by neurocognitive changes and impairment in reality testing.

DESCRIPTION

- Major psychiatric disorder characterized by prodrome, active, and residual psychotic symptoms involving disturbances in appearance, speech, behavior, perception, and thought that last for at least 6 months.
- DSM-5 has eliminated subcategories of schizophrenia (1).
- System(s) affected: central nervous system

EPIDEMIOLOGY

Incidence

- 7.7–43/100,000 (2)
- Predominant sex: male-to-female ratio = 1.4:1.0
- Age of onset: typically <30 years, earlier in males (early to mid-20s) than females (late 20s), with a smaller peak that occurs in women >45 years (3)

Prevalence

- Lifetime (1%): highest prevalence in lower socioeconomic classes and urban settings (2-fold higher risk) (2)
- 1.1% of the population >18 years; similar rates in all countries

ETIOLOGY AND PATHOPHYSIOLOGY

- Stems from a complex interaction between genetic and environmental factors; higher incidence if prenatal infection or hypoxia, winter births, 1st-generation immigrants, advanced paternal age, drug use, and genetic (velocardiofacial) syndromes
- Overstimulation of mesolimbic dopamine D_2 receptors, deficient prefrontal dopamine, and aberrant prefrontal glutamate (NMDA) activity results in perceptual disturbances, disordered thought process, and cognitive impairments (4).

Genetics

If 1st-degree biologic relative has schizophrenia, risk is 8–10%; a 10-fold increase (5).

GENERAL PREVENTION

- Currently, no known preventive measures decrease the incidence of schizophrenia.
- Interventions to improve long-term outcome and associated comorbid conditions are employed during management.

COMMONLY ASSOCIATED CONDITIONS

- Substance use disorders and nicotine dependence are common and lead to significant long-term medical and social complications (6).
- Metabolic syndrome, diabetes mellitus, obesity, and certain infectious diseases, including HIV, hepatitis B, and hepatitis C all occur in higher-than-expected rates in individuals with schizophrenia.

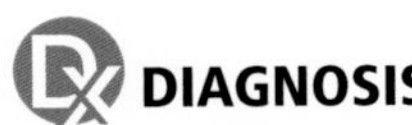

DIAGNOSIS

Focus on identifying an insidious social and functional decline per history with the onset of ≥2 of the following characteristic symptoms on mental status exam:

- Delusions (fixed, false beliefs)
- Hallucinations (auditory>visual perceptual disturbances)
- Disorganized thought (derailed or incoherent speech)
- Grossly disorganized/catatonic behavior (hyper- or hypoactive movements that are often repetitive)
- Negative symptoms (affective flattening, amotivation, avolition, asociality) (1)

PHYSICAL EXAM

No physical findings characterize the illness; however, chronic treatment with neuroleptic agents may result in parkinsonism, tardive dyskinesia, and other extrapyramidal symptoms.

DIFFERENTIAL DIAGNOSIS

- Psychotic disorder due to another medical condition
  - Disorientation, in particular, indicates delirium.
  - Possible medical illnesses include porphyria, TBI, infection, tumor, metabolic, endocrine, and intoxication, including withdrawal states and disorders that affect the CNS (i.e., epilepsy, Huntington disease, Wilson disease, lupus cerebritis, anti-NMDA limbic encephalitis, metachromatic leukodystrophy).
- Substance-induced psychosis: secondary to substance use/abuse, such as cocaine, hallucinogens (amphetamines, LSD, phencyclidine), cannabis (including synthetic), bath salts, alcohol, or prescribed medications including steroids, anticholinergics, and opiates
- Personality disorders (paranoid, schizotypal, schizoid, borderline personality disorder)
- Mood disorders: bipolar disorder, major depressive disorders with psychotic features, or schizoaffective disorder
- Delusional disorder
- Posttraumatic stress disorder
- Cultural belief system

DIAGNOSTIC TESTS & INTERPRETATION

- No tests are available to indicate schizophrenia.
- Imaging and laboratory tests are needed to rule out other causes.

Initial Tests (lab, imaging)

These are needed to rule out a medical etiology of psychotic symptoms and when starting antipsychotic medications; these may include the following:

- Brain MRI, EEG, LP (as clinically indicated)
- CBC, blood chemistries
- Thyroid-stimulating hormone (TSH)
- Blood glucose level, preferably fasting,
- Hemoglobin A1C
- Fasting lipid panel
- Vitamin levels (thiamine, vitamin D, B_{12})
- Drug/alcohol screen of blood and urine
- Urinalysis
- Urine pregnancy test
- Rapid plasma reagin (RPR), HIV
- Heavy-metal exposure: lead, mercury
- Ceruloplasmin, urine porphobilinogen as indicated
- ECG, for baseline QTc

Follow-Up Tests & Special Considerations

Clinical and laboratory tests for routine monitoring, at least yearly, if using antipsychotic medications (7)[A]

- Blood pressure, weight, and waist circumference
- CBC, blood chemistries
- Fasting blood glucose level, hemoglobin A1C
- Lipid panel
- TSH
- Pregnancy test and prolactin level, if indicated
- ECG, monitoring for QTc prolongation

Diagnostic Procedures/Other

- Psychological: not a routine part of assessment
- MRI and EEG to rule out seizure/neurologic disorder
- Lumbar puncture if indicated by clinical presentation

Test Interpretation

No diagnostic pathologic findings; however ventriculomegaly is frequently seen on MRI with whole brain grey matter loss and white matter loss in medial temporal lobe structures preferentially (8)[A].

TREATMENT

MEDICATION

First Line

- Two classes of antipsychotic medications: typical and atypical. 1st-line treatment is with an atypical antipsychotic given lower potential for extrapyramidal side effects.
  - Atypical (2nd generation): risperidone,
  - Olanzapine, ziprasidone, aripiprazole,
  - Quetiapine, paliperidone, iloperidone, asenapine,
  - Lurasidone, clozapine
  - Typical (1st generation): haloperidol, chlorpromazine,
  - Fluphenazine, trifluoperazine, perphenazine,
  - Thioridazine, thiothixene, loxapine
- Medication choice is based on clinical and subjective response and side effect profile (7)[A].
- Sensitivity to extrapyramidal adverse effects: atypical
- For least risk of tardive dyskinesia: quetiapine, clozapine
- For least risk of metabolic syndrome: aripiprazole, ziprasidone, lurasidone
- For poor compliance/high risk of relapse: injectable form of long-acting antipsychotic such as haloperidol, fluphenazine, risperidone, olanzapine, aripiprazole, or paliperidone
- Usual oral daily dose (initial dose may be lower)
  - Chlorpromazine: 200 mg BID
  - Aripiprazole: 10–30 mg/day
  - Asenapine: 5 mg BID (sublingual)
  - Fluphenazine: 5 mg BID
  - Haloperidol: 5 mg BID
  - Lurasidone: 40–80 mg/day
  - Olanzapine: 15–30 mg/day
  - Paliperidone: 3–12 mg/day
  - Perphenazine: 24 mg/day divided BID or TID
  - Quetiapine: 200–300 mg BID
  - Risperidone: 3 mg/day
  - Ziprasidone: 60–80 mg BID (with meal)
  - Clozapine: 200 mg BID
    - Start 12.5 mg/day and increase daily by 25mg until dose of 300 mg/day split into BID dosing; do not exceed 900 mg/day.
    - Effective in treatment of refractory or suicidal patients (7)[A]
    - Serious risk of agranulocytosis mandates registration with National Clozapine Registry and monitoring regular periodic CBC with differential (weekly to once monthly).
    - Significant risk of seizure at higher doses
    - Side effects can include myocarditis, DVT, sialorrhea, tachycardia, and weight gain.

ALERT

All antipsychotics are associated with weight gain and carry the risk of metabolic SE and tardive dyskinesia.

- Managing adverse effects of antipsychotics
  - Dystonic reaction (especially of head and neck): Give diphenhydramine 25–50 mg IM or benztropine 1–2 mg IM.
  - Akathisia: propranolol 10 mg BID or lorazepam 0.5 mg BID
  - Pseudoparkinsonism: trihexyphenidyl 2 mg BID (may be increased to 15 mg/day if needed) or benztropine 0.5 BID (range 1–4 mg/day)
  - Akathisia (restlessness): propranolol (30–60 mg in div doses) or lorazepam (range 1–2 mg/day)
  - Neuroleptic malignant syndrome: hyperthermia, autonomic dysfunction, and extrapyramidal symptoms; requires hospitalization and supportive management (IVF, and cessation of offending neuroleptic)
- Geriatric considerations: All antipsychotics carry a black box warning for increased mortality risk in elderly dementia patients.
- Adjunctive treatments
  - Benzodiazepines
    - May be effective adjuncts to antipsychotics during acute phase of illness
    - Useful for the treatment of catatonia
    - Withdrawal reactions with psychosis or seizures
  - Mood stabilizers (valproic acid lithium, lamotrigine, carbamazepine): may be effective adjuncts for those with agitated/violent behavior (7,9)[A]
  - Antidepressants: if prominent symptoms of depression are present
  - Metformin: helps minimize risk of metabolic SE with use of AP (10)[A]

ISSUES FOR REFERRAL

- Consider in cases of suicidality, coexistence of an addiction, difficulty in engagement, or poor self-care.
- Patients with schizophrenia should receive multidisciplinary care from both a primary care physician and a psychiatrist.
- Family members often benefit from referral to family advocacy organizations such as NAMI (11)[A].

ADDITIONAL THERAPIES

Family and patient education and psychotherapy. These include specific treatments to reduce the impact of psychotic symptoms and to enhance social functioning. Cognitive-behavioral therapy has been shown to be effective for specific symptoms of schizophrenia (12)[C].

COMPLEMENTARY & ALTERNATIVE MEDICINE

No alternative therapies are validated.

SURGERY/OTHER PROCEDURES

- Electroconvulsive therapy (ECT): For patients presenting with catatonic features, the option of ECT should be considered early when insufficient response to benzodiazepines is observed (7)[B].
- Surgical interventions are not available.

INPATIENT CONSIDERATIONS

Initial stabilization focuses on maintaining a safe environment and reducing acute psychotic symptoms and agitation through the initiation of pharmacologic treatment.

Admission Criteria/Initial Stabilization

The decision to admit is usually based on the patient's risk of self-harm or harm to others and the inability to care for self as governed by local legal statute.

Nursing

Monitor for safety concerns and establish a safe and supportive environment.

Discharge Criteria

Based on the patient's ability to remain safe in the community. It reflects a combination of suicide risk, level of psychotic symptoms, support systems, and the availability of appropriate outpatient services.

ONGOING CARE

FOLLOW-UP RECOMMENDATIONS

- Long-term symptom management and rehabilitation depend on engagement in ongoing pharmacologic and psychosocial treatment.
- Monitoring is based on evaluation of symptoms (including safety and psychotic symptoms), looking for the emergence of comorbidities, medication side effects, and prevention of complications.

DIET

- Newer atypical antipsychotics confer a higher risk of metabolic side effects such as diabetes, hypercholesterolemia, and weight gain.
- Although there are no specific dietary requirements, attention should be paid to the high risk of development of obesity and metabolic syndrome in individuals with schizophrenia.

PATIENT EDUCATION

- National Institute of Mental Health: *Schizophrenia*, at www.nimh.nih.gov/health/topics/schizophrenia/index.shtml
- *Helping a Family Member with Schizophrenia*: www.aafp.org/afp/20070615/1830ph.html
- National Alliance on Mental Illness (NAMI): www.NAMI.org

PROGNOSIS

- Typical course is one of remissions and exacerbations. Although uncommon, there are known cases of complete remission and of refractory illness
- Negative symptoms are often most difficult to treat.
- Excessive mortality occurs due to suicide, accidents, coronary artery disease, pulmonary disease, or substance use disorders; guarded prognosis

COMPLICATIONS

- Side effects from antipsychotic medications including tardive dyskinesia, orthostatic hypotension, QTc prolongation, and metabolic syndrome
- Self-inflicted trauma and suicide
- Combative behavior toward others
- Comorbid addictions, including nicotine (13)[A]

REFERENCES

1. American Psychiatric Association. *Diagnostic and Statistical Manual of Mental Disorders*, 5th ed. Arlington, VA: American Psychiatric Association;2013.
2. McGrath JJ. Variations in the incidence of schizophrenia: data versus dogma. *Schizophr Bull.* 2006;32(1):195–197.
3. Riecher-Rössler A, Hafner H. Gender aspects in schizophrenia: bridging the border between social and biological psychiatry. *Acta Psychiatr Scand Suppl*. 2000;102(407):58–62.
4. Laruelle M, Kegeles LS, Abi-Dargham A. Glutamate, dopamine, and schizophrenia: from pathophysiology to treatment. *Ann N Y Acad Sci*. 2003;1003:138–158.
5. Norman RM, Manchanda R, Malla AK, et al. The significance of family history in first-episode schizophrenia spectrum disorder. *J Nerv Ment Dis*. 2007;195(10):846–852.
6. Fagerström K, Aubin HJ. Management of smoking cessation in patients with psychiatric disorders. *Curr Med Res Opin*. 2009;25(2):511–518.
7. Hasan A, Falkai P, Wobrock T, et al. World Federation of Societies of Biological Psychiatry (WFSBP) guidelines for biological treatment of schizophrenia, part 1: update 2012 on the acute treatment of schizophrenia and the management of treatment resistance. *World J Biol Psychiatry*. 2012;13(5):318–378.
8. Shenton ME, Dickey CC, Frumin M, et al. A review of MRI findings in schizophrenia. *Schizophr Res*. 2001;49(1–2):1–52.
9. Essali A, Al-Haj Haasan N, Li C, et al. Clozapine versus typical neuroleptic medication for schizophrenia. *Cochrane Database Syst Rev*. 2009;(1):CD000059.
10. Mizuno Y, Suzuki T, Nakagawa A, et al. Pharmacological strategies to counteract antipsychotic-induced weight gain and metabolic adverse effects in schizophrenia: a systematic review and meta-analysis. *Schizophr Bull*. 2014;40(6)1385–1403.
11. Mojtabai R, Nicholson RA, Carpenter BN. Role of psychosocial treatments in management of schizophrenia: a meta-analytic review of controlled outcome studies. *Schizophr Bull*. 1998;24(4):569–587.
12. Grant PM, Huh GA, Perivoliotis D, et al. Randomized trial to evaluate the efficacy of cognitive therapy for low-functioning patients with schizophrenia. *Arch Gen Psychiatry*. 2012;69(2):121–127.
13. Saha S, Chant D, McGrath J. A systematic review of mortality in schizophrenia: is the differential mortality gap worsening over time? *Arch Gen Psychiatry*. 2007;64(10):1123–1131.

ADDITIONAL READING

Saks E. *The Center Cannot Hold: My Journey Through Madness*. New York, NY: Hyperion; 2007.

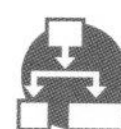

SEE ALSO

Algorithm: Delirium

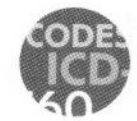

CODES

ICD9

- F20.9 Schizophrenia, unspecified
- F20.0 Paranoid schizophrenia
- F20.1 Disorganized schizophrenia

CLINICAL PEARLS

- A debilitating chronic mental illness that affects all cultures
- Schizophrenia is characterized by positive symptoms, including hallucinations such as voices that converse with/about the patient, delusions that are often paranoid, and negative symptoms, including flattened affect, loss of a sense of pleasure, loss of will/drive, and social withdrawal.
- Multidisciplinary teams to enhance patient and family coping with serious and persistent mental illness, to prevent and treat comorbidities, and to promote recovery

S

SCIWORA SYNDROME (SPINAL CORD INJURY WITHOUT RADIOLOGIC ABNORMALITY)

Patrick M. Carey, DO, MAJ, USA • Jason B. Alisangco, DO, FAAFP

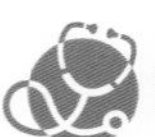

BASICS

Also called spinal cord injury without radiographic evidence of trauma (SCIWORET), spinal cord injury without CT evidence of trauma (SCIWOCTET), or spinal cord injury without neuroimaging abnormality (SCIWONA)

DESCRIPTION

- SCIWORA occurs after trauma; it is an acute spinal cord injury (SCI) and nerve root trauma resulting in transient or permanent sensory, motor, or combined sensorimotor deficits.
- Neural injuries occur without a fracture or misalignment visible on radiographic imaging (x-ray, CT).
- SCIWORA has a broad presentation, from minor neurologic symptoms to complete quadriplegia.

EPIDEMIOLOGY

Incidence

- Variable: reported to be 19–34% of pediatric spinal cord injuries (1)
- Occurs in all populations but is primarily observed in pediatric patients (90%) (1)
- Bimodal: affects children <8 years old and adults >60 years old; rarely occurs between 16 and 36 years old (2)
- There is no association between Chiari malformation type 1 and SCIWORA.

ETIOLOGY AND PATHOPHYSIOLOGY

- Trauma
  - Motor vehicle collision (MVC) (most common cause); either unrestrained passengers, pedestrians, or bicyclists struck by motor vehicles
  - Sports-related injury
  - Significant fall
  - Child abuse
- Mechanism
  - Traumatic neural (edema, hematomyelia, cord disruption) and extraneural (disc injury or ligament disruption) injury occurs after (2,3,4) the following:
    - Hyperextension
    - Hyperflexion
    - Longitudinal distraction
    - Ischemic damage
    - Secondary injury from inflammatory response to tissue damage
- Age: Pediatric patients have a higher incidence of SCIWORA than adults due to anatomic differences and increased mobility and flexibility (1,3,5).
  - Horizontally oriented facet joints, permit more translational motion in the coronal (AP) plane.
  - Anterior wedging of vertebral bodies
  - Elasticity of ligaments and joint capsules permits increased intersegmental movement and disc protrusion.
  - In patients age <8 years, head size-to-trunk ratio is disproportionately large.
  - Weaker nuchal musculature
  - Uncovertebral joints are absent.
  - Pseudosubluxation of C2–C3
- Location
  - Cervical: upper > lower
  - Thoracic: protected and splinted by ribs, preventing forced flexion and extension
  - Lumbar: rare, usually fatal (1)

RISK FACTORS

- History of trauma
- Age <8 years
- Male:female 4:1 (6)
- Improper wear of seatbelt

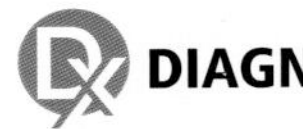

DIAGNOSIS

HISTORY

- MVA
- Sports-related injury
- Fall
- Child abuse

PHYSICAL EXAM

- Assess for sensorimotor deficit.
- Abnormal neurologic findings are not accounted for by known/visible injuries.
- Abnormalities on musculoskeletal exam increases risk of spinal cord injury.

DIFFERENTIAL DIAGNOSIS

- End-plate cartilage fracture
- Transverse myelitis
- Intramedulllary hemorrhage
- Anterior spinal artery syndrome
- Disseminated encephalomyelitis
- Atlantoaxial dislocation
- Central cord syndrome
- Brown-Sequard syndrome

DIAGNOSTIC TESTS & INTERPRETATION

- Radiographic screening with CT of the entire spinal column is recommended (4)[C].
- MRI of the region of suspected neurologic injury (4)[C]
- MRI within 24 hours of injury and consider repeat if normal (6)[C]
- Assessment of spinal stability in a SCIWORA patient is recommended with flexion–extension radiographs in the acute setting and at late follow-up, even in the presence of a magnetic resonance imaging negative for extraneural injury (4)[C].
- Neither spinal angiography nor myelography is recommended in the evaluation of patients with SCIWORA (4)[C].
- CT scan can reliably rule out fracture.

Follow-Up Tests & Special Considerations

- Adult considerations: Adults are less prone to SCIWORA due to decreased flexibility and mobility in comparison to pediatric patients, although SCIWORA is possible in the setting of acute trauma or cervical spondylosis.
- A normal MRI does not rule out SCIWORA (1,2,6).
- MRI abnormalities correlate closely with neurologic injury and prognosis (7)[C].
- MRI may be able to demonstrate neural and extraneural injuries: cartilaginous end-plate fracture, edema, herniation, and interspinous ligamentous injury (1,2).

Diagnostic Procedures/Other

- Diagnosis is based on clinical findings of neurologic dysfunction or MRI abnormality.
- Consider diffusion-weighted MRI and somotosensory-evoked potentials (SSEP) in cases of suspected SCIWORA with normal MRI (4,8)[C].

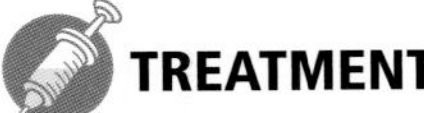

TREATMENT

GENERAL MEASURES

- Immobilize unconscious patients until plain x-ray and CT radiographs are obtained.
- Immobilize until neurologic and pain assessment can be made.
- Transient findings, such as numbness, and a history of trauma should be treated with immobilization following spinal cord injury protocol.
- Supportive care and serial neurologic and musculoskeletal exams
- Blood pressure support (4)[C]
- Corticosteroid use is controversial and is not considered standard practice for pediatric cases (5)[C].

ADDITIONAL THERAPIES

- Rigid external immobilization of the spinal segment for 12 weeks (day and night) (1)
- Immobilization for 12 weeks even after the return of normal neurologic function to minimize SCIWORA recurrence (1,2,4)[C]

- Avoidance of "high-risk" activities for up to 6 months following SCIWORA (2,4)[C]
- Treatment is nonoperative initially. Surgery may be required for spinal cord compression or spine instability secondary to extraneural injury (1,2).
- Surgery for adults is often warranted, as disc and ligamentum flavum pathology is common (2)[C].
- Early discontinuation of external immobilization is recommended for patients who become asymptomatic, and spinal stability is confirmed with flexion and extension radiographs (4)[C].

INPATIENT CONSIDERATIONS

Admission Criteria/Initial Stabilization

- Unexplained neurologic findings (2)[C]
- Neurologic injury found via MRI (2)[C]
- Suspected ligamentous lesion (2)[C]
- Trauma and spinal injury protocol
- Rigid immobilization
- Consultation with a spine surgeon

Discharge Criteria

- Neurologic exam without any deficits
- Resolution of transient neurologic symptoms

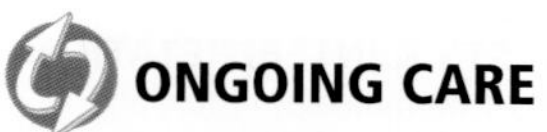

ONGOING CARE

PATIENT MONITORING

- SCIWORA can present with no initial symptoms after trauma followed by subsequent neurologic deterioration.
- Reassess neurologic function within 24–48 hours if patient presents with no initial symptoms after a traumatic event, as there may be a latency period and secondary injury.
- Follow-up MRI before discharge

PROGNOSIS

Initial clinical instability, injury severity, MRI findings, neurologic features, injury location, patient age, and persistence of symptoms have a direct correlation with prognosis.

- Favorable
  - Initial mild to moderate injury
  - Normal or mild edema on initial MRI (1)
  - Resolution of changes as evidenced by follow-up MRI
- Unfavorable
  - Initial severe neural injury
  - MRI findings of spinal cord transection and significant hemorrhage
  - Intramedullary hemorrhage seen on MRI is predictive of complete cord injury (1).
  - Follow-up MRI findings of persistent spinal cord injury
  - Higher cervical injuries
  - Patients age <8 years (1)

COMPLICATIONS

Iatrogenic, delayed, and recurrent SCIWORA have been reported; therefore, careful handling of trauma patients and close follow-up is warranted.

REFERENCES

1. Launay F, Leet AI, Sponseller PD. Pediatric spinal cord injury without radiographic abnormality: a meta-analysis. *Clin Orthop Relat Res*. 2005;(433):166–170.
2. Kasimatis GB, Panagiotopoulos E, Megas P, et al. The adult spinal cord injury without radiographic abnormalities syndrome: magnetic resonance imaging and clinical findings in adults with spinal cord injuries having normal radiographs and computed tomography studies. *J Trauma*. 2008;65(1):86–93.
3. Trigylidas T, Yuh SJ, Vassilyadi M, et al. Spinal cord injuries without radiographic abnormality at two pediatric trauma centers in Ontario. *Pediatr Neurosurg*. 2010;46(4):283–289.
4. Rozzelle CJ, Aarabi B, Dhall SS, et al. Spinal cord injury without radiographic abnormality (SCIWORA). *Neurosurgery*. 2013;72(Suppl 2):227–233.
5. Easter JS, Barkin R, Rosen CL, et al. Cervical spine injuries in children, part II: management and special considerations. *J Emerg Med*. 2011;41(3):252–256.
6. Boese CK, Lechler P. Spinal cord injury without radiographic abnormalities in adults: a systematic review. *J Trauma Acute Care Surg*. 2013;75(2):320–330.
7. Schellenberg M, Islam O, Pokrupa R. Traumatic spinal cord injury without initial MRI abnormality: SCIWORA revisited. *Can J Neurol Sci*. 2011;38(2):364–366.
8. Shen H, Tang Y, Huang L, et al. Application of diffusion-weighted MRI in thoracic spinal cord injury without radiographic abnormality. *Int Orthop*. 2007;31(3):375–383.

ADDITIONAL READING

- Como JJ, Samia H, Nemunaitis GA, et al. The misapplication of the term spinal cord injury without radiographic abnormality (SCIWORA) in adults. *J Trauma Acute Care Surg*. 2012;73(5):1261–1266.
- Kalra V, Gulati S, Kamate M, et al. SCIWORA—spinal cord injury without radiological abnormality. *Indian J Pediatr*. 2006;73(9):829–831.
- Parikh RN, Muranjan M, Karande S, et al. Atlas shrugged: cervical myelopathy caused by congenital atlantoaxial dislocation aggravated by child labor. *Pediatr Neurol*. 2014;50(4):380–383.
- Piatt JH Jr, Campbell JW. Spinal cord injury without radiographic abnormality and the Chiari malformation: controlled observations. *Pediatr Neurosurg*. 2012;48(6):360–363.
- Shah LM, Zollinger LV. Congenital craniocervical anomalies pose a vulnerability to spinal cord without radiographic abnormality (SCIWORA). *Emerg Radiol*. 2011;18(4):353–356.

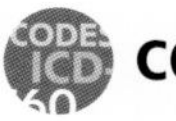

CODES

ICD10

- S14.109A Unsp injury at unsp level of cervical spinal cord, init
- S14.101A Unsp injury at C1 level of cervical spinal cord, init encntr
- S14.102A Unsp injury at C2 level of cervical spinal cord, init encntr

CLINICAL PEARLS

- If a patient presents with a history of trauma and neurologic symptoms but has negative x-ray and CT findings, consider SCIWORA.
- Spinal cord appearance on MRI provides prognostic information (7)[C].
- Treat SCIWORA with early immobilization, continue for 12 weeks, and avoid high-risk activities for an additional 12 weeks (2)[C].
- Immobilization for 12 weeks is superior to 8 weeks (1)[C].
- Consider short-interval follow-up MRI to assess for delayed presentation of pathology (7)[C].

SCLERITIS

Matthew J. Schear, DO, MS • Michael J. Terzella, DO

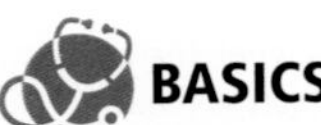

BASICS

DESCRIPTION

- Scleritis is a painful, inflammatory process of the sclera, part of the eye's outer coat.
  - Categorized into anterior or posterior and diffuse, nodular, or necrotizing
  - Commonly associated with systemic disorders
  - Frequently requires systemic antiinflammatory therapy
  - Potentially vision-threatening
- In contrast, episcleritis is a self-limited inflammation of the eye with only mild discomfort.
- System(s) affected: ocular

EPIDEMIOLOGY

- Predominant age: most frequently occurs in 4th and 6th decades; mean age for all types of scleritis is ~52 years.
- Predominant sex: female > male (1.6:1)

Incidence

- Anterior scleritis, ~94% of cases (1)[B]
  - Diffuse anterior scleritis (most common)
- Remaining 6% have posterior scleritis.

Prevalence

Estimated to be 6 cases/100,000 people in the general population

ETIOLOGY AND PATHOPHYSIOLOGY

- Frequently associated with a systemic illness (1)[B]
  - Most commonly associated with rheumatoid arthritis
  - In ~38% of cases, scleritis is the presenting manifestation of an underlying systemic disorder.
  - Necrotizing scleritis has the highest association with systemic disease.
- Other etiologies
  - Proposed pathogenesis is dependent on type of scleritis. In necrotizing scleritis, the predominant mechanism is likely due to the activity of matrix metalloproteinases (2)[C].
  - Drug-induced scleritis has been reported in patients on bisphosphonate therapy.
  - Surgically induced necrotizing scleritis is exceedingly rare and occurs after multiple surgeries.
  - Infectious scleritis occurs most commonly after surgical trauma, and *Pseudomonas aeruginosa* is the most common causative organism (3)[B].

RISK FACTORS

Individuals with autoimmune disorders are most at risk.

COMMONLY ASSOCIATED CONDITIONS

- Rheumatoid arthritis
- Sjögren syndrome
- Ankylosing spondylitis
- Systemic lupus erythematosus
- Reactive arthritis
- Relapsing polychondritis
- Polyarteritis nodosa
- Wegener granulomatosis
- Sarcoidosis
- Inflammatory bowel disease
- Varicella zoster virus
- Syphilis
- Lyme disease
- Tuberculosis

DIAGNOSIS

HISTORY

- Redness and inflammation of the sclera
  - Can be bilateral in about 40% of cases (1)[B]
- Decrease in visual acuity of 2 or more Snellen lines occurred in ~16% of patients (1)[B].
- Photophobia and tearing
- Pain ranging from mild discomfort to extreme localized tenderness (severe pain not a common feature of most inflammatory eye disease)
  - May be described as constant, deep, boring, or pulsating
  - Pain may be referred to the eyebrow, temple, or jaw.
  - Pain may awaken patient from sleep in early hours of morning.
  - Severe pain is most commonly associated with necrotizing scleritis (1)[B].

PHYSICAL EXAM

- Examine sclera in all directions of gaze by gross inspection.
  - A bluish hue may suggest thinning of sclera.
  - Inspect for breadth and degree of injection.
- Check visual acuity.
- Slit-lamp exam using red-free light
  - Episcleritis: conjunctival and superficial vascular plexuses displaced anteriorly
  - Scleritis: Deep episcleral plexus is maximum site of vascular congestion, displaced anteriorly d/t edema of underlying sclera. Characteristic blue or violet color, absent in patients with episcleritis.
- Ocular tenderness
- Dilated fundus exam to rule out posterior involvement
- A complete physical exam, particularly of the skin, joints, heart, and lungs, should be done to evaluate for associated conditions.

DIFFERENTIAL DIAGNOSIS

- Conjunctivitis
- Episcleritis
- Iritis (anterior uveitis)
- Blepharitis
- Trauma
- Ocular rosacea
- Herpes zoster

DIAGNOSTIC TESTS & INTERPRETATION

Consider further tests if warranted by history and physical:

- Routine tests to exclude systemic disease
  - CBC, serum chemistry, urinalysis, ESR, and/or C-reactive protein
- Specific tests for underlying systemic illness
  - Rheumatoid factor, anticyclic citrullinated peptide antibodies, antineutrophil cytoplasmic antibody, and antinuclear antibody may aid in the diagnosis.
- Other tests:
  - Fluorescent treponemal antibody absorption (FTA-ABS), rapid plasma reagin, and Lyme titers
- Further imaging studies, such as a chest x-ray and sacroiliac joint films, may be useful if a specific systemic illness is suspected.
- B-scan US to detect posterior scleritis and thickness of sclera
- If indicated, MRI/CT scan to detect orbital disease

Diagnostic Procedures/Other

Biopsy is not routinely required unless diagnosis remains uncertain after above investigations.

Test Interpretation

Different subtypes of scleritis are associated with varying presentations and distinct findings.

- Diffuse anterior scleritis: widespread inflammation
- Nodular anterior scleritis: immovable, inflamed nodule

- Necrotizing anterior scleritis
  - "With inflammation": Sclera becomes transparent.
  - Scleromalacia perforans without inflammation: painless and only associated with rheumatoid arthritis
- Posterior scleritis: associated with retinal and choroidal complications, adjacent swelling of orbital tissues may occur

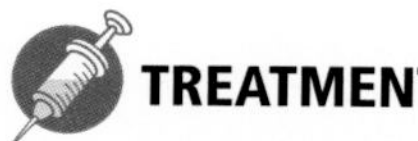

TREATMENT

GENERAL MEASURES

If scleral thinning, glasses/eye shield should be worn to prevent perforation.

MEDICATION

- 1st-line therapies for noninfectious scleritis (4)[C]
  - Oral NSAID therapy, choice based on availability, example is ibuprofen 600–800 mg PO TID–QID provided no contraindications exists. ~37% successful (5)[B]
  - Topical steroids as adjunct, prednisolone acetate 1% ophthalmic suspension
  - Subconjunctival triamcinolone acetonide injection only for nonnecrotizing, 40 mg/mL, 97% improvement after 1 injection. Increased risk of ocular HTN, cataract, and globe perforation (6)[B]
  - Systemic steroids (initial if necrotizing scleritis otherwise use if failure of NSAIDs), prednisone 40–60mg PO QD, taper over 4–6 weeks
  - Antimetabolities including methotrexate, azathioprine, mycophenolate mofetil, cyclophosphamide, and cyclosporine may be used as steroid-sparing agents. They are generally recommended if steroids cannot be tapered below 10 mg PO QD (4)[C].
- 2nd-line therapies (4)[C],(5)[B]
  - Biologics such as infliximab, rituximab, and etanercept may also be used.
- Necrotizing anterior scleritis and posterior scleritis
  - May require immunosuppressive therapy in addition to systemic steroids
  - Treat aggressively due to possible complications if left untreated.
- Infectious
  - Antibiotic therapy resolves about 18% of cases, whereas the remaining often requires surgical intervention such as débridement (3)[B].

ISSUES FOR REFERRAL

- All patients with scleritis should be managed by an ophthalmologist familiar with this condition.
- Rheumatology referral for coexistent systemic disease is helpful for long-term success.

ADDITIONAL THERAPIES

Immunosuppressants used for autoimmune and collagen vascular disorders may be of help in active scleritis.

SURGERY/OTHER PROCEDURES

- In rare cases, scleral biopsy may be indicated to confirm infection or malignancy.
- Ocular perforation requires scleral grafting.

ONGOING CARE

Follow-Up Tests & Special Considerations

- No restrictions
- Avoid contact lens wear only if there is corneal involvement, which is rare.

Patient Monitoring

- Patient in the active stage of inflammation should be followed very closely by an ophthalmologist to assess the effectiveness of therapy.
- Medication use mandates close surveillance for adverse effects.

DIET

No special diet

PATIENT EDUCATION

Scleritis at PubMed Health: http://www.ncbi.nlm.nih.gov/pubmedhealth/PMH0001998/

PROGNOSIS

Scleritis is indolent, chronic, and often progressive.

- Diffuse anterior scleritis (best prognosis)
- Necrotizing anterior scleritis (worst prognosis)
- Recurrent bouts of inflammation may occur.
- Scleromalacia perforans has the highest risk of perforation of the globe.

COMPLICATIONS

- Decrease in vision, anterior uveitis, ocular hypertension, and peripheral keratitis (1)[B]
- Cataract and glaucoma can result from disease or treatment with steroids.
- Ocular perforation can occur in severe stages.

REFERENCES

1. Sainz de la Maza M, Molina N, Gonzalez-Gonzalez LA, et al. Clinical characteristics of a large cohort of patients with scleritis and episcleritis. *Ophthalmology*. 2012;119(1):43–50.
2. Wakefield D, Di Girolamo N, Thurau S, et al. Scleritis: challenges in immunopathogenesis and treatment. *Discov Med*. 2013;16(88):153–157.
3. Hodson KL, Galor A, Karp CL, et al. Epidemiology and visual outcomes in patients with infectious scleritis. *Cornea*. 2013;32(4):466–472.
4. Beardsley RM, Suhler EB, Rosenbaum JT, et al. Pharmacotherapy of scleritis: current paradigms and future directions. *Expert Opin Pharmacother*. 2013;14(4):411–424.
5. Sainz de la Maza M, Molina N, Gonzalez-Gonzalez LA, et al. Scleritis therapy. *Ophthalmology*. 2012;119(1):51–58.
6. Sohn EH, Wang R, Read R, et al. Long-term, multicenter evaluation of subconjunctival injection of triamcinolone for non-necrotizing, noninfectious anterior scleritis. *Ophthalmology*. 2011;118(10):1932–1937.

ADDITIONAL READING

- Doctor P, Sultan A, Syed S, et al. Infliximab for the treatment of refractory scleritis. *Br J Ophthalmol*. 2010;94(5):579–583.
- Fraunfelder FW, Fraunfelder FT. Bisphosphonates and ocular inflammation. *N Engl J Med*. 2003;348(12):1187–1188.
- Iaccheri B, Androudi S, Bocci EB, et al. Rituximab treatment for persistent scleritis associated with rheumatoid arthritis. *Ocul Immunol Inflamm*. 2010;18(3):223–225.
- Rachitskaya A, Mandelcorn ED, Albini TA, et al. An update on the cause and treatment of scleritis. *Curr Opin Ophthalmol*. 2010;21(6):463–467.
- Wakefield D, Di Girolamo N, Thurau S, et al. Scleritis: immunopathogenesis and molecular basis for therapy. *Prog Retin Eye Res*. 2013;35:44–62.

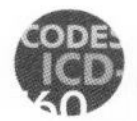

CODES

ICD10

- H15.009 Unspecified scleritis, unspecified eye
- H15.019 Anterior scleritis, unspecified eye
- H15.039 Posterior scleritis, unspecified eye

CLINICAL PEARLS

- Episcleritis is a self-limited inflammation of the eye with mild discomfort. In contrast, scleritis is a painful, severe, and potentially vision-threatening condition, due to the deeper layer of the sclera being involved, for which active treatment is imperative.
- Uveitis, by definition, involves some combination of the iris, ciliary body, and choroid membrane. Scleritis can spread to involve these structures but may not always do so. Both conditions can be associated with underlying inflammatory diseases.
- ~35% of all cases of scleritis are associated with a systemic disease such as rheumatoid arthritis. Necrotizing scleritis has the highest association.

SCLERODERMA

Ann M. Lynch, PharmD, RPh, AE-C • Deborah M. DeMarco, MD

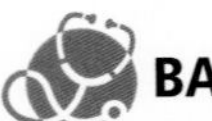

BASICS

DESCRIPTION

- Scleroderma (systemic sclerosis [SSc]) is a chronic disease of unknown cause characterized by diffuse fibrosis of skin and visceral organs and vascular abnormalities.
- Most manifestations have vascular features (e.g., Raynaud phenomenon), but frank vasculitis is rarely seen.
- Can range from a mild disease, affecting the skin, to a systemic disease that can cause death in a few months
- The disease is categorized into 2 major clinical variants (1).
  - Diffuse: distal and proximal extremity and truncal skin thickening
  - Limited
    - Restricted to the fingers, hands, and face
    - CREST syndrome (calcinosis, Raynaud phenomenon, esophageal dysmotility, sclerodactyly, telangiectasia)
- System(s) affected: include, but not limited to skin; renal; cardiovascular; pulmonary; musculoskeletal; gastrointestinal

Geriatric Considerations

Uncommon >75 years of age

Pediatric Considerations

Rare in this age group

Pregnancy Considerations

- Safe and healthy pregnancies are common and possible despite higher frequency of premature births.
- High-risk management must be standard care to avoid complications, specifically renal crisis.
- Diffuse scleroderma causes greater risk for developing serious cardiopulmonary and renal problems. Pregnancy should be delayed until disease stabilizes.

EPIDEMIOLOGY

Incidence

- In the United States: 1–2/100,000/year
- Predominant age
  - Young adult (16–40 years); middle-aged (40–75 years), peak onset 30–50 years
  - Symptoms usually appear in the 3rd–5th decades.
- Predominant sex: female > male (4:1)

Prevalence

In the United States: 1–25/100,000

ETIOLOGY AND PATHOPHYSIOLOGY

Pathophysiology involves both a vascular component and a fibrotic component. Both occur simultaneously. The inciting event is unknown, but there is an increase in certain cytokines after endothelial cell activation that are profibrotic (TGF-β and PDGF).

- Unknown
- Possible alterations in immune response
- Possibly some association with exposure to quartz mining, quarrying, vinyl chloride, hydrocarbons, toxin exposure
- Treatment with bleomycin has caused a scleroderma-like syndrome as has exposure to rapeseed oil.

Genetics

Familial clustering is rare but has been seen.

RISK FACTORS

Unknown

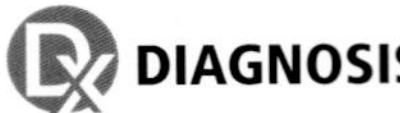

DIAGNOSIS

HISTORY

- Raynaud phenomenon is generally the presenting complaint (differentiated from Raynaud disease, generally affecting younger individuals and without digital ulcers).
- Skin thickening, "puffy hands," pruritus, and gastroesophageal reflux disease (GERD) are often noted early in the disease process.

PHYSICAL EXAM

- Skin
  - Digital ulcerations
  - Digital pitting
  - Tightness, swelling, thickening of digits
  - Hyperpigmentation/hypopigmentation
  - Narrowed oral aperture
  - SC calcinosis
- Peripheral vascular system
  - Telangiectasia
- Joints, tendons, and bones
  - Flexion contractures
  - Friction rub on tendon movement
  - Hand swelling
  - Joint stiffness
  - Polyarthralgia
  - Sclerodactyly
- Muscle
  - Proximal muscle weakness
- GI tract
  - Dysphagia
  - Esophageal reflux due to dysmotility (most common systemic sign in diffuse disease)
  - Malabsorptive diarrhea
  - Nausea and vomiting
  - Weight loss
  - Xerostomia
- Kidney
  - Hypertension
  - May develop scleroderma renal crisis: acute renal failure (ARF)
- Pulmonary
  - Dry crackles at lung bases
  - Dyspnea
- Nervous system
  - Peripheral neuropathy
  - Trigeminal neuropathy
- Cardiac (progressive disease)
  - Conduction abnormalities
  - Cardiomyopathy
  - Pericarditis
  - Secondary cor pulmonale

DIFFERENTIAL DIAGNOSIS

- Mixed connective tissue disease/overlap syndromes
- Scleredema
- Nephrogenic systemic fibrosis
- Toxic oil syndrome (Madrid, 1981, affecting 20,000 people)
- Eosinophilia–myalgia syndrome
- Diffuse fasciitis with eosinophilia
- Scleredema of Buschke

DIAGNOSTIC TESTS & INTERPRETATION

Initial Tests (lab, imaging)

- Nail fold capillary microscopy-drop out is most significant finding.
- CBC
- Creatinine
- Urinalysis (albuminuria, microscopic hematuria)
- Antinuclear antibodies (ANA): positive in >90% of patients
- Anti–Scl-70 (topoisomerase) antibody is highly specific for systemic disease and confers a higher risk of interstitial lung disease (ILD).
- Anticentromere antibody usually associated with CREST variant
- Chest radiograph
  - Diffuse reticular pattern
  - Bilateral basilar pulmonary fibrosis
- Hand radiograph
  - Soft tissue atrophy and acro-osteolysis
  - Can see overlap syndromes such as rheumatoid arthritis
  - SC calcinosis

Follow-Up Tests & Special Considerations

- Pulmonary function tests (PFTs)
  - Decreased maximum breathing capacity
  - Increased residual volume
  - Diffusion defect
- Antibodies to U3-RNP—higher risk for scleroderma-associated pulmonary hypertension
- Anti–PM-Scl antibodies (for myositis) (2)[B]
- Anti-RNA polymerase III—higher risk for diffuse cutaneous involvement and renal crisis (3)[A]
- ECG (low voltage): possible nonspecific abnormalities, arrhythmia, and conduction defects
- Echocardiography: pulmonary hypertension or cardiomyopathy
- Nail fold capillary loop abnormalities
- Upper GI
  - Distal esophageal dilatation
  - Atonic esophagus
  - Esophageal dysmotility
  - Duodenal diverticula
- Barium enema
  - Colonic diverticula
  - Megacolon
- High-resolution CT scan for detecting alveolitis, which has a ground-glass appearance or fibrosis predominant in bilateral lower lobes

Diagnostic Procedures/Other

- Skin biopsy
  - Compact collagen fibers in the reticular dermis and hyalinization and fibrosis of arterioles
  - Thinning of epidermis, with loss of rete pegs, and atrophy of dermal appendages
  - Accumulation of mononuclear cells is also seen.
- Right-sided heart catheterization: Pulmonary hypertension is an ominous prognostic feature.

Test Interpretation

- Skin
  - Edema, fibrosis, or atrophy (late stage)
  - Lymphocytic infiltrate around sweat glands
  - Loss of capillaries
  - Endothelial proliferation
  - Hair follicle atrophy
- Synovium
  - Pannus formation
  - Fibrin deposits in tendons
- Kidney
  - Small kidneys
  - Intimal proliferation in interlobular arteries
- Heart
  - Endocardial thickening
  - Myocardial interstitial fibrosis
  - Ischemic band necrosis
  - Enlarged heart
  - Cardiac hypertrophy
  - Pulmonary hypertension
- Lung
  - Interstitial pneumonitis
  - Cyst formation
  - Interstitial fibrosis
  - Bronchiectasis
- Esophagus
  - Esophageal atrophy
  - Fibrosis

TREATMENT

GENERAL MEASURES

- Treatment is symptomatic and supportive.
- Esophageal dilation may be used for strictures.
- Avoid cold; dress appropriately in layers for the weather; be wary of air conditioning.
- Avoid smoking (crucial).
- Avoid finger sticks (e.g., blood tests).
- Elevate the head of the bed during sleep to help relieve GI symptoms.
- Use softening lotions, ointments, and bath oils to help prevent dryness and cracking of skin.
- Dialysis may be necessary in renal crisis.

MEDICATION

First Line

- ACE inhibitors (ACEIs): for preservation of renal blood flow and for treatment of hypertensive renal crisis
- Corticosteroids: for disabling myositis, pulmonary alveolitis, or mixed connective tissue disease (not recommended in high doses due to increased incidence of renal failure)
- NSAIDs: for joint or tendon symptoms. Caution with long-term concurrent use with ACEIs (potential renal complications)
- Antibiotics: for secondary infections in bowel and active skin infections
- Antacids, proton pump inhibitors: for gastric reflux
- Metoclopramide: for intestinal dysfunction
- Hydrophilic skin ointments: for skin therapy
- Topical clindamycin, erythromycin, or silver sulfadiazine: for prevention of recurrent infectious cutaneous ulcers
- Consider immunosuppressives for treatment of life-threatening or potentially crippling scleroderma or interstitial pneumonitis such as cyclophosphamide for ILD (4)[B].
- Nitrates and dihydropyridine calcium-channel blockers for Raynaud phenomenon
- Avoidance of caffeine, nicotine, and sympathomimetics may ease Raynaud symptoms.
- PDE-5 antagonists (e.g., sildenafil), prostanoids, and endothelin-1 antagonists are changing the management of pulmonary hypertension (5)
- Alveolitis: immunosuppressants and alkylating agents (e.g., cyclophosphamide)

ADDITIONAL THERAPIES

- Anti–TNF-α therapy: Preliminary suggestion is that these may reduce joint symptoms and disability in inflammatory arthritis, but small sample sizes and observational biases lend to the need for further well-designed, adequately powered, longitudinal clinical trials.
- Physical therapy to maintain function and promote strength
- Heat therapy to relieve joint stiffness

SURGERY/OTHER PROCEDURES

- Some success with gastroplasty for correction of GERD
- Limited role for sympathectomy for Raynaud phenomenon
- Lung transplantation for pulmonary hypertension and ILD

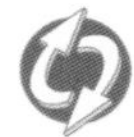

ONGOING CARE

FOLLOW-UP RECOMMENDATIONS

Patient Monitoring

- Monitor every 3–6 months for end-organ and skin involvement and medications. Provide encouragement.
- Echocardiology and PFTs yearly

DIET

Drink plenty of fluids with meals.

PATIENT EDUCATION

- Stay as active as possible, but avoid fatigue.
- Printed patient information available from the Scleroderma Federation, 1725 York Avenue, No. 29F, New York, NY 10128; (212) 427-7040
- Advise the patient to report any abnormal bruising or nonhealing abrasions.
- Assist the patient about smoking cessation, if needed.

PROGNOSIS

- Possible improvement but incurable
- Prognosis is poor if cardiac, pulmonary, or renal manifestations present early.

COMPLICATIONS

- Renal failure
- Respiratory failure
- Flexion contractures
- Disability
- Esophageal dysmotility
- Reflux esophagitis
- Arrhythmia
- Megacolon
- Pneumatosis intestinalis
- Obstructive bowel
- Cardiomyopathy
- Pulmonary hypertension
- Possible association with lung and other cancers
- Death

REFERENCES

1. van den Hoogen F, Khanna D, Fransen J, et al. 2013 classification criteria for systemic sclerosis: an American College of Rheumatology/European League Against Rheumatism collaborative initiative. *Arthritis Rheum*. 2013;65(11):2737–2747.
2. D'Aoust J, Hudson M, Tatibouet S, et al. Clinical and serologic correlates of anti-PM/Scl antibodies in systemic sclerosis: a multicenter study of 763 patients. *Arthritis Rheum*. 2014;66(6):1608–1615.
3. Sobanski V, Dauchet L, Lefevre G, et al. Prevalence of anti-RNA polymerase III antibodies in systemic sclerosis: new data from a French cohort and a systematic review and meta-analysis *Arthritis Rheum*. 2014;66(2):407–417.
4. Roth MD, Tseng CH, Clements PJ, et al. Predicting treatment outcomes and responder subsets in scleroderma-related interstitial lung disease. *Arthritis Rheum*. 2011;63(9):2797–808.
5. Volkmann E, Saggar R, Khanna D, et al. Improved transplant-free survival in patients with systemic sclerosis-associated pulmonary hypertension and interstitial lung disease. *Arthritis Rheum*. 2014:66(7):1900–1908.

ADDITIONAL READING

- Herrick AL. Contemporary management of Raynaud's phenomenon and digits ischemic complications. *Curr Opin Rheum*. 2011;23(6):555.
- Kowal-Bielecka O, Landewé R, Avouac J, et al. EULAR recommendations for the treatment of systemic sclerosis: a report from the EULAR Scleroderma Trials and Research group (EUSTAR). *Ann Rheum Dis*. 2009;68(5):620–628.
- Phumethum V, Jamal S, Johnson SR. Biologic therapy for systemic sclerosis: a systematic review. *J Rheumatol*. 2011;38(2):289–296.
- Steen VD. Pregnancy in scleroderma. *Rheum Dis Clin North Am*. 2007;33(2):345–358, vii.
- Valerio CJ, Schreiber BE, Handler C, et al. Borderline mean pulmonary artery pressure in patients with systemic sclerosis. *Arthritis Reum*. 2013;65(4):1074–1084.

SEE ALSO

Morphea

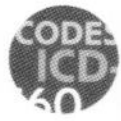

CODES

ICD10

- M34.9 Systemic sclerosis, unspecified
- M34.1 CR(E)ST syndrome
- L94.0 Localized scleroderma [morphea]

CLINICAL PEARLS

- Raynaud phenomenon is frequently the initial complaint.
- Skin thickening, "puffy hands," and GERD are often noted early in disease.
- Patients must be followed proactively for development of pulmonary hypertension or ILD.

SEASONAL AFFECTIVE DISORDER

Christopher White, MD, JD

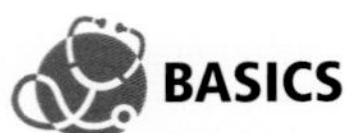

BASICS

DESCRIPTION

- Seasonal affective disorder (SAD) is a heterogeneous mood disorder with depressive episodes usually occurring in winter months, with full remissions in the spring and summer.
- Ranges from a milder form (winter blues) to a seriously disabling illness
- Must separate out patients with other mood disorders (such as major depressive disorder and bipolar affective disorder) whose symptoms persist during spring and summer months

EPIDEMIOLOGY

Incidence

- Affects up to 500,000 people every winter
- Up to 30% of patients visiting a primary care physician (PCP) during winter may report winter depressive symptoms.
- Predominant age: occurs at any age; peaks in 20s and 30s
- Predominant sex: female > male (3:1)

Prevalence

- 1–9% of the general population
- 10–20% of patients identified as having mood symptoms will have a seasonal component.

ETIOLOGY AND PATHOPHYSIOLOGY

The major theories currently involve the interplay of phase-shifted circadian rhythms, genetic vulnerability, and serotonin dysregulation.

- Melatonin produced by the pineal gland at increased levels in the dark has been linked to depressive symptoms; light therapy on the retina acts to inhibit melatonin secretion.
- Serotonin dysregulation because it is secreted less during winter months, must be present for light therapy to work, and treatment with SSRIs appears to reverse SAD symptoms
- Decreased levels of vitamin D, often occurring during low-light winter months, may be associated with depressive episodes in some individuals experiencing SAD symptoms.

Genetics

- Some twin studies and a preliminary study on GPR50 melatonin receptor variants have suggested a genetic component.
- Recent studies indicate an association with the melanopsin gene (OPN4).
- Increased incidence of depression, ADHD, and alcoholism in close relatives

RISK FACTORS

- Most common during months of January and February: Patients frequently visit PCP during winter months complaining of recurrent flu, chronic fatigue, and unexplained weight gain.
- Working in a building without windows or other environment without exposure to sunlight

GENERAL PREVENTION

- Consider use of light therapy at start of winter (if prior episodes begin in October), increase time outside during daylight, or move to a more southern location.
- Bupropion (Wellbutrin) is an FDA-approved antidepressant for the prevention of SAD.

COMMONLY ASSOCIATED CONDITIONS

Some individuals with SAD have a weakened immune system and may be more vulnerable to infections.

DIAGNOSIS

- Carefully document the presence or absence of prior manic episodes.
- Screen for the existence of any suicidal ideation and safety risk factors.
- Remission of symptoms during spring and summer
- Symptoms have occurred for the past 2 years.
- Seasonal episodes associated with winter months substantially outnumber any nonseasonal depressive episodes.
- Under *DSM-5*, SAD is denoted by adding the "with seasonal pattern" specificer to a diagnosis of major depressive disorder, recurrent.

HISTORY

- Symptoms of depression meeting the criteria for major depressive disorder are the following:
  - Sleep disturbance: either too much or too little
  - Lack of interest in life and absence of pleasure from hobbies/activities
  - Guilt: feelings of guilt or worthlessness
  - Energy: fatigue or constantly feeling tired
  - Concentration: difficulty with concentration and memory
  - Appetite: changes in appetite and weight
  - Psychomotor retardation: Patients feel slowed down with decreased activity.
  - Suicidal thoughts: Patients report thoughts of suicide.
- In SAD, hypersomnia, hyperphagia (craving for carbohydrates and sweets), and weight gain usually predominate. Despite sleeping more, patients report daytime sleepiness and fatigue. Cravings may lead to binge eating and weight gains >20 lb.
- Obtain collateral history if patient is unable to provide insight into the seasonal component.

PHYSICAL EXAM

Use exam to exclude other organic causes for symptoms. Focal neurologic deficits, signs of endocrine dysfunction, or stigmata of substance abuse should prompt further testing.

DIFFERENTIAL DIAGNOSIS

- Similar to that of major depression, meaning that organic causes of low energy and fatigue, such as hypothyroidism, anemia, and mononucleosis (or other viral syndromes), need to be considered.
- Other mood disorders without a seasonal component such as major depression, bipolar disorder, adjustment disorder, or dysthymia
- Symptoms should not be better accounted for by seasonal psychosocial stressors, which often accompany the winter holiday seasons.
- Substance abuse

DIAGNOSTIC TESTS & INTERPRETATION

- Thyroid-stimulating hormone to rule out hypothyroidism
- CBC to rule out anemia
- Rule out electrolyte and glucose dysregulation.
- 25-OH vitamin D level
- Pregnancy test for women of childbearing potential
- Urine toxicology screen if substance abuse is a concern
- Imaging not useful unless focal neurologic finding or looking to exclude an organic cause.

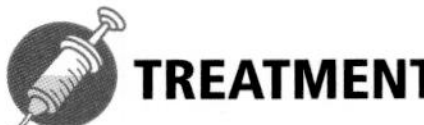

TREATMENT

MEDICATION

Lack of evidence to determine whether light therapy or medication should be the 1st-line agent. Both supported by the literature and in some studies have equal efficacy. Medications have more side effects. Adherence to both remains a critical issue. The ultimate choice depends on the acuity of the patient and the comfort level of the prescribing clinician with each treatment modality (1)[B].

- SSRIs such as sertraline (Zoloft), paroxetine (Paxil), fluoxetine (Prozac), citalopram (Celexa), and escitalopram (Lexapro) in their traditional antidepressant doses (2)[B]
- Bupropion (Wellbutrin) is the only antidepressant currently approved by the FDA for the prevention of SAD (3)[B].

ISSUES FOR REFERRAL

- Patients with a history of ocular disease should be referred for an ophthalmologic exam before phototherapy and for serial monitoring.
- Patients who fail to respond or who develop manic symptoms or suicidal ideation once treatment is initiated should be considered for psychiatric referral.

ADDITIONAL THERAPIES

Phototherapy using special light sources has been shown to be effective in 60–90% of patients, often providing relief with a few sessions (2,4)[B].

- Variables that can regulate effect are the following:
  - Light intensity: Although the minimum light source intensity is under investigation, 2,500 lux is suggested (domestic lights emit, on average, 200–500 lux). There is good evidence for 10,000 lux as the recommended source (2)[B].

– Treatment duration: Exposure time varies based on intensity of light source, with daily sessions of 30 minutes to a few hours.
– Time of treatment: Most patients respond better by using the light therapy early in the morning.
– Color of light source: Emerging data suggest that shorter sessions (20 minutes) of lower intensity (2,500 lux) light-emitting diodes enriched in the blue spectrum have equal efficacy to the traditional white light treatment (30 minutes; 10,000 lux) (5)[B].

- Light box is placed on table several feet away, and the light is allowed to shine onto the patient's eyes (sunglasses should be avoided). Ensure that the light box has an ultraviolet filter.
- Most common side effects are eye strain and headache. Insomnia can result if the light box is used too late in the day. Light boxes also can precipitate mania in some patients.
- Dawn simulation machines gradually increase illumination while the patient sleeps, simulating sunrise while using a significantly less intense light source.

COMPLEMENTARY & ALTERNATIVE MEDICINE

- Work to reduce stress levels through meditation, progressive relaxation exercises, and/or lifestyle modification.
- The potential role of vitamin D supplementation is under investigation. Currently, there is a lack of consistent research to satisfactorily demonstrate that treatment improves SAD symptoms. Reported doses vary widely but typically are between 400 and 800 IU/day (6)[C].

INPATIENT CONSIDERATIONS

Admission Criteria/Initial Stabilization

If the patient develops suicidal ideation as part of his or her depression or mania after treatment is initiated

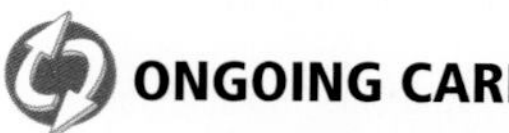

ONGOING CARE

FOLLOW-UP RECOMMENDATIONS

Regular monitoring by PCP or psychiatrist for response to treatment; patients may become manic when treated with SSRIs or light therapy.

Patient Monitoring

Patients should be seen in the outpatient clinic weekly to biweekly when initiating light or pharmacotherapy to monitor treatment results, side effects, and any increased suicidal thoughts if using SSRIs.

DIET

No specific diet modification needed.

PATIENT EDUCATION

- Increase time outdoors during daylight.
- Rearrange home or work environment to get more direct sunlight through windows.

PROGNOSIS

Symptoms, if untreated, generally remit within 5 months with exposure to spring light, only to return in subsequent winters. If treated, patients usually respond within 3–6 weeks.

COMPLICATIONS

Development of suicidal ideation and mania are 2 outcomes the clinician needs to monitor.

REFERENCES

1. Lam RW, Levitt AJ, Levitan RD, et al. The Can-SAD study: a randomized controlled trial of the effectiveness of light therapy and fluoxetine in patients with winter seasonal affective disorder. *Am J Psychiatry*. 2006;163(5):805–812.
2. Kurlansik SL, Ibay AD. Seasonal affective disorder. *Am Fam Physician*. 2012;86(11):1037–1041.
3. Niemegeers P, Dumont GJ, Patteet L, et al. Bupropion for the treatment of seasonal affective disorder. *Expert Opin Drug Metab Toxicol*. 2013;9(9):1229–1240.
4. Terman M, Terman JS. Light therapy for seasonal and nonseasonal depression: efficacy, protocol, safety, and side effects. *CNS Spectr*. 2005;10(8):647–663; quiz 672.
5. Gordijn MC, 't Mannetje D, Meesters Y, et al. The effects of blue-enriched light treatment compared to standard light treatment in seasonal affective disorder. *J Affect Disord*. 2012;136(1–2):72–80.
6. Howland RH. Vitamin D and depression. *J Psychosoc Nurs Ment Health Serv*. 2011;49(2):15–18.

ADDITIONAL READING

- Pail G, Huf W, Pjrek E, et al. Bright-light therapy in the treatment of mood disorders. *Neuropsychobiology*. 2011;64(3):152–162.
- Thaler K, Delivuk M, Chapman A, et al. Second-generation antidepressants for seasonal affective disorder. *Cochrane Database Syst Rev*. 2011;(12):CD008591.

SEE ALSO

- Bipolar I Disorder; Bipolar II Disorder; Depression
- Algorithm: Depressive Episode, Major

CODES

ICD10

- F33.9 Major depressive disorder, recurrent, unspecified
- F33.0 Major depressive disorder, recurrent, mild
- F33.1 Major depressive disorder, recurrent, moderate

CLINICAL PEARLS

- SAD is a subtype of major depressive disorder. Once the patient has a diagnosed mood disorder, such as depression or bipolar, ask whether the symptoms vary in a seasonal pattern to qualify for the diagnosis of SAD. Generally, these patients will report sleeping too much, eating too much (especially carbs and sweets), and gaining weight during winter months.
- As with all psychiatric diagnoses, ensure that the symptoms are not due to an organic process or better explained by substance abuse.
- Lack of good evidence to decide whether light therapy or SSRIs should be the first line agent. Guidelines suggest using SSRIs first if the patient is more acute or has contraindications to light therapy or the clinician is not comfortable with light therapy.
- Light therapy boxes are available from numerous online suppliers but are not extensively regulated; practitioners should take care to ensure that patients are using devices from reputable suppliers.
- If using SSRIs, recent studies indicate that some patients may begin to experience increased suicidal thoughts on therapy; these patients need to be monitored closely as outpatients every 1–2 weeks. Patients on light therapy also should be monitored closely initially in order to adjust treatment. Once stabilized, both groups of patients can be seen every 4–8 weeks during the winter months.
- All patients who demonstrate suicidal ideation or symptoms of mania should be referred for consideration of hospitalization.

SECRETION OF INAPPROPRIATE ANTIDIURETIC HORMONE (SIADH)

Robert A. Baldor, MD, FAAFP

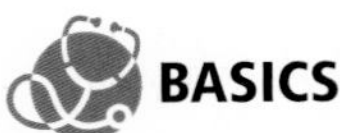

BASICS

DESCRIPTION

- A syndrome of abnormal production of antidiuretic hormone (ADH), despite low serum osmolality, leading to hyponatremia and inappropriately elevated urine osmolality
  - Resulting abnormal urinary free water retention leads to dilutional hyponatremia (total body sodium levels may be normal or near normal, but the patient's total body water is increased).
  - Often secondary to medications but may be associated with an underlying disorder, such as neoplasm, pulmonary disorder, or CNS system disease
- Synonym(s): syndrome of inappropriate secretion of ADH

EPIDEMIOLOGY

Incidence

- Often found in the hospital setting, where incidence can be as high as 35%
- Predominant age: elderly
- Predominate sex: females > males

ETIOLOGY AND PATHOPHYSIOLOGY

- Drugs:
  - Antidepressants (e.g., monoamine oxidase inhibitors [MAOIs], tricyclics, SSRIs)
  - Oral hypoglycemics (e.g., chlorpropamide, metformin)
  - Antineoplastic drugs (e.g., vincristine, vinblastine, cisplatin, cyclophosphamide)
  - Antipsychotic agents (e.g., phenothiazines, thioridazine, haloperidol)
  - Analgesics (e.g., NSAIDs)
  - Antiepileptics (e.g., carbamazepine, oxcarbazepine, valproic acid)
  - Others (e.g., vasopressin, DDAVP, ecstasy, oxytocin, α-interferon)
- Neoplasms (ectopic ADH production):
  - Small cell carcinoma of the lung
  - Hodgkin disease
  - Pancreatic carcinoma
  - Thymoma
  - Mesothelioma
  - Bronchogenic carcinoma
- Infectious diseases:
  - Meningitis
  - Encephalitis
  - Pneumonia
  - Pulmonary tuberculosis (TB)
  - Rocky Mountain spotted fever
  - HIV infection
- Miscellaneous cardiopulmonary conditions:
  - Asthma
  - Atelectasis
  - Myocardial infarction
  - Vascular diseases
- Other:
  - CNS injury
  - Mechanical ventilation
  - Multiple sclerosis
  - Guillain-Barré syndrome
  - Lupus erythematosus
  - Porphyria
  - Hypothyroidism, myxedema
- Idiopathic

Genetics

No known genetic pattern

RISK FACTORS

- Use of predisposing drugs
- Advanced age
- Postoperative status
- Institutionalization

GENERAL PREVENTION

- Search for cause, if unknown.
- Administration of 0.9% sodium chloride in adults during the perioperative period is recommended (if hypernatremia is not present).
- Monitor electrolytes in postoperative patients to determine if fluid intake needs restriction.
- Reduce/change medications, if drug-induced.
- Lifelong restriction of fluid intake

COMMONLY ASSOCIATED CONDITIONS

See "Etiology."

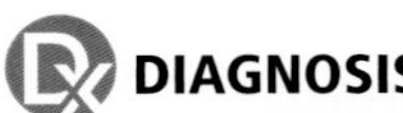

DIAGNOSIS

HISTORY

Early symptoms:

- Fatigue
- Anorexia
- Nausea
- Vomiting
- Diarrhea
- Headaches
- Myalgias
- Increased thirst

PHYSICAL EXAM

Late/severe hyponatremia (serum Na <100–115 mEq/L)

- Altered mental status
- Confusion
- Lethargy
- Seizures
- Psychosis
- Coma
- Death

DIFFERENTIAL DIAGNOSIS

- Postoperative complications:
  - Usually after major abdominal/thoracic surgery
  - Caused by nonosmotic release of ADH, probably mediated by pain afferents
  - ADH increased by pain and narcotics
- Postprostatectomy syndrome
  - Irrigating solution must be nonconducting (i.e., electrolyte-free).
  - D_5W absorbed
- Psychogenic polydipsia
  - Active therapy rarely is needed.
  - Diuresis occurs when intake is stopped.
  - Intake usually >10 L/day
  - Interaction with other psychotropic drugs
- Acute (usually in children)
  - Swallowing water during swimming
  - Diluted formula
  - Tap water enemas
- Endocrine
  - Addison disease
  - Hypothyroidism
- Spurious hyponatremia: caused by increased serum glucose, cholesterol, or proteins
- Appropriate ADH secretion and hyponatremia with decreased effective arterial blood volume (e.g., congestive heart failure [CHF], nephrotic syndrome, cirrhosis)
- Cerebral salt-wasting syndrome (hyponatremia, extracellular fluid depletion, CNS insult)

DIAGNOSTIC TESTS & INTERPRETATION

- Serum Na level: low
- Serum osmolality: low
- Urine osmolality: high
- Urinary Na concentration: high (losing sodium, rather than retaining)
- Serum ADH level: high
- Not usually required for diagnosis but to assess for other concerns:
  - Uric acid
  - Serum glucose; BUN; creatinine
  - Thyroid function
  - Morning cortisol

TREATMENT

GENERAL MEASURES

- Fluid restriction (800–1,000 mL/day) is the main form of treatment (1)[C].
- Mildly symptomatic (serum Na >125 mEq/L [>125 mmol/L]): Restrict fluid to 800–1,000 mL/day.
- Acute (<48 hours duration) or symptomatic (altered mental status, seizure, coma)
  - Hypertonic saline (3% normal saline) bolus
  - Diuresis with loop diuretics
  - Decrease oral free water to maintenance.
  - Increase oral salt.
  - Correct serum Na deficit (mEq Na deficit = [desired Na − actual Na] × 0.5 × body weight [kg]).
  - Increase serum Na slowly with hypertonic saline by 4–6 mEq/L over 4–6 hours (not to exceed 9 mEq/L in a 24-hour period) (2,3).

MEDICATION

- Diuretics: furosemide (Lasix) + hourly NaCl and KCl replacement
  - Requires frequent monitoring (see "Patient Monitoring")
  - Treatment of choice for acute management
- IV saline to increase serum Na cautiously (4) [B]:
  - Goal sodium increase is <9 mEq/L in any 24-period.
  - If serum Na <120 mEq/L or severe neurologic symptoms; consider use of hypertonic saline to increase serum Na by 4–6 mEq/L over the first 4–6 hours.
- Contraindications: Avoid fluids in CHF, nephrotic syndrome, or cirrhosis.
- Precautions: Overly rapid correction (>9–10 mEq/L/day) can increase risk for the following:
  - CHF
  - Subdural and intracerebral hemorrhage
  - Permanent CNS damage, especially with serum Na <120 mEq/L (<120 mmol/L)
  - Demyelination syndrome
- Vasopressin-2 receptor antagonist (the vaptans: tolvaptan, conivaptan) (4),(5)[C]
  - Good efficacy and safety profiles in the treatment of mild to moderate hyponatremia due to SIADH
  - Avoid tolvaptan in patients with liver disease.
- Demeclocycline (second line) (6)[C]
  - Blocks ADH at renal tubule; produces nephrogenic diabetes insipidus
  - Dosage for long-term management: 300–600 mg PO BID
  - Onset of action within 1 week; therefore, not best for acute management

ALERT

Increase Na levels slowly, no more than 9 mEq/L/24 hr, to prevent complications such as central pontine myelinosis (CPM) (7)[C].

ONGOING CARE

FOLLOW-UP RECOMMENDATIONS

Patient Monitoring

- Careful continuous clinical and laboratory monitoring of hyponatremic state during acute phase:
  - Hourly urine output
  - Urine Na
  - Serum Na and potassium (K)
- Chronic management: Monitor underlying cause, as needed.

DIET

May need increased salt/decreased water intake, depending on cause

PATIENT EDUCATION

Diet and fluid restrictions

PROGNOSIS

- Depends on underlying cause; in general, higher morbidity and mortality in hospitalized patients with hyponatremia
- If symptomatic (seizure, coma): high mortality due to cerebral edema if serum Na <120 mEq/L (<120 mmol/L)

COMPLICATIONS

- Osmotic demyelination: central pontine and extrapontine irreversible myelinolysis (2,7)
- Chronic hyponatremia: usually <120 mEq/L (<120 mmol/L)
- Complications of overly rapid correction (see "Treatment," precautions)
- Chronic hyponatremia is associated with osteoporosis (8)[C].

REFERENCES

1. Ellison DH, Berl T. Clinical practice. The syndrome of inappropriate antidiuresis. *N Engl J Med*. 2007;356(20):2064–2072.
2. Adrogué HJ, Madias NE. The challenge of hyponatremia. *J Am Soc Nephrol*. 2012;23(7):1140–1148.
3. Sterns RH, Nigwekar SU, Hix JK. The treatment of hyponatremia. *Semin Nephrol*. 2009;29(3):282–299.
4. Esposito P, Piotti G, Bianzina S, et al. The syndrome of inappropriate antidiuresis: pathophysiology, clinical management and new therapeutic options. *Nephron Clin Pract*. 2011;119(1):c62–c73.
5. Friedman B, Cirulli J. Hyponatremia in critical care patients: frequency, outcome, characteristics, and treatment with the vasopressin V(2)-receptor antagonist tolvaptan. *J Crit Care*. 2013;28(2):219.e1–e12.
6. Sherlock M, Thompson CJ. The syndrome of inappropriate antidiuretic hormone: current and future management options. *Eur J Endocrinol*. 2010;162(Suppl 1):S13–S18.
7. Fleming JD, Babu S. Images in clinical medicine. Central pontine myelinolysis. *N Engl J Med*. 2008;359(23):e29.
8. Verbalis JG, Barsony J, Sugimura Y, et al. Hyponatremia-induced osteoporosis. *J Bone Miner Res*. 2010;25(3):554–563.

SEE ALSO

Hyponatremia

CODES

ICD10

E22.2 Syndrome of inappropriate secretion of antidiuretic hormone

CLINICAL PEARLS

- Fluid restriction to 600–800 mL/day × 2–3 days will result in weight loss and correction of hyponatremia and salt wasting in SIADH. Fluid restriction fails to correct hyponatremia and Na wasting in salt-losing renal disease.
- Cerebral salt wasting is a controversial disease entity and is similar to SIADH. However, patients with SIADH are euvolemic, whereas patients with cerebral salt wasting are hypovolemic. The only real way to establish the diagnosis is through fluid restriction. Serum urate and fractional excretion of urate will be corrected with fluid restriction in SIADH, but will not correct in cerebral salt wasting.
- CPM is a cerebral demyelination syndrome that causes quadriplegia, pseudobulbar palsy, seizures, coma, and death. It is caused by an overly rapid rate of Na correction.
- Safe correction of hyponatremia is important. Online calculators are available: www.medcalc.com/sodium.html.

SEIZURE DISORDER, ABSENCE

Felicia Chu, MD • Puja Vora, MD

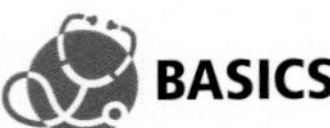

BASICS

DESCRIPTION

An absence seizure is a generalized epileptic seizure characterized by a brief lapse of awareness.

Absence Seizure Types

Absence seizure types according to the International League Again Epilepsy (ILAE) 2010 classification include the following (1):

- Typical absence
  - Formerly called *petit mal seizures*
  - Abrupt-onset behavioral arrest, loss of awareness, and blank staring, sometimes with mild upward eye deviation, repetitive blinking
  - May include automatisms, tonic or atonic features, eyelid or facial clonus, autonomic features
  - Lasts 5–30 seconds
  - Immediate return to normal consciousness
  - Associated with genetic generalized epilepsies, namely, childhood absence epilepsy, juvenile absence epilepsy, and juvenile myoclonic epilepsy
- Atypical absence
  - Onset and offset less abrupt than typical absence seizures
  - Lasts 10–45 seconds
  - Impairment of consciousness often incomplete with continued purposeful activity
  - Postictal confusion sometimes occurs
  - Associated clinical features more pronounced and frequent than in typical absence; atonia most common
  - Associated with syndromic epilepsies, such as Lennox-Gastaut and nonsyndromic epilepsies in patients with developmental delay
- Absence with special features
  - Myoclonic absence
    - Rhythmic clonic jerking at 2–4 Hz, which last 5–10 seconds
    - Unlike myoclonic seizures with no impairment of consciousness, brief lapses of awareness are characteristic of myoclonic absence.
  - Eyelid myoclonia
    - Rhythmic clonic jerking of the eyelids at 5–6 Hz, which last 3–5 seconds
    - Eyelid myoclonia with absence associated with an impairment of consciousness

Epilepsy Diagnoses

Specific diagnoses according to ILAE (2010):

- Childhood absence epilepsy (CAE)
  - Also known as *pyknolepsy*
  - Typical absence seizures are the only seizure type in 90% of children.
  - 10% develop additional generalized tonic–clonic seizures.
  - Seizures last ~10 seconds and often occur hundreds of times per day.
  - Normal neurologic state and development
  - Spontaneous remission occurs in 65–70% of patients during adolescence.
- Juvenile absence epilepsy (JAE)
  - Typical absence seizures are the main seizure type.
  - Seizures last longer than in CAE and occur usually less than once a day.
  - Generalized tonic–clonic seizures occur in most patients, often in the first 1–2 hours after awakening.
  - Seizures often persist into adulthood.

EPIDEMIOLOGY

- Predominant age
  - CAE: onset ages 4–10 years, with peak at ages 5–8 years
  - JAE: onset ages 9–16 years, with peak at ages 10–12 years
- Predominant gender
  - Female > male (3:2–2:1)
  - Absence epilepsy with myoclonus has male predominance.

Incidence

6–8/100,000 per year

Prevalence

5–50/100,000

ETIOLOGY AND PATHOPHYSIOLOGY

- Corticoreticular theory implicates abnormal activity in thalamocortical circuits.
- Thalamic reticular nucleus is responsible for both normal sleep spindles and pathologic slow-wave discharges and contains inhibitory gamma-aminobutyric acid-ergic (GABAergic) neurons.
- These neurons affect low-threshold calcium currents.
- These circuits can fire in oscillatory/rhythmic fashion:
  - Normally, activation of $GABA_A$ receptors causes 10-Hz oscillations in sleep spindle frequency.
  - If $GABA_B$ receptors are strongly activated, oscillation frequency will be 3–4 Hz, similar to spike-and-wave typical absence seizure frequency.

Genetics

- 70–85% concordance occurs in monozygotic twins; 82% share EEG features
- 33% concordance among 1st-degree relatives
- 15–45% have a family history of epilepsy.
- Complex multifactorial inheritance
- For childhood absence, genes/loci implicated include 6q, 8q24, and 5q14.
- Mutations of $GABA_A$ receptor and voltage-gated Ca^{2+} channel are implicated.

COMMONLY ASSOCIATED CONDITIONS

- 3–8% of CAE cases evolve into juvenile myoclonic epilepsy.
- Associated with difficulties in visual attention and visuospatial skills, verbal learning and memory, and reduced language abilities.
- Children with CAE have elevated rates of behavioral and psychiatric comorbidities including attentional deficits, anxiety, depression, isolation, and low self-esteem.
- Large study in 2010 detected overall normal cognition, but 35% of subjects had pretreatment attentional deficits that did not resolve with seizure control.

DIAGNOSIS

Seizures are often so brief that untrained observers are not aware of the occurrence.

HISTORY

- Frequently diagnosed in children being evaluated for poor school performance
- Teachers report that child seems to daydream or zone out frequently.
- Child will forget portions of conversations.
- Child with normal intelligence quotient (IQ) underperforms in school.

PHYSICAL EXAM

- Unless a child has another genetic or acquired abnormality, a neurologic exam usually is normal.
- Seizures may be frequent enough to be observed during physical exam:
  - Manifest by behavioral arrest: Child will stop speaking in mid-sentence, stare blankly, and so forth.
  - Automatisms (repetitive stereotyped behaviors) may be present.
  - Child resumes previous activity.
  - Absence seizures can have a variable effect on respiratory rate, but bradypnea is common.
- Seizures may be induced by hyperventilation:
  - Have child blow on pinwheel or similar exercise to provoke seizure.
  - Alternatively, ask the patient to perform hyperventilation with eyes closed and count. Patient will open eyes at onset of seizure and stop counting.
- Patient manifests unresponsiveness but retains postural tone in a typical absence seizure.

DIFFERENTIAL DIAGNOSIS

- Complex partial seizures
- Psychogenic nonepileptic seizures
- Attention deficit hyperactivity disorder (ADHD)
- Confusional states and acute memory disorders
- Migraine variants
- Panic/anxiety attacks
- Breath-holding spells
- Nonepileptic staring spells: Suggestive features include the following:
  - Events do not interrupt play.
  - Events are first noticed by professional such as schoolteacher, speech therapist, occupational therapist, or physician (rather than parent).
  - During a staring spell, child is responsive to touch or other external stimuli.

DIAGNOSTIC TESTS & INTERPRETATION

- No specific hematologic workup
- Follow blood chemistry, hepatic function, and blood counts specific to drug regimen.
- Drug levels are useful in evaluating symptoms of toxicity or for breakthrough seizures.

Initial Tests (lab, imaging)

- EEG is standard for diagnosis:
  - Typical absence features: 3-Hz spike-and-wave activity on normal EEG background
  - Seizures feature bursts of 34-Hz spike-and-wave activity, which may slow to 2.5–3-Hz during seizure.
  - Seizure usually is evident clinically if bursts last >3 seconds; subtle changes of transient cognitive impairment may be evident with briefer seizures.
  - Hyperventilation and occasionally photic stimulation may induce seizure, thus confirming diagnosis of typical absence epilepsy. In contrast, atypical absence seizures are not susceptible to induction by hyperventilation or photic stimulation.
- Imaging is not routinely indicated in children with typical absence and normal neurologic exam and IQ.
  - Brain MRI is indicated in atypical absence and in children with mixed seizure types when combined with abnormal neurologic exam or low IQ.
  - If imaging is performed, MRI is preferable to CT scan due to higher sensitivity for anatomic abnormalities.

– A review of the brain MRIs of 134 patients with idiopathic generalized epilepsy in 2006 showed 24% with structural abnormalities, 88% of which were nonspecific (2)[B].

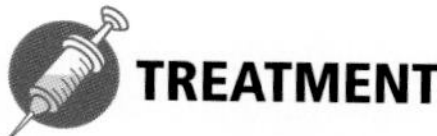

TREATMENT

GENERAL MEASURES

- Review seizure precautions with every patient diagnosed with or suspected to have epilepsy.
- Seizure precautions include bathroom, kitchen, home, driving, outdoors, and sports safety topics as well as special considerations for parents.

MEDICATION

Concern regarding generic medications allowing more breakthrough seizures has not been supported in evidence-based studies (3)[A].

ALERT

Certain common anticonvulsants may exacerbate absence including carbamazepine, oxcarbazepine, phenytoin, phenobarbital, tiagabine, vigabatrin, pregabalin, and gabapentin.

First Line

- Ethosuximide blocks T-type calcium channels:
  - 1st-line, except in absence patients with tonic–clonic seizures (lacks efficacy)
  - High efficacy (4)[A], fastest onset of efficacy (5)[B], and fewer adverse attentional effects compared to valproic acid (4)[A]
  - Side effects: vomiting, diarrhea, abdominal discomfort, hiccups, headache, sedation
  - Adverse effects: rare blood dyscrasias (monitor CBC)
- Valproic acid has multiple mechanisms:
  - 1st choice in absence patients with tonic–clonic, myoclonic, mixed seizure types
  - Very effective, but has highest rate of adverse events leading to treatment discontinuation, including negative attentional effects (4)[A]
  - Side effects: tremor, drowsiness, dizziness, weight gain, alopecia, sedation, vomiting
  - Adverse effects: teratogenicity, pancreatitis, thrombocytopenia, rare fulminant hepatic failure (especially in children <2 years)

Second Line

- Lamotrigine affects sodium channels:
  - Controls seizures but may be less efficacious than ethosuximide or valproic acid (4)[A]
  - May be equally as efficacious for new-onset CAE (5)[B]
  - Side effects: rash, diplopia, headache, insomnia, dizziness, nausea, vomiting, diarrhea
  - Adverse effects: rare Stevens-Johnson rash, more often when coadministered with valproic acid
- Topiramate affects GABA and excitatory neurotransmission:
  - FDA approved for Lennox-Gastaut syndrome
  - Side effects: psychomotor slowing
  - Adverse effects: weight loss, renal stones, myopia, glaucoma (rare), anhidrosis
- Levetiracetam is used off-label:
  - Has been used as both monotherapy and adjunct therapy for absence seizures
  - A small multicenter randomized controlled trial (RCT) showed modest efficacy but not statistically significant versus placebo (6)[C].
- Zonisamide is also used off-label.
- Clonazepam, nitrazepam and clobazam may be effective in the short-term but are not recommended for long-term management due to development of tolerance (few months to a year) and side effects.

Pregnancy Considerations

Anticonvulsants, especially valproic acid, are associated with an increase in fetal malformations. Use of valproic acid in women who are or are likely to become pregnant generally is contraindicated. Obtain specialty consultation.

ADDITIONAL THERAPIES

- Most absence seizure patients respond to a single medication.
- Male sex and an early age at diagnosis are associated with the need for 2 medications to control the disease (7)[B].
- Vagal nerve stimulator (VNS) may be considered as an option for medically refractory absence epilepsy (8)[C].

INPATIENT CONSIDERATIONS

Admission Criteria/Initial Stabilization

- Absence epilepsy rarely requires admission.
- Status epilepticus requires inpatient management.

Discharge Criteria

Resolution of status epilepticus

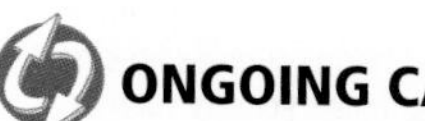

ONGOING CARE

FOLLOW-UP RECOMMENDATIONS

- Patients with associated tonic–clonic seizures should avoid high places and swimming alone.
- Absence rarely persists into adulthood, but affected adults may be restricted from driving, working over open flames, and so forth, as with other generalized and partial epilepsy subtypes.
- Patients should be monitored periodically by a neurologist for evolution of absence epilepsy into tonic–clonic or other seizure types.

PROGNOSIS

- Patient's whose shortest pretreatment EEG seizures are >20 seconds in duration are more likely to achieve seizure freedom, regardless of treatment (9)[A].
- Of those with CAE without tonic–clonic seizures, 90% remit by adulthood.
- 35% of patients with tonic–clonic seizures experience complete remission of absence seizures.
- 15% of patients develop juvenile myoclonic epilepsy.

COMPLICATIONS

Reported frequencies of typical absence status epilepticus range from 5.8 to 9.4% of patients with CAE.

REFERENCES

1. Berg AT, Berkovic SF, Brodie MJ, et al. Revised terminology and concepts for organization of seizures and epilepsies: report of the ILAE Commission on Classification and Terminology, 2005–2009. *Epilepsia* 2010;51(4):676–685.
2. Betting LE, Mory SB, Lopes-Cendes I, et al. MRI reveals structural abnormalities in patients with idiopathic generalized epilepsy. *Neurology*. 2006; 67(5):848–852.
3. Kesselheim AS, Stedman MR, Bubrick EJ, et al. Seizure outcomes following the use of generic versus brand-name antiepileptic drugs: a systematic review and meta-analysis. *Drugs*. 2010;70(5):605–621.
4. Glauser TA, Cnaan A, Shinnar S, et al. Ethosuximide, valproic acid, and lamotrigine in childhood absence epilepsy: initial monotherapy outcomes at 12 months. *Epilepsia*. 2013;54(1):141–155.
5. Hwang H, Kim H, Kim SH, et al. Long-term effectiveness of ethosuximide, valproic acid, and lamotrigine in childhood absence epilepsy. *Brain Dev*. 2012;34(5):344–348.
6. Fattore C, Boniver C, Capovilla G, et al. A multicenter, randomized, placebo-controlled trial of levetiracetam in children and adolescents with newly diagnosed absence epilepsy. *Epilepsia*. 2011;52(4):802–809.
7. Nadler B, Shevell MI. Childhood absence epilepsy requiring more than one medication for seizure control. *Can J Neurol Sci*. 2008;35(3):297–300.
8. Arya R, Greiner HM, Lewis A, et al. Vagus nerve stimulation for medically refractory absence epilepsy. *Seizure*. 2013;22(4):267–270.
9. Dlugos D, Shinnar S, Cnaan A, et al. Pretreatment EEG in childhood absence epilepsy: associations with attention and treatment outcome. *Neurology*. 2013;81(2):150–156.

ADDITIONAL READING

- Glauser TA, Loddenkemper T. Management of childhood epilepsy. *Continuum (Minneap Minn)*. 2013;19(3 Epilepsy);656–681.
- Matricardi S, Verrotti A, Chiarelli F, et al. Current advances in childhood absence epilepsy. *Pediatr Neurol*. 2014;50(3);205–212.
- Tenney, JR. Glauser TA. The current state of absence epilepsy: can we have your attention? *Epilepsy Curr*. 2013;13(3);135–140.
- Vrielynck P. Current and emerging treatments for absence seizures in young patients. *Neuropsychiatr Dis Treat*. 2013;9;963–975.

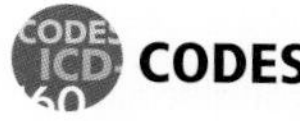

CODES

ICD10

- G40.409 Other generalized epilepsy and epileptic syndromes, not intractable, without status epilepticus
- G40.419 Oth generalized epilepsy, intractable, w/o stat epi
- G40.401 Oth generalized epilepsy, not intractable, w stat epi

CLINICAL PEARLS

- If parents are unable to determine the cause of a staring spell, try suggesting that parents mention something exciting or unexpected like "ice cream" during a spell to get the child's attention rather than calling his or her name.
- To help aid with diagnosis during an exam, try having child blow repetitively on pinwheel (causing hyperventilation) to attempt to trigger absence seizure.
- Ethosuximide and valproic acid are 1st-line agents in treatment of absence seizures. Valproic acid and lamotrigine are recommended for absence patients with tonic–clonic and mixed seizure types.

S

SEIZURE DISORDER, PARTIAL

Ruben Peralta, MD, FACS • Wynne S. Morgan, MD

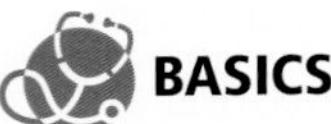

BASICS

DESCRIPTION

- Seizures occur when abnormal synchronous neuronal discharges in the brain cause transient cortical dysfunction.
- Generalized seizures involve bilateral cerebral cortex from the seizure's onset.
- Partial seizures originate from a discrete focus in the cerebral cortex.
- Partial seizures are further divided into simple and complex subtypes:
  - If consciousness is impaired during a partial seizure, it is classified as complex.
  - If consciousness is preserved, it is a simple partial seizure.

EPIDEMIOLOGY

Prevalence

Partial seizures occur in 20/100,000 persons in the United States.

ETIOLOGY AND PATHOPHYSIOLOGY

- Partial seizures begin when a localized seizure focus produces an abnormal, synchronized depolarization that spreads to a discrete portion of the surrounding cortex.
- The area of cortex involved in the seizure determines the symptoms; for example, an epileptogenic focus in motor cortex produces contralateral motor symptoms.
- In some cases, etiology is related to structural abnormalities that are susceptible to epileptogenesis. Most common etiologies vary by life stage:
  - Early childhood: developmental/congenital malformation, trauma
  - Young adults: developmental, infection, trauma
  - Adults 40–60 years of age: cerebrovascular insult, infection, trauma
  - Adults >60 years of age: cerebrovascular insult, trauma, neoplasm
- Complex partial seizures: A common cause is mesial temporal sclerosis.

Genetics

Benign rolandic epilepsy, a form of partial seizure disorder, has an autosomal dominant inheritance pattern with penetrance depending on multiple factors.

RISK FACTORS

- History of traumatic brain injury (1)[B]
- Children exposed to a thiamine-deficient formula (2)[C]

COMMONLY ASSOCIATED CONDITIONS

Epilepsy patients have a higher incidence of depression than the general population.

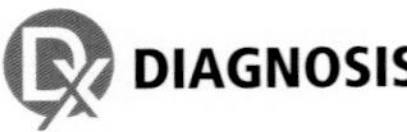

DIAGNOSIS

- Seizure activity usually stereotyped
- Duration: seconds to minutes, unless status epilepticus develops; status epilepticus may present as focal/generalized convulsions/altered mental status without convulsions.
- Simple partial seizures
  - Simple partial seizures are characterized by localized symptoms. The patient is conscious. Symptoms may involve motor, sensory, or psychic systems.
  - Motor: Seizure activity in motor strip causes contraction (tonic) or rhythmic jerking (clonic) movements that may involve 1 entire side of body or may be more localized (i.e., hands, feet, or face).
    - Jacksonian march: As discharge spreads through motor cortex, tonic–clonic activity spreads in predictable fashion (i.e., beginning in hand and progressing up arm and to the face).
  - Sensory/psychic
    - Todd paresis: after motor seizure, residual, temporary weakness in the affected area
    - Parietal lobe: sensory loss/paresthesias, dizziness
    - Temporal lobe: déjà vu, rising sensation in epigastrium, auditory hallucinations/forced memories, unpleasant smell/taste
  - Occipital: visual hallucinations
- Complex partial seizures
  - Impaired consciousness by definition
  - May have aura; this is start of seizure.
- Amnesia for the event, postictal confusion
  - Most often, focus in complex partial seizures is temporal/frontal.
  - Motor manifestations may include dystonic posturing/automatisms (i.e., simple, repetitive movements of face and hands such as lip smacking, picking, or more complex actions such as purposeless walking).
  - Frontal lobe seizure is characterized by brief, bilateral complex movements, vocalizations, often with onset during sleep.

HISTORY

- A detailed description of the seizure should be obtained from an observer.
- Review medication list for drugs that lower seizure threshold (e.g., tramadol, bupropion, theophylline).
- Drugs of abuse (e.g., cocaine) lower seizure threshold.
- History of traumatic brain injury

PHYSICAL EXAM

Include neurologic exam, with attention to lateralizing signs suggestive of structural lesion.

DIFFERENTIAL DIAGNOSIS

- Nonepileptic seizure
- Syncope/postanoxic myoclonus
- Hypoglycemia
- For hemiparesis following event
  - Transient ischemic attack
  - Hemiplegic migraine

DIAGNOSTIC TESTS & INTERPRETATION

EEG: spikes/sharp waves over seizure focus

- Yield of EEG is increased by being obtained in first 24 hours following seizure and by sleep deprivation.
- Frontal lobe seizure focus may be difficult to detect by routine EEG.
- If difficulty with diagnosis, continuous video–EEG monitoring may be appropriate.
- Serum electrolytes, including calcium, magnesium, phosphorus; hepatic function panel; CBC; drugs of abuse
- If measured within 10–20 minutes of suspected seizure, an elevated prolactin level may help to differentiate generalized/complex partial seizure from psychogenic seizure.
- CSF exam if infection is suspected.
- Urinalysis, chest x-ray, levels of antiepileptic drugs for breakthrough seizure
- Technological advances in neuroimaging are usually directed at the diagnosis and prognosis for seizure control (3)[C].
- Emergency evaluation of new seizure: CT scan to screen for hemorrhage and stroke
- After emergency evaluation, MRI with thin cuts through area of interest
- If planning epilepsy surgery, positron emission tomography (PET) scan and/or interictal single-photon emission computed tomography (SPECT) may be of value.
- Magnetoencephalography (MEG) is an evolving technology for localizing seizure focus.

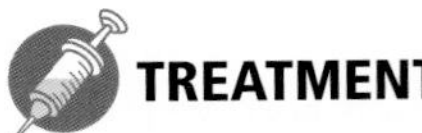

TREATMENT

GENERAL MEASURES

- Ask patient to maintain a seizure diary.
- Note potential triggers, such as stress, sleep deprivation, drug use, discontinuation of alcohol/benzodiazepines, menses.

MEDICATION

- Some physicians do not start medication after a single seizure if EEG and MRI are normal and/or a precipitant is clear and avoidable.
- Antiepileptic drugs (AEDs) act on voltage-gated ion channels, affect neuronal inhibition via enhancement of γ-aminobutyric acid (GABA, an inhibitory neurotransmitter), or decrease neuronal excitation. End result is to decrease the abnormal synchronized firing and to prevent seizure propagation.
- 50% of those with newly diagnosed partial seizures respond to, and tolerate, first AED trial.
- Choose AED based on seizure type, side effect profile, and patient characteristics. Increase dose until seizure control is obtained/side effects become unacceptable.
- Attempt monotherapy, but many patients will require adjunctive agents.
- *Refractory to medications* is defined as failure of at least 3 anticonvulsants to achieve adequate control.
- Several AEDs induce/inhibit cytochrome P450 enzymes (watch for drug interactions).

First Line

- Carbamazepine: affects sodium channels; side effects include GI distress, hyponatremia, diplopia, dizziness, rare pancytopenia/marrow suppression, and exfoliative rash.
- Oxcarbazepine: affects sodium channels; side effects include dizziness, diplopia, hyponatremia, and headache.
- Lamotrigine: affects sodium channels:
  - Side effects include insomnia, dizziness, and ataxia.
  - Risk of Stevens-Johnson reaction (potentially fatal exfoliative rash) especially when given with valproate; requires slow titration
- Levetiracetam: multiple mechanisms; side effects include sedation, ataxia, and irritability.

Second Line

- Phenytoin: affects sodium channels; side effects include ataxia, dizziness, diplopia, tremor, GI upset, gingival hyperplasia, and fever.

- Phenobarbital: multiple mechanisms; side effects include sedation and withdrawal seizures.
- Valproate: multiple mechanisms; side effects include GI upset, weight gain, alopecia, and tremor; less common, thrombocytopenia, hepatitis, pancreatitis
- Topiramate: multiple mechanisms; side effects include anorexia, cognitive slowing, sedation, nephrolithiasis, and anhidrosis.
- Gabapentin: multiple mechanisms; side effects include sedation, dizziness, and ataxia.
- Pregabalin: affects calcium channels; side effects include sedation, dizziness, and weight gain.
- Zonisamide: affects sodium channels
  - Side effects include sedation, anorexia, nausea, dizziness, ataxia, anhidrosis, and nephrolithiasis.
  - Cross-reaction with sulfa allergy

Pregnancy Considerations

- Folate should be prescribed for all women of child-bearing age who are taking AEDs.
- Several AEDs induce hepatic metabolism of oral contraceptives, decreasing their efficacy. AED therapy during 1st trimester is associated with doubled risk for major fetal malformations (6% vs. 3%).
- Phenytoin in pregnancy may result in fetal hydantoin syndrome.
- Valproate is associated with neural tube defects.
- Fetal insult from seizures following withdrawal of therapy also may be severe. Risk-to-benefit balance should be evaluated with high-risk pregnancy and epileptology consultations. Most patients remain on anticonvulsants.
- Consider vagal nerve stimulator during pregnancy (4)[B].

ISSUES FOR REFERRAL

For refractory seizures, consider referral to an epilepsy specialist (5)[B].

ADDITIONAL THERAPIES

- Vagal nerve stimulator: implanted in neck; provides periodic stimulation to vagus nerve; may induce hoarseness, cough, and dysphagia (6)[B]
- New technologies under development include deep brain stimulation.

SURGERY/OTHER PROCEDURES

- For refractory partial complex seizures
- Should have identifiable focus
- Preoperative testing, such as Wada test, should be done to decrease likelihood of inducing aphasia and memory loss.
- Workup also may include MRI, video–EEG monitoring, electrocorticography, MEG, and ictal SPECT.
- 64% will be seizure-free after surgery (with continued medication treatment); 25% will have significant decrease in frequency; 1/3 continue to have disabling seizures.
- Goal of surgical intervention is to reduce reliance on medications; most patients remain on anticonvulsants postoperatively.

INPATIENT CONSIDERATIONS

Admission Criteria/Initial Stabilization

Admit for unremitting seizure (partial/secondary generalized status epilepticus).

ONGOING CARE

FOLLOW-UP RECOMMENDATIONS

- Most states have restrictions on driving for those with seizure disorders.
- Depending on seizure manifestation may recommend against activities such as swimming, climbing to heights, working over open flames, or operating heavy machinery

Patient Monitoring

AED levels if concern over toxicity, noncompliance, or for breakthrough seizures

DIET

Ketogenic or low–glycemic index diet may improve seizure control in some patients.

PATIENT EDUCATION

Avoid potential triggers such as alcohol or drug use and sleep deprivation.

PROGNOSIS

- Risk of seizure recurrence: ~30% after 1st seizure; of these, 50% will occur in the 1st 6 months; 90% in the first 2 years.
- Depends on seizure type; rolandic epilepsy has a good prognosis; temporal lobe epilepsy is more likely to be persistent.
- ~25–30% of all seizures are refractory to current medications.
- AEDs initiated after an initial seizure have been shown to decrease the risk of seizure over the 1st 2 years but are not demonstrated to reduce long-term risk of recurrence.
- Long duration of uncontrolled seizure disorder associated with increased cognitive and functional impairments; early pharmacologic intervention is encouraged.
- The potential for AEDs to confer neuroprotection is under investigation.
- The risk of developing seizure after mild traumatic brain injury remains high for a long period (>10 years) (1)[B].
- Patients with history of military brain injury carry a high risk of intractable posttraumatic epilepsy decades after their injury and, thus, require a long-term medical follow-up (7)[B].

COMPLICATIONS

Risk of accidental injury

REFERENCES

1. Christensen J, Pedersen MG, Pedersen CB, et al. Long-term risk of epilepsy after traumatic brain injury in children and young adults: a population-based cohort study. *Lancet*. 2009;373(9669):1105–1110.
2. Fattal-Valevski A, Bloch-Mimouni A, Kivity S, et al. Epilepsy in children with infantile thiamine deficiency. *Neurology*. 2009;73(11):828–833.
3. Gaillard WD, Cross JH, Duncan JS, et al. Epilepsy imaging study guideline criteria: commentary on diagnostic testing study guidelines and practice parameters. *Epilepsia*. 2011;52(9):1750–1756.
4. Houser MV, Hennessy MD, Howard BC, et al. Vagal nerve stimulator use during pregnancy for treatment of refractory seizure disorder. *Obstet Gynecol*. 2010;115(2):417–419.
5. Hemb M, Velasco TR, Parnes MS, et al. Improved outcomes in pediatric epilepsy surgery: the UCLA experience, 1986–2008. *Neurology*. 2010;74:1768–1775.
6. Siddiqui F, Herial NA, Ali II, et al. Cumulative effect of vagus nerve stimulators on intractable seizures observed over a period of 3 years. *Epilepsy Behav*. 2010;18(3):299–302.
7. Kazemi H, Hashemi-Fesharaki S, Razaghi S, et al. Intractable epilepsy and craniocerebral trauma: analysis of 163 patients with blunt and penetrating head injuries sustained in war. *Injury*. 2012;43(12):2132–2135.

ADDITIONAL READING

- Adams SM, Knowles PD. Evaluation of a first seizure. *Am Fam Physician*. 2007;75(9):1342–1347.
- Auvin S, Vallée L. Febrile seizures: Current understanding of pathophysiological mechanisms [in French]. *Arch Pediatr*. 2009;16(5):450–456.
- Baker MT. The anticonvulsant effects of propofol and a propofol analog, 2,6-diisopropyl-4-(hydroxy-2,2,2-trifluoroethyl)phenol, in a 6 Hz partial seizure model. *Anesth Analg*. 2011;112(2):340–344.
- Cross JH, Jayakar P, Nordli D, et al. Proposed criteria for referral and evaluation of children for epilepsy surgery: recommendations of the Subcommission for Pediatric Epilepsy Surgery. *Epilepsia*. 2006;47:952–959.
- Deprez L, Jansen A, De Jonghe P. Genetics of epilepsy syndromes starting in the first year of life. *Neurology*. 2009;72:273–281.
- Fisher RS, Acevedo C, Arzimanoglou A, et al. ILAE official report: a practical clinical definition of epilepsy. *Epilepsia*. 2014;55(4):475.
- LaFrance WC. Use of serum prolactin in diagnosing epileptic seizures: report of the Therapeutics and Technology Assessment Subcommittee of the American Academy of Neurology. *Neurology*. 2006;84(8):1287–1288; author reply 1287–1288.
- Sankar R, Ramsay E, McKay A, et al. A multicenter, outpatient, open-label study to evaluate the dosing, effectiveness, and safety of topiramate as monotherapy in the treatment of epilepsy in clinical practice. *Epilepsy Behav*. 2009;15(4):506–512.
- Walker LE, Mirza N, Yip VL, et al. Personalized medicine approaches in epilepsy. *J Inter Med*. 2014;277(2):218–234.

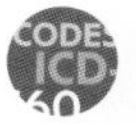

CODES

ICD10

- G40.109 Local-rel symptc epi w simp prt seiz,not ntrct, w/o stat epi
- G40.209 Local-rel symptc epi w cmplx prt seiz,not ntrct,w/o stat epi
- G40.119 Local-rel symptc epi w simple part seiz, ntrct, w/o stat epi

CLINICAL PEARLS

- It is controversial whether AED treatment is indicated after a 1st seizure. Treatment should be strongly considered when a clear structural cause is identified/risk of injury from seizure is high (e.g., osteoporosis, anticoagulation).
- Consider vagus nerve stimulation in pregnancy and in patients with medically refractory seizures.
- Postictal elevation in prolactin levels can help distinguish physiologic from psychogenic seizures.

S

SEIZURE DISORDERS

Allison Hargreaves, MD • Ann M. Lynch, PharmD, RPh, AE-C • Vaishali M. Patel, MD

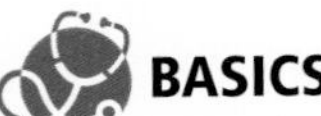

BASICS

DESCRIPTION

- Seizure: sudden change in cortical electrical activity, manifested through motor, sensory, or behavioral changes, and/or an alteration in consciousness
- System(s) affected: nervous
- Synonym(s): epilepsy; convulsion; attacks; spells

Geriatric Considerations

- Epilepsy is the 3rd most common disease of the brain in the elderly, after stroke and dementia.
- Diagnosing epileptic seizures in the elderly may prove difficult, as symptoms such as auras and generalized tonic–clonic seizures are rarer, but status epilepticus is more common.
- Elderly are more sensitive to side effects from AEDs; therefore, target dose should be half of dosing for younger population (1).

Pediatric Considerations

Breastfeeding is not contraindicated. Sedation of the infant should be monitored.

Pregnancy Considerations

- Monitor serum levels of antiepileptic drugs (AEDs).
- There is a 2-fold increase in congenital malformations in children born to mothers taking certain anticonvulsants. Some expectant mothers can stop taking anticonvulsants safely for the 1st trimester or initial 6-week period (organogenesis). Avoid valproate and lamotrigine. Epileptic patients should notify their neurologist before conception, if possible.
- Recommend against use of category C or D AEDs during pregnancy/nursing. Levetiracetam and topiramate are alternatives for women of childbearing potential (2).

EPIDEMIOLOGY

Incidence

- 200,000 new cases of epilepsy are diagnosed in the United States annually, with 45,000 new cases in children <15 years of age.
- Pediatric (<2 years of age) and older adults (>65 years of age) more commonly present with new-onset seizures.
- Predominant sex: male = female

Prevalence

- 2.7 million with seizure disorder
- 4 million people have had ≥1 seizures.
- 326,000 children (≤14 years of age) and 600,000 adults (>65 years of age) have a seizure disorder.

ETIOLOGY AND PATHOPHYSIOLOGY

- Synchronous and excessive firing of neurons, resulting in impairment of normal control of CNS
- True seizures may be triggered by the following metabolic/medical conditions, but seizures occurring due to these conditions do not necessarily define the presence of a seizure disorder (see also "Differential Diagnosis").
  - CNS infection
  - Hyperthyroidism
  - Hypoglycemia or hyperglycemia
  - Hyponatremia
  - Uremia
  - Porphyria
  - Hypoxia
  - Confusional migraine
  - Transient ischemic attack
  - Narcolepsy/sleep disorder
  - Toxins (e.g., lead, picrotoxin, strychnine)
  - Brain tumor
  - Cerebral hypoxia
  - Stroke/cardiovascular accident (CVA)
  - Drug/alcohol overdose/withdrawal
  - Eclampsia
  - Head injury
  - Heat stroke

Genetics

Family history increases risk 3-fold.

RISK FACTORS

Children delivered breech have a prevalence rate of 3.8% compared with 2.2% in vertex deliveries.

GENERAL PREVENTION

Take measures to prevent head injuries. Reduce exposure to lead-containing products. Avoid excessive alcohol/substance use/abuse, hypoglycemia, and sleep deprivation.

COMMONLY ASSOCIATED CONDITIONS

Infections, tumors, drug abuse, alcohol and drug withdrawal, trauma, metabolic disorders

DIAGNOSIS

- Differentiate first between epileptiform seizures and nonepileptiform seizures (NESs).
- NESs are psychogenic and usually associated with a history of psychiatric conditions and often with a history of sexual abuse.
- Physiologic seizures are true cortical events and may require acute intervention.
- Conventional classification of seizures
  - Generalized seizures
    - Tonic–clonic: tonic phase: sudden loss of consciousness; clonic phase: sustained contraction followed by rhythmic contractions of all 4 extremities; postictal phase: headache, confusion, fatigue; clinically hypertensive, tachycardic, and otherwise hypersympathetic
    - Absence: impaired awareness and responsiveness
    - Atonic: abrupt loss of muscle tone
    - Myoclonic: repetitive muscle contractions
  - Febrile seizures
    - Usually ≤6 years
    - Fever without evidence of any other defined cause of seizures
    - Recurrent febrile seizures probably do not increase the risk of epilepsy.
  - Symptomatic focal epilepsies
  - Complex partial seizures
  - Simple partial seizures
  - Nonconvulsive status epilepticus: most commonly seen in ICU patients; no tonic–clonic activity seen so must diagnose with bedside EEG
  - Status epilepticus: repetitive generalized seizures without recovery between seizures; considered a neurologic emergency

HISTORY

- Eyewitness descriptions of event; patient impressions of what occurred before, during, and after the event
- Screen for etiologies, including provoking/ameliorating factors for the event, such as sleep deprivation.
- Ask about bowel/bladder incontinence, tongue biting, other injury, automatisms, or prior seizure activity.

PHYSICAL EXAM

Thorough neurologic exam

DIFFERENTIAL DIAGNOSIS

Below represents a differential diagnosis for the etiology of actual seizures, not for apparent seizures (see also "Etiology," above).

- Idiopathic
- Hippocampal sclerosis and other neurodevelopmental abnormalities of the brain
- Acute infection (meningitis, abscess, encephalitis)
- Metabolic and endocrine disorders
- Trauma
- Drug and alcohol withdrawal
- Tumor
- Vascular disease, including vasculitis
- Familial/genetic, infantile, and pediatric seizure syndromes (e.g., Lennox-Gastaut, benign familial, myoclonic epilepsy of infancy)
- Other etiologies (by age of onset):
  - Infancy (0–2 years)
    - Hypoxic-ischemic encephalopathy/other injury to cerebral cortex
    - Metabolic: hypoglycemia, hypocalcemia, hypomagnesemia, vitamin B_6 deficiency, phenylketonuria
  - Childhood (2–10 years): absence or febrile (usually <6 years) seizure
  - Adolescent (10–18 years): arteriovenous malformation (AVM)
  - Late adulthood (>60 years)
    - Degenerative disease, including dementia
    - Metabolic: hypoglycemia, uremia, hepatic failure, electrolyte abnormality

DIAGNOSTIC TESTS & INTERPRETATION

A negative EEG does not rule out a seizure disorder. Interictal EEG sensitivity may be as low as 20%; multiple EEGs may increase sensitivity to 80%. Prognostically, EEG abnormality may predict likelihood of seizure recurrence.

- Sleep deprivation may be helpful prior to EEG, and hyperventilation and photic stimulation during recording may increase sensitivity for spike wave formations.
- Video EEG monitoring is used to differentiate psychomotor NES from true cortical events.

Initial Tests (lab, imaging)

- Glucose, Na, K, calcium, phosphorus, magnesium, BUN, ammonia. Drug and toxin screens: include alcohol
- AED levels (if patient taking antiepileptic medication)
- CBC and UA: rule out infection
- Imaging is recommended for new-onset seizures when localization-related epilepsy is known/suspected, when the epilepsy classification is in doubt, or when an epilepsy syndrome with remote symptomatic cause is suspected. MRI is preferred to CT because of its superior resolution, versatility, and lack of radiation.
  - CT scan of brain: indicated routinely as initial evaluation, especially in the ER
  - Brain MRI: superior in evaluation of the temporal lobes (e.g., mesial temporal sclerosis)
- Bone scan to determine bone mineral density (BMD): generally done if patients are taking older AEDs such as phenytoin and carbamazepine

Follow-Up Tests & Special Considerations
- Consider an arterial blood gas determination.
- Drugs that may alter lab results: AED therapy may affect the EEG results dramatically.
- Inadequate AED levels: may be altered by many medications such as erythromycin, sulfonamides, warfarin, cimetidine, and alcohol.
- Disorders that may alter lab results: Pregnancy decreases serum concentration.

Diagnostic Procedures/Other
Lumbar puncture (LP) for spinal fluid analysis may be necessary to rule out meningitis if fever and/or impairment of consciousness are present.

Test Interpretation
Pathologic samples are not typically surgically obtained for diagnostic reasons. CT/MRI may be used to identify a nidus for seizure activity.

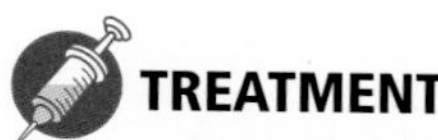

TREATMENT

- 50–60% presenting with an initial unprovoked seizure will not have a recurrence; 40–50% will have a recurrence within 2 years (3).
- Starting antiepileptic medications reduces recurrences of seizures but does not alter long-term outcomes (4)[B].
- Evidence is conflicting whether or not to start AEDs routinely in patients on initial seizure with no focal abnormalities on exam or imaging. Many recommend deferring treatment until a 2nd seizure has occurred (5)[C].

MEDICATION
- AED of choice: Select based on type of seizure, potential adverse effects/drug interactions, and cost.
- Monotherapy is preferred whenever possible. Systematic reviews found insufficient evidence on which to base a 1st- or 2nd-line choice among these drugs in terms of seizure control.
- Treatment options include the following:
  - Carbamazepine (Tegretol): 100–200 mg/day in 1–2 doses; therapeutic range, 4–12 mg/L
  - Phenytoin (Dilantin): 200–400 mg/day in 1–3 doses; therapeutic range, 10–20 mg/L
  - Valproic acid (Depakene): 750–3,000 mg/day in 1–3 doses to begin at 15 mg/kg/day; therapeutic range, 50–150 mg/L
  - Lamotrigine (Lamictal): 25–50 mg/day; adjust in 100-mg increments every 1–2 weeks to 300–500 mg/day in 2 doses
  - Oxcarbazepine (Trileptal): 300 mg BID, increase to 300 mg every 3 days; maintenance, 1,200 mg/day.
  - Topiramate (Topamax): 50 mg/day; adjust weekly to effect; 400 mg/day in 2 doses, max 1,600 mg/day
  - Pregabalin (Lyrica): 150–300 mg/day in 2–3 doses
  - Lacosamide (Vimpat): for refractory seizures; 200–300 mg/day in 2 doses
  - Levetiracetam (Keppra): 1,000 mg/day in 2 doses
  - Eslicarbazepine (Aptiom): 400 mg once/day initially, 800–1200 mg once/day maintenance, adjunctive therapy
- Alternative drugs (in addition to any of the preceding)
  - Phenobarbital: 50–100 mg BID–TID; therapeutic range, 15–40 mg/L
  - Evidence suggests long-term use of phenobarbital may impair cognitive ability.
  - Primidone (Mysoline): 100–125 mg at bedtime; adjust to max of 2,000 mg/day in 2 doses
- Contraindications: Refer to manufacturer's profile of each drug.
- Precautions: Doses should be based on individual's response guided by drug levels.
- Consider cautioning about increased risk of suicide, but risk of untreated seizures is far greater than increased risk of suicide.
- Patients are susceptible to sudden unexpected death in epilepsy, possibly due to cardiac arrhythmia.

ISSUES FOR REFERRAL
Referral and follow-up frequency is based on severity and patient's wishes.

SURGERY/OTHER PROCEDURES
- Resection for seizures that fail traditional therapy
- Vagus nerve stimulation

COMPLEMENTARY & ALTERNATIVE MEDICINE
- No evidence suggests that any complementary medicines reduce seizures, but they may induce serious drug interactions with prescribed AEDs.
- Psychological therapies may be used in conjunction with AED therapy. Cognitive-behavioral therapy, relaxation, biofeedback, and yoga all may be helpful as adjunctive therapy (6)[C].
- Patients with NES should be referred for psychotherapy.

INPATIENT CONSIDERATIONS
Admission Criteria/Initial Stabilization
- Outpatient therapy usually is sufficient, except for status epilepticus.
- Protect the airway and, if possible, protect the patient from physical harm; do not restrain. Administer acute AEDs.

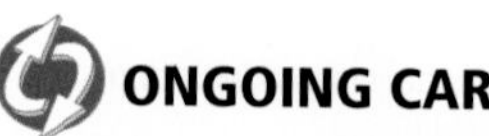

ONGOING CARE

FOLLOW-UP RECOMMENDATIONS
Maintain adequate drug therapy; ensure compliance and/or access to medication. Drug therapy withdrawal may be considered after a seizure-free 2-year period. Expect a 33% relapse rate in the following 3 years.

Patient Monitoring
- Monitor drug levels and seizure frequency.
- CBC and lab values (e.g., calcium, vitamin D) as indicated; BMD
- Monitor for side effects and adverse reactions.
- All patients currently taking any AED should be monitored closely for notable changes in behavior that could indicate the emergence/worsening of suicidal thoughts/behavior/depression.

DIET
Ketogenic diet may be beneficial in children in conjunction with AED therapy and refractory seizures.

PATIENT EDUCATION
- Stress the importance of medication compliance and the avoidance of alcohol and recreational drugs.
- Individuals with uncontrolled seizures should be encouraged to avoid heights and swimming.
- State driving laws: http://www.epilepsyfoundation.org; most states require a minimum of 6 months free of seizures
- http://www.epilepsy.org

PROGNOSIS
- Depends on type of seizure disorder: ~70% will become seizure-free with appropriate initial treatment, 30% will continue to have seizures. The number of seizures within 6 months after first presentation is the most important factor for remission.
- ~90% who are seen for a first unprovoked seizure attain a 1–2-year remission within 4 or 5 years of the initial event (3).
- Life expectancy is shortened in persons with epilepsy.
- The case-fatality rate for status epilepticus may be as high as 20%.

COMPLICATIONS
Drug toxicity

REFERENCES

1. Werhahn KJ. Epilepsy in the elderly. *Dtsch Arztebl Int*. 2009;106(9):135–142.
2. Perucca E, Tomson T. The pharmacological treatment of epilepsy in adults. *Lancet Neurol*. 2011;10(5):446–456.
3. Berg AT. Risk of recurrence after a first unprovoked seizure. *Epilepsia*. 2008;49(Suppl 1):13–18.
4. Geiger WJ, Nievera CC, Musil B, et al. Managing seizures: achieving control while minimizing risk. *J Fam Pract*. 2011;60(8):464–472.
5. Haut SR, Shinnar S. Considerations in the treatment of a first unprovoked seizure. *Semin Neurol*. 2008;28(3):289–296.
6. Marson A, Ramaratnam S. Epilepsy. *Clin Evid*. 2005;(13):1588–1607.

S

ADDITIONAL READING

- Shih JJ, Ochoa JG. A systematic review of antiepileptic drug initiation and withdrawal. *Neurologist*. 2009;15(3):122–131.
- Wiebe S, Téllez-Zenteno JF, Shapiro M. An evidence-based approach to the first seizure. *Epilepsia*. 2008;49(Suppl 1):50–57.

SEE ALSO

Seizures, Febrile; Status Epilepticus

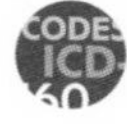

CODES

ICD10
- R56.9 Unspecified convulsions
- P90 Convulsions of newborn
- G40.909 Epilepsy, unsp, not intractable, without status epilepticus

CLINICAL PEARLS

- Switching from brand to generic drug is safe. Monitor seizure activity more closely after switch for 2 months.
- Encourage helmet usage to minimize head injuries.
- To consider driving, patients must be seizure-free for a minimum of 3 months to a year, depending on state requirements.
- Drug initiation after a single seizure will decrease risk of early seizure recurrence but does not affect long-term prognosis of developing epilepsy.

SEIZURES, FEBRILE

Robert A. Baldor, MD, FAAFP

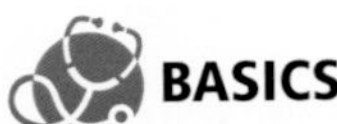

BASICS

DESCRIPTION

- By definition, febrile seizures occur in pediatric patients aged 6 months–5 years with fever ≥100.4°F (38°C). Evidence of an underlying neurologic abnormality, metabolic condition, or intracranial infection excludes this diagnosis.
- Distinguished as simple or complex based on multiple criteria
  - Simple (70–75%; must meet all criteria)
    - Generalized clonic or tonic–clonic seizure activity without focal features
    - Duration <15 minutes
    - Does not recur within 24 hours
    - Resolves spontaneously
    - No history of previous afebrile seizure or seizure disorder
  - Complex (9–35%; only 1 criterion must be met)
    - Partial seizure, focal activity
    - Duration >15 minutes
    - Recurs within 24 hours
    - Requires intervention

EPIDEMIOLOGY

Incidence

- 500,000 febrile seizures occur in the United States annually.
- Most occur in children 6 months–3 years; only 6–15% occur in patients ≥4 years.
- Peak incidence is 18 months of age.
- Risk of recurrence is 32–54%.

Prevalence

- 2–5% of children in United States and Western Europe have at least 1 febrile seizure.
- Cumulative incidence varies in other populations (0.5–10%).

ETIOLOGY AND PATHOPHYSIOLOGY

A variety of mechanisms have been proposed:

- A lower baseline seizure threshold in the age group affected by febrile seizures
- Familial genotypes may result in lower seizure thresholds.
- Fever may alter ion channel activity, resulting in increased circuit excitability.
- Cytokines released secondary to infection, specifically interleukin (IL) 1β, increase neuronal activity.

Genetics

- Evidence for genetic association:
  - Greater concordance in monozygotic than dizygotic twins (56% vs. 14%, respectively)
  - Risk of febrile seizure with a previously affected sibling is increased (10–45% vs. 2–5%).
  - Having 2 affected parents doubles a child's risk of febrile seizure.
- Several rare familial epileptic syndromes present with febrile seizure.

RISK FACTORS

- Family history of febrile seizures; risk increases with the number of affected 1st-degree relatives.
- Any condition causing fever
- Recent vaccination
  - As febrile seizures are a benign entity, the benefits of vaccination outweigh the risk.
  - Risk increases after the administration of all measles-containing vaccines; peak incidence occurs 7–10 days after vaccination.
  - Risk increases on the day of DTaP-IPV-HIB combination vaccine administration.
  - Absolute vaccination-associated risk is very low.
- Prenatal exposure to alcohol and tobacco, iron deficiency anemia, daycare attendance, developmental delay, premature birth, and prolonged NICU stay

GENERAL PREVENTION

Prevention is not usually indicated given the benign nature of this condition, lack of effective interventions, and side effects of prophylactic medications.

COMMONLY ASSOCIATED CONDITIONS

- Viral infections: Frequently implicated pathogens include human herpesvirus 6, influenza, parainfluenza, adenovirus, and respiratory syncytial virus (RSV).
- Bacterial infections: Frequently associated infections include otitis media, pharyngitis, urinary tract infection (UTI), pneumonia, and gastroenteritis.

DIAGNOSIS

HISTORY

- History of present illness:
  - Description of seizure:
    - Febrile seizures are generalized with clonic or tonic–clonic activity.
    - Absence, myoclonic, atonic, and focal seizures are atypical of febrile seizures and warrant further evaluation.
  - Seizure duration
  - Presence of postictal state (consistent with febrile seizure)
  - Number of seizures in previous 24 hours
  - Lethargy, irritability, or decreased level of consciousness as reported by the caretaker
  - Symptoms of underlying infection
  - Symptoms concerning for neurologic deficits
- Past medical history:
  - Existing conditions, including developmental delay, cerebral palsy, and metabolic disorders
  - Recent antibiotic course
  - History of febrile seizures
  - History of afebrile seizures or seizure disorder
  - History of head injury
  - Vaccination status, recent immunization
- Family history: febrile seizures, afebrile seizures, epilepsy, metabolic disorders, and other neurologic conditions
- Social history: factors concerning for child abuse

PHYSICAL EXAM

- Vital signs should be stable and consistent with intercurrent febrile illness; unstable vital signs or toxic appearance warrant further evaluation.
- Identify the presence or absence of focal deficits on a complete neurologic exam.
- Assess for signs of meningitis, including decreased level of consciousness, irritability, meningeal signs, bulging fontanelle, papilledema, and petechiae.
- Identify cause of fever.
- Assess thoroughly for manifestations of child abuse with a careful skin exam, inspection and palpation for occult trauma, and retinal exam if possible.

DIFFERENTIAL DIAGNOSIS

- Seizures due to an etiology other than febrile seizure:
  - Meningitis, encephalitis
  - Primary epilepsy
  - Neonatal seizure
  - Intracranial mass
  - Nonaccidental trauma
  - Electrolyte abnormality
  - Hypoglycemia
  - Metabolic disorder
- Conditions presenting similarly to seizure:
  - Rigors
  - Crying
  - Benign myoclonus of infancy
  - Breath holding spell
  - Choking episode
  - Tic disorder
  - Parasomnia
  - Arrhythmia
  - Metabolic disorder
  - Dystonic reaction

DIAGNOSTIC TESTS & INTERPRETATION

- Routine laboratory tests not recommended to identify an underlying cause of a simple febrile seizure (1)[C]
- Rates of UTI in children with simple febrile seizures and in febrile children without seizure are comparable; consider obtaining urinalysis for susceptible patients (2)[B].
- Blood glucose if the patient is convulsing or is obtunded on presentation (2)[B]
- Lumbar puncture
  - In studies of patients with simple febrile seizures conducted since the initiation of routine infant vaccination against *Haemophilus influenzae*, rates of acute bacterial meningitis were very low (0–0.8%).
  - Seizure is unlikely to be the only presenting symptom of meningitis. Symptoms indicating increased likelihood of meningitis include toxic appearance, altered level of consciousness, meningeal signs, focal neurologic deficits, bulging fontanelle, and petechiae.
  - Cases of bacterial meningitis in children with febrile seizure who return to baseline are rare.
  - Recommendations (1)[B]:
    - Lumbar puncture should be performed in a child with fever and seizure if meningeal signs are present or if there is concern for meningitis or other intracranial pathology based on history and exam.
    - In infants aged 6–12 months, consider lumbar puncture if the child has not been vaccinated against *H. influenzae* or *Streptococcus pneumoniae* according to schedule.

- Consider lumbar puncture for children with fever and seizure who have recently been treated with antibiotics and may thus have partially treated bacterial meningitis.
- The yield of lumbar puncture in children with complex febrile seizure is very low; however, some recommend considering a lumbar puncture in these patients (3)[B].

- Neuroimaging is not routinely recommended for the purposes of identifying the cause of a simple febrile seizure (1)[B].
- Studies have demonstrated limited use of emergent imaging in patients who meet criteria for complex febrile seizure based on multiple episodes in 24 hours; however, imaging may be indicated for focal findings or concerning history or exam (4)[B].

Diagnostic Procedures/Other

- EEG is not recommended in neurologically normal children presenting with simple febrile seizure (1)[B].
- There is mixed evidence for use of EEG after complex febrile seizures; some recommend outpatient EEG on follow-up.

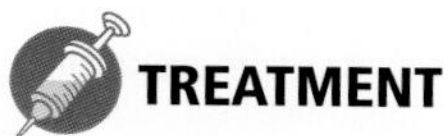

TREATMENT

GENERAL MEASURES

- Acute seizure management
  - Airway: Position the patient laterally, suction secretions, and place a nasopharyngeal airway if necessary.
  - Breathing: Administer oxygen for cyanosis; consider bag-mask ventilation or intubation for inadequate ventilation.
  - Circulation: Establish IV access if 1st-line buccal or nasal midazolam is not effective.
- Antipyretics are helpful for patient comfort but do not prevent seizure recurrence during the initial febrile episode (5)[B].
- Provide supportive care and treat underlying infection if necessary.

MEDICATION

First Line

Treat seizures of ≥5 minutes duration with anticonvulsants:

- Buccal midazolam 0.5 mg/kg or nasal midazolam 0.2 mg/kg (6)[A]
- IV or IM lorazepam 0.1 mg/kg

Second Line

Rectal diazepam is less effective and more commonly associated with respiratory depression than 1st-line treatments 5[B].

ISSUES FOR REFERRAL

Simple febrile seizures do not require referral to a pediatric neurologist.

INPATIENT CONSIDERATIONS

Admission Criteria/Initial Stabilization

- Unstable vital signs
- Concerning findings on history or physical exam
- Prolonged seizure requiring anticonvulsants
- Persistent change in mental status
- Inpatient management of underlying condition is required.

ONGOING CARE

FOLLOW-UP RECOMMENDATIONS

- Anticonvulsant prophylaxis during subsequent febrile episodes (7)[B]
  - The American Academy of Pediatrics recommends against prophylaxis with anticonvulsants due an unacceptable risk–benefit ratio.
  - Phenobarbital is effective but can have serious side effects, including lowering IQ.
  - Prophylaxis with valproic acid may be effective but can cause hepatotoxicity and/or hyperammonemia.
  - Prophylaxis with phenytoin and carbamazepine is ineffective.
  - Oral and rectal diazepam are effective but are not recommended due to the benign nature of febrile seizures.
- Antipyretic prophylaxis during subsequent febrile episodes (7)[B]
  - No study has demonstrated that fever management will prevent recurrence.
  - Ibuprofen and acetaminophen are no more effective than placebo in preventing recurrence.

PATIENT EDUCATION

There is frequently a high degree of parental anxiety associated with febrile seizures. Suggested anticipatory guidance:

- Febrile seizures do not cause brain damage and are associated with a low risk for sequelae.
- The child has a high probability of recurrence:
  - If seizure recurs, position the child safely and do not intervene inappropriately.
  - Time the seizure; call rescue if the child turns blue, has difficulty breathing, or the seizure lasts >5 minutes.
  - If the seizure spontaneously resolves in <5 minutes and the child is well but sleepy, seek immediate attention, but calling rescue is not necessary.

PROGNOSIS

- Recurrence
  - Estimates of recurrence rates vary (32–54%).
  - Factors associated with seizure recurrence include age <12 months at time of 1st episode, 1st-degree relative with history of febrile seizure, and history of complex febrile seizures.
- Intellectual and behavioral outcomes (8)
  - Febrile seizures do not impact cognitive growth or development.
  - Outcomes in children with single and multiple febrile seizures are similar.
- Subsequent development of epilepsy
  - Risk of unprovoked seizure before age 25 is 2.4% in children with a history of simple febrile seizure and 6–8% in children with a history of complex febrile seizure, compared with ~1% in the general population.
  - Factors associated with increased risk include presenting with complex febrile seizure, family history of epilepsy or febrile seizures, cerebral palsy, developmental delay, low birth weight, and prematurity.
- Mortality (8):
  - A slight increase in mortality is attributable in part to underlying neurodevelopmental abnormalities and to the subsequent development of epilepsy.
  - There is not an increased risk for SIDS in siblings of children who have febrile seizures.

COMPLICATIONS

Seizure-related injury, aspiration pneumonia, side effects of prescribed medications or diagnostic procedures, and subsequent parental perception of the child as being vulnerable, especially during subsequent fevers

REFERENCES

1. Subcommittee on Febrile Seizures, American Academy of Pediatrics. Neurodiagnostic evaluation of the child with a simple febrile seizure. *Pediatrics*. 2011;127(2):389–394.
2. Baumer JH. Evidence based guideline for post-seizure management in children presenting acutely to secondary care. *Arch Dis Child*. 2004;89(3):278–280.
3. Kimia A, Ben-Joseph EP, Rudloe T. Yield of lumbar puncture among children who present with their first complex febrile seizure. *Pediatrics*. 2010;126(1):62–69.
4. Hardasmalani MD, Saber M. Yield of diagnostic studies in children presenting with complex febrile seizures. *Pediatr Emerg Care*. 2012;28(8):789–791.
5. Strengell T, Uhari M, Tarkka R. Antipyretic agents for preventing recurrences of febrile seizures: randomized controlled trial. *Arch Pediatr Adolesc Med*. 2009;163(9):799–804.
6. Appleton R, Macleod S, Martland T. Drug management for acute tonic-clonic convulsions including convulsive status epilepticus in children. *Cochrane Database Syst Rev*. 2008;(3):CD001905.
7. Steering Committee on Quality Improvement and Management, Subcommittee on Febrile Seizures American Academy of Pediatrics. Febrile seizures: Clinical practice guideline for the long-term management of the child with simple febrile seizures. *Pediatrics*. 2008;121(6):1281–1286.
8. Jones T, Jacobsen SJ. Childhood febrile seizures: Overview and implications. *Int J Med Sci*. 2007;4(2):110–114.

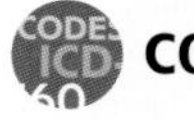

CODES

ICD10

- R56.00 Simple febrile convulsions
- R56.01 Complex febrile convulsions
- G40.901 Epilepsy, unsp, not intractable, with status epilepticus

CLINICAL PEARLS

- Febrile seizures are generally benign, and families can be reassured that children are at low risk of death, subsequent development of epilepsy, and learning or behavioral abnormalities.
- History and physical exam are important tools in identifying children presenting with febrile seizure who may be at greater risk for meningitis or other intracranial pathology.
- For simple febrile seizures, routine labs, lumbar puncture, neuroimaging studies, and EEG are not recommended in the absence of clinical suspicion of serious underlying pathology.
- Prophylaxis with anticonvulsants or antipyretics during subsequent febrile episodes is not recommended due to their lack of effectiveness and the risk of medication-associated side effects.

SEPSIS

Jin Sol Oh, MD • Varun Kumar Bhalla, MD • Steven B. Holsten, Jr., MD, FACS

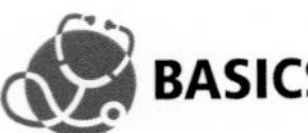

BASICS

DESCRIPTION

- Sepsis is a systemic inflammatory response to infection.
- Synonym(s): septicemia
- Systemic inflammatory response syndrome (SIRS)
  - Temperature >38°C (100.4°F) or <36°C (96.8°F)
  - HR >90 beats/min
  - Respiratory rate >20 breaths/min
  - WBC >12,000 cells/mm^3, or <4,000 cells/mm^3
- Sepsis signs and symptoms
  - General variables
    - Temperature >38.3°C (100.9°F) or <36°C (96.8°F) HR >90 beats/min or >2 standard deviations (SD) above the normal value for age
    - Tachypnea (RR >20 breaths/min or PCO_2 <32 mm Hg)
    - Acute altered mental status (AMS)
    - Significant edema or positive fluid balance (>20 mL/kg over 24 hours)
    - Hyperglycemia (plasma glucose >140 mg/dL or 7.7 mmol/L) in the absence of diabetes
  - Inflammatory variables
    - WBC >12,000 cells/mm^3, or <4,000 cells/mm^3, or normal WBC with >10% bands
    - Plasma C-reactive protein >2 SD above normal
    - Plasma procalcitonin >2 SD above normal
  - Hemodynamic variables
    - Arterial hypotension (SBP <90 mm Hg; MAP <70; or SBP decrease of >40 mm Hg in adults or <2 SD below normal for age)
  - Organ dysfunction variables
    - Arterial hypoxemia (PaO_2/FIO_2 <300)
    - Acute oliguria (urine output <0.5 mL/kg/hr for at least 2 hours)
    - Creatinine increase >0.5 mg/dL or 44.2 μmol/L
    - Coagulation abnormalities (INR >1.5 or aPTT >60 seconds)
    - Ileus (absent bowel sounds)
    - Thrombocytopenia (platelet <100,000)
    - Hyperbilirubinemia (plasma total bilirubin >4 mg/dL or 70 μmol/L)
  - Tissue perfusion variables
    - Hyperlactatemia (>1 mmol/L)
    - Decreased capillary refill or mottling
- Severe sepsis: sepsis-induced hypoperfusion or organ dysfunction
- Septic shock: refractory hypotension unexplained by other causes and despite adequate fluid resuscitation:
  - Hypotension is defined as SAP <90 mm Hg, MAP <70 mm Hg, and reduction in SBP >40 mm Hg from baseline.

Pediatric Considerations

- Definition of sepsis, severe sepsis, septic shock, and multiple organ dysfunctions are similar to definitions for adults but depend on age-specific vital signs and WBC values.
- Drug metabolism is reduced in children with severe sepsis. Monitor drug toxicity labs to prevent adverse effects.

Geriatric Considerations

Often more difficult to diagnose; change in mental status/behavior may be the only early manifestation.

EPIDEMIOLOGY

Incidence

- 3/1,000 population
- Increasing incidence; 750,000 new cases annually in the United States
- 2% of hospitalized patients; ~75% of ICU patients

ETIOLOGY AND PATHOPHYSIOLOGY

- An imbalance between proinflammatory and anti-inflammatory mediators leads to systemic tissue damage.
- Widespread endothelial dysfunction leads to maldistribution of blood flow, causing impaired tissue oxygenation and resultant organ dysfunction.
- Dysregulated nitric oxide production and activation of the coagulation system causes maldistribution of organ blood flow and coagulopathic damage.
- The abnormal inflammatory response can progress to significant immunosuppression.
- Specific etiologic agents
  - Gram-positive (most common) bacteria: *Staphylococcus* sp., *Streptococcus* sp., *Enterococcus* sp.
  - Gram-negative: *Escherichia coli*, *Klebsiella* sp., *Proteus* sp., *Pseudomonas* sp. and anaerobic bacteria
  - Fungi: *Candida* sp. (incidence increased 207% from 1976 to 2000)
- Common sites: lungs (most common), urinary tract, abdomen (biliary tree, intestine, peritonitis), skin (cellulitis, decubitus ulcer, gangrene), heart valves, CNS (meningitis), intravascular catheters
- Unknown site of infection in 20–30% of patients

RISK FACTORS

- Extremes of age (very old or young)
- Ethnicity: African American
- Chronic medical disease: COPD, CHF, cancer, and renal insufficiency/failure
- Immunosuppression
- Bacteremia
- Community-acquired pneumonia
- Indwelling catheters: intravascular, urinary, biliary
- Complicated labor and delivery: premature labor and/or premature rupture of membranes, untreated maternal group B strep colonization

GENERAL PREVENTION

- Vaccination: pneumococcal vaccine in children and also adults who are ≥65 years or with comorbidities placing them at high risk for disease. *Haemophilus influenzae* type B (infants, young children), influenza (H1N1 in pregnant women), meningococcal vaccine
- γ-Globulin for hypo- or agammaglobulinemia
- Treat group B strep carriers during labor.
- Regular hand washing, sterile technique for catheters, appropriate glove use
- Antibiotic prophylaxis for recommended surgical procedures

COMMONLY ASSOCIATED CONDITIONS

- Immunologic: neutropenia, HIV, hypo/agammaglobulinemia, complement deficiency, splenectomy, immunosuppressive medication (corticosteroids, chemotherapy, TNF-α antagonists)
- Diabetes, alcoholism, malignancy, cirrhosis, burns, multiple trauma, IV drug abuse, malnutrition

DIAGNOSIS

HISTORY

- Past medical, surgical, social, occupational, and travel history to identify risk and potential source
- General symptoms
  - Fever, chills, rigors, myalgias
  - Mental status changes: restlessness, agitation, confusion, delirium, lethargy, stupor, coma
- Specific symptoms (relative primary source)
  - Respiratory: cough, sputum production, dyspnea, chest pain
  - Urinary: dysuria, frequency, urgency, flank pain
  - Intra-abdominal: nausea, vomiting, diarrhea, constipation, abdominal pain
  - CNS: stiff neck, headache, photophobia, focal neurologic signs
- End-organ failure symptoms: shortness of breath, oliguria/anuria, mottled skin

PHYSICAL EXAM

- Assess vital signs: hyper/hypothermia, tachycardia, tachypnea, hypotension
- Signs of poor perfusion: delayed capillary refill, cyanosis
- Signs of target organ involvement: jaundice, skin lesions (erythema, petechiae, embolic lesions, purpura)

DIFFERENTIAL DIAGNOSIS

- Bacteremia without sepsis
- Viral, rickettsial, spirochetal, and protozoal diseases
- Collagen vascular diseases, vasculitides, pancreatitis, myocardial infarction, congestive heart failure, pulmonary embolism, thrombotic thrombocytopenic purpura (TTP); hemolytic uremic syndrome (HUS), thyrotoxicosis, adrenal insufficiency, poisoning, drug reaction

DIAGNOSTIC TESTS & INTERPRETATION

Initial Tests (lab, imaging)

- Two sets of blood cultures to document presence of bacteremia (not required for diagnosis; 50% of blood cultures are negative in severe sepsis/septic shock). Obtain cultures before antibiotic therapy. Do not delay the start of antibiotic therapy. Prior antibiotic use may suppress the growth of organisms (1)[B].
- Cultures/Gram stains from potential sites of infection (sputum, urine, pleural fluid, ascites, CSF, wound)
- CBC with differential, C-reactive protein, coagulation profile, comprehensive metabolic profile, lactic acid level, arterial blood gas; urinalysis
- Common findings: leukocytosis, bandemia (>10%), hyperglycemia, metabolic acidosis, mild hyperbilirubinemia, hypoxemia, respiratory alkalosis, proteinuria
- Less common findings (more severe): leukopenia, anemia, thrombocytopenia, prolonged prothrombin time, azotemia, hypoglycemia, lactic acidosis
- Radiographic studies (plain films, ultrasound, CT, or MRI) to confirm source of infection

Diagnostic Procedures/Other

- Aspiration, biopsy, and/or drainage of potentially infected body sites (pleural cavity, peritoneal cavity, biliary tree, CSF, abscess). Interventional radiology techniques to aid in specimen collection as needed.
- Echocardiogram if concern for heart valves as occult source of infection

Test Interpretation

- Inflammation at primary site of infection often with disseminated intravascular coagulation
- Noncardiogenic pulmonary edema

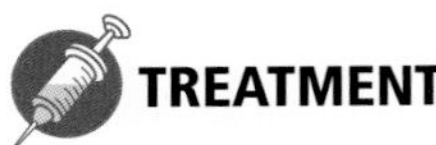

TREATMENT

GENERAL MEASURES

- Assess oxygenation and supplement as needed. Intubate for respiratory failure.

- Invasive monitoring for management of hemodynamic instability using goal-directed therapy.
- Adequate volume resuscitation and vasopressors if required (within first 6 hours). Targets of the following:
  - Central venous pressure (CVP) 8–12 mm Hg, MAP ≥65 mm Hg, urine output ≥0.5 mL/kg/hr (1)[A]
  - Central/mixed venous O_2 saturation ≥70%/65%
    - If goals not met with fluid resuscitation (CVP 8–12 mm Hg) and vasopressors (MAP >65 mm Hg), transfuse packed RBCs to achieve hematocrit >30%; if still <70%, add dobutamine (1)[C].
- Quickly identify source of infection and remove septic foci:
  - Early surgical consultation for acute abdomen, empyema, necrotizing fasciitis
  - Interventional radiology consultation for guided drainage
- Transfuse RBCs, platelets, and/or fresh frozen plasma for coagulopathic complications or in association with planned procedures.
  - Transfuse RBC if Hgb <7.0 to target Hgb of 7.0–9.9 g/dL in absence of tissue hypoperfusion, ischemic coronary artery disease, or acute hemorrhage (1)[B].
- Stress ulcer and DVT prophylaxis (1)[B]
- Glucose control (≥180 mg/dL) (1)[A]

MEDICATION

First Line

- Fluid management
  - Initial therapy: 30 mL/kg of crystalloids (1)[B]
  - Consider adding albumin for patients requiring large volumes of crystalloid (1)[C],(2)[B].
- Vasopressors
  - Norepinephrine (preferred); dopamine (1,3)[B].
  - Low-dose dopamine for renal protection is not recommended (1)[C].
- Broad-spectrum antibiotic (≥1 agents against likely bacterial/fungal pathogens) should be initiated in the first hour after recognition of sepsis or septic shock (1,4)[A]:
  - Adult (*Pseudomonas* not suspected): vancomycin + Gram-negative coverage (3rd-generation cephalosporin, β-lactam/β-lactamase inhibitor, or carbapenem)
  - Adult (*Pseudomonas* suspected): vancomycin + two agents aimed at resistant Gram-negative bacteria ceftazidime/cefepime/carbapenem/piperacillin–tazobactam + either fluoroquinolone (ciprofloxacin) *or* aminoglycoside (gentamicin/amikacin) depending on local hospital sensitivities
  - Nonimmunocompromised child: 3rd-generation cephalosporin
  - Neonate (<7 days old): ampicillin and gentamicin (5)[B]
  - After culture and sensitivity results are available, use organism-specific antibiotic for 7–10 days.
- Antifungals if fungal infection suspected: long-term antibiotic use, TPN, GI surgery
  - Intravenous immunoglobulins (IVIGs) as adjuvant therapy may reduce mortality in adults (6)[B].

ALERT

The European Society of Intensive Care Medicine statement in critically ill patients

- Hydroxyethyl starches (HESs) with MW ≥200 kDA and/or degree of substitution >0.4 are not recommended in severe septic patients (1)[C].
- Albumin may be included in the resuscitation of severe sepsis patients without head injury.
- Hyperoncotic solutions should not be used in fluid resuscitation.

Pregnancy Considerations

β-Lactam antibiotics, macrolides, and metronidazole generally are considered safe.

ALERT

- Adjust doses for renal and/or hepatic impairment.
- Consider narrowing antibiotic regimen at 48–72 hours based on culture results and clinical course (1)[B].
- Possible interactions
  - Aminoglycosides: increased in nephrotoxicity with enflurane, cisplatin, and possibly vancomycin; ototoxicity with loop diuretics; paralysis with neuromuscular-blocking agents

Second Line

- Vasopressors: epinephrine (first alternative), vasopressin, or phenylephrine
- Consider IV hydrocortisone 200 mg per day if the patient is poorly responsive to both IV fluid resuscitation and vasopressors (1)[C].
- Recombinant human-activated protein C (Xigris) was voluntarily withdrawn from the market in 2011.
- Inotropic therapy with dobutamine may benefit patients with myocardial dysfunction or ongoing hypoperfusion despite adequate intravascular volume and MAP (1)[C].

ADDITIONAL THERAPIES

Intermittent hemodialysis or continuous veno-venous hemofiltration

SURGERY/OTHER PROCEDURES

Debride necrotic tissues: Drain or remove abscesses or other foci of infection.

INPATIENT CONSIDERATIONS

Admission Criteria/Initial Stabilization

ICU care

IV Fluids

Aggressive fluid resuscitation with normal saline can result in nongap metabolic acidosis. Not likely with lactated Ringer solution.

ONGOING CARE

FOLLOW-UP RECOMMENDATIONS

Patient Monitoring

- In unstable patients: invasive hemodynamic monitoring, arterial line and central venous catheter placement
- Chem-7 and CBC daily; lactate, mixed venous oxygen saturation q2–4h in initial resuscitation, and daily INR/PTT if DIC is a concern
- Follow antibiotic drug levels (vancomycin, gentamicin).
- Foley catheter placement to monitor urine output

DIET

NPO if intubation being considered; otherwise, enteral feeds are preferred to help preserve mucosal integrity of the GI tract (1)[C].

PATIENT EDUCATION

www.nlm.nih.gov/medlineplus/sepsis.html

PROGNOSIS

Mortality is 10–50% overall. Poor prognostic factors include the inability to mount a fever (>40°C), nonurinary source of infection, nosocomial infection, inappropriate antibiotic coverage, and certain comorbidities (AIDS, cancer, immunosuppression).

COMPLICATIONS

GI hemorrhage, DIC, hyperglycemia, de novo embolic foci of infection, ARDS, multiorgan failure, death

REFERENCES

1. Dellinger RP, Levy MM, Rhodes A, et al. Surviving sepsis campaign: international guidelines for management of severe sepsis and septic shock: 2012. *Crit Care Med*. 2013;41(2):580–637.
2. Raghunathan K, Shaw A, Nathanson B, et al. Association between the choice of IV crystalloid and in-hospital mortality among critically ill adults with sepsis. *Crit Care Med*. 2014;42(7):1585–1591.
3. De Backer D, Biston P, Devriendt J, et al. Comparison of dopamine and norepinephrine in the treatment of shock. *N Engl J Med*. 2010;362(9):779–789.
4. Paul M, Lador A, Grozinsky-Glasberg S, et al. Beta lactam antibiotic monotherapy versus beta lactam-aminoglycoside antibiotic combination therapy for sepsis. *Cochrane Database Syst Rev*. 2014;(1):CD003344.
5. Stockmann C, Spigarelli MG, Campbell SC, et al. Considerations in the pharmacologic treatment and prevention of neonatal sepsis. *Paediatr Drugs*. 2014;16(1):67–81.
6. Alejandria MM, Lansang MA, Dans LF, et al. Intravenous immunoglobulin for treating sepsis, severe sepsis and septic shock. *Cochrane Database Syst Rev*. 2013;(9):CD001090.

ADDITIONAL READING

- Levy MM, Fink MP, Marshall JC, et al. 2001 SCCM/ESICM/ACCP/ATS/SIS International Sepsis Definitions Conference. *Crit Care Med*. 2003;31(4):1250–1256.
- Reinhart K, Perner A, Sprung CL, et al. Consensus statement of the ESICM task force on colloid volume therapy in critically ill patients: authors' reply to comments by Zacharowski et al. *Intensive Care Med*. 2012;38(3):1558–1559.
- Venkataraman R, Kellum JA. Sepsis: update in the management. *Adv Chronic Kidney Dis*. 2013;20(1):6–13.
- Wiener RS, Wiener DC, Larson RJ. Benefits and risks of tight glucose control in critically ill adults: a meta-analysis. *JAMA*. 2008;300(8):933–944.

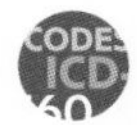

CODES

ICD10

- A41.9 Sepsis, unspecified organism
- R65.10 SIRS of non-infectious origin w/o acute organ dysfunction
- R65.20 Severe sepsis without septic shock

CLINICAL PEARLS

- Appropriate treatment consists of aggressive fluid support with hemodynamic monitoring (pressor support if necessary) along with the early use of broad-spectrum antimicrobial therapy and removal/drainage of foci of infection.
- Despite aggressive treatment, overall mortality rates are still very high (10–50%) in patients with severe sepsis/septic shock.

SEROTONIN SYNDROME

Neela Bhajandas, PharmD • Michael C. Barros, PharmD, BCPS, BCACP • Paul N. Williams, MD

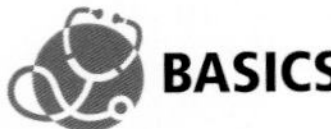

BASICS

DESCRIPTION

- A potentially life-threatening adverse drug reaction that results from excessive stimulation of peripheral and CNS serotonergic receptors
- It is a concentration-dependent toxicity that can develop in any individual who has ingested drug combinations that synergistically increase synaptic 5-HT.
- Serotonin toxicity occurs in 3 main settings: (i) therapeutic drug use, which often results in mild to moderate symptoms; (ii) intentional overdose of a single serotonergic agent, which typically leads to moderate symptoms; and (iii) as the result of a drug interaction between numerous serotonergic agents (most commonly, selective serotonin reuptake inhibitors [SSRIs] and monoamine oxidase inhibitors [MAOIs]), most often associated with severe serotonin toxicity.
- Classically characterized by a triad of symptoms that include mental status change, neuromuscular abnormalities, and autonomic hyperactivity
- Onset is usually within 24 hours, with 60% of cases occurring within 6 hours of exposure to, or change in, dosing of a serotonergic agent. Rarely, cases have been reported weeks after discontinuation of serotonergic agents.

Geriatric Considerations

Elderly are at increased risk given use of multiple meds.

Pediatric Considerations

- Serotonin syndrome has similar manifestations in children and adults.
- General management is unchanged in children, other than medication dosing.

Pregnancy Considerations

- 3rd-trimester exposure to SSRIs has been associated with transient neonatal complications that may reflect either acute drug withdrawal or serotonergic toxicity.
- Symptoms in neonates may include tremors, increased muscle tone, jitteriness, shivering, feeding/digestive disturbances, irritability, agitation, sleep disturbances, increased reflexes, excessive crying, and respiratory disturbances.

EPIDEMIOLOGY

Seen in about 14–16% of SSRI overdose patients

Incidence

- In 2008, there were 106,336 adverse events reported with antidepressant use including 28 deaths. Most of these were associated with SSRIs, either alone or in combination with other drugs. SSRIs alone were responsible for adverse events in 18.8% of cases, with 55.7% due to intentional causes, 39.5% unintentional, and remainder of causes unknown. Of patients reporting adverse effects with SSRIs, 46.6% had symptoms requiring hospitalization, and significant toxic effects occurred in 90 patients with 2 resultant deaths (1)[A].
- The incidence of serotonin syndrome is rising because serotonergic agents are increasingly used in clinical practice and in combination with other serotonergic agents.
- Predominant age: affects all age groups
- Predominant sex: male = female

ETIOLOGY AND PATHOPHYSIOLOGY

- The result of excessive stimulation in peripheral and CNS serotonergic receptors
- Risk is mediated in a dose-related manner to the action of 5-HT/5-HT agonists on 5HT-1a and/or 5HT-2a receptors. The development mechanism of the syndrome is unknown.
- It is hypothesized that the degree of serotonin elevation in blood plasma has to be 10–15%× above baseline levels to result in serotonin toxicity (2)[A].
- A number of drugs are associated with the serotonin syndrome, which usually involves combination with an SSRI. These include SSRIs (e.g., citalopram, escitalopram, fluoxetine, fluvoxamine, paroxetine, sertraline); MAOIs; SNRIs (duloxetine, venlafaxine, desvenlafaxine); tricyclic antidepressants (e.g., amitriptyline); other antidepressants (buspirone, nefazodone, trazodone); lithium; triptans; anticonvulsants (Depakote); analgesics (fentanyl, meperidine, pentazocine, tramadol); antibiotics (linezolid [weak MAOI], ritonavir); over-the-counter (OTC) cough medications (dextromethorphan); some antipsychotics (risperidone, olanzapine); antiemetics (ondansetron, granisetron); other medications, such as metoclopramide, cyclobenzaprine, L-dopa; dietary supplements (tryptophan); herbal supplements (St. John's wort, nutmeg); methylene blue; and drugs of abuse (e.g., MDMA, cocaine, LSD, and amphetamine).
- Initially, patients can develop a peripheral tremor, confusion, and ataxia; systemic signs are next (e.g., agitation, diaphoresis, hyperreflexia, and shivering). If it worsens, the severe signs of fever, jerking, and diarrhea may develop. Serotonin syndrome can last from hours to days after the offending agents are stopped and supportive care is initiated.
- Drug interactions are most often the cause of severe cases of serotonin syndrome. Many of the same classes of medications listed earlier are involved, especially MAOIs (including linezolid) with SSRIs.

Genetics

Unknown

RISK FACTORS

- Serotonergic agents
- Reported following ingestion of a single agent. However, the greatest number of adverse events has been shown to be associated with SSRIs in combination with other substances, and the combination of SSRIs and MAOIs carries the greatest risk for developing serotonin toxicity.

GENERAL PREVENTION

- Consider drug–drug interactions when a multidrug regimen is required and avoid if possible.
- Caution patients about taking SSRIs with OTC medications (e.g., dextromethorphan) or herbal supplements (e.g., St. John wort) prior to consulting a physician.
- Clinician education
- Continual improvement in use of health information technology

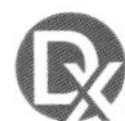

DIAGNOSIS

- Serotonin syndrome is a clinical diagnosis.
- Epidemiologic data suggest that up to 85% of practitioners are unaware of serotonin syndrome.
- *Hunter Toxicity Criteria Decision Rules* aid in the diagnosis of clinically significant serotonin toxicity (sensitivity, 84%; specificity, 97%).
- To fulfill Hunter criteria, a patient must have taken a serotonergic agent and have 1 of the following:
  - Spontaneous clonus
  - Inducible clonus + agitation/diaphoresis
  - Ocular clonus + agitation/diaphoresis
  - Tremor and hyperreflexia
  - Hypertonia
  - Temperature >38°C + ocular clonus/inducible clonus (3)[A]

HISTORY

- Obtain a thorough drug history, including prescription medications, OTC remedies, dietary supplements, herbal supplements, and illicit drugs. Ask about dose, formulation, and recent changes.
- Address possibility of drug overdose, and obtain collateral information if intentional overdose is suspected.
- Elicit description of symptoms, including their onset and progression.

PHYSICAL EXAM

- Vital signs: tachycardia, hypertension, and hyperthermia (severe cases)
- Neuromuscular findings (seen in over half of patients with serotonin syndrome)
  - Hyperreflexia (greater in lower extremities)
  - Clonus (involuntary muscle contractions, most commonly tested by flexing foot upward rapidly; includes ocular)
  - Myoclonus (greater in lower extremities)
  - Tremor (greater in lower extremities)
  - Hypertonia
  - Bilateral Babinski sign
  - Akathisia
  - Tonic–clonic seizures (severe cases)
  - Autonomic signs
    - Diaphoresis
    - Mydriasis
    - Flushing
    - Dry mucous membranes
    - Vomiting, diarrhea, increased bowel sounds
    - Mental status changes: anxiety, disorientation, delirium (4)[A]
    - Severe cases have led to altered level of consciousness, rhabdomyolysis, metabolic acidosis, and disseminated intravascular coagulation (DIC).

DIFFERENTIAL DIAGNOSIS

- Neuroleptic malignant syndrome (NMS)
- Anticholinergic fever (e.g., benztropine, diphenhydramine, oxybutynin, nifedipine, famotidine, atropine, scopolamine; plant poisoning from belladonna/"deadly nightshade," datura, henbane, mandrake, brugmansia)

- Malignant hyperthermia
- Heat stroke
- CNS infection (meningitis, encephalitis)
- Sympathomimetic toxicity
- Nonconvulsive seizures
- Hyperthyroidism
- Tetanus
- Acute baclofen withdrawal

DIAGNOSTIC TESTS & INTERPRETATION

- Serum serotonin levels do not correlate with clinical findings.
- Nonspecific lab findings that may develop include the following:
  - Elevated WBC count
  - Elevated creatine phosphokinase (CK or CPK)
  - Decreased serum bicarbonate
  - Elevated hepatic transaminases
- In severe cases, the following complications may develop:
  - DIC
  - Metabolic acidosis
  - Rhabdomyolysis
  - Renal failure
  - Myoglobinuria
  - Acute respiratory distress syndrome (ARDS) (4)[A]

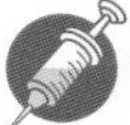

TREATMENT

- Discontinue all serotonergic agents.
- Supportive care is the mainstay of therapy. This includes administration of oxygen and aggressive IV fluids, continuous cardiac monitoring, and correction of vital signs:
  - Benzodiazepines may be effective for the management of agitation in patients with serotonin syndrome.
  - Administration of serotonin antagonists: Cyproheptadine (histamine and serotonin antagonist) may be useful if supportive measures and sedation (benzodiazepines) are unable to control agitation and correct vital signs.
- Mild cases (afebrile, tachycardia, shivering, diaphoresis, mydriasis, hyperreflexia, intermittent tremor or myoclonus)
  - Discontinue precipitating agent(s).
  - Supportive care
  - Sedation
- Moderate cases (temperature >38°C, autonomic instability, mydriasis, hyperactive bowel sounds, diarrhea, diaphoresis, ocular clonus, hyperreflexia, tremor, mild agitation, or hypervigilance)
  - Discontinue precipitating agent(s).
  - Supportive care
  - Sedation
  - Aggressive treatment of autonomic instability
  - Treatment with cyproheptadine should be initiated if agitation and vital sign abnormalities are unimproved with benzodiazepines and supportive care.
  - Hypotension from MAOI interactions should be treated with low doses of direct-acting sympathomimetics (e.g., norepinephrine, phenylephrine, epinephrine); indirect serotonin agonists, such as dopamine, should be avoided.
  - Severe hypertension and tachycardia should be treated with short-acting agents, such as nitroprusside or esmolol.
  - Avoid use of longer acting agents, such as propranolol.
- Severe cases (temperature >41.1°C, autonomic instability, delirium, muscular rigidity, and hypertonicity)
  - Discontinue precipitating agent(s).
  - Immediate sedation
  - Endotracheal intubation as clinically indicated
  - Paralysis as clinically indicated (maintained with nondepolarizing continuous paralytic agents such as vecuronium, cisatracurium, rocuronium)
  - Antipyretic medications are not effective (4)[A]; the increased body temperature is due to muscle activity, not an alteration in the hypothalamic set point.

MEDICATION

- Activated charcoal: may be used in patients who intentionally overdose on serotonergic agents (3)[A]
- Benzodiazepines: may be used to manage agitation in serotonin syndrome and also may correct mild increases in BP and heart rate. Use with caution in patients with delirium, given the known paradoxical effect of exacerbating delirium.
- Cyproheptadine (Periactin): consider use if benzodiazepines and supportive measures are unable to control agitation and correct vital signs:
  - Adults: initial dose 12 mg PO (can also be crushed and given via nasogastric [NG] tube) followed by 2 mg q2h until clinical response observed; 12–32 mg of drug may be required in a 24-hour period.
  - Children
    - <2 years: 0.06 mg/kg q6h
    - 2–6 years: 2 mg q6h
    - 7–14 years: 4 mg q6h
  - Unlikely to be effective in patients who have received activated charcoal.
- Use of antipsychotics with 5-HT2A antagonist activity, such as olanzapine and chlorpromazine, is not recommended (4)[A].

ISSUES FOR REFERRAL

- Psychiatry: for assistance with medication management and follow-up care (inpatient psychiatric care vs. outpatient psychiatric follow-up)
- Toxicology/clinical pharmacology service
- Poison control center

INPATIENT CONSIDERATIONS

Patients with known/suspected serotonin syndrome should be admitted to a medical inpatient unit for observation.

Discharge Criteria

- Mental status has returned to baseline.
- Stable vital signs
- No increase in clonus
- Close patient follow-up ensured

ONGOING CARE

FOLLOW-UP RECOMMENDATIONS

- In mild cases of serotonin toxicity, address risks and benefits of restarting offending agents. Serotonergic medications need to be titrated slowly, and patients must have close outpatient follow-up with physician.
- If patient developed severe serotonin syndrome, the offending agent should likely not be resumed unless precipitant for serotonin syndrome is found (e.g., combination with another serotonin agonist); the patient can be carefully monitored, or there is clear benefit versus risk of restarting the medication.

PROGNOSIS

- Generally favorable with early recognition of the syndrome and prompt initiation of treatment
- Most cases resolve within 24 hours of discontinuation of serotonergic agents; this can be longer depending on the drug's half-life:
  - MAOIs can result in toxicity for several days.
  - SSRIs can result in toxicity for up to several weeks after discontinuation.
- ICU admission is often indicated in severe cases.

COMPLICATIONS

- Adverse outcomes, including death, are usually the consequence of poorly treated hyperthermia.
- Nonhyperthermic patients who survive typically do not have long-term sequelae.

REFERENCES

1. Bronstein AC, Spyker DA, Cantilena LR Jr, et al. 2008 Annual Report of the American Association of Poison Control Centers' National Poison Data System (NPDS): 26th annual report. *Clin Toxicol (Phila)*. 2009;47(10):911–1084.
2. Ables AZ, Nagubilli R. Prevention, recognition, and management of serotonin syndrome. *Am Fam Physician*. 2010;81(9):1139–1142.
3. Dunkley EJ, Isbister GK, Sibbritt D, et al. The Hunter Serotonin Toxicity Criteria: simple and accurate diagnostic decision rules for serotonin toxicity. *QJM*. 2003;96(9):635–642.
4. Boyer EW, Shannon M. The serotonin syndrome. *N Engl J Med*. 2005;352(11):1112–1120.

ADDITIONAL READING

- Isbister GK, Buckley NA, Whyte IM. Serotonin toxicity: a practical approach to diagnosis and treatment. *Med J Aust*. 2007;187(6):361–365.
- McAllen KJ, Schwartz DR. Adverse drug reactions resulting in hyperthermia in the intensive care unit. *Crit Care Med*. 2010;38(6)(Suppl):S244–S252.

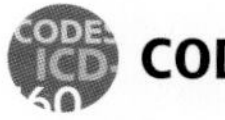

CODES

ICD10

G25.79 Other drug induced movement disorders

CLINICAL PEARLS

Consider serotonin syndrome in patients with recent use of a serotonergic agent (particularly if multiple proserotonergic agents are involved) presenting with unexplained tachycardia, hypertension, hyperthermia, clonus, hyperreflexia, and change in mental status.

SEXUAL DYSFUNCTION IN WOMEN

Amanda M. Carnes, MD • Lisa M. Harris, DO, MAJ, MC, FS

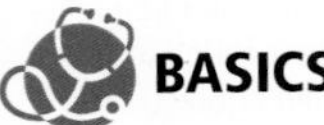

BASICS

- Very common: ~40% of women surveyed in the United States have sexual concerns.
- Includes dissatisfaction with any aspect of sexual experience, including emotional, physical, or relational
- May present as a lack of sexual desire, impaired arousal, pain with sexual activity, or inability to achieve orgasm, and may be lifelong or acquired

DESCRIPTION

- 5 major types
  - Disorders of desire: hypoactive sexual desire with deficient or absent desire for sexual activity or fantasies
  - Disorder of arousal: inability to attain or maintain adequate lubrication/engorgement in response to sexual excitement
  - Disorders of orgasm: delay or absence of orgasm following normal sexual excitement
  - Vaginismus: involuntary contractions of the perineal muscles in response to vaginal penetration
  - Dyspareunia: genital pain associated with intercourse
- *DSM-5* (2013) redefines hypoactive sexual desire disorder and female sexual arousal disorder as female sexual interest/arousal disorder.
- Symptoms must be present for ≥6 months; cause clinically significant distress or impairment; and not be caused by another condition (psychiatric or medical), substance/medication, relationship distress, or other stressor.

ALERT

Take care not to mislabel short-term or possibly adaptive changes in sexual functioning as dysfunction.

- System(s) affected: nervous; reproductive; genitourinary; psychiatric
- Synonym(s): hypoactive sexual desire disorder; sexual aversion disorder; female sexual arousal disorder; inhibited female orgasm

EPIDEMIOLOGY

In two large studies, approximately 40% of women reported sexual problems.

Incidence

Incidence is highest during the postpartum period and perimenopause.

- Postpartum: In a study of >400 primiparous women, 83% reported sexual problems at 3 months postpartum and 64% at 6 months. There was no difference between vaginal and cesarean delivery.
- Perimenopause: Sexual problems are highest in women aged 45–64 years. Although sexual activity decreases with age, so does the distress about sex.

Prevalence

Orgasmic disorders are the most common, followed by desire and arousal disorders.

ETIOLOGY AND PATHOPHYSIOLOGY

The pathophysiology of sexual dysfunction is complex and multifactorial because it can be the result of any etiology that interferes with the normal female sexual response cycle of desire, arousal, orgasm, and resolution.

- Prescription medications
  - SSRIs, MAOIs, and TCAs
  - β-Blockers, ACE inhibitors, and calcium channel blockers
  - GNRH agonists
  - Injectable progestins
  - Antiepileptics
  - Gabapentin
- Disorders of the hypothalamic-pituitary-adrenal system
- Hormonal imbalance/disorders of ovarian function
- Menopause (surgical or natural)
- Anxiety or depression
- Thyroid disease
- Diabetes
- Spinal cord damage
- Maladaptive thoughts/behaviors
- Interrelational difficulties and conflict regarding intimacy
- Control issues in the relationship
- Fear of letting go/fear of negative outcome
- Inability to stay present
- Sexual abuse
- Body image issues
- Drug and alcohol abuse

RISK FACTORS

- Advancing age/menopause
- Previous sexual trauma
- Lack of knowledge about sexual stimulation and response
- Chronic medical problems
  - Depression, anxiety, chronic pain syndromes, and other psychiatric disorders
  - Cardiovascular disease
  - Endocrine disorders
  - Gastrointestinal disorders
  - Neurologic disorders
  - Cancer
- Gynecologic issues
  - Childbirth
  - Pelvic floor or bladder dysfunction
  - Endometriosis
  - Uterine fibroids
  - Chronic vulvovaginal candidiasis/vaginal infections
  - Female genital mutilation
- Relationship factors such as couple discrepancies in expectations and/or cultural backgrounds and attitudes toward sexuality in family of origin
- Medications or substance abuse

COMMONLY ASSOCIATED CONDITIONS

- Marital discord
- Depression

DIAGNOSIS

- Female sexual dysfunction is diagnosed by identifying diagnostic criteria through both a medical and a sexual history.
- The diagnosis requires that the sexual problem be recurrent or persistent and cause personal distress or interpersonal difficulty.

HISTORY

- "Three windows approach" (1)[C]
  - Current situation (relationship problems, poor communication, lack of time)
  - Vulnerability of the individual (negative attitudes, need to maintain self-control, history of sexual abuse/ trauma, propensity to sexual inhibition)
  - Health-related factors that alter sex function (mental health and sexuality, physical health and sexuality, side effects of medication, antidepressants, antipsychotics)
- Nature of the problem
- Degree of distress
- Lifelong versus acquired problem
- Situational versus generalized problem
- Cultural/societal beliefs
- Pregnancy/childbirth history
- Infertility
- Menopausal status (natural, surgical, or post-chemotherapy)
- STIs and vaginitis
- Pelvic surgery, injury, or cancer
- Chronic pelvic pain
- Abnormal genital tract bleeding
- Urinary/anal incontinence
- Marital conflict/partner reaction
- Family dysfunction

PHYSICAL EXAM

- Most commonly, patients have a normal physical exam (1)[C].
  - Assess for anatomic abnormalities.
  - Assess for scars or evidence of trauma.
  - Assess for vaginal atrophy, adequate estrogenization.
  - Assess for infection.
  - Recognize signs of anxiety, apprehension, and pain during the speculum and pelvic exam.
- General physical exam, signs of chronic disease

DIFFERENTIAL DIAGNOSIS

- Medication side effects
- Vaginitis
- Decreased vaginal lubrication secondary to hormonal imbalance
- Decreased sensation secondary to nerve injury
- Multiple sclerosis
- Anatomic abnormalities
- Abdominal surgery (which can interfere with pelvic innervation)
- Depression
- Marital dysfunction, including domestic violence
- Pregnancy
- Pseudodyspareunia (use of complaint of pain to distance self from partner)

DIAGNOSTIC TESTS & INTERPRETATION

Neither estrogen nor androgen levels should be used to determine the cause of the sexual dysfunction because there is no established serum hormone range that correlates with sexual dysfunction.

Initial Tests (lab, imaging)

- As needed to identify infections and other medical causes (1)[C]
- Pap smear, STI testing, Wet prep
- TSH
- Fingerstick blood glucose
- Prolactin
- FSH
- Transvaginal US if indicated

TREATMENT

- Assess patient goals.
- Treatment should address associated chronic conditions.
- Improve diet, exercise, and sleep (1)[C].
- Vaginal moisturizers and lubricants (2)[C]
- Cognitive-behavioral therapy (CBT) to target maladaptive thoughts and behaviors and to disrupt the dysfunctional cycle (1)[C]
- Mindfulness-based CBT (1)[C],(3)[B]
- Education on anatomy, physiology, sexual response, and sexual activities other than intercourse (1)[C]
- Education on communication (1)[C]
- Sex therapy: sensate focus, systematic desensitization exercises, homework exchanging physical touch with partner, or directed masturbation alone (1)[C]
- Physical therapy/biofeedback (1)[C]
- Hormone therapy, alone or in conjunction with other therapies (2)[C],(4)[A]
- Couples therapy for women who have relationship conflicts

MEDICATION

Sexual dysfunction is often a multifactorial psychosocial condition. Using medications does not usually address the cause of the problem and can, in some cases, make the condition worse.

First Line

- Bupropion (1)[C],(5)[A]: adjunct for SSRI-induced sexual dysfunction. Improves sexual arousal and orgasm but not desire. Dose: bupropion SR 150 mg once or twice daily.
- Estrogen replacement with or without progestins (2)[C],(4)[A]: may improve sexual desire, vaginal atrophy, and clitoral sensitivity. Vaginal estrogen therapy is available in cream, vaginal tablet, or ring form.
- Testosterone (1)[C]
  - Use in premenopausal women not supported by data.
  - In naturally or surgically postmenopausal women, adding short-term testosterone to hormone replacement may increase desire.
  - Use >6 months contingent on clear improvement and no adverse effects.
  - Side effects: hirsutism, androgenic alopecia, acne, decreased HDL, liver dysfunction; not FDA approved for sexual dysfunction in women
  - Contraindicated in breast or endometrial cancer, thromboembolic disease, or coronary artery disease
  - Dose: oral methyltestosterone 1.25–2.5 mg/day (1/10 of men's dose) or topical (patch, gel)
- DHEA, selective estrogen receptor modulators (SERMs), and tissue-selective estrogen complexes (TSECs) (1,2)[C],(4)[A]: May improve vaginal atrophy, dryness, and dyspareunia, but not FDA approved, these need additional studies.
- PDE-5 Inhibitors (1)[C]: not recommended

ISSUES FOR REFERRAL

Consider referral for CBT, marriage/couples counseling, or sex therapy.

ADDITIONAL THERAPIES

- Smoking cessation and reduction of alcohol intake
- For childhood trauma: scripting, psychotherapy, cognitive restructuring
- For prescription-drug causes: reduced dosages or change to different medication

COMPLEMENTARY & ALTERNATIVE MEDICINE

- Zestra for Women botanical feminine massage oil: Small trial showed increased arousal, desire, genital sensation, ability to have orgasm, and sexual pleasure.
- Yohimbine: not recommended, potentially dangerous
- Ginseng and St. John's wort: No evidence to support treatment of sexual dysfunction.

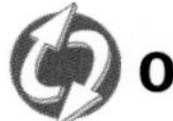

ONGOING CARE

DIET

Weight reduction if overweight or obese

PATIENT EDUCATION

- American Association of Sex Educators, Counselors and Therapists: www.aasect.org.
- National Women's Health Resource Center: www.healthywomen.org
- North American Menopause Society: www.menopause.org
- National Vulvodynia Association: www.nva.org

PROGNOSIS

Lack of desire is most difficult type to treat with <50% success.

REFERENCES

1. Basson R, Wierman ME, van Lankveld J, et al. Summary of the recommendations on sexual dysfunctions in women. *J Sex Med*. 2010;7(1, Pt 2):314–326.
2. Tan O, Bradshaw K, Carr BR, et al. Management of vulvovaginal atrophy-related sexual dysfunction in postmenopausal women: an up-to-date review. *Menopause*. 2012;19(1):109–117.
3. Silverstein RG, Brown AH, Roth HD, et al. Effects of mindfulness training on body awareness to sexual stimuli: implications for female sexual dysfunction. *Psychosom Med*. 2011;73(9):817–825.
4. Nastri CO, Lara LA, Ferriani RA, et al. Hormone therapy for sexual function in perimenopausal and postmenopausal women. *Cochrane Database Syst Rev*. 2013;6:CD009672.
5. Rudkin L, Taylor MJ, Bullemor-Day P, et al. Strategies for managing sexual dysfunction induced by antidepressant medication. *Cochrane Database Syst Rev*. 2013;5:CD003382.

ADDITIONAL READING

- American Psychiatric Association. *Diagnostic and Statistical Manual of Mental Disorders*. 5th ed. Arlington, VA: American Psychiatric Association; 2013.
- Basson R. Review: women's sexual function and dysfunction: current uncertainties, future directions. *Int J Impot Res*. 2008;20(5):466–478.
- Blümel JE, Del Pino M, Aprikian D, et al. Effect of androgens combined with hormone therapy on quality of life in post-menopausal women with sexual dysfunction. *Gynecol Endocrinol*. 2008; 24(12):691.
- Braunstein GD. Safety of testosterone treatment in postmenopausal women. *Fertil Steril*. 2007;88(1):1.
- Carey JC. Pharmacological effects on sexual function. *Obstet Gynecol Clin North Am*. 2006;33(4):599–620.
- Laumann EO, Nicolosi A, Glasser DB, et al. Sexual problems among women and men aged 40–80 y: prevalence and correlates identified in the Global Study of Sexual Attitudes and Behaviors. *Int J Impot Res*. 2005;17(1):39–57.
- Meston CM, Bradford A. Sexual dysfunctions in women. *Annu Rev Clin Psychol*. 2007;3:233–256.
- Modelska K, Cummings S. Female sexual dysfunction in postmenopausal women: systematic review of placebo-controlled trials. *Am J Obstet Gynecol*. 2003;188(1):286–293.
- North American Menopause Society. The role of testosterone therapy in postmenopausal women: position statement of the North American Menopause Society. *Menopause*. 2005;12(5):497.
- Palacios S. Hypoactive sexual desire disorder and current pharmacotherapeutic options in women. *Womens Health (Lond Engl)*. 2011;7(1):95–107.
- Safarinejad MR. Reversal of SSRI-induced female sexual dysfunction by adjunctive bupropion in menstruating women: a double-blind, placebo-controlled and randomized study. *J Psychopharmacol (Oxford)*. 2011;25(3):370–378.
- Safarinejad MR, Hosseini SY, Asgari MA, et al. A randomized, double-blind, placebo-controlled study of the efficacy and safety of bupropion for treating hypoactive sexual desire disorder in ovulating women. *BJU Int*. 2010;106(6):832–839.
- Shifren JL, Davis SR, Moreau M, et al. Testosterone patch for the treatment of hypoactive sexual desire disorder in naturally menopausal women: results of the INTIMATE NM1 study. *Menopause*. 2006;13(5):770–779.
- Shifren JL, Monz BU, Russo PA, et al. Sexual problems and distress in United States women: prevalence and correlates. *Obstet Gynecol*. 2008;112(5):970–978.
- Somboonporn W, Bell RJ, Davis SR. Testosterone for peri and postmenopausal women. *Cochrane Database Syst Rev*. 2005;(4):CD004509.
- Suckling J, Lethaby A, Kennedy R, et al. Local oestrogen for vaginal atrophy in postmenopausal women. *Cochrane Database Syst Rev*. 2006;(4):CD001500.
- Woodis CB, McLendon AN, Muzyk AJ, et al. Testosterone supplementation for hypoactive sexual desire disorder in women. *Pharmacotherapy*. 2012;32(1):38–53.

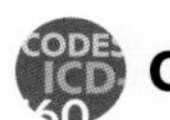

CODES

ICD10

- R37 Sexual dysfunction, unspecified
- F52.0 Hypoactive sexual desire disorder
- N94.1 Dyspareunia

CLINICAL PEARLS

- Female sexual dysfunction is a common, complex, multifactorial problem.
- Most commonly, patients with sexual dysfunction have a normal physical exam.
- Symptoms of sexual dysfunction peak during perimenopause between the ages of 45 and 64 years.
- Several therapies exist for treating sexual dysfunction in women, including behavioral therapy and medications.

SHOULDER PAIN

Nathan Cardoos, MD • J. Herbert Stevenson, MD

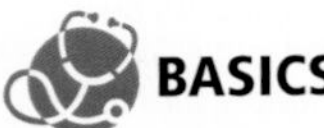

BASICS

DESCRIPTION

Shoulder pain is common and affects patients of all ages:

- Causes include acute trauma or overuse during sports and activities of everyday living.
- Age plays an important role in determining the etiology of shoulder pain.
- Onset and characteristics of pain, weakness, mechanism of injury, and functional limitation help to accurately diagnose shoulder pain.

EPIDEMIOLOGY

- Shoulder pain accounts for 16% of all musculoskeletal complaints.
- The lifetime prevalence of shoulder pain is ~70%.
- Predominant etiology varies with age:
  - <30 years: shoulder instability
  - >30 years: rotator cuff (RTC) disorder
    - 30–50 years: tendinopathy
    - 40–60 years: partial tear
    - >60 years: full-thickness tear
  - >60 years: osteoarthritis (OA) of the glenohumeral joint

Incidence

The incidence of shoulder pain is 7–25 cases/1,000 patients, with a peak incidence in the 4th–6th decades.

ETIOLOGY AND PATHOPHYSIOLOGY

Pathology varies with cause:

- Trauma (fracture, dislocation, ligament/tendon tear, acromioclavicular [AC] separation)
- Overuse (RTC pathology, biceps tenosynovitis, bursitis, muscle strain)
  - RTC disorders most commonly occur from repetitive overhead activity. This leads to impingement of the RTC that progresses through 3 stages:
    - Stage I: tendinopathy
    - Stage II: partial RTC tear
    - Stage III: full-thickness RTC tear
  - Subacromial bursitis can occur with RTC disorders but is rarely an isolated diagnosis.
- Age-related (AC and glenohumeral joint OA, adhesive capsulitis, RTC tear with increasing age; pediatric athletes more commonly have instability and physeal injuries)
- Rheumatologic (rheumatoid arthritis, polymyalgia rheumatica, fibromyalgia)
- Referred pain (neck, gallbladder)

RISK FACTORS

- Repetitive overhead activity
- Overhead and upper extremity weight-bearing sports (baseball, softball, swimming)
- Weight lifting: AC disorders
- Rapid increases in training frequency or load (often associated with improper technique)
- Muscle weakness or imbalance
- Trauma or fall onto the shoulder
- Diabetes, thyroid disorders, female gender, and age 40–60 years are risk factors for adhesive capsulitis.

GENERAL PREVENTION

- Maintenance of necessary shoulder strength and range of motion (ROM)
- Avoid repetitive overhead activities.
- Proper technique (pitching, weight lifting)

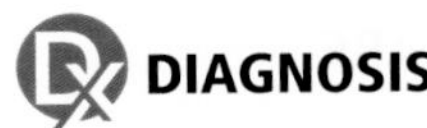

DIAGNOSIS

HISTORY

- Pain characteristics
  - Superior shoulder pain: AC pathology, trapezius strain
  - Lateral/deltoid pain: RTC pathology (RTC pain typically does not extend past elbow.)
  - Diffuse pain: RTC pathology, adhesive capsulitis, glenohumeral OA
  - Night pain: RTC pathology (pain laying on affected side), adhesive capsulitis, glenohumeral OA
  - Stiff shoulder: adhesive capsulitis
  - Pain with cross-body activities: AC pathology
  - Pain with abduction/external rotation (reaching behind): shoulder instability
  - Pain with overhead activity: RTC pathology, AC pathology, labrum pathology
  - Pain with turning neck, pain past elbow: cervical pathology
- Mechanism of injury
  - Fall on outstretched hand: traumatic shoulder instability/dislocation
  - Fall directly onto shoulder: AC joint sprain, clavicle fracture
  - Repetitive overhead activity: RTC pathology
- Age
  - Shoulder instability (subluxation, dislocation, multidirectional instability) is most common cause of shoulder pain in the young athlete (<30 years old).
  - RTC disorders are the most common cause of shoulder pain in patients >30 years old. Severity of RTC disorder increases with age.
  - Older patients (>60 years old) are more likely to have OA.
  - Trauma in a young person <40 years is more commonly associated with dislocation/subluxation; in patients older than 40 years, trauma is more commonly associated with RTC tear.

PHYSICAL EXAM

- Observe as patient disrobes, moves arm, and shakes hand.
- Inspect for malalignment, muscle atrophy, asymmetry, erythema, ecchymosis, or swelling. Scapular winging suggests long thoracic nerve or muscular (trapezius, serratus anterior) dysfunction.
- Palpate for tenderness, warmth, bony step-offs.
- Evaluate active and passive ROM and flexibility:
  - Decreased active AND passive ROM more likely with adhesive capsulitis
  - Mildly decreased active and/or passive ROM may also indicate glenohumeral OA.
- Decreased active, full passive ROM: RTC pathology
- Evaluate for muscle strength including grip, biceps, triceps, and deltoid. Test RTC strength: supraspinatus (empty can test), infraspinatus/teres minor (resisted external rotation), subscapularis (lift-off test, resisted internal rotation). Pain with strength testing of RTC indicates RTC pathology. Weakness could suggest tear.
- Special tests
  - Neer, Hawkin tests: RTC impingement
  - Drop-arm test: RTC tear
  - Cross-arm adduction test: AC joint arthritis
  - Speed, Yergason tests: biceps tendinopathy
  - Apprehension, relocation test: anterior glenohumeral joint instability
  - Sulcus sign: inferior glenohumeral joint instability
  - O'Brien, clunk test: labral pathology
  - Spurling test: cervical pathology

DIFFERENTIAL DIAGNOSIS

- Fracture (clavicle, humerus, scapula), contusion
- RTC disorder: impingement, tear, calcific tendonitis
- Subacromial bursitis
- AC joint pathology (AC separation/OA)
- Biceps tenosynovitis or tear
- Glenohumeral joint OA
- Glenohumeral joint instability (acute dislocation or chronic multidirectional instability)
- Adhesive capsulitis
- Labral tear or associated bony pathology
- Muscle strain (trapezius, deltoid, biceps)
- Cervical radiculopathy
- Other: autoimmune, rheumatologic, referred pain (biliary/splenic, cardiac, pneumonia/lung mass)

DIAGNOSTIC TESTS & INTERPRETATION

- Most shoulder pain can be accurately diagnosed with a careful history and physical exam:
  - Adults with nontraumatic shoulder pain of <4 weeks duration may not require initial imaging.
- History of significant trauma, prolonged symptoms, or red flags (older age, fever, rest pain) suggest need for imaging.
- Plain radiographs are first-line:
  - Assess for fracture, degenerative changes, signs of dislocation (Bankart, Hill-Sachs deformity), signs of large RTC tear (sclerosis, humeral head proximal migration), anatomic deformities contributing to impingement, and occult tumor.
  - Standard views: anteroposterior, scapular Y, axillary

- EMG study of the upper extremity may help differentiate cervical pain referred to the shoulder from a primary shoulder disorder.
- Obtain ECG if any suspicion for cardiac etiology.
- Serologic tests if autoimmune etiology suspected.

Follow-Up Tests & Special Considerations

- CT scan helps rule out occult fracture.
- MRI is gold standard for noninvasive imaging of soft tissue structures, including RTC, biceps tendon.
- MR arthrogram may be necessary to assess for labral tears or small/partial RTC tears.
- Ultrasound (US) is helpful to assess RTC tears, biceps tendinopathies, and AC joint disorders.

Diagnostic Procedures/Other

Diagnostic arthroscopy may be used in the proper setting after noninterventional means have been exhausted and structural injury is suspected.

Test Interpretation

Depends on underlying diagnosis

- Tendinosis rather than tendonitis is often found with stage I impingement.
- Scarring of the shoulder capsule is the hallmark of adhesive capsulitis.
- Calcifications can be found in RTC tendons with calcific tendonitis.

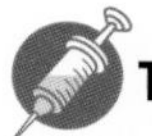

TREATMENT

Treatment is based on underlying diagnosis. In general, conservative therapy includes activity modification, analgesics, and/or anti-inflammatory medicines in association with appropriate rehabilitative strategies.

MEDICATION

First Line

- Analgesics and anti-inflammatory medications may be required for symptomatic relief of shoulder pain:
  - Ibuprofen: 200–800 mg TID
  - Naproxen: 250–500 mg BID
  - Acetaminophen: not to exceed 3 g/day
- Corticosteroid injections (subacromial, glenohumeral) may acutely relieve pain due to RTC pathology, adhesive capsulitis, or OA (1)[A]. This improves ability to engage in rehabilitative activities.
- Corticosteroid injections more likely to be placed accurately if US-guided (2)[A].

ISSUES FOR REFERRAL

Refer for shoulder pain if etiology remains unclear, nonresponsive to conservative care, complicated or displaced fractures, or large RTC tears.

ADDITIONAL THERAPIES

- Physical therapy is beneficial for persistent RTC disorders, adhesive capsulitis, and shoulder instability (3)[A].
- Physical therapy/exercise may improve nonspecific shoulder pain, but it does not generally improve ROM or function (4)[A].
- Manual manipulative therapy by chiropractors, osteopathic physicians, or physical therapists can improve pain with adhesive capsulitis, RTC, and soft tissue disorders (5)[A].

SURGERY/OTHER PROCEDURES

Surgery is necessary for shoulder pain caused by acute displaced fractures, large RTC tears, shoulder dislocation in patients <20 years of age. Surgery may be necessary for shoulder pain unresponsive to conservative measures >3–6 months. Surgery does not appear to be more effective than active nonsurgical treatment in impingement syndrome (6)[A].

COMPLEMENTARY & ALTERNATIVE MEDICINE

Acupuncture may help in the acute setting, although there is no conclusive evidence for its effectiveness.

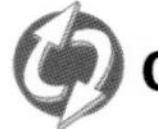

ONGOING CARE

FOLLOW-UP RECOMMENDATIONS

Limiting overhead activity may reduce the symptoms of impingement syndrome.

PATIENT EDUCATION

Refer to specific diagnosis for shoulder pain.

PROGNOSIS

Shoulder pain generally has a favorable outcome with conservative care, but recovery can be slow, with 40–50% with persistent pain or recurrence at 12 months.

REFERENCES

1. Gross C, Dhawan A, Harwood D, et al. Glenohumeral joint injections: a review. *Sports Health*. 2013;(5)2:153–159.
2. Soh E, Li W, Ong KO, et al. Image-guided versus blind corticosteroid injections in adults with shoulder pain: a systematic review. *BMC Musculoskelet Disord*. 2011;12:137.
3. Green S, Buchbinder R, Hetrick SE. Physiotherapy interventions for shoulder pain. *Cochrane Database Syst Rev*. 2003;(2):CD004258.
4. van den Dolder PA, Ferreira PH, Refshauge KM. Effectiveness of soft tissue massage and exercise for the treatment of non-specific shoulder pain: a systematic review with meta-analysis. *Br J Sports Med*. 2014;48(16):1216–1226.
5. Brantingham JW, Cassa TK, Bonnefin D, et al. Manipulative therapy for shoulder pain and disorders: expansion of a systematic review. *J Manipulative Physiol Ther*. 2011;34(5):314–346.
6. Coghlan JA, Buchbinder R, Green S, et al. Surgery for rotator cuff disease. *Cochrane Database Syst Rev*. 2008;(1):CD005619.

ADDITIONAL READING

- Cadogan A, Laslett M, Hing WA, et al. A prospective study of shoulder pain in primary care: prevalence of imaged pathology and response to guided diagnostic blocks. *BMC Musculoskelet Disord*. 2011;12:119.
- Celik D, Sirmen B, Demirhan M. The relationship of muscle strength and pain in subacromial impingement. *Acta Orthop Traumatol Turc*. 2011;45(2):79–84.
- Favejee MM, Huisstede BM, Koes BW. Frozen shoulder: the effectiveness of conservative and surgical interventions—systematic review. *Br J Sports Med*. 2011;45(1):49–56.
- Littlewood C, Ashton J, Chance-Larsen K, et al. Exercise for rotator cuff tendinopathy: a systematic review. *Physiotherapy*. 2012;98(2):101–109.
- Sipola P, Niemitukia L, Kröger H, et al. Detection and quantification of rotator cuff tears with ultrasonography and magnetic resonance imaging—a prospective study in 77 consecutive patients with a surgical reference. *Ultrasound Med Biol*. 2010;36(12):1981–1989.

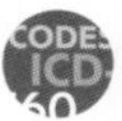

CODES

ICD10

- M25.519 Pain in unspecified shoulder
- S43.429A Sprain of unspecified rotator cuff capsule, init encntr
- M19.019 Primary osteoarthritis, unspecified shoulder

CLINICAL PEARLS

- RTC disorders (tendinopathy, tears) are the most common source of shoulder pain in individuals >30 years of age.
- Shoulder instability (acute dislocation/subluxation or chronic instability) is the most common source of shoulder pain in individuals <30 years of age.
- Patients with diabetes are at increased risk for adhesive capsulitis.

SINUSITIS

Adarsh K. Gupta, DO, MS, FACOFP

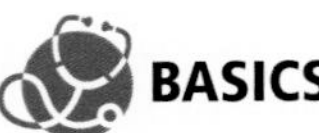

BASICS

DESCRIPTION

- Acute sinusitis is a symptomatic inflammation of $\geq$1 paranasal sinuses of $<$4 weeks' duration resulting from impaired drainage and retained secretions. Because rhinitis and sinusitis usually coexist, "rhinosinusitis" is the preferred term.
- Disease is subacute when symptomatic for 4–12 weeks and chronic when symptomatic for $>$12 weeks.
- System(s) affected: head/eyes/ears/nose/throat (HEENT); pulmonary

EPIDEMIOLOGY

- Affects 31 million individuals in the United States each year
- Diagnosis of acute bacterial rhinosinusitis remains the 5th leading reason for prescribing antibiotics.
- 2% of viral rhinosinusitis episodes have a bacterial superinfection.

Incidence

Incidence highest in early fall through early spring (related to incidence of viral upper respiratory infection [URI]). Adults have 2–3 viral URIs per year; 90% of these colds are accompanied by viral rhinosinusitis. It is 5th most common diagnosis made during family physician visits.

ETIOLOGY AND PATHOPHYSIOLOGY

- Important features
  - Inflammation and edema of the sinus mucosa
  - Obstruction of the sinus ostia
  - Impaired mucociliary clearance
- Secretions that are not cleared become hospitable to bacterial growth.
- Inflammatory response (neutrophil influx and release of cytokines) damages mucosal surfaces.
- Viral: vast majority of cases (rhinovirus; influenza A and B; parainfluenza virus; respiratory syncytial; adeno-, corona-, and enteroviruses)
- Bacterial (complicates 0.2–2% of viral cases)
  - More likely if symptoms worsen after 5–7 days or do not improve $>$10 days
  - *Streptococcus pneumoniae*, *Haemophilus influenzae*, and *Moraxella catarrhalis* are the most common bacterial pathogens.
  - Often overdiagnosed, which leads to overuse of and increasing resistance to antibiotics
  - methicillin-resistant *Staphylococcus aureus* present in 0–15.9% of patients.
- Fungal: seen in immunocompromised hosts (uncontrolled diabetes, neutropenia, use of corticosteroids) or as a nosocomial infection

Genetics

No known genetic pattern

RISK FACTORS

- Viral URI
- Allergic rhinitis
- Asthma
- Cigarette smoking
- Dental infections and procedures
- Anatomic variations
  - Tonsillar and adenoid hypertrophy
  - Turbinate hypertrophy, nasal polyps
  - Cleft palate
- Immunodeficiency (e.g., HIV)
- Cystic fibrosis (CF)

GENERAL PREVENTION

Hand washing to prevent transmission of viral infection

DIAGNOSIS

- History and physical exam suggest and establish the diagnosis but are rarely helpful in distinguishing bacterial from viral causes.
- Use a constellation of symptoms rather than a particular sign or symptom in diagnosis.

HISTORY

- Symptoms somewhat predictive of bacterial sinusitis (1)
  - Worsening of symptoms $>$5–7 days after initial improvement
  - Persistent symptoms for $\geq$10 days
  - Persistent purulent nasal discharge
  - Unilateral upper tooth or facial pain
  - Unilateral maxillary sinus tenderness
  - Fever
- Associated symptoms
  - Headache
  - Nasal congestion
  - Retro-orbital pain
  - Otalgia
  - Hyposomia
  - Halitosis
  - Chronic cough
- Symptoms requiring urgent attention
  - Visual disturbances, especially diplopia
  - Periorbital swelling or erythema
  - Altered mental status

PHYSICAL EXAM

- Fever
- Edema and erythema of nasal mucosa
- Purulent discharge
- Tenderness to palpation over sinus(es)
- Transillumination of the sinuses may confirm fluid in sinuses (helpful if asymmetric; not helpful if symmetric exam).

Pediatric Considerations

- Sinuses are not fully developed until age 20 years. Maxillary and ethmoid sinuses, although small, are present from birth.
- Because children have an average of 6–8 colds per year, they are at risk for developing sinusitis.
- Diagnosis can be more difficult than in adults because symptoms are often more subtle.

DIFFERENTIAL DIAGNOSIS

- Dental disease
- CF
- Wegener granulomatosis
- HIV infection
- Kartagener syndrome
- Neoplasm
- Headache, tension, or migraine

DIAGNOSTIC TESTS & INTERPRETATION

Diagnostic tests are not routinely recommended; no diagnostic tests can adequately differentiate between viral and bacterial rhinosinusitis (2).

- None indicated in routine evaluation
- Routine use of sinus radiography discouraged because of the following:
  - $\geq$3 clinical findings have similar diagnostic accuracy as imaging.
  - Imaging does not distinguish viral from bacterial etiology.
- Limited coronal CT scan can be useful in recurrent infection or failure to respond to medical therapy.

Diagnostic Procedures/Other

Sinus CT if signs suggest extrasinus involvement or to evaluate chronic rhinosinusitis

Test Interpretation

- Inflammation, edema, thickened mucosa
- Impaired ciliary function
- Metaplasia of ciliated columnar cells
- Relative acidosis and hypoxia within sinuses
- Polyps

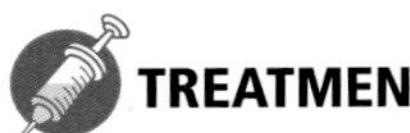

TREATMENT

Most cases resolve with supportive care (treating pain, nasal symptoms). Antibiotics should be reserved for symptoms that persist $>$10 days, onset with severe symptoms (high fever, purulent nasal discharge, facial pain) for at least 3–4 consecutive days, or worsening signs/symptoms that were initially improving (2,3).

GENERAL MEASURES

- Hydration
- Steam inhalation 20–30 minutes TID
- Saline irrigation (Neti pot) or nose drops
- Sleep with head of bed elevated
- Avoid exposure to cigarette smoke or fumes.
- Avoid caffeine and alcohol.
- Antibiotics indicated only when findings suggest bacterial infection.
- Analgesics, NSAIDs
- Acute viral sinusitis is self-limiting; antibiotics should not be used.

MEDICATION

First Line

- Decongestants
  - Pseudoephedrine HCl
  - Phenylephrine nasal spray (limited use)
  - Oxymetazoline nasal spray (e.g., Afrin) (not to be used $>$3 days)
- Analgesics
  - Acetaminophen
  - Aspirin
  - NSAIDs
- Antibiotics
  - Antibiotics have a slight advantage over placebo at 7–14 days (4)[A], yet most improve without therapy.
  - Reserve antibiotic use for patients with moderate to severe disease.
  - Choice should be based on understanding of antibiotic resistance in the community.

- Infectious Disease Society of America recommends the following (1)[B]:
  - Start antibiotics as soon as clinical diagnosis of acute bacterial sinusitis is made.
  - Use amoxicillin-clavulanate rather than amoxicillin alone.
  - Amoxicillin-clavulanate 875/125 mg q12h; 2 g orally BID in geographic regions with high rates of resistant *S. pneumoniae*
  - Doxycycline: 100 mg PO BID an alternative to amoxicillin-clavulanate for initial therapy (adults only)
  - Treat for 5–7 days in adults if uncomplicated bacterial rhinosinusitis (IDSA low-moderate-quality evidence). Treat for 10–14 days in children if uncomplicated bacterial rhinosinusitis (IDSA low-moderate-quality evidence).
- American Academy of Pediatrics recommends the following:
  - Amoxicillin: 45–90 mg/kg/day in 2 divided doses if uncomplicated acute bacterial sinusitis in children
  - Amoxicillin-clavulanate: 80–90 mg/6.4 mg/kg/day in 2 divided doses for children with severe illness, recent antibiotics, or attending daycare
- Initial therapy (narrow-spectrum antibiotics)

- Because allergies may be a predisposing factor, some patients may benefit from use of the following agents:
  - Oral antihistamines
    - Loratadine (Claritin), fexofenadine (Allegra), cetirizine (Zyrtec), desloratadine (Clarinex), or levocetirizine (Xyzal)
    - Chlorpheniramine (Chlor-Trimeton)
    - Diphenhydramine (Benadryl)
  - Leukotriene inhibitors (Singulair, Accolate), especially in patients with asthma
  - Nasal steroids (i.e., fluticasone [Flonase])

Second Line

- Levofloxacin (Levaquin): 750 mg/day for 5 days or moxifloxacin 400 mg/day for 5–7 days (adults only)
- If no response to 1st-line therapy after 72 hours
  - Broaden antibiotic coverage or switch to a different class, evaluate for resistant pathogens or other causes for treatment failure (i.e., noninfectious etiology) fluoroquinolones as above.
- *Note*: Bacteriologic failure rates of up to 20–25% are possible with use of azithromycin and clarithromycin.
- If lack of response to 3 weeks of antibiotics, consider the following:
  - CT scan of sinuses
  - Ear/nose/throat (ENT) referral

ISSUES FOR REFERRAL

Complications or failure of treatment

ADDITIONAL THERAPIES

ALERT

- Meta-analyses have demonstrated no benefit of newer antibiotics over amoxicillin, trimethoprim-sulfamethoxazole (TMP-SMX), or doxycycline.
- Antibiotics recommendations vary with different guidelines. Patients seen by specialists are different from those in a primary care setting. Patients usually do not have complicated sinusitis in primary care setting.
  - American Academy of Otolaryngology—Head and Neck Surgery Foundation (2) recommends the following:
    - Consider watchful waiting without antibiotics in patients with uncomplicated mild illness (mild pain and temperature <101°F) with assurance of follow-up.
- PCV-13 pneumococcal vaccine can be helpful in reducing chronic sinusitis in children (5).
- Use of intranasal steroids produces modest improvement in symptoms when used alone or in combination with antibiotics (6)[B].
- Precautions
  - Decongestants can exacerbate hypertension.
  - Intranasal decongestants should be limited to 3 days to avoid rebound nasal congestion.
  - Significant possible interactions
    - Warfarin (Coumadin): increased INR with macrolides or TMP-SMX
    - Stop statins temporarily with macrolides due to increased risk of myopathy and rhabdomyolysis.

Pregnancy Considerations

- Nasal irrigation with saline, pseudoephedrine, most antihistamines, and some nasal steroids are safe during pregnancy and lactation.
- Antibiotics safe in pregnancy and lactation
  - Amoxicillin, amoxicillin-clavulanate, cephalosporins, azithromycin
- Antibiotic contraindicated: doxycycline, fluoroquinolones
- Antibiotic safe in lactation but not pregnancy: levofloxacin

SURGERY/OTHER PROCEDURES

- If medical therapy fails, consider sinus irrigation.
- Functional endoscopic sinus surgery is the preferred treatment for medically recalcitrant cases.
- Absolute surgical indications
  - Massive nasal polyposis
  - Acute complications: subperiosteal or orbital abscess, frontal soft tissue spread of infection
  - Mucocele or mucopyocele
  - Invasive or allergic fungal sinusitis
  - Suspected obstructing tumor
  - CSF rhinorrhea

INPATIENT CONSIDERATIONS

Hospitalization for complications (e.g., meningitis, orbital cellulitis or abscess, brain abscess)

ONGOING CARE

FOLLOW-UP RECOMMENDATIONS

Return if no improvement after 72 hours or no resolution of symptoms after 10 days of antibiotics.

PATIENT EDUCATION

- http://familydoctor.org
- http://medlineplus.gov

PROGNOSIS

Alleviation of symptoms within 72 hours with complete resolution within 10–14 days

COMPLICATIONS

- Serious complications are rare.
- Meningitis, orbital cellulitis, brain abscess
- Cavernous sinus thrombosis
- Osteomyelitis, subdural empyema

REFERENCES

1. Chow AW, Benninger MS, Brook I, et al. IDSA clinical practice guideline for acute bacterial rhinosinusitis in children and adults. *Clin Infect Dis*. 2012;54(8):e72–e112.
2. Rosenfeld RM, Andes D, Bhattacharyya N, et al. Clinical practice guideline: adult sinusitis. *Otolaryngol Head Neck Surg*. 2007;137(3)(Suppl):S1–S31.
3. Centers for Disease Control and Prevention. Get Smart: homepage. http://www.cdc.gov/getsmart/. Accessed June 27, 2014.
4. Ahovuo-Saloranta A, Rautakorpi UM, Borisenko OV, et al. Antibiotics for acute maxillary sinusitis in adults. *Cochrane Database Syst Rev*. 2014;(2):CD000243.
5. Olarte L, Hulten KG, Lamberth L, et al. Impact of the 13-valent pneumococcal conjugate vaccine on chronic sinusitis associated with Streptococcus pneumoniae in children [published online ahead of print April 25, 2014]. *Pediatr Infect Dis J*.
6. Williamson IG, Rumsby K, Benge S, et al. Antibiotics and topical nasal steroid for treatment of acute maxillary sinusitis: a randomized controlled trial. *JAMA*. 2007;298(21):2487–2496.

ADDITIONAL READING

- American Academy of Pediatrics. Subcommittee on Management of Sinusitis and Committee on Quality Improvement. Clinical practice guideline: management of sinusitis. *Pediatrics*. 2001;108(3):798–808.
- McCoul ED, Jourdy DN, Schaberg MR, et al. Methicillin-resistant *Staphylococcus aureus* sinusitis in nonhospitalized patients: a systematic review of prevalence and treatment outcomes. *Laryngoscope*. 2012;122(10):2125–2131.
- Williams JW Jr, Aguilar C, Cornell J, et al. Antibiotics for acute maxillary sinusitis. *Cochrane Database Syst Rev*. 2003;(2):CD000243.

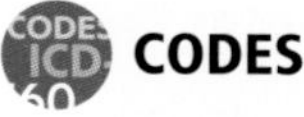

CODES

ICD10

- J01.90 Acute sinusitis, unspecified
- J01.00 Acute maxillary sinusitis, unspecified
- J01.20 Acute ethmoidal sinusitis, unspecified

CLINICAL PEARLS

- When bacterial infection is present, patients recover somewhat more quickly with antibiotics, but the majority will recover with symptomatic treatment alone, and accurate diagnosis of bacterial sinusitis is very difficult.
- Multiple meta-analyses have demonstrated *no* benefit of newer antibiotics over amoxicillin, TMP-SMX, or doxycycline.
- Overall NNT to prevent 1 persistent case at follow-up = 15; harm due to antibiotic-associated diarrhea is similar.
- Significant patient symptom relief with nasal saline spray or drops or irrigation (Neti pot)

SJÖGREN SYNDROME

Katrina Darlene Zedan, MSPAS, PA-C • Vincent F. Honrubia, MD, FACS

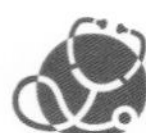

BASICS

- Chronic inflammatory disorder characterized by lymphocytic infiltrates in exocrine organs
- Typically presents with diminished salivary and lacrimal gland function, resulting in sicca symptoms
  - Dry eyes (xerophthalmia), dry mouth (xerostomia), and parotid enlargement
  - Extraglandular symptoms such as arthralgia, arthritis, Raynaud phenomenon, myalgia, pulmonary disease, GI disease, leukopenia, anemia, lymphadenopathy, neuropathy, vasculitis, renal tubular acidosis, and lymphoma
- Primary Sjögren: not associated with other diseases
- Secondary Sjögren: complication of other rheumatologic conditions, most commonly rheumatoid arthritis
- The disease is named after Swedish ophthalmologist Henrik Sjögren (1899–1986), who first described it.

EPIDEMIOLOGY

Incidence

- Annual incidence ~4/100,000.
- People of all races are affected.
- Predominant sex: female > male (9:1)
- Predominant age: can affect patients of any age but is most common in the elderly; onset typically occurs in the 4th–5th decades of life

Prevalence

Sjögren syndrome (SS) affects 1–4 million people in the United States.

ETIOLOGY AND PATHOPHYSIOLOGY

- Multifactorial systemic autoimmune process characterized by infiltration of glandular tissue by CD4 T-lymphocytes
- Theorized that glandular epithelial cells present antigen to the T cells. Cytokine production then occurs, and there is also evidence for B-cell activation, resulting in autoantibody production and increased incidence of B-cell malignancies.
- Etiology is unknown. Estrogen may play a role because SS is more common in women. Exogenous factors such as viral proteins (EBV, HCV, HTLV-1) have also been implicated.

Genetics

SS has a familial tendency suggesting a genetic predisposition, perhaps involving HLA-DR and/or HLA-DQ gene regions.

RISK FACTORS

There are no known modifiable risk factors.

GENERAL PREVENTION

- No known prevention. Complications can be prevented by early diagnosis and treatment.
- Oral health providers play a key role in early detection and management of symptoms resulting from salivary dysfunction (1)[C].

COMMONLY ASSOCIATED CONDITIONS

Secondary SS associated with rheumatoid arthritis, scleroderma, systemic lupus erythematosus (SLE), polymyositis, HIV, hepatitis C

DIAGNOSIS

- Diagnosis is made by presence of compatible clinical signs and symptoms, supported by laboratory data.
- International consensus criteria for SS:
  - Ocular signs and symptoms (at least 1)
    - Troublesome dry eyes daily for >3 months
    - Recurrent sandy/gritty ocular sensation
    - Use of tear substitute >3×/day
  - Oral signs and symptoms (at least 1)
    - Daily symptos of dry mouth for at least 3 months
    - Recurrent feeling of swollen salivary glands
    - Need to drink liquid to help swallow dry foods
  - Objective evidence of dry eyes (at least 1)
    - Schirmer test
    - Rose bengal
    - Lacrimal gland biopsy sample with focus score >1
  - Objective evidence of salivary gland involvement (at least 1)
    - Salivary gland scintigraphy
    - Parotid sialography
    - Unstimulated whole sialometry
  - Laboratory abnormality (at least 1)
    - Anti-SS-A or anti-SS-B
    - Antinuclear antibodies (ANAs)
    - IgM rheumatoid factor (anti-IgG Fc)
- Exclusion criteria: prior head/neck irradiation, HCV infection, AIDS, lymphoma, sarcoidosis, graft-versus-host disease, recent anticholinergic medication use
- Patients who fulfill ≥4 of the criteria likely have SS.

HISTORY

- Decreased tear production, burning, scratchy sensation in eyes
- Difficulty speaking/swallowing, dental caries, xerotrachea
- Enlarged parotid glands or intermittent swelling (bilateral)
- Dyspareunia; vaginal dryness

PHYSICAL EXAM

Common physical exam findings include the following:

- Eye exam: dry eyes (keratoconjunctivitis sicca), decreased tear pool in the lower conjunctiva, dilated conjunctival vessels, mucinous threads, and filamentary keratosis on slit-lamp examination
- Mouth exam: dry mouth (xerostomia); decreased sublingual salivary pool (tongue may stick to the tongue depressor); frequent oral caries, sometimes in unusual locations such as the incisor surface and along the gum line; dark red tongue from prolonged xerostomia
- Ear, nose, and throat exam: bilateral parotid gland enlargement, submandibular gland enlargement
- Skin exam: nonpalpable or palpable vasculitic purpura with lesions that are typically 2–3 mm in diameter and located on the lower extremities
- Other manifestations: chronic arthritis, interstitial nephritis (40%), type I rheumatoid arthritis (20%), vasculitis (25%), vaginal dryness, pleuritis, pancreatitis

DIFFERENTIAL DIAGNOSIS

- Causes of ocular dryness: hypovitaminosis A, decreased tear production unrelated to autoimmune process, chronic blepharitis or conjunctivitis, impaired blinking (i.e., due to Parkinson disease or Bell palsy), infiltration of lacrimal glands (i.e., amyloidosis, lymphoma, sarcoidosis), low estrogen levels
- Causes of oral dryness: anticholinergic medications, sialadenitis due to chronic obstruction, chronic viral infections (i.e., hepatitis C or HIV), irradiation of head and neck
- Causes of salivary gland swelling: unilateral: bacterial infection, neoplasm; bilateral: acute or chronic viral infection (i.e., mumps, Epstein-Barr virus [EBV], coxsackievirus, echovirus, HIV, hepatitis C), granulomatous diseases (i.e., tuberculosis, sarcoidosis), malnutrition, alcoholism, bulimia, acromegaly, diabetes

DIAGNOSTIC TESTS & INTERPRETATION

The following tests can be used to support diagnosis:

- Schirmer test (<5-mm wetness after 5 minutes)
- Rose bengal test (slit lamp)
- Basic labs, special labs (see following text)
- MRI with fat suppression, chest x-ray (CXR), minor salivary gland biopsy
- Most have autoantibodies: +ANAs (95%), +RF (75%)
- In primary SS: +anti-Ro (anti SS-A, 56%) and +anti-La (anti-SS-B, 30%)

Initial Tests (lab, imaging)

Preliminary lab workup

- Basic labs: CBC with differential, BUN/creatinine (Cr), AST/ALT, ESR, C-reactive protein (CRP), urinalysis (UA)
- Special labs: ANA, rheumatoid factor (RF), anti-Ro/SS-A, anti-La/SS-B, anti-Sm, anti-RNP, anti-dsDNA, serum C3 and C4, cryoglobulins, SPEP, UPEP, IgM, IgG, IgA
- Other: HIV, hepatitis C, CXR, minor salivary gland biopsy, MRI with fat suppression
- Initial imaging studies may include the following:
  - Imaging for xerostomia: salivary gland scintigraphy (insensitive but highly specific)
  - Parotid gland sialography (should not be used in acute parotitis)
  - MRI (correlates well with salivary gland biopsy)
  - MRI with fat suppression

Diagnostic Procedures/Other

- Salivary gland biopsy: used to confirm suspected diagnosis of SS or to exclude other causes of xerostomia and bilateral gland enlargement
- Parotid gland biopsy if malignancy is suspected
- Lymph node to rule out pseudolymphoma or lymphoma if suspected

Test Interpretation

Salivary gland biopsy: Histology shows focal collections of lymphocytes; immunocytology shows that most of the lymphocytes are CD4+ T cells.

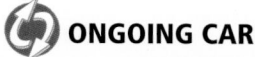

TREATMENT

- Treatment is primarily supportive.
- Treat sicca symptoms—dry eyes, dry mouth.
- Avoid medications that may worsen oral dryness (i.e., anticholinergics).
- Promote good oral hygiene.
- Treat systemic manifestations.
- Address fatigue and pain.

MEDICATION

- Therapy for sicca symptoms: artificial tears and lubricants (2)[C]
- Topical therapy for dry mouth: can be as simple as liberally drinking sips of water, trying sugar-free lemon drops or artificial saliva preparations such as Salivart, Saliment, Xero-Lube, Mouthkote
- Immunosuppressive therapy such as hydroxychloroquine can be used for systemic symptoms; however, it has not shown any benefit in relieving refractory sicca symptoms.
- Evoxac (Cevimeline) may be prescribed for SS-associated xerostomia. It works by stimulating muscarinic cholinergic receptors, increasing salivary gland secretion.
- Dry eyes are graded according to degree of symptoms, conjunctival injection and staining, corneal damage, tear quality, and lid involvement. Artificial tears may be used; however, artificial tears with hydroxymethylcellulose or dextran are more viscous and can last longer.
- Acetaminophen or NSAIDs for arthralgias

First Line

- Xerostomia: sugar-free lozenges, especially malic acid, artificial saliva; pilocarpine 5 mg PO QID or cevimeline 30 mg PO TID
- Keratoconjunctivitis sicca: artificial tears and ocular lubricants for symptomatic relief, topical cyclosporine

Second Line

- Xerostomia: Interferon-alfa lozenges may enhance salivary gland flow.
- Keratoconjunctivitis sicca: topical glucocorticoids or topical NSAIDs (use with caution)
- Immunosuppressive therapy: antimalarials (e.g., hydroxychloroquine) for arthralgias, lymphadenopathies, and skin manifestations; may then consider methotrexate or cyclosporine, which showed subjective improvement but no significant objective improvement
- Early studies show improvement in fatigue with rituximab (3)[B].
- For life-threatening extraglandular manifestations, cyclophosphamide (PO or IV), mycophenolate mofetil, and azathioprine are often used.

ISSUES FOR REFERRAL

- Systemic manifestations or resistant symptoms
- A rheumatologist can help with management.
- Oral health
- Ophthalmology, for grading of severity and management of xerophthalmia

ADDITIONAL THERAPIES

- Patients should use vaginal lubricants, such as Replens, for vaginal dryness. Vaginal estrogen creams can help in postmenopausal women. Be alert for and treat vaginal yeast infections.
- Xerostomia: small sips of water, good dental care
- Keratoconjunctivitis sicca: Conserve tears with side shields or ski/swim goggles, humidifiers, and moist washcloths.
- Dehydroepiandrosterone (DHEA) does not offer improvement in fatigue and well-being above placebo.

SURGERY/OTHER PROCEDURES

Keratoconjunctivitis sicca: If refractory to artificial tears, punctal occlusion is the treatment of choice.

COMPLEMENTARY & ALTERNATIVE MEDICINE

- Some studies show acupuncture benefits saliva production and symptoms of xerostomia.
- There is insufficient evidence to determine the effects of electrostimulation devices on dry mouth symptoms or saliva production in patients with Sjögren syndrome.

INPATIENT CONSIDERATIONS

May be required for extraglandular manifestations, such as cardiopulmonary disease, renal involvement, and CNS manifestations (e.g., optic neuritis, transverse myelitis, vasculitis, or ischemic stroke)

ONGOING CARE

FOLLOW-UP RECOMMENDATIONS

Frequency of follow-up depends on severity.

Patient Monitoring

- Monitor for complications, systemic manifestations, and relief of symptoms.
- Medicolegal pitfalls: Monitor for parotid tumor or lymphoma.

PATIENT EDUCATION

In most cases, simple measures are adequate: humidifiers, sips of water, chewing gum, or artificial tears.

PROGNOSIS

- Hypocomplementemia is an independent risk factor for premature death.
- Primary SS is associated with increased risks of malignancy, non-Hodgkin lymphoma, and thyroid cancer.

COMPLICATIONS

Complications include dental caries, gum disease, dysphagia, salivary gland calculi, keratitis, conjunctivitis, and scarring of the ocular surface.

REFERENCES

1. Mays JW, Sarmadi M, Moutsopoulos NM. Oral manifestations of systemic autoimmune and inflammatory diseases: diagnosis and clinical management. *J Evid Based Dent Pract*. 2012; 12(3)(Suppl):265–282.
2. Aragona P, Spinella R, Rania L, et al. Safety and efficacy of 0.1% clobetasone butyrate eyedrops in the treatment of dry eye in Sjögren syndrome. *Eur J Ophthalmol*. 2013;23(3):368–376.
3. Meijer JM, Meiners PM, Vissink A, et al. Effectiveness of rituximab treatment in primary Sjogren's syndrome: a randomized, double-blind, placebo-controlled trial. *Arthritis Rheum*. 2010;62(4): 960–968.

ADDITIONAL READING

- Dass S, Bowman SJ, Vital EM, et al. Reduction of fatigue in Sjogren's syndrome with rituximab: results of a randomised, double-blind, placebo controlled pilot study. *Ann Rheum Dis*. 2008;67(11): 1541–1544.
- Fischer A, Swigris JJ, du Bois RM, et al. Minor salivary gland biopsy to detect primary Sjogren syndrome in patients with interstitial lung disease. *Chest*. 2009;136(4):1072–1078.
- Fox RI. Sjogren's syndrome. *Lancet*. 2005;366(9482): 321–331.
- Furness S, Bryan G, McMillan R, et al. Interventions for the management of dry mouth: non-pharmacological interventions. *Cochrane Database Syst Rev*. 2013;9:CD009603.
- Hartkamp A, Geenen R, Godaert GL, et al. Effect of dehydroepiandrosterone administration on fatigue, well-being, and functioning in women with primary Sjogren's syndrome: a randomised controlled trial. *Ann Rheum Dis*. 2008;67(1):91–97.
- Liang Y, Yang Z, Qin B, et al. Primary Sjogren's syndrome and malignancy risk: a systematic review and meta-analysis. *Ann Rheum Dis*. 2013;73(6): 1151–1156.
- Miller AV. Sjogren syndrome treatment & management. http://emedicine.medscape.com/article/332125-treatment. Accessed 2014.
- Pan Q, Angelina A, Zambrano A, et al. Autologous serum eye drops for dry eye. *Cochrane Database Syst Rev*. 2013;8:CD009327.
- Ramos-Casals M, Tzioufas AG, Stone JH, et al. Treatment of primary Sjögren syndrome: a systematic review. *JAMA*. 2010;304(4):452–460.
- Stewart CM, Berg KM, Cha S, et al. Salivary dysfunction and quality of life in Sjögren syndrome: a critical oral-systemic connection. *J Am Dent Assoc*. 2008;139(3):291–299.
- von Bültzingslöwen I, Sollecito TP, Fox PC, et al. Salivary dysfunction associated with systemic diseases: systematic review and clinical management recommendations. *Oral Surg Oral Med Oral Pathol Oral Radiol Endod*. 2007;103(Suppl):S57.e1–S57.e15.

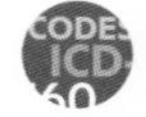

CODES

ICD10

- M35.00 Sicca syndrome, unspecified
- M35.02 Sicca syndrome with lung involvement
- M35.04 Sicca syndrome with tubulo-interstitial nephropathy

CLINICAL PEARLS

- Many symptoms of SS can be treated with simple interventions such as artificial tears and sugar-free lozenges.
- Consider lacrimal duct plugs for dry eyes (placed under local anesthetic by an ophthalmologist).
- Consider minor salivary gland biopsy to confirm diagnosis in the setting of interstitial lung disease.

SLEEP APNEA, OBSTRUCTIVE

Sonya Shipley, MD • John Michael Miller, II, MD

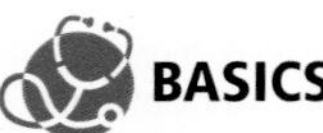

BASICS

DESCRIPTION

- Obstructive sleep apnea (OSA) is defined as repetitive episodes of cessation of airflow (apnea) at the nose and mouth during sleep due to obstruction at the level of the pharynx.
  - Apneas often terminate with a snort/gasp.
  - Repetitive apneas produce sleep disruption, leading to excessive daytime sleepiness.
  - Associated with oxygen desaturation and nocturnal hypoxemia
  - Usual course is chronic.
- System(s) affected: cardiovascular; nervous; pulmonary
- Synonym(s): Pickwickian syndrome; sleep apnea syndrome; nocturnal upper airway occlusion

EPIDEMIOLOGY

Incidence

- Predominant age: middle-aged men and women
- Predominant sex: male > female (2:1)

Prevalence

- Up to 4% in men, 2% in women
- Prevalence is higher in obese/hypertensive patients.

ETIOLOGY AND PATHOPHYSIOLOGY

OSA occurs when the naso- or oropharynx collapses passively during inspiration. Anatomic and neuromuscular factors contribute to pharyngeal collapse.

- Anatomic abnormalities such as increased soft tissue in the palate, tonsillar hypertrophy, macroglossia, and craniofacial abnormalities, predispose the airway to collapse by decreasing the area of the upper airway or increasing the pressure surrounding the airway.
- During sleep, decreased muscle tone in the naso- or oropharynx contributes to airway obstruction and collapse.
- Upper airway narrowing may be due to the following:
  - Obesity, redundant tissue in the soft palate
  - Enlarged tonsils/uvula
  - Low soft palate
  - Large/posteriorly located tongue
  - Craniofacial abnormalities
  - Neuromuscular disorders
  - Alcohol/sedative use before bedtime

RISK FACTORS

- Obesity
- Age >40 years
- Alcohol/sedative intake before bedtime
- Smoking
- Nasal obstruction (due to polyps, rhinitis, or deviated septum)
- Anatomic narrowing of nasopharynx (e.g., tonsillar hypertrophy, macroglossia, micrognathia, retrognathia, craniofacial abnormalities)
- Acromegaly
- Hypothyroidism
- Neurologic syndromes (e.g., muscular dystrophy, cerebral palsy)

GENERAL PREVENTION

Weight control and avoidance of alcohol and sedatives at night can help to prevent airway collapse.

COMMONLY ASSOCIATED CONDITIONS

- Common
  - Hypertension
  - Obesity
  - Daytime sleepiness
  - Metabolic syndrome
- Rare
  - Cardiac arrhythmias
  - Cardiovascular disease
  - Congestive heart failure
  - Pulmonary hypertension
  - Nasal obstructive problems

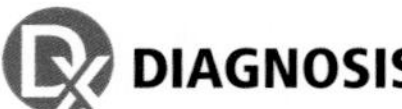

DIAGNOSIS

HISTORY

Elicit a complete history of daytime and nighttime symptoms. Symptoms can be insidious and present for years.

- Daytime symptoms
  - Excessive daytime sleepiness (EDS) or fatigue (cardinal symptom) (1)[A]
    - Mild symptoms occur during quiet activities (e.g., reading, watching television).
    - Severe symptoms occur during dynamic activities (e.g., work, driving).
  - Tired on morning awakening
  - Sore/dry throat
  - Poor concentration, memory problems, irritability, mood changes
  - Morning headaches
  - Decreased libido
  - Depression
- Nighttime symptoms
  - Loud snoring (present in 60% of people with OSA)
  - Snort/gasp that arouses patient from sleep
  - Disrupted sleep
  - Witnessed apneic episodes at night

PHYSICAL EXAM

- OSA is commonly associated with obesity. It is unlikely to be found in those with normal body weight who do not snore (1)[A].
- Focused head and neck exam
  - Short neck with large circumference
  - Oropharynx
    - Narrowing of the lateral airway wall
    - Tonsillar hypertrophy
    - Macroglossia
    - Micrognathia/retrognathia
    - Soft palate edema
    - Long/thick uvula
    - High, arched hard palate
  - Nasopharynx
    - Deviated nasal septum
    - Poor nasal airflow

DIFFERENTIAL DIAGNOSIS

- Other causes of excessive daytime sleepiness such as the following:
  - Narcolepsy
  - Idiopathic daytime hypersomnolence
  - Inadequate sleep time
  - Depressive episodes with excessive daytime sleepiness
  - Periodic limb movements disorder
- Respiratory disorders with nocturnal awakenings such as the following:
  - Asthma
  - Chronic obstructive pulmonary disease
  - Congestive heart failure
- Central sleep apnea
- Sleep-related choking/laryngospasm
- Gastroesophageal reflux
- Sleep-associated seizures (temporal lobe epilepsy)

DIAGNOSTIC TESTS & INTERPRETATION

Initial Tests (lab, imaging)

- When clinically indicated
  - Thyroid-stimulating hormone to evaluate hypothyroidism
  - CBC to evaluate anemia and polycythemia, which can indicate nocturnal hypoxemia
  - Fasting glucose in obesity to evaluate for diabetes
  - Rare: arterial blood gases to evaluate daytime hypercapnia
- Cephalometric measurements from lateral head and neck radiographs aid in surgical treatment.

Diagnostic Procedures/Other

- The gold standard for OSA is polysomnography (PSG), a nighttime sleep study (1)[A].
  - Demonstrates severity of hypoxemia, sleep disruption, and cardiac arrhythmias associated with OSA and elevated end-tidal CO_2
  - Shows repetitive episodes of cessation/marked reduction in airflow despite continued respiratory efforts
  - Apneic episodes must last at least 10 seconds and occur 10–15× per hour to be considered clinically significant.
  - Complete PSG is expensive, and health insurance may not cover the cost.
- Multiple sleep latency testing is a diagnostic tool used to measure the time it takes from the start of a daytime nap period to the first signs of sleep (sleep latency). It provides an objective measurement of daytime sleepiness.
- The apnea/hypoapnea index (AHI) is defined as the total number of apneas and hypoapneas divided by the total sleep time.
  - Mild OSA: AHI = 5–15
  - Moderate OSA: AHI = 15–30
  - Severe OSA: AHI >30
- Drugs that may alter the test results include benzodiazepines and other sedatives that can amplify the severity of apnea seen during the sleep study.
- Early data suggest that home-based diagnosis using portable monitoring devices may be an alternative to laboratory-based PSG if the test is of sufficient duration (2)[B].

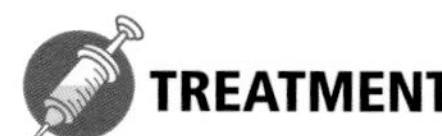

TREATMENT

- Lifestyle modification is the most frequently recommended treatment for mild to moderate OSA. This includes weight loss, exercise, and avoidance of alcohol, smoking, and sedatives, especially before bedtime. Weight loss has been shown to decrease the severity of symptoms in obese patients. Lifestyle modifications should be seen as adjunctive rather than curative therapy (3)[A], and a lack of improvement of symptoms with lifestyle modification should not preclude patients from receiving other therapy such as continuous positive airway pressure (CPAP).

- If OSA is present only when supine, keep the patient off his/her back when sleeping (e.g., tennis ball worn on back of nightshirt or using a sleep position trainer) (4)[B].
- The most effective therapy for mild, moderate, or severe OSA is CPAP (5)[B]. Treatment with CPAP uses a mask interface and a flow generator to prevent airway collapse, thus helping to prevent apnea, hypoxia, and sleep disturbance. Compared with inactive controls, CPAP significantly improves both objective (24-hour systolic and diastolic blood pressures) and subjective measures (Epworth Sleepiness Scale) in OSA patients with symptoms of daytime sleepiness (6)[A]. CPAP may also decrease the risk for atherosclerosis (7)[A] as well as improves insulin resistance in nondiabetic patients (8)[A]. Early data show that these benefits may not be seen in patients who do not have symptoms of daytime sleepiness (9)[B].
- Several types of mask interfaces, including nasal masks, oral masks, and nasal pillows exist for CPAP therapy. Short-term data suggest that nasal pillows are the preferred interface in almost all patients. In patients with compliance difficulty, a different choice of interface may be appropriate (10)[A].
- Oral appliances to treat OSA are available and often subjectively preferred by patients. Although oral appliances have been shown to improve symptoms compared with inactive controls, they are not as effective for reduction of respiratory disturbances as CPAP over short-term data. Treatment with oral appliances may be considered in patients who fail to comply with CPAP therapy (11)[A].

MEDICATION

Medications are yet to be proven effective in treating OSA (12)[A]. Further studies in this area are needed.

First Line

Some short-term data found fluticasone nasal spray, mirtazapine, physostigmine, and nasal lubricant of some benefit; longer-term studies needed.

ISSUES FOR REFERRAL

If sleep apnea is suspected, patient should be referred to a sleep specialist/neurologist for a sleep study evaluation.

SURGERY/OTHER PROCEDURES

Surgical corrections of the upper airway include uvulopalatopharyngoplasty (UPPP), tracheostomy, and craniofacial surgery. Currently no evidence supports the use of surgery for the treatment of OSA (13)[A].

INPATIENT CONSIDERATIONS

On admission, patients should continue to use CPAP/dental devices if they do so at home. They should bring in their own appliance and know their CPAP settings.

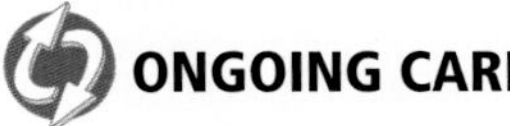

ONGOING CARE

Lifelong compliance with weight loss or CPAP is necessary for successful OSA treatment.

DIET

Overweight and obese patients should be encouraged to lose weight, and all patients must avoid weight gain. Weight loss alone can relieve symptoms of OSA.

PATIENT EDUCATION

- Weight loss and avoidance of alcohol and sedatives can reduce OSA symptoms.
- Significantly sleepy patients should not drive a motor vehicle/operate dangerous equipment.

PROGNOSIS

- EDS is reduced dramatically with appropriate apnea control.
- Lifelong compliance with weight loss or CPAP is necessary for effective treatment of OSA.
- If untreated, OSA is progressive.
- Significant morbidity and mortality with OSA usually are due to motor vehicle accidents or are secondary to cardiac complications, including arrhythmias, cardiac ischemia, and hypertension.

COMPLICATIONS

Untreated OSA may increase the risk for development of hypertension, stroke, myocardial infarction, diabetes, cardiovascular disease, and work-related and driving accidents.

Pediatric Considerations

- The prevalence of pediatric OSA is 1–2% in children 4–5 years of age, and the peak incidence is between 3 and 6 years of age.
- Predominant sex: male = female
- Etiology: The most common cause is tonsillar hypertrophy. Additional causes are obesity and craniofacial abnormalities. OSA is also seen in children with neuromuscular diseases, such as cerebral palsy and spinal muscular atrophy, due to abnormal pharyngeal muscle control.
- Signs and symptoms
  - Nighttime: loud snoring, restlessness, and sweating
  - Daytime: hyperactivity and decreased school performance
  - EDS is not a significant symptom.
- Diagnosis: Gold standard is PSG (PSG may be an even better tool in children due to lessened night-to-night variation. There is a lack of studies showing efficacy of home-based diagnostic studies vs. PSG in children). Abnormal AHI is different in children: >1–2/hr is abnormal.
- Treatment: Surgery is the 1st-line treatment in cases due to tonsillar enlargement (reduces symptoms in 70%). Some data suggest improved academic performance if tonsillectomy is performed for OSA. For cases due to obesity/craniofacial abnormalities, patients can use CPAP treatment (14)[A].

REFERENCES

1. Myers KA, Mrkobrada M, Simel D. Does this patient have obstructive sleep apnea?: the rational clinical examination systemic review. *JAMA*. 2013;310(7):731–741.
2. Wittine LM, Olson EJ, Morgenthaler TI. Effect of recording duration on the diagnostic accuracy of out-of-center sleep testing for obstructive sleep apnea. *Sleep*. 2014;37(5):969–975.
3. Anandam A, Akinnusi M, Kufel T, et al. Effects of dietary weight loss on obstructive sleep apnea: a meta-analysis. *Sleep Breath*. 2013;17(1): 227–234.
4. van Maanen JP, de Vries N. Long-term effectiveness and compliance of positional therapy with the sleep position trainer in the treatment of positional obstructive sleep apnea syndrome. *Sleep*. 2014;37(7):1209–1215.
5. Weaver TE, Mancini C, Maislin G, et al. CPAP treatment of sleepy patients with milder OSA: results of the CATNAP randomized clinical trial. *Am J Respir Crit Care Med*. 2012;186(7): 677–683.
6. Giles TL, Lasserson TJ, Smith BH, et al. Continuous positive airways pressure for obstructive sleep apnoea in adults. *Cochrane Database Syst Rev*. 2008;4:CD001106.
7. Drager LF, Polotsky VY, Lorenzi-Filho G. Obstructive sleep apnea: an emerging risk factor for atherosclerosis. *Chest*. 2011;140(2):534–542.
8. Yang D, Liu Z, Yang H, et al. Effects of continuous positive airway pressure on glycemic control and insulin resistance in patients with obstructive sleep apnea: a meta-analysis. *Sleep Breath*. 2013;17(1):33–38.
9. Barbé F, Durán-Cantolla J, Sánchez-de-la-Torre M, et al. Effect of continuous positive airway pressure on the incidence of hypertension and cardiovascular events in nonsleepy patients with obstructive sleep apnea: a randomized controlled trial. *JAMA*. 2012;307(20):2161–2168.
10. Chai CL, Pathinathan A, Smith B. Continuous positive airway pressure delivery interfaces for obstructive sleep apnoea. *Cochrane Database Syst Rev*. 2006;(4):CD005308.
11. Lim J, Lasserson TJ, Fleetham J, et al. Oral appliances for obstructive sleep apnoea. *Cochrane Database Syst Rev*. 2009;3:CD004435.
12. Mason M, Welsh EJ, Smith I. Drug therapy for obstructive sleep apnoea in adults. *Cochrane Database Syst Rev*. 2013;5:CD003002.
13. Sundaram S, Bridgman SA, Lim J, et al. Surgery for obstructive sleep apnoea. *Cochrane Database Syst Rev*. 2005;(4):CD001004. *Updated 2013*.
14. Marcus C, Brooks L, Draper KA, et al. Diagnosis and treatment of childhood obstructive sleep apnea syndrome. *Pediatrics*. 2012;130(3):e714–e755.

ADDITIONAL READING

- Drager LF, Bortolotto LA, Figueiredo AC, et al. Effects of continuous positive airway pressure on early signs of atherosclerosis in obstructive sleep apnea. *Am J Respir Crit Care Med*. 2007;176(7):706–712.
- Madbouly EM, Nadeem R, Nida M, et al. The role of severity of obstructive sleep apnea measured by apnea-hypopnea index in predicting compliance with pressure therapy, a meta-analysis. *Am J Ther*. 2012;21(4):260–264.
- Rosen CL, Auckley D, Benca R, et al. A multisite randomized trial of portable sleep studies and positive airway pressure autotitration versus laboratory-based polysomnography for the diagnosis and treatment of obstructive sleep apnea: the HomePAP study. *Sleep*. 2012;35(6):757–767.

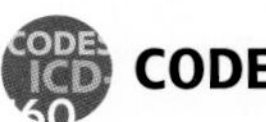

CODES

ICD10

G47.33 Obstructive sleep apnea (adult) (pediatric)

CLINICAL PEARLS

- OSA is characterized by repetitive episodes of apnea at the pharynx, often terminating in a snort/gasp.
- Laboratory polysomnography is the key to diagnosis.
- CPAP is the most effective form of treatment for both mild to moderate and moderate to severe OSA.
- Central sleep apnea may mimic OSA.

SLEEP DISORDER, SHIFT WORK

Ronald G. Chambers, Jr., MD, FAAP • Cindy J. Chambers, MD, MAS, MPH

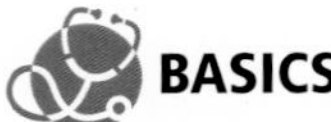

BASICS

DESCRIPTION

- The human system fundamentally relies on a natural circadian rhythm coordinated by the suprachiasmatic nucleus (SCN), an endogenous clock or pacemaker of the hypothalamus, which is responsible for linking the nervous system to the endocrine system (1).
- A shift in work schedule can desynchronize this circadian pacemaker with peripheral cells.
- The major environmental factor that can disrupt or reset the circadian rhythm is light at night (LAN) (1).
- Shift work disorder (SWD), also classified as circadian rhythm sleep disorder, is a sleep disorder caused by a misalignment between the internal circadian rhythm and the required sleep-wake schedule resulting from erratic or nighttime shift work (2).
- Diagnostic criteria for SWD requires that all criteria for circadian rhythm disorders be met in addition to specific SWD criteria (see below).
- Criteria for circadian rhythm disorder:
  - A persistent/recurrent sleep disruption due to either an alteration in the circadian (24-hour) timekeeping system or due to a misalignment between endogenous circadian rhythm and exogenous factors that affect sleep
  - A complaint of insomnia/excessive daytime sleepiness or both
  - An impairment in occupational, educational, or social functioning
  - Insomnia or excessive sleepiness temporarily associated with a recurring work schedule that overlaps with the usual time for sleep
  - Symptoms associated with shift work schedule are present for at least 1 month.
  - Sleep log or actigraphy monitoring (with sleep diaries) for at least 7 days demonstrates disturbed sleep (insomnia) and circadian and sleep time misalignment
  - Sleep disturbance is not due to another current sleep disorder, mental disorder, medical disorder, substance use disorder, or medication use.

EPIDEMIOLOGY

Prevalence

- Shift workers include those who work night shifts, evening shifts, or rotating shifts and comprise approximately 15–25% of the workforce in the United States (2).
- SWD has been estimated to affect 10–23% of the presently 22 million American shift workers, with a prevalence estimate of approximately 2–5% of the general population (14.1% night shift workers and 8.1% of rotating shift workers) (3).

PATHOPHYSIOLOGY

- Circadian rhythms are evident in multiple biologic functions, including body temperature, hormone levels, blood pressure, metabolism, cellular regeneration, sleep/wake cycles, and DNA transcription and translation (2).
- Transcription factors involved in circadian rhythm generation collectively referred to as the "molecular clock" control production of the many proteins that are expressed within a period of approximately 24 hours. This molecular clock is self-sustaining but requires resetting daily or it may become out of sync with environmental cues also called "zeitgebers" (2).
- The most powerful *zeitgeber*, or timekeeper, is light. Light transmitted from the retinohypothalamic tract of the eye to the SCN of the hypothalamus upregulates the production of the "clock gene" (PER) (2).
- Periods of darkness cause the SCN to induce the release of melatonin from the pineal gland, which can also help to reset the molecular clock (2).
- A dysynchrony between the endogenous molecular clock and external cues (most notably light/dark cycles) is responsible for the development of circadian rhythm disorders and can have a severe impact on both physical and mental health (2).

RISK FACTORS

- Shift work, including night shifts, early morning shifts, or rotating shifts
- Younger age and "eveningness"(a.k.a. "night owls" rather than "morning larks") may provide some protection from the development of SWD (2).

Genetics

No genetic predisposition has been described.

GENERAL PREVENTION

- Limit rotating shifts
- Use of bright light during shifts
- Scheduling brief, strategic 10–20-minute naps during shifts, if suitable

COMMONLY ASSOCIATED CONDITIONS

- Shift workers in general have impaired immediate free recall, decreased processing speed, and selective attention, impairments that may worsen with longer duration of shift work (2).
- Shift workers also have been shown to have a much higher risk of vehicular accidents, job-related injuries, absenteeism, and quality control errors (2).
- SWD has been associated with GI disease, specifically peptic ulcer disease, cardiovascular disease (CVD), infertility, mood disorders, and pregnancy complications (2).
- There is also evidence for possible increased risk of breast and prostate cancer. As such, the International Agency for Research on Cancer (IARC) has classified shift work that involves a circadian disruption as a probable carcinogen (1).

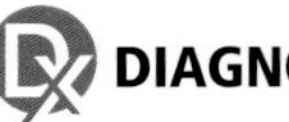

DIAGNOSIS

This is primarily a clinical diagnosis.

HISTORY

- A careful history is critical to assess sleep disturbance including difficulty falling asleep, staying asleep, or nonrestorative sleep.
- Special attention should be paid to the following (4)[C]:
  - Sleep/wake habits
  - Degree of alertness or sleepiness
  - Sleep environment
  - Light exposure before, during, and after shift
  - Job-related factors: length of shift, number of consecutive shifts, commute after shift
  - Medications, as well as over-the-counter (OTC) stimulants such as caffeine and energy drinks
  - Impact on social and domestic responsibilities (including drowsy driving)
- It is also essential to evaluate for symptoms of other sleep disorders, which often coexist and can exacerbate SWD such as the following:
  - Snoring (obstructive sleep apnea [OSA])
  - Sudden sleep attacks and leg symptoms (restless legs syndrome [RLS])
  - Falling asleep at inappropriate times, drop attacks, and daytime fatigue (narcolepsy)

PHYSICAL EXAM

Evaluate for depression, GI, CV, and potential cancer risk as well as signs of OSA such as obesity, a large neck, and a tight oropharynx (4)[C].

DIFFERENTIAL DIAGNOSIS

- Other primary sleep disorders: OSA, RLS, narcolepsy, and psychophysiological insomnia
- Other circadian rhythm sleep disorder such as delayed sleep phase disorder or jet lag syndrome. Distinguishing among these is challenging even for sleep specialists.

DIAGNOSTIC TESTS & INTERPRETATION

- Given possible increased risk for CVD and cancer among shift workers, consider appropriate screenings.

Initial Tests (lab, imaging)

- Fasting lipid panel, fasting glucose, age-appropriate cancer screenings

Diagnostic Procedures/Other

- Evaluation of a sleep/wake diary that records the patient's sleep/wake habits including amount of sleep, naps during the waking hours, and mood (1–2 weeks) (4)[C].
- Consider actigraphy (a mechanical device, often worn on the arm/leg to measure movement): serves as a gross measure of time and amount of activity and rest (4)[C]
- Polysomnography, a measure of sleep duration and quality, is not typically used to diagnose SWD but may be helpful in ruling out other sleep/wake disorders such as sleep apnea and narcolepsy (2)[C].
- Several diagnostic tools are available including the Multiple Sleep Latency Test (MSLT), the Morningness-Eveningness Questionnaire (MEQ), and the Epworth Sleepiness Scale (ESS) to help determine circadian misalignment (2)[C].

Test Interpretation

Typically, sleep diaries and actigraph data reveal the following:

- Increased sleep latency
- Decreased total sleep time
- Frequent awakenings
- Notably, most people revert to nocturnal sleeping on their days off, meaning that every workweek, they start fresh in their attempt to shift their circadian rhythms to align with work schedules.

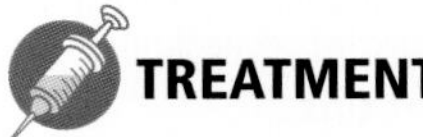

TREATMENT

- The only therapeutic modality deemed as "standard" by the American Academy of Sleep Medicine is planned (or prescribed) sleep schedules (5)[C].
- Other commonly used treatment strategies include optimizing sleep hygiene, bright light, melatonin, caffeine, and other stimulants as well as hypnotics and other medication sleep aids (discussed below).

GENERAL MEASURES

- Sleep hygiene: An important first step in approaching the treatment of sleep disorders is to educate the patient on proper sleep hygiene including minimizing exposure to bright light before and during scheduled sleep periods (maintain a dark sleeping space, wear dark sunglasses following work shift, wearing eye mask to sleep), maintaining a quiet sleep environment (wearing ear plugs to sleep, disconnecting phone, doorbell), retraining core body temperature to shifted sleep/wake schedule (maintain cool sleeping quarters), and avoiding use of stimulants during second half of work shift (2)[C].
- Sleep time: Educate on need of protected time for sleep prior to and following work shifts with strategic use of naps where possible (4)[C].
- Address work/social/domestic factors: Treat psychosocial stress and depression, encourage healthy eating habits, limit substance use, increase exercise to at least 30 minutes 5×/week (not within 2–4 hours of bedtime) (4)[C].
- Work-related interventions: If possible reduce number of consecutive shifts (<4) or reduce shift duration (<12 hours), allow adequate time between shifts (>11 hours), and move heavy workload outside circadian nadir (04:00–07:00) (4)[C].
- Bright light: Several studies have demonstrated that timed bright light and darkness can promote adaptation to night work (6)[C].
- Bright light therapy with conventional light/light boxes (10,000 lux preferable, but >1,000 lux will help) should be given 30 min/day during the night/early morning shift prior to the nadir of the core body temperature rhythm (6)[C].

MEDICATION

First Line

Circadian shift/sleep promoting: Melatonin, 5 mg PO or sublingual, 30 minutes before daytime sleep period. It should be taken only when the patient is home and able to go to bed if the hypnotic effects begin (2)[C].

Sleep promoting medications:

- Melatonin may help shift circadian rhythms and can increase the quality and duration of sleep as well as increase alertness during the work shift.
- Ramelteon (Rozerem), a melatonin receptor agonist, is not FDA-approved for the treatment of SWD but may be helpful in improving daytime sleep (2)[C].
- Antidepressants: Doxepin (tricyclic) and trazodone at low doses can improve sleep without residual daytime impairment (2)[C].
- Intermediate-acting hypnotics zolpidem (Ambien) or eszopiclone (Lunesta) may be used (see below) but can cause postsleep sedation (2)[C].

Second Line

- Wakefulness-promoting agents to reduce daytime sleepiness and improve cognitive performance are as follows (2)[C]:
  - Modafinil (Provigil) 200 mg PO 60 minutes before the shift begins
  - Armodafinil (Nuvigil) 150 mg PO 60 minutes before shift begins
  - Prophylactic caffeine use (200 mg) immediately prior to work shift and during work shift (4)[C].
- Sleep promoting
  - Non-benzodiazepine hypnotics: zolpidem (Ambien) 5–10 mg or eszopiclone (Lunesta) 1–3 mg 30 minutes before desired sleep period. Eszopicolone is the only hypnotic approved for use over 35 days.
  - Antidepressants: doxepin (3–6 mg) and trazodone (25–150 mg) 30-60 minutes prior to bed (2)[C]
  - Benzodiazepines: Estazolam, flurazepam, quazepam, temazepam, and triazolam are FDA-approved for the treatment of insomnia; however, they have high risk of tolerance and withdrawal and should be used cautiously for short-term treatment of insomnia (2)[C].

In general, hypnotics may improve daytime sleep; however, they do not appear to improve sleep maintenance and nighttime alertness and may cause residual sedation during the work hours, potentially worsening SWD symptoms (2)[C].

ISSUES FOR REFERRAL

Refer to a sleep specialist if there is suspicion of other primary sleep disorders and dependence on hypnotics, alcohol, or stimulants.

ONGOING CARE

PATIENT EDUCATION

- Health care providers should discuss good sleep hygiene and advise on how to optimize the sleep environment.
- Shift workers who need to sleep in the daytime must take serious measures to ensure that their sleep environment is cool, dark, and quiet.
- Reserve bedroom for sleeping and intimacy only. Remove all televisions and telephones from bedroom.
- When going to sleep, turn clock away from bed; discourage prolonged reading in bed.
- Blackout shades are usually necessary in order to achieve the proper darkness.

REFERENCES

1. Stevens RG, Hansen J, Costa G, et al. Considerations of circadian impact for defining "shift work" in cancer studies: IARC Working Group Report. *Occup Environ Med*. 2011;68(2):154–162.
2. Morrissette DA. Twisting the night away: a review of the neurobiology, genetics, diagnosis, and treatment of shift work disorder. *CNS Spectr*. 2013;18(Suppl 1):45–53.
3. Roth T. Appropriate therapeutic selection for patients with shift work disorder. *Sleep Med*. 2012;13(4):335–341.
4. Wright KP Jr, Bogan RK, Wyatt JK. Shift work and the assessment and management of shift work disorder (SWD). *Sleep Med Rev*. 2013;17(1):41–54.
5. American Academy of Sleep Medicine. *The International Classification of Sleep Disorders: Diagnostic & Coding Manual*. 2nd ed. Westchester, IL: American Academy of Sleep Medicine; 2005.
6. Bjorvatn B, Pallesen S. A practical approach to circadian rhythm sleep disorders. *Sleep Med Rev*. 2009;13(1):47–60.

ADDITIONAL READING

- Morgenthaler TI, Lee-Chiong T, Alessi C, et al. Practice parameters for the clinical evaluation and treatment of circadian rhythm sleep disorders. An American Academy of Sleep Medicine report. *Sleep*. 2007;30(7):1445–1459.
- Sack RL, Auckley D, Auger RR, et al. Circadian rhythm sleep disorders: part I, basic principles, shift work and jet lag disorders. An American Academy of Sleep Medicine review. *Sleep*. 2007;30(11):1460–1483.
- Sleep Diary: http://www.helpguide.org/misc/sleep-diary.pdf

CODES

ICD10

G47.26 Circadian rhythm sleep disorder, shift work type

CLINICAL PEARLS

- Shift work disorder is associated with shortened and disturbed sleep, fatigue, decreased alertness, cognitive decrements, increased injuries and accidents, reproductive problems, and risks to cardiovascular and gastrointestinal health and has been classified as a carcinogen given possible association with breast and prostate cancer.
- The most important 1st diagnostic step in SWD is to obtain and evaluate a sleep diary.

SMELL AND TASTE DISORDERS

Beth Mazyck, MD • Daniel B. Kurtz, PhD

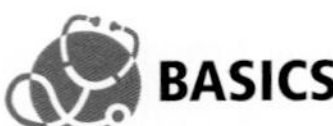

BASICS

DESCRIPTION

- The senses of smell and taste allow a full appreciation of the flavor and palatability of foods and also serve as a warning system against toxins, polluted air, smoke, and spoiled food.
- Physiologically, the chemical senses aid in normal digestion by triggering GI secretions. Smell/taste dysfunction may have a significant impact on quality of life.
- Loss of smell occurs more frequently than loss of taste, and patients frequently confuse the concepts of flavor loss (as a result of smell impairment) with taste loss (an impaired ability to sense sweet, sour, salty, or bitter).
- Smell depends on the functioning of CN I (olfactory nerve) and CN V (trigeminal nerve).
- Taste depends on the functioning of CNs VII, IX, and X. Because of these multiple pathways, total loss of taste (ageusia) is rare.
- Systems affected: nervous, upper respiratory

EPIDEMIOLOGY

Incidence

There are ~200,000 patient visits a year for smell and taste disturbances.

Prevalence

- Predominant sex: male > female. Men begin to lose their ability to smell earlier in life than women.
- Predominant age: Chemosensory loss is age dependent:
  - Age >80 years: 80% have major olfactory impairment; nearly 50% are anosmic.
  - Ages 65–80 years: 60% have major olfactory impairment; nearly 25% are anosmic.
  - Age <65 years: 1–2% have smell impairment.
- Estimated >2 million affected in the United States

ETIOLOGY AND PATHOPHYSIOLOGY

- Smell and/or taste disturbances:
  - Nutritional factors (e.g., malnutrition, vitamin deficiencies, liver disease, pernicious anemia)
  - Endocrine disorders (e.g., thyroid disease, diabetes mellitus, renal disease)
  - Head trauma
  - Migraine headache (e.g., gustatory aura, olfactory aura)
  - Sjögren syndrome
  - Toxic chemical exposure
  - Industrial agent exposure
  - Aging
  - Medications (see below)
  - Neurodegenerative diseases (e.g., multiple sclerosis, Alzheimer disease, cerebrovascular accident, Parkinson disease)
  - Infections (e.g., upper respiratory infection [URI], oral and perioral infections, candidiasis, coxsackievirus, AIDS, viral hepatitis, herpes simplex virus)
- Possible causes of smell disturbance:
  - Nasal and sinus disease (e.g., allergies, rhinitis, rhinorrhea)
  - Cigarette smoking
  - Cocaine abuse (intranasal)
  - Hemodialysis
  - Radiation treatment of head and neck
  - Congenital conditions
  - Neoplasm (e.g., brain tumor, nasal polyps, intranasal tumor)
  - Systemic lupus erythematosus (SLE)
  - Bell palsy
  - Oral/perioral skin lesion
  - Damage to CN I/V
  - Possible association with psychosis and schizophrenia
- Possible causes of taste loss:
  - Oral appliances
  - Dental procedures
  - Intraoral abscess
  - Gingivitis
  - Damage to CN VI, IX, or X
  - Stroke (especially frontal lobe)
- Selected medications that reportedly alter smell and taste:
  - Antibiotics: amikacin, ampicillin, azithromycin, ciprofloxacin, clarithromycin, doxycycline, griseofulvin, metronidazole, ofloxacin, tetracycline, terbinafine, β-lactamase inhibitors
  - Anticonvulsants: carbamazepine, phenytoin
  - Antidepressants: amitriptyline, doxepin, imipramine, nortriptyline
  - Antihistamines and decongestants: zinc-based cold remedies (Zicam)
  - Antihypertensives and cardiac medications: acetazolamide, amiloride, captopril, diltiazem, hydrochlorothiazide, nifedipine, propranolol, spironolactone
  - Anti-inflammatory agents: auranofin, gold, penicillamine
  - Antimanic drugs: lithium
  - Antineoplastics: cisplatin, doxorubicin, methotrexate, vincristine
  - Antiparkinsonian agents: levodopa, carbidopa
  - Antiseptic: chlorhexidine
  - Antithyroid agents: methimazole, propylthiouracil
  - Lipid-lowering agents: statins

Genetics

May be related to underlying genetically associated diseases (Kallmann syndrome, Alzheimer disease, migraine syndromes, rheumatologic conditions, endocrine disorders)

RISK FACTORS

- Age >65 years
- Poor nutritional status
- Smoking tobacco products

GENERAL PREVENTION

- Eat a well-balanced diet, with appropriate vitamins and minerals.
- Maintain good oral and nasal health, with routine visits to the dentist.
- Do not smoke tobacco products.
- Avoid noxious chemical exposures/unnecessary radiation.

Geriatric Considerations

- Elders are at particular risk of eating spoiled food or inadvertently being exposed to natural gas leaks owing to anosmia from aging.
- Anosmia also may be an early sign of degenerative disorders and has been shown to predict increased 5-year mortality (1)[B].

Pediatric Considerations

- Smell and taste disorders are uncommon in children in developed countries.
- In developing countries with poor nutrition (particularly zinc depletion), smell and taste disorders may occur.
- Delayed puberty in association with anosmia (± midline craniofacial abnormalities, deafness, or renal abnormalities) suggests the possibility of Kallmann syndrome (hypogonadotropic hypogonadism).

Pregnancy Considerations

- Pregnancy is an uncommon cause of smell and taste loss or disturbances.
- Many women report increased sensitivity to odors during pregnancy as well as an increased dislike for bitterness and a preference for salty substances.

COMMONLY ASSOCIATED CONDITIONS

URI, allergic rhinitis, dental abscesses

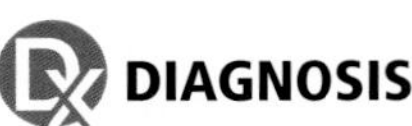

DIAGNOSIS

Smell and taste disturbances are symptoms; it is essential to look for possible underlying causes.

HISTORY

- Symptoms of URI, environmental allergies
- Oral pain, other dental problems
- Cognitive/memory difficulties
- Current medications
- Nutritional status, ovolactovegetarian
- Weight loss or gain
- Frequent infections (impaired immunity)
- Worsening of underlying medical illness
- Increased use of salt and/or sugar to increase taste of food
- Neurodegenerative disease

PHYSICAL EXAM

Thorough HEENT exam

DIFFERENTIAL DIAGNOSIS

- Epilepsy (gustatory aura)
- Epilepsy (olfactory aura)
- Memory impairment
- Psychiatric conditions

DIAGNOSTIC TESTS & INTERPRETATION

Initial Tests (lab, imaging)

Consider (not all patients require all tests)

- CBC
- Liver function tests
- Blood glucose
- Creatinine
- Vitamin B_{12} level
- Thyroid-stimulating hormone (TSH)
- Serum IgE
- CT scanning is the most useful and cost-effective technique for assessing sinonasal disorders and is superior to an MRI in evaluating bony structures and airway patency. Coronal CT scans are particularly valuable in assessing paranasal anatomy (2)[B].

Follow-Up Tests & Special Considerations
Diagnosis of smell and taste disturbances is usually possible through history; however, the following tests can be used to confirm:

- Olfactory tests
  - Smell identification test: evaluates the ability to identify 40 microencapsulated scratch-and-sniff odorants (3)[B]
  - Brief smell identification test (4)[B]
- Taste tests (more difficult because no convenient standardized tests are presently available): Solutions containing sucrose (sweet), sodium chloride (salty), quinine (bitter), and citric acid (sour) are helpful.
- An MRI is useful in defining soft tissue disease; therefore, a coronal MRI is the technique of choice to image the olfactory bulbs, tracts, and cortical parenchyma. Possible placement of an accessory coil (TMJ) over the nose to assist in imaging.

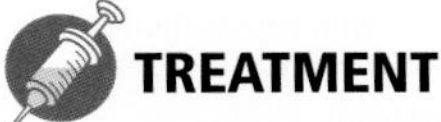

TREATMENT

GENERAL MEASURES

- Appropriate treatment for underlying cause
- Quit smoking (5)[B].
- Treatment of underlying nasal congestion with nasal decongestants and/or nasal/oral steroids (6–9)[B]
- Surgical correction of nasal blockage/nasal polyps (10)[B]
- Some drug-related smell or taste loss or dysgeusias can be reversed with cessation of the offending medication, but it may take many months (11–14)[B].
- Stop repeated oral trauma (e.g., appliances, tongue-biting behaviors).
- Proper nutritional and dietary assessment (2)[C]
- Formal dental evaluation

MEDICATION

- Treat underlying causes as appropriate. Idiopathic cases will often resolve spontaneously.
- Consider trial of corticosteroids topically (e.g., fluticasone nasal spray daily to BID) and/or systemically (e.g., oral prednisone 60 mg daily × 5–7 days) (6)[B].
- Zinc and vitamins (A, B complex) when deficiency is suspected (15)[B]

ISSUES FOR REFERRAL

- Consider referral to an otolaryngologist or neurologist for persistent cases.
- Referral to a subspecialist at a regional smell and taste center when complex etiologies are suspected

SURGERY/OTHER PROCEDURES

If needed for treatment of underlying cause

ONGOING CARE

DIET

- Weight gain/loss is possible because the patient may reject food or may switch to calorie-rich foods that are still palatable.
- Ensure a nutritionally balanced diet with appropriate levels of nutrients, vitamins, and essential minerals.

PATIENT EDUCATION

- Caution patients not to overindulge as compensation for the bland taste of food. For example, patients with diabetes may need help in avoiding excessive sugar intake as an inappropriate way of improving food taste.
- Patients with chemosensory impairments should use measuring devices when cooking and should not cook by taste.
- Optimizing food texture, aroma, temperature, and color may improve the overall food experience when taste is limited.
- Patients with permanent smell dysfunction must develop adaptive strategies for dealing with hygiene, appetite, safety, and health.
- Natural gas and smoke detectors are essential; check for proper function frequently.
- Check food expiration dates frequently; discard old food.

PROGNOSIS

- In general, the olfactory system regenerates poorly after a head injury. Most patients who recover smell function following head trauma do so within 12 weeks of injury.
- Patients who quit smoking typically recover improved olfactory function and flavor sensation.
- Many taste disorders (dysgeusias) resolve spontaneously within a few years of onset.
- Phantosmias that are flow-dependent may respond to surgical ablation of olfactory mucosa.
- Conditions such as radiation-induced xerostomia and Bell palsy generally improve over time.

COMPLICATIONS

- Permanent loss of ability to smell/taste
- Psychiatric issues with dysgeusias and phantosmia

REFERENCES

1. Pinto JM, Wroblewski KE, Kern DW, et al. Olfactory dysfunction predicts 5-year mortality in older adults. *PLOS ONE* 2014;9(9):e107541.
2. Malaty, J, Malaty I. Smell and taste disorders in primary care. *Am Fam Physician*. 2013;88(12):852–859.
3. Doty RL, Shaman P, Dann M. Development of the University of Pennsylvania smell identification test: a standardized microencapsulated test of olfactory function. *Physiol Behav*. 1984;32(3):489–502.
4. Jackman AH, Doy RL. Utility of a three-item smell identification test in detecting olfactory dysfunction. *Laryngoscope*. 2005;115(12):2209–2212.
5. Frye RE, Schwartz BS, Doty RL. Dose-related effects of cigarette smoking on olfactory function. *JAMA*. 1990;263(9):1233–1236.
6. Seiden S, Duncan HL. The diagnosis of a conductive olfactory loss. *Laryngoscope*. 2001;111(1):9–14.
7. Deems DA, Doty RL, Settle RG et al. Smell and taste disorders, a study of 750 patients from the University of Pennsylvania Smell and Taste Center. *Arch Otolaryngol Head Neck Surg*. 1991;117(5):519–528.
8. Apter AJ, Gent JF, Frank ME. Fluctuating olfactory sensitivity and distorted odor perception in allergic rhinitis. *Arch Otolaryngol Head Neck Surg*. 1999;125(9):1005–1010.
9. Mott AE, Cain WS, Lafreniere LG, et al. Topical corticosteroid treatment of anosmia associated with nasal and sinus disease. *Arch Otolarungol Head Neck Surg*. 1977;123(4):367–372.
10. Olsson P, Stjärne P. Endoscopic sinus surgery improves olfacton in nasal polyposi, a multi-center study. *Rhinology*. 2010;48(2):150–155.
11. Naik BS, Shetty N, Maben EV. Drug-induced taste disorders. *Eur J Intern Med*. 2010;21(3):240–243.
12. Ackerman BH, Kasbekar N. Disturbances of taste and smell induced by drugs. *Pharmacotherapy*. 1997;17(3):482–496.
13. Cowart, BJ. Taste dysfunction: a practical guide for oral medicine. *Oral Dis*. 2011;17(1):2–6.
14. Tuccori M, Lapi F, Testi A, et al. Drug-induced taste and smell alterations: a case/non-case evaluation of an Italian database of spontaneous adverse drug reaction reporting. *Drug Saf*. 2011;34(10):849–859.
15. Henkin RI, Martin BM, Agarwal RP. Efficacy of exogenous oral zinc in treatment of patients with carbonic anhydrase VI deficiency. *Am J Med Sci*. 1999;318(6):392–405.

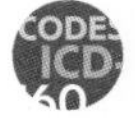

CODES

ICD10

- R43.9 Unspecified disturbances of smell and taste
- R43.1 Parosmia
- R43.2 Parageusia

CLINICAL PEARLS

- Smell disorders are often mistaken as decreased taste by patients.
- Most smell loss is due nasal passage obstruction.
- Actual taste disorders are often related to dental problems or medication side effects.
- Gradual smell loss is very common in the elderly; extensive workup in this population may not be indicated if no associated signs/symptoms are present but may be predictive of 5-year mortality.

S

SOMATIC SYMPTOM (SOMATIZATION) DISORDER

William G. Elder, PhD

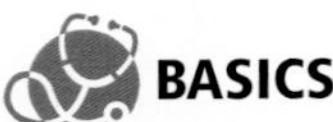

BASICS

DESCRIPTION

- A pattern of one or more somatic symptoms recurring or persisting for more than 6 months that are distressing or result in significant disruption of daily life (1)
- Conceptualization and diagnostic criteria for somatic symptom presentations were significantly modified with the advent of *DSM-5*. Somatic symptom disorder (SSD) is similar in many aspects to the former somatization disorder which required presentation with multiple physical complaints, no longer based on symptoms counts; current diagnosis is based on the way the patient presents and perceives his or her symptoms.
- SSD now includes most presentations that would formerly be considered hypochondriasis. Hypochondriasis has been replaced by illness anxiety disorders, which is diagnosed when the patient presents with significant preoccupation with having a serious illness in the absence of illness-related somatic complaints.
- Somatization increases disability independent of comorbidity and individuals with SSD have health-related functioning that is 2 standard deviations below the mean (1,2).
- Symptoms may be specific (e.g., localized pain) or relatively nonspecific (e.g., fatigue).
- Symptoms sometimes may represent normal bodily sensations or discomfort that does not signify serious disease.
- Suffering is authentic. Symptoms are not intentionally produced or feigned.

EPIDEMIOLOGY

Incidence

- Usually, 1st symptoms appear in adolescence.
- Predominant sex: female > male (10:1) (1)
- Type and frequency of somatic complaints may differ among cultures, so symptom reviews should be adjusted based on culture. More frequent in cultures without Western/empirical explanatory models (3).

Prevalence

- Expected 2% among women and <0.2% among men (4)
- Somatization seen in up to 29% of patients presenting to primary care offices (3)
- Somatic concerns may increase, but other features of the presentation decrease such that prevalence declines after age 65 years (5).

ETIOLOGY AND PATHOPHYSIOLOGY

Unknown

Genetics

Consanguinity studies and single nucleotide polymorphism genotyping indicate that both genetic and environmental factors contribute to the risk of SD (6).

RISK FACTORS

- Child abuse, particularly sexual abuse, has been shown to be a risk factor for somatization.
- Symptoms begin or worsen after losses (e.g., job, close relative, or friend).
- Greater intensity of symptoms often occurs with stress.

COMMONLY ASSOCIATED CONDITIONS

Comorbid with other psychiatric conditions is yet to be determined but is likely to be 20–50% with anxiety, depression, or personality disorders.

DIAGNOSIS

Determining that a somatic symptom is medically unexplained is unreliable, and it is inappropriate to diagnose a mental disorder solely because a medical diagnosis is not demonstrated. Rely on symptoms and presentation rather ruling out medical causes in making the SSD diagnosis.

HISTORY

- One of more somatic complaints, with sometimes a grossly positive review of symptoms
- SSD involves patient excessive thoughts, feelings, or behaviors associated with symptoms or associated health concerns manifested by at least 1 of the following:
  - Disproportionate and persistent thoughts about the seriousness of the symptoms
  - Persistent high level of anxiety about health or symptoms
  - Excessive time or energy devoted to symptoms or health concerns.
- Diagnoses no longer relies on symptom counts, but common symptoms include:
  - Pain symptoms related to different sites such as head, abdomen, back, joints, extremities, chest, or rectum, or related to body functions such as menstruation, sexual intercourse, or urination.
  - GI symptoms such as nausea, bloating, vomiting (not during pregnancy), diarrhea, intolerance of several foods
  - Sexual symptoms such as indifference to sex, difficulties with erection or ejaculation, irregular menses, excessive menstrual bleeding, or vomiting throughout all 9 months of pregnancy
  - Pseudoneurologic symptoms such as impaired balance or coordination, weak or paralyzed muscles, lump in throat or trouble swallowing, loss of voice, retention of urine, hallucinations, numbness (to touch or pain), double vision, blindness, deafness, seizures, amnesia or other dissociative symptoms, loss of consciousness (other than with fainting); none of these is limited to pain
- Patients with SSD frequently use alternative treatments which should be explored for their effects on health and physical functioning (2).

PHYSICAL EXAM

Physical exam remarkable for absence of objective findings to explain the many subjective complaints

DIFFERENTIAL DIAGNOSIS

- Other psychiatric illnesses must be ruled out:
  - Depressive disorders
  - Anxiety disorders
  - Schizophrenia
  - Other somatic disorders: illness anxiety disorder, conversion disorder
  - Factitious disorder
  - Body dysmorphic disorder
- Malingering
- General medical conditions, with vague, multiple, confusing symptoms, must be ruled out.
  - Systemic lupus erythematosus
  - Hyperparathyroidism
  - Hyper- or hypothyroidism
  - Lyme disease
  - Porphyria

DIAGNOSTIC TESTS & INTERPRETATION

Several screening tools are available that help to identify symptoms as somatic:

- Patient Health Questionnaire (PHQ)-15 (screens and monitors symptoms) (7)[B]
- Minnesota Multiphasic Personality Inventory (MMPI) (identifies somatization) (8)[B]

Initial Tests (lab, imaging)

- Laboratory test results do not support the subjective complaints.
- Imaging studies do not support the subjective complaints.

Test Interpretation

None are identified.

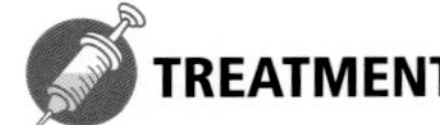

TREATMENT

GENERAL MEASURES

- The goal of treatment is to help the person learn to control the symptoms (9)[B].
- A supportive relationship with a sympathetic health care provider is the most important aspect of treatment:
  - Regularly scheduled appointments should be maintained to review symptoms and the person's coping mechanisms (at least 15 minutes once a month).
  - Acknowledge and explain test results.

- The involvement of a single provider is important because a history of seeking medical attention and "doctor shopping" is common.
- Antidepressant or antianxiety medication and referral to a support group or mental health provider can help patients who are willing to participate in their treatment.
- Patients usually receive the most benefit from primary care providers who accept the limitations of treatment, listen to their patient's concerns, and provide reassurance.
- It is not helpful to tell patients that their symptoms are imaginary.

MEDICATION

Antidepressants (e.g., SSRIs) help to treat comorbid depression and anxiety (10)[C].

ISSUES FOR REFERRAL

- Discourage referrals to specialists for further investigation of somatic complaints.
- Referrals to support groups or to a mental health provider may be helpful.

ADDITIONAL THERAPIES

Treatments have not been evaluated for this recently reformulated disorder. However, there are numerous studies with positive outcomes for patients with various forms of somatization or medically unexplained symptoms.

- Treatment typically includes long-term therapy, which has been shown to decrease the severity of symptoms.
- Individual or group cognitive-behavioral therapy addressing health anxiety, health beliefs, and health behaviors has been shown to be the most efficacious treatment for somatoform disorders (11,12,13)[A].

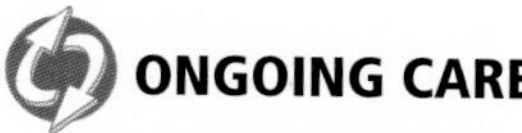

ONGOING CARE

FOLLOW-UP RECOMMENDATIONS

Patients should have regularly scheduled follow-up with a primary care doctor, psychiatrist, and/or therapist.

PATIENT EDUCATION

Encourage interventions that decrease stressful elements of the patient's life:

- Psychoeducational advice
- Increase in exercise
- Pleasurable private time

PROGNOSIS

- Chronic course, fluctuating in severity
- Full remission is rare.
- Individuals with this disorder do not experience any significant difference in mortality rate or significant physical illness.
- Patients with this diagnosis do experience substantially greater functional disability and role impairment than nonsomatizing patients.

COMPLICATIONS

- May result from invasive testing and from multiple evaluations that are performed while looking for the cause of the symptoms
- A dependency on pain relievers or sedatives may develop.

REFERENCES

1. American Psychiatric Association. *Diagnostic and Statistical Manual of Mental Disorders*. 5th ed. Arlington, VA: American Psychiatric Publishing; 2013.
2. Harris AM, Orav EJ, Bates DW, et al. Somatization increases disability independent of comorbidity. *J Gen Intern Med*. 2009;24(2):155–161.
3. Elder WG. Somatoform disorders. In South-Paul J, Matheny SC, Lewis EL, eds. *Current Diagnosis and Treatment in Family Medicine*. 4th ed. New York, NY: Lange-McGraw Hill; 2015.
4. Roca M, Gili M, Garcia-Garcia M, et al. Prevalence and comorbidity of common mental disorders in primary care. *J Affect Disord*. 2009;119(1–3):52–58.
5. Hilderink PH, Collard R, Rosmalen JG, et al. Prevalence of somatoform disorders and medically unexplained symptoms in old age populations in comparison with younger age groups: a systematic review. *Ageing Res Rev*. 2012;12(1):151–156.
6. Koh KB, Choi EH, Lee YJ, et al. Serotonin-related gene pathways associated with undifferentiated somatoform disorder. *Psychiatry Res*. 2011; 189(2):246–250.
7. Kroenke K, Spitzer RL, Williams JB. The PHQ-15: validity of a new measure for evaluating the severity of somatic symptoms. *Psychosom Med*. 2002;64(2):258–266.
8. Wetzel RD, Brim J, Guze SB, et al. MMPI screening scales for somatization disorder. *Psychol Rep*. 1999;85(1):341–348.
9. Heijmans M, Olde Hartman TC, van Weel-Baumgarten E, et al. Experts' opinions on the management of medically unexplained symptoms in primary care. A qualitative analysis of narrative reviews and scientific editorials. *Fam Pract*. 2011;28(4):444–455.
10. Somashekar B, Jainer A, Wuntakal B. Psychopharmacotherapy of somatic symptoms disorders. *Int Rev Psychiatry*. 2013;25(1):107–115.
11. Kroenke K, Swindle R. Cognitive-behavioral therapy for somatization and symptom syndromes: a critical review of controlled clinical trials. *Psychother Psychosom*. 2000;69(4):205–215.
12. Allen LA, Woolfolk RL, Escobar JI, et al. Cognitive-behavioral therapy for somatization disorder: a randomized controlled trial. *Arch Intern Med*. 2006;166(14):1512–1518.
13. Moreno S, Gili M, Magallón R, et al. Effectiveness of group versus individual cognitive-behavioral therapy in patients with abridged somatization disorder: a randomized controlled trial. *Psychosom Med*. 2013;75(6):600–608.

ADDITIONAL READING

- Elder WG Jr, King M, Dassow PL, et al. Managing lower back pain: you may be doing too much. *J Fam Pract*. 2009;58(4):180–186.
- Sharma MP, Manjula M. Behavioural and psychological management of somatic symptom disorders: an overview. *Int Rev Psychiatry*. 2013;25(1):116–124.

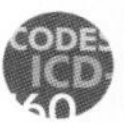

CODES

ICD10

- F45.9 Somatoform disorder, unspecified
- F45.20 Hypochondriacal disorder, unspecified
- F45.22 Body dysmorphic disorder

CLINICAL PEARLS

- A clue is accumulation of more than 13 letter diagnosis (e.g., chronic fatigue syndrome, fibromyalgia syndrome, reflex sympathetic dystrophy, temporomandibular joint syndrome, carpal tunnel syndrome, mitral valve prolapse).
- Inability of more than three physicians to make a meaningful diagnosis suggests somatization.
- Acknowledge the patient's pain, suffering, and disability.
- Do not tell patients the symptoms are "all in their head."
- Emphasize that this is not a rare disorder.
- Discuss the limitations of treatment while providing reassurance that there are interventions that will lessen suffering and reduce symptoms.

S

SPINAL STENOSIS

N. Wilson Holland, MD, FACP, AGSF • Birju B. Patel, MD, FACP, AGSF

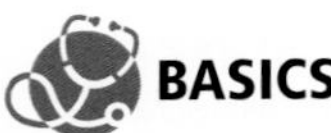

BASICS

DESCRIPTION

Spinal stenosis is narrowing of the spinal canal and foramen occurs:

- Spondylosis or degenerative arthritis is the most common cause of spinal stenosis, resulting from compression of the spinal cord by disc degeneration, facet arthropathy, osteophyte formation, and ligamentum flavum hypertrophy.
- The L4–L5 level is most commonly involved.

EPIDEMIOLOGY

The prevalence of spinal stenosis increases with age due to "wear and tear" on the normal spine.

Incidence

Symptomatic spinal stenosis affects up to 8% of the general population.

Prevalence

- The prevalence of spinal stenosis can be very high if assessed solely by imaging in elderly patients. Not all patients with radiographic spinal stenosis are symptomatic, and the degree of radiographic stenosis does not always correlate with patient symptoms. Lumbar MRI showed significant abnormalities in one study in 22% of asymptomatic patients younger than age 60 years and in 57% of patients older than age 60 years. T2 weighted imaging showed a 98% prevalence of disc degeneration in patients older than 60 years who were asymptomatic (1)[C].
- Predominant age: Symptoms develop in 5th–6th decades (congenital stenosis is symptomatic much earlier) (2)[A].

ETIOLOGY AND PATHOPHYSIOLOGY

- Spinal stenosis can result from congenital or acquired causes. Degenerative spondylosis is the most common cause.
- Disc dehydration leads to loss of height with bulging of the disc annulus and ligamentum flavum into the spinal canal, increasing facet joint loading.
- This leads to reactive sclerosis and osteophytic bone growth, further compressing spinal canal and foraminal neural elements.
- Other causes of acquired spinal stenosis include the following:
  - Trauma
  - Neoplasms
  - Neural cysts and lipomas
  - Postoperative changes
  - Rheumatoid arthritis
  - Diffuse idiopathic skeletal hyperostosis
  - Ankylosing spondylitis
  - Metabolic/endocrine causes such as osteoporosis, renal osteodystrophy, and Paget disease (3)[A]

Genetics

No definitive genetic links

RISK FACTORS

Increasing age and degenerative spinal disease

GENERAL PREVENTION

There is proven prevention for spinal stenosis. Symptoms can be alleviated with flexion at the waist:

- Leaning forward while walking
- Pushing a shopping cart
- Lying in flexed position
- Sitting
- Avoiding provocative maneuvers (back extension, ambulating long distances without resting)

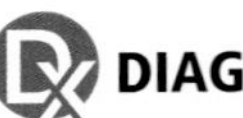

DIAGNOSIS

HISTORY

- The history helps distinguish patients with spinal stenosis from those with other causes of back pain and peripheral vascular disease.
  - Insidious onset and slow progression are typical. Patients complain of discomfort with standing, paresthesias, weakness (often bilateral) (4)[C].
  - Symptoms *worsen with extension* of the spine (prolonged standing, walking downhill, or down stairs).
  - Symptoms *improve with flexion* (sitting, leaning forward while walking, walking uphill or upstairs, lying in a flexed position).
- Neurogenic claudication (i.e., pain, tightness, numbness, and subjective weakness of lower extremities) may mimic arterial insufficiency–related claudication.
- Nocturnal leg cramps may relate to the severity of lumbar spinal stenosis (5)[C].

PHYSICAL EXAM

Neurologic exam may be normal. There may be very few physical findings even in affected patients:

- Examine gait (rule out cervical myelopathy or intracranial pathology)
- Loss of lumbar lordosis
- Evaluate range of motion of lumbar spine
- Pain with extension of the lumbar spine is typical.
- Straight-leg raise test may be positive if nerve root entrapment is present.
- Muscle weakness is usually mild or subtle and involves the L4, L5 and rarely, S1 nerve roots.
- ~1/2 of patients with symptomatic stenosis have a reduced or absent Achilles reflex, and some have reduced or absent patellar reflex.

DIFFERENTIAL DIAGNOSIS

- Vascular claudication. Symptoms of vascular claudication do not improve with leaning forward and usually do not persist with standing.
- Disc herniation
- Cervical myelopathy

DIAGNOSTIC TESTS & INTERPRETATION

Spinal stenosis generally is diagnosed based on of history and physical exam. Imaging (MRI is best) is used to stage severity and plan treatment.

Initial Tests (lab, imaging)

- CBC, ESR, C-reactive protein (if considering infection or malignancy).
- New back pain lasting >2 weeks or back pain accompanied by neurologic findings in patients older than 50 years generally warrants neuroimaging.
- MRI is the modality of choice for the diagnosis of spinal stenosis.
- CT myelography is an alternative to MRI but is invasive and has higher risk of complications.
- Plain radiography helps exclude other causes of new back pain (e.g., malignant lytic lesions) but does not reveal the underlying pathology.
- Radiologic abnormalities in general do not correlate with the clinical diagnosis (6)[C].

Diagnostic Procedures/Other

Surgical decompression is the only definitive treatment in patients who continue to be symptomatic after nonoperative treatment:

- Spinal stenosis generally does not lead to neurologic damage.
- Surgery may be required for pain relief, allowing patients to become more mobile and thus improving overall health and quality of life.

Test Interpretation

- Common radiographic findings included decreased disc height, facet hypertrophy, and spinal canal and/or foraminal narrowing.

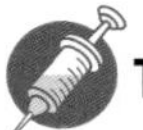

TREATMENT

- In general, nonoperative interventions are preferred unless there are progressive or life-threatening neurologic symptoms:
  - Physical therapy, exercise, weight management, lumbar epidural steroid injections, and medications should all be used prior to consideration for surgery.
  - Recent review of nonoperative treatment options for lumbar spinal stenosis with claudication suggests that there is not enough evidence in the current literature to guide clinical practice.
  - Consider ruling out other forms of neuropathy and peripheral vascular disease.
- If decompressive surgery is performed, it is generally successful in alleviating symptoms of spinal stenosis.
- There is some controversy about whether a fusion should be performed with the decompression because of risk of future spondylolisthesis (7)[A], (8)[C],(9)[A].

MEDICATION

First Line

- Acetaminophen: caution in those with preexisting liver disease; increased warnings for hepatotoxicity; limit daily dose to 3 g in the elderly.
- NSAIDs: Consider potential for GI side effects, fluid retention, and renal failure.

Second Line

- Tramadol—currently a schedule IV controlled substance. Has the potential to cause confusion, dizziness, lower seizure threshold, and increase fall risk in the elderly; should be used with caution
- There is limited evidence for long-term efficacy of lumbar epidural steroid and/or anesthetic injections. Injections maybe less effective in those with more severe stenosis and those with stenosis involving >3 lumbar levels.
- Use opioids judiciously and only when other treatments have failed to control severe pain.

Geriatric Considerations

- Anti-inflammatory medications should be used with caution in the elderly due to the risks of GI bleeding, fluid retention, renal failure, and cardiovascular risks.
- Side effects of opioids, including constipation, confusion, urinary retention, drowsiness, nausea, vomiting, and potential for dependence should be considered.
- >10% of elderly lack Achilles reflexes.

ISSUES FOR REFERRAL

Refer to a spine surgeon when patients are in unremitting pain or have a neurologic deficit.

ADDITIONAL THERAPIES

- General conditioning; patients with spinal stenosis are typically able to ride an exercise bicycle without many problems because leaning forward tends to relieve symptoms.
- Aquatic therapy (helpful for muscle training and general conditioning)
- Back extensor muscle strengthening
- Abdominal muscle strengthening
- Gait training
- A brace or corset may help in the short term but is not recommended for prolonged periods due to development of paraspinal muscle weakness.
- Patients should to continue to be active despite pain to prevent deconditioning.

SURGERY/OTHER PROCEDURES

- Surgery is indicated when symptoms persist despite conservative measures (7)[A].
- Age alone should not be an exclusion factor for surgical intervention. However, cognitive impairment, multiple comorbidities, and osteoporosis may increase the risk of perioperative complications in the elderly.
- Lumbar decompressive laminectomy is the mainstay of treatment. The traditional approach is laminectomy and partial facetectomy.
- Controversy exists about whether the decompression should be supplemented by a fusion procedure:
  - There is evidence that fusion (simple or complex), as opposed to decompression procedure alone, may be associated with higher risk of major complications, increased mortality, and increased resource use in the elderly.
- A less-invasive alternative, known as interspinous distraction (X STOP implant), is also available as a treatment option (10)[B].
- The use of the Aperius interspinous implant device is inconclusive in terms of evidence for efficacy in lumbar spinal stenosis at this time (11,12)[C].
- A unilateral partial hemilaminectomy combined with transmedial decompression may adequately treat stenosis with less morbidity in the elderly population (13)[C].
- Transforaminal balloon treatment may be a viable option for resistant spinal stenosis pain and functional impairment (14)[B].

IN-PATIENT CONSIDERATIONS

Admission Criteria/Initial Stabilization

Unremitting pain that prevents the ability to perform activities of daily living (ADLs). Acute or progressive neurologic deficit

Discharge Criteria

Improved pain or after neurologic deficit has been addressed

ONGOING CARE

FOLLOW-UP RECOMMENDATIONS

- Follow up based on progression of symptoms.
- No limitations to activity; patients may be as active as tolerated. Exercise should be encouraged.

Patient Monitoring

Patients are monitored for improvement of symptoms and development of any complications.

DIET

Nutritional status should be optimized for weight management and for any patients potentially undergoing surgery.

PATIENT EDUCATION

- Activity as tolerated, as long as no other pathology is present (e.g., fractures).
- Patients should alert their physician if they develop progressive motor weakness and/or bladder/bowel dysfunction.
- Patients should know the natural history of the condition and how best to relieve symptoms.

PROGNOSIS

- Spinal stenosis is generally benign, but the pain can lead to limitation in ADLs and progressive disability.
- Surgery is usually successful in improving pain and symptoms in patients who fail nonoperative treatment.
- Clinical outcomes in elderly patients after surgery are similar in terms of pain relief and functional improvement compared with younger patients.

COMPLICATIONS

- Severe spinal stenosis can lead to bowel and/or bladder dysfunction.
- Surgical complications include infection, neurologic injury, chronic pain, and disability.

REFERENCES

1. Baker ADL. Abnormal magnetic resonance scans of the lumbar spine in asymptomatic subjects. A prospective investigation. In: Banaszkiewicz P, Kader DF, eds. *Classic Papers in Orthopedics*. London, England: Springer London; 2014: 245–247.
2. Ammendolia C, Stuber K, de Bruin LK, et al. Nonoperative treatment of lumbar spinal stenosis with neurogenic claudication: a systematic review. *Spine Spine (Phila Pa 1976)*. 2012;37(10): E609–E616.
3. Katz JN, Harris MB. Clinical practice. Lumbar spinal stenosis. *N Engl J Med*. 2008;358(8): 818–825.
4. Suri P, Rainville J, Kalichman L, et al. Does this older adult with lower extremity pain have the clinical syndrome of lumbar spinal stenosis? *JAMA*. 2010;304(23):2628–2636.
5. Ohtori S, Yamashita M, Murata Y. et al. Incidence of nocturnal leg cramps in patients with lumbar spinal stenosis before and after conservative and surgical treatment. *Yonsei Med J*. 2014:55(3): 779–784.
6. Li AL, Yen D. Effect of increased MRI and CT scan utilization on clinical decision-making in patients referred a surgical clinic for back pain. *Can J Surg*. 2011;54(2):128–132.
7. Weinstein JN, Tosteson TD, Lurie JD, et al. Surgical versus nonsurgical therapy for lumbar spinal stenosis. *N Engl J Med*. 2008;358(8):794–810.
8. Deyo RA, Ching A, Matsen L, et al. Use of bone morphogenetic proteins in spinal fusion surgery for older adults with lumbar stenosis: trends, complications, repeat surgery, and charges. *Spine (Phila Pa 1976)*. 2012;37(3):222–230.
9. Deyo RA, Mirza SK, Martin BI, et al. Trends, major medical complications, and charges associated with surgery for lumbar spinal stenosis in older adults. *JAMA*. 2010;303(13):1259–1265.
10. Miller LE, Block JE. Interspinous spacer implant in patients with lumbar spinal stenosis: preliminary results of a multicenter, randomized, controlled trial. *Pain Res Treat*. 2012;2012:823509.
11. Postacchini R, Ferrari E, Cinotti G, et al. Aperius interspinous implant versus open surgical decompression in lumbar spinal stenosis. *Spine J*. 2011;11(10):933–939.
12. Surace MF, Fagetti A, Fozzato S, et al. Lumbar spinal stenosis treatment with Aperius perclid interspinous system. *Eur Spine J*. 2012;21(Suppl 1):S69–S74.
13. Morgalla MH, Noak N, Merkle M, et al. Lumbar spinal stenosis in elderly patients: is a unilateral microsurgical approach sufficient for decompression? *J Neurosurg Spine*. 2011;14(3):305–312.
14. Kim SH, Choi WJ, Suh JH, et al. Effects of transforaminal balloon treatment in patients with lumbar foraminal stenosis: a randomized, controlled, double-blind trial. *Pain Physician*. 2013;16(3):213–224.

SEE ALSO

Algorithm: Low Back Pain, Acute

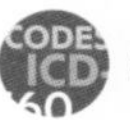

CODES

ICD10

- M48.00 Spinal stenosis, site unspecified
- M48.06 Spinal stenosis, lumbar region
- M48.04 Spinal stenosis, thoracic region

CLINICAL PEARLS

- Spinal stenosis may present as neurogenic claudication (pain, tightness, numbness, and subjective weakness of lower extremities) that mimics vascular claudication.
- Neurogenic claudication (as opposed to vascular claudication) is improved by uphill ambulation and lumbar flexion and is not alleviated by standing.
- Flexion of the spine generally relieves symptoms associated with spinal stenosis.
- Spinal extension (prolonged standing, walking downhill, and walking downstairs) can worsen symptoms of spinal stenosis.
- Urgent surgery should be considered for patients with cauda equina/conus medullaris syndrome or progressive bladder dysfunction. Most other patients with lumbar spinal stenosis can initially be managed conservatively.

SPRAIN, ANKLE

Christine M. Broszko, MD • Nathan Falk, MD

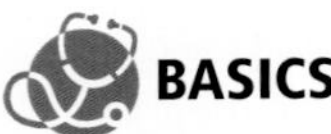

BASICS

DESCRIPTION

Ankle sprains, the most common cause of ankle injury, make up a significant proportion of sports injuries:

- There are several types of ankle sprains: lateral, medial, and syndesmotic (or high ankle sprain).
  - Lateral ankle sprains are the most common, accounting for 85% of all ankle sprains:
    - In lateral ankle sprains, the anterior talofibular ligament (ATFL) is the weakest ligament and most likely to be injured.
    - The calcaneofibular ligament (CFL) is the 2nd most likely ligament to be injured.
    - The posterior talofibular ligament (PTFL) is the least likely to be injured.
  - Medial ankle sprains (5–10%) result from an injury to the deltoid ligament.
  - Syndesmotic (or high ankle) injuries account for 5–10% of ankle sprains.
    - The syndesmosis between tibia and fibula bones consists of the anterior, posterior, and transverse tibiofibular ligaments and the interosseous membrane.
- Ankle sprains can be classified according to the degree of ligamentous disruption:
  - Grade I: mild stretching of a ligament with possible microscopic tears
  - Grade II: incomplete tear of a ligament
  - Grade III: complete ligament tear

Geriatric Considerations

Increased risk of fracture in patients with preexisting bone weakness (osteoporosis/osteopenia)

Pediatric Considerations

- Increased risk of physeal injuries instead of ligament sprain because ligaments have greater tensile strength than physes
- Inversion ankle injuries in children may have a concomitant fibular physeal injury (Salter Harris type I or higher fracture).

EPIDEMIOLOGY

Incidence

- Peak incidence in children (0–12 years old), then adolescents (13–17 years old), and finally adults (≥18 years old) (1)
- 1/2 of all ankle sprains are sports-related; highest incidence in indoor/court sports (basketball, volleyball, tennis)
- Most common sports injury
- More common in males age <30 years and females >30 years old

Prevalence

- 20% of sports injuries in the United States
- 75% of all ankle injuries are sprains.

ETIOLOGY AND PATHOPHYSIOLOGY

- Lateral ankle sprains result from an inversion force with the ankle in plantar flexion.
- Medial ankle sprains are due to forced eversion while in dorsiflexion.
- Syndesmotic sprains result from eversion stress/extreme dorsiflexion along with internal rotation of tibia.

RISK FACTORS

- Previous ankle sprain is the greatest risk factor (3–34% recurrence rate in those with a prior history of an ankle sprain).
- Postural instability, gait alterations (decreased clearance or increased ankle flexion)
- Joint laxity and decreased proprioception are not risk factors.

GENERAL PREVENTION

- Improve overall physical conditioning before participating in sports and throughout the season:
  - Training in agility and flexibility
  - Single-leg balancing
  - Proprioceptive training
- Taping and bracing may help prevent primary injury in selected sports (i.e., volleyball, basketball, football) or reinjury. Taping and bracing do not reduce sprain severity.

COMMONLY ASSOCIATED CONDITIONS

- Contusions
- Fractures
  - Fibula head fracture/dislocation (maisonneuve)
  - Base of the 5th metatarsal fracture
  - Distal fibula physeal fracture (includes Salter-Harris fractures in pediatric patients; most common type of pediatric ankle fracture)

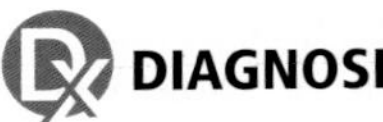

DIAGNOSIS

HISTORY

- Elicit specific mechanism of injury (inversion vs. eversion)
- Popping/snapping sensation during the injury
- Previous history of ankle injuries
- Ability to ambulate immediately after the injury
- Rapid onset of pain and swelling
- Location of pain (lateral/medial)
- Difficulty bearing weight
- Past medical history of systemic/connective tissue disorders

PHYSICAL EXAM

- Timing: Initial assessment for laxity may be insensitive secondary to pain, swelling, and muscle spasm. Repeat exam approximately 5 days after injury may improve sensitivity.
- Compare to uninjured ankle for swelling, ecchymosis, weakness, and laxity.
- Neurovascular exam
- Palpate ATFL, CFL, PTFL, and deltoid ligament for tenderness.
- Palpate lateral and medial malleolus, base of 5th metatarsal, navicular, and entire fibula.
  - High ankle sprain associated with fracture of proximal fibula
- Grade I sprain: mild swelling and pain; no laxity; able to bear weight/ambulate without pain
- Grade II sprain: moderate swelling and pain; mild laxity with end point noted; weight bearing/ambulation painful
- Grade III sprain: severe swelling, pain, and bruising; laxity with no end point; significant instability and loss of function/motion; unable to bear weight/ambulate
  - Swelling less sensitive for grade of tear in pediatric patient
- Special tests:
  - Anterior drawer test to check for ATFL laxity
  - Talar tilt test to check laxity in CFL (with inversion) or deltoid ligament (eversion)
  - Squeeze test of tibia and fibula midcalf to check for syndesmotic injury. Positive test is pain isolated to the syndesmosis; sensitivity 30%, specificity 93.5%
  - Dorsiflexion/external rotation test: Positive test is pain at syndesmosis with rotation; sensitivity 20%, specificity 85%

DIFFERENTIAL DIAGNOSIS

- Tendon injury
  - Tendinopathy/tendon tear
- Fracture and/or dislocation of the ankle/foot
- Hindfoot/midfoot injuries
- Nerve injury
- Contusion

DIAGNOSTIC TESTS & INTERPRETATION

- Ottawa Ankle Rules (nearly 100% sensitive, 30–50% specific) determine whether radiographs are needed to rule out ankle fractures (patient must be 18–55 years; certain patients, e.g., diabetics with diminished sensation, may still need radiographs):
  - Patient reports pain in malleolar zone *AND*
  - Inability to bear weight (walk ≥4 steps) immediately and in the exam room *OR*
  - Bony tenderness at tip/posterior edge of the lateral/medial malleolus
    - Note: Also Ottawa rule for foot imaging series (reported pain in the midfoot zone AND pain with palpation of navicular or base of 5th metatarsal OR inability to bear weight immediately and in the ER/office)
  - Although Ottawa rules are highly sensitive, they should not overrule clinical judgment.
- If radiographs indicated, obtain anteroposterior, lateral, and mortise ankle views.
  - Small avulsion fractures are associated with grade III sprains.
- Consider CT if radiographs are negative but clinical situation suggests occult fracture.
- MRI is gold standard for soft tissue imaging but is expensive and usually unnecessary.
  - Syndesmotic ankle sprains: may see diastasis on radiograph, therefore MRI is more sensitive
- US is a good 2nd-line imaging option with a sensitivity comparable to MRI.

Follow-Up Tests & Special Considerations

If patient condition does not improve in 6–8 weeks, consider CT, MRI, or US.

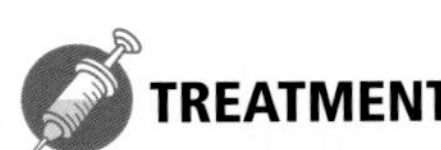

TREATMENT

GENERAL MEASURES

- The majority of grades I, II, and III lateral ankle sprains can be managed conservatively.
- Conservative therapy: PRICE (protection, rest, ice, compression, elevation)
- Protection/compression: For grade I/II sprains, lace-up bracing is superior to air-filled/gel-filled ankle brace, which is superior to elastic bandage/taping alone in providing better support and decreased swelling.
  - Note: The combination of air-filled brace and compression wrap is superior to each individually in terms of return to preinjury joint function at 10 days and 1 month for grades I and II sprains (2)[A].

- Grade III sprains should have short-term immobilization (10 days) with below the knee cast, followed by a semirigid brace (air cast). If a patient refuses casting, a 10-day period of strict non–weight bearing with air cast splint and elastic bandage is a comparable alternative if non–weight bearing is maintained.
- Rest: initially, activity as tolerated. Then, early mobilization and physical therapy may speed recovery/reduce pain:
  - Weight bearing, as tolerated
  - Consider crutches if unable to bear weight.
  - Exercises should be limited to pain-free range of motion. Initiate as early at tolerated.
  - Patients can start mobilization by tracing the alphabet with the foot in the air.
  - Elastic resistance exercises to improve balance
- Ice: Ice for first 3–7 days for pain reduction and decrease recovery time. Do not use heat in an acute injury.
- Elevation: Elevate above heart level to decrease swelling.

MEDICATION

- NSAIDs: preferably oral; however, topical forms (e.g., diclofenac 1% gel) may be used to minimize GI side effects. PRN NSAID dosing has similar outcomes to scheduled dosing with improved safety profile.
  - Naproxen 500 mg BID PRN
- Acetaminophen 650 mg q4–6h (max outpatient therapy dose: 3,250 mg/day)
- Opioids if severe pain

ISSUES FOR REFERRAL

- Malleolar/talar dome fracture
- Syndesmotic sprain
- Dislocation/subluxation
- Tendon rupture
- Ongoing instability
- Uncertain diagnosis

ADDITIONAL THERAPIES

Physical therapy:

- After the acute phase of the injury, all patients with grade II or III sprain should start physical therapy as soon as is feasible to increase range of motion, strength, flexibility, and improve proprioceptive balance (wobble board/ankle disk).
- Functional rehabilitation prevents chronic instability and speeds healing.
- Athletes should go through a sports-specific rehabilitation before returning to play.

SURGERY/OTHER PROCEDURES

- Surgery is typically reserved for treatment of complicated recurrent sprains and certain syndesmotic sprains.
- Patients with chronic ankle instability who fail functional rehabilitation or with poor tissue quality may need anatomic repair/reconstructive surgery.

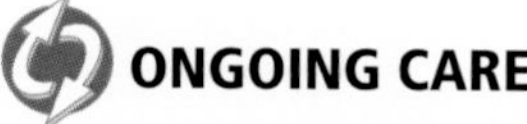

ONGOING CARE

FOLLOW-UP RECOMMENDATIONS

- Ankle-stabilizing orthoses (air stirrup braces, lace-up supports, athletic taping, etc.) should be worn for high-risk sports after a person has sustained an ankle sprain to prevent future ankle sprains.
- Moderate and severe sprains require ankle orthoses for ≥6 months while participating in sports.
- Gradual return to play for athletes with a grade I lateral ankle sprain can generally be accomplished in 1–2 weeks; grade II sprain return to play time is 2–3 weeks; grade III sprain is approximately 4 weeks.
- Syndesmotic sprains can take up to 4 times longer (approx.8–9 weeks) to heal than lateral ankle sprains.

Patient Monitoring

If athletes continue to have symptoms when they return to play or if a patient has pain for 6–8 weeks after injury, repeat examination and consider repeat radiographic imaging or MRI.

PATIENT EDUCATION

- Training on proper use of crutches
- Training on proper use of elastic bandages, brace, and/or orthoses
- Demonstrate mobilization exercises for ankle (alphabet, towel grab).

PROGNOSIS

- Earlier physical therapy and mobilization with bracing allows for faster return to daily living and/or sports.
- Poorer outcomes associated with higher grade of sprain, older patient age, and initial non-weight-bearing status
- Ligamentous strength does not return for months after the injury.

COMPLICATIONS

- Joint instability
- Intermittent swelling/pain if not properly treated
- Accumulation of cartilage damage, leading to degenerative changes
- 5–33% continue to have pain 1 year postinjury.

REFERENCES

1. Doherty C, Delahunt E, Caulfield B, et al. The incidence and prevalence of ankle sprain injury: a systematic review and meta-analysis of prospective epidemiological studies. *Sports Med*. 2014;44(1):123–140.
2. Beynnon B, Renström P, Haugh L, et al. A prospective, randomized clinical investigation of the treatment of first-time ankle sprains. *Am J Sports Med*. 2006;34(9):1401–1412.

ADDITIONAL READING

- Abernethy L. Strategies to prevent injury in adolescent sport: a systematic review. *Br J Sports Med*. 2007;41(10):627–638.
- Bleakley CM, O'Connor SR, Tully MA, et al. Effect of accelerated rehabilitation on function after ankle sprain: randomised controlled trial. *BMJ*. 2010;340:c1964.
- Dizon JM, Reyes JJ. A systematic review on the effectiveness of external ankle supports in the prevention of inversion ankle sprains among elite and recreational players. *J Sci Med Sport*. 2010;13(3):309–317.
- Farwell K, Powden C, Powell M, et al. The effectiveness of prophylactic ankle braces in reducing the incidence of acute ankle injuries in adolescent athletes: a critically appraised topic. *J Sport Rehab*. 2013;22(2):137–142.
- Hiller CE, Nightingale EJ, Lin CW, et al. Characteristics of people with recurrent ankle sprains: a systematic review with meta-analysis. *Br J Sports Med*. 2011;45(8):660–672.
- Jones MH. Acute treatment of inversion ankle sprains: immobilization versus functional treatment. *Clin Orthop Relat Res*. 2007;455:169–172.
- Kerkhoffs GM, Handoll HH, de Bie R, et al. Surgical versus conservative treatment for acute injuries of the lateral ligament complex of the ankle in adults. *Cochrane Database Syst Rev*. 2007;(2):CD000380.
- Kerkhoffs GM, van den Bekerom M, Elders LA, et al. Diagnosis, treatment and prevention of ankle sprains: an evidence-based clinical guideline. *Br J Sports Med*. 2012;46(12):854–860.
- Lamb SE, Marsh JL, Hutton JL, et al. Mechanical supports for acute, severe ankle sprain: a pragmatic, multicentre, randomised controlled trial. *Lancet*. 2009;373(9663):575–581.
- Massey T, Derry S, Moore RA, et al. Topical NSAIDs for acute pain in adults. *Cochrane Database Syst Rev*. 2010;(6):CD007402.
- Mehallo CJ, Drezner JA, Bytomski JR. Practical management: nonsteroidal antiinflammatory drug (NSAID) use in athletic injuries. *Clin J Sport Med*. 2006;16(2):170–174.
- Petersen W, Rembitzki IV, Koppenburg AG, et al. Treatment of acute ankle ligament injuries: a systematic review. *Arch Orthop Trauma Surg*. 2013;133(8):1129–1141.
- Raymond J, Nicholson LL, Hiller CE, et al. The effect of ankle taping or bracing on proprioception in functional ankle instability: a systematic review and meta-analysis. *J Sci Med Sport*. 2012;15(5):386–392.
- Waterman BR, Owens BD, Davey S, et al. The epidemiology of ankle sprains in the United States. *J Bone Joint Surg Am*. 2010;92(13):2279–2284.

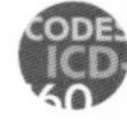

CODES

ICD10

- S96.919A Strain of unsp msl/tnd at ank/ft level, unsp foot, init
- S93.499A Sprain of other ligament of unspecified ankle, init encntr
- S93.419A Sprain of calcaneofibular ligament of unsp ankle, init

CLINICAL PEARLS

- Children are at an increased risk of physeal injuries because ligaments are stronger than physes.
- Conditioning, including proprioceptive training, before participating in sports and throughout the season helps to prevent ankle sprains.
- Functional rehabilitation, rather than total immobilization, is recommended for quicker return to sport and work.
- If patient's condition is not improving in 6–8 weeks, consider advanced imaging with CT, MRI, or US.

SPRAINS AND STRAINS

Nathan Cardoos, MD • J. Herbert Stevenson, MD

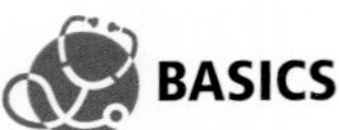

BASICS

DESCRIPTION

- *Sprains* are complete or partial ligamentous injuries either within the body of the ligament or at the site of attachment to bone:
  - Classified as grade I, II, or III (AMA Ligament Injury Classification):
    - Grade I: stretch injury without ligamentous laxity
    - Grade II: partial tear with increased ligamentous laxity but firm endpoint on exam
    - Grade III: complete tear with increased ligamentous laxity and no firm endpoint on exam
  - Usually secondary to trauma (e.g., falls, twisting injuries, motor vehicle accidents)
  - Physical exam is the key to accurate diagnosis.
- *Strains* are partial or complete disruptions of the muscle, muscle-tendon junction, or tendon:
  - Classified as
    - 1st degree: minimal damage to muscle, tendon, or musculotendinous unit
    - 2nd degree: partial tear to the muscle, tendon, or musculotendinous unit
    - 3rd degree: complete disruption of the muscle, tendon, or musculotendinous unit
  - Often associated with overuse injuries

Geriatric Considerations

More likely to see associated bony injuries due to decreased joint flexibility and increased prevalence of osteoporosis and osteopenia

Pediatric Considerations

- Sprains and strains account for 24% of pediatric injuries.
- 3 million pediatric sports injuries occur annually.
- Must be concerned about physeal/apophyseal injuries in the skeletally immature patient

EPIDEMIOLOGY

Incidence

~80% of all U.S. athletes experience a sprain or strain at some point.

Prevalence

- Ankle sprains are among the most common injuries in the primary care setting, accounting for ~30% of sports medicine clinic visits. Most ankle sprains are due to inversion injuries (lateral sprains) involving the anterior talofibular ligament.
- Predominant age
  - Sprains: any age in physically active patient
  - Strains: usually 15–40 years of age
- Predominant sex: male > female for most; female > male for sprain of acromioclavicular ligament

ETIOLOGY AND PATHOPHYSIOLOGY

- Trauma, falls, motor vehicle accidents
- Excessive exercise
- Improper footwear
- Inadequate warm-up and stretching before activity
- Poor conditioning
- Prior sprain or strain

RISK FACTORS

- Prior history of sprain or strain is greatest risk factor for future sprain/strain.
- Change in or improper footwear, protective gear, or environment (e.g., surface)
- Sudden increase in training schedule
- Tobacco use

GENERAL PREVENTION

- Appropriate warm-up and cool-down exercises
- Use proper equipment and footwear.
- Balance training programs improve proprioception and reduce the risk of ankle sprains (1)[B],(2)[A].
- Semirigid orthoses or air casts may prevent ankle sprains during high-risk sports, especially in athletes with history of sprain (3)[A].

COMMONLY ASSOCIATED CONDITIONS

- Effusions, hemarthrosis
- Stress, avulsion, or other fractures
- Syndesmotic injuries
- Contusions
- Dislocations/subluxations

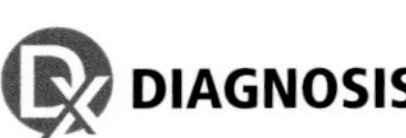

DIAGNOSIS

HISTORY

- May describe feeling or hearing pop or snap
- Obtain thorough description of mechanism of injury including activity, trauma, baseline conditioning, and prior musculoskeletal injuries.

PHYSICAL EXAM

- Gait disturbances
- Inspect for swelling, asymmetry, ecchymosis.
- Palpate for tenderness.
- Evaluate for decreased range of motion (ROM) of joint and joint instability.
- Evaluate for strength.
- Sprains
  - Grade I: tenderness without laxity; minimal pain, swelling; little ecchymosis; can bear weight
  - Grade II: tenderness with increased laxity on exam but firm endpoint; more pain, swelling; often ecchymosis; some difficulty bearing weight
  - Grade III: tenderness with increased laxity on exam and no firm end point; severe pain, swelling; obvious ecchymosis; difficulty bearing weight

DIFFERENTIAL DIAGNOSIS

- Tendonitis
- Bursitis
- Contusion
- Hematoma
- Fracture
- Osteochondral lesion
- Rheumatologic process

DIAGNOSTIC TESTS & INTERPRETATION

- Ankle
  - Anterior drawer test assesses integrity of anterior talofibular ligament.
  - Talar tilt test assesses integrity of calcaneofibular ligament.
  - Squeeze test assesses for syndesmotic injury.
- Knee
  - Lachman test assesses integrity of anterior cruciate ligament. Posterior drawer assesses integrity of posterior cruciate ligament.
  - Valgus/varus stress tests assess integrity of medial and lateral collateral ligaments, respectively.
- Shoulder
  - Positive apprehension test may indicate glenohumeral ligament sprain.
- Radiographs help rule out bony injury; stress views may be necessary. Obtain bilateral radiographs in children to rule out growth plate injuries.
- Use Ottawa foot and ankle rules (age 18–55 years) to determine if radiographs are necessary (4)[A].
- Ankle films: required if pain in the malleolar zone *and*
  - Bone tenderness in posterior aspect distal 6 cm of tibia *or* fibula *or*
  - Unable to bear weight immediately or in emergency department
- Foot films: required if midfoot zone pain is present *and*
  - Bone tenderness at base of 5th metatarsal *or*
  - Bone tenderness at navicular *or*
  - Inability to bear weight immediately or in emergency department

Follow-Up Tests & Special Considerations

- CT scan if occult fracture is suspected.
- MRI is gold standard for imaging soft tissue structures, including muscle, ligaments, and intra-articular structures. If tibiofibular syndesmotic disruption is suspected, MRI is highly accurate for diagnosis (5)[A].

Diagnostic Procedures/Other

Surgery may be required for some partial and complete sprains depending on location, mechanism, and chronicity.

TREATMENT

GENERAL MEASURES

- Acute: PRICEMM therapy (*p*rotection, relative *r*est [activity modification], *i*ce, *c*ompression, *e*levation, *m*edications, *m*odalities)
- Grade I, II ankle sprain: functional treatment with brace, orthosis, taping, elastic bandage wrap
  - Ankle braces (lace-up, stirrup-type, air cast) are a more effective functional treatment than elastic bandages or taping (6)[A].
- Grade III ankle sprain: Short period of immobilization may be needed.
- Refer for early physical therapy (7)[A].
- For high-level athletes with more extensive damage (e.g., biceps or pectoralis disruption), consider surgical referral.

MEDICATION

First Line

- Acetaminophen: not to exceed 3 g/day
- NSAIDs
  - Ibuprofen: 200–800 mg TID
  - Naproxen: 250–500 mg BID
  - Diclofenac: 75 mg BID
- Opioids may be needed acutely for severe pain.
- Acetaminophen and NSAIDs have similar efficacy in reducing pain after ankle sprains (8)[A].
- Topical diclofenac reduces pain in acute ankle sprains (9)[A].
- Platelet-rich plasma injections may aid recovery in treatment of muscle strains, but more studies are needed.

ISSUES FOR REFERRAL

- ACL sprain in athletes/physically active
- Salter-Harris physeal fractures
- Joint instability
- Tendon disruption (i.e., Achilles, biceps)
- Lack of improvement with conservative measures

ADDITIONAL THERAPIES

- Physical therapy is a useful adjunct after a sprain, and early mobilization is crucial (10)[A]:
  - Proprioception retraining
  - Core strengthening
  - Eccentric exercises
  - Theraband exercises
- After hamstring strain, frequent daily stretching and progressive agility and trunk stabilization exercises may speed recovery and reduce risk of reinjury (11)[A].

SURGERY/OTHER PROCEDURES

Casting and surgery are reserved for select partial and complete sprains. Need for surgery depends on the neurovascular supply to the injured area or the ability to attain full ROM and stability of the affected joint. The need for surgery also depends on activity level and patient preference.

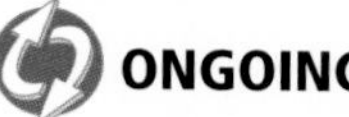

ONGOING CARE

FOLLOW-UP RECOMMENDATIONS

If the affected joint has full strength and ROM, the patient can advance activity as tolerated using pain as a guide for return to activity.

Patient Monitoring

After initial treatment, consider early rehabilitation. Place direct emphasis on limiting swelling and providing pain-free, full ROM.

DIET

Weight loss if obese

PATIENT EDUCATION

- Instructions on how to wrap with elastic bandage
- Injury prevention through proprioceptive training and physical therapy
- ROM and strengthening exercises to restore functional capacity

PROGNOSIS

Favorable with appropriate treatment and rest, 1–8 weeks (or longer) for recovery, depending on the severity of injury

COMPLICATIONS

- Chronic joint instability
- Arthritis
- Muscle contracture

REFERENCES

1. Sefton JM, Yarar C, Hicks-Little CA, et al. Six weeks of balance training improves sensorimotor function in individuals with chronic ankle instability. *J Orthop Sports Phys Ther*. 2011;41(2):81–89.
2. McGuine TA, Keene JS. The effect of a balance training program on the risk of ankle sprains in high school athletes. *Am J Sports Med*. 2006;34(7):1103–1111.
3. Handoll MM, Rowe BH, Quinn KM, et al. Withdrawn: interventions for preventing ankle ligament injuries. *Cochrane Database Syst Rev*. 2011;(5):CD000018.
4. Bachmann LH, Kolb E, Koller MT, et al. Accuracy of the Ottawa ankle rules to exclude fractures of the ankle and mid-foot: a systematic review. *BMJ*. 2003;326(7386):417.
5. Oae K, Takao M, Naito K, et al. Injury of the tibiofibular syndesmosis: value of MR imaging for diagnosis. *Radiology*. 2003;227(1):155–161.
6. Lardenoye S, Theunissen E, Cleffken B, et al. The effect of taping versus semi-rigid bracing on patient outcome and satisfaction in ankle sprains: a prospective, randomized controlled trial. *BMC Musculoskelet Disord*. 2012;13:81.
7. Bleakley CM, O'Connor SR, Tully MA, et al. Effect of accelerated rehabilitation on function after ankle sprain: a randomized control trial. *BMJ*. 2010;340:c1964.
8. Dalton JD Jr, Schweinle JE. Randomized controlled noninferiority trial to compare extended release acetaminophen and ibuprofen for the treatment of ankle sprains. *Ann Emerg Med*. 2006;48(5):615–623.
9. Lionberger DR, Joussellin E, Lanzarotti A, et al. Diclofenac epolamine topical patch relieves pain associated with ankle sprain. *J Pain Res*. 2011;4:47–53.
10. Kerkhoffs GM, Rowe BH, Assendelft WJ, et al. Immobilisation and functional treatment for acute lateral ankle ligament injuries in adults. *Cochrane Database Syst Rev*. 2002;(3):CD003762.
11. Mason DL, Dickens VA, Vail A. Rehabilitation for hamstring injuries. *Cochrane Database Syst Rev*. 2012;(12):CD004575.

ADDITIONAL READING

- Hamilton BH, Best TM. Platelet-enriched plasma and muscle strain injuries: challenges imposed by the burden of proof. *Clin J Sports Med*. 2011;21(1):31–36.
- Pritchard KA, Saliba SA. Should athletes return to activity after cryotherapy? *J Athl Train*. 2014;49(1):95–96.
- Seah R, Mani-Babu S. Managing ankle sprains in primary care: what is the best practice? A systematic review of the last 10 years of evidence. *Br Med Bull*. 2011;97:105–135.

SEE ALSO

Tendinopathy

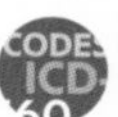

CODES

ICD10

- S93.409A Sprain of unsp ligament of unspecified ankle, init encntr
- S96.919A Strain of unsp msl/tnd at ank/ft level, unsp foot, init
- S43.50XA Sprain of unspecified acromioclavicular joint, initial encounter

CLINICAL PEARLS

For acute injury, remember PRICEMM:

- Protection of the joint
- Relative rest (activity modification)
- Apply ice
- Apply compression
- Elevate joint
- Medications for pain
- Other modalities as needed

S

SQUAMOUS CELL CARCINOMA, CUTANEOUS

Mercedes E. Gonzalez, MD, FAAD • Herbert P. Goodheart, MD

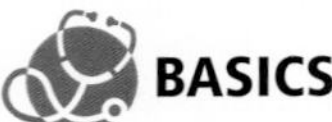

BASICS

- Squamous cell carcinoma (SCC) is a malignant epithelial tumor arising from epidermal keratinocytes. Cutaneous (nonmucous membrane) SCC is the 2nd most common form of skin cancer.
- Lesions most frequently occur on sun-exposed sites of elderly, fair-skinned individuals. Most SCCs arise in actinic keratoses (*solar keratoses*). SCCs that develop from actinic keratoses are slow-growing, minimally invasive, and unaggressive, and the prognosis is usually excellent because distant metastases are extremely rare.
- An SCC may also appear de novo without a preceding actinic keratosis or emerge from a preexisting human papillomavirus (HPV) infection (*verrucous carcinoma*).
- SCCs may develop from causes other than sun exposure such as within an old burn scar or on sites previously exposed to ionizing radiation.
- Metastases are more likely to occur in thicker tumors >6 mm deep (1)[A]. Other risk factors for metastases include lesions that arise on the ears, the vermilion border of the lips, or on mucous membranes. An SCC located on sites that received ionizing radiation on the skin of organ transplant recipients, in chronic inflammatory lesions (e.g., discoid lupus erythematosus), or in long-standing scars or cutaneous ulcers (e.g., venous stasis ulcers), or other nonhealing wounds also have an increased rate of metastasis.
- System(s) affected: skin/exocrine
- Synonym(s): squamous cell carcinoma of the skin; epidermoid carcinoma; prickle cell carcinoma

EPIDEMIOLOGY

- Predominant age: elderly population
- Predominant sex: males > females
- In the United States, 200,000 new cases each year

Incidence

- The escalating incidence in the United States is due to an increase in sun exposure in the general population, aging of the population, earlier and more frequent diagnosis of SCC, and the increase of immunosuppressed patients.
- The incidence is highest in Australia and in the Sun Belt of the United States.

ALERT

Bowen disease (SCC in situ) and frank SCC are 2 of the few skin cancers that should be considered in African Americans. Such non–sun-related SCCs tend to arise on the extremities de novo, in an old scar, or in a lesion of discoid lupus erythematosus.

ETIOLOGY AND PATHOPHYSIOLOGY

- Exact mechanisms are not established; however, SCC is thought to arise from a multistep process that begins with a single mutated keratinocyte.
- UV radiation damages skin cell nucleic acids (DNA), resulting in a mutant clone of the tumor suppressor gene, p53. This leads to an uncontrolled growth of skin cells containing a mutated p53 gene. Additional mutations in genes controlling cellular proliferation and/or death lead to squamous cell dysplasia, which then progresses to SCC in situ and later invasive SCC that has the potential for metastasis.
- Cumulative UV radiation (including tanning salons, and psoralen-UV-A [PUVA] phototherapy) over a lifetime is the major etiologic factor in SCC (2)[A].
- Epidemiologic and experimental evidence suggests other causative agents: ionizing radiation exposure, inorganic arsenic exposure, coal tar, and other oil derivatives.
- Immunosuppression by medications or disease such as HIV/AIDS

Genetics

- Persons of Irish or Scottish ancestry have the highest prevalence of SCC.
- Caucasians with the red hair/fair skin phenotype (associated with certain variant alleles of the human melanocortin-1 receptor [MC1R]) are predisposed to SCC.
- SCC is rare in people of African and Asian descent, although it is the most common form of skin cancer in these populations.

RISK FACTORS

- Older age
- Male sex: However, incidence is increasing in females due to lifestyle changes (e.g., suntan parlors, shorter dresses).
- Chronic sun exposure: SCC is noted more frequently in those with a greater degree of outdoor activity (e.g., farmers, sailors, gardeners).
- Patients with multiple actinic keratoses
- Personal or family history of skin cancer
- Northern European descent
- Fair complexion, fair hair, light eyes
- Poor tanning ability, with tendency to burn
- Organ transplant recipients, chronic immunosuppression
- Exposure to chemical carcinogens (e.g., arsenic, tar) or ionizing radiation
- Smoking (3)[A]
- Therapeutic UV and ionizing radiation exposure
- Defects in cell-mediated immunity related to lymphoproliferative disorders (chronic lymphocytic leukemia [CLL], lymphoma)
- HPV infection
- Chronic scarring and inflammatory conditions
- Specific genodermatoses (e.g., xeroderma pigmentosum, oculocutaneous albinism, and dystrophic epidermolysis bullosa)

GENERAL PREVENTION

Sun-avoidance measures: sunscreens, hats, clothing, and sunglasses with UV protection; tinted windshields and side windows in cars; sun-protective garments

COMMONLY ASSOCIATED CONDITIONS

- Some investigators consider an actinic keratosis to be an early SCC, although relatively few ultimately are found to develop into an SCC.
- Actinic cheilitis and leukoplakia of the mucous membranes of the lips
- Keratoacanthoma
- Cutaneous horn
- Actinic keratoses may be seen in association with the following:
  - Xeroderma pigmentosum, albinism, and vitiligo
  - Immunosuppression
  - Chronic skin ulcers, preexisting scars, burns

DIAGNOSIS

PHYSICAL EXAM

Lesions occur chiefly on chronically sun-exposed areas:

- Face and backs of the forearms and hands
- Bald areas of the scalp and top of ears in men
- The sun-exposed "V" of the neck as well as the posterior neck below the occipital hairline
- In elderly females, lesions tend to occur on the legs and other sun-exposed locations.
- In African Americans, equal frequency in sun-exposed and unexposed areas
- Clinical appearance:
  - Generally slow-growing, firm, hyperkeratotic papules, nodules, or plaques
  - Most SCCs are asymptomatic, although bleeding, pain, and tenderness may be noted.
  - Lesions may have a smooth, verrucous, or papillomatous surface.
  - Varying degrees of ulceration, erosion, crust, or scale
  - Color is often red to brown, tan, or pearly (indistinguishable from basal cell carcinoma).
- Clinical variants of SCC:
  - Bowen disease (SCC in situ): solitary lesion that resembles a scaly psoriatic plaque
  - Invasive SCC: often a raised, firm papule, nodule, or plaque. Lesions may be smooth, verrucous, or papillomatous, with varying degrees of ulceration, erosion, crust, or scale.
  - Cutaneous horn: SCC with an overlying cutaneous horn. A cutaneous horn represents a fingernail plate-like keratinization produced by the SCC. Bowen disease may also produce a cutaneous horn on its surface.
  - Erythroplasia of Queyrat refers to Bowen disease of the glans penis, which manifests as one or more velvety red plaques.
  - Subungual SCC appear as hyperkeratotic lesions under the nail plate or on surrounding periungual skin, often mimicking warts (4)[C].
  - Marjolin ulcer: an SCC evolving from a new area of ulceration or elevation at site of a scar or ulcer
  - HPV-associated SCC: virally induced SCC most commonly as a new or enlarging warty growth on penis, vulva, perianal area, or periungual region
  - Verrucous carcinoma: subtype of SCC that is extremely well differentiated, can be locally destructive, but rarely metastasizes. Lesions are "cauliflower-like" verrucous nodules or plaques.
  - Basaloid SCC: less common than typical SCC; seen more often in men aged 40–70 years.

ALERT

Subungual SCC (4)[C]: Such lesions typically mimic warts.

DIFFERENTIAL DIAGNOSIS

- Solar keratosis: Early SCC lesions may be clinically difficult, if not impossible, to distinguish from a precursor actinic keratosis.
- Basal cell carcinoma may be indistinguishable from an SCC, particularly if the lesion is ulcerated.
- Keratoacanthoma: This lesion also may be clinically and histopathologically impossible to differentiate from an SCC; considered by some to be a low-grade variant of an SCC.
- Verruca vulgaris: The appearance of common warts is often similar to that of SCC lesions.
- Seborrheic keratosis
- Pyoderma gangrenosum
- Venous stasis ulcer
- Chemical or thermal burn

DIAGNOSTIC TESTS & INTERPRETATION

Initial Tests (lab, imaging)

Patients with lymphadenopathy should be evaluated for metastases with CT scanning, MRI, US, or PET.

Diagnostic Procedures/Other
- Surgical biopsy to ensure diagnosis: shave, punch, excisional, incisional biopsy
- Sentinel lymph node biopsy rarely is used to identify micrometastases in patients with high-risk SCC and clinically negative nodes. Whether the early detection of lymph node metastasis leads to enhanced survival in SCC is unknown.

Test Interpretation
- Noninvasive SCC is characterized by an intraepidermal proliferation of atypical keratinocytes. Hyperkeratosis, acanthosis, and confluent parakeratosis are seen within the epidermis. Cellular atypia, including pleomorphism, hyperchromatic nuclei, and mitoses are prominent. Atypical keratinocytes may be found in the basal layer and often extend deeply down the hair follicles, but they do not invade the dermis.
- In the in situ type of SCC (Bowen disease), atypia involves the full thickness of the epidermis but the basement membrane remains intact.
- An invasive SCC penetrates through the basement membrane into the dermis. It has various levels of anaplasia and may manifest relatively few to multiple mitoses and display varying degrees of differentiation, such as keratinization.
- Poorly differentiated tumors are clinically more aggressive. SCCs proliferate 1st by local invasion. Metastases, when they do occur, spread via local lymph ducts to local lymph nodes.

ALERT

Melanoma: An amelanotic melanoma and ulcerated melanoma may also be impossible to distinguish from an SCC.

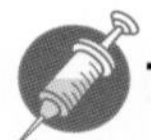

TREATMENT

MEDICATION

First Line
- Total excision: preferred method for SCCs, permitting histologic diagnosis of the tumor margins
- Electrocautery (electrodesiccation) and curettage (ED&C)
  - Best for small lesions (generally <1 cm) on flat surfaces (e.g., forehead, cheek) and SCC in situ (Bowen disease). ED&C may be used to treat superficially invasive SCCs without high-risk characteristics, but it is not appropriate for certain high-risk anatomic locations.
- Cryosurgery with LN_2 in selected lesions, such as SCC in situ
- Micrographic (Mohs) surgery is a microscopically controlled method of removing skin cancers that allows for controlled excision and maximum preservation of normal tissue. It has the highest cure rate (94–99%) of all surgical treatments. Mohs surgery may be indicated for the following:
  - Large, recurrent or invasive SCCs (e.g., to bone or cartilage)
  - Lesions with a poorly delineated clinical border
  - Locations where preservation of normal tissue is extremely important (e.g., tip of the nose, eyelids, ala nasi, ears, lips, and glans penis)
- Radiation therapy is a primary treatment option that is generally restricted to older patients who are physically debilitated or are unable to undergo or refuse to undergo excisional surgery.

Second Line
- Immunotherapy with topical imiquimod (Aldara) 5% cream has been successfully used for the treatment of SCC in situ (Bowen disease), actinic keratoses, genital warts, and superficial basal cell carcinomas (5)[A].
- Topical chemotherapy: topical formulations of 5-fluorouracil (5-FU) (5)[A]
- Intralesional 5-FU and bleomycin has also been used successfully to treat SCCs.
- Photodynamic therapy (PDT): PDT involves application of a photosensitizer (given topically or systemically) followed by exposure to a light source. Used primarily to treat large numbers of solar keratoses not recommended for treatment of invasive SCCs.
- In patients with multiple or recurrent SCCs, or those at high risk, such as organ transplant recipients, chemoprevention with systemic retinoids (6)[C], such as acitretin, may be effective for reducing the number of new SCCs, treating existing SCCs, or at reducing the risk of recurrence after treatment.

ADDITIONAL THERAPIES
For metastatic SCC, oral 5-FU has been used alone or in combination with SC interferon. More recently, epidermal growth factor receptor (EGFR) inhibitors, such as cetuximab, are used in combination with systemic chemotherapy for metastatic disease.

SURGERY/OTHER PROCEDURES
- Complete lymphadenectomy of the draining nodal basin for high-risk tumors
- Metastatic disease requires aggressive management by a multidisciplinary team, involving plastic, ENT/maxillofacial, and general surgeons, or a surgical oncologist.

ONGOING CARE

FOLLOW-UP RECOMMENDATIONS

Patient Monitoring
Skin exam every month for 3 months, 6 months after treatment, and then yearly

PATIENT EDUCATION
Skin self-exam: Encourage sun-avoidance techniques, protective clothing, sunscreens, etc. Artificial tanning devices should be avoided.

PROGNOSIS
- For low-risk SCCs: a 90–95% cure rate with appropriate treatment
- Overall, head and neck lesions have better prognosis; however, lip and ear lesions metastasize more frequently when compared with other sites.
- The ability to produce scale (*keratinization*) indicates a tendency for a lesion to be more differentiated and less likely to metastasize.
- Softer, nonkeratinizing lesions are not as well differentiated and thus are more likely to spread.
- Lesions ≥2 cm are more likely to recur.
- SCCs that arise in areas of non–sun-exposed skin or have a greater tendency to metastasize
- An SCC arising on a mucous membrane or in a chronic ulcer should be regarded as potentially metastatic.
- Recurrence rate and mortality is greater in immunosuppressed patients, especially solid organ transplant recipients.
- SCCs that are deeply invasive (≥6 mm in SC fat), or have perineural involvement are more likely to metastasize.
- When SCC does metastasize, it usually occurs within several years from the time of diagnosis and involves draining lymph nodes.
- Once nodal metastasis of cutaneous SCC has occurred, the overall 5-year survival rate has historically been in the range of 25–35%.

COMPLICATIONS
- Untreated, an SCC becomes indurated, with a tendency to ooze, ulcerate, or bleed.
- Local recurrence
- Metastatic disease

REFERENCES

1. Brantsch KD, Meisner C, Schönfisch B, et al. Analysis of risk factors determining prognosis of cutaneous squamous-cell carcinoma: a prospective study. *Lancet Oncol*. 2008;9(8):713–720.
2. Archier E, Devaux S, Castela E, et al. Carcinogenic risks of psoralen UV-A therapy and narrowband UV-B therapy in chronic plaque psoriasis: a systematic literature review. *J Eur Acad Dermatol Venereol*. 2012;26(Suppl 3):22–31.
3. Leonardi-Bee J, Ellison T, Bath-Hextall F. Smoking and the risk of nonmelanoma skin cancer: systematic review and meta-analysis. *Arch Dermatol*. 2012;148(8):939–946.
4. Riddel C, Rashid R, Thomas V. Ungual and periungual human papillomavirus-associated squamous cell carcinoma: a review. *J Am Acad Dermatol*. 2011;64(6):1147–1153.
5. Micali G, Lacarrubba F, Nasca MR, et al. Topical pharmacotherapy for skin cancer: part II. Clinical applications. *J Am Acad Dermatol*. 2014;70(6): 979.e1–979.e12.
6. Greenberg JN, Zwald FO. Management of skin cancer in solid-organ transplant recipients: a multidisciplinary approach. *Dermatol Clin*. 2011;29(2):231–241.

ADDITIONAL READING

- Martorell-Calatayud A, Sanmartín Jimenez O, Cruz Mojarrieta J, et al. Cutaneous squamous cell carcinoma: defining the high-risk variant. *Actas Dermosifiliogr*. 2013;104(5):367–379.
- Wang J, Aldabagh B, Yu J, et al. Role of human papillomavirus in cutaneous squamous cell carcinoma: a meta-analysis. *J Am Acad Dermatol*. 2014;70(4):621–629.

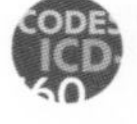

CODES

ICD10
- C44.92 Squamous cell carcinoma of skin, unspecified
- C44.320 Squamous cell carcinoma of skin of unspecified parts of face
- C44.42 Squamous cell carcinoma of skin of scalp and neck

CLINICAL PEARLS
- SCCs that develop from actinic keratoses are generally unaggressive.
- Unlike most basal cell carcinomas, SCCs of the skin are associated with a risk of metastasis, especially those arising on mucous membranes, chronic ulcers, or in immunocompromised patients.
- A subungual SCC can easily be mistaken for a wart.

STEATOHEPATITIS, NONALCOHOLIC

Candace Y. Pau, MD • Theodore X. O'Connell, MD

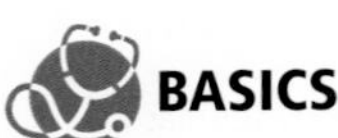

BASICS

DESCRIPTION

- Nonalcoholic steatohepatitis (NASH) is a chronic liver disease causing hepatocellular injury and inflammation due to accumulation of fat within the liver.
- NASH is part of the spectrum of nonalcoholic fatty liver disease (NAFLD), which is defined as the presence of hepatic steatosis (on imaging or histology) without secondary causes for hepatic fat accumulation (pathologic alcohol, use of steatotoxic medications, or hereditary disorders).
- Unlike NAFLD with simple steatosis, NASH is potentially progressive and may result in cirrhosis.

EPIDEMIOLOGY

- NAFLD is the most common form of chronic liver disease in the Western world, and its global prevalence is increasing.
- Most studies of NAFLD prevalence in the United States report rates of 10–35% (1).
- The prevalence of NASH in the United States and other Western countries has been reported as 3–5% (2).
- The prevalence of NAFLD increases with age.
- Age-adjusted prevalence of NAFLD is highest in Mexican Americans, followed by non-Hispanic whites, and was lowest in non-Hispanic blacks (3).
- The incidence of NAFLD is underreported and highly variable (1).

ETIOLOGY AND PATHOPHYSIOLOGY

- NAFLD is the hepatic manifestation of metabolic syndrome.
- Insulin resistance leads to decreased inhibition of lipolysis and increased de novo lipogenesis. Free fatty acids are then inappropriately shifted to nonadipose tissues including the liver.
- Apoptosis and oxidative stress also contribute to the development and progression of NASH.
- Although NAFLD and NASH can remain stable for many years, a second hepatic insult (e.g., cytokine-mediated inflammation, lipid peroxidation, or apoptosis) may trigger the progression to cirrhosis.

RISK FACTORS

- NAFLD occurs in individuals with components of metabolic syndrome.
- Metabolic syndrome increases the risk of NAFLD 4–11-fold.
- Insulin resistance plays a central role in the pathogenesis of NAFLD and the metabolic syndrome.
- Other risk factors
  - Male gender
  - Hypothyroidism, hypopituitarism, sleep apnea, and polycystic ovary syndrome
  - Procedures leading to rapid weight loss (small bowel resections, gastric bypass, and jejunal bypass) may increase risk of NAFLD.
  - Medications: corticosteroids, synthetic estrogens, amiodarone, tamoxifen, methotrexate
  - Other conditions: Wilson disease, hemochromatosis, abetalipoproteinemia, galactosemia, glycogen storage diseases

GENERAL PREVENTION

- Maintain ideal weight, normal lipoprotein, and serum glucose profiles.
- Avoid alcohol.
- Avoid hepatotoxic substances.

COMMONLY ASSOCIATED CONDITIONS

Obesity, type 2 diabetes mellitus, hypertension, hypertriglyceridemia

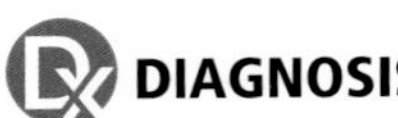

DIAGNOSIS

HISTORY

- Most patients with NAFLD are asymptomatic.
- In symptomatic patients, malaise, fatigue, nausea, and right upper quadrant discomfort are most common.
- Review medical history for comorbid conditions associated with insulin resistance or metabolic syndrome.
- Diagnosis of NAFLD requires no recent or ongoing history of significant alcohol consumption (>21 drinks per week in men, >14 drinks per week in women) (2)[C].

PHYSICAL EXAM

- Hepatomegaly is the most common physical finding in subjects with NAFLD and is present in 75% of patients with NASH.
- Few patients present with peripheral stigmata of chronic liver disease or portal hypertension (palmar erythema, caput medusa, telangiectasias, Dupuytren contracture).

DIFFERENTIAL DIAGNOSIS

Viral hepatitis, alcoholic hepatitis, autoimmune hepatitis, hemochromatosis, Wilson disease, α_1-antitrypsin deficiency

DIAGNOSTIC TESTS & INTERPRETATION

Initial Tests (lab, imaging)

- Liver enzyme tests
  - NAFLD is associated with AST and ALT values under 250 IU/L and/or modest elevation of alkaline phosphatase (4).
  - ALT or AST value >300 IU/L should raise suspicion of alternate pathology (toxins, medications, or infection) (4).
  - AST:ALT ratio <1 suggests NAFLD, whereas AST:ALT ratio >2 suggests alcoholic liver disease. Values between 1 and 2 may be present with either alcoholic liver disease or NASH with advanced fibrosis (4).
- Serum albumin, prothrombin, and bilirubin levels are usually normal.
- Mildly elevated serum ferritin is common (nonspecific inflammatory marker) and does not necessarily indicate increased iron stores.
- Sonographic features of NAFLD are nonspecific and include increased hepatic parenchymal echotexture and vascular blurring (PPV 62%) (2).
- Hepatic steatosis can be diagnosed with CT imaging (decreased hepatic parenchymal attenuation relative to the spleen, PPV 76%) or MRI. Noninvasive imaging cannot distinguish between fatty liver and steatohepatitis, and the stage of fibrosis cannot be determined unless features of portal hypertension are present (4).
- The NAFLD fibrosis score (http://nafldscore.com) is based on 6 variables (age, body mass index [BMI], hyperglycemia, platelet count, albumin, AST:ALT ratio) and is clinically useful for identifying patients with bridging fibrosis and/or cirrhosis (2)[B].

Follow-Up Tests & Special Considerations

- Exclude coexisting etiologies for liver disease: viral hepatitis, hemochromatosis, autoimmune liver disease, and Wilson disease.

Diagnostic Procedures/Other

- Liver biopsy is the gold standard for characterizing liver histology in patients with suspected NAFLD.
- Consider biopsy in patients with NAFLD who are at increased risk of steatohepatitis and advanced fibrosis or in whom competing etiologies for hepatic steatosis and coexisting chronic liver disease cannot otherwise be excluded (2)[B].

Test Interpretation

- Histologic diagnosis of NASH is based on a composite pattern of injury rather than a single defining feature.
- The NAFLD Activity Score (NAS) is based on the presence/severity of the following histologic features:
  - Steatosis (0–3)
  - Lobular inflammation (0–3)
  - Ballooning (0–3)
- Most patients with NASH have an NAS of 5 or greater, whereas NAS of 2 or less is usually not associated with a diagnosis of NASH (5)[B].

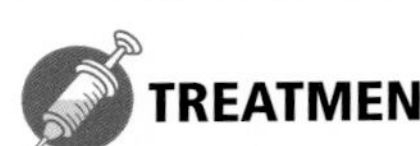

TREATMENT

Treatment entails the following: 1) maximizing control of associated comorbidities, 2) avoiding factors that promote progression of liver disease, and 3) specific treatment for NASH.

GENERAL MEASURES

- Weight loss of at least 3–5% of body weight improves steatosis. Greater weight loss (up to 10%) appears necessary to improve necroinflammation (2)[B].
- Avoid alcohol and hepatotoxic substances.

MEDICATION

No firmly established evidence-based treatment exists for NASH.

First Line

- Intensive lifestyle changes leading to weight loss consistently show the most benefit.

- Vitamin E administered at daily doses of 800 IU/day improves liver histology in nondiabetic adults with biopsy-proven NASH and should be considered as 1st therapy (2)[B].
- Vitamin E is not recommended to treat NASH in diabetic patients, NAFLD without liver biopsy, NASH cirrosis, or cryptogenic cirrhosis (2)[C].
- HMG CoA reductase inhibitors (statins) can be used to treat dyslipidemia in patients with NAFLD and NASH but should not be used specifically to treat NASH (2)[B].

Second Line

- Pharmacologic treatment of obesity may be considered in those with a BMI >30 kg/m^2 or a BMI >27 kg/m^2 with associated obesity-related comorbidities (4).
- Pioglitazone can be used to treat steatohepatitis in patients with biopsy-proven NASH, but the long-term safety and efficacy of pioglitazone in patients with NASH is not established, and most patients in this trial were nondiabetic (2)[B].
- The use of metformin and ursodeoxycholic acid are not recommended for treatment of NAFLD/NASH (2)[A,B].

Pediatric Considerations

- NAFLD has been reported in children as early as 2 years of age and NASH-related cirrhosis as early as age 8 years (2).
- Screening for NAFLD in overweight and obese children is controversial. A recent expert committee recommends biannual screening with liver enzyme measurements in overweight children (2)[B].
- Children with fatty liver who are very young or who are not overweight should be tested for other causes of liver disease, such as fatty acid oxidation defects, lysosomal storage diseases, peroxisomal disorders, hepatitis, Wilson disease, and autoimmune diseases (2)[C].
- Liver biopsy in children with suspected NAFLD should be performed when the diagnosis is unclear, where there is possibility of multiple diagnoses, or before starting therapy with potentially hepatotoxic medications (2)[B].
- 1st-line treatment for children with NAFLD is weight loss and lifestyle modifications (2)[B].

ISSUES FOR REFERRAL

Referral to a hepatologist with/without liver biopsy helps with staging and prognosis.

SURGERY/OTHER PROCEDURES

- The lack of randomized clinical trials precludes assessment of the benefits and harms of bariatric surgery as a therapeutic approach for patients with NASH (6)[A].
- Although abdominal weight loss surgery coupled with rapid weight loss has been implicated as contributing to development of NASH, it is not contraindicated in otherwise eligible obese patients (2)[A].

COMPLEMENTARY & ALTERNATIVE MEDICINE

- Probiotic therapies can reduce liver aminotransferases, total cholesterol, and TNF-α and improve insulin resistance in NAFLD patients (7)[A].
- Omega-3 fatty acids may be used to treat hypertriglyceridemia in patients with NAFLD (2,8)[B].

ONGOING CARE

FOLLOW-UP RECOMMENDATIONS

- All patients should be tested for hepatitis A and B and vaccinated, if appropriate.
- Patients with NASH cirrhosis should be considered for hepatocellular carcinoma screening according to the AASLD/ACG practice guidelines (http://www.aasld.org/practiceguidelines/Documents/Bookmarked%20Practice%20Guidelines/HCCUpdate2010.pdf) (2)[B].
- Current evidence does not support routinely repeat liver biopsies in patients with NAFLD or NASH (2)[C].

Patient Monitoring

Patients with fatty liver disease should be seen regularly to detect disease progression through the following:

- Patient complaints (encephalopathy, ascites, fatigue)
- Physical exam findings (spider telangiectasia, palmar erythema, splenomegaly)
- Laboratory findings (changes in liver enzyme tests, decreasing platelets, elevated bilirubin, decreasing albumin)
- Incidental imaging study findings (cirrhotic liver, splenomegaly, varices, ascites)

DIET

Restrictions of total calories, simple carbohydrates, and alcohol are required to control diabetes, weight, and lipids.

PATIENT EDUCATION

Ongoing follow-up and motivational interviewing to assess lifelong changes in diet, exercise, and alcohol use

PROGNOSIS

- 25–35% of NASH patients develop fibrosis, whereas 9–20% develop cirrhosis (3).
- Patients with NAFLD have greater all-cause mortality. The most common causes of death are cardiovascular disease, malignancy, and hepatic failure.

COMPLICATIONS

Steatohepatitis may progress to cirrhosis, with complications including variceal bleeding, ascites, encephalopathy, liver failure, and development of hepatocellular carcinoma.

REFERENCES

1. Vernon G, Baranova A, Younossi ZM. Systematic review: the epidemiology and natural history of non-alcoholic fatty liver disease and non-alcoholic steatohepatitis in adults. *Aliment Pharmacol Ther*. 2011;34(3):274–285.
2. Chalasani N, Younossi Z, Lavine JE, et al. The diagnosis and management of non-alcoholic fatty liver disease: practice guideline by the American Association for the Study of Liver Diseases, American College of Gastroenterology, and the American Gastroenterological Association. *Hepatology*. 2012;55(6):2005–2023.
3. Schneider AL, Lazo M, Selvin E, et al. Racial differences in nonalcoholic fatty liver disease in the U.S. population. *Obesity (Silver Spring)*. 2014;22(1):292–299.
4. Ramesh S, Sanyal AJ. Evaluation and management of non-alcoholic steatohepatitis. *J Hepatol*. 2005;42(Suppl 1):S2–S12.
5. Bondini S, Kleiner DE, Goodman ZD, et al. Pathologic assessment of non-alcoholic fatty liver disease. *Clin Liver Dis*. 2007;11(1):17–23, vii.
6. Chavez-Tapia NC, Tellez-Avila FI, Barrientos-Gutierrez T, et al. Bariatric surgery for non-alcoholic steatohepatitis in obese patients. *Cochrane Database of Syst Rev*. 2010;(1):CD007340.
7. Ma YY, Li L, Yu CH, et al. Effects of probiotics on nonalcoholic fatty liver disease: a meta-analysis. *World J Gastroenterol*. 2013;19(40):6911–6918.
8. Dasarathy S, Dasarathy J, Khiyami A, et al. Double-blind randomized placebo-controlled clinical trial of omega 3 fatty acids for the treatment of diabetic patients with nonalcoholic steatohepatitis. *J Clin Gastroenterol*. 2015;49(2):137–144.

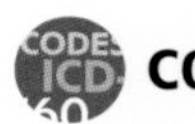

CODES

ICD10

- K75.81 Nonalcoholic steatohepatitis (NASH)
- K76.0 Fatty (change of) liver, not elsewhere classified

CLINICAL PEARLS

- Prevalence of NAFLD and NASH is higher in patients with metabolic syndrome or any one of its components (diabetes, obesity, hypertriglyceridemia).
- Liver biopsy is the gold standard for diagnosis.
- Lifestyle changes to treat components of the metabolic syndrome are central to the treatment of NAFLD.
- Vitamin E should be considered as 1st-line therapy in nondiabetic patients with biopsy-proven NASH.
- Statins should be considered in patients who have NAFLD with dyslipidemia.

STRESS FRACTURE

Nandhini Veeraraghavan, MD

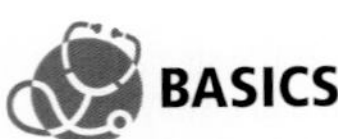

BASICS

DESCRIPTION

- Stress fractures are overuse injuries caused by cumulative microdamage from repetitive bone loading.
- Stress fractures occur in different situations:
  - Fatigue fracture: abnormal stress applied to normal bone (e.g., young college athletes or new military recruits with increased physical activity demands and inadequate conditioning)
  - Insufficiency fracture: normal stress applied to structurally abnormal bone (e.g., femoral neck fracture in osteopenic bone)
  - Combination fracture: abnormal stress applied to abnormal bone (e.g., female long-distance runners with premature osteoporosis from female athletic triad)
- Weight-bearing bones of the lower extremity are most commonly affected at the following sites:
  - Tibia
  - Metatarsal bones
  - Fibula
  - Navicular
  - Femoral neck
  - Pars interarticularis
- Less commonly affected sites:
  - Pelvis
  - Calcaneus
  - Ribs
  - Ulna
- High-risk stress fractures occur in zones of tension or areas with poor blood supply and are more likely to result in fracture displacement and/or nonunion. High-risk sites include the following:
  - Tension side of femoral neck
  - Anterior tibial diaphysis
  - Sesamoids
  - Pars interarticularis of lumbar spine (L4, L5)
  - 5th metatarsal at metaphyseal–diaphyseal junction
  - Proximal 2nd metatarsal
  - Medial malleolus
  - Tarsal navicular
  - Patella
  - Talar neck
- Synonym(s): march fracture; fatigue fracture

EPIDEMIOLOGY

Incidence

- Greatest incidence in 15–27-year-old patients
- Females more commonly affected than males
- Affects 9–21% of track and field athletes annually
- Accounts for as many as 8% of visits to sports medicine and orthopedic clinics
- Occurs in <1% of general population

Prevalence

- Affects 5% of military recruits
- Affects 1–3% of college athletes

ETIOLOGY AND PATHOPHYSIOLOGY

- Bone is a dynamic tissue that is constantly remodeling in response to applied physiologic stress.
- Repetitive loading or overuse causes microfractures that can't heal due to imbalance between bone resorption and bone formation.
- If microdamage accumulates in excess of reparation, bony fatigue leads to stress fracture.

RISK FACTORS

- Intrinsic
  - Female athlete triad (low energy availability with or without disordered eating, menstrual dysfunction, and low bone mineral density)
  - History of previous stress fracture
  - History of osteoporosis, osteomalacia, rheumatoid arthritis, corticosteroid therapy
  - Skeletal malalignment: pes cavus, pes planus, leg length discrepancies, excessive forefoot varus, tarsal coalitions, prominent posterior calcaneal process, tight heel cords
  - Increased vertical loading rate (e.g., heel-to-toe running instead of forefoot striking)
  - Muscle fatigue and decreased lean muscle mass
  - Extremes of body size and composition
  - Previous inactivity or low aerobic fitness
- Extrinsic
  - Type of exercise—running, track and field, basketball, gymnastics, soccer, and dance are highest risk.
  - Rapid increase in mileage, running pace, or training cycles
  - Inappropriate footwear
  - Hard training surface
  - Inadequate recovery or rest and training with fatigued muscle
- Tobacco use

GENERAL PREVENTION

- Avoid abrupt increases in physical activity (no more than 10% increase in load per week).
- Reduce intensity and duration of activity if new-onset pain.
- Proper footwear
- Increasing dynamic physical activity (jumping; plyometric training) increases bone density and resistance to mechanical stress.
- Decrease vertical loading rate either by switching to forefoot strike style running or (if continuing with heel-to-toe strike) by using a heel pad insert.
- Shock-absorbing foot inserts may help.
- Increasing calcium and vitamin D (skim milk and low-fat dairy product) intake may reduce the rate of stress fractures in female runners/military recruits.

COMMONLY ASSOCIATED CONDITIONS

- Osteoporosis/osteopenia
- Female athlete triad
- Metabolic bone disorders

DIAGNOSIS

HISTORY

- Insidious onset of vague bony pain over period of weeks worsened with physical activity
- Rest initially relieves pain.
- If untreated, pain progresses and may occur earlier during training sessions or even at rest. Pain also becomes more localized.
- History of recent change in training intensity, alteration in training terrain, and/or footwear
- Assess dietary practices: energy availability, disordered eating, and weight fluctuations.
- Assess menstrual history: menarche, oligomenorrhea, or amenorrhea.

PHYSICAL EXAM

- Height, weight, BMI, and any stigmata of disordered eating (cold extremities, hypercarotenemia, lanugo hair, calluses on back of fingers, poor oral hygiene, parotid gland hypertrophy, bradycardia, or orthostatic hypotension)
- Antalgic gait
- Point tenderness or percussion tenderness over injury site
- Placing a vibrating tuning fork over the fracture site may intensify pain.
- Swelling may be present.
- Specific tests:
  - Hop test for tibial stress fracture: cannot hop on one leg 10 times; if able to perform test, consider shin splints (medial tibial stress syndrome)
  - Fulcrum test for femoral stress fracture: With patient seated, provoke pain by applying downward force on the distal femur while other hand uses the midthigh as fulcrum on femoral shaft.
  - Single-leg hyperextension (Stork) test for pars interarticularis fracture of lumbar spine: Stand on leg of symptomatic side and extend lumbar spine. Positive if painful.
- Anatomic malalignment may be present (leg length discrepancy, pes planus/cavus).

DIFFERENTIAL DIAGNOSIS

- Shin splints (medial tibial stress syndrome—pain resolves with rest; stress fracture pain does not)
- Infection (osteomyelitis)
- Soft tissue injury (sprain, tendonitis, and periostitis)
- Compartment syndrome
- Bony fracture
- Neoplasm (osteoid osteoma)
- Entrapment syndromes
- Intermittent claudication

DIAGNOSTIC TESTS & INTERPRETATION

- None unless clinically indicated for suspected disease (e.g., female athlete triad, hyperparathyroidism, and vitamin D deficiency)
- Plain films:
  - First line in suspected stress fracture
  - Findings typically seen 2–8 weeks after onset of pain.
  - Sensitivity during early stages (1–2 weeks) may be as low as 10%.
  - May see periosteal callus, "gray cortex sign" (region of decreased cortical intensity), osteopenia, endosteal reaction, or ill-defined cortical margin
  - Severe cases may show discrete fracture.

Follow-Up Tests & Special Considerations

- MRI:
  - Gold standard for imaging stress fractures
  - Very sensitive
  - Better evaluation of exact anatomic location and extent of injury
- Bone scan:
  - Sensitive but nonspecific for stress fracture
  - Should not be used to assess healing process

- CT scan:
  - Less sensitive than MRI or bone scan for early stress fractures but has an important role in evaluating occult fractures of foot, tibia, carpal scaphoid, and pars interarticularis
  - Can distinguish diseases (osteoid osteoma, malignancy, and osteomyelitis) that mimic stress fracture on bone scan
  - Bony detail provided by CT scan allows differentiation of complete versus incomplete fracture especially when MRI is equivocal.
- US:
  - Not routinely used but may be of particular use in the evaluation of metatarsal stress fracture to distinguish from other causes of metatarsalgia (e.g., Morton neuroma)
- Classification by radiographic grading (1)
  - Grade I: normal x-ray, positive STIR short time inversion recovery (STIR) MRI
  - Grade II: normal x-ray, positive STIR + positive T2-weighted MRI
  - Grade III: discrete line or discrete periosteal reaction on x-ray, positive T1/T2-weighted MRI but with no definite cortical break
  - Grade IV: fracture or periosteal reaction on x-ray, positive T1/T2-weighted fracture line

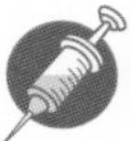

TREATMENT

- Protection, rest, ice, compression, and elevation (PRICE) for acute pain and edema
- Decrease activity to the level of pain-free functioning.
- Pain at rest or with gentle range of motion (ROM) may require temporary immobilization.
- Painful ambulation is criterion for crutches with periodic walking trial.
- Pneumatic leg brace is effective in decreasing the return-to-play time for tibial shaft stress fracture (2)[C].
- For low-risk stress fracture, slowly increase impact loading once ambulation and daily activities are pain free. Progression of activity depends on the individual and should be modified according to symptoms (3,4).
- High-risk fractures often require immediate immobilization and a period of non–weight-bearing. Many patients will require early surgical intervention to avoid nonunion and facilitate earlier return to sport (5,6).
- In bisphosphonate-associated femoral stress fracture, prophylactic nail fixation may avoid fracture completion, shorten hospital stay, and decrease subsequent morbidity (7)[C].

MEDICATION

First Line

- Calcium and vitamin D supplementation should be initiated when dietary intake is inadequate or deficiencies are found.
- Acetaminophen
- NSAIDs are beneficial for pain and inflammation but may adversely affect fracture healing and should, therefore, be used sparingly.
- Bisphosphonates theoretically could treat stress fractures by suppressing bone remodeling. There is no conclusive evidence to prove that this improves fracture healing in humans. Currently, only case reports have shown benefit (8)[A].

ISSUES FOR REFERRAL

Orthopedic consultation for high-risk fractures, failure to improve with standard treatment, evidence of nonunion within 3–4 weeks, or inability to tolerate rehabilitation

ADDITIONAL THERAPIES

- Electrical stimulator may be an adjunct for delayed union and nonunion.
- Extracorporeal shock wave therapy (ESWT) and pulsed US may have some potential benefits but require additional study (9)[A].
- Physical therapy:
  - Correct training errors and inappropriate mechanics predisposing to stress fracture.
  - Strengthen muscles around the site of stress fracture.
  - Encourage cross training to maintain cardiovascular fitness.
  - Correct anatomic variations.
  - Antigravity treadmills

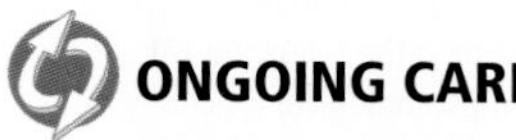

ONGOING CARE

FOLLOW-UP RECOMMENDATIONS

- Once the patient is pain free, low-impact training can start and be advanced gently as tolerated.
- Once running has resumed, increase mileage slowly.

Patient Monitoring

Radiographs every 4–6 weeks to document healing progress

PATIENT EDUCATION

- Gradually increase activity as tolerated as long as patient is pain free.
- Rest and reevaluate if there is a recurrence of pain.
- Correct mechanical and training errors.
- Strengthen core muscles.

PROGNOSIS

- Stress fractures in young people have a good prognosis.
- Older patients or those with metabolic bone disease often develop insufficiency fractures in other bones.
- Time to return to full activity:
  - Grade I: 3+ weeks
  - Grade II: 5+ weeks
  - Grade III: 11+ weeks
  - Grade IV: 14+ weeks

COMPLICATIONS

- Completion of fracture
- Delayed union
- Nonunion
- May require surgery with internal fixation

REFERENCES

1. Beck BR, Bergman AG, Miner M, et al. Tibial stress injury: relationship of radiographic, nuclear medicine bone scanning, MR imaging, and CT severity grades to clinical severity and time to healing. *Radiology*. 2012;263(3):811–818.
2. Matheson GO, Brukner P. Pneumatic leg brace after tibial stress fracture for faster return to play. *Clin J Sport Med*. 1998;8(1):66.
3. Mayer SW, Joyner PW, Almekinders LC, et al. Stress fractures of the foot and ankle in athletes. *Sports Health*. 2014;6(6):481–491. doi:10.1177/1941738113486588.
4. Pegrum J, Crisp T, Padhiar N. Diagnosis and management of bone stress injuries of the lower limb in athletes. *BMJ*. 2012;344:e2511. doi:10.1136/bmj.e2511.
5. Shindle MK, Endo Y, Warren RF, et al. Stress fractures about the tibia, foot, and ankle. *J Am Acad Orthop Surg*. 2012;20(3):167–176.
6. Behrens SB, Deren ME, Matson A, et al. Stress fractures of the pelvis and legs in athletes: a review. *Sports Health*. 2013;5(2):165–174.
7. Ward WG, Carter CJ, Wilson SC, et al. Femoral stress fractures associated with long term bisphosphonate treatment. *Clin Orthop Relat Res*. 2012;470(3):759–765.
8. Shima Y. Use of bisphosphonates for the treatment of stress fractures in athletes. *Knee Surg Sports Traumatol Arthrosc*. 2009;17(5):542–550.
9. Griffin XL, Smith N, Parsons N, et al. Ultrasound and shockwave therapy for acute fractures in adults. *Cochrane Database Syst Rev*. 2012;2:CD008579. doi:10.1002/14651858 .CD008579.pub2.

S

ADDITIONAL READING

- Chen YT, Tenforde AS, Fredericson M. Update on stress fractures in female athletes: epidemiology, treatment, and prevention. *Curr Rev Musculoskelet Med*. 2013;6(2):173–181. doi:10.1007/s12178-013-9167-x.
- Ross AC, Manson JE, Abrams SA, et al. The 2011 report on dietary reference intakes for calcium and vitamin D from the Institute of Medicine: what clinicians need to know. *J Clin Endocrinol Metab*. 2011;96(1):53–58.

SEE ALSO

Algorithm: Foot Pain

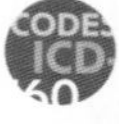

CODES

ICD10

- M84.38XA Stress fracture, other site, initial encounter for fracture
- M84.369A Stress fracture, unsp tibia and fibula, init for fx
- M84.376A Stress fracture, unspecified foot, init encntr for fracture

CLINICAL PEARLS

- Diagnosis requires a high index of suspicion because x-rays are often negative initially.
- Identification and treatment of female athletic triad helps prevent stress fractures.
- Progressing activity levels gradually and avoiding sudden increases in activity or running mileage also help prevent stress fractures.
- Identify high-risk fractures, as they often require immobilization and surgery.

STROKE REHABILITATION

Aaron Hauptman, MD • Jordan Eisenstock, MD

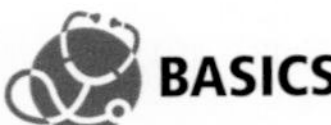

BASICS

DESCRIPTION

- Stroke is a compromise in blood supply to an area of the nervous system, secondary to hemorrhage or occlusion, with resultant infarction of nervous tissue.
- 3rd leading cause of death and the leading cause of long-term disability in the United States (1)
- Rehabilitation refers to the process of restoring a debilitated person toward baseline functionality.
- Specific rehabilitation techniques should be used depending on the individual and based on particular deficits and brain regions impacted.
- Rehabilitation involves cycling through the following (2):
  - Assessment of patient with the goal of identification and quantification needs of the individual
  - Setting of objectives that are realistic, concrete, and attainable
  - Repetition of assessment to gauge changes in status, with subsequent alteration of techniques as necessary
- Motor impairment is the most commonly recognized impairment secondary to stroke.
- Speech and language, swallowing, vision, sensation, and cognition are also commonly impaired.

EPIDEMIOLOGY

Incidence

- Each year, ~795,000 people suffer stroke; ~610,000 are 1st attacks, and 185,000 are recurrent attacks (3).
- ~14% of stroke survivors reach full recovery in physical function; 25–50% need assistance poststroke (1).
- According to the WHO, 15 million people suffer stroke worldwide each year. Of these, 5 million die, and another 5 million are permanently disabled.

Prevalence

- ~7 million Americans ≥20 years old have had a stroke (~3%) (3).
- ~50 million stroke survivors worldwide (4)
- >1/2 of strokes in people <65 years result in death within 8 years (1).

ETIOLOGY AND PATHOPHYSIOLOGY

Stroke involves a compromise in blood supply to an area, usually by either rupture or blockage of a vessel. Of all strokes, 87% are ischemic, 10% intracerebral hemorrhage, and 3% subarachnoid hemorrhage (3).

Neural Mechanisms of Remodeling

Poststroke remodeling changes provide some degree of recovery that varies considerably between individuals. Outcomes are greatest when remodeling mimicks normal organization to the greatest degree possible. Neurophysiologic changes involved in spontanous recovery include the folllowing (5)[B]:

- Augmented excitability in areas of cortex functionally connected to injured brain
- Increased activity contralateral to traumatized cortex
- Changes in somatotopic map in other regions

Research suggests a critical window for neurophysiologic changes, further understanding of which may facilitate neurorehabilitation by augmenting endogenous healing. Animal studies suggest promising strategies for enhancing rehabilitative efforts including growth factors, hormones, proteins, cytokines, stem cells, etc. Studies are ongoing exploring combinations of plasticity-promoting factors, rehabilitative training, and imaging/biomarker modalities together with carefully timed neurorehabilitation that takes advantage of endogenous plasticity timing. Such work is complicated by the vast heterogeneity of stroke insults but offers promising options for future multimodal treatments.

RISK FACTORS

Risk factors for stroke are discussed in the topics "Stroke, Acute" and "Atherosclerosis."

GENERAL PREVENTION

See "Stroke, Acute."

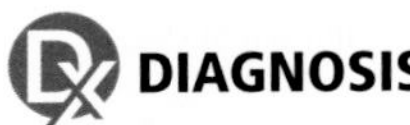

DIAGNOSIS

HISTORY

- For acute stroke symptoms, see "Stroke, Acute."
- A wide variety of systems and functions are commonly impacted by stroke, depending on type, severity, location, etc. including the following (2):
  - Consciousness and psychological functions
    - Orientation, arousal, alertness, attention, intellect, personality, sleep, memory, cognition, perception, behavior, temperament, psychomotor functions, etc.
  - Perceptual functions, most commonly
    - Vision, proprioception, touch sensation
  - Communication, excretory, and sexual functions
    - Vocal control and articulation; intake of food (chewing, swallowing), urinary and bowel functions; sexual function
  - Neuromuscular and ADLs
    - Muscle strength, stability, endurance, reflexes, tone, gait, voluntary movement

PHYSICAL EXAM

- Neurologic manifestations should be examined based on location of stroke when known but should include investigation of the following:
  - Sensory or motor deficits, especially unilaterally (i.e., hemiparesis/hemiplegia)
  - Dysarthria or aphasia
  - Visual field deficits (i.e., hemianopsia)
  - Dysphagia
  - Apraxia
  - Unilateral facial palsy
- Neuropsychiatric evaluation should be undertaken to assess cognitive, intellectual, personality, memory, psychomotor, and other system changes that may benefit from treatment during rehabilitation.

DIFFERENTIAL DIAGNOSIS

- Differential diagnosis in stroke rehabilitation should take into account acute changes that are inconsistent with general trend in the individual patient's status.
- New changes in motor function, mental status, etc. could represent new stroke.
- Subacute changes could include a wide range of neuromuscular, neuropsychiatric, or psychiatric diseases that could be related or unrelated to the initial stroke event.

DIAGNOSTIC TESTS & INTERPRETATION

A wide range of standardized, quantifiable scales have been used to track outcomes in stroke rehabilitation. These include the following (2):

- Neurologic scales
  - Glasgow coma scale, Mini-Mental State Examination, NIH stroke scale among others
- Global ADL scales
  - Including, but not limited to, Barthel index, functional independence measure, modified Rankin scale, Frenchay activities index, trunk control test, timed up-and-go, stair-climbing test, Toronto bedside swallowing screening test, etc.
- Family and caretaker contextual factors are very important to stroke rehabilitation and have been shown to impact outcomes, so thorough assessment should include testing such as the following:
  - Caregiver Strain Index, Family Assessment Device
- See topic "Stroke, Acute."

Follow-Up Tests & Special Considerations

Monitor the coagulation profile of patients on anticoagulants.

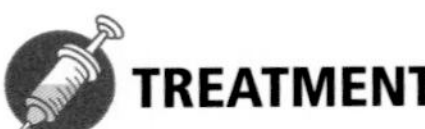

TREATMENT

- Tailor to specific stroke-related sequelae.
- The 3 major stroke rehabilitation goals are as follows (1):
  - Prevent/treat prolonged inactivity complications.
  - Prevent recurrent stroke and cardiovascular events.
  - Increase aerobic fitness.

GENERAL MEASURES

- Prevention and/or treatment of the complications associated with stroke (4)[C]
- Aspiration
  - Immediately after stroke, up to 50% of patients have dysphagia; this improves in many.
  - Remain NPO until bedside swallow assessment.
  - Prevention of aspiration involves postural changes, increased sensory input, swallowing maneuvers, active exercise programs, diet modifications, nonoral feeding (if indicated), psychological support, and supportive nursing
- Pulmonary embolism/deep venous thrombosis
  - Risk highest during first 3–120 days post stroke
  - Pneumatic compression devices and compression stockings
  - Ambulation as soon as possible
- Skin breakdown
  - Increased risk due to loss of sensation, impaired circulation, older age, decreased level of consciousness, inability to move due to paralysis, and incontinence of urine or stool
  - Frequent repositioning (at least q2h) with special care to avoid excessive friction
  - Keep skin clean and dry.
- Spasticity
  - Occurs in ~35% of stroke survivors; treat with combination of modalities:
    - Range of motion exercises
    - Heat, cold, or electric stimulation
    - Splinting
    - Oral medications for spasticity of cerebral origin (e.g., dantrolene, tizanidine); phenol or botulinum toxin injections for targeting specific muscles or muscle groups
- Malnutrition
  - Nutritional assessment with a diet history and monitoring by a dietician
- Seizures
  - More common after hemorrhagic stroke (11%) than after ischemic stroke (9%)
  - Antiepileptic drugs and elimination of disturbances (i.e., toxins, metabolic) that may lower seizure threshold

- Falls
  - Lifestyle changes
    - Avoid loose rugs; maintain a clear path without obstruction.
    - Avoid slippery surfaces (such as wet floors).
    - Maintain good lighting.
    - Shoes with nonskid soles
    - Slow down movements for transfers or walking.
- Severe sleep apnea
  - Lifestyle changes
    - Stop smoking; lose weight.
    - Sleep on side versus back.
    - Mouthpieces and breathing devices (CPAP)
    - Surgery
- Neurocognitive (7)
  - Wide range of deficit patterns that can be focal (e.g., aphasia) or diffuse (general cognitive slowing)
    - Most broadly effected are orientation, language, attention, and memory.
    - Common particular deficits: aphasia, neglect, cognitive slowing, memory/executive deficits
    - Assessment, treatment, and outcomes vary markedly based on stroke type, location, severity, timing, and additional factors.
    - Cognitive rehabilitation has some success in focal deficits but less in diffuse changes.
    - Pharmacology: evidence of efficacy for escitalopram and rivastigmine
    - Additional modalities under investigation: therapies such as rTMS and prism adaptation have sown some benefit in driving plasticity and functional brain changes
- Depression
  - May be organic secondary to stroke or reactive to the stroke itself
- Poststroke depression has been found to cause higher mortality, poorer functional recovery, and less activity socially (1)[C].
  - Treat with a combination of pharmacotherapy and psychotherapy:
    - Evidence suggests heterocyclic antidepressants are effective in the setting of poststroke depression but must be closely monitored in older adults due to side effects.
    - SSRIs are also effective in treating poststroke depression.
    - All stroke patients should be assessed for depression and treated with the appropriate antidepressant for 6 months.

MEDICATION

First Line

- Management of controllable risk factors, including BP reduction, diabetes, and cholesterol (Initiate statin therapy, if history of TIA or stroke with evidence of atherosclerosis, LDL $\geq$100, and no CHD.)
- Anticoagulation with warfarin for patients with mechanical prosthetic heart valves and ischemic stroke or TIA (dosage varies depending on optimum INR for patient in setting of comorbidities)
- Note potential medication interactions (e.g., warfarin and SSRIs due to liver enzyme metabolism).
- Antiplatelet drugs (aspirin, aspirin/dipyridamole, clopidogrel) decrease relative risk of stroke, MI, or death by ~22% (7)[C].

ISSUES FOR REFERRAL

For stroke survivors who require 24-hour care of medical comorbidities, close physician supervision, and specialized nursing care (RN with specialized training or rehabilitation experience), an inpatient rehabilitation facility (IRF) can offer hospital-level care.

ADDITIONAL THERAPIES

Physical, occupational, speech, and recreational therapy

INPATIENT CONSIDERATIONS

Admission Criteria/Initial Stabilization

- For stroke survivors requiring 24-hour care, close physician supervision, and specialized nursing care (RN with specialized training or rehabilitation experience), an inpatient rehabilitation facility (IRF) can offer hospital-level care.
- Such patients must also require and receive a minimum of 3 hours daily occupational or physical therapy for no less than 5 days each week; this can be combined with other skilled modalities, such as speech–language or prosthetic–orthotic services) to meet the 3-hour per day requirement.
- Either the aforementioned is required, or an IRF is the only reasonable setting in which a low-intensity rehab program may be executed.
- An alternative setting is a skilled nursing facility for residents needing daily rehab or nursing care on an inpatient basis.
- See "Stroke, Acute."

IV Fluids

Avoid D5W in acute setting to avoid hyperglycemia and its secondary effects.

Nursing

An alternative inpatient setting is a skilled nursing facility that provides nursing care or rehabilitation to residents needing daily rehab or nursing care on an inpatient basis.

ONGOING CARE

FOLLOW-UP RECOMMENDATIONS

Patient should follow-up regularly with primary care physician for management of risk factors for stroke.

Patient Monitoring

Continue to monitor risk factors. Lab studies monitored periodically may include hemoglobin A1c (and finger-stick glucose testing in diabetics), lipid panel, CBC including platelets, lipid profile, coagulation studies (PT/INR—of special importance in patients on anticoagulation).

DIET

Low salt, low calorie, low saturated and trans fat, low cholesterol.

PATIENT EDUCATION

National Stroke Association: www.stroke.org

PROGNOSIS

- Strong evidence suggests an organized, interdisciplinary stroke care team of physicians, nurses, therapists, family, and patient can reduce mortality rates and the likelihood of institutional care and long-term disability. It can also enhance recovery and increase ADL independence.
- Aggressive rehabilitation beyond the time window of the 1st poststroke months, including treadmill with or without body weight support, can increase aerobic capacity and sensorimotor functionality.

COMPLICATIONS

- Aspiration
- Pulmonary embolism/deep venous thrombosis
- Muscle atrophy
- Osteoporosis
- Skin breakdown
- Spasticity
- Malnutrition
- Seizures
- Severe sleep apnea

REFERENCES

1. Gordon NF, Gulanick M, Costa F, et al. Physical activity and exercise recommendations for stroke survivors: an American Heart Association scientific statement from the Council on Clinical Cardiology, Subcommittee on Exercise, Cardiac Rehabilitation, and Prevention; the Council on Cardiovascular Nursing; the Council on Nutrition, Physical Activity, and Metabolism; and the Stroke Council. *Circulation*. 2004;109(16):2031–2041.
2. Langhorne P, Bernhardt J, Kwakkel G. Stroke rehabilitation. *Lancet*. 2011;377(9778):1693–1702.
3. Roger VL, Go AS, Lloyd-Jones DM, et al. Heart disease and stroke statistics–2011 update: a report from the American Heart Association. *Circulation*. 2011;123(4):e18–e209.
4. Miller EL, Murray L, Richards L, et al. Comprehensive overview of nursing and interdisciplinary rehabilitation care of the stroke patient: a scientific statement from the American Heart Association. *Stroke*. 2010;41:2402–2448.
5. Wahl AS, Schwab ME. Finding an optimal paradigm after stroke: enhancing fiber growth and training of the brain at the right moment. *Front Hum Neurosci*. 2014;8(1):1–13.
6. Cumming TB, Marshall RS, Lazar RM. Stroke, cognitive deficits, and rehabilitation: still an incomplete picture. *Int J Stroke*. 2013;8(1):38–45.
7. Furie KL, Kasner SE, Adams RJ, et al. Guidelines for the prevention of stroke in patients with stroke or transient ischemic attack: a guideline for healthcare professionals from the American Heart Association/American Stroke Association. *Stroke*. 2011;42(1):227–276.

SEE ALSO

- Brain Injury—Post Acute Care Issues; Stroke, Acute; Dementia; Delirium
- Algorithm: Stroke

CODES

ICD10

- I63.9 Cerebral infarction, unspecified
- I69.10 Unsp sequelae of nontraumatic intracerebral hemorrhage
- I69.11 Cognitive deficits following nontraumatic intcrbl hemorrhage

CLINICAL PEARLS

- Stroke is the 3rd leading cause of death and the leading cause of long-term disability in the United States.
- An essential part of poststroke management is the treatment of controllable risk factors, including BP reduction and cholesterol control (initiate statin therapy, if history of TIA or stroke with evidence of atherosclerosis, LDL $\geq$100).
- Strong evidence suggests an organized, interdisciplinary stroke care team of physicians, nurses, therapists, family, and patient can reduce mortality rates and the likelihood of institutional care and long-term disability. It can also enhance recovery and increase ADL independence.

S

STROKE, ACUTE

Nihal Patel, MD • Marc Fisher, MD

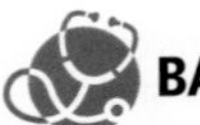 ## BASICS

A cerebrovascular accident (CVA) is an infarction or hemorrhage in the brain.

DESCRIPTION

Stroke is the sudden onset of a focal neurologic deficit(s) resulting from either infarction or hemorrhage within the brain.

- 2 broad categories: ischemic (thrombotic or embolic; 87%) and hemorrhagic (13%)
- Hemorrhage can be intracerebral or subarachnoid.
- System(s) affected: neurologic; vascular
- Synonym(s): CVA; cerebral infarct; brain attack
- Related terms: transient ischemic attack (TIA), a transient episode of neurologic dysfunction due to focal ischemia without permanent infarction on imaging (see topic "Transient Ischemic Attack [TIA]")

Pediatric Considerations

- Cardiac abnormalities (congenital heart disease, paradoxical embolism, rheumatic fever, bacterial endocarditis)
- Metabolic: homocystinuria, Fabry disease

EPIDEMIOLOGY

Incidence

Annual incidence in the United States is ~795,000.

Prevalence

- Prevalence in the United States: 550/100,000
- Predominant age: Risk increases >45 years of age and is highest during the 7th and 8th decades.
- Predominant sex: male > female at younger age, but higher incidence in women with age ≥75 years

ETIOLOGY AND PATHOPHYSIOLOGY

- 87% of stroke is ischemic, 3 main subtypes for etiology: thrombosis, embolism, and systemic hypoperfusion. Large vessel artherothrombotic strokes are commonly related to the origin of the internal carotid artery. Small vessel lacunar strokes are commonly due to lipohyalinotic occlusion. Embolic strokes are largely from a cardiac source (due to left atrial thrombus, atrial fibrillation, recent MI, valve disease or mechanical valves) or ascending aortic atheromatous disease (>4 mm).
- 13% of stroke is hemorrhagic; most commonly due to HTN. Other causes include intracranial vascular malformations (cavernous angiomas, AVMs), cerebral amyloid angiopathy (lobar hemorrhages in elderly), and anticoagulation.
- Other causes include fibromuscular dysplasia (rare), vasculitis, or drug use (cocaine, amphetamines).

Genetics

Stroke is a polygenic multifactorial disease, with some clustering within families.

RISK FACTORS

- Uncontrollable: age, gender, race, family history/genetics, prior stroke or TIA
- Controllable/modifiable/treatable
  - Metabolic: diabetes, dyslipidemia
  - Lifestyle: smoking, cocaine use, amphetamine use
  - Cardiovascular: hypertension, atrial fibrillation, valvular heart disease, endocarditis, recent MI, severe carotid artery stenosis, hypercoagulable states, and patent foramen ovale

GENERAL PREVENTION

Smoking cessation, regular exercise, weight control to maintain nonobese BMI and prevent type 2 diabetes, use alcohol in moderation, control BP, and manage hyperlipidemia; use of antiplatelet agent such as aspirin, in high-risk persons; treatment of nonvalvular atrial fibrillation with dose-adjusted warfarin or dabigatran, apixiban, and rivoroxiban

COMMONLY ASSOCIATED CONDITIONS

Coronary artery disease is the major cause of death during the first 5 years after a stroke.

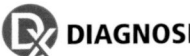

 ## DIAGNOSIS

HISTORY

Acute onset of focal arm/leg weakness, facial weakness, difficulty with speech or swallowing, vertigo, visual disturbances, diminished consciousness; presence of vomiting and severe headache favor diagnosis of hemorrhagic stroke.

PHYSICAL EXAM

- Anterior (carotid) circulation: hemiparesis/hemiplegia, neglect, aphasia, visual field defects
- Posterior (vertebrobasilar) circulation: diplopia, vertigo, gait and limb ataxia, facial paresis, Horner syndrome, dysphagia, dysarthria, alternating sensory loss

DIFFERENTIAL DIAGNOSIS

- Migraine (complicated)
- Postictal state (Todd paralysis)
- Systemic infection, including meningitis or encephalitis (infection also may uncover or enhance previous deficits)
- Toxic or metabolic disturbance (hypoglycemia, acute renal failure, liver failure, drug intoxication)
- Brain tumor, primary or metastases
- Head trauma
- Other types of intracranial hemorrhage (epidural, subdural, subarachnoid)
- Trauma, septic emboli

DIAGNOSTIC TESTS & INTERPRETATION

Primarily used to narrow differential and identify etiology of stroke

Initial Tests (lab, imaging)

- ECG
- Serum glucose level, including fingerstick testing (exclude hypo- and hyperglycemia)
- CBC, including platelets
- Electrolytes, including BUN and creatinine
- Coagulation studies: PT, PTT, INR
- Markers of cardiac ischemia
- Emergent brain imaging with noncontrast CT (or brain MRI with diffusion weighted [DW]-MRI) to exclude hemorrhage can be lifesaving.
- Subsequent multimodal CT (perfusion CT, CTA, unenhanced CT) or MRI to improve diagnosis of acute ischemic stroke

Follow-Up Tests & Special Considerations

Consider LFT, tox screen, blood alcohol, ABG, lumbar puncture if suspected subarachnoid hemorrhage (SAH), EEG if suspect seizures, blood type and cross

- DW-MRI is more sensitive than CT for acute ischemic stroke; however, MRI also is better than CT for diagnosis of posterior fossa lesions (1)[B].
- Emergent treatment (IV thrombolysis) should not be delayed to obtain advanced imaging studies.
- Follow-up imaging of carotid vessels with Doppler ultrasound, CTA, or MRA of head and neck should be completed.

Diagnostic Procedures/Other

Echocardiogram (transthoracic and/or transesophageal) in patients with increased suspicion for cardioembolic source. In cryptogenic stroke patients, prolonged ECG monitoring should be performed with a 30-day event monitor.

Test Interpretation

Early CT findings: hyperdense MCA sign (increased attenuation of proximal portion of the MCA; is associated with thrombosis of MCA), loss of gray-white differentiation in cortical ribbon, sulcal effacement, loss of insular ribbon

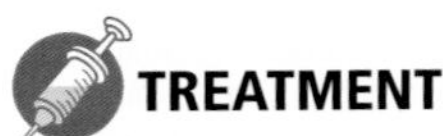

TREATMENT

- BP closely monitored in the first 24 hours (2)[A]
  - Antihypertensives should be withheld unless systolic BP >220 mm Hg or diastolic BP >120 mm Hg, with a goal to lower BP by ~15% during first 24 hours if treatment is indicated. If thrombolytic therapy is to be initiated, BP must be <185/110 prior to thrombolytics.
  - In acute spontaneous intracranial hemorrhagic stroke, goal for BP control is 160/90 or target MAP 110 (see topic on "Subarachnoid Hemorrhage" for details on BP management). With suspicion for elevated ICP, BP should be reduced with goal to keep cerebral perfusion pressure between 61 and 80 mm Hg.
  - Antihypertensive medications should be restarted 24 hours after stroke onset for patients with a history of hypertension who are neurologically stable.

ALERT

Thrombolysis: IV thrombolysis should be started in patients with measurable neurologic deficits that do not clear spontaneously, presenting within 3–4.5 hours of stroke symptom onset.

- Exclusion criteria for thrombolysis within 3 hours of onset include:
  - Symptoms suggestive of SAH
  - Head trauma or prior stroke within 3 months
  - MI within 3 months
  - GI or gastric ulcer hemorrhage within 21 days
  - Major surgery within 14 days
  - Arterial puncture at noncompressible site within 7 days
  - Any history of intracranial hemorrhage
  - Elevated BP (systolic >185 mm Hg and diastolic >110 mm Hg)
  - Active bleeding or acute trauma on examination
  - Taking anticoagulant and INR ≥1.7
  - Activated PTT not in normal range if heparin received during previous 48 hours; platelet count <100,000 mm^3
  - Blood glucose concentration <50 mg/dL
  - Seizure with postictal residual neurologic impairment
  - Multilobar infarction on CT (hypodensity >1/3 cerebral hemisphere)
  - Patient or family members not able to weigh and understand potential risks and benefits of treatment

- Extended exclusion criteria for thrombolysis within 4.5 hours include per AHA/ASA guidelines:
  - Age >80 years
  - All patients taking oral anticoagulants regardless of INR
  - National Institute of Health (NIH) Stroke Scale >25
  - History of stroke and diabetes
- Antiplatelet agents: Oral aspirin (initial dose, 325 mg) should be started within 24–48 hours.

MEDICATION

First Line

- BP management: antihypertensive options include:
  - Labetalol 10–20 mg IV over 1–2 minutes, which may be repeated once
  - Nicardipine infusion 5 mg/hr, titrate up by 2.5 mg/hr at 5–15-minute intervals to maximum of 15 mg/hr; reduce to 3 mg/hr when target BP is reached
- Thrombolysis, IV administration of rtPA: Infuse 0.9 mg/kg, maximum dose 90 mg over 60 minutes with 10% of dose given as bolus over 1 minute.
  - Admit to ICU or stroke unit, with neurologic exams every 15 minutes during infusion, every 60 minutes for next 6 hours, then hourly until 24 hours after treatment.
  - Discontinue infusion and obtain emergent CT scan if severe headache, angioedema, acute hypertension, or nausea and vomiting develop.
  - Measure BP every 15 minutes for first 2 hours, every 30 minutes for next 6 hours, then every hour until 24 hours after treatment. Maintain BP <185/105. Follow-up CT at 24 hours before starting anticoagulants or antiplatelet agents.
- Antiplatelet: aspirin 325 mg/day within 48 hours, or 24–48 hours after thrombolytic therapy

Second Line

Carotid endarterectomy (CEA) for carotid artery stenosis rarely is indicated emergently. CEA is indicated for stenosis >70% ipsilateral to TIA or incomplete stroke lesion, and may be indicated for 50–69% stenosis in carefully selected patients, depending on risk factors.

ISSUES FOR REFERRAL

Follow-up with neurologist 1 week after discharge, with subsequent follow-up based on individual circumstances.

ADDITIONAL THERAPIES

- Prophylactic antibiotics are *not* recommended.
- Deep vein thrombosis (DVT) prophylaxis should be instituted for immobilized patients.
- Corticosteroids are *not* recommended for cerebral brain edema.
- Statin use should be continued without interruption following acute stroke.
- At discharge, patient should be referred for physical therapy, occupational therapy, and speech therapy, as necessary.

SURGERY/OTHER PROCEDURES

- Ventricular drain may be placed for patients with acute hydrocephalus secondary to stroke (most commonly due to cerebellar stroke).
- Decompressive surgery is recommended for major cerebellar infarction; it should be considered for malignant middle cerebral artery infarction, especially if the patient is <60 years of age.
- Consider mechanical embolus removal with a cerebral infarction device in carefully selected patients, with evidence of potentially salvageable tissue on advanced imaging.

COMPLEMENTARY & ALTERNATIVE MEDICINE

Acupuncture starting within 30 days from stroke onset may improve neurologic functioning.

INPATIENT CONSIDERATIONS

Admission Criteria/Initial Stabilization

- Observe closely within first 24 hours for neurologic decline, particularly due to brain swelling.
- Keep head of bed at least 30 degrees when elevated ICP is suspected. Patients with ischemic stroke may benefit from a horizontal bed position during the acute phase.
- Monitor cardiac rhythm for at least first 24 hours to identify any arrhythmias.
- Airway support and ventilatory assistance may be necessary due to diminished consciousness or bulbar involvement; supplemental oxygen should be reserved for hypoxic patients. Consider elective intubation for patients with malignant edema.
- Correct hypovolemia with normal saline.
- All patients should be kept NPO until a formal swallow evaluation has been performed; to reduce risk of aspiration pneumonia, maintain elevated head of bed to 30 degrees.
- Hypoglycemia can cause neurologic dysfunction; rapidly correct during initial evaluation.
- Hyperglycemia within first 24 hours after stroke is associated with poor functional outcomes and AHA/ASA guidelines: insulin treatment for patients with glucose levels >140–185 mg/dL.
- In patients with ICH secondary to anticoagulant use, correction of an elevated INR is necessary with use of IV vitamin K and fresh frozen plasma or prothrombin concentrate complex. Factor VII infusion should be used in patients needing urgent surgical intervention (i.e., those with cerebellar hemorrhage who are neurologically deteriorating).
- DVT prophylaxis

IV Fluids

IV hydration with maintenance amounts of normal saline until swallowing status is assessed; monitor fluid balance closely

Nursing

- Regular neurologic exams more frequent in first 24 hours (every 1–2 hours)
- Fall precautions; frequent repositioning to prevent skin breakdown

Discharge Criteria

Medically stable, adequate nutritional support, neurologic status stable or improving

ONGOING CARE

FOLLOW-UP RECOMMENDATIONS

- Secondary prevention of stroke with aggressive management of risk factors
- Platelet inhibition using aspirin, clopidogrel, or aspirin plus extended-release dipyridamole (Aggrenox) based on physician and patient preference

Patient Monitoring

Follow-up every 3 months for 1st year, then annually.

DIET

Patients with impaired swallowing should receive nasogastric or percutaneous endoscopic gastrostomy feedings to maintain nutrition and hydration.

PATIENT EDUCATION

National Stroke Association (800-STROKES or http://www.stroke.org)

PROGNOSIS

Variable, depending on subtype and severity of stroke; NIH stroke scale may be used for prognosis

COMPLICATIONS

- Acute: brain herniation, hemorrhagic transformation, MI, congestive heart failure, dysphagia, aspiration pneumonia, UTI, DVT, pulmonary embolism, malnutrition, pressure sores
- Chronic: falls, depression, dementia, orthopedic complications, contractures

REFERENCES

1. Chalela JA, Kidwell CS, Nentwich LM, et al. Magnetic resonance imaging and computed tomography in emergency assessment of patients with suspected acute stroke: a prospective comparison. *Lancet*. 2007;369(9558):293–298.
2. Adams HP Jr, del Zoppo G, Alberts MJ, et al. Guidelines for the early management of adults with ischemic stroke: a guideline from the American Heart Association/American Stroke Association Stroke Council, Clinical Cardiology Council, Cardiovascular Radiology and Intervention Council, and the Atherosclerotic Peripheral Vascular Disease and Quality of Care Outcomes in Research Interdisciplinary Working Groups: the American Academy of Neurology affirms the value of this guideline as an educational tool for neurologists. *Stroke*. 2007;38(5):1655–1711.

ADDITIONAL READING

Yew KS, Cheng E. Acute stroke diagnosis. *Am Fam Physician*. 2009;80(1):33–40.

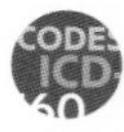

CODES

ICD10

- I63.9 Cerebral infarction, unspecified
- I61.9 Nontraumatic intracerebral hemorrhage, unspecified
- I63.50 Cereb infrc due to unsp occls or stenos of unsp cereb artery

CLINICAL PEARLS

- Unless stroke is hemorrhagic or patient is undergoing thrombolysis, BP should not be lowered acutely to maintain perfusion of penumbric region.
- IV thrombolysis should be considered in eligible patients with neurologic deficits that do not clear spontaneously within 3–4.5 hours of symptom onset.
- DW-MRI is more sensitive than conventional CT for acute ischemic stroke. MRI is also better than CT for diagnosis of posterior fossa lesions.

SUBCONJUNCTIVAL HEMORRHAGE

Cara Marshall, MD

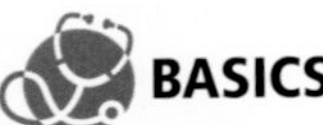

BASICS

DESCRIPTION

- Subconjunctival hemorrhage (SCH) is bleeding from small blood vessels underneath the conjunctiva, the thin clear skin covering the sclera of the eye.
- SCH is diagnosed clinically:
  - Flat, well-demarcated areas of extravasated blood can be seen just under the surface of the conjunctiva of the eye (red patch of blood sign).
  - SCH is more common in the inferior and temporal regions (1).
- Typically, SCH resolves spontaneously within 1–2 weeks.

EPIDEMIOLOGY

- Male = female, no gender predilection found.
- Common. 3% rate of diagnosis in outpatient eye clinic (2)

Incidence

Incidence increases

- With increasing age
- In contact lens wearers (5% of cases) (3)
- With systemic diseases such as diabetes, hypertension (HTN), and coagulation disorders
- During summer months, possibly due to trauma (2)

ETIOLOGY AND PATHOPHYSIOLOGY

- Direct trauma to the blood vessels of the conjunctiva from blunt or penetrating trauma
- Direct trauma to the conjunctiva from improper contact lens placement or improper cleaning
- Increased BP in the vessels of the conjunctiva from hypertension or from the temporary increase in BP from a Valsalva type maneuver (e.g., vomiting)
- Damaged vessels from diabetes and atherosclerotic disease
- Increased bleeding tendencies from either thrombocytopenia or elevated PT/elevated INR (4)
- Trauma to the eye
- Valsalva maneuvers causing sudden severe venous congestion such as coughing, sneezing, vomiting, straining, severe asthma or COPD exacerbation, weightlifting or childbirth/labor (1)
- Hypertension
- Atherosclerotic disease and diabetes
- Bleeding factors such as thrombocytopenia or elevated PT (from either disease or medication side effects)
- In patients age >60 years, HTN is the most common etiology.
- In patients <40 years, trauma/Valsalva and contact lens use are the most common etiologies.
- In patients >40 years, conjunctivochalasis (redundant conjunctival folds) and presence of pinguecula are strongly associated (3).

RISK FACTORS

- Age
- Contact lens wearer
- Systemic diseases
- Bleeding disorders (5)
- Recent cataract surgery

GENERAL PREVENTION

- Correct cleaning and maintenance of contact lenses
- Protective eyewear in sports and hobbies
- Control of high BP
- Optimizing control of systemic diseases such as diabetes and atherosclerotic disease
- Control of prothrombin time (PT)/international normalized ratio (INR) in patients on Coumadin therapy (6)

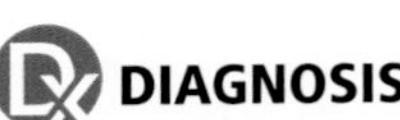

DIAGNOSIS

HISTORY

- Generally asymptomatic; usually the patient notices the redness in the mirror or another person mentions it to the patient.
- There should be little to no pain involved (6)[C].
- Obtain history of trauma. Subconjunctival hemorrhage can occur 12–24 hours after orbital fracture (1).
- Obtain history of contact lens usage or recent cataract, laser-assisted in situ keratomileusis (LASIK), or other ocular surgery (5)[C].
- Comprehensive past medical history to evaluate if at risk for systemic diseases or taking medications that might increase risk
- Obtain history for current systemic symptomatology.

PHYSICAL EXAM

- Evaluate BP to assess control (2)[C].
- Measure visual acuity; this should be normal in a simple SCH (6)[C].
- Verify that the pupils are equal and reactive to light and accommodation; this should be normal with an SCH (6)[C].
- There should be no discharge or exudate noted (6)[C].
- Look at sclera for a bright red demarcated patch.
  - Demarcated area is most often on inferior aspect of eye due to gravity (3)[C].
- If penetrating trauma is a consideration, do a gentle digital assessment of the integrity of the globe (4)[C].
- Slit lamp exam should be performed if there is a history of trauma (1).

Geriatric Considerations

In older adults, the area of SCH will be more widespread across the sclera (3). Elastic and connective tissues are more fragile with age, and underlying conditions such as HTN and diabetes may contribute.

DIFFERENTIAL DIAGNOSIS

- Viral, bacterial, allergic, or chemical conjunctivitis (enterovirus and coxsackie virus most common) (1)[B]
- Foreign body to conjunctiva
- Penetrating trauma
- Acute angle glaucoma

- Iritis
- Recent ocular surgery
- Contact lens induced
- Child abuse (particularly if bilateral in an infant or toddler) (1)
- May occur in newborns after vaginal delivery

DIAGNOSTIC TESTS & INTERPRETATION

If a foreign body is suspected, perform a fluorescein exam.

- Fluorescein exam of a patient with a SCH should show no uptake of staining (6)[C].
- Typically none; SCH is a clinical diagnosis.
- If an orbital fracture is suspected, may obtain plain facial bone films or CT scan (4)[C]

Follow-Up Tests & Special Considerations

If history and physical exam suggest a bleeding etiology (6)[C]

- CBC
- PT/INR

ALERT
If a penetrating injury is suspected, may obtain a CT scan of the orbits but not an MRI (if object may be metal) (4)[C]

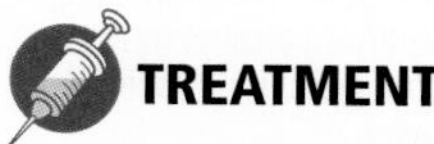

TREATMENT

GENERAL MEASURES

- Control BP.
- Control blood glucose.
- Control INR.
- Wear protective eyewear.

MEDICATION

No prescription medications are useful in treatment of SCH.

ISSUES FOR REFERRAL

- If a penetrating eye injury is suspected, send the patient to the emergency room for emergent ophthalmology consultation.
- If the patient complains of any decreased visual acuity or visual disturbances, refer to an ophthalmologist as soon as possible.
- If there is no resolution of SCH within 2 weeks, patient may need referral to an ophthalmologist.

ADDITIONAL THERAPIES

- Warm compresses
- Eye lubricants (6)[C]

ONGOING CARE

FOLLOW-UP RECOMMENDATIONS

- Follow up only if the area does not resolve within 2 weeks.
- If SCH recurs, then work up patient for systemic sources such as bleeding disorders (6)[C].

PATIENT EDUCATION

- Reassurance of the self-limited nature of the problem and typical time frame for resolution
- Education to return to clinic if the area does not heal or recurs.
- Correct cleaning and maintenance of contact lenses.
- Instructions on causes, self-care, and warning signs are available at PubMed Health: Subconjunctival Hemorrhage at www.ncbi.nlm.nih.gov/pubmed health/PMH0002583/.

PROGNOSIS

Excellent

COMPLICATIONS

Rare

REFERENCES

1. Tarlan B, Kiratli H. Subconjunctival hemorrhage: risk factors and potential indicators. *Clin Ophthalmol.* 2013;7:1163–1170.
2. Fukuyama J, Hayasaka S, Yamada K, et al. Causes of subconjunctival hemorrhage. *Ophthalmologica.* 1990;200(2):63–67.
3. Mimura T, Yamagami S, Mori M, et al. Contact lens-induced subconjunctival hemorrhage. *Am J Ophthalmol.* 2010;150(5):656–665.e1.
4. Wirbelauer C. Management of the red eye for the primary care physician. *Am J Med.* 2006;119(4):302–306.
5. Mimura T, Usui T, Yamagami S, et al. Recent causes of subconjunctival hemorrhage. *Ophthalmologica.* 2010;224(3):133–137.
6. Cronau H, Kankanala RR, Mauger T, et al. Diagnosis and management of red eye in primary care. *Am Fam Physician.* 2010;81(2):137–144.

ADDITIONAL READING

- Mimura T, Usui T, Yamagami S, et al. Subconjunctival hemorrhage and conjunctivochalasis. *Ophthalmology.* 2009;116(10):1880–1886.
- Mimura T, Yamagami S, Usui T, et al. Location and extent of subconjunctival hemorrhage. *Ophthalmologica.* 2010;224(2):90–95.

CODES

ICD10

- H11.30 Conjunctival hemorrhage, unspecified eye
- H11.31 Conjunctival hemorrhage, right eye
- H11.32 Conjunctival hemorrhage, left eye

CLINICAL PEARLS

- SCH is a clinical diagnosis. The condition is typically asymptomatic and will resolve spontaneously in 1–2 weeks.
- Always check BP in a patient with SCH, as HTN is a risk factor.
- Indications for immediate referral to an ophthalmologist are eye pain, change in vision, lack of pupil reactivity, and/or penetrating eye trauma.
- Reassurance and comfort measures are key.
- Contact lens wearers should not wear contacts until the SCH resolves completely.

SUBSTANCE USE DISORDERS

S. Lindsey Clarke, MD, FAAFP

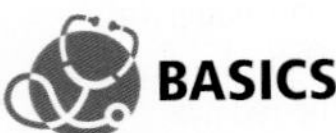

BASICS

DESCRIPTION

A substance use disorder manifests as any pattern of substance use causing significant physical, mental, or social dysfunction.

- Substances of abuse include the following:
  - Alcohol
  - Tobacco
  - Cannabinoids (marijuana)
  - Synthetic marijuana (Spice, K2)
  - Prescription medications
    - CNS depressants (barbiturates, benzodiazepines, hypnotics)
    - Opioids and morphine derivatives (codeine, fentanyl, hydrocodone, hydromorphone, meperidine, methadone, morphine, oxycodone)
    - Stimulants (amphetamines, methylphenidate)
    - Dextromethorphan
  - Stimulants (cocaine, amphetamines, methamphetamines)
  - Club drugs (MDMA, flunitrazepam, γ-hydroxybutyrate or GHB)
  - Opioids (heroin, opium)
  - Dissociative drugs (ketamine, phencyclidine [PCP])
  - Hallucinogens (lysergic acid diethylamide [LSD], salvia)
  - Bath salts (synthetic cathinones)
  - Inhalants (glue, paint thinners, nitrous oxide)
  - Anabolic steroids
- See also www.drugabuse.gov/drugs-abuse.
- System(s) affected: cardiovascular; endocrine/metabolic; CNS
- Synonym(s): drug abuse; drug dependence; substance abuse

Geriatric Considerations

- Alcohol is the most commonly abused substance, and abuse often goes unrecognized.
- Higher potential for drug interactions

Pregnancy Considerations

Substance abuse may cause fetal abnormalities, morbidity, and fetal or maternal death.

EPIDEMIOLOGY

Incidence

- Predominant age: 16–25 years
- Predominant sex: male > female

Prevalence

- 23.9 million (9.2%) Americans reported current illicit drug use in 2012.
- 9.5% for age 12–17 years; 21.3% for age 18–25 years
- Nearly 1 in 5 young adult men use marijuana.

ETIOLOGY AND PATHOPHYSIOLOGY

Multifactorial, including genetic, environmental

Genetics

Substances of abuse affect dopamine, acetylcholine, γ-aminobutyric acid, norepinephrine, opioid, and serotonin receptors. Variant alleles may account for susceptibility to disorders.

RISK FACTORS

- Male gender, young adult
- Depression, anxiety
- Other substance use disorders
- Family history
- Peer or family use or approval
- Low socioeconomic status
- Unemployment
- Accessibility of substances of abuse
- Family dysfunction or trauma
- Antisocial personality disorder
- Academic problems, school dropout
- Criminal involvement

GENERAL PREVENTION

Early identification and aggressive early intervention improve outcomes.

COMMONLY ASSOCIATED CONDITIONS

- Depression
- Personality disorders
- Bipolar affective disorder

ALERT

Prescription narcotic overdose is the leading cause of accidental death between the ages of 25 and 45 years in the United States; this correlates with increased prescribing of long-acting oxycodone (see www.cdc.gov/injury/wisqars/pdf/leading_causes_of_death_by_age_group_2011-a.pdf).

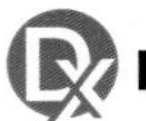

DIAGNOSIS

Substance use disorder (*DSM-5* criteria): ≥2 of the following in past year, with severity based on number of criteria present:

- Missed work or school
- Use in hazardous situations
- Continued use despite social or personal problems
- Craving
- Tolerance (decreased response to effects of drug due to constant exposure)
- Withdrawal upon discontinuation
- Using more than intended
- Failed attempts to quit
- Increased time spent obtaining, using, or recovering from the substance
- Interference with important activities
- Continued use despite health problems

HISTORY

- History of infections (e.g., endocarditis, hepatitis B or C, TB, STI, or recurrent pneumonia)
- Social or behavioral problems, including chaotic relationships and/or employment
- Frequent visits to emergency department
- Criminal incarceration
- History of blackouts, insomnia, mood swings, chronic pain, repetitive trauma
- Anxiety, fatigue, depression, psychosis

PHYSICAL EXAM

- Abnormally dilated or constricted pupils
- Needle marks on skin
- Nasal septum perforation (with cocaine use)
- Cardiac dysrhythmias, pathologic murmurs
- Malnutrition with severe dependence

DIFFERENTIAL DIAGNOSIS

- Depression, anxiety, or other mental states
- Metabolic delirium (hypoxia, hypoglycemia, infection, thiamine deficiency, hypothyroidism, thyrotoxicosis)
- ADHD
- Medication toxicity

DIAGNOSTIC TESTS & INTERPRETATION

ALERT

Screening: a single question: "How many times in the past year have you used an illegal drug or used a prescription medication for nonmedical reasons?": in primary care setting, resulted in sensitivity of 100% and specificity of ~75% (1)[B]

- CRAFFT questionnaire is superior to CAGE (cut down, annoyed by criticism, guilty about drinking, eye-opener drinks) for identifying alcohol use disorders in adolescents and young adults; sensitivity is 94% with ≥2 "yes" answers.
  - C: Have you ever ridden in a *c*ar driven by someone (including yourself) who was "high" or who had been using alcohol or drugs?
  - R: Do you ever use alcohol or drugs to *r*elax, feel better about yourself, or fit in?
  - A: Do you ever use alcohol or drugs while you are *a*lone?
  - F: Do you ever *f*orget things you did while using alcohol or drugs?
  - F: Do your family or *f*riends ever tell you that you should cut down on your drinking or drug use?
  - T: Have you gotten into *t*rouble while you were using alcohol or drugs?
- Blood alcohol concentration
- Urine drug screen (UDS) (order qualitative UDS and, if specific drug is in question, a quantitative analysis for specific drug; order confirmatory serum tests if you suspect false positive)
- Approximate detection limits
  - Alcohol: 6–10 hours
  - Amphetamines and variants: 2–3 days
  - Barbiturates: 2–10 days
  - Benzodiazepines: 1–6 weeks
  - Cocaine: 2–3 days
  - Heroin: 1–1.5 days
  - LSD, psilocybin: 8 hours
  - Marijuana: 1 day–4 weeks
  - Methadone: 1 day–1 week
  - Opioids: 1–3 days
  - PCP: 7–14 days
  - Anabolic steroids: oral, 3 weeks; injectable, 3 months; nandrolone, 9 months
- Liver transaminases
- HIV, hepatitis B and C screens
- Echocardiogram for endocarditis
- Head CT scan for seizure, delirium, trauma

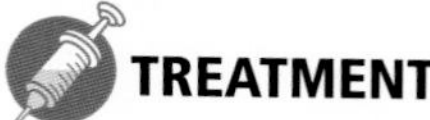

TREATMENT

Determine substances abused early (may influence disposition).

GENERAL MEASURES

- Nonjudgmental, medically oriented attitude
- Motivational interviewing and brief interventions can overcome denial and promote change.
- Behavioral and cognitive therapy
- Community reinforcement
- Interventional counseling
- Self-help groups to aid recovery (Alcoholics Anonymous, other 12-step programs)
- Support groups for family (Al-Anon and Alateen)

MEDICATION

- Alcohol withdrawal: See "Alcohol Abuse and Dependence" and "Alcohol Withdrawal."
- Benzodiazepine or barbiturate withdrawal
  - Gradual taper preferable to abrupt discontinuation
  - Substitution of longer acting benzodiazepine or phenobarbital
- Nicotine withdrawal: See "Tobacco Use and Smoking Cessation."
- Opioid withdrawal
  - Methadone: 20 mg/day PO; use restricted to inpatient settings and specially licensed clinics (2)[A]
  - Clonidine: 0.1–0.2 mg PO TID for autonomic hyperactivity (3)[A]
  - Buprenorphine: 8–16 mg/day sublingually; may precipitate a more severe withdrawal if initiated too soon; use restricted to licensed clinics and certified physicians (4)[A]
- Stimulant withdrawal
  - No agent with clear benefit for cocaine.
  - Anti-cocaine vaccine in development
  - Naltrexone: 50 mg PO twice weekly reduces amphetamine use in dependent patients (5)[B].
  - Methylphenidate ER: titrated up to 54 mg/day PO might enhance abstinence in amphetamine-dependent patients
- Adjuncts to therapy
  - Use all medications in conjunction with psychosocial behavioral interventions.
  - Antiemetics, nonaddictive analgesics for opioid withdrawal
  - Nonhabituating antidepressants, mood stabilizers, anxiolytics, and hypnotics for comorbid mood and anxiety disorders and insomnia that persist after detoxification
- Contraindications
  - Buprenorphine in lactation
  - Naltrexone in pregnancy, liver disease
- Precautions: Clonidine can cause hypotension.
- Significant possible interactions
  - Buprenorphine and ketoconazole, erythromycin, or HIV protease inhibitors
  - Naltrexone and opioid medications (may precipitate or exacerbate withdrawal)

ISSUES FOR REFERRAL

- Consider addiction specialist, especially for opioid and polysubstance abuse.
- Maintenance therapy for opioid dependence (e.g., methadone) only in licensed clinics
- Psychiatrist for comorbid psychiatric disorders
- Social services

INPATIENT CONSIDERATIONS

Admission Criteria/Initial Stabilization

- Indications for inpatient detoxification
  - History of withdrawal symptoms (e.g., seizures)
  - Disorientation
  - Threat of harm to self or others
  - Obstacles to close monitoring (follow-up)
  - Comorbid medical illness
  - Pregnancy
- For narcotic addiction and withdrawal
- Look for signs of severe infection (e.g., bacterial endocarditis).

IV Fluids

Maintenance until patient is taking fluids well by mouth

Nursing

- Take frequent vital signs during withdrawal.
- Monitor for signs of drug use in the hospital.

Discharge Criteria

Detoxification complete

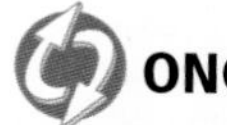

ONGOING CARE

FOLLOW-UP RECOMMENDATIONS

Restricted if dangerous, psychotic, or disoriented

Patient Monitoring

Verify patient's compliance with the substance abuse treatment program.

DIET

Patients often are malnourished.

PATIENT EDUCATION

- Substance Abuse and Mental Health Services Administration: http://samhsa.gov or 800-662-HELP for information, treatment facility locator
- Alcoholics Anonymous: www.aa.org
- Narcotics Anonymous: www.na.org

PROGNOSIS

- Patients in treatment for longer periods (≥1 year) have higher success rates.
- Behavioral therapy and pharmacotherapy are most successful when used in combination.

COMPLICATIONS

- Serious harm to self and others: accidents, violence
- Overdoses resulting in seizures, arrhythmias, cardiac and respiratory arrest, coma, death
- Hepatitis, HIV, tuberculosis, syphilis
- Subacute bacterial endocarditis
- Malnutrition
- Social problems, including arrest
- Poor marital adjustment and violence
- Depression, schizophrenia
- Sexual assault (alcohol, flunitrazepam, GHB)

REFERENCES

1. Smith PC, Schmidt SM, Allensworth-Davies D, et al. A single-question screening test for drug use in primary care. *Arch Intern Med*. 2010;170(13):1155–1160.
2. Amato L, Davoli M, Minozzi S, et al. Methadone at tapered doses for the management of opioid withdrawal. *Cochrane Database Syst Rev*. 2013;2:CD003409.
3. Gowing L, Farrell MF, Ali R, et al. Alpha2-adrenergic agonists for the management of opioid withdrawal. *Cochrane Database Syst Rev*. 2014;3:CD002024.
4. Gowing L, Ali R, White JM. Buprenorphine for the management of opioid withdrawal. *Cochrane Database Syst Rev*. 2009;(3):CD002025.
5. Jayaram-Lindström N, Hammarberg A, Beck O, et al. Naltrexone for the treatment of amphetamine dependence: a randomized, placebo-controlled trial. *Am J Psychiatry*. 2008;165(11):1442–1448.

ADDITIONAL READING

- Patterson DA, Morris GW Jr, Houghton A. Uncommon adverse effects of commonly abused illicit drugs. *Am Fam Physician*. 2013;88(1):10–16.
- Shapiro B, Coffa D, McCance-Katz EF. A primary care approach to substance misuse. *Am Fam Physician*. 2013;88(2):113–121.
- Standridge JB, Adams SM, Zotos AP. Urine drug screening: a valuable office procedure. *Am Fam Physician*. 2010;81(5):635–640.
- Substance Abuse and Mental Health Services Administration. *Results from the 2012 National Survey on Drug Use and Health: Summary of National Findings* (NSDUH Series H-46, HHS Publication No. [SMA] 13-4795). Rockville, MD: Substance Abuse and Mental Health Services Administration; 2013. http://www.samhsa.gov/data/NSDUH.aspx.

SEE ALSO

Alcohol Abuse and Dependence; Alcohol Withdrawal; Tobacco Use and Smoking Cessation

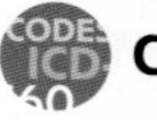

CODES

ICD10

- F19.10 Other psychoactive substance abuse, uncomplicated
- F10.10 Alcohol abuse, uncomplicated
- F12.10 Cannabis abuse, uncomplicated

CLINICAL PEARLS

- Substance use disorders are prevalent, serious, and often unrecognized in clinical practice. Comorbid psychiatric disorders are common.
- Substance abuse is distinguished by family, social, occupational, legal, or physical dysfunction that is caused by persistent use of the substance.
- Dependence is characterized by tolerance, withdrawal, compulsive use, and repeated overindulgence.
- Motivational interviewing, brief interventions, and a nonjudgmental attitude can help to promote a willingness to change behavior.Research shows the benefit of referring patients with alcohol dependence to an addiction specialist or treatment program (4)[A].

S

SUDDEN INFANT DEATH SYNDROME

Fern R. Hauck, MD, MS • Kim Michal Stein, MD

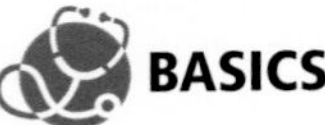

BASICS

- Leading cause of death in infants 1–12 months of age
- 3rd leading cause of infant mortality overall
- SIDS deaths have been reduced by >50% in the United States and other countries that have introduced risk-reduction campaigns, heavily focused on back sleeping for infants.
- The condition still remains mysterious, and the exact cause is unknown.

DESCRIPTION

- The sudden death of an infant <1 year of age that remains unexplained after a thorough case investigation, including performance of a complete autopsy, examination of the death scene, and review of the clinical history
- Sudden infant death syndrome (SIDS) was first formally defined in 1969. The definition was revised in 1989.
- In past 20 years there has been a shift in classifying sleep-related deaths as accidental suffocation and asphyxia in bed or unknown cause rather than SIDS, which has created increased confusion about how to define and study these deaths. Several classification systems have been proposed that attempt to address this problem (1).
- System(s) affected: cardiovascular; endocrine/metabolic; nervous; pulmonary
- Synonym(s): crib death; cot death

EPIDEMIOLOGY

- SIDS can affect any infant, but some infants are at higher risk than others, including African Americans and American Indians/Native Americans, males, infants whose mothers smoked/used illegal drugs during pregnancy, and several others described below.
- There is a characteristic age pattern, with deaths peaking at 2–4 months, and more deaths occurring during the colder seasons.

Incidence

- For 2010: all races: 0.52/1,000 live births (2,058 cases/year)
  - White non-Hispanic: 0.50/1,000 live births (1,077 cases/year)
  - African American non-Hispanic: 0.98/1,000 live births (577 cases/year)
  - Hispanic: 0.31/1,000 live births (297 cases/year)
  - Native American: 0.90/1,000 live births (42 cases/year)
  - Asian/Pacific Islander: 0.22/1,000 live births (55 cases/year)
- Predominant age: uncommon in 1st month of life; peak occurs between 2 and 4 months of age; 90% of deaths occur by 6 months of age
- Predominant sex: male > female (52–60% male)

Pediatric Considerations

Occurs only in infants

ETIOLOGY AND PATHOPHYSIOLOGY

Strong evidence for a respiratory pathway that includes the following stages:

- A life-threatening event causes severe asphyxia and/or brain hypoperfusion. This can include rebreathing exhaled carbon dioxide in a facedown position.
- The vulnerable infant does not wake up or turn his or her head in response to asphyxia, resulting in further rebreathing and inability to recover from apnea.
- Progressive apnea leads to hypoxic coma.
- Bradycardia and hypoxic apnea occur.
- Autoresuscitation fails, resulting in prolonged apnea and death (2).
- There are many theories. There may be subtle developmental abnormalities resulting from pre- and/or perinatal brain injury, which make the infant vulnerable to SIDS.
- Possible causes
  - Abnormalities in respiratory control and arousal responsiveness
  - Central and peripheral nervous system abnormalities
  - Cardiac arrhythmias
  - Rebreathing in facedown position on soft surface, leading to hypoxia and hypercarbia
  - SIDS may occur when ≥1 environmental risk factors interact with ≥1 genetic risk factors.

Genetics

Emerging evidence for genetic risk factors, especially related to impaired brainstem regulation of breathing or other autonomic control, impaired immune responses, and cardiac ion channelopathies associated with long QT syndrome and fatal arrhythmia

RISK FACTORS

- Although some infants may die from SIDS who have no apparent risk factors, most have ≥1 of the following risk factors associated with SIDS:
  - Race: African Americans and Native Americans have highest incidence.
  - Season: late fall and winter months
  - Time of day: between midnight and 6 AM
  - Activity: during sleep
  - Low birth weight; intrauterine growth retardation (IUGR)
  - Poverty
- Maternal factors
  - Younger age
  - Decreased education
  - Maternal use of cigarettes/drugs (e.g., cocaine, opiates) during pregnancy
  - Higher parity
  - Inadequate prenatal care
- Respiratory/GI infection in recent past
- Sleep practices
  - Prone and side sleep positions
  - Overheating from heavy clothing and bedding and/or elevated room temperature
  - Soft bedding
  - Bed sharing, independent of other factors (3)[B]
  - Parental smoking, alcohol, and drug use greatly increase the risk associated with bed sharing (3)[B].
  - No room sharing
- Passive cigarette smoke exposure after birth
- Not using pacifier; not breastfeeding

GENERAL PREVENTION

Because a SIDS death is sudden and the cause is unknown, SIDS cannot be "treated." However, some measures may be effective in reducing the risk of SIDS (4)[B].

- Maternal avoidance of cigarette smoking and illicit drug use during pregnancy
- Avoidance of passive cigarette smoke exposure
- Avoidance of the prone (facedown) and side sleep positions, excessive bed clothing, and soft bedding such as pillows, comforters, and bumper pads or a soft mattress. Bumper pads of any kind are not recommended.
- Avoidance of overheating
- A crib, bassinet, or cradle conforming to federal safety standards is the recommended sleeping location.
- Avoidance of bed sharing with the infant, particularly by adults other than the parent(s) or by other children. Bed sharing should be avoided if the mother/father has used cigarettes, drugs, or alcohol. Bed sharing on couches is very dangerous and should never be done.
- Infants who sleep in the same room, as their parents (without bed sharing) have a lower risk of SIDS. It is recommended that infants sleep in a crib/bassinet in their parents' bedroom, which when placed close to their bed will allow for more convenient breastfeeding and contact.
- Breastfeeding is associated with a decreased risk of SIDS and is recommended for all infants (5)[B].
- Pacifier use is associated with a reduced risk of SIDS.
  - Consider offering a pacifier at bedtime and nap time (6)[B].
  - Delay the introduction of the pacifier among breastfed infants until 3–4 weeks of age.
  - Pacifier use has not been found to be detrimental to breastfeeding if it is introduced after the baby is 3–4 weeks of age, when breastfeeding is well established (7)[A].
- Avoid commercial devices marketed to reduce the risk of SIDS.
- It is critical that all people caring for infants, including daycare providers, be instructed in these risk-reduction measures.
- Newborn nurseries should implement these recommendations well before discharge, so parents see appropriate practices modeled.
- The guidelines related to safe infant sleep environment are also effective in reducing the risk of other sleep-related infant deaths (4).

COMMONLY ASSOCIATED CONDITIONS

Infants are generally well, or may have had a mild febrile illness (i.e., gastroenteritis or an upper respiratory infection) prior to death.

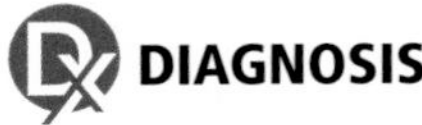

DIAGNOSIS

The diagnosis of SIDS is made by trained medical examiners/coroners when the death is believed to be from natural causes and after thorough reviews of the medical history, death scene investigation, and postmortem examination do not produce an explanation of the death.

HISTORY

Infant usually found unresponsive by parent/other caregiver without any warning

PHYSICAL EXAM

- These babies generally appear healthy or may have had a minor upper respiratory/GI infection in the last 2 weeks before death.
- Complete postmortem exam to look for signs of possible trauma/child abuse or other cause of death

DIFFERENTIAL DIAGNOSIS

- Accidental suffocation/asphyxia
- Abnormalities of fatty acid metabolism (e.g., deficiency of medium-chain acyl-coenzyme A dehydrogenase or of carnitine)
- Dehydration/electrolyte disturbance
- Homicide

DIAGNOSTIC TESTS & INTERPRETATION

Standardized postmortem protocols have been proposed. Although testing varies across sites, common diagnostic tests include electrolytes, toxicology, and microbiology.

- Postmortem laboratory tests are performed to rule out other causes of death (e.g., electrolytes to rule out dehydration and electrolyte imbalance). No consistently abnormal laboratory tests are found.
- Pneumocardiograms have been abandoned in the workup.
- X-rays to rule out possible child abuse

Diagnostic Procedures/Other

Because the diagnosis of SIDS is often one of "exclusion," it is crucial to do a thorough death scene investigation and case review in addition to the autopsy and laboratory tests.

Test Interpretation

Characteristic findings on postmortem examination

- Frothy discharge, sometimes blood tinged, from nostrils and mouth
- Petechiae on surface of lungs, heart, and thymus gland in 50–85% (but not unique to SIDS)
- Pulmonary congestion and edema often present
- Morphologic markers of hypoxia: increased gliosis in brain stem, retention of periadrenal brown fat, and hematopoiesis in the liver
  - Present to varying degrees; not confirmed by all studies

ONGOING CARE

General recommendations for positioning infants

- Infants frequently should be placed on their bellies when awake and observed by responsible adults to prevent head flattening (plagiocephaly) that can result from infants sleeping supine.
- Avoid placing infants for extended periods in car seat carriers or "bouncers."
- Upright "cuddle time" should be encouraged.
- Alter the side to which the infant places his or her head during sleep.
- Swaddling infants may aid in sleeping more comfortably in the supine position. Infants should never be swaddled if sleeping in the prone or side position. Swaddling should be discontinued when the infant starts to roll over, or when the infant reaches the age of 3–4 months.

FOLLOW-UP RECOMMENDATIONS

- Safe sleep and SIDS risk-reduction messages should be delivered at all well-child checks and by all health professionals in a consistent manner.
- Parents often change from the recommended practices as the baby gets older, often during the peak SIDS incidence period. Thus, it is important to ask about infant care practices at each well-child check.

Patient Monitoring

Although some authorities recommend cardiopulmonary monitoring in siblings of prior SIDS victims, no evidence indicates that the use of monitors prevents SIDS, and they should not be prescribed for that purpose (8)[B].

PATIENT EDUCATION

- Family counseling (see "Prognosis")
- Safe to Sleep: InformationLine (800) 505-CRIB (2742); Web site: http://www.nichd.nih.gov/sts/Pages/default.aspx
- Centers for Disease Control and Prevention: Web site: http://www.cdc.gov/SIDS/
- First Candle, Bel Air, MD (800) 221-SIDS (7437); Web site: http://www.firstcandle.org/
- CJ Foundation for SIDS, Hackensack, NJ (888) 8CJ-SIDS (825-7437); Web site: http://www.cjsids.org/
- Cribs for Kids, Pittsburgh, PA (888) 721-CRIB (2742); Web site: http://www.cribsforkids.org/

PROGNOSIS

- SIDS deaths have a powerful impact on families and their functioning. Physicians play an important role in providing immediate information about SIDS and sensitive counseling to limit parents' misinformation and feelings of guilt.
- Counseling needs of families vary from the short term to long term.
  - Support groups are helpful to many couples.
  - Physicians need to be familiar with resources available in their communities to help families mourning a SIDS death.
- Follow-up counseling, including review of the autopsy report with the family after some time has passed, is important to help with understanding this condition and to alleviate the tremendous guilt these families experience.
- Parents need to be counseled about subsequent pregnancies.
  - Genetic testing and counseling may be indicated to rule out a metabolic/other genetically acquired disorder.
  - Parents need to be advised of the most current recommendations regarding sleep position and other infant care practices during subsequent pregnancies.

REFERENCES

1. Shapiro-Mendoza, CK, Camperlengo L, Ludvigsen R, et al. Classification system for the Sudden Unexpected Infant Death Case Registry and its application. *Pediatrics*. 2014;134(1):e210–e219.
2. Kinney HC, Thach BT. The sudden infant death syndrome. *N Engl J Med*. 2009;361(8):795–805.
3. Carpenter R, McGarvey C, Mitchell E, et al. Bed sharing when parents do not smoke: is there a risk of SIDS? An individual level analysis of five major case-control studies. *BMJ Open*. 2013;3(5):e002299. doi:10.1136/bmjopen/2012/002299.
4. Task Force on Sudden Infant Death Syndrome, Moon RY. Policy Statement. SIDS and other sleep-related infant deaths: expansion of recommendations for a safe infant sleeping environment. *Pediatrics*. 2011;128(5):1030–1039.
5. Hauck FR, Thompson JM, Tanabe KO, et al. Breastfeeding and reduced risk of sudden infant death syndrome: a meta-analysis. *Pediatrics*. 2011;128(1):103–110.
6. Hauck FR, Omojokun OO, Siadaty MS. Do pacifiers reduce the risk of sudden infant death syndrome? A meta-analysis. *Pediatrics*. 2005;116(5):e716–e723.
7. O'Connor NR, Tanabe KO, Siadaty MS, et al. Pacifiers and breastfeeding: a systematic review. *Arch Pediatr Adolesc Med*. 2009;163(4):378–382.
8. Committee on Fetus and Newborn; American Academy of Pediatrics. Apnea, sudden infant death syndrome, and home monitoring. *Pediatrics*. 2003;111(4, Pt 1):914–917.

ADDITIONAL READING

Task Force on Sudden Infant Death Syndrome, Moon RY. Technical Report. SIDS and other sleep-related infant deaths: expansion of recommendations for a safe infant sleeping environment. *Pediatrics*. 2011;128(5):e1341–e1367.

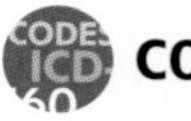

CODES

ICD10

R99 Ill-defined and unknown cause of mortality

CLINICAL PEARLS

- Although the exact cause of SIDS is unknown, several risk-reduction measures will significantly reduce an infant's chance of dying from SIDS.
- SIDS incidence has decreased by >50% just by placing infants in a supine position to sleep.
- Breastfeeding is recommended for all infants.
- Safe sleeping arrangements and pacifier use are other ways to reduce the risk of SIDS.

SUICIDE

Irene C. Coletsos, MD • Harold J. Bursztajn, MD

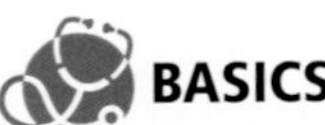

BASICS

DESCRIPTION

Suicide and attempted suicide are significant causes of morbidity and mortality.

EPIDEMIOLOGY

- Predominant sex:
  - Women *attempt* suicide 1.5× more often than men. Men *complete* suicide 4× more often than women. Men are more likely to choose a means with high lethality.
- Predominant age: adolescent (2nd leading cause of death, per 2012 CDC statistics [latest available]); geriatric population
- Predominant race: 84% of people who complete suicides are white, non-Hispanic. Native Americans have the next highest rate in the United States. Whites have twice the risk of suicide compared with African Americans.
- Marital status: single > divorced; widowed > married
- Worldwide, in of all countries, youths (ages 10–24 years) are the highest risk group.

Incidence

- In 2010, 10th leading cause of death in adults in the United States. Military service (not specifically active duty) is associated with increased risk. In 2009, 2010, 2012, and 2013, more soldiers died of suicide than in active duty, according to a congressional study and the National Center for Veterans.
- Worldwide, the 3rd leading cause of death

RISK FACTORS

- "Human understanding is the most effective weapon against suicide. The greatest need is to deepen the awareness and sensitivity of people to their fellow man" (Shneidman, American Association of Suicidology).
- Be alert to a combination of "perturbation" (increased emotional disturbance) and "lethality" (having the potential tools to cause death).
- 80% who complete suicides had a previous attempt.
- 90% who complete suicide meet *Diagnostic and Statistical Manual* criteria for Axis I or II disorders: major depression; bipolar disorder; anorexia nervosa; panic disorder; borderline and antisocial personality disorders. Schizophrenia or acute onset of psychosis are also risk factors, due to command hallucinations or even the negative affect or hopelessness that can accompany these states.
- Substance use (alcohol; "bath salts" and other hallucinogens; opioids)
- Family history of suicide
- Physical illness
- Despair: feeling unendurable emotional pain *and* has "given up" on self, feels without hope and, consciously or unconsciously, unworthy of help
- Among teenagers: not feeling "connected" to their peers or family; being bullied; poor grades
- Psychosocial: recent loss: What may seem to be a small loss (to a medical provider) may be a devastating loss to the patient. *Patient-specific* factors need to be taken into account; social isolation; anniversaries and holidays. Patients who attempt suicide also seem to have impaired decision-making skills and risk awareness, and increased impulsivity, compared with patients who have never attempted suicide (1).
- If a patient is incompetent (e.g., too delusional) to inform providers about the potential for suicide, that puts the patient at increased risk; consider hospitalization.
- Access to lethal means: firearms, poisons (including prescription and nonprescription drugs)

GENERAL PREVENTION

- Know how to access resources 24/7 within and outside of the health care institution.
- Screen for risk factors, and consider the overall clinical picture. Screening instruments include the Patient Health Questionnaire-9 (PHQ-9), the Columbia Suicide Severity Rating Scale, Beck's Scale for Suicidal Ideation, Linehan's Reasons for Living Inventory, and Risk Estimator for Suicide.
- Treat underlying mental illness and substance abuse. Screen for possession of means of harm, including prescription and nonprescription drugs and firearms (encourage these patients to remove guns from their homes and to relinquish gun licenses).
- Women being treated for cancer, chronic obstructive pulmonary disease (COPD), heart disease, osteoporosis, or stroke were found to be at higher risk for suicide (even without a history of depression).
- Create a safety plan for patients at risk for suicide and their families, including education about how to access emergency care 24 hours a day.
- Public education about how to help others access emergency psychiatric care. Suicidal people may 1st confide in those they trust outside health care (e.g., family members, religious leaders, community elders, "healers," hairdressers, and bartenders).
- For the military: multiple resources: www.realwarriors.net. Suggested treatments include cognitive restructuring techniques (that their experience with adversity can be a sources of strength) and help with problem-solving (so the service member does not feel like a "burden").
- For teens, young adults, and their educators: suggestions and advice for students/families and educators: www.cdc.gov/healthyyouth/adolescenthealth; www.stopbullying.gov
- In developing world countries, pesticide ingestion is a common method of suicide. Limiting free access has led to reduced suicide rates.

DIAGNOSIS

HISTORY

- Depressed patients should be asked about ideation and about a plan:
  - "Have you ever felt that life isn't worth living? Do you ever wish you could go to sleep and not wake up? Are you having thoughts about killing yourself?"
- Use psychodynamic formulation, which combines mental-state exam (i.e., behavior, mood, mental content, judgment), past history (i.e., what resources has the patient used in the past for support, and are they currently available?), and history of current illness. If the patient is experiencing a loss, is under stress, and does not have access to a previously sustaining resource (e.g., a significant other, a pet, sports ability, a job), that patient is under increased risk for suicide.
- Prior attempts: precipitants, lethality, intent to die, precautions taken to avoid being rescued, reaction to survival (a patient who is upset that the suicide was not completed is at increased risk)
- History of psychiatric symptoms, substance abuse. Also note strengths, such as reasons to live, hopes for future, social supports. A patient without these is at increased risk.
- Collateral history is important (from friends, family, physicians). It may be appropriate to break confidentiality if patient is at imminent risk of suicide.

PHYSICAL EXAM

- Medical conditions: delirium, intoxication, withdrawal, medication side effects
- Psychosis: Observe for signs of/ask about command auditory hallucinations to kill oneself, delusional guilt, and persecutory delusions.
- In adults: Observe for signs of hopelessness/despair (see "Risk Factors").
- In teens: Screen for risk factors: substance abuse, bullying, poor grades, social isolation, because teens may not appear depressed.

DIFFERENTIAL DIAGNOSIS

Differentiate between patients and pseudopatients (i.e., those who are using suicide threats and gestures to manipulate others).

DIAGNOSTIC TESTS & INTERPRETATION

Diagnostic Procedures/Other

Brief tests that could be part of any medical/mental health assessment:

- PHQ-9: http://www.med.umich.edu/1info/FHP/practiceguides/depress/phq-9.pdf and www.teenscreen.org
- Columbia Suicide Severity Rating Scale, clinical instructions: www.cssrs.columbia.edu/c-ssrs_Triage_guidelines.pdf
- Suicide Trigger Scale-version 3, (STS-3), which measures a patient's "ruminative flooding" (self-critical, repetitive thoughts) and "frantic hopelessness" (feeling trapped, suicide is the only choice): http://www.ncbi.nlm.nih.gov/pmc/articles/PMC3443232/

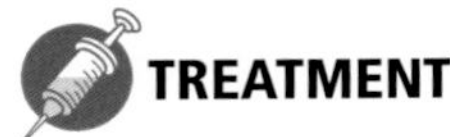

TREATMENT

GENERAL MEASURES

- Patients expressing active suicidal thoughts or who made an attempt require immediate evaluation for risk factors, mental status, and capacity (to determine if they are able/or willing to inform treaters about suicidal intentions), as well as a formal psychiatric consultation. Careful primary care screening can be as effective at identifying risk as a psychological assessment.
- Cognitive therapy decreased reattempt rate in prior suicide attempters by half. 1) Establish therapeutic alliance. Have patient tell a story about recent suicidal thought or action. 2) Help patient develop the skills needed to deal with the thoughts or feelings that trigger suicidal crises. 3) Have patient imagine being in the situation that brought on the earlier crisis, but this time, guide that patient to practice problem-solving strategies—reinforcing the use of coping skills, rather than suicidal actions (2,3).
- Psychotherapy with suicidal patients is a challenge even for the most experienced clinicians. The countertransference, a clinician's feelings toward a patient, can evolve into wanting to be rid of the patient. If the patient detects this, the risk of suicide is heightened. The clinician can avoid this by recognizing countertransference and bearing it within so that the patient remains unaware (4).

- Among military personnel: ACE campaign: Ask about suicidal thoughts; care for the person, including removing access to lethal weapons; "escort" the soldier to help: an emergency room, to calling 911 or a support hotline such as (800) 273-TALK (8255)

MEDICATION

- Psychopharmacology "is not a substitute for getting to know the patient"(5).
- Patients are at increased risk of suicide at the outset of antidepressant treatment and when it is discontinued. Consider tapering/switching medical therapies rather than sudden discontinuation. Monitor carefully at these times.
- Anxiety, agitation, and delusions increasing in intensity are risk factors for suicide and should be treated aggressively.
- In patients with mood disorders, a meta-analysis of randomized, controlled trials found that lithium reduced the risk of death by suicide by 60% (5)[A].
- Agitated or combative patients may require sedation with IV or IM benzodiazepines and/or antipsychotics. Clinical response is typically seen within 20–30 minutes if given IM/IV.

Pediatric Considerations

FDA posted black box warning for antidepressant use in the pediatric population after increased suicidality was noted. If risk of untreated depression is sufficient to warrant treatment with antidepressants, children must be monitored closely for suicidality.

First Line

ECGs before prescribing or continuing antidepressants or antipsychotics to look for QT prolongation

ISSUES FOR REFERRAL

Consider a psychiatric consult. All decisions regarding treatment must be carefully documented and communicated to all involved health care providers

INPATIENT CONSIDERATIONS

Admission Criteria/Initial Stabilization

- Inpatient hospitalization if patient is suicidal with a plan to act or is otherwise at high risk; if immediate risk for self-harm, may be hospitalized involuntarily
- Immediately after a suicide attempt, treat the medical problems resulting from the self-harm before attempting to initiate psychiatric care.
- Order lab work (e.g., solvent screen, blood and urine toxicology screen, aspirin and acetaminophen levels). Patients may not disclose ingestions if they wish to succeed in their attempt or if they are undergoing mental status changes.
- Risk for self-harm continues even in hospital setting. Immediate search for and remove potentially dangerous objects, 1-to-1 constant observation, medication. Mechanical restraints only if necessary for patient safety.
- The period after transfer from involuntary to voluntary hospitalization is also a time of high risk.

Discharge Criteria

- No longer considered a danger to self/others
- Clinicians should be aware that a patient may *claim* that he or she is no longer suicidal in order to facilitate discharge—and complete the act. Look for clinical and behavioral signs that the patient truly is no longer in despair and is hopeful, such as improved appetite, sleep, engagement with staff, and group therapy. Clinicians should check with family and ancillary staff because patients may share more information with them than with doctors.
- Provide information about 24/7 resources.

ONGOING CARE

FOLLOW-UP RECOMMENDATIONS

Patient Monitoring

- Increase monitoring at the beginning of treatment, when changing medications, and on discharge.
- Educate family members and other close contacts/confidants to the warning signs of suicidality. For adults: despair/hopelessness, isolation, discussing suicide, stating that the world would be a "better place" without them, losses in areas key to the patient's self-worth. For youths: may exhibit the same signs and symptoms, but one should be aware of these additional risks: history of abuse (e.g., sexual, physical), bullying in person or via electronic media (e.g., text messages or social Web sites), family stress, changes in eating and sleeping patterns, suicidality of friends, and giving away treasured items
- Make sure that the patient is willing to accept the type of follow-up offered. Do not assume that just setting it up is sufficient protection.
- Curtail access to firearms.
- Limiting the number of pills may be appropriate for an impulsive patient. However, clinicians may believe that by simply limiting the number of pills they prescribe, they are preventing further suicide attempts, an example of "magical thinking." Clinicians who find themselves thinking this way can take it as a warning sign that their patients may actually be at increased risk of suicide.

PATIENT EDUCATION

Patients who feel they are in danger of hurting themselves should consider one or several of these options:

- Call 911.
- Go directly to an emergency room.
- If already in counseling, contact that therapist immediately.
- Call the National Suicide Prevention Hotline at (800) 273-TALK (8255).
- Servicemen and servicewomen and their families can call (800) 796-9699; if there is no immediate answer, call (800) 273-TALK (8255).

PROGNOSIS

The key to a favorable course and prognosis is early recognition of risk factors, early diagnosis and treatment of a psychiatric disorder, and appropriate intervention and follow-up.

COMPLICATIONS

- According to the American Association of Suicidality (AAS), the grief process for significant others of suicide victims can be lifelong and can be expressed in emotions ranging from anger to despair. Survivors often attempt to shoulder the burden on their own because of the added guilt and shame of the nature of the attempted death or death.
- The AAS recommends the following:
  - Counseling: could include short-term behavioral therapy as well as psychotherapy; some therapy should focus on the survivors' relationships to their current and future significant others. Survivors often seek out life partners as "replacements" for those they lost—could interfere with mourning (6).
  - Sympathetic listening by friends
  - Support during holidays
  - More self-help strategies: www.survivorsofsuicide.com

REFERENCES

1. Jollant F, Bellivier F, Leboyer M, et al. Impaired decision making in suicide attempters. *Am J Psychiatry.* 2005;162(2):304–310.
2. Brown GK, Ten Have T, Henriques GR, et al. Cognitive therapy for the prevention of suicide attempts: a randomized controlled trial. *JAMA.* 2005;295(5):563–570.
3. Ghahramanlou-Holloway M, Neely L, Tucker J. A cognitive behavioral strategy for preventing suicide. *Current Psychiatry.* 2014;13(8):19–28.
4. Maltsberger JT, Buie DH. Countertransference hate in the treatment of suicidal patients. *Arch Gen Psychiatry.* 1974;30(5):625–633.
5. Cipriani A, Pretty H, Hawton K, et al. Lithium in the prevention of suicidal behavior and all-cause mortality in patients with mood disorders: a systematic review of randomized trials. *Am J Psychiatry.* 2005;162(10):1805–1819.
6. Massicotte WJ. Faculty, Canadian Institute of Psychoanalysis; Chair, National Scientific Program Committee. Correspondence, April 24, 2009.

ADDITIONAL READING

- Bryan CJ, Jennings KW, Jobes DA, et al. Understanding and preventing military suicide. *Arch Suicide Res.* 2012;16(2):95–110.
- Gutheil TG, Bursztajn H, Brodsky A. The multidimensional assessment of dangerousness: competence assessment in patient care and liability prevention. *Bull Am Acad Psychiatry Law.* 1986;14(2):123–129.
- O'Connor E, Gaynes BN, Burda BU, et al. Screening for and treatment of suicide risk relevant to primary care: a systematic review for the U.S. Preventive Services Task Force. *Ann Intern Med.* 2013;158(10):741–754.

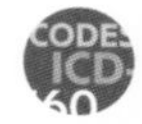

CODES

ICD10

- R45.851 Suicidal ideations
- T14.91 Suicide attempt
- Z91.5 Personal history of self-harm

CLINICAL PEARLS

- Key preventative measure is to listen to a patient and take steps to keep him or her safe. This could include immediate hospitalization. Questions to explore include, "Are you thinking of killing yourself?," "Who do you have to live for?," and "What should change so that you could live with your suffering?"
- Clozapine, lithium, and cognitive-behavioral therapy are associated with a reduction in the risk of suicide.
- Family members and contacts of people who have attempted or committed suicide suffer from reactions ranging from rage to despair. Their grief is often longer lasting and less well-treated because of the shame and guilt associated with the act. Encourage them to discuss this and consider counseling.
- Resources for clinicians: www.suicidology.com; www.suicideassessment.com

SUPERFICIAL THROMBOPHLEBITIS

Jeremy Golding, MD, FAAFP

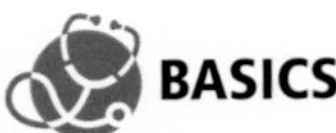

BASICS

DESCRIPTION

- Superficial thrombophlebitis is venous inflammation with secondary thrombosis.
- Traumatic thrombophlebitis types:
  - Injury
  - IV catheter related
  - Intentional (i.e., sclerotherapy)
- Septic (suppurative) thrombophlebitis types:
  - Iatrogenic, long-term IV catheter use
  - Infectious, mainly syphilis and psittacosis
- Aseptic thrombophlebitis types:
  - Primary hypercoagulable states: disorders with measurable defects in the proteins of the coagulation and/or fibrinolytic systems
  - Secondary hypercoagulable states: clinical conditions with a risk of thrombosis
- Mondor disease
  - Rare presentation of anterior chest/breast veins of women
- System(s) affected: cardiovascular
- Synonym(s): phlebitis; phlebothrombosis

Geriatric Considerations

Septic thrombophlebitis is more common; prognosis is poorer.

Pediatric Considerations

Subperiosteal abscesses of adjacent long bone may complicate the disorder.

Pregnancy Considerations

- Associated with increased risk of aseptic superficial thrombophlebitis
- NSAIDs are contraindicated.

EPIDEMIOLOGY

- Predominant age
  - Traumatic/IV related has no predominate age/sex.
  - Aseptic primary hypercoagulable state
    - Childhood to young adult
- Aseptic secondary hypercoagulable state
  - Mondor disease: women, ages 21–55 years
  - Thromboangiitis obliterans onset: ages 20–50 years
- Predominant sex
  - Suppurative: male = female
  - Aseptic
    - Mondor: female > male (2:1)
    - Thromboangiitis obliterans: female > male (1–19% of clinical cases)

Incidence

- Septic
  - Incidence of catheter-related thrombophlebitis is 88/100,000 persons.
  - Develops in 4–8% if cutdown is performed
- Aseptic primary hypercoagulable state: antithrombin III and heparin cofactor II deficiency incidence is 50/100,000 persons.
- Aseptic secondary hypercoagulable state
  - In pregnancy, 49-fold increased incidence of phlebitis
  - Superficial migratory thrombophlebitis in 27% of patients with thromboangiitis obliterans

Prevalence

- Superficial thrombophlebitis is common.
- 1/3 of patients in a medical ICU develop thrombophlebitis that eventually progresses to the deep veins.

ETIOLOGY AND PATHOPHYSIOLOGY

- Similar to deep venous thrombosis. Virchow triad of vessel trauma, stasis, and hypercoagulability (genetic, iatrogenic, or idiopathic)
- Mondor disease pathophysiology not completely understood
- Septic
  - *Staphylococcus aureus*, *Pseudomonas*, *Klebsiella*, *Peptostreptococcus* sp.
  - *Candida* sp.
- Aseptic primary hypercoagulable state
  - Due to inherited disorders of hypercoagulability
- Aseptic secondary hypercoagulable states
  - Malignancy (Trousseau syndrome: recurrent migratory thrombophlebitis): most commonly seen in metastatic mucin or adenocarcinomas of the GI tract (pancreas, stomach, colon, and gallbladder), lung, prostate, and ovary
  - Pregnancy
  - Oral contraceptives
  - Behçet, Buerger, or Mondor disease

Genetics

Not applicable other than hypercoagulable states

RISK FACTORS

- Nonspecific
  - Immobilization
  - Obesity
  - Advanced age
  - Postoperative states
- Traumatic/septic
  - IV catheter (plastic > coated)
  - Lower extremity IV catheter
  - Cutdowns
  - Cancer, debilitating diseases
  - Burn patients
  - AIDS
  - Varicose veins
- Aseptic
  - Pregnancy
  - Oral contraceptives
  - Surgery, trauma, infection
  - Hypercoagulable state (i.e., factor V, protein C or S deficiency, others)
- Thromboangiitis obliterans: persistent smoking
- Mondor disease
  - Breast cancer or breast surgery

GENERAL PREVENTION

- Avoid lower extremity cannulations/IV.
- Insert catheters under aseptic conditions, secure cannulas, and replace every 3 days.
- Avoid stasis and use usual deep vein thrombosis (DVT) prophylaxis in high-risk patients (i.e., ICU, immobilized)

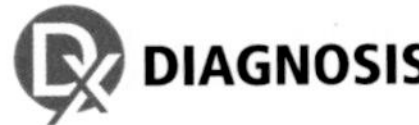

DIAGNOSIS

HISTORY

Pain along the course of a vein

PHYSICAL EXAM

- Swelling, tenderness, redness along the course of a vein or veins
- May look like localized cellulitis or erythema nodosum
- Fever in 70% of patients in septic phlebitis
- Sign of systemic sepsis in 84% of suppurative cases

DIFFERENTIAL DIAGNOSIS

- Cellulitis
- DVT
- Erythema nodosum
- Cutaneous polyarteritis nodosa

DIAGNOSTIC TESTS & INTERPRETATION

Initial Tests (lab, imaging)

Often none necessary if afebrile, otherwise healthy

- Small or distal veins (i.e., forearms or below the knee): no recommended imaging
- If concern for more proximal extension: venous Doppler US to assess extent of thrombosis and rule out DVT

Follow-Up Tests & Special Considerations

- If suspicious for sepsis
  - Blood cultures (bacteremia in 80–90%)
  - Consider culture of the IV fluids being infused.
  - CBC demonstrates leukocytosis.
- Aseptic: evaluation for coagulopathy if recurrent or without another identifiable cause (e.g., protein C and S, lupus anticoagulant, anticardiolipin antibody, factor V and VIII, homocysteine)
- In migratory thrombophlebitis, have a high index of suspicion for malignancy.
- Repeat venous ultrasound to assess effectiveness of therapy.
  - If thrombosis is extending, more aggressive therapy required.

Test Interpretation

The affected vein is enlarged, tortuous, and thickened with endothelial damage and necrosis.

TREATMENT

GENERAL MEASURES

- Suppurative: consultation for urgent surgical venous excision
- Local, mild
  - Conservative management, antibiotics not useful
  - For varicosities
    - Compression stockings, maintain activities
  - Catheter/trauma associated
    - Immediately remove IV and culture tip.
    - Elevate with application of warm compresses.
    - If slow to resolve, consider LMWH.
- Large, severe, or septic thrombophlebitis
  - Inpatient care or bed rest with elevation and local warm compress
  - When the patient is ambulating, then start compression stockings or Ace bandages.

MEDICATION

First Line

- Best medication(s) and duration of treatment are not well-defined (1)[A].
- Localized, mild thrombophlebitis (usually self-limited)
  - NSAIDs and ASA for inflammation/pain reduce symptoms and local progression (1).

Second Line

- Septic/suppurative
  - May present or be complicated by sepsis
  - Requires IV antibiotics (broad spectrum initially) and anticoagulation
- Large veins or involving long saphenous vein are at risk for progression into DVT; consider pharmacologic preventive therapies.
  - To prevent venous thromboembolism (VTE), 4 weeks of LMWH; such as enoxaparin
  - 45 days of fondaparinux was found to reduce DVT and VTE by 85% (relative risk reduction) in 1 large study (2)[B].
- Superficial thrombophlebitis related to inherited or acquired hypercoagulable states is addressed by treating the related disease.

ISSUES FOR REFERRAL

Severely inflamed or very large phlebitis should be evaluated for excision.

SURGERY/OTHER PROCEDURES

- Septic
  - Surgical consultation for excision of the involved vein segment and involved tributaries
  - Drain contiguous abscesses
  - Remove all associated cannula and culture tips.
- Aseptic: Manage underlying conditions.
  - Evaluate for saphenous vein ligation to prevent deep vein extension.
  - Consider referral for varicosity excision.

INPATIENT CONSIDERATIONS

Admission Criteria/Initial Stabilization

- Septic: inpatient
- Aseptic: outpatient

ONGOING CARE

FOLLOW-UP RECOMMENDATIONS

Patient Monitoring

- Septic: routine WBC count and differential. Target treatment based on culture results.
- Severe aseptic
  - Repeat venous Doppler US in 1–2 weeks to ensure no DVT and assess treatment effectiveness: Do not expect resolution, just nonprogression.
  - Repeat clotting studies.
- Local, mild thrombophlebitis typically resolves with conservative therapy and does not require specific monitoring unless there is a failure to resolve.

DIET

No restrictions

PATIENT EDUCATION

Review local care, elevation, and use of compression hose for acute treatment and prevention of recurrence.

PROGNOSIS

- Septic/suppurative
  - High mortality (50%) if untreated
  - Depends on treatment delay or need for surgery
- Aseptic
  - Usually benign course; recovery in 2–3 weeks
  - Depends on development of DVT and early detection of complications
  - Aseptic thrombophlebitis can be isolated, recurrent, or migratory.
  - Recurrence likely if related to varicosity or if severely affected vein not removed

COMPLICATIONS

- Septic: systemic sepsis, bacteremia (84%), septic pulmonary emboli (44%), metastatic abscess formation, pneumonia (44%), subperiosteal abscess of adjacent long bones in children
- Aseptic: DVT, VTE, thromboembolic phenomena

REFERENCES

1. Di Nisio M, Wichers IM, Middeldorp S. Treatment for superficial thrombophlebitis of the leg. *Cochrane Database Syst Rev*. 2013;4:CD004982.
2. Decousus H, Prandoni P, Mismetti P, et al. Fondaparinux for the treatment of superficial-vein thrombosis in the legs. *N Engl J Med*. 2010; 363(13):1222–1232.

ADDITIONAL READING

- Gillet JL, Ffrench P, Hanss M, et al. Predictive value of D-dimer assay in superficial thrombophlebitis of the lower limbs [in French]. *J Mal Vasc*. 2007;32(2): 90–95.
- Samlaska CP, James WD. Superficial thrombophlebitis. I. Primary hypercoagulable states. *J Am Acad Dermatol*. 1990;22(6, Pt 1):975–989.
- Samlaska CP, James WD. Superficial thrombophlebitis. II. Secondary hypercoagulable states. *J Am Acad Dermatol*. 1990;23(1):1–18.
- Wichers IM, Di Nisio M, Büller HR, et al. Treatment of superficial vein thrombosis to prevent deep vein thrombosis and pulmonary embolism: a systematic review. *Haematologica*. 2005;90(5):672–677.

SEE ALSO

Deep Vein Thrombophlebitis (DVT)

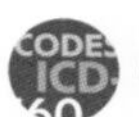

CODES

ICD10

- I80.9 Phlebitis and thrombophlebitis of unspecified site
- I80.00 Phlbts and thombophlb of superfic vessels of unsp low extrm
- I80.8 Phlebitis and thrombophlebitis of other sites

CLINICAL PEARLS

- Mild superficial thrombophlebitis is typically self-limiting and responds well to conservative care
- Lower extremity disease benefits from anticoagulation to prevent DVT.
- Septic thrombophlebitis requires admission for antibiotics and anticoagulation. If severe, consider surgical consultation for venous excision.

SURGICAL COMPLICATIONS

Nathaniel J. Walsh, MD • James R. Yon, MD • Edward James Kruse, DO

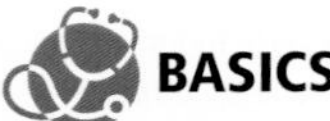

BASICS

DESCRIPTION

- Any negative outcome in operative or postoperative period; no consensus on definition
- Multiple classification systems exist based on severity.

EPIDEMIOLOGY

Incidence

Incidence varies with type of operation, operative time, hospital, surgeon, and patient comorbidities.

- Emergent cases associated with more complications than nonemergent cases (22.8% vs. 14.2%) and have higher mortality rate (6.5% vs. 1.4%) (1)
- Mortality rate in general and vascular surgery is 3.5–6.9% (2).
- Overall complication rate in general and vascular surgery is 24.6–26.9%.
- Postoperative fever is very common. Incidence ranges 14–91% (3).
- Rate of venous thromboembolic events: 3/1,000 surgical discharges in the United States
- Complications after bariatric surgery: anastomotic leak (0–5.6%), internal hernia (3–4.5%), marginal ulcer (1–16%), GI bleeding (0.6–4%), and acute distention of distal stomach
- Rate of ventral hernia after laparotomy: 2–25% (4)
- Surgical site infection (SSI) incidence varies with type of operation
  - 1–2% clean operative site (e.g., hernia repair)
  - 5–15% clean contaminated site (e.g., cholecystectomy)
  - 10–20% contaminated site (e.g., colectomy)
  - 50% dirty operative site

ETIOLOGY AND PATHOPHYSIOLOGY

- Fever caused by pyrogens (mediated by IL-1, IL-6, TNF, interferon- γ): bacteria, viruses, antigen–antibody complexes
- Most common noninfectious causes of postoperative fever: DVT, gout, transfusion reaction, alcohol withdrawal, hematoma, medication, pancreatitis (3)
- Wound dehiscence: poor wound healing, malnutrition, excessive tension, poor surgical technique, diabetes, obesity
- Deep vein thrombosis (DVT): blood clot formation incited by Virchow triad
  - Hypercoagulability
  - Hemodynamic changes (stasis, turbulence)
  - Endothelial injury/dysfunction
- Neurologic: delirium (hypoactive, hyperactive, or mixed)
- Renal failure
  - Drug toxicity (commonly antibiotics)
  - Inadequate resuscitation leading to poor perfusion (catecholamine release during surgery and activation of renin-angiotensin-aldosterone system) results in acute tubular necrosis (ATN).
- Respiratory
  - Pulmonary mechanics are compromised postoperatively. Precipitating factors include pain and altered mental status.
  - Decreased vital capacity leads to atelectasis, pneumonitis or pneumonia, and acute respiratory distress syndrome (ARDS).
  - Aspiration can occur at any time. Stomach acid/particulate matter causes an inflammatory reaction in airway, leading to respiratory distress or death.
  - Pulmonary edema due to fluid transudation to alveolus from fluid overload or heart failure
- Cardiac
  - Postoperative MI occurs within 3 days of surgery; caused by anesthetics and blood loss (loss of as little as 500 mL can cause shock).
  - Arrhythmia is due to destabilization of cardiac membranes or prolongation of conduction.
- Small bowel obstruction: Adhesive bands cause bowel torsion or constriction at any time after intra-abdominal procedures.
- Urinary retention: more frequent in men than women; impaired coordination between α-receptors in the bladder neck and parasympathetic stimulation to the bladder due to anesthetic agents
- Fever in the first 24 hours is usually due to atelectasis. Consider the 5 Ws.
  - Wind—atelectasis, pulmonary nodular amyloidosis (PNA), aspiration (24–48 hours)
  - Water—UTI (72 hours)
  - Walking—deep venous thrombosis (7 days)
  - Wound—SSI (4–5 days typically but anytime)
  - Wonder drugs—drug fever (anytime)
- Emergent causes of early postoperative fever (24–48 hours): necrotizing infection, pulmonary embolus, anastomotic leak, adrenal insufficiency, alcohol withdrawal, and malignant hyperthermia (3)
- *Staphylococcus aureus* is the most common cause of wound infection. Others include *Streptococcus*, *Pseudomonas*, *Proteus*, and *Klebsiella*.
- Hematoma: usually from inadequate hemostasis
- Seroma: disruption of small blood vessels and inflammation
- UTI: related to indwelling catheter
- Renal failure: hypovolemia, drug toxicity (commonly due to antibiotics or IV contrast)
- Respiratory: volume overload, aspiration, and decreased vital capacity lead to decreased diffusion capacity. Pulmonary embolism formation is another possible postoperative etiology.
- Pulmonary embolism: generally due to thromboembolism from the deep veins of the legs or pelvis; more rarely from air, fat, or amniotic fluid
- Cardiac: Arrhythmia occurs due to electrolyte abnormalities, catecholamine release (from pain), hypercapnia, and digitalis.
- Fistula/intestinal leak: generally occurs at the site of bowel anastomosis due to suture line or staple line breakdown
- Stomal complications
  - More common in obese patients
  - Include fibrosis of bowel at stoma, necrosis, retraction, skin breakdown, parastomal hernia, prolapsed of stoma, and stomal stricture
  - Most complications are due to technical errors at the time of operation.

Genetics

- Malignant hyperthermia syndrome (MHS): autosomal dominant inheritance with incomplete penetrance; a skeletal muscle disorder; hypermetabolic crisis following administration of halogenated inhalational anesthetic agents or succinylcholine
- Incidence: 1/50–100,000; treated with dantrolene
- No practical screening tests for general population.

RISK FACTORS

- People at increased operative risk include the following:
  - Poorly controlled diabetes/obesity
  - Heart disease (especially myocardial infarction [MI] and heart failure)
  - Bleeding disorders
  - Malnutrition
  - Renal failure
  - Liver and pulmonary disease
  - Smoking—current smokers have increased rates of major respiratory complications and SSI regardless of surgical specialty, complexity of case, or operative time (5).
  - Immunosuppression
  - Malignancy
  - Increased preoperative frailty as defined by measureable baseline frailty traits (6).
- Other risk factors:
  - Prolonged surgery
  - Immobility following surgery
  - Emergency surgery
- Bleeding disorders, including hemophilia

GENERAL PREVENTION

Preventive measures span entire perioperative period.

- Clip hair instead of shaving preoperatively, although data unclear (7).
- Smoking cessation (pulmonary complications decrease with increasing time after cessation) (8)
- Imaging
- Appropriate fluid/blood resuscitation
- Assessment of underlying risk factors
- Preoperative antibiotics, when appropriate
- Sterile technique
- Warming during surgery

COMMONLY ASSOCIATED CONDITIONS

- Adrenal insufficiency steroids preoperatively
- Arrhythmia
- Liver failure in patients with preexisting disease
- Renal insufficiency
- Delirium tremens in alcoholics/delirium
- Thyroid storm in patients with undiagnosed hyperthyroidism
- Depression

Pediatric Considerations

Operative procedures can lead to severe anxiety in children aged 1–2 years, with lasting emotional disturbance in 20%.

Geriatric Considerations

90% of patients >65 years of age experienced depression after surgery, with ADLs impaired in 50%. Increase human contact to prevent withdrawal and reduce symptoms.

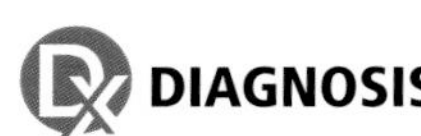

DIAGNOSIS

HISTORY

- Wound infection: history of surgery several days prior to presentation with pain, warmth, redness, or drainage at site of incision.
- Expanding mass is consistent with seroma or hematoma. Hematoma more likely if surgery within 2–3 days; seroma more likely if interval is longer.
- Dehiscence/hernia: Patients may feel sutures "pop" and sense a palpable bulge. Attributed to increased abdominal pressure (e.g., coughing, Valsalva maneuver) or excessive tension on wound
- DVT: pain, swelling, and redness of leg in immobilized patient or with hypercoagulability
- Renal failure: oliguria or anuria, fatigue, electrolyte abnormalities, elevated creatinine and BUN

- Pulmonary: lack of incentive spirometry, narcotics, fluid retention, age >65 years, shortness of breath
- Cardiac: elderly, cardiac dysfunction; chest pain in 27% of perioperative MI (most are pain free)
- Ileus or small bowel obstruction: progressive nausea, bilious vomiting, inability to tolerate PO intake, abdominal pain, cessation of flatus
- Fistula or intestinal leak: severe abdominal pain (leak), fever, nausea/vomiting, drainage at skin
- Stomal complications: pain at stoma site, change in color of stoma, decreased output, increased amount of bowel above skin level (prolapsed or hernia)
- Urinary retention: inability to void, suprapubic pain

PHYSICAL EXAM

- Low fevers are not significant until 48 hours postoperative. Wound infection is most common cause of fever after 72 hours.
- High fever, mental status changes, hypotension, and rigors are associated with severe wound complications or intestinal leak.
- Fascial dehiscence is a surgical emergency.
- Detection of intra-abdominal complications more challenging in obese patients due to body habitus
- Dolor, tumor, rubor, and calor may indicate a wound infection, fever, pus or foul-smelling discharge.
- Hematoma: expanding, tender mass. Seroma: slowly expanding, nontender mass
- Dehiscence/hernia: salmon-colored drainage on postoperative days 4–5, evisceration, or later as ventral hernia; may see open incision or palpable fascial edge, rarely tender
- Renal failure: persistent oliguria; can have pericardial rub, bleeding/hematoma if uremic
- Pulmonary: dyspnea, cough, fever, basilar crackles or rhonchi, poor inspiratory effort, dullness to percussion at bases
- Cardiac: peripheral edema, irregularly irregular heartbeat, tachycardia
- Ileus/small bowel obstruction: "tinkling" or absent bowel sounds, tympanitic abdomen, distention, tenderness to palpation, occasionally guarding
- Fistula/intestinal leak: enteric or bilious contents draining from skin opening, acute/firm abdomen, fever, guarding, peritoneal signs, hypotension
- Stomal complications are evident when the ostomy appliance is removed: skin irritation, black/discolored intestinal mucosa, retracted or prolapsed ostomy
- Urinary retention: suprapubic pain, palpable bladder
- Anastomotic leak: may manifest as isolated tachycardia or patient anxiety in after gastric bypass

DIAGNOSTIC TESTS & INTERPRETATION

Initial Tests (lab, imaging)

- CBC with differential, blood culture and sensitivity (C/S), chemistries, BUN/creatinine, urinalysis (UA), urine C/S, ABG, chest x-ray (CXR)
- Blood cultures within 48 hours of surgery are usually unnecessary (negative most of the time) (3)[B].
- Obtain blood culture from any central venous access (central line, port, etc.).
- Elevated WBC count with wound infections, atelectasis, pneumonia, infected hematoma/seroma, bowel leak, and stomal complications
- Renal failure: BUN, creatinine, urine chemistries, FENa
- Pulmonary: hypoxia, hypercarbia on ABG
- Cardiac: elevated troponins, creatinine kinase (CK), CK-MB, electrocardiogram (ECG)
- UTI: UA, urine C/S
- Subcutaneous gas can be seen in necrotizing infection on x-ray or CT.
- CT or ultrasound can be used to diagnose hernia or fascial disruption.
- Small bowel obstruction/ileus: Abdominal series with chest 1 view shows air–fluid levels, dilated small bowel.
- Fistula: Fistulogram aids in diagnosis and is critical for treatment planning.
- Intestinal leak: CXR reveals free air under the diaphragm; CT shows fluid collection in abdomen.
- Bladder scan can help diagnose urinary retention if diagnosis in doubt.
- DVT: duplex ultrasound; image iliac veins if possible
- Pulmonary: CXR, CT pulmonary angiography more sensitive test for suspected pulmonary embolism

Diagnostic Procedures/Other

- Exploratory laparotomy/laparoscopy if extremely ill/septic and diagnosis is unknown.
- Intra-abdominal abscesses frequently can be drained percutaneously.
- Cardiac: ECG shows signs of ischemia or dysrhythmia.

TREATMENT

MEDICATION

- Opiates and NSAIDs for pain control
- VTE prophylaxis as appropriate
- Serotonin antagonists (i.e.,—ondansetron) for PONV
- Broad-spectrum antibiotics for sepsis or severe infection (piperacillin/tazobactam and vancomycin)
- Simple wound infections and stomal complications: 1st- or 2nd-generation cephalosporins, trimethoprim/sulfamethoxazole, or clindamycin
- Intestinal leak: gram-negative, anaerobic, and gram-positive coverage (levofloxacin plus metronidazole)
- Pneumonia should be treated empirically with antibiotics appropriate for health care–associated pneumonia and ventilator-associated pneumonia.

SURGERY/OTHER PROCEDURES

- Wound infections may need surgical débridement.
- Hematomas may need reexploration and hemostasis.
- Dehiscence/hernia should be repaired. Evisceration is a surgical emergency.
- Small bowel obstruction that fails to resolve or improve with nasogastric decompression in 48 hours should be explored.
- Intestinal leak is a surgical emergency for immediate exploration and repair. Fistulas may need surgical intervention to resolve.
- Some stomal complications (necrosis, retraction, parastomal hernia) need surgical revision.

INPATIENT CONSIDERATIONS

Admission Criteria/Initial Stabilization

Hemodynamic instability, respiratory distress, need for IV fluids/antibiotics, or nasogastric decompression

- Fluid resuscitation, as needed
- Broad-spectrum antibiotics, if the patient is septic
- IV antibiotics for infections

Discharge Criteria

Able to tolerate PO intake, voiding, return of bowel function, afebrile, good wound healing, and pain controlled

Nursing

- Teaching for drain maintenance and wound care/dressing change prior to discharge
- Close follow-up (1–2 weeks)
- NPO with tube feeds or TPN for patients with fistula upon discharge

REFERENCES

1. Becher RD, Hoth JJ, Miller PR, et al. A critical assessment of outcomes in emergency versus nonemergency general surgery using the American College of Surgeons National Surgical Quality Improvement Program database. *Am Surg*. 2011;77(7):951–959.
2. Ghaferi A, Birkmeyer JD, Dimick JB. Variation in hospital mortality associated with inpatient surgery. *N Engl J Med*. 2009;361(14):1368–1375.
3. Pile JC. Evaluating postoperative fever: a focused approach. *Cleve Clin J Med*. 2006;73(Suppl 1):S62–S66.
4. Fischer JP, Wink JD, Nelson JA, et al. Among 1,706 cases of abdominal wall reconstruction, what factors influence occurrence of major operative complications? *Surgery*. 2014;155(2):311–319.
5. Hawn MT, Houston TK, Campagna EJ, et al. The attributable risk of smoking on surgical complications. *Ann Surg*. 2011;254(6):914–920.
6. Robinson TN, Wu DS, Pointer L, et al. Simple frailty score predicts postoperative complications across surgical specialties. *Am J Surg*. 2013;206(4):544–550.
7. Tanner J, Norrie P, Melen K. Preoperative hair removal to reduce surgical site infection. *Cochrane Database Syst Rev*. 2011;(11):CD004122.
8. Gronkjaer M, Eliasen M, Skov-Ettrup LS, et al. Preoperative smoking status and postoperative complications: a systematic review and meta-analysis. *Ann Surg*. 2014;259(1):52–71.
9. Thomsen T, Tonnesen H, Moller AM. Effect of preoperative smoking cessation interventions on postoperative complications and smoking cessation. *Br J Surg*. 2009;96(5):451–461.

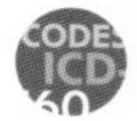

CODES

ICD10

- R50.82 Postprocedural fever
- T81.4XXA Infection following a procedure, initial encounter
- T81.31XA Disruption of external operation (surgical) wound, not elsewhere classified, initial encounter

CLINICAL PEARLS

- Smoking is associated with increased risk for general morbidity, wound complications, general infections, pulmonary complications, neurologic complications, and admission to the intensive care unit (8).
- Smoking cessation at any interval prior to surgery decreases postoperative complications (9).
- Appropriate antibacterial preparation should be used to decrease bacterial counts.
- Treatment of some complications related to hospitalization will no longer be reimbursed by payers, including wrong-site surgery and central venous catheter infections.
- Respiratory complications are the most costly surgical complications related to surgical episode of care (4).

S

SYNCOPE

Santiago O. Valdes, MD, FAAP

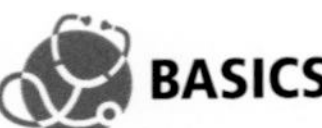

BASICS

DESCRIPTION

- Transient loss of consciousness characterized by unresponsiveness, loss of postural tone, and spontaneous recovery; usually caused by cerebral hypoxemia
- System(s) affected: cardiovascular; nervous

EPIDEMIOLOGY

Incidence

- Up to 20% of adults will have ≥1 episode by age 75 years; 15% of children <18 years of age
- Accounts for 1–6% of hospital admissions and ~3% of emergency room visits
- Annually, prevalence of fainting spells resulting in medical evaluation was 9.5/1,000 inhabitants (1).

Prevalence

In institutionalized elderly (>75 years of age), 6%

ETIOLOGY AND PATHOPHYSIOLOGY

- In some cases, vagal response leads to decreased heart rate.
- Systemic hypotension secondary to decreased cardiac output and/or systemic vasodilation leads to a drop in cerebral perfusion and resulting loss of consciousness.
- Cardiac (obstruction to outflow)
  - Aortic stenosis
  - Hypertrophic cardiomyopathy
  - Pulmonary embolus
- Cardiac arrhythmias
  - Sustained ventricular tachycardia (VT)
  - Supraventricular tachycardia (SVT) (atrial fibrillation, atrial flutter, reentrant SVT)
  - 2nd- and 3rd-degree AV block
  - Sick sinus syndrome
- Noncardiac
  - Reflex-mediated vasovagal (neurocardiogenic/neurally mediated), situational (micturition, defecation, cough, hair combing)
  - Orthostatic hypotension
  - Drug induced
  - Neurologic: seizures; transient ischemic attack (can in theory cause syncope but presentation usually markedly clinically different from pure syncope)
  - Carotid sinus hypersensitivity
  - Psychogenic

Genetics

Specific cardiomyopathies and arrhythmias may be familial (i.e., long QT syndrome, catecholaminergic polymorphic VT, hypertrophic cardiomyopathy).

RISK FACTORS

- Heart disease
- Dehydration
- Drugs
  - Antihypertensives
  - Vasodilators (including calcium channel blockers, ACE inhibitors, and nitrates)
  - Phenothiazines
  - Antidepressants
  - Antiarrhythmics
  - Diuretics

GENERAL PREVENTION

See "Risk Factors."

COMMONLY ASSOCIATED CONDITIONS

See "Etiology."

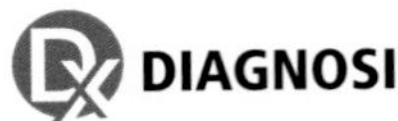

DIAGNOSIS

HISTORY

- Careful history, physical exam, and an ECG are more important than other investigations in determining the diagnosis (2)[A]. Syncope associated with physical exertion suggests a potential cardiac etiology.
- Make sure that the patient or witness (if present) is not talking about vertigo (i.e., sense of rotary motion, spinning, and whirling), seizure, or causes of fall without loss of consciousness.
- Even after careful evaluation, including diagnostic procedures and special tests, the cause will be found in only 50–60% of the patients.
- Onset of syncope is usually rapid, and recovery is spontaneous, rapid, and complete. Duration of episodes are typically brief (<60 seconds). The presence of underlying cardiac or neurologic conditions provides the key to diagnosis.
- Ask for family history of long QT syndrome, hypertrophic cardiomyopathy, or unexplained sudden cardiac death in young family members.

PHYSICAL EXAM

- BP and pulse, both lying and standing
- Check for cardiac murmur or focal neurologic abnormality.

DIFFERENTIAL DIAGNOSIS

- Drop attacks
- Coma
- Vertigo
- Seizure disorder

DIAGNOSTIC TESTS & INTERPRETATION

History and physical examination should guide laboratory testing.

Initial Tests (lab, imaging)

Consider (not all indicated in all individuals) the following:

- CBC
- Electrolytes, BUN, creatinine, glucose (rarely helpful: <2% have hyponatremia, hypocalcemia, hypoglycemia, or renal failure causing seizures)
- Cardiac enzymes (only if history suggestive of cardiac ischemia)
- D-dimer (for pulmonary embolism workup)
- hCG
- Lung scan or helical CT scan of thorax if history and physical exam suggest pulmonary embolism (PE)

Follow-Up & Special Considerations

- If history and physical suggest ischemic, valvular, or congenital heart disease (3)
  - ECG
  - Exercise stress test (if syncope with exertion) (3)[C]
  - Echocardiogram (3)[B]
  - Cardiac catheterization
- If CNS disease suspected (3)[C]
  - EEG
  - Head CT scan
  - Head MRI/MRA when vascular cause is suspected
  - Do not order these tests without hints of CNS disease on history or physical exam.
- ECG monitoring, either in hospital or ambulatory (Holter) (3)[C]
  - Useful in 4–15% of patients
  - Should be done in patients with heart disease or recurrent syncope
  - Arrhythmias frequently documented but not always associated with syncope
- Electrophysiologic studies (3,4)[C]
  - Have been positive in 18–75% of patients
  - Induction of VT and dysfunction of His-Purkinje system are the 2 most common abnormalities.
  - Should be done in patients with heart disease and recurrent syncope, although they may not show whether arrhythmia noted or induced during study is cause of syncope
- Carotid hypersensitivity evaluation (3,4)[C]
  - Carotid hypersensitivity should be considered in patients with syncope during head turning, especially while wearing tight collars, and with neck tumors and neck scars.
  - The technique is not standardized; 1 side at a time is compressed gently at a time for 20 seconds with constant monitoring of pulse and BP/ECG.
  - Atropine should be readily available.
- Tilt-table testing ± isoproterenol infusion (3)[B],(4)[C]
  - Provocative test for vasovagal syncope
  - Perform if cardiac causes have been excluded; role in workup of patients with syncope of unknown origin
  - Protocol is not standardized but has been reported positive (symptomatic hypotension and bradycardia) in 26–87% of patients; also positive in up to 45% of control subjects.
- Psychiatric evaluation (3)[C]: Anxiety, depression, and alcohol and drug abuse can be associated with syncope.

Diagnostic Procedures/Other

Patient-activated implantable loop recorders can record 4–5 minutes of retrograde ECG rhythm. Helpful in selective patients with recurrent syncope, with yield of 32–80% (3,4)[B].

Test Interpretation

Depends on etiology and presence of underlying cardiac or neurologic conditions

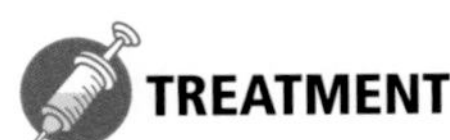

TREATMENT

Maintaining good hydration status and normal salt intake are initial therapy. Educate patients of the premonitory signs of syncope (5)[B].

GENERAL MEASURES

- Elderly patients without previously recognized heart disease should be admitted if the physician thinks that the cause of syncope is likely cardiac.
- Patients without heart disease, especially young patients (age <60 years), can be worked up safely as outpatients.

- Prescribe antiarrhythmics for documented arrhythmias occurring simultaneously with syncope or symptoms of presyncope. Asymptomatic arrhythmias do not necessarily require treatment.
- The decision to treat patients on basis of arrhythmias or conduction abnormalities provoked or detected during EPS is even more problematic: Does the arrhythmia or conduction abnormality have anything to do with the patient's symptoms?
- Most would treat patients with provoked sustained VT with an antiarrhythmic drug that suppressed arrhythmia during study.
- Rationale for such treatment: Recurrent syncope is less frequent in patients with positive EPS who are treated than it is in those who have negative EPS.

MEDICATION

First Line

- Geared toward specific underlying cardiac or neurologic abnormalities
- In cases of recurrent vasovagal/neurocardiogenic/neurally mediated syncope (6)[B]
  - α-Adrenergic agonists (midodrine)
  - Mineralocorticoids (fludrocortisone)
  - β-Adrenergic blockers

Second Line

- SSRIs (paroxetine, sertraline, fluoxetine)
- Vagolytics (disopyramide)

ISSUES FOR REFERRAL

When cardiac or neurologic etiologies are suspected, obtain appropriate consultation, as indicated.

ADDITIONAL THERAPIES

For vasovagal/neurocardiogenic/neurally mediated syncope:

- Counterpressure maneuvers, orthostatic training, and exercise have improved vasovagal symptoms and recurrence (3,5)[C].
- Head-up tilt sleeping (3)[C]
- Abdominal binders and/or support stockings (3)[C]

SURGERY/OTHER PROCEDURES

- Implantable cardioverter-defibrillator (ICD) placement for patients with cardiac conditions with high risk of sudden death and/or recurrent syncope on medications (i.e., long QT syndrome, catecholaminergic polymorphic VT, hypertrophic cardiomyopathy) (3)[B]
- Many recommend pacemaker implantation in patients with the following:
  - 2nd- (Mobitz type II) and 3rd-degree heart block
  - H-V intervals $>$100 ms
  - Pacing-induced infranodal block
  - Sinus node recovery time $\geq$3 seconds

INPATIENT CONSIDERATIONS

Admission Criteria/Initial Stabilization

Patients with benign etiologies of syncope with negative ED workups are associated with benign outcomes, even in the presence of other risk factors (7)[B].

Patients with suspected cardiac or neurologic cause for syncope should be admitted to the hospital for evaluation.

- Support ABCs.
- Stabilize heart rate and BP, typically with IV fluids.

IV Fluids

Use isotonic crystalloid fluids for fluid resuscitation, if needed.

Nursing

Close monitoring of BP and heart rate during initial presentation

Discharge Criteria

- Attainment of hemodynamic stability
- Satisfactory completion of workup for etiology
- Adequate control of specific arrhythmia or seizure, if present

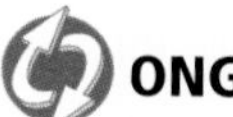

ONGOING CARE

FOLLOW-UP RECOMMENDATIONS

Patient Monitoring

- Frequent follow-up visits for patients with cardiac causes of syncope, especially patients on antiarrhythmics
- Patients with an unknown cause of syncope rarely (5%) are diagnosed during the follow-up.

DIET

- No specific diet unless the patient has heart disease.
- Increased fluid and salt intake to maintain intravascular volume in cases of recurrent vasovagal syncope

PATIENT EDUCATION

- Reassure the patient that most cardiac causes of syncope can be treated, and patients with noncardiac causes do well, even if the cause of syncope is never discovered.
- Physical counterpressure maneuvers can prevent recurrences of vasovagal syncope.
- Physician and patient should carefully consider whether the patient should continue to drive while syncope is being evaluated. Physicians should be aware of pertinent laws in their own states.

PROGNOSIS

- Cumulative mortality at 2 years
  - Low: young patients ($<$60 years of age) with noncardiac or unknown cause of syncope
  - Intermediate: older patients ($>$60 years of age) with noncardiac or unknown cause of syncope
  - High: patients with cardiac cause of syncope
- Independent predictors of poor short-term outcomes (8,9)[B]
  - Abnormal ECG
  - Shortness of breath
  - Systolic BP $<$90 mm Hg
  - Hematocrit $<$30%
  - Congestive heart failure

COMPLICATIONS

- Trauma from falling
- Death (see "Prognosis")

REFERENCES

1. Malasana G, Brignole M, Daccarett M, et al. The prevalence and cost of the faint and fall problem in the state of Utah. *Pacing Clin Electrophysiol*. 2011;34(3):278–283.
2. Kessler C, Tristano JM, De Lorenzo R. The emergency department approach to syncope: evidence-based guidelines and prediction rules. *Emerg Med Clin North Am*. 2010;28(3):487–500.
3. Task Force for the Diagnosis and Management of Syncope, European Society of Cardiology, European Heart Rhythm Association, et al. Guidelines for the diagnosis and management of syncope (version 2009). *Eur Heart J*. 2009;30(21): 2631–2671.
4. Brignole M, Hamdan MH. New concepts in the assessment of syncope. *J Am Coll Cardiol*. 2012;59(18):1583–1591.
5. Romme JJ, Reitsma JB, Go-Schön IK, et al. Prospective evaluation of non-pharmacological treatment in vasovagal syncope. *Europace*. 2010;12(4):567–573.
6. Kuriachan V, Sheldon RS, Platonov M. Evidence-based treatment for vasovagal syncope. *Heart Rhythm*. 2008;5(11):1609–1614.
7. Grossman SA, Fischer C, Kancharla A, et al. Can benign etiologies predict benign outcomes in high-risk syncope patients? *J Emerg Med*. 2011;40(5):592–597.
8. Quinn JV, Stiell IG, McDermott DA, et al. Derivation of the San Francisco Syncope Rule to predict patients with short-term serious outcomes. *Ann Emerg Med*. 2004;43(2):224–232.
9. Saccilotto RT, Nickel CH, Bucher HC, et al. San Francisco Syncope Rule to predict short-term serious outcomes: a systematic review. *CMAJ*. 2011;183(15):E1116–E1126.

ADDITIONAL READING

- Parry SW, Tan MP. An approach to the evaluation and management of syncope in adults. *BMJ*. 2010; 340:c880.
- Reed MJ, Newby DE, Coull AJ, et al. The ROSE (risk stratification of syncope in the emergency department) study. *J Am Coll Cardiol*. 2010;55(8): 713–721.
- Strickberger SA, Benson DW, Biaggioni I, et al. AHA/ACCF scientific statement on the evaluation of syncope: from the American Heart Association Councils on Clinical Cardiology, Cardiovascular Nursing, Cardiovascular Disease in the Young, and Stroke, and the Quality of Care and Outcomes Research Interdisciplinary Working Group; and the American College of Cardiology Foundation in Collaboration with the Heart Rhythm Society. *J Am Coll Cardiol*. 2006;47(2):473–484.

SEE ALSO

- Aortic Valvular Stenosis; Atrial Septal Defect (ASD); Carotid Sinus Hypersensitivity; Hypertrophic cardiomyopathy; Patent Ductus Arteriosus; Pulmonary Arterial Hypertension; Pulmonary Embolism; Seizure Disorders; Stokes-Adams Attacks
- Algorithms: Syncope; Transient Ischemic Attack

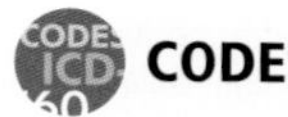

CODES

ICD10

R55 Syncope and collapse

CLINICAL PEARLS

- A careful history and physical exam are key to a diagnosis.
- Use the ECG/event-recorder to evaluate for cardiac conditions.
- True neurologic causes of syncope are very rare; by far, cardiac causes are more common.
- $<$2% of cases are caused by hyponatremia, hypocalcemia, hypoglycemia, or renal failure causing seizures.

SYNCOPE, REFLEX (VASOVAGAL SYNCOPE)

Melinda Y. Kwan, DO, MPH • Norton Winer, MD

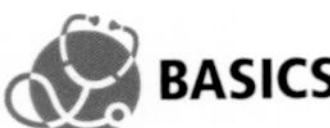

BASICS

Syncope is a reversible loss of consciousness and postural tone secondary to systemic hypotension and cerebral hypoperfusion due to vasodilation and/or bradycardia (rarely, tachycardia) with spontaneous recovery and no neurologic sequelae. The term syncope excludes seizures, coma, shock, or other states of altered consciousness.

DESCRIPTION

- Derived from the Greek term "syncopa," meaning "to cut short"
- Sudden, transient loss of consciousness characterized by unresponsiveness, falling, and spontaneous recovery
- Common cause of syncope in all age groups, especially in patients with no evidence of neurologic or cardiac disease
- 4 types: vasovagal or neurocardiogenic syncope, situational syncope, orthostatic hypotension, carotid sinus hypersensitivity, and glossopharyngeal/trigeminal neuralgia syncope (uncommon) (1)

EPIDEMIOLOGY

- Mortality: cardiac-related syncope 20–30% and 5% in idiopathic syncope
- Age: any age

Incidence

- Ranges from 7.5% in children age <18 years to 15% in adults age >70 years
- 36–62% of all syncopal episodes
- 30% recurrence rate

Prevalence

22% in the general population

ETIOLOGY AND PATHOPHYSIOLOGY

Cause: an abnormal interaction of the normal mechanisms for maintaining BP and upright posture

- In normal individuals, upright posture results in venous pooling and transient decrease in BP.
- Neurally induced syncope may result from a cardioinhibitory response, a vasodepressor response, or a combination of the 2.
- Increased cardiovagal tone leads to bradycardia or asystole, and decreased peripheral sympathetic activity leads to venodilation and hypotension (2).
- Vasovagal syncope usually has a precipitating event, often related to fright, pain, panic, exercise, noxious stimuli, or heat exposure (2).
- Carotid sinus syncope is precipitated by position change, turning head, or wearing a tight collar. (Possible neck tumors or surgical scarring)
- Situational syncope is related to micturition, defecation, postexercise, postprandial, cough, or phobia of needle or blood (3).
- Glossopharyngeal syncope is related to throat or facial pain (4).

Genetics

Vasovagal syncope: strong heritable component to the etiology of >20% of cases

RISK FACTORS

- Low resting BP
- Age: older age
- Prolonged supine position with resulting deconditioning of autonomic control

GENERAL PREVENTION

Avoidance of precipitating events or situations, prevent hypoglycemic events for diabetics, elastic stockings, adequate hydration. Limited evidence suggests that polydipsia may reduce recurrences.

COMMONLY ASSOCIATED CONDITIONS

- Cardiopulmonary disorders: CHF, MI, arrhythmias, hypertrophic obstructive cardiomyopathy, HTN, pulmonary embolism
- Neurologic disorders: autonomic dysfunction, Shy-Drager, Parkinson disease, multiple system atrophy, transient ischemic attack, vertebrobasilar insufficiency, peripheral neuropathy
- Psychiatric disorders
  - Generalized anxiety disorder
  - Panic disorder
  - Major depression
  - Alcohol dependence

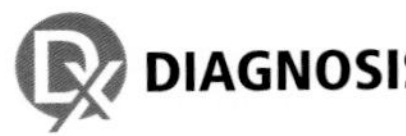

DIAGNOSIS

HISTORY

- Evaluation of syncope and presyncope are the same.
- Important first to rule out cardiac syncope
- Neurally mediated syncope is preceded by blurred vision, palpitations, nausea, warmth, diaphoresis, or light-headedness, or there may be history of nausea, warmth, diaphoresis, or fatigue *after* syncope (5)[C].
- Vasovagal syncope
  - 3 phases: prodrome, loss of consciousness, and postsyncope
  - Precipitating event or stimulus is usually identified, such as panic, fright, pain, or exercise.
  - Athletes may have after exertion (diagnosis of exclusion).
  - Position: *can be preceded by prolonged standing but can occur from any position; generally resolves when the patient becomes supine*
    - Preceding events: as discussed earlier
    - Prodrome: as listed earlier for neurally mediated syncope
  - Duration: generally brief (seconds–minutes)
  - Recovery: may be prolonged with persistent nausea, pallor, and diaphoresis but without neurologic change or confusion
- Carotid sinus syncope is precipitated by position change, after turning head, or wearing a tight collar.
- Situational syncope is related to micturition, defecation, or coughing.
- Glossopharyngeal syncope (less common) is related to throat or facial pain (4)[C].
  - Precipitating events or situations may include panic, pain, exercise, micturition, defecation, coughing, or swallowing.

PHYSICAL EXAM

- Vital signs, including orthostatics and bilateral BP
- Cardiac exam: volume status, murmurs, rhythm, carotid bruits
- Neurologic exam: signs of focal deficit
- Assess for occult blood loss, including guaiac.
- Dix-Hallpike to rule out benign paroxysmal vertigo

DIFFERENTIAL DIAGNOSIS

- Seizure
- Hypoglycemia
- Cardiac syncope
- Cerebrovascular syncope
- Orthostatic hypotension
- Drop attacks
- Psychiatric illness

DIAGNOSTIC TESTS & INTERPRETATION

As indicated by history and physical exam, includes basic tests to rule out the 3 main reasons for syncope: hypoglycemia, arrhythmia, and anemia

Initial Tests (lab, imaging)

- Blood sugar
- ECG should be ordered for all patients. Abnormal ECG findings are common in patients with cardiac syncope.
- CBC to rule out anemia
- Head CT, MRI/MRA, carotid ultrasound only in patients whose history or physical exam suggests a neurologic cause of syncope
  - The 2007 American College of Emergency Physicians (ACEP) Guidelines for diagnostic testing for syncope are as follows (6):
    - *Level A recommendations:* standard 12-lead ECG
    - *Level B recommendations:* none specified
    - *Level C recommendations:* laboratory testing and investigations, including echocardiography or head CT, to be performed only if indicated by specific findings in the history or physical examination

Follow-Up Tests & Special Considerations

- 24-hour Holter monitoring only in patients with a high probability of cardiac cause of syncope and/or abnormal ECG findings
- A low hemoglobin without obvious cause of bleed would warrant a guaiac, CT head to rule out subarachnoid hemorrhage (SAH), CT abdomen to rule out retroperitoneal bleed.
- Stroke, bleed, or carotid stenosis will require appropriate disease-oriented management.
- EEG only when history or physical exam is very suggestive of seizure activity
- Implantable loop recorder

Diagnostic Procedures/Other

- Head-up tilt table testing
  - Contraindicated in patients with known cardiac or neurovascular disease or in pregnancy
  - Indicated for recurrent syncope or single episode accompanied by injury or risk to others (e.g., pilots, surgeons)
  - Uses positional changes to reproduce symptoms
  - Positive tests are diagnostic for vasovagal syncope.
- Carotid sinus massage, only in a monitored setting (i.e., BP and HR monitoring, IV access)
  - Contraindicated in patients with carotid disease (careful auscultation prior to massage is essential)
  - Pressure at the angle of the jaw for 5 seconds with simultaneous ECG monitoring
  - Positive tests (causing syncope or cardiac pause >3 seconds) are diagnostic of carotid sinus syncope.
- Psychiatric evaluation: to rule out anxiety, depression, and alcohol abuse

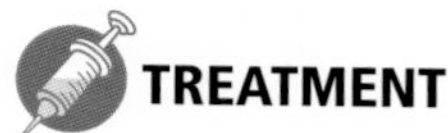

TREATMENT

Therapy is primarily for recurrent syncope. Situational syncope will not warrant any treatment.

GENERAL MEASURES

Recognition and avoidance of precipitating events. Medical management is based on small, nonrandomized clinical trials.

First Line

- Nonpharmacologic treatment
  - Includes patient counseling
    - Development of coping skills
    - Increased salt and fluid intake
  - Moderate exercise training
  - Tilt table training
    - Progressively prolonged periods of enforced upright posture
  - Intense gripping of the hands and tensing of the arms for 2 minutes at the onset of tilt-induced symptoms raised systolic BP (7)[C].

Second Line

- α-agonists are mainly used for orthostatic hypotension.
  - Midodrine is commonly used. It increases peripheral vascular resistance and venous return. Side effects include HTN, paresthesia, urinary retention, "goose bumps," hyperactivity, dizziness, tremor, and nervousness.
- SSRIs: Paroxetine, fluoxetine, and sertraline are SSRIs useful in treating neurocardiogenic/vasovagal syncope.
  - Serotonin induces vagally mediated bradycardia and hypotension.
  - Side effects include weight gain, nausea, anxiety, sexual dysfunction, and insomnia.
- Mineralocorticoids: Fludrocortisone has been found helpful mainly in orthostatic hypotension.
  - Helpful in renal sodium absorption and increasing the vasoconstrictive peripheral vascular response
  - Adverse reactions include fluid retention, HTN, HF, peripheral edema, and hypokalemia.
- β-Blockers: Metoprolol, atenolol, or pindolol are mainly used for postural tachycardia syndrome (POTS).
  - Block peripheral vasodilators and ventricular mechanoreceptor stimulation
  - Stabilization of HR and BP
  - Side effects: hypotension and bradycardia (with worsening of syncope), fatigue, depression, and sexual dysfunction
  - Contraindicated in asthma

ISSUES FOR REFERRAL

Neurology or cardiology, as needed

ADDITIONAL THERAPIES

- Increased salt and fluid intake: may include salt tablets or electrolyte/sports drinks
- Moderate exercise training
- Tilt-table training: involves periods of prolonged, forced upright posture
- Use of support/pressure stockings
- Leg crossing, hand grip, or arm tensing

COMPLEMENTARY & ALTERNATIVE MEDICINE

These include treatments for underlying heart disease or precipitating factors like anxiety. None of these are proven therapies.

- Nutrition and supplements: omega-3 fatty acids, multivitamin, CoQ10, acetyl-L-carnitine, alpha-lipoic acid, and L-arginine
- Herbs: green tea (*Camellia sinensis*), bilberry (*Vaccinium myrtillus*), and ginkgo (*Ginkgo biloba*)
- Homeopathy: Carbo vegetabilis, opium, sepia
- Acupuncture: An analysis of 102 serious cases showed improvement in most. It may precipitate fainting.

SURGERY/OTHER PROCEDURES

Pacemaker placement may be of use in patients with frequent neurocardiogenic/vasovagal syncope that is refractory to other therapies (7)[C].

- Prevents prolonged bradycardia or asystole during syncopal episodes
- Long-term effect
- Invasive placement procedure

INPATIENT CONSIDERATIONS

Admission Criteria/Initial Stabilization

2007 ACEP Guidelines mandate that the patient be admitted if (6):

- *Level B recommendations*
  - Admit patients with syncope and evidence of heart failure or structural heart disease.
  - Admit patients with syncope and high-risk factors.
- High-risk stratification is based on following factors:
  - Older age and associated comorbidities
  - Abnormal ECG, hematocrit (Hct) 30 (if obtained)
  - History or presence of heart failure, coronary artery disease, or structural heart disease
- Additional causes to admit
  - Syncope occurring during exercise
  - Syncope causing severe injury
  - Family history of sudden death

IV Fluids

IV fluids to stabilize HR and BP: isotonic crystalloids, as needed

Nursing

Vital sign monitoring

Discharge Criteria

Hemodynamically stable and workup satisfactory

ONGOING CARE

DIET

- Increased salt intake may be helpful if not contraindicated (2)[C].
- Maintain fluid intake.

PATIENT EDUCATION

- To identify and avoid precipitating events or situations
- Avoid dehydration, alcohol consumption, warm environments, tight clothing, and long periods of standing motionless.
- Recognize presyncopal symptoms.
- Use behaviors, such as lying down, to avoid syncope.

PROGNOSIS

May be recurrent but not life-threatening

COMPLICATIONS

May result in injury from fall

REFERENCES

1. Angaran P, Klein GJ, Yee R, et al. Syncope. *Neurol Clin*. 2011;29(4):903–925.
2. Raj S, Coffin ST. Medical therapy and physical maneuvers in the treatment of the vasovagal syncope and orthostatic hypotension. *Prog Cardiovasc Dis*. 2013;55(4):425–433.
3. Gauer RL. Evaluation of syncope. *Am Fam Physician*. 2011;84(6):640–650.
4. Chen-Scarabelli C, Scarabelli TM. Neurocardiogenic syncope. *BMJ*. 2004;329(7461):336.
5. Chen LY, Benditt DG, Shen WK. Management of syncope in adults: an update. *Mayo Clin Proc*. 2008;83(11):1280–1293.
6. Huff S, Decker W. Clinical policy: critical issues in the evaluation and management of adult patients presenting to the emergency department with syncope. *Ann Emerg Med*. 2007;49(4):431–444.
7. Grubb BP. Clinical practice. Neurocardiogenic syncope. *N Engl J Med*. 2005;352(10):1004–1010.

ADDITIONAL READING

- Lelonek M. Genetics in neurocardiogenic syncope [in Polish]. *Prz Lek*. 2006;63(12):1310–1312.
- Márquez MF, Urias-Medina K, Gómez-Flores J, et al. Comparison of metoprolol vs clonazepam as a first treatment choice among patients with neurocardiogenic syncope [in Spanish]. *Gac Med Mex*. 2008;144(6):503–507.

SEE ALSO

Algorithms: Syncope; Transient Ischemic Attack and Transient Neurologic Defects

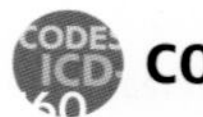

CODES

ICD10

R55 Syncope and collapse

CLINICAL PEARLS

- History should include a careful analysis of the events preceding the attack.
- It is important to rule out cardiologic or neurologic pathology.
- Prodrome is often present.
- Recovery may be prolonged, with persistent symptoms but no neurologic deficit or confusion.
- Patient counseling to avoid precipitating situations or events is 1st-line treatment.
- Pregnant females can have reflex syncope when moving from supine to lateral decubitus or upright positions.

SYPHILIS

Melissa Badowski, PharmD • Mahesh C. Patel, MD

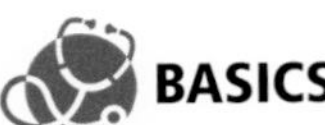

BASICS

DESCRIPTION

- A chronic, systemic infectious disease caused by *Treponema pallidum*
- Transmitted sexually, vertically (maternal–fetal) by direct contact with an active lesion and via blood transfusions
- Untreated disease includes 4 overlapping stages.
  - Primary: usually single painless chancre at point of entry; appears in 10–90 days; chancre heals without treatment in 3–6 weeks
  - Secondary: appears 2–8 weeks after primary chancre. Nonpruritic rash on palms or soles of feet, mucous membrane lesions, headache, fever, lymphadenopathy, alopecia
  - Latent: seroreactive without evidence of disease
    - Early latent: acquired within the last year
    - Late latent: exposure >12 months prior to diagnosis
  - Tertiary (late): Serology may be negative (fluorescent treponemal antibody absorption [FTA-ABS] test typically positive).
    - Gumma, cardiovascular, and late neurosyphilis; may be fatal
  - Neurosyphilis: *any* type of CNS involvement; can occur at *any* stage
    - Psychosis, delirium, dementia
- Syphilis can affect nearly every organ/tissue in the body leading to moniker "the great imitator."

Pediatric Considerations

In noncongenital cases, consider child abuse.

Pregnancy Considerations

- All pregnant patients should be screened with VDRL or rapid plasma reagin (RPR) test early in pregnancy. If high exposure risk, repeat at 28 weeks and at delivery (1,2)[A].
- The same nontreponemal test used for initial screening should be used for follow-up (1,2)[A].

EPIDEMIOLOGY

Incidence

- Syphilis rate decreased until 2000. Has increased (primarily in men) since (3)[A]
- In 2013: 5.3/100,000. Highest for men aged 25–29 years and women aged 20–24 years (3)[A]
  - Men: 9.8/100,000
  - Women: 0.9/100,000
- Congenital: 8.7 cases/100,000 live births (4)[A]
- Race/ethnicity (3)[A]
  - Male (per 100,000 population)
    - White, non-Hispanic: 5.4
    - Black, non-Hispanic: 27.9
    - Hispanic: 11.6.6
    - Asian/Pacific Islander: 4.6
    - American Indian/Alaska native: 4.7
  - Female (per 100,000 population)
    - White, non-Hispanic: 0.3
    - Black, non-Hispanic: 4.0
    - Hispanic: 0.8
    - Asian/Pacific Islander: 0.2
    - American Indian/Alaska native: 1.0

Prevalence

- Predominant sex: male (91%) > female (9%) (3)[A]
- Greatest increase in men having sex with men (MSM) (3)[A]

ETIOLOGY AND PATHOPHYSIOLOGY

T. pallidum subspecies *pallidum*, spirochete. Can enter through intact mucous membranes or breaks in skin. Highly infectious individuals to as few as 60 spirochetes have ~50% chance of infection.

RISK FACTORS

MSM, multiple sexual partners, exposure to infected body fluids, IV drug use, transplacental transmission, adult inmates, high-risk sexual behavior, HIV positive

GENERAL PREVENTION

Education regarding safe sex; condoms reduce but do not eliminate transmission (5)[A]

COMMONLY ASSOCIATED CONDITIONS

HIV infection, hepatitis B, other STIs

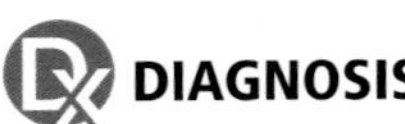

DIAGNOSIS

HISTORY

Previous sexual contact with partner with known infection/partner or high-risk sexual behavior

PHYSICAL EXAM

Signs/symptoms depend on stage.

- Primary: single (occasionally multiple), usually painless ulcer (chancre) in groin or at other point of entry
- Secondary
  - Rash: skin/mucous membranes
    - Rough, red-brown macules, usually on palms and soles
    - May appear with chancre or after it has healed
  - Nonspecific symptoms: fever, adenopathy, malaise, headache, hair loss

DIFFERENTIAL DIAGNOSIS

- Primary: chancroid, lymphogranuloma venereum, granuloma inguinale, condyloma acuminata, herpes simplex, Behçet syndrome, trauma, carcinoma, mycotic infection, lichen planus, psoriasis, fungal infection
- Secondary: pityriasis rosea, drug eruption, psoriasis, lichen planus, viral exanthema, Stevens-Johnson syndrome
- Positive serology, asymptomatic: previously treated syphilis/other spirochetal disease (yaws, pinta)

DIAGNOSTIC TESTS & INTERPRETATION

Initial Tests (lab, imaging)

- Dark-field microscopy demonstrating *T. pallidum* spirochetes in lesion exudate/tissue biopsy: gold standard but difficult and not very sensitive (6)[A]
- Nontreponemal tests (VDRL/RPR) (3,6)[A]
  - Primary screening test: positive within 7 days of exposure
  - Nonspecific, false-positive results common; must confirm diagnosis with treponemal tests
  - Positive test should be quantified, and titers followed regularly after treatment.
    - Titers usually correlate with disease activity; 4-fold change is clinically significant.
    - Titers decrease with time/treatment; following adequate treatment for primary/secondary disease, a 4-fold decline is typically seen after 6–12 months.
    - Absence of a 4-fold decline suggests potential treatment failure.
    - ~15% of appropriately treated patients do not have a 4-fold decline in titer 12 months after treatment. Management is unclear, repeat HIV testing and/or CSF examination and continue to follow titers.
    - With appropriate treatment, titers should eventually be negative (see serofast reaction).
    - Titers of patients treated in latent stages decline more gradually.
  - Prozone phenomenon: negative results from high titers of antibody; test diluted serum
  - Serofast reaction: persistently positive results years after successful treatment; new infection diagnosed by 4-fold rise in titer
  - Conditions that may alter treponemal testing (all stages of syphilis can have a false-negative RPR result, especially in primary syphilis)
    - Pregnancy, autoimmune disease, mononucleosis, malaria, leprosy, viral pneumonia, cardiolipin antigens, injection drug use, acute febrile illness, HIV infection; elderly can have false-positive results
- Treponemal tests (*confirmatory test after positive nontreponemal screening test*): FTA-ABS, TP-PA (*T. pallidum* particle agglutination) (6)[A]:
  - Confirmatory test; not used for screening
  - Usually positive for life after treatment
  - Titers of no benefit
  - 15–25% of patients treated during primary stage revert to serologic nonreactivity after 2–3 years.
- Lumbar puncture (6)[A]
  - Indicated if clinical evidence of neurologic or ocular/auditory manifestations
  - Some experts advise in all secondary and early latent cases—even without neurologic symptoms.
  - HIV-positive patients with late latent/latent of unknown duration
  - In patients with late latent/latent of unknown duration if nonpenicillin therapy planned
  - In treatment failures
  - If other evidence of active tertiary syphilis is present (e.g., aortitis, gumma, iritis)
  - In children to rule out neurosyphilis
  - VDRL, not RPR, used on CSF; may be negative in neurosyphilis; highly specific but insensitive.
  - Send CSF for protein, glucose, and cell count.
  - Monitor resolution by cell count at 6 months along with serologies as recommended (see "Patient Monitoring").
  - Negative FTA-ABS or microhemagglutination (MHA)-TP on CSF excludes neurosyphilis (highly sensitive).
  - Positive FTA-ABS or MHA-TP on CSF not diagnostic because of high false-positive rate.
  - Traumatic tap, tuberculosis (TB), pyogenic/aseptic meningitis can all result in false-positive VDRL.

TREATMENT

GENERAL MEASURES

- Advise patients to avoid intercourse until treatment is complete, and track partners (6)[A].
- Test concurrently for HIV (3,6)[A].
- Management of sexual contacts (6)[A]
  - Presumptively treat partners exposed within 90 days of diagnosis.
  - Treat those exposed >90 days before diagnosis presumptively if serologic results are not available immediately and follow-up is uncertain.
  - Treat those exposed to a patient diagnosed with syphilis of unknown duration and who have high treponemal titers (>1:32) presumptively also.
  - Long-term sex partners of patients with latent infection should be evaluated clinically and serologically and treated accordingly.

MEDICATION

ALERT

Bicillin L-A should be used and *not* Bicillin C-R (combination benzathine–procaine penicillin) when penicillin G benzathine is indicated.

First Line

Parenteral penicillin G is drug of choice. Particular formulation is determined by the disease stage and clinical presentation.

- Primary, secondary, and early latent <1 year (6)[A]
  - Benzathine penicillin G 2.4 million units IM × 1
  - Penicillin-allergic patients: doxycycline 100 mg PO BID × 2 weeks, or tetracycline 500 mg PO QID × 2 weeks, or ceftriaxone 1 g IM or IV daily × 10–14 days
    - Azithromycin 2 g PO × 1 dose (early syphilis only; should not be used in MSM or pregnancy)
    - Resistance and treatment failures have been noted in several geographical locations in the United States.
- Late latent/latent of unknown duration and tertiary without evidence of neurosyphilis (6)[A]
  - Benzathine penicillin G 2.4 million units IM weekly × 3 doses
  - Penicillin-allergic patients: Attempt desensitization and treatment with penicillin or doxycycline 100 mg PO 2 BID × 28 days, *or* tetracycline 500 mg PO QID × 28 days; compliance may be an issue.
- Neurosyphilis (6)[A]
  - Aqueous crystalline penicillin G 3–4 million units IV q4h or continuous infusion × 10–14 days
  - Procaine penicillin G 2.4 million units IM daily in conjunction with probenecid 500 mg PO QID × 10–14 days (if compliance can be ensured)
  - Penicillin-allergic patients: Attempt desensitization and treat with penicillin; ceftriaxone 2 g/day IM or IV × 10–14 days.
  - If late latent, latent of unknown duration, or tertiary in addition to neurosyphilis, consider also treating as recommended for late latent after completion of neurosyphilis treatment.
- Congenital (6)[A]
  - Aqueous crystalline penicillin G 50,000 U/kg/dose IV q12h × first 7 days of life and q8h thereafter for a total of 10 days, or procaine penicillin G 50,000 U/kg/dose IM daily × 10 days
  - If negative CSF serologies, normal physical exam, and titer: Maternal titer, then 50,000 U/kg benzathine penicillin G IM in single dose is also alternative.
  - If >1 day of drug is missed, restart course.
  - Children (after newborn period): aqueous crystalline penicillin G 50,000 U/kg/dose IV q4–6h × 10 days; late latent, 50,000 U/kg IM as 3 doses at 1-week intervals
  - Epidemiologic treatment for contacts without symptoms: Treat as primary after serologies.
  - HIV-infected and pregnant patients may show poor response to recommended IM doses. Use IV therapy for all treatment failures in these patients.
  - Do not give benzathine or procaine penicillins IV.
- Children (after newborn period) (6)[A]: aqueous crystalline penicillin G 50,000 U/kg/dose IV q4–6h × 10 days; late latent, 50,000 U/kg IM as 3 doses at 1-week intervals
- Pregnancy (6)[A]
  - Treatment same as for nonpregnant patients
  - Some recommend 2nd dose of 2.4 million units benzathine penicillin G 1 week after initial dose in 3rd trimester or with primary, secondary, or early latent syphilis.
  - Penicillin sensitivity: No proven alternatives to penicillin exist for treatment during pregnancy.
  - Consider desensitization to treat with penicillin.
  - HIV-infected and pregnant patients may show poor response to recommended IM doses. Use IV therapy for all treatment failures in these patients.

- Epidemiologic treatment for contacts without symptoms: Treat as primary after serologies.

- Precautions (6)[A]
  - HIV-infected and pregnant patients may show poor response to recommended IM doses. Use IV therapy for all treatment failures in these patients.
  - Do not give benzathine or procaine penicillins IV.

ONGOING CARE

FOLLOW-UP RECOMMENDATIONS

- Clinical and serologic evaluation at 6 and 12 months after treatment; if >1 year duration, check at 24 months (6)[A]
- In HIV-infected persons, clinical and serologic evaluation at 3, 6, 9, 12, and 24 months after therapy (6)[A]

Patient Monitoring

- Use VDRL or RPR test to monitor therapy: 4-fold rise in titer indicates new infection, whereas failure to decrease 4-fold in 6–12 months may indicate treatment failure (although definitive criteria for cure not established); always use same test (preferably same lab) as initial screening test (6)[A].

- Strongly consider retreatment for persistent clinical signs or recurrence, 4-fold rise in titers, or failure of initially high titer to decrease 4-fold by 6–12 months.

- Neurosyphilis: Repeat lumbar puncture every 6 months to check for normalization of CSF cell count (± CSF-VDRL and protein evaluation) (6)[A].

PATIENT EDUCATION

No intimate contacts until 4-fold titer drop

PROGNOSIS

- Excellent in all cases except patients with late syphilis complications and with HIV infection
- Syphilis in HIV-infected patient
  - Treatment same as for HIV-negative patients
  - More often false-negative treponemal and nontreponemal tests or unusually high titers
  - Response to therapy less predictable
  - Early syphilis: increased risk of neurosyphilis and higher rates of treatment failure
  - Late neurosyphilis: harder to treat; can occur up to 20+ years after infection

COMPLICATIONS

- Membranous glomerulonephritis
- Paroxysmal cold hemoglobinemia
- Meningitis and tabes dorsalis
- Cardiovascular aneurysms; valvular damage
- Irreversible organ damage
- Jarisch-Herxheimer reaction
  - Fever, chills, headache, myalgias, new rash
  - Common when starting treatment (of primary/secondary disease; less common with tertiary) owing to lysis of treponemes
  - Should not be confused with drug reaction
  - Managed with analgesics and antipyretics

S

REFERENCES

1. Gomez GB, Kamb ML, Newman LM, et al. Untreated maternal syphilis and adverse outcomes of pregnancy: a systematic review and meta-analysis. *Bull World Health Org*. 2013;91(3):217–226.
2. U.S. Preventive Services Task Force. Screening for syphilis infection in pregnancy: U.S. Preventive Services Task Force reaffirmation recommendation statement. *Ann Intern Med*. 2009;150(10):705–709.
3. Patton ME, Su JR, Nelson R, et al; Centers for Disease Control and Prevention. Primary and secondary syphilis—United States, 2005–2013. *MMWR Morb Mortal Wkly Rep*. 2014;63(18):402–406.
4. Centers for Disease Control and Prevention. *Sexually Transmitted Disease Surveillance 2012*. Atlanta, GA: U.S. Department of Health and Human Services; 2013.
5. Koss CA, Dunne EF, Warner L. A systematic review of epidemiologic studies assessing condom use and risk of syphilis. *Sex Transm Dis*. 2009;36(7):401–405.
6. Workowski KA, Berman S; Centers for Disease Control and Prevention. Sexually transmitted diseases treatment guidelines, 2010. *MMWR Recomm Rep*. 2010;59(RR-12):1–110.

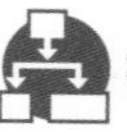

SEE ALSO

Chlamydia Infection (Sexually Transmitted); Gonococcal Infections

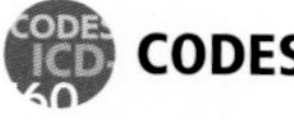

CODES

ICD10

- A53.9 Syphilis, unspecified
- A51.0 Primary genital syphilis
- A53.0 Latent syphilis, unspecified as early or late

CLINICAL PEARLS

- All patients with high-risk activity or HIV-positive status should be screened for syphilis.
- Penicillin remains the treatment of choice for syphilis.
- Syphilis rates are rising—particularly among men having sex with men (MSM).

TARSAL TUNNEL SYNDROME

Tara Futrell, MD • J. Herbert Stevenson, MD

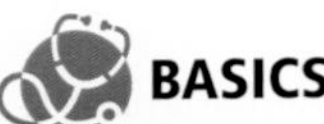

BASICS

DESCRIPTION

Tarsal tunnel syndrome is a compression neuropathy of the posterior tibial nerve as it passes behind the medial malleolus and under the flexor retinaculum (laciniate ligament) in the medial ankle, through a region commonly known as the tarsal tunnel.

Pregnancy Considerations

- Tarsal tunnel syndrome can occur during pregnancy, typically secondary to local compression caused by fluid retention and volume changes (1).
- Care usually is supportive until after delivery because many cases resolve after pregnancy.

EPIDEMIOLOGY

- Women are slightly more affected than men (56%).
- All postpubescent ages are affected.

ETIOLOGY AND PATHOPHYSIOLOGY

- The posterior tibial nerve passes through the tarsal tunnel, which is formed by 3 osseus structures—sustentaculum tali, medial calcaneus, and medial malleolus—and covered by the laciniate ligament
- Compression of the posterior tibial nerve within the confined space of the tarsal tunnel results in decreased blood flow, ischemic damage, and resultant symptoms (1).
- Chronic compression can destroy endoneurial microvasculature, leading to edema and (eventually) fibrosis and demyelination (2).
- Increased pressure in the tarsal tunnel can be caused by a variety of mechanical and biochemical mechanisms. The specific cause for compression is identifiable in only 60–80% of patients (1).
- 3 general categories of conditions leading to tarsal tunnel syndrome: trauma, space-occupying lesion, and deformity (1)
  - Trauma including displaced fractures, deltoid ligament sprains, or tenosynovitis
  - Varicosities
  - Hindfoot varus or valgus
  - Fibrosis of the perineurium
- Other causes of compression include the following:
  - Osseous prominences
  - Ganglia
  - Lipoma
  - Neurolemmoma
  - Inflammatory synovitis
  - Pigmented villonodular synovitis
  - Tarsal coalition
  - Accessory musculature
- In patients with systemic disease (e.g., diabetes), the "double crush" syndrome refers to the development of a 2nd compression along the same nerve at a site of anatomic narrowing in patients with previous proximal nerve damage (3).
- Tarsal tunnel decompression may improve sensory impairment and restore protective sensation in diabetic peripheral neuropathies if there is nerve entrapment at the tarsal tunnel.

RISK FACTORS

- Tarsal tunnel syndrome has been associated with certain occupations and activities involving repetitive weight bearing on the foot and ankle (jogging, dancing).
- Other possible risk factors include the following (4):
  - Diabetes
  - Systemic inflammatory arthritis
  - Connective tissue disorders
  - Obesity
  - Varicosities
  - Heel varus or valgus
  - Bifurcation of the posterior tibial nerve into medial and lateral plantar nerves proximal to the tarsal tunnel

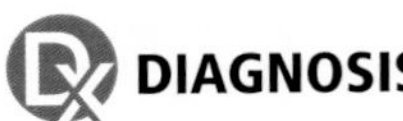

DIAGNOSIS

Tarsal tunnel syndrome is largely a clinical diagnosis, characterized by pain and paresthesias in a predictable distribution along the medial aspect of the ankle and plantar surface of the foot (1).

HISTORY

- History of trauma (may be trivial) to the foot precipitating pain
- Pain behind medial malleolus radiating to the longitudinal arch and plantar aspect of foot including the heel
- Sensation of tightness, burning, tingling, and numbness are usually present (1).
- Pain usually worsens during standing or activity.
- Pain radiates proximally up the medial leg (Valleix phenomenon) in 33% of patients with severe compression.
- Some patients have substantial night pain, which may be related to venostasis.
- Symptoms improve with rest, wearing loose footwear, and elevation.
- In advanced nerve compression, motor involvement may cause weakness, atrophy, and digital contractures of the intrinsic foot muscles (4).

ALERT

Other neuropathies due to systemic causes, such as diabetes, alcoholism, HIV, or drug reactions, present with similar symptoms.

PHYSICAL EXAM

- Foot alignment
  - Examine for hindfoot varus or valgus deformity.
  - Exaggerating heel dorsiflexion, inversion, or eversion may reproduce symptoms by stretching or compressing the posterior tibial nerve.
- Palpate the tarsal tunnel and the course of the tibial nerve for the following:
  - Tenderness
  - Swelling (space-occupying lesion)
- Tinel sign: Percussion over the course of the tibial nerve may reproduce paresthesias that radiate distally.
- Valleix sign: Percussion over the course of the tibial nerve may produce paresthesias that radiate proximally.
- Cuff test: Inflating a pneumatic cuff engorges varicosities and reproduces symptoms.
- Compression test: Applying pressure to the tarsal tunnel for 60 seconds may reproduce symptoms.
- Sensory examination
  - The medial calcaneal nerve usually is spared, but numbness and altered sensation may be present in the distribution of the medial or lateral plantar nerve.
  - Vibratory sensation and 2-point discrimination are decreased early in the disease process.
- Motor examination
  - Intrinsic foot weakness is difficult to assess.
  - Rarely, weakness of toe plantar flexion may be present.
  - Atrophy of the abductor hallucis or abductor digiti minimi may be seen late in the disease process.

DIFFERENTIAL DIAGNOSIS

- Peripheral neuropathies (diabetes, alcoholism, HIV, or drug related)
- Inflammatory arthritis (rheumatoid arthritis)
- Morton neuroma
- Metatarsalgia
- Subtalar joint arthritis
- Tibialis posterior tendinitis/dysfunction
- Plantar fasciitis
- Plantar callosities
- Peripheral vascular disease
- Lumbar radiculopathy
- Proximal injury or compression of the tibial branch of the sciatic nerve

DIAGNOSTIC TESTS & INTERPRETATION

Initial Tests (lab, imaging)

Routine lab tests help rule out other conditions that may mimic tarsal tunnel syndrome, including diabetic neuropathy, rheumatoid arthritis, thyroid dysfunction, or other systemic illnesses (5).

- Routine weight-bearing radiographs, followed by CT if necessary to assess for fracture or structural abnormality
- Consider evaluation of lumbar spine x-ray if double crush (injury to lumbar nerve results in compensatory injury to posterior tibial nerve) is suspected (5).
- MRI: can be helpful in assessing the tarsal tunnel for soft tissue masses or other sources of nerve compression before surgery (1).
- Ultrasound: Can be used to assess for tenosynovitis, ganglia, varicose veins, or lipomas (1)

Pediatric Considerations

MRI is recommended for evaluating pediatric tarsal tunnel syndrome to exclude neoplastic mass.

Diagnostic Procedures/Other

Electrodiagnostic studies

- Electromyography (EMG) of the intrinsic muscles of the foot can be used to confirm the diagnosis of tarsal tunnel syndrome (6). However, a normal EMG does not exclude the diagnosis, as there is a false-negative rate of around 10% (1).
- Nerve conduction studies may reveal slowed conduction of the tibial nerve.
- Evaluate for proximal nerve compression, including a lumbar radiculopathy or a double crush phenomenon.

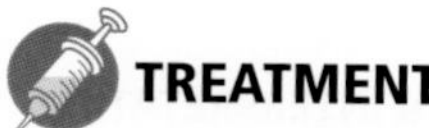

TREATMENT

Conservative management is recommended, except for tarsal tunnel syndrome of acute onset or in the setting of a known space-occupying lesion (excluding synovitis).

MEDICATION

First Line

- Analgesics and anti-inflammatory medications
- Local corticosteroid injection
- Medications that alter neurogenic pain (tricyclic antidepressants, antiepileptic drugs, nerve blockers)

ADDITIONAL THERAPIES

- Rest/immobilization
- Taping and bracing
- Orthotics or shoe modification
- Physical therapy to strengthen the intrinsic and extrinsic muscles of the foot and to restore the medial longitudinal arch
- Other modalities (stretching, US, massage, icing)
- Compression stockings to decrease swelling
- Weight loss for obese patients

SURGERY/OTHER PROCEDURES

- Surgery is indicated (1,2,7).
  - If nonoperative measures fail following a 3–6-month trial
  - In the setting of acute tarsal tunnel syndrome
  - If a space-occupying lesion is identified
- The surgical outcome is dependent on technique and postoperative management. 50–95% of cases have a good to excellent outcome.
- At the time of surgical exploration, assess for the following:
  - Focal swelling, scarring, or nerve abnormalities
  - A pathologic source of compression
- Postoperative management includes the following:
  - Non–weight-bearing splint until incision heals (2–3 weeks), followed by progressively increased weight-bearing and range of motion exercises
  - RICE protocol (rest, ice, compression, elevation) to limit swelling

ONGOING CARE

PATIENT EDUCATION

- Discuss conservative and surgical options based on individual patient circumstance and preference.
- A decision about surgical intervention should be made with a clear understanding risks, benefits, and potential adverse outcomes.

PROGNOSIS

The most symptomatic improvement with surgery is expected for the following:

- Patients with a positive Tinel sign (3)[B]
- Young patients
- Short duration of symptoms <1 year.
- Localized space-occupying lesion (1)
- No motor neuron involvement

COMPLICATIONS

- The main adverse outcome is an unsuccessful surgical intervention characterized by lack of improvement, partial/incomplete improvement, or temporary improvement with recurrence of symptoms (1).
- Causes for a failed tarsal tunnel release include the following:
  - Incorrect diagnosis
  - Incomplete release
  - Adhesive neuritis (external scar formation)
  - Intraneural damage (systemic disease, direct nerve injury)
  - Failure to treat all sources of nerve compression in a double crush phenomenon
- Electrodiagnostic studies are rarely helpful in determining the cause of a failed tarsal tunnel release.
- Results with surgical revision are poorer than those for the primary surgical release.

REFERENCES

1. Ahmad M, Tsang K, MacKenney PJ, et al. Tarsal tunnel syndrome: a literature review. *Foot Ankle Surg*. 2012;18(3):149–152.
2. Dellon AL. The four medial ankle tunnels: a critical review of perceptions of tarsal tunnel syndrome and neuropathy. *Neurosurg Clin North Am*. 2008;19(4):629–648.
3. Dellon AL, Muse VL, Scott ND, et al. A positive Tinel sign as predictor of pain relief or sensory recovery after decompression of chronic tibial nerve compression in patients with diabetic neuropathy. *J Reconstr Microsurg*. 2012;28(4):235–240.
4. Reade BM, Longo DC, Keller MC. Tarsal tunnel syndrome. *Clin Podiatr Med Surg*. 2001;18(3):395–408.
5. Franson J, Baravarian B. Tarsal tunnel syndrome: a compression neuropathy involving four distinct tunnels. *Clin Podiatr Med Surg*. 2006;23(3):597–609.
6. Patel AT, Gaines K, Malamut R, et al. Usefulness of electrodiagnostic techniques in the evaluation of suspected tarsal tunnel syndrome: an evidence-based review. *Muscle Nerve*. 2005;32(2):236–240.
7. Sung KS, Park SJ. Short-term operative outcome of tarsal tunnel syndrome due to benign space-occupying lesions. *Foot Ankle Int*. 2009;30(8):741–745.

ADDITIONAL READING

- Abouelela AA, Zohiery AK. The triple compression stress test for diagnosis of tarsal tunnel syndrome. *Foot*. 2012;22(3):146–149.
- Allen JM, Greer BJ, Sorge DG, et al. MR imaging of neuropathies of the leg, ankle, and foot. *Magn Reson Imaging Clin N Am*. 2008;16(1):117–131.
- Campbell WW, Landau ME. Controversial entrapment neuropathies. *Neurosurg Clin N Am*. 2008;19(4):597–608.
- Gondring WH, Tarun PK, Trepman E. Touch pressure and sensory density after tarsal tunnel release in diabetic neuropathy. *Foot Ankle Surg*. 2012;18(4):241–246.
- Imai K, Ikoma K, Imai R, et al. Tarsal tunnel syndrome in hemodialysis patients: a case series. *Foot Ankle Int*. 2013;34(3):439–444.
- Kennedy JG, Baxter DE. Nerve disorders in dancers. *Clin Sports Med*. 2008;27(2):329–334.
- Shapiro BE, Preston DC. Entrapment and compressive neuropathies. *Med Clin North Am*. 2009;93(2):285–315.

SEE ALSO

Algorithm: Foot Pain

CODES

ICD10

- G57.50 Tarsal tunnel syndrome, unspecified lower limb
- G57.51 Tarsal tunnel syndrome, right lower limb
- G57.52 Tarsal tunnel syndrome, left lower limb

CLINICAL PEARLS

- Tarsal tunnel typically presents with pain and tingling of the medical ankle and plantar foot.
- Tinel sign is the most sensitive and specific test for diagnosing tarsal tunnel on physical examination.
- EMG cannot be used to independently diagnose tarsal tunnel syndrome, it can only be used to confirm the clinical diagnosis.
- Conservative management is recommended, except for patients with an acute onset or known space-occupying lesion.

TEETHING

Dana Nguyen, MD, FAAFP • Katrina E. Walters, MD, FAAFP, FM

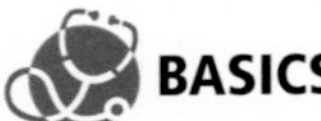

BASICS

DESCRIPTION

- Teething is the eruption of the primary or deciduous teeth, which most children experience without difficulty. It is a natural, gradual, and predictable process, with normal variation among infants (1,2).
- Primary (deciduous) teeth
  - Primary tooth eruption usually begins at 5–7 months of age.
  - The order of primary tooth eruption and average age is the following:
    - Central mandibular incisors (5–7 months)
    - Central maxillary incisors (6–8 months)
    - Lateral mandibular incisors (7–10 months)
    - Lateral maxillary incisors (8–11 months)
    - Cuspids (16–20 months)
    - 1st molars (10–16 months)
    - 2nd molars (20–30 months)
  - Delayed eruption may be familial or due to systemic syndromes or nutritional deficiencies. Delayed eruption may also be seen with cleft palate and lower birth weight (3,4,5).
  - Tooth eruption in premature infants occurs according to postconceptual age rather than age since birth (chronologic age) (2).
  - Natal/neonatal teeth
    - Natal teeth (present at birth) occur in 1/2,000 neonates.
    - Neonatal teeth erupt in the 1st month of life.
    - Natal/neonatal teeth are most often prematurely erupted primary (deciduous) teeth but may be supernumerary.
    - 15–20% of cases are familial; also may be secondary to a syndrome or congenital anomalies of the head and neck.
    - Natal/neonatal teeth may be loose, but most are the normal deciduous lower central incisors and can persist.
    - Natal/neonatal teeth may be removed if there is an aspiration risk or if they cause trauma to the infant or to the mother (breastfeeding) (2).

EPIDEMIOLOGY

Incidence

Predominant age: birth–3 years of age

ETIOLOGY AND PATHOPHYSIOLOGY

Teething symptoms are more common with eruption of the primary incisors (6).

Genetics

Both premature and delayed tooth eruption may be familial. Primary failure of eruption has been linked to mutations of the *PTHR1* gene (5).

COMMONLY ASSOCIATED CONDITIONS

Teething may be coincident with other common childhood conditions, causing local or systemic signs and symptoms (e.g., fever, GI disturbance, fussiness, drooling, rash, and sleep disturbance). No pattern of symptoms that distinguishes teething from any other cause. Other possible causes of systemic symptoms should be ruled out prior to attributing them to teething (7).

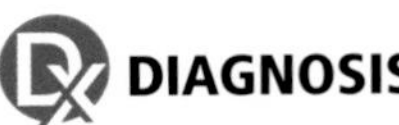

DIAGNOSIS

HISTORY

- Biting
- Drooling
- Rubbing of gingivae
- Sucking
- Irritability
- Wakefulness
- Ear rubbing
- Facial rash
- Decreased appetite for solid foods
- Loose stools
- Temperature elevation <38.3°C
- Many infants do not have any symptoms.

- Symptoms most often occur 4 days before eruption and resolve by 3 days after eruption and are more common in ages 4–24 months (6,8–10)[B].

PHYSICAL EXAM

- Infants may have no signs or symptoms of teething, although symptoms are present in most children.
- Excessive drooling and chewing on fingers begins at 3–4 months of age. This is also the time that normal hand–mouth stimulation increases salivation.

- Discomfort may be observed more commonly with the eruption of the 1st tooth, the molars, and/or with the simultaneous eruption of multiple teeth (11)[B].
- Minor signs and symptoms of biting or chewing, drooling, irritability, facial rash, and low-grade fever (<101.9°F; 38.9°C) have been reported in association with teething, although no evidence identifies specific signs/symptoms caused by teething (9)[B].
- Serious signs and symptoms (e.g., fever >101.9°F; 38.9°C, dehydration) are not caused by teething and warrant evaluation for organic disease (7)[A].

- A small red or white spot may appear over the swollen gingivae just prior to tooth eruption.
- Local inflammation, swelling, or hematoma (bluish swelling) can be found on the involved gingivae overlying the erupting tooth. Gingival irritation was present in 96% of infants in one study (11)[B].

DIFFERENTIAL DIAGNOSIS

Herpetic gingivostomatitis: Infants with fever, irritability, sleeplessness, and difficulty feeding may have underlying infection caused by herpes simplex virus. Some infants with positive culture may not have evidence of inflammation or ulceration expected in gingivostomatitis.

DIAGNOSTIC TESTS & INTERPRETATION

Imaging

Radiographs can distinguish prematurely erupted primary teeth from supernumerary teeth.

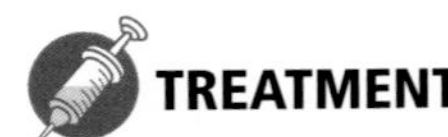

TREATMENT

GENERAL MEASURES

- Education of mothers regarding common symptoms of teething and management options resulted in decreased use of pharmacologic treatment and increased use of other methods such as rubbing the gums (12)[B].

- Treatment includes reassurance and symptomatic treatment.
- Provide the infant with a safe, 1-piece teething ring, clean cloth, or pacifier for gumming.
- Apply pressure over involved swollen gingivae with a clean finger or piece of wet gauze.
- May use cool (but not frozen) fluids, cold teething rings, or cold vegetables such as a peeled cucumber
- Avoid the use of alcohol (historically rubbed on gingivae for an analgesic effect).
- Gingival hematomas that erupt appear as blue cysts. Most do not require medical intervention. Be sure there are no other signs of a bleeding disorder.
- Avoid the following:
  - Dipping a pacifier or teething ring in sugar or honey
  - Giving an infant a bottle in bed
  - Using fluid-filled teething rings (contents may leak)
  - Using frozen foods or teething rings (these could cause thermal damage to the tissues)
  - Tying a teething ring around infant's neck (13)[C]

MEDICATION

First Line

For an infant with low-grade fever, irritability, and/or inflamed gingivae (where other comforting measures have not been of help), acetaminophen in proper doses (15 mg/kg/dose q4–6h PRN) can be used.

Second Line

ALERT

Over-the-counter preparations for teething, such as lidocaine (Xylocaine 2%), or benzocaine (Baby Ora-Gel, Num-Zit Gel, Num-Zit Liquid, Baby Anbesol), should be AVOIDED. Misuse, overuse, toxicity, and sensitivity have been reported.

- These are of questionable benefit because they are washed off quickly by saliva, and the benefit may be due in part to the pressure placed on the gingivae when applied.
  - FDA issued a warning about possible serious harm, to include death (14)[A].

ISSUES FOR REFERRAL

- Parents should establish a dental home for infants by 12 months of age. Dental caries remain the most prevalent infectious disease in children in the United States. Preventative care and anticipatory guidance offered in a dental home help prevent early childhood caries (15)[A].
- Other medical problems may delay tooth eruption. It is reasonable to refer a child who has not erupted a tooth by 18 months of age to a dentist, if he or she is not seeing one already (5)[C].

ADDITIONAL THERAPIES

Infants who bite or chew while breastfeeding can be trained not to bite by withdrawing the child from the breast for a moment, and then resume. Resist urge to startle the infant.

COMPLEMENTARY & ALTERNATIVE MEDICINE

Homeopathy is used to treat teething. Chamomilla is one reported treatment, but no efficacy or safety studies have been published (16)[C].

INPATIENT CONSIDERATIONS

Admission Criteria/Initial Stabilization

Outpatient

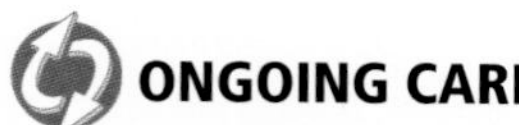

ONGOING CARE

FOLLOW-UP RECOMMENDATIONS

No restrictions

DIET

Breastfeeding can continue during and after teething. Otherwise, no special diet required.

PATIENT EDUCATION

- Parents should be cautioned not to misinterpret teething as the cause of any systemic manifestation. The health provider should be consulted for any systemic complaints.
- American Dental Association, Mouth Healthy Web site: http://www.mouthhealthy.org/en/babies-and-kids/
- Teething Tots: http://kidshealth.org/parent/pregnancy_newborn/common/teething.html

PROGNOSIS

Normal progression through the teething process without illness

REFERENCES

1. Aktoren O, Tuna EB, Guven Y, et al. A study on neonatal factors and eruption time of primary teeth. *Community Dent Health*. 2010;27(1):52–56.
2. Cunha RF, Boer FA, Torianni DD, et al. Natal and neonatal teeth: review of the literature. *Pediatr Dent*. 2001;23(2):158–162.
3. Kobayashi TY, Gomide MR, Carrara CF. Timing and sequence of primary tooth eruption in children with cleft lip and palate. *J Appl Oral Sci*. 2010;18(3):220–224.
4. Sajjadian N, Shajari H, Jahadi R, et al. Relationship between birth weight and time of first deciduous tooth eruption in 143 consecutively born infants. *Pediatr Neonatol*. 2010;51(4):235–237.
5. Stellzig-Eisenhauer A, Decker E, Meyer-Marcotty P, et al. Primary failure of eruption (PFE)—clinical and molecular genetics analysis [in English, German]. *J Orofac Orthop*. 2010;71(1):6–16.
6. Noor-Mohammed R, Basha S. Teething disturbances: prevalence of objective manifestations in children under age 4 months to 36 months. *Med Oral Patol Oral Cir Bucal*. 2012;17(3):e491–e494.
7. Tighe M, Roe MF. Does a teething child need serious illness excluding? *Arch Dis Child*. 2007;92(3):266–268.
8. Feldens CA, Faraco IM, Ottoni AB, et al. Teething symptoms in the first year of life and associated factors: a cohort study. *J Clin Pediatr Dent*. 2010;34(3):201–206.
9. Macknin ML, Piedmonte M, Jacobs J, et al. Symptoms associated with infant teething: a prospective study. *Pediatrics*. 2000;105(4, Pt 1):747–752.
10. Wake M, Hesketh K, Lucas J. Teething and tooth eruption in infants: a cohort study. *Pediatrics*. 2000;106(6):1374–1379.
11. Kiran K, Swati T, Kamala BK, et al. Prevalence of systemic and local disturbances in infants during primary teeth eruption: a clinical study. *Eur J Paediatr Dent*. 2011;12(4):249–252.
12. Plutzer K, Spencer AJ, Keirse MJ. How first-time mothers perceive and deal with teething symptoms: a randomized controlled trial. *Child Care Health Dev*. 2012;38(2):292–299.
13. McIntyre GT, McIntyre GM. Teething troubles? *Br Dental J*. 2002;192(5):251–255.
14. U.S. Food and Drug Administration. FDA Drug Safety Communication: FDA recommends not using lidocaine to treat teething pain and requires new Boxed Warning. http://www.fda.gov/Drugs/DrugSafety/ucm402240.htm. Published June 26, 2014. Updated October 9, 2014. Accessed 2014.
15. American Academy of Pediatric Dentistry. Clinical Affairs Committee—Infant Oral Health Subcommittee. Guideline on infant oral health care. *Pediatr Dent*. 2012;34(5):148–152.
16. Thompson E, Bishop J, Northstone K. The use of homeopathic products in childhood: data generated over 8.5 years from the Avon Longitudinal Study of Parents and Children (ALSPAC). *J Altern Complement Med*. 2010;16(1):69–79.

ADDITIONAL READING

- American Academy of Pediatrics. Children's Oral Health website: http://www2.aap.org/commpeds/dochs/oralhealth/index.html. Accessed 2014.
- American Academy of Pediatrics Oral health initiative. Protecting all children's teeth (PACT): a pediatric oral health training program: http://www2.aap.org/oralhealth/pact/pact-home.cfm. Accessed 2014.
- Williams GD, Kirk EP, Wilson CJ, et al. Salicylate intoxication from teething gel in infancy. *Med J Aust*. 2011;194(3):146–148.

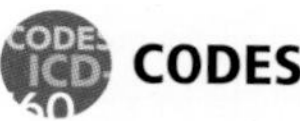

CODES

ICD10

K00.7 Teething syndrome

CLINICAL PEARLS

- Parents and caregivers should follow the American Academy of Pediatrics' recommendations for treating teething pain.
  - Use a teething ring chilled in the refrigerator (not frozen).
  - Gently rub or massage the child's gums with your finger to relieve the symptoms.
  - Topical pain relievers and medications that are rubbed on the gums are not necessary or even useful because they wash out of the baby's mouth within minutes, and they can be harmful.
- Teething may cause discomfort but does not cause significant fevers.
- Teething babies can still breastfeed. Babies can be taught not to bite, and breastfeeding may continue past 12 months of age without difficulty.

T

TELOGEN EFFLUVIUM

Adarsh K. Gupta, DO, MS, FACOFP

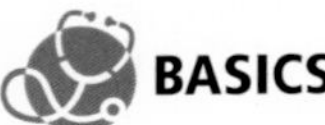

BASICS

Diffuse hair loss or hair thinning; most often an acute self-limited process

DESCRIPTION

Telogen effluvium (TE) is a transient condition in which there is a premature conversion of a significant proportion of anagen (growth phase) hairs into telogen (resting phase) hairs resulting in increased shedding of these resting hair follicles and the clinical appearance of moderate to severe hair thinning.

- 5 proposed types of TE (1)
  - Immediate anagen release: a highly common form, lasting 3–4 weeks, in which follicles meant to remain in anagen phase enter telogen prematurely due to a signal, including high fever, drug induced, or stress
  - Delayed anagen release: occurs most often postpartum, in which a large group of hair follicles that have remained in the anagen phase for an extended period all together enter the telogen phase, resulting in hair loss
  - Short anagen: a somewhat speculative type, in which at least 50% of the hair follicles have an idiopathic shortening of the anagen phase, resulting in a corresponding doubling of the follicles in the telogen phase
  - Immediate telogen release: Normal resting club hairs remain within the hair follicle until an unknown signal causes their release, initiating the anagen stage to begin. In this type, the resting club hairs are prematurely released, ending the telogen phase abruptly and causing diffuse shedding.
  - Delayed telogen release: In this type, the presence of increased visible light, whether it be a seasonal or environmental change, is thought to end a prolonged telogen phase and initiate the anagen phase, resulting in diffuse shedding of hair follicles.

EPIDEMIOLOGY

Incidence

2nd most common cause of alopecia

Prevalence

Unknown

ETIOLOGY AND PATHOPHYSIOLOGY

- The hair cycle consists of 2 predominant phases. The anagen (growth phase) and the telogen (resting phase), lasting ~3 years and 3 months, respectively. On the scalp, ~10–15% of hairs are in the telogen phase normally. Due to the presence of some types of external/internal stress, there may be an increase in the percentage of telogen hairs. As new anagen hairs emerge, these telogen hair follicles are forced out. The preceding event usually occurs 2–3 months prior to the appearance of hair loss.
- It is hypothesized that substance P plays a key role in the pathogenesis of TE through various mechanisms (2,3). Studies have been conducted on human hair follicles in vitro and mice hair follicles in vivo, which support this theory.
- Role of substance P includes the following (4):
  - Upregulation of substance P receptor, NK1, at the gene and protein level, leading to premature catagen development and hair growth inhibition
  - Upregulation of nerve growth factor (NGF) and subsequently its hair apoptosis–producing receptor, p75NTR
  - Downregulation of hair-growth–promoting receptor, TrkA
  - Upregulation of major histocompatibility class (MHC) I and β_2-microglobulin resulting in loss of hair follicle immune-privilege
  - Increase in tumor necrosis factor-α release by mast cells resulting in hair keratinocyte apoptosis
- Decreased cortisol levels in chronic stress states may also enhance the effects of substance P (5).

RISK FACTORS

- Infection
- Trauma
- Major surgery
- Thyroid disorder
- Febrile illness
- Malignancy
- Allergic contact dermatitis (6)
- Iron deficiency anemia (7)
- Excess vitamin A (1)
- Protein-calorie restriction (1)
- End-stage liver or renal disease
- Hormonal changes (including pregnancy, delivery, and estrogen-containing medications) (1)
- Chronic stress
- Drug induced (β-blockers, anticonvulsants, antidepressants, anticoagulants, retinoids, ACE-inhibitors, etc.) (1)
- Immunizations

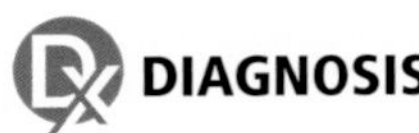

DIAGNOSIS

HISTORY

- Commonly, an inciting event 2–6 months previous
- Fear of becoming bald
- Patients often present with bags of hair to emphasize the severity of their hair loss.

PHYSICAL EXAM

- Decreased density of hair on the scalp, most commonly involving the crown
- In rare cases of chronic TE, there is hair loss of eyebrows and pubic region.
- May be able to demonstrate diffuse shedding of hair when running fingers through scalp
- Shed hairs are telogen hairs, which have a small bulb of unpigmented or pigmented keratin on the root end.
- May effect nail growth, resulting in the appearance of Beau lines, which are transverse grooves on the nails of the hands and feet

DIFFERENTIAL DIAGNOSIS

- Hypothyroidism
- Hyperthyroidism
- Alopecia areata (diffuse pattern)
- Androgenetic alopecia
- Drug-induced alopecia
- Systemic lupus erythematosus
- Secondary syphilis
- Trichotillomania

DIAGNOSTIC TESTS & INTERPRETATION

Most often, TE is a clinical diagnosis of exclusion.

Blood work may be collected primarily to rule out other possible causes of hair loss and/or to identify a possible cause for TE.

Initial Tests (lab, imaging)

If indicated

- CBC, ferritin
- TSH
- Creatinine
- Consider hepatic enzymes.
- Consider RPR/VDRL.

Diagnostic Procedures/Other

- Hair pull test: unreliable; performed by gently pulling 25–30 hairs from various sites on a patient's scalp. Each pull should elicit <5 normal club hairs; increased quantity may indicate possibility of TE (1).
- Hair clip test: Performed by cutting 25–30 hairs from the patient's scalp and examining them under a microscope. A negative test (not indicative of TE) will demonstrate <10% of hair shafts of small diameter. A positive test will demonstrate >10% of hair shafts of small diameter (1).
- Trichogram: ~50 hairs are plucked from the patient's scalp, and the number of telogen and anagen hairs present are counted. In TE, there will be >10% of hairs in the telogen phase.
- Scalp biopsy: rarely needed; it is recommended that several 4-mm punch biopsies be obtained, all horizontally embedded to determine an accurate anagen-to-telogen ratio. Histologically, catagen-to-telogen hairs have numerous apoptotic cells in the outer sheath epithelium. >12–15% of hair follicles in telogen phase is consistent with TE (1,8).

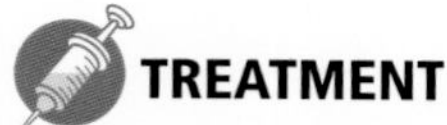

TREATMENT

TE is a benign, self-limited process. Identify and correct underlying cause. Patient should be reassured that full hair growth will occur in ~6 months–1 year. No treatment is required.

MEDICATION

- Minoxidil: stimulates hair regrowth via arteriolar smooth muscle vasodilation; not effective in TE
- Oral zinc therapy: New medication that may have benefits for patients with TE through various mechanisms all essential to hair growth, including the following (9)[C] :
  - Cofactor for enzymes needed in nucleic acid and protein synthesis and cell division
  - Inhibition of the catagen phase by blocking certain enzymes involved in hair apoptosis
  - Involved in hair growth regulation via hedgehog signaling

COMPLEMENTARY & ALTERNATIVE MEDICINE

A nutritionist may be consulted to help evaluate the deficiencies or excess vitamin and mineral intake in a patient's diet. Rarely, cause of hair loss in well-nourished individuals

REFERENCES

1. Headington JT. Telogen effluvium. New concepts and review. *Arch Dermatol*. 1993;129(3):356.
2. Grover C, Khurana A. Telogen effluvium. *Indian J Dermatol Venereol Leprol*. 2013;79(5):591–603.
3. Hadshiew IM, Foitzik K, Arck PC, et al. Burden of hair loss: stress and the underestimated psychosocial impact of telogen effluvium and androgenetic alopecia. *J Invest Dermatol*. 2004;123(3):455–457.
4. Peters EMJ, Liotiri S, Bodó E, et al. Probing the effects of stress mediators on the human hair follicle: substance P holds central position. *Am J Pathol*. 2007;171(6):1872–1886.
5. Katayama I, Bae SJ, Hamasaki Y, et al. Stress response, tachykinin, and cutaneous inflammation. *J Investig Dermatol Symp Proc*. 2001;6(1):81–86.
6. Tosti A, Piraccini BM, van Neste DJ. Telogen effluvium after allergic contact dermatitis of the scalp. *Arch Dermatol*. 2001;137(2):187–190.
7. Trost LB, Bergfeld WF, Calogeras E. The diagnosis and treatment of iron deficiency and its potential relationship to hair loss. *J Am Acad Dermatol*. 2006;54(5):824–844.
8. Sinclair R, Jolley D, Mallari R, et al. The reliability of horizontally sectioned scalp biopsies in the diagnosis of chronic diffuse telogen hair loss in women. *J Am Acad Dermatol*. 2004;51(2):189–199.
9. Karashima T, Tsuruta D, Hamada T, et al. Oral zinc therapy for zinc deficiency-related telogen effluvium. *Dermatol Ther*. 2012;25(2):210–213.

ADDITIONAL READING

Mounsey AL, Reed SW. Diagnosing and treating hair loss. *Am Fam Physician*. 2009;80(4):356–362.

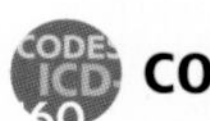

CODES

ICD10

L65.0 Telogen effluvium

CLINICAL PEARLS

- TE is a self-limited form of nonscarring alopecia; most often acute.
- TE is due to a premature conversion of a significant proportion of anagen (growth phase) hairs into telogen (resting phase) hairs, resulting in increased shedding of these resting hair follicles and the clinical appearance of moderate to severe hair thinning and loss when growth resumes.
- There are many potential causes of TE, both emotional and physiologic. Often it is hard to determine the etiology, but eliminating the stressor often is the key to resolving TE and stimulating new hair growth.
- No treatment is needed. Patient should be reassured that complete hair regrowth will occur in 6 months–1 year.

TEMPOROMANDIBULAR JOINT DISORDER (TMD)

Benjamin N. Schneider, MD • Scott A. Fields, MD, MHA

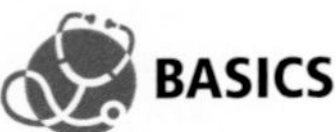

BASICS

DESCRIPTION

- Syndrome characterized by
  - Pain and tenderness involving the muscles of mastications and surrounding tissues
  - Sound, pain, stiffness, or grating in the temporomandibular joint (TMJ) with movement
  - Limitation of mandibular movement with possible locking or dislocation
  - Recent research suggests that TMD is a complex disorder with multiple causes consistent with a biopsychosocial model of illness (1)[B].
- System(s) affected: musculoskeletal
- Synonym(s): temporomandibular joint syndrome; temporomandibular joint dysfunction; myofascial pain–dysfunction syndrome; bruxism; orofacial pain

EPIDEMIOLOGY

Incidence

- Symptoms more common in ages 30–50 years
- Predominant sex: female > male (4:1)

Prevalence

Up to 1/2 the population has at least 1 sign or symptom of TMD, but most are not limited by symptoms, and <1:4 seek medical or dental treatment.

ETIOLOGY AND PATHOPHYSIOLOGY

- Pathophysiology is multifactorial, involving anatomic, behavioral, emotional, and cognitive factors.
- The American Academy of Orofacial Pain categorizes TMD according to anatomic origins of pain and the change in name from TMJ to TMD emphasizes that many patients suffer from muscular and not articular pain.
- Articular disorders of the joint
  - Congenital disorders
  - Inflammatory disorders: synovitis, arthritides, capsulitis
  - TMJ disk derangement
  - Hyper- or hypomobile TMJ
  - TMJ trauma: condylar fractures, dislocation
- Muscle disorders involving the muscles of mastication
  - Occlusomuscular dysfunction (bruxism)
  - Masticatory muscle spasm
  - Myositis
  - Myofibrosis
  - Neoplasia
  - Poorly fitting dentures

Genetics

Research is ongoing in gene polymorphisms associated with TMD and other pain disorders. These include the catechol O-methyltransferase gene (COMT), which is thought to be associated with changes in pain responsiveness.

RISK FACTORS

- Macrotrauma to the face, jaw and neck, including cervical whiplash injuries
- Rheumatologic and degenerative conditions involving the TMJ
- Psychosocial stress and poor adaptive capabilities
- Repetitive microtrauma from dental malocclusion, including inappropriate dental treatment
- Link with bruxism and jaw/teeth clenching is inconsistent.

GENERAL PREVENTION

- Elimination of tension-causing oral habits
- Reduction in overall muscle tension

COMMONLY ASSOCIATED CONDITIONS

Craniomandibular disorders, somatization disorder, somatoform pain disorder, other chronic pain syndromes, fibromyalgia, tension headache

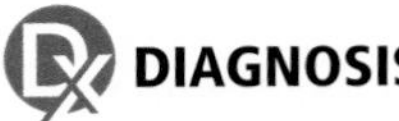

DIAGNOSIS

- TMD is a clinical diagnosis, and localized pain is the unifying feature.
- Several research classification systems exist. Most share several of the history and physical findings listed below.

HISTORY

- Facial and/or TMJ pain
- Locking/catching of jaw; decreased range of motion
- TMJ noises: clicking, grinding, popping
- Headache, earache, neck pain

PHYSICAL EXAM

- Test jaw range of motion (opening, closing, lateral, protrusive) and masticatory muscle strength.
  - Maximal (pain-free) jaw opening with interincisal distance <40 mm is suggestive if accompanied by other signs and symptoms (normal 35–55 mm)
  - Deviation to the affected side is common.
- There may be tenderness over the TMJ.
- Palpation of muscles of mastication may produce tenderness.
- Clicking of jaw with opening

DIFFERENTIAL DIAGNOSIS

- Condylar fracture/dislocation
- Trigeminal neuralgia
- Dental or periodontal conditions
- Neoplasm of the jaw, orofacial muscles, or salivary glands
- Acute, nondental infection: parotitis, sialadenitis, otitis, mastoiditis
- Jaw claudication: giant cell arteritis
- Migraine or tension type headache
- Ramsay-Hunt syndrome (zoster auricular syndrome)

DIAGNOSTIC TESTS & INTERPRETATION

- There are no labs to rule in TMD.
- Blood work may be useful to rule out other conditions (CBC, CMP, ESR, CRP).

Imaging

- TMD is a clinical diagnosis based primarily on history and physical exam.
- Often, a poor correlation is found between pain severity and pathologic changes seen in joint or muscle tissues. Consider the following for severe or treatment-resistant cases, with MR or CT more useful as part of surgical workup:
  - Panoramic dental radiographs are a good 1st-line screen.
  - CT scan allows fine detail of bony structures.
  - US: Effusion and findings correlate with MRI and subjective pain.
  - MRI: noninvasive study for disc position; more sensitive than US; can help determine need for surgical management

Diagnostic Procedures/Other

- Local anesthetic nerve block can differentiate orofacial pain of articular versus muscular origins.
- Arthroscopy can be diagnostic for cartilage and bony pathology.

Test Interpretation

- Condylar head displacement
- Anterior disc displacement
- Posterior capsulitis
- Loosening of disc and capsular attachments
- Chondroid metaplasia of disc leading to disc perforation and degeneration

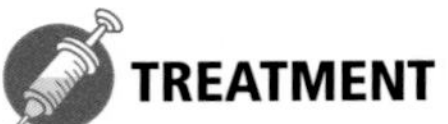

TREATMENT

Signs and symptoms will abate without intervention in most patients. 50% report improvement in 1 year and 85% by 3 years. With conservative therapy, symptoms resolve in 75% of cases within 3 months.

- Therapeutic exercises, especially if displacement is present, included formal physical therapy.
- Psychosocial interventions, including cognitive-behavioral therapy with or without biofeedback (2)[A]
- Behavior modification to eliminate tension-relieving oral habits (2)[A]
- Occlusal adjustment cannot be recommended for the management or prevention of TMD, as there is an absence of evidence from RCTs that occlusal adjustment treats or prevents TMD (3)[A].
- Insufficient evidence exists either for or against the use of stabilization splint therapy for the treatment of TMD (4)[A].

- The American Dental Association recommends a "less is often best" stepwise approach and offers the following stepwise progression for therapy:
  - Eating softer foods
  - Avoiding chewing gum and nail biting
  - Modifying pain with heat
  - Relaxation techniques including meditation and biofeedback
  - Exercises to strengthen jaw muscles
  - Medications
  - Night guards and orthotics

MEDICATION

First Line

- Naproxen
- Topical methylsalicylate
- Gabapentin
- Ibuprofen, if osteoarthritis is suspected (5)[B]

Second Line

- Muscle relaxants
- Tricyclic antidepressants
- Botulinum neurotoxin
- Acupuncture
- Opiates should be reserved for perioperative or severe or recalcitrant cases (5)[B].
- Ineffective medications (5)[B]
  - The following medications when compared with placebo in RCTs were shown to be ineffective in improving pain and should not be used for the treatment of TMD:
    - Benzodiazepines
    - Topical capsaicin
    - Diclofenac
    - Celecoxib

ADDITIONAL THERAPIES

Joint and muscle injections

- There is very limited evidence to recommend for or against injections into or around the TMJ. Proposed therapies include steroids, hyaluronic acid, local anesthetics, and, recently, botulinum toxin.
- Steroids given >3 times annually may accelerate degenerative changes.
- Recent studies suggest that botulinum toxin type A (Botox) injections may be successful in cases that have failed 1st-line pharmacologic therapy (6)[B].

COMPLEMENTARY & ALTERNATIVE MEDICINE

- Glucosamine may be effective if pain is secondary to osteoarthritis of the TMJ (5)[B].
- Multiple electronic diagnostic and treatment modalities are currently marketed to patients; however, the scientific literature does not support the use of electronic diagnostic and treatment devices for TMD at this time.

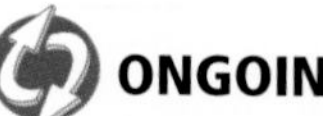

ONGOING CARE

FOLLOW-UP RECOMMENDATIONS

- Relax jaw by disengaging teeth.
- Avoid wide, uncontrolled opening, such as yawning.
- Stress management and behavior-modification counseling may be helpful.
- Be aware of any teeth-clenching or grinding habits.

Patient Monitoring

- Ongoing assessment of clinical response to conservative therapies (NSAIDs, behavior modification, occlusal splints) is necessary.
- Surgical procedure to correct disc displacement or replace a damaged disc may be indicated only if the patient has not responded to conservative treatment.

DIET

Soft diet to reduce chewing

PROGNOSIS

- With conservative therapy, symptoms resolve in 75% of cases within 3 months.
- Patients benefit most from a comprehensive treatment approach including the following:
  - Restoration of normal muscle function
  - Pain control
  - Stress management
  - Behavior modification

COMPLICATIONS

- Secondary degenerative joint disease
- Chronic TMJ dislocation
- Loss of joint range of motion
- Depression and chronic pain syndromes

REFERENCES

1. Slade GC, Fillingim RB, Sanders AE, et al. Summary of findings from the OPPERA prospective cohort study of incidence of first-onset temporomandibular disorder: implications and future directions. *J Pain*. 2013;14(12)(Suppl):T116–T124.
2. Aggarwal VR, Lovell K, Peters S, et al. Psychosocial interventions for the management of chronic orofacial pain. *Cochrane Database Syst Rev*. 2011;(11):CD008456.
3. Koh H, Robinson PG. Occlusal adjustment for treating and preventing temporomandibular joint disorders. *Cochrane Database Syst Rev*. 2009;(1):CD003812.
4. Al-Ani MZ, Davies SJ, Gray RJ, et al. Stabilisation splint therapy for temporomandibular pain dysfunction syndrome. *Cochrane Database Syst Rev*. 2004;(1):CD002778.
5. Mujakperuo HR, Watson M, Morrison R, et al. Pharmacological interventions for pain in patients with temporomandibular disorders. *Cochrane Database Syst Rev*. 2010;(10):CD004715.
6. Ihde SK, Konstantinovic VS. The therapeutic use of botulinum toxin in cervical and maxillofacial conditions: an evidence-based review. *Oral Surg Oral Med Oral Pathol Oral Radiol Endod*. 2007;104(2):e1–e11.

ADDITIONAL READING

- American Dental Association. Patient Information. http://www.ada.org/en/Home-MouthHealthy/az-topics/t/tmj. Accessed 2014.
- Haketa T, Kino K, Sugisaki M, et al. Randomized clinical trial of treatment for TMJ disc displacement. *J Dent Res*. 2010;89(11):1259–1263.
- Scrivani SJ, Keith DA, Kaban LB. Temporomandibular disorders. *N Engl J Med*. 2008;359(25):2693–2705.

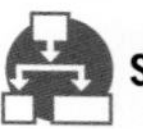

SEE ALSO

Headache, Tension

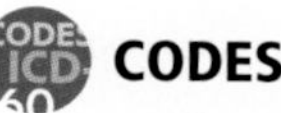

CODES

ICD10

- M26.60 Temporomandibular joint disorder, unspecified
- M26.69 Other specified disorders of temporomandibular joint
- M26.62 Arthralgia of temporomandibular joint

CLINICAL PEARLS

- The condition called TMD actually designates a number of potential underlying joint and muscle conditions involving the jaw.
- Characteristics of all are pain and functional limitation.
- Cognitive-behavioral therapy reduces pain, depression, and limitation of function.
- Exercises may improve function and pain.
- Evidence is lacking to support occlusion correction or splinting.
- Naproxen, gabapentin, topical methylsalicylate, glucosamine, amitriptyline, acupuncture, and botulinum toxin injections have some evidence of efficacy.

T

TESTICULAR MALIGNANCIES

Huy Tan Tran, MD, LCDR, MC, USN • Moses H. Cheng, MAJ, MC, USA

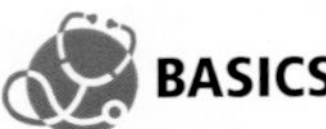

BASICS

DESCRIPTION

- Testicular cancer accounts for 1% of all cancers in men; it is the most common solid malignancy in men aged 15–34 years (1).
- An estimated 8,820 new cases were diagnosed and an estimated 380 deaths occurred in the United States in 2014 (2).
- Treatment produces an overall 5-year survival of 95.3%; for African American patients, this 5-year survival rate is alarmingly lower but has improved from 86% to 90% (2).

ETIOLOGY AND PATHOPHYSIOLOGY

95% of all malignant tumors arising in the testes are germ cell tumors (GCTs), which are subclassified as follows:

- Seminomatous GCTs: most common type overall
- Nonseminomatous GCTs (NSGCTs): These include embryonal cell carcinoma, choriocarcinoma, yolk sac tumor, teratomas, or often multiple cell types; these are more clinically aggressive tumors.

RISK FACTORS

- Cryptorchidism is the most firmly established risk factor: Relative risk of testicular cancer in all patients with cryptorchidism is 3–8, with a lower relative risk of 2–3 in those undergoing orchiopexy by age 12 years; in patients with unilateral cryptorchidism, the relative risk of testicular cancer in the contralateral normally descended testis is negligible (3).
- Personal history of testicular cancer
- Positive family history for testicular cancer
- Testicular dysgenesis
- Klinefelter syndrome
- Caucasian race
- HIV infections

GENERAL PREVENTION

No evidence that screening for testicular cancer is effective (4).

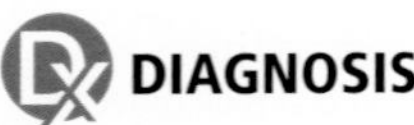

DIAGNOSIS

HISTORY

- A painless solid testicular mass is pathognomonic for testicular cancer.
- Clinical symptoms of epididymitis or orchitis that do not respond to treatment warrant further evaluation.
- Gynecomastia can be a rare systemic endocrine manifestation of testicular neoplasm.

PHYSICAL EXAM

- Testicular exam: Palpate for size, consistency, and nodules; masses do not transilluminate; a firm, hard, or fixed area should be considered suspicious.
- Lymph node and abdominal exam: Evaluate for masses.
- Gynecomastia

DIAGNOSTIC TESTS & INTERPRETATION

Initial Tests (lab, imaging)

- α-Fetoprotein (AFP), β-human chorionic gonadotropin (β-hCG), lactate dehydrogenase (LDH), creatinine, chemistry profile, complete blood count, liver enzymes, chest x-ray (CXR), and testicular US
- Tumor markers AFP, β-hCG, and LDH are used to assist with diagnosis, prognosis, assessing treatment outcome, and monitoring for relapse:
  - AFP
    - Produced by nonseminomatous testicular cancer and is therefore associated with this histologic type
    - Those with a histologically "pure" testicular seminoma and an elevated AFP are assumed to possess an undetected focus of nonseminoma tumor.
  - β-hCG
    - May be associated with both seminomatous or nonseminomatous tumors
    - Hypogonadism and marijuana use may cause benign elevations of β-hCG.
  - LDH is less specific than AFP.
- Testicular US is the initial study.
- If an intratesticular mass is identified, measure serum AFP, LDH and β-hCG and order a CXR.
- CT scan of the abdomen/pelvis, positron emission tomography (PET) scan, MRI of the brain, and bone scan are used for staging and metastases evaluation as clinically indicated.

Diagnostic Procedures/Other

- Radical inguinal orchiectomy is the primary procedure for diagnosis and treatment.
- Testicular biopsy may be rarely considered if a suspicious intratesticular abnormality is identified on US; however, testicular microcalcification on US without any other abnormality can simply be observed and does not demand a biopsy.
- For those with unilateral testicular cancer, contralateral testicular biopsy is not routinely performed but should be considered when there is a cryptorchid testis, marked testicular atrophy, or a suspicious US for intratesticular abnormalities.

Test Interpretation

Clinical staging (5):

- Stage 0: carcinoma in situ
- Stage IA: tumor limited to testis and epididymis without vascular/lymphatic invasion; tumor may invade into the tunica albuginea but not the tunica vaginalis; normal serum tumor markers
- Stage IB: tumor limited to testis and epididymis with vascular/lymphatic invasion or tumor extending through tunica albuginea with involvement of tunica vaginalis; tumor invades the spermatic cord with or without vascular/lymphatic invasion; tumor invades the scrotum with or without vascular/lymphatic invasion; no lymph node involvement or distant metastasis; normal serum tumor markers
- Stage IS: any tumor with elevated serum tumor markers but no nodal involvement or metastasis
- Stage IIA: any tumor with lymph node mass/masses $<$2 cm
- Stage IIB: any tumor with lymph node mass/masses 2–5 cm
- Stage IIC: any tumor with lymph node mass $>$5 cm
- Stage IIIA: any tumor/lymph node presence; with nonregional nodal or pulmonary metastasis; either serum tumor markers normal or with mild elevation
- Stage IIIB: any tumor/lymph node presence; no distant metastasis or nonregional nodal involvement or pulmonary metastasis; with moderately elevated serum tumor markers
- Stage IIIC: any tumor/lymph node presence; with or without any metastasis; with greatly elevated serum tumor markers

DIFFERENTIAL DIAGNOSIS

Epidermoid cyst, epididymitis, hernia, hydrocele, hematoma, lymphoma, orchitis, spermatocele, testicular torsion, varicocele

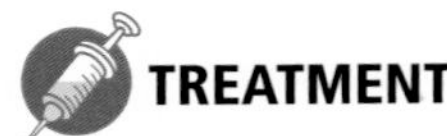

TREATMENT

GENERAL MEASURES

- Seminoma
  - Stages IA, IB: Options may include surveillance (for low tumor load malignancy, i.e., pT1 or pT2), single-agent carboplatin, or radiotherapy.
  - Stage IS: radiotherapy
  - Stages IIA, IIB: radiotherapy to include para-aortic and ipsilateral iliac lymph nodes or primary chemotherapy regimen for selected patients with stage IIB
  - Stages IIC, III
    - Good risk (any primary site and no nonpulmonary visceral metastases and normal AFP with any β-hCG or LDH): primary etoposide and cisplatin (EP) or bleomycin, etoposide, and cisplatin (BEP) chemotherapy
    - Intermediate risk (any primary site and nonpulmonary visceral metastases and normal AFP with any β-hCG or LDH): primary BEP chemotherapy
- Nonseminoma: Tumors with both seminomatous and nonseminomatous histology are managed as nonseminomatous:
  - Stage IA: nonseminomatous surveillance protocol or nerve-sparing retroperitoneal lymph node dissection (RPLND)
  - Stage IB: nerve-sparing RPLND or primary chemotherapy; for T2 only can enter nonseminomatous surveillance protocol
  - Stage IS: primary chemotherapy followed by response evaluation:
    - Complete response, negative tumor markers: nonseminomatous surveillance protocol or nerve-sparing RPLND
    - Partial response, negative tumor markers: surgical resection of all residual masses
    - Incomplete response: consider 2nd-line therapy
  - Stage IIA
    - Negative tumor markers: nerve-sparing RPLND or primary chemotherapy
    - Persistent marker elevation: primary chemotherapy followed by response evaluation
      - Complete response, negative tumor markers: nonseminomatous surveillance protocol or nerve-sparing RPLND
      - Partial response, negative tumor markers: surgical resection of all residual masses
      - Incomplete response: consider 2nd-line therapy
  - Stage IIB
    - Negative tumor markers: nerve-sparing RPLND or primary chemotherapy
    - Persistent marker elevation: primary chemotherapy followed by response evaluation
      - Complete response, negative tumor markers: nonseminomatous surveillance protocol or nerve-sparing RPLND
      - Partial response, negative tumor markers: surgical resection of all residual masses
      - Incomplete response: consider 2nd-line therapy
  - Stage IIC: primary chemotherapy followed by response evaluation:
    - Complete response, negative tumor markers: nonseminomatous surveillance protocol or nerve-sparing RPLND

- Partial response, negative tumor markers: surgical resection of all residual masses
- Incomplete response: consider 2nd-line therapy
- Stages IIIA, IIIB, IIIC: primary chemotherapy or clinical trial, depending on risk profile, which is based on tumor, metastases, and postorchiectomy serum tumor markers
- Brain metastases: primary chemotherapy + radiotherapy and the consideration of surgery, as clinically indicated

MEDICATION

First Line

Primary chemotherapy regimens for GCTs:

- EP: etoposide 100 mg/m^2/day IV on days 1–5, cisplatin 20 mg/m^2/day IV on days 1–5; repeat every 21 days (1)[A]
- BEP: etoposide 100 mg/m^2/day IV on days 1–5, cisplatin 20 mg/m^2/day IV on days 1–5; bleomycin 30 U/dose IV weekly on days 1, 8, and 15 or days 2, 9, and 16; repeat every 21 days (1)[A]
- VIP: etoposide 75 mg/m^2/day IV on days 1–5; mesna 120 mg/m^2 slow IV push before ifosfamide on day 1, then mesna 1,200 mg/m^2 IV continuous infusion on days 1–5; ifosfamide 1,200 mg/m^2/day on days 1–5; cisplatin 20 mg/m^2/day IV on days 1–5, repeat every 21 days (1)[A]

Second Line

- These agents are considered in patients who do not respond to 1st-line therapy or those who experience a recurrence: carboplatin, cisplatin, etoposide, ifosfamide, mesna, paclitaxel, and vinblastine (1)[A]
- Gemcitabine, oxaliplatin, and paclitaxel are used in palliative chemotherapy regimens (1)[A]

ADDITIONAL THERAPIES

Consider sperm banking before treatment that may compromise fertility; rarely covered by insurance

SURGERY/OTHER PROCEDURES

- Radical inguinal orchiectomy: primary treatment for testicular cancer for all patients; prosthesis can be inserted at this time.
- RPLND identifies nodal metastases and provides accurate pathologic staging of the retroperitoneum.

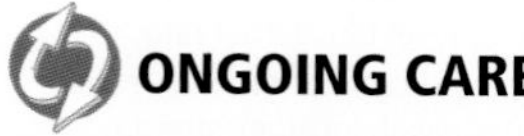

ONGOING CARE

FOLLOW-UP RECOMMENDATIONS

- Pure seminoma: Specifics are noted in the National Comprehensive Cancer Network guidelines (1):
  - Stages IA, IB: in general, H&P, AFP, β-hCG, LDH every 3–4 months for years 1–2, every 6–12 months for years 3–4, then annually; abdominal/pelvic CT every 6–12 months for years 1–3, then annually for years 3–10; CXR, as clinically indicated
  - Stage IS: H&P, AFP, β-hCG, LDH every 4 months for years 1–2, then annually for years 3–10; abdominal/pelvic CT annually for 3 years; CXR, as clinically indicated
  - Stages IIA, IIB (select): in general, H&P, AFP, β-hCG, LDH every 3 months for year 1, every 6 months for years 2–5, then annually for years 6–10; abdominal/pelvic CT every 6–12 months for years 1–2, then annually for year 3; CXR every 6 months for years 1–2; certain select stages differ in follow-up
  - Stages IIB (select), IIC, III: Check all serum tumor markers along with chest, abdominal, and pelvic CT:
    - Residual mass 0–3 cm and normal serum tumor markers: H&P, AFP, β-hCG, LDH, CXR every 2 months for year 1, every 3 months for year 2, every 6 months for years 3–4, then annually; abdominal/pelvic CT scans, and PET scans, as clinically indicated
    - Residual mass >3 cm and normal serum tumor markers: PET scan 6 weeks after chemotherapy
      - Negative PET scan: H&P, AFP, β-hCG, LDH, CXR every 2 months for year 1, every 3 months for year 2, every 6 months for years 3–4, then annually; abdominal/pelvic CT scans, and PET scans, as clinically indicated
      - Positive PET scan: Consider RPLND or 2nd-line chemotherapy or radiotherapy; then H&P, AFP, β-hCG, LDH, CXR every 2 months for year 1, every 3 months for year 2, every 6 months for years 3–4, then annually; abdominal/pelvic CT scans, and PET scans, as clinically indicated
  - Any recurrence: Treat according to extent of disease at relapse.
- Nonseminoma: Specifics are noted in the National Comprehensive Cancer Network guidelines (1):
  - Stages IA, IB on surveillance only: H&P, AFP, β-hCG, LDH, CXR every 1–2 months for year 1, every 2 months for year 2, every 3 months for year 3, every 4 months for year 4, every 6 months for year 6, annually thereafter; abdominal/pelvic CT every 3–4 months for year 1, every 4–6 months for year 2, every 6–12 months for years 3–4, annually for year 5, and every 1–2 years thereafter
  - Follow-up after complete response to chemotherapy and RPLND: H&P, AFP, β-hCG, LDH, CXR every 2–3 months for years 1–2, every 3–6 months for year 3, every 6 months for year 4, every 6–12 months for year 5, annually thereafter; abdominal/pelvic CT every 6 months for year 1, every 6–12 months for year 2, every 12 months for years 3–5, as clinically indicated thereafter
  - Follow-up after RPLND only: H&P, AFP, β-hCG, LDH, CXR every 2–3 months for years 1–2, every 3– 6 months for year 3, every 6 months for year 4, every 6–12 months for year 5, annually thereafter; abdominal/pelvic CT at baseline and, as clinically indicated, thereafter

PROGNOSIS

>90% of patients diagnosed are cured, including 70–80% with advanced tumors (1).

COMPLICATIONS

- Surgical: hematoma, hemorrhage, infection, and infertility
- Radiotherapy: radiation enteritis and infertility
- Late complications (6):
  - Cardiovascular toxicity and 2nd malignancies each have a 25-year risk of about 16% in those treated with chemotherapy and/or radiotherapy.
  - Risk for secondary malignancies remains increased for at least 35 years after treatment.
  - Increased incidence of metabolic syndrome occurs and is likely associated with lower testosterone levels.
  - Other late complications associated with chemotherapy, depending on the regimen, include chronic neurotoxicity, ototoxicity, renal function impairment, and pulmonary fibrosis.
- The incidence of late relapse in treated testicular cancer is now estimated to be 2–6%; the time to late relapse ranges from 2 to 32 years, with a median of 6 years (6).

REFERENCES

1. Motzer RJ, Agarwal N, Beard C, et al. Testicular cancer. *J Natl Compr Canc Netw*. 2012;10(4):502–535.
2. Howlader N, Noone AM, Krapcho M, et al, eds. *SEER Cancer Statistics Review, 1975–2011*. Bethesda, MD: National Cancer Institute. http://seer.cancer.gov/csr/1975_2011/. Accessed 2014.
3. Lip SZ, Murchison LE, Cullis PS, et al. A meta-analysis of the risk of boys with isolated cryptorchidism developing testicular cancer in later life. *Arch Dis Child*. 2013;98(1):20-6.
4. Ilic D, Misso ML. Screening for testicular cancer. *Cochrane Database Syst Rev*. 2011;(2):CD007853.
5. Testis. In: Edge SB, Byrd DR, Compton CC, et al, eds. *AJCC Cancer Staging Manual*. 7th ed. New York, NY: Springer; 2010:469–478.
6. Efstathiou E, Logothetis CJ. Review of late complications of treatment and late relapse in testicular cancer. *J Natl Compr Canc Netw*. 2006;4(10):1059–1070.

ADDITIONAL READING

- Siegel R, Naishadham D, Jemal A. Cancer statistics, 2012. *CA Cancer J Clin*. 2012;62(1):10–29.
- Society for Adolescent Health and Medicine, Marcell AV, Bell DL, et al. The male genital examination: a position paper of the Society for Adolescent Health and Medicine. *J Adolesc Health*. 2012;50(4):424–425.
- U.S. Preventive Services Task Force. Screening for testicular cancer: U.S. Preventive Services Task Force reaffirmation recommendation statement. *Ann Intern Med*. 2011;154(7):483–486.
- Wood HM, Elder JS. Cryptorchidism and testicular cancer: separating fact from fiction. *J Urol*. 2009;181(2):452–461.

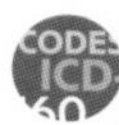

CODES

ICD10

- C62.90 Malig neoplasm of unsp testis, unsp descended or undescended
- C62.00 Malignant neoplasm of unspecified undescended testis
- C62.10 Malignant neoplasm of unspecified descended testis

CLINICAL PEARLS

- Testicular cancer is the most common solid organ tumor in men aged 15–34 years.
- Testicular US is initial imaging of choice for testicular pathology.
- Radical inguinal orchiectomy is used for both diagnosis and treatment.
- 96% overall survival at 10 years after diagnosis and treatment
- Cardiovascular toxicity and secondary malignancies are concerning late-term complications of chemotherapy and/or radiotherapy.

The views expressed in this article are those of the author(s) and do not necessarily reflect the official policy or position of the Department of the Navy, Department of Defense, or the U.S. Government.

T

TESTICULAR TORSION

Jonathan Green, MD • Michael P. Hirsh, MD

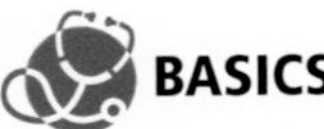

BASICS

DESCRIPTION

- Twisting of testis and spermatic cord, resulting in acute ischemia and loss of testis if unrecognized.
  - Intravaginal torsion: occurs within tunica vaginalis, only involves testis and spermatic cord
  - Extravaginal torsion: involves twisting of testis, cord, and processus vaginalis as a unit. Typically seen in neonates
- System(s) affected: reproductive

Geriatric Considerations

Rare in this age group

Pediatric Considerations

Peak incidence at age 14 years (1)

EPIDEMIOLOGY

Incidence

- ~1/4,000 males before age 25 years
- Predominant age
  - Occurs from newborn period to 7th decade
  - 65% of cases occur in 2nd decade, with peak at age 14 years (1).
  - 2nd peak in neonates (in utero torsion usually occurs around week 32 of gestation) (1)

ETIOLOGY AND PATHOPHYSIOLOGY

- Twisting of spermatic cord causes venous obstruction, edema of testis, and arterial occlusion.
- "Bell clapper" deformity is most common anatomic anomaly predisposing to intravaginal torsion.
  - High insertion of the tunica vaginalis on the spermatic cord, resulting in increased testicular mobility within tunica vaginalis (2)
  - Bilateral in ~80% of patients (1,2)
- No clear anatomic defect is associated with extravaginal testicular torsion.
  - In neonates, the tunica vaginalis is not yet well attached to scrotal wall, allowing torsion of entire testis including tunica vaginalis (1).
- Usually spontaneous and idiopathic (1)
- 20% of patients have a history of trauma.
- 1/3 have had prior episodic testicular pain.
- Contraction of cremasteric muscle or dartos may play a role and is stimulated by trauma, exercise, cold, and sexual stimulation.
- Increased incidence may be due to increasing weight and size of testis during pubertal development.
- Possible alterations in testosterone levels during nocturnal sex response cycle; possible elevated testosterone levels in neonates (1)
- Testis must have inadequate, incomplete, or absent fixation within scrotum (1,2).
- Torsion may occur in either clockwise or counterclockwise direction (3).

Genetics

- Unknown
- Familial testicular torsion, although previously rarely reported, may involve as many as 10% of patients (4).

RISK FACTORS

- May be more common in winter
- Paraplegia
- Previous contralateral testicular torsion

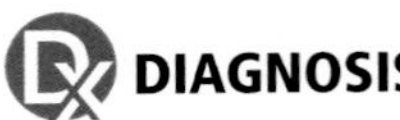

DIAGNOSIS

HISTORY

- Acute onset of pain, often during period of inactivity.
- Onset of pain usually sudden but may start gradually with subsequent increase in severity (1,2,3).
- Nausea and vomiting are common.
  - Presence may increase the likelihood of testicular torsion versus other differential diagnoses (1,2,5).
- Prior history of multiple episodes of testicular pain with spontaneous resolution in an episodic crescendo pattern may indicate intermittent testicular torsion (6).

PHYSICAL EXAM

- Scrotum is enlarged, red, edematous, and painful (1,2).
- Testicle is swollen and exquisitely tender (1,2).
- Testis may be high in scrotum with a transverse lie.
- Absent cremasteric reflex (1,2,3)

DIFFERENTIAL DIAGNOSIS

- Torsion appendix testis (this may account for 35–67% of acute scrotal pain cases in children) (2)
- Epididymitis (8–18% of acute scrotal pain cases) (2)
- Orchitis
- Incarcerated or strangulated inguinal hernia
- Acute hydrocele
- Traumatic hematoma
- Idiopathic scrotal edema
- Acute varicocele
- Epididymal hypertension (venous congestion of testicle or prostate due to sexual arousal that does not end in orgasm)
- Testis tumor
- Henoch-Schönlein purpura
- Scrotal abscess
- Leukemic infiltrate

DIAGNOSTIC TESTS & INTERPRETATION

- Doppler US may confirm testicular swelling but is diagnostic by demonstrating lack of blood flow to the testicle; positive predictive value (PPV) of 89.4% (5,7)[B].
- In boys with intermittent, recurrent testicular torsion, both Doppler US and radionuclide scintigraphy findings will be normal (7)[B].

Diagnostic Procedures/Other

- Doppler US flow detection demonstrates absent or reduced blood flow with torsion and increased flow with inflammatory process (reliable only in first 12 hours) (7)[B].
- Radionuclide testicular scintigraphy with technetium-99m pertechnetate demonstrates absent/decreased vascularity in torsion and increased vascularity with inflammatory processes (including torsion of appendix testes) (8)[C].

Test Interpretation

- Venous thrombosis
- Tissue edema and necrosis
- Arterial thrombosis
- Decreased Doppler flow also seen in hydrocele, abscess, hematoma, or scrotal hernia (7).
- Sensitivity of radionuclide testicular scintigraphy is decreased relative to ultrasonography because hyperemia in the torsed testicle can mimic flow (8).

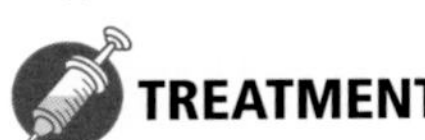

TREATMENT

- Manual reduction: best performed by experienced physician; may be successful, facilitated by lidocaine 1% (plain) injection at level of external ring
  - Difficult to determine success of manual reduction, especially after giving local anesthesia.
  - Manual reduction might require sedation, and the entire process may delay definitive treatment.
  - Even if successful, must always be followed by surgical exploration, urgently but not emergently (6)[C]

- Surgical exploration via scrotal approach with detorsion, evaluation of testicular viability, orchidopexy of viable testicle, orchiectomy of nonviable testicle (5)[B]
- In boys with a history of intermittent episodes of testicular pain, scrotal exploration is warranted with testicular fixation if abnormal testicular attachments are confirmed (5)[B].

GENERAL MEASURES
Early exam is crucial because necrosis of the testicle can occur after 6–8 hours (1,9)[C].

SURGERY/OTHER PROCEDURES
Operative testicular fixation of the torsed testicle after detorsion and confirmation of viability

- At least 3- or 4-point fixation with nonabsorbable sutures between the tunica albuginea and the tunica vaginalis (5)[B]
- Excision of window of tunica albuginea with suture to dartos fascia (5,10)[B]
- Any testis that is not clearly viable should be removed (5)[B].
- Testes of questionable viability that are preserved and pexed invariably atrophy (5)[B]
- Bilateral testicular fixation is recommended by many surgeons (5)[B].
- Contralateral testicle frequently has similar abnormal fixation and should be explored (5)[B],(6)[C].

ONGOING CARE

FOLLOW-UP RECOMMENDATIONS

Patient Monitoring
- Postoperative visit at 1–2 weeks
- Yearly visits until puberty may be needed to evaluate for atrophy.

DIET
Regular

PATIENT EDUCATION
Possibility of testicular atrophy in salvaged testis with depressed sperm counts. Importantly, fertility rates in patients with 1 testicle remain excellent.

PROGNOSIS
- Testicular salvage
  - Salvage is related directly to duration of torsion (85–97% if within 6 hours, 20% after 12 hours <10% if >24 hours) (9).
  - The degree of torsion is related to testicular salvage.
    - The median degree of torsion is <360 in patients who are explored and orchidopexy performed.
    - The median degree of torsion is 540 in patients who undergo exploration and require orchiectomy (3).
- 80–94% may have depressed spermatogenesis related to duration of ischemic injury (possibly related to autoimmune-mediated injury) (9).
- Up to 45% of patients undergoing orchiopexy for testicular torsion will develop atrophy of testicle.

COMPLICATIONS
- Possible testicular atrophy
- Abnormal spermatogenesis
- Infertility
  - Fertility rates with 1 testicle remain excellent.
  - Nearly, 36% of patients who experience torsion have sperm counts <20 million/mL (8).

REFERENCES

1. Boettcher M, Bergholz R, Krebs TF, et al. Clinical predictors of testicular torsion in children. *Urology*. 2012;79(3):670–674.
2. Edelsberg JS, Surh YS. The acute scrotum. *Emerg Med Clin North Am*. 1988;6(3):521.
3. Sessions AE, Rabinowitz R, Hulbert WC, et al. Testicular torsion: direction, degree, duration and disinformation. *J Urol*. 2003;169(2):663–665.
4. Cubillos J, Palmer JS, Friedman SC, et al. Familial testicular torsion. *J Urol*. 2011;185(Suppl 6): 2469–2472.
5. Van Glabeke E, Khairouni A, Larroquet M, et al. Acute scrotal pain in children: results of 543 surgical explorations. *Pediatr Surg Int*. 1999;15(5–6): 353–357.
6. Eaton SH, Cendron MA, Estrada CR, et al. Intermittent testicular torsion: diagnostic features and management outcomes. *J Urol*. 2005;174(4): 1532–1535; discussion 1535.
7. Yagil Y, Naroditsky I, Milhem J, et al. Role of doppler ultrasonography in the triage of acute scrotum in the emergency department. *J Ultrasound Med*. 2010;29(1):11–21.
8. Saleh O, El-Sharkawi MS, Imran MB. Scrotal scintigraphy in testicular torsion: an experience at a Tertiary Care Centre. *Int Med J Malaysia*. 2012; 11(1):9–14.
9. Kapoor S. Testicular torsion: a race against time. *Int J Clin Pract*. 2008;62(5):821–827.
10. Figueroa V, Pippi Salle JL, Braga LH, et al. Comparative analysis of detorsion alone versus detorsion and tunica albuginea decompression (fasciotomy) with tunica vaginalis flap coverage in the surgical management of prolonged testicular ischemia. *J Urol*. 2012;188(Suppl 4): 1417–1422.

CODES

ICD10
- N44.00 Torsion of testis, unspecified
- N44.03 Torsion of appendix testis
- N44.01 Extravaginal torsion of spermatic cord

CLINICAL PEARLS
- The diagnosis of testicular torsion is usually made by physical exam. Patients with suspected torsion should be taken to the OR without delay. If diagnosis is in question, a testicular Doppler US may be done to evaluate blood flow.
- Although testicular necrosis may be present within 6–8 hours of torsion, this is highly variable.
- Infertility can be a problem even if the testicle is viable. Autoimmune antibodies may be produced, and they may affect subsequent fertility.

T

TESTOSTERONE DEFICIENCY

Robert A. Baldor, MD, FAAFP • Jeremy Golding, MD, FAAFP

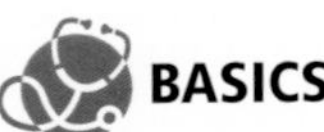

BASICS

DESCRIPTION

- FDA definition: testosterone <300 ng/dL (in men)
- Testosterone is essential for normal sexual development and function.
- Testosterone levels may decline with aging and in certain disease states.
- Low androgen levels increase the risk of low-trauma fractures and are associated with a decline in sexual function, sense of well-being, muscle mass, and strength.
- System(s) affected: body composition and strength, bone, cardiovascular, reproductive, mood, central nervous system, hematologic
- Synonym(s): hypogonadism; hypoandrogenism; androgen deficiency in the aging male syndrome

EPIDEMIOLOGY

Incidence

- 12.3/1,000 person-years in the United States
- Late-onset hypogonadism: 481,000 new cases in the United States, men 40–69 years of age

Prevalence

- 2–4 million men in United States; because of problems of definition, the prevalence in women is undetermined.
- 12% of men in their 50s; 28% between 70 and 79 years of age; 49% in men ≥80 years of age

ETIOLOGY AND PATHOPHYSIOLOGY

- Normal hypothalamic–pituitary–testis axis
  - Hypothalamus produces GnRH, which stimulates pituitary to produce follicle-stimulating hormone (FSH) and luteinizing hormone (LH).
  - LH stimulates the testis to produce testosterone.
  - Testosterone inhibits production of LH through negative feedback.
- Primary testosterone deficiency: Testes produces insufficient amount of testosterone; FSH/LH levels are elevated.
- Secondary testosterone deficiency (also known as *hypogonadotropic hypogonadism*): low testosterone from inadequate production of LH
- Congenital syndromes: undescended testicles
- Orchiectomy; testicular trauma
- Infectious: mumps orchitis, HIV/AIDS, tuberculosis
- Systemic
  - Cushing syndrome
  - Hemochromatosis
  - Autoimmune
  - Granulomatous
  - Severe illness (e.g., renal disease, cirrhosis)
  - Sickle cell disease
- Obesity; obstructive sleep apnea
- Drugs that decrease production: corticosteroids, ethanol, ketoconazole, spironolactone, marijuana, opioids, cimetidine
- Elevated prolactin
  - Prolactinoma
  - Dopamine antagonists block inhibitory dopamine effects on prolactin secretion: neuroleptics, metoclopramide, etc.
- Idiopathic hypogonadotropic hypogonadism
- Chemotherapy
- Radiation to the testis

Genetics

Some chromosomal disorders are inherited:

- Klinefelter: XXY karyotype (small testis, eunuchoid body habitus, gynecomastia)
- Kallmann: abnormal gonadotropin-releasing hormone (GnRH) secretion due to abnormal hypothalamus development (micropenis, anosmia)

RISK FACTORS

- Obesity, type 2 diabetes, COPD
- Medications that affect testosterone production or metabolism
- Stress
- Undescended testicles
- Trauma; infection; radiation or tumors of testis, pituitary, hypothalamus; chemotherapy
- Exposure to environmental endocrine modulators
- Chronic infections or inflammatory disease

GENERAL PREVENTION

General health maintenance, such as prevention and treatment of obesity

COMMONLY ASSOCIATED CONDITIONS

- Infertility, low sperm count, erectile dysfunction
- Osteopenia/osteoporosis
- Diabetes, dyslipidemia, depression: increased incidence and shorter time to diagnosis
- Increased ratio of fat to lean body mass
- Free testosterone levels are lower in those with Alzheimer disease.

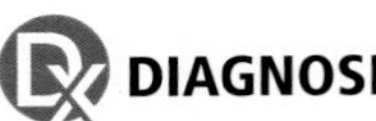

DIAGNOSIS

Test populations who may be at increased risk of testosterone deficiency due to congenital conditions or environmental exposures; broad-based population screening for testosterone deficiency is not recommended.

HISTORY

- Congenital and developmental abnormalities
- Infertility
- Sexual function issues, including decreased libido, erectile dysfunction
- Depression, fatigue, difficulty with concentration/attention
- Decreased beard growth (increased interval between shaving), decreased muscle strength, energy level
- Increase in body fat, development of diabetes
- Bone fractures from relatively minor trauma
- Testicular trauma, infection, radio- or chemotherapy
- Decrease in testicle size or consistency
- Headaches or vision changes suggesting pituitary dysfunction
- Use of medications for associated conditions increases risk of low testosterone.

PHYSICAL EXAM

- Infancy: ambiguous genitalia
- Puberty
  - Impaired growth of penis, testicles
  - Lack of secondary male characteristics
  - Gynecomastia, eunuchoid habitus
- Adulthood
  - Note whether muscular development, hair patterns on face and body, and fat distribution are consistent with age.
  - Presence of gynecomastia
  - Dermatologic changes to suggest hemochromatosis, corticosteroid excess
  - Eunuchoid habitus: lower body >2 cm longer than upper, arm span >2 cm longer than height
  - Kyphosis, loss of height, especially more than expected for age
- Testicular exam on Prader orchidometer
  - Normal testis: 20–30 cc
  - Normal volume but soft and atrophic suggests postpubertal hypogonadism
  - Volume <5 cc suggests prepubertal causes.
  - Small and firm testis suggests Klinefelter.

DIFFERENTIAL DIAGNOSIS

- Ambiguous genitalia; micropenis
- Cryptorchidism
- Delayed puberty
- Obesity (lower total testosterone; assess bioavailable testosterone to confirm)
- Normal aging

DIAGNOSTIC TESTS & INTERPRETATION

An accurate diagnosis is based on the level of *bioavailable* testosterone; with aging, illness, or certain other exposures (e.g., tobacco smoke), levels of sex hormone–binding globulin may increase and total testosterone level may not reflect hormone that is actually available to the tissues.

Initial Tests (lab, imaging)

- In symptomatic individuals, morning total testosterone level as initial test (1)[B]. Morning timing is more important for younger men in whom there is more diurnal variation than in older men.
- Opinions differ regarding use and whether to measure or calculate free testosterone value:
  - Total testosterone reference range: 300–1,200 ng/dL (350 in younger men); free, 9–30 ng/dL; bioavailable testosterone at least 70 ng/dL
  - Repeat the test in the morning if screening results are low.
  - Diagnosis should not be made during an acute or subacute illness.
- Imaging is not helpful in the initial diagnosis of testosterone deficiency.

Follow-Up Tests & Special Considerations

- If testosterone is low or low-normal, check LH:
  - High LH level: primary hypogonadism
  - Low or normal LH: secondary hypogonadism
    - Check prolactin: High level inhibits GnRH.
    - Check TSH: hypothyroidism
    - Transferrin saturation: hemochromatosis
    - Dexamethasone suppression test (Cushing)
- Karyotype if Klinefelter suspected
- If pituitary causes are suspected, CT or MRI may be used to evaluate structural lesions.

Diagnostic Procedures/Other

Dual-emission x-ray absorptiometry bone scan to evaluate bone density

TREATMENT

Testosterone replacement is recommended for symptomatic men with low testosterone levels.

GENERAL MEASURES

- Pretreatment labs: CBC, lipid profile, liver function tests, and prostate-specific antigen (PSA)
- Baseline physical exam (including digital rectal exam and prostate exam)
- For secondary testosterone deficiency, correction of underlying cause may be necessary.
- If fertility is not an issue, testosterone replacement therapy is recommended in symptomatic men with androgen deficiency who have low testosterone levels to induce and maintain secondary sex characteristics and to improve their sexual function, sense of well-being, muscle mass and strength, and bone mineral density (1)[B].
- Testosterone therapy is contraindicated in patients with breast or prostate cancer, palpable prostate nodule or induration, PSA >3 ng/mL without further urologic evaluation, hematocrit >50, hyperviscosity, untreated obstructive sleep apnea, severe lower urinary tract symptoms with an International Prostate Symptom Score >19, or class III or IV heart failure.
- Testosterone therapy is not recommended for
  - Mood or strength improvement in otherwise healthy older men
  - Asymptomatic men with low testosterone measurements (1)[B]
- Testosterone-deficient men with HIV infection or receiving high doses of glucocorticoid treatment may benefit from short-term testosterone therapy to promote preservation of lean body mass and bone density (1)[B].
- Carefully weigh risks and benefits (2)[A] in men at elevated cardiovascular risk.

MEDICATION

First Line

- Testosterone gels/pumps/solutions (AndroGel, Testim, Fortesta, Axiron)
  - Typical dose of 50–100 mg testosterone applied daily
  - Improvements in sexual function, mood, lean body mass, and bone density have been reported (3)[B].

ALERT

- Must avoid transfer of testosterone gel to female partner or children
- Oral therapy is not recommended:
  - May cause liver toxicity
  - Physiologic levels are difficult to maintain.
  - Not beneficial in older men

Second Line

- Delatestryl (testosterone enanthate) or Depo-Testosterone (testosterone cypionate) injection
  - 100 mg/week or 200 mg every 2 weeks
  - Inexpensive
  - Levels high immediately after injection; fall to very low before next injection is due; may cause mood swings
- Transdermal patch (Androderm)
  - More expensive
  - May cause skin irritation
  - Nonscrotal patch: 1–2 patches daily
  - Rotate sites to avoid irritation.
- Transbuccal bioadhesive tablets (Striant)
  - 30 mg BID applied to gum region above incisor tooth
  - Gum-related events in 16% of men
- SC pellets (Testopel) or compounded
  - Last 3–6 months
  - May be difficult to adjust dose; easier to customize with compounded formulation
  - Requires surgical insertion, which can be done in the office with local anesthesia

ISSUES FOR REFERRAL

- In prepubertal patients, starting hormonal therapy at the appropriate age is of paramount importance:
  - In hypogonadotropic hypogonadism, testosterone therapy does not confer fertility or stimulate testicular growth.
  - Pulsatile LH-releasing hormone or human chorionic gonadotropin therapy is an option.
- Elevated PSA; abnormal prostate exam

COMPLEMENTARY & ALTERNATIVE MEDICINE

Dehydroepiandrostenedione supplementation has not been studied adequately in humans to define potential risks versus benefits (4)[C].

ONGOING CARE

Monitoring the effectiveness of therapy, as well as surveillance for adverse effects of replacement, is necessary every 6–12 months.

FOLLOW-UP RECOMMENDATIONS

Patient Monitoring

Monitor replacement therapy for 2–4 months initially and then 6–12 months thereafter:

- Digital prostate exam, PSA, lipid profile, CBC, serum glutamic pyruvic transaminase before initiating therapy and at least annually thereafter
- Testosterone levels until stabilized

DIET

- Calcium 1,200 mg/day, vitamin D 800 IU/day
- Hypocaloric diet to reduce weight if obese

PATIENT EDUCATION

- Testosterone deficiency is a chronic condition that is likely to need lifelong replacement therapy.
- Women and children must not be allowed to come in contact with testosterone replacement products.

PROGNOSIS

- Sustained reversal of symptoms is the goal of therapy when adequate serum levels of testosterone are achieved.
- Hypogonadotropic hypogonadism may be reversed successfully in 10% of patients.
- Androgen supplementation does not seem to improve any aspects of age-related frailty.

COMPLICATIONS

- Decreased sexual desire, muscle mass, bone density, loss of secondary sexual characteristics
- Complications of testosterone replacement:
  - Benign prostate hyperplasia exacerbation
  - Gynecomastia
  - Acne
  - Aggressive behavior
  - Polycythemia
  - Exacerbation of sleep apnea
  - Possible increased risk for cardiovascular events (2)[A]
  - Hepatotoxicity with prolonged use
  - Exacerbation of metastatic prostate cancer

REFERENCES

1. Bhasin S, Cunningham GR, Hayes FJ, et al. Testosterone therapy in adult men with androgen deficiency syndromes: an Endocrine Society clinical practice guideline. *J Clin Endocrinol Metab*. 2010;95(6):2536–2559.
2. Xu L, Freeman G, Cowling BJ, et al. Testosterone therapy and cardiovascular events among men: A systematic review and meta-analysis of placebo-controlled randomized trials *BMC Med*. 2013;11:108. doi:10.1186/1741-7015-11-108.
3. Wang C, Cunningham G, Dobs A, et al. Long-term testosterone gel (AndroGel) treatment maintains beneficial effects on sexual function and mood, lean and fat mass, and bone mineral density in hypogonadal men. *J Clin Endocrinol Metab*. 2004;89(5):2085–2098.
4. Muller M, van den Beld AW, van der Schouw YT, et al. Effects of dehydroepiandrosterone and atamestane supplementation on frailty in elderly men. *J Clin Endocrinol Metab*. 2006;91(10):3988–3991.

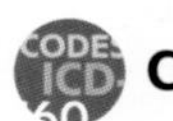

CODES

ICD10

- E29.1 Testicular hypofunction
- E89.5 Postprocedural testicular hypofunction

CLINICAL PEARLS

- Every man presenting with a complaint of erectile dysfunction or with a low-trauma fracture should be assessed for the presence of hypogonadism.
- Initial test of choice is a morning total testosterone; if low, repeat morning total testosterone.
- Testosterone replacement therapy in aging men is likely of little benefit and may be associated with harms.

THALASSEMIA

Herbert L. Muncie, Jr., MD

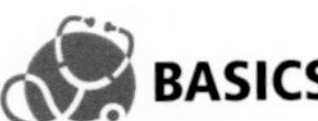

BASICS

DESCRIPTION

- A group of inherited hematologic disorders that affect the synthesis of adult hemoglobin tetramer (HbA) (1,2)[C]
- α-Thalassemia is due to a deficient synthesis of α-globin chain, whereas β-thalassemia is due to a deficient synthesis of β-globin chain:
  - The synthesis of the unaffected globin chain proceeds normally.
  - The unbalanced globin chain production causes unstable hemoglobin tetramers, which leads to hypochromic, microcytic RBCs, and hemolytic anemia.
- α-Thalassemia is more common in persons of Mediterranean, African, and Southeast Asian descent, whereas β-thalassemia is more common in patients of African and Southeast Asian descent.
- Types
  - Thalassemia (minor) trait (α or β): absent or mild anemia with microcytosis and hypochromia
  - α-Thalassemia major with hemoglobin Barts usually results in fatal hydrops fetalis (fluid in $\geq$2 fetal compartments secondary to anemia and fetal heart failure).
  - α-Thalassemia intermedia with hemoglobin H (hemoglobin H disease): hemolytic anemia and splenomegaly
  - β-Thalassemia major: severe anemia, growth retardation, hepatosplenomegaly, bone marrow expansion, and bone deformities. Transfusion therapy is necessary to sustain life. Patients require >8 transfusion events per year. An event may be multiple transfused units.
  - β-Thalassemia intermedia: milder form; transfusion therapy may not be needed or may be needed later in life.
- Other variants include hemoglobin E/β-thalassemia in Southeast Asians, which often mimics the severity of α-thalassemia major.
- System(s) affected: hematologic/lymphatic/immunologic; cardiac; hepatic
- Synonym(s): Mediterranean anemia; hereditary leptocytosis; Cooley anemia

Pediatric Considerations

- β-Thalassemia major causes symptoms during early childhood, usually starting at 6 months of age, and requires periodic transfusions to sustain life.
- Newborn's cord blood or heel stick should be screened for hemoglobinopathies with hemoglobin electrophoresis or comparably accurate test, although this primarily detects sickle cell disease.

Pregnancy Considerations

- Preconception genetic counseling is advised for couples at risk for having a child with thalassemia and for parents or other relatives of a child with thalassemia (3)[A].
- Once pregnant, a chorionic villus sample at 10–11 weeks' gestation or an amniocentesis at 15 weeks' gestation can be done to detect point mutations or deletions with polymerase chain reaction (PCR) technology.

EPIDEMIOLOGY

Incidence

- Occurs in ~4.4/10,000 live births
- Predominant age: Symptoms start to appear 6 months after birth with β-thalassemia major.
- Predominant sex: male = female

Prevalence

- Worldwide, ~200,000 people are alive with β-thalassemia major and <1,000 patients are in the United States.
- In the worldwide population, an estimated 1.5% are β-thalassemia carriers and 5% α-thalassemia carriers (4).

ETIOLOGY AND PATHOPHYSIOLOGY

Unknown; it is unclear how the imbalance of α-globin in β-thalassemia and β-globulin in α-thalassemia results in ineffective red cell genesis and hemolysis.

Genetics

- Inherited in an autosomal recessive pattern
- α-Thalassemia results from a deletion of $\geq$1 of the 4 genes, 2 on each chromosome 16, responsible for α-globin synthesis. 1-gene deletion is a silent carrier state, 2-gene deletion is the trait, 3-gene deletion results in hemoglobin H, and 4-gene deletion results in hemoglobin Bart, causing fatal hydrops fetalis.
- Nondeletional forms do occur rarely. Hemoglobin H Constant Spring is the most common nondeletional form.
- β-Thalassemia is caused by any of >200-point mutations and, very rarely, deletions on chromosome 11, although 20 alleles account for >80% of the mutations.
- Significantly disparate phenotype with the same genotype occurs because β-globin chain production can range from near-normal to absent.

RISK FACTORS

Family history of thalassemia

GENERAL PREVENTION

- Prenatal information: genetic counseling regarding partner selection and information on the availability of diagnostic tests during the pregnancy
- Complication prevention
  - For offspring of adult thalassemia patients, an evaluation for thalassemia by 1 year of age
  - Severe forms
    - Avoid exposure to sick contacts.
    - Keep immunizations up to date.
  - Promptly treat bacterial infections. (After splenectomy, patients should maintain a supply of an appropriate antibiotic to take at the onset of symptoms of a bacterial infection.)
  - Dental checkups every 6 months
  - Avoid activities that could increase the risk of bone fractures.

COMMONLY ASSOCIATED CONDITIONS

See "Complications."

DIAGNOSIS

Thalassemia (minor) trait has no signs or symptoms.

HISTORY

- Poor growth
- Excessive fatigue
- Cholelithiasis
- Pathologic fractures
- Shortness of breath

PHYSICAL EXAM

- Pallor
- Splenomegaly
- Jaundice
- Maxillary hyperplasia/frontal bossing due to massive bone marrow expansion
- Dental malocclusion

DIFFERENTIAL DIAGNOSIS

- Iron deficiency
- Other microcytic anemias: lead toxicity, sideroblastic
- Other hemolytic anemias
- Hemoglobinopathies

DIAGNOSTIC TESTS & INTERPRETATION

Special tests

- Bone marrow aspiration to evaluate for causes of microcytic anemia is rarely needed.
- Multiple indices have been evaluated to discriminate β-thalassemia trait from iron deficiency anemia, yet none is sensitive enough to exclude β-thalassemia trait.
- Hemoglobin: usual range 10–12 g/dL with thalassemia trait and 3–8 g/dL with β-thalassemia major before transfusions
- Hematocrit
  - 28–40% in thalassemia trait
  - May fall to <10% in β-thalassemia major
- Peripheral blood
  - Microcytosis (MCV <70 fl)
  - Hypochromia (MCH <20 pg)
  - High percentage of target cells
  - Reticulocyte count elevated
- Red cell distribution width (RDW)
  - A normal RDW with a microcytic hypochromic anemia is almost always thalassemia trait.
  - Although the RDW is usually normal, it can be elevated in ~50% of thalassemia trait patients. This is in contrast to iron deficiency anemia, where the RDW is almost always elevated (90%).
- Hemoglobin electrophoresis
  - In α-thalassemia trait, no recognizable electrophoretic pattern occurs in adults.
  - However, in the neonatal period, 3–10% of trait patients will have hemoglobin H or hemoglobin Bart at birth, which would confirm α-thalassemia.
  - If HbA_2 is below normal (<2.5%) with a normal HbF level, the diagnosis is α-thalassemia intermedia (HbH disease).
  - In the neonatal period with β-thalassemia trait, the electrophoresis is normal. However, in adults, elevated HbA_2 levels (>4%) may be present but are usually normal (5).
  - β-Thalassemia major or intermedia has elevated HbA_2, elevated HbF, and reduced or absent HbA.
- DNA analysis
  - α-Thalassemia can definitively be diagnosed with genetic testing of hemoglobin A1 and A2 (for deletions and point mutations), but this is not routinely done due to the high cost.

Pediatric Considerations

For children, calculate Mentzer index (mean corpuscular volume/RBC count).

- <13: suggests thalassemia
- >13: suggests iron deficiency test interpretation
- Liver iron concentrations can be assessed with MRI (FerriScan).

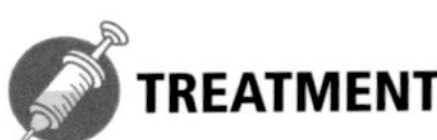

TREATMENT

- Outpatient for mild cases
- Inpatient for transfusion therapy

GENERAL MEASURES
- Mild cases (trait or minor) require no therapy.
- Thalassemia intermedia: Normally, no therapy is necessary unless hemoglobin falls to a level that causes symptoms; then transfusion therapy may be needed. Decision is based primarily on patient's quality of life.
- Iron supplements should not be given unless iron deficiency is confirmed. Supplements can increase the risk of iron overload.
- Thalassemia major
  - A regular transfusion schedule to increase post-transfusion hemoglobin to 13.0–14.0 g/L and maintain a mean hemoglobin level of at least 9.3 g/dL (1.4 mmol/L)
  - Iron overload (6)[C]
    - Patients receiving transfusion therapy increase total body iron 4× over the normal amount.
    - Therapy is iron chelation. (See "Medication.")

MEDICATION
Thalassemia intermedia and major: folic acid supplements (1 mg/day)

First-Line Chelation
β-Thalassemia major
- Iron chelation with deferoxamine (Desferal)
  - Usually continuous SC or IV infusion
  - Acute toxicity: initial—1,000 mg IV, may be followed by 500 mg every 4 hours for 2 doses; subsequent doses of 500 mg every 4–12 hours based on response (max 6,000 mg/day)
  - Chronic: 20–40 mg/kg over 8–12 hours daily
  - Usually started by 5–8 years of age
  - Treatment lasts 3–5 years to reach serum ferritin <1,000 ng/mL.
- Deferasirox (Exjade): 20–30 mg/kg/day PO acceptable alternative (7); approved for transfusion- and non–transfussion-dependent patients with hepatic iron concentrations ≥5 mg/g of dry weight and serum ferritin >300 μg/L ; renal and hepatic monitoring is recommended.

Second-Line
Chelation with deferiprone (Ferriprox) 25 mg/kg TID PO initially is an acceptable alternative for patients who have not responded to deferoxamine; may provide more cardioprotection. A drawback is weekly CBC because ~1% of patients develop agranulocytosis.

ISSUES FOR REFERRAL
Thalassemia major usually requires hematology consult.

ADDITIONAL THERAPIES
β-Thalassemia intermedia
- Hydroxyurea may improve hemoglobin 1–2 g/dL.
- Psychological support seems appropriate for this chronic disease. However, no conclusions can be made regarding specific psychological therapies.

SURGERY/OTHER PROCEDURES
- Splenectomy
  - May be needed if hypersplenism causes an increase in the transfusion requirements (>180–200 mL/kg/year) (8)
  - Defer surgery until patient is at least 4 years of age (due to increased infection risk).
  - Administer pneumococcal polyvalent-23 vaccine 1 month before splenectomy. Children should complete their pneumococcal conjugate vaccine series before surgery.
  - Daily penicillin prophylaxis, 250 mg BID, after splenectomy for 2 years for all patients and for children until age 16 years.
- Bone marrow transplantation with HLA-identical related donor stem cells in children before developing hepatitis or iron overload has high likelihood of remission but may impair fertility.

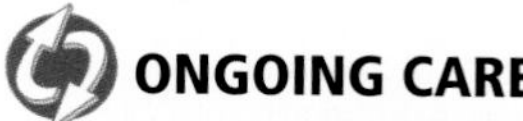

ONGOING CARE

FOLLOW-UP RECOMMENDATIONS
- Thalassemia trait requires no restrictions.
- β-Thalassemia major
  - Avoid strenuous activities (e.g., football, soccer).
  - Acceptable activity levels will be determined on an individual basis depending on the severity of the disorder.

Patient Monitoring
- Thalassemia-trait patients require no special follow-up.
- For β-thalassemia major, lifelong monitoring is necessary because the therapy and disease progression have numerous potential complications.

DIET
- Thalassemia trait requires no restrictions.
- β-Thalassemia major
  - Limit intake of iron-rich foods (e.g., red meats such as liver and some cereals).

PATIENT EDUCATION
Printed patient information available from Cooley Anemia Foundation, 330 7th Ave. Suite 900, New York, NY 10001; http://www.thalassemia.org or http://www.cooleysanemia.org

PROGNOSIS
- Outlook varies depending on type.
- Thalassemia-trait patients live a normal lifespan.
- β-Thalassemia major patients live an average of 17 years and usually die by age 30 years.
- Iron overload causes most of the morbidity and mortality:
  - Cardiac events are the primary cause of death.
  - Myocardial iron deposition is best assessed with MRI T2 (9).
  - Effective iron chelation is improving longevity.

COMPLICATIONS
- Chronic hemolysis
- Susceptibility to infections after splenectomy
- Infections from blood transfusion
- Jaundice
- Leg ulcers
- Cholelithiasis
- Osteoporosis and low-trauma fractures
- Impaired growth rate
- Delayed or absent puberty
- Hypogonadism
- Hepatic siderosis
- Splenomegaly
- Cardiac disease from iron overload
- Thromboembolic phenomenon
- Aplastic and megaloblastic crises

REFERENCES

1. Muncie HL Jr, Campbell J. Alpha and beta thalassemia. *Am Fam Physician*. 2009;80(4):339–344.
2. Higgs DR, Engel JD, Stamatoyannopoulos GI. Thalassaemia. *Lancet*. 2012;379(9813):373–383.
3. Tamhankar PM, Agarwal S, Arya V, et al. Prevention of homozygous beta thalassemia by premarital screening and prenatal diagnosis in India. *Prenat Diagn*. 2009;29(1):83–88.
4. Peters M, Heijboer H, Smiers F, et al. Diagnosis and management of thalassaemia. *BMJ*. 2012;344:e228.
5. Mosca A, Paleari R, Ivaldi G, et al. The role of haemoglobin A(2) testing in the diagnosis of thalassaemias and related haemoglobinopathies. *J Clin Pathol*. 2009;62(1):13–17.
6. Fleming RE, Ponka P. Iron overload in human disease. *N Engl J Med*. 2012;366(4):348–359.
7. Taher A, El-Beshlawy A, Elalfy MS, et al. Efficacy and safety of deferasirox, an oral iron chelator, in heavily iron-overloaded patients with beta-thalassaemia: the ESCALATOR study. *Eur J Haematol*. 2009;82(6):458–465.
8. Galanello R, Origa R. Beta-thalassemia. *Orphanet J Rare Dis*. 2010;5:11.
9. Pennell DJ, Udelson JE, Arai AE, et al. Cardiovascular function and treatment in β-thalassemia major. a consensus statement from the American Heart Association. *Circulation*. 2013;128(3):281–308.

ADDITIONAL READING

- Borgna-Pignatti C. Modern treatment of thalassaemia intermedia. *Br J Haematol*. 2007;138(3):291–304.
- Dussiot M, Maciel TT, Fricot A, et al. An activin receptor IIA ligand trap corrects ineffective erythropoiesis in beta-thalassemia. *Nat Med*. 2014;20(4):398–407.
- Paulson RF. Targeting a new regulator of erythropoiesis to alleviate anemia. *Nat Med*. 2014;20(4):334–3350.

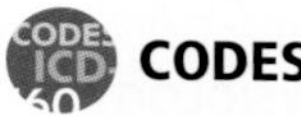

CODES

ICD10
- D56.9 Thalassemia, unspecified
- D56.1 Beta thalassemia
- D56.0 Alpha thalassemia

CLINICAL PEARLS

- Thalassemia (group of inherited hematologic disorders that affect the synthesis of adult hemoglobin tetramer) is a genetic condition; hemoglobin will not improve over time.
- α-Thalassemia is due to a deficient synthesis of the α-globin chain, whereas β-thalassemia is due to a deficient synthesis of the β-globin chain.
- Hemoglobin electrophoresis is needed for genetic counseling but not to make the diagnosis of thalassemia minor when evaluating a patient with mild hypochromic, microcytic anemia, and normal serum ferritin.
- Anemia from thalassemia minor is not due to inadequate iron availability or iron storage. Therefore, iron supplements will not improve the anemia and could be harmful due to GI distress and iron overload. If coexisting iron deficiency is proven, then iron therapy is appropriate.

T

THORACIC OUTLET SYNDROME

Muhammad Imran Khan, MD • Najm Hasan Siddiqui, MD

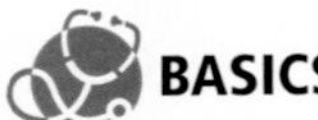

BASICS

DESCRIPTION

- A constellation of symptoms that affect the head, neck, shoulders, and upper extremities caused by compression of the neurovascular structures (i.e., brachial plexus and subclavian vessels) at the thoracic outlet, specifically in the area superior to the 1st rib and posterior to the clavicle
- 3 forms of thoracic outlet syndrome (TOS) have been described: neurogenic, vascular (containing venous and arterial symptoms), and nonspecific (includes traumatic and secondary to certain provocative movements).
- Synonym(s): scalenus anticus syndrome; cervical rib syndrome; costoclavicular syndrome

Pregnancy Considerations

Generalized tissue fluid accumulations and postural changes may aggravate symptoms.

EPIDEMIOLOGY

Incidence

- Predominant age
  - Neurogenic type (95%): 20–60 years
  - Venous type (4%): 20–35 years
  - Arterial type (1%; atherosclerosis): young adult or >50 years
- Predominant sex
  - Neurogenic type: female > male (3.5:1)
  - Venous type: male > female
  - Arterial type: male = female
- No objective confirmatory tests available to measure true incidence.
- Estimated 3–8/1,000 cases for neurogenic type
- Incidence of other TOS types is unclear.

ETIOLOGY AND PATHOPHYSIOLOGY

The interscalene triangle area is reduced in TOS and may become smaller during certain shoulder and arm movements. Fibrotic bands, cervical ribs, and muscle variations may further narrow the triangle. Trauma or provocative movements affecting the lower brachial plexus have strong implications in TOS pathogenesis.

- 3 known causes of TOS: anatomic, traumatic/repetitive movement activities, and neurovascular entrapment
- Anatomic: Variations in the anatomy of the neck scalene muscles may be responsible for presentations of the neurologic type of TOS and may involve the superior border of the 1st rib. Cervical ribs also have been implicated as a cause of neurologic TOS, with subsequent neuronal fibrosing and degeneration associated with arterial hyalinization in the lower trunk of the brachial plexus. Fibrous bands to cervical ribs are often congenital.
- Trauma or repetitive movement activities: motor vehicle accidents with hyperextension injury and resulting fibrosis, including fibrous bands to the clavicle; musicians who maintain prolonged positions of shoulder abduction or extension may be at increased risk
- Neurovascular entrapment: occurring in the costoclavicular space between the 1st rib and the head of the clavicle

RISK FACTORS

- Trauma, especially to the shoulder girdle
- Presence of a cervical rib
- Posttraumatic, exostosis of clavicle or 1st rib, postural abnormalities (e.g., drooping of shoulders, scoliosis), body building with increased muscular bulk in thoracic outlet area, rapid weight loss with vigorous physical exertion and/or exercise, pendulous breasts
- Occupational exposure: computer users; musicians; repetitive work involving shoulders, arms, hands
- Young, thin females with long necks and drooping shoulders

GENERAL PREVENTION

Consider observation or further evaluation in patients with cervical ribs.

COMMONLY ASSOCIATED CONDITIONS

- Paget–von Schrötter syndrome: thrombosis of subclavian vein
- Gilliatt-Sumner hand: neurogenic atrophy of abductor pollicis brevis

DIAGNOSIS

HISTORY

- Neurologic type, upper plexus (C4–C7)
  - Pain and paresthesias in head, neck, mandible, face, temporal area, upper back/chest, outer arm, and hand in a radial nerve distribution
  - Occipital and orbital headache
- Neurologic type, lower plexus (C8–T1)
  - Pain and paresthesias in axilla, inner arm, and hand in an ulnar nerve distribution, often nocturnal
  - Hypothenar and interosseous muscle atrophy
- Venous type: arm claudication, cyanosis, swelling, distended arm veins
- Arterial type: digital vasospasm, thrombosis/embolism, aneurysm, gangrene

PHYSICAL EXAM

- Positive Adson maneuver (head rotation to the affected side with cervical extension and then deep inhalation); test is positive if paresthesias occur or if radial pulse is not palpable during maneuver.
- Tenderness to percussion or palpation of supraclavicular area
- Worsening of symptoms with elevation of arm, overhead extension of arms, or with arms extended forward (e.g., driving a car, typing, carrying objects); prompt disappearance of symptoms with arm returning to neutral position
- Morley test
  - Brachial plexus compression test in the supraclavicular area from the scalene triangle
  - Positive with reproduction of an aching sensation and typical localized paresthesia
- Hyperabduction test: diminishment of radial pulse with elevation of arm above the head
- Military maneuver (i.e., costoclavicular bracing): When patient elevates chin and pushes shoulders posteriorly in an extreme "at-attention" position, symptoms are provoked.
- 1-minute Roos test
  - A thoracic outlet shoulder girdle stress test
  - Shoulders and arms are braced in a 90-degree abducted and externally rotated position; patient is required to clench and relax fists repetitively for 1 minute.
  - A positive test reproduces the symptom.

DIFFERENTIAL DIAGNOSIS

- Cervical disk or carpal tunnel syndrome
- Orthopedic shoulder problems (shoulder strain, rotator cuff injury, tendonitis)
- Cervical spondylitis
- Ulnar nerve compression at elbow and hand
- Multiple sclerosis
- Spinal cord tumor/disease
- Angina pectoris
- Migraine
- Complex regional pain syndromes
- C3–C5 and C8 radiculopathies

DIAGNOSTIC TESTS & INTERPRETATION

Initial Tests (lab, imaging)

CBC, ESR, and C-reactive protein (CRP) determination may rule out underlying inflammatory conditions.

- Radiograph (chest, C-spine, shoulders) [1][C] may reveal elongated C7 transverse process or a cervical rib, Pancoast tumor, or healed clavicle fracture.
- Nerve conduction studies and electromyography (EMG)
- CT scan or MRI, although MRI is the method of choice when searching for nerve compression
- Contrast-enhanced 3D MRA using provocative arm positioning allows excellent imaging of the arteries and veins on both sides and thus provides a noninvasive imaging alternative to digital subtraction angiography in patients with suspected vascular TOS [2][B].
- Doppler and duplex US if vascular obstruction is suspected
- Arteriogram and venogram have limited roles; useful when symptoms suggestive of arterial insufficiency or ischemia, or in planning surgical intervention [3][C].

Diagnostic Procedures/Other

No indicated procedures; anesthetic anterior scalene block may relieve pressure by scalene muscles on the brachial plexus, making this type of block diagnostic and potentially therapeutic, but it poses the risk of procedural damage to the brachial plexus.

Test Interpretation

Systematic results of biopsy have not been reported. There is no indication for biopsy unless to investigate another underlying condition.

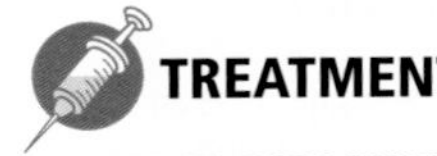

TREATMENT

GENERAL MEASURES

- Conservative management usually involves approaches to reduce and redistribute pressure and traction through the use of physiotherapy or prosthesis.

- Interscalene injections of botulinum toxin have been shown to decrease symptoms of TOS (4)[C]. A single, CT-guided Botox injection into the anterior scalene muscle may offer an effective, minimally invasive treatment for NTOS [5][A].
- Physical therapy will develop strength in pectoral girdle muscles and achieve normal posture (1)[C].
- Severe cases may use taping, adhesive elastic bandages, moist heat, TENS, or US but should not substitute active exercise and correction of posture and muscle imbalance [6][B].

MEDICATION

- No firm evidence exists for any approach to the 4 types of TOS.
- Physical therapy is 1st-line treatment [6][B].
- Anti-inflammatory (ibuprofen)
  - Adult dose: 400–800 mg PO q8h; not to exceed 3,200 mg/day
  - Pediatric dose
    - <12 years: 10 mg/kg/dose every 6–8 hours
    - >12 years: as in adults
  - Contraindications: documented hypersensitivity, active PUD, renal or hepatic impairment, recent use of anticoagulants, hemorrhagic conditions
- Neuropathic pain: Tricyclic antidepressants, carbamazepine, gabapentin, phenytoin, pregabalin; muscle relaxants such as baclofen, metaxalone, or tizanidine may be helpful.
- Severe pain: Consider opiates for brachial plexus nerve block, steroid injections.

ISSUES FOR REFERRAL

- Neurologic, anesthesiologic, orthopedic, vascular surgery referral(s) may be indicated depending on the type of pathologic condition.
- Physical and rehabilitation physicians

SURGERY/OTHER PROCEDURES

- Operative if vascular involvement is present and/or loss of function or lifestyle occurs secondary to severity of symptoms and if conservative therapy fails after 2–3 months (1)[C]
- Transaxillary 1st rib resection (TFRR) may provide better pain relief than supraclavicular neuroplasty of the brachial plexus (SNBP), although, overall, both treatment options have generally positive outcomes (7)[B].
- Resection of 1st rib or cervical ribs via transaxillary (preferred with good to excellent outcome 80% of patients), supraclavicular (good to excellent outcome 80% of patients), posterior approaches (reserved for complicated TOS due to necessity of large muscle incision)
- Transaxillary approach provides a good exposure and cosmesis in patients with TOS. It should be considered as the gold standard in the management of TOS (8)[B].
- Supraclavicular scalenectomy (9)[C]
- Isolated pectoral minor tenotomy (PMT) is a low-risk outpatient procedure that is effective for the treatment of selected patients with disabling NTOS, with early outcomes similar to supraclavicular decompression + PMT (10)[A].
- Excision of adhesive bands, anterior scalenectomy (11)[B]

INPATIENT CONSIDERATIONS

Admission Criteria/Initial Stabilization

Conservative, outpatient, nonpharmacologic treatment is reasonable 1st-line therapy except in cases of thromboembolic phenomena and acute ischemia, symptoms of chronic vascular occlusion, stenosis, arterial dilatation, or progressive neurologic deficit (6)[B].

ONGOING CARE

FOLLOW-UP RECOMMENDATIONS

Correct improper posture, practice proper posture, exercises to strengthen shoulder elevator and neck extensor muscles, stretching exercises for scalene muscles, support bra for women with pendulous breasts, breast reduction surgery in selected cases; sleep with arms below chest level, avoid/reduce prolonged hyperabduction.

Patient Monitoring

Office follow-up visits every 3–4 weeks

PATIENT EDUCATION

Physical therapy, postural exercises, ergonomic workstation

PROGNOSIS

Follow-up from surgery at mean of 7.5 years showed that functional results were excellent, good, fair, and poor in 87 (49.4%), 61 (34.6%), 14 (8%), and 14 (8%) procedures, respectively (12).

Durable long-term functional outcomes can be achieved predicated on a highly selective approach to the surgical management of patients with TOS. A majority of operated patients will not require adjunctive procedures or chronic narcotic use (13).

COMPLICATIONS

- Postoperative shoulder, arm, hand pain, and paresthesias in 10%
- Patients who will have symptomatic recurrences at 1 month–7 years postoperatively (usually within 3 months): 1.5–2%
- Patients who will have brachial plexus injury, probably due to intraoperative traction: 0.5–1%
- Reoperation is indicated for symptomatic recurrence with long posterior remnant of 1st rib (posterior approach) or with disrupted fibrous adhesions (transaxillary approach).
- Venous obstruction or arterial emboli; usually responds to thrombolytics

REFERENCES

1. Huang JH, Zager EL. Thoracic outlet syndrome. *Neurosurgery*. 2004;55(4):897–902; discussion 902–903.
2. Ersoy H, Steigner ML, Coyner KB, et al. Vascular thoracic outlet syndrome: protocol design and diagnostic value of contrast-enhanced 3D MR angiography and equilibrium phase imaging on 1.5- and 3-T MRI scanners. *AJR Am J Roentgenol*. 2012;198(5):1180–1187.
3. Sanders RJ, Hammond SL, Rao NM. Diagnosis of thoracic outlet syndrome. *J Vasc Surg*. 2007;46(3):601–604.
4. Lee GW, Kwon YH, Jeong JH, et al. The efficacy of scalene injection in thoracic outlet syndrome. *J Korean Neurosurg Soc*. 2011;50(1):36–39.
5. Christo PJ, Christo DK, Carinci AJ, et al. Single CT-guided chemodenervation of the anterior scalene muscle with botulinum toxin for neurogenic thoracic outlet syndrome. *Pain Med*. 2010;11(4):504–511.
6. Vanti C, Natalini L, Romeo A, et al. Conservative treatment of thoracic outlet syndrome. A review of the literature. *Eura Medicophys*. 2007;43(1):55–70.
7. Sheth RN, Campbell JN. Surgical treatment of thoracic outlet syndrome: a randomized trial comparing two operations. *J Neurosurg Spine*. 2005;3(5):355–363.
8. Lattoo MR, Dar AM, Wani ML, et al. Outcome of trans-axillary approach for surgical decompression of thoracic outlet: a retrospective study in a tertiary care hospital. *Oman Med J*. 2014;29(3):214–216.
9. Glynn RW, Tawfick W, Elsafty Z, et al. Supraclavicular scalenectomy for thoracic outlet syndrome—functional outcomes assessed using the DASH scoring system. *Vasc Endovascular Surg*. 2012;46(2):157–162.
10. Vemuri C, Wittenberg AM, Caputo FJ, et al. Early effectiveness of isolated pectoralis minor tenotomy in selected patients with neurogenic thoracic outlet syndrome. *J Vasc Surg*. 2013;57(5):1345–1352.
11. Urschel HC, Kourlis H. Thoracic outlet syndrome: a 50-year experience at Baylor University Medical Center. *Proc (Bayl Univ Med Cent)*. 2007;20(2):125–135.
12. Degeorges R, Reynaud C, Becquemin JP. Thoracic outlet syndrome surgery: long-term functional results. *Ann Vasc Surg*. 2004;18(5):558–565.
13. Scali S, Stone D, Bjerke A, et al. Long-term functional results for the surgical management of neurogenic thoracic outlet syndrome. *Vasc Endovascular Surg*. 2010;44(7):550–555.

ADDITIONAL READING

- Aralasmak A, Cevikol C, Karaali K, et al. MRI findings in thoracic outlet syndrome. *Skeletal Radiol*. 2012;41(11):1365–1374.
- Demondion X, Herbinet P, Van Sint Jan S, et al. Imaging assessment of thoracic outlet syndrome. *Radiographics*. 2006;26(6):1735–1750.
- Povlsen B, Belzberg A, Hansson T, et al. Treatment for thoracic outlet syndrome. *Cochrane Database Syst Rev*. 2010;(1):CD007218.

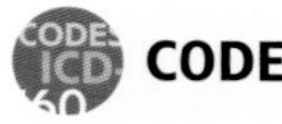

CODES

ICD10

G54.0 Brachial plexus disorders

CLINICAL PEARLS

- Consider breast reduction for patients with pendulous breasts.
- Avoid opiate dependence.
- Consider pain clinic referral if there are nonsurgical causes.

T

THROMBOPHILIA AND HYPERCOAGULABLE STATES

Christopher Hogan, MD

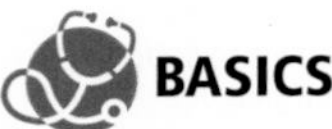

BASICS

DESCRIPTION

- An inherited or acquired disorder of the coagulation system predisposing an individual to thromboembolism (the formation of a venous, or less commonly, an arterial blood clot) (1).
- Venous thrombosis typically manifests as deep venous thrombosis (DVT) of the lower extremity in the legs or pelvis and pulmonary embolism (PE) (1).
- System(s) affected: cardiovascular; nervous; pulmonary; reproductive; hematologic
- Synonym(s): hypercoagulation syndrome, prothrombotic state

EPIDEMIOLOGY

- An inherited thrombophilic defect or risk can be detected in up to 50% of patients with venous thromboembolism (VTE).
- Factor V Leiden is the most common inherited thrombophilia (1/2 of all currently characterizable inherited thrombophilia cases involve the factor V Leiden mutation), and it is present in its heterozygous form in up to ~20% of patients with a 1st VTE.
- Heterozygous prothrombin G20210A mutation, the 2nd most common inherited thrombophilia, is present in up to ~8% of patients with VTE.

Incidence

1st-time thromboembolism

- ~100/100,000/year among the general population
- <1/100,000/year in those age <15 years
- ~1,000/100,000/year in those age ≥85 years

Prevalence

- 40–80% of lower extremity orthopedic procedures can result in DVT if prophylaxis is not used.
- VTE accounts for ~1.2–4.7 deaths per 100,000 pregnancies.

ETIOLOGY AND PATHOPHYSIOLOGY

- Virchow triad as a cause of VTE includes blood stasis, vascular endothelial injury, and abnormalities in circulating blood constituents (i.e., hypercoagulability).
- An imbalance between the hemostatic and fibrinolytic pathways leads to thrombus formation.
- VTE is considered to be the result of genetic tendencies with other acquired risks.
- Upper extremity DVT: >60% are associated with venous catheters. Malignancy is an additional significant risk (2).

Genetics

- The most common genetic thrombophilias (factor V Leiden, prothrombin G20210A, proteins C and S, and antithrombin III deficiency) are inherited in an autosomal dominant pattern.
- Homozygous mutations generally have a higher risk of VTE.
- Factor V Leiden/activated protein C (aPC) resistance is the most common inherited thrombophilia.
  - 2–5% prevalence among Caucasians; rare in African Americans or Asians
  - aPC does not cleave factor Va, so thrombin formation continues.
  - Other acquired risks are synergistic (3).
- Prothrombin gene mutation G20210A: prevalence 6% among Caucasians. Heterozygous carriers have increased risk of thrombosis.
- Hyperhomocysteinemia: 5–6% among the general population. Increases risk of coronary artery disease/myocardial infarction, cerebrovascular accident, and DVT/PE. Acquired in those with folate, vitamin B_{12}, and vitamin B_6 deficiencies
- Antithrombin deficiency: <0.2% among the general population; produced in the liver; acquired deficiency in disseminated intravascular coagulation (DIC), sepsis, liver disease, nephrotic syndrome
- Protein C and S deficiencies: 0.5% and 1% incidences, respectively, among the general population. Homozygotes and heterozygotes are hypercoagulable. Vitamin K–dependent, produced in the liver. Protein C inactivates Va and VIIIa. Protein C may become an acquired deficiency in liver disease, sepsis, DIC, acute respiratory distress syndrome, and after surgery. Protein S is a cofactor for protein C, and it may become an acquired deficiency with oral contraceptive pill (OCP) use, pregnancy, liver disease, sepsis, DIC, HIV, and nephrosis.

RISK FACTORS

- Acquired risk factors:
  - Immobilization or prolonged travel
  - Trauma
  - Surgery, especially orthopedic
  - Malignancies (especially pancreatic, ovarian, brain, and lymphoma)
  - Pregnancy
  - Acute medical illness
  - Exogenous female hormones/oral contraceptives
  - Obesity
  - Nephrotic syndrome
  - Antiphospholipid syndrome (APS) and lupus anticoagulant
  - Myeloproliferative disorders (polycythemia vera, essential thrombocythemia)
  - Hyperviscosity syndromes (sickle cell, paraproteinemias)
  - Hyperhomocysteinemia secondary to vitamin deficiencies (B_6, B_{12}, folic acid)
  - Tamoxifen, thalidomide, lenalidomide, bevacizumab, L-asparaginase, erythropoietic stimulating agents
  - Previous thromboembolism
- Established genetic factors:
  - Factor V Leiden
  - Prothrombin G20210A mutation
  - Protein C deficiency
  - Protein S deficiency
  - Antithrombin III deficiency
- Rare genetic factors:
  - Dysfibrinogenemia
  - Hyperhomocysteinemia (methylene tetrahydrofolate reductase mutation)
- Indeterminate factors:
  - Elevated factor VIII
- Age: >60 years
- Gender: men
- Race: Incidence is higher among African Americans.

GENERAL PREVENTION

- Consider prophylaxis with medications in any hospitalized patient with VTE risk factors; hospitalized patients should be encouraged to ambulate as soon as possible (4)[A].
- Consider mechanical prophylaxis in patients at low risk for VTE or those in whom anticoagulation may be contraindicated.
- Consider prophylaxis with low-molecular-weight heparin (LMWH) + aspirin in pregnant patients with APS or other thrombophilia.
- Prophylaxis with unfractionated heparin or LMWH should be considered in patients with genetic or acquired risks of thrombosis and an anticipated additional risk, such as the immobilization associated with surgery.
- Use caution with procoagulant medicines (e.g., OCPs) in asymptomatic individuals who have a known hereditary predisposition.

COMMONLY ASSOCIATED CONDITIONS

Advanced age, cancer, pregnancy, obesity, prior history of thrombosis, surgery, immobilization

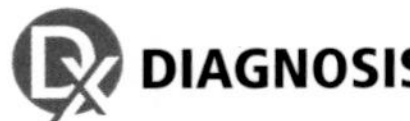

DIAGNOSIS

HISTORY

Consider prothrombotic assessment for the following:

- Unprovoked thrombosis at age <45–50 years
- Thrombosis at an unusual anatomic site or recurrent thromboses
- Family history suggesting multiple individuals affected with VTE
- Recurrent pregnancy loss or thrombosis with OCP use

PHYSICAL EXAM

- DVT: swelling, pain, warmth, and redness, usually of one extremity
- PE: dyspnea, pleurisy, hemoptysis, hypoxia, tachycardia
- Superficial phlebitis: red, painful cord palpable along the path of thrombosed vein
- Postthrombotic syndrome: pain, swelling, pigmentation, and/or ulceration

DIAGNOSTIC TESTS & INTERPRETATION

Testing for heritable thrombophilia in all patients with a 1st episode of VTE is not required (2,5)[B].

Initial Tests (lab, imaging)

- CBC
- aPC profile: ≤2.0 implies factor V Leiden mutation; 95–100% are factor V Leiden positive; false-positive finding in pregnancy or with use of OCPs, confirm with factor V Leiden mutation testing or consider factor V Leiden mutation testing up front.
  - aPC resistance may be unreliable while taking LMWH or unfractionated heparin (UFH).
- Prothrombin G20210A genetic assay
- ATIII functional assay
  - Will be low with acute thrombosis and on heparin therapy
- Protein C functional assay
  - May be low with acute thrombosis; will be lower on warfarin
- Protein S antigen and functional assay and free S
  - May be low with acute thrombosis; will be lower on warfarin
- Antiphospholipid antibodies: phospholipid-dependent tests and anticardiolipin antibodies, lupus anticoagulant
  - May be unreliable on heparin
- Consider evaluation for subclinical malignancy in an unprovoked thrombosis in those >50 years of age or at greater risk.
- Consider homocysteine level, although treatment of hyperhomocysteinemia (vitamins B_{12} and B_6, folate) does not alter the thrombophilic risk.

Follow-Up Tests & Special Considerations
Dysfibrinogenemia and plasminogen deficiency are very rare causes of thrombophilia.

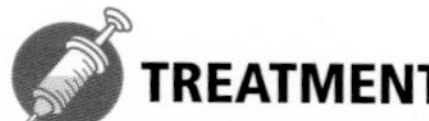

TREATMENT

MEDICATION

First Line

- Parenteral anticoagulation: LMWH has largely replaced UFH as 1st-line therapy for VTE.
  - Enoxaparin (Lovenox): 1 mg/kg SC BID for at least 5 days (with concomitant warfarin) until international normalized ratio (INR) has reached 2 for at least 24 hours
    - Enoxaparin is preferred in patients with active cancer for a minimum of 3 months (can dose at 1.5 mg/kg SC daily), after which time the patient can be reevaluated to continue enoxaparin or transition to warfarin.
    - Adverse reactions: bleeding, heparin-induced thrombocytopenia (HIT) <0.5% incidence, bone loss (uncommon)
    - Reversal: Stop LMWH.
  - UFH: 80 U/kg or 5,000-unit IV bolus, then 18 U/kg/hr or 1,300 U/hr to target the activated partial thromboplastin time (aPTT) to a corresponding anti-Xa level of 0.3–0.7 U/mL. The 1st aPTT should be checked 6 hours after initial therapy and adjusted per standard heparin nomograms, aiming for an adequate level within 24 hours. Transition to warfarin is similar to the recommendations for enoxaparin.
    - SC UFH is an alternative and can be given as 5,000 U IV (once) followed by 250 U/kg SC BID, or 250 U/kg bolus followed by 250 U/kg BID (monitored as for IV UFH), or 333 U/kg once followed by 250 U/kg SC BID (unmonitored).
    - Adverse reactions: bleeding, HIT 3% incidence, bone loss (long-term use)
    - Reversal: Stop heparin, protamine.
- Oral anticoagulation:
  - Warfarin (Coumadin): 5 mg/day initially and adjust to INR 2–3 for at least 3 months, potentially indefinitely in those with high risk of recurrence, recurrent or unprovoked VTE
    - Warfarin requires careful and frequent monitoring because of many drug–drug and drug–diet (e.g., vitamin K) interactions.
    - Adverse reactions: bleeding, skin necrosis (rare and early in course)
    - Reversal: four-factor prothrombin complex concentrate (PCC); fresh frozen plasma and/or vitamin K
- Pregnancy (controversial): low-dose aspirin and/or LMWH or UFH; warfarin is contraindicated.
- Several other newly approved anticoagulant medications are indicated for acute management. Their main benefit is the decreased need for frequent testing. However, most of the new medications do not have a reversal agent.

Second Line

Usually indicated when contraindication to heparin or LMWH, such as heparin-associated thrombosis and thrombocytopenia, if there is an inability to use IV drugs, or renal failure

- Factor Xa inhibitors:
  - Fondaparinux: efficacious for prevention and treatment of acute VTE, postoperative prophylaxis, PE (FDA-approved indications)
    - Dose: acute VTE/PE. Weight <50 kg: 5 mg/day SC; weight 50–100 kg: 7.5 mg/day SC; weight >100 kg: 10 mg/day SC; use for 5–9 days until oral anticoagulation is therapeutic.
    - Prophylaxis: 2.5 mg/day SC
    - Dose adjustments: needed for renal insufficiency; if creatinine clearance is <30 mL/min, use is contraindicated.
- Rivaroxaban: oral factor Xa inhibitor, FDA-approved for postoperative thromboprophylaxis after hip/knee replacement, treatment of DVT/PE, and for thromboembolic prophylaxis in patients with nonvalvular atrial fibrillation (6)[C]
- Direct thrombin inhibitors: most commonly used for anticoagulation in HIT. Representative drugs include the following:
  - Lepirudin: excreted by kidneys, crosses the placenta; dosing based on creatinine clearance; therapeutic dose based on aPTT
  - Argatroban: liver metabolized; may be dose-adjusted in liver dysfunction; therapeutic dose based on aPTT
  - Dabigatran: oral direct thrombin inhibitor, FDA-approved for treatment of DVT/PE after parenteral anticoagulant and for thromboembolic prophylaxis in patients with nonvalvular atrial fibrillation (noninferior to warfarin). Currently no known antidote to anticoagulant effect. May be dialyzable (6)[C]

SURGERY/OTHER PROCEDURES

- Catheter extraction/thrombectomy for extreme emergencies (e.g., massive PE where thrombolysis not feasible)
- Inferior vena cava filter
  - Reduces short-term risk of PE in those with contraindications to anticoagulation (e.g., GI bleeding, cerebral hemorrhage)
  - May increase long-term risk of recurrent DVT
  - Use for patients with multiple episodes of recurrent thromboembolism despite therapeutic anticoagulation and contraindication to anticoagulation.

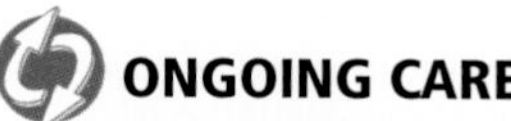

ONGOING CARE

FOLLOW-UP RECOMMENDATIONS

Avoid significant risk for trauma (e.g., contact sports, climbing a ladder).

Patient Monitoring

Monitor warfarin as frequently as needed to maintain an INR goal of 2–3.

DIET

Vitamin K–stable diet if patient is taking warfarin

PATIENT EDUCATION

- Assume that any drug may enhance or attenuate the warfarin effect.
- Increase the frequency of monitoring following any medication change to ensure therapeutic anticoagulation and to avoid overanticoagulation, especially with antibiotics.
- Many drugs may modulate warfarin effect: alcohol, antibiotics, aspirin, NSAIDs, acetaminophen.

PROGNOSIS

- Patients with a provoked VTE (i.e., surgery, hospitalization) not receiving chronic anticoagulation have a risks of recurrence of 7% (year 1), 16% (year 5), and 23% (year 10).
- Patients with an unprovoked VTE not receiving chronic anticoagulation have risks of recurrence of 15% (year 1), 41% (year 5), and 53% (year 10).
- Currently, there are no data from randomized, controlled trials or controlled clinical trials about the benefits of thrombophilia testing to decrease the risk of recurrent VTE (1).

COMPLICATIONS

Venous or arterial thrombosis; bleeding in anticoagulated patients

REFERENCES

1. Cohn DM, Vansenne F, de Borgie CA, et al. Thrombophilia testing for prevention of recurrent venous thromboembolism. *Cochrane Database Syst Rev*. 2012;12:CD007069.
2. Baglin T, Gray E, Greaves M, et al. Clinical guidelines for testing for heritable thrombophilia. *Br J Haematol*. 2010;149(2):209–220.
3. Anderson JA, Weitz JI. Hypercoagulable states. *Clin Chest Med*. 2010;31(4):659–673.
4. Hill J, Treasure T; National Clinical Guideline Centre for Acute and Chronic Conditions. Reducing the risk of venous thromboembolism in patients admitted to hospital: summary of NICE guidance. *BMJ*. 2010;340:c95.
5. National Clinical Guideline Centre. The management of venous thromboembolic diseases and the role of thrombophilia testing. *NICE Clinical Guidelines*. 2012:144.
6. Schulman S, Crowther MA. How I treat with anticoagulants in 2012: new and old anticoagulants, and when and how to switch. *Blood*. 2012;119(13):3016–3023.

ADDITIONAL READING

Hirsh J, Bauer KA, Donati MB, et al. Parenteral anticoagulants: American College of Chest Physicians Evidence-Based Clinical Practice Guidelines (8th edition). *Chest*. 2008;133(6)(Suppl):141S–159S.

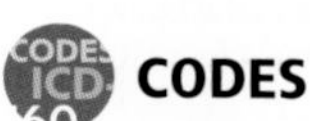

CODES

ICD10

- D68.59 Other primary thrombophilia
- D68.51 Activated protein C resistance
- D68.2 Hereditary deficiency of other clotting factors

CLINICAL PEARLS

- Factor V Leiden (resistance to aPC) is the most common inherited thrombophilia, with a prevalence of 2–7% in the U.S. Caucasian population.
- Test patients <50 years of age with a history of venous thrombosis, and consider testing 1st-degree relatives.
- Rule out malignancy, especially in those >50 years of age.

T

THROMBOTIC THROMBOCYTOPENIC PURPURA

Kellie A. Sprague, MD

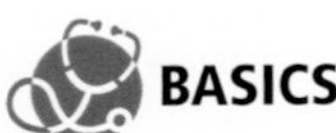

BASICS

DESCRIPTION

- An acute syndrome of microangiopathic hemolytic anemia (MAHA) and consumptive thrombocytopenia with deposition of hyaline thrombi in terminal arterioles and capillaries leading to ischemic multiorgan damage
- Thrombotic thrombocytopenic purpura (TTP) is characterized by MAHA and thrombocytopenia, with or without the following signs and symptoms (1):
  - Neurologic symptoms
  - Renal dysfunction
  - Fever
  - Most patients do not show the historic pentad of MAHA, thrombocytopenia, renal dysfunction, neurologic abnormalities, and fever because treatment is initiated before the pentad can develop.

EPIDEMIOLOGY

Incidence

- Predominant age: 30–60 years
- Predominant sex: female > male
- Incidence ratio in blacks to whites is 3:1.
- The age–sex–race standardized incidence of clinically suspected TTP is 6/million/year in the United States (2).

ETIOLOGY AND PATHOPHYSIOLOGY

- In TTP, the aggregating agent responsible for platelet thrombi is unusually large von Willebrand factor (UL vWF) multimers, which are far larger than those found in normal plasma.
- A metalloproteinase, ADAMTS13, which normally enzymatically cleaves UL vWF multimers to prevent clumping within vessels, is deficient, defective, or absent, allowing UL vWF to react with platelets. This leads to the endothelial cell damage and disseminated thrombi characteristic of TTP.
- Arterioles most often affected are in the brain, kidney, pancreas, heart, and adrenal glands. Lungs and liver are relatively spared.
- In familial TTP, patients have an inherited deficiency of ADAMTS13 (1).
- In acquired idiopathic TTP, autoantibodies are directed against the metalloproteinase ADAMTS13 (1,3).
- Endothelial injury, either directly from a drug/toxin or indirectly via platelet/neutrophil activation has been proposed as a cause of secondary TTP especially in those without ADAMTS13 deficiency.
  - Drug-induced (see "Risk Factors")
  - Hematopoietic cell transplantation

Genetics

TTP is most often an acquired disorder. A congenital form of inherited TTP (Schulman-Upshaw syndrome) is due to a mutation at the ADAMTS13 metalloproteinase gene locus on chromosome 9q34. This rare form of TTP has an autosomal-recessive pattern of inheritance (4).

RISK FACTORS

- Pregnancy and oral contraceptives
- AIDS and early symptomatic HIV infection
- Autoimmune disease
  - Antiphospholipid antibody syndrome
  - Systemic lupus erythematosus
  - Scleroderma
- Cancer
- Hematopoietic stem cell transplantation
- Drug toxicity
  - Cancer chemotherapy
    - Mitomycin C and gemcitabine
    - Bleomycin and cisplatin
  - Calcineurin inhibitors
    - Tacrolimus and cyclosporine
  - Immune-mediated
    - Quinine and quinidine
    - Ticlopidine and clopidogrel

COMMONLY ASSOCIATED CONDITIONS

- TTP/HUS/atypical HUS (hemolytic uremic syndrome) have similar presentations with MAHA and thrombocytopenia and multiorgan involvement.
- TTP generally presents with minimal renal involvement and may have neurologic abnormalities, whereas the opposite tends to be more characteristic of HUS/atypical HUS.
- However, patients with HUS and TTP may have both prominent renal and neurologic manifestations, often making the distinction unclear, thus leading to the hybrid name "TTP-HUS."
- ADAMTS13 levels are diminished in adults with familial or acquired idiopathic TTP but are normal in children diagnosed with HUS following infection with *Escherichia coli* (particularly type O157:H7), so-called typical HUS. Atypical HUS is due to complement dysregulation.

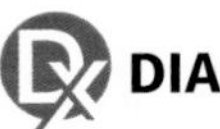

DIAGNOSIS

- Most common symptoms are nonspecific: nausea, vomiting, weakness, abdominal pain, fatigue, fever
- Related to thrombocytopenia
  - Easy bruising, purpura, or petechiae
  - Epistaxis, menorrhagia, bleeding gums
  - GI bleeding
  - Intracranial hemorrhage
  - Visual symptoms due to retinal hemorrhage
- Related to hemolytic anemia (MAHA): jaundice, fatigue
- Related to end-organ ischemia
  - Neurologic: CNS symptoms occur in 50%.
    - Often fluctuating symptoms
    - Headache
    - Altered mental status: Spectrum runs from behavioral/personality changes to obtundation/stupor/coma.
    - Seizures
    - Stroke
  - Renal: hematuria, oliguria, or anuria
  - Cardiac: arrhythmia, myocardial infarction, heart failure

HISTORY

- Generally acute onset of symptoms but subacute in about 1/4 of patients
- It is important to assess for potential underlying causes or risk factors (see discussion earlier).

PHYSICAL EXAM

- Fever
- Mental status/neurologic: confusion, coma, stupor, weakness
- HEENT: retinal hemorrhage, scleral icterus, epistaxis
- Abdomen/GI: nonspecific tenderness
- Skin: jaundice, petechiae, purpura, ecchymoses

DIFFERENTIAL DIAGNOSIS

- HUS and atypical HUS: See "Commonly Associated Conditions."
- Antiphospholipid antibody syndrome: prolonged partial thromboplastin time (PTT) and presence of lupus anticoagulant
- Systemic lupus erythematosus
- Malignant hypertension (HTN): diastolic >130 mm Hg, papilledema, retinal hemorrhages
- Pregnancy-associated preeclampsia/eclampsia or HELLP levels: low ATIII levels
- Disseminated intravascular coagulation
  - Prolonged prothrombin time (PT)/PTT, low fibrinogen
  - Low factors V and VIII
  - Secondary to sepsis/shock or widely disseminated malignancy
- Idiopathic TTP
  - No hemolysis, normal lactate dehydrogenase (LDH) and bilirubin
  - Presence of antiplatelet antibodies
- Malignancy-associated microangiopathy
- Evan syndrome (autoimmune hemolytic anemia and thrombocytopenia): positive direct Coombs test
- Sclerodermal kidney

DIAGNOSTIC TESTS & INTERPRETATION

Initial Tests (lab, imaging)

- CBC
  - Hemoglobin (decreased): average is 8–10 g/dL
  - Platelets decreased: typically in the 10–30,000 range
- Reticulocyte count (increased)
- Haptoglobin decreased (hemolysis)
- Peripheral smear
  - Schistocytes (prominent, >1% of RBCs)
  - Helmet cells, RBC fragments
  - Nucleated RBCs
  - Polychromasia (reticulocytosis)
- Coagulation studies
  - Normal in most; mild elevation in 15%
  - Fibrinogen normal
- Coombs test: negative direct Coombs test
- Electrolytes, BUN/creatinine: mild elevation of BUN and creatinine (creatinine <3 mg/dL)
- Liver function studies: increased indirect bilirubin (hemolysis)
- LDH: 5–10× normal
- Urinalysis
  - Proteinuria, microscopic hematuria
  - Positive dipstick for large blood, but minimal RBCs on microscopic exam
- ECG: sinus tachycardia, heart block
- Troponin: increased if cardiac involvement
- HIV, hepatitis A, B, C testing: Exclude underlying viral precipitant.
- Pregnancy test
- Pretreatment ADAMTS13 activity level of <10% is useful in distinguishing acquired or familial TTP from other disorders.
- Head CT/MRI scan: performed if mental status changes are present to rule out possible intracranial hemorrhage or ischemic changes

Test Interpretation

Biopsy of affected organs shows platelet thrombi within or beneath damaged endothelium. However, biopsy is rarely obtained because the diagnosis is made on clinical grounds and laboratory findings.

TREATMENT

- Prompt treatment of TTP is necessary due to the high mortality (90%).
- In the absence of another apparent cause, the dyad of MAHA and thrombocytopenia is sufficient to begin treatment for TTP while the workup proceeds (1,3):
  - Plasma exchange transfusion (PEX) is the cornerstone of treatment of classic TTP (3)[A].
  - PEX replaces deficient or defective metalloproteinase (ADAMTS13) and removes UL vWF and antimetalloproteinase antibodies.
  - PEX should be begun immediately and continued daily.
  - Optimal PEX duration is unknown. Convention is to continue for 2 days after platelet count is ≥150,000 (5)[C].
  - Fresh frozen plasma: temporary measure until PEX can be initiated (3)[B]

MEDICATION

First Line

- Glucocorticoids may be of benefit in some patients. British guidelines recommend its use for all patients (5)[B]:
  - Steroids may work by suppressing the autoantibodies inhibiting ADAMTS13 activity.
  - Use may be in patients with severe ADAMTS13 deficiency, in the setting of exacerbation when PEX is stopped or in relapse after remission.
  - Little benefit of steroids when used as monotherapy
  - Doses: prednisone 1 mg/kg/day and taper once in remission or methylprednisolone 1 g/day IV × 3 days
- Rituximab, an anti-CD20 antibody that deletes B cells, may reduce relapse when given in conjunction with PEX and steroids (6).
  - Dose: 375 mg/m^2 IV weekly × 4 weeks

Second Line

The following medications are used in refractory cases:

- Rituximab (5)[B]
- Vincristine, cyclophosphamide cyclosporine
- Intravenous immunoglobulin (IVIG) (3)

ISSUES FOR REFERRAL

- Hematology or blood bank for plasma exchange transfusion
- Nephrology for dialysis
- Cardiology for presence of significant heart block or ischemia
- Neurosurgery for intracranial hemorrhage

SURGERY/OTHER PROCEDURES

Splenectomy is reserved for severe, refractory cases (7).

INPATIENT CONSIDERATIONS

Admission Criteria/Initial Stabilization

- ABCs, oxygen, IV access, telemetry
- Volume resuscitation if hypotensive/actively bleeding
- Packed RBCs can be transfused safely.
- Platelet transfusion may be used for the treatment of hemorrhage.

Discharge Criteria

On normalization and stabilization of neurologic symptoms, LDH, platelets, and renal function

ONGOING CARE

FOLLOW-UP RECOMMENDATIONS

- No maintenance therapy is required. After PEX is discontinued, blood counts should be monitored over a few months. If testing results remain normal, testing interval can be lengthened.
- Promptly evaluate any symptoms of relapse.

PATIENT EDUCATION

- On discharge, advise patients to self-monitor for signs of relapse (e.g., fever, headache, bruising).
- Patients should be advised about prolonged periods of fatigue following the acute phase.
- See National Heart, Lung and Blood Institute Web site: http:www.nhlbi.nih.gov/health/dci/Diseases/ttp/TTP_WhatIs.html.

PROGNOSIS

- Most patients recover fully from idiopathic TTP when treated promptly:
  - 30-day mortality is 10% in those who receive PEX.
  - 70% respond within 14 days; 90% respond within 28 days.
  - 80% survival in patients with idiopathic TTP treated with PEX (8)
- Initial LDH and platelet counts are not predictive of the patient's response to treatment.
- Final platelet count and LDH or the length or intensity of treatment does not predict relapse.
- Low levels of ADAMTS13 activity during remission are associated with higher risk of relapse (9).
- In patients with severe ADAMTS13 deficiency, the risk of relapse is estimated to be 41% at 7.5 years, with the greatest risk being in the 1st year.

COMPLICATIONS

- Patients may experience mild cognitive impairments in attention, concentration, and memory following ≥1 episodes of TTP.
- Complications of PEX include the following:
  - Central line infections and hemorrhage
  - Citrate toxicity
  - Hypersensitivity reactions to frequent plasma

REFERENCES

1. Sadler JE. Von Willebrand factor, ADAMTS13, and thrombotic thrombocytopenic purpura. *Blood*. 2008;112(1):11–18.
2. Terrell DR, Williams LA, Vesley SK, et al. The incidence for thrombotic thrombocytopenic purpura-hemolytic uremic syndrome: all patients, idiopathic patients, and patients with severe ADAMTS13 deficiency. *J Thromb Heamost*. 2005;3(7):1432–1436.
3. George JN. Clinical practice. Thrombotic thrombocytopenic purpura. *N Engl J Med*. 2006;354(18):1927–1935.
4. Levy GG, Nicholas WC, Lian EC, et al. Mutations in a member of the ADAMTS gene family cause thrombotic thrombocytopenia purpura. *Nature*. 2001;413(6855):488–494.
5. Scully M, Hunt B, Benjamin S, et al. Guidelines on the diagnosis and management of thrombotic thrombocytopenic purpura and other thrombotic microangiopathies. *Br J Haematol*. 2012;158(3):323–355.
6. Scully M, McDonald V, Cavenagh J, et al. A phase 2 study of the safety and efficacy of rituximab with plasma exchange in acute acquired thrombotic thrombocytopenic purpura. *Blood*. 2011;118(7):1746–1753.
7. Beloncle F, Buffet M, Coindre JP, et al; Thrombotic Microangiopathies Reference Center. Splenectomy and/or cyclophosphamide as salvage therapies in thrombotic thrombocytopenic purpura: the French TMA Reference Center experience. *Transfusion*. 2012:52(11):2436–2444.
8. Kremer Hovigna JA, Vesley SK, Terell DR, et al. Survival and relapse in patients with thrombotic thrombocytopenic purpura. *Blood*. 2010;115(8):1500–1511.
9. Peyvandi F, Lavoretano S, Palla R, et al. ADAMTS13 and anti-ADAMTS13 antibodies are markers for recurrence or acquired thrombotic thrombocytopenia purpura during remission. *Haematologica*. 2008;93(2):232–239.

ADDITIONAL READING

Tsai HM. Thrombotic thrombocytopenic purpura and the atypical hemolytic uremic syndrome: an update. *Haematol Oncol Clin N Am*. 2013;27(3):565–584.

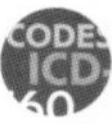

CODES

ICD10

- M31.1 Thrombotic microangiopathy
- D69.42 Congenital and hereditary thrombocytopenia purpura
- D69.3 Immune thrombocytopenic purpura

CLINICAL PEARLS

- The diagnosis of TTP is made clinically; common symptoms are nonspecific: nausea, vomiting, weakness, abdominal pain, fatigue, fever, and easy bruising, purpura, or petechiae.
- The historical pentad of fever, neurologic symptoms, renal dysfunction, MAHA, and thrombocytopenia is not present in most patients.
- The dyad of MAHA and thrombocytopenia is sufficient to initiate treatment with PEX.
- Do not wait for results of ADAMTS13 determination to initiate therapy.

THYROID MALIGNANT NEOPLASIA

James P. Miller, MD

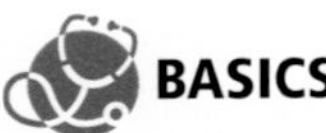

BASICS

DESCRIPTION

Thyroid malignant neoplasia is an autologous growth of thyroid nodules with potential for metastases.

- Papillary carcinoma
  - Most common variety, 60–70% of thyroid tumors
  - Peak incidence in the 3rd–4th decades
  - 3× more common in women
  - May be associated with radiation exposure
  - Tumor contains psammoma bodies, 50%.
  - Metastasizes by lymphatic route (30% at time of diagnosis)
  - Multicentric in ≥20%, especially in children
  - Higher risk in patients with Hashimoto thyroiditis
- Follicular carcinoma
  - 10–20% of thyroid tumors
  - Peak incidence in 5th decade of life
  - Incidence has been decreasing since the addition of dietary iodine.
  - Metastasizes by the hematogenous route
- Hürthle cell carcinoma (variant of follicular with poorer prognosis)
  - 2–3% of thyroid malignancies
  - Usually in patients >60 years
  - No gender difference
  - Radioresistant
  - Composed of distinct large eosinophilic cells with abundant cytoplasmic mitochondria
  - Variant of follicular carcinoma with worse prognosis
- Medullary thyroid carcinoma (MCT)
  - Arises from parafollicular cells, C cells
  - Multiple endocrine neoplasia (MEN) syndromes (MEN2A, MEN2B, FMTC). Prevalence of MEN2 is 1:30,000.
  - MCT associated with MEN2B occur in childhood, those with MEN2A occur in young adults, and those with FMTC occur at middle age.
  - 3–4% of all thyroid tumors
  - 25–35% are associated with MEN syndromes (2A more common than 2B), which can be familial or sporadic.
  - Calcitonin is a chemical marker.
  - *RET* proto-oncogene mutation is screen; family members who carry the *RET* gene should consider early prophylactic thyroidectomy.
- Anaplastic carcinoma
  - 3% of thyroid tumors
  - Most aggressive form of thyroid neoplasia
  - More common in females
  - Usually in patients >60 years
- Other: lymphoma, sarcoma, or metastatic (renal, breast, or lung)
- System(s) affected: endocrine/metabolic
- Synonym(s): follicular carcinoma of the thyroid; papillary carcinoma of the thyroid; Hürthle cell carcinoma of the thyroid; anaplastic cell carcinoma of the thyroid

Geriatric Considerations

Risk of malignancy increases at >60 years.

Pediatric Considerations

- >60% of thyroid nodules are malignant.
- <2% of thyroid malignancies occur in children and adolescents.

EPIDEMIOLOGY

Incidence

- 12.9/100,000 per year in the United States
- Deaths: 0.5/100,000 per year in the United States
- In 2014, estimated 62,980 new cases and 1,890 deaths from thyroid cancer in the United States
- Predominant age: usually >40 years
- Predominant sex: female > male (2.6:1) prevalence
- Lifetime risk of developing thyroid cancer is 1.1%.
- In 2011, 566,708 patients living with thyroid cancer in the United States

ETIOLOGY AND PATHOPHYSIOLOGY

Unknown

Genetics

- Familial polyposis of the colon, Turcot syndrome, and Gardner syndrome with the *APC* gene (5q21)
- Medullary: autosomal dominant with MEN syndrome
- *BRAF* mutation
- *RET* oncogene

RISK FACTORS

- Family history
- Neck irradiation (6–2,000 rads): papillary carcinoma
- Iodine deficiency: follicular carcinoma
- MEN2: medullary carcinoma; autosomal dominant
- Previous history of subtotal thyroidectomy for malignancy: anaplastic carcinoma
- Asian race
- Female gender

GENERAL PREVENTION

- Physical exam in high-risk group
- Calcium infusion or pentagastrin stimulation test screening in high-risk MEN patients
- Screen for *RET* proto-oncogene in groups at-risk for MCT.

COMMONLY ASSOCIATED CONDITIONS

Medullary carcinoma: pheochromocytoma, hyperparathyroidism, ganglioneuroma of the GI tract, neuromata of mucosal membranes

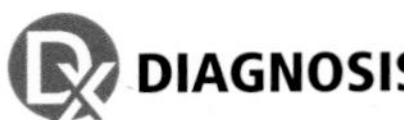

DIAGNOSIS

HISTORY

- Change in voice (hoarseness)
- Positive family history
- Neck mass
- Dysphagia
- Dyspnea
- Cough
- Difficulty swallowing

PHYSICAL EXAM

- Neck mass: If fixed to surrounding tissue, this finding suggests advanced disease.
- Cervical adenopathy

DIFFERENTIAL DIAGNOSIS

- Multinodular goiter
- Thyroid adenoma
- Thyroglossal duct cyst
- Thyroiditis
- Thyroid cyst
- Ectopic thyroid
- Dermoid cyst

DIAGNOSTIC TESTS & INTERPRETATION

- Medullary carcinoma: calcitonin level (normal <30 pg/mL [300 ng/L]), pentagastrin stimulation test and *RET* proto-oncogene
- Thyroglobulin (TG) level: postoperative tumor marker
- DNA content of tumors from biopsy specimen: Diploid content has a better prognosis.
- Thyroid function tests usually normal
- Thyroid scan: 12–15% of cold nodules are malignant; rate is higher in patients <40 years of age and those with microcalcifications on US.
- US: Solid mass and microcalcifications are more suspicious of malignancy.
- CT scan and MRI can be useful to evaluate large substernal masses and recurrent soft tissue masses.
- ^{18}F-FDG positron-emission tomographic scan can help if the cytology is inconclusive; helpful with recurrent disease when patient has a negative ^{131}I scan and an elevated TG level

Diagnostic Procedures/Other

- Fine-needle aspiration (FNA)
- Surgical biopsy/excision
- Laryngoscopy if vocal cord paralysis is suspected

Test Interpretation

- Papillary: psammoma bodies, anaplastic epithelial papillae
- Follicular: anaplastic epithelial cords with follicles
- Hürthle cell: large eosinophilic cells with granular cytoplasm
- Medullary: large amounts of amyloid stroma
- Anaplastic: small cell and giant cell undifferentiated tumors

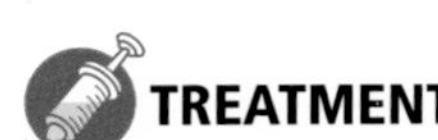

TREATMENT

MEDICATION

Postoperatively, will require thyroid hormone replacement: goal is to keep TSH <0.1 mU/L

- Levothyroxine (T_4, Synthroid) 100–200 μg/day, *or*
- Liothyronine (T_3, Cytomel) 50–100 μg/day

GENERAL MEASURES

- Papillary/follicular: ^{131}I thyroid remnant ablation
- Medullary: Vandetanib has been tried in patients with advanced disease (1)[B].
- Anaplastic: Doxorubicin and cisplatin have achieved partial remission in some patients (2)[B].
- Recurrent tumor: Sorafenib has been used in patients with recurrent disease.

ADDITIONAL THERAPIES

- External beam radiation for advanced disease
- I^{131} is used in high-risk patients with papillary and follicular tumors. The role is to ablate remnant thyroid tissue to improve specificity of future TG assays (3)[C].

SURGERY/OTHER PROCEDURES

- Papillary carcinoma: lobectomy with isthmectomy (if lesion <1 cm) or total thyroidectomy and removal of suspicious lymph nodes. Total thyroidectomy for tumors >1 cm (4)[B]
- Follicular carcinoma and Hürthle cell: total thyroidectomy and removal of suspicious lymph nodes
- Medullary carcinoma: total thyroidectomy with central node dissection; unilateral or bilateral modified radical neck dissection if lateral nodes are histologically positive
- Anaplastic carcinoma: aggressive en bloc thyroidectomy; tracheostomy often required; not responsive to ^{131}I

ONGOING CARE

FOLLOW-UP RECOMMENDATIONS

Patient Monitoring

- 10–30% of initially disease-free patients will develop recurrence and/or metastases. 80% recur in neck and 20% with distant metastases. Lung is most common site of distant metastases.
- Thyroid scan at 6 weeks and administration of ^{131}I for any visible uptake; any evidence of residual thyroid tissue (after total thyroidectomy) or lymph node disease noted on scan is treated with radioactive iodine.
- At 6 months and then yearly, the patient should have a thyroid scan and chest x-ray.
- Papillary and follicular: A TG level should be done yearly. Recombinant human thyroid-stimulating hormone (rhTSH)–stimulated TG level may be more sensitive.
- Medullary: Calcitonin level should be done yearly with pentagastrin stimulation.
- The thyroid scan and TG level should be done with the patient in the hypothyroid state induced by 6-week withdrawal of levothyroxine or 2–3-week withdrawal of liothyronine.
- Decreased incidence of recurrence when TSH is suppressed

DIET

Avoid iodine deficiency.

PATIENT EDUCATION

National Cancer Institute: (301) 496-5583; http://www.cancer.gov

PROGNOSIS

- Taken together: 5-year survival of thyroid cancer is 97.8%.
- Favorable factors: female, multifocality, regional LN involvement
- Adverse factors: age >45 years, follicular histology, primary tumor >4 cm, extrathyroid extension, distant metastases
- Papillary carcinoma: 10-year overall survival is 93%; 30-year cancer-related death rate of 6%
- Follicular carcinoma: 10-year overall survival is 85%; histologically, microinvasive tumors parallel papillary tumor results, whereas grossly invasive tumors do far worse. 30-year cancer-related death rate of 15%
- Hürthle cell carcinoma: 93% 5-year survival rate and 83% survival rate overall; grossly invasive tumor survival <25%
- Medullary carcinoma: negative nodes, 90% 5-year survival rate and 85% 10-year survival rate; with positive nodes, 65% 5-year survival rate and 40% 10-year survival rate. Prognosis worse for MEN2B compared to MEN2A. Overall 10-year survival is 75%.
- Anaplastic carcinoma: survival unexpected. Long-term survivors should have original pathology reexamined.

COMPLICATIONS

- Recurrence of tumor is 10–30%. 80% recur in neck, and 20% recur distally.
- Hoarseness from tumor invasion or operative injury to recurrent laryngeal nerve
- Hypoparathyroidism from operative injury to parathyroid glands

REFERENCES

1. Wells SA Jr, Robinson BG, Gagel RF, et al. Vandetanib in patients with locally advanced or metastatic medullary thyroid cancer: a randomized, double-blind phase III trial. *J Clin Oncol*. 2012;30(2):134–141.
2. Shimaoka K, Schoenfeld DA, DeWys WD, et al. A randomized trial of doxorubicin versus doxorubicin plus cisplatin in patients with advanced thyroid carcinoma. *Cancer*. 1985;56(9):2155–2160.
3. Mazzaferri EL, Jhiang SM. Long-term impact of initial surgical and medical therapy on papillary and follicular thyroid cancer. *Am J Med*. 1994;97(5):418–428.
4. Bilimoria KY, Bentrem DJ, Ko CY, et al. Extent of surgery affects survival for papillary thyroid cancer. *Ann Surg*. 2007;246(3):375–381.

ADDITIONAL READING

- Blamey S, Barraclough B, Delbridge L, et al. Using recombinant human TSH for the diagnosis of recurrent thyroid cancer. *ANZ J Surg*. 2005;75(1–2):10–20.
- Burns WR, Zeiger MA. Differentiated thyroid cancer. *Semin Oncol*. 2010;37(6):557–566.
- Cox AE, LeBeau SO. Diagnosis and treatment of differentiated thyroid carcinoma. *Radiol Clin North Am*. 2011;49(3):453–462, vi.
- Haugen BR, Pacini F, Reiners C, et al. A comparison of recombinant human thyrotropin and thyroid hormone withdrawal for the detection of thyroid remnant or cancer. *J Clin Endocrinol Metab*. 1999;84(11):3877–3885.
- Marsh DJ, Gimm O. Multiple endocrine neoplasia: types 1 and 2. *Adv Otorhinolaryngol*. 2011;70:84–90.
- Pitt SC, Moley JF. Medullary, anaplastic, and metastatic cancers of the thyroid. *Semin Oncol*. 2010;37(6):567–579.
- Wang W, Larson SM, Fazzari M, et al. Prognostic value of [18F]fluorodeoxyglucose positron emission tomographic scanning in patients with thyroid cancer. *J Clin Endocrinol Metab*. 2000;85(3):1107–1113.

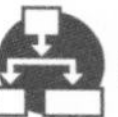

SEE ALSO

Multiple Endocrine Neoplasia (MEN) Syndromes

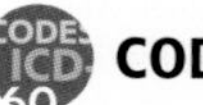

CODES

ICD10

C73 Malignant neoplasm of thyroid gland

CLINICAL PEARLS

- Standard workup for a patient suspected of having a thyroid cancer is a physical exam, TSH level, neck US, and FNA.
- Thyroglobulin levels can be elevated in several thyroid disorders. Its usefulness comes once the diagnosis of cancer has been made. It serves as a better marker for recurrent disease.
- ~2% of the normal population will have a positive ^{18}F-FDG positron-emission tomographic scan, so it is more useful for postresection follow-up.

T

THYROIDITIS

Robert A. Baldor, MD, FAAFP

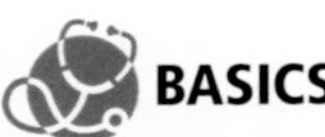

BASICS

DESCRIPTION

Inflammation of the thyroid gland that may be painful or painless

- Thyroiditis with thyroid pain
  - Subacute granulomatous thyroiditis (nonsuppurative thyroiditis, de Quervain thyroiditis, or giant cell thyroiditis): self-limited; viral URI prodrome, symptoms and signs of thyroid dysfunction (variable)
  - Infectious/suppurative thyroiditis
    - Bacterial, fungal, mycobacterial, or parasitic infection of the thyroid
    - Most commonly associated with *Streptococcus pyogenes*, *Staphylococcus aureus*, and *Streptococcus pneumoniae*.
  - Radiation-induced thyroiditis: from radioactive iodine therapy (1%) or external irradiation for lymphoma and head/neck cancers
- Thyroiditis with no thyroid pain
  - Hashimoto (autoimmune) thyroiditis (chronic lymphocytic thyroiditis): most common etiology of chronic hypothyroidism; autoimmune disease; 90% of patients with high-serum antithyroid peroxidase (TPO) antibodies
  - Postpartum thyroiditis: episode of thyrotoxicosis, hypothyroidism, or thyrotoxicosis followed by hypothyroidism in the 1st year postpartum or after spontaneous/induced abortion in women who were without clinically evident thyroid disease before pregnancy
  - Painless (silent) thyroiditis (subacute lymphocytic thyroiditis): mild hyperthyroidism, small painless goiter, and no Graves ophthalmopathy/pretibial myxedema
  - Riedel (fibrous) thyroiditis: rare inflammatory process involving the thyroid and surrounding cervical tissues; associated with various forms of systemic fibrosis; presents as a firm mass in the thyroid commonly associated with compressive symptoms (dyspnea, dysphagia, hoarseness, and aphonia) caused by local infiltration of the advancing fibrotic process with hypocalcemia and hypothyroidism
  - Drug-induced thyroiditis: interferon-α, interleukin-2, amiodarone, or lithium

EPIDEMIOLOGY

- Subacute granulomatous thyroiditis: most common cause of thyroid pain; peaks during summer; incidence: 3/100,000/year; female > male (4:1); peak age: 40–50 years
- Suppurative thyroiditis: commonly seen with preexisting thyroid disease/immunocompromise
- Hashimoto thyroiditis: peak age of onset, 30–50 years; can occur in children; primarily a disease of women; female > male (7:1)
- Postpartum thyroiditis: female only; occurs within 12 months of pregnancy in 8–11% of pregnancies; occurs in 25% with type 1 diabetes mellitus; incidence is affected by genetic influences and iodine intake.
- Painless (silent) thyroiditis: female > male (4:1) with peak age 30–40 years; common in areas of iodine sufficiency
- Reidel thyroiditis: female > male (4:1); highest prevalence age 30–60 years

ETIOLOGY AND PATHOPHYSIOLOGY

- Hashimoto disease: Antithyroid antibodies may be produced in response to an environmental antigen and cross-react with thyroid proteins (molecular mimicry). Precipitating factors include infection, stress, sex steroids, pregnancy, iodine intake, and radiation exposure.
- Subacute granulomatous thyroiditis: probably viral
- Postpartum thyroiditis: autoimmunity-induced discharge of preformed hormone from the thyroid
- Painless (silent) thyroiditis: autoimmune

Genetics

Autoimmune thyroiditis is associated with the CT60 polymorphism of cytotoxic T-cell lymphocyte–associated antigen 4. Also associated with HLA-DR4, -DR5, and -DR6 in whites

RISK FACTORS

- Hashimoto disease: family history of thyroid/autoimmune disease, personal history of autoimmune disease (type 1 diabetes, celiac disease), high iodine intake, cigarette smoking, selenium deficiency
- Subacute granulomatous thyroiditis: recent viral respiratory infection
- Suppurative thyroiditis: congenital abnormalities (persistent thyroglossal duct/piriform sinus fistula), greater age, immunosuppression
- Radiation-induced thyroiditis: high-dose irradiation, younger age, female sex, preexisting hypothyroidism
- Postpartum thyroiditis: smoking, history of spontaneous/induced abortion
- Painless (silent) thyroiditis: iodine-deficient areas

GENERAL PREVENTION

Selenium may decrease inflammatory activity in pregnant women with autoimmune hypothyroidism and may reduce postpartum thyroiditis risk in those positive for TPO antibodies.

COMMONLY ASSOCIATED CONDITIONS

Postpartum thyroiditis: family history of autoimmune thyroid disease; HLA-DRB, -DR4, and -DR5

DIAGNOSIS

HISTORY

- Hypothyroid symptoms (e.g., constipation, heavy menstrual bleeding, fatigue, weakness, dry skin, hair loss, cold intolerance)
- Hyperthyroid symptoms (e.g., irritability, heat intolerance, increased sweating, palpitations, loose stools, disturbed sleep, and lid retraction)
- Subacute granulomatous thyroiditis: sudden/gradual onset, with preceding upper respiratory infection/viral illness (fever, fatigue, malaise, anorexia, and myalgia are common); pain may be limited to thyroid region or radiate to upper neck, jaw, throat, or ears.
- Classic triphasic course (thyrotoxic, hypothyroid, recovery) but variable in the following: subacute, silent, and postpartum thyroiditis (1)[C]

PHYSICAL EXAM

- Examine thyroid size, symmetry, and nodules.
  - Hashimoto disease: 90% have a symmetric, diffusely enlarged, painless gland, with a firm, pebbly texture; 10% have thyroid atrophy.
  - Postpartum thyroiditis: painless, small, nontender, firm goiter (2–6 months after delivery)
  - Reidel thyroiditis: rock-hard, wood-like, fixed, painless goiter, often accompanied by symptoms of esophageal/tracheal compression (stridor, dyspnea, a suffocating feeling, dysphagia, and hoarseness)
- Signs of hypothyroid: delayed relaxation phase of deep tendon reflexes, nonpitting edema, dry skin, alopecia, bradycardia
- Signs of hyperthyroid: moist palms, hyperreflexia, tachycardia/atrial fibrillation

DIFFERENTIAL DIAGNOSIS

Simple goiter; iodine-deficient/lithium-induced goiter; Graves disease; lymphoma; acute infectious thyroiditis; oropharynx and trachea infections; thyroid cancer; amiodarone; contrast dye; amyloid

DIAGNOSTIC TESTS & INTERPRETATION

- Thyroid-stimulating hormone (TSH), anti-TPO antibodies
- Hashimoto disease
  - High titers of anti-TPO antibodies
  - New subtype: IgG4 thyroiditis, which is histopathologically characterized by lymphoplasmacytic infiltration, fibrosis, increased numbers of IgG4-positive plasma cells, and high serum IgG4 levels; more closely associated with rapid progress, subclinical hypothyroidism, higher levels of circulating antibodies, and more diffuse low echogenicity (2)[C]
- Subacute granulomatous thyroiditis
  - High T_4, T_3; low TSH during early stages and elevated later; TSH varies with phase (1)[C].
  - High thyroglobulin; normal levels of anti-TPO and antithyroglobulin antibodies (present in 25%, usually low titers)
  - Elevated erythrocyte sedimentation rate (ESR) (usually >50 mm/hr) and C-reactive protein; mild anemia and slight leukocytosis; LFTs frequently abnormal during initial hyperthyroid phase and resolve over 1–2 months.
- Suppurative thyroiditis
  - In the absence of preexisting thyroid disease, thyroid function normal, but hyper-/hypothyroidism may occur.
  - Elevated ESR and WBC with marked increase in left shift
  - Fine-needle aspiration (FNA) of the lesion with Gram stain and culture is the most useful diagnostic test.
- Postpartum thyroiditis (3)[B]
  - Anti-TPO antibody positivity is the most useful marker for the prediction of postpartum thyroid dysfunction.
  - Women known to be anti-TPO-Ab+ should have TSH measured at 6–12 weeks' gestation and at 6 months postpartum or as clinically indicated.
  - Thyrotoxic phase occurs 1 and 6 months postpartum (most commonly at 3 months) and usually lasts only 1–2 months.
  - Hypothyroidism occurs between 3 and 8 months (most commonly at 6 months).
  - Most patients (80%) have normal thyroid function at 1 year; 30–50% of patients develop permanent hypothyroidism within 9 years.
  - High thyroglobulin, normal ESR
- Painless (silent) thyroiditis
  - Hyperthyroid state in 5–20%: averages 3–4 months, and total duration of illness is <1 year, followed by hypothyroidism and then a return to normal state; some have primary/subclinical hypothyroidism.
  - ~50% have anti-TPO antibodies (1)[C].

- Reidel thyroiditis (4)[C]
  - Hypothyroidism due to extensive replacement of the gland by scar tissue. Anti-TPO antibodies are present in 2/3 of patients along with low radioactive iodine uptake (RAIU).
- Drug-induced thyroiditis
  - Hyper-/hypothyroidism, low RAIU, and variable presence of anti-TPO antibodies
- US: shows variable heterogeneous texture, hypoechogenic in subacute, painless (silent), and postpartum thyroiditis
- Thyroid RAIU scan: decreased in all forms of thyroiditis but not helpful in establishing diagnosis of Hashimoto disease. High RAIU in hashitoxicosis, Graves disease
- Random urine iodine measurement may be helpful to distinguish from other causes of low RAIU.
  - Urine iodine <500 μg/L (subacute granulomatous thyroiditis)
  - Urine iodine >1,000 μg/L (in patients with exposure to excess exogenous iodine/radiocontrast material)

Diagnostic Procedures/Other

- Hashimoto with a dominant nodule should have FNA to rule out thyroid carcinoma.
- Open biopsy is necessary for a definitive diagnosis of Reidel thyroiditis.

Test Interpretation

- Hashimoto disease: lymphocytic infiltration with formation of Askanazy (Hürthle) cells, oxyphilic changes in follicular cells, fibrosis, thyroid atrophy
- Subacute granulomatous thyroiditis: giant cells, mononuclear cell (granulomatous) infiltrate
- Postpartum thyroiditis: lymphocytic infiltration, occasional germinal centers, disruption and collapse of thyroid follicles
- Painless (silent) thyroiditis: lymphocytic infiltration, but without fibrosis, Askanazy cells, and extensive lymphoid follicle formation

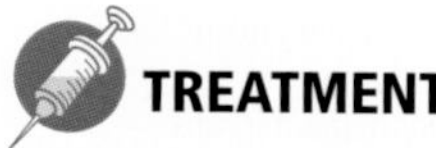

TREATMENT

GENERAL MEASURES

Analgesics for pain; corticosteroids for severe granulomatous thyroiditis

MEDICATION

- Hashimoto disease (2)[C]
  - If hypothyroid/goitrous: levothyroxine (1.7 μg/kg/day for adults <50 years of age). If no cardiac complications and no adrenal insufficiency, 1/2 replacement dose and increase to full replacement in 10 days.
    - If >50 years of age or heart disease and/or adrenal insufficiency, begin with 25 μg/day and titrate to TSH of lower limit normal range.
- If thyrotoxic and symptomatic: propylthiouracil and propranolol
- An elevated TSH level in a woman who is pregnant or attempting to become pregnant is an indication for thyroid replacement.
- Subacute granulomatous thyroiditis
  - Anti-inflammatory agents for 2–8 weeks (NSAIDs or aspirin)
  - Pain with no improvement in 2–3 days after NSAID use: prednisone 40 mg/day; should result in pain relief in 1–2 days; if not, question diagnosis.
  - Severe pain: prednisone 40–60 mg/day discontinued over 4–6 weeks. If pain recurs, increase dose for several weeks and then taper.
  - Symptomatic hyperthyroidism: β-Blockers while thyrotoxic (propranolol 40–120 mg/day)
  - Symptomatic hypothyroid phase: Levothyroxine, as above, target TSH in the normal range.
- Suppurative thyroiditis
  - Parenteral empiric, broad-spectrum antibiotics, and surgical drainage
- Painless (silent) thyroiditis
  - No treatment needed.
  - If symptomatic during hyperthyroid state, treat with β-blocker (propranolol 40–120 mg/day).
  - Prednisone shortens the period of hyperthyroidism. Monitor TSH every 4–8 weeks to confirm resolution.
  - Treat hypothyroid symptoms and asymptomatic patients with TSH >10 mU/L with levothyroxine (50–100 μg/day), to be discontinued after 3–6 months.
- Postpartum thyroiditis (5)[C]
  - Treat symptomatic hyper-/hypothyroid state. Most do not need treatment.
  - Caution in breastfeeding mothers because β-blockers are secreted into breast milk.
  - For symptomatic hypothyroidism, treat with levothyroxine. Otherwise, remonitor in 4–8 weeks. Taper replacement hormone after 6 months if thyroid function has normalized.
- Reidel thyroiditis (4)[C]
  - Corticosteroids in early stages but controversial thereafter. Prednisone 10–20 mg/day for 4–6 months, possibly continued thereafter if effective
  - Long-term anti-inflammatory medications to arrest progression and maintain a symptom-free course
  - Tamoxifen 10–20 mg twice daily as monotherapy or in conjunction with prednisone reduces mass size and clinical symptoms.
  - Methotrexate is used with some success.
  - Reduction of goiter seen with a combination of mycophenolate mofetil (1 g BID) and 100 mg/day prednisone.
  - Debulking surgery is limited to isthmusectomy to relieve constrictive pressure when total thyroidectomy is not possible.
- Drug-induced thyroiditis
  - Discontinue offending drug.

SURGERY/OTHER PROCEDURES

Enlarged painful thyroid or tracheal compression

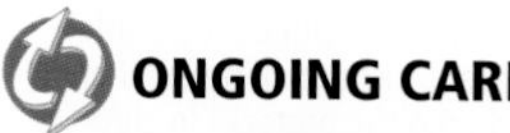

ONGOING CARE

FOLLOW-UP RECOMMENDATIONS

Patient Monitoring

- Hashimoto disease: Repeat thyroid function tests every 3–12 months.
- Subacute granulomatous thyroiditis: Repeat thyroid function tests every 3–6 weeks until euthyroid, then every 6–12 months.
- Postpartum thyroiditis: Check TSH annually.
- Reidel thyroiditis: CT of cervical mediastinal region is recommended.
- TSH every 6 months in patients on amiodarone

Pregnancy Considerations

- Avoid radioisotope scanning if possible.
- Keep TSH maximally suppressed.
- If using RAIU scan, discard breast milk for 2 days because RAI is secreted in breast milk.

PROGNOSIS

- Hashimoto disease: persistent goiter; eventual thyroid failure
- Subacute granulomatous thyroiditis: 5–15% hypothyroid beyond a year: some with eventual return to normal; remission may be slower in the elderly; recurrence rate: 1–4% after a year
- Painless (silent) thyroiditis: 10–20% hypothyroid beyond a year; recurrence rate 5–10% (much higher in Japan)
- Postpartum thyroiditis: 15–50% hypothyroid beyond a year; women may be euthyroid/continue to be hypothyroid at the end of 1st postpartum year. 70% recurrence rate in subsequent pregnancies; substantial risk exists for later development of hypothyroidism/goiter.

REFERENCES

1. Samuels MH. Subacute, silent, and postpartum thyroiditis. *Med Clin North Am*. 2012;96(2):223–233.
2. Li Y, Nishihara E, Kakudo K. Hashimoto's thyroiditis: old concepts and new insights. *Curr Opin Rheumatol*. 2011;23(1):102–107.
3. De Groot L, Abalovich M, Alexander EK, et al. Management of thyroid dysfunction during pregnancy and postpartum: an Endocrine Society clinical practice guideline. *J Clin Endocrinol Metab*. 2012;97(8):2543–2565. doi:10.1210/jc.2011-2803
4. Hennessey JV. Clinical review: Riedel's thyroiditis: a clinical review. *J Clin Endocrinol Metab*. 2011;96(10):3031–3041.
5. Reid SM, Middleton P, Cossich MC, et al. Interventions for clinical and subclinical hypothyroidism in pregnancy. *Cochrane Database Syst Rev*. 2010;(7):CD007752.

ADDITIONAL READING

Duntas LH. Selenium and the thyroid: a close-knit connection. *J Clin Endocrinol Metab*. 2010;95(12): 5180–5188.

SEE ALSO

Hyperthyroidism; Hypothyroidism, Adult

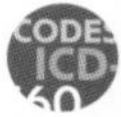

CODES

ICD10

- E06.9 Thyroiditis, unspecified
- E06.1 Subacute thyroiditis
- E06.0 Acute thyroiditis

CLINICAL PEARLS

- TSH elevation above the normal range indicates a hypothyroid state; suppressed TSH indicates hyperthyroid state. Follow up with free T_3/T_4 determination.
- Follow patients on thyroid replacement with periodic TSH level.

T

TINEA (CAPITIS, CORPORIS, CRURIS)

Elisabeth L. Backer, MD

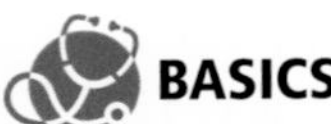

BASICS

DESCRIPTION

- Superficial fungal infections of the skin/scalp; various forms of dermatophytosis; the names relate to the particular area affected (1).
  - Tinea cruris: infection of crural fold and gluteal cleft
  - Tinea corporis: infection involving the face, trunk, and/or extremities; often presents with ring-shaped lesions, hence the misnomer *ringworm*.
  - Tinea capitis: infection of the scalp and hair; affected areas of the scalp can show characteristic black dots resulting from broken hairs.
- Dermatophytes have the ability to subsist on protein, namely keratin.
- They cause disease in keratin-rich structures such as skin, nails, and hair.
- Infections result from contact with infected persons/animals
  - Zoophilic infections are acquired from animals.
  - Anthropophilic infections are acquired from personal contact (e.g., wrestling) or fomites.
  - Geophile infections are acquired from the soil.
- System(s) affected: skin; exocrine
- Synonym(s): jock itch; ringworm

EPIDEMIOLOGY

Incidence

- Tinea cruris
  - Predominant age: any age; rare in children
  - Predominant sex: male > female
- Tinea corporis
  - Predominant age: all ages
  - Predominant sex: male = female
- Tinea capitis
  - Predominant age: 3–9 years; almost always occurs in young children
  - Predominant sex: male = female

Prevalence

Common

Pediatric Considerations

- Tinea cruris is rare prior to puberty.
- Tinea capitis is common in young children.

Geriatric Considerations

Tinea cruris is more common in the geriatric population due to an increase in risk factors.

Pregnancy Considerations

Tinea cruris and capitis are rare in pregnancy.

ETIOLOGY AND PATHOPHYSIOLOGY

Superficial fungal infection of skin/scalp

- Tinea cruris: Source of infection is usually the patient's own tinea pedis, with agent being transferred from the foot to the groin via the underwear when dressing; most common causative dermatophyte is *Trichophyton rubrum*; rare cases caused by *Epidermophyton floccosum* and *T. mentagrophytes*.
- Tinea corporis: most commonly caused by *T. rubrum*; *T. tonsurans* most often found in patients with tinea gladiatorum
- Tinea capitis: *T. tonsurans* found in 90% and *Microsporum* sp. in 10% of patients

Genetics

Evidence suggests a genetic susceptibility in certain individuals.

RISK FACTORS

- Warm climates; summer months and/or copious sweating; wearing wet clothing/multiple layers (tinea cruris)
- Daycare centers/schools/confined quarters (tinea corporis and capitis)
- Depression of cell-mediated immune response (e.g., individuals with atopy or AIDS)
- Obesity (tinea cruris and corporis)
- Direct contact with an active lesion on a human, an animal, or rarely, from soil; working with animals (tinea corporis)

GENERAL PREVENTION

- Avoidance of risk factors, such as contact with suspicious lesions
- Fluconazole or itraconazole may be useful in wrestlers to prevent outbreaks during competitive season.

COMMONLY ASSOCIATED CONDITIONS

Tinea pedis, tinea barbae, tinea manus

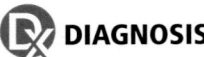

DIAGNOSIS

HISTORY

- Lesions range from asymptomatic to pruritic.
- In tinea cruris, acute inflammation may result from wearing occlusive clothing; chronic scratching may result in an eczematous appearance.
- Previous application of topical steroids, especially in tinea cruris and corporis, may alter the overall appearance causing a more extensive eruption with irregular borders and erythematous papules. This modified form is called *tinea incognito*.

PHYSICAL EXAM

- Tinea cruris: well-marginated, erythematous, half-moon–shaped plaques in crural folds that spread to upper thighs; advancing border is well defined, often with fine scaling and sometimes vesicular eruptions. Lesions are usually bilateral and do not include scrotum/penis (unlike with *Candida* infections) but may migrate to perineum, perianal area, and gluteal cleft and onto the buttocks in chronic/progressive cases. The area may be hyperpigmented on resolution.
- Tinea corporis: scaling, pruritic plaques characterized by a sharply defined annular pattern with peripheral activity and central clearing (ring-shaped lesions); papules and occasionally pustules/vesicles present at border and, less commonly, in center.
- Tinea capitis: commonly begins with round patches of scale (alopecia less common). In its later stages, the infection frequently takes on patterns of chronic scaling with either little/marked inflammation or alopecia. Less often, patients will present with multiple patches of alopecia and the characteristic black-dot appearance of broken hairs. Extreme inflammation results in kerion formation (exudative, pustular nodulation).

DIFFERENTIAL DIAGNOSIS

- Tinea cruris
  - Intertrigo: inflammatory process of moist opposed skin folds, often including infection with bacteria, yeast, and fungi; painful longitudinal fissures may occur in skin folds.
  - Erythrasma: diffuse brown, scaly, noninflammatory plaque with irregular borders, often involving groin; caused by bacterial infection with *Corynebacterium minutissimum;* fluoresces coral red with Wood lamp
  - Seborrheic dermatitis of groin
  - Psoriasis of groin ("inverse psoriasis")
  - Candidiasis of groin (typically involves the scrotum)
  - Acanthosis nigricans
- Tinea capitis
  - Psoriasis
  - Seborrheic dermatitis
  - Pyoderma
  - Alopecia areata and trichotillomania
  - Aplasia cutis congenital
- Tinea corporis
  - Pityriasis rosea
  - Eczema (nummular)
  - Contact dermatitis
  - Syphilis
  - Psoriasis
  - Seborrheic dermatitis
  - Subacute systemic lupus erythematosus (SLE)
  - Erythema annulare centrifugum
  - Erythema multiforme; erythema migrans
  - Impetigo circinatum
  - Granuloma annulare

DIAGNOSTIC TESTS & INTERPRETATION

Wood lamp exam reveals no fluorescence in most cases (*Trichophyton* sp.); 10% of infections, those caused by *T. rubrum* will fluoresce with a green light.

Initial Tests (lab, imaging)

- Potassium hydroxide (KOH) preparation of skin scrapings from dermatophyte leading border shows characteristic translucent, branching, rod-shaped hyphae.
- Arthrospores can be visualized within hair shafts. Spores and/or hyphae may be seen on KOH exam.

Follow-Up Tests & Special Considerations

- Reevaluate to assess response, especially in resistant/extensive cases
- Fungal culture using Sabouraud dextrose agar/dermatophyte test medium

Test Interpretation

- Skin scrapings show fungal hyphae in epidermis.
- Arthrospores found in hair shafts; spores and/or hyphae seen on KOH exam.

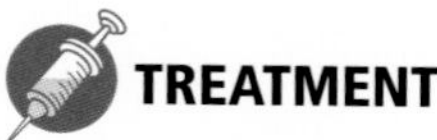

TREATMENT

GENERAL MEASURES

- Careful handwashing and personal hygiene; laundering of towels/clothing of affected individual; no sharing of towels/clothes/headgear
- Evaluate other family members, close contacts, or household pets.
- Avoid predisposing conditions such as hot baths and tight-fitting clothing (boxer shorts are better than briefs).
- Keep area as dry as possible (talcum/powders may be beneficial).
- Itching can be alleviated by OTC preparations such as Sarna or Prax.
- Topical steroid preparations should be avoided (see "Tinea Incognito"), unless absolutely needed to control itching and only after definitive diagnosis and initiation of antifungal treatment.
- Nystatin should be avoided in tinea infections but is indicated for cutaneous candidal infections.
- Avoid contact sports (e.g., wrestling) temporarily while starting treatment.

MEDICATION

First Line

- Tinea cruris/corporis (2)[C]
  - Topical azole antifungal compounds
    - Econazole 1% (Spectazole), ketoconazole (Nizoral): usually applied BID × 2–3 weeks
    - Terbinafine 1% (Lamisil): OTC compound; can be applied once or BID × 1–2 weeks
    - Butenafine 1% (Mentax): applied once daily × 2 weeks; also very effective
  - To prevent relapse, use for 1 week after resolution.
- Tinea capitis (3)[A]
  - PO griseofulvin for *Trichophyton* and *Microsporum* sp.; microsized preparation available; dosage 10–20 mg/kg/day (max 1,000 mg); taken BID or as a single dose daily × 6–12 weeks
  - PO terbinafine can be used for *Trichophyton* sp. at 62.5 mg/day in patients weighing 10–20 kg; 125 mg/day if weight 20–40 kg; 250 mg/day if weight >40 kg; use for 4–6 weeks.
  - PO itraconazole can be used for *Microsporum* sp. and matches griseofulvin efficacy while being better tolerated. Dosage of 3–5 mg/kg/day, but most studies have used 100 mg/day × 6 weeks in children >2 years of age.

Second Line

Tinea cruris/corporis

- Oral antifungal agents are effective but not indicated in uncomplicated tinea cruris/corporis cases. They can be used for resistant and extensive infections or if the patient is immunocompromised. If topical therapy fails, consider possible oral therapy. Griseofulvin can be given 500 mg/day for 1–2 weeks.
- The following oral regimens have been reported in medical literature as being effective but currently are not specifically approved by the FDA for tinea cruris:
  - PO terbinafine (Lamisil): 250 mg/day × 1 week
  - PO itraconazole (Sporanox): 100 mg BID once and repeated 1 week later
  - PO fluconazole (Diflucan): 150 mg once/week × 4 weeks
- Topical terbinafine 1% solution has been studied recently and appears effective as a once-daily application for 1 week.
- Oral antifungals have many interactions including warfarin, OCPs, and alcohol; advise checking for drug interactions prior to use; contraindicated in pregnancy. Monitor for liver toxicity when using oral antifungals.

ISSUES FOR REFERRAL

Refer if disease is nonresponsive/resistant, especially in immunocompromised host.

ADDITIONAL THERAPIES

Treatment of secondary bacterial infections

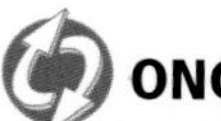

ONGOING CARE

FOLLOW-UP RECOMMENDATIONS

Reevaluate response to treatment.

Patient Monitoring

Liver function testing prior to therapy and at regular intervals during course of therapy for patients requiring oral terbinafine, fluconazole, itraconazole, and griseofulvin

PATIENT EDUCATION

Explain the causative agents, predisposing factors, and prevention measures.

PROGNOSIS

- Excellent prognosis for cure with therapy in tinea cruris and corporis.
- In tinea capitis, lesions will heal spontaneously in 6 months without treatment but scarring is more likely.

COMPLICATIONS

- Secondary bacterial infection
- Generalized, invasive dermatophyte infection

REFERENCES

1. Ameen M. Epidemiology of superficial fungal infections. *Clin Dermatol*. 2010;28(2):197–201.
2. Gupta AK, Cooper EA. Update in antifungal therapy of dermatophytosis. *Mycopathologia*. 2008;166(5–6):353–367.
3. Gupta AK, Drummond-Main C. Meta-analysis of randomized, controlled trials comparing particular doses of griseofulvin and terbenafine for the treatment of tinea capitis. *Pediatr Dermatol*. 2013:30(1):1–6.

ADDITIONAL READING

- Akinwale SO. Personal hygiene as an alternative to griseofulvin in the treatment of tinea cruris. *Afr J Med Sci*. 2000;29(1):41–43.
- Bonifaz A, Saúl A. Comparative study between terbinafine 1% emulsion-gel versus ketoconazole 2% cream in tinea cruris and corporis. *Eur J Derm*. 2000;10(2):107–109.
- Gonzalez U, Seaton T, Bergus G, et al. Systemic antifungal therapy for tinea capitis in children. *Cochrane Database Sys Rev*. 2007;(4):CD004685.
- Lesher JL Jr, Babel DE, Stewart DM, et al. Butenafine 1% cream in the treatment of tinea cruris: a multicenter, vehicle-controlled, double-blind trial. *J Am Acad Dermatol*. 1997;36(2)(Pt 1):S20–S24.
- Nozickova M, Koudelkova V, Kulikova Z, et al. A comparison of the efficacy of oral fluconazole, 150 mg/week versus 50 mg/day, in the treatment of tinea corporis, tinea cruris, tinea pedis, and cutaneous candidosis. *Int J Dermatol*. 1998;37(9):703–705.
- Seebacker C, Bouchara JP, Mignon B. Updates on the epidemiology of dermatophyte infections. *Mycopathologia*. 2008;166(5–6):335–352.
- Tey HL, Tan AS, Chan YC. Meta-analysis of randomized, controlled trials comparing griseofulvin and terbinafine in the treatment of tinea capitis. *J Am Acad Dermatol*. 2011;64(4):663–670.

T

CODES

ICD10

- B35.0 Tinea barbae and tinea capitis
- B35.4 Tinea corporis
- B35.6 Tinea cruris

CLINICAL PEARLS

- Tinea corporis is characterized by scaly plaque, with peripheral activity and central clearing.
- Tinea cruris is characterized by erythematous plaque in crural folds usually sparing the scrotum.
- Tinea capitis is a fungal infection of the scalp affecting hair growth. Topical therapy is ineffective for this infection.

TINEA PEDIS

Elisabeth L. Backer, MD

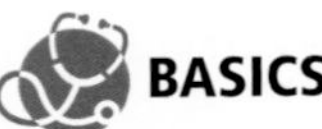

BASICS

DESCRIPTION

- Superficial infection of the feet caused by dermatophytes
- Most common dermatophyte infection encountered in clinical practice
- Often accompanied by tinea manuum, tinea unguium, and tinea cruris
- Two clinical forms: acute and chronic; both are contagious
- System(s) affected: skin/exocrine
- Synonym(s): athlete's foot

EPIDEMIOLOGY

- Predominant age: 20–50 years, although can occur at any age (1)[C]
- Predominant gender: male > female

Prevalence

4% of population

Pediatric Considerations

Rare in younger children; common in teens

Geriatric Considerations

Elderly are more susceptible to outbreaks because of immunocompromise and impaired perfusion of distal extremities.

ETIOLOGY AND PATHOPHYSIOLOGY

Superficial infection caused by dermatophytes that thrive only in nonviable keratinized tissue.

- *Trichophyton mentagrophytes* (acute)
- *Trichophyton rubrum* (chronic)
- *Trichophyton tonsurans*
- *Epidermophyton floccosum*

Genetics

No known genetic pattern.

RISK FACTORS

- Hot, humid weather
- Sweating
- Occlusive/tight-fitting footwear
- Immunosuppression
- Prolonged application of topical steroids

GENERAL PREVENTION

- Good personal hygiene
- Wearing rubber or wooden sandals in community showers, bathing places, locker rooms
- Careful drying between toes after showering or bathing; blow-drying feet with hair dryer may be more effective than drying with towel.
- Changing socks and shoes frequently
- Applying drying or dusting powder
- Applying topical antiperspirants
- Putting on socks before underwear to prevent infection from spreading to groin

COMMONLY ASSOCIATED CONDITIONS

- Hyperhidrosis
- Onychomycosis
- Tinea manuum/unguium/cruris/corporis

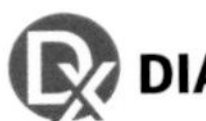

DIAGNOSIS

HISTORY

- Itchy, scaly rash on foot, usually between toes; may progress to fissuring/maceration in toe web spaces.
- May be associated with onychomycosis and other tinea infections

PHYSICAL EXAM

- Acute form: self-limited, intermittent, recurrent; scaling, thickening, and fissuring of sole and heel; scaling or fissuring of toe webs; or pruritic vesicular/bullous lesions between toes or on soles
- Chronic form: most common; slowly progressive, pruritic erythematous erosion/scales between toes, in digital interspaces; extension onto soles, sides/dorsum of feet (moccasin distribution); if untreated, may persist indefinitely
- Other features: strong odor, hyperkeratosis, maceration, ulceration
- Tinea pedis may occur unilateral or bilateral.

DIFFERENTIAL DIAGNOSIS

- Interdigital type: erythrasma, impetigo, pitted keratolysis, candidal intertrigo
- Moccasin type: psoriasis vulgaris, eczematous dermatitis, pitted keratolysis
- Inflammatory/bullous type: impetigo, allergic contact dermatitis, dyshidrotic eczema (negative KOH examination of scrapings), bullous disease

DIAGNOSTIC TESTS & INTERPRETATION

Wood lamp exam will not fluoresce unless complicated by another fungus, which is uncommon; *Malassezia furfur* (yellow to white), *Corynebacterium* (red), or *Microsporum* (blue-green).

Initial Tests (lab, imaging)

Testing is not needed in typical presentation.

- Direct microscopic exam (potassium hydroxide) of scrapings of the lesions
- Culture (Sabouraud medium)

Test Interpretation

- Potassium hydroxide preparation: septate and branched mycelia
- Culture: dermatophyte

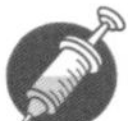

TREATMENT

Treatment is generally with topical antifungal medications for up to 4 weeks and is more effective than placebo:

- Acute treatment
  - Aluminum acetate soak (Burow solution; Domeboro, one pack to one quart warm water) to decrease itching and acute eczematous reaction
  - Antifungal cream of choice BID after soaks
- Chronic treatment:
  - Antifungal creams BID, continuing for 3 days after the rash is resolved: terbinafine 1% (possibly most effective topical), clotrimazole 1%, econazole 1%, ketoconazole 2%, tolnaftate 1%, etc. (2)[A]
  - May try systemic antifungal therapy; see below (consider if concomitant onychomycosis or after failed topical treatment).

GENERAL MEASURES

- Soak with aluminum chloride 30% or aluminum subacetate for 20 minutes BID.
- Careful removal of dead/thickened skin after soaking or bathing
- Chronic or extensive disease or nail involvement requires oral antifungal medication and systemic therapy.

MEDICATION

For use when topical therapy has failed

First Line

- Systemic antifungals (4)[A]:
  - Itraconazole (Sporanox): 200 mg PO BID for 14 days (cure rate >90%)
  - Terbinafine (Lamisil): 250 mg/day PO for 14 days
- If concomitant onychomycosis:
  - Itraconazole: 200 mg PO BID for 1st week of month for 3 months. Liver function testing is recommended.
  - Terbinafine: 250 mg/day PO for 12 weeks, or pulse dosing: 500 mg/day PO for 1st week of month for 3 months. Not recommended if creatinine clearance <50 mL/min.
- Pediatric dosing options:
  - Griseofulvin: 10–15 mg/kg/day or divided
  - Terbinafine:
    - 10–20 kg: 62.5 mg/day
    - 20–40 kg: 125 mg/day
    - >40 kg: 250 mg/day
- Itraconazole: 5 mg/kg/day
- Fluconazole: 6 mg/kg/week
- Contraindications: itraconazole, pregnancy Category C

- Precautions: All systemic antifungal drugs may have potential hepatotoxicity.
- Significant possible interactions: Itraconazole requires gastric acid for absorption; effectiveness is reduced with antacids, H_2 blockers, proton pump inhibitors, etc. Take with acidic beverage such as soda if on antacids.

Second Line

- Systemic antifungals: griseofulvin 250–500 mg of microsize BID daily for 21 days
- Contraindications (griseofulvin):
  - Patients with porphyria, hepatocellular failure
  - Patients with history of hypersensitivity to griseofulvin
- Precautions (griseofulvin):
  - Should be used only in severe cases
  - Periodic monitoring of organ-system functioning, including renal, hepatic, and hematopoietic
  - Possible photosensitivity reactions
  - Lupus erythematosus, lupus-like syndromes, or exacerbation of existing lupus erythematosus has been reported.
- Significant possible interactions (griseofulvin):
  - Decreases activity of warfarin-type anticoagulants
  - Barbiturates usually depress griseofulvin activity.
  - May potentiate effect of alcohol, producing tachycardia and flush

ISSUES FOR REFERRAL

If extensive or resistant disease, especially in immunocompromised host

ADDITIONAL THERAPIES

- Treatment of secondary bacterial infections
- Treatment of eczematoid changes

ONGOING CARE

FOLLOW-UP RECOMMENDATIONS

Avoid sweating feet.

Patient Monitoring

Evaluate for response, recognizing that infections may be chronic/recurrent.

DIET

No restrictions

PATIENT EDUCATION

See "General Prevention."

PROGNOSIS

- Control but not complete cure
- Infections tend to be chronic with exacerbations (e.g., in hot weather).
- Personal hygiene and preventive measures such as open-toed sandals, careful drying, and frequent sock changes are essential.

COMPLICATIONS

- Secondary bacterial infections (common portal of entry for streptococcal infections, producing lymphangitis/cellulitis of lower extremity)
- Eczematoid changes

REFERENCES

1. Ameen M. Epidemiology of superficial fungal infections. *Clin Dermatol*. 2010;28:197.
2. Crawford F, Hollis S. Topical treatments for fungal infections of the skin and nails of the foot. *Cochrane Database Syst Rev*. 2007;(3):CD001434.
3. Rotta I, Sanchez A, Gonçalves PR, et al. Efficacy and safety of topical antifungals in the treatment of dermatomycosis: a systematic review. *Br J Dermatol*. 2012;166(5):927–933.
4. Bell-Syer SE, Hart R, Crawford F, et al. Oral treatments for fungal infections of the skin of the foot. *Cochrane Database Syst Rev*. 2002;(2):CD003584.

ADDITIONAL READING

Gupta AK, Cooper EA. Update in antifungal therapy of dermatophytosis. *Mycopathologia*. 2008;166(5–6):353.

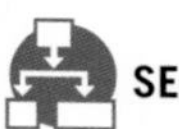

SEE ALSO

Dermatitis, Contact; Dyshidrosis

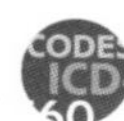

CODES

ICD10

B35.3 Tinea pedis

CLINICAL PEARLS

- Treatment is generally with topical antifungal medications for up to 4 weeks.
- Often is recurrent/chronic in nature
- Careful drying between toes after showering or bathing helps prevent recurrences. (Blow drying feet with hair dryer may be more effective than drying with towel.)
- Socks should be changed frequently. Put on socks before underwear to prevent infection from spreading to groin (tinea cruris).
- Dusting and drying powders (containing antifungal agents) may prevent recurrences.

TINEA VERSICOLOR

Elisabeth L. Backer, MD

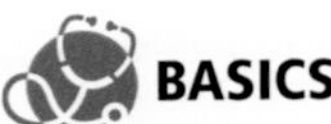

BASICS

DESCRIPTION

- Rash due to a common superficial mycosis with a variety of colors and changing shades of color, predominantly present on trunk and proximal upper extremities; macules usually hypopigmented, light brown, or salmon-colored; fine scale often apparent. It is not a dermatophyte infection.
- System(s) affected: skin/exocrine
- Synonym(s): pityriasis versicolor

EPIDEMIOLOGY

Incidence

- Common, occurs worldwide, especially in tropical climates
- Predominant age: teenagers and young adults
- Predominant sex: male = female

Pediatric Considerations

Usually occurs after puberty (except in tropical areas); facial lesions are more common in children.

Geriatric Considerations

Not common in the geriatric population

ETIOLOGY AND PATHOPHYSIOLOGY

Inhibition of pigment synthesis in epidermal melanocytes, leading to hypomelanosis; in the hyperpigmented type, the melanosomes are large and heavily melanized (1)[C].

- Saprophytic yeast: *Pityrosporum orbiculare* (also known as *P. ovale, Malassezia furfur*, or *M. ovalis*), which is a known colonizer of all humans
- Development of clinical disease associated with transformation of *Malassezia* from yeast cells to pathogenic mycelial form due to host and/or external factors.

Genetics

Genetic predisposition may exist.

RISK FACTORS

- Hot, humid weather
- Use of topical skin oils
- Hyperhidrosis
- HIV infection/immunosuppression
- High cortisol levels (Cushing, prolonged steroid administration)
- Pregnancy
- Malnutrition
- Oral contraceptives

GENERAL PREVENTION

- Recheck and treat again each spring prior to tanning season.
- Avoid skin oils.

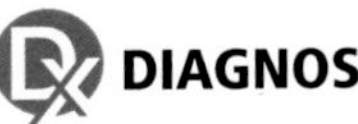

DIAGNOSIS

HISTORY

- Asymptomatic scaling macules on trunk
- Possible mild pruritus
- More prominent in summer
- Sun tanning accentuates lesions because infected areas do not tan.
- Periodic recurrences common

PHYSICAL EXAM

- *Versicolor* refers to the variety and changing shades of colors. Color variations can exist between individuals and also between lesions.
- Sun-exposed areas: lesions usually white/hypopigmented
- Covered areas: lesions often brown or salmon-colored
- Distribution (sebum-rich areas): chest, shoulders, back (also face and intertriginous areas)
  - Face more likely to be involved in children
- Appearance: small individual macules that frequently coalesce
- Scale: fine, more visible with scraping

DIFFERENTIAL DIAGNOSIS

Other skin diseases with discolored macules and plaques, including the following:

- Pityriasis alba/rosea ("Christmas tree-like" distribution visible in *P. rosea*)
- Vitiligo (presents without scaling)
- Seborrheic dermatitis (more erythematous; thicker scale)
- Nummular eczema
- Secondary syphilis
- Erythrasma
- Mycosis fungoides

DIAGNOSTIC TESTS & INTERPRETATION

Wood lamp: yellow to yellow-green fluorescence or pigment changes

Initial Tests (lab, imaging)

- Direct microscopy of scales with 10% potassium hydroxide (KOH) preparation to visualize hyphae and spores ("spaghetti and meatballs" pattern)
- Routine lab tests usually not necessary
- Fungal culture not useful

Test Interpretation

- Short, stubby, or Y-shaped hyphae
- Small, round spores in clusters on hyphae

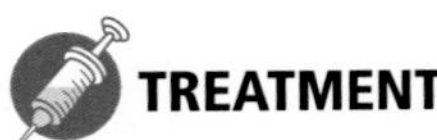

TREATMENT

GENERAL MEASURES

- Apply prescribed topical medications to affected skin with cotton balls.
- Pigmentation may take months to fade or fill in.
- Repeat treatment each spring prior to sun exposure; some may require repeated treatment during the summer as prophylaxis.
- Patients who fail topical treatment can be treated with an oral/systemic medication.

MEDICATION

Topical antifungal therapy is the treatment of choice in limited disease. Evidence is generally of poor quality, but data suggest that longer durations of treatment and higher concentrations of active agents produce greater cure rates (2)[A].

First Line

- Ketoconazole 2% shampoo applied to damp skin and left on for 5 minutes × 1–3 days *or*
- Selenium sulfide shampoo 2.5% (Selsun):
  - Allowed to dry for 10 minutes prior to showering: daily × 1 week *or*
  - Allowed to remain on body for 12–24 hours prior to showering: once a week × 4 weeks *or*

- Clotrimazole 1% topical (Lotrimin) BID × 2–4 weeks *or*
- Miconazole 2% (Micatin, Monistat) BID × 2–4 weeks *or*
- Ketoconazole 2% (Nizoral) cream BID × 2–4 weeks *or*
- Terbinafine (Lamisil) 1% solution BID × 1 week *or*
- Terbinafine (Lamisil Derm Gel) once daily × 1 week
- Cure rates of topical antiyeast preparations typically 70–80%; healing continues after active treatment. Resumption of even pigmentation may take months.
- Contraindications: Ketoconazole is contraindicated in pregnancy.
- Newer preparations: 2.25% selenium sulfide foam; ketoconazole 2% gel

Second Line
- Use for extensive disease or nonresponders
- Oral fluconazole 300 mg once weekly for 2 weeks
- Itraconazole 200 mg/day PO × 1 week; cure rate >90% (3)[C].
- Oral ketoconazole (rarely needed and has significant adverse reactions) 400 mg in single dose or 200 mg/day for 1 week; cure rate >90%
- Oral terbinafine or griseofulvin not effective
- Pramiconazole has been studied but is not yet available for clinical use.

ISSUES FOR REFERRAL
- If resistant to treatment
- If extensive disease occurs in immunocompromised host.

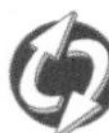

ONGOING CARE

- Ketoconazole 2% or selenium sulfide 2.5% shampoo can be used weekly for maintenance or monthly for prophylaxis.
- Itraconazole 400 mg once monthly during the warmer months of the year can also reduce recurrences.

FOLLOW-UP RECOMMENDATIONS
Warn patients that whiteness will remain for several months after treatment.

Patient Monitoring
- Recheck and treat again each spring prior to tanning season.
- Failure to respond should prompt reassessment or dermatology referral.
- Resistance to treatment, frequent recurrences, or widespread disease may point to immunodeficiency.

PATIENT EDUCATION
For patient education materials favorably reviewed on this topic, contact American Academy of Dermatology, 930 N. Meacham Road, P.O. Box 4014, Schaumberg, IL 60168-4014; (708) 330-0230.

PROGNOSIS
- Duration of lesions months/years
- Recurs almost routinely because this yeast is a known human colonizer

REFERENCES

1. Morishita N, Sei Y. Microreview of pityriasis versicolor and *Malassezia* species. *Mycopathologia*. 2006;162(6):373–376.
2. Hu SW, Bigby M. Pityriasis versicolor: a systematic review of interventions. *Arch Dermatol*. 2010;146(10):1132.
3. Bhogal CS, Singal A, Baruah MC. Comparative efficacy of ketoconazole and fluconazole in the treatment of pityriasis versicolor: a one year follow-up study. *J Dermatol*. 2001;28(10):535–539.

ADDITIONAL READING

- Faergemann J, Todd G, Pather S, et al. A double-blind, randomized, placebo-controlled, dose-finding study of oral pramiconazole in the treatment of pityriasis versicolor. *J Am Acad Dermatol*. 2009;61(6):971.
- Güleç AT, Demirbilek M, Seçkin D, et al. Superficial fungal infections in 102 renal transplant recipients: a case-control study. *J Am Acad Dermatol*. 2003;49(2):187–192.
- Gupta AK, Batra R, Bluhm R, et al. Pityriasis versicolor. *Dermatol Clin*. 2003;21(3):413.
- Köse O, Bülent Tatan H, Riza Gür A, et al. Comparison of a single 400 mg dose versus a 7-day 200 mg daily dose of itraconazole in the treatment of tinea versicolor. *J Dermatolog Treat*. 2002;13(2):77–79.

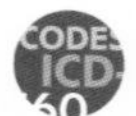

CODES

ICD10
B36.0 Pityriasis versicolor

CLINICAL PEARLS

- Noncontagious macules of varying colors, with fine scale
- Recurrence in summer months
- More apparent after tanning. Skin areas with fungal infection do not tan; thus, hypopigmented areas become more visible.
- Warn patients that whiteness will remain for several months after treatment.

TINNITUS

Donna I. Meltzer, MD

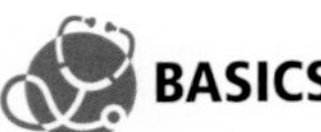

BASICS

DESCRIPTION

- Tinnitus is a perceived sensation of sound in the absence of an external acoustic stimulus; often described as a ringing, hissing, buzzing, or whooshing
- Derived from the Latin word *tinnire*, meaning "to ring" (1)
- May be heard in one or both ears or centrally within the head (2)
- Two types: subjective (most common) and objective tinnitus
- Subjective tinnitus: perceived only by the patient; can be continuous, intermittent, or pulsatile
- Objective tinnitus: can be heard by the examiner; usually pulsatile; <1% cases (3)

EPIDEMIOLOGY

Prevalence

- Tinnitus reported by 35–50 million adults in United States; although underreported, 12 million seek medical care (4).
- Affects 10–15% of adults
- Prevalence increases with age and peaks between ages of 60 and 69 years (5).
- Prevalence of 13–53% in general pediatric population (6)
- Ethnic: whites > blacks and Hispanics (4)
- Gender: males > females

Incidence

- Incidence increasing in association with excessive noise exposure
- Higher rates of tinnitus in smokers and hypertensives (5)

ETIOLOGY AND PATHOPHYSIOLOGY

- Precise pathophysiology is unknown; numerous theories have been proposed. Cochlear damage from ototoxic agents or noise exposure damage hair cells so that the central auditory system compensates, resulting in hyperactivity in cochlear nucleus and auditory cortex. Animal models have identified brain abnormalities resulting in increased firing and synchrony in auditory cortex (7).
- Subjective tinnitus causes the following:
  - Otologic: hearing loss, cholesteatoma, cerumen impaction, otosclerosis, Ménière disease, vestibular schwannoma
  - Ototoxic medications: anti-inflammatory agents (aspirin, NSAIDs); antimalarial agents (quinine, chloroquine); antimicrobial drugs (aminoglycosides); antineoplastic agents, loop diuretics, miscellaneous drugs (antiarrhythmics, antiulcer, anticonvulsants, antihypertensives, psychotropic drugs; anesthetics (3,5)
  - Somatic: temporomandibular joint (TMJ) dysfunction, head or neck injury
  - Neurologic: multiple sclerosis, spontaneous intracranial hypertension, vestibular migraine, type I Chiari malformation
  - Infectious: viral, bacterial, fungal
- Objective tinnitus causes the following:
  - Patulous eustachian tube
  - Vascular: aortic or carotid stenosis, venous hum, arteriovenous fistula or malformation, vascular tumors, high cardiac output state (anemia)
  - Neurologic: palatal myoclonus, idiopathic stapedial muscle spasm

Genetics

Minimal genetic component

RISK FACTORS

- Hearing loss (but can have tinnitus with normal hearing)
- High level noise exposure
- Advanced age
- Use of ototoxic medications
- Otologic disease (otosclerosis, Ménière disease, cerumen impaction)

GENERAL PREVENTION

- Avoid loud noise exposure and wear appropriate ear protection to prevent hearing loss.
- Monitor ototoxic medications and avoid prescribing more than one ototoxic agent concurrently.

COMMONLY ASSOCIATED CONDITIONS

- Sensorineural hearing loss caused by presbycusis (age associated hearing loss) or prolonged loud noise exposure
- Conductive hearing loss due to cerumen, otosclerosis, cholesteatoma
- Psychological disorders: depression, anxiety, insomnia, suicidal ideation
- Despair, frustration, interference with concentration and social interactions, work hindrance

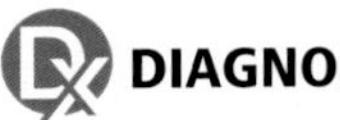

DIAGNOSIS

HISTORY

- Onset gradual (presbycusis) or abrupt (following loud noise exposure)
- Timing: can be continuous (hearing loss) or intermittent (Ménière disease)
- Pattern: nonpulsatile >> pulsatile (often vascular cause)
- Location: bilateral > unilateral (vestibular schwannoma, cerumen, Ménière disease)
- Pitch: high pitch (with sensorineural hearing loss)> low pitch (Ménière disease)
- Associated symptoms: hearing loss, headache, noise intolerance, vertigo, TMJ dysfunction, neck pain
- Exacerbating factors: loud noise; jaw, head, or neck movements
- Alleviating factors: hearing aid, position change, medications
- Medication use (prescription, OTC, supplements)
- Hearing and past noise exposure (occupational, military, recreational)
- Psychosocial history (depression, sleep habits)
- Impact of tinnitus: Tinnitus Handicap Inventory, Tinnitus Functional Index

PHYSICAL EXAM

- HEENT, neck, neurologic, and vascular examinations
- Ear: cerumen impaction, effusion, cholesteatoma
- Check hearing; air and bone conduction testing with 512- or 1,024-Hz tuning fork (Weber and Rinne tests)
- Eye: funduscopic exam for papilledema (intracranial hypertension) or visual field change (mass)
- TMJ: palpate for tenderness and crepitus with movement
- Cranial nerve, Romberg test (equilibrium), finger to nose, gait
- Auscultate for bruits or murmurs over ear canal, periauricular areas, orbit, neck, chest.

DIFFERENTIAL DIAGNOSIS

Pulsatile tinnitus: carotid stenosis, aortic valve disease, AV malformation, high cardiac output state (anemia, hyperthyroidism), paraganglioma (glomus tumor)

Nonpulsatile tinnitus: auditory hallucinations (8)

DIAGNOSTIC TESTS & INTERPRETATION

- Tinnitus is a symptom; no objective test to confirm diagnosis
- Pure tone audiometry (air and bone conduction)
- Speech discrimination testing
- Tympanometry
- Auditory brainstem response (ABR); less sensitive and specific than MRI for diagnosis of vestibular schwannoma (3)
- Carotid Doppler ultrasonography (neck bruit)

Initial Tests (lab, imaging)

Little evidence to support lab testing other than targeted lab studies based on history and physical exam. Lab investigation is not indicated in all patients; use clinical judgment. Consider the following:

- CBC
- BUN/creatinine, fasting glucose, lipid panel
- Thyroid-stimulating hormone
- Clinical evaluation should precede radiologic studies.
- Nonpulsatile tinnitus: MRI with or without contrast
- Pulsatile tinnitus: Contrast-enhanced temporal bone CT, MRI, MRA/ MRV, CTA/ CTV, carotid ultrasound, and conventional angiography all have been used to work up pulsatile tinnitus.
- CTA/ CTV; CTA evaluates middle ear and arterial causes (carotid artery stenosis, aberrant ICA, persistent stapedial artery); CTV evaluates venous causes (sinus thrombosis, sinus stenosis, dehiscent jugular bulb) (9)[C].
- No studies have compared sensitivity and specificity of MRA/V with CTA/V in the evaluation of pulsatile tinnitus.
- Cerebral angiography is gold standard for diagnosis of suspected dural arteriovenous fistula.

Follow-Up Tests & Special Considerations

Consider HIV, RPR, autoimmune panel, Lyme test, Vitamin B_{12} level.

Diagnostic Procedures/Other

Electronystagmography (vestibular testing for Ménière disease)

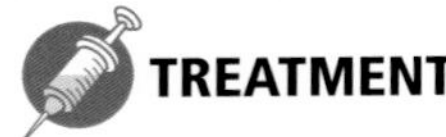

TREATMENT

GENERAL MEASURES

- Individualize treatment based on the severity of tinnitus and impact on function.
- Reassure patient.
- Manage treatable pathology.
- Education, relaxation therapy, cognitive-behavioral therapy (CBT)
- Hearing aids (corrects hearing and might mask tinnitus); can be tried even if there is minimal hearing loss. No evidence to support or refute the use of hearing aids (10)[B].
- Protect hearing against future loud noise.
- Masking sound devices or generators; on discontinuation might have decreased tinnitus (residual inhibition)
- Discontinue ototoxic medications.

MEDICATION

No pharmacologic agent has been shown to cure or consistently alleviate tinnitus.

First Line

- Antidepressants (SSRIs or TCAs): probably help with psychological distress. Newer review states insufficient evidence that antidepressant drug therapy improves tinnitus (11)[B].

- Melatonin decreases tinnitus intensity and improves sleep quality; most effective in men, those without depression or prior treatment, and those with more severe bilateral tinnitus (12)[B]

Second Line

- Anticonvulsants (carbamazepine): used to treat tinnitus for years. Recent studies indicate that they may have a small effect (of doubtful clinical significance) on tinnitus (13)[A].
- Benzodiazepines help reduce tinnitus distress, but regular use discouraged.
- Vitamin B_{12} supplements may improve tinnitus in some patients.
- No difference between gabapentin and control group in patients with isolated tinnitus (14)[B].
- Higher caffeine intake associated with lower incidence of tinnitus in women (15)[B]

ISSUES FOR REFERRAL

- Audiologist for comprehensive hearing evaluation and management
- Otolaryngologist, neurologist, or neurosurgeon depending on pathology
- Dental referral for TMJ treatment and dental orthotics (splint, night guard)
- Therapists for CBT cognitive behavioral therapy (CBT), biofeedback, education, and relaxation techniques

ADDITIONAL THERAPIES

- Sound therapy (masking): Patients wear low-level noise generators to mask the tinnitus noise; commonly used, but no strong evidence for its efficacy (16)[B].
- CBT employs relaxation exercises, coping strategies, and deconditioning techniques to reduce arousal levels and reverse negative thoughts about tinnitus. Depression and severity of tinnitus improved with CBT (17)[A].
- Tinnitus retraining therapy (TRT) combines counseling, education, and acoustic therapy (soft music, sound machine) to minimize bothersome nature of tinnitus. Often requires a team approach and up to 2 years of therapy. Might be more effective than sound masking (18)[B]
- Transcranial magnetic stimulation (TMS): A noninvasive method to stimulate neurons in the brain by rapidly changing magnetic fields. Safe for short-term use; insufficient data to support long term safety of repetitive TMS (19)[B]
- Neurofeedback: a method to help patients regulate abnormal oscillatory brain activity and reduce intensity of tinnitus
- Hyperbaric oxygen therapy: no beneficial effect on tinnitus (20)[A]

SURGERY/OTHER PROCEDURES

- Cochlear implants (for severe sensorineural hearing loss)
- Ablation of cochlear nerve (destroys hearing)
- Epidural stimulation of secondary auditory cortex with implanted electrodes suppressed tinnitus in small subset of patients.
- Otosclerosis: stapedectomy surgery with implantation of ossicular prosthesis
- Severe Ménière disease not alleviated by medications: installation of endolymphatic shunt, labyrinthectomy, or vestibular neurectomy
- Auditory neoplasms: surgical resection/radiation
- Pulsatile tinnitus due to atherosclerotic carotid artery disease: carotid endarterectomy

COMPLEMENTARY & ALTERNATIVE MEDICINE

- Zinc supplements might improve tinnitus in those with zinc deficiency. One study in elderly did not demonstrate effectiveness of zinc treatment (21)[B].
- Ginkgo biloba has potential benefit, but recent reviews question the effectiveness (22)[B].
- Botulinum toxin (for palatal myoclonus)
- Acamprosate (used to treat alcohol dependence): Small studies noted improvement in tinnitus severity.
- Hypnosis (unknown effectiveness)
- Acupuncture (unknown effectiveness)
- Low-power laser to mastoid bone (unknown effectiveness)

INPATIENT CONSIDERATIONS

Admission Criteria/Initial Stabilization

Not applicable

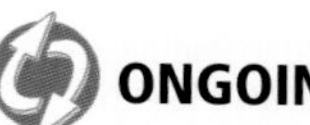

ONGOING CARE

FOLLOW-UP RECOMMENDATIONS

- Audiologist: for hearing evaluation and therapy
- Counseling as needed for psychological distress
- Family physician: as needed for support and guidance

PATIENT EDUCATION

- Help patients understand the relatively benign nature of tinnitus.
- Self-help groups
- American Tinnitus Association: (800) 634-8978; www.ata.org
- National Institute on Deafness and Other Communication Disorders: (800) 241-1044; www.nidcd.nih.gov
- American Academy of Family Physicians: http://familydoctor.org

PROGNOSIS

- Tinnitus persisted in 80% of older patients and increased in severity in 50% (3).
- Focus on managing tinnitus and reducing severity, not curing.

REFERENCES

1. Baguley D, McFerran D, Hall D. Tinnitus. *Lancet*. 2013;382(9904):1600–1607.
2. Langguth B, Kreuzer PM, Kleinjung T, et al. Tinnitus: causes and clinical management. *Lancet Neurol*. 2013;12(9):920–930.
3. Yew KS. Diagnostic approach to patients with tinnitus. *Am Fam Physician*. 2014;89(2):106–113.
4. Shargorodsky J, Curhan GC, Farwell WR. Prevalence and characteristics of tinnitus among US adults. *Am J Med*. 2010;123(8):711–718.
5. Zimmerman E, Timboe A. Tinnitus: steps to take, drugs to avoid. *J Fam Pract*. 2014;63(2):82–88.
6. Bae SC, Park SN, Park JM, et al. Childhood tinnitus: clinical characteristics and treatment. *Am J Otolaryngol*. 2014;35(2):207–210.
7. Galazyuk AV, Wenstrup JJ, Hamid MA. Tinnitus and underlying brain mechanisms. *Curr Opin Otolaryngol Head Neck Surg*. 2012;20(5):409–415.
8. Smith GS, Romanelli-Gobbi M, Gray-Karagrigoriou E, et al. Complementary and integrative treatments: tinnitus. *Otolaryngol Clin North Am*. 2013;46(3):398–408.
9. Sajisevi M, Weissman JL, Kaylie DM. What is the role of imaging in tinnitus? *Laryngoscope*. 2014;124(3):583–584.
10. Hoare DJ, Edmondson-Jones M, Sereda M, et al. Amplification with hearing aids for patients with tinnitus and co-existing hearing loss. *Cochrane Database Syst Rev*. 2014;1:CD010151.
11. Baldo P, Doree C, Molin P, el al. Antidepressants for patients with tinnitus. *Cochrane Database Syst Rev*.2012;9:CD003853.
12. Hurtuk A, Dome C, Holloman CH, et al. Melatonin: can it stop the ringing? *Ann Otol Rhinol Laryngol*. 2011;120(7):433–440.
13. Hoekstra C, Rynja SP, van Zanten GA, et al. Anticonvulsants for tinnitus. *Cochrane Database Syst Rev*. 2011;(7):CD007960.
14. Dehkordi MA, Abolbashari S, Taheri R, et al. Efficacy of gabapentin on subjective idiopathic tinnitus: a randomized, double-blind, placebo-controlled trial. *Ear Nose Throat J*. 2011;90(4):150–158.
15. Glicksman JT, Curhan SG, Curhan GC. A prospective study of caffeine intake and risk of incident tinnitus. *Am J Med*. 2014;127(8):739–743.
16. Hobson J, Chisholm E, El Refaie A. Sound therapy (masking) in the management of tinnitus in adults. *Cochrane Database Syst Rev*. 2012;11:CD006371.
17. Martinez-Devesa P, Perera R, Theodoulou M, et al. Cognitive behavioural therapy for tinnitus. *Cochrane Database Syst Rev*. 2010;(9):CD005233.
18. Phillips JS, McFerran D. Tinnitus retraining therapy (TRT) for tinnitus. *Cochrane Database Syst Rev*. 2010;(3):CD007330.
19. Meng Z, Liu S, Zheng Y, et al. Repetitive transcranial magnetic stimulation for tinnitus. *Cochrane Database Syst Rev*. 2011;(10):CD007946.
20. Bennett MH, Kertesz T, Perleth M, et al. Hyperbaric oxygen for idiopathic sudden sensorineural hearing loss and tinnitus. *Cochrane Database Syst Rev*. 2012;10:CD004739.
21. Coelho C, Witt SA, Ji H, et al. Zinc to treat tinnitus in the elderly: a randomized placebo controlled crossover trial. *Otol Neurotol*. 2013;34(6):1146–1154.
22. Hilton MP, Zimmermann EF, Hunt WT. Ginkgo biloba for tinnitus. *Cochrane Database Syst Rev*. 2013;3:CD003852.

ADDITIONAL READING

- Hoare DJ, Kowalkowski VL, Kang S, et al. Systematic review and meta-analyses of randomized controlled trials examining tinnitus management. *Laryngoscope*. 2011;121(7):1555–1564.
- Kim JI, Choi JY, Lee DH, et al. Acupuncture for the treatment of tinnitus: a systematic review of randomized clinical trials. *BMC Complement Altern Med*. 2012;12:97.
- Newman CW, Sandridge SA, Bea SM, et al. Tinnitus: patients do not have to "just live with it." *Cleve Clinic J Med*. 2011;78(5):312–319.

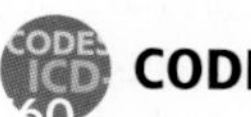

CODES

ICD10

- H93.19 Tinnitus, unspecified ear
- H93.11 Tinnitus, right ear
- H93.12 Tinnitus, left ear

CLINICAL PEARLS

- People have different levels of tolerance to tinnitus. It may affect sleep, concentration, and emotional state. Many patients with chronic tinnitus have depression.
- To keep tinnitus from worsening, avoid loud noises and minimize stress.
- Optimal management may involve multiple strategies.

TOBACCO USE AND SMOKING CESSATION

Felix B. Chang, MD, DABMA, ABIHM

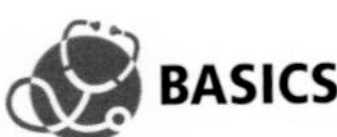

BASICS

DESCRIPTION

- Use of tobacco of any form
- *Smokeless tobacco* refers to tobacco products that are sniffed, sucked, or chewed.
- Nicotine sources: cigars, pipes, waterpipes, hookahs, and cigarettes

EPIDEMIOLOGY

Incidence

- 2.4 million new smokers annually in the United States (2.6% initiation rate)
- 58.8% of new smokers are <18 years of age (5.8% initiation rate for teens).

Prevalence

- 443,000 deaths annually in the United States
- Cigarette smoking among adults in the United States: 21.3% of adults in 2012–2013
- Highest among those aged 18–25 (40.8%)
- Adults aged >25 years (28.5%)
- Race: highest among whites (22.1%) and African Americans (21.3%) and is lower among Hispanics (14.6%) and Asians (12%)
- Gender: male > female (21.5% vs. 17.3%)
- Inversely proportional to education level
- 31% in men >15 years old from 187 countries in 2012

ETIOLOGY AND PATHOPHYSIOLOGY

- Addiction due to nicotine's rapid stimulation of the brain's dopamine system (teenage brain especially susceptible)
- Atherosclerotic risk due to adrenergic stimulation, endothelial damage, carbon monoxide, and adverse effects on lipids
- Direct airway damage from cigarette tar
- Carcinogens in all tobacco products

RISK FACTORS

- Presence of a smoker in the household
- Easy access to cigarettes
- Perceived parental approval of smoking
- Comorbid stress and psychiatric disorders
- Low self-esteem/self-worth
- Poor academic performance
- Boys: high levels of aggression and rebelliousness
- Girls: preoccupation with weight and body image

GENERAL PREVENTION

- Most 1st-time tobacco use occurs before high school graduation, so educational interventions should target students in grade and middle schools and must address health consequences and psychosocial aspects of smoking (1)[A].
- The AAFP's Tar Wars program has targeted 4th and 5th graders successfully.
- Other helpful measures include the following:
  - Smoking bans in public areas and workplaces
  - Restriction of minors' access to tobacco
  - Restrictions on tobacco advertisements
  - Raising prices through taxation
  - Media literacy education
  - Tobacco-free sports initiatives

COMMONLY ASSOCIATED CONDITIONS

- Coronary artery disease
- Cerebrovascular disease
- Peripheral vascular disease
- Abdominal aortic aneurysm (AAA)
- COPD
- Cancer of the lip, oral cavity, pharynx, larynx, lung, esophagus, stomach, pancreas, kidney, bladder, cervix, and blood
- Pneumonia
- Osteoporosis
- Periodontitis
- Alcohol use
- Depression and anxiety
- Reduced fertility

Pregnancy Considerations

Women who smoke or are exposed to 2nd-hand smoke during pregnancy have increased risks of miscarriage, placenta previa, placental abruption, premature rupture of membranes, preterm delivery, low-birth-weight infants, and stillbirth.

Pediatric Considerations

- 2nd-hand smoke increases the risk of the following in infants and children:
  - Sudden infant death syndrome
  - Acute upper and lower respiratory tract infections
  - More frequent and more severe exacerbations of asthma
  - Otitis media and need for tympanostomies
- Nicotine passes through breast milk, and its effects on the growth and development of nursing infants are unknown.

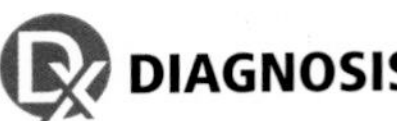

DIAGNOSIS

HISTORY

- Ask about tobacco use and 2nd-hand smoke exposure at every physician encounter.
- Type and quantity of tobacco used
- Pack years = packs/day × years
- Awareness of health risks
- Assess interest in quitting.
- Identify triggers for smoking.
- Prior attempts to quit: method, duration of success, reason for relapse

PHYSICAL EXAM

- General: tobacco smoke odor
- Skin: premature face wrinkling
- Mouth: nicotine-stained teeth; inspect for suspicious mucosal lesions
- Lungs: crackles, wheezing, increased or decreased volume
- Vessels: carotid or abdominal bruits, abdominal aortic enlargement, peripheral pulses, stigmata of peripheral vascular disease

DIAGNOSTIC TESTS & INTERPRETATION

- CXR for patients with pulmonary symptoms or signs of cancer but not for screening
- The USPSTF recommends 1-time screening US for AAA in men ≥65 years of age who ever smoked (number needed to screen to prevent 1 AAA = 500).

Diagnostic Procedures/Other

PFTs for smokers with chronic pulmonary symptoms, such as wheezing and dyspnea

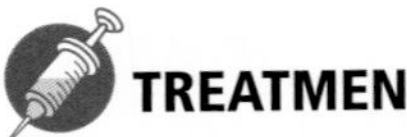

TREATMENT

Both behavioral counseling and pharmacotherapy benefit patients who are trying to quit smoking especially when use in combination.

ALERT

Provider recommending smoking cessation at *every clinical visit* improves cessation rates. Nonpharmacologic approaches are appropriate for pregnant women and patients who smoke <10 cigarettes/day.

GENERAL MEASURES

- Behavioral counseling includes the 5 As of promoting smoking cessation:
  - Ask about tobacco use at every office visit.
  - Advise all smokers to quit.
  - Assess the patient's willingness to quit.
  - Assist the patient in his or her attempt to quit.
  - Arrange follow-up.
- Patients ready to quit smoking should set a quit date within the next 2 weeks. No difference in success rates between patients who taper prior to their quit date and those who stop abruptly.
- It might help for patients to have a quitting partner, such as a spouse, friend, or coworker, to provide mutual encouragement.
- Patients desiring to quit should dispose of all smoking paraphernalia (such as lighters) on their quit dates to make relapse more difficult.
- Patients must anticipate and avoid social/environmental triggers for smoking and should have a plan for dealing with the urge to smoke.

MEDICATION

First Line

- Varenicline (Chantix): 0.5 mg/day PO × 3 days, then 0.5 mg BID × 4 days, then 1 mg BID for 11 weeks (2)[A]:
  - Start 1–4 weeks prior to smoking cessation and continue for 12–24 weeks
  - Superior to placebo and to bupropion; number needed to treat = 7
  - S/E: nausea, insomnia, headache, depression, suicidal ideation; safety not established in adolescents or patients with psychiatric or cardiovascular disease; pregnancy Category C
- Bupropion SR (Zyban): 150 mg PO × 3 days, then 150 mg BID:
  - Start 1 week prior to smoking cessation, and continue for 7–12 weeks
  - Twice as effective as placebo
  - Drug of choice for patients with depression or schizophrenia
  - S/E: tachycardia, headache, nausea, insomnia, dry mouth; contraindicated in patients who have seizure disorders or anorexia/bulimia; pregnancy Category C (2)(3)[A]

- Nicotine replacement therapy (e.g., patch, gum, lozenge, inhaler, nasal spray) (2)(3)[A]:
  - Improves quit rates by 50–70% versus placebo
  - Over-the-counter
  - Patch (NicoDerm CQ 21, 14, and 7 mg):
    - 1 patch q24h
    - Start with 21 mg if smoking ≥10 cigarettes/day; otherwise, start with 14 mg.
    - 6 weeks on initial dose, then taper
    - 2 weeks each on subsequent doses
    - No proven benefit beyond 8 weeks
  - E-cigarettes
    - Contain less nicotine than cigarette
    - Considered less "dangerous" than tobacco but not as well studied as other NRT (4)[B]
    - Conflicting data on whether teen use increases or decreases risk to cigarette progression
  - Gum (Nicorette, 2 and 4 mg):
    - Use 4 mg if smoking ≥25 cigarettes/day.
    - Chew 1 piece q1–2h × 6 weeks, then 1 q2–4h × 3 weeks, then 1 q4–8h × 3 weeks.
  - May use in combination with bupropion; monitor for hypertension
  - S/E: headache, pharyngitis, cough, rhinitis, dyspepsia; all mainly with inhaler and spray forms
  - Pregnancy Category D

Second Line

- Nortriptyline: 25–75 mg/day PO or in divided doses:
  - Start 10–14 days prior to smoking cessation and continue for at least 12 weeks.
  - Efficacy similar to bupropion, but side effects more common; pregnancy Category D
  - The antidepressants bupropion and nortriptyline aid long-term smoking cessation (5)[A].
- Clonidine: 0.1 mg PO BID or 0.1 mg/24 hr transdermal patch weekly (2):
  - Side effects: hypotension, bradycardia, depression, fatigue; pregnancy Category C

ADDITIONAL THERAPIES

The following interventions have been shown to be effective in helping patients quit smoking:

- Advice from nurses, especially in hospital
- Individual counseling/group therapy
- Telephone counseling/web-based cessation programs
- Exercise (not conclusive, ineffective) (6)[A]
- Acupuncture: short-term effects (7)[A]
- Naltreoxone. No evidence (8)[A]
- Opiates antagonist. No evidence (2)[A]

COMPLEMENTARY & ALTERNATIVE MEDICINE

Acupuncture, aversive therapy, and hypnosis have not been proven to enhance long-term smoking cessation.

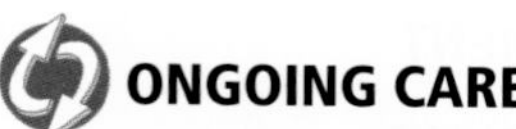

ONGOING CARE

FOLLOW-UP RECOMMENDATIONS

- Follow up 3–7 days after scheduled quit date and at least monthly for 3 months thereafter.
- Telephone follow-up if office visits not feasible
- Refraining from tobacco products for first 2 weeks is critical to long-term abstinence.
- Encourage patients who relapse to try again. Most smokers experience ≥1 failed attempts before quitting permanently. Reinforce behavioral interventions.

Patient Monitoring

- Short-term withdrawal symptoms include dysphoria, depressed mood, irritability, anxiety, insomnia, increased appetite, and poor concentration.
- Longer term risks of smoking cessation include weight gain (4–5 kg on average) and depression.
- Quitting also is associated with exacerbations of ulcerative colitis and worsening of cognitive function in patients with schizophrenia.
- Nicotine withdrawal syndrome: dysphoric or depressed mood, insomnia, irritability, frustration, or anger; anxiety, difficulty concentrating, restlessness, and increased appetite or weight gain
- Lung cancer risk by smoking status: heavy smokers 1.00, light smokers 9.44(0.35–056), ex-smokers 0.17(0.13–0.23), never smoker 0.09(0.06–0.13); adjusted hazard ratio (95% CI) (9)

DIET

Healthy eating for limiting weight gain following smoking cessation

PATIENT EDUCATION

1-800-QUIT-NOW: free counseling, resources, and support for quitting

PROGNOSIS

- Measurable cardiovascular benefits of smoking cessation begin as early as 24 hours after quitting and continue to mount until the risk is reduced to that of nonsmokers by 5–15 years.
- People who quit smoking after a heart attack or cardiac surgery reduce their risk of death by 1/3.
- Relapse rates initially >60% but decrease to 2–4% per year after completing 2 years of abstinence.

COMPLICATIONS

- Disability and premature death due to heart attack, stroke, cancer, COPD
- Smoking more than doubles the risk of coronary artery disease and doubles the risk of stroke.
- Smokers are 12–22× more likely than nonsmokers to die from lung cancer.

REFERENCES

1. Moyer VA, U.S. Preventive Services Task Force. Primary care interventions to prevent tobacco use in children and adolescents: U.S. Preventive Services Task Force recommendations statement. *Ann Intern Med*. 2013;159(8):552–557.
2. Cahill K, Stevens S, Perera R, et al. Pharmacological interventions for smoking cessation: an overview and network meta-analysis. *Cochrane Database Syst Rev*. 2013;5:CD009329. doi:10.1002/14651858.CD009329.pub2.
3. National Guideline Clearinghouse. *Guideline Synthesis: Treatment of Tobacco Dependence*. Rockville, MD: Agency for Healthcare Research and Quality; 2001.
4. Bhatnagar A, Whitsel LP, Ribisl KM,et al. Electronic cigarettes: a policy statement from the American Heart Association. *Circulation*. 2014;130(16):1418–1436.
5. Huges J, Stead L, Hartmann-Boyce J, et al. Antidepressants for smoking cessation. *Cochrane Database Syst Rev*. 2014;1:CD000031. doi:10.1002/14651858.CD000031.pub4.
6. Ussher M, Taylor A, Faulkner G. Exercise interventions for smoking cessation. *Cochrane Database Syst Rev*. 2012;1:CD002295. doi: 10.1002/14651858.CD002295.pub5.
7. White A. Rampes H, Liu JP, et al. Acupuncture and related interventions for smoking cessation. *Cochrane Database Syst Rev*. 2014;1:CD000009. doi:10.1002/14651858.CD000009.pub4.
8. David S, Lancaster T, Stead L, et al. Opiates antagonist for smoking cessation. *Cochrane Database Syst Rev*. 2013;6:CD003086. doi:10.1002/14651858 .CD003086.pub3.
9. Godtfredsen N, Prescott E, Osler M. Effect of smoking reduction on lung cancer risk. *JAMA* 2005;294(12):1505–1510.

T

ADDITIONAL READING

- Larzelere MM, Williams DE. Promoting smoking cessation. *Am Fam Physician*. 2012;85(6):591–598.
- Quitnet: www.quitnet.com

SEE ALSO

Nicotine Addiction; Substance Use Disorders

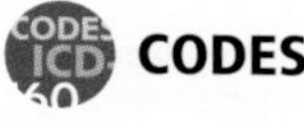

CODES

ICD10

- F17.210 Nicotine dependence, cigarettes, uncomplicated
- F17.213 Nicotine dependence, cigarettes, with withdrawal
- F17.211 Nicotine dependence, cigarettes, in remission

CLINICAL PEARLS

- Quitting smoking has both immediate and long-term health benefits.
- Every patient who uses tobacco should be offered smoking cessation.
- Use the 5 As: ask, advise, assess, assist, and arrange.
- Behavioral counseling and medication are most effective for helping patients to quit smoking when they are used in combination.
- Depression with suicidal ideations is a contraindication to use varenicline.

TORCH INFECTIONS

Katrina E. Walters, MD, FAAFP, FM • Michael Tarpey, MD

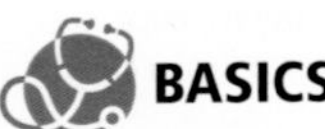

BASICS

DESCRIPTION

- An acronym describing a group of infections that are acquired prenatally or during the birth process and have similar physical findings, including skin and ocular manifestations
  - *T*oxoplasmosis: protozoan parasite, *Toxoplasma gondii*
  - *O*ther (syphilis): Spirochete, *Treponema pallidum*
  - *R*ubella: virus
  - *C*MV: cytomegalovirus
  - *H*erpes: herpes simplex virus (HSV)
- System(s) affected: skin/exocrine, HEENT, nervous, GI, lymphatic/heme, renal, cardiac, pulmonary
- Synonym(s): CMV infection, also known as cytomegalic inclusion disease (CID) or cytoplasmic inclusion body disease

EPIDEMIOLOGY

- Predominant age: prenatal to infants
- Predominant sex: male = female

Incidence

- Toxoplasmosis: 1.1/1,000 live births
- Syphilis: 10.1/100,000 live births
- Rubella: no longer endemic in the United States; rare cases seen with immigrant mothers
- CMV: 1/100 live births; defects present in 10% of infected infants
- Herpes: 1/5,000 live births

ETIOLOGY AND PATHOPHYSIOLOGY

- All infections transmitted vertically, either transplacentally or through maternal genital tract.
- Toxoplasmosis: *T. gondii* protozoan results in cyst dissemination throughout tissues and host cell death; maternal infection acquired via fecal–oral route
- Syphilis: Spirochetes cause inflammatory damage to most organ systems; maternal infection sexually transmitted
- Rubella: mechanism of damage unclear, possibly secondary to vasculitis; maternal infection through inhalation of aerosol particles
- CMV: Immunosuppressive virus replicates in leukocytes, secretory glands, and kidneys; maternal infection through close contact with infected body fluids (1–2-year-old children most common source)
- Herpes: Virus replicates in sensory ganglion; inability to control replication results in disseminated infection; maternal infection sexually transmitted

RISK FACTORS

- General: inadequate prenatal care
- Toxoplasmosis: risk of transmission highest in 3rd trimester: Effects are more severe with 1st- or 2nd-trimester infection; syphilis: congenital infection most likely with maternal early syphilis
- Rubella: inadequate maternal vaccination
- CMV: care for preschool-aged children during pregnancy; maternal age <25 years; risk of transmission highest in 3rd trimester and with primary maternal infection; effects more severe with 1st trimester infection
- Herpes: initial episode of HSV; active genital lesions at delivery; positive HSV serology at delivery *and* vaginal delivery; invasive monitoring; prolonged rupture of membranes; premature labor

GENERAL PREVENTION

- Toxoplasmosis: Avoid handling of cat litter and raw meat; avoid consumption of raw meat and unpasteurized goat milk; wear rubber gloves for meat preparation and gardening.
- Syphilis: Screen with VDRL or rapid plasma reagin (RPR) test at 1st prenatal visit and again in 3rd trimester and delivery for high-risk mothers; confirm with fluorescent treponemal antibody absorption (FTA-ABS). Give infected, previously untreated pregnant women penicillin G IM, dose 2.4 million units once for primary, secondary, or early latent; 2.4 million units weekly every 3 weeks for late latent and tertirary. Desensitize penicillin-allergic patients.

ALERT

- Treatment may provoke early labor or fetal distress (Jarisch-Herxheimer reaction) but should not be delayed (1)[A].
- Rubella: Test IgG titers to determine immunity at initial prenatal visit. Vaccinate nonimmune postpartum.
- CMV: Avoid prolonged exposure to young children during pregnancy; hand washing; insufficient evidence for immunoglobulin or vaccine use (2)[A]
- Herpes: Cesarean delivery for active genital lesions decreases transmission; insufficient evidence for antiviral prophylaxis decreasing neonatal herpes incidence, although it does decrease viral shedding, clinical lesions, and number of cesarean sections. Prophylactic treatment with acyclovir 200 mg QID or 400 mg TID or valacyclovir 500 mg BID starting at 36 weeks' gestation. Recommend treatment with acyclovir of the asymptomatic neonate delivered to mother with active lesions until neonatal PCR and viral cultures are negative and maternal serology and PCR indicate a recurrent episode (3)[A],(4)[C].

DIAGNOSIS

HISTORY

- Toxoplasmosis: no maternal symptoms or history of flulike syndrome
- Syphilis, rubella, and CMV: maternal history of fever and rash
- Herpes: 60–80% of newborn infections occur in mother with no known prior genital lesions.

PHYSICAL EXAM

- Common features: microcephaly, intracranial calcifications, rash, intrauterine growth restriction, jaundice, hepatosplenomegaly, hepatitis, and thrombocytopenia
- Toxoplasmosis: hydrocephalus, intracranial calcifications, chorioretinitis
- Syphilis: most infants asymptomatic; early signs are snuffles (rhinitis), poor feeding, retinitis, jaundice and hepatosplenomegaly; rash varies from red macular to bullous; chronic infection may present with neurosyphilis (tabes dorsalis, deafness), Hutchinson incisors, mulberry molars, saddle nose deformity, or uveitis.
- Rubella: Classic triad involves sensorineural hearing loss, ocular abnormalities (cataracts, glaucoma, retinopathy), and congenital heart disease (patent ductus arteriosus [PDA]).
- CMV: Most infected infants are asymptomatic; 10% with symptoms including common features mentioned earlier and petechiae and purpura (blueberry muffin rash), deafness, chorioretinitis
- Herpes: vesicular lesions on skin, eyes, or mouth; fever; irritability; focal neurologic symptoms

DIFFERENTIAL DIAGNOSIS

- Congenital lymphocytic choriomeningitis virus
- Encephalopathies
- Meningitis
- Parvovirus B19
- Bacterial sepsis
- HIV
- Varicella
- Epstein-Barr virus
- Enteroviruses
- Hepatitis B

DIAGNOSTIC TESTS & INTERPRETATION

Initial Tests (lab, imaging)

- Toxoplasmosis: Isolation of organism from serum/CSF is definitive but difficult; newborn serum testing of IgM and IgA antibodies; maternal blood enzyme linked immunoassay (EIA); head CT (ring-enhancing lesions, diffuse calcifications (5)
- Syphilis: newborn screen with VDRL or RPR test, confirm with FTA-ABS; CSF for VDRL, cell count, and protein; chest x-ray (CXR) (pneumonia alba); long bone x-ray (onion-skinning, rat bite tibia) (6)
- Rubella: viral isolation by polymerase chain reaction (PCR) preferred over serologic testing.
- CMV: DNA PCR or viral culture from urine or saliva in first 3 weeks of life; PCR on dried blood spot available for retrospective testing but low sensitivity (34–100%); cranial ultrasound (intracranial calcifications, white matter loss, ventriculomegaly, microgyria) (2,7)[A]
- Herpes: HSV culture of vesicle, mucosal surfaces; CSF PCR; MRI brain if concern for encephalitis

Follow-Up Tests & Special Considerations

- Rubella: echocardiography to diagnose heart defects; head CT may show intracranial calcifications.
- CMV: brain MRI for symptomatic newborns or if abnormalities on cranial ultrasound
- HSV: If CSF PCR positive, repeat LP until PCR DNA negative prior to discontinuing antibiotics (4)[C]

Diagnostic Procedures/Other

- Toxoplasmosis: opthalmic exam
- Rubella and CMV: ophthalmic and audiology evaluation
- Herpes: ophthalmic exam

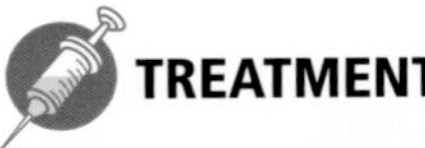

TREATMENT

GENERAL MEASURES

- Nutritional and respiratory support
- Phototherapy for hyperbilirubinemia

MEDICATION

First Line

- Toxoplasmosis: Pyrimethamine (1 mg/kg/day PO daily for 6 months, then Monday, Wednesday, Friday for 6 months; max 25 mg/day) and sulfadiazine (100 mg/kg/day PO q12h) for 12 months in both symptomatic and asymptomatic infants. Folinic acid (5–10 mg 3×/week) to reduce hematologic toxicity (7)[B]
- Syphilis: aqueous crystalline penicillin G 50,000 U/kg IV q12h for 7 days, then q8h for total treatment of 10 days. Desensitize patient if penicillin-allergic (1)[A].
- Rubella: No specific antiviral agent indicated.
- CMV: Ganciclovir 6 mg/kg IV q12h for 6 weeks for severe disease or CNS symptoms (8)[A]
- Herpes: insufficient evidence to evaluate antiviral use in neonates; recommended treatment is acyclovir 20 mg/kg IV q8h for 14–21 days (4)[C],(9)[A].

Second Line

- Syphilis: procaine penicillin G 50,000 U/kg IM daily for 10 days (1)[A]
- CMV: valganciclovir 15 mg/kg PO BID for 6 weeks (off-label use) (8)[A]

ISSUES FOR REFERRAL

Consider consultation based on organ systems involved (ophthalmology, cardiology, neurology, orthopedics).

SURGERY/OTHER PROCEDURES

- Possibility of gastrostomy placement based on nutritional needs
- Rubella: repair of congenital heart defects

INPATIENT CONSIDERATIONS

Admission Criteria/Initial Stabilization

Infected neonates to remain inpatient from birth; respiratory support

IV Fluids

Indicated if oral feeding is inadequate; determined by weight-based calculations

Discharge Criteria

Once stable and treatment is completed or arranged on outpatient basis; infants infected with rubella must remain hospitalized in isolation until 2 cultures taken 1 month apart are negative.

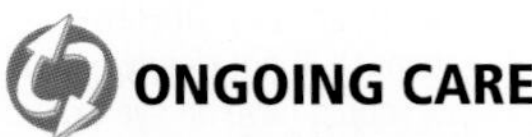

ONGOING CARE

FOLLOW-UP RECOMMENDATIONS

Patient Monitoring

- Continue to follow neurologic and developmental status.
- Toxoplasmosis: follow-up every 2 weeks until stable, then monthly while being treated; CBC every week for 1 month, then every 2 weeks
- Syphilis: serologic testing every 2–3 months until nonreactive or 4-fold titer decrease (should occur by 6 months of age, otherwise, repeat LP and treatment). If CSF is abnormal, repeat LP every 6 months until normal (1)[A].
- Rubella: vision and hearing screens
- CMV: hearing screens every 2–3 months until age 3 years, then annually until age 6 years; annual eye exam until age 5 years for symptomatic newborns; CBC and LFTs weekly during treatment (risk of pancytopenia/hepatitis toxicity) (2)[A]

DIET

Normal diet, as tolerated

PATIENT EDUCATION

- An infected mother should be informed of potential harm to the fetus.
- Pregnant women should avoid contact with those infected with rubella.

PROGNOSIS

- Toxoplasmosis: development and behavior normal with adequate treatment; chorioretinitis in 26% of treated infants
- Syphilis: 6.4% mortality rate; poor if symptomatic in first few weeks of life
- Rubella: poor outcome with significant organ damage
- CMV: normal development if 12-month exam within normal limits; chorioretinitis untreatable
- Herpes: 30% mortality of treated disseminated disease; good outcome with treated mucocutaneous infections.

COMPLICATIONS

- Toxoplasmosis: meningoencephalitis with hydrocephalus, seizure disorder, vision impairment, deafness, mental retardation
- Syphilis: pneumonia alba, stillbirth, multiple organ damage
- Rubella: deafness, vision impairment, skeletal defects, congenital heart defects
- CMV: progressive, delayed hearing loss, chorioretinitis, pancytopenia
- Herpes: seizures, pneumonia, adrenal involvement, respiratory distress, liver dysfunction, eczema herpeticum

REFERENCES

1. Workowski KA, Berman S; Centers for Disease Control and Prevention. Sexually transmitted diseases treatment guidelines, 2010. *MMWR Recomm Rep*. 2010;59(RR-12):1–110.
2. Goderis J, De Leenheer E, Smets K, et al. Hearing loss and congenital CMV infection: a systematic review. *Pediatrics*. 2014;134(5):972–982.
3. Hollier LM, Wendel GD. Third trimester antiviral prophylaxis for preventing maternal genital herpes simplex virus (HSV) recurrences and neonatal infection. *Cochrane Database Syst Rev*. 2008;(1):CD004946. doi:10.1002/14651858.cd004946.pub2.
4. Kimberlin DW, Baley J; Committee on Infectious Diseases and Committee on Fetus and Newborn. Guidance on management of asymptomatic neonates born to women with active genital lesions. *Pediatrics*. 2013;131(2):e635–e646.
5. Del Pizzo J. Focus on diagnosis: congenital Infections (TORCH). *Pediatr Rev*. 2011;32(12):537–542.
6. Cohen SE, Klausner JD, Engelman J, et al. Syphilis in the modern era: an update for physicians. *Infect Dis Clin North Am*. 2013;27(4):705–722.
7. Mcleod R, Boyer K, Karrison T, et al. Outcome of treatment for congenital toxoplasmosis, 1981–2004: the National Collaborative Chicago-Based, Congenital Toxoplasmosis Study. *Clin Infect Dis*. 2006;42(10):1383–1394.
8. Kadambari S, Williams EJ, Luck S, et al. Evidence based management guidelines for the detection and treatment of congenital CMV. *Early Hum Dev*. 2011;87(11):723–728.
9. Jones CA, Walker KS, Badawi N. Antiviral agents for treatment of herpes simplex virus infection in neonates. *Cochrane Database Syst Rev*. 2009;(3):CD004206. doi:10.1002/14651858.CD004206.pub2.

ADDITIONAL READING

- Anzivino E, Fioriti D, Mischitelli M, et al. Herpes simplex virus infection in pregnancy and in neonate: status of art of epidemiology, diagnosis, therapy and prevention. *Virol J*. 2009;6:40.
- Control and prevention of rubella: evaluation and management of suspected outbreaks, rubella in pregnant women, and surveillance for congenital rubella syndrome. *MMWR Recomm Rep*. 2001;50(RR-12):1–23.
- de Jong EP, Vossen AC, Walther FJ, et al. How to use . . . neonatal TORCH testing. *Arch Dis Child Educ Pract Ed*. 2013;98(3):93–98.

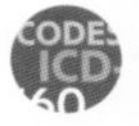

CODES

ICD10

- P00.2 Newborn affected by maternal infec/parastc diseases
- P37.1 Congenital toxoplasmosis
- P35.1 Congenital cytomegalovirus infection

CLINICAL PEARLS

- Adequate prenatal care is paramount for prevention of TORCH infections.
- TORCH infections may present similarly, but targeted diagnostic workups are indicated based on clinical presentation. Providers should remain diligent to possible neonatal HSV given the majority of cases occur in mothers with no prior history of genital lesions.
- Sequelae of TORCH infections may have delayed presentations and infants require regular monitoring.

T

TORTICOLLIS

Bryan C. Bordeaux, DO, MPH • Tisamarie B. Sherry, MD, PhD

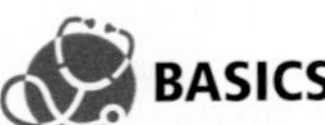

BASICS

DESCRIPTION

- Torticollis is a spectrum of disorders characterized by head tilt with rotation or involuntary movement.
- Pediatric disorders include the following:
  - Congenital muscular torticollis (CMT): seen at birth or in early infancy—accounts for 80% of torticollis cases presenting in infancy. Results from unilateral fibrosis and shortening of the sternocleidomastoid (SCM) muscle
  - Acquired torticollis
- Adult disorders include the following:
  - Acquired torticollis (also known as "wryneck")—usually self-limited.
  - Spasmodic torticollis, (cervical dystonia) caused by recurrent involuntary muscular contractions
  - Other less common forms of torticollis include oculogyric, gastroesophageal reflux–induced, arthritis-related, scoliosis-related, and hysterical torticollis.
- System(s) affected: musculoskeletal; nervous
- Synonym(s): acute wryneck; idiopathic generalized torticollis; SCM torticollis; neonatal torticollis; idiopathic cervical dystonia; focal dystonia; nuchal dystonia

EPIDEMIOLOGY

- ~90% of cases occur in individuals aged 31–60 years.
- Predominant age: CMT: newborn and infants; pediatric acquired torticollis, <10 years; adult acquired torticollis, 30–60 years; spasmodic torticollis, 30–50 years (mean age 40–43 years)
- Predominant sex: spasmodic torticollis, female > male (1.6:1); CMT, male > female (3:2)

Incidence

Congenital: up to 1/250 births; spasmodic: 1/100,000; overall incidence for torticollis is 24/1 million persons.

Prevalence

All focal dystonias combined: 295/1 million persons; no reliable data for acquired torticollis.

ETIOLOGY AND PATHOPHYSIOLOGY

- CMT
  - Intrauterine malpositioning may lead to foreshortening and fibrosis of the SCM.
  - Birth trauma (e.g., clavicular fracture) can lead to CMT as well.
- Pediatric acquired torticollis
  - CNS disorders, increased intracranial pressure
  - Ocular disorders—abnormal head/neck positioning as visual compensation
  - Bony abnormalities, soft tissue pathologies
  - Gastrointestinal disease
  - Drug induced
  - Conversion disorder
- Adult acquired torticollis
  - Emotional stress, postural factors (e.g., work, sleep, lying while reading or watching TV, prolonged unusual positioning of neck), or exposure to cold. Many cases are idiopathic.
  - Medication reactions (most commonly anticholinergics, amphetamines, and certain anesthetic agents)
- Spasmodic torticollis
  - Muscular spasm secondary to traumatic, infectious or inflammatory insult
  - Cervical spine injuries and spondylosis, ocular disorders, organic CNS disorders, psychogenic causes, certain tumors and vestibular dysfunction can all contribute to cervical dystonia.

Genetics

Spasmotic torticollis may also have a genetic basis.

RISK FACTORS

- CMT: intrauterine crowding, breech presentation, ischemia, birth injury
- Pediatric acquired torticollis: soft tissue inflammation or infection, neurologic disease, visual disturbances, trauma
- Adult acquired torticollis: stress, unusual neck position (particularly when sleeping), exposure to cold, medications, trauma, infection
- Spasmodic: family history of dystonia, soft tissue inflammation or infection, neurologic conditions, visual disturbances, trauma

Pediatric Considerations

CMT: without treatment becomes a fibrous cord and may be associated with persistent craniofacial deformities and persistent torticollis

COMMONLY ASSOCIATED CONDITIONS

- >80% of infants with CMT present with craniofacial asymmetry, deformational plagiocephaly, and developmental dysplasia of the hip (DDH).
- CMT and pediatric acquired torticollis: Consider Klippel-Feil syndrome (congenital fusion of cervical vertebrae).
- Pediatric and adult acquired torticollis: Consider spinal abnormalities, tumors.
- Spasmodic torticollis often accompanied by behavioral health conditions

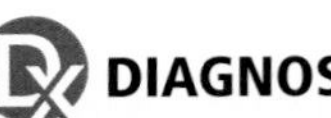

DIAGNOSIS

HISTORY

- Abnormal head posture, neck pain, headache, neck muscle stiffness, restricted neck range of motion, neck mass or swelling
- Birth history in children
- Family history of dystonias
- Medication history
- Recent cervical spine trauma

PHYSICAL EXAM

- Normal ROM: flexion 60 degrees; extension 75 degrees; rotation 90 degrees; side-bending 45 degrees
- Torticollis presents as rotational (twisting), anterocollis (flexion), laterocollis (side bending), and retrocollis (extension) with the head tilting to the affected side (80%, to right side) and the chin rotating to the opposite side.
- Spasm of trapezius, SCM, and other neck muscles
- Tenderness over the affected SCM
- Neck mass, lymphadenopathy
- Craniofacial asymmetry (plagiocephaly) consistent with congenital or chronic torticollis
- Phasic jerking or tremor of antagonist muscles
- Physical gesturing (*geste antagoniste*) such as touching face or chin to reduce dystonia (pathognomonic for spasmodic torticollis)
- Ocular irregularities (e.g., diplopia)
- Spinal abnormality: Short neck with low posterior hairline may indicate occipitocervical synostosis.
- Structural abnormalities of the hips or feet
- Common physical findings in different types of torticollis
  - CMT: Firm, nontender, palpable enlargement of the SCM may appear from birth or develop over weeks.
  - Pediatric and adult acquired torticollis: unilateral neck stiffness, pain, spasm, or decreased ROM without trauma
  - Spasmodic torticollis may initially present with neck stiffness progressing to pain, head jerking, and neck spasms.

DIFFERENTIAL DIAGNOSIS

- Osseous
  - Atlantoaxial rotatory subluxation
  - Atlanto-occipital subluxation
  - Posttraumatic fracture or dislocation
  - Cervical disc disease
  - Congenital scoliosis
  - Klippel-Feil syndrome
  - Occipitocervical synostosis
  - Grisel syndrome
  - Syringomyelia
  - Arnold-Chiari malformation
- Nonosseous
  - Myositis involving cervical muscles
  - Soft tissue trauma
  - Neoplastic: spinal cord tumor, acoustic neuroma, osteoblastoma, orbital tumor, fibromatosis, metastasis
  - Infection: upper respiratory infection, cervical lymph node abscess, epidural abscess, retropharyngeal abscess, vertebral osteomyelitis
  - Vestibular disorders
  - Essential head tremor
  - Basal ganglion diseases
  - Cranial nerve palsy
  - Psychiatric disorders
  - Drugs or toxins
  - Down syndrome
  - Sandifer syndrome
  - Myasthenia gravis

DIAGNOSTIC TESTS & INTERPRETATION

Lab studies are only needed to exclude underlying disease.

- Radiographs should be taken to rule out spinal pathology in traumatic and congenital cases.
- Consider MRI or CT scan of cervical spine for patients with neurologic deficits.
- CMT can be confirmed with US of involved SCM.

Follow-Up Tests & Special Considerations

Infants with CMT should be screened for DDH by physical exam and subsequent US if not clearly normal (1)[C]. All pediatric patients should have an eye exam.

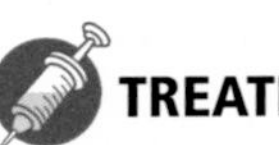

TREATMENT

GENERAL MEASURES

- CMT
  - >90% of children achieve good outcome with conservative treatment if initiated by age 1 year.
  - Conservative treatment includes positioning, environmental adaptations, passive and active stretching of the tight SCM muscle, strengthening of weak neck and trunk muscles, and movement therapy.
  - Physical therapy (PT) and stretching should be started before ages 3–6 months (2)[B].
  - Place toys on opposite side of bed from rotational deformity to encourage use of affected muscles.
  - Surgery is indicated for refractory cases, a tight muscular band, or SCM mass.

- Pediatric acquired torticollis
  - Place a television on opposite side of bed from rotational deformity.
  - Some patients respond well to low-dose levodopa (100–300 mg) with carbidopa.
- Adult and pediatric acquired torticollis
  - Conservative management includes soft cervical collar, intermittent heat or ice, bed rest, and analgesics for pain relief.
- Spasmodic
  - Conservative: soft cervical collar, heat or ice, bed rest
  - Selective peripheral nerve denervation
  - Pallidal deep brain stimulation can achieve lasting improvements in medication-resistant cases (3)[B].

MEDICATION

First Line

- Treatment for spasms
  - Botulinum toxin injections may be more effective than anticholinergic drugs for cervical dystonia (4)[B],(5)[A]. Major predictors of treatment success are correct dosing and identification of affected muscles. Note that the recommended doses are general guidelines and must be individualized to the patient. EMG (6)[A] or PET-CT (7)[B] may help guide the injection site. Immunoresistance can develop but is rare (8)[A]:
    - Botulinum toxin types A and B have been found effective and safe for treating adults (≥16) with cervical dystonia (9)[A].
    - CMT: botulinum toxin type A was found effective in a case series (2)[C].
  - Botox: botulinum toxin type A
    - Adult: initial 1.25–2.5 units (0.05–0.1 mL) IM into most active neck muscles; repeat every 3–4 months; not to exceed 200 units cumulative dose in 1-month period
    - Pediatric: <12 years of age, not established; >12 years, administer as for adults
    - Xeomin (botulinum toxin type A free from complexing proteins) has shown comparable safety and efficacy to Botox (10)[B].
  - Myobloc: botulinum toxin type B
    - Adult: 2,500–5,000 units IM divided among affected muscles in patients treated previously with any type of botulinum toxin; use lower dose in untreated patients.
    - Pediatric: not established
  - Diazepam
    - Adult: 2–10 mg PO TID/QID
    - Pediatric: 1–2.5 mg PO TID/QID; increase gradually as needed or tolerated.
  - Diphenhydramine or diazepam can be used for torticollis caused by medications (4)[C]:
    - Diphenhydramine
      - Adult: 25–50 mg PO q6–8h PRN, not to exceed 400 mg/day; 10–50 mg IV/IM q6–8h PRN, not to exceed 400 mg/day
      - Pediatric: 12.5–25 mg PO TID/QID or 5 mg/kg/day or 150 mg/m^2/day divided TID/QID. PRN, not to exceed 300 mg/day; 5 mg/kg/day IV/IM or 150 mg/m^2/day, divided QID. PRN, not to exceed 300 mg/day
  - Anticholinergics may relieve acute muscle spasms (4)[C], but high doses are usually necessary and benefit is often delayed.
  - Carbidopa-levodopa (4)[C] for focal dystonia of unknown cause: Trial might be warranted although some non–dopa-responsive dystonias improve, equal numbers have symptoms worsen.
- Treatment for pain
  - NSAIDs and acetaminophen; consider opiates for only the most severe pain.

ISSUES FOR REFERRAL

- Refer prolonged symptoms of idiopathic spasmodic torticollis to a neurologist.
- Fixed deformities in children may require surgical consultation.
- CMT: Refer if visual dysfunction (ophthalmology), failed hip screen (orthopedics), abnormal neurologic exam (neurology), plagiocephaly (plastic surgery), or patient presents with bony prominence (orthopedics).

ADDITIONAL THERAPIES

- Osteopathic manipulation may be useful:
  - Direct myofascial stretching of cervical region with attention to the SCM
  - Occipital-atlantal release
  - V-spread of the occipitomastoid suture on the side of restriction
  - Muscle energy and/or functional positional release at the cervical region
- PT may be beneficial for acquired childhood and adult torticollis (11)[B].
- If detected early, 90% of CMT responds to stretching exercises.

SURGERY/OTHER PROCEDURES

CMT: Surgical release if PT is unsuccessful by age 1 year

COMPLEMENTARY & ALTERNATIVE MEDICINE

Acupuncture may also provide benefit.

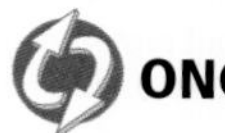

ONGOING CARE

FOLLOW-UP RECOMMENDATIONS

- Monitor infants with CMT every 2–4 weeks until resolved.
- Depression is common in protracted cases, screen accordingly.

PROGNOSIS

- CMT: good for correctable pathologies
  - 50–70% resolve spontaneously by 1st year
  - >90% of children achieve good to excellent outcomes with conservative treatment when therapy is instituted by age 1 year.
- Pediatric acquired torticollis: good when the underlying pathology is discovered and treated
- Adult acquired torticollis: excellent; generally resolves in a few days to weeks
- Spasmodic: may wax and wane for years, even with treatment

COMPLICATIONS

- Facial asymmetry in CMT; possibly an increased risk of developmental delay/disorders
- Dental malocclusion
- Degenerative osteoarthritis of the cervical spine, hypertrophy of the SCM muscle, and paresthesia due to compressed nerve roots
- Depression

REFERENCES

1. Joiner ERA, Andras LM, Skaggs DL. Screening for hip dysplasia in congenital muscular torticollis: is physical exam enough? *J Child Orthop*. 2014;8(2):115–119.
2. Do TT. Congenital muscular torticollis: current concepts and review of treatment. *Curr Opin Pediatr*. 2006;18(1):26–29.
3. Walsh RA, Sidiropoulos C, Lozano AM, et al. Bilateral pallidal stimulation in cervical dystonia: blinded evidence of benefit beyond 5 years. *Brain*. 2013;136(Pt 3):761–769.
4. Tarsy D, Simon DK. Dystonia. *N Engl J Med*. 2006;355(8):818–829.
5. Patel S, Martino D. Cervical dystonia: from pathophysiology to pharmacotherapy. *Behav Neurol*. 2013;26(4):275–282.
6. Nijmeijer SW, Koelman JH, Kamphuis DJ, et al. Muscle selection for treatment of cervical dystonia with botulinum toxin—a systematic review. *Parkinsonism Relat Disord*. 2012;18(6):731–736.
7. Lee HB, An YS, Lee HY, et al. Usefulness of (18)f-fluorodeoxyglucose positron emission tomography/computed tomography in management of cervical dystonia. *Ann Rehabil Med*. 2012;36(6):745–755.
8. Coleman C, Hubble J, Schwab J, et al. Immunoresistance in cervical dystonia patients after treatment with abotulinum toxin A. *Int J Neurosci*. 2012;122(7):358–362.
9. Simpson DM, Blitzer A, Brashear A, et al. Assessment: botulinum neurotoxin for the treatment of movement disorders (an evidence-based review): report of the Therapeutics and Technology Assessment Subcommittee of the American Academy of Neurology. *Neurology*. 2008;70(19):1699–1706.
10. Dressler D, Paus S, Seitzinger A, et al. Long-term efficacy and safety of incobotulinumtoxinA injections in patients with cervical dystonia. *J Neurol Neurosurg Psychiatry*. 2013;84(9):1014–1019.
11. Queiroz MA, Chien HF, Sekeff-Salem FA, et al. Physical therapy program for cervical dystonia: a study of 20 cases. *Funct Neurol*. 2012;27(3):187–192.

ADDITIONAL READING

- Consky EA. Clinical assessments of patients with cervical dystonia. In: Jancovic J & Hallett M, eds. *Therapy with Botulinum Toxin*. New York, NY: Marcel Dekker; 1994:211–237.
- Jankovic J. Treatment of cervical dystonia with botulinum toxin. *Mov Disord*. 2004;19(Suppl 8):S109–S115.
- Tomczak KK, Rosman NP. Torticollis. *J Child Neurol*. 2013;28(3):365–378.

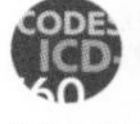

CODES

ICD10

- M43.6 Torticollis
- Q68.0 Congenital deformity of sternocleidomastoid muscle
- G24.3 Spasmodic torticollis

CLINICAL PEARLS

- Suspect torticollis in patients with head tilt, chin lift, and restricted movement of the neck.
- Consider secondary causes, and rule out as necessary based on history and physical exam.
- Most adult cases are self-limiting and resolve within days to weeks.
- In congenital and acquired pediatric cases, placing items of interest to the child (e.g., TV, toys) on the opposite side of the bed helps to speed resolution.

T

TOURETTE SYNDROME

Evan R. Horton, PharmD • Brendan P. Kelly, MD

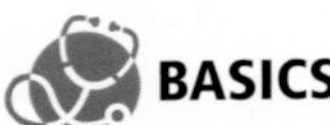

BASICS

DESCRIPTION

- A childhood-onset neurobehavioral disorder characterized by the presence of multiple motor and at least 1 phonic tic (see "Physical Exam")
  - Tics are sudden, brief, repetitive, stereotyped motor movements (motor tics) or sounds (phonic tics) produced by moving air through the nose, mouth, or throat.
  - Tics tend to occur in bouts.
  - Tics can be simple or complex.
    - Motor tics precede vocal tics.
    - Simple tics precede complex tics.
  - Tics often are preceded by sensory symptoms, especially a compulsion to move.
  - Patients are able to suppress their tics, but voluntary suppression is associated with an inner tension that results in more forceful tics when suppression ceases.
  - System(s) affected: nervous

EPIDEMIOLOGY

Incidence

- Predominant age
  - Average age of onset: 7 years (3–8 years)
  - Tic severity is greatest at ages 7–12 years.
    - 96% present by age 11 years
  - Of children with Tourette syndrome (TS), 50% will experience complete resolution of symptoms by age 18 years (based on self-reporting).
- Predominant sex: male > female (3:1)
- Predominant race/ethnicity: clinically heterogeneous disorder, but non-Hispanic whites 2:1 compared with Hispanics and/or blacks

Prevalence

0.77% overall in children

- 1.06% in boys
- 0.25% in girls

ETIOLOGY AND PATHOPHYSIOLOGY

Abnormalities of dopamine neurotransmission and receptor hypersensitivity, most likely in the ventral striatum, play a primary role in the pathophysiology.

- Abnormality of basal ganglia development
- Mechanism is uncertain; may involve dysfunction of basal ganglia–thalamocortical circuits, likely involving decreased inhibitory output from the basal ganglia, which results in an imbalance of inhibition and excitation in the motor cortex
- Controversial pediatric autoimmune neuropsychiatric disorder association with *Streptococcus* (PANDAS)
  - TS/obsessive-compulsive disorder (OCD) cases linked to immunologic response to previous group A β-hemolytic streptococcal infection (GABHS)
  - Thought to be linked to 10% of all TS cases
  - 5 criteria
    - Presence of tic disorder and/or OCD
    - Prepubertal onset of neuropsychosis
    - History of sudden onset of symptoms and/or episodic course with abrupt symptom exacerbation, interspersed with periods of partial/complete remission
    - Evidence of a temporal association between onset/exacerbation of symptoms and a prior streptococcal infection
    - Adventitious movements during symptom exacerbation (e.g., motor hyperactivity)

Genetics

- Predisposition: frequent familial history of tic disorders and OCD
- Precise pattern of transmission and genetic origin unknown. Recent studies suggest polygenic inheritance with evidence for a locus on chromosome 17q; sequence variants in *SLITRK1* gene on chromosome 13q also are associated with TS.
- Higher concordance in monozygotic compared with dizygotic twins; wide range of phenotypes

RISK FACTORS

- Risk of TS among relatives: 9.8–15%
- 1st-degree relatives of individuals with TS have a 10–100-fold increased risk of developing TS.
- Low birth weight, maternal stress during pregnancy, severe nausea and vomiting in 1st trimester

COMMONLY ASSOCIATED CONDITIONS

- OCD (28–67%)
- ADHD (50–60%)
- Conduct disorder
- Depression/anxiety including phobias, panic attacks, and stuttering
- Learning disabilities (23%)
- Impairments of visual perception, sleep disorders, restless leg syndrome, and migraine headaches

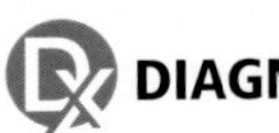

DIAGNOSIS

HISTORY

Diagnosis of TS is based on history and clinical presentation (i.e., observation of tics with/without presence of coexisting disorders). Identify comorbid conditions.

PHYSICAL EXAM

- Typically, the physical exam is normal.
- Motor and vocal tics are the clinical hallmarks.
- Tics fluctuate in type, frequency, and anatomic distribution over time.
- Multiple motor tics include facial grimacing, blinking, head/neck jerking, tongue protruding, sniffing, and touching.
- Vocal tics include grunts, snorts, throat clearing, barking, yelling, and hiccupping.
- Tics are exacerbated by anticipation, emotional upset, anxiety, or fatigue.
- Tics subside when patient is concentrating/absorbed in activities.
- Motor and vocal tics may persist during all stages of sleep, especially light sleep.
- Blink reflex abnormalities may be observed.
- No known clinical measures reliably predict children who will continue to express tics in adulthood; severity of tics in late childhood is associated with future tic severity.
- *Diagnostic and Statistical Manual of Mental Disorders* (5th ed.; *DSM-5*) criteria (1)[C]:
  - A. Both multiple motor and one or more vocal tics have been present at some time during the illness, although not necessarily concurrently.
  - B. The tics may wax and wane in frequency but have persisted for more than 1 year since first tic onset.
  - C. Onset is before age 18 years.
  - D. The disturbance is not attributable to the physiologic effects of a substance (e.g., cocaine) or another medical condition (e.g., Huntington disease, postviral encephalitis).

DIFFERENTIAL DIAGNOSIS

- Chronic motor/vocal tic disorder
- Transient tic disorder
- Tic disorder not otherwise specified
- Huntington disease
- Stroke
- Lesch-Nyhan syndrome
- Wilson disease
- Sydenham chorea
- Multiple sclerosis
- Postviral encephalitis
- Head injury
- Seizures
- Toxin exposure (e.g., carbon monoxide)
- Drug effects (e.g., dopamine agonists, fluoroquinolones)

DIAGNOSTIC TESTS & INTERPRETATION

Initial Tests (lab, imaging)

- No definitive lab tests diagnose TS.
- Thyroid-stimulating hormone (TSH) should be measured because of association of tics with hyperthyroidism.
- No imaging studies diagnose TS.
- EEG shows nonspecific abnormalities; useful only to differentiate tics from epilepsy

Test Interpretation

- Smaller caudate volumes in patients with TS
- Striatal dopaminergic terminals are increased, as is striatal dopamine transporter (DAT) density.

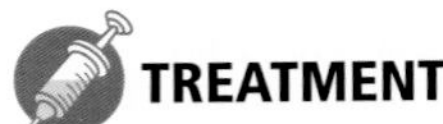

TREATMENT

GENERAL MEASURES

- Treatment assessment
  - Yale Global Tic Severity Score
  - Tourette Syndrome Severity Scale
  - Global Assessment of Functioning Scale
  - Gilles de la Tourette Syndrome Quality of Life Scale
- Educate that tics are neither voluntary nor psychiatric.
- Many patients require no treatment; patient should play an active role in treatment decisions.
- Educate patient, family, teachers, and friends to identify and address psychosocial stressors and environmental triggers.
- No cure for tics: Treatment is purely symptomatic, and multimodal treatment usually is indicated.
- Neurologic and psychiatric evaluation may be useful for other primary disorders and comorbid conditions (especially ADHD, OCD, and depression).
- TS clusters with several comorbid conditions; each disorder must be evaluated for associated functional impairment because patients often are more disabled by their psychiatric conditions than by the tics; choice of initial treatment depends largely on worst symptoms (tics, obsessions, or impulsivity).
- When pharmacotherapy is employed, monotherapy is preferred to polytherapy.

MEDICATION

First Line

- Atypical antipsychotics
- Risperidone: now recommended for standard therapy (2)[A]
  - Initiate 0.25 BID; titrate to 0.25–6 mg/day
  - As effective as haloperidol and pimozide for tics with fewer side effects
  - Effective against comorbidities such as OCD
  - Side effects may limit use: sedation, weight gain, and fatigue.
- α_2-Adrenergic receptor agonists (3)[B]
  - Historically, 1st-line agents due to favorable side-effect profile, but suboptimal efficacy in limited clinical trials
  - Side effects: sedation and hypotension common
    - Initiate therapy gradually and taper when discontinuing to avoid cardiac adverse events.
  - Clonidine 0.1–0.3 mg/day given BID to TID
    - Maximum dose: 0.5 mg/day
    - 25–50% of patients report at least some reduction in tics.
  - Guanfacine 1–3 mg/day given daily or BID
    - Less sedating and longer duration of action compared with clonidine
    - Improves motor/vocal tics by 30% in some studies; no better than placebo in others

Second Line

- Neuroleptics
  - Typical antipsychotics
    - High risk for extrapyramidal symptoms (EPS)
    - Haloperidol: initiate 0.5 mg/day and titrate 0.5 mg/week up to 1–4 mg at bedtime (2)[B]
      - FDA-approved for treating tics
      - Considered last option of typical antipsychotics due to lower efficacy and increased side effects compared to similar medications
    - Pimozide: initiate 0.5 mg/day and titrate 0.5 mg/week up to 1–4 mg at bedtime (4)[A]
      - FDA-approved for treating tics
      - Risk of cardiac toxicity (prolonged Q–T interval and arrhythmias); must be given under ECG monitoring; long-term use may induce sedation, weight gain, depression, pseudoparkinsonism, and akathisia.
      - Found to work better in long-term control of tics versus acute exacerbations
    - Fluphenazine: 2.5–10 mg/day
      - Effective but less favored due to side effects
  - Atypical antipsychotics (2)[C]
    - Olanzapine: initiate 2.5–5.0 mg/day; titrate up to 20 mg/day
      - Equally effective as haloperidol and pimozide
      - May cause metabolic disturbances and weight gain
    - Quetiapine: initiate 100–150 mg/day; titrate to 100–600 mg/day
      - Well tolerated but limited data exists
    - Ziprasidone: 5–40 mg/day
    - Aripiprazole: initiate 2 mg/day; titrate up to 20 or 30 mg/day
      - Few studies but favorable side-effect profile
- Alternative treatments
  - Topiramate: 25–200 mg/day (3)[A]; promising data but not sufficient efficacy so far to recommend as first or second line
  - Tetrabenazine
  - Baclofen
- Treatment of ADHD in patients with tics (5)[A]
  - Stimulants
    - Comorbid tic disorder is not a serious contraindication, as previously held; exacerbation of tics is neither clinically significant nor common.
    - Methylphenidate: 2.5–30 mg/day
    - Dextroamphetamine: 5–30 mg/day
  - α_2-Adrenergic agonists
    - Guanfacine
    - Clonidine
      - The combination of methylphenidate and clonidine has shown superior efficacy in treating both ADHD and tic symptoms compared to monotherapy with either agent in 1 trial.
  - Other medications
    - Atomoxetine
    - Desipramine
- Treatment of OCD in patients with tics (6)[B]
  - SSRIs
    - 1st-line treatment of OCD
    - Side effects include nausea, insomnia, sexual dysfunction, headache, and agitation.
    - Comorbid tic disorder not a contraindication; exacerbation of tics neither clinically significant nor common.
    - Black box warning for suicidality with SSRIs Fluoxetine: 10–80 mg/day
    - Fluvoxamine: 50–300 mg/day
    - Sertraline: 50–200 mg/day
  - Tricyclic antidepressants
    - Clomipramine: 25–200 mg/day
      - Can be used in patients refractory to SSRIs or to augment SSRIs in partial responders
      - Side effects: weight gain, dry mouth, lowered seizure threshold, and constipation; ECG changes, including Q–T prolongation and tachycardia

ADDITIONAL THERAPIES

- Botulinum toxin injections in severe cases or where chronic medication therapy is not preferred
- Habit-reversal training provides a viable tic suppression treatment: works equally for motor and vocal tics.

SURGERY/OTHER PROCEDURES

Thalamic ablation and deep brain stimulation have been used experimentally (7)[C].

COMPLEMENTARY & ALTERNATIVE MEDICINE

Nonpharmacologic therapy

- Reassurance and environmental modification
- Identification and treatment of triggers
- Behavioral therapy: awareness/assertiveness training, relaxation therapy, habit-reversal therapy, and self-monitoring has shown to significantly decrease tic severity.
- Hypnotherapy
- Biofeedback
- Acupuncture
- Cannabinoids: insufficient evidence to recommend; small trials show small positive effects in some parameters (8)[A].

ONGOING CARE

FOLLOW-UP RECOMMENDATIONS

Patient Monitoring

Observe for associated psychiatric disorders.

PATIENT EDUCATION

- Reassurance that many patients with tics do not need medication; often education and/or therapy is all that is required.
- National Tourette Syndrome Association: http://www.tsa-usa.org

PROGNOSIS

- Symptoms will fluctuate throughout illness.
- Tic severity typically stabilizes by age 25 years.
- 60–75% of young adults show some improvement in symptoms.
- 10–40% of patients will exhibit full remission.

REFERENCES

1. American Psychiatric Association. *Diagnostic and Statistical Manual of Mental Disorders*. 5th ed. Arlington, VA: American Psychiatric Association; 2013.
2. Huys D, Hardenacke K, Poppe P, et al. Update on the role of antipsychotics in the treatment of Tourette syndrome. *Neuropsychiatr Dis Treat*. 2012;8:95–104.
3. Roessner V, Plessen KJ, Rothenberger A, et al. European clinical guidelines for Tourette syndrome and other tic disorders. Part II: pharmacological treatment. *Eur Child Adolesc Psychiatry*. 2011;20(4):173–196.
4. Pringsheim T, Marras C. Pimozide for tics in Tourette's syndrome. *Cochrane Database Syst Rev*. 2009;(2):CD006996.
5. Pringsheim T, Steeves T. Pharmacological treatment for attention deficit hyperactivity disorder (ADHD) in children with comorbid tic disorders. *Cochrane Database Syst Rev*. 2011;(4):CD007990.
6. Lombroso PJ, Scahill L. Tourette syndrome and obsessive-compulsive disorder. *Brain Dev*. 2008;30(4):231–237.
7. Savica R, Stead M, Mack KJ. Deep brain stimulation in Tourette syndrome: a description of 3 patients with excellent outcome. *Mayo Clin Proc*. 2012;87(1):59–62.
8. Curtis A, Clarke CE, Rickards HE. Cannabinoids for Tourette's syndrome. *Cochrane Database Syst Rev*. 2009;(4):CD006565.

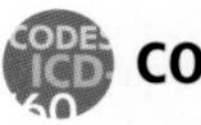

CODES

ICD10

F95.2 Tourette's disorder

CLINICAL PEARLS

- TS is diagnosed by history and witnessing tics; have parent video patient's tics if not present on exam in your office.
- Nearly 50% of children with tics also have ADHD. Stimulants may be used as 1st-line treatment for ADHD (tics are not a contraindication, as previously believed).

TOXIC EPIDERMAL NECROLYSIS

John W. Faught, MD • David H. Yun, MD

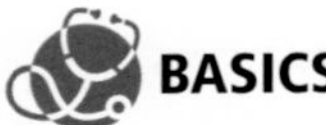

BASICS

A severe T-cell–mediated immunologic reaction resulting in extensive epidermal detachment that requires immediate drug withdrawal (if inciting medication present) and admission to a burn/ICU unit

DESCRIPTION

- Toxic epidermal necrolysis (TEN) is a severe dermatologic condition marked clinically by extensive epidermal detachment of skin and mucous membranes.
- On the same spectrum as Stevens-Johnson syndrome (SJS) with TEN defined as >30% body surface area (BSA) epidermal detachment. SJS is <10% BSA involvement, whereas SJS/TEN overlap is 10–30% BSA involvement.
- Most often the result of an adverse drug reaction: secondary to inappropriate immune response/activation to drug or drug metabolites
- System(s) affected: skin/mucosa; respiratory; gastrointestinal (GI); genitourinary; ocular involvement
- Synonym(s): toxic erythema necrosis, Lyell syndrome (1)

EPIDEMIOLOGY

Incidence

- Incidence of 0.4–1.9 cases per million per year worldwide; with the highest incidence in Africa, Asia, and India
- Affects all ages, males and females affected equally.
- Special consideration in the geriatric population, immunosuppressed and HIV patients (risk 1:1,000), and those with malignancy TEN has an average mortality rate of 25–30% (1).

ETIOLOGY AND PATHOPHYSIOLOGY

- TEN is characterized by widespread keratinocyte apoptosis that leads to epidermal detachment from the dermis.
- Pathologic mechanism has not been fully established, although immune mechanisms and altered drug metabolism have been suggested:
  - Recognition of offending drug triggers HLA class 1 molecule-initiated CD8+ cytotoxic T-cell activation (CD 8+ T cells). T-cell and natural killer (NK) cell induce damage via perforin/granzyme/granulysin damage or Fas/Fas ligand (FasL) interaction.
  - Tumor necrosis factor-α (TNF-α) and reactive nitric oxide have also been implicated in keratinocyte damage (2).
- >80–90% of TEN is drug-induced. >100 drugs have been found to cause SJS/TEN. Commonly implicated medications include the following:
  - Antibacterial and antifungal agents (sulfonamides, penicillins, cephalosporins, tetracycline, terbinafine)
  - Anticonvulsants (hydantoins, barbiturates, carbamazepine, lamotrigine)
  - Nonantibiotic sulfonamides (sulfasalazine)
  - Analgesics, oxicam-NSAIDs
  - Allopurinol
  - Nevirapine

Genetics

Certain HLA haplotypes predispose to increased susceptibility to SJS/TEN with particular drug use:

- *HLA-B*1502* has been associated with carbamazepine-induced SJS in the Han Chinese population; the FDA recommends genotyping of all Asian patients for *HLA-B*1502* before initiating carbamazepine treatment.
- *HLA-B*5801* has been linked to allopurinol-induced SJS; *HLA-B85701*, *HLADR7*, and *HLA-DQ3* are associated with abacavir-induced hypersensitivity.
- *HLA-A*0206 and HLA-B12* may be a marker of increased ocular complications in SJS/TEN in Japanese and Caucasian patients, respectively (1).

RISK FACTORS

- Immunosuppression, including HIV/AIDS, specific HLA haplotypes, and malignancy (1)
- Multiple concurrent medications increase risk.

GENERAL PREVENTION

- Always ask patients about prior adverse drug events.
- Be aware of medications with higher incidence of cutaneous drug reactions.

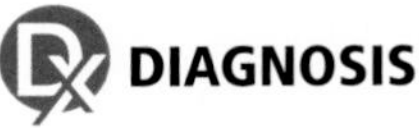

DIAGNOSIS

HISTORY

- Onset typically 1–3 weeks after initiation of drug.
- Prodrome of fever, malaise, headache, sore throat, and conjunctivitis followed by skin lesions after 1–3 days (detailed below in "Physical Exam")

PHYSICAL EXAM

- Lesions start as painful erythematosus macules followed by development of atypical target lesions with dusky center that progress to vesicles and bullae with surrounding erythema:
  - Vesicles coalesce, forming flaccid bullae that slough and result in full-thickness epidermal necrosis/detachment.
  - Start on face and trunk but spread to include palms and soles
- Positive Nikolsky sign: Gentle lateral pressure causes epidermal separation.
- Involvement of the eyes, oral, and genital mucosa are often seen.

DIFFERENTIAL DIAGNOSIS

Acute generalized exanthematous pustulosis (AGEP) and staphylococcal scalded skin syndrome (SSSS) can resemble TEN. Bullous formation in TEN can appear similar to blistering diseases, including pemphigus (3).

DIAGNOSTIC TESTS & INTERPRETATION

TEN is mostly diagnosed clinically and confirmed by histopathology of skin lesions.

- No specific lab tests
- Anemia, leukopenia, thrombocytopenia, neutropenia may be present; elevated BUN, erythrocyte sedimentation rate (ESR), and transaminases
- Granulysin found to be elevated in skin blisters; serum granulysin and FasL also found to be elevated before the development of skin and mucosal lesions. Development of a rapid immunochromatographic test to measure serum granulysin is in progress (3).
- SCORTEN:
  - Validated TEN-specific severity of illness score based on the following variables evaluated during first 24 hours of hospital admission. Each factor assigned 1 point:
    - Age ≥40 years
    - Presence of malignancy
    - Detached BSA ≥10%
    - Tachycardia ≥120/min
    - Serum urea >10 mmol/L
    - Serum glucose >14 mmol/L
    - Serum bicarbonate <20 mmol/L
- Score of 0–1 has a predictive mortality of 3.2%, whereas score of ≥5 has mortality of 90% (4)[B].

Test Interpretation

- Evaluation of skin biopsy specimen provides definitive diagnosis.
- H/E and frozen section specimens enable visualization of apoptotic keratinocytes in early lesions and dermoepidermal separation, dermal lymphocytic infiltrate, and widespread epidermal necrosis in late lesions. Dermal infiltrate density and adnexal, follicular, and eccrine gland necrosis on pathology were not associated with worse prognosis.

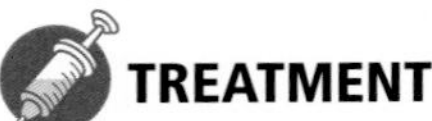

TREATMENT

- Supportive care is still the mainstay of TEN treatment; withdrawal of offending drug agent, if known, is imperative.
- Early transfer to an ICU/burn unit is critical, as patients can rapidly deteriorate:
  - Aggressive management of fluid and electrolyte balance, temperature, prevention and treatment of infection, analgesia, nutrition, and respiratory support. Fluid replacement depends on extent of skin and mucosa involvement and may be 5–7 L in first 24 hours; special consideration in pediatric population
  - Antibiotics should be avoided unless a proven infection exists.
  - Debate on role of débridement; use of wound dressing on exposed dermis to promote reepithelialization and prevent infection
- Ophthalmologic consult to assess severity of ocular involvement (4)[C]

MEDICATION

- Lack of randomized controlled clinical trials in evaluating efficacy of various treatments
- Role of systemic corticosteroids in the treatment of TEN is controversial:
  - Systemic steroid pulse therapy (methylprednisolone) and topical betamethasone early in TEN before widespread skin detachment prevented ocular complications in a small case series with SJS and TEN (5)[C].

– Other studies have found no benefit in the use of systemic corticosteroids or IVIG over supportive care (6)[B].
- IVIG shown to inhibit Fas–FasL interaction and cell death in vitro. In humans, IVIG doses >2 g/kg (3–4 g/kg total) within 4 days of onset of skin lesions may have earlier cessation of disease progression but no overall effect on mortality except in the pediatric population (7)[B].
- Anti–TNF-α agents, cyclosporine, and etanercept have demonstrated benefit in small case series, but controlled studies are needed to define their role in treatment (8)[C],(9)[B],(10)[C].

INPATIENT CONSIDERATIONS

- Transfer to a burn center capable of multidisciplinary care early in course improves outcomes.
- Aggressive management of fluid resuscitation, nutritional supplementation, and wound care
- Ocular complications occur in the majority of patients and may include synechiae, corneal ulcers, xerophthalmia, symblepharon, Meibomian gland dysfunction, panophthalmitis, and blindness (11)[C].
- With severe TEN, patient may have respiratory, GI, hepatic, or renal complications.

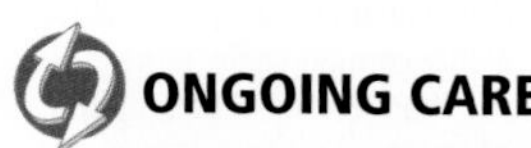

ONGOING CARE

FOLLOW-UP RECOMMENDATIONS

- Avoidance of inciting drug or drug class in the future
- Monitoring of dermatologic and ocular sequelae

PROGNOSIS

- Skin reepithelialization usually occurs within 1–3 weeks after epidermal detachment.
- There may be residual skin and ocular sequelae.

COMPLICATIONS

- Skin sequelae include scarring, hypo- and hyperpigmentation, nail loss, and stricture formation (vaginal, urethral, anal).
- Ocular complications may include persistent xerophthalmia and photophobia with possible corneal opacity.

REFERENCES

1. Schwartz RA, McDonough PH, Lee BW. Toxic epidermal necrolysis: part I. Introduction, history, classification, clinical features, systemic manifestations, etiology, and immunopathogenesis. *J Am Acad Dermatol*. 2013; 69(2):173.e1–173.e13.
2. Viard-Leveugle I, Gaide O, Jankovic D, et al. TNF-α and IFN-γ are potential inducers of Fas-mediated keratinocyte apoptosis through activation of inducible nitric oxide synthase in toxic epidermal necrolysis. *J Invest Dermatol*. 2013;133(2):489–498.
3. Schwartz RA, McDonough PH, Lee BW. Toxic epidermal necrolysis: part II. Prognosis, sequelae, diagnosis, differential diagnosis, prevention, and treatment. *J Am Acad Dermatol*. 2013;69(2): 187.e1–187.e16.
4. Firoz BF, Henning JS, Zarzabal LA, et al. Toxic epidermal necrolysis: five years of treatment experience from a burn unit. *J Am Acad Dermatol*. 2012;67(4):630–635.
5. Araki Y, Sotozono C, Inatomi T, et al. Successful treatment of Stevens-Johnson syndrome with steroid pulse therapy at disease onset. *Am J Ophthalmol*. 2009;147(6):1004–1011, 1011.e1.
6. Lee HY, Dunant A, Sekula P, et al. The role of prior corticosteroid use on the clinical course of Stevens-Johnson syndrome and toxic epidermal necrolysis: a case-control analysis of patients selected from the multinational EuroSCAR and RegiSCAR studies. *Br J Dermatol* 2012;167(3):555–562.
7. Huang YC, Li YC, Chen TJ. The efficacy of intravenous immunoglobulin for the treatment of toxic epidermal necrolysis: a systematic review and meta-analysis. *Br J Dermatol*. 2012;167(2): 424–432.
8. Valeyrie-Allanore L, Wolkenstein P, Brochard L, et al. Open trial of ciclosporin treatment for Stevens-Johnson syndrome and toxic epidermal necrolysis. *Br J Dermatol* 2010;163(4):847–853.
9. Kirchhof MG, Miliszewski MA, Sikora S, et al. Retrospective review of Stevens-Johnson syndrome/toxic epidermal necrolysis treatment comparing intravenous immunoglobulin with cyclosporine. *J Am Acad Dermatol*. 2014;71(5):941–947.
10. Paradisi A, Abeni D, Bergamo F, et al. Etanercept therapy for toxic epidermal necrolysis. *J Am Acad Dermatol*.2014;71(2):278–283.
11. Abela C, Hartmann CE, De Leo A, et al. Toxic epidermal necrolysis (TEN): the Chelsea and Westminster Hospital wound management algorithm. *J Plast Reconstr Aesthet Surg*. 2014:67(8):1026–1032.

ADDITIONAL READING

- Valeyrie-Allanore L, Bastuji-Garin S, Guégan S, et al. Prognostic value of histologic features of toxic epidermal necrolysis. *J Am Acad Dermatol*. 2013;68(2):e29–e35.
- Vélez NF, Saavedra-Lauzon AP. Toxic exanthems in the adult population. *Am J Med*. 2010;123(4): 296–303.
- Zhu QY, Ma L, Luo XQ, et al. Toxic epidermal necrolysis: performance of SCORTEN and the score-based comparison of the efficacy of corticosteroid therapy and intravenous immunoglobulin combined therapy in China. *J Burn Care Res*. 2012;33(6):e295–e308.

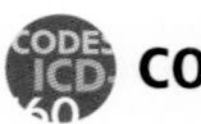

CODES

ICD10

L51.2 Toxic epidermal necrolysis [Lyell]

CLINICAL PEARLS

- SJS and TEN are on a spectrum, with TEN the more severe disease.
- Expert care in burn centers improves outcomes.

TOXOPLASMOSIS

Jonathan MacClements, MD, FAAFP

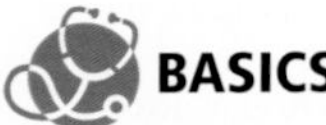

BASICS

- Obligate intracellular protozoan parasite *Toxoplasma gondii*
- Most common latent protozoan infection
- Clinically significant disease typically manifests only in pregnancy or in an immunocompromised patient.

DESCRIPTION

- Acute self-limited infection in immunocompetent
- Acute symptomatic or reactivated latent infection in immunocompromised persons
- Congenital toxoplasmosis (acute primary infection during pregnancy)
- Ocular toxoplasmosis

Pediatric Considerations

- The earlier fetal infection occurs, the more severe.
- Risk of perinatal death is 5% if infected in 1st trimester.

Pregnancy Considerations

- Pregnant immunocompromised and HIV-infected women should undergo serologic testing.
- Seronegative pregnant women should receive preventive counseling.
- Serologic testing during pregnancy remains controversial.

EPIDEMIOLOGY

Incidence

- Prevalence of congenital toxoplasmosis in the United States: 10–100/100,000 live births
- Predominant sex: male > female

Prevalence

- Present in every country and seropositivity rates range from <10% to >90% (1)[A].
- In the United States, 11% aged 6–49 years are seropositive. Age-adjusted prevalence in the United States is 22.5%.
- Seroprevalence among women in the United States is 15%.

ETIOLOGY AND PATHOPHYSIOLOGY

Transmission of *T. gondii*, an obligate intracellular sporozoan, to humans

- Ingestion of raw or undercooked meat, food, or water containing tissue cysts or oocytes; usually from soil contaminated with feline feces
- Transplacental passage from infected mother to fetus; risk of transmission is 30% on average.
- Blood product transfusion and solid-organ transplantation
- Ingested *T. gondii* oocysts enter host gastrointestinal tract where bradyzoites/tachyzoites are released, penetrate contiguous cells, replicate, and are transported to susceptible tissues where clinical disease manifests.

Genetics

Human leukocyte antigen (HLA) DQ3 is a genetic marker of susceptibility in AIDS.

RISK FACTORS

- Immunocompromised states, including HIV infection with CD4 cell count <100/μL
- Primary infection during pregnancy; risk of transmitting infection to the fetus increases with gestational age at seroconversion. Transmission in the 1st trimester is associated with more severe consequences.
- Chronically infected pregnant women who are immunocompromised also have an increased risk of congenital toxoplasmosis.

GENERAL PREVENTION

Prevention is important in seronegative pregnant women and immunodeficient patients.

- Avoid eating undercooked meat: Cook to 152°F (66°C) or freeze for 24 hours at ≤−12°C.
- Avoid drinking unfiltered water.
- Wash produce thoroughly.
- Strict hand hygiene after touching soil
- Wear gloves and wash hands after handling raw meat or cat litter.
- Avoid shellfish; (*Toxoplasma* cysts)

COMMONLY ASSOCIATED CONDITIONS

- Chorioretinitis; self-limiting, febrile lymphadenopathy; mononucleosis-like illness
- An unclear association exists between schizophrenia and several infectious agents including *T. gondii*.

DIAGNOSIS

HISTORY

- Congenital toxoplasmosis
  - Clinical presentation varies widely; 80% of patients are asymptomatic at birth.
  - Classic triad *uncommon:* chorioretinitis, hydrocephalus, cerebral calcifications
  - Manifestations may include prematurity, intrauterine growth retardation (IUGR).
  - Jaundice, rash accompanying a mononucleosis-like illness
  - Mental retardation, seizures, visual defects, spasticity, sensorineural hearing loss
- Ocular toxoplasmosis
  - Chorioretinitis: focal necrotizing retinitis
  - Yellowish-white elevated cotton patch
  - Congenital disease usually bilateral; acquired, unilateral
  - Symptoms include blurred vision, scotoma, pain, and photophobia.
- Acute toxoplasmosis (immunocompetent host)
  - ~90% of patients are asymptomatic.
  - Most common manifestation is bilateral, symmetric, nontender cervical lymphadenopathy.
  - Constitutional symptoms such as fever, chills, and sweats are usually mild.
  - Headaches, myalgias, pharyngitis, hepatosplenomegaly, and diffuse nonpruritic maculopapular rash may occur.
  - Pregnant women are often asymptomatic. Acute or reactivation in immunocompromised host.
  - Most common site is CNS with toxoplasmic encephalitis.
  - Headache; focal neurologic deficits and seizures
  - Fever usually present
  - Extracerebral toxoplasmosis: pneumonitis, chorioretinitis; rarely: GI system, liver, musculoskeletal system, heart, bone marrow, bladder, and orchitis

PHYSICAL EXAM

- In adults: fever, lymphadenopathy, nonpruritic rash
- In newborns: hydrocephalus, neurologic abnormalities, hepatosplenomegaly, chorioretinitis, microcephaly, mental retardation

DIFFERENTIAL DIAGNOSIS

Syphilis, lymphoma, progressive multifocal leukoencephalopathy, cryptococcal meningitis, congenital TORCH infections, *Listeria* infection, tuberculosis (TB), erythroblastosis fetalis

DIAGNOSTIC TESTS & INTERPRETATION

- CBC: atypical lymphocytosis, anemia, thrombocytopenia
- Serology interpretation
  - In acute infection, IgM antibodies appear within the 1st week.
  - Diagnosis can be made if initial test demonstrates positive IgM and negative IgG, with both tests being positive 2 weeks later.
  - If follow-up IgG remains negative 2–4 weeks later but IgM is still positive, it is likely a false positive.
  - Negative IgG rules out prior infection (remains detectable for life).
- Types of serologic tests
  - ELISA: most commonly used
  - Sabin-Feldman dye test: gold standard against which all other serologic assays are compared
  - IFA test: more readily available in commercial labs
  - ISAGA: widely available commercially; more sensitive and specific than IFA for detecting IgM
  - Avidity testing: confirmatory test to establish whether positive IgM/IgG reflects recent or chronic infection
- PCR: *T. gondii* DNA amplification in blood or amniotic fluid; used for diagnosis of fetal infection
- Culture (rarely necessary): Organism can be isolated either by cell culture or by mouse inoculation.

Initial Tests (lab, imaging)

- Diagnosis of primary infection is typically based on history and confirmed by serology.
- Serum *Toxoplasma*-specific IgG and IgM are first step.
- According to the result of IgM test, the avidity of IgG may be determined.
- Diagnosis of maternal infection and congenital toxoplasmosis.
  - Pregnant women who have mononucleosis-like illness but negative heterophile test should be tested for toxoplasmosis.
  - Maternal infection accurately diagnosed when based on 2 blood samples at least 2 weeks apart showing seroconversion
  - High avidity of IgG during 1st trimester argues against maternal primary infection.
  - Real-time PCR analysis for *T. gondii* on amniotic fluid predicts fetal infection and is a good means for deciding appropriate treatment and surveillance.
  - Fetal ultrasound is useful for prognosis.
  - Routine screening for toxoplasmosis is not recommended.
- Diagnosis of congenital toxoplasmosis after birth
  - Serology requires several serum samples for IgM and IgA antibodies.
  - Sampling of the cord or peripheral blood should be done within the first 2 weeks.
  - Ophthalmologic, auditory, and neurologic examinations; lumbar puncture; and head CT should be performed.
- Diagnosis of toxoplasmic encephalitis
  - Serology for IgG
  - Imaging: MRI more sensitive than CT scan for identification of characteristic ring-enhancing brain lesions

- MRI: for identifying multiple ring-enhancing brain lesion in AIDS patients with cerebral toxoplasmosis
- SPECT and PET scans: can be useful in distinguishing toxoplasmosis from CNS lymphoma

Diagnostic Procedures/Other
- Lymph node biopsy
- Brain biopsy in CNS disease
- Amniocentesis with PCR (risk of false negatives and false positives)
- Placental isolation of *Toxoplasma* is diagnostic.

Test Interpretation
- Confirmatory, meningocerebritis ± abscesses with necrosis, Giemsa
- Lymph node histology shows triad of the following:
  - Reactive follicular hyperplasia
  - Irregular clusters of epithelioid histiocytes on and blurring margins of germinal centers
  - Distension of sinuses with monocytoid cells
- Sensitivity of triad 62.5%, specificity 91.3%

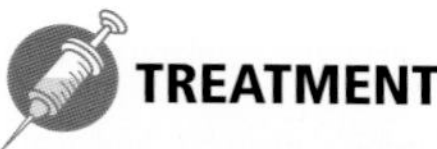

TREATMENT

GENERAL MEASURES
Immunocompetent patients usually require no treatment.

MEDICATION
First Line

ALERT
Important: All pyrimethamine-containing regimens should include leucovorin (folinic acid 10–25 mg/day PO) during and 1 week after completion of pyrimethamine therapy to prevent drug-induced hematologic toxicity (2)[A].

- Treatment in immunocompromised hosts
  - Initial drug regimen of choice is pyrimethamine 200 mg loading dose PO, followed by 50 mg/day plus sulfadiazine 4–6 g/day PO in 4 divided doses; for those intolerant or allergic to sulfadiazine, clindamycin 600–1,200 mg IV or 450 mg PO QID can be used instead.
  - Alternative regimens for patients intolerant to sulfadiazine and clindamycin include the following:
    - Pyrimethamine: 200 mg loading dose PO, followed by 50 mg/day plus azithromycin 900–1,200 mg PO once daily
    - Pyrimethamine: 200 mg loading dose PO, then 50 mg/day + atovaquone 1500 mg PO BID
    - Sulfadiazine: 1,000-1,500 mg QID plus atovaquone 1,500 mg BID
    - Trimethoprim-sulfamethoxazole: 10/50 mg/kg/day PO or IV divided BID (for 30 days) may be an effective alternative in resource-poor settings.
  - Duration of therapy: typically 6 weeks, which decrease to lower doses for secondary prophylaxis (2,3)[A]
  - Adjunctive steroids should be used in patients with signs of increased intracranial pressure.
  - Anticonvulsants, if there is a history of seizures
- Prophylaxis in immunocompromised patients
  - Primary prophylaxis: indicated for patients with HIV infection and CD4 count <100 cells/μL who are *T. gondii* IgG–positive
    - Trimethoprim-sulfamethoxazole-DS: 1 tablet PO daily. Alternative for sulfa allergy is dapsone 50 mg/day PO *plus* pyrimethamine 50 mg PO weekly *plus* leucovorin 25 mg PO weekly *or* atovaquone 1,500 mg PO daily.
  - Secondary prophylaxis: Following 6 weeks of therapy, administer lower doses of drugs:
    - Sulfadiazine 2–4 g/day in 2–4 divided doses *plus* pyrimethamine 25–50 mg/day is the 1st choice.
    - Alternative regimens include clindamycin 600 mg PO q8h *plus* pyrimethamine 25–50 mg/day PO *or* atovaquone 750 mg PO BID–QID ± pyrimethamine 25 mg PO daily.
- Pregnant women (3)[A]
  - Prenatal treatment in pregnant women diagnosed with toxoplasmosis: lack of evidence on whether antenatal treatment reduces congenital transmission; however, prenatal treatment is usually offered.
  - If <18 weeks' gestation: Spiramycin 1 g PO q8h without food until delivery if amniotic fluid PCR is negative. Does not treat infection in the fetus
  - If >18 weeks' gestation: Pyrimethamine and sulfadiazine should be considered only if fetal infection is documented by positive amniotic fluid PCR (pyrimethamine is teratogenic):
    - Pyrimethamine: 50 mg PO q12h for 2 days, then 50 mg/day plus sulfadiazine 75 mg/kg PO × 1 dose, then 50 mg/kg q12h (max 4 g/day)
- Treatment of infected newborns: Treat regardless of clinical manifestations:
  - Pyrimethamine 2 mg/kg/day (max 50 mg) × 2 days, then 1 mg/kg/day (max 25 mg) × 2–6 months, then 1 mg/kg (max 25 mg) on Monday, Wednesday, and Friday, sulfadiazine 100 mg/kg/day divided BID, and leucovorin 10 mg three times per week during pyrimethamine and one week after discontinuation
- Treatment in immunocompetent nonpregnant patients: generally do not require treatment unless symptoms are severe or prolonged; 1 of the following 2 regimens can be used:
  - Pyrimethamine: 100 mg loading dose PO, followed by 25–50 mg/day *plus* sulfadiazine 2–4 g/day in 4 divided doses
  - Pyrimethamine: 100 mg loading dose PO, followed by 25–50 mg/day *plus* clindamycin 300 mg PO QID

Second Line
- Clindamycin: 900–1,200 mg TID IV used for ocular and CNS toxoplasmosis alone and in combination with pyrimethamine; as effective as the sulfadiazine-pyrimethamine, but fewer adverse effects
- Corticosteroids (prednisone 1–2 mg/kg/day) are added for macular chorioretinitis or CNS infection.
- Alternatives: atovaquone (Mepron), azithromycin (Zithromax), clarithromycin (Biaxin), or dapsone *plus* pyrimethamine and leucovorin
- Trimethoprim-sulfamethoxazole appears to be equivalent to pyrimethamine-sulfadiazine in AIDS patients with CNS disease.

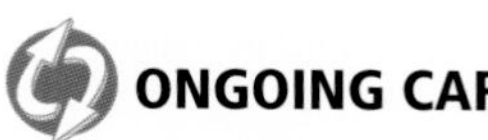

ONGOING CARE

FOLLOW-UP RECOMMENDATIONS
Patient Monitoring
Precautions
- Monitor for bone marrow, renal, or liver toxicity.
- Good hydration: Sulfadiazine is poorly soluble and may crystallize in the urine.
- Watch for antibiotic-associated diarrhea Sulfonamides may alter phenytoin and warfarin levels or interfere with oral hypoglycemic agents.

PATIENT EDUCATION
- See "General Prevention."
- www.aafp.org/afp/20030515/2145ph.html
- http://familydoctor.org/familydoctor/en/diseases-conditions/toxoplasmosis.html

PROGNOSIS
- Immunodeficient patients often relapse if treatment/suppression therapy is stopped.
- Treatment may prevent the development of untoward sequelae in infants with congenital toxoplasmosis.

REFERENCES

1. Torgerson PR, Mastroiacovo P. The global burden of congenital toxoplasmosis: a systematic review. *Bull World Health Organ*. 2013;91(7):501–508.
2. Montoya JG, Liesenfeld O. Toxoplasmosis. *Lancet*. 2004;363(9425):1965–1976.
3. Montoya JG, Remington JS. Management of *Toxoplasma gondii* infection during pregnancy. *Clin Infect Dis*. 2008;47(4):554–566.

ADDITIONAL READING

- Bodaghi B, Touitou V, Fardeau C, et al. Toxoplasmosis: new challenges for an old disease. *Eye (Lond)*. 2012;26(2):241–244.
- Garweg JG, Stanford MR. Therapy for ocular toxoplasmosis–the future. *Ocul Immunol Inflamm*. 2013;21(4):300–305.
- Kaplan JE, Benson C, Holmes KH, et al. Guidelines for prevention and treatment of opportunistic infections in HIV-infected adults and adolescents: recommendations from CDC, the National Institutes of Health, and the HIV Medicine Association of the Infectious Diseases Society of America. *MMWR Recomm Rep*. 2009;58(RR–4):1–207; quiz CE1–CE4.
- Wallon M, Franck J, Thulliez P, et al. Accuracy of real-time polymerase chain reaction for *Toxoplasma gondii* in amniotic fluid. *Obstet Gynecol*. 2010;115(4):727–733.

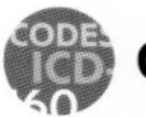

CODES

ICD10
- B58.9 Toxoplasmosis, unspecified
- P37.1 Congenital toxoplasmosis
- B58.2 Toxoplasma meningoencephalitis

CLINICAL PEARLS
- Newborn screening for congenital toxoplasmosis not currently recommended
- Primary prevention is most important, particularly for seronegative pregnant women and immunodeficient patients.
- Immunologically normal patients typically do not need treatment.
- Most common manifestation of acute toxoplasmosis in immunocompetent host is bilateral, symmetric, nontender cervical lymphadenopathy.

T

TRACHEITIS, BACTERIAL

Mary Cataletto, MD, FAAP, FCCP

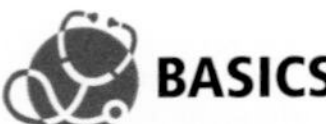

BASICS

DESCRIPTION

- Acute, potentially life-threatening infraglottic bacterial infection following a primary viral infection, usually parainfluenzae or influenza viruses
  - Direct laryngoscopy reveals marked subglottic edema and thick mucopurulent secretions, sometimes causing pseudomembranes.
- System(s) affected: pulmonary
- Synonym(s): laryngotracheobronchitis; pseudomembranous croup; bacterial croup

EPIDEMIOLOGY

Incidence

- Estimated annual incidence: 0.1/100,000
- 1st cases described prior to 1950; resurgence of cases has been noted since 1979.
- Peak incidence in children: fall and winter
- Predominant age: 6 months to 8 years; mean age 4 years (similar to croup)
- Infections in adolescents and adults have been reported.
- Predominant sex: male > female (2:1)
- Accounts for 5–14% of upper airway obstruction in children requiring critical care services

Prevalence

- Rare illness
- Most common potentially life-threatening upper airway infection in children
- Methicillin-resistant *Staphylococcus aureus* (MSRA) may contribute to changing epidemiology and virulence.

ETIOLOGY AND PATHOPHYSIOLOGY

- *Staphylococcus aureus* (most common pediatric cause): consider MRSA
- *Haemophilus influenzae* type B
- *Streptococcus pyogenes* group A
- *Streptococcus pneumoniae*
- *Moraxella catarrhalis* (associated with higher intubation rate; more frequent in younger children)
- Often polymicrobial

Genetics

No known genetic predisposition

RISK FACTORS

- Periods of increased seasonal activity of respiratory viruses
- Reports following adenoidectomy, with chronic tracheal aspiration, with evidence of other concurrent infections, including sinusitis, otitis, pneumonia, or pharyngitis

GENERAL PREVENTION

- Standard precautions, with scrupulous attention to hand washing, especially when caring for tracheostomy patients
- Vaccination against viruses that may predispose to bacterial tracheitis

COMMONLY ASSOCIATED CONDITIONS

- Consider anatomic abnormalities or foreign body as well as recent pharyngeal or laryngeal surgery.
- Predisposing: Down syndrome, immunodeficiency, subglottic hemangioma, tracheoesophageal fistula repair, tracheobronchomalacia
- Viral coinfection may occur.

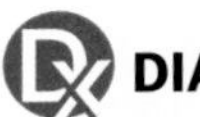

DIAGNOSIS

- May present with fever and systemic toxicity or as more localized disease
- Careful history and physical exam are the best methods to distinguish bacterial tracheitis from croup and other rare causes of upper airway obstruction.

HISTORY

- Prodromal upper respiratory tract symptoms
- Gradual progression of mild upper airway symptoms over 1 hour to 6 days to acute, febrile phase of rapid respiratory decompensation
- No drooling
- No response to aerosolized epinephrine

PHYSICAL EXAM

FEVER >38°C (100.4°F)

- Child usually lying flat
- Toxic appearance
- Variable degree of respiratory distress (1)
  - Tachypnea
  - Inspiratory stridor (1)
- Voice and cry usually normal
- Drooling uncommon

DIFFERENTIAL DIAGNOSIS

- Severe croup (viral)
- Spasmodic croup
- Diphtheria
- Retropharyngeal abscess
- Epiglottitis
- Pneumonia
- Foreign body aspiration

DIAGNOSTIC TESTS & INTERPRETATION

- Routine laboratory studies are not required to make the diagnosis.
- Radiographs are neither definitive nor diagnostic.
- Tracheal endoscopy provides a definitive diagnosis (2).

Initial Tests (lab, imaging)

- Bacterial cultures of tracheal secretions are required for culture isolates and sensitivities.
- Rapid antigen or polymerase chain reaction (PCR)–based testing for respiratory viruses may be helpful.
- Routine laboratory studies may not be helpful.
- Blood cultures rarely positive
- CBC results may vary.
  - WBC count may show marked leukocytosis or may be normal.
  - Increased band cell count
- Radiographs may be normal, but exudates may mimic the findings in foreign body aspiration.
- Pneumonic infiltrates are common.
- Anteroposterior (AP) and lateral neck x-rays show subglottic and tracheal narrowing (i.e., steeple sign on AP film) with haziness and radiopaque linear or particulate densities (crusts).
- In patients with risk of acute respiratory obstruction, either do not obtain x-rays or monitor carefully.

Follow-Up Tests & Special Considerations

Follow chest film if suspect pneumonia.

Diagnostic Procedures/Other

- Direct laryngoscopy and tracheoscopy is diagnostic and demonstrates
  - Normal supraglottic structures
  - Marked subglottic erythema and edema
  - Ulcerations
  - Epithelial sloughing
  - Copious mucopurulent secretions ± plaques or pseudomembranes
- Obtain Gram stain and aerobic, anaerobic, and viral cultures of tracheal secretions during the procedure.

Test Interpretation

- Tracheal biopsy is rarely indicated but may be considered in immunodeficient child or child with ulcerative colitis.
- Diffuse inflammation of larynx, trachea, and bronchi
- Mucopurulent exudate; microabscesses may be present.
- Semiadherent membranes (containing numerous neutrophils and cellular debris) may be identified within the trachea.

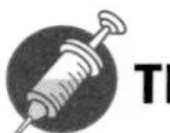

TREATMENT

- Treat as potentially life-threatening airway emergency
- Children with suspected or actual bacterial tracheitis should be cared for in a pediatric ICU.
- Assess and monitor respiratory status; supplemental oxygen may be required.
- Airway protection and support, as necessary (at least 50% require intubation; some studies report up to 100%)
- Ventilatory support may be required.
- Suctioning
- Different clinical course in previously healthy children compared with those with artificial airway

MEDICATION

- Empiric therapy should cover the most common pathogens until sensitivities are available: antistaphylococcal agent (vancomycin or clindamycin) and a 3rd-generation cephalosporin (e.g., ceftriaxone or cefotaxime) (2)[C].
- In the case of technology-dependent children with tracheostomy, make initial antibiotic choices based on previous tracheal culture.

- Narrow regimen when pathogens and sensitivities available
- Contraindications: Refer to the manufacturer's literature for each drug.
- Precautions: Refer to the manufacturer's literature for each drug. Avoid aminoglycosides in patients with previous hearing loss.
- Significant possible interactions: Refer to the manufacturer's literature for each drug.

ISSUES FOR REFERRAL

All children with suspected or actual bacterial tracheitis should be cared for in a pediatric ICU by a pediatric critical care team that may include the following subspecialists: pediatric intensivist, infectious disease specialist, pulmonologist, and/or otolaryngologist.

ADDITIONAL THERAPIES

- At present, evidence is lacking to establish the effect of heliox inhalation in the treatment of croup in children.
- For technology-dependent children with artificial airway:
  - Initial antibiotic choices should cover most recent tracheal aspirate isolates and then be refined according to culture and sensitivity results.
  - Adjunctive aerosol therapy may be helpful, particularly when multidrug-resistant organisms are present.

SURGERY/OTHER PROCEDURES

- Tracheostomy may be necessary.
- Therapeutic bronchoscopy may be necessary to facilitate removal of inspissated secretions.
- Tracheal membranes may require removal.

INPATIENT CONSIDERATIONS

- Aggressive supportive care and airway protection are paramount.
- Initial treatment of choice for bacterial tracheitis is broad-spectrum antibiotic coverage.
- Children with tracheitis and artificial airways present unique challenges: Tracheoscopy is important in establishing diagnosis in this population.
- Be vigilant for possible MRSA.

Pediatric Considerations

- True pediatric emergency
- Admission to ICU
- Maintain airway: often difficult due to copious secretions
  - Endotracheal or nasotracheal intubation usually needed, especially in infants and children <4 years of age
  - Much less likely to need intubation if child >8 years of age
  - Advantage of intubation is ability to clear trachea and bronchi of secretions and pseudomembranes.
- Vigorous pulmonary toilet to clear airway of secretions
- Hydration, humidification, antibiotics

Admission Criteria/Initial Stabilization

- Suspected or confirmed diagnosis of tracheitis
- Respiratory distress
- Artificial airway

Nursing

- Provide calm, quiet environment for child once endoscopy and cultures are done.
- Airway monitoring
- Frequent suctioning
- Monitor fluid balance.
- Establish and maintain open lines of communication with child and parents.

Discharge Criteria

No longer in need of acute care

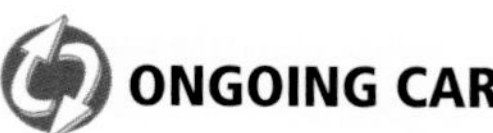

ONGOING CARE

FOLLOW-UP RECOMMENDATIONS

Patient Monitoring

Children with artificial airways will require ongoing follow-up.

DIET

Varies with clinical situation

PATIENT EDUCATION

Keep immunizations up to date.

PROGNOSIS

- Intubation generally 3–11 days
- Usually requires 3–7 days of hospitalization
- With effective early recognition and management, complete recovery can be expected.
- Cardiopulmonary arrest and death have occurred.

COMPLICATIONS

- Cardiopulmonary arrest
- Hypotension
- Acute respiratory distress syndrome (ARDS)
- Pneumonia
- Formation of pseudomembranes

REFERENCES

1. Tebruegge M, Pantazidou A, Thorburn K, et al. Bacterial tracheitis: a multi-centre perspective. *Scand J Infect Dis*. 2009;41(8):548–557.
2. American Academy of Pediatrics. *Pediatric Pulmonology*. Elk Grove Village, Illinois: American Academy of Pediatrics; 2011:955.

ADDITIONAL READING

- Bjornson CL, Johnson DW. Croup. *Lancet*. 2008;371(9609):329–339.
- Graf J, Stein F. Tracheitis in pediatric patients. *Semin Pediatr Infect Dis*. 2006;17(1):11–13.
- Hopkins A, Lahiri T, Salerno R, et al. Changing epidemiology of life-threatening upper airway infections: the reemergence of bacterial tracheitis. *Pediatrics*. 2006;118(4):1418–1421.
- Huang YL, Peng CC, Chiu NC, et al. Bacterial tracheitis in pediatrics: 12 year experience at a medical center in Taiwan. *Pediatr Int*. 2009;51(1):110–113.
- Loftis L. Acute infectious upper airway obstructions in children. *Semin Pediatr Infect Dis*. 2006;17(1): 5–10.
- Rotta AT, Wiryawan B. Respiratory emergencies in children. *Respir Care*. 2003;48(3):248–258; discussion 258–260.
- Salamone FN, Bobbitt DB, Myer CM, et al. Bacterial tracheitis reexamined: is there a less severe manifestation? *Otolaryngol Head Neck Surg*. 2004;131(6):871–876.
- Shah S, Sharieff GQ. Pediatric respiratory infections. *Emerg Med Clin N Am*. 2007;25(4):961–979, vi.
- Vorwerk C, Coats T. Heliox for croup in children. *Cochrane Database Syst Rev*. 2010;(2):CD006822.

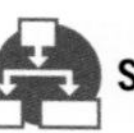

SEE ALSO

Croup (Laryngotracheobronchitis); Epiglottitis

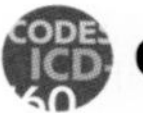

CODES

ICD10

- J04.10 Acute tracheitis without obstruction
- J04.11 Acute tracheitis with obstruction
- J05.0 Acute obstructive laryngitis [croup]

CLINICAL PEARLS

- Bacterial tracheitis is an acute, potentially life-threatening, infraglottic bacterial infection following a primary viral infection that accounts for 5–14% of upper airway obstructions in children requiring critical care services.
- Children with suspected or actual bacterial tracheitis should be cared for in a pediatric ICU.
- Endoscopy provides a definitive diagnosis (2).
- Initial treatment of choice for bacterial tracheitis is broad-spectrum antibiotic coverage, aggressive airway protection, and supportive care (2).

T

TRANSIENT ISCHEMIC ATTACK (TIA)

Emilio A. Russo, MD • Elizabeth M. Cain, MD, FAAFP

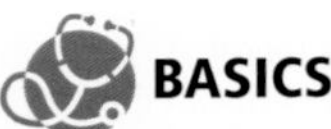

BASICS

DESCRIPTION
- A transient episode of neurologic dysfunction due to focal brain, retinal, or spinal cord ischemia without acute infarction
- No longer diagnosed based on timeframe of symptoms.
- Most important predictor of stroke: 7–40% of patients with stroke report previous TIA.
- Synonym(s): ministroke

EPIDEMIOLOGY
- Incidence of TIA underestimated because some patients do not report symptoms.
- 200,000–500,000 new TIA cases reported each year
  - 83 cases/100,000 people/year in the United States
  - 400–800 cases/100,000 persons aged 50–59 years
- Prevalence of TIA in general population: ~2.3%
- Predominant age: risk increases >60 years; highest in 7th and 8th decades
- Predominant sex: male > female (3:1)
- Predominant race/ethnicity: African Americans > Hispanics > Caucasians. The difference in African Americans is exaggerated at younger ages.

ETIOLOGY AND PATHOPHYSIOLOGY
Temporary reduction/cessation of cerebral blood flow adversely affecting neuronal function
- Carotid/vertebral atherosclerotic disease
  - Artery-to-artery thromboembolism
  - Low-flow ischemia
- Small, deep vessel disease associated with HTN
  - Lacunar infarcts
- Cardiac diseases
  - 1–6% of patients with MI develop stroke.
- Embolism secondary to the following:
  - Valvular (mitral valve) pathology
  - Mural hypokinesias/akinesias with thrombosis (acute anterior MI/congestive cardiomyopathies)
  - Cardiac arrhythmia (atrial fibrillation accounts for 5–20% incidence)
- Hypercoagulable states
  - Antiphospholipid antibodies
  - Deficiency of protein S, protein C
  - Presence of antithrombin III
  - Oral contraceptives
  - Pregnancy and parturition
- Arteritis
  - Noninfectious necrotizing vasculitis
  - Drugs
  - Irradiation
  - Local trauma
- Sympathomimetic drugs (e.g., cocaine)
- Other causes: spontaneous and posttraumatic (e.g., chiropractic manipulation) arterial dissection
- Fibromuscular dysplasia

Genetics
Inheritance is polygenic, with tendency to clustering of risk factors within families.

RISK FACTORS
- Hypertension (HTN)
- Cardiac diseases (A-fib, MI, valvular disease)
- Diabetes
- Hyperlipidemia
- Atherosclerotic disease (carotid/vertebral stenosis)
- Cigarette smoking
- Thrombophilias

GENERAL PREVENTION
- Lifestyle changes: smoking cessation, diet modification, weight loss, regular aerobic exercise, and limited alcohol intake
- Use of ASA and statins as primary prevention may be considered in certain populations.
- Strict control of medical risk factors: *Diabetes* (glycemic control), *HTN* (thiazide and/or ACE/ARB), *Hyperlipidemia* (statins), anticoagulation when high risk of cardioembolism (e.g., atrial fibrillation, mechanical valves)

ALERT
10–20% of patients with TIA have CVA within 90 days; 25–50% of those occur within the first 48 hours.

Geriatric Considerations
- Older patients have a higher mortality rate than younger patients—highest in 7th and 8th decades.
- Atrial fibrillation is a frequent cause among the elderly.

Pediatric Considerations
- Congenital heart disease is a common cause among pediatric patients.
- Other causes include the following:
  - Metabolic: homocystinuria, Fabry disease
  - Central nervous system (CNS) infection
  - Clotting disorders
  - Marfan syndrome
  - Moyamoya disease

Pregnancy Considerations
- Preeclampsia, eclampsia, and HELLP
- TTP and hemolytic uremic syndrome
- Postpartum angiopathy
- Cerebral venous thrombosis
- Hypercoagulable states related to pregnancy

COMMONLY ASSOCIATED CONDITIONS
- Atrial fibrillation
- Uncontrolled HTN
- Carotid stenosis

DIAGNOSIS

HISTORY
- Obtain witness accounts with emphasis on symptom onset, progression, and recovery.
- Carotid circulation (hemispheric): monocular visual loss, hemiplegia, hemianesthesia, neglect, aphasia, visual field defects (amaurosis fugax); less often, headaches, seizures, amnesia, confusion
- Vertebrobasilar (brain stem/cerebellar): bilateral visual obscuration, diplopia, vertigo, ataxia, facial paresis, Horner syndrome, dysphagia, dysarthria; also headache, nausea, vomiting, and ataxia
- Past medical history, baseline functional status

- ABCD2 score: predicts risk of CVA within 48 hours (1)[A]
  - Score of 0–1:0%; 2–3: 1.3%; 4–5: 4.1%; 6–7:8.1%
  - **A**ge >65 years: 1 point
  - **B**P 140/90 mm Hg: 1 point
  - Symptoms of focal weakness: 2 points
  - Speech impaired without weakness: 1 point
  - **D**uration >60 minutes: 2 points
  - **D**uration 10–59 minutes: 1 point
  - **D**iabetes: 1 point

PHYSICAL EXAM
- Vital signs, oxygen saturation
- Thorough neurologic and cardiac exams

DIFFERENTIAL DIAGNOSIS
- Evolving stroke
- Migraine (hemiplegic)
- Focal seizure (Todd paralysis)
- Hypoglycemia
- Bell palsy
- Neoplasm of brain
- Subarachnoid hemorrhage
- Intoxication
- Electrolyte abnormalities

DIAGNOSTIC TESTS & INTERPRETATION

Initial Tests (lab, imaging)
- Patients with TIA should undergo neuroimaging evaluation within 24 hours of symptom onset.

- MRI, including diffusion-weighted imaging is the preferred brain diagnostic modality; if not available then noncontrast head CT (2)[B].
- Noninvasive imaging of the cervicocephalic vessels should be performed routinely as part of the evaluation of suspected TIA (2)[A].
- Initial assessment of the extracranial vasculature may involve carotid US/TCD, MRA, or CTA depending on the availability and expertise and characteristics of the patient (2)[B].
- Routine blood tests (CBC, chemistry, PT/PTT, UPT, and fasting lipid panel) are reasonable in evaluation of patient with TIA (2)[B].

Follow-Up Tests & Special Considerations
- If only noninvasive testing is performed prior to CEA, it is reasonable to pursue 2 concordant noninvasive findings; otherwise, catheter angiography should be considered (2)[B].
- Echo is reasonable in evaluation of patients with suspected TIA especially when no other cause is noted (2)[B].
- TEE is useful in identifying PFO, aortic arch atherosclerosis, and valvular disease and is reasonable when this will alter management (2)[B].
- Prolonged cardiac monitoring is useful in patients with an unclear etiology after initial brain imaging and ECG (2)[B].

- EEG: if seizure suspected

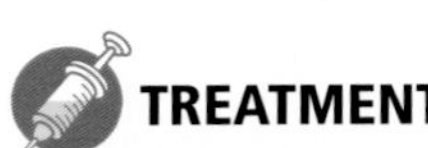

TREATMENT

GENERAL MEASURES
- TIA is a neurologic emergency. Immediate medical attention should be sought within 24 hours of symptom onset.
- Current evidence suggests that patients with high-risk TIAs require rapid referral and 24-hour admission (see ABCD2 scoring).
- Acute phase
  - Inpatient for surgery and high-risk groups
  - Outpatient investigations may be considered based on patient's stroke risk, arrangement of follow-up, and social circumstances.
- Antiplatelet therapy to prevent recurrence or future CVA
- Treatment/control of underlying associated conditions

MEDICATION

- For patients with TIA, the use of antiplatelet agents rather than oral anticoagulation is recommended to reduce risk of recurrent stroke and other cardiovascular events, with the exception of cardioembolic etiologies (2)[A].
- *Uncertain* if switching agent in patients who have additional ischemic attacks while on antiplatelet therapy is beneficial (3)[C].

First Line

- Enteric-coated aspirin: 160–325 mg/day in the acute phase (4)[A] followed by long-term antiplatelet therapy for noncardioembolic TIA and anticoagulation for cardioembolic etiology
- Combined therapy if started within 24 hours of symptom onset has shown decrease in ischemic stroke with no change in bleeding risk in Chinese populations: clopidogrel 300 mg on day 1 followed by 75 mg daily for 90 days plus ASA 75–300 mg on day 1 then 75 mg daily for 21 days.
- Antiplatelet therapy
  - ER dipyridamole–ASA (Aggrenox): 25/200 mg BID (3,5)[B]
  - Combined therapy with dipyridamole and ASA is better than ASA alone (4,6)[A].
  - More expensive than ASA alone and may have more side effects.
  - Aspirin 50–325 mg/day (3)[A]
    - Contraindications: active PUD and hypersensitivity to ASA or NSAIDs
    - Precautions: may aggravate preexisting peptic ulcer disease; may worsen symptoms of asthma
    - Significant possible interactions: may potentiate effects of anticoagulants and sulfonylurea analogues
  - Clopidogrel 75 mg/day (3)[B]
    - Can be used in patients who are allergic to ASA (3)[B]
    - Precautions: Thrombotic thrombocytopenic purpura (TTP) can occur and increases risk of bleeding when combined with aspirin.
    - May be very slightly more effective than aspirin alone (4)[B]; more expensive and more side effects than aspirin
- Anticoagulation therapy
  - Factor Xa inhibitors (rivaroxaban, apixaban), direct thrombin inhibitor (dabigatran) (7)[B]
    - Noninferior to warfarin in nonvalvular AF
    - Precautions: avoid in CKD (CrCl <30 mL/min)
    - Expensive
  - Warfarin (INR-adjusted dose) (3,8)[A]
    - Contraindications: intolerance/allergy, active liver disease, active bleeding, pregnancy
    - Significant possible interactions: antibiotics, antiepileptics, antifungals, and many others
  - ASA 325 mg/day or ASA 81/clopidigrel 75 mg/day (3)[A]
    - Patients who cannot take anticoagulation for reasons other than bleeding risk

Second Line

Ticlopidine (Ticlid): 250 mg PO BID

- For patients who cannot tolerate other agents
- Contraindications: hypersensitivity, presence of hematopoietic/hemostatic disorders, conditions associated with bleeding, severe liver dysfunction
- Precautions: neutropenia (0.8% severe), which is reversible with cessation of the drug. Monitor blood counts every 2 weeks for first 3 months. TTP can occur.
- Significant possible interactions: Digoxin plasma levels decreased 15%; theophylline half-life increased from 8.6 to 12.2 hours.

ISSUES FOR REFERRAL

- Neurology for ongoing workup and treatment
- Cardiology if cardiac cause suspected
- Vascular surgery if carotid endarterectomy appropriate

ADDITIONAL THERAPIES

- Secondary prevention of TIA should be initiated. Venous thromboembolism (VTE) prophylaxis
- Patients with TIA or ischemic stroke should be started on a statin (9,10)[A].
- BP should be reduced when appropriate after 24 hours. ACE inhibitors/thiazide have shown to be of benefit (9)[A].

SURGERY/OTHER PROCEDURES

- Consider carotid endarterectomy in patients with a high degree of carotid artery stenosis (9)[A].
- When CEA is indicated for patients with TIA, surgery within 2 weeks is reasonable if there are no contraindications to early revascularization (9)[B].

INPATIENT CONSIDERATIONS

Admission Criteria/Initial Stabilization

- Symptoms <72 hours and the following (11)[C]:
  - ABCD2 score of ≥3
  - ABCD2 score of 0–2 and uncertainty that dx workup can be completed within 2 days as outpatient.
  - ABCD2 score of 0–2 and evidence that indicates the patient's event was caused by focal ischemia.
- Correct fluid and electrolyte imbalances.

Discharge Criteria

Consider safety at home if another incident occurs.

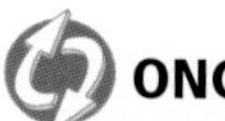

ONGOING CARE

FOLLOW-UP RECOMMENDATIONS

Patient Monitoring

- Follow-up every 3 months for 1st year then annually
- Close attention to recurrent or subsequent CVA

DIET

As appropriate for underlying medical problems

PROGNOSIS

- The risk of stroke on the ipsilateral side within 90 days and cumulative thereafter is 10–20%.
- Frequency increases with the addition of multiple risk factors and severity of carotid stenosis.
- Patients with larger artery occlusion or cardioembolic etiology are at increased risk of recurrence.
- The major cause of death in the first 5 years is cardiac disease.

COMPLICATIONS

- Stroke
- Functional impairment

REFERENCES

1. Tsivgoulis G, Stamboulis E, Sharma VK, et al. Multicenter external validation of the ABCD2 score in triaging TIA patients. *Neurology*. 2010;74(17):1351–1357.
2. Adams RJ, Albers G, Alberts MJ, et al. Update to the AHA/ASA recommendations for the prevention of stroke in patients with stroke and transient ischemic attack. *Stroke*. 2008;39(5):1647–1652.
3. Lansberg MG, O'Donnell MJ, Khatri P, et al. Antithrombotic and thrombolytic therapy for ischemic stroke: antithrombotic therapy and prevention of thrombosis, 9th ed.: American College of Chest Physicians Evidence-Based Clinical Practice Guidelines. *Chest*. 2012;141(2 Suppl):e601S–e636S.
4. Albers GW, Amarenco P, Easton JD, et al. Antithrombotic and thrombolytic therapy for ischemic stroke: American College of Chest Physicians Evidence-Based Clinical Practice Guidelines (8th edition). *Chest*. 2008;133(6 Suppl):630S–669S.
5. De Schryver EL, Algra A, van Gijn J. Dipyridamole for preventing stroke and other vascular events in patients with vascular disease. *Cochrane Database Syst Rev*. 2007;(3):CD001820.
6. Yip S, Benavente O. Antiplatelet agents for stroke prevention. *Neurotherapeutics*. 2011;8(3):475–487.
7. Nagarakanti R, Ellis CR. Dabigatran in clinical practice. *Clin Ther*. 2012;34(10):2051–2060.
8. Aguilar MI, Hart R, Pearce LA. Oral anticoagulants versus antiplatelet therapy for preventing stroke in patients with non-valvular atrial fibrillation and no history of stroke or transient ischemic attacks. *Cochrane Database Syst Rev*. 2007;(3):CD006186.
9. Furie KL, Kasner SE, Adams RJ, et al. Guidelines for the prevention of stroke in patients with stroke or transient ischemic attack: a guideline for healthcare professionals from the American Heart Association/American Stroke Association. *Stroke*. 2011;42(1):227–276.
10. Manktelow BN, Potter JF. Interventions in the management of serum lipids for preventing stroke recurrence. *Cochrane Database Syst Rev*. 2009;(3):CD002091.
11. Adams HP Jr, del Zoppo G, Alberts M, et al. Guidelines for the early management of adults with ischemic stroke. *Circulation*. 2007;115(20):e478–e534.

ADDITIONAL READING

Wang Y, Wang Y, Zhao X, et al. Clopidogrel with aspirin in acute minor stroke or transient ischemic attack. *N Engl J Med*. 2013;369(1):11–19.

SEE ALSO

Algorithms: Stroke; TIA and Transient Neurologic Deficit

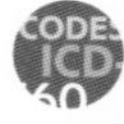

CODES

ICD10

- G45.9 Transient cerebral ischemic attack, unspecified
- G45.1 Carotid artery syndrome (hemispheric)
- G45.0 Vertebro-basilar artery syndrome

CLINICAL PEARLS

- Primary/secondary prevention is important, stressing smoking cessation, exercise, weight loss, limited ETOH intake, and control of HTN, hyperlipidemia, and diabetes.
- Antiplatelet therapy (e.g., aspirin or clopidogrel or aspirin-dipyridamole) should be initiated.
- Warfarin should be initiated in patients with atrial fibrillation or cardioembolic risk factors.
- A 30% risk of stroke exists within 5 years of a TIA.

TRANSIENT STRESS CARDIOMYOPATHY

Timothy P. Fitzgibbons, MD, PhD • Gerard P. Aurigemma, MD

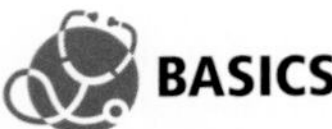

BASICS

DESCRIPTION

- Transient stress cardiomyopathy (TSC) is a unique cause of reversible left ventricle (LV) dysfunction with a presentation indistinguishable from the acute coronary syndromes (ACS), particularly ST-segment elevation myocardial infarction (MI) (1)[A],(2).
- Typically, the patient is a postmenopausal woman who presents with acute chest pain or dyspnea after an identifiable "trigger" (i.e., an acute emotional or physiologic stressor).
- First reported by authors from Japan, TSC was known initially as the *takotsubo syndrome* because the typical LV morphology (i.e., apical ballooning) resembled that of a Japanese octopus trap or *takotsubo* (3)[B].
- Presenting clinical features include the following:
  - Chest symptoms and/or dyspnea
  - ECG changes, including ST-segment elevations or diffuse T-wave inversions
  - Mild elevation in cardiac biomarkers (creatine kinase [CK], troponin)
  - Transient wall motion abnormalities that may involve the base, midportion, and/or lateral walls of the LV
  - The apex of the right ventricle (RV) may be affected in up to 25% of cases (4)[B].
- Clinical features may vary on a case-by-case basis, and formal diagnostic criteria have not been established.
- Authors from the Mayo Clinic have proposed that 3 of the 4 following criteria establish the diagnosis (1)[A]:
  - Transient akinesis or dyskinesis of the LV apical and midventricular segments with regional wall motion abnormalities extending beyond a single epicardial vascular distribution
  - Absence of obstructive coronary artery disease (CAD) or angiographic evidence of acute plaque rupture
  - New ECG abnormalities, either ST-segment elevation or T-wave inversion
  - Absence of
    - Recent significant head trauma
    - Intracranial bleeding
    - Pheochromocytoma
    - Obstructive epicardial CAD
    - Myocarditis
    - Hypertrophic cardiomyopathy
- Synonym(s): takotsubo cardiomyopathy; apical ballooning syndrome; stress cardiomyopathy; broken heart syndrome; ampulla cardiomyopathy

EPIDEMIOLOGY

Incidence

- TSC accounts for a small percentage (1–3%) of ACS.
- In a recent prospective evaluation of patients admitted to the ICU, as many as 28% had apical ballooning, often in association with sepsis.
- Predominant sex: 82–100% of cases occur in women.
- Predominant age: Mean age of patients is 62–75 years.

Prevalence

2.2% of patients presenting to a referral hospital with ST-segment MIs were found to have TSC.

ETIOLOGY AND PATHOPHYSIOLOGY

- The exact pathophysiology is not known.
- It has been speculated that overwhelming activation of the sympathetic nervous system incites a cascade of events, including the following:
  - Catecholamine-induced LV dysfunction: "biased agonism" of epinephrine for β_2-adrenergic receptors, located predominantly at the cardiac apex (5)
  - Endothelial dysfunction and vasospasm: Prolonged TIMI frame counts and diffuse multivessel spasm have been observed in the acute phase, but more recent studies do not support this mechanism.
  - Cellular metabolic injury
    - Myocardial norepinephrine release
    - Calcium overload
    - Contraction band necrosis

Genetics

No genetic associations have been described to date.

RISK FACTORS

- Female sex
- Postmenopausal state
- Emotional stress (i.e., argument, death of family member)
- Physiologic stress (i.e., acute medical illness)

COMMONLY ASSOCIATED CONDITIONS

Death from TSC is rare, and most cases resolve rapidly, within 2–3 days. Reported complications include the following:

- Left-sided heart failure
- Pulmonary edema
- Cardiogenic shock and hemodynamic compromise
- Dynamic LV outflow tract gradient complicated by hypotension
- Mitral regurgitation
- Ventricular arrhythmias
- LV thrombus formation
- LV free wall rupture
- Death (rare, 0–8%)

DIAGNOSIS

Because TSC often is indistinguishable from an ACS, it should be treated initially as such:

- Activate emergency medical services or report to emergency department.
- Oxygen, IV access, and ECG monitoring
- Urgent cardiology consultation

HISTORY

- Exposure to a "trigger event"
  - Emotional stress: argument, death of family member, divorce, public speaking, etc.
  - Physiologic stress: acute medical condition such as head trauma, asthma attack, seizure, etc.
- Acute onset of dyspnea or chest pain
- Palpitations
- Syncope

PHYSICAL EXAM

Exam may be unremarkable or may include any of the following:

- Tachypnea
- Tachycardia
- Hypotension
- Jugular venous distension
- Bibasilar rales
- S_3 gallop
- Systolic ejection murmur due to dynamic LV outflow tract gradient
- Holosystolic murmur of mitral regurgitation

DIFFERENTIAL DIAGNOSIS

- Acute ST-segment elevation MI
- Pulmonary embolism
- Myopericarditis
- Pheochromocytoma
- Hypertrophic cardiomyopathy
- Subarachnoid hemorrhage or stroke

DIAGNOSTIC TESTS & INTERPRETATION

- ECG should be done urgently and may show the following:
  - Diffuse ST-segment elevations
  - Diffuse and often dramatic T-wave inversions
  - QTc interval prolongation (6)[B]
  - Q waves
- Laboratory tests typically reveal a mild elevation in cardiac biomarkers such as
  - CK (rarely >500 U/mL)
  - Troponin I
  - B-type natriuretic peptide (BNP)
  - Markers of high filling pressures (e.g., BNP) tend to be higher than markers of necrosis (e.g., CK, troponin).
  - TSC can be distinguished from AMI with 95% specificity using a BNP/TnT ratio ≥1,272 (sensitivity 52%) (7)[B].
- Chest radiograph
  - Cardiomegaly
  - Pulmonary edema
- Echocardiogram
  - Reduced LV systolic function
  - Abnormal diastolic function, including evidence of increased filling pressures
  - Regional wall motion abnormalities in one of the following patterns:
    - Classic or "takotsubo-type" ballooning of the apex with a hypercontractile base
    - "Reverse takotsubo": apical hypercontractility with basal akinesis
    - "Midventricular" akinesis with apical and basal hypercontractility
    - Focal or localized akinesis of an isolated segment
  - Dynamic intracavitary LV gradient
  - Mitral regurgitation
  - Variable involvement of the right ventricle
- Cardiac MRI
  - Reduced LV function
  - Wall motion abnormalities as described for transthoracic echocardiography
  - Absence of delayed hyperenhancement with gadolinium

Diagnostic Procedures/Other

- Because ST-segment elevation MI is the diagnosis of exclusion, patients typically are referred for urgent cardiac catheterization.
- Coronary angiography
  - Nonocclusive CAD
  - Rarely, epicardial coronary spasm
  - Endothelial dysfunction as measured by fractional flow reserve or TIMI frame counts
- Left-sided heart catheterization: increased LV end-diastolic pressure to a similar degree as AMI (8)[B]
- Ventriculography: wall motion abnormalities as described for transthoracic echocardiography
- Right-sided heart catheterization
  - Increased pulmonary capillary wedge pressure
  - Secondary pulmonary hypertension
  - Increased right ventricular filling pressures
  - Reduced cardiac output or cardiogenic shock (cardiac index <2 and mean arterial pressure [MAP] <60 mm Hg)

Test Interpretation

Characteristic pathologic findings of involved myocardium have not been described.

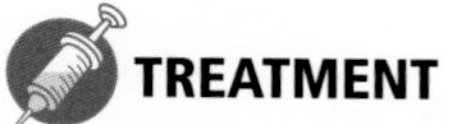

TREATMENT

- Activation of emergency medical services
- Advanced cardiac life support therapies as needed
- Oxygen
- IV access
- ECG monitoring

MEDICATION

After diagnostic cardiac catheterization, empirical treatment goals are as follow:

- Management of hypotension: differentiation between cardiogenic shock or dynamic LV cavity gradient
- Management of increased filling pressures and congestive states
- Attenuation of sympathetic drive

First Line

- There are no evidence-based treatment recommendations for TSC. The following are based on heart failure treatment guidelines.
- Consideration should be given to β-blockers in all patients (e.g., metoprolol 12.5–75 mg PO BID or carvedilol 6.25–25 mg PO BID) if tissue perfusion is adequate (9)[C].
- If there is evidence of left ventricular systolic dysfunction or pulmonary edema, consider the following:
  - Furosemide: 20–40 mg IV/PO BID as needed to reduce LV filling pressures and dyspnea (9)
  - ACE inhibitors: lisinopril 10–40 mg/day PO or equivalent (9)

Second Line

Short-term anticoagulation should be considered in patients with severely reduced LV function to prevent LV thrombus formation. Unfractionated heparin 80 U/kg IV bolus followed by 18 U/kg/hr IV or Lovenox 1 mg/kg SC BID.

ISSUES FOR REFERRAL

All patients with TSC generally should be comanaged with cardiology while inpatient and referred to cardiology as an outpatient.

ADDITIONAL THERAPIES

- Urgent cardiology consultation and consideration of cardiac catheterization
- Hypotension may require the following:
  - Vasopressors (e.g., dopamine or Levophed) if there is no LV outflow tract gradient (9)[C]
  - Phenylephrine and IV fluids to increase afterload in the presence of an LV outflow tract gradient (9)[C]
  - Cardiogenic shock that is not due to an LV outflow tract gradient may require placement of an intra-aortic balloon pump.

INPATIENT CONSIDERATIONS

Admission Criteria/Initial Stabilization

- 12-lead ECG
- Chest radiograph
- Laboratory testing
- Echocardiography
- Patients with TSC usually are admitted for observation because the differential diagnosis includes ACS.

IV Fluids

Normal saline infusion to support BP, if necessary, and no evidence of heart failure

Discharge Criteria

Generally considered after exclusion of ACS and resolution of

- Congestive state
- Hypotension
- Profound impairments of systolic function

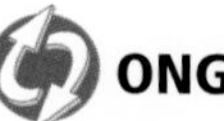

ONGOING CARE

FOLLOW-UP RECOMMENDATIONS

- Impairments in systolic function typically resolve in 2–3 days but may last as long as 1 month.
- Patients should follow up with cardiology and serial echocardiography to document improved LV function.

PROGNOSIS

- Prognosis is excellent. Inpatient mortality is rare and ranges from 0 to 8%.
- Recurrence is rare; it also has been reported in 0–8% of patients.

REFERENCES

1. Bybee KA, Kara T, Prasad A, et al. Systematic review: transient left ventricular apical ballooning: a syndrome that mimics ST-segment elevation myocardial infarction. *Ann Intern Med.* 2004;141(11):858–865.
2. Bybee KA, Prasad A. Stress-related cardiomyopathy syndromes. *Circulation.* 2008;118(4):397–409.
3. Dote K, Sato H, Tateishi H, et al. Myocardial stunning due to simultaneous multivessel coronary spasms: a review of 5 cases [in Japanese]. *J Cardiol.* 1991;21(2):203–214.
4. Fitzgibbons TP, Madias C, Seth A, et al. Prevalence and clinical characteristics of right ventricular dysfunction in transient stress cardiomyopathy. *Am J Cardiol.* 2009;104(1):133–136.
5. Paur H, Wright PT, Sikkel MB, et al. High levels of circulating epinephrine trigger apical cardiodepression in a β2-adrenergic receptor/Gi dependent manner: a new model of takotsubo cardiomyopathy. *Circulation.* 2012;126(6): 697–706.
6. Madias C, Fitzgibbons TP, Alsheikh-Ali AA, et al. Acquired long QT syndrome from stress cardiomyopathy is associated with ventricular arrhythmias and torsades de pointes. *Heart Rhythm.* 2011;8(4):555–561.
7. Randhawa MS, Dhillon AS, Taylor HC, et al. Diagnostic utility of cardiac biomarkers in discriminating takotsubo cardiomyopathy from acute myocardial infarction. *J Card Fail.* 2014;20(1):2–8.
8. Medeiros K, O'Connor MJ, Baicu CF, et al. Systolic and diastolic mechanics in stress cardiomyopathy. *Circulation.* 2014;129(16):1659–1667.
9. Hunt S, Abraham WT, Chin MH, et al. 2009 Focused update incorporated into the ACC/AHA 2005 guidelines for the diagnosis and management of heart failure in adults: a report of the American College of Cardiology Foundation/American Heart Association Task Force on Practice Guidelines developed in collaboration with the International Society for Heart and Lung Transplantation. *J Am Coll Cardiol.* 2009;53(15):e1–e90.

SEE ALSO

Algorithm: Chest Pain/Acute Coronary Syndrome

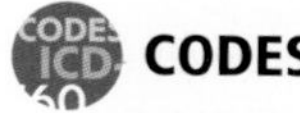

CODES

ICD10

I51.81 Takotsubo syndrome

CLINICAL PEARLS

- TSC is a cause of reversible LV dysfunction with a clinical presentation indistinguishable from the ACS's, particularly ST-segment elevation MI.
- Echocardiography may strongly suggest the diagnosis.
- Treatment is supportive and should include β-blockers in most patients, and diuretics and ACE inhibitors in patients with CHF.

TRICHOMONIASIS

Adriana C. Linares, MD, MPH, DrPH

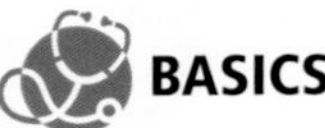

BASICS

DESCRIPTION

- Sexually transmitted urogenital infection caused by a pear-shaped, parasitic protozoan
- A cause of nongonococcal urethritis (NGU) in men
- System(s) affected: genitourinary
- Synonym(s): trich; trichomonal urethritis

EPIDEMIOLOGY

Incidence

- Affects >120 million women worldwide. It is considered to be the most common curable sexually transmitted infection worldwide (1).
- Estimated 7.4 million new cases annually in the United States among men and women
- 10–25% of vaginal infections
- 1–17% of cases of NGU; reported prevalence rates among men without urethritis have ranged from 0% to 8%.
- Predominant age: young and middle-aged adults
  - Rare until onset of sexual activity
  - Not uncommon in postmenopausal women; age is not protective, and long-term carriage is possible.
- Predominant sex: Male = female, but women are more commonly symptomatic.

Pediatric Considerations

Rare in prepubertal children; confirmed diagnosis should raise concern of sexual abuse.

Prevalence

- 2.3% of young adults
  - 2.8% of women
  - 1.7% of men
- 3.1% of all U.S. women
- Racial disparity exists:
  - 1.3% of white, non-Hispanic women
  - 1.8% of Mexican American women
  - 13.3% of black, non-Hispanic women (2)

ETIOLOGY AND PATHOPHYSIOLOGY

- *Trichomonas vaginalis*: a pear-shaped, flagellated, parasitic protozoan
- Grows best at 35°–37°C in anaerobic conditions at pH of 5.5–6
- STI
- Transmission via a nonvenereal route is possible because the organism survives for several hours in a moist environment.

Genetics

No known genetic considerations

RISK FACTORS

- Multiple sexual partners
- Unprotected intercourse
- Lower socioeconomic status
- Other STIs
- Untreated partner with previous infection

GENERAL PREVENTION

- Use of male or female condoms
- Reducing exposure by limiting numbers of partners
- Male circumcision may be protective (3)[B].

COMMONLY ASSOCIATED CONDITIONS

- Other STIs, including HIV (4)
- Bacterial vaginosis

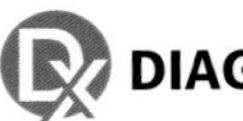

DIAGNOSIS

HISTORY

- Women
  - Yellow-green, malodorous vaginal discharge
  - Vulvovaginal pruritus
  - Dysuria
  - 50–75% are asymptomatic.
- Men
  - Dysuria
  - Urethral discharge
  - 80% are asymptomatic.

PHYSICAL EXAM

- Women
  - Vaginal erythema
  - Yellow-green, frothy, malodorous vaginal discharge
  - Petechiae on cervix (strawberry cervix; seen in ~10% of patients)
  - Basic medium: usually pH >4.5; however, it is not very specific because pH is also elevated in bacterial vaginosis
- Men: penile discharge, spontaneous and with expression

DIFFERENTIAL DIAGNOSIS

- Women (other vaginitides)
  - Bacterial vaginosis
  - Vaginal candidiasis
  - Chlamydial infection
  - Gonorrheal infection
  - Mixed vaginitis
- Men (other urethritides)
  - Chlamydial infection
  - Gonorrheal infection

DIAGNOSTIC TESTS & INTERPRETATION

Initial Tests (lab, imaging)

- Wet mounts of vaginal or urethral discharge: direct visualization of motile trichomonads
  - Sensitivity: 60–70%
  - Specificity: 99.8%
- Gram stain
- Culture: sensitivity: >95%; can take 4–7 days
  - ELISA and direct fluorescent antibody tests: sensitivity of 80–90%
  - Rapid diagnostic kits using polymerase chain reaction DNA probes: sensitivity, 97%; specificity, 98%

Follow-Up Tests & Special Considerations

Detection on Papanicolaou smear

- Sensitivity: 57–98%
- Specificity: 97%

Diagnostic Procedures/Other

Detection on self-obtained sample

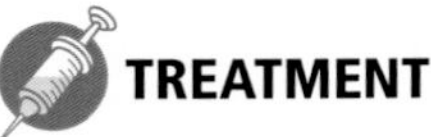

TREATMENT

- Symptomatic individuals require treatment.
- Asymptomatic partners should be treated presumptively.
- Complete screening for other STIs, including HIV, gonorrhea, chlamydia, syphilis, hepatitis B, and hepatitis C, should be considered part of required treatment.
- Patients should abstain from sexual intercourse during treatment and until they are asymptomatic.

GENERAL MEASURES

If metronidazole resistance is suspected, use tinidazole. (5)[A]

MEDICATION

First Line

- Metronidazole: 2 g PO, 1 dose (6)[A]
  - FDA pregnancy risk Category B
  - American Association of Pediatrics recommends abstaining from breastfeeding during treatment and for 12–24 hours after last dose, but this is an old recommendation not supported by current evidence. Avoid alcohol during treatment and for 24 hours after completion.

- Tinidazole: 2 g PO, 1 dose
  - FDA pregnancy risk Category C
  - Abstain from breastfeeding during treatment and for 3 days after the dose.
  - Avoid alcohol during treatment and for 72 hours after completion.

Second Line
- Only if still symptomatic after initial treatment
- Metronidazole: 500 mg PO BID for 7 days

Pregnancy Considerations
Metronidazole is effective against a trichomoniasis infection during pregnancy but may increase the risk of preterm and low-birth-weight babies.

ISSUES FOR REFERRAL
- Multidrug-resistant organism
- Patient allergy to metronidazole: Desensitization to metronidazole is possible.

ADDITIONAL THERAPIES
- Men
  - None currently available in the United States
- Women
  - Clotrimazole: 1% vaginal cream daily HS for 7 days
  - Sulfanilamide-aminacrine-allantoin vaginal suppositories BID for 7 days
  - Nonoxynol 9
  - Povidone-iodine douche

COMPLEMENTARY & ALTERNATIVE MEDICINE
Not sufficiently investigated to be recommended

INPATIENT CONSIDERATIONS

Admission Criteria/Initial Stabilization
Admission may be necessary for resistant organisms because IV therapy provides higher tissue concentrations.

Discharge Criteria
Clearance of infection

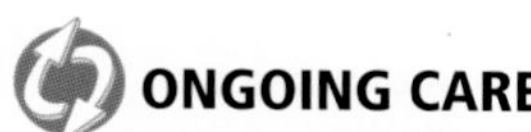

ONGOING CARE

FOLLOW-UP RECOMMENDATIONS
- If symptoms persist after initial treatment, reculture and/or repeat wet mount.
- Test of cure in asymptomatic individuals is controversial at this point (6).

DIET
Abstain from alcohol while being treated with 5-nitroimidazole derivatives, such as metronidazole, due to disulfiram-like reaction.

PATIENT EDUCATION
Educate about the sexually transmitted aspect of the infection:
- Inform partner so that partner can be treated.
- Discuss safe sex during health maintenance visits.
- Abstain from intercourse while undergoing treatment; use condoms if abstention is not feasible/possible.
- Avoid alcohol during treatment with metronidazole or tinidazole.
- Condom use can prevent recurrence.

PROGNOSIS
- Excellent
- Usually treated after 1 course, but increasing number of metronidazole-resistant cases

COMPLICATIONS

Pregnancy Considerations
Linked to low birth weight, preterm/premature rupture of membranes, and preterm birth

REFERENCES

1. Silver BJ, Guy RJ, Kaldor JM, et al. *Trichomonas vaginalis* as a cause of perinatal morbidity: a systematic review and meta-analysis. *Sex Trans Dis*.2014;41(6):369–376.
2. Sutton M, Sternberg M, Koumans EH, et al. The prevalence of *Trichomonas vaginalis* infection among reproductive-age women in the United States, 2001–2004. *Clin Infect Dis*. 2007;45(10):1319–1326.
3. Sobngwi-Tambekou J, Taljaard D, Nieuwoudt M, et al. Male circumcision and *Neisseria gonorrhoeae, Chlamydia trachomatis* and *Trichomonas vaginalis*: observations after a randomised controlled trial for HIV prevention. *Sex Transm Infect*. 2009;85(2):116–120.
4. Fastring DR, Amedee E, Gatski M, et al. Co-occurrence of *Trichomonas vaginalis* and bacterial vaginosis and vaginal shedding of HIV-1 RNA. *Sex Transm Dis*. 2014;41(3):173–179.
5. Seña AC, Bachmann LH, Hobbs MM. Persistent and recurrent *Trichomonas vaginalis* infections: epidemiology, treatment and management considerations. *Expert Rev Anti Infect Ther*. 2014;12(6):673–685.
6. Workowski KA, Berman S; Centers for Disease Control and Prevention. Sexually transmitted diseases treatment guidelines, 2010. *MMWR Recomm Rep*. 2010;59(RR-12):1–110.

ADDITIONAL READING

- Allsworth JE, Ratner JA, Peipert JF, et al. Trichomoniasis and other sexually transmitted infections: results from the 2001–2004 National Health and Nutrition Examination Surveys. *Sex Transm Dis*. 2009;36(12):738–744.
- Forna F, Gülmezoglu AM. Interventions for treating trichomoniasis in women. *Cochrane Database Syst Rev*. 2003;(2):CD000218.
- Gülmezoglu AM, Azhar M. Interventions for trichomoniasis in pregnancy. *Cochrane Database Syst Rev*. 2011;(5):CD000220.
- Hale T. *Medications and Mothers' Milk: A Manual of Lactational Pharmacology (Medications and Mother's Milk)*. 14th ed. Amarillo, TX: Pharmasoft Medical; 2010.
- Helms DJ, Mosure DJ, Secor WE, et al. Management of *Trichomonas vaginalis* in women with suspected metronidazole hypersensitivity. *Am J Obstet Gynecol*. 2008;198(4):370.e1–e7.
- Klebanoff MA, Carey JC, Hauth JC, et al. Failure of metronidazole to prevent preterm delivery among pregnant women with asymptomatic *Trichomonas vaginalis* infection. *N Engl J Med*. 2001;345(7):487–493.
- McClelland RS, Sangare L, Hassan WM, et al. Infection with *Trichomonas vaginalis* increases the risk of HIV-1 acquisition. *J Infect Dis*. 2007;195(5):698–702.
- Miller M, Liao Y, Gomez AM, et al. Factors associated with the prevalence and incidence of *Trichomonas vaginalis* infection among African American women in New York City who use drugs. *J Infect Dis*. 2008;197(4):503–509.
- Saperstein AK, Firnhaber GC. Clinical inquiries. Should you test or treat partners of patients with gonorrhea, chlamydia, or trichomoniasis? *J Fam Pract*. 2010;59(1):46–48.
- Wendel KA, Workowski KA. Trichomoniasis: challenges to appropriate management. *Clin Infect Dis*. 2007;44(Suppl 3):S123–S129.
- Wiese W, Patel SR, Patel SC, et al. A meta-analysis of the Papanicolaou smear and wet mount for the diagnosis of vaginal trichomoniasis. *Am J Med*. 2000;108(4):301–308.

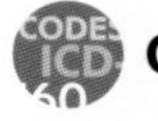

CODES

ICD10
- A59.9 Trichomoniasis, unspecified
- A59.03 Trichomonal cystitis and urethritis
- A59.01 Trichomonal vulvovaginitis

CLINICAL PEARLS
- Both partners need to be treated for trichomoniasis.
- Test of cure is controversial. Emergence of resistance to metronidazole may increase need for repeat testing, but evidence is not yet clear.
- Avoid alcohol during treatment with standard agents.
- Treatment does not reduce risk of adverse pregnancy outcomes.
- Male circumcision may be protective.

TRICHOTILLOMANIA

Carol Hustedde, PhD • William G. Elder, PhD

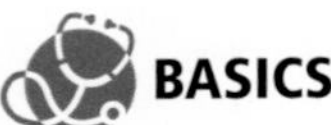

BASICS

- Trichotillomania (TTM) is a hair-pulling disorder characterized by self-induced, repeated, and often noticeable hair loss. It can become severe and difficult to control.
- TTM is currently conceptualized as a compulsive behavior related to obsessive-compulsive disorder (OCD). Tension or boredom typically play a significant role, and the individual may be conscious or unconscious that they are pulling hair.

DESCRIPTION

- TTM causes uncontrollable hair pulling from anywhere on the body, although the scalp is the most common area followed by the eyelashes, eyebrows, pubic/perirectal area, axilla, and face. It usually results in variable degrees of alopecia.
- TTM usually presents in childhood or early adolescence.
- Denial and hiding of hair pulling is common.
- Recurrence or worsened hair pulling is associated with increased stress/anxiety, but TTM can also occur at times of relaxation and distraction, such as when reading.
- The 3 subtypes of TTM: early onset, automatic, and focused.
- When TTM is associated with trichophagia, it may also result in GI complaints secondary to bezoars.
- TTM has frequent comorbidity with other psychiatric diagnoses.

EPIDEMIOLOGY

- It is difficult to assess the exact number of individuals affected by TTM because of the social stigma associated with it. Small studies have estimated a range of 1–3.5% for late adolescents and young adults.
- It is possible that up to 1 of 50 individuals are affected by TTM at least once in their lifetime.
- The mean age of onset is at 13 years.
- During childhood, males and females are equally affected by TTM. During adulthood, females are far more affected than males.

ETIOLOGY AND PATHOPHYSIOLOGY

- Serotonin deficiency
- Tension relief
- Habitual behavior
- There is currently a significant flux in the conceptualizations of the mechanisms and causes of impulse control, behavior, anxiety, and OCDs. Brain imaging and biochemical and neuropsychological studies should help to resolve this issue. It can be expected that there will be increased differentiation as well as redefinitions of disorders that are based on neurophysiology and brain circuitry.

Genetics

Genetics appears to contribute to the development of TTM as demonstrated by a higher rate of concordance in monozygotic twins (38.1%) versus dizygotic twins (0%). Genetic involvement is multifaceted and not clearly understood at this time.

RISK FACTORS

- Positive family history
- Other psychiatric disorders: depression, OCD, anxiety, posttraumatic stress disorder (PTSD), eating disorders, nail biting, skin picking

COMMONLY ASSOCIATED CONDITIONS

- Depression
- Anxiety
- OCD
- Eating disorders

DIAGNOSIS

- TTM may be difficult to diagnose because individuals may deny it because of the social stigma and embarrassment.
- Several TTM-specific assessment tools have been developed that further understanding about psychopathology of TTM.
- Assessment should include multiple sources of information to provide understanding of TTM in context.

HISTORY

- TTM most commonly manifests as hair pulling from any part of the body, resulting in alopecia of variable severity.
- The scalp is the most common area from which hair is pulled but can also involve other parts of the body, such as eyebrows and eyelashes.
- Individuals will conceal hair pulling because of embarrassment. However, when asked about it by a medical professional, they will divulge extent of problem and their efforts to control it.
- TTM may also cause social isolation because individuals may withdraw from friends and family to engage in hair-pulling behavior.
- If TTM is associated with trichophagia (compulsive eating of hair), it may present with various GI symptoms with variable severity, from acute generalized abdominal pain to a bowel obstruction secondary to a trichobezoar.
- TTM is not always associated with anxiety and stress, but it is commonly precipitated by highly stressful situations. The action of hair pulling may be associated with tension relief.

PHYSICAL EXAM

- The most common manifestation of TTM is alopecia.
- The severity of the alopecia is variable, from isolated areas of hair loss to complete baldness.
- Hair loss can be from any part of the body.
- The Friar Tuck sign may be seen, which consists of hair loss seen in a circular pattern with varying lengths of broken hairs.
- There is also a lack of dermatologic abnormalities associated with the hair loss.
- In addition to the hair loss, hair abnormalities consisting of damaged hair follicles, broken hairs of varying lengths
- When TTM is associated with trichophagia and, consequently, trichobezoars, there may be symptoms of abdominal pain, nausea, vomiting, obstructive jaundice, bowel obstruction symptoms, and anemia.
- Patients with TTM may also pull hairs from other people and pets, sometimes surreptitiously. They may also pull fibers from carpets and fabrics.

DIFFERENTIAL DIAGNOSIS

- Alopecia areata
- Tinea capitis
- Traction alopecia
- Loose anagen syndrome
- OCD
- Schizophrenia or other psychotic disorders
- Stereotypic movement disorders
- Factitious behaviors

DIAGNOSTIC TESTS & INTERPRETATION

US or CT scan for trichobezoar detection

Diagnostic Procedures/Other

- Trichotillomania Scale for Children
- Trichotillomania Diagnostic Interview
- National Institute of Mental Health Trichotillomania Questionnaire
- Premonitory Urge for Tics Scale

Test Interpretation

- Punch biopsy: high frequency of telogen hairs; deformed, noninflamed catagen hairs; melanin pigment casts
- Trichogram
- Referrals
  - Some diagnostic procedures may require a dermatology referral. In the presence of missing hair follicles or other hair disorder, a dermatology consult will allow for visual and/or microscopic (trichogram) analysis to determine structure and cycle of the hair disorder.
  - A referral to a psychiatrist, psychologist, or psychopharmacologist who specializes in impulse control and OCD may be helpful. He or she will have access to the specialized symptoms scales described above and also is likely to have professional relationships with psychotherapists who can provide specific therapies, such as habit reversal training. Such referral may also allow for stepped treatment including aggressive use of SSRIs and other antidepressants with combinations of 2nd-line pharmacologic options sometimes tried for impulse control and OCD disorders.

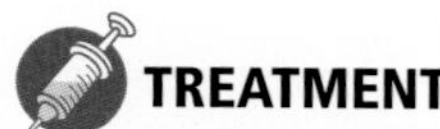

TREATMENT

- Treatment of TTM involves both psychological methods that include specific psychotherapies, pharmacologic treatment, and combined approaches.
- Psychological treatment of TTM may be the primary treatment and is almost always needed in addition to medications.
  - Habit reversal training (HRT) has the strongest empirical support in adults (1)[B]:
    - HRT is a behavioral therapy that is effective in reducing troublesome behaviors associated with TTM. It consists of 4 main components: awareness training, development of a competing response, building motivation, and generalization of skills.
  - Principles of cognitive-behavior therapy can be adjusted to developmental age to treat young children (2)[B].
  - Relaxation training (when stress is high)
  - Support groups to deal with stigma and denial
  - Treatment of comorbid psychiatric condition
  - Unlikely to be helpful
    - Undifferentiated, nonspecific psychotherapy
    - Hypnosis
    - Acupuncture
  - A nutritional supplement, N-acetylcysteine (1,200–2,400 mg/day), shows some benefit for adults but not for children and adolescents.

MEDICATION

First Line

- SSRIs remain the 1st-line pharmacologic option, with a dosing strategy similar to that for OCD.
- SSRIs
  - Fluoxetine (Prozac): 20–80 mg/day
  - Sertraline (Zoloft): 50–200 mg/day
  - Paroxetine (Paxil): 10–50 mg/day
  - Citalopram (Celexa): 20–40 mg/day
  - Escitalopram (Lexapro): 10–20 mg/day

Second Line

- Tricyclic antidepressants
- Atypical antipsychotics
- Opioid blockers
- Glutamate modulators

SURGERY/OTHER PROCEDURES

Surgery is only warranted for removal of trichobezoars.

INPATIENT CONSIDERATIONS

Inpatient admission is usually not due to TTM itself but either treatment of comorbid psychiatric conditions or a bowel obstruction secondary to trichobezoar.

ONGOING CARE

DIET

No special diet required for TTM

PATIENT EDUCATION

- TTM is a multifactorial condition. Not only do medications aid in the treatment of TTM, but also psychological therapies may have a significant benefit as well.
- Online resources: www.trich.org; www.stoppulling.com

PROGNOSIS

TTM tends to be a chronic disorder; however, it can be transient in childhood.

COMPLICATIONS

- Trichobezoars
- Alopecia

REFERENCES

1. Morris S, Zickgraf H, Dingfelder H, et al. Habit reversal training in trichotillomania: guide for the clinician. *Expert Rev Neurother*. 2013;13(9):1069–1077.
2. Tompkins M. Cognitive-behavior therapy for pediatric trichotillomania. *J Rat-Emo Cognitive-Behav Ther*. 2014;32:98–109.

ADDITIONAL READING

- Chattopadhyay K. The genetic factors influencing the development of trichotillomania. *J Genet*. 2011;91(2):259–262.
- Duke DC, Keeley ML, Geffken GR, et al. Trichotillomania: a current review. *Clin Psychol Rev*. 2010;30(2):181–193.
- Franklin ME, Zagrabbe K, Benavides KL. Trichotillomania and its treatment: a review and recommendations. *Expert Rev Neurother*. 2011;11(8):1165–1174.
- Grant J, Odlaug B, Kim S. N-acetylcysteine, a glutamate modulator, in the treatment of trichotillomania. *Arch Gen Psychiatry*. 2009;66(7):756–763.
- Harrison JP, Franklin ME. Pediatric trichotillomania. *Curr Psychiatry Rep*. 2012;14(3):188–196.
- Novak CE, Keuthen NJ, Stewart SE, et al. A twin concordance study of trichotillomania. *Am J Med Genet B Neuropsychiatr Genet*. 2009;150B(7):944–949.
- Springer K, Brown M, Stulberg DL, et al. Common hair loss disorders. *Am Fam Physician*. 2003;68(1):93–102.
- Tolin DF, Franklin ME, Diefenbach GJ, et al. Pediatric trichotillomania: descriptive psychopathology and an open trial of cognitive behavioral therapy. *Cogn Behav Ther*. 2007;36(3):129–144.
- Trichotillomania Learning Center. Expert consensus guidelines on treatment of trichotillomania, skin picking and other body-focused repetitive behaviors. www.trich.org/dnld/ExpertGuidelines_000.pdf. Accessed 2014.

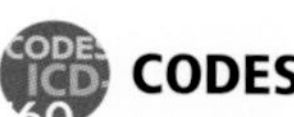

CODES

ICD10

F63.3 Trichotillomania

CLINICAL PEARLS

- Etiology of TTM is multifactorial and differs among individuals. It is important to distinguish between different etiologies.
- Patients may benefit from psychotherapy and medications.
- It is important to realize that TTM is underreported and underdiagnosed because of the social stigma.
- TTM can have a significant impact on psychological, social, academic, and occupational functions.

TRIGEMINAL NEURALGIA

Noah M. Rosenberg, MD • Stacy Potts, MD, MEd

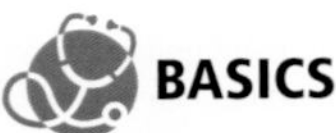

BASICS

DESCRIPTION

- Disorder of the sensory nucleus of the trigeminal nerve (cranial nerve [CN] V) that produces episodic, paroxysmal, severe, lancinating facial pain lasting seconds to minutes in the distribution of ≥1 divisions of the nerve
- Often precipitated by stimulation of well-defined, ipsilateral trigger zones: usually perioral, perinasal, and, occasionally, intraoral (e.g., by washing, shaving)
- System(s) affected: nervous
- Synonym(s): tic douloureux; Fothergill neuralgia; trifacial neuralgia; prosopalgia

EPIDEMIOLOGY

Incidence

- Women: 5.9/100,000/year
- Men: 3.4/100,000/year
- >70 years of age: ~25.6/100,000/year
- Predominant age:
  - >50 years; incidence increases with age.
  - Rare <35 years of age (consider another primary disease; see "Etiology")
- Predominant sex: female > male (~2:1)

Prevalence

16/100,000

Pediatric Considerations

Unusual during childhood

Pregnancy Considerations

Teratogenicity limits therapy for 1st and 2nd trimesters.

ETIOLOGY AND PATHOPHYSIOLOGY

- Demyelination around the compression site seems to be the mechanism by which compression of nerves leads to symptoms.
- Demyelinated lesions may set up an ectopic impulse generation, causing erratic responses: hyperexcitability of damaged nerves and transmission of action potentials along adjacent, undamaged, unstimulated sensory fibers.
- Compression of trigeminal nerve by anomalous arteries or veins of posterior fossa, compressing trigeminal root
- Etiologic classification:
  - Idiopathic (classic)
  - Secondary: cerebellopontine angle tumors (e.g., meningioma); tumors of CN V (e.g., neuroma, vascular malformations), trauma, demyelinating disease (e.g., multiple sclerosis [MS])

RISK FACTORS

Unknown

COMMONLY ASSOCIATED CONDITIONS

- Sjögren syndrome; rheumatoid arthritis
- Chronic meningitis
- Acute polyneuropathy
- MS
- Hemifacial spasm
- Charcot-Marie-Tooth neuropathy
- Glossopharyngeal neuralgia

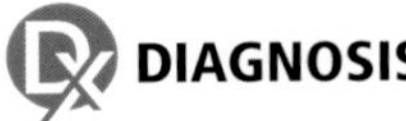

DIAGNOSIS

HISTORY

Paroxysms of pain in the distribution of the trigeminal nerve

PHYSICAL EXAM

All exam findings typically are negative due to the paroxysmal nature of the disorder.

DIFFERENTIAL DIAGNOSIS

- Other forms of neuralgia usually have sensory loss. Presence of sensory loss nearly excludes the diagnosis of TN (if younger patient, frequently MS).
- Neoplasia in cerebellopontine angle
- Vascular malformation of brainstem
- Demyelinating lesion (MS is diagnosed in 2–4% of patients with trigeminal neuralgia.)
- Vascular insult
- Migraine, cluster headache
- Giant cell arteritis
- Postherpetic neuralgia
- Chronic meningitis
- Acute polyneuropathy
- Atypical odontalgia
- SUNCT syndrome (short-lasting, unilateral, neuralgiform pain with conjunctival injection, and tearing)

DIAGNOSTIC TESTS & INTERPRETATION

- The International Headache Society diagnostic criteria for classic trigeminal neuralgia (TN) are as follows:
  - Paroxysmal attacks of pain lasting from a fraction of 1 second to 2 minutes, affecting ≥1 divisions of the trigeminal nerve
  - Pain has at least an intense, sharp, superficial, or stabbing characteristic or is precipitated from trigger areas or by trigger factors.
  - Attacks are stereotyped in the individual patient.
  - No clinically evident neurologic deficit found.
  - Not attributed to another disorder
- Secondary trigeminal neuralgia is characterized by pain that is indistinguishable from classic TN but is caused by a demonstrable structural lesion other than vascular compression.
  - Indicated in all 1st-time presenting patients to rule out secondary causes
- MRI versus CT scan: MRI, with and without contrast, offers more detailed imaging and is preferred, if not contraindicated.
- Routine head imaging identifies structural causes in up to 15% of patients.
- No positive findings are significantly correlated with diagnosis.

Test Interpretation

- Trigeminal nerve: inflammatory changes, demyelination, and degenerative changes
- Trigeminal ganglion: hypermyelination and microneuromata

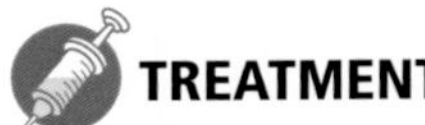

TREATMENT

GENERAL MEASURES

- Outpatient
- Drug treatment is first approach.
- Invasive procedures are reserved for patients who cannot tolerate, fail to respond to, or relapse after chronic drug treatment.
- Avoid stimulation (e.g., air, heat, cold) of trigger zones, including lips, cheeks, and gums.

MEDICATION

First Line

- Carbamazepine (Tegretol) (1)[A]: Start at 100–200 mg BID; effective dose usually 200 mg QID; max dose 1,200 mg/day:
  - 70–90% of patients respond initially.
  - By 3 years, 30% are no longer helped (number needed to treat [NNT] = 1.7) (1)[A].
  - Most common side effect: sedation
- Contraindications: concurrent use of monoamine oxidase inhibitors (MAOIs)
- Precautions: caution in the presence of liver disease
- Significant possible medication interactions: macrolide antibiotics, oral anticoagulants, anticonvulsants, tricyclics, oral contraceptives, steroids, digitalis, isoniazid, MAOIs, methyprylon, nabilone, nizatidine, other H_2 blockers, phenytoin, propoxyphene, benzodiazepines, and calcium channel blockers
- Oxcarbazepine (Trileptal): Start at 150–300 mg BID; effective dose usually 375 mg BID; max dose 1,200 mg/day:
  - Efficacy similar to carbamazepine
  - Faster, with less drowsiness and fewer drug interactions than carbamazepine
  - Decreases serum sodium
  - Most common side effect: sedation

Second Line

- Antiepileptic drugs: insufficient evidence from randomized, controlled trials to show significant benefit from antiepileptic drugs in trigeminal neuralgia (2)[A]
- Phenytoin (Dilantin): 300–400 mg/day (synergistic with carbamazepine):
  - Potent P450 inducer (enhanced metabolism of many drugs)
  - Various CNS side effects (sedation, ataxia)
- Baclofen (Lioresal): 10–80 mg/day; start at 5–10 mg TID with food (as an adjunct to phenytoin or carbamazepine); side effects: drowsiness, weakness, nausea, vomiting

- Gabapentin (Neurontin): Start at 100 mg TID or 300 mg at bedtime; can increase dose up to 300–600 mg TID–QID. Can be used as monotherapy or in combination with other medications and reduces the cost of illness
- Lamotrigine: Titrate up to 200 mg BID over weeks; side effect: 10% experience rash.
- Antidepressants, including amitriptyline, fluoxetine, trazodone:
  - Used especially with anticonvulsants
  - Particularly effective for atypical forms of trigeminal neuralgia
- Clonazepam (Klonopin) frequently causes drowsiness and ataxia.
- Sumatriptan (Imitrex) 3 mg SC reduces acute symptoms and may be helpful after failure of conventional medical therapy.
- Capsaicin cream topically
- Botulinum toxin injection into zygomatic arch
- Valproic acid (Depakene, Depakote)

ISSUES FOR REFERRAL
Initial treatment failure or positive findings on imaging studies

ADDITIONAL THERAPIES
- Radiotherapy
- Stereotactic radiosurgery, such as gamma knife radiosurgery, has been shown to be effective after drug failure:
  - Produces lesions with focused gamma knife radiation
  - Therapy aimed at the proximal trigeminal root
  - Minimal clinically effective dose: 70 Gy
  - ~60–80% of patients achieve complete relief within 1 year; by 3 years, ~30–40% maintain complete relief (3)[B].
  - Most common side effect: sensory disturbance (facial numbness)
  - Failure rates are higher in patients with past TN-related invasive procedures.

SURGERY/OTHER PROCEDURES
- Microvascular decompression of CN V at its entrance to (or exit from) brainstem:
  - 98% of patients achieve initial pain relief; by 20 months, 86% maintain complete relief (NNT = 2) (4)[B].
  - Surgical mortality across studies was 0.3–0.4%.
  - Most common side effect: transient facial numbness and diplopia, headache, nausea, vomiting
  - Pain relief after procedure strongly correlates with the type of TN pain: Type 1 (shocklike pain) results in better outcomes than type 2 (constant pain).
- Peripheral nerve ablation (multiple methods):
  - Higher rates of failure and facial numbness than decompression surgery
  - Radiofrequency thermocoagulation
  - Neurectomy
  - Cryotherapy: high relapse rate
  - Partial sensory rhizotomy
- 4% tetracaine dissolved in 0.5% bupivacaine nerve block (only a few case reports to date; ropivacaine)
- Alcohol block or glycerol injection into trigeminal cistern: unpredictable side effects (dysesthesia and anesthesia dolorosa); temporary relief
- Peripheral block or section of 5th nerve proximal to Gasserian ganglion
- Balloon compression of Gasserian ganglion
- Evidence supporting destructive procedures for benign pain conditions remains limited (5)[A].

COMPLEMENTARY & ALTERNATIVE MEDICINE
Acupuncture, moxibustion (herb): weak evidence for efficacy (6)[B]

ONGOING CARE

FOLLOW-UP RECOMMENDATIONS
Regular outpatient follow-up to monitor symptoms and therapeutic failure

Patient Monitoring
- Carbamazepine and/or phenytoin serum levels
- If carbamazepine is prescribed: CBC and platelets at baseline, then weekly for a month, then monthly for 4 months, then every 6–12 months if dose is stable (regimens for monitoring vary)
- Reduce drugs after 4–6 weeks to determine whether condition is in remission; resume at previous dose if pain recurs. Withdraw drugs slowly after several months, again to check for remission or if lower dose of drugs can be tolerated.

DIET
No special diet

PATIENT EDUCATION
- Instruct patient regarding medication dosage and side effects, risk-to-benefit ratios of surgery or radiation therapy.
- Support organizations:
  - The Facial Pain Association (formerly the Trigeminal Neuralgia Association): www.fpa-support.org
  - Living with Trigeminal Neuralgia: www.livingwithtn.org

PROGNOSIS
- 50–60% eventually fail pharmacologic treatment.
- After having microvascular decompression surgery, most patients wish they had undergone the procedure sooner.
- Of those, relapse is seen in ~50% of stereotactic radiosurgeries and ~27% of surgical microvascular decompressions.

COMPLICATIONS
- Mental and physical sluggishness; dizziness with carbamazepine
- Paresthesias and corneal reflex loss with stereotactic radiosurgery
- Surgical mortality and morbidity associated with microvascular decompression

REFERENCES

1. Wiffen PJ, Derry S, Moore RA, et al. Carbamazepine for chronic neuropathic pain and fibromyalgia in adults. *Cochrane Database Syst Rev*. 2014;(4):CD005451.
2. Zhang, J, Yang M, Zhou M, et al. Non-antiepileptic drugs for trigeminal neuralgia. *Cochrane Database Syst Rev*. 2013;12:CD004029.
3. Karam SD, Tai A, Wooster M, et al. Trigeminal neuralgia treatment outcomes following Gamma Knife radiosurgery with a minimum 3-year follow-up. *J Radiat Oncol*. 2014;3:125–130.
4. Sekula RF Jr, Frederickson AM, Jannetta PJ, et al. Microvascular decompression for elderly patients with trigeminal neuralgia: a prospective study and systematic review with meta-analysis. *J Neurosurg*. 2011;114(1):172–179.
5. Zakrzewska JM, Akram H. Neurosurgical interventions for the treatment of classical trigeminal neuralgia. *Cochrane Database Syst Rev*. 2011;(9):CD007312.
6. Liu H, Li H, Xu M, et al. A systematic review on acupuncture for trigeminal neuralgia. *Altern Ther Health Med*. 2010;16(6):30–35.

T

ADDITIONAL READING

- Attal N, Cruccu G, Baron R, et al. EFNS guidelines on the pharmacological treatment of neuropathic pain: 2010 revision. *Eur J Neurol*. 2010;17(9):e1113–e1188.
- Gronseth G, Cruccu G, Alksne J, et al. Practice parameter: the diagnostic evaluation and treatment of trigeminal neuralgia (an evidence-based review): report of the Quality Standards Subcommittee of the American Academy of Neurology and the European Federation of Neurological Societies. *Neurology*. 2008;71(15):1183–1190.
- Miller JP, Acar F, Burchiel KJ. Classification of trigeminal neuralgia: clinical, therapeutic, and prognostic implications in a series of 144 patients undergoing microvascular decompression. *J Neurosurg*. 2009;111(6):1231–1234.

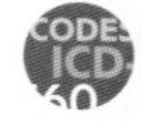

CODES

ICD10
G50.0 Trigeminal neuralgia

CLINICAL PEARLS
- Patients with TN typically have a normal physical exam.
- The long-term efficacy of pharmacotherapy for TN is 40–50%.
- If pharmacotherapy fails, stereotactic radiosurgery or surgical microvascular decompression often is successful.

TRIGGER FINGER (DIGITAL STENOSING TENOSYNOVITIS)

Alan M. Ehrlich, MD • Robert A. Yood, MD

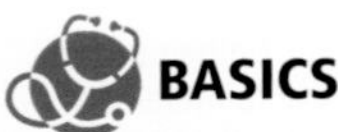

BASICS

DESCRIPTION

Trigger finger is a clicking, snapping, or locking of a finger/thumb with extension movement (after flexion) ± associated pain.

EPIDEMIOLOGY

Incidence

- Adult population: 28/100,000/year
  - Rare in children
- Diabetics have ~4× the risk of the general population (1)[B].
- Predominant age
  - Childhood form typically involves thumb.
  - Adult form typically presents in the 5th and 6th decades of life and involves thumb/digits.
- Predominant sex
  - Children: female = male
  - Adults: female > male (6:1)

Prevalence

Lifetime prevalence in the general population is 2.6%.

PEDIATRIC CONSIDERATIONS

- The thumb is more commonly involved in children.
- When children have a trigger finger instead of a trigger thumb, surgery is often more complicated.
- Release of the A1 pulley alone is often insufficient, and other procedures may be necessary at the time of surgery.

ETIOLOGY AND PATHOPHYSIOLOGY

- Narrowing around the A1 pulley usually is due to either thickening from inflammation, protein deposition, or thickening of the tendon itself. With prolonged inflammation, fibrocartilaginous metaplasia of the tendon sheath occurs.
- The flexor tendon may become nodular, which can exacerbate triggering because the nodule has difficulty passing under the A1 pulley.
- Because intrinsic flexor muscles are stronger than extensors, the finger can stick in the flexed position.
- No clear association with repetitive movements

RISK FACTORS

- Diabetes mellitus
- Rheumatoid arthritis
- Hypothyroidism
- Mucopolysaccharide disorders
- Amyloidosis

GENERAL PREVENTION

Most cases are idiopathic, and no known prevention exists. No clear association with repetitive movements

COMMONLY ASSOCIATED CONDITIONS

- De Quervain tenosynovitis
- Carpal tunnel syndrome
- Dupuytren contracture (usually occurs in 4th/5th digit; thickening of palmar connective tissue results in a flexion contracture of the distal digit)
- Diabetes mellitus
- Rheumatoid arthritis
- Hypothyroidism
- Amyloidosis

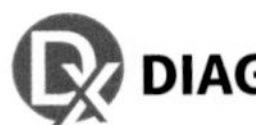

DIAGNOSIS

Diagnosis is based on clinical presentation.

HISTORY

History of clicking, snapping, or locking of a finger/thumb when attempting to extend thumb or finger after flexion ± associated pain

PHYSICAL EXAM

- A palpable nodule may be present.
- Snapping/locking may be present, but neither is necessary for the diagnosis.
- Tenderness to palpation is variable.

DIAGNOSTIC TESTS & INTERPRETATION

Test Interpretation

- Thickening of the A1 pulley with fibrocartilaginous metaplasia
- Thickening/nodule formation of flexor tendon

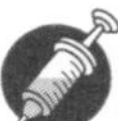

TREATMENT

- Splinting the metacarpophalangeal (MCP) joint at 10–15 degrees of flexion for 6 weeks with the distal joints free to move has been reported to be effective:
  - Splinting is more effective for treating fingers than thumbs (70% vs. 50%).
  - Less effective with severe symptoms, symptoms >6 months, and multiple digits involved (1)[B]
- Long-acting corticosteroids may be injected to achieve symptom relief. Subsequent injections are less likely to work.
- Surgery has high success rate for patients unresponsive to splinting/corticosteroid injections.

GENERAL MEASURES

Splinting/steroid injection should be tried before surgery. Splinting may be more effective for preventing recurrence than as initial treatment (2)[B].

MEDICATION

First Line

- Steroid injection of the tendon sheath/surrounding SC tissue has 57–90% success rate.
- Injection in surrounding tissues is as efficacious as injecting into the tendon sheath (1,3)[B]. Injection into the palmar surface at the midproximal phalanx is associated with less pain than injection of tendon sheath at MCP joint (4)[B].
- Corticosteroid injection has higher success rate than splinting. Higher success rates are associated with a shorter duration of symptoms (2)[B].

Second Line

- Oral NSAIDs may reduce pain and discomfort, but they have not been shown to reduce the underlying cause. They do not reduce symptoms of snapping/locking.
- Injection with diclofenac may be an alternative to corticosteroid for patients with diabetes mellitus where increase in blood sugar may be a concern.
- Corticosteroids appear more effective during the 1st 3 weeks postinjection, but efficacy appears similar to other modalities by 3 months postinjection (5)[B].

ISSUES FOR REFERRAL
Refer to a hand surgeon for release if the patient is not responding to splinting and/or steroid injections.

ADDITIONAL THERAPIES
Physiotherapy has been used in the treatment of trigger digits in children.

SURGERY/OTHER PROCEDURES
- Surgical release can be done as an open procedure or percutaneously.
- Success rates with either procedure are high; no apparent differences in terms of treatment success or rates of complications (5)[A].
- Surgery has a lower rate of recurrence of trigger finger than corticosteroid injection (5)[A].
- Most hand surgeons still prefer the open release because of concern about avoiding nerve injury with the blind procedure.

INPATIENT CONSIDERATIONS
Admission Criteria/Initial Stabilization
Day surgery for trigger finger release

Discharge Criteria
Absence of complications

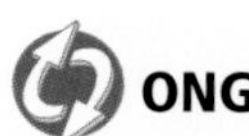

ONGOING CARE

FOLLOW-UP RECOMMENDATIONS
- Follow-up is needed only if symptoms persist or if complications of surgery develop.
- Splinting of the affected digit to minimize flexion/extension of the MCP joint helps with symptom resolution (1)[B],(6)[C].

PROGNOSIS
Prognosis is excellent with either conservative or surgical intervention. Recurrence following corticosteroid injection is more likely for patients with type 1 diabetes mellitus, younger patients, involvement of multiple digits, and patients with a history of other upper extremity tendinopathies (7)[B].

COMPLICATIONS
- Complications from surgery include infection, bleeding, digital nerve injury, and persistent pain and loss of range of motion of the affected finger. The rate of major complications is low (3%), but the rate of minor complications (including loss of range of motion) can be significantly higher (up to 28%).
- Injury to the A2 pulley may result in bowstringing, which is a bulging of the flexor tendon in the palm with flexion. This can be associated with pain.
- Diabetic patients may have increased blood sugar levels for up to 5 days following steroid injection.

REFERENCES

1. Akhtar S, Bradley MJ, Quinton DN, et al. Management and referral for trigger finger/thumb. *BMJ*. 2005;331(7507):30–33.
2. Salim N, Abdullah S, Sapuan J, et al. Outcome of corticosteroid injection versus physiotherapy in the treatment of mild trigger fingers. *J Hand Surg Eur Vol*. 2012;37(1):27–34.
3. Kazuki K, Egi T, Okada M, et al. Clinical outcome of extrasynovial steroid injection for trigger finger. *Hand Surg*. 2006;11(1–2):1–4.
4. Pataradool K, Buranapuntaruk T. Proximal phalanx injection for trigger finger: randomized controlled trial. *Hand Surg*. 2011;16(3):313–317.
5. Shakeel H, Ahmad TS. Steroid injection versus NSAID injection for trigger finger: a comparative study of early outcomes. *J Hand Surg Am*. 2012;37(7): 1319–1323.
6. Ryzewicz M, Wolf JM. Trigger digits: principles, management, and complications. *J Hand Surg Am*. 2006;31(1):135–146.
7. Rozental TD, Zurakowski D, Blazar PE. Trigger finger: prognostic indicators of recurrence following corticosteroid injection. *J Bone Joint Surg Am*. 2008;90(8):1665–1672.

ADDITIONAL READING

- Cardon LJ, Ezaki M, Carter PR. Trigger finger in children. *J Hand Surg Am*. 1999;24(6):1156–1161.
- Fleisch SB, Spindler KP, Lee DH. Corticosteroid injections in the treatment of trigger finger: a level I and II systematic review. *J Am Acad Orthop Surg*. 2007;15(3):166–171.
- Guler F, Kose O, Ercan EC, et al.. Open versus percutaneous release for the treatment of trigger thumb. Orthopedics. 2013 Oct 1;36(10):e1290–e1294.
- Moore JS. Flexor tendon entrapment of the digits (trigger finger and trigger thumb). *J Occup Environ Med*. 2000;42(5):526–545.
- Wang J, Zhao JG, Liang CC. Percutaneous release, open surgery, or corticosteroid injection, which is the best treatment method for trigger digits? *Clin Orthop Relat Res*. 2013;471(6):1879–1886.
- Will R, Lubahn J. Complications of open trigger finger release. *J Hand Surg Am*. 2010;35(4):594–596.

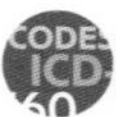

CODES

ICD10
- M65.30 Trigger finger, unspecified finger
- M65.319 Trigger thumb, unspecified thumb
- M65.329 Trigger finger, unspecified index finger

CLINICAL PEARLS

- Trigger finger is caused by narrowing of the A1 flexor tendon pulley.
- Splinting the MCP joint at 10–15 degrees flexion for 6 weeks can be used as initial conservative treatment.
- Splinting is more effective for fingers than thumbs (70% vs. 50%). Splinting is less effective with severe symptoms, symptoms >6 months, and multiple digits involved.
- Long-acting corticosteroid injections are another effective treatment for trigger finger.
- Open and percutaneous surgical release has high success rates.

TROCHANTERIC BURSITIS (GREATER TROCHANTERIC PAIN SYNDROME)

David W. Kruse, MD • Joann Y. Chang, MD

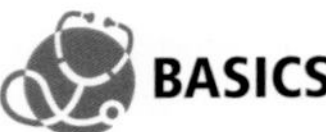

BASICS

Trochanteric bursitis is the historical term referring to lateral hip pain and tenderness over the greater trochanter. Because many patients lack an inflammatory process within the trochanteric bursa, this condition has been more recently referred to as *greater trochanteric pain syndrome* (GTPS) (1).

DESCRIPTION

- Bursae are fluid-filled sacs found primarily at tendon attachment sites with bony protuberances:
  - Multiple bursae are in the area of the greater trochanter of the femur.
  - These bursae are associated with the tendons of the gluteus muscles, iliotibial band (ITB), and tensor fasciae latae.
  - The subgluteus maximus bursa is implicated most commonly in lateral hip pain (1).
- Other structures of the lateral hip include the following:
  - ITB; tensor fasciae latae; gluteus maximus tendon; gluteus medius tendon; gluteus minimus tendon; quadratus femoris muscle; vastus lateralis tendon; piriformis tendon
- *Bursitis* refers to bursal inflammation.
- *Tendinopathy* refers to any abnormality of a tendon, inflammatory or degenerative. *Enthesopathy* refers to abnormalities of the zones of attachment of ligaments and tendons to bones.

EPIDEMIOLOGY

Incidence

- 1.8 patients/1,000 persons/year
- Peak incidence in 4th–6th decades

Prevalence

- Predominant sex: female > male
- More common in running and contact athletes
  - Football, rugby, soccer

ETIOLOGY AND PATHOPHYSIOLOGY

- Acute: abnormal gait or poor muscle flexibility and strength lead to the following:
  - Bursal friction and secondary inflammation
  - Tendon overuse and inflammation
  - Direct trauma from contact or frequently lying with body weight on hip can cause an inflammatory response ("hip pointer").
- Chronic
  - Fibrosis and thickening of bursal sac due to chronic inflammatory process
  - Tendinopathy due to chronic overuse and degeneration: gluteus medius and minimus (1,2)

Genetics

No known genetic factors

RISK FACTORS

Multiple factors have been implicated (1,3):

- Female gender
- Obesity
- Tight hip musculature (including ITB)
- Direct trauma
- Total hip arthroplasty
- Abnormal gait or pelvic architecture
  - Leg length discrepancy
  - Sacroiliac (SI) joint dysfunction
  - Knee or hip osteoarthritis
  - Abnormal foot mechanics (e.g., pes planus, overpronation)
  - Neuromuscular disorder: Trendelenburg gait

GENERAL PREVENTION

- Maintain ITB, hip, and lower back flexibility and strength.
- Avoid direct trauma (use of appropriate padding in contact sports).
- Avoid prolonged running on banked or crowned surfaces.
- Wear appropriate shoes.
- Maintain appropriate body weight loss.

COMMONLY ASSOCIATED CONDITIONS

- Biomechanical factors (1)
  - Tight ITBs; leg length discrepancy; SI joint dysfunction; pes planus
  - Width of greater trochanters greater than width of iliac wings (4)[B]
- Other associated pathology (1):
  - Low back pain
  - Knee and hip osteoarthritis
  - Obesity

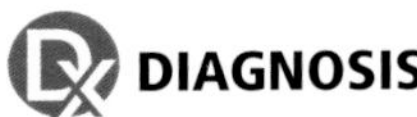

DIAGNOSIS

HISTORY

General history (1)

- Pain localized to the lateral aspect of the hip or buttock
- Pain may radiate to groin or lateral thigh (pseudoradiculopathy).
- Pain exacerbated by the following:
  - Prolonged walking or standing
  - Rising after prolonged sitting
  - Sitting with legs crossed
  - Lying on affected side
- Other historical features:
  - Direct trauma to affected hip
  - Chronic low back pain
  - Chronic leg/knee/ankle/hip pain
  - Recent increase in running distance or intensity
  - Change in running surfaces

PHYSICAL EXAM

- Observe gait.
- Point tenderness with direct palpation over the lateral hip is characteristic of GTPS (1)[B].
- Other exam features have lower sensitivity (1)[B]:
  - Pain with extremes of passive rotation, abduction, or adduction
  - Pain with resisted hip abduction and external or internal rotation
  - Trendelenburg sign
- Other tests to rule out associated conditions:
  - Patrick-FABERE (flexion, abduction, external rotation, extension) test for SI joint dysfunction
  - Ober test for ITB pathology
  - Flexion and extension of hip for osteoarthritis
  - Leg length measurement
  - Foot inspection for pes planus or overpronation
  - Lower extremity neurologic assessment for lumbar radiculopathy or neuromuscular disorders
  - Hip lag sign (5)

DIFFERENTIAL DIAGNOSIS

- ITB syndrome
- Osteoarthritis or avascular necrosis of the hip
- Lumbosacral osteoarthritis/disc disease with nerve root compression
- Fracture or contusion of the hip or pelvis—particularly in setting of trauma
- Stress reaction/fracture of femoral neck—particularly in female runners
- Septic bursitis/arthritis

DIAGNOSTIC TESTS & INTERPRETATION

No routine lab testing is recommended.

Initial Tests (lab, imaging)

- Diagnosis can be made by history and exam, but radiologic imaging can be helpful based on history and physical exam to rule out specific bony pathology (stress fracture, etc).
- If imaging is ordered
  - Anteroposterior and frog-leg views of affected hip
  - Consider lumbar spine radiographs if back pain is thought to be a contributing factor.
  - US can be helpful to define anatomy and guide aspiration or injection.
  - MRI is image of choice in recalcitrant pain or to formally exclude stress fracture.

Follow-Up Tests & Special Considerations
- If there is a concern for a septic bursitis, then aspiration or incision and drainage may be necessary.
- Advanced imaging rarely necessary; detection of abnormalities on MRI is a poor predictor of GTPS (6)[B].

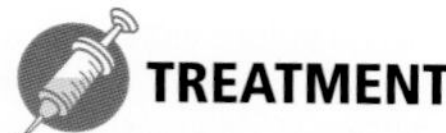

TREATMENT

GENERAL MEASURES
- Physical therapy to address underlying dysfunction and rebuild atrophic muscle mass
- Correct pelvic/hip instability.
- Correct lower limb biomechanics.
- Low-impact conditioning and aquatic therapy
- Gait training
- Weight loss (if applicable)
- Minimize aggravating activities such as prolonged walking or standing.
- Avoid lying on affected side.
- Runners
  - May need to decrease distance and/or intensity of runs during treatment period of 2–4 weeks
  - May need a period of cessation of running; amount of time is case specific but may range from 2–4 weeks.
  - Should avoid banked tracks or roads with excessive tilt

MEDICATION
First Line
- NSAIDs (1)[B]: Treat for 2–4 weeks.
  - Naproxen: 500 mg PO BID
  - Ibuprofen: 800 mg PO TID
- Corticosteroid injection is effective for pain relief (7)[C]. In certain cases, injection can be considered 1st-line therapy:
  - Dexamethasone: 4 mg/mL *or*
  - Kenalog: 40 mg/mL 1–2 mL
  - Consider adding a local anesthetic (short- and/or long-acting) for more immediate pain relief.
  - Can be repeated for recurrence with similar effect if original treatment showed a strong response
  - Goal is acute or subacute pain relief (8)[A].

ISSUES FOR REFERRAL
- Septic bursitis
- Recalcitrant bursitis

ADDITIONAL THERAPIES
- Ice
- Low-energy shock wave therapy has been shown to be superior to other nonoperative modalities (8)[A].
- Focus on achieving flexibility of hip musculature, particularly the ITB.
- Address contributing factors:
  - Low back flexibility
  - If leg length discrepancy, may need heel lift
  - If pes planus or overpronation, may need arch supports or custom orthotics

SURGERY/OTHER PROCEDURES
- Surgery rare but effective in refractory cases (9)[A]
- If surgery is indicated, potential options include the following:
  - Arthroscopic bursectomy
  - Release of the ITB
  - Gluteus medius tendon repair

COMPLEMENTARY & ALTERNATIVE MEDICINE
- Acupuncture
- Prolotherapy
- Growth factor injection techniques
- Platelet-rich plasma injection

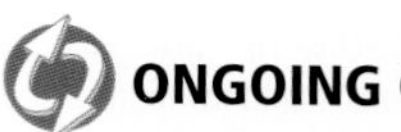

ONGOING CARE

FOLLOW-UP RECOMMENDATIONS
4 weeks posttreatment, sooner if significant worsening

PATIENT EDUCATION
- Maintain hip musculature flexibility, including ITB.
- Correct issues that may cause abnormal gait:
  - Low back pain
  - Knee pain
  - Leg length discrepancy (heel lift)
  - Foot mechanics (orthotics)
- Gradual return to physical activity

PROGNOSIS
Depends on chronicity and recurrence, with more acute cases having an excellent prognosis

COMPLICATIONS
Bursal thickening and fibrosis

REFERENCES

1. Williams BS, Cohen SP. Greater trochanteric pain syndrome: a review of anatomy, diagnosis and treatment. *Anesth Analg.* 2009;108(5):1662–1670.
2. Domb BG, Carreira DS. Endoscopic repair of full-thickness gluteus medius tears. *Arthrosc Tech.* 2013;2(2):e77–e81.
3. Farmer KW, Jones LC, Brownson KE, et al. Trochanteric bursitis after total hip arthroplasty: incidence and evaluation of response to treatment. *J Arthroplasty.* 2010;25(2):208–212.
4. Viradia NK, Berger AA, Dahners LE. Relationship between width of greater trochanters and width of iliac wings in trochanteric bursitis. *Am J Orthop.* 2011;40(9):E159–E162.
5. Kaltenborn A, Bourg CM, Gutzeit A, et al. The hip lag sign—prospective blinded trial of a new clinical sign to predict hip abductor damage. *PLoS ONE.* 2014;9(3):e91560.
6. Blankenbaker DG, Ullrick SR, Davis KW, et al. Correlation of MRI findings with clinical findings of trochanteric pain syndrome. *Skeletal Radiol.* 2008;37(10):903–909.
7. Stephens MB, Beutler AI, O'Connor FG. Musculoskeletal injections: a review of the evidence. *Am Fam Physician.* 2008;78(8):971–976.
8. Brinks A, van Rijn RM, Willemsen SP, et al. Corticosteroid injections for greater trochanteric pain syndrome: a randomized controlled trial in primary care. *Ann Fam Med.* 2011;9(3):226–234.
9. Lustenberger DP, Ng VY, Best TM, et al. Efficacy of treatment of trochanteric bursitis: a systematic review. *Clin J Sport Med.* 2011;21(5):447–453.

ADDITIONAL READING

- Baker CL Jr, Massie RV, Hurt WG, et al. Arthroscopic bursectomy for recalcitrant trochanteric bursitis. *Arthroscopy.* 2007;23(8):827–832.
- Barnthouse NC, Wente TM, Voos JE. Greater trochanteric pain syndrome: Endoscopic treatment options. *Oper Tech Sports Med.* 2012;20:320–324.
- Hugo D, de Jongh HR. Greater trochanteric pain syndrome. *SA Orthopaedic Journal.* 2012;11(1):28–33.
- McMahon SE, Smith TO, Hing CB. A systematic review of imaging modalities in the diagnosis of greater trochanteric pain syndrome. *Musculoskeletal Care.* 2012;10(4):232–239.
- Pretell J, Ortega J, García-Rayo R, et al. Distal fascia lata lengthening: an alternative surgical technique for recalcitrant trochanteric bursitis. *Int Orthop.* 2009;33(5):1223–1227.

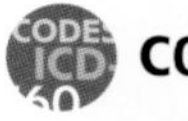

CODES

ICD10
- M70.60 Trochanteric bursitis, unspecified hip
- M70.62 Trochanteric bursitis, left hip
- M70.61 Trochanteric bursitis, right hip

CLINICAL PEARLS
- Patients with GTPS often present inability to lie on the affected side.
- Femoral neck stress fractures are a do-not-miss diagnosis, particularly in young female runners.
- Corticosteroid injection often helpful as initial therapy, particularly for pain relief to allow for aggressive physical therapy.
- Physical therapy is treatment mainstay for correcting biomechanical imbalances and restoring proper function.

TUBERCULOSIS

Carlos Atore, MD • Swati B. Avashia, MD, FAAP

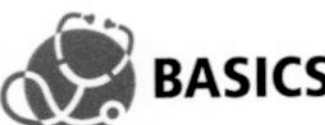

BASICS

DESCRIPTION

- Active tuberculosis
  - Occurs from primary infection or reactivation of latent infection
  - Affects 10% of infected individuals without preventive therapy
  - Risk increases with immunosuppression: highest the first 2 years after infection.
  - Well-described forms: pulmonary (85% of cases), miliary (disseminated), meningeal, abdominal
- Usually acquired by inhalation of airborne bacilli from a person with active tuberculosis (TB). Bacilli multiply in alveoli and spread via macrophages, lymphatics, and blood. 3 possible outcomes:
  - Eradication: Tissue hypersensitivity halts infection within 10 weeks.
  - Primary infection
  - Latent infection: (See "Tuberculosis, Latent [LTBI].")

Pediatric Considerations

- In children, the rate of progression to disease is faster, the risk of progression to disease is higher, and severe disease is more common.
- Most children with pulmonary TB are asymptomatic.
- Treatment of pediatric TB should involve 4 drugs and be directly observed (DOT).

EPIDEMIOLOGY

Incidence

- Worldwide (2012): 8.6 million (13% HIV coinfected)
- United States (2012): 9,951 (3.2/100,000), 127 MDR, and 107 of those were foreign born (1)

Prevalence

Worldwide (2011): 170 cases/100,000 population (36% decrease since 1990); highest burden in Asia and Africa (1)

ETIOLOGY AND PATHOPHYSIOLOGY

- *Mycobacterium tuberculosis*, *Mycobacterium bovis*, or *Mycobacterium africanum* are causative organisms.
- Cell-mediated response by activated T lymphocytes and macrophages forms a granuloma that limits bacillary replication. Destruction of the macrophages produces early "solid necrosis." In 2–3 weeks, "caseous necrosis" develops, and latent tuberculosis infection (LTBI) ensues. In immunocompetent, granuloma undergoes "fibrosis" and calcification. In immunocompromised patients, primary progressive TB develops.

RISK FACTORS

- For infection: homeless, ethnic minorities, close quarters (correctional facilities, nursing homes, barracks); close contact with infected individual; persons from areas with high incidence of active TB (Asia, Africa, Latin America, former Soviet Union states); health care workers; medically underserved, low income, substance abuse
- For development of disease once infected: HIV; lymphoma; silicosis; diabetes mellitus; chronic renal failure; cancer of head, neck, or lung; children <5 years of age; malnutrition; systemic corticosteroids, immunosuppressive drugs; IV drug abuse, alcohol abuse, cigarette smokers; <2 years since infection with *M. tuberculosis*; history of gastrectomy or jejunal bypass; <90% of ideal body weight

GENERAL PREVENTION

- Screening and treatment of LTBI. Active cases must be reported to health department for identification; test and treat all close contacts.
- Bacille Calmette-Guérin (BCG) vaccine: Live attenuated *M. bovis*, prevents 50% of pulmonary disease and 80% of meningitis and miliary disease in children. Use more common in countries with endemic TB. In the United States, consider BCG for high-risk children with negative PPD and HIV tests or for health workers at risk for drug-resistant infection.

COMMONLY ASSOCIATED CONDITIONS

Immunosuppression; HIV-coinfection; malignancy

DIAGNOSIS

HISTORY

- Known exposure to case of active TB
- Underlying medical conditions: immunosuppression
- Tobacco use. Recreational drug use
- Signs and symptoms:
  - General: fever, night sweats, weight loss, malaise, painless adenopathy
  - Pulmonary TB: cough, hemoptysis
  - Abdominal TB: presents acutely as surgical abdomen; chronic abdominal TB varies in presentation, vague abdominal symptoms, abdominal mass, "doughy" abdomen.
  - Meningitis: See "Tuberculosis, CNS."
  - Miliary: See "Tuberculosis, Miliary."

PHYSICAL EXAM

- Often entirely normal. Specific findings depend on organs involved: adenopathy, rales, or hepatosplenomegaly.
- Late findings: renal, bone, or CNS disease

DIFFERENTIAL DIAGNOSIS

- Pulmonary TB: pneumonia (bacterial fungal, atypical), malignancy, tularemia, actinomycosis
- Extrapulmonary TB: syphilis, cat-scratch disease, leishmaniasis, leprosy; rheumatoid disease; erythema nodosum, erythema induratum, syphilis, other mycobacterial infections

DIAGNOSTIC TESTS & INTERPRETATION

Initial Tests (Immunogenesis)

To determine if someone has developed an immune response to mycobacterium

- Tuberculin skin test (TST) (e.g., PPD): 5 U (0.1 mL) intermediate-strength intradermal injection into volar forearm. Measure induration at 48–72 hours:
  - PPD positive if induration
    - >5 mm and HIV infection, recent TB contact, immunosuppressed, disease on x-ray
    - >10 mm and age <4 years or other risk factors
    - >15 mm and age >4 years and no risk factors
    - 2-step test if no recent PPD, age >55 years, nursing home resident, prison inmate, or health care worker. 2nd test 1–3 weeks after initial test; interpret as usual.
  - Context of PPD results:
    - False positive: BCG (unreliable, should not affect decision to treat)
    - False negative: HIV, steroids, gastrectomy, alcoholism, renal failure, sarcoidosis, malnutrition, hematologic or lymphoreticular disorder, very recent exposure
    - If positive once, not necessary to repeat
    - No need for control with *Candida*/other
- Interferon-γ release assays (IGRAs) measure interferon release after stimulation in vitro by *M. tuberculosis* antigens (2)[A]:
  - Lack of cross-reaction with BCG and most nontuberculous mycobacteria
    - Preferred (better specificity) for testing persons who have had BCG (vaccine or for cancer therapy)
  - TST is preferred in children age <5 years (3)[A].

Initial Tests-Active TB (lab, imaging)

- 3 consecutive sputum samples (8–24-hour intervals with at least 1 in early AM) for acid-fast bacilli (AFB) stain and culture by aerosol induction, gastric aspirate (children), or bronchoalveolar lavage
- Positive AFB: Treat immediately. Culture and sensitivity ultimately guide treatment.
- Chest radiograph
  - Primary TB: infiltrate with or without effusion, atelectasis, or adenopathy. Ghon lesion: calcified tuberculous caseating granuloma (tuberculoma); If associated with calcified ipsilateral hilar lymph node then Ghon (or Ranke) complex.
  - Recrudescent TB: cavitary lesions and upper-lobe disease with hilar adenopathy
  - HIV: atypical findings with primary infection, right upper-lobe atelectasis
- CT chest: good sensitivity, tree-in-bud (centrilobular nodules with branching linear opacities)

Follow-Up Tests & Special Considerations

- Baseline CBC, creatinine, AST, ALT, bilirubin, alkaline phosphatase, visual acuity, and red–green color discrimination (regimens involving ethambutol)
- HIV: If positive, get baseline CD4 count.
- High risk: Check hepatitis B and C (injection drug users, Africa or Asia born, HIV infected).
- Extrapulmonary: urine, CSF, bone marrow, and liver biopsy for culture as indicated
- Nonspecific laboratory findings: anemia, monocytosis, thrombocytosis, hypergammaglobulinemia, SIADH, sterile pyuria

Diagnostic Procedures/Other

Culture: TB traditionally takes several weeks for definitive culture results. New (faster) techniques such as the MGIT, Xpert MTB/RIF, and MODS assay are becoming more widely available, allowing for more rapid identification of TB infection (and MDR strains).

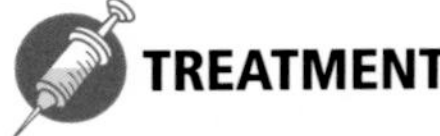

TREATMENT

GENERAL MEASURES

- If clinical suspicion, treat immediately. Prescribing physician is responsible for treatment completion.
- Respiratory and droplet precautions
- Not infectious if favorable clinical response after 2–3 weeks of therapy and 3 negative AFB smears

MEDICATION

Ideal body weight used for dosing. Directly observed therapy (DOT) strongly recommended for all, but required for children, institutionalized patients, nonadherent patients, and nondaily regimens (4)[C].

First Line

- LTBI
  - Isoniazid (INH) for 9 months at 5 mg/kg/day (max of 300 mg) *or* 15 mg/kg (max of 900 mg) 2×/week (5)[A] *or*

– INH 15 mg/kg + rifapentine 300–900 mg weekly for 12 weeks given by DOT for patients age ≥12 years (5,6)[A]

- Active TB infection
  – Regimen 1 (preferred) (7)[A]:
    ○ Initial phase:
      ▪ INH 5 mg/kg, rifampin (RIF) 10 mg/kg (max 600 mg), pyrazinamide (PZA) 15–30 mg/kg, and ethambutol (EMB) 15–20 mg/kg daily for 8 weeks, *or*
      ▪ INH/RIF/PZA/EMB 5 day/week for 8 weeks
  – Continuation phase:
    ○ INH/RIF daily for 18 weeks; or, if DOT, INH/RIF 5 days/week for 18 weeks (recommended for HIV+ with CD4 <100 cells/mm^3 due to increased risk of resistance), *or*
    ○ INH/RIF 2–3×/week for 18 weeks (not used if HIV+ with CD4 <100; may have increased risk of relapse), *or*
    ○ INH/rifapentine once weekly for 18 weeks (acceptable only for HIV-patients without cavitary disease, may have increased risk of relapse) (7)[A]
  – Regimen 2:
    ○ Initial phase:
      ▪ INH/RIF/PZA/EMB daily for 2 weeks, then twice weekly for 6 weeks, *or*
      ▪ INH/RIF/PZA/EMB 5 d/week for 2 weeks, then twice weekly for 6 weeks
    ○ Continuation phase:
      ▪ INH/RIF 2–3×/week for 18 weeks (not recommended if HIV+ with CD4 <100; may have increased risk of relapse), *or*
      ▪ INH/rifapentine once weekly for 18 weeks (acceptable only for HIV-patients without cavitary disease; may have increased risk of relapse) (7)[A]
      ▪ Treat TB in pregnancy with INH, RIF, and EMB; add pyridoxine 25 mg/day.

Pregnancy Considerations

- Streptomycin: ototoxic and nephrotoxic; do not use in pregnancy. Pyrazinamide not used in pregnant women in the United States
- Congenital infection: from maternal miliary or endometrial TB. If suspected, get PPD, CXR, lumbar puncture, and culture placenta. Start treatment promptly.
- Breastfeeding: ok while taking TB drugs; supplement with pyridoxine 25 mg/day.

Pediatric Considerations

- Children: Ethambutol is not used.
- Children on medication may attend school.

ALERT

- Maximum drug doses: RIF 600 mg all regimens, PZA 2,000 mg/day or 4,000 mg 2×/week, EMB, 600 mg/day or 4,000 mg 2×/week
- If patient does not receive PZA during entire first 2 months, extend treatment to 9 months.
- *Mycobacterium bovis* is resistant to PZA; must be treated 9 months
- Continue EMB until organism susceptibility to INH+RIF is determined (7)[A].

Second Line

Include fluoroquinolones and injectable aminoglycosides. Use when MDR is suspected or patient intolerance (see "Tuberculosis, MDR").

ISSUES FOR REFERRAL

ALERT

Public health authorities should be notified for all cases of active TB. Consult infectious disease specialist for cases of drug-resistant TB and for cases involving HIV-positive patients on antiretroviral therapy.

ADDITIONAL THERAPIES

- Pyridoxine: 50 mg may prevent INH-associated peripheral neuropathy, especially for those who are malnourished or have comorbidities that increase risk of neuropathy (6)[A].
- Steroids: recommended for TB meningitis or pericarditis, use concomitant anti-TB therapy (4)[B]

SURGERY/OTHER PROCEDURES

For extrapulmonary complications (spinal cord compression, bowel obstruction, constrictive pericarditis)

COMPLEMENTARY & ALTERNATIVE MEDICINE

Vitamin D deficiency may increase susceptibility to TB and development of active TB (8)[C].

INPATIENT CONSIDERATIONS

- Negative pressure isolation with personal respirators and droplet precautions
- 3 consecutive negative sputum AFB smears for release from isolation

Discharge Criteria

Once TB has been excluded or the patient has 1) effective therapy, is clinically improving, and is not an infectious risk; 2) arrange outpatient follow-up with a provider comfortable managing TB; 3) and coordinate case management with the local public health department.

ONGOING CARE

FOLLOW-UP RECOMMENDATIONS

Patient Monitoring

- Assess monthly for treatment adherence and adverse medication effects. CXR at 3rd month.
- For HIV+: CD4 count, CBC, and liver enzymes q3mo
- Liver enzymes monthly if chronic liver disease, alcohol use, pregnant, or postpartum. Temporarily discontinue medications if asymptomatic and enzymes ≥5× normal or if symptomatic and enzymes ≥3× normal.
- Visual acuity and red–green color monthly if on ethambutol >2 months or doses >20 mg/kg/day
- If culture-positive after 2 months of therapy, reassess drug sensitivity, initiate DOT, coordinate care with public health authorities, and consider infectious disease consultation if not already involved.

PATIENT EDUCATION

- Emphasize importance of medication adherence.
- Screen and treat close contacts.
- Alert patient that health authorities must be notified.
- Tuberculosis General Information, 2011: http://www.cdc.gov/tb/publications/factsheets/general/tb.htm

PROGNOSIS

Few complications and full resolution of infection if drugs taken for full course as prescribed

COMPLICATIONS

- Cavitary lesions can become secondarily infected.
- Risk for drug resistance increases with HIV-positive, treatment nonadherence, or residence in area with high incidence of resistance.
- MDR-TB: resistance to INH and rifampicin
- XDR-TB: resistant to fluoroquinolones (9% of MDR)

REFERENCES

1. World Health Organization. *WHO global tuberculosis report 2013*. http://www.who.int/tb/publications/global_report/en/. Accessed 2014.
2. Mazurek GH, Jereb J, Vernon A, et al. Updated Guidelines for using interferon gama release assays to detect *Mycobacterium tuberculosis* infection: United States. *MMWR Recomm Rep*. 2010;59(RR-5):1–25.
3. Centers for Disease Control and Prevention. National shortage of purified-protein derivative tuberculin products. *MMWR Morb Mortal Wkly*. 2013;62(16):312.
4. Golden MP, Vikram HR. Extrapulmonary tuberculosis: an overview. *Am Fam Physician*. 2005;72(9):1761–1768.
5. Drugs for tuberculosis. *Treat Guidel Med Lett*. 2012;10(116):29–36; quiz 37–38.
6. Centers for Disease Control and Prevention. Recommendations for use of an isoniazid-rifapentine regimen with direct observation to treat latent *Mycobacterium tuberculosis* infection. *MMWR Morb Mortal Wkly Rep*. 2011;60(48):1650–1653.
7. Hall RG, Leff RD, Gumbo T. Treatment of active pulmonary tuberculosis in adults: current standards and recent advances. *Pharmacotherapy*. 2009;29(12):1468–1481.
8. Luong KVQ, Nguyen LTH. Impact of vitamin D in the treatment of tuberculosis. *Am J Med Sci*. 2011;341(6):493–498.

ADDITIONAL READING

- Centers for Disease Control and Prevention. Trends in tuberculosis: United States 2012. *MMWR Morb Wkly Rep*. 2013;62(11):201–205.
- World Health Organization. *Guidelines for Treatment of Tuberculosis*. 4th ed. Geneva, Switzerland: World Health Organization; 2010. http://www.who.int/tb/publications/2010/9789241547833/en/. Accessed 2014.

SEE ALSO

- Tuberculosis, CNS; Tuberculosis, Latent (LTBI); Tuberculosis, Miliary
- Algorithm: Weight Loss, Unintentional

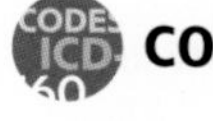

CODES

ICD10

- A15.9 Respiratory tuberculosis unspecified
- A15.0 Tuberculosis of lung
- A19.9 Miliary tuberculosis, unspecified

CLINICAL PEARLS

- Have high suspicion for TB in patients with chronic cough and 1 additional risk factor.
- TB is fully curable when diagnosed and treated appropriately.
- Children and elderly clinically exhibit fewer classic features of TB.

T

TUBERCULOSIS, LATENT (LTBI)

Kay A. Bauman, MD, MPH

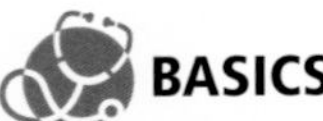

BASICS

DESCRIPTION

- Tuberculosis (TB) is a common infection transmitted by inhaling airborne bacilli from a person with active TB. The bacilli multiply in the alveoli and are carried by macrophages, lymphatics, and blood to distant sites (e.g., lung, pleura, brain, kidney, bone).
- Latent TB infection (LTBI) is an asymptomatic, noninfectious condition that follows exposure to an active case of TB. It is usually detected by a positive skin test (i.e., purified protein derivative [PPD]), positive interferon-γ release assay (IGRA) test. In LTBI, acid-fast bacilli smear and culture are negative, and CXR does not suggest active TB.
- TB: Active disease occurs in 5–10% of infected individuals not receiving preventive therapy. Chance of active TB increases with immunosuppression and is highest for all individuals within 2 years of infection; 85% of the cases are pulmonary, which can spread by person-to-person aerosol route.
- The majority of active TB cases occur in foreign-born persons as a result of reactivation of LTBIs.
- LTBI treatment is a key component of the TB elimination strategy of the United States. An estimated 4,000–11,000 cases of active TB were prevented by LTBI treatment in 2002.

ALERT

Test for LTBI (PPD or IGRA), and treat latent infection in high-risk populations (1).

EPIDEMIOLOGY

- High-risk groups include immigrants from Asia, Latin America, Africa, and the Pacific basin; homeless persons; persons with a history of drug use or history of incarceration; HIV-infected individuals; and health care workers.
- Also at high risk are those newly exposed, particularly children.
- In 2013, Asians had the highest active TB case rate of all groups, 26 times the rate in whites. The rate of TB in Hispanics is 7 times that in whites, and for non-Hispanic blacks, the rate of TB is 8 times higher than for whites (1).
- Of active TB cases in 2013 in ethnic minorities, 95% of Asian cases, 75% of Hispanic cases, 40% of black cases, and 23% of white cases were foreign-born (1), further emphasizing the need to screen foreign-born persons for latent TB and treat those whose screening tests are positive.
- In 2013, 7% of active TB cases in the United States were in HIV-positive individuals, and 6% were homeless (1).

Prevalence

- 4% of the U.S. population has LTBI.
- Worldwide, it is estimated that 1/3 of the population harbors latent TB.
- Predominant gender: male > female

ETIOLOGY AND PATHOPHYSIOLOGY

Mycobacterium tuberculosis, *Mycobacterium bovis*, and *Mycobacterium africanum*

RISK FACTORS

- HIV infection, immunosuppression
- Immigrants (from Asia, Africa, Latin America, Pacific Islands, or area with high rate of TB), including migrant workers
- Close contact with infected individual
- Institutionalization (e.g., prison, nursing home)
- Use of illicit drugs
- Lower socioeconomic status or homeless
- Health care workers
- Chronic medical disease such as diabetes mellitus (DM), end-stage renal disease, cancer, or silicosis; organ transplant (immunosuppression)
- Persons with fibrotic changes on CXR consistent with previous TB infection (2)
- Recent TB skin test (TST) converters (2)
- Laboratory personnel working with mycobacteria

GENERAL PREVENTION

Screen for LTBI, and treat individuals with positive tests.

COMMONLY ASSOCIATED CONDITIONS

- HIV infection (see "Inital Tests")
- Immunosuppression

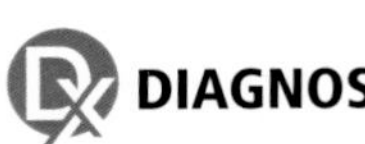

DIAGNOSIS

HISTORY

LTBI: Assess risk. History of immigration from a high-risk area, history of IV drug use and/or drug treatment, HIV, homelessness, recent incarceration, immunosuppression

PHYSICAL EXAM

No signs of infection

DIFFERENTIAL DIAGNOSIS

Fungal infections; atypical mycobacteria or *Nocardia*

DIAGNOSTIC TESTS & INTERPRETATION

Initial Tests (lab, imaging)

- None routinely recommended
- In higher risk patients: liver profile, hepatitis C virus (HCV) and hepatitis B virus (HBV) screening
- HIV test recommended to assess risk for active TB in men who have sex with men or persons with a history of IV drug use
- CXR required to rule out TB in asymptomatic infected persons
- CT scan of the chest has good sensitivity.

Diagnostic Procedures/Other

- PPD: 5 U (0.1 mL) intermediate-strength intradermal volar forearm. Measure induration at 48–72 hours:
  - Positive if induration is
    - >5 mm and patient has HIV infection (or suspected) (2), is immunosuppressed, had recent close TB contact, or has clinical evidence of active or old disease on CXR
    - >10 mm and patient age <4 years or has other risk factors noted earlier
    - >15 mm and patient age >4 years and has no risk factors (2)
  - Negative if induration <5 mm on initial test and, if indicated, on second test.
  - Use the 2-step test (administer a second intradermal test 1–3 weeks after initial test; measure and interpret as usual) if patient has had no recent PPD and is age >55 years or is a nursing home resident, prison inmate, or health care worker.
- The interferon blood test or QuantiFERON-TB and QuantiFERON-TB GOLD measure the release of interferon by sensitized lymphocytes when exposed to antigens of *M. tuberculosis*. It is unaffected by prior BCG vaccination, requires only one patient visit, and has improved sensitivity and specificity but is costly (3).
- Special considerations
  - Steroids: false-negative skin test
  - Measles vaccine: may suppress tuberculin activity; simultaneous PPD and measles vaccine recommended; if not simultaneous, defer PPD 4–6 weeks after measles vaccine.
  - The multiple-puncture tine test is not recommended.
  - Do not use history of BCG vaccination as a reason to ignore a positive PPD in adults and forego recommendation for treatment.
  - Disorders that may alter results and give a false-negative skin test:
    - Recent viral infection
    - New (<10 weeks) infection
    - Severe malnutrition
    - HIV
    - Anergy
    - Age <6 months
    - Overwhelming TB

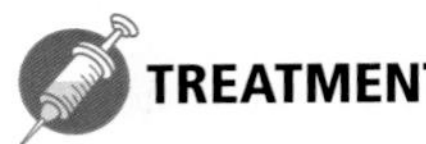

TREATMENT

GENERAL MEASURES

- Must exclude active TB
- Treatment for LTBI is crucial to control and eliminate TB disease in the United States because it both decreases the risk of active TB in those treated and decreases risks to those potentially infected by those same people (2).
- Treat LTBI at any age if patient has HIV, has had close TB contact, is a recent converter (<2 years), is an IV drug user, has an abnormal CXR, has a high-risk medical condition, or is in another high-risk group:
- Directly observed therapy (DOT) is recommended if patient adherence is not assured.
  - Use isoniazid (INH) (for 9 months).
  - Acceptable alternative: INH × 6 months
  - Use INH 900 mg and rifapentine 900 mg weekly for 12 weeks.
- Treat LTBI during pregnancy if patient has recent infection or is HIV positive (use INH with pyridoxine, and monitor liver enzymes); otherwise, treatment may be postponed until postpartum (2).
- Special considerations for HIV infection and suspected INH resistance (2)

- *Note:* Because of severe liver injury and death associated with rifampin and pyrazinamide, these medications are less often recommended for LTBI (2).
- Exclusions: cirrhosis, active hepatitis, history of excessive alcohol consumption (2)

MEDICATION

- INH alone
  - INH-scored tablets: 100 mg, 300 mg, or syrup 10 mg/mL
    - Daily: adult 300 mg; pediatric 10–15 mg/kg (maximum 300 mg)
    - Twice weekly: adult 900 mg; pediatric 20–30 mg/kg (maximum 900 mg)
    - Treatment for 9 months; typical completion rates of ≤60%
    - Precautions
      - Follow liver function if the patient has history of alcoholism, HBV, HCV, or other liver dysfunction or new signs of liver injury.
      - INH: Peripheral neuritis and hypersensitivity are possible. Consider pyridoxine.
      - INH: An idiosyncratic drug reaction that results in INH-associated severe liver injury has been reported by the CDC in 17 patients in years 2004–2008. These included 15 adults and 2 children; 5 underwent liver transplantation and 5 subsequently died (1 of the liver transplant recipients). Thus, monitoring of patients while on treatment is recommended, looking for symptoms of liver injury (all were symptomatic!), and not be limited to laboratory monitoring. The rate of this reaction is difficult to calculate, as unknown numbers of patients are treated for LTBI, but one estimate is 291,000–433,000/year in the United States (4).
- INH and rifapentine
  - Patients >12 years: rifapentine, a rifampin-like drug used to treat LTBI, 900 mg weekly (if patient >50 kg) and INH, 15–25 mg/kg weekly (rounded to nearest 50 or 100 mg; 900 mg max) for 12 weeks given as direct observation therapy. This new and shorter treatment has increased rates of completion compared with 9 months of INH (82% compared with 69% in one trial), slightly more adverse effects (4.9% vs. 3.7%), and is more costly (approximately $160 vs. $6 for course of treatment):
    - Contraindications to INH/rifapentine: HIV patients receiving antiretroviral therapy, pregnancy. Rifapentine may cause hyperuricemia and hematuria (5).
- Alternative: rifampin alone
  - Adults 600 mg/day for 4 months; children 10–20 mg/kg/day for 6 months (max 600 mg/day). Fewer data exist for efficacy of this regimen but can be considered for contacts of INH-resistant TB or patient with INH contraindications. In one study, the 4-month course increased compliance from 62.6% with INH to 71.6% with rifampin (6).

ADDITIONAL THERAPIES

Pediatric Considerations

- Protocol for newborn with mother/household contact with infection or disease
- If mother or household contact has LTBI, skin test all household contacts, and treat any with positive PPD.
- If contact has abnormal CXR, separate infant until infectious status known; if not contagious, monitor infant PPD (7).
- If mother has disease and is possibly contagious, evaluate infant for congenital TB, and test for HIV; separate newborn until mother is noninfectious (7).
- If congenital TB is suspected, treat.
- If no congenital disease, start INH, and repeat PPD after 3–4 months. If positive, reassess infant, and finish 9 months of INH. If PPD is negative and source is noninfectious, stop INH and monitor infant (7).
- BCG vaccine, live-attenuated *M. bovis*: used more commonly in developing countries in children to prevent complications of TB

INPATIENT CONSIDERATIONS

Geriatric Considerations

- Before entering a chronic-care facility, patients should have a PPD using 2-step protocols.
- INH side effects are more pronounced.

Discharge Criteria

- Activity, as tolerated
- No isolation required

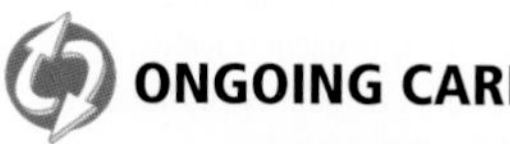

ONGOING CARE

FOLLOW-UP RECOMMENDATIONS

Patient Monitoring

- During preventive therapy for LTBI: initial monthly visits to assess adherence to regimen and to monitor for hepatitis and neuropathy; if stable, can monitor less frequently
- If patient remains asymptomatic, repeat CXR is not needed.
- Check liver enzymes if patient is symptomatic, is HIV positive, has chronic liver disease, uses alcohol, or is pregnant or postpartum, and modify drugs, if needed.

DIET

Regular; consider pyridoxine supplement, 10–50 mg/day.

PROGNOSIS

- Generally, there are few complications and treatment is effective if drugs are taken for full course as prescribed.
- Retreatment is not necessary.

COMPLICATIONS

Recrudescent TB

REFERENCES

1. Alami NN, Yuen CM, Miramontes R, et al; Centers for Diesase Control and Prevention. Trends in tuberculosis—United States, 2013. *MMWR Morb Mortal Wkly Rep*. 2014;63(11):229–233.
2. Jensen PA, Lambert LA, Iademarco MF, et al. Guidelines for preventing the transmission of *Mycobacterium tuberculosis* in health-care settings, 2005. *MMWR Recomm Rep*. 2005;54(RR-17):1–141.
3. Campos-Outcalt D. When, and when not, to use the interferon-gamma TB test. *J Fam Pract*. 2005;54(10):873–875.
4. Centers for Disease Control and Prevention. Severe isoniazid-associated liver injuries among persons being treated for latent tuberculosis infection—United States, 2004–2008. *MMWR Morb Mortal Wkly Rep*. 2010;59(8):224–229.
5. Centers for Disease Control and Prevention. Recommendations for use of an isoniazid-rifapentine regimen with direct observation to treat latent *Mycobacterium tuberculosis* infection. *MMWR Morb Mortal Wkly Rep*. 2011;60(48):1650–1653.
6. Page KR, Sifakis F, Montes de Oca R, et al. Improved adherence and less toxicity with rifampin vs isoniazid for treatment of latent tuberculosis: a retrospective study. *Arch Intern Med*. 2006;166(17):1863–1870.
7. American Academy of Pediatrics. *Red Book: 2003 Report of the Committee on Infectious Diseases*. Elk Grove Village, IL: American Academy of Pediatrics; 2003.

ADDITIONAL READING

- Centers for Disease Control and Prevention; American Thoracic Society. Update: adverse event data and revised American Thoracic Society/CDC recommendations against the use of rifampin and pyrazinamide for treatment of latent tuberculosis infection—United States, 2003. *MMWR Morb Mortal Wkly Rep*. 2003;52(31):735–739.
- Young DB, Gideon HP, Wilkinson RJ. Eliminating latent tuberculosis. *Trends Microbiol*. 2009;17(5):183–188.

SEE ALSO

Tuberculosis; Tuberculosis, Miliary

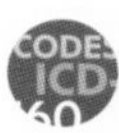

CODES

ICD10

- R76.11 Nonspecific reaction to skin test w/o active tuberculosis
- R76.12 Nonspecific reaction to cell mediated immunity measurement of gamma interferon antigen response without active tuberculosis

CLINICAL PEARLS

- Treatment for LTBI is crucial to control and eliminate TB disease in the United States; an estimated 4% of the U.S. population has LTBI.
- Test household contacts of PPD-positive patients.
- History of BCG vaccination, especially >10 years before PPD testing, should not be considered as the cause of a positive PPD. The interferon-γ blood test is unaffected by prior BCG vaccination.
- Treat all HIV-positive patients with LTBI with a prophylactic regimen.
- Screen foreign-born persons for latent TB, and treat those who are positive.

TYPHOID FEVER

Douglas W. MacPherson, MD, MSc(CTM), FRCPC

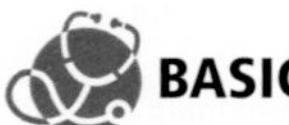

BASICS

- Typhoid fever is a common enteric bacterial disease around the world transmitted by ingestion of contaminated food or water.
- Most cases in the United States are imported from endemic areas of South or Southeast Asia and Latin America.

DESCRIPTION

- Typhoid fever is an acute systemic illness in humans caused by *Salmonella typhi*.
  - Classic example of enteric fever caused by *Salmonella* bacterium
- Enteric fevers due to *Salmonella paratyphi* can present in a manner similar to classic typhoid fever.
- Typhoid is endemic in developing nations with poor sanitation. Most cases in North America and other developed nations are acquired after travel to disease-endemic areas.
- Travelers visiting family or friends may be at greater risk of typhoid.
- Mode of transmission is fecal–oral through ingestion of contaminated food (commonly poultry or milk) or water.
- Incubation period varies from 7 to 21 days.
- System(s) affected: gastrointestinal; pulmonary; skin/exocrine
- Synonym(s): typhoid; typhus abdominalis; enteric fever; nervous fever; slow fever

Geriatric Considerations

Disease is more serious in the elderly.

Pediatric Considerations

Disease is more serious in infants but may be milder in children.

EPIDEMIOLOGY

Although typhoid outbreaks have been described in the United States, most cases are reported in international travelers returning from endemic transmission areas.

- Predominant age: all ages
- Predominant sex: male = female

Incidence

In the United States, 300–500 new cases per year

ETIOLOGY AND PATHOPHYSIOLOGY

- Historically, typhoid fever (untreated) occurs in several week-long stages.
- The initial infection is transmitted via the fecal–oral route, with a GI source of the bacterium resulting in bacteremia and sepsis. Involvement of the bowel wall (Peyer patch) rarely may be associated with bleeding from the bowel or bowel perforation.
- The first stage involves fluctuations in temperature with relative bradycardia (Faget sign). Other symptoms include headache, cough, malaise, epistaxis, and abdominal pain.
- The second stage involves much higher fever (with persistent relative bradycardia). Mental status changes are possible (agitation—"nervous fever"). Rose spots appear in some patients on the chest and abdomen. Abdominal pain is common as is constipation or diarrhea (with characteristic malodorous "pea soup" appearance).
- The 3rd week is when most complications occur due to intestinal hemorrhage or encephalitis.
- The final week is characterized by defervescence and recovery.
- *S. typhi* chronic carrier state may occur with shedding of the bacterium in the stools. Potential person-to-person transmission may occur. In a chronic carrier state, *S. typhi* locates in the biliary tract and gallbladder. Chronic suppressive antimicrobials may clear a carrier state. In extreme cases, cholecystectomies have been performed to attempt to clear carriage of *S. typhi*.

RISK FACTORS

Must be considered in any patient presenting with fever after tropical travel or exposure to a chronic carrier

GENERAL PREVENTION

- Food and water precautions help prevent all enteric infections, including typhoid fever.
- Avoid tap water, salad/raw vegetables, unpeeled fruits, and dairy products in tropical travel.
- Avoid undercooked poultry or poultry products left unrefrigerated for prolonged periods.
- Wash hands before and after food preparation.
- For high-risk travel to an endemic area, consider vaccination against typhoid.
  - Parenteral ViCPS or capsular polysaccharide typhoid vaccine (Typhim Vi) *or*
  - Ty21a or live oral typhoid vaccine (Vivotif Berna), particularly if traveler will be at prolonged risk (>4 weeks)
- Consider vaccination for workers exposed to *S. typhi* or those with household or intimate exposure to a carrier of *S. typhi*.
- Occupational health and safety precautions, including screening of domestic and commercial food handlers, may be considered in some situations.

DIAGNOSIS

Assess the clinical presentation and exposure history, including travel and known exposures to chronic *S. typhi* carriers. The stages of untreated typhoid fever are described in "Etiology and Pathophysiology."

HISTORY

Patient presentation

- Travel history to an endemic region and exposure to contaminated food or water
- Exposure to a chronic *S. typhi* carrier
- Fever, headache
- Malaise
- Abdominal discomfort/bloating/constipation
- Diarrhea (less common)
- Dry cough
- Confusion/lethargy

PHYSICAL EXAM

- Fever
- Relative bradycardia
- Cervical adenopathy
- Conjunctivitis
- Rose spot (transient erythematous maculopapular rash in anterior thorax or upper abdomen)
- Splenomegaly
- Hepatomegaly

DIFFERENTIAL DIAGNOSIS

- Malaria
- "Enteric fever–like" syndrome caused by *Yersinia enterocolitica*, pseudotuberculosis, and *Campylobacter* spp.
- Enteric fever caused by nontyphoid *Salmonella* spp.
- Infectious hepatitis
- Dengue
- Atypical pneumonia
- Infectious mononucleosis
- Subacute bacterial endocarditis
- Tuberculosis
- Brucellosis
- Q fever
- Toxoplasmosis
- Typhus
- Viral infections: Epstein-Barr virus (EBV), cytomegalovirus (CMV), viral hemorrhagic agents

DIAGNOSTIC TESTS & INTERPRETATION

Due to the rarity of enteric fevers/typhoid syndromes in the United States, a high level of clinical suspicion is necessary for accurate diagnosis.

- Definitive diagnosis is by culture of *S. typhi* from blood or other sterile body fluid.
- Isolation of *S. typhi* in sputum, urine, or stool leads to a presumptive diagnosis in typical clinical presentation.
- Serology is nonspecific and typically not useful.
- If there are multiple negative blood cultures, or in patients with prior antibiotic therapy, diagnostic yield is better with bone marrow culture.
- Anemia, leukopenia (neutropenia), thrombocytopenia, or evidence of disseminated intravascular coagulopathy. Elevated liver enzymes are common.
- Have a high clinical suspicion for intestinal perforation or consider serial plain abdominal films looking for evidence of perforation in ill patients complaining of persistent abdominal tenderness.

Diagnostic Procedures/Other

- Bone marrow aspirate for culture of *S. typhi* is more sensitive than blood cultures but rarely indicated as a primary investigation.
- Bone marrow aspiration may be done for evaluation of a persistent fever in a clinically suspect situation with negative cultures or as part of an investigation of fever of unknown origin.

Test Interpretation

Classically, pathology of the bowel shows mononuclear proliferation involving lymphoid tissue of intestinal tract, especially Peyer patches of the terminal ileum.

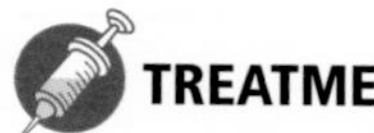

TREATMENT

Indications and contraindications for specific treatment of typhoid disease and chronic carrier states must be determined on an individual basis. Factors to be considered are age, public health and occupational health risk (e.g., food handler, chronic care facilities, medical personnel), intolerance to antibiotics, and evidence of biliary tract disease.

Awareness of emerging drug-resistant *S. typhi* strains globally and the epidemiology of the patient's exposure may direct primary therapy. Knowledge of local resistance patterns for presumptive treatment or laboratory sensitivity should guide therapy. Fluoroquinolone-resistant *S. typhi* is common in Asia.

GENERAL MEASURES

- Fluid and electrolyte support
- Strict isolation of patient's linen, stool, and urine
- Consider serial plain abdominal films for evidence of perforation, usually in the 3rd–4th week of illness.
- For hemorrhage: blood transfusion and management of shock

MEDICATION

First Line

- Chloramphenicol: pediatric 50 mg/kg/day PO QID × 2 weeks; adult dose 2–3 g per day PO divided q6h for 2 weeks *or*
- Ampicillin: pediatric 100 mg/kg/day (max 2 g) QID PO × 2 weeks; adults 500 mg q6h for 2 weeks *or*
- Ciprofloxacin: 500 mg PO BID × 2 weeks, *indicated in multiple-drug-resistant typhoid*
  - Has been used successfully and safely in children; WHO recommends as first line in areas with drug resistance to older 1st-line antibiotics.
  - Fluoroquinolones may prevent clinical relapse better than chloramphenicol (1)[A].
- Ceftriaxone: pediatric 100 mg/kg/day × 2 weeks; adult dose: 1–2 g IV once daily × 2 weeks *or*
- Azithromycin: pediatric 10–20 mg/kg (max 1 g) PO daily × 5–7 days; adult dose: 1 g PO once followed by 500 mg PO daily × 5–7 days
- Chronic carrier state
  - Ampicillin: 4–5 g/day plus probenecid 2 g/day QID × 6 weeks (for patients with normally functioning gallbladder without evidence of cholelithiasis)
  - Ciprofloxacin: 500 mg PO BID for 4–6 weeks is also efficacious. Chloramphenicol resistance has been reported in Mexico, South America, Central America, Southeast Asia, India, Pakistan, Middle East, and Africa.
- Contraindications: Refer to manufacturer's profile for each drug.
- Precautions: Rarely, Jarisch-Herxheimer reaction appears after antimicrobial therapy.
- Significant possible interactions: Refer to manufacturer's profile for each drug.

Second Line

Trimethoprim–sulfamethoxazole

- Furazolidone: 7.5 mg/kg/day PO × 10 days; in uncomplicated multidrug-resistant typhoid; safe in children; efficacy >85% cure

Pregnancy Considerations

Ciprofloxacin therapy is relatively contraindicated in children and in pregnant patients.

ISSUES FOR REFERRAL

Complications of sepsis, bowel perforation

SURGERY/OTHER PROCEDURES

- Complications: bowel perforation
- Cholecystectomy may be warranted in carriers with cholelithiasis, relapse after therapy, or intolerance to antimicrobial therapy.

INPATIENT CONSIDERATIONS

Admission Criteria/Initial Stabilization

- Inpatient if acutely ill
- Outpatient for less ill patient or for carrier

Nursing

Observe enteric precautions.

ONGOING CARE

FOLLOW-UP RECOMMENDATIONS

Bed rest initially, then activity as tolerated

Patient Monitoring

See "General Measures."

DIET

NPO if abdominal symptoms are severe. With improvement, begin normal low-residue diet, with high-calorie supplementation if malnourished.

PATIENT EDUCATION

- Discuss chronic carrier state and its complications.
- For family members, travelers, or workers at risk, provide education about food/water hygiene and vaccination.
- Educate patients that the typhoid vaccines do not protect against *S. paratyphi* infection.
- Typhoid vaccines protect 50–80% of recipients (not 100%) with diminishing effectiveness over 2–4 years.
- CDC patient handout: www.cdc.gov/vaccines/pubs/vis/downloads/vis-typhoid.pdf

PROGNOSIS

Overall prognosis is good with therapy, <2% mortality rate, 15% relapse rate with some antibiotic treatments, and 3% bowel perforation.

COMPLICATIONS

- Intestinal hemorrhage and perforation in distal ileum
- Patients (up to 3%) may become chronic carriers-persistent stool excretor of *S. typhi* for >1 year.
- Seeding of the biliary tract may become a focus for relapse of typhoid fever: most common in females and older patients (>50 years of age).
- Osteomyelitis is more common in patients with sickle cell anemia, systemic lupus erythematosus, and hematologic neoplasms, as well as in immunosuppressed hosts.
- Endovascular infection in the elderly and in patients with a history of bypass operation or aneurysm
- Rarely, endocarditis or meningitis

REFERENCES

1. Thaver D, Zaidi AK, Critchley J, et al. A comparison of fluoroquinolones versus other antibiotics for treating enteric fever: meta-analysis. *BMJ*. 2009;338:b1865.

ADDITIONAL READING

- Basnyat B. Typhoid fever in the United States and antibiotic choice. *JAMA*. 2010;303(1):34; author reply 34–35.
- Butler T. Treatment of typhoid fever in the 21st century: promises and shortcomings. *Clin Microbiol Infect*. 2011;17(7):959–963.
- Centers for Disease Control and Prevention. Travelers' safety. Chapter 3. Infectious diseases related to travel. Typhoid and paratyphoid fever. http://wwwnc.cdc.gov/travel/yellowbook/2014/chapter-3-infectious-diseases-related-to-travel/typhoid-and-paratyphoid-fever. Accessed 2014.
- Centers for Disease Control and Prevention. Typhoid fever. *National Center for Emerging and Zoonotic Diseases*. http://www.cdc.gov/nczved/divisions/dfbmd/diseases/typhoid_fever/. Accessed 2014.
- Chalya PL, Mabula JB, Koy M, et al. Typhoid intestinal perforations at a university teaching hospital in Northwestern Tanzania: a surgical experience of 104 cases in a resource-limited setting. *World J Emerg Surg*. 2012;7:4.
- Clark TW, Daneshvar C, Pareek M, et al. Enteric fever in a UK regional infectious diseases unit: a 10 year retrospective review. *J Infect*. 2010;60(2):91–98.
- Crump JA, Mintz ED. Global trends in typhoid and paratyphoid fever. *Clin Infect Dis*. 2010;50(2):241–246.
- Effa EE, Lassi ZS, Critchley JA, et al. Fluoroquinolones for treating typhoid and paratyphoid fever (enteric fever). *Cochrane Database Syst Rev*. 2011;(10):CD004530.
- Kaurthe J. Increasing antimicrobial resistance and narrowing therapeutics in typhoidal salmonellae. *J Clin Diagn Res*. 2013;7(3):576–579.
- Kroger AT, Atkinson WL, Marcuse EK, et al. General recommendations on immunization: recommendations of the Advisory Committee on Immunization Practices (ACIP). *MMWR*. 2006;55(RR-15):1–48.
- Sánchez-Vargas FM, Abu-El-Haija MA, Gómez-Duarte OG. Salmonella infections: an update on epidemiology, management, and prevention. *Travel Med Infect Dis*. 2011;9(6):263–277.

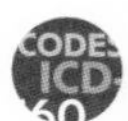

CODES

ICD10

- A01.00 Typhoid fever, unspecified
- Z22.0 Carrier of typhoid
- A01.03 Typhoid pneumonia

CLINICAL PEARLS

- Consider typhoid (along with malaria, dengue, and other travel-associated infections) in febrile travelers returning from endemic areas such as Latin America, sub-Saharan Africa, or South Asia.
- Routine blood cultures detect *S. typhi* but may be negative if antibiotics administered prior to testing.
- A history or documentation of vaccination against *S. typhi* does not exclude the diagnosis of typhoid fever.

T

TYPHUS FEVERS

Douglas W. MacPherson, MD, MSc(CTM), FRCPC

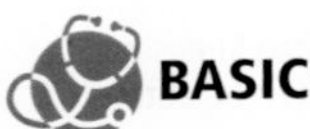

BASICS

Typhus is an infectious disease syndrome caused by several rickettsial bacterial organisms resulting in acute, chronic, and recurrent disease (1)[C].

DESCRIPTION

- Acute infection caused by 3 species of *Rickettsia*
  - Epidemic typhus: human-to-human transmission by body louse; primarily in setting of refugee camps, war, famine, and disaster. Recrudescent disease occurs years after initial infection and can be a source of human outbreak. Flying squirrels are a reservoir.
  - Endemic (murine) typhus: spread to humans by rat flea bite
  - Scrub typhus: infection and infestation of chiggers and of rodents to humans by the chigger; primarily in Asia and western Pacific areas
- System(s) affected: endocrine/metabolic; hematologic/lymphatic/immunologic; pulmonary; skin/exocrine
- Synonym(s): louse-borne typhus; Brill-Zinsser disease; murine typhus

EPIDEMIOLOGY

- Epidemic and endemic typhus: rare in the United States (outside of South Texas)
- Scrub typhus: travelers returning from endemic areas only (rare)

Incidence

Endemic typhus: $<$100 cases annually, primarily in states around the Gulf of Mexico, especially South Texas; underreporting suspected

ETIOLOGY AND PATHOPHYSIOLOGY

- Epidemic typhus by *Rickettsia prowazekii*
- Endemic typhus by *Rickettsia typhi*
- Scrub typhus by *Rickettsia tsutsugamushi*

RISK FACTORS

- Vector exposure
- Travel to endemic countries

Geriatric Considerations

Elderly may have more severe disease.

GENERAL PREVENTION

Vector control:

- Scrub typhus: Wear protective clothing and use insect repellents.
- Endemic typhus: Practice ectoparasite and rodent control.
- Epidemic typhus: delousing and cleaning of clothing; vaccine for those at high risk of exposure (typhus vaccine production has been discontinued in the United States)

DIAGNOSIS

Typhus syndromes are rare in the United States. A high level of clinical suspicion is necessary to make the diagnosis.

HISTORY

Travel or other risk exposure

- Fever, chills
- Intractable headache
- Myalgias, malaise
- Cough, rash, ocular pain

PHYSICAL EXAM

- General
  - Fever
  - Relative bradycardia (scrub typhus)
- Epidemic typhus
  - Incubation period $\sim$1 week
  - Macular or maculopapular rash beginning on trunk $\sim$5th day of illness
  - Nonproductive cough
  - Pulmonary infiltrates
- Endemic typhus
  - Incubation period 1–2 weeks
  - Macular or maculopapular rash beginning on trunk 3rd–5th day of illness
- Scrub typhus
  - Incubation period 1–3 weeks
  - Eschar at bite site
  - Regional lymphadenopathy
  - Generalized lymphadenopathy
  - Splenomegaly
  - Macular or maculopapular rash beginning on trunk approximately 5th day of illness
  - Relative bradycardia early in disease
  - Ocular pain
  - Conjunctival injection

DIFFERENTIAL DIAGNOSIS

- Other rickettsial disease: Rocky Mountain spotted fever; ehrlichiosis; Mediterranean spotted fever (boutonneuse fever) (*Rickettsia conorii*)
- Bacterial meningitis; meningococcemia
- Measles
- Rubella
- Toxoplasmosis
- Leptospirosis
- Typhoid fever
- Dengue
- Malaria
- Relapsing fever
- Secondary syphilis
- Viral syndromes: mononucleosis, acute retroviral syndrome

DIAGNOSTIC TESTS & INTERPRETATION

- Specific serologies with rising antibody titer
- If suspected, isolate *Rickettsia* in qualified laboratory to minimize the risk of laboratory-acquired infection.
- CDC Rickettsial Zoonoses Branch 404-639-1075.

Initial Tests (lab, imaging)

- CBC often normal
- Weil-Felix serologic reaction may be positive; test value hampered to mid-illness or after and by low sensitivity and nonspecificity; epidemic and endemic typhus, 4-fold titer rise or titer $>$1/320 to OX-19; scrub typhus, 4-fold rise in titer to OX-K
- Hyponatremia in severe cases
- Hypoalbuminemia in severe cases
- Recent antibiotic exposure may alter lab results.

Test Interpretation

Diffuse vasculitis on skin biopsy

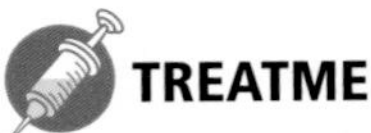

TREATMENT

Initiate treatment based on epidemiologic risk and clinical presentation.

GENERAL MEASURES

- Skin and mouth care
- Supportive care for the severely ill, directed at complications

MEDICATION

First Line

- Begin treatment when diagnosis is likely, and continue until the clinical state improves and the patient is afebrile for at least 48 hours; usual course is 5–7 days.
- Children $\geq$8 years of age and adults
  - Doxycycline IV/PO: adults 100 mg q12h, children $\leq$45 kg: 5 mg/kg/day divided twice daily (max of 200 mg/24 hr); $>$45 kg: Refer to adult dosing.
  - Children $\leq$8 years of age: Risk of dental staining from tetracyclines is minimal if short courses are administered.
  - Tetracycline: 25 mg/kg PO initially, then 25 mg/kg/day in equally divided doses q6h
- Children $\leq$8 years of age, pregnant women, or if typhoid fever is suspected
  - Chloramphenicol: 50 mg/kg PO initially, then 50 mg/kg/day in equally divided doses q6h
  - If severely ill, chloramphenicol sodium succinate: 20 mg/kg IV initially, infused over 30–45 minutes, then 50 mg/kg/day infused in equally divided doses q6h until orally tolerable
  - Azithromycin, fluoroquinolones, and rifampin may be alternatives depending on the clinical scenario.

- Precautions: Refer to the manufacturer's profile for each drug.
- Significant possible interactions: Refer to the manufacturer's profile for each drug.

Second Line

- Doxycycline: single oral dose of 100 or 200 mg for those in refugee camps, victims of disasters, or in the presence of limited medical services
- Isolated reports indicate that erythromycin and ciprofloxacin are effective.
- Azithromycin 3-day course is effective for scrub typhus; better tolerated than doxycycline but more expensive
- Rifampin may be effective in areas where scrub typhus responds poorly to standard antirickettsial drugs.

ISSUES FOR REFERRAL

Infectious disease consultation is recommended. Contact with CDC and local public health authorities.

- One study has suggested that treatment of Mediterranean spotted fever with a fluoroquinolone may result in a more severe clinical course.

INPATIENT CONSIDERATIONS

Admission Criteria/Initial Stabilization

- Outpatient care unless severely ill
- Severely ill or constitutionally unstable (e.g., shock)

ONGOING CARE

FOLLOW-UP RECOMMENDATIONS

Patient Monitoring

- Admit severely ill patients.
- If outpatient treatment, ensure regular follow-up to assess clinical improvement and resolution.

DIET

As tolerated

PATIENT EDUCATION

Travel advice (minimize exposure risks, vector avoidance)

PROGNOSIS

- Recovery is expected if treatment is instituted promptly.
- Relapses may follow treatment, especially if initiated within 48 hours of onset (this is *not* an indication to delay treatment). Relapses are treated the same as primary disease.
- Without treatment, the mortality rate of typhus is 40–60% for epidemic, 1–2% for endemic, and up to 30% for scrub disease.
- Mortality is higher among the elderly.

COMPLICATIONS

Organ-specific complications (particularly in the 2nd week of illness): azotemia, meningoencephalitis, seizures, delirium, coma, myocardial failure, hyponatremia, hypoalbuminemia, hypovolemia, shock and death

REFERENCES

1. Centers for Disease Control and Prevention. Chapter 3. Infectious diseases related to travel. Rickettsial (spotted and typhus fevers) and related infections (anaplasmosis and ehrlichiosis). http://wwwnc.cdc.gov/travel/yellowbook/2014/chapter-3-infectious-diseases-related-to-travel/rickettsial-spotted-and-typhus-fevers-and-related-infections-anaplasmosis-and-ehrlichiosis. Accessed 2014.

ADDITIONAL READING

- Adjemian J, Eremeeva ME, Dasch GA. Rickettsial (spotted and typhus fevers) and related infections (anaplasmosis and ehrlichiosis). Chapter 5. Other infectious disease related to travel. wwwnc.cdc.gov/travel/yellowbook/2010/chapter-5/rickettsial-and-related-infections.htm. Accessed 2014
- Botelho-Nevers E, Raoult D. Host, pathogen and treatment-related prognostic factors in rickettsioses. *Eur J Clin Microbiol Infect Dis*. 2011;30(10):1139–1150.
- Botelho-Nevers E, Rovery C, Richet H, et al. Analysis of risk factors for malignant Mediterranean spotted fever indicates that fluoroquinolone treatment has a deleterious effect. *J Antimicrob Chemother*. 2011;66(8):1821–1830.
- Botelho-Nevers E, Socolovschi C, Raoult D, et al. Treatment of *Rickettsia* spp. infections: a review. *Expert Rev Anti Infect Ther*. 2012;10(12):1425–1437.
- Graham J, Stockley K, Goldman RD. Tick-borne illnesses: a CME update. *Pediatr Emerg Care*. 2011;27(2):141–147; quiz 148–150.
- Green JS, Singh J, Cheung M, et al. A cluster of pediatric endemic typhus cases in Orange County, California. *Pediatr Infect Dis J*. 2011;30(2):163–165.
- Hendershot EF, Sexton DJ. Scrub typhus and rickettsial diseases in international travelers: a review. *Curr Infect Dis Rep*. 2009;11(1):66–72.
- Jensenius M, Fournier PE, Raoult D. Rickettsioses and the international traveler. *Clin Infect Dis*. 2004;39(10):1493–1499.
- Molina N. Borders, laborers, and racialized medicalization Mexican immigration and US public health practices in the 20th century. *Am J Public Health*. 2011;101(6):1024–1031.
- Panpanich R, Garner P. Antibiotics for treating scrub typhus. *Cochrane Database Syst Rev*. 2002;(3):CD002150.
- Phimda K, Hoontrakul S, Suttinont C, et al. Doxycycline versus azithromycin for treatment of leptospirosis and scrub typhus. *Antimicrob Agents Chemother*. 2007;51(9):3259–3263.
- Walker DH, Paddock CD, Dumler JS, et al. Emerging and re-emerging tick-transmitted rickettsial and ehrlichial infections. *Med Clin North Am*. 2008;92(6):1345–1361, x.

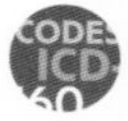

CODES

ICD10

- A75.9 Typhus fever, unspecified
- A75.0 Epidemic louse-borne typhus fever d/t Rickettsia prowazekii
- A75.2 Typhus fever due to Rickettsia typhi

CLINICAL PEARLS

- Consider typhus (along with malaria and dengue) in febrile travelers from endemic areas.
- Rickettsial infections typically present within 2–14 days. Febrile illnesses presenting with onset >18 days after travel are unlikely to be rickettsial.
- Routine blood cultures do not detect *Rickettsia*.
- Prior vaccination does not exclude the diagnosis of typhus.

ULCER, APHTHOUS

Elise Mikaloff, DO, CPT, MC • Paul Savel, MD

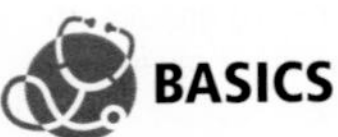

BASICS

DESCRIPTION

- Self-limited, painful ulcerations of the nonkeratinized oral mucosa, which are often recurrent
- Synonyms: canker sores; aphthae; aphthous stomatitis
  - Comes from *aphth* meaning "ulcer" in Greek; first used by Hippocrates between 460 and 370 BC to categorize oral disease (1)
- Categorization
  - Minor aphthous ulcers (2)
    - Usually <10 mm in diameter
    - Self-limited, healing within 4–14 days
    - Rarely affect the dorsum of the mouth
    - Nonscarring
  - Major aphthous ulcers (Sutton disease) (2)
    - Usually >10 mm in diameter
    - Can affect the dorsum of the mouth
    - May take weeks to months to heal
    - Generally more painful than minor aphthous ulcers
    - May cause scarring
  - Herpetiform ulcers (2)
    - Usually 2–3 mm in diameter, may coalesce to form larger ulcerations
    - Unrelated to viral-caused herpetic stomatitis
    - Occur in small clusters numbering 10s–100s, lasting 1–4 weeks
    - Generally more painful than minor aphthous ulcers
    - May cause scarring

EPIDEMIOLOGY

- Most frequent chronic disease of the oral cavity, affecting 5–25% of the population (3)
- More common in patients between 10 and 40 years of age, women, Caucasians, nonsmokers, and those of higher socioeconomic status (3)
- Minor aphthous ulcers
  - Most common: 70–85% of all aphthae
- Major aphthous ulcers
  - 10–15% of all aphthae
- Herpetiform
  - Least common: 10% of all aphthae

Prevalence

Lifetime prevalence of 5–60% (3)

ETIOLOGY AND PATHOPHYSIOLOGY

Likely multifactorial; exact etiology unknown

RISK FACTORS

- Genetic factors: Offspring of those with recurrent aphthous ulcers (RAS) have a 90% chance of developing RAS (4)[C].
- Local trauma: sharp teeth, dental treatments, or mucosal injury secondary to toothbrushing
- Increased stress and anxiety
- Nutritional deficiencies: iron, vitamin B, and folate
- Immunodeficiency
- Recent cessation of tobacco use
- Food sensitivity: to benzoic acid/cinnamaldehyde
- Medications
  - NSAIDS
  - β-Blockers
  - Alendronate
  - Methotrexate
- Neutropenia
- Endocrine alterations (i.e., menstrual cycle) (2)

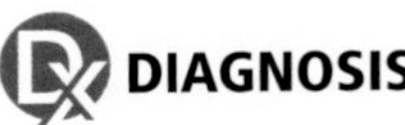

DIAGNOSIS

Diagnosis is made by history and clinical presentation. Lab work is rarely helpful to diagnose aphthous ulcers (2)[A].

HISTORY

- May experience prodrome of burning sensation of oral mucosa 1–2 days prior to appearance of ulcers
- Patients typically complain of oral ulcerations, which are painful and exacerbated by movement of the mouth. Exacerbation may also be reported with certain foods (hot, spicy, acidic, or carbonated foods or drinks) (2)[A].
- Ask about ulcerative lesions of other anatomic areas, family history, or prior history of aphthous ulcers (2)[A].

PHYSICAL EXAM

- Round or ovoid ulcerations generally <10 mm in size. Covered with a grayish-white pseudomembrane surrounded by an erythematous halo (3)[A]
- Ulcers are typically found in the buccal or lip mucosa, ventral tongue, soft palate, or oral vestibule. Rarely on the dorsum of the mouth/lips
- Evaluate for signs of secondary infection: elevated temperature, increased surrounding edema, or pus drainage.

DIFFERENTIAL DIAGNOSIS

- Oral trauma
  - Biting
  - Dentures
- Infection
  - Herpes virus (herpetic stomatitis): vesicular lesions on keratinized tissue (dorsal tongue, vermillion border). Generally not present on mucosa (4)[C]
  - HIV: Ulcerations have lengthened healing time and tend to be more painful (4)[C].
- Mucocutaneous disease; especially if chronic or nonhealing
  - Lichen planus
  - Pemphigus
- Malignancy: Investigate and closely monitor nonhealing lesions, especially those with ipsilateral cervical lymphadenopathy.
- Important to evaluate for underlying systemic disease, causing aphthous-like ulcerations
  - Highest suspicion in adult patients with their initial episode or in individuals with additional lesions elsewhere in the body (3)[A],(4)[C].
  - Behçet syndrome: autoimmune systemic vasculitis usually involving mucous membranes
    - Genital and oral ulceration
    - Uveitis
  - Reiter syndrome: reactive arthritis, preceded by infection, usually of the genital tract (2)[A]
    - Uveitis
    - Urethritis
    - HLA-B27–associated arthritis
  - Sweet syndrome: acute neutrophilic dermatitis (4)[C]
    - Fever, sudden onset
    - Erythematous skin plaques/papules, well-demarcated
    - Leukocytosis
    - 50% of patients have an associated malignancy.
    - Most often in middle-aged females
  - Inflammatory bowel disease (IBD): Crohn disease, ulcerative colitis
    - 10% of patients with Crohn disease experience recurrent oral ulcers (4)[C].
    - Bloody or persistent diarrhea
    - Weight loss
  - Cyclic neutropenia (4)[C]
    - Recurrent fevers associated with infections, occasionally occurring intraorally.
    - Begins in childhood
  - Systemic lupus erythematosus (SLE): autoimmune vascular collagen disease
    - Oral lesions have great variability, including recurrent ulceration.
  - Gluten-sensitive enteropathy (celiac disease)
    - Weight loss and signs of malabsorption
    - Bloating and diarrhea

DIAGNOSTIC TESTS & INTERPRETATION

May consider complete blood count, folic acid, ferritin, vitamin B_{12} to evaluate for systemic causes based on presentation (2)[A]

Follow-Up Tests & Special Considerations

- HIV is associated with increased amount of ulcers and increased healing time.
- Biopsy and viral cultures for nonhealing ulcers or atypical presentations
- Rheumatologic serology if underlying systemic disease is suspected

TREATMENT

GENERAL MEASURES

- Management is symptomatic. Goal is to reduce inflammation and relieve pain.
- Avoid potentially irritating food or drink:
  - Spicy
  - Acidic
  - Hot
  - Carbonated beverages.
  - Abrasive/hard foods (i.e., chips, nuts, etc.)
- Behavior modification to reduce dental trauma with toothbrush or bruxism

MEDICATION

In general, the goals of treatment depend on the extent of ulceration and frequency of outbreaks.

First Line

- Topical corticosteroids (to improve healing time and symptoms) (2)[A]
  - Adverse effects: may increase risk of oral candidiasis (more likely with higher potency formulations)
  - Preparations
    - Triamcinolone 0.1% dental paste
      - Apply sparingly to ulcers three times daily for up to 2 weeks or until ulcer resolution.
    - Hydrocortisone pellets
      - 2.5-mg pellets applied to ulcer four times daily for up to 2 weeks or until ulcer resolution
      - Not available in United States
    - Fluocinonide 0.05% gel or ointment
      - Apply sparingly to ulcer four times daily for up to 2 weeks or until ulcer resolution.
    - Dexamethasone 5 mg/5 mL elixir
      - Rinse for 3 minutes and spit four times daily until ulcer resolution.
- Topical anesthetics (to reduce symptoms only) (2)[A]
  - Adverse effects: may cause initial stinging
  - Preparations
    - Lidocaine 2% gel
      - Apply four times daily or prior to eating as needed for pain, for up to 2 weeks or until ulcer resolution.
- Antimicrobial mouth rinses (improve healing time and prevent recurrence)
  - Adverse effects: may cause superficial tooth staining
  - Preparations
    - Chlorhexidine aqueous mouthwash 0.12% or 0.2%
      - Use four times daily for up to several months.
- Topical immunomodulators (improves healing time, reduces symptoms, and prevents recurrence when used in prodromic phase) (2)[A]
  - Adverse effects: may cause stinging sensation
  - Preparation
    - Amlexanox 5% oral paste
      - Apply to ulcers four times daily for up to 2 weeks or until ulcer resolution.

Second Line

- Systemic corticosteroids–rescue therapy in acute, severe, recurrent outbreaks (2,3)[A]
  - Prednisone 25 mg/day, then tapered over 2 months (3)[A]
- Colchicine and dapsone have been used with limited success but should be used with caution due to side effects (2,3)[A].

ISSUES FOR REFERRAL

Otolaryngology or dental referral if lesions have not resolved as expected

ADDITIONAL THERAPIES

Vitamin B_{12} supplementation has been shown to decrease burden of outbreaks and recurrence, independent of preexisting deficiency in one small study (5)[B]. Multivitamins have not been shown to be effective (6)[B].

SURGERY/OTHER PROCEDURES

Chemical cautery with silver nitrate (reduces ulcer pain but not healing time) (7)[B]

COMPLEMENTARY & ALTERNATIVE MEDICINE

Some small cohort studies show clinical improvement with minimal side effects of several herbal and alternative treatments (3)[A].

- *Glycyrrhiza* (licorice) (8)[B]
- *Myrtus communis* (myrtle) (9)[B]
- Bee propolis (3)[A]

REFERENCES

1. Preeti L, Magesh K, Rajkumar K, et al. Recurrent aphthous stomatitis. *J Oral Maxillofac Pathol*. 2011;15(3):252–256.
2. Belenguer-Guallar J, Jiménez-Soriano Y, Claramunt-Lozano A. Treatment of recurrent aphthous stomatitis. A literature review. *J Clin Exp Dent*. 2014;6(2):e168–e174.
3. Brocklehurst P, Tickle M, Glenny AM, et al. Systemic interventions for recurrent aphthous stomatitis (mouth ulcers). *Cochrane Database Syst Rev*. 2012;9:CD005411.
4. Chavan M, Jain H, Diwan N, et al. Recurrent aphthous stomatitis: a review. *J Oral Pathol Med*. 2012;41(8):577–583.
5. Carrozzo M. Vitamin B12 for the treatment of recurrent aphthous stomatitis. *Evid Based Dent*. 2009;10(4):114–115.
6. Lalla RV, Choquette LE, Feinn RS, et al. Multivitamin therapy for recurrent aphthous stomatitis: a randomized, double-masked, placebo-controlled trial. *J Am Dent Assoc*. 2012;143(4):370–376.
7. Soylu Özler G. Silver nitrate cauterization: a treatment option for aphthous stomatitis. *J Craniomaxillofac Surg*. 2014;42(5):e281–e283.
8. Martin MD, Sherman J, van der Ven P, et al. A controlled trial of a dissolving oral patch concerning glycyrrhiza (licorice) herbal extract for the treatment of aphthous ulcers. *Gen Dent*. 2008;56(2):206–210; quiz 211–212, 224.
9. Babaee N, Mansourian A, Momen-Heravi F, et al. The efficacy of a paste containing *Myrtus communis* (myrtle) in the management of recurrent aphthous stomatitis: a randomized controlled trial. *Clin Oral Investig*. 2010;14(1):65–70.

ADDITIONAL READING

- Hopper SM, Babl FE, McCarthy M, et al. A double blind, randomised placebo controlled trial of topical 2% viscous lidocaine in improving oral intake in children with painful infectious mouth conditions. *BMC Pediatr*. 2011;11:106.
- Kozlak ST, Walsh SJ, Lalla RV. Reduced dietary intake of vitamin B12 and folate in patients with recurrent aphthous stomatitis. *J Oral Pathol Med*. 2010;39(5):420–423.
- Liu C, Zhou Z, Liu G, et al. Efficacy and safety of dexamethasone ointment on recurrent aphthous ulceration. *Am J Med*. 2012;125(3):292–301.
- Pakfetrat A, Mansourian A, Momen-Heravi F, et al. Comparison of colchicine versus prednisolone in recurrent aphthous stomatitis: a double-blind randomized clinical trial. *Clin Invest Med*. 2010;33(3):e189–e195.

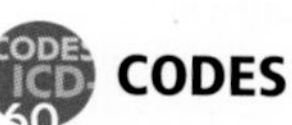

CODES

ICD10

K12.0 Recurrent oral aphthae

CLINICAL PEARLS

- Aphthous ulcers are the most common chronic disease of the oral cavity.
- Most cases are mild, self-limited episodes.
- Appropriate treatment should be aimed at symptom control and promotion of healing.
- If lesions are nonhealing, simultaneously occur elsewhere in the body, or when patients present with a sudden initial episode in adulthood, it is imperative to rule out secondary causes.

ULCERATIVE COLITIS

Jason E. Domagalski, MD, FAAFP

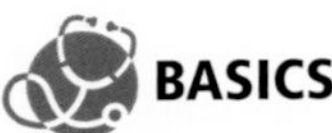

BASICS

DESCRIPTION

- Idiopathic inflammatory disease of the colonic mucosa that can affect any section of the colon from the rectum to the cecum
- >95% of patients have rectal involvement, 50% limited to rectum and sigmoid; 20% have pancolitis.

EPIDEMIOLOGY

Incidence

- United States: 9–12 new cases/100,000 persons/year
- Predominant age: 15–35 years; 2nd and smaller peak in the 7th decade
- Predominant sex: female > male (slight)

Prevalence

205–240/100,000 persons

Pregnancy Considerations

- Increased risk of preterm delivery and small for gestational age birth.
- 30% with inactive disease relapse in pregnancy.
- Treatment with sulfasalazine does not seem to affect pregnancy outcome. Supplement with folate (2 mg daily) to prevent neural tube defects.
- Patients should delay pregnancy until disease is inactive for minimum of 3 months.

ETIOLOGY AND PATHOPHYSIOLOGY

Unknown; hypotheses include allergy to dietary components and abnormal immune responses to bacterial or "self" antigens; final common path is mucosal inflammation secondary to immune cell infiltration.

Genetics

- Family history in 5–10% in population surveys and 20–30% in referral-based studies
- 50–60% concordance rate in identical twin studies
- Associations with interleukin 23/Th17 pathway as well as interleukin 10 and interferon gamma genes

RISK FACTORS

- Better sanitation, indoor work environments, and fatty foods increase risk.
- NSAIDs can activate disease.
- Appendectomy protects against late disease onset.
- Negative association with smoking: Relative risk of smokers is 40% of nonsmokers.

GENERAL PREVENTION

- Increased risk for colon cancer w/o colectomy.
- Aspirin (≥300 mg/day) and ursodeoxycholic acid (10 mg/kg/day) are preventive.

Pediatric Considerations

- Breastfeeding may be protective for pediatric inflammatory bowel disease (IBD).
- More likely pancolonic at onset and shorter time from diagnosis to colectomy (median 11.1 years)

COMMONLY ASSOCIATED CONDITIONS

- Extracolonic manifestations in 10–15%
- Arthritic conditions, including large joint arthritis, sacroiliitis, and ankylosing spondylitis
- Pyoderma gangrenosum
- Episcleritis and uveitis
- Asymptomatic fatty liver (common)
- Primary sclerosing cholangitis: 1–4%
- Cirrhosis of liver: 1–5%
- Bile duct carcinoma
- Thromboembolic disease: 1–6%

DIAGNOSIS

HISTORY

Bloody diarrhea; tenesmus; abdominal pain; rectal urgency, occasional fecal incontinence; weight loss; arthralgias

PHYSICAL EXAM

- Arthralgias and arthritis: 15–40%
- Spondylitis: 3–6%
- Ocular: 4–10%; includes uveitis, cataracts, keratopathy, and central serous retinopathy
- Erythema nodosum
- Pyoderma gangrenosum
- Aphthous ulcers of mouth: 5–10%

DIFFERENTIAL DIAGNOSIS

- Hemorrhoids, neoplasms, colonic diverticula, arteriovenous malformation, Crohn disease
- Infectious diarrhea, including bacterial (enterotoxigenic *Escherichia coli*), *Clostridium difficile* colitis, and parasitic (*Entamoeba histolytica*)
- Herpes simplex, *Chlamydia trachomatis, Cryptosporidium, Isospora belli*, cytomegalovirus
- Radiation proctitis; ischemic colitis

DIAGNOSTIC TESTS & INTERPRETATION

- Anemia (chronic disease ± iron deficiency)
- Leukocytosis during exacerbation
- Elevated ESR and CRP
- Electrolyte abnormalities, especially hypokalemia
- Hypoalbuminemia, elevated LFTs
- Perinuclear antineutrophil cytoplasmic antibody (pANCA) is elevated in 60–70% of cases, also found in 40% of pts with Crohn.

Initial Tests (lab, imaging)

- Plain abdominal films
  - Obtain immediately if significant abdominal tenderness, fever, and leukocytosis for early diagnosis of toxic megacolon and perforation
- Upper GI series with small bowel follow-through to rule out Crohn disease
- Ultrasound, MRI, scintigraphy, and CT may have similar accuracy in diagnosis of IBD (1)[A].
- Stool culture and stool testing for parasites to rule out infectious colitis (2)[C].
- *C. difficile* antigen if recent antibiotics.

Diagnostic Procedures/Other

- Sigmoidoscopy (may include biopsy) is often sufficient to make initial diagnosis.
- Colonoscopy (may include biopsy)
  - Evaluate premalignant features; differentiate from Crohn disease; investigate stricture/mass; define extent and location of disease
- Full colonoscopy contraindicated in severe, active disease/colonic dilatation (risk of perforation)

Test Interpretation

Inflammation of the colonic mucosa with ulcerations:

- Ulcerations are hyperemic and hemorrhagic.
- Mucosal separation, distortion, and atrophy of the crypts on histology (2)[C]
- Rectum is involved 95% of the time.
- Extends proximally, without skips
- May affect terminal ileum, so-called backwash ileitis

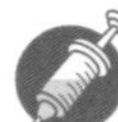

TREATMENT

Management involves acute treatment of inflammatory symptoms, followed by maintenance of remission; therapeutic approach determined by symptom severity and the extent of colonic involvement: topical therapies most effective for disease distal to the descending colon.

- 5-aminosalicylic acid (5-ASA) is effective in inducing remission in mild to moderate disease (number needed to treat [NNT] = 6) and preventing relapse in quiescent disease (NNT = 4) (3)[A]:
  - Topical mesalamine may be superior to oral aminosalicylates or topical steroids for proctitis but often have systemic side effects (3)[A].
  - Combination of oral and topical aminosalicylates is more effective than either alone.
- Corticosteroid therapies are effective at inducing remission in active disease (NNT = 3).
- Azathioprine or 6-mercaptopurine (6-MP) are not recommended for inducing remission in active disease but reduce relapse in patients with quiescent disease (NNT = 4) (3)[A].
- Maintenance of remission in mild to moderate distal disease with the following: mesalamine suppositories for proctitis or enemas for distal colitis, sulfasalazine, balsalazide, or combination oral and topical mesalamine (3)[A]
- Maintenance of remission in mild to moderate extensive disease with sulfasalazine, olsalazine, mesalamine, and balsalazide (3)[A]
- Infliximab is effective at inducing remission in ambulatory patients with moderate to severely active disease (NNT = 4) (3)[A].

GENERAL MEASURES

Control inflammation, prevent complications, and replace nutritional losses and blood volume.

MEDICATION

First Line

- Sulfasalazine
  - Uncoated tablets. Adults: initial: 1 g PO q6–8h; maintenance: 500 mg PO q6h; children ≥6 years: initial: 40–60 mg/kg/day PO in 3–6 divided doses; maintenance: 30 mg/kg/day PO divided q6h (max 2 g/day)
  - Enteric-coated tablets. Adults: initial: 3–4 g/day PO in divided doses q6–8h; maintenance: 2 g/day PO in divided doses; children ≥6 years: initial: 40–60 mg/kg/day PO in 3–6 divided doses; maintenance: 30 mg/kg/day PO in 4 divided doses (max 2 g/day)
- Mesalamine
  - Oral delayed-release tablets (Asacol) to induce remission; adults: 800 mg PO TID × 6 weeks
  - Oral controlled-release tablets (Pentasa) for maintenance of remission; adults: 1 g PO QID
  - Single daily dose available for mesalamine under brand Lialda (acute therapy 4.8 g once daily or 2.4 g once daily for maintenance) and brand Apriso (1.5 g once daily; approved in the United States ONLY for maintenance)
  - Once daily dosing is as effective as conventional TID dosing for mild to moderately active UC treatment and to maintain remission (5)[A].
- 5-ASA (e.g., mesalamine) enemas and suppositories can be used to treat proctitis/proctosigmoiditis:
  - Suppositories: (Canasa) adults: 1,000 mg per rectum at bedtime
  - Enemas: adults: 4 g per rectum, retained for 8 hours each night; use for 3–6 weeks or until remission is achieved.

- Balsalazide: adults: 2.25 g PO TID for total daily dose of 6.75 g for 8–12 weeks; children/adolescents: 2.25 g PO TID for total daily dose of 6.75 g or 750 mg PO TID for total daily dose of 2.25 g for 8 weeks
- Olsalazine: adults: 500 mg PO BID (up to 3 g/day); children $>$2 years old: 30 mg/kg/day in 2 divided doses (up to 2 g/day), primarily used for maintenance

Second Line

- Prednisone for severe exacerbations: adult dosage: initial: 40–60 mg/day PO (max 1 mg/kg/day) × 7–10 days; taper over 2–3 months; can be given IV in hospitalized patients
- Infliximab is effective in patients whose disease is refractory to conventional treatment (3,4)[A]:
  - Adult dose: 5 mg/kg IV at weeks 0, 2, and 6 for induction, then maintenance of 5 mg/kg IV is given every 8 weeks
- Adalimumab: for moderate to severe ulcerative colitis refractory to steroids and azathioprine/6-MP. Initial dose: 160 mg SQ (given as 4 injections on day one or two injections daily over two consecutive days; limit injections to 40 mg per injection); 2nd dose 2 weeks later: 80 mg, and maintenance: 40 mg every other week thereafter. Should only be continued if evidence of remission by 8 weeks (4).

Pediatric Considerations

- Infliximab can increase the risk of cancer in children and adolescents; weigh risks versus benefits.
- Immunomodulators can be used in patients unresponsive to steroids and aminosalicylates or who cannot be weaned from high-dose steroids:
  - Daily abdominal plain films until improvement.
  - If dilatation of colon increases/treatment has failed to attain reversal in 72 hours, emergency colectomy is indicated.

SURGERY/OTHER PROCEDURES

- Indicated for medically refractory disease or if treatment side effects are unacceptable (particularly with high-dose steroids)
- May be emergent for massive hemorrhage, perforation, and toxic dilatation of the colon. The surgery of choice for emergency is total or subtotal abdominal colectomy with end ileostomy.
- Surgery also indicated for cancer/multisite mucosal dysplasia.
- Total colectomy with ileostomy is *curative*.
- Total proctocolectomy with ileal pouch anal anastomosis (IPAA) is the most common surgery and an appropriate alternative to ileostomy. Common complications include pouchitis (50%) and need for reoperation in up to 30% (2).
- Regular proctoscopic surveillance is required if a colonic mucosal cuff is retained.

COMPLEMENTARY & ALTERNATIVE MEDICINE

- Insufficient evidence exists to support the efficacy of probiotics to maintain remission (6)[A].
- Encouraging results but limited studies for aloe vera gel, wheat grass juice, *Andrographis paniculata* extract (HMPL-004), topical Xilei-san, curcumin, *Boswellia serrata* gum resin, *Plantago ovata* seeds, evening primrose oil, wormwood, and *Tripterygium wilfordii* (7)[A]

INPATIENT CONSIDERATIONS

Admission Criteria/Initial Stabilization

- Obtain imaging studies to assess disease activity
- Initiate IV corticosteroids and rule out infectious etiologies (*C. difficile*, cytomegalovirus, shigella/ameba).

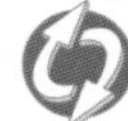

ONGOING CARE

FOLLOW-UP RECOMMENDATIONS

Patient Monitoring

- Surveillance colonoscopy. Recommendations vary. Most begin a surveillance program after 8 years of disease with involvement beyond the splenic flexure with total colonoscopy every 1–2 years including multiple random biopsies or targeted biopsies using chromoendoscopy.
- Magnification chromoendoscopy may detect significantly more intraepithelial neoplasias than conventional colonoscopy.
- There are no prospective studies to determine the optimal number of biopsy specimens.
- Nonadenomatous dysplasia lesions or masses are associated with cancer in 33–83% of cases and warrant total colectomy according to recent recommendations.
- Annual LFTs and cholangiography for cholestasis: patients on long-term mesalamine need annual BUN/creatinine due to risk of nephrotoxicity.

Pediatric Considerations

Cancer surveillance is important because cumulative risk of cancer increases with duration of disease.

DIET

- NPO during acute exacerbations
- Lactose-free diet is often recommended.
- Omega-3 fatty acids, seal and cod liver oil, dietary lactulose, wheat grass juice, vitamin D, and diets with decreased meat and alcohol have been recommended to reduce relapses and improve systemic symptoms (evidence inconsistent) (7)[A].

PATIENT EDUCATION

- Discuss the importance of adherence to drug therapy to induce and maintain remission.
- Self-help organizations such as Crohn and Colitis Foundation of America (CCFA): www.ccfa.org

PROGNOSIS

- Variable; mortality for initial attack is $\sim$5%; 75–85% experience relapse; and up to 20% require colectomy.
- Colon cancer risk is the single most important risk factor affecting long-term prognosis.
- Primary sclerosing cholangitis increases the risk of colon cancer in patients with ulcerative colitis.
- Left-sided colitis and ulcerative proctitis have favorable prognoses with probable normal lifespan.

Geriatric Considerations

- Increased mortality if 1st presentation occurs after 60 years of age.
- Consider lower medication dosages and slower titration due to risks of polypharmacy.

COMPLICATIONS

Perforation; toxic megacolon; liver disease; stricture formation (<Crohn disease); colon cancer

REFERENCES

1. Horsthuis K, Bipat S, Bennink RJ, et al. Inflammatory bowel disease diagnosed with US, MR, scintigraphy, and CT: meta-analysis of prospective studies. *Radiology*. 2008;247(1):64–79.
2. Kornbluth A, Sachar DB, Practice Parameters Committee of the American College of Gastroenterology. Ulcerative colitis practice guidelines in adults: American College of Gastroenterology, Practice Parameters Committee. *Am J Gastroenterol*. 2010;105(3):501–523.
3. Talley NJ, Abreu MT, Achkar JP, et al. An evidence-based systematic review on medical therapies for inflammatory bowel disease. *Am J Gastroenterol*. 2011;106(Suppl 1):S2–S2.
4. Sandborn WJ, van Assche G, Reinisch W, et al. Adalimumab induces and maintains clinical remission in patients with moderate-to-severe ulcerative colitis. *Gastroenterology*. 2012;142(2):257–265.e1–e3.
5. Feagan BG, MacDonald JK. Once daily oral mesalamine compared to conventional dosing for induction and maintenance of remission in ulcerative colitis: a systematic review and meta-analysis. *Inflamm Bowel Dis*. 2012;18(9):1785–1794.
6. Jonkers D, Penders J, Masclee A, et al. Probiotics in the management of inflammatory bowel disease: a systematic review of intervention studies in adult patients. *Drugs*. 2012;72(6):803–823.
7. Ng SC, Lam YT, Tsoi KK, et al. Systematic review: the efficacy of herbal therapy in inflammatory bowel disease. *Aliment Pharmacol Ther*. 2013;38(8):854–863.

ADDITIONAL READING

- Huang X, Lv B, Jin HF, et al. A meta-analysis of the therapeutic effects of tumor necrosis factor-α blockers on ulcerative colitis. *Eur J Clin Pharmacol*. 2011;67(8):759–766.
- Soetikno RM, Lin OS, Heidenreich PA, et al. Increased risk of colorectal neoplasia in patients with primary sclerosing cholangitis and ulcerative colitis: a meta-analysis. *Gastrointest Endosc*. 2002;56(1):48–54.
- Targan SR, Landers CJ, Yang H, et al. Antibodies to CBIR1 Flagellin define a unique response that is associated independently with complicated Crohn's disease. *Gastroenterology*. 2005;128(8):2020–2028.

SEE ALSO

Algorithm: Hematemesis (Bleeding, Upper GI)

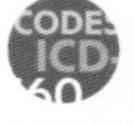

CODES

ICD10

- K51.90 Ulcerative colitis, unspecified, without complications
- K51.919 Ulcerative colitis, unspecified with unspecified complications
- K51.80 Other ulcerative colitis without complications

CLINICAL PEARLS

- Treat proctitis with 5-ASA suppositories.
- Normal screening labs (ESR, hemoglobin, platelets, and albumin) do NOT rule out IBD.
- The low sensitivity of pANCA limits its use as an isolated diagnostic tool.
- Colectomy is curative.
- 6–47% of UC patients have extracolonic disease manifestations.
- Routine surveillance colonoscopy is recommended every 1–2 years after patients have had UC for 8 years (the point at which the risk of colorectal cancer in UC patients increases significantly, particularly for those with disease beyond the splenic flexure).
- UC always involves the colon and has continuous areas of inflammation with shallow mucosal ulcerations and crypt granulomas are not seen on biopsy (differentiating features from Crohn colitis).

UPPER RESPIRATORY INFECTION (URI)

Lisa M. Schroeder, MD • Alysha M. Rahman, MD

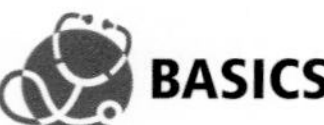

BASICS

Upper respiratory infections (URIs) are one of the most common medical diagnoses, contributing to ~30 million office visits annually and resulting in missed days from work/school.

DESCRIPTION
- Inflammation of nasal passages resulting from infection with multiple respiratory viruses
- Most cases are mild to moderate in severity, self-limited, and amenable to self-treat.
- System(s) affected: ENT; pulmonary

EPIDEMIOLOGY
- Each virus has different seasonal peaks (e.g., rhinovirus: late spring, fall); most infections occur during the winter months.
- Symptoms usually peak in 1–3 days and can last up to 2 weeks.
- Transmission:
  - Contact with contaminated skin/surface followed by contact with mucous membranes (hand-to-face contact)
  - Aerosolized particles from sneezing and coughing
- Viruses may last up to 2 hours on skin and even longer on environmental surfaces.

Incidence
- Predominant age: children > adults
  - Preschool children: 5–7 URI/year
  - Kindergarten: 12 URI/year
  - Schoolchildren: 7 URI/year
  - Adolescents/adults: 2–3 URI/year
- Predominant sex: male = female

ETIOLOGY AND PATHOPHYSIOLOGY
Rhinoviruses infect the ciliated epithelial mucosa of the upper airway, resulting in edema and hyperemia and mucous production.
- Histology: Edema of subepithelial connective tissue and a scanty cellular infiltrate containing neutrophils, plasma cells, lymphocytes, and eosinophils results in exudation of serous and mucinous fluid.
- Rhinovirus causes a "nondestructive" inflammation of the mucous membranes.
- Influenza and parainfluenza viruses denude respiratory epithelium to the basement membrane.
- Usually due to 1 of several hundred viral strains from different families; spread within geographic region and groups with close contact
  - Rhinovirus (>100 serotypes): 30–50%; incubation period 1–5 days
  - Influenzavirus types A, B, C: 10–15%; incubation period 1–4 days
  - Coronaviruses: 10–15%
  - Parainfluenza, respiratory syncytial virus (RSV): 5%; more common in children; incubation period 1 week
  - Enteroviruses, adenoviruses: <10%
- *In many cases, no specific pathogen is identified.*

RISK FACTORS
- Exposure to infected people
- Touching one's face with contaminated fingers
- Allergic disorders
- Smoking
- Immunosuppression
- Stress

GENERAL PREVENTION
- Frequent hand washing, especially in children (1,2)[A]
- Limiting exposure to infected persons/children

COMMONLY ASSOCIATED CONDITIONS
- Pharyngitis
- Sinusitis
- Otitis media
- Bronchitis
- Bronchiolitis
- Pneumonia
- Croup
- Asthma

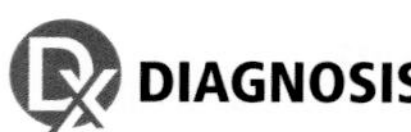

DIAGNOSIS

- Nasal congestion: 80–100%
- Sneezing: 50–70%
- Throat irritation: 50%
- Cough: 40%
- Hoarseness: 30%
- Malaise: 20–25%
- Headache: 25%
- Fever >100°F (37.7°C): 0–1%

PHYSICAL EXAM
- Low-grade temperature; mild tachycardia common with fever; tachypnea if significant respiratory involvement
- Rhinorrhea (clear, yellow, or green)
- Mucosal edema and/or inflammation
- Postnasal drainage
- Pharyngeal erythema
- Dull tympanic membranes

DIFFERENTIAL DIAGNOSIS
- Allergic rhinitis
- Acute sinusitis
- Strep pharyngitis
- Infectious mononucleosis
- Influenza
- Pertussis
- Otitis media

DIAGNOSTIC TESTS & INTERPRETATION

Initial Tests (lab, imaging)
- No routine lab testing is typically needed, as diagnosis is based on clinical findings.
- In cases of pharyngitis, rapid streptococcal antigen testing with reflex culture can be used to rule out group A streptococcal infection.
- Rapid influenza antigen testing if influenza suspected
- Heterophile antibody testing if infectious mononucleosis is suspected
- Imaging not routinely indicated

Follow-Up Tests & Special Considerations
Patients should consider contacting a physician's office for fever >101°F associated with systemic symptoms, difficulty breathing, or purulent drainage >2 days.

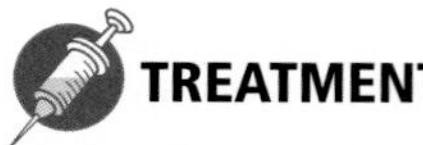

TREATMENT

GENERAL MEASURES
- Smoking cessation
- Vaporizer/humidifier: no consistent benefit proven

MEDICATION
Most cases of URI resolve spontaneously without specific intervention. Treatment is symptom-driven and for patient comfort.

First Line
- Saline nasal irrigation is safe for adults and children.
- *Antibiotics are not recommended. They produce minimal to no reduction in symptoms or duration, with greater risk of side effects from usage* (3)[A].
- Analgesics: acetaminophen, and NSAIDs for relieving aches and pains associated with URI (4,5)[A]

Second Line
- Many mouthwashes, gargles, and lozenges are promoted to relieve the pain of sore throat. The demulcent effects of hard candy, gargling with warm saline, and products with anesthetics (benzocaine/phenol) may provide pain relief.
- Aromatic oils (menthol, camphor, eucalyptus), in topical/lozenge form, produce a sensation of increased airflow in the absence of a significant change in airflow resistance.
- Topical decongestants (sympathomimetics) reduce nasal mucosa swelling and airflow resistance, promote drainage. Sprays preferred over drops in patients >6 years of age:
  - *Limit use to 3 days*, as rebound congestion may occur after 72 hours of use with resultant rhinitis medicamentosa.
    - Oxymetazoline
      - Adults and children aged 6–12 years: 0.05% solution, 2–3 sprays in each nostril BID
- Oral decongestants (sympathomimetic) have some advantages over topical decongestants: longer duration of action, lack of local irritation, and no risk of rebound congestion (6)[B].
  - Pseudoephedrine: potential for abuse/misuse or diversion for methamphetamine production
  - Use with caution for patients with cardiovascular disease, HTN, and BPH:
    - Adults: 60 mg q4–6h (120 mg sustained-release q12h) superior to placebo in short-term use (6)
    - Children aged 6–12 years: 30 mg q4–6h; 2–5 years: 15 mg q4–6h
- Acute cough, postnasal drip, and throat clearing associated with the common cold can be treated with a 1st-generation antihistamine/decongestant preparation (brompheniramine and sustained-release pseudoephedrine) (7)[A].

- Antihistamines: minimal benefit when used as monotherapy. Only 1st-generation (sedating) antihistamines show any symptomatic relief, but sedation may be worse than relief (8)[B]:
  - Chlorpheniramine
    - Adults: 4 mg QID, 8 mg TID, 12 mg BID
    - Children age 6–12 years: 2 mg q4–6h
  - Diphenhydramine
    - Adults: 25–50 mg q4–6h PRN
    - Children age 6–12 years 12.5–25mg q4–6h PRN

Pediatric Considerations

In 2007, the FDA issued a warning on all cough and cold preparations for children age ≤2 years due to risk of overdose (9,10)[A].

COMPLEMENTARY & ALTERNATIVE MEDICINE

- Zinc prevents viral replication in vitro:
  - Avoid intranasal preparations of zinc: risk of potential permanent loss of smell (11)[C]
  - Has shown moderate benefit in reducing symptoms and duration, but proper dosing has not been determined
- Echinacea has not proven effective for treatment of common cold symptoms (12)[C].
- Probiotics may decrease severity and duration of URIs and possibly reduce episodes (13)[B].
- Vitamin C (ascorbic acid) (14)[C]
  - Regular supplementation trials have shown that vitamin C may reduce the duration of colds.
  - Vitamin C prophylaxis *not* recommended for general use but may be beneficial in those exposed to severe physical exertion and cold environments.

Geriatric Considerations

Cold medications, especially decongestants and antihistamines, commonly produce adverse effects in older people and should not be used routinely in this setting.

Pregnancy Considerations

- Decongestants: Most are Category B or C.
- Antihistamines: Most are Category B or C.

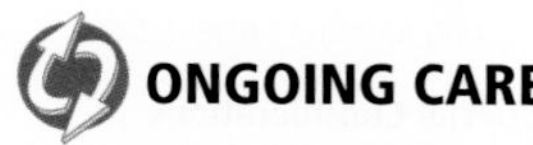

ONGOING CARE

FOLLOW-UP RECOMMENDATIONS

Contact a physician's office for prolonged fever, difficulty breathing, or concern for secondary complications.

DIET

Encourage fluids and adequate hydration.

PATIENT EDUCATION

- Discuss with patients the difference between viral and bacterial infections; instruct about appropriate antibiotic use.
- Good hand hygiene
- Symptomatic treatment; no cure
- Reinfection is possible with reexposure.
- Patient information: www.niaid.nih.gov/factsheets/cold.htm

PROGNOSIS

- Excellent; expect full recovery. Usual duration 5–7 days but may last up to 2 weeks. For smokers, 3–4 additional days
- Cough may persist after other symptoms have resolved.

COMPLICATIONS

Small percentage may develop worsening symptoms leading to secondary otitis media, sinusitis, bronchitis, or pneumonia.

REFERENCES

1. Centers for Disease Control and Prevention. Treatment guidelines for upper respiratory tract infections. www.cdc.gov. Accessed 2014.
2. Jefferson T, Del Mar CB, Dooley L, et al. Physical interventions to interrupt or reduce the spread of respiratory viruses. *Cochrane Database Syst Rev*. 2011;(7):CD006207.
3. Kenealy T, Arroll B. Antibiotics for the common cold and acute purulent sinusitis. *Cochrane Database Syst Rev*. 2013;6:CD000247.
4. Li S, Yue J, Dong BR, et al. Acetaminophen (paracetamol) for the common cold in adults. *Cochrane Database Syst Rev*. 2013;7:CD008800.
5. Kim SY, Chang YJ, Cho HM, et al. Non-steroidal anti-inflammatory drugs for the common cold. *Cochrane Database Syst Rev*. 2013;6:CD006362.
6. Horak F, Zieglmayer P, Zieglmayer R, et al. A placebo-controlled study of the nasal decongestant effect of phenylephrine and pseudoephedrine in the Vienna Challenge Chamber. *Ann Allergy Asthma Immunol*. 2009;102(2):116–120.
7. Pratter MR. Cough and the common cold: ACCP evidence-based clinical practice guidelines. *Chest*. 2006;129(1)(Suppl):72S–74S.
8. Sutter AI, Lemiengre M, Campbell H, et al. Antihistamines for the common cold. *Cochrane Database Syst Rev*. 2003;(3):CD001267.
9. U.S. Food and Drug Administration. Public health advisory: nonprescription cough and cold medicine use in children. http://www.fda.gov/cder/drug/advisory/cough_cold.htm. Accessed August 15, 2007.
10. Centers for Disease Control and Prevention. Infant deaths associated with cough and cold medications—United States, 2005. *MMWR Morb Mortal Wkly Rep*. 2007;56(1):1–4. http://www.cdc.gov/od/oc/media/mmwrnews/2007/n070111.htm. Accessed 2014.
11. Singh M, Das RR. Zinc for the common cold. *Cochrane Database Syst Rev*. 2013;6:CD001364.
12. Linde K, Barrett B, Wolkart K, et al. Echinacea for preventing and treating the common cold. Cochrane Acute Respiratory Infections Group. *Cochrane Database Syst Rev*. 2006;(1):CD000530.
13. Hao Q, Lu Z, Dong BR, Et al. Probiotics for preventing acute upper respiratory tract infections. *Cochrane Database Syst Rev*. 2011;(9):CD006895.
14. Hemilä H, Chalker E. Vitamin C for preventing and treating the common cold. *Cochrane Database Syst Rev*. 2013;1:CD000980.

ADDITIONAL READING

- Rosenfeld RM, Andes D, Bhattacharyya N, et al. Clinical practice guideline: adult sinusitis.*Otolaryngol Head Neck Surg*. 2007;137(3)(Suppl):S1–S31.
- Simasek M, Blandino DA. Treatment of the common cold. *Am Fam Physician*. 2007;75(4):515–520.
- Walder ER, Applegate KE, Bordley C, et al. Clinical practice guideline for diagnosis and management of acute bacterial sinusitis in children aged 1–18 years. *Pediatrics*. 2013;132(1):e262–e280.

U

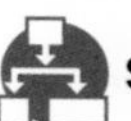

SEE ALSO

Bronchitis, Acute; Pharyngitis; Rhinitis, Allergic

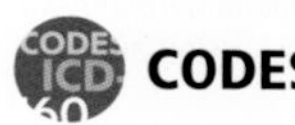

CODES

ICD10

- J06.9 Acute upper respiratory infection, unspecified
- J11.1 Influenza due to unidentified influenza virus with other respiratory manifestations
- B97.4 Respiratory syncytial virus causing diseases classd elswhr

CLINICAL PEARLS

- Supportive therapy is mainstay; most commonly recommended treatments lack medical evidence.
- If pharyngitis is the primary complaint, rule out group A *Streptococcus* with point of care testing.
- Limit unnecessary use of antibiotics.
- Smokers have symptoms that last 3–4 more days than nonsmokers.

URETHRITIS

Karen Cherian, MD • David O. Parrish, MD

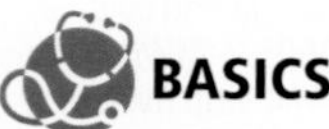

BASICS

DESCRIPTION
- Urethral inflammation marked by dysuria, pruritus, mucopurulent discharge, and/or hematuria
- Usually a result of an STI or, less commonly, autoimmune disorders (Reiter syndrome), trauma, or chemical irritation
- Complications include epididymitis, endocarditis, meningitis, or disseminated gonococcal infection.
  - Risk factors
  - Women and men <25 years of age
  - Patients with history of prior STIs
  - Patients with new and/or multiple sexual partners
  - Sex workers
  - Drug users
  - African Americans
  - Men who have sex with men
  - Patients with inconsistent condom use

EPIDEMIOLOGY

Incidence
- In 2011, 1.4 million new cases of chlamydia and 321,000 cases of gonorrhea were reported by the CDC. Prevalence varies by region, with highest incident in southern United States; racial discrepancies include an 8× higher rate for African Americans and a 2.7× higher rate for Hispanic patients compared with whites.
- Predominant age: 15–24 years, sexually active, following trends for STI
- Predominant sex: Men report symptoms more frequently, but similar incidence is likely.

ETIOLOGY AND PATHOPHYSIOLOGY
- Predominantly, *Neisseria gonorrhoeae* and *Chlamydia trachomatis* infection increased transmission among HIV-positive persons.
- Less common infectious agents include the following:
  - *Ureaplasma urealyticum*
  - *Trichomonas vaginalis*
  - Herpesvirus
  - *Mycoplasma genitalium*
  - Viral: conflicting data on HPV, herpes simplex
- Noninfectious causes (generally rare): foreign bodies, soaps, shampoos, douches, spermicides, urethral instrumentation

RISK FACTORS
- Multiple sexual partners and unprotected intercourse
- African American, Native American, or Hispanic ethnicity
- History of STIs, bacterial vaginosis, recurrent candidiasis
- Excessive use of chemical lubricants or powders

GENERAL PREVENTION
- Safer sex techniques and treatment of all partners
- Abstinence
- Avoidance of excessive lubricants, powders, or chemical irritants

COMMONLY ASSOCIATED CONDITIONS

ALERT
- Patients with any suspected STI should undergo testing for syphilis, hepatitis B and C, *Trichomonas*, and HIV.
- Gonorrhea and chlamydia are reportable to the Health Department.

DIAGNOSIS
- Important to take detailed sexual and travel history; increased incidence seen with travel to some regions with resistance to cephalosporins in Asian countries
- In men
  - Abrupt onset of dysuria symptoms 3–14 days after exposure to an infected sexual partner
  - Urethral discharge: may be profuse and purulent in acute gonorrhea
  - Urethral itching or tenderness
  - Proctitis, pharyngitis, and conjunctivitis also may be present (sexual history is important).
- In women: Classic urethral syndrome often is not present.
  - Tenderness, edema, and inflammation of the urethral meatus, especially in women
  - Dyspareunia
  - Vaginitis, cystitis, cervicitis
- Fever is not part of the syndrome and usually suggests another diagnosis.
- Bloody discharge: rarely seen and suggests another diagnosis
- Suprapubic or abdominal pain suggests another diagnosis or the emergence of complications (e.g., PID, prostatitis, or cystitis).
- Key physical exam points:
  - Expression of purulent urethral discharge
  - Palpate scrotum to check for epididymitis or orchitis.
  - Check for ulcers.
  - Check for inguinal lymphadenopathy.

Pediatric Considerations
In pediatric patients, proven cases of gonorrhea, chlamydia, and trichomoniasis require evaluation for sexual abuse.

DIFFERENTIAL DIAGNOSIS
- Other genitourinary tract diseases:
  - Cystitis/urinary tract infection
  - Epididymitis
  - Prostatitis
  - PID
  - Pyelonephritis
- Vaginal atrophy, especially in postmenopausal women
- Stevens-Johnson syndrome
- Reiter syndrome: uveitis, urethritis, arthritis (can't see, can't pee, can't climb a tree)
- Wegener granulomatosis

DIAGNOSTIC TESTS & INTERPRETATION
- For patients who present without symptoms and state that a sexual partner was treated for this problem, obtain specimens for lab tests and provide immediate treatment.
- Check culture and antibiotic susceptibilities in patients suspected of having resistant infections.
- Evidence is insufficient to recommend for or against screening in asymptomatic men at increased risk.

ALERT
The U.S. Preventive Services Task Force recommends screening all sexually active women until age 25 years and all women at increased risk of infection.
- Gram stain of discharge: ≥5 WBCs per high-power field (HPF) indicates urethritis. Intracellular gram-negative diplococci strongly indicate gonorrhea.
- Cultures of the intraurethral/endocervical swabs
  - Gonorrhea and chlamydia cultures should be obtained in all symptomatic patients.
  - Culture may be performed on urethral exudates if they are present.
- Nucleic acid amplification test (NAAT) using polymerase chain reaction assay on urine is very sensitive and specific but costly. Also test for other, less common pathogens if negative.
- Urinalysis
  - Usually normal in cases of simple urethritis
  - First-void urine often is positive for leukocyte esterase and should have 10 WBCs per HPF in urethritis.
  - Men should not have urinated for at least 4 hours prior.
- Urine culture: performed only if Gram stain of discharge is unremarkable or unobtainable
- Wet prep: may reveal *Trichomonas*; trichomoniasis, bacterial vaginosis, and *Candida* infection; need to be evaluated for persistent symptoms after antibiotic course
- Syphilis, HIV, and hepatitis B serology as indicated to rule out concomitant STIs

Initial Tests (lab, imaging)

ALERT
When an STI is suspected, provide informed consent and recommend HIV testing at initial presentation.

Follow-Up Tests & Special Considerations
Test of cure for chlamydia and gonorrhea is recommended in pregnant women or when treatment noncompliance is suspected.

Diagnostic Procedures/Other
Urethrocystoscopy for cases with suspected foreign body, intraurethral warts, urethral stricture

Test Interpretation
Urethral strictures (untreated gonorrhea), intraurethral lesions (venereal warts, congenital anomalies), PID, or tubo-ovarian abscesses possible

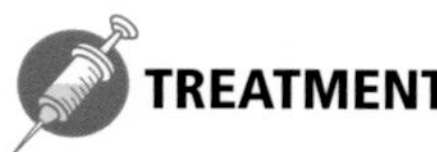

TREATMENT

GENERAL MEASURES
All sexual partners who came in contact with the patient within 60 days should be evaluated, tested, and treated for both gonorrhea and chlamydia.

MEDICATION

First Line

- Most cases can be treated in the outpatient setting.
- Single-dose regimens, directly observed in office for noncompliant or high-risk patients
- Antibiotics should not be withheld from symptomatic patients until culture results are known if there is a convincing clinical presentation.
- Treatment should cover both gonorrhea and chlamydia and any other suspected pathogens (1)[A].
- Gonorrhea
  - Ceftriaxone 250 mg IM *and* either doxycycline 100 mg PO BID for 7 days *or* azithromycin 1 g PO single dose
  - For children ≤45 kg: ceftriaxone 125 mg IM single dose
  - If ceftriaxone is not an option: cefixime 400 mg PO single dose *and* either doxycycline 100 mg PO BID × 7 days *or* azithromycin 1 g PO followed by a test of cure in 1 week
  - If patient has high-risk allergy to cephalosporins, azithromycin 2 g PO can be given, followed by a test of cure in 1 week. This should be limited due to increasing resistance.
- Chlamydia
  - Doxycycline: 100 mg PO BID for 7 days *or*
  - Azithromycin: 1 g PO single dose
- Trichomoniasis
  - Metronidazole: 2 g PO single dose *or* metronidazole 250 mg TID for 7 days
- Recurrent and resistant urethritis
  - Metronidazole: 2 mg PO single dose *or* tinidazole 2 g PO single dose *and* azithromycin 1 g PO single dose, if not already used for initial episode
  - Erythromycin 500 mg PO QID for 7 days *and* acyclovir 400 mg PO TID for 5 days if suspicious for herpes simplex virus (HSV)
- Contraindications: sensitivity to any of the indicated medications
- Precautions: Patients taking tetracyclines may have increased photosensitivity.
- Significant possible interactions
  - Tetracyclines should not be taken with milk products or antacids.
  - Oral contraceptives may be rendered less effective by oral antibiotics. Patients and partners should use a backup method of birth control for the remainder of the cycle.

Pregnancy Considerations

- Tetracyclines and quinolones are contraindicated.
- Avoid erythromycin estolate because of an increased risk of cholestatic jaundice; otherwise, use the standard treatment recommendations.
- Single-dose therapy is recommended.

Second Line

- Gonorrhea
  - Fluoroquinolones were previously considered 2nd-line treatment options; however, due to reported worldwide resistance, they are no longer recommended by the CDC.
  - Resistance to penicillin and tetracycline has been reported in up to 1/3 of isolates of *N. gonorrhoeae*.
  - Gonococcal treatment resistance noted to be more common among men who have sex with men, when compared to men who have sex with women.
- Chlamydia
  - Ofloxacin 300 mg PO BID for 7 days *or*
  - Levofloxacin 500 mg/day PO for 7 days *or*
  - Erythromycin base 500 mg PO QID for 7 days *or* erythromycin ethylsuccinate 800 mg PO QID for 7 days
- Patients with persistent symptoms and signs after adequate treatment should be evaluated for other causes of urethritis.
  - Resistant strains of *U. urealyticum* or *M. genitalium*
  - *T. vaginalis*
  - Herpes simplex virus
  - Adenovirus
  - Enteric bacteria
  - Chronic nonbacterial prostatitis
  - Chronic pelvic pain syndrome

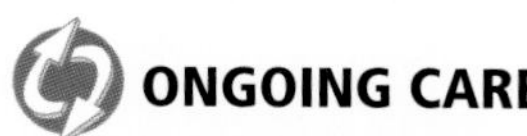

ONGOING CARE

FOLLOW-UP RECOMMENDATIONS

- Full activity
- Sexual activity should be avoided until both partners complete treatment and are symptom-free or 7 days after single-dose therapy.
- Patients should refer their sexual partners for evaluation if they had sexual contact within 60 days of symptom onset. If the last sexual encounter was >60 days prior to symptom onset, the last sex partner should still be referred for diagnosis.
- If sexual partner is unlikely to follow-up, consider giving the patient antibiotic therapy to give to the partner.

Patient Monitoring

Instruct patients to return if symptoms persist or recur after completing treatment. Test of cure cultures usually are not required unless the patient is pregnant.

DIET

Avoid alcohol when taking metronidazole.

PATIENT EDUCATION

Most important to emphasize the need for compliance with therapy, treatment of sexual partners, and use of safer sex practices; patients should be urged to undergo screening for other STIs.

PROGNOSIS

If the diagnosis is firmly established, appropriate medications are prescribed, and the patient is compliant with treatment, relief of symptoms occurs within days and the problem will resolve without sequelae.

COMPLICATIONS

- Stricture formation
- Epididymitis
- Prostatitis
- Proctitis
- PID in women
- Disseminated gonococcal infection
- Gonococcal meningitis
- Gonococcal endocarditis
- Perinatal transmission (chlamydial conjunctivitis, chlamydial pneumonia, ophthalmia neonatorum)
- Reiter syndrome

REFERENCES

1. Centers for Disease Control and Prevention. Sexually transmitted diseases treatment guidelines, 2010. *MMWR Morb Mortal Wkly Rep*. 2010;59(RR-12):1–110.

ADDITIONAL READING

- Ansart S, Hochedez P, Perez L, et al. Sexually transmitted diseases diagnosed among travelers returning from the tropics. *J Travel Med*. 2009;16(2):79–83.
- Centers for Disease Control and Prevention. *Sexually Transmitted Disease Surveillance, 2007*. Atlanta, GA: U.S. Department of Health and Human Services; 2008.
- Centers for Disease Control and Prevention, Workowski KA, Berman SM. Sexually transmitted diseases treatment guidelines. *MMWR Recomm Rep*. 2006;55(RR-11):1–94.
- Kirkcaldy RD, Zaidi A, Hook EW III, et al. *Neisseria gonorrhoeae* antimicrobial resistance among men who have sex with men and men who have sex exclusively with women: the Gonococcal Isolate Surveillance Project, 2005–2010. *Ann Intern Med*, 2013;158(5, Pt 1):321–328.
- U.S. Preventive Services Task Force. Screening for chlamydia infections: recommendations and rationale. *Am J Prev Med*. 2001;20(3)(Suppl):90–94.
- Wetmore CM, Manhart LE, Lowens MS, et al. *Ureaplasma urealyticum* is associated with nongonococcal urethritis among men with fewer lifetime sexual partners: a case-control study. *J Infect Dis*. 2011;204(8):1274–1282.
- Workowski KA, Berman S; Centers for Disease Control and Prevention. Sexually transmitted diseases treatment guidelines, 2010. *MMWR Recomm Rep*. 2010:59(RR-12):1–110.

SEE ALSO

- Chlamydia Infection (Sexually Transmitted); Epididymitis; Gonococcal Infections; Pelvic Inflammatory Disease (PID); Prostatitis; Urinary Tract Infection (UTI) in Females; Urinary Tract Infection (UTI) in Males; Vulvovaginitis, Estrogen Deficient; Vulvovaginitis, Prepubescent
- Algorithms: Dysuria; Genital Ulcers; Urethral Discharge

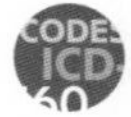

CODES

ICD10

- N34.2 Other urethritis
- A56.01 Chlamydial cystitis and urethritis
- A54.01 Gonococcal cystitis and urethritis, unspecified

CLINICAL PEARLS

- Urethral inflammation marked by painful urination, pruritus, hematuria, and/or discharge
- Usually, a result of an STI or, less commonly, autoimmune disorders (Reiter syndrome), trauma, or chemical irritation
- Complications such as urethral stricture in men or PID in women may occur if untreated.

URINARY TRACT INFECTION (UTI) IN FEMALES

Akhil Das, MD, FACS

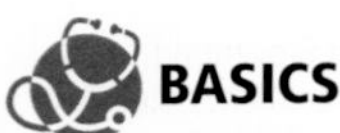

BASICS

DESCRIPTION

- Urinary tract infection (UTI) is the presence of pathogenic microorganisms within the urinary tract with concomitant symptoms.
- This topic refers primarily to infectious cystitis; other complicated UTIs, such as pyelonephritis, are discussed elsewhere.
- Uncomplicated UTI: occurs in patients who have a normal, unobstructed urinary tract, who have no history of recent instrumentation, and whose symptoms are confined to the lower urinary tract. Uncomplicated UTIs are most common in young, sexually active women.
- Complicated UTI: an infection of the lower or upper urinary tract in the presence of an anatomic abnormality, a functional abnormality, or a urinary catheter
- Recurrent UTI: symptomatic UTIs that follow resolution of an earlier episode, usually after appropriate treatment
  - No single definition of the frequency of recurrent UTI exists, but a pragmatic definition is ≥3 infections per year.
  - Most recurrences are thought to represent reinfection rather than relapse.
  - No evidence indicates that recurrent UTIs lead to health problems such as hypertension or renal disease in the absence of anatomic or functional abnormalities of the urinary tract (1)[A].
- System(s) affected: renal/urologic
- Synonym(s): cystitis; infectious cystitis

EPIDEMIOLOGY

Incidence

- Accounts for 8 million doctor visits and 1 million emergency room visits, and contributes to >100,000 hospital admissions each year
- 11% of women have UTIs in any given year.
- Predominant age: young adults and older
- Predominant sex: female > male

Prevalence

- >50% of females have at least 1 UTI in their lifetime.
- 1 in 4 women have recurrent UTIs.

ETIOLOGY AND PATHOPHYSIOLOGY

- Bacteria and subsequent infection in the urinary tract arise chiefly via ascending bacterial movement and propagation (1).
- Pathogenic organisms (*Escherichia coli*) possess adherence factors and toxins that allow initiation and propagation of genitourinary infections:
  - Type 1 and *P. pili* (*pyelonephritis-associated pili*)
  - Lipopolysaccharide
- Most UTIs are caused by bacteria originating from bowel flora:
  - *E. coli* is the causative organism in 80% of cases of uncomplicated cystitis.
  - *Staphylococcus saprophyticus* accounts for 15% of infections.
  - Enterobacteriaceae (i.e., *Klebsiella, Proteus, Enterobacter,* and *Pseudomonas)* also contribute.
- *Candida* is associated with nosocomial UTI (2).

Genetics

Women with human leukocyte antigen 3 (HLA-3) and nonsecretor Lewis antigen have an increased bacterial adherence, which may lead to an increased risk in UTI.

RISK FACTORS

- Previous UTI
- Diabetes mellitus (DM)
- Pregnancy
- Sexual activity
- Use of spermicides or diaphragm
- Underlying abnormalities of the urinary tract such as tumors, calculi, strictures, incomplete bladder emptying, urinary incontinence, neurogenic bladder
- Catheterization
- Recent antibiotic use
- Poor hygiene
- Estrogen deficiency
- Inadequate fluid intake

GENERAL PREVENTION

- Maintain good hydration.
- Women with frequent or intercourse-related UTI should empty bladder immediately before and following intercourse; consider postcoital antibiotic.
- Avoid feminine hygiene sprays and douches.
- Wipe urethra from front to back.
- Cranberry juice (not cranberry juice cocktail) consumption may prevent recurrent infections.

COMMONLY ASSOCIATED CONDITIONS

See "Risk Factors."

Geriatric Considerations

- Elderly patients are more likely to have underlying urinary tract abnormality.
- Acute UTI may be associated with incontinence or mental status changes in the elderly.

DIAGNOSIS

HISTORY

Note: Any or all may be present:

- Burning during urination
- Pain during urination (dysuria)
- Urgency (sensation of need to urinate often)
- Frequency
- Sensation of incomplete bladder emptying
- Blood in urine
- Lower abdominal pain or cramping
- Offensive odor of urine
- Nocturia
- Sudden onset of urinary incontinence
- Dyspareunia

PHYSICAL EXAM

- Suprapubic tenderness
- Urethral and/or vaginal tenderness
- Fever or costovertebral angle tenderness indicates upper UTI.

DIFFERENTIAL DIAGNOSIS

- Vaginitis
- Asymptomatic bacteriuria
- STDs causing urethritis or pyuria
- Hematuria from causes other than infection (e.g., neoplasia, calculi)
- Interstitial cystitis
- Psychological dysfunction

DIAGNOSTIC TESTS & INTERPRETATION

Initial Tests (lab, imaging)

- No lab testing is necessary in women with high likelihood of lower UTI based on classic symptoms.
- Urinalysis
  - Pyuria (>10 neutrophils/high-power field [HPF])
  - Bacteriuria (any amount on unspun urine, or 10 bacteria/HPF on centrifuged urine)
  - Hematuria (>5 RBCs/HPF)
- Dipstick urinalysis
  - Leukocyte esterase (75–96% sensitivity, 94–98% specificity, when >100,000 colony-forming units [CFU])
  - Nitrite tests useful with nitrite-reducing organisms (e.g., enterococci, *S. saprophyticus, Acinetobacter*)
- Urine culture: *only* indicated if diagnosis is unclear or patient has recurrent infections and resistance is suspected
  - Presence of 100,000 CFU/mL of organism indicates infection.
  - Identification of a single organism at lower CFU/mL likely also represents infection in the presence of appropriate symptoms.
  - Suspect a contaminated specimen when culture shows multiple types of bacteria.
- Imaging studies are often not required in most cases of UTI.

Follow-Up Tests & Special Considerations

- In nonpregnant, premenopausal women with symptoms of UTI, positive urinalysis, and no risks for complicated infection, empirical treatment may be given without obtaining a urine culture.
- Dipstick urinalysis may be helpful but not necessary in patients with characteristic symptoms (i.e., high pretest probability).
- Imaging may be indicated for UTIs in men, infants, immunocompromised patients, febrile infection, signs or symptoms of obstruction, failure to respond to appropriate therapy, and in patients with recurrent infections.
- CT scan and MRI provide the most complete anatomic data in adults.

Pediatric Considerations

For infants and children, obtain US; if ureteral dilatation is detected, obtain either voiding cystourethrogram or isotope cystogram to evaluate for reflux.

Diagnostic Procedures/Other

- Urethral catheterization maybe necessary to obtain a urine specimen from children and adults if the voided urine is suspected of being contaminated.
- Suprapubic bladder aspiration or urethral catheterization techniques can be used to obtain specimens from infants.
- Cystourethroscopy can be used for patients with recurrent UTIs and previous anti-incontinence surgery or hematuria (3)[A].

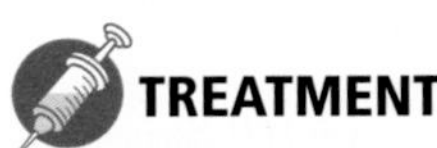

TREATMENT

GENERAL MEASURES

- Maintain good hydration.
- Maintain good hygiene.
- 1/4 of women with uncomplicated UTI experience a 2nd UTI within 6 months and 1/2 at some time during their lifetime.

MEDICATION

First Line

- The urinary tract topical analgesic phenazopyridine 100–200 mg TID produces rapid relief of symptoms and should be offered to patients with more than minor discomfort; it is available over the counter. This medication is not a substitute for definitive treatment. This medication also may alter urinalysis but not the urine culture.
- Uncomplicated UTI (adolescents and adults who are nonpregnant, nondiabetic, afebrile, immunocompetent, and without genitourinary anatomic abnormalities)
  - Trimethoprim-sulfamethoxazole (TMP-SMZ; Bactrim): 160/800 mg PO BID × 3 days, best where resistance of *E. coli* strains <20%
  - 5-day course of nitrofurantoin or 3-day fluoroquinolone course should be used in patients with allergy to TMP-SMZ and in areas where *E. coli* resistance to TMP-SMZ >20%.
  - Fosfomycin (Monurol): 3 g PO single dose (expensive)
- Lower UTI in pregnancy
  - Nitrofurantoin (Macrobid): 100 mg PO BID × 7 days
  - Cephalexin (Keflex): 500 mg PO BID × 7 days
- Postcoital UTI: single-dose TMP-SMX or cephalexin may reduce frequency of UTI in sexually active women.
- Complicated UTI (pregnancy, diabetes, febrile, immunocompromised patient, recurrent UTIs): Extend course to 7–10 days of treatment with antibiotic chosen based on culture results; may begin with fluoroquinolone, TMP-SMX, or cephalosporin while awaiting results (avoid using nitrofurantoin for complicated UTI)
  - Fluoroquinolones are not safe during pregnancy and are usually avoided in treatment of children.
  - TMP-SMX use in pregnancy is not desirable (especially in 3rd trimester) but is appropriate in some circumstances (3)[A].

Second Line

- Uncomplicated UTI
  - Ciprofloxacin: 250 mg PO BID × 3 days; should be reserved for complicated UTIs
  - Beta-lactams (amoxicillin/clavulanate, cefdinir, cefpodoxime proxetil) for 3–7 days
- Chronic UTIs
  - Women with recurrent symptomatic UTIs can be treated with continuous or postcoital prophylactic antibiotics. Treatment duration guided by the severity of patient symptoms and by physician and patient preference: Consider 6 months of therapy, followed by observation for reinfection after discontinuing prophylaxis:
    - Continuous antimicrobial prophylaxis involves daily administration of low-dose TMP-SMX 40/200 mg or nitrofurantoin 50–100 mg, among others.
- Another treatment option is self-started antibiotics.

Pediatric Considerations

Long-term antibiotics appear to reduce the risk of recurrent symptomatic UTI in susceptible children, but the benefit is small and must be considered together with the increased risk of microbial resistance.

ISSUES FOR REFERRAL

Men with uncomplicated UTI and most other patients with complicated UTI should be referred to a urologist for evaluation.

Pediatric Considerations

UTI in children, especially <1 year of age, should prompt workup for urinary tract anomalies.

SURGERY/OTHER PROCEDURES

- Urinary tract obstruction with urosepsis requires urgent drainage of the obstructed system.
- Patients with emphysematous pyelonephritis or pyonephrosis may need immediate surgical intervention.

COMPLEMENTARY & ALTERNATIVE MEDICINE

- Preliminary studies indicate that *Vaccinium macrocarpon* (cranberry) juice may help to prevent and treat UTIs by inhibiting bacterial adherence to the bladder epithelium.
- Cranberry juice may decrease the number of symptomatic UTIs over a 1-year period, particularly for women with recurrent UTIs. The optimal dosage or method of administration (e.g., juice, tablets, or capsules) is still unclear.

INPATIENT CONSIDERATIONS

Inpatient evaluation is reserved for patients with complicated or upper tract UTI's. Majority of UTI's are managed in an outpatient setting.

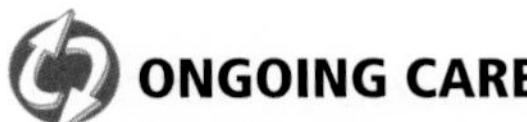

ONGOING CARE

FOLLOW-UP RECOMMENDATIONS

- 1st or rare UTI: Young or middle-aged, nonpregnant adult females require no follow-up if UTI is clinically cured after 3-day therapy.
- If symptoms persist after 2–3 days of therapy, obtain culture/sensitivity and change antibiotic accordingly.

Pregnancy Considerations

- UTI during pregnancy always requires culture/sensitivity and usually requires a 7–14-day treatment.
- Following the treatment of acute infection, pregnant women warrant surveillance urine cultures every trimester. They may receive prophylactic antibiotics for the remainder of pregnancy for recurrent or upper tract disease.

PATIENT EDUCATION

- Although no controlled studies support this intervention, postcoital voiding is commonly advised.
- FamilyDoctor Web site: http://familydoctor.org/online/famdocen/home/women/gen-health/190.html

PROGNOSIS

Symptoms resolve within 2–3 days of antibiotic treatment in almost all patients.

COMPLICATIONS

- Pyelonephritis or sepsis
- Renal abscess
- Acute urinary outlet obstruction

Pregnancy Considerations

Pregnant females, infants, and young children with cystitis are at higher risk of pyelonephritis.

REFERENCES

1. Kodner CM, Thomas Gupton EK. Recurrent urinary tract infections in women: diagnosis and management. *Am Fam Physician*. 2010;82(6):638–643.
2. Hooten TM. Clinical practice. Uncomplicated urinary tract infection. *N Engl J Med*. 2012;366(11):1028–1037.
3. Zalmanovici Trestioreanu A, Green H, Paul M, et al. Antimicrobial agents for treating uncomplicated urinary tract infection in women. *Cochrane Database Syst Rev*. 2010;(10):CD007182.

ADDITIONAL READING

- Gupta K, Hooton TM, Naber KG, et al. International clinical practice guidelines for the treatment of acute uncomplicated cystitis and pyelonephritis in women: a 2010 update by the Infectious Diseases Society of America and the European Society for Microbiology and Infectious Diseases. *Clin Infect Dis*. 2011;52(5):e103–e120.
- Jepson RG, Craig JC. Cranberries for preventing urinary tract infections. *Cochrane Database Syst Rev*. 2008;(1):CD001321.
- Litza JA, Brill JR. Urinary tract infections. *Prim Care*. 2010;37(3):491–507, viii.
- Mehnert-Kay SA. Diagnosis and management of uncomplicated urinary tract infections. *Am Fam Physician*. 2005;72(3):451–456.
- Mody L, Juthani-Mehta M. Urinary tract infections in older women: a clinical review. *JAMA* 2014;311(8):844–854.
- Stapleton A, Stamm WE. Prevention of urinary tract infection. *Infect Dis Clin N Am*. 1997;11(3):719–733.
- Williams G, Craig JC. Long-term antibiotics for preventing recurrent urinary tract infection in children. *Cochrane Database Syst Rev*. 2011;(3):CD001534.

SEE ALSO

Algorithm: Dysuria

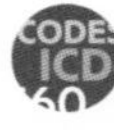

CODES

ICD10

- N39.0 Urinary tract infection, site not specified
- N30.90 Cystitis, unspecified without hematuria
- N30.91 Cystitis, unspecified with hematuria

CLINICAL PEARLS

- Uncomplicated UTIs cause significant morbidity but generally do not cause renal damage.
- Treatment of uncomplicated UTIs reduces morbidity, but the risk of recurrence stays the same.
- Bacteria originating from intestinal tract cause most UTIs, especially *E. coli*.
- Imaging studies are not required for most women with UTIs.
- Uncomplicated UTIs should be treated for 3 days (TMP-SMX) or 5 days (nitrofurantoin).
- All pregnant women with bacteriuria should be treated.

URINARY TRACT INFECTION (UTI) IN MALES

Amy L. Wiser, MD • Holly Milne Hofkamp, MD • Scott A. Fields, MD, MHA

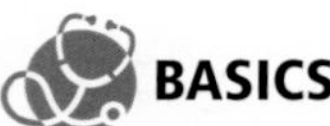

BASICS

DESCRIPTION
- Cystitis is an infection of the lower urinary tract, usually resulting from a single gram-negative enteric bacteria. (See also "Prostatitis," "Pyelonephritis," and "Urethritis.")
- System(s) affected: renal/urologic
- Synonym(s): urinary tract infection (UTI); cystitis
- Conventional consideration of UTI in male newborn, infant, and elderly men as complicated, with associated functional/structural mechanisms.
- In otherwise healthy males ages 15–50 years, UTI is uncommon and considered uncomplicated.

EPIDEMIOLOGY
Incidence
- Approximately 20% of UTIs occur in men (1).
- Predominant age: increases with age
- Uncommon in men <50 years of age
- 6–8 infections/10,000 men aged 21–50 years (2)

Prevalence
Lifetime prevalence approximately 14% (1)

ETIOLOGY AND PATHOPHYSIOLOGY
- *Escherichia coli* (majority of infections)
- *Klebsiella*
- *Enterobacter*
- *Enterococcus*
- *Proteus*
- *Serratia*
- *Citrobacter*
- *Providencia*
- *Streptococcus faecalis* and *Staphylococcus* sp.
- *Pseudomonas* and *Morganella* (more common in elderly and catheterized patients)
- Pathogenesis—bacterial entry into urinary tract via ascension or bladder instrumentation

Genetics
Not applicable

RISK FACTORS
- Age
- Obesity (3)
- History of prior UTI
- Outlet obstruction
  - Benign prostatic hypertrophy (BPH)—incidence of 33% of men with UTIs (4)
  - Urethral stricture
  - Calculi
- Cognitive impairment
- Fecal incontinence
- Urinary incontinence
- Anal intercourse
- Recent urologic surgery
- Infection of the prostate/kidney
- Urinary tract instrumentation, catheterization
- Immunocompromised host
- Diabetes
- Bladder diverticula
- Neurogenic bladder
- Institutionalization
- Uncircumcised
- Engaging in sex with an infected female partner (2)

GENERAL PREVENTION
- Prompt treatment of predisposing factors
- Use a catheter only when necessary; if needed, use aseptic technique and closed system and remove as soon as possible.
- Currently, cranberry products are not recommended for preventing UTIs in men (5).

COMMONLY ASSOCIATED CONDITIONS
- Acute bacterial pyelonephritis
- Chronic bacterial pyelonephritis
- Urethritis
- Prostatitis
- Prostatic hypertrophy
- Prostate cancer

Geriatric Considerations
Bacteriuria is common among the elderly; may be related to functional status and usually is transient. Of men older than 65 years of age, 5–10% have asymptomatic bacteriuria (ASB). If ASB is noted, no treatment is needed (6,7).

Pediatric Considerations
Can be associated with obstruction to normal flow of urine, such as vesicoureteral reflux. Unique diagnostic criteria and evaluation recommendations exist (see below) (8).

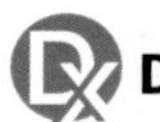

DIAGNOSIS

HISTORY
- Urinary frequency
- Urinary urgency
- Dysuria
- Hesitancy
- Slow urinary stream
- Dribbling of urine
- Nocturia
- Suprapubic discomfort or perineal pain
- Low back pain
- Hematuria
- Systemic symptoms (chills, fever) or flank pain, nausea, vomiting present with concomitant pyelonephritis or prostatitis (9).

PHYSICAL EXAM
- Suprapubic tenderness
- Costovertebral angle (CVA) tenderness and/or fever may be present with concomitant pyelonephritis/prostatitis/epididymitis.

DIFFERENTIAL DIAGNOSIS
- Anatomic/functional pathology of the urinary tract
- Urethritis/STIs
- Infections in other sites of the genitourinary tract (e.g., epididymis, prostatitis). More than 90% of men with febrile UTI have concomitant prostate infection (9).

DIAGNOSTIC TESTS & INTERPRETATION
Initial Tests (lab, imaging)
- Urine dipstick/manual microscopy of clean catch midstream void showing the following:
  - Pyuria (>10 WBCs)
  - Bacteriuria
  - Positive leukocyte esterase (in males: sensitivity, 78%; specificity, 59%; positive predictive value [PPV], 71%; negative predictive value [NPV], 67%)
  - Positive nitrite (in males: sensitivity, 47%; specificity, 98%; PPV, 96%; NPV, 59%)
  - In general, leukocyte esterase is more sensitive and nitrite is more specific in detecting UTI (10).
- Automated microscopy/flow cytometry that measures cell counts and bacterial counts can be used to improve screening characteristics (sensitivity, 92%; specificity, 55%; PPV, 47%; NPV, 97%). The high NPV of these screening tests allows for more judicious use of urine culture (11).
- Urine culture: >100,000 colony-forming units (CFU; >10^5 CFU) of bacteria/mL of urine confirm diagnosis. Lower counts, such as >10^3 CFU, also may be indicative of infection, especially in the presence of pyuria. Diagnosis in infants and children <24 months made on the basis of both pyuria and 50,000 CFU on culture.
- Renal and bladder ultrasound recommended in infants and young children after first confirmed UTI.

Follow-Up Tests & Special Considerations
- Consider assessing for risk factors for STIs, as chlamydial/gonococcal urethritis can mimic a UTI. If risk factors are present, use urine nucleic acid amplification tests to identify gonococcal and *Chlamydia* infections and treat as necessary.
- Further urologic evaluation is warranted to rule out other disorders in men with recurrent UTI, febrile UTI, or pyelonephritis. This may include the following:
  - Ultrasound
  - Cystoscopy
  - Urodynamics
  - IV pyelography
- Value of a urologic evaluation in a single uncomplicated UTI has not been determined (9).
- Antibiotics prior to culture or phenazopyridine prior to urine dipstick can alter results.

Test Interpretation
Depends on site of infection

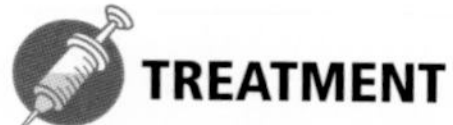

TREATMENT

GENERAL MEASURES

- Hydration
- Analgesia, if required
- Patient with indwelling catheters
  - If asymptomatic bacterial colonization, no need to treat (sterilization of urine is not possible, and resistant organisms may take up residence).
  - If symptomatic of acute infection, institute treatment.

MEDICATION

First Line

- Acute, uncomplicated cystitis
  - Treat empirically; strongly consider if nitrite positive, using local resistance patterns or based on culture and sensitivity results for 7 days (9)[B]. For empirical therapy, a fluoroquinolone or trimethoprim-sulfamethoxazole DS usually used to treat the most likely pathogens (9).
- Complicated, febrile, or recurrent infection
  - Prescribe a minimum of 2 weeks antibiotics based on antimicrobial sensitivities with repeat urine check after the treatment. In men with febrile UTI or pyelonephritis, prostatic involvement also has to be considered. Treatment of concomitant prostatitis requires antimicrobials with good prostatic tissue and fluid penetration (fluoroquinolones) (9)[B].

Second Line

According to culture and sensitivity results and patient's history

ISSUES FOR REFERRAL

Further urologic evaluation and referral are warranted to rule out other disorders in men with recurrent UTI, febrile UTI, or pyelonephritis.

INPATIENT CONSIDERATIONS

Admission Criteria/Initial Stabilization

- Inability to tolerate oral medications
- Acute renal failure
- Suspected sepsis

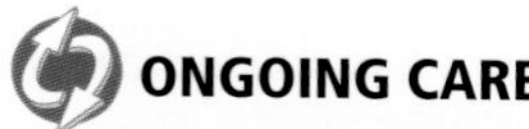

ONGOING CARE

FOLLOW-UP RECOMMENDATIONS

Patient Monitoring

Close follow-up until clinically well

DIET

Encourage adequate fluid intake.

PATIENT EDUCATION

For patient education materials about this topic that have been reviewed favorably, contact the National Kidney Foundation, 30 E. 33rd Street, Suite 1100, New York, NY 10016; 212-889-2210.

PROGNOSIS

Clearing of infections with appropriate antibiotic treatment

COMPLICATIONS

- Pyelonephritis
- Ascending infection
- Recurrent infection
- Prostatitis

REFERENCES

1. Griebling T. Urological Diseases in America Project: trends in the resource use for urinary tract infections in men. *J Urol*. 2005;173(4):1288–1294.
2. Wagenlehner FM, Weidner W, Pilatz A, et al. Urinary tract infections and bacterial prostatitis in men. *Curr Opin Infect Dis*. 2014;27(1):97–101.
3. Semins MJ, Shore AD, Makary MA, et al. The impact of obesity on urinary tract infection risk. *Urology*. 2012;79(2):266–269.
4. Drekonja DM, Rector TS, Cutting A, et al. Urinary tract infection in male veterans: treatment patterns and outcomes. *JAMA Intern Med*. 2013;173(1):62–68.
5. Jepson R, Williams G, Craig J. Cranberries for preventing urinary tract infections. *Cochrane Database Syst Rev*. 2012;10:CD001321.
6. Rowe TA, Juthani-Mehta M. Diagnosis and management of urinary tract infection in older adults. *Infect Dis Clin N Am*. 2014;28(1):75–89.
7. Matthews SJ, Lancaster JW. Urinary tract infections in the elderly population. *Am J Geriatr Pharmacother*. 2011;9(5):286–309.
8. Subcommittee on Urinary Tract Infection, Steering Committee on Quality Improvement and Management, Robert KB. Urinary tract infection: clinical practice guideline for the diagnosis and management of the initial UTI in febrile infants and children 2 to 24 months. *Pediatrics*. 2011;128(3):595–610.
9. Grabe M, Bishop MC, Bjerklund-Johansen TE, et al. Uncomplicated urinary tract infections in adult. In: *Guidelines on Urological Infections*. Arnhem, The Netherlands: European Association of Urology; 2013:15–25.
10. Koeijers JJ, Kessels AG, Nys S, et al. Evaluation of the nitrite and leukocyte esterase activity tests for the diagnosis of acute symptomatic urinary tract infection in men. *Clin Infec Dis*. 2007;45(7):894–896.
11. Evans R, Davison M, Sim L, et al. Testing by Sysmex UF-100 flow cytometer and with bacterial culture in a diagnostic laboratory: a comparison. *J Clin Pathol*. 2006;59(6):661–662.

ADDITIONAL READING

- Coupat C, Pradier C, Degand N, et al. Selective reporting of antibiotic susceptibility data improves the appropriateness of intended antibiotic prescriptions in urinary tract infections: a case-vignette randomised study. *Eur J Clin Microbiol Infect Dis*. 2013;32(5):627–636.
- Foxman B. Urinary tract infection syndromes: occurrence, recurrence, bacteriology, risk factors, and disease burden. *Infect Dis Clin N Am*. 2014;28(1):1–13.
- Gerber GS, Brendler CB. Evaluation of the urologic patient: history, physical examination, and urinalysis. In: Walsh PC, Retik AB, Vaughn ED Jr, eds. *Campbell's Urology*. 8th ed. Philadelphia, PA: Saunders; 2002:107.
- Koeijers JJ, Verbon A, Kessels AG, et al. Urinary tract infection in male general practice patients: uropathogens and antibiotic susceptibility. *Urology*. 2010;76(2):336–340.

SEE ALSO

- Prostate Cancer; Prostatic Hyperplasia, Benign (BPH); Prostatitis; Pyelonephritis; Urethritis
- Algorithms: Dysuria; Urethral Discharge

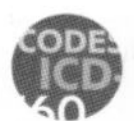

CODES

ICD10

- N39.0 Urinary tract infection, site not specified
- N30.90 Cystitis, unspecified without hematuria
- B96.20 Unsp Escherichia coli as the cause of diseases classd elswhr

CLINICAL PEARLS

- Cystitis is an infection of the lower urinary tract, usually resulting from a single gram-negative enteric bacteria.
- Risk factors/causes: age, history of UTI, obesity, BPH, cognitive impairment, fecal incontinence, urinary incontinence, anal intercourse, recent urologic surgery, catheterization, infection of the prostate/kidney, urinary tract instrumentation, immunocompromised host, diabetes, neurogenic bladder, outlet obstruction, sex with infected female partner
- Evaluation: urinalysis, urine culture, STI testing (e.g., gonorrhea, *Chlamydia* by culture/DNA probe)
- Treat empirically with fluoroquinolones or trimethoprim-sulfamethoxazole DS for 7 days.

UROLITHIASIS

Phillip Fournier, MD

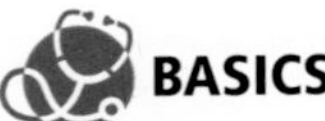

BASICS

DESCRIPTION

- Stone formation within the urinary tract: Urinary crystals bind to form a nidus which grows to form a calculus (stone).
- Range of symptoms: asymptomatic to obstructive; febrile morbidity if result of infection

EPIDEMIOLOGY

- The worldwide epidemiology differs according to both geographic area (higher prevalence in hot, arid, or dry climates) and socioeconomic conditions (dietary intake and lifestyle). Radiolucent stones and stones secondary to infection are less influenced by environmental conditions.
- Vesical calculosis (bladder stones) due to malnutrition during early life is frequent in Middle East and Asian countries.
- Incidence in industrialized countries seems to be increasing, probably due to improved diagnostics as well as to increasingly rich diets.
- Increased incidence in patients with surgically induced absorption issues, such as Crohn disease and gastric bypass surgery (1)[B]

Incidence

- In industrialized countries: 100–200/100,000/year (2)
- Predominant age: mean age is 40–60 years.
- Predominant sex: male > female (~2:1) (3)

ETIOLOGY AND PATHOPHYSIOLOGY

- Supersaturation and dehydration lead to high salt content in urine which congregates.
- Stasis of urine
  - Renal malformation (e.g., horseshoe kidney, ureteropelvic junction obstruction)
  - Incomplete bladder emptying (e.g., neurogenic bladder, prostate enlargement, multiple sclerosis)
- Crystals may form in pure solutions (homogeneous) or on existing surfaces, such as other crystals or cellular debris (heterogeneous).
- Balance of promoters and inhibitors: organic (Tamm-Horsfall protein, glycosaminoglycan, uropontin, nephrocalcin) and inorganic (citrate, pyrophosphate)
- Calcium oxalate and/or phosphate stones (80%)
  - Hypercalciuria
    - Absorptive hypercalciuria: increased jejunal calcium absorption
    - Renal leak: increased calcium excretion from renal proximal tubule
    - Resorptive hypercalciuria: mild hyperparathyroidism
  - Hypercalcemia
    - Hyperparathyroidism
    - Sarcoidosis
    - Malignancy
    - Immobilization
    - Paget disease
- Hyperoxaluria
  - Enteric hyperoxaluria
    - Intestinal malabsorptive state associated with irritable bowel disease, celiac sprue, or intestinal resection
    - Bile salt malabsorption leads to formation of calcium soaps.
  - Primary hyperoxaluria: autosomal recessive, types I and II
  - Dietary hyperoxaluria: overindulgence in oxalate-rich food
- Hyperuricosuria
  - Seen in 10% of calcium stone formers
  - Caused by increased dietary purine intake, systemic acidosis, myeloproliferative diseases, gout, chemotherapy, Lesch-Nyhan syndrome
  - Thiazides, probenecid
- Hypocitraturia
  - Caused by acidosis: renal tubular acidosis, malabsorption, thiazides, enalapril, excessive dietary protein
- Uric acid stones (10–15%): hyperuricemia causes as discussed earlier
- Struvite stones (5–10%): infected urine with urease-producing organisms (most commonly *Proteus* sp.)
- Cystine stones (<1%): autosomal-recessive disorder of renal tubular reabsorption of cystine
- Bladder stones: seen with chronic bladder catheterization and some medications (indinavir)
- In children: usually due to malnutrition

Genetics

- Up to 20% of patients have a family history. However, spouses of those who form stones have higher calcium excretion rates than controls, suggesting strong dietary–environmental factors.
- Autosomal dominant: idiopathic hypercalciuria
- Autosomal recessive
  - Cystinuria, Lesch-Nyhan syndrome, hyperoxaluria types I and II
  - Ehlers-Danlos syndrome, Marfan syndrome, Wilson disease, familial renal tubular acidosis

RISK FACTORS

- White > African American in regions with both populations
- Family history
- Previous history of nephrolithiasis
- Diet rich in protein, refined carbohydrates, and sodium
- Occupations associated with a sedentary lifestyle or with a hot, dry workplace
- Incidence rates peak during summer secondary to dehydration.
- Obesity
- Surgically/medically induced malabsorption (Crohn disease, gastric bypass, celiac)

GENERAL PREVENTION

- Hydration (4)[A]
- Decrease salt and meat intake
- Avoid oxalate-rich foods.

Pediatric Considerations

Rare: more common in men with low socioeconomic status

Pregnancy Considerations

- Pregnant women have the same incidence of renal colic as do nonpregnant women.
- Most symptomatic stones occur during the 2nd and 3rd trimesters, heralded by symptoms of flank pain/hematuria.
- Most common differential diagnosis is physiologic hydronephrosis of pregnancy. Use ultrasound to avoid irradiation. Noncontrast-enhanced CT scan also is diagnostic.
- Treatment goals
  - Control pain and avoid infection, and preserve renal function until birth or stone passage.
  - 30% require intervention, such as stent placement.

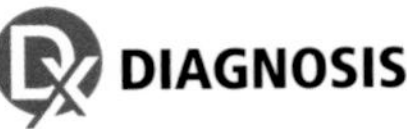

DIAGNOSIS

HISTORY

- Pain
  - Renal colic: cute onset of severe groin and/or flank pain
  - Distal stones may present with referred pain in labia, penile meatus, or testis.
- Microscopic/gross hematuria occurs in 95% of patients.
- Nonspecific symptoms of nausea, vomiting, tachycardia, diaphoresis
- Low-grade fever without signs of infection
- Infectious origin: associated with high-grade fevers require more urgent treatment (see the following text)
- Frequency and dysuria especially occur with stones at the vesicoureteric junction (VUJ).
- Asymptomatic: nonobstructing stones within the renal calyces

PHYSICAL EXAM

Tender costovertebral angle with palpation/percussion and/or iliac fossa

DIFFERENTIAL DIAGNOSIS

- Appendicitis
- Ruptured aortic aneurysm
- Musculoskeletal strain
- Pyelonephritis (upper UTI)
- Pyonephrosis (obstructed upper UTI; emergency)
- Perinephric abscess
- Ectopic pregnancy
- Salpingitis

DIAGNOSTIC TESTS & INTERPRETATION

- Urinalysis for RBCs, leukocytes, nitrates, pH (acidic urine <5.5 is associated with uric acid stones; alkaline >7 with struvite stones)
- Midstream urine for microscopy, culture, and sensitivity
- Blood: urea, creatinine, electrolytes, calcium, and urate; consider CBC.
- Parathyroid hormone only if calcium elevated
- Stone analysis if/when stone passed

Initial Tests (lab, imaging)

- Noncontrast-enhanced helical CT scan of the abdomen and pelvis has replaced IV pyelogram as the investigation of choice (5)[A].
  - Stone is found most commonly at levels of ureteric luminal narrowing: pelviureteric junction, pelvic brim, and VUJ
  - Acute obstruction: Proximal ureter and renal pelvis are dilated to the level of obstruction, and perinephric stranding is possible on imaging.

- X-ray of kidneys, ureter, and bladder to determine if stone is radiopaque or lucent
  - Calcium oxalate/phosphate stones are radiopaque.
  - Uric acid stones are radiolucent.
  - Staghorn calculi (that fill the shape of the renal calyces) are usually struvite and opaque.
  - Cystine stones are faintly opaque (ground-glass appearance).
- Ultrasound has low sensitivity and specificity but is often the first choice for pregnant women.

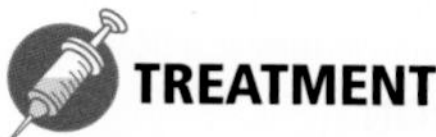

TREATMENT

GENERAL MEASURES

- 75% of patients are successfully treated conservatively and pass the stone spontaneously.
- Stones that do not pass usually require surgical intervention.
- 30–50% of patients will have recurrent stones.
- Increased fluid intake; eliminate carbonated drinks

MEDICATION

- Medical expulsive therapy: α_1-antagonists (e.g., tamsulosin) and calcium channel blockers (e.g., nifedipine) improve likelihood of spontaneous stone passage with a number needed to treat (NNT) of ~5 (6).
- Class C in pregnancy

ISSUES FOR REFERRAL

- Urgent referral of patients with UTI/sepsis or acute renal failure/solitary kidney
- Early referral of pregnant patients, large stones (>8 mm), chronic renal failure, children
- Refer patients if no passage at 2–4 weeks or poorly controlled pain.

ADDITIONAL THERAPIES

- Uric acid stone dissolution therapy
  - Alkalinize urine with potassium citrate; keep pH >6.5.
  - Allopurinol 100–300 mg/day PO (for those who continue to form stones despite alkalinization of urine)
- Cystine stone dissolution/prevention
  - Alkalinize urine with potassium citrate; keep pH >6.5.
  - Chelating agents: captopril, α-mercapto propionylglycine, D-penicillamine
- Consider altering medications that increase risk of stone formation: probenecid, loop diuretics, salicylic acid, salbutamol, indinavir, triamterene, acetazolamide.
- Vitamin D supplementation has not been proven to induce stone formation.
- Treat hypercalciuria with thiazides on an acute basis only
- Treat hypocitraturia with potassium citrate and high-citrate juices (e.g., orange, lemon).
- Treat enteric hyperoxaluria with oral calcium/magnesium, cholestyramine, and potassium citrate.

SURGERY/OTHER PROCEDURES

- Immediate relief of obstruction is required for patients with the following conditions:
  - Sepsis
  - Renal failure (obstructed solitary kidney, bilateral obstruction)
  - Uncontrolled pain, despite adequate analgesia
- Emergency surgery for obstruction
  - Placement of a retrograde stent (i.e., endoscopic surgery, usually requires an anesthetic)
  - Radiologic placement of a percutaneous nephrostomy tube
- Elective surgery for stone treatment
  - Extracorporeal shock wave lithotripsy
  - Ureteroscopy with basket extraction/lithotripsy (laser/pneumatic)
  - Percutaneous nephrolithotomy
- Open surgery is uncommon.

INPATIENT CONSIDERATIONS

Admission Criteria/Initial Stabilization

- Analgesia
  - Combination of NSAIDs (ketorolac 30–60 mg) and oral opiate
  - Parenteral opioid if vomiting or if preceding fails to control pain (morphine 5–10 mg IV or IM q4h)
  - Antiemetic if required or prophylactically with parenteral narcotics
- Septic patients with urosepsis or pyonephrosis may require IV antibiotics (once blood and urine cultures are taken), IV fluids, and, in severe cases, cardiorespiratory support in intensive care during recovery.

ONGOING CARE

FOLLOW-UP RECOMMENDATIONS

- Patients with ureteric stones who are being treated conservatively should be followed until imaging is clear or stone is visibly passed.
  - Strain urine and send stone for composition.
  - Tamsulosin and nifedipine in selected patients to speed passage
  - Present to the hospital if pain worsens/signs of infection.
  - If pain management is suboptimal or stone does not progress or pass within 2–4 weeks, patient should be referred to a urologist and imaging should be repeated.
- Patients with recurrent stone formation should have follow-up with a urologist for metabolic workup: 24-hour urine for volume, pH, creatinine, calcium, cystine, phosphate, oxalate, uric acid, and magnesium.

DIET

ALERT

- Increased fluid intake for life cannot be overemphasized for decreasing recurrence. Encourage intake of 2–3 L/day; advise patient to have clear urine rather than yellow.
- Decrease or eliminate carbonated drinks.
- Patients who form calcium stones should minimize high-oxalate foods such as green leafy vegetables, rhubarb, peanuts, chocolates, and beer.
- Decrease protein and salt intake.
- Lowering calcium intake is inadvisable and even may increase urine calcium excretion.

PROGNOSIS

- Spontaneous stone passage depends on stone location (proximal vs. distal) and stone size (<5 mm, 90% pass; >8 mm, 10% pass).
- Stone recurrence: 50% of patients at 10 years

REFERENCES

1. Matlaga BR, Shore AD, Magnuson T, et al. Effect of gastric bypass surgery on kidney stone disease. *J Urol*. 2009;181(6):2573–2577.
2. Tiselius HG. Epidemiology and medical management of stone disease. *BJU Int*. 2003;91(8):758–767.
3. Scales, CD Jr, Curtis LH, Norris RD, et al. Changing gender prevalence of stone disease. *J Urol* 2007;177(3):979–982.
4. Qiang W, Ke Z. Water for preventing urinary calculi. *Cochrane Database Sys Rev*. 2004;(3):CD004292.
5. Worster A, Preyra I, Weaver B, et al. The accuracy of noncontrast helical computed tomography versus intravenous pyelography in the diagnosis of suspected acute urolithiasis: a meta-analysis. *Ann Emerg Med*. 2002;40(3):280–286.
6. Hollingsworth JM, Rogers MA, Kaufman SR, et al. Medical therapy to facilitate urinary stone passage: a meta-analysis. *Lancet*. 2006;368(9542);1171–1179.

ADDITIONAL READING

Penniston KL, Jones AN, Nakada SY, et al. Vitamin D repletion does not alter urinary calcium excretion in healthy postmenopausal women. *BJU Int*. 2009;104(10): 1512–1516.

SEE ALSO

Algorithms: Dysuria; Renal Calculi; Urethral Discharge

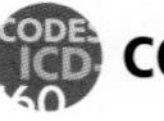

CODES

ICD 10

- N20.9 Urinary calculus, unspecified
- N20.0 Calculus of kidney
- N20.1 Calculus of ureter

CLINICAL PEARLS

- Incidence in industrialized countries seems to be increasing, probably due to improved diagnostics as well as to increasingly rich diets.
- Vesical calculosis (bladder stones) due to malnutrition during early life is frequent in Middle East and Asian countries.
- Medical expulsive therapy: α_1-Antagonists (e.g., terazosin) and calcium channel blockers (e.g., nifedipine) improve likelihood of spontaneous stone passage with NNT of ~5.
- Increased fluid intake for life cannot be overemphasized for decreasing recurrence. Encourage 2–3 L/day intake; advise patient to have clear urine rather than yellow.
- Patients who form calcium stones should minimize high-oxalate foods such as green leafy vegetables, rhubarb, peanuts, chocolates, and beer.
- Decrease protein and salt intake.
- Lowering calcium intake is inadvisable and even may increase urine calcium excretion.

URTICARIA

Phung Dinh Phan, DO, CPT, USA • Lloyd A. Runser, MD, MPH, FAAFP

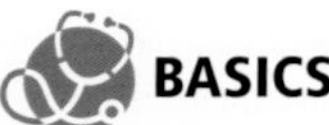

BASICS

DESCRIPTION

- A cutaneous lesion involving transient edema of the epidermis and/or dermis characterized by the acute onset of a polymorphic lesion with central pallor of varying sizes and edema with an erythematous flare associated with itching and sometimes burning sensation; lesions are fleeting with return to normal skin appearance within 24 hours.
- Pathophysiology is primarily mast cell degranulation and subsequent histamine release.
- Angioedema may occur with urticaria although characterized by sudden pronounced erythematous edema of the lower dermis and subcutis; may take up to 72 hours to remit.
- Pruritus and burning are more commonly associated with urticaria; pain more often with angioedema.
  - Spontaneous urticaria: acute: persists <6 weeks
- Specific extrinsic triggers commonly are the cause, although a vast number of possible causes exist (e.g., drugs, foods, infections [especially streptococci], envenomation, allergens, and autoimmune).
- Underlying etiology may be difficult to pinpoint.
  - Chronic spontaneous urticaria: persists >6 weeks with >2 episodes/week off-treatment.
- Unlike acute urticaria, 80% of cases have no obvious external stimulus.
- If symptoms occur less than twice a week, this is more likely recurrent acute urticaria and should be approached as such.
- For those with chronic urticaria, 40% have concurrent angioedema.
- Chronic infection, pseudoallergy, malignancy including mastocytosis, autoimmunity (especially thyroid), and medications may underlie the remaining 20% (1).
- 1/2 of those with chronic idiopathic urticaria have sera positive for IgG that releases histamine through binding of IgE or its receptor.
- Inducible urticaria
  - Dermatographism: "skin writing" or the appearance of linear wheals at the site of friction, scratching, or any type of irritation. This is the most common physical urticaria.
  - Cold urticaria: Wheals occur within minutes of rewarming after cold exposure; 95% idiopathic but can be due to infections (mononucleosis, HIV), neoplasia, or autoimmune diseases.
  - Delayed pressure urticaria: Urticaria occurs 0.5–12 hours after pressure to skin (e.g., from elastic or shoes), may be pruritic and/or painful, and may not subside for several days.
  - Solar urticaria: from sunlight exposure, usually UV; onset in minutes; subsides within 2 hours
  - Heat urticaria: from direct contact with warm objects or air; rare
  - Vibratory urticaria/angioedema: very rare; secondary to vibrations (e.g., motorcycle)
  - Cholinergic urticaria: due to brief increase of core body temperature from exercise, baths, or emotional stress; small pin-sized (5–10-mm) wheals surrounded by an erythema but also can have larger wheals. This is the second most common form.
  - Adrenergic urticaria: also caused by stress; extremely rare; vasoconstricted, blanched skin around pink wheals as opposed to cholinergic's erythematous surrounding
  - Contact urticaria: wheals at sites where chemical substances contact the skin, may be either IgE-dependent (e.g., latex) or IgE-independent (e.g., stinging nettle)
  - Aquagenic and solar urticaria: small wheals after contact with water of any temperature or UV light, respectively; rare
- System(s) affected: integumentary
- Synonym(s): hives; wheals

EPIDEMIOLOGY

Incidence

- Equally distributed across all ages: children more likely to have acute, whereas adults and elderly predisposed to chronic urticaria
- Predominant gender: female > male (2:1 in chronic urticaria)
- In 20% of patients, chronic urticaria lasts >10 years (1).

Prevalence

- Affects anywhere from 5 to 25% of the population
- Of people with urticaria, 40% have no angioedema, 40% have urticaria and angioedema, and 20% have angioedema with no urticaria.
- Up to 3% of the population at some point has chronic idiopathic urticaria.
- Chronic urticaria affects only 0.1–3% of children.

ETIOLOGY AND PATHOPHYSIOLOGY

- Mast cell degranulation with release of inflammatory reactants, which leads to vascular leakage, inflammatory cell extravasation, and dermal (angioedema) and/or epidermal (wheals/hives) edema
- Histamine, cytokines, leukotrienes, and proteases are main active substances released.
- Mast cell degranulation may be caused by allergen cross-linkage of IgE, autoimmune activation of FcϵRI (IgE receptor), substance P, C5a, opiates, or physical stimuli.
- Spontaneous acute urticaria
  - Bacterial infections: strep throat, sinusitis, otitis, urinary tract
  - Viral infections: rhinovirus, rotavirus, hepatitis B, mononucleosis, herpes
  - Foods: peanuts, tree nuts, seafood, milk, soy, fish, wheat, and eggs; tend to be IgE-mediated; pseudoallergenic foods such as strawberries, tomatoes, preservatives, and coloring agents contain histamine.
  - Drugs: IgE-mediated (e.g., penicillin and other antibiotics), direct mast cell stimulation (e.g., aspirin, NSAIDs, opiates)
  - Inhalant, contact, ingestion, or occupational exposure (e.g., latex, cosmetics)
  - Parasitic infection; insect bite/sting
  - Transfusion reaction
- Spontaneous chronic urticaria
  - Chronic subclinical allergic rhinitis, eczema, and other atopic disorders
  - Chronic indolent infections: *Helicobacter pylori*, fungal, parasitic (*Anisakis simplex*, strongyloidiasis), and chronic viral infections (hepatitis)
  - Collagen vascular disease (cutaneous vasculitis, serum sickness, lupus)
  - Thyroid autoimmunity, especially Hashimoto
  - Hormonal: pregnancy and progesterone
  - Autoimmune antibodies to the IgE receptor α chain on mast cells and to the IgE antibody
  - Chronic medications (e.g., NSAIDs, hormones, ACE inhibitors)
  - Malignancy
  - Physical stimuli (cold, heat, vibration, pressure) in physical urticaria

Genetics

No consistent pattern known: Chronic urticaria has increased frequency of HLA-DR4 and HLA-D8Q MHC II alleles.

RISK FACTORS

- Atopic diseases, asthma, allergic rhinitis, other allergies
- Of patients, >50% possess an atopic disease, >40% with allergic rhinitis, and >15% have atopic dermatitis or allergic asthma in chronic urticaria.

GENERAL PREVENTION

Treatment of any underlying atopic or other disease; avoidance of known triggers

COMMONLY ASSOCIATED CONDITIONS

- Angioedema
- Anaphylaxis

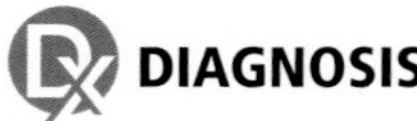

DIAGNOSIS

HISTORY

- Duration, timing (onset/offset), and distribution of lesions; exacerbating and alleviating factors and history of atopy and/or autoimmune diseases
- Potential trigger exposure
- Concomitance of angioedema: pruritus in urticarial wheals versus pain in angioedema
- Urticaria may be an initial symptom of a generalized anaphylactic reaction.
- Fast onset; resolves in <24–48 hours

PHYSICAL EXAM

- Single/multiple raised, polymorphic indurated plaques with central pallor and edema with an erythematous flare
- Variably sized: ≥1–20 cm
- Evaluate for underlying conditions including thyroid abnormalities (nodules), bacterial, viral, or fungal infection (e.g., fever).
- Often, lesions have cleared and patient's photographs may be useful.

DIFFERENTIAL DIAGNOSIS

- Anaphylaxis (may present with urticaria)
- Morbilliform or fixed drug eruptions
- Erythema multiforme
- Systemic lupus erythematous (SLE), vasculitis, and polyarteritis
- Angioedema without urticaria
- Urticaria pigmentosa/systemic mastocytosis
- Bullous pemphigoid (urticarial stage)
- Arthropod bite
- Atopic/contact dermatitis
- Viral exanthem

DIAGNOSTIC TESTS & INTERPRETATION

- Acute urticaria: Testing should be directed by clinical suspicion of underlying cause:
  - Full lab workups provide little, except in cases of a failed trial of antihistamines, lesions that last >24 hours, lesions that do not blanch on pressure or leave pigmentary changes.
  - Allergy skin tests and radioallergosorbent test (RAST) for inhaled allergens, insects, drugs, or foods
  - Infection: Consider pharyngeal culture, LFTs, mononucleosis test, urinalysis in appropriate setting.

- Chronic urticaria: Extensive lab testing is not indicated and has not proven to improve outcome nor is it cost-effective. Limit lab testing according to clinical history and indication. Skin or IgE testing should be limited to specific history of provoking allergen (2)[C].
  - CBC with differential, ESR, and/or CRP is recommended by most guidelines.
  - Thyroid function tests, LFTs, and urinalysis are recommended by several guidelines.
  - Consider allergy skin tests and RAST for inhaled allergens, insects, drugs, or foods; total IgE level.
  - Autoimmune: ESR, ANA, RF, complement (e.g., CH50, C3, C4), cryoglobulins in urticarial vasculitis
  - Tests for *H. pylori* (e.g., antibodies) in dyspeptic patients. Consider stool for ova and parasites in at-risk individuals.
  - Autologous serum skin testing: injection of serum under skin to test for presence of IgE receptor–activating antibodies
  - Consider malignancy workup, including serum protein electrophoresis and immunofixation in the proper setting.

    Indicated only if clinical suspicion for underlying indolent infections/malignancy.
- Use the Urticaria Activity Score (UAS7) for assessing CSU.

Diagnostic Procedures/Other

- Food and drug reactions: elimination of (or challenges with) suspected agents
- Physical and special forms of urticaria: challenge tests:
  - Dermatographism: Stroke skin lightly with rounded object and observe for surrounding urticaria.
  - Cold urticaria: ice cube test: Place ice cube on skin for 5 minutes; observe for 10–15 minutes.
  - Cholinergic: Exercise to the point of sweating/partial immersion in 42°C bath for 10 minutes.
  - Solar: exposure to different wavelengths of light
  - Delayed pressure: Apply 5-lb sandbag to back for 20 minutes; observe 6 hours later.
  - Aquagenic: Apply water at various temperatures.
  - Vibratory: Apply vibration 4–5 minutes with a lab mixing device; observe.
- Skin biopsy to rule out urticarial vasculitis in cases of lesions lasting >24 hours

Test Interpretation

- Early lesions: dermal edema with intravascular margination of neutrophils
- Late lesions: scant polymorphous perivascular and interstitial infiltrate, with no expansion of cell walls/fibrin deposition

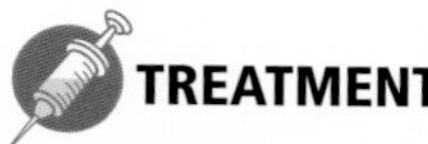

TREATMENT

GENERAL MEASURES

- Calamine or 1% topical menthol may be useful.
- Avoid the eliciting stimulus (e.g., diet modification, pressure, temperature changes/extremes).
- NSAIDs and alcohol may exacerbate symptoms.

ISSUES FOR REFERRAL

Referral to an allergist, immunologist, or dermatologist for recalcitrant cases, complex management, testing for potential triggers, and anaphylaxis

MEDICATION

First Line

- Second-generation antihistamine (H_1) blockers are the first-line treatment of any urticaria in which avoidance of stimulus is impossible or not feasible (3,4)[A]:
  - Fexofenadine (Allegra): 180 mg/day
  - Loratadine (Claritin): 10 mg/day, increasing to 30mg/day if needed; only medication studied for safe use in pregnancy
  - Desloratadine (Clarinex): 5 mg/day (5,6)[A]
  - Cetirizine (Zyrtec): 10 mg/day, increasing to 30 mg per day if needed
  - Levocetirizine (Xyzal): 5 mg/day; requires weight-based dosing in children (6)[A]
  - Rupatadine: novel H_1 antagonist with antiplatelet-activating factor activity
- First-generation antihistamines (H_1; for patients with sleep disturbed by itching):
  - Older children and adults: hydroxyzine or diphenhydramine 25–50 mg q6h
  - Children <6 years of age: diphenhydramine 12.5 mg q6–8h (5 mg/kg/day) or hydroxyzine (10 mg/5 mL) 2 mg/kg/day divided q6–8h
- Precautions and notes: drowsiness and dry mouth and eyes in first-generation H_1 blockers (elderly)

Second Line

Doubling the typical second-generation H_1 blocker dosages should be attempted before adding first-generation H_1 or H_2 blockers (3,4,6)[A].

- H_2-specific antihistamines (beneficial as adjuvants): cimetidine, ranitidine, nizatidine, famotidine

Third Line

- Corticosteroids: prednisolone 20–50 mg/day for max of 10 days; best used only for exacerbations; avoid chronic use (3,4)[C].
- Doxepin: tricyclic antidepressant with strong H_1- and H_2-blocking properties; 10–30 mg at bedtime; sedation limits usefulness (3)[C].
- Leukotriene antagonists (montelukast, zileuton, and zafirlukast): safe and worth trying in chronic, unresponsive cases; useful alone but best used in addition to antihistamines; limited data on use in treating acute urticaria (7)[A]
- Refractory symptoms
  - Omalizumab: anti-IgE; effective, expensive. 150–300 mg SQ q2–4wk. Restrict to allergists (3,4,8)[A].
  - Cyclosporine: well-studied, effective (2.5–5 mg/kg/day); best used in combination with antihistamines; significant renal side effects (3,4)[C]
  - Methotrexate: antifolate; proven useful in recalcitrant cases; GI upset most common complaint; long-term requires LFT monitoring.
  - UV therapy decreases number of mast cells; has shown promise in the treatment of mastocytosis-induced urticaria (4)[C].

INPATIENT CONSIDERATIONS

Admission Criteria/Initial Stabilization

Educating patient on use of EpiPen as pathophysiology similar. If the airway is threatened, immediate consult to evaluate for laryngeal edema and need for airway access

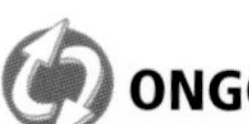

ONGOING CARE

FOLLOW-UP RECOMMENDATIONS

Patient Monitoring

A diary of potential triggers (e.g., foods, activities) may help in recalcitrant/persistent cases.

PROGNOSIS

Resolution of acute symptoms: 70% <72 hours. Of patients with chronic urticaria, 35% will be symptom-free in a year; another 30% will see symptom reduction. Not life-threatening, but 18% will have decreased quality of life.

REFERENCES

1. Leru P. Urticaria—an allergologic, dermatologic or multidisciplinary disease? *Rom J Intern Med*. 2013;51(3–4):125–130.
2. Choosing Wisely initiative of ABIM: American Academy of Allergy, Asthma & Immunology recommendation. http://choosingwisely.org/wp-content/uploads/2012/04/5things_12_factsheet_aaaai.pdf. Accessed 2014.
3. Zuberbier T, Aberer W, Asero R, et al. The EAACI/GA(2) LEN/EDF/WAO guideline for the definition, classification, diagnosis, and management of urticaria: the 2013 revision and update. *Allergy*. 2014;69(7):868–887.
4. Bernstein J, Lang D, Khan D, et al. The diagnosis and management of acute and chronic urticaria: 2014 update. *J Allergy Clin Immunol*. 2014;133(5):1270–1277.
5. Grob J, Auquier P, Dreyfus I, et al. Quality of life in adults with chronic idiopathic urticaria receiving desloratadine: a randomized, double-blind, multicentre, placebo-controlled study. *J Eur Acad Dermatol Venereol*. 2008;22(1):87–93.
6. Staevska M, Popov TA, Kralimarkova T, et al. The effectiveness of levocetirizine and desloratadine in up to 4 times conventional doses in difficult-to-treat urticaria. *J Allergy Clin Immunol*. 2010;125(3):676–682.
7. Di Lorenzo G, Pacor ML, Mansueto P, et al. Randomized placebo-controlled trial comparing desloratadine and montelukast in monotherapy and desloratadine plus montelukast in combined therapy for chronic idiopathic urticaria. *J Allergy Clin Immunol*. 2004;114(3):619–625.
8. Maurer M, Rosén K, Hsieh HJ, et al. Omalizumab for the treatment of chronic idiopathic or spontaneous urticaria. *N Engl J Med*. 2013;368(10):924–935.

ADDITIONAL READING

- Maurer M, Weller K, Bindslev-Jensen C, et al. Unmet clinical needs in chronic spontaneous urticaria. A GA²LEN task force report. *Allergy*. 2011;66(3):317–330.
- Poonawalla T, Kelly B. Urticaria: a review. *Am J Clin Dermatol*. 2009;10(1):9–21.
- Zuberbier T, Balke M, Worm M, et al. Epidemiology of urticaria: a representative cross-sectional survey. *Clin Exp Dermatol*. 2010;35(8):869–873.

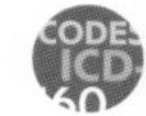

CODES

ICD10

- L50.9 Urticaria, unspecified
- L50.1 Idiopathic urticaria
- L50.8 Other urticaria

CLINICAL PEARLS

- "Chronic urticaria" with <2 episodes/week should be approached as acute.
- Antihistamines are the best studied and most efficacious therapy but may require higher-than-normal doses for efficacy.
- Lesions lasting >24 hours should be evaluated for urticarial vasculitis.

U

UTERINE AND PELVIC ORGAN PROLAPSE

Maryse A. Pedoussaut, MD • John Delzell, Jr., MD, MSPH • Suzanne Minor, MD, FAAFP

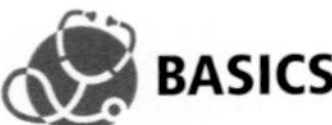

BASICS

DESCRIPTION

- Symptomatic descent of one or more of (1,2)
  - the anterior vaginal wall (bladder or cystocele)
  - the posterior vaginal wall (rectum or rectocele)
  - the apex of the vagina (uterine cervix descent and prolapse)
  - the vault (cuff) after hysterectomy (vault prolapse)
- Prolapses above or to the hymen are not symptomatic (2).
- Associated symptoms (2):
  - Feeling of vaginal or pelvic pressure
  - Heaviness
  - Bulging
  - Bowel or bladder symptoms
- Cost associated with treatment is more than $1 billion annually (~200,000 surgeries/year) (2).

EPIDEMIOLOGY

Incidence

Pelvic organ prolapse (POP) is common but not always symptomatic. It does not always progress with time. In a 3-year prospective cohort study of 249 women, prolapse increased by at least 2 cm in 11% and regressed by 2 cm in 3% (2).

Prevalence

- A national survey of 7,924 women (over 20 years of age) found a prevalence of 25% for one or more pelvic floor disorders (including urinary incontinence, fecal incontinence, and POP). Prevalence of POP was 2.9% (3).
- The prevalence of lower urinary tract symptoms is as high as 50% in parous women. 11% of all women have surgery for POP or lower urinary tract symptoms by 80 years old (4).
- 3–6% of women who present for gynecologic care have a prolapse beyond hymen (2).

ETIOLOGY AND PATHOPHYSIOLOGY

- Insidious process begins long before symptoms develop.
- There is a complex interaction between the pelvic floor musculature, connective tissue, and the vaginal wall, which provides support from the perineum to the sacrum (2). Integrity of levator ani is essential to this support system by providing a platform on which the pelvic organs rest (2).
- Symptomatic women typically have multiple defects, including laxity of supporting tissue and damage to the levator ani (2).
- Half of anterior prolapse can be attributed to apical descent of the vagina (2).

RISK FACTORS

- Vaginal childbirth (2): Women who have delivered two children vaginally have a relative risk of 8.4 and every additional child (up to five deliveries) increases the risk of prolapse by 10–20% (2).
- Age: Every 10 years of age increases the risk of prolapse by 40% (2). POP will become more prevalent, as the elderly population is expected to double by 2030 (5).
- Obesity: BMI >25 may increase the risk of developing prolapse (2).
- Constipation: independent risk factor in a survey of more than 2,000 women (2)
- Race: White and Hispanic women may be at higher risk than black or Asian women (2).
- Occupation (heavy lifting): variable support in the literature (2)
- Hysterectomy: variable support in the literature (2)
- Obstetric factors (operative delivery, infant weight, length of pushing in second stage of labor): variable support in the literature (2)

GENERAL PREVENTION

There is some evidence that pelvic floor muscle training ("Kegel exercises") may decrease the risk of symptomatic POP (6)[B]. Weight loss and proper management of conditions that cause increase in intra-abdominal pressure may help prevent the problem.

COMMONLY ASSCIATED CONDITIONS

- Urinary incontinence
- Other urinary symptoms (4):
  - Urgency
  - Frequency

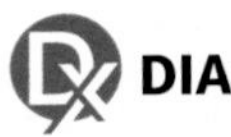

DIAGNOSIS

HISTORY

- Less than half of women discuss symptoms with PCP. Only 10–12% seek medical attention. Barriers include embarrassment, social stigma, ability to cope, belief that POP is part of the aging process, belief that treatment options are limited, and fear of surgery (4).
- Common symptoms include the following:
  - Feeling a bulge in vagina
  - Something "falling out" of vagina
  - Pelvic pressure
  - Difficulty with voiding or defecation
  - Urgency
  - Frequency
  - Incontinence (urinary or fecal)
  - Constipation
- Document the presence, duration, and severity of urinary, bowel, or prolapse symptom. Assess impact on sexual function and quality of life with validated questionnaires (PISQ 9 OR 12) (1,7).
- Assess past medical history:
  - Gravity and parity/obstetric history
  - History of ascites
  - Chronic constipation
  - Document physical impairment (mobility, dexterity, or visual acuity), as this may affect management (1).
  - Document the patient's desire, goals, and expectation (1).

PHYSICAL EXAM

- Abdominal examination to document any distention or masses
- Complete pelvic and rectal examination. Have patient cough or strain, particularly in an upright (standing) position while examining the distal vagina.
- The GOLD STANDARD is to measure vaginal decent using the Pelvic Organ Prolapse Quantification (POPQ) scale, which is a scale that describes the prolapse in relationship to the vaginal hymen (2). The validated simplified version has four measurements with classification in 4 stages. Patient is supine with the head of the bed at 45 degrees, performing Valsalva.
  - Stage 1: prolapse in which the distal point is superior or equal to 1 cm above hymen
  - Stage 2: prolapse in which the distal point is between 1 cm above and 1 cm below hymen
  - Stage 3: prolapse in which the distal point is superior or equal to 1 cm below the hymen, but some vaginal mucosa is not everted
  - Stage 4: complete vaginal vault eversion ("procidentia"). Entire vaginal mucosa everted (2)
- A split speculum can be used to observe anterior, posterior, and apical parts of the vagina successively.
- Patient should be standing for maximum decent (2).

DIFFERENTIAL DIAGNOSIS

- Rectal prolapse
- Hemorrhoids
- Bartholin cyst
- Cervical elongation

DIAGNOSTIC TESTS & INTERPRETATION

Initial Tests (lab, imaging)

- Urinalysis if symptomatic POP (1)
- Renal function (serum creatinine) if urinary incontinence and probability of renal impairment (1)
- Imaging: not routinely recommended (1)

Follow-Up Tests & Special Considerations

- Postvoid residual if patient has urinary incontinence
- Urodynamic testing prior to invasive treatment or after treatment failure to plan further therapy (1)
- Imaging of upper urinary tract if hematuria or back pain (1)
- Cystoscopy recommended if patient has hematuria, pain, or discomfort suggesting bladder lesion (1)
- Colonoscopy or sigmoidoscopy if patient has fecal incontinence (1)
- Colonoscopy, air contrast barium enema, and/or computed tomography if change in bowel habits or rectal bleeding (1)

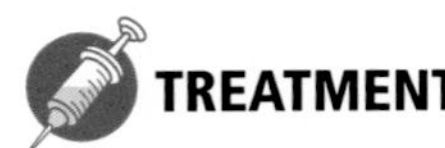

TREATMENT

GENERAL MEASURES

- Treatment should take into account type and severity of symptoms, patient's age, other comorbid conditions, sexual function, infertility, and risk of recurrence.
- Treatment for asymptomatic patients:
  - Stage 1 or 2: clinical observation (2)
  - Stage 3 or 4: regular follow-up and evaluation (every 6–12 months) (2)
- Treatment is indicated when there is urinary/bowel obstruction or hydronephrosis regardless of the degree of prolapse (2).

- A vaginal pessary should be considered in all women presenting with symptomatic prolapse (8)[B].
  - There are more than 13 types of silicone devices that may be inserted into the vagina to support the pelvic organs.
  - The most commonly used pessaries are the ring pessary and Gellhorn (8).
  - They may prevent prolapse progression and may prove to be an appropriate prevention strategy in the future because the surgical failure rate is around 30% (2).
  - Most women can be successfully fitted with a pessary (8)[B].
  - Satisfaction rate for patients using pessaries is very high (8)[B].
- Complications may be seen with neglected pessaries, such as erosions, abrasions, ulcerations, and vaginal bleeding. Minor complications such as vaginal discharge and odor can be treated without discontinuing pessary use (8)[B]. Vaginal erosion can be treated by removal of pessary and optional vaginal estrogen supplementation.

MEDICATION

First Line

- Treatment of vaginal atrophy with topical estrogens may be beneficial for symptomatic POP (9)[B] if there are no contraindications. Suggested to use in conjunction with pelvic floor muscle training (9)
- Vaginal creams
  - Estradiol cream 0.01% (Estrace)
  - Conjugated estrogens 0.625 mg/day (Premarin)
- Vaginal tablet
  - Estradiol 10 μg (Vagifem)
- Vaginal ring
  - Estradiol 2 mg (Estring)

ISSUES FOR REFERRAL

Referral when pessary or surgery is necessary

ADDITIONAL THERAPIES

Pelvic floor muscle training: may reduce the symptoms of POP (1). Pelvic floor muscle training does not affect the degree of prolapse, only the symptoms (1).

SURGERY/OTHER PROCEDURES

- Reconstructive procedures are done with the goal of restoration of vaginal anatomy.
- Reconstructive surgery is associated with a high rate of failure (1 in 3 lifetime risk of repeat surgery). New procedures, using surgical mesh and graft material, have higher success rates but limited follow-up or comparative data (2).
- Abdominal procedures such as sacral colpopexy using graft material have a higher success rate but a longer operating time, longer time to return to normal activity levels, and an increased cost (10)[B]. There may be resulting problems with sexual function and bladder/bowel complaints (2).

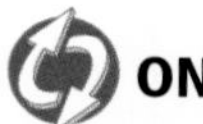

ONGOING CARE

PATIENT EDUCATION

- Patients should be educated about pessary complications and possible symptoms of POP if they are still asymptomatic.
- Limit caffeine product and bladder irritants if urinary symptoms.
- Using insoluble fibers may help patients with bowel complaints such as constipation.

COMPLICATIONS

- There is a risk of vaginal mesh extrusion, erosions, dyspareunia, and pelvic pain after surgical repair (11).
- Delays in diagnosis (4)[B]:
  - 61% reported POP symptoms to a physician.
  - 65.9% blamed themselves for the delay (fear of surgery, embarrassment).
  - 1/3 of women blame their physician for the delay in diagnosis.

REFERENCES

1. Abrams P, Andersson KE, Birder L, et al. Fourth International Consultation on Incontinence recommendations of the International Scientific Committee: evaluation and treatment of urinary incontinence, pelvic organ prolapse, and fecal incontinence. *Neurourol Urodyn*. 2010;29(1):213–240.
2. Abed H, Rogers RG. Urinary incontinence and pelvic organ prolapse: diagnosis and treatment for the primary care physician. *Med Clin North Am*. 2008;92(5):1273–1293.
3. Wu J, Vaughan, C, Goode P, et al. Prevalence and trends of symptomatic pelvic floor disorders in US women. *Obstet Gynecol*. 2014;123(1):141–148.
4. Krissi H, Eitan R, Peled Y. The role of primary physicians in the diagnostic delay of lower urinary tract and pelvic organ prolapse symptoms. *Eur J Obstet Gynecol Reprod Biol*. 2012;161(1):102–104.
5. Chow D, Rodríguez LV. Epidemiology and prevalence of pelvic organ prolapse. *Curr Opin Urol*. 2013;23(4):293–298.
6. Hagen S, Stark D. Conservative prevention and management of pelvic organ prolapse in women. *Cochrane Database Syst Rev*. 2011;(12):CD003882.
7. Aschkenazi S, Rogers R, Beaumont J, et al. The modified short pelvic organ prolapse/urinary incontinence sexual questionnaire, the PISQ-9 for use in a general female population. http://www.ics.org/Abstracts/Publish/46/000201.pdf. Accessed 2014.
8. Robert M, Schulz JA, Harvey MA, et al. Technical update on pessary use. *J Obstet Gynaecol Can*. 2013;35(7):664–674.
9. Ismail SI, Bain C, Hagen S. Oestrogens for treatment or prevention of pelvic organ prolapse in postmenopausal women. *Cochrane Database Syst Rev*. 2010;(9):CD007063.
10. Maher C, Feiner B, Baessler K, et al. Surgical management of pelvic organ prolapse in women. *Cochrane Database Syst Rev*. 2013;4:CD004014.
11. Chermansky CJ, Winters JC. Complications of vaginal mesh surgery. *Curr Opin Urol*. 2012;22(4):287–291.

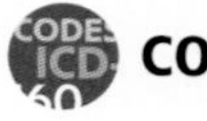

CODES

ICD10

- N81.9 Female genital prolapse, unspecified
- N81.10 Cystocele, unspecified
- N99.3 Prolapse of vaginal vault after hysterectomy

CLINICAL PEARLS

- Many women do not discuss POP with their doctor—ask routinely.
- Vaginal pessary should be considered in all patients with symptomatic prolapse.
- Traditional surgical treatment has a high long-term failure rate (1 in 3).

UTERINE MYOMAS

Laura K. Randolph, DO, MS • Michael P. Hopkins, MD, MEd

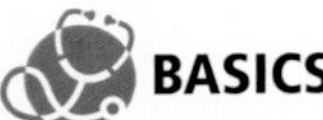

BASICS

DESCRIPTION

- Uterine leiomyomas are well-circumscribed, pseudoencapsulated, benign monoclonal tumors composed mainly of smooth muscle with varying amounts of fibrous connective tissue (1,2).
- 3 major subtypes
  - Subserous: common; external; may become pedunculated
  - Intramural: common; within myometrium; may cause marked uterine enlargement
  - Submucous: ~5% of all cases; internal, evoking abnormal uterine bleeding and infection; occasionally protruding from cervix
- Rare locations: broad, round, and uterosacral ligaments
- System affected: reproductive
- Synonym(s): fibroids; myoma; fibromyoma; myofibroma; fibroleiomyoma

EPIDEMIOLOGY

Incidence

- Cumulative incidence up to 80%
  - 60% in African American women by age 35 years; 80% by age 50 years
  - 40% in Caucasian women by age 35 years; 70% by age 50 years (1,3)
- Incidence increases with each decade during reproductive years.
- Rarely seen in premenarchal females
- Predominant sex: females only

ETIOLOGY AND PATHOPHYSIOLOGY

- Enlargement of benign smooth muscle tumors that may lead to symptoms affecting the reproductive, GI, or genitourinary system
- Complex multifactorial process involving transition from normal myocyte to abnormal cells and then to visibly evident tumor (monoclonal expansion)
  - Hormones (1): Increases in estrogen and progesterone are correlated with myoma formation (i.e., rarely seen before menarche). Estrogen receptors in myomas bind more estradiol than normal myometrium (2).
  - Growth factors (1)
    - Increased smooth muscle proliferation (transforming growth factor β [TGF-β], basic fibroblast growth factor [bFGF])
    - Increase DNA synthesis (epidermal growth factor [EGF], platelet-derived growth factor [PDGF], activin, myostatin)
    - Stimulate synthesis of extracellular matrix (TGF-β)
    - Promote mitogenesis (TGF-β, EGF, insulin-like growth factor [IGF], prolactin)
    - Promote angiogenesis (bFGF, vascular endothelial growth factor [VEGF])
  - Vasoconstrictive hypoxia (1): proposed, but not confirmed, mechanism of myometrial injury during menstruation

Genetics

- A variety of somatic chromosomal rearrangements have been described in 40% of uterine myomas.
  - Mutations in the gene encoding mediator complex subunit 12 (MED12) on the X chromosome were found in 70% of myomas in one study (3).
- Higher levels of aromatase and therefore estrogen have been found in myomas in African American women (3).

RISK FACTORS

- African American heritage
  - 2.9× greater risk than Caucasian women; occur at a younger age, are more numerous, larger, and more symptomatic (1)
- Early menarche (<10 years)
- Nulliparous
- Hypertension
- Familial predisposition
  - 2.5× more likely in women with a 1st-degree relative with myomas (1)
- Obesity
  - Risk increases by 21% with each 10 kg of weight gain (1).
- Alcohol

COMMONLY ASSOCIATED CONDITIONS

Endometrial and breast cancer also associated with high unopposed estrogen stimulation

DIAGNOSIS

HISTORY

- Usually asymptomatic, 30% present with abnormal symptoms (2).
- Symptoms include the following:
  - Abnormal uterine bleeding, usually heavy/prolonged menses
  - Pain: infrequent, usually associated with torsion of pedunculated myoma, degeneration, or cervical dilation by submucous myoma near cervical os
  - Pressure on bladder: suprapubic discomfort, urinary frequency/obstruction
  - Pressure on rectosigmoid: may cause low back pain, constipation
  - Infertility: rare, estimated 1–2.5% (2); usually from submucous myoma distorting the uterine cavity or interference with implantation

ALERT

Rapid growth, particularly in perimenopausal/postmenopausal patients, may indicate sarcoma. Extremely rare, 0.1–0.3% of cases (2)

PHYSICAL EXAM

- Usually incidental finding on abdominal and pelvic exam
- Firm, smooth nodules/masses arising from uterus
- Masses are mobile without tenderness.

DIFFERENTIAL DIAGNOSIS

- Intrauterine pregnancy
- Cancer, including ovarian, uterine, or leiomyosarcoma
- Cecal/sigmoid tumor
- Appendiceal abscess
- Diverticulitis
- Pelvic kidney
- Urachal cyst

DIAGNOSTIC TESTS & INTERPRETATION

Initial Tests (lab, imaging)

- Pregnancy test
- Hemoglobin
- Pelvic ultrasound: shows characteristic hypoechoic appearance (4)
- Saline infusion hysterosonography: helps to distinguish submucosal myomas
- Hysterosalpingogram: evaluates the contour of the endometrial cavity (4)
- CT scan or MRI: may help to differentiate complex cases or used when uterine artery embolization is planned (4)[B]

Follow-Up Tests & Special Considerations

Consider cancer antigen 125 (CA-125): may be slightly elevated in some cases of uterine myoma but generally more useful in differentiating myomas from various gynecologic adenocarcinomas

- IV pyelogram: if suspect ureteral distortion (4)
- Barium enema

Diagnostic Procedures/Other

- Fractional dilation and curettage: aids in ruling out cervical/uterine carcinomas when clinically suspicious
- Hysteroscopy: helps to diagnose submucosal/intracavitary myomas
- Laparoscopy: useful in complex cases and to rule out other pelvic diseases/disorders

Test Interpretation

- Myomas are usually multiple and vary in size and location; have been reported up to 100 lb
- Gross pathology: firm tumors with characteristic whorl-like trabeculated appearance; a thin pseudocapsular layer is present.
- Microscopic: bundles of smooth muscle mixed with varying amounts of connective tissue elements running in different directions
- Cellular variant has a preponderance of muscle cells. Mitoses are rare.
- May undergo various types of degeneration
  - Hyaline degeneration: very common
  - Calcification: late result of circulatory impairment to myomas
  - Infection and suppuration: most common with submucosal myomas
  - Necrosis: most common with pedunculated myomas secondary to torsion

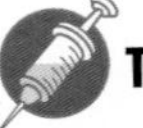

TREATMENT

- Treatment must be individualized.
- Medical therapy may be of benefit.
- Patients with minimal symptoms may be treated with iron preparations and analgesics.
- Conservative management of asymptomatic myomas
  - Pelvic exams and ultrasounds at ≥3-month intervals if size remains stable
  - Substantial regression usually occurs after menopause.
- Surgical options should be considered if symptomatic or worrisome myomas are unresponsive to conservative/medical management.

GENERAL MEASURES

Patients not desiring pharmacologic therapy or surgery may consider the following:

- Uterine artery embolization: averages 50% shrinkage of myomas (4)[A]; painful and may cause ovarian failure (1–2%), amenorrhea, or other complications; shorter hospital stay and quicker recovery but no difference in satisfaction compared with hysterectomy (2,5)[B]

- MRI-guided focused ultrasound (MRgFUS): noninvasive, ultrasound transducer passes through abdominal wall and causes coagulative necrosis of fibroid; up to 98% reduction in myoma volume and symptoms. Not appropriate for some types of myomas (2)[B]. Efficacy may be comparable with other hysterectomy-sparing procedures (6)[B]. Fertility has been shown to be preserved (7)[A].

MEDICATION

- Progestins may reduce overall uterine size (4)[B].
  - Norethindrone 10 mg/day
  - Medroxyprogesterone 200 mg IM monthly
  - Levonorgestrel intrauterine device (2)[B]
- Combination oral contraceptives: may help prevent development of new fibroids
  - Contraindications: history of thromboembolic events
- Gonadotropin-releasing hormone agonists
  - Nafarelin (nasal spray), goserelin acetate, and leuprolide
  - Induces abrupt artificial menopause; may reduce myoma symptoms dramatically; induces atrophy of myomas by up to 40% in 2–3 months (4)[B]
  - May be valuable as preoperative adjunct to myomectomy/hysterectomy by allowing recovery of anemia, donation of autologous blood, and possibly converting abdominal to vaginal hysterectomy (4)[B]
  - Not recommended for use >6 months because of osteoporosis risk
  - Following discontinuation, myomas return within 60 days to pretherapy size.
- Antiprogesterones
  - Mifepristone
    - Shown to have similar reduction in myoma size as gonadotropin-releasing hormone agonists (6)[B]
  - Selective progesterone receptor modulator (SPRM)
    - Ulipristal acetate: may be as effective as gonadotropin-releasing hormones with fewer side effects (8)[B]

ISSUES FOR REFERRAL

- Medical therapy may be initiated by a primary care physician/gynecologist after adequate pelvic examination.
- Surgical considerations may be pursued with gynecologic consultation.
- Uterine embolization may be discussed with an interventional radiologist.

SURGERY/OTHER PROCEDURES

- Surgical management is indicated in the following situations (4)[B]:
  - Excessive uterine size or excessive rate of growth (except during pregnancy)
  - Submucosal myomas when associated with hypermenorrhea
  - Pedunculated myomas that are painful or undergo torsion, necrosis, and hemorrhage
  - If a myoma causes symptoms from pressure on bladder/rectum
  - If differentiation from ovarian mass is not possible
  - If associated pelvic disease is present (endometriosis, pelvic inflammatory disease)
  - If infertility/habitual abortion is likely due to the anatomic location of the myoma
- Surgical procedures
  - Preliminary pelvic examination, Pap smear, and endometrial biopsy should be performed to rule out malignant/premalignant conditions.
  - Hysterectomy: may be performed vaginally, laparoscopically, robotically, or by laparotomy
    - Effective in relieving symptoms and improving quality of life (6)[B]
    - Similar fertility and live birth rates between laparoscopic and abdominal myomectomy (2)[B]
    - FDA discourages the use of laparoscopic power morcellation during hysterectomy or myomectomy for uterine fibroids given the risk of spreading an occult malignancy (9).
  - Abdominal, laparoscopic, or robotic myomectomy may be performed in younger women who want to maintain fertility (4)[B].
  - Hysteroscopic/laparoscopic cautery/laser myoma resection can be performed in selected patients.
  - Endometrial ablation: for small submucosal myomas

INPATIENT CONSIDERATIONS

Admission Criteria/Initial Stabilization

- Usually outpatient
- Inpatient for some surgical procedures

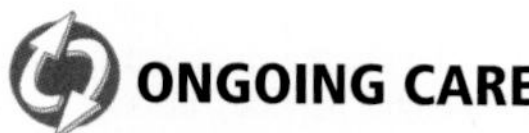

ONGOING CARE

FOLLOW-UP RECOMMENDATIONS

Patient Monitoring

- Pelvic examination and ultrasound: every 2–3 months for newly diagnosed symptomatic/excessively large myomas
- Hemoglobin and hematocrit: if uterine bleeding is excessive
- Once uterine size and symptoms stabilize, monitor every 6–12 months.

DIET

No restrictions

PATIENT EDUCATION

- Society of Interventional Radiology: http://sirweb.org/patients/uterine-fibroids/
- U.S. Department of Health and Human Services: http://womenshealth.gov/faq/uterine-fibroids.cfm
- American Congress of Obstetricians and Gynecologists: http://www.acog.org

PROGNOSIS

- Resection of submucosal fibroids has been associated with increased fertility (6)[B].
- At least 10% of myomas recur after myomectomy; however, most women will not require further treatment (6)[B].

COMPLICATIONS

- May mask other gynecologic malignancies (e.g., uterine sarcoma, ovarian cancer)
- Degenerating fibroids may cause pain and bleeding.
- May rarely prolapse through the cervix

Pregnancy Considerations

- Rapid growth of fibroids is common.
- Pregnant women may need additional fetal testing if placenta is located over or near fibroid.
- Complications during pregnancy: abortion, premature labor, 2nd-trimester rapid growth leading to degeneration and pain, and 3rd-trimester fetal malpresentation and dystocia during labor and delivery
- Cesarean section is recommended if the endometrial cavity was entered during myomectomy due to increased risk of uterine rupture.

Geriatric Considerations

In postmenopausal patients with newly diagnosed uterine myoma/enlarging uterine myomas, have a high suspicion of uterine sarcoma/other gynecologic malignancy.

REFERENCES

1. Parker WH. Etiology, symptomatology, and diagnosis of uterine myomas. *Fertil Steril*. 2007;87(4):725–736.
2. Duhan N, Sirohiwal D. Uterine myomas revisited. *Eur J Obstet Gynecol Reprod Biol*. 2010;152(2):119–125.
3. Bulun SE. Uterine fibroids. *N Engl J Med*. 2013:369(14);1344–1355.
4. Wallace EE, Vlahos NF. Uterine myomas: an overview of development, clinical features, and management. *Obstetrics Gynecol*. 2004;104(2):393–406.
5. Freed MM, Spies JB. Uterine artery embolization for fibroids: a review of current outcomes. *Semin Reprod Med*. 2010;28(3):235–241.
6. Parker WH. Uterine myomas: management. *Fertil Steril*. 2007;88(2):255–271.
7. Hesley GK, Gorny KR, Woodrum DA. MR-guided focused ultrasound for the treatment of uterine fibroids. *Cardiovasc Intervent Radiol*. 2013;36(1):5–13.
8. Donnez J, Tomaszewski J, Vázquez F, et al. Ulipristal acetate versus leuprolide acetate for uterine fibroids. *N Engl J Med*. 2012;366(5):421–432.
9. U.S. Food and Drug Administration. Laparoscopic uterine power morcellation in hysterectomy and myomectomy: FDA safety communication. http://www.fda.gov/MedicalDevices/Safety/AlertsandNotices/ucm393576.htm. Accessed 2014.

ADDITIONAL READING

Laughlin SK, Schroeder JC, Baird DD. New directions in the epidemiology of uterine fibroids. *Semin Reprod Med*. 2010;28(3):204–217.

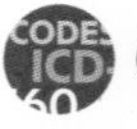

CODES

ICD10

- D25.9 Leiomyoma of uterus, unspecified
- D25.2 Subserosal leiomyoma of uterus
- D25.1 Intramural leiomyoma of uterus

CLINICAL PEARLS

- Uterine myomas are benign smooth muscle tumors composed mainly of fibrous connective tissue.
- Usually incidental finding on pelvic exam or ultrasound but may cause pelvic pain and pressure, abnormal uterine bleeding, and/or infertility
- Management ranges from conservative to medical to surgical.

UVEITIS

Shailendra K. Saxena, MD, PhD • Mikayla Spangler, PharmD, BCPS • Laura K. Klug, PharmD

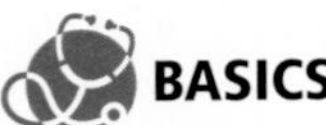

BASICS

DESCRIPTION

- A nonspecific term used to describe any intraocular inflammatory disorder
- Symptoms vary, depending on depth of involvement and associated conditions
- The uvea is the middle layer of the eye between the sclera and retina. The anterior part of the uvea includes the iris and ciliary body. The posterior part of the uvea is the choroid.
  - Anterior uveitis: refers to ocular inflammation limited to the iris (iritis) alone or iris and ciliary body (iridocyclitis)
  - Intermediate uveitis: refers to inflammation of the structures just posterior to the lens (pars planitis or peripheral uveitis)
  - Posterior uveitis: refers to inflammation of the choroid (choroiditis), retina (retinitis), or vitreous near the optic nerve and macula
- System(s) affected: nervous
- Synonym(s): iritis; iridocyclitis; choroiditis; retinochoroiditis; chorioretinitis; anterior uveitis; posterior uveitis; pars planitis; panuveitis. Synonyms are anatomic descriptions of the focus of the uveal inflammation.

Geriatric Considerations

The inflammatory response to systemic disease may be suppressed.

Pediatric Considerations

- Infection should be the primary consideration.
- Allergies and psychological factors (depression, stress) may serve as a trigger.
- Trauma is also a common cause in this population.

Pregnancy Considerations

May be of importance in the selection of medications

EPIDEMIOLOGY

- Predominant age: all ages
- Predominant sex: male = female, except for human leukocyte antigen B27 (HLA-B27) anterior uveitis: male > female

Incidence

- Overall prevalence is 38–714 cases/100,000 annual incidence
- Anterior uveitis most common

Prevalence

Iritis is 4× more prevalent than posterior uveitis.

ETIOLOGY AND PATHOPHYSIOLOGY

- Infectious: may result from viral, bacterial, parasitic, or fungal etiologies
- Suspected immune-mediated: possible autoimmune or immune-complex–mediated mechanism postulated in association with systemic (especially rheumatologic) disorders
  - Autoimmune uveitis (AIU) patients should be referred to an ophthalmologist for local treatment
- Isolated eye disease
- Idiopathic (~25%)
- Some medications may cause uveitis. The most causative medications include rifabutin, bisphosphonates, sulfonamides, metipranolol, topical corticosteroids, brimonidine, prostaglandin analogs, anti–vascular endothelial growth factor (VEGF) agents, bacillus Calmette-Guerin (BCG) vaccination, and systemic and intraocular cidofovir.
- Masquerade syndromes: diseases such as malignancies that may be mistaken for primary inflammation of the eye

Genetics

- No specific pattern for uveitis in general
- Iritis: 50–70% are HLA-B27–positive.
- Predisposing gene for posterior uveitis associated with Behçet disease may include HLA-B51.

RISK FACTORS

- No specific risk factors
- Higher incidence seen with specific associated conditions

COMMONLY ASSOCIATED CONDITIONS

- Viral infections: herpes simplex, herpes zoster, HIV, cytomegalovirus
- Bacterial infections: brucellosis, leprosy, leptospirosis, Lyme disease, propionibacterium infection, syphilis, tuberculosis (TB), Whipple disease
- Parasitic infections: acanthamebiasis, cysticercosis, onchocerciasis, toxocariasis, toxoplasmosis
- Fungal infections: aspergillosis, blastomycosis, candidiasis, coccidioidomycosis, cryptococcosis, histoplasmosis, sporotrichosis
- Suspected immune-mediated: ankylosing spondylitis, Behçet disease, Crohn disease, drug or hypersensitivity reaction, interstitial nephritis, juvenile rheumatoid arthritis, Kawasaki disease, multiple sclerosis, psoriatic arthritis, Reiter syndrome, relapsing polychondritis, sarcoidosis, Sjögren syndrome, systemic lupus erythematosus, ulcerative colitis, vasculitis, vitiligo, Vogt-Koyanagi (Harada) syndrome
- Isolated eye disease: acute multifocal placoid pigmentary epitheliopathy, acute retinal necrosis, bird-shot choroidopathy, Fuchs heterochromatic cyclitis, glaucomatocyclitic crisis, lens-induced uveitis, multifocal choroiditis, pars planitis, serpiginous choroiditis, sympathetic ophthalmia, trauma
- Masquerade syndromes: leukemia, lymphoma, retinitis pigmentosa, retinoblastoma

DIAGNOSIS

HISTORY

- Decreased visual acuity
- Pain, photophobia, blurring of vision (1)[C]
  - Usually acute
- Anterior uveitis (~80% of patients with uveitis) (1)[C]
  - Generally acute in onset
  - Deep eye pain
  - Photophobia (consensual)
- Intermediate and posterior uveitis (2)
  - Unresolving floaters
  - Generally insidious in onset
  - More commonly bilateral

PHYSICAL EXAM

Slit-lamp exam and indirect ophthalmoscopy are necessary for precise diagnosis (1)[C].

- Anterior uveitis (~80% of patients with uveitis)
  - Conjunctival vessel dilation
  - Perilimbal (circumcorneal) dilation of episcleral and scleral vessels (ciliary flush)
  - Small pupillary size of affected eye
  - Hypopyon or hyphema (WBCs or RBCs pooled in the anterior chamber)
  - Frequently unilateral (95% of HLA-B27–associated cases); if first occurrence and otherwise asymptomatic, no further diagnostic testing needed (1)[C]
  - Bilateral involvement and systemic symptoms (fever, fatigue, abdominal pain) may be associated with interstitial nephritis (1)[C].
  - Systemic disease is most likely to be associated with anterior uveitis (in 1 study, 53% of patients were found to have systemic disease) (1)[C].
- Intermediate and posterior uveitis
  - More commonly bilateral
  - Posterior inflammation will generally cause minimal pain or redness unless associated with an iritis.

DIFFERENTIAL DIAGNOSIS

- Acute angle-closure glaucoma
- Conjunctivitis
- Episcleritis
- Keratitis
- Scleritis

DIAGNOSTIC TESTS & INTERPRETATION

No specific test for the diagnosis of uveitis. Tests for etiologic factors or associated conditions should be based on history and physical exam (1)[C].

Initial Tests (lab, imaging)

- CBC, BUN, creatinine (interstitial nephritis) (1)[C]
- HLA-B27 typing (ankylosing spondylitis, Reiter syndrome) (1)[C]
- Antinuclear antibody, ESR (systemic lupus erythematosus, Sjögren syndrome) (1)[C]
- Venereal disease research laboratory (VDRL) test, fluorescent titer antibody (syphilis) (1)[C]
- Fluorescent treponemal antibosy absorption (FTA-ABS) or microhemagglutination assay for antibodies to *Treponema pallidum* (MHA-TP) (1)[C]
- Purified protein derivative (PPD) tuberculin skin test (TB) (1)[C]
- Lyme serology (Lyme disease) (1)[C]
- Disorders that may alter lab results: immunodeficiency
- Chest x-ray (sarcoidosis, histoplasmosis, TB, lymphoma) (1)[C]
- Sacroiliac radiograph (ankylosing spondylitis) (1)[C]

Diagnostic Procedures/Other

Slit-lamp exam (1)[C]

Test Interpretation

- Keratic precipitates
- Inflammatory cells in anterior chamber or vitreous
- Synechiae (fibrous tissue scarring between iris and lens)
- Macular edema
- Perivasculitis of retinal vessels

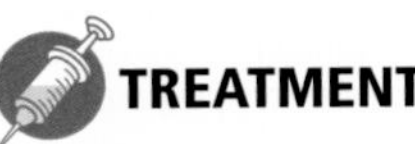

TREATMENT

GENERAL MEASURES

- Outpatient care with urgent ophthalmologic consultation
- Medical therapy best initiated following full ophthalmologic evaluation

- Treatment of underlying cause, if identified
- Anti-inflammatory therapy

MEDICATION

First Line

- The treatment depends on the etiology, location, and severity of the inflammation.
- Prednisolone acetate 1% ophthalmic suspension: two drops to the affected eye q1h initially, tapering to once a day with improvement
  - Contraindications
    - Hypersensitivity to the medication or component of the preparation
    - Topical corticosteroid therapy is contraindicated in uveitis secondary to infectious etiologies, unless used in conjunction with appropriate anti-infectious agents.
  - Precautions
    - Topical corticosteroids may increase intraocular pressure, increase susceptibility to infections, impair corneal or scleral wound healing, or cause corneal epithelial toxicity, or crystalline keratopathy. Prolonged use may cause cataract formation and exacerbate existing herpetic keratitis, which may masquerade as iritis.
  - Significant possible interactions
- Systemic corticosteroids are useful for maintenance therapy for patients with noninfectious uveitis. These should always be used with other immunosuppressive medications for steroid-sparing effects; prednisone 5–10 mg daily (3,4)[B]
- Cycloplegic agents may be used to dilate the eye and relieve pain. Agents include scopolamine hydrobromide 0.25% (Isopto Hyoscine) or atropine 1% 1–2 drops up to QID or homatropine hydrobromide (Isopto) 2% or 5% 1–2 drops BID or as often as q3h if necessary (1)[C].
  - Contraindications
    - Cycloplegia is contraindicated in patients known to have, or be predisposed to, glaucoma.
  - Precautions
    - Use extreme caution in infants, young children and elderly because of increased susceptibility to systemic effects.

Second Line

- Anti-inflammatory: prednisolone sodium phosphate 1%, dexamethasone sodium phosphate 0.1%, dexamethasone suspension, rimexolone 1% (Vexol), and loteprednol etabonate 0.5% (Lotemax), difluprednate (Durezol) 0.05% (1,4)[C]
  - Rimexolone 1% (Vexol) may be equally effective as prednisolone acetate 1% for short-term treatment of anterior uveitis (1)[C].
  - Loteprednol etabonate (Lotemax) may not be as effective as prednisolone acetate 1% but may be less likely to increase intraocular pressure in cases of acute anterior uveitis.
- Periocular corticosteroids may be injected with triamcinolone acetonide being most commonly used. 40 mg/1 mL (5)[C].
- Intravitreous corticosteroid deposits may also be used for long-term maintenance. Fluocinolone acetonide (Retisert) 590 μg released over 30 months, dexamethasone (Ozurdex) 0.7 mg released slowly over 3–6 months (4,5)[B].
  - Retisert has caused all patients to develop cataracts and significant increases in intraocular pressure in about 2/3 of patients, whereas Ozurdex had only 1/4 of patients require medication for increased intraocular pressure and 15% develop cataracts (5)[C].
- Intravitreal corticosteroid injections are used only in severe cases of recurrence; triamcinolone acetonide 4–20 mg/0.1 mL, dexamethasone phosphate 0.4 mg/0.1 mL, dexamethasone implant (Ozurdex)
  - Ozurdex has a longer effect than triamcinolone acetonide.
- Immunosuppressive agents including antimetabolites (methotrexate, azathioprine and mycophenalate mofetil), T-cell inhibitors (cyclosporine, tacrolimus, and sirolimus), and alkylating agents (cyclophosphamide, chlorambucil) may be employed in cases resistant to initial treatment but close monitoring is required (4,5)[C].
- Although biologic therapy has been used for refractory uveitis, the sparsity of randomized clinical trials as well as high cost and adverse effect potential of these agents limit their use (3,4)[C].
- Systemic and ophthalmic preparations of NSAIDs may provide some symptom relief (1)[C].

ISSUES FOR REFERRAL

Caution should be used when using empiric treatment; referral to an ophthalmologist is recommended in most cases.

SURGERY/OTHER PROCEDURES

Various surgical procedures may be used therapeutically for visual rehabilitation, diagnostically, or to manage complications associated with uveitis (6).

ONGOING CARE

FOLLOW-UP RECOMMENDATIONS

Patient Monitoring

- Complete history and physical to evaluate for associated systemic disease
- Ophthalmologic follow-up as recommended by consultant

PATIENT EDUCATION

- Instruct on proper method for instilling eye drops.
- Wear dark glasses if photophobia is a problem.

PROGNOSIS

- Depends on the presence of causal diseases or associated conditions
- Uveitis resulting from infections (systemic or local) tends to resolve with eradication of the underlying infection.
- Uveitis associated with seronegative arthropathies tends to be acute (lasting <3 months) and frequently recurrent.

COMPLICATIONS

- Cycloplegia: paralysis of the ciliary muscle of the eye, resulting in a loss of accommodation
- Loss of vision as a result of the following:
  - Keratic precipitate deposition on the corneal or lens surfaces (1)
  - Increased intraocular pressure, acute angle-closure glaucoma (1)
  - Formation of synechiae
  - Cataract formation (1)
  - Vasculitis with vascular occlusion, retinal infarction
  - Macular edema (1)
  - Optic nerve damage

REFERENCES

1. American Optometric Association. Optometric clinical practice guideline: care of the patient with anterior uveitis. http://www.aoa.org/documents/CPG-7.pdf. Accessed 2014.
2. Selmi C. Diagnosis and classification ofautoimmune uveitis. *Autoimmunity Rev*. 2014;13(4–5):591–594.
3. De Smet MD, Taylor SR, Bodaghi B, et al. Understanding uveitis: the impact of research on visual outcomes. *Prog Retin Eye Res*. 2011;30:452–470.
4. Babu K, Mahendradas P. Medical management of uveitis—current trends. *Indian J Opthalmol*. 2013;61(6):277–283.
5. Gallego-Pinazo R, Dolz-Marco R, Martinez-Castillo S, et al. Update on the principles and novel local and systemic therapies for the treatment of non-infectious uveitis. *Inflamm Allergy Drug Targets*. 2013;12(1):38–45.
6. Murthy SI, Pappuru RR, Latha KM, et al. Surgical management in patient with uveitis. *Indian J Opthalmol*. 2013;61(6):284–290.

ADDITIONAL READING

- Levy RA, de Andrade FA, Foeldvari I, et al. Cutting-edge issues in autoimmune uveitis. *Clin Rev Allergy Immunol*. 2011;41(2):214–223.
- Majumder PD, Biswas J. Pediatric uveitis: an update. *Oman J Ophthalmol*. 2013;6(3):140–150.
- Pan J, Kapur M, McCallum R. Noninfectious immune-mediated uveitis and ocular inflammation. *Curr Allergy Asthma Rep*. 2014;14(1):409.
- Yang MM, Lai TY, Luk FO, et al. The roles of genetic factors in uveitis and their clinical significance. *Retina*. 2014;34(1):1–11.

SEE ALSO

Conjunctivitis, Acute; Glaucoma, Primary Closed-Angle; Scleritis

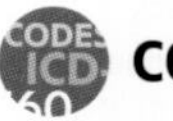

CODES

ICD10

- H20.9 Unspecified iridocyclitis
- H30.90 Unspecified chorioretinal inflammation, unspecified eye
- H20.019 Primary iridocyclitis, unspecified eye

CLINICAL PEARLS

- Symptoms vary depending on depth of involvement and associated conditions but should be suspected when eye pain is associated with visual changes.
- Severe or unresponsive uveitis may require therapy, including periocular injection of corticosteroids, sustained-release corticosteroid implants, systemic corticosteroids, cytotoxic agents, immunosuppressive agents, immunomodulatory agents, or tumor necrosis factor inhibitors.

VAGINAL ADENOSIS

Laura K. Randolph, DO, MS • Michael P. Hopkins, MD, MEd

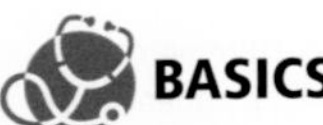

BASICS

DESCRIPTION

- The normal vagina is lined with squamous epithelium. Adenosis is characterized by the presence of columnar epithelium or glandular tissue in the wall of the vagina.
- At about the 15th week of embryologic development, the müllerian system, which forms the upper 2/3 of the vagina, fuses with the invaginating cloaca or urogenital sinus to form the lower 1/3 of the vagina. Squamous metaplasia from the cloacal region then produces a squamous epithelium through the vagina.
- Adenosis occurs when this squamous epithelium fails to epithelialize the vagina completely.
- 3 main types of adenosis epithelium described
  - Endocervical
  - Endometrial
  - Tubal
- System(s) affected: reproductive

Geriatric Considerations

- Adenosis is a disorder of the young female. By menopause, the vagina and cervix should be completely epithelialized.
- The presence of glandular epithelium in the postmenopausal patient is an indication for excision and close evaluation for the possibility of a well-differentiated adenocarcinoma.

Pregnancy Considerations

Pregnancy produces a wide eversion of the transformation zone of the cervix. This occasionally will become so widely everted that it will extend onto the vaginal fornices, leading to the impression of adenosis. This will resolve after the pregnancy is completed.

EPIDEMIOLOGY

Incidence

- Although the cumulative incidence of vaginal adenosis is unknown, the incidence of cloacal malformations is 1/20,000–1/25,000 live births.
- Although spontaneous vaginal adenosis appears to be fairly common (10% of adult women), it is mostly an insignificant coincidental finding. Widespread symptomatic involvement is rare (1).

Prevalence

- In the United States: Adenosis is relatively common, affecting 10–20% of young females studied. As maturation progresses with puberty, epithelialization occurs (2).
- Predominant age
  - Age <1 month: 15%
  - Prepubertal: typically absent
  - Age 13–25 years: 13%
  - Age >25 years: decreasing prevalence, uncommon beyond age 30 years (1)

ETIOLOGY AND PATHOPHYSIOLOGY

- In most young females, the etiology is incomplete squamous metaplasia or epithelialization. This occurs as a natural phenomenon and resolves with age.
- Described as congenital or acquired (3)
  - Congenital: proliferation of the remnant müllerian epithelium in the vagina due to exposure to diethylstilbestrol (DES) in utero (DES daughters)
  - Transformation-related protein 63 (TRP63/p63) marks the cell fate decision of müllerian duct epithelium to become squamous epithelium in the cervix and vagina. DES disrupts the TRP63 expression and induces adenosis lesions (4).
  - Acquired: trauma and inflammation causing spontaneous de novo changes or changes in an acquired lesion in the vaginal epithelium
    - Trauma: carbon dioxide laser, 5-fluorouracil, vaginal packs, chronic pessary use
    - Proliferation of the glandular cells in the remnant müllerian epithelium of the vagina due to sex hormones
    - Idiopathic spontaneous change in epithelium; no cause has been identified.

RISK FACTORS

Adenosis of the vagina/cervix may arise in up to 90% of DES daughters, and there is a 40-fold increased risk of the subsequent development of clear cell adenocarcinoma (5).

GENERAL PREVENTION

None: last DES exposure in the 1970s

COMMONLY ASSOCIATED CONDITIONS

DES exposure

- Adenosis from DES exposure should lead to an evaluation of other DES-related abnormalities.
- Müllerian tract anomalies associated with DES exposure include cervical hood, cervical ridge, shortened cervix, incompetent cervix, and T-shaped uterine cavity.
- Patients with known DES exposure should have their reproductive tract evaluated prior to conception.
- Most patients with adenosis have not been DES-exposed and do not require evaluation of the reproductive system.
- DES is a synthetic, nonsteroidal estrogen that was used to prevent spontaneous abortions or premature deliveries from 1938 to 1971 (5). An estimated 5 million women were prescribed DES during this period (4).
- The FDA issued a drug bulletin in 1971 advising physicians to stop prescribing DES to pregnant women because of its link to vaginal clear cell adenocarcinoma in DES daughters (5).

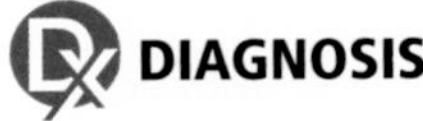

DIAGNOSIS

HISTORY

- Maternal DES exposure
- Complaints of
  - Profuse mucoid vaginal discharge from the glandular epithelium
  - Pruritus
  - Pain/soreness of the vaginal introitus
  - Postcoital bleeding
  - Dyspareunia

PHYSICAL EXAM

On pelvic exam, adenosis appearance is varied: patchy or diffuse red stippling, granularity or nodularity, single or multiple cysts, erosions, ulcers, or warty protuberances that may even extend to the vulva (1).

DIFFERENTIAL DIAGNOSIS

- Erosive lichen planus
- Fixed drug eruption
- Erythema multiforme

- Bullous skin disease
- Adenocarcinoma
  - A thorough evaluation for adenocarcinoma of the vagina arising in adenosis should be done.
  - A biopsy may be necessary to ensure that the process represents only benign adenosis.

DIAGNOSTIC TESTS & INTERPRETATION

Initial Tests (lab, imaging)

4-quadrant Pap smear should be used liberally to isolate quadrants of the vagina that may contain abnormalities. None, unless diagnosed with underlying malignancy

Follow-Up Tests & Special Considerations

Pap smear can be followed by colposcopy and biopsy.

Diagnostic Procedures/Other

Colposcopy should be used to outline areas of adenosis to ensure that no malignancy is present.

Test Interpretation

- Biopsy will show benign glandular epithelium.
- Biopsies in the areas of ongoing squamous metaplasia will be typical for this process (3).

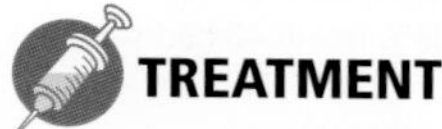

TREATMENT

GENERAL MEASURES

- Unless malignancy is present, conservative treatment is indicated.
- In most young females with this condition, it will resolve with expectant management (1)[C].
- Treatment is warranted in women with severe subjective symptoms that impair the quality of life (6).

ISSUES FOR REFERRAL

Malignancy found on biopsy warrants referral to gynecologic oncology specialist.

SURGERY/OTHER PROCEDURES

- Aggressive therapy, such as laser or surgical excision, is necessary if premalignant or malignant changes arise (3)[C].
- Symptomatic treatment with carbon dioxide laser coagulation, unipolar coagulation, or, lastly, vaginal resection (1)

INPATIENT CONSIDERATIONS

Admission Criteria/Initial Stabilization

Outpatient management

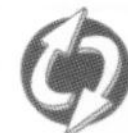

ONGOING CARE

FOLLOW-UP RECOMMENDATIONS

Patient Monitoring

If the initial colposcopy is normal, a yearly 4-quadrant Pap smear of the vagina and of the cervix is all that is necessary.

DIET

No special diet

PATIENT EDUCATION

- No limitations
- It is not necessary to avoid intercourse or placing objects in the vagina.
- The patient should be educated to keep annual pelvic and Pap smear appointments. In most situations, this is benign, and expectant management is all that is necessary.
- www.acog.org

PROGNOSIS

- It is expected that most patients will have squamous metaplasia and epithelialization with complete resolution of the adenosis.
- The rare patient, 1/1,000–1/10,000, may develop adenocarcinoma in the adenosis and will require definitive therapy as for vaginal cancer.
  - Cumulative incidence of progression of adenosis to adenocarcinoma is 1.5/1,000 for DES daughters (5).

COMPLICATIONS

- Infertility with DES association
- Adverse pregnancy outcome with DES association
- Adenocarcinoma of vagina

REFERENCES

1. Kranl C, Zelger B, Kofler H, et al. Vulval and vaginal adenosis. *Br J Dermatol*. 1998;139(1):128–131.
2. Sandberg EC. The incidence and distribution of occult vaginal adenosis. *Am J Obstet Gynecol*. 1968;101(3):322–334.
3. Chattopadhyay I, Cruickshan DJ, Packer M. Non diethylstilbestrol induced vaginal adenosis—a case series and review of literature. *Eur J Gynaecol Oncol*. 2001;22(4):260–262.
4. Laronda MM, Unno K, Butler LM, et al. The development of cervical and vaginal adenosis as a result of diethylstilbestrol exposure in utero. *Differentiation*. 2012;84(3):252–260.
5. National Toxicology Program, Department of Health and Human Services. Diethylstilbestrol. *Report on Carcinogens*, 12th ed. 2011:159–161.
6. Cebesoy FB, Kutlar I, Aydin A. Vaginal adenosis successfully treated with simple unipolar cauterization. *J Natl Med Assoc*. 2007;99(2):166–167.

ADDITIONAL READING

Bamigboye AA, Morris J. Oestrogen supplementation, mainly diethylstilbestrol, for preventing miscarriages and other adverse pregnancy outcomes. *Cochrane Database Syst Rev*. 2003;(3):CD004353.

SEE ALSO

Vaginal Malignancy

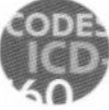

CODES

ICD10

- Q52.4 Other congenital malformations of vagina
- N89.8 Other specified noninflammatory disorders of vagina
- T38.5X5A Adverse effect of other estrogens and progestogens, initial encounter

CLINICAL PEARLS

- Adenosis is characterized by the presence of columnar epithelium or glandular tissue in the wall of the vagina.
- Adenosis is more common among women exposed to DES daughters.
- Adenosis is rarely associated with an underlying vaginal malignancy.

VAGINAL BLEEDING DURING PREGNANCY

Virginia Van Duyne, MD

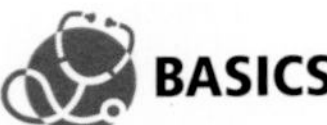

BASICS

DESCRIPTION

- Vaginal bleeding during pregnancy has many causes and ranges in severity from benign with normal pregnancy outcome to life threatening for both infant and mother.
- Etiology can be from the vagina, cervix, uterus, fetus, or placenta. The differential diagnosis is guided by the gestational age of the fetus.

EPIDEMIOLOGY

Prevalence

- In early pregnancy: 7–25% of patients
- In late pregnancy: 0.3–2% of patients

ETIOLOGY AND PATHOPHYSIOLOGY

- Many times the cause is unknown.
- Anytime in pregnancy:
  - Cervicitis (infectious or noninfectious)
  - Vaginal or cervical trauma (including postcoital)
  - Cervical lesion or neoplasia
  - Hyperemia of cervix (increased blood flow from pregnancy)
- Early pregnancy:
  - For up to 50% of early pregnancy bleeding, no cause is ever found.
  - Ectopic pregnancy: leading cause of 1st-trimester maternal death in the United States. Risk factors: previous ectopic, trauma to fallopian tubes (tubal surgery, infection, tumor), congenital anomaly of tubes, in utero diethylstilbestrol (DES) exposure, current use of IUD, history of infertility, tobacco use
  - Spontaneous abortion: risk factors: advanced maternal age (AMA), alcohol use, tobacco use, anesthetic gas, heavy caffeine use, cocaine use, chronic maternal diseases (poorly controlled diabetes mellitus [DM], celiac disease, autoimmune diseases such as antiphospholipid syndrome), short interconception time (3–6 months), current use of IUD, maternal infection (e.g., herpes simplex virus [HSV], gonorrhea, chlamydia, toxoplasmosis, listeriosis, HIV, syphilis, malaria), medications (e.g., retinoids, methotrexate, NSAIDs), multiple previous therapeutic abortions, previous spontaneous abortion, toxins (arsenic, lead, polyurethane), uterine abnormalities (congenital, adhesions, fibroids)
  - Implantation bleeding: benign, about 6 days after fertilization
  - Uterine fibroids
  - Subchorionic bleed: in late 1st trimester
  - Low-lying placenta
  - Gestational trophoblastic disease: hydatidiform mole (most common), choriocarcinoma, or placental-site trophoblastic tumors
- Late pregnancy:
  - Bloody show of labor (mucus plug)
  - Placenta previa: painless bleeding; occurs in 0.4% deliveries in the United States. Risk factors: previous history of placenta previa, previous uterine surgery (cesarean section, D&C), chronic hypertension, multiparity, multiple gestation, tobacco use, AMA
  - Placental abruption: painful bleeding; occurs in 1–2% deliveries in the United States. Risk factors: previous placental abruption, 1st-trimester bleeding, hypertension, preeclampsia, multiple gestation, tobacco, cocaine or methamphetamine use, unexplained elevated maternal α-fetoprotein, poly- or oligohydramnios, AMA, trauma to abdomen, premature rupture of membranes, thrombophilia, short umbilical cord, male fetus, chorioamnionitis, nutritional deficiency
  - Vasa previa: minimal bleeding with fetal distress; rare (1:2,500 deliveries). Risk factors: in vitro fertilization, multiple gestation, placental abnormalities (low-lying position, bilobate, succenturiate lobe, velamentous insertion of umbilical cord)
  - Placenta accreta, increta, percreta: risk factors: uterine scar (e.g., from cesarean section, endometrial ablation, or D&C), current placenta previa, AMA, tobacco use, multiparity, uterine anomalies, uterine fibroids, hypertension
  - Uterine rupture: vaginal bleeding, abnormal fetal heart rate, and disordered or hypertonic uterine contractions with or without pain. Risk factors: previous cesarean section (most common), trauma, use of oxytocin or prostaglandins, multiparity, external cephalic version, placental abruption, shoulder dystocia, placenta percreta, müllerian duct anomalies, history of pelvic radiation

RISK FACTORS

See specific etiologies in earlier discussion.

GENERAL PREVENTION

- Address modifiable risk factors such as domestic violence and tobacco and drug use.
- If placenta or vasa previa, nothing per vagina

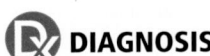

DIAGNOSIS

HISTORY

- Anytime in pregnancy: quality of pregnancy dating, context (e.g., following bowel movement, during voiding, after intercourse, drug use, or trauma including domestic violence), amount of bleeding, obstetrical history, personal or family history of inherited bleeding disorders
- Early pregnancy: severe nausea/vomiting (can be associated with molar pregnancy); amount of bleeding, pelvic pain, or suprapubic cramping (e.g., spontaneous abortion, ectopic) complications in previous pregnancies (e.g., spontaneous abortion, abruption, 1st-trimester vaginal bleeding)
- Late pregnancy: contractions (labor), abdominal pain especially between contractions (abruption, uterine rupture), presence or absence of fetal movement, rupture of membranes
- See "Etiology and Pathophysiology" for additional pertinent history.

PHYSICAL EXAM

- Vital signs: When present, signs of hemodynamic instability are first tachycardia and tachypnea, then hypotension and thready pulse.
- Abdomen: uterine tenderness, fundal height (increasing fundal height may be associated with placental abruption)
- Speculum: Visualize cervix and identify source of bleeding (from cervical os or from within vagina).
- Cervix: assess for dilation; required to assess for labor but should not be performed until placenta previa ruled out via ultrasound
- Fetal monitoring: Doppler heart tones in early pregnancy; external fetal monitoring for gestational age >26 weeks

DIFFERENTIAL DIAGNOSIS

- Hematuria (UTI, kidney stones)
- Rectal bleeding

DIAGNOSTIC TESTS & INTERPRETATION

Initial Tests (lab, imaging)

- CBC
- Blood type and screen; if significant hemorrhage, type and cross-match
- Quantitative β-human chorionic gonadotropin (β-hCG):
  - Prior to 12 weeks, levels can be followed serially every 2 days with following trends:
    - Doubles or at least 66% rise in 48 hours in normal pregnancy
    - Falls in spontaneous abortion
    - Extremely high in molar pregnancy
    - Rises gradually (<50% in 48 hours) or plateaus in ectopic pregnancy

- Transvaginal ultrasound should be used to confirm an intrauterine pregnancy (IUP) when the quantitative β-hCG >2,000 (1)[A].

- Other lab tests based on clinical scenario:
  - Wet mount, gonorrhea/chlamydia, Pap smear
  - Progesterone level occasionally used to determine viability in threatened abortion (<5 indicates not viable, >25 indicates viability, 5–25 is equivocal).
  - Bleeding time, fibrinogen, and fibrin split products: if suspect coagulopathy or abruption
  - Kleihauer-Betke: low sensitivity and specificity for abruption; helpful for dosing Rho(d) immune globulin (RhoGAM)
- Ultrasound is the preferred imaging modality:
  - Early pregnancy:
    - Gestational sac seen at 5–6 weeks; fetal heartbeat observed by 8–9 weeks
    - Diagnostic of ectopic with nearly 100% sensitivity when β-hCG level 1,500–2,000 mIU/mL. If no IUP is present and ultrasound does not confirm ectopic pregnancy, serial quantitative β-hCG values should be followed (2)[C].
  - Late pregnancy:
    - Proceed to rule out placenta previa with ultrasound, labor with serial cervical exams, and abruption with external fetal monitoring.

ALERT

Confirm fetal presentation and placental position prior to cervical exam.

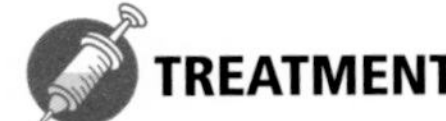

TREATMENT

MEDICATION

First Line

- Treat underlying cause of bleeding, if identified.
- If mother is Rh negative, give RhoGAM to prevent autoimmunization. In late pregnancy, dose according to the amount of estimated fetomaternal hemorrhage.

- If cause of bleeding is preterm labor, consider betamethasone for fetal lung maturity if <34 weeks' gestation. Tocolytics may be used to prolong pregnancy to allow for course of steroids.
- If threatened abortion: Consider progesterone (relative risk 0.53) (3)[A].
- If mother has an inherited bleeding disorder or if bleeding is severe, consider recombinant or donor blood products.

SURGERY/OTHER PROCEDURES

- Cesarean section may be indicated for recurrent or uncontrolled bleeding with placenta or vasa previa.
- If ectopic is diagnosed, immediate surgical treatment may be needed. Some early ectopic pregnancies can be treated medically if certain criteria are met (2)[C].
- Surgical uterine evacuation is necessary for molar pregnancy due to malignant potential (4)[C].
- Incomplete or inevitable spontaneous abortion: Management is patient centered. In the absence of infection, patient may elect expectant, medical, or surgical management. If expectant management, typically wait 2 weeks for patient to complete abortion; most complete by 9 days. If at 2 weeks abortion is not completed or medical management has failed, surgical intervention (D&C or aspiration) is generally indicated (5)[A]. May send tissue to pathology to confirm.

INPATIENT CONSIDERATIONS

Admission Criteria/Initial Stabilization

- In early pregnancy: based on quantity of bleeding, need for surgical treatment for ectopic pregnancy, or presence of infection in case of spontaneous abortion
- In late pregnancy, if significant bleeding and/or presence of maternal or fetal compromise
- In late pregnancy with trauma, if ≥2 contractions/10 minutes

Discharge Criteria

- In late pregnancy, may discharge when bleeding has stopped; labor, previa, and abruption have been ruled out; and fetal heart tracing is normal.
- After trauma in late pregnancy, may discharge home if normal fetal heart tracing for ≥4 hours with <2 contractions/10 minutes

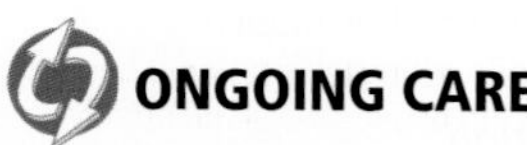

ONGOING CARE

PATIENT MONITORING

- Patient should be instructed to report any increase in the amount or frequency of bleeding and to seek immediate care if experiencing fever, abdominal pain, or sudden increased bleeding. Patient should save any tissue passed vaginally for examination.
- Frequency of outpatient follow-up as indicated based on etiology of bleeding

PATIENT EDUCATION

- American Academy of Family Physicians (AAFP): www.familydoctor.org
- American College of Obstetricians & Gynecologists (ACOG): www.acog.org

PROGNOSIS

- Prognosis depends on the etiology of vaginal bleeding, severity of bleeding, and rapidity of diagnosis.
- Maternal mortality is 31.9 deaths/100,000 ectopic pregnancies.
- 1/2 of patients with early pregnancy bleeding miscarry. If fetal heart activity (ultrasound) present in 1st-trimester bleed, <10% chance of pregnancy loss.
- Heavy bleeding in early pregnancy, particularly when accompanied by pain, is associated with higher risk of spontaneous abortion. Spotting and light episodes are not, especially if lasting only 1–2 days.
- Subchorionic hemorrhage has about 2–3-fold increased risk of spontaneous abortion. Smaller hemorrhage and presence of viable fetal heart rate confer lower risk of loss. Most resolve spontaneously.
- Women with early pregnancy bleeding have an increased risk of preterm delivery, premature rupture of membranes, manual removal of placenta, placental abruption, elective cesarean delivery, and term labor induction later in the same pregnancy. These women also have an increased risk of adverse pregnancy outcomes, including hyperbilirubinemia, congenital anomalies, NICU admission, and reduced neonatal birth weight. Finally, there is an increased risk in subsequent pregnancies of recurrence of early pregnancy bleeding.
- Bed rest has not been shown to affect the outcome of bleeding in early pregnancy but may be indicated for bleeding in late pregnancy with placenta or vasa previa or with maternal hypertension.

REFERENCES

1. Crochet JR, Bastian LA, Chireau MV. Does this woman have an ectopic pregnancy? The rational clinical examination systematic review. *JAMA*. 2013;209(16):1722–1729.
2. Deutchman M, Tubay AT, Turok D. First trimester bleeding. *Am Fam Physician*. 2009;79(11):985–994.
3. Wahabi HA, Fayed AA, Esmaeil SA, et al. Progestogen for treating threatened miscarriage. *Cochrane Database Syst Rev*. 2011;(12):CD005943.
4. Snell BJ. Assessment and management of bleeding in the first trimester of pregnancy. *J Midwifery Womens Health*. 2009;54(6):483–491.
5. Nanda K, Lopez LM, Grimes DA, et al. Expectant care versus surgical treatment for miscarriage. *Cochrane Database Syst Rev*. 2012;3:CD003518.

ADDITIONAL READING

- Chi C, Kadir RA. Inherited bleeding disorders in pregnancy. *Best Pract Res Clin Obstet Gynaecol*. 2012;26(1):103–117.
- Dadkhah F, Kashanian M, Eliasi G. A comparison between the pregnancy outcome in women both with or without threatened abortion. *Early Hum Dev*. 2010;86(3):193–196.
- Griebel CP, Halvorsen J, Golemon TB, et al. Management of spontaneous abortion. *Am Fam Physician*. 2005;72(7):1243–1250.
- Grimes DA. Estimation of pregnancy-related mortality risk by pregnancy outcome, United States, 1991 to 1999. *Am J Obstet Gynecol*. 2006;194(1):92–94.
- Hasan R, Baird DD, Herring AH, et al. Association between first-trimester vaginal bleeding and miscarriage. *Obstet Gynecol*. 2009;114(4):860–867.
- Lykke JA, Dideriksen KL, Lidegaard O, et al. First-trimester vaginal bleeding and complications later in pregnancy. *Obstet Gynecol*. 2010;115(5):935–944.
- Magann EF, Cummings JE, Niederhauser A, et al. Antepartum bleeding of unknown origin in the second half of pregnancy: a review. *Obstet Gynecol Surv*. 2005;60(11):741–745.
- Mercier FJ, Van de Velde M. Major obstetric hemorrhage. *Anesthesiol Clin*. 2008;26(1):53–66.
- Mukul LV, Teal SB. Current management of ectopic pregnancy. *Obstet Gynecol Clin North Am*. 2007;34(3):403–419.
- Oyelese Y, Ananth CV. Placental abruption. *Obstet Gynecol*. 2006;108(4):1005–1016.
- Publications Committee, Society for Maternal-Fetal Medicine, Belfort MA. Placenta accrete. *Am J Obstet Gynecol*. 2010;203(5):430–439.
- Sakornbut E, Leeman L, Fontaine P. Late pregnancy bleeding. *Am Fam Physician*. 2007;75(8):1199–1206.
- Walfish M, Neuman A, Wlody D. Maternal haemorrhage. *Br J Anaesth*. 2009;103(Suppl 1):i47–i56.
- Wijesiriwardana A, Bhattacharya S, Shetty A, et al. Obstetric outcome in women with threatened miscarriage in the first trimester. *Obstet Gynecol*. 2006;107(3):557–562.

SEE ALSO

Abnormal Pap and Cervical Dysplasia; Abortion, Spontaneous (Miscarriage); Abruptio Placentae; Cervical Malignancy; Cervical Polyps; Cervicitis, Ectropion, and True Erosion; Chlamydial Sexually Transmitted Diseases; Ectopic Pregnancy; Placenta Previa; Preterm Labor; Trichomoniasis; Vaginal Malignancy

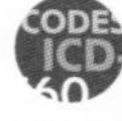

CODES

ICD10

- O20.9 Hemorrhage in early pregnancy, unspecified
- O46.90 Antepartum hemorrhage, unspecified, unspecified trimester
- O20.0 Threatened abortion

CLINICAL PEARLS

- Obtain blood type and screen on all women presenting with vaginal bleeding in pregnancy and administer RhoGAM to all Rh-negative patients.
- For up to 50% of early pregnancy bleeding, no cause is ever found.
- Always consider ectopic pregnancy in 1st-trimester bleeding.
- Do not perform digital exam in late pregnancy bleeding until placenta has been located on ultrasound.

VAGINAL MALIGNANCY

Laura K. Randolph, DO, MS • Michael P. Hopkins, MD, MEd

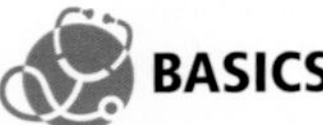

BASICS

DESCRIPTION

- Carcinomas of the vagina are uncommon: 3% of gynecologic malignancies.
- Vaginal intraepithelial neoplasia (VAIN), defined by squamous cell atypia, is classified by the depth of epithelial involvement:
  - VAIN 1: 1/3 thickness
  - VAIN 2: 2/3 thickness
  - VAIN 3 and carcinoma in situ (CIS): more than 2/3 with CIS, designating full-thickness neoplastic changes without invasion through the basement membrane
- Invasive malignancies: Vaginal malignancies include squamous cell carcinoma (85–90%), adenocarcinoma (5–10%), sarcoma (2–3%), and melanoma (2–3%). Clear cell carcinoma is a subtype of adenocarcinoma. Invasive squamous cell carcinoma has the potential for metastasis to the lungs and liver.
- To be classified as a vaginal malignancy, only the vagina can be involved. If the cervix or vulva is involved, then the tumor is classified as a primary cancer arising from the cervix or the vulva.
- Most vaginal malignancies are metastatic (e.g., cervix, vulva, endometrium, breast, ovary).

Pregnancy Considerations

This malignancy is not associated with pregnancy.

EPIDEMIOLOGY

Incidence

- An estimated 3,170 new cases will be diagnosed in 2014 with 880 resulting deaths (1).
- Predominant age
  - CIS: mid-40–60 years
  - Invasive squamous cell malignancy: mid-60–70 years
  - Adenocarcinoma: any age; 50 years is mean age. Peak incidence is between 17–21 years of age.
  - Clear cell adenocarcinoma occurs most often in females <30 years with a history of exposure to diethylstilbestrol (DES) in utero.
  - Mixed müllerian sarcomas and leiomyosarcomas in the adult population: mean age 60 years

Pediatric Considerations

Vaginal tumors are extremely rare. Rhabdomyosarcoma (botryoid and embryonal subtype) is the most common malignant neoplasm of the vagina. Less common entities are germ cell tumor and clear cell adenocarcinoma.

Prevalence

In the United States, it is 1 of the rarest of all gynecologic malignancies (3%).

ETIOLOGY AND PATHOPHYSIOLOGY

- Women with a history of cervical malignancy have a higher probability of developing squamous cell malignancy in the vagina even after hysterectomy.
- Human papillomavirus (HPV) is found in 80–93% of patients with vaginal CIS and 50–65% of the patients with invasive vaginal carcinoma (2,3).
- HPV-16 is the most common, found in 66% of CIS and 55% of invasive vaginal cancers.
- Smokers have a higher incidence.
- Clear cell adenocarcinoma of the vagina in young women has been associated with DES exposure. The incidence, however, is exceedingly rare, estimated at 1/1,000–1/10,000 exposed females.
- Metastatic lesions can involve the vagina, spreading from the other gynecologic organs.
- Although rare, renal cell carcinoma, lung adenocarcinoma, GI cancer, pancreatic adenocarcinoma, ovarian germ cell cancer, trophoblastic neoplasm, and breast cancer can all metastasize to the vagina.

Genetics

No known genetic pattern

RISK FACTORS

- Similar risk factors as cervical cancer
- Age
- African American
- Smoking
- Multiple sex partners, early age of 1st sexual intercourse
- History of squamous cell cancer of the cervix or vulva
- HPV infection
- Vaginal adenosis
- Vaginal irritation
- DES exposure in utero

COMMONLY ASSOCIATED CONDITIONS

Due to the field effect, patients with vaginal cancer are more likely to develop malignancy in the cervix or vulva and should be followed closely.

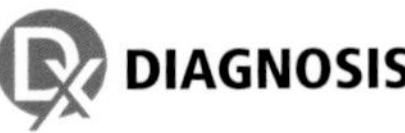

DIAGNOSIS

HISTORY

- Abnormal bleeding is the most common symptom.
- Postcoital bleeding can result from direct trauma to the tumor.
- Vaginal discharge
- Dyspareunia
- Urinary symptoms, including hematuria and increased frequency
- Constipation
- Pain along with symptoms and signs of hydroureter are late findings when the tumor has spread into the paravaginal tissues and extends to the pelvic sidewall.

Pediatric Considerations

In children, sarcomas can present either as a mass protruding from the vagina or as abnormal genital bleeding.

PHYSICAL EXAM

Pelvic examination

- The vagina, uterus, adnexa (fallopian tubes and ovaries), bladder, and rectum should be evaluated for unusual changes.
- Vaginal malignancies are found most commonly on the posterior wall in the upper 1/3 of the vagina.

DIFFERENTIAL DIAGNOSIS

- Premalignant changes: VAIN 1, 2, 3, and CIS
- Adequate biopsies ensure that invasive lesions are not overlooked. Invasive lesions penetrate the basement membrane and cannot be treated conservatively.
- Other malignancies, such as endometrial, cervix, bladder, or colon cancer, can invade directly into the vagina or metastasize to the vagina.
- In the childbearing years, trophoblastic disease should be considered:
  - The vagina is a common site of metastases; however, biopsy should typically be avoided because the implants are very vascular and may hemorrhage if sampled.
  - The clinical presentation is typically obvious so histopathologic confirmation before treatment is not required.

DIAGNOSTIC TESTS & INTERPRETATION

Initial Tests (lab, imaging)

- Pap smear may incidentally detect asymptomatic lesions.
- Biopsy suspicious lesions.
- Chest x-ray (CXR): to evaluate for metastatic disease
- IV pyelogram (IVP): to evaluate for ureteral obstruction
- CT scan and MRI: to evaluate the liver and retroperitoneum, especially the lymph nodes in the pelvic and periaortic area
- Barium enema to rule out rectal invasion
- PET scan detects primary and secondary metastatic lesions more often than CT scan.

ALERT

PET scan correlation with CT scan lesions strongly suggests malignancy.

Follow-Up Tests & Special Considerations

- Lymphoscintigraphy as part of the pretreatment evaluation can result in a change in the radiation fields and improve comprehensive treatment planning in women with vaginal cancer.
- HPV vaccination: Implementation of prophylactic HPV vaccination could prevent ~2/3 of the intraepithelial lesions in the lower genital tract but is yet unproven.

Diagnostic Procedures/Other

- Colposcopy with directed biopsies for small lesions
- Wide excision under anesthesia of superficial disease may be necessary to ensure that invasive cancer is not present.
- Cystoscopy to rule out bladder invasion
- Sigmoidoscopy to rule out rectal invasion

Test Interpretation

Tumors are staged clinically:

- Stage 0: VAIN and CIS
- Stage I: carcinoma limited to the vaginal wall (26%)
- Stage II: involves the subvaginal tissues but has not extended to the pelvic wall (37%)
- Stage III: extends to the pelvic wall (24%)
- Stage IV: extends beyond the true pelvis (13%)
  - IVa: Tumor invades bladder and/or rectal mucosa and/or direct extension beyond the true pelvis.
  - IVb: spread to distant organs

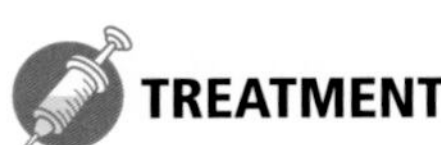

TREATMENT

GENERAL MEASURES

Treatment methods for VAIN and CIS include the following:

- Wide local excision
- Partial or total vaginectomy

- Intravaginal chemotherapy with 5% fluorouracil cream
- Laser therapy
- Intracavitary radiation therapy

MEDICATION

- Imiquimod
  - In a review of the effectiveness of 5% imiquimod cream in the treatment of VAIN, the following results were reported (4)[C]:
    - 26–100% of patients had complete regression.
    - 0–60% of patients had partial regression.
    - 0–37% experienced recurrence.
- Contraindications
  - The diagnosis must be established with certainty prior to treatment.
  - If there is any doubt that a process beyond in situ disease exists, vaginectomy must be performed. These patients are often elderly, and aggressive therapy is limited by the patient's performance status and ability to tolerate radical surgery, chemotherapy, or radiation.

ISSUES FOR REFERRAL

Patients should be treated by a gynecologic oncologist and/or a radiation oncologist.

ADDITIONAL THERAPIES

- Treatment with radiotherapy depends on the stage of disease. This treatment option should be discussed with physicians experienced with this malignancy.
- It is common to use radiotherapy and chemotherapy (chemoradiation) for better cancer control.
- Early-stage primary squamous cell carcinoma treated with radiation alone has shown good results (5)[A].
- Stage III vaginal cancer may benefit from combined radiation and hyperthermia (6)[C].
- Patients with advanced squamous cell carcinoma or adenocarcinoma receive concurrent irradiation and cisplatin-based chemotherapy (7)[B].
- Neoadjuvant chemotherapy followed by radical surgery may benefit select patients (8)[C].
- In most tumor types, metastatic disease from the vagina to other sites is only minimally responsive to chemotherapy.
- With one exception, no chemotherapeutic agents have shown a survival advantage. The exception is childhood sarcomas, which have been treated with combinations of the following:
  - Vincristine
  - Dactinomycin (actinomycin-D)
  - Cyclophosphamide (Cytoxan)
  - Cisplatin
  - Etoposide (VP-16)

SURGERY/OTHER PROCEDURES

- Whenever there is a doubt as to the presence or absence of invasive disease, vaginectomy must be performed.
- Invasive lesions usually are treated by radiation therapy, but stage I lesions can be treated with radical hysterectomy or radical vaginectomy with pelvic lymph node dissection (9)[A].
- If the lesion involves the lower vagina, inguinal node dissection also must be done because cancer involving the lower vagina can metastasize to the groin region.
- Premenopausal women who desire to retain ovarian function are better candidates for radical surgery for early-stage disease, with vaginal reconstruction possible afterward.
- Patients who have not completed their family can occasionally be treated with limited resection and localized radiation to the area.
- Sarcomas are treated by radiation therapy followed by pelvic exenteration if persistent disease is present.

Pediatric Considerations

The treatment of vaginal tumors today mainly consists of neoadjuvant chemotherapy followed by local control with surgery or radiotherapy.

Geriatric Considerations

Older patients, many with a long history of smoking, are at a higher risk for malignancies requiring surgical treatments.

ONGOING CARE

FOLLOW-UP RECOMMENDATIONS

- Patients are usually ambulatory and able to resume full activity by 6 weeks after surgery.
- Most patients are fully active while receiving chemotherapy and radiation therapy.

Patient Monitoring

- Pelvic examination and Pap smear every 3 months for 2 years, then every 6 months for the next 3 years and then yearly thereafter
- Annual CXR

PATIENT EDUCATION

- Printed patient information available from American College of Obstetricians and Gynecologists, 409 12th St., SW, Washington, DC 20024-2188; 800-762-ACOG: http://www.acog.org
- American Cancer Society: http://www.cancer.gov
- Medline Plus: http://www.nlm.nih.gov/medlineplus/vaginalcancer.html

PROGNOSIS

Stage and 5-year survival (10)

- I: 77.6%
- II: 52.2%
- III: 42.5%
- IVA: 20.5%
- IVB: 12.9%

COMPLICATIONS

- Those typically associated with major abdominal surgery or radiation therapy
- Common complications of treatment include rectovaginal or vesicovaginal fistulas, rectal/vaginal strictures, radiation cystitis, and/or proctitis.

REFERENCES

1. Siegel R, Ma J, Zou Z, et al. Cancer statistics, 2014. *CA Cancer J Clin*. 2014;64(1):9–29.
2. Daling J, Madeleine MM, Schwartz SM, et al. A population-based study of squamous cell vaginal cancer: HPV and cofactors. *Gynecol Oncol*. 2002;84(2):263–270.
3. Smith JS, Backes DM, Hoots BE, et al. Human papillomavirus type-distribution in vulvar and vaginal cancers and their associated precursors. *Obstet Gynecol*. 2009;113(4):917–924.
4. Iavazzo C, Pitsouni E, Athanasiou S, et al. Imiquimod for treatment of vulvar and vaginal intraepithelial neoplasia. *Int J Gynaecol Obstet*. 2008;101(1):3–10.
5. Tran PT, Su Z, Lee P, et al. Prognostic factors for outcomes and complications for primary squamous cell carcinoma of the vagina treated with radiation. *Gynecol Oncol*. 2007;105(3):641–649.
6. Franckena M, van der Zee J. Use of combined radiation and hyperthermia for gynecological cancer. *Curr Opin Obstet Gynecol*. 2010;22(1):9–14.
7. Dalrymple JL, Russell AH, Lee SW, et al. Chemoradiation for primary invasive squamous carcinoma of the vagina. *Int J Gynecol Cancer*. 2004;14(1):110–117.
8. Benedetti Panici P, Bellati F, Plotti F, et al. Neoadjuvant chemotherapy followed by radical surgery in patients affected by vaginal carcinoma. *Gynecol Oncol*. 2008;111(2):307–311.
9. Tjalma WA, Monaghan JM, de Barros Lopes A, et al. The role of surgery in invasive squamous carcinoma of the vagina. *Gynecol Oncol*. 2001;81(3):360–365.
10. Beller U, Benedet JL, Creasman WT, et al. Carcinoma of the vagina. FIGO 26th annual report on the results of treatment in gynecological cancer. *Int J Gynaecol Obstet*. 2006;95(Suppl 1):S29–S42.

ADDITIONAL READING

- Creasman WT. Vaginal cancers. *Curr Opin Obstet Gynecol*. 2005;17(1):71–76.
- Fernandez-Pineda I, Spunt SL, Parida L, et al. Vaginal tumors in childhood: the experience of St. Jude Children's Research Hospital. *J Pediatr Surg*. 2011;46(11):2071–2075.
- Frumovitz M, Gayed IW, Jhingran A, et al. Lymphatic mapping and sentinel lymph node detection in women with vaginal cancer. *Gynecol Oncol*. 2008;108(3):478–481.
- Gray HJ. Advances in vulvar and vaginal cancer treatment. *Gynecol Oncol*. 2010;118(1):3–5.
- Hampl M, Sarajuuri H, Wentzensen N, et al. Effect of human papillomavirus vaccines on vulvar, vaginal, and anal intraepithelial lesions and vulvar cancer. *Obstet Gynecol*. 2006;108(6):1361–1368.

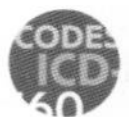

CODES

ICD10

- C52 Malignant neoplasm of vagina
- D07.2 Carcinoma in situ of vagina
- N89.3 Dysplasia of vagina, unspecified

CLINICAL PEARLS

- Vaginal cancer is rare; 85–90% of vaginal cancers are squamous cell.
- Vaginal malignancies are found most commonly on the posterior wall in the upper 1/3 of the vagina.
- Most vaginal malignancies are metastatic (from cervix, vulva, endometrium, breast, or ovary).

VAGINITIS AND VAGINOSIS

Jeremy Golding, MD, FAAFP

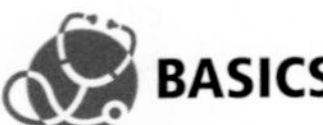

BASICS

DESCRIPTION

- Vulvovaginal candidiasis (VVC): inflammation of the vagina and vulva caused by infection with *Candida* species
- Bacterial vaginosis (BV): a polymicrobial syndrome in which the hydrogen peroxide–producing lactobacilli normally found in the vagina are replaced by other bacteria. VVC and BV are not generally considered STIs.
- Desquamative vaginitis (DV): a rare inflammatory vaginitis of unknown etiology
- Other causes of vaginitis include allergic and contact dermatitis from feminine hygiene products (fragrances, creams, douches, lubricants, and their preservatives). Atrophic vaginitis is caused by estrogen deficiency.
- A number of dermatoses, such as lichen planus, lichen sclerosus, and psoriasis, may mimic vaginitis symptoms.
- System(s) affected: reproductive; skin/exocrine
- Synonym(s): VVC: Monilial vulvovaginitis; vaginal yeast infection; BV: *Gardnerella* vaginosis; nonspecific vaginitis; *Haemophilus* vaginitis; *Corynebacterium* vaginitis

EPIDEMIOLOGY

- Both VVC and BV are common among reproductive-age females, whereas DV is more common in postmenopausal women.
- Most cases of VVC are related to *Candia albicans*, but may be caused by other *Candida* sp. (e.g., *Candida glabrata and Candida krusei*).

Prevalence

- VVC: 2nd most common cause of vaginitis after BV
  - 75% of women diagnosed at least once with VVC; up to 45% diagnosed more than once
  - <5% of females are diagnosed with recurrent VVC (defined as ≥4 episodes of VVC in 1 year).
  - Studies have shown that up to 72% of women may be colonized with *Candida* but do not exhibit symptoms of vaginitis.
- BV: Prevalence varies based on age, race/ethnicity, and socioeconomic status:
  - Most common vaginal infection among reproductive-aged women
  - The National Health and Nutrition Examination Survey (NHANES) data reported an overall prevalence of 29%, with the highest rates (50%) among black women.

Pediatric Considerations

VVC and BV are less common before the onset of puberty and after menopause.

ETIOLOGY AND PATHOPHYSIOLOGY

- VVC: Overgrowth of yeast in the vagina
- BV: Shift from a healthy lactobacilli-based endogenous flora to an anaerobically based endogenous flora, including *Gardnerella vaginalis*, *Mobiluncus* sp., *Mycoplasma hominis*, *Peptostreptococcus*, *Prevotella*, *Bacteroides*, and *Atopobium vaginae*; the rectum may be a reservoir of organisms leading to autoinfection.
- Aerobic vaginitis has been described in which lactobacilli are decreased in number and aerobic organisms including *Escherichia coli*, group B streptococci, and *Staphylococcus aureus* predominate.
- Newer data suggest that BV in not a single entity; at least 4 different microbiologic profiles have been identified.

RISK FACTORS

- VVC: diabetes mellitus (DM) with poor glycemic control, antibiotic therapy, immunosuppression (e.g., corticosteroid therapy, HIV infection), high-estrogen states (e.g., pregnancy, oral contraceptive use, hormone-replacement therapy); *C. albicans* accounts for 85–90% of vaginitis cases in pregnancy.
- BV: Black race, lower socioeconomic status, smoking, new or multiple sex partner(s), female sex partners, spermicide use, vaginal douching

GENERAL PREVENTION

- Vulvar hygiene (see "General Measures"); avoid implicated feminine hygiene products.
- Maintenance therapy for recurrent cases
- Treatment of sexual partners generally is not recommended but may be considered in recurrent cases.

COMMONLY ASSOCIATED CONDITIONS

- STIs
- Balanitis may rarely occur among male partners of females with VVC.
- Research is limited in same-sex partners. Symptomatic partners should be evaluated.

DIAGNOSIS

HISTORY

- VVC: vaginal and vulvar pruritus, vulvar pain, external dysuria, and dyspareunia; thick, curd-like vaginal discharge
- BV: 50% of women are asymptomatic. Unpleasant musty or fishy vaginal odor, exacerbated by intercourse. 10–30% may have vaginal/vulvar irritation; thin gray-white or frothy vaginal discharge
- DV: vaginal pain or burning with yellow to gray discharge, and pruritus

PHYSICAL EXAM

- VVC: thick, curd-like vaginal discharge; vulvar erythema and edema; vulvar fissures and excoriations; normal vaginal pH (<4.5)
- BV: 10–30% may have vaginal/vulvar irritation. Thin gray–white vaginal discharge is mildly adherent to vaginal walls; 10% have frothy discharge; pH >4.5
- DV: Diffuse exudative vaginitis with epithelial exfoliation without vulvar or perineal disease; pH >4.5

DIFFERENTIAL DIAGNOSIS

- Physiologic discharge and cervical ectropion
- Trichomoniasis
- Contact dermatitis
- Mechanical/chemical irritation
- Cervicitis (chlamydial or gonococcal)
- Urinary tract infection (UTI)
- Atrophic vaginitis
- Dermatoses: lichen sclerosus, lichen planus, seborrheic dermatitis, psoriasis

DIAGNOSTIC TESTS & INTERPRETATION

- Wet mount: Prepare 2 slides, both with fresh vaginal discharge: 1 with sodium chloride (NaCl) and 1 with 10% potassium hydroxide (KOH):
  - The presence of budding yeasts and hyphae consistent with VVC (may be more easily seen on KOH prep)
  - Clue cells: At least 20% of total epithelial cells considered clinically significant for diagnosis of BV (saline).
  - WBCs are not numerous in BV but may be present in large numbers in candidiasis.
  - Increased parabasal and inflammatory cells indicative of DV
- Amsel's diagnostic criteria for BV (need 3 out of 4): clue cells, characteristic vaginal discharge, vaginal pH >4.5, and positive "whiff test" (transient but potent amine or fishy odor with the addition of 10% KOH); vaginal pH also may suggest need for testing for *Trichomonas*. In cases of aerobic vaginitis, clue cells may be <20%.
- Diagnosis of DV requires all of the following: symptoms (discharge, dyspareunia, pruritus, burning, or irritation), vaginal inflammation, pH >4.5, and appropriate wet prep findings.
- Consider vaginal culture for VVC when characteristic symptoms are present, vaginal pH is normal, and no yeast are present on wet mount or to identify species if no improvement with treatment or relapse occurs within 2 months.
- Positive culture for *Candida* sp. or other yeast species may only indicate colonization; clinical correlation is required.
- VVC or BV: may be noted on cytology but must be correlated with clinical symptoms; asymptomatic women generally do not need treatment.
- DNA probe–based tests are available (Affirm VP III, Becton Dickinson, Sparks, MD), but it is unclear whether identification of the presence of yeast (or low numbers of *G. vaginalis*) indicates that the organism is the cause of symptoms. Routine use is likely not cost-effective.
- Over-the-counter tests are available that may suggest the diagnosis of BV or VVC.

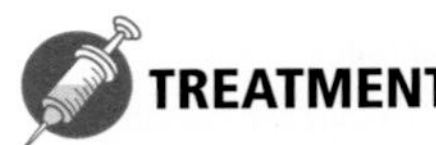

TREATMENT

GENERAL MEASURES

- Avoid douching, use of panty liners, pantyhose, occlusive pants, and undergarments.
- Regular use of condoms may help to prevent BV, as exposure to alkaline semen may trigger symptoms for some women.

MEDICATION

First Line

- VVC (1)
  - Fluconazole 150 mg PO once; use with caution in patients with liver disease and with coadministration of other drugs.
    - Short-course therapy with topical azoles is effective in 80–90% of patients.
  - Many topical therapies are available over the counter:
    - Butoconazole 2% cream 5 g intravaginally × 3 days
    - Clotrimazole 1% cream 5 g intravaginally daily × 7–14 days *or* 2% cream 5 g intravaginally daily × 3 days
    - Miconazole 2% cream 5 g intravaginally daily × 7 days; *or* 4% cream 5 g intravaginally daily × 3 days; *or* 100 mg vaginal suppository, 1 suppository daily × 7 days; *or* 200 mg vaginal suppository, 1 suppository daily × 3 days; *or* 1,200 mg vaginal suppository, 1 suppository × 1 day
    - Tioconazole 6.5% ointment 5 g intravaginally in a single application

- Prescription therapies include the following:
  - Butoconazole 2% cream (single-dose bioadhesive) 5 g intravaginally × single application
  - Nystatin 100,000-unit vaginal tablet, 1 tablet daily × 14 days
  - Terconazole 0.4% cream 5 g intravaginally daily × 7 days; *or* 0.8% cream 5 g intravaginally daily × 3 days; *or* 80 mg vaginal suppository, 1 suppository daily × 3 days
- BV
  - Metronidazole (Flagyl) 500 mg PO BID × 7 days *or*
  - Metronidazole 0.75% vaginal gel 5 g intravaginally daily × 5 days
    - 85–90% of women respond to initial treatment; however, recurrence rates may be as high as 80%.
  - Clindamycin 300 mg PO BID × 7 days
    - Antibiotic resistance against clindamycin and metronidazole has been reported and may be responsible for some cases of recurrent BV.
- DV (2)
  - Clindamycin 2% vaginal gel 4–5 g daily × 4–6 weeks
  - Hydrocortisone 10% 3–5 g daily × 4–6 weeks

ALERT
Oil-based preparations may weaken latex condoms.

Second Line

- VVC
  - Recurrent VVC: Obtain cultures. Infections associated with *C. glabrata* (5–15%) are less responsive to 1st-line therapies.
  - Consider longer duration therapy (7–14 days of topical or oral fluconazole every 3rd day for a total of 3 doses).
  - Suppressive maintenance therapy (oral fluconazole weekly × 6 months or topical treatments weekly)
  - Women with recurrent candidiasis may benefit from fluconazole 150 mg/week plus cetirizine 10 mg/day for allergy or itching.
  - Boric acid: 600 mg gelatin capsule inserted vaginally daily × 2 weeks (indicated for non-*albicans* disease; 70% clinical and mycologic cure rate)
- BV
  - Metronidazole 2 g PO single dose (less effective than alternative regimens)
  - Clindamycin cream 2%, 5g intravaginally HS × 7days
  - Clindamycin ovules 100 mg intravaginally at bedtime × 3 days
  - Tinidazole 2 g PO daily for 2 days or 1 g PO once daily for 5 days are options for patients who do not tolerate metronidazole or have difficulty with compliance.
  - Regimens for treating recurrent BV involve use of metronidazole PO × 7 days and vaginal boric acid 600 mg × 21 days.

ALERT
Avoid any alcohol-containing product while taking metronidazole.

Pregnancy Considerations

- VVC: Topical therapy preferred over oral therapy
- BV: Associated with preterm delivery; however, it is unclear whether the treatment of BV prevents preterm delivery. All symptomatic women should be treated; screening is reserved for women at high risk for preterm delivery. Avoid creams; metronidazole 500 mg PO BID × 7 days or clindamycin 300 mg PO BID × 7 days. Package labeling of metronidazole indicates that it is contraindicated in the 1st trimester of pregnancy, but this is not supported by recent meta-analyses of available data.

ISSUES FOR REFERRAL

Treating male sexual partners does not reduce symptoms or prevent recurrence, but this may be considered in patients who have recurrent infection.

COMPLEMENTARY & ALTERNATIVE MEDICINE

- A Cochrane analysis reviewed the use of probiotics for BV and found inconclusive evidence to recommend probiotics as primary treatment or as a preventive strategy (3)[A]. Further study was recommended.
- Acidification of the vagina has not been proven beneficial.

ONGOING CARE

FOLLOW-UP RECOMMENDATIONS

- Delay sexual relations until symptoms clear/discomfort resolves.
- Use of condoms may reduce recurrence of BV.

Patient Monitoring

- Generally, no specific follow-up needed; if symptoms persist or recur within 2 months, repeat pelvic exam and culture.
- Consider suppressive therapy for women with recurrent infection.

DIET

Reduction of sugar intake has been recommended but is not supported by evidence.

PATIENT EDUCATION

- American College of Obstetricians and Gynecologists (ACOG), 409 12th St., SW, Washington, DC 20024-2188; 800-762-ACOG: www.acog.org
- American Academy of Family Physicians: www.familydoctor.org

PROGNOSIS

VVC: 80–90% of uncomplicated cases cured with appropriate treatment; 30–50% of recurrent infections return after discontinuation of maintenance therapy; there is a relatively high spontaneous remission rate of untreated symptoms as well.

COMPLICATIONS

- VVC may occur following treatment of BV.
- BV has been associated with an increased risk of acquisition and transmission of STIs, including HIV.
- BV has been associated with increased risk of pregnancy complications, including preterm birth, chorioamnionitis, postpartum and postabortal endometritis, and pelvic inflammatory disease.

REFERENCES

1. Hainer BL, Gibson MV. Vaginitis. *Am Fam Physician*. 2011;83:807–815.
2. Sobel JD, Reichman O, Misra D, et al. Prognosis and treatment of desquamative inflammatory vaginitis. *Obstet Gynecol*. 2011;117(4):850–855.
3. Senok AC, Verstraelen H, Temmerman M, et al. Probiotics for the treatment of bacterial vaginosis. *Cochrane Database Syst Rev*. 2009;(4):CD006289.

ADDITIONAL READING

- American Congress of Obstetricians and Gynecologists (ACOG) FAQ028, Aug. 2011. www.acog.org/~/media/For%20Patients/faq028.pdf?dmc=1&ts=20131111T1039456914
- Donders G. Diagnosis and management of bacterial vaginosis and other types of abnormal vaginal bacterial flora: a review. *Obstet Gynecol Surv*. 2010;65(7):462–473.
- Li J, McCormick J, Bocking A, et al. Importance of vaginal microbes in reproductive health. *Reprod Sci*. 2012;19(3):235–242.
- Pappas PG, Kauffman CA, Andes D, et al. Clinical practice guidelines for the management of candidiasis: 2009 update by the Infectious Disease Society of America. *Clin Infect Dis*. 2009;48(5):503–535.
- Ray D, Goswami R, Banerjee U, et al. Prevalence of *Candida glabrata* and its response to boric acid vaginal suppositories in comparison with oral fluconazole in patients with diabetes and vulvovaginal candidiasis. *Diabetes Care*. 2007;30(2):312–317.
- Workowski KA, Berman S, Centers for Disease Control and Prevention (CDC), et al. Sexually transmitted diseases treatment guidelines, 2010. *MMWR Recomm Rep*. 2010;59(RR-12):1–110.

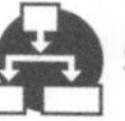

SEE ALSO

Algorithm: Discharge, Vaginal

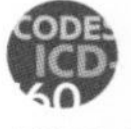

CODES

ICD10

- N76.0 Acute vaginitis
- B37.3 Candidiasis of vulva and vagina
- N95.2 Postmenopausal atrophic vaginitis

CLINICAL PEARLS

- Clinical symptoms, signs, and microscopy have relatively poor performance compared with so-called gold standards such as culture and DNA probe assays, but these more sensitive assays can detect organisms that may not be causing symptoms.
- Most women experience relief of symptoms with therapy chosen without such gold standard tests, even when the treatment does not correspond with the underlying infection.
- Vaginal pH is underused as a diagnostic tool for evaluation of vaginitis.
- Treatment of sexual partners is not currently the standard of care for either BV or VVC.

VARICOSE VEINS

Joseph A. Florence, MD • Thomas R. Avonda, MD

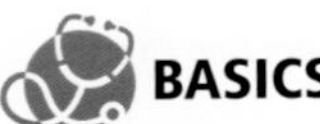

BASICS

DESCRIPTION

- Superficial venous disease causing a permanent dilatation and tortuosity of superficial veins, usually occurring in the legs and feet; caused by systemic weakness in the vein wall and may result from congenitally incomplete valves or valves that have become incompetent
- Affects legs where reverse flow occurs when dependent
- Truncal varices involve the great and small saphenous veins; branch varicosities involve the saphenous vein tributaries.
- Categorized as the following:
  - Uncomplicated (cosmetic)
  - With local symptoms (pain confined to the varices, not diffuse)
  - With local complications (superficial thrombophlebitis, may rupture causing bleeding)
  - Complex varicose disease (diffuse limb pain, swelling, skin changes/ulcer)
- System(s) affected: cardiovascular; skin

ALERT

Ulceration of varicose veins has a high rate of infection, which can lead to sepsis.

Geriatric Considerations

- Common; usually valvular degeneration but may be secondary to chronic venous deficiency
- Elastic support hose and frequent rests with legs elevated rather than ligation and stripping

Pregnancy Considerations

- Frequent problem
- Elastic stockings are recommended for those with a history of varicosities or if prolonged standing is involved.

EPIDEMIOLOGY

Incidence

- Predominant age: middle age
- Predominant gender: female > male (2:1)
- National Women's Health Information Center estimates that 50% of women have varicose veins.

ETIOLOGY AND PATHOPHYSIOLOGY

- Varicose veins are caused by venous insufficiency from faulty valves in ≥1 perforator veins in the lower leg, causing secondary incompetence at the saphenofemoral junction (valvular reflux).
- Valvular dysfunction causing venous reflux and subsequently venous hypertension (HTN)
- Failed valves allow blood to flow in the reverse direction (away from the heart), from deep to superficial and from proximal to distal veins.
- Deep thrombophlebitis
- Increased venous pressure from any cause
- Congenital valvular incompetence
- Trauma (consider arteriovenous fistula; listen for bruit)
- Presumed to be due to a loss in vein wall elasticity with failure of the valve leaflets
- An increase in venous filling pressure is sufficient to promote varicose remodeling of veins by augmenting wall stress and activating venous endothelial and smooth muscle cells (1).

Genetics

Autosomal dominant with incomplete penetrance

RISK FACTORS

- Increasing age
- Pregnancy, especially multiple pregnancies
- Prolonged standing
- Obesity
- History of phlebitis (postthrombotic syndrome)
- Family history
- Female sex
- Increased height
- Congenital valvular dysfunction

COMMONLY ASSOCIATED CONDITIONS

- Stasis dermatitis
- Large varicose veins may lead to skin changes and eventual stasis ulceration.

DIAGNOSIS

HISTORY

- Symptoms range from minor annoyance/cosmetic problem to a lifestyle-limiting problem.
- Localized symptoms: pain, burning, itching
- Generalized symptoms
  - Leg muscular cramp, aching
  - Leg fatigue/swelling
- Pain if varicose ulcer develops
- Symptoms often worse at the end of the day, especially after prolonged standing
- Women are more prone to symptoms due to hormonal influences: worse during menses.
- No direct correlation with the severity of varicose veins and the severity of symptoms

PHYSICAL EXAM

- Inspect lower extremities while the patient is standing. Varicose veins in the proximal femoral ring and distal portion of the legs may not be visible when the patient is supine.
- Varicose veins are the following:
  - Dilated, tortuous, superficial veins, chiefly in the lower extremities
  - Dark purple/blue in color, raised above the surface of the skin
  - Often twisted, bulging, and can look like cords
  - Most commonly found on the posterior/medial lower extremity
- Edema of the affected limb may be present.
- Skin changes may include the following:
  - Eczema
  - Hyperpigmentation
  - Lipodermatosclerosis
- Spider veins (idiopathic telangiectases)
  - Fine intracutaneous angiectasis
  - May be extensive/unsightly
- Neurologic sensory and motor exam
- Peripheral arterial vasculature; pulses
- Musculoskeletal exam for associated rheumatologic/orthopedic issues

DIFFERENTIAL DIAGNOSIS

- Nerve root compression
- Arthritis
- Peripheral neuritis
- Telangiectasia: smaller, visible blood vessels that are permanently dilated
- Deep vein thrombosis
- Inflammatory liposclerosis

DIAGNOSTIC TESTS & INTERPRETATION

Duplex ultrasound: Noninvasive imaging duplex ultrasound will confirm the etiology, anatomy, and pathophysiology of segmental venous reflux. The severity of both symptoms and signs tends to correlate with the degree of venous reflux, which is identified by duplex ultrasound as retrograde or reversed flow of greater than 0.5 seconds duration (2).

Diagnostic Procedures/Other

Duplex scanning, venous Doppler study, photoplethysmography, light-reflection rheography, air plethysmography, and other vascular testing should be reserved for patients who have venous symptoms and/or large (>4 mm in diameter) vessels or large numbers of spider telangiectasia indicating venous HTN.

Test Interpretation

A clinical classification illustrating the current physical state is useful in clinical practice (1).

- 0: no visible or palpable signs of venous disease
- 1: spider veins or telangiectasias
- 2: varicose veins
- 3: edema
- 4: skin changes (pigmentation, eczema, lipodermatosclerosis, atrophie blanche)
- 5: healed ulcer
- 6: active ulcer

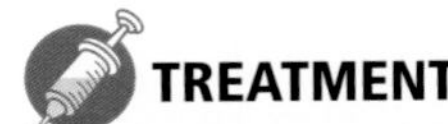

TREATMENT

- Conventional wisdom suggests conservative therapy (e.g., elevation, external compression, weight loss) as being helpful; however, there is insufficient, high-quality evidence to determine whether or not compression stockings are effective as the sole and initial treatment of varicose veins in people without healed or active venous ulceration, or whether any type of stocking is superior to any other type (3)[A].
- All the current modalities of endoluminal and open surgical treatment have similar short-term outcomes and risks (4)[A].
- Appropriate surgical treatment has the best long-term outcomes and evidence base (4)[A].
- Treatment of choice, however, depends on many factors, including local expertise (4)[A].
- When comparing quality of life, pain relief, and long-term relief, surgery is favored (5)[A].
- Endovenous laser ablation (EVLA); radiofrequency ablation, foam sclerotherapy, and surgical stripping for great saphenous varicose veins are all efficacious (6)[A].
- Endovenous ablation (radiofrequency and laser) is at least as effective as surgery in the treatment of great saphenous varicose veins; however, ultrasound-guided foam sclerotherapy has insufficient support from available data (6)[A].
- The ambulatory conservative hemodynamic correction of venous insufficiency method (cure conservatrice et hémodynamique de l'insuffisance veineuse en ambulatoire [CHIVA]) is a less-invasive approach based on venous hemodynamics with deliberate preservation of the superficial venous system. The CHIVA method reduces recurrence of varicose veins and produces fewer side effects than vein stripping (7)[A].

GENERAL MEASURES

Patients with unsightly varicose veins often seek treatment for cosmetic reasons.

MEDICATION

Superficial thrombophlebitis is not an infective condition and does not require antibiotic treatment.

ISSUES FOR REFERRAL

- Emergency: bleeding from a varicosity that has eroded the skin
- Urgent: varicosity that has bled and is at risk for bleeding again
- Soon: ulcer that is progressive/painful despite treatment
- Routine
  - Active/healed ulcer/progressive skin changes that may benefit from surgery
  - Recurrent superficial thrombophlebitis
  - Troublesome symptoms attributable to varicose veins or patient and provider feel that the extent, site, and size of the varicosities are having a severe impact on quality of life.

ADDITIONAL THERAPIES

- Apply elastic stockings before lowering legs from the bed.
- Activity
  - Frequent rest periods with legs elevated
  - If standing is necessary, frequently shift weight from side to side.
  - Appropriate exercise routine as part of conservative treatment
  - Walking regimen after sclerotherapy is important to help promote healing.
  - Never sit with legs hanging down.
- Physical therapy

SURGERY/OTHER PROCEDURES

- Surgery
  - Improved quality-adjusted life-years and symptoms compared to conservative management at 2 years (1)[A]
  - Surgery is indicated if there is pain, recurrent phlebitis, or skin changes/ulceration or for cosmetic improvement for severe cases.
  - Minimally invasive techniques include the following:
    - Radiofrequency ablation (RFA): compared with surgery provides a faster return to work; less pain, better short-term quality of life; less bruising and tenderness compared with endovenous laser therapy (1)[A]
    - Endovenous microwave ablation (EMA) is an effective new technique for the treatment of varicose veins and had a more satisfactory clinical outcome than high ligation and stripping (HLS) in the short term (8)[A].
    - EVLA is as effective as conventional surgery (CS) and superior to ultrasound-guided foam sclerotherapy (UGFS), according to occlusion on ultrasound duplex (9)[B].
    - Quality of life improves after treatment in all groups (EVLA, CS, UGFS), significantly (9)[B].
    - There is no significant difference between EVLA and open surgery in patients with great saphenous vein incompetence (10)[A].
- Sclerotherapy is a simple, safe, and particularly effective for smaller, early varicosities and also for residual veins after surgery (11)[C].
- Radiotherapy
  - RFA takes longer to perform but has better early outcome than CS in patients with great saphenous varicose veins.
  - Radiofrequency and laser treatments replace "stripping"; however, most varicosities still require phlebectomy/sclerotherapy.

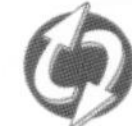

ONGOING CARE

DIET

- No special diet
- Weight-loss diet is recommended if obesity is a problem.

PATIENT EDUCATION

- Avoid long periods of standing and crossing legs when sitting.
- Exercise (walking, running) regularly to improve leg strength and circulation.
- Maintain an appropriate weight.
- Wear elastic support stockings.
- Avoid clothing that constricts legs.
- Surgery/sclerotherapy may not prevent development of varicosities, and the procedure may need to be repeated in later years.
- National Heart, Lung and Blood Institute, Communications and Public Information Branch, National Institutes of Health, Building 31, Room 41–21, 9000 Rockville Pike, Bethesda, MD 20892; 301-496-4236. www.nhlbi.nih.gov

PROGNOSIS

- Usual course: chronic
- Favorable with appropriate treatment
- Surgery has a nonsignificant reduction in the risk of varicose vein recurrence compared with liquid sclerotherapy and endoluminal interventions (6)[A].
- Increasing disease severity by venous clinical severity score (VCSS) is associated with reductions in quality of life (12)[B].

COMPLICATIONS

- Complications with sclerotherapy include hyperpigmentation, matting, local urticaria, cutaneous necrosis, microthrombi, accidental intra-arterial injection, phlebitis, deep vein thrombosis, thromboembolism, scintillating scotomas, nerve damage, and allergic reactions.
- Petechial hemorrhages
- Chronic edema
- Superimposed infection
- Varicose ulcers
- Pigmentation
- Eczema
- Recurrence after surgical treatment
- Scarring/nerve damage from stripping technique
- Neurologic complications after sclerotherapy are rare (6)[B].

REFERENCES

1. Hamdan A. Management of varicose veins and venous insufficiency. *JAMA*. 2012;308(24):2612–2621.
2. Coleridge-Smith P, Labropoulos N, Partsch H, et al. Duplex ultrasound investigation of the veins in chronic venous disease of the lower limbs—UIP consensus document. Part I. Basic principles. *Eur J Vasc Endovasc Surg*. 2006;31(1):83–92.
3. Shingler S, Robertson L, Boghossian S, et al. Compression stockings for the initial treatment of varicose veins in patients without venous ulceration. *Cochrane Database Syst Rev*. 2013;(12):CD008819.
4. Wright N, Fitridge R. Varicose veins—natural history, assessment and management. *Aust Fam Physician*. 2013;42(6):380–384.
5. Kistner RL, Eklof B, Masuda EM. Diagnosis of chronic venous disease of the lower extremities: the "CEAP" classification. *Mayo Clin Proc*. 1996;71(4):338–345.
6. Nesbitt C, Eifell RK, Coyne P, et al. Endovenous ablation (radiofrequency and laser) and foam sclerotherapy versus conventional surgery for great saphenous vein varices. *Cochrane Database Syst Rev*. 2011;(10):CD005624.
7. Bellmunt-Montoya S, Escribano JM, Dilme J, et al. CHIVA method for the treatment of chronic venous insufficiency. *Cochrane Database Syst Rev*. 2013;(7):CD009648.
8. Yang L, Wang XP, Su WJ, et al. Randomized clinical trial of endovenous microwave ablation combined with high ligation versus conventional surgery for varicose veins. *Eur J Vasc Endovasc Surg*. 2013;46(4):473–479.
9. Biemans AA, Kockaert M, Akkersdijk GP, et al. Comparing endovenous laser ablation, foam sclerotherapy, and conventional surgery for great saphenous varicose veins. *J Vasc Surg*. 2013;58(3):727–734.e1.
10. Rasmussen L, Lawaetz M, Bjoern L, et al. Randomized clinical trial comparing endovenous laser ablation and stripping of the great saphenous vein with clinical and duplex outcome after 5 years. *J Vasc Surg*. 2013;58(2):421–426.
11. Subbarao NT, Aradhya SS, Veerabhadrappa NH. Sclerotherapy in the management of varicose veins and its dermatological complications. *Indian J Dermatol Venereol Leprol*. 2013;79(3):383–388.
12. Lozano Sánchez FS, Sánchez Nevarez I, González-Porras JR, et al. Quality of life in patients with chronic venous disease: influence of the socio-demographical and clinical factors. *Int Angiol*. 2013;32(4):433–441.

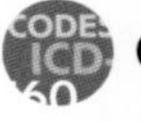

CODES

ICD10

- I83.90 Asymptomatic varicose veins of unspecified lower extremity
- I83.009 Varicose veins of unsp lower extremity w ulcer of unsp site
- I83.10 Varicose veins of unsp lower extremity with inflammation

CLINICAL PEARLS

- Long-term safety and efficacy of surgery for the treatment of varicose veins is supported by low-quality evidence. Less-invasive treatments, which are associated with less periprocedural disability and pain, are supported by short-term studies (3)[A].
- Endovascular treatment of varicose veins is safe and effective and has a rapid recovery (6)[A]. Insufficient evidence exists to prefer sclerotherapy over surgery (5)[A].
- The efficacy of sclerotherapy is not significantly affected by the choice of sclerosant, dose, formulation (foam vs. liquid), local pressure dressing, or degree and length of compression (5)[A].

V

VASCULITIS

Irene J. Tan, MD, FACR

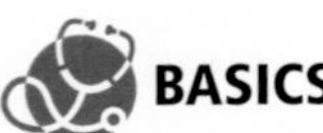

BASICS

DESCRIPTION

Vasculitis is an inflammatory disease of the blood vessels.

- Clinical features result from the destruction of blood vessel walls with subsequent thrombosis, ischemia, bleeding, and/or aneurysm formation.
- Vasculitis consists of a large, heterogeneous group of diseases classified by the predominant size, type, and the location of involved blood vessels (1).
  - Small-vessel vasculitis
    - Microscopic polyangiitis (MPA)
    - Granulomatosis with polyangiitis (GPA, formerly Wegener granulomatosis)
    - Eosinophilic granulomatosis with polyangiitis (EGPA; formerly Churg-Strauss syndrome)
    - Antiglomerular basement membrane disease (anti-GBM)
    - Cryoglobulinemic vasculitis
    - IgA vasculitis (Henoch-Schönlein purpura [HSP])
    - Hypocomplementemic urticarial vasculitis
  - Medium-vessel vasculitis
    - Polyarteritis nodosa (PAN)
    - Kawasaki disease (KD)
  - Large-vessel vasculitis
    - Takayasu arteritis (TAK)
    - Giant cell arteritis (GCA)
- Vasculitis occurs as a primary disorder or secondary to infection, a drug reaction, malignancy, or connective tissue disease.
  - Variable vessel vasculitis
    - Behçet disease
    - Cogan syndrome
  - Single-organ vasculitis
    - Cutaneous leukocytoclastic angiitis
    - Cutaneous arteritis
    - Primary CNS vasculitis
  - Vasculitis associated with systemic disease
    - Lupus vasculitis
    - Rheumatoid vasculitis
    - Sarcoid vasculitis
  - Vasculitis associated with other etiology
    - Hepatitis C–associated cryoglobulinemic vasculitis
    - Hepatitis B–associated vasculitis
    - Syphilis-associated aortitis
    - Drug-induced immune complex vasculitis
    - Drug-associated antineutrophil cytoplasmic antibodies (ANCA)–associated vasculitis
    - Cancer-associated vasculitis
- Protean features often delay definitive diagnosis.

EPIDEMIOLOGY

Highly variable, depending on the vasculitic syndrome

- *Hypersensitivity vasculitis is the most commonly encountered vasculitis in clinical practice.*
- KD, IgA vasculitis, and dermatomyositis are more common in children.
- TAK is most prevalent in young Asian women. GPA, MPA, and EGPA are more common in middle-aged males.
- GCA occurs exclusively in those >50 years of age and is rare in the African American population.

Incidence

The annual incidence in adults unless otherwise specified:

- IgA vasculitis: 200–700/1 million in children <17 years of age
- GCA: 170/1 million
- KD: depends on race/age; ~170/1 million
- PAN: 2–33/1 million
- GPA: 4–15/1 million
- MPA: 1–24/1 million
- EGPA: 1–3/1 million
- TAK: 2/1 million
- Hypersensitivity vasculitis: depends on drug exposure patterns
- Viral-/retroviral-associated vasculitis: unknown; >90% of cases of cryoglobulinemic vasculitis are associated with hepatitis C.
- Connective tissue disorder–associated vasculitis: variable

ETIOLOGY AND PATHOPHYSIOLOGY

- 3 major immunopathogenic mechanisms
  - Immune-complex formation: systemic lupus erythematosus (SLE), IgA vasculitis (HSP), and cryoglobulinemic vasculitis
  - ANCAs: GPA, MPA, and EGPA
  - Pathogenic T-lymphocyte response: giant cell arteritis and Takayasu arteritis
- Pathophysiology best understood where known drug triggers have been identified (e.g., antibiotics, sulfonamides, and hydralazine)

Genetics

- A number of the vasculitic syndromes have been linked to candidate genes.
- No single gene has been found to cause vasculitis.
- Angiotensin-converting enzyme insertion/deletion polymorphism is associated with susceptibility to vasculitis, especially in Behçet disease and IgA vasculitis.

RISK FACTORS

A combination of genetic susceptibility and environmental exposure most likely to trigger onset of vasculitis.

GENERAL PREVENTION

- None
- Early identification is the key to prevent irreversible organ damage in severe forms of systemic vasculitis.

COMMONLY ASSOCIATED CONDITIONS

Hepatitis C (cryoglobulinemic vasculitis), hepatitis B (PAN), cytomegalovirus (CMV), Epstein-Barr virus (EBV), HIV (viral-/retroviral-associated vasculitis), SLE, rheumatoid arthritis (RA), Sjögren syndrome, mixed connective tissue disease (MCTD), dermatomyositis, ankylosing spondylitis, Behçet disease, relapsing polychondritis (CTD-associated vasculitis), respiratory tract methicillin-resistant *Staphylococcus aureus* (MRSA) (GPA)

DIAGNOSIS

HISTORY

- Consider patient's age, sex, and ethnicity.
- Comprehensive medication history
- Family history of vasculitis
- Constitutional symptoms: fever, weight loss, malaise, fatigue, diminished appetite, sweats
- CNS: mononeuritis multiplex, polyneuropathy, headaches, visual loss, tinnitus, stroke, seizure, encephalopathy
- Heart/lung: myocardial infarction, cardiomyopathy, pericarditis, cough, chest pain, hemoptysis, dyspnea
- Renal: hematuria
- GI: abdominal pain, hematochezia, perforation
- Musculoskeletal: arthralgia, myalgia
- Miscellaneous: unexplained ischemic or hemorrhagic events, chronic sinusitis, and recurrent epistaxis
- Note the organs affected and estimate the size of blood vessels involved.
- Demographics, clinical features, and the predominant vessel size/organ involvement help identify specific type of vasculitis.

PHYSICAL EXAM

- Vital signs: blood pressure (hypertension) and pulse (regularity and rate)
- Skin: palpable purpura, livedo reticularis, nodules, ulcers, gangrene, nail bed capillary changes
- Neurologic: cranial nerve exam, sensorimotor exam
- Ocular exam: visual fields, scleritis, episcleritis
- Cardiopulmonary exam: rubs, murmurs, arrhythmias
- Abdominal exam: tenderness, organomegaly

DIFFERENTIAL DIAGNOSIS

- Fibromuscular dysplasia
- Embolic disease (atheroma, cholesterol emboli, atrial myxoma, mycotic aneurysm with embolization)
- Vasospasm, drug-induced (cocaine, amphetamines, ergots)
- Thrombotic thrombocytopenic disorders (disseminated intravascular coagulation [DIC], thrombotic thrombocytopenic purpura [TTP], antiphospholipid syndrome, heparin- or warfarin-induced thrombosis)
- Systemic infection (infective endocarditis, fungal infections, disseminated gonococcal infection, Lyme disease, syphilis, Rocky Mountain spotted fever [RMSF], bacteremia)
- Malignancy (lymphomatoid granulomatosis, angioimmunoblastic T-cell lymphoma, intravascular lymphoma)
- Miscellaneous (Goodpasture syndrome, sarcoidosis, amyloidosis, Whipple disease, congenital coarctation of aorta)

DIAGNOSTIC TESTS & INTERPRETATION

ALERT

- Renal involvement is often clinically silent. Therefore, routine serum creatinine and urinalysis with microscopy are needed to identify underlying glomerulonephritis.
- Initial tests to exclude alternate diagnosis and guide appropriate therapy
- Routine tests
  - CBC
  - Liver enzymes
  - Serum creatinine
  - Urinalysis with microscopy
- Specific serology
  - Antinuclear antibodies (ANA)
  - Rheumatoid factor (RF)
  - Rapid plasma reagin/venereal disease reaction level (RPR/VDRL)
  - RMSF titer
  - Lyme test
  - Complements C3, C4
  - ANCA
  - Anti–proteinase 3 antibodies (anti-PR3)
  - Antimyeloperoxidase antibodies (anti-MPO)
  - Hepatitis screen for B and C
  - Cryoglobulin

- Antiglomerular basement membrane titer
  - HIV
  - Serum protein electrophoresis
- Miscellaneous
  - Drug screen
  - ESR
  - C-reactive protein
  - Creatine kinase (CK)
  - Blood culture
  - ECG
- CXR, CT scan, MRI, and arteriography may be required to delineate extent of organs involved.

Diagnostic Procedures/Other

- Electromyography with nerve conduction studies may be useful for documenting neuropathy and to target affected nerve for biopsy.
- Biopsy of affected site confirms diagnosis (e.g., temporal artery, sural nerve, renal biopsy).
- If biopsy is not practical, angiography may be diagnostic for large- and medium-vessel vasculitides.
- Bronchoscopy may be required to differentiate pulmonary infection from potentially life-threatening hemorrhagic vasculitis in patients with hemoptysis.

Test Interpretation

Blood vessel biopsy shows immune cell infiltration into vessel wall layers with varying degrees of necrosis and granuloma formation, depending on the type of vasculitis.

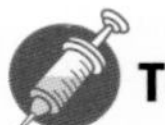

TREATMENT

GENERAL MEASURES

- Discontinue the offending drug for hypersensitivity vasculitis.
- Simple observation for mild cases of IgA vasculitis

MEDICATION

First Line

Corticosteroids are the initial systemic anti-inflammatory of choice.

Second Line

Cytotoxic medications, immunomodulatory, or biologic agents (e.g., cyclophosphamide (2)[B],(4,5)[A] methotrexate (3,5)[A], azathioprine (3,5)[A], leflunomide (5)[A], mycophenolate mofetil (2)[B],(5)[A], and rituximab (4,5)[A], are often required in combination with corticosteroids for rapidly progressive vasculitis with significant organ involvement or inadequate response to corticosteroids.

ISSUES FOR REFERRAL

- Rheumatology referral for complicated cases where newer or more toxic treatments are required
- Nephrology referral for persistent hematuria or proteinuria, rising creatinine, or a positive ANCA titer
- Pulmonary referral for persistent pulmonary infiltrate unresponsive to antibiotic therapy or gross hemoptysis

ADDITIONAL THERAPIES

- IVIG and aspirin for KD, but corticosteroids are contraindicated
- Plasma exchange appears to improve recovery of patients with severe acute renal failure secondary to vasculitis and pulmonary hemorrhage (5)[A].

SURGERY/OTHER PROCEDURES

Rarely, corrective surgery is required to repair tissue damage as a result of aggressive vasculitis.

INPATIENT CONSIDERATIONS

Admission Criteria/Initial Stabilization

- Hemoptysis, acute renal failure, intestinal ischemia, any organ-threatening symptoms or signs, and/or need for biopsy
- Initial therapy is guided by the organ system involved.
  - If pulmonary hemorrhage is present, life-saving measures may include mechanical ventilation, plasmapheresis, and immunosuppression.
  - If acute renal failure is present, electrolyte and fluid balance, as well as plasma exchange and immunosuppression should be considered.
  - If signs of intestinal ischemia are present, patient should be NPO and be considered for plasmapheresis, immunosuppression, and parenteral nutrition.

Discharge Criteria

Stabilization or resolution of potential life-threatening symptoms

ONGOING CARE

FOLLOW-UP RECOMMENDATIONS

If significant coronary artery disease is involved in KD, moderate activity restriction may be of benefit.

Patient Monitoring

Frequent clinical follow-up supported by patient self-monitoring to identify disease relapse

DIET

Diets should be specifically altered for patients with renal involvement or those with hyperglycemia/dyslipidemia as a result of therapeutic corticosteroids.

PROGNOSIS

Prognosis is good for those patients with vasculitis and limited organ involvement. Relapsing courses, renal, intestinal, or extensive lung involvement have a poorer prognosis.

COMPLICATIONS

- Persistent organ dysfunction may be the result of the disease, medications, or inflammation/scarring in the more serious forms of vasculitis.
- Early morbidity/mortality is due to active vasculitic disease; delayed morbidity/mortality may also be secondary to complications of chronic therapy with cytotoxic medications.

REFERENCES

1. Jennette JC, Falk RJ, Bacon PA, et al. 2012 revised International Chapel Hill Consensus Conference nomenclature of vasculitides. *Arthritis Rheum*. 2013;65(1):1–11.
2. Appel GB, Contreras G, Dooley MA, et al. Mycophenolate mofetil versus cyclophosphamide for induction treatment of lupus nephritis. *J Am Soc Nephrol*. 2009;20(5):1103–1112.
3. Bosch X, Guilabert A, Espinosa G, et al. Treatment of antineutrophil cytoplasmic antibody associated vasculitis: a systematic review. *JAMA*. 2007;298(6):655–669.
4. Stone JH, Merkel PA, Spiera R, et al. Rituximab versus cyclophosphamide for ANCA-associated vasculitis. *N Engl J Med*. 2010;363(3):221–232.
5. Walters GD, Willis NS, Craig JC. Interventions for renal vasculitis in adults. A systematic review. *BMC Nephrol*. 2010;11:12.

ADDITIONAL READING

- Bertsias G, Ioannidis JP, Boletis J, et al. EULAR recommendations for the management of systemic lupus erythematosus. Report of a Task Force of the EULAR Standing Committee for International Clinical Studies Including Therapeutics. *Ann Rheum Dis*. 2008;67(2):195–205.
- Gatto M, Iaccarino L, Canova M, et al. Pregnancy and vasculitis: a systematic review of the literature. *Autoimmun Rev*. 2012;11(6–7):A447–A459.
- Lee YH, Choi SJ, Ji JD, et al. Associations between the angiotensin-converting enzyme insertion/deletion polymorphism and susceptibility to vasculitis: a meta-analysis. *J Renin Angiotensin Aldosterone Syst*. 2012;13(1):196–201.
- National Heart Lung and Blood Institute Diseases and Conditions Index: Vasculitis: http://www.nhlbi.nih.gov/health/health-topics/topics/vas. Accessed 2014.
- Vasculitis Foundation: www.vasculitisfoundation.org/
- Walters GD, Willis NS, Craig JC. Interventions for renal vasculitis in adults. A systematic review. *BMC Nephrol*. 2010;11:12.
- Weiss PF, Feinstein JA, Luan X, et al. Effects of corticosteroid on Henoch-Schönlein purpura: a systematic review. *Pediatrics*. 2007;120(5):1079–1087.
- Wood L, Tulloh R. Kawasaki disease: diagnosis, management and cardiac sequelae. *Expert Rev Cardiovasc Ther*. 2007;5(3):553–561.

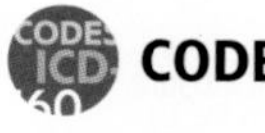

CODES

ICD10

- I77.6 Arteritis, unspecified
- M31.30 Wegener's granulomatosis without renal involvement
- M30.0 Polyarteritis nodosa

CLINICAL PEARLS

- Suspect vasculitis in patients with a petechial rash, palpable purpura, glomerulonephritis, pulmonary-renal syndrome, intestinal ischemia, or mononeuritis multiplex.
- Exclude silent renal involvement by obtaining serum creatinine and urinalysis with microscopy.
- Vasculitis has "skip" lesions, which may complicate diagnostic biopsy.
- In patients with vasculitis, look for a primary process such as infection, thrombosis, or malignancy.

VENOUS INSUFFICIENCY ULCERS

Barbara J. Provo, MSN, FNP-BC, CWON • Rishi Esvy Subbarayan, MD

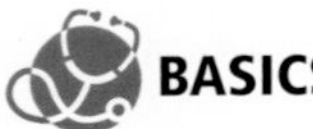

BASICS

- Venous insufficiency disorders include simple spider veins, varicose veins, and leg edema.
- In the United States, 23% of adults have varicose veins, an estimated 22 million women and 11 million men.
- Venous leg ulcers are the most serious consequence of venous insufficiency.
- 500,000 people in the United States have chronic venous ulcers, with an estimated treatment cost of >$3 billion per year.

DESCRIPTION

- Full-thickness skin defect with surrounding pigmentation and dermatitis
- Most frequently located in ankle region of lower leg ("gaiter region")
- Present for >30 days and fails to heal spontaneously
- May only have mild pain unless infected
- Other signs of chronic venous insufficiency include edema/brawny edema and chronic skin changes (i.e., hyperpigmentation and/or fibrosis).

EPIDEMIOLOGY

Up to 80% of leg ulcers are caused by venous disease; arterial disease accounts for 10–25%, which may coexist with venous disease.

Incidence

- Overall incidence of venous ulcers is 18/100,000 persons.
- Prevalent sex: women > men (20.4 vs. 14.6 per 100,000 for venous ulcer); increased with age for both sexes

Prevalence

- Seen in ~1% of adult population in industrialized countries, increased to 5% in patients ≥80 years old
- Prevalence studies only available for Western countries
- Point prevalence underestimates the extent of the disease because ulcers often recur.
- 70% of ulcers recur within 5 years of closure.

ETIOLOGY AND PATHOPHYSIOLOGY

- In a diseased venous system, venous pressure in the deep system fails to fall with ambulation, causing venous hypertension.
- Venous hypertension comes from the following:
  - Venous obstruction
  - Incompetent venous valves in the deep or superficial system
  - Inadequate muscle contraction (e.g., arthritis, myopathies, neuropathies) so that the calf pump is ineffective
- Venous pressure transmitted to capillaries leading to venous hypertensive microangiopathy and extravasation of RBCs and proteins (especially fibrinogen)
- Increased RBC aggregation leads to reduced oxygen transport, slowed arteriolar circulation, and ischemia at the skin level, contributing to ulcers.
- Leukocytes aggregate to hypoxic areas and increase local inflammation.
- Factors promoting persistence of venous ulcers
  - Prolonged chronic inflammation
  - Bacterial infection, critical colonization

RISK FACTORS

- History of leg injury
- Obesity
- Congestive heart failure (CHF)
- History of deep venous thrombosis (DVT)
- Failure of calf muscle pump (e.g., ankle fusion, inactivity) is a strong independent predictor of poorly healing wounds.
- Previous varicose vein surgery
- Family history

GENERAL PREVENTION

- Primary prevention after symptomatic DVT: Prescribe compression hose to be used as soon as feasible for at least 2 years (≥20–30 mm Hg compression).
- Secondary prevention of recurrent ulceration includes compression, correction of the underlying problem, and surveillance. Circumstantial evidence from 2 RCTs showed those who stopped wearing compression hose were more likely to recur.
- Compression hose reduces rates of recurrence compared with no compression.
- Because most ulcers develop following some type of trauma, avoiding lower leg trauma may help to prevent ulceration.

COMMONLY ASSOCIATED CONDITIONS

Up to 50% of patients have allergic reactions to topical agents commonly used for treatment.

- Contact sensitivity was more common in patients with stasis dermatitis (62% vs. 38%).

- Avoid neomycin sulfate in particular (including triple antibiotic ointment) (1)[A].

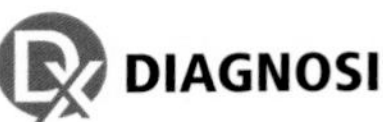

DIAGNOSIS

A diagnosis of venous reflux or obstruction must be established by an objective test beyond the routine clinical examination of the extremity.

HISTORY

- Family history of venous insufficiency and ulcers
- Recent trauma
- Nature of pain: achy (better with leg elevation)
- Wound drainage
- Duration of wound and over-the-counter (OTC) treatments already attempted
- History of DVTs (especially factor V Leiden mutation; strongly associated with ulceration)
- History of leg edema that improves overnight
- Edema that does not improve overnight is more likely lymphedema.

PHYSICAL EXAM

- Look for evidence of venous insufficiency:
  - Pitting edema
  - Hemosiderin staining (red and brown spotty or diffuse pigment changes)
  - Stasis dermatitis
  - White skin lesions (atrophie blanche)
  - Lipodermatosclerosis ("bottle neck" narrowing in the lower leg from fibrosis and scarring)
- Look for evidence of significant lymphedema (i.e., dorsal foot or toe edema, edema that does not resolve overnight or with elevation). This may require referral for special comprehensive lymph therapy.
- Examine for palpable pulses.

ALERT

- Examine wound for the following:
  - Length, width, depth, to monitor wound healing rate
  - Presence of necrotic tissue
  - Presence of biofilms or infection: purulent material in the wound, increased amount odorous exudate, spreading cellulitis, fever, and chills
- Get initial and interim girth measurements (at ankle and midcalf) to monitor edema.
- Important to rule out poor arterial circulation:
  - Compression dressings cannot be used in patients with ankle brachial index (ABI) <0.8

DIFFERENTIAL DIAGNOSIS

- Arterial insufficiency ulcer
- Neuropathic ulcer
- Malignancy
- Sickle cell ulcer
- Vasculitic ulcer
- Calciphylaxis
- Cryoglobulinemia
- Pyoderma gangrenosum
- Collagen vascular disease
- Leishmaniasis
- Cutaneous tuberculosis

DIAGNOSTIC TESTS & INTERPRETATION

- Consider prothrombin time (PT)/international normalization ratio (INR) and partial thromboplastin time (PTT) if patient is anticoagulated.
- Consider biopsy of leg ulcers that fail to heal or have atypical features.
- Consider factor V Leiden mutation; strongly associated with venous ulcers.
- Test for diabetes as necessary with fasting glucose.
- Use duplex imaging to diagnose anatomic and hemodynamic abnormalities with venous insufficiency. It will also identify any DVT present.

Diagnostic Procedures/Other

- Check ABI for evidence of arterial disease.
- An ABI <0.8 is a relative contraindication to compression therapy.
- Duplex imaging for evaluation of superficial and deep venous reflux and incompetent perforator veins.
- With concomitant severe arterial insufficiency, refer to a vascular surgeon for revascularization.

Test Interpretation

Strongly consider biopsy on wounds with atypical locations, failure to heal, or any suspicion of malignancy.

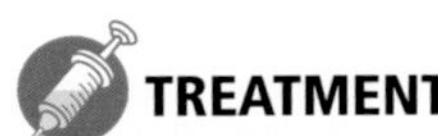

TREATMENT

GENERAL MEASURES

Dressings: All wounds need some kind of a dressing underneath the compression system.

- Wound dressings: no single type of dressing proved superior (2)[B]

- Maintain semimoist wound environment: not excessively wet or dry
- Wounds are often exudative until edema is decreased: Use absorptive dressings (calcium alginate or absorptive pads). Both superabsorbent diapers and female protection pads are cost-effective alternatives.
- Consider using barrier ointment/cream to prevent maceration of surrounding skin.

- If wound tends to be dry, use a hydrogel.
- A hydrocolloid dressing may be used with minimal exudate, if skin adhesive is tolerated.

MEDICATION

- Effective compression management is the cornerstone of therapy.
- Diuretics may help to reduce edema, but compression is the mainstay.
- Pentoxifylline 400 mg PO TID, in addition to local care and compression, improves cure rates. There is some response even without compression. GI side effects are common (3)[A].
- Aspirin 300 mg PO daily; effective when used with compression therapy

ISSUES FOR REFERRAL

- With prominent toe or foot edema, consider lymphedema. Refer to certified lymphedema therapist (CLT).
- Refer to a wound clinic for complex or poorly healing ulcers
- Refer to a vein clinic or vascular specialist for recurrent ulcers
- Use home health nurses to help with immobile patients needing frequent wrapping/dressing changes

ADDITIONAL THERAPIES

- Edema management: Reduce venous hypertension and improve venous return to reduce inflammation, pain, and improve healing (4)[A].
  - Compression therapy for edema management is the cornerstone of treatment for venous insufficiency with or without ulcers.
  - Short-stretch multilayer bandages are ideal for acute phase, until edema is stable, and the patient can be fitted for compression hose.
  - Long-term compression hose (fit once edema is reduced). Aim for a minimum pressure 20–30 mm Hg, preferably 30–40 mm Hg.
  - Elevation of legs to heart level for 30 minutes 3–4 times per day.
  - Exercise to strengthen calf muscle pump is also effective.
- Infection control
  - Débride necrotic tissue.
  - Treat cellulitis (usually Gram-positive bacteria) with bactericidal systemic antibiotics. Suspect local infection when there is pain or no improvement in the wound after 2 weeks of compression. Consider deep quantitative swab, after thorough cleansing, or tissue biopsy for culture.
  - Treat critical colonization with topical antimicrobials, such as cadexomer iodine (silver dressings and honey are widely used, but definitive data are lacking) (5)[B].
- For venous ulcers resistant to healing with wound care and compression, consider adding an intermittent compression pump 1–4 hours/day.
- Encourage exercise (e.g., activation of calf muscle pump with ankle flexion and extension) in conjunction with leg compression and elevation.
- Vacuum-assisted closure (VAC) dressings may be beneficial, but no clear benefit over optimal traditional wound care.

SURGERY/OTHER PROCEDURES

- Necrotic tissue impedes healing.
  - Consider sharp debridement.
  - Other methods include enzymatic ointments (collagenase), low-frequency ultrasound, and wet-to-dry dressings.
  - Avoid using collagenase with silver dressings because silver inactivates the enzyme.
- Allografts made of synthetic skin bilayered with living keratinocytes and fibroblasts improve healing at 6 months; insufficient evidence to support use of autografts.
- In patients with ulcers refractory to conservative therapy, a variety of endovenous and surgical options exist. Consultation with a vascular surgeon is recommended.
- Endovenous ablation of incompetent superficial and perforator veins has shown to reduce the size and recurrence of ulcers in those who have failed conventional compression therapy (6)[A].
- A subset of patients with nonhealing ulcers have stenosis and obstruction of the deep venous system. Venous angioplasty and stenting is emerging as an important adjunct to compression and other medical therapy (7)[A].

COMPLEMENTARY & ALTERNATIVE MEDICINE

- Chestnut seed extract (50 mg BID) is effective for venous insufficiency but not ulceration.
- Topical medicinal honey used on wounds shows no evidence of improved healing.
- Oral zinc has not been shown to be beneficial

INPATIENT CONSIDERATIONS

For those with acute significant cellulitis

Admission Criteria/Initial Stabilization

Infected wounds requiring IV antibiotics, especially in diabetics

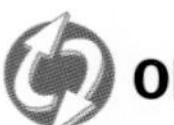

ONGOING CARE

- Venous insufficiency is a lifelong issue.
- After resolution of an ulcer, edema management must be maintained lifelong.

FOLLOW-UP RECOMMENDATIONS

When ulcers are nearly healed and edema is controlled, switch from compression bandages to compression hose.

- Insurance may not reimburse for compression hose unless an ulcer is present.
- Referral for hose fitting must be done just prior to the ulcer being healed.

Patient Monitoring

Monitor the ulcer for healing by measuring its area. Expect at least 10% reduction every 2 weeks.

DIET

- Obese patients may benefit from weight loss.
- Low-salt diets help fluid retention.

PATIENT EDUCATION

- Patient education for understanding of underlying mechanism is important for long-term management.
  - Develop long-term plan for edema management and instruction on compression therapy.
  - Instruct the patient on topical wound therapy.
  - Teach early recognition and treatment of new ulcers or cellulitis.

PROGNOSIS

- Ulcers recur frequently. Early identification and immediate treatment are essential.
- Ongoing diligence, with edema control, avoiding infections, and avoiding trauma are important.

REFERENCES

1. Machet L, Couche C, Perrinaud A, et al. A high prevalence of sensitization still persists in leg ulcer patients: a retrospective series of 106 patients tested between 2001 and 2002 and a meta-analysis of 1975-2003 data. *Br J Dermatology*. 2004;150(5):929–935.
2. Palfreyman SJ, Nelson EA, Lochiel R, et al. WITHDRAWN: Dressings for healing venous leg ulcers. *Cochrane Database Syst Rev*. 2014;(5):CD001103.
3. Jull AB, Arroll B, Parag V, et al. Pentoxifylline for treating venous leg ulcers. *Cochrane Database Syst Rev*. 2012;(3):CD001733.
4. O'Meara S, Cullen NA, Nelson EA, et al. Compression for venous leg ulcers. *Cochrane Database Syst Rev*. 2012;(11):CD000265.
5. O'Meara S, Al-Kurdi D, Ologun Y, et al. Antibiotics and antiseptics for venous leg ulcers. *Cochrane Database Syst Rev*. 2014;(1):CD003557.
6. Harlander-Locke M, Lawrence AA, Jimenez JC, et al. The impact of ablation of incompetent superficial and perforator veins on ulcer healing rates. *J Vasc Surg*. 2012;55(2):458–464.
7. Raju S, Darcey R, Neglen P. Unexpected major role for venous stenting in deep reflux disease. *J Vasc Surg*. 2010;51(2):401–408.

ADDITIONAL READING

- Hamdan A. Management of varicose veins and venous insufficiency. *JAMA*. 2012;208:2612–2621.
- Kearon C, Kahn SR, Agnelli G, et al. Antithrombotic therapy for venous thromboembolic disease: American College of Chest Physicians Evidence-Based Clinical Practice Guidelines (8th Edition). *Chest*. 2008;133(Suppl 6):454S–545S.
- Metcalf DG, Bowler PG. Biofilm delays wound healing: a review of the evidence. *Burns Trauma*. 2013;1(1):5–12.
- Nelson EA, Bell-Syer SE. Compression for preventing recurrence of venous ulcers. *Cochrane Database Syst Rev*. 2014;(9):CD002303.

SEE ALSO

Algorithm: Leg Ulcer

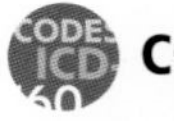

CODES

ICD10

- I87.2 Venous insufficiency (chronic) (peripheral)
- I83.009 Varicose veins of unsp lower extremity w ulcer of unsp site
- I89.0 Lymphedema, not elsewhere classified

CLINICAL PEARLS

- Initial diagnostic workup should include venous duplex scan and arterial evaluation.
- Refer patients with ABI <0.8 to vascular surgery specialist.
- Refer patients with recurrent or poor healing venous ulcers to venous specialist or wound specialist.
- Compression is essential for edema management with or without wounds.
- Treat critical colonization with topical antimicrobials (avoid neomycin).
- Make sure that the diagnosis is correct, and biopsy when in doubt.

VENTRICULAR SEPTAL DEFECT

Natalie S. Shwaish, MD • Brent J. Barber, MD

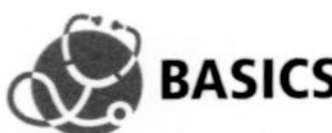

BASICS

DESCRIPTION

- Congenital or acquired defect of the interventricular septum that allows communication of blood between the left and the right ventricles
- Other than bicuspid aortic valve, it is the most common congenital heart malformation reported in infants and children. It also occurs as a complication of acute myocardial infarction (MI).
- Severity of the defect is correlated with its size, with large defects being the most severe.
- Blood flow across the defect typically is left to right, depending on defect size and pulmonary vascular resistance (PVR).
- Prolonged left to right shunting of blood can lead to pulmonary hypertension (HTN). Eventually, there will be reversal of flow across the defect and cyanosis (Eisenmenger complex).

Geriatric Considerations

Almost entirely associated with MI

Pediatric Considerations

Congenital defect

ALERT

- Pregnancy may exacerbate symptoms and signs of a ventricular septal defect (VSD).
- Can be tolerated during pregnancy if VSD is small
- May be associated with an increased risk of preeclampsia in women with an unrepaired VSD

EPIDEMIOLOGY

Incidence

- Congenital defect: no gender predilection, occurs in ~2/1,000 live births
- Post-MI: males are affected more than females

Prevalence

In the US:

- Congenital defect: lowered prevalence in adults due to spontaneous closure
- Post-MI: estimated to complicate 1–3%

ETIOLOGY AND PATHOPHYSIOLOGY

- Congenital
- In adults, complication of MI

Genetics

Multifactorial etiology; autosomal dominant and recessive transmissions have been reported

RISK FACTORS

- Congenital:
  - Risk of sibling being affected: 4.2%
  - Risk of offspring being affected: 4%
  - Prematurity
- Complication of MI:
  - First MI
  - HTN
  - Most frequently within 1st week after MI
  - Occurs in 1–3% of MIs, most commonly after anterior MI

GENERAL PREVENTION

For adults, avoid risk factors for MI and obtain evaluation before pregnancy.

COMMONLY ASSOCIATED CONDITIONS

- Congenital:
  - Tetralogy of Fallot
  - Aortic valvular deformities, especially aortic insufficiency and bicuspid aortic valve
  - Down syndrome (trisomy 21), endocardial cushion defect
  - Transposition of great arteries
  - Coarctation of aorta
  - Tricuspid atresia
  - Truncus arteriosus
  - Patent ductus arteriosus
  - Atrial septal defect
  - Pulmonic stenosis
  - Subaortic stenosis
- Adult: coronary artery disease

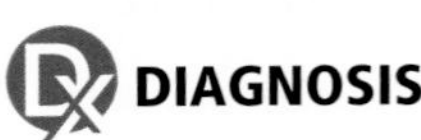

DIAGNOSIS

HISTORY

- Presentation depends on the degree of shunting across the defect; may be completely asymptomatic with small defects
- Respiratory distress, tachypnea, tachycardia
- Diaphoresis with feeds, poor weight gain in infants

PHYSICAL EXAM

- Small defect:
  - Harsh holosystolic murmur loudest at left lower sternal border
  - Detected after PVR drops at 4–8 weeks of life
- Moderate defect:
  - Harsh holosystolic murmur at left lower sternal border associated with a thrill
  - Forceful apical impulse with lateral displacement
  - Increased intensity of P_2
  - Diastolic rumble at apex due to increased flow across the mitral valve
- Large defect:
  - Holosystolic murmur heard throughout the precordium with diastolic rumble at apex with precordial bulge and hyperactivity, although large defects may have little or no murmur initially
  - If congestive heart failure (CHF) exists: tachycardia, tachypnea, and hepatomegaly
  - If pulmonary HTN exists: cyanosis with exertion
  - If Eisenmenger complex is present: cyanosis and clubbing

DIFFERENTIAL DIAGNOSIS

- Any defect with left-to-right shunt, such as patent ductus arteriosus, atrial septal defect
- Children: tetralogy of Fallot
- Adults: mitral regurgitation

DIAGNOSTIC TESTS & INTERPRETATION

Initial Tests (lab, imaging)

- A 12-lead ECG may suggest severity of VSD. Initially, left ventricular hypertrophy and left atrial enlargement may be evident. With pulmonary HTN, right ventricular hypertrophy and right atrial enlargement may be seen.
- A chest x-ray (CXR) may demonstrate increased pulmonary vascularity and/or cardiomegaly.
- A 2D echocardiogram for visualization of location and size of defect
- Color flow Doppler for direction and velocity of VSD jet; may be used to estimate right ventricular pressure

Follow-Up Tests & Special Considerations

- Weight and hematocrit check
- Cardiac catheterization performed occasionally for perioperative planning or to assess need for closure of defect

Diagnostic Procedures/Other

- Cardiac catheterization (left and right sides of heart) can confirm the diagnosis, document number of defects, quantify ratio of pulmonary blood flow to systemic blood flow (Qp/Qs), and determine PVR.
- Demonstration of an oxygen saturation step up from the right atrium to the distal pulmonary artery

Test Interpretation

- Congenital VSD (4 major anatomic types)
  - Membranous (70%)
  - Muscular (20%)
  - Atrioventricular canal type (5%)
  - Supracristal (5%; higher in Asians)
- Post-MI VSD predominantly involves muscular septum.
- After surgical repair, right bundle branch block is common.

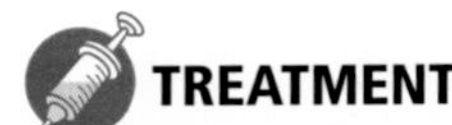

TREATMENT

- Start diuretic therapy if overload signs present (1)[A].
- Minimize IV fluids.
- Consider ACE inhibitor and/or digoxin.
- Nasogastric feeds for neonates
- Correct anemia via iron supplementation or a possible RBC transfusion.

GENERAL MEASURES

- Appropriate health care maintenance
- Outpatient, until surgical repair is indicated
- Inpatient in setting of acute MI
- Inpatient for treatment of severe CHF

MEDICATION

First Line

- Per the 2007 American Heart Association guidelines, endocarditis antibiotic prophylaxis is not recommended for most VSDs. It is recommended for VSDs associated with complex cyanotic heart disease, during the first 6 months after surgical repair, or for residual VSDs located near the patch following surgery (2)[A]. However, recent reports suggest that patients with a left ventricle to right atrium VSD (Gerbode defect) are at higher risk for endocarditis and thus may also need antibiotic prophylaxis (3)[C].
- Pediatric: Medications aim to control pulmonary edema, decrease work of breathing, and allow for growth:
  - Furosemide 1–2 mg/kg PO/IV once to twice a day
  - Digoxin: infants <2 years of age, 10 μg/kg/day PO divided BID; children, 2–10 years of age, 5–10 μg/kg/day PO divided BID; children >10 years of age, 2–5 μg/kg/day PO divided BID
  - Spironolactone 1–2 mg/kg/day divided BID
  - Captopril 0.1–0.4 mg/kg PO given q6–24h (maximum 6 mg/kg/24 hr)

- Adults: Digoxin and diuretics may be beneficial in some circumstances (1)[A].
- Side effects:
  - Drugs that increase systemic vascular resistance may increase left-to-right shunting and cause signs and symptoms of pulmonary overcirculation.
  - HTN

Second Line

- Surgical closure is generally indicated if the pulmonic-to-systemic flow is >2:1 or with poorly controlled pulmonary overcirculation despite maximal medical and dietary interventions.
- If an infant with a VSD has persistent pulmonary HTN or failure to grow, surgical repair generally is recommended prior to 6 months of age even if patient is otherwise asymptomatic.
- For post-MI VSDs, afterload reduction, inotropic support, intra-aortic balloon pump, and left ventricular assist device may be used to stabilize the patient prior to surgery. Surgical repair includes septal debridement and patch placement.

ISSUES FOR REFERRAL

Close follow-up of a congenital VSD is necessary until primary intracardiac repair is performed to ensure that significant pulmonary HTN does not develop.

ADDITIONAL THERAPIES

- Infant caloric requirements up to 150 kcal/kg/day for adequate weight gain
- Treatment of iron-deficiency anemia to increase oxygen-carrying capacity

SURGERY/OTHER PROCEDURES

- Surgical correction with either a VSD patch or repair is commonly used. Postsurgical outcomes for isolated VSD are excellent. Complications are rare and include reoperation for residual VSD, extended hospital stay, arrhythmias, valve injury, depressed ventricular function, and heart block (4)[B].
- Percutaneous transcatheter device closure has become a safe and effective option for some children with small to moderate VSDs. There is a greater risk of conduction abnormality with this technique compared to surgical closure; however, recent studies have shown steroids may decrease this risk. Complications include embolization of the device, residual defects, and complete heart block (5)[A].
- Periventricular device closure of isolated VSDs without cardiopulmonary bypass is feasible and safe under transesophageal echocardiographic (TEE) guidance. However, further evaluation of intermediate and long-term results is necessary (6)[A].

INPATIENT CONSIDERATIONS

Admission Criteria/Initial Stabilization

- Failure to thrive
- Pulmonary overcirculation/CHF
- Stabilize airway
- Reduce temperature stress

Nursing

Frequent vital sign monitoring; daily weight and calorie counts

Discharge Criteria

CHF stabilization, weight gain, or successful repair

ONGOING CARE

FOLLOW-UP RECOMMENDATIONS

- Small VSDs without evidence of CHF or pulmonary HTN generally can be followed every 1–5 years after the neonatal period.
- Moderate to large VSDs require more frequent follow-up.
- Potential complications of VSDs include right ventricular outflow obstruction and aortic valve prolapse.

Patient Monitoring

- Physical growth and development monitoring
- Influenza vaccine for children >6 months of age
- Palivizumab to children <12 months of age with hemodynamically significant lesions. Children with small VSDs do not need RSV prophylaxis (7)[A].

DIET

- Low sodium in heart failure
- High calorie in failure to thrive

PATIENT EDUCATION

- No activity restriction in absence of pulmonary HTN
- Parents need support and instructions for prevention of complications until the child is ready for surgery.

PROGNOSIS

- Congenital:
  - Course is variable depending on the size of the VSD.
  - Small VSD: 25–45% will close spontaneously by age 3 years. Muscular defects are more likely to close spontaneously.
  - Large VSD: CHF or failure to thrive in infancy necessitating surgical repair.
  - 20-year survival rate for isolated VSD: 98.3%
  - Progressive pulmonary vascular disease and pulmonary HTN are the most feared complications of VSD caused by left-to-right shunting and may eventually lead to reversal of the shunt (Eisenmenger complex). Death usually occurs in the 4th decade of life if untreated.
- Post-MI:
  - With medical management alone, 80–90% mortality in the first 2 weeks
  - Prognosis worse with inferior MI compared with anterior MI

COMPLICATIONS

- CHF
- Aortic insufficiency
- Sudden death
- Hemoptysis
- Cerebral abscess
- Paradoxical emboli
- Cardiogenic shock
- Heart block rarely may accompany surgical closure.
- Pulmonary HTN

REFERENCES

1. Faris RF, Flather M, Purcell H, et al. Diuretics for heart failure. *Cochrane Database Sys Rev*. 2012;2:CD003838.
2. Wilson W. Prevention of infective endocarditis. Guidelines from the American Heart Association. A guideline from the American Heart Association Rheumatic Fever, Endocarditis, and Kawasaki Disease Committee, Council on Cardiovascular Disease in the Young, and the Council on Clinical Cardiology, Council on Cardiovascular Surgery and Anesthesia, and the Quality of Care and Outcomes Research Interdisciplinary Working Group. *Circulation*. 2007;116(15):1736–1754.
3. Lax D, Bhatt RD, Klewer SE, et al. Are all ventricular septal defects created equal?. *J Am Soc Echocardiogr*. 2010;23(7):791.e5–791.e7.
4. Scully BB, Morales DL, Zafar F, et al. Current expectations for surgical repair of isolated ventricular septal defects. *Ann Thorac Surg*. 2010;89(2):544.
5. Yang L, Tai BC, Khin LW, et al. Systematic review on the efficacy and safety of transcatheter device closure of ventricular septal defects (VSD). *J Interven Cardiol* 2014;27(3):260–272.
6. Yin S, Zhu D, Lin K, et al. Perventricular device closure of congenital ventricular septal defects. *J Card Surg*. 2014;29(3):390–400.
7. Committee on Infectious Diseases and Bronchiolitis Guidelines Committee. Updated guidance for palivizumab prophylaxis among infants and young children at increased risk of hospitalization for respiratory syncytial virus infection. *Pediatrics*. 2014;134(2):415-420.

ADDITIONAL READING

Penny DJ, Vick GW III. Ventricular septal defect. *Lancet*. 2011;377(9771):1103–1112.

SEE ALSO

Down Syndrome; Myocardial Infarction, Myocardial Infarction, ST-Segment Elevation (STEMI); Non–ST-Segment Elevation (NSTEMI); Tetralogy of Fallot

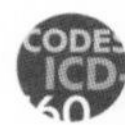

CODES

ICD10

- Q21.0 Ventricular septal defect
- I23.2 Ventricular septal defect as current comp following AMI
- Q21.3 Tetralogy of Fallot

CLINICAL PEARLS

- A loud 2–3/6 low-pitched harsh holosystolic murmur at the left lower sternal border is typical.
- A diastolic rumble at the apex indicates moderate to large VSD or Qp:Qs >2:1, which likely will require surgical or percutaneous closure.
- Disappearance of the murmur could be secondary to spontaneous closure of the defect or the development of pulmonary HTN.
- Development of a new murmur of semilunar valve insufficiency should be further evaluated. Pulmonary regurgitation may occur as PVR increases, and the development of aortic regurgitation usually will require early surgery.

V

VERTIGO

Amy Okpaku, DO

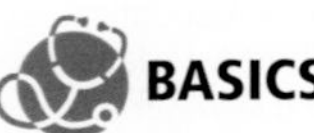

BASICS

DESCRIPTION

- Sensation of movement ("room spinning") when no movement is actually occurring; results from peripheral/central causes or may be induced by medications/anxiety disorders
- Important to distinguish between vertigo, presyncope (patient feels like they are going to black out; vision and hearing may become obscured), disequilibrium (off balance), and light-headedness (vague, inconsistent symptoms, no rotational component)
- System(s) affected: nervous
- Synonym(s): dizziness; acute vestibular neuronitis; labyrinthitis; benign paroxysmal positional vertigo (BPPV)

EPIDEMIOLOGY

Incidence

- Vertigo accounts for 54% of cases of dizziness reported in primary care; >90% of these patients are diagnosed with peripheral causes such as BPPV (1).
- Predominant sex: female = male; women are more likely to experience central causes, particularly vertiginous migraine.

Geriatric Considerations

Patients who are elderly and have risk factors for cerebrovascular disease (CVD) are more likely to experience central causes.

Prevalence

- Ranges from 5 to 10% within the general population
- Lifetime prevalence for BPPV is 2.4%.

ETIOLOGY AND PATHOPHYSIOLOGY

- Dysfunction of the rotational velocity sensors of the inner ear results in asymmetric central processing.
  - This is related to the combination of sensory disturbance of motion and malfunction of the central vestibular apparatus.
- Peripheral causes: acute labyrinthitis, acute vestibular neuronitis, BPPV, herpes zoster oticus, cholesteatoma, Ménière disease, otosclerosis (1)
- Central causes: cerebellar tumor, CVD, migraine, multiple sclerosis (1)
- Drug causes: psychotropic agents (antipsychotics, antidepressants, anxiolytics, anticonvulsants, mood stabilizers), aspirin, aminoglycosides, furosemide (diuretics), amiodarone, alpha-/beta blockers, nitrates, urologic medications, muscle relaxants, phosphodiesterase inhibitors (sildenafil), excessive insulin
  - Other causes: cervical, psychological

Genetics

Family history of CVD/migraines may indicate higher risk of central causes.

RISK FACTORS

- History of migraines
- History of CVD/risk factors for CVD
- Use of ototoxic medications
- Trauma/barotrauma
- Perilymphatic fistula
- Heavy weight bearing
- Psychosocial stress/depression
- Exposure to toxins

GENERAL PREVENTION

- Precautions to avoid injuries from falls that may occur secondary to imbalance
- If due to motion sickness, consider pretreatment with anticholinergics, such as scopolamine.

DIAGNOSIS

HISTORY

- Determine if true vertigo or other cause. Spinning is indicative of true vertigo (1,2).
- Ask about the presence of the following symptoms: dizziness, rotary illusions, nystagmus, nausea and vomiting, hearing loss, diaphoresis, pain, and neurologic symptoms (e.g., ataxia) (1,2).
- Obtain other medical and medication history (1,2).
  - Recent use of ototoxic medications (e.g., aminoglycosides)
  - History of alcohol, nicotine, and caffeine use
  - Sexual history
  - History of CVD/risk factors for CVD
- Symptoms that help distinguish between common causes (does not include all, see differential diagnoses) (2)
  - Vertigo
    - With *hearing loss*: Consider Ménière disease, acoustic neuroma, labyrinthitis, herpes zoster oticus (Ramsay Hunt syndrome), transient ischemic attack (TIA), cholesteatoma.
    - Without *hearing loss*: Consider BPPV, migrainous vertigo, vestibular neuritis, infection.
  - Presyncope: cerebral vascular disease, CAD, arrhythmia, medication, orthostatic hypotension
  - Disequilibrium (off balance): medication, orthostatic hypotension, peripheral neuropathy, cerebellar disorders, Parkinson disease
  - Light-headedness: medications, orthostatic hypotension, anxiety/stress, infection

PHYSICAL EXAM

- Neurologic: cranial nerves for signs of palsies, nystagmus
- Balance
  - Peripheral: mild to moderate, able to walk
  - Central: severe, unable to walk
- Dix-Hallpike maneuver performed by rapidly moving the patient from a sitting position to the supine position with the head turned 45 degrees to the right. After waiting 20–30 seconds, observe for nystagmus, the patient is returned to the sitting position. If no nystagmus was observed, the procedure then is repeated on the left side.
  - The presence of nystagmus indicates a positive test, implying that peripheral causes should be investigated.
  - If induced nystagmus does not subside, consider central causes.
- Head and neck: tympanic membranes
  - Vesicles: herpes zoster oticus
  - Cholesteatoma
  - Infection
- Cardiovascular: orthostatic changes in BP, dehydration/autonomic dysfunction

DIFFERENTIAL DIAGNOSIS

- Acoustic neuroma
- Anxiety disorder
- Arrhythmia
- BPPV
- Cerebellar degeneration, hemorrhage, or tumor
- Dehydration
- Eustacean tube dysfunction/middle ear effusion
- Hypoglycemia
- Labyrinthitis/labyrinthine concussion
- Ménière disease
- Multiple sclerosis
- Orthostatic hypotension
- Perilymphatic fistula
- Parkinson disease
- Peripheral neuropathy
- Syphilis
- Vascular ischemia
- Vertiginous migraine
- Vestibular neuronitis/ototoxicity

DIAGNOSTIC TESTS & INTERPRETATION

Initial Tests (lab, imaging)

- Consider CBC/chemistry panel in the absence of clinical findings pointing to a specific cause. Not routinely necessary
- Consider MRI in the presence of other neurologic symptoms, risk factors for CVD, or progressive unilateral hearing loss.

Diagnostic Procedures/Other

Audiometry if acoustic neuroma or Ménière disease is suspected

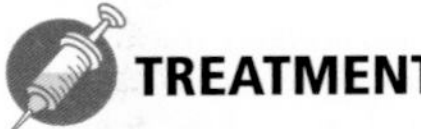

TREATMENT

GENERAL MEASURES

Treatments depend on cause.

- BPPV: Epley maneuver (2),(3)[A]/modified Epley maneuver (2),(3)[B] (www.youtube.com)
- Vestibular neuronitis and labyrinthitis
  - Vestibular-suppressant medications (1)[C],(2,4)
  - Vestibular rehabilitation exercises (1)[B],(2,4)
  - No evidence to support improvement of symptoms with corticosteroid use (5).
- Ménière disease (see separate topic) (1)[B],(2,4)
  - Low-salt diet (<1–2 g/day)
  - Diuretics such as hydrochlorothiazide
- Vascular ischemia: prevention of future events through BP reduction, lipid lowering, smoking cessation, antiplatelet therapy, and anticoagulation, if necessary. MRI or CT if suspected (1)[C],(2)

- Vertiginous migraines: dietary and lifestyle modifications, vestibular rehabilitation exercises, prophylactic and migraine abortive medications (1)[B],(2,4,6)
- Psychological: SSRIs, benzodiazepines for severe associated anxiety. Longer acting medications recommended over benzodiazepines because of side effects. Monitor for worsening of vertigo from medication used (1)[B],(2,4).

MEDICATION

Avoid use of medication in mild cases. Use for acute phase only (few days at most), as longer term use may impair adaptation/compensation by the brain (1,4). Medications not recommended for BPPV (1,2).

- Meclizine: 12.5–50 mg PO q4–8h (1)
- Dimenhydrinate: 25–100 mg PO, IM, or IV q4–8h (1)
  - Precautions: concomitant use of CNS depressants, prostatic hyperplasia, glaucoma
  - Adverse effects: sedation, xerostomia
  - Interactions: CNS depressants
  - Prochlorperazine: 5–10 mg PO or IM q6–8h; 25 mg rectally q12h; 5–10 mg by slow IV over 2 minutes (1)
    - Contraindications: blood dyscrasias, age <2 years, severe hypotension
    - Precautions: children with acute illness, glaucoma, history of breast cancer, impaired cardiovascular function, pregnancy, prostatic hyperplasia
    - Adverse effects: sedation, xerostomia, hypotension, extrapyramidal effects
    - Interactions: phenothiazines, tricyclic antidepressants
  - Metoclopramide: 5–10 mg PO q6h, 5–10 mg slow IV q6h (1)
    - Contraindications: concomitant use of drugs with extrapyramidal effects, seizure disorders
    - Precautions: history of depression, Parkinson disease, hypertension
    - Adverse effects: sedation, fluid retention, constipation
    - Interactions: linezolid, cyclosporine, digoxin, levodopa
  - Psychiatric causes (1)
    - SSRIs for depression and anxiety
    - Lorazepam (Ativan) 0.5–2 mg orally, IM, or IV every 4–8 hours for more severe anxiety
    - Diazepam (Valium) 2–10 mg orally or IV every 4–8 hours for more severe anxiety

Geriatric Considerations

Use vestibular-suppressant medications with caution due to increased risk of falls and urinary retention.

Pregnancy Considerations

Meclizine and dimenhydrinate are pregnancy Category B.

ISSUES FOR REFERRAL

Consider referral to otolaryngologist, ENT specialist, vestibular rehabilitation therapist, or neurologist if patient requires further care.

ADDITIONAL THERAPIES

- Epley maneuver/modified Epley maneuver for BPPV to displace calcium deposits in the semicircular canals (1–3)
  - Effective for short-term symptomatic improvement and for converting patient from positive to negative Dix-Hallpike maneuver
  - Contraindications: carotid stenosis, unstable cardiac disease, severe neck disease
- Vestibular rehabilitation exercises: ball toss, lying-to-standing, target-change, thumb-tracking, tightrope, walking turns

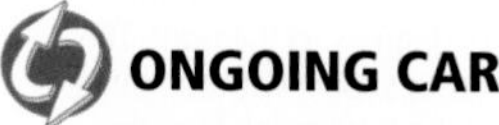

ONGOING CARE

FOLLOW-UP RECOMMENDATIONS

Balance exercises should be adhered to for symptom reduction and return to normal activities of daily living (ADLs).

Patient Monitoring

After 1–2 weeks, assess for the following:

- Recurrence of symptoms
- New-onset symptoms
- Medication-related adverse effects
- Relief from vestibular rehabilitation exercises

DIET

- Restricted salt intake for Ménière disease
- Dietary modifications for vertiginous migraine

PATIENT EDUCATION

- Reduce sodium intake (Ménière disease).
- Avoid triggers such as caffeine/alcohol (vertiginous migraine).

PROGNOSIS

Depends on diagnosis and response to treatment

COMPLICATIONS

- Anxiety
- Depression
- Disability
- Injuries from falls

REFERENCES

1. Swartz R, Longwell P. Treatment of vertigo. *Am Fam Physician*. 2005;71(6):1115–1122.
2. Post R, Dickerson L. Dizziness: a diagnostic approach. *Am Fam Physician*. 2010;82(4): 361–368, 369.
3. Hunt WT, Zimmermann EF, Hilton MP. Modifications of the Epley (canalith repositioning) manoeuvre for posterior canal benign paroxysmal positional vertigo (BPPV). *Cochrane Database Syst Rev*. 2012;4:CD008675.
4. Hain TC, Uddin M. Pharmacological treatment of vertigo. *CNS Drugs*. 2003;17(2):85–100.
5. Fishman JM, Burgess C, Waddell A. Corticosteroids for the treatment of idiopathic acute vestibular dysfunction (vestibular neuritis). *Cochrane Database Syst Rev*. 2011;(5):CD008607.
6. Fotuhi M, Glaun B, Quan SY, et al. Vestibular migraine: a critical review of treatment trials. *J Neurol*. 2009;256(5):711–716.

ADDITIONAL READING

- Bhattacharyya N, Baugh RF, Orvidas L. Clinical practice guideline: benign paroxysmal positional vertigo. *Otolaryngol Head Neck Surg*. 2008;139(5) (Suppl 4):S47–S81.
- Fife TD, Iverson DJ, Lempert T, et al. Practice parameter: therapies for benign paroxysmal positional vertigo (an evidence-based review): report of the Quality Standards Subcommittee of the American Academy of Neurology. *Neurology*. 2008;70(22):2067–2074.
- Hilton M, Pinder D. The Epley (canalith repositioning) maneuver for benign paroxysmal positional vertigo. *Cochrane Database Syst Rev*. 2004;(2):CD003162.
- Labuguen RH. Initial evaluation of vertigo. *Am Fam Physician*. 2006;73(2):244–251.

SEE ALSO

- Ménière Disease; Motion Sickness
- Algorithm: Vertigo

CODES

ICD10

- R42 Dizziness and giddiness
- H81.10 Benign paroxysmal vertigo, unspecified ear
- H81.49 Vertigo of central origin, unspecified ear

CLINICAL PEARLS

- Risk factors include history of migraines, history of CVD/CVD risk factors, use of ototoxic medications, trauma/barotrauma, perilymphatic fistula, heavy weight bearing, psychosocial stress, and exposure to toxins.
- The presence of nystagmus indicates a positive Dix-Hallpike test, implies a peripheral causes. If nystagmus persists, investigate a central cause.
- The Epley maneuver is recommended for the treatment of BPPV; this maneuver repositions calcium debris within the semicircular canals to provide relief from vertigo; a modified version of the maneuver can be performed at home.
- Medications are not recommended for BPPV.

VERTIGO, BENIGN PAROXYSMAL POSITIONAL (BPPV)

Janet O. Helminski, PT, PhD

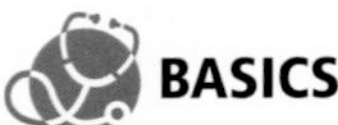

BASICS

DESCRIPTION

- Benign paroxysmal positional vertigo (BPPV) is a mechanical disorder of the inner ear characterized by a brief period of vertigo experienced when the position of the patient's head is changed relative to gravity.
- The brief period of vertigo is caused by abnormal stimulation of ≥1 of the 3 semicircular canals of the inner ear, with the posterior canal most commonly affected.
- BPPV is the single most common cause of vertigo.

EPIDEMIOLOGY

- The lifetime prevalence of BPPV is 2.4%, and the 1-year incidence is 0.6%. The age of onset is most commonly between the 5th and 7th decades of life, and the incidence of BPPV increases with each decade of life, peaking in the 6th and 7th decades (1).
- Prevalent sex: female > male (1)
- BPPV affects the quality of life of elderly patients and is associated with reduced activities of daily living scores, falls, and depression (2).

Prevalence

Common

ETIOLOGY AND PATHOPHYSIOLOGY

- In BPPV, calcite particles (otoconia) that normally weight the sensory membrane of the maculae become dislodged and settle into the semicircular canal, changing the dynamics of the canal. Reorientation of the canal relative to gravity causes the otoconia to move to the lowest part of the canal, causing displacement of the endolymph, deflection of the cupula, and activation of the primary afferent. This results in the generation of nystagmus and the associated sensation of vertigo.
- BPPV may be idiopathic, posttraumatic, or associated with viral neurolabyrinthitis.

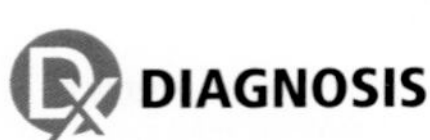

DIAGNOSIS

The diagnosis is established based on history and findings on positional testing (2,3)[A]. Positional tests place the plane of the canal being tested into the plane parallel with gravity.

HISTORY

- Brief episodes of vertigo (sensation that the room is spinning) associated with
  - Rolling over in bed
  - Getting out of bed
  - Looking up (referred to as "top-shelf syndrome")
  - Bending forward
  - Quick head movements
- Patients may also complain of light-headedness or feeling "off balance."
- Frequently, patients complain of nausea and, if severe enough, vomiting.

PHYSICAL EXAM

- The Dix-Hallpike Test (DHT) is used to diagnose BPPV (2,3)[A]. The test provokes the characteristic nystagmus associated with the symptoms of vertigo. For the DHT, the estimated sensitivity is 79% (95% CI 65–94) and specificity is 75% (95% CI 33–100) (4)[B].
- To perform the DHT, the patient is positioned in long-sitting on the exam table with the knees extended. If testing the right posterior canal, the head is rotated 45 degrees to the right. The patient is then lowered to supine with the head 30–40 degrees below the horizontal, over the edge of the exam table. The position is maintained for a minimum of 45 seconds. The patient is then returned to the seated position. The procedure is repeated toward the left.
- For each position, the clinician notes the direction of the fast phase of the nystagmus and the latency and duration of the nystagmus. For posterior canal BPPV, in the head hanging position, the otoconia move away from the ampullary organ resulting in an upbeating and torsional nystagmus. The superior poles of the eyes beat up toward the forehead and rotate toward the lower-most ear, the involved ear—consistent with excitation of the posterior canal ampullary organ. On return to the seated position, the otoconia move toward the ampullary organ resulting in the nystagmus reversing direction—consistent with inhibition of the posterior canal ampullary organ. The latency of onset of nystagmus is 1–45 seconds, and the duration is usually <1 minute. The nystagmus fatigues (reduction in the severity of symptoms) with repeated positioning. For anterior canal BPPV, in the head-hanging position toward the right and left, the eyes will beat primarily down toward the chin. In 50% of patients, a small rotation of the eyes toward the involved ear will be observed. For lateral canal BPPV, a directional-changing positional nystagmus is observed in the test positions; the eyes will beat linear-horizontal toward the ground (geotropic nystagmus) or beat toward the sky (apogeotropic nystagmus). For example, with geotropic lateral canal BPPV, the nystagmus observed would be right beating in the right head-hanging position and left beating in the left head-hanging position. In most patients with lateral canal BPPV, there is one position in which the nystagmus is more intense. The side with the nystagmus of the greatest intensity indicates the side involved with geotropic lateral canal BPPV and the uninvolved side with apogeotropic lateral canal BPPV. Alternative positional tests are available if the patient is unable to assume the DHT positions (side-lying test) or if the lateral canal is involved (supine roll test) (3)[A],(4)[B].
- No further testing is indicated unless the diagnosis is uncertain, or there are additional symptoms and signs unrelated to BPPV that warrant testing (3)[A].

DIFFERENTIAL DIAGNOSIS

- Orthostatic hypotension and other disorders that cause low BP; symptoms usually occur when the patient stands up.
- Damage to the brainstem or cerebellum can cause positional vertigo but is accompanied by other neurologic signs and usually has a different pattern of nystagmus.
- Low spinal fluid pressure may cause positional symptoms that are better when the patient lies down.
- Migraine-associated vertigo

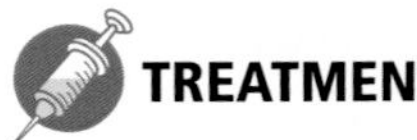

TREATMENT

- The Canalith Repositioning Procedure (CRP) or Epley maneuver is effective in the treatment of posterior canal BPPV (2,3)[A]. Using a particle repositioning maneuver, the clinician moves the patient through a series of positions. With each position, the otoconia settles to the lowest part of the canal. The debris is moved around the arc of the canal into the vestibule. In randomized controlled trials, the average short-term success rate of the CRP following 1 treatment session is 80 ± 9% (2)[A]. Contraindications are carotid stenosis, unstable cardiac disease, and severe neck disease. If the CRP is ineffective, self-administered CRP is performed at home (2,3)[A]. The patient performs the CRP on the bed with the head extended over the edge of a pillow. Better outcomes are achieved with a combination of CRP with self-administered CRP (2,3)[A].
- CRP illustrated for right posterior canal BPPV. The clinician moves the patient through a series of 4 provoking positions, starting with the placement of the right posterior canal (involved canal) in the right head-hanging position of the DHT. The head is then rotated a total of 90 degrees toward the left (uninvolved side) into 45 degrees of left head rotation. Maintaining 45 degrees of left head rotation, the patient is rolled onto the left side (uninvolved side) with the head slightly elevated from the supporting surface. The patient then sits up and flexes the neck 36 degrees. Each position is maintained for a minimum of 45 seconds or as long as the nystagmus lasts. The procedure is repeated 3 times.
- Postmaneuver activity restrictions are often advocated (2)[A]. For 1 week following the maneuver, patients should avoid lying on the involved side, use 2 pillows to sleep slightly elevated, and avoid up-and-down movements of the head. Patients sleeping on their affected side have a higher recurrence rate than those sleeping in other positions (5)[B].

MEDICATION

- Vestibular suppressant medications are not recommended for treatment of BPPV, other than for the short-term management of vegetative symptoms (3)[A].
- Antiemetics such as ondansetron (Zofran) may be considered for prophylaxis for patients who have had severe nausea or vomiting with the DHT.
- Vestibular suppressants such as benzodiazepines and antihistamines should be avoided because they may suppress nystagmus during the DHT and treatment.

ISSUES FOR REFERRAL

Consider a referral to a specialist if BPPV is unresponsive to treatment or if the patient is diagnosed with atypical BPPV involving the anterior or lateral canal. Other maneuvers are available for treatment of typical and atypical BPPV. Consider referring to a physical therapist, otolaryngologist, or neurologist.

ADDITIONAL THERAPIES

- Brandt-Daroff exercises, habituation exercises, are not as effective as self-administered CRP. At 1 week, the average success rate for the Brandt-Daroff exercise is 23–24% compared with 90% for self-administered CRP (2,6)[A].
- Surgical intervention is rarely indicated, except for refractory BPPV, and includes posterior canal occlusion and singular neurectomy.

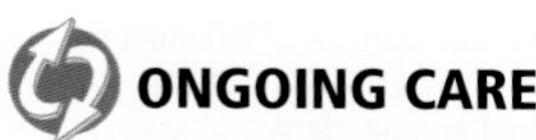

ONGOING CARE

FOLLOW-UP RECOMMENDATIONS

The patient should follow up within a week after treatment to ensure resolution.

PATIENT EDUCATION

A number of illustrative videos are available at www.youtube.com.

PROGNOSIS

- 30% of patients diagnosed with BPPV will spontaneously resolve within 1 week (3)[A].
- BPPV often recurs. Of patients treated successfully, 25% redevelop BPPV within 1 year and 44% redevelop BPPV within 2 years (2)[A].

COMPLICATIONS

During the maneuvers, a canal conversion may occur. The debris from the canal being treated may reflux into another canal.

REFERENCES

1. von Brevern M, Radtke A, Lezius F, et al. Epidemiology of benign paroxysmal positional vertigo: a population based study. *J Neurol Neurosurg Psychiatry*. 2007;78(7):710–715.
2. Helminski JO, Zee DS, Janssen I, et al. Effectiveness of particle repositioning maneuvers in the treatment of benign paroxysmal positional vertigo: a systematic review. *Phys Ther*. 2010;90(5):663–678.
3. Bhattacharyya N, Baugh RF, Orvidas L, et al. Clinical practice guideline: benign paroxysmal positional vertigo. *Otolaryngol Head Neck Surg*. 2008;139(5)(Suppl 4):S47–S81.
4. Halker RB, Barrs DM, Wellik KE, et al. Establishing a diagnosis of benign paroxysmal positional vertigo through the dix-hallpike and side-lying maneuvers: a critically appraised topic. *Neurologist*. 2008;14(3):201–204.
5. Li S, Tian L, Han Z, et al. Impact of postmaneuver sleep position on recurrence of benign paroxysmal positional vertigo. *PLoS One*. 2013;8(12):e83566.
6. Amor-Dorado JC, Barreira-Fernandez MP, Aran-Gonzalez I, et al. Particle repositioning maneuver versus Brandt-Daroff exercise for treatment of unilateral idiopathic BPPV of the posterior semicircular canal: a randomized prospective clinical trial with short- and long-term outcome. *Otol Neurotol*. 2012;33(8):1401–1407.

ADDITIONAL READING

- Fife TD, Iverson DJ, Lempert T, et al. Practice parameter: therapies for benign paroxysmal positional vertigo (an evidence-based review): report of the Quality Standards Subcommittee of the American Academy of Neurology. *Neurology*. 2008;70(22):2067–2074.
- Oghalai JS, Manolidis S, Barth JL, et al. Unrecognized benign paroxysmal positional vertigo in elderly patients. *Otolaryngol Head Neck Surg*. 2000;122(5):630–634.
- Radtke A, von Brevern M, Tiel-Wilck K, et al. Self-treatment of benign paroxysmal positional vertigo: Semont maneuver vs Epley procedure. *Neurology*. 2004;63(1):150–152.

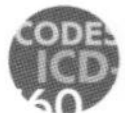

CODES

ICD10

- H81.10 Benign paroxysmal vertigo, unspecified ear
- H81.12 Benign paroxysmal vertigo, left ear
- H81.11 Benign paroxysmal vertigo, right ear

CLINICAL PEARLS

- The diagnosis of BPPV is based on history and findings on positional testing (DHT).
- The typical presentation is reports of brief episodes of vertigo (sensation that the room is spinning) associated with a change in position of the head relative to gravity.
- BPPV may be treated effectively with particle-repositioning maneuvers.
- Vestibular suppressant medications are not recommended for treatment of BPPV, other than for the short-term management of symptoms.

VINCENT STOMATITIS

Steven A. House, MD, FAAFP

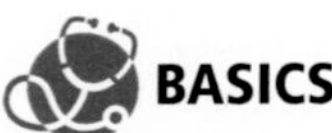

BASICS

DESCRIPTION
- Inflammatory oral infection of the gingiva, characterized by gingival necrosis, bleeding, and pain
- Disease caused by *Fusobacterium, Prevotella intermedia,* spirochetes, and heavy growth of oral flora
- Concomitant infection with Epstein-Barr virus, herpes simplex virus, and type 1 human cytomegalovirus is common.
- Organisms invade gingiva and oral papillae with the formation of a pseudomembranous exudate.
- Clinical presentation includes ulceration, halitosis, pain, bleeding, and necrosis. It is differentiated from other periodontal diseases in that onset is rapid, papillae are ulcerated and appear "punched out," and there is interdental necrosis (1).
- Synonym(s): Vincent angina; trench mouth; acute necrotizing ulcerative gingivitis

EPIDEMIOLOGY

Incidence
- Predominant age: 18–30 years in developed countries
- 3–14 years of age among malnourished children

Prevalence
- A Chilean study of 9,203 students aged 12–21 years revealed a prevalence of 6.7%.
- Overall prevalence decreases with age.

ETIOLOGY AND PATHOPHYSIOLOGY
- Impaired host immunologic response due to immunocompromise or malnutrition
- Loss of integrity of the oral mucosa
- Increased bacterial attachment with herpesvirus active infection

RISK FACTORS
- Poor oral hygiene
- Orthodontics (2)
- Infrequent or absent dental care
- Malnutrition
- Tobacco use
- Herpesvirus infection
- Immunosuppression
- Psychological stress
- Diabetes, especially if uncontrolled (3)
- Down syndrome
- Pregnancy (3)

GENERAL PREVENTION
- Regular dental care
- Proper oral hygiene
- Appropriate nutrition
- Prompt recognition and institution of therapy
- Stress management

COMMONLY ASSOCIATED CONDITIONS
- Bacteremia
- Osteomyelitis
- Tooth loss
- Noma/Cancrum oris, which can be life-threatening
- Aspiration pneumonia

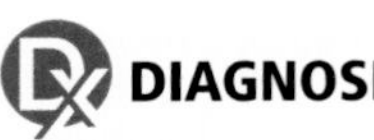

DIAGNOSIS

HISTORY
- Acute onset of gingival ulcer
- Halitosis
- Painful, bleeding, and inflamed gingiva
- Fever
- Malaise
- History of immunosuppression chemotherapy, HIV infection
- History of herpesvirus infection

PHYSICAL EXAM
- Ulceration of the oral papillae
- Inflamed, erythematous gingiva
- Formation of gray, pseudomembranous exudate
- Necrotic tissue on gingiva and surrounding structures
- Cervical lymphadenopathy

DIFFERENTIAL DIAGNOSIS
- Herpes simplex virus
- Periodontitis
- Pericoronitis
- Medication side effects
- Oral malignancy
- Xerostomia
- Diphtheria
- Lymphoma / leukemia
- Primary syphilis
- Ascorbic acid deficiency
- Gingivitis
- Behçet disease

DIAGNOSTIC TESTS & INTERPRETATION

Initial Tests (lab, imaging)
- Diagnosis is primarily based on clinical exam, but if systemic illness or localized spread to surrounding tissues is suspected, the following studies should be considered:
  - Aerobic and anaerobic cultures of inflamed or debrided tissue
  - Group A strep rapid antigen detection assay
  - Group A strep throat culture
  - Blood cultures if systemic involvement
  - Dental radiographs
  - Facial radiographs or CT of the neck and sinuses if infection has progressed

TREATMENT

MEDICATION

- Decision regarding locus of treatment (outpatient or inpatient) and route (PO or IV) depends on the degree of systemic illness present and on the involvement of structures in the neck.
- Medication regimens provided below are for outpatient treatment.

First Line

- Penicillin V K 500 mg q6h for 7–10 days (4)[C] *or*
- Amoxicillin 500 mg TID for 7 days *or*
- Amoxicillin-clavulanate 875 mg q12h for 7–10 days if more concerned regarding complications

Second Line

- Metronidazole 500 mg q8h for 7–10 days *or*
- Erythromycin 500 mg BID for 7 days (if PCN allergy) (4)[C] *or*
- Clindamycin 450 mg q8h for 7–10 days (if PCN allergy)(1)[C]

ISSUES FOR REFERRAL

Patients can be evaluated and treated by oral surgeon, dentist/periodontist, or ear, nose, and throat specialist depending on patient preference and severity of infection.

ADDITIONAL THERAPIES

- Chlorhexidine gluconate 0.12% BID or salt water rinses (2)[C]
- Pain management with NSAIDs (5)[C]

SURGERY/OTHER PROCEDURES

- Débridement of inflamed and necrotic tissue
- Dental extraction

INPATIENT CONSIDERATIONS

Admission Criteria/Initial Stabilization

- Failure of oral antibiotics and disease progression
- Need for parenteral antibiotics and analgesia
- Inability to meet nutritional and/or hydration needs

IV Fluids

May be required if patient is unable to tolerate oral fluids

Discharge Criteria

- Arrest of disease progression and improvement at site
- Ability to tolerate oral antibiotics and fluids
- Oral analgesia is effective.

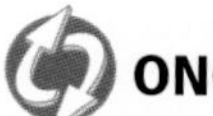

ONGOING CARE

FOLLOW-UP RECOMMENDATIONS

Frequent dental cleanings and examinations

DIET

- Proper nutrition
- Multivitamin supplementation

PATIENT EDUCATION

- Proper nutrition
- Appropriate oral hygiene
- Tobacco cessation
- Stress management

COMPLICATIONS

- Malnutrition
- Pain
- Poor dentition, tooth loss
- Systemic infection
- Involvement of soft tissues and structures of the neck

REFERENCES

1. Atout NA, Todescan S. Managing patient with necrotizing ulcerative gingivitis. *J Can Dent Assoc*. 2013;79:d46.
2. Sangani I, Watt E, Cross D. Necrotizing ulcerative gingivitis and the orthodontic patient: a case series. *J Orthod*. 2013;40(1):77–80.
3. Silk H. Diseases of the mouth. *Prim Care*. 2014;41(1):75–90.
4. Edwards PC, Kanjirath P. Recognition and management of common acute conditions of the oral cavity resulting from tooth decay, periodontal disease, and trauma: an update for the family physician. *J Am Board Fam Med*. 2010;23(3):285–294.
5. Hodgdon A. Dental and related infections. *Emerg Med Clin North Am*. 2013;31(2):465–480.

ADDITIONAL READING

- Carlson JA, Dabiri G, Cribier B, et al. The immunopathobiology of syphilis: the manifestations and course of syphilis are determined by the level of delayed-type hypersensitivity. *Am J Dematopathol*. 2011;33(5):433–460.
- Lopez R, Fernandez O, Jara G, et al. Epidemiology of necrotizing ulcerative gingival lesions in adolescents. *J Periodontal Res*. 2002;37(6):439–444.
- Marik PE. Pulmonary aspiration syndromes. *Curr Opin Pulm Med*. 2011;17(3):148–154.
- Porter SR. Diet and halitosis. *Curr Opin Clin Nutr Metab Care*. 2011;14(4):463–468.
- Slots J. Herpesviral-bacterial synergy in the pathogenesis of human periodontitis. *Curr Opin Infect Dis*. 2007;20(3):278–283.

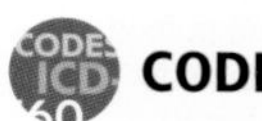

CODES

ICD10

A69.1 Other Vincent's infections

CLINICAL PEARLS

- Poor oral hygiene and immunosuppression are key factors in infection.
- Early recognition and institution of therapy decrease complications.
- Penicillin is the drug of choice for patients not systemically ill.

VITAMIN B_{12} DEFICIENCY

Yadira E. Acevedo, MD

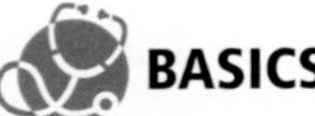

BASICS

- Vitamin deficiency related to inadequate intake or absorption of cobalamin (vitamin B_{12})
- Cobalamin is critical for CNS functioning.
- Deficiency can cause a multitude of symptoms and disorders including megaloblastic anemia, bone marrow dysfunction, and diverse and potentially irreversible neuropsychiatric changes.
- Neuropsychiatric disorders are due to demyelination of cervical, thoracic dorsal, and lateral spinal cords; demyelination of white matter; and demyelination of cranial and peripheral nerves (1)[C].
- Low vitamin B_{12} level can lead to elevated methylmalonic acid (MMA) and homocysteine levels.
- Elevated MMA causes abnormality in fatty acid synthesis affecting neuronal membrane.
- Elevated homocysteine is neurotoxic through overstimulation of the *N*-methyl-D-aspartate (NMDA) receptor and toxic to vasculature through activation of coagulation system and effects on endothelium.

DESCRIPTION

Normal B_{12} absorption

- B_{12} present in animal-source foods (meat, fish, eggs, milk) and foods fortified with B_{12}
- Dietary vitamin B_{12} (cobalamin) bound to food is cleaved by acids in stomach and bound to haptocorrin (commonly known as R-factor).
- Duodenal proteases cleave B_{12} from haptocorrin.
- In duodenum, B_{12} uptake depends on binding to intrinsic factor (IF) secreted by gastric parietal cells.
- B_{12}-IF complex is absorbed by terminal ileum into portal circulation.
- Body's B_{12} stored in liver = 50–90%
  - B_{12} secreted into bile from liver recycled via enterohepatic circulation
  - Delay 5–10 years from onset of B_{12} deficiency to clinical symptoms due to hepatic stores and enterohepatic circulation
- Typical Western diet: 5–30 μg/day; however, only 1–5 μg/day is effectively absorbed.
  - Recommend 2.4 μg/day for adults and 2.6 μg/day during pregnancy and 2.8 μg/day during lactation (most prenatal vitamins contain B_{12})

EPIDEMIOLOGY

Prevalence

- Endemic area: northern Europe, including Scandinavia; more common in those of African ancestry
- Prevalence 5–20% in developed countries
  - 12% in elderly living in community
  - 30–40% in elderly in institutions, sick, or malnourished
  - 5% patients in tertiary reference hospitals
- Prevalence by age group
  - 20–39 years old: prevalence 3%
  - 40–59 years old: prevalence 4%
  - >70 years old: prevalence 6%

ETIOLOGY AND PATHOPHYSIOLOGY

- Decreased oral intake
  - Vegetarians and vegans: B_{12} is found in animal-source foods; however, strict vegetarians uncommonly develop deficiency because only 1 mg/day is needed, with adequate amounts present in legumes.
- Decreased intrinsic factor
  - Pernicious anemia (PA): can be associated with autoantibodies directed against gastric parietal cells and/or IF
  - Chronic atrophic gastritis: autoimmune attack on gastric parietal cells causing autoimmune gastritis and leading to decreased IF production
  - Gastrectomy: Removal of entire or part of stomach decreases amount of parietal cells.
- Decreased ileal absorption
  - Crohn disease: Terminal ileal inflammation decreases body's ability to absorb B_{12}.
  - Chronic alcoholism: decreases body's ability to absorb B_{12}
  - Ileal resection
  - Pancreatic insufficiency: Pancreatic proteases are required to cleave the vitamin B_{12}-haptocorrin bond to allow vitamin B_{12} to bind to intrinsic factor.
  - *Helicobacter pylori* infection: impairs release of B_{12} from bound proteins
- Medications: Proton pump inhibitors (PPIs), H_2 antagonists, and antacids decrease gastric acidity, inhibiting B_{12} release from dietary protein; metformin
- Hereditary (rare)
  - Imerslund-Grasbeck disease (juvenile megaloblastic anemia)
  - Congenital deficiency of transcobalamin
  - Severe methylene tetrahydrofolate reductase deficiency
  - Abnormalities of methionine synthesis

Causes:

- Food-cobalamin malabsorption syndrome
  - As many as 60–70% of cases
  - Primary cause in elderly
  - Pathophysiology: inability to release cobalamin from food or binding protein, especially if in the setting of hypochlorhydria
  - Seen in atrophic gastritis, long-term ingestion of antacids and biguanides, possible relationship to *H. pylori* infection
- PA
  - 15–30% of all cases; most frequent cause of severe disease. Neurologic disorders are common presenting complaints.
  - Common in elderly, as high as 20%, with mild atrophic gastritis, hypochlorhydria, and impaired release of dietary vitamin B_{12}
  - Autoimmune disease with destruction of gastric fundal mucosa cells via a cell-mediated process
  - Anti-gastric parietal cell antibodies: sensitivity >90%, specificity 50%; use for screening test
  - Anti-intrinsic factor antibodies: sensitivity 50%
  - Associated with other autoimmune diseases
- Insufficient dietary intake: 2% of cases; vegans or long-standing vegetarians
- Infants born to vitamin B_{12}–deficient mothers may have deficiency or develop it if breastfed exclusively.
- Intestinal causes:
  - 1% of cases; prevalence depends on risk factors, such as surgical conditions
  - Gastrectomy: due to decreased production of intrinsic factor
  - Gastric bypass: appears 1–9 years after surgery, prevalence 12–33%
  - Ileal resection or disease
  - Fish tapeworm
  - Severe pancreatic insufficiency
- Undetermined etiology
  - 1/10 of cases

Genetics

Imerslund-Grasbeck disease (juvenile megaloblastic anemia) caused by mutations in the amnionless (AMN) or cubilin (CUBN) genes with autosomal recessive pattern of inheritance; inadequate ileal uptake of B_{12}-IF complex and B_{12} renal protein reabsorption

GENERAL PREVENTION

Risk factors: vegan diet, age >65 years, female, chronic atrophic gastritis, Crohn disease or other ileal disorders, chronic medication use including PPI, metformin, H_2 antagonists

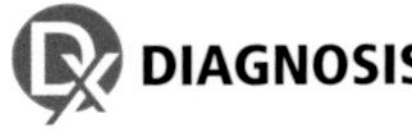

DIAGNOSIS

Symptoms and physical exam findings:

- Asymptomatic patients may be diagnosed by the incidental finding of anemia or an elevated mean corpuscular volume (MCV) during routine testing or evaluation of unassociated disorders.
- Hematologic
  - Frequent: macrocytosis, neutrophil hypersegmentation, spinal cord medullar megaloblastosis (blue spinal cord)
  - Rare: isolated thrombocytopenia and neutropenia, pancytopenia
  - Very rare: hemolytic anemia, thrombotic microangiopathy with schistocytes
- Neuropsychiatric
  - Frequent: sensory polyneuritis, paresthesias, positive Babinski sign, weakness, gait unsteadiness, loss of proprioception (impaired vibratory sensation, positive Romberg, ataxia, hyperreflexia)
  - Classic, but uncommon: subacute combined degeneration of spinal cord associated with PA; myelin degeneration in the lateral and posterior columns; ataxia, proprioception and vibration loss, bowel and bladder incontinence, orthostatic hypotension, decreased memory, mania, delirium, psychosis, depression
- Digestive
  - Classic: Hunter glossitis, jaundice, and high lactate dehydrogenase and bilirubin
  - Possible: abdominal pain, dyspepsia, nausea, vomiting, diarrhea
  - Rare: mucocutaneous ulcers
- Other
  - Frequent: pallor, edema, jaundice
  - Under investigation: chronic vaginal and urinary infections, atrophy of vaginal mucosa, hypofertility, venous thromboembolism, angina, miscarriages
  - Commonly insidious and nonspecific; thus, delay in diagnosis is common.

HISTORY

- Underlying disease associated with vitamin B_{12} deficiency
- Fatigue, anorexia
- Depression
- Falls (due to diminished proprioception)
- Loss of sensation in "stocking-glove" distribution
- Glossitis/loss of sense of taste, and other subtle, nonspecific neurologic symptoms

DIAGNOSTIC TESTS & INTERPRETATION

- Measurement of vitamin B_{12}, CBC (MCV)
- Measurement of B_{12} may be low or low normal depending on institution's cutoff value.
  - 65–95% sensitivity levels <200 pg/mL
  - May need additional tests such as MMA and homocysteine if vitamin B_{12} level is low normal (<350 pg/mL) and no evidence of anemia depending on clinical suspicion
- If high suspicion on normal B_{12} with high/normal MCV, consider testing MMA and homocysteine levels.
- MCV often increased
- Measurement of MMA
  - 98% sensitive
  - Levels increased in renal failure and volume depletion
- Measurement of homocysteine
  - 96% sensitive
  - Levels increased in folate deficiency, renal failure, and homocystinuria
- Other tests: folate and other markers of anemia (iron studies)
- MCV may be normal, decreased, or increased if vitamin B_{12} deficiency coexists with other forms of anemia, such as iron deficiency or hemolysis. Thus, RBCs may be normochromic, normocytic, or hypochromic microcytic.

ALERT

- Low levels of vitamin B_{12} are seen in folate deficiency, HIV, and multiple myeloma.
- Elevated levels of vitamin B_{12} are seen in renal disease, occult malignancy, and alcoholic liver disease and as a result of technical error.
- Macrocytosis may be due to folate deficiency, reticulocytosis, medications, bone marrow dysplasia, and hypothyroidism or be masked by concomitant microcytic anemia.
- Serum homocysteine and MMA
  - Elevated in B_{12} deficiency secondary to decreased metabolism
  - If both are normal, B_{12} deficiency is effectively ruled out.
  - If MMA is normal and homocysteine is increased, think folate deficiency.
- PA
  - Check antibody to intrinsic factor; positive test is confirmatory for PA, but sensitivity is only 50–70%.
  - Anti-parietal cell antibody positivity indicates pernicious anemia.
  - For patients who are antibody positive, consider screening for autoimmune thyroid disease.

Pregnancy Considerations

Because B_{12} crosses the placenta, pregnant women with low levels of B_{12} are at higher risk of having children with neural tube defects, congenital heart defects, developmental delay, and failure to thrive. Exclusively breastfed infants of mothers who are B_{12} deficient are at risk of developing B_{12} deficiency.

Diagnostic Procedures/Other

- Bone marrow exam is usually unnecessary in the evaluation of B_{12} deficiency because of the inability to differentiate from folate deficiency.
- Spinal cord imaging is not standard; MRI in selected cases, especially with severe myelopathy

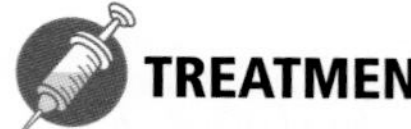

TREATMENT

MEDICATION

- Parenteral cyanocobalamin replacement recommended in patients with severe neurologic symptoms: IM cyanocobalamin (2)[C]
  - 1,000 μg/day for 7 days, *then*
  - 1,000 μg weekly for 4 weeks, *then*
  - 1,000 μg monthly for life
- High-dose, daily oral cyanocobalamin at doses of 1,000–2,000 μg are as effective as monthly intramuscular injection and is the preferred route of initial therapy in most circumstances because it is cost-effective and convenient (3)[A]. Requires greater patient compliance. Transnasal and buccal preparations of cyanocobalamin are also available; however, further study is needed.

ALERT

Folic acid without vitamin B_{12} in patients with PA is contraindicated; it will not correct neurologic abnormalities.

INPATIENT CONSIDERATIONS

Admission Criteria/Initial Stabilization

- Consider blood transfusion for severe anemia.
- Draw blood for hematologic parameters before transfusing.

ONGOING CARE

FOLLOW-UP RECOMMENDATIONS

Patient Monitoring

- Hematologic
  - Reticulocytosis in 1 week
  - Rise in hemoglobin beginning at 10 days; usually will return to normal in 6–8 weeks
  - Monitor potassium in profoundly anemic patients (hypokalemia due to potassium use).
  - Serum MMA decreases with replacement therapy.
- Neurologic: can note improvement within 3 months of treatment; however, maximum improvement noticed at 6–12 months. Some symptoms may be irreversible.

DIET

Meat, animal protein, and legumes unless contraindicated

REFERENCES

1. Lachner C, Steinle NI, Regenold WT. The neuropsychiatry of vitamin B_{12} deficiency in elderly patients. *J Neuropsychiatry Clin Neurosci*. 2012;24(1):5–15. AQ1
2. Stabler SP. Clinical practice. Vitamin B_{12} deficiency. *N Engl J Med*. 2013;368(2):149–160.
3. Vidal-Alaball J, Butler C, Cannings-John R, et al. Oral vitamin B_{12} versus intramuscular B_{12} for vitamin B_{12} deficiency. *Cochrane Database Syst Rev*. 2005;(3):CD004655.

ADDITIONAL READING

- Allen LH. How common is vitamin B_{12} deficiency? *Am J Clin Nutr*. 2009;89(2):693S–696S.
- Bizzaro N, Antico A. Diagnosis and classification of pernicious anemia. *Autoimmun Rev*. 2014;13(4–5):565–568.
- Fernández-Bañares F, Monzón H, Forné M. A short review of malabsorption and anemia. *World J Gastroenterol*. 2009;15(37):4644–4652.
- Langan RC, Zawistoski KJ. Update on vitamin B_{12} deficiency. *Am Fam Phys*. 2011;83(12):1425–1430.
- Mazokopakis EE, Starakis IK. Recommendations for diagnosis and management of metformin-induced vitamin B_{12} (Cbl) deficiency. *Diabetes Res Clin Pract*. 2012;97(3):359–367.
- Oberley MJ, Yang DT. Laboratory testing for cobalamin deficiency in megaloblastic anemia. *Am J Hematol*. 2013;88(6):522–526.

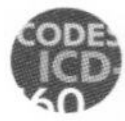

CODES

ICD10

- E53.8 Deficiency of other specified B group vitamins
- D51.0 Vitamin B_{12} defic anemia due to intrinsic factor deficiency
- D51.3 Other dietary vitamin B_{12} deficiency anemia

CLINICAL PEARLS

- Consider screening for B_{12} deficiency in high-risk patients including the elderly and monitoring B_{12} levels annually if on metformin or on chronic PPIs.
- Correcting folate deficiency without treating with cyanocobalamin in megaloblastic anemia may correct hematologic but not neurologic disorders.
- Vitamin B_{12} deficiency can coexist with other causes of anemia, including iron deficiency or hemolysis; thus, MCV can be normal, decreased, or increased.
- For patients with PA, cyanocobalamin replacement must be lifelong.
- Patients with PA are at increased risk for other autoimmune conditions as well as gastric malignancy.

VITAMIN D DEFICIENCY

Frank J. Domino, MD • Samir Malkani, MD, MRCP (UK)

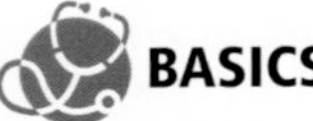

BASICS

This topic covers the commonly acquired vitamin D deficiency and not type II vitamin D–resistant rickets/type I pseudovitamin D–resistant rickets (both rare autosomal recessive disorders).

DESCRIPTION

- Vitamin D is both a hormone and a vitamin.
- Cholecalciferol (D_3) is synthesized in the skin by exposure to ultraviolet B (UV-B) radiation. Ergocalciferol (D_2) and D_3 are present in foods.
- D_2 and D_3 are hydroxylated in the liver to 25 vitamin D (calcidiol), its major circulating form.
- Calcidiol is further hydroxylated in the kidney to the active metabolite 1,25 vitamin D (calcitriol).
- Hypocalcemia stimulates parathyroid hormone (PTH) to be secreted, which prompts the increased conversion of 25 vitamin D to 1,25 vitamin D.
  - 1,25 vitamin D decreases renal calcium and phosphorus excretion, increases intestinal calcium and phosphorus absorption, and increases osteoclast activity. These effects increase serum calcium.

EPIDEMIOLOGY

- Unclear in general population
- In the community, a cohort study of asymptomatic adolescents in Boston found 24.1% were deficient, with 4.6% severely deficient.
- A study of hospitalized patients in Massachusetts found 57% vitamin D–deficient (VDD).
- Women with history of osteoporosis/osteoporotic fracture have high prevalence of vitamin D deficiency.
- A cross-sectional study of patients with persistent, nonspecific pain in an urban Minneapolis primary care clinic found 93% deficient and 28% severely deficient.
- A cohort study in Arizona found >25% of adults were VDD; highest rates among African Americans and Hispanics
- Prevalence of vitamin D Deficiency is increased in obese individuals.

Pediatric Considerations

NHANES data found 70% of children did not have sufficient 25-OH vitamin D serum levels (9% deficient and 61% insufficient), which was associated with an increase in BP and decrease in high-density lipoprotein (HDL) cholesterol.

ETIOLOGY AND PATHOPHYSIOLOGY

- Insufficient dietary intake of vitamin D and/or lack of UV-B exposure (in sunlight) results in low levels of vitamin D.
  - This limits calcium absorption, causing excess PTH to be released.
- PTH stimulates osteoclast activity, which helps to normalize calcium and phosphorous, but results in osteomalacia.
- Dietary deficiency
  - Inadequate vitamin D intake
- Inadequate sunlight exposure
  - Institutionalized/hospitalized patients
- Chronic illness: liver/kidney disease
- Malabsorptive states

Genetics

Vitamin D–dependant rickets type 1 occurs due to inactivating mutation of the 1 alpha hydroxylase gene; as a result, calcidiol is autosomal recessive not hydroxylated to calcitriol.

RISK FACTORS

- Inadequate sun exposure
- Female
- Dark skin
- Immigrant populations
- Low socioeconomic status
- Latitudes higher than 38 degrees
- Elderly
- Institutionalized
- Depression
- Medications (phenobarbital, phenytoin)
- Gastric bypass surgery
- Obesity

GENERAL PREVENTION

- Adequate exposure to sunlight and dietary sources of vitamin D (plants, fish); many foods are fortified with vitamin D_2 and D_3.
- Recommended daily allowance from the 2010 Institute of Medicine Report is minimally 600 IU/day for those 1–70 years of age and 800 IU/day for those >70 years of age. Up to 4,000 IU/day is safe in healthy adults without risk of toxicity.
- Higher intake of vitamin D recommended for age >50 years
- 2005 and 2009: Meta-analysis demonstrated for ages 51–70 years, minimally recommended supplementation is 800 IU/day to prevent nonvertebral fractures.

Pediatric Considerations

The American Academy of Pediatrics recommends all breast-fed babies receive 400 IU/day of vitamin D beginning "within the 1st few days of life."

Pregnancy Considerations

ACOG recommends data insufficient to screen all pregnancies; only those "at risk" and states it is safe to take 1,000–2,000 IU/day during pregnancy (1)[B]

Geriatric Considerations

U.S. Preventive Services Task Force recommends seniors take at least 800 IU/day vitamin D to reduce risk of falls in community-dwelling older adults (2)[A].

COMMONLY ASSOCIATED CONDITIONS

- Osteomalacia, osteoporosis
- Premenstrual syndrome
- Rickets
- Celiac disease
- Gastric bypass
- Chronic renal disease
- Bacterial vaginosis in pregnant women
- Hypertension

ALERT

VDD is associated with risk of myocardial infarction (MI) and all-cause mortality (3)[A].

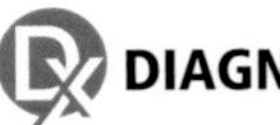

DIAGNOSIS

- Nonspecific musculoskeletal complaints
- Weak antigravity muscles
- Fracture with minimal trauma

HISTORY

- Senior citizens at risk of falling
- Renal disease
- GI (malabsorption) disorders
- Liver dysfunction
- Immigration from tr autosomal recessive opical to colder climates
- Dark-skinned/veiled individuals
- Housebound patients
- Women at perimenopause

PHYSICAL EXAM

- Vague neurologic signs: numbness, proximal myopathy, paresthesias, muscle cramps, laryngospasm
- Chvostek sign: contraction of the facial muscles by tapping along the facial nerve
- Trousseau phenomenon: carpal spasms and paraesthesia produced by pressure on nerves and vessels of the upper arm, by inflation of a BP cuff
- Tetany, seizures

DIAGNOSTIC TESTS & INTERPRETATION

Initial Tests (lab, imaging)

- 25-OH vitamin D (most sensitive measure of vitamin D status)
- Vitamin D deficiency
  - <20 ng/mL
- PTH elevation: not routinely obtained unless severe deficiency
- Low-normal/low calcium and phosphorous
- Elevated alkaline phosphatase (in later disease)
- Plain radiographs: If atypical fracture, radiographs may show osteomalacia (pseudofractures/looser zones) in pelvis, femur, and fibula.
- Osteoporosis screen
  - Women ≥65 years with no risk factors
  - Women ≥60 years at risk: body weight <70 kg (best predictor)
  - Less evidence: smoking, low body mass index, family history, decreased activity, alcohol or caffeine use
  - African American women have higher bone density than Caucasians.

TREATMENT

- Treatment goals remain unclear, but current "normal" 25-OH vitamin D levels are based on suppression of PTH.
- Obesity: Treatment of VDD in obesity, especially those who are obese and depressed, improves outcomes (4)[B].
- Hypertension: Vitamin D supplementation, especially those with dark skin, lowers BP in those with hypertension.

ALERT

All-cause mortality: Cochrane Systematic Review found vitamin D supplementation lowers all-cause mortality (5)[A].

Geriatric Considerations

In senior citizens, serum 25-OH vitamin D of 20 ng/mL resulted in improved physical performance scores; recent data suggests supplementation may not improve fracture risk and remains unclear about a true benefit.

MEDICATION

- Vitamin D sufficient (25-OH vitamin D ≥20 ng/mL)
  - Vitamin D 800–4,000 IU/day D_2/D_3 (6)[A]
  - D_3 (animal derived) may be slightly more effective than D_2 (plant derived), but clinical significance is uncertain.
  - Calcium supplementation: Unclear benefit and may increase some CHD risk in patients. No supplementation currently required (see below).
- Vitamin D deficiency (25-OH vitamin D <20 ng/mL)
  - D_2 50,000 IU/week for 8–12 weeks, followed by 800–2,000 IU/day of vitamin D_3 (6)[A]
- Calcium: meta-analysis data support
  - Dietary intake of ~700 mg/day leads to best outcomes; higher doses did NOT decrease risk of osteoporotic fractures.
  - Dietary calcium may be more beneficial than calcium supplementation.
  - Supplementary calcium associated with an increased risk of MI, especially in women (7)[A], but this data remains controversial (8)[C].

ISSUES FOR REFERRAL

Endocrinology if no response to treatment

ADDITIONAL THERAPIES

Aggressive calcium in ICU patients with ionized calcium <3.2 mg/dL or if symptomatic (tetany, seizures, QT prolongation, bradycardia, or hypotension, or ventilated patient with decreased diaphragmatic function)

INPATIENT CONSIDERATIONS

Admission Criteria/Initial Stabilization

- Symptoms of severe hypocalcemia *or*
- Malabsorption syndromes

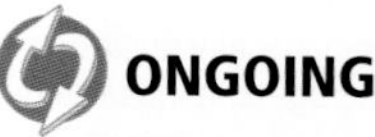

ONGOING CARE

FOLLOW-UP RECOMMENDATIONS

Follow-up of abnormal 25-OH vitamin D not required

DIET

- Cod liver oil is most potent source of vitamin D and has ~1,300 IU vitamin D/tablet/tablespoon.
- Fatty fish (tuna, salmon)
- Fortified milk (100 IU/8 oz), cereal, and foods

PROGNOSIS

- Systematic review of 63 observational studies found adequate 25 vitamin D levels correlate with lower rates of colon, breast, and prostate cancer.
- Cohort study found that vitamin D deficiency is correlated with increased risk of all-cause mortality.

ALERT

Meta-analysis data support supplementation of >500 IU/day lowered the risk of all-cause mortality (5,9)[A] but remains controversial.

REFERENCES

1. American Congress of Obstetricians and Gynecologists Committee on Obstetric Practice. Vitamin D: screening and supplementation during pregnancy. Committee Opinion No. 495. American College of Obstetricians and Gynecologists. *Obstet Gynecol*. 2011;118(1):197–198.
2. Moyer VA; U.S. Preventive Services Task Force. Prevention of falls in community-dwelling older adults: U.S. Preventive Task Force recommendation statement. *Ann Intern Med*. 2012;157(3):197–204.
3. Correia IC, Sodre F, Garcia G, et al. Relationship of severe deficiency of vitamin D to cardiovascular mortality during acute coronary syndromes. *Am J Cardiol*. 2013;111(3):324–327.
4. Maleswaran KS, Berry DJ, Lu C, et al. Causal relationship between obesity and vitamin D status: bi-directional Mendelian randomization analysis of multiple cohorts. *PLoS Med*. 2013;10(2):e1001383.
5. Bjelakovic G, Gluud LL, Nikolova D. Vitamin D supplementation for prevention of mortality in adults. *Cochrane Database Syst Rev*. 2011;(7):CD007470.
6. Holick MF, Binkley NC, Bischoff-Ferrari HA, et al. Evaluation, treatment, and prevention of vitamin D deficiency: an Endocrine Society clinical practice guideline. *J Clin Endocrinol Metab*. 2011;96(7):1911–1930.
7. Bolland MJ, Avenell A, Baron JA, et al. Effect of calcium supplements on risk of myocardial infarction and cardiovascular events: meta-analysis. *BMJ*. 2010;341:c3691.
8. Chrysant SG, Chrysant GS. Controversy regarding the association of high calcium intake and increased risk for cardiovascular disease. *J Clin Hypertens (Greenwich)*. 2014;16(8):545–550.
9. Chowdhury R, Kunutsor S, Vitezova A, et al. Vitamin D and risk of cause specific death: systematic review and meta-analysis of observational cohort and randomised intervention studies. *BMJ*. 2014;348:g1903.

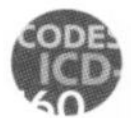

CODES

ICD10

- E55.9 Vitamin D deficiency, unspecified
- M83.8 Other adult osteomalacia

CLINICAL PEARLS

- Risk factors for VDD: senior citizen, renal disease, GI (malabsorption) disorders, liver dysfunction, immigration from tropical to colder climates, dark-skinned/veiled individuals, housebound patients, perimenopause
- Diagnosis: 25-OH vitamin D (most sensitive measure of vitamin D status)
- Vitamin D deficiency: <20 ng/mL
- Up to 4,000 IU/day is safe in healthy adults without risk of toxicity.
- 2005 and 2009: Meta-analysis demonstrated for ages 51–70 years minimally recommended supplementation is 800 IU/day to prevent nonvertebral fractures.
- The American Academy of Pediatrics recommends all breast-fed babies receive 400 IU/day of vitamin D beginning within a few days of birth.

VITAMIN DEFICIENCY

Stella O. King, MD, MHA

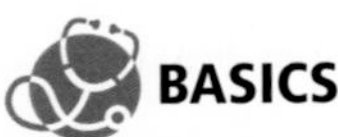

BASICS

DESCRIPTION

- Vitamins are essential micronutrients required for normal metabolism, growth, and development.
- Specific vitamin deficiencies can lead to medical conditions and health complications.
- Deficiencies are rarely diagnosed or documented in the Western world. Regulations mandating vitamin supplementation in food products, adequate food supply, availability of vitamin supplements, and lack of physician awareness all play a role.
- Fat-soluble vitamins (A, D, E, K)

EPIDEMIOLOGY

Incidence

- Predominant age
  - Geriatric population and vulnerable populations: pregnant women, chronic disease states
- Travelers with extended stays in developing nations
- Individuals from Africa and Southeast Asia are at increased risk.
- Vitamin deficiencies in Western world uncommon
- Vitamin levels are rarely measured (exceptions include vitamin B_{12} [risk increases >50 year of age] and folate [risk increases with specific states: pregnancy, antiepileptic drugs, neoplastic processes, alcoholism]).

Prevalence

Varies by age groups, comorbid conditions, geography, and setting (i.e., urban, rural)

ETIOLOGY AND PATHOPHYSIOLOGY

- Deficiencies usually related to disease can develop under healthy conditions and generally occur by 1 of 5 mechanisms:
  - Reduced intake
  - Diminished absorption
  - Increased use
  - Increased demand
  - Increased excretion
- Chronic disease states: HIV, malabsorption, chronic liver and kidney disease, alcoholism, pernicious anemia
- Gastric surgeries: gastric bypass, gastrectomy, small or large bowel resection
- Predisposition related to certain medicines: prednisone, phenytoin, isoniazid, protease inhibitors, proton pump inhibitors, chronic antibiotic use, penicillamine, hydralazine
- Malnutrition, imbalanced nutrition, eating disorders: obesity, bulimia/anorexia, fad diets, extreme vegetarianism
- Dialysis
- Parasitic infestation

Genetics

- Cystic fibrosis
- Rare genetic predisposition
  - Autoimmune disease (e.g., pernicious anemia)
  - Congenital enzyme deficiencies (e.g., biotinidase deficiency)
  - Transcobalamin II deficiency
  - Ataxia and vitamin E deficiency (AVED)
- A-β-lipoproteinemia

RISK FACTORS

Poverty, malnutrition, chronic disease states, advanced age, dietary restrictions, bariatric surgery, and exclusively breastfed infants

GENERAL PREVENTION

- No data exist that demonstrate that use of a multivitamin decreases the risk of any disease.
- Ingesting large and varied amounts of vitamins increases risk of toxicity and drug–drug interactions.
- Antioxidant use has not been shown to impact cancer incidence and, in some studies, has *increased* risk of death.
- Balanced diet: avoidance of fad diets
- Vitamin supplementation, when appropriate

ALERT

Use of multivitamins has not resulted in decreased risk of cancer, heart disease, stroke, or all-cause mortality.

Geriatric Considerations

U.S. Preventive Services Task Force recommends at least 800 IU/day of vitamin D to lower risk of falls, fractures.

COMMONLY ASSOCIATED CONDITIONS

Osteoporosis, anemia, neuropathies, Hartnup disease

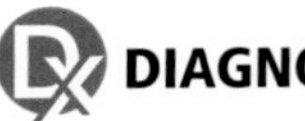

DIAGNOSIS

HISTORY

- Dietary intake (1)[A]
- Night blindness (2)[A]
- Decreased visual acuity (2)[A]
- Poor wound healing (3)[A]
- Hyperkeratosis of skin (2,3)
- Neuropathy (1)[A]
- Abnormal food cravings (pica) (4)[B]
- Osteomalacia or history of fracture (5)[A]
- Spina bifida (6)[A]
- Previous GI or gastric bypass surgery (7)[A]
- Prior or current medical conditions
  - Tuberculosis (TB), HIV infection, hepatitis, neoplasm
  - Hypermetabolic state
    - Thyrotoxicosis
    - 2nd- or 3rd-degree burns
    - Wound healing
    - Any systemic infection
- Chronic disease requiring steroids or immunosuppressants
- Malabsorptive or chronic GI disorder: celiac disease, sprue, Crohn disease, ulcerative colitis
- Parenteral or enteral nutrition via tube feeding
- Pregnancy
- Medications, supplements
- Food allergies or intolerances

PHYSICAL EXAM

- Breakdown of skin integrity (3)
- Coarse or thinning hair
- Reduced visual acuity (2)
- Beefy, red tongue
- Angular cheilitis (perlèche)
- Poor dentition and gingivitis (3)
- Cognitive impairment (1)
- Bruising and/or petechiae (3)
- Sensory and motor neuropathies (1)
- Ataxic gait (1)
- Rash (3)

DIFFERENTIAL DIAGNOSIS

Several medical conditions may mimic symptoms and signs of vitamin deficiencies.

- Diabetes mellitus (DM), thyroid disorders, hyperparathyroidism, heart failure, Alzheimer disease, multiple sclerosis, substance abuse, toxic ingestions, and hematologic disorders/malignancies

DIAGNOSTIC TESTS & INTERPRETATION

Initial Tests (lab, imaging)

- No routine screening indicated.
- Test if symptomatic or history indicates at high risk.
- CBC
- If clinical characteristics are present, consider the following:
  - 25 OH vitamin D (5)[A]
  - Prothrombin time (PT)/partial thromboplastin time (PTT)
  - Vitamin B_{12} and folate levels (1)[A]
  - Serum homocysteine and methylmalonic acid levels if high suspicion of vitamin B_{12} deficiency with normal serum B_{12} level (1)[A]
  - Retinol serum level, retinol binding protein (2)[A]
- Ancillary tests include the following:
  - BUN, calcium, phosphorus, magnesium
  - Albumin, liver function tests
- X-ray of long bones and spine (8)[A]
- Bone densitometry: indicated in the following (5)[A]:
  - Women >65 years of age, men >70 years of age
  - Patients with chronic steroids or immunosuppressants, thyroid medicine, or on antiepileptics (see topic "Osteoporosis")

Follow-Up Tests & Special Considerations

Bariatric surgery patients at risk for deficiencies (7)[A]

- Cyanocobalamin, thiamine, folic acid, calcium, vitamin D, iron, zinc, vitamin A

Test Interpretation

- Vitamin A (retinol) (2)[A]
  - Decreased visual acuity, Bitot spots
  - Advanced disease: keratomalacia and blindness
- Vitamin B_1 (thiamine)
  - Wernicke encephalopathy: memory disturbance, truncal ataxia, nystagmus, ophthalmoplegia
  - Korsakoff syndrome: anterograde and retrograde amnesia, confabulation
  - Dry beriberi: symmetric motor and sensory peripheral neuropathy, paresthesias, loss of reflexes
  - Wet beriberi: cardiovascular symptoms of peripheral vasodilation, high-output failure, dyspnea, and tachycardia
- Vitamin B_2 (riboflavin): glossitis, stomatitis, cheilitis
- Vitamin B_3 (niacin): pellagra: dermatitis, dementia, and diarrhea
- Vitamin B_6 (pyridoxine): dermatitis, cheilitis, atrophic glossitis, neuropathy
- Vitamin B_{12} (cobalamin): pernicious anemia, subacute combined degeneration, gait disturbance, cognitive impairment, neuropathy
- Vitamin C (ascorbic acid): scurvy: ecchymoses, bleeding gums (3)[A]
- Vitamin D (calciferol): rickets, osteomalacia, osteopenia/osteoporosis
- Vitamin K: ecchymosis, mucosal bleeding (9)[A]

TREATMENT

MEDICATION

- Encourage patients to bring in vitamin and supplement bottles for review.
- Folic acid and vitamin B_6/B_{12} therapy has been shown to lower homocysteine levels; however, no data show benefit regarding cognitive impairment or developing diabetic nephropathy, retinopathy, and coronary heart disease (CHD)/vascular diseases.

COMPLEMENTARY & ALTERNATIVE MEDICINE

- Ask patients about herbal and dietary supplements.
- Assess for potential adverse drug effects/reactions.

INPATIENT CONSIDERATIONS

Admission Criteria/Initial Stabilization

- Daily B-vitamin complex (folate, B_6, B_{12}), including thiamine supplementation (dose = 100 mg) via oral or parenteral route, for admitted or postoperative patients with chronic medical conditions (10)[A]
- Patients with alcohol dependence should be administered thiamine, folic acid, and multivitamin.
- Treat thiamine deficiency with thiamine replacement prior to IV fluids containing glucose to prevent precipitation of Korsakoff psychosis (10)[A].
- Consider obtaining prealbumin/albumin levels and a dietary consult for the malnourished patient.
- No consensus practice guidelines for supplement dosing regimens after bariatric surgery. Recommend B vitamins, vitamin D, and minerals.

Geriatric Considerations

- Vitamin B_{12} deficiency exists in 25% of the general population ≥65 years of age necessitating supplementation. Treatment of symptomatic or severe deficiency: cyanocobalamin 1,000 μg/day IM × 1 week and then weekly for 1 month. Prevention of recurrence or treatment of mild deficiency: regimen of oral B_{12} 1,000–2,000 μg/day or IM B_{12} 100–1,000 μg every 3 months (1)[A].
- >40% of elderly in United States are vitamin D deficient.
- Deficiency is defined as serum 25 OH vitamin D level <20 ng/mL (5)[A].
- Treatment for vitamin D deficiency = 50,000 IU of oral ergocalciferol for 8 weeks (5)[A]

Pediatric Considerations

- Hemorrhagic disease of the newborn (9)[A]
  - Neonates may exhibit vitamin K deficiency because they require 1 week of life to establish their intestinal flora (which manufacture vitamin K); breast milk is a poor source.
  - Condition peaks 2–10 days after birth; signs: bleeding from the umbilical stump and/or circumcision site along with generalized bruising and GI hemorrhage
  - Prevention: routine injection of newborns with vitamin K (1 mg)
  - Vitamin D deficiency: Vitamin D supplementation (400 IU/day) is recommended in all exclusively breastfed infants starting in the 1st few days of life (American Academy of Pediatrics [AAP]) to prevent rickets (8)[A].
- Morbidly obese and minority children are at increased risk for vitamin D deficiency (11)[A].
- Vitamin A deficiency is significant in the developing world in children (2)[A].
- In children age >6 months in developing countries, vitamin A supplementation has been shown to decrease mortality (2)[A].
- Vitamin deficiency is a risk factor for developmental delay.
- Supplemental vitamins in otherwise healthy children are not mandated by medical authorities.

Pregnancy Considerations

All pregnant women and women of childbearing age considering pregnancy should be strongly encouraged to take a multivitamin containing 0.4 mg folic acid daily to prevent neural tube defects (6)[A].

ONGOING CARE

DIET

Monitor nutrient intake and consider supplementation with enteral nutrition (e.g., Boost, Ensure, Sustacal) if patient is anorexic or exhibits dysphagia.

PATIENT EDUCATION

- Multivitamins are generally safe but have limited value in a patient with adequate diet.
- Drug–drug interactions may occur between vitamins and some medications.
- Risk of vitamin toxicity can occurs most commonly with the fat-soluble vitamins (A, D, E, K). Refer to the Recommended Dietary Allowance (RDA) for specific intake guidelines.

PROGNOSIS

- Most vitamin deficiencies are fully reversible if treated without undue delay.
- Vitamin repletion or supplementation may be <3 months or greater, depending on cause of deficiency.

COMPLICATIONS

Vitamin toxicities

- Liver failure (vitamins A, D, E, K)
- Desquamation of skin (vitamin A)
- Neuropathy (vitamin B_6)
- Kidney stones (vitamin C)
- Hypercoagulability (vitamin K)
- Pseudohyperparathyroidism (vitamin D)
- Masking of pernicious anemia (folic acid)

REFERENCES

1. Stabler SP. Clinical practice. Vitamin B12 deficiency. *N Engl J Med*. 2013;368(2):149–160.
2. Rotondi MA, Khobzi N. Vitamin A supplementation and neonatal mortality in the developing world: a meta-regression of cluster-randomized trials. *Bull World Health Organ*. 2010;88(9):697–702.
3. Al-Dabagh A, Milliron BJ, Strowd L, et al. A disease of the present: scurvy in "well-nourished" patients. *J Am Acad Dermatol*. 2013;69(5):e246–e247.
4. Advani S, Kochhar G, Chachra S, et al. Eating everything except food (PICA): a rare case report and review. *J Int Soc Prev Community Dent*. 2014;4(1):1–4.
5. Bordelon P, Ghetu MV, Langan RC. Recognition and management of vitamin D deficiency. *Am Fam Physician*. 2009;80(8): 841–846.
6. U.S. Preventive Services Task Force. Folic acid for the prevention of neural tube defects: U.S. Preventive Services Task Force recommendation statement. *Ann Intern Med*. 2009;150(9):626–631.
7. Ramos-Leví AM, Pérez-Ferre N, Sánchez-Pernaute A, et al. Severe vitamin A deficiency after malabsortive bariatric surgery. *Nutr Hosp*. 2013;28(4):1337–1340.
8. Wagner CL, Greer FR; American Academy of Pediatrics Section on Breastfeeding, et al. Prevention of rickets and vitamin D deficiency in infants, children, and adolescents. *Pediatrics*. 2008;122(5):1142–1152.
9. Puckett RM, Offringa M. Prophylactic vitamin K for vitamin K deficiency bleeding in neonates. *Cochrane Database Syst Rev*. 2000;(4):CD002776.
10. Thomson AD, Marshall EJ. The treatment of patients at risk of developing Wernicke's encephalopathy in the community. *Alcohol Alcohol*. 2006;41(2):159–167.
11. Turer CB, Lin H, Flores G. Prevalence of vitamin D deficiency among overweight and obese US children. *Pediatrics*. 2013;131(1):e152–e161.

ADDITIONAL READING

- Bjelakovic G, Nikolova D, Gluud LL, et al. Antioxidant supplements for prevention of mortality in healthy participants and patients with various diseases. *Cochrane Database Syst Rev*. 2008;(2):CD007176.
- Haller CA. Clinical approach to adverse events and interactions related to herbal and dietary supplements. *Clin Toxicol (Phila)*. 2006;44(5):605–610.
- House AA, Eliasziw M, Cattran DC, et al. Effect of B-vitamin therapy on progression of diabetic nephropathy: a randomized controlled trial. *JAMA*. 2010;303(16):1603–1609.
- Kunadian V, Ford GA, Bawamia B, et al. Vitamin D deficiency and coronary artery disease: a review of the evidence. *Am Heart J*. 2014;167(3):283–291.
- Neuhouser ML, Wassertheil-Smoller S, Thomson C, et al. Multivitamin use and risk of cancer and cardiovascular disease in the Women's Health Initiative cohorts. *Arch Intern Med*. 2009;169(3):294–304.
- Rosen CJ. Clinical practice. Vitamin D insufficiency. *N Engl J Med*. 2011;364(3):248–254.
- Sesso HD, Christen WG, Bubes V, et al. Multivitamins in the prevention of cardiovascular disease in men: the Physicians' Health Study II randomized controlled trial. *JAMA*. 2012;308(17):1751–1760.
- U.S. Preventive Services Task Force. Vitamin D and calcium supplementation to prevent fractures: preventive medication. http://www.uspreventiveservicestaskforce.org/uspstf/uspsvitd.htm. Accessed February 2013.

CODES

ICD10

- E56.9 Vitamin deficiency, unspecified
- E56.0 Deficiency of vitamin E
- E55.9 Vitamin D deficiency, unspecified

CLINICAL PEARLS

- Obtain a thorough dietary history.
- All pregnant women and women of childbearing age should be counseled to take a multivitamin with 0.4 mg folic acid (6)[A].
- All exclusively breastfed infants should be given 400 IU vitamin D supplementation starting in the 1st few days of life and continued until weaned to formula or, if >12 months, taking 32 oz of fortified cow's milk daily (8)[A].

VITILIGO

Cindy England Owen, MD

BASICS

DESCRIPTION

- An acquired depigmentation of skin, which correlates with a loss of epidermal melanocytes. There are 3 clinical variants, each with subtypes.
- Localized: often in childhood, rapid onset then stabilizes. Involvement of hair is common early in the course. Lacks associated autoimmune diseases.
  - Focal: few lesions, random distribution
  - Segmental: Lesions occur within a dermatome (mostly trigeminal) or may follow Blaschko lines. Lesions usually stop abruptly at the midline (1).
  - Mucosal: only mucosal surfaces involved.
- Generalized/nonsegmental (most common variant): progressive, with flares, commonly associated with autoimmunity. Common locations are acral, periorificial, and in sites sensitive to pressure/friction (Koebner phenomenon) (1).
  - Vulgaris: most common subtype. Scattered macules, often symmetric, wide distribution, mostly hands, axillae, and groin
  - Acrofacial: on distal extremities and face
  - Mixed: coexistence of above
- Universal: involves >80% of the body surface area (BSA). Most likely to have family history; comorbidities are common and associated with poorest quality-of-life (QOL) scores.
- Other rare variants
  - Ponctué: discrete confetti-like macules (1)
  - Inflammatory: peripheral erythematous rim (1)
  - Trichrome: tan zone is present between normal and depigmented skin (1).
  - Quadrichrome: as above but with marginal/perifollicular hyperpigmentation (1)
  - Blue: Dermal melanophages give blue hue, in areas affected by prior postinflammatory hyperpigmentation (1).
- System(s) affected: skin, mucous membranes
- Synonym(s): leukoderma

EPIDEMIOLOGY

- 50% begin before age 20 years, peak in females: 1st decade; males: 5th decade. Onset earlier with positive family history; can appear as early as 6 weeks (1).
- Predominance: male = female; however, females are more likely to seek treatment (1).
- No race or socioeconomic predilection

Prevalence

~1% in the United States and Europe; 0.1–8% in the world; highest in Gujarat, India, at 8.8% (1)

ETIOLOGY AND PATHOPHYSIOLOGY

Most likely a spectrum of disorders with a common phenotype, and multiple mechanisms contribute to the pathology (convergence theory).

- Genetic: see above.
- Autoimmune: humoral autoantibodies and skin-homing T cells (1)
- Neural: local or systemic dysregulation leading to excess neurotransmitters (1)
- Viral: direct melanocyte toxicity, cytomegalovirus (CMV), hepatitis C, and Epstein-Barr virus (EBV) found in lesional biopsies (1)
- Oxidative stress from elevated H_2O_2 and NO and decreased catalase and erythrocyte glutathione (1)

Genetics

- Polygenic/multifactorial inheritance
- 20% of patients report affected relative, but monozygotic twins have only 23% concordance.
- HLA haplotypes, small nucleotide polymorphisms, and specific genes are all possible contributors (1).

RISK FACTORS

- Family history of vitiligo/autoimmune disorders
- Personal history of associated conditions

COMMONLY ASSOCIATED CONDITIONS

- Most common
  - Endocrine: thyroid disease (hypothyroidism/hyperthyroidism), hypoparathyroidism, Addison disease, insulin-dependent diabetes
  - Dermatologic: psoriasis, atopic dermatitis, alopecia areata, chronic urticaria, halo nevi, ichthyosis
  - Pernicious anemia
  - Hypoacusis, rheumatoid arthritis
  - Ocular abnormalities in up to 40%
  - Elevated antinuclear antibodies in up to 40%
  - Elevated thyroperoxidase antibodies in 50%
- Less common
  - Systemic lupus erythematosus
  - Inflammatory bowel disease
  - Melanoma (may be a sign of positive outcome of melanoma) and other skin cancers
  - Syndromes: Alezzandrini; mitochondrial encephalomyopathy, lactic acidosis, and stroke-like episodes (MELAS); Schmidt; and autoimmune polyendocrinopathy candidiasis ectodermal dysplasia (APCED)
- Age >50 years at onset should prompt investigation for associated conditions.

Pediatric Considerations

Associated with Hashimoto thyroiditis in a significant portion of children. Screening at onset and possibly annually may be beneficial.

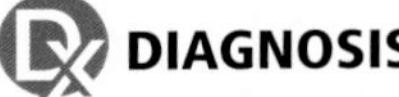

DIAGNOSIS

HISTORY

- Inquire about recent history of sunburns, pregnancy, skin trauma, or emotional stress (1).
- Family history of premature graying, vitiligo, and autoimmune disorders
- Review of systems for related associated conditions
- Ascertain psychological impact on QOL, Dermatology Life Quality Index (DLQI).

PHYSICAL EXAM

- Full-body skin exam with Wood lamp to accentuate lesions and distinguish depigmentation from hypopigmentation (1)
- Lesions are well-demarcated, uniform white macules and patches.
- Look for evidence of repigmentation (most commonly around hair follicles).

DIFFERENTIAL DIAGNOSIS

- Infectious: tinea versicolor, leprosy, leishmaniasis, onchocerciasis, treponematoses (pinta/syphilis)
- Postinflammatory hypopigmentation: psoriasis, atopic dermatitis, pityriasis alba, systemic lupus erythematosus, scleroderma
- Inherited hypomelanoses: piebaldism, tuberous sclerosis, Waardenburg, hypomelanosis of Ito, Vogt-Koyanagi-Harada
- Malformations: nevus anemicus, nevus depigmentosus
- Paraneoplastic: mycosis fungoides, melanoma-associated leukoderma
- Occupational and chemical induced
  - Occupational: phenolic/catechol derivatives and arsenic-containing compounds
  - Chemical: numerous, including cosmetics, cleansers, insecticides, and even medications (imatinib, potent topical corticosteroids [TCS])(1)
- Melasma: Normal skin may be confused as vitiligo in the setting of surrounding hyperpigmentation.
- Halo nevi
- Lichen sclerosis et atrophicus
- Idiopathic guttate hypomelanosis
- Progressive acquired macular hypomelanosis

DIAGNOSTIC TESTS & INTERPRETATION

Initial Tests (lab, imaging)

- TSH, CBC, ANA (1)
- Consider antithyroid peroxidase, antithyroglobulin antibodies, hemoglobin, vitamin B_{12} levels if family/patient history of autoimmune disease (1).

Follow-Up Tests & Special Considerations

- Monitor for disease progression/flares.
- Monitor for symptoms of related conditions.

Diagnostic Procedures/Other

- Skin biopsy rarely needed. Highest yield is with comparison of lesional/perilesional biopsies.
- Consider ophthalmologic and audiologic evaluation.

Test Interpretation

Few or no epidermal melanocytes. At margins, melanocytes may be larger, vacuolated, and dendritic. Early lesions show inflammation, and later, degeneration, including of adnexa and nerves.

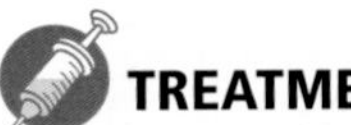

TREATMENT

The variant of vitiligo may affect response.

- If untreated, progression is the natural course for those with mucosal involvement, family history, koebnerization, and nonsegmental variants.
- Lesions that respond best are on the face, of recent onset, in darker skin type, and in younger patients.

GENERAL MEASURES

- Sunscreen to decrease sunburn and prevent accentuation of uninvolved skin
- Corrective camouflage as coverup (Cover FX, Dermablend)

MEDICATION

- Individualize therapy depending on age, extent, distribution, and rate of progression.
- Many therapies are considered "off-label" and not FDA approved for vitiligo, although they are often considered 1st-line therapy.
- Corticosteroids: Mid-potency topical corticosteroids (mometasone furoate, fluticasone propionate) applied daily as monotherapy are considered 1st-line treatments. Do not use on face/axilla/groin; do not occlude except under close monitoring. Pediatric: as above, for children >12 years of age. Consider decreased potency. Local side effects including atrophy, telangiectasia, hypertrichosis, acneiform eruptions, and striae limit treatment; regular steroid holidays are recommended (2). The combination of light therapy and TCS is the most effective treatment overall (3). Most efficacious on sun-exposed areas: face/neck, dark skinned patients, newer lesion (3). Addition of tretinoin 0.025–0.05% BID is effective and can decrease potential skin atrophy (4). Systemic corticosteroids can be helpful, but dosage and safety parameters have not been fully evaluated (2,5)[A].

- Topical calcineurin inhibitors: slightly inferior to TCS as monotherapy but better side effect profile (3,6,7)[B]; can be used as adjunctive to light therapy; carries a controversial black box warning for a theoretical risk of lymphoma or skin cancer. Extensive safety profiling has not revealed any evidence for this in children or adults using topical calcineurin inhibitors. Local reactions include burning sensation, pruritus, erythema, and rare transient hyperpigmentation (3).
  - Tacrolimus 0.03% or 0.1% ointment BID (2). Pediatric: 0.03% ointment BID, for children >2 years of age (7).
  - Pimecrolimus 1% cream BID (2). Pediatric: as adults, for children >2 years of age (7).
- Topical vitamin D_3 analogs: less effective than TCS alone, but in combination with TCS or phototherapy can shorten time until, and improve stability of, repigmentation 7[B].
  - Calcipotriene ointment 1–2 × per day. Pediatric: not defined.
  - Available as a combination formulation, betamethasone dipropionate 0.064%/calcipotriene 0.005% ointment daily, max dose of 100 g/week for 4 weeks, not for >30% BSA, and not for face/axilla/groin. Pediatric: not defined.
- Oral vitamin D_3: reported to induce repigmentation. Oral vitamin D_3 35,000 units once daily plus low-calcium diet for 6 months. Pediatric: not defined.
- Phototherapy: Narrow band UVB (NBUVB) is superior to UVA and indicated for lesions involving more than 15–20% BSA (7,8)[A]. Psoralen and khellin enhance the effect of light. Psoralen plus UVA (PUVA) may increase the incidence of skin cancers. Khellin may have reduced cross-linking of DNA, may be less carcinogenic, however, it is associated with increased liver toxicity (8). L-phenylalanine can be used topically and orally as a photosensitizer for natural or artificial light. Pediatric: Oral PUVA is contraindicated.
- Laser therapy: Excimer laser (308 nm) is superior to other light therapy. Helium neon laser works for segmental vitiligo (7)[A].
- Antioxidants: may have protective role in preventing melanocyte degradation from reactive oxygen species. Options include vitamin C, vitamin E, Vitix, *Polipodium leucotomos* extracts, and *Ginkgo biloba* (6)[B].
- Surgical therapy: See later discussion.
- New concepts: Tumor necrosis factor-α inhibitors, cyclosporine, cyclophosphamide, azathioprine, minocycline, and immunosuppressants are currently being evaluated (8).

First Line

- Recommended: avoidance of triggering factors plus TCS alone or in combination with NBUVB
- Alternatively
  - Topical calcineurin inhibitors (preferred for face, neck, axilla, and groin)
  - NBUVB
  - PUVA in adults
  - Camouflage and psychotherapy should be offered to all patients at any stage (8).

Second Line

- Recommended: photochemotherapy with psoralens or vitamin D analogues
- Alternatively
  - Topical vitamin D analogues
  - Targeted phototherapy
    - 308-nm laser in combination with topical steroids, topical calcineurin inhibitors, or vitamin D analogues
  - Oral corticosteroids (pulse therapy)
  - Surgical treatments indicated for stable 2–3-cm lesions, refractory to other treatments
    - Mini-punch graft (pretreat with cryotherapy/dermabrasion or posttreat with phototherapy) (9)[B]
    - Suction blister graft (9)[B]
    - Autologous melanocyte suspension transplant (6)[B]

ISSUES FOR REFERRAL

- Dermatologist: for facial/widespread vitiligo or when advanced therapy necessary
- Ophthalmologist: for ocular symptoms or monitoring of TCS near eyes
- Endocrinologist: evaluation/management of associated conditions
- Psychologist: for severe distress
- Medical geneticist for associated conditions

ADDITIONAL THERAPIES

- Depigmentation therapy with monobenzone, hydroquinone, or Q-switched ruby laser: for extensive vitiligo recalcitrant to therapy (9)
- Pseudocatalase with addition of NBUVB (2)[B]
- Prostaglandin E for short-duration disease and localization to face and scalp (2)[B]
- Cosmetic tattooing for localized stable vitiligo

SURGERY/OTHER PROCEDURES

- Goal is to transport melanocytes from other areas of the skin. Methods include punch, blister, or split-thickness skin grafting, or transplantation of autologous melanocytes.
- Dermabrasion and curettage alone or in combination with 5-fluorouracil may induce follicular melanocyte reservoirs (7)[B].
- Patients who koebnerize or form keloids may be worse, and permanent scarring is a risk for all patients.

COMPLEMENTARY & ALTERNATIVE MEDICINE

- *Ginkgo biloba* 60 mg PO daily may significantly improve extension and spreading of lesions (8)[B].
- *Polipodium leucotomos* may help with repigmentation with NBUVB and aid in reducing phototoxic reactions (7,8)[B].

ONGOING CARE

FOLLOW-UP RECOMMENDATIONS

- Monitor for symptoms of related conditions.
- With topical steroids, follow at regular intervals to avoid steroid atrophy, telangiectasia, and striae distensae.

DIET

No restrictions

PATIENT EDUCATION

- Discussion of disease course, progression, and cosmesis
- Education regarding trauma/friction and Koebner phenomenon

PROGNOSIS

- Vitiligo may remain stable or slowly or rapidly progress.
- Spontaneous repigmentation is uncommon.
- Generalized vitiligo is often progressive, with flares. Focal vitiligo often has rapid onset, then stabilizes.

COMPLICATIONS

- Adverse effects of each treatment modality
- Psychiatric morbidity: depression, adjustment disorder, low self-esteem, sexual dysfunction, and embarrassment in relationships (1)
  - Different cultures may have different perceptions/social stigmas about vitiligo. Some believe it to be contagious or related to infection. Women with vitiligo may have difficulty finding a marriage partner and have low self-esteem.

REFERENCES

1. Alikhan A, Felsten LM, Daly M, et al. Vitiligo: a comprehensive overview Part I. Introduction, epidemiology, quality of life, diagnosis, differential diagnosis, associations, histopathology, etiology, and work-up. *J Am Acad Dermatol*. 2011;65(3):473–491.
2. Colucci R, Lotti T, Moretti S. Vitiligo: an update on current pharmacotherapy and future directions. *Expert Opin Pharmacother*. 2012;13(13):1885–1899.
3. Felsten LM, Alikhan A, Petronic-Rosic V. Vitiligo: a comprehensive overview Part II: treatment options and approach to treatment. *J Am Acad Dermatol*. 2011;65(3):493–514.
4. Kwon HB, Choi Y, Kim HJ, et al. The therapeutic effects of a topical tretinoin and corticosteroid combination for vitiligo: a placebo-controlled, paired-comparison, left-right study. *J Drugs Dermatol*. 2013;12(4):e63–e67.
5. Njoo MD, Spuls PI, Bos JD, et al. Nonsurgical repigmentation therapies in vitiligo. Meta-analysis of the literature. *Arch Dermatol*. 1998;134(12):1532–1540.
6. Lepe V, Moncada B, Castanedo-Cazares JP, et al. A double-blind randomized trial of 0.1% tacrolimus vs 0.05% clobetasol for the treatment of childhood vitiligo. *Arch Dermatol*. 2003;139(5):581–585.
7. Whitton ME, Pinart M, Batchelor J, et al. Interventions for vitiligo. *Cochrane Database Syst Rev*. 2010;(1):CD003263.
8. Taieb A, Alomar A, Böhm M, et al. Guidelines for the management of vitiligo: the European Dermatology Forum consensus. *Br J Dermatol*. 2013;168(1):5–19.
9. Patel NS, Paghdal KV, Cohen GF. Advanced treatment modalities for vitiligo. *Dermatol Surg*. 2012;38(3):381–391.

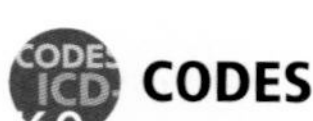

CODES

ICD10

L80 Vitiligo

CLINICAL PEARLS

- Vitiligo can be a psychologically devastating skin disease.
- Screen for associated diseases, particularly if onset occurs later in life.
- Treatment should be individualized based on BSA, skin type, and patient goals.
- Dermatology consultation when extensive disease, facial involvement, and when advanced treatments are considered.

VOCAL CORD DYSFUNCTION

Ileana Bembenek, MD • Chris Wheelock, MD

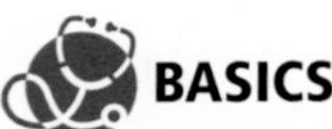

BASICS

DESCRIPTION

- A breathing disorder in which vocal cords adduct inappropriately mostly during inspiration. This may result in wheezing, stridor, and upper airway obstruction.
- Synonym(s): paradoxical vocal fold motion (PVFM)

EPIDEMIOLOGY

Incidence

Not well defined

Prevalence

- Also not well defined, likely uncommon in the general population.
- Mostly diagnosed in patients evaluated for asthma and exercise induced dyspnea
- Likely female predominance (2:1–3:1)
- 71% of patients were adults and 29% of patients were <18 years of age. It has, however, been diagnosed in young children.
- Suspected in approximately 3% of the highly athletic intercollegiate athletes population with exercise-induced asthma (1)

ETIOLOGY AND PATHOPHYSIOLOGY

- Likely multifactorial—exact etiology unclear
- Possible laryngeal hyperresponsiveness to irritants, for example, allergic rhinitis with postnasal drip, smoke, or other irritants
- Gastroesophageal reflux disease can cause mucosal damage or can cause symptoms as an irritant (2).
- Noncompetitive and competitive exercise—unknown mechanism (3)
- Psychological stresses such as competitive sports

Genetics

None defined

RISK FACTORS

See "Commonly Associated Conditions."

COMMONLY ASSOCIATED CONDITIONS

- Asthma
- Gastroesophageal reflux disease
- Rhinosinusitis
- Psychological conditions such as posttraumatic stress disorder, anxiety, depression, and panic disorder

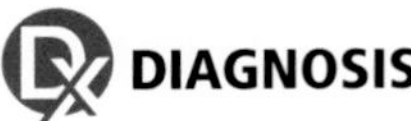

DIAGNOSIS

HISTORY

- Recurrent episodes of "difficulty breathing in," wheezing, throat or chest tightness, chocking sensation
- Some elite athletes describe wheezing as often inspirational or rarely expirational stridor; however, it may resolve spontaneously when activity ceases.
- Sense of panic and agitation
- The stridor is often mistaken for wheezing and, therefore, patients are commonly diagnosed with asthma.
- The symptoms tend to be relatively mild but can be prolonged and severe.
- Exercise is a common cause of vocal cord dysfunction and often leads to the mistaken diagnosis of exercise induced asthma.
- Patients who do not respond to bronchodilator therapy should be evaluated for the possibility of vocal cord dysfunction.

PHYSICAL EXAM

- Inspiratory stridor
- Cough
- Wheezing (especially if unresponsive to bronchodilators)
- Mild respiratory distress

DIFFERENTIAL DIAGNOSIS

- Asthma: primary differential diagnosis because wheezing is a big component—although PVFM can also be seen concomitantly with asthma (1,2). The key differences between the two are the following:
  - Asthma not typically associated with a sensation of chocking
  - Vocal cord dysfunction produces more difficulty breathing with inspiration as opposed to expiration.
  - PVFM not responsive to asthma treatment (unless coexisiting) (1)
- Laryngeal angioedema
- Epiglottitis
- Vocal cord polyps/tumor
- Vocal cord paralysis
- Croup
- Tracheal stenosis or masses
- Laryngomalacia (2)

DIAGNOSTIC TESTS & INTERPRETATION

Initial Tests (lab, imaging)

- Flexible laryngoscopy—gold standard (1)[C]
  - Allows for direct visualization of abnormal adduction of the vocal cords
  - May allow for diagnosis in more than half of asymptomatic patients; however, provocation tests such as methacholine (4), exercise (3),and histamine may be needed for diagnosis (3,4)[C].
- Pulmonary function testing with flow volume loop
  - Most commonly used test
  - Positive findings consist of normal expiratory volume loop with a flattened inspiratory volume loop. This is consistent with extrathoracic upper airway obstruction (5)[C].
  - May require exercise testing for patients in whom exercise is the trigger
  - Useful for distinguishing from asthma, as in that case, the expiratory loop would be affected instead
- Arterial blood gases
  - Useful to rule out other causes of severe respiratory distress

TREATMENT

GENERAL MEASURES

- Short term
  - Reassurance and supportive care; controlling asthma if coexisting
  - Breathing instruction, which include the following:
    - Panting (breath rapidly and shallow)
    - Diaphragmatic breathing
    - Breathing through the nose
    - Breathing through a straw or through pursed lips
    - Exhaling with a hissing sound
    - Administration of helium and oxygen combination has been reported in one case series to reduce airway resistance resulting in improvement of symptoms (1,2)[C].
- Long term
  - Avoid triggers.
  - Behavioral speech/voice therapy (6)[B]
  - Treat underlying conditions.

MEDICATION

First Line

No medications are specifically helpful. Exercise-induced PVFM may respond to anticholinergics in addition to speech therapy; thus, consider a trial of ipratropium if symptoms are exercise induced (7)[C].

ISSUES FOR REFERRAL

- Diagnosis and treatment may require assistance of pulmonologist, otolaryngologists, allergist, psychiatrist, and/or psychologist.
- Speech therapy is the mainstay of long-term treatment for patients with ongoing symptoms. It helps reduce recurrence.

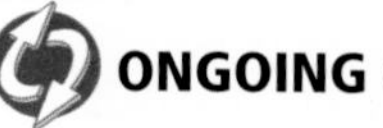

ONGOING CARE

PROGNOSIS

Spontaneous resolution is common.

REFERENCES

1. Ibrahim WH, Gheriani HA, Almohamed AA, et al. Paradoxical vocal cord motion disorder: past present and future. *Postgrad Med J*. 2007;83(977):164–172.
2. Morris MJ, Allan PF, Perking PJ. Vocal cord dysfunction: aetiologies and treatment. *Clin Pulm Med*. 2006;13:73–86.
3. Chiang T, Marcinow AM, deSilva BW, et al. Exercise-induced paradoxical vocal fold motion disorder: diagnosis and management. *Laryngoscope*. 2013;123(3):727–731.
4. Perkins PJ, Morris MJ. Vocal cord dysfunction induced by methacholine challenge testing. *Chest*. 2002;122(6):1988–1993.
5. Mobeireek A, Alhamad A, Al-Subaei A, et al. Psychogenic vocal cord dysfunction simulating bronchial asthma. *Eur Respir J*. 1995;8(11):1978–1981.
6. Sullivan MD, Heywood BM, Beukelman DR. A treatment for vocal cord dysfunction in female athletes: an outcome study. *Laryngoscope*. 2001;111(10):1751–1755.
7. Doshi DR, Weinberger MM. Long-term outcome of vocal cord dysfunction. *Ann Allergy Asthma Immunol*. 2006;96(6):794–799.

ADDITIONAL READING

- Deckert J, Deckert L. Vocal cord dysfunction. *Am Fam Physician*. 2010;81(2):156–159.
- Jain S, Bandi V, Zimmerman J, et al. Incidence of vocal cord dysfunction in patients presenting to emergency room with acute asthma exacerbation. *Chest*. 1997;116(Suppl 2):243S.
- Newsham KR, Klaben BK, Miller NJ, et al. Paradoxical vocal-cord dysfunction: management in athletes. *J Athl Train*. 2002;37(3):325–328.
- Nolan PK, Goodman D, Chrysler M, et al. Spirometry coupled with pulse oximetry in the emergency department to rule out status asthmaticus and suggest vocal cord dysfunction. *Chest*. 2006;130:241S–242S.
- Pargeter NJ, Mansur AH. The effectiveness of speech and language therapy in vocal cord dysfunction. *Thorax*. 2006;61(Suppl 2):ii126.
- Pitchenik AE. Functional laryngeal obstruction relieved by panting. *Chest*. 1991;100(5):1465–1467.
- Weir M. Vocal cord dysfunction mimics asthma and may respond to heliox. *Clin Pediatr (Phila)*. 2002;41(1):37–41.

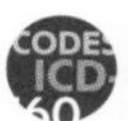

CODES

ICD10

- J38.3 Other diseases of vocal cords
- J38.00 Paralysis of vocal cords and larynx, unspecified
- J38.1 Polyp of vocal cord and larynx

CLINICAL PEARLS

- Always consider vocal cord dysfunction in poorly controlled asthmatics.
- A multidisciplinary approach may be required for diagnosis and treatment.
- Speech therapy is the mainstay of long-term treatment.

V

VON WILLEBRAND DISEASE

Aneel A. Ashrani, MD, MS • Ewa M. Wysokinska, MD

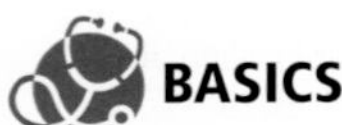

BASICS

DESCRIPTION

- von Willebrand disease (vWD) is a bleeding disorder caused by deficiency or a defect of *von Willebrand factor* (vWF) protein.
- vWF is critical to the initial stages of blood clotting, acting as a bridge for platelet adhesion; it also acts as a carrier for factor VIII (FVIII).
- vWD primarily manifests as mucocutaneous or perioperative bleeding.
- vWD is an inherited condition but rarely can be acquired (1,2).

EPIDEMIOLOGY

Prevalence

- Prevalence of the inherited forms of vWD is ~1–2% of the general population with 2:1 female to male ratio.
- Exact prevalence of the acquired forms of vWD (AvWD) is unknown but is estimated to be up to 0.1% of the general population.

Pediatric Considerations

Many cases of vWD are diagnosed in childhood, often during initial years of menstruation.

Pregnancy Considerations

Although levels of vWF increase during pregnancy, women with vWD are more likely to experience an increased incidence of obstetric complications that manifest with bleeding.

ETIOLOGY AND PATHOPHYSIOLOGY

- vWF is a large, multimeric protein that is released from endothelial cells and is also carried within platelets in alpha granules.
- vWF binds to collagen at sites of vascular injury and creates a surface for platelet adhesion through GP1b receptor. This results in platelet plug formation.
- vWF is also a carrier for FVIII and stabilizes this factor from degradation. A deficiency in vWF may result in lower levels of FVIII.
- When vWF is deficient or dysfunctional, primary hemostasis is compromised, resulting in increased mucocutaneous and postprocedural bleeding.
- 3 major categories of vWD exist:
  - Type 1, the most common and mildest form, represents 60–80% of cases.
    - Mild to moderate quantitative deficiency of vWF and concordant deficiency of FVIII
    - Generally, a mild bleeding disorder
  - Type 2 caused by qualitative defect in vWF accounts for 10–30% of cases and is divided into the following multiple subtypes.
    - Type 2A is noted for loss of hemostatically active large multimers, with low ristocetin cofactor/vWF activity.
    - Type 2B, noted for increased binding affinity for platelets, is associated with thrombocytopenia, low ristocetin cofactor/vWF activity, abnormal ristocetin-induced platelet aggregation (RIPA) and loss of large multimers.
    - Type 2M is noted for defective platelet or collagen binding without loss of large multimers.
    - Type 2N demonstrates defective binding to FVIII, which results in increased clearance of FVIII and hemophilia A–like picture
  - Type 3 represents 1–5% of cases:
    - Most severe form characterized by markedly decreased-to-undetectable levels of vWF and FVIII
    - Manifests as Hemophilia A with hemarthroses
- Acquired form of vWD may be due to cardiovascular, hematologic, or autoimmune conditions, as well as tumors and medications.
- The pathophysiology of AvWD is related to the underlying cause and may result from shear induced cleaving of VWF in cardiovascular conditions, increased adsorption of vWF by certain tumor cells or activated platelets, or presence of anti-vWF autoantibodies detected in hematologic disorders.

Genetics

- The 175-kb gene for vWF is located on short arm of chromosome 12.
- Type 1 follows an autosomal dominant inheritance pattern, with variable expressivity.
- Type 2 varies but primarily follows an autosomal dominant inheritance pattern.
- Type 3 follows an autosomal recessive inheritance pattern.

COMMONLY ASSOCIATED CONDITIONS

AvWD may be found in patients with hematologic disorders such as MGUS and myeloproliferative neoplasms. Commonly associated cardiovascular conditions include aortic stenosis and LVAD placement.

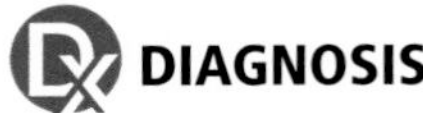

DIAGNOSIS

HISTORY

- Most patients with vWD have a positive family history of bleeding disorder; however, patients with mild forms of vWD and their families may be unaware of their disease. Those with acquired vWD often have no family history of this disorder.
- The most important component of diagnosis is the hemostatic history.
- Common symptoms are those of mucocutaneous (recurrent epistaxis, menorrhagia, ecchymosis) or postprocedural bleeding. Hemarthroses are a rare presentation, mostly associated with type 2N and 3.

PHYSICAL EXAM

- Physical exam may be entirely normal, although there may be some ecchymoses.
- Findings suggestive of other causes of increased bleeding should be sought (liver disease, skin laxity, or telangiectasias).

DIFFERENTIAL DIAGNOSIS

- Primary hemostatic disorders: congenital thrombocytopenia or qualitative platelet defects, coagulation factor deficiencies
- Secondary hemostatic disorders: liver disease, uremia, connective tissue disorders, coagulation factor inhibitors

DIAGNOSTIC TESTS & INTERPRETATION

Initial Tests (lab, imaging)

- The specific tests for vWD include vWF antigen (VWF:Ag), vWF activity/ristocetin cofactor activity (VWF:RCo) (if available: collagen-binding activity [VWF:CB]) and FVIII activity; these tests should be ordered when suspicion for vWD is high. Additional specific tests include RIPA, vWF multimer analysis, and vWF propeptide (vWFpp).
- Other tests include CBC, PT/INR, aPTT, platelet function analyzer assay (PFA-100).
  - Platelet count is often normal, except in type 2B or in AvWD when there is an underlying myeloproliferative disorder.
  - Platelet function assays via PFA-100 (i.e., collagen/epinephrine and collagen/ADP closure time) are usually prolonged but may be normal in mild disease.
  - PT/INR is normal, unless there is concurrent liver disease or warfarin/Coumadin use.
  - Activated PTT may be prolonged if a decrease in FVIII accompanies vWD.
- Specific tests for vWD
  - vWF antigen testing is done via immunologic methods:
    - vWF antigen testing has a positive predictive value (PPV) of 33% for detecting significant FVIII deficiency and a PPV of 80% for detecting ristocetin cofactor activity abnormalities.
    - vWF antigen may be normal in type 2 vWD.
  - Ristocetin cofactor activity is a functional assessment of vWF. Ristocetin promotes binding of platelets to vWF, and this activity is disproportionately reduced compared to vWF antigen in most forms of type 2 vWD.
  - Ratio of VWF:RCo to VWF:Ag <0.5–0.7 may be used to differentiate type 1 from type 2 vWD.
  - Alternatively, latex particle–enhanced immunoassay may be used to quantify vWF activity. A specific monoclonal anti-vWF antibody directed against platelet GP1b–binding site of vWF adsorbed onto the latex reagent reacts with plasma vWF proportional to the vWF activity.
  - Collagen-binding activity, another functional assessment of vWF, is reduced in most forms of vWD.
  - FVIII activity may be normal or mildly decreased in most types of vWD (in 2N and type 3, levels are markedly decreased).
  - vWFpp is useful in accelerated clearance variants of vWD.
  - vWF multimer analysis is performed by electrophoresis on agarose gel. This test differentiates patients with type 2 vWD.
  - RIPA is useful in diagnosing type 2B vWD.
  - FVIII-vWF binding assay activity is low in patients with type 2N vWD.
  - Genotype testing may also be used especially for types 2 and 3 (1,2).

Follow-Up Tests & Special Considerations

- Unless patients have severe forms of vWD or are undergoing treatment, follow-up laboratory studies are not usually obtained.
- Patients with blood group O have 20–30% baseline lower levels of vWF antigen and ristocetin cofactor activity.
- vWF is an acute-phase reactant, so elevations may be seen in inflammatory conditions, liver disease, pregnancy (which may correct mild deficits), or with estrogen use.

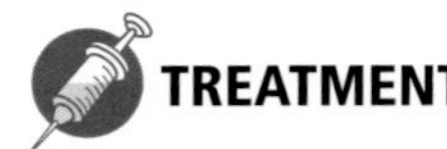

TREATMENT

GENERAL MEASURES

- Most patients with type 1 vWD do not require activity restrictions.
- Patients with type 3 vWD should avoid contact sports.
- An emergency ID bracelet may be useful.

MEDICATION

First Line

- Desmopressin (DDAVP)
  - Enhances release of vWF from endothelial cells
  - Primarily effective for type 1 vWD; not to be used in type 2B
  - Typically raises vWF by 2- to 3-fold from baseline levels (3)[B]
  - Not effective in severe deficiencies, in types of vWD with defective vWF, or for prophylaxis prior to major procedures
  - Dosed 0.3 μg/kg (max 20 μg) IV/SC; intranasal (high concentration) spray: <50 kg: 150 μg/day; >50 kg: 300 μg/day (Stimate)
  - Common side effects: flushing, tachycardia, water retention, hyponatremia
  - Obtain repeat testing of ristocetin cofactor activity and FVIII 1 and 4 hours after infusion to evaluate peak response and clearance of DDAVP.
  - Tachyphylaxis may develop with prolonged dosing; limit use to 3–5 days.
- vWF and FVIII concentrates
  - Plasma-derived vWF and FVIII concentrates of various purity such as Humate-P, Alphanate, Wilate, or Fandhi (not available in United States) are commercial concentrates of vWF and FVIII that are given in doses of 25–60 IU/kg/day based on clinical situation (4,5)[B]:
    - Administration of 1 IU/kg vWF:RCo concentrate raises the plasma RCo activity by approximately 2%.
    - Dose of vWF concentrate may be adjusted for FVIII levels and ristocetin cofactor activity.
    - FVIII levels should be monitored to avoid supranormal levels and possible venous thromboembolism (VTE).
    - Contraindicated if patient develops alloantibodies to vWF
  - New recombinant form of vWF concentrate is effective in clinical trials but not yet available for clinical use (6)[B].
  - In patients with severe bleeding phenotype, prophylactic treatment is used.
- Cryoprecipitate
  - Cryoprecipitate contains FVIII, fibrinogen, vWF, factor XIII, and fibronectin.
  - Not considered as safe as the virus-inactivated plasma concentrates listed above and should not be used unless those are unavailable
- Antifibrinolytics
  - Useful for mucosal bleeding
  - Contraindicated in patients with hematuria due to risk of retention of large blood clots in the renal collecting system
  - Given as adjunct to DDAVP
  - Aminocaproic acid may be given at 50–70 mg/kg q4–6h IV or PO.
  - Tranexamic acid may be given at 10–15 mg/kg IV or 25 mg/kg (1300 mg) PO q8–12h.
- Recombinant FVIIa/Novoseven
  - Used for patients who develop alloantibodies to vWF
  - Given as IV bolus of 90 μg/kg q2h or 20 μg/kg every hour until hemostasis is achieved

Second Line

- Oral contraceptives raise vWF/FVIII levels and have a role in the treatment of chronic menorrhagia.
- Platelets may be given as an adjunct to factor concentrates if hemostasis has not been achieved.
- IVIG has been useful in some patients with AvWD associated with monoclonal gammopathy (7).
- Recombinant FVIIa has been used effectively in patients with type 3 vWD.

ISSUES FOR REFERRAL

The diagnosis and management of vWD is not always straightforward; consider consultation with hematologist.

SURGERY/OTHER PROCEDURES

Valve replacement or correction may be curative for patients with AvWD associated with underlying cardiovascular conditions.

INPATIENT CONSIDERATIONS

Admission Criteria/Initial Stabilization

- For patients with major bleeding or those undergoing major surgical procedures, levels of ristocetin cofactor/vWF activity and FVIII need to be restored to 80–100 IU/dL for 1st 2 days and then maintained >50 IU/dL for 5–7 days.
- For patients undergoing minor surgical procedures, maintain FVIII levels >50 IU/dL for 5–7 days.
- For patients delivering or in need of epidural anesthesia, obtain FVIII levels >50 IU/dL.

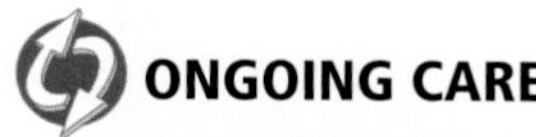

ONGOING CARE

FOLLOW-UP RECOMMENDATIONS

Patients should be seen by a hematologist prior to invasive procedures for determination of perioperative management or advice regarding delivery.

PATIENT MONITORING

Patients with mild disease do not require monitoring.

DIET

No dietary restrictions are recommended. However, aspirin and other NSAIDs should be avoided due to their antiplatelet effects, which can exacerbate the bleeding phenotype.

PATIENT EDUCATION

National Hemophilia Foundation: www.hemophilia.org/NHFWeb/MainPgs/MainNHF.aspx?menuid=182&contentid=47&rptname=bleeding

PROGNOSIS

Most patients with vWD have a normal life expectancy.

COMPLICATIONS

- Significant perioperative bleeding may occur.
- Patients with type 3 vWD and type 2N can have bleeding complications similar to patients with hemophilia A such as hemarthrosis and intracranial hemorrhage.
- Patients with aortic stenosis and AvWD are known to have higher rates of GI bleeding.
- Multiple transfusions may result in alloantibodies against vWF.
- Venous thromboembolism may result from supranormal levels of FVIII.

REFERENCES

1. Lillicrap D. von Willebrand disease: advances in pathogenetic understanding, diagnosis, and therapy. *Blood*. 2013;122(23):3735–3740.
2. Nichols WL, Hultin MB, James AH, et al. von Willebrand disease (VWD): evidence-based diagnosis and management guidelines, the National Heart, Lung, and Blood Institute (NHLBI) Expert Panel report (USA). *Haemophilia*. 2008;14(2):171–232.
3. Hanebutt FL, Rolf N, Loesel A, et al. Evaluation of desmopressin effects on haemostasis in children with congenital bleeding disorders. *Haemophilia*. 2008;14(3):524–530.
4. Mannucci PM, Chediak J, Hanna W, et al. Treatment of von Willebrand disease with a high-purity factor VIII/von Willebrand factor concentrate: a prospective, multicenter study. *Blood*. 2002;99(2):450–456.
5. Thompson AR, Gill JC, Ewenstein BM, et al. Successful treatment for patients with von Willebrand disease undergoing urgent surgery using factor VIII/VWF concentrate (Humate-P). *Haemophilia*. 2004;10(1):42–51.
6. Mannucci PM, Kempton C, Millar C, et al. Pharmacokinetics and safety of a novel recombinant human von Willebrand factor manufactured with a plasma-free method: a prospective clinical trial. *Blood*. 2013;122(5):648–657.
7. Tiede A, Rand JH, Budde U, et al. How I treat acquired von Willebrand syndrome. *Blood*. 2011;117(25):6777–6785.

ADDITIONAL READING

- Kessler CM. Diagnosis and treatment of von Willebrand disease: new perspectives and nuances. *Haemophilia*. 2007;13(Suppl 5):3–14.
- Kumar S, Pruthi RK, Nichols WL. Acquired von Willebrand disease. *Mayo Clin Proc*. 2002;77(2):181–187.
- Lippi G, Franchini M, Salvagno GL, et al. Correlation between von Willebrand factor antigen, von Willebrand factor ristocetin cofactor activity and factor VIII activity in plasma. *J Thromb Thrombolysis*. 2008;26(2):150–153.
- Mannucci PM. Treatment of von Willebrand's disease. *N Engl J Med*. 2004;351(7):683–694.
- Robertson J, Lillicrap D, James PD. Von Willebrand disease. *Pediatr Clin North Am*. 2008;55(2):377–392, viii–ix.
- Sciscione AC, Mucowski SJ. Pregnancy and von Willebrand disease: a review. *Del Med J*. 2007;79(10):401–405.

SEE ALSO

Algorithms: Bleeding Gums; Ecchymosis

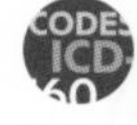

CODES

ICD10

D68.0 Von Willebrand's disease

CLINICAL PEARLS

- vWD varies from a minor to severe bleeding disorder; affects 1–2% of the U.S. population
- It is important to determine the exact type of vWD (1, 2, or 3) to guide treatment.
- AvWD should be considered in patients with acquired bleeding disorder if they have underlying predisposing conditions.

VULVAR MALIGNANCY

Radhika Sharma, MD • Michael P. Hopkins, MD, MEd

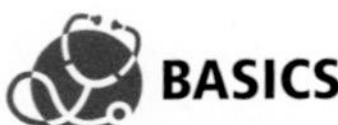

BASICS

DESCRIPTION

- Premalignant lesions of the vulva are collectively known as vulvar intraepithelial neoplasia (VIN). Exposure to human papillomavirus (HPV) has been linked to >70% of VIN (1).
- Invasive squamous cell carcinoma is the most common malignancy involving the vulva (90% of patients). Can be well, moderately, or poorly differentiated and derives from keratinized skin covering the vulva and perineum.
- Melanoma is the second most common type of vulvar malignancy (8%) and sarcoma is the third (1).
- Other invasive cell types include basal cell carcinoma, Paget disease, adenocarcinoma arising from Bartholin gland or apocrine sweat glands, adenoid cystic carcinoma, small cell carcinoma, verrucous carcinoma, and sarcomas.
- Sarcomas are usually leiomyosarcoma and probably arise at the insertion of the round ligament in the labium major; however, sarcoma can arise from the any structure of the vulva, including blood vessels, skeletal muscle, and fat.
- Rarely, breast carcinoma has been reported in the vulva and is thought to arise from ectopic breast tissue.
- System(s) affected: reproductive

Geriatric Considerations

- Older patients with associated medical problems are at high risk from radical surgery. The surgery, however, is usually well tolerated.
- Patients who are not surgical candidates can be treated with combination chemotherapy and/or radiation.
- In the very elderly, palliative vulvectomy provides relief of symptoms for ulcerating symptomatic advanced disease.

EPIDEMIOLOGY

Incidence

- In 2013, 4,305 women were diagnosed with vulvar cancer and 925 women died from vulvar cancer in the United States (2).
- Ethnic distribution: more common in Caucasian women than in any other race
- Surveillance, epidemiology, and end result (SEER) data showed that the incidence of in situ vulvar carcinoma increased by >400% between 1973 and 2000.
- Mean age at diagnosis 65 years; in situ disease: mean age 40 years; invasive malignancy: mean age 60 years (2)

ETIOLOGY AND PATHOPHYSIOLOGY

- Patients with cervical cancer are more likely to develop vulvar cancer later in life, secondary to "field effect" phenomenon with a carcinogen involving the lower genital tract (2).
- HPV has been associated with squamous cell abnormalities of the cervix, vagina, and vulva; 55% of vulvar cancers are attributable to oncogenic HPV, predominantly HPV 16 and 33; 92% of VIN 2/3, vaginal intraepithelial neoplasia (VAIN) 2/3, and anal intraepithelial neoplasia (AIN) are attributable to HPV.
- Squamous cell carcinoma
  - The warty basaloid type, also known as bowenoid type, is related to HPV infection and occurs in younger women. Although traditionally graded in a three-level system, the International Society for the Study of Vulvovaginal Disease voted not to use a grading system for VIN in 2004. This system eliminated VIN 1 and combined VIN 2 and VIN 3. This is based on the fact that VIN 1 is not reproducible. VIN 2 and VIN 3 were combined because VIN 2 is rare and carries the same risk of progression to malignancy as VIN 3 (1).
  - The more common variant is simplex or differentiated and does not appear to be related to HPV, occurs in older age groups, and associated with lichen sclerosus and chronic venereal diseases; it is thought to carry a higher risk of progression to malignancy.
  - Melanoma, second most common histology, often identified in postmenopausal women; often pigmented but can be amelanotic, arising de novo, often found on clitoris or labia minora (1).
- Cases not associated with HPV infection are typically associated with vulvar dystrophies, such as lichen sclerosus or squamous cell hyperplasia.
- Smoking is associated with squamous cell disease of the vulva, possibly from direct irritation of the vulva by the transfer of tars and nicotine on the patient's hands or from systemic absorption of carcinogen.

Genetics

No known genetic pattern

RISK FACTORS

- VIN or cervical intraepithelial neoplasia (CIN)
- Smoking
- Lichen sclerosus (vulvar dystrophy)
- HPV infection
- Autoimmune processes
- Immunodeficiency syndromes or immunosuppression
- Northern European ancestry

GENERAL PREVENTION

- HPV vaccination has the potential to decrease vulvar cancer by 60% (3,4).
- Abstinence from smoking/smoking cessation counseling (1)

COMMONLY ASSOCIATED CONDITIONS

- Patients with invasive vulvar cancer are often elderly and have associated medical conditions.
- High rate of other gynecologic malignancies

DIAGNOSIS

HISTORY

Complaints of pruritus or raised lesion in the vaginal area

PHYSICAL EXAM

- In situ disease: a small raised area associated with pruritus, single vulvar plaque, ulcer, or mass on labia majora, perineum, clitoris
- Vulvar bleeding, dysuria, enlarged lymph nodes less common symptomatology
- Invasive malignancy: an ulcerated, nonhealing area; as lesions become large, bleeding occurs with associated pain and foul-smelling discharge; enlarged inguinal lymph nodes indicative of advanced disease.

DIFFERENTIAL DIAGNOSIS

- Infectious processes can present as ulcerative lesions and include syphilis, lymphogranuloma venereum, and granuloma inguinale.
- Disorder of Bartholin gland, seborrheic keratosis, hidradenomas, lichen sclerosus, epidermal inclusion cysts
- Crohn disease can present as an ulcerative area on the vulva.
- Rarely, lesions can metastasize to the vulva.

DIAGNOSTIC TESTS & INTERPRETATION

Initial Tests (lab, imaging)

- Hypercalcemia can occur when metastatic disease is present.
- Squamous cell antigen can be elevated with invasive disease.

Follow-Up Tests & Special Considerations

- Upon examination, any suspicious lesions should be biopsied.
- Diagnosis based on histologic findings following vulvar biopsy (5)
- The vulva can be washed with 3% acetic acid to highlight areas and visualized with a colposcope, allows for visualization of acetowhite lesions and vascular lesions (5).
- For patients with new onset of pruritus, the area of pruritus should be biopsied.
- Liberal biopsies must be used to diagnose in situ disease prior to invasion and to diagnose early invasive disease.
- The patient should not be treated for presumed benign conditions of the vulva without full exam and biopsy, including Pap smear and colposcopy of cervix, vagina, and vulva.
- When symptoms persist, reexamine and rebiopsy.
- Treatment of benign condyloma of the vulva has not been shown to decrease the eventual incidence of in situ or invasive disease of the vulva.
- CT scan to evaluate pelvic and periaortic lymph node status if tumor >2 cm or if suspicion of metastatic disease (5)[A].

Diagnostic Procedures/Other

Office vulvar biopsy is done to establish the diagnosis.

Test Interpretation

A surgical staging system is used for vulvar cancer (International Federation of Obstetrics and Gynecology Classification)

- Stage I: tumor confined to the vulva
  - Stage IA: lesions ≤2 cm in size, confined to the vulva or perineum and with stromal invasion ≤1 mm, no node metastasis
  - Stage IB: lesions >2 cm in size or with stromal invasion >1 mm, confined to the vulva or perineum, with negative nodes
- Stage II: tumor of any size with extension to adjacent perineal structures (1/3 lower urethra, 1/3 lower vagina, anus) with negative nodes
- Stage III: tumor of any size with or without extension to adjacent perineal structures (1/3 lower urethra, 1/3 lower vagina, anus) with positive inguinofemoral lymph nodes
  - Stage IIIA
    - With 1 lymph node metastasis (≥5 mm), or
    - 1–2 lymph node metastases (<5 mm)
  - Stage IIIB
    - With ≥2 lymph node metastases (≥5 mm), or
    - ≥3 lymph node metastases (<5 mm)
  - Stage IIIC: with positive nodes with extracapsular spread
- Stage IV: tumor invades other regional (2/3 upper urethra, 2/3 upper vagina) or distant structures
  - Stage IVA: tumor invades any of the following:
    - Upper urethral and/or vaginal mucosa, bladder mucosa, rectal mucosa, or fixed to pelvic bone
    - Fixed or ulcerated inguinofemoral lymph nodes
  - Stage IVB: any distant metastasis, including pelvic lymph nodes (6)[B]

TREATMENT

GENERAL MEASURES

- Wide excision can be performed for carcinoma in situ, and any suspicious lesion should be excised for definitive diagnosis.
- Cystoscopy and sigmoidoscopy should be performed if there is a question of invasion into the urethra, bladder, or rectum.

MEDICATION

- As an adjuvant therapy, fluorouracil (Efudex) cream for in situ disease can produce occasional results but is not well tolerated because of irritation of the vulva (7)[A].
- Chemoradiotherapy with cisplatin and 5-fluorouracil (5-FU) has been successful in advanced or recurrent disease, although local morbidity is increased (7)[A].
- Contraindications: elderly patients: If chemotherapeutic agents are used, pay close attention to the patient's performance status and ability to tolerate aggressive chemotherapy.

ISSUES FOR REFERRAL

Patients may need care from a gynecologic oncologist and/or a radiation oncologist.

ADDITIONAL THERAPIES

- Preoperative radiation therapy can be used in those with advanced vulvar cancer (5)[B].
- Adjuvant radiation should be considered with tumor size >4 cm, evidence of lymphovascular invasion, positive surgical margins, or lymph node involvement.
- Preoperative chemoradiation allows for a less radical surgical procedure in patients who are not surgical candidates (7)[A].
- Postoperative radiation decreases recurrence frequency and may improve survival (7)[A].
- Radiation is contraindicated with verrucous carcinoma because it induces anaplastic transformation and increases metastases.

SURGERY/OTHER PROCEDURES

- In situ disease can be treated with wide excision or laser vaporization of the affected area. Laser vaporization is preferable in the younger patient, whereas wide excision is preferable in the elderly patient, in whom the risk of invasive disease is also higher (5)[A].
- If tumor extension within <1 cm from structures that will not be removed, preoperative radiation to prevent inadequate surgical margins prior to excision
- Inguinofemoral lymphadenectomy removal of superficial inguinal and deep femoral lymph nodes
- 1 cm tumor free margin is required because smaller margin would increase risk of recurrence (7)[A].
- Stage IA: radical local excision without lymph node dissection if <1 mm invasion, >1 mm invasion ipsilateral lymph node excision
- Stage IB: radical local excision with ipsilateral inguinofemoral lymph node dissection because the risk of metastases is greater than 8%
- Stage II: modified radical vulvectomy and/or chemoradiation and groin node dissection
- Stages III and IV: neoadjuvant chemoradiation and less radical surgery
- Pelvic exenteration after radiation provides effective therapy for advanced or recurrent malignancies involving the bladder or rectum.
- More limited surgery
  - Has been undertaken for early invasive lesions, especially in young patients, to preserve the clitoris and sexual function
  - Sentinel lymph node biopsy (SLNB) also has been advocated for early invasive lesion; however, it requires operator expertise.
  - Radical vulvectomy with bilateral groin node dissection through separate incisions provides better cosmetic results than en bloc technique.
  - Unilateral lymphadenectomy should be considered when lesion <2 cm, lateral lesion >2 cm from vulvar midline, or no palpable groin nodes (6)[B].

INPATIENT CONSIDERATIONS

Typically inpatient for treatment

Admission Criteria/Initial Stabilization

In advanced malignancy involving the urethra and rectum, concomitant cisplatin/5-FU chemotherapy with radiation produces a significant decrease in size of the primary tumor, usually obviating the need for pelvic exenteration.

ONGOING CARE

FOLLOW-UP RECOMMENDATIONS

Patient Monitoring

- Early stage, treated with surgery alone: clinical exam of the groin nodes and vulvar area every 6 months for 2 years; then annually
- Following chemoradiation, assessment for further treatment within 6–12 weeks of therapy completion
- Advance stage, clinical exam of the groin nodes and vulvar area every 3 months for 2 years; then every 6 months for 3 years, and then annually (8)[B]
- Cervical and/or vaginal cytology annually
- Majority of relapses occur within first year.

DIET

As tolerated and according to comorbid conditions

PATIENT EDUCATION

- American College of Obstetricians and Gynecologists (ACOG), 409 12th St. SW, Washington, DC 20024-2188; (800) 762-ACOG; www.acog.org
- American Cancer Society: www.cancer.org

PROGNOSIS

The 5-year survival is based on stage:

- Stage I: 78.5%
- Stage II: 58.8%
- Stage III: 43.2%
- Stage IV: 13.0%
- Inguinal and/or femoral node involvement is most important determinant of survival (9)[A].

COMPLICATIONS

- The major complications from radical vulvectomy and groin node dissection are wound breakdown, lymphedema, urinary stress incontinence, and psychosexual consequences.
- Two common complications with radical vulvectomy and bilateral groin node dissection
  - In the immediate postoperative period, ~50% of patients experience breakdown of the wound. This requires aggressive wound care by visiting nurses as often as twice a day. The wounds usually granulate and heal over a period of 6–10 weeks.
  - ~15–20% of patients experience some form of mild-to-moderate lymphedema after the groin node dissection. These patients should be instructed in the use of leg elevation and support hose. <1% of patients experience severe, debilitating lymphedema.

REFERENCES

1. Crosbie EJ, Slade RJ, Ahmed AS. The management of vulval cancer. *Cancer Treat Rev*. 2009;35(7):533–539.
2. U.S. Cancer Statistics Working Group. *United States Cancer Statistics: 1999–2010 Incidence and Mortality Web-based Report*. Atlanta, GA: Department of Health and Human Services, Centers for Disease Control and Prevention, and National Cancer Institute; 2013.
3. Hampl M, Sarajuuri H, Wentzensen N, et al. Effect of human papillomavirus vaccines on vulvar, vaginal, and anal intraepithelial lesions and vulvar cancer. *Obstet Gynecol*. 2006;108(6):1361–1368.
4. Markowitz LE, Dunne EF, Saraiya M, et al. Quadrivalent human papillomavirus vaccine: recommendations of the Advisory Committee on Immunization Practices (ACIP). *MMWR Recomm Rep*. 2007;56(RR-2):1–24.
5. de Hullu JA, van der Zee AG. Surgery and radiotherapy in vulvar cancer. *Crit Rev Oncol Hematol*. 2006;60(1):38–58.
6. Radziszewski J, Kowalewska M, Jedrzejczak T, et al. The accuracy of the sentinel lymph node concept in early stage squamous cell vulvar carcinoma. *Gynecol Oncol*. 2010;116(3):473–477.
7. Shylasree TS, Bryant A, Howells RE. Chemoradiation for advanced primary vulval cancer. *Cochrane Database Syst Rev*. 2011;(4):CD003752.
8. Stuckey A, Schutzer M, Rizack T, et al. Locally advanced vulvar cancer in elderly women: is chemoradiation beneficial? *Am J Clin Oncol*. 2013;36(3):279–282.
9. Salani R, Backes FJ, Fung MF, et al. Posttreatment surveillance and diagnosis of recurrence in women with gynecologic malignancies: Society of Gynecologic Oncologists recommendations. *Am J Obstet Gynecol*. 2011;204(6):466–478.

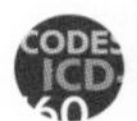

CODES

ICD10

- C51.9 Malignant neoplasm of vulva, unspecified
- D07.1 Carcinoma in situ of vulva
- C51.0 Malignant neoplasm of labium majus

CLINICAL PEARLS

- 60% of vulvar cancers are attributable to oncogenic HPV, and 92% of all VIN 2/3, VAIN 2/3, and AIN are attributable to HPV. Therefore, HPV vaccination has the potential to decrease vulvar cancer by 1/3.
- Biopsy all suspicious or nonhealing vulvar lesions.

VULVODYNIA

Tara J. Neil, MD

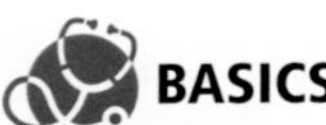

BASICS

DESCRIPTION

- Vulvar discomfort, often described as burning. Occurs in the absence of relevant visible findings, relevant lab abnormalities, or a clinically identifiable neurologic disorder
- Classification is based on whether pain is generalized or localized and whether it is provoked (by physical contact), spontaneous, or mixed.
  - Generalized: involvement of majority of the vulva; usually persistent or spontaneous pain
  - Localized: severe pain of certain vulvar areas such as the vestibule (formerly known as *vestibulodynia*), usually provoked with touch or attempted vaginal entry; thought to be the leading cause of painful intercourse among premenopausal women
    - Primary: introital dyspareunia from 1st episode of intercourse or 1st insertion of tampon or vaginal speculum
    - Secondary: introital dyspareunia developing after a period of painless intercourse, tampon use, or speculum exams

EPIDEMIOLOGY

- Most women diagnosed between the ages of 20 and 80 years
- Patients are psychologically comparable with asymptomatic controls and have similar marital satisfaction.

Incidence

- Recent retrospective study estimates annual rate of new onset vulvodynia to be 1.8% (1).
- Evidence indicates lifetime cumulative incidence approaches 15%, suggesting nearly 14 million U.S. women will experience persistent vulvar discomfort at some point in their lives (2).

Prevalence

- Reports between 3.1% and 15%; non–clinical-based studies approximate a prevalence of 7% with validation by exam.
- Studies show Hispanics are 80% more likely to present with vulvar pain compared with Caucasians and African Americans (3).

ETIOLOGY AND PATHOPHYSIOLOGY

- Vulvodynia is likely to be neuropathically mediated:
  - Allodynia and hyperalgesia are thought to result from neurogenic inflammation, leading to sensitization of primary afferents by inflammatory peptides, prostaglandins, and cytokines. Impulses transmitted to the CNS, where reinforcing signals sustain pain loop
  - In recent investigations of vulvar biopsy specimens, increased neuronal proliferation and branching in vulvar tissue are evident when compared with tissue of asymptomatic women.
- Pelvic floor pathology also should be considered: In one study, the vulvodynia group showed an increase in pelvic floor hypertonicity at the superficial muscle layer, less vaginal muscle strength with contraction, and decreased relaxation of pelvic floor muscles after contraction (2).
- No cause of vulvodynia has been established. It is most likely a neuropathic pain caused by the following:
  - Recurrent vulvovaginal candidiasis or other infections
  - Chemical exposure (trichloroacetic acid) or physical trauma
  - Reduced estrogen receptor expression/changes in estrogen concentration
  - CNS etiology, similar to other regional pain syndromes

RISK FACTORS

- Vulvovaginal infections, specifically candidiasis. Unclear if infection, treatment, or underlying hypersensitivity is the cause (4)
- Hormonal factors: Controversial evidence proposes increased risk with use of oral contraception pills (OCPs); early age at 1st use of OCPs and longer duration of use has been associated with increased risk.
- Pelvic floor dysfunction: Increased instability of pelvic floor muscles may perpetuate vulvar tissue inflammation, leading to vascular changes and histamine release.
- Comorbid interstitial cystitis and painful bladder syndrome; potentially related to common embryologic origin of structures
- Abuse: increased risk of vulvodynia if childhood physical or sexual abuse by a primary family member; causal relationship remains unclear (2).
- Depression and anxiety (4)
- Other neuropathic disorders, including regional pain syndrome

Genetics

Proposed genetic deficiency impairing one's ability to stop the inflammatory response triggered by infection or chemicals; homozygosity of the 2 alleles of the interleukin-1 receptor antagonist occurs in 25–50% of vestibulodynia patients, compared with <10% in controls (5).

GENERAL PREVENTION

- Wear 100% cotton underwear in the daytime and no underwear to sleep.
- Avoid douching and other vulvar irritants such as perfumes, dyes, detergents.
- Avoid abrasive activities and tight, synthetic clothing.
- Avoid panty liners.
- Clean the vulva with water only, and pat area dry after bathing.
- Avoid use of hair dryers in the vulvar area.

COMMONLY ASSOCIATED CONDITIONS

Higher incidence of chronic pain syndromes associated with vulvodynia, including chronic cystitis, irritable bowel syndrome (IBS), fibromyalgia, migraines, depression, endometriosis, low back pain

DIAGNOSIS

- Vulvodynia is a clinical diagnosis and should be suspected in any women with chronic pain at the introitus and vulva (5)[B].

- Pain should be characterized using a standard measure such as the McGill Pain Questionnaire; duration and nature of the pain should be established. Use physical exam to rule out other causes of vulvovaginal pain. Negative fungal culture, along with relevant history and positive cotton swab test (see below), confirm diagnosis.

HISTORY

Adequate sexual, social, and pain history should be taken to assess degree of symptoms. Visual pain scales and pain diaries may be helpful (6)[B]:

- Specifically ask about bowel and bladder habits, history of trauma or abuse, history of infections including herpes, and personal hygiene.
- Onset of vulvodynia often sudden and without precedents
- Pain often described as generalized, unprovoked.
- Specific skin complaints may suggest alternate diagnosis; a history of allergies may suggest vulvar dermatitis.
- Assess for precipitants of vulvar pain: tight garments, bicycle riding, tampon use, prolonged sitting, perfumed or deodorant soaps, douching.
- Assess for complaints of dyspareunia:
  - Presence of vaginismus (involuntary vaginal muscle spasm), adequate lubrication, anorgasmia, partner problems, abuse
  - Psychosexual morbidity significantly higher in patients with vulvodynia; counseling may complement medical interventions.

PHYSICAL EXAM

- Ask patient to show where pain is localized or most painful.
- Mouth and skin exams to assess for lesions suggestive of lichen planus or lichen sclerosus
- Vaginal exam should be done to exclude other causes of vulvovaginal pain, including external inspection; palpation; and single digit, speculum, and bimanual exams:
  - The vulva may be erythematous, especially at the vestibule. Discomfort with separation of the labia minora is common.
  - Spontaneous or elicited pain at the lower 1/2 of anterior vaginal wall suggests bladder etiology.
- Bulbocavernosus and anal wink reflexes should be checked to assess for peripheral neuropathy.

DIFFERENTIAL DIAGNOSIS

- Infections: candidiasis, herpes, human papillomavirus (HPV), bacterial vaginosis, trichomoniasis, dermatophytes
- Inflammation: lichen planus, immunobullous disorder, allergic vulvitis, lichen sclerosus, atrophic vaginitis
- Neoplasia: Paget disease, vulvar or vaginal intraepithelial neoplasia, squamous cell carcinoma
- Neurologic/muscular: herpes neuralgia, spinal nerve compression, vaginismus

DIAGNOSTIC TESTS & INTERPRETATION

Cotton swab or Q-tip test: Vulva tested for localized areas of pain beginning at thighs and continuing medially toward vestibule using the soft end and broken sharp end of the cotton swab. 5 distinct positions (2, 4, 6, 8, and 10 o'clock) surveyed using light palpation. Pain rated on a scale from 0 (none) to 10 (most severe). Posterior introitus and posterior hymenal remnants most common sites of increased sensitivity

Initial Tests (lab, imaging)

- Vaginal pH, wet mount, and yeast culture are recommended to rule out vaginitis.
- Gonorrhea and chlamydia testing done at physician's discretion
- HPV screening is unnecessary; no association has been identified between HPV and vulvodynia.

Follow-Up Tests & Special Considerations
- Varicella-zoster and herpes simplex virus should be considered if ulcers or vesicular eruptions are present.
- Biopsy should be considered if concerned about neoplasm or dermatophyte infection or if the patient is resistant to treatment.

Diagnostic Procedures/Other
Colposcopy can be helpful if epidermal abnormalities are present. This should be done with caution because acetic acid worsens vulvar pain.

Test Interpretation
No specific histologic features are associated with vulvodynia, although reactive squamous atypia has been observed. Biopsies are unnecessary for diagnosis. Presence of rash/altered mucosa is not consistent with vulvodynia; this requires further evaluation (6)[C].

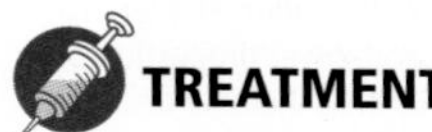

TREATMENT

A trial of several medications for at least 3 months is usually needed.

GENERAL MEASURES
- Combining treatments should be encouraged when treating women with vulvodynia (6)[C]: Various reports on use of a combination of medical treatments, psychotherapy, and dietary intervention reveal women on these combinations do significantly better compared with those who receive medication only.

MEDICATION
- Oral therapies
  - Tricyclic antidepressants (TCAs): 1st-line treatment for unprovoked vulvodynia (6)[B]; do not stop use abruptly; contraindicated in patients with cardiac abnormalities and those taking MAOIs; fatigue, constipation, sweating, palpitations, and weight gain are most common side effects:
    - Amitriptyline, nortriptyline: most widely studied; start at 10 mg daily; dose should be titrated to pain control. Average effective dose is 60 mg daily. In 1 study, a 47% complete response rate was recorded (7)[B]. Nortriptyline may be preferred due to less anticholinergic adverse effects.
  - Gabapentin: Started at 300 mg daily at HS and increased by 300 mg every 3 days. Maximum recommended dose is 3,600 mg daily divided into 3 doses. Dosing regimen limits popularity.
  - SSNRIs: not commonly used; however, have been helpful in those who cannot tolerate TCAs
    - Venlafaxine may be helpful in some patients.
    - Duloxetine has also been used.
  - Opioids/NSAIDs: not consistently helpful in relieving vulvar pain
- Topical therapies
  - Lidocaine 5% ointment: for provoked vestibulodynia; application advised 15–20 minutes prior to intercourse. Penile numbness and possible toxicity with ingestion can occur:
    - A trial of local anesthetics may be recommended for all patients who present with vulvodynia. Use judiciously to avoid increased irritation (6)[C].
    - In 1 study, lidocaine 5% ointment was left in vestibule overnight (average of 8 hours) for a period of 6–8 weeks; at follow-up, up to 76% of women reported no discomfort with intercourse (2)[C].
  - Cromolyn 4% cream: decreases mast cell degranulation in vulvar tissue; recommended application TID (4)[C]
  - Capsaicin 0.025%: decreases in discomfort and increases in frequency of intercourse with 20-minute daily application (2)[B]
  - Topical amitriptyline 2% combined with baclofen 2% is helpful in patients with comorbid vaginismus.
  - Topical corticosteroids and testosterone creams have not been shown to alleviate symptoms of vulvodynia.
  - Gabapentin 3% ointment or gabapentin 6% (must be compounded)
  - Topical nitroglycerin may be helpful but may cause headaches.
  - Topical estrogen
- Injectable therapies
  - Triamcinolone acetonide: No more than 40 mg should be injected monthly; is best when combined with 0.25–0.5% bupivacaine
  - Submucosal methylprednisone and lidocaine: reports of up to 68% response rate with weekly injections (6)[B]
  - Interferon-α: useful in treatment of vestibulodynia. Side effects (myalgias, fever, malaise) limit use.
  - Botulinum toxin A injectable

ISSUES FOR REFERRAL
A team approach is recommended for most effective management. Triage to psychosexual medicine, psychology, and pain management teams should be strongly considered (6)[B].

ADDITIONAL THERAPIES
- Biofeedback/physical therapy: useful with concomitant vaginismus. Treats both generalized and localized vulvar pain; treatment value for unprovoked pain remains unclear. Most studies report an average of 12–16-week treatment time.
- Surface electromyography (sEMG): efficacious for pelvic floor rehabilitation. Patients are more likely to experience pain-free sexual intercourse after sEMG. Significant reductions seen on pain measures at long-term follow-up.
- Cognitive-behavioral therapy (CBT): One randomized trial revealed that CBT is associated with a 30% decrease in vulvar discomfort with sexual intercourse. CBT is the recommended treatment for patients who present with dyspareunia as a main complaint (5)[B].

COMPLEMENTARY & ALTERNATIVE MEDICINE
Acupuncture: Small studies of women with unprovoked vulvodynia who did not respond to conventional treatment reported significant decreases in pain severity with acupuncture; treatment value with provoked pain is unknown (6)[C].

SURGERY/OTHER PROCEDURES
- Surgery may be considered for patients who have failed to respond to other measures. Use of surgical treatment is not recommended for generalized vulvodynia (6)[B].
- 60–80% of women who undergo surgery report a significant reduction in pain symptoms; however, when surveyed, patients prefer behavioral therapies to surgical intervention.
- A 3-armed randomized trial in 2001 found that women who underwent surgical intervention were more satisfied than those treated with biofeedback or CBT (5)[B].
- All patients who are considering surgical intervention should be tested for vaginismus. Vestibulectomy is less successful in this subgroup.
- Surgical approaches
  - Local excision: precise localization of painful areas; tissue closed in elliptical fashion
  - Total vestibulectomy: Incision is made and tissue is removed from Skene ducts to perineum. The vagina is then brought down to cover defect.
  - Perineoplasty: vestibulectomy plus removal of perineal tissue; incision usually terminated above the anal orifice; reserved for severe cases (5)[B]

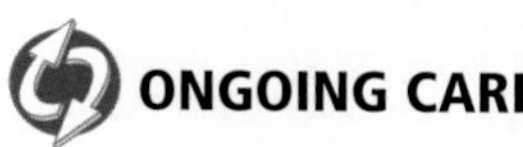

ONGOING CARE

PATIENT EDUCATION
Patients should be reassured that this condition is neither infectious nor does it predispose to cancer (6)[C]. Emphasize self-hygiene. Encourage treatment with home remedies, including ice packs, sitz baths, and barrier cream to preserve moisture after bathing.

PROGNOSIS
Traditionally viewed as a chronic pain disorder, new evidence of remission has been documented; recent 2-year follow-up study revealed 1 in 10 vulvodynia patients reported remission.

REFERENCES

1. Reed B, Haefner H, Sen A, et al. Vulvodynia incidence and remission rates among adult women: a 2-year follow-up study. *Obstet Gynecol*. 2008; 112(2, Pt 1):231–237.
2. Boardman L, Stockdale C. Sexual pain. *Clin Obstet Gynecol*. 2009;52(4):682–690.
3. Harlow BL, Stewart EG. A population-based assessment of chronic unexplained vulvar pain: have we underestimated the prevalence of vulvodynia? *J Am Med Womens Assoc*. 2003;58(2):82–88.
4. Groysman V. Vulvodynia: new concepts and review of the literature. *Dermatol Clin*. 2010;28(4): 681–696.
5. Reed B. Vulvodynia: diagnosis and management. *Am Fam Physician*. 2006;73(7):1231–1238.
6. Nunns M, Mandal D, Byrne J, et al. Guidelines for the management of vulvodynia. *Br J Dermatol*. 2010;162(6):1180–1185.
7. Haefner H, Collins M, Davis G, et al. The vulvodynia guideline. *J Low Genit Tract Dis*. 2005;9(1): 40–51.

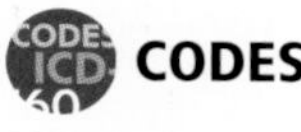

CODES

ICD10
- N94.819 Vulvodynia, unspecified
- N94.818 Other vulvodynia
- N94.810 Vulvar vestibulitis

CLINICAL PEARLS

Vulvodynia is a clinical diagnosis; it should be suspected in any woman with chronic pain at the introitus and vulva.

V

VULVOVAGINITIS, ESTROGEN DEFICIENT

Maria De La Luz Nieto, MD

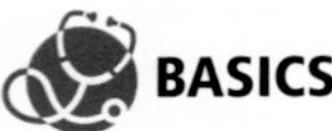

BASICS

DESCRIPTION

- Vaginal atrophy is due to decreased blood flow to vaginal epithelium, resulting in thinning of the female genital tissues.
- Estrogen deficiency affects all tissues in the female body; however, the genital tissues are especially hormone-responsive and are most affected, leading to atrophy.
- Patients with estrogen-deficient vulvovaginitis may present with urinary incontinence, vaginal burning and itching, dyspareunia, increased urinary frequency, or recurrent UTIs.
- System(s) affected: reproductive

EPIDEMIOLOGY

Incidence

- Predominant age: postmenopausal females. The average age of menopause in the United States is 51.3 years but ranges from 45 to 55 years old.
- May affect lactating women
- Predominant sex: female only
- May occur in younger women with premature ovarian failure

Prevalence

- Most postmenopausal women are affected to some degree.
- Up to 40% of postmenopausal women experience symptoms severe enough to seek treatment.

ETIOLOGY AND PATHOPHYSIOLOGY

- Decreased estrogen levels in the vagina and vulva result in decreased blood flow and decreased lubrication of vaginal and vulvar tissue.
- Vaginal and vulvar tissues become thin secondary to decreased vaginal cell maturation.
- Decreased cellular maturation results in decreased glycogen stores, which affects the normal vaginal flora and pH.
- Estrogen deficiency due to the following:
  - Menopause (surgical or natural)
  - Premature ovarian failure (chemotherapy, irradiation, autoimmune, anorexia, genetic)
  - Postpartum, lactation
  - Medications that alter hormonal concentration, such as gonadotropin-releasing hormone agonists, and antiestrogens, such as tamoxifen and danazol
  - Elevated prolactin from hypothalamic–pituitary disorders

Genetics

No known pattern

RISK FACTORS

Estrogen-deficient states

COMMONLY ASSOCIATED CONDITIONS

- Urge and stress urinary incontinence
- Pelvic organ prolapse
- Frequent UTIs
- Bacterial vaginosis or yeast infections

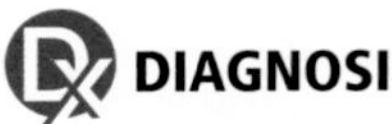

DIAGNOSIS

HISTORY

- All female patients should be asked about symptoms because many women are embarrassed to discuss these issues with their health care providers (1)[C].
  - Vaginal dryness
  - Dyspareunia
  - Pruritus
  - Burning
  - Pressure
  - Tenderness
  - Malodorous discharge
  - Urinary symptoms: dysuria, hematuria, frequency, infections, stress, and urge urinary incontinence
- Ask about self-treatment and products used.
- Determine exposure to irritants (e.g., soaps, feminine sprays, lotions, lubricants, constant pad use).

PHYSICAL EXAM

Evidence for the diagnosis includes the following:

- Loss of pubic hair
- Decreased vulvar and vaginal fullness
- Decreased vulvar subcuticular fat and moisture
- Pale-appearing, shiny, smooth vaginal and urethral epithelium
- Vaginal shortening, intolerance to speculum exams
- Loss of vaginal rugation
- Pelvic organ prolapse
- Shorten urethra

DIFFERENTIAL DIAGNOSIS

- Malignancy
- Dermatologic conditions of vulva and vagina:
  - Dermatitis
  - Lichen sclerosis
  - Lichen planus
- Bacterial or yeast vulvovaginitis

DIAGNOSTIC TESTS & INTERPRETATION

Because vulvovaginitis is a clinical diagnosis, labs are not always necessary, but if suspect dermatologic or oncologic condition, biopsy is recommended (2)[A].

Initial Tests (lab, imaging)

However, the following labs may be obtained as corroborative of clinical impression:

- Check follicle-stimulating hormone (FSH) and estrogen levels. FSH rises and estrogen drops with menopause.
- Evaluate for infections via wet preparation and vaginal pH (usually >5).
- Urine dip and urinalysis if suspected concomitant UTI
- Perform cytology for maturation index: Higher proportion of parabasal cells and lower proportion of intermediate and superficial cells indicate decreased maturation index.

Follow-Up Tests & Special Considerations

Drugs that may alter lab results:

- Estrogen therapy will alter the maturation index.
- Digoxin has estrogen-like properties.
- Tamoxifen may produce menopausal-type symptoms but also may act on genital tissues as a weak estrogen agonist.
- Progestins, danazol, and gonadotropin-releasing hormone agonists may produce a reversible pseudomenopause state.

Test Interpretation

- Thinning of the cornified squamous layer of both the vulva and the vagina
- Increased parabasal cells
- Compact underlying collagenous tissue

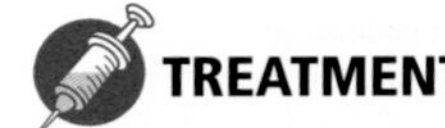

TREATMENT

GENERAL MEASURES

- Wear loose-fitting, undyed cotton underwear.
- Avoid prolonged pad use, especially scented pads.
- Avoid feminine deodorant sprays and douching.
- Use over-the-counter water-based lubricants, as needed.
- Symptomatic relief, if needed (e.g., cool baths or compresses)

MEDICATION

- Vaginal estrogen can reverse atrophic changes and help to alleviate symptoms (3)[A].
  - Vaginal cream 1 g (conjugated equine estrogens or estradiol cream): Insert via applicator each night × 14 days and then 2–3× per week.
  - Vaginal estradiol 10-μg tablet: Insert via pre-loaded applicator each night × 14 days and then 2–3× per week.
  - Estradiol-containing vaginal ring 2 mg: Insert into vagina, and replace every 3 months.
- Estrogen therapy should be used in the lowest possible dose for the shortest duration of time (4)[B].
- Long-term therapy may be necessary owing to the chronic nature of estrogen-deficient vulvovaginitis (5)[A].

- Systemic therapy typically is used as hormonal treatment of vasomotor symptoms and not for the primary treatment of estrogen-deficient vulvovaginitis.
- Contraindications:
  - Breast or estrogen-dependent carcinoma
  - Undiagnosed vaginal bleeding
  - Thromboembolic disorders
  - Thrombophlebitis
  - Pregnancy
- Precautions: Any abnormal vaginal bleeding must be evaluated.

- Nonestrogen therapy: estrogen agonist/antagonist (6)[B]
  - Ospemifene (Osphena) 60 mg tablet daily

- Contraindications:
  - Breast or estrogen-dependent carcinoma
  - Undiagnosed vaginal bleeding
  - Thromboembolic disorders
  - Thrombophlebitis
  - Hepatic impairment
- Precautions: Any abnormal vaginal bleeding must be evaluated, monitor for DVT and stroke.

ISSUES FOR REFERRAL

- Refer to urogynecologist for evaluation if symptomatic due to pelvic organ prolapse and/or stress and urge urinary incontinence.
- Recurrent UTIs should be referred to urogynecology and/or urology for evaluation.

INPATIENT CONSIDERATIONS

Admission Criteria/Initial Stabilization

Outpatient treatment

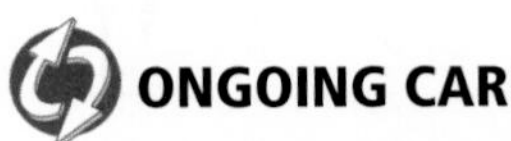

ONGOING CARE

FOLLOW-UP RECOMMENDATIONS

No restrictions

Patient Monitoring

Instruct the patient that symptoms should improve within 30–60 days. If they do not, reevaluate and reexamine for other causes.

DIET

No special diet

PATIENT EDUCATION

- American College of Obstetricians and Gynecologists (ACOG), 409 12th St., SW, Washington, DC 20024-2188; 800-762-ACOG: www.acog.org
- Lactating postpartum women with high levels of prolactin are in a hypoestrogenic state. These women should be instructed to use lubrication for symptoms of dyspareunia and reassured that the symptoms will resolve when they are no longer breastfeeding.

PROGNOSIS

The prognosis is excellent. Most symptoms will be alleviated with vaginal estrogen replacement therapy.

COMPLICATIONS

- Recurrent UTIs may occur in women with vaginal atrophy.
- Vaginal atrophy predisposes patients to vaginal infections.

REFERENCES

1. Mehta A, Bachmann G. Vulvovaginal complaints. *Clin Obstet Gynecol*. 2008;51(3):549–555.
2. Johnston SL, Farrell SA, Bouchard C, et al. The detection and management of vaginal atrophy [in English, French]. *J Obstet Gynaecol Can*. 2004;26(5):503–515.
3. Farquhar CM, Marjoribanks J, Lethaby A, et al. Long-term hormone therapy for perimenopausal and postmenopausal women. *Cochrane Database Syst Rev*. 2005;(3):CD004143.
4. Ibe C, Simon JA. Vulvovaginal atrophy: current and future therapies (CME). *J Sex Med*. 2010;7(3): 1042–1050; quiz 1051.
5. Suckling J, Lethaby A, Kennedy R. Local oestrogen for vaginal atrophy in postmenopausal women. *Cochrane Database Syst Rev*. 2006;(4):CD001500.
6. Constantine G, Graham S, Portman DJ, et al. Female sexual function improved with ospemifene in postmenopausal women with vulvar and vaginal atrophy: results of a randomized, placebo-controlled trial [published online ahead of print September 25, 2014]. *Climacteric*. 2014:1–7.

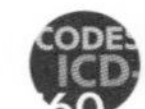

CODES

ICD10

- N95.2 Postmenopausal atrophic vaginitis
- E28.39 Other primary ovarian failure

CLINICAL PEARLS

- Estrogen-deficient vulvovaginitis affects virtually all postmenopausal women to some degree.
- This disorder is often associated with urinary incontinence, increased urinary frequency, and recurrent UTIs.
- Lab tests are generally unnecessary to make the diagnosis.
- Vaginal estrogen preparations, rather than systemic preparations, should be 1st-line therapy in a woman whose primary complaint is associated with vaginal atrophy.

VULVOVAGINITIS, PREPUBESCENT

Katherine M. Callaghan, MD

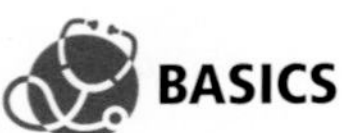

BASICS

DESCRIPTION

- Vulvitis is inflammation of the external genitals.
- Vaginitis, often associated with vaginal discharge, is inflammation involving the vaginal mucosa.
- In premenarchal girls, vulvitis is usually primary with secondary extension into the vagina.
- System(s) affected: reproductive, skin/exocrine
- Synonym(s): vaginitis; vulvitis

EPIDEMIOLOGY

Incidence

Unknown

Prevalence

Most common gynecologic problem in prepubertal girls

ETIOLOGY AND PATHOPHYSIOLOGY

- In the prepubertal child, the levels of estrogen are low.
- Due to the low levels of estrogen, the vaginal epithelium is thin, immature, and fragile.
- Absence of pubic hair and a well-developed labia, as well as close proximity of the anus and vagina, make contamination more likely.
- The prepubertal child also has an absence of lactobacilli, creating a neutral to alkaline vaginal pH.
- Neutral pH, atrophic mucosa, and moist environment of the vagina increase the risk of infection.
- Most cases of pediatric vulvovaginitis are nonspecific inflammation.
- Specific infections that occur are typically respiratory, enteric, or sexually transmitted.
- Nonspecific vulvovaginitis
- Poor perineal hygiene
- Nonspecific chemical irritants (bubble baths, scented soaps, shampoos)
- Tight-fitting clothing

Genetics

Understudied

RISK FACTORS

- Prepubertal girls are particularly susceptible due to behavioral and anatomic reasons:
  - Inadequate hand washing or perineal cleansing after urination and defecation
  - Tight-fitting clothing
  - Proximity of the vagina to the anus, lack of protective hair, and labial fat pads
  - Trauma
- Obese girls are also susceptible to nonspecific vulvovaginitis (1).

GENERAL PREVENTION

- Good perineal hygiene (including wiping from front to back)
- Urination with legs spread apart and labia separated
- Avoidance of tight-fitting clothing and nonabsorbent underwear
- Avoidance of irritants such as harsh soaps and bubble baths
- The most common respiratory pathogen is *Streptococcus pyogenes*. Vulvitis may occur in the absence of respiratory symptoms.
- *Shigella* vaginitis is associated with mucopurulent bloody discharge and likewise is not always accompanied by a history of diarrhea.

Etiologies

Streptococcus pyogenes	*Yersinia enterocolitica*
Staphylococcus aureus	*Neisseria gonorrhoeae*
Haemophilus influenzae	*Chlamydia trachomatis*
Moraxella catarrhalis	*Trichomonas vaginalis*
Streptococcus pneumoniae	*Papilloma virus*
Neisseria meningitidis	*Herpes virus*
Shigella	

- *Enterobius vermicularis* (pinworms)
  - Very common in young children and certain populations
  - Should be considered in children with vaginal itching and irritation
  - Most common symptom is nocturnal perineal itching
- Foreign body
  - Presents with foul-smelling, bloody, or brown discharge from the vagina
  - Should be considered with recurrent vulvovaginitis where other causes have been eliminated
- Other
  - With chronic vulvovaginitis, anatomic abnormalities or systemic disease should be considered:
    - Anatomic abnormalities include double vagina with fistula, ectopic ureter, and urethral prolapse.
- Systemic disease (inflammatory diseases)
- Other conditions, such as lichen sclerosus, vitiligo, psoriasis, and atopic dermatitis, should be considered.

ALERT

Cultures of sexually transmitted organisms in prepubertal children warrant investigations of sexual abuse.

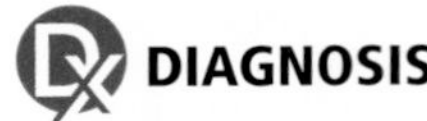

DIAGNOSIS

HISTORY

- Irritation and erythema of vulva
- Itching
- Bleeding
- Vaginal discharge
- Unpleasant odor
- Dysuria
- Soreness

PHYSICAL EXAM

- Look for evidence of chronic illness or dermatologic disease.
- Look for trauma or other signs that may correlate with abuse.
- Inspect the genital area in the supine position:
  - Excoriation of the genital area
  - Inflammation (erythema, swelling) of the introitus
  - Inspect the vagina and cervix in the knee–chest position.
  - Perform rectal exam if vaginal bleeding or abdominal pain.

DIFFERENTIAL DIAGNOSIS

- Contact dermatitis
- Eczema
- Psoriasis
- Lichen sclerosus

DIAGNOSTIC TESTS & INTERPRETATION

Initial Tests (lab, imaging)

- Culture for bacteria, fungi (yeast), or viruses (herpes).
- Urinalysis, urine culture, and urine for STI (via nucleic acid amplification test)
- Tape exam for pinworms
- Potassium hydroxide and saline smears of vaginal discharge, if present
- If an anatomic abnormality is suspected, imaging may be necessary to confirm.
- Consider consultation with a pediatric or adult gynecologist to determine the most appropriate imaging study.

Follow-Up Tests & Special Considerations

Exploration of the vagina for a foreign body may be necessary in cases of persistent, recurrent vulvitis.

Diagnostic Procedures/Other

If blood or foul-smelling discharge is present, visualization is mandatory:

- Place the child in the knee–chest position for best results. Hold the buttocks apart and slightly upward.
- Visualization of the vagina may be necessary by using a nasal speculum or infant laryngoscope.
- If available, consider referral to a provider with specific training/experience in this specialized exam.

TREATMENT

- The definitive diagnosis of bacterial vulvitis requires a culture of vulva and vaginal secretions.
- The typical colony count and bacterial mix are unknown in prepubescent girls. Antibiotic use should be directed against the species with the highest colony count.
- General hygiene should always be recommended, particularly in cases of a retained foreign body (e.g., toilet paper).
- When no cause is identified, treatment should focus on hygiene as well as minimizing soap exposure and tight-fitting clothes (2).

GENERAL MEASURES

- Appropriate health care: outpatient (except where systemic illness requires hospital care)
- Soak the vulva/perineum in a small amount of clear, warm water for 15 minutes BID.
- If smegma is present in the labial folds, clean the area gently with a mild soap.

MEDICATION

First Line

- To break the itching–scratching–infection cycle, use a low-dose topical hydrocortisone cream for a limited time.
- Estrogen deficiency with labial adhesion/agglutination: estrogen cream 0.625 mg to fused area nightly for 2 weeks
- Antibiotic use should be restricted to cases of bacterial infection only (3).
- Specific organisms on culture
  - Group A *Streptococcus*, *S. pneumoniae*: penicillin V (Pen Vee K) 250 mg PO BID–TID for 10 days
  - *H. influenzae*: amoxicillin, 20–40 mg/kg/day PO divided TID for 7 days
  - *S. aureus*: cephalexin, 25–50 mg/kg/day PO divided QID for 7–10 days *or* dicloxacillin, 25 mg/kg/day divided QID for 7–10 days *or* amoxicillin-clavulanate, 20–40 mg/kg/day PO divided BID for 7–10 days
  - *S. pyogenes*: amoxicillin, 50 mg/kg/day PO divided into 3 doses/day for 10 days
  - *Candida* sp.: topical nystatin (Mycostatin), miconazole, clotrimazole, or terconazole
  - *Shigella*: trimethoprim/sulfamethoxazole or ampicillin for 5 days
  - Pinworms: mebendazole, 100 mg PO, repeated in 2 weeks
  - *C. trachomatis*: ≤45 kg: erythromycin, 50 mg/kg/day QID for 14 days; ≥45 kg and <8 years old: azithromycin, 1 g PO single dose; ≥45 kg and ≥8 years old: azithromycin, 1 g PO single dose or doxycycline 100 mg BID for 7 days
  - *N. gonorrhoeae*: ≤45 kg: ceftriaxone, 125 mg IM plus medication for chlamydia; >45 kg: ceftriaxone, 250 mg IM × 1 plus medication for chlamydia
  - *Trichomonas*: metronidazole, 15 mg/kg/day PO divided TID (max 250 mg TID) for 7 days
- Contraindications: allergy to proposed treatment
- Precautions: Avoid potential allergens and topical sensitizers if possible.

ISSUES FOR REFERRAL

- Suspected sexual abuse
- Suspected anatomic abnormality (except minor labial agglutination)
- Persistent, severe, or recurrent infections

ONGOING CARE

FOLLOW-UP RECOMMENDATIONS

Patient Monitoring

Monitor for fever, pruritus, and vaginal discharge.

DIET

- Healthy balanced diet, high in fiber to prevent constipation
- Adequate fluid intake

PATIENT EDUCATION

Hygiene

- Wipe front to back after elimination.
- Avoid bubble baths and other irritating products.
- Clean daily with mild soap and water and dry gently with soft towel or cool hair dryer.
- Apply bland ointments for skin protection, if necessary.

PROGNOSIS

Excellent

COMPLICATIONS

- If an STI is identified and not treated effectively, the patient is at risk for pelvic inflammatory disease (PID).
- Vaginismus

REFERENCES

1. Van Eyk N, Allen L, Giesbrecht E, et al. Pediatric vulvovaginal disorders: a diagnostic approach and review of the literature. *J Obstet Gynaecol Can*. 2009;31(9):850–862.
2. Delago C, Finkel MA, Deblinger E. Urogenital symptoms in premenarchal girls: parents' and girls' perceptions and associations with irritants. *J Pediatr Adolesc Gynecol*. 2012;25(1):67–73.
3. Dei M, DiMaggio F, DiPaolo G, et al. Vulvovaginitis in childhood. *Best Pract Res Clin Obstet Gynaecol*. 2010;24(2):129–137.

ADDITIONAL READING

- Emans JS. Vulvovaginal problems in the prepubertal child. In: Emans SJ, Laufer MR, Goldstein DP, eds.: *Pediatric and Adolescent Gynecology*. 5th ed. Philadelphia: Lippincott Williams & Wilkins; 2005:83–99.
- Joishy M, Ashtekar CS, Jain A, et al. Do we need to treat vulvovaginitis in prepubertal girls? *BMJ*. 2005;330(7484):186–188.
- Merkley K. Vulvovaginitis and vaginal discharge in the pediatric patient. *J Emerg Nurs*. 2005;31(4):400–402.
- Rome ES. Vulvovaginitis and other common vulvar disorders in children. *Endocr Dev*. 2012;22:72–83.
- Sticker T. Vulvovaginitis. *Ped Child Health*. 2009;20:143–145.
- Velander MH, Mikkelsen DB, Bygum A. Labial agglutination in a prepubertal girl: effect of topical oestrogen. *Acta Derm Venereol*. 2009;89(2):198–199.

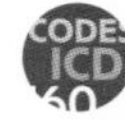

CODES

ICD10

- N76.0 Acute vaginitis
- N77.1 Vaginitis, vulvitis and vulvovaginitis in dis classd elswhr

CLINICAL PEARLS

- Vulvovaginitis is the most common gynecologic problem in prepubescent girls.
- The hypoestrogenic state and prepubescent anatomy may increase susceptibility to vulvar and vaginal infection.
- Treatment is typically supportive (avoid scratching, warm soaks) but may require antibiotics if a bacterial infection is suspected.
- Isolating an infection with known sexual transmission should prompt further investigation.
- Recurrent or persistent vulvitis, especially with foul-smelling discharge, should prompt a skilled exam of the vagina for a retained foreign body.
- Good perineal hygiene will limit this condition.

WARTS

Mercedes E. Gonzalez, MD, FAAD • Herbert P. Goodheart, MD

BASICS

- Warts (verrucae) are benign growths that are confined to the epidermis. All warts are caused by the human papillomavirus (HPV). Warts can appear on any area of the skin or mucous membranes. Common warts are predominantly seen in children and young adults.
- Clinically, warts are rather arbitrarily described as the following:
  - Common warts (verrucae vulgaris)
  - Plantar warts (verrucae plantaris)
  - Flat warts (verrucae plana)
  - Venereal warts (condyloma acuminatum)
  - Epidermodysplasia verruciformis is a rare, lifelong hereditary disorder characterized by chronic infection with HPV.
- System(s) affected: skin/exocrine

DESCRIPTION

- Common warts are most often found at sites subject to frequent trauma, such as the hands and feet. Because warts often vary widely in shape, size, and appearance, the various descriptive names for them generally reflect their clinical appearance, location, or both.
- For example, filiform (fingerlike) warts are threadlike, planar warts are flat, and plantar warts are located on the plantar surfaces (soles) of the feet.
- Genital warts, or condyloma acuminata, may be large and cauliflower-like, or they may consist of small papules.
- Warts on mucous membranes (mucosal papillomas), such as those in the mouth or vagina, tend to be white in color due to moisture retention.

EPIDEMIOLOGY

Incidence

- Predominant age: young adults and children
- Predominant sex: female = male

Prevalence

- ~7–10% of the U.S. population
- Common warts appear 2 times as frequently in whites as in blacks or Asians.

ETIOLOGY AND PATHOPHYSIOLOGY

- HPV is a double-stranded, circular, supercoiled DNA virus.
- The virus infects epidermal keratinocytes, stimulating cell proliferation.
- Various strains of DNA HPV: To date, >150 different subtypes have been identified.
- Common warts: HPV types 2 and 4 (most common), followed by types 1, 3, 27, 29, and 57
- Palmoplantar warts: HPV type 1 (most common), followed by types 2, 3, 4, 27, 29, and 57
- Flat warts: HPV types 3, 10, and 28
- Butcher warts: HPV type 7
- The virus is passed primarily through skin-to-skin contact or from the recently shed virus kept intact in a moist, warm environment.

RISK FACTORS

- HIV/AIDS and other immunosuppressive diseases (e.g., lymphomas)
- Immunosuppressive drugs that decrease cell-mediated immunity (e.g., prednisone, cyclosporine, and chemotherapeutic agents)
- Pregnancy
- Handling raw meat, fish, or other types of animal matter in one's occupation (e.g., butchers)
- Previous wart infection

GENERAL PREVENTION

There is no known way to prevent warts.

DIAGNOSIS

- Most often made on clinical appearance
- Skin biopsy, if necessary

PHYSICAL EXAM

- Distribution of warts is generally asymmetric, and lesions are often clustered or may appear in a linear configuration due to scratching (autoinoculation).
- Common wart: rough-surfaced, hyperkeratotic, papillomatous, raised, skin-colored to tan papules, 5–10 mm in diameter; several may coalesce into a larger cluster (mosaic wart); most frequently seen on hands, knees, and elbows; usually asymptomatic but may cause cosmetic disfigurement or tenderness
- Filiform warts: These are long, slender, delicate, fingerlike growths, usually seen on the face around the lips, eyelids, or nares.
- Plantar warts often have a rough surface and appear on the plantar surface of the feet in children and young adults:
  - Can be tender and painful; extensive involvement on the sole of the foot may impair ambulation, particularly when present on a weight-bearing surface.
  - Most often seen on the metatarsal area, heels, and toes in an asymmetric distribution (pressure points)
  - Pathognomonic "black dots" (thrombosed dermal capillaries); punctate bleeding becomes more evident after paring with a no. 15 blade.
  - Both common and plantar warts generally demonstrate the following clinical findings:
    - A loss of normal skin markings (dermatoglyphics) such as finger, foot, and hand prints
    - Lesions may be solitary or multiple, or they may appear in clusters (mosaic warts).
- Flat warts: slightly elevated, flat-topped, skin-colored or tan papules, small (1–3 mm) in diameter
  - Commonly found on the face, arms, dorsa of hands, shins (women)
  - Sometimes exhibit a linear configuration caused by autoinoculation
  - In men, shaving spreads flat warts.
  - In women, they often occur on the shins, where leg shaving spreads lesions.
- Epidermodysplasia verruciformis (rare): Widespread flat, reddish brown pigmented papules and plaques that present in childhood with lifelong persistence on the trunk, hands, upper and lower extremities, and face are characteristic.

DIFFERENTIAL DIAGNOSIS

- Molluscum contagiosum
- Seborrheic keratosis
- Epidermal nevus
- Acrochordon (skin tag)
- Solar keratosis and cutaneous horn
- Acquired digital fibrokeratoma
- Squamous cell carcinoma (SCC)
- Keratoacanthoma
- Subungual SCC can easily be misdiagnosed as a subungual wart or onychomycosis.
- Corns/calluses
  - Corns (clavi) are sometimes difficult to distinguish from plantar warts. Like calluses, corns are thickened areas of the skin and most commonly develop at sites subjected to repeated friction and pressure, such as the tops and the tips of toes and along the sides of the feet.
    - Corns are usually hard and circular, with a polished or central translucent core, like the kernel of corn from which they take their name.
    - Corns do not have "black dots," and skin markings are retained except for the area of the central core.

ALERT

- A melanoma on the plantar surface of the foot can mimic a plantar wart.
- Verrucous carcinoma, a slow-growing, locally invasive, well-differentiated SCC, also may be easily mistaken for a common or plantar wart.

DIAGNOSTIC TESTS & INTERPRETATION

Diagnosis

- HPV cannot be cultured, and lab testing is rarely necessary.
- Definitive HPV diagnosis can be achieved by the following:
  - Electron microscopy
  - Viral DNA identification employing Southern blot hybridization is used to identify the specific HPV type present in tissue
  - Polymerase chain reaction may be used to amplify viral DNA for testing.

Follow-Up Tests & Special Considerations

Skin biopsy if unusual presentation or if diagnosis is unclear

Test Interpretation

- Histopathologic features of common warts include digitated epidermal hyperplasia, acanthosis, papillomatosis, compact orthokeratosis, hypergranulosis, dilated tortuous capillaries within the dermal papillae, and vertical tiers of parakeratotic cells with entrapped red blood cells above the tips of the digitations.
- In the granular layer, HPV-infected cells may have coarse keratohyaline granules and vacuoles surrounding wrinkled-appearing nuclei. These koilocytic (vacuolated) cells are pathognomonic for warts.

TREATMENT

- The abundance of therapeutic modalities described below is a reflection of the fact that none of them is uniformly or even clearly effective in trials. Placebo treatment response rate is significant and quality of evidence in general is poor. Beyond topical salicylates, there is no clear evidence-based rationale for choosing 1 method over another (1)[A].
- The choice of method of treatment depends on the following:
  - Age of the patient
  - Cosmetic and psychological considerations
  - Relief of symptoms

- Patient's pain threshold
- Type of wart
- Location of the wart
- Experience of the physician

GENERAL MEASURES

- There is no ideal treatment.
- In children, most warts tend to regress spontaneously.
- In many adults and immunocompromised patients, warts are often difficult to eradicate.
- Painful, aggressive therapy should be avoided unless there is a need to eliminate the wart(s).
- For surgical procedures, especially in anxious children, pretreat with anesthetic cream such as EMLA (emulsion of lidocaine and prilocaine).

MEDICATION

First Line

- Self-administered topical therapy
  - Keratolytic (peeling) agents: The affected area(s) should be hydrated first by soaking in warm water for 5 minutes before application. Most over-the-counter agents contain salicylic acid and/or lactic acid; agents such as Duofilm, Occlusal-HP, Trans-Ver-Sal, and Mediplast
- Office-based
  - Cantharidin 0.7%, an extract of the blister beetle that causes epidermal necrosis and blistering
  - Combination cantharidin 1%, salicylic acid 30%, and podophyllin resin 5% in flexible collodion; applied in a thin coat, occluded 4–6 hours, then washed off

Second Line

Home-based

- Imiquimod 5% (Aldara) cream, a local inducer of interferon, is applied at home by the patient. It is approved for external genital and perianal warts and is used off-label and may be applied to warts under duct tape occlusion. It is applied at bedtime and washed off after 6–10 hours. Applied to flat warts without occlusion.
- Topical retinoids (e.g., tretinoin 0.025–0.1% cream or gel) for flat warts

Office-based

- Immunotherapy: induction of delayed-type hypersensitivity with the following:
  - Diphenylcyclopropenone (DCP) (2)[A]
  - Dinitrochlorobenzene (DNCP)
  - Squaric acid dibutylester (SADBE): There is possible mutagenicity and side effects with this agent.
- Intralesional injections
  - Mumps or *Candida* antigen
  - Bleomycin: Intradermal injection is expensive and usually causes severe pain.
  - Interferon-α-2b
- Oral therapy
  - Oral high-dose cimetidine: possibly works better in children
  - Acitretin (an oral retinoid)
- Other treatments (all have all been used with varying results)
  - Dichloroacetic acid, trichloroacetic acid, podophyllin, formic acid, aminolevulinic acid in combination with blue light, 5-fluorouracil, silver nitrate, formaldehyde, levamisole, topical cidofovir (3)[B] or IV cidofovir for recalcitrant warts in the setting of HIV, and glutaraldehyde

COMPLEMENTARY & ALTERNATIVE MEDICINE

- Duct tape: Cover wart with waterproof tape (e.g., duct tape). Leave the tape on for 6 days, and then soak, pare with emery board, and leave uncovered overnight; then reapply tape cyclically for 8 cycles; 85% resolved compared with 60% efficacy with cryotherapy (4)[A].
- Hyperthermia: safe and inexpensive approach; immerse affected area into 45°C water bath for 30 minutes 3 × per week
- Hypnotherapy
- Raw garlic cloves have demonstrated some antiviral activity.
- Vaccines are currently in development.

Pregnancy Considerations

The use of some topical chemical approaches may be contraindicated during pregnancy or in women who are likely to become pregnant during the treatment period.

SURGERY/OTHER PROCEDURES

- Cryotherapy with liquid nitrogen (LN_2) may be applied with a cotton swab or with a cryotherapy gun (Cryogun). Aggressive cryotherapy may be more effective than salicylic acid (5)[A], but it is associated with increased adverse effects (blistering and scarring):
  - Best for warts on hands; also during pregnancy and breastfeeding
  - Fast; can treat many lesions per visit
  - Painful; not tolerated well by young children
  - Freezing periungual warts may result in nail deformation.
  - In darkly pigmented skin, treatment can result in hypo- or hyperpigmentation.
- Light electrocautery with or without curettage
  - Best for warts on the knees, elbows, and dorsa of hands
  - Also good for filiform warts
  - Tolerable in most adults
  - Requires local anesthesia
  - May cause scarring
- Photodynamic therapy: Topical 5-aminolevulinic acid is applied to warts followed by photoactivation (6)[B].
- CO_2 or pulse-dye laser ablation: expensive and requires local anesthesia
- For filiform warts: Dip hemostat into LN_2 for 10 seconds, then gently grasp the wart for 10 seconds and repeat. Wart sheds in 7–10 days.

ONGOING CARE

FOLLOW-UP RECOMMENDATIONS

Patient Monitoring

1/3 of the warts of epidermodysplasia may become malignant.

PROGNOSIS

- More often than not (especially in children), warts tend to "cure" themselves over time.
- In many adults and immunocompromised patients, warts often prove difficult to eradicate.
- Rarely, certain types of lesions may transform into carcinomas.

COMPLICATIONS

- Autoinoculation (pseudo-Koebner reaction)
- Scar formation
- Chronic pain after plantar wart removal or scar formation
- Nail deformity after injury to nail matrix

REFERENCES

1. Kwok CS, Gibbs S, Bennett C, et al. Topical treatments for cutaneous warts. *Cochrane Database Syst Rev*. 2012;12;9:CD001781.
2. Choi Y, Kim Do H, Jin SY, et al. Topical immunotherapy with diphenylcyclopropenone is effective and preferred in the treatment of periungual warts. *Ann Dermatol*. 2013;25(4):434–439.
3. Fernández-Morano T, del Boz J, González-Carrascosa M, et al. Topical cidofovir for viral warts in children. *J Eur Acad Dermatol Venereol*. 2011;25(12):1487–1489.
4. Wenner R, Askari SK, Cham PM, et al. Duct tape for the treatment of common warts in adults: a double-blind randomized controlled trial. *Arch Dermatol*. 2007;143(3):309–313.
5. Kwok CS, Holland R, Gibbs S. Efficacy of topical treatments for cutaneous warts: a meta-analysis and pooled analysis of randomized controlled trials. *Br J Dermatol*. 2011;165(2):233–246.
6. Ohtsuki A, Hasegawa T, Hirasawa Y, et al. Photodynamic therapy using light-emitting diodes for the treatment of viral warts. *J Dermatol*. 2009;36(10):525–528.

ADDITIONAL READING

- Dasher DA, Burkhart CN, Morrell DS. Immunotherapy for childhood warts. *Pediatr Ann*. 2009;38(7):373–379.
- Simonart T, de Maertelaer V. Systemic treatments for cutaneous warts: a systematic review. *J Dermatolog Treat*. 2012;23(1):72–77.

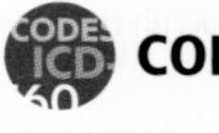

CODES

ICD10

- B07.9 Viral wart, unspecified
- B07.0 Plantar wart
- A63.0 Anogenital (venereal) warts

CLINICAL PEARLS

- No single therapy for warts is uniformly effective or superior; thus, treatment involves a certain amount of trial and error.
- Because most warts in children tend to regress spontaneously within 2 years, benign neglect is often a prudent option.
- Conservative, nonscarring, least painful, least expensive treatments are preferred.
- Freezing and other destructive treatment modalities do not kill the virus but merely destroy the cells that harbor HPV.

WILMS TUMOR

John K. Uffman, MD, MPH

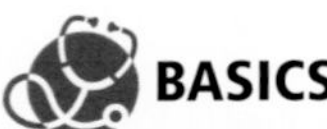

BASICS

DESCRIPTION

- An embryonal renal neoplasm containing blastemal, stromal, or epithelial cell types, usually affecting children <5 years of age
- Most common renal tumor in children; 5th most common pediatric malignancy
- Staging: In the United States, National Wilms Tumor Study Group (NWTSG) staging is done pretreatment based on radiographic imaging and surgery, whereas in Europe/Asia, Société Internationale d'Oncologie Pédiatrique (SIOP) staging is done *after* neoadjuvant chemotherapy is administered (1):
  - I: tumor limited to kidney; completely excised
  - II: tumor extends beyond kidney; completely excised
  - III: residual nonhematogenous tumor confined to abdomen (lymph nodes positive, spillage of tumor, peritoneal implants, extension beyond resection region)
  - IV: hematogenous metastases
  - V: bilateral renal involvement
- System(s) affected: renal/urologic
- Synonym(s): nephroblastoma

Pediatric Considerations

- Occurs only in children
- Most common renal malignancy in childhood

EPIDEMIOLOGY

Incidence

- Frequency rare in East Asian populations than whites
- Frequency higher in black children than in whites
- Predominant age: median age of 36.5 months
- Predominant sex: female > male (1.1:1)
- Represents 6–7% of all childhood cancers
  - >80% are diagnosed before 5 years of age (median age is 3.5 years at diagnosis).
  - Wilms tumor makes up 95% of all renal cancers in children <15 years (2).

Prevalence

United States: 0.69/100,000; 7.6 cases/1 million children <15 years

ETIOLOGY AND PATHOPHYSIOLOGY

- Hereditary or sporadic forms of genetic mutation
- Familial form: autosomal dominant trait with incomplete penetrance (1%)
- Potential of parental occupational exposure (machinists, welders, motor vehicle mechanics, auto body repairmen)

Genetics

- Several congenital anomalies are known to be associated with Wilms tumor. A 2-stage mutational model has been proposed: occurrence in either hereditary form or sporadic form. Patients with aniridia have a deletion of the short arm of chromosome 11 (11p13).
- Abnormalities of chromosome 11 at the 11p15 locus are associated with Beckwith-Wiedemann syndrome. Wilms tumor-suppressor gene (*WT1*) has been identified as well as additional candidates for another suppressor gene (*WT2*). Chromosome band 17q12–21 has been linked to 2 kindreds with Wilms tumor, and other kindred are associated with a Wilms tumor predisposition gene at 19q13.3–q13.4. Loss of heterozygosity at chromosomes 16q and 1p is associated with adverse outcome (1)[C].
- p53 is associated with anaplastic Wilms tumors (2).

RISK FACTORS

- Familial occurrence (5%) (2)
  - These patients tend to have earlier age of onset.
  - Familial patients have greater risk of bilateral disease.
- Parental occupation (machinists, welders, motor vehicle mechanics, auto body repairmen)
- Maternal exposure to pesticides prior to child's birth (3)
- High birth weight or preterm birth (3)
- Compared with firstborn, being a 2nd or later birth may be associated with significantly decreased risk of Wilms tumor (3).

GENERAL PREVENTION

- Routine surveillance in patients with syndromes associated with Wilms tumor
- Routine screening with serial renal US at 3–4-month intervals has been recommended in children who have syndromes associated with an incidence of Wilms tumor >5% (4)[C].
- Routine screening with serial renal US also recommended for infants born to kindreds with familial Wilms (every 3–4 months until age 7 years) (4)[C]

COMMONLY ASSOCIATED CONDITIONS

- Aniridia (partial or complete absence of iris) 600× normal risk
- Hemihypertrophy (100× normal risk)
- Cryptorchidism
- Hypospadias
- Duplicated renal collecting systems
- Denys-Drash syndrome (nephropathy, renal failure, male pseudohermaphroditism, Wilms tumor)
- Klippel-Trenaunay syndrome
- WAGR complex (Wilms tumor, aniridia, genitourinary malformations, and mental retardation)
- Beckwith-Wiedemann syndrome (visceromegaly, macroglossia, omphalocele, hyperinsulinemic hypoglycemia)

DIAGNOSIS

- Symptoms of pain, anorexia, vomiting, malaise in 30% (1)
- >90% present with asymptomatic abdominal mass (5)

HISTORY

- History of increasing abdominal size
- Usually asymptomatic; may have fever, abdominal pain

PHYSICAL EXAM

- Palpable upper abdominal mass
- Fever, hepatosplenomegaly
- Rarely, signs of acute abdomen with free intraperitoneal rupture
- Cardiac murmur
- Ascites, prominent abdominal wall veins, varicocele
- Gonadal metastases
- Aniridia (present in 1.1% of Wilms tumor patients)
- Hypertension (20–65%) (1)

DIFFERENTIAL DIAGNOSIS

- Neuroblastoma
- Hepatic tumor
- Sarcoma
- Rhabdoid tumor
- Cystic nephroma
- Renal cell carcinoma (generally occurs in older children)
- Mesoblastic nephroma: distinguished only by histology. Age usually <6 months, essentially benign, although metastases have been reported; tend to be locally invasive
- Nephroblastomatosis: considered premalignant; may present as nodularity of 1 or both kidneys

DIAGNOSTIC TESTS & INTERPRETATION

- Urinalysis (occasional hematuria, proteinuria)
- CBC (anemia)
- Lactate dehydrogenase
- Plasma renin (rarely helpful)
- Urine catecholamines
- Serum creatinine and calcium
- Coagulation factors
- Chest radiograph
- Abdominal US (with Doppler imaging): best initial test. Gives best information about tumor and extension into inferior vena cava
- CT scan (with IV and oral contrast material) of chest and abdomen. Allows anatomic visualization and excludes synchronous bilateral disease with a high degree of sensitivity (2)
- CT may have high sensitivity and specificity for atriocaval thrombus and obviate the needs for US (2).
- Chest lesions only identified on CT have improved event-free survival with 3 drug treatment regimens (6)[B].

Diagnostic Procedures/Other

Occasionally, bone marrow aspiration is necessary to distinguish from neuroblastoma.

Test Interpretation

- Favorable findings (mortality of 7%)
  - Bulky lesion, well encapsulated
  - Focal areas of hemorrhage and necrosis
  - Absence of anaplasia and sarcomatous cell types
  - Presence of blastemal, stomal, and epithelial elements (5)
    - Predominance of epithelial elements usually are less aggressive when diagnosed early but tend to be resistant to treatment when diagnosed late.
    - Predominance of blastemal elements indicate more aggressive tumors.
- Unfavorable histology (mortality rate of 57%)
  - Anaplasia: markedly enlarged and multipolar mitotic figures, 3-fold enlargement of nuclei in comparison with adjacent similar nuclei, hyperchromasia of enlarged nuclei; anaplasia may be diffuse or focal.
  - Sarcomatous changes: now considered to be separate from Wilms, not subtypes (mortality 64%)
  - Rhabdoid tumor of the kidney: now considered to be separate tumor from Wilms
- Nephroblastomatosis: considered premalignant
- Nephrogenic rests (5): These are precursor lesions found in 25–40% of Wilm; found in 1% of infants at autopsy, but most do not develop into malignancy.

TREATMENT

GENERAL MEASURES

- Appropriate health care: inpatient workup and treatment until stable postoperatively and induction chemotherapy completed
- Chemotherapy; some recommend pretreatment with neoadjuvant chemotherapy (1).
  - May decrease incidence of intraoperative tumor rupture (debatable)
  - May result in inappropriate treatment with chemotherapeutic agents of non-Wilms tumors (5%) or benign lesions (1.6%)
  - Results in the inability to directly compare treatment results worldwide
- Radiation therapy in stage II (unfavorable histology), stage III, and stage IV

MEDICATION

First Line

- Children typically treated with protocols based on staging, histology, and other variables as part of a multimodal therapy approach (chemotherapy, radiation, surgery). The following medications may be used as part of a protocol:
  - Dactinomycin (Actinomycin-D)
  - Vincristine
  - Doxorubicin
  - Cyclophosphamide (Cytoxan)
  - Ifosfamide
  - Etoposide
  - Topotecan
  - Irinotecan

Second Line

- Doxorubicin (Adriamycin)
- Cyclophosphamide

SURGERY/OTHER PROCEDURES

- Exploration of contralateral kidney no longer required if adequate CT done preoperatively
- Radical nephroureterectomy and lymph node sampling is needed to provide precise staging information.
- Renal sparing resection
  - Tumors usually too large, but 10–15% may be amenable to partial nephrectomy if given preoperative chemotherapy (4)[C].
  - May be recommended for patients with high risk of bilateral disease or renal failure (4)[C]
- Sampling of any enlarged lymph nodes (absence of any lymph nodes in the surgical specimen mandates treatment as stage III disease) (5)[B]
- Identification of any retained tumor with titanium clips
- Tumor should be given to pathologist fresh, not in formalin.
- Vertical midline incision if tumor extension to right atrium—increased morbidity (2)
- Bilateral Wilms tumors (represent 4–6% of Wilms) (5)[B]
  - Preoperative chemotherapy with reevaluation by CT or MRI after 6 weeks (some are biopsied prior to chemotherapy)
  - Renal sparing operation at 6 weeks if good response to chemotherapy:
    - Partial nephrectomy or wedge excision of tumor preferred but only if it does not compromise tumor resection
    - Kidney with lowest tumor burden is addressed first. If successful resection accomplished, radical nephrectomy can be done on the contralateral kidney. Bilateral partial nephrectomy may be possible in some cases.
- Preoperative treatment also generally is accepted in a solitary kidney, horseshoe kidneys, intravascular extension of tumor above the intrahepatic vena cava, and in the case of respiratory distress from extensive metastatic tumor.
- Treatment of patients with relapsed Wilms (7)[B]: Current treatment is either with chemotherapy with or without radiation therapy alone or high-dose chemotherapy followed by autologous stem cell rescue.

ONGOING CARE

FOLLOW-UP RECOMMENDATIONS

Patient Monitoring

- Multidrug chemotherapy every 3–4 weeks for 16 weeks–15 months depending on stage
- Every 4 months for 1 year, every 6 months for 2nd to 3rd year; yearly after that
- CBC, CT of chest and abdomen with each visit
- Patients at high risk for developing Wilms tumor should be monitored with renal US every 3–4 months until 5 years of age. Patients with Beckwith-Wiedemann syndrome or Simpson-Golabi-Behmel syndrome should have yearly US until 7 years of age (8)[C].

PATIENT EDUCATION

- Possibility of 2nd malignancy (up to 12% by age 50 years)
- Side effects of chemotherapy, radiation therapy

PROGNOSIS

- With favorable histology (1)
  - Children <2 years of age and stage I, favorable histology: 98% survival in NWTSG 1–3 studies
  - Children with stage III, favorable histology tumor: overall survival of 89% in NWTSG 3–4 studies
- With diffuse anaplasia (1)
  - Children with stage I, diffuse or focal anaplasia: overall survival 82.6%
  - Stage II tumors with anaplasia: overall survival 81.5%
  - Stage III tumors with anaplasia: overall survival 66.7%
  - Stage IV tumors with anaplasia: overall survival 33.3%
- With bilateral involvement (stage V): 4-year survival 81.7% (1)
- With rhabdoid features: 19% 3-year survival
- Survival of patients with relapsed Wilms tumor is 40–70% (8)[B]:
  - Patients with pulmonary relapse only had higher 4-year survival rate (77.7%) compared to other sites (41.6%).

COMPLICATIONS

- Complication rate of 6–10%
- 1–2% will develop 2nd malignant neoplasms (leukemia, lymphoma, hepatocellular carcinoma, soft tissue sarcoma): 12.2% by 50 years of age
- High risk of delivering low-birth-weight infants, perinatal mortality in offspring of female survivors of Wilms tumor
- Chest is usual site of recurrence.
- Occurrence of 2nd malignant neoplasms in 2% of patients 7–34 years after treatment
  - Bone and soft tissue sarcomas, breast cancer, hepatocellular carcinoma, lymphoma, gastrointestinal tract tumors, melanoma, leukemias
- Surgical complications
  - Postoperative small bowel obstruction (5–7%)
  - Tumor rupture with spillage in 15.3% according to NWTSG-5; this may be spontaneous or surgical and results in upstaging the tumor. Only 2.7% of spills are considered avoidable. Incidence of tumor spillage is reported at 2.2% by SIOP following preoperative neoadjuvant chemotherapy (5)[B].
- Local tumor recurrence
  - Abdominal tumor recurrence after tumor spillage is reduced by radiation therapy (10 or 20 Gy).
- Renal failure
- Cardiomyopathy (usually related to doxorubicin and radiation therapy)
- Impaired pulmonary function (radiation therapy)

REFERENCES

1. Sonn G, Shortliffe LM. Management of Wilms tumor: current standard of care. *Nat Clin Pract Urol*. 2008;5(10):551–560.
2. Davidoff AM. Wilms tumor. *Adv Pediatr*. 2012;59(1): 247–267.
3. Chu A, Heck JE, Ribeiro KB, et al. Wilms' tumour: a systematic review of risk factors and meta-analysis. *Paediatr Perinat Epidemiol*. 2010;24(5):449–469.
4. Nakamura L, Ritchey M. Current management of Wilms' tumor. *Curr Urol Rep*. 2010;11(1):58–65.
5. Ko EY, Ritchey ML. Current management of Wilms' tumor in children. *J Pediatr Urol*. 2009;5(1):56–65.
6. Grundy PE, Green DM, Dirks AC, et al. Clinical significance of pulmonary nodules detected by CT and not CXR in patients treated for favorable histology Wilms tumor on national Wilms tumor studies-4 and -5: a report from the children's oncology group. *Pediatr Blood Cancer*. 2012;59(4):631–635.
7. Presson A, Moore TB, Kempert P. Efficacy of high-dose chemotherapy and autologous stem cell transplant for recurrent Wilms' tumor: a meta-analysis. *J Pediatr Hematol Oncol*. 2010;32(6):454–461.
8. Scott RH. Surveillance for Wilms tumor in at-risk children: pragmatic recommendations for best practice. *Arch Dis Child*. 2006;91(12):995–999.

CODES

ICD10

- C64.9 Malignant neoplasm of unsp kidney, except renal pelvis
- C64.1 Malignant neoplasm of right kidney, except renal pelvis
- C64.2 Malignant neoplasm of left kidney, except renal pelvis

CLINICAL PEARLS

- Wilms is most common renal tumor in children; it is an embryonal renal neoplasm containing blastemal, stromal, or epithelial cell types, usually affecting children <5 years of age.
- Risks include parental occupation (machinists, welders, motor vehicle mechanics, auto body repairmen) and maternal exposure to pesticides prior to child's birth.
- Nephrectomy performed as soon as possible after completing radiographic evaluation is the major component in tumor staging.

ZOLLINGER-ELLISON SYNDROME

Douglas S. Parks, MD

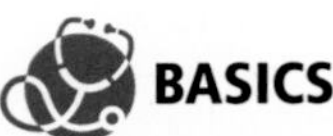

BASICS

DESCRIPTION

- Zollinger-Ellison syndrome triad
  - Markedly elevated gastric acid secretion
  - Peptic ulcer disease
  - A gastrinoma or non-β islet cell tumor of the pancreas or duodenal wall that produces gastrin
    - Gastrinomas (at the time of diagnosis) may be single or multiple (1/2–2/3), large or small, benign or malignant (2/3), sporadic (70–75%) or associated with MEN1 (*multiple endocrine neoplasia type 1*) (25–30%).
- System(s) affected: endocrine/metabolic; gastrointestinal
- Synonym(s): Z-E syndrome; pancreatic ulcerogenic tumor syndrome; multiple endocrine neoplasia, partial; ulcerogenic islet cell tumor

EPIDEMIOLOGY

Incidence

- 1–3 per million per year in the United States
- Predominant age: middle age (30–65 years)
- Predominant sex: male > female (1.3:1)

Pediatric Considerations

Aggressive cases have been reported in teenagers.

Pregnancy Considerations

Rare, pregnancy alters medication choices and surgical timing.

ETIOLOGY AND PATHOPHYSIOLOGY

- Gastrinoma is equally distributed between the head of the pancreas and the 1st or 2nd portion of the duodenum; if in the pancreas, the lesion is more likely to metastasize to the liver.
- Also may be found rarely in the mesentery, peritoneum, spleen, skin, or mediastinum (possibly metastasis with primary not identified)

Genetics

~25–30% of cases occur in association with the MEN1 syndrome—tumors of pancreas, pituitary, and parathyroid.

RISK FACTORS

- MEN1
- Family history of ulcer disease

GENERAL PREVENTION

Screen 1st-degree relatives of patients with MEN1.

COMMONLY ASSOCIATED CONDITIONS

- MEN1
- Insulinoma
- Carcinoid tumors

DIAGNOSIS

HISTORY

Average of 5 years of symptoms, including recurrent ulcers before diagnosis is made

- Abdominal pain is most common symptom (80%).
- Diarrhea (postprandial and fasting) (70%)
- Heartburn (60%)
- Nausea (30%)
- Reflux esophagitis
- Vomiting that is unresponsive to standard therapy
- Weight loss

PHYSICAL EXAM

- Hepatomegaly with metastasis
- Conjunctival pallor if anemic
- Complications of severe peptic ulcer disease, including hemorrhage, perforation, and obstruction
- Signs of MEN1 are hypercalcemia, hyperparathyroidism, and Cushing syndrome.

Geriatric Considerations

Consider the diagnosis in a patient with persistent or recurring peptic ulcer disease; it is a less aggressive disease if it appears after 65 years.

DIFFERENTIAL DIAGNOSIS

- Elevated serum gastrin with hypochlorhydria/achlorhydria
  - Atrophic gastritis
  - Drug-induced (associated with proton pump inhibitors [PPIs])
  - Gastric cancer
  - Pernicious anemia
  - Postvagotomy
- Elevated serum gastrin with normal or increased gastric acid
  - Antral G-cell hyperfunction
  - Chronic renal failure
  - *Helicobacter pylori* infection
  - Gastric outlet obstruction
  - Retained gastric antrum
- Consider gastrinoma in all patients with the following symptoms:
  - Recurrent or refractory ulcer disease
  - Gastric hypertrophy and ulcers
  - Duodenal and jejunal ulcers
  - Ulcers and diarrhea
  - Ulcers and kidney stones
  - Hypercalcemia and ulcers
  - Pituitary disease
  - Family history of ulcer disease or endocrine tumors suggestive of MEN1

DIAGNOSTIC TESTS & INTERPRETATION

- Preferred test is secretion stimulation test: gastrin level >100 pg/mL (>100 ng/L) (1)[A],(2)[B].
- Some gastrin assays undermeasure serum gastrin. If have strong index of suspicion but gastrin levels low, may need to repeat with a different lab (3)[B].

- Gastric secretory studies: basal acid output
- Alternative test is calcium infusion test: gastrin level >400 pg/mL (test is less specific and more dangerous because of IV calcium infusion).
- Elevated serum gastrin fasting level: >1,000 pg/mL with ulcers diagnostic; >200 pg/mL with ulcers is suggestive.
- Elevated basal gastric acid output: >15 mEq/hr (>15 mmol/hr)
- Gastric pH <2 with elevated gastrin
- Check serum calcium, phosphorus, cortisol, and prolactin to rule out MEN1.
- Drugs may alter lab results:
  - Histamine (H_2) blockers and PPIs may increase gastric pH and serum gastrin.
  - Hold PPIs 7 days and H_2 blockers 2 days prior to drawing gastrin level.
- Endoscopic US: finds 24–38% of primary tumors
- Endoscopic findings, including esophagitis, duodenal ulceration with multiple ulcers, and prominent gastric and duodenal folds
- Used to localize tumor for possible resection

- Much more likely to find tumors >3 cm (95%) than <1 cm (<15%) (4)[B]

- Abdominal CT scan: most useful for pancreatic tumors and metastasis >3 cm
- Abdominal US, MRI, and angiography are not typically useful except in large tumors.
- Somatostatin receptor scintigraphy (SRS): more sensitive than radiologic studies but still only finds 30% of small tumors
- Portal venous sampling and selective venous sampling for gastrin can localize the area of tumor and metastasis (80–90% sensitivity).
- Brain imaging (MRI) is useful if MEN1 is suspected.

- Because pancreatic tumors are most likely to be large and to metastasize to the liver (worse prognosis), SRS and an abdominal CT scan are suggested to look for resectable tumors. Surgical resection may improve prognosis (5)[B].

Diagnostic Procedures/Other

Endoscopy may reveal tumors in the duodenal wall; multiple ulcers, including jejunal ulcers; and prominent gastric and duodenal folds.

Test Interpretation

- 90% of gastrinomas are found in the gastric triangle (the borders are the bile duct, the junction of 2nd and 3rd portions of the duodenum, and the junction of the head and body of pancreas).
- ~50% of gastrinomas are in the head of the pancreas (more likely >3 cm, metastasis to liver).
- ~50% of gastrinomas are in the wall of the 1st or 2nd portion of duodenum (more likely to be small, solitary).
- 2/3 of gastrinomas are malignant.
- 50% of gastrinomas stain positive for adrenocorticotropic hormone (ACTH), vasoactive intestinal polypeptide, insulin, or neurotensin.
- 1/3 of patients have metastasis on presentation: regional nodes > liver > bone, > peritoneum, spleen, skin, and mediastinum.
- Biopsy shows hyperplasia of antral gastrin-producing cells and histology is similar in appearance to carcinoid.

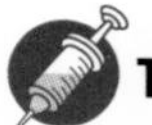

TREATMENT

GENERAL MEASURES

- Advanced imaging initially to evaluate for resection
- Surgical removal when primary tumor can be identified and as adjunct to control symptoms
- Medical treatment for symptom control when primary tumor is not found or metastasis on initial diagnosis

MEDICATION

- PPIs are the 1st-line treatment; H_2 blockers can be added.
- Medications heal 80–85% of ulcers, most of which recur. Lifelong medication use should be anticipated.
- 4–8-fold higher PPI dose often necessary
  - Start at a lower dose, and titrate to symptoms (or maximum recommended dosage).
- If hyperparathyroidism is present (MEN1), correct hypercalcemia.

First Line

- PPIs
  - Omeprazole 60–120 mg/day
  - Lansoprazole 60–180 mg/day (doses >120 mg need to be divided BID)
  - Rabeprazole 60–100 mg/day up to 60 mg BID
  - Pantoprazole 40–240 mg/day PO; 80–120 mg q12h IV
- H_2 blockers
  - Cimetidine 300 mg q6h up to 2.4 g/day
  - Ranitidine 150 mg q12h up to 6 g/day
  - Famotidine 20 mg q6h; up to 640 mg/day
- Contraindications
  - Known hypersensitivity to the drug
  - H_2 blockers: antiandrogen effects, drug interactions due to cytochrome P450 inhibition
  - PPIs: none
- Precautions
  - Adjust doses for geriatric patients and patients with renal insufficiency.
  - Gynecomastia has been reported with high-dose cimetidine (>2.4 g/day).
  - PPIs may induce a profound and long-lasting effect on gastric acid secretion, thereby affecting the bioavailability of drugs depending on low gastric pH (e.g., ketoconazole, ampicillin, iron).
- Significant possible interactions: Consider drug–drug interactions and consult prescribing materials accordingly.

Second Line

- Octreotide may slow growth of liver metastases, or (occasionally) promote regression. Octreotide LAR can be given every 28 days (4)[B].

- Chemotherapy regimens using streptozocin, 5-fluorouracil, and doxorubicin shows limited response.
- Interferon shows a limited response but may be useful in combination with octreotide.

SURGERY/OTHER PROCEDURES

- Laparotomy may be necessary to search for resectable tumors unless patient has liver metastasis on presentation or MEN1; surgery improves outcomes (6)[B].

- Definitive therapy: removal of identifiable gastrinomas (95% of tumors are found at the time of surgery; 5-year cure is 40% when all are removed)
- Total gastrectomy is rarely indicated.
- In MEN1, parathyroidectomy, by lowering calcium, may also decrease acid production and decrease antisecretory drug use. Gastrinomas in MEN1 are generally small, benign, and multiple, and surgery is not usually curative in this situation.

INPATIENT CONSIDERATIONS

Admission Criteria/Initial Stabilization

- Titrate medication to symptom control
- Appropriate surveillance postoperatively to look for metastasis

ONGOING CARE

FOLLOW-UP RECOMMENDATIONS

Patient Monitoring

- Longitudinal follow-up to evaluate for metastases
- Titrate medical therapy to control symptoms.

- Advise patients of potential danger of stopping antisecretory treatment. Rare cases have been reported of severe adverse outcomes within 2 days of stopping PPIs for testing (7)[B]. Gastric acid analysis can be used to help guide medical therapy to maintain basal gastric acid output at <10 mEq/hr (<2 mEq/hr if patient has complications such as perforation or esophagitis).

DIET

Restrict foods that aggravate symptoms.

PATIENT EDUCATION

Inform patients as to the nature of disease and prognosis.

PROGNOSIS

- Overall survival rate: 5–10 years: 69–94%
- The prognosis improves if complete surgical removal of the tumor is possible.
- If liver metastasis is present on initial surgery, 5-year survival is 30–40%; 10-year survival is 25%.

- Mortality is directly related to liver metastasis tumor size and presence of pancreatic tumors (4,5)[B].

COMPLICATIONS

- Complications of peptic ulcer disease (bleeding, perforation, obstruction)
- 2/3 of gastrinomas are malignant with metastasis.
- Paraneoplastic phenomena (e.g., production of ACTH with resulting Cushing syndrome) is possible.

- Decrease in vitamin B_{12} levels is possible with long-term PPI use (8)[A].

REFERENCES

1. Berna MJ, Hoffmann KM, Long SH, et al. Serum gastrin in Zollinger-Ellison syndrome: II. Prospective study of gastrin provocative testing in 293 patients from the National Institutes of Health and comparison with 537 cases from the literature evaluation of diagnostic criteria, proposal of new criteria, and correlations with clinical and tumoral features. *Medicine (Baltimore)*. 2006;85(6):331–364.
2. Kuiper P, Biemond I, Masclee AA, et al. Diagnostic efficacy of the secretin stimulation test for the Zollinger-Ellison syndrome: an intra-individual comparison using different dosages in patients and controls. *Pancreatology*. 2010;10(1):14–18.
3. Rehfeld JF, Bardram L, Hilsted L, et al. Pitfalls in diagnostic gastrin measurements. *Clin Chem*. 2012;58(5):831–836.
4. Hoffmann KM, Furukawa M, Jensen RT. Duodenal neuroendocrine tumors: classification, functional syndromes, diagnosis and medical treatment. *Best Pract Res Clin Gastroenterol*. 2005;19(5):675–697.
5. Jensen RT. Gastrinomas: advances in diagnosis and management. *Neuroendocrinology*. 2004; 80(Suppl 1):23–27.
6. Morrow EH, Norton JA. Surgical management of Zollinger-Ellison syndrome; state of the art. *Surg Clin North Am*. 2009;89(5):1091–1103.
7. Poitras P, Gingras MH, Rehfeld JF. The Zollinger-Ellison syndrome: dangers and consequences of interrupting antisecretory treatment. *Clin Gastroenterol Hepatol*. 2012;10(2):199–202.
8. Thomson AB, Sauve MD, Kassam N, et al. Safety of the long-term use of proton pump inhibitors. *World J Gastroenterol*. 2010;16(19):2323–2330.

ADDITIONAL READING

- Hirschowitz BI, Fineberg N, Wilcox CM, et al. Costs and risks in the management of patients with gastric acid hypersecretion. *J Clin Gastroenterol*. 2010;44(1):28–33.
- Mortellaro VE, Hochwald SN, McGuigan JE, et al. Long-term results of a selective surgical approach to management of Zollinger-Ellison syndrome in patients with MEN-1. *Am Surg*. 2009;75(8):730–733.
- Smallfield GB, Allison J, Wilcox CM, et al. Prospective evaluation of quality of life in patients with Zollinger-Ellison syndrome. *Dig Dis Sci*. 2010;55(11): 3108–3112.

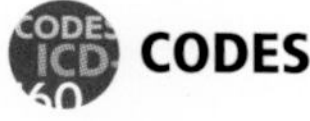

CODES

ICD10

E16.4 Increased secretion of gastrin

CLINICAL PEARLS

- ~25–30% of cases of Z-E syndrome occur in association with MEN1.
- Once Z-E is diagnosed, it is important to hunt for gastrinomas in the head of the pancreas and the 1st or 2nd portion of the duodenum.
- PPIs heal ulcers in cases of Z-E; lifelong therapy should be anticipated.
- Z-E syndrome should be considered if peptic ulcers recur or if high doses of PPI are needed to control symptoms/ulcers.

INDEX

C

Q

R

S

W

X

Y

Z